W9-BHV-859

Haddad and Winchester's
Clinical Management of Poisoning and Drug Overdose

Haddad and Winchester's Clinical Management of Poisoning and Drug Overdose

FOURTH EDITION

MICHAEL W. SHANNON, MD, MPH

Chief and CHB Chair
Division of Emergency Medicine
Children's Hospital Boston
Professor of Pediatrics
Harvard Medical School
Senior Toxicologist
MA/RI Regional Center for Poison Control and Prevention
Boston, Massachusetts

STEPHEN W. BORRON, MD, MS

Clinical Professor of Emergency Medicine (Surgery)
University of Texas Health Science Center at San Antonio
Consultant in Toxicology
South Texas Poison Center
San Antonio, Texas
Associate Clinical Professor of Emergency Medicine, Medicine, and Occupational and Environmental Health
The George Washington University
Washington, DC

MICHAEL J. BURNS, MD

Assistant Professor of Medicine
Harvard Medical School
Co-Director, Division of Medical Toxicology
Department of Emergency Medicine
Beth Israel Deaconess Medical Center
Boston, Massachusetts

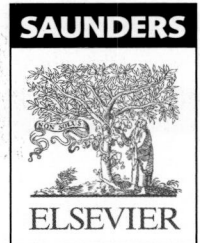

SAUNDERS

ELSEVIER

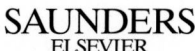

SAUNDERS
ELSEVIER

1600 John F. Kennedy Boulevard
Suite 1800
Philadelphia, PA 19103-2899

HADDAD AND WINCHESTER'S CLINICAL MANAGEMENT
OF POISONING AND DRUG OVERDOSE, FOURTH EDITION
Copyright © 2007 by Saunders, an imprint of Elsevier Inc.

ISBN: 978-0-7216-0693-4

All rights reserved. No part of this publication may be reproduced or transmitted in any form or by any means, electronic or mechanical, including photocopying, recording, or any information storage and retrieval system, without permission in writing from the publisher.
Permissions may be sought directly from Elsevier's Health Sciences Rights Department in Philadelphia, PA, USA: phone: (+1) 215 239 3804, fax: (+1) 215 239 3805, e-mail: healthpermissions@elsevier.com. You may also complete your request on-line via the Elsevier homepage (http://www.elsevier.com), by selecting "Customer Support" and then "Obtaining Permissions."

Notice

Knowledge and best practice in this field are constantly changing. As new research and experience broaden our knowledge, changes in practice, treatment, and drug therapy may become necessary or appropriate. Readers are advised to check the most current information provided (i) on procedures featured or (ii) by the manufacturer of each product to be administered, to verify the recommended dose or formula, the method and duration of administration, and contraindications. It is the responsibility of the practitioner, relying on their own experience and knowledge of the patient, to make diagnoses, to determine dosages and the best treatment for each individual patient, and to take all appropriate safety precautions. To the fullest extent of the law, neither the Publisher nor the Editors assume any liability for any injury and/or damage to persons or property arising out or related to any use of the material contained in this book.

Previous editions copyrighted 1998, 1990, 1983.

Library of Congress Cataloging-in-Publication Data
Haddad and Winchester's clinical management of poisoning and drug overdose / [edited by]
Michael Shannon, Stephen W. Borron, Michael Burns. — 4th ed.
  p. ; cm.
  Rev. ed. of: Clinical management of poisoning and drug overdose / [edited by] Lester M. Haddad, Michael W. Shannon, James F. Winchester. 3rd ed. c1998
  Included bibliographical references and index.
  ISBN 978-0-7216-0693-4
  1. Poisoning. 2. Medication abuse. 3. Drugs — Overdose. I. Haddad, Lester M. II. Shannon, Michael W. III. Borron, Stephen W. IV. Burns, Michael, MD. V. Clinical management of poisoning and drug overdose. VI. Title: Clinical management of poisoning and drug overdose.
  [DNLM: 1. Poisoning—therapy. QV 601 H126 2007]

RA1211.C584 2007
615.9'08—dc22

2006037454

Acquisitions Editor: Todd Hummel
Developmental Editor: Melissa Dudlick
Publishing Services Manager: Joan Sinclair
Design Direction: Steven Stave
Text Designer: Melissa Olson

Printed in China

Last digit is the print number: 9 8 7 6 5 4 3 2 1

Working together to grow
libraries in developing countries

www.elsevier.com | www.bookaid.org | www.sabre.org

ELSEVIER   BOOK AID International   Sabre Foundation

To Elaine, Evan, and Lila, whose patience made this book possible; to Drs. Fred Lovejoy and Gary Fleisher for their mentorship; and to all the toxicology fellows with whom I've had the pleasure of working. Thank you.

Michael W. Shannon

To Dr. Edward (Mel) Otten, who first encouraged me to study the management of chemical and radiological emergencies; to Drs. James Lockey, James R. Roberts and Suman Wason, who mentored me in my unconventional approach to occupational medicine and toxicology training; to Professors Chantal Bismuth and Frédéric Baud, who afforded me the opportunity to expand my knowledge of toxicology in an international environment; to my family and colleagues, without whose constant support my participation would not have been possible.

Stephen W. Borron

I am forever grateful to my wife, Maureen, and children, Ryan, Liam, and Riley, whose unwavering love, support, and understanding during the editing process greatly contributed to the success of this work.

Michael J. Burns

CONTRIBUTORS

Cynthia K. Aaron, MD, FACMT, FACEP
Associate Professor of Medicine and Pediatrics
Wayne State University School of Medicine
Director, Clinical and Medical Toxicology Education
Children's Hospital of Michigan Regional Poison
    Center
Detroit Medical Center
Detroit, Michigan

Jawaid Akhtar, MD
Assistant Professor
Department of Emergency Medicine
University of Pittsburgh Medical Center
Medical Toxicologist
Pittsburgh Poison Center
Children's Hospital of Pittsburgh
Pittsburgh, Pennsylvania

Steven E. Aks, DO
Associate Professor of Emergency Medicine
Rush University
Director, The Toxikon Consortium
Chief, Section of Toxicology
Department of Emergency Medicine
Cook County Hospital
Chicago, Illinois

Timothy E. Albertson, MD, MPH, PhD
Professor of Medicine, Pharmacology/Toxicology,
    Emergency Medicine, and Anesthesiology
University of California–Davis
VA Northern California Hospitals and Clinics
Chief, Division of Pulmonary/Critical Care Medicine
Medical Director, Sacramento Division
California Poison Control System
University of California–Davis Medical Center
Sacramento, California

Alfred Aleguas, Jr., RPH, BSPharm, PharmD
Adjunct Faculty
University of Rhode Island College of Pharmacy
Kingston, RI
Clinical Manager
MA/RI Regional Center for Poison Control and
    Prevention
Boston, Massachusetts
Staff Pharmacist
The Westerly Hospital
Westerly, Rhode Island

Linda G. Allison, MD, MPH
Professor, Physician Assistant Studies
Le Moyne College
Syracuse, New York

Angela C. Anderson, MD, FAAP
Associate Professor
Departments of Emergency Medicine and Pediatrics
Brown University Medical School
Attending Physician
Department of Pediatric Emergency Medicine
Rhode Island and Hasbro Children's Hospitals
Providence, Rhode Island

Juan C. Arias, MD
Postdoctoral Fellow
Department of Surgery
Division of Emergency Medicine
The University of Texas Health Science Center at
    San Antonio
San Antonio, Texas

Alexander B. Baer, MD
Clinical Instructor
Department of Emergency Medicine
University of Virginia
Charlottesville, Virginia
Attending Physician
Rockingham Memorial Hospital
Harrisonburg, Virginia

Frédéric J. Baud, MD
Professor of Critical Care Medicine
Hôpital Lariboisière
Université Paris VII
Paris, France

Carl R. Baum, MD, FAAP, FACMT
Associate Professor of Pediatrics
Yale University School of Medicine
Attending Physician, Pediatric Medicine
Director, Toxicology Service
Director, Center for Children's Environmental
    Toxicology (toxikid.org)
Yale–New Haven Children's Hospital
New Haven, Connecticut

Martin Belson, MD
Medical Toxicologist
National Center for Environmental Health
Pediatric Emergency Medicine
Children's Healthcare of Atlanta
Atlanta, Georgia

John G. Benitez, MD, MPH, FACMT, FACPM
Associate Professor of Emergency Medicine,
    Environmental Medicine, and Pediatrics
University of Rochester
Managing Director and Associate Medical Director
Ruth A. Lawrence Poison and Drug Information Center
University of Rochester Medical Center
Rochester, New York

Neal L. Benowitz, MD
Professor of Medicine, Psychiatry, and
    Biopharmaceutical Sciences
University of California-San Francisco
Chief of Clinical Pharmacology
San Francisco General Hospital
San Francisco, California

David P. Betten, MD
Assistant Clinical Professor
Department of Emergency Medicine
Michigan State University College of Human Medicine
East Lansing, Michigan
Attending Physician
Sparrow Health System
Lansing, Michigan

Brian Christopher Betts, MD
Chief Resident
Internal Medicine Department
University of Minnesota
Minneapolis, Minnesota

Lawrence Stilwell Betts, MD, PhD, CIH, FACOEM
Professor
Family and Community Medicine
Associate Clinical Professor of Physiological Sciences
Eastern Virginia Medical School
Norfolk, Virginia
President, Lawrence Stilwell Betts, MD, PhD, P.C.
Poquoson, Virginia
Consultant
SafetyCall and International Poison Center
Bloomington, Minnesota

Michael Beuhler, MD
Clinical Instructor of Emergency Medicine
University of North Carolina at Chapel Hill
Chapel Hill, North Carolina
Medical Director, Carolinas Poison Center
Carolinas Medical Center
Charlotte, North Carolina

Steven B. Bird, MD
Assistant Professor of Emergency Medicine
Division of Medical Toxicology
University of Massachusetts Medical School
Worcester, Massachusetts

Carolyn M. Blume-Odom, RN, BSN
RN, Certified Specialist in Poison Information
Missouri Regional Poison Control Center
St. Louis, Missouri

Stephen W. Borron, MD, MS
Clinical Professor of Emergency Medicine (Surgery)
University of Texas Health Science Center at San
    Antonio
Consultant in Toxicology
South Texas Poison Center
San Antonio, Texas
Associate Clinical Professor of Emergency Medicine,
    Medicine, and Occupational and Environmental
    Health
The George Washington University
Washington, DC

Edward W. Boyer, MD, PhD
Associate Professor of Emergency Medicine
University of Massachusetts Medical School
Worcester, Massachusetts
Lecturer in Pediatrics
Harvard Medical School
Assistant in Medicine
Children's Hospital Boston
Boston, Massachusetts
Chief, Division of Medical Toxicology
UMass Memorial Medical Center
Worcester, Massachusetts

Sally M. Bradberry, BSc, MB, ChB, MRCP
Assistant Director
National Poison Information Service (Birmingham
    Unit)
City Hospital
Birmingham, United Kingdom

Jeffrey Brent, MD, PhD
Clinical Professor of Medicine and Pediatrics
University of Colorado Health Sciences Center
Denver, Colorado

D. Eric Brush, MD
Assistant Professor
Department of Emergency Medicine
Division of Medical Toxicology
University of Massachusetts Medical Center
Worcester, Massachusetts

Michael J. Burns, MD
Assistant Professor of Medicine
Harvard Medical School
Co-Director, Division of Medical Toxicology
Department of Emergency Medicine
Beth Israel Deaconess Medical Center
Boston, Massachusetts

Javier R. Caldera, MD
Clinical Instructor
University of Texas Southwestern Medical Center
Toxicology Fellow
Parkland Memorial Hospital
Dallas, Texas

Thomas R. Caraccio, PharmD, RPH, DABAT
Associate Professor
Department of Emergency Medicine
State University of New York at Stony Brook
Stony Brook, New York
Managing Director
Long Island Regional Poison Control Center
Winthrop University Hospital
Mineola, New York

Edward W. Cetaruk, MD
Assistant Clinical Professor of Medicine
Department of Medicine
Section of Clinical Pharmacology and Toxicology
University of Colorado Health Sciences Center
Toxicology Associates, PLLC
Denver, Colorado

Andrew Chan, MB ChB, FRCP (Ldn), FCCP
Associate Professor
University of California–Davis
Sacramento, California
VA Northern California Health Care System
Mather, California

Peter B. Chase, MD, PhD
Assistant Professor
Clinical Emergency Medicine
University of Arizona College of Medicine
Director, Medical Toxicology Residency Program
University Medical Center
Consultant
Arizona Poison and Drug Information Center
Tucson, Arizona

James Cisek, MD, MPH
Virginia Commonwealth University
University of Richmond
Medical Director
Community Commitment
Bon Secours Health System
VCU Medical Center
Richmond, Virginia

Richard F. Clark, MD
Professor of Medicine
University of California–San Diego
Director, Division of Medical Toxicology
UCSD Medical Center
San Diego, California

Kirk L. Cumpston, DO, FACEP
Assistant Professor
Department of Emergency Medicine
Assistant Medical Director, Virginia Poison Center
Medical College of Virginia Hospital
Virginia Commonwealth University Health Science
    Center
Richmond, Virginia

Steven C. Curry, MD
Department of Medical Toxicology
Banner Good Samaritan Regional Medical Center
Department of Medicine
University of Arizona College of Medicine
Phoenix, Arizona

Paul I. Dargan, MBBS, MD, MRCP
Consultant Physician and Clinical Toxicologist
Guy's & St. Thomas Poisons Unit
Guy's & St. Thomas NHS Foundation Trust
London, UK

G. Patrick Daubert, MD
Assistant Professor
Director, Clinical and Medical Toxicology Education
Assistant Director, California Poison Control System,
    Sacramento Division
University of California–Davis
Sacramento, California

João Delgado, MD
Assistant Professor of Emergency Medicine
University of Connecticut School of Medicine
Divisions of Emergency Medicine and Medical
    Toxicology
Hartford Hospital
Hartford, Connecticut

Valerie A. Dobiesz, MD, FACEP
Associate Professor of Emergency Medicine
Associate Residency Director
Education Director
University of Illinois College of Medicine
Chicago, Illinois

J. Ward Donovan, MD, FACMT, FACEP
Professor Emeritus
Emergency Medicine
Pennsylvania State University College of Medicine
Hershey, Pennsylvania
Medical Director, PinnacleHealth Toxicology Center
Chief, Section of Medical Toxicology
PinnacleHealth System Hospitals
Harrisburg, Pennsylvania

Robert P. Dowsett, BM, BS, FACEM
Department of Emergency Medicine
Westmead Hospital
Westmead, New South Wales, Australia

Antonio Dueñas-Laita, MD, PhD
Professor of Clinical Toxicology
University of Valladolid School of Medicine
Head of Regional Toxicology Unit
Río Hortega Hospital
Valladolid, Spain

Judith M. Eisenberg, MD, MS
Medical Officer
Hazard Evaluations and Technical Assistance Branch
Division of Surveillance, Hazard Evaluations and Field
    Studies
Centers for Disease Control and Prevention
Cincinnati, Ohio

Timothy B. Erickson, MD, FACEP, FACMT, FAACT
Professor of Emergency Medicine
Director, Division of Clinical Toxicology
Residency Program Director
Department of Emergency Medicine
University of Illinois College of Medicine
Chicago, Illinois

Michele Burns Ewald, MD
Department of Pediatrics
Harvard University Medical School
Attending Physician
Children's Hospital Boston
Director, Harvard Medical Toxicology Fellowship
Medical Director
MA/RI Regional Center for Poison Control and
    Prevention
Boston, Massachusetts

Susan Farrell, MD
Assistant Professor of Medicine
Harvard Medical School
Director of Student Programs
Department of Emergency Medicine
Brigham and Women's Hospital
Boston, Massachusetts

Tania M. Fatovich, MD, MS-HES
Department of Emergency Medicine
Brigham and Women's Hospital
The Gilbert Program in Medical Simulation
Harvard Medical School
Boston, Massachusetts

Miguel C. Fernández, MD
Associate Professor/Clinical
Division of Emergency Medicine
Department of Surgery
Medical and Managing Director
The South Texas Poison Center
University of Texas Health Science Center at San Antonio
San Antonio, Texas

J.W. Fijen, MD, PhD
Senior Lecturer in Intensive Care
University Medical Center Utrecht
Utrecht, Netherlands
Senior Medical Consultant
National Institute for Public Health and the Environment
Bilthoven, Netherlands

Chris Foley, MD
Internist
Minnesota Natural Medicine
Vadnais Heights, Minnesota

R. Brent Furbee, MD
Associate Clinical Professor
Division of Medical Toxicology
Department of Emergency Medicine
Indiana University School of Medicine
Medical Director
Indiana Poison Center
Indianapolis, Indiana

Ann-Jeannette Geib, MD
Medical Toxicologist
PinnacleHealth Toxicology Center
Harrisburg Hospital
Emergency Physician
PinnacleHealth Hospitals
Harrisburg, Pennsylvania

Robert J. Geller, MD
Associate Professor of Pediatrics
Emory University School of Medicine
Medical Director, Georgia Poison Center
Grady Health System
Director, Emory Southeast Pediatric Environmental
    Health Specialty Unit
Chief of Pediatrics
Emory Service at Grady Health System
Atlanta, Georgia

Carl A. Germann, MD
Emergency Physician
Maine Medical Center
Portland, Maine

Melissa L. Givens, MD, MPH
Clinical Assistant Professor
University of Washington School of Medicine
Seattle, Washington
Attending Physician
Madigan Army Medical Center
Tacoma, Washington

Ronald E. Goans, PhD, MD, MPH
Clinical Associate Professor
Tulane School of Public Health and Tropical Medicine
New Orleans, Louisiana
Senior Medical Consultant
MJW Corporation
Amherst, New York

Nora Goldschlager, MD
Professor of Clinical Medicine
University of California–San Francisco
Associate Director, Cardiology Division
Director, SFGH Coronary Care Unit, ECG Laboratory,
    and Pacemaker Clinic
San Francisco General Hospital
San Francisco, California

Andis Graudins, MBBS (Hons), PhD
Conjoint Senior Lecturer
Faculty of Medicine
University of New South Wales
Kensington, New South Wales, Australia
Senior Staff Specialist
Clinical Toxicology and Emergency Medicine
Prince of Wales Hospital
Randwick, New South Wales, Australia

Michael I. Greenberg, MD, MPH
Professor of Emergency Medicine
Drexel University College of Medicine
Wayne, Pennsylvania

Tee L. Guidotti, MD, MPH, DABT
Professor and Chair
Department of Environmental and Occupational
    Health
School of Public Health and Health Services
Professor and Director, Division of Occupational
    Medicine and Toxicology
Department of Medicine
School of Medicine and Health Sciences
The George Washington University Medical Center
The George Washington University Hospital
Washington, DC

Alan H. Hall, MD
Clinical Assistant Professor of Preventive Medicine and
    Biometrics
University of Colorado Health Sciences Center
Denver, Colorado
President and Chief Medical Toxicologist
Toxicology Consulting and Medical Translating
    Services, Inc.
Elk Mountain, Wyoming

Christine A. Haller, MD
Assistant Professor of Medicine and Clinical
    Pharmacology
Division of Clinical Pharmacology
Department of Medicine and Laboratory Medicine
San Francisco General Hospital
University of California, San Francisco
San Francisco, California

Daniel A. Handel, MD, MPH
Resident in Emergency Medicine
University of Cincinnati Medical Center
Cincinnati, Ohio

Philippe Hantson, MD, PhD
Professor of Toxicology
Catholic University of Louvain
Head, Center for Clinical Toxicology
Cliniques St.-Luc
Brussels, Belgium

Matthew W. Hedge, MD
Assistant Professor
Department of Emergency Medicine
Wayne State University School of Medicine
Associate Medical Director
Children's Hospital of Michigan Regional Poison Center
Detroit Receiving Hospital
Detroit, Michigan

Fred M. Henretig, MD
Professor of Pediatrics and Emergency Medicine
University of Pennsylvania School of Medicine
Director, Section of Clinical Toxicology
Children's Hospital of Philadelphia
Philadelphia, Pennsylvania

Michael G. Holland, MD, FACMT, FACOEM, FACEP
Clinical Assistant Professor of Emergency Medicine
SUNY Upstate Medical University
Syracuse, New York
Attending Physician
Department of Occupational Medicine
Glen Falls Hospital
Glen Falls, New York

Knut Erik Hovda, MD, PhD
Department of Acute Medicine
Ulleval University Hospital
Oslo, Norway

Dag Jacobsen, MD, PhD, FAACT
Professor of Medicine and Clinical Toxicology
University of Oslo
Director, Department of Acute Medicine
Division of Medicine
Ulleval University Hospital
Oslo, Norway

Alison L. Jones, BSc, MD, FRCP, FRCPE, FiBIOL
Professor of Medicine and Clinical Toxicology
Faculty of Health
University of Newcastle
Callaghan, New South Wales, Australia

David N. Juurlink, BPhm, MD, PhD, FRCPC
Assistant Professor
Departments of Medicine, Pediatrics, and Health Policy,
    Management, and Evaluation
University of Toronto
Division Head
Division of Clinical Pharmacology and Toxicology
Staff Physician
Division of General Internal Medicine
Sunnybrook Health Sciences Centre
Consultant Toxicologist
Ontario Regional Poison Information Centre
The Hospital for Sick Children
Toronto, Ontario, Canada

Ziad N. Kazzi, MD, FAAEM
Assistant Professor
Co-Director, Center for Emerging Infections and
    Emergency Preparedness
Department of Emergency Medicine
University of Alabama at Birmingham
Birmingham, Alabama

Nicholas J. Kenyon, MD
Assistant Professor of Medicine
University of California–Davis
Davis, California

Fergus Kerr, MBBS, MPH, FACEM
Clinical Toxicologist
Statewide Toxicology Service
Deputy Director
Emergency Department
Austin Health
Melbourne, Victoria, Australia

Daniel C. Keyes, MD, MPH, FACMT
Physician Advisor
Concentra Health Services
Carrollton, Texas
Clinical Associate Professor
Division of Toxicology, Emergency Medicine
Department of Surgery
University of Texas Southwestern Medical Center
Dallas, Texas

Edwin M. Kilbourne, MD
Chief Medical Officer
National Center for Environmental Health and the
    Agency for Toxic Substances and Disease Registry
Centers for Disease Control and Prevention
Atlanta, Georgia

Richard Kingston, PharmD
Professor
Department of Experimental and Clinical
    Pharmacology
College of Pharmacy
University of Minnesota
Minneapolis, Minnesota
President and Senior Toxicologist
Regulatory and Scientific Affairs
SafetyCall International Poison Center
Bloomington, Minnesota

Mark A. Kirk, MD
Assistant Professor
Division of Medical Toxicology
Department of Emergency Medicine
University of Virginia
Charlottesville, Virginia

Laura J. Klein, MD
Volunteer Clinical Faculty
Department of Psychiatry
University of Colorado Health Sciences Center
Denver, Colorado

Kurt C. Kleinschmidt, MD
Division of Emergency Medicine
Department of Surgery
Chief, Section of Toxicology
Director, Toxicology Fellowship Program
University of Texas Southwestern Medical Center
Associate Medical Director
Emergency Services Department
Parkland Memorial Hospital
Dallas, Texas

Wendy Klein-Schwartz, PharmD, MPH
Associate Professor
University of Maryland School of Pharmacy
Coordinator of Research and Education
Maryland Poison Center
Baltimore, Maryland

Edward P. Krenzelok, PharmD
Professor of Pharmacy and Pediatrics
University of Pittsburgh
Director, Pittsburgh Poison Center
University of Pittsburgh Medical Center
Pittsburgh, Pennsylvania

Melisa W. Lai, MD
Department of Pediatrics
Harvard Medical School
Boston, Massachusetts

Frédéric Lapostolle, MD, DMC
Emergency Medicine
SAMU 93, EA3409
Hôpital Avicenne
Université Paris XIII
Bobigny, France

Eric J. Lavonas, MD
Division of Medical Toxicology
Department of Emergency Medicine
Director, Medical Toxicology Hospital Services
Medical Director, Hyperbaric Medicine
Carolinas Medical Center
Charlotte, North Carolina

Michael Levine, MD
Resident, Emergency Medicine
Harvard Affiliated Emergency Medicine Residency
Harvard Medical School
Resident, Emergency Medicine
Massachusetts General Hospital/Brigham & Women's
    Hospital Residency in Emergency Medicine
Boston, Massachusetts

William J. Lewander, MD
Professor of Pediatrics
Brown University School of Medicine
Director, Pediatric Emergency Medicine
Hasbro Children's Hospital
Rhode Island Children's Hospital
Providence, Rhode Island

Ivan E. Liang, MD
Assistant Professor of Emergency Medicine
Tufts University Medical School
Attending Physician
St. Elizabeth's Hospital
Boston, Massachusetts

Erica L. Liebelt, MD, FACMT
Associate Professor of Pediatrics and Emergency Medicine
University of Alabama at Birmingham School of Medicine
Director, Medical Toxicology Services
UAB Hospital and Children's Hospital
Birmingham, Alabama

James G. Linakis, PhD, MD
Associate Professor of Emergency Medicine and Pediatrics
Brown University School of Medicine
Associate Director, Pediatric Emergency Medicine
Hasbro Children's Hospital
Rhode Island Hospital
Providence, Rhode Island

Christopher H. Linden, MD
Professor
Division of Medical Toxicology
Department of Emergency Medicine
University of Massachusetts Medical School
Worcester, Massachusetts

Richard Lynton, MD
Assistant Clinical Professor
Department of Internal Medicine
University of California School of Medicine
Davis, California
Attending Physician
VA Northern California Health Care System
VA Medical Center Sacramento
Mather, California

Rebekah C. Mannix, MD
Instructor in Pediatrics
Staff Physician, Division of Emergency Medicine
Children's Hospital Boston
Boston, Massachusetts

Jack Maypole, MD
Assistant Professor of Pediatrics
Boston University School of Medicine
Department of Pediatrics
Boston Medical Center
Director of Pediatrics
South End Community Health Center
Boston, Massachusetts

R.B. McFee, DO, MPH
Assistant Professor
Department of Preventive Medicine
State University of New York at Stony Brook
Stony Brook, New York
Consultant
Long Island Regional Poison and Drug Information Center
Winthrop University Hospital
Mineola, New York

Charles McKay, MD, FACMT, FACEP, ABIM
Associate Professor of Emergency Medicine
University of Connecticut School of Medicine
Farmington, Connecticut
Section Chief
Division of Medical Toxicology
Department of Traumatology and Emergency Medicine
Hartford Hospital
Hartford, Connecticut

Jude McNally, BSPharm, RPH, DABAT
College of Pharmacy
University of Arizona
Tucson, Arizona

Bruno Mégarbane, MD, PhD
Assistant Professor
Université Paris VII
Physician in Critical Care Medicine
Medical and Toxicological Critical Care Department
Hôpital Lariboisière
Paris, France

J. Meulenbelt, MD, PhD
Senior Lecturer in Intensive Care and Clinical Toxicology
University Medical Center Utrecht
Utrecht, Netherlands
Director, National Poisons Information Center
National Institute for Public Health and the Environment
Bilthoven, Netherlands

Dana B. Mirkin, MD
Occupational Health Physician
St. David's Occupational Health Services
Austin, Texas

Brent W. Morgan, MD
Associate Professor
Emory University
Georgia Poison Center
Atlanta, Georgia

Brian Morrissey, MD
Assistant Professor of Medicine
University of California—Davis School of Medicine
Davis, California
University of California—Davis Medical Center
Sacramento, California

Allison A. Muller, BS, PharmD
Adjunct Faculty
University of Pennsylvania School of Veterinary Medicine
Adjunct Assistant Professor
Temple University School of Pharmacy
Adjunct Assistant Professor
University of the Sciences
Philadelphia College of Pharmacy
Clinical Managing Director
The Children's Hospital of Philadelphia Poison Control
   Center
Philadelphia, Pennsylvania

Nancy G. Murphy, MD
Lecturer
Department of Emergency Medicine
Dalhousie University
Medical Director
IWK Regional Poison Centre
Halifax, Nova Scotia, Canada

Kristine A. Nañagas, MD
Assistant Professor
Division of Medical Toxicology
Department of Emergency Medicine
Indiana University School of Medicine
Indiana Poison Center
Indianapolis, Indiana

Jeffrey B. Nemhauser, MD
Medical Officer
Radiation Studies Branch
Centers for Disease Control and Prevention
Atlanta, Georgia

Heikki Erik Nikkanen, MD
Instructor in Medicine
Harvard Medical School
Attending Physician
Department of Emergency Medicine
Brigham & Women's Hospital
Attending Physician
Division of Medical Toxicology
Children's Hospital
Boston, Massachusetts

Kent R. Olson, MD, FACEP, FAACT, FACMT
Clinical Professor of Medicine, Pediatrics, and Pharmacy
Division of Clinical Pharmacology
University of California, San Francisco
Medical Director, San Francisco Division
California Poison Control System
San Francisco, California

John D. Osterloh, MD, MS
Chief Medical Officer and Toxicologist
Centers for Disease Control and Prevention
Atlanta, Georgia

Wesley Palatnick, MD, FRCPC, DABEM, DABMT
Professor and Head
Section of Emergency Medicine
University of Manitoba
Medical Director
Department of Emergency Medicine
Health Sciences Centre
Winnipeg, Manitoba, Canada

Robert B. Palmer, PhD, DABAT
Toxicologist
Toxicology Associates, Prof LLC
Assistant Clinical Professor
University of Colorado School of Medicine
Denver, Colorado
Adjunct Associate Professor
University of Wyoming
Laramie, Wyoming

Alberto Perez, MD, FACEP, ABMT
Assistant Clinical Professor
University of Connecticut School of Medicine
Farmington, Connecticut
Emergency Physicion/Medical Toxicologist
Windham Community Memorial Hospital
Willimantic, Connecticut

Holly E. Perry, MD
Assistant Professor of Pediatrics
University of Connecticut School of Medicine
Consultant
Connecticut Regional Poison Control Center
Farmington, Connecticut
Staff Physician
Connecticut Children's Medical Center
Hartford, Connecticut

Scott D. Phillips, MD, FACP, FACMT
Associate Clinical Professor
Department of Medicine
University of Colorado Health Sciences Center
Attending Faculty
Rocky Mountain Poison and Drug Center
Denver, Colorado

David C. Pigott, MD
Residency Program Director
Associate Professor and Vice Chair for Education
Department of Emergency Medicine
University of Alabama at Birmingham
Birmingham, Alabama

Heidi Pinkert, MD
Clinical Assistant Professor of Emergency Medicine
Weill Medical College of Cornell University
New York, New York
Attending Physician
Lincoln Medical and Mental Health Center
Bronx, New York

Alex T. Proudfoot, BSc, MB, FRCPE, FRCP
Consultant Clinical Toxicologist
National Poison Information Service (Birmingham Unit)
Birmingham, United Kingdom

Rouhollah Prueitt, MD
Clinical Instructor
University of Texas Southwestern Medical Center
Toxicology Fellow
Parkland Memorial Hospital
Dallas, Texas

Lawrence S. Quang, MD
Assistant Professor of Pediatrics
Case Western Reserve University School of Medicine
Medical Director
Greater Cleveland Poison Control Center
Attending Physician
Division of Pediatric Emergency Medicine and the Mary Ann Swetland Center for Environmental Health
Rainbow Babies and Children's Hospital
University Hospitals Case Medical Center
Cleveland, Ohio

James W. Rhee, MD
Assistant Professor
Section of Emergency Medicine
The University of Chicago
Chicago, Illinois

William H. Richardson, MD
Medical Director
Palmetto Poison Center
Palmetto Health Richland Medical Center
Clinical Assistant Professor
University of South Carolina
South Carolina College of Pharmacy
Columbia, South Carolina

Jon C. Rittenberger, MD
Instructor
Department of Emergency Medicine
University of Pittsburgh School of Medicine
Pittsburgh, Pennsylvania

Steven D. Salhanick, MD
Staff Toxicologist
Children's Hospital Boston
Boston, Massachusetts

Anthony J. Scalzo, MD, FAAP, FACMT, FAACT
Professor and Director
Division of Toxicology
St. Louis University School of Medicine
Medical Director
Missouri Regional Poison Control Center
St. Louis, Missouri

Heather K. Schuller, PharmD
Clinical Toxicologist
SafetyCall International Poison Center
Bloomington, Minnesota

Michael D. Schwartz, MD
Medical Toxicologist
Division of Toxicology
Agency for Toxic Substances and Disease Registry
Centers for Disease Control and Prevention
Georgia Poison Center
Atlanta, Georgia

Donna Seger, MD, FAACT, FACEP, ABMT
Associate Professor of Medicine and Emergency Medicine
Department of Medicine and Emergency Medicine
Medical Director
Tennessee Poison Center
Vanderbilt University Medical Center
Nashville, Tennessee

Michael W. Shannon, MD, MPH, FAAP, FACEP, FAACT, FACMT
Chief and CHB Chair
Division of Emergency Medicine
Children's Hospital Boston
Professor of Pediatrics
Harvard Medical School
Senior Toxicologist
MA/RI Regional Center for Poison Control and Prevention
Associate Director
The Pediatric Environmental Health Center
Boston, Massachusetts

Mahesh Shrestha, MD
Adjunct Professor of Medicine and Surgery
University of Texas Southwestern Medical School
Dallas, Texas
Emergency Department Physician
Crozer-Chester Medical Center
Upland, Pennsylvania

Leo J. Sioris, PharmD
Professor
Department of Experimental and Clinical Pharmacology
College of Pharmacy
University of Minnesota
Minneapolis, Minnesota
Senior Clinical Toxicologist
SafetyCall International Poison Center
Bloomington, Minnesota

Marco L. Sivilotti, MD, MSc, FRCPC, FACEP, FACMT
Associate Professor
Departments of Emergency Medicine and Pharmacology and Toxicology
Queen's University
Kingston, Ontario, Canada
Consultant
Ontario Regional Poison Information Center
Hospital for Sick Children
Toronto, Ontario, Canada

Sara Skarbek-Borowska, MD
Assistant Professor
Department of Emergency Medicine
University of New Mexico School of Medicine
Assistant Professor
Department of Emergency Medicine
The University of New Mexico Health Sciences Center
Albuquerque, New Mexico

Susan C. Smolinske, PharmD, DABAT
Associate Professor
Department of Pediatrics
Wayne State University
Managing Director
Children's Hospital of Michigan Regional Poison
   Control Center
Detroit, Michigan

Curtis P. Snook, MD, FACEP, FACMT
Consultant
Cincinnati Drug and Poison Information Center
Cincinnati Children's Hospital Medical Center
Cincinnati, Ohio

David G. Spoerke, MS, RPH
Freelance Pharmacognosy Writer
Lakewood, Colorado

Jeffrey R. Suchard, MD, FAECP, FACMT
Associate Professor of Clinical Emergency Medicine
Director of Medical Toxicology
Department of Emergency Medicine
University of California–Irvine Medical Center
Orange, California

Young-Jin Sue, MD
Department of Pediatrics
Division of Pediatric Emergency Medicine
Clinical Associate Professor of Pediatrics
Albert Einstein College of Medicine
Attending Physician
Pediatric Emergency Services
Children's Hospital at Montefiore
Bronx, New York

Matthew D. Sztajnkrycer, MD, PhD
Assistant Professor of Emergency Medicine
Mayo Medical School
Consultant
Department of Emergency Medicine
Mayo Clinic
Rochester, Minnesota
Staff Toxicologist
Hennepin Regional Poison Center
Minneapolis, Minnesota

Sharon Ternullo, BS, PharmD, CSPI
Adjunct Faculty
Albany College of Pharmacy
Albany, New York
Coordinator of Drug Information
Certified Poison Information Specialist
Ruth A. Lawrence Regional Poison and Drug
   Information Center
University of Rochester Medical Center
Rochester, New York

Dung Thai, MD, PhD
Medical Director
Medical Sciences
Amgen, Inc.
South San Francisco, California

R. Steven Tharratt, MD, MPVM
Professor of Clinical Internal Medicine
School of Medicine
University of California–Davis
Sacramento Division
California Poison Control System
Kaiser Permanente North
Sacramento, California

Jerry D. Thomas, MD
Assistant Professor of Emergency Medicine
Emory University School of Medicine
Toxicologist
Georgia Poison Center
Atlanta, Georgia

Karen E. Thomas, MPH
Consulting Epidemiologist
Georgia Poison Center
Atlanta, Georgia

Josef G. Thundiyil, MD, MPH
Assistant Clinical Professor of Emergency Medicine
Orlando Regional Medical Center
Orlando, Florida

Anthony J. Tomassoni, MD, MS, FACEP, FACMT
Associate Professor
University of Vermont College of Medicine
Burlington, Vermont
Medical Director
Northern New England Poison Center
Maine Medical Center
Portland, Maine

Stephen J. Traub, MD
Assistant Professor of Medicine
Harvard Medical School
Co-Director
Division of Toxicology
Beth Israel Deaconess Medical Center
Boston, Massachusetts

John Harris Trestrail III, BSPharm, RPh, FAACT, DABAT
Managing Director
DeVos Children's Hospital Regional Poison Center
Grand Rapids, Michigan

J. Allister Vale, MD, FRCP, FRCPS, FFOMFAACT, FCBTS
National Poison Information Service (Birmingham
  Unit) and West Midlands Poison Unit
City Hospital
Birmingham, United Kingdom

Jason Vena, MD
Fellow in Medical Toxicology
University of Connecticut
Hartford Hospital
Hartford, Connecticut

Frank G. Walter, MD, FACEP, FACMT, FAACT
Associate Professor of Emergency Medicine
Chief, Division of Medical Toxicology
University of Arizona College of Medicine
Director of Clinical Toxicology
University Medical Center
Tucson, Arizona

Richard Y. Wang, DO
Senior Medical Officer
Organic Analytical Toxicology Branch
Division of Laboratory Sciences
National Center for Environmental Health
Centers for Disease Control and Prevention
Atlanta, Georgia

Sharita E. Warfield, MD, MS
Associate Clinical Professor
Department of Emergency Medicine/Toxicology
Wayne State University
Detroit, Michigan
Attending Physician/Medical Toxicologist
Department of Emergency Medicine/Toxicology
Detroit Medical Center
Detroit, Michigan

Paul M. Wax, MD
Clinical Professor of Surgery (Emergency Medicine)
University of Texas Southwestern
Dallas, Texas

Suzanne R. White, MD
Dayanandan Professor and Chair
Department of Emergency Medicine
Wayne State University School of Medicine
Medical Director
Children's Hospital of Michigan Regional Poison
  Control Center
Detroit Medical Center
Detroit, Michigan

James F. Wiley II, MD, MPH
Professor of Pediatrics and Emergency Medicine/
  Traumatology
University of Connecticut School of Medicine
Consultant
Connecticut Regional Poison Control Center
Farmingham, Connecticut

Saralyn R. Williams, MD
Associate Professor of Clinical Medicine
Department of Medicine
Department of Emergency Medicine
Vanderbilt University
Nashville, Tennessee

Alan David Woolf, MD, MPH
Associate Professor of Pediatrics
Harvard Medical School
Program Director
Environmental Health
Children's Hospital Boston
Boston, Massachusetts

Mark Yarema, MD, FRCPC
Division Chief, Research
Department of Emergency Medicine
Calgary Health Region
Calgary, Alberta, Canada

Luke Yip, MD, FACMT
Clinical Assistant Professor
School of Pharmacy
Department of Pharmaceutical Sciences
University of Colorado Health Sciences Center
Attending Staff Physician
Consultant Clinical Toxicologist
Department of Medicine
Division of Medical Toxicology
Denver Health Medical Center
Attending Faculty
Consultant Clinical Toxicologist
Rocky Mountain Poison and Drug Center
Denver, Colorado

PREFACE

This fourth edition of *Clinical Management of Poisoning and Drug Overdose*, is re-titled to include the name of its creators, Lester Haddad and Jim Winchester. While neither of them was formally trained in medical toxicology, Lester and Jim were visionary in recognizing the need for a comprehensive toxicology textbook. From the first edition in 1983 to the 3rd edition in 1998, Haddad and Winchester compiled the key information that clinicians who manage poisoned patients would need; they were successful in their goal of providing a resource that was clear, succinct, and evidence-based, without expansive discussions of underlying molecular biology or exhaustive literature reviews. Equally important, with each edition, Haddad and Winchester recruited medical toxicologists as authors, in order to present recommendations from those who were recognized experts in the field. With plans to write a fourth edition, Drs. Haddad and Winchester entrusted us to continue their vision for this textbook. We are honored to assume this responsibility and hope that we have been successful in maintaining its value. As with previous editions, we write *Haddad and Winchester's Clinical Management of Poisoning and Drug Overdose* for emergency physicians, pediatricians, internists, occupational/environmental medicine physicians, and public health officials, as well as medical toxicology fellows, house officers, and medical students.

The subspecialty of medical toxicology continues to evolve rapidly. For example, since the last edition of the textbook, no less than 4 new antidotes have entered clinical practice. The number of board certified medical toxicologists now exceeds 300 with these experts providing consultation to poison centers, academic medical centers, emergency departments, laboratories, and government agencies. With the growth of medical toxicology as a subspecialty has also come the same maturation that all new clinical fields undergo. Included in the process of maturation is greater rigor in medical toxicology research, the development of basic science research niches by medical toxicologists, and success with receiving extramural funding from NIH and other agencies that support the principles of high-quality research that advances human health.

The establishment of medical toxicology as a distinct clinical subspecialty has greatly benefited poisoned patients. Gone is the era in which there was debate about whether there was a well-defined body of knowledge about poisonings that called for the creation of a distinct subspecialty; medical toxicologists are now recognized as possessing expertise that truly makes a difference in patient outcome after a poisoning. The U.S. Department of Health and Human Services, in acknowledgement of the importance of poison centers and the medical toxicologists who direct them, has begun to fund poison centers as a vital part of public health.

In order to meet the needs of clinicians, this 4th edition of *Haddad and Winchester's Clinical Management of Poisoning and Drug Overdose* has added several new features. First, to make this edition as authoritative as possible, we recruited practicing toxicologists to write each chapter. Parenthetically, this is also the first edition in which all the editors are medical toxicologists, who have primary practices in pediatrics, emergency medicine, and occupational/environmental medicine. Second, along with Elsevier, we have attempted to create a textbook with international appeal and value. Contributors to this edition include medical toxicologists in England, Australia, and elsewhere. Our hope is that clinicians from all countries will find each chapter useful and relevant to their practice. Finally, in an era of frequent acts of terrorism and other disasters, we have created a new section, *Disasters and Terrorism*. New chapters, including *Principles of Children's Environmental Health, Ill-Defined Toxic Syndromes* and *Performance Enhancers*, reflect new medical issues that clinicians regularly face.

The three of us thank our superb group of contributors who provided their thorough and conscientious expertise in each chapter. We thank the supportive staff of Elsevier, particularly Todd Hummel, who helped us navigate the project from beginning to end. We thank our families and loved ones, who permitted us to devote the many hours needed to create a work such as this. Finally, we extend to our readers the hope that this text will benefit them in their pursuit of knowledge about principles of poison management and in the care of their patients.

MICHAEL W. SHANNON, MD, MPH
STEPHEN W. BORRON, MD, MS
MICHAEL J. BURNS, MD

CONTENTS

PART I

General Information

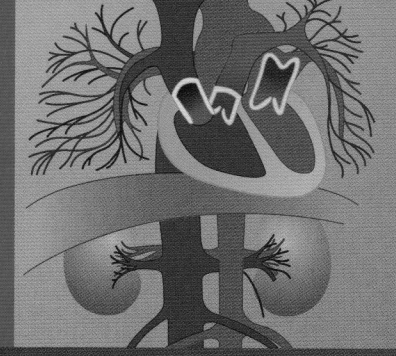

1

The History of Toxicology

MICHAEL W. SHANNON, MD, MPH

Although it is difficult to provide a strict definition of *poison*, in its broadest definition the term denotes any substance that has the ability to harm a living organism from either the plant or animal kingdom. However, in the discipline of clinical toxicology, poison generally refers to any agent that can kill, injure, or impair normal physiologic function in humans.[1,2]

The history of toxicology, including its writers, poisons, and poisoners, is extensive and colorful; the field can clearly claim a lineage that traces back more than 10,000 years. Over these millennia, the science (and art) of poisons and poisoning has been punctuated by events that provide a useful perspective. This chapter provides an overview of select events that have shaped the practice of medical toxicology.

HISTORICAL TIMELINE

Ancient Times

Throughout these early years of recorded history, the use of poisons was well described. The Sumerians of Mesopotamia are given credit for chronicling (circa 1400 BC) the world of poisons in their descriptions of the spirit Gula, who was "the mistress of charms and spells." The ancient Greeks were familiar with the toxicities of metals, particularly arsenic, and the poisonous plant hemlock (*Conium maculatum*). Developed as a tool for capital punishment, hemlock was used to execute Socrates in 402 BC. The ancient Romans also developed and utilized poisons; homicide with agents including amygdalin (cyanide) and belladonna were favored. Papyri from the period around 300 BC provide evidence that ancient Egyptians understood and exploited the toxic properties of arsenic, copper, lead, and antimony. Dioscorides (AD 40–90), a physician and pharmacologist, is credited with creating the first treatise of toxicology, the *Materia Medica* (Fig. 1-1).[3] In his text, which remained an authoritative reference for the next 15 centuries, he created a classification scheme for poisons, distinguishing between those of plant, animal, and mineral origin. Another important figure of this era was Mithradates VI, King of Turkey during the period 114–63 BC (Fig. 1-2). Mithradates lived in constant fear of being poisoned.[4] He therefore studied antidotes extensively and can be considered a pioneer in the development of antidotal therapy. Mithradatum was the name given to one of his famous antidotes.

The Medieval Era

This period of clinical toxicology also contains unique chapters. During this time, apothecaries, corresponding to modern-day pharmacists, provided both "potions and poisons." Commonly used poisons of this era included arsenic and other heavy metals, amygdalin, strychnine, belladonna, and aconite.

The Renaissance

By the Middle Ages, toxicology had reached great prominence. Italian alchemists often devoted their careers to

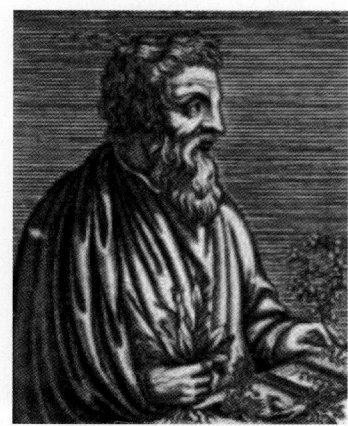

FIGURE 1-1 Dioscorides. (From Wikipedia: Pedanius Dioscorides.)

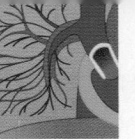

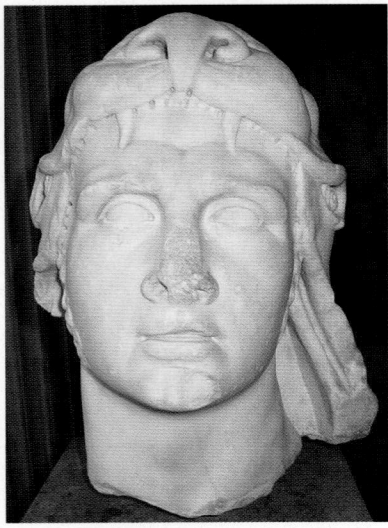

FIGURE 1-2   King Mithradates. (From Anonymous: C. Julius Caesar.)

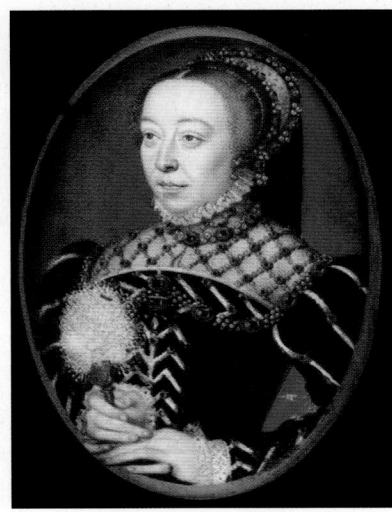

FIGURE 1-4 Catherine De Medici. (From Anonymous: Who's Who in Tudor history.)

developing lethal agents. Famous names during this period were the Borgias, a family of reputed poisoners, and Paracelsus. Born Theophrast von Hohenheim, Paracelsus (1493–1541) was an alchemist, physician, and astrologer (Fig. 1-3).[5] He is considered one of the "fathers of toxicology." A committed student of toxicology, Paracelsus is credited with making the famous statement, "All things are poison and nothing is without poison; only the dose makes that a thing which [sic] is no poison." One of the most important publications of the era was *Neopoliani Magioe Naturalis,* written in 1589 by Giovanni Battista Porta. This book described different methods of poisoning the unsuspecting.

The 16th through 18th Centuries

Throughout the 16th century, the development of poisoning techniques spread rampantly across Europe as Italian alchemists migrated to France. Catherine de

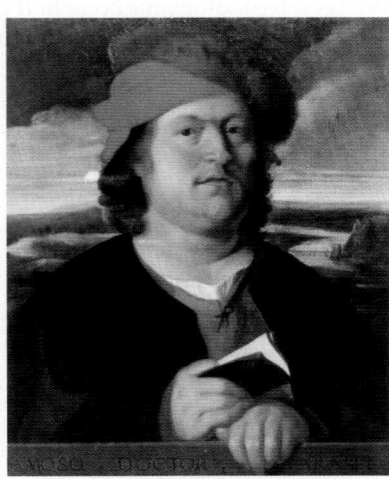

FIGURE 1-3 Paracelsus, painted by a student of Rubens. (From The Alchemy Web Site: Paracelsus.)

Médici is credited with bringing many of the Italian techniques of poisoning to France (Fig. 1-4).[6] During this era, the French School of Poisoners became hugely popular. In an effort to contain the growing epidemic of poisoning, King Louis XIV began to limit the availability of toxic agents; for example, he forbade apothecaries from selling arsenic and required purchasers to sign a register. The king ultimately created the Chambre Ardente, a council that was responsible for investigating poisonings. Many members of nobility (e.g., Queen Elizabeth) appointed food tasters to ensure that no poison had been surreptitiously placed in their food. By the 17th century, poisoning had become a scientific discipline; schools of toxicology were established in both Venice and Rome.[7]

The 19th through 21st Centuries

During these centuries, toxicology took several new paths. First, during the Victorian period (19th century), forensic toxicology was developed in an effort to apprehend poisoners. Important techniques of investigation, including postmortem analysis, began to appear. This was also a period of remarkable drug discovery and development, with many pharmaceutical agents proving, as Paracelsus said, to be both beneficial and harmful. Many infamous drugs were developed during this era, including ipecac, cocaine, opium (laudanum), and barbiturates. While all had great therapeutic value, their toxicity was at the same time discovered and eventually feared.

Another important aspect of this period was, in parallel with the industrial revolution, the birth of occupational toxicology. As many valuable but toxic consumer products were developed, the need to protect workers from toxicologic threats ushered in a new scientific and public health field. One of the most important figures of this period was Dr. Alice Hamilton (Fig. 1-5).[8,9] Dr. Hamilton (1869–1970) was the first U.S. physician to

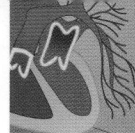

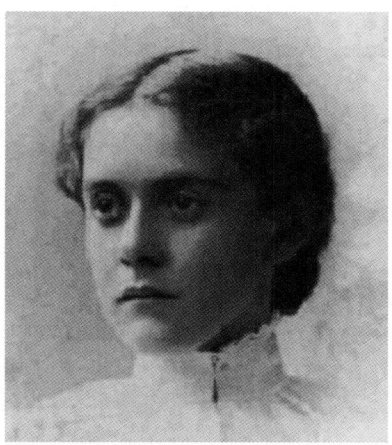

FIGURE 1-5 Alice Hamilton, MD.

name and residence. Authorities eventually discovered her and accused her of being an accomplice to more than 600 homicides. She was arrested and ultimately tortured and strangled in prison.

Mary Ann Cotton (1832–1873) is considered one of the most prolific serial killers in English history (Fig. 1-6).[10] She is suspected of murdering more than 21 unsuspecting victims before she was caught, convicted, and hanged. Victims of Mary Cotton usually succumbed to a severe gastrointestinal disorder ("gastric fever"), ultimately traced to her penchant for using arsenic to poison her victims.

Harold Shipman (1946–2004) was one of the most prolific serial killers in modern history (Fig. 1-7). A British physician, he is estimated to have killed 250 patients between 1970 and 1988. Dr. Shipman's modus operandi was to prey on the elderly, particularly elderly

devote herself to research in industrial medicine. Writing her first article on the topic in 1908, she went on to become the first woman on the faculty of Harvard University.

The 20th and 21st centuries have been filled with many more events and accomplishments in medical toxicology. Perhaps the most important of these has been the development of a mammoth pharmaceutical industry, which can be credited with creating new drugs at a remarkable pace. With the development and use of many drugs has come, often tragically, the discovery of unanticipated toxicities. The study of drug toxicity has also led to important new principles of pharmacology (e.g., drug interactions). Finally, in the current "era of the gene," pharmacology has added the disciplines of pharmacogenomics, which explores the ways in which an individual's genetic makeup predetermines how he or she will respond to a medication or even a toxin (e.g., both lead and mercury toxicity are now known to be modulated by several key genes).

Another important aspect of 20th and 21st century toxicology has been the focus on poisoning management. Over the past 50 years, poison centers have been created around the world, assisting clinicians and the public in poisoning management; prevention has become an equally important part of the poison control mission.

FAMOUS POISONERS, POISONS, AND POISONINGS

Poisoners

A 17th century Neapolitan woman known simply as Toffana (1653–1723) invented an arsenic-based face paint called Acqua Toffana. This potion was primarily marketed as a cosmetic; female customers would consult with Toffana to learn the proper uses of the makeup. Reportedly, many women became rich widows after wearing the cosmetic on their cheeks when in the presence of their spouses. Because of her dread of being revealed as a poisoner, Toffana continually changed her

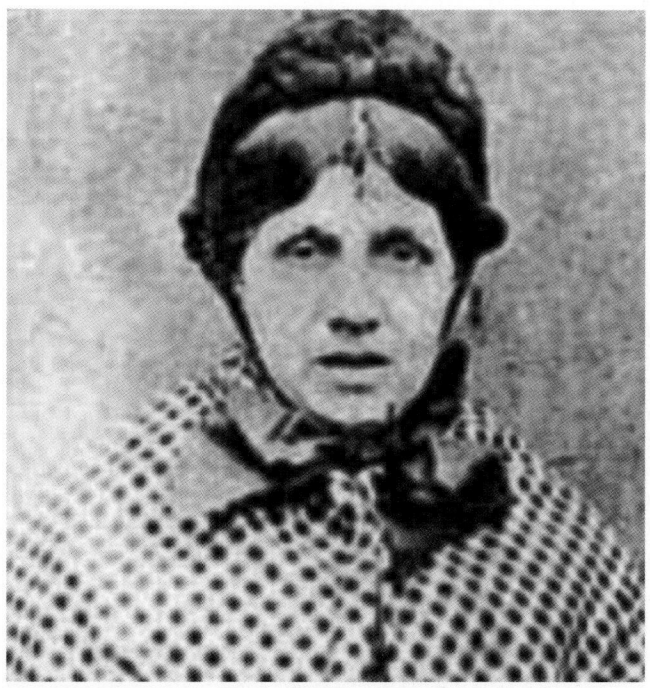

FIGURE 1-6 Mary Ann Cotton. (From Anonymous: The poisoners—Mary Ann Cotton.)

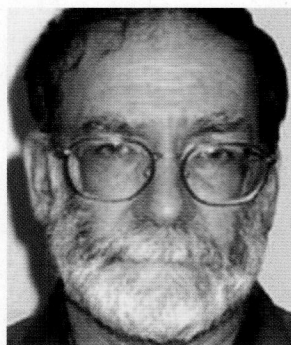

FIGURE 1-7 Dr. Harold Shipman. (From British Broadcasting Corporation: Shipman Draws 7.3M viewers.)

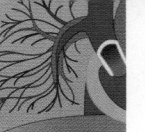

women. During home visits he would inject his victims with morphine, giving the appearance that they died from the complications of their advanced years; he was also usually the signatory on the victims' death certificates. Dr. Shipman was ultimately arrested and convicted of killing 15 men and women. In 2004, while imprisoned, he committed suicide.

Shoko Asahara (born Chizuo Matsumoto [1955–]) was the founder of the religious group Aum Shinrikyo (Fig. 1-8).[11] In March 1995, on a Monday morning (intentionally timed to produce the greatest number of casualties), he and his followers orchestrated the release of the nerve agent sarin in multiple subway cars carrying Tokyo commuters. In the process, he became the architect of one of the most important events of domestic terrorism in history. Asahara's apocalyptic efforts actually began in 1994, when his cult first released sarin in a small residential area within the city of Matsumoto; this resulted in injury to more than 600 residents; 7 died in that incident.[12,13] In the sarin release in 1995, however, multiple cult members effectively coordinated the widespread release of the poison. Victims developed cholinergic toxicity that was sometimes severe, consisting of miosis, vomiting, abdominal pain, respiratory distress, seizures, and respiratory failure. Ultimately 5500 casualties were produced, of which 984 were moderately affected; at least a dozen victims died.[12]

Poisons

ARSENIC

As a poison, arsenic has a long and infamous history. Ancient documents suggest this heavy metal was recognized as early as 500 BC; its first use as a poison is thought to date back to the 8th century. While arsenic was used medicinally (e.g., Fowler's solution was a widely used 18th and 19th century medication prescribed for dermatitis and for asthma), its primary use was as a poison. Stories of homicidal arsenic poisoning are found

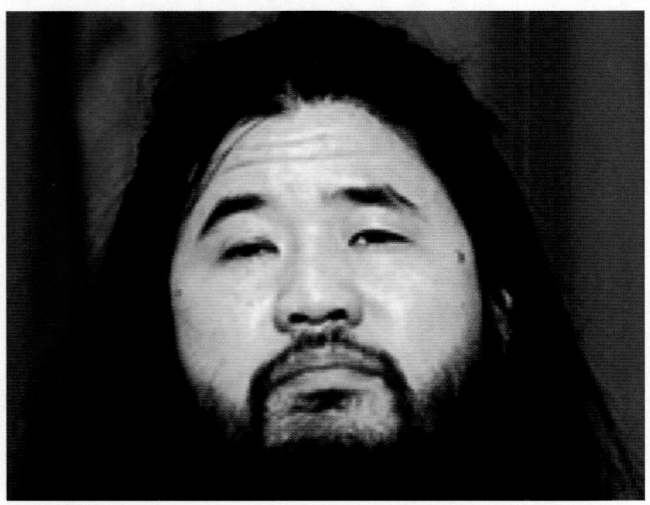

FIGURE 1-8 Shoko Asahara. (From Wikipedia: Profile: Shoko Asahara.)

throughout history. The metal's toxicity was exploited during World War II with development of the arsenic-based chemical weapon lewisite. The Allies, working diligently, were able to develop an antidote against lewisite, British anti-lewisite (BAL).[14] BAL, also known as dimercaprol, proved to be a very valuable chelator; it is still used to treat poisoning by arsenic, lead, and other metals. Other details of arsenic's history are found in Chapter 74.

COCAINE

The alkaloid derived from erythroxylon coca is a toxic medicinal that has also enjoyed a long and illustrious history. Coca chewing dates back to 3000 BC; cocaine was isolated and used as a medication in the 19th century. A popular substance, it was added to wine and other beverages, well into the 20th century.[15] As a therapeutic agent, cocaine was unique because (1) it had great therapeutic value; (2) it had a very narrow therapeutic window, with toxicity, sometimes life-threatening, appearing even in those who were taking it in appropriate doses; and (3) it was highly addictive. A long list of individuals, including Sigmund Freud, Robert Louis Stevenson, and the legendary American surgeon William Halstead, became addicted to cocaine during their careers. In the 1980s, cocaine alkaloid (first known as "free-base" and then "crack") appeared, creating an even more addictive drug. Through the 1990s, crack use in the United States became epidemic, producing an extraordinarily large population of cocaine abusers. Cocaine remains one of the most widely abused drugs in the world. Chapter 42 describes cocaine and its history in greater detail.

OPIUM (LAUDANUM)

The discovery of opium dates back to ancient civilization; Hippocrates wrote of the virtues of poppy wine for medicinal purposes. In the 15th century, Paracelsus mixed it with alcohol, producing "tincture of laudanum." Through the 17th and 18th centuries, use of opium by people of all socioeconomic strata spread quickly. Like cocaine, the drug was found to have remarkable therapeutic value, which often came at the cost of hopeless addiction. In much of the 19th and early 20th centuries, the opium derivative known as laudanum was widely used to treat a range of illnesses. Heroin succeeded laudanum and equally addicted historical figures such as Elizabeth Barret Browning, Lenny Bruce, Charlie Parker, William Borroughs, and Janis Joplin.

CYANIDE

The toxicity of bitter almonds, ground peach pits, and cassava were known well before cyanide was specifically identified in 1782. Once isolated and synthesized, the toxin, being a potent pesticide, was a boon to the agriculture industry. However, its lethal effects on those who were inadvertently exposed after improper handling were also quickly discovered. Cyanide's greatest infamy, however, is associated with its use during the Hitler regime when, as part of his ethnic cleansing campaign ("The Final Solution"), millions were executed with Zyklon-B, a cyanide-based substance used in the gas

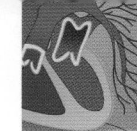

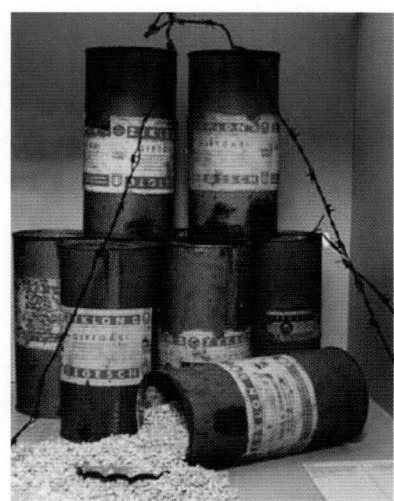

FIGURE 1-9 Zyklon B, a cyanide-containing substance used during the Holocaust. (From Anonymous: Judaism.)

chambers of occupation camps (Fig. 1-9). Cyanide continues to be used as a homicidal agent, in gas chamber executions that are part of capital punishment. The agent is discussed further in Chapter 88.

Poisonings

History records many poisoning events made infamous by the large number of individuals affected. Large scale poisonings have included:

> War-related events (e.g., the use of chemical weapons during both World Wars)
>
> Industrial catastrophes (e.g., Minamata Bay, Japan, and Bhopal, India)
>
> Climactic/geological events (e.g., the London smog and Lake Nyos "eruption")
>
> Pharmaceutical disasters (e.g., eosinophilia-myalgia syndrome, gasping baby syndrome, and thalidomide disasters)
>
> Food-borne poisonings (e.g., "St. Anthony's fire" and aflatoxin epidemics)
>
> Domestic terrorism (e.g., sarin release in Tokyo subways)

A brief description of several of these events is described below.

EOSINOPHILIA-MYALGIA SYNDROME

In 1989, an illness appeared in the United States, characterized by the onset of myalgia, arthralgia, weakness, rash, and scleroderma-like skin changes. Associated laboratory findings included evidence of rhabdomyolysis and a striking eosinophilia.[16,17] Known as *eosinophilia-myalgia syndrome* (EMS), the disease rapidly spread throughout the United States. Epidemiologic investigation quickly traced the disease to use of the dietary supplement L-tryptophan, which had become a popular remedy for insomnia, premenstrual syndrome, depression, and other maladies. Further investigation linked the development of EMS to use of L-tryptophan from specific

manufacturing lots.[18,19] By March 1990, the Centers for Disease Control and Prevention (CDC) had identified almost 1500 cases of EMS with at least 38 deaths. Ultimately, the L-tryptophan produced by a single manufacturer was incriminated.[20,21] Careful inspection of the manufacturing site revealed that a significant production change had recently occurred; the former technique, in which tryptophan was produced by a fermentation process involving the bacterium *Bacillus amyloliquefaciens,* was altered by the introduction of a new strain of *B. amyloliquefaciens.* As a result, there appeared to be increased synthesis of several tryptophan intermediates. A specific chemical contaminant, di-tryptophan aminal of acetaldehyde (DTAA) was specifically incriminated (Fig. 1-10) in the development of EMS.[22,23] Closure and immediate changes in the manufacturing process led to the disappearance of this disorder as quickly as it began. However, many victims were left with enduring health problems.[24]

GASPING BABY SYNDROME

In spring 1981, an unusual illness appeared in neonatal intensive care units (NICUs). NICU staff noted that newborns who had been clinically stable would suddenly develop multisystem disease, severe metabolic acidosis, and a haunting gasp, which signaled their death. Known as *gasping baby syndrome,* the illness spread across NICUs nationally. In June 1981, a New Orleans neonatologist, Dr. Juan Gershanik, noted in a postmortem urine analysis for organic acids that large amounts of hippuric acid, a known metabolite of benzyl alcohol, were found. Noticing that vials of bacteriostatic water containing 0.9% benzyl alcohol were present throughout the NICU, Dr. Gershanik reported his suspicion that gasping baby syndrome was the result of excessive benzyl alcohol administration secondary to the liberal use of bacteriostatic saline.[25] Other pediatricians began to report similar suspicions.[26,27] The Food and Drug

A

B

FIGURE 1-10 Di-tryptophan aminal of acetaldehyde (DTAA), incriminated in the etiology of the eosinophilia-myalgia syndrome. Original (*A*) and revised (*B*) structures are shown.

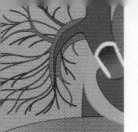
Administration and American Academy of Pediatrics soon recommended that bacteriostatic saline no longer be used in NICUs. When this occurred, neonatal mortality rates around the country fell dramatically; reports of mortality rates falling from 50% to 2% appeared.[28,29] There was also a noticeable fall in the incidence of kernicterus and intraventricular hemorrhage among ill neonates.[28,30] Ultimately, conservative estimates were that benzyl alcohol was responsible for more than 300 neonatal deaths and thousands of permanent neurologic disabilities.

THE THALIDOMIDE DISASTER

Thalidomide was developed as a sedative-hypnotic; it became popular soon after it was first marketed in 1957. Known as Contergan in Germany, Distaval in England, and Kevadon in Canada, thalidomide quickly became the third-largest selling drug in Europe; by 1960, it was being sold around the world. Its reported efficacy in the treatment of hyperemesis gravidarum led to even greater use of the drug by pregnant women. However, when the Merrell Company of Cincinnati submitted a New Drug Application to market Kevadon in the United States on September 12, 1960, a young, new FDA scientist, Dr. Frances O. Kelsey, was assigned to perform the review (Fig. 1-11). Dr. Kelsey was dissatisfied with the safety data submitted for thalidomide and denied approval of the drug.[31] In the midst of FDA battles with Merrell, in November 1961, McBride and Lenz, working independently of each other, both published reports suggesting a link between the use of thalidomide and development of phocomelia and other limb abnormalities (Fig. 1-12).[32] As little as one dose of thalidomide, taken during a critical period of gestation, was found to produce a range of devastating birth defects. The drug was withdrawn in 1962, but not before it had produced more than 10,000

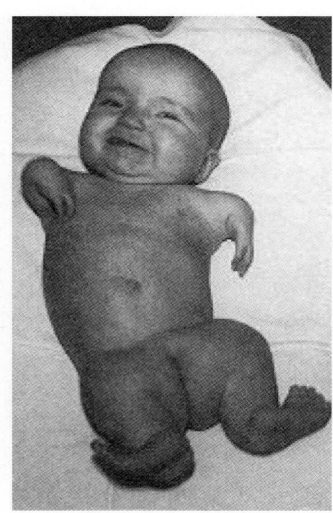

FIGURE 1-12 Thalidomide-associated phocomelia.

children with limb abnormalities. Dr. Kelsey, credited with preventing the thalidomide disaster from occurring in the United States, was awarded the Gold Medal Award for Distinguished Federal Civilian Service by President John F. Kennedy.

MINAMATA BAY

From 1932 to 1968, the Chisso Corporation near Minamata Bay, Japan, dumped an estimated 27 tons of mercury compounds into Minamata Bay. In 1956, four inhabitants of Minamata Bay were noted to have an unusual neurologic disease, thought initially to be infectious.[12] Investigation quickly led to the discovery that many people of the region had similar symptoms of diffuse numbness, slurred speech, and tunnel vision. Ultimately more than 50,000 were affected, with more than 2000 unequivocally having what became known as Minamata disease. The range of symptoms in adults included tingling sensations, muscle weakness, ataxia, tunnel vision, slurred speech, hearing loss, and abnormal behavior. Approximately 30 offspring of the inhabitants were born with severe, devastating neurologic disease, which included spasticity, mental retardation, seizures, and visual disturbances (Fig. 1-13).[33]

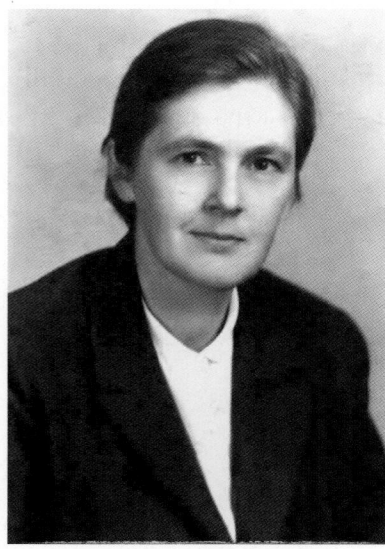

FIGURE 1-11 Food and Drug Administration scientist Frances O. Kelsey, credited with preventing the sale of thalidomide in the United States.

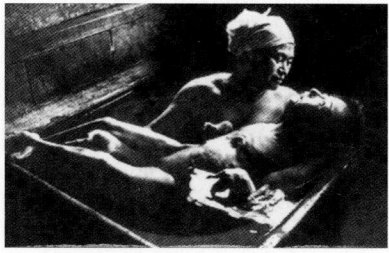

FIGURE 1-13 Childhood victim of Minamata disease. (Photo by W. Eugene Smith. From McCann HG: Mercury found in midwest rain.)

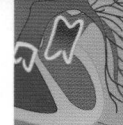

LONDON SMOG

On December 4, 1952, an unusual temperature inversion struck London. This climatic event trapped the polluted air that was being regularly discharged from the millions of coal fires that burned daily.[34] For the subsequent week, concentrations of smog became so thick, visibility fell to a few yards; concentrations of ambient particulate matter were as high as 400 μg/m³.[34] Thousands of Londoners developed respiratory ailments, including pneumonia, bronchitis, and asthma. An estimated 12,000 citizens died from respiratory problems produced by "The Great London Smog" (Fig. 1-14).

LAKE NYOS

On August 21, 1986, Lake Nyos, a large volcanic lake located in Cameroon, released a massive cloud of carbon dioxide. Being heavier than air, the carbon dioxide descended on the villages located in a valley 250 m below. Witnesses described loud rumbling sounds made by the lake followed by the appearance of an enormous white cloud; an estimated 10^9 m³ of volcanic gas was released.[12] Victims succumbed quickly to the anesthetic effects of high-concentration carbon dioxide. Upon arrival of the medical teams, 1700 humans and all animal and insect life in the region were dead.[12]

BHOPAL

One of the most significant industrial disasters in history occurred on the morning of December 3, 1984, at a large chemical plant in Bhopal, India. The plant, owned by Union Carbide, contained large storage tanks of methyl isocyanate gas (the compound was used as a precursor to the pesticide carbaryl). Without warning, during the dark hours of early morning, a methyl isocyanate tank ruptured, spreading the toxic gas across the streets of Bhopal. Wakened by suffocation, large numbers of victims arrived to local hospitals with sudden blindness and respiratory distress. More than 200,000 were affected by the gas; the death toll was estimated to be approximately 2500.[12] Many Bhopal survivors were left with chronic, disabling lung disease.[35,36]

JONESTOWN, GUYANA

The Reverend Jim Jones was a religious zealot who in 1977, after creating the People's Temple in San Francisco, created the township of Jonestown in Guyana, South America, bringing with him more than 1000 followers (Fig. 1-15). Initial reports from Jonestown indicated that

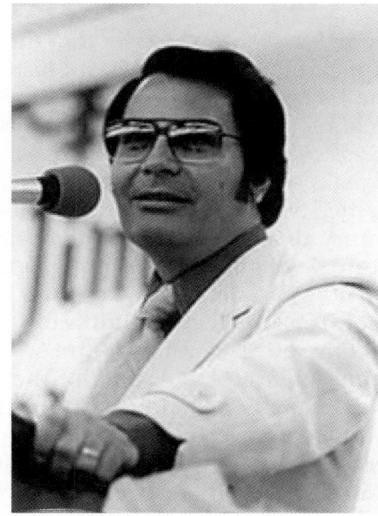

FIGURE 1-15 Reverend Jim Jones.

Jones's disciples lived in apparent happiness. However, when several residents sent reports of cruel treatment, coercion, and bondage to relatives in the United States, Congressman Leo Ryan went to Jonestown to investigate abuse allegations, bringing with him an 18-member party of officials, reporters, and members of "Concerned Relatives of Peoples Temple Members." Arriving in Jonestown in November 1978, Congressman Ryan was prevented from interviewing inhabitants and carrying out his planned investigation. When he attempted to leave Jonestown, he was gunned down at an airstrip by Jones disciples. On November 18, 1978, fearing that additional authorities would soon come and possibly close Jonestown, Reverend Jones called for the mass suicide of his disciples. All drank or were forced to drink a grape flavored beverage that contained Valium and cyanide. The 276 children were killed first; a total of 914 died, including Reverend Jones, who died of a self-inflicted gunshot wound (Fig. 1-16).[37]

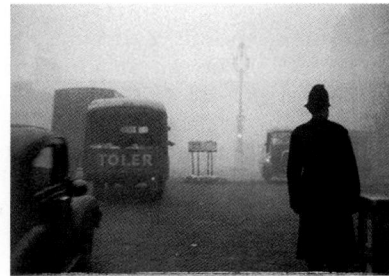

FIGURE 1-14 London smog, 1952. (From National Public Radio: London during the killer smog.)

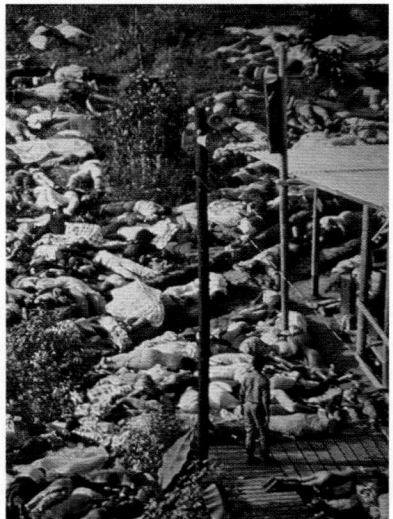

FIGURE 1-16 The mass suicide at Jonestown, Guyana, 1978.

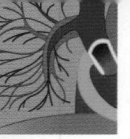

ST. ANTHONY'S FIRE

Described by a 9th century writer, St. Anthony's fire, which has appeared several times in history, was the popular name for epidemic ergotism that resulted from the ingestion of rye that had been contaminated with the fungus *Claviceps purpurea*. Also referred to as "dancing mania," outbreaks of St. Anthony's fire appeared repeatedly between the 13th and 16th centuries. It was not until the 17th century that its cause was identified. The last reported outbreak occurred in France in 1951.[38] There are also beliefs that women accused of witchcraft in the Salem trials of 1692 had ergot-induced psychosis and seizures.[39] Victims of St. Anthony's fire would typically develop burning pain and gangrene of the extremities, convulsions, hallucinations, and psychosis; death would often ensue. Ergot's powerful vasocontrictive properties were responsible for the severe extremity vasospasm that produced pain and gangrene. Central nervous system effects were the apparent result of the alkaloid's effects on serotonin receptors. Interestingly, the study of ergot alkaloids led to the development of the hallucinogen lysergic acid diethylamide (LSD), as well as therapeutic agents including ergotamine, dihydroergotamine, methysergide, and others.

THE DEVELOPMENT OF MEDICAL TOXICOLOGY

Since the early 20th century, organized efforts in poisoning management and prevention have led to the development of medical toxicology as a clinical discipline that is distinct from other medical subspecialties. Key events in this process were the establishment of poison control centers, followed by the creation of important supporting organizations.

Poison Control Centers

By the 1930s, childhood poisoning had become a common cause of unintentional injury to children, accounting for almost 50% of significant childhood accidents. Household products (e.g., lye) were a particularly common source of severe and often fatal poisoning. However, there was little information on the toxicity of household products that could be used in prompt and effective management of childhood poisoning. In the 1930s, Dr. Jay Arena, a pediatrician at Duke University, began to compile data on the household products, providing advice to local clinicians. Dr. Arena is credited with writing one of the first modern textbooks on poisoning management.

Prior to the 1950s, there was no formal system for poisoning treatment in the United States.[40] By this time, there were well over 250,000 different brand name products on the market. Health care professionals presented with cases of acute poisoning usually had little knowledge of what ingredients were contained in these new products, making it difficult to treat these patients. A Chicago pharmacist, Louis Gdalman, began recording information on the toxicity of various products on small cards; he also developed a data collection form that he would use when he provided consultations. In November 1953, he helped to establish the first poison center in the United States at Presbyterian-St Luke's Hospital. In 1958, the American Association of Poison Control Centers (AAPCC) was formed. From here, poison centers proliferated: By 1970, there were almost 600 centers nationally. At the same time, poisoning fatalities in children dropped dramatically. The AAPCC was instrumental in creating multiple preventive efforts, including the establishment of National Poison Prevention Week and enactment of the Poison Prevention Packaging Act. As poison centers increasingly served the function of a public health agency, the AAPCC developed a means for monitoring and reporting epidemiologic data, known as the Toxic Exposure Surveillance System (TESS). Annual data from TESS are now published by the AAPCC for use by those who are interested in tracking the epidemiology of poisoning (www.aapcc.org). In 2002, a universal telephone number for access to poison control centers (800-222-1222) was established, simplifying access to poison centers.

The Subspecialty of Medical Toxicology

As principles of poisoning management and prevention established themselves, several organizations were created to support the clinicians who provided this care. In 1968, the American Academy of Clinical Toxicology (AACT) was formed. Consisting of physicians, pharmacists, scientists, and veterinarians, the AACT began to expand the focus of poisoning beyond childhood exposures to adult poisonings, including intentional exposures (attempted suicides), workplace exposures, drug interactions, envenomations, and environmental toxicology. Around the world, similar organizations were established, including the European Association of Poison Centres and Clinical Toxicologists (EAPCCT), the Canadian Association of Poison Control Centers (CAPCC), and the Australian Society of Clinical and Experimental Pharmacologist and Toxicologist (ASCEPT).

As these efforts evolved, it became clear that toxicology had evolved into a well-defined medical specialty. As such, standards for training and certification were needed. In 1974 the AACT created the American Board of Medical Toxicology (ABMT), a physician-only organization responsible for establishing fellowship training guidelines and creating a certifying examination. Medical toxicology fellowships began to appear; the first board examination in medical toxicology was given in 1974. However, the field of medical toxicology suffered from ABMT's position as an independent certifying organization, rather than a member of the American Board of Medical Specialties (ABMS) which, by this time, had established itself as an umbrella organization that housed the specialties and subspecialties recognized by the American Medical Association. The ABMT and medical toxicology therefore struggled to gain the same stature as ABMS specialties and subspecialties. This led to efforts by ABMT leaders to find parent organizations within the ABMS who would sponsor medical toxicology as a new, defined clinical subspecialty. These efforts culminated in

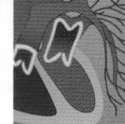

1992 with three ABMS boards—the American Board of Pediatrics, the American Board of Emergency Medicine, and the American Board of Preventive Medicine—agreeing to make medical toxicology a jointly supported subspecialty. The Subboard in Medical Toxicology was formed, providing the first ABMS certifying examination in 1994. Simultaneously, the ABMT was reestablished as the American College of Medical Toxicology (ACMT), with the goal of being a scientific organization that provides support to the medical toxicology community.

Currently, there are approximately 300 practicing, board-certified medical toxicologists, indicating the relative youth of the field. These individuals have vital roles in medicine and public health, being in federal agencies (e.g., the Food and Drug Administration, and Centers for Disease Control), medical directors of poison control centers (a requirement for poison center certification), directors of occupational health programs, and physician-scientists.

CONCLUSION

Throughout recorded time, toxicology has been part of the fabric of society. While its history has been dark at times, the evolving clinical specialty of poisoning management/prevention and the establishment of medical toxicology as a subspecialty have provided important public health advances. The science of toxicology will undoubtedly continue to provide both important discoveries and other memorable events in future years.

REFERENCES

1. Gallo MA: History and scope of toxicology. In Klaassen CD (ed): Toxicology—The Basic Science of Poisons, 5th ed. New York, McGraw-Hill, 1996.
2. Shannon M, Haddad L: Emergency management of poisoning. In Shannon M, Haddad L, Winchester J (eds): Clinical Management of Poisoning and Drug Overdose. Philadelphia, Saunders, 1998, pp 2–31.
3. Anonymous: Pedanius Dioscorides. Wikipedia, http://en.wikipedia.org/wiki/Pedanius_Dioscorides. Accessed May 22, 2006.
4. Lendering J: C. Julius Caesar. http://www.livius.org/caa-can/caesar/caesar02.html, accessed May 21, 2006.
5. McLean A: Portraits of Paracelsus. The Alchemy Web Site, http://www.levity.com/alchemy/paracelsus_portraits.html, accessed May 21, 2006.
6. Eakins LE: Who's Who in Tudor History. http://tudorhistory.org/people/medici. Accessed May 21, 2006.
7. Holdworth T, Tasker K, Thompson A, et al: The history of poisoning—timeline. In *Poisoning Through the Ages.* http://www.portfolio.mvm.ed.ac.uk/studentwebs/session2/group12/contents.html, accessed May 21, 2006.
8. Anonymous: Dr. Alice Hamilton. Chemical Achievers—The Human Face of the Chemical Sciences. The Chemical Heritage Foundation, http://www.chemheritage.org/classroom/chemach/environment/hamilton.html, accessed May 22, 2006.
9. Centers for Disease Control and Prevention: Alice Hamilton, MD. MMWR 1999; 48:462. http://www.cdc.gov/mmwr/preview/mmwrhtml/MM4822bx.htm, accessed May 22, 2006.
10. Anonymous: The poisoners—Mary Ann Cotton. The Crime Library—Criminal Minds and Methods. http://www.crimelibrary.com/criminal_mind/forensics/toxicology/5.html, accessed May 22, 2006.
11. Anonymous: Profile: Shoko Asahara. Wikipedia, http://en.wikipedia.org/wiki/Shoko_Asahara, accessed May 22, 2006.
12. Langford N, Ferner R: Episodes of environmental poisoning worldwide. Occup Environ Med 2002;59:855–860.
13. Morita H, Yanagisawa N, Nakajima T, et al: Sarin poisoning in Matsumoto, Japan. Lancet 1995;356:290–293.
14. Vilensky JA, Redman K: British anti-lewisite (dimercaprol): an amazing history. Ann Emerg Med 2003;41:378–383.
15. Anonymous: Written Testimonials in the History of Advertising. Wikipedia, http://en.wikipedia.org/wiki/Testimonial, accessed May 22, 2006.
16. Shapiro S, Kilbourne EM, Eidson M, et al: L-tryptophan and eosinophilia-myalgia syndrome. Lancet 1994;344:817–819.
17. Hertzman PA, Clauw DJ, Kaufman LD, et al: The eosinophilia-myalgia syndrome: status of 205 patients and results of treatment 2 years after onset. Ann Intern Med 1995;122:851–855.
18. Hertzman PA, Blevins WL, Mayer J, et al: Association of the eosinophilia-myalgia syndrome with the ingestion of tryptophan. N Engl J Med 1990;322:869–873.
19. Kamb ML, Murphy JJ, Jones JL, et al: Eosinophilia-myalgia syndrome in L-tryptophan-exposed patients. JAMA 1992;267:77–82.
20. Slutsker L, Hoesly FC, Miller L, et al: Eosinophilia-myalgia syndrome associated with exposure to tryptophan from a single manufacturer. JAMA 1990;264:213–217.
21. Belognia EA, Hedberg CW, Gleich GJ, et al: An investigation of the cause of the eosinophilia-myalgia syndrome associated with tryptophan use. N Engl J Med 1990;323:357–365.
22. Larkin M: Contaminant found in over-the-counter 5-hydroxy-L-tryptophan. Lancet 1998;352:791.
23. Centers for Disease Control and Prevention: Analysis of L-tryptophan for the etiology of eosinophilia-myalgia syndrome. MMWR 1990;39:589–591.
24. Sullivan EA, Kamb ML, Jones JL, et al: The natural history of eosinophilia-myalgia syndrome in a tryptophan-exposed cohort in South Carolina. Arch Intern Med 1996;156:973–975.
25. Gershanik J, Boecler G, Ensley H, et al: The gasping syndrome and benzyl alcohol poisoning? N Engl J Med 1982;307:1385–1388.
26. Lovejoy FH: Fatal benzyl alcohol poisoning in neonatal intensive care units—a new concern for pediatricians. Am J Dis Child 1982;136:974–975.
27. Brown WJ, Buist NRM, Gipson H, et al: Fatal benzyl alcohol poisoning in a neonatal intensive care unit. Lancet 1982;1:1250.
28. Hiller JL, Benda GI, Rahatzad M, et al: Benzyl alcohol toxicity: impact on mortality and intraventricular hemorrhage among very low birth weight infants. Pediatrics 1986;77:500–506.
29. Committee on Fetus and Newborn and Committee on Drugs: Benzyl alcohol: toxic agent in neonatal units. Pediatrics 1983;72:356–358.
30. Jardine DS, Rogers K: Relationship of benzyl alcohol to kernicterus, intraventricular hemorrhage, and mortality in preterm infants. Pediatrics 1989;83:153–160.
31. McFadyen RE: Thalidomide in America: a brush with tragedy. Clio Med 1976;2:79–93.
32. Lenz W: Thalidomide and congenital abnormalities. Lancet 1962;1:45–46.
33. Tsubaki T, Irukayama K: Minamata Disease. Amsterdam, Elsevier Scientific, 1977.
34. Donaldson K: The biological effects of coarse and fine particulate matter. Occup Environ Med 2003;60:313–314.
35. Cullinan P, Acquilla S, Dhara VR: Respiratory morbidity 10 years after the Union Carbide gas leak at Bhopal: a cross sectional survey. BMJ 1997;314:338.
36. Desikan P: Bhopal: the lingering tragedy. BMJ 2004;329:1410.
37. Anonymous: Jonestown. Wikipedia, http://en.wikipedia.org/wiki/Jonestown, accessed May 21, 2006.
38. Fuller JG: The Day of St. Anthony's Fire. New York, McMillan, 1968.
39. Caporael L: Ergotism: the Satan loosed in Salem? Science 1976;192:21–26.
40. Burda A, Burda N: The nation's first poison control center: taking a stand against accidental childhood poisoning in Chicago. Vet Hum Toxicol 1997;39:115–119.

2 *Emergency Management of Poisoning*

A A General Approach to Poisoning

MICHAEL W. SHANNON, MD, MPH

Medical toxicology is one of the most important and dynamic fields in medicine today, since the practicing physician is continually faced with the management of poisoning, drug overdose, and adverse drug effects. The abuse of both prescription and illicit drugs in the United States continues unabated. Because the process of drug approval is more rapid, it is often not until the agent has been in use for some time, during the postmarketing period, before its toxicity is fully appreciated.

Defining the incidence of human poisoning is not easy. There are multiple sources of data on drug overdose and substance abuse. The Toxic Exposure Surveillance System (TESS) of the American Association of Poison Control Centers tabulates referrals for human poisoning called into the nation's poison centers. In 2004, it recorded 2,395,582 exposures, with 1106 deaths; analgesics were the most common cause of a fatal outcome.[1] The National Institute of Drug Abuse surveys emergency department visits through its Drug Abuse Warning Network (DAWN), and in 2002 reported that a total of 4427 deaths resulted from drug abuse, with cocaine being the most commonly implicated agent.[1,2]

However, these sources vastly underestimate the number of toxic events in humans. For example, reports of intoxicated patients who die from trauma, drowning, and fires are not consistently included in any national data set, nor are those of patients with medical complications from therapy, such as chemotherapy or anesthetics. Morbidity that results from chronic abuse (e.g., heart disease from cocaine or nicotine abuse and cirrhosis from alcohol abuse) or industrial exposures, and the long-term effects of environmental hazards, is not rigorously compiled and is probably impossible to quantify.

The most common causes of poisoning-related death in the United States have been carbon monoxide poisoning, cocaine use, and tricyclic antidepressant overdose.[1] Poisoning with analgesics, aspirin, and acetaminophen also remains a leading cause of death. Calcium channel blocker overdose has surpassed digitalis overdose as the most common cause of cardiovascular drug-related death.

DEFINITION

To poison means to injure or kill with a substance that is known or discovered to be harmful. Thus, the term *poisoning* connotes clinical symptomatology. It also implies that the toxic exposure is unintentional (e.g., in the case of an elderly patient who misreads a drug label). In contrast, the term *overdose* implies intentional toxic exposure, either in the form of a suicide attempt or as inadvertent harm secondary to purposeful drug abuse. The terms *poisoning* and *drug overdose* often are used interchangeably, especially when prescription drugs are the agents, even though by definition a drug overdose does not produce poisoning unless it causes clinical symptoms.

Poisoning has a bimodal incidence, occurring most commonly in children who are 1 to 5 years of age and in the elderly. Overdose, whether motivated by suicidal intent or the result of abuse, occurs through adulthood. Toxic exposure in those between the ages of 6 and 12 years is uncommon; when it occurs, the patient must be assessed carefully to ensure that psychiatric follow-up is provided when indicated.[1]

THE GENERAL APPROACH TO POISONING

The general approach to the poisoned patient can be divided into six phases: (1) stabilization; (2) laboratory assessment; (3) decontamination of the gastrointestinal tract, skin, or eyes; (4) administration of an antidote; (5) elimination enhancement of the toxin; and (6) observation and disposition.

Emergency Management

Because overdose patients are often clinically unstable when discovered, resuscitation with establishment of the airway, adequate support of ventilation and perfusion, and maintenance of all vital signs (including temperature) must be accomplished first. Continuous cardiac and pulse oximetry monitoring is essential. Rapid-sequence intubation (RSI) may be indicated in patients with an airway in jeopardy. Naloxone, 2 mg intravenously (IV); thiamine, 100 mg intravenously (IV); and 50% dextrose, 50 mL IV (if patients are shown on Dextrostix testing to be hypoglycemic) are generally given to all adults in coma, once an IV line has been established and appropriate blood studies have been performed.[3,4] Maintenance of blood pressure and tissue perfusion may require the provision of volume, correction of acid-base disturbance, administration of pressor agents, and antidotal therapy. Table 2A-1 lists the common emergency antidotes.

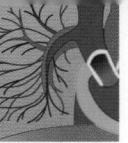

TABLE 2A-1 Common Emergency Antidotes

POISON	ANTIDOTE	DOSE*	COMMENTS
Acetaminophen	N-acetylcysteine	140 mg/kg initial oral dose, followed by 70 mg/kg every 4 hr × 17 doses or intravenously as 150 mg/kg × 15 minutes then 50 mg/kg × 4 hr then 100 mg/kg × 16 hr	Most effective within 16–24 hr; may be useful after chronic intoxication
Atropine, anticholinergics	Physostigmine	Initial dose 0.5–2 mg (IV); children, 0.02 mg/kg	Can produce convulsions, bradycardia
Benzodiazepines	Flumazenil	0.2 mg (2 mL) (IV) over 15 sec; repeat 0.2 mg (IV) as necessary; initial dose not to exceed 1 mg	Limited indications; recommended only for reversal of pure benzodiazepine sedation
β blockers	Glucagon	Adult: 5–10 mg (IV) initially Child: 50–150 ug/kg (IV) initially Continuous infusion as needed	Stimulates cAMP synthesis, increasing myocardial contractility
Calcium channel blockers	Calcium chloride 10%	1 g (10 mL) (IV) over 5 min as initial dose; repeat as necessary in critical patients; doses up to 10 g may be necessary to restore blood pressure	Avoid extravasation; tissue destructive
	Insulin/glucose	0.5–1.0 U/kg initially then 0.5–1.0 U/kg/hr as needed to maintain systolic blood pressure	Monitor serum potassium and glucose
Carbon monoxide	Oxygen	1–3 atmospheres	Hyperbaric oxygen may be indicated
Cyanide	Amyl nitrite, then sodium nitrite, then sodium thiosulfate	Administer pearls every 2 min Adult: 10 mL of 3% solution over 3 min (IV) Child: 0.33 mL (10 mg of 3% solution)/kg over 10 minutes Adult: 25% solution, 50 mL (IV) over 10 minutes Child: 25% solution, 1.65 mL/kg	
Digitalis	Digoxin antibody fragments	Varies by patient weight, serum digoxin concentration, and/or dose ingested	
Hydrofluoric acid	Calcium	Topical exposure: Apply calcium gluconate gel; if pain is not relieved, administer 10% calcium gluconate 10 mL in 40 mL D₅W via IV (Bier block) infusion; if pain is not relieved, administer calcium gluconate by intra-arterial infusion over 4 hr Ingestion: 10% calcium gluconate (IV)	Monitor for hypocalcemia; treat electrolyte disturbances aggressively
Iron	Deferoxamine mesylate	Initial dose: 40–90 mg/kg (IV or IM), not to exceed 1 g; Infusion: 15 mg/kg hr (IV)	Higher infusion doses may be needed in severe overdose to achieve chelant excess; monitor and treat hypotension
Metals Mercury Arsenic Gold	British antilewisite (BAL), also known as dimercaprol	4-6 mg/kg IM, every 4–8 hr	Contraindicated if patient has a peanut allergy or G6PD deficiency
Lead	DMSA (succimer), CaNa₂ EDTA	10 mg/kg/dose, bid × 28 days 35–50 mg/kg/day (maximum 1.0–1.5g), bid or as a continuous infusion	Monitor liver function tests, add BAL if lead level > 70 µg/dL in children, > 100 µg/dL in adults
Methanol	Ethyl alcohol	500 mg/kg of 10% ethanol, then continuous infusion of 100 mg/kg/hr	Watch for hypoglycemia, hypothermia, and lethargy in children; solution is hyperosmolar, requiring central venous catheter in children; maintain serum ethanol concentration at 100 mg/dL
	Fomepizole	15 mg/kg loading dose, 10 mg/kg every 12 hr IV	Significantly safer than ethanol
Nitrites (and other methemoglobin formers)	Methylene blue	1–2 mg/kg of 1% solution (IV) over 5 min	Can produce hemolysis in high dose; give no more than 7 mg/kg/day in adults, 4 mg/kg/day in children; severe or resistant cases may require exchange transfusion

Continued

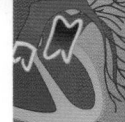

TABLE 2A-1 Common Emergency Antidotes (*Cont'd*)

POISON	ANTIDOTE	DOSE*	COMMENTS
Opiates and opioids	Naloxone	Adults: 0.4–2.0 mg (IV or IM) Child: 0.01–0.1 mg/kg (IV or IM)	Larger doses may be necessary after severe overdose or overdose of synthetic agent, e.g., propoxyphene
	Nalmafene	Adult: 1 mg (IV) Child: 0.25 ug/kg (IV)	
Organophosphates, nerve agents Carbamates (severe exposure)	Atropine	Adult: 0.5–2 mg IV Child: 0.05 mg/kg Child: 0.05 mg/kg	Enormous doses of atropine may be needed in severe cases
	Pralidoxime (2-PAM)	Adult: 1 g (IV) then 500–1000 mg/hr as needed Child 15–40 mg/kg then 15–40 mg/kg/hr	Must be added to atropine if nicotinic or central symptoms are present
Tricyclic antidepressants	Sodium bicarbonate	Sodium bicarbonate 1–2 ampules (IV), bolus or infusion	Administer if QRS interval is ≥ 100 msec; maintain serum pH at 7.45–7.55; avoid severe alkalosis

cAMP, cyclic adenosine monophosphate; DMSA, dimercaptosuccinic acid; EDTA, ethylenediaminetetraacetic acid; G6PD, glucose-6-phosphate deficiency; IM, intramuscularly; IV, intravenously.
*Dosage listed may require modification or adjunctive therapy according to specific clinical conditions; see each specific chapter for details.

BOX 2A-1 CLINICAL CONDITIONS AND EXAMPLE AGENTS IN THE POISONED PATIENT THAT MAY NECESSITATE ENDOTRACHEAL INTUBATION

Corrosive ingestion (sodium hydroxide, sulfuric acid)
Corrosive inhalation (ammonia, chlorine)
Envenomation (hymenoptera, crotalid)
Anaphylaxis (hymenoptera)
Pulmonary edema (opioids, chemical weapons [e.g., choking agents])
Bronchorrhea (organophosphates or nerve agents)
Severe central nervous system (CNS) depression (ethanol, opioids, barbiturates)
Cerebrovascular accident (cocaine)
Seizures (isoniazid, theophylline)
Aspiration (hydrocarbons)
Hypercarbia (CNS depressants, nerve agents, botulism)

ADVANCED AIRWAY MANAGEMENT

In addition to basic airway management, many victims of poisoning require advanced management that includes endotracheal intubation. Clinical situations in which endotracheal intubation may be necessary in poisoned patients are numerous (Box 2A-1). Intubation offers the advantages of complete airway control, protection from aspiration of gastric contents, provision of a route for suctioning of secretions, and a means of optimizing both oxygenation and ventilation. However, the process of intubating an awake patient is difficult and is associated with potential adverse effects, including coughing, gagging, vomiting, tachycardia or bradycardia, hypertension, hypoxia, and increased intracranial pressure. Moreover, emergency intubation can be challenged by vocal cords that are obscured by secretions, unusual airway anatomy, a full stomach, or active vomiting.

Therefore, this task requires a thorough understanding of advanced airway management principles and of their application in a manner that prevents worsening of the clinical situation. RSI is a method of rapidly obtaining airway control with minimal physiologic disturbance. The process of RSI involves a patterned sequence of preparation, drug administration, intubation, and postintubation management.[5-7]

In the emergency department, RSI has historically had its greatest role in the patient with severe head trauma in whom intubation could exacerbate already increased intracranial pressure. However, because it is designed to blunt or prevent all adverse responses associated with endotracheal intubation, RSI is the ideal method of intubation in the poisoned patient. With the use of drugs having a short duration of action, RSI also is advantageous because it is a measure that permits temporary airway control for the patient with mildly compromised airway reflexes who requires gastrointestinal decontamination (lavage followed by activated charcoal administration) but who does not require prolonged intubation. RSI requires several essential steps that include the use of pharmacologic agents (Table 2A-2). To be performed safely, RSI must occur in the following sequence.

Evaluation

The clinician must first evaluate the patient's airway to determine the necessary equipment and the best technique for safe intubation. Particular attention should be directed to abnormalities in the cervical spine and temporomandibular joint because these will significantly impede rapid and uncomplicated intubation. If there is any question about the stability of the cervical spine, immobilization must be maintained. The oral cavity should be closely examined for the presence of foreign bodies.

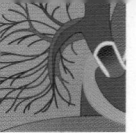

TABLE 2A-2 Pharmacotherapy Used in Rapid Sequence Intubation

AGENT	DOSE*	
Pretreatment Agents		
Atropine	0.01–0.02 mg/kg (minimum, 0.1 mg; maximum, 1.0 mg)	
Lidocaine	1–2 mg/kg	
Sedatives and Anesthetics		
BARBITURATES		
Sodium thiopental	3–5 mg/kg	
Methohexital	1 mg/kg	
BENZODIAZEPINES		
Midazolam	0.1 mg/kg	
ETOMIDATE	0.1–0.3 mg/kg	
KETAMINE	1–2 mg/kg	
OPIOIDS		
Fentanyl	2–5 μg/kg	
PROPOFOL	2–4 mg/kg	
Skeletal Muscle Relaxants		
DEPOLARIZING AGENTS		
Succinylcholine	1–2 mg/kg	
NONDEPOLARIZING AGENTS		
	DEFASCICULATING DOSE	FULL DOSE
Pancuronium	0.01–0.05 mg/kg	0.1 mg/kg
Vecuronium	0.01–0.05 mg/kg	0.1–0.2 mg/kg
Atracurium		0.5 mg/kg
Rocuronium		0.5–1.0 mg/kg

*Doses listed are for intravenous administration.

BOX 2A-2   EQUIPMENT NEEDED FOR ENDOTRACHEAL INTUBATION

Syringe for endotracheal cuff inflation
100% oxygen
Face mask
Bag-valve apparatus
Suction equipment
Catheter
Yankauer suction tube
Stylet
Magill forceps
Oral airway
Nasopharyngeal airway ("trumpet")
Laryngoscope handle and blades
Endotracheal tubes
Tongue depressors
Syringe for endotracheal cuff inflation
Tape
Tincture of benzoin

TABLE 2A-3 Age-Specific Endotracheal Tube Sizes

AGE	INTERNAL DIAMETER (mm)
Infant	
Premature	2.5
Full term	3.0
1–6 mo	3.5
6–12 mo	4.0
Child	
2 yr	4.5
4 yr	5.0
6 yr	5.5
8 yr	6.5
10 yr	7.0
Adolescent and Adult	
12 yr	7.5
≥14 yr	8.0–9.0

Accompanying principles:
1. Small sizes are necessary for nasotracheal intubation.
2. Endotracheal tubes two sizes smaller than age appropriate should be immediately available.

Preparation

Before intubation, all necessary equipment must be present so that serious delays or unforeseen complications can be prevented. An IV line should be established and the patient connected to a cardiac monitor and pulse oximeter. The equipment necessary for endotracheal intubation is outlined in Box 2A-2. The proper functioning of all equipment should be ensured before it is used. Appropriate endotracheal tube size also should be determined (Table 2A-3). Unanticipated difficulties with intubation are common; "difficult airway" equipment (e.g., illuminated or fiberoptic-directed endotracheal tubes) should be kept close at hand.

Preoxygenation

Oxygen should be administered for 2 to 3 minutes before intubation; this produces a washout of nitrogen from the lungs, replacing this gas with an oxygen reservoir. The oxygen reservoir allows several minutes of apnea during which intubation can be performed without the risk of producing hypoxia. Assisted ventilation with bag-valve-mask apparatus should only be provided if the patient's own respiratory efforts are inadequate because it risks inflation of the stomach, which increases the likelihood of vomiting. Patients who are breathing spontaneously should be given 100% oxygen by face mask for several minutes before intubation.

Pretreatment

Pretreatment involves the administration of pharmacologic agents that prevent adverse physiologic changes that may occur during intubation. Agents included in this category are lidocaine and atropine.

IV administration of the anesthetic lidocaine appears to blunt the increase in intracranial pressure that

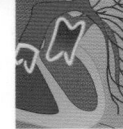

accompanies intubation. Although scientific proof of lidocaine's efficacy is sparse, it is appropriate—particularly in the patient with suspected intracranial hypertension—to administer lidocaine, 1.0 to 2.0 mg/kg IV, 3 to 4 minutes before intubation.[8-10]

Bradycardia can accompany RSI in two circumstances. In young children, both posterior pharyngeal stimulation and administration of succinylcholine can result in severe bradycardia. Therefore, in children younger than 5 years, atropine should be administered before induction. The dose of atropine is 0.01 to 0.02 mg/kg (maximum, 1.0 mg). No less than 0.1 mg of atropine should be administered because smaller doses can produce paradoxical bradycardia.

Severe bradycardia can also occur in patients of any age who have been exposed to medications or toxins with negative chronotropic actions. For example, in patients who have ingested β antagonists (e.g., propranolol), calcium channel blockers, and digoxin, RSI can produce an abrupt decrease in heart rate or frank cardiac arrest. Therefore, in patients who are undergoing RSI after exposure to these agents, atropine should either be administered prophylactically or kept immediately available should emergency administration become necessary.

Induction

Induction consists of two components: administration of a sedative/anesthetic agent to produce unconsciousness, and the subsequent administration of an agent that produces complete skeletal muscle relaxation (paralysis); both actions facilitate intubation. Because administration of these drugs leads to apnea and paralysis, it is essential that induction proceed quickly and efficiently; this underscores the importance of having all intubation equipment immediately available and in working order.

A number of medications of different pharmacologic classes are used to produce sedation before skeletal muscle relaxation (see Table 2A-2). These drugs include benzodiazepines, opioids, barbiturates, propofol, etomidate, and ketamine. Among the benzodiazepines, midazolam, when given in a dose of 0.1 mg/kg IV (up to a range of 5 to 6 mg in an adult), is ideal because its effects are rapid in onset and short in duration. The drug also offers the advantage of producing muscle relaxation and amnesia. Opioids are another class of drugs that can be used; however, many opioids, such as morphine, may prompt histamine release, with resultant hemodynamic changes. Fentanyl in a dose of 2 to 5 μg/kg is highly effective at producing rapid sedation and relaxation with minimal cardiovascular change. Several barbiturates can produce rapid sedation and relaxation. The most popular of these is sodium thiopental (dose 3 to 5 mg/kg). Equally effective but with a shorter duration of action are methohexital, propofol, and etomidate. Finally, ketamine is a dissociative anesthetic that can produce rapid onset of a state in which the patient is insensitive to pain but maintains an awake appearance and continues to have protective airway reflexes. The typical IV induction dose of ketamine is 1 to 2 mg/kg. Unlike other sedatives/anesthetics, ketamine can produce significant elevations in pulse, blood pressure, intracranial pressure, and myocardial oxygen consumption, and such an increase in any of these could worsen the patient's clinical condition. Because ketamine has a potent bronchodilating effect, it retains its important role as an induction agent in the patient with severe bronchospasm.[11-13]

After administration of a sedative/anesthetic, skeletal muscle relaxation is performed. Skeletal muscle relaxants, all of which interrupt acetylcholine function at the myoneural junction, are typically divided into depolarizing and nondepolarizing categories. Depolarizing agents, of which succinylcholine is the model drug, produce muscle depolarization before paralysis; this results in initial generalized muscle fasciculation. Nondepolarizing relaxants produce paralysis without initial depolarization. The nondepolarizing skeletal muscle relaxants include pancuronium, vecuronium, atracurium, and rocuronium.

Succinylcholine is the most popular muscle relaxant because it has several desirable properties, including a rapid onset of action (less than 1 minute) and an extremely short duration of action. Customary paralyzing doses of succinylcholine are 1 to 2 mg/kg IV.

Despite its efficacy and popularity, succinylcholine can produce several adverse effects. These include hyperkalemia, prolonged paralysis, malignant hyperthermia, and hemodynamic changes. Hyperkalemia, which can be severe, has been most commonly associated with administration of succinylcholine to those with burns, crush injuries, select neuropathies (e.g., Guillain-Barré syndrome), and myopathies (e.g., childhood muscular dystrophies). Prolonged paralysis can occur in those who have a genetic deficiency in serum cholinesterase, the enzyme that inactivates the drug. Prolonged paralysis may also occur in patients with liver disease, the elderly, and those who have ingested anticholinesterase insecticides (carbamates or organophosphates). Malignant hyperthermia is a syndrome characterized by muscle rigidity, hyperthermia, autonomic disturbances, acidosis, rhabdomyolysis, myoglobinuria, renal failure, and coagulopathy. Occurring in genetically predisposed individuals, malignant hyperthermia may appear without warning in those who are given inhalation anesthetics or succinylcholine. The mortality rate associated with this syndrome is approximately 5% to 10%. A malignant hyperthermia-like picture can also occur in children with skeletal muscular disorders (e.g., muscular dystrophy) who are given succinylcholine. Finally, succinylcholine-induced muscle depolarization can lead to transient increases in intracranial and intra-abdominal pressure, with accompanying changes in cardiac output.[14] Because of these potential adverse effects, nondepolarizing muscle relaxants are often recommended as adjuncts to or substitutes for succinylcholine use. As adjuncts, nondepolarizing agents, when given before succinylcholine, can prevent muscle fasciculation and its attendant physiologic effects. The so-called "defasciculating dose" of a nondepolarizing agent is approximately one tenth the full dose of that agent. For example, pancuronium can be given in a dose of 0.01 mg/kg IV before the

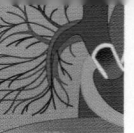

administration of succinylcholine to prevent fasciculation. Nondepolarizing agents can also be used solely for skeletal muscle relaxation. However, they generally have a much slower onset of action (as long as 3 to 5 minutes) and produce a longer duration of paralysis. Also, many nondepolarizing agents stimulate histamine release, producing significant hemodynamic changes. Therefore, they are not ideal agents for RSI. Rocuronium appears to have the most rapid onset of all nondepolarizing agents, approaching that of succinylcholine with regard to time to complete muscle relaxation in the less than ideal conditions generally found during emergency intubation.[15] Significant warnings to succinylcholine use in the pediatric population have been recently added, based on the possibility of life-threatening cardiac arrhythmias. According to these new warnings, children with undiagnosed myopathies (e.g., a muscular dystrophy) could develop hyperkalemia sufficient to produce a cardiac disturbance.[16]

Intubation

Suction must be immediately available when intubation is performed. The patient undergoing emergency intubation often has a full stomach; the risk for vomiting and aspiration is therefore significant. This risk is minimized both by the RSI technique and by the direct application of pressure on the cricoid cartilage (Sellick's maneuver), which occludes the esophagus. Adequate preoxygenation and limiting the duration of the intubation attempt to less than 20 to 30 seconds should prevent significant hypoxia.

The differences between the airway of the child and that of the adult have important implications for endotracheal intubation.

1. The child has a relatively large tongue; this makes direct visualization of the larynx difficult.
2. The child has larger tonsils, which also obscure visualization.
3. The infant's larynx is located more cephalad than that of the adult. As a result, the angle between the tongue and the glottis is more acute, and visualization of the larynx is impaired.
4. The subglottic area of the infant is the narrowest part of the larynx and may impede the passage of an endotracheal tube passed through the vocal cords.

Postintubation Management

Immediately after successful endotracheal intubation, placement of the endotracheal tube must be confirmed by detection of bilateral equal breath sounds on chest auscultation, end-tidal carbon dioxide monitoring, or chest radiography; of these, chest auscultation is the least sensitive method and should never be used in isolation to confirm endotracheal tube placement. After confirmation, the tube should be secured either with a strap or with benzoin and adhesive tape. Inflation of the endotracheal tube cuff should be performed to minimize aspiration of gastric contents (although aspiration of activated charcoal around cuffed endotracheal tubes is a

frequent occurrence). Until recently, because the airway of the young child has an area of narrowing ("physiologic cuffing"), cuffed endotracheal tubes were not used in the pediatric patient. Pediatric cuffed tubes are now available; their use is encouraged in most circumstances. If long-term intubation is necessary, sedatives/anesthetics and nondepolarizing muscle relaxants should continue to be administered.

In unskilled or unprepared hands, emergency endotracheal intubation can have disastrous consequences. Even when performed by the most experienced hands, this complex procedure can have complications that should be anticipated so that they can be quickly recognized and treated. These complications include:

Dental or oral cavity trauma
Gagging and vomiting
Hypoxia
Hypercarbia
Bradycardia
Tachycardia
Hypertension
Hypotension
Increased intracranial pressure
Pneumomediastinum
Pneumothorax
Cardiac arrhythmias
Myocardial ischemia or infarction
Aspiration
Laryngospasm
Esophageal intubation
Tracheal injury

Circulatory Support

Poisoned patients often present to the emergency department with hypotension or frank shock. Provision of circulatory support through interventions that may include volume expansion, vasopressor therapy, antidote administration, and correction of electrolyte and acid-base disturbances is essential in initial management.

Many medications and toxins produce hypotension (Box 2A-3). Depending on the ingested substance, the low blood pressure may have a number of causes. For example, blood pressure depressions may occur from direct depression of myocardial contractility (e.g., quinidine), disturbances of central nervous system cardiorespiratory centers (e.g., clonidine), severe gastrointestinal fluid losses (e.g., acetaminophen, iron, arsenic, ricin, mushrooms), peripheral vasodilation (e.g., angiotensin-converting enzyme inhibitors), or a combination of these effects (e.g., theophylline, calcium channel blockers, tricyclic antidepressants). Hypotension also can result from the secondary effects of toxins (e.g., cocaine-induced myocardial infarction). Finally, blood pressure disturbances in the poisoned patient may represent accompanying trauma (e.g., severe spinal cord injury or internal hemorrhage). With the multitude of possible causes, the clinician, on the basis of the known pathophysiology of a particular drug and after having performed a thorough physical assessment, should determine, if at

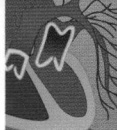

BOX 2A-3	INTOXICATIONS COMMONLY ASSOCIATED WITH HYPOTENSION

Pharmaceuticals

α Antagonists
Angiotensin-converting enzyme (ACE) inhibitors
Barbiturates
β Blockers
Calcium-channel blockers
Clonidine
Digoxin
Monoamine oxidase inhibitors
Opioids
Phenothiazines
Quinidine
Theophylline
Tricyclic antidepressants

Metals and Minerals

Arsenic
Iron

Envenomations

Marine (scombroid, ciguatera, coelenterates)
Reptile (crotalid)
Hymenoptera

Chemical Weapons

Ricin

all possible, the probable cause of hypotension if he or she is to provide a specific intervention.

VOLUME EXPANSION

Appropriate cardiac output relies on the adequacy of intravascular volume. After poisoning, intravascular volume may decrease abruptly. This decrease can be absolute, occurring as a result of a direct loss of intravascular volume (e.g., pulmonary edema, gastrointestinal pooling), or relative, resulting from severe peripheral vasodilation (e.g., angiotensin-converting enzyme inhibitor or α-antagonist overdose). In either case, hypotension should first be treated with the administration of volume-expanding agents.[17]

Many fluids are acceptable for emergency volume expansion. Normal saline and lactated Ringer's solution are generally the most readily available isotonic agents. Adults should receive up to 500- to 1000-mL boluses of isotonic fluid while blood pressure is monitored; children should be given 10 to 40 mL/kg. After the administration of each bolus, the patient should be reassessed for improvements in cardiac output.

Alternative fluids that can be used for volume expansion in the poisoned patient include albumin and whole blood. Each of these fluids has a role that is best determined by the pathophysiologic mechanism responsible for the hypotension. Being colloid rather than crystalloid in nature, these fluids in theory maintain intravascular volume better than saline solutions do. In clinical situations in which a "leaky capillary syndrome"

is mechanistically the source of intravascular volume loss, the use of colloid solutions may be preferred. Whole blood is most valuable in situations in which there is frank blood loss. With severe hemolysis (e.g., after arsine or stibine exposure), exchange transfusion with whole blood may be necessary.

Usually, the adequacy of volume expansion is determined clinically by an increase in blood pressure. Other clinical signs of improved cardiac output include resolution of cyanosis and normalization of capillary refill time. Central venous pressure and Swan-Ganz catheter monitoring, although invasive, provide the best evidence of appropriate intravascular volume.

Fluid overload is a potential complication of volume expansion. This is most likely to occur in patients who receive excess fluids over a short period of time. Also, after an overdose of a myocardial depressant such as tricyclic antidepressants or quinidine, a fluid bolus that could be tolerated by a healthy individual can produce pulmonary edema in the overdose patient. Therefore, administration of modest boluses of fluid is generally recommended; if cardiac output remains inadequate after fluids have been given, vasopressor therapy should be initiated.

VASOPRESSOR THERAPY

In the patient with severe hypotension, vasopressor therapy is necessary if blood pressure is not satisfactorily improved after volume expansion. Vasopressors are drugs that can be administered to maintain cardiac output. These agents have specific effects on the heart or blood vessels, augmenting myocardial function or increasing vasomotor tone, or both. With rare exception, vasopressors used in the acute management of hypotension are short-acting drugs that must be given by continuous IV infusion.[17]

Vasopressors generally act at adrenergic (α and β), D (dopamine), or glucagon receptors (Table 2A-4). The adrenergic system has been further defined with the recognition of two major α-adrenergic receptor subtypes (α_1 and α_2) and three β-adrenergic receptor subtypes (β_1, β_2, and β_3). Coupled with intracellular G proteins, these membrane-bound receptors effect an intracellular chain of events that includes changes in the activity of adenylate cyclase. This action goes on to modulate the level of intracellular cyclic adenosine monophosphate (cAMP), which in turn alters phospholipase activity or opens gated calcium channels. Although the cellular mechanisms of this system have become much better defined, the general principles of vasopressor action remain unchanged. For example, α-adrenergic receptor agonists produce vascular smooth muscle contraction. β_1-Adrenergic receptor agonists produce increased heart rate and contractility, whereas β_2-adrenergic receptor agonists promote generalized smooth muscle relaxation (including bronchial and vascular). Vasopressor therapy is designed to improve cardiac output through manipulation of the specific receptor most appropriate for the clinical situation. A number of vasopressors can be used to provide blood pressure support (see Table 2A-4). The

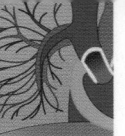

TABLE 2A-4 Common Vasopressors by Dose Range and Mechanism of Action

AGENT	α-ADRENERGIC	β₁-ADRENERGIC	β₂-ADRENERGIC	DOPAMINERGIC
		RECEPTOR TYPE		
Epinephrine (0.1–0.5 µg/kg/min)				
Low-dose		+++	+++	
Moderate-dose	+	+++	+++	
High-dose	+++	++		
Norepinephrine (0.1–0.5 µg/kg/min)	+++	++		
Dopamine (2–20 µg/kg/min)				
Low-dose				+++
Moderate-dose		+++		
High-dose	+++			
Dobutamine (2–20 µg/kg/min)	+	+++	+	
Phenylephrine (0.1–0.5 µg/kg/min)	+++			
Nonadrenergic agents				
Amrinone (5–15 µg/kg/min)				
Glucagon (50–150 µg/kg/hr)				
Calcium chloride				

+, Mild effect; ++, moderate effect; +++, major effect.

indications for the use of these drugs vary slightly, depending on the clinical circumstance.

Epinephrine

Epinephrine elevates blood pressure primarily through its α-adrenergic-stimulating properties. This effect also is valuable in improving myocardial and cerebral blood flow. Because it also has prominent β-adrenergic agonist effects, epinephrine is variably effective at producing marked increases in blood pressure. Epinephrine therapy is initiated at a dose of 0.1 to 0.5 µg/kg/min. Epinephrine is particularly effective in intoxications associated with hypotension and bronchospasm (e.g., Hymenoptera envenomation and anaphylactic reactions).

Norepinephrine

Norepinephrine stimulates both α- and β-adrenergic receptors, with slightly greater stimulation of α-adrenergic receptors. The effect is improved vasomotor tone in conjunction with increased myocardial chronotropy and inotropy. Norepinephrine infusions are typically initiated in a dose of 0.1 to 0.5 µg/kg/min.

Dopamine

Dopamine is a precursor of norepinephrine. The most popular of vasopressors, dopamine appears to have at least three mechanisms of action: (1) promotion of norepinephrine synthesis, (2) a tyramine-like effect that stimulates release of preformed norepinephrine, and (3) direct stimulation of vascular dopamine receptors.

The cardiovascular effects of dopamine are variable, depending on the infusion rate. At relatively low doses (1 to 2 µg/kg/min), the drug dilates renal and mesenteric vessels without marked increases in heart rate or blood pressure. At doses of 2 to 10 µg/kg/min, β-adrenergic receptor stimulation predominates, producing significant increases in cardiac output. Finally, at doses greater than 10 µg/kg/min, α-adrenergic receptor stimulation is the primary action, resulting in marked peripheral vasoconstriction. The general dose range for dopamine infusion is 2 to 20 µg/kg/min.

Dopamine is safe and effective for any type of drug-induced hypotension. In the past, there have been theoretic concerns that dopamine's β-adrenergic effect in the face of phenothiazine or tricyclic antidepressant intoxication would increase the peripheral vasodilatation associated with overdose, exacerbating hypotension. However, experimental data and clinical experience have failed to confirm this adverse effect from dopamine use. Also, with hypotension after monoamine oxidase inhibitor overdose, dopamine's effects are somewhat unpredictable; it may be relatively ineffective (owing to the lack of pre-formed norepinephrine), or it can produce an exaggerated response (because of its tyramine-like action).

Dobutamine

Dobutamine is a synthetic catecholamine with almost exclusive β-adrenergic receptor-stimulating effects. Its primary mechanism of blood pressure improvement is direct myocardial inotropy; thus, reflex peripheral vasodilation may occur with its use. Unlike dopamine, dobutamine does not release preformed norepinephrine. The usual dosage range for dobutamine is 2 to 20 µg/kg/min, although doses as high as 40 µg/kg/min have been used. High-dose infusions often increase myocardial oxygen demands, which, if unmet, can result in myocardial ischemia. Nonetheless, dobutamine is extremely effective in syndromes of heart failure.

Phenylephrine

Phenylephrine has both α- and β-adrenergic receptor-stimulating properties, although its α-adrenergic receptor actions predominate. Phenylephrine is a potent stimulator of vasomotor tone; it is therefore very effective in patients in hypotensive states resulting from severe peripheral vasodilation (e.g., following overdose with an α-adrenergic antagonist, such as prazocin or a phenothiazine neuroleptic, e.g., chlorpromazine). Phenylephrine

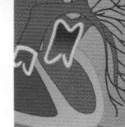

infusions are given in a typical dose range of 0.1 to 0.5 µg/kg/min.

Amrinone

Amrinone is a novel, nonadrenergic cardiac stimulant that improves myocardial contractility while inducing vasodilation. Its mechanism of action appears to be direct inhibition of phosphodiesterase; the result of this is increased intracellular cAMP activity, an action that increases transmembrane calcium flux, potentiating cardiac chronotropy and inotropy. Amrinone's effects have been compared with those of dobutamine and nitroprusside combination therapy. Amrinone may be particularly valuable in the treatment of calcium channel blocker intoxication; its inhibition of cAMP breakdown results in greater phosphorylation of L-type calcium channels, potentially increasing their permeability. Experimental data support its role in this specific poisoning.[18] Amrinone can be used to treat syndromes of left ventricular failure but should not be administered in the presence of myocardial ischemia; like dobutamine, it may increase myocardial demands, resulting in infarction. Because of its potent vasodilating action, amrinone may cause a hypotensive response in those with low intravascular volume. The usual dosage range for this agent is 5 to 15 µg/kg/min; the total daily dose should not exceed 10 mg/kg per day.

Glucagon

Glucagon is a single-chain pancreatic polypeptide that is an effective inotropic and chronotropic agent. Its mechanism of action is direct stimulation of myocardial glucagon receptors; these receptors, when stimulated, increase the formation of myocardial cAMP. The resultant effect is positive inotropy and, to a lesser degree, positive chronotropy. Glucagon is theoretically most effective after β blocker overdose, in which decreased β-adrenergic receptor activation leads to diminished cAMP production. The hormone may also provide therapeutic benefit in hypotension after calcium channel blocker overdose.[18] Glucagon is given in an initial dose of 1 to 10 mg (50 to 150 µg/kg in children). If effective in augmenting blood pressure, it can be given as a continuous infusion of 5 to 10 mg/hr (100 µg/kg/hr in children). Some preparations of glucagon are marketed as a lyophilized compound with a 0.2% phenol-based diluent for reconstitution. While single doses of such a product can be given after standard reconstitution, glucagon for continuous infusion should be reconstituted with saline to prevent phenol toxicity. Adverse effects from glucagon include hyperglycemia, nausea, vomiting, and ileus.

Calcium

Calcium plays a key role in regulating cardiac inotropy through its binding to troponin C, an action that permits interaction between actin and myosin. Although most of the calcium that produces this change resides in an intracellular calcium pool, extracellular calcium does diffuse into cells and contributes to increased contractility. Although diffusion of calcium into the myocardium is "gated"—that is, it is tightly controlled—high con-

centrations of extracellular calcium, particularly in the face of channel blockade (e.g., after overdose of calcium-channel blockers), sometimes improve contractility. Administration of IV calcium chloride is indicated in the management of hypotension resulting from calcium channel blocker overdose (see Table 2A-1), hyperkalemia, and hypocalcemia.

Clinical Evaluation

A thorough history taking and physical examination are essential to the diagnosis of the toxic patient. Poisoning should be suspected in any patient who presents with multisystem disturbance until proven otherwise. Although the initial manifestations of poisoning are myriad, a patient with acute poisoning often presents with coma, cardiac arrhythmia, seizures, metabolic acidosis, or gastrointestinal disturbance, either together as symptom complexes or as isolated events. Symptom complexes, or toxidromes (Table 2A-5), may give clues to an unknown poisoning. For example, a patient with a history of depression who presents with coma, seizures, a widened QRS complex or evidence of dysrhythmia on electrocardiography, and dilated pupils has likely taken a tricyclic antidepressant. Hepatic, renal, respiratory, and hematologic disturbances are generally delayed manifestations of poisoning.

The clinical evaluation, in addition to the history taking and physical examination, includes an assessment of major signs of toxicity presented by the patient and evaluation of the laboratory data.

HISTORY

When one suspects poisoning or drug overdose, the primary goal of history taking is identification of the toxic agent. Sometimes diagnosis is easy, as in the case of the toddler who ingests iron tablets in the mother's presence. Sometimes it is difficult, as in the case of the patient who is hiding a history of drug abuse and passes out at work or who has an unexpected seizure. Prior medical or psychiatric history, current medications, and allergies should be obtained from family or friends if the patient is unable to relate the information. The following questions may be revealing:

What other medicines are in the house?
What was the patient doing that day?
Does the patient live alone, did he or she just lose a job, or have there been recent emotionally traumatic events?
Is the patient eating a special diet or taking a new health food, alternative medication, or performance enhancer?
Could the patient inadvertently have taken too much of a prescribed medication?
If it can be identified, is the substance nontoxic? (See Box 2A-4.)

PHYSICAL EXAMINATION

The physical examination can help in determining the extent of poisoning and may reveal the presence of a

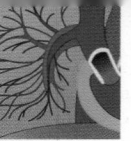

TABLE 2A-5 Examples of Symptom Complexes, or Toxidromes

TOXIDROME OR COMPLEX	CONSCIOUSNESS	RESPIRATIONS	PUPILS	OTHER	POSSIBLE TOXIC AGENT/MECHANISM
Cholinergic	Coma	↑↓	Pinpoint	Fasciculations Incontinence Salivation Wheezing Lacrimation Bradycardia	Organophosphate insecticides, carbamates, nicotine
Anticholinergic	Agitation, hallucinations, or coma	↑	Dilated	Fever, flushing Dry skin and mucous membranes Urinary retention	Anticholinergics (atropine, Jimson weed, antihistamines)
Opioid	Coma	↓	Pinpoint	Track marks Hypothermia Hypotension	Opiates, opioids
Extrapyramidal	Wakefulness	↑	—	Torsion of head/neck	Phenothiazines, haloperidol risperidol
Tricyclic antidepressant	Coma (initially, agitation)	↓	Dilated	Cardiac arrhythmia Convulsions Hypotension Prolonged QRS interval	Tricyclic antidepressants
Sedative/hypnotic	Coma	↓	Midsize or small	Hypothermia Decreased reflexes Hypotension	Sedatives, barbiturates
Salicylates	Agitation or lethargy	↑	Midsize or small	Diaphoresis Tinnitus Alkalosis (early) Acidosis (late)	Aspirin, oil of wintergreen
Sympathomimetic	Agitation, hallucinations	↑	Dilated	Seizures Tachycardia Hypertension Diaphoresis Metabolic acidosis Tremor Hyperreflexia	Cocaine Theophylline Amphetamines Caffeine

---

BOX 2A-4   NONTOXIC INGESTIONS

Abrasives
Adhesives
Antacids
Antibiotics
Baby product cosmetics
Ballpoint pen inks
Bath oil (castor oil and perfume)
Bathtub floating toys
Birth control pills
Bleach (<5% sodium hypochlorite)
Body conditioners
Bubble bath soaps (detergents)
Calamine lotion
Candles (beeswax or paraffin)
Chalk (calcium carbonate)
Colognes
Cosmetics
Crayons marked AP, CP
Dehumidifying packets (silica or charcoal)
Deodorants
Deodorizers, spray and refrigerator

Elmer's glue
Fabric softeners
Fish bowl additives
Glues and pastes
Hand lotions and creams
3% hydrogen peroxide
Incense
Indelible markers
Ink (black, blue)
Iodophil disinfectant
Laxatives
Lipstick
Lubricant
Magic Markers
Makeup (eye, liquid, facial)
Matches
Mineral oil
Modeling clay
Newspaper
Pencil (graphite lead, coloring)
Perfumes

Petroleum jelly (Vaseline)
Play-Doh
Polaroid picture coating fluid
Putty (less than 2 oz)
Rubber cement
Sachets (essential oils, powder)
Shampoos (liquid)
Shaving creams and lotions
Soap and soap products
Spackles
Suntan preparations
Sweetening agents (aspartame)
Teething rings
Thermometers (mercury)
Toothpaste with or without fluoride
Toy pistol caps (potassium chlorate)
Vitamins with or without fluoride
Watercolors
Zinc oxide
Zirconium oxide

Nontoxic is defined as producing little to no toxicity when ingested in small amounts.

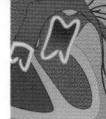

TABLE 2A-6 Important Clues on Physical Examination	
CLINICAL FINDING	**DIAGNOSTIC EXAMPLE**
Needle tracks	Intravenous drug abuse
Characteristic odor of breath	Gasoline
Destruction of nasal mucosa/cartilage	Cocaine abuse
New significant heart murmur	Infective endocarditis
Pulmonary edema	Heroin abuse
Boardlike abdomen	Black widow spider bite
Salivation and lacrimation	Organophosphates
"Boiled lobster" skin	Boric acid poisoning

toxic syndrome, of any underlying disease, or concomitant trauma. Repeated assessment, especially of vital signs and of cardiac, pulmonary, and neurologic status, is critical to proper management of the toxicologic patient. The physical examination also can provide valuable clues as to the particular toxin involved (Table 2A-6).

Vital Signs

As part of the initial evaluation, complete determination of vital signs, including measurement of body temperature initially and throughout the emergency department assessment, is mandatory. Obtaining a core body temperature measurement may be necessary. Hyperthermia can occur with a number of ingestions and in infectious illness, but it is characteristic of poisoning with salicylates, anticholinergics, monoamine oxidase inhibitors, and dinitrophenol; it is occasionally also seen after intoxication with phencyclidine, LSD, or cocaine, especially following seizures. Life-threatening malignant hyperthermia following drug overdose may occur. Hypothermia is common and may occur because of exposure to cold, hypoglycemia, or overdose of a number of sedatives, especially barbiturates, ethanol, carbamazepine, narcotics, and phenothiazines. Bradycardia can be seen with overdose of digitalis, cholinergic agents, β blockers, and calcium channel blockers, but it also may be seen with hypothermia or spinal cord trauma. Hypertension is characteristic of intoxication with cocaine, amphetamines, phencyclidine, and sympathomimetics.

Skin

The skin should be examined for needle tracks, burns, bruises, or lacerations. Needle tracks may be confined to the groin or other areas that are not readily visible. A "boiled lobster" appearance suggests ingestion of a boric acid–containing roach powder insecticide. Generalized flushing suggests an allergic reaction, niacin overdose, anticholinergic poisoning, scombroid fish poisoning, or an alcohol-disulfiram reaction.

Diaphoresis suggests hypoglycemia, salicylate or organophosphate poisoning, hyperthyroidism, drug or alcohol withdrawal, or shock from cardiac or other etiology. Jaundice may follow overdose of acetaminophen, aspirin, iron, carbon tetrachloride, mushrooms, copper, or phosphorus. Petechiae and ecchymoses suggest coumadin overdose. Bullae may be secondary to skin hypoxia or prolonged pressure and are seen after sedative-hypnotic overdoses (especially barbiturate overdose), carbon monoxide poisoning, and thermal burns. Bullae may also follow rattlesnake envenomation. Bullous lesions or soft tissue swelling should prompt evaluation for rhabdomyolysis, an occasional finding in patients following prolonged coma or severe hyperthermia, such as in cocaine abuse.

Breath

It is important to smell the patient's breath. Alcohol is the most common odor detected on the breath of an intoxicated patient in the emergency department. The accurate identification of other odors varies greatly among physicians. A fruity odor may be detectable in the patient with diabetic ketoacidosis. Cyanide poisoning can be associated with the smell of almonds. The smell of cleaning fluid suggests carbon tetrachloride poisoning. Gasoline, camphor, hydrogen sulfide, ether, turpentine, methyl salicylate, paraldehyde, phenol, and organophosphate insecticides all have characteristic odors. Arsenic and tellurium intoxication is associated with the odor of garlic.

Ear, Nose, and Throat

A nasal examination may reveal chronic insufflation of cocaine. An edematous, often elongated uvula may be seen with marijuana use or exposure to corrosive agents.

Lungs

Auscultation of the lungs may provide diagnostic clues. In narcotic or tricyclic antidepressant overdose, pulmonary edema may be a complication, leading to the appearance of adventitious noises. In all overdose patients, aspiration pneumonitis, the result of a depressed gag reflex, is a possibility. Inhalation of toxic gases may produce wheezing and pulmonary compromise. Pneumothorax may be detected in patients who smoke cocaine, methamphetamine, or any other heated, impure substance. Mediastinal emphysema from marijuana or crack cocaine smoking also may be detected by auscultation.

Heart

Examination of the heart may reveal a new murmur, which in an intravenous drug abuser suggests endocarditis. Bradycardia is common after the overdose of four classes of cardiac agents: calcium channel blocker, β blocking agents, digitalis preparations, and central α_2 antagonists (e.g., clonidine or guanfacine). A ventricular arrhythmia on electrocardiography in a young patient suggests cocaine toxicity. An irregularly irregular heartbeat that is new in a patient on an alcoholic binge suggests atrial fibrillation—the so-called "holiday heart" syndrome.

Abdomen

A boardlike abdomen in a patient with a history of spider bite is characteristic of black widow envenomation. Examination of the abdomen in an overdose patient often reveals an adynamic ileus. In patients with abdominal pain, a surgical abdomen must be ruled

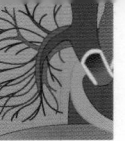

out. Hepatomegaly suggests liver congestion (e.g., with pyrrolizidine toxicity).

Neurologic Assessment

All patients should undergo a careful neurologic examination. Issues of major concern are concomitant head trauma and spinal cord trauma in comatose patients. Serial neurologic examinations are key to proper assessment (see discussion of coma in section on Level of Consciousness).

Extremities

The extremities should be evaluated to detect thrombophlebitis, fracture or dislocation, or vascular insufficiency. Rhabdomyolysis and the compartment syndrome are definite concerns in overdose patients, especially in those with prolonged coma or underlying trauma.

ASSESSMENT OF MAJOR SIGNS OF TOXICITY

The toxicologic patient presenting in the acute setting often exhibits the following, either alone or in combination: coma, cardiac arrhythmia, metabolic acidosis, gastrointestinal disturbance, and seizures.

Level of Consciousness

Consciousness is defined as an awareness of self and the environment. Coma is unarousable unresponsiveness. Wakefulness implies the ability to be aroused. These three functional states are mediated by the ascending reticular activating system, a tract that courses through the diencephalon, midbrain, and pons. Diseases produce coma either by diffusely affecting the brain or by encroaching upon the brainstem. Coma may be produced by (1) a supratentorial mass lesion, such as a subdural hematoma; (2) a brainstem lesion (uncommon); or (3) metabolic disorders that widely depress or interrupt brain function.

One of the most common manifestations of acute poisoning is coma. The principles of coma management are relatively straightforward. Patients in coma must be stabilized initially by establishment of an airway, proper oxygenation with continuous pulse oximetry, insertion of an IV line with normal saline, and resuscitation, if necessary (see earlier section on Emergency Management). The clinical evaluation of the comatose patient is invaluable not only in determining the depth of coma and assessing for trauma, but also in providing a baseline for repeated clinical assessment. Coma can be assessed either using the simple AVPU (*A*lert, responsive only to *V*erbal stimuli, responsive only to *P*ainful stimuli, *U*nresponsive) or Glasgow coma scales.

The major causes of coma in patients seen in the emergency department include poisoning (e.g., carbon monoxide poisoning), drug overdose, head trauma, cerebrovascular accident, anoxia, infection (e.g., meningitis), and diabetes and other systemic disorders such as renal failure, hepatic coma, and cardiac arrhythmia. The physician must rule out each condition before establishing the diagnosis of poisoning.

Supratentorial structural lesions are suggested by a rapid progression of signs, including changes in respiratory pattern, disconjugate gaze, lateralizing signs, or loss of doll's eyes movements.

A metabolic cause of coma may be indicated by the persistence of the pupillary light reflex; a depression of respiration and consciousness more pronounced than other neurologic signs; preceding altered mental states; asterixis or fasciculations, or both; the presence of a ciliospinal reflex; and extracranial signs, such as jaundice. Repeated assessment of the comatose patient is critical to proper management of poisoning.

Pupils

Evaluation of the patient's pupils is most helpful. Midpoint fixed pupils or a unilateral dilated pupil suggests a structural lesion. Pinpoint pupils suggest overdose of opiates, clonidine, organophosphate insecticides, nerve agents (e.g., sarin), chloral hydrate, phenothiazines, or nicotine. Dilated pupils are nonspecific.

Ocular Movements

A disturbance of ocular movements (e.g., loss of doll's eyes movements) suggests a structural lesion. *Nystagmus* suggests intoxication with phenytoin, phencyclidine, carbamazepine, and, occasionally, ethanol.

Respirations

It is important to note abnormal patterns of breathing. Posthyperventilation apnea, Cheyne-Stokes respirations, and apneustic breathing strongly suggest that a structural lesion is the cause of the patient's coma. Central neurogenic hyperventilation is a classic presentation of brainstem injury. Kussmaul breathing can occur after salicylate or dinitrophenol poisoning. Compensatory hyperventilation may accompany methanol or ethylene glycol poisoning or other toxin-producing metabolic acidosis. Respiratory arrest is a common presentation in the patient who has taken a central nervous system depressant and may lead to multisystemic dysfunction resulting from severe hypoxic injury.

Motor Function

Decorticate and decerebrate posturing suggests a structural lesion. It is important to realize that patients with poisoning or drug overdose (e.g., tetrodotoxin intoxication) may appear brain dead; have fixed, dilated pupils; be in an unresponsive coma; and lack the cold caloric response, yet recover fully in time.

CARDIAC ARRHYTHMIA

A 12-lead electrocardiogram and continuous cardiac monitoring are essential for any patient with significant poisoning. Evidence of an arrhythmia or other important diagnostic clues may be present on electrocardiography, such as a widened QRS complex in cyclic antidepressant overdose or a prolonged QT interval in trazadone or arsenic poisoning overdose. Box 2A-5 lists common toxic causes of cardiac arrhythmia.

The patient with life-threatening cardiac arrhythmia or cardiac arrest should be managed on the basis of the general principles of resuscitation and the American Heart Association's advanced cardiac life support

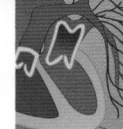

BOX 2A-5	COMMON TOXIC CAUSES OF CARDIAC DISTURBANCES

Conduction Disturbances

Prolonged PR Interval
Digoxin and other digitalis compounds
Lithium

Prolonged QRS Interval
Chloroquine, quinine, quinidine, and related compounds
Diphenhydramine
Plant cardiac glycosides (e.g., lily of the valley)
Tricyclic antidepressants

Prolonged QT Interval
Arsenic
Cisapride
Disopyramide
Droperidol
Erythromycin
Haloperidol
Hypocalcemia (after hydrofluoric acid exposure)
Pentamidine
Phenothiazines
Sotalol
Thioridazine

Rhythm Disturbances (Ventricular or Supraventricular)

β blockers
Calcium channel blockers
Carbon monoxide
Clonidine
Cocaine
Theophylline

BOX 2A-6	CAUSES OF A HIGH–ANION GAP METABOLIC ACIDOSIS

Alcoholic ketoacidosis
Cyanide
Diabetic ketoacidosis
Ethylene glycol
Iron
Isoniazid
Lactic acidosis
Metformin
Methanol
Salicylates
Uremia

METABOLIC ACIDOSIS AND DISTURBANCES IN SERUM OSMOLALITY

Causes of a high-anion gap metabolic acidosis are listed in Box 2A-6. The assessment of metabolic acidosis includes not only arterial (or, less ideally, venous) blood gas analysis, but also studies of serum sodium, potassium, chloride, carbon dioxide, blood urea nitrogen (BUN), creatinine, glucose, acetone, serum osmolality, and urine pH, as well as urinalysis. Determination of the anion gap is helpful in the diagnosis and management of poisoning.

The clinician can measure serum osmolality either directly by determining the freezing point (osmometry) or by calculation. The formula for calculating osmolality is

$$\text{Serum osmolality} = 2 \times Na^+ \ (mEq/L) + BUN \ (mg/dL)/2.8 + Glucose \ (mg/dL)/18$$

When laboratory data are expressed in international (SI) units, the formula for calculation of serum osmolality simply equals $2 \times Na + BUN + glucose$. The normal serum osmolality is 280 to 295 mOsm/L. An osmometer measurement indicating a serum osmolality that is more than 10 mOsm/L greater than the calculated osmolality is termed an osmolar gap; it suggests the presence of an osmotically active substance that is not accounted for by the calculated osmolality. Causes of an osmolar gap are listed in Box 2A-7. The most common cause of an osmolar gap is consumption of an alcohol. The osmolar gap can be used to estimate the serum concentration of an alcohol, based on that alcohol's molecular weight (Table 2A-7). A substance contributes to osmolality only if it achieves relatively high blood levels and has a low molecular weight. Most drugs or intoxicants cannot be detected with use of the osmolar gap.

GASTROINTESTINAL DISTURBANCE

The causes of toxic gastrointestinal disturbance are many. The patient with iron, arsenic, or ricin poisoning has severe, repeated episodes of vomiting and may develop gastrointestinal hemorrhage. Theophylline overdose also causes persistent retching. Acute lithium and arsenic poisoning characteristically produce massive diarrhea. Patients with acute mercury poisoning have a mucous-type diarrhea, with the subsequent development

(ACLS) guidelines. If cyclic antidepressant overdose is suspected, administration of IV sodium bicarbonate is indicated for correction of ventricular arrhythmia or conduction disturbances. Sodium bicarbonate may also be effective in the treatment of other overdose by other agents associated with prolongation of the QRS interval, including diphenhydramine and cocaine. Administration of IV calcium chloride is the primary therapeutic measure for calcium channel blocker overdose. Use of digoxin antibody fragments is indicated for digitalis poisoning, and glucagon for β blocker overdose (see Table 2A-1). In referred patients who have already been hospitalized elsewhere, ventricular arrhythmia may be due to hyperkalemia because renal failure may have ensued; in such patients, IV sodium bicarbonate, glucose/insulin, and, if necessary, calcium chloride administration may be warranted. Magnesium has a singular role in the treatment of drug-induced prolongation of the QT interval, a conduction disturbance that is often the prelude to torsades de pointes and other life-threatening disturbances.[19] In all intoxicated patients, correction of hypoxia, metabolic acidosis, and fluid and electrolyte disturbance serves to reduce the incidence of cardiac arrhythmias.

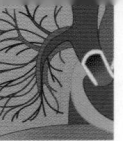

BOX 2A-7	CAUSES OF AN OSMOLAR GAP

Diseases or Conditions

Hyperproteinemia
Hyperlipidemia

Alcohols

Acetone
Ethanol
Ethylene glycol
Isopropyl alcohol
Methanol

Pharmaceuticals

Propylene glycol (an excipient in parenteral medications)
Intravenous contrast
Mannitol

BOX 2A-8	COMMON TOXIC CAUSES OF SEIZURES

Anticholinergics (e.g., diphenhydramine)
Bupropion
Camphor
Carbon monoxide
Cocaine
Insulin
Isoniazid
Lindane
Lithium
Oral hypoglycemics
Propoxyphene
Strychnine
Theophylline
Tramadol
Tricyclic antidepressants

TABLE 2A-7 Molecular Weight of Alcohols and Their Contribution to the Osmolar Gap

	MOLECULAR WEIGHT (DALTONS)	OSMOLAL GAP (mOsm/kg) AT 100 mg/dL
Ethanol	46	22
Ethylene glycol	62	16
Isopropyl alcohol	60	17
Methanol	32	31

of hemorrhagic colitis. One of the most striking presentations is caused by phosphorus poisoning, which produces luminescent vomitus and flatus. The early presentation of organophosphate or nerve agent exposure is similar to that of acute gastroenteritis and is characterized by abdominal cramps, vomiting, and diarrhea, with subsequent development of neurologic signs. Poisoning from mushrooms (see Chapter 23), toxic marine life (see Chapter 25), botulism, and food (see Chapter 26) should be included in the differential diagnosis. Chemotherapeutic agents (see Chapter 56) are well-known causes of toxic gastroenteritis.

The management of gastrointestinal disturbance in the toxic patient includes following the general principles of blood, fluid, and electrolyte resuscitation, when indicated; judicious use of parenteral antiemetics to control persistent vomiting; specific measures such as antidotal therapy (e.g., in iron or organophosphate poisoning); or interventional therapy, such as charcoal hemoperfusion (in theophylline overdose) or hemodialysis (in lithium overdose), when indicated.

SEIZURES

Common agents that cause seizures are listed in Box 2A-8. Almost any drug or toxin is capable of producing a seizure. Delayed seizures occurring during a recovery period may be a sign of sedative-hypnotic or alcohol withdrawal.

Seizures should be managed first with establishment of an airway and oxygenation. Patients with a simple isolated seizure may require only observation and supportive care, whereas repetitive seizures or status epilepticus, which can be life threatening, must be managed aggressively. Some seizures are particularly difficult to control, such as those seen with theophylline or cocaine overdose.

The standard regimen for seizure control in overdose of an unknown agent is use of the full therapeutic dosages of benzodiazepines (e.g., diazepam or lorazepam), followed by administration of phenytoin or a barbiturate (e.g., phenobarbital or pentobarbital). In patients with status epilepticus, RSI may be necessary and the use of thiopental is indicated, with electroencephalographic monitoring to ensure control of electrical seizure activity; the use of additional paralytics, such as pancuronium bromide, may be warranted.

Specific measures to control seizures may be indicated, such as administration of pyridoxine for isoniazid-induced seizures.

LABORATORY EVALUATION

Box 2A-9 lists specific blood studies whose results may be used for diagnosis and to direct therapy of the overdose patient. In every significant poisoning, routine studies include a complete blood count; determination of serum electrolytes, glucose, BUN, creatinine, and calcium; urinalysis; prothrombin time; pulse oximetry; end-tidal CO_2 monitoring, and 12-lead electrocardiography. Arterial blood gas analysis is necessary for evaluating respiratory status and acid-base abnormalities, particularly in the comatose or seizure patient. The measurement of serum salicylate and acetaminophen levels is generally added in the case of the patient with overdose of an unknown substance, because these agents are often co-ingestants or are contained in combination drugs. Measurement of hepatic enzymes is important in the evaluation of acetaminophen toxicity. The advantage of a toxicologic drug screen in initial management is equivocal. Box 2A-10 gives a partial list of drugs and toxins not commonly

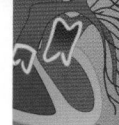

BOX 2A-9	TOXICOLOGIC BLOOD STUDIES THAT MAY DIRECT THERAPY

Acetaminophen
Carboxyhemoglobin
Digoxin
Ethanol
Ethylene glycol
Iron
Lithium
Methanol
Salicylate
Theophylline

BOX 2A-10	A PARTIAL LIST OF DRUGS AND TOXINS NOT COMMONLY DETECTED WITH ROUTINE DRUG SCREENING

Antihypertensives
Organophosphates
Antiarrhythmics
Carbon monoxide
Cyanide
Digitalis
Ethylene glycol
Heavy metals
Hydrocarbons
Oral hypoglycemics
Iron
Isoniazid
Lithium
LSD
Methanol
Mushrooms
Venoms

BOX 2A-11	RADIOPAQUE TOXINS

Drugs
Chloral hydrate
Enteric-coated preparations
Phenothiazines
Sustained-release products

Metals and Minerals
Arsenic
Calcium
Iron
Lithium
Lead
Potassium

Foreign Bodies
Crack vials
Drug packets

pH monitoring is helpful in the management of salicylate overdose. Urine is the best specimen to use for "drug screening" purposes. A urinalysis is also useful in the early identification of acute renal failure or rhabdomyolysis with myoglobinuria.

The intravenous drug abuser requires special blood testing, such as evaluation for human immunodeficiency virus, a hepatitis profile, a blood culture to identify bacteremia, and evaluation for rhabdomyolysis.

Chest radiography is an aid for diagnosing aspiration pneumonia or pulmonary edema. Box 2A-11 lists agents that are radiopaque on plain film radiography of the abdomen. Computed tomography may be useful if underlying trauma is suspected. Finally, lumbar puncture may be indicated for ruling out meningitis in a patient with fever and coma.

Decontamination of the Eyes, Skin, and Gastrointestinal Tract

OCULAR DECONTAMINATION
See Chapter 15.

DERMAL DECONTAMINATION
Being the largest and most superficial organ in the body, the skin is often subject to exposure to toxins and is affected in 7.9% of reported cases. At least 50% of occupational illnesses involve the skin. The effects of these exposures can be local or systemic (Box 2A-12).

The skin provides many barriers to the absorption of toxins. The stratum corneum forms an important first barrier and is highly effective when it is completely intact. However, when skin wounds are present, when the wounds are wet, and when exposure is to certain highly lipophilic substances (e.g., organophosphate insecticides), significant absorption of toxin through the skin can occur. The skin of infants is notable for being more permeable than that of adults to substances of all classes.

detected with routine drug screening. Further laboratory blood studies are tailored to assess the individual diagnostic and therapeutic needs of the patient.

It is extremely important to remember to "treat the patient, not the lab." One should never withhold therapy while waiting for a confirmatory drug level in a critical patient, such as a patient with tricyclic antidepressant overdose who is exhibiting a widened QRS complex. In contrast, performing hemodialysis on a completely asymptomatic patient with lithium overdose on the basis of one test result indicating an elevated serum lithium concentration would be equally unwise.

Serial blood level determinations are often helpful in guiding therapy in patients undergoing hemodialysis; in patients in whom concretions have formed, such as those with barbiturate, iron, salicylates, or meprobamate intoxication; or in patients receiving antidotal therapy (e.g., serial measurement of lead level is useful in patients receiving IV CaNa$_2$ EDTA for management of lead poisoning).

A urinalysis is necessary. Performing a urine pregnancy test is wise in all women of childbearing age. Urine

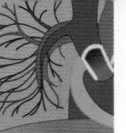

BOX 2A-12	TOXINS ASSOCIATED WITH SYSTEMIC TOXICITY AFTER DERMAL ABSORPTION

Aniline dyes
Camphor
Dinitrophenol
Hexachlorophene
Hydrofluoric acid
Lindane (γ-benzene hydrochloride)
Organophosphate insecticide
Nerve agents
Nitrobenzene
Organic mercury
Phenol
Thallium

TABLE 2A-8 Specific Interventions for Toxic Dermal Exposure

TOXIN	THERAPEUTIC INTERVENTION
Hydrofluoric acid	Calcium gluconate
Instant-bonding adhesive ("Super Glue")	Polyoxyethylene sorbitan (Neosporin)
Elemental sodium	Mineral oil
Organophosphate insecticide	Protected decontamination

The range of dermal toxins is broad. Most of these substances are corrosive agents capable of producing burns that may become full thickness (i.e., third degree). Other types of agents are irritants, sensitizers (including photosensitizers), allergens, vesicants, and exfoliants.

Management

As with ocular exposures, the general principles of management after exposure to dermal toxins are many. As soon as a toxic dermal exposure is recognized, decontamination efforts should begin. If the victim is immersed in a toxic fluid, the first step in management is his or her extrication without injury to the assistant. The victim should disrobe him- or herself at the scene. If the victim requires assistance, undressing should be done as safely as possible. Protective gear should be donned before assistance with decontamination is rendered. Unless the agent is highly reactive (e.g., elemental sodium), it is appropriate to wash the victim thoroughly with water, preferably in a nearby decontamination shower. Generally speaking, water should not be used to decontaminate skin in exposures to sodium, phosphorus, calcium oxide, chlorosulphonic acid, and titanium tetrachloride. When emergency medical personnel arrive to the scene, they should continue skin decontamination. Again, if the agent is known to have significant dermal absorption, emergency medical personnel should provide themselves every available level of self-protection. Certain toxins such as organophosphates can contaminate the air within the ambulance and produce ill effects among personnel if prehospital decontamination efforts are inadequate.

Upon arrival at a health care facility, the victim may require quarantine, depending on the nature of the agent. Skin decontamination in a decontamination shower should continue. Particular caution should be exercised in the decontamination of victims of organophosphate insecticide or organophosphate-based nerve gas exposure; health care personnel have been overcome secondarily by contaminants on victims when they assisted in their care without donning proper protective gear.

Water is the most commonly used skin decontaminant and is highly effective for most dermal exposures. In select cases, specific agents should be used to assist in management (Table 2A-8).

Without exception, toxin-induced skin burns should be treated according to existing burn management guidelines. These include wound débridement and dressing, monitoring for infection, fluid management, and surgical consultation when appropriate.

ELIMINATION OF POISON FROM THE GASTROINTESTINAL TRACT

After the ingestion of a toxic substance, with the exception of agents that have a direct toxic effect on the gastrointestinal tract (e.g., iron or corrosives), that substance must be systemically absorbed and circulated before it reaches a target organ and exerts clinical toxicity. Preventing the absorption of toxin is therefore the foundation of treatment after ingestion of a toxin has occurred. The term *gastrointestinal decontamination* (GID) has been coined to describe those interventions that are useful in preventing toxin absorption. With the exception of rare interventions such as gastroscopy, GID is considered to have only three components: (1) gastric evacuation, (2) administration of adsorbent, and (3) catharsis. Gastric evacuation is accomplished through gastric lavage. Syrup of ipecac, once used as an emetic for treatment of toxic ingestions, is no longer routinely recommended for this purpose. There are several agents that can adsorb toxic substances, reducing their systemic absorption and subsequent toxicity (Table 2A-9). Of these, activated charcoal is the most important adsorbent; there are few substances that activated charcoal will not adsorb (Box 2A-13). Catharsis, once an integral part of management, also has a diminishing role in the treatment of poisoned patients.

Gastrointestinal decontamination is discussed in greater detail in Chapter 2B.

ANTIDOTES

With the development of sophisticated new antidotes and the changing spectrum of clinical poisoning, the use of emergency antidotes is assuming an increasing role in clinical toxicology. However, antidotes are useful in only a fraction of poisonings.[1] Table 2A-1 lists the common emergency antidotes. In poisoning with a known substance, early antidote use is indicated for emergency stabilization, often within the first hour.

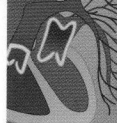

TABLE 2A-9 Adsorbents Used in the Management of Toxic Ingestions	
ADSORBENT	**TOXIN**
Activated charcoal	Pharmaceuticals, organic agents
Cholestyramine	Organochlorines (chlordecone, lindane)
Sodium phosphorsulfonate (Kayexalate)	Lithium, potassium
Fuller's earth, bentonite	Paraquat
Starch	Iodine
Potassium ferricyanate (Prussian blue)	Thallium

TABLE 2A-10 Additional Treatment Methods for Enhanced Elimination of Absorbed Substance	
TREATMENT	**DRUG**
Hemodialysis	Lithium
	Ethylene glycol
	Methanol
	Salicylate
	Theophylline
	Valproate (in severe overdose)
Hemoperfusion	Theophylline
	Phenobarbital
Alkalinization of urine	Phenobarbital
	Salicylates

BOX 2A-13	SUBSTANCES NOT WELL ADSORBED TO ACTIVATED CHARCOAL

Alcohols

Acetone
Ethanol
Isopropyl alcohol
Methanol
Glycols (ethylene glycol, propylene glycol, diethylene glycol)

Hydrocarbons

Petroleum distillates
Plant hydrocarbons (e.g., pine oil)

Metals and Inorganic Minerals

Arsenic
Boric acid
Fluoride
Iron
Lead
Sodium

Corrosives

Sodium hydroxide
Sulfuric or nitric acid

ELIMINATION ENHANCEMENT OF ABSORBED SUBSTANCES

There are multiple methods by which agents in the systemic circulation, whether ingested or administered parenterally, can be removed. The four most clinically useful means of elimination enhancement are (1) multiple-dose activated charcoal, (2) hemodialysis, (3) hemoperfusion, and (4) urine alkalinization. Potential roles for these interventions are found in Table 2A-10 and Box 2A-14. Further discussion of elimination of a substance that has already been absorbed is provided in Chapter 2C.

OBSERVATION AND SUPPORTIVE CARE

Observation and supportive care are the mainstays of therapy for the poisoned patient. Indiscriminate use of gastric lavage, antidotes, and drugs should be avoided. All too often, the toxic agent is unknown, multiple drugs have been taken, or the patient is too unstable to undergo an aggressive therapy such as hemodialysis. Monitoring of vital signs, cardiac telemetry, and oxygen saturation is mandatory.

Hospitalization in an intensive care unit is generally indicated for the patient with serious poisoning. Multisystem monitoring with blood studies and assessment of other parameters are indicated, and upon detection of any specific system disturbance, appropriate subspecialty consultation is warranted.

Some agents such as iron, mercury, acetaminophen, paraquat, carbon tetrachloride, and *Amanita phalloides* toxin have a latent phase, in which the patient appears to recover from the initial insult, only to decompensate 24 to 72 hours postingestion. Patients with overdose of sustained-release capsules, such as calcium channel blocker or theophylline preparations, also may have delayed manifestation of poisoning. Rarely, the tricyclic antidepressants have been known to cause fatal arrhythmia up to 3 days following ingestion. Some effects are not seen until later, such as hypertension following phencyclidine ingestion, hemorrhagic colitis following mercury ingestion, and disseminated intravascular coagulation following snakebite. One must also watch for the delayed pulmonary (see Chapter 9), hepatic (see Chapter 11), renal (see Chapter 12), and hematologic (see Chapter 14) manifestations of poisoning.

Hyperbaric oxygen can provide oxygen at pressures greater than normal atmospheric pressure, which is given as 1 atmosphere (atm) or 760 mm Hg. Three atmospheres is the maximal pressure humans can tolerate over a reasonable period of time; hyperbaric units generally do not exceed 2.5 to 2.8 atm. The use of hyperbaric oxygenation is becoming standard therapy for patients with significant carbon monoxide poisoning, and it is becoming more available (see Chapter 87) for carbon tetrachloride poisoning, and possibly for cyanide and hydrogen sulfide poisoning.

Admission to an intensive care unit following antidotal therapy for further management and observation is generally indicated. Further discussion of each antidote and its use is provided in the chapter on the specific poison.

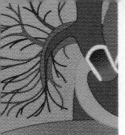

| BOX 2A-14 | EFFICACY OF MULTIPLE-DOSE ACTIVATED CHARCOAL IN ENHANCING DRUG ELIMINATION |

Effective

Phenobarbital
Theophylline
Carbamazepine
Salicylates
Digitoxin
Dapsone

Questionably Effective

Anticholinergic/antihistaminic agents
Sustained-release pharmaceuticals
Thyroid hormone
Valproate

Unlikely to Be Effective

Aminoglycoside antibiotics
Anticholinergic/antihistaminic agents
Calcium channel blockers
Phenothiazines
Propoxyphene
Tricyclic antidepressants

Patients may require observation because of an underlying disease that may be exacerbated because of the overdose, such as diabetes, congestive heart failure, cardiac rhythm disturbances, or chronic lung disease. Observation may be necessary to evaluate or treat complications, such as in a patient with an overdose who fell and sustained trauma or in a patient who develops aspiration pneumonitis or interstitial pulmonary edema.

The IV use of illicit drugs is associated with multiple complications; observation is especially indicated for patients experiencing these complications, which include bacterial endocarditis, rhabdomyolysis, and neurologic sequelae.

DISPOSITION

The disposition of the patient with intoxication may involve medical and psychiatric care as well as social follow-up. All patients admitted to the hospital with intentional overdose warrant close observation and the institution of suicide precautions. These patients may need appropriate restraint or observation if further injury or additional overdose attempts are to be prevented. Overt or subtle attempts or gestures indicate the need for psychiatric evaluation. Often, outpatient follow-up is necessary; for example, a child with kerosene ingestion

may require further examination and chest radiography, and a child who has ingested anticoagulant rat poison may require serial outpatient monitoring of prothrombin times. The issue of child abuse or neglect may need consideration whenever a pediatric patient is treated. Finally, long-term follow-up may be indicated; for example, hepatitis and HIV testing may be needed in the IV drug abuser.

REFERENCES

1. Watson WA, Litovitz TL, Klein-Schwartz W, et al: 2003 Annual report of the American Association of Poison Control Centers Toxic Exposure Surveillance System. Am J Emerg Med 2004; 22(5):335–404.
2. Drug Abuse Warning Network, U.S. Department of Health and Human Services, 2004. Retrieved October 28, 2004, from http://dawninfo.samhsa.gov/pubs_94_02/mepubs/default.asp.
3. Littlejohn C: Management of intentional overdose in A&E departments. Nurs Times 2004;100(33):38–43.
4. Merigian KS, Blaho K: Diagnosis and management of the drug overdose patient. Am J Ther 1997;4(2–3):99–113.
5. Bledsoe GH, Schexnayder SM: Pediatric rapid sequence intubation: a review. Pediatr Emerg Care 2004;20(5):339–344.
6. Bush S, Gray A, McGowan A, Nichol N: Rapid sequence intubation. J Accid Emerg Med 2000;17(4):309.
7. Dronen S: Rapid-sequence intubation: a safe but ill-defined procedure. Acad Emerg Med 1999;6(1):1–2.
8. Frakes MA: Rapid sequence induction medications: an update. J Emerg Nurs 2003;29(6):533–540.
9. Robinson N, Clancy M: In patients with head injury undergoing rapid sequence intubation, does pretreatment with intravenous lignocaine/lidocaine lead to an improved neurological outcome? A review of the literature. Emerg Med J 2001;18(6):453–457.
10. Walls RM: Lidocaine and rapid sequence intubation. Ann Emerg Med 1996;27(4):528–529.
11. Chugh K: Acute asthma in emergency room. Indian J Pediatr 2003;70(Suppl 1):28–33.
12. Lau TT, Zed PJ: Does ketamine have a role in managing severe exacerbation of asthma in adults? Pharmacotherapy 2001;21(9):1100–1106.
13. Petrillo TM, Fortenberry JD, Linzer JF, Simon HK: Emergency department use of ketamine in pediatric status asthmaticus. J Asthma 2001;38(8):657–664.
14. Clancy M, Halford S, Walls R, Murphy M: In patients with head injuries who undergo rapid sequence intubation using succinylcholine, does pretreatment with a competitive neuromuscular blocking agent improve outcome? A literature review. Emerg Med J 2001;18(5):373–375.
15. Perry J, Lee J, Wells G: Rocuronium versus succinylcholine for rapid sequence induction intubation. Cochrane Database Syst Rev 2003;(1):CD002788.
16. Succinylcholine. Lexi-comp Online, 2004. Retrieved November 1, 2004, from http://www.crlonline.com/crlsql/servlet/crlonline.
17. Tabaee A, Givertz MM: Pharmacologic management of the hypotensive patient. In Irwin RS, Rippe JM (eds): Intensive Care Medicine. Philadelphia, Lippincott Williams & Wilkins, 2004, pp 295–302.
18. Salhanick SD, Shannon MW: Management of calcium channel antagonist overdose. Drug Saf 2003;26:65–79.
19. Roden DM: Drug-induced prolongation of the QT interval. N Engl J Med 2004;350(10):1013–1022.

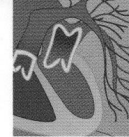

B Decontamination

STEPHEN W. BORRON, MD, MS

CONTROVERSY AND CONSENSUS

The treatment of toxic exposures by application of decontamination procedures has a long history. Logic suggests that removing even a portion of a toxic dose of a substance before it can act on the organism should improve outcomes. However, clinical and experimental studies have often failed to demonstrate the anticipated benefits. As a consequence, a number of consensus conferences and position statements have been developed to address various decontamination methods. The most recent iterations of these documents are briefly reviewed here. It should be recalled in the decision-making process that the conclusions of an expert panel are limited by the quality of the available evidence base. A number of case series and randomized clinical trials examining decontamination methods have been published, with numbers of patients in the range of 300 to 1000 or more.[1-4] Unfortunately, most of the randomized clinical trials investigating decontamination methods have lacked sufficient statistical power to discern important differences for outcomes involving any specific toxicant. In fact, there are noteworthy basic obstacles to performing reproducible, informative decontamination studies. Overdose patients frequently misrepresent or are ignorant of what dose of a compound they have taken or when the exposure occurred. Clearly, decontamination procedures should have greater effect when applied early, before significant absorption has taken place. Yet many studies include patients who are already significantly poisoned (i.e., symptomatic due to absorption), in whom decontamination measures would be expected to have little impact, unless the exposure is ongoing. Enrolling a large number of patients with similar clinical presentations (single drug, similar quantity of drug ingested and time since ingestion) is very difficult in a single center or even multiple centers. Confirmation of exposure by laboratory studies is often unavailable, requiring the clinician to depend on the history (which may be inaccurate) and physical findings (which may be nonspecific) in arriving at the diagnosis of poisoning. There are likewise problems with randomization schemes,[5] and basic inclusion and exclusion criteria.

In addition, there are problems with the process of evidence-based reviews themselves. Language bias occurs in some evidence-based reviews,[6] such that non–English language publications, potentially of good quality, are often excluded from consideration. In addition, the premises on which the evidence review is based may not be universally applicable. The conclusions reached, based on studies performed in urban tertiary care centers where hospitals are capable of providing state-of-the-art intensive care, may not apply equally to a remote hospital in a rural area, or even less so to a clinic in a developing country. Thus, while careful consideration should be given to position papers and consensus conference proceedings, individual judgment will necessarily enter into the decision to employ any decontamination method for a given case of exposure. Unfortunately, an unintended consequence of the publication of position papers is that they may in fact squelch further research.[5]

METHODS OF DECONTAMINATION

A number of methods of decontamination exist and may be employed depending on the circumstances of exposure. Decontamination of the skin and eyes, as well as the gastrointestinal tract, will be discussed. Extracorporeal methods of purification (hemodialysis, charcoal filtration, etc.) are covered in Chapter 2C.

SKIN AND EYE DECONTAMINATION

Decontamination of the skin and eyes is employed to reduce local tissue injury (chemical burns or irritation) and/or absorption that may result in systemic consequences. The decision to perform skin and eye decontamination is often based on the presence of symptoms, such as burning or itching. This is an insensitive evaluation method; thus, decontamination of these organs should primarily depend on careful consideration of the circumstances of exposure and the physical and toxicologic properties of the compound. Protection of personnel during eye and skin decontamination is important to avoid secondary contamination of health care providers. The choice of personal protective equipment is beyond the scope of this chapter. The reader is referred to Chapter 103 and to the recent Occupational Safety and Healthy Administration (OSHA) best practices document.[7]

Choice of Decontamination Methods Based on Physical Properties of the Toxicant

In almost all cases, clothing, jewelry, and shoes should be rapidly and completely removed prior to washing. It has been suggested in studies of radionuclide contamination that this process alone can remove the majority of a contaminant. This will, of course, depend on the physical properties of the toxicant but is a logical first step. Solids and dust should be gently brushed away before decontamination with a solution. In this way, the heat generated from water reactive compounds can be diminished, as is caking of solids.

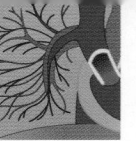

In some cases, water or other decontamination solutions may be unavailable or in short supply. In such cases, dry decontamination, using an absorbent material (charcoal, flour, earth) followed by brushing or wiping may be attempted.

Choice of Decontamination Solutions

The selection of skin decontamination solutions has historically been a choice between water for polar (water-soluble) compounds and water plus a mild soap or detergent for nonpolar compounds. Water alone is typically employed for initial eye decontamination. Physiologic saline and other saline-based eye washes are often employed for eye decontamination in health care and industrial settings. The use of these solutions has been largely empiric and practical, based on widespread availability rather than on critical evaluation of their efficacy. Yano and colleagues studied water irrigation of burns involving 1 mol/L HCl in rats, measuring subcutaneous pH as a measure of penetration of the acid and efficacy of decontamination. These investigators found that maximal subcutaneous pH depression had occurred by 7 minutes following application of the acid. Animals undergoing water irrigation at 1 or 3 minutes postexposure demonstrated some benefit; however, animals irrigated at 10 minutes had no appreciable improvement in pH, compared with control.[8] These investigators had previously demonstrated lack of efficacy of water irrigation after 10 minutes in a 2N NaOH burn model.[9] Clearly time is of the essence in irrigation of corrosive exposures. With regard to eye exposures, Kuckelkorn and colleagues[10] pointed out that water is hypotonic to corneal stroma, allowing edema and increased penetration by chemicals. They recommend use of amphoteric solutions to avoid these problems.

In recent years, a number of novel decontamination solutions have come to market. Diphoterine (Prevor Laboratories, Moulin de Verville, France), an amphoteric solution has been proposed for use in both acid and alkali exposures of eyes and skin, with emphasis on immediate irrigation (at the scene of the incident) rather than for hospital treatment. A recent article[11] that compared Diphoterine to physiological saline in alkaline eye burns demonstrated more rapid healing of grade 1 and 2 burns with Diphoterine than with saline. The study suffers from a number of deficiencies, including lack of randomization and significant delays and variability in initial irrigation (in the field) and secondary irrigation in hospital (with either Diphoterine or saline). Nonetheless, the time to corneal reepithelialization was approximately six times as long after saline for grade 1 burns and almost twice as long for grade 2 burns, compared with Diphoterine-treated eyes. There were an insufficient number of grade 3 burns to detect any significant difference between groups. Despite its shortcomings, this study suggests the potential for improved healing using Diphoterine in alkaline eye burns and warrants further investigation. The same study group had previously shown in a study of ammonia burns

in New Zealand albino rabbit eyes that early application (within 10 minutes) of Diphoterine rapidly corrected pH, whereas saline irrigation did not. Furthermore, saline-treated eyes had stromal edema, whereas Diphoterine-treated eyes did not.[12] The need for early irrigation is emphasized by this experimental study; however, the cited clinical study demonstrates some benefit even with delayed treatment (mean 4.7 hours).[11] Cavallini and Casati studied Diphoterine in experimental skin burns in rats involving 52% hydrochloric acid. Skin flushing with Diphoterine reduced substance P release during the first 48 hours after burn and was associated with better wound healing and higher concentrations of β-endorphin 7 days later when compared with normal saline or 10% calcium gluconate.[13] Hall and colleagues[14] have reviewed the chemical and physical properties and proposed uses of Diphoterine. Hexafluorine, manufactured by the same company, is proposed for treatment of exposures to hydrogen fluoride. Both Diphoterine and Hexafluorine are indicated for skin and eye decontamination.*

The National Nuclear Security Administration's Sandia National Laboratories has developed decontamination foam, referred to as EasyDECON 200 or DF 200. This product is purported to be effective against a variety of chemical and biological warfare agents, including cyanide, phosgene, mustard, VX, G agents, anthrax, *Yersinia pestis*, and corona viruses. The Illinois Institute of Technology and the Southwest Research Institute have performed tests of the ability of the compound to neutralize chemical and biological agents. While there is mention on the laboratory's website of seeking U.S. Food and Drug Administration (FDA) approval of DF 200 for personal decontamination, no peer-reviewed studies of its use in humans were identified. As such, this product cannot be currently recommended for human use.

Most authors recommend against neutralization of acid and base burns due to the risk for exothermic reaction leading to thermal burns. Simple dilution with water or milk after oral ingestion of corrosives is uncommon in Europe, but the norm after ingestions in the United States. Penner demonstrated in an ingestion model that dilution of concentrated sulfuric acid with an equivalent volume of water results in a temperature elevation of approximately 80°C. Neutralization results in even greater heat production. He suggested that vigorous gastric aspiration (likewise considered controversial given the risk for esophageal or gastric perforation) prior to cold fluid lavage is the treatment of choice in patients treated immediately following acid ingestion.[15] A recent experimental study involving irrigation of rat skin exposed to 2N NaOH with 5% acetic acid suggests that neutralization may not always be contraindicated. The investigators demonstrated more rapid correction of pH, no difference in peak temperatures, and improved outcomes in animals treated with 5% acetic acid rather than water. These findings cannot

---

*Diphoterine and Hexafluorine are proprietary products without generic equivalents. Use of the trade name in this chapter does not constitute an endorsement.

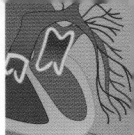

be generalized, but indicate the need to readdress current dogma regarding neutralization.[16]

Duration of Decontamination

The ideal duration of eye and skin decontamination is yet to be determined. Recommendations for copious irrigation are common, without further precision. Fifteen minutes is probably the most commonly recommended duration for eye irrigation. Kuckelkorn and colleagues have recommended a minimum of 30 minutes for eye irrigation after chemical exposures.[17] One retrospective study of 172 eye burn victims suggested that outcomes were better among those who had prolonged (1 to 2 hours) irrigation.[18] Irrigating to a relatively neutral pH is often attempted. If this is employed, it is helpful to remember that the pH of saline for intravenous injection (often employed for eye irrigation) is appreciably acidic (approximately 4.5) so that one should wait a few minutes after irrigation to measure the pH in order to allow the patient's own tears to replace the saline irrigation fluid in the conjunctival sac.

Temperature

The appropriate temperature for decontamination fluids has also been poorly studied. While increasing temperature of decontamination liquids reduces the likelihood of hypothermia in inclement climes and improves water solubility, heat also dilates skin pores and blood vessels, which may lead to increased absorption. If excessive, it may aggravate chemical or thermal burns. OSHA's recently published *Best Practices Guide for First Receivers*[7] recommends a 5-minute wash with tepid water, based on recommendations from the U.S. Army for chemical decontamination.[19] Mcintyre and colleagues recommend "warm, but not excessively warm" water for decontamination.[20] Eye irrigation should be performed with room temperature solutions. Careful thought should be given to environmental conditions and risk for exposure when decontamination must be done out of doors.

MASS CASUALTIES

The duration and type of skin and eye decontamination performed in mass casualty situations may vary from that in cases involving single patients based on triage considerations. Management of mass casualties is covered in Chapter 103.

Decontamination Systems

A great number of options have been developed in recent years for skin decontamination, due to the increased interest in hazardous materials and chemical terrorism issues. Examples of decontamination stretchers and facilities are shown in Figures 2B-1 to 2B-3. Many others exist. One of the overriding considerations in determining the kind of decontamination facilities and equipment to purchase should be their capacity for rapid deployment. The experience with the sarin terrorist attack in Tokyo revealed that hospitals may be rapidly

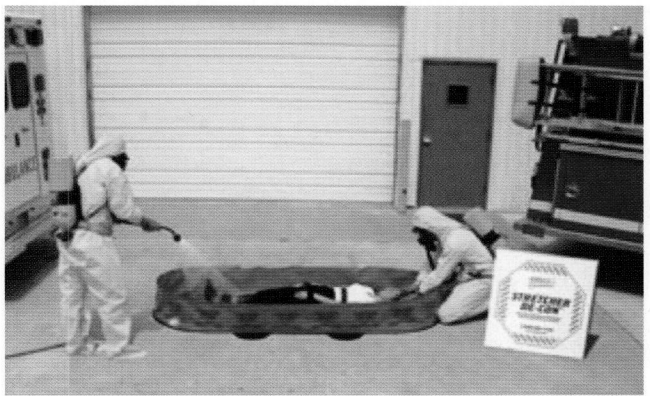

FIGURE 2B-1 Portable decontamination stretcher.

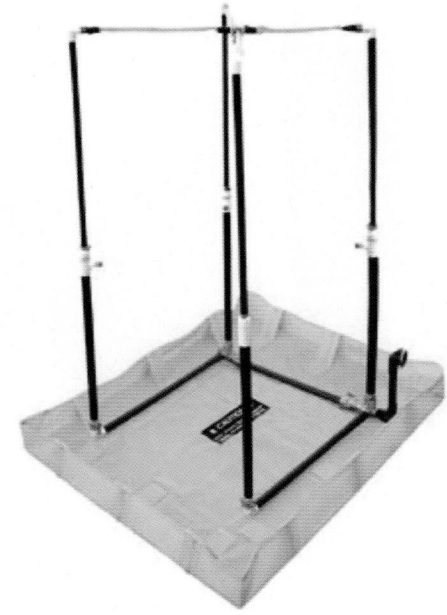

FIGURE 2B-2 Portable decontamination shower.

inundated with contaminated casualties. Decontamination protocols that are not deployable within minutes (preferably 5 to 10 minutes) after an incident may serve little purpose in protecting the facility and health care providers from contamination. Serious consideration should be given to the complexity of the setup process, one that typically will not be employed frequently. One example of a locally developed immediate deployment sheltered outdoor decontamination unit is shown in Figure 2B-4. This unit can be deployed in less than 2 minutes and provides for decontamination of both ambulatory and stretcher patients.

Personnel

It is common practice to utilize physicians, nurses, and other critical emergency department (ED) staff to do decontamination. This is probably not advisable for a number of reasons. First, decontamination does not require great technical skill, and very little stabilization

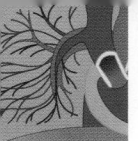

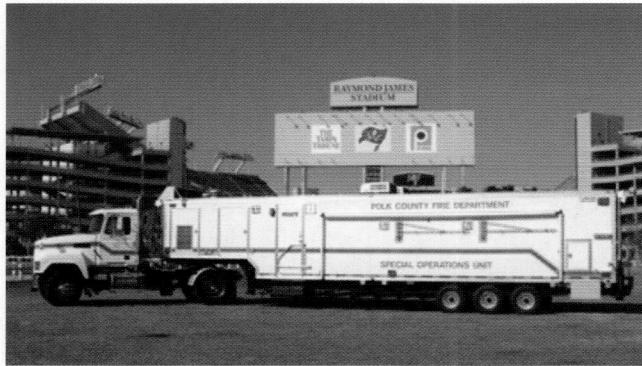

A

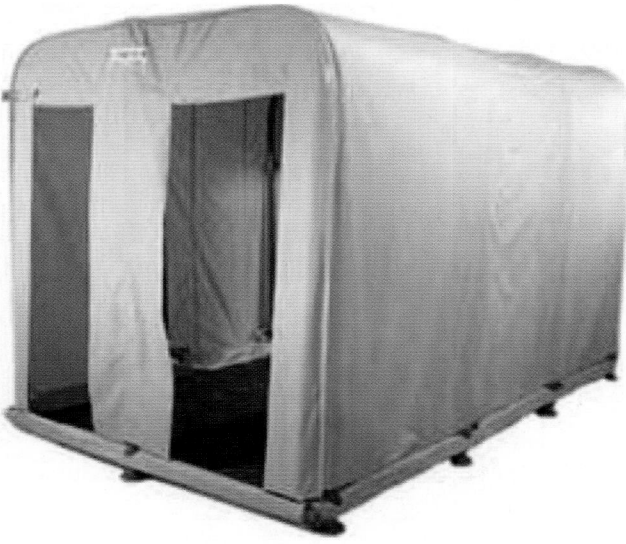

B

FIGURE 2B-3 **A,** Portable decontamination trailer. **B,** Portable decontamination tent.

can be performed during the decontamination process. Furthermore, if there are problems and decontaminating personnel are unable to continue, such a practice results in incapacitation of primary emergency care providers. Neither should security personnel, in general, be tasked with this responsibility, since a mass casualty situation will require their services for security itself. A number of alternatives have been suggested. Some hospitals train housekeeping staff to perform decontamination. Others have nurses from other units (burn units have extensive experience in wound care and cleaning) don protective clothing and prepare for decontamination while the ED staff prepares the decontamination facility and the ED proper to receive casualties.

SPECIAL SITUATIONS

Radionuclides

Decontamination of radionuclides from the skin may be performed in a manner analogous to chemical exposures. Uranium hexafluoride exposures should be treated in a manner analogous to that for hydrofluoric acid burns. Wounds heavily contaminated with radionuclides may require surgical débridement and should be covered after initial decontamination. See Chapter 104 regarding radiation emergency management for further information.

Fluorides

Hydrogen fluoride, ammonium biflouride, and other soluble fluorides may pose a unique case in terms of decontamination. While an initial quick flush with water is appropriate, the patient may benefit from rapid decontamination with a substance that can bind the fluoride. Hexafluorine has been reported to prevent significant skin burns in both humans and experimental animals when applied immediately after exposure.[21,22] Two randomized studies in rats found, however, that Hexafluorine was no better than water in preventing electrolyte disturbances caused by fluoride[23,24] and perhaps less effective than water or water plus calcium gluconate in reducing burn injury.[24] Thus, Hexafluorine's efficacy in fluoride injury remains controversial.[25] Researchers in hydrogen fluoride manufacturing facilities frequently recommend skin irrigation with benzalkonium chloride solution based on studies performed in pigs.[26,27] Calcium gluconate irrigation of skin[28] and eyes[29] has also been recommended to bind fluoride and prevent further injury. Other investigators have found calcium gluconate to be no more effective than water or saline and perhaps detrimental in eye irrigation.[30,31] In summary, the ideal decontamination of hydrogen fluoride burns to skin and eyes remains to be determined.

Phenol

Phenol is unique in its capacity to cause nonpainful burns and systemic toxicity. Water irrigation may increase phenol absorption.[32] Generally accepted skin irrigation therapy consists of isopropanol[32,33] or polyethylene glycol solutions.[32,34]

Flammable Metals and Other Water-Reactive Materials

White phosphorus is pyrophoric (i.e., it burns in the presence of air). It is thus indispensable to provide adequate copious irrigation with water. The application of copper sulfate has been recommended,[35] but an experimental study in rats demonstrated increased lethality in animals receiving topical treatment with 1% copper sulfate.[36] Eldad and colleagues have evaluated various phosphorus burn treatment recommendations and have concluded that copious water irrigation is superior to other treatments.[37]

HIGH-PRESSURE INJECTION INJURIES

High-pressure injection injuries should be mentioned here due to their requirement for special care and high

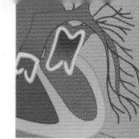

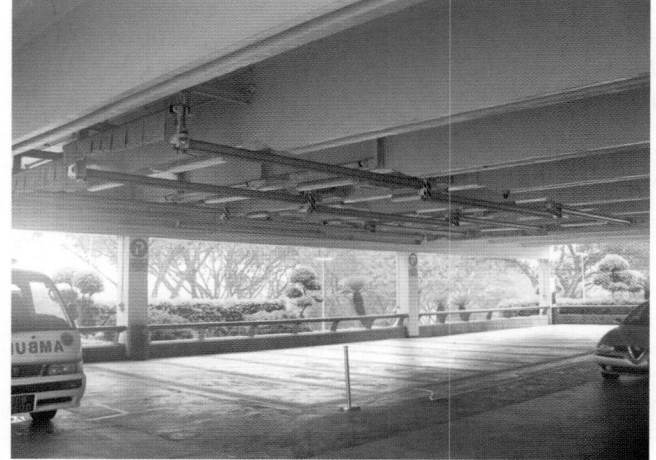

A

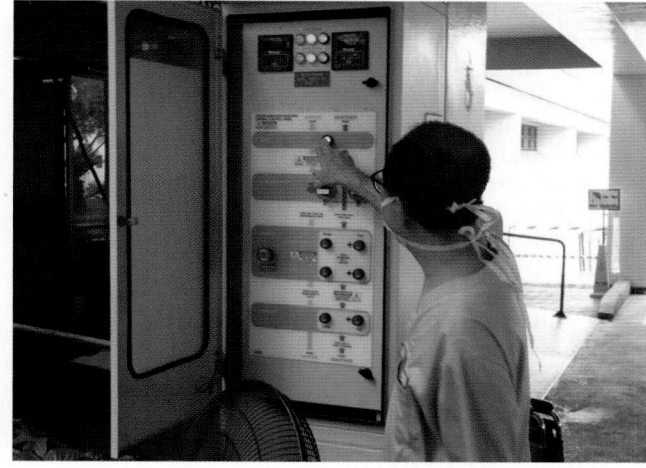

B

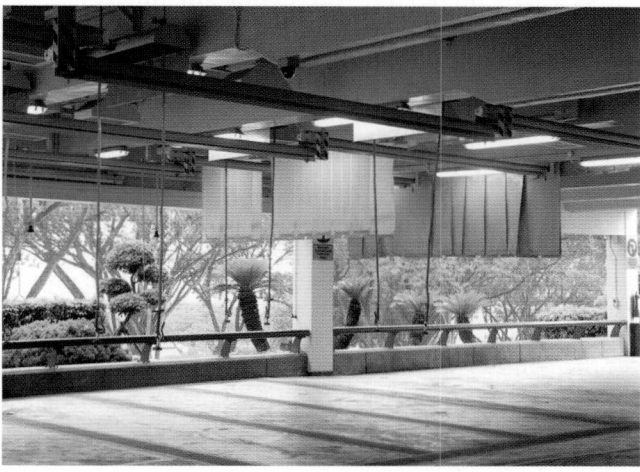

C

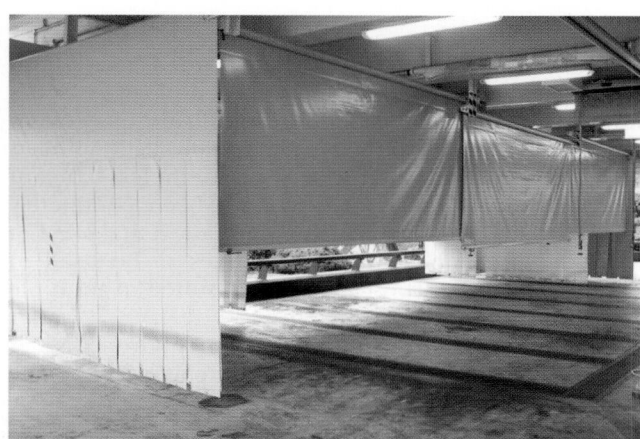

D

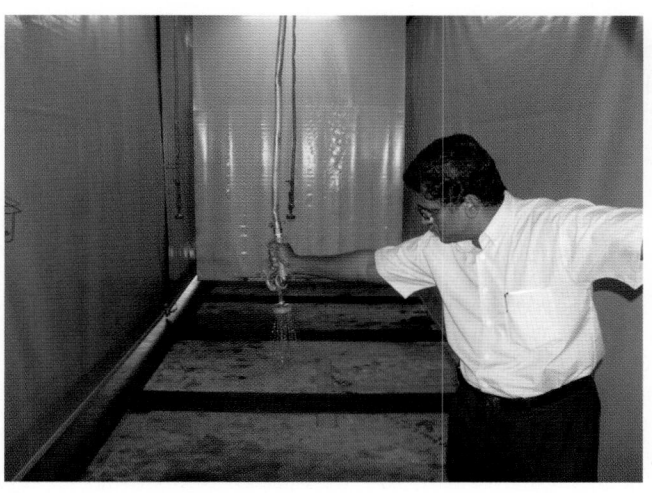

E

FIGURE 2B-4 A, Fixed immediate deployment decontamination facility at Singapore General Hospital and Drug and Poisons Information Centre. The unit is located in the drive-through ambulance bay in front of the emergency department. This shows the unit in predeployment position. **B,** Deployment of the unit requires turning on a few switches, which control descent of the shower heads, flexible walls, and temperature control. The unit is ready for operation in approximately 2 minutes. **C,** Shower heads drop out of the ceiling for self- or assisted irrigation. **D,** Flexible walls drop from the overhead frame, providing easy ingress, egress, and protection from elements, as well as privacy. **E,** The unit is ready for use. Floor drains collect the water for appropriate disposal. (Photographs courtesy of Dr. Gaerpo Ponampalam and the Singapore Drug and Poisons Information Centre.)

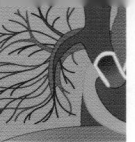

risk for morbidity. Wounds inflicted by pressurized paint guns or grease guns are often deceivingly benign appearing on the surface. The temptation is to simply decontaminate the overlying skin and wash the puncture wound (if visible) from the surface. Such an approach may result in loss of function or even complete loss of a limb. Such wounds need to be explored thoroughly, perhaps best done in the operating room, for evidence of subcutaneous contamination.[38,39]

TETANUS PROPHYLAXIS

All eye and skin exposures resulting in violation of the epithelium should prompt consideration of the need for tetanus toxoid administration.

GASTRIC EMPTYING

Emetics

The only emetic currently recommended for use in humans is syrup of ipecac. Previously employed emetics continue to be responsible for significant pathology, however. The administration of table salt has long been condemned in the literature[40]; nonetheless, recent reports illustrate that its use has not been completely abandoned and that it remains potentially lethal.[41,42] Liu reported that copper sulfate continues to be used in China for emetic purposes and has resulted in multiple fatalities in recent years.[43]

The dose of ipecac is 5 to 10 mL in children 6 to 12 months of age or 15 mL in children 1 to 12 years of age. This should be followed by 10 to 20 mL water per kg body weight. Older children and adults should receive 30 mL ipecac followed by 200 to 300 mL of water. Ipecac is contraindicated in the following situations:

> Ingestion of petroleum distillates
> Ingestion of strong acids or bases
> Ingestion of strychnine or other proconvulsants
> Unconsciousness or absence of gag reflex

Ipecac has a number of potential adverse effects, including lethargy, cramps, and diarrhea. When taken chronically, it may induce muscle cramps and both skeletal[44] and cardiac myopathy.[45] It is subject to frequent abuse by patients with eating disorders, a factor that led to a review of the product's safety by the FDA in 2003.

The American Academy of Clinical Toxicology (AACT) and the European Association of Poisons Centres and Clinical Toxicologists (EAPCCT) reviewed the medical literature regarding the use of ipecac in 1997.[46] This combined task force more recently examined their previous findings and literature that had appeared since their earlier review. In brief, they concluded that syrup of ipecac should not be administered routinely in the management of poisoned patients. They pointed out that in experimental studies the amount of marker removed by ipecac was highly variable and diminished with time. Furthermore they concluded that there is no evidence from clinical studies that ipecac improves the outcome of poisoned patients and recommended that its routine administration in the ED be abandoned. Finally, they signaled the absence of data to support or exclude ipecac administration soon after poison ingestion, the administration of ipecac potentially reducing the effectiveness of activated charcoal, oral antidotes, and whole bowel irrigation (WBI).[47]

There are indications that the use of syrup of ipecac has dramatically declined in recent years, and it is likely that this trend will continue.[48,49] Bond examined the evolving use of ipecac in U.S. poison centers, comparing rates of referral to the ED and moderate or greater outcomes in patients younger than 6 years with unintentional ingestions. This comparison was carried out according to the frequency with which centers recommended use of ipecac. Overall, use of ipecac was extremely rare (1.8%) and significant adverse outcomes even lower (0.6%). Comparing the two groups of 32 centers each, there were no significant differences in referral rates or adverse outcomes. Bond concluded that there was no reduction in resource utilization (ED referral) or improvement in patient outcome from the use of syrup of ipecac at home and that while the data could not exclude a benefit in a very limited set of poisonings, such a benefit remained to be proven. Shannon, in an editorial in the same issue, sounded the demise of ipecac on the basis of lack of proven efficacy, changing patterns in poison center approaches to the management of pediatric ingestions (including preference for activated charcoal when decontamination is indicated), and the move by the FDA to rescind ipecac's over-the-counter status.[50] This prediction was prescient, since the American Academy of Pediatrics, based on Bond's article and the factors cited by Shannon, revised its position statement on ipecac use, calling for abandonment of the regular stocking of it in the home.[51]

More recently, a U.S. government–convened review panel of experts published their conclusions regarding ipecac use.[52] The panel concluded that the use of ipecac syrup might have an acceptable benefit-to-risk ratio when:

> There is no contraindication to the use of ipecac syrup.
> There is substantial risk of serious toxicity to the victim.
> There is no alternative therapy available or effective to decrease gastrointestinal absorption (e.g., activated charcoal).
> There will be a delay of more than 1 hour before the patient will arrive at an emergency medical facility.
> Ipecac syrup can be administered within 30 to 90 minutes of the ingestion.
> Ipecac syrup administration will not adversely affect more definitive treatment that might be provided at a hospital.

Given these restrictions, rural residents might consider keeping ipecac on hand for home use under poison center direction. Otherwise, these recommendations sharply limit the applicability of the drug and, thus, the induction of vomiting in general.

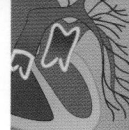

Gastric Lavage

The employment of gastric lavage is controversial and varies markedly depending on geographic area and the background and training of the practitioner. Gastric lavage involves blind placement of a large-bore gastric tube into the stomach, in a patient who can either protect his or her own airway or in whom the airway has been protected by an endotracheal tube, with the goal of removing toxicant remaining in the stomach through a combination of instillation of water or physiological saline, followed by suction or gravity-induced drainage. This cycle of instillation/drainage is repeated until the effluent is clear or until several liters of water/saline have been passed through the tube. This procedure has been widely popular in the past and continues to be employed in many EDs around the world. It is, however, a largely unproven therapy.

INDICATIONS

The indications for gastric lavage are recent ingestion (generally less than 1 hour, unless the ingestion involves agents that decrease gastric motility, such as anticholinergics) of a substance of sufficient quantity to be likely to cause serious harm in the absence of removal. The procedure should be given greater consideration in ingestions for which inadequate treatment modalities exist (paraquat) or in cases where delivery of proven effective therapy (antidotes or extracorporeal removal) is likely to be delayed.

CONTRAINDICATIONS

Ingestion of low-viscosity petroleum products, corrosives (acids and alkalis) and inability to protect the airway (unless tracheal intubation has been performed beforehand) are contraindications to gastric lavage.

ADVERSE EFFECTS

Serious adverse effects of gastric lavage are relatively rare but may be significant. The procedure may induce hypoxia,[53] perforation of the gastrointestinal tract or pharynx,[54,55] fluid and electrolyte abnormalities,[56] inadvertent tracheal intubation, as well as aspiration pneumonitis.[57] Tracheal intubation is not completely protective against aspiration.

EFFICACY

The AACT/EAPCCT recently reviewed the animal and clinical literature regarding gastric lavage and published a position statement,[58] which states in part that gastric lavage should not be employed routinely, if ever, in the management of poisoned patients. The study group pointed out that in experimental studies, the amount of marker removed by gastric lavage is highly variable and diminishes with time and that few clinical studies have demonstrated a beneficial effect on outcome.

The quality of the gastric lavage literature is, for the most part, lacking. Few studies have the power to detect significant differences in outcome for a single toxicant, and it seems unscientific to compare outcomes after ingestion of widely varying products. Furthermore, there are many unknowns in any clinical trial, the most significant of these being the time between ingestion and treatment and the amount of toxicant ingested. It is fair to say that the evidence for efficacy is currently deficient, but that lack of efficacy has not been proven either.

Endoscopy

The use of endoscopy in the diagnosis of caustic injuries is addressed in Chapter 98. Its use in the retrieval of foreign objects, such as batteries,[59] firearm cartridges,[60] and various pill fragments[61-66] has been reported in humans and studied in animals,[67] but has not been systematically addressed in humans. Faigel and colleagues report that endoscopic use of the Roth net was most effective in removal of button batteries.[67] Like other forms of decontamination, endoscopy to retrieve tablet fragments has been associated with significant complications; thus, the decision to perform endoscopy in these circumstances should be carefully weighed against the risks.[62]

Surgical Laparotomy for Decontamination

Surgical gastrointestinal decontamination has been employed for button battery ingestions,[68-70] cocaine and narcotic drug packets,[71-77] and bezoars of iron[78] and theophylline,[79] among others. Batteries passing the esophagus usually are expelled in the feces and are generally believed to require no intervention, although recent reports of early battery leakage have called the "wait and see" approach into question.[80,81] Button batteries, when impacted in the esophagus, should generally be removed by endoscopy unless perforation is suspected.[59,67,82] The trend toward use of smaller batteries by manufacturers has decreased the incidence of this problem. In the case of cocaine and heroin bodypackers/stuffers, many cases can be managed conservatively with WBI or other purgatives. Most researchers agree, however, that acute toxicity (drug leakage) and bowel obstruction are indications for immediate laparotomy.[71,73,75]

ABSORBANTS

Activated Charcoal

Charcoal binds to diverse substances, rendering them less available for systemic absorption from the gastrointestinal tract. It is obtained as a product of pyrolysis of numerous organic compounds (petroleum, wood, peat) and "activated" by heating it to 600° F to 900° F, in the presence of steam, carbon dioxide, or air. This gives the product a small particle size and large surface area. While charcoal adheres to many substances, a significant number of compounds and classes of compounds are poorly absorbed by charcoal. These include metals (lithium, sodium, iron, potassium) and alcohols. Thallium appears to be an exception, being relatively well absorbed by charcoal.[83]

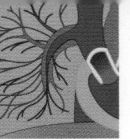

Activated charcoal products containing sorbitol should be avoided where possible because (1) the efficacy of cathartics is lacking (see below); (2) sorbitol is emetogenic and can increase the risk for vomiting the charcoal; and (3) sorbitol administration in infants is associated with dehydration and other life-threatening events.

Single-Dose Activated Charcoal

Activated charcoal is administered as a slurry, either in water or sorbitol, orally or via a nasogastric tube. Dose recommendations vary, but generally a larger dose is considered better, to assure that binding capacity exceeds the amount of toxicant present. The recommended dose is 0.5 to 1 g/kg in children or 25 to 100 g in adults.

INDICATIONS

In general, to be maximally effective, charcoal should be administered as soon as possible after ingestion of the toxicant, preferably within 1 hour. Green and colleagues studied this issue in healthy volunteers in a randomized crossover study. After giving 4 g (the equivalent of eight extra-strength tablets) of acetaminophen to patients, then giving charcoal at 1, 2, or 3 hours after ingestion, they found no differences in the area under the curve of plasma acetaminophen. The investigators stated that "data do not support the administration of activated charcoal as a gastrointestinal decontamination strategy beyond 1 hour after drug overdose."[84] While there are obvious problems in extrapolating toxicokinetic results from a study involving a nontoxic dose to all overdoses, the results do suggest that benefit clearly decreases over time.

As for most decontamination measures, the indications for single dose activated charcoal are controversial. The recently released revision of the Single-dose Activated Charcoal Position Statement of the AACT/EAPCCT states that single-dose activated charcoal should not be administered routinely in the management of poisoned patients, but that it may be considered if a patient has ingested a potentially toxic amount of a poison (which is known to be adsorbed to charcoal) up to 1 hour previously. The researchers state that the potential for benefit after 1 hour cannot be excluded. Finally, they emphasize that there is no evidence that the administration of activated charcoal improves clinical outcome.[85]

CONTRAINDICATIONS

Charcoal administration is generally considered contraindicated in ingestions of caustics, since it is probably ineffective in reducing their potential for harm and furthermore makes endoscopy difficult. Charcoal generally should not be administered when there is a high risk for gastrointestinal hemorrhage or perforation. Charcoal is likewise contraindicated in any patient in whom the airway protection is not assured. It should not be administered in the presence of hydrocarbons with high aspiration potential. Charcoal should not be administered in the case of ileus or mechanical bowel obstruction.

ADVERSE REACTIONS AND COMPLICATIONS

One of the most common adverse events associated with charcoal administration is vomiting, which occurs in approximately 7% to 15% of patients. Abdominal bloating is also quite common. Both diarrhea and constipation may occur. Complications have been described, including pulmonary aspiration and direct administration into the lungs via misplaced nasogastric tube. Aspiration appears to be relatively rare, but may have serious consequences.[57,86-89]

Multiple-Dose Activated Charcoal

Multiple-dose activated charcoal (MDAC) has been proposed for use in the case of drugs that undergo extensive enterohepatic or enteroenteric circulation. Drugs with small volumes of distribution are particularly susceptible to removal by adsorption to charcoal in the gut, which has sometimes been referred to as "gastrointestinal dialysis." Although experimental and volunteer studies have demonstrated that MDAC increased elimination of a number of compounds, there is little proof of clinical benefit.

INDICATIONS

The AACT/EAPCCT has concluded that although many studies in animal and volunteer studies have demonstrated MDAC increases drug elimination significantly, there are no controlled studies in poisoned patients that demonstrate MDAC reduces morbidity and mortality. Pending further evidence of direct benefits, the study group recommended that MDAC be considered only if a patient has ingested a life-threatening amount of carbamazepine, dapsone, phenobarbital, quinine, or theophylline.[90]

CONTRAINDICATIONS

The contraindications for MDAC are essentially those of single-dose activated charcoal. The admonition for use in intestinal obstruction is of even greater import in the case of MDAC. The presence of decreased peristalsis (often associated with anticholinergic drugs and opiates) should provoke extreme caution in the administration of MDAC.

Prussian Blue

Prussian blue is an effective absorbent for the management of thallium and cesium intoxications. See Chapters 75 and 104 for further information.

Fuller's Earth

Fuller's earth is often recommended for gastrointestinal decontamination of paraquat (see Chapter 78). Although effective for this purpose, this substance is found in few hospitals. Activated charcoal is an effective absorbent of paraquat and should be employed when Fuller's earth is not available.[91]

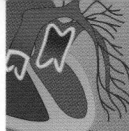

ACCELERATION OF GASTROINTESTINAL TRANSIT

Cathartics

Cathartics comprise another group of compounds recommended since ancient times for the purpose of eliminating toxicants from the gastrointestinal tract. The two most common categories of cathartics are the magnesium salts (e.g., magnesium citrate, magnesium sulfate) and nondigestible carbohydrates (e.g., sorbitol). Despite their long history of use, there is virtually no evidence of their efficacy. On the contrary, cathartics may induce significant harm in certain groups of patients, particularly children and those with renal disease.

INDICATIONS

There are no evident indications for the use of a cathartic alone in the treatment of poisoning.[92] An AACT/EAPCCT position statement concluded that experimental data are conflicting regarding the use of cathartics in combination with activated charcoal. The study group found no published clinical studies that investigated the ability of a cathartic, with or without activated charcoal, to reduce the bioavailability of drugs or to improve the outcome of poisoned patients. They went on to say that based on available data, the routine use of a cathartic in combination with activated charcoal is not endorsed and that if a cathartic is used, it should be limited to a single dose in order to minimize adverse effects of the cathartic.

DOSE

The dose of sorbitol is approximately 1 to 2 g/kg.[92] When given in combination with activated charcoal for single dose-activated charcoal therapy, the dose should be determined on the basis of charcoal dosing. If multiple doses of charcoal are to be administered, repeated use of sorbitol is not recommended. For magnesium citrate, the dose is 4 to 6 mL/kg in children and 300 to 480 mL in adults.

CONTRAINDICATIONS

Cathartics are contraindicated in the presence of bowel obstruction, in the absence of bowel sounds, or in the case of recent bowel surgery or intestinal perforation. They should likewise not be employed in the case of corrosive ingestions or when significant electrolyte disturbances, dehydration, or hemodynamic instability are present. Magnesium-containing cathartics must be avoided in patients with renal insufficiency and heart block. Caution should be employed in patients at extremes of age.

COMPLICATIONS

Cathartics frequently cause cramping, nausea, and vomiting. Significant dehydration may occur if catharsis is excessive, with resultant hypotension. Cathartic-related hypermagnesemia may result in cardiac dysrhythmias. Elderly patients and those with renal dysfunction are at particular risk.[93-95] Massive doses of cathartics may result in cardiopulmonary arrest.[93]

Whole Bowel Irrigation

WBI involves the administration, by mouth or nasogastric tube, of large amounts of an iso-osmotic polyethylene glycol electrolyte solution (Go-Lytely [Braintree Laboratories, Braintree, MA], Co-Lyte [Schwarz Pharma, Mequon, WI], and others) with the goal of removing unabsorbed toxicant from the gastrointestinal tract as rapidly as possible by rectal expulsion. One rationale for its use includes the fact that some compounds are poorly absorbed by charcoal, particularly iron and lithium. WBI may be of particular interest in the case of sustained-release or enteric-coated compounds and in the case of drug packets (body packers). The AACT/EAPCCT's consensus panel concluded that WBI should not be used routinely and that there is no conclusive evidence that it improves the outcome of poisoned patients. Based on evidence from volunteer studies, the group recommended that WBI be considered for potentially toxic ingestions of sustained-release or enteric-coated drugs, particularly in those patients who present more than 2 hours after drug ingestion. They more strongly endorsed WBI for patients who have ingested substantial amounts of iron because the morbidity is high and there are no other effective options for gastrointestinal decontamination. Another potential indication cited for the use of WBI is expulsion of ingested packets of illicit drugs.[96]

DOSE

Polyethylene glycol electrolyte solution (e.g., Go-Lytely, Co-Lyte, NuLytely [Braintree Laboratories, Braintree, MA]) is administered by mouth or nasogastric tube at 25 to 40 mL/kg/hr until the rectal effluent is clear or until the desired effect is otherwise demonstrated (e.g., passage of drug packets demonstrated by imaging studies). Computed tomography (CT) with contrast has often been used to identify retained packets, but a recent case report demonstrated incomplete sensitivity of CT to detect all unexpelled drug packets.[72]

CONTRAINDICATIONS

WBI is contraindicated in the presence of mechanical or functional (ileus) bowel obstruction or perforation and in the presence of significant gastrointestinal hemorrhage. It should likewise be avoided if the patient is hemodynamically unstable.

COMPLICATIONS

Nausea and vomiting are not uncommon. Abdominal bloating and cramping may occur. Vomiting in the case of an unprotected airway may result in pulmonary aspiration.

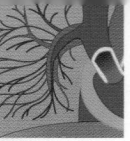

DECISION ANALYSIS FOR DECONTAMINATION

The decision to employ decontamination methods in an individual case must be determined based on the factors present in that individual case.

Dose Assessment

First and foremost in the decision to attempt decontamination is a determination of whether a significant exposure has occurred. This is critical for numerous reasons: (1) needless decontamination procedures may delay other definitive therapy for systemic toxicity; (2) conversely, failure to adequately decontaminate the skin may increase morbidity of contaminated patients and result in secondary contamination of health care providers and facilities; and (3) decontamination, as discussed, is not without risks. It is vital to recall Hippocrates' admonition: *Primum non nocerum.* Dose/exposure assessment is extremely difficult on an acute basis due to the great number of unknowns. Young children cannot recount the quantity or quality of what they have ingested. Self-harm attempts are often accompanied by attempts to conceal or, conversely, to exaggerate the consumption of potentially toxic compounds. It is rare that contemporaneous exposure information (air concentrations or even product identification) is available after environmental exposures associated with hazardous materials releases or acts of terror. Fear associated with these events may result in psychogenic illness at times indistinguishable from that of the toxic exposure. When doubt exists, it may be safer to decontaminate, but this should be a considered decision.

Toxic Potential

Once it is established that an exposure has occurred (or if exposure cannot be excluded) and some attempt has been made to determine the magnitude of the exposure, one must examine the toxic potential of the compound(s) in question, keeping in mind that the toxicity of combined substances is not always equal to the sum of their individual toxicities. Approaches to the treatment of poisoning are deeply rooted in personal experience and colored by bias in the literature. Recent studies have reexamined the need to decontaminate victims of certain exposures that were previously approached aggressively from a therapeutic standpoint.[97,98]

An Integrated Approach to Decontamination Procedures

Decisions around decontamination must be individualized. A suggested approach is found in Figure 2B-5. This nonvalidated algorithm should simply be considered a pathway for considering options. There are numerous potential exceptions to the general suggestions in the figure.

WHEN SHOULD GASTRIC LAVAGE BE PERFORMED ALONE?

One might consider gastric lavage alone in the case of presentation of poisoning within 1 hour of ingestion by a highly toxic compound that is not readily absorbed by charcoal. Lithium is one such example.

WHEN IS GASTRIC LAVAGE FOLLOWED BY CHARCOAL APPROPRIATE?

Reiterating, gastric lavage is most likely to be effective in an early-presenting, potentially lethal ingestion. Cyanide is an example of a highly toxic compound that might be removed by lavage, but is also readily absorbed by charcoal.

IS THERE A ROLE FOR CHARCOAL FOLLOWED BY WHOLE BOWEL IRRIGATION?

Yes. Illicit drug packets containing cocaine or heroin may leak. A dose of activated charcoal given prophylactically (in the absence of symptoms) could theoretically absorb eventual leakage, while WBI accelerates passage of the packets. As a reminder, clinical evidence of toxicity (leakage) is an indication for laparotomy. Similarly, charcoal followed by WBI may be indicated for ingestions of enteric coated tablets.

WHEN SHOULD WHOLE BOWEL IRRIGATION BE UTILIZED?

In cases in which ingestion of a substance known to be effectively eliminated by WBI (such as lead, zinc, or iron) is not recent (and thus not likely to benefit from gastric lavage) and when the substance is not readily absorbed by charcoal, WBI alone may be indicated.

CONSULTATION

It should be clear from the discussion that the previously common "reflex arc" of ingestion-decontamination should not apply. The decision to apply a particular procedure or combination may not be simple. For this reason, consultation with a regional poison center and/or medical toxicologist is strongly suggested in cases of uncertainty.

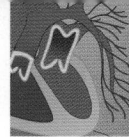

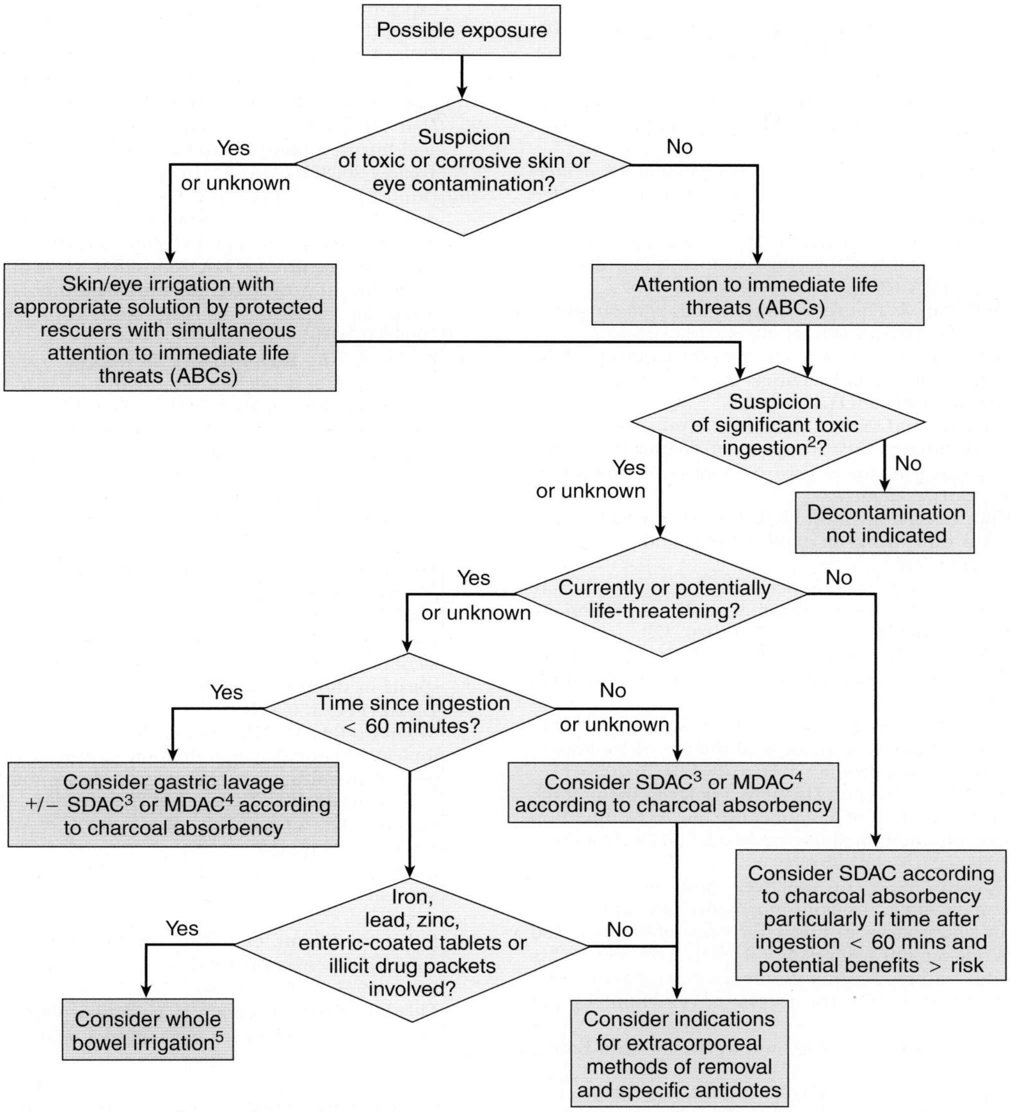

```
                        ┌─────────────────┐
                        │ Possible exposure│
                        └────────┬────────┘
                                 ↓
                           ╱───────────╲
        Yes              ╱  Suspicion    ╲              No
    or unknown         ╱  of toxic or corrosive skin or ╲
    ◄─────────────────┤    eye contamination?          ├─────────────►
                       ╲                              ╱
                        ╲───────────╱
```

Possible exposure

Suspicion of toxic or corrosive skin or eye contamination?

Yes or unknown → **Skin/eye irrigation with appropriate solution by protected rescuers with simultaneous attention to immediate life threats (ABCs)**

No → **Attention to immediate life threats (ABCs)**

Suspicion of significant toxic ingestion²?

No → **Decontamination not indicated**

Yes or unknown → **Currently or potentially life-threatening?**

Yes or unknown → **Time since ingestion < 60 minutes?**

No → **Consider SDAC³ or MDAC⁴ according to charcoal absorbency**

No → **Consider SDAC according to charcoal absorbency particularly if time after ingestion < 60 mins and potential benefits > risk**

Yes → **Consider gastric lavage +/− SDAC³ or MDAC⁴ according to charcoal absorbency**

No or unknown → **Consider SDAC³ or MDAC⁴ according to charcoal absorbency**

Iron, lead, zinc, enteric-coated tablets or illicit drug packets involved?

Yes → **Consider whole bowel irrigation⁵**

No → **Consider indications for extracorporeal methods of removal and specific antidotes**

FIGURE 2B-5 This flow diagram is essentially based on the current recommendations of the American Academy of Clinical Toxicologists and the European Association of Poisons Centres and Clinical Toxicologists. These recommendations are based on weight of evidence in the published literature, but this algorithm has not been validated. See text for details on individual decontamination procedures, indications, and contraindications.

1. Irritants, corrosives, and substances toxic by skin absorption should be removed. Liquids with high volatility and potential for secondary contamination (organic solvents) should likewise be removed. When in doubt, decontamination is appropriate; however, life-saving interventions (ABCs) take precedence over decontamination. Personnel should wear protective garments appropriate to the hazard.

2. If the history is reliable and the ingestion is clearly nontoxic, no decontamination is required. The urge to "do something" should be weighed against the maxim to "first, do no harm."

3. Single-dose activated charcoal (SDAC) is considered most effective when administered less than 1 hour after ingestion of a toxic substance. There is insufficient evidence to support or condemn its use with toxic ingestions presenting more than 1 hour later. In general, metals (lithium, iron, but not thallium) and alcohols are poorly absorbed.

4. Multiple-dose activated charcoal (MDAC) should be considered primarily if a patient has ingested a life-threatening amount of carbamazepine, dapsone, phenobarbital, quinine, or theophylline. Multiple-dose activated charcoal increases the elimination of amitriptyline, dextropropoxyphene, digitoxin, digoxin, disopyramide, nadolol, phenylbutazone, phenytoin, piroxicam, and sotalol, but evidence is insufficient to support its use in these ingestions.

5. Whole bowel irrigation should not be performed in the presence of ileus or bowel obstruction.

6. If uncertainty exists about the need for decontamination procedures, contact the regional poison control center and/or a medical toxicologist.

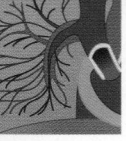

REFERENCES

1. Merigian KS, Blaho KE: Single-dose oral activated charcoal in the treatment of the self-poisoned patient: a prospective, randomized, controlled trial. Am J Ther 2002;9(4):301–308.
2. Merigian KS, Woodard M, Hedges JR, et al: Prospective evaluation of gastric emptying in the self-poisoned patient. Am J Emerg Med 1990;8(6):479–483.
3. Kulig K, Bar-Or D, Cantrill SV, et al: Management of acutely poisoned patients without gastric emptying. Ann Emerg Med 1985;14(6):562–567.
4. Pond SM, Olson KR, Osterloh JD, Tong TG: Randomized study of the treatment of phenobarbital overdose with repeated doses of activated charcoal. JAMA 1984;251(23):3104–3108.
5. Buckley NA, Eddleston M: The revised position papers on gastric decontamination. Clin Toxicol (Phila) 2005;43(2):129–130.
6. Gregoire G, Derderian F, Le Lorier J: Selecting the language of the publications included in a meta-analysis: is there a Tower of Babel bias? J Clin Epidemiol 1995;48(1):159–163.
7. Occupational Health and Safety Administration: OSHA Best Practices for Hospital-based First Receivers of Victims from Mass Casualty Incidents Involving the Release of Hazardous Substances. Washington, DC, OSHA, 2005.
8. Yano K, Hosokawa K, Kakibuchi M, et al: Effects of washing acid injuries to the skin with water: an experimental study using rats. Burns 1995;21(7):500–502.
9. Yano K, Hata Y, Matsuka K, et al: Experimental study on alkaline skin injuries—periodic changes in subcutaneous tissue pH and the effects exerted by washing. Burns 1993;19(4):320–323.
10. Kuckelkorn R, Schrage N, Keller G, Redbrake C: Emergency treatment of chemical and thermal eye burns. Acta Ophthalmol Scand 2002;80(1):4–10.
11. Merle H, Donnio A, Ayeboua L, et al: Alkali ocular burns in Martinique (French West Indies). Evaluation of the use of an amphoteric solution as the rinsing product. Burns 2005;31(2):205–211.
12. Gerard M, Josset P, Louis V, et al: [Is there a delay in bathing the external eye in the treatment of ammonia eye burns? Comparison of two ophthalmic solutions: physiological serum and Diphoterine]. J Fr Ophtalmol 2000;23(5):449–458.
13. Cavallini M, Casati A: A prospective, randomized, blind comparison between saline, calcium gluconate and diphoterine for washing skin acid injuries in rats: effects on substance P and beta-endorphin release. Eur J Anaesthesiol 2004;21(5):389–392.
14. Hall AH, Blomet J, Mathieu L: Diphoterine for emergent eye/skin chemical splash decontamination: a review. Vet Hum Toxicol 2002;44(4):228–231.
15. Penner GE: Acid ingestion: toxicology and treatment. Ann Emerg Med 1980;9(7):374–379.
16. Andrews K, Mowlavi A, Milner SM: The treatment of alkaline burns of the skin by neutralization. Plast Reconstr Surg 2003;111(6):1918–1921.
17. Kuckelkorn R, Kottek A, Schrage N, Reim M: Poor prognosis of severe chemical and thermal eye burns: the need for adequate emergency care and primary prevention. Int Arch Occup Environ Health 1995;67(4):281–284.
18. Saari KM, Leinonen J, Aine E: Management of chemical eye injuries with prolonged irrigation. Acta Ophthalmol Suppl 1984;161:52–59.
19. U.S. Army Center for Health Promotion and Preventive Medicine (USACHPPM): Personal Protective Equipment Guide for Military Medical Treatment Facility Personnel Handling Casualties from Weapons of Mass Destruction and Terrorism Events. Report No. Technical Guide 275. Aberdeen Proving Ground, MD, USACHPPM, 2003.
20. Macintyre AG, Christopher GW, Eitzen E Jr, et al: Weapons of mass destruction events with contaminated casualties: effective planning for health care facilities. JAMA 2000;283(2):242–249.
21. Hall AH, Blomet J, Gross M, Nehles J: Hexafluorine for emergent decontamination of hydrofluoric acid eye/skin splashes. Semicond Saf Assoc J 2000;14:20–33.
22. Mathieu L, Nehles J, Blomet J, Hall AH: Efficacy of hexafluorine for emergent decontamination of hydrofluoric acid eye and skin splashes. Vet Hum Toxicol 2001;43(5):263–265.
23. Hulten P, Hojer J, Ludwigs U, et al: Hexafluorine vs. standard decontamination to reduce systemic toxicity after dermal exposure to hydrofluoric acid. J Toxicol Clin Toxicol 2004;42(4):355–361.
24. Hojer J, Personne M, Hulten P, Ludwigs U: Topical treatments for hydrofluoric acid burns: a blind controlled experimental study. J Toxicol Clin Toxicol 2002;40(7):861–866.
25. Hall AH, Blomet J, Mathieu L: Topical treatments for hydrofluoric acid burns: a blind controlled experimental study. J Toxicol Clin Toxicol 2003;41(7):1031–1034.
26. Dunn BJ, MacKinnon MA, Knowlden NF, et al: Hydrofluoric acid dermal burns. An assessment of treatment efficacy using an experimental pig model. J Occup Med 1992;34(9):902–909.
27. Dunn BJ, MacKinnon MA, Knowlden NF, et al: Topical treatments for hydrofluoric acid dermal burns. Further assessment of efficacy using an experimental piq model. J Occup Environ Med 1996;38(5):507–514.
28. Burkhart KK, Brent J, Kirk MA, et al: Comparison of topical magnesium and calcium treatment for dermal hydrofluoric acid burns. Ann Emerg Med 1994;24(1):9–13.
29. Bentur Y, Tannenbaum S, Yaffe Y, Halpert M: The role of calcium gluconate in the treatment of hydrofluoric acid eye burn. Ann Emerg Med 1993;22(9):1488–1490.
30. Beiran I, Miller B, Bentur Y: The efficacy of calcium gluconate in ocular hydrofluoric acid burns. Hum Exp Toxicol 1997;16(4):223–228.
31. McCulley JP: Ocular hydrofluoric acid burns: animal model, mechanism of injury and therapy. Trans Am Ophthalmol Soc 1990;88:649–684.
32. Hunter DM, Timerding BL, Leonard RB, et al: Effects of isopropyl alcohol, ethanol, and polyethylene glycol/industrial methylated spirits in the treatment of acute phenol burns. Ann Emerg Med 1992;21(11):1303–1307.
33. Monteiro-Riviere NA, Inman AO, Jackson H, et al: Efficacy of topical phenol decontamination strategies on severity of acute phenol chemical burns and dermal absorption: in vitro and in vivo studies in pig skin. Toxicol Ind Health 2001;17(4):95–104.
34. Stewart CE: Chemical skin burns. Am Fam Physician 1985;31(6):149–157.
35. Kaufman T, Ullmann Y, Har-Shai Y: Phosphorus burns: a practical approach to local treatment. J Burn Care Rehabil 1988;9(5):474–475.
36. Eldad A, Simon GA: The phosphorous burn—a preliminary comparative experimental study of various forms of treatment. Burns 1991;17(3):198–200.
37. Eldad A, Wisoki M, Cohen H, et al: Phosphorous burns: evaluation of various modalities for primary treatment. J Burn Care Rehabil 1995;16(1):49–55.
38. Valentino M, Rapisarda V, Fenga C: Hand injuries due to high-pressure injection devices for painting in shipyards: circumstances, management, and outcome in twelve patients. Am J Ind Med 2003;43(5):539–542.
39. Gutowski KA, Chu J, Choi M, Friedman DW: High-pressure hand injection injuries caused by dry cleaning solvents: case reports, review of the literature, and treatment guidelines. Plast Reconstr Surg 2003;111(1):174–177.
40. Moder KG, Hurley DL: Fatal hypernatremia from exogenous salt intake: report of a case and review of the literature. Mayo Clin Proc 1990;65(12):1587–1594.
41. Casavant MJ, Fitch JA: Fatal hypernatremia from saltwater used as an emetic. J Toxicol Clin Toxicol 2003;41(6):861–863.
42. Turk EE, Schulz F, Koops E, et al: Fatal hypernatremia after using salt as an emetic—report of three autopsy cases. Leg Med (Tokyo) 2005;7(1):47–50.
43. Liu J, Kashimura S, Hara K, Zhang G: Death following cupric sulfate emesis. J Toxicol Clin Toxicol 2001;39(2):161–163.
44. Lacomis D: Case of the month. June 1996—anorexia nervosa. Brain Pathol 1996;6(4):535–536.
45. Ho PC, Dweik R, Cohen MC: Rapidly reversible cardiomyopathy associated with chronic ipecac ingestion. Clin Cardiol 1998;21(10):780–783.
46. Krenzelok EP, McGuigan M, Lheur P: Position statement: ipecac syrup. American Academy of Clinical Toxicology; European Association of Poisons Centres and Clinical Toxicologists. J Toxicol Clin Toxicol 1997;35(7):699–709.

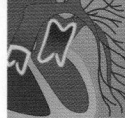

47. Position paper: ipecac syrup. J Toxicol Clin Toxicol 2004;42(2): 133–143.

48. Bond GR: Home syrup of ipecac use does not reduce emergency department use or improve outcome. Pediatrics 2003;112: 1061–1064.

49. Krenzelok EP: Ipecac syrup-induced emesis . . . no evidence of benefit. Clin Toxicol (Phila) 2005;43(1):11–12.

50. Shannon M: The demise of ipecac. Pediatrics 2003;112(5): 1180–1181.

51. American Academy of Pediatrics Committee on Injury, Violence, and Poison Prevention: Poison treatment in the home. Pediatrics 2003;112(5):1182–1185.

52. Manoguerra AS, Cobaugh DJ: Guideline on the use of ipecac syrup in the out-of-hospital management of ingested poisons. Clin Toxicol (Phila) 2005;43(1):1–10.

53. Jorens PG, Joosens EJ, Nagler JM: Changes in arterial oxygen tension after gastric lavage for drug overdose. Hum Exp Toxicol 1991;10(3):221–224.

54. Mariani PJ, Pook N: Gastrointestinal tract perforation with charcoal peritoneum complicating orogastric intubation and lavage. Ann Emerg Med 1993;22(3):606–609.

55. Wald P, Stern J, Weiner B, Goldfrank L: Esophageal tear following forceful removal of an impacted oral-gastric lavage tube. Ann Emerg Med 1986;15(1):80–82.

56. Leclerc F, Martin V, Gaudier B: [Water intoxication following gastric lavage]. Nouv Presse Med 1981;10(14):1149–1150.

57. Liisanantti J, Kaukoranta P, Martikainen M, Ala-Kokko T: Aspiration pneumonia following severe self-poisoning. Resuscitation 2003;56(1):49–53.

58. Vale JA, Kulig K: Position paper: gastric lavage. J Toxicol Clin Toxicol 2004;42(7):933–943.

59. Yardeni D, Yardeni H, Coran AG, Golladay ES: Severe esophageal damage due to button battery ingestion: can it be prevented? Pediatr Surg Int 2004;20(7):496–501.

60. McNutt TK, Chambers-Emerson J, Dethlefsen M, Shah R: Bite the bullet: lead poisoning after ingestion of 206 lead bullets. Vet Hum Toxicol 2001;43(5):288–289.

61. Saeki S, Shimoda T, Sakai H, et al: Successful treatment of theophylline toxicity by upper gastrointestinal endoscopy. Respir Med 2003;97(6):734–735.

62. Lapostolle F, Finot MA, Adnet F, et al: Radiopacity of clomipramine conglomerations and unsuccessful endoscopy: report of 4 cases. J Toxicol Clin Toxicol 2000;38(5):477–482.

63. Warren JB, Griffin DJ, Olson RC: Urine sugar reagent tablet ingestion causing gastric and duodenal ulceration. Arch Intern Med 1984;144(1):161–163.

64. Wobser E, Hoppe A: [Endoscopic removal of carbamide-containing tablet conglomerates]. Dtsch Med Wochenschr 1977; 102(49):1825–1826.

65. Rackwitz R, Lani K, Kiefhaber P, et al: [Radiological evidence and removal of tablet conglomerates in intoxication with bromide-containing hypnotics (author's translation)]. Dtsch Med Wochenschr 1977;102(33):1181–1184, 1186.

66. Conso F, Celerier M, Maury D, Dubost C: [Letter: Ingestion of potassium permanganate tablets]. Nouv Presse Med 1974; 3(34):2184–2185.

67. Faigel DO, Stotland BR, Kochman ML, et al: Device choice and experience level in endoscopic foreign object retrieval: an in vivo study. Gastrointest Endosc 1997;45(6):490–492.

68. Steib A, Steiner F, Abbass A, Flesch F: [Accidental ingestion of a battery]. Ann Fr Anesth Reanim 1984;3(5):385–387.

69. Temple DM, McNeese MC: Hazards of battery ingestion. Pediatrics 1983;71(1):100–103.

70. Studley JG, Linehan IP, Ogilvie AL, Dowling BL: Swallowed button batteries: is there a consensus on management? Gut 1990;31(8): 867–870.

71. Schaper A, Hofmann R, Ebbecke M, et al: [Cocaine-body-packing. Infrequent indication for laparotomy]. Chirurg 2003;74(7): 626–631.

72. Olmedo R, Nelson L, Chu J, Hoffman RS: Is surgical decontamination definitive treatment of "body-packers"? Am J Emerg Med 2001;19(7):593–596.

73. Aldrighetti L, Paganelli M, Giacomelli M, et al: Conservative management of cocaine-packet ingestion: experience in Milan, the main Italian smuggling center of South American cocaine. Panminerva Med 1996;38(2):111–116.

74. Malbrain ML, Neels H, Vissers K, et al: A massive, near-fatal cocaine intoxication in a body-stuffer. Case report and review of the literature. Acta Clin Belg 1994;49(1):12–18.

75. Utecht MJ, Stone AF, McCarron MM: Heroin body packers. J Emerg Med 1993;11(1):33–40.

76. Suarez CA, Arango A, Lester JL 3rd: Cocaine-condom ingestion. Surgical treatment. JAMA 1977;238(13):1391–1392.

77. McCarron MM, Wood JD: The cocaine 'body packer' syndrome. Diagnosis and treatment. JAMA 1983;250(11):1417–1420.

78. Barsky P: Surgical removal of iron tablets. J Pediatr 1982; 101(6):1038.

79. Cereda JM, Scott J, Quigley EM: Endoscopic removal of pharmacobezoar of slow release theophylline. BMJ 1986;293(6555):1143.

80. Rebhandl W, Steffan I, Schramel P, et al: Release of toxic metals from button batteries retained in the stomach: an in vitro study. J Pediatr Surg 2002;37(1):87–92.

81. Mallon PT, White JS, Thompson RL: Systemic absorption of lithium following ingestion of a lithium button battery. Hum Exp Toxicol 2004;23(4):193–195.

82. Chan YL, Chang SS, Kao KL, et al: Button battery ingestion: an analysis of 25 cases. Chang Gung Med J 2002;25(3):169–174.

83. Hoffman RS, Stringer JA, Feinberg RS, Goldfrank LR: Comparative efficacy of thallium adsorption by activated charcoal, prussian blue, and sodium polystyrene sulfonate. J Toxicol Clin Toxicol 1999;37(7):833–837.

84. Green R, Grierson R, Sitar DS, Tenenbein M: How long after drug ingestion is activated charcoal still effective? J Toxicol Clin Toxicol 2001;39(6):601–605.

85. Chyka PA, Seger D, Krenzelok EP, Vale JA: Position paper: single-dose activated charcoal. Clin Toxicol (Phila) 2005;43(2):61–87.

86. Osterhoudt KC, Alpern ER, Durbin D, et al: Activated charcoal administration in a pediatric emergency department. Pediatr Emerg Care 2004;20(8):493–498.

87. Dorrington CL, Johnson DW, Brant R: The frequency of complications associated with the use of multiple-dose activated charcoal. Ann Emerg Med 2003;41(3):370–377.

88. Graff GR, Stark J, Berkenbosch JW, et al: Chronic lung disease after activated charcoal aspiration. Pediatrics 2002;109(5): 959–961.

89. Moll J, Kerns W 2nd, Tomaszewski C, Rose R: Incidence of aspiration pneumonia in intubated patients receiving activated charcoal. J Emerg Med 1999;17(2):279–283.

90. American Academy of Clinical Toxicology; European Association of Poisons Centres and Clinical Toxicologists: Position statement and practice guidelines on the use of multi-dose activated charcoal in the treatment of acute poisoning. J Toxicol Clin Toxicol 1999;37(6):731–751.

91. Idid SZ, Lee CY: Effects of Fuller's earth and activated charcoal on oral absorption of paraquat in rabbits. Clin Exp Pharmacol Physiol 1996;23(8):679–681.

92. Position paper: cathartics. J Toxicol Clin Toxicol 2004;42(3): 243–253.

93. Qureshi T, Melonakos TK: Acute hypermagnesemia after laxative use. Ann Emerg Med 1996;28(5):552–555.

94. Kontani M, Hara A, Ohta S, et al: Hypermagnesemia induced by massive cathartic ingestion in an elderly woman without pre-existing renal dysfunction. Intern Med 2005;44(5):448–452.

95. Smilkstein MJ, Smolinske SC, Kulig KW, Rumack BH: Severe hypermagnesemia due to multiple-dose cathartic therapy. West J Med 1988;148(2):208–211.

96. Position paper: whole bowel irrigation. J Toxicol Clin Toxicol 2004;42(6):843–854.

97. Ingels M, Lai C, Tai W, et al: A prospective study of acute, unintentional, pediatric superwarfarin ingestions managed without decontamination. Ann Emerg Med 2002;40(1):73–78.

98. Shepherd G, Klein-Schwartz W, Anderson BD: Acute, unintentional pediatric brodifacoum ingestions. Pediatr Emerg Care 2002;18(3):174–178.

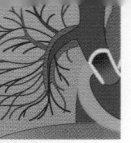

C Principles of Elimination Enhancement

CURTIS P. SNOOK, MD ■ DANIEL A. HANDEL, MD, MPH

Once a drug or toxin has been absorbed, a number of means exist to enhance its elimination. Chapter 2D addresses extracorporeal techniques of toxin removal from the blood (e.g., hemodialysis and hemoperfusion), which, when performed on an emergency short-term basis such as for poisoning, are done intermittently using a large double-lumen catheter in a central vein with flow through the circuit driven by a pump. Other types of dialysis exist that also usually do not require arterial access and are more versatile in that they do not pose as great a hemodynamic stress to the patient; however, they also are generally much slower in their rates of clearance. One of these alternatives, multiple-dose activated charcoal (MDAC), involves use of the patient's own gastrointestinal mucosa as a dialyzer.

All of these techniques share in common with dialysis the underlying principle of filtering a toxin from the blood using a semipermeable membrane in order to enhance its clearance. A number of substance-related factors affect the clearance rates that can be achieved by dialysis techniques. First, a toxin must distribute primarily into the intravascular compartment—that is, have a low volume of distribution, in order to be removed by a dialysis technique at a clinically significant rate. Second, molecular size is important, with low molecular weight substances crossing the dialysis membrane from an area of high concentration (blood) to an area of low concentration (dialysate). Even higher molecular weight substances can cross and thus be removed from the blood by convection when dialysis is supplemented with ultrafiltration, which relies on a membrane with a high permeability coefficient and a high transmembrane pressure. Finally, high protein binding presents a large molecular size to the membrane (i.e., a protein-bound drug), thus limiting the rate of clearance, unless the toxin is adsorbed from the serum proteins such as with the use of a charcoal cartridge in hemoperfusion.

MULTIPLE-DOSE ACTIVATED CHARCOAL

Preabsorptive Elimination Enhancement

Delayed absorption may occur after toxic ingestion: (1) with sustained-release preparations, (2) if tablet conglomerates form in the gastrointestinal tract, (3) if the substance delays gastrointestinal motility. or, (4) if a poorly absorbed substance (e.g., phenytoin) is ingested. Multiple doses of activated charcoal have been used in these situations to enhance preabsorptive elimination. Whole bowel irrigation, the other treatment modality used to enhance preabsorptive elimination, appears to provide no additional benefit when administered to treat a drug overdose for which activated charcoal is an effective adsorbent[1]; it may even limit the adsorptive capacity of activated charcoal.[2]

Postabsorptive Elimination Enhancement

Two theories have been advanced to account for the observed acceleration of drug clearance associated with the use of MDAC after the drug's absorption from the gastrointestinal tract. One theory explains this acceleration by charcoal's interruption of the enterohepatic recirculation of hepatically metabolized drugs. The other is aptly called "gastrointestinal dialysis," a term coined by Levy in an editorial that accompanied the seminal work on this topic by Berg and colleagues.[3,4] Using an animal model of intravenous theophylline poisoning, Kulig and colleagues measured bile theophylline concentrations and were able to demonstrate that the observed increase in theophylline clearance with MDAC was not due to interruption of enterohepatic recirculation of the drug.[5] Arimori and colleagues demonstrated in an experimental model that the exsorption rate of theophylline into the intestinal lumen increased in proportion to the administered dose of theophylline, suggesting that the gastrointestinal dialysis effect may increase with escalating dose for some toxins.[6]

Indications

Given that overall mortality from overdose is low, that the efficacy of gastrointestinal decontamination techniques declines significantly with advancing time after ingestion, and that significant delay to clinical presentation occurs in the majority of ingestions, elimination enhancement techniques, including MDAC, have come under recent scrutiny.[7] Tenenbein cited case reports of complications from MDAC with a lack of proven clinical benefit in arguing that its role in the treatment of poisoning required reassessment.[8]

These cautions notwithstanding, review of the available evidence suggests that MDAC can accelerate drug clearance, achieving rates comparable to more invasive techniques such as hemodialysis. Moreover, a recent study of complications associated with MDAC use found that they occurred infrequently.[9] There are also data suggesting that MDAC improves outcome in selected poisoning cases. One report describes two presentations of the same patient with phenytoin toxicity, one in which MDAC was not used and a second in which it was; the second hospitalization was 3 days shorter despite the patient having a higher serum phenytoin level.[10] A recent single-blind, randomized, placebo-controlled trial performed in Sri Lanka demonstrated a significant reduction in mortality from yellow oleander poisoning

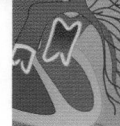

BOX 2C-1	TOXINS FOR WHICH MDAC INCREASES CLEARANCE

Acetaminophen[68]
Carbamazepine[69-71]
Dapsone[13]
Dextropropoxyphene[72]
Digitoxin[73,74]
Phenytoin[75-77]
Phenobarbital[35,78,79]
Piroxicam[80]
Thallium[81]
Theophylline[5,6,12,82]
Yellow oleander[11]

_____

MDAC, multiple-dose activated charcoal.

BOX 2C-2	TOXINS FOR WHICH MDAC'S EFFECTS ON CLEARANCE ARE EQUIVOCAL

Digoxin[12,14,15,73,83,84]
Salicylate[86-90]
Tricyclic Antidepressants[91-94]
Vancomycin[36,95]

_____

MDAC, multiple-dose activated charcoal.

with MDAC therapy when compared with treatment with single-dose activated charcoal.[11]

Further study is needed to define the circumstances in which the benefits of MDAC appear to justify its risks. However, some predictions can be made based on available data. MDAC has been demonstrated to accelerate the clearance of a number of toxins (Box 2C-1). Chyka and colleagues found in a porcine model that MDAC enhanced elimination of acetaminophen, digoxin, and theophylline but not valproic acid.[12] Drugs with relatively lower intrinsic clearance (digoxin, theophylline) were cleared with MDAC more rapidly than were drugs with higher intrinsic clearance (acetaminophen). Interestingly, volume of distribution, half-life, and protein binding were not significantly correlated with MDAC enhancement of clearance. However, therapeutic doses were administered in this study, limiting application of these results to the overdose setting. A volunteer study of dapsone ingestion using a randomized crossover design along with data from two overdose cases showed a doubling of elimination with MDAC in healthy volunteers and a greater increase in the overdose patients, again suggesting that the effectiveness of MDAC also may be a function of dose for a given toxin.[13]

Contraindications

Significant adverse effects with MDAC preclude its use in patients for which no significant clinical benefit is expected. There are some drugs or drug classes for which data are conflicting (Box 2C-2). For example, the available studies suggest that MDAC likely would not be beneficial in unselected cases of digoxin poisoning. However, one volunteer study of MDAC for enhancement of digoxin clearance applied kinetic predictions to suggest that greater clearance with MDAC would occur in patients with renal impairment[14]; animal data support this assertion.[12] In a case of chronic digoxin poisoning, MDAC effectively accelerated drug clearance when digoxin antibody fragments were unavailable and hemodialysis had been unsuccessful.[15] Box 2C-3 lists the

drugs investigated for which MDAC has not been shown to accelerate clearance.

MDAC often is poorly tolerated. Virtually all patients in one study complained of poor palatability and bloating with MDAC, with one patient withdrawing because of repeated vomiting.[14] Transient constipation may occur with MDAC use in susceptible patients. Protracted vomiting also has been reported to limit the usefulness of MDAC in theophylline poisoning.[16]

Aspiration of charcoal is another well-recognized complication of MDAC. In one published case, an unintubated patient treated for phenobarbital and carbamazepine overdose with gastric lavage followed by MDAC vomited and aspirated 12 hours after therapy was initiated, eventually dying on hospital day 15.[17] Another reported patient with theophylline overdose was treated with ipecac followed by MDAC. He went on to develop convulsions followed by aspiration, eventuating in his death.[18] In the most sobering case, a patient aspirated activated charcoal despite airway control.[19] This patient received MDAC after intubation and gastric lavage for desipramine and thiothixene overdose. After extubation the next day, the patient vomited, aspirated charcoal, and had a cardiorespiratory arrest from which he could not be resuscitated. In a similar case, a patient who ingested thioridazine and imipramine underwent endotracheal intubation and gastric lavage after he had a seizure. He received 50 g of activated charcoal by nasogastric tube followed by 25 g and then 50 g with sorbitol every hour for 6 hours.[20] When the nasogastric tube was removed, the patient vomited, became cyanotic and had a respiratory arrest. Charcoal was suctioned from the patient's lungs until hospital day seven. Rau

BOX 2C-3	TOXINS FOR WHICH MDAC DOES NOT INCREASE CLEARANCE

Amiodarone[96]
Astemizole[97]
Chlorpropamide[98]
Chloroquine[96]
Diltiazem[99]
Pholcodine[100]
Valproate[101]
Tobramycin[102]

_____

MDAC, multiple-dose activated charcoal.

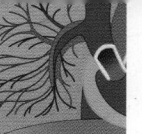

and colleagues described three deaths from charcoal aspiration among 15 patients treated with charcoal for central nervous system–depressant overdose without airway protection. Their subsequent six overdose patients were intubated prior to charcoal administration and no cases of aspiration occurred.[21] In light of this experience, any patient at risk for aspiration (i.e., one in whom diminished consciousness, depressed airway reflexes, or seizures are present or anticipated), should have a firm indication for MDAC and a protected airway before undertaking the procedure. Equally important, there appears to be a ceiling effect for charcoal adsorption such that increasing dose or frequency beyond a certain point results in no additional therapeutic benefit.[22]

Overdose victims with decreased gastrointestinal motility may develop bowel obstruction with use of MDAC. A number of cases have reported MDAC resulting in small bowel obstruction, abdominal distension, constipation, rectal bleeding, and even intestinal perforation when either the overdose itself or the therapy for the overdose involved anticholinergic drugs.[23-28] Appendicitis in association with MDAC use has been reported.[29] Another patient with chronic theophylline toxicity treated with MDAC developed small bowel obstruction and was found on laparotomy to have adhesions at the ileocecal valve secondary to a previous hysterectomy; multiple pieces of charcoal were found in the bowel at the site of obstruction measuring 4.5 × 5 × 3 cm in aggregate.[30]

Cathartics are ineffective as a means of elimination enhancement after poisoning.[31] However, to avoid constipation and charcoal inspissation, cathartics often are coadministered. Sorbitol is the usual choice because of its rapid onset and palatability. Sorbitol is typically marketed in a 70% concentration with activated charcoal because it is bacteriostatic at this concen-tration.[32,33] Using excessive or multiple doses of sorbitol with activated charcoal in poisoning is associated with significant morbidity, including hypernatremia resulting in death, and should be avoided.[34] Magnesium citrate or sulfate occasionally are used instead of sorbitol. Patients with premorbid magnesium abnormalities or those receiving excessive doses of magnesium cathartic can suffer serious morbidity, including hypermagnesemia, which can be fatal.[34]

Dosing

The optimal dosing for activated charcoal in MDAC is unknown. The commonly accepted dose is 1 g/kg (maximum of 50 g) of activated charcoal initially, followed by 0.5 g/kg (maximum 25 g) every 4 hours thereafter. Others have suggested a dose of 1 g/kg of activated charcoal in 4.3 mL/kg body weight of 70% sorbitol every 4 hours until the first charcoal stool appears. In children, the same weight-based dose of activated charcoal is recommended.[33] A third set of published guidelines for adults has suggested an initial dose of 50 to 100 g, with additional doses given at a rate of at least 12.5 g/hr until the patient is improving clinically and by relevant laboratory parameters. This latter set of recommendations includes lower dosing (10 to 25 g) for children younger than 5 years of age, smaller doses more frequently along with antiemetic use in vomiting patients, and no use of cathartics, particularly in young children.[7] MDAC has been used safely in infants and neonates[35,36]; it has even been used to treat neonatal hyperbilirubinemia.[37]

Patients receiving MDAC should be intubated, ideally with a cuffed endotracheal tube, if they are obtunded or have diminished airway reflexes or seizures. The charcoal should be diluted with at least 8 mL of water per gram of charcoal. MDAC should not be administered in the presence of ileus or bowel obstruction. Coadministration of anticholinergic agents should be avoided during MDAC. Charcoal should be withheld 4 hours prior to extubation. Gastric contents should be aspirated with a nasogastric tube prior to extubation to avoid the complications previously discussed. Magnesium cathartics should be used with caution, particularly in patients with decreased renal function, and are best avoided in such patients given that safer alternatives are available. It is a common practice to give the first dose of charcoal with a cathartic, usually sorbitol, and to give subsequent doses without cathartic. The availability of only sorbitol-charcoal preparations can be problematic in hospitals with such rigid stocking patterns.[38] Electrolytes should be closely monitored if more than one dose of cathartic is administered.

Box 2C-4 summarizes the indications, contraindications, and dosing guidelines for MDAC use in poisoning.

BOX 2C-4   MDAC: INDICATIONS, CONTRAINDICATIONS, AND DOSING GUIDELINES

Indication

Life-threatening ingestion of substance adsorbable by activated charcoal
Evidence or anticipation of ongoing absorption (rising drug levels later than expected, sustained-release preparations)

Contraindication

Anticipation or presence of decreased mental status, anticipation or presence of seizures, or decreased gag reflex without a cuffed endotracheal tube in place for airway protection
Ileus or bowel obstruction

Dosing Guidelines

Activated charcoal:
1 g/kg followed by 0.5g/kg every 4 hr
Sorbitol: If used with the first dose of AC:
   adult: 4.3 mL/kg body weight of 70% sorbitol;
   child: 4.3 mL/kg body weight of 35% sorbitol;
   subsequent doses in aqueous suspension of 8 mL water/g AC

AC, activated charcoal; MDAC, multiple-dose activated charcoal.

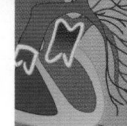

CONTINUOUS VENO-VENOUS HEMOFILTRATION

Continuous veno-venous hemofiltration (CVVH) and similar modalities used for what is termed "continuous renal replacement therapy" increasingly are being used in the therapy of critically ill patients, including those suffering from poisoning. CVVH offers a number of useful advantages over traditional dialysis techniques. First, it can be used in patients with renal failure who are hemodynamically unstable and require large volumes of parenteral nutrition. In CVVH isotonic fluid is removed from the femoral vein slowly and continuously rather than in 1- to 4-L increments over a 2- to 4-hour treatment session, the typical pattern for hemodialysis (HD). Also, the diffusion clearance inherent to HD results in the return of a hypo-osmolar fluid to the intravascular space, resulting in a further loss of intravascular volume in comparison with CVVH. The latter restores volume losses with isotonic replacement fluid and fluid refilling from the overhydrated body parenchyma.[39] Second, trained nursing staff can administer CVVH, though it requires their continuous attention. Finally, the typical rebound in serum drug levels from redistribution observed after HD are not seen with continuous modalities such as CVVH.

The main disadvantage of CVVH in comparison with HD is the slower rate of toxin removal it can achieve. This disadvantage is significant if rapid toxin removal is critical to the patient's survival, which often is the case. Thus, the use of CVVH for a toxin whose elimination is enhanced by dialysis techniques should be considered only when hemodynamic instability precludes the use of HD, when HD is not available, or if the inherently slower rate of toxin removal is clinically acceptable.

CVVH does not require arterial access—a pump is used to provide the pressure gradient necessary for filtration. Anticoagulation is required to optimize the lifespan of the apparatus (which requires replacement when it becomes clotted). However, the need for anticoagulation is less than for arteriovenous techniques because of the controlled blood flow provided by the pump, particularly in smaller pediatric circuits.[40] Animal data demonstrate that CVVH can achieve adequate flow rates with pediatric-sized filters and circuits.[41] The blood is passed through a highly permeable hemofilter, forming an ultrafiltrate made up of plasma and filtered solutes. Hemodiafiltration refers to the use of a dialysate fluid on the opposite side of the filter from the blood flowing in a counter current direction. Table 2C-1 summarizes the relative advantages and disadvantages of CVVH, continuous arterial-venous hemofiltration (CAVH), HD and peritoneal dialysis (PD).

Indications

Box 2C-5 lists the toxins for which CVVH has been shown to speed elimination. Toxin-related factors determining clearance by CVVH include the sieving coefficient (dependent upon molecular weight and protein binding)

TABLE 2C-1 Advantages and Disadvantages of CAVH, CVVH, HD, and PD[40]

TECHNIQUE	ADVANTAGES	DISADVANTAGES
CAVH	Less hemodynamic instability Ease of administration	Slower clearance rates Systemic anticoagulation Highest risk of clotting and air emboli
CVVH	Less hemodynamic instability Ease of administration	Slower clearance rates Systemic anticoagulation Higher risk of clotting and air emboli
HD	Faster clearance rates	More hemodynamic instability

PD	Faster clearance rates	More hemodynamic instability
		Peritoneal complications:
		  Increased abdominal pressure
		  Decrease in ventilation
		Peritoneal plural leaks
		Peritonitis
		Contraindicated if recent abdominal surgery

CAVH, continuous arterial-venous hemofiltration; CVVH, continuous veno-venous hemofiltration; HD, hemodialysis; PD, peritoneal dialysis.

BOX 2C-5 TOXINS FOR WHICH CVVH INCREASES CLEARANCE

Amrinone[103]
Barium[104]
Ceftriaxone[105]
Ethylene glycol[106]
Imipenem[107]
Lithium[108]
Metformin[109]
Salicylate[110]
Tobramycin[111]
Vancomycin[42,111]

CVVH, continuous veno-venous hemofiltration.

---

and the volume of distribution.[42] CVVH has been useful in a number of poisoning-related complications and in one condition that can result from poisoning. Hepatic and renal failure from acetaminophen have been managed successfully with CVVH in conjunction with aggressive supportive measures.[43] CVVH has been used for hyperphosphatemia from tumor lysis syndrome in conjunction with hemodialysis.[44] Myoglobin in an animal study and in humans from drug- and exercise-induced rhabdomyolysis has been removed successfully by CVVH.[45-47] Severe lactic acidosis induced by propofol improved significantly with the use of CVVH.[48] CVVH has been shown to be safe and effective in treating radiocontrast-induced acute renal failure after percu-

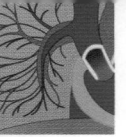

taneous coronary interventions.[39] Hypothermia is associated with poisoning, particularly when central nervous system depressants result in excessive exposures to cold ambient temperatures. CVVH has been used with success in rewarming a patient with severe accidental hypothermia.[49]

Contraindications

Toxins for which CVVH has not been shown to speed elimination are listed in Box 2C-6. One patient treated with a lorazepam infusion developed toxicity from the propylene glycol diluent, despite receiving CVVH with dialysis (CVVHD), suggesting that the glycol was not effectively removed.[50] Care should be exercised in choosing the replacement fluid; lactate-buffered solutions have been reported to induce hyperlactatemia.[51] Since CVVH requires systemic anticoagulation, contraindications include recent surgery and gastrointestinal or intracranial hemorrhage. However, regional heparinization can be used with those patients for whom CVVH is necessary but who cannot tolerate systemic heparinization.[40] Trisodium citrate is a useful alternative to heparin as a regional anticoagulant with CVVHD to minimize the risk of hemorrhage and thrombocytopenia. However, caution should be exercised in patients with decreased hepatic function as use of trisodium citrate in this context is associated with severe hypercalcemia.[52]

A summary of the indications and contraindications for CVVH in poisoning are listed in Box 2C-7.

PERITONEAL DIALYSIS

Though the first use of peritoneal dialysis PD dates back to 1923,[53] experiments with peritoneal lavage were carried out as early as 1877.[54] Numerous advances have been made since this early work was done, including the addition of substrates to the dialysate to enhance the elimination of certain drugs. Given the ease in most medical centers of obtaining HD, PD has fallen out of favor in most instances for the treatment of acute intoxication, although it continues to be used as a bridge when HD is not available or as an adjunct to enhance elimination. Because of its "second-tier" status, recent literature and research on its use in poisoning are sparse.

Method

The peritoneal surface area of an adult has been estimated to be 22,000 cm²,[55] allowing this structure to serve as an excellent semipermeable membrane for dialysis. PD involves in principle the passive movement of drug or toxin down its concentration gradient from the intravascular space in capillaries dispersed throughout the lining of the peritoneum into the dialysis solution infused into this cavity. As with other dialysis techniques, PD is particularly effective in removing drugs with small volumes of distribution and low protein binding.[56] The intermittent method of PD involves the use of one

---

BOX 2C-6	TOXINS FOR WHICH CVVH DOES NOT INCREASE CLEARANCE

Amikacin[112]
Arsenic[113]
Valproate[114]

CVVH, continuous veno-venous hemofiltration.

BOX 2C-7	CONTINUOUS VENO-VENOUS HEMOFILTRATION: INDICATIONS AND CONTRAINDICATIONS

Indications	Contraindications

Dialyzable toxin
  low volume of distribution
  low protein binding
  molecular weight < 10,000
  daltons
Hemodynamically unstable
  patient or hemodialysis not
  available or impractical
  (small children)
Drug-induced rhabdomyolysis
Drug-related hypothermia
Hyperphosphatemia
Toxin-induced lactic acidosis
Radiocontrast-induced acute
  renal failure
	Hemodynamically stable enough
	  for dialysis (relative)
	Underlying contraindication to
	  anticoagulation (relative)
	High toxin clearance critical to
	  patient survival
	Absence of adequate nursing care

---

catheter to introduce the dialysate by gravity, removing it at a later time through the same access.[54] This process also can be carried out using two catheters.[56] Two liters of fluid (1200 mL/m² or 50 mL/kg in children) are used per exchange, with the fluid typically left in the peritoneal cavity for 45 to 60 minutes.[55] In contrast, during continuous ambulatory peritoneal dialysis (CAPD), dialysate is left in the peritoneum for much longer periods of time. Extending this period beyond 72 hours or leaving the catheter in place between courses of PD increases the risk of infection.

Various additives, such as glucagon, albumin, prostaglandin E_2 (PGE_2), lipids, furosemide, streptokinase, and chelating agents, have been added to dialysis fluid in the attempt to enhance elimination with varying degrees of success.[57-59] A mildly hypo-osmolar solution is used to prevent water removal during dialysis, with electrolyte concentrations similar to that of extracellular fluid.[54] When the osmolality of the dialysate is increased, increased solute removal occurs at the expense of a negative fluid balance with each exchange.[55]

Disadvantages and Complications

Whereas PD can be a continuous process, its elimination rate is significantly less than that of HD and other more invasive methods of extracorporeal therapy. Blood flow via mesenteric circulation in PD cannot be adjusted as it can in HD, and the mechanics of instilling and draining

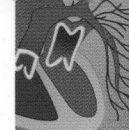

dialysate into and from the peritoneum limit achievable clearance rates.[57] The time required to eliminate a given amount of toxin is three to six times greater with PD than with HD, depending on the properties of the agent. The elimination of small molecules that are highly membrane permeable is rate-limited by blood and dialysate flow rates, whereas the elimination rate of large molecules depends primarily on membrane surface area.[60] In severe poisoning from a dialyzable toxin, the difference in achievable clearance rates between HD and PD can have enormous clinical significance, as one case series of methanol poisoning illustrates.[61] Thus, PD should not be substituted for HD in such cases unless the latter is absolutely inaccessible. If HD is not available in one treating facility but patient transfer is possible, the patient should be transferred. PD may be used as an adjunct during the transfer to speed toxin elimination.

Similar to other methods of extracorporeal elimination enhancement, PD can produce electrolyte shifts and loss of serum proteins. Pulmonary complications, including bronchitis/pneumonia, pleural effusions, and atelectasis, also are known adverse effects.[54] Bowel perforation from catheter misplacement occurs with an incidence of 1.3% according to one report.[62] The other major complication of PD, especially CAPD, is peritonitis, which usually limits the long-term use of this technique.[55] The dialysate additive icodextrin has been reported to cause a blistering skin reaction that resolves upon cessation of the use of the substance.[63]

Indications

PD can be used for toxins of up to 10,000 daltons in molecular weight and when a filtration rate of no greater than 15 mL/min is required.[64] It can be used when HD is not currently available and the patient's clinical status is critical. It can be used also when anticoagulation is contraindicated due to comorbidities.[65] PD has been more widely used in the pediatric population, especially in the contexts of acute renal failure seen in hemolytic-uremic syndrome, congestive heart failure, chronic renal failure, and hyperkalemia.[55,62] Because of the difficulties of vascular access in small children as well as the difficulty in removing excess fluid gained between courses of dialysis without causing profound hypotension, PD offers distinct advantages in this population.

The toxins for which PD hastens clearance and those for which its effects on clearance have been equivocal are listed in Boxes 2C-8 and 2C-9, respectively. Note that there are toxins listed in Box 2C-7 that are eliminated by the kidneys, such as baclofen, for which PD has been found useful in poisoning accompanied by renal failure even though PD effects on clearance are small when renal function is normal. Also, PD has proven useful in treating toxin-induced renal failure apart from effects on toxin clearance. Hypercalcemia from overadministration of vitamin D in an anephric child has been effectively

BOX 2C-8	TOXINS FOR WHICH PD INCREASES CLEARANCE

Achrocidin[115]
Amatoxins[116]
Amikacin[117]
Chromium (hexavalent)[118]
Copper (PD with salt-poor albumin)[119,120]
Ethylene glycol[121,122]
Glutethimide[123-125]
Isopropanol[126]
Lithium[127-129]
Meprobamate[130-134]
Methamphetamine[135]
Methanol[61,136-138]
Phenobarbital[135]
Salicylates[63,139]
Sodium chloride[140]
Vancomycin[141]

PD, peritoneal dialysis.

BOX 2C-9	TOXINS FOR WHICH PD'S EFFECTS ON CLEARANCE ARE EQUIVOCAL

Amphetamine[142]
Baclofen[143]
Boric acid[144-147]
Bromate[148,149]
Caffeine[150]
Chromium[151,152]
Gentamicin[153]
Mercury[154,155]
Methyprylon[156,157]
Propoxyphene[158-160]
Quinine[161-163]

PD, peritoneal dialysis.

treated with PD.[66] PD does not effectively remove the digoxin-Fab complex in the treatment of digoxin poisoning in the context of renal failure.[67]

Contraindications

In the pediatric population, PD is contraindicated when there is severe intraperitoneal hemorrhage that is sometimes seen in hemolytic-uremic syndrome with thrombocytopenia.[55] The presence of focal peritonitis, a fecal fistula or colostomy, abdominal adhesions, and recent abdominal surgery with use of a prosthetic material, a major vascular anastomosis, or an open wound, are relative contraindications for PD.[65]

Box 2C-10 lists the toxins for which peritoneal dialysis has not been found effective in accelerating clearance. A summary of the indications and contraindications for peritoneal dialysis in poisoning are listed in Box 2C-11.

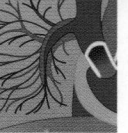

BOX 2C-10   TOXINS FOR WHICH PD DOES NOT INCREASE CLEARANCE

Amitriptyline[163]
Chloroquine[164]
Chlorpropamide[165]
Isoniazid[166]
Methaqualone[167,168]
Phenol[169]
Rifampicin[166]
Thallium[170]
Valacyclovir[171]

PD, peritoneal dialysis.

BOX 2C-11   PERITONEAL DIALYSIS: INDICATIONS AND CONTRAINDICATIONS

Indications	Contraindications

Dialyzable toxin
  low volume of distribution
  low protein binding
  molecular weight < 10,000
    daltons
Hemodynamically unstable
  patient or hemodialysis not
  available or impractical
  (small children)
Drug excretion impaired by
  hepatic or renal failure
	Severe intraperitoneal hemorrhage
	Hemodynamically stable enough
	  for dialysis (relative)
	High toxin clearance critical to
	  patient survival
	Absence of adequate nursing care
	Focal peritonitis, fecal fistula,
	  colostomy, undiagnosed
	  abdominal disease, extensive
	  adhesions, recent abdominal
	  surgery with prosthetic
	  material, vascular anastomosis
	  or open wound (relative)

REFERENCES

1. Burkhart KK, Wuerz RC, Donovan JW: Whole-bowel irrigation as adjunctive treatment for sustained-release theophylline overdose. Ann Emerg Med 1992;21:1316–1320.
2. Kirshenbaum LA, Sitar DS, Tenenbein M: Interaction between whole-bowel irrigation solution and activated charcoal: implications for the treatment of toxic ingestions. Ann Emerg Med 1990;19:1129–1132.
3. Berg MJ, Berlinger WG, Goldberg MJ, et al: Acceleration of the body clearance of phenobarbital by oral activated charcoal. Ann Emerg Med 1982;307:642–644.
4. Levy G: Gastrointestinal clearance of drugs with activated charcoal. N Engl J Med 1982;307:676–678.
5. Kulig K, Bar-Or D, Rumack BH: Intravenous theophylline poisoning and multiple-dose charcoal in an animal model. Ann Emerg Med 1987;16:842–846.
6. Arimori K, Nakano M: Dose-dependency in the exsorption of theophylline and the intestinal dialysis of theophylline by oral activated charcoal in rats. J Pharm Pharmacol 1988;40:101–105.
7. American Academy of Clinical Toxicology, European Association of Poisons Centres and Clinical Toxicologists: Position statement and practice guidelines on the use of multi-dose activated charcoal in the treatment of acute poisoning. Clin Toxicol 1999;37:731–751.
8. Tenenbein M: Multiple doses of activated charcoal: time for reappraisal? Ann Emerg Med 1991;20:529–531.
9. Dorrington CL, Johnson DW, Brant R, et al. The frequency of complications associated with the use of multiple-dose activated charcoal. Ann Emerg Med 2003;41:370–377.
10. Howard CE, Roberts RS, Ely DS, Moye RA: Use of multiple-dose activated charcoal in phenytoin toxicity. Ann Pharmacother 1994;28:201–203.
11. de Silva HA, Fonseka MM, Pathmeswaran A, et al. Multiple-dose activated charcoal for treatment of yellow oleander poisoning: a single-blind, randomized, placebo-controlled trial. Lancet 2003; 361:1935–1938.
12. Chyka PA, Holley JE, Mandrell TD, Sugathan P: Correlation of drug pharmacokinetics and effectiveness of multiple-dose activated charcoal therapy. Ann Emerg Med 1995;25:356–362.
13. Neuvonen PJ, Elonen E, Mattila MJ: Oral activated charcoal and dapsone elimination. Clin Pharmacol Ther 1980;27:823–827.
14. Lalonde RL, Deshpande R, Hamilton PP, et al: Acceleration of digoxin clearance by activated charcoal. Clin Pharmacol 1985; 37:367–371.
15. Critchley JA, Critchley LA: Digoxin toxicity in chronic renal failure: treatment by multiple dose activated charcoal intestinal dialysis. Hum Exp Toxicol 1997;16:733–735.
16. Amitai Y, Lovejoy FH: Characteristics of vomiting associated with acute sustained release theophylline poisoning: implications for management with oral activated charcoal. Clin Toxicol 1987; 25:539–554.
17. Menzies DG, Busuttil A, Prescott LF: Fatal pulmonary aspiration of oral activated charcoal. Br Med J 1988;297:459–460.
18. Benson B, VanAntwerp M, Hergott T: A fatality resulting from multiple dose activated charcoal therapy (abstract). Vet Hum Toxicol 1989;31:335.
19. Harsch HH: Aspiration of activated charcoal (letter). N Engl J Med 1986;314:318.
20. Givens T, Holloway M, Wason S: Pulmonary aspiration of activated charcoal: a complication of its misuse in overdose management. Pediatr Emerg Care 1992;8:137–140.
21. Rau NR, Nagaraj MV, Prakash PS, Nelli P: Fatal pulmonary aspiration of oral activated charcoal (letter). Br Med J 1988; 297:918–919.
22. Ilkhanipour K, Yealy DM, Krenzelok EP: Activated charcoal surface area and its role in multiple-dose charcoal therapy. Am J Emerg Med 1993;11:583–585.
23. Watson WA, Cremer KF, Chapman JA: Gastrointestinal obstruction associated with multiple-dose activated charcoal. J Emerg Med 1986;4:401–407.
24. Ray MJ, Radin, DR, Condie JD, et al: Charcoal bezoar. small bowel obstruction secondary to amitriptyline overdose therapy. Dig Dis Sci 1988;33:106–107.
25. Mizutani T, Naito H, Oohashi N: Rectal ulcer with massive hemorrhage due to activated charcoal treatment in oral organophosphate poisoning. Hum Exp Toxicol 1991; 10:385–386.
26. Longdon P, Henderson A: Intestinal pseudo-obstruction following the use of enteral charcoal and sorbitol and mechanical ventilation with papaveretum sedation for theophylline poisoning. Drug Saf 1992;7:74–77.
27. Gomez HF, Brent JA, Munoz DC, et al: Charcoal stercolith with intestinal perforation in a patient treated for amitriptyline ingestion. J Emerg Med 1994;12:57–60.
28. Atkinson SW, Young Y, Trotter GA: Treatment with activated charcoal complicated by gastrointestinal obstruction requiring surgery. Br Med J 1992;305:563.
29. Eroglu A, Kucuktulu U, Erciyes N, Turgutalp H: Multiple dose-activated charcoal as a cause of acute appendicitis. J Toxicol Clin Toxicol 2003;41:71–73.
30. Goulbourne KB, Cisek JE: Small-bowel obstruction secondary to activated charcoal and adhesions. Ann Emerg Med 1994;24: 108–110.
31. Barceloux D, McGuigan M, Hartigan-Go K: Position statement: cathartics. American Academy of Clinical Toxicology; European Association of Poisons Centres and Clinical Toxicologists. J Toxicol Clin Toxicol 1997;35:743–752.
32. Cooney DO: Palatability of sucrose-, sorbitol-, and saccharin-sweetened activated charcoal formulations. Am J Hosp Pharm 1980;37:237–239.
33. Minocha A, Krenzelok EP, Spyker DA: Dosage recommendations for activated charcoal-sorbitol treatment. Clin Toxicol 1985;23: 579–587.

34. Mauro LS, Nawarskas JJ, Mauro VF: Misadventures with activated charcoal and recommendations for safe use. Ann Pharmacother 1994;28:915–924.

35. Amitai Y, Degani Y: Treatment of phenobarbital poisoning with multiple dose activated charcoal in an infant. J Emerg Med 1990;8:449–450.

36. Kucukguclu S, Tuncok Y, Ozkan H, et al: Multiple-dose activated charcoal in an accidental vancomycin overdose. Clin Toxicol 1996;34:83–86.

37. Amitai Y, Regev M, Arad I, et al: Treatment of neonatal hyperbilirubinemia with repetitive oral activated charcoal as an adjunct to phototherapy. J Perinat Med 1993;21:189–194.

38. Wax PM, Wang RY, Hoffman RS, et al: Prevalence of sorbitol in multiple-dose activated charcoal regimens in emergency departments. Ann Emerg Med 1993;22:1807–1812.

39. Marenzi GC, Bartorelli AL, Lauri G, et al: Continuous veno-venous hemofiltration for the treatment of contrast-induced acute renal failure after percutaneous coronary interventions. Cathet Cardiovasc Intervent 2003;58:59–64.

40. Bunchman TE, Donckerwolcke RA: Continuous arterial-venous diahemofiltration and continuous veno-venous diahemofiltration in infants and children. Pediatr Nephrol 1994;8:96–102.

41. Werner HA, Herbertson MJ, Seear MD: Functional characteristics of pediatric veno-venous hemofiltration. Crit Care Med 1994;22:320–325.

42. Shah M, Quigley R: Rapid removal of vancomycin by continuous veno-venous hemofiltration. Pediatr Nephrol 2000;14:912–915.

43. Agarwal R, Farber MO: Is continuous veno-venous hemofiltration for acetaminophen-induced acute liver and renal failure worthwhile? Clin Nephrol 2002;2:167–170.

44. Sakarcan A, Quigley R: Hyperphosphatemia in tumor lysis syndrome: the role of hemodialysis and continuous veno-venous hemofiltration: Pediatr Nephrol 1994;8:351–353.

45. Nicolau D, Feng YS, Wu AH, et al: Myoglobin clearance during continuous veno-venous hemofiltration with or without dialysis. Int J Artif Organs 1998;21:205–209.

46. Yen TH, Chang CT, Wu MS, Huang CC: Acute rhabdomyolysis after gemfibrozil therapy in a pregnant patient complicated with acute pancreatitis and hypertriglyceridemia while receiving continuous veno-venous hemofiltration therapy. Ren Fail 2003;25:139–143.

47. Bastani B, Frenchie D: Significant myoglobin removal during continuous veno-venous haemofiltration using F80 membrane (letter). Nephrol Dial Transplant 1997;12:2035–2036.

48. Cray SH, Robinson BH, Cox PN: Lactic academia and bradyarrhythmia in a child sedated with propofol. Crit Care Med 1998;26:2087–2092.

49. van der Maten J, Schrijver G: Severe accidental hypothermia: rewarming with CVVHD. Neth J Med 1996;49:160–163.

50. Al-Khafaji AH, Dewhirst WE, Manning HL: Propylene glycol toxicity associated with lorazepam infusion in a patient receiving continuous veno-venous hemofiltration with dialysis. Anesth Analg 2002;94:1583–1585.

51. Tan HK, Uchino S, Bellomo R: The acid-base effects of continuous hemofiltration with lactate or bicarbonate buffered replacement fluids. Int J Artif Organs 2003;26:477–483.

52. Nowak MA, Campbell TE: Profound hypercalcemia in continuous veno-venous hemofiltration dialysis with trisodium citrate anticoagulation and hepatic failure (letter). Clin Chem 1997;43:412–413.

53. Ganter G: Ueber die beseitgung giftiger stoffe aus blute durch dialyse, Munchen Med Wochenschr 1923;70:1478.

54. Mattocks AM, El-Bassiouni EA: Peritoneal dialysis: a review. J Pharm Sci 1971;60:1767–1782.

55. Fine RN: Peritoneal dialysis update. J Pediatr 1982;100:1–7.

56. Holazo AA, Colburn WA: Pharmacokinetics of drugs during various detoxification procedures for overdose and environmental exposure. Drug Metab Rev 1982;13:715–743.

57. Blye E, Lorch J, Cortell S: Extracorporeal therapy in the treatment of intoxication. Am J Kidney Dis 1984;3:321–338.

58. Maher JF: Interactions of drugs and peritoneal dialysis. Proc Clin Dial Transplant Forum 1978;8:168–170.

59. Knepshield JH, Schreiner GE, Lowenthal DT, Gelfand CM: Dialysis of poisons and drugs—annual review. Amer Soc Artif Intern Organs 1973;19:590–633.

60. Babb AL, Popovich RP, Christopher TG, et al: The genesis of the square meter-hour hypothesis. Trans Am Soc Artif Intern Organs 1971;17:81–91.

61. Keyvan-Larijarni H, Tannenberg AM: Methanol intoxication: comparison of peritoneal dialysis and hemodialysis treatment. Arch Intern Med 1974;134:293–296.

62. Chan JC, Campbell RA: Peritoneal dialysis in children: survey of its indications and applications. Clin Pediatr 1973:12:131–139.

63. Goldsmith D: Jayewardene S, Sabharwal N, Cooney K: Allergic reactions to the polymeric glucose-based peritoneal dialysis fluid icodextrin in patients with renal failure. Lancet 2000;355:897.

64. Heath A: Pharmacokinetic evaluation of forced diuresis, dialysis, and hemoperfusion. Dev Toxicol Environ Sci 1986;12:339–345.

65. Miller RB, Tassistro CR: Current concepts: peritoneal dialysis. N Eng J Med 1969;281:945–949.

66. Counts SJ, Baylink DJ, Shen FH, et al: Vitamin D intoxication in an anephric child. Ann Intern Med 1975;82:196–200.

67. Berkovitch M, Akilesh MR, Gerace R, et al:. Acute digoxin overdose in a newborn with renal failure: use of digoxin immune Fab and peritoneal dialysis. Ther Drug Monitor 1994;16:531–533.

68. Montoya-Cabrera MA, Escalante-Galindo P, Nava-Juarez A, et al: [Evaluation of the efficacy of N-acetylcysteine administered alone or in combination with activated charcoal in the treatment of acetaminophen overdoses]. Gac Med Mex 1999;135:239–243.

69. Wason S, Baker RC, Carolan P, et al: Carbamazepine overdose—the effects of multiple dose activated charcoal. Clin Toxicol 1992;30:39–48.

70. Montoya-Cabrera MA, Sauceda-Garcia JM, Escalante-Galindo P, et al: Carbamazepine poisoning in adolescent suicide attempters. Effectiveness of multiple-dose activated charcoal in enhancing carbamazepine elimination. Arch Med Res 1996;27:485–489.

71. Stremski ES, Brady WB, Prasad K, Hennes HA: Pediatric carbamazepine intoxication. Ann Emerg Med 1995;25:624–630.

72. Karkkainen S, Neuvonen PJ: Effect of oral charcoal and urine pH on dextropropoxyphene pharmacokinetics. Int J Clin Pharmacol Ther Toxicol 1985;23:219–225.

73. Pond S, Jacobs M, Marks J, et al: Treatment of digitoxin overdose with oral activated charcoal. Lancet 1981;21:1177–1178.

74. Park GD, Goldberg MJ, Spector R, et al: The effects of activated charcoal on digoxin and digitoxin clearance. Drug Intell Clin Pharm 1985;19:937–941.

75. Mauro LS, Mauro VF, Brown DL, Somani P: Enhancement of phenytoin elimination by multiple-dose activated charcoal. Ann Emerg Med 1987;16:1132–1135.

76. Weichbrodt GD, Elliott DP: Treatment of phenytoin toxicity with repeated doses of activated charcoal. Ann Emerg Med 1987;16:1387–1389.

77. Ros SP, Black LE: Multiple-dose activated charcoal in management of phenytoin overdose. Pediatr Emerg Care 1989;5:169–170.

78. Frenia ML, Schauben JL, Wears RL, et al: Multiple-dose activated charcoal compared to urinary alkalinization for the enhancement of phenobarbital elimination. Clin Toxicol 1996;34:169–175.

79. Ebid AH, Abdel-Rahman HM: Pharmacokinetics of phenobarbital during certain enhanced elimination modalities to evaluate their clinical efficacy in management of drug overdose. Ther Drug Monit 2001;23:209–216.

80. Laufen H, Leitold M: The effect of activated charcoal on the bioavailability of piroxicam in man. Int J Clin Pharmacol Ther Toxicol 1986;24:48–52.

81. Rusyniak DE, Furbee RB, Kirk, MA: Thallium and arsenic poisoning in a small midwestern town. Ann Emerg Med 2002;39:307–311.

82. Arimori K, Nakano M: Accelerated clearance of intravenously administered theophylline and phenobarbital by oral doses of activated charcoal in rats. A possibility of the intestinal dialysis. J Pharmacobiodyn 1986;9:437–441.

83. Reissell P, Manninen V: Effect of administration of activated charcoal and fibre on absorption, excretion and steady state blood levels of digoxin and digitoxin. Evidence for intestinal excretion of the glycosides. Acta Med Scand Suppl 1982;668:88–90.

84. Boldy DA, Smart V, Vale JA: Multiple doses of charcoal in digoxin poisoning. Lancet 1985;2:1076–1077.

85. Ibanez C, Carcas AJ, Frias J, Abad F: Activated charcoal increases digoxin elimination in patients. Int J Cardiol 1995;48:27–30.

86. Barone JA, Raia JJ, Huang YC: Evaluation of the effects of multiple-dose activated charcoal on the absorption of orally administered salicylate in a simulated toxic ingestion model. Ann Emerg Med 1988;17:34–37.

87. Ho JL, Tierney MG, Dickinson GE: An evaluation of the effect of repeated doses of oral activated charcoal on salicylate elimination. J Clin Pharmacol 1989;29:366–369.

88. Kirshenbaum LA, Mathews SC, Sitar DS, Tenenbein M: Does multiple-dose charcoal therapy enhance salicylate excretion? Arch Intern Med 1990;150:1281–1283.

89. Mayer AL, Sitar DS, Tenenbein M: Multiple-dose charcoal and whole-bowel irrigation do not increase clearance of absorbed salicylate. Arch Intern Med 1992;152:393–396.

90. Johnson D, Eppler J, Giesbrecht E: Effect of multiple-dose activated charcoal on the clearance of high-dose intravenous aspirin in a porcine model. Ann Emerg Med 1995;26:569–574.

91. Crome P, Dawling S, Braithwaite RA, et al: Effect of activated charcoal on absorption of nortriptyline. Lancet 1977;2:1203–1205.

92. Scheinin M, Virtanen R, Iisalo E: Effect of single and repeated doses of activated charcoal on the pharmacokinetics of doxepin. Int J Clin Pharmacol Ther Toxicol 1985;23:38–42.

93. Goldberg MJ, Park GD, Spector R, et al: Lack of effect of oral activated charcoal on imipramine clearance. Clin Pharmacol Ther 1985;38:350–353.

94. Kärkkäinen S, Neuvonen PJ: Pharmacokinetics of amitriptyline influenced by oral charcoal and urine pH. Int J Clin Pharmacol Ther Toxicol 1986;24:326–332.

95. Davis RL, Roon RA, Koup JR, Smith AL: Effect of orally administered activated charcoal on vancomycin clearance. Antimicrob Agents Chemother 1987;31:720–722.

96. Laine K, Kivistö KT, Neuvonen PJ: Failure of oral activated charcoal to accelerate the elimination of amiodarone and chloroquine. Hum Exp Toxicol 1992;11:491–494.

97. Laine K, Kivistö KT, Neuvonen PJ: The effect of activated charcoal on the absorption and elimination of astemizole. Hum Exp Toxicol 1994;13:502–505.

98. Neuvonen PJ, Kärkkäinen S: Effects of charcoal, sodium bicarbonate, and ammonium chloride on chlorpropamide kinetics. Clin Pharmacol Ther 1983;33:386–393.

99. Roberts D, Honcharik N, Sitar DS, Tenenbein M: Diltiazem overdose: pharmacokinetics of diltiazem and its metabolites and effect of multiple dose charcoal therapy. Clin Toxicol 1991;29:45–52.

100. Laine K, Kivistö KT, Ojala-Karlsson P, Neuvonen PJ: Effect of activated charcoal on the pharmacokinetics of pholcodine, with special reference to delayed charcoal ingestion. Ther Drug Monit 1997;19:46–50.

101. al-Shareef A, Buss DC, Shetty HG, et al: The effect of repeated-dose activated charcoal on the pharmacokinetics of sodium valproate in healthy volunteers. Br J Clin Pharmacol 1997;43:109–111.

102. Davis RL, Koup JR, Roon RA, et al: Effect of oral activated charcoal on tobramycin clearance. Antimicrob Agents Chemother 1988;32:274–275.

103. Hellinger A, Wolter K, Marggraf G, et al: Elimination of amrinone during continuous veno-venous haemofiltration after cardiac surgery. Eur J Clin Pharmacol 1995;48:57–59.

104. Koch M, Appoloni O, Haufroid V, et al: Acute barium intoxication and hemodiafiltration. J Toxicol Clin Toxicol 2003;41:363–367.

105. Kroh UF, Lennartz H, Edwards DJ, Stoeckel K: Pharmacokinetics of ceftriaxone in patients undergoing continuous veno-venous hemofiltration. J Clin Pharmacol 1996;36:1114–1119.

106. Walder AD, Tyler CK: Ethylene glycol antifreeze poisoning. Anaesthesia 1994;49:964–967.

107. Tegeder I, Bremer F, Oelkers F, et al: Pharmacokinetics of imipenem-cilastatin in critically ill patients undergoing continuous venovenous hemofiltration. Antimicrob Agents Chemother 1997;41:2640–2645.

108. Hazouard E, Ferrandiere M, Rateau H, et al: Continuous veno-venous haemofiltration versus continuous veno-venous haemodialysis in severe lithium self-poisoning:a toxicokinetics study in an intensive care unit. Nephrol Dial Transplant 1999;14:1605–1606.

109. Barrueto F, Meggs WJ, Barchman MJ: Clearance of metformin by hemofiltration in overdose. Clin Toxicol 2002;40:177–180.

110. Wrathall G, Sinclair R, Moore A, Pogson D: Three case reports of the use of haemodiafiltration in the treatment of salicylate overdose. Hum Exp Toxicol 2001;20:491–495.

111. Armstrong DK, Hidalgo HA, Eldadah M: Vancomycin and tobramycin clearance in an infant during continuous hemofiltration. Ann Pharmacother 1993;27:224–227.

112. Robert R, Rochard E, Malin F, et al: Amikacin pharmacokinetics during continuous veno-venous hemofiltration (letter). Crit Care Med 1991;19:588–589.

113. Hantson P, Haufroid V, Buchet JP, Mahieu P: Acute arsenic poisoning treated by intravenous dimercaptosuccinic acid (DMSA) and combined extrarenal epuration techniques. J Toxicol Clin Toxicol 2003;41:1–6.

114. Kay TD, Playford HR, Johnson DW: Hemodialysis versus continuous veno-venous hemodiafiltration in the management of severe valproate overdose. Clin Nephrol 2003;59:56–58.

115. Morton KC: Peritoneal dialysis in acute poisoning: successful treatment of a 15-month-old child ingesting 30 times the adult dose of Achrocidin. Clin Pediatr 1966;5:565–567.

116. Langer M, Vesconi S, Iapichina G, et al: [The early removal of amatoxins in the treatment of amanita phalloides poisoning (author's translation)] Klin Wochenschr 1980;58:117–123.

117. Green FJ, Lavelle KJ, Aronoff GR, et al: Management of amikacin overdose. Am J Kidney Dis 1981;1:110–112.

118. Kaufman DB, DiNicola W, McIntosh R: Acute potassium dichromate poisoning: treated by peritoneal dialysis. Amer J Dis Child 1970;119:374–376.

119. Cole DE: Peritoneal dialysis for removal of copper. Br Med J 1978;1:50–51.

120. Cole DE, Lirenman DS: Role of albumin-enriched peritoneal dialysate in acute copper poisoning. J Pediatrics 1978;92:955–957.

121. Vale JA, Prior JG, O'Hare JP, et al: Treatment of ethylene glycol poisoning with peritoneal dialysis. Br Med J 1982;284:557.

122. Sabeel AI, Kurkus J, Lindholm T: Intensified dialysis treatment of ethylene glycol intoxication. Scand J Urol Nephrol 1995;29:125–129.

123. DeMyttenaere M, Schoenfeld L, Maher JF: Treatment of glutethimide poisoning: a comparison of forced diuresis and kinetics. JAMA 1968;203:165–167.

124. Ozdemir AI, Tannenberg AM: Peritoneal and hemodialysis for acute glutethimide. N Y State J Med 1972;72:2076–2079.

125. von Hartitzsch B, Pinto MH, Mauer SM, et al: Treatment of glutethimide intoxication: an in vivo comparison of lipid, aqueous, and peritoneal dialysis with albumin. Proc Dial Transplant Forum 1973;3:102–106.

126. Mecikalski MB, Depner TA: Peritoneal dialysis for isopropanol poisoning. West J Med 1982;137:322–325.

127. Wilson JH, Donker AJ, VanDerHem GK, Wientjes J: Peritoneal dialysis for lithium poisoning. Br Med J 1971;2:749–750.

128. Brown EA, Pawlikowski TR: Lithium intoxication treated by peritoneal dialysis. Br J Clin Pract 1981;35:90–91.

129. Rose SR, Klein-Schwartz W, Oderda GM, et al: Lithium intoxication with acute renal failure and death. Drug Intell Clin Pharm 1988;22:691–694.

130. Dyment PG, Curtis DD, Gourrich GE: Meprobamate poisoning treated by peritoneal dialysis. J Pediatr 1965;67:124–126.

131. Graae J, Ladefoged J: [Severe meprobamate poisoning treated by hemodialysis and peritoneal dialysis]. Nordisk Medicin 1969;8:601–603.

132. Castell DO, Sode J: Meprobamate intoxication treated with peritoneal dialysis. Ill Med J 1967;131:298–299.

133. Mouton DE, Cohen RJ, Barrett O: Meprobamate poisoning: successful treatment with peritoneal dialysis. Am J Med Sci 1967;253:706–709.

134. Laroche B, Dan PH, Lapandry C, et al: [Acute meprobamate poisoning. Efficacy of peritoneal dialysis]. Cah Anesthesiol Cahiers d'Anesthesiologie 1984;37:677–679.

135. Wallace HE, Neumayer F, Gutch CF: Amphetamine poisoning and peritoneal dialysis: a case report. Am J Dis Child 1964;108:657–661.

136. Stinebaugh BJ: The use of peritoneal dialysis in acute methyl alcohol poisoning. Arch Intern Med 1960;105:145–149.

137. Wenzl JE, Mills SD, McCall JT: Methanol poisoning in an infant: successful treatment with peritoneal dialysis. Amer J Dis Child 1968;116:445–447.

138. Keyvan-Larijarni H, Tannenberg AM: Comparison of peritoneal and hemodialysis: treatment of methanol intoxication. Proc Dial Transplant Forum 1973;3:107–109.

139. Schlegel RJ, Altstatt LB, Canales L, et al: Peritoneal dialysis for severe salicylism: an evaluation of indications and results. J Pediatr 1966;69:553–562.

140. El-Dahr S, Gomez RA, Campbell FG, Chevalier RL: Rapid correction of acute salt poisoning by peritoneal dialysis. Pediatr Nephrol 1987;1:602–604.

141. Hekster YA, Vree TB, Weemaes CM, Rotteveel JJ: Toxicologic and pharmacokinetic evaluation of a case of vancomycin intoxication during continuous ambulatory peritoneal dialysis. Pharm Weekbl Sci 1986;8:293–297.

142. Zalis EG, Cohen RJ, Lundberg GD: Use of peritoneal dialysis in experimental amphetamine poisoning. Proc Soc Exp Biol Med 1965;120:278–281.

143. Chen, YC, Chang CT, Fang JT, Huang CC: Baclofen neurotxicity in uremic patients: is continuous ambulatory peritoneal dialysis less effective than intermittent hemodialysis? Ren Fail 2003;25:297–305.

144. Segar WE: Peritoneal dialysis in the treatment of boric acid poisoning. N Engl J Med 1960;262:798–800.

145. Baliah T, MacLeish H, Drummond KN: Acute boric acid poisoning: report of an infant successfully treated by peritoneal dialysis. Can Med Assoc J 1969;101:166–168.

146. Martin GI: Asymptomatic boric intoxication: value of peritoneal dialysis. N Y State J Med 1971;71:1842–1844.

147. Baker MD, Bogema SC: Ingestion of boric acid by infants. Am J Emerg Med 1986;4:358–361.

148. Lichtenberg R, Zeller WP, Gatson R, Hurley RM: Bromate poisoning. J Pediatr 1989;114:891–894.

149. Warshaw BL: Treatment of bromate poisoning (letter). J Pediatr 1989;115:660–661.

150. Walsh I, Wasserman GS, Mestad P, Lanman RC: Near-fatal caffeine intoxication treated with peritoneal dialysis. Pediatr Emerg Care 1987;3:244–249.

151. Schiffl H, Widmann P, Weiss M, Massry SG: Dialysis treatment of acute chromium intoxication and comparative efficacy of peritoneal versus hemodialysis in chromium removal. Miner Electrolyte Metab 1982;7:28–35.

152. Matey P, Allison KP, Sheehan TM, Gowar JP: Chromic acid burns: early aggressive excision is the best method to prevent systemic toxicity. J Burn Care Rehabil 2000;21:241–245.

153. Fuquay D, Koup J, Smith AL: Brief clinical and laboratory observations: management of neonatal gentamicin overdosage. J Pediatr 1981;99:473–476.

154. Lowenthal DT, Chardo F, Reidenberg MM: Removal of mercury by peritoneal dialysis. Arch Intern Med 1974;134:139–141.

155. Yoshida M, Satoh H, Igarashi M, et al: Acute mercury poisoning by intentional ingestion of mercuric chloride. Tohku J Exp Med 1997;182:347–352.

156. Polin RA, Henry D, Pippinger CE: Peritoneal dialysis for severe methyprylon intoxication. J Pediatr 1977;90:831–833.

157. Collins JM: Peritoneal dialysis for severe methyprylon intoxication (letter). J Pediatr 1978;92:519–520.

158. McCarthy WH, Keenan RL: Propoxyphene hydrochloride poisoning: report of the first fatality. JAMA 1964;187:460–461.

159. Karliner JS: Propoxyphene hydrochloride poisoning: report of a case treated with peritoneal dialysis. JAMA 1967;199:152–155.

160. Gary NE, Maher JF, DeMyttenaere MH, et al: Acute propoxyphene hydrochloride intoxication. Arch Intern Med 1968;121:453–457.

161. Markham TN, Dodson VN, Eckberg DL: Peritoneal dialysis in quinine sulfate intoxication. JAMA 1967;202:1102–1103.

162. Donadio JV, Whelton A, Gilliland PF, Cirksena WJ: Peritoneal dialysis in quinine intoxication. JAMA 1968;204:182.

163. Brooks MH, Hano JE, Clayton LE, et al: Quinine extraction during peritoneal dialysis: the role of nonionic diffusion. Invest Urol 1970;7:510–516.

164. Sabto J, Pierce RM, West H, Gurr FW: Hemodialysis, peritoneal dialysis, plasmapheresis and forced diuresis for the treatment of quinine overdose. Clin Nephrol 1981;16:264–268.

165. Halle MA, Collipp PJ: Amitriptyline hydrochloride poisoning: unsuccessful treatment by peritoneal dialysis. N Y State J Med 1969;69:1434–1436.

166. McCann WP, Permisohn R, Palmisano PA: Fatal chloroquine poisoning in a child: experience with peritoneal dialysis. Pediatrics 19754;55:536–538.

167. Graw RG, Clarke RR: Chlorpropamide intoxication-treatment with peritoneal dialysis. Pediatrics 1970;45:106–109.

168. Kumar L, Singhi PD, Pereira BJ, et al: Accidental poisoning with isoniazid and rifampicin in an infant: role of peritoneal dialysis. Nephrol Dial Transplant 1989;4:156–157.

169. Proudfoot AT, Noble J, Nimmo J, et al: Peritoneal dialysis and haemodialysis in methaqualone (Mandrax) poisoning. Scott Med J 1967;13:232–236.

170. DeMarco V, Bear R, Kapur BM: Peritoneal dialysis in methaqualone overdose. Can Med Assoc J 1975;113:823.

171. Thomas BB: Peritoneal dialysis and Lysol poisoning. Br Med J 1969;3:720.

172. Koshy KM, Lovejoy FH: Thallium ingestion with survival: ineffectiveness of peritoneal dialysis and potassium chloride diuresis. Clin Toxicol 1981;18:521–525.

173. Okada T, Nakao T, Matsumoto H, et al: Valacyclovir neurotoxicity in a patient with end-stage renal disease treated with continuous ambulatory peritoneal dialysis. Clin Nephrol 2002;58:168–170.

D   Hemodialysis and Hemoperfusion

JUAN C. ARIAS, MD ■ STEPHEN W. BORRON, MD, MS

Chapter 2C addresses the use of peritoneal dialysis, various forms of hemofiltration, and multiple-dose activated charcoal (MDAC) as so-called "gastrointestinal dialysis." This chapter discusses the more classic methods for extracorporeal removal of toxicants, namely, hemodialysis (HD) and hemoperfusion (HP). In addition, we briefly discuss a newer methodology, the molecular adsorbents recirculating system (MARS, also referred to as albumin dialysis), which was developed primarily for the treatment of fulminant liver failure (FLF), but has recently been employed in the treatment of a variety of poisonings.

As has been pointed out in previous chapters, extracorporeal methods for toxicant removal should be viewed as important adjuncts rather than as primary approaches to specific poisonings. The most effective method of removal of toxicants from the body in most cases is maintenance of properly functioning kidneys, liver, and lungs through excellent supportive care. The ultimate evaluation of efficacy of extracorporeal methods is in fact through direct comparison with spontaneous elimination by the body.[1] In the absence of careful attention to resuscitation and supportive care, these adjuncts may be of little use; they may even be dangerous. Further-

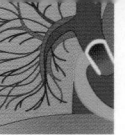
more, while dozens of toxicants have been shown to be removed by HD or HP,[2] evidence-based support for significant clinical improvement from these procedures is often lacking. As will be shown, each of these procedures has benefits and risks, which must be carefully weighed against other methods of treatment.

It is difficult to ascertain the frequency with which HD and HP are employed in the treatment of poisoning. Based on the most recent Toxic Exposure Surveillance Survey,[3] it would appear that use of HD ($N = 1730$) largely exceeds that of HP ($N = 30$). Both procedures were far more commonly performed in adults older than 19 years (93% of HD cases and 90% of HP cases) than in children. Use of these extracorporeal removal techniques in children younger than 6 years was rare (seven cases of HD, one case of HP). These figures are undoubtedly underestimates of real use, since reporting to poison centers by physicians is voluntary and incomplete. Nonetheless, they suggest that extracorporeal purification therapies have a limited role in management of poisoning in the United States.

METHODOLOGY

Hemodialysis

HD requires the passage of blood from the body through an external circuit, in which it is anticoagulated and placed in sustained contact with a selectively permeable membrane prior to being returned to the patient. Opposite the membrane and flowing in countercurrent direction is a heated dialysate, the composition of which can be varied according to the indications for dialysis. The variation of electrolyte concentrations, addition of buffers, and sometimes other additives allow the operator to manipulate the passage of these elements from one side of the membrane to the other. HD operates on the basis of three principles: diffusion, osmosis, and ultrafiltration.[4] Diffusion relies on concentration gradients, with solutes moving from an area of higher concentration to an area of lower concentration, ultimately resulting in equilibration. Osmotic pressure results in the movement of water from one side of a semipermeable membrane to the other, dependent on a higher concentration of solutes on the other side. Manipulation of plasma sodium concentrations (sodium profiling) during dialysis can induce a net flow of water from cells into the plasma, allowing for its ultimate removal from the plasma. Ultrafiltration involves movement of fluid across the membrane due to the presence of a pressure gradient. This principle allows control of fluid loss during dialysis and can be manipulated via varying dialysate pressure (pressure control) or by variation of dialysate flow volumes (volumetric control). Volumetric control is more common in modern dialysis machines. In the case of toxicants, diffusion into the dialysate is the primary end point, although amelioration of acid-base and electrolyte conditions is often an important additional goal.

Dialyzer specifications (blood flow rate, surface area, and membrane construction) determine, in part, the efficacy of drug or chemical removal from the blood. Pharmacodynamic and pharmacokinetic factors (molecular weight, lipid solubility, protein binding, toxicant concentration gradient, and volume of distribution [Vd]) are equally critical factors which will be discussed in further detail below.[2]

Hemoperfusion

HP implies the passage of blood through a device containing absorbent particles.[2] It may be performed alone or in combination with HD and has been employed for a number of years in the management of poisonings. Resin HP with variants of Amberlite XAD (Rohm & Haas, Philadelphia, PA) was viewed as promising in the 1970s and 1980s. However, very few recent reports of resin HP have been published.[5-10] This is likely in part due to unavailability of medical-grade resin cartridges in many geographic areas. Activated charcoal appears to be the most commonly used absorbent material based on published reports, but hospital availability of even these cartridges appears to be limited. A recent survey of New York City 911-receiving hospitals revealed that only about one third of those surveyed had charcoal hemoperfusion (CHP) cartridges readily available (only one hospital had pediatric cartridges). Just 3 of 34 responding hospitals had used CHP within the previous 5 years. Reasons cited by the authors for limited cartridge availability and use of CHP were decreasing clinical use of phenobarbital and theophylline and improved efficacy of HD.[11]

CHP irreversibly binds water- and lipid-soluble drugs and chemicals in the molecular weight range of 113 to 40,000 Da, a much larger range than that for HD (<~300 Da). Plasma drug extraction ratios for HP are superior to those for HD for acetaminophen (paracetamol), digoxin, glutethimide, paraquat, phenobarbital, and theophylline.[2] However, further examination of this list may reveal, in part, why HP is seldom employed in the United States. N-acetylcysteine is effective for acetaminophen poisoning, widely available, and less invasive. Digoxin Fab fragments are far more effective than HP in binding and eliminating digitalis glycosides. Glutethimide is rarely prescribed in the United States. Paraquat poisonings are rather rare in the United States, and HP has not been shown to alter outcomes, despite of reduction of plasma concentrations.[12] As mentioned previously, phenobarbital and theophylline have largely been replaced in clinical use by other agents, and the less invasive MDAC has been shown to be effective in reducing plasma concentrations of these agents, although it has not been proven to alter outcomes.[13]

Molecular Adsorbents Recirculating System

The Molecular Adsorbents Recirculating System (MARS) is a relatively new method of extracorporeal decontamination, which employs dialysis across a membrane impregnated with albumin and a 20% albumin dialysate,

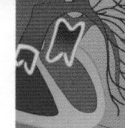

thus attracting highly protein-bound substances. In addition, charcoal and anion exchange resin cartridges are employed to filter the dialysate, regenerating it for continued use.[14] MARS may be of interest in the setting of poisons that have a predilection for liver toxicity, as the system is capable not only of removing certain hepatotoxins, but also reducing hyperbilirubinemia, restoring hemodynamics, diminishing hepatic encephalopathy, and improving renal function.[14] MARS has been used to maintain patients in liver failure during the peritransplant period.[15-18] The existing data for MARS in general are encouraging, but the evidence base is limited.[19] This caveat is even truer in the setting of poisoning.

GENERAL PRINCIPLES FOR EXTRACORPOREAL DECONTAMINATION

Modalities and Susceptible Substances

A number of factors determine the suitability of use of HD or HP as extracorporeal methods of removal of a given toxicant. In the case of HD, chemical and drug removal are determined by factors as blood flow rate, dialysate flow rate, dialyzer surface area, and pore structure of the chosen membrane and by pharmacodynamic and pharmacokinetic factors such as molecular size (usually <300 Da), lipid solubility, protein binding, Vd, and concentration gradient. For HP, the selection of filter material has historically been important (charcoal vs. resin cartridges). With scarce availability of resin cartridges, the choice has essentially reverted to charcoal. HP is typically reserved for drugs with a low Vd and high protein binding,[20] but as mentioned previously, compounds of larger molecular weight may be removed. HD frequently causes hypotension, whereas this is reportedly less often a problem in HP. As such, in instances where hemodynamic instability after poisoning is an issue, HP may be preferable even if less efficacious for a particular toxicant. Vasopressors such as dopamine and norepinephrine are absorbed by the cartridges and therefore should be administered in the circuit after the sorbent. A definite role for MARS therapy in poisoning has not yet been established. In general, substances that are highly bound to albumin and poorly susceptible to other forms of treatment, including HD and HP, should prompt consideration of MARS, particularly in the setting of liver failure.

Molecular Weight

In order to be effectively hemodialyzed, toxicants should ideally be of low molecular weight (<300 Da).[21] Examples of toxicants of low molecular weight are methanol (32.04 Da), ethanol (46.07 Da), ethylene glycol (62.07 Da), lithium carbonate (73.89 Da), butoxyethanol (118.20 Da), aspirin (180.15 Da), and theophylline (180.17 Da).[21]

Volume of Distribution

A low molecular weight alone is not sufficient, however, to assure effective dialyzability. For example, nortripty-

line has a molecular weight of 299.85 Da, but is poorly removed by HD. This is due to its very large Vd.[22] The Vd is the theoretical volume into which a drug distributes in the body and is generally expressed in liters or liters/kg body weight. Substances with a small Vd (<1 L/kg) reside to a greater extent in the bloodstream and can generally be effectively removed by using extracorporeal methods. The Vd of a drug is the most important determinant of the efficacy of HP.[20] Even when extracorporeal methods are very efficient in removing toxicants from the blood, if the theoretical Vd is high, the pharmodynamic effect achieved is likely to be minimal, as the concentration at the drug target tissue may be virtually unchanged.

Protein Binding

A third critical factor in predicting efficacy of extracorporeal methods is protein binding. HD is of limited value for substances that are highly protein bound. CHP, on the other hand, remains effective in cases of drug overdose with substances of high protein binding capacity.[20] A study conducted in 12 patients treated with HP, with drug overdoses involving 20 different drugs, showed that the efficacy of drug removal through absorption by activated charcoal was dependent on the binding affinity, which is related to the protein binding percentage. This study concluded that drugs that are protein bound at levels of up to 95% are effectively removed from the blood with HP.[20] Following HD or HP, substances with a higher Vd and high protein binding percentage tend to redistribute from storage tissues to plasma. For this reason, a single extracorporeal substance removal session may be insufficient.[21]

Water Solubility

Water solubility is also an important factor in determining dialyzability. Water-soluble substances like ethanol, methanol, ethylene glycol, salicylates, theophylline, lithium, and valproate tend to have limited distribution in adipose tissues, thus limiting their Vd. This property makes them ideal for extracorporeal drug removal.

WHEN SHOULD HEMODIALYSIS OR HEMOPERFUSION BE CONSIDERED?

Poisoning by a substance susceptible to extracorporeal removal is not in itself an adequate justification for the procedure.[2] In general, extracorporeal methods should be reserved for poisonings for which toxic metabolic activation is anticipated (e.g., methanol, ethylene glycol), for which blood concentrations or the amount of toxicant absorbed foretell very serious toxicity, and for patients who have not improved despite of appropriate supportive care (volume repletion, acid-base correction, use of vasopressors, ion-trapping diuresis, and administration of specific antidotes). Winchester[2] identifies six clinical considerations for HD or HP in poisoning: (1) progressive deterioration; (2) depression of midbrain function leading to hypoventilation, hypothermia, and hypotension;

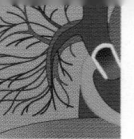

(3) development of, or predisposition to, complications of coma, such as pneumonia or septicemia; (4) impairment of drug excretion; (5) poisoning of substances possessing metabolic and/or delayed effects; and (6) poisons extractable at a rate exceeding endogenous elimination. These considerations could be condensed to (1) patients who are very sick or likely to become so and (2) toxicants for which HD/HP are effective in removal and known to make a clinical difference in outcome.

Toxicant Blood Concentrations

Blood concentrations of certain toxicants (e.g., methanol and ethylene glycol) have been proposed as indicators for HD. Historically, a plasma concentration of 50 mg/dL has been used as a threshold for the need for dialysis in both ethylene glycol[23] and methanol[24] poisonings. The availability of fomepizole, a safe and effective inhibitor of alcohol dehydrogenase, has altered the indications for HD.[25-28] While HD continues to be a useful and often necessary adjunct in the treatment of toxic alcohol poisonings, an elevated blood concentration of the alcohol alone is no longer considered sufficient to require HD.

Metabolic Acidosis

Severe metabolic acidosis accompanying methanol and ethylene glycol, as well as other toxic alcohol poisonings, is a clear indication for HD, regardless of blood concentration. In these cases, HD not only effectively removes the toxicants and their acidic metabolites, but helps in directly correcting the acid-base balance of the patient. Even when the toxicant's molecular weight, protein binding, or Vd do not conform to the criteria necessary for dialyzability, HD should be considered in the setting of severe metabolic acidosis and/or renal failure. An example of this can be found in overdoses by metformin. Metformin would be expected to be poorly dialyzable on the basis of its very large Vd. However, metformin toxicity results in severe metabolic acidosis, which may be ameliorated by application of HD techniques.[29,30]

SPECIAL POPULATIONS

Children

Both HD and HP may be performed in children, but both pose greater challenges than in adults. Vascular access is obviously more difficult in small children. For this reason, peritoneal dialysis has been historically used more often in children. However, use of peritoneal dialysis for acute renal failure in children appears to be decreasing and use of HD increasing over time.[31] As mentioned before, availability of CHP cartridges suited to use in children may be extremely limited, even in major metropolitan areas.[11] However, it appears that if antidotal therapy for ethylene glycol is administered before the onset of renal insufficiency, HD, even in

children, may be safely avoided.[32] Given the long half-life of methanol, HD is still considered advisable in children after treatment with fomepizole.[33]

Chronic Renal Failure

Obviously, poisonings by substances normally eliminated by the kidneys may require HD or HP in patients with chronic renal failure.[34]

COMPLICATIONS OF HEMODIALYSIS AND HEMOFILTRATION

Both HD and HP are associated with potential serious complications (Box 2D-1). The most serious complications associated with HD include hypotension (which by extension may lead to myocardial or brain infarction) and bleeding associated with anticoagulation. An addi-

---

BOX 2D-1	POTENTIAL ACUTE COMPLICATIONS OF HD AND HP

Catheter-Related Issues

Hemorrhage
Thrombosis
Infection
Central vein stenosis

Anticoagulation-Related Issues

Gastrointestinal hemorrhage
Intracerebral hemorrhage
Cardiac tamponade
Heparin-induced
   thrombocytopenia
Heparin-related thrombosis

Hypotension-Related Issues

Mesenteric ischemia
Ischemic pancreatitis
Myocardial infarction
Transient ischemic attack
Cerebral infarction

Dialysate-Related Issues

Electrolytemias
Acid-base disorders
Treatment water contamination

Charcoal Cartridge–Related Issues

Electrolytemias
Thrombocytopenia
Leukopenia
Hypocalcemia

Multiple Etiology Issues

Pulmonary embolism/air
   embolism
Disequilibrium syndrome*
Cardiac arrhythmias
Angina
Cardiac arrest
Fever (bacteria, contaminated
   dialysis water)
Muscle cramps
Anaphylactoid reactions to
   membranes
Severe hemolysis
Hypoglycemia

---

*Nausea, vomiting, headache, blurred vision, confusion, and fatigue potentially leading to seizures, coma, and arrhythmias.
Adapted from Rahman MH: Acute hemolysis with acute renal failure in a patient with valproic acid poisoning treated with charcoal hemoperfusion. Hemodial Int 2006;10(3):256–259; Himmelfarb J: Hemodialysis complications. Am J Kidney Dis 2005;45(6):1122–1131; and Davenport A: Intradialytic complications during hemodialysis. Hemodial Int 2006;10(2):162–167.

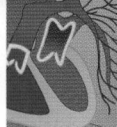

tional significant consequence is reduction of therapeutic levels of drugs, which may result in unmasking of conditions protected by these agents. Complications appear to be relatively fewer in HP, but may nonetheless be important. HP is associated with the destruction of platelets, such that significant thrombocytopenia and bleeding may occur. This complication has been reduced by coating of the sorbent particles with a polymer solution.[2] Hypocalcemia likewise may occur.[35] Rahman and colleagues recently reported on the case of a patient treated with CHP for valproate poisoning. Despite of the use of coated charcoal, the patient developed severe hemolysis, which the researchers attributed to mechanical damage to red cells by the high flow rate through the cartridge. The patient required packed red blood cells, platelets, and fibrin transfusions, developing oliguric-anuric renal failure that required 23 days of HD over a period of several weeks. She ultimately regained her normal renal function.[36]

RISK AND COST-BENEFIT CONSIDERATIONS

Transfer

HD and HP are not universally available. Thus, transfer to centers capable of performing these procedures may at times be required. The decision to transfer a patient for these therapies should rest on evaluation of several elements: (1) Is the patient stable for transport? (2) Will the patient's outcome likely be significantly better if the procedure is undertaken? (3) Are there acceptable alternatives to HD or HP? Each of these issues should be studied prior to committing a patient to prolonged and expensive or potentially hazardous transport to another facility for extracorporeal decontamination procedures.

As mentioned above, HD and HP have significant potential for complications. In certain poisonings, such as ethylene glycol and methanol intoxications, where HD was formerly routinely prescribed in the presence of high blood concentrations, recent improvements in specific antidotes have led to therapeutic alternatives. For example, if a patient with significant ethylene glycol poisoning arrives at the hospital before the onset of acidosis and renal failure, early treatment with fomepizole alone may preempt the need for HD.[25,26,28] Even in the case of methanol, HD may be avoided in selective cases after early treatment with fomepizole.[28] Methanol's elimination half-life is much greater than that of ethylene glycol, however, and may require prolonged antidotal treatment in the absence of HD.

Intensive Care Unit Admission

Requirement for acute HD and/or HP generally implies costly intensive care unit (ICU) admission. As mentioned above, early administration of fomepizole may forego the need for HD and ICU admission in ethylene glycol and selected methanol poisonings, if administered prior to the onset of acidosis and end-organ damage (renal failure or visual disturbances). While fomepizole is relatively expensive, a multiple-day ICU admission and HD might exceed drug costs. In other situations, HD or HP may shorten ICU or hospital stays and be cost conscious procedures. A formal cost-benefit analysis of these various treatment options would be useful.

EVALUATION OF EFFICACY

The evaluation of efficacy of extracorporeal methods of blood purification should ultimately rest on improvement in patient outcomes. However, a good outcome after HD or HP is not equivalent to established efficacy. Indeed, the literature is replete with case reports of the "successful use" of HD and HP in cases of poisoning in which the procedure may have had little impact at all on outcome. As mentioned in the beginning, the efficacy of extracorporeal purification procedures must be compared with the efficacy of elimination of the substance in question by the kidneys, liver, and lungs. Thus, one cannot estimate the utility by simply measuring blood concentrations before and after HD/HP.[1] Rather, the amount of extracted drug should be measured directly in the dialysate or via elution from the cartridge, or alternatively, indirectly from hourly differences in simultaneously arterial (inlet)–venous (outlet) concentrations multiplied by the purification system blood flow.[1] These amounts can then be compared to the concentrations in urine (determination of spontaneous renal clearance) and to the quantity believed to have been absorbed to determine efficacy. Before and after blood concentrations give some idea of the combined efficacy of corporeal and extracorporeal elimination, but the interpretation may be clouded by ongoing intestinal absorption or redistribution of the toxicant. Elimination by other routes (pulmonary, sweat) should be likewise considered.

TOXIC SUBSTANCES AMENABLE TO EXTRACORPOREAL ELIMINATION

The list of toxic substances that have been subjected to HD and/or HP is quite long. Winchester[2] provides a list of more than 200 substances removed with dialysis and HP. As already mentioned, the ability to remove a toxic substance by HP or HD is not equivalent to an indication for these procedures. One must take into account the patient's underlying health (renal or hepatic insufficiency), the toxicity of the absorbed substance, the presence of or likelihood of advancing to severe illness, the availability of these procedures, and the availability of acceptable alternatives (good supportive care, antidotes). A list of a few substances that have frequently been subjected to extracorporeal removal follows (Table 2D-1). The list is not comprehensive and does not necessarily imply an indication for HD/HP. The reader is referred to individual chapters for detailed indications for these and other forms of therapy.

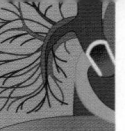

TABLE 2D-1 "COP, I'VE STUMBLED"			
SUBSTANCE	**SEE CHAPTER**	**HEMODIALYSIS (REFERENCES)**	**HEMOPERFUSION (REFERENCES)**
Carbamazepine	40	(39–42)	(42–44)
Osmolal gap, increased	31, 32	(45–47)	
Propylene glycol	32	(47,48)	
Isopropanol	32	(49,50)	
Valproic acid	40	(51–58)	(51,57,58)
Excess acids (severe metabolic acidosis of toxic origin)	64, 90, 98	(29,59–61)	
Salicylates	48	(62–64)	
Theophylline	65	(11,65,66)	(65,66)
Uremia due to nephrotoxic drugs	12		
Methanol (formate)	32	(27,28,33,46, 67,68)	
Barbiturates/ butoxyethanol	40 32	(69–71) (72,74)	(69,74,75)
Lithium	30	(76,77)	
Ethylene glycol/ ethanol	32, 31	(68,78,79)/(80)	
Diethylene glycol/ triethylene glycol	32	(81,82)	

This mnemonic serves as a reminder of some common substances encountered in poisonings potentially subject to removal by extracorporeal purification methods. Selected references are provided. Presence of a substances in this chart does not imply that extracorporeal methods are necessary or advisable. Clinical judgment is required.

SPECIFIC SUBSTANCES REMOVED BY CONVENTIONAL HEMODIALYSIS AND HEMOPERFUSION

Toxic Alcohols and Glycols

The alcohol and glycols generally have toxicity that is inversely related to molecular weight. This, along with limited protein binding, small volumes of distribution, and relatively high water solubility, makes them particularly amenable to removal by HD. Ethylene glycol (see Chapter 32B) has a molecular weight of 62 Da, it has no significant protein binding, and it distributes primarily in total body water (Vd = 0.6–0.8 L/kg), rendering it readily removable by HD.[21,83] Additionally, glycolate, the toxic by-product of ethylene glycol responsible for acidosis, is effectively removed by HD.[59,60] The indications for HD in ethylene glycol poisoning have been reviewed.[26,28,49] Pizon and Brooks have stated that an extremely high ethylene glycol level should be considered an indication for HD regardless of the patient's acid-base status or renal function due to hyperosmolarity.[78]

Methanol (see Chapter 32A) is likewise small (32 Da), with minimal protein binding and a Vd of 0.6 L/kg.

Formic acid, the toxic by-product of methanol responsible for acidosis and retinal toxicity, is removed by HD.[61] Hovda and colleagues have suggested that HD may be performed on an "elective" basis in selected methanol poisonings if patients are rapidly treated with bicarbonate and fomepizole.[27,84] Several researchers have recently reviewed the indications for HD after methanol poisoning.[24,28,85]

Isopropanol (see Chapter 32C) may also be removed by HD, although the indications for HD are limited, due to generally good outcomes with supportive care.[49,86] HD has been proven to be effective in removing both isopropanol and acetone from the plasma.[49] Lacouture and colleagues have recommended HD in cases where the blood isopropanol concentration exceeds 400 mg/dL.[87]

Salicylates

Salicylates (see Chapter 48) are compounds of low molecular weight. They are moderately to highly protein bound (50%–90%), with very small volumes of distribution. Although salicylates are highly protein bound at therapeutic concentrations, the fraction of unbound drug increases in the setting of overdose, rendering it amenable to removal by HD or HP. Early HD is recommended due to the high propensity of salicylates to cause serious toxicity and death.[64] The importance of concurrent alkalinization of the urine has been underscored by Higgins and colleagues.[63] Because of acid-base and electrolyte abnormalities associated with salicylate poisoning, acute HD, rather than HP, is generally preferred.[21]

Theophylline

Theophylline (see Chapter 65) has a low molecular weight and small Vd with moderate protein binding. Shannon addressed the use of HD and HP in theophylline poisoning in a 10-year prospective, observational study.[66] The study included acute, chronic, and acute-on-therapeutic poisonings. The incidence of major toxicity was significantly greater in those undergoing HD. Shannon concluded that while HP provides a higher theophylline clearance rate than HD, the latter appears to have comparable efficacy in reducing the morbidity of severe theophylline intoxication and is associated with a lower rate of procedural complications.[66]

Lithium

Lithium carbonate (see Chapter 30) remains a commonly used therapeutic agent in the treatment of bipolar disorder. While its Vd is low, it concentrates in brain matter, rendering effective treatment more difficult. It has minimal protein binding and a very small molecular weight, and thus is amenable to treatment with HD. Indications for dialysis remain controversial.[88] Recently, newer forms of extracorporeal purification for lithium poisoning have been proposed[89] (see Chapter 2C) which allow slower removal of lithium without rebound levels.

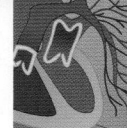

Carbamazepine

Carbamazepine has a relatively low molecular weight (236 Da), but a fairly large Vd (1–2 L/kg) and is about 80% protein bound at therapeutic levels. Its active metabolite 10,11-epoxide (CBZE), is approximately 50% protein bound.[42,44] Because of the high protein binding, activated charcoal and CHP have generally been favored in treatment; however, high-efficiency dialysis may also be effective.[40]

Valproic Acid

Valproic acid (see Chapter 40) is a low molecular weight (144 Da) anticonvulsant with a small Vd and saturable protein binding. At therapeutic concentrations, 90% to 95% of valproic acid is protein bound, but in overdose the degree of protein binding is relatively less (i.e., there is more unbound drug available for extracorporeal purification). Saturation of protein binding sites occurs at levels greater than 150 μg/mL, at which 54% to 70% of the drug is protein bound. At a level of 300 μg/mL, 35% of valproic acid is protein bound,[51,57,58] rendering it amenable to extracorporeal drug removal techniques.[55,90] Both HP and HD, alone and in combination, have been used in cases of valproate toxicity. Valproic acid elimination has been shown to be enhanced about tenfold by the use of extracorporeal methods.[57] While the half-life of the drug is effectively diminished, the precise role of these procedures in valproate toxicity remains to be established.[58]

SUBSTANCES REMOVED BY MARS

A nonexhaustive list of substances for which MARS has been used in poisoning includes theophylline,[91] cytotoxic mushrooms,[92-97] phenytoin,[98] acetaminophen (paracetamol),[99] and a copper-chromium-containing solution.[100] MARS appears to improve liver failure from multiple causes, but further prospective studies are needed to determine the role this technique should play in patient care.[14]

SUMMARY

In conclusion, HD and HP remain important, but secondary methods of treatment in poisoning by specific substances. These modalities cannot be substituted for excellent supportive care, and in some cases the need for them has been supplanted by effective antidotes. Both HD and HP are associated with complications and are not universally available. Careful evaluation of individual cases should guide the decision to use extracorporeal circulation. MARS or albumin dialysis may be of clinical benefit in selected poisonings.

REFERENCES

1. Bismuth C: Biological valuation of extra-corporeal techniques in acute poisoning. Acta Clin Belg Suppl 1990;13:20–28.
2. Winchester JF: Dialysis and hemoperfusion in poisoning. Adv Ren Replace Ther 2002;9(1):26–30.
3. Lai MW, Klein-Schwartz W, Rodgers GC, et al: 2005 Annual Report of the American Association of Poison Control Centers' national poisoning and exposure database. Clin Toxicol (Phila) 2006; 44(6–7):803–932.
4. Toltec International Inc: How hemodialysis (dialysis) works. December 20, 2006. Available at http://www.toltec.biz/how_hemodialysis_works.htm
5. Durakovic Z: Combined hemoperfusion and hemodialysis treatment of poisoning with cholinesterase inhibitors. Korean J Intern Med 1993;8(2):99–102.
6. Durakovic Z, Gasparovic V: [Use of extracorporeal circulation in the treatment of 2,4-dichlorophenoxyacetic acid poisoning]. Acta Med Iugosl 1990;44(1):65–73.
7. Koppel C, Thomsen T, Heinemeyer G, Roots I: Acute poisoning with bromofosmethyl (bromophos). J Toxicol Clin Toxicol 1991; 29(2):203–207.
8. Mydlik M, Derzsiova K, Mizla P, Beno P: [Hemoperfusion in mushroom poisoning. Clinical analysis of 58 patients]. Cas Lek Cesk 1993;132(15):464–467.
9. Mydlik M, Derzsiova K, Smolko P, et al: [Hemoperfusion with Amberlite XAD-4 in acute theophylline poisoning]. Cas Lek Cesk 1995;134(5):145–146.
10. Mydlik M, Mizla P, Klimcik J, et al: [Use of hemoperfusion and cholinesterase in acute poisoning with organophosphate cholinesterase inhibitors—clinical analysis of 50 patients]. Vnitr Lek 1991;37(7–8):645–651.
11. Shalkham AS, Barbara MK, Robert SH, et al: The availability and use of charcoal hemoperfusion in the treatment of poisoned patients. Am J Kidney Dis 2006;48(2):239–241.
12. Bismuth C, Schermann JM, Garnier R, et al: Elimination of paraquat. Dev Toxicol Environ Sci 1986;12:347–356.
13. Bradberry SM, Vale JA: Multiple-dose activated charcoal: a review of relevant clinical studies. J Toxicol Clin Toxicol 1995;33(5): 407–416.
14. Sen S, Jalan R: The role of the Molecular Adsorbents Recirculating System (MARS) in the management of liver failure. Perfusion 2004;19(Suppl 1):43–48.
15. Choi JY, Bae SH, Yoon SK, et al: Preconditioning by extracorporeal liver support (MARS) of patients with cirrhosis and severe liver failure evaluated for living donor liver transplantation—a pilot study. Liver Int 2005;25(4):740–745.
16. Hommann M, Kasakow LB, Geoghegan J, et al: Application of MARS artificial liver support as bridging therapy before split liver retransplantation in a 15-month-old child. Pediatr Transplant 2002;6(4):340–343.
17. Kellersmann R, Gassel HJ, Buhler C, et al: Application of Molecular Adsorbent Recirculating System in patients with severe liver failure after hepatic resection or transplantation: initial single-centre experiences. Liver 2002;22(Suppl 2):56–58.
18. Steiner C, Mitzner S: Experiences with MARS liver support therapy in liver failure: analysis of 176 patients of the International MARS Registry. Liver 2002;22(Suppl 2):20–25.
19. Brown RS Jr. MARS preconditioning for living donor liver transplantation: panacea or placebo? Liver Int 2005;25(4):692–695.
20. Kawasaki CI, Nishi R, Uekihara S, et al: How tightly can a drug be bound to a protein and still be removable by charcoal hemoperfusion in overdose cases? Clin Toxicol (Phila) 2005;43(2): 95–99.
21. Borkan SC: Extracorporeal therapies for acute intoxications. Crit Care Clin 2002;18(2):393–420, vii.
22. Kvist EE, Al-Shurbaji A, Dahl ML, et al: Quantitative pharmacogenetics of nortriptyline: a novel approach. Clin Pharmacokinet 2001;40(11):869–877.
23. Brent J: Fomepizole for the treatment of ethylene glycol poisoning. Methylpyrazole for Toxic Alcohols Study Group. N Engl J Med 1999;340(11):832–838.
24. Brent J: Fomepizole for the treatment of methanol poisoning. N Engl J Med 2001;344(6):424–429.
25. Borron SW: Fomepizole in treatment of uncomplicated ethylene glycol poisoning. Lancet 1999;354(9181):831.
26. Brent J: Current management of ethylene glycol poisoning. Drugs 2001;61(7):979–988.

27. Hovda KE: Fomepizole may change indication for hemodialysis in methanol poisoning: prospective study in seven cases. Clin Nephrol 2005;64(3):190–197.

28. Megarbane B: Current recommendations for treatment of severe toxic alcohol poisonings. Intens Care Med 2005;31(2):189–195.

29. Guo PYF: Severe lactic acidosis treated with prolonged hemodialysis: recovery after massive overdoses of metformin. Semin Dial 2006;19(1):80–83.

30. Panzer U: Combination of intermittent haemodialysis and high-volume continuous haemofiltration for the treatment of severe metformin-induced lactic acidosis. Nephrol Dial Transplant 2004; 19(8):2157–2158.

31. Williams DM: Acute kidney failure: a pediatric experience over 20 years. Arch Pediatr Adolesc Med 2002;156(9):893–900.

32. Caravati EM: Treatment of severe pediatric ethylene glycol intoxication without hemodialysis. J Toxicol Clin Toxicol 2004;42(3): 255–259.

33. Brown MJ: Childhood methanol ingestion treated with fomepizole and hemodialysis. Pediatrics 2001;108(4):e77.

34. Chen L-L: Chronic renal disease patients with severe star fruit poisoning: hemoperfusion may be an effective alternative therapy. Clin Toxicol 2005;43(3):197–199.

35. Pond SM: Extracorporeal techniques in the treatment of poisoned patients. Med J Aust 1991;154(9):617–622.

36. Rahman MH: Acute hemolysis with acute renal failure in a patient with valproic acid poisoning treated with charcoal hemoperfusion. Hemodial Int 2006;10(3):256–259.

37. Himmelfarb J: Hemodialysis complications. Am J Kidney Dis 2005; 45(6):1122–1131.

38. Davenport A: Intradialytic complications during hemodialysis. Hemodial Int 2006;10(2):162–167.

39. Kielstein JT: High-flux hemodialysis—an effective alternative to hemoperfusion in the treatment of carbamazepine intoxication. Clin Nephrol 2002;57(6):484–486.

40. Schuerer DJE, Brophy PD, Maxvold NJ, et al: High-efficiency dialysis for carbamazepine overdose. J Toxicol Clin Toxicol 2000; 38(3):321–323.

41. Koh KH: High-flux haemodialysis treatment as treatment for carbamazepine intoxication. Med J Malaysia 2006;61(1):109–111.

42. Spiller HA: Management of carbamazepine overdose. Pediatr Emerg Care 2001;17(6):452–456.

43. Cameron RJ: Efficacy of charcoal hemoperfusion in massive carbamazepine poisoning. J Toxicol Clin Toxicol 2002;40(4): 507–512.

44. Deshpande G: Repeat charcoal hemoperfusion treatments in life threatening carbamazepine overdose. Pediatr Nephrol 1999; 13(9):775–777.

45. Barnes BJ: Osmol gap as a surrogate marker for serum propylene glycol concentrations in patients receiving lorazepam for sedation. Pharmacother 2006;26(1):23–33.

46. Hunderi OH, Knut EH, Dag J: Use of the osmolal gap to guide the start and duration of dialysis in methanol poisoning. Scand J Urol Nephrol 2006;40(1):70–74.

47. Parker MG: Removal of propylene glycol and correction of increased osmolar gap by hemodialysis in a patient on high dose lorazepam infusion therapy. Intens Care Med 2002;28(1):81–84.

48. Jorens PG: Unusual D-lactic acid acidosis from propylene glycol metabolism in overdose. J Toxicol Clin Toxicol 2004;42(2): 163–169.

49. Abramson S: Treatment of the alcohol intoxications: ethylene glycol, methanol and isopropanol. Curr Opin Nephrol Hypertens 2000;9(6):695–701.

50. Trullas JC: Life-threatening isopropyl alcohol intoxication: is hemodialysis really necessary? Vet Hum Toxicol 2004;46(5): 282–284.

51. Al Aly Z: Extracorporeal management of valproic acid toxicity: a case report and review of the literature. Semin Dial 2005; 18(1):62–66.

52. Eyer F, Felgenhauer N, Gempel K, et al: Acute valproate poisoning: pharmacokinetics, alteration in fatty acid metabolism, and changes during therapy. J Clin Psychopharmacol 2005;25(4): 376–380.

53. Guillaume CPE: Successful use of hemodialysis in acute valproic acid intoxication. J Toxicol Clin Toxicol 2004;42(3):335–336.

54. Johnson LZ: Successful treatment of valproic acid overdose with hemodialysis. Am J Kidney Dis 1999;33(4):786–789.

55. Kane SL: High-flux hemodialysis without hemoperfusion is effective in acute valproic acid overdose. Ann Pharmacother 2000;34(10):1146–1151.

56. Kielstein JT, Woywodt A, Schumann G, et al: Efficiency of high-flux hemodialysis in the treatment of valproic acid intoxication. J Toxicol Clin Toxicol 2003;41(6):873–876.

57. Singh SM: Extracorporeal management of valproic acid overdose: a large regional experience. J Nephrol 2004;17(1):43–49.

58. Sztajnkrycer MD: Valproic acid toxicity: overview and management. J Toxicol Clin Toxicol 2002;40(6):789–801.

59. Moreau CL: Glycolate kinetics and hemodialysis clearance in ethylene glycol poisoning. META Study Group. J Toxicol Clin Toxicol 1998;36(7):659–666.

60. Jacobsen D: Glycolate causes the acidosis in ethylene glycol poisoning and is effectively removed by hemodialysis. Acta Med Scand 1984;216(4):409–416.

61. Hantson P: Formate kinetics in methanol poisoning. Hum Exp Toxicol 2005;24(2):55–59.

62. Dargan PI: An evidence based flowchart to guide the management of acute salicylate (aspirin) overdose. Emerg Med J 2002; 19(3):206–209.

63. Higgins RM: Alkalinization and hemodialysis in severe salicylate poisoning: comparison of elimination techniques in the same patient. Clin Nephrol 1998;50(3):178–183.

64. Yip L: Concepts and controversies in salicylate toxicity. Emerg Med Clin 1994;12(2):351–364.

65. Higgins RM: Severe theophylline poisoning: charcoal haemoperfusion or haemodialysis? Postgrad Med 1995;71(834):224–226.

66. Shannon MW: Comparative efficacy of hemodialysis and hemoperfusion in severe theophylline intoxication. Acad Emerg Med 1997;4(7):674–678.

67. Chebrolu SB: Phosphorus-enriched hemodialysis for the treatment of patients with severe methanol intoxication. Int J Artif Organs 2005;28(3):270-274.

68. Youssef GM: Validation of a method to predict required dialysis time for cases of methanol and ethylene glycol poisoning. Am J Kidney Dis 2005;46(3):509–511.

69. Lindberg MC: Acute phenobarbital intoxication. South Med J 1992;85(8):803–807.

70. Palmer BF: Effectiveness of hemodialysis in the extracorporeal therapy of phenobarbital overdose. Am J Kidney Dis 2000;36(3): 640–643.

71. Jacobs F: Conventional haemodialysis significantly lowers toxic levels of phenobarbital. Nephrol Dial Transplant 2004;19(6): 1663–1664.

72. Burkhart KK: Hemodialysis following butoxyethanol ingestion. J Toxicol Clin Toxicol 1998;36(7):723–725.

73. Gualtieri JF: Repeated ingestion of 2-butoxyethanol: case report and literature review. J Toxicol Clin Toxicol 2003;41(1):57–62.

74. Bentley C: The treatment of severe drug intoxication with charcoal hemoperfusion in series with hemodialysis. J Dial 1979;3(4):337–348.

75. Lin JL: Critical, acutely poisoned patients treated with continuous arteriovenous hemoperfusion in the emergency department. Ann Emerg Med 1995;25(1):75–80.

76. Jaeger A: When should dialysis be performed in lithium poisoning? A kinetic study in 14 cases of lithium poisoning. J Toxicol Clin Toxicol 1993;31(3):429–447.

77. Meyer RJ: Hemodialysis followed by continuous hemofiltration for treatment of lithium intoxication in children. Am J Kidney Dis 2001;37(5):1044–1047.

78. Pizon AF: Hyperosmolality: another indication for hemodialysis following acute ethylene glycol poisoning. Clin Toxicol 2006; 44(2):181–183.

79. Porter WH, Rutter PW, Bush BA, et al: Ethylene glycol toxicity: the role of serum glycolic acid in hemodialysis. J Toxicol Clin Toxicol 2001;39(6):607–615.

80. Atassi WA: Hemodialysis as a treatment of severe ethanol poisoning. Int J Artif Organs 1999;22(1):18–20.

81. Borron SW: Intravenous 4-methylpyrazole as an antidote for diethylene glycol and triethylene glycol poisoning: a case report. Vet Hum Toxicol 1997;39(1):26–28.

82. Brophy PD: Childhood diethylene glycol poisoning treated with alcohol dehydrogenase inhibitor fomepizole and hemodialysis. Am J Kidney Dis 2000;35(5):958–962.

83. Goodman JW, Goldfarb DS: The role of continuous renal replacement therapy in the treatment of poisoning. Semin Dial 2006;19(5):402–407.

84. Hovda KE: Methanol and formate kinetics during treatment with fomepizole. Clin Toxicol 2005;43(4):221–227.

85. Kostic MA: Rethinking the toxic methanol level. J Toxicol Clin Toxicol 2003;41(6):793–800.

86. Zaman F, Pervez A, Abreo K: Isopropyl alcohol intoxication: a diagnostic challenge. Am J Kidney Dis 2002;40(3):E12.

87. Lacouture PG: Acute isopropyl alcohol intoxication. Diagnosis and management. Am J Med 1983;75(4):680–686.

88. Scharman EJ: Methods used to decrease lithium absorption or enhance elimination. J Toxicol Clin Toxicol 1997;35(6):601–608.

89. Menghini VV: Treatment of lithium intoxication with continuous venovenous hemodiafiltration. Am J Kidney Dis 2000;36(3):E21.

90. Matsumoto J: Successful treatment by direct hemoperfusion of coma possibly resulting from mitochondrial dysfunction in acute valproate intoxication. Epilepsia 1997;38(8):950–953.

91. Korsheed S, Selby NM, Fluck RJ: Treatment of severe theophylline poisoning with the molecular adsorbent recirculating system (MARS). Nephrol Dial Transplant 2006 December 12 [Epub ahead of print].

92. Sein Anand J, Chodorowsk Z, Hydzik P. Molecular adsorbent recirculating system—MARS as a bridge to liver transplantation in amanita phalloides intoxication. Przegl Lek 2005;62(6):480–481.

93. Lionte C, Sorodoc L, Simionescu V: Successful treatment of an adult with Amanita phalloides-induced fulminant liver failure with molecular adsorbent recirculating system (MARS). Rom J Gastroenterol 2005;14(3):267–271.

94. Rubik J, Pietraszek-Jezierska E, Kaminski A, et al: Successful treatment of a child with fulminant liver failure and coma caused by Amanita phalloides intoxication with albumin dialysis without liver transplantation. Pediatr Transplant 2004;8(3):295–300.

95. Wu BF, Wang MM: Molecular adsorbent recirculating system in dealing with maternal Amanita poisoning during the second pregnancy trimester: a case report. Hepatobiliary Pancreat Dis Int 2004;3(1):152–154.

96. Covic A, Goldsmith DJ, Gusbeth-Tatomir P, et al: Successful use of Molecular Absorbent Regenerating System (MARS) dialysis for the treatment of fulminant hepatic failure in children accidentally poisoned by toxic mushroom ingestion. Liver Int 2003;23 (Suppl 3):21–27.

97. Shi Y, He J, Chen S, et al: MARS: optimistic therapy method in fulminant hepatic failure secondary to cytotoxic mushroom poisoning—a case report. Liver 2002;22(Suppl 2):78–80.

98. De Schoenmakere G, De Waele J, Terryn W, et al: Phenytoin intoxication in critically ill patients. Am J Kidney Dis 2005; 45(1):189–192.

99. Koivusalo AM, Yildirim Y, Vakkuri A, et al: Experience with albumin dialysis in five patients with severe overdoses of paracetamol. Acta Anaesthesiol Scand 2003;47(9):1145–1150.

100. Prokurat S, Grenda R, Lipowski D, et al: MARS procedure as a bridge to combined liver-kidney transplantation in severe chromium-copper acute intoxication: a paediatric case report. Liver 2002;22(Suppl 2):76–77.

3 *Laboratory Diagnoses and Drug Screening*

JOHN D. OSTERLOH, MD, MS ■ CHRISTINE A. HALLER, MD

Clinical laboratory tests that indicate the effects or presence of drugs can be useful in the emergency evaluation of the patient with an overdose. However, the majority of toxicologic diagnoses and therapeutic decisions are made on the basis of clinical findings, even though advances in technology have provided the potential ability to measure many toxins. It is easy to extol the technologic virtues of new toxicologic measurement techniques, but the application of these laboratory techniques is limited by practical considerations. The time required for analysis is often longer than the critical time course of an overdose case. Also, laboratories cannot support the cost of performing the variety of procedures, maintaining the instruments, supporting the regulatory and administrative infrastructure, and providing the training and specialized labor needed for analyzing every toxin.

The interpretation of laboratory toxicologic measurements requires that the relationship between the presence or the concentration of a toxin and its pharmacologic or toxicologic effects be known. For most toxins, our knowledge of such relationships is limited or unstudied, precluding the meaningful use of advanced technologic measures in direct clinical evaluations. Even when well studied, no clear relationship may exist. For example, a toxin at an effector site may not be in rapid equilibrium with the sampled fluid (e.g., lithium in the serum is not representative of lithium in the brain during the first 24 hours of an acute overdose); or the measured toxin may be metabolized to an unknown, unmeasured, and active metabolite. Occasionally, limited information about pharmacologic relationships for common drug toxins has been derived from the monitoring of low-dose therapeutic situations. However, predictions based on pharmacokinetics or pharmacodynamics of drugs administered in the therapeutic range do not always extrapolate to overdose (e.g., theophylline elimination is first order at therapeutic doses and zero order in overdose).

Although the utility of many toxicologic measurements may be limited, the proper use of certain laboratory tests (both drug tests and biochemistry tests) in the emergency setting can be applied to many toxicologic presentations. A consensus paper on use of toxicologic tests for emergency evaluation of the overdosed patient was recently published.[1] This chapter reviews the utility, reliability, and application of toxicologic testing in the emergency evaluation of the intoxicated patient. Other situations are delimited, such as toxicologic testing for forensic cause of death, driving while intoxicated, methadone compliance programs, and surveillance drug screening (employee, athlete). Throughout this chapter, it is emphasized that appropriate use of such testing should be considered in the context of the clinical presentation of the patient. Frequently, intoxicated patients are diagnosed by signs and symptoms, or recognition of specific toxidromes. Common laboratory tests used in selected toxidromes are listed in Table 3-1.

TABLE 3-1 Selected Toxicologic Syndromes by Class of Drugs and Common Tests Ordered

CLASS OF DRUG	SIGNS	POSSIBLE CLINICAL, LABORATORY, AND TOXICOLOGIC TEST
Opiates and opioids	CNS depression (somnolent → coma)	Naloxone
	Slowed respiratory rate	ABG
	T° normal or low	GLU
	If BP decreased, pulse may not increase	DAU
	Miosis	
	DTR usually decreased	
Alcohols, barbiturates	CNS depression (stuporous → coma)	Calorics, thiamine
	Ataxia	ABG
	T° usually decreased	ALT, PT
	DTR decreased	OG, AG
	Metabolic acidosis with ethanol, methanol	Ca, Mg
	and ethylene glycol	GLU
	If BP decreased, pulse may increase	DAU
		Serum or breath ethyl alcohol
Anticholinergics	Delirium	ABG
	Increased pulse, increased T°	EKG
	Skin is flushed, warm, dry (no sweating)	CK, K
	Decreased bowel sounds	Cr/BUN
	Urinary retention	CDS
	Blurred vision	
	Arrhythmias, prolonged QT	

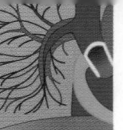

TABLE 3-1 Selected Toxicologic Syndromes by Class of Drugs and Common Tests Ordered—(*Cont'd*)

CLASS OF DRUG	SIGNS	POSSIBLE CLINICAL, LABORATORY, AND TOXICOLOGIC TEST
Stimulants	Acute psychosis (nonreality) Increased pulse, increased BP, 　increased T° Increased respiratory rate Agitation Increased muscle tone/activity Dilated pupils Sweating Seizures	ABG EKG CK GLU K Cr/BUN DAU
Tricyclic antidepressants	Anticholinergic syndrome Hypotension Coma Seizures Sinus tachycardia Supraventricular tachycardia (early) Widened QRS, QT Ventricular arrhythmias	ABG EKG K DAU or CDS TCIS
Benzodiazepines	CNS depression Mild (if any) respiratory depression BP, pulse, T° are not greatly affected DTR intact	ABG DAU
Phenothiazines	Decreased BP, decreased T° Rigidity, dystonias, torticollis Miosis Anticholinergic syndrome (see above) Seizures	ABG CDS EKG
Salicylates	Nausea, vomiting, abdominal pain Respiratory alkalosis Metabolic acidosis Confusion Diaphoresis Hypoglycemia	ABG GLU K, AG Quant
Theophylline	Tachycardia Hypokalemia Hypotension Seizures	ABGs K Quant GLU
Iron	Nausea, vomiting, abdominal pain GI bleeding Hypotension Hypovolemia Acidosis Renal failure Cardiovascular collapse	ABGs K Hgb GLU TIBC Quant ALT, PT
Lithium	Tremor, chorea Ataxia, rigidity, hyperreflexia Abdominal pain Lethargy, confusion Seizures	Na, K, Cr CK EKG Quant
Isoniazid	Metabolic acidosis Seizures Hepatitis	ABG, K, ALT, CK
Oral hypoglycemics	Hypoglycemia Coma Diaphoresis	GLU Ketones
β blockers	Bradycardia Hyperglycemia Hypotension with slowed cardiac 　conduction	EKG GLU K CDS
Acetaminophen	Increased ALT, PT	ALT PT BILI Quant
Hydrocarbon inhalants	Stupor, confusion, headache Ataxia Liver injury Respiratory depression Cardiac arrhythmias	ABG ALT Chest x-ray EKG

ABGs, arterial blood gases; AG, anion gap; ALT, alanine aminotransferase; BP, blood pressure; BILI, bilirubin; BUN, urea nitrogen; CDS, comprehensive drug screen; CK, creatine kinase; CNS, central nervous system; Cr, creatinine; DAU, drugs of abuse screen; DTR, deep tendon reflex; EKG, electrocardiogram; GLU, glucose; K, potassium; Na, sodium; OG, osmolal gap; PT, prothrombin time; Quant, quantitative drug determination; T°, temperature; TCIS, tricyclic immunoassay screen.
Blood glucose analysis may be ordered in any of the above syndromes involving altered mental status.

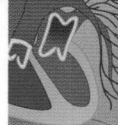

USE OF MEDICAL AND TOXICOLOGIC TESTS

Medical tests can be categorized as belonging to one of three types: monitoring, diagnostic testing, and screening.[2] For each type, there is a different purpose for applying the test and a different prior probability that the test condition exists (Table 3-2). This prior probability dramatically affects the reliability of a test for each of these situations (see later section on Toxicologic Screens). In the monitoring of a patient, the change in a highly prevalent test condition—such as blood pressure, body temperature, or therapeutic drug concentrations—is being followed. The most important requisite for this type of test is precision or the ability to detect change. Thus, therapeutic drug monitoring and quantitative toxicologic tests that follow drug concentrations over time (e.g., lithium) must be precise. Diagnostic tests are applied in situations in which the presence of one of several test conditions is highly likely or suspected. Because various alternative disease conditions would have moderate probabilities of existing based on the diagnostician's evaluation, specificity is the more important attribute for "rule-in" diagnostic testing (i.e., no misidentification of a test condition). Diagnostic tests aid in making choices from a limited set of alternatives or confirming a highly likely diagnosis. For example, a patient with chest pain may have a myocardial infarction, esophagitis, neurologic or musculoskeletal injury. Electrocardiography findings and troponin testing can be applied to increase or decrease the probability of myocardial infarction as the cause of the symptoms. Occasionally, diagnostic tests are used to rule out other diseases. In this special case, the necessary attribute of the test is sensitivity. Often ruling out is not the original intent of a particular diagnostic test, representing the potential for clinical misapplication. Toxicologic panel testing or screening (e.g., comprehensive drug screen or coma panel) can be considered a diagnostic test when overdose is considered in the differential diagnosis and when the initial medical evaluation does not provide a clear picture of what is causing the signs or symptoms. Such testing may help answer the question, Is the patient's condition due to drugs or a disease, and secondarily, which drug(s) are involved? Screening tests must have good sensitivity (finding all cases) if they are to detect the test condition in a low-prevalence situation. An example of this is screening for phenylketonuria in newborns. In the application of this test, there is no prior suspicion or preselection, and all newborns are tested. Nonspecificity arising from the screening tests can be corrected with subsequent, more specific testing.

The prior probability of a test condition (e.g., drugs present) will strongly influence the reliability (i.e., predictive value of a positive or negative test result, also known as posterior probabilities) at given values of sensitivity and specificity.[3] In employee drug screening programs (low prior probability of drugs being present), toxicologic methods are adapted in order to improve sensitivity for finding low concentrations of drugs, or for detecting only a few drugs in unselected populations.[2,4] Without such adaptations, the ratio of false-positive results to true-positive results would be high in this low-prevalence setting. In emergency toxicologic testing, procedures are designed to detect a larger number of drugs at high concentrations in patients clinically suspected of overdose (i.e., high prior probability, diagnostic situations). Thus, with regard to these definitions, the term *toxicologic screen* is a misnomer.

This raises the issue of what types of laboratories perform these tests. The development and use of toxicologic methods have evolved from a number of varied situations. Medical examiners investigating cause of death have other forensic evidence that often suggests a drug-related cause (raising the prior probability that the test condition exists in those forensic specimens). The concentrations of drugs or toxins are frequently very high, so analytic sensitivity is often not an issue; however, the type of tissue examined may frequently alter the ability of the analytic technique to detect a toxin. In surveillance drug screening (e.g. employee, athlete), low concentrations of drugs are expected for a small group of selected drugs of abuse, but these tests are applied to populations in which the prevalence of persons abusing drugs is low. So, additional confirmatory procedures are often necessary. Compliance programs (e.g., criminal justice, substance abuse) also test individuals for drug use. However, the prevalence of drug use in this selected population is much greater than in surveillance programs, as are the concentrations of the few drugs monitored. In each of these situations, the toxicologic methods are tailored to specific needs.

TABLE 3-2 Types of Medical and Toxicologic Test Situations

TYPE OF MEDICAL APPLICATION	PURPOSE	PRESELECTION OF POPULATION	PRIOR PROBABILITY (OR PREVALENCE) OF TEST CONDITION	PRIMARY ATTRIBUTE REQUIRED OF TEST	CLINICAL EXAMPLE	TOXICOLOGIC EXAMPLE
Monitoring	Measure change	Yes	85%–100%	Precision	BP, T°	TDM
Diagnostic	Categorize, confirm	Yes	30%–85%	Specificity*	Troponin	Tox "screen"
Screening	Find	No	0%–30%	Sensitivity	PKU	Employee drug testing

BP, blood pressure; PKU, phenylketonuria; T°, temperature; TDM, therapeutic drug monitoring.
*Specificity is the primary attribute for the commonly used "rule-in" or confirmatory diagnostic tests. Most diagnostic tests are not "rule-out" by design. If used this way, sensitivity is the primary attribute required.

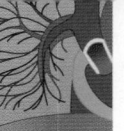

The laboratory performing emergency toxicologic testing must consider the prevalence and the types of drugs that must be tested and should adapt methods to the sensitivity, specificity, accuracy, and precision required in their locale (see later section on Analytic Accuracy of Toxicologic Screens).[1,2] Also, before any test is applied, it must be (1) analytically valid (i.e., defined and tested for detection limits, the calibration-response relationship, precision, referenced accuracy, dynamic range, interferences), (2) reliable (i.e., have appropriate clinical sensitivity, specificity, and predictive value), and (3) demonstrate utility (i.e., the test result will assist the clinician in making a diagnosis or in effecting a change in the course of therapy or disposition of the patient).

DRUG TESTING TECHNIQUES

The techniques for detecting the presence of drugs include a variety of chromatographic methods, immunoassays, chemical tests, and spectrometric techniques. Each of these general techniques can be developed or adapted so that they detect a large number of drugs and chemicals, or they can be focused specifically to detect and quantitate only certain drugs. The analysis of drugs, chemicals, or toxins is predicated on the matching of the properties or behavior (e.g., chemical, chromatographic, or light absorption) of a substance with that of a valid reference compound; that is, the analysis is comparative. For a laboratory to be able test for a particular drug, it must possess that drug for the comparative process. Because the biologic sample matrix may contain components that can interfere with the detection of a drug, isolation of the drug from the biologic matrix is often necessary before characterization procedures are applied. With regard to usefulness, immunoassays and gas or liquid chromatographic techniques have the widest applications for single and multiple drug screens, respectively, or for quantitation. The major techniques have been compared for their sensitivity and specificity to commonly screened illicit drugs.[5,6] Most broad screening methods are limited by the range of drugs detectable at one time or by sensitivity. In addition, methods can vary considerably with respect to individual drugs. For example, without application of derivatization techniques, ease of detection for morphine would be ranked as follows: immunoassay > thin-layer chromatography > gas chromatography. In contrast, in the detection of trazodone, the order may be reversed.

Chemical spot tests have been used in the past as initial quick screening tests for certain drugs. They rely on the chemical reactivity of the drug in the presence of specific reagents. These tests are usually not applied in settings in which a high degree of sensitivity or specificity is required (e.g., not in employee drug testing). A few of these tests (e.g. Trinder's for salicylate, ferric-perchlorate-nitrate [FPN] test for phenothiazines) offer rapid application and adequate accuracy when applied in emergency settings in which high drug concentrations are present.[7]

Spectrometric assays may require a chemical reaction (direct or enzymatic) that converts the target drug into a light-absorbing species. These assays were commonly used in the distant past for the routine determination of barbiturates, acetaminophen, salicylates, quinidine, methaqualone, and chlordiazepoxide. Still in use today are the spectrometric assays for carboxyhemoglobin, methemoglobin, and cyanide. In uncomplicated cases, these three methods have adequate accuracy for quantifying spectrometric chemicals in overdose situations. However, spectrometric methods are prone to interference. For example, sulfhemoglobin and the antidote for methemoglobin, methylene blue, cause false elevation of methemoglobin levels with the co-oximetry method (see other examples in Tables 3-3 and 3-4). Many spectrometric assays have been replaced by enzymatic or immunologic assays, which can be performed on automated analyzers that perform a variety of other laboratory tests.

Immunoassays are available for rapid identification of about a dozen individual classes or specific drugs in urine and for quantitation of about a dozen drugs in serum. Most immunoassay methods are easily adapted to automated analyzers used in the general hospital laboratory for performing other clinical diagnostic tests. Any immunoassay relies on the ability of a drug-specific antibody to bind to either labeled drug (which may be bound to a fluorescent molecule, to an enzyme, or attached to a solid matrix) or to the free drug in a sample. Immunoassay techniques are available with a variety of analytic end points based on aggregation-light transmission, enzyme product formation, fluorescent polarization, and other principles. The most common immunoassay techniques used for the detection of drugs are the enzyme immunoassay (Fig. 3-1), fluorescent polarization immunoassay, and immunoaggregation assay. Each specific drug assay is commercially available as a kit, but kits are available for only a limited number of drugs. Usually such assays have analytic sensitivity in excess of that needed for the detection of overdose concentrations and use preassigned cutoff values that determine positive versus negative results. When immunoassays are used as initial screens; their results may require confirmation by a second method, depending on the pretest probabilities, sensitivity, and specificity. For example, employee drug testing with an immunoassay will require confirmatory testing. When a testable drug is suspected in an intoxicated patient (high prior probability), confirmatory testing is not usually needed, excepting immunoassays for the amphetamine class of drugs, which have many cross-reacting substances (see Table 3-3).[8,9] If the clinician is applying the test as a screening type test (rather than confirming a diagnosis), then confirmation should be requested.

Point-of-care testing is now widely available because advances in technology have resulted in an increasing number of commercial hand-held test kits for rapid qualitative screening for drugs of abuse. These are immunoassay based. Products such as Triage (Biosite Diagnostics, San Diego, CA) and OnTrak Testcup-er (Roche Laboratories, Nutley, NJ) incorporate various immunoassay systems into a single-use unit with premade reagents and preset thresholds for detection of select

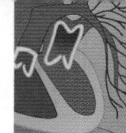

TABLE 3-3 Qualitative Toxicologic Methods Used in Urine, Detection Intervals, and Interferences

DRUG/GROUP	REAGENT/METHOD NAME	TYPE OF METHOD	DOSAGE DETECTABLE* (DETECTON INTERVAL)	INTERFERENCES, NONSPECIFICITY[†]
Salicylate	Trinder's	SC	TD (<1 day), OD	Salicylamide, diflunisal, ketonuria, phenylketonuria, proteinuria, sulfonamides, hippuric acids (toluene, xylene)[‡]
Acetaminophen (p-aminophenol)	Ortho-cresol (rarely used)	SC	TD (<1 day), OD	N-acetyl cysteine, phenols from throat lozenges and mouthwashes,[‡] proteinuria)
Phenothiazines (metabolites)	Forrest or FPN (ferric-perchlorate-nitric)	SC	TD for some (<3 days) OD	Salicylates, ketonuria,[‡] proteinuria
Ethchlorvynol	Diphenylamine (rarely used)	SC	OD (<3 days)	
Phencyclidine, methadone, tricyclics	Tetrabromophenophthalein ethyl ester (rarely used)	SC	OD	Other narcotics, antihistamines, antipsychotics[‡]
Chloral hydrate (trichloroethanol)	Fujiwara	SC	OD (<2 days)	Other chlorinated hydrocarbons
Opiates (morphine, codeine)	EMIT, FPIA, KIMS, CEDIA, RIA, CMI	IA	RD (<3 days), OD	Other opiates (hydrocodone, hydromorphone, oxycodone, dihydrocodeine), morphine from poppy seeds, adulterants,[§] rifampin, ofloxacin
Barbiturates	EMIT, FPIA, KIMS, CEDIA, RIA, CMI	IA	RD (<4 days), OD	Other less used barbiturates, NSAIDs[ǁ] adulterants[§]
Benzodiazepines (as oxazepam metabolite)	EMIT, FPIA, KIMS, CEDIA, RIA, CMI	IA	TD for some, OD (days to weeks)	Other less used benzodiazepines,[§] NSAID's[ǁ] less sensitive to triazolam, lorazepam, clonazepam, alprazolam, flunitrazepam (diazepam, nordiazepam, chlordiazepoxide, temazepam, midazolam, oxazepam are typically detected)
Amphetamines (amphetamine/methamphetamine)	EMIT, FPIA, KIMS, CEDIA, RIA, CMI	IA	RD (<2 day), OD	Newer generation assays react with MDA, MDMA, STP, and l-methamphetamine (in Vlck's inhaler). Older assays cross-reacted with many adrenergic amines,[¶] chlorpromazine[‡]
Marijuana (11-nor-9-carboxyl-tetrahydrocannabinol)	EMIT, FPIA, KIMS, CEDIA, CMI	IA	RD (<1 wk single use, <2 mo if chronic use), OD	Dronabilol, hemp products, pantoprazole (?); adulterants[§]
Cocaine (benzoylecgonine)	EMIT, FPIA, KIMS, CEDIA, CMI	IA	RD (<2 days), OD	Few, teas made from coca leaf, adulterants[§]
Phencyclidine	EMIT, FPIA, KIMS, CEDIA, CMI	IA	RD (<1 wk), OD	PCP analogues, ketamine, chlorpromazine, diphenhydramine, dextromethophan, venlafaxine
Ethanol	Enzymatic	SC	RD (<1 day), OD	Microbiologic production of ethanol in poorly stored urine
Tricyclics	CMI, others	IA	TD, OD	Quetiapine, diphenhydramine, atomoxetine, carbamazepine

CEDIA, cloned enzyme donor immunoassay; CMI, colloidal gold microparticle immunoassay; EMIT, enzyme multiplied immunoassay technique; FPIA, fluorescent polarization immunoassay; IA, immunoassay; KIMS, kinetic interaction of microparticle spheres; MDA, methylenedioxyamphetamine; MDMA, methylenedioxymethamphetamine ("Ecstasy"); NSAID, nonsteroidal anti-inflammatory drug; PCP, phencyclidine; RIA, radioimmunoassay; SC, spectrochemical (color change); STP, 2,5-dimethoxy-4-methylamphetamine.
*Method sensitive to overdose dosage (OD), therapeutic dosage (TD), or recreational dosage (RD) for window of time detectable in parentheses.
[†]Not all reagent/methods cross-react to the same extent.
[‡]Requires large amounts.
[§]Adulterants; see text.
[ǁ]Negative interference.
[¶]Adrenergic amines such as phenylpropanolamine, ephedrine, pseudoephedrine, fenfluramine, phenteramine, isometheptene, and propylhexidrine. Also ranitidine, ritodrine, methylphenidate, labetolol, sertraline, trimethobenzamide, and others in the past. Also drugs metabolized to amphetamine: famprofazone, seligiline.

drugs in urine. Several studies have demonstrated excellent concordance of point-of-care devices with central laboratory analyzers.[9,10] These devices may be advantageous in smaller clinical laboratories receiving small numbers of toxicology samples. However, because of limitations in specificity and sensitivity with immunoassays, these products should be utilized as preliminary tests that require clinical correlation or confirmation by standard laboratory methods.

Chromatographic assays are widely used in emergency toxicology because a large number of drugs can be detected on a single chromatogram. Sensitivity is adequate for detecting the presence of many common pharmaceuticals at concentrations seen in overdose. For most

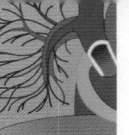

TABLE 3-4 Potential Interferences for Quantitative Serum Drug and Chemistry Tests Used in Emergency Toxicology

DRUG OR TOXIN	METHOD*	CAUSES OF FALSELY INCREASED BLOOD LEVEL
Acetaminophen	SC (rare use)	Salicylate, salicylamide, methyl salicylate (each will increase acetaminophen level by 10% of its level in mg/L); bilirubin; phenols; renal failure (each 1 mg/dL increase in creatinine = 30 mg/L acetaminophen)
Amitriptyline	HPLC, GC	Cyclobenzaprine, diphenhydarmine
	IA	Cyclobenzaprine, thioridazine, chlorpromazine, atomoxetine
Carboxyhemoglobin	SC	Fetal hemoglobin (lipemia or high methemoglobin also may falsely decrease on some instruments)
Chloride	SC, EL	Bromide (0.8–1.0 mEq/L Cl = 1 mEq/L Br)
Creatinine	SC (rare use)	Ketoacidosis (may increase creatinine up to 2–3 mg/dL); cephalosoporins; creatine (e.g., with rhabdomyolysis)
	EZ	Lidocaine metabolite, 5-fluorouracil
Digoxin	IA	Endogenous digoxin-like natriuretic substances in newborns and in patients with renal failure (up to 1 ng/mL), pregnancy, and liver failure. Oleander and bufotoxin glycosides cross-react as digoxin.
		Elevations after digoxin antibody (Fab) administration. Rarely, human antimouse antibodies in patient.
Ethanol	SC (rare use)	Other alcohols and ketones in oxidation methods.
	EZ	Isopropanol from venipunture disinfectant. Patients with elevated LDH and lactate.
Ethylene glycol	SC	Other glycols; elevated triglycerides
Iron	SC	Deferoxamine causes 15% lowering of total iron-binding capacity (TIBC). Lavender-top Vacutainer tube contains EDTA, which lowers total iron.
Isopropanol	GC	Skin disinfectant containing isopropyl alcohol used before venipuncture (highly variable, usually trivial, but up to 40 mg/dL).
Lithium	F, EL	Green-top Vacutainer specimen tube (contains lithium heparin) may cause marked elevation (up to 6–8 mEq/L)
	SC	Quinidine, procainamide
Methemoglobin	SC	Sulfhemoglobin (cross-positive, 10% by oximeter); methylene blue (2 mg/kg dose gives transient false-positive up to 15% methemoglobin level); hyperlipidemia (triglyceride > 6000 mg/dL, may give false methemoglobin up to 28.6%)
		Falsely decreased level with in vitro spontaneous reduction to hemoglobin in Vacutainer tube (~10% of value/hr). Analyze within 1 hr.
Osmolality	Osm	Lavender-top (EDTA) Vacutainer specimen tube (15 mOsm/L); gray-top (fluoride-oxalate) tube (150 mOsm/L); blue-top (citrate) tube (10 mOsm/L); green-top (lithium heparin) tube (theoretically, up to 6–8 mOsm/L)
		Falsely normal if vapor pressure method used (alcohols are volatilized)
Salicylate	SC	Diflunisal, ketosis, salicylamide. Accumulated salicylate metabolites in patients with renal failure (~10% increase).
	IA	Diflunisal
	SC	Decreased or altered salicylate level; bilirubin; phenylketones
Theophylline	HPLC	Rarely, acetazolamide, cephalosporins. Endogenous xanthines and accumulated theophylline metabolites in renal failure (minor effect).
	IA	Caffeine. Accumulated theophylline metabolites in renal failure.

EDTA, ethylenediaminetetraacetic acid; EL, electrochemical; EZ, enzymatic; F, flame emission; GC, gas chromatography; HPLC, high-pressure liquid chromatography; IA, immunoassay; LDH, lactate dehydrogenase; SC, spectrochemical; TLC, thin-layer chromatography.

chromatographic procedures, drugs first must be extracted from serum or urine. In many cases, further chemical derivatization is necessary for making drugs compatible with the chromatographic phase or detection system. For example, in the detection of morphine by gas chromatography, the extracted morphine may be *N*-acetylated (or other derivative) to decrease its polarity, increase its volatility, and enhance its detectability. The partially isolated drug (extract) is separated from other solutes during its interaction with the chromatographic stationary phase. There are three general types of chromatography used in toxicologic analyses: thin-layer chromatography, gas chromatography, and high-performance liquid chromatography.

In thin-layer chromatography (TLC), extracted drugs are dried onto silica gel–coated plates. During the migration of a solvent up the plate, separation of the components and drugs in the extract is achieved by their differential interaction with the silica gel and solvent (Fig. 3-2). Chemical reactants sprayed on the plate localize (detect) the drugs, and the drugs' locations are compared with the locations of reference drugs migrated parallel to the unknown extract. Usually a series of different chemical reactions are used in this process. The "staining" sequence and the ability to specify the migration distance of each drug endow TLC with the specificity that often is unachievable with the use of more elaborate procedures. However, with TLC, the analytical sensitivity for most drugs is limited to about 1.0 mg/L or greater, varying with the drug being tested, the detection method, and the amount of starting sample material. Many potent drugs may not be detectable with this technique (e.g., digoxin, lysergic acid diethylamide [LSD]) because of extremely low concentrations. TLC for drug detection in emergency situations has become standardized owing to the availability of commercially

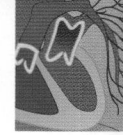

No drug in sample

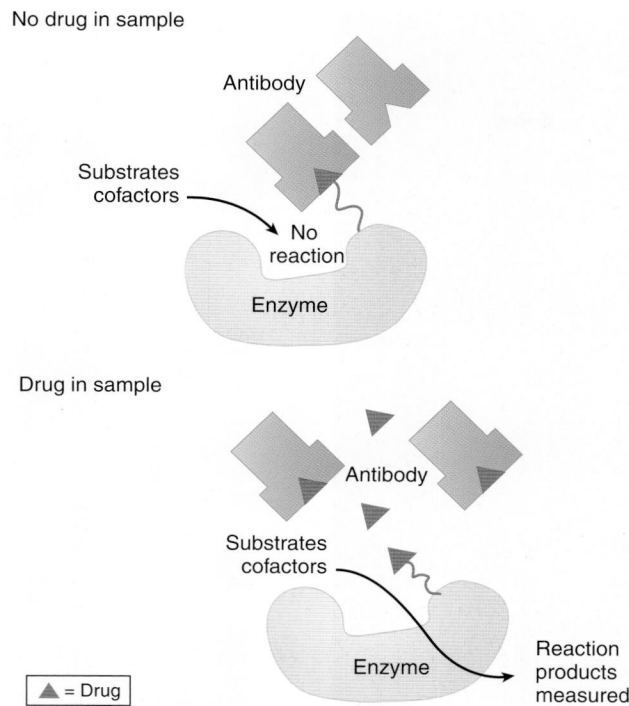

FIGURE 3-1 Principle of an enzyme immunoassay. A drug-specific antibody inhibits an enzymatic reaction because of a drug label on the enzyme. The greater the amount of free drug in the sample, the less the inhibition by the antibody and the faster the reaction of the enzyme system.

prepared TLC systems (e.g., ToxiLab, Ansys, Inc., Irvine, CA). This has allowed expertise in the TLC identification of drugs to be less technologist dependent and results to be similar from laboratory to laboratory (see Fig. 3-2). Comigration of 30 or more drugs can be carried out on a single plate, allowing for drug identification with the use of information in a reference compendium. TLC will probably remain a common technique when testing for a broad range of unknown drugs.

High-performance liquid chromatography (HPLC) is similar in many respects to TLC. Drugs are separated within tightly packed columns, and high pressure is applied to the columns to elute the drugs. Column materials for HPLC may be silica gel, as with TLC, or nonpolar phases (e.g., alkyl groups) bonded to small particles. With the former, the drug is eluted with organic solvents, and with the latter, solvents miscible in aqueous buffers are used. Often, drugs eluting from the end of the column are detected on the basis of their absorption of ultraviolet light. Other detection techniques are based on refractometry, conductivity, electrochemical (redox) reactions, and mass spectrometry. Drugs are identified only by the time that it takes for each to be eluted from the column (retention time). HPLC systems have not been widely used in broad drug screening partly because of the narrow range of drug polarity that can be analyzed in one run. However, systems that change the composition of eluting solvent during a single run (gradient systems) or those that use multiple-column processing can broaden the detection window. Certain

automated instruments have been shown to be useful in screening for a wide variety of drugs of overdose,[11,12] as well as the use of HPLC/mass spectrometry. Because of this high selectivity (resolution or separation of similar drugs), much HPLC work is directed toward the screening for classes of similar compounds, confirming the presence of selected agents or for quantitating specified drugs. Quantitation involves the measurement of the sizes of peaks relative to those of a standard compound added in a fixed quantity to all samples (internal standard). With extraction and evaporation of the extracting solvent, detection limits of 0.01 to 1.0 mg/L often are achieved with HPLC.

Gas chromatography (GC) requires that the extracted drug be volatile at the temperatures inside the GC column (80° C to 300° C). Drugs and toxins can be chemically modified to make them more volatile. During injection onto the beginning of the column, the solvated drugs are heated. Drugs in the gas phase are separated from each other by interaction with the "liquid" stationary phase (at high temperatures) on the column. Drugs eluting from the column can be detected on the basis of their thermal conductivity, combustibility, ability to donate electrons or capture β-particle beams, ionization, and other characteristics. The range of selective detectors for GC is quite broad. One mode of detection that merits discussion is gas chromatography/mass spectrometry (GC-MS). A portion of the effluent gases from GC are ionized by bombardment in an electron beam or other methods. The detected molecular fragments that result are characteristic of the eluting drug. When only unique fragments are monitored, the sensitivity can extend into the nanogram-per-liter range.

For both GC and GC-MS, the range of drugs that can be run on a single column is wide, but it is also limited by volatility and polarity. Current GC applications for screening of the many drugs seen in overdose cases are derived from methods developed in the 1970s.[13] With the introduction of capillary columns and MS detection, many similar drug molecules can be screened with good resolution (specificity).[6] An example of a chromatogram of standards used in emergency urine screening is shown in Figure 3-3. After extraction, evaporation of solvent, and reconstitution, the mixture is injected and volatilized into the gas stream of the column. As with other similar systems, about 0.05 to 0.5 mg/L of a large number of drugs is detectable. A common simple GC application is the determination of volatile alcohols, in which ethanol, methanol, isopropanol, and other volatile solvents can be identified and quantitated quickly.

EMERGENCY SERUM QUANTITATION OF OVERDOSED DRUGS

Rationale and Use

Serum quantitation of drugs or toxins in overdose are used for (1) diagnosis; (2) monitoring the course of the patient; (3) determining whether toxicity is occurring but not yet clinically apparent; (4) satisfying criteria for

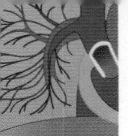

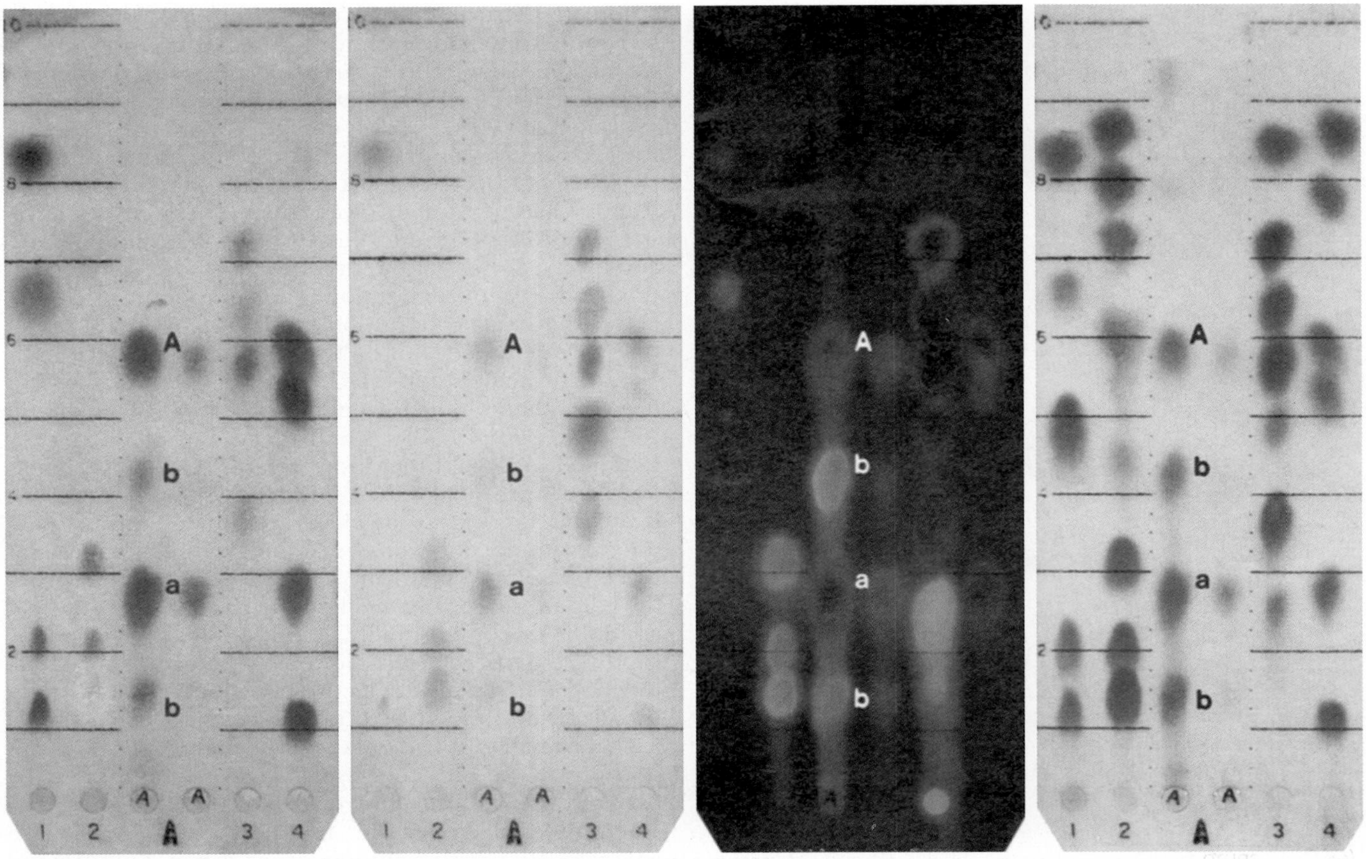

FIGURE 3-2 Diagram of a standardized thin-layer chromatography system for identification of a wide spectrum of drugs (ToxiLab). Drugs from urine were extracted and plated in the middle of lane A and chromatographed. Lanes 1 to 4 are standard drugs comigrated with lane A. Sequential staining with chemical reagents (phases I through IV) and migration distance aid in the identification of the unknown drug in lane A. Amitriptyline (A) and its metabolite nortriptyline (a) are detected. Other metabolites (b) are also detected. (Courtesy of ToxiLab, Ansys, Inc., Irvine, CA.)

therapeutic interventions (e.g., dialysis); and (5) evaluating the efficacy of those interventions.[2,14,15] In the emergency setting, relatively few quantitative drug measurements meet these goals. These drugs include acetaminophen, salicylates, theophylline, digoxin, ethanol, methanol, valproic acid, ethylene glycol, iron, carbon monoxide, and lithium (Table 3-5).[1,2]

Two criteria must be satisfied in order for drug quantitation to be useful. First, clinical indicators that would otherwise reveal the status or condition of the patient must be absent. If the suspected toxin is known or its presence highly probable and if toxicity is apparent (i.e., clinical effects are observed), knowledge of drug concentration is of limited utility, except in patients with an overdose of any drugs listed in the previous paragraph. For most patients with drug intoxication, clinical indicators provide immediate evidence of the severity of the poisoning and are of greater value than measurements of drug concentration. For example, the clinical manifestations in the patient with an overdose of a tricyclic antidepressant indicate the course and severity of the ingestion. The second criterion that must be satisfied for measurements of drug concentrations to be useful is evidence of a concentration-effect relationship.

Unfortunately, only a few drugs have established concentration-effect relationships, and many more remain unstudied.[15] In therapeutic drug monitoring, concentration-effect relationships may be clearly established for the end points of efficacy or low-level toxicity. These therapeutic relationships cannot simply be extrapolated to the overdose setting. For instance, carbamazepine has anticonvulsant properties at therapeutic concentrations of 5 to 10 mg/L, but may cause seizures when taken in overdose. Similarly, a therapeutic dose of theophylline may have a half-life of six hours, but in overdose amounts, the half-life may be much longer.

Quantitation of drug concentrations is indicated for drugs that may require hemoperfusion (e.g., theophylline, phenobarbital) or hemodialysis (e.g., salicylates, methanol, valproic acid), either as a criterion to initiate the therapy or to assess its efficacy (see Table 3-5). Quantitation of drug concentrations may also be required when a clinician is deciding whether to treat a patient with certain antidotes (e.g., Fab fragments for digoxin overdose) and when chelation therapy is being considered (e.g., deferoxamine for iron poisoning). Certainly, other clinical data may alter how the balance of clinical management is carried out. For example, it is well known that hypo-

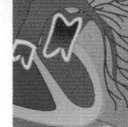

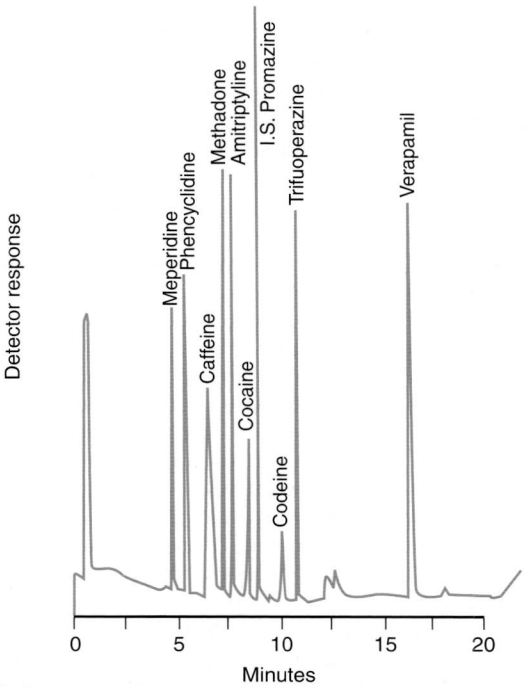

FIGURE 3-3 Chromatogram of a quality control urine sample containing 10 drugs after extraction from urine and detection by capillary gas chromatography with nitrogen-phosphorus detection. The concentration of caffeine and verapamil is 2.0 mg/L; that of each other drug is 0.5 mg/L. The limit of detection is about 0.05 mg/L.

magnesemia, hypokalemia, and underlying atherosclerotic heart disease are factors in the manifestation of digoxin toxicity.

Availability and Accuracy

With the increased use of quantitative serum immunoassays performed on rapid chemistry analyzers, most large hospital laboratories are able to provide a drug measurement that would usually be available as therapeutic drug monitoring assays. However, of all hospitals (N = 5402) capable of performing routine chemistry tests, only 63% performed assays for iron, 38% for lithium, 79% for theophylline, 51% for salicylate, and 51% for acetaminophen.[16]

Many emergency department (ED) physicians and medical toxicologists would like to see greater availability of serum quantitation for ethylene glycol to guide clinical management of suspected ingestions of this chemical. Because of the availability of a new antidote, fomepizole (Antizol [Jazz Pharmaceuticals, Palo Alto, CA]), the toxic effects of ethylene glycol and methanol can often be avoided, but the decision for hemodialysis is frequently made on the basis of concentrations that are greater than 25 to 50 mg/dL. Regionalized toxicology centers have been proposed as a means to increase the availability of rapid turnaround testing for a larger spectrum of toxins like ethylene glycol.

TABLE 3-5 Quantitation of Toxins: Guidance for Therapeutic Interventions

DRUG/TOXIN	MINIMAL CLINICAL PRESENTATION FOR CONSIDERATION OF INTERVENTION	CONCENTRATION GUIDANCE	THERAPY	RATIONALE FOR INTERVENTION
Acetaminophen	History of ingestion	>150 mg/L @ 4 hr, >50 mg/L @ 12 hr	NAC	Prevent hepatotoxicity
Theophylline	Hypotension Tachycardia	>100 µg/mL (acute OD only)	HP/HD esmolol	Prevent seizures
Phenobarbital	Coma	>100 µg/mL	HP/HD	Shorten coma time
Lithium (chronic)	Altered mental status, or tremor (greater concern if preexisting renal insufficiency)	>2.5–4 mEq/L (chronic OD only)	HD	Minimize CNS effects, prevent seizures
Methanol	AG metabolic acidosis + osmolar gap	History and CP for antidote >50 mg/dL for HD	4MP, ethanol, HD	Avoid blindness, fatality
Ethylene glycol	AG metabolic acidosis + osmolar gap	History and CP for antidote >50 mg/dL for HD	4MP, ethanol, HD	Reduce acidosis and avert renal injury
Salicylate	AG metabolic acidosis, respiratory alkalosis	>30 mg/dL to initiate intervention	Bicarb, HD	Promote salicylate elimination, prevent pulmonary and cerebral edema
Digoxin (acute)	AV block, hyperkalemia, bradycardia (acute)	>2.5–4 ng/mL (acute OD only)	Fab	Avoid cardiovascular failure
Iron	History of ingestion	>500 µg/dL	Deferoxamine	Avoid cardiovascular collapse, renal and hepatic failure
Carbon monoxide	Headache, dizziness, nausea, confusion, coma	Carboxy hemoglobin >5%	Oxygen, possibly hyperbaric therapy	Prevent neurologic sequelae

AG, anion gap; AV, atrioventricular; CNS, central nervous system; CP, clinical presentation; Fab, digoxin-specific antibodies; HD, hemodialysis; HP, hemoperfusion; 4MP, 4-methylpyrazole; NAC, N-acetylcysteine.
*For additional clinical effects, see Table 3-1.

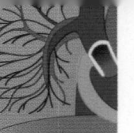

The interassay imprecision for quantitative serum assays that are used in emergency toxicology is generally less than 5%. Not only must serum quantitation techniques be adequately precise to recognize a change occurring from one time point to another, but they should also be accurate (i.e., near to a true value) so that management decisions may be made relative to predetermined decision values. The accuracy and interlaboratory variability of quantitative serum measurements may be assessed on the basis of results from proficiency testing programs.[16] In general, accuracy and agreement of results obtained by different laboratories are favorable for drugs measured commonly and by uniform techniques (e.g., antiepileptic drugs). For drugs that are measured infrequently and by more diverse methods, the results obtained are more diverse. Currently, interlaboratory coefficients of variation less than 8% and biases less than 15% have been demonstrated for the quantitation of most therapeutic drug monitoring–type drugs.[16]

Altered Analytic, Pharmacokinetic, and Pharmacodynamic Relationships in Overdosage

Serum drug quantitations must be evaluated with respect to each patient's clinical condition, drug pharmacokinetics, and timing of the specimen. The variation from person to person in the metabolism of medications and toxic chemicals (Fig. 3-4), the interactions of disease processes and medications, the altered pharmacologic properties of drugs at overdose concentrations, and the potential for interference in assays may affect how a measured drug concentration is interpreted.[2,15] For example, when taken in overdose, salicylates are more toxic than the linear extrapolation of effects of therapeutic concentrations would predict. This difference is the result of the elevation of free (unbound) concentrations with increasing serum concentrations, an increase in central nervous system penetration at acidic blood pH, and the saturation of metabolic pathways in the presence of the higher concentrations.

Interpretation of drug levels may be altered by the consideration of several factors together. For instance, a renal failure patient receiving normal doses of digoxin may have no digoxin-related symptoms even though the patient has a serum digoxin level of 4 ng/mL. Falsely measured digoxin-like substances in renal failure may raise the patient's measured "digoxin" level by up to 1 ng/mL. In addition, cross-reaction of accumulated metabolites due to poor renal clearance may falsely elevate the measured level an additional 2 ng/mL. While quantitative measurements tend to be highly specific, other drugs and disease states can produce analytical interferences, leading to false results (see Table 3-4). In contrast, a different patient with a measured digoxin level of 2 ng/mL may exhibit digoxin-related toxicity that is due to a coexisting hypokalemia.

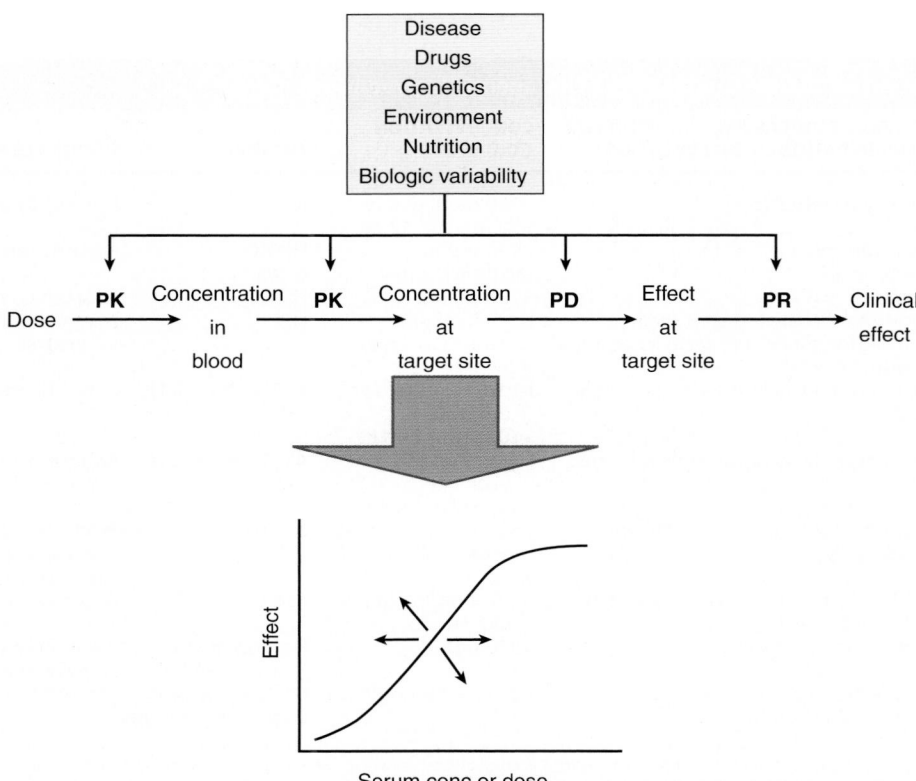

FIGURE 3-4 Factors producing altered pharmacologic relationships. PD, pharmacodynamics; PK, pharmacokinetics; PR, physiologic response to pharmacologic effect.

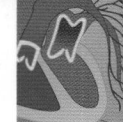

When drug levels are ordered from the laboratory, they must be interpreted with an understanding of the drug's pharmacokinetics and sample timing. For instance, lithium and digoxin exhibit slow distribution from the central blood compartment into peripheral tissues, and an elevated level soon after ingestion may not be a reliable predictor of toxicity. Postdistributional (equilibrated) levels better reflect concentrations associated with toxicity at peripheral target sites. In addition, some drugs exhibit significant delays in reaching peak levels after overdose due to erratic absorption profiles (e.g. carbamazepine), slowing of gut motility (acetaminophen combined with diphenhydramine), or slow dissolution due to sustained-release formulations (lithium, divalproate). In these situations, repeated quantitative measurements may be required.

TOXICOLOGIC SCREENS

Types of Screens

A toxicologic screen is a combination of many different laboratory procedures that is aimed at identifying the drugs most commonly encountered in emergency toxicology. Screens may include as many different assays as are necessary for the identification of target drugs. Alternatively, to shorten turnaround times, screens can be focused or abbreviated so that they test for only a few common, critical, or difficult-to-recognize drugs. The numbers and types of drugs on the screen can be adapted somewhat to reflect regional differences in drug prevalence.[1,17] Ultimately, the availability of accurate, inexpensive commercial methods is often the greater determinant.

COMPREHENSIVE SCREENING

Comprehensive screening may include spot tests, immunoassays, TLC, and GC-MS procedures and may require 3 to 4 hours of intensive labor. Such broad screens or searches are applied to urine specimens and may include 80 to 200 target drugs or toxins. Because the search is wide and the prior probability is low for detection of a particular toxin, many laboratories will not report a drug's presence unless the agent has been detected on two procedures or unless the single method is known to be highly specific for a highly prevalent intoxicant (e.g., GC for ethanol). For instance, initial identification of codeine by immunoassay would be considered only presumptive and not reportable. Subsequent confirmation (e.g., by TLC or GC-MS) would make the result reportable. Lack of confirmation or the absence of initial identification would be reported as "not detected." Confirmation is not always a requirement in clinical testing, depending on clinical prior probability, the specificity of the single test used, and the implications of a positive test result.

A comprehensive approach to screening with multiple complementary methods will detect most common drugs used in overdose concentrations,[18] yet only 6% of hospital or clinic laboratories are enrolled in proficiency testing for comprehensive screening. This fact suggests that the capability to perform such comprehensive testing is not widespread.[16] Drugs that are typically included on a comprehensive toxicologic screen are listed in Box 3-1, and toxins that are not usually detectable in such toxicologic screens are listed in Box 3-2. Many of these undetectable drugs are either not very prevalent or not very toxic, but many important toxins are not routinely detected in comprehensive screening procedures (e.g.,

---

BOX 3-1   TYPES OF COMMON DRUGS INCLUDED ON MOST CHROMATOGRAPHICALLY BASED COMPREHENSIVE "TOX SCREENS"

Volatiles: ethanol, methanol, isopropanol, acetone
Barbiturates/sedatives: amobarbital, secobarbital, pentobarbital, butalbital, butabarbital, phenobarbital, glutethimide, methaqualone
Antiepileptics: phenytoin, carbamazepine, phenobarbital
Benzodiazepines: as parent drugs or metabolites, chlordiazepoxide, oxazepam diazepam, alprazolam, lorazepam, temazepam
Antihistamines: diphenhydramine, chlorpheniramine, brompheniramine, tripennelamine, trihexiphenidyl, doxylamine, pyrilamine
Antidepressants: amitriptyline, nortriptyline, doxepin, imipramine, desimipramine, trazedone, amoxapine, sertraline, fluoxetine
Antipsychotics: trifluoperazine, perphenazine, prochlorperazine, chlorpromazine, olanzepine, risperidone
Stimulants: amphetamine, methamphetamine, phenylpropanolamine, ephedrine, methylenedioxyamphetamine (MDA), methylenedioxymethamphetamine (MDMA, or "Ecstasy")
Narcotics analgesics: morphine, codeine, oxycodone, hydrocodone, hydromorphone, meperidine, pentazocine, propoxyphene, methadone
Other analgesics: salicylates, acetaminophen
Cardiovascular drugs: lidocaine, propranolol, metoprolol, quinidine, procainamide, verapamil
Others: caffeine, cyclobenzaprine, hydroxyzine, nicotine, oral hypoglycemics, strychnine

---

BOX 3-2   TOXINS NOT DETECTABLE BY CHROMATO-GRAPHICALLY BASED EMERGENCY TOX SCREENS, CLASSFIED BY AREA OF DIFFICULTY

Too polar: antibiotics, diuretics, isoniazid, ethylene glycol, lithium, lead, iron
Too nonpolar: steroids, Δ^9-tetrahydrocannabinol (THC)
Too nonvolatile: plant and fungal alkaloids, some phenothiazines
Too volatile: aromatic and halogenated hydrocarbon solvents, anesthetic gases, noxious gases (hydrogen sulfide, nitrogen dioxide, carbon monoxide)
Concentration too low: (Potent drugs or drugs with large volumes of distribution): clonidine, fentanyl, colchicine, ergot alkaloids, LSD, dioxin, digoxin, THC
Toxic anions (too polar): thiocyanate, cyanide, fluoride, bromide, borate, nitrite
New drugs: e.g., buspirone, aripiprazole

Nonchromatographically based tests may be available for some toxins as separate tests.

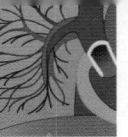

ethylene glycol, γ-hydroxybutyrate [GHB], isoniazid, and cyanide). Assays for drugs not included in the toxicologic screen can often be requested as separate quantitative tests. Clinicians can help reduce clinical false-negative results (which can occur when a test is ordered that is not capable of detecting the suspected agent) by knowing which drugs and toxins are not included on the screens at their hospitals. Clinical laboratories should inform ED staff when method changes are made that affect test specificity, or when drug assays are added or dropped from toxicologic screens.

DRUGS-OF-ABUSE SCREENS

A smaller screen for illicit drugs also is commonly offered and available with a rapid turn-around time. A drugs-of-abuse screen typically consists of six to eight immunoassays for common illicit substances tested in urine, with confirmation procedures performed as needed or requested by the clinician. The drugs-of-abuse screen might include such drugs as opiates (morphine, codeine), amphetamines, cocaine, and propoxyphene and is typically most used by the emergency and psychiatric services. Drugs-of-abuse screens are based on immunoassays that have been developed and primarily marketed for use by drug surveillance programs and not for overdose diagnostic use. Hence the cutoff concentrations used for determination of a positive or negative may be inappropriately low for use in assessing an overdose patient. For an assay with a low-level cutoff, the positive detection of the drug may be due to earlier drug use that is unrelated to the current clinical condition (see Table 3-3 for detection intervals). Communication between the laboratory and the treating physician is essential for selection of the appropriate sequence and choice of tests, clinical correlation of results, to speed analysis, and to help the laboratory make the best use of its resources.

CONFIRMATORY TESTING

In testing for illicit drug use, it is recommended that preliminary results be confirmed by a second specific test, whether at the time of the report or later, because false-positive documentation in the clinical record may have negative consequences for the patient. Also, the clinical laboratory should include a list of major cross-reacting substances (see Table 3-3) when a positive result is reported if not confirmed by a second method.[1,2] The detection and reporting of some highly prevalent and nonillicit drugs may not require confirmation because this higher prior probability combined with a test of fairly good specificity allows for adequate confidence in the test result (e.g., predictive value of the positive test is high). Also, because some drugs often are present in drug-using populations that may be seen in the ED, or because they contribute little to the clinical picture, no testing may be needed. For example, although some hospital laboratories test for marijuana, it is not recommended in emergency situations because (1) it is highly prevalent in the drug-using population that may overdose on more serious drugs, (2) it is rarely considered responsible for serious toxicologic effects,

and (3) it is excreted in urine for long periods of time after use and thus may not be temporally related to the acute clinical picture.

SPECIMEN REQUIREMENTS

Urine specimens submitted for toxicologic analysis should be collected in a preservative-free container and transported to the clinical laboratory as soon as feasible. A specimen volume of approximately 30 mL will be adequate for most toxicologic analyses. Stability of most drugs is expected for 24 hours in urines stored at 25°C, for as long as 2 weeks for specimens refrigerated at 2° C to 8° C, and for years in specimens frozen at −20° C to −80° C. Generally, urine is analyzed for diagnostic testing and serum is analyzed for quantitative determinations. Other specimen types are used in other toxicologic testing situations (Table 3-6).

Rationale and Use of Toxicologic Screens

In the emergency setting, urine and blood can be obtained as soon as a toxicologic etiology is considered in the differential diagnosis. Drugs-of-abuse screens can confirm the clinical suspicion of a few common drugs relatively quickly. It is unlikely that comprehensive screening will produce results that will affect early diagnosis or emergency management (see later section on Clinical Utility of Toxicologic Screens), but if the initial diagnosis remains unclear, a comprehensive screen may help determine the etiology in a small percentage of cases. Testing of urine specimens identifies the greatest number of drugs in easily detectable quantities. When compared with assays using serum or gastric aspirates, urine yielded the highest rate of positive findings.[18-20] Comprehensive screening of serum or blood is not widely available, although it is possible with the application of newer techniques. The analytical limitations of serum screening include lower concentrations of drugs found in serum, small sample size, and the incompatibilities of serum with some testing methodologies. In some cases, however, drugs may not have reached the urine in measurable quantities soon after ingestion, allowing earlier detection in the plasma. Also, some drugs are highly metabolized, and thus little of the parent drug may be detectable in the urine. Although gastric samples often contain high concentrations of the parent drugs, testing of gastric aspirates should not be performed routinely. In one study, patients who had undergone gastric lavage for initial management had the following proportion of positive results for the presence of drugs on analyses of specimens: urine, 93%; serum, 54% (samples screened for sedative-hypnotics and ethanol); and gastric aspirate or lavage effluent, 38%.[20]

When ordering a toxicologic screen, the clinician should write suspected drugs or drug classes and the key symptoms or the working diagnosis on the requisition. This facilitates both the screening process and the communication of results back to the ordering physician. For instance, if a toxicologic screen is ordered and

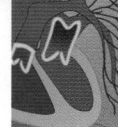

TABLE 3-6 General Advantages and Disadvantages of Some Common Specimen Types for Use in Drug Monitoring and Toxicologic Testing

TISSUE OR FLUID	ADVANTAGES	DISADVANTAGES
Whole blood or red cells	May reflect tissue levels or body burdens Concentration-effect relationships may exist Available	Harder to process than serum Sampling time in relation to dose must be known Requires some distribution into red cells
Serum or plasma	May reflect dynamically active fraction of drug Concentration-effect relationships may exist Available	Easier to process than blood Sampling time in relation to dose must be known In overdose, less sensitive detection than for many drugs found in urine Less useful and often not possible for toxins concentrated in red cells due to variability or sensitivity issues
Saliva	May reflect serum concentrations or unbound (free) concentrations Usually available	Variable acquisition of a reliable specimen Requires additional method validation (vs. serum-based methods)
Urine	When quantitated, may reflect daily exposure or intake of short half-life drugs that are eliminated by kidneys In overdose, a wider number of drugs in higher concentrations are present for detection Usually available	Less direct relation to tissue concentrations or effects than serum or blood Collection interval may be important May not be applicable to drugs that are highly lipophilic, highly metabolized, or not renally eliminated
Gastric aspirate fluid	In overdose, high concentrations of parent drug may be present without metabolites	Little relation to tissue concentration or effect, but may identify some intoxicants
Hair	When quantitated, may represent an accumulative dose May indicate timing or history of exposure per segment of hair	Use not established for most drugs or toxins Potential for external contamination Potential effect of hair treatments
Meconium	May reflect maternal (and fetal) exposures to drugs during last 2 months of pregnancy	Limited to sampling only the first day of newborn life Difficult specimen to process

clonidine is specified as the drug suspected of causing pinpoint pupils and respiratory depression, the laboratory can inform the clinician that the screening methods would be unlikely to detect clonidine, but that testing for opiates could be performed. In another case, a physician may order only a test for amphetamines in urine because the patient is "acting bizarrely." In this case, a comprehensive screen may be recommended by the laboratory since several other drug classes, including antihistamines, belladonna alkaloids, and dextromethorphan, can cause altered behavior. The best method of communication is the use of a requisition form containing adequate prompts and sufficient space for written comments. In a survey addressing the use of these forms, only 48% had space for the listing of suspected drugs.[21]

Drugs Found in Drug Overdose

Two and one quarter million cases of accidental (85.2%) or intentional (11.6%) poison exposures, with about 800 deaths, are reported annually by poison control centers in the United States.[22] The number of recorded poisoning deaths occurring in the United States in 1995 was 18,549 as reported by the National Center for Health Statistics.[23] Since only 5% of intoxication deaths are reported to poison control centers, the total number of poison exposures in the United States may be underestimated.[24] The low incidence of fatality reflects the low toxicity of exposure in the majority of cases and

the effect of medical treatment; however, drug ingestions (i.e., not other toxins) accounted for 77% of poison-related deaths. The drug categories responsible for the deaths reported by poison control centers in order of frequency were analgesics (narcotic and non-narcotic), sedative-hypnotics/antipsychotics, antidepressants, stimulants (including amphetamines, cocaine, and phencyclidine), cardiovascular drugs, and alcohol.[22] The top five drugs found in various situations are listed in Table 3-7.[22,23,25,26] The incidence of detection of barbiturates and ethanol has decreased, while that of benzodiazepines, other sedative-hypnotic drugs, and stimulants, particularly cocaine, has increased. A retrospective review of records from an inner city ED from 1988 to 1997 found that cocaine was the most common drug presentation, accounting for 33% of drug-related visits.[25] In contrast (see Table 3-7), poisoning mortality data from the National Center for Health Statistics report a slightly different spectrum of toxic exposures associated with death, listing opiates, motor vehicle exhaust gas (carbon monoxide), cocaine, psychotropic drugs, analgesics, and ethanol as the more common causes.[23] Although exposure to a single drug is implicated in 92% of reports, 48% of fatal cases involved two or more substances.[22] Unintentional exposures account for the majority of pediatric poisonings and usually involve single substances. Drugs are responsible for only a minority of all exposures in children (27%), but they account for a large portion of intoxications, hospital admissions, and deaths, particularly among

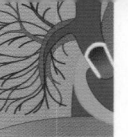

TABLE 3-7 Top Five Drugs Involved in Emergency Department (ED) Visits and Poisoning Deaths

RANK	POISON CONTROL DEATH REPORTS (AAPCC 2001)	POISONING DEATHS NATIONAL CENTER FOR HEALTH STATISTICS (NCHS 1995)	HOSPITAL/ED CHART REVIEW RUSH-PRESBYTERIAN-ST. LUKE'S HOSPITAL (1988–1997)	DRUG-RELATED ED VISITS (DAWN 2001)
1	Analgesics	Opiates	Cocaine	Ethanol
2	Sedative-hypnotics/ antipsychotics	Motor vehicle exhaust gas	Opiates	Cocaine
3	Antidepressants	Cocaine	Marijuana	Marijuana
4	Stimulants street drugs	Tranquilizers/psychotropics	Benzodiazepines	Benzodiazepines
5	Cardiovascular agents	Analgesics/antipyretics	Phencyclidine (PCP)	Analgesics

Drug Abuse Warning Network (DAWN) data are underreported and only a small fraction of ED cases are reported to the American Association of Poison Control Centers (AAPCC). Poison Control Center deaths represent only 5% of deaths seen in the NCHS database.

teenagers.[22,27-29] Drugs found on emergency toxicologic screens mimic these trends, but vary by report because of regional differences, ordering patterns, and the composition of the screens.[30] However, comprehensive screening can detect up to 84% of the fatal drugs and around 90% of drugs involved in ED visits.[18,31]

Analytic Accuracy of Toxicologic Screens

Currently, testing in emergency hospital laboratories can be assessed by hospital laboratories' participation in proficiency testing programs administered by the College of American Pathologists.[16] For immunoassay-based drugs-of-abuse screening, the proportion of false-positive results is generally low (less than 1% for 12 drug classes), and false-negative results also account for less than 1% of results among the 2900 laboratories responding, with some notable exceptions (35% false-negative results on one barbiturate challenge, 27% false-negative results on one marijuana challenge). Although other surveys indicate higher false-negative rates, these low rates are due in part to the restricted nature of this testing, in that the laboratories expect that only these few classes of drugs are present or absent in these samples. In actual clinical practice, the occurrence of false-positive results is higher due to cross-reactive drugs and other interferences (see Table 3-3), especially when confirmation is omitted.

In comprehensive toxicologic screening, the incidence of false-negative results on testing for an infrequently tested drug, such as ethchlorvynol, can be as high as 52%, compared with about 6% for a common drug such as codeine.[16] The false-negative rate for these less commonly tested drugs is due to poor validation of analytical parameters for these agents, particularly cutoff concentrations or the limits of detection. Also, false-negative results may be due to a problem of the proficiency testing survey, in that the laboratory fails to state it has no method for detecting the drug in question. The occurrence of false-positive results is lower in part because of high drug concentrations seen in cases of overdose and because of the use of complementary confirmatory techniques. However, even when using several methods, including GC-MS technology, misidentification of drugs can occur. Many false-positive and some false-negative

results on these surveys may also be due to misidentification within a drug class (i.e., pentobarbital for amobarbital). Thus, the impact of this error on clinical diagnosis would be small.

Testing accuracy will vary depending on the purpose of the testing program (e.g., forensic cause of death, surveillance, compliance) and the analytical strategies employed. For instance, adulteration detection is particularly important in urine drug surveillance programs; methods include visual scrutiny of the sample for abnormal foaming, color or odor, alterations in specific gravity, creatinine concentration, temperature, pH, and tests measuring specific adulterants (nitrites, glutaraldehyde, pyridinium chlorochromate). False-negative results due to interference from intentional adulteration are much less likely in emergency toxicologic screening. Common adulteration techniques include dilution (by ingestion or direct addition of water), substitution (with purchased urine or the urine of another person or animal), ingestion of weak acids or bases (e.g., vinegar or bicarbonate, respectively) to influence the excretion of basic or acidic drugs, the use of interfering substances to alter test results (e.g., benzalkonium chloride), and the addition of strong chemicals (e.g., soap, bleach, or glutaraldehyde) to impair biologically based immunoassays.[32-34]

Accuracy of the Clinical Diagnosis

Although several early studies indicated that information on drug ingestion was unreliable or unavailable in 75% of 167 drug overdose cases,[35,36] numerous studies indicate that the correct drug or class of drug could be identified in 80% to 85% of the cases by recognition of toxidromes,[37] or by consideration of the patient history, physical examination, basic laboratory tests, and a few quantitative drug tests.[38] Generally, diagnoses are incorrect or unknown in less than 15% of cases when initial findings were compared with data collected during extensive follow-up and other toxicologic testing.[37-39]

Clinical Reliability of Toxicologic Screens

Overall, clinical reliability of toxicologic screens depends on (1) analytic sensitivity and specificity, (2) whether a particular laboratory routinely tests for the expected

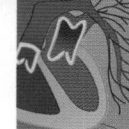

drugs, and (3) the prior probability of overdose. The prevalence of positive results on drug screens in overdose cases is about 50% to 80%. Prevalence of positive screens will show regional and temporal variability reflecting changes in patterns of drug abuse. In addition, prevalence of drug use differs with patient demographics. For example, dextromethorphan is an increasingly commonly abused substance among adolescents, and may be more prevalent than substances such as cocaine or methylene-dioxymethamphetamine (MDMA, or "ecstasy"), which are detected in increased frequency in young adults. If it is assumed that the prior probability of drugs being present in a patient who appears to have an overdose is 50% and if the comprehensive toxicologic screen has a sensitivity of 70% to 90%, then the predictive value of a negative test result is 63% to 83%. If the specificity is from 90% to 100%, then the predictive value of a positive test result is 83% to 100%. Thus, in this case, the rule-in value of the toxicologic screen is better than its rule-out value. Kellerman and associates[19] indicated that most physicians tend to use toxicologic screens to rule out drug toxicity as a diagnosis and are less likely to use these screens for rule-in purposes. Such use is disconcerting if the positive predictive value of toxicologic screens is higher than their negative predictive value in high-prevalence settings. On the other hand, when diagnostic choices are few and the working diagnosis is unlikely to be drug intoxication, rule-out testing is reasonable. For example, if a patient was highly suspected to have a non-drug-induced metabolic coma, the prior probability of involvement of detectable drugs might be considered very low (e.g., 5%) in light of other data indicating metabolic causes (e.g., liver failure). With this prior probability and the same specificity and sensitivity of the toxicologic screen, the predictive value of a negative test result is from 76% to 90%, and the predictive value of a positive test result is 33%; hence, the rule-out value is better (see discussion in the ensuing section on Clinical Utility of Toxicologic Screens).

Clinical Utility of Toxicologic Screens

Do the results of toxicologic screens alter the diagnosis or change patient management? Toxicologic screens may have limited utility for the following reasons:

1. Diagnostic and management decisions are made before toxicologic test results are returned.
2. Benign diagnostic intervention may preclude the need for these tests (e.g., response to naloxone in opiate intoxication).
3. Few specific interventions or antidotal therapies depend on toxicologic test outcomes.[40]
4. The incidence of overall morbidity is low (less than 1%[22,41]), in the setting of optimal patient management, including decontamination and supportive therapy.
5. Toxicity is often apparent on presentation.
6. There is a lack of rapid commercial assays for some drugs commonly involved in emergency room evaluations (e.g. oxycodone, ketamine, GHB).

Clinical features allow for identification of a toxic syndrome and also can be prognostic of outcome.[39] Alternatively, the drugs that cause most of the deaths (see Drugs Found in Drug Overdose) are frequently detectable by screening, including some drugs unsuspected by the physician. Studies from the 1970s and 1980s assessed the utility of toxicologic screens with retrospective chart reviews to find alteration in management or diagnosis, and some used prospective assessment with the completion of questionnaires by physicians receiving drug test results. These studies indicated that the impact of screening on clinical diagnosis and management is low (less than 15%).[39,42-45] Kellerman and associates[45] had examined the utility of toxicologic screens most carefully. In prospective evaluations before and after the return of toxicologic screen results, they showed that diagnostic certainty increased by a mean value of 16.5% (the prior probability of drug toxicity was 75.5% and increased to a posterior probability or post-test probability of 92.0%) and that these changes in diagnostic certainty occurred in 66% of the 183 cases evaluated. These researchers concluded that other clinical information obtained by physicians may have inflated the estimated utility of toxicologic screens in the diagnostic process. More recent studies using current technology for pediatric intoxications have confirmed these impressions.[46,47] In a retrospective review, Belson and Simon found that in 227 of 234 comprehensive drugs screens done on children in the ED, the diagnosis was suspected by clinical presentation, was found by limited serum drug quantitation, or the detected intoxicant was considered clinically insignificant.[46] For differentiating drug-induced from functional psychosis in psychiatric evaluations, the utility of toxicologic screening has also been examined,[48,49] both indicating that the disposition of the patient within the hospital was unaltered by test results. However, one study found that the diagnosis was aided in 82% and clinical management was changed in 25% when point-of-care drug testing was used. Many of the studies cited have focused only on positive toxicologic screen results. The impact of a negative test result is difficult to assess, but may also be considered contributory to the diagnostic and treatment process, if an intervention is avoided.

OTHER TOXICOLOGIC TESTING SITUATIONS

Surveillance Testing

Outside the realm of emergency toxicology testing are specialized applications of toxicologic testing in selected populations, including (1) workplace or employee drug surveillance programs (see http://workplace.samhsa.gov/), (2) program compliance testing (e.g., methadone maintenance or addiction rehabilitation programs), and (3) athletic drug testing for adherence to antidoping rules and regulations of amateur and professional sports organizations. Generally, the aim of these types of testing is to detect substances of low prior probability that may

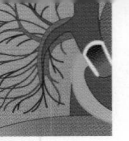

indicate physical or mental impairment or violation of an established drug use policy. Often these testing circumstances have legal ramifications. In addition, there are mandated procedures and policies to follow, such as reporting requirements and chain-of-custody documentation. Therefore, the ED is not a good venue for the collection of such specimens. The specific use and combination of methods applied in emergency toxicology testing is different and should not be misapplied to these specialized situations.

Sexual Assault

ED staff may be required to obtain urine or blood specimens in situations of suspected drug-facilitated sexual assault or by order of arresting officers. Such testing will require specific procedures for collection and submission to a reference laboratory or program. For example, "date rape" agents such as flunitrazepam and GHB require send-out testing to a specialized reference laboratory. Urine and serum specimens of this type should be frozen and retained until such analysis is requested.

Maternal and Infant Drug Screening

Testing mothers and infants for the presence of drugs is sometimes useful in explaining the clinical state of the infant, if the drug is still present in pharmacologically active amounts. However, most often this type of testing is performed as a component of an overall more comprehensive assessment of the infant's home environment or parental care by social services. In some cases, custody decisions can hinge on the overall picture, which may include a urinary drugs-of-abuse screen.

Brain Death

Outside the ED, usually on the wards or intensive care unit, the determination of brain death may involve the exclusion of the presence of drugs that may mimic or interfere with the determination of brain death. Certain drugs, such as barbiturates, known to affect brain function at certain concentrations, may require serum quantitation in some circumstances. In other situations, the patient's history, the time for clearance of potential drugs from the body, or a noncontributory comprehensive toxicologic screen may provide sufficient evidence that drugs are not a factor.

Environmental and Occupational Exposure Assessment

Guidelines for interpreting concentrations in chemical exposures (e.g., to metals or hydrocarbons) are usually based on timed or chronic exposure. These guidelines and cutoffs are often used for discerning excessive (but not necessarily toxic, as in workplace monitoring) exposure, rather than for identifying amounts associated with effects (i.e., for diagnosis). Although not the topic of this chapter, background levels and laboratory methods for determining a narrow selection of commonly encountered inorganic substances (e.g., lead, mercury, cadmium, arsenic trichloroethylene, benzene, toluene, hexane, and polychlorinated biphenyls) are available. The reader is directed to other reference texts on these topics.[50,51]

Testing for Nondrug Toxins

Few tests in this area have been developed or studied mainly due to limited commercial potential. Toxins from plants, animals, microorganisms, and chemical sources are numerous, but exposures are less frequent than drugs. Although potent and deadly toxins in these categories are many, most exposures tend to result in minimal or short-lived toxicity. Certain plant toxins such as nicotine, strychnine, and atropine can be identified on comprehensive toxicologic screens. Specific tests for digoxin (e.g., oleander), cyanide (from cyanogenic glycoside-containing plants, fire exposure, or ingestion), and carboxyhemoglobin can be ordered from the laboratories of larger hospitals. Few other specific plant and fungal toxins can be measured, and the clinician must rely on history and physical examination information to guide diagnosis and management. However, most regional poison centers have contacts with a wide variety of agencies that can help in identifying materials from plants, mushrooms, and chemicals used in agriculture.

SUMMARY

Emergency physicians who use toxicologic testing should learn the capabilities of their institutions' laboratories: What is detectable? What is not detectable? What are the expected turnaround times? Do pharmacologic relationships exist? With regard to requests for testing, the laboratory should allow the physician to order limited test combinations. The physician can assist the laboratory in conducting the appropriate toxicologic testing by providing the differential diagnosis and a list of suspected drugs. Only a few drugs require serum quantitation for making therapeutic decisions (Box 3-3). Urine drug screening is useful in confirming drug-related presentations and may infrequently reveal the presence of other unsuspected drugs. The impact of the results of emergency drug screening on diagnosis and therapy may be minimal. Although in most applications the positive predictive (rule-in) value of comprehensive drug screening in the emergency setting is greater than its negative (rule-out) predictive value, toxicologic screening may be useful as a rule-out test when drug-related effects are of low probability in the differential diagnosis.

Future directions in the laboratory diagnosis of the intoxicated patient are likely to include additional applications of new immunoassays in point-of-care testing applications, particularly in the ED. Development of commercial assays for highly prevalent drugs of abuse such as semisynthetic opioids, GHB, and designer

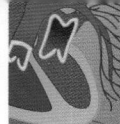

BOX 3-3	SUMMARY: SITUATIONS IN WHICH TOX TESTING IS USEFUL

Overdoses That Require Serum Drug Concentration to Confirm the Diagnosis or Monitor Course and Severity

Acetaminophen	Antiepileptics and barbiturates
Salicylate	Methanol
Theophylline	Ethylene glycol
Valproate	Ethanol
Iron	

Overdoses That Require Serum or Blood Drug Concentrations as Criteria for Therapy or to Assess Effectiveness of Therapy

All drugs above	Carbon monoxide
Lithium	Lead, mercury
Digoxin	Methemoglobin
Long-acting sedatives	

Situations in Which Qualitative Tox Screens Have Utility

"Ruling in" (confirmation) a moderately probable working diagnosis of drug intoxication
"Ruling out" drug intoxication when it is highly unlikely anyway
Not for screening

stimulant amines would likely be of clinical benefit in overdose situations.

REFERENCES

1. Wu AHB, McKay C, Broussard LA, et al: National Academy of Clinical Biochemistry Laboratory Medicine Practice Guidelines: recommendations for the use of laboratory tests to support poisoned patients who present to the emergency department. Clin Chem 2003;49:357–379.
2. Osterloh JD: Utility and reliability of emergency toxicologic testing. Emerg Med Clin North Am 1990;8:693–723.
3. Griner PF, Mayewski RJ, Mushlin AI, Greenland P: Selection and interpretation of diagnostic tests and procedures—principles and applications. Ann Intern Med 1981;94:553–600.
4. Spiehler VR, O'Donnell CM, Gokhale DV: Confirmation and certainty in toxicologic screening. Clin Chem 1988;34:1535–1539.
5. Ferrara SD, Tedeschi L, Frison G, et al: Drugs-of-abuse testing in urine: statistical approach and experimental comparison of immunochemical and chromatographic techniques. J Anal Toxicol 1994;18:278–291.
6. Levine B: Principles of Forensic Toxicology. Washington, DC, American Association of Clinical Chemistry, 1999.
7. Flanagan RJ, Braithwaite RA, Brown SS, et al: International Programme on Chemical Safety. Geneva, World Health Organization, 1995.
8. Dasgupta A, Saldana S, Kinnaman G, et al: Analytical performance evaluation of EMIT II monoclonal amphetamine/methamphetamine assay: more specificity than EMIT d.a.u. monoclonal amphetamine/methamphetamine assay. Clin Chem 1993;39: 104–108.
9. Taylor EH, Oertli EH, Wolfgang JW, Mueller E: Accuracy of five on-site immunoassay drugs of abuse testing devices. J Anal Toxicol 1999;23:119–124.
10. Peredy TR, Powers RD: Bedside diagnostic testing of body fluids. Am J Emerg Med 1997;15:400–407.
11. Binder SR, Regalia M, Biaggi-McEachern, Mazhar M: Automated liquid chromatographic analysis of drugs in urine by on-line cleanup and isocratic multi-column separation. J Chromatogr 1989;473:325–341.
12. Sadeg N, Francois G, Petit B, et al: Automated liquid-chromatographic analyzer used for toxicology screening in a

general hospital: 12 months experience. Clin Chem 1997;43: 498–504.
13. Forester EH, Hatchett D, Garriott JC: A rapid, comprehensive screening procedure for basic drugs in blood or tissues by gas chromatography. J Anal Toxicol 1978;2:50–55.
14. Prescott LF: Limitations of hemodialysis and forced diuresis. In Curry AS (ed): Symposium on the Poisoned Patient—Role of the Laboratory. CIBA Foundation Symposium. New York, Elsevier Science, 1974.
15. Rosenberg J, Benowitz NL, Pond S: Pharmacokinetics of drug overdose. Clin Pharmacokinet 1981;6:161–192.
16. College of American Pathologists: Urine Toxicology Survey 1999 Sets UDS-A and UT-C; Therapeutic Drug Monitoring Survey 1995 Set Z-B; and Chemistry Survey 1999 Sets UDS-A and UT-C. Chicago, IL, College of American Pathologists, 1995.
17. Lasky FD, Wesley JF, Marx AJ: Changes in the pattern of drugs detected in a toxicology screen in an upstate New York hospital. Pathol Annu 1985;20:161–187.
18. Hepler BR, Sutheimer CA, Sunshine I: The role of the toxicology laboratory in emergency medicine. II. Study of an integrated approach. Clin Toxicol 1984–1985;22:503–528.
19. Kellerman AL, Fihn SD, Logerfro JP, et al: Utilization and yield of drug screening in the emergency department. Am J Emerg Med 1988;6:14–20.
20. Auerbach PS, Osterloh J, Braun O, et al: Efficacy of gastric emptying: gastric lavage vs. emesis induced with ipecac. Ann Emerg Med 1986;15:692–698.
21. Fligner CL, Robertson WO: Request and report forms in toxicology screening [Abstract]. In: Proceedings of the American Association of Poison Control Centers (AACT/AAPCC/ABMT/CAPCC) Annual Scientific Meeting, Kansas City, KS, August 4–9, 1985.
22. Watson WA, Litovitz TL, Rodgers GC Jr, et al: 2002 Annual report of the American Association of Poison Control Centers Toxic Exposure Surveillance System. Am J Emerg Med 2003;21:353–421.
23. Fingerhut LA, Cox CS: Poisoning mortality 1985–1995. Public Health Rep 1998;113:218–233.
24. Hoppe-Roberts JM, Lloyd LM, Chyka PA: Poisoning mortality in the United States: comparison of national mortality statistics and poison control center reports. Ann Emerg Med 2000;35:440–448.
25. Leikin JB, Morris RW, Warren M, Erickson T: Trends in a decade of drug abuse presentation to an inner city ED. Am J Emerg Med 2001;19:37–39.
26. U.S. Substance Abuse and Mental Health Services Administration: Drug Abuse Warning Network (DAWN) 2001 Annual Report. Rockville, MD, U.S. Substance Abuse and Mental Health Services Administration, 2001.
27. Fazen LE, Lovejoy FH, Crone RK, et al: Acute poisoning in a children's hospital: a 2-year experience. Pediatrics 1986;77:144–151.
28. Jacobsen D, Halvorsen K, Marstrander J, et al: Acute poisonings of children in Oslo. Acta Paediatr Scand 1983;72:553–557.
29. Trinkoff AM, Baker SP: Poisoning hospitalizations and deaths from solids and liquids among children and teenagers. Am J Public Health 1986;76:657–660.
30. Schwartz JG, Stuckey JH, Prihoda TJ, et al: Hospital-based toxicology: patterns of use and abuse. Tex Med 1990;86:44–51.
31. Linder MW: Report reveals trends in drugs seen in poisonings. Clin Forensic Toxicol News 1999;June:2–4.
32. Mikkelsen SL, Ash KO: Adulterants causing false negatives in illicit drug testing. Clin Chem 1988;34:2333–2336.
33. Jambor L: Adulterants continue to challenge laboratories. Clin Forensic Toxicol News 2000;January:8–10.
34. Wu AHB, Bristol B, Sexton K, et al: Adulteration by "urine luck." Clin Chem 1999;45:1051–1057.
35. Bury RW, Mashford ML: Use of a drug-screening service in an inner-city teaching hospital. Med J Aust 1981;1:132–133.
36. Teitelbaum DT, Morgan J, Gray G: Nonconcordance between clinical impression and laboratory findings in clinical toxicology. Clin Toxicol 1977;10:417–422.
37. Nice A, Leikin JB, Maturen A, et al: Toxidrome recognition to improve efficiency of emergency urine drug screens. Ann Emerg Med 1988;17:676–680.
38. Rygnestad T, Berg KJ: Evaluation of benefits of drug analysis in the routine clinical management of acute self-poisoning. Clin Toxicol 1984;22:51–61.

39. Brett AS: Implications of discordance between clinical impression and toxicology analysis in drug overdose. Arch Intern Med 1988;148:437–441.

40. Brett AS, Rothschild N, Gray R, et al: Predicting the clinical course in intentional drug overdose: implications for use of the intensive care unit. Arch Intern Med 1987;147:133–137.

41. Jacobsen D, Fredericksen PS, Knutsen KM, et al: A prospective study of 1212 cases of acute poisoning: general epidemiology. Hum Toxicol 1984;3:93–106.

42. Wiltbank TB, Sine HE, Brody BB: Are emergency toxicology measurements really used? Clin Chem 1974;20:116–118.

43. Mahoney JD, Gross PL, Stern TA: The use of the toxic screen in the management of overdosed patients [Abstract]. In: Proceedings of the AACT/AAPCC/ABMT/CAPCC Annual Scientific Meeting, September 27 to October 2, 1987, Vancouver, BC, 1987, p 29.

44. Helliwell M, Hampel G, Sinclair E: Value of emergency toxicological investigations in differential diagnosis of coma. BMJ 1979;2:819–821.

45. Kellerman AL, Fihn SD, Logerfro JP, et al: Impact of drug screening in suspected overdose. Ann Emerg Med 1987;16:1206–1216.

46. Belson MG, Simon HK: Utility of comprehensive toxicologic screens in children. Am J Emerg Med 1999;17:221–224.

47. Stephan M, Prybys K, Snook C: Utility of the pediatric toxicology screen [Abstract]. In North American Congress of Clinical Toxicology Annual Scientific Meeting, Rochester, NY, September 16–19, 1995. Clin Tox 1995;33:519.

48. Schiller MJ, Shumway M, Batki SL: Utility of routine drug screening in a psychiatric emergency setting. Psychiatr Serv 2000;51:474–478.

49. Buck C, Write D, Brunner D, et al: Evaluation of rapid urine toxicological testing in patients with altered mental status in the emergency department [Abstract]. In North American Congress of Clinical Toxicology Annual Scientific Meeting, La Jolla, CA, September 28 to October 4, 1999. Clin Tox 1999;37:597.

50. Lauwery RR, Hoet P: Industrial Chemical Exposure—Guidelines for Biological Monitoring. Boca Raton, FL, Lewis Publishers, 2001.

51. Centers for Disease Control and Prevention: Second National Report on Human Exposure to Environmental Chemicals. Atlanta, GA, National Center for Environmental Health Publication No. 02-0716, 2003.

4

Principles of Pharmacology

DAVID N. JUURLINK, BPHM, MD, PHD ■ MARCO L. SIVILOTTI, MD, MSC

Pharmacology is the science that deals with the interactions between living systems and externally derived chemicals (xenobiotics), especially drugs used for the prevention, treatment, or diagnosis of disease. An understanding of basic pharmacologic principles is essential to allow a rational approach to commonly encountered problems in clinical toxicology. This chapter outlines many fundamental concepts of pharmacology and how those concepts relate to the care of poisoned patients.

DISPOSITION OF DRUGS AND TOXINS

Exposure to toxins can occur through environmental contamination, by intentional means (with or without the intent to cause harm), or during the course of medical treatment. Intoxication or poisoning results when a substance is present in a sufficient quantity, in the right place, and at the right time to influence one or more physiologic processes in a deleterious way. Before exerting such an effect, however, the drug or toxin must first be delivered to the target tissues. Although this may sometimes be immediate, as in the case of a caustic dermal exposure, for most drugs the rapidity, intensity, and duration of effect are heavily influenced by four related aspects of drug movement within the body: absorption, distribution, biotransformation (also called *metabolism*), and elimination.

These processes typically require passage across cell membranes. Drugs and other substances pass through membranes by a variety of mechanisms, the most important of which are passive diffusion and active transport. *Diffusion* is a passive process driven by differences in concentration, whereby drugs move down a gradient from areas of higher concentration to areas of lower concentration. Diffusion may involve movement across intercellular junctions, through transmembrane channels (pores), or directly across membranes themselves. *Active transport,* as the term implies, is an energy-dependent process in which substances usually are transported by a transmembrane carrier protein against a concentration gradient. Active transport processes differ from passive diffusion not only in their requirement for metabolic energy but also in their selectivity for a single chemical entity or group of related compounds, their saturability, and their susceptibility to inhibition. *Facilitated diffusion processes* are similar to active transport in that they demonstrate selectivity, saturability, and potential for inhibition, but they do not require energy and do not operate against concentration gradients.

Absorption

Absorption refers to movement of a substance from site of administration into the blood space. Of the various sites from which absorption can take place, the gastrointestinal tract is the most important because the majority of acute poisonings involve ingestion. Passive diffusion from the gastrointestinal tract occurs most readily with lipid-soluble, low-molecular-weight, nonionized compounds such as alcohols. The absorption of these compounds is limited only by the absorptive surface area and factors that reduce the surface interface with intestinal epithelium, such as the presence of food.

Drug absorption also may be influenced by the pH at the site of absorption. In general, absorption is reduced by ionization, because the presence of a charge decreases a drug's lipid solubility and hampers its transmembrane flux. The degree to which a drug is ionized at a given pH depends on its ionization constant (pK). The pK of an acid or base is the pH at which 50% of a compound exists in ionized form and 50% in nonionized form (Fig. 4-1). Because it is on a logarithmic scale, pH changes of a single unit can cause up to a tenfold change in concentration of either the ionized or nonionized form.

Many drugs are either weak acids or weak bases. Weakly acidic drugs (HA) (e.g., acetylsalicylic acid) can release a proton in aqueous solution, resulting in the formation of an anion (A$^-$), as shown in the usual Brønsted-Lowry expression below:

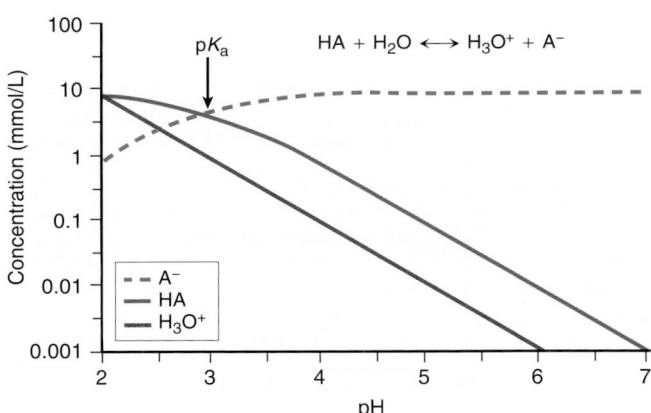

FIGURE 4-1 In aqueous solution, salicylic acid (HA) ionizes to yield salicylate anion (A$^-$) and a proton (H$^+$), which combine with water to form hydronium (H$_3$O$^+$). The pK_a of salicylate (3.0) is the pH at which 50% exists as HA and 50% exists as A$^-$. As the pH rises, more A$^-$ is formed, although little additional ionization takes place above pH 5.0, when virtually no un-ionized salicylate remains.

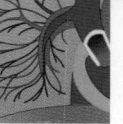

$$HA + H_2O \leftrightarrow H_3O^+ + A^-$$

Such drugs are less ionized (and therefore better absorbed) in an acidic milieu such as the stomach, which favors the left side of the above formula. Conversely, weak bases are more readily absorbed in an alkaline environment, such as when intraluminal pH is elevated by the use of antacids or gastric acid–suppressing medications. The influence of pH on drug absorption is illustrated in Figure 4-2.

The rate-limiting step for absorption of solid xenobiotics from the gastrointestinal tract is usually dissolution, a process that can be altered by changes in pH, the rate of gastric emptying, the presence of food, and the formulation. These complex relationships are relevant particularly in the setting of acute poisoning, because decisions regarding gastrointestinal decontamination (see Chapter 2B) are influenced by the likelihood that a product remains in the gastrointestinal tract. Many liquid drugs are absorbed very rapidly following ingestion, reducing the likelihood that gastrointestinal decontamination will effect a significant reduction in the overall amount of drug absorbed. Drugs formulated as capsules or tablets dissolve more slowly and may be more amenable to interventions aimed at limiting absorption. This is particularly true of drugs with modified release systems, such as enteric coatings or polymer matrices, which may release contents over 12 hours or longer.

Gastrointestinal motility also can influence the rate and extent of drug absorption. For most drugs, absorption from the stomach is minimal, and the drug gains access to the systemic circulation only after passing the pylorus. The presence of food in the stomach increases pyloric tone, slowing the delivery of drug to the duodenum. Similarly, many drugs, including opioids, salicylates, and drugs with antimuscarinic activity (i.e., cyclic antidepressants and antihistamines), can slow gastric emptying. Reduced gastric emptying leads to delayed drug absorption and lower peak drug levels, because the drug is presented to the absorptive surface of the small intestine more slowly. In acutely poisoned patients, delayed gastric emptying may extend the window of opportunity for gastrointestinal decontamination maneuvers.[1]

In the small intestine, the presence of microvilli on the luminal epithelium increases the absorptive surface area markedly. In fact, the surface area available for absorption is so much larger than the stomach that for many drugs the effects of pH on ionization are rendered insignificant. Following absorption from the small intestine, drugs enter the portal circulation and then the liver prior to reaching the systemic circulation. Many drugs undergo significant metabolic inactivation during this migration, a process variably referred to as *first pass metabolism* or *presystemic extraction*.

In recent years, it has become recognized that the small intestinal epithelium functions as an active barrier to drug absorption.[2] Specifically, many drugs are metabolized within the small intestine enterocyte, actively transported back into the intestinal lumen, or both. Moreover, these processes can be inhibited or induced by drugs and diet. For example, grapefruit contains bergamottin, naringin, and other flavonoids that may inhibit oxidative drug metabolism of a large number of drugs in the enterocyte.[3,4] Consequently, absorption may increase dramatically for drugs that normally have a high degree of presystemic extraction (e.g., nifedipine and simvastatin). Conversely, St. John's wort and other compounds can both induce the oxidative metabolism of the same drugs and promote active transfer back into the lumen.[5] This can lead to dramatic reductions in the blood levels of drugs such as cyclosporine and tacrolimus, sometimes with dramatic clinical consequences.[6,7] A more detailed discussion of these interactions is given later in this chapter.

ABSORPTION BY OTHER ROUTES
Parenteral Absorption
Intravenous injection is the most common route by which drugs are administered parenterally and avoids first pass hepatic metabolism and other barriers to oral absorption. Because serum drug concentrations rise much more rapidly, the rate of infusion of some drugs must be carefully regulated to avoid toxicity.

Direct intramuscular injection is possible for some drugs soluble in aqueous solutions or, occasionally, as long-acting depot injections intended to minimize the need for frequent injections. Before an intramuscularly administered drug can exert an effect, absorption into the blood compartment is necessary. This rate is highly dependent on tissue perfusion and on the chemical properties of the drug and its formulation. Drugs given by subcutaneous injection may be absorbed into the blood rapidly, but this process can be purposefully slowed by the nature of the formulation. For example, Lente insulin (insulin zinc suspension) is a mixture of crystallized and amorphous insulins in a buffer that

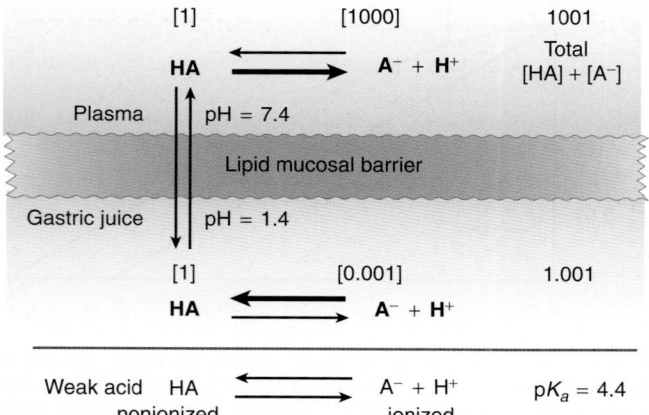

FIGURE 4-2 For a weak acid with a pK_a of 4.4, the low pH of gastric juice favors the undissociated species (HA). Following absorption across the lipid mucosal barrier, equilibrium favors the dissociated species (A^-) because plasma pH is 7.4. (From Wilkinson GR: Pharmacokinetics. In Hardman JG, Limbrid LE, Gilman AG [eds]: Goodman and Gilman's The Pharmacological Basis of Therapeutics, 10th ed. New York, McGraw-Hill, 2001, p 4.)

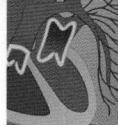

decreases their solubility. Although this precludes intravenous administration of Lente insulin, it leads to slower dissolution in the subcutaneous tissue, resulting in more gradual absorption and a longer duration of action (see Chapter 64)[8].

Sublingual Absorption

Some drugs can be absorbed directly into the venous capillary network of the oral mucosa. Absorption from the sublingual route generally is rapid and avoids first pass metabolism by the liver. Examples of drugs administered by the sublingual route include captopril, nicotine, nifedipine, and nitroglycerin.

Pulmonary Absorption

The lungs also serve as an important site for the absorption of certain drugs (e.g., volatile anesthetics) and many toxins (e.g., nicotine, cyanide, and carbon monoxide). Because the lungs receive essentially all of the cardiac output and because the alveoli offer an enormous surface area for absorption, many gases and very small particles (<1 μm) that enter the lower airways can be dissolved rapidly into blood.

Dermal Absorption

The stratum corneum consists of flattened, nonviable corneocytes filled with hydrophilic keratin proteins and separated by hydrophobic lamellar lipids, providing an effective barrier to the absorption of most drugs and toxins. Penetration of xenobiotics through intact skin is determined by the lipid solubility of the drug, the thickness of the stratum corneum, and the concentration gradient. Drug penetration can be enhanced by the use of an organic solvent vehicle such as carbon tetrachloride, methanol, and dimethyl sulfoxide, provided the xenobiotic partitions into the vehicle rather than escaping into the stratum corneum. Xenobiotics larger than about 1000 daltons do not penetrate adult skin easily. Inflamed, denuded, or immature skin provides a much more permeable barrier to absorption.

Distribution

Following absorption, chemicals circulate throughout the body within the blood space and translocate into other tissues in a process called *distribution*. In general, the amount of the drug or toxin at the site of action represents only a small proportion of the total amount absorbed, whereas the rest of the drug distributes in other tissues such as muscle and fat. A given drug distributes in a relatively predictable way that is governed by its chemical properties, including lipid solubility, molecular weight, and charge.

It is helpful to characterize the extent to which various drugs distribute into different body tissues. The *volume of distribution* of a drug reflects this apparent space in the body available to contain the absorbed drug, as estimated by the concentration in the blood or plasma:

$$\text{Vd (volume units)} = \frac{\text{amount of drug in body (mass)}}{\text{concentration (mass per volume)}}$$

Importantly, Vd is a theoretical construct rather than an actual volume of fluid; hence the term *apparent volume of distribution*. Molecules that are very large (i.e., heparin and the volume expander hetastarch) are generally confined to the vascular space and have a volume of distribution approaching that of plasma, or about 40 mL/kg in adults. Drugs that are hydrophilic (i.e., lithium and neuromuscular junction blocking agents) tend to distribute throughout total body water and have a Vd on the order of 0.6 L/kg body weight. Other drugs are bound to body tissues extensively, such that only a small fraction is present in the blood. One example is amiodarone, with a volume of distribution that is highly variable but can exceed more than 100 L/kg body weight.

Typically, drugs with large volumes of distribution are highly lipophilic chemicals that concentrate within tissue compartments such as muscle or fat. Sometimes it is helpful to view these tissues as "reservoirs." This concept illustrates why drugs with large volumes of distribution (i.e., those that preferentially distribute outside the vascular compartment) are not readily removed by extracorporeal methods such as hemodialysis. The time course of a drug's distribution into these various compartments usually is determined by the blood flow into the compartment and the exchange kinetics between the circulation and the compartment (see Pharmacokinetics, later).

When the V_d and administered dose of a xenobiotic are known, the formula shown earlier can be used to estimate peak serum concentration. Use of the formula as written, however, presumes that all of the drug is absorbed and none is yet eliminated. It will, therefore, often overestimate serum concentration of a xenobiotic, particularly after ingestion. It is clinically useful, however, to estimate "worst case scenario" peak serum concentrations after ingestion with a known maximal quantity available of a toxicant.

The blood-brain barrier (BBB) and placenta are special barriers to drug distribution. The BBB is a specialized system of capillary endothelial cells that, unlike those in the peripheral vasculature, limits the entry of drugs and toxins into the central nervous system by a combination of physical barriers (intercellular tight junctions) and active transport processes.[9] However, several drugs pass the BBB freely, and its permeability can be increased significantly by inflammatory processes such as meningitis. Transplacental drug passage is relevant particularly for drugs that may harm the fetus (i.e., warfarin, phenytoin, and ethanol) or, if given immediately prior to delivery, the neonate (i.e., opiate analgesics). Nearly all drugs administered during pregnancy cross the placenta to some degree, but the process is far more efficient for nonionized, lipid-soluble drugs. Like the BBB, the placenta is capable of active drug efflux and oxidative drug metabolism (discussed later in this chapter), both of which serve to minimize fetal drug exposure.[10]

Protein Binding

Many drugs and poisons are bound to some extent to plasma proteins, particularly albumin and α_1-acid

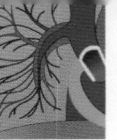

glycoprotein. Binding to plasma proteins limits the extent to which drugs can traverse capillary walls and enter tissues, effectively sequestering a drug because the drug-protein complex is too large to diffuse from the vascular space. Only the unbound ("free") fraction can do so, and as such only this portion can exert a physiologic effect. The binding involves reversible, weak electrostatic, hydrophobic, or van der Waals forces, and the extent of protein binding varies considerably among drugs. Some highly lipophilic organic compounds are very tightly bound to albumin. One such example is the anticoagulant warfarin, which is almost completely bound; only the free fraction is able to exert a biologic effect. Albumin binds weak acids more strongly than weak bases, and it generally does not bind drugs that are either hydrophilic or neutral.

When two drugs that both bind to albumin are given simultaneously, they may compete for available binding sites, increasing the free fraction of the other. Although this displacement from plasma proteins often is cited as an important mechanism by which drug interactions can be mediated, this is not the case for the vast majority of protein-bound drugs, since the free fraction generally is metabolized and eliminated relatively quickly.[11] Drugs and toxins also can bind to other proteins, including α_1-acid glycoprotein, an acute phase reactant that binds to many acidic drugs (i.e., cyclic antidepressants, methadone, some local anesthetics, and antimalarial drugs).[12,13]

Biotransformation

Most xenobiotics undergo chemical transformation before they are eliminated from the body. This process is called *biotransformation* or *metabolism*, and its products are called *metabolites*. Biotransformation generally yields products that are more polar and therefore more water-soluble. These metabolites are less able to pass through biologic membranes, are more restricted in their tissue distribution, and are more readily eliminated in the bile and urine. Biotransformation occasionally converts drugs into more toxic compounds in a process termed *bioactivation*; common examples include acetaminophen (converts to *N*-acetyl-*p*-benzoquinone imine), methanol (converts to formic acid), and chloral hydrate (converts to trichloroacetic acid).

Although biotransformation reactions can occur in many organs, the liver is quantitatively the most important site. Drug metabolizing enzymes are present in various parts of the hepatocyte; by convention, their location is indicated by the in vitro fraction of homogenized liver tissue in which the enzymatic activity is found. Drug metabolizing enzymes are therefore referred to as *soluble* (found principally in the cytosol), *mitochondrial*, or *microsomal* (found principally in the endoplasmic reticulum).

Biotransformation reactions generally are categorized as one of two types: phase I or phase II. Many drugs undergo sequential metabolism in phase I and phase II processes. Commonly, the small structural change imparted by phase I metabolism is necessary for phase II metabolism to proceed. Specific examples of phase I and phase II reactions are shown in Table 4-1.

PHASE I METABOLISM

Phase I metabolism is characterized by reactions involving oxidation, reduction, or hydrolysis. The result is a less dramatic chemical alteration of the parent compound than what occurs with phase II metabolism, but the clinical consequences often are very significant, resulting in complete or partial drug inactivation or, in some instances, production of a biologically active or toxic compound.

Microsomal oxidative reactions are quantitatively the most important of the phase I metabolic processes. Most of these involve the cytochrome P-450 (CYP450) enzyme system, previously called the *mixed function oxidase system*.[14] Once thought to consist of a few proteins, it is now recognized that CYP450 represents a large family of related heme-containing enzymes. The system draws its name from the maximal spectral absorbance at 450 nm when the enzymes are bound to carbon monoxide. Although more than 60 different CYP isoenzymes exist, most are relatively unimportant in humans.

By convention, the nomenclature of CYP isoenzymes involves a number (the *family*), an uppercase letter (the *subfamily*), and another number (the *form*). CYP enzymes exhibit a high degree of structural homology, which is greatest for enzymes within the same family (e.g., CYP2C9 and CYP2C19). Despite this homology, each enzyme form has a distinctive pattern of drugs they metabolize (termed *substrates*) and a distinctive pattern

TABLE 4-1	Subtypes and Sites of Drug Metabolism	
PHASE	**METABOLIC PATHWAY**	**LOCATION OF ENZYMES**
Phase I	*Oxidation*	
	Hydroxylation	M
	Dealkylation	M
	Epoxidation	M
	S- and N-oxidation	M
	Desulfuration	M
	Dehalogenation	M
	Deamination	M, mitochrondria
	Alcohol oxidation	M, S
	Aldehyde oxidation	S
	Reduction	
	Aldehyde reduction	S
	Azoreduction	M
	Nitroreduction	M, S
	Hydrolysis	
	De-esterification	M, S, plasma
	Deamidation	M, S
Phase II	*Conjugation*	
	Glucuronidation	M
	Sulfation	S
	Glutathione conjugation	S
	Methylation, acetylation	S
	Acylation	S

M, microsomes (endoplasmic reticulum); S, soluble fraction (cytosol).

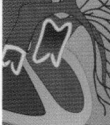

Reduction	Hydrolysis
Aldehyde Reduction	**De-esterification**

<table>
<tr><td>

$Cl_3C—CH—OH \rightleftharpoons Cl_3C—\overset{O}{C}—H \longrightarrow Cl_3C—CH_2—OH$

|

Chloral hydrate   Chloralaldehyde   Trichloroethanol
</td><td>

Cocaine → Methylecgonine
</td></tr>
</table>

Conjugation	
Glucuronide Conjugation	**Amino Acid (Glycine) Conjugation**

Morphine → Morphine glucuronide

Salicylic acid → Salicyluric acid

| **Acetylation** |

Isoniazid → Acetylisoniazid

Sulfate Conjugation	**Glutathione Conjugation**

Acetaminophen →

Acetaminophen → [reactive intermediate] →

Conjugates formed from the drug–glutathione complex in a multistep process are actually N-acetyl cysteine conjugates, called mercapturic acids.

B

FIGURE 4-4 *Continued.* **B,** Reductions and other reactions.

urine, but other routes include elimination via the intestine, lungs, bile, and sweat.

RENAL ELIMINATION

Many drugs depend on the kidney either largely or exclusively for elimination. The kidney is a highly vascular organ that normally receives about 25% of cardiac output. With the exception of very large molecules (>20,000 daltons) and drugs that are bound extensively to plasma proteins, most drugs undergo passive glomerular filtration, a process driven primarily by the pressure gradient between the afferent and efferent arterioles.

Once in the lumen, drugs may be reabsorbed through tubular epithelial cells into the peritubular blood or eliminated in the urine. The degree of reabsorption is heavily influenced by lipid solubility, with poor reabsorption of drugs that carry an electrostatic charge. This feature sometimes can be exploited in the management of poisoned patients by therapeutic manipulation of urinary pH. The urinary excretion of weak acids (e.g., salicylic acid, phenobarbital, or chlorpropamide) is enhanced by alkalinization of the urine. Raising the intraluminal pH by the administration of sodium bicarbonate favors the formation of the ionized species, effectively "trapping" the compound in the urine and enhancing elimination. Although acidification of the urine with ascorbic acid or ammonium chloride can enhance the elimination of weak bases (i.e., amphetamine, phencyclidine, and quinidine), this rarely is done in practice because of the associated risk of metabolic acidosis and myoglobinuria. Importantly, manipulation

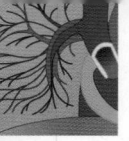
BOX 4-1	**SUBSTRATES, INHIBITORS, AND INDUCERS OF P-GLYCOPROTEIN**	
Substrate	**Inhibitor**	**Inducer**
Amiodarone	Amiodarone	Dexamethasone
Colchicine	Clarithromycin, erythromycin	Rifampin
Cyclosporine	Cyclosporine	Hypericum (St. John's wort)
Digoxin	Itraconazole, ketoconazole	
Erythromycin	Quinidine	
HIV protease inhibitors	Ritonavir	
Loperamide	Verapamil	
Lovastatin		
Morphine		
Tacrolimus		
Various anticancer agents (e.g., doxorubicin, etoposide, paclitaxel, teniposide, vincristine)		
Verapamil		

of urinary pH does not significantly influence the elimination of strong acids or bases, which are ionized throughout the physiologic range of urinary pH.

In addition to glomerular filtration, many drugs are actively transported into the lumen of the nephron. This generally is accomplished by one of three processes. The multidrug efflux pump P-glycoprotein (P-gp) is localized on the apical surface of proximal tubular epithelial cells and transports a wide variety of lipophilic compounds (Box 4-1), such as digoxin, colchicine, and many chemotherapeutic agents. It is encoded by the multidrug resistance protein (MDR1), named for the resultant resistance of tumor cells to vinca alkaloids and anthracyclines. Inhibition of P-gp by macrolide antibiotics, calcium channel antagonists, quinidine, and other compounds can lead to digoxin accumulation and toxicity. A variety of organic anion transport proteins (OATPs) have been characterized that nonselectively transport endogenous uric acid as well as benzyl penicillin, 3-hydroxy-3-methylglutaryl (HMG) coenzyme A inhibitors, and methotrexate. The OATPs can be inhibited by probenecid and nonsteroidal anti-inflammatory agents.[10,20] Similarly, organic cation transport

proteins (OCTPs) transport procainamide, triamterene, and the endogenous bases choline and histamine, and they are inhibited by quinidine.[21,22]

For drugs that are highly dependent on the kidney for elimination, the presence of renal disease hampers drug excretion and is a significant risk factor for the development of toxicity during therapeutic use. Appropriate dose adjustment and, when appropriate, selection of therapeutic alternatives can minimize the likelihood of this occurrence.

PHARMACOKINETICS

Clinical pharmacokinetics is the mathematical description of the time-dependent fate of a drug, toxin, or metabolite in the body. In other words, it is the study of "what the body does to the drug" as a function of time. Conversely, pharmacodynamics (discussed later in this chapter) describes "what a drug does to the body" as a function of dose or exposure.

The concentration of most drugs that are predominantly eliminated by the kidney can be considered to follow a "two compartment" pharmacokinetic model (Fig. 4-5). Following absorption, the drug distributes first into the *central compartment*, which includes the blood space and the richly perfused organs such as the heart, lungs, and kidneys. Once there, it may be eliminated by the kidney or undergo distribution into the peripheral compartment, which includes less well-perfused organs and tissues such as muscle and fat. A set of differential equations can be used to estimate changes in concentration and movement between compartments over time.

To illustrate, serum digoxin concentrations can be modeled using typical two-compartment pharmacokinetics. Following the oral administration of a single dose, a concentration-time curve of a drug can be generated, as shown in Figure 4-6. From the figure, three phases are apparent: an absorption phase, a distribution (α) phase, and an elimination (β) phase. The two latter phases can be described mathematically by the *half-life* (denoted as $t_{1/2\alpha}$ and $t_{1/2\beta}$, respectively). The elimination half-life ($t_{1/2\beta}$) is frequently reported in pharmacokinetic studies and reflects the time required for the drug concentration to decline by 50% after the drug is stopped.

The clinical applicability of the compartment concept is also illustrated by lithium, which is easily removed

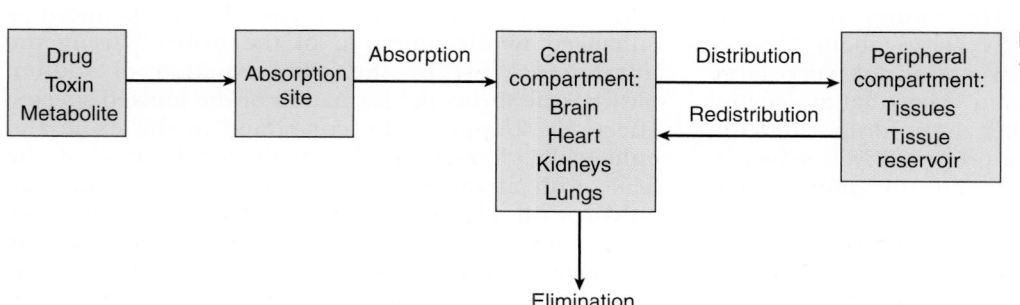

FIGURE 4-5 Example of a two-compartment model.

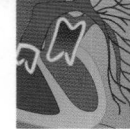

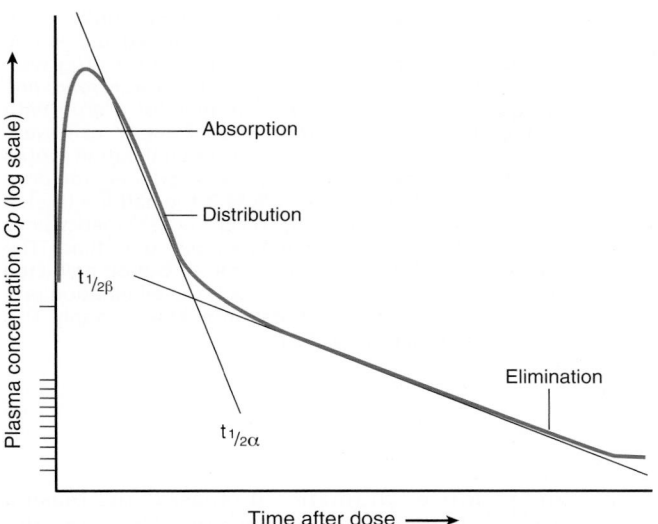

FIGURE 4-6 Phases of drug movement in a two-compartment model.

from the plasma compartment by hemodialysis. However, plasma concentrations rebound thereafter because lithium distributes slowly back into the vascular space from the tissue water compartment (Fig. 4-7). Similarly, the access of acetylsalicylic acid to the brain and other tissue compartments is strongly influenced by pH, and acidemia facilitates the movement of the nonionized acid across cellular membranes.

Other Types of Pharmacokinetic Models

Although compartmental models with first order transfer between compartments are widely used, they are mathematically abstract and have limited anatomical and physiologic relevance. *Physiologic pharmacokinetic models* use basic physiologic and biochemical data to describe the processes affecting chemical distribution and disposition. These models use a lumped *compartmental approach,* separating the body into a series of biologically relevant anatomical compartments of defined volumes, such as eliminating organ compartments (e.g., kidney and liver) and noneliminating tissue compartments (e.g., adipose tissue). All compartments are then connected in anatomical order based on the blood circulatory system to form an integrated model in which the transfer of drugs between compartments is governed by actual blood flow rates and tissue solubilities (partition coefficients). In contrast, *noncompartmental* pharmacokinetic models permit direct influx of drug into a central pool and indirect entry from a noncentral pool, as well as removal from either a central or a noncentral pool. The most significant advantage of noncompartmental models is that they do not assume specific compartments for chemicals or metabolites.

Types of Pharmacokinetic Processes

The elimination kinetics observed for a drug in vivo is generally described as either *first order* or *zero order.*

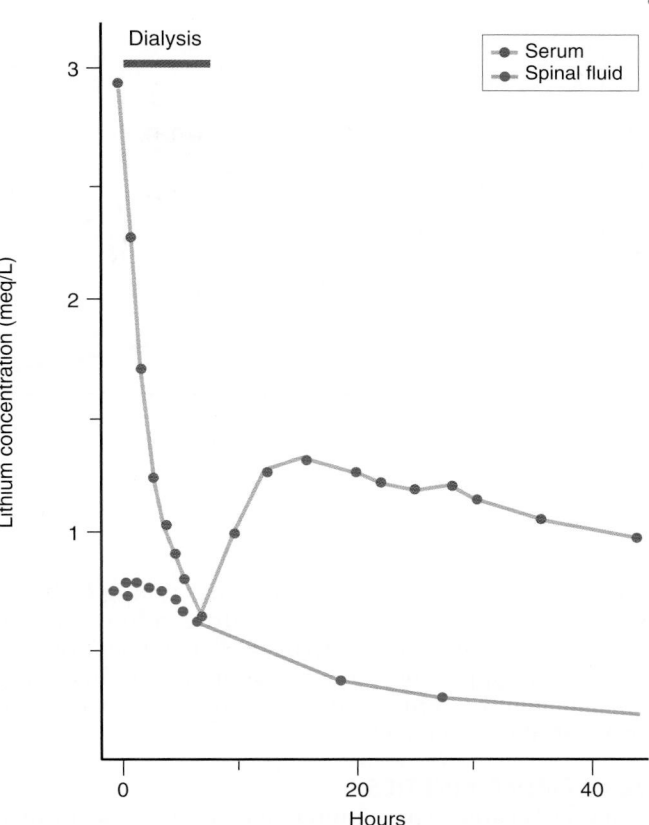

FIGURE 4-7 Serum and spinal fluid lithium levels in a 48-year-old lithium-intoxicated man who was anuric. Serum levels decline rapidly with dialysis and rise again as lithium redistributes from tissues. Spinal fluid levels respond slowly to changes in serum level. (From Amdisen A, Skoldborg H: Haemodialysis for lithium poisoning. Lancet 1969;2:213.)

Although the terms may at first seem confusing, they are conceptually straightforward.

FIRST ORDER KINETICS

Most drugs follow first order kinetics at therapeutic dosing, meaning that the rate at which they are eliminated from the body is directly proportional to the blood concentration. In other words, a constant proportion of the drug is eliminated per unit time. The concentration-time curve of first order drug elimination is curvilinear, but when plotted on a semilogarithmic graph (i.e., a graph with a logarithmic Y axis) yields a straight line (Fig. 4-8).

In an acutely poisoned patient, plotting serum concentrations against time allows for estimation of $t_{1/2\beta}$ after the calculation of the elimination rate constant (k_e), which is the fraction of drug eliminated per unit time, given by:

$$k_e = \frac{(\ln C_1 - \ln C_2)}{(t_2 - t_1)}$$

where C_1 and C_2 reflect drug concentration at different times t_1 and t_2, respectively. The elimination half-life is, therefore, inversely proportional to the first order elimination rate constant, given by:

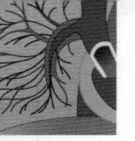

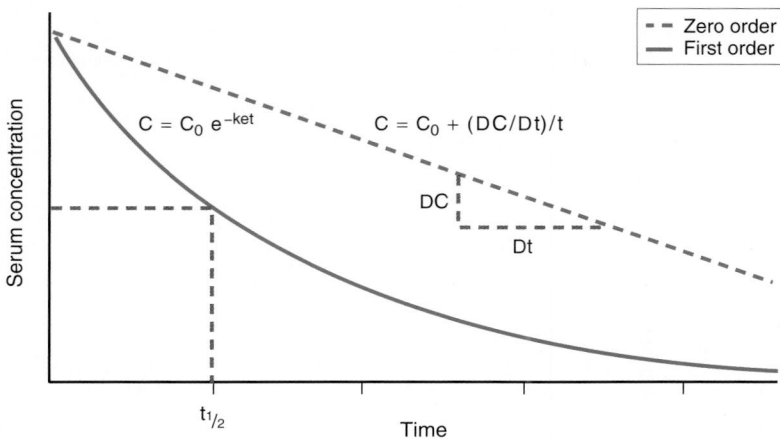

FIGURE 4-8 *Concentration-time curves under zero order and first order kinetics. The* dashed upper line *illustrates the concentration-time plot for a drug with zero order elimination, whereas the* lower solid line *illustrates the concentration-time plot for a drug with first order elimination. Note that if the Y axis were expressed logarithmically, first order elimination would appear as a straight line. The time required for drug concentration to decrease by 50% is the half-life ($t_{1/2}$), a concept that does not apply in zero order kinetics since a constant amount is eliminated per unit time. The concentration (C) at any given time (t) can be predicted from the formulas shown, although the elimination rate constant must be known if first order kinetics apply. This value is equivalent to $0.693 / t_{1/2}$.*

$$t_{1/2\beta} = \frac{\ln 2}{k_e} = \frac{0.693}{k_e}$$

Miscalculation of $t_{1/2\beta}$ occurs when the timing of blood samples is inaccurate or when drug administration (including absorption) is ongoing. The concept of half-life is only applicable under conditions of first order kinetics and represents the time needed for concentrations to fall by half.

ZERO ORDER KINETICS

Some medications are eliminated from the body in such a way that a constant amount (rather than a constant proportion) is removed per unit time. This sort of elimination is called *zero order kinetics* or *nonlinear pharmacokinetics* because a plot of concentration versus time is not described by a straight line on a semi-logarithmic graph. Important examples of drugs that exhibit zero order kinetics following typical doses include ethanol and acetylsalicylic acid. The rate of elimination is simply expressed as the fall in concentration per unit time.

MICHAELIS-MENTEN KINETICS

All active processes can be saturated, but they will appear not to be if the concentrations involved are below the limit of the saturable process. The rate of metabolism, therefore, depends on the substrate concentration in plasma (C_p), and is given by:

$$\text{Rate} = \frac{V_{max} \times C_p}{(K_m + C_p)}$$

where V_{max} is the maximum rate of metabolism (i.e., metabolic capacity) in mass per unit time and K_m is a constant with a value equal to the plasma concentration (mass per unit volume) at which the metabolic rate is half maximal. This is often referred to as *Michaelis-Menten kinetics.*

Because the metabolism of most drugs takes place at concentrations well below this threshold ($C_p \ll K_m$), these drugs exhibit first order kinetics. For some drugs however, saturation occurs at or near therapeutic concentrations. Above this threshold ($C_p > K_m$), elimination becomes zero order, and small increases in dose can produce dramatic increases in plasma concentrations. This concept is especially relevant in the setting of drug overdose, in which concentrations are often much higher than the normal therapeutic range.

Phenytoin is perhaps the best example of a drug exhibiting Michaelis-Menten kinetics, since its K_m values often overlap with therapeutic levels.[23] For phenytoin, values of V_{max} and K_m generally vary in adults from 100 to 1000 mg/day and 1 to 15 mg/L, respectively.[23,24]

Clearance

Drugs are eliminated from the body at varying rates. An important kinetic concept is the *clearance* of a drug, which is the rate of its elimination by all routes relative to its concentration in a biological fluid, given by:

$$\frac{\text{CL}}{\text{(volume per time)}} = \frac{\text{mass rate of elimination (mass per time)}}{\text{concentration (mass per volume)}}$$

Most often, the fluid of interest is blood or plasma, and these concentrations constitute the denominator of this equation. It follows that clearance can also be estimated from the slope of the elimination phase of the concentration versus time (k_e) when the volume of distribution is known:

$$\text{CL (volume per time)} = k_e \text{ (per time)} \times \text{Vd (volume)}$$

The rate of infusion or dosing of a medication can be substituted for mass rate of elimination in the equation above under steady-state conditions, to target a therapeutic serum concentration at steady state:

$$\frac{\text{Target concentration}}{\text{(mass per volume)}} = \frac{\text{dosing rate (mass per time)}}{\text{CL (volume per time)}}$$

By mass balance and integrating the definition of CL given above over time:

$$\text{CL (volume per time)} = \frac{\text{dose (mass)}}{\text{AUC (mass} \times \text{time/volume)}}$$

where AUC is the area under the concentration-time curve. Like Vd, clearance can sometimes assume very large

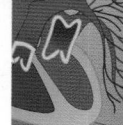

values that do not appear to be physiologic. For example, the clearance of transdermally administered nitroglycerin from venous blood may exceed 30 L per minute.

Clearance also may be thought of as the hypothetical volume of a fluid from which a substance is totally and irreversibly removed per unit time. However, because some drugs rely heavily on other organs such as the liver or bile, total body clearance (CL_{total}) is actually the sum of the clearance by all routes (i.e., CL_{kidney} + CL_{liver} + CL_{other}).

The clearance of a drug by an organ (or system) can be calculated if one knows the blood flow and drug concentrations in the afferent and efferent blood, using the following formula:

$$CL_{organ} = \frac{Q \times (C_{IN} - C_{OUT})}{C_{IN}}$$

where Q is blood flow (volume per time) and C_{IN} and C_{OUT} are the concentrations in incoming (often arterial) and outgoing (often venous) blood. The expression $(C_{IN} - C_{OUT}) / C_{IN}$ is sometimes termed the *extraction ratio*. If a drug is efficiently removed by an organ (typically the liver), the concentration of drug in efferent blood will be far lower than that in afferent blood and the extraction ratio will approach 1. Lidocaine, verapamil, and propranolol are examples of drugs with high hepatic extraction ratios.

The clearance of drugs and toxins can sometimes be markedly increased by hemodialysis. This is most effective with small, water-soluble molecules with minimal protein binding and a low V_d (i.e., do not partition extensively to tissues in the extravascular space), such as methanol. The clearance of drugs by a dialysis membrane can be calculated by sampling concentrations in both limbs of the dialysis circuit in a similar fashion, as outlined above.

Bioavailability

Bioavailability, denoted in pharmacokinetic equations by the symbol *F*, is the proportion of drug that reaches the systemic circulation. Following absorption, orally administered drugs entering the portal circulation may be partly metabolized by the liver. For some drugs, such as propranolol, this "first pass" metabolism is extensive and explains why oral doses often are much higher than intravenous doses. Inasmuch as it influences absorption (above), solubility also is an important determinant of bioavailability, with very hydrophilic drugs having limited absorption because they cannot easily pass through lipid membranes. Finally, some drugs are unstable at gastric pH (e.g., penicillin G), which significantly limits their bioavailability.

By definition, drugs administered by intravenous injection have F = 1, since all drug enters the blood space. The bioavailability of an orally administered drug can be determined experimentally by plotting serial measurements of drug concentration against the time from administration. Integrating the total area under this curve and multiplying by the clearance indicates the quantity of drug absorbed, which may then be compared

to the amount administered. For example, if 100 mg of a drug whose CL = 1 L/hour is administered by mouth and the calculated AUC is 75 mg × hour/L, then F = 0.75.

PHARMACODYNAMICS

Pharmacodynamics describes the effects of drugs and toxins on human physiology mediated by interactions with molecules within the patient. Such effects are a function of dose and duration of exposure to drugs, a relationship that can be expressed using dose-response curves. The quantitative relationship between the dose of a xenobiotic and the magnitude of its biological effect as it relates to poisoning often is termed *toxicodynamics*.

Targets of Drug Action

In most instances, drugs interact with specialized cellular proteins in ways that alter the function of the macromolecule and, consequently, the cell itself. These target proteins often involve enzymes, ion channels, carrier molecules, and receptors. Receptors can be located at various locations in a cell, including on its surface, within the cytoplasm, or in the nucleus. The endogenous compounds that bind to these receptors are termed *ligands* and include neurotransmitters, hormones, and other autacoids. Drug-receptor interactions mediate the biological effects of the vast majority of drugs. Notable exceptions include ethanol and the volatile anesthetics, such as halothane and enflurane, which may exert their effects by altering the physical chemistry of cell membranes.

The formation of a drug-receptor complex generates a biological response, which is a function of the number of drug-receptor complexes formed:

Drug + Receptor ↔ Drug-Receptor Complex → Response

This reaction is governed by the law of mass action, and the clinical effect is therefore proportional to drug dose. A *dose-response curve* describes the theoretical relationship between receptor occupancy and the clinical effect of a drug. The typical sigmoidal dose-response curve is shown in Figure 4-9. The X axis usually is expressed in logarithmic units and may represent a single administered dose, a serum concentration, an infusion rate at steady-state, or a more complex measure of exposure such as inhaled gas concentration multiplied by duration of exposure. The Y axis may represent the proportion that experiences a binary outcome, such as death in an animal study, or a continuous outcome, such as analgesia or fractional decrease in mean arterial pressure measured in a single individual.

RELATIONSHIP BETWEEN DOSE AND RESPONSE

A *graded dose-response curve* permits inference regarding the important concepts of *potency* and *efficacy*. Potency refers to the location of the curve along the X axis and describes the concentration of a drug needed to exert a specific physiologic effect. The potency of an agonist

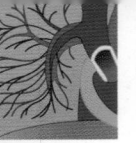

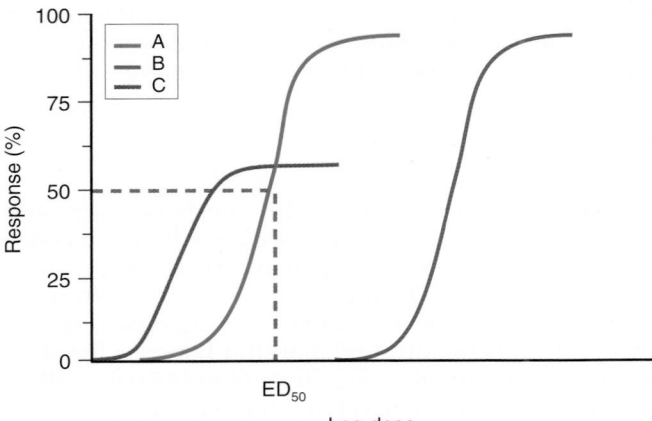

FIGURE 4-9 Dose-response curves of various agonists. Y axis represents degree of drug response, and X axis represents logarithm of dose. The dose-response curve for a strong agonist (drug A) shows that half-maximal effect occurs at dose ED_{50}. Drug B is a weaker agonist (i.e., a higher dose is required for the same effect as occurred with drug A) but has equal efficacy. This curve could also represent the dose-response curve for drug A in the presence of a noncompetitive antagonist. Drug C is a partial agonist, and, although it is more potent than drug C (which has a higher ED_{50}), it is less efficacious because it has a lower maximal efficacy.

often is expressed in terms of the concentration producing a half-maximal response (the EC_{50}). For example, hydromorphone is a more potent analgesic than morphine, and it therefore has a lower EC_{50} and a dose-response curve to the left of that produced by morphine. Efficacy, on the other hand, reflects the maximum effect that can be achieved with a drug and is reflected in the height of the dose-response curve. Hydromorphone and morphine have equal analgesic efficacy despite differences in potency.

Quantal dose-effect curves differ in that the Y axis reflects the percentage of individuals with a dichotomous event (e.g., seizure, systolic blood pressure < 80 mm Hg, or death). Such curves often are expressed in terms of the *median effective dose* (ED_{50}), the dose at which 50% of individuals exhibit the specified beneficial effect. If the quantal end point is death of a group of experimental animals, the *median lethal dose* (LD_{50}) is often reported. Assuming the threshold for attaining the response is normally distributed in the population, then the shape of the dose-response curve is described by the sigmoidal probit function, which is the cumulative area under a Gaussian normal distribution.

Agonists and Antagonists

Drugs that modulate receptor function can be characterized according to their effects relative to the endogenous ligand. An *agonist* elicits cellular and physiologic effects similar to those of an endogenous ligand. Agonists may be further classified according to the mechanism by which they produce this effect. Agonists that bind to and stimulate the receptor are termed *direct agonists*. Examples include pentobarbital at γ-aminobutyric acid

(GABA) receptors; phenylephrine and isoproterenol, which mimic the effects of norepinephrine and epinephrine at α- and β-adrenergic receptors, respectively; and methacholine, which mimics the actions of acetylcholine at muscarinic receptors. *Indirect agonists* have little or no inherent activity at receptors themselves, but they can enhance the activity of endogenous ligands by increasing the amount of ligand available for binding, either by enhancing its release, impeding its removal, or impairing its catabolism at or near the effector site. An example is physostigmine, which indirectly augments the activity of acetylcholine at muscarinic and nicotinic receptors by inhibiting its metabolism by acetylcholinesterase.

Conversely, *antagonists* reduce or abolish the effects of a drug or ligand. Antagonism can be mediated by a variety of processes. Most often, antagonists act by occupying receptor sites and preventing the binding of agonists. Common examples include naloxone (an opioid receptor antagonist), pancuronium and related compounds (which block the activity of acetylcholine at nicotinic receptors in the neuromuscular junction), and flumazenil (a benzodiazepine receptor antagonist).

Chemical antagonism describes the process whereby one agent hinders the effect of another by reacting or binding to it directly. The antidotes succimer (see Chapters 71, 73, and 74), dimercaprol (see Chapter 73), and hydroxycobalamin (see Chapter 88) are examples of chemical antagonists commonly encountered in clinical toxicology. *Pharmacokinetic antagonism* assumes special importance in toxicology. It refers to instances in which one drug reduces the effect of another by decreasing its absorption (e.g., activated charcoal),[25] enhancing its elimination (e.g., sodium bicarbonate for salicylate intoxication), or hastening its degradation or inactivation (rarely employed in clinical toxicology but typified experimentally by the use of butyrylcholinesterase as an antagonist of cocaine toxicity and hydrolase enzymes in the treatment of organophosphate poisoning).[26,27]

Agonists and antagonists can be classified further according to whether their effects are reversible (sometimes termed *surmountable*) or irreversible. The former is more common in clinical medicine, where agonists and antagonists often "compete" for the same receptors, and the clinical result reflects the balance of these processes. For example, 0.1 mg of naloxone is generally adequate to reverse the unwanted effects of morphine in many clinical settings, but a 50- to 100-fold higher dose may be needed in a patient with a large overdose of a more potent synthetic opioid. Irreversible agonists and antagonists are characterized by receptor dissociation that occurs very slowly or not at all, and is a characteristic feature of interactions involving covalent binding. Some clinically relevant examples include phenoxybenzamine, an irreversible inhibitor of catecholamine activity at α-adrenergic receptors, and soman, which irreversibly inhibits acetylcholinesterase (following dealkylation).

Whereas the number of available receptors for a given ligand or drug can be considered static in the acute setting, changes in receptor density can occur over time as part of an adaptive response. *Up-regulation* (or sensitization) refers to an increase in receptor density

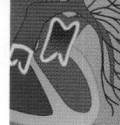

resulting from low levels of the endogenous ligand or chronic exposure to an antagonist, while *down-regulation* (or desensitization) denotes a decrease in receptor density with prolonged exposure to large amounts of ligand or persistent exposure to another agonist. *Up-regulation* and *down-regulation* also may result from alterations in postreceptor processes (i.e., downstream signaling protein changes) and occur independently of changes in receptor density. In general, when *down-regulation* has occurred, a decreased effect is noted with continued or subsequent exposure to the same concentration of a xenobiotic.

The term *toxicodynetics* has been proposed to describe the time course of toxic effects in poisoned patients. Increasingly complicated mechanistic or empirical mathematical models are being used to estimate when such toxicity is likely to occur and how long it should last, as in the example of circulating blood cell counts following chemotherapy. The models build upon pharmacokinetic concepts, but they describe the drug effect (rather than the serum drug concentration) as a function of time.[28]

GENETIC VARIABILITY IN DRUG RESPONSE

One of the most rapidly developing areas in pharmacology is the burgeoning appreciation of the determinants of individual variability in drug response. Genetic variation can influence any aspect of a drug's absorption, metabolism, distribution, or excretion, and it can also modulate its effects at the site of action.[16]

Genetic Differences in Drug Response

Pharmacogenomics is the study of the many different genes that influence drug response, whereas *pharmacogenetics* denotes the study of inherited variations in drug metabolism and response. Like other hereditary traits, genetically determined differences in drug response are subject to significant ethnic and geographic variability, with clustering in specific populations. In most instances, variability results from single-nucleotide polymorphisms (SNPs) that can yield a gene product with only one different amino acid residue but a dramatically less functional protein. Less commonly, genetic polymorphisms or multiple allelic duplication can result in increased functional activity of the resultant protein.[29]

The influence of genetic variability on drug absorption and excretion is perhaps best illustrated by polymorphisms in the multidrug efflux pump P-glycoprotein (P-gp). The C/C genotype is associated with greater P-gp activity and is present in 83% of individuals from West Africa but only 26% of Caucasians.[30,31] This polymorphism confers decreased bioavailability as well as enhanced renal and biliary clearance of P-gp substrates such as digoxin, cyclosporine, and protease inhibitors (see Box 4-1), and it conversely imparts greater clinical relevance to P-gp inhibition by drugs such as macrolide antibiotics and azole antifungals.[9,32]

Genetic variability also influences the biotransformation of many drugs and can involve either phase I or phase II metabolism.[16] Polymorphisms in the CYP450 system (Table 4-3) can have dramatic effects on the safety and efficacy of treatment. For example, the antihypertensive agent debrisoquine is no longer in clinical use today because approximately 7% of Caucasian patients who took the drug experienced a profound hypotensive response. Originally labeled "debrisoquine sensitive," these patients were later found to have no functional debrisoquine hydroxylase, an enzyme now referred to as CYP2D6. Polymorphisms of CYP2C9 also are common, and they can dramatically enhance the hypoglycemic effects of glyburide and the hypoprothrombinemic response to warfarin, two common drugs that rely heavily on CYP2C9 for inactivation.[33-35]

Genetic variation in phase II metabolism is perhaps best illustrated by variation in the metabolism of isoniazid and other drugs containing aromatic amines or

		TABLE 4-3 Selected Pharmacogenetic Variants of Drug Metabolizing Enzymes	
ENZYME	**APPROXIMATE FREQUENCY OF POOR METABOLIZER PHENOTYPE**	**EXAMPLES OF CLINICALLY RELEVANT SUBSTRATE DRUGS**	**CLINICAL CONSEQUENCE OF POOR METABOLIZER PHENOTYPE**
CYP2C9	15% of Caucasians*	(S)-warfarin	Heightened sensitivity to anticoagulant effect
CYP2D6	4% of Africans/Asians* 7%–10% of Northern Europeans 1% in Asians, Indians	Glyburide and other sulfonylureas Codeine Cyclic antidepressants Methamphetamine, MDMA Metoprolol	Enhanced hypoglycemic response Decreased conversion to morphine; reduced analgesic effect Enhanced drug effect Enhanced drug effect/toxicity Slightly enhanced drug effect
Butyrylcholinesterase (pseudocholinesterase)	1 in 3500 Caucasians	Succinylcholine	Markedly prolonged paralysis
N-Acetyltransferase-2	40%–70% in Caucasians 18% in Japanese	Isoniazid Hydralazine Procainamide	Enhanced drug effect
Thiopurine *S*-Methyltransferase	1 in 300 Caucasians 1 in 2500 Asians	Azathioprine Mercaptopurine	Enhanced drug effect

*Frequency of genetic polymorphisms conveying at least moderate reductions in metabolic capacity.

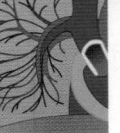

hydrazine moieties, such as procainamide, dapsone, and hydralazine. The expression of *N*-acetyltransferase 2 (*NAT2*) in liver and gut mucosa is highly polymorphic, resulting in a bimodal distribution of plasma isoniazid concentrations. Patients with the slow acetylator phenotype (approximately 40% to 70% of Caucasians and 10% to 30% of Asians) exhibit reduced presystemic extraction (i.e., higher bioavailability) and slower elimination of isoniazid. Slow acetylator status may enhance the effectiveness of therapy yet increase the risk of isoniazid-associated complications such as neuropathy and hepatitis.[36,37]

Future Applications of Pharmacogenomics

As the many genetic variations within the human genome are more completely characterized, anticipating the response of a patient to a drug before treatment is initiated will become increasingly possible.[38] To accomplish this, an individual's DNA would be sequenced for the presence of specific SNPs. Whereas this was previously a laborious, expensive process, DNA microarrays are increasingly available as a tool for the rapid identification of thousands of SNPs in an individual patient's genome within a few hours.[38]

Such technology may predict not only a drug's efficacy but also the likelihood of toxicity. For example, several polymorphisms in the β_2-adrenergic receptor have been described.[39] These polymorphisms significantly influence the clinical response to albuterol and may modulate its arrthymogenicity.[40] Indeed, in the near future it is probable that the enrollment of patients in clinical trials will be governed by whether they will experience benefit or harm from a drug, as determined by their genetic makeup. Although this will make it easier for clinical trials to identify treatment effects, it will also likely hamper the generalizability of results to patients whose genetic makeup is different or not known.

ACKNOWLEDGMENT

Drs. B. C. Metts, Jr., W. J. Hunter, and J. Ambre wrote previous editions of this chapter.

REFERENCES

1. Green R, Sitar DS, Tenenbein M: Effect of anticholinergic drugs on the efficacy of activated charcoal. J Toxicol Clin Toxicol 2004;42:267–272.
2. Wacher VJ, Salphati L, Benet LZ: Active secretion and enterocytic drug metabolism barriers to drug absorption. Adv Drug Deliv Rev 2001;46:89–102.
3. Dresser GK, Bailey DG: The effects of fruit juices on drug disposition: a new model for drug interactions. Eur J Clin Invest 2003;33 (Suppl 2):10–16.
4. Bailey DG, Dresser GK: Interactions between grapefruit juice and cardiovascular drugs. Am J Cardiovasc Drugs 2004;4:281–297.
5. Markowitz JS, DeVane CL: The emerging recognition of herb-drug interactions with a focus on St. John's wort (Hypericum perforatum). Psychopharmacol Bull 2001;35:53–64.
6. Ruschitzka F, Meier PJ, Turina M, et al: Acute heart transplant rejection due to Saint John's wort. Lancet 2000;355:548–549.
7. Breidenbach T, Kliem V, Burg M, et al: Profound drop of cyclosporin A whole blood trough levels caused by St. John's wort (Hypericum perforatum). Transplantation 2000;69:2229–2230.
8. Gualandi-Signorini AM, Giorgi G: Insulin formulations—a review. Eur Rev Med Pharmacol Sci 2001;5:73–83.
9. Fromm MF: P-glycoprotein: a defense mechanism limiting oral bioavailability and CNS accumulation of drugs. Int J Clin Pharmacol Ther 2000;38:69–74.
10. Kim RB: Organic anion-transporting polypeptide (OATP) transporter family and drug disposition. Eur J Clin Invest 2003;33(Suppl 2):1–5.
11. Benet LZ, Hoener BA: Changes in plasma protein binding have little clinical relevance. Clin Pharmacol Ther 2002;71:115–121.
12. Rodriguez M, Ortega I, Soengas I, et al: Alpha-1-acid glycoprotein directly affects the pharmacokinetics and the analgesic effect of methadone in the rat beyond protein binding. J Pharm Sci 2004;93:2836–2850.
13. Israili ZH, Dayton PG: Human alpha-1-glycoprotein and its interactions with drugs. Drug Metab Rev 2001;33:161–235.
14. Guengerich FP: Role of cytochrome P450 enzymes in drug-drug interactions. Adv Pharmacol 1997;43:7–35.
15. Michalets EL: Update: clinically significant cytochrome P-450 drug interactions. Pharmacotherapy 1998;18:84–112.
16. Weinshilboum R: Inheritance and drug response. N Engl J Med 2003;348:529–537.
17. Dresser GK, Bailey DG: A basic conceptual and practical overview of interactions with highly prescribed drugs. Can J Clin Pharmacol 2002;9:191–198.
18. Mitchell JR, Nelson SD, Thorgeirsson SS, et al: Metabolic activation: biochemical basis for many drug-induced liver injuries. Prog Liver Dis 1976;5:259–279.
19. Eyer F, Meischner V, Kiderlen D, et al: Human parathion poisoning. A toxicokinetic analysis. Toxicol Rev 2003;22:143–163.
20. Mikkaichi T, Suzuki T, Tanemoto M, et al: The organic anion transporter (OATP) family. Drug Metab Pharmacokinet 2004;19:171–179.
21. Perri D, Ito S, Rowsell V, Shear NH: The kidney—the body's playground for drugs: an overview of renal drug handling with selected clinical correlates. Can J Clin Pharmacol 2003;10:17–23.
22. Lee W, Kim RB: Transporters and renal drug elimination. Annu Rev Pharmacol Toxicol 2004;44:137–166.
23. Levy RH: Phenytoin: biopharmacology. Adv Neurol 1980;27:315–321.
24. Richens A: Clinical pharmacokinetics of phenytoin. Clin Pharmacokinet 1979;4:153–169.
25. Buckley NA, Whyte IM, O'Connell DL, Dawson AH: Activated charcoal reduces the need for *N*-acetylcysteine treatment after acetaminophen (paracetamol) overdose. J Toxicol Clin Toxicol 1999;37:753–757.
26. Sun H, Shen ML, Pang YP, et al: Cocaine metabolism accelerated by a re-engineered human butyrylcholinesterase. J Pharmacol Exp Ther 2002;302:710–716.
27. Petrikovics I, Hong K, Omburo G, et al: Antagonism of paraoxon intoxication by recombinant phosphotriesterase encapsulated within sterically stabilized liposomes. Toxicol Appl Pharmacol 1999;156:56–63.
28. Krzyzanski W, Jusko WJ: Multiple-pool cell lifespan model of hematologic effects of anticancer agents. J Pharmacokinet Pharmacodyn 2002;29:311–337.
29. Kirchheiner J, Henckel HB, Meineke I, et al: Impact of the CYP2D6 ultrarapid metabolizer genotype on mirtazapine pharmacokinetics and adverse events in healthy volunteers. J Clin Psychopharmacol 2004;24:647–652.
30. Kurata Y, Ieiri I, Kimura M, et al: Role of human MDR1 gene polymorphism in bioavailability and interaction of digoxin, a substrate of P-glycoprotein. Clin Pharmacol Ther 2002;72:209–219.
31. Schaeffeler E, Eichelbaum M, Brinkmann U, et al: Frequency of C3435T polymorphism of MDR1 gene in African people. Lancet 2001;358:383–384.
32. Yu DK: The contribution of P-glycoprotein to pharmacokinetic drug-drug interactions. J Clin Pharmacol 1999;39:1203–1211.
33. Taube J, Halsall D, Baglin T: Influence of cytochrome P-450 CYP2C9 polymorphisms on warfarin sensitivity and risk of over-

anticoagulation in patients on long-term treatment. Blood 2000;96:1816–1819.

34. Niemi M, Cascorbi I, Timm R, et al: Glyburide and glimepiride pharmacokinetics in subjects with different CYP2C9 genotypes. Clin Pharmacol Ther 2002;72:326–332.

35. Kirchheiner J, Brockmoller J: Clinical consequences of cytochrome P450 2C9 polymorphisms. Clin Pharmacol Ther 2005;77:1–16.

36. Clark DW: Genetically determined variability in acetylation and oxidation. Therapeutic implications. Drugs 1985;29:342–375.

37. Huang YS, Chern HD, Su WJ, et al: Polymorphism of the N-acetyltransferase 2 gene as a susceptibility risk factor for anti-tuberculosis drug-induced hepatitis. Hepatology 2002;35:883–889.

38. Evans WE, McLeod HL: Pharmacogenomics—drug disposition, drug targets, and side effects. N Engl J Med 2003;348:538–549.

39. Dishy V, Sofowora GG, Xie HG, et al: The effect of common polymorphisms of the beta2-adrenergic receptor on agonist-mediated vascular desensitization. N Engl J Med 2001;345:1030–1035.

40. Israel E, Chinchilli VM, Ford JG, et al: Use of regularly scheduled albuterol treatment in asthma: genotype-stratified, randomised, placebo-controlled cross-over trial. Lancet 2004;364:1505–1512.

5

Drug Interactions

MICHAEL W. SHANNON, MD, MPH

Over the past 5 years there has been an explosion of interest in the causes of adverse drug effects and potential mechanisms for preventing them. In the monograph *To Err is Human*, The Institute of Medicine identified medication-related adverse events as a leading cause of preventable death.[1] One area of concern has been adverse effects that result from drug-drug interactions, particularly since many of these effects are predictable.

The modification of drug effects has the potential to reduce the effectiveness of a drug, enhance the drug's toxicity, or both. Also, adverse interactions do not occur only between drugs; they can occur between drugs and diet (e.g., potentiation of calcium channel blockers by grapefruit juice), drugs and environmental agents (e.g., photosensitivity eruptions in those exposed to sunlight while taking sulfonamides or tetracyclines), drugs and alternative remedies (e.g., potentiation of Coumadin-induced anticoagulation by tonka beans), and between drugs and substances of abuse (e.g., serotonin syndrome in those taking monoamine oxidase inhibitors who use methylenedioxymethamphetamine [Ecstasy]).[2]

Drugs may interact with each other through a number of different mechanisms, which may be classified as pharmaceutical, pharmacokinetic, or pharmacodynamic (Box 5-1). Interactions through any of these mechanisms may result in unpredictable clinical effects or toxicologic responses. Pharmaceutical interactions include those that produce drug inactivation when compounds are physically mixed together before administration. For example, aminoglycosides are inactivated by certain β-lactam antibiotics when these drugs are mixed together in the same intravenous fluid. Pharmacokinetic interactions can occur when the disposition characteristics of one compound (i.e., absorption, distribution, metabolism, or excretion) are influenced by those of another. This type of interaction may involve one or more specific aspects of a drug's pharmacokinetic profile. For example, a compound may displace a drug from its protein-binding sites, consequently increasing its elimination from the body. Finally, drugs may interact pharmacodynamically (i.e., compete for the same receptor or physiologic system), altering a patient's response to drug therapy.[3] A small group of drugs is involved in serious drug interactions with some frequency (Box 5-2).

The number of known, clinically important drug interactions, combined with the ever-increasing number of available pharmacologic agents underscores the need to understand the pharmacologic basis of drug interactions. This chapter reviews the pharmacokinetic and pharmacodynamic basis of drug interactions, using clinically important interactions as examples.

EPIDEMIOLOGY

The prevalence of adverse drug interactions has been estimated to range between 2.2% and 30% in hospitalized patients and 9.2% and 70.3% in ambulatory patients.[4-7] The emergency department is a focal point for the diagnosis or development of adverse drug reactions; emergency department surveillance data suggest that adverse drug events account for 7 per 1000

BOX 5-1	PRIMARY MECHANISMS OF CLINICALLY IMPORTANT DRUG INTERACTIONS

Pharmaceutical
Drug compatibility
Drug stability

Pharmacokinetic
Absorption
Distribution
Metabolism
Excretion

Pharmacodynamic
Receptor binding
Receptor reactivity
Enzyme inhibition
   Competitive
   Noncompetitive

BOX 5-2	DRUGS COMMONLY INVOLVED IN SERIOUS DRUG INTERACTIONS

Cyclosporine
Erythromycin
Fluconazole
Itraconazole
Ketoconazole
Monoamine oxidase inhibitors
Meperidine
Phenytoin
Protease inhibitors
Rifampin
Selective serotonin reuptake inhibitors (SSRIs)
Theophylline
Warfarin

Adapted from Kohn LT, Corrigan JM, Donalson MS (eds): To Err is Human: Building a Safer Health System. Washington, DC, The Institute of Medicine, National Academy Press, 1999.

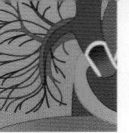
visits.[8] The events take on multiple origins. First, patients may present to the emergency department with manifestations of an adverse drug reaction. In cases in which the diagnosis of drug interaction is not obvious, the emergency physician may be unsuspecting; the patients may even be discharged without the diagnosis being made. For example, serotonin syndrome, which often is the result of a drug interaction, is commonly overlooked by clinicians from all specialties.[9] Additionally, an estimated 70% to 85% of emergency department encounters result in prescription therapy.[10] The emergency physician therefore has a significant role in making therapeutic decisions that do not result in a predictable drug interaction.

PHARMACOKINETIC MECHANISMS OF DRUG INTERACTIONS

Gastrointestinal Absorption

Absorption is defined as the translocation of drug from its site of administration into the systemic circulation. Drugs administered extravascularly, by the oral, sublingual, or intramuscular routes, must cross several membranes to reach the systemic circulation before distribution to their sites of action. The process of absorption can be divided into and influenced by two distinct domains: rate and extent. Both domains are influenced by the physico-chemical properties of the drug as well as various host factors. The physicochemical properties of a drug that affect absorption include molecular weight, degree of lipid solubility, extent of ionization at physiologic pH, and type of formulation (e.g., tablet, capsule, or liquid).

Several potential types of interactions between two or more compounds can influence the rate or amount of drug absorption from the gut (Box 5-3). For example, foods or drugs capable of altering gastrointestinal pH could theoretically modify the absorption characteristics of a compound by altering the proportion of drug that is in its ionized, less lipid-soluble state. Thus, coadministra-tion of antacids, histamine-2 (H_2) receptor antagonists, or proton pump inhibitors, all which alter gastro-intestinal pH, could substantially influence the amount of drug—particularly a weak base—that is absorbed from

TABLE 5-1 Selected Clinically Important Interactions Due to Alteration of Drug Absorption	
DRUG	**COMPOUND AFFECTED**
Antacids	Captopril
	Ketoconazole
	Isoniazid
Cholestyramine	Digitalis glycosides
	Thyroid hormone
Sucralfate	Ciprofloxacin
	Digoxin
	Ketoconazole
	Phenytoin
	Quinolone antibiotics
	Tetracycline
	Theophylline
	Valproic acid

the stomach.[11] Conversely, these drugs, by decreasing gastric acid secretion, might promote an increase in the absorption of acid-labile drugs (e.g., penicillin G). Concomitant administration of antacids with other medications can lead to clinically important interactions arising from the gastrointestinal and chemical effects of the aluminum, calcium, and magnesium ions liberated from the antacid preparation.[11] For example, a clinically relevant interaction occurs between antacids and quinolone antibiotics (Table 5-1). Other agents may affect drug absorption. Cholestyramine resin also has been shown to reduce the systemic absorption of common pharmaceuticals. Sucralfate, another treatment for gastritis, can lower the absorption of digoxin, phenytoin, and quinolone antibiotics significantly.

Drugs that affect gastrointestinal motility may influence the gastrointestinal absorption of orally administered drugs by controlling the rate of drug delivery to the major absorptive surfaces, as well as the duration of contact with these surfaces.[12] For example, coadministration of an anticholinergic agent has been shown to increase the rate and extent of digoxin absorption; conversely, digoxin absorption appears to decrease after metoclopramide administration.[13] Co-administration of gastric promotility agents (e.g., metoclopramide) has been shown to decrease the time to peak serum drug concentration (T_{max}) and increase the peak serum drug concentration (C_{max}), but in general it has no appreciable effect on the drugs' overall extent of bioavailability.[12] Consequently, the clinical significance of this drug interaction is unclear. Interestingly, the magnitude of the effect of gastro-intestinal promotility agents on the T_{max} and C_{max} of orally administered drugs appears to be more common and much greater when the motility agent is administered intravenously rather than orally.

Distribution

Drug distribution describes the movement of a pharma-cologically or toxicologically active moiety from the systemic circulation into various body compartments,

BOX 5-3	MECHANISMS INVOLVED IN INTERACTIONS THAT AFFECT DRUG ABSORPTION FROM THE GASTROINTESTINAL TRACT

Alteration of gastric emptying rate or gastrointestinal motility
Modification of volume, composition, or viscosity of gastrointestinal secretions
Effects of pH on drug ionization and dissolution
Effects of mucosal and bacterial drug metabolism
Interactions with active transport systems
Alterations of splanchnic blood flow
Complexation and chelate formation
Toxic effects on gastrointestinal mucosa

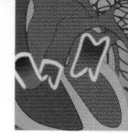

tissues, and cells. The pharmacokinetic parameter estimate, volume of distribution (Vd), is an apparent value that attempts to describe the relationship between the amount of drug in the body, including the blood. The process of distribution depends on the partition coefficient of a drug between blood and tissue, regional blood flow, and the extent of binding to plasma protein or tissues.

Alterations in drug distribution most commonly result from the displacement of bound drug from circulating plasma proteins. Acidic compounds typically bind albumin whereas basic compounds bind predominantly to α_1-acid glycoprotein.[3,14] The free or unbound fraction of a compound is the pharmacologically active moiety, capable of traversing cellular membranes, diffusing into tissues, and binding to receptors. As such, changes in drug binding that result in an increase in the amount of free drug may increase the amount of drug available for tissue distribution, increasing the drug's concentration at the site of action and amplifying its effect. For example, the displacement of Coumadin from serum albumin-binding sites by other highly protein-bound compounds (e.g., aspirin) represents a classic example of such an interaction.[3] This traditional view of simple competitive displacement of drug from circulating proteins, however, is based on a number of assumptions, many of which have not been clinically validated.[3,14]

A number of variables may directly influence the physiologic impact of a drug displacement interaction. For such reactions to be important clinically, both compounds must be at least 80% bound to the same protein species. In addition, the displaced compound must exhibit capacity-limited body clearance or have a relatively small apparent Vd (<0.15 L/kg).[3,14] This last factor is likely to be the most important, because as the Vd increases, less of the total amount of drug in the body is present in the plasma compartment. Thus, with proportionately less compound to displace and a larger "space" in which to distribute, the effect of a displacement interaction would be minimal. Finally, it is important to recall that increasing the amount of free drug concurrently increases the amount of compound available for metabolism or excretion and can result in an accelerated elimination rate for the displaced drug.[3]

The physiologic impact of drug-drug protein displacement reactions clearly depends on the balance among a large number of variables. Importantly, after a drug overdose there is great uncertainty about the impact of a single large dose of a displacing agent on the overall biodisposition of the displaced agent. Moreover, the magnitude and duration of the interaction are determined by the normal saturability of the drug-plasma protein complex. In some cases, protein binding for some highly protein-bound drugs has clinical significance in overdose. For example, an increase in free valproic acid concentration appears to make the drug easier to remove by extracorporeal drug removal techniques, such as hemodialysis.[15,16] These preliminary reports confirm the importance of identifying potential changes in the extent of protein binding for highly protein-bound drugs; any significant change in the amount of free, unbound drug could affect the timing and severity of clinical manifestations and the approach to treatment.

Changes in a drug's Vd that result from altered tissue binding, although rare, are exemplified by the now well-known interaction between digoxin and quinidine.[17] The decrease observed in quinidine Vd and the concurrent increase in serum digoxin concentrations most likely are due to digoxin tissue-binding displacement by quinidine. These changes in digoxin pharmacokinetics have been noted to occur after administration of a single dose of quinidine. In addition to causing tissue displacement, quinidine also decreases the renal and nonrenal clearance of digoxin. Quinine, the S-isomer of quinidine, also has been shown to interfere with nonrenal clearance of digoxin.[18]

Metabolism

Drug metabolism is divided into the two general categories of phase I and phase II transformation reactions.[19] Phase I reactions involve structural alteration of drug, typically by processes including oxidation, hydrolysis, and reduction. Phase II reactions most commonly involve conjugation of a water-soluble moiety to the parent drug. Phase II reactions include glucuronidation, sulfation, and methylation.[20] Most phase I reactions are performed by the cytochrome P-450 family of isoenzymes.

The cytochrome P-450 (CYP450) enzymes are found primarily in the gut and liver. Their name is derived from the characteristic of maximal absorption at a wavelength of 450 nm. According to current nomenclature, the cytochrome isoenzymes are grouped into families (1, 2, and 3), divided into subfamilies (A through E), and specified by number.

The cytochrome isoenzymes have many features that give them great variability in action, both within and among individuals. As a result, they and their activity are a common cause of drug interactions, particularly drug-drug interactions.[21] The four most important variables that affect CYP450 activity are genetic heterogeneity, age-related changes, enzyme induction, and enzyme inhibition.

The genes encoding for each drug-metabolizing enzyme can develop mutations that result in the production of a protein that has decreased, increased, or absent enzymatic activity.[22] Examples of CYP450 isoenzymes with clinically important genetic polymorphisms include CYP2D6 and CYP2E1. Such polymorphisms can lead to unexpected drug responses.[23] However, over the last decade, technology that permits both genotypic and phenotypic probing of the cytochrome enzymes has greatly improved the ability to identify individuals with abnormal activity. This growing field of pharmacogenetics has greatly increased the ability to reduce the risk of developing adverse drug reactions by identifying susceptible individuals before their receipt of the drug.[24-29]

The development of CYP450 enzyme activity occurs progressively in postnatal life and undergoes additional changes throughout life. Consequently, the risk of devel-

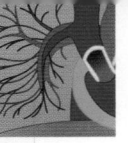

oping a drug interaction often is a function of patient age. As an example, CYP1A2 has negligible activity in the newborn[30]; after reaching peak activity in adults, it appears to have waning activity in the elderly years.

Induction refers to an increase in enzyme activity. Induction results either from increased production of enzyme (through enhanced transcription and translation) or through a reduction in the natural rate of enzyme breakdown.[29] Not all cytochrome enzymes are inducible; of the major isoenzymes, CYP1A2, CYP2C9, CYP2E1, and CYP3A are best known for having clinically relevant inducers.

CYP450 enzyme inhibition is classified as either reversible or irreversible. The most common type, *reversible inhibition*, occurs when a second substrate competes with the primary drug for the active site of the enzyme. This process also may be referred to as *competitive inhibition*. An example of such inhibition occurs after the coadministration of diltiazem and cyclosporine. Diltiazem is a reversible inhibitor of CYP3A4, the enzyme responsible for the elimination of cyclosporine. Diltiazem coadministration interferes with cyclosporine clearance, resulting in higher serum cyclosporine concentrations. Competitive inhibition is transient with the enzyme returning to normal activity once the inhibitor has been cleared. In *irreversible inhibition*, a substrate binds to a CYP450 enzyme, sometimes altering the enzyme structure and producing permanent enzyme inactivation. With irreversible inhibition, only synthesis of new enzyme can restore its normal physiologic function. Monoamine oxidase inhibitors produce such permanent effects on the enzyme.

Drugs used to treat HIV infection have a significant propensity for drug-drug interaction via the CYP450 isoenzymes.[31]

The six cytochrome isoenzymes of greatest importance are described in more detail below and are summarized in Table 5-2. Many reviews of CYP450 function and drug interactions have been recently published.[19,20,29]

CYP1A2

Many commonly used medications, including caffeine, theophylline, tricyclic antidepressants, and warfarin, are metabolized by CYP1A2. Activity of CYP1A2 can be induced by tobacco smoke, charbroiled foods, and cruciferous vegetables. Several medications induce CYP1A2 activity, including phenytoin, phenobarbital, and rifampin. Omeprazole and ritonavir simultaneously may induce CYP1A2 and inhibit one or more other CYP isoenzymes. Inhibitors of CYP1A2 include erythromycin, ciprofloxacin, fluvoxamine, and grapefruit juice.

CYP2C9

CYP2C9 is responsible for the metabolism of medications including ibuprofen, phenytoin, and warfarin. Rifampin is a powerful inducer of CYP2C9 activity and therefore decreases serum concentrations of its substrates. Amiodarone, fluoxetine, and fluconazole are among several drugs known to inhibit CYP2C9 activity. Genetic polymorphisms occur in 1% to 3% of Caucasians, contributing to abnormally decreased enzyme activity in these individuals.

CYP2C19

Medications metabolized by CYP2C19 include several benzodiazepines, citalopram, tricyclic antidepressants, and omeprazole. Rifampin induces CYP2C19 activity, whereas fluvoxamine, fluoxetine, and ritonavir inhibit this enzyme. Genetic polymorphisms are responsible for

---

TABLE 5-2 Substrates, Inducers, and Inhibitors of Major Human Cytochromes

CYTOCHROME	SUBSTRATES	INDUCERS	INHIBITORS
CYP1A2	Caffeine, theophylline, tricyclic antidepressants, warfarin	Charbroiled food, omeprazole, phenobarbital, phenytoin, tobacco smoke	Erythromycin, fluvoxamine, grapefruit juice, quinolone antibiotics
CYP2C9	Diclofenac, glipizide, ibuprofen, phenytoin, tolbutamide, warfarin,	Phenobarbital, Rifampin	Amiodarone, cimetidine, fluconazole, fluoxetine, itraconazole, ketoconazole, metronidazole, ritonavir
CYP2C19	Diazepam, imipramine, nelfinavir, omeprazole, pantroprazole, propranolol,	Rifampin	Fluoxetine, fluvoxamine, omeprazole, ritonavir, sertraline
CYP2D6	Codeine, dextromethorphan, flecainide, fluoxetine, haloperidol, metoprolol, paroxetine, perphenazine, propranolol, sertraline, timolol, tricyclic antidepressants, venlafaxine		Cimetidine, dextromethorphan, fluoxetine, haloperidol, paroxetine, sertraline
CYP2E1	Acetaminophen, ethanol	Disulfiram	Ethanol, isoniazid
CYP3A	Alprazolam, astemizole, atorvastatin, carbamazepine, cisapride, cyclosporine, diltiazem, losartan, lovastatin, midazolam, nifedipine, simvastatin, terfenadine, theophylline verapamil	Carbamazepine, ethanol, phenobarbital, phenytoin, rifampin, St. John's wort	Cimetidine, clarithromycin, cyclosporine, diltiazem, erythromycin, fluoxetine, fluvoxamine, grapefruit juice, HIV protease inhibitors, itraconazole, ketoconazole, nifedipine, verapamil

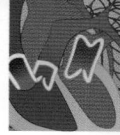

significant interpatient variability in CYP2C19 activity. The enzyme is absent in 13% to 23% of Asians and 3% of Caucasians.[29]

CYP2D6

CYP2D6 comprises a relatively small percentage (2% to 6%) of the total cytochrome P-450 in the liver but is involved in the metabolism of many medications (up to 25%). Multiple tricyclic antidepressants, β blockers, haloperidol, sertraline, paroxetine, and thioridazine are among the common drugs metabolized by CYP2D6. Interestingly, the conversion of codeine to the active form, morphine, is catalyzed by CYP2D6; patients with low CYP2D6 activity demonstrate a poor analgesic response to codeine.[32] There are no significant inducers of this activity. However, several medications inhibit CYP2D6, the most potent being cimetidine, fluoxetine, haloperidol, and paroxetine. Genetic polymorphisms play a significant role in determining CYP2D6 activity. Approximately 1% to 3% of African American and Asian patients and 5% to 10% of Caucasians lack this enzyme, placing them at risk for increased toxicity from medications that are metabolized by CYP2D6.[32] A subpopulation with higher than usual activity also has been described ("extensive and ultrarapid metabolizers").[25,26,33]

CYP2E1

Although CYP2E1 metabolizes a relatively small fraction of medications, it plays a significant role in the activation and inactivation of many agents. CYP2E1 metabolizes small organic molecules (e.g., ethanol, carbon tetrachloride) as well as acetaminophen and dapsone. Although only a small percentage of acetaminophen is metabolized by CYP2E1, the drug's hydroxylation produces N-acetyl-p-benzoquinone imine (NAPQI), the putative molecule responsible for acetaminophen hepatotoxicity. Chronic ethanol use can induce CYP2E1 activity, leading to a greater percentage of acetaminophen metabolized to NAPQI, increasing the risk of hepatotoxicity from acetaminophen use. Many scientists question the existence of an important ethanol-acetaminophen interaction.[34,35]

CYP3A

CYP3A is the most abundant, clinically significant group of cytochrome P-450 isoenzymes. The CYP3A group is composed of four major isoenzymes: CYP3A3, CYP3A4, CYP3A5, and CYP3A7. CYP3A4 is the most common and is implicated in the majority of drug interactions. However, since these enzymes are so closely related (having as much as 97% sequence homology), they often are referred to collectively by the subfamily name, CYP3A. Up to 60% of the liver's total cytochrome P-450 is CYP3A, and nearly 50% of all clinically relevant medications are metabolized by CYP3A. The presence of CYP3A in the small intestine results in decreased bioavailability of many ingested drugs. CYP3A inducers include the glucocorticoids, rifampin, carbamazepine, phenobarbital, and phenytoin. Among the many significant CYP3A inhibitors are grapefruit juice, erythromycin, ketoconazole, clarithromycin, and verapamil.

NONMICROSOMAL DRUG METABOLISM ENZYMES

A number of compounds can impair or directly inhibit hepatic drug metabolism by interacting with non-CYP450 (nonmicrosomal) enzymes. Disulfiram (Antabuse) is a potent inhibitor of the nonmicrosomal enzyme acetaldehyde dehydrogenase, which is responsible for the metabolism of ethanol to acetic acid. Concurrent ethanol consumption and disulfiram administration leads to acetaldehyde accumulation and the classic Antabuse reaction, characterized by unpleasant symptoms that include facial flushing, throbbing headache, nausea, vomiting, sweating, palpitations, hypotension, and syncope. Another important nonmicrosomal reaction is the serotonin syndrome that results from administration of agents such as meperidine by patients who are taking monoamine oxidase inhibitors.[9]

Acetylation by the enzyme N-acetyltransferase (NAT) is another important, non-CYP pathway of drug metabolism. Dapsone, hydralazine, isoniazid, procainamide, and the sulfonamides are examples of drugs metabolized via acetylation. Acetylation polymorphisms are well described. Variants in the alleles coding for NAT occur in 50% of Americans, Caucasian and black, resulting in slow acetylator status. Slow acetylator phenotypes occur in 60% to 70% of Northern Europeans and 5% to 10% of Asians. Slow acetylators have an increased risk of drug toxicity, but they also experience longer drug effectiveness. Those with the fast acetylator phenotype may fail to experience the desired therapeutic response to treatment as a result of the rapid metabolism of drug.

Elimination

The most common pathway by which drugs or their metabolites are eliminated from the body is via the kidneys. Interactions that influence renal clearance of a compound primarily alter the physiologic processes of glomerular filtration, tubular reabsorption, or active tubular secretion. Additionally, agents that alter renal blood flow also may influence renal elimination. Nevertheless, for such interactions to be of clinical importance, the overall elimination of active drug must depend primarily on renal mechanisms. For example, as discussed earlier, displacement interactions may transiently increase the amount of free drug in the vascular compartment, resulting in an increase in the amount of drug available to be filtered by the glomeruli and excreted.

In contrast to displacement interactions, a number of drugs can directly influence glomerular filtration through other mechanisms. The nonsteroidal anti-inflammatory drugs (NSAIDs)—aspirin, ibuprofen, indomethacin, naproxen, and others—all have been shown to reversibly depress renal function. This drug-induced decrease in renal function most likely is a result of NSAIDs' inhibition of renal prostaglandin synthesis and can result in increased side effects because of accumulation of other concurrently administered drugs (e.g., lithium).

Modification of the passive distal tubular reabsorption of weak acids and bases is another mechanism by which

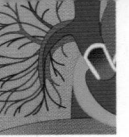

drugs may interact and represents a potentially important therapeutic modality in the treatment of certain intoxications. An inverse relationship exists between the compound's degree of ionization and the overall amount of a compound reabsorbed from the urine—that is, the greater the amount of compound present in the urine in the un-ionized, more lipid-soluble state, the greater the amount reabsorbed. In general, for renal clearance to be sensitive to changes in urine pH, acidic and basic drugs must have pK_a values that range between 3 to 7.5 and 7 to 11, respectively. This principle of altering urinary pH has been used in the management of a number of drug intoxications, particularly those by salicylates and phenobarbital. Alkalization of urine by either intermittent or continuous intravenous infusion of sodium bicarbonate can significantly decrease distal tubular reabsorption of both of these drugs. Intra-luminal trapping of acids in their ionized form appears to be greatest when urine pH exceeds 7.5.[36] Although the manipulation of urinary pH to promote ion trapping and to augment renal clearance appears desirable, it is not without risk. Rapidly raising urinary pH requires an increase in blood pH, a change that may be undesirable and possibly detrimental in certain instances.[36,37] Furthermore, clinicians must weigh carefully the associated risks of pH manipulation and the time necessary to achieve effective changes in urinary pH with the effectiveness of other therapeutic modalities and, most important, with the anticipated duration of serious symptoms.[36]

Finally, biliary secretion represents an often over-looked but relatively important means for the elimination of a number of drugs and substrates, and a pathway with which drug interactions may occur. Parent compounds or their metabolites excreted via the bile may be reabsorbed into the systemic circulation from the distal ileum. This process of enterohepatic circulation is an important mechanism responsible for delayed and prolonged drug absorption and elimination of a number of commonly used drugs (e.g., carbamazepine). Increasing the total body clearance of such compounds by interfering with the enterohepatic circulation is the basis for administering repeated doses of oral activated charcoal as a therapeutic intervention to patients who experience intoxications involving compounds that undergo substantial enterohepatic circulation.[38]

Drug–Nutrient Interactions

Nutritional habits may influence dramatically the response to pharmacologic intervention. The type and quantity of food consumed as well as the overall nutritional status of a patient may directly or indirectly alter drug disposition characteristics. For example, there is an extensive list of nutrients that interact with warfarin action (Box 5-4). The specific composition of a meal can markedly alter drug absorption. The most notable example of food-associated inhibition of drug absorption involves the complexation of tetracycline compounds when coadministered with divalent cation-containing compounds (e.g., milk, cheese, antacids, vitamins). However, it is unusual for such an interaction to result in significantly decreased systemic bioavailability. What occurs more frequently is that the rate but not the overall extent of drug absorption is decreased when the drug is administered in the presence of food. The intestinal absorption of some commonly administered drugs, such as acetaminophen, digoxin, many penicillin and cephalosporin analogs, and phenytoin, may be delayed or reduced when these agents are given in the presence of food.[39] Conversely, the bioavailability of some orally administered drugs, including spironolactone, griseo-fulvin, and cefuroxime axetil, can be increased when the drugs are administered in the presence of food.

Coadministration of certain medications with enteral nutrition formulas may result in altered drug absorption and poor therapeutic effect. Subtherapeutic patient responses have been noted in patients receiving carbamazepine or phenytoin when these drugs are co-administered with enteral formulas.[39,40] The mechanism of this drug-nutrient interaction is unknown but clearly exceeds simple drug adherence to the feeding tubing. To minimize the effect that enteral nutrition formulas may have on the bioavailability of these drugs, the tube feeding should be stopped and the tubing flushed approximately 1 to 2 hours before drug administration. Tube feeding can be resumed 1 to 2 hours later.

BOX 5-4	FOODS THAT INTERACT WITH WARFARIN

Vegetables

Alfalfa
Asparagus
Broccoli
Brussels sprouts
Cabbage
Cauliflower
Kale
Lettuce
Onions
Spinach
Turnip greens
Watercress

Herbal Products

Ginseng
Green teas
Melilot
Tonka beans
Woodruff

Miscellaneous

Avocado
Fish oils
Liver
Soybeans
Papain

From Manzi S, Shannon M: Drug interactions—a review. Clin Ped Emerg Med 2005;6:93–102.

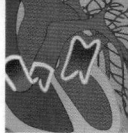

Both hepatic drug metabolism and renal elimination can be influenced by the type and quantity of nutrient consumed. Cabbage, Brussels sprouts, and cauliflower all have been shown to contain bioactive indoles that are potent inducers of intestinal and hepatic drug-metabolizing enzymes. Conversely, compounds present in grapefruit juice are capable of inhibiting the activity of both cytochrome and noncytochrome enzymes.[41] Diets high in protein (e.g., >40% of total calories) have been shown to increase the metabolic capacity of the hepatic mixed-function oxidase system; this results in increased clearances of a number of drugs (e.g., propranolol). This increase in body clearance is not observed when similar quantities of either carbohydrate or fat are substituted for protein. In addition, diets deficient in protein are associated with altered renal hemodynamics, a condition that leads to marked decreases in glomerular filtration, which further influences a drug's body clearance and pharmacodynamics.

Pharmacodynamic Mechanisms of Drug Interactions

In patients receiving multiple drugs, the overall effects manifested are a summation of the similar or opposing but independent actions of these multiple agents on a given cell or organ system. These interactions historically have not been considered drug interactions, yet many are of extreme clinical importance. These interactions are properly termed *pharmacodynamic drug interactions* and are thought to involve drug-receptor interactions, either directly or indirectly.

The types of interactions that might occur at the receptor level are varied. Moreover, the understanding of these interactions often is confounded because simple potentiation or antagonism is distinctly uncommon. Most of these interactions occur through an interplay of receptor mechanisms controlling the function of a given tissue or organ system. In a similar fashion, drugs may interact with physiologic or biochemical control loops, a process that leads to alterations in response to normal stimuli and input signals. Finally, one drug may prevent access of another to its site of action, and thus the pharmacodynamic process is abrogated.

Direct Receptor Effects

In a few instances, drug interactions occur through direct receptor site antagonism. Consider, for example, an asthmatic patient receiving the β_2-adrenergic agonist bronchodilator albuterol who develops angina and is treated with propranolol. The nonselective blocker propranolol clearly has the potential to inhibit the bronchodilator effect of the β_2-adrenergic agonist drug. The use of specific receptor agonists or antagonists (e.g., naloxone, phentolamine) represents desired interactions at the receptor level that are of immense clinical importance in the treatment of poisoned patients.

Another example of direct pharmacodynamic interaction can occur during therapy with the warfarin anticoagulants. Quinidine appears to augment the cellular uptake of warfarin, increasing warfarin's effective concentration at the site of action.

Indirect Receptor Effects

Pharmacodynamic interactions associated with indirect receptor effects are side effects of one drug that mimic the pharmacologic effects of another. Augmentation of the hypoglycemic effects of insulin and oral hypoglycemic agents by nonselective β-blocking agents is an example of agents with differing mechanisms of action that produce the same clinical effects.

The use of drugs with actions on the myocardium, cardiac conduction system, or capacitance and resistance vessels predisposes to a large number of pharmacodynamic interactions. Calcium channel blockers and β-adrenergic receptor antagonists often augment the myocardial depressant, bradycardiac, and hypotensive effects of one another when used in concert. Other effects augmented by the simultaneous administration of vasoactive drugs and β-adrenergic blocking agents include exacerbation of first-dose hypotensive effects of prazosin and enhancement of the hypertensive response during clonidine withdrawal.

The proliferation of NSAIDs (prescription and over-the-counter) have focused attention on a number of serious interactions that may occur with these agents. The sodium and water retention that result from long-term use of these agents may blunt the antihypertensive effects of angiotension-converting enzyme inhibitors (e.g., captopril, enalapril, and others), thiazide diuretics, and β-adrenergic blocking agents. These effects also may offset the benefits of diuretic therapy in mild to moderate congestive heart failure.

SUMMARY

Drug interactions remain an important consequence of pharmacologic intervention. It is clear that the pharmacologic response of a drug can be markedly influenced by concurrent administration of another therapeutic agent or food. These interactions may result in a decreased therapeutic effect or in an increase in the amount and extent of untoward reactions. Despite the well-described and real clinical consequences of certain drug interactions, this aspect of patient care often continues to be overlooked.

Drugs can interact via a number of pharmaceutical, pharmacokinetic, or pharmacodynamic mechanisms. These interactions may occur as a result of concurrently prescribed therapeutic modalities, environmental variables, or the patient's specific habits, such as diet, alcohol use, and tobacco use. The increasingly predictable nature of drug interactions underscores how important it is for all health care practitioners to understand the mechanisms of drug interactions, anticipate the possibility of their occurrence, and, ideally, prevent them.

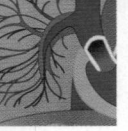

REFERENCES

1. Kohn LT, Corrigan JM, Donalson MS (eds): To Err is Human: Building a Safer Health System. Washington, DC, The Institute of Medicine, National Academy Press, 2000.
2. Parrott AC: Recreational Ecstasy/MDMA, the serotonin syndrome, and serotonergic neurotoxicity. Pharmacol Biochem Behav 2002;71:837–844.
3. Frazee LA, Reed MD: Warfarin and nonsteroidal antiinflammatory drugs: why not? Ann Pharmacother 1995;29:1289–1291.
4. Gosney M, Tallis R: Prescription of contraindicated and interacting drugs in elderly patients admitted to the hospital. Lancet 1984;2:564–567.
5. Kinney EL: Expert system detection of drug interactions: results in consecutive inpatients. Comput Biomed Res 1986;19:462–467.
6. Dambro MR, Kallgren MA: Drug interactions in a clinic using COSTAR. Comput Biol Med 1988;18:31–38.
7. Shinn AF, Shrewsbury RP, Anderson KW: Development of a computerized drug interaction database (MEDICOM) for use in a patient specific environment. Drug Inf J 1983;17:205–210.
8. Budnitz DS, Pollock DA, Mendelsohn AB, et al: Emergency department visits for outpatient adverse drug events: demonstration for a national surveillance system. Ann Emerg Med 2005;45:197–206.
9. Boyer EW, Shannon M: The serotonin syndrome. N Engl J Med 2005;352:1112–1120.
10. Manzi S, Shannon M: Drug therapy in the pediatric emergency department. In Yaffe SJ, Aranda JV (eds): Neonatal and Pediatric Pharmacology. Philadelphia, Lippincott Williams & Wilkins, 2005 pp 278–307.
11. Sadowski DC: Drug interactions with antacids. Mechanisms and clinical significance. Drug Saf 1994;11:395–407.
12. Greiff JM, Rowbotham D: Pharmacokinetic drug interactions with gastrointestinal motility modifying agents. Clin Pharmacokinet 1994;27:447–461.
13. Kirch W, Janisch AD, Santos SR, et al: Effect of cisapride and metoclopramide on digoxin bioavailability. Eur J Drug Metab Pharmacokinet 1986;11:249–250.
14. Sansom LN, Evans AM: What is the true clinical significance of plasma protein binding displacement interactions? Drug Saf 1995;12:227–233.
15. Guillaume CP, Stolk L, Dejagere TF, Kooman JP: Successful use of hemodialysis in acute valproic acid intoxication. J Toxicol Clin Toxicol 2004;42:335–336.
16. Kielstein JT, Woywodt A, Schumann G, et al: Efficiency of high-flux hemodialysis in the treatment of valproic acid intoxication. J Toxicol Clin Toxicol 2003;41:873–876.
17. Schenck-Gustafsson K, Jogestrand T, Nordlander R, Dahlqvist R: Effect of quinidine on digoxin concentration in skeletal muscle and serum in patients with atrial fibrillation. Evidence for reduced binding of digoxin in muscle. N Engl J Med 1981;305:209–211.
18. Wandell M, Powell JR, Hager WD, et al: Effect of quinine on digoxin kinetics. Clin Pharmacol Ther 1980;28:425–430.
19. Manzi S, Shannon M: Drug interactions—a review. Clin Ped Emerg Med 2005;6:93–102.
20. Shannon M: Drug-drug interactions and the cytochrome P450 system: an update. Ped Emerg Care 1997;13:350–353.
21. Zhou S, Yung Chan S, Cher Goh B, et al: Mechanism-based inhibition of cytochrome P450 3A4 by therapeutic drugs. Clin Pharmacokinet 2005;44:279–304.
22. Ingelman-Sundberg M: Polymorphism of cytochrome P450 and xenobiotic toxicity. Toxicology 2002;181–182:447–452.
23. Pirmohamed M, Park BK: Cytochrome P450 enzyme polymorphisms and adverse drug reactions. Toxicology 2003;192:23–32.
24. Phillips KA, Veenstra DL, Oren E, et al: Potential role of pharmacogenomics in reducing adverse drug reactions: a systematic review. JAMA 2001;286:2270–2279.
25. Ma MK, Woo MH, McLeod HL: Genetic basis of drug metabolism. Am J Health Syst Pharm 2002;59:2061–2069.
26. Caraco Y: Genes and the response to drugs. N Engl J Med 2004;351:2867–2869.
27. Tsai YJ, Hoyme HE: Pharmacogenomics: the future of drug therapy. Clin Genet 2002;62:257–264.
28. Rogers JF, Nafziger AN, Bertino JS Jr: Pharmacogenetics affects dosing, efficacy, and toxicity of cytochrome P450-metabolized drugs. Am J Med 2002;113:746–750.
29. Sikka R, Magauran B, Ulrich A, Shannon M: Bench to bedside: pharmacogenomics, adverse drug interactions, and the cytochrome P450 system. Acad Emerg Med 2005;12:1227–1235.
30. Tateishi T, Asoh M, Yamaguchi A, et al: Developmental changes in urinary elimination of theophylline and its metabolites in pediatric patients. Pediatr Res 1999;45:66–70.
31. Piscitelli SC, Gallicano KD: Interactions among drugs for HIV and opportunistic infections. N Engl J Med 2001;344:984–996.
32. Cascorbi I: Pharmacogenetics of cytochrome p4502D6: genetic background and clinical implication. Eur J Clin Invest 2003;33 (Suppl 2):17–22.
33. Gasche Y, Daali Y, Fathi M, et al: Codeine intoxication associated with ultrarapid CYP2D6 metabolism. N Engl J Med 2004; 351:2827–2831.
34. Rumack BH: Acetaminophen misconceptions. Hepatology 2004;40:10–15.
35. Rumack BH: Acetaminophen hepatotoxicity: the first 35 years. J Toxicol Clin Toxicol 2002;40:3–20.
36. Proudfoot AT, Krenzelok EP, Vale JA: Position paper on urine alkalinization. J Toxicol Clin Toxicol 2004;42:1–26.
37. Albertson TE, Dawson A, de Latorre F, et al: TOX-ACLS: toxicologic-oriented advanced cardiac life support. Ann Emerg Med 2001;37(4 Suppl):S78–S90.
38. American Academy of Clinical Toxicology, European Association of Poisons Centres and Clinical Toxicologists: Position statement and practice guidelines on the use of multi-dose activated charcoal in the treatment of acute poisoning. J Toxicol Clin Toxicol 1999;37:731–751.
39. Doak KK, Haas CE, Dunnigan KJ, et al: Bioavailability of phenytoin acid and phenytoin sodium with enteral feedings. Pharmacotherapy 1998;18:637–645.
40. Clark-Schmidt AL, Garnett WR, Lowe DR, Karnes HT: Loss of carbamazepine suspension through nasogastric feeding tubes. Am J Hosp Pharm 1990;47:2034–2037.
41. Bailey DG, Dresser GK: Interactions between grapefruit juice and cardiovascular drugs. Am J Cardiovasc Drugs 2004;4:281–297.

6

Acid–Base, Fluid, and Electrolyte Balance

MICHAEL SHANNON, MD, MPH

The poisoned patient commonly presents with acid–base, volume, and electrolyte disturbances. The purpose of this chapter is to discuss the basic principles of acid–base balance, the regulation of body fluid volumes, intracellular and extracellular fluid, and electrolyte composition. Aberrations of these are common among intoxicated patients; an understanding of their basis and the rationale for certain intervention strategies are key in management.

ACID–BASE DISORDERS

Acid–base homeostasis may be affected by a toxic substance or its metabolite (primary disturbance) or by dysfunction or failure of various organ systems (secondary disturbance). In addition, disorders may arise because of an intervention (e.g., gastric lavage that leads to metabolic alkalosis or the use of cathartics that leads to hypernatremic dehydration).

Fundamental Concepts of Acid–Base Homeostasis

The pH of body fluids is regulated within a narrow range because of the participation and interplay of several regulatory systems. The most important systems are the lungs and the respiratory control center of the central nervous system (CNS), the kidney, and the body's buffer systems. The most important buffer system is the *bicarbonate-carbonic acid system,* which regulates extracellular bicarbonate level and partial pressure of carbon dioxide (pCO_2), the pCO_2 is regulated by the respiratory center and pulmonary system. Endogenous production of carbon dioxide leads to an increase in its concentration, which, in combination with water, forms carbonic acid; carbonic acid then readily dissociates to hydrogen ion and bicarbonate:

$$CO_2 + H_2O \rightarrow H_2CO_3 \rightarrow H^+ + HCO_3^-$$

From this equation, the Henderson-Hasselbalch derivation is made, which states that

$$pH = pK_a + \log (HCO_3^-)/(pCO_2)$$

where pH is the logarithm of hydrogen ion concentration, reflecting plasma acidity and representing the balance between serum bicarbonate level and pCO_2 (the respiratory component). The normal serum bicarbonate level is 24 to 28 mEq/L, and the normal PCO_2 is 36 to 44 mm Hg.

Definitions

ACIDEMIA VERSUS ALKALEMIA

When serum pH is less than 7.36, the patient has acidemia; when serum pH is greater than 7.44, the patient has alkalemia. The pH itself indicates neither the origin of the disorder nor whether there is physiologic compensation in response to the initial disorder. In contrast, acidosis and alkalosis are disease states that, if left unopposed, can change the plasma pH. If the initial change in bicarbonate level or PCO_2 is severe enough to override the body's buffer and defense mechanisms, then acidemia or alkalemia ensues. Acidosis or alkalosis can be present without concomitant acidemia and alkalemia, particularly if there is secondary compensation (e.g., in respiratory alkalosis accompanying a severe lactic metabolic acidosis secondary to septicemia, such that the pH is normal or even alkalemic despite the presence of metabolic acidosis).

METABOLIC VERSUS RESPIRATORY DISTURBANCES

A *metabolic acid–base disorder* is a disturbance caused by a change in serum bicarbonate level. *Metabolic acidosis* is defined as a decrease in serum bicarbonate level to less than 24 mEq/L, whereas *metabolic alkalosis* is defined as an increase in the serum bicarbonate level to more than 28 mEq/L. In contrast, a *respiratory acid–base disorder* refers to a disorder caused by a change in the PCO_2. *Respiratory acidosis* is defined as a PCO_2 greater than 44 mm Hg, and *respiratory alkalosis* is defined as a decrease in PCO_2 to less than 36 mm Hg. Physiologically, when these disturbances occur, secondary defenses, or compensatory mechanisms, are set into play with a goal of minimizing any change in serum pH. In the normal host, metabolic acidosis results in hyperventilation and a decrease in PCO_2, whereas metabolic alkalosis leads to secondary hypoventilation and an increase in PCO_2. These respiratory changes, particularly hyperventilation, may be blunted or absent in severely intoxicated patients. Respiratory acidosis leads to increased renal reabsorption of bicarbonate and net acid excretion, increasing the serum bicarbonate level, whereas respiratory alkalosis leads to an increase in the renal excretion of bicarbonate accompanied by a decrease in the serum bicarbonate level. These physiologic responses are proportional to the magnitude of the initial disorder and tend to return pH toward normal—but never completely to normal.

SIMPLE/MIXED ACID–BASE DISORDERS

A *simple acid–base disorder* is defined as a single disturbance with an appropriate accompanying secondary physiologic response. A response that is disproportionate in magnitude to the appropriate response—for instance, marked respiratory acidosis accompanied by only a mild increase in serum bicarbonate level—implies the coexistence of another primary disorder and therefore is a *mixed acid–base disorder.* Mixed acid–base disorders are common particularly in critically ill poisoned patients,

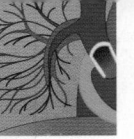

such as those with salicylate poisoning who have both metabolic acidosis and respiratory alkalosis and those with ethanol intoxication who have a lactic acidosis with a concomitant respiratory acidosis occurring because of the drug's CNS depressant effect.

METABOLIC ACIDOSIS

Metabolic acidosis, characterized by a serum bicarbonate level of less than 24 mEq/L usually, but not always, is accompanied by a decrease in bicarbonate level to give a pH of less than 7.36, and thus results in acidemia. Four general mechanisms produce metabolic acidosis: a loss of extracellular bicarbonate greater than extracellular chloride (e.g., with diarrhea or renal tubular acidosis); gain of hydrogen ions exogenously or endogenously, with subsequent metabolic consumption of extracellular bicarbonate (e.g., as with formic acid production after methanol ingestion or lactic acidosis from metformin use); failure to excrete the body's obligatory daily acid load (e.g., as in renal failure); and dilution of extracellular bicarbonate. With the initial decrease in serum bicarbonate level and subsequent acidemia, secondary mechanisms initiate the return of pH toward normal. These mechanisms include extracellular buffering, intracellular buffering, the renal excretion of the acid load, and the respiratory compensatory response. Following an acid load, bicarbonate, the most important extracellular buffer, is called into action to buffer acid loss, milliequivalent for milliequivalent. After several hours, intracellular buffers also participate and buffer approximately 55% to 60% of the acid load. Excess extracellular hydrogen ions then enter the cell in exchange for sodium and potassium ions. In general, metabolic disorders such as metabolic acidosis tend to cause a greater shift of intracellular potassium to the extracellular space than do respiratory disorders. Bicarbonate itself can cause shifts of potassium ions without changes in pH. In organic acidosis, the organic acid ions (i.e., keto acids or lactic acid) can enter cells with the excess hydrogen ions, whereas chloride cannot. Therefore, organic acidosis does not cause significant potassium redistribution when compared with mineral acidosis. Although the described mechanisms act in concert to minimize drastic changes in pH, the kidney alone possesses the ability to generate new bicarbonate by excreting the excess hydrogen ions. This process begins early but takes several days and occurs due to an increase in both ammonium excretion and titratable acidity.

An initial decrease in pH stimulates the ventilatory response mediated both by peripheral chemoreceptors and the medullary receptors in the CNS, which respond to changes in cerebral interstitial pH. A characteristic of the ventilatory response is an increase in tidal volume more so than in respiratory rate. Although occurring within minutes to hours, the maximum ventilatory response to metabolic acidosis may take 12 to 24 hours and probably reflects slow movement of hydrogen ions across the relatively impermeable blood-brain barrier. The ventilatory protective effect lasts only several days,

probably because P_{CO_2} lowers renal bicarbonate reabsorption and results in an appropriate bicarbonate loss. Secondary hyperventilation is a physiologic response to an initial aberration in homeostasis and should be proportional to the initial decrease in serum bicarbonate level. Mathematically, the appropriate P_{CO_2} response is determined by the following equation:

$$P_{CO_2} = 1.5(HCO_3^-) + 8$$

which defines a predictable relationship between P_{CO_2} and bicarbonate for any degree of metabolic acidosis. Any P_{CO_2} responses outside the predicted range would imply the presence of a secondary primary disturbance—that is, a mixed acid–base disturbance. For example, in severe metabolic acidosis, the serum bicarbonate of 10 mEq/L would have an expected P_{CO_2} response of approximately 23 mm Hg; a P_{CO_2} greater than this would suggest concomitant respiratory acidosis along with metabolic acidosis. Conversely, if P_{CO_2} were less than 23 mm Hg, respiratory alkalosis with concomitant metabolic acidosis would occur. Metabolic acidosis is described as either high or normal anion-gap acidosis. The anion gap equals the serum sodium level minus the sum of the serum chloride and serum bicarbonate levels, and it represents other unmeasured anions not accounted for by chloride and bicarbonate, such as plasma proteins and albumin, needed to maintain electric neutrality. The normal anion gap is 12 ± 2 (range, 8 to 16 mEq/L). If serum albumin is less than 4 g/dL, a corrective addition of 3 for each gram of albumin below 4 must be added.

Elevated Anion-Gap Metabolic Acidosis

Metabolic acidosis with a high anion gap results from an accumulation of organic and inorganic acids and a subsequent decrease in extracellular bicarbonate level. Common causes of metabolic acidosis are listed in Box 6-1. Patients with elevated anion-gap acidosis frequently have multiple severe electrolyte disorders, a greater frequency of admission to intensive care units, and a greater

BOX 6-1	**CAUSES OF ELEVATED ANION-GAP METABOLIC ACIDOSIS**

Cyanide
Ethylene glycol
Formaldehyde
Ibuprofen
Inborn errors of metabolism
Ketoacidosis
   Diabetic ketoacidosis
   Alcohol ketoacidosis
   Starvation
Lactic acidosis
Metabolic acidosis
Methanol
Renal failure
Salicylate
Toluene

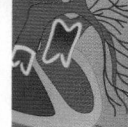

mortality rate compared with those with a normal anion gap. Most often, elevated anion-gap acidosis is accompanied by identifiable increases in organic acids levels (e.g., as in salicylate, ethylene glycol, and methanol ingestions and in lactic acidosis). Severe salicylate ingestions are associated with anion gaps in the range of 15 to 20 mEq/L, whereas ethylene glycol and methanol ingestions and lactic acidosis are associated with anion gaps greater than 30 mEq/L. Although an anion gap is most commonly associated with metabolic acidosis, it also may be present in metabolic alkalosis. This can be explained on the basis of coexisting elevated anion-gap acidosis and metabolic alkalosis (the mixed metabolic disorder), an alkalemia-induced increase in lactic acid production, or an increase in the negative charges on plasma proteins. Other causes are dehydration, therapy with sodium salts, strong acids, and certain antibiotics. Occasionally, organic acidosis (e.g., ketoacidosis) may be associated with a normal anion-gap metabolic acidosis if the organic acid excretion in catabolism equals the rate of organic acid production. Because excess organic acids are buffered milliequivalent for milliequivalent by extracellular bicarbonate, any elevation in anion gap is accompanied by a proportional decrease in serum bicarbonate level. Therefore, examination of both the decrease in serum bicarbonate level and the increase in the anion gap may suggest a mixed metabolic disorder. For instance, if the decrease in serum bicarbonate concentration is greater than the increment in the anion gap, another mechanism other than the elevated anion-gap acidosis is causing a decrease in serum bicarbonate (e.g., hyperchloremic metabolic acidosis), which therefore constitutes the mixed elevated-normal anion-gap acidosis. On the other hand, an increase in the anion gap exceeding the decrement in serum bicarbonate level suggests that another mechanism is responsible for an increase in serum bicarbonate level (i.e., metabolic alkalosis), which now constitutes a mixed elevated anion-gap metabolic acidosis/metabolic alkalosis. In lactic acidosis, the ratio of change in the anion gap to the change in serum bicarbonate is approximately 1.6 to 1.24, owing to buffering of much of the acidosis in the intracellular space.

The osmolal gap also may be helpful in establishing the diagnosis of an elevated anion-gap acidosis. The osmolal gap is the difference between the measured and the calculated plasma osmolality and is given by the following formula:

$$\text{Serum osmolality} = 1.8 \times Na^+ + \text{blood glucose (mg/dL)}/18 + \text{BUN (mg/dL)}/2.8$$

If the measured osmolality exceeds the calculated osmolality by 10 mOsm/kg or greater, then other osmotically active substances such as ethanol, methanol, ethylene glycol, isopropanol, and mannitol are present (see Chapters 1 and 32 for further discussion of the osmolal gap).

RENAL FAILURE

Acute renal failure and chronic renal failure are common causes of elevated anion-gap acidosis. The metabolic acidosis of renal failure is the result of the inability to excrete the acid load. The anions contributing to the elevated anion gap are predominantly sulfate, phosphate, and other unmeasured ions. In chronic renal failure, the anion gap usually is normal until the glomerular filtration rate decreases to below 30 mL/min and is accompanied by an anion-gap increase to 17 to 23 mEq/L. Drug-induced causes of acute renal failure are discussed in Chapter 12.

LACTIC ACIDOSIS

Conversion of lactic acid back to pyruvate and in turn to glucose (via the Cori cycle) or to carbon dioxide (via the Krebs cycle) is the metabolic fate of lactic acid. However, conversion of lactic acid to pyruvate would release extracellular bicarbonate initially consumed during the generation of lactic acidosis. The normal serum lactic acid level is 1 mEq/L (range, 0.5 to 1.5 mEq/L). In most cases of lactic acidosis, there are components of increased production and decreased catabolism of lactic acid. It results most often from anaerobic metabolism whereby the cellular delivery of oxygen or its utilization is impaired, and anaerobic glycolysis with production of lactic acid results. Lactic acidosis is a common feature of severely poisoned patients and may be seen alone or superimposed on other forms of acidosis, such as alcoholic ketoacidosis, methanol intoxication, and salicylate poisoning. Lactic acidosis is associated with a profound illness that includes weakness, anorexia, impaired mentation, hypotension, tachycardia, and hyperventilation. Blood lactate levels are uniformly elevated, and the higher they are, the worse the prognosis. In the absence of renal failure, lactic acidosis is accompanied by a phosphate-to-creatinine ratio in blood greater than 3 and may be associated with hyperuricemia because lactate and urate compete for the same secretory pathways in the renal tubule. As mentioned earlier, potassium shifts from intracellular to extracellular compartments do not occur, and any associated hyperkalemia is due to another cause. Drug-induced causes of lactic acidosis are shown in Table 6-1 along with the proposed mechanisms responsible for the lactic acid production.

In the treatment of lactic acidosis, attention should be directed toward the underlying cause. In addition, cardiovascular function and ventilation must be improved, and hypovolemia and hypoxemia corrected. Although intravenous sodium bicarbonate has been standard therapy, its use in the treatment of lactic acidosis is controversial. Dichloroacetate, which stimulates pyruvate dehydrogenase, the catalyst for oxidation of lactate to pyruvate, may be helpful in its treatment, particularly if volume overload or renal failure is present.

KETOACIDOSIS

Alcohol ketoacidosis is a common clinical entity and must be considered in the differential diagnosis of elevated anion-gap metabolic acidosis in the alcoholic. Depleted glycogen storage, poor caloric intake, and the direct effect of alcohol in suppressing gluconeogenesis can lead to hypoglycemia. Hypoglycemia along with volume depletion suppresses insulin release and stimulates the release of glucagon, which predisposes to ketosis. In

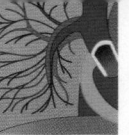

TABLE 6-1 Drug or Chemical Causes of Lactic Acidosis

DRUG OR CHEMICAL	MECHANISM
Acetaminophen	Acute liver failure
Biguanides	Decreased utilization and increased production of lactate
Carbon monoxide	Tissue hypoxia
Cocaine	Seizures, vasoconstriction
Cyanide	Anaerobic metabolism
Ethanol	Acetate-induced increase in NADH/NAD, inhibition or conversion of lactate to glucose, thiamine deficiency, liver disease, seizures
Ethylene glycol	Seizures, acute renal failure, ethanol, cardiovascular collapse
Isoniazid	Seizures
Methanol	Acidemia, decreased lactate utilization, formic acid, hypotension
Salicylates	Uncoupled oxidative phosphorylation
Papaverine, nalidixic acid, iron, streptozotocin, strychnine, chloramphenicol, sorbitol, xylitol	Unknown

addition, alcohol can stimulate lipolysis to produce acetaldehyde and, ultimately, acetate, which allows for increased keto production. Alcohol increases the NADH/NAD ratio in its metabolism; this, in turn, favors the conversion of acetoacetate to β-hydroxybutyrate, and an increase in the β-hydroxybutyrate-to-acetoacetate ratio is a characteristic feature of alcoholic ketoacidosis. Lactic acidosis also may accompany the ketoacidosis as a result of hypotension, sepsis, or gastrointestinal bleeding or as a consequence of ethanol intoxication. Blood glucose level usually is normal; however, if it is in the hyperglycemic range, it suggests the presence of diabetes mellitus. The treatment is volume resuscitation, and this treatment usually effects reversal of ketosis within hours. Any accompanying electrolyte abnormalities should be corrected; also, the administration of bicarbonate is required, as is the use of insulin.

SALICYLATE INTOXICATION

The metabolic acid–base disturbance characteristic of salicylate intoxication typically is a primary mild to moderate metabolic acidosis accompanied by a primary (not compensatory) respiratory alkalosis, the result of the drug's potent respiratory stimulant action. These findings are invariable in severe aspirin toxicity unless the victim has ingested an agent that depresses respiratory drive. The origin of the acidosis is multifactorial but includes uncoupling of oxidative metabolism and salicylate stimulation of organic acid (lactic acid and ketoacid) production. Ketone products may be found in 25% of cases and may contribute to false elevations in serum creatinine.

The importance of recognizing the complex acid–base disturbances of salicylate intoxication cannot be overemphasized. Salicylate overdose is prominent among the agents and conditions that produce a mixed metabolic acidosis and respiratory alkalosis. In patients with a P_{CO_2} less than 30 to 35 mm Hg and/or a serum bicarbonate level of 18 mEq/L or less, a serum salicylate level should be obtained if these abnormal findings are unexplained. Salicylates are discussed further in Chapter 48.

METHANOL

Methanol intoxication is accompanied by the production of formaldehyde and formic acid; production of the latter leads to a profoundly elevated anion gap, which usually develops 12 to 24 hours after ingestion. Although controversial, formic acid seems to be the earliest cause of anion-gap elevation, although lactic and other organic acids may contribute to this disturbance. Additionally, multiple-organ failure results in decreased hepatic lactate utilization. In untreated patients, as methanol is metabolized, an early osmolal gap and normal or slightly elevated anion gap is followed by a decrease in the osmolal gap with an increase in the anion gap. Treatment includes correction of the profound academia with bicarbonate administration, use of fomepizole or ethanol to inhibit the metabolism of methanol, and hemodialysis to correct the profound acidemia and remove the toxic compounds. Methanol is further discussed in Chapter 32.

ETHYLENE GLYCOL

Ethylene glycol intoxication leads to serious, life-threatening anion-gap acidosis. The decrease in serum bicarbonate level is due to buffering of excess glycolic acid, which contributes primarily to the elevation of the anion gap. However, increases in lactic acid and β-hydroxybutyrate also occur with ethylene glycol intoxication, adding to the metabolic acidosis. Lactic acidosis usually occurs in the later stages of ethylene glycol intoxication; its etiology is not completely understood. Hyperchloremic metabolic acidosis may occur also from accompanying proximal renal tubular dysfunction. As with methanol, ethylene glycol is associated with an increased osmolal gap; also like methanol, the metabolism of ethylene glycol produces a reciprocal change in the osmolal and anion gaps. Treatment includes aggressive correction of metabolic acidosis and administration of fomepizole or ethanol. Hemodialysis removes ethylene glycol and its breakdown products in addition to correcting the acidosis. Ethylene glycol is further discussed in Chapter 32B.

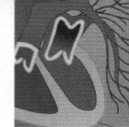

PARALDEHYDE

Paraldehyde is a pungent, colorless liquid used primarily for the treatment of seizures; it has been supplanted by safer and more effective agents and rarely is used today. Paraldehyde is metabolized predominantly to acetaldehyde and acetic acid and ultimately to carbon dioxide and water. The drug produces an elevated anion-gap metabolic acidosis by ill-defined mechanisms, possibly by increasing the NADH/NAD ratio, which favors the conversion of acetoacetate to β-hydroxybutyrate.

TOLUENE

Toluene is metabolized to benzoic acid and hippuric acid, which accumulate to yield an elevated anion-gap metabolic acidosis accompanied by hepatic and renal failure. Long-term toluene exposure can lead to type I distal tubular acidosis and type II proximal tubular acidosis associated with Fanconi's syndrome with a normal anion gap.

MISCELLANEOUS CAUSES OF ELEVATED ANION-GAP METABOLIC ACIDOSIS

The miscellaneous causes of elevated anion-gap metabolic acidosis include ingestion of formaldehyde, ibuprofen, cocaine, theophylline, phencyclidine, cyanide, or iron.

Historically, the commonly used mnemonic for metabolic acidosis has been MUDPILES (methanol, uremia, diabetic ketoacidosis, phenformin or paraldehyde, lactate, ethanol or ethylene glycol, and salicylates). However, this mnemonic has four shortcomings: not all of its elements are toxic agents; the toxins phenformin and paraldehyde rarely are used clinically, if at all; newer agents are associated with metabolic acidosis (e.g., metformin); and common and important agents (e.g., cyanide and ibuprofen) are not included. The mnemonic therefore no longer has great clinical value.

METABOLIC ACIDOSIS WITH A NORMAL ANION GAP (HYPERCHLOREMIC METABOLIC ACIDOSIS)

Metabolic acidosis with normal anion gap results from a loss of fluid with a bicarbonate concentration greater than chloride concentration, the addition of acids with chloride as their associated anion, or the transient dilution of extracellular bicarbonate with nonbicarbonate solutions. To maintain electroneutrality, the decrease in serum bicarbonate is associated with a proportionate increase in the serum chloride level. For example, in diarrhea, bicarbonate loss is greater than chloride loss; thus, hyperchloremia develops. Accompanying this is extracellular volume contraction, which stimulates renal retention of sodium with chloride, rather than of bicarbonate, because of the increased availability of chloride. This, in turn, leads to the development of hyperchloremic metabolic acidosis. Normal anion-gap metabolic acidosis can be divided into hypochloremic and hyperchloremic forms. Box 6-2 lists the causes of normal anion-gap metabolic acidosis.

In the context of poisoning, diarrhea may occur after ingestion of many agents, including colchicine, arsenic, antibiotics, and iron. Drug-induced renal tubular acidosis (Box 6-3) may be seen with the use of ampho-

tericin, lithium, toluene, vitamin D, and analgesics (all of which produce type I renal tubular acidosis). In contrast, type II renal tubular acidosis may be caused by tetracycline, carbonic anhydrase inhibitors, cadmium, mercury, lead, uranium, toluene, and 6-mercaptopurine. Type II renal tubular acidosis usually is accompanied by a greater than 15% fractional excretion of bicarbonate, along with aminoaciduria, phosphaturia, glycosuria, and uricosuria (Fanconi's syndrome). Type IV renal tubular acidosis may be induced by tubular interstitial disease caused by ingestion of spironolactone, triamterene, lithium, nonsteroidal anti-inflammatory drugs (NSAIDs),

---

BOX 6-2	**CAUSES OF NORMAL ANION-GAP METABOLIC ACIDOSIS**

Ammonium chloride
Anion exchange resins
Arginine hydrochloride
Diarrhea
Primary hyperparathyroidism
Parenteral alimentation
Post hypocapnia
Renal tubular acidosis
Small bowel/pancreatic drainage
Ureterosigmoidostomy/obstructed ileal conduit

BOX 6-3	**CAUSES OF DRUG-RELATED RENAL TUBULAR ACIDOSIS**

Type I

Amphotericin
Analgesics
Lithium
Toluene
Vitamin D

Type II

Acetazolamide
Cadmium
Lead
Mafenide acetate
6-Mercaptopurine
Mercury
Outdated tetracycline
Streptozotocin
Toluene
Uranium

Type IV

Amiloride
Angiotensin-converting enzyme inhibitors
β blockers
Cyclosporine
Lithium
Nonsteroidal anti-inflammatory drugs
Spironolactone
Triamterene

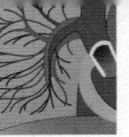
angiotensin-converting enzyme inhibitors, and cyclosporine. A normal anion-gap metabolic acidosis also may be seen in ingestions of elemental sulfur and of the sulfur-containing amino acids, methionine, cystine, and cysteine. Similarly, chlorine gas inhalation and intoxication with hydrochloric acid, ammonium chloride, lysine hydrochloride, arginine hydrochloride, calcium chloride, and magnesium chloride—all of which contribute to generation of chloride ions—lead to normal anion-gap acidosis.

Clinical Features, Consequences, and Treatment of Metabolic Acidosis

Acidemia and metabolic acidosis produce several cardiovascular effects. Acidemia directly impairs myocardial contractility, although it also possesses some positive inotropic action, the secondary result of catecholamine release. As pH decreases to less than 7.2, negative inotropic effects predominate and heart rate increases; as pH decreases to less than 7.1, the heart rate also may fall. Acidemia also predisposes to life-threatening ventricular arrhythmias and to arterial vasodilation and venoconstriction, both of which increase central blood volume. In combination with its negative inotropic effects, acidemia can lead to pulmonary edema. The hemodynamic consequences of acidemia lead to a vicious cycle of decreased myocardial contractility that produces tissue hypoxia and lactic acidosis, which in turn increase acidemia, further impairing myocardial contractility. All of these factors produce shock.

Acidemia induces an increase in both respiratory rate and tidal volume. Because of the Bohr effect, academia produces a rightward shift of the oxyhemoglobin dissociation curve. In the CNS, acidemia induces a spectrum of altered consciousness—from confusion to coma—probably as a result of changes in cerebrospinal fluid pH and, in the case of respiratory acidosis, a direct CNS depressant effect of carbon dioxide (CO_2 narcosis). Respiratory acidosis tends to have a greater effect than metabolic acidosis on mental status.

Gastrointestinal effects of acidosis include abdominal pain, nausea, and vomiting, particularly in the setting of ketoacidosis. Changes in serum potassium levels depend on the form of the acidosis (metabolic or respiratory) and the specific types of metabolic acidosis (mineral or organic), as well as other factors, including changes in serum osmolality and changes in plasma insulin, aldosterone, and catecholamine levels. Acidemia mobilizes skeletal calcium, leading to an increase in ionized calcium concentration.

The principal treatment is directed at the underlying cause of the metabolic acidosis. Factors to be considered are not only the etiology but also the magnitude of the metabolic acidosis and the rate at which it develops. The management of rapidly developing severe metabolic acidosis secondary to ethylene glycol poisoning with cardiovascular collapse is far more important than the treatment of a patient with a mildly elevated anion-gap metabolic acidosis after a seizure.

Controversy surrounds the use of sodium bicarbonate in the treatment of metabolic acidosis. Proponents recommend the use of bicarbonate sufficient to maintain a blood pH greater than 7.20 because a systemic pH less than 7.20 is associated with adverse hemodynamic effects, including reduced cardiac output, arterial vasodilation, and arrhythmias. Conversely, critics argue that bicarbonate is not helpful and might be detrimental because, in models of lactic acidosis, exogenous alkali can increase lactic acid production. Therefore, it would seem prudent to use sodium bicarbonate judiciously in the treatment of metabolic acidosis, particularly if the pH is less than 7.2 and the bicarbonate level is less than 10 to 12 mEq/L. Several formulas have been suggested to express the bicarbonate deficit. They are based on body weight and volume distribution of bicarbonate. However, these formulas should be used only as guides, especially because acidemia increases the volume of distribution of bicarbonate (e.g., at a pH of 7.1, the volume of distribution of bicarbonate is approximately 80% of total body weight). Because rapid bolus administration of bicarbonate is dangerous, large amounts should be infused slowly over 30 to 60 minutes. "Overshoot alkalosis" may be seen in lactic acidosis and in ketoacidosis when the lactic acid and keto acids are oxidized to bicarbonate under severe reductive conditions in response to exogenous bicarbonate. Bicarbonate administration also may cause hypokalemia and hypocalcemia, which present their own risks. Similarly, volume and sodium overload from sodium bicarbonate may be seen; when the presence of volume overload precludes the use of sodium bicarbonate, hemodialysis should be considered.

METABOLIC ALKALOSIS

Metabolic alkalosis is defined as an increase in the serum bicarbonate level to greater than 28 mEq/L. Usually, but not always, this is accompanied by an increase in pH to greater than 7.40. Metabolic alkalosis is quite common in hospitalized patients and is associated with significant morbidity and mortality. It develops from a net gain of extracellular bicarbonate or of one of its precursors, a net loss of hydrogen ions from the extracellular space, or a loss of fluid containing more chloride than bicarbonate from the extracellular space. Metabolic alkalosis is maintained by a decrease in the glomerular filtration rate, a decrease in the real or effective extracellular volume, hypokalemia, hypochloremia, and hypercapnia, and an increase in mineralocorticoid effects. The initial increase in serum bicarbonate level produces alkalemia, which initiates secondary mechanisms to prevent drastic changes in pH. These include extracellular and intracellular buffering, increased renal excretion of excess alkali, and a respiratory compensatory response. The initial increase in pH depresses central and peripheral chemoreceptors and leads to hypoventilation and hypercapnia, which minimize the initial increase in pH. However, the respiratory response is not as predictable as

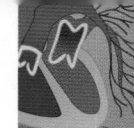

it is in metabolic acidosis and is limited by the development of hypoxemia, which occurs as a result of hypoventilation. Any decrease in P_{O_2} to below 70 to 80 mm Hg stimulates ventilation, which counterbalances the effects of metabolic alkalosis—hence, the respiratory response to metabolic alkalosis is more variable. Rarely does P_{CO_2} increase to greater than 55 to 60 mm Hg as a response to simple metabolic alkalosis. Hypoxemia is a result of hypoventilation and, therefore, the alveolar-arterial oxygen gradient is normal. P_{CO_2} increases by 0.5 to 0.7 mm Hg for each milliequivalent per liter increase in serum bicarbonate level. A P_{CO_2} that is less than predicted suggests the presence of respiratory alkalosis along with metabolic alkalosis, whereas a P_{CO_2} that is greater than predicted suggests respiratory acidosis along with the metabolic alkalosis.

Causes of Metabolic Alkalosis

Metabolic alkalosis is divided into three categories: sodium chloride–responsive metabolic alkalosis, sodium chloride–resistant metabolic alkalosis, and miscellaneous. In sodium chloride–responsive metabolic alkalosis, there is a decrease in real or effective extracellular volume and hypochloremia accompanied by avid renal reabsorption of sodium chloride and a urine chloride concentration of less than 10 mEq/L (although, in diuretic-induced metabolic alkalosis, urine chloride level may be greater than 10 mEq/L) due to an increase in mineralocorticoid activity. Characteristically, there is an increase in the distal reabsorption of sodium and an increase in potassium and hydrogen ion excretion with urinary chloride levels greater than 20 mEq/L. Hypovolemia is not responsible, and administration of sodium chloride does not correct the alkalosis; rather, treatment is directed at inhibiting excess mineralocorticoid activity. Box 6-4 summarizes the causes of metabolic alkalosis that do not fall into the categories already discussed.

Metabolic Alkalosis in Poisoning and Drug Overdose

Metabolic alkalosis is a fairly uncommon acid–base disorder in the poisoned patient, but it may occur in those with eating disorders, diuretic abusers, and those with drug-induced Bartter's syndrome. The latter may be caused by administration of aminoglycosides. Chewing tobacco and imported licorice that contains glycyrrhizic acid have potent mineralocorticoid activity; use of these products leads to metabolic alkalosis. Ingestion of excess bicarbonate may lead to metabolic alkalosis only if the kidney is unable to excrete the excess alkali or if renal failure is present. Overshoot alkalosis may occur in response to the correction of organic acidosis by excess bicarbonate.

Clinical Features of Metabolic Alkalosis

The features of metabolic alkalosis are in large part related to the specific cause; however, alkalemia per se

BOX 6-4	CAUSES OF METABOLIC ALKALOSIS

Sodium Chloride–Responsive

Cystic fibrosis
Diuretics
Posthypercapnia
Villous adenoma
Vomiting

Sodium Chloride–Resistant

Adrenogenital syndrome
Bartter's syndrome
Capreomycin
Carbenoxolone
Chewing tobacco
Cushing's syndrome
Gentamicin
Licorice ingestion
Liddle syndrome
Primary aldosteronism
Renal artery stenosis
Severe potassium depletion

Miscellaneous

Antacid–sodium polystyrene in renal failure
Bicarbonate administration
Hypomagnesemia
Milk-alkali syndrome
Nonparathyroid hypercalcemia
Overshoot alkalosis
Penicillin, carbenicillin, ticarcillin
Poststarvation refeeding

may produce neuromuscular irritability along with seizures, tetany, delirium, and hyperreflexia. Oxygen delivery to tissues is reduced because metabolic alkalosis shifts the oxyhemoglobin dissociation curve to the left. Concomitant with the alkalosis, there may be hypokalemia, hypocalcemia, decreased ionized calcium, hypomagnesemia, hypophosphatemia, and hypoxemia, which can further complicate the clinical picture.

Treatment

The primary treatment of metabolic alkalosis is to identify and manage the underlying cause. Sodium chloride is administered for sodium chloride–responsive metabolic alkalosis, and volume expansion will correct it. Sodium-resistant metabolic acidosis may respond to measures to increase the glomerular filtration rate and to correction of mineralocorticoid activity. In patients with metabolic alkalosis who are volume overloaded, such as in those with congestive heart failure, acetazolamide—a carbonic anhydrase inhibitor—may be helpful and can lead to increased renal bicarbonate excretion. In the patient undergoing continuous nasogastric suction or with protracted vomiting, the histamine-2 blockers reduce hydrochloric acid secretion and can be used as therapy. In the patient with renal failure who has significant

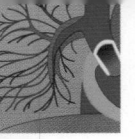

metabolic alkalosis, dialysate with a low bicarbonate or low acetate concentration and a low chloride concentration may be used in correcting the metabolic alkalosis.

RESPIRATORY ACIDOSIS

Respiratory acidosis generally is defined as an increase in the P_{CO_2} to greater than 44 mm Hg. The increase in P_{CO_2} and subsequent acidemia initiate changes aimed at preventing drastic changes in pH. Intracellular buffering via red cell hemoglobin, phosphate, and protein exchange intracellular sodium and potassium for the excess extracellular hydrogen ions. CO_2 retention, also known as hypercapnia, leads to increased renal hydrogen ion secretion and net acid excretion, as well as to increased bicarbonate reabsorption. Although beginning early, the maximum effect of these actions takes several days. For each 10 mm Hg increase in P_{CO_2}, serum bicarbonate level increases by 1 to 2 mEq/L; in chronic respiratory acidosis, for every 10 mm Hg in P_{CO_2}, the bicarbonate level increases 3 to 4 mEq/L. Any changes in P_{CO_2} or serum bicarbonate concentration outside those predicted indicate coexisting metabolic alkalosis as well as respiratory acidosis; likewise, bicarbonate levels less than those predicted imply the existence of metabolic acidosis as well as respiratory acidosis. Respiratory acidosis usually is the result of impaired ventilation secondary to CNS depression. It is one of the most common acid–base disturbances in the poisoned patient and may result from the drugs listed in Box 6-5.

Features and Treatment of Respiratory Acidosis

Altered states of consciousness are common in respiratory acidosis, as are abnormal ventilatory patterns, tachycardia, arrhythmias, diaphoresis, visual disturbances, headache, delirium, and coma. Many of the CNS effects are related to increased cerebral blood flow secondary to hypercapnia and subsequently increased cerebrospinal fluid pressure. The acidemia itself can have significant adverse hemodynamic effects. Treatment of the condition, therefore, is directed at improving ventilation.

RESPIRATORY ALKALOSIS

Respiratory alkalosis is defined as an acid–base disturbance characterized by a P_{CO_2} less than 36 mm Hg; the secondary changes it produces are brought about to prevent drastic changes in pH. Intracellular hydrogen ions are exchanged for sodium and potassium to neutralize the excess bicarbonate and, thus, minimize the increased P_{CO_2}. The kidney decreases net acid excretion and bicarbonate reabsorption and, thus, tends to return pH toward normal. Although this process begins early, maximal response does not occur for several days. Serum bicarbonate level decreases by 1 to 3 mEq/L for each 10 mm Hg decrease in P_{CO_2}, whereas

BOX 6-5	CAUSES OF RESPIRATORY ACIDOSIS

Central Causes

Drugs
Anesthetics
Barbiturates
Ethanol
Ethylene glycol
Methanol
Opiates
Sedatives

Central Nervous System Lesions
Infection
Trauma
Tumor
Vascular accidents

Neuromuscular Causes

Botulism
Guillain-Barré syndrome
Hypokalemia
Myasthenia gravis
Pickwickian syndrome
Primary hypoventilation

Thoracic/Pulmonary Causes

Aspiration pneumonia
Chronic obstructive pulmonary disease
Pneumonia
Pneumothorax
Pulmonary embolism
Pulmonary edema
Smoke inhalation

Airway Obstruction

Bronchoconstriction
Foreign body
Epiglottal/laryngeal edema (e.g., phencyclidine poisoning)

in chronic respiratory alkalosis, bicarbonate level decreases by 3 to 5 mEq/L for every 10 mm Hg decrease in P_{CO_2}. Values outside this prediction indicate a metabolic alkalosis as well as respiratory alkalosis (when serum bicarbonate level is greater than predicted) and metabolic acidosis as well as respiratory alkalosis (when the serum bicarbonate is less than predicted). Rarely does serum bicarbonate decrease to less than 14 to 16 mEq/L in compensation. Respiratory alkalosis is the most common acid–base disorder encountered in intensive care, and the greater the degree of hypocapnia and alkalemia, the worse the prognosis. Box 6-6 lists the causes of respiratory alkalosis, of which salicylate ingestion is the most common.

Features and Treatment of Respiratory Alkalosis

The main features are related to neuromuscular irritability, with certain oral and digital paresthesias, carpopedal spasm, tetany, seizures, and altered consciousness. Significant hypocapnia leads to a decrease in

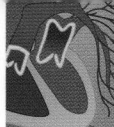

BOX 6-6	CAUSES OF RESPIRATORY ALKALOSIS

General

Anxiety
Brainstem lesions
Encephalitis and meningitis
Fever
Encephalopathy
Pain
Pregnancy
Salicylates
Thyrotoxicosis
Tumors

Peripheral

Congestive heart failure
Hypotension
Hypoxemia
Interstitial lung disease
Pneumonia
Pulmonary embolism

Miscellaneous

Cirrhosis
Mechanical ventilation
Sepsis

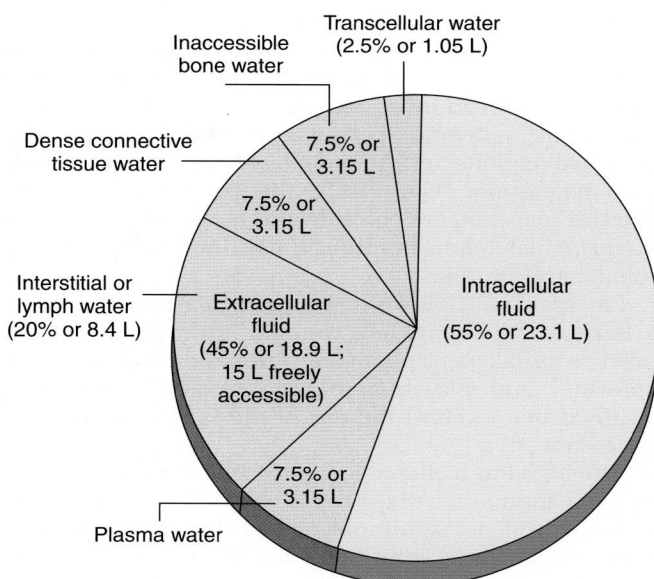

FIGURE 6-1 Distribution of whole body water in a 70-kg human adult. Men = 42 L; women = 35 L. Most values shown are for men.

cerebral blood flow and is linked to the CNS manifestations. The small increase in anion gap may be observed secondary to an increase in lactic acid production due to an increase in tissue anaerobic glycolysis brought on by alkalemia. Treatment is directed at the primary disorder; raising the P_{CO_2} by administering enriched inhaled carbon dioxide or by a rebreathing mask, or simply by having the patient breathe into a bag, may hasten the recovery from this disorder.

MIXED ACID–BASE DISORDERS

Drug intoxication may result in mixed acid–base disorders (i.e., the presence of two or more primary acid-base disorders). These are common in the overdose situation, either as a result of the primary ingestant or as a result of the therapeutic interventions used to correct the poisoning.

REGULATION OF BODY FLUID VOLUMES AND TONICITY

The body fluid, or *whole body water*, in an average 70-kg man consists of about 42 L of water. The fluid is divided into two distinct subgroups: the intracellular fluid and the extracellular fluid (Fig. 6-1).

Except for bone, tissues that do not contain fat (the lean body mass) are 60% to 85% water; muscle and the gray matter of brain are the "wettest" tissues of the body, being 70% to 85% water. Connective tissue and erythrocytes are the driest nonadipose tissues (60%

water). Fatty tissue, in contrast, is 20% water; therefore, an obese person contains proportionately less water by weight than does a thin person. In obese individuals, whole body water decreases to closer to 40%. In general, women possess more fat than men; consequently, the water content of women is relatively less than that of men.

The water content of the body is relatively high in infancy, decreases to adult levels by late childhood, and thereafter decreases slowly but progressively with age. The gender difference in body water content develops at puberty and continues throughout life.

Intracellular water constitutes some 55% to 60% of whole body water. Excluding the relatively inaccessible bone water, total extracellular fluid water (plasma, as well as interstitial and transcellular water) makes up the difference. For an average man, total extracellular fluid water is 15 L (or approximately 20% to 25% of the body weight). The extravascular or interstitial fluid space accounts for 12 L of the extracellular fluid, whereas 3 L are present as plasma within the circulation. In an average young man, total blood volume is 6% to 8% of body weight (70 mL/kg); this gives absolute values for blood and plasma volumes of 5 L and 3 L, respectively.

Intracellular and extracellular fluid compartments are separated by cell membranes that selectively control passage of ions and nutrients but are freely permeable to water; although ionic gradients may exist across cell membranes, movement of water establishes an osmotic equilibrium, and any osmotic gradients are corrected rapidly.

INTRACELLULAR FLUID COMPOSITION

The ionic composition of body fluids can be discussed in terms of chemical equivalents. Concentrations of all ionic constituents are expressed as the sum of con-

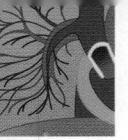

centrations of the positive ions (cations) and negative ions (anions). Ionic balance is obligatory in order to maintain the electrical neutrality of the body fluids. The principal cations in extracellular fluid are sodium, potassium, calcium, and magnesium, whereas the principal cations in intracellular fluid are potassium and magnesium. Conversely, the principal anions in extracellular fluid are chloride and bicarbonate, whereas the principal anions in intracellular fluid are phosphate, sulfate, and proteins.

Electrical neutrality is maintained in all body fluids by a balance of cations and anions; however, in clinical practice, usually only plasma or serum sodium, potassium, chloride, and bicarbonate are measured, and it is assumed that levels of the rest of the cations and anions are balanced.

The high intracellular–low extracellular concentration of potassium and the reverse for sodium favor the movement of potassium out of and that of sodium into cells. Such ionic gradients are maintained by the presence of sodium-potassium pumps in the cell membrane and are critical in protecting cell volume. High concentrations of osmotically active anionic protein within cells, relative to the interstitial fluid, establish a Donnan equilibrium that increases the osmotic activity within the cell. Any movement of water into cells is prevented by the act of extrusion of sodium, whereas interference with the potassium-sodium pump mechanism results in cellular accumulation of sodium and chloride, with loss of potassium and resultant cellular edema.

Transcellular fluids are predominantly products of cell secretion. The composition of the fluids varies according to their cellular origin. Under physiologic conditions, secreted fluids tend to be recirculated or reabsorbed, but under pathologic (or treatment) conditions, failure to reabsorb continuously secreted fluids may lead to significant losses of volume and electrolytes, as seen with diarrhea, vomiting, and nasogastric suction. Drainage of intestinal fluids may result in considerable losses of chloride and bicarbonate (e.g., in the presence of small intestinal fistulae or with extreme diarrhea, such as that seen in cholera). Similarly, drainage of gastric and salivary juices may result in loss of considerable quantities of hydrogen ions as well as chloride. Diarrhea produced by cholera also results in massive sodium and water loss, which produces not only hypovolemia but also hyponatremia. *Third space fluid loss* refers to sequestration of fluids within cavities (e.g., pleural, pericardial, and intraperitoneal).

MOVEMENT OF WATER BETWEEN INTRACELLULAR AND EXTRACELLULAR FLUID SPACES: OSMOLARITY AND OSMOLALITY

Water moves freely across cell membranes, and an osmotic disequilibrium cannot be sustained. Thus, distribution of total body water depends on the number of active particles in the intracellular and extracellular spaces. The osmotically driven "shifts" of body water adjust intracellular and extracellular osmolality to maintain osmotic neutrality. One osmole is the mass of a solute (or mixture of a solute) that, when dissolved in 1 L, gives a solution that has an osmotic pressure of 22.4 atm at 0°C. Osmolar concentrations generally are determined indirectly by measuring changes of the physical function of solutions, such as depression of the freezing point below that of water. Osmolality determined in this fashion (or osmoles per 100 g of plasma water) is obtained. The term *osmolality* is preferred to the commonly misused term *osmolarity* (osmoles per liter of whole plasma) and is more appropriate in considering physiologic relationships.

In practice, plasma osmolality mainly reflects plasma sodium concentration, and it must be remembered that water added to or removed from any fluid compartment behaves as though it were added to or removed from whole body water. Second, sodium added to or removed from extracellular fluid alters sodium concentration, as though it had been added to or removed from whole body water. Third, sodium concentration in plasma does not necessarily reflect changes in extracellular fluid volume because hypernatremia may exist with low, normal, or increased extracellular fluid. The same remarks apply to hyponatremia or normal serum sodium concentrations. Fourth, changes in the volume of intracellular fluid and extracellular fluid usually are proportional (and in the same direction) with a gain or loss of water, with intracellular and extracellular fluid volumes changing in opposite directions with gains or losses of restricted solutes, such as sodium and potassium. Other important solutes that contribute to plasma osmolality are glucose and blood urea nitrogen.

CELLULAR RESPONSES TO REDISTRIBUTION OF FLUID

Changes in extracellular osmolality can bring about major swelling or contraction of cells, but the primary effects are seen in the brain. Hyponatremia induced in animals causes brain swelling initially, with diminishing changes occurring within several hours. Correction of brain swelling is complete usually at 24 hours, with the brain responding to extracellular hypotonicity by losing potassium and chloride. In experimental models of hypernatremia, brain water is initially lost, with gains of sodium, potassium, and chloride soon achieved by brain cells. Between 4 hours and several days, brain water content returns to normal, and an increased osmotic activity is sustained through the generation and accumulation of organic solutes such as amino acids. Hypoglycemia also can cause an acute loss of brain water, with a return to normal levels within a few hours, principally because of changes in the concentration of ions and organic solutes. Similarly, mannitol removes water from the brain but does not result in the generation of new intracellular organic molecules (idiogenic osmoles). For this reason, mannitol is not associated with effective adaptive changes in the regulation of intracellular

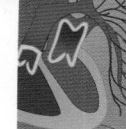

volume of the brain, and, consequently, brain volume decreases.

REGULATION OF BODY FLUID VOLUMES AND DAILY FLUID BALANCE

Because sodium is the dominant cation of extracellular fluid, it is the critical determinant of extracellular fluid volume by virtue of its osmotic activity, and by virtue of its effect on renal sodium chloride reabsorption. It is the major determinant of renal water reabsorption. It is through the reabsorption of sodium and water that the kidney regulates extracellular fluid volume. The reabsorption of sodium by the kidney is an intensely and finely regulated process for the conservation of sodium and water, and also for its secondary effects on hydrogen ion excretion through bicarbonate reabsorption; it is also linked to potassium secretion. A detailed discussion of sodium reabsorption by the kidney is beyond the scope of this text, but two major mechanisms in sodium homeostasis are worth discussing in relationship to the diagnosis and management of poisoned patients.

Sodium is freely filtered at the glomerulus and is reabsorbed isotonically at the proximal convoluted tubule, with 60% to 70% of filtered sodium being proximally reabsorbed. Consequently, the glomerular filtrate volume is reduced by 60% to 70% in the proximal tubule; this provides substantial control of fluid balance. In the descending limb of the loop of Henle, the tubule is less permeable to sodium and urea but more permeable to water; consequently, the glomerular filtrate passing through the loop of Henle increases in sodium concentration, with consequent increases in osmolality. The thin ascending limb of the loop of Henle is permeable to sodium and urea but relatively impermeable to water, whereas in the thick ascending limb of the loop of Henle there is active transport of chloride, which also facilitates sodium reabsorption. Subsequently, the ascending limb of the loop of Henle accounts for 20% to 25% of sodium reabsorption. In the distal nephron (the distal convoluted tubule and collecting duct), 5% to 10% of sodium is reabsorbed, facilitating potassium secretion, and is in part responsive to aldosterone.

Because the renal excretion of sodium is variable and, under physiologic conditions, equal to sodium intake, the kidney must vary its excretion of sodium in the wide range encountered in humans (i.e., one to several hundred milliequivalents every 24 hours). It follows that regulatory mechanisms closely govern sodium excretion. These mechanisms include: glomerular filtration; physical factors, such as postglomerular protein oncotic pressure; aldosterone; antidiuretic hormone; and atrial natriuretic peptide. These substances all are coordinated to maintain the balance of extracellular fluid volume. It is well known that infusion of saline increases glomerular filtration rate and reduces renin excretion, thereby reducing aldosterone secretion; such actions promote natriuresis, increasing urinary sodium excretion. The reverse occurs when volume contraction is present with

sodium being retained by the kidney. Compensatory mechanisms, principally mediated by antidiuretic hormone secretion, are initiated to conserve water, whereas a reduction in renal blood flow probably leads to conservation of sodium.

Antidiuretic hormone (ADH) is an octapeptide produced in the supraoptic and paraventricular nuclei of the hypothalamus. It is transported in the nerves from the hypothalamus in the posterior hypophysis and median eminence, where it is stored. In response to a variety of stimuli, ADH is released, altering the permeability of the distal tubule and collecting duct to water; the renal tubular cell contains receptors for ADH. A resultant increase in the water permeability of the distal tubule and collecting duct occurs, and, if there is hypertonicity of the medullary interstitium (brought about by the countercurrent concentration mechanism in the loop of Henle), water reabsorption occurs. The prime factor in producing ADH secretion is the plasma osmolality. A change in osmolality as small as 1% produces ADH secretion; a 1% to 2% change in osmolality initiates thirst. In contrast, a 6% change in the extracellular fluid volume is required to produce the same effect on ADH. Dehydration and hypernatremia lead to reduced renal perfusion and increased ADH secretion. The result is the excretion of small amounts of urine that are low in sodium and highly concentrated. Replacement of free water corrects the problem in patients with pure insensible water loss. In the syndrome of diabetes insipidus, water loss arises either because of a central defect in ADH production or release, or because of renal insensitivity to ADH (nephrogenic diabetes insipidus). Because of the action of ADH on the most distal sites of the nephron, it is possible for the patient to retain sodium maximally but still excrete volumes of water equal to 10% to 50% of the glomerular filtration rate. The loss of water in diabetes insipidus results in 10 to 15 L of dilute urine with a low total sodium excretion. The result is concentration of plasma and stimulation of the thirst mechanism, which leads to the ingestion of large quantities of water for replacement of water losses. Drugs known to have an effect on ADH status are shown in Box 6-7.

Detailed discussion of the factors involved in the production of hypernatremia and hyponatremia and of hyperkalemia and hypokalemia is beyond the scope of this text. However, the principal disorders associated with abnormalities of these cations in poisoned patients are shown in Table 6-2. The management of derangements of both sodium and potassium is outlined in Table 6-2.

ASSESSMENT AND MANAGEMENT OF FLUID AND ELECTROLYTE IMBALANCE

The two important clinical disturbances in fluid balance are volume overload and volume contraction. *Volume overload* is manifested by the presence of peripheral edema, ascites, and/or pulmonary edema. As a general rule, a 4% increase in whole body water is required to produce clinical signs of peripheral edema. Other signs

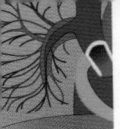

| BOX 6-7 | DRUG-INDUCED ALTERATIONS IN ANTIDIURETIC HORMONE (ADH) RELEASE AND ACTIVITY |

Central Reduction in ADH Secretion

Ethanol
Phenytoin/diphenylhydantoin
Glucocorticoids
Chlorpromazine
Reserpine
Morphine*

Central Stimulation of ADH Release

Clofibrate
Chlorpropamide
Nicotine
Vincristine
Cyclophosphamide
Tolbutamide
Carbamazepine
Acetylcholine
Carbachol
Methacholine
Barbiturates
Meperidine
Prostaglandin E_1
Isoproterenol

Peripheral Reduction in ADH Activity

Lithium
Demeclocycline
Acetohexamide
Tolazamide†
Glyburide†
Propoxyphene†
Amphotericin
Methoxyflurane
Colchicine
Vinblastine
Norepinephrine

Peripheral Enhancement of ADH Activity

Chlorpropamide
Acetaminophen
Indomethacin

*Mechanism not fully elucidated; raises threshold for osmotically induced ADH secretion.
†Mechanism not fully elucidated; not due to reduction in ADH secretion.

In the syndrome of inappropriate ADH (SIADH) secretion, urine sodium concentration is high, urine osmolality is high, and the blood urea nitrogen level is low; the condition is best treated with water restriction. Because of the risk of central pontine myelinolysis, serum sodium concentration in SIADH and other conditions associated with severe hyponatremia should be corrected slowly (at a rate of no more than 1 mEq/L).

In intoxicated patients, especially those with exposures producing fluid and electrolyte disturbances, body weight should be measured daily; fluid intake and output should be recorded accurately. Using these measurements, the clinician can identify significant changes in fluid and electrolyte balance.

Day-to-day management of fluid and electrolytes depends on multiple factors, including the total body deficits or excesses prior to institution of intravenous fluid therapy, the planned therapeutic interventions such as forced diuresis or hemodialysis, and the toxin. In the absence of complicating factors, one can assume the normal fluid and electrolyte requirements for a 70-kg person, which are defined as "basal" requirements, as outlined in Table 6-3.

MANAGEMENT OF RELATIVE HYPOVOLEMIA IN POISONING

In acute poisoning due to barbiturates, opioids, theophylline, tricyclic antidepressants, sedative-hypnotics, and many other drugs, an abrupt increase in the venous capacitance occurs, with a relative deficit of plasma volume. The relative hypovolemia due to increased venous capacitance also may be compounded by decreased venous return and extravascular fluid loss. These factors can result in significant hypotension. Such vasodilation often responds to augmentation of plasma volume by volume expansion. In some instances the use of vasopressor drugs may be necessary (see Chapter 2). However, improvement in central venous pressure may remain inadequate. In these circumstances a flow-directed pulmonary arterial catheter (Swan-Ganz) may be useful in assessing both central venous pressure and pulmonary capillary wedge pressure, serving as a more accurate guide to fluid replacement.

In some ingestions, aggressive volume expansion with the use of crystalloid solutions may be disadvantageous because these solutions may reduce the osmotic hydrostatic gradient, thereby increasing pulmonary capillary water. This occurrence has been implicated in the development of adult respiratory distress syndrome ("shock lung") in severely hypotensive patients. In view of the potential adverse effects of crystalloid solutions, colloid solutions such as albumin may be preferred for the treatment of hypovolemic shock in patients who might develop pulmonary edema.

of volume overload are distended neck veins and congestive heart failure, manifested by tachycardia, and a gallop on cardiac auscultation. In contrast, *volume contraction* is manifested by diminished skin turgor; dry, cracked lips; and sunken eyes. Resting or orthostatic tachycardia and hypotension also may be seen with volume contraction.

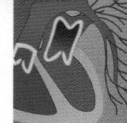

TABLE 6-2 Principal Disorders of Sodium and Potassium in Intoxicated Patients

		DISORDER AND EXAMPLES	TREATMENT
Hypernatremia	Normal body Na$^+$	Drug-induced diabetes insipidus	Diuretics and water replacement
		Sweating (salicylates, organophosphates)	
	High body Na$^+$	Steroids	Water replacement
		Hypertonic saline, NaCl, NaHCO$_3$	
		Saline emetics	
	Low body Na$^+$	Osmotic diuretics (mannitol)	Hypotonic saline
		Sweating (salicylates)	
		Diarrhea (organophosphates, antibiotics)	
Hyponatremia	↓ ECF volume	Diuretics (tubular and osmotic)	Isotonic saline
		Rhabdomyolysis	
		Steroid deficiencies	
		Vomiting/diarrhea/pancreatitis	
	↑ ECF volume (nonedematous)	Steroid deficiency	Water restriction
		Hypothyroidism	
		Beer-drinker's hyponatremia	
		Drugs (see Box 6-3)	
	↑↑ ECF volume (edematous)	Drug-induced	Water restriction
		Hepatic, renal, cardiac failure	
		ACE inhibitors	
Hyperkalemia	↑ True K$^+$	Acidosis	Correct
		Arginine hydrochloride	
		Digitalis intoxication	Stop drug
		Geophagia	
		K$^+$-sparing diuretics	Glucose/insulin
		Steroid deficiency	
		NSAIDs	
		Hemolysis	Ion exchange resins
		Rhabdomyolysis	Dialysis
		Salt substitutes	
		Penicillin	
		β blockers	
		Heparin	
Hypokalemia	Without K$^+$ deficit	Respiratory alkalosis (salicylate or respirator induced)	K$^+$ replacement
	With K$^+$ deficit	Nasogastric suction, vomiting	K$^+$ replacement
		Alcoholism	
		Inadequate K$^+$ replacement	
		Laxative abuse	
		Drug-induced diarrhea	
		Excessive steroids	
		Licorice abuse	
		Osmotic diuretics (mannitol, glucose)	
		Diuretics	
		Carbenicillin/penicillin/aminoglycosides	

ACE, angiotensin-converting enzyme; ECF, extracellular fluid.

TABLE 6-3 Daily Basal Fluid, Electrolyte, and Caloric Requirements

WATER/ELECTROLYTE REQUIREMENTS	BASAL REQUIREMENTS	METABOLIC REQUIREMENTS	CALORIC REQUIREMENTS
Water	1.5–2.0 L*	100 mL/100 cal	0–10 kg: 100 cal/kg
Sodium	75 mEq	2–3 mEq/100 cal	11–20 kg: 1000 cal plus 50 cal/kg over 10 kg
Potassium	60 mEq	2–3 mEq/100 cal	>20 kg: 1500 cal plus 20 cal/kg over 20 kg
Magnesium	8 mEq	—	
Chloride	—	4–6 mEq/100 cal	

*Insensible losses (approximately 700 mL) plus volume equivalent to urine volume.

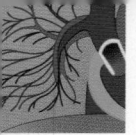
FURTHER READING

Ayus JC, Krothapalli RK, Arieff AL: Treatment of symptomatic hyponatremia and its relation to brain damage. N Engl J Med 1987;317:1190.

Brenner BM (ed): Brenner & Rector's The Kidney, 7th ed. Philadelphia: Elsevier, 2004.

Ganong WF: Review of Medical Physiology, 21st ed. New York; McGraw-Hill, 2003.

Irwin RS, Rippe JM: Intensive Care Medicine, 5th ed. Philadelphia: Lippincott Williams & Wilkins, 2003.

Levin ER, Gardner DG, Samson WK: Natriuretic peptides. N Engl J Med 1998;339:321–328.

Marx JA, Hockberger RS, Walls RM (eds): Rosen's Emergency Medicine: Concepts and Clinical Practice, 5th ed. St. Louis, Mosby, 2002.

Stein JH: Stein's Internal Medicine, 5th ed. St. Louis, Mosby, 1998.

7

Forensic Toxicology

A General Principles

JOHN HARRIS TRESTRAIL III, BSPHARM, RPH

At a Glance...

- The real science of forensic toxicology began in 1814, with the work of physician M.J.B. Orfila.
- Poisoners are nonconfrontational, and the majority of known poisoners are male.
- All things are potentially poisonous; it all depends on the dose.
- Analytical toxicology can tell you that a poison is present, but not why it is there.
- Approximately 41% of known poisoners have multiple victims.
- To prove death was due to a poison, it must have been absorbed and in systemic circulation.
- Every death with no visible signs of violence is a poisoning until facts prove otherwise.
- The Center for the Study of Criminal Poisoning is an organization that assists investigators on an international level.

> While toxicology admits of being extensively applied to other medical sciences, it is in medical jurisprudence that its power and extent are most evident.
>
> *Sir Robert Christison, British toxicologist*

A relatively new area for clinical toxicologists to enter, as consultants or expert witnesses, is for the use of their knowledge of poisons in the investigation of crimes in which these agents have played a role. The two major examples of this activity are in cases of product tampering, and murder by poison. It is the attempt of this chapter to review some of the principles of the forensic sciences as they apply to the area of toxicology. For brevity in these discussions, the author has used the term *he* in the description of the poisoner, but the reader can correctly substitute the term *he/she* without being in error.

WHAT IS FORENSIC TOXICOLOGY?

Forensic toxicology is that branch of the science that deals with the application of the study of poisons to the law. In this respect it overlaps into many other important forensic areas such as pathology, analytical chemistry, criminal investigation, and litigation.

However, forensic toxicology as a science is still relatively young, going back only a few hundred years, and it is certainly true today that we stand upon the shoulders of giants in this field.

HISTORICAL DEVELOPMENT OF FORENSIC TOXICOLOGY

Poison is one of the oldest weapons for murder known to man. As were the stick and the stone, poisons were used long before the development of arrows, spears, and gunpowder. Even though it is an old tool for murder, writings on the subject began to appear only in the relatively recent past.

Some of the earliest writings on the subject of criminal poisoning, and its investigation, were from India. Two of these early works are the *Charaka Samhita*, and the *Susruta Samhita*, which date from around 600 to 100 BC. Another early Indian work, known as the *Veda*, provided physicians with specific directions in the detection of poisoners based on their demeanor.

The beginning of the real modern scientific investigation of toxicology, and its application to forensics, started with the work of French physician Mathieu Joseph Bonaventure Orfila (1787–1853), who was to hold the chair of Legal Medicine at the Sorbonne in Paris. With respect to forensic toxicology, Orfila was to play an important role in the famous 1840 Paris poisoning case of Marie LaFarge, by adopting the then relatively new Marsh test for arsenic.

Through his early animal experimentations, Orfila was able to determine the toxic dosages and physical effects produced by a number of poisonous compounds. His studies eventually led to the publication, in 1814, of his monumental two-volume work, *Traité des Poisons: Tirés des Règnes Minéral, Végétal et Animal; ou Toxicologie Générale* [*Dissertation of Poisons: Covering the Relevant Mineral, Vegetable and Animal; or General Toxicology*]. In his work, Orfila divided the then known poisons into the following six classifications: corrosives, astringents, acrids, stupefying or narcotics, narcotico-acids, and septics or petreficants. This pioneering work in toxicology has garnered him the title "Father of Forensic Toxicology." Translations of Orfila's popular work soon appeared in Spanish, German, and Italian. An English translation of his work first appeared in 1816, and American editions were published in 1817 and 1826. The four augmented and corrected French editions of his work were published in 1818, 1826, 1843, and 1852. Other great toxicologists studied the works of Orfila and eventually wrote their own texts on the subject of poison and its application to the law.

One of these early toxicologists was the Scottish physician Robert Christison (1797–1882), who published

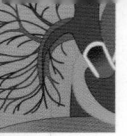

his first work, *A Treatise on Poisons*, in 1829. Christison was appointed Medical Advisor to the Crown in Scotland, and from 1829 to 1866 he was the medical witness in almost every important toxicologic case in Scotland, and many in England. Further editions of his work appeared in 1832, 1836, and 1845.

Another of the British toxicologists was the physician Alfred Swaine Taylor (1806–1880), who published his work *On Poisons, in Relation to Medical Jurisprudence and Medicine* in 1848. Taylor was the leading author on the subject of medical jurisprudence in the 19th century. In his books on medical jurisprudence and poisons, which were the standard works throughout the world, he codified the legal precedents, judicial rulings, and anatomic and chemical data that bore on his special subject of study. His second British edition was published in 1859. The works of both Christison and Taylor were subsequently published in America, and became the standard references for physicians and scientists up until the beginning of the 1900s.

America did not see a book published by one of its native sons until the publication of *Microchemistry of Poisons, Including Their Physiological, Pathological, and Legal Relations: Adapted to the Use of the Medical Jurist, Physician, and General Chemist* in 1869, by physician Theodore George Wormley (1826–1897). This book was considered his highest lifetime work, as never before in America had toxicologic subjects been handled with the high degree of literary skill and with such care to detail. The steel engravings of the images of microscopic poison residues, done by Wormley's wife, remain a marvel of the steel engraver's art. His work went on to a second edition in 1885.

The first book that was dedicated totally to the criminal investigation of poisoners and their use of poison as a weapon for murder, was *Criminal Poisoning: Investigational Guide for Law Enforcement, Toxicologists, Forensic Scientists, and Attorneys*, by forensic toxicologist John Harris Trestrail III (1944–), published in 2000. In this work, the epidemiology of criminal poisoning, the characteristics and advantages of ideal poisons, pathologic aspects of poisons, techniques for investigating murder by poisons, and trial strategies for attorneys when prosecuting a case involving poisons as weapons are discussed.

For the expert consultant to be effective in the determination of the possible toxicologic consequences of exposure to a poison, he or she must be aware of both the qualitative and quantitative toxicologic information that is determined by the application of analytical toxicology to the body in question.

HISTORICAL DEVELOPMENT OF ANALYTICAL TOXICOLOGY

It is probably safe to assume that the development of the science of general toxicology closely followed along with the developments in the field of chemistry. The beginnings of analytical toxicology were not to be seen until well into the 1800s.

The individual who first made it very difficult for the poisoner to get away with his murder by utilizing the then popular poison arsenic was Scottish chemist James Marsh (1794–1846). In 1836, Marsh developed and published a chemical test—that was to bear his name—that made it possible to detect the presence of arsenical compounds in food as well as in biologic specimens. Marsh observed that by taking a sample that contained arsenic and mixing it with zinc and sulfuric acid, the chemical reaction resulted in the production of arsine gas. The arsine gas produced by the chemical reaction, when heated, deposited a mirror of metallic arsenic on a cold surface. This test was so sensitive that it was able to detect the presence of arsenic in very minute concentrations. It now became possible to prove in court the presence of arsenical compounds, and thus the probable cause of the death of an individual. For the poisoner, the Marsh test was a definite setback. Soon after Marsh's contribution, other analytical test enhancements came into being.

Hugo Reinsch developed a test that allowed for the detection of arsenic at a level of approximately 0.00002 parts of a substance. Other analytical tests used during the first half of the 1900s included Bittendorf's test, the Gutzeit test, Hefti tests, and the Kage modification.

Over the years, with the development of more specific chemical testing and sensitive electronic instrumentation, the science of analytical toxicology has proven its invaluable role in aiding the forensic toxicologists in their work.

With the combined expertise of the forensic and analytical toxicologists, they become effective aids for the criminal investigator when dealing with a possible case of criminal poisoning.

CRIMINAL POISONING: INVESTIGATIVE ISSUES

A lack of witnesses and a crime surrounded by secrecy make the investigations of poisoning crimes very difficult. As stated by professor of forensic medicine John Glaister in his work *The Power of Poison*, "The very fact that the poisoner does not prepare his poison in the presence of the victim or before witnesses, but that the process is carried out in great secrecy, is the principal reason why the bringing home of the guilt of the criminal concerned becomes even more involved."[1]

The basic tenet in investigating a possible homicidal poisoning begins with considering it in the first place. If one does not look for the possibility of a poisoning, one will never be able to find it. Basically, the poisoner does not worry about disposing of his victim, for he counts on the medical establishment to do it for him. As a murderer, the poisoner wants his victim's death to appear most natural, which will result in the issuing of a death certificate and will not raise suspicion. This lack of suspicion will eventually lead to the burial or cremation of the remains, and thus the hiding of the most important evidence of the crime: the body. The body of the victim is the major source of important clues that tell the tale of what happened.

If poison is found in the body of a victim, the first question that is raised is why the substance is there at all.

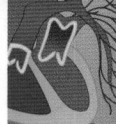

One must always remember that analytical toxicology only tells one that a poison is there; it does not answer the question of why the poison is there.

SOURCES OF POISON IN THE VICTIM

There can be many reasons why there may be a quantity of a potential poison found in an individual.

The source was accidental. Toxic levels of poisons can enter the body from such sources as the environment (e.g., arsenic in the ground water), or the exposure may have been occupational (e.g., lead from shooting ranges, automobile battery recycling, or other occupational sources).

The source was natural. Poisons can be found in the body after the consumption of certain food sources (e.g., arsenic after a large seafood meal or from the consumption of contaminated herbal remedies). High levels of a suspected poison can also be found in the body due to a medical condition (e.g., copper from Wilson's disease).

The source was self-administered. The victim might have received a toxic amount of a substance from a source that was administered by the victim himself (e.g., from misuse of a product, from substance abuse like a "hot shot," or from suicidal intent).

The source was administered by another individual. The victim might have received a toxic amount of a substance from a source that was administered by another individual (e.g., substance abuse, product tampering, or homicidal intent).

If it is determined that the source of the poison was administered by another individual with homicidal intent, then the question arises for the investigators as to who might be a suspect they should begin to investigate. What are some characteristics of the homicidal poisoner that could guide their investigation?

THE HOMICIDAL POISONER'S CHARACTERISTICS

To date no major scientific studies have been conducted that would allow one to create the criminal investigative analysis (sometimes erroneously referred to as a psychological profile) of the homicidal poisoner. However, some of the commonalities thought to be exhibited by this group of criminals include the following: non-confrontational, cowardly, greedy, fantasist, artistic, immature, possession of vanity (think they will not be discovered), and possessing a limited mind without sympathy.[1,2] Because of the nature of the crime, it is very possible that a poisoner shares some commonalities with a bomber, whose commonality has been worked on by the U.S. Federal Bureau of Investigation.

In 1996, criminal investigators Westveer, Trestrail, and Pinizzotto[3] published the results of the first epidemiologic study of criminal poisoning in the United States. Their study group results came from an analysis of criminal poisonings reported to the Department of Justice through the Uniform Crime Report program. Their investigation found that during the decade 1980 to 1989, in the 202,785 homicides reported, there were a total of 292 poisoning cases, in which there was a single offender associated with a single victim. This represented 14 poisonings per 100,000 reported homicides. Some of the information that was revealed in this study group of 292 poisoning murders is listed below.

Gender Relationships

Victims were equally divided between male and female.

If the victim was female, the offender was usually a male.

If the victim was a male, the offender was equally a male or female.

Offenders were male twice as often as female.

Racial Relationships

Victim and offender were usually of the same race.

Victims were mostly white.

If the victim was white, the offender was usually a male.

If the victim was black, the offender was equally a male or female.

Black victims were males twice as often as females.

White victims were equally male or female.

For both black and white offenders, there were twice as many males as females.

Age Characteristics

Victims were most numerous in the 25 to 29 year age range.

Offenders were most numerous in the 20 to 34 year age range.

Other Findings

Poisonings averaged 1.47 per million population per year.

The unknown offender rate for poisonings was 20 to 30 times higher than in nonpoisoning homicides!

An analysis of 900 cases of known criminal poisonings collected by the author of this chapter found the following:

Sex of offender: male (45%), female (38%), unknown (17%), showing that the majority of known poisoners are male. It is assumed that males perpetrate most murders, but poison is probably the preferred weapon of females. It is very possible that females are better at getting away with their crime due to their almost universal domestic roles: preparation of meals, taking care of the sick, and cleaning up the home.

Background of offender: dentist (1%), general public (68%), minister (1%), nurse (5%), juvenile (2%), pharmacist (1%), physician (7%), political (3%),

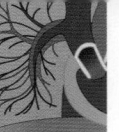

scientist (1%), unknown (11%). This seems to indicate that the vast majority of known poisoners are members of the general public, with no specific medical or scientific background.

Poison used: arsenic (26%), cyanide (9%), strychnine (6%). These top three agents represented 41% of the poisons used.

Number of victims: single (59%), multiple (41%). This shows that in known cases, poisoners were able to carry out multiple homicides before their crimes were eventually detected.

Motive for the crime: individual profit (23%), personal cause (10%), domestic (9%), nonspecific motive (5%), political extremism (6%). Most of the time, the motive for a poisoning murder revolves around money or the elimination of a significant other due to abuse or to obtain another significant other.

Location of the crime: United States (42%), Great Britain/England (21%), France (6%), Italy (4%). This analysis is naturally biased by the literature and news media available for analysis.

Overall, these studies seem to once again support the hypothesis that murder by poison is one of the easiest homicides to remain undetected. There is no other form of homicide that produces a serial killer rate as high as the 41% found in the poisoner group, as well as an unknown offender rate, which is 20 to 30 times higher than other forms of homicide.[1]

Certainly, further studies are warranted to try and determine if there are any commonalities found among the criminal poisoners. However, these studies await a focus of determination from interested parties, along with adequate funding to support this important research. Interviews of convicted poisoners whose cases are without appeal could be conducted in a manner similar to those studies already carried out that have looked for commonalities in convicted offenders of serial rape or serial murder.

With all of the unknown offenders and lack of witnesses, is there anything that could guide the investigators as they look into who might have caused the death of the victim? The answer is yes. There are observable clues that might indicate that something untoward might have happened to the victim.

WHEN SHOULD AN INVESTIGATOR'S SUSPICION BE AROUSED?

Here are some questions regarding signs that should quickly arouse suspicion in the toxicologist or criminal investigators that something in the "natural death" is not what it initially appears:

1. Was there a sudden death in a normally healthy individual?
2. Was there any interference in getting medical attention for the victim?
3. Was there the failure of a "natural disease" to respond to standard treatment?
4. Were relatives or friends not sent for during the victim's illness?
5. Are there no visible signs of violence?
6. Was there any history of a "cyclical illness" (in which the victim was ill at home, got better in a medical facility, then returned home and became ill again)?
7. Were there any common symptoms in a group of individuals?
8. Is there anyone around the victim with knowledge of poisons?
9. Was anyone anxious to dispose of food, drink, or medications?
10. Was a request made that there be no autopsy?
11. Was a request made for a rapid cremation?
12. Is the cause of death being vehemently insisted on by anyone in a possible suspect group?
13. Is anyone in a possible suspect group attempting to guide the investigation?

Certainly, the presence of one or more of these signs does not indicate that there was definitely a poisoning, or point the finger at the murderer, but all in all, any of these observed signs should make the investigator pause and ask the question, "Am I dealing with a possible homicidal poisoning in this case?" The prime mandate is that every death with no visible signs of violence is a poisoning until facts prove otherwise. Only through the constant practice of this rule will the victims of poisonings be found and given justice.

When it has been determined that a possible poisoning has occurred, what agencies or groups can an investigator turn to for assistance in the investigation of criminal poisoning?

ORGANIZATIONS AND RESOURCES FOR FORENSIC TOXICOLOGY

National and international organizations dealing with the specialty of forensic toxicology include the following: Society of Forensic Toxicologists (SOFT), The International Association of Forensic Toxicologists (TIAFT), and the toxicology section of the American Academy of Forensic Sciences (AAFS). These organizations deal mostly with the area of analytical toxicology, and more information on these organizations can be found at their individual websites.

There is also an organization that specializes mainly on the aspects of the investigation of criminal poisoning. The Center for the Study of Criminal Poisoning (CSCP) was founded in 1997 in order to provide an international mechanism for the exchange of information on homicidal poisonings. To these ends, the CSCP carries out the following activities:

1. Maintaining a database on criminal poisoning cases.
2. Providing training workshops on the investigation of murder by poison.
3. Conducting forensic research projects.
4. Encouraging international communications on criminal poisonings.

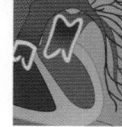

The CSCP has developed a reporting tool to be used in the sharing of information on homicidal poisoning cases and tampering incidents, and has made it available internationally to law enforcement agencies as well as forensic pathologists. This homicidal poisoning case registry reporting form is provided in Figure 7A-1 for duplication and submission of reports to the CSCP.

Once the investigation has proven that there is sufficient proof that a criminal poisoning has occurred, and that there is a suspect, the strategy for trial planning must begin.

CRIMINAL POISONING: LEGAL ISSUES

Murder by poison is one of the most difficult types of crime to take to litigation. One of the major problems is that in the vast majority of poisoning cases, there are no witnesses to the criminal action. This makes almost all of the available evidence indirect, or as it is otherwise termed, *circumstantial.*

The main question to be resolved by the court is whether the accused killed the deceased by poison. As stated by Wigmore,[4] the main question for the prosecution

---

Homicidal Poisoning Case Registry
(Please type or print, and use one form per VICTIM)

About the Victim

Victim's name: _____   Victim's age: _____

Victim's gender: _____   Victim's race: _____

About the Offender

Offender's name: _____   Offender's age: _____

Offender's gender: _____   Offender's race: _____

Offender's relationship to victim: _____

Offender's motive: _____

Offender's conviction status: _____

Additional offender information: _____

About the Poison

Poison(s) used: _____

Route of poison administration: _____

Source of the poison: _____

Location of the poisoning: _____
(home, public place, etc)

About Your Reporting Agency

Your case #: _____   Date: _____

Your name: _____   Your title: _____

Your address: _____

_____

_____

Telephone (voice): _____   Telephone (FAX): _____

E-mail address: _____

Please mail or FAX this completed form, and any supporting materials to:

John H. Trestrail, III RPb, FAACT, DABAT
CENTER for the STUDY of CRIMINAL POISONING
1840 Wealthy, S.E. Grand RapIds
MI 49506-2968 USA
Telephone: (616) 391-9099 (voice)
Fax: (616) 391-8417
E-mail: venomous@iserv.net

FIGURE 7A-1   Homicidal poisoning case registry.

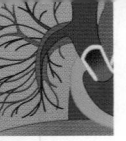

really resolves into three component questions of fact, each of which must be proved:

1. That the deceased's death was caused by poison.
2. That the poison was administered to the deceased by the accused.
3. That the accused was aware of the lethal nature of the administered substance.

Unless it can be proved by pathologic examination and/or analytical toxicology evidence that the deceased died from a poison, it is futile to inquire as to who might have murdered the person by this method. In attempting to prove that the poison was administered by the accused, one must be able to prove that the accused had an opportunity to administer the toxic agent. Lack of opportunity to administer the poison is one of the strongest arguments used for the accused by defense council. It is also important for the prosecution to be able to prove that the accused had possession of the poison and that no other person could possibly or probably have administered the poison. In proving that the accused had knowledge of the lethal nature of the compound in question, it is important for one to look at the educational background of the accused, references in his possession, and his possible access to information through vocation or avocation. One must always remember to consider access to information by computer from various Internet resources.

One of the difficulties in court is getting all the parties to agree on whether the agent in question is really a poison, by the acceptable definition of a poison.

Definition of Poison

Although it sounds easy, it is often very difficult to come up with an acceptable legal definition of what is a *poison*. The definitions of *poison* may differ by the laws of various states. Some of the definitions found in the legal literature include the following:

"Poison: is any substance, where introduced into the system, either directly or by absorption, produces violent, morbid or fatal changes, of which destroys living tissue with which it comes in contact." [Watkins vs. National Elec. Products Corp., C.C.A. Pa., 165, F.2d 980,982.]
"Poison: any substance which, when relatively small amounts are ingested, inhaled, absorbed, or applied to, injected into, or developed within the body, has chemical action that may cause damage to structure or disturbance of function producing symptomatology, illness, or death." [*Stedman's Medical Dictionary*, 26th ed., Williams & Wilkins, Baltimore, MD, 1995.]
"Poison: any substance which when ingested, inhaled, or absorbed, or when applied to, injected into, or developed within the body, in relatively small amounts, by its chemical action may cause damage to structure or disturbance of function." [*The*

Sloane-Dorland Annotated Medical-Legal Dictionary, West Publishing Co., New York, NY, 1987.]

What is really the major factor in defining a poison? To almost all toxicologists, the statement made by the famous 16th-century alchemist Phillippus Theophrastus Aureolus Bombastus von Hohenheim, also known as Paracelsus (1493–1541), comes about as close to the concept of poison as can be made. In his 1564 "Third Defense," he wrote, "What is there that is not poison, all things are poison and nothing (is) without poison. Solely the dose determines that a thing is not a poison." Just like the saying "everyone has his or her price," every substance has its dose at or beyond which lethality can occur. One can kill with water just as well as drugs; the only difference is the amount (dependent on the factors of concentration and time duration of exposure) to which the victim is exposed.

CRIMINAL POISONING: TRIAL STRATEGIES

In order to be able to prove "murder by poison," the following must be absolutely locked into place:

1. The "chain of evidence" was maintained. Being able to absolutely prove who had possession of the case evidence and when he or she took possession of it.
2. Presence of the poison has been proven by analysis. Utilizing information gained from both pathologic observations and chemical testing.
3. The poison was absorbed systemically and in circulation. For a poison to kill, it has to get to the right target organ or system in a concentration that would cause damage to the site and result in a fatality.

The prosecution will also have to be able to prove the following:

1. The death was caused by the poison. This fact will be proved through a combination of information gained from the death scene investigation, pathologic examination, and chemical analyses.
2. The accused administered the poison. Proving that the defendant had the opportunity and possession of the substance, and that it was not possible or probable that any other person could have given it.
3. The accused was aware of the poison's lethality. This is done by proving the possession of knowledge gained by conversation or research from reading.

CASE EXAMPLES

The following examples of actual homicidal poisoning cases show the effective results of a combined team of individuals from the specialties of forensic pathology, forensic toxicology, analytical toxicology, death investigators, and attorneys, working together to bring justice to the victim of this heinous type of crime.

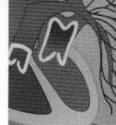

The Joanne Curley Case

Beginning in 1990, Joanne Curley of Wilkes-Barre, Pennsylvania, began administering the toxic metallic rodenticide thallium to her husband, Robert. Her motive was the $300,000 life insurance policy on her spouse. She slowly began to administer the poison to him in his food and drink and also brought thallium-laced iced tea to him as he lay near death in the hospital. In order to throw investigators off the trail, she also administered small amounts of the poison to herself and her daughter. In 1994, under pressure from concerned family members, authorities exhumed the body of the deceased. Analysis of his hair gave a chronological time line of the administration of the poison and linked his wife as the only possible perpetrator of the occurrences. Faced with the solid evidence of analytical and forensic toxicology, and in order to avoid a trial and a possible death penalty, she pled guilty to her husband's murder.

The Ronald Clark O'Bryan Case

On October 31, 1974, the children in Pasadena, Texas, were going about their normal Halloween activities. Eight-year-old Timothy Marc O'Bryan celebrated the evening by consuming some of his holiday candy. Shortly after consuming the powdery contents of a Giant Pixy Stick, he collapsed and died. Since it was the death of a normally healthy individual, suspicion centered on the product he had consumed. Subsequent analytical toxicology tests found that the product contained not a candy powder but potassium cyanide. Tampered treats were also found in the bags of four other children, who fortunately had not consumed any of the "candy." Panic ensued around the area that a demented tamperer had struck in their community! On physical examination, it was found that the treats had been opened and crudely stapled shut. Investigation soon centered on the dead boy's father, Ronald Clark O'Bryan, a Houston, Texas, optician. Investigators found that the suspect had recently taken out $65,000 worth of life insurance on his two children (motive), and witnesses stated that he had been making inquiries about the lethal dosage of cyanide and had attempted to purchase the same poison. At trial, without ever admitting to the crime, but with the damning forensic evidence, O'Bryan was found guilty. Ronald O'Bryan, whom the public dubbed the "Candy Man" and who nationally changed Halloween festivities forever, was executed by lethal injection on March 31, 1984.

CONCLUSION

Although the study of toxicology can be applied to all areas of living—environmental, occupational, clinical, and many others—it is in the area of its forensic application where the need for this special knowledge clearly cries out. It is with the application of our knowledge of poisons, their kinetics, toxicology, and analysis that one day the chances of success of the poisoner will hopefully begin to diminish and the chances of law enforcement's success will increase, to bring justice to the victims of this sinister and almost invisible crime.

DISCLAIMER

The information contained in this chapter is intended to serve the reader with general background information representing various aspects of toxicology as it applies to modern litigation. However, this is not intended to serve as a substitute for intensive research respecting various issues, as each case must be approached on a case-by-case basis. Some cases will require intensive research independent of this work.

REFERENCES

1. Glaister J: The Power of Poison. New York, William Morrow, 1954, p 12.
2. Rowland J: Poisoner in the Dock: Twelve Studies in Poisoning. London, Arco, 1960.
3. Westveer AE, Trestrail JH, Pinizzotto J: Homicidal poisonings in the United States: an analysis of the Uniform Crime Reports from 1980 through 1989. Am J Forensic Med Pathol 1996;17(4): 282–298.
4. Wigmore JH: Circumstantial evidence in poisoning cases. Clinics 1943;1(6):1507–1519.

SUGGESTED READING

Browne GL, Stewart CG: Reports of Trials for Murder by Poisoning. London, Stevens and Sons, 1883.
Farrell M: Poisons and Poisoners: An Encyclopedia of Homicidal Poisonings. London, Robert Hale, 1992.
Furst A: The Toxicologist as Expert Witness: A Hint Book for Courtroom Procedure. Washington, DC, Taylor & Francis, 1997.
Jones RG: Poison! The World's Greatest True Murder Stories. Secaucus, NJ, Lyle Stuart, 1987.
McLaughlin T: The Coward's Weapon. London, Robert Hale, 1980.
Thompson CJS: Poison Mysteries Unsolved. London, Hutchinson & Co., 1937.
Thompson CJS: Poisons and Poisoners. New York, Macmillan, 1931.
Thorwald J: Proof of Poison. London, Thames and Hudson, 1966.
Trestrail JH: Criminal Poisoning: Investigational Guide for Law Enforcement, Toxicologists, Forensic Scientists, and Attorneys. Totowa, NJ, Humana, 2000.

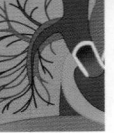

B   Clinical Issues

PHILIPPE E. HANTSON, MD, PHD

At a Glance...

- The major obstacle to organ transplantation is the lack of suitable donors, but poisoned patients are often overlooked as potential organ donors.
- Extremely strict brain death criteria have to be applied in this particular setting.
- Experience with grafts obtained from intoxicated donors is limited, but the results appear similar to those observed with nonpoisoned donors. To date, no failure has been related to a toxic origin.
- Each case needs to be evaluated on an individual basis according to the clinical, biologic, and morphologic findings in the donor, and to the knowledge of the toxicologic properties of the compound.

INTRODUCTION AND EPIDEMIOLOGY

Postmortem studies are particularly important in cases of fatal poisoning, not only to determine the cause of death but also to collect data on the target organs of some specific poisonings. They usually combine a morphologic analysis and a study of the toxicokinetics of the substance. This question is essential when organ donation is considered from a donor declared brain dead after acute poisoning. Even though this occurrence seems exceptional, poisoned donors should not be systematically overlooked as potential organ donors.[1,2] Current data available from the transplant coordination organizations indicate that poisoned patients represent less than 1% of all organ donors.

The purpose of this chapter is to present the experience of organ donation after fatal poisoning and to discuss organ acceptability criteria.

In 1994, Leikin and colleagues published a series of 17 poisoned patients who were accepted as organ donors.[3] The toxicants involved were ethanol (n = 8), cocaine (n = 5), carbon monoxide (n = 5), barbiturates (n = 2), cannabis (n = 1), lead (n = 1), and phenylpropanolamine (n = 1), with six patients having had multidrug involvement. There were 41 recipients, including 32 kidney transplantations and 9 liver transplantations. There were two fatalities in the early postoperative phase in the liver group, but it was concluded that death was definitely not related to the toxic origin of the graft. In the kidney group, renal function immediately after the procedure was good in 28 of 32 patients (1 graft loss occurred on day 5 due to thrombosis, 3 had transient dysfunction) and remained satisfactory at 8-month follow-up in 31 of 32 cases.

The experience of a single center in Belgium was described in a series of 21 poisoned donors collected over an 8-year period.[4-6] In this center, poisoned donors in brain death status represented 7% of all the organ donors for this time period. The toxicants involved were benzodiazepines (n = 2), tricyclic antidepressants (n = 1), benzodiazepines and tricyclic antidepressants (n = 1), barbiturates (n = 2), insulin (n = 2), carbon monoxide (n = 3), cyanide (n = 1), methaqualone (n = 1), paracetamol (acetaminophen) (n = 1), and methanol (n = 7). On the whole, 58 grafts were obtained: 39 kidneys, 6 hearts, 2 lungs, 9 livers, and 2 pancreases. Overall recipient survival rates at 1 year and 5 years were, respectively, 100% and 88% in the kidney group, 100% and 100% in the pancreas group, 67% and 67% in the liver group, 50% and 33% in the heart group, and 100% and 100% in the single case of lung transplantation. One liver graft and one kidney graft failed to function after 1 month. Two additional kidney grafts and one liver graft failed after a longer delay. The analysis of the causes of mortality or morbidity (graft loss) did not reveal any correlation with the toxic origin of the grafts.

CRITERIA FOR ORGAN AND DONOR ACCEPTABILITY

Several criteria have to be met when organ donation is considered after fatal poisoning[7]:

1. The first crucial issue is the accuracy of the brain death diagnosis in the presence of drugs influencing the central nervous system.[8] Even if brain death is basically a clinical diagnosis, confirmatory tests may be required. The confirmatory tests may demonstrate the absence of cerebral blood flow (four-vessel angiography, radioisotope technique, and transcranial Doppler) or the absence of cerebral electrical activity (electroencephalography [EEG], multimodality evoked potentials). Cerebral four-vessel angiography is the gold standard in this condition; however, this test is invasive and cannot be easily repeated at the bedside. There are several limitations to the use of EEG because this technique is very sensitive to hypothermia, drugs, and metabolic disorders. In experienced hands, multimodality evoked potentials investigations were found to be extremely helpful in this particular setting.[8]
2. The patient considered as a potential organ donor should not be exhibiting any clinical sign of toxicity associated with the toxic exposure.
3. The possible damages to the organs to be harvested are to be carefully evaluated. Direct toxic injuries may be found in the target organs of poisoning, while indirect injury due to anoxia or metabolic disorders may be noted in the other organs. Usually, the same methodology as for nonpoisoned donors can be applied. This is mainly based on routine

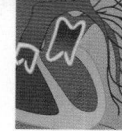

laboratory analysis (biologic markers) and on morphologic examination; tissue biopsies after organ harvesting are then particularly helpful.

4. Due to tissue storage with some substances, there is a theoretical risk for secondary poisoning of the recipient. This risk should be limited by a perfect understanding of the toxicokinetics of the concerned toxin.

5. The problem of organ donation from nonintravenous drug abusers remains an open issue.[1,9] It is important that, particularly in the drug abuse population, all potential organ donors undergo a thorough infectious disease screening prior to transplantation to exclude as far as possible the transmission of an infectious agent (hepatitis B and C, human immunodeficiency virus). Such screening, however, will not detect the donors who are still in the window of infectivity.

SPECIFIC SUBSTANCES

Psychotropic Drugs

Multiple organ procurements have been performed after fatalities due to benzodiazepine or barbiturate overdoses.[4-6] Heart donation after barbiturate poisoning is possible provided hemodynamic disturbances have been corrected.

Theoretically, with tricyclic antidepressants (TCAs), there is a risk of accumulation of the toxic substance in some tissues (lung, kidney, heart, liver). The literature includes at least one case that describes the possible transmission to the recipient of TCAs stored in the liver graft.[10] The heart is obviously a target organ of TCA poisoning, and heart donation is contraindicated; moreover, extremely high TCA concentrations can be found in the myocardium at postmortem analysis. For the other organs, it seems advisable to wait until the donor plasma TCA concentration falls well below 2000 ng/mL. This cannot always be achieved because sustained high blood concentrations are sometimes observed after massive TCA overdose. Furthermore, quantitative analyses of TCAs are not universally available.

Few data with regard to the more recent selective serotonin reuptake inhibitors (SSRIs) exist. Mortality directly due to SSRI overdose is low, but severe serotonin syndrome may rapidly progress to cardiac arrest, coma, seizures, or multi-organ failure with disseminated intravascular coagulation. Cardiotoxicity due to SSRIs is usually low and can be identified on the electrocardiogram (ECG) (conduction abnormalities, prolonged QT interval). Death may exceptionally result from malignant arrhythmias. This obviously contraindicates heart donation. In a single case report, the heart was procured from a donor who died from ventricular fibrillation following venlafaxine and fluoxetine overdose.[11] High doses of vasopressors were initially required in the donor before the heart was finally accepted. The recipient suffered multiple episodes of supraventricular arrhythmias during the postoperative phase, and it was speculated that SSRI accumulation in heart tissue might have played a role.

Before considering organ donation, it must be remembered that some SSRIs (e.g., fluoxetine) and their metabolites have a prolonged elimination half-life, suggesting the possibility of tissue storage (e.g., in the lung) with these agents.

ACETAMINOPHEN

Surprisingly, a relatively few number of heart or kidney transplantations have been reported from donors who died from acetaminophen poisoning.[9] Both oliguric and nonoliguric acute renal failure has been described following acetaminophen overdose, mostly as a component of multi-organ failure complicating fulminant hepatic failure.[12] It occurs rarely in the absence of clinical or biochemical evidence of liver damage. Histologic findings are consistent with acute tubular necrosis. Kidney donation may be considered in fatal acetaminophen poisoning according to the laboratory data and the results of renal biopsy. There is no direct evidence that acetaminophen causes cardiotoxicity.[13] Nonspecific ECG changes have been noted in patients with acetaminophen overdose. Postmortem studies revealed histological features in some cases that were consistent with toxic myocarditis, such as diffuse myocardial damage with interstitial edema or bands of necrosis and hemorrhage. It is very likely that other factors contributed to toxicity, because such lesions have been widely observed in fulminant hepatic failure not due to acetaminophen poisoning. At least three cases of uncomplicated heart transplantations have been reported in this setting.[13] The lung is also not directly damaged in case of acetaminophen poisoning, and lung donation is possible. Finally, pancreatitis seems also to be extremely rare after acetaminophen overdose.

CARBON MONOXIDE

Fatalities due to accidental exposure to carbon monoxide (CO) are still quite common, but it should be noted that few of these fatalities could result in organ procurement. CO reduces both the oxygen-carrying capacity of hemoglobin and oxygen delivery to tissues. CO binds to the cytochrome oxidase system to reduce cellular utilization of oxygen. As expected, tissues most sensitive to oxygen deprivation (central nervous system, myocardium) are most sensitive to CO toxicity. The pathologic substrate for myocardial toxicity from CO poisoning is the subendocardial region, characterized by scattered areas of necrosis, hemorrhage, and muscle fiber degeneration; these lesions are similar to those observed in anoxia from another origin.

There are many case reports of successful kidney, pancreas, lung, or liver transplantation from CO-poisoned donors.[14,15] The possibility of heart donation still remains controversial, in spite of the positive experience that has frequently been published (Table 7B-1).[16-25] Of concern are the reports of impaired cardiac contractility during the postoperative phase where the role of CO toxicity can be at least suspected.[21] This is in agreement with an isolated report showing a

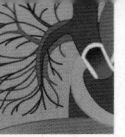
TABLE 7B-1 Experience with Heart Procurement from CO-Poisoned Donors

AGE (YR)/ SEX	COHb	CPR	ECG	CARDIAC ENZYMES	ECHO	INOTROPIC DRUGS	OUTCOME	REFERENCES
		DONORS				RECIPIENTS		
29/M	14.7%	No	NI	CK-MM↑	NI	No	+	17
27/F	43%	Yes	NI	CK-MM↑	NI	No	+	17
30/M	>29%	No	Abn	No	—	—	+	18
25/M	—	No	Abn	—	—	—	+ but X after 1 yr (rejection)	19
5 cases	16.4%– 20%	3	NI	CK-MM↑	NI (2)	Dopamine < 4 µg/kg/min, dobutamine < 1.5 µg/kg/min	2+,3X	20
31/F	36%	Yes	NI	CK-MB↑	NI	Postoperative biventricular assist device	+	21
25/F	—	Yes	NI	—	NI	Dopamine 10 µg/kg/min	+	22
46/M	—	Yes	NI	—	NI	No	+	22
40/F	—	—	NI	—	NI	Dobutamine	X	23
14/F	—	—	NI	—	NI	Dobutamine	+	23
20/M	—	—	NI	—	NI	No	+	23
25/M	—	—	NI	—	NI	—	+	23
15/M	—	—	NI	—	NI	No	+	23
47/M	—	—	NI	—	NI	Epinephrine	+	23
17/M	48%	Yes	Abn	—	NI	Dopamine	X	24
30/M	10%	Yes	—	—	—	No	X	25
17/M	8%	Yes	NI	No	—	No	X	16

Abn, abnormal; COHb, carboxyhemoglobin; CPR, cardiopulmonary resuscitation; ECG, electrocardiogram; Echo: echocardiography; NI, normal; —, not available; ↑, increased; +, alive; X, deceased.

depression of myocardial contractility following acute CO poisoning in a patient who had no electrocardiographic, angiographic, or biologic evidence of myocardial infarction; electron microscopy of the endomyocardial biopsy showed ultrastructural changes in the mitochondria that are a primary target of CO intracellular toxicity. Some donors described in the literature had received prolonged resuscitation and vasopressors before the harvesting procedure. Some had an abnormal ECG or echocardiography, with increased cardiac enzymes. Therefore, it seems of utmost importance to exclude from heart donation the donors presenting these features. The determination of CO blood levels is not helpful for the decision to remove or not remove the heart, although myocardial ischemia following CO poisoning is usually seen with carboxyhemoglobin levels above 25%.

Theoretically, lung donation is possible after pure CO poisoning.[23] When CO intoxication occurs following smoke inhalation, there is an increased risk for chemical or thermal injury to the lung.

CYANIDE

Acute pure cyanide poisoning is rare. Cyanide inhibits mitochondrial cytochrome-*c* oxidase activity. This results in a shift of aerobic to anaerobic metabolism, eventually leading to adenosine triphosphate depletion and lactic acidosis. Cyanide is distributed to all the tissues via the blood; its concentration in red cells is much greater than that in plasma. Cyanide is metabolized in the liver by an endogenous enzyme, rhodanase, to thiocyanate. Half-life for the conversion of cyanide to thiocyanate from a nonlethal dose in humans is between 20 minutes and 1 hour. As expected, the brain and the heart are particularly sensitive to cyanide-induced hypoxia. Collapse of the cardiovascular system requires cyanide doses higher than those necessary for injury to the central nervous system. This explains why brain death may be observed in patients who underwent successful cardiopulmonary resuscitation after cyanide exposure. The experience with organ donation following fatal cyanide exposure is summarized in Table 7B-2. At least two cases of successful heart transplantation have been described in the literature.[26-28] In addition, there are numerous reports of cornea, kidney, pancreas, or liver transplantations.[29-34] There is a theoretical risk for transmission of poisoning to the recipient. However, the elimination half-life of cyanide in patients treated with antidotes is usually much less than 24 hours. In forensic medicine, a blood cyanide of greater than or equal to 1.0 mg/L (38.5 µmol/L) is generally considered to represent a potentially toxic concentration.[35] No clinical symptoms develop with whole blood concentrations below 0.2 mg/L (7.7 µmol/L), and organ harvesting may then be proposed. It has also been shown that, during the course of pure cyanide poisoning, a plasma lactate concentration of at least 8 mmol/L was indicative of a toxic blood cyanide concentration (at least 1.0 mg/L). It seems therefore imperative to achieve the correction of lactic acidosis before any procedure.

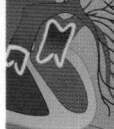

TABLE 7B-2 Literature Data on Organ Procurement from Cyanide-Poisoned Donors

ORGANS PROCURED	TOTAL NUMBER OF GRAFTS	CYANIDE BLOOD LEVEL (ADMISSION) (μmol/L)	CYANIDE BLOOD LEVEL (PROCUREMENT) (μmol/L)	IMMEDIATE OUTCOME	LATE OUTCOME (1 YEAR)	REFERENCES
Heart	1	Thiocyanate: 0.34		Good	Good (3 mo)	28
	1	—	0.95 (postmortem)	Good	Good	26,27
Liver	1	—	0.95 (postmortem)	Good	Good	26,27
Kidney	2	804	8	Dialysis (transient)	Good	32
	2	4.2	1.8	Good	Good	31
	2	—	0.95 (postmortem)	Good (1 acute rejection)	Good	26,27
	2	Thiocyanate: 0.34		Good	Good (3 mo)	28
	2	—	—	Good	1 acute rejection	29
	2	261	23	Good	Good (9 mo)	30
Pancreas	1	4.2	1.8	Good	Good	31
Cornea	2	—	—	Good	Good	33
	2	Thiocyanate: 0.34	—	Good	Good (3 mo)	28
	2	—	0.95 (postmortem)	Good	Good	26,27
	2	261	23	Good	Good (9 mo)	30

—, unavailable.

ORGANOPHOSPHATES

The liver and kidneys were harvested from a 17-year-old boy who was declared brain dead 5 days after the voluntary ingestion of an unknown amount of malathion.[36] Blood and tissue concentrations of malathion were not obtained. At the time of organ removal, there was no sign of hepatotoxicity or renal toxicity. No further cholinergic toxicity was evident after discontinuation of atropine and pralidoxime. These data cannot be extrapolated to other organophosphate compounds. Organophosphates are generally lipophilic and initially concentrate in the liver; redistribution may also occur to fatty tissues. Malathion can be activated to malaoxon but is rapidly hydrolyzed to nontoxic metabolites and excreted primarily by the kidney. Due to differences in disposition, each organophosphate compound should be analyzed on an individual basis before considering organ donation.

METHANOL

Methanol poisoning might still be regarded by some transplant physicians as an absolute or relative contra-indication to organ donation. However, the experience with organ procurement from patients poisoned by methanol is growing, as illustrated by some recent publications (Table 7B-3).[22,37-45] In contrast to the relatively rapid metabolism of ethylene glycol, methanol is slowly metabolized into formaldehyde and formate by alcohol and aldehyde dehydrogenases. Formic acid accumulation may reflect the severity of methanol poisoning. While variable concentrations of formic acid have been found in different tissues (e.g., heart, liver, kidney) at postmortem studies, it seems unlikely that a significant toxicity could be transferred to the organ recipient. The brain and the retina are the main target organs of poisoning. Brain death may be the consequence of diffuse brain edema or of hemorrhagic lesions mainly originating in the basal ganglia. The largest experience exists now with kidney donation. Kidney graft biopsies performed before transplantation revealed minor tubulointerstitial lesions as usually seen in grafts and ascribable to an ischemia-reperfusion sequence or, in some cases, minor hydropic changes.[38] No glomerular or vascular lesions were observed. Fatty changes and microvesicular fat have been described in the hepatocytes in an autopsy study. However, it should be recalled that the patients poisoned by methanol are often chronic ethanol abusers. The liver can be safely procured after methanol poisoning provided that liver function tests are normal with absence of steatosis at the biopsy. The incidence of pancreatic injury (increase of pancreatic enzymes or clinically severe acute necrotizing pancreatitis) after methanol poisoning probably has been underestimated.[46] The pathophysiology remains unclear. Here also, the pancreas injury may be at least triggered by chronic ethanol consumption or ethanol administration as an antidote for methanol poisoning. This suggests that successful pancreatic transplantation may be difficult.[37] Experience with lung or heart transplantation is far more limited.[22,43,44] The lung is not a target organ of methanol poisoning and trans-plantation is acceptable. As for the heart, it seems also that methanol poisoning is not an absolute contra-indication to organ donation. There is no clear evidence that methanol or its toxic metabolites may provoke direct injury to the myocardium. Cardiac dysfunction in fatal cases of methanol poisoning is usually related to the severity of metabolic acidosis. Heart donation should only be considered when no inotropic support is required in the donor.

Before starting any harvesting procedure, it is essential to have achieved the correction of metabolic acidosis and to wait until methanol has completely disappeared from blood.

ETHYLENE GLYCOL

Ethylene glycol, due to its metabolism to glycoaldehyde, glycolic acid, and glyoxalate, causes severe metabolic acidosis. Most deaths occur during this period of metabolic acidosis, which is associated with cerebral edema, seizures, and multi-organ failure. Glyoxalate is

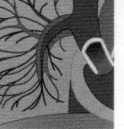

TABLE 7B-3 Organ Donation after Fatal Methanol Poisoning

ORGANS PROCURED	TOTAL NUMBER OF GRAFTS	IMMEDIATE OUTCOME	LATE OUTCOME (SURVIVAL RATE OR GRAFT FUNCTION)		REFERENCES
			1 YEAR	5 YEARS	
Heart	4	1 death	NI function in 3 cases	—	43
	1	Good	NI function	NI function	41,42
	3	Postoperative complications in 2 cases	NI death after 18 mo; NI function in 2 cases	NI function (4–7 yr) in 2 cases	22
	2	1 death	—	—	37
Lung	1 double	Good	NI function	NI function	44
	2	Good	—	—	37
Liver	5	1 death	NI function in 4 cases	—	43
	1	Good	NI function after 5 mo	—	45
	4	1 death	—	—	37
	3	Good	NI function	NI function	39,41,42
Kidney	29	Good	100% survival	83% survival	43
	13	Good	100% survival	100% survival with NI function	42
	2	—	—	—	45
	9 + 1 kidney and pancreas	1 death	—	—	37
	4	Good	NI function after 2 yr	—	40
	4	1 death	NI function	—	38

Fatalities and postoperative complications were not related to methanol poisoning.
—, not available; NI, normal.

converted to oxalate, which precipitates as calcium oxalate crystals in body tissues. Oxalate crystal deposition has been described not only in the kidney, but also in the brain and other organs. Renal failure usually occurs within 24 to 48 hours after ingestion. Because the kidney is clearly a major target organ, kidney donation remains contraindicated even though positive experiences have been reported. In contrast, there is no report of significant hepatic damage directly related to ethylene glycol poisoning, and successful liver procurement has been reported.[47] As for the heart, no transplant data are available. Cardiocirculatory failure may be a terminal event in presence of severe metabolic acidosis; heart donation should only be considered in patients with a normal ECG and echocardiography who do not require inotropic drugs.

The same precautions (correction of metabolic acidosis, absence of detectable toxicant) should be observed as in methanol poisoning.

ILLICIT SUBSTANCES

Leikin and colleagues have reported successful kidney and liver transplantations from donors who were positive for cocaine on the toxicology screen.[3] However, the possibility of heart donation remains debatable.[48,49] Cocaine is an increasing cause of intracerebral bleeding in young people and is more and more frequently identified in the biologic fluids of patients presenting with traumatic brain death. It can be assumed that the incidence of nonintravenous cocaine use is increasing among the potential organ donors in the general population. Some transplant teams have suggested liberalization of donor acceptability criteria in order to increase the heart donor pool.[49] They claim that the

outcome of patients who received transplanted hearts obtained from nonintravenous cocaine users was not significantly different from that observed with grafts procured from donors who had no history of cocaine use. This conclusion is not fully supported by some clinical observations and by our knowledge of the possible cardiotoxicity following acute or chronic cocaine use. At autopsy, cocaine-associated findings include myocarditis and myocyte and contraction band necrosis; left ventricular hypertrophy may occur after several years of cocaine abuse. For these reasons, heart donation should only be considered with extreme caution. In contrast, it does not seem that inhalation of cocaine or marijuana contraindicates lung procurement.[50]

Published experience is now also appearing with the drug Ecstasy (3,4-methylenedioxymethamphetamine). Multi-organ procurements (heart, liver, kidney, kidney-pancreas, lung) were obtained from two donors who died from brain edema following ecstasy use.[51] Two fatalities were observed among the eight recipients, but they were not related to a toxic origin.

UNUSUAL SUBSTANCES

Successful transplantations have been reported from donors who died from complications of long-acting anticoagulant therapy. Fatal fulminant hepatic failure due to *Amanita* poisoning led to heart and kidney donation.

CONCLUSION

Successful organ transplantation is possible with grafts coming from brain-dead donors following acute

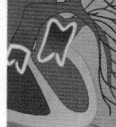

poisoning. A thorough examination of each individual case should be performed jointly by the members of the transplant team and medical toxicologists.

REFERENCES

1. Wood DM, Dargan PI, Jones AL: Poisoned patients as potential organ donors: postal survey of transplant centres and intensive care units. Critical Care 2003;7:147–154.
2. Hantson P, Mahieu P: Organ donation after fatal poisoning. QJM 1999;92:415–418.
3. Leikin JB, Heyn-Lamb R, Erickson T, Snyder J: The toxic patient as a potential organ donor. Am J Emerg Med 1994;12:151–154.
4. Hantson Ph, Vekemans MC, Squifflet JP, Mahieu P: Outcome following organ removal from poisoned donors: experience with 12 cases and a review of the literature. Transplant Int 1995; 8:185–189.
5. Hantson P, Mahieu P, Hassoun A, Otte JB: Outcome following organ removal from poisoned donors in brain death status: a report of 12 cases and review of the literature. J Toxicol Clin Toxicol 1995;33:709–712.
6. Hantson P, Vekemans MC, Vanormelingen P, et al: Organ procurement after evidence of brain death in victims of acute poisoning. Transplant Proc 1997;29:3341–3342.
7. Hantson P: The poisoned donors. Curr Opin Organ Transplant 1999;4:125–129.
8. Hantson P, Mahieu P, de Tourtchaninoff M, Guérit JM: The problem of "brain death" and organ donation in poisoned patients. In Machado C (ed): Recent Developments in Neurology "Brain Death." Amsterdam, Elsevier, 1995, pp 119–126.
9. Jones AL, Simpson KJ: Drug abusers and poisoned patients: a potential source of organs for transplantation. QJM 1998;91: 589–592.
10. Fattinger KE, Rentsch KM, Meier PJ, et al: Safety of liver donation after fatal intoxication with the tricyclic antidepressant trimipramine. Transplantation 1996;62:1259–1262.
11. Tenderich G, Dagge A, Schulz U, et al: Successful use of cardiac allograft from serotonin antagonist intoxication. Transplantation 2001;72:529.
12. Jones AL, Prescott LF: Unusual complications of paracetamol poisoning. QJM 1997;90:161–168.
13. Hantson P, Vekemans MC, Laterre PF, et al: Heart donation after fatal acetaminophen poisoning. J Toxicol Clin Toxicol 1997;35:325–326.
14. Verran D, Chui A, Painter D, et al: Use of liver allografts from carbon monoxide poisoned cadaveric donors. Transplantation 1996;62:1514–1515.
15. Hebert MJ, Boucher A, Beaucage G, et al: Transplantation of kidneys from a donor with carbon monoxide poisoning. N Engl J Med 1992;326:1571.
16. Hantson P, Vekemans MC, Squifflet JP, Mahieu P: Organ transplantation from victims of carbon monoxide poisoning. Ann Emerg Med 1996;27:673–674.
17. Smith JA, Bergin PJ, Williams TJ, Esmore DS: Successful heart transplantation with cardiac allografts exposed to carbon monoxide poisoning. J Heart Lung Transplant 1992;11:698–700.
18. Iberer F, Königsrainer A, Wasler A, et al: Cardiac allograft harvesting after carbon monoxide poisoning. Report of a successful orthotopic heart transplantation. J Heart Lung Transplant 1993;12:499–500.
19. Roberts JR, Bain M, Klachko MN, et al: Successful heart transplantation from a victim of carbon monoxide poisoning. Ann Emerg Med 1995;26:652–655.
20. Koerner MM, Tenderich G, Minami K, et al: Extended donor criteria: use of cardiac allografts after carbon monoxide poisoning. Transplantation 1997;63:1358–1360.
21. Rodrigus IE, Conraads V, Amsel BJ, Moulijn AC: Primary cardiac allograft failure after donor carbon monoxide poisoning treated with biventricular assist device. J Heart Lung Transplant 2001; 20:1345–1348.
22. Bentley MJ, Mullen JC, Lopushinsky SR, Modry DL: Successful cardiac transplantation with methanol or carbon monoxide-poisoned donors. Ann Thorac Surg 2001;71:1194–1197.
23. Luckraz H, Tsui SS, Parameshwar J, et al: Improved outcome with organs from carbon monoxide poisoned donors for intrathoracic transplantation. Ann Thorac Surg 2001;72:709–713.
24. Karwande SV, Hopfenbeck JA, Renlund DG, et al: The Utah transplantation program. An avoidable pitfall in donor selection for heart transplantation. J Heart Transplant 1989;8:422–424.
25. Shennib H, Adoumie R, Fraser R: Successful transplantation of a lung allograft from a carbon monoxide-poisoning victim. J Heart Lung Transplant 1992;11:68–71.
26. Snyder JW, Unkle DW, Nathan HM, Yang S-L: Successful donation and transplantation of multiple organs from a victim of cyanide poisoning. Transplantation 1993;55:425–427.
27. Swanson-Biearman B, Krenzelok EP, Snyder JW, et al: Successful donation and transplantation of multiple organs from a victim of cyanide poisoning. J Toxicol Clin Toxicol 1993;31:95–99.
28. Barkoukis TJ, Sarbak CA, Lewis D, Whittier FC: Multiorgan procurement from a victim of cyanide poisoning. A case report and review of the literature. Transplantation 1993;55: 1434–1436.
29. Puig JM, Lloveras J, Knobel H, et al: Victims of cyanide poisoning make suitable organ donors. Transplant Int 1996;9:87–88.
30. Ravishankar DK, Kashi SH: Organ transplantation from donor who died of cyanide poisoning: a case report. Clin Transplant 1998;12:142–143.
31. Hantson P, Squifflet JP, Vanormelingen P, Mahieu P: Organ transplantation after fatal cyanide poisoning. Clin Transplant 1999;13:72–73.
32. Brown P, Buckels J, Jain A, McMaster P: Successful cadaveric renal transplantation from a donor who died from cyanide poisoning. BMJ 1987;294:1325.
33. Lindquist TD, Oiland D, Weber K: Cyanide poisoning victims as corneal transplant donors. Am J Ophthalmol 1988;106:354–355.
34. Hantson P, Vekemans MC, Squifflet JP, et al: Successful pancreas-renal transplantation after cyanide poisoning. Clin Transplant 1991;5:419–421.
35. Baud FJ, Borron SW, Megarbane B, et al: Value of lactic acidosis in the assessment of the severity of acute cyanide poisoning. Crit Care Med 2002;30:2044–2050.
36. Dribben WH, Kirk MA: Organ procurement and successful transplantation after malathion poisoning. J Toxicol Clin Toxicol 2001;39:633–636.
37. Chari RS, Hemming AW, Cattral M: Successful kidney pancreas transplantation from donor with methanol intoxication. Transplantation 1998;66:674–675.
38. Friedlaender MM, Rosenmann E, Rubinger D, et al: Successful renal transplantation from two donors with methanol intoxication. Transplantation 1996;61:1549–1552.
39. Hantson P, Kremer Y, Lerut J, et al: Successful liver transplantation with a graft coming from a methanol-poisoned donor. Transplant Int 1996;9:437.
40. Zavala A, Nogue S: Methanol poisoning and renal transplant. Rev Esp Anestesiol Reanim 1986;33:373.
41. Hantson P, Vanormelingen P, Lecomte C, et al: Fatal methanol poisoning and organ donation: experience with seven cases in a single center. Transplant Proc 2000;32:491–492.
42. Hantson P, Vanormelingen P, Squifflet JP, et al: Methanol poisoning and organ transplantation. Transplantation 1999;68:165–166.
43. Lopez-Navidad A, Caballero F, Gonzalez-Segura C, et al: Short- and long-term success of organs transplanted from acute methanol poisoned donors. Clin Transplant 2002;16:151–162.
44. Evrard P, Hantson P, Ferrant E, et al: Successful double lung transplantation with a graft obtained from a methanol poisoned donor. Chest 1999;115:1458–1459.
45. Zota V, Popescu I, Ciurea S, et al: Successful use of the liver of a methanol-poisoned, brain dead donor. Transplant Int 2003;16: 444–446.
46. Hantson P, Mahieu P: Pancreatic injury following acute methanol poisoning. J Toxicol Clin Toxicol 2000;38:297–303.
47. Dy-Liacco MS, Tuttle-Newhall EJ, Collins BH, Kuo PC: Liver transplantation from a cadaver donor with ethylene-glycol-induced brain death. Transplantation 2003;75:1056.
48. Houser SL, MacGillivray T, Aretz HT: The impact of cocaine on the donor heart: a case report. J Heart Lung Transplant 2000;19:609–611.

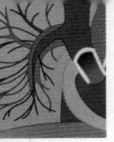

49. Freimark D, Czer LS, Admon D, et al: Donors with a history of cocaine use: effect on survival and rejection frequency after heart transplantation. J Heart Lung Transplant 1994;13:1138–1144.

50. Bhorade SM, Vigneswaran W, McCabe MA, Garrity ER: Liberalization of donor criteria may expand the donor pool without adverse consequence in lung transplantation. J Heart Lung Transplant 2000;19:1199–1204.

51. Caballero F, Lopez-Navidad A, Cotorruelo J, Txoperena G: Ecstasy-induced brain death and acute hepatocellular failure: multiorgan donor and liver transplantation. Transplantation 2002;74:532–537.

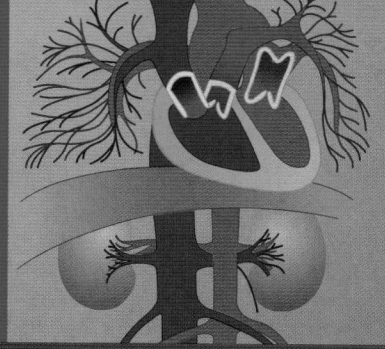

SECTION B
EFFECTS OF POISONING BY ORGAN SYSTEM

8

Cardiovascular Toxicology

NANCY G. MURPHY, MD ■ NEAL L. BENOWITZ, MD ■ NORA GOLDSCHLAGER, MD

Cardiovascular complications account for a substantial proportion of the morbidity and mortality in cases of drug overdose. Drug- or toxin-induced cardiovascular syndromes include hypotension and circulatory shock, hypertension, arrhythmias, and pulmonary edema. This chapter focuses on disturbances of cardiac function, particularly circulatory failure and arrhythmias. Patho-physiology, recognition of specific types of overdose, and principles of management are discussed.

HYPOTENSION AND CIRCULATORY SHOCK

Mechanisms

Hypotension occurs after overdosage with many different types of drugs. The mechanisms of hypotension are diverse, and hemodynamic patterns vary with different drugs in different stages of overdose and according to the presence and nature of underlying medical illness. Cardiac output may be reduced as a result of drug-induced myocardial depression, relative hypovolemia resulting from venous pooling, or true hypovolemia resulting from vascular injury and fluid loss from the vascular space. Peripheral vascular resistance may be reduced because of drug-induced vascular relaxation, adrenergic receptor blockade, or depression of central vasomotor tone. Myocardial and vascular dysfunction resulting from hypoxia, acidosis, and hypotension may complicate the picture.

The importance of hypotension is that it warns the physician of possible circulatory insufficiency; blood pressure also is one of several indicators of response to treatment. The diagnosis of circulatory shock depends on evidence of tissue hypoperfusion. Urine output and markers of cellular metabolism, such as lactate, are useful indicators of hypoperfusion, but they must be interpreted in the context of physical findings, hemodynamic variables, and other metabolic parameters (arterial blood gas, glucose).[1] In patients with underlying coronary artery or cerebrovascular disease, the development of cardiac or cerebral ischemia may limit the tolerable extent of hypotension.

Management

Hypotensive patients should be placed in an intensive care unit where vital signs, fluid intake and output, body weight, and other parameters of circulatory function can be monitored continuously. Because indirect measurements of arterial blood pressure are difficult to obtain and often do not reflect true intra-arterial pressure in hypotensive states, direct measurement of intra-arterial blood pressure is preferred.

If a patient has hypotension without signs of tissue hypoperfusion, fluids should be administered at sufficient rates to maintain urine output and to compensate for insensible losses. Fluids should be of appropriate composition to provide electrolyte needs. In many patients with signs of hypoperfusion of tissues, correction of acid-base and electrolyte disturbances and modest fluid therapy are sufficient to increase perfusion to adequate levels. However, increased pulmonary vascular permeability complicates many cases of drug overdose, and fluid therapy may cause pulmonary edema. For this reason, fluids must be administered cautiously. A reasonably safe way to administer fluids is by short infusions of small volumes (100 to 200 mL) of normal saline solution. If the clinical response is inadequate and if the patient has no evidence of pulmonary edema, the short infusions should be repeated but should not exceed a total of 1000 to 2000 mL over 1 to 2 hours. Evidence of pulmonary edema includes worsening hypoxia, decreasing lung compliance (manifested by increasing pressure necessary to ventilate a patient with a given tidal volume), and development of pulmonary rales.

If shock persists despite fluid challenge, catheterization of the pulmonary artery and measurement of pulmonary artery and pulmonary capillary wedge

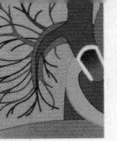

pressure, cardiac output, and mixed venous oxygen saturation from the pulmonary artery is useful to monitor subsequent fluid therapy and to optimize drug therapy. The goal of fluid therapy is to reestablish adequate tissue perfusion without producing fluid overload and/or pulmonary edema. As long as the pulmonary capillary wedge pressure remains low (<12 mm Hg), further fluid can be administered. If evidence of tissue hypoperfusion persists when pulmonary capillary wedge pressures have been restored to normal or pulmonary edema is evident, pressor or inotropic agents should be administered to restore adequate perfusion. In persons with chronic cardiac failure, higher pressures (≥20 mm Hg) may be necessary to maintain an adequate cardiac output, and fluid therapy must be managed more on the basis of clinical assessment of pulmonary edema than on filling pressures per se.

Hemodynamic monitoring aids in the selection of pressor or inotropic drugs. For example, if circulatory failure is associated with low or low-normal peripheral vascular resistance, norepinephrine or dopamine should be selected. Both agents primarily are vasoconstrictors with some inotropic effects. Normalization of vascular resistance is a useful end point for titration of infusion rate. The renal vasodilatory effect of low dose dopamine has made it the preferred vasopressor; however, there is no evidence that "renal dose" dopamine provides any benefit to patients with impending renal failure or with concomitant vasoconstrictor therapy. In cases of overdose with drugs that have α-adrenergic receptor–blocking effects, such as phenothiazines or tricyclic antidepressants, more selective α-adrenergic agonists, such as norepinephrine or phenylephrine, may be required.[2] In vasodilatory shock refractory to standard high dose vasopressors, vasopressin as an adjunctive therapy may be helpful, although this agent has been studied primarily in septic shock and postcardiotomy shock.[3]

If vascular resistance is normal or high and depressed cardiac output is the determining factor in circulatory failure, drugs or interventions that increase cardiac output should be selected. Isoproterenol is useful particularly when myocardial depression is associated with bradyarrhythmias, although it may be arrhythmogenic; dobutamine, a dopamine analog with relatively selective inotropic activity and less arrhythmogenic potential, is useful when heart rate is already adequate. In some patients, the addition of the phosphodiesterase inhibitor amrinone to other vasopressors has resulted in hemodynamic improvement. Amrinone is both an inotropic and a vasodilating agent and should not be used when peripheral vascular resistance is low. In patients with both myocardial depression and low vascular resistance, epinephrine or combinations of norepinephrine or dopamine and isoproterenol may be useful. Specific agents that may improve myocardial contractility are calcium and insulin/dextrose in calcium channel blocker overdose and glucagon in β-blocker overdose. If fluid replacement, vasopressors, and other inotropic agents do not reverse drug-induced shock, circulatory assist devices should be used, such as intra-aortic balloon pump or cardiopulmonary bypass.

Pressor therapy has potential risks: pressor-induced venoconstriction can increase venous return and worsen pulmonary edema, and arteriolar constriction can further reduce tissue perfusion. However, in studies of the effects of infusion of norepinephrine in patients who overdosed with sedative drugs, the positive effects of norepinephrine on cardiac output outweighed the vasoconstrictor effects, and blood pressure increased without an increase in vascular resistance.[4]

ARRHYTHMIAS

General Mechanisms

Three basic mechanisms are involved in the production and maintenance of arrhythmias: abnormal impulse formation, abnormal impulse conduction, and abnormal triggering.

ABNORMAL IMPULSE FORMATION

The sinus node is the normal pacemaker since it has the fastest intrinsic firing rate. This intrinsic firing rate is influenced by the resting membrane potential, the threshold potential, and the slope of the diastolic depolarization (phase 4). Conditions or agents that increase the slope of phase 4, lower the threshold potential toward the resting potential, or raise the resting membrane potential so that it approaches the threshold potential result in an increase in sinus rate as well as generation of automatic impulses from cells that do not normally manifest automaticity. A new site of pacing results when the rate generated by this abnormal focus exceeds the sinus pacemaker rate. Conversely, conditions or agents that decrease the rate of diastolic depolarization, raise the threshold potential toward 0, or lower the resting membrane potential so that it takes longer to reach threshold potential result in a decrease in the spontaneous firing rate.

ABNORMAL IMPULSE CONDUCTION

Delays in conduction or block of conduction of electrical impulses, together with differential refractoriness of myocardial tissues, may lead to reentry tachyarrhythmias. Such arrhythmias are initiated by early impulses that encounter refractory tissue or anatomic obstacles (e.g., scar), through which they cannot propagate because of their prematurity; thus, they travel down alternate slowly conducting pathways. If the impulses return to the area originally refractory but now excitable, the tissue is able to conduct them. This particular set of electrophysiologic circumstances (unilateral conduction delay and slow impulse transmission in alternate pathways) can lead to paroxysmal or sustained arrhythmias (Fig. 8-1).

TRIGGERED RHYTHMS

Triggered rhythms are abnormal initiations of impulses that occur as a result of afterdepolarizations, which are oscillations of the action potential during phases 2 to 4. Two types of afterdepolarizations are distinguished from each other by their temporal relationship within the

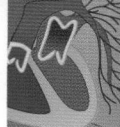

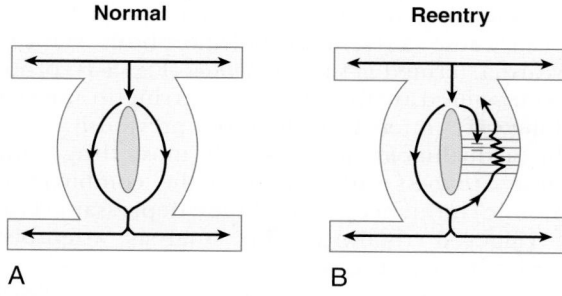

Normal   **Reentry**

A   B

FIGURE 8-1 Drug-induced reentry: Schema of Purkinje's tissue or ventricular muscle through which impulse transmission occurs. **A,** Normal depolarization of a muscle segment. Impulses spread simultaneously down various conduction pathways to depolarize distal areas. Depolarization and repolarization proceed homogeneously. **B,** Reentry. The *hatched area* represents a local area with depressed conduction, which might be produced by a membrane-depressant drug. An impulse traveling anterogradely in an area of depressed conduction is blocked (*dark horizontal lines*); impulses traveling in adjacent pathways, however, can pass through the area of conduction delay in retrograde fashion. If tissue proximal to the depressed area is repolarized already and is now excitable, restimulation (reentry) occurs.

repolarization phase: early and delayed afterdepolarizations (EADs and DADs). EADs are the most common foci for triggered rhythms in the poisoned patient and are caused by blockade of outward potassium channels. The surplus of intracellular cations result in delay of return of the action potential to its baseline and upward oscillations of the action potential above threshold. Torsades de pointes and ventricular tachycardias often are precipitated by these triggered responses. DADs occur at the end of repolarization and result from intracellular calcium overload, as seen in digitalis toxicity or excess catecholamine states. Although triggered rhythms have not been incontrovertibly proved to be responsible for specific arrhythmias in patients, many rhythm disturbances, particularly if they are pause or bradycardia dependent or occur in association with a prolonged QTU interval, are likely due to this underlying mechanism.

Arrhythmogenesis in Poisoned Patients

In the setting of drug overdose, cardiac arrhythmias can be caused by direct or indirect sympathomimetic effects, anticholinergic effects, the effects of altered central nervous system (CNS) regulation of peripheral autonomic activity, and myocardial membrane depression. Contributing factors to arrhythmogenesis during the course of drug overdose include hypotension, hypoxia, and disturbances in acid–base and electrolyte balance.

SYMPATHETIC INFLUENCES
The action of many drugs involves the autonomic nervous system, so it is useful to understand the effects of sympathetic and parasympathetic activity on cardiac electrophysiology. β-Adrenergic stimulation accelerates spontaneous diastolic depolarization, thereby increasing the sinus rate; enhancement of automaticity in other

pacemaker tissues (atrial, atrioventricular [AV] junctional, Purkinje) may result in accelerated ectopic rhythms. β-Adrenergic stimulation also increases conduction velocity in slow (calcium-dependent) channel fibers, thus leading to more rapid sinoatrial and AV nodal conduction of impulses. The effect of catecholamines on fast channel fibers such as normal Purkinje fibers is to accelerate repolarization and shorten the action potential duration and refractory period, although effects on conduction velocity are relatively negligible. Finally, β-adrenergic stimulation enhances afterdepolarization magnitude, thereby increasing the potential for triggered tachyarrhythmias. $β_1$-receptor blockade causes blunting of chronotropic, dromotropic, and inotropic effects of endogenous and exogenous catecholamines.

PARASYMPATHETIC INFLUENCES
Parasympathetic stimulation slows the rate of spontaneous diastolic depolarization, resulting in slowing of the firing rates of pacemaker tissues. Slowing of the sinus rate may result in the emergence of an escape rhythm originating in supraventricular or ventricular tissue. Delay in impulse transmission through the AV node as a result of parasympathetic stimulation may produce AV block; this "vagotonic block" usually occurs in the presence of sinus slowing and can take the form of progressive delay in impulse conduction through the AV node (Figs. 8-2 and 8-3). The effects of cholinergic stimulation on ventricular conduction tissue include the raised electric threshold necessary for induction of ventricular fibrillation, particularly in the presence of high sympathetic activity. Inhibition of cholinergic receptors results in unopposed sympathetic stimulation, which results in sinus tachycardia (rate usually < 150 beats per minute) and a modest rise in blood pressure.

An interesting arrhythmia resulting from increased parasympathetic tone has been recognized. It is characterized by supraventricular tachyarrhythmias, especially atrial fibrillation, occurring during periods of high vagal tone, such as sleep, and is not found during exercise or stress. Drugs such as digitalis or β-adrenergic blocking agents tend to precipitate or worsen these arrhythmias. These arrhythmias can be treated effectively (suppressed) by oral theophylline, if not otherwise contraindicated, or by cardiac pacing to eliminate the pause or bradycardia dependence. The underlying mechanism of production of this arrhythmia may be acetylcholine-mediated shortening and dispersion of atrial refractory periods, resulting in inhomogeneous atrial repolarization and depolarization sequences. Because these arrhythmias do not connote underlying heart disease, their recognition is important. Anticholinergic effects also may rarely predispose to AV nodal reentrant tachyarrhythmias via differential effects on nodal conduction velocity and refractoriness of reentrant pathways.

MEMBRANE DEPRESSION
In a drug-overdosed patient, a direct effect on myocardial membranes is another important mechanism contribut-

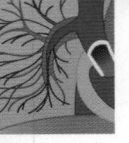

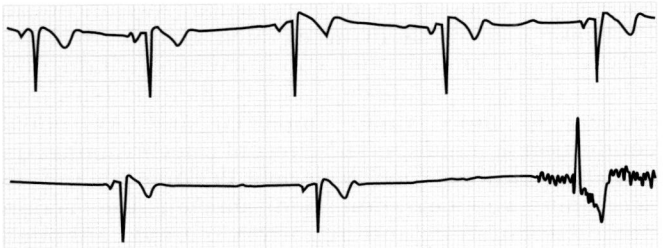

FIGURE 8-2 MCL$_1$ tracing recorded during ipecac-induced emesis in a patient with alleged barbiturate overdose. During the Valsalva maneuver of vomiting, marked slowing of sinus rate with prolongation of the PR interval occurs, resulting in a prolonged pause in rhythm terminated by a ventricular escape beat. Sinus slowing with or without concomitant AV block, such as depicted here, is due to hypervagotonia, and the arrhythmia is known as *vagotonic block*. This has no prognostic significance for underlying heart disease. The arrhythmia usually is transient and requires no specific treatment.

ing to arrhythmogenesis. Depressant effects on membrane responsiveness are exemplified by quinidine, which inhibits the fast sodium current, so that for a given resting membrane potential depolarization is associated with a reduced rate of voltage change and a reduced maximum achieved voltage. As a result, impulse conduction is slowed. In addition, membrane depressants shift the threshold potential toward 0, thus requiring stimuli of greater intensity to initiate the action potential. Additional effects of quinidine include prolongation of the action potential duration and refractory period, which prolong repolarization time. These electrophysiologic effects result in slowed repolarization and depolarization times, especially in His-Purkinje tissue. These events are reflected in the surface electrocardiogram (ECG) as a prolongation of the QT interval and, in toxic doses, of the QRS duration. With severe intoxication, intraventricular block and asystole supervene, with inability to generate a response for any stimulus strength; this is manifested clinically by failure to respond to cardiac pacing at high stimulus voltage.

The basis for the arrhythmogenic effect of quinidine lies in part in its ability to produce disparate depolarization and repolarization times in His-Purkinje tissue and to delay impulse transmission. The production of unidirectional conduction block and the delay in impulse propagation in other areas enable reentry

tachycardias to occur. Quinidine and quinidine-like agents also can cause a form of polymorphous ventricular tachycardia, termed *torsades de pointes* (Fig. 8-4), probably due to triggered rhythms when occurring in the setting of a long QTU interval, as discussed previously.

The arrhythmogenic effects of most drugs during overdose are best understood as the combination of autonomic influences, membrane-depressant effects, and triggered rhythms. Our analysis attempts to categorize them in this way.

Management of Arrhythmias

Hypotension, hypoxia, and acid–base and electrolyte disturbances occurring during the course of drug overdose may contribute to arrhythmia production and should be corrected (Table 8-1).

SUPRAVENTRICULAR ARRHYTHMIAS

Sinus tachycardia and other supraventricular arrhythmias usually respond to supportive therapy and subside as the offending drug is excreted, but if they are associated with hemodynamic compromise, especially in patients with preexisting coronary or cerebrovascular disease, specific therapy is warranted. For excess sympathetic activity, benzodiazepines and a β_1-selective blocker, such as esmolol or metoprolol, are appropriate. Physostigmine may be indicated for anticholinergic drug ingestions. However, with concomitant evidence of cardiac membrane depression, as occurs with overdose of tricyclic antidepressants, such an approach may itself be hazardous, as discussed later. If the supraventricular tachycardia is due to theophylline toxicity, administration of esmolol or metoprolol is useful in slowing a rapid ventricular response to atrial fibrillation or flutter without significant compromise in blood pressure. Electrical cardioversion is an acceptable alternative when arrhythmias are life threatening and fail to respond to pharmacologic treatment.

VENTRICULAR ARRHYTHMIAS

Pharmacologic therapy for drug-induced ventricular arrhythmias is similar to that used in the setting of acute myocardial ischemia. An important exception exists in cases of overdose of membrane-depressant drugs such as quinidine or tricyclic antidepressants; in these instances, similar sodium channel blocking agents such as

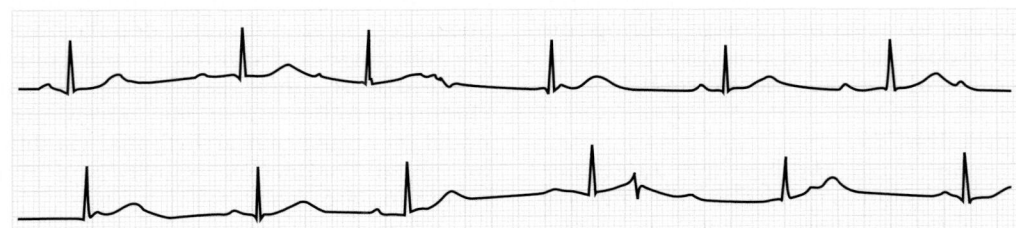

FIGURE 8-3 A 13-year-old girl ingested 325 mg of phenylpropanolamine and presented with a headache and blood pressure of 130/100 mm Hg. The electrocardiogram showed sinus arrhythmia with Wenckebach-type AV block, reflecting surges of vagal tone. The vagal discharge is a reflex response to phenylpropanolamine-induced vasoconstriction and hypertension.

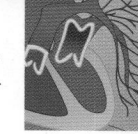

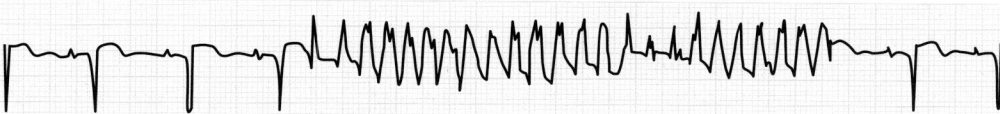

FIGURE 8-4 V_1 rhythm strip showing polymorphous ventricular tachycardia occurring abruptly and without warning. This particular arrhythmia often is referred to as *torsades de pointes*, reflecting a twisting of the QRS complexes around the electrocardiographic baseline. It occurs in association with prolongation of the QT interval due to any cause (including idiopathic) and may be seen also in acute ischemic heart disease. In this tracing, the QT interval, measured from other leads, was 0.56 seconds.

TABLE 8-1 Arrhythmias and Their Management

TYPE	COMMENT	TREATMENT
Tachyarrhythmias		
All		Correct hypotension and acid–base and electrolyte disturbances
Sinus tachycardia	Usually can be made to vary with respiration, exercise, carotid sinus massage	No specific treatment indicated. If hemodynamic compromise, β blockade
Ectopic atrial tachycardia	If 2:1 AV conduction ratio, suspect digitalis toxicity	If hemodynamic compromise, β blockade, sotalol, amiodarone, or calcium channel blockade. If digitalis toxic, withdraw digitalis
Atrial flutter	Adenosine produces sufficient AV block to discern atrial activity. If QRS rhythm is regular and slow (<100), suspect AV block, which might be due to digitalis toxicity and/or β- and calcium entry blocker overdosage	Direct current cardioversion (low energy levels usually suffice); pace termination; IV verapamil, diltiazem, esmolol, or metoprolol will slow ventricular rate; procainamide IV ibutilide for pharmacologic conversion
Atrial fibrillation	May appear to be regular at more rapid rates. Distinguish from multifocal atrial tachycardia by lack of defined atrial activity	Intravenous diltiazem, verapamil, esmolol, and/or metoprolol or amiodarone to slow ventricular response (if necessary). Direct current cardioversion if an accessory pathway is known or suspected and ventricular response is rapid
Junctional tachycardia	No variation in rate with respiration, exercise. Distinguish from sinus tachycardia with long PR interval or ventricular tachycardia (if QRS complex is wide). May be due to digitalis toxicity	If rate is rapid, β blockade, physostigmine,* pace termination; direct current cardioversion
Ventricular ectopy (couplets, triplets, multiform complexes, sustained tachycardia, fibrillation)	If due to membrane-depressant drugs, other drugs in this class are to be avoided. If due to bradycardia, increase basic rate	IV lidocaine, β blockade, isoproterenol, magnesium, and/or cardiac pacing if due to bradycardia or associated with long QT. Direct current cardioversion or defibrillation. Procainamide IV if sustained monomorphic ventricular tachycardia in ischemic setting. IV amiodarone if hemodynamically destabilizing rapid ventricular tachycardia
Bradyarrhythmias		
Sinus bradycardia, including sinus arrest, sinoatrial block, and vagotonic bradycardia		No specific therapy. If hemodynamic decompensation, IV atropine, isoproterenol, cardiac pacing
Vagotonic AV block	AV block with varying PR intervals is associated with slowing of sinus rates. Seen in states with high vagal tone, including sleep and specific situations such as suctioning or endoscopy	No specific therapy. Atropine, oral theophylline, if sustained. Note: Atropine should not be administered if vagotonic rhythm is a reflex response to drug-induced hypertension, because it will aggravate the hypertension
AV block type I (Wenckebach)		If hemodynamic compromise, atropine, IV isoproterenol, cardiac pacing
Type II (Mobitz II) high-degree or complete block	If atrial rate is increased by atropine or isoproterenol, increase in degree of AV block may occur	Cardiac pacing

AV, atrioventricular; IV, intravenous.
*May be hazardous if associated with membrane-depressant drug overdose.

procainamide and disopyramide are contraindicated. Selection of secondary drugs depends on the particular overdose; thus, benzodiazepines and a β₁ blocker might be indicated for sympathomimetic drug overdose, magnesium or digitalis antibodies for digitalis overdose, and high dose magnesium (1 to 2 g over 1 to 2 minutes) and overdrive pacing or isoproterenol for polymorphous ventricular tachycardia with a long QT interval (torsades de pointes).[5] Sustained ventricular tachycardia and fibrillation require electrical conversion or defibrillation; intravenous administration of amiodarone can be used to attempt to prevent recurrence.

WIDE COMPLEX TACHYCARDIA OF UNCERTAIN ORIGIN

The ECG occasionally shows a regular wide complex QRS rhythm without readily discernible atrial activity; the origin of the QRS rhythm may thus be uncertain. Rate alone is not a useful criterion in distinguishing ventricular tachycardia from supraventricular tachycardia with intraventricular aberration, especially in a patient suffering from a drug overdose. QRS morphology, on the other hand, can be helpful. Ventricular tachycardia is suggested by very bizarre QRS complexes; superior deviation of the mean frontal plane QRS axis; qR, RR′, or R waves in leads aVr and V₁; rS or QS in leads aVL and V₆; or concordance (similarity) of QRS morphology in the precordial leads. Supraventricular tachycardia with intraventricular aberration is suggested by QRS morphology that closely resembles typical bundle branch block patterns. Past ECGs with which to compare current ones may be helpful if they have shown a previously present bundle branch block pattern or ventricular premature complexes that resemble the present rhythm (Fig. 8-5).

The relationship of ventricular to atrial activity may afford another clue to the origin of the QRS rhythm. Establishing this relationship when atrial activity is not easily seen on the surface ECG often requires placing an electrode catheter in the esophagus or right atrium to register atrial electrical signals. The simultaneous recording of a surface ECG lead and intracardiac or intraesophageal electrogram permits recognition of atrial activity. If this activity occurs independently of (is dissociated from) the regular ventricular rhythm, the QRS rhythm is almost certainly ventricular tachycardia. If atrial activity occurs irregularly at rates faster than the regular ventricular rhythm, the rhythm is atrial fibrillation. Atrial activity that is dissociated from the regular ventricular rhythm suggests a junctional or ventricular tachycardia. If atrial activity occurs at a rate that is a multiple of the QRS rate, atrial flutter or atrial tachycardia with some degree of block is suggested. If a 1:1 relationship between atrial and ventricular activity is demonstrated, the direction of impulse transmission (AV or ventriculoatrial) is not known; only by changing the conduction ratios may the correct diagnosis be made. For example, if carotid sinus massage is applied in a patient with regular wide complex tachycardia and 1:1 AV relationship and ventricular asystole occurs despite persistence of atrial activity, the rhythm was supraven-

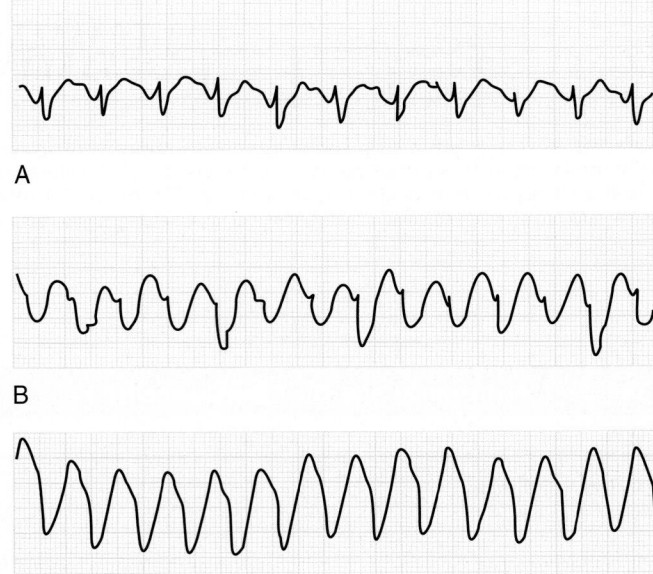

A

B

C

FIGURE 8-5 These lead I rhythm strips were obtained from a 40-year-old woman who ingested 6 g of amitriptyline (Elavil). In **A**, the rhythm is sinus with a long PR interval. In strips **B** and **C**, recorded within a 20-minute period, no P waves are seen and the QRS complexes are broad and bizarre. Close scrutiny reveals that the QRS complexes in strips **B** and **C** resemble those in strip **A** except that they are more aberrant. The value of previously recorded tracings when evaluating a wide complex tachycardia, as in strip **C**, is illustrated by these electrocardiograms.

tricular in origin (Fig. 8-6). Some patients with hyperkalemia have a wide QRS complex rhythm without discernible P waves, in which the QRS complexes are nevertheless stimulated via the His-Purkinje system by the sinus node. This rhythm is termed *sinoventricular conduction.* The absence of P waves is due to hyperkalemia-related atrial arrest, and treatment of the hyperkalemia results in restoration of atrial muscle depolarization and appearance of P waves.

Management of hemodynamically significant wide complex tachycardia while the diagnosis is being established should include carotid sinus massage as a readily applied initial maneuver but should be directed toward the potentially most life-threatening arrhythmia. Thus, intravenous lidocaine should be used for presumed ventricular tachycardia as the agent of first choice. When the nature of the overdose is unknown, however, electrical cardioversion may be the procedure of choice to avoid compounding the problem of arrhythmia and hemodynamic instability, provided there is reasonable certainty that the rhythm is not sinus in origin. Failure to convert a wide complex tachycardia to another rhythm after direct current cardioversion should suggest that sinus tachycardia may indeed be present. Certain antiarrhythmic agents, notably flecainide, can cause monomorphic ventricular tachycardia refractory to cardioversion attempts. Amiodarone, although not well studied in the context of toxicologic emergencies, may be used for refractory ventricular arrhythmias.

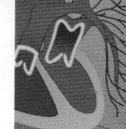

Surface lead V$_1$

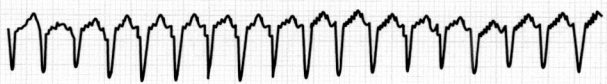

Intracardiac electrogram

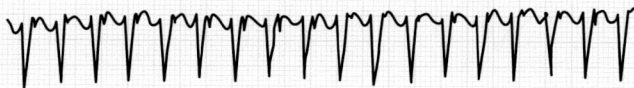

Intracardiac electrogram during carotid sinus massage

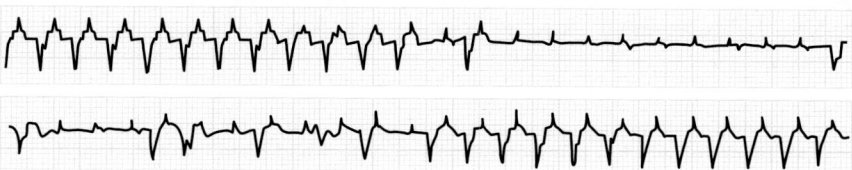

FIGURE 8-6 The patient is a 67-year-old man with chronic obstructive pulmonary disease. He developed tachycardia during treatment with aminophylline. The surface electrocardiographic V$_1$ lead (*top*) shows a QRS duration of 0.12 seconds and no clearly discerned atrial activity. Intracardiac electrography (*middle*) reveals a 1:1 relationship between ventricular (the broad, large deflections) and atrial (the sharp, small deflections) activity. The direction of impulse transmission is not known. Carotid sinus massage (*bottom*) shows no change in atrial activity, whereas ventricular response is blocked, probably at the AV node. The change in the AV conduction ratio produced by carotid massage allows the diagnosis of atrial tachycardia to be made.

BRADYARRHYTHMIAS

Bradyarrhythmias, particularly AV block, may occur unpredictably and may require temporary transvenous cardiac pacing. Before pacemaker insertion, transcutaneous pacing and pharmacologic therapy may be necessary in an attempt to maintain heart rate, blood pressure, and cardiac output. Intravenous administration of atropine should be tried to treat sinus or junctional bradycardia, except if hypertension is present (reflex bradycardia); intravenous administration of isoproterenol may be used for unresponsive sinus or junctional or ventricular bradycardias. These agents should be used with caution, however, because both may cause significant sinus or junctional tachycardia, and isoproterenol may cause ventricular extrasystolic activity, including ventricular tachycardia. If the bradycardia is corrected but the hypotension is persistent, inotropic agents and toxin-specific agents should be used (e.g., glucagon for β-blocker poisoning).

CARDIAC PACING IN DRUG OVERDOSE

Pacemaker-related difficulties encountered in drug-overdosed patients may be related to inability to sense a suboptimal intracardiac signal or to capture (depolarize) the atria or ventricles. To be sensed properly by a pacemaker generator, an intracardiac signal must have certain characteristics: adequate amplitude, rapid rate of change of voltage, and optimal signal duration. In patients overdosed with agents that alter impulse conduction or cause or contribute to myocardial ischemia or failure, the intracardiac signal often is of too poor a quality to be sensed, leading to improper demand pacemaker function. The resulting earlier-than-expected pacing stimulus that follows unsensed spontaneous beats may cause repetitive atrial or ventricular rhythms, including ventricular tachycardia and fibrillation.

Another problem encountered in drug-overdosed patients is failure of the pacing stimulus to depolarize sufficient amounts of myocardial tissue to cause ventricular activation, resulting in failure to pace. This can come about as a result of myocardial intercellular or intracellular edema or as a result of failure of pacing stimulus propagation throughout the muscle due to hyperkalemia, hypoxia, acidosis, or membrane-depressant agents. The failure to pace may be total, with all pacing stimuli failing to depolarize the ventricles, or intermittent, in which various degrees of pacemaker exit block may occur, including Wenckebach-type conduction (Fig. 8-7).

Because transcutaneous pacing is not effective over time, it should not be used except in emergencies and should be followed by transvenous pacing to ensure stable heart rate support.

Some patients in whom failure to pace is life threatening may require cardiopulmonary bypass or intra-aortic balloon (triggering off the pacing stimulus) support to maintain circulatory function.

PULMONARY EDEMA

Pulmonary edema frequently complicates overdose with drugs such as narcotics, sedatives/hypnotics, salicylates, and sympathomimetic agents. Acute inhalational noncardiogenic pulmonary edema can be caused by smoke, ammonia, chlorine, nitrous oxide, and phosgene. The pathophysiology of drug-induced pulmonary edema involves increased pulmonary capillary permeability, as evidenced by normal or low pulmonary capillary wedge pressures and pulmonary edema fluid with a protein concentration similar to that of plasma. In contrast, cardiogenic pulmonary edema is characterized by increased capillary hydrostatic pressure and pulmonary wedge pressures of greater than 20 mm Hg.

The mechanisms by which sedative-hypnotic drugs produce capillary endothelial damage are not fully understood. Depression of respiration may lead to hypoxemia, precapillary pulmonary hypertension, increased vascular permeability, and, finally, extravasation of fluid. An analogy has been made to cases of pulmonary edema at high altitude, in which hypoxia

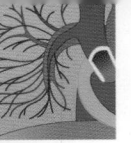

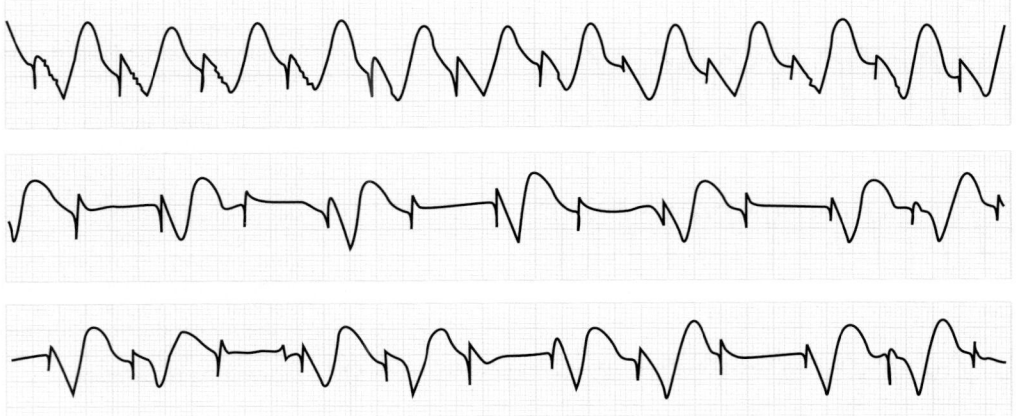

FIGURE 8-7 The patient was a 76-year-old man who had chronic congestive heart failure, recurrent ventricular tachycardia for which he was being treated with procainamide, paroxysmal AV block for which a transvenous pacing system had been implanted, and renal failure. He was admitted to the hospital with acute pulmonary edema. His serum potassium level was 5.0 mEq/L, and his serum procainamide level was 19 ng/mL. The *top* MCL$_1$ rhythm strip shows a paced QRS rhythm with extremely wide QRS complexes; atrial activity is not discerned. The *bottom two* continuous MCL$_1$ rhythm strips, recorded shortly after the top strip, show episodic failure of ventricular capture by the pacing stimuli, with a pattern suggesting Wenckebach's block of the pacing stimuli. Because there was no evidence of pacemaker generator malfunction, the failure to capture in this clinical setting was considered to result from myocardial stimulation threshold elevation and failure of impulse conduction owing to the membrane-depressant effects of the procainamide. Treatment with low-dose isoproterenol and intravenous steroids was without effect, and the patient died.

produces a similar picture, which is rapidly reversed by oxygen therapy. Ethchlorvynol, when injected intravenously, is an example of a drug that directly injures the alveolocapillary membrane. Infused salicylate, possibly by effects on prostaglandin synthesis, increases microvascular permeability. Pulsatile lymphatic activity is reduced and lymphatic drainage is retarded during barbiturate anesthesia. This also might contribute to the net accumulation of fluid in the lungs after drug overdose.

Neurogenic pulmonary edema, possibly mediated by massive sympathetic discharge, has been well described after brain injury and has been suggested to occur after overdoses of drugs such as narcotics and salicylates. Sympathomimetic drugs can cause pulmonary edema owing to severe hypertension and diastolic noncompliance. This is most common after intravenous administration. By the time such a patient is evaluated by a physician, blood pressure may be normal or even low, with evidence of hypovolemia due to sequestration of fluid into the lungs and other extravascular sites. Direct depression of myocardial function by drugs may aggravate pulmonary edema caused by pulmonary capillary damage or, in the context of fluid therapy for hypotension, may result in cardiogenic pulmonary edema in the absence of pulmonary capillary damage.

Drug-induced pulmonary edema can be present on admission or may develop subsequently during the clinical course; in either case, it complicates management of shock states. Fluid filtration into the lungs depends in part on pulmonary capillary pressure and, therefore, on left atrial pressure. A difficult clinical situation may arise in which intracardiac filling pressures adequate to maintain cardiac output may result in pulmonary transudation. Suggestions about fluid therapy and the use of pulmonary capillary wedge pressures have been discussed. Diuretics may not be effective in treating drug-induced pulmonary edema because filling pressures are already normal or low, and further diuresis can potentiate hypotension. Infusions of albumin have been proposed to increase plasma oncotic pressure and to draw fluid from the lungs. This is not useful because the protein content of the edema fluid is of similar composition to that of plasma, and this indicates that albumin passes through vascular endothelium as freely as water.

Mechanical ventilation with positive end-expiratory pressure is an important tool used in the management of drug-induced pulmonary edema. Positive end-expiratory pressure increases functional residual capacity, reduces intrapulmonary shunting, and increases pulmonary compliance. Supplemental oxygen usually is necessary to maintain arterial oxygen tension at 60 to 70 mm Hg. Placing the patient in the prone position and using inverse ratio ventilation may improve ventilation-perfusion mismatches and oxygenation, respectively. The ventilatory technique of high-frequency oscillatory ventilation maximizes gas exchange while minimizing the complication of barotrauma.[6]

RECOGNITION AND MANAGEMENT OF CARDIAC DISTURBANCES CAUSED BY SPECIFIC DRUGS

Sedative-Hypnotic Drugs

PATHOPHYSIOLOGY

Sedative-hypnotic drugs are involved in many cases of drug overdose. Although cardiac complications per se

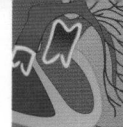

are uncommon, it is important to understand how this class of drugs might influence cardiovascular disturbances caused by coingested drugs. The major action of sedative-hypnotic drugs is on the CNS and results in reduced sympathetic and increased parasympathetic peripheral autonomic tone. Barbiturates have been shown to depress myocardial function in animals, but severe myocardial depression is uncommon in humans. Cardiac output is commonly reduced because of relative hypovolemia caused by increased venous capacitance and absolute hypovolemia due to fluid loss into tissues, the latter a consequence of increased vascular permeability.[7] Cardiac output and heart rate may be lower than normal as a result of hypothermia and reduced metabolic demands. As a consequence of inhibition of sympathetic function, heart rate frequently is less than expected for the degree of hypotension.

An important complication of sedative-hypnotic drug overdose is pulmonary edema, which results from increased pulmonary vascular permeability, as just discussed. As a consequence, hypoxia and metabolic acidosis develop, and they may worsen myocardial performance and potentiate arrhythmias.

The management of hypotension and shock due to sedative-hypnotic overdose includes judicious use of fluids and pressor drugs. Because venous pooling contributes to reduced cardiac output, the Trendelenburg position (head down, legs up) may substantially increase venous return, cardiac output, and blood pressure. Infusion of modest amounts of colloid or crystalloid fluids is sufficient to correct hypovolemia and to increase cardiac output and tissue perfusion to adequate levels in many patients. Failure to achieve adequate tissue perfusion despite increased cardiac filling pressure or evidence of pulmonary edema is an indication for the use of pressor drugs, as discussed.

Sympathomimetics

GENERAL CONSIDERATIONS

Sympathetic overactivity can be caused by a number of drugs and toxins, as well as by sedative-drug withdrawal syndromes (Box 8-1). The typical manifestations are sinus or atrial tachycardia (Fig. 8-8), hypertension, seizures, hyperthermia, and, in massive ingestions, cardiovascular collapse and respiratory failure. Occasionally, ventricular irritability and, rarely, ventricular fibrillation with death are observed.

Cocaine

Cocaine is a potent sympathomimetic drug that is well known for its cardiovascular complications. It is abused for its euphoric effects but tolerance to CNS effects develops rapidly. Thus, the duration of euphoria is much shorter than the presence of the drug in the body. Repeated doses may result in accumulation of drug and cardiovascular toxicity at a time when the user exhibits neither euphoria nor a sympathomimetic toxidrome.

Cocaine is a potent inhibitor of neuronal catecholamine uptake, which is a major mechanism of limiting the action of norepinephrine. In addition to its

---

BOX 8-1   CARDIAC DISTURBANCES DUE TO SYMPATHOMIMETIC DRUGS AND TOXINS

Drugs

Amphetamines
Cocaine
Phencyclidine
Monoamine oxidase inhibitors
Phenylpropanolamine and other over-the-counter
   sympathomimetics
Theophylline
Caffeine
Δ^9-tetrahydrocannabinol
Lysergic acid diethylamide and other hallucinogens
Chloral hydrate*
Ethanol
Hydrocarbon solvents* (such as toluene)
Freon* (and other fluorocarbon aerosols)
Sedative drug abstinence

Cardiovascular Disturbances

Sinus tachycardia
Atrial tachycardia
Sinus bradycardia[†]
Ventricular premature beats
Ventricular tachycardia
Ventricular fibrillation
Hypertension
Hypotension[‡]

Other Common Manifestations

Dilated pupils[§]
Diaphoresis
Fever
Excitement, anxiety, psychosis (often paranoid)[‖]
Tremor
Seizures
Hypokalemia
Metabolic acidosis

---

*Sensitizes myocardium to catecholamines.
[†]Reflex response to vasoconstrictors such as phenylpropanolamine.
[‡]Late manifestation, usually severe overdose.
[§]Excepting phencyclidine and alcohols.
[‖]Phencyclidine, alcohols, and solvents may cause ataxia, lethargy, or coma.

---

potent sympathomimetic action, in high doses cocaine blocks fast sodium channels in the myocardium; the result is depression of depolarization and slowing of conduction velocity. This is manifested on ECG as prolonged PR, QRS, and QT intervals, similar to that seen with type IA antiarrhythmics.[8]

Other effects of cocaine include coronary artery vasoconstriction that is mediated by α-adrenergic stimulation and possibly by release of endothelium-derived vasoconstrictors, such as endothelin.[9] A procoagulant effect of cocaine may predispose to in situ coronary artery thrombosis. The sympathomimetic effects of cocaine lead to increased myocardial oxygen demand and, in context of both the procoagulant effect and vasoconstriction, may result in myocardial ischemia, acute myocardial infarction, and arrhythmias.[10]

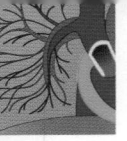

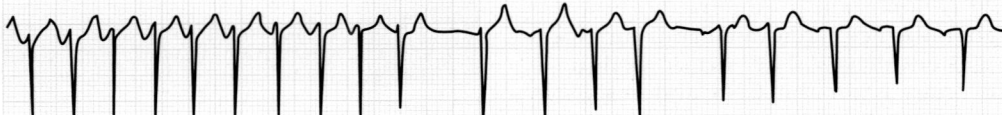

FIGURE 8-8 The patient, a 27-year-old cocaine user, was admitted to the coronary care unit for electrocardiographic monitoring after having had two syncopal spells. The MCL$_1$ rhythm strip shows bursts of atrial tachycardia, which terminate spontaneously, and atrial premature beats, some of which are not conducted.

Long-term cocaine use has been associated with left ventricular hypertrophy and diastolic dysfunction, systolic dysfunction, and dilated cardiomyopathy. Patchy myocardial necrosis with contraction band necrosis has been observed at autopsy and is believed to be the result of intense catecholamine stimulation of the heart. Arrhythmogenesis is thought to occur secondary to sympathomimetic activity and sodium channel blockade in the presence of myocardial ischemia, metabolic derangements, and anatomic abnormalities, as described earlier.

Management depends on specific manifestations of toxicity (Table 8-2). Hypertension is typically managed with benzodiazepines and vasodilators such as nitroglycerin and nitroprusside. Phentolamine, an α-antagonist, also can be used to counteract the vasoconstriction. Arrhythmias result primarily from β-adrenergic stimulation. β$_1$-specific blockers, such as esmolol or metoprolol, should be selected rather than nonselective β blockers to avoid antagonizing the β$_2$-mediated arteriolar dilation that may be opposing the α-mediated vasoconstriction. Nonselective β$_2$ blockade can worsen the hypertension. If the arrhythmia is a wide complex tachycardia, sodium bicarbonate should be used to counteract the sodium channel blockade effect of cocaine. Lidocaine also has been used safely in this context. Other type I antiarrhythmic drugs should be avoided.

Myocardial ischemia and infarction are important manifestations of cocaine toxicity. Treatment should include oxygen, aspirin, nitrates, and benzodiazepines. Because vasospasm is a mechanism of myocardial ischemia in this context, calcium channel blockers should be used. Other treatment options for coronary vasoconstriction include phentolamine and labetalol (the latter in the presence of tachycardia). Propranolol should be avoided because of the potential harmful effects of β$_2$ blockade, as discussed previously. The decision to administer fibrinolytics in cocaine intoxication requires extreme caution because of the risk of hypertension-related complications (i.e., cerebral hemorrhage), associated trauma, and high frequency of misleading ECGs. Early repolarization variant (J point and ST elevation) is a common cause of abnormal ECG in young patients with cocaine-associated chest pain. If available, coronary angiography and revascularization with angioplasty, if required, is the preferred method of treatment of cocaine-induced acute myocardial infarction. If this is unavailable, and the patient has classic symptoms and signs of acute myocardial infarction and no contraindications, fibrinolytics can be given.

Hyperthermia results from increased muscular activity due to agitation, seizures (increasing heat generation), and intense vasoconstriction (impairing heat dissipation).[11] Immediate cooling and sedation are necessary to reduce morbidity and mortality. First-line agents are benzodiazepines, which treat both agitation and seizures. Haloperidol and other dopamine antagonists should be avoided because they may lower the seizure threshold,

TABLE 8-2 Treatment of Cardiovascular Complications of Sympathomimetic Drug Poisoning	
MANIFESTATIONS	**TREATMENT**
Tachyarrhythmias	Reduce environmental stimulation,* benzodiazepines
Sinus or atrial	None, metoprolol, esmolol, verapamil, diltiazem
Ventricular	Metoprolol, lidocaine, cardioversion
Hypertension	Reduce environmental stimulation,* benzodiazepines
	Phentolamine
	Nitroprusside
	β blocker (β$_1$-specific if possible) if associated with tachycardia
Convulsions	Lorazepam, diazepam, phenytoin, phenobarbital
Hyperthermia	Stop seizures
	Pancuronium if seizures uncontrollable
	External cooling
	High inspired oxygen
Myocardial ischemia/infarction	Nitrates, calcium channel blockers, thrombolysis–esmolol/metoprolol
Cardiovascular collapse	Fluids (may require massive amounts in presence of hyperthermia)
	Pressors (unpredictable sensitivity)

*Especially phencyclidine and hydrocarbons.

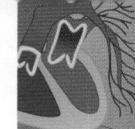

further impair heat dissipation and/or potentiate cardiac arrythmias.[8] External cooling measures and paralysis to reduce heat generation may be necessary to control hyperthermia. Even when muscle hyperactivity is prevented by paralysis, persistent seizure activity may cause brain injury. Therefore, electroencephalograms should be used to monitor paralyzed patients, and seizures should be controlled with anticonvulsant drugs or general anesthesia, if necessary. Ventilation with high oxygen concentrations is indicated in hyperthermia to meet the resultant extreme metabolic demands on organ systems. Acute renal failure may result from hypovolemia, hypotension, and rhabdomyolysis with myoglobinuria and may be prevented by vigorous fluid replacement, alkalinization of the urine, and, possibly, the use of mannitol.

Amphetamine-Like Drugs and Over-the-Counter Products

Many amphetamine-like drugs, such as ephedrine (ma huang) and related alkaloids, are available without prescription as herbal products advertised for their weight loss and athletic performance–enhancing effects. Caffeine usually is present in these supplements and may increase the risk of adverse cardiovascular events due to potentiation of sympathomimetic effects of ephedrine. Over-the-counter medications, such as decongestants, often contain sympathomimetic agents (phenylephrine, pseudoephedrine, or ephedrine) that have the potential to cause adverse cardiovascular events. Phenylpropanolamine, which has a direct agonist effect on α-adrenergic receptors, has been removed from the U.S. market due to its association with hemorrhagic stroke in previously healthy young women.[12] Illicitly obtained amphetamines (methamphetamine, 3,4-methylenedioxymethamphetamine/MDMA) and their derivatives are widely abused for their euphoric effects. The euphoria is associated with CNS and adrenomedullary sympathetic activation, producing the sympathomimetic toxidrome. Chronic use can lead to dilated cardiomyopathy, and these patients may present in frank congestive heart failure.[13]

Amphetamines displace and release catecholamines stored in neurons, directly stimulate postsynaptic adrenergic receptors, and may inhibit monoamine oxidase, the enzyme responsible for intraneuronal degradation of catecholamines. As a result of these actions, adverse cardiovascular events have been reported in temporal association with the use of amphetamines and amphetamine-like substances. These effects include acute myocardial infarction, severe hypertension, myocarditis, and lethal cardiac arrhythmias.[14] Other amphetamine-induced effects include cerebrovascular events, seizures, hyperthermia, and rhabdomyolysis. The management of amphetamine toxicity is similar to that discussed in the section on cocaine toxicity, as both the pathophysiology and manifestations of amphetamine toxicity are similar to that of cocaine (see Table 8-2).

Monoamine Oxidase Inhibitors

Clinical manifestations of monoamine oxidase (MAO) inhibitor toxicity resemble those of other sympathomimetic drugs: restlessness, hyperactivity, confusion or stupor, neuromuscular irritability, hypertension, seizures, and hyperpyrexia. Hypertension, which most often occurs after ingestion of tyramine-containing foods or beverages or after taking other sympathomimetic drugs but can also occur after an overdose, may be severe, often is associated with severe headache, and has been associated with intracerebral hemorrhage. Hypotension also can occur after overdose.

Understanding the pathophysiology of MAO inhibitor reactions requires understanding of the role of MAO in the body. MAO is located within adrenergic neurons, where it metabolizes catecholamines and related monoamines, and in the gastrointestinal mucosa and liver, where it metabolizes dietary monoamines, such as tyramine. Inhibition of MAO within the adrenergic neuron results in accumulation of both active and relatively inactive (such as octopamine) monoamines. Octopamine and other relatively inactive monoamines act as false neurotransmitters in that they are released by neuronal stimulation into nerve endings, where they do not effectively activate vascular receptors. As a consequence, MAO inhibitors, when taken continually, may lower blood pressure. However, MAO inhibitors, by slowing monoamine metabolism, also may increase pressor responses to catecholamines released by other drugs. Most important in causing hypertension is that MAO inhibitors in the gut and liver increase the bioavailability of tyramine, which in turn releases catecholamines stored in adrenergic neurons. Ingestion of foods rich in tyramine can lead to massive catecholamine release and hypertensive crisis.[15]

Tranylcypromine is an MAO inhibitor that causes catecholamine release itself and, among the MAO inhibitor class of drugs, has been implicated most commonly in cardiovascular toxicity. The newer, selective MAO inhibitors have less potential to cause hypertensive crises due to drug interactions or tyramine-containing foods. However, severe adverse effects have been described with moclobemide, a reversible inhibitor of MAO-A and selegiline, an irreversible MAO-B inhibitor.[16] It is important also to recognize the potential interaction between meperidine and MAO inhibitors. The combination has resulted in severe hypertension, hyperthermia, and seizures. The mechanism is thought to be related to excess serotonin effect in the brain. Therapy for MAO toxicity is similar to that of other sympathomimetic drugs.

Serotonin reuptake inhibitors (e.g., fluoxetine) do not cause direct cardiovascular toxicity but do interact with MAO inhibitors and other serotonergic medications to produce the so-called serotonin syndrome. This syndrome is associated with confusion, fever, diaphoresis, hyperreflexia, and myoclonus and usually is self-limited with supportive care.[17]

Theophylline and Caffeine

Cardiac toxicity of theophylline occurs in a different context from that of stimulant drugs. The most common circumstance is overdosage during therapy for obstructive airway disease, often as a result of hepatic dysfunction, which reduces the rate of theophylline metabolism. Accidental or suicidal overdose occurs often in persons

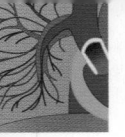
with underlying medical illnesses. The nature and severity of these medical conditions have a strong impact on the course and severity of cardiac toxicity.

The typical cardiovascular manifestations of theophylline overdose result from β-adrenergic stimulation and include tachycardia and arrhythmias (Fig. 8-9). Hypotension (rather than hypertension, as occurs with most other sympathomimetic drugs) is encountered in severe intoxications. Like amphetamines, theophylline causes systemic and local vascular catecholamine release. In addition, theophylline at high concentrations may inhibit phosphodiesterase, an enzyme that degrades intracellular cyclic adenosine monophosphate (cAMP), which, in turn, mediates β-adrenergic actions. Theophylline also directly relaxes vascular smooth muscle and acts as an adenosine antagonist. Convulsions typically occur with an overdose, and cardiac and respiratory arrest are the usual causes of death.

Management of cardiac toxicity due to theophylline ingestion in persons with chronic lung disease may be difficult. β-Adrenergic blocking agents are logical and effective treatment for supraventricular and ventricular arrhythmias, but they also may worsen airway obstruction. Relatively cardiospecific β blockers, such as esmolol or metoprolol, can be tried and the antiarrhythmic effects closely titrated against evidence of worsening airway obstruction. Esmolol is useful particularly in this instance because of its short half-life.[18]

Hypotension due to theophylline use usually results from peripheral vasodilation, at least early in the course of overdose. However, with prolonged β-sympathetic stimulation (many hours or even days), myocarditis with reduced ventricular function may occur late in the course of theophylline overdose. In addition, many older patients with chronic lung disease have ischemic heart disease. Extreme tachycardia (150 to 180 beats per minute, depending on myocardial function) and hypotension may reduce cardiac output and therefore myocardial perfusion, resulting in impaired myocardial function.

Management of theophylline-induced hypotension includes correction of metabolic disturbances and arrhythmias and administration of fluids and pressor agents. If pressor drugs are to be used, it is useful to know the cardiac output and to be able to compute the systemic vascular resistance. If cardiac output is high and systemic vascular resistance is low, as in many cases of theophylline overdose, administration of vasoconstrictors such as norepinephrine and selective β-adrenergic antagonists, such as esmolol or metoprolol, are indicated. If cardiac output is low despite adequate cardiac filling pressures and systemic vascular resistance is normal or high as sometimes occurs late in the case of theophylline overdose and in persons with preexisting myocardial disease, inotropic agents such as dobutamine might be selected.

In the presence of severe toxicity, particularly in a patient with serious underlying medical disease, the persistence of theophylline in the body and the time course of toxicity may be prolonged (≥24 hours), and acceleration of drug removal by hemoperfusion should be undertaken.[19]

Caffeine is widely consumed in beverages such as coffee and colas, in over-the-counter stimulants, and in various other combination analgesic and cold medications. Caffeine has pharmacologic actions similar to those of theophylline. Caffeine potentiates the effects of sympathomimetic drugs and might contribute to stimulant-induced adverse cardiac events. For example, ephedra-containing dietary supplements often contain

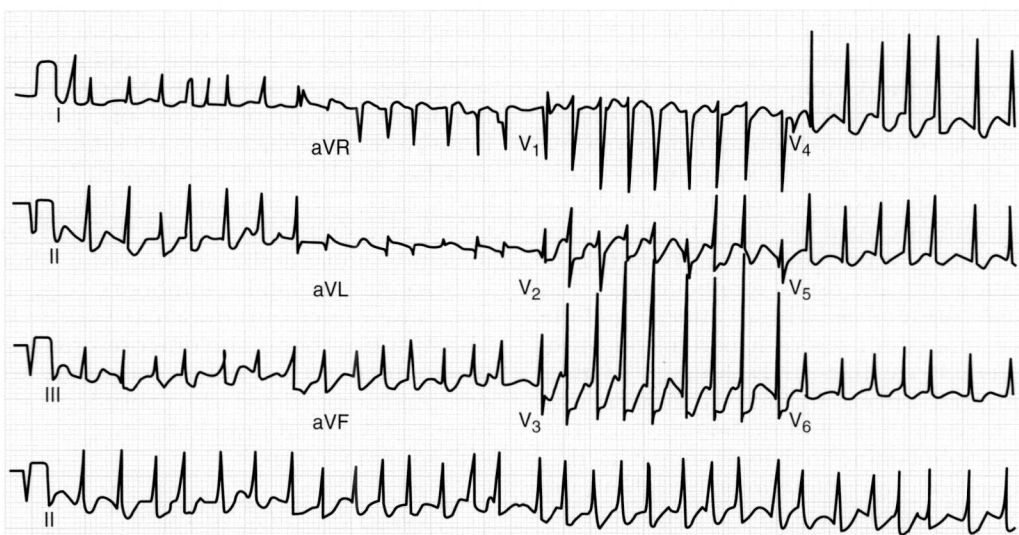

FIGURE 8-9 A 56-year-old female ingested an unknown amount of theophylline in a suicide attempt. She presented in atrial fibrillation with rapid ventricular rate (180 beats per minute) and a blood pressure of 60 mm Hg. She was treated successfully with esmolol, which immediately slowed the heart rate and increased the blood pressure. The initial theophylline level was 125 mg/L, which was treated with multiple-dose activated charcoal. Dialysis was recommended but was not performed, because the second level 4 hours later was 78 mg/L. Serial cardiac enzymes revealed an elevated troponin level, indicating myocardial injury as a complication. The patient recovered uneventfully thereafter.

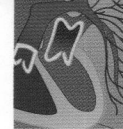

caffeine as well. Caffeine alone rarely causes severe cardiac toxicity, although cases of supraventricular tachycardias are reported. Patients with ischemic heart disease and preexisting ventricular arrhythmias may be particularly susceptible to these adverse events.[13] Severe caffeine intoxication with tachyarrhythmias followed by cardiovascular collapse and death has occurred in children. We treated an adult who had ingested a massive amount of caffeine (NoDoz) and who had sinus tachycardia with a rate of 190 beats per minute, hypokalemia, hyperglycemia, metabolic acidosis, and rhabdomyolysis (Fig. 8-10).

Δ⁹-Tetrahydrocannabinol and Hallucinogens

The usual cardiovascular effects of Δ^9-tetrahydrocannabinol (THC), the principal psychoactive component in marijuana and other cannabis products, are tachycardia,

a slight increase in recumbent blood pressure, and, with large doses or in susceptible persons, orthostatic hypotension. THC acts on widely distributed cannabinoid receptors and endocannabinoid systems. The effects of THC on heart rate result from centrally mediated sympathetic activation and reduced parasympathetic activity and systemic release of catecholamines. Orthostatic hypotension results from impaired sympathetic reflex responses and, in particular, deficient venoconstriction.

Sinus tachycardia can reach rates of 140 to 150 beats per minute or higher and, manifested as palpitations, can contribute to the anxiety reaction occasionally reported by novice users or those consuming marijuana containing unusually large amounts of THC. In otherwise healthy persons, no specific treatment other than reassurance is necessary. Patients with ischemic

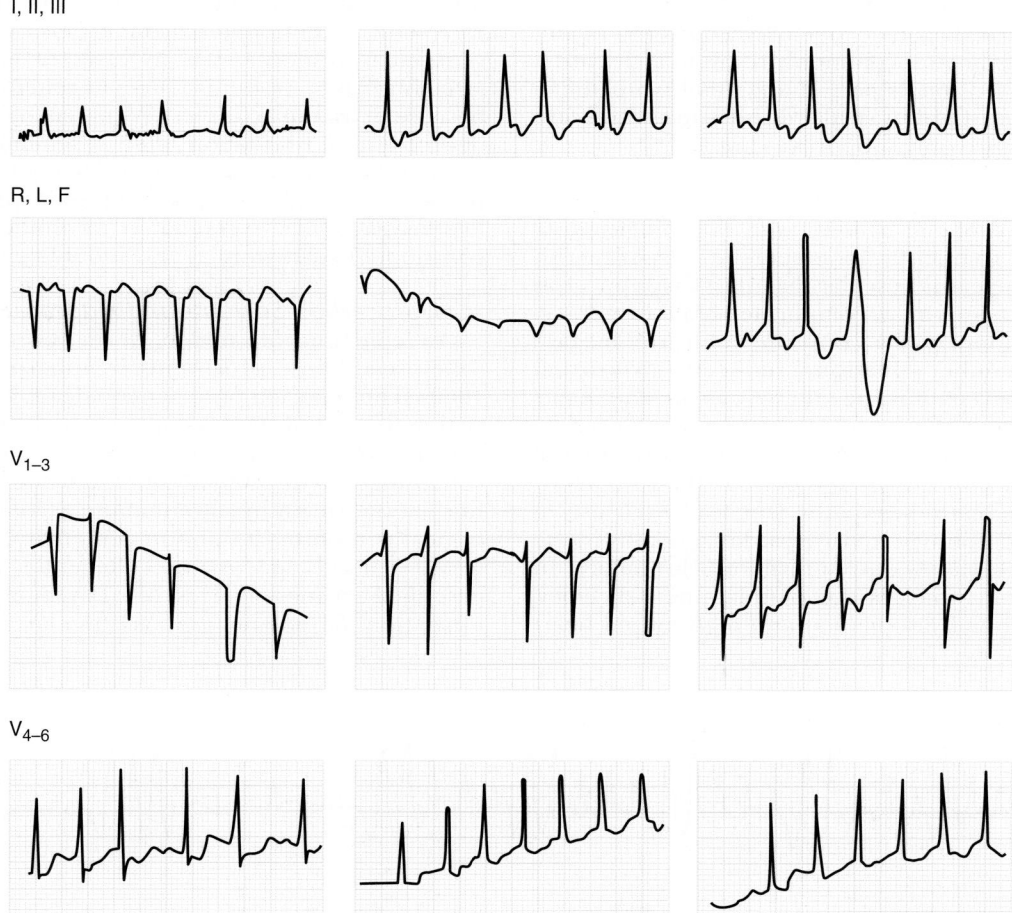

FIGURE 8-10 The patient is a 30-year-old schizophrenic woman who allegedly ingested the contents of four bottles of the over-the-counter preparation NoDoz, each containing 60 100-mg caffeine tablets. She was brought to the emergency room awake but mute and apparently hallucinating. Blood pressure was 112/74 mm Hg; heart rate, 180 to 200 beats per minute; serum potassium level, 2.2 mEq/L; and serum caffeine level, 200 µg/mL.

This admission electrocardiogram shows a supraventricular tachycardia at a rate of about 180 to 190/min. The tachycardia is probably sinus in origin, judging from the P wave configurations. AV nodal Wenckebach's block is present and probably the result of the tachycardia rate (and the inability of the AV node to respond) rather than of the pharmacologic effects of caffeine. Ventricular ectopic complexes also are present.

The patient was treated with potassium and fluids, with prompt initial slowing of the sinus rate to 150 beats per minute, then with gradual return to normal during the next 48 hours.

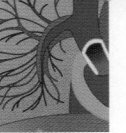
heart disease are at greater risk from the effects of THC, although myocardial infarction is a rare occurrence. The combination of increased myocardial oxygen demand due to the tachycardia and increased myocardial contractility as well as decreased myocardial oxygen delivery due to effects of carbon monoxide derived from marijuana smoke may aggravate the ischemia. Persons with angina pectoris are not able to exercise as long after smoking marijuana. Ischemia combined with systemic release of catecholamines also might result in potentially severe arrhythmias. Orthostatic dizziness occasionally is reported by recreational users of cannabis, particularly after eating larger than usual quantities of THC in cookies or brownies. Patients receiving THC as an adjunct to cancer chemotherapy may exhibit orthostatic hypotension, particularly when they are dehydrated because of their disease. Hypotension responds well to placing the patient into a horizontal or Trendelenburg position and administering fluids; administration of pressors is rarely necessary.[20]

Lysergic acid diethylamide, phenylcyclidine, psilocybin, and other hallucinogens commonly result in tachycardia and mild hypertension as part of a general sympathetic arousal syndrome. Cardiovascular disturbances rarely are serious and require only supportive care.

Ethanol

Chronically alcoholic patients with toxicologic problems are seen frequently in emergency departments. Chronic or acute cardiovascular disorders may appear as primary problems or may complicate other overdoses. Alcoholic cardiomyopathy consisting of cardiomegaly, ventricular chamber dilation, reduced myocardial contractility, and pathologic alterations in the heart muscle involving both ventricles can be diagnosed in patients in whom the sole causative agent is ethanol consumption of more than 80 g per day for 10 years or more. Alcoholic cardiomyopathy is a leading cause of nonishemic and nonhypertensive cardiomyopathy in the United States. It is a low output form of heart failure. In contrast, beriberi, which is due to thiamine deficiency, results in peripheral vasodilation and high output heart failure. Alcoholic cardiomyopathy may result in low cardiac output, pulmonary congestion, diverse arrhythmias, or sudden death, and is treated medically like other types of congestive failure.[13]

Heavy binge drinkers may present with a sudden onset of arrhythmias, particularly atrial fibrillation or flutter with rapid ventricular response but also atrial or junctional tachycardia and ventricular arrhythmias (alcohol-induced atrial fibrillation has been termed *holiday heart*) (Fig. 8-11). The arrhythmias may be due to preclinical cardiomyopathy, electrolyte abnormalities (including deficiency of potassium, phosphate, or magnesium), or early stages of alcohol withdrawal.

Abstinence from ethanol (and other sedative drugs) may be associated with intense sympathetic hyperactivity, hypertension, and many types of tachyarrhythmias, usually supraventricular but also ventricular arrhythmias, and sudden death.

Lidocaine and β-adrenergic antagonists have been used to treat arrhythmias caused by ethanol. β blockers, verapamil, or diltiazem may be necessary to control the ventricular response rate in cases of alcohol-induced atrial fibrillation or flutter. Digoxin generally is not useful because it is not a direct AV nodal blocker. Alcohol-induced atrial fibrillation often is self-limited, resolving spontaneously in 24 to 36 hours. Metabolic disturbances, particularly hypokalemia, hypophosphatemia, and hypomagnesemia, common in alcoholic persons, may contribute to arrhythmias and should be corrected.

Hydrocarbon Solvents and Fluorocarbon Aerosols

An epidemic of sudden death was associated with widespread abuse of solvents by inhalation in the late 1960s. The reported prodrome to death was described as victims becoming increasingly excited or panicky after sniffing or inhaling the solvent, exercising, then collapsing. The presumed cause of death was ventricular fibrillation. Death by solvent abuse accounted for 12.2% of deaths reported to poison centers in 2000 in the 13- to 19-year-old age group.[21] Recently, a case report described a witnessed arrest of a 15-year-old girl following inhalation of butane gas. Ventricular fibrillation was

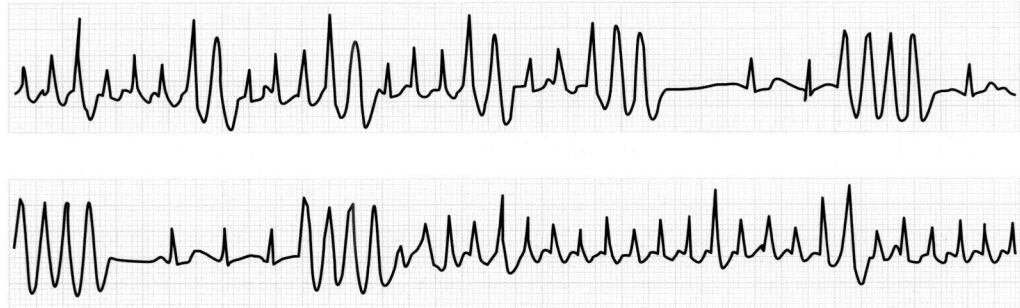

FIGURE 8-11 These two continuous lead II rhythm strips were recorded in a 48-year-old alcoholic man admitted to the hospital after a syncopal spell preceded by palpitations. Sinus rhythm is interrupted by atrial tachycardia. Frequent premature ventricular complexes also are present, as well as bursts of ventricular tachycardia, which occasionally interrupt the atrial tachyarrhythmia. The rhythm was treated with intravenous lidocaine, which abolished the bursts of ventricular tachycardia but had no effect on the atrial arrhythmia. All arrhythmias resolved within 12 hours of admission. Work-up for organic heart disease was nondiagnostic, and 24-hour ambulatory electrocardiographic monitoring before hospital discharge failed to reveal any rhythm abnormalities.

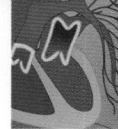

documented by paramedics and treated with defibrillation and then epinephrine for the ensuing asystole. The patient survived the cardiac arrest but was left with significant neurologic impairment.[22] Animal studies have shown that many solvents, such as toluene, benzene, chloroform, trichloroethane, trichloroethylene, trifluoroethane, and other fluoroalkenes (Freons), potentiate arrhythmias due to infused epinephrine. Thus, doses of epinephrine that usually produce no arrhythmias may cause ventricular tachycardia or fibrillation after solvent or fluorocarbon exposure. Solvent inhalation, even in the presence of normal oxygenation, may cause sinoatrial slowing followed by escape junctional or ventricular rhythms. The combination of depressed sinoatrial automaticity and myocardial sensitization to catecholamines, released by exercise or emotional stimuli, possibly accounts for the fatal ventricular arrhythmias. Toluene sniffing also causes renal tubular dysfunction as well as severe hypokalemia,[23] hypophosphatemia, and metabolic acidosis, which might aggravate arrhythmias. Ingestion of hydrocarbons typically is associated with a chemical pneumonitis and CNS depression; however, arrhythmias with ECG changes and elevation in cardiac enzymes suggestive of myocardial necrosis have been reported.

Obviously, little can be done to treat "sudden sniffing deaths." However, in persons who are intoxicated with solvents or fluorocarbons, steps can be taken to lessen the risk of arrhythmias, at least according to the current hypothesis of pathogenesis. Before hospital evaluation, patients should be advised to avoid strenuous exercise. Once in hospital, they should be placed in a quiet, nonthreatening environment and sedated, if necessary. Sympathomimetic drugs such as pressors and bronchodilators should be avoided. Ventricular arrhythmias are best treated with β-blocking agents.

Sympathetic-Inhibiting Drugs

Cardiac disturbances caused by sympathetic-inhibiting drugs are listed in Box 8-2.

β-ADRENERGIC RECEPTOR BLOCKERS

Cardiac disturbances caused by β-adrenergic receptor blockers result from receptor blockade, which all drugs in this class demonstrate, and other actions such as membrane-depressant or sympathomimetic effects, which differ among drugs within the class. β-Adrenergic blockade itself is associated with AV block (usually first degree), sinus bradycardia, and the emergence of ectopic escape pacemakers in healthy hearts.[24] In persons with underlying cardiac conduction disease, advanced AV block with slow ventricular rates can occur. Occasionally, in the presence of severe underlying myocardial disease in which contractility depends on sympathetic activity, acute β-adrenergic receptor blockade can result in hypotension or cardiac failure, including shock or acute pulmonary edema and death. With gradual dose escalation, however, most patients with severe cardiac failure are able to tolerate β blockers with beneficial effects on mortality.

BOX 8-2	CARDIAC DISTURBANCES CAUSED BY SYMPATHETIC-INHIBITING DRUGS

Drugs

Propranolol and other β blockers
Methyldopa
Clonidine and other imidazoline derivatives
Reserpine
Guanethidine
Prazosin and other α blockers

Cardiovascular Disturbances

Sinus bradycardia
Atrioventricular block
Hypotension
Cardiac failure*

Other Common Manifestations

Sedation†
Small pupils‡
Diarrhea
Seizures§
Hyperkalemia
Bronchoconstriction‖

---

*Usually in patients with underlying myocardial disease.
†Except guanethidine and prazosin.
‡Particularly clonidine and prazosin.
§Propranolol and other membrane-depressant β blockers; rarely clonidine.
‖Usually in patients with previous asthma.

In previously healthy persons, drugs such as propranolol, with membrane-depressant effects, can in large doses directly depress myocardial function and result in hypotension caused by reduced cardiac output.[25] Drugs such as pindolol, with intrinsic sympathomimetic activity, can cause tachycardia and hypertension despite concurrent β-blockade after an overdose. Sotalol, a β blocker with type III antiarrhythmic activity, is associated with QT prolongation and the development of torsades de pointes. QT prolongation and arrhythmogenesis is dose related and occurs both with therapeutic dosing (especially in the presence of renal insufficiency) and in overdose.

Therapy is summarized in Table 8-3. Sinus bradycardia usually is well tolerated and requires no specific therapy. If sinus bradycardia results in hemodynamic compromise, atropine, glucagon, or temporary transvenous pacing should be considered. AV block resulting in hemodynamic compromise is an indication for temporary transvenous pacing, with dual-chamber preferred, if feasible.

Hypotension usually can be managed with fluids and correction of bradyarrhythmias. In the presence of myocardial depression, glucagon, which activates adenylate cyclase by a nonadrenergic mechanism, may enhance myocardial contractility and increase cardiac output.[26] Epinephrine, dobutamine, amrinone, and milrinone potentially are useful inotropic agents, although the doses may need to be higher than usual because of β blockade. Calcium chloride has been

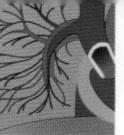

TABLE 8-3 Treatment of Cardiovascular Complications of Sympathetic-Inhibiting Drug Poisoning

MANIFESTATION	TREATMENT
Bradyarrhythmias	
Sinus or atrial	None, glucagon,* atropine, pacing, isoproterenol
Junctional and ventricular	Isoproterenol, pacing, glucagon*
Ventricular tachyarrhythmias	Lidocaine
	Cardioversion
Hypotension	Trendelenburg's position
	Treat bradyarrhythmias if present
	Fluids (invasive hemodynamic monitoring advised with preexisting cardiac disease)
	Glucagon, dobutamine* (if normal or high systemic vascular resistance)
	Dopamine, norepinephrine (if low systemic vascular resistance)
Hypertension†	Phentolamine
	Nitroprusside

*Particularly when related to β-blocker overdose.
†Clonidine, methyldopa, guanethidine; note hypertension is often *transient* and is followed by hypotension.

reported to increase blood pressure after propranolol overdose that is unresponsive to other medications.[27]

Sympatholytic Antihypertensive Drugs and Other Centrally Acting α_2-Adrenergic Agonists

Clonidine is used in the treatment of hypertension, narcotic or alcohol withdrawal, perimenopausal hot flashes, and attention deficit hyperactivity disorder. Over-the-counter topical decongestants commonly contain imidazoline derivatives (naphazoline, tetrahydrozoline, oxymetazoline, and xylometazoline), which can cause systemic toxicity after either topical exposure or ingestion, particularly in children.

Most patients who have ingested excessive doses of sympatholytic antihypertensive drugs have sinus bradycardia and hypotension when first seen by a physician.[28] Drugs such as methyldopa, clonidine, and reserpine, which are active in the CNS, commonly cause sedation or coma. After an overdose of clonidine or imidazoline derivatives, miosis and respiratory depression resembling narcotic overdose also may ensue. However, hypotension and bradycardia usually are more prominent than respiratory depression after clonidine or imidazoline poisoning. The reverse is true for narcotics. Clonidine and imidazoline derivatives, by direct α-adrenergic receptor agonist activity, and methyldopa, reserpine, and guanethidine, through systemic release of catecholamines, also have been associated with transient and sometimes severe hypertension (Fig. 8-12)

Naloxone has been used in clonidine overdose with variable success and should not be relied on as the primary therapy for cardiovascular toxicity from this drug. Naloxone is recommended for cases of clonidine poisoning with severe respiratory depression and may be considered in patients with severe alteration of mental status and cardiovascular compromise. Naloxone use in topical imidazoline toxicity has not been studied.[29]

In most cases, hypotension due to antihypertensive drug overdose is not severe and can be managed by the legs up, head down position and intravenous fluids.

When hypotension is severe in the presence of bradycardia, atropine or cardiac pacing increases heart rate and cardiac output and usually increases blood pressure. Although often not necessary, modest doses of dopamine and norepinephrine usually are effective. Hypertension resulting from use of clonidine or other sympatholytic drugs is best treated with the short-acting α-adrenergic receptor antagonist phentolamine and, if necessary, vasodilators such as nitroprusside. The hypertensive phase after clonidine overdose is relatively brief, and antihypertensive treatment should be tapered before the subsequent hypotensive effects become manifested.

Anticholinergic Drugs and Toxins

Cardiac disturbances caused by anticholinergic drugs and toxins are listed in Box 8-3.

The various anticholinergic drugs or toxins that may be ingested are too numerous to list separately. In most cases, they cause sinus tachycardia with mild hypertension. Serious arrhythmias resulting from purely anticholinergic compounds are uncommon unless a patient has underlying ischemic heart disease. For example, by increasing myocardial oxygen demand owing to tachycardia, atropine has caused ventricular tachycardia and fibrillation in patients after myocardial infarction. Many patients with anticholinergic signs have ingested antihistamine-sympathomimetic combinations or drugs such as tricyclic antidepressants or neuroleptics with both anticholinergic and membrane-depressant effects that result in more serious cardiovascular disturbances.

If treatment is necessary because of hypotension, organ ischemia, severe hypertension, or severe central anticholinergic syndrome (i.e., delirium, coma) due to use of anticholinergic drugs, the most specific therapy is administration of cholinesterase inhibitors. Physostigmine is used because it enters the brain and antagonizes the CNS and peripheral autonomic effects. Although benzodiazepines are used more commonly for treatment of agitation due to anticholinergic poisoning, physostigmine may be more effective and result in fewer

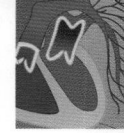

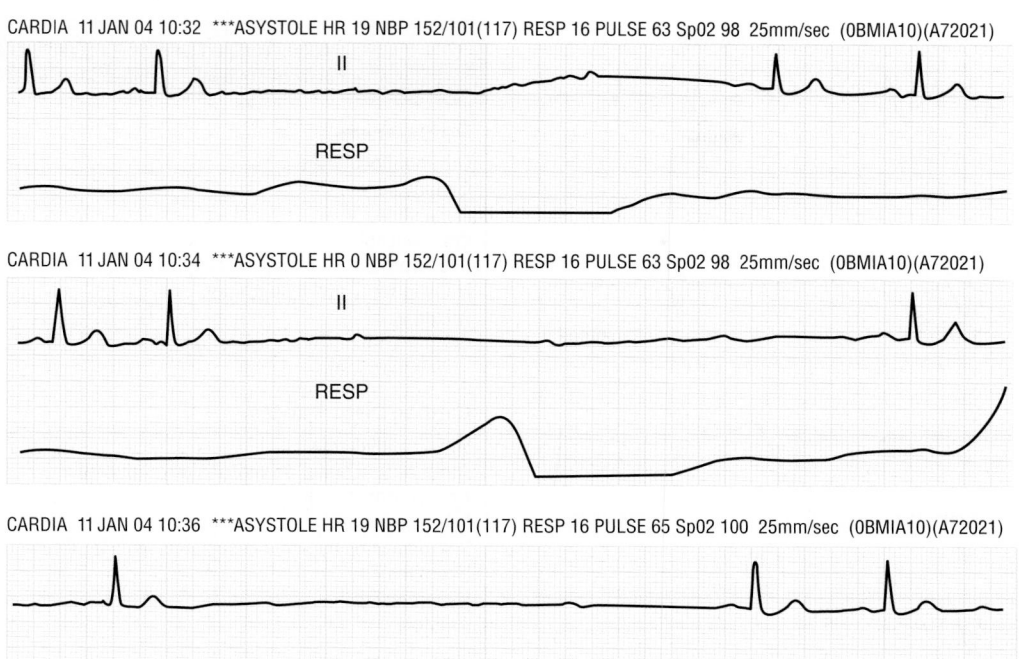

FIGURE 8-12 A 54-year-old man allegedly took an overdose of clonidine. Presenting vital signs included a pulse of 60 beats per minute and a blood pressure of 165/110 mm Hg. While in the emergency department, he complained of sudden onset of black spots in his visual field in association with this rhythm. He did not lose consciousness and his blood pressure remained in the normal range. The cardiac monitor revealed an irregular sinus bradycardia followed by sinus slowing and arrest accompanied by complete AV block. The occurrence of AV block with sinus slowing/arrest is described as "vagotonic AV block" and is consistent with both the sympatholytic and vagotonic effects of clonidine. The arrhythmia resolved spontaneously and did not recur.

BOX 8-3	**CARDIAC DISTURBANCES CAUSED BY ANTICHOLINERGIC DRUGS AND TOXINS**

Drugs

Atropine, belladonna, scopolamine
Antihistamines (including most over-the-counter hypnotics)
Tricyclic antidepressants
Plants (such as jimsonweed)
Mushrooms (such as *Amanita muscaria**)
Antipsychotics[†]

Cardiac Disturbances

Sinus tachycardia
Atrial tachycardia
Ventricular premature beats
Hypertension

Other Common Manifestations

Sedation
Delirium, coma
Fever
Dry, flushed skin
Dilated pupils
Dry mucous membranes
No sweating
Hypoactive or absent bowel sounds
Urinary retention

---

*May have muscarinic as well as anticholinergic activity.
[†]Especially phenothiazines.

complications.[30] Alternatively, because anticholinergic drugs result in an imbalance between sympathetic and parasympathetic activity with a predominance of the former, β-blockers also may be effective in treating sinus and other supraventricular tachyarrhythmias. Both physostigmine and β-blockers may be hazardous when given to persons with depressed myocardial contractility; depressed AV conduction, such as after a tricyclic antidepressant overdose; or both (Fig. 8-13).

Cholinomimetic Toxins and Drugs

Cardiac disturbances and other common manifestations of poisoning by cholinomimetic drugs and toxins are listed in Box 8-4. The most common type of cholinomimetic poisoning is that due to exposure to organophosphate or carbamate insecticides resulting in excess cholinesterase inhibition.[31] The cardiovascular effects of organophosphates are unpredictable and often change over the time course of the poisoning. Early in the course, acetylcholine stimulates nicotinic receptors at sympathetic ganglia and causes tachycardia and mild hypertension. Later it stimulates muscarinic receptors or blocks ganglionic transmission by hyperpolarization, and bradycardia and hypotension result. The most common cardiac finding in organophosphate poisoning is sinus tachycardia. In severe poisonings, however, advanced AV block, bradyarrhythmias with hypotension, and asystole may occur.

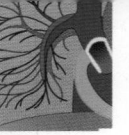
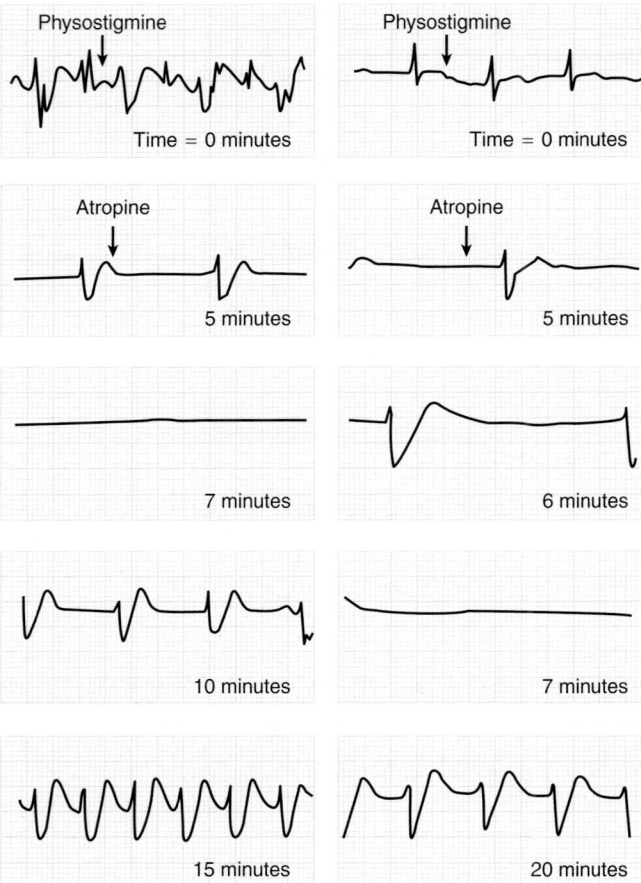

FIGURE 8-13 The strips in the *left panel* are from a 32-year-old man who had ingested 2300 mg of amitriptyline and who received physostigmine, 2 mg intravenously, for treatment of status epilepticus. Subsequently, junctional bradycardia developed and was unresponsive to atropine, and asystole occurred. Junctional rhythm was restored after treatment with epinephrine and bicarbonate. Sinus rhythm returned, the QRS narrowed during the next 12 hours, and the patient recovered fully.

The strips in the *right panel* are from a 25-year-old man who ingested 5000 mg of imipramine and 150 mg of propranolol. He received two doses of physostigmine, 2 mg intravenously, for recurrent motor seizures. After the second dose, sinus bradycardia developed and was unresponsive to atropine, and asystole occurred. After 10 minutes of closed chest cardiac massage and treatment with epinephrine and bicarbonate, sinus rhythm returned, although severe hypotension persisted. This patient's electrocardiogram results and blood pressure eventually became normal, but he died as a result of irreversible brain damage.

Delayed ventricular tachycardia of the torsades de pointes type may occur as late as 5 days after acute intoxication with organophosphates. The mechanism is believed to be a persistent imbalance between sympathetic and parasympathetic influences on the heart. The result is nonhomogeneous repolarization (associated with a long QT interval) and a predisposition to ventricular arrhythmias.

Bradyarrhythmias, if hemodynamically significant, usually can be treated effectively by administration of atropine or glycopyrrolate. Atropine or glycopyrrolate must compete with excess acetylcholine at the receptor

BOX 8-4	CARDIAC DISTURBANCES DUE TO CHOLINOMIMETIC DRUGS AND TOXINS

Drugs

Organophosphates
Carbamates
Physostigmine
Bethanechol
Pilocarpine
Neostigmine, pyridostigmine
Nicotine
Central cholinesterase inhibitors (donopezil, rivastigmire, galantamine)

Cardiac Disturbances

Sinus bradycardia
Atrial or junctional or ventricular bradycardia
Atrioventricular block
Sinus tachycardia*
Ventricular tachycardia associated with QT interval prolongation†
Hypotension
Hypertension*
Asystole

Other Common Manifestations

Pulmonary secretions and/or edema
Small pupils
Diaphoresis
Lacrimation
Salivation
Urinary frequency and/or incontinence
Abdominal cramps
Diarrhea
Fasciculations
Convulsions
Muscle weakness and paralysis
Respiratory failure

---

*May be seen in the early stages of cholinesterase inhibition and nicotine poisoning due to ganglionic stimulation.
†May be delayed up to several days after initial intoxication.

site; thus, extremely large doses are required. Doses should be increased until cholinergic signs such as salivation, diaphoresis, and bronchorrhea are reversed.[32] When anticholinergic drugs are not effective, cardiac pacing is indicated. Sinus or atrial tachycardia causing hemodynamic compromise is a greater problem to treat because drugs such as propranolol that might slow the rate might also worsen bronchoconstriction or aggravate conduction disturbances later in the course of the overdose. Patients with clinical signs of cholinesterase inhibition or an abnormal ECG (including QT interval prolongation) should have continuous cardiac monitoring for the possibility of developing ventricular tachycardia. The ECG findings may remain abnormal for several days. Treatment of ventricular tachycardia is similar to that previously described for torsades de pointes, except that anticholinergic drugs also may be used to normalize autonomic influences on the heart. Pulmonary secretions (sometimes presenting as apparent acute pulmonary edema) or respiratory failure also may

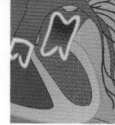

result in hypoxia and acidosis, which aggravate arrhythmias and hypotension; anticholinergic drugs are the treatment of choice for bronchorrhea. Pralidoxime may be effective in reversing the neuromuscular-blocking effects of organophosphates, but it has little effect on cardiovascular toxicity.

Reversible acetylcholinesterase inhibitors, such as donepezil, rivastigmine, and galantamine, are used in the treatment of mild to moderate Alzheimer's disease. Experience with toxicity is very limited and has occurred in the context of dosing errors and unintentional overdose. These agents have a relatively high selectivity for neuronal acetylcholinesterases and a higher affinity for acetylcholinesterases than pseudocholinesterases but can, in overdose, cause peripheral cholinomimetic effects. In case reports and anecdotal experience with donepezil toxicity, presenting symptoms have consisted of nausea, vomiting, sinus bradycardia, and increased bronchial secretions.[33] Treatment should include supportive care, gastrointestinal decontamination with activated charcoal, and atropine. There is no known role for pralidoxime.

Membrane-Depressant Drugs and Toxins

TYPE I ANTIARRHYTHMIC DRUGS

Type IA, B, and C antiarrhythmic agents affect phase 0 (upstroke velocity of the action potential) and action potential durations to various degrees in different portions of the conduction system and in ventricular and atrial muscle. These differences are reflected in varying effects on the ECG (Table 8-4).

The cardiac disturbances caused by membrane-depressant drugs and toxins are listed in Box 8-5.

Quinidine is the prototypical membrane-depressant drug. Quinidine and other type IA antiarrhythmic drugs (including procainamide and disopyramide) impede the fast sodium current across cardiac cell membranes and slow conduction, particularly in the His-Purkinje system.[34] In toxic doses, slowed conduction and prolonged repolarization are demonstrated by progressively marked QT prolongation, QRS widening, or AV block. Loss of atrial activity and slow ventricular rhythm owing to a failure to depolarize pacemaker cells may be observed (Fig. 8-14). Ventricular tachycardia and fibrillation may occur after therapeutic doses ("quinidine syncope") as well as after overdose. Ventricular tachycardia in the presence of a long QT interval usually is of the polymorphous (torsades de pointes) type, and it is characterized by undulation of the QRS polarity about an isoelectric point (Fig. 8-15; see also Fig. 8-8).

In addition to its electrophysiologic effects, quinidine in large doses depresses myocardial contractility and relaxes blood vessels, resulting in hypotension. In cases of massive overdose, this may produce shock. Disopyramide, and quinidine to a lesser extent, also has anticholinergic effects that may result in sinus tachycardia after a mild overdose. Similarly, overdoses of type IC antiarrhythmic drugs, such as flecainide and propafenone, may result in bradyarrhythmias, conduction delays, and depressed cardiac contractility with shock. These drugs may have a significant proarrhythmic action and can cause ventricular tachycardia, even at therapeutic doses in people with left ventricular dysfunction.

Therapeutic options for ventricular tachycardia due to quinidine or quinidine-like drugs include use of magnesium, overdrive pacing to shorten the QTU interval, lidocaine, phenytoin, and possibly amiodarone[35] (Table 8-5). Treatment of conduction disturbances and hypotension is discussed in the section on tricyclic antidepressant toxicity.

CALCIUM CHANNEL BLOCKERS

Calcium channel blockers (CCBs) block intracellular entry of calcium by binding L-type calcium channels located primarily in cardiac and vascular smooth muscle. The result is decreased cardiac inotropy and chronotropy and decreased vascular tone. Verapamil has depressive effects predominantly on sinoatrial (SA)/AV nodal conduction and myocardial contractility. Diltiazem is similar in action to verapamil but produces less cardiac depression at therapeutic doses. Nifedipine and other dihydropyridines act preferentially on vascular smooth muscle, resulting in vasodilation; their effect on cardiac conduction is nil in therapeutic doses.

The cardiac manifestations of toxicity are essentially an extension of the therapeutic effects. However, in overdose, the selectivity of specific agents may be lost. Serious toxicity can occur even with therapeutic doses of CCBs in persons with underlying cardiac disease, and similar effects are observed in healthy people after overdose.

Hypotension is a common feature of CCB overdose and results from different mechanisms. Vasodilation can result in hypotension due to decreased systemic vascular resistance; this is an effect of all CCBs. Other mechanisms of hypotension are negative inotropy and chronotropy that lead to decreased cardiac output, bradyarrhythmias, and shock. Inhibition of calcium entrance into the myocardial cell, which is necessary for muscle contraction, results in depressed myocardial contractility. Verapamil- and diltiazem-induced depression of slow-response cardiac cells also can result in sinus bradycardia or arrest and AV block, particularly in the setting of preexisting cardiac conduction disease.

Management should be directed at the mechanism of toxicity. For bradycardia refractory to atropine, glucagon can be used first, followed by cardiac pacing. Hypotension may be due to vasodilation or negative inotropy or both. Vasodilation should be treated with fluids and vasopressors. There are a number of treatments that counteract the negative inotropy. Calcium chloride or gluconate is recommended, particularly for the treatment of hypotension. Calcium can completely reverse the negative inotropic effects of CCBs, and it may partially reverse the electrophysiologic toxicity but appears to have no effect in reversing vasodilation. The effective dose of calcium has been debated. In general, initial bolus doses of calcium salts followed by continuous infusion with monitoring of serum calcium is a reasonable approach, using the hemodynamic profile

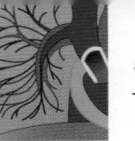

TABLE 8-4 Electrophysiologic Differences Among Antiarrhythmic Agents

CLASS	CLASS NAME	EXAMPLES	DEPRESS PHASE 0 SODIUM CHANNEL BLOCKADE	PROLONG ACTION POTENTIAL DURATION	SYMPATHOLYTIC EFFECT	DEPRESS SLOW RESPONSE CALCIUM ENTRY BLOCKADE	DEPRESS PHASE 4 DEPOLARIZATION	PROLONGATION OF SURFACE ECG INTERVALS			
								PR	QRS	QT	JT
IA	Membrane anesthetics	Quinidine Procainamide, Disopyramide	2+	1+	0/+	0	1+	0/+	0/+	2+	2+
IB	Same	Lidocaine Mexiletine	2+	—	0	0	—	0	0	0	0
IC	Same	Flecainide Propafenone	2+	0/–	0/+	0/+	1+	2+	2+	1+	0
II	β blockers	Propranolol Metoprolol Esmolol	0/+	0/–	2+	0	1+	0/+	0	0	0
III	—	Amiodarone Sotalol Dofetilide Ibutilide	1+	2+	1+	0	1+	1+	0	2+	2+
IV	Calcium blockers	Verapamil Diltiazem	0	1+	1+	2+	1+	0/+	0	0	0/+

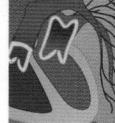

BOX 8-5	CARDIAC DISTURBANCES CAUSED BY MEMBRANE-DEPRESSANT DRUGS AND TOXINS

Drugs

Quinidine
Procainamide
Disopyramide
Flecainide
Tricyclic antidepressants
Diphenhydramine (high dose)
Phenothiazines and related neuroleptics
Propafenone
Propranolol (and other membrane-depressant β blockers)*
Cocaine (high dose)

Cardiac Effects and Disturbances

QT interval prolongation†
Intraventricular conduction delay (QRS interval prolongation)
Atrioventricular block
Junctional or ventricular bradycardia
Ventricular tachycardia (often polymorphous)‡
Ventricular fibrillation‡
Asystole
Hypotension

Other Common Manifestations
No syndromes about which one can generalize, although many agents in this group have anticholinergic effects

*Membrane depression seen with massive overdose; this is *not* a manifestation of β blockade.
†Among β blockers, only sotalol is reported to increase the QT interval. Flecainide usually does not increase the QT interval.
‡In the case of β blockers, usually occurs in association with bradyarrhythmia.

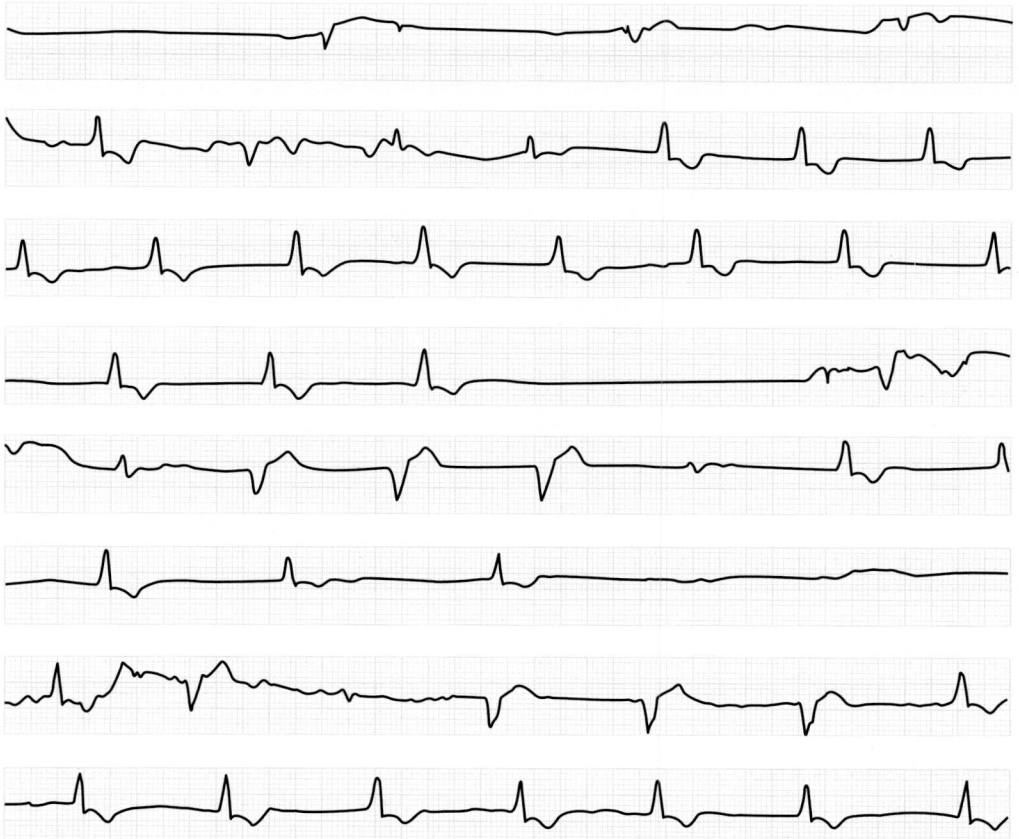

FIGURE 8-14 These strips are from a 76-year-old woman who was admitted to the coronary care unit with syncopal spells. She had been taking digoxin and quinidine for congestive heart failure and ventricular arrhythmias. Serum levels of both these agents were in the toxic range (serum digoxin level was 3.4 ng/mL, quinidine 10 mg/mL). This continuously recorded V₁ rhythm strip demonstrates absence of atrial activity and prolonged pauses in QRS rhythm, which are terminated by different ventricular escape foci at different rates. Despite aggressive medical management, the patient died within 48 hours with electromechanical dissociation.

as a guide for dosing. High-dose calcium administration has been described in CCB overdose resulting in serum levels as high as 23.8 mg/dL with no adverse effect.[36] Glucagon also has positive inotropic effects and should be administered. There is evidence also that therapy with high-dose insulin and glucose in severe CCB poisoning can improve myocardial contractility significantly when standard therapies have failed.[37] Finally, therapies such

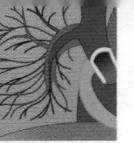

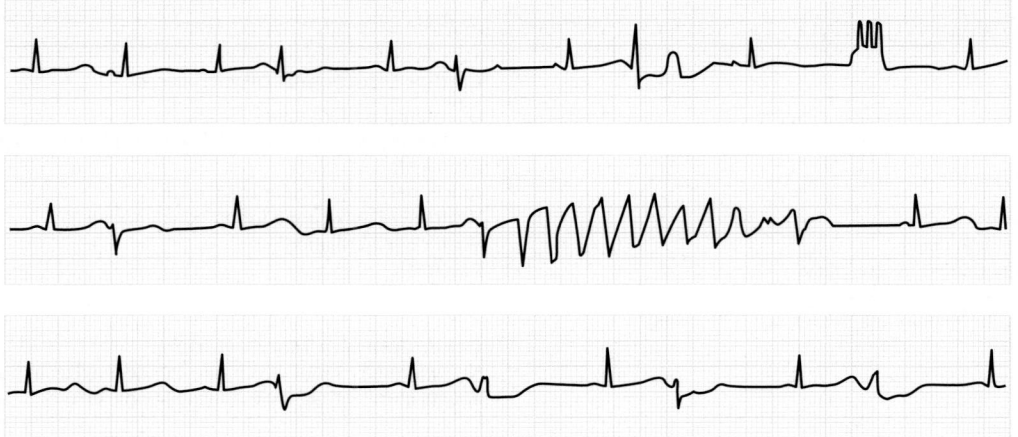

FIGURE 8-15 The patient is a 64-year-old woman who was begun on oral quinidine therapy for frequent premature ventricular beats associated with palpitations. These continuous lead II rhythm strips were recorded after the third 200-mg dose and show a markedly prolonged QT interval, frequent multiform ventricular ectopic beats, and a self-terminating burst of polymorphous ventricular tachycardia. The serum level of quinidine obtained after the recording of these tracings was 3.6 mg/mL. Quinidine was withdrawn and oral procainamide substituted without further complications.

TABLE 8-5 Treatment of Cardiovascular Complications of Membrane-Depressant Drug Poisoning	
MANIFESTATION	**TREATMENT**
QRS prolongation	Sodium bicarbonate
Arrhythmias	
Sinus tachycardia	None, esmolol or metoprolol
Atrial tachycardia or fibrillation	Same as above plus cardioversion
Ventricular premature beats and tachycardia	Magnesium, lidocaine, isoproterenol (with long QT only)
	Overdrive pacing
Bradyarrhythmias	Atropine
	Isoproterenol
	Pacemaker*
Hypotension	Fluids (hemodynamic monitoring advised in evidence of cardiac failure or myocardial depression)
	Treat bradyarrhythmias
	Dopamine, norepinephrine (low systemic vascular resistance)
	Dobutamine, isoproterenol (low cardiac output)
	Intra-aortic balloon pump or cardiopulmonary bypass (if intractable cardiogenic shock)
*May require high-voltage output to ensure capture.	

as pacing, intra-aortic balloon pump, and extracorporeal bypass have been used successfully in refractory shock in this setting.

TRICYCLIC ANTIDEPRESSANTS AND ANTIPSYCHOTIC DRUGS

At one time, tricyclic antidepressants (TCAs) accounted for more cardiac morbidity and mortality than any other class of drugs. With the introduction of selective serotonin reuptake inhibitors, the incidence of TCA overdose has declined but the morbidity and mortality remains high. The mechanisms of TCA action include a strong anticholinergic effect, inhibition of neuronal uptake of catecholamines, membrane depression, peripheral α-adrenergic blockade, and CNS-mediated inhibition of sympathetic reflexes.

In mild and moderate cases of TCA overdose, anticholinergic effects and increased circulating cate-cholamines result in sinus tachycardia, increased cardiac output, and normal or increased blood pressure. In severe cases, impaired His-Purkinje and intraventricular conduction and depressed myocardial contractility predominate, and hypotension is observed. Prolongation of the QRS duration is present in most cases of serious TCA toxicity. The finding of a rightward terminal 40-ms frontal plane QRS vector (130 to 270 degrees) is reported to be more sensitive than QRS widening in detecting tricyclic poisoning in adults, but not in children (who may normally have a rightward axis). In one study, the finding of a terminal R wave in aV_R greater than 3 mm was shown to be the only ECG finding that significantly predicted the development of seizures and dysrhythmias (Fig. 8-16).[38,39] Bundle branch block, AV block with a slow ventricular rhythm, and asystole may occur in the most severe poisonings (see Fig. 8-15; see also Figs. 8-5 and 8-13). Responsiveness to electrical

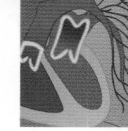

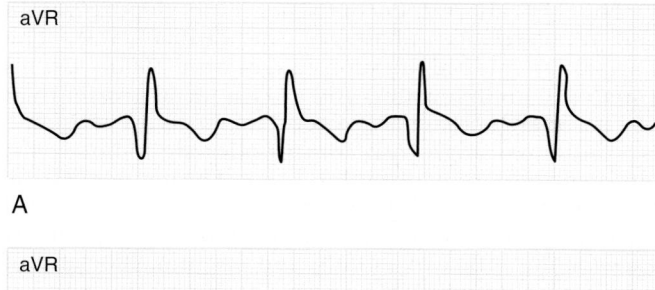

A

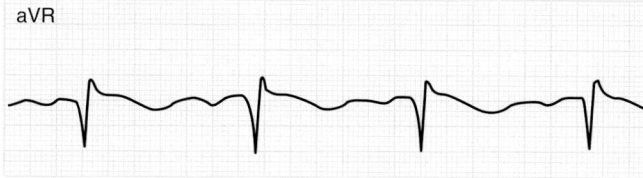

B

FIGURE 8-16 A 14-year-old girl with a suicidal ingestion of amitriptyline presented with altered mental status. **A,** Her initial ECG revealed a QRS of 110 and a prominent R wave in aVR. The patient seized just as preparations for intubation were being made. **B,** Subsequent to termination of the seizure with lorazepam, sodium bicarbonate boluses were administered with resolution of the tall R wave in aVR and narrowing of the QRS interval to 90 ms. The patient subsequently recovered uneventfully and was transferred to the psychiatric service on hospital day 3.

stimulation is decreased so that pacing thresholds are often higher than normal; in extreme cases, the myocardium does not respond at all to pacing. Hypotension usually results from depressed cardiac output. Cardiac output may be reduced as a result of venous pooling with inadequate cardiac filling (associated with low pulmonary capillary wedge pressure) or, in more severe poisoning, as a result of myocardial depression (associated with normal or high wedge pressure).

Therapy for TCA overdoses should be tailored to the particular cardiovascular disturbance. Sinus tachycardia is the most common cardiac disturbance in TCA toxicity and usually is not associated with hemodynamic instability. Sinus tachycardia and supraventricular arrhythmias, if associated with hemodynamic disturbances (either excessive hypertension or hypotension), can, in theory, be controlled with physostigmine or propranolol. These drugs can depress cardiac conduction and their use in the past has resulted in significant toxicity, such as severe bradyarrhythmias and asystole (see Fig. 8-13). Their use is therefore not advocated in the setting of TCA overdose.

The administration of sodium bicarbonate achieves both an increased extracellular sodium concentration, overcoming the sodium channel blockade, and an increased extracellular pH, which facilitates sodium conductance (Fig. 8-17). Sodium bicarbonate also results in a decreased extracellular potassium concentration. All of these effects may result in improved membrane responsiveness and increased conduction velocity in fast-response (His-Purkinje) cells.[40] Therefore, any intraventricular conduction delay (QRS > 0.10, R in aVr > 3 mm, right bundle branch block), wide complex tachycardia, or hypotension should be treated with sodium loading and serum alkalinization. Alkalinization can be achieved also with hyperventilation but results in hypocapnia, which

may lower the seizure threshold, and seizures are a common and serious complication of tricyclic antidepressant overdose.

After sodium bicarbonate, lidocaine is the treatment of choice for ventricular arrhythmias. Other type IA or IC sodium channel blocking antiarrhythmic drugs (quinidine, procainamide, disopyramide, propafenone, flecainide), which have additive membrane-depressant effects, should be avoided. Overdrive pacing has been used successfully to treat torsades de pointes ventricular tachycardia caused by type IA drugs or long QT syndrome and would likely be useful in treating TCA overdose as well. Amiodarone could be considered for ventricular tachycardia or fibrillation unresponsive to lidocaine, but this has not been studied. Amiodarone impairs conduction via weak calcium channel and β-blocker effects and could worsen TCA-induced atrioventricular block.

Because both tachycardia and intraventricular conduction delay are characteristic and ventricular tachycardia is not uncommon, the diagnostic problem of a wide complex tachycardia of uncertain origin is common; diagnosis and treatment of this arrhythmia were discussed in detail in an earlier section of this chapter.

Intracardiac pacing is indicated in patients with high-grade AV block. If intraventricular conduction is worsening (i.e., if the QRS complex is widening) early in the clinical course, when the extent of ultimate myocardial depression is not yet known, prophylactic insertion of a transvenous pacemaker is advised because of the chance of sudden deterioration. The presence of sinus or ventricular bradycardia rather than the usual supraventricular tachycardia indicates severe toxicity and warrants pacing as well.

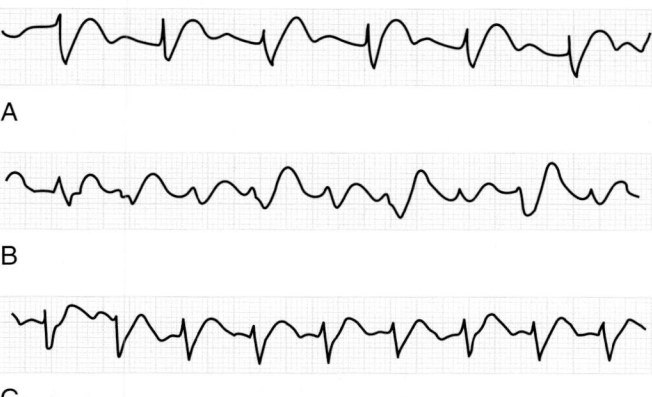

A

B

C

FIGURE 8-17 Lead II electrocardiograms recorded in a 40-year-old woman who ingested 6 g of amitriptyline (Elavil). The top strip (**A**), recorded on admission, shows a wide QRS rhythm and markedly prolonged QTU interval; atrial activity is not clearly discernible. Strips **B** and **C** were recorded 30 and 60 minutes, respectively, after intravenous administration of 44 mEq of NaHCO₃. In **B**, the QRS rate increased and alternation of QRS complexes is present. The QT interval remains prolonged, but the U wave is less prominent, and the QRS duration of alternate complexes has narrowed. Atrial activity still is not readily seen. In **C**, P waves precede each QRS complex and QRS duration remains prolonged, but the QT interval has shortened. This series of tracings suggests a supraventricular origin of the rhythm in strips **A** and **B**.

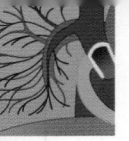

Hypotension is common after a TCA overdose. In many patients, hypotension can be managed successfully with fluids. If pressors are required, α-adrenergic agonists such as norepinephrine or dopamine are preferred. Dobutamine may prove to be useful in managing myocardial depression with normal or increased vascular resistance. Profound cardiogenic shock resulting from TCA overdose often is unresponsive to medical treatment and has a poor prognosis. In these cases, extracorporeal membrane oxygenation and cardiopulmonary bypass may be the only means of sustaining life until the body can eliminate the drug. Intra-aortic balloon pumping for drug intoxication associated with intractable shock has been successful.

Phenothiazines and other antipsychotic drugs have pharmacologic properties similar to those of TCAs, but arrhythmias are generally not as difficult to control, and cardiogenic shock is uncommon. Hypotension is more likely due to peripheral α₁-adrenergic blockade and usually responds well to recumbent posture and intravenous fluids. Differences between TCAs and antipsychotic drugs probably reflect dissimilar potencies with respect to membrane actions and different concentrations in cardiac tissue. The TCAs and their potentially toxic demethylated and hydroxylated metabolites are concentrated in the myocardium to a much greater extent than are the phenothiazines. Atypical antipsychotics produce less cardiotoxicity than traditional agents. Most commonly, sinus tachycardia is the only cardiac manifestation of toxicity; supraventricular and ventricular arrhythmias have been described in overdose. Although repolarization abnormalities such as prolonged QT can occur, and sudden death has occurred in overdose, there have been no reports of torsades de pointes in the setting of overdose with atypical antipsychotic overdose.[41]

Drug-Induced QT Prolongation and Torsades de Pointes

Numerous medications, such as antiarrhythmics, antipsychotics, antibiotics, and antihistamines, have the potential to cause QT prolongation and thus increase the risk of arrhythmias, specifically torsades de pointes ventricular tachycardia (VT).

The QT interval encompasses both depolarization and repolarization phases of the cardiac cycle. The normal QT interval duration ranges from 300 to 450 ms (up to 470 ms in females) and a QT interval greater than 500 ms or an increase of greater than 60 ms over baseline is considered high risk for torsades de pointes VT, although the predictive value is low. During depolarization, there is a rapid influx of positive ions (sodium) and during repolarization, efflux of potassium gradually exceeds the influx of sodium and calcium. Blocking of this potassium outflow current prolongs the plateau phase of the action potential, which is manifested as QT prolongation on the ECG. Therapeutically, the resultant lengthened refractory period suppresses arrhythmias. However, blocking the outward potassium current allows excessive inward current and may result in early afterdepolarizations, which are seen on the ECG as prominent U waves (Fig. 8-18). These early afterdepolarizations eventually can reach threshold amplitude and trigger torsades de pointes VT.[5]

Torsades de pointes is a form of polymorphic VT associated with a long QT interval and a twisting polarity of the QRS. It tends to terminate and recur spontaneously with syncope, presyncope, or no symptoms. It can deteriorate into ventricular fibrillation and death.

Risk factors for torsades de pointes VT among patients treated with medications that prolong the QT interval include female gender, heart disease, hypokalemia, hypomagnesemia, bradycardia, excessive medication dose, drug interactions, and preexisting long QT or a family history of long QT. The majority of cases of torsades de pointes VT induced by noncardiac drugs had at least two of these risk factors in one study.[42]

Treatment of drug-induced QT prolongation depends on the circumstance. Incidental finding of QT prolongation in the setting of both therapeutic use and overdose should prompt a detailed review of the above risk factors and discontinuation of the offending agent. Electrolyte abnormalities should be corrected, if present, and the patient should be monitored until the QT interval normalizes. If the patient presents with torsades de pointes VT, management should include discontinuation of the offending drug and suppression of early afterdepolarizations with magnesium, potassium, and

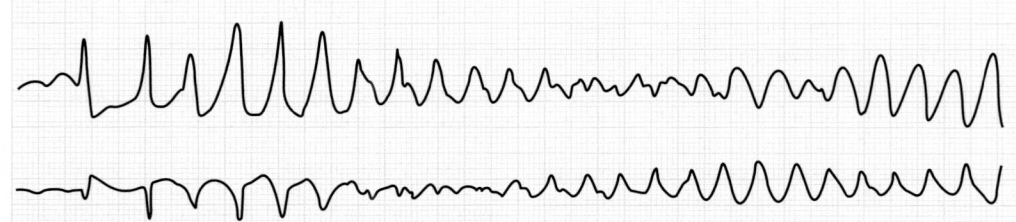

FIGURE 8-18 A 54-year-old man on methadone (140 mg PO daily) presented after an alleged overdose of clonazepam with mild lethargy and a sinus bradycardia of 50 beats per minute. Serum levels of potassium and magnesium were 4.4 and 1.6 mEq/L, respectively. Early in the course of his emergency department stay, he developed torsades de pointes ventricular tachycardia (**A**). He was defibrillated and intravenous magnesium was administered. A 12-lead ECG after resolution of the arrhythmia revealed a significantly prolonged QT interval with presence of "giant" U waves, attributed to the high dose of methadone. The prolonged QT interval resolved over 3 days and the patient was discharged with no further sequelae.

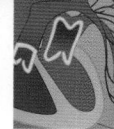

BOX 8-6	DRUGS WITH DEFINITE QT PROLONGATION AND TORSADES DE POINTES VENTRICULAR TACHYCARDIA*

Antiarrhythmics
   Disopyramide
   Dofetilide
   Flecainide
   Ibutilide
   Procainamide
   Quinidine
   Sotalol
Other cardiac medications
   Bepridil
Tricyclic antidepressants
   Citalopram
Antipsychotics
   Thioridazine
   Haloperidol
   Droperidol
Antihistamines
   Astemizole
   Terfenadine
Anti-infectives
   Chloroquine
   Erythromycin
   Halofantrine
   Pentamidine
Gastrointestinal agents
   Cisapride (restricted indications)
   Droperidol
Opioids
   Levomethadyl
   Methadone
Arsenic
Organophosphate poisoning

*This list is not exhaustive.

lidocaine. Increasing the heart rate to shorten the QT interval can be accomplished with overdrive pacing. If this is unavailable, isoproterenol may be used to accelerate the heart rate. Defibrillation is necessary when torsades de pointes VT degenerates into ventricular fibrillation. Please see Box 8-6 for a list of drugs that cause torsades de pointes. There is a website that lists all current drugs associated with torsades de pointes VT: www.torsades.org.

Miscellaneous Drugs and Toxins

Cardiovascular disturbances due to miscellaneous drugs and toxins are listed in Table 8-6.

DIGITALIS

Mortality and major morbidity due to digitalis overdose result from tachyarrhythmias, heart block, and hyperkalemia. Digitalis inhibits the sodium-potassium adenosine triphosphatase (ATPase) pump located on the cell membrane. In the therapeutic situation, this results in greater intracellular calcium concentrations, which is believed to account for increased myocardial contrac-

tility. After an overdose, disruption of sodium and potassium movement across membranes results in depressed conduction velocity, as described for membrane-depressant drugs. In addition, automaticity of previously nonautomatic tissue is enhanced due to increased rate of diastolic depolarization and possibly to spontaneous afterdepolarizations ("triggered" rhythms). Digitalis also may increase sympathetic and parasympathetic neural activity. Sympathetic stimulation enhances automaticity and excitability, whereas parasympathetic stimulation further decreases conduction velocity. Thus, an overdose with digitalis is characterized by arrhythmias demonstrating both increased automaticity and depressed atrioventricular and/or intraventricular conduction.[43]

Tachyarrhythmias due to digitalis intoxication typically include ectopic atrial tachycardia with AV block (generally and classically 2:1), AV junctional tachycardia, and ventricular tachycardia (classically bidirectional) or fibrillation (Figs. 8-19 and 8-20). Ventricular arrhythmias are reported to occur more commonly in persons with underlying heart disease. Bradyarrhythmias include sinus bradycardia, sinoatrial block, second-degree and complete AV block, slow ventricular response in patients with atrial fibrillation, idioventricular rhythm, and asystole (Fig. 8-21). Digitalis rarely causes atrial fibrillation or flutter. Severe hyperkalemia due to inhibition of sodium-potassium exchange in skeletal muscle can contribute to AV block and depressed myocardial excitability (Fig. 8-22).

Digoxin-specific Fab fragments are the main treatment for severe digitalis toxicity. Digoxin-specific Fab fragments are the definitive treatment for life-threatening ventricular arrhythmias or hyperkalemia. The antibodies bind free digoxin and may completely reverse digitalis toxicity within 15 to 30 minutes.

In the event that this treatment modality is either unavailable or ineffective, therapy is directed at the specific arrhythmia and normalization of serum potassium level. Supraventricular arrhythmias rarely require specific treatment because the ventricular response is reasonably slow. Patients who have been taking diuretics may be depleted of potassium and magnesium, and supraventricular tachyarrhythmias may respond to potassium or magnesium supplementation. However, potassium may depress AV conduction, and, as described earlier, in extreme overdoses life-threatening hyperkalemia may be present.

Ventricular tachyarrhythmias may respond to lidocaine; quinidine-like membrane-depressant drugs should be avoided. Phenytoin has been reported to be effective in treating arrhythmias, because it may enhance AV conduction while depressing automaticity, but its effect is inconsistent and unpredictable. Esmolol also has been used to treat ventricular arrhythmias; however, β blockers may also worsen conduction disturbances. Cardioversion is relatively contraindicated since it may result in ventricular fibrillation or asystole.[44]

Sinus bradycardia and AV conduction block, in light of the vagal actions of digitalis, may respond to administration of atropine. Cardiac pacing is indicated in patients with complete AV block or second-degree

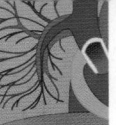

TABLE 8-6 Cardiovascular Disturbances—Miscellaneous Drugs and Toxins

DRUG/TOXIN	MECHANISMS OF ACTION	CARDIOVASCULAR DISTURBANCES	OTHER COMMON MANIFESTATIONS
Digitalis (including foxglove, oleander, lily of the valley, and toad venom [bufotoxin])	Inhibits Na$^+$-K$^+$ ATPase-dependent pump, increases automaticity, afterdepolarizations, decreases atrioventricular conduction velocity, increases vagal and ? sympathetic activity	Atrial tachycardia with atrioventricular block Junctional tachycardia Ventricular ectopy, tachycardia, fibrillation Sinus bradycardia Sinoatrial block High-grade atrioventricular block Slow ventricular response to atrial fibrillation or flutter Asystole	Nausea, vomiting Hypokalemia (with diuretic use) Hyperkalemia (severe intoxication)
Opiates	Central nervous system–mediated increase in parasympathetic and decrease in sympathetic tone	Bradycardia Atrial fibrillation Hypotension Long QT (methadone)	Miosis Respiratory depression Coma Pulmonary edema
Lithium	Disturbed cardiac potassium metabolism	Sinus bradycardia ST-T abnormalities Ventricular ectopy	Tremor, ataxia Confusion, stupor, coma Neuromuscular irritability, convulsions Azotemia
Ergot derivatives	Constriction of vascular smooth muscle	Cardiac ischemia (angina, coronary spasm with possible myocardial infarction) Peripheral vasospasm Gangrene	Headache (reason for excessive use of ergots)
Carbon monoxide, hydrogen sulfide	Binds to hemoglobin, preferentially to oxygen, causing chemical asphyxia	Cardiac ischemia (electrocardiographic abnormalities, myocardial infarction) Hypotension	Headache Coma Metabolic acidosis (with normal oxygen tension) Pulmonary edema
Cyanide	Binds to cytochrome oxidase, causing chemical asphyxia	Hypotension	
Arsenic	Interferes with cellular respiration	Cardiac ischemia Myocarditis ST-T abnormalities QT prolongation Polymorphous ventricular tachycardia Hypotension	Abdominal pain Vomiting, diarrhea Hepatitis Skin rash Renal failure Peripheral neuropathy (late) Chills, fever
Arsine	Hemolysis, anemia	Cardiac ischemia Peaked T waves Pulmonary edema	Hyperkalemia Hemoglobinuria Renal failure
Phosphorus	"Protoplasmic poison"	ST-T abnormalities QT prolongation Ventricular tachycardia/fibrillation Asystole Hypotension	Corrosive burns of skin and gastrointestinal tract Severe gastroenteritis "Smoking" luminescent vomitus and stool
Iron	Cellular membrane injury	ST-T wave abnormalities Hypovolemia Myocardial necrosis Hypotension	Nausea, vomiting, diarrhea Gastrointestinal bleeding Hyperglycemia Leukocytosis Metabolic acidosis Hepatic necrosis
Fluoride	Hypocalcemia Hyperkalemia	QT interval prolongation Peaked T waves Ventricular fibrillation Sudden death	Nausea, vomiting, diarrhea Tetany, hyperreflexia Respiratory depression
Organic mercury (chronic)		ST-T abnormalities QT prolongation	Sore mouth, metallic taste, vomiting, diarrhea, tremor, dysarthria, ataxia
Lead		Chest pain Cardiac failure ST-T abnormalities Hypertension	Anorexia Abdominal pain, constipation Anemia Peripheral neuropathy Encephalopathy

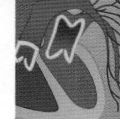

TABLE 8-6 Cardiovascular Disturbances—Miscellaneous Drugs and Toxins (*Cont'd*)

DRUG/TOXIN	MECHANISMS OF ACTION	CARDIOVASCULAR DISTURBANCES	OTHER COMMON MANIFESTATIONS
Scorpion and spider venom	? Massive catecholamine release; myocarditis	Hypertension Tachycardia ST-T abnormalities QT prolongation Atrial and ventricular arrhythmias Pulmonary edema Hypotension	Pain at site of envenomation Anxiety Diaphoresis, fasciculations, and/or muscle spasm Abdominal pain and rigidity Paresthesias, convulsions
Ciguatera fish poisoning	Increased membrane sodium permeability	Bradycardia Hypotension	Paresthesias Abdominal pain, nausea, vomiting, diarrhea Respiratory depression
Emetine (syrup of ipecac)	Inhibition of protein synthesis Disrupts oxidative phosphorylation	ST wave abnormalities QT interval prolongation Cardiomyopathy (biventricular cardiac failure) Ventricular arrhythmias	Recurrent vomiting Cachexia Skeletal myopathy
Colchicine	Cellular microtubular toxin	Myocardial injury ST segment abnormalities Hypovolemia Hypotension Pulmonary edema Sudden death	Nausea, vomiting, abdominal pain Respiratory failure Pancytopenia, leukopenia Coagulopathy Myopathy Polyneuropathy
γ-Hydroxybutyrate (GHB)	GABA$_B$ agonism	Bradycardia Hypotension	Coma Myoclonus
Aconite (Chinese herbs—fuzi, chuanwu, cauwu)	Aconatine and related alkaloids block sodium channel	Bradycardia Ventricular tachycardia (may be monomorphic or polymorphic)	Paresthesias Ataxia

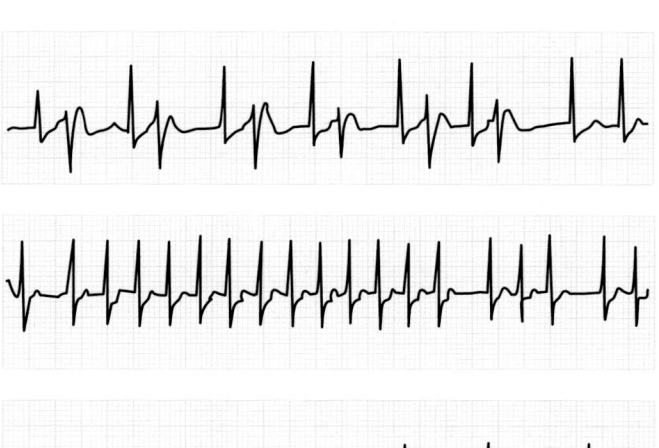

FIGURE 8-19 Three lead II rhythm strips were recorded during a period of several hours in a 30-year-old patient who intentionally ingested 24.8 mg of digoxin. The *top strip* shows atrial fibrillation and R-on-T ventricular bigeminy. The *middle strip* shows a run of atrial tachycardia that terminates spontaneously to sinus rhythm and resumes immediately. The *bottom strip* illustrates high-degree AV block that, because of the morphology of the QRS complexes, is considered to be originating in the AV node or the His bundle. Because all these rhythms occurred and recurred within short periods, treatment was difficult and consisted of only transvenous cardiac pacing for bradyarrhythmias. All bradyarrhythmias disappeared by 22 hours, and all arrhythmias by 1 week.

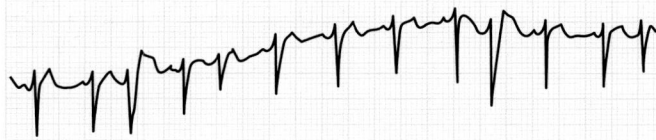

FIGURE 8-20 The patient is a 69-year-old man who was admitted to the hospital with acute congestive heart failure 7 weeks after having suffered an anterior wall myocardial infarction. This MCL$_1$ rhythm strip was recorded after administration of 1.5 mg of intravenous digoxin during an 18-hour period. The atrial rate is somewhat irregular at about 150 beats per minute. Periods of AV nodal Wenckebach's block are present, with the second QRS complex of the period conducted aberrantly. Episodes of 2:1 AV block also are present. The serum digoxin level at this time was 4 ng/mL. The rhythm was restored to sinus after withdrawal of digoxin.

heart block or when bradyarrhythmias result in hemodynamic compromise. Correction of hyperkalemia may in itself reverse AV block.

Ingestion of plant-derived cardiac glycosides (oleander leaves, foxglove, lily of the valley, ouabain) or toad venom (bufotoxin) also can cause digitalis-like poisoning. Toad venom sold as an aphrodisiac ("Love Stone," "Rock Hard") and Chinese herbal medications (Chan Su, kyushin) have been banned in the United States by the Food and Drug Administration (FDA). Anecdotal reports suggest that poisonings from naturally occurring cardiac glycosides may respond to digoxin-specific Fab fragments.[45]

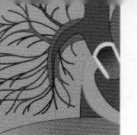

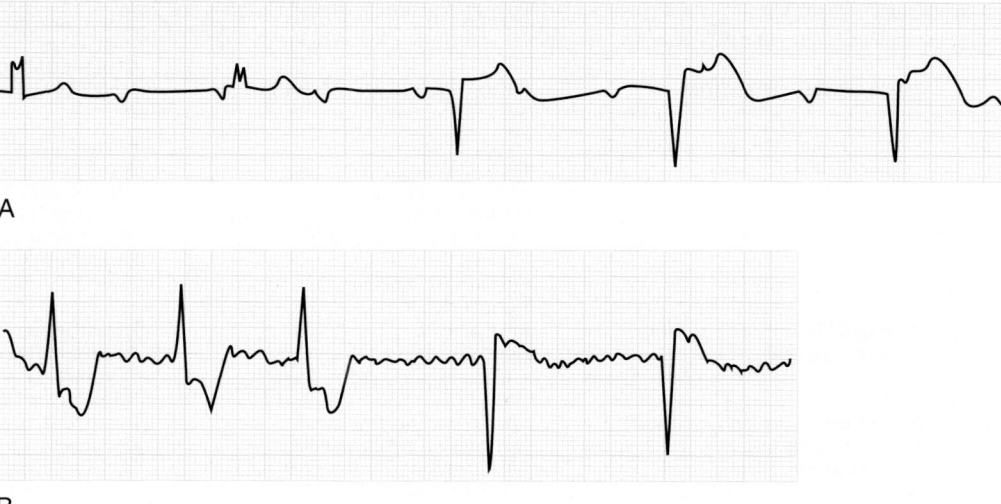

FIGURE 8-21 These two MCL₁ rhythm strips depict examples of AV block in the setting of digitalis toxicity. **A,** Sinus rhythm and complete AV block are present. The QRS complexes are of two types: The first two have a right bundle branch block pattern, and the last three have a left bundle branch block pattern; they occur at two different rates. The long duration of the QRS complexes as well as their very slow rate suggests that the origin of these escape beats is in the distal His-Purkinje system. In this situation, atropine may not result in improved AV conduction, and temporary cardiac pacing often is required. **B,** The atrial rhythm is fibrillation. High-grade AV block is present, as evidenced by the slow ventricular response. The QRS complexes have two morphologies: right and left bundle branch block patterns. The first three complexes occur at a nearly regular rate, suggesting a ventricular escape focus. The last two complexes occur at a slower escape interval and rate, suggesting instability of the origin of the first three complexes and emergence of a yet more distal pacemaker. Again, atropine may not be of benefit in this situation, and cardiac pacing may be required.

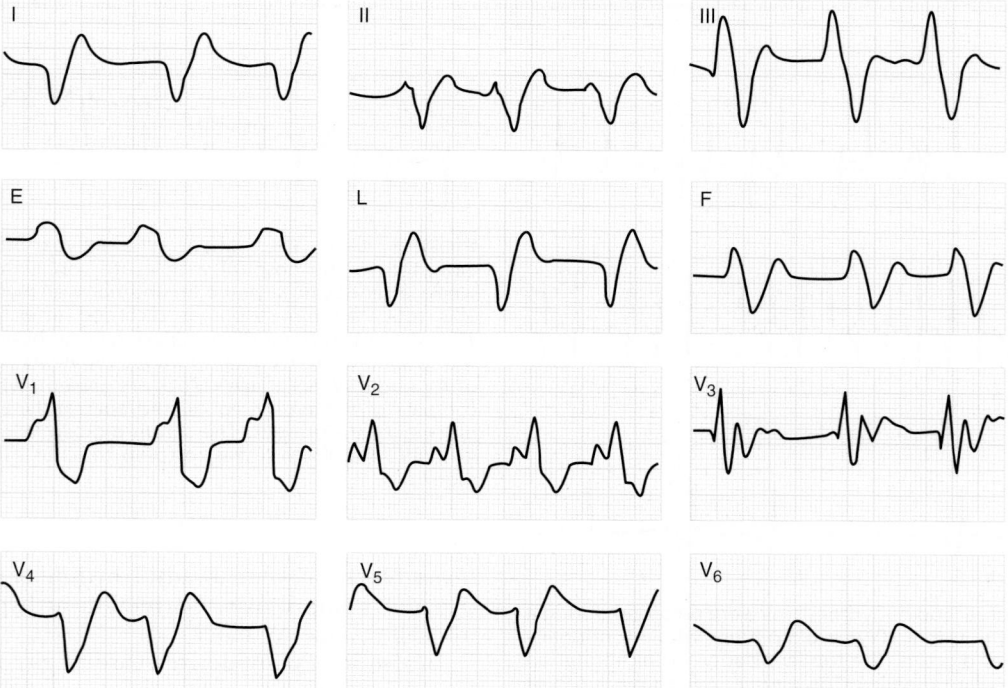

FIGURE 8-22 The patient was a 68-year-old man who was admitted to the hospital in moribund condition. He had long-standing congestive heart failure and was being treated with oral digoxin and diuretics. His serum potassium level on admission was 10.0 mEq/L, and his serum digoxin level was 5.2 ng/mL. He died shortly after this 12-lead electrocardiogram was obtained, with electromechanical dissociation. The electrocardiogram shows absence of discernible atrial activity and an irregular, wide complex QRS rhythm having a right bundle branch block configuration. The markedly increased QRS duration suggests hyperkalemia, which in this patient may have been due in part to digitalis toxicity.

OPIATES

Although toxicity from acute opiate overdose is related primarily to respiratory depression, opiates may have significant cardiac and vascular effects. They generally have little effect on the myocardium, although norpropoxyphene, a major metabolite of propoxyphene, may be cardiotoxic. CNS effects of narcotics result in increased vagal activity. Narcotics dilate peripheral veins and arterioles, presumably through a CNS-mediated effect on sympathetic tone. Consequently, hypotension and relative bradycardia are common. Arrhythmias occur occasionally, most commonly atrial fibrillation. Quinidine and procaine, as well as other local anesthetics, commonly adulterate heroin sold on the street and may themselves contribute to myocardial depression or even cardiac arrest.

Noncardiogenic pulmonary edema is a common and serious complication of narcotic overdose. Although pulmonary edema usually occurs after injection of narcotics, it may not become evident until naloxone has been administered. Sudden reversal of narcotic-induced venodilation and venous pooling combined with pulmonary capillary injury causing fluid to enter the lungs at relatively low cardiac filling pressures most likely accounts for naloxone-induced pulmonary edema.

Therapy for opiate overdose in general includes administration of naloxone and supportive care. No specific therapy for arrhythmias usually is necessary. Naloxone may convert coarse atrial fibrillation to fine atrial fibrillation with a faster ventricular response rate rather than to normal sinus rhythm. If atrial fibrillation persists, the use of verapamil, diltiazem, or metoprolol is indicated to slow the rate. Intermittent positive expiratory pressure is beneficial in the treatment of pulmonary edema, as discussed previously.[46]

LITHIUM

Cardiac toxicity of lithium overdose usually is not prominent. Administration of lithium in usual therapeutic doses produces flattening or inversion of the T wave in nearly all patients. Sinus node disturbances, manifested by sinus bradycardia or sinoatrial block, sometimes associated with ventricular ectopy, and junctional or ventricular escape rhythms have been reported in patients with lithium intoxication and during long-term therapy.[47] Ventricular tachyarrhythmias in association with lithium therapy have been reported but are uncommon. Hypotension may complicate lithium overdose, but this appears to be related to dehydration or pulmonary complications in the course of prolonged coma rather than caused by direct cardiovascular toxicity. A mechanism for the cardiac effects of lithium has been suggested by animal studies. Lithium enters myocardial cells and displaces intracellular cations, predominantly potassium. Lithium then leaves the cell more slowly than does potassium and thereby disturbs the usual transmembrane ionic currents.

Treatment is directed toward the specific arrhythmia, as described in Table 8-1, and toward acceleration of lithium elimination, as discussed in Chapter 30.

ERGOT AND TRIPTAN DERIVATIVES

Ergotamine and other ergot derivatives are used widely in the treatment of migraine headache and have resulted in significant cardiac and vascular toxicity. The basic action of ergot drugs is constriction of vascular smooth muscle (both α-adrenergic agonist and nonadrenergic effects), although many of the drugs also have α-adrenergic receptor-blocking activity. Intense constriction of peripheral arteries, with resultant coolness, pallor, or cyanosis of the extremity, sometimes progressing to gangrene, is a typical manifestation of ergotism. Intermittent claudication occurs initially, and then ischemic rest pain develops with progression of vasospasm. In addition, ergot derivatives have been reported to worsen angina or cause myocardial infarction, presumably owing to coronary vasoconstriction, particularly but not exclusively in persons with underlying coronary artery disease.[48] Intravenous administration of ergonovine was used diagnostically at one time during cardiac catheterization to provoke coronary vasospasm, but it is no longer used due to deaths related to refractory coronary spasm. We treated a patient who took excessive quantities of ergotamine tablets for severe migraine headaches; the patient had chest pain and diffuse, reversible ST segment elevation indicating coronary vasospasm (Fig. 8-23).

Amphetamine-like drugs also can produce vascular spasm similar to that produced by ergot derivatives. In particular, 4-bromo-2,5-dimethoxyamphetamine injection has produced severe vascular insufficiency and in one case led to a bilateral lower extremity amputation.

Therapy for ergot-induced vasospasm includes anticoagulation with heparin, the use of direct vasodilators such as sodium nitroprusside for peripheral vasospasm, nitroglycerin for coronary vasospasm, and α-adrenergic blockers. Rapid dilation of vessels in an intensely vasoconstricted patient results in relative hypovolemia and hypotension; thus, fluid replacement must be anticipated. If a specific vessel is affected, vasodilators should be infused intra-arterially into that vessel to allow maximal local vasodilation to be achieved without effecting excessive systemic hypotension. Nifedipine or other CCBs may prove useful also in treating ergot-induced coronary vasospasm. Other treatments with varying results have included anticoagulants, epidural anesthesia, low-molecular-weight dextran, hyperbaric oxygen, and surgical sympathectomy.

The triptans (5-hydroxytryptamine [5-HT] agonists) have eclipsed the use of other abortive migraine agents. Their therapeutic action is believed to result from constriction of extracerebral blood vessels and reduction of neurogenic inflammation. Serotonin receptors are abundant in the coronary arteries and, when stimulated, may cause vasoconstriction. Serious adverse cardiac events, such as myocardial infarction, have been described during therapeutic use of these agents. Despite their widespread use, complications associated with the triptans are rare and can be further minimized by careful selection of patients who have symptoms or risk factors suggestive of cardiovascular disease.[49] Treatment of toxicity mainly is supportive with specific

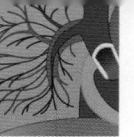

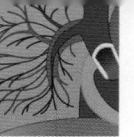

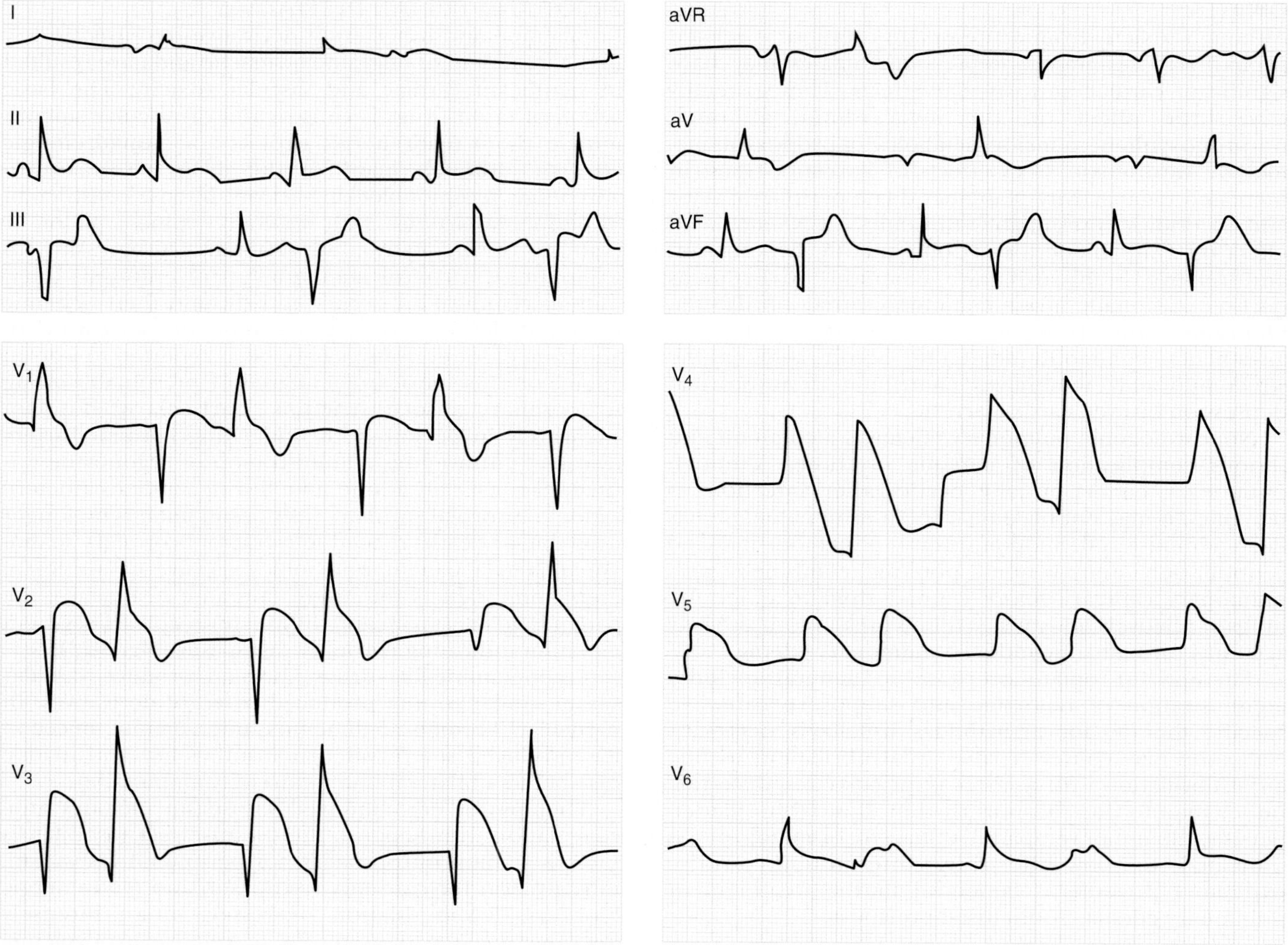

FIGURE 8-23 The patient is a 50-year-old man who was taking ergotamine for cluster headaches. When the headaches worsened, he ingested up to 10 mg/hr, developed severe substernal chest pain, and had an episode of syncope. This 12-lead electrocardiogram was recorded on admission to the coronary care unit. The rhythm is sinus with ventricular bigeminy; diffuse ST segment elevation is present, consistent with coronary artery spasm. After large oral and intravenous doses of nitrates, chest pain and ST segment elevation resolved, but recurrent episodes of pain were associated with return of ST elevation, ventricular ectopy, and bursts of ventricular tachycardia. Myocardial infarction was not documented. Selective coronary arteriography documented coronary spasm during a spontaneous attack of chest pain. Pain and ST segment elevation resolved over 2 weeks coincidentally with oral nifedipine therapy.

cardiac treatment being dependent on the presence of ECG or cardiac enzyme abnormalities.

CHEMICAL ASPHYXIANTS

Carbon monoxide, hydrogen sulfide, and cyanide inhibit oxygen transport to tissues or use of oxygen within tissues, resulting in tissue hypoxia. The usual presentation in severe cases of poisoning is coma or metabolic acidosis or both. Tachypnea (with evidence of respiratory alkalosis), tachycardia, and hypotension are common, although carbon monoxide poisoning in particular can be associated with hypertension. ECG changes, including T wave flattening or inversion, ST segment depression or elevation, and conduction disturbances, frequently are observed, and myocardial necrosis or infarction may occur. Premature ventricular contractions and atrial

fibrillation are noted occasionally. ECG abnormalities may be a misleading index of the severity of carbon monoxide poisoning, however, because ST-T abnormalities and arrhythmias are nonspecific and may not reflect the magnitude of impairment of the myocardium. Echocardiography is a useful adjunct in assessment of carbon monoxide–induced cardiac damage, especially in comatose patients or those with underlying cardiopulmonary disease.[50] ECG or echocardiographic abnormalities after carbon monoxide poisoning may persist for days or even weeks after treatment, possibly as a result of focal myocardial injury.[51]

Pulmonary edema may complicate acute carbon monoxide poisoning, and noncardiogenic versus cardiogenic edema resulting from myocardial damage must be differentiated. Even mild exposure to carbon monoxide

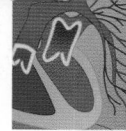

can have significant effects in persons with underlying vascular disease. With carboxyhemoglobin concentrations as low as 3%, the duration of exercise to the onset of chest pain in persons with angina pectoris, or leg pain in persons with intermittent claudication, is significantly reduced. Therapy is directed toward improving tissue oxygenation, as described in Chapter 87.

ARSENIC AND OTHER METALS

Acute arsenic poisoning, by interfering with cellular respiration, may produce an ECG picture of myocardial ischemia and may be associated with focal myocardial hemorrhage, although patients who recover have no cardiac symptoms. Acute and chronic arsenic poisoning can be associated with T wave changes and QT prolongation and with ventricular tachycardia and fibrillation. Arsenic-induced torsades de pointes VT has been reported.[52]

Arsine gas, by causing massive hemolysis and severe anemia, also results in ECG abnormalities, most commonly peaked T waves (possibly related to hyperkalemia), but myocardial ischemia (due to severe anemia and possibly myocardial effects of arsine) also is evident. Death due to arsine exposure in patients who reach the hospital often is secondary to cardiac failure; pathology shows myocardial degeneration. Treatment should include correction of hyperkalemia, transfusion, and therapy of cardiac failure.

Elemental phosphorus and organic mercury poisonings have been associated with ST-T wave abnormalities, QT prolongation, and various arrhythmias (including ventricular tachycardia). After elemental phosphorus ingestion, shock resulting from depressed myocardial contractility and abnormally low systemic vascular resistance occurs and often is difficult to treat. Death in the early phase of phosphorus poisoning is due to shock, ventricular fibrillation, or asystole.

Although uncommon, chronic lead poisoning may be associated with myocarditis characterized by chest pain (angina pectoris saturnina), sinus tachycardia, ventricular gallop, pulmonary congestion, hypertension, ST-T abnormalities, and premature ventricular contractions on the ECG. Autopsy of children dying of lead encephalopathy has shown chronic myocarditis. Clinical features usually subside after treatment with chelating agents.

Acute severe iron (and other heavy metal) poisoning causes shock owing to vasodilation and hypovolemia, the latter resulting from vascular damage and fluid loss. Myocardial injury and dysfunction may also contribute. ECG abnormalities, including T wave inversion, may be present.

SCORPIONS, SPIDERS, AND HYMENOPTERA

Patients with poisonous scorpion stings typically show anxiety, profuse diaphoresis, and hypertension. Myocarditis, characterized by sinus tachycardia, conduction abnormalities, and ST-T abnormalities, including tall peaked T waves, QT prolongation, and atrial and ventricular arrhythmias, may be evident. In severe poisoning, pulmonary edema, hypotension, and ECG changes suggesting myocardial infarction occur. Death is due to congestive heart failure or shock or both; sudden

deaths presumably due to arrhythmias also are reported.[53] The clinical and myocardial histologic manifestations of scorpion sting resemble those of massive catecholamine infusion, and urinary catecholamine excretion has been noted to be increased in scorpion sting victims. Although there is little published experience in this regard, the use of α- and β-adrenergic blocking drugs for treatment of hypertension and arrhythmias is logical. Treatment of cardiac failure and shock is supportive.

Labile blood pressure, atrial arrhythmias, and cardiovascular collapse occasionally are observed in patients after black widow spider bites. Increased urinary catecholamine metabolite excretion also has suggested a role of excess catecholamines in this syndrome, and adrenergic blockers may be useful in management.

Hymenoptera (bees and wasps) stings are well known to cause anaphylaxis, manifested by hypotension, cyanosis, bronchospasm, and collapse in allergic patients. Chest pain and myocardial infarction, probably resulting from profound hypotension, occasionally occur as well.[54]

GAMMA-HYDROXY BUTYRIC ACID

γ-Hydroxybutyric acid (GHB) is a naturally occurring analog of γ-aminobutyric acid (GABA), which has FDA approval for treatment of narcolepsy. GHB also has been abused as a nutritional supplement for bodybuilding, a drug of abuse for euphoria, a sexual enhancer, and a drug to facilitate sexual assault. In overdose, the typical presentation is profound CNS depression, respiratory depression, sinus bradycardia, and, occasionally, hypotension. ECG abnormalities other than sinus bradycardia, such as conduction disturbances, are not typical of GHB intoxication and should prompt investigation for the presence of other cardiotoxic substances. Treatment usually is supportive with attention to airway protection. Sinus bradycardia is responsive to atropine, if necessary, and hypotension responds to intravenous fluids. GHB-induced hypotension generally does not require pressors.[55]

Withdrawal syndromes after chronic GHB use can occur after frequent use within 6 hours of the last dose. The withdrawal syndrome is characterized by nausea, vomiting, anxiety, and tremor, initially followed by autonomic instability and severe delirium. Treatment is supportive; benzodiazepines, usually in high doses, have been effective. Barbiturates and propofol have been used in refractory cases.[56]

SOME OTHER NATURAL PRODUCTS

Many natural products have cardiovascular effects, and a comprehensive review of these is beyond the scope of this chapter. Three toxins have become of particular interest to poison centers and are mentioned briefly.

Ciguatera fish poisoning, caused by ingestion of fish contaminated with ciguatera toxins, produces cardiovascular toxicity as well as gastrointestinal and neurologic symptoms. Patients often experience bradycardia and hypotension, which may be quite severe. Detailed autonomic studies of one such patient revealed that the bradycardia and hypotension were due to both excessive

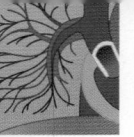
vagal tone and depression of sympathetic nervous responses.[57,58] Hypotension usually responds to volume expansion and anticholinergic drug therapy.

Scombroid fish poisoning occurs after ingestion of fish that contains high levels of histamine and possibly other bioactive amines. Histamine is produced in the fish when bacteria metabolize the amino acid histidine. This elevated histamine level causes a syndrome of flushing, urticaria, diaphoresis, palpitations, gastrointestinal distress, and headache. There have been case reports of hypotension and bradycardia associated with scombroid toxicity, although these are rare manifestations. Treatment is supportive with use of antihistamines and corticosteroids, when indicated. Hypotension refractory to intravenous fluids may respond to epinephrine.[59]

Aconite poisoning can occur after ingestion of Chinese herbs or teas that contain *Aconitum carmichaelii* or *Aconitum kusnezoffii*. The herbal preparations that contain these herbs include fuzi, chuanwu, and cauwu. If these herbs are not boiled for an adequate time, the alkaloids aconitine, mesaconitine, and others, which are extremely potent toxins, may be ingested. Cardiovascular manifestations include shock with bradycardia or ventricular tachycardia (either monomorphic or polymorphic) or ventricular fibrillation.[60] Several fatalities have been reported. Amiodarone and flecainide have been suggested as first-line antiarrhythmic agents for ventricular tachycardia due to aconite poisoning.

REFERENCES

1. Kellum JA, Pinsky MR: Use of vasopressor agents in critically ill patients. Curr Opin Crit Care 2002;8:236–241.
2. European Resuscitation Council: Part 8: advanced challenges in resuscitation. Section 2: toxicology in ECC. Resuscitation 2000;46:261–266.
3. Landry DW, Oliver JA: The pathogenesis of vasodilatory shock. N Engl J Med 2001;345:588–595.
4. Shubin H, Weil MH: The mechanism of shock following suicidal doses of barbiturate, narcotics and tranquilizing drugs, with observations on the effects of treatment. Am J Med 1965;38:853.
5. Viskin S, Justo D, Halkin A, Zeltser D: Long QT syndrome caused by noncardiac drugs. Prog Cardiovasc Dis 2003;45:415–427.
6. Perina DG: Noncardiogenic pulmonary edema. Emerg Med Clin North Am 2003;21:385–393.
7. Shubin H, Weil MH: Shock associated with barbiturate intoxication. JAMA 1971;215:263.
8. Hahn IH, Hoffman RS: Cocaine use and acute myocardial infarction. Emerg Med Clin North Am 2001;19:493–509.
9. Vasica G, Tennant CC: Cocaine use and cardiovascular complications. Med J Aust 2002;177:260–262.
10. Lange RA, Hillis LD: Cardiovascular complications of cocaine use. N Engl J Med 2001;345:351–358.
11. Shanti CM, Lucas CE: Cocaine and the critical care challenge. Crit Care Med 2003;31:1851–1859.
12. Kernan WN, Viscoli CM, Brass LM, et al: Phenylpropanolamine and the risk of hemorrhagic stroke. N Engl J Med 2000; 343:1826–1832.
13. Frishman W, et al: Cardiovascular manifestations of substance abuse: part 2: alcohol, amphetamines, heroin, cannabis, and caffeine. Heart 2003;5:253–271.
14. Haller CA, Benowitz NL: Adverse cardiovascular events and central nervous system events associated with dietary supplements containing ephedra alkaloids. N Engl J Med 2000;343:1833–1838.
15. Livingston MG, Livingston HM: Monoamine oxidase inhibitors: an update on drug interactions. Drug Saf 1996;14:219–227.
16. Jacob JE, Wagner ML, Sage JI: Safety of selegiline with cold medications. Ann Pharmacother 2003;37:438–441.
17. Birmes P, Coppin D, Schmitt L, Lauque D: Serotonin syndrome: a brief review. CMAJ 2003;168:1439–1442.
18. Minton NA, Henry JA: Treatment of theophylline toxicity. Am J Emerg Med 1996;14:606–612.
19. Cooling DS: Theophylline toxicity. J Emerg Med 1993;11:415–426.
20. Jones RT: Cardiovascular system effects of marijuana. J Clin Pharm 2002;42:58S–63S.
21. Lorenc JD: Inhalant abuse in the pediatric population: a persistent challenge. Curr Opin Ped 2003;15:204–209.
22. Williams DR, Cole SJ: Ventricular fibrillation following butane gas inhalation. Resuscitation 1998;37:43–45.
23. Baskerville JR, Tichenor GA, Rosen PB: Toluene-induced hypokalemia: case report and literature review. Emerg Med J 2001;18:514–516.
24. Love JN, Enlow B, Howell JM, et al: Electrocardiographic changes associated with beta blocker toxicity. Ann Emerg Med 2002;40:603–610.
25. Love JN, Howell JM, Litovitz TL, et al: Acute beta blocker overdose: factors associated with the development of cardiovascular morbidity. J Toxicol Clin Toxicol 2000;38:275–281.
26. Bailey B: Glucagon in blocker and calcium channel blocker overdoses: a systematic review. J Toxicol Clin Toxicol 2003;41:595–602.
27. Brimacombe JR, Scully M, Swainston R: Propranolol overdose—a dramatic response to calcium chloride. Med J Aust 1991;155:267.
28. Musshof F, Gerschlauer A, Madea B: Naphazoline intoxication in a child—a clinical and forensic toxicological case. Forensic Sci Int 2003;134:234–237.
29. Eddy O, Howell JM: Are one or two dangerous? Clonidine and topical imidazolines exposure in toddlers. J Emerg Med 2003;25:297–302.
30. Burns MJ, Linden CH, Graudins A, et al: A comparison of physostigmine and benzodiazepines for treatment of anticholinergic poisoning. Ann Emerg Med 2000;35:374–381.
31. Kwong TC: Organophosphate pesticides: biochemistry and clinical toxicology. Ther Drug Mon 2002;24:144–149.
32. Choi PT, Quinonez LG, Cook DJ, et al: The use of glycopyrrolate in a case of intermediate syndrome following acute organophosphate poisoning. Can J Anesth 1998;45:337–340.
33. Shepherd G, Klein-Schwartz W, Edwards R: Donepezil overdose: a tenfold dosing error. Ann Pharmacother 1999;33:812–815.
34. Caron J, Libersa C: Adverse effects of class I antiarrhythmic drugs. Drug Saf 1997;17:8–36.
35. Benowitz NL: Antiarrhythmics. In Descotes J (ed): Human Toxicology. Amsterdam, Elsevier, 1996.
36. Salhanick SD, Shannon MW: Management of calcium channel antagonist overdose. Drug Saf 2003;26:65–79.
37. Yuan TH, Kerns WP, Tomaszewski CA, et al: Insulin-glucose as adjunctive therapy for severe calcium channel antagonist poisoning. J Toxicol Clin Toxicol 1999;37:463–474.
38. Harrigan RA, Brady WJ: ECG abnormalities in tricyclic anti-depressant ingestion. Am J Emerg Med 1999;17:387–393.
39. Singh N, Singh HK, Khan IA: Serial electrocardiographic changes as a predictor of cardiovascular toxicity in acute tricyclic antidepressant overdose. Am J Ther 2002;9:75–79.
40. Shannon M, Liebelt EA: Toxicology reviews: targeted management strategies for cardiovascular toxicity from tricyclic antidepressant overdose: the pivotal role for alkalinization and sodium loading. Ped Emerg Care 1998;14:293–298.
41. Burns MJ: The pharmacology and toxicology of atypical antipsychotic agents. J Toxicol Clin Toxicol 2001;39:1–14.
42. Zeltser D, Justo D, Halkin A, et al: Torsades de pointes due to noncardiac drugs; most patients have easily identifiable risk factors. Medicine 2003;82:282–290.
43. Hauptman PJ, Kelly RA: Digitalis. Circulation 1999;99:1265–1270.
44. Ma G, Brady WJ, Pollack M, Chan TC: Electrocardiographic manifestations: digitalis toxicity. J Emerg Med 2001;20:145–152.
45. Gowda RM, Cohen RA, Khan IA: Toad venom poisoning: resemblance to digoxin toxicity and therapeutic implications. Heart 2003;89:e14.
46. Sporer KA: Acute heroin overdose. Ann Intern Med 1999;130:584–590.
47. Moltedo JM, Porter GA, State MW, Snyder CS: Sinus node dysfunction associated with lithium therapy in a child. Tex Heart Inst J 2002;29:300–202.

48. Galer BS, Lipton RB, Solomon S, et al: Myocardial ischemia related to ergot alkaloids: a case report and review of the literature. Headache 1991;31:446–450.

49. Nappi G, Sandrini G, Sances G: Tolerability of the triptans: clinical implications. Drug Saf 2003;26;93–107.

50. Corya BC, Black MJ, McHenry PL: Echocardiographic findings after acute carbon monoxide poisoning. Br Heart J 1976;38:712.

51. Gandini C, Castoldi AF, Candura SM, et al: Carbon monoxide cardiotoxicity. J Toxicol Clin Toxicol 2001;39:15–44.

52. Unnikrishan D, Dutcher JR, Varshneya N, et al: Torsades de pointes in 3 patients with leukemia treated with arsenic trioxide. Blood 2001;97:1514–1516.

53. Kumar EB, Soomro RS, al Hamdani A, el Shimy N: Scorpion venom cardiomyopathy. Am Heart J 1992;123:725–729.

54. Gueron M, Illa R, Margulis G: Arthropod poisons and the cardiovascular system. Am J Emerg Med 2000;18:708–714.

55. Mason PE, Kerns WP II: Gamma-hydroxybutyric acid intoxication. Acad Emerg Med 2002;9:730–739.

56. Dyer JE, Roth B, Hyma BA: Gamma-hydroxybutyrate withdrawal syndrome. Ann Emerg Med 2001;37:147–153.

57. Geller RJ, Benowitz NL: Orthostatic hypotension in ciguatera fish poisoning. Arch Intern Med 1992;152:2131.

58. Mines D, Stahmer S, Shepherd SM: Poisonings; food fish, shellfish. Emerg Med Clin North Am 1997;15:157–177.

59. Hall M: Something fishy: six patients with an unusual cause of food poisoning! Emerg Med (Fremantle) 2003;15;293–295.

60. Tai YT, But PP, Young K, et al: Cardiotoxicity after accidental herb-induced aconite poisoning. Lancet 1992;340:1254.

9
Pulmonary Toxicology

MICHAEL G. HOLLAND, MD

Acute care toxicology usually involves management of ingested toxicants. However, health care providers in occupational medicine rarely encounter toxic ingestions and are most concerned with inhalational or dermal exposures. This chapter organizes and gives a basic introduction to the toxicology of pulmonary exposures and the response of the pulmonary system to these toxicants, as well as discusses pulmonary manifestations of systemic adverse drug reactions and toxicants.

Any discussion of pulmonary toxicology would be incomplete without covering the worst industrial catastrophe in history: the Bhopal disaster. On December 4, 1984, the Union Carbide plant in Bhopal, India, released 80,000 pounds (40 tons) of methyl isocyanate (MIC). MIC is a very hygroscopic compound that is known to be quite reactive: Pressure and heat build up rapidly when it is mixed with water. MIC was used at this plant as a chemical intermediate in the production of carbamate pesticides. Somehow, water entered the vessel that contained the compound. Hours later, when the pressure within the storage tank exceeded the relief valve, the MIC vapor escaped. When the MIC was released into the ambient air, thousands of people close to the plant were immediately exposed to very high concentrations, causing severe injuries, and many victims died in their sleep. As the cloud of this irritant gas spread to the populous city of Bhopal 1 mile away, many thousands more were afflicted, and more than 15,000 people were seen in the hospital that night. Over the next several days, more than 100,000 people sought medical care. The final official death toll at the time was estimated to be greater than 2500; more recently, the deaths attributed to that single accident exceed 6000. Because of the nature of the injuries to the respiratory tract, many of those injured remain disabled today.[1,2]

SCOPE OF THE PROBLEM

Pulmonary exposures are very common. The American Association of Poison Control Centers (AAPCC) data from 2002 reveal that inhalation exposure was involved in 154,167 cases reported to poison centers, or 6.5% of the total number of poison center cases. Inhalation exposure accounted for 103 deaths or 8.9% of the total number of fatalities. The majority of these deaths were due to carbon monoxide exposure. The AAPCC data also reveal that occupational or environmental exposures accounted for a total of 42 deaths or 3.6% of the total cases reported. Most of these were from inhalation exposure.[3]

Many toxic gases are produced by small specialty industries, and many of these workplaces may not have a safety officer or an industrial hygiene department that ensures worker safety. Historically, workers in these situations have been at increased risk of having significant exposures to toxic gases and vapors, because air monitoring or engineering controls are expensive and time-consuming. With the passage of the Occupational Safety and Health Act in 1972, this situation has improved in the United States, but it remains a significant problem in less regulated, developing nations. However, a significant portion of American workers have the potential exposure to respiratory irritants. For instance, the number one chemical produced in the United States is sulfuric acid, mists or vapors of which are highly irritating to the pulmonary system. Many of the top 50 chemicals produced in the United States are toxic or irritant gases. The National Institute for Occupational Safety and Health (NIOSH) estimates that over 500,000 U.S. workers have the potential to be exposed to anhydrous ammonia alone.[4]

Firefighters and first responders may be exposed to numerous hazards, since structural fires produce many toxic gases, such as hydrogen cyanide (HCN), carbon monoxide (CO), hydrogen chloride (HCl), acrolein, sulfur dioxide (SO_2), and phosgene. The latest AAPCC data suggest that toxic gas exposure is responsible for 4.9% of workplace deaths in the United States. Of these, the major lethal gas is the colorless and odorless carbon monoxide.

When the Aum Shinrikyo cult released sarin vapors in a Tokyo subway in 1995, the world became acutely aware of the possibility of military nerve agents being used in civilian arenas. With the terrorist attacks of September 11, 2001, Americans finally became cognizant of the fact that no country is immune to terrorist acts. However, people have been using gaseous warfare agents against their enemies for centuries. For example, a mixture of pitch and sulfur was burned and the smoke used as a gas warfare agent in the war between Athens and Sparta in 428 BC. World War I was the first large-scale conflict that saw regular use of chemical warfare agents, most notably mustard gas, chlorine, and phosgene. Phosgene alone was responsible for up to 80% of deaths due to chemical agents during that war. More recently, Iraq used mustard gas against Iranian soldiers in 1988 and various chemical agents against the Kurds in the 1990s.

Most of the danger of ingested toxicants comes from the effects of systemic absorption. However, when a caustic poison such as lye is ingested, the gastrointestinal tract is the site of local toxicity/injury. Conversely, most irritant gases injure the respiratory tract, but numerous toxicants in the gaseous phase can be absorbed rapidly into the systemic circulation via the large alveolar surface area and the rich pulmonary capillary blood supply. In fact, the inhalation route approaches the rapidity of intravenous administration.

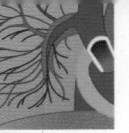

In addition to gaseous or vapor exposures causing lung injury, certain toxicants affect the lung after systemic absorption from another route, the most notable being the dication herbicide paraquat (PQ^{++}). Paraquat is actively transported and concentrated in the lung, where it is reduced by nicotinamide adenine dinucleotide phosphate (NADPH) to a monocation radical, $^{\bullet}$PQ^{+}. This reactive radical rapidly reacts with molecular O$_2$ to form a superoxide radical, $^{\bullet}$O$_2$, which then also regenerates the original PQ^{++}. The cycle can repeat itself, due to the abundant supply of NADPH and molecular oxygen in the lung. The superoxide radicals then cause lipid peroxidation and pneumocyte cell death. This seems to occur more readily when victims are treated with high fractions of inspired oxygen (FIO$_2$). The pulmonary injury is then followed by a proliferative phase leading to pulmonary fibrosis. Antioxidants are being investigated as treatment options.[5]

Numerous therapeutic drugs also can induce interstitial pneumonitis, such as amiodarone, tocainide, flecainide, nitrofurantoin, and hydrochlorothiazide. Cytotoxic chemotherapeutic agents typically can cause interstitial pneumonitis as well as interstitial fibrosis. Angiotensin-converting enzyme inhibitors commonly cause cough as a side effect. Pulmonary edema is well known to occur after opiate overdose, but it also can be seen with salicylates, phenothiazines, butyrophenones, and tricyclic antidepressants. The ergot derivative bromocriptine is associated mainly with pleural effusion, whereas methysergide has been associated with pleural effusion and fibrosis. Asthmatic reactions can be induced by nonsteroidal anti-inflammatory drugs (NSAIDs) and aspirin, as well as by β blockers, calcium antagonists, and dipyridamole. Leukotriene antagonists are linked to the development of Churg-Strauss syndrome, and penicillamine and certain antibiotics can cause bronchiolitis obliterans. Anorectic agents have been linked to the development of primary pulmonary hypertension.[6]

Many toxicants, such as sedative-hypnotics, cyclic antidepressant agents, or opiates, alone or in combination, cause hypoventilation and a subsequent hypoxemia seen on arterial blood gas analysis or via pulse oximetry. If this condition does not improve after administration of appropriate reversal agent, such as naloxone for opiates or flumazenil for benzodiazepines, then intubation is necessary. Any drug or toxicant that causes enough sedation to affect respiratory drive also can cause loss of protective reflexes. Aspiration of gastric contents into the airway can cause an aspiration pneumonitis and subsequent acute respiratory distress syndrome and respiratory failure. Chest radiograph examinations should be performed in all cases in which aspiration is suspected by the history of a patient with a decreased level of consciousness that has vomited. Similarly, when physical examination findings suggest aspiration (rales on auscultation of the chest, or vomitus seen on face or in airway), or when there is an alveolar-arterial (A-a) gradient (oxygenation does not improve after increasing the respiratory rate or by increasing the FIO$_2$), aspiration pneumonitis must be considered and chest radiograph performed. Finally, with ingestion of hydrocarbon (e.g., gasoline, kerosene, mineral seal oil) there is a high incidence of aspiration of the hydrocarbon into the airway owing to its low viscosity, especially when vomiting occurs. Hydrocarbon aspiration causes acute lung injury via depletion of surfactant, which causes alveolar collapse and intrapulmonary shunting. Many of these patients can have minimal findings initially on chest radiograph, but they may be very symptomatic with respiratory distress with coughing and wheezing. Subsequent chest radiograph examinations can show an ARDS-type pattern. Please see Chapters 33, 34, and 93 for a detailed discussion of these toxicants.

PULMONARY ANATOMY AND PHYSIOLOGY

The lung, like the skin, is an organ that consists of a very large epithelial surface that is continuously exposed to the outside world. Unlike the skin, the lung cannot make use of multiple layers of relatively impermeable cells as a barrier, because the gas exchange function of the lung requires thin gas-permeable cell membranes between the alveolar air and the blood. Instead, the lung uses specialized mucus secretions produced by the airway goblet cells to trap and remove inhaled environmental toxicants and debris.[7]

The pulmonary system can be divided into the upper airway, the lower airway, and the lung parenchyma. The glottis is the dividing point separating the upper airway and lower airway. The lung parenchyma functional gas exchange unit, or acinus, begins at the respiratory bronchiole. The upper airway surface anatomy includes the nasal mucosa, the tongue and oral mucosa, and naso- and oropharynx. Because of similar exposures to ambient airborne gases and toxicants, the ocular mucosa is closely linked with the upper airway. The surface area of the upper airway is small, measuring a few hundred square centimeters of total area. However, because of the multiple divisions of the alveoli, the total surface area of the lower airways and lung parenchyma is huge, measuring over 70 square meters, approximately the size of a tennis court.

The cartilaginous lower airway, which consists of the trachea and the bronchi and their subdivisions, are lined with ciliated epithelial cells and goblet cells. These ciliated cells sweep the respiratory mucus (produced by goblet cells) upward, where particulates that are trapped in this mucus can be coughed out or swallowed. This upward removal system is known as the *mucociliary escalator*. Alveolar macrophages that have phagocytosed inhaled antigens and debris are removed by this system as well. The lower airways distal to the terminal bronchioles lack cartilaginous support. The acinus, or terminal respiratory unit, consists of the respiratory bronchiole, the alveolar duct, and the alveolus; this is where gas exchange takes place.

There are numerous important cell types in the lung parenchyma: alveolar epithelial cells (types I and II), interstitial cells, capillary endothelial cells, alveolar

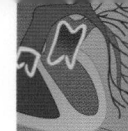

macrophages, and Clara cells. Type 1 alveolar epithelial cells account for 90% of the total alveolar surface area and are the chief structural cells of the alveolar wall. These type I cells maintain the alveolar-blood barrier and are responsible for gas exchange. They are thin and flat, with a paucity of intracellular organelles. This structure facilitates gas exchange, but it renders them quite fragile and very susceptible to injury when exposed to inhaled toxicants or irritant gases. Type II alveolar epithelial cells are cuboidal cells that cover the remaining 10% of the alveolar surface. They are responsible for manufacturing pulmonary surfactant. Surfactant is composed of phospholipid bound to lecithin, and it maintains inflation of the alveolus by reducing surface tension, which stabilizes the alveolus, thereby increasing lung compliance, and reduces the work of breathing. Type II cells also are able to differentiate into type I cells to replace those fragile cells that are damaged from inhaled or systemic toxicants.[8]

Capillary endothelial cells are the most abundant parenchymal lung cells, accounting for almost one third of the cell population. They are the interface between the vascular space and the lung interstitium. They can be damaged by both inhaled irritants and systemic toxicants. When endothelial cells are injured, the resultant capillary leakage of fluid into the interstitium, and subsequently the alveolus, can cause decreased compliance, decreased diffusing capacity, and even noncardiogenic pulmonary edema.

Interstitial cells, which account for more than one third of the lung cells, are located in the area between the alveolar epithelium and the vascular endothelium. These include fibroblasts, mast cells, macrophages, and plasma cells; they perform various functions including immune response and injury repair. Exaggerated fibroblast stimulation after acute lung injury can lead to pulmonary fibrosis.

Alveolar macrophages are the first line of defense against inhaled organisms, foreign antigens, or particles that reach the alveoli. They phagocytose foreign material, and then migrate to the mucous layer to be expelled via the mucociliary escalator. They also can move into the interstitial space and gain access to the pulmonary lymphatic system. There they can release cytokines that direct further immune responses and cell recruitment. This cytokine response has implications in various pulmonary disease processes such as asthma, hypersensitivity pneumonitis, silicosis, and asbestosis.

Clara cells, which are nonciliated bronchiolar cells, contain P-450 enzymes and perform most of the metabolic activity of the lungs. Clara cells can differentiate into goblet cells, which secrete mucus, and they also can differentiate into ciliated cells to replace those lost to injury.

Because the respiratory system is directly exposed to the external environment, the lungs contain more lymphatics than does any other organ. This rich lymphatic system is responsible for manufacturing antibodies against inhaled foreign antigens, as well as initiating cell-mediated immune responses. The pulmonary lymphatic response to injury or antigenic exposures also includes release of cytokines. Cytokines are small proteins having a molecular weight of less than 30 kD that act as chemical messengers between cells and are known to play a pivotal role in the inflammatory cascade. This has implications in the development of occupational lung diseases such as asthma, hypersensitivity pneumonitis, and organic dust toxic syndrome.

PARTICLE DEPOSITION

The pulmonary tree is assaulted constantly by particulates in the air. Whether these particulates deposit on the airway walls, reach the alveoli, or simply remain in the air stream to be exhaled depends on many factors. The factors related to the type of particle include size, electrostatic charge, and aerodynamics (i.e., whether it is a particle or a fiber). Small particles have irregular shapes, but their motion is determined largely by their aerodynamic diameter, which depends on their inertial and gravitational motion in air.

In vitro experimentation reveals that particle deposition in the airways occurs via five mechanisms: impaction, gravitational sedimentation, brownian diffusion, electrostatic deposition, and interception. Impaction occurs primarily at airway bifurcations and is most important for particles having an aerodynamic diameter of more than 1 μm. Gravitational sedimentation occurs primarily in long airway segments. Brownian diffusion affects smaller particles (<0.5 μm). Electrostatic deposition refers to particles with a charge that have been recently generated by mechanical dispersion. Finally, interception in an airway segment occurs primarily with fibers, which are defined as any particle with a length-to-width ratio of more than 3:1.[9]

In vivo, the depth and rate of respiration also affect deposition. Slow, deep respirations favor simple gravitational sedimentation, which distribute the particle more evenly in the pulmonary tree. Conversely, rapid shallow respiration favors impaction of the particles against larger central airways or at bifurcations. All this being equal, the aerodynamic diameter, or size of the particle, influences the primary location of deposition in the pulmonary tree. Larger particles (>10 μm) primarily deposit in the upper airways. Particles between 2.5 and 6 μm deposit in the lower airways, and particles smaller than 2.5 μm deposit primarily in the lung parenchyma (alveolar ducts and alveoli). Very small particles (<0.1 μm) often remain in the air stream and are exhaled.

CONTROL OF RESPIRATIONS

Efficient gas exchange depends on adequate respiratory drive, an intact and patent airway, strong muscles of respiration (diaphragm and chest wall), normal alveolar architecture, and adequate pulmonary capillary blood flow. Abnormalities among any of these components can cause respiratory compromise.

Respiratory drive is controlled by peripheral chemoreceptors located in the carotid body, as well as

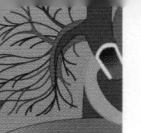

central chemoreceptors located in the brainstem. The peripheral receptors detect hypoxia, whereas the central receptors detect lowered CSF pH due to increases in CO_2. Both respond to these signals by increasing the depth and rate of respiration. Toxicants that cause a decrease in these responses to respiratory drive can induce hypoxemia. Central nervous system depressants, such as barbiturates, can cause respiratory depression by blunting the normal physiologic response to stimulation of these chemorecpetors. Opioids interact at multiple receptor sites in the body. The μ-opioid receptors are responsible for most of the clinical effects seen with available opioids, and agents acting at the μ receptors show little or no selectivity between the two subtypes, designated $μ_1$ and $μ_2$. Stimulation of the $μ_1$-opioid receptor causes analgesia and the pleasurable euphoria sought by abusers. Overstimulation at the $μ_2$-opioid receptor is responsible for the respiratory depression seen in opioid overdoses.

Airway compromise can be caused by ingestion of local irritants, such as caustics or dieffenbachia, or airway swelling induced by allergic angioedema seen in anaphylaxis or the angioedema seen with angiotensin-converting enzyme inhibitors. Chest wall rigidity induced by fentanyl, as well as respiratory muscular weakness caused by organophosphates, carbamates, and botulinum toxin, can cause respiratory failure.

Acute lung injury, formerly known as noncardiogenic pulmonary edema, can be caused by a multitude of inhaled or ingested toxicants (see later). This condition causes pulmonary capillary fluid to leak into the alveolar space, disrupting efficient gas exchange and decreasing the normal pulmonary compliance. Late sequelae of acute lung injury can include bronchiolitis obliterans fibrosa, which permanently impairs gas exchange and causes a restrictive defect. Other pulmonary reactions, such as hypersensitivity pneumonitis and certain pneumoconiosis, can induce permanent pulmonary fibrosis with impairment of gas exchange and restrictive lung disease. Aspiration of gastric contents and subsequent pneumonia/pneumonitis can impair efficient gas exchange by inducing a ventilation-perfusion mismatch, in which blood flows to an area of the lung incapable of gas exchange.

Finally, impairment of pulmonary capillary blood flow can cause ventilation-perfusion mismatch, in which ventilated areas cannot perform gas exchange due to inadequate perfusion. This can occur with any drug causing pulmonary embolus (e.g., estrogen, oral contraceptives), as well as inert substances and debris injected intravenously by drug abusers (e.g., talc, vegetable matter, cotton). Septic emboli can occur in this setting from inadvertent injection of microorganisms.

DEFINITION OF TERMS

Most laypersons and many medical professionals misuse or interchange the terms *gas*, *fume*, and *vapor*. For instance, most complaints of noxious "fumes" in the workplace actually refer to an objectionable odor of the vapors of liquids that are in use at the time. By convention, a *gas* is defined as a substance that normally is in the vapor phase at room temperature, which occupies an enclosed space, and can be changed into a liquid by a decrease in temperature or an increase in pressure. In the strict sense, a *vapor* therefore is the gaseous phase of a substance normally in the liquid state at room temperature but that also can be changed into a liquid by a decrease in temperature or increase in pressure. *Aerosols*, of which there are two types, are dispersions of solid or liquid particles in a gaseous medium (usually air). A *fume* is an aerosol of solid particles generated by heating, usually of metals, and often is accompanied by oxidation of these metals (e.g., zinc oxide fumes form when welding galvanized metals). An aerosol of liquid particles is a *mist* that is generated by mechanical dispersion, whereas a *fog* is a mist generated by condensation. Other airborne contaminants are dusts and smoke. *Dusts* are solid particles generated either by disintegration of organic or inorganic materials, or by mechanical dispersion such as sanding or grinding, and are capable of temporary dispersion in air. *Smoke* usually is a mixture of gases, vapors, and aerosols of solids generated by incomplete combustion.[10]

Acute Lung Injury and Acute Respiratory Distress Syndrome

Acute lung injury (ALI) is the term given to the pathophysiologic presentation of diffuse alveolar injury. It may be a result of inhalational injury or a consequence of systemic disease, such as sepsis or severe hypovolemic shock. This disorder is defined as a syndrome of inflammation and increased pulmonary membrane permeability with multiple manifestations (radiographic, physiologic, clinical) that cannot be explained by cardiogenic pulmonary edema. *Acute respiratory distress syndrome* (ARDS) is the most severe form of ALI and is distinguished by the severity of the oxygenation deficit. Clinically, ALI syndrome is established when criteria in four categories are met:

1. *Timing*: The disorder is acute by definition; therefore, manifestations must occur within a few days of the insult.
2. *Pulmonary physiology*: The pulmonary edema is *non*cardiogenic; therefore, the pulmonary capillary wedge pressure must be less than 18 mm Hg and the edema fluid found in the alveolus and interstitium must be protein-rich, indicating endothelial and epithelial membrane exudates rather than a transudate from congestive heart failure.
3. *Radiography*: Chest radiographs must demonstrate diffuse bilateral infiltrates.
4. *Oxygenation*: Low ratio of partial pressure of arterial oxygen (PaO_2) to FIO_2; in other words, a large A-a gradient must be present. Specifically, ALI is present when PaO_2/FIO_2 is less than 300 mm Hg; ARDS is present when this ratio is less than 200 mm Hg.[11]

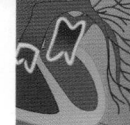

Bronchiolitis Obliterans Fibrosa and Bronchiolitis Obliterans Organizing Pneumonia

Bronchiolitis obliterans fibrosa (BOF), also known as obliterative bronchiolitis, is a response to small airway injury where inflammation and epithelial disruption subsequently are followed by an ingrowth of granulation tissue into the airway lumen, resulting in partial or complete obstruction. The granulation tissue then organizes with resultant fibrosis, which can completely obliterate the airway lumen. BOF occurs as a result of inhalational injury to the small airways after exposure to irritant gases, mineral dusts, toxic metal fumes, or crack cocaine or from paraquat ingestion. BOF also can result from drug-induced pulmonary injury due to a wide variety of therapeutic agents, such as gold salts, sulfasalazine, and amiodarone. It also is seen in chronic rejection after lung transplantation and after certain viral infections (e.g., cytomegalovirus, respiratory syncytial virus). BOF is manifested as an obstructive defect with no response to bronchodilator therapy. Patients often have cough and significant dyspnea. Corticosteroid treatment after acute lung injury due to toxic inhalation can be effective when given acutely in large doses for 1 month. Once fibrosis has occurred, treatment largely is ineffective.[10]

Bronchiolitis obliterans organizing pneumonia (BOOP), also known as proliferative bronchiolitis obliterans, is characterized by an organizing intraluminal exudate. Fibrotic buds known as Masson bodies are seen in respiratory bronchioles, alveolar ducts, and alveoli. Foamy alveolar macrophages are present in alveolar spaces and inflammatory changes are seen in alveolar walls. BOOP can be caused by inhalational exposures, especially to water-soluble gases. It has been reported also after exposure to irritant gases, postinfection, in transplant rejection, as well as in many systemic inflammatory disorders such as ulcerative colitis. Chest radiographs show diffuse infiltrates and spirometry reveals a restrictive defect. Treatment is directed at the underlying cause; removal from exposure is essential, and corticosteroid treatment has shown considerable success.[12]

Interstitial Pneumonitis and Diffuse Alveolar Damage

Interstitial pneumonitis refers to interstitial collections of inflammatory cells, mild fibrosis, and reactive type II pneumocytes. This can be seen after numerous pulmonary injuries and toxic exposures, both via the inhalational route as well as systemic exposure. The healing phase can result in fibrosis and honeycombing.

Diffuse alveolar damage (DAD) is a pulmonary toxic reaction, most commonly caused by cytotoxic chemotherapeutic agents such as bleomycin, busulfan, carmustine, cyclophosphamide, melphalan, and mitomycin; it also has been reported with gold salts. The damage results from necrosis of type II pneumocytes and alveolar capillary endothelial cells. DAD has an early exudative phase (1 week after injury) characterized by alveolar and interstitial edema and hyaline membrane formation. The late proliferative phase (2 weeks later) shows proliferation of type II pneumocytes and interstitial fibrosis. Depending on the severity of the initial injury, DAD can improve significantly after withdrawal of the drug, progress to interstitial fibrosis, and, in severe cases, may progress to honeycomb lung.[13]

HYPERSENSITIVITY REACTIONS

Asthma

Asthma is a common disorder characterized by variable airflow obstruction, airway inflammation, and airway hyper-responsiveness to various stimuli. The airflow usually is fully reversible, either spontaneously or with treatment. The definition of occupational asthma varies depending on the author, but it can be thought of as a work-related variable airway obstruction or airway hyper-responsiveness owing to an exposure in the workplace. The broadest definition includes both asthma that is *caused by* the workplace exposure and a worker's preexisting asthma that is *aggravated by* workplace exposures. This extremely broad definition might be better termed *work-related asthma*, and it is estimated that up to 33% of all asthma cases may be considered work-related using this definition, but not necessarily work-induced. Most authorities reserve the term *occupational asthma* for cases that are actually caused by the workplace exposure, and place the incidence at approximately 5%. Not surprisingly, occupational disease surveillance data indicate that occupational asthma is the most common occupational respiratory disease in industrialized nations.[14-16]

The two major types of occupational asthma are *irritant-induced* and *sensitizer-induced*. Exposure to a significant dose of an irritating gas, dust, mist, or fume can cause irritant-induced asthma (IIA) without an intervening latent period. Classically, IIA was described as only being caused by a single isolated intense exposure; more recently, it has also been described as a result of lower-level exposures that have occurred over a period of months to years. The resulting asthmatic condition may be termed *IIA* or *reactive airways dysfunction syndrome* (RADS). The condition may be short-lived or cause lifelong IIA/RADS and disability. In these cases, there is generalized airway hyper-responsiveness but no specific responsiveness to any particular agent or antigen. Treatment in these cases can be quite difficult, and long-term disability is possible.

The classic form of occupational asthma is sensitizer-induced asthma. In this type, the worker becomes sensitized to the offending agent and requires a variable amount of time between the first exposure and onset of illness. Once sensitized, however, even minute quantities of the agent may trigger a significant asthmatic response. Most cases of sensitizer-induced asthma are caused by exposure to high-molecular-weight organic compounds that are considered "complete allergens." These high-molecular-weigh compounds are proteins with a molecular

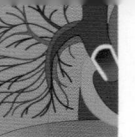

weight of more than 500 d and include traditional allergens such as animal dander, microbial spores, and plant proteins. The asthma is a type I, immunoglobulin E (IgE)–mediated immediate hypersensitivity reaction. Common names often are applied to this form of sensitizer-induced occupational asthma, such as bakers' asthma (due to wheat flour exposure) and mushroom picker's asthma (due to spore exposures).

One of the most prevalent forms of sensitizer-induced asthma is latex allergy, which can affect 2% to 17% of health care workers. Natural rubber latex gloves can induce an immediate, type I hypersensitivity reaction to the protein allergens. These latex protein allergens adhere to the cornstarch powders used as donning agents. They can then become airborne and are inhaled, causing systemic exposures and sensitization. Using gloves with higher protein contents correlates with higher allergenicity. Using powder-free, low-protein gloves has been effective in reducing symptoms and decreasing markers of systemic sensitization.[17]

Low-molecular-weight compounds (<500 d) such as antibiotics or metals also can cause sensitizer-induced asthma, by acting as incomplete allergens or haptens that then bind to serum proteins such as albumin and become complete antigens. Other low-molecular-weight compounds, such as toluene diisocyanate and trimellitic anhydride, sensitize by other mechanisms that are poorly understood. Increased secretion of monocyte chemoattractant protein-1 by mononuclear cells may be a major mechanism in isocyanate-induced asthma. Isocyanate exposure also has been shown to induce an overproduction of matrix metalloproteinase-9, and Trimellitic anhydride also may have a direct effect on airways even in subjects who are not sensitized to the agents. In the guinea pig model, nonsensitized animals exposed to trimellitic anhydride developed airflow limitation and eosinophilic airway inflammation.[18]

The chemical structure of the low-molecular-weight agent seems to be an important factor in its ability to sensitize. The presence of at least two reactive groups that can then form bonds with native human macromolecules, such as albumin, conveys the ability of these agents to induce asthma in exposed workers.[15] Hundreds of low-molecular-weight compounds have been implicated in inducing occupational asthma, the most well known being plicatic acid in western red cedar, toluene diisocyanate in polyurethane foam and urethane coatings industries, and abietic acid in colophony pine rosin used in soldering fluxes in the electronics industry.[19]

Some agents, such as organophosphate and carbamate insecticides, have a direct pharmaceutical action of stimulating cholinergic receptors, which causes bronchoconstriction. These agents can induce airflow obstruction without prior sensitization and do not require binding to native proteins or cellular mediators. Additionally, byssinosis is a variable airflow obstruction seen in textile workers that resembles occupational asthma. The etiologic agent is unclear: it is due either to a pharmacologic reaction to the cotton, flax, or soft hemp dusts or to endotoxin from fungal or bacterial contamination of the cotton. Tolerance seems to develop, because workers' cough and chest tightness are worse in the beginning of the workweek (Monday cough) but become milder as the week progresses. The disease occurs only in workers with longer exposure histories, or in those with higher total dust exposures. Allergic mechanisms are not active in this disorder, but a direct release of histamine and induction of inflammation are probably responsible. Recent studies suggest that chronic obstructive disease may develop in long-term workers.[20]

When evaluating a patient who presents with significant respiratory symptoms with bronchoconstriction, the possibility of work-related asthma always must be in the differential diagnosis, especially in patients with no prior history of asthma, with asthma of recent onset, or with acute exacerbations of previously stable asthma. Careful questioning regarding the temporal relationship between the onset of symptoms as they relate to exposures at work can be helpful. Sensitizer-induced asthma can have a biphasic or dual response, in which exposure to the allergen may induce an immediate bronchoconstriction (known as the early response) and a delayed or late response some 4 to 8 hours later. The early response usually is self-limited and often resolves without specific bronchodilator therapy. This is primarily mediated by mast cell degranulation and histamine release. The late response often follows with airway inflammation, hyper-responsiveness, and obstruction. The pathophysiology of the late response is complex and not completely understood. There is a pivotal role for numerous chemoattractant substances. A specialized type of CD4+ lymphocyte, known as the T-helper 2 (T_H-2) lymphocyte, seems to be responsible for the chronic inflammation that is present in sensitizer-induced asthma. Cytokines such as IL-4, IL-5, and IL-13 (which are produced by T_H-2 cells) and chemokines attract neutrophils and eosinophils into the airway epithelium. The eosinophils then cause airway epithelial injury by releasing proteins, lipid mediators, and oxygen radicals. Lymphocytes are also active, and they release cytokines that activate mast cells and eosinophils.[21]

As the airway inflammatory cascade continues, the increased mucus secretion and capillary endothelial and alveolar epithelial permeability all contribute to mucosal edema and narrowing of the airway caliber. The reduced caliber causes the airflow obstruction and the resultant signs and symptoms of an acute attack.

Some workers may exhibit only the late response, becoming ill hours after leaving the workplace, when the causal relationship may not be apparent. The presence of the dual response may hinge on factors such as the type of compound, dose, length of exposure time, and concomitant use of medication. Low-molecular-weight agents generally seem more likely to induce an isolated late response, whereas high-molecular-weight "complete" allergens more commonly cause a dual response. There is, however, considerable overlap.[10,16]

The mechanism by which chronic airway inflammation occurs in IIA/RADS is poorly understood. Direct chemical injury to airway cells causes an inflammatory response and release of cytokines and inflammatory mediators.

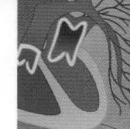

Neurogenic pathways are probably involved also, with the end result being airflow obstruction.

Acute treatment of occupational asthma is no different than that of conventional asthma, which consists of inhaled β agonists, supplemental oxygen, and systemic corticosteroids, as condition dictates. Severe exacerbations associated with hypoxia and/or CO_2 retention require treatment in the intensive care unit. Long-term management hinges on identifying the sensitizer, when possible, and removing the patient from further exposure. Irritant-induced RADS may have significant long-term sequelae that do not improve with removal from the workplace. Tables 9-1 and 9-2 list the exposures and occupations known to be associated with occupational asthma.[16,18,19,22]

Hypersensitivity Pneumonitis (Extrinsic Allergic Alveolitis)

Hypersensitivity pneumonitis (HP) is an interstitial lung disease caused by a combination of type III (humoral or IgG-mediated) and type IV (cell-mediated) delayed hypersensitivity reactions that usually occur after inhalational exposure to a wide variety of organic dusts, antigens, and some chemicals. Most commonly, HP has been associated with occupations having exposures to moldy organic materials, such as moldy hay in farmer's lung and moldy grain in grain worker's lung. It can be seen also in animal handlers due to exposure to animal proteins and excreta (pigeon breeder's lung). Exposures

to various chemicals that also cause occupational asthma, such as toluene diisocyanate (TDI), trimellitic anhydride (TMA), and heated phenolic resins containing phthalic anhydride, also have been implicated in HP.[23] Some therapeutic drugs have been implicated as causing HP, such as simvastatin, dapsone, penicillamine, paclitaxel, mesalamine, gold, and chemotherapeutic agents (Table 9-3).

The pathophysiology of HP involves immune complex deposition in the lung of sensitized individuals, with the resultant release of immune mediators and cytokines, as well as inflammatory cell infiltration. Acutely this involves neutrophils, but later lymphocytes predominate. The typical presentation occurs 4 to 6 hours after an intense inhalation exposure (in an appropriate occupational setting) to the responsible antigen, and patients commonly have fever, chills, malaise, cough, and dyspnea. Chest radiographs are abnormal in greater than 80% of cases, and they often have a reticulonodular pattern or reveal patchy infiltrates. High-resolution CT scanning (HRCT) is more sensitive and has been suggested as the preferred imaging study (see later). HRCT may show reticulonodular infiltrates or ground-glass opacities. There usually is hypoxia, and patients have crepitant rales upon auscultation of the chest. Pulmonary function testing can be normal or may show a restrictive defect and a decreased diffusion capacity. The acute episode usually resolves within 1 to 3 days, and corticosteroid treatment may be of some benefit. Repeated exposures often cause a worsening of the presentation; tolerance,

TABLE 9-1 High-Molecular-Weight (HMW) Sensitizing Agents and Job Titles Associated with Occupational Asthma[16,22]	
HMW SENSITIZING AGENTS	**ASSOCIATED OCCUPATIONS/INDUSTRIES**
Animal Products	
Animal dander	Animal handlers, veterinary workers, farmers
Pigeons (e.g., excreta, feathers)	Pigeon breeders
Chickens, turkeys	Poultry processing
Mice	Laboratory technicians
Guinea pigs	Laboratory technicians
Wool	Wool workers, sorters
Marine organisms: prawns, crabs, oysters	Prawn workers, oyster processing, crab processing
Plant Products	
Raw Tobacco	Tobacco industry
Flours (wheat, rye)	Bakers, food processing
Enzymes	
Bacillus subtilis	Detergent manufacturing
Papain	Meat processing
Trypsin, Pepsin	Pharmaceuticals
Foods (spices, grains, flours)	Chefs, food industry, food preparers
Natural rubber latex	Health care workers, rubber industry
Gums (acacia, arabic, tragacanth, karaya)	Pharmaceuticals, printing
Coffee beans, tea leaves	Coffee production, tea workers
Castor beans	Castor oil production
Seeds: flaxseed, cottonseed, linseed, psyllium seed	Bakers, oil extraction, seed workers
Woods (e.g., oak, mahogany, California redwood)	Sawmills, carpenters, woodworkers
Hops	Brewery workers, farmers
Microorganisms	
Fungi, molds	Farmers, bakers, various other industries

Adapted from Holland MG: Critically injured workers. In Brent J, Wallace KL, Burkhart KK, et al (eds): Critical Care Toxicology. Philadelphia, Mosby, 2005, used with permission.

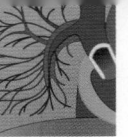

TABLE 9-2 Low-Molecular-Weight (LMW) Sensitizing Agents and Job Titles Associated with Occupational Asthma[16,18,19]

LMW SENSITIZING AGENTS	ASSOCIATED OCCUPATIONS/INDUSTRIES
Antibiotics	
Penicillins, cephalosporins, tetracyclines	Pharmaceuticals
Drugs	
α-Methyldopa, cimetidine, hydralazine, opiates, penicillamine, others	Pharmaceuticals
Inorganic Chemicals	
Ammonium persulfate	Beauticians, chemical production workers
Fluoride	Aluminum pot-room workers
Metals	
Aluminum	Aluminum smelting
Chromium salts	Leather tanning, metal plating, hard metal
Cobalt	Tungsten carbide hard metal workers
Nickel	Metal plating
Palladium	Metal plating, jewelers
Platinum	Platinum refining, electroplating, fluorescent screen manufacturing, jewelers
Vanadium	Ferrovanadium workers (hard metal workers)
Zinc	Metal plating
Organic Chemicals	
Abietic acid (colophony pine rosin)	Soldering, electronics manufacturing
Acrylates	Glues
Aldehydes:	
Formaldehyde	Hospital workers, laboratory technicians
Gluteraldehyde	
Amines (ethanolamine)	Soldering, paint application, machining metal
Anhydrides:	
Trimellitic anhydride (TMA)	Plastics, epoxy resins
Phthalic anhydride	
Dyes	Dye industry, fabrics
Insecticides (pyrethrins, OPs)	Farmers, insecticide applicators
Isocyanates:	
Toluene diisocyanate (TDI)	Polyurethane foam manufacturing
Diphenylmethane diisocyanate (MDI)	Foundries, paint application
Plicatic acid (western red cedar)	Lumber, logging, carpenters, cabinet makers
Paraphenylenediamine	Fur dyer, chemical worker
Phenol	Chemical worker, laboratory worker
Piperazine	Chemical processing
Styrene	Chemical production, polymer industry

Adapted from Holland MG: Critically injured workers. In Brent J, Wallace KL, Burkhart KK, et al (eds): Critical Care Toxicology. Philadelphia, Mosby, 2005, used with permission.

such as that seen in inhalation fevers, does not occur. In fact, repeated low-level exposures cause a progressive, often irreversible pulmonary fibrosis. These patients may present from a typical occupational setting with the insidious onset of a constellation of signs and symptoms, including dyspnea, cough, weight loss, and fatigue. Chest radiographs may reveal increased interstitial markings and fibrosis, and pulmonary function testing usually shows restrictive disease and decreased diffusion capacity.

The diagnosis of HP can be difficult, if not controversial. Diagnosis traditionally has relied on various nonspecific clinical symptoms and signs, with demonstration of interstitial markings on chest radiographs, the presence of serum precipitating antibodies against appropriate antigens, a lymphocytic alveolitis on bronchoalveolar lavage (BAL), and/or a granulomatous reaction on lung biopsies. However, when considered separately, none of these findings is pathognomonic for HP. Specifically, chest radiographs are normal in 20% of acute cases. Serum precipitins document exposure to the offending antigen but don't imply disease, because many co-workers with similar exposures but without disease demonstrate serum precipitins. BAL can be helpful, because a normal lymphocyte BAL count rules out all but residual disease, but an alveolar lymphocytosis is not specific to HP. Transbronchial biopsies are of limited usefulness, even when granulomas are found, because these are present in other diseases. HP gives a typical, albeit nonspecific, pattern of bilateral ground glass or poorly defined centrilobular nodular opacities on HRCT.

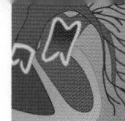

TABLE 9-3   Exposures Reported to Cause Hypersensitivity Pneumonitis (HP)

DISEASE	USUAL SOURCE	PROBABLE ANTIGENS	COMMENTS
Plant Products			
Farmer's lung	Moldy hay	Thermophilic actinomycetes: *Faenia rectivirgula, Thermoactinomyces vulgaris; Aspergillus* spp	Primary antigens are not molds but thermophilic bacteria
Bagassosis	Moldy pressed sugarcane	Thermophilic actinomycetes: *F. rectivirgula, T. vulgaris*	Bagasse is pressed sugarcane
Mushroom worker's disease	Moldy compost	Thermophilic actinomycetes: *F. rectivirgula, T. vulgaris*	
Malt worker's lung	Contaminated barley	*Aspergillus clavatus*	
Maple bark stripper's disease	Contaminated maple logs	*Cryptostroma corticale*	
Humidifier lung	Contaminated humidifier water	Thermophilic actinomycetes: *T. vulgaris, T. candidus; Penicillium* spp, *Cephalosporium* spp; Amoeba	Related exposures also can cause humidifier fever
Familial HP	Contaminated wood dust in walls	*Bacillus subtilis*	
Compost lung	Compost	*Aspergillus*	
Cheese washer's disease	Cheese casings	*Penicillium* spp	
Cephalosporium HP	Contaminated basements	*Cephalosporium*	Seen when sewage contaminates basement
Sauna taker's disease	Sauna water	*Pullularia* spp	Hot tub lung caused by atypical mycobacterium
Detergent worker's disease	Detergent	*Bacillus subtilis* enzymes	
Japanese summer-type HP	Contaminated house dust, tatami mats	*Trichosporon cutaneum*	*T. cutaneum* is an imperfect yeast
Dry rot lung	Rotting wood	*Merulius lacrymans*	
Office worker's HP	Contaminated dusts from HVAC systems	?	Multiple fungal and bacterial antigens may be responsible
Potato riddler's disease	Moldy straw around potatoes	Thermophilic actinomycetes: *F. rectivirgula, T. vulgaris, Aspergillus* spp	
Tobacco worker's disease	Moldy tobacco	*Aspergillus* spp	
Hot tub lung	Contaminated hot tub water	Atypical mycobacterium, *Cladosporium* spp	
Wine grower's lung	Moldy grapes	*Botrytis cinerea*	
Grain worker's lung	Grain dust	*Erwinia herbicola*	
Pyrethrin alveolitis	Pesticides	Pyrethrins	Pyrethrins are natural insecticides derived from chrysanthemum flowers; also a cause of occupational asthma
Animal Products			
Pigeon breeder's disease	Pigeon droppings	Altered pigeon serum	
Duck fever	Duck feathers	Duck proteins	
Turkey handler's lung	Turkey products	Turkey proteins	
Bird fancier's lung	Bird products	Bird proteins	
Dove pillow's lung	Bird feathers	Bird proteins	
Laboratory worker's HP	Rat fur	Male rat urine	
Pituitary snuff taker's disease	Pituitary powder	Bovine and porcine proteins	
Mollusk shell HP	Mollusk shells	Animal proteins	
Chemicals			
Toluene diisocyanate (TDI) HP	TDI	TDI-albumin complex	Also most common industrial chemical asthma inducer
Trimellitic anhydride (TMA) HP	TMA	TMA-albumin complex	Can also cause occupational asthma, and TMA-pulmonary hemorrhage-anemia syndrome
Diphenylmethane diisocyanate (MDI) HP	MDI	MDI-albumin complex	Can also cause occupational asthma
Epoxy resin lung	Heated epoxy resin	Phthalic anhydride	
Pauli's HP	Pauli's reagent	Sodium diazobenzene-sulfonate	

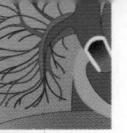

Lacasse and coworkers recently formulated diagnostic criteria for HP, relying on BAL and HRCT as the "gold standard," and, if needed, other diagnostic procedures. BAL lymphocytosis (>30% for non- and ex-smokers; >20% for smokers) and the typical HRCT findings were required for a diagnosis of HP to be accepted without resorting to additional diagnostic procedures, such as open lung biopsy. Six significant predictors of HP were identified: exposure to a known offending antigen, positive precipitating antibodies to the offending antigen, recurrent episodes of symptoms, inspiratory crackles on physical examination, symptoms occurring 4 to 8 hours after exposure, and weight loss. The likelihood of HP in any given patient increased as more predictors were present, with a 98% probability of HP when all six were present.[24]

Treatment of acute episodes consists of administering oxygen and admission to hospital when necessary. Corticosteroids are the only useful medications in the treatment of HP. They have benefit in the acute attacks at a dose of 1 mg/kg/day of prednisolone. However, the mainstay of treatment is withdrawal from exposures and prevention of any further contact with the inciting antigen or chemical.[23,25]

TOXIC INHALANT INJURY

Many occupations have potential exposure to gases, and, as a result, often these have significant potential for lung injury or systemic toxicity. Gases of toxicologic importance can be divided into three major categories: simple asphyxiants, toxic or chemical asphyxiants, and irritant gases.

Simple Asphyxiants

Simple asphyxiants have no inherent toxicity other than displacing oxygen from ambient air, thereby inducing anoxia. This is especially important in confined spaces, where the lack of air movement and ventilation may allow these gases to replace oxygen. Also, many are heavier than air and tend to accumulate in low areas. In the case of the chemical production worker, confined spaces such as reactor vessels may contain no oxygen; entry for vessel cleaning requires self-contained breathing apparatus or other supplied air respirators.

The simple asphyxiants commonly encountered by workers include nitrogen, simple hydrocarbons (e.g., propane, butane), and carbon dioxide. When encountered in confined spaces, a simple asphyxiant can cause anoxic central nervous system injury due to oxygen deprivation. The degree of injury depends on the extent and duration of anoxia. Additionally, the hydrocarbon simple asphyxiant (e.g., ethylene, propylene, butadiene, isobutylene, methane, ethane) also pose a significant explosive hazard. These confined space exposures usually occur in the situation of inadequate safety training and/or lack of proper supervision; often this occurs in newly hired workers who are unfamiliar with the inherent dangers. Treatment of simple asphyxiant

exposure involves removal from the source, adequate ventilation, and supplemental O_2.

Toxic or Chemical Asphyxiants

The gases considered to be chemical asphyxiants act by either decreasing the oxygen-carrying capacity of the blood (carbon monoxide, methemoglobin producers) or by interfering with cellular use of oxygen (cyanide, hydrogen sulfide). These toxicants are covered in detail in other chapters of this text (see Chapters 88, 89, and 91).

Irritant Gases

Irritant gases cause injury patterns that are directly related to their water solubility. Highly soluble gases such as HCl, NH_3, SO_2, and formaldehyde (CH_2O) and acid vapors cause immediate irritation of the mucous membranes of the upper respiratory tract because they easily dissolve in the moisture of these tissues. They cause direct tissue injury via burning by extremes of pH in the cases of acids and bases, or by forming an acid or base quickly upon dissolution in the physiologic fluids. Ammonia reacts with water to form ammonium hydroxide, a strong alkali, with the ability to cause airway injury and sloughing. Airway injury also may be caused by a more chemically reactive substance. For example, toxic cadmium fumes can cause a pneumonitis and acute lung injury due to inhibition of cellular and enzymatic function by the metal.

Highly water-soluble irritant gases cause immediate burning in the mucous membranes of the eyes, nose, mouth, and throat. The primary site of injury, therefore, is the upper respiratory tract, for two reasons. First, this immediate onset of symptoms tends to limit the exposure; the victim does not tolerate exposures long enough for significant lower airway injury and rapidly exits the area causing the symptoms. Second, these soluble gases first deposit in the upper airways, making less concentration available to the lower respiratory tract. When exposures occur in confined spaces, or when victims have associated injuries that inhibit their ability to escape, prolonged exposures can result in lower respiratory tract and pulmonary parenchymal injury. Significant symptoms of upper tract burning and irritation with signs of mucosal and conjunctival inflammation, when accompanied by laryngeal symptoms and cough, indicates a possibility of lower respiratory tract injury and the need for admission and observation. Delayed pulmonary injury has been observed, with the onset of noncardiogenic pulmonary edema due to ARDS hours later. Long-term sequelae may include RADS/IIA, restrictive or obstructive defects, bronchiectasis, or bronchial stenosis. Conversely, the lack of upper respiratory signs or symptoms rules out any significant exposure of a highly soluble irritant gas and obviates the need for prolonged observation.[10,23,26]

Phosgene, oxides of nitrogen (e.g., NO_2, N_2O_4; commonly designated NO_x), and ozone are poorly water-soluble gases. These insoluble gases cause little or no upper respiratory tract symptoms. In fact, the only

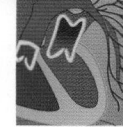

warning may be a nonobjectionable odor, such as freshly mown hay in the case of phosgene, or bleach-like odor of nitrogen dioxide. Because there is no initial irritation, employees often are unaware of ongoing exposure. Thus, longer exposures can be tolerated, and the concentration reaching the lower airways is higher due to lack of deposition in the upper airway mucosa. Eventually, a significant amount dissolves in the water of the lower airway and alveolus. Often, injury is then caused by formation of a new compound, usually an acid, base, or free radical. In these cases, delayed alveolar injury is possible, and onset of lower respiratory tract injury and pulmonary edema occurs 6 to 12 hours after a significant exposure.

Phosgene (carbonyl chloride) is encountered in chemical synthesis as an intermediate for isocyanate and pesticides, or as a by-product when chlorinated hydro-carbons are burned or heated. This can occur when Freon refrigerants burn in fires or when metals that had previously been cleaned with chlorinated hydrocarbon degreasers are welded or torch-cut. Phosgene also has historical significance as a World War I gaseous warfare agent, responsible for almost 80% of the deaths by chemical warfare gases. It is greater than three times heavier than air and accumulates in lower areas, making it an ideal agent for the trench warfare that was common during that campaign. Nitrogen dioxide is found in recently stored silage, especially corn grown during drought conditions, and is the agent responsible for silo filler's disease. It reacts with water in the lung to produce nitric and nitrous acids, which are likely responsible for the acute lung injury. The oxides of nitrogen begin to form within 12 hours of storage and can continue for 2 weeks. Oxides of nitrogen also form as by-products of combustion of fossil fuels or use of explosives, from lightning, and from oxidation of ambient nitrogen during high temperature arc welding. Nitric acid production workers can be exposed to NO_2 gas (the bubbles in fuming nitric acid are NO_2).

The initial alveolar injury usually results in alveolar-capillary leak, with edema and inflammation of the airway epithelium and submucosa. The fragile alveolar type I pneumocytes are particularly susceptible to injury, and irritant gases that reach the alveolus cause inflammation of the respiratory bronchioles and subsequent pulmonary edema and development of hyaline membranes and ARDS. The injury to the alveoli can be diffuse, and type II pneumocytes and fibroblast proliferate in an attempt to repair alveolar damage. In the recovery phase, resorption of hyaline membranes and exudates occurs. In some patients, the collagen deposition that follows can lead to long-term pulmonary fibrosis, whereas in others, recovery is complete.[27]

Due to the lack of upper respiratory tract irritation associated with exposure to low solubility irritant gases, patients often go home and develop these symptoms remote from the worksite. Without a detailed occupational history, the connection to the workplace exposure may go unnoticed. The clinical picture may present as ARDS, and sepsis or some other nonoccupational cause may be suspected. Treatment consists of O_2 and ventilatory support as dictated by the clinical picture. Recent evidence suggests that lower tidal volumes and lower airway pressures in ventilated patients may improve survival.[28] Depending on the severity of injury, mortality rates from severe ARDS may be significant, and patients who recover may be left with permanent pulmonary impairment. Corticosteroids probably are useful to prevent the late sequelae of BOF that is seen after nitrogen dioxide exposures. Their value in other toxic inhalation injuries is suggested by animal studies, but it is not proven in humans.[10]

The spectrum of water solubility is wide, and many gases do not fit neatly into categories of high, medium, or low water solubility (Table 9-4).[29] Medium solubility gases, like chlorine, have dissolution rates in the upper airway moisture that is midway between the highly soluble and the poorly soluble irritant gases. Significant chlorine gas exposures can cause upper airway symptoms of burning and irritation, but these may be milder than with the highly soluble gases. Exposures may be tolerated longer than that of the highly soluble gases and, there-fore, may progress to lower airway injury and delayed pulmonary edema. Chlorine exerts its toxic effect by formation of hydrochloric acid and hypochlorous acid once it dissolves in the water of the respiratory tract. Clinical suspicion and careful evaluation are necessary when making disposition decisions following exposures to the medium solubility gases. When in doubt, 24 hours of observation in hospital is warranted.

Chronic Obstructive Pulmonary Disease

Chronic obstructive pulmonary disease (COPD) is defined as a condition of airflow obstruction that is not fully reversible (as opposed to asthma in which the airflow generally is reversible). COPD is quite prevalent, with more than 16 million patients with the disease in the United States and probably even more who fit the criteria but remain undiagnosed due to the insidious onset of mild symptoms. The overwhelmingly predom-inant cause of COPD is tobacco smoking; however, exposures to irritating dusts, gases, and fumes probably have the capacity to induce this disorder.[30] Plausible evidence for this exists when considering IIA. There likely is overlap between IIA and COPD. Many IIA patients have airflow obstruction that is not fully reversible, and their disease often is more persistent than sensitizer-induced occupational asthma, as well as more difficult to treat. Other evidence is from the developing world, where exposure to smoke generated from the use of wood or fossil fuels for indoor cooking and heating that is not properly ventilated may be of importance comparable to tobacco smoking for COPD development.[31] The American Thoracic Society has estimated that the population-attributed risk for COPD was estimated to be 15% to 20% due to occupational exposures.[32] Several more recent studies lend further support to the theory that occupational exposures can increase the risk of COPD. Some of the industries with increased risk include rubber, plastics, and leather manufacturing; utilities; textile manufacturing; the

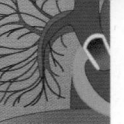

TABLE 9-4 Relative Solubilities of Common Irritant Gases[29]

GAS, CHEMICAL FORMULA	RELATIVE VAPOR DENSITY (AIR = 1)	SOLUBILITY IN WATER	RELATIVE SOLUBILITY
Hydrogen fluoride, HF	1.86	Freely soluble in water	Very high
Hydrogen chloride, HCl	1.27	82.3 g/100 mL water	Very high
Chloramine: NH_2Cl (Bleach + NH_3)	N/A (liquid)	Freely soluble in water	Very high
Formaldehyde	1.04	55 g/100 mL water	High
Ammonia, NH_3	0.59	47 g/100 mL water	High
Fluorine, F_2	1.31	Reactive	Medium high
Acrolein (C=C-C=O)	1.9	21 g/100 mL water	Medium high
Sulfur dioxide, SO_2	2.263	17.7 g/100 mL water	Medium high
Methyl isocyanate (MIC), CH_3NCO	1.42	10 g/100 mL water	Medium high
Chlorine, Cl_2	2.47	1.46 g/100 mL water	Medium
Phosgene (Carbonyl chloride, $COCl_2$)	3.48	0.9 g/100 mL water	Low
Chlorine dioxide, ClO_2	2.33	0.3 g/100 mL water	Low
Nitrogen dioxide, NO_2	2.62	0.3 g/100 mL water	Low
Ozone, O_3	1.66	0.001 g/100 mL water	Very low

Adapted from Holland MG: Critically injured workers. In Brent J, Wallace KL, Burkhart KK, et al (eds): Critical Care Toxicology. Philadelphia, Mosby, 2005, used with permission.

armed forces; chemical, petroleum, and coal manufacturing; and the construction industry.[33] These exposures to dusts, gases, and fumes may cause COPD independent from cigarette smoking; when combined with cigarette smoking, the effects appear to be more than additive.[34]

INHALATION FEVERS

Metal fume fever (MFF) is the classic example of an inhalational fever, but inhalational fever syndromes can occur after inhaling a wide variety of organic and inorganic materials. The same occupational settings also can give rise to HP, so it must be included in the differential diagnosis. In contradistinction to HP, these exposures can cause a self-limited, flulike illness consisting of fever, chills, generalized body aches, and malaise. Patients frequently complain of headache, sore throat, chest pain, and cough, and they may have some dyspnea. There often is an elevated white blood cell count, but generally there are no other laboratory abnormalities. Usually, there is no hypoxemia, chest radiograph abnormalities, or pulmonary infiltrates. The syndrome usually arises within a few hours after exposure and resolves within 1 day, with no residual effects. The mechanism appears to be a nonimmunologic reaction in the alveolus, causing release of cytokines and inflammatory mediators. Specifically, alveolar macrophages release cytokines interleukin (IL)-4, IL-6, and tumor necrosis factor α (TNF-α), which are known endogenous pyrogens. Complement may be activated, and T lymphocytes can release other inflammatory mediators. Repeated exposures cause a "desensitization," or tachyphylaxis, whereby symptoms are worse at the beginning of the work week (Monday morning fever), and after repeated exposures may elicit no symptoms at all. There are no residual defects seen on spirometric evaluation.

Diagnosis is made based on the above criteria, after ruling out influenza or other infectious causes. A good occupational history is essential, as infections usually are higher up on the diagnostic list when isolated patients present with these symptoms. A group of workers presenting with similar symptoms from the same occupational exposure setting makes it easier to consider. Treatment for the inhalation fevers is supportive, as this clinical entity is entirely self-limited. Proper education of the worker regarding the exposures that lead to this syndrome and appropriate engineering controls or fitting with appropriate respiratory protection can prevent further episodes.

Many of the occupational settings where inhalation fevers occur also harbor risks of other acute lung injuries. For instance, welding of galvanized steel produces zinc oxide fumes responsible for MMF, but welding metal with cadmium can produce acute lung injury and death; and high-temperature arc welding in a confined space can cause significant NO_2 exposure leading to ARDS. Farmers who unload silos may be exposed to silage that is contaminated with thermophilic bacteria and molds that can cause inhalation fever (silo unloader's disease), but exposure to freshly stored silage can cause silo filler's disease due to liberation of NO_2 (acute lung injury). Moreover, farmers with moldy hay exposure may induce hypersensitivity pneumonitis due to exposure to the fungi and thermophilic bacteria that grow in wet hay.

In contrast to inhalation fevers, the acute episode of HP often is accompanied by hypoxemia and pulmonary infiltrates on chest radiographs. Although fever is required for the diagnosis of inhalation fevers, it also may be present in HP or acute lung injury. The key distinguishing features in inhalation fevers are that chest radiographs show no abnormalities and there usually is no hypoxia, whereas these features are prominent in ARDS and HP. Repeated exposures to the causative agents of inhalation fevers causes a tolerance or significantly diminished response. Symptoms may be prominent when starting work or resuming after a vacation period. By the end of a workweek, exposures may cause no symptoms, and no permanent pulmonary sequelae develop. However, repeated insults of HP and acute lung injury after irritant

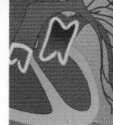

gas exposures often cause pulmonary function abnormalities and can lead to fibrosis and restrictive lung disease. Attack rates after typical exposures for the inhalation fevers can be high, often higher than 80% in one report of organic dust toxic syndrome, whereas HP occurs only in a small percentage of those exposed. Sensitization is required for the development of HP but not for inhalation fever. Repeated bouts of inhalation fevers due to certain exposures (humidifier fever) may predispose individuals to the development of HP, because these exposures settings also contain antigens responsible for HP (Table 9-5).[35,36]

Metal Fume Fever

Heating metals to a greater temperature than their melting point, such as while welding, causes formation of solid aerosols (fumes), often with accompanying oxidation. The resultant particle size of 0.1 to 1.0 μm reaches the alveoli easily, where an acute inflammatory cell response causes release of cytokines, producing a constellation of symptoms. The classic syndrome of MFF involves a metallic taste in the mouth, fever, rigors, headache, chest pain, and dyspnea, with an abrupt onset 4 to 12 hours after exposure. Clinical tolerance to these effects occurs after regular exposure.[37] Zinc oxide fumes are the classic cause of MFF, and in the 18th century was predominantly seen in brass foundries, where copper and zinc are heated to form the alloy brass. This gave rise to the then-common name given to what we now know as MFF: brasser's flu or brass founder's ague. More recently it has been seen after welding galvanized steel, in which the heating of zinc in the galvanized coatings forms zinc oxide fumes.[38] There is some limited epidemiological evidence that other metal fumes, such as those produced when magnesium and copper are heated, can cause MFF.[39,40]

Polymer Fume Fever

Teflon (polytetrafluoroethylene [PTFE]) can form pyrolysis degradation products when heated. Inhaling these products can lead to an inhalational fever known as polymer fume fever (PFF). PFF commonly occurs when Teflon-coated metals are welded or flame cut. Demolition of buildings with torch cutting of polymer coated wires, for example, also may cause the syndrome. It has been described in PTFE workers after smoking cigarettes that are contaminated with PTFE resins from their hands. This usually self-limited, flulike illness presents similarly to MFF, and diagnosis is based on the history of appropriate exposure. With prolonged exposures, or when higher temperatures are involved, pulmonary involvement with accompanying chest radiograph findings of consolidation are possible.[41] There even has been a case of PFF from burning of the PTFE coating of a nonstick frying pan.[42]

Humidifier Fever

Humidifier fever is an inhalation fever syndrome caused by exposure to air contaminated by humidifier water that has excessive growth of microorganisms, most notably

Pseudomonas and other gram-negative bacteria, as well as amoeba. It is a self-limited syndrome with features remarkably similar to MFF, and diagnosis usually is made after several workers from the same building present with the appropriate signs and symptoms. It occurs more often during winter months, when heated winter air is dry and these humidification systems are in common use. Nonsmokers are more susceptible than smokers. Humidifier fever is not to be confused with humidifier lung, which is a type of hypersensitivity pneumonitis that occurs after repeated exposure to humidifier contaminants. There can be considerable overlap of these entities, with both syndromes occurring in different workers with the same exposure.[43]

Pontiac Fever

Pontiac fever is simply a type of humidifier fever caused by exposure to water contaminated by *Legionella pneumophila*. In contrast with Legionnaires' disease caused by the same organism, Pontiac fever is a self-limited, flulike illness that was first described in 1968 in workers at the County Health Department Building in Pontiac, Michigan. It occurred after common source exposure to the air-conditioning system that was contaminated with *L. pneumophila*. Various other indoor water sources such as fountains, whirlpools, and spas have been implicated in causing Pontiac fever after contamination with *Legionella* species.[44,45]

Organic Dust Toxic Syndrome

Organic dust toxic syndrome (ODTS) is a catch-all term applied to a variety of inhalation fever syndromes that occur after exposure to many different organic dust mixtures.[38,39] Many of these dusts are associated with agricultural industries and include bacteria, fungi, grains, silage, hay, animal dander, pollen, and other complex mixtures. There seems to be a dose-response relationship, whereby higher dust concentrations and longer exposures increase the likelihood of developing the syndrome. In most instances, dust concentrations have been described as being so thick that is was difficult to see across the room. These conditions normally only occur in the agricultural setting, hence the common name "silo unloader's disease." Symptoms include fever, malaise, chest tightness, cough, and generalized aches. Hypoxia and chest radiograph abnormalities typically are absent, and the syndrome usually resolves without sequelae. However, there is a strong overlap with the causative agents of HP, and in these exposure settings HP must be ruled out.[35,46]

PNEUMOCONIOSES

Coal Workers Pneumoconiosis and Silicosis

Fibrotic lung diseases can develop after heavy mineral dust exposures to silica quartz (silicosis), coal (coal

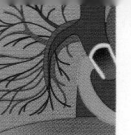

TABLE 9-5 Comparison of Acute Inhalation Syndromes

SYNDROME	PRIOR SENSITIZATION REQUIRED	SIGNS AND SYMPTOMS	PHYSICAL EXAM FINDINGS	PFT	CHEST RADIOGRAPHY/ HRCT FINDINGS	ABG/DL$_{CO}$ OTHER LABS	COMMENTS
Hypersensitivity pneumonitis (HP), acute	Yes	Fever, chills, malaise, cough, chest pains, dyspnea, headache	Rales on exam	Restrictive, clears upon resolution	Reticulonodular infiltrates, ground-glass opacities	Hypoxia, reduced DL$_{CO}$	Farmer's lung, many other terms; avoidance of further exposures and corticosteroids mainstays of treatment
HP, chronic	Yes	Insidious onset of dyspnea, weight loss	Rales	Restrictive	Fibrosis	Hypoxia; Reduced DL$_{CO}$	Occurs from repeated exposures, which if unnoticed and chronic may be misdiagnosed as idiopathic pulmonary fibrosis
Metal fume fever (MFF)	No	Fever, chills, malaise, cough, chest pains, dyspnea, headache; "metallic taste"	Usually normal, may have dry crackles on exam	Normal	Normal	Normal ABG, normal DL$_{CO}$, leukocytosis, elevated LDH	Brasser's flu; continued exposures cause less severe reactions
Organic dust toxic syndrome (ODTS)	No	Fever, chills, malaise, cough, chest pains, dyspnea, headache	Usually normal, may have dry crackles on exam	Normal	Normal	Normal	Silo unloader's disease
Pontiac fever	No	Fever, flulike illness	Usually normal, may have dry crackles on exam	Normal	Normal	Normal	Due to exposure to *Legionella pneumophila* from contaminated indoor water sources (e.g., HVAC systems, spas)
Polymer fume fever (PFF)	No	Fever, chills, malaise, cough, chest pains, dyspnea, headache	Usually normal, may have dry crackles on exam	Normal	Normal	Normal	Continued exposures cause less severe reactions; in severe cases of overwhelming exposure a chemical pneumonitis may develop
Byssinosis	Probably	Chest tightness, cough, dyspnea, onset 1–2 hr after exposure	Wheezes	Obstructive	Normal	Usually normal	Continued exposures cause less severe reactions
Asthma, sensitizer-induced	Yes	Chest tightness, dyspnea, cough; onset usually immediate, can be delayed or both (dual response)	Wheezes	Obstructive	Usually normal, can have hyperinflation	Normal DL$_{CO}$, normal ABG, severe attacks may have hypoxia	Continued exposures causes increased sensitization and more severe reactions

TABLE 9-5 Comparison of Acute Inhalation Syndromes (Cont'd)

SYNDROME	PRIOR SENSITIZATION REQUIRED	SIGNS AND SYMPTOMS	PHYSICAL EXAM FINDINGS	PFT	CHEST RADIOGRAPHY/ HRCT FINDINGS	ABG/DL_{CO} OTHER LABS	COMMENTS
Asthma, irritant-induced (IIA, RADS)	No	Chest tightness, dyspnea, cough; onset usually immediate, can be delayed	Wheezes	Obstructive	Usually normal, can have hyperinflation	Normal DL_{CO}; normal ABG, severe attacks may have hypoxia	May have persistent airway hyper-responsiveness to many environmental stimuli (e.g., cold, dusts); can be difficult to treat

ABG, arterial blood gas; DL_{CO}, single breath carbon monoxide lung diffusion capacity; HRCT, high-resolution computerized tomography scanning; LDH, lactate dehydrogenase; PFT, pulmonary function tests; RADS, reactive airways dysfunction syndrome.

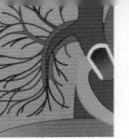

worker's pneumoconiosis [CWP]), and asbestos fibers (asbestosis), among others. These diseases are decreasing in incidence in the United States, owing to increased awareness, regulatory changes, and improved industrial hygiene practices. Due to the long latencies from exposure to development of disease, new cases from exposure that ceased 20 to 30 years ago are still being diagnosed. However, the exposure levels necessary to cause many of these pneumoconioses are still occurring in developing nations.

Exposure to coal mine dust and/or crystalline silica results in pneumoconiosis with initiation and progression of pulmonary fibrosis. In a recent NIOSH review, Castranova and Vallyathan describe in vitro and animal studies, as well as data obtained from exposed workers, which show that four basic mechanisms are operative in the initiation and progression of these pneumoconioses:

- Coal dust and silica have direct cytotoxic effects. The resulting lung cell damage causes release of proteolytic enzymes and lipases, which then leads to pulmonary fibrosis.
- Inhaled dusts are engulfed by pulmonary phagocytic cells that produce oxidants to destroy the dusts. This can exceed the amount of antioxidants present and cause lipid peroxidation, protein nitrosation, cell injury, and further lung scarring.
- Numerous cell mediators are released from alveolar macrophages and epithelial cells, which leads to infiltration of inflammatory cells like polymorphonuclear leukocytes and macrophages. Proinflammatory cytokines and various reactive species are subsequently produced, again leading to further lung injury and fibrotic scarring.
- These same alveolar macrophages and epithelial cells can secrete growth factors after initial healing from injury, which stimulates fibroblast proliferation and eventual scarring.[47]

Classic findings of silicosis include restrictive lung disease associated with silicotic nodules in the hilar nodes and parenchyma, with a predilection for the upper lobes. The silicotic nodule in the hilar lymph nodes occasionally may calcify in its periphery, leading to the pathognomonic egg-shell appearance on chest radiograph. In a small portion of chronic silicosis cases, the silicotic nodules coalesce and form larger fibrotic masses, known as progressive massive fibrosis (PMF). With PMF, pulmonary architecture becomes distorted and vessels, bronchioles, and alveoli may be destroyed, and the end result is respiratory failure. These cases are caused by large amounts of dust exposures in an occupational setting that occurred over many years. They are primarily of historical interest, because dust exposures necessary to cause silicosis this severe rarely occur today, and current cases are a result of exposures that occurred decades ago.[48]

Certain occupations, such as sandblasting, still can lead to chronic silicosis, and current regulatory standards and personal protective equipment may not be adequate to prevent this disease. However, the reduction in incidence of severe silicosis has lead to the use of HRCT scans to detect more subtle, early, subclinical findings such as micronodules and calcifications that are not evident on plain chest radiographs. Patients with silicosis have a high incidence of pulmonary mycobacterial infections (both tuberculosis and atypical mycobacterium), as well as fungal diseases such as cryptococcosis, blastomycosis, and coccidioidomycosis. This is likely due to an impairment of the normal pulmonary immune response by silica dust exposure that is not well understood. Silicosis has also been epidemiologically linked with systemic connective tissue diseases (CTD), such as scleroderma (termed *Erasmus syndrome*) and rheumatoid arthritis (*Caplan syndrome*). Some authors have estimated that the risk of these CTD is 2.5 to 15 times higher in silicosis patients than in those without silicosis.[48] However, more recent clinical studies have failed to show the same risks seen in older studies of miners.[49-51]

Asbestos and Man-Made Vitreous Fibers

Asbestos is probably the best-studied occupational and environmental inhalation health hazard in humans. It is generally accepted that all six asbestos fiber types can cause pleural plaques, pleural fibrosis, interstitial fibrosis (asbestosis) of the lung parenchyma, carcinoma of the lung, and mesothelioma, but potency and risk vary with fiber type and exposure history. Dust control regulations in developed nations have become progressively more demanding compared with the 10 to 100 fiber/cc exposure concentrations of the mid-20th century.

Man-made vitreous fibers (MMVFs) are synthetic, vitreous silicate fibers widely used in present-day insulation and construction industries in industrialized nations due to the decline in the use of asbestos materials. MMVFs can be categorized into insulation wools (rock wool and slag wool), glass fibers (glass wool, continuous glass filaments and microfibers), and refractory ceramic fibers (RCFs, kaolin-wool and other high-temperature insulating fibers). There are more than 70 varieties of synthetic inorganic fibers in use today.

Respirable fibers of concern have a length-to-width ratio of at least 3:1 and an aerodynamic diameter less than 10 μm, corresponding to a measured physical diameter of less than approximately 3 to 4 μm. The current U.S. Department of Labor Occupational and Safety Health Organization (OSHA) permissible exposure limit is 0.1 fibers/cc, time-weighted average (TWA), for all six asbestos fiber types. There are no U.S. standards for MMVFs at this time.

Fibrosis from asbestos appears to arise when pulmonary macrophages, neutrophils, and other inflammatory cells release mediators such as lysosomal enzymes, arachidonic acid intermediates, proteases, cytokines, growth factors, and reactive oxygen species. This results in a chronic inflammatory process that stimulates fibroblast proliferation, causing excess collagen to be deposited in the area of the offending fiber. Continued exposure, which allows diffuse deposition of these fibers, leads to generalized

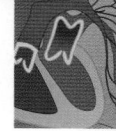

fibrosis, or asbestosis, which has a predilection for the lower lobes. Chest radiograph findings of lower lobe irregular fibrotic densities are typical, with indistinct cardiac and pericardial borders. Pleural or pericardial calcifications (plaques) are virtually pathognomonic for asbestos exposure. HRCT scanning is more sensitive than conventional radiographs for detection of pleural and parenchymal disease. The increased risk of lung cancer and mesothelioma seen in asbestos exposures may be due to the reactive oxygen species, which can cause DNA damage to critical genes coding for detoxifying enzymes.

MMVFs have been in use since the 1800s, with very few reports of pulmonary disease due to MMVF exposure, but pleural plaques have been reported in a cohort of refractory ceramic fibers (RCF) manufacturing workers in the United States. MMVFs are less durable and less respirable than asbestos fibers. Although there is some evidence that RCFs are capable of inducing lung tumors in rats and mesotheliomas in hamsters, current data do not show an excess risk of lung cancer in humans. Recent studies have shown RCF workers can develop pleural plaques without concomitant interstitial fibrosis. It is unknown whether these pleural changes signify a future risk for human mesothelioma. Long-term follow-up studies of the RCF worker cohorts are needed. At the present time, whether inhaled MMVFs represent a human carcinogenic risk is unknown.[52]

Metal Pneumoconioses[48,53]

Inhalation of metal dusts and fumes can induce a wide range of lung pathology, including airway disorders, cancer, and parenchymal diseases. Metal inhalation can cause granulomatous disease, giant cell interstitial pneumonitis, chemical pneumonitis, and interstitial fibrosis, among other disorders. The major offending metals are aluminum, beryllium, cadmium, cobalt, copper, iron, mercury, and nickel.

Beryllium and nickel exposure induce an immunologic reaction in the lung. Beryllium probably acts as an incomplete antigen, or hapten, and is presented by antigen-presenting cells to CD4+ T cells, which then react with the hapten via specific receptors. Only about 15% of workers exposed to beryllium develop chronic beryllium disease, which suggests that genetic factors play an important role. Other metals such as cadmium and mercury induce nonspecific damage, probably by initiating production of reactive oxygen species. Additionally, there is genetic susceptibility associated with increased risk in developing hard metal disease from cobalt exposure.

ALUMINUM
Occupational exposures to aluminum dusts and fumes have been associated with parenchymal lung disorders such as pneumoconiosis, fibrosis, and granulomatous lung disease. The prevalence of disease in exposed workers is relatively low when compared with beryllium exposure. The mechanisms by which aluminum causes parenchymal disease are unknown.

BERYLLIUM
Due to its light weight, low density, high melting point, and high tensile strength, beryllium has been used in the nuclear power industry and other high-technology applications. Beryllium acts as an incomplete antigen, or hapten, and is presented by antigen-presenting cells to CD4+ T cells, which possess receptors on their surface capable of recognizing the antigen. Workplace exposure to beryllium results in three possible outcomes: (1) workers who show no evidence of an immune response or sensitization to beryllium and do not develop chronic beryllium disease (CBD); (2) workers who become sensitized to beryllium, as demonstrated by skin testing or the blood beryllium lymphocyte proliferation test (BeLPT), but who do not have any evidence of CBD; and (3) workers who have become sensitized, as demonstrated by blood lymphocyte test or skin patch tests, and have developed CBD—a granulomatous or mononuclear cell infiltration of the lung and other tissues that is clinically indistinguishable from sarcoidosis. There is some evidence of a dose-response relationship for the development of CBD, but even nonproduction employees working nearby (e.g., secretaries, front office personnel) have developed the disease from trivial exposures. There is good evidence that the current OSHA standard of 2 µg/m^3 8-hour TWA is not protective. Workers exposed to levels below this have become sensitized and developed CBD. The U.S. Department of Energy (DOE) recognized this and, in 1999, developed its own action level of 0.2 µg/m^3, which is also the American Conference of Governmental Industrial Hygienists's threshold limit value for beryllium.[54] The DOE requires medical monitoring and BeLPT for all beryllium-associated workers. The safe level at which no worker becomes sensitized is unknown. Workers with exposures below 0.1 µg/m^3 have become sensitized.[55] Sensitization can occur in 1% to 16%, and chronic beryllium disease occurs in approximately 2% to 6% of exposed workers, through the refining of beryllium-containing ores as well as manufacturing and use of beryllium metals, oxides, alloys, ceramics, and beryllium-containing products. However, attack rates for CBD can be as high as 17% in some highly exposed cohorts, lending evidence for some dose-response relationship. Workers who are involved in machining or grinding beryllium metal have higher exposures to beryllium dusts, and have a higher rate of CBD. Workers with evidence of sensitization or CDB must be removed completely from further beryllium exposure.

CADMIUM
Exposure to cadmium occurs in production of nickel cadmium (Ni-Cd) batteries, electroplating, and manufacture of pigments or cadmium alloys. Nonoccupational exposures occur from tobacco smoking. Cadmium has a low boiling point and, therefore, forms toxic metal fumes readily when heated, such as when soldering, welding, or making alloys. Acute inhalation of cadmium fumes can cause a syndrome initially similar to MFF. However, cadmium is toxic to the alveolar epithelium and endothelium, the mechanism of which may be an

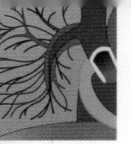

oxidant-induced cytotoxicity. Consequences of acute exposures are a delayed chemical pneumonitis, pulmonary edema, and death. Long-term sequelae such as pulmonary fibrosis and emphysema can result. Epidemiologic studies suggest chronic exposures that do not cause an acute pulmonary injury pattern also are associated with emphysema and pulmonary fibrosis.

COBALT

Hard metal is a mixture of predominantly cobalt metal and tungsten carbide particles, with smaller quantities of other alloys (e.g., titanium, molybdenum, chromium). Cobalt alloys have great strength, hardness, and resistance to oxidation. These properties make hard metal ideal for use in drilling and grinding tools. Worker exposure to hard metal dusts occurs in the manufacturing and use of these hard metal tools.

The term *hard metal disease* (HMD) is used to refer to all the respiratory diseases that result from exposure to hard metal dust, which include reactive airways disease and the parenchymal diseases—giant cell interstitial pneumonitis, bronchiolitis obliterans, hypersensitivity pneumonitis, and interstitial fibrosis.

Workers with hard metal parenchymal diseases can have resolution of symptoms when removed from exposure early in the course of the disease, but symptoms often recur upon return to exposures at work. With long-term exposure, increasing dyspnea, restrictive lung disease, reduced diffusing capacity, and eventual interstitial fibrosis can develop. This fibrosis may continue to progress even after removal from exposure. Bizarre, cannibalistic, giant, multinucleated cells obtained via BAL typically are considered a hallmark of HMD.

Cobalt is a known sensitizer, and the pathogenic mechanism of HMD most likely is immunologic. Only a small percentage of exposed workers are affected, and there is a reversal of the helper/suppressor T-cell ratios seen on BAL specimens. Sensitized workers have positive results on skin patch tests and lymphocyte proliferation tests to cobalt salts. Genetic susceptibility also is evident in the development of HMD.

COPPER

Exposure to copper fumes may cause MFF (see earlier), as well as upper respiratory irritation and nasal septal ulceration or perforation. However, despite its widespread use, respiratory illness is reported infrequently with copper exposure and longitudinal study of copper refinery workers show no increase in respiratory diseases. Exposure to Bordeaux mixture, a solution of copper sulfate used as an antimildew agent in vineyards, has caused an interstitial lung disease in some workers.

IRON

Siderosis generally is considered a benign pneumoconiosis resulting from the inhalation of iron oxide dust. Workers may be exposed to this dust in the manufacture of iron oxide, the preparation of emery rock for grinders, and the use of these grinding tools. Siderosis also can develop due to exposure to iron oxide fumes while welding. Although clinical symptoms usually are minimal or nonexistent, the findings on chest radiography in siderosis are often striking, with diffuse reticulonodular densities. A minority of patients can develop both restrictive disease and reduced diffusing capacity.

MERCURY

Elemental mercury is a liquid that is easily volatilized, especially when heated. Pulmonary toxicity occurs primarily from the accidental inhalation of elemental mercury vapor, usually in the home setting. It can cause an acute airway irritation and rare episodes of pulmonary edema, chronic interstitial fibrosis, or death. The pathogenesis is due to mercury's propensity to bind to sulfhydryl groups of cellular enzymes, as well as the formation of mercury-protein adducts. Once these enzymes are inactivated, subsequent oxidant injury and secondary destruction of pulmonary epithelial cells can occur. Exposure to high-dose elemental mercury vapor causes severe airway irritation, leading to tracheobronchitis, bronchiolitis, and, occasionally, pulmonary edema and death. Most cases of mercury vapor exposure do not result in permanent lung damage; severe cases may develop chronic interstitial fibrosis.

NICKEL

Nickel is a potent sensitizer, and roughly 10% of the U.S. population is dermally sensitized to nickel, with higher rates reported in women, possibly from more exposure to nickel-containing jewelry. Occupational exposure to nickel compounds is associated with IgE-mediated sinusitis, dermatitis, and asthma. High-dose exposures can cause chemical pneumonitis, pulmonary edema, and, rarely, pulmonary fibrosis. In the upper airway, nickel exposure is associated with rhinitis and sinusitis, anosmia, nasal septal perforation, and nasal carcinoma. In the lower airway, nickel exposure can lead to epithelial dysplasia and lung cancer. High-dose exposure to nickel carbonyl causes chemical pneumonitis and pulmonary edema. Although pulmonary fibrosis may result, complete recovery is the usual course. Response or tolerance to nickel, as in other metals, depends on genetic susceptibility and cytokine responses.

NEWER OCCUPATIONAL LUNG DISEASES

Microwave Popcorn Workers and Bronchiolitis Obliterans

Bronchiolitis obliterans, a rare, severe lung disease characterized by cough, dyspnea on exertion, and airway obstruction that does not respond to bronchodilators, can occur after certain occupational exposures. Inhalation exposure to agents such as nitrogen dioxide, sulfur dioxide, anhydrous ammonia, chlorine, phosgene, and certain mineral and organic dusts can cause irreversible damage to small airways known as bronchiolitis obliterans. Patients show an obstructive ventilatory defect without chest radiograph diffusing capacity abnormalities.

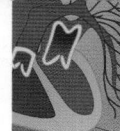

In May 2000, eight persons who had formerly worked at a plant that produces microwave popcorn were reported to the Missouri Department of Health to have bronchiolitis obliterans. Epidemiologic evidence and exposure monitoring have suggested that diacetyl (2,3-butanedione), a di-ketone used as an artificial butter flavor, is the causative agent. Workers in other plants that use artificial butter flavorings also have developed bronchiolitis obliterans.[56,57]

Nylon Flock Worker's Lung

Even materials previously thought to be inert and innocuous can subsequently cause disease when their physical properties are altered. This is apparently the case with nylon flock worker's lung, a newly described interstitial lung disease. Flocking is a widely used industrial process in which nylon polyamide fibers are cut into short lengths and then glued to a backing fabric to produce plush, velvet-like material. The flocked material is then used to produce clothing, upholstery, and plush toys and novelty items. The majority of the industry uses a guillotine-type cutter that produces precise fiber length (called precision-cut flock), but it is slow and therefore more costly. Rotary cutters are much faster but produce more variable fiber lengths, called random-cut flock. In addition, when these rotary cutter blades become dull, they heat up and can melt the nylon or produce very small fragments that can become airborne. These small fragments have an aerodynamic diameter of less than 10 μm and cause a respirable dust found in these workplaces. This nylon respirable dust has been shown in animal models to cause an intense inflammatory reaction.[58] All cases of nylon flock worker's lung reported to date have been from the only two plants that use rotary cutters and produce random-cut flock.

A comprehensive survey of workers at these plants showed a high frequency of eye and throat irritation, respiratory symptoms, and systemic symptoms during the workday. Workers with the interstitial lung disease experienced progressive dry, nonproductive cough, and dyspnea. The mean latency from time of hire to onset of symptoms was 6 years, and the latency from onset of symptoms to diagnosis was 1 year. Most chest radiographs were normal, but some showed reticulonodular or patchy infiltrates. HRCT scans, the imaging study of choice, showed patchy ground-glass opacity, scattered areas of consolidation, diffuse micronodularity, or peripheral honeycombing. Pulmonary function testing was variable, usually showing restrictive defects, but occasionally obstructive defects or normal spirometry was seen. BAL revealed eosinophilia (>25%) or lymphocytosis (>30%), with or without neutrophilia. The biopsy specimens from affected patients revealed a characteristic lymphocytic bronchiolitis and peribronchiolitis with lymphoid hyperplasia. All those affected had improvement in symptoms as well as radiographic and functional improvement after leaving the workplace. However, complete recovery was not seen.[59,60]

PULMONARY TOXICITY OF THERAPEUTIC MEDICATIONS

Many therapeutic medications can affect the pulmonary system. These effects include a wide spectrum of disorders such as hypoventilation due to any central nervous system depressant drugs like opioids and sedative/hypnotics and bronchoconstriction and bronchospasms from inhaled medications or any drug that can induce anaphylaxis or anaphylactoid reactions. Inflammatory and fibrotic changes in the lung can be caused by a variety of medication classes, as well as ARDS from any overdose situation resulting in prolonged hypotension and/or multi-organ failure. Also, any drug that causes enough central nervous system depression and lack of protective reflexes can lead to aspiration hazard and subsequent pneumonitis.

Pulmonary toxicity from therapeutic drug administration is reported most commonly with the chemotherapeutic agents, occurring in up to 10% of all patients receiving certain drugs. The likelihood of developing pulmonary toxicity from these agents increases with increasing age of the patient, higher cumulative dose, concurrent radiation therapy, concurrent O_2 therapy, concurrent chemotherapy, and preexisting pulmonary disease. The clinical signs and symptoms are similar regardless of the type of chemotherapeutic agent, often showing restrictive defects on spirometry and decreased diffusion capacity for single breath carbon monoxide (DL_{co}).

The common pulmonary manifestations of chemotherapeutic agents are interstitial pneumonitis, BOOP, and DAD. Tables 9-6 and 9-7 illustrate representative drugs and the toxicities seen with therapeutic use.[13,61-70] Chest radiographs frequently have normal results despite clinical signs and symptoms and changes in pulmonary function testing. HRCT scans are very helpful in identifying parenchymal abnormalities, guiding proposed biopsy sites, and monitoring response to therapy.[6,61-64,70,71]

SUMMARY

The fragile pulmonary system is in direct contact with airborne dusts and toxicants, and, as such, is susceptible to numerous acute and chronic effects from these exposures. This has been most prominently demonstrated in the occupational setting, where acute inhalation syndromes such as MFF, PFF, and ODTS were first described. Exposure to various antigens and/or chemical agents in the occupational setting has led to our understanding of hypersensitivity syndromes such as HP and occupational asthma. Occupational exposures to airborne dusts and fibers have caused workers to develop the historically well-known pneumoconioses such as CWP, asbestosis, silicosis, and CBD, as well as newer syndromes such as popcorn worker's lung and nylon flock worker's lung.

Pulmonary manifestations of other toxic exposures are evident in the nonoccupational settings when

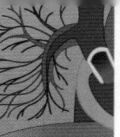

TABLE 9-6 Therapeutic and Abused Drugs and Their Pulmonary Toxicities[55-57,61]

THERAPEUTIC DRUG CLASS	REPRESENTATIVE DRUGS	TYPE OF PULMONARY TOXICITY SEEN	COMMENTS
β-Adrenergic blockers	Nonselective β blockers: nadolol, propranolol, timolol	Bronchoconstriction; IP, pleurisy, and PF have been reported	Timolol ophthalmic administration can cause exacerbation of asthma
	Cardioselective β blockers: betaxolol, atenolol, bisoprolol, esmolol, metoprolol	Bronchoconstriction; IP, pleurisy, and PF have been reported	
Calcium channel blockers	Verapamil, nifedipine	Bronchoconstriction (rare)	Evidence mainly from single case reports
Angiotensin-converting enzyme (ACE) inhibitors	Captopril, lisinopril	Cough, dyspnea, bronchospasms	Incidence of cough high, necessitating cessation of therapy in 10% of cases; mechanism appears to be kallikrein-prostaglandin system, with build-up of proinflammatory mediators such as substance P and bradykinin
Angiotensin II receptor antagonists	Losartan, candesartan, others	Cough	Incidence much less than ACE inhibitors; these agents have little effect on kallikrein-prostaglandin system
Antiarrhythmic agents	Amiodarone	IP, PF, ARDS, RF	Dose and time-dependent effects, lower doses much less incidence
	Flecainide	IP, ARDS	
	Tocainide	IP, PF	PF incidence 0.3%
	Dipyridamole	Bronchoconstriction	Incidence as high as 0.15% after IV use for dipyridamole-thallium imaging
Anti-inflammatory agents	Aspirin	Therapeutic: asthma, bronchospasms / Overdose: hyperpnea ARDS, RF	High incidence of bronchospasms in asthmatics with nasal polyps; asthma related to increases in leukotrienes, decrease in prostaglandins due to co-ox enzyme inhibition
	Ketorolac	Anaphylactoid reactions	
	NSAIDs	Bronchoconstriction, anaphylactoid	Most NSAIDs cause exacerbations in aspirin-sensitive individuals
	Gold salts	HP, IP, PF, BOOP	Incidence < 1%; BAL shows lymphocyte predominance; also drug-induced SLE
	Penicillamine	Alveolitis, HP, SLE, pleural effusions, Goodpasture's syndrome, eosinophilic pneumonia	Occurs in sensitized individuals; also drug-induced SLE
Leukotriene antagonists	Zafirlukast, montelukast	Churg-Strauss syndrome (CSS)	CSS: allergic granulomatous vasculitis with asthma, pulmonary infiltrates
Antibiotics	Nitrofurantoin	Acute and chronic IP, eosinophilic pneumonitis	One of the most common drug-induced pulmonary diseases; acute: onset in hours to days; chronic: after years of Rx; also drug-induced SLE
	Isoniazid (INH)	HP	HP with peripheral eosinophilia; also drug-induced SLE
	Penicillin	HP, pleural effusions	Also drug-induced SLE
	Sulfasalazine	Pulmonary infiltrates, eosinophilic pneumonia, eosinophilia, BOF	Rare; effects due to metabolites 5-aminosalicylic acid and sulfapyridine
	Aminoglycosides	Respiratory muscle weakness	Occurs after excessive serum levels, ? reversible with physostigmine
	Aminosalicylic acid	Hypersensitivity reactions, pleural effusions, alveolar infiltrates, cough	Incidence up to 5%; associated fever, rash, lymphadenopathy, hepatomegaly
	Amphotericin B	Decreased PFT, BO	
	Pentamidine	Bronchospasms	Seen after nebulized or IV
	Polymyxin	Respiratory muscle weakness	Occurs after excessive serum levels, ? reversible with physostigmine
	Streptomycin	Pleural effusions	Also drug-induced SLE
	Tetracycline	Pulmonary infiltrates, pleural effusions	Also drug-induced SLE
Antiasthmatic medications	Ipratropium bromide	Bronchoconstriction	Paradoxical, likely due to benzalkonium in nebulizer solution
	Hydrocortisone succinate	Bronchoconstriction	Paradoxical; not seen with other steroid preparations
	Cromolyn sodium	Bronchoconstriction, pulmonary edema, pulmonary infiltrates with eosinophilia	Hypersensitivity reaction, may be IgE-mediated

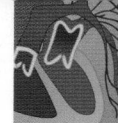

TABLE 9-6 Therapeutic and Abused Drugs and Their Pulmonary Toxicities[55-57,61] *(Cont'd)*

THERAPEUTIC DRUG CLASS	REPRESENTATIVE DRUGS	TYPE OF PULMONARY TOXICITY SEEN	COMMENTS
Nebulizer and metered dose inhaler solutions	Preservatives: sulfites, alcohol, metabisulfites, benzalkonium chloride, ascorbic acid	Bronchospasms	Most have been removed; metabisulfite probably works through SO_2 stimulation of irritant receptors; benzalkonium through release of mast cell mediators
	Emulsifiers: soy lecithin, oleic acid	Bronchospasms	
	Diluents: sorbitan	Bronchospasms	Hypertonicity may cause bronchospasms
	Propellants	Bronchospasms	Accounts for 58%–99% of MDIs
Diuretics	Hydrochlorothiazide (HCTZ)	IP, noncardiogenic pulmonary edema	Rare occurrence, onset within hours of administration
Chemotherapeutic agents	Bleomycin	IP, HP, BOOP	Pulmonary toxicity in 10% of all patients, death in 1%–2%
	Carmustine	IP, PF	PF onset can be delayed many years
	Cyclophosphamide	PF, BOF, BOOP	Incidence < 1%
	Azathioprine	IP	Incidence < 1%
	Cytarabine	NCPE	Has been fatal
	Busulfan	PF	Up to 4% incidence, insidious onset, can be delayed for years
	Chlorambucil	IP, PF	Rare case reports
	Doxorubicin	IP, PF	
	Melphalan	IP, PF	Rare case reports
	Methotrexate	IP, HP, RF, BOOP, pulmonary edema	HP incidence up to 7%, reversible
	Mercaptopurine	IP, PF	
	Mitomycin	Nonspecific pulmonary toxicity, PF	Incidence < 10%, higher in combination chemotherapy
	Nitrogen mustards	Pleural effusions, pulmonary edema	
	Nitrosoureas	PF, pulmonary hypertension	
	Vinca alkaloids	PF, RF, pulmonary edema	Usually only with combination chemotherapy
	Procarbazine	PF	
	Teniposide,	PF	
	Chlorozotocin	PF	
Drugs of abuse	Heroin (diacetyl morphine)	A, PF, NCPE	NCPE mechanisms: direct alveolar type II cell toxicity, neurogenic, hypersensitivity, acute hypoxic effect
	Cocaine	IP, HP, BOF, BOOP, A, pulmonary edema, RF, pneumothorax, pneumomediastinum	Inhaled crack cocaine most common form; direct toxicity, hypersensitivity, and impurities are all likely mechanisms; Rx with corticosteroids
Opioids	Methadone, d-propoxyphene	NCPE	Isolated case reports
Stimulants	Methylphenidate	Abnormal PFT, hemoptysis	Seen with abuse only
Psychotropics	Phenothiazines	Pulmonary edema	Rare, single case reports
	Butyrophenones	Pulmonary edema	Rare, single case reports
	Tricyclic antidepressants (TCA)	ARDS	Due to aspiration pneumonitis and/or NCPE
	Trazodone	Eosinophilic pneumonia, RF	
Anticonvulsants	Carbamazepine	IP	Hypersensitivity reactions
HMG Co A Inhibitors "Statins"	Simvastatin, pravastatin, lovastatin	HP, IP, PF	Rare case reports only; also myalgias, drug-induced SLE seen
β-Adrenergic agonists	Ritodrine, albuterol, terbutaline	Pulmonary edema, alveolar infiltrates, bronchospasms, pulmonary embolus	Seen when given IV for tocolysis
Ergot alkaloids	Methysergide, bromocriptine	Pleural effusion, pleural fibrosis	Retroperitoneal fibrosis also seen
Anorectic agents	Fenfluramine, amphetamine derivatives	Pulmonary hypertension	

A, asthma; ARDS, acute respiratory distress syndrome; BO, bronchiolitis obliterans; BOF, bronchiolitis obliterans fibrosa; BOOP, bronchiolitis obliterans organizing pneumonia; HP, hypersensitivity pneumonitis; IP, interstitial pneumonitis; IV, intravenously; NCPE, noncardiogenic pulmonary edema; PF, pulmonary fibrosis; PFT, pulmonary function tests; RF, respiratory failure, SLE, systemic lupus erythematosus.

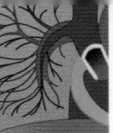

TABLE 9-7 Pulmonary Toxic Manifestations of Therapeutic Medications

PULMONARY TOXICITY/CONDITION	ASSOCIATED DRUGS	COMMENTS
Pulmonary eosinophilia[65]	**Occasionally associated:** acetylsalicylic acid, carbamazepine, granulocyte-macrophage colony-stimulating factor, minocycline nilutamide, penicillamine, propylthiouracil, sulfa-containing antibiotics, sulfasalazine **Rarely associated:** beclomethasone, chloroquine, cocaine, dapsone, desipramine, diclofenac, erythromycin, heroin, imipramine, IL-2, isoniazid, isotretinoin, mesalamine, methylphenidate, paclitaxel, para-(4)-aminosalicylic acid, penicillins, phenylbutazone, procarbazine, propranolol, ranitidine, trimipramine, zafirlukast	
Bronchospasms[66]	**Frequent:** ACE inhibitors, amiodarone, amphotericin B, antidepressants, phenelzine, tranylcypromine, isocarboxazid, aspirin, β blockers (propranolol labetalol, atenolol, timolol), carbamazepine, cyclophosphamide, D-tubocurarine, D-penicillamine ergots, erythromycin, gemcitabine, heroin, iodine radiocontrasts, isoflurane, melphalan, mesalamine, methotrexate, nitrofurantoin, NSAIDs, suxamethonium, sulfonamides, vinblastine **Drugs of abuse:** inhaled cocaine, marijuana, heroin **Occasional:** acetylcysteine, adenosine, aminoglycoside antibiotics, betahistine, cephalosporins, cytokines, desensitization extracts, hydrocortisone, interferon-α, interferon-β, isotretinoin L, asparaginase, melphalan, mesalamine, methylprednisolone, paclitaxel, penicillins, propofol, prostaglandin-F2α polyethylene glycol, rifampicin, risperidone, verapamil, vindesine, zanamivir	
Cough[70]	ACE inhibitors, angiotensin receptor blockers, bucillamine, desflurane, dirithromycin, fentanyl, IL-2, isoflurane, ketobemidone, L-tryptophan, methotrexate, morphine, mycophenolate, mofetil, nitrofurantoin, paroxetine, propofol, sertraline, steroids, streptokinase, sufentanil, sulfonamides	Also, virtually any medication delivered by the inhalational route, i.e., via nebulizers or metered-dose inhaler
Pulmonary edema[67]	**Antineoplastic and immunosuppressant agents:** cytarabine arabinoside, gemcitabine, immune globulin, interleukin, methotrexate, mitomycin, muromonab-CD3, pentostatin, tretinoin **Cardiovascular agents:** calcium channel blockers (amlodipine, nifedipine, nisoldipine, verapamil), epinephrine, phenylephrine, propranolol **Respiratory agents:** epoprostenol, nitric oxide renal agents: acetazolamide chlorothiazide/hydrochlorothiazide **Neuropsychiatric agents:** ethchlorvynol, phenothiazines, tricyclic antidepressants **Analgesic agents:** aspirin, methadone, morphine, propoxyphene, heroin **Obstetric agents:** ergonovine, tocolytics, oxytocin **Miscellaneous agents:** protamine, contrast agents	
Bronchiolitis obliterans organizing pneumonia[68] (BOOP)	**Antimicrobials:** amphotericin-B, cephalosporin, minocycline, nitrofurantoin **Anti-inflammatory agents:** gold, sulfasalazine **Cardiovascular agents:** amiodarone, acebutolol **Chemotherapeutic agents:** busulfan, bleomycin, doxorubicin, methotrexate, mitomycin-C **Miscellaneous:** carbamazepine, phenytoin, ticlopidine, interferons-α, -β, -γ; L-tryptophan, FK 506, cocaine (illicit use)	Usually resolves when condition is recognized and drug withdrawn; steroid Rx often helpful
Parenchymal lung diseases[69]	**Antirheumatic drugs:** methotrexate, penicillamine, gold salts, aspirin (overdose only), **Opiates:** heroin, methadone, codeine, morphine, buprenorphine **Thiazides:** hydrochlorothiazide	Parenchymal diseases include pneumonitis/fibrosis, NCPE (DAD), hypersensitivity pneumonitis, eosinophilic pneumonia, BOOP

environmental exposures occur as a result of hazardous materials incidents in communities, the worst example being the Bhopal disaster where an MIC release resulted in thousands of deaths and permanent injuries. The particular area of the pulmonary system injured depends largely on the water solubility of the gas involved: highly water-soluble gases affect the upper airways primarily, whereas low water-soluble gases tend to cause deeper, alveolar injury.

The generous pulmonary capillary network that allows gas exchange also provides an excellent delivery system for inhaled medications, the most common therapeutic use being administration of inhalational general anesthetics. This also is the route of administration of various drugs of abuse such as crack cocaine, marijuana, and abused inhalants. Likewise, this is the mechanism for systemic poisoning after exposure to asphyxiants, especially CO, which happen frequently in the workplace and home environments, both as accidental exposures and in suicide attempts. This generous blood supply also makes the lungs susceptible to injury by some systemically administered therapeutic medications, most notably the antineoplastic agents. A sound knowledge of inhalational effects of various agents and pulmonary effects from systemic drugs and toxicants is critical to the proper management of patients in both the occupational arena and more traditional clinical settings.

REFERENCES

1. Melius JM: The Bhopal disaster. In Rom WN (ed): Environmental and Occupational Medicine, 2nd ed. Boston, Little, Brown, 1992, pp 921–926.
2. Davra VR, Dhara R: The Union Carbide disaster in Bhopal: a review of health effects. Arch Environ Health 2002;57:391–404.
3. Watson W, Litovitz T, Rodgers G, et al: 2002 annual report of the American Association of Poison Control Centers Toxic Exposure Surveillance System. Am J Emerg Med 2003;21:353–421.
4. Ammonia. Hazardous Subtances Data Bank. http://toxnet. nlm.nih.gov/cgi-bin/sis/search/f?./temp/~s08Rxr:1 Accessed December 17, 2003.
5. Suntres ZE: Role of antioxidants in paraquat toxicity. Toxicology 2002;180:65–77.
6. Ben-Noun L: Drug-induced respiratory disorders: incidence, prevention and management. Drug Saf 2000;23:143–164.
7. Samet JM, Cheng PW: The role of airway mucus in pulmonary toxicology. Environ Health Perspect 1994;102(Suppl 2):89–103.
8. Ware LB, Matthay MA: Medical progress: the acute respiratory distress syndrome. N Engl J Med 2000;342:1334–1349.
9. Lippman M: Particle deposition and pulmonary defense mechanisms. In Rom W (ed): Environmental and Occupational Medicine, 3rd ed. Philadelphia, Lippincott-Raven, 1998, pp 245–261.
10. Smith DC: Acute inhalation injury. Clin Pulm Med 1999;6:224–235.
11. Kimmel EC, Still KR: Acute lung injury, acute respiratory distress syndrome and inhalation injury: an overview. Drug Chem Toxicol 1999;22:1–128.
12. Epler GR: Bronchiolitis obliterans organizing pneumonia. Arch Intern Med 2001;161:158–64.
13. Rossi SE, Erasmus JJ, McAdams HP, et al: Pulmonary drug toxicity: radiologic and pathologic manifestations. Radiographics 2000; 20:1245–1259.
14. Tarlo SB, Leung K, Broder I, et al: Asthmatic subjects symptomatically worse at work: prevalence and characterization among a general asthma clinic population. Chest 2000;118:1309–1314.
15. Banks DE, Wang ML: Occupational asthma: "the big picture." Occup Med 2000;15:335–358.
16. Malo JL: How much asthma can be attributed to occupational factors (revisited)? Chest 2000;118:1232–1234.
17. Ahmed SM, Aw TC, Adisesh A: Toxicological and immunological aspects of occupational latex allergy. Toxicol Rev 2004;23:123–134.
18. Malo JL, Lemiere C, Gautrin D, Labrecque M: Occupational asthma. Curr Opin Pulm Med 2004;10:57–61.
19. Chan-Yeung M, Malo JL: Current concepts: occupational asthma. N Engl J Med 1995;333:107–112.
20. Christiani DC, Wang XR: Respiratory effects of long-term exposure to cotton dust. Curr Opin Pulm Med 2003;9:151–155.
21. Busse WW, Lemanske RF: Advances in immunology: asthma. N Engl J Med 2001;344:350–362.
22. Rabatin JT, Cowl CT: A guide to the diagnosis and treatment of occupational asthma. Mayo Clin Proc 2001;76:633–640.
23. Beckett WS: Current concepts: occupational respiratory diseases. N Engl J Med 2000;342:406–413.
24. Lacasse Y, Selman M, Costabel U, et al: Clinical diagnosis of hypersensitivity pneumonitis. Am J Respir Crit Care Med 2003;168:952–958.
25. Cormier Y, Desmeules M: Treatment of hypersensitivity pneumonitis (HP): comparison between contact avoidance and corticosteroids. Can Respir J 1994;1:223–228.
26. Taylor AJ: Respiratory irritants encountered at work. Thorax 1996;51:541–545.
27. Maier LA: Clinical approach to chronic beryllium disease and other nonpneumoconiotic interstitial lung diseases. J Thorac Imaging 2002;17:273–284.
28. Ware LB, Matthay MA: The acute respiratory distress syndrome. N Engl J Med 2000;342:1334–1349.
29. Hazardous Substances Data Bank.
30. Balmes JR: Occupational contribution to the burden of chronic obstructive pulmonary disease. J Occup Environ Med 2005; 47:154–160.
31. Chronic bronchitis and emphysema. In Mun JF, Nadel JA, Mason RJ, Boushay HA (eds): Murray & Nadel's Textbook of Respiratory Medicine, 3rd ed. Philadelphia, WB Saunders, 2000.
32. Balmes J, Becklake M, Blanc P, et al: Occupational contribution to the burden of airway disease (an official statement of the American Thoracic Society). Am J Respir Crit Care Med 2003;167:787–797.
33. Trupin L, Earnest G, San Pedro M, et al: The occupational burden of chronic obstructive pulmonary disease. Eur Respir J 2003; 22:462–469.
34. Hnizdo E, Sullivan PA, Bang KM, Wagner G: Association between chronic obstructive pulmonary disease and employment by industry and occupation in the U.S. population: a study of data from the Third National Health and Nutrition Examination Survey. Am J Epidemiol 2002;156:738–746.
35. Seifert SA, Von Essen S, Jacobitz K, et al: Organic dust toxic syndrome: a review. J Toxicol Clin Toxicol 2003;41:185–193.
36. Singh N, Davis GS: Review: occupational and environmental lung disease. Curr Opin Pulm Med 2002;8:117–125.
37. Fine JM, Gordon T, Chen LC, et al: Characterization of clinical tolerance to inhaled zinc oxide in naïve subjects and sheet metal workers. J Occup Environ Med 2000;42:1085–1091.
38. Barceloux DG: Zinc. Clin Toxicol 1999;37:279–292.
39. Barceloux DG: Copper. Clin Toxicol 1999;37:217–230.
40. Nemery B: Metal toxicity and the respiratory tract. Eur Respir J 1990;3:202–219.
41. Shusterman DJ: Polymer fume fever and other fluorocarbon pyrolysis-related syndromes. Occup Med 1993;8:519–531.
42. Blandford TB, Seamon PJ, Hughes R, et al: A case of polytetrafluoroethylene poisoning in cockatiels accompanied by polymer fume fever in the owner. Vet Rec 1975;96:175–178.
43. Nordness ME, Zacharisen MC, Schlueter DP, Fink JN: Occupational lung disease related to Cytophaga endotoxin exposure in a nylon plant. J Occup Environ Med 2003;45:385–392.
44. Fang GD, Yu VL, Vickers RM: Disease due to Legionellaceae (other than Legionella pneumophila). Historical, microbiological, clinical, and epidemiological review. Medicine 1989;68:116–132.
45. Fields BS, Haupt T, Davis JP, et al: Pontiac fever due to Legionella micdadei from a whirlpool spa: possible role of bacterial endotoxin. J Infect Dis 2001;184:1289–1292.
46. Von Essen S, Fryzek J, Nowakowski B, Wampler M: Respiratory symptoms and farming practices in farmers associated with an acute febrile illness after organic dust exposure. Chest 1999; 116:1452–1458.

47. Castranova V, Vallyathan V: Silicosis and coal workers' pneumoconiosis. Environ Health Perspect 2000;108(Suppl 4):675–684.

48. De Vuyst P, Camus P: The past and present of pneumoconioses. Curr Opin Pulm Med 2000;6:151–156.

49. Steen V: Occupational scleroderma. Curr Opin Rheum 1999; 11:490.

50. Silman AJ, Jones S: What is the contribution of occupational environmental factors to the occurrence of scleroderma in men? Ann Rheum Dis 1992;51:1322–1324.

51. Burns CJ, Laing TJ, Gillespie BW, et al: The epidemiology of scleroderma among women: assessment of risk from exposure to silicone and silica. J Rheumatol 1996;23(11):1994–1911.

52. Osinubi OY, Gochfeld M, Kipen HM: Health effects of asbestos and nonasbestos fibers. Environ Health Perspect 2000;108(Suppl 4):665–674.

53. Kelleher P, Pacheco K, Newman LS: Inorganic dust pneumonias: the metal-related parenchymal disorders. Environ Health Perspect 2000;108 (Suppl 4):685–696.

54. Chronic Beryllium Disease Prevention Program. Office of Environment, Safety and Health, Department of Energy. Final rule. Fed Regist 1999;64:68854–68914.

55. Henneberger PK, Cumro DC, Deubner DD, et al: Beryllium sensitization and disease among long-term and short-term workers in a beryllium ceramics plant. Int Arch Occup Environ Health 2001;74:167–176.

56. Centers for Disease Control and Prevention (CDC): Fixed obstructive lung disease in workers at a microwave popcorn factory—Missouri, 2000–2002. MMWR Morb Mortal Wkly Rep 2002;51:345–347.

57. Kreiss K, Gomaa A, Kullman G, et al: Clinical bronchiolitis obliterans in workers at a microwave-popcorn plant. N Engl J Med 2002;347:330–338.

58. Porter DW, Castranova V, Robinson VA, et al: Acute inflammatory reaction in rats after intratracheal instillation of material collected from a nylon flocking plant. J Toxicol Environ Health 1999; 57:25–45.

59. Kern DG, Kuhn C III, Ely EW, et al: Flock worker's lung: broadening the spectrum of clinicopathology, narrowing the spectrum of suspected etiologies. Chest 2000;117:251–259.

60. Centers for Disease Control and Prevention (CDC): Chronic interstitial lung disease in nylon flocking industry workers—Rhode Island, 1992-1996. MMWR Morb Mortal Wkly Rep 1997;46:897–901.

61. Lantuejoul S, Brambilla E, Brambilla C, Devouassoux G: Statin-induced fibrotic nonspecific interstitial pneumonia. Eur Respir J 2002;19:577–580.

62. Liscoet-Loheac N, Andre N, Couturaud F, et al: [Hypersensitivity pneumonitis in a patient taking pravastatin] Rev Mal Respir 2001;18(4 Pt 1):426–428.

63. Liebhaber MI, Wright RS, Gelberg HJ, et al: Polymyalgia, hypersensitivity pneumonitis and other reactions in patients receiving HMG-CoA reductase inhibitors: a report of ten cases. Chest 1999;115:886–889.

64. Foucher P, Camus P: The Drug-Induced Lung Diseases. Available at: http://www.pneumotox.com/.

65. Allen J: Drug-induced eosinophilic lung disease. Clin Chest Med 2004;25:77.

66. Babu K, Marshall BG: Drug-induced airway diseases. Clin Chest Med 2004;25:113.

67. Lee-Chiong T: Drug-induced pulmonary edema and acute respiratory distress syndrome. Clin Chest Med 2004;25:95.

68. Epler G: Drug-induced bronchiolitis obliterans organizing pneumonia. Clin Chest Med 2004;25:89.

69. Lock BJ, Eggert M, Cooper JA: Infiltrative lung disease due to noncytotoxic agents. Clin Chest Med 2004;25:47.

70. Rossi SE, Erasmus JJ, McAdams HP, et al: Pulmonary drug toxicity: radiologic and pathologic manifestations. Radiographics 2000; 20:1245–1259.

71. Cleverley JR, Screaton NJ, Hiorns MP, et al: Drug-induced lung disease: high-resolution CT and histological findings. Clin Radiol 2002;57:292–299.

10 *Clinical Neurotoxicology*

JAWAID AKHTAR, MD ■ JON C. RITTENBERGER, MD

A wide variety of neurologic syndromes results from toxic exposures. Some neurotoxins produce specific and characteristic syndromes (see Chapter 10A), whereas others may produce conditions that are insidious or diagnosed as other common illnesses. Many toxins share common mechanisms and therefore manifest similar toxicities. This chapter provides a general review of neurotoxicology based on the physiologic actions of drugs and neurotoxins. It begins with a brief review of synaptic neurotransmission, because many toxins disrupt steps in this multifaceted process (Box 10-1). Each neurotransmitter system is then individually reviewed, and the toxins that disrupt its action and the syndromes that result are highlighted. Finally, a review of toxin-induced neuropathies is presented.

SYNAPTIC NEUROTRANSMISSION

Neurons are specialized cells involved with communication and information processing[1] (Fig. 10-1). The main structural features of nerve terminals are synaptic vesicles, mitochondria, elements of the smooth endoplasmic reticulum, cytoskeletal structures, and the plasma membrane that surrounds the axon. The nerve terminal (presynaptic) plasma membrane is separated from the plasma membrane of the postsynaptic neuron by a thin cleft called the synapse. Neuronal communication is neurohumoral and occurs at the synapse via the exocytotic release of small chemicals called neurotransmitters, for which specific receptors exist on postsynaptic neurons (Box 10-2).[2,3]

Neurotransmitters are stored in synaptic vesicles. Synaptic vesicles tend to cluster at discrete regions underneath the presynaptic plasma membrane, and each cluster behaves as an anatomic and functional unit composed of equivalent elements of neurotransmitters. Presynaptic plasma membrane shows areas of structural specialization at areas of synaptic clustering, and it is at these "active zones" that exocytosis of classic neurotransmitters occur. The neurotransmitter, on release into the synaptic cleft, binds to specific postsynaptic receptors to initiate postsynaptic activity. Synaptic vesicles, after exocytosis, are recycled and used in subsequent secretory cycles (see Box 10-2).

The activity of neurotransmitters is defined by and mediated through their interaction with pre- and postsynaptic receptors. Receptors are specialized

BOX 10-1	**CELLULAR TARGETS AND POTENTIALLY NEUROTOXIC AGENTS**
Adrenergic receptors:	Clonidine and imidazolines, sympathomimetics, sympatholytics, ergot alkaloids, antipsychotic agents (chlorpromazine, clozapine), yohimbine
Cannabinoid receptor:	Cannabinoid (marijuana, hashish)
Cholinesterase:	Organophosphates, carbamates, nerve gas agents, physostigmine
Dopamine receptors:	Apomorphine, bromocriptine, antipsychotic drugs
GABA receptors:	Benzodiazepine, cyclopyrrolones (zopiclone), imidazopyridines (zolpidem), barbiturates, ethanol, penicillin, muscimol (*Amanita muscaria*), bicuculline, neuroactive steroids (alphaxalone), flumazenil, baclofen
Glycine receptors:	Strychnine, brucine
Histamine receptors:	Antihistamines, TCAs
Membrane lipid:	General anesthetic drugs (e.g., halothane)
MAO:	MAO inhibitors (iproniazid, phenelzine, isocarboxazid)
Muscarinic receptors:	Curare, *A. muscaria*, *Atropa belladonna*, scopolamine, certain antipsychotics and antihistamines
Nicotinic receptors:	Nicotine, neuromuscular blocking drugs, α-bungarotoxin
NMDA receptor:	Arylcyclohexylamine (phencyclidine, ketamine), ethanol, domoic acid
Norepinephrine reuptake:	TCAs, reserpine, amphetamine, cocaine
Opioid receptors:	Opioid agonists (heroin, morphine, opium, meperidine, methadone) and antagonists (naloxone, naltrexone)
Potassium channel:	Barium, 4-aminopyridine, tetraethylammonium ion, cesium, polypeptide toxins from scorpion (charybdotoxin), bee (apamin), snake (dendrotoxin)
Purine receptors:	Adenosine, caffeine, theophylline
Serotonin receptor:	Atypical neuroleptics, buspirone, ondansetron, granisetron, LSD, mescaline, psilocybin, cyproheptadine, methysergide
Serotonin reuptake:	TCAs, selective serotonin reuptake inhibitors, nefazodone, venlafaxine
Sodium channel:	Local anesthetics, TCAs, tetrodotoxin (puffer fish), saxitoxin (paralytic shellfish), frog-skin poison (batrachotoxin), aconitine, veratridine, scorpion and anemone toxins

GABA, γ-aminobutyric acid; LSD, lysergic acid diethylamide; MAO, monoamine oxidase; NDMA, *N*-methyl-D-aspartate; TCA, tricyclic antidepressants.

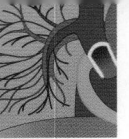

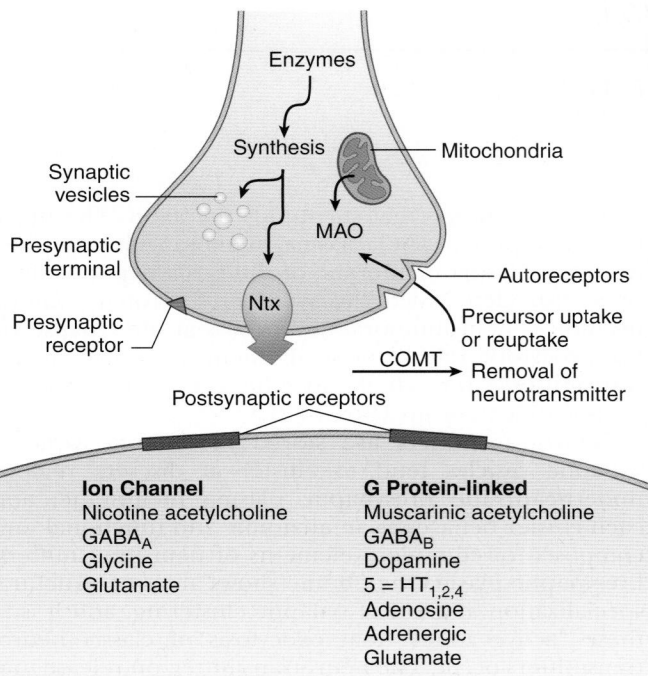

Ion Channel
Nicotine acetylcholine
$GABA_A$
Glycine
Glutamate

G Protein-linked
Muscarinic acetylcholine
$GABA_B$
Dopamine
$5 = HT_{1,2,4}$
Adenosine
Adrenergic
Glutamate

FIGURE 10-1 A schematic representation of a synapse showing the principal structures and sites of drug action. This synapse is a hybrid for the purpose of visualization; as outlined in the text, a neuron is typically highly specialized for a specific neurotransmitter system. COMT, catechol O-methyl transferase; GABA, γ-aminobutyric acid; 5-HT, 5-hydroxytryptamine; MAO, monoamine oxidase; Ntx, neurotransmitter.

BOX 10-2   SYNAPTIC NEUROTRANSMITTERS

Biogenic Amines

Catecholamines
 Epinephrine
 Norepinephrine
 Dopamine
Indolamines
 Serotonin
 Histamine

Ester

Acetylcholine

Purines

Adenosine

Amino Acids

Excitatory
 Glutamate
 Aspartate
Inhibitory
 γ-Aminobutyric acid
 Glycine

Peptides

Enkephalins

structures that have the ability to uniquely recognize a drug, hormone, or neurotransmitter. Receptors may be ligand-gated ion channels that are coupled to ion flow, G protein–coupled receptors, growth factors with tyrosine kinase activity that cause tyrosine phosphorylation, or steroid receptors that transport steroids into the nucleus.

Ligand-gated ion channels mediate fast-excitatory and -inhibitory synaptic neurotransmission in the central nervous system (CNS). The family of ligand-gated ion channels now comprises nicotinic acetylcholine, γ-aminobutyric acid (GABA) types A and C, glycine, serotonin 5-HT₃, and kainate, N-methyl-D-aspartate (NMDA) and α-amino-3-hydroxy-5-methyl-4-isoxazolepropionic acid (AMPA) glutamate receptors. Activation of ligand-gated ion channels results in a conformational change and opening of a pore (ionopore) in the membrane of the postsynaptic cells. This allows the passage of ions, to which the membrane was previously impermeable. The prototypic member of this receptor family is the nicotinic cholinergic receptor; stimulation of this receptor by acetylcholine allows sodium ion (sometimes calcium ion) influx and membrane depolarization. Ionopores for other ions such as chloride ions are associated with inhibitory transmission in the CNS. Excitatory neurotransmitters commonly result in postsynaptic increased sodium or calcium ion influx, or decreased potassium efflux to result in membrane depolarization and trigger an action potential. Inhibitory neurotransmitters often produce an increase in postsynaptic chloride influx or potassium efflux to stabilize or hyperpolarize the membrane and prevent membrane depolarization.

The G protein family of receptors (so named because it binds guanosine triphosphate [GTP]) is not linked to ionopores but to enzymes that are located within the membrane of the postsynaptic cell.[4] These enzymes act as transducers for the action of the neurotransmitter (first messenger) from the outside of the cell to the inside and produce second messengers. G protein receptors are able to regulate the rate of second messenger production and degradation via control of the activity of a number of effector enzymes. These include isoenzymes of adenylate cyclase, phospholipase C, and cyclic guanosine monophosphate (cGMP) phosphodiesterase families. G protein–coupled receptors also regulate ionic flux through ion channels either by direct G protein regulation or via second messenger–mediated phosphorylation events.

Binding of GTP to a G protein changes the activity of adenylate cyclase. Increased formation of cyclic adenosine monophosphate (cAMP) activates specific protein kinases by phosphorylation, and these in turn phosphorylate other proteins. At some receptors, however, stimulation of the receptors causes inhibition of adenylate cyclase and a decrease in intracellular cAMP. Some receptors are linked to the enzyme guanylate cyclase, which converts guanosine triphosphate to cGMP, which in turn acts as a second messenger in a manner analogous to that of cAMP. Phosphorylation of the membrane proteins cAMP and cGMP results in changes

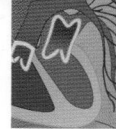

in membrane permeability to specific ions and in others to activation of further enzyme systems, which then mediate the biologic response. Termination of the signal involves hydrolysis of cAMP and cGMP by phosphodiesterase enzymes. Response of the postsynaptic cell can thus be influenced by drugs acting on the enzymes involved (i.e., adenylate cyclase, guanylate cyclase, and phosphodiesterase). Phosphatidylinositol breakdown, which is stimulated by phospholipase C located in cell membranes, represents another type of second messenger system. The breakdown of phosphatidylinositol 4,5-bisphosphate leads to the release of inositol triphosphate and diacylglycerol. Diacylglycerol is an activator of kinase C, whereas inositol triphosphate in turn stimulates other intracellular messengers such as calcium or calmodulin.

Calcium ions are necessary for transmission at synaptic junctions and have a dual role in neuronal secretion. Calcium influx following the action potential triggers synaptic vesicle exocytosis and regulates the amount of vesicles released. The action potential, caused by a depolarizing stimulus, begins with a transient, voltage-gated opening of sodium channels that allows sodium to enter the fiber and depolarize the membrane fully. This is followed by a transient voltage-gated opening of potassium channels that allows potassium to leave and repolarize the membrane.

Presynaptic neurotransmitter release is modulated by presynaptic receptors called autoreceptors.[2] Autoreceptors often are inhibitory and prevent further release of neurotransmitter from the same neuron. These receptors, however, also may be excitatory. In addition, these receptors may influence the release of neurotransmitters from neighboring neurons (heteroreceptors). Autoreceptors often are coupled to G proteins. They prevent further neurotransmitter release by increasing potassium efflux or limiting calcium ion influx, effects that hyperpolarize the membrane.

THE NEUROTRANSMITTER SYSTEM AND NEUROTOXICITY

The neurotransmitter system has many components, and toxins may interact with, augment, or disrupt any step in neurotransmission. A toxin can disrupt ionic channels, block or stimulate presynaptic or postsynaptic receptors, alter presynaptic neurotransmitter reuptake, or block neurotransmitter degradation. Many of these substances are used as pharmaceutical agents in clinical practice, and some are naturally occurring biologic toxins or manmade chemicals. The details of the processes involved in synaptic transmission vary from one transmitter to another and are discussed as the individual neurotransmitter system is reviewed.

A drug that produces a response and mimics the effect of an endogenous regulatory compound is known as an agonist. Antagonists bind to the receptor site with zero intrinsic regulatory activity to initiate a response and, therefore, cause inhibition of the agonist. Certain drugs are able to reduce the activity of receptor systems that are active in the absence of agonists. Agonists increase the activity of receptor systems, and this opposite or negative activity is known as inverse agonism.

The Purinergic System

Adenosine and adenosine triphosphate (ATP) are purines that are released from neurons and other cells and produce widespread effects on many organ systems by binding to cell-surface purinergic receptors. ATP also is released from non-neuronal sources including platelets, mast cells, and, possibly, endothelial cells. Receptors for both adenosine and ATP are widely distributed in the nervous system and in other tissues such as the heart, intestine, and bladder. Receptors that bind adenosine or ATP are designated P_1 and P_2 purinergic receptors, respectively.[5] Adenosine and some adenosine analogues activate adenosine receptors but not ATP receptors, and some ATP analogues activate ATP receptors but not adenosine receptors.

Four P_1 receptors, designated A_1, A_{2A}, A_{2B} and A_3, have been pharmacologically characterized and all are members of the G protein–coupled receptor superfamily. A_1 adenosine receptors are widely distributed in the CNS. Central A_1 receptor activity includes sedation, analgesia, neuroprotection, and anticonvulsant activity. Adenosine potentiates the antinociceptive action of norepinephrine in the spinal cord. Many of the central effects of adenosine are attributed to the modulation of neurotransmitter release in the CNS. Opiates have been shown to induce the release of adenosine, and some effects of opiates are blocked by adenosine receptor antagonists. In the periphery, adenosine A_1 receptors are found in the heart, where they produce negative inotropic, chronotropic, and dromotropic responses. In adipose tissue, they inhibit lipolysis and enhance insulin-stimulated glucose transport. In the kidneys, they reduce glomerular filtration pressure and produce antidiuresis.

A_1 receptor activation produces effects by inhibiting adenylate cyclase (decreased cAMP) and by increasing or decreasing phospholipase activity. Presynaptic A_1 receptor activation results in decreased calcium conductance and decreased exocytosis of neurotransmitter. Presynaptic A_1 autoreceptors antagonize norepinephrine release in the sympathetic nervous system. In addition, A_1 receptor agonists result in decreased release of epinephrine and norepinephrine from adrenal glands. In the heart, there is an increase in atrioventricular nodal refractoriness and inhibition of delayed afterdepolarizations. Postsynaptic A_1 receptor stimulation increases potassium channel conductance to produce membrane depolarization. These effects counteract those of the sympathetic nervous system and augment the actions of the parasympathetic nervous system. In the heart, adenosine activates the acetylcholine-sensitive potassium current in the atrium and sinoatrial and atrioventricular nodes. This results in shortening of the action potential duration and slowing of normal automaticity.

The A_2 receptors are classified further into A_{2A} and A_{2B} subtypes, depending on their affinity for adenosine. A_2 receptors present on sensory nerves in the carotid

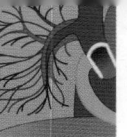
body, aortic body, and pulmonary circulation, and elsewhere produce excitatory sensory input. A_{2A} receptor activation in the vascular bed classically is associated with vasodilation and hypotension. These effects are mediated in part by the elevation of intracellular cAMP and by activation of ATP-dependent potassium channels. Activation of the A_{2A} receptor on platelet membranes elevates intracellular cAMP levels, resulting in inhibition of platelet aggregation. The A_3 receptors are found throughout the brain and are heavily expressed in the pineal body, lungs, and spleen. A_3 receptor activation decreases adenylate cyclase activity and increases phospholipase C. Although the central effects of A_3 receptors are not fully elucidated, their activation appears to potentiate ischemic cellular injury.

Activation of adenosine receptors is largely neuroprotective. A_2 receptor activation preserves tissue oxygen and substrate delivery via cerebral vasodilation. A_1 receptor activation decreases tissue oxygen requirements and raises the seizure threshold. Adenosine, an adenosine agonist, is an effective antiepileptic agent in experimental animals. Similarly, drugs that are A_1 receptor system agonists have anticonvulsant properties. Conversely, drugs that antagonize the effects of A_1 receptors lower the seizure threshold. Agents that antagonize A_2 receptors produce cerebral vasoconstriction and may potentiate neurotoxicity during seizures or other conditions that limit oxygen delivery to the brain. Carbamazepine is an A_1 receptor antagonist, which may partly explain seizures that occur with overdose of this psychotropic.[6] Caffeine, theophylline, and theobromine are three important alkaloids derived from xanthine. Methylxanthines are competitive antagonists at A_1 and A_2 receptors and may produce seizures with acute and chronic overdose. Methylxanthine-associated seizures have a reported mortality of up to 50% (see Chapter 65). The reason for this high mortality results from A_1 antagonism and consequent impaired self-termination of seizure activity.[7] In addition, neurologic morbidity is enhanced from concurrent A_2 receptor antagonism, which produces cerebral vasoconstriction during seizures. $GABA_A$ receptor agonism, especially by barbiturates, is most effective in preventing and terminating methylxanthine-induced seizures. Intravenous adenosine may attenuate theophylline-induced seizures by receptor antagonism or from nonspecific adenosine actions.[8] Phenytoin remains ineffective in treating theophylline-induced seizures and may increase mortality.[9] Dipyramidole inhibits adenosine reuptake and inhibits adenosine deaminase, actions that result in raised adenosine concentrations. Benzodiazepines partly inhibit adenosine uptake, which may account for some of their anticonvulsant properties.[10]

ATP receptors have a wide tissue distribution. In the autonomic nervous system, ATP is released as a cotransmitter from both sympathetic and parasympathetic neurons. ATP that is released is broken down rapidly by widely distributed 5'-nucleotidases; this results in the formation of adenosine. ATP has a biphasic or inhibitory effect due to its breakdown to adenosine. The physiologic and pharmacologic actions of ATP are mediated through activation of P_2 purinergic receptors, of which at least five subtypes (P_{2U}, P_{2T}, P_{2X}, P_{2Y}, and P_{2Z} purinergic receptors) have been identified. It is now known that the P_{2X} receptor is a ligand-gated ion channel, whereas the P_{2Y} receptor is G protein activated.[11] The receptors are classified largely on the basis of the relative agonist potencies of ATP and a number of structural analogues. The role of these receptors in neurotoxicity is yet to be defined.

The Catecholaminergic System

Three distinct catecholamines—dopamine, norepinephrine, and epinephrine—are involved in neurotransmission. Norepinephrine is the predominant catecholamine in peripheral tissue and sympathetic nerves. Epinephrine, formed by N-methylation of norepinephrine, is released from the adrenal glands and stimulates catecholamine receptors in various organs. Small amounts of epinephrine are found also in the CNS, particularly in the brainstem.[12] A few sympathetic fibers release acetylcholine (e.g., those serving sweat glands). Dopamine, the precursor of norepinephrine, also has biologic activity in the periphery, especially in the kidneys.

The amino acid L-tyrosine is hydroxylated to dihydroxy-L-phenylalanine (L-dopa) by tyrosine hydroxylase, a mixed-function oxidase located in the cytoplasm and on cell membranes. Tyrosine hydroxylase also hydroxylates phenylalanine to form tyrosine, which is then converted to L-dopa. Dopa decarboxylase, a pyridoxine-dependent enzyme, catalyzes the removal of the carboxyl group from dopa to form dopamine.[3] In neurons that synthesize epinephrine or norepinephrine, dopamine diffuses into synaptic vesicles, where the enzyme dopamine-β-hydroxylase hydroxylates dopamine, forming norepinephrine. In chromaffin cells that synthesize epinephrine, the final step in the pathway is catalyzed by the enzyme phenylethanolamine N-methyltransferase. Catecholamines are concentrated in the synaptic vesicles and also are found free in the cytoplasmic fluid. The action of catecholamines released at the synapse is terminated by reuptake. The excess catecholamine is repackaged in storage vesicles or degraded by mitochondrial monoamine oxidase (MAO). These isoenzymes are integral flavoproteins on outer mitochondrial membranes. The MAO enzymes exist in two forms, A and B. MAO-A preferentially deaminates norepinephrine and serotonin and is selectively inhibited by clorgyline or moclobemide, whereas MAO-B acts on dopamine and is selectively inhibited by deprenyl (see Chapter 29). Catechol O-methyltransferase acts on extraneuronal catecholamine and is responsible for inactivation of catecholamine that is not effectively removed from the synaptic cleft.

The effects of catecholamines are mediated by cell-surface receptors.[13] All adrenergic neurons contain G protein–coupled receptors.[3] Adrenergic receptors are subdivided into two types, α and β receptors. α-Adrenergic receptor activation inhibits adenylate cyclase and decreases cellular cAMP levels, whereas β receptor

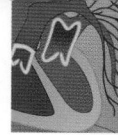

activation increases adenylate cyclase activity and increases cellular cAMP concentrations. α-Adrenergic receptors have the following order of potency for agonists: epinephrine ≥ norepinephrine >> isoproterenol. β-Adrenergic receptors have the following order of potency for agonists: isoproterenol > epinephrine ≥ norepinephrine.[3] The α-adrenergic receptors are responsible for the excitatory actions of norepinephrine and mediate the contraction of most smooth muscles, particularly vascular smooth muscles, resulting in vasoconstriction. An exception is the gut, where α-adrenergic receptor activation relaxes smooth muscle cells. β-Adrenergic receptor activation increases the rate and contractility of the heart, relaxes smooth muscles in the bronchioles and the uterus, and causes vasodilation.

α-Adrenoceptors are divided into two types, α_1 and α_2 receptors. In peripheral tissues, α_1 adrenoceptors are located on the postsynaptic membrane, whereas α_2 adrenoceptors are located on both presynaptic and postsynaptic membranes. Stimulation of postsynaptic α receptors (α_1 and α_2) results in vasoconstriction. Stimulation of presynaptic α_2 autoreceptors, however, decreases norepinephrine release. Stimulation of postsynaptic α_2 adrenoceptors in the brainstem inhibits sympathetic nervous system output and results in sedation.

β Adrenoceptors are divided into three types, β_1, β_2, and β_3 receptors. Peripheral β_1 receptors are found predominantly in the myocardium. Epinephrine and norepinephrine are equivalent in potency as agonists at this receptor. Peripheral β_2 receptors are found on smooth muscle, the myocardium, and numerous other tissues. Epinephrine is 10- to 50-fold more potent at β_2 receptors than norepinephrine.[2,3] When present, presynaptic β_2-adrenergic receptors facilitate the release of norepinephrine from sympathetic nerves. β_3-Adrenergic receptors are found in fat, skeletal muscle, and other peripheral tissues. Norepinephrine is 10-fold more potent at the β_3 receptor compared with epinephrine.[2] The physiologic role of this receptor is not fully known.

Five subtypes of the dopamine receptor have been identified. The D_1 and D_5 receptors are coupled to stimulation of adenylate cyclase. D_2, D_3, and D_4 receptors have an opposing effect on adenylate cyclase.[14] In the brain, the principal functions mediated by dopamine are the control of movements of behavior, including motivation, cognitive function, and emotion. Newer antipsychotic agents target D_2 receptors, and the evidence suggests that patients experience fewer extrapyramidal side effects (see Chapter 38).[15] In the pituitary gland, dopamine controls the release of prolactin and α-melanocyte–stimulating hormone. In the cardiovascular system, it is important in the regulation of blood pressure. Dopamine receptors have therefore been identified functionally in tissues related to these effects (e.g., pituitary gland and certain blood vessels). The antihypertensive effects of fenoldopam are mediated by D_1 receptor activation in the kidney.[16] The largest concentrations of dopamine receptors, however, are in the basal ganglia and the limbic system.

Numerous drugs affect catecholamine neurotransmission. Tyrosine analogues such as metyrosine (α-methyl-*p*-tyrosine) impair the synthesis of dopamine and norepinephrine by blocking the enzyme tyrosine hydroxylase. Disulfiram and diethyldithiocarbamate inhibit dopamine β-hydroxylase and can produce sympatholytic effects by interfering with the production of norepinephrine from dopamine. Reserpine and tetrabenazine inhibit the uptake of dopamine and other catecholamines into vesicles, causing depletion of endogenous neuronal catecholamines. α-Methyldopa causes dopamine depletion by replacement of dopamine with a relatively inactive false transmitter, α-methyldopamine; this causes hypotension and sedation. Other false neurotransmitters include metaraminol and octopamine. Peripheral presynaptic antiadrenergic drugs such as guanethidine and bretylium inhibit norepinephrine release from the presynaptic terminal by depleting the nerve endings of noradrenaline. The neurotoxin 6-hydroxydopamine is taken up by an active uptake mechanism and accumulates in catecholamine-containing neurons, destroying them through the autooxidative liberation of hydrogen peroxide or from formation of a quinone. Indirect-acting agents are agonists or sympathomimetics that cause release of cytoplasmic norepinephrine in the absence of adrenergic receptor binding and presynaptic vesicle exocytosis. These drugs enter the presynaptic terminals and displace stores of norepinephrine from storage vesicles (e.g., amphetamine and tyramine) or inhibit reuptake of catecholamine already released (e.g., cocaine and tricyclic antidepressants) (Box 10-3).[3] Indirect agents typically bind to the amine transport proteins (uptake-1 system) and interfere with uptake of endogenous catecholamines while facilitating reverse transport of cytoplasmic catecholamines into the synaptic cleft.[2] Indirect agents exhibit tachyphylaxis—that is, their effects diminish on repeated administration as the catecholamine pools become depleted. Tricyclic antidepressants principally interfere with norepinephrine and serotonin reuptake; dopamine reuptake is affected to a lesser degree (see Chapter 27). Amphetamine also can inhibit reuptake, whereas lithium facilitates reuptake. The MAO inhibitors block metabolism of biogenic amines (norepinephrine, serotonin, dopamine), increasing the synaptic concentration of these neurotransmitters (see Chapter 29). MAO inhibitors also act as indirect agents.

Direct-acting agents are agonists that produce their sympathomimetic effects by direct binding to and activation of α- or β-adrenergic receptors (e.g., norepinephrine, epinephrine, and isoproterenol) (see Box 10-3).[3] Mixed-acting agents (e.g., phenylpropanolamine, dopamine, and pseudoephedrine) produce sympathomimetic effects both directly and indirectly. For instance, phenylpropanolamine (PPA) is a direct agonist on α-adrenergic receptors but also acts indirectly to promote release of norepinephrine from sympathetic nerve terminals. The toxicity of PPA is characterized by hypertension and a reflex bradycardia. Ingestion of α_2-adrenergic agonists such as clonidine or other imidazolines (e.g., oxymetazoline and tetrahydrozoline) may

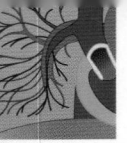

BOX 10-3   SYMPATHOMIMETICS

Direct Acting

α-Adrenergic Agonists
Norepinephrine
Metaraminol
Phenylephrine
Epinephrine
Midodrine
Dobutamine
Methoxamine
Ergot alkaloids

β-Adrenergic Agonists
Dobutamine
Epinephrine
Isoproterenol
Albuterol/levalbuterol/
 salbutamol
Metaproterenol
Pirbuterol
Bitolterol
Fenoterol
Formoterol
Salmeterol
Ritodrine
Ethylnorepinephrine
Prenalterol
Isoetharine
Terbutaline
Clenbuterol

Indirect Acting

Amphetamine
MAO inhibitors
Methylphenidate
Pemoline
Tricyclic antidepressants
Tramadol
Phencyclidine
Phenmetrazine
Tyramine
Propylhexedrine

Mixed Acting

Dopamine
Ephedrine
Phenylpropanolamine
Pseudoephedrine
Cocaine
Mephentermine

MAO, monoamine oxidase.
Data from Kandel ER, Schwartz JH, Jessel TM (eds): Principles of Neural Science, 3rd ed. New York, Elsevier Science, 1991; and Hoffman TT, Taylor P: Neurotransmission: the autonomic and somatic motor nervous systems. In Hardman JG, Limbird LE, Gilman AG (eds); Goodman & Gilman's The Pharmacological Basis of Therapeutics, 10th ed. New York, McGraw-Hill, 2001, pp 115-153.

produce a mixed clinical picture; stimulation of central α_2-adrenergic receptors in the brain decreases central sympathetic outflow, whereas stimulation of peripheral α_1-adrenergic receptors results in vasoconstriction and transient hypertension (see Chapter 62). Peripheral postsynaptic α-adrenergic antagonists (e.g., phenoxybenzamine, phentolamine, prazosin, hydralazine, and minoxidil) compete with endogenous catecholamines for binding to α_1- and α_2-adrenergic receptors. The α-adrenergic receptors (primarily α_1) also are blocked by tricyclic antidepressants (e.g., amitriptyline and imipramine), certain antipsychotic agents (e.g., phenothiazines, clozapine, and risperidone), antiarrhythmic agents (e.g., quinidine), and certain β blockers (e.g., labetalol and carvedilol). β Blockers primarily antagonize the effects of catecholamines at β-adrenergic receptors (see Chapter 60). β-Blocking drugs occupy β-adrenergic receptors and competitively block receptor occupancy by catecholamines and other β-adrenergic agonists. Most β-blocking drugs are pure antagonists; however, a few are partial agonists (e.g., pindolol and acebutolol) and may produce intrinsic sympathomimetic activity.

Similar to sympathomimetics, dopamine agonists can be direct, indirect, or mixed. Direct agonists bind to and activate various dopamine receptors directly, whereas indirect agents block dopamine uptake and/or stimulate presynaptic dopamine release. Direct dopamine receptor agonists include apomorphine, bromocriptine, fenoldopam, and pergolide. Indirect agonists include agents that cause dopamine release (e.g., benztropine, diphenhydramine, orphenadrine) and those that block dopamine reuptake (e.g., cocaine, amphetamines, methylphenidate, amantadine, benztropine, bupropion, diphenhydramine, and pemoline). Dopamine antagonists include specific receptor antagonists (e.g., antipsychotics, buspirone, metoclopramide, and amoxapine), agents that block synthesis (e.g., metyrosine), agents that prevent vesicle storage (e.g., reserpine and tetrabenazine) or cause dopamine depletion (e.g., α-methyldopa), or agents that destroy dopaminergic neurons (e.g., 1-methyl-4-phenyl-1,2,3,6-tetrahydropyridine (MPTP).[2]

Sympathomimetic toxicity often leads to CNS and cardiovascular complications. Cocaine (see Chapter 42) and amphetamines (see Chapter 44) produce their clinical effects predominantly from reuptake blockade and enhanced presynaptic release of catecholamines (e.g., norepinephrine and dopamine), serotonin, acetylcholine, and excitatory amino acids (e.g., aspartate and glutamate) from central and peripheral nerve terminals. Amphetamine and cocaine toxicity often includes psychostimulatory (e.g., euphoria, restlessness, excessive speech and motor activity, tremor, and insomnia) and sympathomimetic (e.g., tachycardia, hypertension, hyperthermia, and diaphoresis) effects. Intracerebral and subarachnoid hemorrhage may occur as a result of malignant hypertension and cerebral vasculitis. The actions of pemoline and methylphenidate are similar to those of amphetamine. Many of the phenylamphetamines and amphetamines may produce hallucinations. 5-Methoxy-3,4-methylenedioxyamphetamine (MMDA) can be formed in vivo from myristicin, present in the dried seeds of the nutmeg tree (*Myristica fragrans*) and can produce psychomimetic effects when consumed in large amounts. Mescaline is an alkaloid component of the peyote cactus and produces psychotomimetic activity by its amphetamine-like actions (see Chapter 45). Cathinone, cathine, and methcathinone, related natural alkaloids found in the leaves and stems of Catha edulis, or khat, produces effects indistinguishable from those of amphetamines. Ephedrine is both an α- and β-adrenergic agonist; in addition, it enhances release of norepinephrine from sympathetic neurons. It is a naturally occurring drug found in various species of the plant Ephedra (ma huang), indigenous to China.

Blockade of the nigrostriatal dopamine receptors (primarily D_2 receptors) produces extrapyramidal symptoms such as parkinsonism, akathisia, and dystonia (see Chapter 38). Cholinergic input to the caudate and putamen appears to be unaffected, with resultant cholinergic excess. Neuroleptics and drugs such as metoclopramide cause parkinsonism through such a mechanism. Chronic manganese poisoning damages the

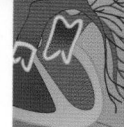

globus pallidus, leading to permanent neurologic damage.[17] "Manganese madness" is characterized by emotional lability, hallucinations, irritability, and aggressiveness (see Chapter 75). Carbon disulfide, a volatile, lipid-soluble industrial solvent, and carbon monoxide inhalation produce parkinsonian features owing to damage to the globus pallidus. Although acute carbon monoxide poisoning has a high mortality, a delayed extrapyramidal syndrome can develop in those who recover from the acute effects. Carbon monoxide produces symmetric necrosis of the globus pallidus with demyelination of the subcortical white matter.[18] Methanol poisoning produces optic atrophy and low-density lesions on computed tomography in the region of the putamen, and putaminal necrosis has been confirmed histologically.[19] A plant and fungal neurotoxin, 3-nitropropionic acid, found in mildewed sugar cane, is a succinate dehydrogenase inhibitor that produces basal ganglion injury.[20] In 1983, some intravenous drug abusers injected MPTP, a compound produced during illicit synthesis of a narcotic related to meperidine.[21] MPTP selectively destroys dopaminergic neurons in the substantia nigra, producing a condition indistinguishable from idiopathic Parkinson's disease. Treatment of these side effects attempts to re-establish the dopamine/acetylcholine balance required for smooth motor movements.

A central hyperexcitation syndrome with fever, delirium, and hypertension occurs when MAO inhibitors such as phenelzine, isocarboxazid, or tranylcypromine are coadministered with phenothiazines, tricyclic antidepressants, serotonergic reuptake inhibitors, and sympathomimetic amines (amphetamine, methamphetamine, ephedrine, phenylpropanolamine) (see Chapters 10A and 29). Sympathomimetic amines commonly are found in some nasal sprays, nose drops, and over-the-counter cold preparations. MAO in the gastrointestinal tract and liver prevents access to the general circulation of ingested, indirectly acting agents such as tyramine and phenylethylamine, contained in foods such as aged cheese, yeast, chicken liver, and pickled herring. However, individuals taking MAO inhibitors do not have this protection and can suffer severe hypertensive crises after eating a large amount of tyramine-containing food. An exaggerated response to the usual dose of meperidine also has been observed.

Neuroleptic malignant syndrome (NMS) is an uncommon but life-threatening disorder that occurs in those who are sensitive to the extrapyramidal effects of antipsychotics (see Chapters 10A and 38). However, it is important to consider the diagnosis of NMS in any patient who has recently received medications that affect CNS dopaminergic pathways. Lithium, carbamazepine, and cocaine may predispose patients to the development of NMS. The syndrome may begin from a few days to a few weeks after initiation or alteration of neuroleptic drug therapy. NMS is thought to be mediated by a reduction in D_2 dopaminergic activity in certain areas of the CNS (e.g., basal ganglia and hypothalamus).[22] Rigidity, catatonia, and fluctuating consciousness associated with autonomic hyperactivity, including hyperpyrexia, and elevated serum creatinine kinase concentrations are typical features of NMS.

The Serotonergic System

Serotonin (5-HT or 5-hydroxytryptamine) is an indolealkylamine that functions as a neurotransmitter in the CNS. 5-HT also is present in many cells outside the CNS. Peripherally, 5-HT has a major role in gastrointestinal motility and is involved in platelet aggregation. 5-HT does not cross the blood-brain barrier; thus, neurons must synthesize their own transmitters. L-Tryptophan readily crosses the blood-brain barrier and is taken up into serotonergic nerve terminals via an active transport process. Hydroxylation to 5-hydroxytryptophan (5-HTP) occurs by the enzyme tryptophan hydroxylase and the cofactor tetrahydrobiopterin. This is the rate-limiting step, because the enzyme tryptophan hydroxylase is not saturated under normal conditions. Diets high in L-tryptophan can result in increased synthesis of 5-HT in the CNS. The 5-HTP is decarboxylated by the nonspecific aromatic L-amino acid 5-HTP decarboxylase to 5-HT. The mechanism of sequestration of 5-HT in storage granules is similar to that of catecholamines. 5-HT is then packaged into storage vesicles that protect it from cytosolic degradation by MAO. It is released by an exocytotic mechanism and acts on both presynaptic and postsynaptic receptors. Serotonergic transmission is terminated primarily by reuptake of the amine by a specific 5-HT transporter. After reuptake, the free indolamine is either repackaged or metabolized by MAO and aldehyde dehydrogenase to 5-hydroxyindoleacetic acid.

Several serotonin receptors have been cloned and are identified as $5-HT_1$, $5-HT_2$, $5-HT_3$, $5-HT_4$, $5-HT_5$, $5-HT_6$, and $5-HT_7$. All 5-HT receptors interact with G proteins except $5-HT_3$ receptors; the latter are transmitter-gated ion channels. Within the $5-HT_1$ group there are subtypes $5-HT_{1A}$, $5-HT_{1B}$, $5-HT_{1D}$, $5-HT_{1E}$, and $5-HT_{1F}$. There are three $5-HT_2$ subtypes, $5-HT_{2A}$, $5-HT_{2B}$, and $5-HT_{2C}$, and two $5-HT_5$ subtypes, $5-HT_{5A}$ and $5-HT_{5B}$. Some serotonin receptors are presynaptic and others are postsynaptic.

Serotonin is involved in feeding, control of sleep and wakefulness, sexual behavior, mood and emotion, thermoregulation, circadian rhythmicity, drug-induced hallucinatory states, and neuroendocrine function in the CNS. It also serves as a precursor for the pineal hormone melatonin. Drugs that alter serotonin neurotransmission may have a wide array of clinical effects; the effects largely depend on the specific body area and serotonin receptor subtype affected.

Inhibition of 5-HT uptake has both an antidepressant and anxiolytic effect. Serotonin reuptake is blocked by some of the tricyclic antidepressants; however, the selective serotonin reuptake inhibitors (SSRIs), such as sertraline, fluoxetine, and venlafaxine, are more potent inhibitors of serotonin uptake than of norepinephrine and increase serotonin concentrations in the presynaptic cleft. Trazodone and nefazodone are weak cyclic antidepressants that weakly block 5-HT reuptake and antagonize $5-HT_2$ receptors. The antidepressant effects

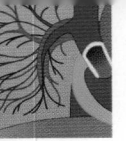

of MAO inhibitors are partly mediated by their prevention of 5-HT catabolism. Buspirone represents a new class of antianxiety agent whose anxiolytic action is related to agonism at the 5-HT_{1A} receptor in the brain. 3,4-Methylenedioxyamphetamine (MDMA ["Ecstasy"]), an amphetamine derivative, produces clinical effects primarily by causing the release of serotonin and blocking its reuptake. Other amphetamines and cocaine also promote 5-HT neuronal release and block reuptake. Certain opioids (e.g., dextromethorphan, meperidine) and psychotropics (e.g., amoxapine, tramadol) also inhibit 5-HT reuptake to produce effects.

Partial agonist activity at 5-HT_{2A} receptors mediates the psychedelic effects of central hallucinogens of the indoleamine (e.g., lysergic acid diethylamide [LSD] and psilocybin) and phenylethylamine (e.g., mescaline) class (see Chapter 45). LSD also has agonistic activity at 5-HT_{1A} and 5-HT_{1C} receptors. Lysergic acid, which is an agonist at many 5-HT receptors, is found in the seeds of several species of the morning glory family (*Rivea corymbosa, Ipomoea violacea*) and is produced by the fungus *Claviceps purpurea*, which grows on grain. The hallucinogenic mushrooms of the *Psilocybe* genus contain the thermostabile indole-alkylamine psilocybin and its dephosphorylated congener, psilocin. These substances are structurally related to serotonin and are about 100 times less potent than LSD. Bufotenin is the hallucinogenic indole derivative similar to serotonin found in cohoba snuff and in the skin and parotid glands of the toad *Bufo marinus*. Recently, new drugs of abuse have surfaced. 5-MeO-DIPT or "Foxy Methoxy" and alpha-methyltryptamine or AMT have similar hallucinogenic effects as psilocybin and are being seen at clubs in large metropolitan areas.[23] Metoclopramide and cisapride are 5-HT_4 receptor agonists that stimulate gut motility.[24]

Tryptophan hydroxylase can be blocked by *p*-chlorophenylalanine, thus decreasing the concentration of 5-HT. Drugs such as reserpine that disrupt the storage of catecholamines also impair the storage of 5-HT. Atypical neuroleptics (e.g., risperidone, clozapine), in contrast with conventional agents, strongly block serotonin 5-HT_2 receptors in the frontal cortex and striatal system in addition to their antagonism of adrenergic and dopamine receptors; antagonism at 5-HT_{2A} receptors produces independent antipsychotic effects and decreases the risk for developing extrapyramidal movement disorders (see Chapter 38). A new antipsychotic, aripiprazole, has partial agonist activity at both 5-HT_{1A} and 5-HT_{2A} receptors. Mirtazapine is an antidepressant that has numerous receptor effects; part of its activity is mediated by antagonism at 5-HT_2 and 5-HT_3 receptors. The antiemetic effects of ondansetron, granisetron, and metoclopramide are mediated through 5-HT_3 receptor antagonism, and agonists at 5-HT_{1D} and 5-HT_{1B} receptors such as sumatriptan are effective in treating migraine headaches.[24] Ergot alkaloids are nonspecific, partial 5-HT receptor agonists/antagonists. For instance, dihydroergotamine is thought to produce its antimigraine effects via agonist activity at 5-HT_{1B} and 5-HT_{1D} activity.[24] Methysergide produces its effects from 5-HT_1 and 5-HT_2 receptor antagonism. Like methysergide, cyproheptadine also is an antagonist at 5-HT_1 and 5-HT_2 receptors.

Concurrent use of two or more serotonergic drugs may result in a marked increase of serotonin in the synapses and may produce the "serotonin syndrome" (see Chapters 10A and 29).[25] This important pharmacodynamic interaction has been commonly reported when fluoxetine or one of the SSRIs is used in the presence of an MAO inhibitor. Moreover, other combinations seem just as capable of producing this syndrome. The SSRIs have been implicated in combination with tryptophan, dextromethorphan, and lithium.

Opioids

The term *opiate* was used originally to designate narcotic drugs derived from opium—that is, morphine and codeine and their many semisynthetic derivatives prepared from the seed capsules of the poppy *Papaver somniferum* (see Chapter 33). Later, the term *opioid* was coined to refer in a generic sense to all drugs, natural and synthetic, that have morphine-related actions, as well as to the endogenous peptides (e.g., dynorphin A, endorphin, enkephalin) later discovered to have such actions. Opioid receptors differ in their regional distribution in the CNS.[26] The opioids induce their biologic effects by interacting with three major classes of receptors, the δ, κ, and μ receptors. More recently an "orphan" receptor has been identified and named ORL (opioid receptor-like) because of a high degree of homology to the "classical" opioid receptors. The σ receptor, however, is no longer regarded as an opioid receptor.

Morphine and β-endorphin are potent μ receptor agonists, whereas the enkephalins are less potent. μ Receptors mediate supraspinal analgesia, respiratory depression, miosis, euphoria, and physical dependence. Most of the clinically used opiates such as morphine, methadone, and codeine selectively interact with the μ opioid receptor. Naloxone and naltrexone are more potent antagonists at μ receptors than at δ or κ receptors. The κ receptor mediates spinal analgesia and sedation but not respiratory depression. Agonists at the κ receptor are less addictive and do not produce respiratory depression as severely as do μ agonists. Tramadol is a centrally-acting, partial μ-opioid receptor agonist that is structurally similar to morphine. It also inhibits the uptake of norepinephrine and 5-HT, which suggests that its antinociceptive property is mediated by both opioid and nonopioid mechanisms.

The opioid receptors work by activation of G proteins, subsequent inhibition of adenyl cyclase, and activation of receptor-operated potassium channels or suppression of receptor-operated calcium channels.[27] Binding to the μ and δ receptors leads to opening of the potassium channel, whereas binding to κ sites results in closing of calcium channels. As a result, membrane hyperpolarization and neuronal suppression occurs. Opioid receptors function primarily by exerting inhibitory modulation of synaptic transmission in both the CNS

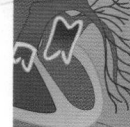

and the myenteric plexus. Often they are found on presynaptic nerve terminals, where their action results in decreased release of excitatory neurotransmitters. All three major receptor sites are involved in pain modulation. δ Receptors have been implicated in cardiovascular effects, whereas κ receptors seem to have a role in salt and water balance. Both μ and δ receptors mediate the decreased gastrointestinal motility effects observed with opioids. A given opioid drug may interact to a variable extent with all three types of receptors and can act as an agonist, a partial agonist, or an antagonist at each.

Opiates and opioids in overdose cause sedation and respiratory depression. Death usually is due to respiratory failure, generally as a result of apnea or pulmonary aspiration. The respiratory depression is complicated by bradycardia and hypotension. Pinpoint pupils usually are considered to be the classic sign of narcotic poisoning. Miosis is the result of μ and κ receptor activation, which results in an excitatory action on the parasympathetic nerve innervating the pupil. Normeperidine, the metabolite of meperidine, a synthetic opioid structurally different from morphine, is known to produce seizures on multiple dosing.[28] The neurotoxicity of normeperidine is manifested by signs of CNS stimulation that include tremors, twitching, myoclonus, and seizures. Treatment consists of administering benzodiazepines to reduce CNS excitation. Naloxone is contraindicated because it may increase the incidence of seizures. Propoxyphene causes delusions, hallucinations, and seizures, often with naloxone-resistant cardiodepression.

Opioid-associated depression of respiration and mental status can be reversed by administration of opioid antagonists. Most opioid antagonists compete for binding with agonists at the μ receptor and reverse the effects of endogenous or exogenous ligands by eliciting no postreceptor activity. Opioid receptor antagonists have variable potency and clinical half-lives; the dose administered also determines the duration of antagonist effects.[27] The half-life of naloxone is shorter than that of most opioids, and patients may again manifest signs of toxicity after the effect of naloxone wears off. Nalmefene is a new injectable methylene analogue of naltrexone with a half-life of about 11 hours, which is much longer than naloxone's half-life of 1 to 2 hours. Naltrexone is an opioid receptor antagonist with effects that last up to 48 hours after oral dosing.[27] Numerous synthetic agents have been developed that are partial agonist/antagonists (e.g., buprenorphine, pentazocine, butorphanol, meptazinol, and nalbuphine). Opioid reversal in opioid-dependent patients poses a risk of precipitating withdrawal symptoms. Reversal and withdrawal symptoms can be produced following the administration of either a pure antagonist or partial agonist/antagonist to the opiate-addicted or intoxicated patient.

The Cholinergic System

Acetylcholine is a neurotransmitter distributed throughout the CNS and peripheral nervous system (PNS). In the PNS, acetylcholine is found in somatic motor nerves, autonomic ganglia, all parasympathetic postganglionic nerves, and a small number of sympathetic postganglionic nerves. In the PNS, the action of acetylcholine is responsible for mediating parasympathetic nerve stimulation.

The enzyme choline acetyltransferase catalyzes the acetylation of choline by acetyl coenzyme A to form acetylcholine in the motor nerve terminals. Acetylcholine is sequestered in synaptic vesicles and is released when extracellular calcium enters the neuron after depolarization. The released acetylcholine diffuses through the synaptic cleft to interact with the cholinergic receptor. The action of acetylcholine is terminated by hydrolysis by acetylcholinesterase, which is present in high concentrations in the synapse. Metabolism produces acetate and choline, and the breakdown products are used for resynthesis of acetylcholine. The enzyme acetylcholinesterase is widely distributed throughout the body in both neuronal and non-neuronal tissues. It is known as *true* or *specific cholinesterase*, unlike pseudocholinesterase, which is made primarily in the liver and appears in plasma. It has a lower affinity for acetylcholine and metabolizes some drugs, including cocaine and succinylcholine.

Nicotinic and muscarinic receptors are the two major cholinergic receptors that mediate the effects of acetylcholine. Both nicotinic and muscarinic receptors are present in the brain, and their properties are similar to those of peripheral receptors. Five muscarinic receptors, glycoproteins designated M_1 through M_5, have been molecularly cloned and described. Many drugs with actions at peripheral cholinergic receptors are without central effects because they do not cross the blood-brain barrier. Peripheral nicotinic receptors are found in autonomic ganglia (postsynaptic neurons of both sympathetic and parasympathetic neurons) and the neuromuscular junction of skeletal muscles.[29] Peripheral muscarinic receptors are responsible for postganglionic parasympathetic neurotransmission; however, some sympathetic responses such as piloerection and sweating also are mediated through muscarinic receptors. Muscarinic receptors also are found in visceral smooth muscle, cardiac muscle, secretory glands, and the endothelial cells of the vasculature.

The muscarinic receptors belong to the family of the G protein–coupled receptor. The postsynaptic response initiated by acetylcholine binding to muscarinic receptors is varied and depends on receptor subtype. For instance, stimulation of M_1 and M_3 receptors results in hydrolysis of polyphosphoinositides and release of intracellular calcium.[30] In contrast, stimulation of M_2 and M_4 receptors is linked to adenyl cyclase inhibition and subsequent increased potassium efflux and membrane hyperpolarization. The decreased heart rate observed from vagus nerve stimulation is mediated by M_2 receptors.[30] Nicotinic receptors are part of a ligand-gated channel composed of five polypeptide subunits. Nicotinic neuronal receptors show ligand specificity distinct from receptors in the neuromuscular junction (NMJ). Stimulation of these nicotinic channels at the NMJ by acetylcholine results in sodium influx, membrane depolarization, and a triggered action potential. At some

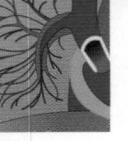

nicotinic receptors in the PNS and CNS, calcium influx may accompany sodium influx to generate postsynaptic excitatory potentials.

The cholinergic receptor agonists and the cholinesterase inhibitors comprise a large group of drugs that mimic the effects of acetylcholine. Direct cholinergic agonists are divided into esters of choline (e.g., acetylcholine and methacholine) and alkaloids (e.g., muscarine, nicotine, pilocarpine, bethanechol, and carbachol). Most cholinergic agonists bind to both muscarinic and nicotinic receptors, but a few are highly selective. Their spectrum of action depends on the receptor type stimulated—that is, muscarinic or nicotinic. The immediate peripheral clinical effects of excessive muscarinic stimulation include salivation, vomiting, diarrhea, sweating, cutaneous vaso-dilation, miosis, and bronchial vasoconstriction, whereas excessive nicotinic stimulation leads to muscle fascicu-lation, weakness, paralysis, hypertension, tachycardia, vomiting, and diarrhea (see Chapter 76). Central muscarinic agonist effects include sedation, coma, extrapyramidal movement disorders, and seizures. Central nicotinic agonist effects include seizures. Muscarinic antagonists block the actions of acetylcholine at muscarinic sites and block responses evoked by stimulation of parasympathetic nerves (see Chapter 39). At therapeutic doses, muscarinic antagonists do not bind to nicotinic receptors and neuromuscular blockers do not bind to muscarinic receptors. Ganglion blockers such as hexamethonium, mecamylamine, and trimethaphan block the action of acetylcholine and similar agonists at the nicotinic receptors of both parasympathetic and sympathetic ganglia. They are seldom used clinically.

Jimson weed (*Datura stramonium*) and deadly night-shade (*Atropa belladonna*) contain the alkaloids atropine, hyoscyamine, and hyoscine. These alkaloids also are found in other plants belonging to the Solanaceae family. These alkaloids are competitive muscarinic receptor antagonists and in toxic amounts produce the anticholinergic (antimuscarinic) syndrome charac-terized by hot dry skin, hyperthermia, hyperactivity, confusion, delirium and hallucinations, and eventually coma, respiratory depression, and cardiovascular collapse (see Chapter 39). Neuroleptics, tricyclic antidepressants, antiparkinson drugs, and certain antihistamines, skeletal muscle relaxants, and glaucoma medications also have antimuscarinic activity, and overdoses may mimic atropine poisoning. Physostigmine is used as an antidote in anticholinergic poisoning. It is a tertiary amine compound that crosses the blood-brain barrier and acts as a reversible inhibitor of acetylcholinesterase.

Direct-acting muscarinic receptor agonists such as pilocarpine and choline esters produce predictable signs of muscarinic excess when given in overdose. *Amanita muscaria* contains clinically insignificant amounts of muscarine, a cholinergic agonist, but mushrooms of the genera *Inocybe*, *Clitocybe*, and *Omphalotus* contain muscarine and usually are responsible if cholinergic symptoms dominate. Peripheral effects are recognized clinically as the "SLUDGE" phenomenon of salivation, lacrimation, urination, defecation, gastrointestinal

cramping, and emesis. All the effects are blocked by atropine and its congeners. Cholinesterase inhibitors are used as insecticides and nerve gas poisons (see Chapters 76 and 105A). Nerve agents are organophosphorus compounds that are similar to but much more potent than organophosphorus insecticides. They lead to accumulation of acetylcholine, with hyperactivity at both muscarinic and nicotinic receptors and stimulation of the CNS. Atropine blocks the action of excess acetylcholine primarily at muscarinic sites, decreasing secretions, bronchoconstriction, and intestinal motility. Oximes such as pralidoxime work by reactivating phosphorylated cholinesterase enzyme and protecting the enzyme from further inhibition. They act primarily at nicotinic sites with reversal of skeletal muscle weakness and should be used in conjunction with atropine. Pralidoxime's action on muscarinic symptoms is less pronounced than that of atropine. However, early administration of the oximes after poisoning is essential because nerve agents binding to the active site of acetylcholinesterase undergo a rapid process of "aging" (i.e., the chemical bond between the nerve agent and acetylcholinesterase becomes progressively resistant to deactivators, starting minutes after nerve agent poisoning). An "intermediate syndrome" has been described 1 to 4 days after the acute phase of organophosphate toxicity, presenting with sudden respiratory paralysis, cranial nerve palsy, and weakness of neck flexors and proximal limb muscles, but this may be related to inadequate pralidoxime therapy.[31,32] In addition, some organophos-phates such as tri-ortho-cresyl phosphate cause a peripheral neuropathy associated with axonal demyeli-nation that usually appears 2 to 3 weeks after exposure. Preceding cholinergic symptoms may be mild or even absent. These axonal effects are independent of cholinesterase inhibition and are due to inhibition of a second enzyme known as neuropathy target esterase.

Acetylcholine is also the neurotransmitter found at the NMJ. A number of biologic toxins produce effects at the NMJ. Cessation of toxic exposure usually results in complete recovery. A number of toxins disrupt neuromuscular transmission by altering the release of acetylcholine or by producing receptor blockade. The heat-labile neurotoxin botulinum produced by the anaerobic bacterium *Clostridium botulinum* produces muscle paralysis by preventing the release of acetyl-choline from nerve terminals (see Chapter 26). Venoms of snakes, such as the Mojave rattlesnake, impair neuromuscular transmission by postsynaptic receptor blockade, which may be irreversible or partially reversible, in addition to inhibiting acetylcholine release (see Chapter 21B).[33] The black widow spider (*Latrodectus mactans*) and some species of tarantula produce a venom (α-latrotoxin) that causes presynaptic release and depletion of acetylcholine from presynaptic vesicles through both calcium dependent and calcium inde-pendent mechanisms (see Chapter 22A).[34,35] Other arachnids that produce neurotoxins include ticks, funnel-web spiders, and scorpions. The funnel-web spider toxin (atraxotoxin) contains calcium channel inhibitors that can produce neuromuscular blockade. A

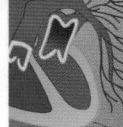

toxin found in the salivary glands of pregnant North American ticks (*Dermacentor andersoni* and *D. variabilis*) causes presynaptic block of acetylcholine release but can also affect conduction in small-diameter motor and sensory axons.[36] Removal of the tick often is curative, leading to complete clinical recovery. Drugs called *hemicholiniums* can block transmission at the neuromuscular junction by blocking the uptake of choline. Cholinesterase inhibitors such as the organophosphate compounds and carbamates inactivate acetylcholinesterase by phosphorylation, preventing acetylcholine degradation to produce a syndrome of cholinergic excess. Direct nicotinic receptor antagonists competitively block activity at the NMJ and result in weakness or muscle paralysis. NMJ blocking agents may block nicotinic receptors without activity (e.g., nondepolarizing) or may initially stimulate activity and subsequently block activity due to persistent binding (e.g., depolarizing blockade). Nondepolarizing agents include d-tubocurarine, atracurium, pancuronium, vecuronium, and rocuronium. Depolarizing blockers include succinylcholine and decamethonium. Many therapeutic drugs produce NMJ blockade by multiple presynaptic and postsynaptic actions. These agents include inhalational anesthetics (e.g., halothane, isoflurane), antibiotics (e.g., aminoglycosides, tetracyclines), magnesium salts, local anesthetics (e.g., lidocaine), corticosteroids, and calcium channel blockers.[37]

The sodium channel of cholinergic neurons is the target of several potent poisons. Venoms of the *Centruroides* genus of scorpions of Arizona and Mexico and *Leiurus quinquestriatus* are neurotoxic (see Chapter 22B). They affect sodium channels with resultant prolongation of action potentials as well a spontaneous depolarization of nerves of both the adrenergic and parasympathetic nervous systems. Tetrodotoxin found in the puffer fish species, suborder Tetraodontoidea, selectively blocks fast sodium channels in nerves and muscle membranes (see Chapter 25). It is found in fish (Echinodermata), the California newt (*Taricha*), blue-ringed octopus (*Hapalochlaena maculosa*), frogs (*Atelopus*), and marine bacteria. Tetrodotoxin relaxes vascular smooth muscle and blocks preganglionic cholinergic motor, sensory, and sympathetic neurotransmission. Saxitoxin, produced by the dinoflagellate *Protogonyaulax catenella* and by some bacteria, is found in plankton-eating shellfish (clams, oysters, mussels, scallops) and has an action similar to that of tetrodotoxin. Ciguatoxin, a toxin elaborated by the dinoflagellate *Gambierdiscus toxicus*, enhances quantal acetylcholine release at the neuromuscular junction by prolonging the duration of sodium channel opening. Batrachotoxin, found in the skin of a South American frog (*Phyllobates aurotaenia*), and the plant alkaloids aconitine and veratridine prevent closure or inactivation of voltage-dependent sodium channels. A second important class of sodium channel blockers includes local anesthetics such as lidocaine and related antiarrhythmic agents. This quinidine-like membrane-stabilizing effect is shared with the tricyclic antidepressants and is responsible for the cardiotoxicity. Potassium channel blockers such as 4-aminopyridine are convulsants, and polypeptide toxins from scorpion (charybdotoxin), bee (apamin), or snake (dendrotoxin) venoms also interfere with potassium channel activity.

The Histaminergic System

The histaminergic system functions in the regulation of arousal, body temperature, locomotor activity, analgesia, regulation of biologic rhythms, feeding, drinking, and vascular dynamics.[38] Many of the psychotropic drugs interact with histamine receptors.

Histamine in the brain is formed from L-histidine by decarboxylation by histidine and L-amino acid decarboxylase. Unlike with the monoamines and amino acid transmitters, there does not appear to be an active reuptake process for histamine after its release. Histamine is metabolically inactivated by histamine methyltransferase.

Histamine receptors are divided into four subtypes, H_1, H_2, H_3, and H_4, and belong to the family of G protein-coupled receptors. H_1 receptor agonism leads to activation of phospholipase C, formation of diacylglycerol and inositol-1,4,5-triphosphate and subsequent activation of protein kinases, phospholipase A_2, and release of intracellular calcium.[39] H_1 receptors are found in the smooth muscle of the intestines, bronchi, and blood vessels. H_1 receptor activation results in smooth muscle contraction in these organ systems. H_2 receptor agonism leads to activation of adenyl cyclase, increased cAMP, and activation of protein kinases.[39] H_2 receptors are found in gastric parietal cells and in the vascular system and CNS. H_2 receptor activation leads to gastric acid secretion and vascular smooth muscle relaxation. Activation of H_1 receptors on vascular endothelial cells also results in vascular smooth muscle relaxation (vasodilation). Activation of H_1 receptors on vascular endothelial cells leads to local production of nitric oxide or endothelial-derived relaxing factor and prostacyclin (PGI_2), both potent mediators of vasodilation.[39] H_3 receptors are found in the brain and the periphery and regulate histamine release. Recent evidence suggests that the H_3 receptor regulates the release of several important neurotransmitters (e.g., acetylcholine, dopamine, GABA, norepinephrine, serotonin), in both the PNS and CNS. The H_4 receptor is highly expressed in peripheral blood leukocytes and intestinal tissue.

Antihistamines (see Chapter 39) are related structurally to histamine and competitively antagonize the effects of histamine on H_1 and H_2 receptor sites. H_1 receptor antagonists block the bronchoconstrictive, large vessel vasoconstrictive, small vessel vasodilatory, enhanced gut motility, and increased permeability effects of histamine. H_2 receptor antagonists block gastric acid secretory and vasodilatory effects of histamine. Many first-generation H_1 receptor antagonists (e.g., diphenhydramine and pyrilamine) also possess anticholinergic effects, and the major signs of acute overdose are similar to those caused by classic antimuscarinic agents and are treated accordingly. They also may stimulate or depress the CNS, and some agents such as diphenhydramine possess local anesthetic and membrane-depressant effects when they are taken in large doses.

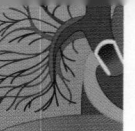

The Glutaminergic System

Amino acids found in the brain can function as neurotransmitters and be either excitatory or inhibitory. Glutamic acid and aspartic acid are excitatory, and the main inhibitory transmitters are GABA and glycine.

Glutamates are present in high concentration in the CNS. They do not cross the blood-brain barrier and are synthesized from glucose, glutamine, aspartate, and other precursors. The synthesis of glutamate is mediated by the enzyme glutamate dehydrogenase. Glutamate is released from nerve terminals by a calcium-dependent exocytosis mechanism similar to other neurotransmitters. Glutamate is inactivated by reuptake; several uptake transporters remove glutamate from the synaptic cleft into both neuronal and glial cells. Glutamate that is taken up into glial cells is oxidized through the Krebs cycle or converted to glutamine by the enzyme glutamine synthetase. Glutamine subsequently is released back into the synapse and then recycled back into the nerve terminal to be converted to glutamate. Glutamate is stored in vesicles for subsequent release.

Receptors for glutamate have a wide distribution in the CNS and are present on neurons that receive input from other neurotransmitter systems.[40] Glutamate receptors convey most of the fast excitatory neurotransmission in the CNS and act through both *ligand-gated ion channels* (ionotropic) and G protein–coupled receptors (metabotropic). The ionotropic glutamate receptors are named after the agonists kainate, AMPA, and NMDA. The AMPA and the kainate receptor are collectively known as the non-NMDA receptor.[41] The non-NMDA receptors predominantly mediate sodium influx with activation, whereas NMDA receptor activation primarily promotes calcium ion influx. These channels also allow sodium ion influx and potassium ion efflux with activation. Metabotropic glutamate (mGlu) receptors are G protein–coupled receptors that have been subdivided into three groups, based on sequence similarity, pharmacology, and intracellular signaling mechanisms. These receptors may be excitatory or inhibitory to postsynaptic membranes. When excitatory, activation of the receptor often is associated with impaired potassium ion efflux. When inhibitory, activation of the receptor often is associated with enhanced potassium ion efflux.

At least five distinct sites of pharmacologic or regulatory significance have been identified on the NMDA receptor.[42] There are two different agonist recognition sites for glutamate and glycine: a polyamine regulatory site that promotes receptor activation, and separate recognition sites for magnesium and zinc that act to inhibit flux through agonist-bound receptors. The NMDA receptor requires simultaneous binding of glutamate and glycine for activation.[43] They are known as coagonists because neither glycine nor glutamate alone can open the channel. The glycine site on the NMDA receptor is pharmacologically distinct from the classic spinal inhibitory glycine receptor in that it is not blocked by strychnine. Polyamines such as spermine and spermidine increase the ability of glutamate and glycine

to open ion channels by binding on their modulatory sites.[44] Thus, glutamate, glycine, and certain polyamines act in concert to open NMDA ion channels. Zinc and magnesium are endogenous blockers of the NMDA receptor and bind to different receptor sites. Magnesium, unlike zinc, exerts a voltage-dependent block on the open ion channel. Other voltage-dependent blockers of the NMDA receptor channels include dizocilpine (MK-801), phencyclidine, ketamine, and dextrorphan. Ethanol acts as an allosteric inhibitor at the NMDA receptor, and it is suggested that the behavioral disinhibition produced by ethanol is mediated by an action on the NMDA receptor and that the ataxia, somnolence, and CNS depression are mediated through other receptors.[45] Acute alcohol withdrawal is accompanied by excessive NMDA activity and is thought to explain some of the characteristic agitation, hallucinations, and convulsions.[46]

AMPA receptors are widely distributed in the CNS, and in the absence of other excitatory activity, AMPA receptors may mediate fast depolarizing responses at most excitatory synapses in the CNS. Kainate receptors activate neuronal membrane channels that are distinguishable from those associated with NMDA and AMPA receptors on the basis of their conductance and desensitization properties. Distinct kainate receptors are involved in some neuropathologic events mediated by excitatory amino acids in the CNS.

Glutamate receptors may have a role in acute neuronal death in response to various insults to the nervous system, including anoxia, hypoglycemia, seizures, and mechanical trauma. The non-NMDA receptors also may be involved in neuropathologic processes. Glutamate receptor activation can cause seizures, and excitatory amino acid receptor antagonists may be of primary value for the treatment of epilepsy. Postischemic neuronal damage is attributed in part to overactivity of the excitatory amino acid neurotransmitter systems. Elevated extracellular glutamate levels result in glutamate receptor–mediated increase in postsynaptic intracellular calcium levels. Excitotoxicity, the "excitation to death" of neurons, results mainly from the intracellular calcium increase subsequent to overexcitation of neurons. This translocation of calcium leads to a cascade of events with formation of free radicals, activation of nitric oxide synthetase, and cell death. Nitric oxide is produced after stimulation of the enzyme nitric oxide synthetase. Nitric oxide is a novel neuronal messenger that acts with surrounding neurons, not by synaptic transmission but by diffusion between cells. In excess, nitric oxide is toxic to neurons. This toxicity is mediated largely by an interaction with the superoxide anion, presumably through the generation of the oxidant peroxynitrite. This cascade can be halted by administration of NMDA receptor antagonists.[47] Studies show that NMDA antagonists are more effective in reducing penumbral damage after cerebral arterial occlusion. Chronic neurodegenerative disorders such as olivopontocerebellar atrophy and Huntington's chorea are associated with disorders of excitatory amino acid transmission, as is amyotrophic lateral sclerosis. The role that NMDA receptors play in ischemic and nonischemic

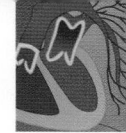

neurotoxicity is not completely understood and under investigation.

Domoic acid was identified as the toxin in a major outbreak of food poisoning in Canada in 1987.[48] The alga *Nitzschia pungens* was found to be the source of the toxin, which contaminated blue mussels. Domoic acid is a glutamate analogue and produces neurotoxicity by overstimulation of the glutaminergic system. Dietary consumption of the chickling (not chick) pea *Lathyrus sativus* or other potentially neurotoxic *Lathyrus* species is associated with lathyrism characterized by spastic paraparesis. The offending agent in the pea is thought to be β-N-oxalyl-amino-L-alanine (BOAA). The cycad *Cycas circinalis* has a BOAA-like constituent, β-N-methylamino-L-alanine (BMAA), and may be the cause of the motor neuron disease that occurs in Guam. Phencyclidine and ketamine are known as *dissociative anesthetics* because they produce a feeling of being apart from one's environment. They are antagonists at the N-methyl-D-aspartate subtype of the glutamate receptor and act by blocking the ion channel (see Chapter 43). The primary antiepileptic action of felbamate is believed to be at the strychnine-insensitive glycine binding site at the NMDA receptor. It is shown also to weakly potentiate GABA receptor binding. Lamotrigine, another antiepileptic drug, is thought to act by inhibiting the release of glutamate. Nimodipine inhibits release of glutamate by blockade of voltage-gated calcium channels.

The GABAergic and Glycinergic Systems

The amino acids GABA and glycine are the primary inhibitory neurotransmitters that mediate fast postsynaptic inhibition in the nervous system. Their action is to bind specifically to GABA and glycine receptors, respectively.

Glucose is the principal precursor for GABA production, although glutamate, pyruvate, and other amino acids can act as precursors. Glutamic acid is formed from the transamination of α-ketoglutarate, formed from glucose metabolism in the Krebs cycle by GABA α-oxoglutarate transaminase. Glutamic acid decarboxylase catalyzes the decarboxylation of glutamic acid to form GABA. The cofactor is pyridoxal phosphate. Pyridoxal phosphate is synthesized from pyridoxine (vitamin B_6) by the enzyme pyridoxine kinase. The action of GABA released into the synaptic cleft is inactivated by a high-affinity, sodium-dependent uptake process. Enzymatic breakdown entails transamination to succinic semialdehyde by GABA transaminase. The next step is oxidation to succinic acid by succinic semi-aldehyde dehydrogenase, with the succinic acid then entering the Krebs cycle.

GABA receptors predominate in the brain, where they have a widespread distribution.[49] Three types of receptors for GABA have been characterized. $GABA_A$ receptors open chloride channels, causing hyperpolarization and inhibition of the recipient neuronal cell. $GABA_A$ receptors are multimembered, with five subunits assembled into a functional complex. The five major binding sites are for GABA, benzodiazepines, barbiturates, picrotoxin, and the anesthetic steroid.

These binding domains serve to modulate the receptors to GABA stimulation. The binding of GABA is enhanced by benzodiazepines, barbiturates, certain steroids, etomidate, propofol, chloral hydrate, meprobamate, ethanol, and zolpidem (see Chapters 34, 35, and 36); these agents serve as indirect receptor agonists. The binding of GABA is inhibited indirectly by flumazenil, penicillins, aztreonam, MAO inhibitors, tricyclic antidepressants, maprotiline, amoxapine, and organochlorine insecticides. $GABA_B$ receptors belong to the G protein–coupled receptor superfamily. Activation of $GABA_B$ receptors results in presynaptic inhibition by impairing calcium ion influx and neurotransmitter release or postsynaptic inhibition by increasing potassium ion efflux and cellular hyperpolarization. $GABA_B$ receptors are activated by baclofen and γ-hydroxybutyrate (GHB) and antagonized by phaclofen and saclofen (see Chapters 37 and 46). $GABA_C$ receptors are the newly identified member of the GABA receptor family. They are also linked to chloride channels, with distinct physiologic and pharmacologic properties. In contrast with the fast and transient responses elicited from $GABA_A$ receptors, $GABA_C$ receptors mediate slow and sustained responses. Pharmacologically, $GABA_C$ receptors are bicuculline- and baclofen-insensitive, and they are not modulated by many $GABA_A$ receptor modulators (such as benzodiazepines and barbiturates).

A number of agonists bind to the binding site and elicit GABA-like responses. Muscimol is a naturally occurring GABA analogue isolated from the hallucinogenic mushrooms *A. muscaria* and *A. pantherina* that acts as a potent, direct receptor agonist (see Chapter 23).[50] Benzodiazepines enhance GABAergic transmission indirectly. Benzodiazepine binding results in an increased affinity of GABA for its receptor and an increased frequency of chloride channel opening (see Chapter 35).[49] A wide variety of nonbenzodiazepines, such as β-carbolines, cyclopyrrolones (zopiclone), and imidazopyridines (zolpidem), also bind to the benzodiazepine site to enhance GABAergic transmission.[51] Pure benzodiazepine overdoses usually are not fatal. However, the newer, short-acting agents may increase greatly the frequency of complication, especially when benzodiazepines are combined with other CNS depressant drugs and alcohol. The benzodiazepine antagonist flumazenil is one of several 1,4-benzodiazepine derivatives that binds with high affinity to the benzodiazepine receptor and acts as a competitive antagonist at this receptor. Thus, flumazenil is an indirect $GABA_A$ antagonist. Caution in flumazenil administration is warranted in mixed overdoses, when benzodiazepine may provide a neuroprotective or cardioprotective action.

Barbiturates facilitate GABA-mediated synaptic transmission by increasing the duration of chloride channel opening with GABA binding (see Chapter 36).[49,52] At pharmacologic concentrations, some barbiturates (e.g., pentobarbital) are known to allosterically increase binding of benzodiazepine and GABA to their binding sites. At high concentrations, certain barbiturates (e.g., pentobarbital) act as direct agonists and directly open

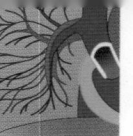

chloride channels.[52] The allosteric regulation of GABA$_A$ receptor function by neuroactive steroids is well known, and the steroid recognition site provides a potentially important target in the development of new therapeutic agents.[53] General anesthetics, including barbiturates, volatile gases, steroids, and alcohols, enhance GABA-mediated chloride conductance.[54] Gabapentin, an amino acid structurally related to GABA, is being used currently in the treatment of epilepsy. Gabapentin appears to have GABA-mimetic properties; it may increase GABA concentrations by stimulating glutamic acid decarboxylase, the enzyme that produces GABA from glutamate (see Chapter 40). The anticonvulsant valproic acid is an indirect GABA agonist; it increases GABA concentrations by increasing activity of glutamic acid decarboxylase and inhibiting GABA transaminase and succinic semialdehyde dehydrogenase, enzymes that degrade GABA. Vigabatrin (γ-vinyl-GABA), an anti-epileptic, is an irreversible inhibitor of GABA transaminase and increases GABA concentration. Topiramate and tiagabine, both anticonvulsants, are indirect GABA agonists. Alcohol is known to augment GABA-mediated chloride flux, and ethanol may exert some of its effect by enhancing the function of the GABA receptor.[55]

Bicuculline, a plant alkaloid, is a competitive GABA antagonist and is selective for the GABA$_A$ receptor that controls chloride permeability. Picrotoxin found in the berries of the shrub *Anamirta cocculus* is a GABA$_A$ receptor channel blocker. The active principle picrotoxin works on the gating process of the channel. Penicillin is a chloride channel blocker with a net negative charge that occludes the chloride channel by interacting with the positively charged amino acid residues within the channel pore. Pyridoxal phosphate antagonists such as isoniazid and other hydrazines, such as monomethyl-hydrazine in the mushroom *Gyromitra (Helvella) esculenta*, produce seizures by impairing GABA synthesis (see Chapter 23).[56] Intravenous pyridoxine is used to combat the toxicity. Cyanide inhibits glutamic acid decarboxylase, thereby decreasing GABA, and it may partly account for seizures occurring in cyanide toxicity.[57] The chlorinated hydrocarbons inhibit the action of GABA by binding to the picrotoxin site on the GABA$_A$ receptor to produce seizures.[58] Baclofen is an orally active GABA-mimetic agent and acts as a GABA$_B$ agonist.[59] It causes hyperpolarization by increasing potassium conductance and has presynaptic inhibitory functions. Baclofen in an overdose produces drowsiness, coma, seizures, respiratory depression, and arrhythmias (see Chapter 37). The sedative/hypnotic effect of GHB is mediated by GABA$_B$ receptor and specific GHB receptor agonism (see Chapter 46). Similarly, the sedative/hypnotic effects of γ-butyrolactone and 1,4-butanediol, which both are readily bioconverted to GHB, are mediated by these receptors.

Glycine is another inhibitory neurotransmitter that mediates fast postsynaptic inhibition in the nervous system. Like GABA$_A$, the postsynaptic glycine receptor is linked to a chloride channel. Activation of the glycine receptor causes chloride channel opening, hyper-polarization of the postsynaptic membrane, and inhibition of neuronal firing.[60] The glycine receptors are predominantly found in the spinal cord and the brainstem. Glycine also is likely the inhibitory neurotransmitter in the reticular formation. Glycine is present in the forebrain, where it functions as a coagonist of the NMDA glutamate receptor. At this receptor, glycine promotes the actions of glutamate, the major excitatory neurotransmitter in the CNS. The pharmacology of the glycine receptor is known less extensively than that of the GABA receptors. They are defined by their antagonism by the convulsive alkaloid, strychnine, in contrast to the strychnine-insensitive glycine-binding site that is associated with the excitatory NMDA subclass of the glutamate receptor. This explains why strychnine's effect is localized to the medulla and spinal cord only.

Strychnine, an alkaloid found in the seeds of the tree *Strychnos nux-vomica*, increases the level of neuronal excitability by selective antagonism at glycine receptors (see Chapter 24). The clinical picture simulates that of generalized seizures and is characterized by diffuse skeletal muscle contraction, muscular rigidity, opisthotonus, trismus, rhabdomyolysis, myoglobinuria, and acute respiratory and renal failure. Strychnine is used primarily as a rodenticide and is found sometimes as an adulterant in illicit drugs such as cocaine or heroin. Barbiturates and diazepam are effective antagonists of strychnine. *Calycanthus* species (Carolina allspice) contain the strychnine-like toxin calycanthine, which may produce convulsions. Tetanus toxin inhibits the release of glycine from nerve endings in the brainstem and spinal cord.

TOXICITY SPECIFIC TO THE PERIPHERAL NERVOUS SYSTEM

Neurotoxins almost invariably produce polyneuropathy and rarely are implicated in focal neuropathy. Neurologic dysfunction usually occurs as part of a systemic toxicity.[61] The neurotoxicity may occur in isolation, however, and then need to be differentiated from other nontoxic causes of neuropathies. The development of a neuropathy is directly related to continued exposure to a particular toxin. The neuropathy often improves when the exposure is discontinued. If the neuropathy progresses after removal of a suspected toxin, then other causes should be considered (Box 10-4).

Diseases of the peripheral nervous system can be classified in two ways. The first categorization depends on the distribution: focal, multifocal, diffuse, proximal, distal, symmetric, or segmental. The second system depends on the anatomic location of the pathologic process: muscle, neuromuscular junction, or peripheral nerve. Further differentiation is based on involvement of the neuron, axon, or myelin.

Symmetric Generalized Neuropathies

The most common form of drug- or toxin-induced neuropathy is a symmetric distal axonopathy. The neuropathy reflects failure of axonal transport and begins distally, where the axons are most vulnerable, and

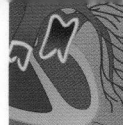

BOX 10-4	CHARACTERISTIC FEATURES OF TOXIC NEUROPATHY

Consistent pattern of neurologic dysfunction
Reproducible pathophysiologic or pathologic findings
Temporal relationship between exposure and onset of the clinical finding
Nonfocal disorder
Neurotoxicity improves with cessation of exposure

predominantly affects long and large-diameter axons, progressing proximally. Axonopathies usually have a subacute onset with gradual progression and clinically are reflected by a symmetric, distal, diffuse, stocking and glove–type sensorimotor loss. Sensory signs and symptoms initially predominate over motor deficits. Withdrawal of the toxic insult is necessary for recovery, which often is prolonged and slow. Axonal regeneration occurs at a rate of 2 mm/day, with recovery in an order reverse to that of the initial loss (i.e., proximal before distal).

Demyelinating neuropathy is characterized by lesions that occur in the myelin sheath or Schwann cells. The axons usually are spared. The onset usually is subacute, and the involvement in myelinopathy, unlike in axonopathy, is predominantly distal and motor because the heavily myelinated large motor fibers are more severely affected than the small-diameter myelinated and unmyelinated sensory fibers. The demyelination may be patchy, however, with early proximal involvement. Areflexia is characteristic, and sensory symptoms are minimal. Recovery from a myelinopathy usually is rapid, early, and complete when compared with that from an axonopathy. The buckthorn toxin, found in high concentrations in the endocarp of the fruit of *Karwinskia humboldtiana*, and perhexiline are the few toxins causing a peripheral myelinopathy.

Toxic injury to the cell body directly is termed a *neuropathy*. The dorsal root ganglions are especially involved. This vulnerability is because of a poorly formed nerve-blood barrier and the fenestrated blood vessels with increased vascular perfusion. Neuronopathies rarely are the cause of toxic insults. Neuronopathies are characterized by the rapid or subacute onset of motor or sensory deficits. The neurologic defect mirrors the nerve root involved and can occur anywhere. Recovery is variable and often incomplete because of incomplete neuronal recovery. Toxic neuronopathies can be caused by mercury, pyridoxine, and doxorubicin.

Acute and chronic heavy metal exposure may produce neuropathies. Metal compounds tend to be stored in bones, from where they may be gradually released into the circulation, subsequently delaying recovery time. Other system (i.e., hematopoietic, renal, and gastrointestinal) dysfunctions usually accompany the neuropathy. Arsenic produces a generalized axonal peripheral neuropathy with predominant sensory involvement (see Chapter 74). Symptoms of toxicity usually appear 5 to 10 days after ingestion, with painful dysesthesias and numbness in the feet and hands. Arsenic reacts with the sulfhydryl groups on various enzymes necessary for cellular metabolism. Both inorganic and organic lead is neurotoxic. Lead intoxication produces a demyelinating neuropathy with predominantly motor involvement (see Chapter 73). Lead intoxication in children, unlike that in adults, may produce an encephalopathy rather than a peripheral neuropathy. Mercury exposure causes a subacute, diffuse, predominantly motor neuropathy (see Chapter 71). Thallium compounds have been used as rodenticides, and toxicity produces an axonal neuropathy with prominent systemic features that include alopecia and autonomic dysfunction (see Chapter 75). Aluminum has been implicated in the causation of dialysis encephalopathy, a progressive acute syndrome found in patients undergoing dialysis (see Chapter 75).

A number of organic compounds also produce neuropathies. The rodenticide Vacor causes a severe, rapid-onset distal axonopathy with associated autonomic dysfunction and diabetes mellitus due to necrosis of pancreatic β cells (see Chapter 79).[62] The neuropathy can be prevented by nicotinamide, and Vacor may inhibit nicotinamide dinucleotide–dependent enzyme with disruption of an axonal-dependent process. Peripheral neurotoxic organic solvents include *n*-hexane and methyl-*N*-butyl ketone, carbon disulfide, and trichlorethylene.[63] *n*-Hexane and methyl-*N*-butyl ketone are metabolized to 2,5-hexanedione, the active agent that damages the peripheral nerves. Methyl ethyl ketone enhances the neurotoxic effects of *n*-hexane and methyl-*N*-butyl ketone without itself being neurotoxic. Trichloroethylene may cause trigeminal neuropathy through its breakdown product, dichloroacetylene. Allyl chloride, used in the manufacture of epoxy resin, produces a characteristic distal axonopathy with sensory loss and loss of ankle jerks. Acrylamide monomer, unlike its polymer, is neurotoxic and produces a distal axonopathy involving large myelinated fibers. Ethylene oxide, commonly used as a sterilizing agent, produces a distal sensorimotor axonopathy with numbness, weakness, and areflexia (see Chapter 80). Residual ethylene oxide in dialysis tubing after the sterilization process may contribute to peripheral neuropathy in patients undergoing long-term hemodialysis.[64] Methyl bromide exposure causes a distal symmetric axonopathy with involvement of the pyramidal tracts and cerebellum. Polychlorinated biphenyls have been associated with outbreaks of neuropathy when cooking oil has been contaminated with tetrachlorobiphenyl (Table 10-1).[65]

CONCLUSION

An exciting future lies ahead in neurotoxicology. The knowledge of normal brain physiology and its response to insult has grown tremendously. The number of new antidepressants has greatly increased. Clinical trials of drugs that treat ischemic and traumatic brain injury are under way. The results of these studies will further expand the understanding of neurotoxicity and lead to the development of better therapies.

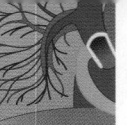

TABLE 10-1 Selected Neurotoxins That Produce Neuropathy

TOXINS	EXPOSURE RISK	PATHOLOGIC FINDING	CLINICAL FEATURES
Arsenic	Metallurgy, pesticides, wood preservatives, pigments, ant stakes, weed killers	Axonopathy (S > M)	GI distress, psychosis, hyperkeratosis, hyperpigmentation, Mees' lines, anemia
Lead	Lead production, solders, batteries, pigment, insecticides, auto radiators, moonshine, construction workers, folk medicine (*azarcon* and *greta*)	Axonopathy (M > S)	GI distress, microcytic anemia, basophilic stippling, encephalopathy, acute tubular dysfunction, gout, hyperuricemia
Mercury	Gold and silver extraction, dental amalgams, fungicides, environmental contamination, thermometers	Axonopathy (M > S)	GI distress, tremor, ataxia, gingivostomatitis, neuropsychiatric disturbances
Thallium	Manufacture of optical lenses, photoelectric cells, and costume jewelry; rodenticide	Axonopathy (M > S)	GI distress, delirium, seizures, coma, alopecia, choreoathetosis, ataxia, tremor, Mees' lines
Carbon disulfide	Insecticides, rayon fiber production	Axonopathy (MS)	Encephalopathy, parkinsonian syndromes, nystagmus, psychosis
Acrylamide	Production of acrylamide resins	Axonopathy (MS)	Irritant, contact dermatitis, ataxia
Allyl chloride	Epoxy resin and glycerin production	Axonopathy (S > M)	Irritant, pulmonary edema
Ethylene oxide	Sterilizing agent, solvent, plasticizer, chemical intermediate	Axonopathy (MS)	Convulsions, arrhythmias, leukemia
Hexacarbons (e.g., hexane)	Solvents	Axonopathy (SM)	GI dysfunction, hyperhidrosis, autonomic dysfunction
Methyl bromide	Insecticidal fumigant, fire extinguisher ingredient	Axonopathy (MS)	Irritant, dermatitis, tremor, seizure, coma, dementia, psychosis, extrapyramidal symptoms
Trichloroethylene	Typewriter correction fluid, insecticides, spot removers, paint removers	Myelinopathy	Extrapyramidal dysfunction, degreaser's flush
Polychlorinated biphenyls (PCBs)	High-temperature insulators, transformers, carbonless copy papers	Myelinopathy	Chloracne, hepatic transaminitis, porphyria
Organophosphates	Pesticides	Axonopathy (M > S)	Cholinergic symptoms, agitation, seizures, coma
Vacor (PNU)	Rodenticides	Axonopathy (M > S)	Nausea, vomiting, autonomic dysfunction, insulin-dependent diabetes mellitus

GI, gastrointestinal; M, motor; S, sensory.

REFERENCES

1. Kandel ER, Schwartz JH, Jessel TM (eds): Principles of Neural Science, 3rd ed. New York, Elsevier Science, 1991.
2. Hoffman TT, Taylor P: Neurotransmission: the autonomic and somatic motor nervous systems. In Hardman JG, Limbrid LE, Gilman AG (eds): Goodman & Gilman's The Pharmacological Basis of Therapeutics, 10th ed. New York, McGraw-Hill, 2001, pp 115–153.
3. Hoffman BB: Catecholamines, sympathomimetic drugs, and adrenergic receptor antagonists. In Hardman JG, Limbrid LE, Gilman AG (eds): Goodman & Gilman's The Pharmacological Basis of Therapeutics, 10th ed. New York, McGraw-Hill, 2001, pp 1215–1268.
4. Bourne HR, Sanders DA, McCormick F: The GTPase superfamily: conserved structure and molecular mechanism. Nature 1991; 349:117–129.
5. Palmer TM, Stiles GL: Adenosine receptor. Neuropharmacology 1995;34:683–694.
6. Clark M, Post RM: Carbamazepine, but not caffeine, is highly selective for adenosine A1 binding sites. Eur J Pharmacol 1989;164:399–401.
7. Eldridge FL, Paydarfar D, Scott C, et al: Role of endogenous adenosine in recurrent generalized seizures. Exp Neurol 1989;103:179–185.
8. Shannon MW, Maher TJ: Anticonvulsant effects of intracerebroventricular adenosine in theophylline-induced seizures. Vet Hum Toxicol 1994;36:350.
9. Blake KV, Massey KL, Hendes L, et al: Relative efficacy of phenytoin and phenobarbital for the prevention of theophylline-induced seizures in mice. Ann Emerg Med 1988;17:1024–1028.
10. Phyllis JW, O'Regan MH: The role of adenosine in the central actions of the benzodiazepines. Prog Neuropsychopharmacol Biol Psychiatry 1988;12:389–404.
11. Mackenzie AB, Suprenant A, North AB: Functional and molecular diversity of purinergic ion channel receptors. Ann NY Acad Sci 1999;868:716–729.
12. Molinoff PB, Axelrod J: Biochemistry of catecholamines. Annu Rev Biochem 1971;40:465–500.
13. Caron MG, Lefkowitz RJ: Catecholamines receptors: structure, function, and regulation. Recent Prog Horm Res 1993;48:277.
14. Felder RA, Eisner GM, Jose PA: D1 dopamine receptor signaling defect in spontaneous hypertension. Acta Physiol Scand 2000;68:245–250.
15. Hartman DS, Civelli O: Molecular attributes of dopamine receptors: new potential for antipsychotic drug development. Ann Med 1996;28:211–219.
16. Murphy MB, Murray C, Shorten GD: Drug therapy: fenoldopam—a selective peripheral dopamine-receptor agonist for the treatment of severe hypertension. N Engl J Med 2001;345:1548–1557.

17. Mena I: Manganese poisoning. In Vinken PJ, Bruyn GW (eds): Handbook of Clinical Neurology, vol 21. New York, Elsevier Science, 1977, pp 821–823.

18. Ginsberg MD: Carbon monoxide. In Spencer PS, Schaumburg HH (eds): Experimental and Clinical Neurotoxicology. Baltimore, William & Wilkins, 1980, pp 374–394.

19. Aquilonius SM, Asmark H, Enoksson P, et al: Computerised tomography in severe methanol intoxication. BMJ 1978;2:929.

20. He FS: Extrapyramidal lesions induced by mildewed cane poisoning (with report of three cases). Chung Hua I Hsueh Tsa Chih 1987;67:395–396.

21. Tanner CM, Langston JW: Do environmental toxins cause Parkinson's disease? A critical review. Neurology 1990;322:1781–1787.

22. Granner MA, Wooten GF: Neuroleptic malignant syndrome or parkinsonism hyperpyrexia syndrome. Semin Neurol 1991; 11:228–335.

23. DEA Intelligence Division. (2002, October). Trippin' on tryptamines: the emergence of foxy and AMT as drugs of abuse. Accessed January 6, 2004, at http://www.usdoj.gov/dea/pubs/intel/02052/02052p.html.

24. Sanders-Bush E, Mayer SE: 5-Hydroxytryptamine (serotonin): receptor agonists and antagonists. In Hardman JG, Limbrid LE, Gilman AG (eds): Goodman & Gilman's The Pharmacological Basis of Therapeutics, 10th ed. New York, McGraw-Hill, 2001, pp 269–290.

25. Mill KC: Serotonin syndrome. Am Fam Med 1995;52:1475–1482.

26. Reisine T: Opiate receptors. Neuropharmacology 1995;34:463–472.

27. Gutstein HB, Akil H: Opioid analgesics. In Hardman JG, Limbrid LE, Gilman AG (eds): Goodman & Gilman's The Pharmacological Basis of Therapeutics, 10th ed. New York, McGraw-Hill, 2001, pp 569–619.

28. Kaiko RF, Foley KM, Grabinski PY, et al: Central nervous system excitatory effects of meperidine in cancer patients. Ann Neurol 1983;13:180–185.

29. Galzi JL, Changeux JP: Molecular organization and regulations. Neuropharmacology 1995;34:563–582.

30. Brown JH, Taylor P: Muscarinic receptor agonists and antagonists. In Hardman JG, Limbrid LE, Gilman AG (eds): Goodman & Gilman's The Pharmacological Basis of Therapeutics, 10th ed. New York, McGraw-Hill, 2001, pp 155–173.

31. Benson BJ, Tolo D, McIntire M: Is the intermediate syndrome in organophosphate poisoning the result of insufficient oxime therapy? J Toxicol Clin Toxicol 1992;30:347–349.

32. Haddad LM: Organophosphate poisoning: intermediate syndrome? J Toxicol Clin Toxicol 1992;30:331–332.

33. Kitchens CS, Van Mierop LH: Envenomation by the eastern coral snake (*Micrurus fulvius*). JAMA 1987;258:1615–1618.

34. Rauber A: Black widow spider bites. J Toxicol Clin Toxicol 1983–84;21:473.

35. Nicholson GM, Graudins A: Spiders of medical importance in the Asia-Pacific: Atracogoxin, latrotoxin and related spider neuro-toxins. Clin Exp Pharmacol Physiol 2002;29:785–794.

36. Kincaid JC: Tick bite paralysis. Semin Neurol 1990;10:32–34.

37. Taylor P: Agents acting at the neuromuscular junction and autonomic ganglia. In Hardman JG, Limbrid LE, Gilman AG (eds): Goodman & Gilman's The Pharmacological Basis of Therapeutics, 10th ed. New York, McGraw-Hill, 2001, pp 193–213.

38. Hough LB: Cellular localization and possible functions for brain histamine: recent progress. Prof Neurobiol 1987;30:469–505.

39. Brown NJ, Roberts II LJ: Histamine, bradykinin, and their antagonists. In Hardman JG, Limbrid LE, Gilman AG (eds): Goodman & Gilman's The Pharmacological Basis of Therapeutics, 10th ed. New York, McGraw-Hill, 2001, pp 645–667.

40. Pin JP, Duvoisin R: The metabotrophic glutamate receptors: structure and functions. Neuropharmacology 1995;34:1219–1237.

41. Bettler B, Mulle C: AMPA and kainate receptors. Neuro-pharmacology 1995;34:123–139.

42. Mori H, Mishina M: Structure and function of the NMDA receptor channel. Neuropharmacology 1995;34:1219–1237.

43. Kleckner NW, Dingledine R: Requirements for glycine in activation of NMDA receptors expressed in *Xenopus* oocyte. Science 1988;241:835–837.

44. Williams K, Romano C, Dichter MA, et al: Modulation of the NMDA receptor by polyamines. Life Sci 1991;48:469–498.

45. Weight FF, Lovinger DM, White G, et al: Alcohol and anaesthetic actions on excitatory amino acid-activated ion channels. Ann N Y Acad Sci 1990;625:97–107.

46. Hoffman PL, Grant KA, Snell LD, et al: NMDA receptors: role in ethanol withdrawal seizures. Ann N Y Acad Sci 1992;654:52–60.

47. Olney JW: Excitatory amino acids and neuropsychiatric disorders. Ann Rev Pharmacol Toxicol 1990;30:47–71.

48. Perl TM, Bedard L, Kosatsky T, et al: An outbreak of toxic encephalopathy caused by eating mussels contaminated with domoic acid. N Engl J Med 1990;322:1775–1780.

49. Luddens H, Korpi ER, Seeburg PH: GABA$_A$/benzodiazepine receptor heterogeneity: neurophysiological implications. Neuro-pharmacology 1995;34:245–254.

50. Krogsgaard-Larsen P, Brehm L, Schaumburg K: Muscimol, a psychoactive constituent of Amanita muscaria, as a medicinal chemical model structure. Acta Chem Scand [B] 1981;35:311–324.

51. Mohler H, Okada T: Benzodiazepine receptor: demonstration in the central nervous system. Science 1977;198:849–851.

52. Korpi ER, Mattila MJ, Wisden W, Luddens H: GABA-A receptor subtypes: clinical efficacy and selectivity of benzodiazepine site ligands. Ann Med 1997;29:275–282.

53. Majewska MD, Harrison NL, Schwartz RD, et al: Steroid hormone metabolites are barbiturate-like modulators of the GABA receptor. Science 1986;232:1004–1007.

54. Allan AM, Harris RA: Anesthetic and convulsant barbiturates alter γ-aminobutyric acid-stimulated chloride flux across brain mem-branes. J Pharmacol Exp Ther 1986;238:763–768.

55. Suzdak PD, Schwartz RD, Skolnick P, et al: Ethanol stimulates γ-aminobutyric acid receptor-mediated chloride transport in rat brain synaptoneurosomes. Proc Natl Acad Sci U S A 1986;83:4071–4075.

56. William HL, Killah MS, Jenny EH, et al: Convulsant effects of isoniazid. JAMA 1951;152:1317–1321.

57. Gosselin RE, Smith RP, Hodge HC: Clinical Toxicology of Commercial Products, 5th ed. Baltimore, Williams & Wilkins, 1984.

58. Lummis SC, Buckinham SD, Rauh JJ, et al: Blocking actions of heptachlor at an insect central nervous system GABA receptor. Proc R Soc Lond Biol Sci 1990;240:97–106.

59. Ogata N: Pharmacology and physiology of GABA$_B$ receptors. Gen Pharmacol 1990;21:395–402.

60. Langosch D, Becker CM, Betz H: The inhibitory glycine receptor: a ligand-gated chloride channel of the central nervous system. Eur J Biochem 1990;194:1–8.

61. Schaumberg HH, Spencer PS, Thomas PK (eds): Disorder of Peripheral Nerves. Philadelphia, F. A. Davis, 1983.

62. LeWitt P: The neurotoxicity of the rat poison vacor. N Engl J Med 1980;302:73–77.

63. Spencer PS, Schaumberg HH, Sabri M, et al: The enlarging view of hexacarbon neurotoxicity. Crit Rev Toxicol 1980;7:279–356.

64. Windebank AJ, Blexrud MD: Residual ethylene oxide in hollow fiber hemodialysis units is neurotoxic in vitro. Ann Neurol 1989;26:63–68.

65. Murai Y, Kuroiwa Y: Peripheral neuropathy in chlorobiphenyl poisoning. Neurology 1971;21:1173–1176.

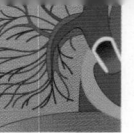

A   Drug-Associated Neuromuscular Syndromes

MICHAEL BEUHLER, MD

A "neuromuscular disorder" refers to a pathophysiologic state created by an abnormal interaction between nerve and muscle. In toxicology, most neuromuscular disorders relate to an abnormal interaction between the central or peripheral nervous systems (CNS or PNS) and the motor innervation of skeletal muscles. Drug-associated neuromuscular disorders are typically adverse effects that occur during therapeutic, occupational, or recreational use or overuse of various xenobiotics. These disorders may be dose related or idiosyncratic, mild or severe, reversible or irreversible, and can occur early or late following exposure. Three drug-associated neuromuscular disorders will be extensively reviewed in this chapter. For discussion of other drug-associated neuromuscular disorders, you should refer to the specific chapter covering a particular drug. For instance, extrapyramidal movement disorders are discussed in Chapter 38, the Antipsychotic Agents.

When exposure to a xenobiotic produces, with some regularity, a specific constellation of neuromuscular physical signs and symptoms, they are referred to as syndromes. Syndrome designations are often reserved for disorders that are associated with significant patient morbidity. The majority of drug-associated neuromuscular syndromes are manifested by exaggerated muscular tone and resultant hyperthermia. Although the pathophysiologic mechanisms underlying the neuromuscular hyperactivity are frequently unique, clinical signs and symptoms often have significant overlap, thus making accurate diagnosis difficult. Recognition of the unique clinical features of each syndrome will facilitate diagnosis and assist treatment. In this chapter, the neuroleptic malignant syndrome (NMS), serotonin syndrome, and malignant hyperthermia (MH) will be reviewed and the similarities and differences of their etiology, pathophysiology, clinical findings, and treatment will be highlighted.

NEUROLEPTIC MALIGNANT SYNDROME

Please also see Chapter 38.

Introduction, History, and Epidemiology

This syndrome was first described in 1960 when fever and rigidity were associated with haloperidol therapy.[1] During the 1960s, the syndrome was increasingly recognized as a separate entity from lethal catatonia. By the 1980s, NMS had become widely accepted as a complication of neuroleptic use. During the past 10 to 15 years, the mortality rate from NMS has declined due to a wider recognition of patients at risk, earlier diagnosis, decreases in neuroleptic dosing, the use of newer and safer atypical antipsychotics, and improvements in critical care.

From retrospective studies, the incidence of NMS has been estimated to occur in 0.02% to 3% in patients treated with neuroleptics.[2] Prospective studies estimate an incidence of 0.07% to 0.9%.[3-5] The incidence of NMS appears to be decreasing. This is likely due to the use of lower doses of neuroleptics, the use of atypical agents (see Chapter 38), and earlier recognition with prevention of full syndrome development. Stricter criteria for diagnosis may now limit the reporting of NMS. In addition, new cases are less likely to be published in the current literature now that the syndrome is well characterized.

There does not appear to be a gender or age preference for NMS, but it is more common in men and adults due to greater frequency of neuroleptic use in these patient populations. Patients with neuropsychiatric disorders such as Parkinson's disease and catatonia and those with severe forms of functional psychiatric disorders are at greater risk for developing NMS.[2] Patients with preexisting organic brain syndrome appear to have a higher risk for mortality and morbidity from NMS.

NMS has been reported with several types of medications that result in decreased CNS dopamine tone. The high-potency neuroleptics such as haloperidol, fluphenazine, and thiothixene are probably more likely to cause the syndrome, but it has been reported with lower-potency neuroleptics as well. Although haloperidol has been associated with more documented cases of NMS, this may reflect more widespread use of this antipsychotic rather than greater absolute risk with this particular agent. Even the newer, atypical agents, which have a decreased propensity to produce extrapyramidal side effects (EPS) (e.g., risperidone, clozapine, olanzapine, and quetiapine), have been associated with NMS.[2,6,7] Non-neuroleptic dopamine antagonists (e.g., amoxapine and metoclopramide) have caused episodes of NMS. Drugs that result in lower levels of dopamine (e.g., reserpine, tetrabenazine, and α-methyl tyrosine) have been associated with NMS. NMS has also been reported following the abrupt cessation of dopamine agonists (e.g., levodopa/carbidopa and amantadine) used for the treatment of Parkinson's disease.[8,9]

There are several purported risk factors for developing NMS. They include large doses of neuroleptics and/or rapid dose escalation, a positive history of NMS, antecedent agitated behavior, dehydration or infection (e.g., pneumonia or sepsis), the presence of electrolyte disorders (e.g., hypo- or hypernatremia), and concomitant treatment with other psychotropic agents (e.g., lithium, anticholinergic agents). Lithium is thought to decrease striatal dopamine synthesis, thus theoretically predisposing to NMS.[10] Lithium is associated with its own neurotoxicity that may be mistaken for NMS. Thus, the diagnosis of NMS should be made with caution for

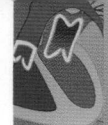

patients who are treated with lithium and neuroleptics simultaneously.[11,12]

NMS is an idiosyncratic reaction to neuroleptic therapy and is not the result of overdose. For patients with NMS, serum levels of neuroleptics are typically in the normal range. Overdose of certain traditional neuroleptics (e.g., chlorpromazine, thioridazine) may occasionally produce short-lived patient agitation and hyperthermia. The clinical course (abrupt onset over minutes to hours and duration of 1 to 2 days) is distinctly different from that of NMS (gradual onset over days and duration of 1 to 2 weeks).

NMS-like symptoms had been reported for years prior to the initial use of neuroleptics. This separate syndrome with similar clinical characteristics is called lethal catatonia (or malignant catatonia). In its final or advanced stages, lethal catatonia is clinically indistinguishable from NMS. The patient often has gradual worsening of psychiatric symptoms that include moodiness and melancholia for several days preceding the full syndrome. Typically, 1 to 2 days prior to developing lethal catatonia patients develop severe agitation and mania. Following this period, they develop catatonia, labile blood pressure, muscular rigidity, and mottled skin, similar to NMS. It is often difficult to differentiate lethal catatonia from NMS. The absence of a change in antecedent antidopamine drug therapy by history and presence of prodromal psychiatric symptoms suggest a diagnosis of lethal catatonia.[13]

Pathophysiology of Neuroleptic Malignant Syndrome

The pathophysiology of NMS has been investigated for decades but has not yet been fully elucidated. NMS is theorized to be the result of a relative dopamine blockade (specifically D_2-receptor blockade) in the mesolimbic, mesocortical, nigrostriatal, and hypothalamic brain regions.[2] This is largely based on the observation that the syndrome occurs in the presence of dopamine depletion or antagonist therapy, is associated with temperature abnormalities (controlled by preoptic anterior hypothalamic dopamine tracts), and motor symptoms are exaggerations of extrapyramidal neuroleptic side effects. However, there are some limitations to the dopamine antagonist or hypofunction theory.

The syndrome has been reported to occur at therapeutic serum neuroleptic levels, and effects last much longer then expected based on the elimination kinetics of neuroleptics. The syndrome has been reported to continue despite a subtherapeutic concentration or absence of neuroleptic in the CNS. This is partly explained by the counterhypothesis that NMS effects persist due to dopamine receptor hypersensitivity or increased number of dopamine receptors. However, one would expect the patient to manifest signs and symptoms often associated with dopamine excess (i.e., choreoathetoid movements, hallucinations), when CNS dopamine receptors are no longer occupied and activated due to drug metabolism. Such stigmata are not commonly reported with NMS. There does, however,

seem to be some temporal relationship between the duration of symptoms and the triggering agent's half-life, as demonstrated by depot injections generally being implicated in longer clinical courses than immediate-release oral or intramuscular formulations.

There is a link between serotonin (5-HT) and dopamine activity. The newer antidepressants have 5-HT_{2A} antagonism, which is thought to increase dopamine tone in the striatum and prefrontal cortex (by disinhibition). This 5-HT antagonism is thought to limit adverse effects (e.g., EPS) and contribute to the antipsychotic drug effects. Selective serotonin reuptake inhibitors (SSRIs) aggravate haloperidol-induced dystonia and parkinsonism in monkeys (by a decrease in brain dopamine).[14] Treatment of rats with agents that increase 5-HT enhances catalepsy after blockade of dopamine receptors.[15] This suggests a dopamine-serotonin relationship, with increased 5-HT tone causing decreased dopamine tone.[16] There are several cases of EPS and NMS triggered by SSRIs in the literature.[17,18]

Clinical Manifestations of Neuroleptic Malignant Syndrome

NMS is most often characterized by fever, muscular rigidity, altered mental status, and autonomic dysfunction.[2,19] Fever and muscular rigidity are usually present but not required for diagnosis. The reported signs and symptoms of NMS syndrome are listed in Table 10A-1. Increased muscle tone is often present (97%), being described as "lead pipe rigidity," usually by those familiar with that phrase's linkage to NMS. The rigidity may have a cog-wheeling component. Other EPS symptoms (dystonia, dysphagia, gait abnormalities) may be present. Tremor (mild to severe, fine or coarse) has been reported. Mutism may be part of the syndrome and is occasionally described associated with fearful facial expressions. Elevated temperatures are common (98%) although not universal.[2,20] Other symptoms associated with NMS include diaphoresis, tachypnea, tachycardia, and altered mental status (97%).[2] Urinary incontinence is uncommonly reported. Seizures are rarely reported, and should prompt investigation for another diagnosis.

Diagnosis of Neuroleptic Malignant Syndrome

The diagnosis of NMS is clinical and based on suggestive history and physical findings along with a high level of suspicion in the appropriate clinical setting. By history, the patient must have recently had a dopaminergic agent started, the dose increased, or an intervention that decreased CNS dopamine tone.

Several clinical diagnostic criteria are available to facilitate the diagnosis of NMS. The disadvantage of applying rigid diagnostic criteria is that borderline or atypical cases will be excluded, possibly delaying proper therapy. This is particularly important since NMS is a heterogeneous disorder that exists along a severity continuum from moderate to very severe cases. Atypical cases may not have rigidity or elevated temperature and

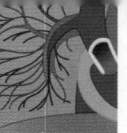

TABLE 10A-1 Signs and Symptoms of Neuroleptic Malignant Syndrome (NMS)/Serotonin Syndrome/Malignant Hyperthermia

CLINICAL FEATURES	NMS	SEROTONIN SYNDROME	MALIGNANT HYPERTHERMIA
Triggering agent	Neuroleptic	Proserotonergic agent	Succinylcholine or inhaled anesthetic
Onset	Slow (hours to days)	Fast (minutes to hours)	Very fast to fast (minutes to hours)
Duration	Long (days to weeks)	Short (1–2 days)	Short (1–3 days)
Agitation	Sometimes	Yes	No
Confusion	Yes	Sometimes	Unusual
Hyperactivity	No	Yes	No
Bradykinesia/stupor	Yes	No	Unusual
Myoclonus	No	Yes	No
Shivering	No	Yes/sometimes	No
Tremor	Sometimes	Yes	No
Pupils	Mid-sized	Large	Not specific
Hyperreflexia	No	Yes (especially lower extremities)	No
Rigidity	Severe	Sometimes	Severe
Rigidity type	Extrapyramidal (leadpipe)	Pyramidal (clasp-knife)	Generalized
Hyperpyrexia	Yes	Yes	Severe
Tachypnea	Yes	Yes	Yes
Tachycardia	Yes	Yes	Yes (severe)
Hypertension	Sometimes	Yes	Sometimes
Leukocytosis	Yes	Uncommon	Not typical
Elevated creatine phosphokinase	Severe	Mild	Severe

Adapted from Gillman PK: The serotonin syndrome and its treatment. J Psychopharmacol 1999;13:100–109; Gillman K: Serotonin toxicity. www.psychotropical.com/SerotoninToxicity.doc, accessed January 15, 2005; and Wappler F, Fiege M, Schulte am Esch J: Pathophysiological role of the serotonin system in malignant hyperthermia. Br J Anaesth 2001;87(5):794–798.

can make diagnosis difficult. A flexible definition is probably in the patient's best interest to allow for initiation of aggressive supportive treatment. In general, it is important to initially exclude any alternative diagnoses (e.g., infection) (see later section on Differential Diagnosis).

There are no laboratory studies that confirm the diagnosis of NMS. The laboratory abnormalities that have been associated with NMS are relatively nonspecific. They include markedly elevated creatine phosphokinase (CPK), increased white blood cell (WBC) count, myoglobinuria, and occasionally, diffuse slowing on electroencephalography (EEG). Serum iron levels have been reported to be low with NMS and have been suggested as a useful marker. Serum iron, however, appears to decrease with inflammatory responses, and thus has no prognostic significance.[21,22]

There is significant variation in the time between the administration of the "triggering" medication and the onset of NMS. Reports range from days to weeks from the addition or change in the medication to development of signs and symptoms of NMS. Once the illness begins, symptoms progress slowly and peak over a period of 24 to 72 hours. The total duration of the illness varies greatly. The duration of illness appears to be longer for patients who received depot neuroleptics as compared with oral or immediate release intramuscular formulations. The disease often has a fluctuating clinical course, irrespective of the treatment. Improvement is usually observed within 48 to 96 hours of discontinuation of the triggering medication. Full recovery, however, is slow and often takes 10 or more days. Full recovery may occasionally take several weeks, and some NMS signs and symptoms improve while others persist.[2] For example,

patients can have improvement of their rigidity and resolution of elevated serum CPK, but still have altered mental status and hyperthermia.

Mortality appears to be related to the severity of hyperthermia and the degree of alteration of consciousness. Mortality from NMS usually results from renal failure, pulmonary embolism, respiratory failure, acute respiratory distress syndrome, cardiovascular collapse, or disseminated intravascular coagulation (DIC). This stresses the need for aggressive supportive care. Postmortem examination is unlikely to demonstrate specific CNS findings.

Persistent neurologic sequelae have been reported following episodes of NMS. These persistent neurologic findings include cognitive dysfunction, catatonia, continued rigidity, dystonia, and amnesic symptoms.[23,24] Medical complications (such as hypoxic encephalopathy) can result in prolonged symptomatology. The patient may also have exacerbations of underlying psychiatric illness after removal of neuroleptics and/or treatment with dopamine agonists.

SEROTONIN SYNDROME

Please also see Chapter 29.

Introduction, History, and Epidemiology

Although not initially recognized as a distinct clinical entity, serotonin syndrome has existed for over half a century. The first published description of the syndrome occurred in 1955 when a fatal case of "toxic encephalitis"

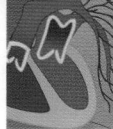

was noted after meperidine was administered to a patient taking iproniazid for pulmonary tuberculosis.[25] The use of L-tryptophan in conjunction with monoamine oxidase inhibitors (MAOIs) in the 1960s caused a similar illness marked by hyperactivity that was due to excess CNS serotonin levels.[26,27] It was not until 1982, however, that the syndrome was fully characterized and the term *serotonin syndrome* appeared in the literature.[28]

Several studies have attempted to estimate the frequency of serotonin syndrome; all of them suffer from varying degrees of methodologic problems. Despite these study limitations, the incidence of severe serotonin syndrome is quite low during therapeutic dosing of non-MAOI agents. There have only been approximately 200 cases of serotonin syndrome reported in the literature since it was initially characterized. This low reporting, however, may not reflect a true incidence. This illness, like NMS, has a continuum of severity. Thus, the incidence of the syndrome will depend on the flexibility of clinical criteria used for diagnosis. It is likely that mild signs and symptoms of serotonin excess occur frequently with many different proserotonergic agents. The severity of these symptoms, however, is mild enough to be overlooked by both patients and treating physicians and thus will not be diagnosed as serotonin syndrome. A recent surge in popularity of SSRIs over traditional antidepressants as well as increased education (and thus recognition) of the signs and symptoms of serotonin syndrome may lead to an increased incidence of syndrome diagnosis. In addition, the recent increased use of psychoactive medications in children is expected to increase the incidence of serotonin syndrome in this age group.

There does not appear to be an age or gender preference for the development of serotonin syndrome. Underlying organic brain disease may be a risk factor that predisposes patients to the development of the syndrome. The incidence of serious morbidity and mortality associated with serotonin syndrome varies greatly and is related to individual host factors (i.e., comorbid illness), drug combinations (i.e., the "dose" of serotonin stimulation), and the timeliness of diagnosis and treatment.

Most cases of serotonin syndrome occur with combination therapy of more than one proserotonergic agent, but it has been reported with serotonergic monotherapy and recreational use of indoleamine and phenylethylamine derivatives (e.g., "Ecstasy"). Although serotonin syndrome is usually an adverse drug interaction that follows the combination of therapeutic doses of proserotonergic agents, it will also occur following proserotonergic drug overdose.

Pathophysiology of Serotonin Syndrome

Serotonin syndrome is caused by increased CNS 5-HT receptor activation. Usually, increased 5-HT receptor activation is due to significantly elevated CNS levels of 5-HT, which occurs as a result of proserotonergic agent activity. It is helpful to think of serotonin syndrome not as an on/off phenomenon, but as a continuous spectrum of toxicity caused by increased CNS 5-HT levels. This is

similar to the spectrum of illness severity that exists for NMS. Unlike NMS, however, serotonin syndrome is not an idiosyncratic reaction but a dose-effect phenomenon caused by the combination of proserotonergic agents. Some investigators have advocated calling it serotonin toxicity, which is a more accurate description of the phenomenon. In many well-documented cases of serotonin syndrome, however, serum drug levels are often in the therapeutic range. Serum levels of proserotonergic drugs, however, may not correlate with end-organ concentrations or, more importantly, elevated CNS serotonergic activity.

There are several different groups of 5-HT receptors found in the CNS. Most of the symptoms seen in serotonin syndrome are believed to be caused by stimulation of the postsynaptic $5\text{-}HT_{2A}$ receptor.[29-32] This receptor is a G protein linked to phosphoinositide-specific phospholipase C as well as a K^+ channel (causes depolarization).[33] Although stimulation of the $5\text{-}HT_{1A}$ receptor generates stereotypical behavior in mice once thought to be analogous to serotonin syndrome in humans, it is not believed to contribute significantly to the pathologic consequences of serotonin toxicity, and specific antagonists do not provide protection against serotonin syndrome lethality in a rat model.[30,31]

The stimulation of $5\text{-}HT_{2A}$ receptors may occur in several different ways: increased 5-HT synthesis (e.g., L-tryptophan); increased 5-HT release (e.g., amphetamines); decreased 5-HT catabolism (e.g., MAOIs); decreased 5-HT reuptake (e.g., SSRIs); direct 5-HT receptor stimulation (e.g., 5-methoxy-*N,N*-dimethyltryptamine [DMT]); and increased postsynaptic 5-HT response by secondary messenger systems (e.g., lithium). Serotonin syndrome may also be precipitated following the withdrawal of an agent with $5\text{-}HT_{2A}$ antagonist effects in a patient with 5-HT receptor up-regulation/hypersensitivity or in a patient on an SSRI.[34]

The propensity of an agent to cause serotonin syndrome is often directly correlated with its ability to increase brain serotonin levels or to directly stimulate $5\text{-}HT_{2A}$ receptors. Usually a combination of pharmaceutical agents is required to elicit serotonin syndrome, but it has been reported following overdose of single agents.[35,36] For instance, serotonin syndrome was noted to occur in 14% to 16% of patients who overdosed on SSRIs in one study. In addition, overdose of MAOIs produces a toxic syndrome that significantly overlaps with serotonin syndrome. It is much more common for serotonin syndrome to occur when two agents are combined that raise brain serotonergic tone by two different mechanisms. For example, many of the severe or fatal serotonin syndrome episodes have been due to an MAOI interaction with a selective serotonin uptake inhibitor.

Serotonin reuptake inhibition appears to be a very commonly encountered cause of serotonin syndrome. The SSRIs paroxetine, clomipramine (a tricyclic antidepressant [TCA]), sertraline, fluoxetine, and venlafaxine (a serotonin norepinephrine reuptake inhibitor [SNRI]) have all been implicated as causes of serotonin syndrome. Besides clomipramine, the other TCAs (e.g., imipramine, dothiepin, and amitriptyline) have a much

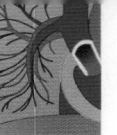

lower affinity for the 5-HT reuptake transporter.[37,38] These TCAs have rarely caused serotonin syndrome but do not usually cause significant morbidity unless combined with an MAOI. It has been hypothesized that chlorpheniramine and, possibly, brompheniramine can contribute to serotonin syndrome due to SSRI properties of these drugs.[37,39] Duloxetine, a novel SSRI, is also likely capable of causing serotonin syndrome.

Certain synthetic opiates have SSRI activity and have been implicated as agents capable of precipitating serotonin syndrome when combined with other proserotonergic agents. These opiates include tramadol, meperidine, dextromethorphan, methadone, and pentazocine.[40] Tramadol may have serotonin-releasing properties in addition to being an SSRI.[41]

Traditional, irreversible, nonselective MAOIs (e.g., tranylcypromine, phenelzine, and clorgyline) and the newer, reversible, nonselective MAOIs (e.g., moclobemide) are readily capable of precipitating serotonin syndrome when combined with other proserotonergic agents (see Chapter 29).[40,42] Selegiline, a selective, irreversible MAOI-B inhibitor, may cause serotonin syndrome at higher doses since MAO selectivity is lost at supratherapeutic doses.[43,44] Linezolid, a newer antibiotic that has reversible MAO activity, has the potential to cause a serotonin syndrome.

Several drugs of abuse (e.g., hallucinogenic amphetamines, alklytryptamines, and lysergamides) can potentiate 5-HT CNS activity and result in serotonin syndrome–like toxicity, either alone or in combination with other agents. The direct serotonin receptor agonists (e.g., lysergic acid diethylamide (LSD), 2,5 dimethoxy-4 methylamphetamine (DOM), DMT, and serotonin-releasing agents (e.g., cocaine and 3,4-methylenedioxymethamphetamine [MDMA]) may produce serotonin syndrome–like toxicity.[45-47] L-tryptophan is converted to serotonin in the CNS and has caused serotonin syndrome when combined with an MAOI or SSRI.

Several substances have been implicated in causing serotonin syndrome whose contributing mechanism is not well understood. Lithium is believed to contribute to serotonin syndrome because it causes an inhibition of phosphatases, thus resulting in increased intracellular inositol phosphates and potentiating the secondary messenger effects of serotonin.[33,48] Trazadone and nefazodone have been implicated in several cases of serotonin syndrome, even though they appear to have 5-HT$_{2A}$ antagonistic properties and are not particularly potent 5-HT uptake inhibitors.[37,40,49] Buspirone is a direct 5-HT$_{1A}$ agonist and has been implicated in causing serotonin syndrome, although its effect appears weak.[46,50] Sumatriptan (a 5-HT$_{1D}$ agonist) has been implicated as a cause of serotonin syndrome through uncertain mechanisms.[39,51] It appears that 5-HT$_3$ antagonists (e.g., ondansetron and similar antiemetics) are unlikely to cause serotonin syndrome, although this is controversial.[52] Bromocriptine and L-dopa increase brain serotonin levels and can theoretically facilitate the development of serotonin syndrome.[53]

It is important to understand the pharmacokinetic and pharmacodynamic characteristics of certain proserotonergic agents. For example, fluoxetine and its active metabolite, norfluoxetine, have long elimination half-lives.[40] This means that there will be significant serotonin uptake inhibition long after the agent is stopped. Thus, a "washout" period of 4 weeks is recommended after drug discontinuation. Another example is the use of irreversible MAOIs. Patients will require 4 to 5 weeks for the effect of these enzyme inhibitors to completely resolve. Significant P-450 interactions (and the effect of genetic polymorphisms) are observed with several of the psychiatric medications and can result in potentiation and prolongation of their effect. For example, paroxetine has significant CYP2D6 inhibition, which can increase serum levels of other medications metabolized by CYP2D6.

Clinical Manifestation of Serotonin Syndrome

There is a great range in the severity of the clinical signs and symptoms of serotonin toxicity. It can manifest as unpleasant side effects reported with routine SSRI use to a hyperthermic, life-threatening syndrome. Typical signs and symptoms include CNS changes (i.e., agitation, confusion, anxiety, headache, mydriasis, hallucinations, insomnia, and dizziness), autonomic hyperactivity (i.e., hypertension, hyperthermia, tachycardia, tachypnea, flushing, diaphoresis, and shivering) gastrointestinal effects (i.e., nausea, vomiting, abdominal pain, and diarrhea), and neuromuscular abnormalities (i.e., clonus, myoclonus, tremor, sweating, trismus, hyperreflexia, ocular clonus, and muscular rigidity).[54-56] Although not pathognomonic, hyperreflexia, clonus (myoclonus and ocular clonus), and/or symmetric rigidity (more prominent in the lower extremities) are characteristic findings associated with serotonin syndrome.

Diagnosis of Serotonin Syndrome

As with NMS, the diagnosis of serotonin syndrome is clinical and based on suggestive history and physical findings. There are no laboratory tests that confirm the diagnosis. Diagnosis is best made by excluding other etiologies (see later section on Differential Diagnosis) and application of preestablished criteria. The use of strict diagnostic criteria is not recommended because it will not allow the inclusion of atypical cases of serotonin syndrome. Absolute frequency of symptoms is impossible to determine due to the limited nature of case reports. Of note, serotonin syndrome is not a manifestation of EPS and should not be associated with dyskinesis or cogwheeling.

One of the marked differences between serotonin syndrome and NMS is the time course of symptom onset and duration of illness. With serotonin syndrome, symptom onset often occurs rapidly or within minutes to hours after introduction of or an increase in dose of the proserotonergic agent. In contrast, with NMS, symptom onset occurs gradually and insidiously over days following the introduction of an antidopaminergic agent. One of the diagnostic criteria for serotonin syndrome is that

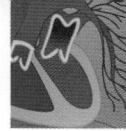

symptoms should begin soon after starting a serotonergic agent, and in almost all situations they have started within 24 hours of the addition of the medication. The majority of episodes are mild, and relatively short-lived. Most patients recover from serotonin syndrome within 24 hours, but patients with a severe syndrome may have signs and symptoms for 2 to 3 days.

Laboratory analysis is not useful for making a specific diagnosis; it appears to be better suited for eliminating alternative diagnoses. Nonspecific findings include elevated WBC count, increased CPK, and mild metabolic acidosis. In general, the CPK elevation is not usually as severe as what is observed with NMS or MH, but significant elevation is occasionally seen with critically ill individuals. Laboratory analysis may help identify drugs of abuse as well as assisting in the identification and treatment of complications associated with serotonin syndrome (e.g., hypoxia, pneumonia, rhabdomyolysis, renal failure, hepatic transaminitis, and DIC). Life-threatening complications of serotonin syndrome commonly occur in patients with severe and prolonged neuromuscular hyperactivity and resultant hyperthermia.

MALIGNANT HYPERTHERMIA

Introduction, History, and Epidemiology

Malignant hyperthermia (MH) was first described in 1962.[57] It is an idiosyncratic drug reaction triggered by inhaled anesthetics and/or by the depolarizing paralytic succinylcholine. It is a disease that primarily occurs in the operating room, with an incidence of about 1 in 12,000 to 1 in 40,000 general anesthetic cases.[58] It is believed that the number of susceptible patients is likely higher since 50% of patients in whom the syndrome develops have had prior anesthesia without manifesting MH.[59,60] It is thought that those of African descent have a much lower rate of the genetic defect than whites.[61] There are several different proteins linked to the disease and several different genetic differences within each gene. For example, there have been more than 20 different abnormal ryanodine receptor genes (RYR1) identified alone.

MH is different from the other two "neuromuscular" syndromes in that the pathology is maintained without further stimulation at the neuromuscular junction. It is a disease of abnormal cytosolic calcium physiology that occurs in skeletal muscle cells and results in a cascade of pathophysiologic changes that culminate in a hypermetabolic state. When it was first recognized and reported, MH was associated with significant mortality (approximately 80%). Fortunately, the mortality rate has fallen to about 5% with aggressive, early treatment with dantrolene. There is a swine model (porcine stress syndrome [PSS]) that has allowed significant research in the field. The PSS model, however, is limited; unlike humans, the genetic defect in the swine model is limited to one specific change in the ryanodine receptor.

A syndrome of excessive susceptibility to stress resulting in morbidity clinically similar to MH has been reported, without any of the usual MH triggers.[62] In this MH-like syndrome, individuals experience elevations in temperature, labile blood pressure, acrocyanosis, muscle cramping, fasciculations and elevated CPK with certain environmental "stressors." These "stressors" have included long car rides, bad news, increased external temperatures, medical illness and excessive activity. There may be a family history of mysterious sudden death, or of muscle cramps and easy fatigability with exercise. This has been termed the human stress syndrome, and individuals may be at higher risk for exertional heat stroke. This syndrome is believed to share a similar pathology with MH, but without the antecedent exposure to anesthetic/paralytic agents.[62,63] MH gene abnormalities have been found in some patients with this stress-induced syndrome and exercise-induced rhabdomyolysis.[64-66]

Pathophysiology of Malignant Hyperthermia

Under normal physiologic conditions, elevated intracellular calcium levels trigger contraction. The ryanodine receptor of the sarcoplasmic reticulum is associated with the dihydropyridine receptor (DHPR, L-type calcium channel) of the cellular membrane, and a structural change of the DHPR (which occurs during depolarization) is believed to open the ryanodine receptor. This elevated intracellular calcium stimulates more calcium release from the sarcoplasmic reticulum (calcium-induced calcium release). An increase in inositol-1,4,5-triphosphate is also responsible for mobilizing stored calcium through its own sarcoplasmic reticulum receptor (InsP$_3$).

MH is caused by a cascade of biochemical changes in skeletal muscle, culminating in markedly increased metabolic rates within muscle cells. Sustained muscle contraction and rigidity typically occur. Acute toxicity is marked by elevated intracellular calcium levels. Many MH patients (and the heat-intolerant swine) have a defect in this ryanodine receptor that is believed to trigger excessive calcium release from the sarcoplasmic reticulum. The specific defect may be attributed to increased rates of calcium-induced calcium release. Some (but not all) studies have hypothesized that there are higher basilar intracellular calcium concentrations within MH-prone muscle cells.[67,68] This increased intracellular calcium concentration would cause increased metabolic rate and increased activity of the sarcoplasmic Ca^{2+}/ATPase. The increased metabolic rate can occur without having contracture.[58] Higher levels of cyclic adenosine monophosphate (cAMP) are found in MH patients during exercise when compared with control patients, providing additional evidence for an alteration in the secondary messenger system.[69] The cell membrane sodium channel populations are different between MH patients and controls, possibly as a result of chronically elevated intracellular Ca^{2+} levels.[70]

The initial trigger that leads to elevated intracellular calcium concentrations is not well understood. For the inhaled anesthetics, it has been hypothesized that these

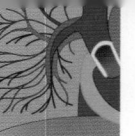

agents interact with the ryanodine channel and lower the threshold for release of calcium from the sarcoplasmic reticulum.[58] For succinylcholine, cellular depolarization from motor end-plate stimulation leads to elevated intracellular calcium concentrations. Phosphodiesterase inhibitors have rarely been reported to cause MH; elevated intracellular calcium concentrations may occur from these agents' effects on cAMP levels and the secondary messenger system.

Several genetic mutations have been found to be associated with MH, but only about half of malignant hyperthermia–sensitive (MHS) families have documented RYR1 mutations.[71] Another gene that has been recently implicated is the dihydropyridine receptor gene; other gene abnormalities have been suggested.[72] Cases of MH have been associated with various myopathic, metabolic, and mitochondrial genetic disorders.[73] Of interest, persistent CPK elevations are frequently found in asymptomatic MH individuals.[72]

The administration of 5-HT agonists to skeletal muscle from MH patients can trigger contractures.[74-77] This suggests a link between MH and serotonin. It is believed, however, that the increase in circulating 5-HT is a secondary response to (like catecholamine increase) and not a primary cause of contractures. The use of 5-HT receptor antagonists has not prevented morbidity from triggered MH in the PSS model.[78,79] It has been observed that 5-HT$_2$ antagonists reduce the MH response in human biopsies, possibly by causing hyperpolarization or modifying IP$_3$ levels.[33,76,80] Serotonin antagonists (such as cyproheptadine) have not been used in humans for MH.

Although similar to NMS in clinical appearance, MH syndrome has markedly different pathophysiology. Key differences between MH and NMS are the rapid onset of symptoms with MH versus the slower onset with NMS, and the shorter duration of illness in MH. In addition, patients with episodes of NMS have been successfully treated with inhaled anesthetics. Although it has been suggested previously that neuroleptics might be able to trigger MH, subsequent study has shown this not to be true. There is no apparent link between NMS and MH.[81]

Clinical Manifestation of Malignant Hyperthermia

MH often begins rapidly after administration of the triggering agent (inhaled anesthetic or succinylcholine). Most of the inhaled anesthetics can trigger MH, including halothane, enflurane, isoflurane, methoxyflurane, desflurane, and servoflurane.[82] Synergy between the two classes of agents has been reported. MH has also been reported to be caused by enoximone, a phosphodiesterase inhibitor.[83-85] One should also consider stressors (such as trauma or procedures) as potential triggers for the syndrome. There are "safer" alternative agents that may be used for anesthesia in patients at risk for MH. These agents include propofol, benzodiazepines, nitrous oxide, and narcotics.[59,86]

The signs and symptoms of MH are reflective of a greatly increased metabolic rate. The earliest, most sensitive, and specific signs of MH are increased rate of CO$_2$ production (as either expired CO$_2$ or partial pressure of CO$_2$ in arterial blood [PaCO$_2$]). Other early findings include a rapid rise in core temperature (as fast as 1° F every 5 minutes), diffuse muscle rigidity, and acidosis.[58] Temperature often rapidly increases and may not be initially noticed if the patient began at a subnormal temperature. Tetanic muscle contraction within 20 minutes after the muscle relaxants are administered is often reported. Symptoms of the full syndrome include tachycardia, rigidity, poor chest wall compliance, acidosis, cyanosis, mottling, hypotension, ventricular arrhythmias, increased ventricular rate, and elevated CPK. Hyperkalemia and marked hyperthermia carry a poor prognosis. As for other hyperthermic syndromes, the incidence of secondary complications and mortality is directly correlated with the severity and duration of hyperthermia. Sometimes the initial symptoms are subtle, such as increased masseter muscle tone during intubation; masseter rigidity may make intubation difficult. Generalized rigidity shortly following the administration of inhaled anesthetics or succinylcholine is virtually pathognomonic for MH. Generalized muscle rigidity, however, may not be present. Clinical rigidity may be relatively mild compared with subsequent CPK elevation, lactate, and myoglobinuria. In some patients, particularly those with delayed or atypical cases, the only symptoms might be muscle cramping and urinary color change reflective of ongoing rhabdomyolysis seen postoperatively.[87,88]

While the majority of cases have rapid onset, there are reports of delayed onset (especially with desflurane). The onset of the signs and symptoms of MH may not occur until the time of paralytic reversal or later in the recovery room.[89] When succinylcholine is used, it is believed to accelerate the onset of the episode. The use of nondepolarizing paralytics are believed to slow the onset of the MH episode.[82] Isolated rhabdomyolysis may sometimes occur and is associated with a delayed presentation and diagnosis.[90] Recurrence of symptoms is not uncommon (see later section on Malignant Hyperthermia Management).

Complications of MH include electrolyte abnormalities (i.e., hyperkalemia, hypercalcemia, hypocalcemia), ventricular fibrillation, DIC, rhabdomyolysis, hypoxia, hyperthermia, pulmonary edema, cerebral edema, and encephalopathy. These complications are ultimately responsible for the mortality and morbidity of MH. Autopsy findings (other than muscle biopsies) are nonspecific. Weakness and fatigue may last for months following an episode.[62]

DIAGNOSIS OF HYPERTHERMIC SYNDROMES

The initial diagnosis for all three syndromes is made clinically and based on a suggestive history and physical findings. Although confirmatory laboratory tests do not exist for NMS and serotonin syndrome, the diagnosis of MH can be confirmed by the in vitro halothane or caffeine contracture test. In general, specific laboratory

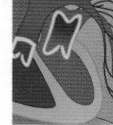

and other ancillary tests are obtained to rule out other illnesses that may be confused with these hyperthermic syndromes. For instance, during the initial patient evaluation, a diligent investigation for all sources of infection should be made, including blood, urine, and cerebrospinal fluid cultures. In addition, recommended laboratory tests include CBC, electrolytes, serum creatine phosphokinase (CPK), and urinalysis. An EEG may be obtained to exclude seizure activity.

The gold standard for diagnosis of MH is a muscle biopsy specimen that is then exposed to halothane and caffeine; the basis for this test is that contractions are seen at much lower concentrations of the triggering agents than in normal muscle tissue. There are two significantly different protocols in use for testing the muscle tissue: the North American Malignant Hyperthermia Group Protocol and the European Malignant Hyperthermia Group Protocol. Either of these protocols may be utilized but they have differing reported sensitivities and specificities.[91,92] Both protocols have a sensitivity close to 100%, whereas the specificity for the European protocol is 82% to 93% but only 78% for the North American protocol.[92] These protocols will categorize patients into one of three different groups: malignant hyperthermia negative, malignant hyperthermia sensitive (MHS), and malignant hyperthermia equivocal (MHE). Positive in vitro muscle contraction to both halothane and caffeine results in an MHS designation, whereas a positive contraction to only one agent results in an MHE designation. For maximum clinical safety, MHE is treated as MHS. The concentration of halothane and caffeine used as well as the strength of contraction should be reported.

There are some significant limitations of the halothane-caffeine contracture test. Caffeine is believed to increase calcium release from the sarcoplasmic reticulum.[58] The test requires an open biopsy; this combined with its poor specificity makes it ineffective as a screening test. There is a significant difference in outcome between the two protocols,[91] and significant intralaboratory variability as well as variability within the same biopsy.[93] False-positive results have been reported in patients with myopathies, but these patients may be at higher risk for developing MH. Abnormal in vitro muscle contraction similar to MH has also been observed in some patients that have suffered exertional heat stroke, suggesting a common pathology. The muscle biopsy has no utility in diagnosis of NMS. Although there are reports of abnormal contractions of muscle fibers to fluphenazine, this was performed at very high concentrations and has not been replicated.[94] In addition, patients who have suffered from NMS have undergone general anesthesia without any problems, and no familial link has been found between the two diseases.

DIFFERENTIAL DIAGNOSIS

Although these three neuromuscular syndromes are all characterized by alterations in mental status, autonomic dysfunction, and neuromuscular hyperactivity, they are often readily distinguishable by history, temporal profile, and the presence of unique physical findings. The clinical signs and symptoms that can be used to differentiate these syndromes are listed in Table 10A-1. The presence of clonus (myoclonus and ocular clonus), hyperreflexia, and tremors are unique to serotonin syndrome and not present with the other two neuromuscular syndromes. Rigidity is lead pipe type and diffuse with NMS, rigor mortis–like and diffuse with MH, and clasp-knife type and more prominent in the lower extremities with serotonin syndrome.

These three hyperthermic syndromes must be differentiated from other conditions associated with fever and neuromuscular hyperactivity. These include the anticholinergic and sedative-hypnotic withdrawal syndromes; poisoning by hallucinogens, salicylates, and other uncouplers (e.g., dinitrophenol), lithium, MAOIs, strychnine, nicotine, and sympathomimetics; and nontoxic etiologies, such as intracranial hemorrhage, brain tumors, CNS infections (e.g., meningoencephalitis, brain abscess), CNS vasculitis, thyrotoxicosis, addisonian crisis, heat stroke, pheochromocytoma, hypocalcemia, hypomagnesemia, tetanus, and lethal catatonia.

EPS can occasionally look like early NMS, and some clinicians have proposed a spectrum of basal ganglia dopamine dysfunction, with NMS being the extreme manifestation along a continuum. The presence of EPS that are persistent and resistant to or exacerbated by anticholinergic treatment may suggest early NMS.

MANAGEMENT OF HYPERTHERMIC SYNDROMES

Management of NMS, serotonin syndrome, and MH involves immediate termination of any precipitating drugs, the provision of aggressive supportive care, and the administration of adjunctive pharmacotherapies for each syndrome. Aggressive supportive care entails the control of patient agitation and neuromuscular hyperactivity, intravenous rehydration, treatment of hyperthermia, and treatment of associated complications. Gastrointestinal decontamination is not useful for NMS, MH, or serotonin syndrome due to the delay of onset of symptoms and the route of administration of the precipitating agents. The decrease in mortality observed for NMS and serotonin syndrome is most likely due to early recognition and better critical care medicine, not due to specific antidotes. In contrast, the timeliness of initiation of the antidote, dantrolene, is critical to effect a good survival for those with MH.

Complications of these syndromes are similar and can include rhabdomyolysis, renal failure, aspiration pneumonitis, respiratory failure, thromboembolism, deep venous thrombosis, infection, electrolyte imbalance, DIC, hepatic dysfunction, and cardiovascular collapse. Supportive care should be aggressive and directed at preventing or treating these complications. Special attention should be directed to ventilator status (especially if there is chest wall rigidity preventing ventilation),

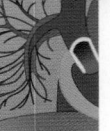
hydration, temperature, electrolytes, and possible seizures. Aggressive fluid hydration is usually warranted; if comorbidities are present, then central monitoring for fluid status may be required. Hydration and possible alkalinization of the urine will help treat the rhabdomyolysis and myoglobinuria that often results. Vasopressor support should be given as needed for hypotension, assuming that fluid resuscitation is complete.

Many of the complications of these syndromes occur largely as a result of neuromuscular hyperactivity and secondary hyperthermia. Attention should be directed to careful temperature monitoring and should always rely on core temperature readings because peripheral measurements can be erroneous. Cooling measures may initially include intravenous (IV) benzodiazepines (diazepam 0.1 to 0.3 mg/kg or lorazepam 0.05 to 0.1 mg/kg), antipyretics, evaporative cooling, ice packs, cooled IV fluids, and adjunctive pharmacotherapies specific to each syndrome. For those patients with NMS and serotonin syndrome who develop severe or protracted hyperthermia (i.e., temperature greater than 40° C), the use of nondepolarizing paralytics (e.g., pancuronium) is strongly recommended.[95] Neuromuscular blockade will achieve rapid, predictable, and effective reduction of rigidity and fever. In contrast, for patients with MH, treatment with dantrolene is the key to minimizing mortality from severe hyperthermia. Neuromuscular blockade will not achieve muscle relaxation with MH.

Neuroleptic Malignant Syndrome Management

There are many opinions as to the "correct" treatment for NMS. Most of what we know about treatment for this syndrome is from collections of case reports, case series, or retrospective, noncontrolled studies. There have been no prospective, controlled treatment studies. Immediate discontinuation of the offending agent is central to successful treatment. One should also ensure that other non-neuroleptic dopamine-blocking agents (e.g., metoclopramide) and other syndrome-potentiating medications (e.g., lithium, anticholinergic agents) are stopped as well. Supportive care is often overlooked in a rush to use the most "up to date" treatment. Because the natural course of the illness is often characterized by waxing and waning symptoms, initial improvement may be mistakenly interpreted as a positive response to a specific treatment.

Benzodiazepines and barbiturates have been used successfully in individual cases and retrospective, uncontrolled studies. In one retrospective study of 16 patients with NMS, clinical improvement was noted within 24 to 72 hours of benzodiazepine treatment initiation (e.g., lorazepam).[96] Regardless, it is uncertain if benzodiazepines hasten the recovery from NMS over supportive care alone. Benzodiazepine therapy has the advantage of being generally safe with minimal side effects. The alternative sedating agents, barbiturates, may lower the blood pressure when administered rapidly, which limit their utility with the unstable patient.

Theoretically there should be some CNS benefit for either drug due to increased γ-aminobutyric acid (GABA) tone limiting central neurologic excitation and possible injury. Standard initial IV doses of benzodiazepines (diazepam 0.1 to 0.3 mg/kg or lorazepam 0.05 to 0.1 mg/kg) should be employed. Additional doses may be administered as needed to achieve the desired level of sedation and sympatholysis. Another GABA agonist, propofol (2,6 diisopropylphenol), might be effective for the short-term treatment of those patients with severe agitation and muscular rigidity. In this setting, propofol should only be administered to patients that are intubated. Propofol is complicated by potential hypotension due to its negative inotropic effects.

Due to the similarity of NMS to MH, dantrolene has been utilized for the treatment of fever and muscle rigidity associated with NMS. Dantrolene is a direct skeletal muscle relaxant; it prevents calcium release from skeletal muscle sarcoplasmic reticulum by acting on the ranitidine receptor. It has very little affect on smooth and cardiac muscle. It is very effective for MH, but its efficacy in NMS has not been firmly established. Anecdotal experience suggests occasional efficacy, but case control studies have had mixed results. Dantrolene will not terminate muscular rigidity and hyperthermia as rapidly as nondepolarizing paralytic therapy. Doses utilized have ranged from 25 mg to more then 300 mg per day. It is available in an oral and IV form; a starting IV dose of 1 to 2.5 mg/kg every 6 to 12 hours is recommended, titrating the dose upward as needed. A maximum dose of 10 mg/kg/day is recommended. Side effects of dantrolene include dizziness, headache, fatigue, drowsiness, and weakness (rarely clinically significant).[97] Idiosyncratic reactions from chronic use that have been reported include hepatic dysfunction and a pleuropericardial reaction. Dantrolene has not been shown (and would not be expected) to correct a central disorder of thermoregulation.[98] It should probably be reserved for NMS patients with rigidity who have failed other treatments.

Bromocriptine has been used at a dose of 2.5 to 15 mg given three times a day. Bromocriptine is a partial dopamine agonist/antagonist. In rat studies, it can reverse the catatonia induced by neuroleptics. Data on its efficacy are mixed; studies have been done showing both benefit and lack thereof (see Chapter 38). Some retrospective studies have demonstrated a significant reduction in mortality from NMS in those patients treated with bromocriptine as compared with supportive care alone.[99,100] In addition, some patients who were treated with bromocriptine for NMS experienced recurrence of NMS symptoms when this therapy was suddenly discontinued. It has some mild side effects, namely nausea, vomiting, limited vasospasm, dyskinesias, hallucinations, and worsening psychosis. Bromocriptine does have a mild stimulatory effect on 5-HT receptors and does reduce brain serotonin turnover.[101] Its indiscriminate use should be tempered with the knowledge that it might theoretically worsen serotonin syndrome.[53] It should be strongly considered for treatment of unequivocal cases of NMS.

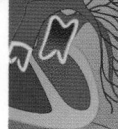

Amantadine is a parkinsonian drug reported to be successfully used for NMS in only a few cases, making firm conclusions about its efficacy impossible.[102] It has minimal dopamine agonistic properties and its benefit may actually arise from its N-methyl-D-aspartate, glutamate receptor antagonist properties.[103] It has been used in divided doses from 200 to 400 mg a day. L-dopa/carbidopa has been tried with mixed success. There is evidence that L-dopa can cause serotonin release, which could worsen serotonin syndrome. In general, other dopaminergic agents should be considered before amantadine or L-dopa are initiated.

For treatment of EPS from neuroleptic use, anticholinergic agents are often employed. The theory is that decreasing cholinergic tone increases dopamine tone, thus alleviating the symptoms of dopamine receptor antagonism. However, in general, anticholinergic agents have not been shown to be of benefit for NMS. They are likely to be detrimental when the dose is increased due to their effect on heat dissipation and CNS effects. They should be stopped or possibly tapered if the patient has been on them for a prolonged period.

Electroconvulsive therapy (ECT) has been reported as effective for the treatment of NMS, although controlled studies are lacking.[104] Some of the early cases had morbidity associated with the procedure, but with closer monitoring these events have not recurred. ECT increases brain catecholamine (i.e., dopamine) levels, which is believed to be the reason for its successful use. The successful use of ECT for NMS utilizing general anesthesia is additional evidence that MH and NMS are different syndromes. One should consider the use of ECT for patients with protracted signs and symptoms of NMS or those with catatonia after the illness has resolved.[24]

The best treatment for NMS is probably early recognition, immediate discontinuation of the precipitating agent, and vigilant supportive care in an intensive care unit setting. Adjunctive pharmacologic agents may be added.

Once the episode of NMS has resolved, there is often a need to restart medication in patients with mental illness. Ideally, one should wait at least 2 weeks prior to restarting neuroleptics. Doses should be given orally, initiated at the lowest possible dose, and titrated up very slowly. Atypical or low-potency antipsychotics should be utilized. Patients should be in a setting where their temperature and clinical status can be closely monitored. Risk factors such as dehydration and agitation should be addressed and treated with IV fluids and sedation with benzodiazepines.

Serotonin Syndrome Management

Because serotonin toxicity exists as a disease spectrum, it is difficult to give unifying or all-inclusive treatment recommendations. As for NMS, good supportive care and immediate discontinuation of the offending/triggering agent are the most important aspects of treatment and will achieve a good outcome in the vast majority of patients. Depending on the pharmacokinetics and severity of the reaction, treatment decisions range from outpatient to intensive care unit admission. The severe serotonin reactions are usually due to MAOI interactions with another proserotonergic agent. These patients should probably be admitted to the intensive care unit due to the potential severity of the syndrome.

Serotonin syndrome is due to excessive stimulation at certain CNS 5-HT receptors (most likely 5-HT$_{2A}$ and possibly some 5-HT$_{1A}$). Treatment with 5-HT$_{2A}$ receptor antagonists have been effective in animal models of serotonin syndrome and in case series of patients with serotonin syndrome. Cyproheptadine, an antihistamine with serotonin antagonist effects, has been effective for the treatment of serotonin syndrome.[35,105] There are no randomized, controlled trials that have demonstrated the efficacy of cyproheptadine or other 5-HT$_{2A}$ receptor antagonists (e.g., chlorpromazine, olanzapine, risperidone, methysergide) for the treatment of serotonin syndrome. Efficacy for these pharmacotherapies is difficult to establish since serotonin syndrome is often self-limited and has a relatively short duration. Cyproheptadine is only available as an oral formulation; the usual dose in adults is 4 to 8 mg every 1 to 4 hours, up to a maximum of 32 mg/day.[48] For children, the cyproheptadine dose is 1 to 2 mg every 1 to 4 hours, up to a maximum of 12 mg/day. There often is a positive response after a single dose, but larger doses may be necessary for those with serotonin syndrome as a complication of a serotonin agonist overdose. Cyproheptadine has some sedating and anticholinergic side effects, which may become problematic at the higher recommended doses. Methysergide has blockade at 5-HT$_1$ and 5-HT$_2$ receptors and has been infrequently used for serotonin syndrome; it has less 5-HT$_{2A}$ affinity than cyproheptadine.[53] The recommended methysergide dose is 2 to 6 mg orally; it is not available for parenteral use. For either agent, if charcoal was given, larger doses may be required or this treatment may need to be abandoned due to adsorption of the antidote to charcoal.

Chlorpromazine has been used as treatment for serotonin syndrome with positive results. In addition to its dopamine receptor antagonist effects, chlorpromazine is a potent 5-HT$_{2A}$ receptor antagonist with similar potency to cyproheptadine. It has the advantage of having a parenteral formulation and can be administered either IV or intramuscularly (IM).[106] A starting dose might be 50 mg IM with a repeat dose in 4 hours if necessary; dosing is usually every 6 hours.[29] Hypotension is common following larger doses of chlorpromazine. Thus, intravenous fluid administration should accompany or precede this therapy. Chlorpromazine is associated with numerous side effects (sedation, anticholinergic effects, dopaminergic blockade, potential to induce seizures, cardiac conduction effects). Use of this agent, while potentially effective, may also be associated with adverse effects and complicate patient treatment. Chlorpromazine should not be used if there is any concern for NMS.

Other pharmacologic agents have been used for serotonin syndrome with mixed results. Benzodiazepines have been tried with mixed results. These agents are best reserved for patients with significant muscle rigidity

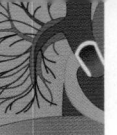

and hyperthermia. Diazepam or lorazepam may be administered in the same doses as recommended for NMS.[107] The central GABA receptors are believed to have an inhibitory influence on serotonin syndrome.[46] Very limited data exist for propranolol, which has been used to treat some of the hypertensive symptoms. Propranolol is a 5-HT$_{1A}$ antagonist and, thus, is not expected to reverse all the signs and symptoms of the syndrome.[46,108] Due to its potential for adverse hemodynamic effects, propranolol must be used with considerable caution and cannot be recommended for first-line use. Mirtazapine has been used for the treatment of serotonin syndrome and theoretically may be efficacious via its 5-HT$_{2A}$ antagonistic properties.[109,110] Nitroglycerin has been used and has resulted in some clinical improvement anecdotally.[111] There is the theoretical possibility of exacerbating serotonin syndrome if treated with bromocriptine; this drug can increase brain 5-HT levels.[53,112] Animal experimental data support the use of memantine (and possibly risperidone) for serotonin syndrome, but no human experience exists.[113,114] Dantrolene has been used for serotonin syndrome without documented benefit. Dantrolene may cause increased CNS 5-HT tone and, thus, its use is not recommended for treatment of serotonin syndrome.[115] Intubation and paralysis should be employed as they are for NMS if muscular rigidity or hyperthermia is severe and not initially responsive to alternative measures.

Restarting medications should be done after a sufficient recovery time has been allowed. Exactly how long depends on the half-life of the drug and its metabolites and the duration of ongoing drug effect. With irreversible MAOI therapy, MAO is permanently inhibited and adequate time should be allowed (3 to 5 weeks) for regeneration of the enzyme prior to reinitiation of another proserotonergic agent.[48,116] When medications are restarted, they should be restarted one at a time at the lowest effective dose and slowly advanced to the target level. Additional medications can subsequently be added as needed. A reevaluation of the need for MAOI treatment and the most potent serotonin reuptake inhibitors should be performed. Agents with less proserotonergic effect should be tried initially and started at low doses.

Malignant Hyperthermia Management

This syndrome has a radically different pathophysiology from NMS and serotonin syndrome. The pathology is within the skeletal muscle itself and is not secondary to enhanced nerve activity and motor end-plate stimulation. No benefit is derived from benzodiazepines and nondepolarizing paralytics. As for the other hyperthermic syndromes, when MH is suspected, the precipitating agents must be discontinued immediately. For MH, aggressive supportive care includes hyperventilation, IV fluid administration, correction of electrolyte abnormalities (e.g., hyperkalemia, hypocalcemia, hypercalcemia), rapid cooling, and treatment of associated complications as they occur (e.g., rhabdomyolysis, renal failure, respiratory failure). Bicarbonate has been

advocated, and that combined with dextrose should be beneficial to treat associated hyperkalemia.

The treatment of choice is dantrolene. There is a direct correlation between survival and early administration of dantrolene in patients with MH.[117] Dantrolene is believed to interact with the ryanodine skeletal muscle receptor, preventing further release of calcium from the sarcoplasmic reticulum, halting the pathologic cascade operative in MH. The starting dose of dantrolene is 2.5 mg/kg IV. This dose can be repeated every 2 to 3 minutes until a maximum of 10 mg/kg has been administered. The IV formulation is preferred in all situations of MH due to uncertain levels achieved with oral dosing. Dantrolene is occasionally used as prophylaxis for patients with a previous history of MH or with a very strong family history of anesthetic-associated deaths. In this situation it is given as a 2.5 mg/kg dose prior to anesthesia; but despite this pretreatment, patients can still develop MH, so there should be strong consideration for using "safer" agents in such patients.

Once a patient has developed MH, dantrolene should be continued every 6 hours until symptoms completely resolve, because dantrolene has a half-life of 12 hours.[118] When repeated doses are used, patients are much less likely to have a recurrence of symptoms. Sufficient dosing is recommended because subtherapeutic amounts of dantrolene may paradoxically open the ryanodine channel, possibly exacerbating illness.[119] The use of calcium channel blockers (e.g., verapamil) with dantrolene has been associated with hyperkalemia and hypotension. The use of calcium channel antagonists for arrhythmias is thus not recommended, even though this synergistic toxicity has not been demonstrated in a dog model.[120] Short-term side effects of dantrolene have included weakness, dizziness, and fatigue; clinically significant weakness appears to be rare.[97]

REFERENCES

1. Delay J, Pichot P, Lemperiere T, et al: Un neuroleptique majeur nonphenothiazine et non-reserpinique, l'haloperidol, dans le traitement des psychoses. Ann Med Psychol 1960;118:145–152.
2. Caroff SN, Mann SC: Neuroleptic malignant syndrome. Med Clin North Am 1993;77(1):185–202.
3. Keck PE, Pope HG, McElroy SL: Declining frequency of neuroleptic malignant syndrome in a hospital population. Am J Psychiatry 1991;148:880–882.
4. Gelenberg AJ, Bellinghansen B, Wojcik JD, et al: A prospective survey of neuroleptic malignant syndrome in a short-term psychiatric hospital. Am J Psychiatry 1988;145:517–518.
5. Keck PE, Sebastianelli J, Pope HG, et al: Frequency and presentation of neuroleptic malignant syndrome in a state psychiatric hospital. J Clin Psychiatry 1989;50:352–355.
6. Farver DK: Neuroleptic malignant syndrome induced by atypical antipsychotics. Expert Opin Drug Saf 2003;2(1):22–35.
7. Karagianis FL, Phillips LC, Hogan KP, LeDrew KK: Clozapine-associated neuroleptic malignant syndrome: two new cases and a review of the literature. Ann Pharmacother 1999;33:623–630.
8. Friedman JH, Feinberg SS, Feldman RG: A neuroleptic malignant-like syndrome due to levodopa therapy withdrawal. JAMA 1985;254(19):2792–2795.
9. Hermesh H, Sirota P, Eviatar J: Recurrent neuroleptic malignant syndrome due to haloperidol and amantadine. Biol Psychiatry 1989;25:962–965.
10. Friedman E, Gershon S: Effect of lithium on brain dopamine. Nature 1973;243:520–521.

11. Spring G, Frankel M: New data on lithium and haloperidol incompatibility. Am J Psychiatry 1981;138(6):818–821.

12. Davis JM, Caroff SN, Mann SC: Treatment of neuroleptic malignant syndrome. Psychiatr Ann 2000;30(5):325–331.

13. Carroll BT, Taylor RE: The nondichotomy between lethal catatonia and neuroleptic malignant syndrome. J Clin Psychopharmacol 1997;17(3):235–236.

14. Korsgaard S, Gerlach J, Christensson E: Behavioral aspects of serotonin-dopamine interaction in the monkey. Eur J Pharmacol 1985;118:245–252.

15. Carter CJ, Pycock CJ: Possible importance of 5-hydroxytryptamine in neuroleptic induced catalepsy in rats [proceedings]. Br J Pharmacol 1977;60(2):267P–268P.

16. Kapur S, Remington G: Serotonin-dopamine interaction and its relevance to schizophrenia. Am J Psychiatry 1996;153(4):466–476.

17. Halman M, Goldbloom DS: Fluoxetine and neuroleptic malignant syndrome. Biol Psychiatry 1990;28:518–521.

18. Caley CF: Extrapyramidal reactions and the selective serotonin-reuptake inhibitors. Ann Pharmacother 1997;31:1481–1489.

19. Addonizio G, Susman VL, Roth SD: Neuroleptic malignant syndrome: review and analysis of 115 cases. Biol Psychiatry 1987;22:1004–1020.

20. Totten V, Hirschenstein E, Hew P: Neuroleptic malignant syndrome presenting without initial fever: a case report. J Emerg Med 1994;12(1):43–47.

21. Taylor C, Rogers G, Goodman C, et al: Hematologic, iron-related, and acute-phase protein responses to sustained strenuous exercise. J Appl Physiol 1987;62(2):464–469.

22. Rosebush PI, Mazurek MF: Serum iron and neuroleptic malignant syndrome. Lancet 1991;338:149–150.

23. Van Harten PN, Kemperman CJF: Organic amnestic disorder: a long-term sequel after neuroleptic malignant syndrome. Biol Psychiatry 1991;29:407–410.

24. Caroff S, Mann SC, Keck PE Jr, Francis A: Residual catatonic state following neuroleptic malignant syndrome. J Clin Psychopharmacol 2000;20(2):257–259.

25. Mitchell RS: Fatal toxic encephalitis occurring during iproniazid therapy in pulmonary tuberculosis. Ann Intern Med 1955;42:417–424.

26. Oates JA, Sjoerdsma A: Neurologic effects of tryptophan in patients receiving a monoamine oxidase inhibitor. Neurology 1960;10:1076–1078.

27. Grahame-Smith DG: Studies in vivo on the relationship between brain tryptophan, brain 5-HT synthesis and hyperactivity in rats treated with a monoamine oxidase inhibitor and L-tryptophan. J Neurochem 1971;18:1055–1066.

28. Insel TR, Roy BF, Cohen RM, et al: Possible development of the serotonin syndrome in man. Am J Psychol 1982;139:954–955.

29. Gillman PK: The serotonin syndrome and its treatment. J Psychopharmacol 1999;13:100–109.

30. Nisijima K, Shioda K, Yoshino T, et al: Diazepam and chlormethiazole attenuate the development of hyperthermia in an animal model of the serotonin syndrome. Neurochem Int 2003;43:155–164.

31. Nisijima K, Yoshino T, Yui K, Katoh S: Potent serotonin (5-HT)$_{2A}$ receptor antagonists completely prevent the development of hyperthermia in an animal model of the 5-HT syndrome. Brain Res 2001;890:23–31.

32. Mazzola Pomietto P, Aulakh CS, Wozniak KM, et al: Evidence that 1-(2,5-dimethoxy-4-iodophenol)-2-aminopropane (DOI)-induced hyperthermia in rats is mediated by stimulation of 5-HT$_{2A}$ receptors. Psychopharmacology 1995;117:193–199.

33. Siegel GJ (ed): Basic Neurochemistry. Philadelphia, Lippincott Williams & Wilkins, 1999.

34. Zerjav-Lacombe S, Dewan V: Possible serotonin syndrome associated with clomipramine after withdrawal of clozapine. Ann Pharmacother 2001;35:180–182.

35. Horowitz Z, Mullins ME: Cyproheptadine for serotonin syndrome in an accidental pediatric sertraline ingestion. Pediatr Emerg Care 1999;15(5):325–327.

36. Isbister GK, Bowe SJ, Dawson A, Whyte IM: Relative toxicity of selective serotonin reuptake inhibitors (SSRIs) in overdose. J Toxicol Clin Toxicol 2004;42:277–285.

37. Tatsumi M, Groshan K, Blakely RD, Richelson E: Pharmacological profile of antidepressants and related compounds at human monoamine transporters. Euro J Pharmacol 1997;340:249–258.

38. Whyte IM, Dawson AH, Buckley NA: Relative toxicity of venlafaxine and selective serotonin reuptake inhibitors in overdose compared to tricyclic antidepressants. QJM 2003;96:369–374.

39. Gillman PK: Serotonin syndrome: history and risk. Fundam Clin Pharmacol 1998;12:482–491.

40. Gillman K: Serotonin toxicity. Accessed January 15, 2005, at www.psychotropical.com/SerotoninToxicity.doc.

41. Bamigbade TA, Davidson C, Langford RM, Stamford JA: Actions of tramadol, its enantiomers and principle metabolite, O-desmethyltramadol, on serotonin (5-HT) efflux and uptake in the rat dorsal raphe nucleus. Br J Anaesth 1997;79:352–356.

42. Brodribb TR, Downey M, Gilbar PJ: Efficacy and adverse effects of moclobemide. Lancet 1994;343:475.

43. Zornberg GL, Bodkin JA, Cohen BM: Severe adverse interaction between pethidine and selegiline. Lancet 1991;337:246.

44. Hinds NP, Hiller CE, Wiles CM: Possible serotonin syndrome arising from an interaction between nortriptyline and selegiline in a lady with parkinsonism. J Neurol 2000;247:811.

45. Francis E, Harchelroad F: LSD/fluoxetine-induced serotonin syndrome. J Toxicol Clin Toxicol 1996;34(5):560.

46. Marsden CA, Heal DJ (ed): Central Serotonin Receptors and Psychotropic Drugs. Oxford, Blackwell Scientific, 1992.

47. Brush ED, Bird SB, Boyer EW: Monoamine oxidase inhibitor poisoning resulting from Internet misinformation on illicit substances. J Toxicol Clin Toxicol 2004;42(2):191–195.

48. Hardman JG, Limbird LE (eds): Goodman & Gillman's The Pharmacological Basis of Therapeutics, 9th ed. New York, McGraw-Hill, 1996.

49. John L, Perreault MM, Tao T, Blew PG: Serotonin syndrome associated with nefazodone and paroxetine. Ann Emerg Med 1997;29(2):287–289.

50. Baetz M, Malcolm D: Serotonin syndrome from fluvoxamine and buspirone. Can J Psychiatry 1995;40(7):428–429.

51. Mathew NT, Tietjen GE, Lucker C: Serotonin syndrome complicating migraine pharmacotherapy. Cephalalgia 1996;16:323–327.

52. Turkel SB, Nadala JG, Wincor MZ: Possible serotonin syndrome in association with 5-HT$_3$ antagonist agents. Psychosomatics 2001;42(3):258–260.

53. Sandyk R: L-Dopa induced "serotonin syndrome" in a parkinsonian patient on bromocriptine. J Clin Psychopharmacol 1986;6(3):194.

54. Kuisma MJ: Fatal serotonin syndrome with trismus. Ann Emerg Med 1995;26(1):108.

55. Mills KC: Serotonin syndrome: a clinical update. Crit Care Clin 1997;13(4):763–783.

56. Sternbach H: The serotonin syndrome. Am J Psychiatry 1991;148:705–813.

57. Denborough MA, Forster JF, Lovell RR, et al: Anaesthetic deaths in a family. Br J Anaesth 1962;34:395–396.

58. Mickelson JR, Louis CF: Malignant hyperthermia: excitation-contraction coupling, Ca^{2+} release channel, and cell Ca^{2+} regulation defects. Physiol Rev 1996;76(2):537–592.

59. Nelson TE, Flewellen EH: The malignant hyperthermia syndrome. N Engl J Med 1983;309(7):416–418.

60. Britt BA, Kalow W: Malignant hyperthermia: a statistical review. Can Anaesth Soc J 1970;17(4):293–315.

61. Lane JE, Brooks AG, Logan MS, et al: An unusual case of malignant hyperthermia during desflurane anesthesia in an African-American patient. Anesth Analg 2000;91:1032–1034.

62. Jardon OM: Physiologic stress, heat stroke, malignant hyperthermia—a perspective. Milit Med 1982;147:8–14.

63. Bendahan D, Kozak-Ribbens G, Confort-Gouny S, et al: A noninvasive investigation of muscle energetics supports similarities between exertional heat stroke and malignant hyperthermia. Anesth Analg 2001;93:683–689.

64. Wappler F, Fiege M, Steinfath M, et al: Evidence for susceptibility to malignant hyperthermia in patients with exercise-induced rhabdomyolysis. Anesthesiology 2001;94:95–100.

65. Wappler F, Fiege M, Antz M, Schulte am Esch J: Hemodynamic and metabolic alterations in response to graded exercise in a

patient susceptible to malignant hyperthermia. Anesthesiology 2000;92:268–272.

66. Tobin JR, Jason DR, Challa VR, et al: Malignant hyperthermia and apparent heat stroke. JAMA 2001;286(2):168–169.

67. Bendahan D, Kozak-Ribbens G, Rodet L, et al: 31Phosphorus magnetic resonance spectroscopy characterization of muscular metabolic anomalies in patients with malignant hyperthermia: application of diagnosis. Anesthesiology 1998;88(1):96–107.

68. Lopez JR, Contreras J, Linares N, Allen PD: Hypersensitivity of malignant hyperthermia-susceptible swine skeletal muscle to caffeine is mediated by high resting myoplasmic [Ca^{2+}]. Anesthesiology 2000;92:1799–1806.

69. Standec A, Stefano G: Cyclic AMP in normal and malignant hyperpyrexia susceptible individuals following exercise. Br J Anaesth 1984;56:1243–1246.

70. Fletcher JE, Wieland SJ, Karan SM, et al: Sodium channel in human malignant hyperthermia. Anesthesiology 1997;86(5): 1023–1032.

71. Ball SP, Johnson KJ: The genetics of malignant hyperthermia. J Med Genet 1993;30(2):89–93.

72. Gurrera RJL: Is neuroleptic malignant syndrome a neurogenic form of malignant hyperthermia? Clin Neuropharmacol 2002;25(4):183–193.

73. Lambert C, Blanloeil Y, Horber RK, et al: Malignant hyperthermia in a patient with hypokalemic periodic paralysis. Anesth Analg 1994;79:1012–1014.

74. Wappler F, Scholz J, von Richthofen V, et al: Attenuation of serotonin-induced contractures in skeletal muscle from malignant hyperthermia-susceptible patients with dantrolene. Acta Anesthesiol Scand 1997;41:1312.

75. Wappler F, Scholz J, Oppermann S, et al: Ritanserin attenuates the in vitro effects of the 5-HT2 receptor agonist DOI on skeletal muscles from malignant hyperthermia susceptible patients. J Clin Anesth 1997;9:306–311.

76. Wappler F, Fiege M, Schulte am Esch J: Pathophysiological role of the serotonin system in malignant hyperthermia. Br J Anaesth 2001;87(5):794–798.

77. Wappler F, Roewer N, Kochling A, et al: Effects of the serotonin 2 receptor agonist DOI on skeletal muscle specimens from malignant hyperthermia-susceptible patients. Anesthesiology 1996;84(6):1280–1287.

78. Richter A, Scholz J, Loscher W, et al: Effects of the 5-HT$_2$ receptor antagonist ritanserin on halothane-induced increase of inositol phosphates in porcine malignant hyperthermia. Arch Pharmacol 1996;354:593–597.

79. Löscher W, Gerdes C, Richter A: Lack of prophylactic or therapeutic efficacy of 5-HT2A receptor antagonists in halothane induced porcine malignant hyperthermia. Arch Pharmacol 1994;350:365–374.

80. Wappler F, Scholz J, Fiege M, et al: 5-HT$_2$ receptor antagonist-mediated inhibition of halothane-induced contractures in skeletal muscle specimens from malignant hyperthermia susceptible patients. Naunyn Schmiedebergs Arch Pharmacol 1999;360:376–381.

81. Hermesh H, Aizenberg D, Lapidot M, Munitz H: Risk of malignant hyperthermia among patients with neuroleptic malignant syndrome and their families. Am J Psychiatry 1988; 145(11):1431–1434.

82. Allen GC, Brubaker CL: Human malignant hyperthermia associated with desflurane anesthesia. Anesth Analg 1998;86(6): 1328–1331.

83. Fiege M, Wappler F, Weisshorn R, et al: In vitro and in vivo effects of the phosphodiesterase-iii inhibitor enoximone on malignant hyperthermia-susceptible swine. Anesthesiology 2003;98:944–949.

84. Riess FC, Fiege M; Moshar S, et al: Rhabdomyolysis following cardiopulmonary bypass and treatment with enoximone in a patient susceptible to malignant hyperthermia. Anesthesiology 2001;94:355–357.

85. Fiege M, Wappler F, Scholz J, et al: Effects of the phospho-diesterase-III inhibitor enoximone on skeletal muscle specimens from malignant hyperthermia susceptible patients. J Clin Anesth 2000;12:123–128.

86. McKenzie AJ, Couchman KG, Pollock N: Propofol is a "safe" anesthetic agent in malignant hyperthermia susceptible patients. Anaesth Intensive Care 1992;20(2):165–168.

87. Fierobe L, Nivoche Y, Mantz J, et al: Perioperative severe rhabdomyolysis revealing susceptibility to malignant hyper-thermia. Anesthesiology 1998;88(1):263–265.

88. Harwood T, Nelson TE: Massive postoperative rhabdomyolysis after uneventful surgery: a case report of subclinical malignant hyperthermia. Anesthesiology 1998;88(1):265–268.

89. Hoenemann CW, Halene-Holtgraeve TB, Booke M, et al: Delayed onset of malignant hyperthermia in desflurane anesthesia. Anesth Analg 2003;96:165–167.

90. Wohlfeil ER, Woehlck HJ, McElroy ND: Malignant hyperthermia triggered coincidentally after reversal of neuromuscular blockade in a patient from the Hmong people of Laos. 1998;88(6): 1667–1668.

91. Islander G, Twetman ER: Comparison between the European and North American protocols for diagnosis of malignant hyper-thermia susceptibility in humans. Anesth Analg 1999;88(5): 1155–1160.

92. Allen GC, Larach MG, Kunselman AR: The sensitivity and specificity of the caffeine-halothane contracture test: a report from the North American malignant hyperthermia registry. Anesthesiology 1998;88(3):579–588.

93. Ørding H, Islander G, Bendixen D, Ranklev-Twetman E: Between-center variability of results of the in vitro contracture test for malignant hyperthermia susceptibility. Anesth Analg 2000;91(2): 452–457.

94. Caroff S, Rosenberg H, Gerber JC: Neuroleptic malignant syndrome and malignant hyperthermia. Lancet 1983;1(8318):244.

95. Sangal R, Dimitrijevic R: Neuroleptic malignant syndrome successful treatment with pancuronium. JAMA 1985;254(19): 2795–2796.

96. Francis A, Koch M, Chandragiri S, et al: Is lorazepam a treatment for neuroleptic malignant syndrome? CNS Spectrum 2000;5:54–57.

97. Wedel DJ, Quinlan JG, Iaizzo PA: Clinical effects of intravenously administered dantrolene. Mayo Clin Proc 1995;70:241–246.

98. Amsterdam JT, Syverud SA, Barker WJ, et al: Dantrolene sodium for treatment of heatstroke victims: lack of efficacy in a canine model. Am J Emerg Med 1986;4:399–405.

99. Sakkas P, Davis JM, Hua J, et al: Pharmacotherapy of neuroleptic malignant syndrome. Psychiatr Ann 1991;21:157–164.

100. Sakkas P, Davis JM, Janicak PG, et al: Drug treatment of the neuroleptic malignant syndrome. Psychopharmacol Bull 1991;27:381–384.

101. Hutt CS, Snider SR, Fahn S: Interaction between bromocriptine and levodopa. Neurology 1977;27:505–510.

102. McCarron MM, Boettger ML, Peck JJ: A case of neuroleptic malignant syndrome successfully treated with amantadine. J Clin Psychiatry 1982;43(9):381–382.

103. Kornhuber J, Weller M: Psychotogenicity and N-methyl-D-aspartate receptor antagonism: implications for neuroprotective pharmacotherapy. Biol Psychiatry 1997;41:135–144.

104. Nisijima K, Ishiguro T: Electroconvulsive therapy for the treatment of neuroleptic malignant syndrome with psychotic symptoms: a report of five cases. J ECT 1999;15(2):158–163.

105. Graudins A, Stearman A, Chan B: Treatment of the serotonin syndrome with cyproheptadine. J Emerg Med 1998;16(4):615–619.

106. Gillman PK: Serotonin syndrome treated with chlorpromazine. J Clin Psychopharmacol 1997;17:128–129.

107. Cano-Munoz JL, Montejo-Iglesias ML, Yanez-Saez RM, Galvez-Borrero IM: Possible serotonin syndrome following the combined administration of clomipramine and alprazolam. J Clin Psychiatry 1995;56(3):122.

108. Guze BH, Baxter LR: The serotonin syndrome: case responsive to propranolol. J Clin Psychopharmacol 1986;6(2):119–120.

109. Hoes MJAJM: Mirtazapine as treatment for serotonin syndrome. Pharmacopsychiatry 1996;29:81.

110. de Boer T: The pharmacologic profile of mirtazapine. J Clin Psychiatry 1996;57:19–25.

111. Brown TM: Nitroglycerine in the treatment of the serotonin syndrome. Ann Pharmacother 1996;30:191.

112. Kline SS, Mauro LS, Scala-Barnett DM, Zick D: Serotonin syndrome versus neuroleptic malignant syndrome as a cause of death. Clin Pharm 1989;8:510–514.

113. Nisijima K, Shioda K, Yoshino T, et al: Memantine, an NMDA antagonist, prevents the development of hyperthermia in an

animal model for serotonin syndrome. Pharmacopsychiatry 2004;37:57–62.

114. Hamilton S, Malone K: Serotonin syndrome during treatment with paroxetine and risperidone. J Clin Psychopharmacol 2000;20(1):103–105.

115. Nisijima K, Ishiguro T: Does dantrolene influence central dopamine and serotonin metabolism in the neuroleptic malignant syndrome? A retrospective study. Biol Psychiatry 1993;33:45–48.

116. Kolecki P: Venlafaxine induced serotonin syndrome occurring after abstinence from phenelzine for more than two weeks. J Toxicol Clin Toxicol 1997;35:211–212.

117. Kolb ME, Horne ML, Martz R: Dantrolene in human malignant hyperthermia: a multicenter study. Anesthesiology 1982;56:254–262.

118. Ward A, Chaffman MO, Sorkin ME: Dantrolene, a review of its pharmacodynamic and pharmacokinetic properties and therapeutic use in malignant hyperthermia, the neuroleptic malignant syndrome and an update on its use in muscle spasticity. Drugs 1986;32:130–168.

119. Nelson T, Lin M, Zapata-Sudo G, Sudo RT: Dantrolene sodium can increase or attenuate activity of skeletal muscle ryanodine receptor calcium release channel: clinical implications. Anesthesiology 1996;84(6):1368–1379.

120. San Juan AC, Wong KC, Port JD: Hyperkalemia after dantrolene and verapamil-dantrolene administration in dogs. Anesth Analg 1988;67:759–762.

11 *Hepatic Toxicology*

ALISON L. JONES, BSc, MD ■ PAUL I. DARGAN, MBBS, MD

INTRODUCTION AND IMPORTANCE

Many potentially toxic substances enter the body via the gastrointestinal tract. As the blood supply from the gastrointestinal tract (through the portal vein) drains into the liver, the liver comes into contact with them, and this exposure often is at a higher concentration than that received by other tissues. The liver is essential for the metabolic disposal of virtually all xenobiotics. This process is achieved mostly without injury to the liver itself or to other organs.

Some compounds, such as carbon tetrachloride, are toxic themselves and/or produce metabolites that cause liver injury in a dose-dependent fashion. Most agents, however, cause liver injury only under special circumstances when toxins accumulate. Factors contributing to the build-up of such toxic substances include genetic enzyme variants (metabolizing enzymes with altered function due to gene defects), which allow greater formation of the harmful metabolite, and induction (greater production) of an enzyme, which produces more than the usual quantity of toxic substance. There also may be accumulation of toxic substances by interference with regular nontoxic metabolic pathways by substrate competition for enzymes (e.g., ethanol and trichloroethylene) or depletion of substrates used to metabolize the toxins or prevent toxic injury (e.g., glutathione). In addition there are a number of other factors that can potentially increase the risk of drug-related hepatotoxicity. Generally, women are more susceptible to drug-induced hepatotoxicity (with the exception of azathioprine hepatotoxicity, which is more common in men).[1,2] Being older than 60 years of age is associated with a greater risk of drug-induced hepatotoxicity (particularly with nonsteroidal anti-inflammatory drugs [NSAIDs]), whereas children appear to be more susceptible to salicylate and valproate-related hepatotoxicity.[1,3,4] Nutritional status also can be important—malnutrition probably is associated with liver glutathione depletion and a greater risk of hepatotoxicity in acetaminophen overdose.[5,6] Conversely, the risk of halothane hepatotoxicity is greater in obese patients.[7]

Hepatocytes near the portal tract branches (zone 1) receive blood that is rich in oxygen and nutrients, but those near the hepatic vein branches (zone 3) receive blood that has lost much of its nutrients and oxygen (Fig. 11-1). Therefore, zone 3 of the liver is sensitive particularly to damage from toxic compounds. Zone 3 cells also have a higher level of some metabolic enzymes and higher lipid synthesis than zone 1, which may also explain why zone 3 tends to be the most damaged and why lipid accumulation is a common response to this damage (see the carbon tetrachloride example later).

Allyl alcohol (2-propen-l-ol), however, causes zone 1 necrosis partly because this is the first area exposed to the compound in the blood and partly because of the presence of the enzyme alcohol dehydrogenase in zone 1, which produces reactive toxic metabolites (see Fig. 11-1).

Toxic substances can damage cells in target organs in many ways. The eventual pattern of response may be reversible injury or an irreversible change leading to the death (necrosis) of the cell or perhaps to carcinogenesis (cancer). Molecular mechanisms of liver injury are shown in Box 11-1.[8]

Toxin-induced liver injury is a major challenge, because its difficult to differentiate from hepatic disease due to other causes, including hepatic drug reactions, which may mimic almost any kind of liver disease.[9,10] Failure to recognize hepatic injury that is caused by a toxin may lead to worsening of hepatic injury or even hepatic failure.

EPIDEMIOLOGY OF DRUG-RELATED HEPATOTOXICITY

The epidemiology of drug hepatotoxicity is relatively poorly documented.[11] There are a number of reasons for this, including the difficulty encountered in making a definitive diagnosis of drug hepatotoxicity.[12] Many cases are subclinical and are never detected or detected only by chance as part of a routine biochemical workup, and many cases are not correctly identified as drug related. Clinical studies during the premarketing phase of drug

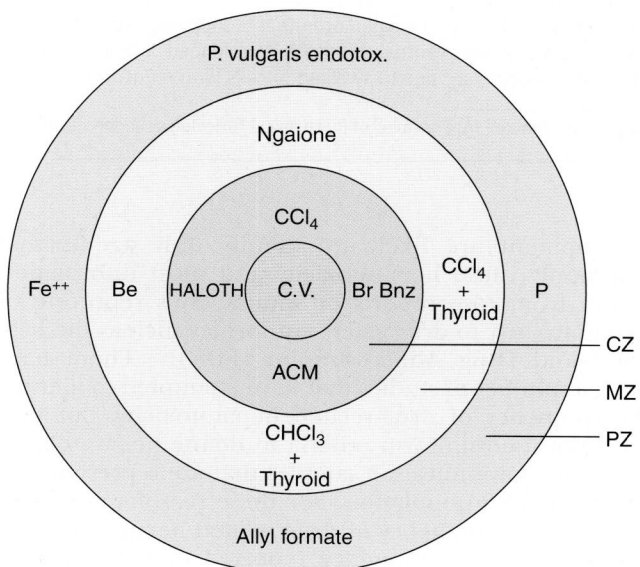

FIGURE 11-1 Hepatic zones. ACM, anticentromere; C.V., centrallvein; CZ, centrilobular zone (zone 3); MZ, midlobular zone (zone 2); PZ, periportal zone (zone 1).

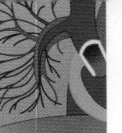

BOX 11-1   MOLECULAR MECHANISMS OF LIVER INJURY

Covalent binding: Free radicals have an unpaired electron centered on a carbon, nitrogen, sulfur, or oxygen atom and hence are extremely reactive, electrophilic species, which can react with a variety of cellular components. Free radicals and other reactive intermediates may be produced by metabolism, which interact with proteins and other macromolecules binding covalently to them. There is a correlation between the amount of binding and tissue damage, though this may reflect production of other damaging species. Binding to critical sites on proteins alters their function by, for example, inhibiting an enzyme or damaging a membrane, but binding could be to noncritical sites, and therefore be of no toxicologic importance.

Lipid peroxidation: Lipid peroxidation is caused by the attack of a free radical on unsaturated lipids (particularly polyunsaturated fatty acids found in cell membranes), the reaction being terminated by the production of lipid alcohols, aldehydes, or malondialdehyde. Therefore, there is a cascade of peroxidative reactions, which leads to the destruction of lipid unless stopped by a protective mechanism or a chemical reaction such as disproportionation, which gives rise to a nonradical product. The structural integrity of membrane lipids is adversely affected, leading to alterations in fluidity or permeability of membranes, destabilization of lysosomes, and altered function of the endoplasmic reticulum and mitochondria. Such mechanisms are thought to be involved in liver damage caused by carbon tetrachloride and white phosphorus.

Thiol group changes: Glutathione is responsible for cellular protection and if depleted, a cell is made more vulnerable to toxic substances. Reactive intermediates of toxic substances can react with glutathione either by a direct chemical reaction or by a glutathione transferase–mediated reaction. If excessive, these reactions can deplete cellular glutathione and leave essential proteins vulnerable to attack by oxidation, cross-linking, formation of disulfides, or covalent adducts.

Enzyme inhibition: Sometimes inhibition of an enzyme may lead to cell death; for example, cyanide inhibits cytochrome aa_3, leading to blockage of cellular respiration. This results in depletion of intracellular adenosine triphosphate (ATP)—ATP is produced by mitochondria and is the main energy source within the cell—and other vital endogenous molecules.

Ischemia: Reduction of oxygen or nutrients supplied to cells results in cell damage and eventual cell death if prolonged. Ischemia may be a secondary event due to swelling of cells with reduction of blood flow. As a result changes in subcellular skeleton and organelles may occur. This may result in ATP depletion, changes in Ca^{2+} concentration, damage to intracellular organelles, and DNA damage, and stimulation of apoptosis (programmed cell death) may occur. For example, phalloidin (a toxin from toxic mushrooms) causes centrilobular necrosis (see discussion on toxic mushrooms).

Depletion of ATP: Depletion of ATP may be caused by many toxic substances, usually by the uncoupling of mitochondrial oxidative phosphorylation or by DNA damage that causes activation of poly(ADP-ribose) polymerase. Depletion of ATP in the cell means that active transport in and out of the cell is altered or stopped and changes in electrolytes, particularly Ca^{2+}, lead to changes in biosynthesis within the cell, such as protein synthesis, production of glucose, and lipid synthesis. A very important mechanism of cellular damage is alteration of the intracellular Ca^{2+} concentration. Changes in the intracellular distribution of this ion have been implicated in the cytotoxicity of many toxic substances including carbon tetrachloride. Interference with Ca^{2+} homeostasis may occur as a result of inhibition of Ca^{2+} ATPs, direct damage to the plasma cell membrane allowing leakage of Ca^{2+}, or depletion of intracellular ATP.

Damage to intracellular organelles: Damage to intracellular organelles can result from the above mechanisms of injury; for example, carbon tetrachloride damages both smooth and rough endoplasmic reticulum, leading to disruption of protein synthesis of the whole cell. Mitochondrial damage may occur, for example, after exposure to hydrazine, leading to functional changes and rupture of mitochondria. The mitochondria are crucial to the cell, and inhibition of their electron transport chain leads to rapid cell death.

DNA damage: DNA damage may result from compounds such as alkylating agents; for example, dimethyl sulphate can cause single-strand breaks in DNA, resulting in the activation of poly(ADP-ribose) polymerase, which catalyses post-translational protein modification and is involved in polymerization reactions and DNA repair. Severe DNA damage may result from its activation and be sufficient to lead to cell death or carcinogenesis.

Apoptosis: Apoptosis is programmed cell death. Some foreign compounds may stimulate such cell death by the influx of calcium into a cell. In other cases, cell death may be mediated by cytokines (e.g., interleukin-6), chemicals produced by activated white blood cells capable of mediating tissue injury.

Data from Timbrell JA: Principles of Biochemical Toxicology. London, Taylor & Francis, 1992.

---

development are likely to identify only agents that commonly cause hepatotoxicity and most information comes from case reports or spontaneous reporting of hepatotoxicity to drug safety authorities such as the U.S. Food and Drug Administration (FDA).[11] There have been a number of studies that have attempted to identify the frequency of drug-related hepatotoxicity, but they have not used uniform criteria to define hepatotoxicity and many have not used samples that are representative of the general population. For these reasons it is likely that the true frequency of drug-related hepatotoxicity is greater than the frequency reported in the following studies. It has been estimated that drugs account for 3% to 5% of cases of jaundice admitted to hospitals and 10% of cases of acute liver failure.[13-16]

In a French study, all cases of symptomatic drug-related hepatotoxicity were collected for an area with a population of 81,301 inhabitants.[1] Over the 3 years studied, 34 cases were identified, 82% occurring in outpatients, with the diagnosis being made in primary care in approximately half of the cases. Two deaths were attributed to drug-related acute liver failure, whereas the other 32 patients recovered fully. The most common drugs implicated were antibiotics, psychtropics, hypolipemic agents, and NSAIDs. The crude annual incidence rate was 13.9 ± 2.4 per 100,000 and standardized annual incidence rate 8.1 ± 1.5, with a female-to-male ratio of 0.86 until 49 years of age and 2.62 at older than 50 years of age.[1] When these figures were compared with spontaneous reporting figures it was estimated that

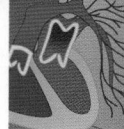

16 times more cases were identified.[1] In a retrospective cohort study in the United Kingdom, using a primary care database, the incidence rate of drug-related hepatotoxicity varied from greater than 100 per 100,000 users of isoniazid to less than 10 per 100,000 for users of omeprazole, ranitidine, NSAIDs, and amoxicillin; amoxicillin-clavulanic acid and cimetidine were associated with an intermediate risk of between 10 and 100 per 100,000.[17] A further two epidemiologic studies in France suggested that the overall incidence of drug-related hepatotoxicity has not changed significantly in the last 10 years; however, for the reasons discussed previously, these data may not be reliable.[18,19]

There is relatively little published information on the long-term outcome of drug-induced liver disease.[12] A recent study looked at the natural history of patients with drug-induced liver disease proven through liver biopsy.[20] The most common agents involved were antibiotics, NSAIDs, phenytoin, and halothane. At a median follow-up of 5 years (range, 1 to 19 years) 39% of patients had persistent significant abnormalities in liver blood tests and/or scans.[20] Factors predicting persistence or development of chronic liver disease were fibrosis at the time of the initial biopsy and continued exposure to the drug.[20]

DIAGNOSIS OF TOXIN- OR DRUG-INDUCED LIVER INJURY

Determining the Etiological Agent(s)

When assessing a patient with virtually any kind of liver disease, the best policy is to systematically evaluate the possibility of drug- or toxin-induced liver disease. The first step is to establish clearly and meticulously any drugs the patient has been taking, including over-the-counter and herbal or traditional medicine preparations. The patient may not disclose use of certain compounds for fear of admitting to their use or misuse (e.g., Ecstasy [3,4-methylenedioxy-methamphetamine, MDMA], cocaine, hypnotics, antidepressants, anabolic agents, or neuroleptic drugs). It is estimated that greater than 1000 drugs have the potential for hepatotoxicity,[21] and space limitations here preclude their complete tabulation. Any list of hepatotoxic drugs represents only a soon outdated snapshot, because new drugs are released into the market constantly and the nature of the premarketing studies is that they are small and hence potential for hepatotoxicity is seldom recognized until the postmarketing stage when a larger population is exposed to the drug. The reader is referred to Stricker's book for an exhaustive list.[21] However, a list of common drugs and toxins in overdose-causing hepatotoxicity is provided below and discussed in more detail later in this chapter.

In addition, poisoning may result from ingestion of natural toxins or synthetic chemicals in food or drink.[9,22] These also are detailed later in this chapter.

Occupational exposure to hepatotoxic agents also occurs as agents with hepatotoxic potential have been used in various industries (Table 11-1). The number of occupations that give exposure to hepatotoxic agents is large and includes the manufacture of munitions, rubber, rocket fuels, cosmetics, processed foods, paints, insecticides, herbicides, pharmaceuticals, and chemical products (Box 11-2). The risk, however, is largely hypothetical and a clear history of exposure taking place is required to make the diagnosis. However, many instances of poisoning from exposure to carbon tetrachloride (CCl_4) have resulted from the use of this volatile solvent as a dry-cleaning agent in a poorly ventilated room, particularly by those who drink ethanol to excess.[22]

A large number of chemicals are found in the home as components of household products (Table 11-2) or as pesticides (Table 11-3). Household products likely to contain hepatotoxic chemicals are those used for cleaning clothes and furniture and for paint removal. Despite the potential hepatotoxicity of some household products, the number of reported instances is very low. There is little evidence that hepatic injury has occurred as a result of correct use of pesticides.

In contrast, accidental or deliberate overdose of a known drug or chemical (e.g., CCl_4, acetaminophen [paracetamol], iron) is a very common cause of hepatotoxicity. Ingestion of organochlorine insecticides, herbicides, fungicides, copper salts, or compounds of trivalent arsenic also can lead to hepatotoxicity. Ingestion of rodenticides containing phosphorus has led to numerous cases of severe liver injury.[23] Occasionally, liver damage has been caused by ingestion of rodenticides containing thallium or warfarin.[9] In general, acute hepatic injury due to ingestion of pesticides has been very rare.[22]

Evidence must also be gathered that may point to an alternative diagnosis (e.g., alcohol intake, blood transfusions, high-risk sexual activity, intravenous drug misuse, arrhythmias). Viral serology (hepatitis A, B, C, and E, HIV, cytomegalovirus, Epstein-Barr virus) and ultrasonography often are required, particularly in cases in which the liver function tests indicate cholestasis. Other liver disease (autoimmune chronic active hepatitis, hemochromatosis, primary biliary cirrhosis, Wilson's disease) must be excluded.[24]

Chronology

Once the list of toxins to which the patient has been exposed has been compiled, the chronology of each treatment should be compared with that of the liver disease. As a general rule, toxins or drugs introduced within the last 6 to 12 weeks should be most suspect, although a shorter duration (1 to 7 days) may be observed in patients who have been exposed previously to the drug/chemical and have been sensitized. It is important not to exclude any that have been withdrawn before the onset of the liver injury; for example, with the amoxicillin and clavulanic acid combination, jaundice may not become apparent until 2 weeks after the treatment. Amiodarone may continue to cause liver damage long after it has been stopped. Information that strengthens the case for an iatrogenic reaction includes previous adverse effects with the drug or related analogs and presence of immunoallergic manifestations, such as drug-induced rash.

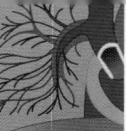

TABLE 11-1 Partial List of Agents Likely To Be Encountered Occupationally, with Indication of Hepatotoxic Effects in Experimental Animals and Humans

	EXPERIMENTAL ANIMALS	HUMANS	LESION*
Organic, Nonhalogenated			
Alcohols and glycols			
Allyl alcohol	+	?	Necrosis, zone 1
Dioxane	+	+	Necrosis, zone 3
Ethyl alcohol	+	+	See Chapter 32B
Ethylene glycol	±	±	
Methyl alcohol	±	±	
Isopropyl alcohol	0	0	
Aldehydes, acetyls, acetates, esters	0	0	
Amines, aliphatic			
Ethanolamine	+	?	Degeneration
Ethylenediamine	+	?	Degeneration
Amines aromatic			
4,4′-Diaminodiphenylmethane (methylene dianiline)	+	+	Cholestasis
4-Dimethylaminobenzene	+	?	Degeneration, CA[†]
Cyanides and nitriles			
Acetonitrile	±	?	Degeneration
Acrylonitrile	±	?	Degeneration
Hydrogen cyanide	0	0	
Hydrocarbons, aliphatic			
Alicyclic	±	0	
Cyclopropane	±	0	
Cyclohexane	±	0	
Gasoline (C8–C10)	±	0	
n-Heptane	±	0	
Hexane	±	0	
Turpentine	±	0	
Hydrocarbons, aromatic			
Benzene	±	±	Trivial steatosis
Diphenyl	+	+	Necrosis
Naphthalene	0	0	
p-Terbutyl toluene	±	0	
Styrene	+	0	Degeneration, steatosis
Tetraline	+	0	Steatosis, necrosis
Toluene	±	±	Trivial steatosis
Xylene	±	±	Steatosis, necrosis in fatal poisoning after ingestion
Nitroaliphatic compounds			
Nitroethane	+	+	Necrosis
Nitromethane	+	+	Necrosis
2-Nitropropane	+	+	Necrosis
1-Nitropropane	+	+	Steatosis, necrosis
Nitroaromatic compounds			
Dinitrobenzene	+	+	Necrosis
Dinitrophenol	±	±	?Cholestasis
2,6-Dinitrotoluene	+	+	Necrosis, CA[†]
Nitrobenzene	+	±	Degeneration
Nitrodiphenyl	±	±	
Picric acid (2,4,6-trinitrophenol)	+	+	Necrosis
Tetryl	+	+	Necrosis
Trinitrotoluene (TNT)	+	+	Necrosis
Organic, Halogenated			
Haloaliphatic compounds			
Bromoform	+	+	Necrosis, zone 3
Bromoethene (vinyl bromide)	+	?	Degeneration, CA[†]
Carbon tetrachloride	+	+	Necrosis, zone 3, fat, CA[†]
Carbon tetrabromide	+	+	Necrosis, zone 3
Chloroform	+	+	Necrosis, zone 3, fat
Chloroethane (vinyl chloride)	+	+	Degeneration, CA[†], angiosarcoma hepatoportal sclerosis
Chloroprene	±	?	Degeneration
1,2-Dibromoethane	+	+	Necrosis, zone 3, CA[†]
1,2-Dichloroethane	+	+	Necrosis, CA[†]
Fluoroethane	?	?	

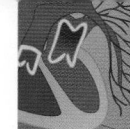

TABLE 11-1 Partial List of Agents Likely To Be Encountered Occupationally, with Indication of Hepatotoxic Effects in Experimental Animals and Humans (*Cont'd*)

	EXPERIMENTAL ANIMALS	HUMANS	LESION*
Haloaliphatic compounds (*Continued*)			
Halothane	+	+	Necrosis, zone 3
Methyl chloride	±	±	Degeneration
Methylene chloride	±	±	Degeneration
Propylene chloride	+	+	Necrosis
Tetrachloroethane	+	+	Necrosis
Tetrachloroethylene	+	±	Steatosis, degeneration, necrosis only with severe exposure
1,1,2-Trichloromethane	+	+	Necrosis, steatosis
1,1,1-Trichloromethane	+	±	Steatosis, degeneration, necrosis only with severe exposure
Haloaromatic compounds			
2-Acetylaminofluorine	+	+	Degeneration, CA[†]
Benzyl chloride	±	±	
Brominated biphenyls	+	±	Steatosis, necrosis in animals
Brominated benzenes	+	+	Necrosis, zone 3
Chlordecone	+	±	Steatosis, CA[†]
Chlorinated biphenyls	+	±	Steatosis, necrosis in animals Steatosis in humans
3,3'-Dichlorobenzidine	+	?	Degeneration, CA[†]
4,4'-Methylenebis (2-chloroaniline)	+	?	Necrosis, CA[†]
O-Dichlorobenzene	+	?	Necrosis, zone 3[‡]
p-Dichlorobenzene	+	?	Degeneration, CA[†]
Chlorinated benzenes	+	+	Necrosis, zone 3
Chlorinated naphthalanes	+	+	Necrosis
Pentachlorophenol	+	±	Degeneration, CA[†]
Nitrochloroaliphatics	+	+	Necrosis
Nitrochloroaromatics	+	+	Necrosis, CA[†]
Organic miscellaneous			
β-Propiolactone	+	?	Necrosis
Carbon disulfide	±	?	Steatosis
Decalin	+	0	Steatosis, necrosis
Dimethyl sulfate	0	0	
Dimethylacetamide	+	+	Degeneration
Dimethylformamide	+	+	Steatosis, necrosis
Diphenyl oxide	+	+	Necrosis
Ethyleneimine	+	?	CA[†]
Furans	±	±	
Hydrazine	+	+	Steatosis, necrosis
Mercaptans	−	0	
N-Nitrosodimethylamine (dimethylnitrosamine)	+	+	Necrosis, CA[†]
Pyridine	+	+	Necrosis
Bipyridyls			
Paraquat	+	+	Necrosis early, bile duct injury and cholestasis later
Diquat	+	+	Necrosis
Inorganic			
Arsenic	+	+	Steatosis, necrosis angiosarcoma, CA[†]
Arsine	0	0	
Beryllium	+	+	Granuloma in humans
Boronhydrides	+	+	Zone 2 necrosis in exposed animals Granulomas, hepatoportal
Bordeaux mixture (copper salts and lime as spray)	?	+	Steatosis Sclerosis, cirrhosis, angiosarcoma
Cadmium	+	?	Necrosis, cirrhosis
Chromium	+	±	Degeneration
See Table 11-3			

0, no known injury; ±, trivial injury, i.e., minor degeneration or steatosis; +, definite hepatic injury.
*Ability to cause injury on ingestion or injection, not in ordinary ocupational exposure.
[†]Hepatocarcinogenic in experimental animals.
[‡]2-Chloro-2-bromo, 1,1,1, trifluoroethane. Injury is due to idiosyncrasy.

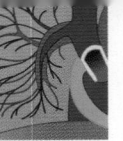

BOX 11-2	SOME OCCUPATIONS THAT ENTAIL EXPOSURE TO HEPATOTOXIC CHEMICALS

Airplane makers	Lacquer makers and lacquerers
Airplane pilots	Leather workers
Airplane hangar employees	Linoleum makers
Artificial pearl makers	Lithographers
Burnishers	Paint remover makers and users
Cement (rubber, plastic) makers	Painters, paint makers
Cementers (rubber)	Paraffin workers
Chemical industry workers	Perfume makers
Chemists	Petroleum refiners
Chlorinated rubber makers	Pharmaceutical workers
Cobblers	Photographic material workers
Color makers	Polish (metal) makers and users
Degreasers	Printers
Dry cleaners	Pyroxylen-plastics workers
Dye makers	Rayon makers
Dyers	Refrigerator workers
Electric transformer and condenser makers	Resins (synthetic) makers
Electroplaters	Rubber workers
Enamel makers and enamelers	Scourers (metal)
Extractors, oil and fats	Shoe factory workers
Fillers (plastics)	Soap makers
Fire extinguisher makers	Spreaders (rubber works)
Galvanizers	Straw hat makers
Garage workers	Tapers (airplanes)
Gardeners (insecticides)	Thermometer makers
Gas (illuminating) workers	Tobacco denicotinizers
Glass (safety) makers	Varnish makers and users
Glue workers	Varnish removers
Ink makers	Waterproofers
Insecticide sprayers/makers	Wax makers
Insulators (wire)	

From Zimmerman HJ: Hepatotoxicity: Adverse Effects of Drugs and Other Chemicals on the Liver. New York, Appleton-Century-Crofts, 1978, with permission of copyright holder.

Diversity and Classification of Drug- and Toxin-Induced Liver Disease

The next step in diagnosis relies on comparison of the patient's liver disease with the types of liver disease known to be associated with the drugs or toxins to which he or she has been exposed. Stricker is very useful for identifying likely therapeutic drugs causing hepatotoxicity,[21] and once suspected they should be withdrawn immediately. The ultimate step in diagnosis of therapeutic drug-induced liver disease is based on the improvement in the liver disease, which usually occurs within a few days or weeks following cessation of exposure to drug.

A differential white count may show eosinophilia and nonspecific autoantibodies (antinuclear, antismooth muscle) at relatively low titers that regress after interruption of the treatment, which may strengthen a diagnosis of immune-mediated drug-induced liver disease. However, specific serologic markers are available for only a minority of drugs (Table 11-4).[25-29]

A liver biopsy is not necessary in most cases of acute liver injury. In rare cases, it is helpful either to eliminate other causes of liver injury or to show lesions suggestive of drug-induced hepatotoxicity, and it can be carried out even in the presence of significant coagulopathy by the transjugular approach if necessary. The standard transabdominal route is the most common, though it also can be done under laparoscopic control. This has advantages in being able to see the biopsied area and photocoagulate any bleeding points.[30]

The pattern of liver damage from the mechanisms in Box 11-1 shows that the liver's response to injury is limited and includes fatty liver, necrosis (cell death), cholestasis, cirrhosis, and carcinogenesis.

FATTY LIVER

This is the accumulation of triglycerides (fats) in the liver cells. Fatty liver is a common response to toxicity, often occurring as a result of interference with protein synthesis in hepatocytes, such as after exposure to hydrazine (H_2N-NH_2), for example.[31] Normally it is a reversible process that does not lead to cell death, although it can occur in combination with liver cell death (necrosis), as is the case with CCl_4 exposure.[32] Two types of fatty liver or steatosis can occur. Tetracycline and

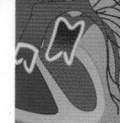

TABLE 11-2 Household Products That Might Be Hepatotoxic

PRODUCT	TOXIC AGENT
Antifreeze	Chlorobenzene
Carburetor cleaner	Chlorobenzene
Christmas tree lights (bubbling)	Methylene chloride
Drug-cleaning fluids	Chlorinated aliphatic compounds
Drugs hepatotoxic in overdose	Acetaminophen
	Aspirin
	Ethanol
	Ferrous salts
	Phenylbutazone
Furniture polishes and waxes	Antimony (trivalent)
	Nitrobenzene
	Cellosolve
Mothballs	Chlorobenzenes
Paint products	
Brush cleaners	Cresols
Paints	Arsenic (trivalent)
Plasticizers, lacquers, resins	Varied
Removers, paint, wax, etc.	Chlorinated aliphatic compounds
Pesticides	See Table 11-3
Plastic menders, greasers, plasticizers, glues	Ethylenedichloride, phthalates
Shoe cleaners	Aniline
	Nitrobenzene
Spray repellent	Vinyl chloride
Stamping inks	Phenol
Toilet bowl blocks	Paradichlorobenzene

Any unknown product should be considered potentially hepatotoxic, and all halogenated ones should be considered hepatotoxic until otherwise determined.

hypoglycin A produce microvesicular steatosis—the fat droplets are small, there are many in each hepatocyte, and the nucleus is in the center of the cell. Other substances (e.g., ethanol, methotrexate) lead to macrovesicular steatosis. Individual large fat droplets within each cell displace the nucleus to the periphery. See Box 11-3 for examples of drugs and toxins that cause steatosis.[33-39] Repeated exposure to compounds that cause fatty liver, such as ethanol, may lead to cirrhosis.

TABLE 11-3 Specific Uses of Various Potentially Hepatotoxic Pesticides

	HALOGEN COMPOUNDS	As	Cu	DIOXINS*	P,Th, WARFARIN
Fumigants	+	−	−	−	−
Fungicides	+	+	+	−	−
Herbicides	+	−	−	+	−
Insecticides	+	+	+	−	−
Rodenticides	−	+	−	−	+

As, inorganic arsenic derivatives; Cu, copper compounds; P, white allomorph of phosphorus; Th, thallium compunds.
*Dioxins present in herbicides as contaminants.

TABLE 11-4 Serologic Markers for Immunologically Mediated Drug- or Toxin-Induced Liver Disease

SPECIFIC SEROLOGIC MARKER	DRUG
Antitrifluoroacetylated proteins	Halothane hepatitis[25]
Antimitochondrial type 6 (anti-M6) autoantibody	Iproniazid hepatitis[26]
Antiliver kidney microsomal type 2 (anti-LKM2) autoantibody	Tienilic acid hepatitis[27]
Antiliver microsomal autoantibody	Dihydralazine hepatitis[28]
Lymphocyte proliferation assays	Immunoallergic drug-induced hepatitis[29]

BOX 11-3   DRUGS AND TOXINS THAT CAUSE STEATOSIS

Amiodarone[33]
Aspirin and Reye's syndrome[34,35]
Dideoxynucleoside antiviral agents[36]
Ethanol[37]
Methotrexate[38]
Perhexilene[38]
Tetracycline[39]
Valproate[39]

ACUTE HEPATITIS

Acute hepatitis is the most common drug- or toxin-induced lesion. A liver biopsy is rarely necessary for the diagnosis. These cases tend to be diagnosed from the maximal increase in serum alanine aminotransferase (ALT), a marker of hepatocyte damage, and alkaline phosphatase (AP), a marker of "cholestasis," and from the ratio of ALT/AP, with each activity being expressed in multiples of the upper limit of normal (N) (Table 11-5).[40]

Hepatitis may occur by direct cell injury (necrosis), with disruption of intracellular function, or by indirect injury by immune-mediated membrane damage.

TABLE 11-5 Liver Function Test Criteria for Diagnosis of Acute Hepatitis[40]

INJURY TYPE	CRITERIA
Hepatocellular	If only ALT is increased (>2 N) or when both activities are increased, if the ALT/AP ratio is ≥ 5 (reference 6). NB: Many other medical differential diagnoses (e.g., viral hepatitis, Budd-Chiari syndrome, microvesicular steatosis, low output cardiac failure) may also give such a liver test profile.
Mixed	ALT and AP are increased and the ALT/AP ratio is between 2 and 5.
Cholestatic	AP is increased > 2 N or when both ALT and AP are increased, if the ALT/AP ratio is ≤ 2.

ALT, alanine aminotransferase; AP, alkaline phosphatase; N, normal.

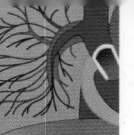
As mentioned previously, allyl alcohol causes peri-portal (zone 1) necrosis partly because alcohol dehydrogenase is present in zone 1 and partly because this is the first area exposed to the compound in the blood (see Fig. 11-1). Conversely, CCl₄ and bromobenzene cause zone 3 (centrilobular) necrosis as a result of metabolic activation in that region (Fig. 11-2). Mid-zonal (zone 2) necrosis is less common than the other two types of necrosis, but it occurs with beryllium toxicity (see Fig. 11-1). The explosive trinitrotoluene (TNT) can cause massive liver necrosis involving all zones. Ischemia (impaired blood supply to the liver) also may contribute to necrosis; for example, phalloidin, a toxic substance present in poisonous mushrooms, may cause swelling of the cells lining the sinusoids and therefore reduce the oxygen and nutrients supplied to hepatocytes. Hepatitis due to direct toxicity is not associated clinically with hypersensitivity manifestations. The liver injury may have relatively high frequency, consistent with direct toxicity.

Hepatitis due to immune mechanisms has a low frequency, but this may also be true in idiosyncratic hepatitis due to direct toxicity. The frequency of immunologically mediated hepatitis (as that of hepatitis due to direct toxicity) may be influenced by either genetic or acquired metabolic factors (such as microsomal enzyme induction). Immunoallergic hepatitis frequently is associated clinically with hypersensitivity manifestations, such as fever, rash, and blood eosinophilia, and a marked inflammatory infiltrate in the liver with sometime eosinophils, or granulomas. Immunoallergic hepatitis promptly recurs after inadvertent drug rechallenge. In some cases (halothane, tienilic acid, clometacin, α-methyldopa) the patient's sera have been shown to contain antibodies directed against hepatic neoantigens (see Table 11-4).

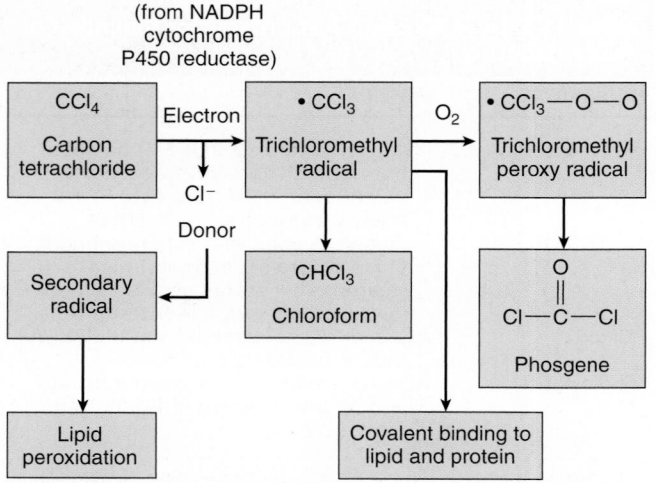

FIGURE 11-2 Metabolic activation of carbon tetrachloride (CCl₄).

DRUGS THAT CAUSE ACUTE HEPATOCELLULAR HEPATITIS AND THEIR MECHANISMS OF HEPATOTOXICITY

Acetaminophen (Paracetamol)

Recent reports have raised the possibility of toxicity from acetaminophen given in therapeutic doses.[41,42] In most cases of apparent therapeutic toxicity in children, the patterns of liver function tests, clinical course, and plasma concentrations represent those of acetaminophen overdose (see Fig. 11-1).[42] The confusion often is between therapeutic intent to treat fever or pain and therapeutic dose.[42] Often parents are tempted to give extra doses of pediatric acetaminophen preparations, and the apparent therapeutic toxicity in children is probably due to overdosage.[42] In adults, unlike the pediatric population, not all the cases are clear-cut overdoses.[42] Other factors, such as timing, stated dose, stated product, other products/drugs (particularly those that delay gastric emptying), glutathione depletion, and enzyme induction, may be operating, not to mention inadequate treatment with N-acetylcysteine.[42] This causes confusion, but the possibility remains that a few people might be more susceptible to acetaminophen at therapeutic doses.

Acetaminophen overdose is discussed in detail in Chapter 47. Poisoning with acetaminophen is characterized by liver damage, though a variety of less common manifestations, including pancreatitis, renal failure, and thrombocytopenia, also can be seen.[43]

The mechanism of toxicity in early acetaminophen poisoning (within 15 hours) has been well understood since the 1970s, and it depends on the metabolism of acetaminophen by cytochrome P-450 mixed-function oxidases (CYP2E1 and CYP3A4 in humans) to the active N-acetyl-p-benzoquinone imine metabolite.[42,44] This metabolite then causes cell death by covalent binding to hepatic proteins and enzymes once intracellular glutathione is depleted.[45] Centrizonal necrosis tends to occur first.[46] The antidote, N-acetylcysteine, if given at an early enough stage, particularly within the first 8 to 12 hours of ingestion, prevents hepatic cell damage by production of cysteine, which acts as a glutathione donor.[45,47] The standard treatment line indicating when N-acetylcysteine should be given is lowered by 50% for chronic alcoholics and users of enzyme-inducing drugs (such as phenytoin, carbamazepine, phenobarbital, primidone, and rifampicin) because such patients are at increased risk of toxicity due to increased production of the active metabolite, which is due to CYP enzyme induction.[48] Alcohol (ethanol) is actually protective if coingested with an acetaminophen overdose, but whether chronic excessive use increases the risk of hepatotoxicity when an acetaminophen overdose is taken remains controversial.[49,50] In animals chronic ethanol administration causes induction of hepatic microsomal enzymes (especially CYP2E1) and so increases formation of the toxic metabolite and increases acetaminophen hepatotoxicity.[49] However, because of dose-dependence and species differences in expression, activity, and inducibility of isoenzymes, it is not justifiable to extrapolate these

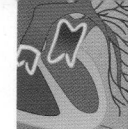

results to humans.[49,50] In a recent series of 553 patients with acetaminophen hepatotoxicity at a regional liver unit, there was no association between chronic alcohol consumption and the severity of hepatotoxicity.[51]

Factors that lead to depletion of intrahepatic glutathione probably also potentiate acetaminophen hepatotoxicity in overdose. Fasting decreased glucuronidation of acetaminophen in rats; hence, more active metabolite was present, potentiating acetaminophen-induced hepatic necrosis.[52] Fasting has been claimed to predispose to toxicity in humans, and a few cases suggest that patients with glutathione depletion are at increased risk of acetaminophen poisoning.[5,6] The mean half-life of acetaminophen is significantly longer in infants and children with protein-energy malnutrition.[53] Patients with HIV and AIDS have been shown to have systemic glutathione deficiency[54,55] and probably also have hepatic glutathione deficiency. Patients with advanced HIV have been shown to have reduced acetaminophen glucuronidation and increased formation of hepatotoxic oxidative acetaminophen metabolites.[56] It therefore seems a reasonable precaution to treat malnourished patients and patients who are seropositive for HIV who have taken an overdose with N-acetylcysteine at a lower acetaminophen level using the lower treatment line.

In contrast, little is known about the mechanisms of injury in late acetaminophen poisoning. Recently, a significant role of macrophages and Kupffer cells in production of cytokines and chemokines and activation of hepatic sinusoidal cells and neutrophils has been established.[57,58] In addition, activated macrophages and Kupffer cells produce potentially toxic reactive oxygen species such as superoxide and peroxynitrite, capable of directly mediating tissue injury.[58,59] Nitric oxide is proposed as a hepatoprotective mechanism against oxidative injury.[60,61] Many studies have tried to evaluate which of many hundreds of cytokines and chemokines are important in the pathogenesis of liver injury by acetaminophen without a clear result.[62,63] Such studies are complicated by the fact that the presence of cytokines does not mean they are directly involved in the pathogenesis; they may just be an epiphenomena of injury.[63] Nuclear transcription factors NF-κB and IL-6 are negative regulators of hepatocyte inflammatory cytokines.[64] The current hypothesis is that toxicity occurs when the tumor necrosis factor pathway is activated but only in the absence of activation of the protective negative modulating NF-κB pathway.[64] In addition to their role in the pathogenesis of cell injury, tumor necrosis factor-α and other cytokines facilitate the process of regeneration and repair.[65,66] Knowledge of the mechanisms of liver injury, at the cellular level, is important in the development of new treatments for acetaminophen overdose, particularly in late presenting patients who are at greatest risk of hepatotoxicity.

Cocaine

It is estimated that 22 million Americans have used cocaine at least once and that 5 million Americans use it regularly.[67] Fifteen percent of cocaine-use inpatients

(not administered intravenously) have mild elevations of liver enzymes.[67] Most addicts take cocaine intranasally rather than orally, as it had been assumed that the stomach hydrolyses cocaine. However, oral cocaine produces dose-related hepatotoxicity in male mice.[68] Acute cocaine hepatotoxicity is caused by hyperpyrexia, hypotension, and direct toxicity of the cocaine and can cause severe hepatic dysfunction.[69,70] Cocaine is metabolized by cytochrome P-450 to norocaine, which is further oxidized to N-hydroxynorocaine, norocaine nitroxide, and norocaine nitrosonium ion.[71] These metabolites cause an oxidant stress and lipid peroxidation in hepatocytes.[70,72] Mouse studies suggest that a hydroxyl radical produced by the reaction of nitric oxide and superoxide via peroxynitrite may be involved in the pathogenesis of cocaine hepatotoxicity.[73,74] In animals, toxicity is enhanced by inducers (phenobarbital, ethanol) of cytochrome P-450 and prevented by cytochrome P-450 inhibitors (particularly CYP2A).[70,71,75,76] The presence of noninjurious doses of lipopolysaccharide (LPS) appears to potentiate the hepatotoxicity of cocaine in mouse models,[77] and pretreatment with N-acetylcysteine prevents this.[78] Cotreatment with adrenergic antagonist drugs appears to reduce the hepatotoxicity of cocaine.[79]

Cocaine-induced hepatotoxic patients have a huge rise in ALT activity with 48 hours,[69,80] and liver lesions are in the centrilobular zone, extending into the midlobular zone.[71,81] Hepatocytes adjacent to the central vein are spared,[71] although hepatic enzyme-inducing and -inhibiting agents affect the site of necrosis.[82]

Ecstasy (3,4-methylenedioxymethamphetamine)

The social use of Ecstasy and amphetamines is widespread in Europe and the United States.[83] Recreational use of this drug presents an important but often concealed cause of hepatitis or acute liver failure, particularly in young people.[83] Hepatotoxicity has featured in several hundreds of cases of intoxication with Ecstasy in the literature and it is probable that many are subclinical and go undetected.[84-88] The evidence to date suggests there is more than one pattern of hepatotoxicity, in which different mechanisms may be responsible. The clinical pattern varies from asymptomatic hepatitic liver function tests to acute hepatic failure due to hepatocellular necrosis, from which some patients recover but others die or require liver transplantation.[83-87] Some present with cholestasis.[83] Rarely, accelerated panacinar fibrosis has been observed.[89] Subacute hepatitic toxicity, with cumulative damage on recurrent exposure, has been reported after recurrent ingestions over a period of time.[87,89,90] Hepatotoxicity may be variously manifest at histological level as a microvesicular fatty change, small foci, or cell necrosis or massive hepatic necrosis,[84,87,91] but it is most commonly due to necrosis.

In humans, oxidation is the main metabolic pathway for Ecstasy,[92] and this reaction is catalyzed by cytochrome P-450 CYP2D6 in yeast[93] and CYP2D in rats.[94] Thus, methylenedioxyamphetamine (MDA) is a main MDMA metabolite.[95]

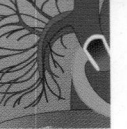

In humans, the molecular mechanisms involved in the hepatotoxicity of MDMA remain poorly understood. Immune-mediated mechanisms have been hypothesized to play a part in Ecstasy- or amphetamine-induced liver damage, as a result of the observation that rechallenge with ecstasy produced greater liver damage, and this has occurred in some patients in the absence of hyperthermia.[87,96] Liver biopsy in one patient suggested an autoimmune hepatitis-like injury, which resolved spontaneously on withdrawal of the drug.[96] However, a dose-dependent effect can be seen.[97]

Many patients with hepatotoxicity have been hyperpyrexic for several hours,[86,87,98] although this has not occurred in every case. Rat livers perfused by hyperthermic solutions show oxidative stress with superoxide formation.[99] Animals normally react to hyperthermia by the rapid transcription and translation of heat shock proteins, which help the cell survive thermal stress.[100-102] Administration of amphetamine to rats caused hyperthermia but no induction of heat shock protein in the liver, which suggests the liver may have impaired thermotolerance when amphetamine is present.[83,103] In mice (and probably in humans), high ambient temperature contributes to hepatotoxicity.[97,104,105] It is also postulated that apoptosis may occur.[106]

Incubation of hepatocytes with d-amphetamine induced a concentration-dependent glutathione depletion, which was prevented by pretreatment with the P-450 enzyme inhibitor metyrapone in rats.[94] Glutathione depletion most likely contributes to hepatotoxicity of amphetamines and ecstasy.

Hepatic damage has followed the intravenous use of methamphetamine and amphetamine,[107-109] but this is probably a result of viral infection by hepatitis B or C due to contaminated needles.[109]

Iron

After overdose of iron, the amount absorbed is probably about 10%.[110] All of the absorbed iron goes to the liver via the portal vein and enters cells via a receptor mediated endocytosis of transferrin-bound iron.[110,111] Acute hepatic necrosis (mid zone necrosis) can result from the ingestion of large amounts of iron,[23,112] particularly if there is failure to recognize the severity of poisoning and delay in administration of the antidote deferoxamine (see Chapter 72). Shortly after ingestion, evidence of severe gastrointestinal injury is noted, with nausea, vomiting, diarrhea, and melena. Symptoms may abate for a short period followed within 1 to 3 days by the third phase in which evidence of hepatic injury, jaundice, elevated aspartate transaminase (AST) and ALT and striking hypothrombinemia appear, with periportal necrosis.[113,114] Evidence from case reports and animal studies suggests hepatotoxicity occurs early in the clinical course (within the first 24 to 48 hours) and has relatively high mortality.[114] The lowest serum iron concentration associated with hepatotoxicity is 304 μM/L (1700 μg/dL), although it was not clear at what time post-ingestion this sample was taken.[112]

It has long been suspected that free radicals play a part in metal-induced hepatotoxicity because of the powerful pro-oxidant action of iron and copper salts in vitro, which catalyze free radical reactions.[115] The resulting oxyradicals have the potential to damage cellular lipids, nucleic acids, proteins, and carbohydrates, and this impairs cellular function and integrity.[115] Kupffer cells have enhanced respiratory bursts.[116,117] Cells have cytoprotective mechanisms (antioxidants, scavenging enzymes, repair processes) that act to counteract free radicals, thus the extent of damage depends on the balance between free radical generation and cytoprotective systems. Iron overload in vivo can result in oxidative damage to lipids in vivo, once the plasma concentration of metal exceeds a threshold level. In the liver, this lipid peroxidation is associated with impairment of membrane-dependent functions of mitochondria (oxidative metabolism) and lysosomes (membrane integrity, fluidity, pH). Although these findings do not prove causality, lipid peroxidation likely is involved, since similar functional defects are produced by metal-induced lipid peroxidation in these organelles in vitro.[110] Iron impairs hepatic mitochondrial respiration, primarily through a decrease in cytochrome c oxidase activity. In iron overload, hepatocellular calcium homeostasis may be impaired through damage to mitochondrial and microsomal calcium sequestration.[110] Reduced cellular adenosine triphosphate (ATP) levels, lysosomal fragility, impaired cellular calcium homeostasis, and damage to DNA all may contribute to hepatocellular injury in iron overload. Deferoxamine is the treatment of choice in significant iron poisoning, in addition to acting as an iron chelating agent it also has antioxidant properties and can reverse or arrest iron-induced lipid peroxidation.[118,119]

Unlike most other hepatotoxins, the periportal areas of the hepatic lobule are the primary sites of injury. This is the site for hepatic regeneration, which probably accounts for the relatively high mortality.[110]

Halothane

Halothane is a general anesthetic that causes mild hepatotoxicity in 20% of individuals.[25,120] In contrast, a very small subset of individuals develops severe halothane hepatitis, which is thought to have an immunologic basis.[25,120] Halothane is transformed by cytochrome P-450 via both oxidative and reductive pathways to reactive metabolites. The reductive pathway (via CYP2A6 and CYP3A4)[121] forms a radical, CF_3CHCl, which under certain conditions (microsomal enzyme induction and hypoxia) may lead to direct hepatotoxicity in animals. The oxidative pathway (via CYP2E1)[121] forms reactive acyl chloride (CF_3COCl) that binds covalently to hepatic proteins, including plasma membrane proteins. These trifluoroacetylated proteins can lead to immunization and to the severe form of hepatitis seen in rare subjects. This occurs in 1 out of every 10,000 subjects after first anesthesia within 2 weeks of the procedure. In one study, 25 (45%) of 56 patients with halothane hepatitis had autoantibodies against CYP2E1.[122]

Jaundice is more frequent after repeated exposure and occurs sooner; 12 days after first exposure, 7 days after second exposure, and 5 days after third exposure. Jaundice frequently is associated with fever (75%) and

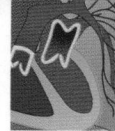

eosinophilia (40%). Sera from patients with severe halothane hepatitis contain antibodies against trifluoroacetylated plasma membrane proteins such as protein disulfide isomerase, microsomal carboxylesterase, calreticulin, Erp72, GRP 78, and Erp99.[25,123,124] Halothane hepatitis is hepatocellular. It is best avoided by avoiding repeated exposure, especially over short intervals.[125] Halothane was the most frequent cause of hepatotoxicity resulting in death over a 21-year period in New Zealand.[126]

Isoniazid (with or without Rifampicin)

Major adverse reactions to antituberculosis drugs can cause significant morbidity and compromise treatment regimens for tuberculosis, and antituberculosis drug-induced hepatitis is one of the most prevalent drug-induced liver injuries.[127] Most cases of antituberculous drug-induced hepatitis have been attributed to isoniazid. Isoniazid given alone increases serum transaminase activity in 10% of patients and causes clinical hepatotoxicity in 1%.[128] Peak risk is in the second month of therapy.[128] Hepatocellular damage without hypersensitivity manifestations take place. Isoniazid is metabolized to a reactive toxic metabolite in the liver.[129] Isoniazid is first acetylated into acetylisoniazid by hepatic N-acetyltransferase, which is hydrolyzed into acetylhydrazine. Acetylhydrazine may be either acetylated again, into the nontoxic diacetylhydrazine, or transformed by cytochrome P-450 CYP2E1[129] into the reactive acetyl radical that binds covalently to hepatic proteins.[130] Approximately 40% of Caucasians and blacks, but 90% of Japanese, are rapid acetylators of isoniazid.[131] Rapid acetylators form acetylhydrazine at a faster rate, but at the same time, detoxify it to diacetylhydrazine at a faster rate. Thus, slow acetylators have a higher risk of hepatotoxicity than do rapid acetylators.[127,131] In addition, slow acetylators are prone to develop more severe hepatotoxicity than rapid acetylators[127,132] CYP2E1 genetic polymorphism may be associated with susceptibility to antituberculous drug-induced hepatitis.[129]

Rifampicin in therapeutic doses when given alone is seldom hepatotoxic and mainly produces cholestatic liver injury. However, in patients receiving both isoniazid and rifampicin, the incidence of hepatitis is 5% to 8%, mainly during the first month of therapy.[133] Acute hepatic failure due to the combination tends to develop even earlier, after about 1 week of treatment.[133] Pessayre and Mazel[134] suggest that rifampicin, a microsomal enzyme inducer, increases the formation of the reactive isoniazid metabolite.

Liver function tests should be monitored in patients receiving antituberculosis drugs in the first few days, within the first week, and once a month thereafter. Isoniazid should be withdrawn if ALT exceeds three times the upper limit of normal.

Nonsteroidal Anti-inflammatory Drugs

Hepatotoxicity is an uncommon but potentially lethal complication of therapy with nonsteroidal anti-inflammatory drugs (NSAIDs). Clinically apparent liver injury occurs in 1 to 8 cases per 100,000 patient years of NSAID use.[135-138] Hepatotoxicity can occur with all NSAIDs but appears to be more common with diclofenac and sulindac,[137,139] and most commonly within 6 to 12 weeks of initiation of therapy. Patients who have experienced hepatotoxicity to one NSAID often have the same reaction if the drug is restarted or a sister drug is given. Female patients older than 50 years of age who have autoimmune disease and those on potentially hepatotoxic drugs appear to be particularly susceptible, but whether this merely represents the population taking NSAIDs remains to be established.[135] Liver function test abnormalities usually settle within 4 to 6 weeks of stopping the causative drug. However, some patients may develop liver failure and require liver transplantation.[139,140] Several NSAIDs have been withdrawn from clinical use because of associated hepatotoxicity.[141-143] The new more selective cyclooxygenase 2 (COX-2) inhibitors (e.g., celecoxib, rofecoxib) also are associated with hepatotoxicity.[144-147]

Two main mechanisms are responsible for injury, hypersensitivity and metabolic aberration. Hypersensitivity reactions often have significant antinuclear factor (ANF) or anti–smooth muscle antibody titers, lymphadenopathy, and eosinophilia. Rechallenge results in an increase in ANF titers.[148] Metabolic aberrations can occur as genetic polymorphisms and alter susceptibility. It may account for the incidence of 1 to 8 in every 100,000 prescriptions. In vitro metabolism of aceclofenac reflects phenotypic variability among donor liver cells.[149]

Recent in vitro animal studies have shown that the mechanism of diclofenac toxicity relates both to impairment of ATP synthesis by mitochondria and to production of active metabolites, particularly n,5-dihydroxydiclofenac, which causes direct cytotoxicity.[150,151] Mitochondrial permeability transition also has been shown to be important in diclofenac-induced liver injury, resulting in generation of reactive oxygen species, mitochondrial swelling, and oxidation of nicotinamide adenine dinucleotide phosphate (NADP) and protein thiols.[152] Other studies have shown that ferrous iron release from rat liver microsomes contributes to naproxen-induced microsomal lipid peroxidation.[153] Toxicity thus relates both to impairment of ATP synthesis by mitochondria and to drug metabolism. Nearly all of the NSAIDs have been implicated in causing liver injury, and they tend to be hepatocellular in nature.[139,154,155]

Patients who develop NSAID-induced hepatotoxicity must be advised to stop taking NSAIDs permanently. Acetaminophen remains the analgesic of choice for these patients, even if they are jaundiced.[156,157] They also may safely switch to aspirin use because the toxicity of NSAIDs relates to their diphenylamine ring molecular structure, which aspirin does not have.[142]

Phenytoin

Phenytoin is a microsomal enzyme inducer. Its administration to patients commonly causes a rise in γ-glutamyltransferase and may cause a small rise in ALT and AP in some patients.[158] Clinical hepatitis is much less common (serious idiosyncratic reactions occur in approximately 1% of patients[159]) and occurs within 6 weeks of therapy,

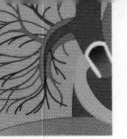

usually associated with fever, rash, lymphadenopathy, lymphocytosis, hepatomegaly, splenomegaly, and eosinophilia, suggesting an allergic mechanism. Phenytoin is metabolized to a 3,4-epoxide.[160] An autoantibody against a 53-kD microsomal protein has been reported.[158] Hepatitis is predominantly hepatocellular, but sometimes it is mixed.

Thiazolidinediones

These drugs act as insulin-sensitizing agents and are used in the management of type 2 diabetes mellitus. Troglitazone was the first agent in this class to be used clinically, but it has now been withdrawn after being implicated in more than 100 cases of hepatotoxicity, including a number of deaths and cases of acute liver failure that required liver transplantation.[161-172] Significant hepatotoxicity was more common in women and obese patients, but concurrent use of other drugs and pre-existing liver disease did not appear to increase the risk of troglitazone-induced liver disease.[165] The onset of hepatotoxicity often was delayed (mean, 4 months; range, 8 days to 12 months), but progression to acute liver failure once hepatotoxicity developed often was rapid and, in some cases, liver injury continued to progress after discontinuation of troglitazone.[167-170,173]

Troglitazone is metabolized by CYP3A4 and CYP2C8 to a quinine metabolite, which may cause hepatotoxicity similar to that seen with antimalarials and quinolone antibiotics.[174] The hypotoxicity of troglitazone is predominantly hepatocellular, but in addition, the sulfate metabolite of troglitazone inhibits hepatobiliary transport of bile acids by competing with the bile acid export pump, so there may also be a cholestatic element.[171]

The other thiazolidinediones (pioglitazone and rosiglitazone) are similar structurally to troglitazone, but their metabolic pathways differ and they do not appear to have the same hepatotoxic potential as troglitazone. In large clinical trials the incidence of liver enzyme elevations with these two drugs did not differ from placebo.[175,176] There have been two reports of hepatotoxicity with rosiglitazone and one related to pioglitazone; all of these patients recovered.[177-179] In one case of troglitazone-related hepatotoxicity, the patient was successfully treated with rosiglitazone with no recurrence of hepatotoxicity.[180]

Many other drugs cause acute hepatocellular hepatitis and some of these are listed in Box 11-4.[181-205]

MUSHROOMS THAT CAUSE ACUTE HEPATOCELLULAR HEPATITIS

Hepatotoxic mushrooms may be mistaken for edible mushrooms. Several hundred deaths per year are attributable to hepatotoxic mushrooms, especially in Europe,[206] and the amount ingested need not be great (see Chapter 23). There are more than 21,000 published cases of amatoxin poisoning.[201,207] Fatal mushroom poisoning is relatively rare in North America. There are many thousands of species of mushrooms, but the number of poisonous species is small. Most fatal poisonings are due to the ingestion of *Amanita phalloides* or the

closely related *A. verna* or *A. virosa*.[206] Amatoxins are bicyclic octapeptides that bind eukaryotic DNA-dependent RNA polymerase II and inhibit transcription.[208,209] A single mushroom has been estimated to contain a fatal dose.[206] The toxicity results from thermostable toxins (amatoxins and phallotoxins) present in the mushroom. They cause a syndrome of hepatorenal failure similar to that caused by CCl_4 and white phosphorus. The lesion produced by mushroom poisoning is steatosis and centrizonal (zone 3) necrosis. Degenerative changes of the gastrointestinal tract, kidneys, heart, and central nervous system also occur.[210]

The syndrome consists of a latent period of 6 to 20 hours after ingestion of poisonous mushrooms followed by extremely severe gastrointestinal symptoms, including abdominal cramps/pain, vomiting, and diarrhea. These symptoms usually are promptly followed by cyanosis and shock. Within 1 to 2 days, hepatocellular jaundice and uremia are noted. Central nervous system abnormalities such as confusion, coma, and convulsions may occur during the first 3 days after ingestion.[206] Electrocardiogram evidence of myocardial involvement may include bundle branch block and premature ventricular beats.[206] Hemolytic anemia may occur. AST and ALT levels are strikingly elevated, as with those of CCl_4 poisoning.[210]

Mortality rate is 10% to 25%.[210] Death within 4 to 8 days results from hepatic failure, severe dehydration, and collapse or central nervous system complications. Death also may occur during the first 48 hours from choleriform diarrhea,[210] of which children are more at risk.

No specific antidote is available, but several agents have been tried, including penicillins, silymarin, thioctic acid, and antioxidants. Benzylpenicillin, *N*-acetylcysteine, and silymarin all are effective in animal models of *Amanita* poisoning.[207,211-215] However, in a recently published review of 2108 patients treated for *Amanita* poisoning, benzylpenicillin did not appear to offer a significant benefit, whereas *N*-acetylcysteine and silymarin were associated with a modest benefit; these data need to be interpreted with caution as the review was retrospective and uncontrolled.[207]

CHEMICALS THAT CAUSE ACUTE HEPATOCELLULAR HEPATITIS

Carbon Tetrachloride Poisoning

Careless use or sniffing of the solvent carbon tetrachloride (CCl_4) leads to centrilobular necrosis,[216-221] usually accompanied by renal tubular epithelial necrosis. Alcoholic individuals are particularly susceptible. The syndrome consists of renal and hepatic failure, usually preceded by transient neurological and gastrointestinal symptoms. Immediately after exposure, dizziness, headache, visual disturbances, and confusion occur, reflecting the anesthetic properties of haloalkenes.[22,216,218] Nausea, vomiting, and abdominal pain with diarrhea occur also during the first 24 hours, especially if ingestion has occurred. Evidence of hepatic disease

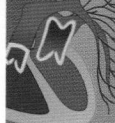

| **BOX 11-4** | **OTHER COMMON DRUGS THAT CAUSE ACUTE HEPATOCELLULAR HEPATITIS** |

Amoxicillin-clavulanic acid: Hepatocellular or cholestatic hepatitis.[181]

Allopurinol: Patients on diuretics or those with compromised renal function are most susceptible. Hepatitis occurs most frequently during the first month of treatment and is hepatocellular. Granulomas, fever, rashes, and eosinophilia suggest an allergic/hypersensitivity mechanism.[182]

Amodiaquine: Hepatocellular jaundice and even acute liver failure. Amodiaquine undergoes autoxidation into a reactive quinoneimine.[183,184]

Aspirin: Hepatitis occurs after one to several weeks of treatment. This is a dose-related phenomenon related to intrinsic salicylate hepatotoxicity and generally occurs only when aspirin is used in full anti-inflammatory doses. Plasma salicylate concentrations greater than 25 mg/L are likely to lead to hepatic injury, whereas concentrations less than 15 mg/L rarely do. Hepatic injury often is silent, or, at least, anicteric. However, a few cases with hepatic encephalopathy have been described. Use of aspirin during viral infections favors the secondary development of Reye's syndrome in children.[185]

Cyproterone acetate: Often produces mild abnormalities in liver function tests. However, it has also produced acute liver failure in elderly patients. It may also lead to hepatocellular carcinoma.[186]

Dantrolene: Prolonged administration of dantrolene increases serum transaminase activity in 1% to 8% of recipients and produces jaundice in 0.6%. Hepatitis usually occurs between month 2 and 5 of treatment, with a fatality rate of 28%. Hypersensitivity is uncommon.[187]

Dihydralazine and hydralazine: Hepatitis occurs weeks to months after treatment and is hepatocellular. Some cases of associated fever or blood eosinophilia have been described. Anti–smooth muscle, antimitochondrial, and antimicrosomal antibodies have been observed. The antimicrosomal antibodies are directed against the cytochrome P-450 1A2 isoenzyme, which transforms dihydralazine into reactive radicals. Slow acetylators are at increased risk of developing hepatitis.[188,189]

Disulfiram: Disulfiram is converted into reactive metabolites and causes abnormal liver biochemistry in 25% of recipients during the first few weeks of treatment, which represents direct toxicity. However, clinically relevant effects accompanied by hypersensitivity manifestations occur within 2 months of treatment and at least 10 cases of acute liver failure have been reported.[190,191]

Enflurane: Hepatitis closely resembles halothane hepatitis. Enflurane is transformed into reactive acyl halide metabolites, which cause immune-mediated hepatitis.[192]

Fipexide: Has produced acute liver failure in three patients.[193]

Ketoconazole: Overt hepatitis on rechallenge with drug. May produce cirrhosis.[194,195]

Lamotrigine: Acute hepatitis has been reported in six patients (acute liver failure in two of these), with onset between 2 and 3 weeks of starting therapy. Liver function tests normalized in five patients when lamotrigine was stopped; the other patient had mildly abnormal liver function tests.[196-198]

Methyldopa: Hepatitis seen in pregnancy, sometimes with hemolytic anemia.[199]

Nicotinic acid/Niacin: Hepatotoxicity.[200]

Nifedipine: Acute hepatotoxicity accompanied by eosinophilia.[201-203]

Pyrazinamide: The incidence of pyrazinamide-induced hepatotoxicity is higher than that of other first-line antituberculosis drugs.[204]

Tacrine: Half of patients treated have abnormal liver functions tests. One case of fatal hepatic necrosis has been documented.[205]

---

usually follows the exposure by 2 to 4 days, but it can occur at 24 hours. Jaundice develops in 50% of cases of poisoning; it is hepatocellular and rapid in evolution. Renal failure begins a few days after the liver damage and peaks in the second week. It may be heralded by oliguria between the second and fourth day after exposure. Continued oliguria or anuria beyond day 4 and rising blood urea during the first and second weeks indicates the presence of tubular necrosis. Renal failure is the cause of death in most fatal cases.[22,216] Pulmonary edema is observed in most patients who survive for longer than 1 week. Laboratory features include a low hemoglobin concentration and a neutrophil leucocytosis. Toward the end of the first week frank uremia secondary to renal tubular necrosis develops. There are striking elevations of AST and ALT[22,222] and prolongation of the prothrombin ratio. Mortality rate was 25% prior to hemodialysis.[22] N-acetylcysteine has been used successfully to treat the hepatotoxicity of CCl4.[223] With chronic exposure, like in the case of ethanol, CCl4 causes micronodular and macronodular cirrhosis.

White Phosphorus Poisoning

Suicide by deliberate ingestion of phosphorus in cockroach powder, rat poison, or firecrackers often takes place in the developing world. It causes mid-zone necrosis and periportal steatosis.[224] Mortality rate is high (50%), and renal tubular necrosis is common in such cases. Initially, there are severe, irritant effects on the gastrointestinal tract: nausea, vomiting, abdominal pain and diarrhea, and even hematemesis and shock. The vomitus and feces are phosphorescent and have a strong garlic odor, as does the breath. One third of patients die during this 8- to 24-hour stage. One third of patients recover and one third go to the next stage, which is a latent, symptom-free period for 1 to 3 days.[225] The third stage is characterized by hepatic failure, renal failure, and recurrent central nervous system involvement, including restlessness, coma, and toxic psychosis. Jaundice is apparent between days 3 and 5 after poisoning and renal failure is apparent between days 1 and 4. AST and ALT levels are only moderately elevated (compared with CCl4 poisoning) and coagulopathy occurs.[22,226-228]

Inorganic Arsenicals, Thallium, and Borates

These compounds can cause neurological, muscular, renal, and gastrointestinal manifestations. Hepatic injury (necrosis and steatosis) is a regular feature of the intoxication, but it has only a contributory role in

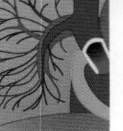

determining the outcome. Jaundice and other evidence of hepatic failure are rare, and they can be recognized only in patients who survive for a few days. Prolonged exposure causes cirrhosis.[22,23,229]

Sniffing of Chloroform, Trichloroethylene, or Perchloroethylene

Often users who develop jaundice have histological features of necrosis and fat deposition in the liver. Features of toxicity include a syndrome usually of lesser severity than that due to CCl₄ poisoning.[22,230,231]

Copper

Clinical features of copper poisoning are similar to those of iron overdose. Even dermal application has been associated with hepatotoxicity. Copper salt ingestion causes gastrointestinal erosions, centrizonal necrosis, and renal tubular necrosis. The course resembles that of other forms of hepatorenal failure. Severe nausea, vomiting, diarrhea, and abdominal pain, accompanied by metallic taste, are followed by jaundice, high aminotransferase activities, and hepatomegaly by the second or third day after ingestion.[232,233]

Other chemicals associated with hepatocellular hepatitis are shown in Box 11-5.[234-240]

DRUGS AND TOXINS THAT CAUSE MIXED HEPATITIS

Mixed hepatitis reflects both hepatocellular necrosis and cholestasis in the same patient from direct necrosis or by adverse immune response against the liver[241] and causing the liver function tests abnormalities shown in Box 11-6.[242-264]

HMG-CoA Reductase Inhibitors ("Statins")

Hepatotoxicity from a mixed hepatocellular-cholestatic mechanism has been reported with atorvastatin, fluvastatin, lovastatin, cerivastatin (predominantly hepatocellular mechanism, now removed because of frequent rhabdomyolysis), simvastatin, and pravastatin.[256-262] Elevation of liver enzymes up to three times the upper limit of normal occurs in up to 3% of patients who take these agents and is usually dose dependent and occurs within 3 months of initiating therapy.[256-262] The incidence of severe hepatotoxicity is low (0.2 per 100,000), although there are a number of published cases of acute liver failure due to statins.[257] There is conflicting evidence on the cross-toxicity of these agents (e.g., in one patient with simvastatin-related toxicity, pravastatin also caused hepatotoxicity but atorvastatin was not associated with hepatotoxicity).[263] Although rhabdomyolysis commonly is associated with statin-fibrate combination therapy, concurrent liver injury with this combination does not appear to be more common than with statin therapy alone.[264]

> ### BOX 11-5   OTHER CHEMICALS ASSOCIATED WITH HEPATOCELLULAR HEPATITIS
>
> **Polychlorinated biphenyls:** In 1968, hepatic injury developed in 11% of more than 1000 people in Japan who ate food prepared with cooking oil contaminated with polychlorinated biphenyl.[234-236]
> **Nitrites and nitrates:** Caused hepatic necrosis due to reaction of nitrites with secondary amines in the fish to form dimethylnitrosamine. They may be used as food preservatives.[9]
> **Beryllium:** Central zone necrosis.[237]
> **Toluene:** Subacute necrosis.[238]
> **Tetrachloroethane:** Subacute necrosis in industrially exposed humans. Ingestion or inhalation of high concentration, however, leads to acute disease similar to that induced by CCl₃.[239]
> **Insecticide poisoning (e.g., DDT and paraquat):** A number of insecticides are chlorinated hydrocarbons. Ingestion of large amounts of DDT ($\approx$6 g) and paraquat (20 g) has led to zone 3 centrizonal hepatic necrosis. Paraquat also is associated with a later selective destruction of bile ducts and cholestasis.[240]

> ### BOX 11-6   DRUGS THAT CAUSE MIXED HEPATOCELLULAR AND CHOLESTATIC HEPATITIS IN THERAPEUTIC DOSES
>
> Angiotensin-converting enzyme inhibitors[242]
> Carbamazepine[243]
> Chlorpropamide[244]
> Cimetidine[245]
> Clozapine[246]
> Haloperidol[247]
> Methimazole[248]
> Nitrofurantoin[249]
> Dextropropoxyphene[250]
> Quinidine[251]
> Ranitidine[252]
> Sulfonamides[249,253]
> Tamoxifen[254]
> Terbinafine[255]
> HMG-CoA reductase inhibitors (e.g., pravastatin, simvastatin, atorvastatin)[256-264]

ANGIOTENSIN-CONVERTING ENZYME (ACE) INHIBITORS AND ANGIOTENSIN II RECEPTOR INHIBITORS

There have been a number of reports of pure cholestatic jaundice, hepatocellular hepatitis, and a mixed hepatotoxicity with all of the angiotensin-converting enzyme (ACE) inhibitors and reports of acute liver failure associated with lisinopril and enalapril.[265-272] Onset of hepatotoxicity can be delayed up to 1 to 3 years, but it generally occurs within the first 3 to 4 months and is more common after a dose increase.[266,271]

There is little published data on the newer angiotensin II receptor antagonists, but there have been published case reports of hepatotoxicity associated with candesartan (hepatocellular), irbesartan (cholestatic), and losartan (hepatocellular).[273-277]

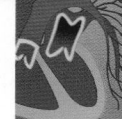

DRUGS AND TOXINS THAT CAUSE ACUTE CHOLESTATIC HEPATITIS

Because of the close interrelation between bile ducts and hepatocytes, damage to bile ducts may be accompanied by damage to hepatocytes by the build-up of bile, which damages cell membranes in excess. A list of common agents that cause acute cholestatic hepatitis is shown in Box 11-7.[278-284] Cholestasis can result from direct bile duct necrosis or by adverse immune response against the liver.[241] Clinically, cholestasis presents as jaundice, pruritus, and dark urine. Biochemically, in pure cholestasis there is an increase in AP, conjugated bilirubin and γ-glutamyl transpeptidase; in mixed cholestatic-hepatitis the ALT also increases but the ALT/AP ratio is between 2 and 5.

DRUGS AND TOXINS THAT CAUSE PURE CHOLESTASIS WITHOUT HEPATITIS

Bile duct injury may result from exposure to a number of compounds, particularly those that are concentrated in bile. The result of the damage is cholestasis due to debris from necrotic cells blocking the ductules.

Accidental contamination of food by industrial chemicals can lead to domestic hepatotoxicity. Epping jaundice occurred in the United Kingdom after contamination of flour by a leaking container of 4,4′-diaminodiphenylmethane (methylenedianiline).[9] Similar injuries have been acquired occupationally with this chemical.[285]

Drugs that cause pure cholestasis are listed in Box 11-8.[286-292]

CIRRHOSIS

Cirrhosis is characterized by regenerative nodules (clumps of new cells) within fibrotic tissue (amorphous tissue) forming an irregular lobulated (defined) pattern. Any repetitive injury resulting in cell death (necrosis) followed by repair mechanisms may lead to cirrhosis. This happens because the liver has only a limited capacity to regenerate.[293]

BOX 11-7	DRUGS THAT CAUSE ACUTE CHOLESTATIC HEPATITIS IN THERAPEUTIC DOSES

Amoxicillin-clavulanic acid (can also get acute hepatocellular hepatitis)[181,278,279]
Azathioprine[280]
Chlorpromazine[281]
Erythromycin[282]
Flucloxacillin[282]
Gold salts[283]
Penicillamine[28]

BOX 11-8	DRUGS AND TOXINS THAT CAUSE PURE CHOLESTASIS WITHOUT HEPATITIS IN THERAPEUTIC DOSES

Estrogens and oral contraceptives[286]
Anabolic steroids[287]
Cyclosporin[288]
4,4′-methylenedianiline (Epping jaundice)[289,290]
Rapeseed oil-aniline (Spanish toxic oil syndrome)[291,292]

The classic and most common agent that causes cirrhosis is ethanol.[293,294] In addition, compounds that do not appear to cause acute necrosis, such as ethionine, may cause cirrhosis after chronic exposure.[295]

Other drugs or chemicals that have been reported to cause cirrhosis include ketoconazole, amiodarone, and floxuridine.[296-299]

The main problems with cirrhosis are portal hypertensive complications (i.e., variceal bleeding) and ascites, together with encephalopathy when the liver cell mass becomes insufficient to cope.[300-303]

VENO-OCCLUSIVE DISEASE

Rarely, a toxin may damage sinusoids and endothelial cells directly; for example, monocrotaline, a plant alkaloid, which is metabolized to a reactive molecule, causes damage and blockage of the venous return to the liver and secondary ischemic death of hepatocytes.[304]

DRUG- OR TOXIN-INDUCED HEPATIC TUMORS

Liver tumors may be benign[305] (grow in situ) or malignant (able to metastasize to other tissues). They may arise from any cell type within the liver (e.g., adenoma,[305] hepatocellular carcinoma [aflatoxin,[306,307] dimethylnitrosamine,[308] ethanol,[309] hepatitis C[310]], or hemangiosarcoma [vinyl chloride[311,312]]).

Among the various mycotoxins (toxins produced by molds on nuts, oil seeds, and grains), the aflatoxins have been the subject of intensive research because they are potent carcinogens. Aflatoxin B_1 is a very reactive compound (Fig. 11-3). Its carcinogenicity is associated with its biotransformation to a highly reactive, electrophilic oxide, which forms covalent bonds, adducts with DNA, ribonucleic acid (RNA), and protein (see Fig. 11-3).[306,307] Damage to DNA is thought to induce tumor growth. There may be species differences due to differences in biotransformation and susceptibility to the initial biochemical lesion.

Dimethylnitrosamine is evenly distributed throughout the body, but exposure to single doses causes centrilobular hepatic necrosis indicating that metabolism is an important factor in its toxicity.[308] One metabolite is a highly reactive alkylating agent that methylates nucleic

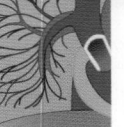
Aflatoxin B₁

2,3-Epoxyaflatoxin B₁

FIGURE 11-3 Aflatoxin B₁.

acids and proteins. The degree of methylation of DNA in vivo correlates with the risk of tumor induction in those tissues.

Vinyl chloride (or vinyl chloride monomer) is the starting point in the manufacture of poly(vinyl chloride). Chronic exposure leads to a "vinyl chloride disease," which includes skin changes, changes to the bones of the hands, and liver damage. Hemangiosarcoma is a tumor of sinusoidal cells (not hepatocytes) that also may result from chronic exposure to vinyl chloride.[311,312] This again appears to occur because the epoxide intermediate and fluoroacetaldehyde bind to DNA and proteins respectively within the cell. Hemangiosarcoma has been associated also with arsenite exposure, although the mechanism is still unclear. It should be stressed that the experience in humans with carcinogenicity has not been replicated in animal models.

HERBAL AND PLANT CAUSES OF HEPATOTOXICITY

Hepatic impairment from use of conventional drugs is widely acknowledged but there is less awareness of the potential hepatotoxicity of herbal preparations. Plants and herbs are considered to be harmless and commonly are used for self-medication without supervision. However, many plants and herbs can cause severe hepatotoxicity, including acute and chronic abnormalities and even cirrhotic transformation and acute liver failure (Box 11-9).[313-356] This list probably represents the tip of an emerging iceberg.

The diagnosis of herbal hepatotoxicity often is delayed because patients may not readily give a history of their use of herbals, so it is important that a detailed history be taken of exposure to drugs (prescribed, over the counter, and illicit/recreational), chemicals, plants, and traditional medicines in all patients with hepatotoxicity. There has been reports of hepatotoxicity related to Chinese herbal medicine (CHM), including at least three cases of acute liver failure.[357-364] As discussed below, it can be difficult to identify the specific component of the CHM that is responsible for hepatotoxicity, but the genus *Paeonia* has been present in at least four cases of severe hepatotoxicity.[357,359,361] Two studies have looked at the incidence of hepatotoxicity in patients taking these agents.[362,363] In a review of 1265 patients taking CHM, one developed acute hepatitis and 106 (8.4%) developed an increase in ALT up to three times normal, which returned to normal in 95% of patients.[362] In a study of 1507 patients using CHM for chronic pain, 14 had a reversible increase in ALT greater than two times normal, the risk being greater with use of *glycyrrhizae radix* and *atractylodis macrophalae*.[364] Prescriptions of CHM often contain up to 25 different ingredients, so if hepatotoxicity develops it can be difficult to identify which agent is responsible.

PRINCIPLES OF MANAGEMENT FOR DRUG- OR TOXIN-INDUCED LIVER DISEASE

General Management

Drug- or toxin-induced hepatotoxicity must be considered in the differential diagnosis of all patients presenting with a spectrum of disease that ranges from isolated deranged liver function tests in an otherwise well patient to acute liver failure. The degree and extent of liver injury should be monitored by serial prothrombin time estimations and liver function tests, including bilirubin, aminotransferases, alkaline phosphatase, and albumin. As discussed earlier it is important to exclude all other nondrug causes of liver disease. Liver biopsy should be considered if the extent of liver damage or etiology is in doubt. Accurate clinical assessment of renal function—that is, more than simply monitoring plasma urea and electrolytes—is also required.

Patients who develop hepatotoxicity must be advised to stop taking the drug or stop exposure to the toxin. Acetaminophen is the analgesic of choice for these patients, even if they are jaundiced.[156,157] Meticulous supportive care is critical to good outcome. Systemic hypotension, which may reduce liver blood flow, should be avoided with judicious fluid and inotropic support.[365]

Hyperthermia, if present (e.g., MDMA hepatotoxicity), should be treated aggressively with cold fluids, but care should be taken to avoid provocation of hyponatremia due to antidiuretic hormone (ADH) release.[366,367] The role of dantrolene is controversial.[368] It acts to control calcium release at the sarcoplasmic reticulum and thus reduce "muscular" source of heat. However, hyperthermia from amphetamines or Ecstasy also is attributed to a central hyperthermic effect, and there is no evidence that dantrolene has any action on the central nervous system. There may be a role for specific 5-hydroxytryptamine (5-HT) drugs, such as cyproterone, to reduce central nervous system–induced hyperthermia.

The development of acute liver failure is characterized by cerebral edema, circulatory shock, coagu-

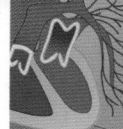

BOX 11-9 PLANTS AND HERBALS ASSOCIATED WITH HEPATOTOXICITY

Germander (*Teucrium chamaedrys*): The diterpenoids of the plant are transformed by cytochromes P-450 3A into hepatotoxic epoxide metabolites. Mixed hepatocellular and cholestatic or acute cholestatic hepatitis results. Several cases have occurred, mainly in France, Spain, and Canada.[313-316]

Pyrrolizidine alkaloids: Use of plants that contain unsaturated pyrrolizidine alkaloids (PAs), such as *Symphytum officinale* (comfrey), *Tussilago farfara, Heliotropium, Senecio,* and t'u-san-ci'l (Compositae), is associated with hepatotoxicity due to veno-occlusive disease. This is due to the conversion of PAs to cytotoxic pyrroles, which damage hepatic sinusoidal and endothelial cells, resulting in ischemic damage and centrilobular necrosis. Liver failure can occur in the acute phase with mortality of 20% to 40%, but complete recovery is also reported. Chronic PA veno-occlusive disease has a poor prognosis.[314-323]

Pennyroyal oil: Pulegone is the main component that has been shown to deplete hepatic glutathione. It is metabolized to menthofuran, which is directly toxic to hepatocytes. Both pulegone and menthofuran are metabolized via CYP2E1. Administration of *N*-acetylcysteine is recommended in all cases of ingestion of more than 10 mL of pennyroyal oil.[324-328]

Skullcap: Diterpenoid containing metabolite-mediated hepatotoxicity.[329]

Teucrium polium: One reported case of acute liver failure requiring liver transplantation.[330]

Chaparral leaf (creosote bush, *Larrea tridentata*): Nineteen reported cases of hepatotoxicity (mixed-cholestatic hepatitis), occurring 3 to 52 weeks after ingestion, with resolution over 1 to 17 weeks in most patients. However, there have been two cases of acute liver failure with successful liver transplant and four cases of chronic liver disease progressing to cirrhosis.[331-334]

Kava (*Piper methysticum*): There have been at least 22 cases of acute hepatitis, including 18 cases of acute liver failure. Generally, the hepatotoxicity settles within 8 weeks, but two patients with ALF have required liver transplantation. Liver histology shows extensive hepatocellular necrosis, and additional cholestasis was identified in two cases. In one report, two patients with kava hepatotoxicity were poor metabolizers of debrisoquine, and so it is possible that CYP2D6 deficiency may increase the risk of kava hepatotoxicity.[335-338]

Senna fruit extracts: Commonly used as laxatives and stool softeners. Metabolite rhein anthrane is thought to cause hepatotoxicity.[339]

Fruit of the cycad tree: Found on Guam, contains a potent hepatotoxin that can also lead to hepatic injury when eaten.[340]

Senecio, Heliotropium, Crotalaria: More than 100 alkaloids have been identified and these cause centrizonal necrosis and veno-occlusive disease. The clinical picture is of relatively acute or subacute hepatic failure, with ascites, jaundice, and a mortality rate of 20%.[341]

Camphor: Hepatitis.[342,343]

Mediterranean glue thistle (*Atractylis gummifera*): Hepatic necrosis, possibly due to interference with hepatic ADP and ATP transport inhibiting oxidative phosphorylation and induction of the mitochondrial membrane permeability transition pore resulting in apoptosis.[344]

Impila (*Callilepsis laureola*): The carboxyatractyloside component produces an acute illness with abdominal pain, vomiting, convulsions, and acute renal and liver failure (centrizonal necrosis) with profound hypoglycemia. Up to 63% patients die within 24 hours, with an overall mortality rate of 91% at 5 days.[345]

Cascara sagrada: Cholestatic hepatitis.[346]

Isabgol: Giant cell hepatitis.[347]

Venencapsan (horse chestnut leaf): Steatosis.[348,349]

Prostata: Hepatic fibrosis.[350]

Ma Huang (*Ephedra* species): There have been two case reports of severe acute hepatitis in patients using ma huang for weight loss. However, the contents of the products were not formally analyzed to confirm botanical identity.[351,352]

Jin Bu Huan: There have been 10 reported cases of acute hepatitis and one case of chronic hepatitis related to jin bu huang use. Levo-tetrahydropalmatine is the active agent and probably responsible for the hepatotoxicity, which developed at a mean of 20 weeks (range, 6 days to 52 weeks) in the reported cases. Liver biopsy in one case showed eosinophilic infiltrates and cholestasis.[353-355]

Greater celandine (*Chelidonium majus*): Ten reported cases of reversible mixed cholestasis-hepatitis within 3 months, one unintentional rechallenge resulting in a recurrence of hepatotoxicity. Commercial extracts of greater celandine contain more than 20 alkaloids and the toxic component has not been identified.[356]

---

lopathy, and renal failure, as well as liver failure with encephalopathy.[369] Conservative management focuses on invasive hemodynamic monitoring and prevention of complications such as cerebral edema, infection, renal failure, and coagulopathy.[369] A common cause of death from acute liver failure is cerebral edema due to raised intracranial pressure.[370] Intracranial pressure may increase rapidly and waiting for clinical signs such as pupil abnormalities, bradycardia, or hypertension may result in brain death before treatment can be started. Therefore, intracerebral pressure monitoring ideally should be undertaken in all patients who fulfill liver transplant criteria.[369] Controlled hypothermia has been proposed as a treatment for patients with acetaminophen-related acute liver failure.[371] Jalan and coworkers actively cooled (to 32°C–33°C) seven patients with acetaminophen-related acute liver failure and increased intracranial pressure unresponsive to treatment with mannitol and ultrafiltration. All seven showed a decrease in intracranial pressure with cooling (from 45 mm Hg [25 to 49] to 16 mm Hg [13 to 17]).[371] In addition, in some reports, hypothermia associated with acetaminophen overdose appears to have provided additional protection by slowing metabolic activation of acetaminophen.[372,373]

Specific Therapies

STEROIDS

The role of steroids in cases postulated to have an immune component has not been properly evaluated, although steroids probably have rationale in cases in which rechallenge with the drug produces significant hepatotoxicity.[83] Once a viral etiology has been excluded, a therapeutic trial with high-dose steroids (e.g.,

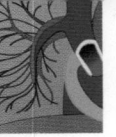

prednisolone 40 mg/day) is worthy of consideration in such patients.

N-ACETYLCYSTEINE

N-acetylcysteine (NAC; see Chapter 47) is used routinely for the management of early and late acetaminophen poisoning. Its mechanism of action is well understood in early poisoning, where it replenishes intracellular glutathione by acting as a cysteine donor.[45] In late acetaminophen poisoning NAC has been shown to alter cytokine concentrations, such as interleukin-1 and tumor necrosis factor.[374-376] Chemopreventive properties of NAC include reduction of oxidized thiol groups in key enzymes that permits reestablishment of calcium homeostasis, which plays a key role in apoptosis.[377] NAC blocks electrophiles and scavenges reactive oxygen species, and it can restore the capacity of the intracellular proteolytic system to degrade toxic arylated proteins.[378] The catheter study by Harrison and coworkers reporting that NAC acts by hemodynamic action together with prostaglandin E_1 (PGE_1) to increase cardiac output, oxygen delivery, and utilization has recently been challenged.[379,380] Using end-tidal CO_2 as a measure of oxygen uptake, Walsh and colleagues demonstrated that NAC administration alone did not lead to an increase in oxygen utilization.[380] The increase in cardiac output seen was transient, lasting, at most, 20 to 30 minutes. Whether regional hyperemia in one or multiple circulations is likely to benefit patients with acute liver failure remains a critical but unanswered question.[369]

N-acetylcysteine also is used for CCl_4 poisoning,[223] and it may have a role in amatoxin mushroom poisoning.[207]

LIVER TRANSPLANTATION

The role of liver transplantation in acute liver failure is controversial and emotive. Orthotopic or auxiliary liver transplantation has been performed successfully in patients with acute liver failure due to acetaminophen,[381] Ecstasy,[83,382] NSAIDs (e.g., diclofenac),[383,384] iron,[385] A. phalloides,[386] isoniazid,[387] and many other drugs and chemicals.[386,387]

In the United Kingdom, the presence of non–acetaminophen drug–induced acute liver failure is considered to be a poor prognostic feature. Association with two of the following four features is considered to be an indicator for emergency liver transplantation[388]: jaundice to encephalopathy developing over more than 1 week; age younger than 10 years or older than 40 years; serum bilirubin greater than 300 μM/L; prothrombin time greater than 50 seconds. Different criteria are used in the United Kingdom for transplantation for acetaminophen-induced liver failure.[389] Ninety-two percent of patients whose peak prothrombin time exceeded 180 seconds died.[390] Ninety-three percent of patients with an increasing prothrombin time between day 3 and day 4 died.[390] In clinical practice, if a patient's prothrombin time starts to improve, full recovery occurs. The O'Grady criteria (arterial blood pH of less than 7.3 or H+ of more than 50 nmol/L or prothrombin time of more than 100 seconds and serum creatinine more than

300 μM/L in patients with grade III or grade IV encephalopathy) currently provides the best guide for when to transplant for acetaminophen poisoning in the United Kingdom.[391] It therefore follows that in the care of patients prior to transplantation it is important to avoid giving fresh frozen plasma (unless there is life-threatening bleeding), vitamin K, or sedative drugs.[391] Recently, the O'Grady criteria have been modified to include the post-resuscitation serum lactate concentration, and this has increased the sensitivity from 76% to 91%.[392] A threshold value of 3.0 mmol/L after resuscitation even when used alone has a sensitivity of 76% and a specificity of 97% in predicting nonsurvival.[392]

Contraindications to transplantation may vary between transplant centers, but in the United Kingdom they include HIV-positive status, acute alcoholism (i.e., delirium tremens), serious sepsis, acute intravenous drug abuse, serious chronic psychiatric illness associated with high risk of repeat suicide attempts, and extrahepatic malignancy.[391]

A report of 7 years' experience of treating acetaminophen-induced liver failure at Kings College, London, found survival rate improved from less than 50% in 1987 to 78% in 1993.[393] Meticulous supportive care and transplants were believed to be responsible, among other factors.

MOLECULAR ADSORBENTS RECIRCULATIONS SYSTEM

Water-soluble drugs can be removed by hemodialysis or hemofiltration. However, kinetically this method of elimination is unsuitable for protein-bound drugs. The molecular adsorbents recirculations system (MARS) offers particular promise in removal of highly protein-bound drugs and in the management of acute liver failure.[394] Severe phenytoin toxicity has been successfully treated with the MARS system.[395]

REFERENCES

1. Sgro C, Clinard F, Ouazir K: Incidence of drug-induced hepatic injuries: a French population based study. Hepatology 2002;36:451–455.
2. Romagnuolo J, Sadowski DC, Lalor E, et al: Cholestatic hepatocellular injury with azathioprine: a case report and review of the mechanisms of hepatotoxicity. Can J Gastroenterol 1998;12:479–483.
3. Halpin TJ, Holtzhauer F, Campbell RJ, et al: Reye's syndrome and medication use. JAMA 1982;248:678–681.
4. Powell-Jackson PR, Jackson JM, Williams R, et al: Hepatotoxicity to sodium valproate. Gut 1984;25:673–681.
5. Whitcomb DC, Block GD: Association of acetaminophen hepatotoxicity with fasting and ethanol use. JAMA 1994;272: 1845–1850.
6. McClements BM, Hyland M, Calander ME, Blair TL: Management of paracetamol poisoning complicated by enzyme induction due to alcohol or drugs. Lancet 1990;335:1526.
7. Brown BR: Halogenated anaesthetics and hepatotoxicity. S Afr Med J 1981;59:422–424.
8. Timbrell JA: Principles of Biochemical Toxicology. London, Taylor & Francis, 1992.
9. Zimmerman HJ: Chemical hepatic injury. In Haddad LM, Winchester JF (eds): Clinical Management of Poisoning and Drug Overdose, 3rd ed. Philadelphia, WB Saunders, 1998.
10. Farrell GC: Drug-induced liver injury. New York, Churchill Livingstone, 1994.

11. Larrey D: Drug-induced hepatitis: epidemiologic, clinical, diagnostic and physiopathologic aspects in 1995. Rev Med Interne 1995;16:752–758.

12. Danan G: Causality assessment of drug-induced liver injury. J Hepatol 1988;7:132–136.

13. Dossing M, Andreasen PB: Drug-induced liver disease in Denmark. An analysis of 572 cases of hepatotoxicity reported to Danish Board of Adverse Reactions to Drugs. Scan J Gastroenterol 1982;17:205–211.

14. Friss H, Andreasen PB: Drug-induced hepatic injury. An analysis of 1100 cases reported to the Danish committee on Adverse Drug Reactions between 1978 and 1987. J Intern Med 1992;232:113–118.

15. Hoofnagle JH, Carithers RL Jr, Shapiro C, Ascher N: Fulminant hepatic failure: summary of a workshop. Hepatology 1995; 21:240–252.

16. Dossing M, Sonne J: Drug-induced hepatic disorders. Incidence, management and avoidance. Drug Saf 1993;9:441–449.

17. Garcia Rodriguez LA, Ruigomez A, Jick H: A review of epidemiologic research on drug-induced acute liver injury using the general practice research database in the UK. Pharmacotherapy 1997;17:721–728.

18. Biour M, Poupon R, Calmus Y, et al: Hepatotoxicity of drugs. A data bank of hepatic involvement and responsible drugs. Gastroenterol Clin Biol 1987;11:56–67.

19. Biour M, Poupon R, Grange JD, Chazouilleres O: Drug-induced hepatotoxicity. The 13th updated edition of the bibliographic database of drug-related liver injuries and responsible drugs. Gastroenterol Clin Biol 2000;24:1052–1091.

20. Aithal PG, Day CP: The natural history of histologically proved drug-induced liver disease. Gut 1999;44:731–735.

21. Stricker BH: Drug-induced hepatic injury, 2nd ed. Amsterdam, Elsevier, 1992.

22. Zimmerman JH: Hepatotoxicity: The Adverse Effects of Drugs and Other Chemicals on the Liver. New York, Appleton-Century-Crofts, 1978.

23. Arena JM, Drew RH (eds): Poisoning: Toxicology-Symptoms-Treatment, 5th ed. Springfield, IL, Charles C Thomas, 1986.

24. Benichou C: Criteria of drug-induced liver disorders. Report of an international consensus meeting. J Hepatol 1990;11:272–276.

25. Gut J, Christen U, Huwyler J: Mechanisms of halothane toxicity: novel insights. Pharmacol Ther 1993;58:133–155.

26. Pons C, Dansette PM, Gregeois J, et al: Human anti-mitochondria autoantibodies appearing in iproniazid-induced immunoallergic hepatitis recognize human liver monoamine oxidase B. Biochem Biophys Res Commun 1996;218:118–124.

27. Lecoeur S, Andre C, Beaune PH: Tienilic acid-induced autoimmune hepatitis: anti-liver and -kidney microsomal type 2 autoantibodies recognize a three-site conformational epitope on cytochrome P4502C9. Mol Pharmacol 1996;50:326–333.

28. Dalekos GN, Zachou K, Liaskos C, et al: Autoantibodies and defined target autoantigens in autoimmune hepatitis: an overview. Eur J Intern Med 2002;13:293–303.

29. Maria VA, Pinto L, Victorino RM: Lymphocyte reactivity to ex-vivo drug antigens in drug-induced hepatitis. J Hepatol 1994;21:151–158.

30. Helmreich-Becker I, Meyer zum Buschenfelde KH, Lohse AW: Safety and feasibility of a new minimally invasive diagnostic laparoscopy technique. Endoscopy 1998;30:756–762.

31. Sarich TC, Youssefi M, Zhou T, et al: Role of hydrazine in the mechanism of isoniazid hepatotoxicity rabbits. Arch Toxicol 1996;70:835–840.

32. Weber LW, Boll M, Stampfl A: Hepatotoxicity and mechanism of action of haloalkanes: carbon tetrachloride as a toxicological model. Crit Rev Toxicol 2003;33:105–136.

33. Richer M, Roberts S: Fatal hepatotoxicity following oral administration of amiodarone. Ann Pharmacother 1995;29:582–586.

34. Kaneda M, Kashiwamura S, Ueda H, et al: Inflammatory liver steatosis caused by IL-12 and IL-18. J Interferon Cytokine Res 2003;23:155–162.

35. Trost LC, Lemasters JJ: Role of the mitochondrial permeability transition in salicylate toxicity of cultured rat hepatocytes: implications for the pathogenesis of Reye's syndrome. Toxicol Appl Pharmacol 1997;147:431–441.

36. Koch RO, Graziadei IW, Zangerle R, et al: Acute hepatic failure and lactate acidosis associated with antiretroviral treatment for HIV. Wien Klin Wochenschr 2003;115:135–140.

37. Maher JJ: Alcoholic steatosis and steatohepatitis. Semin Gastrointest Dis 2002;13:31–39.

38. Farrell GC: Drugs and steatohepatitis. Semin Liver Dis 2002;22:185–194.

39. Hautekeete ML, Degott C, Benhamou JP: Microvesicular steatosis of the liver. Acta Clin Belg 1990;45:311–326.

40. Pessayre D, Larrey D, Biour M: Drug-induced liver injury. In Bircher J, Benhamou J-P, McIntyre N, et al (eds): Oxford Textbook of Clinical Hepatology. Oxford, Oxford University Press, 1999, pp 1261–1315.

41. Bridger S, Henderson K, Glucksman E, et al: Deaths from low dose paracetamol poisoning. BMJ 1998;316:1724–1725.

42. Prescott LF: Therapeutic misadventure with paracetamol: fact or fiction? Am J Ther 2000;7:99–114.

43. Jones AL, Prescott LF: Unusual complications of paracetamol poisoning. QJM 1997;90:161–168.

44. Corcoran GB, Mitchell JR, Vaishnav YN, Horning EC: Evidence that acetaminophen and N-hydroxyacetaminophen for a common arylating intermediate, N-acetyl-p-benzoquinoneimine. Mol Pharmacol 1980;18:536–542.

45. Mitchell JR, Thorgeirsson SS, Potter WZ, et al: Acetaminophen-induced hepatic injury: protective role of glutathione in man and rationale for therapy. Clin Pharmacol Ther 1974;16:676–684.

46. Lesna M, Watson AJ, Douglas AP, et al: Evaluation of Paracetamol-induced damage in liver biopsies. Acute changes and follow-up findings. Virchows Arch A Pathol Anat Histol 1976;370: 333–344.

47. Prescott LF, Illingworth RN, Critchley JA, et al: Intravenous N-Acetylcysteine: the treatment of choice for paracetamol poisoning. BMJ 1979;2:1097–1100.

48. Management of acute paracetamol poisoning. Guidelines agreed by the UK National Poisons Information Service 1998. Supplied to Accident and Emergency Centres in the United Kingdom by the Paracetamol Information Centre in collaboration with the British Association for Accident and Emergency Medicine. Norfolk, UK, Paracetamol Information Centre, 1998.

49. Prescott LF: Paracetamol, alcohol and the liver. Br J Clin Pharmacol 2000;49:291–301.

50. Jones AL, Dargan PI: Should a lower treatment line be used when treating paracetamol poisoning in chronic ethanol users: the case against. Drug Saf 2002;25:625–632.

51. Makin A, Williams R: Paracetamol hepatotoxicity and alcohol consumption in deliberate and accidental overdose. QJM 2000;93:341–349.

52. Price VF, Miller MG, Jollow DT: Mechanism of fasting-induced potentiation of acetaminophen hepatotoxicity in the rat. Biochem Pharmacol 1987;36:427–433.

53. Mehta S, Nain CK, Yadav D, et al: Disposition of acetaminophen in children with protein calorie malnutrition. Int J Clin Pharmacol Ther Toxicol 1985;23:311–315.

54. Buhl R, Jaffe HA, Holroyd KA, et al: Systemic glutathione deficiency in symptom-free HIV-seropositive individuals. Lancet 1989;2:1294–1298.

55. Helbling B, von Overbeck J, Lauterburg BH: Decreased release of glutathione into the systemic circulation of patients with HIV infection. Eur J Clin Invest 1996;26:38–44.

56. Esteban A, Perez-Mateo M, Boix V, et al: Abnormalities in the metabolism of acetaminophen in patients infected with the human immunodeficiency virus (HIV). Methods Find Exp Clin Pharmacol 1997;19:129–132.

57. Laskin DL, Pendino KJ: Macrophages and inflammatory mediators in tissue injury. Ann Rev Pharmacol Toxicol 1995;35:655–677.

58. Lawson JA, Farhood A, Hopper RD, et al: The hepatic inflammatory response after acetaminophen overdose: role of neutrophils. Toxicol Sci 2000;54:509–516.

59. Tapia G, Cornejo P, Ferreira J, et al: Acetaminophen-induced liver oxidative stress and hepatotoxicity: influence of Kupffer cell activity assessed in the isolated perfused rat liver. Redox Rep 1997;3:213–218.

60. Kuo PC, Slivka A: Nitric oxide decreases oxidant-mediated hepatocyte injury. J Surg Res 1994;56:594–600.

61. Kuo PC, Schroeder RA, Loscalzo J: Nitric oxide and acetaminophen-mediated oxidative injury: modulation of interleukin-1-induced nitric oxide synthesis in cultured rat hepatocytes. J Pharmacol Exp Ther 1997;282:1072–1083.

62. Takada H, Mawet E, Shiratori Y, et al: Chemotactic factors released from hepatocytes exposed to acetaminophen. Dig Dis Sci 1995;40:1831–1836.

63. Jones AL, Simpson KJ: Proinflammatory and chemokine concentrations are raised in plasma of patients with late paracetamol poisoning. J Accid Emerg Med 2000;17:69.

64. Blazka ME, Germolec DR, Simeonova P, et al: Acetaminophen-induced hepatotoxicity is associated with early changes in NF-kB and NF-IL6 DNA binding activity. J Inflamm 1996;47:138–150.

65. Devalarja R, Barve S, Hill D, McClain C: Acetaminophen hepatotoxicity: new insights. Gastroenterology 1998;114:A1234.

66. Hogaboam CM, Bone-Larson CL, Steinhauser ML, et al: Novel CXCR2-dependent liver regenerative qualities of ELR-containing CXC chemokines. FASEB J 1999;13:1565–1574.

67. Kothur R, Marsh F, Posner G: Liver function tests in non-parenteral cocaine users. Arch Intern Med 1991;151:1126–1128.

68. Labib R, Turkall R, Abdel-Rahman MS: Oral cocaine produces dose-related hepatotoxicity in male mice. Toxicol Lett 2001;125:29–37.

69. Silva MP, Roth D, Reddy KR, et al: Hepatic dysfunction accompanying acute cocaine intoxication. J Hepatol 1991;12:312–315.

70. Mallat A, Dhumeaux D: Cocaine and the liver. J Hepatol 1991;12:275–278.

71. Ndikum-Moffor FM, Schoeb TR, Roberts SM: Liver toxicity from norcocaine nitroxide, an N-oxidative metabolite of cocaine. J Pharmacol Exp Ther 1998;284:413–419.

72. Devi BG, Chan AW: Impairment of mitochondrial respiration and electron transport chain enzymes during cocaine-induced hepatic injury. Life Sci 1997;60:849–855.

73. Aoki K, Ohmori M, Takimoto M, et al: Cocaine-induced liver injury in mice is mediated by nitric oxide and reactive oxygen species. Eur J Pharmacol 1997;336:43–49.

74. Boelsterli UA, Wolf A, Goldlin C: Oxygen free radical production mediated by cocaine and its ethanol-derived metabolite, cocaethylene, in rat hepatocytes. Hepatology 1993;18:1154–1161.

75. Bornheim LM: Effect of cytochrome P450 inducers on cocaine-mediated hepatotoxicity. Toxicol Appl Pharmacol 1998;150:158–165.

76. Aoki K, Takimoto M, Ota H, et al: Participation of CYP2A in cocaine-induced hepatotoxicity in female mice. Pharmacol Toxicol 2000;87:26–32.

77. Labib R, Turkall R, Abdel-Rahman MS: Endotoxin potentiates cocaine-mediated hepatotoxicity by nitric oxide and reactive oxygen species. Int J Toxicol 2003;22:305–316.

78. Labib R, Abdel-Rahman MS, Turkall R: N-acetylcysteine pretreatment decreases cocaine and endotoxin induced hepatotoxicity. J Toxicol Environ Health A 2003;66:223–239.

79. Roberts SM, DeMott RP, James RC: Adrenergic modulation of hepatotoxicity. Drug Metab Rev 1997;29:329–353.

80. Perino LE, Warren GH, Levine JS: Cocaine-induced hepatotoxicity in humans. Gastroenterology 1987;93:176–180.

81. Kanel GC, Cassidy W, Shuster L, et al: Cocaine-induced liver cell injury: comparison of morphological features in man and in experimental models. Hepatology 1990;11:646–651.

82. Roth L, Harbison RD, James RC, et al: Cocaine hepatotoxicity: influence of hepatic enzyme inducing and inhibiting agents on the site of necrosis. Hepatology 1992;15:934–940.

83. Jones AL, Simpson KJ: Mechanisms and management of hepatotoxicity in ecstasy (MDMA) and amphetamine intoxications. Aliment Pharmacol Ther 1999;13:129–133.

84. Henry JA, Jeffreys KJ, Dawling S: Toxicity and deaths from 3,4-methylenedioxymethamphetamine ("ecstasy"). Lancet 1992;340:384–387.

85. De Man RA, Wilson JH, Tjen HS: Acute liver failure caused by methylenedioxymethamphetamine ("ecstasy"). Ned Tijdschr Geneeskd 1993;137:727–729.

86. Jones AL, Jarvie DR, MacDermid G, et al: Hepatocellular damage following amphetamine intoxication. Clin Toxicol 1994;32:435–444.

87. Ellis AJ, Wendon JA, Portmann B, et al: Acute liver damage and ecstasy ingestion. Gut 1996;38:454–458.

88. Andreu V, Mas A, Bruguera M, et al: Ecstasy: a common cause of severe acute hepatotoxicity. J Hepatol 1998;29:394–397.

89. Khakoo SI, Coles CJ, Armstrong JS, et al: Hepatotoxicity and accelerated fibrosis following 3,4-methylenedioxymethamphetamine ("ecstasy") usage. J Clin Gastroenterol 1995;20:244–247.

90. Ijzermans JN, Tilanu HW, de Man RA, et al: Ecstasy and liver transplantation. Ann Med Intern 1993;144:568.

91. Milroy CM, Clark JC, Forrest AR: Pathology of deaths associated with "ecstasy" and "eve" misuse. J Clin Pathol 1996;49:149–153.

92. Maurer HH, Moeller MR, Roesler M, et al: On the metabolism of 3,4-methylenedioxymethamphetamine (MDMA) in man. Ther Drug Monti 1993;14:148.

93. Tucker GT, Lennard MS, Ellis SW, et al: The demethylenation of methylenedioxymethamphetamine ("Ecstasy") by debrisoquine hydroxylase (CYP2D6). Biochem Pharmacol 1994;47:1151–1156.

94. Carvalho F, Remiao F, Amado F, et al: D-Amphetamine interaction with glutathione in freshly isolated rat hepatocytes. Chem Res Toxicol 1996;9:1031–1036.

95. Carvalho M, Milhazes N, Remiao F, et al: Hepatotoxicity of 3,4-methylenedioxyamphetamine and alpha methyldopamine in isolated rat hepatocytes: formation of glutathione conjugates. Arch Toxicol 2004;78:16–24.

96. Fidler H, Dhillon A, Gertner D, et al: Chronic ecstasy (3,4-methylenedioxymethamphetamine) abuse: a recurrent and unpredictable cause of severe acute hepatitis. J Hepatol 1996;25:563–566.

97. Greene SL, Dargan PI, O'Connor N, et al: Multiple toxicity from 3,4-methylenedioxymethamphetamine "ecstasy." Am J Emerg Med 2003;21:121–124.

98. Willis EJ, Findlay JM, McManus JP: Effects of hyperthermia therapy on the liver. II. Morphological observations. J Clin Pathol 1976;29:1–10.

99. Skibba JL, Stadnicka A, Kalbfleisch JH: Hyperthermic liver toxicity: a role of oxidative stress. J Surg Oncol 1989;42:103–112.

100. Cairo G, Bardella L, Schiaffonati L, et al: Synthesis of heat shock proteins in rat liver after ischaemia and hyperthermia. Hepatol 1985;5:357–361.

101. Lindquist S, Craig EA: The heat-shock proteins. Annu Rev Genet 1988;22:631–677.

102. Subjeck JR, Sciandra JJ, Chao CF, et al: Heat shock proteins and biological response to hyperthermia. Br J Cancer Suppl 1982;45:127–131.

103. Lu D, Das DK: Induction of differential heat shock gene expression in heart, lung, liver, brain and kidney by a sympathomimetic drug amphetamine. Biochem Biophys Res Comm 1993;192:808–812.

104. Carvalho M, Carvalho F, Bastos ML: Is hyperthermia the triggering factor for hepatotoxicity induced by 3,4-methylenedioxymethamphetamine (ecstasy)? An in vitro study using freshly isolated mouse hepatocytes. Arch Toxicol 2001;74:789–793.

105. Carvalho M, Carvalho F, Remião F, et al: Effect of 3,4-methylenedioxymethamphetamine ("ecstasy") on body temperature and liver antioxidant status in mice: influence of ambient temperature. Arch Toxicol 2002;76:166–172.

106. Montiel-Duarte C, Varela-Rey M, Oses-Prieto JA, et al: 3,4-Methylenedioxymethamphetamine ("Ecstasy") induced apoptosis of cultured rat liver cells. Biochim Biophys Acta 2002;1588:26–32.

107. Harvey JK, Todd CW, Howard JW: Fatality associated with Benzedrine ingestion: a case report. Del Med J 1949;21:537–540.

108. Kalant H, Kalant OJ: Death in amphetamine users: causes and rates. Can Med Assoc J 1975;112:299–304.

109. Smith DE, Fischer CM: An analysis of 310 cases of acute high-dose methamphetamine toxicity in Haight-Ashbury. Clin Toxicol 1970;3:117–124.

110. Tenenbein M: Toxicokinetics and toxicodynamics of iron poisoning. Toxicol Lett 1998;102–103:653–656.

111. Brown RJ, Gray JD: The mechanisms of acute ferrous sulphate poisoning. Can Med Assoc J 1955;73:192–197.

112. Strom RL, Schiller P, Seeds AE, Ten Bensel R: Fatal iron poisoning in a pregnant female. Minn Med 1976;59:483–489.

113. Gleason WA, de Mellow DE, De Castro FJ, Connors JJ: Acute hepatic failure in severe iron poisoning. J Pediatr 1979;95:138–140.

114. Tenenbein M: Hepatotoxicity in acute iron poisoning. J Toxicol Clin Toxicol 2001;39:721–726.

115. Britton RS: Metal-induced hepatotoxicity. Semin Liver Dis 1996;16:3–12.

116. Videla LA, Fernandez V, Tapia G, Varela P: Oxidative stress-mediated hepatotoxicity of iron and copper: role of Kupffer cells. Biometals 2003;16:103–111.

117. Tapia G, Troncoso P, Galleano M, et al: Time course study of the influence of acute iron overload on Kupffer cell functioning and hepatotoxicity assessed in the isolated perfused rat liver. Hepatology 1998;27:1311–1316.

118. Tenenbein M: Benefits of parenteral deferoxamine for acute iron poisoning. J Toxicol Clin Toxicol 1996;34:485–489.

119. Khan S, Ramwani JJ, O'Brien PJ: Hepatocyte toxicity of mechloroethane and other alkylating anticancer drugs: role of lipid peroxidation. Biochem Pharmacol 1992;43:1963–1967.

120. Ray DC, Drummond GB: Halothane hepatitis. Br J Anaesth 1991;67:84–99.

121. Spracklin DK, Thummel KE, Kharasch ED: Human reductive halothane metabolism in vitro is catalyzed cytochrome P450 2A6 and 3A4. Drug Metab Dispos 1996;24:976–983.

122. Bourdi M, Chen W, Peter RM, et al: Human cytochrome P450 2E1 is a major autoantigen associated with halothane hepatitis. Chem Res Toxicol 1996;9:1159–1166.

123. Kenna JG, Satoh H, Christ DD, et al: Metabolic basis for a drug hypersensitivity: antibodies in sera from patients with halothane hepatitis recognize liver neoantigens that contain the trifluoroacetyl group derived from halothane. J Pharmacol Exp Ther 1988;245:1103–1109.

124. Vergani D, Mieli-Vergani G, Alberti A et al: Antibodies to the surface of halothane-altered rabbit hepatocytes in patients with severe halothane-associated hepatitis. N Engl J Med 1980;303:66–71.

125. Davis P, Holdsworth CD: Jaundice after multiple halothane anaesthetics administered during the treatment of carcinoma of the uterus. Gut 1973;14:566–568.

126. Pillans PI: Drug associated hepatic reactions in New Zealand: 21 years experience. N Z Med J 1996;109:315–319.

127. Huang YS, Chern HD, Su WJ, et al: Polymorphism of the N-acetyltransferase 2 gene as a susceptibility risk factor for anti-tuberculosis drug-induced hepatitis. Hepatology 2002;35:883–889.

128. Black M, Mitchell JR, Zimmerman HJ, et al: Isoniazid-associated hepatitis in 114 patients. Gastroenterology 1975;69:289–302.

129. Huang YS, Chern HD, Su WJ, et al: Cytochrome P450 2E1 genotype and the susceptibility to antituberculosis drug-induced hepatitis. Hepatology 2003;37:924–930.

130. Timbrell JA, Wright JM, Baillie TA: Monoacetylhydrazine as a metabolite of isoniazid in man. Clin Pharmacol Ther 1977;22:602–608.

131. Ellard GA: Variations between individuals and populations in the acetylation of isoniazid and its significance for the treatment pulmonary tuberculosis. Clin Pharmacol Ther 1976;19:610–625.

132. Ohno M, Yamaguchi I, Yamamoto I, et al: Slow N-acetyltransferase 2 genotype affects the incidence of isoniazid and rifampicin-induced hepatotoxicity. Int J Tuberc Lung Dis 2000;4:256–261.

133. Pessayre D, Bentata M, Degott C, et al: Isoniazid-rifampin fulminant hepatitis. A possible consequence of the enhancement of isoniazid hepatotoxicity by enzyme induction. Gasteroenterology 1977;72:284–289.

134. Pessayre D, Mazel P: Induction and inhibition of hepatic drug metabolizing enzymes by rifampin. Biochem Pharmacol 1976;25:943–949.

135. Garcia-Rodriguez LA, Williams R, Derby LE, et al: Acute liver injury associated with nonsteroidal anti-inflammatory drugs and the role of risk factors. Arch Int Med 1994;154:311–316.

136. Manoukian AV, Carson JL: Nonsteroidal anti-inflammatory drug-induced hepatic disorders. Incidence and prevention. Drug Saf 1996;15:64–71.

137. Walker AM: Quantitative studies of the risk of serious hepatic injury in persons using nonsteroidal anti-inflammatory drugs. Arthritis Rheum 1997;40:201–208.

138. Sgro C, Clinard F, Ouazir K, et al: Incidence of drug-induced hepatic injuries: a French population-based study. Hepatology 2002;36:451–455.

139. O'Connor N, Dargan PI, Jones AL: Hepatocellular damage from non-steroidal anti-inflammatory drugs. QJM 2003;96:787–791.

140. Rodriguez-Gonzalez FJ, Montero JL, Puente J, et al: Orthotopic liver transplantation after subacute lvier failure induced by therapeutic doses of ibuprofen. Am J Gastroenterol 2002;97:2476–2477.

141. Koff RS: Liver disease induced by nonsteroidal anti-inflammatory drugs. In Borda IT, Koff RS (eds): A Profile of Adverse Effects. Philadelphia, Hanley and Belfus, 1992, pp 133–145.

142. Boelsterli UA, Zimmerman HJ, Kretz-Rommel A: Idiosyncratic liver toxicity of nonsteroidal anti-inflammatory drugs: molecular mechanism and pathology. Crit Rev Toxical 1995;25:207–235.

143. Rabkin JM, Smith MJ, Orloff SL, et al: Fatal fulminant hepatitis associated with bromofenac use. Ann Pharmacother 1999;33:945–947.

144. Nachimuthu S, Volfinzon L, Gopal L: Acute hepatocellular and cholestatic injury in a patient taking celecoxib. Postgrad Med 2001;77:548–550.

145. Merlani G, Fox M, Oehen HP, et al: Fatal hepatotoxicity secondary to nimesulide. Eur J Clin Pharmacol 2001;57:321–326.

146. Alegria P, Lebre L, Chagas C: Celecoxib-induced cholestatic hepatotoxicity in a patient with cirrhosis. Ann Intern Med 2002;137:75.

147. Huster D, Schubert C, Berr F, et al: Rofecoxib-induced cholestatic hepatitis: treatment with molecular adsorbent recycling system (MARS). J Hepatol 2002;37:413.

148. Greaves RR, Agarwal A, Patch D, et al: Inadvertent diclofenac rechallenge from generic and non-generic prescribing, leading to liver transplantation for fulminant liver failure. Eur J Gastroenterol Hepatol 2001;13:71–73.

149. Ponsoda X, Pareja E, Gomez-Lechon MJ, et al: Drug biotransformation by human hepatocytes. In vitro/in vivo metabolism by cells from the same donor. J Hepatol 2001;34:19–24.

150. Masubuchi Y, Yamada S, Horie T: Possible mechanisms of hepatocyte injury induced by diphenylamine and its structurally related NSAIDS. J Pharmacol Exp Ther 2000;292:982–987.

151. Bort R, Ponsoda X, Jover R, et al: Diclofenac toxicity to hepatocytes: a role for drug metabolism in cell toxicity. J Pharmacol Exp Ther 1999;288:65–72.

152. Masubuchi Y, Nakayama S, Horie T: Role of mitochondrial permeability transition in diclofenac-induced hepatotoxicity in rats. Hepatology 2002;35:544–551.

153. Ji B, Masubuchi Y, Horie T: A possible mechanism of naproxen-induced lipid-peroxidation in rat liver microsomes. Pharmacol Toxicol 2001;89:43–48.

154. Zimmerman HJ: Update on hepatotoxicity due to classes of drugs in common clinical use: non-steroidal drugs, antiflammatory drugs, antibiotics, antihypertensives and cardiac and psychotropic agents. Semin Liver Dis 1990;10:322–338.

155. Rabinovitz M, Van Thiel DH: Hepatotoxicity of non-steroidal anti-inflammatory drugs. Am J Gastroenterol 1992;87:1696–1704.

156. Prescott LJ: Effect of non-narcotic analgesics on the liver. Drugs 1986;32:129–147.

157. Jones AL: Recent advances in the management of late Paracetamol poisoning. Emerg Med 2000;12:14–21.

158. Leeder JS: Mechanisms of idiosyncratic hypersensitivity reactions to antiepileptic drugs. Epilepsia 1998;39(Suppl 7):S8–S16.

159. Smythe MA, Umstead GS: Phenytoin hepatotoxicity: a review of the literature. DICP 1989;23:13.

160. Moustafa MA, Claesen M, Adline J, et al: Evidence for an arene-3,4-oxide as a metabolic intermediate in the meta- and para-hydroxylation of phenytoin in the dog. Drug Metab Dispos 1983;11:574–580.

161. Watkins PB, Whitcomb RW: Hepatic dysfunction associated with troglitazone. N Engl J Med 1998;338:916–917.

162. Murphy EJ, Davern TJ, Shakil O: Troglitazone-induced fulminant hepatic failure. Dig Dis Sci 2000;45:549–553.

163. Gitlin N, Julie NL, Spurr CL: Two cases of severe clinical and histologic hepatotoxicity associated with troglitazone. Ann Intern Med 1998;129:36–38.

164. Neuschwander-Tetri A, Isley WL, Oki JC: Troglitazone induced hepatic failure leading to liver transplantation. Ann Intern Med 1998;129:38–41.

165. Kohlroser J, Mathai J, Reichheld J: Hepatotoxicity due to troglitazone: report of two cases and review of adverse events reported to the US FDA. Am J Gastroenterol 2000;95:272–276.

166. Schiano T, Dolehide K, Hart J, Baker AL: Severe but reversible hepatitis induced by troglitazone. Did Dis Sci 2000;45:1039–1042.

167. Bell DS, Ovalle F: Late onset troglitazone-induced hepatic dysfunction. Diabetes Care 2000;2:128–129.

168. Jagannath S, Rai R: Rapid onset subfulminant liver failure associated with troglitazone. Ann Intern Med 2000;132:677.
169. Menon KV, Angulo P, Lindor KD: Severe cholestatic hepatitis from troglitazone in a patient with non-alcoholic steatohepatitis and diabetes mellitus. Am J Gastroenterol 2001;96:1631–1634.
170. Iwase M, Yamaguchi M, Yoshinari M: A Japanese case of liver dysfunction after 19 months of troglitazone treatment. Diabetes Care 1999;22:1382–1384.
171. Funk C, Ponelle C, Scheuermann G, Pantze M: Cholestatic potential of troglitazone as a possible factor contributing to troglitazone-induced hepatotoxicity: in vivo and in vitro interaction at the cacalicular bile salt export pump in the rat. Mol Pharmacol 2001;59:627–635.
172. Shibuya M, Watanabe M, Yoshikuni F: An autopsy case of troglitazone induced fulminant hepatitis. Diabetes Care 1998;21;2140–2143.
173. Sitruk V, Mohib S, Grando-Lemiare V, et al: Acute cholestatic hepatitis induced by glimepride. Gastroenterol Clin Biol 2000;24: 1233–1234.
174. Bloomgarden ZT: American Diabetes Association 60th Scientific Sessions, 2000: thiazolidinediones, obesity and related topics. Diabetes Care 2001;24:162–166.
175. Lebovitz HE, Salzman A: Rosiglitazone liver safety update. Diabetes 2000;49:123.
176. Rubin CJ, Schneider RL: Pioglitazone liver enzyme profile is similar to placebo in US controlled clinical trials. Diabetes 2000;49:39.
177. Maeda K: Hepatocellular injury in a patient receving pioglitazone. Ann Intern Med 2001;135:306.
178. Forman LM, Simmons DA, Diamond RH: Hepatic failure in patient taking rosiglitazone. Ann Intern Med 2000;132:118–121.
179. Al-salman J, Arjomand H, Kemp DG, Mittal M: Hepatocellular injury in a patient receiving rosiglitazone. Ann Intern Med 2000;132:121–124.
180. Lenhard MJ, Funk WB: Failure to develop hepatic injury fom rosiglitazone in a patient with a history of troglitazone-induced hepatitis. Diabetes Care 2001;24:168–169.
181. Zaidi SA: Hepatitis associated with amoxicillin/clavulanic acid and/or ciprofloxacin. Am J Med Sci 2003;325:31–33.
182. Knowles SR, Shapiro LE, Shear NH: Reactive metabolites and adverse drug reactions: clinical considerations. Clin Rev Allergy Immunol 2003;24:229–238.
183. Taylor WR, White NJ: Antimalarial drug toxicity: a review. Drug Saf 2004;27:25–61.
184. Raymond JM, Dumas F, Baldit C, et al: Fatal acute hepatitis due to amodiaquine. J Clin Gastroenterol 1989;11:602–603.
185. Prescott LF: Effects of non-narcotic analgesics on the liver. Drugs 1986;32(Suppl 4):129–147.
186. Friedman G, Lamoureux E, Sherker AH: Fatal fulminant hepatic failure due to cyproterone acetate. Dig Dis Sci 1999;44:1362–1363.
187. Chan CH: Dantrolene sodium and hepatic injury. Neurology 1999;40:1427–1432.
188. Beaune PH, Lecoeur S: Immunotoxicology of the liver: adverse reactions to drugs. J Hepatol 1997;26(Suppl 2):37–42.
189. Roschlau G, Baumgarten R, Fengler JD: Dihydralazine hepatitis. Morphologic and clinical criteria for diagnosis. Zentralbl Allg Pathol 1990;136:127–134.
190. Chick J: Safety issues concerning the use of disulfiram in treating alcohol dependence. Drug Saf 1999;20:427–435.
191. Eliasson E, Stal P, Oksanen A, et al: Expression of autoantibodies to specific cytochromes P450 in case of disulfiram hepatitis. J Hepatol 1998;29:819–825.
192. Reichle FM, Conzen PF: Halogenated inhalational anaesthetics. Best Pract Res Clin Anaesthesiol 2003;17:29–46.
193. Durand F, Samuel D, Bernuau J, et al: Fipexide-induced fulminant hepatitis. Report of three cases with emergency liver transplantation. J Hepatol 1992;15:144–146.
194. Chien RN, Sheen IS, Liaw YF: Unintentional rechallenge resulting in a causative relationship between ketoconazole and acute liver injury. Int J Clin Pract 2003;57:829–830.
195. Kim TH, Kim BH, Kim YW, et al: Liver cirrhosis developed after ketoconazole-induced acute hepatic injury. J Gastroenterol Hepatol 2003;18:1426–1429.
196. Makin AJ, Fitt S, Williams R, Duncan JS: Fulminant hepatic failure induced by lamotrigine. BMJ 1995;311:292.

197. Sauve G, Bresson-Hadni S, Prost P: Acute hepatitis after lamotrigine administration. Drug Dis Sci 2000;45:1874–1877.
198. Arnon R, DeVivo D, Defelice AR, Kazlow PG: Acute hepatic failure in a child treated with lamotrigine. Pediatr Neurol 2000;18:251–252.
199. Breland BD, Hicks GS Jr: Hepatitis and hemolytic anemia associated with methyldopa therapy. Drug Intell Clin Pharm 1982;16:489–492.
200. Dalton TA, Berry RS: Hepatotoxicity associated with sustained-release niacin. Am J Med 1992;93:102–104.
201. Shaw DR, Misan GM, Johnson RD: Nifedipine hepatitis. Aust N Z J Med 1987;17:447–448.
202. Dorn-Beineke A, Hassan AW, Brautigam J, et al: Phenprocoumon-induced hepatitis as an immunologically mediated drug allergic complication of antithrombotic therapy. Thromb Haemost 2003;90:1210–1213.
203. Hinrichsen H, Luttges J, Kloppel G, et al: Idiosyncratic drug allergic phenprocoumon-induced hepatitis with subacute liver failure initially misdiagnosed as autoimmune hepatitis. Scand J Gastroenterol 2001;36:780–783.
204. Yee D, Valiquette C, Pelletier M, et al: Incidence of serious side effects from first-line antituberculos drugs among patients treated for active tuberculosis. Am J Respir Crit Care Med 2003;167: 1472–1477.
205. Blackard WG Jr, Sood GK, Crowe DR, et al: Tacrine. A cause of fatal hepatotoxicity? J Clin Gastroenterol 1998;26:57–59.
206. Spoerke DG, Rumack BH (eds): Handbook of Mushroom Poisoning. Diagnosis and Treatment. Baca Raton, FL, CRC Press, 1994.
207. Enjalbert F, Rapoir S, Nouguier-Soule J, et al: Treatment of amatoxin poisoning: 20-year retrospective analysis. J Toxicol Clin Toxicol 2002;40:715–757.
208. Enjalbert F, Gallion C, Jehl F, et al: Amatoxins and phallatoxins in amanita species. HPLC determination. Mycologica 1993;85: 579–584.
209. Wieland T: The toxic peptides from amanita mushrooms. Int J Pept Protein Res 1983;22:257–276.
210. Herold R, Straub PW: Acute hepatic necrosis of hepatitis and mushroom poisoning. The value of coagulation tests in their differentiation, prognostic assessment and pathogenesis. Helv Med Acta 1978;37:5.
211. Floersheim GL, Schneeberger J, Bucher K: Curative potencies of penicillin in experimental amanita phalloides poisoning. Agents Actions 1971;2:138–141.
212. Floersheim GL, Eberhard M, Tschumi P, Duckert P: Effects of penicillin and silymarin on liver enzymes and blood clotting factors in dogs given a boiled preparation of amanita phalloides. Toxicol Appl Pharmacol 1978;46:455–462.
213. Bogle G, Tuchweber B, Trost W, Mengs U: Protection by silibinin against Amanita phalloides intoxication in beadles. Toxicol Appl Pharmacol 1984;73:355–362.
214. Locatelli C, Maccarini D, Ferruzi M, et al: Intossicazioni acute da Amanita phalloides: proposta di terapia con N-Acetilcisteina. Ann Mus Civ Rovereto 1989;4:211–212.
215. Locatelli C, Travaglia A, Sala G, et al: The role of N-acetylcysteine and forced diuresis in the treatment of phalloidea poisoning. Minerva Anestesiol 1990;56:1361–1363.
216. Dossing M, Skinhoj P: Occupational liver injury. Present state of knowledge and future perspectives. Int Arch Occup Environ Health 1985;56:11.
217. Zimmerman HJ: Effects of alcohol on other hepatotoxins. Alcohol Cin Exp Res 1986;10:3.
218. Ruprah M, Mont TG, Flannagan RJ: Acute carbon tetrachloride poisoning in 19 patients: implications for diagnosis and treatment. Lancet 1985;1:107.
219. Simmons JE, McDonald A, Seely JC, et al: Potentiation of carbon tetrachloride hepatotoxicity by inhaled methanol: time course of injury and recovery. J Toxicol Environ Health 1995;46:203–216.
220. Shibayama Y: Potentiation of carbon tetrachloride hepatotoxicity of hypoxia. Br J Exp Pathol 1986;67:909–914.
221. Slater TF, Cheeseman KH, Ingold KU: Carbon tetrachloride toxicity as a model for studying free-radical mediated liver injury. Philos Trans R Soc Lond B Biol Sci 1985;311:633–645.
222. Wroblewski F: Clinical significance of alterations in transaminase activities in serum and other body fluids. Adv Clin Chem 1958;1:313.

223. Mathieson PW, Williams G, MacSweeney JE: Survival after massive ingestion of carbon tetrachloride treated by intravenous infusion of acetylcysteine. Hum Toxicol 1985;4:627–631.

224. Greenberger NJ, Robinson WL, Isselbacher KJ: Toxic hepatitis after the ingestion of phosphorus with subsequent recovery. Gastroenterol 1964;47:179–183.

225. Fletcher GF, Galambos JT: Phosphorus poisoning in humans. Arch Int Med 1963;112:846–852.

226. Brewer E, Haggerty RJ: Toxic hazards. Rat poisons. II. Phosphorus. N Engl J Med 1958;258:147.

227. Rodriguez-Iturbe B: Acute yellow phosphorus poisoning. N Engl J Med 1971;284:157.

228. Simon FA, Pickering LK: Acute yellow phosphorus poisoning. Smoking stool syndrome. JAMA 1976;235:1343.

229. Poklis A, Saady J: Arsenic poisoning: Acute or chronic. Suicide or murder. Am J Forensic Med Pathol 1990;11:226.

230. Clearfield JR: Hepatorenal toxicity from sniffing spot remover (metchloroethylene). Am J Dig Dis 1970;15:851.

231. Tucker SC, Patterson TE: Hepatitis and halothane sniffing. Ann Intern Med 1974;30:667.

232. Goyer RA: Toxic effects of metals. In Klaassen CD (ed): Casarette and Doull's Toxicology: The Basic Science of Poisons, 5th ed. New York, Macmillan, 1996, pp 691, 736.

233. Jantsch W, Kulig K, Rumack BH: Massive copper sulfate ingestion resulting in hepatotoxicity. J Toxicol Clin Toxicol 1984;22:585.

234. Kimbrough RD: The toxicity of polychlorinated polycyclic compounds and related chemicals. CRC Crit Rev Toxicol 1974;2:445.

235. Kuratsune M, Yoshimura T, Matsuzaka J, et al: Epidemiologic study of oil contaminated with a commercial brand of polychlorinated biphenyls. Environ Health Perspect 1972;1:119.

236. Safe S: Toxicology, structure-function relationship, and human and environmental health impacts of polychlorinated biphenyls: progress and problems. Environ Health Perspect 1993;100:259–268.

237. Skilleter D, Cain K, Dinsdale D, et al: Biochemical mechanisms and morphological selectivity in hepatotoxicity: studies in cultures of hepatic-parenchymal and non-parenchymal cells. Xenobiotica 1985;15:687–693.

238. Brautbar N, Williams J II: Industrial solvents and liver toxicity: risk assessment, risk factors and mechanisms. Int J Hyg Environ Health 2002;205:479–491.

239. Paolini M, Sapigni E, Mesirca R, et al: On the hepatotoxicity of 1,1,2,2-tetrachloroethane. Toxicology 1992;73:101–115.

240. Tomiyama N, Watanabe M, Takeda M, et al: A comparative study on the reliability of toxicokinetic parameters for predicting hepatotoxicity of DDT in rats receiving a single or repeated administration. Toxicol Sci 2003;28:403–413.

241. Liu ZX, Kaplowitz N: Immune-mediated drug-induced liver disease. Clin Liver Dis 2002;6:467–486.

242. Yeung E, Wong FS, Wanless IR, et al: Ramipril-associated hepatotoxicity. Arch Pathol Lab Med 2003;127:1493–1497.

243. Kalapos MP: Carbamazepine-provoked hepatotoxicity and possible aetiopathological role of glutathione in the events. Retrospective review of old data and call for new investigation. Adverse Drug React Toxicol Rev 2002;21:123–141.

244. Schneider HL, Hornbach KD, Kniaz JL: Chlorpropamide hepatotoxicity: report of a case and review of the literature. Am J Gastroenterol 1984;79:721–724.

245. Fisher AA, Le Couteur DG: Nephrotoxicity and hepatotoxicity of histamine H2 receptor antagonists. Drug Saf 2001;24:39–57.

246. Hummer M, Kurz M, Kurzthaler I, et al: Hepatotoxicity of clozapine. J Clin Psychopharmacol 1997;17:314–317.

247. Munyon WH, Salo R, Briones DF: Cytotoxic effects of neuroleptic drugs. Psychopharmacology (Berl) 1987;91:182–188.

248. Woeber KA: Methimazole-induced hepatotoxicity. Endocr Pract 2002;8:222–224.

249. Thiim M, Friedman LS: Hepatotoxicity of antibiotics and antifungals. Clin Liver Dis 2003;7:381–399.

250. Bergeron L, Guy C, Ratrema M, et al: Dextropropoxyphene hepatotoxicity: four cases and literature review. Therapie 2002;57:464–472.

251. Slezak P: Quinidine hepatotoxicity. Med J Aust 1981;1:139.

252. Devuyst O, Lefebvre C, Geubel A, et al: Acute cholestatic hepatitis with rash and hypereosinophilia associated with ranitidine treatment. Acta Clin Belg 1993;48:109–114.

253. Zaman F, Ye G, Abreo KD, et al: Successful orthotopic liver transplantation after trimethoprim-sulfamethoxazole associated fulminant liver failure. Clin Transplant 2003;17:461–464.

254. Lasso Vega MC, Zapater P, Such J, et al: Toxic hepatitis associated with tamoxifen use. A case report and literature review. Gastroenterol Hepatol 2002;25:247–250.

255. Ajit C, Suvannasankha A, Zaeri N, et al: Terbinafine-associated hepatotoxicity. Am J Med Sci 2003;325:292–295.

256. Farmer JA, Torre-Amione G: Comparative tolerability of the HMG-CoA reductase inhibitors. Drug Saf 2000;23:197–213.

257. Ballare M, Xampanini M, Airoldi G: Hepatotoxicity of HMG-CoA reductase inhibitors. Minerva Gastroenterol Dietol 1992;38:41–44.

258. Grimbert S, Pessayre D, Degott C: Acute hepatitis induced by the HMG-CoA reductase inhibitor lovastatin. Drug Dig Sci 1999;39:2032–2033.

259. Hartleb M, Rymarczyk C, Januszewski K: Acute cholestatic hepatitis associated with pravastatin. Am J Gastroenterol 1999;94:1388–1390.

260. Huchzermeyer H, Munzenmaier R: Lovastatin-induced acute cholestatic hepatitis. Dtsch Med Wochenschr 1995;120:252–256.

261. Gascon A, Zabala S, Iglesias E: Acute cholestasis during long term treatment with fluvastatin in a nephritic patient. Nephrol Dial Transpl 1999;14:1038.

262. Punthakee Z, Scully LJ, Guindi MM, Ooi TC: Liver fibrosis attributed to lipid-lowering medications: two cases. J Intern Med 2001;250:249–254.

263. Nakad A, Bataille L, Hamoir V: Atorvastatin-induced acute hepatitis with absence of cross-toxicity with simvastatin. Lancet 1999;53:1763–1764.

264. Athyros VG, Papageorgiou AA, Hatzikonstandinou HA: Safety and efficacy of long-term statin-fibrate combinations in patients with familial combined hyperlipidaemia. Am J Cardiol 1997;80:608–613.

265. Rosellini SR, Costa PL, Gaudio M, et al: Hepatic injury related to enalapril. Gastroenterology 1989;97:810.

266. Hagley MT, Hulisz DT, Burns CM: Hepatotoxicity associated with angiotensin-converting enzyme inhibitors. Ann Phamacother 1993;27:228–231.

267. Larrey D, Babany G, Bernau J, et al: Fulminant hepatitis after lisinopril administration. Gastroenterology 1990;99:1832–1833.

268. Nunes AC, Amaro P, Mac F, et al: Fosinopril induced prolonged cholestatic jaundice and pruritis: first case report. Eur J Gastroenterol Hepatol 2001;13:279–282.

269. Rahmat J, Gelfand RL, Gelfand M, et al: Captopril-associated cholestatic jaundice. Ann Intern Med 1985;102:56–58.

270. Hagley MT, Benak RL, Hulisz DT: Suspected cross-reactivity of enalapril and captopril induced hepatotoxicity. Ann Pharmacother 1992;26:780–781.

271. Jeserich M, Ihling C, Allgaier HP, et al: Acute liver failure due to enalapril. Herz 2000;25:689–693.

272. Todd P, Levison D, Farthing MJ: Enalapril related acute cholestatic jaundice. J R Soc Med 1990;83:271–272.

273. Andrade RJ, Lucena MI, Santella F: Hepatic injury associated with losartan. Ann Pharmacother 1998;32:1371.

274. Hariraj R, Stoner E, Jader S, et al: Drug points: prolonged cholestasis associated with irbesartan. BMJ 2000;321:547.

275. Vallejo I, Garcia Morillo S, Pamies E: Acute hepatitis induced by candesartan. Med Clin (Barc) 2000;1115:719.

276. See S, Stirling AL: Candesartan cilexitil: an angiotensin II receptor blocker. Am J Health Syst Pharm 2000;57:739–746.

277. Gonzalez-Jiminez D, Varela JM, Calderon E, et al: Candesartan and acute liver injury. Eur J Clin Pharmacol 2000;56:769–770.

278. Yap I, Gwee KA, Wee A: Augmentin-induced cholestatic jaundice—a case report. Singapore Med J 1993;34:464–465.

279. O'Donohue J, Oien KA, Donaldson P, et al: Co-amoxiclav jaundice: clinical and histological features and HLA class II association. Gut 2000;47:717–720.

280. Romagnuolo J, Sadowski DC, Lalor E, et al: Cholestatic hepato-cellular injury with azathioprine: a case report and review of the mechanisms of hepatotoxicity. Can J Gastroenterol 1998;12:479–483.

281. Knodell RG: Effects of chlorpromazine on bilirubin metabolism and biliary secretion in the rat. Gastroenterology 1975;69:965–972.

282. Hautekeete ML: Hepatotoxicity of antibiotics. Acta Gastroenterol Belg 1995;58:290–296.

283. Basset C, Vadrot J, Denis J, et al: Prolonged cholestasis and ductopenia following gold salt therapy. Liver Int 2003;23:89–93.
284. Rosenbaum J, Katz WA, Schumacher HR: Hepatotoxicity associated with use of D-penicillamine in rheumatoid arthritis. Ann Rheum Dis 1980;39:152–154.
285. Bastian PG: Occupational hepatic caused by methylenedianiline. Med J Aust 1984;141:533.
286. Kaplowitz N, Aw TY, Simon FR, et al: Drug-induced hepatotoxicity. Ann Intern Med 1986;104:826–839.
287. Hepatic effects of 17 alpha-alkylated anabolic-androgenic ster. HIV Hotline 1998;8:2–5.
288. Stone BG, Udani M, Sanghvi A, et al: Cyclosporin A-induced cholestasis. The mechanism in a rat model. Gastroenterology 1987;93:344–351.
289. Hall AJ, Harrington JM, Waterhouse JA: The Epping jaundice outbreak: a 24 year follow up. J Epidemiol Community Health 1992;46:327–328.
290. Kopelman H, Robertson MH, Sanders PG, et al: The Epping jaundice. BMJ 1966;5486:514–516.
291. Doll R: Spanish toxic oil syndrome. Med Hist 2003;47:99.
292. A search for an animal model of the Spanish toxic oil syndrome. Food Chem Toxicol 2002;40:1551–1567.
293. Leiber CS: Alcoholic liver injury: pathogenesis and therapy in 2001. Pathol Biol (Paris) 2001;49:738–752.
294. Ugarte G, Iturriaga H, Insunza I: Some effects of ethanol on normal and pathologic livers. Prog Liver Dis 1970;3:355–370.
295. Kurihara T, Akimoto M, Kurokawa K, et al: Effects of a gastric mucosal protecting agent in rats with liver cirrhosis. J Gastroenterol Hepatol 1992;7:405–410.
296. Harrison RF, Elias E: Amiodarone-associated cirrhosis with hepatic and lymph node granulomas. Histopathology 1993;22:80–82.
297. Bach N, Schultz BL, Cohen LB, et al: Amiodarone hepatotoxicity: progression from steatosis to cirrhosis. Mt Sinai J Med 1989;56:293–296.
298. Pettavel J, Gardiol D, Bergier N, Schnyder P: Fatal liver cirrhosis associated with long-term arterial infusion of floxuridine. Lancet 1986;2:1162–1163.
299. Kim TH, Kim BH, Kim YW, et al: Liver cirrhosis developed after ketoconazole-induced acute hepatic injury. J Gastroenterol Hepatol 2003;18:1426–1429.
300. Arteel G, Marsano L, Mendez C, et al: Advances in alcoholic liver disease. Best Pract Res Clin Gastroenterol 2003;17:625–647.
301. Comar KM, Sanyal AJ: Portal hypertensive bleeding. Gastroenterol Clin North Am 2003;32:1079–1105.
302. Thalheimer U, Mela M, Patch D, et al: Prevention of variceal rebleeding. Lancet 2003;361:2244–2245.
303. Vilstrup H: Cirrhosis and bacterial infections. Rom J Gastroenterol 2003;12:297–302.
304. Copple BL, Ganey PE, Roth RA: Liver inflammation during monocrotaline hepatotoxicity. Toxicology 2003;190:155–169.
305. Biecker E, Fischer HP, Strunk H, et al: Benign hepatic tumours. Z Gastroenterol 2003;41:191–200.
306. Rogers AE: Toxicity and carcinogenicity of aflatoxins in experimental animals. In Pollack JD (ed): Reye's Syndrome. New York, Grune & Stratton, 1974, p 135.
307. Wogan GN: Aflatoxins as risk factors for hepatocellular carcinoma in humans. Cancer Res 1992;52:1145.
308. Sell S: Cellular origin of hepatocellular carcinomas. Semin Cell Dev Biol 2002;13:419–424.
309. Naccarato R, Farinati F: Hepatocellular carcinoma, alcohol, and cirrhosis: facts and hypotheses. Dig Dis Sci 1991;36:1137–1142.
310. Blum HE: Molecular therapy and prevention of hepatocellular carcinoma. Hepatobiliary Pancreat Dis Int 2003;2:11–22.
311. Kielhorn J, Melber C, Wahnschaffe U, et al: Vinyl chloride: still a cause for concern. Environ Health Perspect 2000;108:579–588.
312. Ward E, Boffetta P, Andersen A, et al: Update of the follow-up of mortality and cancer incidence among European workers employed in the vinyl chloride industry. Epidemiology 2001;12:710–718.
313. Larrey D, Vial T, Pauwels A: Hepatitis after germander (Teucrium chamaedrys) administration: another instance of herbal medicine toxicity. Ann Intern Med 1992;117:129–132.
314. Fau D, Lekehal M, Farrell G: Diterpenoids from germander, an herbal medicine, induce apoptosis in isolated rat hepatocytes. Gastroenterology 1997;113:1334–1346.
315. Lekehal M, Pessayre D, Lereau JM: Hepatotoxicity of the herbal medicine germander: metabolic activation of its furano diterpenoids by cytochrome P4503A depletes cytoskeleton-associated protein thiols and forms plasma membrane blebs in rat hepatocytes. Hepatology 1996;24:212–218.
316. De Berardinis V, Moulis C, Maurice M: Human microsomal epoxide hydrolase is the target of germander-induced autoantibodies on the surface of human hepatocytes. Mol Pharmacol 2000;58:542–551.
317. Mattocks AR, Driver HF, Barbour RH, Robins DJ: Metabolism and toxicity of synthetic analogues of macrocyclic diester pyrrolizidine alkaloids. Chem Biol Interact 1986;58:95–108.
318. Winship KA: Toxicity of comfrey. Adverse Drug React Toxicol Rev 1991;10:47–59.
319. Weston CF, Cooper BT, Davies JD: Veno-occlusive disease of the liver secondary to ingestion of comfrey. BMJ 1987;295:183.
320. Steenkamp V, Stewart M, Zuckerman M: Clinical and analytical aspects of pyrrolizidine alkaloid poisoning caused by South African traditional medicines. Ther Drug Monit 2000;22:302–306.
321. Stickel F, Egerer G, Seitz HK: Hepatotoxicity of botanicals. Public Health Nutr 2000;3:113–124.
322. DeLeve LD, McCuskey RS, Wang X: Characterization of a reproducible rat model of hepatic veno-occlusive disease. Hepatology 1999;29:1779–1791.
323. Wang X, Kanel GC, DeLeve LD: Support of sinusoidal endothelial cell glutathione prevents hepatic veno-occlusive disease in the rat. Hepatology 2000;31:428–434.
324. Anderson IB, Mullen WH, Meeker JE: Pennyroyal toxicity: measurement of toxic metabolites in two cases and review of the literature. Ann Intern Med 1996;124:726–734.
325. Bakerink JA, Gosper SM, Dimand RJ, Eldridge MW: Multiple organ failure after ingestion of pennyroyal oil from herbal tea in two infants. Pediatrics 1996;98:944–947.
326. Khojasteh-Bakht SC, Chen W, Koenigs LL: Metabolism of (R)+-pulegone and (R)+-menthofuran by human liver cytochrome P450s: evidence for formation of a furan epoxide. Drug Metab Dispos 1999;27:574–580.
327. Sullivan JB Jr, Rumack BH, Thomas H Jr, et al: Pennyroyal oil poisoning and hepatotoxicity. JAMA 1979;242:2873–2874.
328. Sztajnkrycer MD, Otten EJ, Bond GR, et al: Mitigation of pennyroyal oil hepatotoxicity in the mouse. Acad Emerg Med 2003;10:1024–1028.
329. Haouzi D, Lekehal M, Moreau A, et al: Cytochrome P450-generated reactive metabolites cause mitochondrial permeability transition, caspase activation, and apoptosis in rat hepatocytes. Hepatology 2000;32:303–311.
330. Mattei A, Rucay P, Samuel D: Liver transplantation for acute liver failure after herbal medicine (Teucrium polium) administration. J Hepatol 1995;22:597.
331. Batchelor WB, Heathcote J, Wanless IR: Chaparral-induced hepatic injury. Am J Gastroenterol 1995;90:831–833.
332. Sheikh NM, Philen RM, Love LA: Chaparral-associated hepatotoxicity. Arch Intern Med 1997;157:913–919.
333. Batchelor WB, Heathcote J, Wanless IR: Chaparral-induced hepatic injury. Am J Gastroenterol 1995;90:831–832.
334. Smith BC, Desmond PV: Acute hepatitis induced by ingestion of the herbal medicine chaparral. Aust N Z J Med 1993;23:526.
335. Escher M, Desmeales J, Giostra E, Mentha G: Hepatitis associated with Kava, a herbal remedy for anxiety. BMJ 2001;322:139.
336. Kraft M, Spahn TW, Menzel J: Fulminant liver failure after administration of the herbal antidepressant Kava-Kava. Dtsch Med Wochenschr 2001;126:970–972.
337. Russmann S, Lauterburg BH, Helbling A: Kava hepatotoxicity. Ann Intern Med 2001;135:68–69.
338. Strahl S, Ehret V, Dahm HH, Maier KP: Necrotizing hepatitis after taking herbal remedies. Dtsch Med Wochenschr 1998;123:1410–1414.
339. Xing JH, Soffer EE: Adverse effects of laxatives. Dis Colon Rectum 2001;44:1201–1209.
340. Fukunishi R: Acute hepatic lesions induced by cycasin. Acta Pathol 1973;23:639.
341. Atal CK: Semisynthetic derivatives of pyrrolizidine alkaloids of pharmacodynamic importance: a review. Lloydia 1978;41:312–326.

342. Uc A, Bishop WP, Sanders KD: Camphor hepatotoxicity. South Med J 2000;93:596–598.

343. Jimenez JF, Brown AL, Arnold WC, Byrne WJ: Chronic camphor ingestion mimicking Reye's syndrome. Gastroenterology 1983;84:394–398.

344. Stewart MJ, Steenkamp V: The biochemistry and toxicity of atractyloside: a review. Ther Drug Monit 2000;22:641–649.

345. Popat A, Shear NH, Malkiewicz I: The toxicity of Callilepis laureola, a South African traditional herbal medicine. Clin Biochem 2001;34:229–236.

346. Nadir A, Reddy D, Van Thiel DH: Cascara sagrada-induced intrahepatic cholestasis causing portal hypertension: case report and review of herbal hepatotoxicity. Am J Gastroenterol 2000;95:3634–3637.

347. Fraquelli M, Colli A, Cocciolo M, Conte D: Adult syncytial giant cell chronic hepatitis due to herbal remedy. J Hepatol 2000;33:505–508.

348. De Smet PA, Van den Eertwegh AJ, Lesterhuis W, et al: Hepatotoxicity associated with herbal tablets. BMJ 1996;313:92.

349. Takegoshi K, Tohyama T, Cox D: A case of Venoplant-induced hepatic injury. Gastroenterol Japan 1986;21:62–65.

350. Hamid S, Rojter S, Vierling J: Protracted cholestatic hepatitis after the use of Prostata. Ann Intern Med 1997;127:169–170.

351. Nadir A, Sangeeta A, King P, Marshall JB: Acute hepatitis associated with the use of a Chinese herbal product, Ma-Huang. Am J Gastroenterol 1996;91:1436–1438.

352. Borum ML: Fulminant exacerbation of autoimmune hepatitis after the use of ma-huang. Am J Gastroenterol 2001;96:1654–1655.

353. Picciotto A, Campo N, Brizzolara R: Chronic hepatitis induced by Jin Bu Huan. J Hepatol 1998;28:165–167.

354. Horowitz RS, Feldhaus K, Dart RC: The clinical spectrum of Jin Bu Huan toxicity. Arch Intern Med 1996;156:899–903.

355. Woolf GM, Petrovic LM, Rojter SE: Acute hepatitis associated with the Chinese herbal product Jin Bu Huan. Ann Intern Med 1994;121:729–735.

356. Benninger J, Schneider HT, Schuppan D: Acute hepatitis induced by greater celandine (Chelidonium majus). Gastroenterology 1999;117:1234–1237.

357. Yoshida EM, McLean CA, Cheng ES: Chinese herbal medicine, fulminant hepatitis and liver transplantation. Am J Gastroenterol 1996;91:2647–2648.

358. Perharic-Walton L, Murray V: Toxicity of Chinese herbal remedies. Lancet 1992;340:674.

359. Gorey JD, Wahlqvist ML, Boyce NW: Adverse reaction to a Chinese herbal remedy. Med J Aust 1992;157:484–486.

360. Pillans PI: Herbal medicines and toxic hepatitis. N Z Med J 1994;107:432–433.

361. Kane JA, Kane SP, Jain S: Hepatitis induced by traditional Chinese herbs; possible toxic components. Gut 1995;36:146–147.

362. Al-Khafaji M: Monitoring of liver enzymes in patients on Chinese medicines. JCM 2000;62:6–10.

363. McRae CA, Agarwal K, Mutimer D, Bassedine MF: Hepatitis associated with Chinese herbs. Eur J Gastroenterol Hepatol 2002;14:559–562.

364. Melchart D, Linde K, Hager S: Monitoring of liver enzymes in patients treated with traditional Chinese drugs. Complement Ther Med 1999;7:208–216.

365. Lautt WW: Intrinsic regulation of hepatic blood flow. Can J Physiol Pharmacol 1996;74:223–233.

366. Holden R, Jackson MA: Near-fatal hyponatraemia coma due to vasopressin over-secretion after "ecstasy" (3,4 MDMA). Lancet 1996;347:1052.

367. Box SA, Prescott LF, Freestone S: Hyponatraemia at a rave. Postgrad Med J 1997;73:53–54.

368. Denborough MA, Hopkinson KC: Dantrolene and "ecstasy." Med J Aust 1997;166:165–166.

369. Ellis A, Wendon J: Circulatory, respiratory, cerebral and renal derangements in acute liver failure: pathophysiology and management. Semin Liver Dis 1996;16:379–388.

370. Lee WM: Acute liver failure. Am J Med 1994;96:S3–S9.

371. Jalan R, Damink SW, Deutz NE, et al: Moderate hypothermia for uncontrolled intracranial hypertension in acute liver failure. Lancet 1999;354:1164–1168.

372. Kritharides L, Fasset R, Singh B: Paracetamol-associated coma, metabolic acidosis, renal and hepatic failure. Intensive Care Med 1988;14:439–440.

373. Block R, Jankowski JA, Lacoux P, Pennington CR: Does hypothermia protect against the development of hepatitis in paracetamol overdose? Anaesthesia 1992;47:789–791.

374. Aruoma OI, Halliwell B, Hey BM, Butler J: The antioxidant action of N-acetylcysteine. Its reaction with hydrogen peroxide, hydroxyl radical, superoxide and hypochlorous acid. Free Radic Biol Med 1989;6:593–597.

375. Bernuau J, Benhamou JP: Fulminant and subfulminant liver failure. In McIntyre NM, Benhamou JP, Rodes J (eds): The Oxford Textbook of Clinical Hepatology. Oxford, Oxford University Press, 1991, pp 923–942.

376. Gressier B, Cabanis A, Lebegue S, et al: Comparison of in vitro effects of two thiol-containing drugs on human neutrophils hydrogen peroxide production. Methods Find Exp Clin Pharmacol 1993;15:101–105.

377. Tee LG, Boobis AR, Davies DS: N-acetylcysteine for paracetamol overdose. Lancet 1986;1:331–332.

378. Chyka PA, Butler AY, Holliman BJ, Herman MI: Utility of acetylcysteine in treating poisonings and adverse drug reactions. Drug Saf 2000;22:123–148.

379. Harrison PM, Wendon JA, Gimson AE, et al: Improvement by acetylcysteine of haemodynamics and oxygen transport in fulminant hepatic failure. N Engl J Med 1991;324:1852–1857.

380. Walsh TS, Hopton P, Lee A: A comparison between the Fick method and indirect calorimetry for determining oxygen consumption in patients with fulminant hepatic failure. Crit Care Med 1998;26:1200–1207.

381. Bailey B, Amre DK, Gaudreault P: Fulminant hepatic failure secondary to acetaminophen poisoning: a systematic review and meta-analysis of prognostic criteria determining the need for liver transplantation. Crit Care Med 2003;31:299–305.

382. De Carlis L, De Gasperi A, Slim AO, et al: Liver transplantation for ecstasy-induced fulminant hepatic failure. Transplant Proc 2001;33:2743–2744.

383. Greaves BR, Agarwal A, Patch D, et al: Inadvertent diclofenac rechallenge from generic and non-generic prescribing leading to liver transplantation for ulminant liver failure. Eur J Gastroenterol Hepatol 2001;13:71–73.

384. Jones AL, Latham T, Shallcross TM, Simpson KJ: Fulminant hepatic failure due to diclofenac treaeted successfully by orthotopic liver transplant. Transplant Proc 1998;30:192–194.

385. Kozaki K, Egawa H, Garcia-Kennedy R, et al: Hepatic failure due to massive iron ingestion successfully treated with liver transplantation. Clin Transplant 1995;9:85–87.

386. Jackson N, Ellis A, Rhodes A, et al: Non-paracetamol drug induced acute liver failure in a specialist liver intensive care unit: a seven year experience. Hepatology 1998;28:496.

387. Bernal W: Changing patterns of causation and the use of transplantation in the UK. Semin Liver Dis 2003;23:227–237.

388. O'Grady JG, Alexander GJ, Hayllar KM, et al: Early indicators of prognosis in fulminant hepatic failure. Gastroenterology 1989;97:439–445.

389. Harrison PM, O'Grady JG, Keays RT, et al: Serial prothrombin time as prognostic indicator in paracetamol induced fulminant hepatic failure. BMJ 1990;301:964–966.

390. O'Grady JG, Wendon J, Tan KC, et al: Liver transplantation after paracetamol overdose. BMJ 1991;303:221–223.

391. Jones AL: Recent advances in the management of late paracetamol poisoning. Emerg Med 2000;12:14–21.

392. Bernal W, Donaldson N, Wyncoll D, Wendon J: Blood lactate as an early predictor of outcome in paracetamol-induced acute liver failure: a cohort study. Lancet 2002;16:558–563.

393. Makin AJ, Wendon J, Williams R: A 7-year experience of severe acetaminophen-induced hepatotoxicity, 1987–1993. Gastroenterology 1995;109:1907–1916.

394. Sen S, Ytrebo LM, Rose C, et al: Albumin dialysis: a new therapeutic strategy for intoxication from protein-bound drugs. Intensive Care Med 2004;30:496–501.

395. Sen S, Ratnaraj N, Davies NA, et al: Treatment of phenytoin toxicity by the molecular adsorbents recirculating system (MARS). Epilepsia 2003;44:265–267.

12 *Renal Toxicology*

A Acute Renal Failure

MIGUEL C. FERNÁNDEZ, MD

Acute renal failure (ARF) is one of the most common and serious consequences of poisoning or drug overdose. ARF is a clinical syndrome of diverse causes (Box 12A-1) in which a relatively sudden deterioration of renal function results in the inability of the kidneys to regulate normal homeostasis. Its importance stems from the acuteness and severity of the clinical manifestations that develop and the potential for reversibility of the condition, particularly if it is recognized early and the appropriate preventive and therapeutic measures are instituted promptly. ARF can be a self-limited condition and is one example of organ failure that is totally reversible and for which replacement therapy is available. Nevertheless, ARF is principally associated with a high mortality rate because of the seriousness of the underlying conditions that lead to its onset, which are in turn aggravated by the loss of renal regulatory functions.[1]

Much of what we know about ARF was relatively recently elucidated.[2] Human activity has often led to infection, crush injury, dehydration, massive hemorrhage, and other causes of shock and tissue injury. Historically, acute anuria was attributed to obstruction or associated with edema, earlier known as dropsy. Nonobstructive suppression or retention of urine was termed *ischuria renalis* in the Age of Enlightenment, which came to be attributed to either inflammation or "paralysis of the kidneys."[3] In 1909, Osler classified ARF under the general heading of acute Bright's disease. He described a broad and vague group of cases of ARF related to burns, other trauma, and the toxicants turpentine, potassium chlorate, and carbolic acid (phenol). Acute renal lesions that affected crushed or wounded soldiers were described in the German literature during and immediately after World War I.[4] In 1923, Muir used the term *war nephritis* and others used the term *field* or *trench nephritis* in describing variations of ARF.[5] Sporadic reports of ARF in traumatized civilians began to appear in the literature thereafter and were soon followed by reports of cases of ARF that ensued after prolonged, complicated, and infected surgical procedures.[6] In 1926, Haas described his poorly accepted hemodialysis invention for treatment of uremia.[7] In 1941 Bywaters, and Beall reported on four patients who sustained crush injuries during the bombing of London in the Battle of Britain and developed ARF, and although they did not make a clear etiologic connection, they made the first modern description of rhabdomyolysis.[8] In 1945 nephritis following mite-borne rickettsial scrub typhus infection was described by several researchers.[9,10] Detailed studies of ARF developed during efforts to elucidate the mechanism of shock in battle injuries.[11] This, coupled with the further development of hemodialysis and renal replacement therapy by Kolff and Beck in 1944, led to a rapid expansion of knowledge about ARF, while hemodialysis became better accepted as further studies led to improvements of outcome in the 1950s.[12-14] Literature in the 1960s concerning patients whose kidneys had failed because of the acute renal toxicity

---

BOX 12A-1 MAJOR CAUSES OF ACUTE RENAL FAILURE

Prerenal Failure

Extracellular circulating fluid volume contraction
 Gastrointestinal losses: vomiting, diarrhea
 Fluid sequestration: burns, pancreatitis, peritonitis, crush injury, venous ligation
 Renal losses: diuretics, diabetic ketoacidosis
Blood loss
Central or cardiac shock: congestive heart failure, myocardial infarction, tachyarrhythmias, central nervous system injury
Septicemia: endotoxic shock
Anoxia (requires salt depletion)

Postrenal Failure

Prostatic hypertrophy, tumors, calculi, blood clots, ureteral edema, retroperitoneal fibrosis, inadvertent ureteral ligation, papillary necrosis

Renal Failure

Primary damage to tubular epithelium
 Ischemia
 Nephrotoxic
  Drugs: aminoglycosides, methoxyflurane, cytolytic agents, phenytoin, cisplatin, bismuth, rifampin
  Radiopaque contrast agents
  Respiratory pigments: hemoglobin, myoglobin
  Poisons: heavy metals, carbon tetrachloride, animal toxins
  Intratubular precipitation: uric acid, myeloma proteins, mucoprotein, sulfas, calcium, xanthine, oxalate
Primary damage to glomeruli and small renal vasculature
 Acute glomerulonephritis, collagen vascular disease, malignant hypertension, serum sickness, thrombotic microangiopathy
Primary damage to major renal vessels
 Thrombosis, embolization, atheroembolism
Parenchymal necrosis
 Cortical, papillary

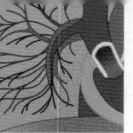

of drugs and poisons emphasized removal through renal replacement therapy.[13]

Presently, ARF is classified into three general categories: that caused by renal hypoperfusion (prerenal), that caused by intrinsic parenchymal lesions of the kidneys (renal, or intrinsic), and that caused by obstruction of the urinary outflow passages (postrenal, or obstructive uropathy). These categories and their relative prevalence as a cause of ARF are shown in Figure 12A-1.

PATHOPHYSIOLOGY

The hallmarks of ARF are the onset of progressive oliguria and azotemia, typically over a period of hours to days, stemming from a sudden decrease in glomerular filtration rate (GFR) and leading to an acute rise in blood urea nitrogen (BUN) and serum creatinine (Cr) concentrations.[15] Daily urine volume less than the volume necessary to excrete the waste products of the body is termed oliguria. Azotemia exists when the blood contains a higher than normal quantity of urea or other nitrogen-containing substances. Normal human kidneys are able to maximally concentrate the urine to 1200 mOsm/L of water. To maintain normal homeostasis, an adult must excrete about 600 mOsm of solute, with urea constituting 40% to 50% of this obligatory solute load. Therefore, the daily urine excretion necessary to maintain homeostasis is about 400 to 500 mL in an adult with normal renal function who is concentrating the urine maximally and consuming a normal diet, and oliguria is said to be present if urine production is less than this amount. Normal daily urine output of 1000 to 1500 mL reflects the intake of water in excess of the amount necessary to maintain homeostasis, thus allowing the excretion of less concentrated urine. This is a desirable consequence since concentrating the urine maximally entails added work and energy consumption by the kidneys, rendering them more susceptible to injury.[16]

Urea excretion is diminished in individuals with low dietary intake of protein or in those unable to metabolize protein to urea (hepatic cirrhosis). Because urea constitutes half of the normal solute load, the daily urine output to maintain balance in these individuals is reduced to about 300 mL. By the same token, in individuals on restricted salt intake or patients whose kidneys are in a sodium retention state (congestive heart failure, nephrotic syndrome, hepatic cirrhosis), the urine output necessary to maintain balance is also reduced to the extent that the load of sodium excreted and, therefore, the amount of water obligated to it are now reduced. Conversely, in a hypercatabolic state (trauma, burn, or sepsis), when urea production is increased, or in conditions in which diuretics are used to inhibit sodium reabsorption, a proportionately larger urine volume is necessary to clear the solute load.[17]

Injured kidneys that are unable to absorb and maximally concentrate urine require a larger volume of water to excrete the daily load of solutes. Thus, in kidneys only able to concentrate urine to 600 mOsm, 1000 mL of urine would have to be excreted to maintain homeostasis, whereas in kidneys only able to concentrate to 300 mOsm, 2000 mL of urine would have to be excreted. This would be the case of chronically diseased kidneys, but much more important for purposes of this chapter is the situation in the early stages of acute renal injury. One of the first structural consequences of injured tubular cells appears to be a loss of the polar distribution of the sodium-potassium-adenosine triphosphatase (Na-K-ATPase) pump, with consequent impairment of the capacity to absorb filtered sodium and, hence, the subsequent natriuresis and inability to achieve medullary hypertonicity necessary to concentrate the urine maximally.[1,18] The duration of this otherwise invariable phase of early acute renal injury varies, depending on the magnitude and severity of the insult to the kidneys. This stage when the urine output is high at a time that the GFR is declining has been termed nonoliguric ARF (Fig. 12A-2). Its early detection, by noting increasing BUN and Cr concentrations, is important because removal of the insult may prevent progression to oliguric ARF, with its graver prognosis.

In terms of laboratory values, ARF is commonly defined as an increase in Cr concentration of 0.5 mg/dL, an increase in BUN of 10 to 15 mg/dL, or an increase of more than 50% over the baseline levels of either one. The early identification of progressive incremental changes in BUN and Cr concentrations are key to making an early diagnosis of ARF.[19] An acute reduction in the normal regulatory function of the kidneys can occur in the presence of reduced, normal, or high urine

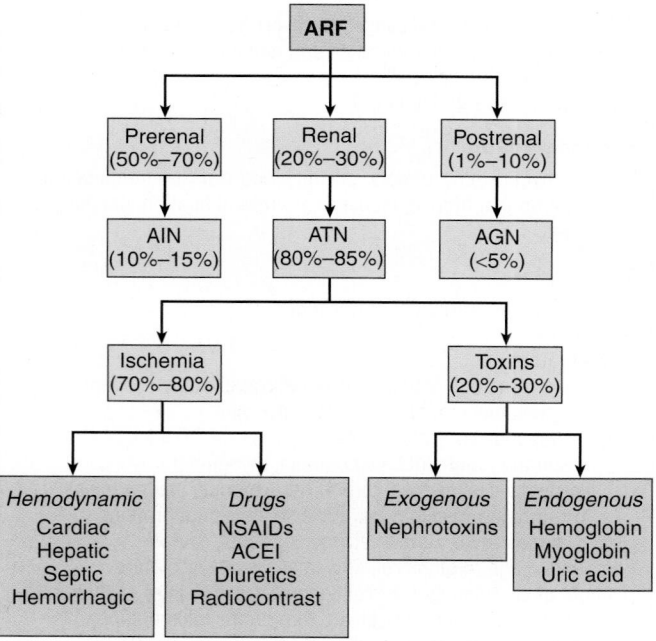

FIGURE 12A-1 Prevalence and principal forms of acute renal failure. ACEI, angiotensin-converting enzyme inhibitors; AGN, acute glomerulonephritis; AIN, acute interstitial nephritis; ARF, acute renal failure; ATN, acute tubular necrosis; NSAIDS, nonsteroidal anti-inflammatory drugs.

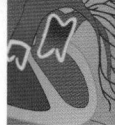

TABLE 12A-1 Range of Daily Urine Composition					
				ACUTE RENAL FAILURE	
		NORMAL	**PRERENAL FAILURE**	**OLIGURIC**	**NONOLIGURIC**
Volume	(mL/24 hr)	300–1500	<400	<400	1500+
Urea	(g/24 hr)	20	15	5	10
	(mM/24 hr)	350	250	85	170
Creatinine	(g/24 hr)	1–1.5	>1.0	<1.0	<1.0
Sodium	(mEq/24 hr)	100	5	25	100
Potassium	(mEq/24 hr)	50–79	10	>50	>50

flow rates (Table 12A-1). The clinical jargon of "good urine output" is a misnomer that provides a false sense of security and should be abandoned.

TOXIC ACUTE RENAL FAILURE

Strictly defined, toxic ARF is acute tubular cell injury and ultimate acute tubular necrosis (ATN) due to dose-dependent direct cell damage caused by a toxic agent that is usually limited to a specific part of the tubule. More broadly defined, in the general context of ARF, the renal injury may be induced by a host of agents that exert a detrimental effect at various sites within the entire nephron by mechanisms other than direct cell injury and that are not necessarily dose dependent (Fig. 12A-3).[20,21]

Injury due to exogenous poisons, such as mercuric chloride ($HgCl_2$), formerly the best-characterized form of toxic ATN, is now rare. Much of the ARF currently encountered is due to drugs,[22-24] whose increased availability and wider use have been associated with a host of undesirable side effects. The kidneys as the principal organs for the excretion of drugs and their metabolites are particularly prone to their side effects. The renal factors that render the kidneys particularly susceptible to injury are listed in Box 12A-2. Volume depletion is extremely important to recognize and correct early, because the associated increase in renal vascular resistance and consequent ischemia is central to much of the

nephrotoxicity encountered in clinical practice.[1,18,25] The nonrenal factors that contribute to increased drug-induced injury are listed in Box 12A-3. Clearly, the physician-related factors noted in Box 12A-3 can be circumvented. By the same token, of the patient-related factors, recognition of reduced renal function allows the physician to avert renal hypoperfusion and can prevent renal injury through appropriate adjustments of drug dosage and correction of volume depletion.

Furthermore, although strictly defined acute renal toxicity is a result of toxic effects on the renal parenchyma, several toxic agents exert their effect by causing impaired perfusion of the kidneys (prerenal) or their direct renal toxicity (renal) is magnified in the presence of reduced extracellular circulating fluid volume (ECFV). As such, it is essential to fully appreciate the sequence of events that characterize prerenal ARF.

PRERENAL FAILURE

Prerenal failure is usually present in patients with vascular collapse or circulatory insufficiency (see Box 12A-1). In their attempt to preserve ECFV, the kidneys sustain functional changes without demonstrable organic or structural damage (Fig. 12A-4). The most important of these is severe but reversible renal vasoconstriction with a preferential renal cortical hypoperfusion.[26] The resultant reduction in renal blood flow may be associated with reduced glomerular filtration and thus a decreased filtration of solute. In addition, a greater fraction of this filtrate (urea, water, sodium) is reabsorbed under the influence of volume-stimulated factors. Simultaneous stimulation of antidiuretic hormone secretion usually occurs in response to volume changes. Thus, the oliguria that results is associated with urine that is characteristically highly concentrated and low in sodium content. The azotemia that may be present is the result of increased reabsorption of urea and may develop in the absence of an actual decline in GFR. When renal circulation is restored, these patients respond with a prompt diuresis with correction of the azotemia and oliguria.[27] An important aspect of prerenal ARF is that it represents an earlier and reversible change in renal circulation that, if left uncorrected, may ultimately lead to organic renal damage (see Fig. 12A-2). At the very

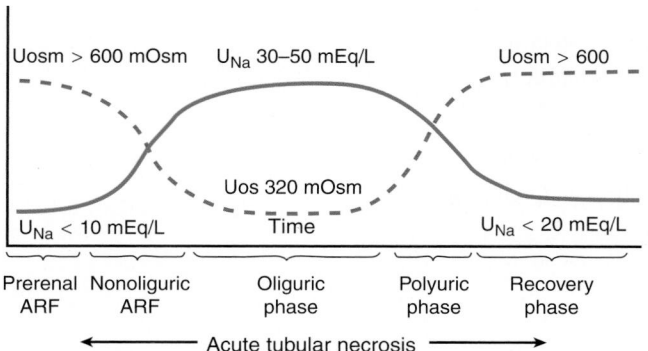

FIGURE 12A-2 Changes in urine osmolality and sodium concentration during the various phases of acute renal failure.

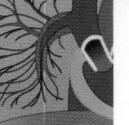

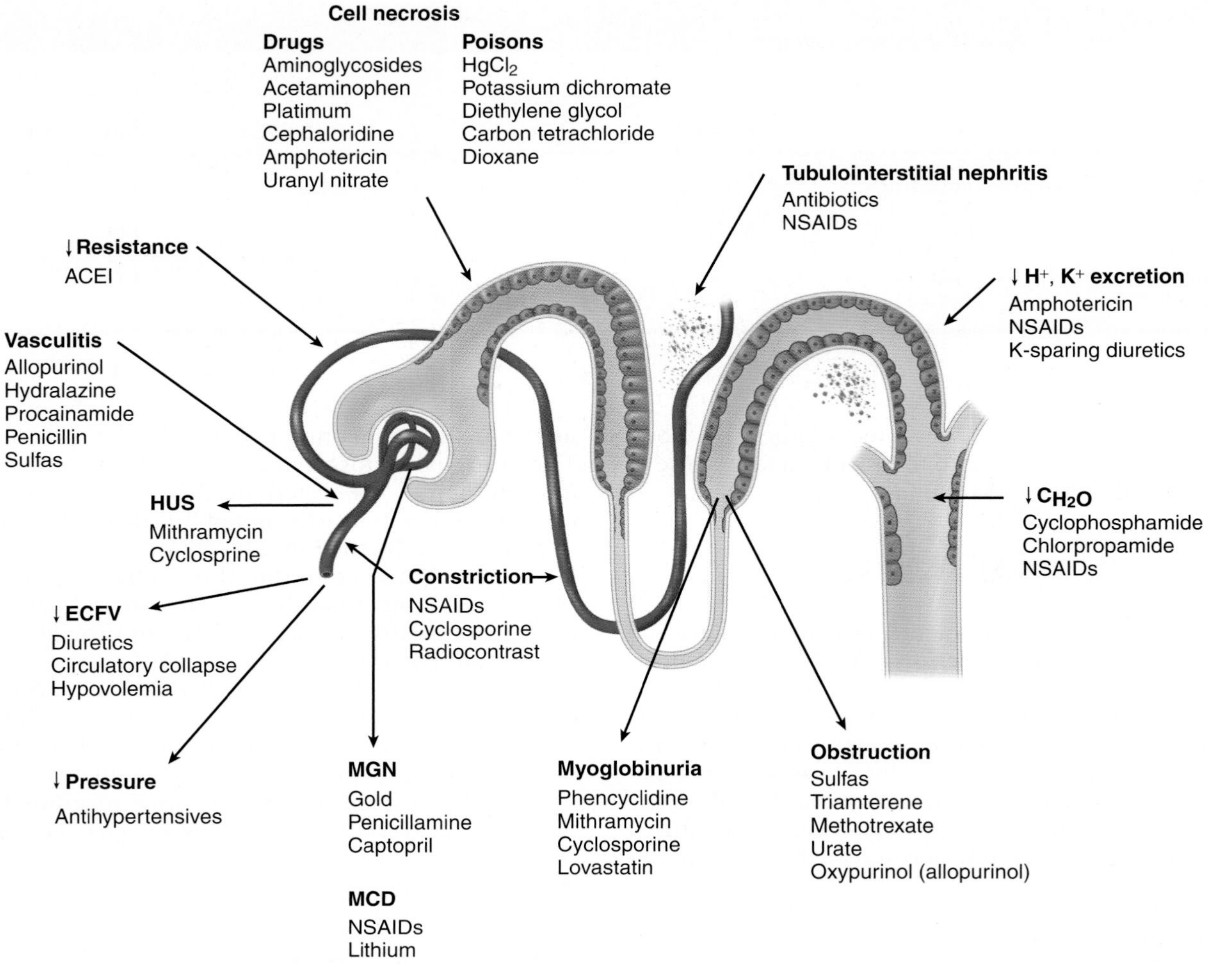

Cell necrosis

Drugs
Aminoglycosides
Acetaminophen
Platinum
Cephaloridine
Amphotericin
Uranyl nitrate

Poisons
$HgCl_2$
Potassium dichromate
Diethylene glycol
Carbon tetrachloride
Dioxane

Tubulointerstitial nephritis
Antibiotics
NSAIDs

↓ H^+, K^+ excretion
Amphotericin
NSAIDs
K-sparing diuretics

↓ Resistance
ACEI

Vasculitis
Allopurinol
Hydralazine
Procainamide
Penicillin
Sulfas

HUS
Mithramycin
Cyclosprine

↓ ECFV
Diuretics
Circulatory collapse
Hypovolemia

Constriction→
NSAIDs
Cyclosporine
Radiocontrast

↓ CH_2O
Cyclophosphamide
Chlorpropamide
NSAIDs

↓ Pressure
Antihypertensives

MGN
Gold
Penicillamine
Captopril

MCD
NSAIDs
Lithium

Myoglobinuria
Phencyclidine
Mithramycin
Cyclosporine
Lovastatin

Obstruction
Sulfas
Triamterene
Methotrexate
Urate
Oxypurinol (allopurinol)

FIGURE 12A-3 Schematic representation of the mechanisms and sites of injury within the nephron of the major nephrotoxic drugs. ^CH_2O, free water clearance; ECFV, extracellular fluid volume; HUS, hemolytic-uremic syndrome; MCD, minimal change disease; MGN, membranous glomerulopathy.

least, it renders the underperfused kidneys much more susceptible to toxic injury.

Although this category of ARF may be identified by the usual accompanying signs of peripheral circulatory failure and low ECFV, the composition of the urine is the main clue to its diagnosis (see Figs. 12A-2 and 12A-4). The urine is characteristically low in sodium content (<10 mEq/L, fractional sodium excretion <1%) and high in concentration (urine osmolarity >500 $mOsm/KgH_2O$).

A number of drugs exert their detrimental effects on the kidneys by inducing or aggravating prerenal ARF

BOX 12A-2 FACTORS PREDISPOSING THE KIDNEYS TO DRUG TOXICITY

High blood flow
Tubular transport and metabolism of drugs
Tubular fluid concentration in the medulla
Distal tubular fluid acidification

BOX 12A-3 FACTORS AFFECTING DRUG-RELATED NEPHROTOXICITY

Patient Related

Kidney disease
↓ Extracellular circulating fluid volume/↑ renal vascular resistance
Abuse/dependence

Drug Related

Nephrotoxicity
Immunogenicity
Vasoconstrictive
Hypersensitivity

Physician Related

Dosing
Monitoring
Duration
Mixing

↓, decreased; ↑, increased.

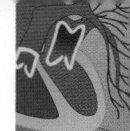

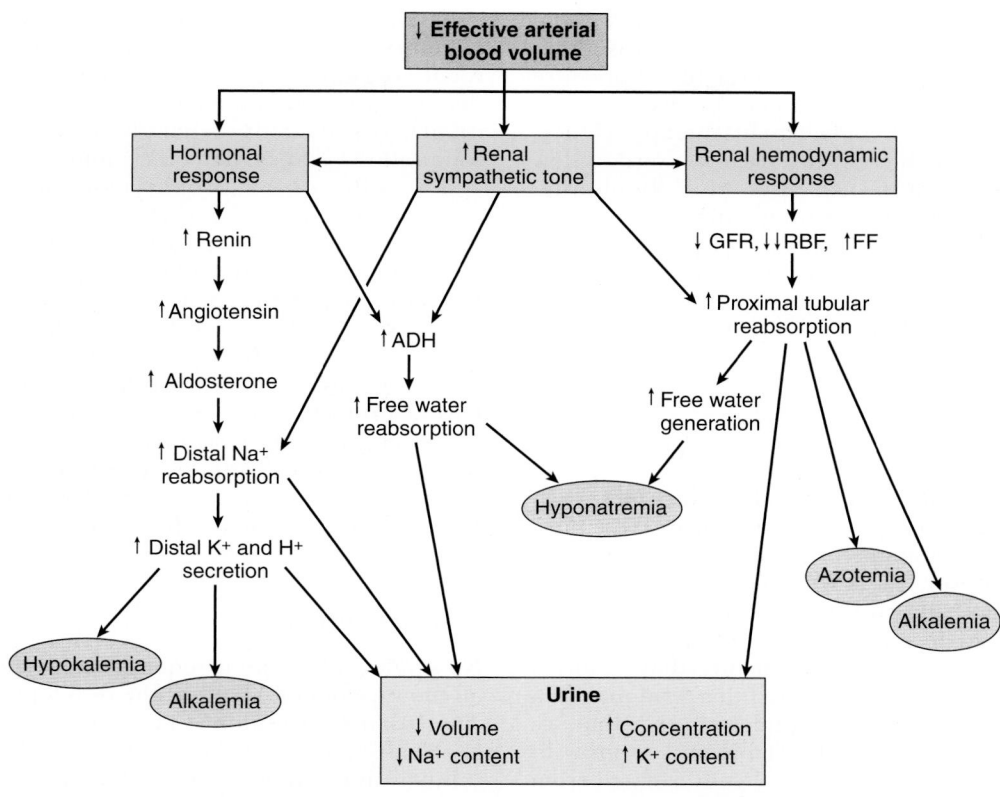

FIGURE 12A-4 Pathogenetic pathways implicated in prerenal failure. The arrows reflect the directional changes in the parameters depicted. The legends enclosed in the ovals indicate the changes in the blood chemistries that might be expected. ADH, antidiuretic hormone; FF, filtration fraction; GFR, glomerular filtration rat; RBF, renal blood flow.

(see Fig. 12A-3). Most notable among these are diuretics, whose injudicious and nondiscriminating use accounts for most cases of ARF in the hospital setting.[27,28] A second and common cause is nonsteroidal inflammatory drugs (NSAIDs).[28,29] By inhibiting cyclooxygenase, the principal enzyme in prostaglandin synthesis, NSAIDs deprive the kidneys of the protective vasodilatory prostaglandins and thereby aggravate any existing vasoconstriction and initiate a hemodynamically mediated ARF. This is usually a mild and reversible effect but on occasion results in severe oliguric ARF requiring renal replacement therapy.[29] Patients with preexisting ineffective ECFV and decreased renal perfusion (congestive cardiomyopathy, cirrhosis, sepsis, or diuretic therapy) or those with preexisting renal disease (nephrotic syndrome, chronic renal failure) are at risk for NSAID-induced ARF. A third group of drugs that inhibit the protective effect of efferent arteriolar vasoconstriction on maintaining GFR in the presence of reduced renal perfusion are the angiotensin-converting enzyme (ACE) inhibitors. The vasodilatory effect of these agents on the afferent arteriole is potentially salutary but essentially modest; by contrast, their effect on the postcapillary efferent arterioles is greater and results in a sudden decline in the glomerular intracapillary hydrostatic pressure (P_{GC}) necessary for filtration. Unless blood flow (Qa) to the kidneys is increased by the afferent dilatation, the result is a sudden reduction in GFR. As is

the case with NSAIDs, the renal effects of ACE inhibition are usually modest and reversible but on occasion result in severe oliguric ATN necessitating renal replacement therapy.[30] The detrimental effect of ACE inhibitors is most evident in patients who have severe congestive cardiomyopathy, renal artery stenosis, or reduced ECFV; they are unable to compensate for the loss of P_{GC} by increasing Qa. Given the role of diuretics in causing ECFV depletion, it is not unexpected that most cases of ACE inhibitor–induced ARF observed clinically are in patients who have severe congestive cardiomyopathy and who are diuresed aggressively. The combined nephrotoxic effect of NSAIDs and diuretics is associated with a several-fold increase in the development of ARF.[31] Additionally, the use or abuse of medications and dietary or herbal supplements or drugs that either directly or indirectly lead to increased sympathetic tone, agitation, or muscle activity and heat production can lead to rhabdomyolysis and ARF.[32]

Notable among the causes of prerenal ARF are those due to antihypertensive agents, which, even in the absence of decreased ECFV, induce a reduction in renal perfusion pressure that can result in ARF. Not unexpectedly, this is most evident in individuals who have accelerated or malignant hypertension and in whom the endothelial swelling caused by the preexisting severe hypertension results in a narrowed lumen with a high renal vascular resistance that requires high pressure

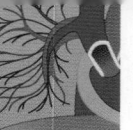

levels to perfuse the narrowed and constricted renal vasculature.[33] It is in these individuals that the sudden and severe reduction in the mean arterial blood pressure (>25 mm Hg) can result in the onset of progressive ARF, often necessitating renal replacement therapy. Hence, gradual titration of the blood pressure downward in slow increments is important in such cases, while monitoring renal function and maintaining adequate ECFV. Although the inducement of renal hypoperfusion may induce ARF, calcium channel blockers have been shown to protect against acute renal injury at both the vascular and tubular epithelial level in both ARF and chronic renal failure.[34]

RENAL FAILURE

The broad definition of renal failure includes such diverse entities as acute glomerulonephritis, vasculitis, thrombotic microangiopathy, and papillary necrosis (see Box 12A-1). However, the vast majority of ARF cases encountered clinically are most commonly due to ischemia, nephrotoxic agents, or a combination of both (see Fig. 12A-1).[24,35] The ultimate picture that results is that of ATN, although strictly defined this term may be a misnomer because the apparently necrotic cells that are excreted have been shown to be viable and to grow in vitro in cultures of tubular epithelial cells isolated from the urine.[36] Their shedding into the urine is one of the consequences of cell injury, rather than actual necrosis, which in addition to the loss of their polarity sustain a loss of cell wall integrins and a decomposition of their attachment to the basement membrane and to each other. This accounts for the loss of their anchorage and ultimate shedding into the urine.[1,25,37] In addition to microscopic examination of the urine for tubular epithelial cells that are shed, analysis of the urine is extremely valuable in the diagnosis (see Figs. 12A-2 and 12A-4), showing a characteristically high sodium (>50 mEq/L, fractional sodium excretion > 1%) and literally isosmotic concentration (320 to 350 mOsm/kg of water).

Should the patient survive, in the absolute majority of cases regeneration of tubular cells sets in and restores renal function. The regenerative and repair process of the injured tubules is an early event that is activated at the very start of injury, culminates during the ensuing days, and results in the ultimate restoration of normal renal structure and function.[38,39] The clinical course that ATN follows has been divided into four phases that correspond to the various phases of epithelial cell injury, necrosis, and regeneration. They are of variable duration and have considerable overlap.

Initial Phase

The initial phase is the period of ischemia or exposure to the nephrotoxic agent; it continues until oliguria develops (see Fig. 12A-2). The importance of identifying this phase stems from the fact that it represents a potentially reversible stage. Its length varies and depends largely on the causative agent (may last 5 to 7 days). In

general, an abnormal sediment (cylindruria), tubular proteinuria (β₂-microglobulins), lysozymuria, and a renal concentrating defect precede by several days any decrease in GFR caused by nephrotoxic agents. Other tubular dysfunctions (renal glycosuria, tubular acidosis, sodium loss) may be detectable and should be sought.

The efficacy of prophylactic measures that on occasion are effective during this phase (mannitol, loop diuretics, dopamine) relates to their ability to increase renal blood flow and solute excretion. These measures may also have the capacity to convert oliguric to nonoliguric renal failure (see Fig. 12A-2 and Table 12A-1). As a rule, their efficacy in preventing ARF clinically is questionable.[24] On the other hand, prostaglandins have a protective role in the renal autoregulation that is associated with vasoconstricting insults. Inhibitors of prostaglandin synthesis (NSAIDs) or inhibitors of efferent constriction (ACE inhibitors), used during this phase, can accentuate the ischemia and precipitate oliguria.[28-30,40]

Oliguric Phase

No single pathogenetic sequence appears to account for all the varieties of ATN and the development of oliguria. The balance of evidence favors the view that excessive backleak across the damaged tubular epithelium and tubular obstruction by the sloughed cells are important. Changes in glomerular permeability and filtration rate also appear to be contributing mechanisms.[1,25] The degree of involvement of any of these potential pathogenetic mechanisms varies and depends on the nature, severity, and duration of the initial nephrotoxic insult.

Oliguria is present in 60% to 70% of cases encountered clinically; another 30% to 40% are diagnosed earlier and are associated with a nonoliguric ARF (see Fig. 12A-2 and Table 12A-1). The average duration of the oliguria is 1 to 2 weeks, and daily urine volume averages 150 mL. Anuria (urine output <50 to 75 mL/day) is uncommon. If oliguria continues for longer than 4 weeks, more likely diagnostic entities to rule out are cortical necrosis, acute glomerulonephritis, and vasculitis. The duration of oliguria is of some prognostic significance, with a longer duration portending a greater likelihood of complications and undesirable outcomes.

Diuretic Phase

The diuretic phase begins when the 24-hour urine volume exceeds 500 mL/day. Classically, at the onset of this phase, urine volume doubles on successive days until a volume of 2000 to 3000 mL is reached. This phase lasts from 7 to 14 days. With the onset of diuresis, the renal blood flow and GFR gradually increase. The urine is at first isosmotic and literally appears to be pure plasma filtrate. As the regenerating tubular cells recover some ability to reabsorb sodium and concentrate urea, the urine gradually contains less sodium and more urea than plasma. Thus, blood chemistry values do not begin to correct with the onset of the diuretic phase, and days may pass before these values begin to normalize. As

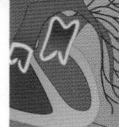

diuresis continues, however, the azotemia gradually diminishes. Factors contributing to the diuresis observed in this phase include (1) osmotic diuresis resulting from mobilization of the urea accumulated during the oliguric phase, (2) functional inadequacy of the regenerating tubular cells to reabsorb the glomerular filtrate and concentrate the urine, and (3) pushing intravenous fluids, because overzealous replacement of urine output maintains a patient in a continuous state of volume expansion. Thus, one ends up "chasing" the urine output by infusing gradually larger volumes of fluid.[25,41]

Although apparently similar to nonoliguric ARF, the diuretic phase of ATN is a totally different entity in that unlike the increasing BUN and Cr of the former, the BUN and Cr levels gradually decline during the diuretic phase. Although the decrement is modest during the first few days, it gradually increases in pace as cellular function matures and the GFR is restored. It is important to remember that many drugs are still poorly excreted during the diuretic phase, and dosage adjustments may be necessary if further drug toxicity is to be avoided.

Convalescent Phase

BUN and Cr levels are usually normal within 5 to 60 days after the onset of the diuretic phase. GFR, however, increases more slowly and may be 70% to 80% of normal within months. The ability to elaborate a maximally concentrated urine will return but may take several months. The principal renal symptoms during this phase are nocturia and polyuria, which gradually subside as the ability to concentrate urine improves. As a rule, there is no convincing evidence of progressive renal disease in recovered patients.

Although urinary tract infection is common during the oliguric phase because of prior urethral catheterization, evidence of persistent chronic infection is rare.

TOXIC ACUTE TUBULAR NECROSIS

The principal agents associated with toxic ATN are listed in Box 12A-4. The exact incidence of nephrotoxicity for

BOX 12A-4	AGENTS ASSOCIATED WITH TOXIC ACUTE TUBULAR NECROSIS

Antibiotics: Aminoglycosides, cephalosporin, amphotericin, vancomycin, pentamidine, sulfas, acyclovir, foscarnet, penicillin, tetracycline
Antineoplastic agents
   Alkylating agents: Cisplatin, carboplatin, ifosfamide
   Antimetabolites: Methotrexate, ara-C, 5-fluorouracil, 5-azacitidine, 6-thioguanine
Metals: Mercury, bismuth, cadmium, chromium, lead, gold, platinum, uranium, lithium
Organic solvents: Ethylene glycol, diethylene glycol, carbon tetrachloride
Miscellaneous: Radiocontrast agents, heroin, phencyclidine, cocaine, mannitol

any of these agents is not known, but the sequence in which they are listed parallels that with which they are encountered.[23,24,28,33,42,43]

Antibiotics

Aminoglycosides are among the most widely prescribed antibiotics. Nephrotoxicity develops in 10% to 15% of persons who use these drugs and depends on the total dose, the duration of treatment, and the frequency of administration. These highly water-soluble agents are freely filtered and absorbed in the proximal tubule. It is their accumulation within the epithelial cells that accounts for their nephrotoxicity. The variations in degree of nephrotoxicity observed remain unexplained but have been attributed to a number of risk factors, such as age, gender, reduced renal function, volume depletion, potassium and magnesium depletion, and hepatic failure. As a rule, toxicity results in nonoliguric ARF, with recovery from mild renal failure if the drug is discontinued, but it can lead to oliguric ARF if the insult remains undetected and drug administration is continued. The role of monitoring drug levels to predict nephrotoxicity is equivocal because the antibiotic levels actually increase when nephrotoxicity is already established.[42,44,45]

The increased availability of cephalosporins has been associated with an increasing incidence of reported cases of ARF, some of which are due to their nephrotoxic effect, particularly evident with use of cephaloridine, whereas others are a result of a hypersensitivity reaction and are due to acute interstitial nephritis.[46]

The vast number of antibiotics used in the treatment of human immunodeficiency virus (HIV)-infected patients renders this group of patients particularly susceptible to toxic ATN.[47,48] Incriminated agents include pentamidine, foscarnet, amphotericin, acyclovir, and sulfas. Approximately one third of patients receiving pentamidine and two thirds of those receiving foscarnet have clinical evidence of ARF due to tubular injury. By contrast, the sulfas and acyclovir exert their detrimental effect by intratubular precipitation, and amphotericin exerts its detrimental effect by complexing with the plasma membrane and increasing the cellular aqueous pores (see Fig. 12A-3). The latter accounts for the early polyuria and distal renal tubular acidosis, which with continued therapy result in a dose-dependent toxic ATN.[24,33,42]

Antineoplastic Agents

The nephrotoxicity associated with antimetabolites is generally cumulative and chronic, although acute injury can result in the presence of severe volume compromise, excessive dosing, and multiple-drug use.[49] Cancer is the underlying disease in as many as one fifth of cases of ARF in some series, not because of the nephrotoxic effect of antimetabolites alone but rather because of the antimicrobials and analgesics used in their management. Yet another cause of ARF is that of acute massive tumor tissue necrosis, particularly in lymphoproliferative

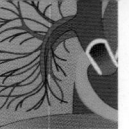

disorders, with resultant acute urate nephropathy, a potentially preventable lesion with adequate hydration, alkalization of the urine, and inhibition of uric acid synthesis with prophylactic allopurinol.[49-51] Thrombotic microangiopathy is a rare cause of ARF that has been associated with mithramycin, cyclosporine, and 5-fluorouracil therapy.[52,53]

Heavy Metals

Exposure to heavy metals is usually chronic in nature and results in various renal abnormalities that are primarily tubular in nature, ranging from proximal tubular dysfunction to oliguric ARF and chronic tubulointerstitial nephritis. Of the metals listed in Box 12A-4, mercuric chloride is the one that is most typically associated with toxic ATN, but this cause of toxicity has literally vanished. Uranium also gives rise to a toxic ATN that closely resembles that of mercuric chloride nephrotoxicity. A similar picture has been reported after excessive doses of bismuth and chromium.[13,24] Lead exposure, such as lead stabilizers used plastics manufacturing, may lead to reversible azotemia or chronic toxicity,[54] and chronic environmental lead exposure, even at low levels, is associated with progressively impaired renal function.[55]

Organic Solvents

Cases of accidental ingestion or attempted suicide with the antifreeze solution ethylene glycol are not rare. Oxalate, one of the metabolites of ethylene glycol, accounts for much of its nephrotoxicity owing to the intratubular precipitation of cytotoxic calcium oxalate monohydrate crystals that readily form in the presence of calcium (see Fig. 12A-3).[56] Diethylene glycol, an organic chemical solvent, causes tubular necrosis and recently was the cause of an epidemic of toxic ATN in children in Haiti. Carbon tetrachloride, another industrial solvent, causes direct, dose-dependent renal and hepatic toxicity, which is much less commonly encountered nowadays.[13,24]

Biologic Agents

Animal venoms, including those from snakes and arthropods (particularly arachnids and hymenopterans), may cause both obstructive and toxic acute renal failure, in part due to hemolysis and rhabdomyolysis, resulting in the release of myoglobin and hemoglobin from myocytes and erythrocytes, respectively.[57,58] Additionally, some infectious diseases, such as those caused by *Brucella* species and malaria infection by *Plasmodium* species, may also cause hemolysis and rhabdomyolysis leading to ARF.[59,60] Myoglobin and hemoglobin dissociate into globin and hematin as well as free iron, iron complexes, and reactive oxygen species. Globin can precipitate in the renal tubules, causing obstructive nephropathy, while hematin causes direct damage to renal tubular cells, also known as pigment nephropathy. Oxygen radicals, iron, and hemoglobin itself may also play a role in the cytotoxicity due to venoms or other toxins or toxicants.[61]

Many botanical species and some fungus species are associated with acute renal failure. Botanical nephrotoxins are found in medicinal herbs, both identified and misidentified, and in common edible plants such as djenkol beans (*Pithecolobium lobatum*, Southeast Asia) and medicinal herbs such as root of impila (*Callilepis laureola*, South Africa) and *uña de gato*, or cat's claw (*Uncaria* species, South and Central America, Asia).[62-64] One of the most infamous cases of mistaken herbal medicine identification, poorly termed Chinese herbal nephropathy, occurred in Belgium in the 1990s. A weight reduction herbal preparation that was said to contain *Stephania tetrandra* and *Magnolia officinalis* actually contained at least one *Aristolochia* species herb that has been shown to be nephrotoxic and carcinogenic, and its ingestion resulted in an outbreak of rapidly progressive renal fibrosis among over 100 patients.[65]

Mushrooms of several genera are associated with renal failure that may be caused by volume depletion or renal cytotoxicity. Species of *Amanita*, *Galerina*, and *Lepiota* containing the cyclopeptide amatoxin can lead to acute renal failure. Ingestion of *Cortinarius* species containing the toxin orellanine can cause latent toxicity with an onset of symptoms that may be from 2 to 21 days. In cases of amatoxin or orellanine poisoning, renal pathology includes tubular necrosis prominent in the proximal tubules with interstitial edema and no glomerular changes. In severe *Cortinarius* cases, renal tubular necrosis develops that may result in death several weeks after the poisoning in up to 15% of cases. Acute renal failure occurs in 30% to 55% of patients who may go on to develop chronic renal insufficiency and who may end up requiring long-term hemodialysis or renal transplant. Recovery is likely for most patients within a month to several months in less severe cases.[66]

Amatoxin-containing species ingestion involves fulminant hepatic necrosis and carries a higher mortality rate. Whereas hemodialysis may be useful in severe mushroom-induced renal failure cases, plasmapheresis, hemofiltration, venovenous charcoal hemoperfusion, and hemodialysis have not been efficacious in treating cyclopeptide-induced hepatic failure.[67] Other Amanita species that do not contain amatoxin, *Amanita smithiana* (found in the Pacific Northwest), *Amanita proxima* (Europe), and *Amanita pseudoporphyria* Hongo (Japan), are also associated with delayed-onset acute renal failure that may be due to allenic norleucine by an unknown mechanism.[68] Venovenous charcoal hemoperfusion or hemodialysis may be useful in these cases.

OTHER FORMS OF PARENCHYMAL ACUTE RENAL FAILURE

Of the renal parenchymal forms of ARF, other than ATN, both acute interstitial nephritis (AIN) and acute glomerulonephritis can be a side effect of a number of drugs (see Fig. 12A-3). By far the more common of these two is that of AIN, which although first identified as being due to infection in the preantibiotic era is now

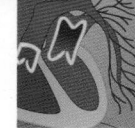

most commonly encountered with the very drugs used to treat infections.[46,69]

The principal drugs that have been associated with AIN are listed in Box 12A-5. Unlike toxic ATN, AIN is not dose dependent, develops in only some individuals, and is usually associated with the classic findings of a hypersensitivity reaction (fever, eosinophilia, elevated immunoglobulin E levels) that are often transient and on occasion with eosinophiluria. The impairment in renal function begins with discrete abnormalities of tubular function and progresses to ARF. The renal failure is nonoliguric in the early stages of the disease and is usually accompanied by findings of tubular dysfunction (renal glycosuria, hypouricemia, and β_2-microglobinuria due to their decreased tubular reabsorption). If renal failure is undetected and administration of the incriminated agent continues, oliguric ARF ensues and is severe enough to require renal replacement therapy. Renal failure is more common in the elderly and more severe in those who become oliguric. In most, the renal failure is reversible and its course can be shortened by brief use (2 to 4 weeks) of steroid therapy. In some (10% to 15%) of those with severe renal failure, irreversible renal failure may persist.

Among the agents that produce AIN, that due to NSAIDs is unique in that it generally presents with renal failure that is accompanied by the nephrotic syndrome.[70] Oxidative stress and mitochondrial dysfunction occur in the kidney in response to these drugs, and these effects may be mediated by free radicals and activation of phospholipases.[71] The onset after initiation of therapy with NSAIDs is usually longer than that observed with other agents and takes longer (months) to subside after discontinuation. In addition, no beneficial effect of steroids has been noted in cases of AIN due to NSAIDs.[29,46]

Iodinated radiocontrast agents are a cause of acute renal toxicity. The injury that results ranges from modest tubular dysfunction, which may remain undetected, to severe ARF with ATN, which may require renal replacement therapy. In patients who sustain renal injury, the ARF is generally nonoliguric and develops within 2 to 4 days of the procedure, although a sudden onset of oliguric ARF can ensue on occasion. Proposed mechanisms of radiocontrast-induced ARF include renal ischemia due to intrarenal vasoconstriction, particularly in the presence of volume depletion, tubular obstruction, and oxygen-free-radical-mediated direct tubular

toxicity induced by iodinated contrast. Of the several predisposing factors incriminated, that of decreased ECFV, reduced renal function (Cr > 2 mg/dL), diabetes mellitus, and total dose of radiocontrast agent injected are especially important. Adequate volume expansion with a brisk diuresis initiated before and maintained well after the procedure, coupled with use of N-acetylcysteine, and limitation of the dose of radiocontrast agents administered, is effective in circumventing the undesirable side effect of these agents.[72-74] N-acetylcysteine may provide tissue protection through its antioxidative effects and by increasing intracellular glutathione concentrations.[75-77]

Rhabdomyolysis consequent to the overuse of many drugs, including sedative hypnotics and opiates and opioids, can result in ARF. Myoglobinuria and hyperuricosuria, due to muscle injury, in a setting of severely compromised ECFV account for the ARF that develops. Prompt recognition, with restoration of intravascular volume and alkalization of urine, can prevent progression to oliguric ARF. A similar picture can occur after overdosage with sympathetic stimulating drugs, such as cocaine, amphetamines, and phencyclidine or therapeutic use of gemfibrozil, particularly when used in combination with statin drugs.[78,79]

Lithium can induce renal tubular acidosis resulting in polyuria, volume depletion, and water and electrolyte abnormalities. Severe lithium poisoning can lead to acute tubular necrosis and altered renal function, albuminuria, copper metabolism, and urinary enzyme abnormalities.[80]

Other less common forms of ARF are due to glomerular lesions that result from a vasculitis that has been reported in association with the use of allopurinol, hydralazine, procainamide, penicillin, and sulfas. The thrombotic microangiopathy associated with certain antineoplastic agents has been mentioned. Finally, membranous glomerulopathy has been noted with the use of gold, penicillamine, and captopril.[24,33,42]

TREATMENT

Renal replacement therapy has greatly simplified the management of ARF. Nevertheless, certain principles governing fluid and electrolyte management are important to monitor and correct in order to avoid the invasive nature of dialysis, when possible.[20,81]

Prerenal Failure

Prompt recognition of the manifestations of prerenal ARF is extremely important.[38,82] Prerenal ARF represents an early and reversible change in renal hemodynamics that if left uncorrected can lead to ATN. It is characterized by symptoms of peripheral circulatory failure (low blood pressure, rapid pulse, orthostatic hypotension, dry mucous membranes); urine that is low in volume, sodium content (<10 to 20 mEq/L), and fractional sodium excretion (<1%) but highly concentrated (urine osmolarity >500 mOsm/kg of water); and rising levels of BUN and Cr (see Figs. 12A-2 and 12A-4).

BOX 12A-5	PRINCIPAL AGENTS ASSOCIATED WITH ACUTE INTERSTITIAL NEPHRITIS

Antimicrobials
Penicillins, cephalosporins, sulfonamides, rifampin

Nonsteroidal Anti-inflammatory Drugs
Propionic acid derivatives, others

Miscellaneous
Phenindione, phenytoin, thiazide diuretics, allopurinol, cimetidine

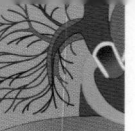

Apart from discontinuing drugs that aggravate the effects of decreased ECFV discussed previously (diuretics, antihypertensives, ACE inhibitors, NSAIDs), the principal effort should be directed at judiciously restoring ECFV.

If the diagnosis is in doubt in the presence of cardiac disease, direct measurement of pulmonary arterial wedge pressure may be indicated prior to initiating volume replacement. If no response to volume replacement therapy is evident, several therapies may be initiated, either alone or in combination, although each has potential risks and controversial benefits. Low-dose dopamine (0.5–2.0 µg/kg/min) has been advocated to enhance renal perfusion and diuresis. However, several clinical studies have shown questionable benefit and numerous potential deleterious multisystemic effects from dopamine therapy at even low doses despite the theoretical potential benefits in critically ill patients.[83,84] Therefore, it is recommended that it should be used in this manner only after critical care specialist consultation. Although administration of mannitol (12.5–25 g) or furosemide after volume replacement may induce diuresis, whether or not this effect is renoprotective is controversial, as is their use in conjunction with dopamine. The salutory effect of these pharmacologic maneuvers is, at best, transient and equivocal, particularly once oliguric ARF is established.[39] In fact, mannitol itself can induce ARF.[85] If there is no observed response to their initial administration, their continued use would be contraindicated. Again, it is advised that these therapies be used with caution and in consultation with critical care specialists.

Renal Failure

During the initial phase of ARF, efforts to restore intravascular volume outlined for prerenal ARF should be continued. Appropriate antibiotics for coexistent infection or sepsis should be initiated at the full loading dose, but any subsequent dosing should be modified for a GFR of less than 20 mL/min until this usually reversible phase is actually reversed or its progression to oliguric ARF is ruled out. The use of potentially aggravating and nephrotoxic agents (NSAIDs, ACE inhibitors, antihypertensives, diuretics) should be avoided and the use of radiocontrast agents minimized and restricted to those that are absolutely essential for a definitive diagnosis.

During the oliguric phase of ARF, in well-managed cases without serious complications, the BUN level rises 10 to 20 mg/dL per day and Cr level 0.5 to 1 mg/dL per day. In hypercatabolic patients (trauma, rhabdomyolysis), Cr concentration may increase by more than 2 mg/dL per day. In patients without complications, plasma potassium values can increase by 0.5 mEq/L per day; in catabolic states, it may increase by as much as 1 to 2 mEq/L in hours. Weight losses of 0.2 to 0.5 kg/day are expected because of catabolism; in complicated hypercatabolic states, weight loss may be 1 kg/day. Hypocalcemia (6 to 8 mg/dL) is common, reflecting hypoalbuminemia, hyperphosphatemia, and skeletal resistance to parathyroid hormone.

Water replacement should be restricted to a volume equivalent to urine volume plus extrarenal losses (gastric suction, diarrhea, wound drainage). Insensible losses (800 mL/day) should be restored by 400 to 500 mL of fluid only, because endogenous water production is 300 to 400 mL/day. Water requirements increase in the presence of high ambient temperature, fever, and low relative humidity. Adequate fluid replacement can best be monitored by the following:

1. Daily weight measurement. ARF is a catabolic state, and a daily weight loss of 0.5 kg or 1 pound should be expected. Any weight gain can represent only excess fluid administration.
2. Measuring serum sodium concentration. An increase in serum sodium level (>145 mEq/L) would indicate insufficient water replacement, whereas a decline in serum sodium level (<135 mEq/L) would reflect excess water replacement.

The administration of *sodium chloride* should be restricted once the initial volume replacement during the prerenal ARF or the initial phase of ARF has been accomplished. The guiding principles of sodium chloride replacement are as follows:

1. Body weight losses in excess of 300 g/day in the presence of a normal serum sodium level should be replaced, 1 mL of isotonic saline for each gram of weight loss.
2. Gastrointestinal losses, wound drainage, and estimated sequestered fluid require replacement with isotonic sodium chloride.
3. If acidosis develops, salt losses should be replaced with sodium bicarbonate. Available forms of sodium bicarbonate are concentrated (7.5% $NaHCO_3$) and hypertonic (890 mOsm). They must not be administered as a bolus or added to isotonic saline solution. They should be restored to isotonicity in glucose or half normal saline solution.

Potassium intake must be restricted. Small deficits need not be replaced. Hypokalemia, unless severe (<3 mEq/L), should not be corrected. Hyperkalemia, if present, can be best treated with correction of acidosis and with sodium polystyrene sulfonate ion exchange resin (Kayexalate, Sanofi-Aventis, Bridgewater, NJ; Kionex, Paddock Labs, Minneapolis, MN; Marlexate, Marlex Pharmaceuticals, Inc., Newcastle, DE). The exchange resins are most effective when used as retention enemas. Hyperkalemia is always an indication to consider dialysis.

Caloric requirements (30 kcal/kg body weight per day) must be met to avoid increased catabolism. In the presence of sepsis, surgery, or burns, the usual caloric requirements are increased by as much as 50%. Caloric intake can be given as glucose (20% to 70%) and fat emulsions (10% to 20%). Any protein given should consist of high-biologic-value essential amino acids and should not exceed 0.5 g/kg of body weight per day.

The potential for upper gastrointestinal bleeding is high in ARF. H_2-receptor blocking agents should be used.

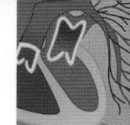

Antacids, if used, represent added loads of aluminum and calcium. The use of magnesium-containing antacids is contraindicated.

Dialysis should be started early and performed daily. Continuous renal replacement seems to have a distinct advantage in the dialysis management of these patients.[86] The dialysis bath should be adjusted to the level of serum potassium and should be bicarbonate based. Convincing evidence for the advantage of biocompatible membranes in ARF has been presented.[87] Dialyzers used should have a biocompatible membrane.

The onset of the diuretic phase requires continued vigilance. Dialysis must be continued through this phase until predialysis BUN levels begin to diminish well below 100 mg/dL and patients have no problems with elevated potassium levels. The serum sodium level must be monitored by measurements of body weight and sodium concentration as outlined for the oliguric phase. Although urinary losses must be replaced, pushing fluids must be avoided. This can best be accomplished by replacing urine output no more frequently than every 8 to 12 hours, depending on the previous urine volume, in order to avoid the continued overexpansion of ECFV that is often present. It is unusual for patients to have urine volumes greater than 3 to 4 L/day during this phase unless too much fluid is being administered. It is important to remember that renal function remains compromised, and many drugs are still poorly excreted during the diuretic phase. Dosage adjustment should remain in effect if drug toxicity is to be avoided.

REFERENCES

1. Thadhani R, Pascual M, Bonventre JV: Acute renal failure [see comment] [Review]. N Engl J Med 1996;334(22):1448–1460.
2. Eknoyan G: Emergence of the concept of acute renal failure. Am J Nephrol 2002;22(2–3):225–230.
3. Dickinson WH: On renal and urinary affections. New York, William Wood & Co, 1885.
4. Minami S: Uber Nierenveranderrungen nach Verschuttung. Virchows Arch Pathol Anat 1923;245:247.
5. Muir R, Dunn JS: War nephritis. In: History of the Great War: Medical Services: Pathology. London, His Majesty's Stationery Office, 1923, pp 541–565.
6. Husfeldt E, Bjering T: Renal lesions for traumatic shock. Acta Med Scand 1937;91:279.
7. Haas G: Uber Versuche der Blutauswaschung am Lebenden mit Hilfe der Dialyse. Arch Exp Pathol Pharmakol 1926;116:158–172.
8. Bywaters EGL, Beall D: Crush injuries and renal function. BMJ 1941;1:427.
9. Settle EB, Pinkerton H, Corbett AJ: Pathologic study of Tsutsugamushi disease (scrub typhus) with notes on clinico-pathologic correlation. J Lab Clin Med 1945;30:639–661.
10. Yeomans A, Snyder JC, Murray ES, et al: Azotemia in typhus fever. Ann Intern Med 1945;23:711–753.
11. Van Slyke DD: The effects of shock on the kidney. Ann Intern Med 1948;28:701.
12. Kolff W, Berk H: The artificial kidney: a dialyser with a great area. Acta Med Scand 1944;117:121–134.
13. Schreiner GE, Maher JF: Toxic nephropathy. Am J Med 1965;38:409–449.
14. Swann RC, Merrill JP: The clinical course of acute renal failure. Medicine 1953;32(2):215–292.
15. Safirstein RL: Acute renal failure. In Greenberg A, Cheung AK Coffman TM, et al (eds): Primer on Kidney Diseases, 4th ed. Philadelphia, WB Saunders, 2005, pp 280–286.
16. Brezis M, Rosen S: Hypoxia of the renal medulla—its implications for disease [Review]. N Engl J Med 1995;332(10):647–655.
17. Bonventre J: Pathophysiology of ischemic acute renal failure. In Ronco C, Bellomo R, Brendolan A (eds): Sepsis, Kidney and Multiple Organ Dysfunction. Basel, Switzerland, Karger, 2004, pp 19–30.
18. Fish EM, Molitoris BA: Alterations in epithelial polarity and the pathogenesis of disease states [Review]. N Engl J Med 1994;330(22):1580–1588.
19. Perrone RD, Madias NE, Levey AS: Serum creatinine as an index of renal function: new insights into old concepts [see comment] [Review]. Clin Chem 1992;38(10):1933–1953.
20. Albright RC Jr: Acute renal failure: a practical update [Review]. Mayo Clin Proc 2001;76(1):67–74.
21. Perazella MA: Drug-induced renal failure: update on new medications and unique mechanisms of nephrotoxicity. Am J Med Sci 2003;325(6):349–362.
22. Biradar V, Urmila A, Renuka S, Pais P: Clinical spectrum of hospital acquired renal failure: a study from tertiary care hospital. Indian J Nephrol 2004;14:93–96.
23. Mathew TH: Drug-induced renal disease [Review]. Med J Aust 1992;156(10):724–728.
24. Swan SK, Bennett WM: Nephrotoxic acute renal failure. In Lazarus JM, Brenner B (eds): Nephrotoxic Acute Renal Failure. New York, Churchill Livingstone, 1993, pp 357–392.
25. Paller MS, Cheung AK, Coffman TM: Pathophysiology of acute renal failure. In National Kidney Foundation Primer on Kidney Diseases. San Diego, CA, Academic, 1994, pp 126–133.
26. Lameire N: The pathophysiology of acute renal failure. Crit Care Clin 2005;21(2):197–210.
27. Eknoyan G: Diagnosis of disturbances. In Seldin DW, Giebisch GH (eds): The Regulation of Sodium and Chloride Balance. New York, Raven, 1990, pp 237–259.
28. Davidman M, Olson P, Kohen J, et al: Iatrogenic renal disease. Arch Intern Med 1991;151(9):1809–1812.
29. Palmer BF, Henrich WL: Clinical acute renal failure with nonsteroidal anti-inflammatory drugs [Review]. Semin Nephrol 1995;15(3):214–227.
30. Toto RD, Mitchell HC, Lee HC, et al: Reversible renal insufficiency due to angiotensin converting enzyme inhibitors in hypertensive nephrosclerosis [see comment]. Ann Intern Med 1991;115(7):513–519.
31. Huerta C, Castellsague J, Varas-Lorenzo C, Garcia Rodríguez LA: Nonsteroidal anti-inflammatory drugs and risk of ARF in the general population. Am J Kidney Dis 2005;45(3):531–539.
32. Sandhu RS, Como JJ, Scalea TS, et al: Renal failure and exercise-induced rhabdomyolysis in patients taking performance-enhancing compounds. J Trauma 2002;53(4):761–764.
33. Garella S: Drug-induced renal disease: a clinical approach to its detection. AFK Nephrol Lett 1990;4:32.
34. Schrier RW, Burke TJ: Role of calcium-channel blockers in preventing acute and chronic renal injury. J Cardiovasc Pharmacol 1991;18(Suppl 6):38–43.
35. Esson ML, Schrier RW: Diagnosis and treatment of acute tubular necrosis [see comment] [Review]. Ann Intern Med 2002;137(9):744–752.
36. Racusen LC, Fivush BA, Li YL, et al: Dissociation of tubular cell detachment and tubular cell death in clinical and experimental "acute tubular necrosis." Lab Invest 1991;64(4):546–556.
37. Goligorsky MS, DiBona GF: Pathogenetic role of arg-gly-asp recognizing integrins in acute renal failure. Proc Natl Acad SCi U S A 1993;90:5700.
38. Humes HD: Recovery phase of acute renal failure: the cellular and molecular biology of regenerative repair. Kidney 1991;24:1.
39. Toback FG: Regeneration after acute tubular necrosis [Review]. Kidney Int 1992;41(1):226–246.
40. Whelton A: Nephrotoxicity of nonsteroidal anti-inflammatory drugs: physiologic foundations and clinical implications. Am J Med 1999;106(5B, Suppl):13–24.
41. Hutchinson FN: Management of acute renal failure. In Greenberg A, Cheung AK, Coffman TM, et al (eds): National Kidney Foundation Primer on Kidney Diseases. San Diego, CA, Academic, 1994, pp 157–162.
42. Cooper K, Bennett WM: Nephrotoxicity of common drugs used in clinical practice [Review]. Arch Intern Med 1987;147(7):1213–1218.

43. Gill N, Nally JV Jr, Fatica RA: Renal failure secondary to acute tubular necrosis: epidemiology, diagnosis, and management. Chest 2005;128(4):2847–2863.

44. Rougier F, Claude D, Maurin M, Maire P: Aminoglycoside nephrotoxicity. Curr Drug Targets Infect Disord 2004; 4(2):153–162.

45. Tune BM: Renal tubular transport and nephrotoxicity of betalactam antibiotics: structure-activity relationships. Miner Electrolyte Metab 1994;20:221.

46. Eknoyan G: Acute tubulointerstital nephritis. In Schrier RW, Gottschalk CW (eds): Diseases of the Kidney. Boston, Little, Brown, 1996, pp 1249–1272.

47. Berns JS, Cohen RM, Stumacher RJ, Rudnick MR: Renal aspects of therapy for human immunodeficiency virus and associated opportunistic infections [Review]. J Am Soc Nephrol 1991;1(9):1061–1080.

48. Rao TK, Friedman EA: Outcome of severe acute renal failure in patients with acquired immunodeficiency syndrome. Am J Kidney Dis 1995;25(3):390–398.

49. Cobos E, Hall RR: Effects of chemotherapy on the kidney [Review]. Semin Nephrol 1993;13(3):297–305.

50. Curry SC, Chang D, Connor D: Drug- and toxin-induced rhabdomyolysis [Review]. Ann Emerg Med 1989;18(10):1068–1084.

51. Simmonds HA, Cameron JS, Morris GS, Davies PM: Allopurinol in renal failure and the tumor lysis syndrome. Clin Chim Acta 1986;160:189–195.

52. Jackson AM, Rose BD, Graff LG, et al: Thrombotic microangiopathy and renal failure associated with antineoplastic chemotherapy. Ann Intern Med 1984;101(1):41–44.

53. Poch E, Gonzalez-Clemente JM, Torres A: Silent renal microangiopathy after mitomycin C therapy. Am J Nephrol 1990;10:514.

54. Coyle P, Kosnett MJ, Hipkins K: Severe lead poisoning in the plastics industry: a report of three cases. Am J Ind Med 2005;47(2):172–175.

55. Yu CC, Lin JL, Lin-Tan DT: Environmental exposure to lead and progression of chronic renal diseases: a four-year prospective longitudinal study. J Am Soc Nephrol 2004;15(4):1016–1022.

56. Guo C, McMartin KE: The cytotoxicity of oxalate, metabolite of ethylene glycol, is due to calcium oxalate monohydrate formation. Toxicology 2005;208(3):347–355.

57. Betten DP, Richardson WH, Tong TC, Clark RF: Massive honey bee envenomation-induced rhabdomyolysis in an adolescent. Pediatrics 2006;117(1):231–235.

58. Kamiguti AS, Theakston RD, Sherman N, Fox JW: Mass spectrophotometric evidence for P-III/P-IV metalloproteinases in the venom of the Boomslang (Dispholidus typus). Toxicon 2000; 38(11):1613–1620.

59. Reynaud F, Mallet L, Lyon A, Rodolfo JM: Rhabdomyolysis and acute renal failure in Plasmodium falciparum malaria. Nephrol Dial Transplant 2005;20(4):847.

60. Toprak O, Kaptan F, Cirit M, et al: Recurrent rhabdomyolysis and mild acute renal failure associated with acute Brucella infection. Nephrol Dial Transplant 2005;20(4):848–849.

61. Yoo YM, Kim KM, Kim SS, et al: Hemoglobin toxicity in experimental bacterial peritonitis is due to production of reactive oxygen species. Clin Diagn Lab Immunol 1999;6(6):938–945.

62. Hilepo JN, Bellucci AG, Mossey RT: Acute renal failure caused by "cat's claw" herbal remedy in a patient with systemic lupus erythematosus. Nephron 1997;77(3):361.

63. Jha V, Chugh KS: Nephropathy associated with animal, plant, and chemical toxins in the tropics. Semin Nephrol 2003;23(1):49–65.

64. Steenkamp V, Stewart MJ: Nephrotoxicity associated with exposure to plant toxins, with particular reference to Africa [Review]. Ther Drug Monit 2005;27(3):270–277.

65. Greensfelder L: Alternative medicine. Herbal product linked to cancer. Science 2000;288(5473):1946.

66. Berger KJ, Guss DA: Mycotoxins revisited: Part II. J Emerg Med 2005;28(2):175–183.

67. Diaz JH: Syndromic diagnosis and management of confirmed mushroom poisonings [Review]. Crit Care Med 2005;33(2): 427–436.

68. Iwafuchi Y, Morita T, Kobayashi H, et al: Delayed onset acute renal failure associated with Amanita pseudoporphyria Hongo ingestion. Intern Med 2003;42(1):78–81.

69. Markowitz GS, Perazella MA: Drug-induced renal failure: a focus on tubulointerstitial disease [Review]. Clin Chim Acta 2005; 351(1–2):31–47.

70. Gambaro G, Perazella MA: Adverse renal effects of anti-inflammatory agents: evaluation of selective and nonselective cyclooxygenase inhibitors [Review] [62 refs]. J Intern Med 2003;253(6):643–652.

71. Basivireddy J, Jacob M, Balasubramanian KA: Indomethacin induces free radical-mediated changes in renal brush border membranes. Arch Toxicol 2005;79(8):441–450.

72. Krinloosky FA, Simon N, Santhanam S: Acute renal failure: association with administration of radiographic contrast material. JAMA 1993;239:125.

73. Oudemans-van Straaten HM: Contrast nephropathy, pathophysiology and prevention. Int J Artif Organs 2004;27(12):1054–1065.

74. Porter GA: Contrast-associated nephropathy: presentation, pathophysiology and management. Miner Electrolyte Metab 1994;20:232.

75. Goldenberg I, Matetzky S: Nephropathy induced by contrast media: pathogenesis, risk factors and preventive strategies [Review]. Can Med Assoc J 2005;172(11):1461–1471.

76. Lin J, Bonventre JV: Prevention of radiocontrast nephropathy. Curr Opin Nephrol Hypertens 2005;14(2):105–110.

77. Liu R, Nair D, Ix J, et al: N-acetylcysteine for the prevention of contrast-induced nephropathy. A systematic review and meta-analysis. J Gen Intern Med 2005;20(2):193–200.

78. Roth D, Alarcon FJ, Fernandez JA, et al: Acute rhabdomyolysis associated with cocaine intoxication. N Engl J Med 1988; 319(11):673–677.

79. Layne RD, Sehbai AS, Stark LJ: Rhabdomyolysis and renal failure associated with gemfibrozil monotherapy. Ann Pharmacother 2004;38(2):232–234.

80. Chmielnicka J, Nasiadek M: The trace elements in response to lithium intoxication in renal failure. Ecotoxicol Environ Saf 2003;55(2):178–183.

81. Gambaro G, Bertaglia G, Puma G, D'Angelo A: Diuretics and dopamine for the prevention and treatment of acute renal failure: a critical reappraisal [Review]. J Nephrol 2002;15(3):213–219.

82. Better OS, Stein JH: Early management of shock and prophylaxis of acute renal failure in traumatic rhabdomyolysis [see comment] [Review]. N Engl J Med 1990;322(12):825–829.

83. Dorman HR, Sondheimer JH, Cadnapaphornchai P: Mannitol-induced acute renal failure [Review]. Medicine 1990;69(3): 153–159.

84. Mehta RL: Therapeutic alternatives to renal replacement for critically ill patients in acute renal failure [Review]. Semin Nephrol 1994;14(1):64–82.

85. Hakim RM, Wingard RL, Parker RA: Effect of the dialysis membrane in the treatment of patients with acute renal failure [see comment]. N Engl J Med 1994;331(20):1338–1342.

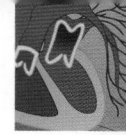

B | Chronic Renal Toxicity

MICHAEL W. SHANNON, MD, MPH

Chronic renal toxicity may be defined as a persistent and progressive functional and structural defect in the kidneys. This chapter addresses those drugs and toxins that cause renal injury over a period of months to years. Nephrotoxins that cause acute renal dysfunction are discussed in Chapter 12A; common causes of drug-induced acute renal failure are listed in Box 12A-1. Common causes of chronic renal toxicity are listed in Box 12B-1 and have been reviewed in recent articles.[1-3]

Chronic renal failure is commonly classified as prerenal, intrinsic, or postrenal, depending on the underlying pathophysiologic etiology.[4] Prerenal dysfunction is typically the result of renal hypoperfusion, produced by conditions including hypovolemia, low cardiac output, and renal vasoconstriction. Prolonged hypoperfusion can secondarily lead to intrinsic renal injury. Drugs and toxins can produce primary intrinsic injury, for example, by precipitating within renal cells or the tubular lumen. Postrenal dysfunction is commonly the result of obstruction (e.g., myoglobin precipitation) and rarely the primary result of drugs or toxins.

CLINICAL PRESENTATION

The diagnosis of chronic renal toxicity is based almost exclusively on a decrease in renal function. Unlike acute renal failure, in which urine output may abruptly decrease, chronic renal toxicity is by nature insidious and clinically difficult to recognize.

A decrease in renal function is determined by the measurement of serum creatinine concentration. Serum creatinine determination is most informative when considered in the context of total body muscle mass and gender. Serum creatinine is derived from the metabolism of creatinine in muscle and therefore reflects total muscle mass. Dietary meat intake also affects serum creatinine but to a lesser extent. Parenthetically, serum creatinine concentration can be artifactually elevated by acetone, cephalosporins, and other drugs when measured by the Jaffe reaction.[5-7] Moreover, drugs can increase serum creatinine concentration without alterations in overall renal function via other means; cimetidine can significantly reduce renal tubular secretion of creatinine, without alterations in glomerular filtration or other aspects of renal function.[7]

Creatinine is eliminated from the body predominantly by glomerular filtration, with a small contribution from renal secretion. Cockcroft and Gault first proposed an empirical formula that uses serum creatinine value (in mg/dL) to assess glomerular filtration rate (GFR) (Equation 12B-1):

Creatinine clearance = $(140 - \text{age}) \times \text{Weight in kg}/72 \times \text{Scr}$

Their formula is as accurate a determinant of GFR as the more arduous procedure of 24-hour urine collection for creatinine clearance determination.[1,4,8] Note that this equation for predicting GFR includes a term for age, representing age-associated changes in renal function. For women, the result is multiplied by 0.85. GFR decreases by approximately 1 mL/min per year after the age of 40 years. However, the serum creatinine value does not concomitantly increase with age because of the almost equivalent decrease in muscle mass. Using the Cockcroft-Gault equation yields a more accurate

---

BOX 12B-1   COMMON CAUSES OF CHRONIC RENAL FAILURE

Nontoxicologic
Chronic interstitial nephritis
    Metabolic (hypercalcemia, hypokalemia)
    Hematologic/oncologic (multiple myeloma)
Diabetic nephropathy
Glomerulonephritis
Hereditary renal disease (polycystic kidney disease)
Hypertensive nephrosclerosis
Ischemic nephropathy
Obstructive, reflux nephropathy

Toxicologic
Analgesics
Angiotensin-converting enzyme (ACE) inhibitors
Angiotensin II receptor blockers

Antimicrobials
    Acyclovir
    Cedofivir

Immunosuppressives
    Cyclosporine
    Tacrolimus (FK-506)

Lithium

Chemotherapeutic agents
    Cisplatinim
    Carboplatin
    Chloroethylnitrosoureas
    Metotrexate
    Interferon-α

Drugs of abuse
    Heroin
    Cocaine

Environmental and occupational toxins
    Lead
    Cadmium
    Mercury
    Tobacco smoke

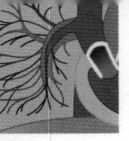

estimate of renal function than does serum creatinine determination. Some form of renal disease should therefore be suspected when the GFR is less than the age-appropriate value.

The differential diagnosis of chronic renal failure is extensive (see Box 12B-1). The four most common causes of chronic progressive renal disease are diabetes mellitus, hypertension, glomerulonephritis, and polycystic kidney disease. Therefore, chronic renal disease due to drugs and environmental toxins represents a small subset of the large population of such patients. Patients with chronic renal toxicity generally have the histologic lesion of chronic interstitial nephritis, a description that is also useful as a disease category. Compared with patients having other categories of chronic renal failure, those with chronic interstitial nephritis tend to have low-grade proteinuria (<1.5 g per 24 hours), urinary sediment with few cells or casts, infrequent or mild hypertension, preserved or increased urine volume with a tendency toward sodium wasting, elevated uric acid level, hyperchloremic metabolic acidosis, and anemia disproportionately severe for the degree of renal failure. These abnormalities are a consequence of injury to renal epithelial cells throughout the nephron.

Proximal tubule cells reabsorb filtered sodium, chloride, bicarbonate, glucose, calcium, phosphate, amino acids, and low-molecular-weight proteins, and secrete organic anions. Proximal epithelial cell injury

can therefore result in impaired reabsorption (increased urinary excretion) of these substances. Fanconi's syndrome is the clinical term for defective proximal tubule dysfunction resulting in urinary loss of these substances. Distal tubule epithelial cells secrete hydrogen ions and potassium. Injury to these cells may lead to metabolic acidosis and hyperkalemia. Collecting tubule epithelial cells are responsible for concentrating the urine by water reabsorption. Injury of these cells produces nephrogenic diabetes insipidus, which in minor form may be manifested simply as an increase in urine volume and urinary frequency.

Epithelial cell injury also leads to the appearance in urine of proteins that are normal cellular constituents, mainly brush border membrane and lysosomal proteins. Alanine aminopeptidase, alkaline phosphatase, γ-glutamyl transpeptidase, N-acetylglucosaminidase, and β-galactosidase may appear; these have been proposed as markers for identifying early or mild renal injury before the occurrence of a detectable reduction in GFR.

A CLINICAL APPROACH TO PATIENTS WITH CHRONIC RENAL FAILURE

A useful guideline for the clinical approach to patients with increased serum creatinine concentration (or a decrease in GFR) is shown in Figure 12B-1. The presence

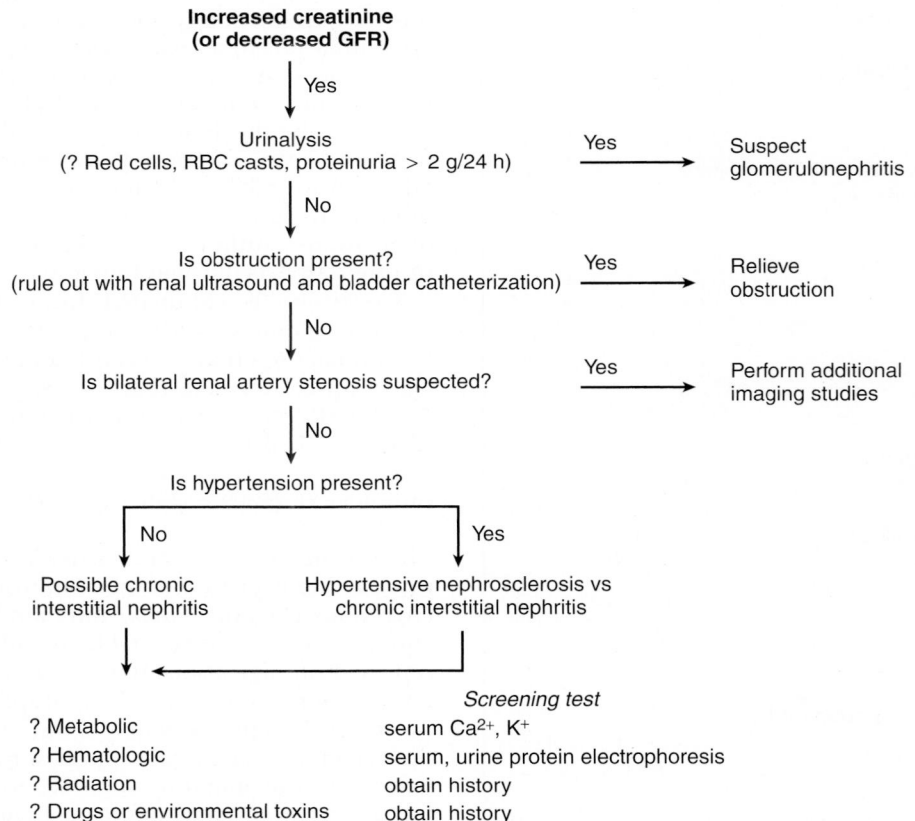

FIGURE 12B-1 Approach to the patient with chronically decreased renal function. GFR, glomerular filtration rate; RBC, red blood cell.

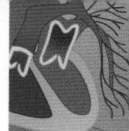

of numerous red blood cells or red blood cell casts should lead one to suspect glomerulonephritis. Similarly, urinary protein in excess of 2 g per 24 hr is more characteristic of glomerular disease than chronic interstitial disease. The possibility that the renal disease is caused by multiple myeloma or another monoclonal gammopathy can be ruled out by serum and urine protein electrophoresis and immunofixation. If a patient has an unremarkable urinalysis result, the possibility of obstruction should be ruled out with bladder catheterization and renal ultrasonography. In patients with diffuse atherosclerosis or risk factors for atherosclerosis, the possibility of bilateral renal artery stenosis should be considered. Metabolic factors should be considered when chronic interstitial nephritis is diagnosed. At a minimum, the serum potassium and calcium levels should be measured.

Investigation for toxicologic causes of chronic interstitial nephritis should be initiated first by careful history taking of drug ingestion (prescription, over-the-counter drugs, and alternative remedies[9]; see Box 12B-1), and assessment for environmental exposure, including occupational and nonoccupational exposures. In many cases of chronic renal toxicity, it is not possible to firmly establish a toxicologic origin, although the circumstantial evidence may be very convincing.

No unique pathophysiologic process is responsible for the development of chronic renal toxicity. Therefore, disease-specific descriptions are most informative.

THERAPEUTIC AGENTS

Nonsteroidal Anti-Inflammatory Agents

EPIDEMIOLOGY

Nonsteroidal anti-inflammatory drugs (NSAIDs) have long been suspected to be a cause of chronic renal disease.[9-12] The full impact of NSAIDs on renal function is unknown because it is typically difficult to accurately measure their use over long periods.[9] Most studies have suggested that a cumulative intake of more than 1 to 3 kg of an NSAID is required to produce chronic renal disease. Therefore, clinical disease would not be recognized until a patient had consumed large daily doses of NSAIDs for several years. Conservative estimates are that between 1% and 3% of patients with end-stage renal disease in the United States have "analgesic" nephropathy. Throughout the world, a striking variation is noted in the incidence of analgesic nephropathy, with areas of greater frequency being found in Belgium, Australia, Scotland, and Switzerland.[9,12]

NSAIDs are commonly divided into conventional agents (e.g., aspirin, acetaminophen, naproxen, and ibuprofen) and cyclooxygenase-2 (COX-2) inhibitors. All NSAIDs inhibit cyclooxygenase. However, conventional NSAIDs possess the theoretical disadvantage of inhibiting both COX-1 and COX-2. COX-1 is generally associated with the production of prostaglandins responsible for beneficial, homeostatic body functions; for example, COX-1 appears to play a key role in maintenance of the

integrity of the gastric mucosa. In contrast, COX-2 produces the prostaglandins that most directly mediate inflammation. NSAIDs and COX-2 inhibitors both markedly decrease production of renal prostaglandin E_2 (PGE_2). PGE_2 has a number of functions, including dilation of the renal bed. Inhibition of PGE_2 is associated with reductions in renal blood flow, along with other adverse effects. Consequently, conditions associated with decreased circulating volume (e.g., congenital heart failure and cirrhosis) can further compromise renal blood flow, placing patients at greater risk for developing NSAID- or COX-2-associated renal failure. COX-2 inhibitors are significantly less likely than NSAIDs to produce renal injury. Moreover, some NSAIDs (e.g., sulindac) are less nephrotoxic than other NSAIDs, presumably because they have less effect on PGE_2 and PGI_2.

Phenacetin was the earliest recognized nephrotoxic NSAID. Because of its association with renal disease, it is no longer marketed. Phenacetin was linked not only to the development of renal disease but also to hypertension, cardiovascular disease, and cancer. In a 20-year prospective study of women who were identified as regular users of phenacetin, the relative risk for death due to urologic or renal disease was 16.1.[13]

Acetaminophen, the major metabolite of phenacetin, is another NSAID associated with the development of chronic interstitial nephritis and renal failure. In a case-control study of subjects hospitalized with a new diagnosis of chronic renal disease, the odds ratio of end-stage renal disease was 3.21 when daily users of acetaminophen were compared with infrequent users.[14] Another case-control study using a similar experimental design found the odds ratio of end-stage renal disease to be 2.1 for subjects who took 366 or more acetaminophen pills for a year, compared with those who consumed fewer than 104 pills per year.[15] This study further estimated that between 8% and 10% of all cases of end-stage renal disease were attributable to acetaminophen use.

PATHOPHYSIOLOGY

NSAIDs can produce chronic interstitial nephritis and papillary necrosis. Although nephritis typically resolves after discontinuation of NSAID use, it occasionally becomes chronic. The precise mechanism of analgesic injury is unclear but probably includes effects produced by the analgesic's toxic metabolite. Acetaminophen accumulates in the renal medulla and papilla, where it is further metabolized by conjugation or oxidation.[9,12] Conjugation is the usual mechanism of metabolism, although under toxicologic conditions oxidation predominates. Acetaminophen oxidation is catalyzed by cytochrome P-450 and results in generation of the free radical intermediate N-acetyl-p-benzoquinone imine. Acetaminophen can also be deacetylated to yield p-aminophenol, which is then oxidized by cytochrome P-450 to p-benzoquinone imine. Glutathione preferentially reacts with these metabolites to protect intrinsic renal macromolecules. When renal glutathione is depleted, renal injury occurs. This proposed mechanism is similar to the mechanism proposed for acetaminophen-induced liver injury.

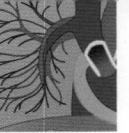

NSAIDs can also produce important electrolyte disturbances. For example, because NSAIDs both inhibit renin secretion and compete with aldosterone for binding sites, hyperkalemia can occur in those who chronically use NSAIDs. This effect can become life threatening in the elderly or those with preexisting chronic renal disease.

CLINICAL PRESENTATION

Analgesic nephropathy occurs more frequently in women than men. The prototypical patient is one who has suffered chronically from headache or low back pain. Some of these patients also have chronic gastrointestinal symptoms caused by chronic use of NSAIDs. The majority of patients have consumed a mixture of analgesic agents rather than drugs of a single category.

An early sign of analgesic-produced renal insufficiency is impaired renal concentrating ability; patients may also have sterile pyuria. During episodes of papillary necrosis, patients can have flank pain, pyuria, and hematuria. Acute ureteral obstruction may result, and necrotic papillary tissue is often passed in the urine. Intravenous pyelography reveals the characteristic ring sign, which is actually contrast agent surrounding the sloughed papilla. Renal ultrasonography reveals small, irregularly contoured kidneys with irregular thinning of the renal cortex. Past papillary necrosis produces triangular papillary calcifications.[16] The presence of papillary calcification on computed tomography is probably the most sensitive indicator of analgesic nephropathy (Fig. 12B-2).[17] On renal biopsy, the kidneys have interstitial infiltrates and fibrosis.

Long-term use of analgesics also increases the risk for developing transitional cell carcinoma of the urinary collecting system and bladder.[18,19] This risk may continue even after cessation of analgesic use. Therefore, hematuria that develops in a patient with a history of chronic analgesic abuse should prompt a thorough search for bladder and collecting system tumors.

OUTCOME AND TREATMENT

The natural history of analgesic nephropathy is often the development of end-stage renal disease. Renal function may stabilize in patients who discontinue analgesic use or switch to a nontoxic drug, even when they already have substantial renal impairment. Once chronic renal insufficiency has developed as a result of analgesic use, any additional NSAID, even one unlikely to cause chronic interstitial nephritis (e.g., aspirin) may impair renal function.

Antimicrobials

Several antimicrobials, particularly antibiotics and antivirals, are associated with both acute and chronic renal injury (see Box 12B-1). What many of these agents have in common is the ability to produce "crystal nephropathy."[9,11] The most common members of this group include acyclovir, sulfadiazine, and indinavir. Volume contraction is an important contributor to the development of crystal nephropathy, making conditions such as diarrhea, nausea/vomiting, ascites, or heart failure high-risk preexisting conditions when these drugs are administered. Specific agents are discussed earlier in this chapter.

IMMUNOSUPPRESSIVES

Cyclosporine

EPIDEMIOLOGY

With the widespread use of cyclosporine as an immunosuppressant agent in solid organ transplantation, bone marrow transplantation, and immune-mediated diseases, it has become apparent that chronic renal disease is an unavoidable consequence of long-term cyclosporine use.[9,20,21] The incidence and severity of cyclosporine-mediated renal disease are debated and depend in large part on the dose of cyclosporine administered and the presence of other risk factors for impaired renal function. However, even in patients without preexisting renal disease, long-term use of cyclosporine results in depressed glomerular filtration and renal blood flow and a high incidence of hypertension. In some patients, these renal effects are reversible as soon as use of the drug is discontinued. In other patients, however, structural injury that is not immediately reversible occurs. Among this latter group of patients, some may develop progressive renal insufficiency; others maintain stable renal function for a number of years.

PATHOPHYSIOLOGY

Acute administration of cyclosporine causes selective renal vasoconstriction in both experimental animals and humans.[9,22] Renal vasoconstriction causes a decrease in

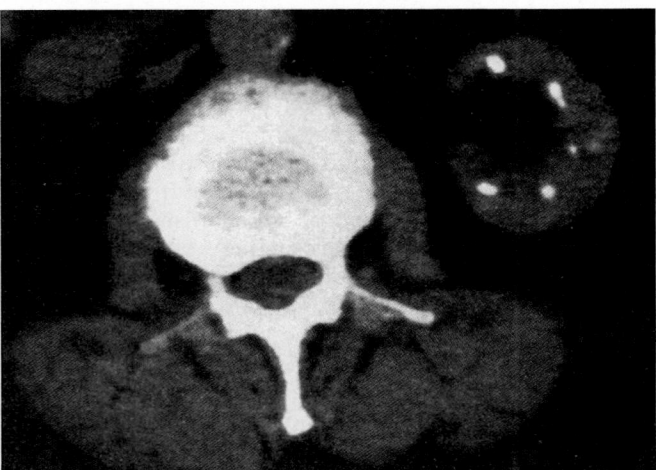

FIGURE 12B-2 Analgesic nephropathy. This computed tomography (CT) scan demonstrates papillary calcification characteristic of analgesic nephropathy. Calcifications appear as triangular, ringlike, or polygonal calcifications on the papillary line. Other CT findings in analgesic nephropathy include a decrease in renal volume and irregular contour. (From Elseviers MM, De Schepper A, Corthouts R, et al: High diagnostic performance of CT scan for analgesic nephropathy in patients with incipient to severe renal failure. Kidney Int 1995;48:1316; reprinted with permission of Blackwell Scientific.)

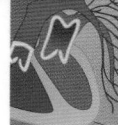

renal blood flow and a consequent decrease in GFR. While these effects are immediately reversible, they occur repeatedly in patients after administration of each dose of cyclosporine. Multiple mediators for renal vasoconstriction have been proposed and include activation of the sympathetic nervous system, with participation of endothelin as a second messenger, alterations in the balance of vasoconstrictor and vasodilator prostaglandins, and activation of the renin-angiotensin system.

The relationship between acute and chronic nephrotoxicity after cyclosporine use has not been clarified. It is likely that recurrent or persistent vasoconstriction causes chronic ischemic injury of the kidneys; chronic cyclosporine-related nephropathy is characterized by the same physiologic alterations of reduced renal plasma flow and GFR as well as by the development of histologic indicators of chronic renal injury. Both preglomerular and glomerular vessels are involved, as is the renal parenchyma. Cyclosporine arteriopathy is characterized by arterial hyalinosis and, in severe cases, myocyte degeneration and thrombosis of the arteriole (Fig. 12B-3). Glomerular injury is characterized by focal segmental sclerosis. Renal parenchymal disease is characterized by tubular atrophy and interstitial fibrosis, which is often described as patchy or striped in appearance (Fig. 12B-4).[23]

Arteriopathy and interstitial fibrosis have been reproduced in rodents after administration of cyclosporine for 2 to 4 or more weeks. In rodents, salt depletion markedly enhances the development of these lesions. The earliest vascular change observed was eosinophilic granular transformation of smooth muscle cells in the glomerular afferent arterioles.[24] The renal parenchymal lesion of interstitial fibrosis is preceded by tubular and interstitial cell proliferation and macrophage infiltration.[25] Increased accumulation of type I and type IV collagen eventually results in fibrosis.

CLINICAL PRESENTATION

Cyclosporine produces a number of adverse effects, including neurotoxicity, hypertrichosis, and gingival hyperplasia, but its most common and severe complication is chronic nephrotoxicity.[9,26] Renal dysfunction often appears in the absence of other problems and is recognized only by an increase in serum creatinine values. Cyclosporine toxicity has no other specific renal or clinical markers, although 60% to 100% of patients also develop hypertension. Chronic cyclosporine toxicity is associated with the use of higher doses of cyclosporine (>5 mg/kg per day) and may be more common in patients who have had episodes of acute nephrotoxicity.[27,28] Attempts to correlate the development of chronic nephrotoxicity with blood levels of cyclosporine or its metabolites have largely been unsuccessful. The diagnosis of chronic cyclosporine nephrotoxicity is usually made when all other potential contributing factors have been

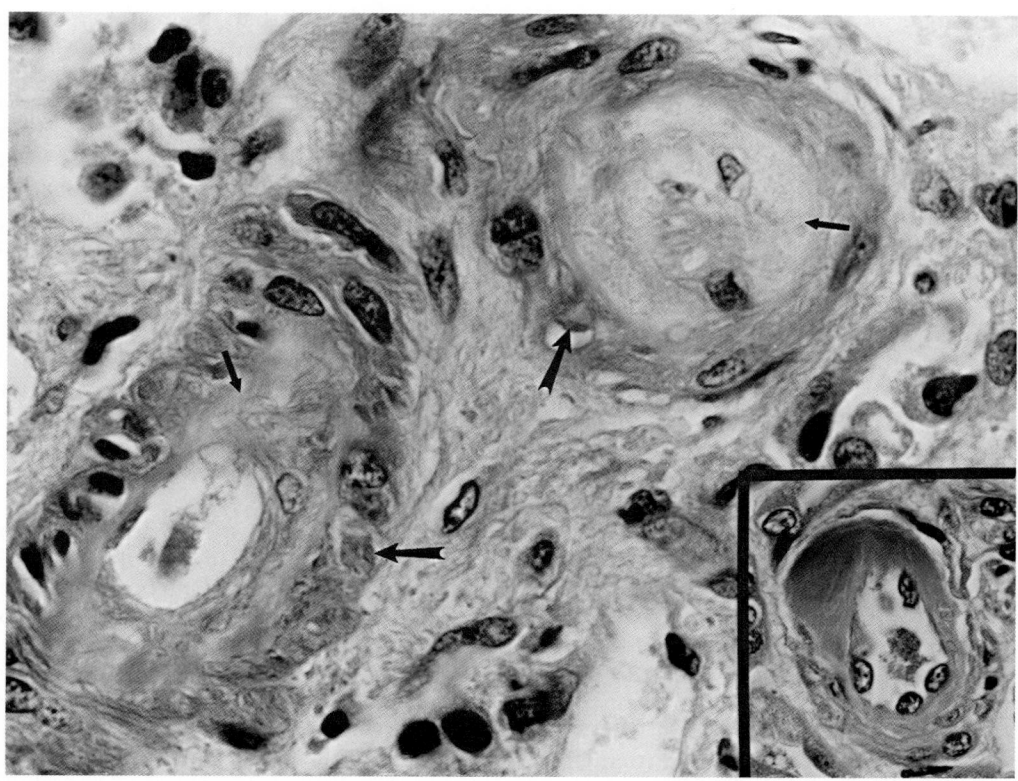

FIGURE 12B-3   Acute cyclosporine arteriopathy is characterized by focal smooth muscle degeneration (*large arrows*) and mucoid intimal thickening (*short arrows*). Note the loss of smooth muscle cells in the lower right quadrant of the vessel on the left. *Inset:* Chronic cyclosporine arteriopathy. The myocytes are replaced by hyaline deposits that protrude toward the outer aspect of the media.

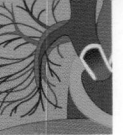
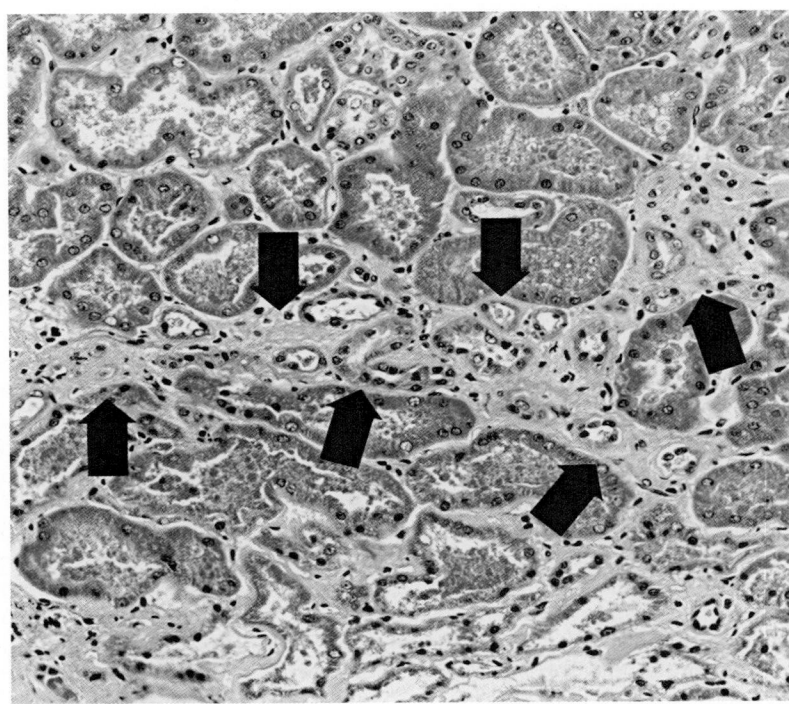

FIGURE 12B-4 Interstitial fibrosis resulting from cyclosporine toxicity. Bandlike "striped" areas of fibrosis and tubular atrophy are seen between the arrows. This interstitial fibrosis is not fundamentally different from that seen with other causes of chronic nephrotoxicity.

eliminated and renal function remains impaired. Functional and pathologic involvement may be dissociated, and some patients with well-preserved renal function have shown arteriopathy and interstitial fibrosis on renal biopsy.[29]

OUTCOME AND TREATMENT

The long-term outcome of chronic cyclosporine nephrotoxicity is unclear. Initial reports of cardiac transplant recipients receiving high doses of cyclosporine suggested that long-term administration of cyclosporine resulted in the development of end-stage renal disease that necessitated the use of dialysis in a substantial portion of patents.[23,30] Many other studies, however, have suggested that after the initial decrease in GFR, renal function stabilizes for many years.[9,31,32] Some have cautioned that despite stabilization in renal function, progressive glomerulosclerosis and interstitial fibrosis may occur and may ultimately result in further impairment of renal function and possible development of end-stage renal disease.

Most would agree that cessation of cyclosporine use leads to stabilization or improvement in renal function. However, many patients being treated with cyclosporine do not have this option (e.g., heart or liver transplant recipients). Avoiding high doses of cyclosporine is recommended but must be balanced against the possibility that too low a dose may result in ineffective immunosuppression with partial loss of therapeutic efficacy. When cyclosporine use can be discontinued in patients with severe nephrotoxicity, eventual improve-

ment may occur. Even severe cyclosporine arteriopathy has been observed to reverse with discontinuation or lowering of the dose of cyclosporine.[33] Various renal vasodilators have been demonstrated to reduce the acute vasoconstriction induced by cyclosporine; calcium channel blockers improve renal blood flow and GFR in patients receiving long-term cyclosporine therapy.[34-38] However, it is not known whether these agents can prevent the development of chronic renal disease in patients exposed to cyclosporine for prolonged periods.

Tacrolimus

Tacrolimus produces chronic renal failure via the same mechanism as cyclosporine, that is, by producing renal vasoconstriction.

Lithium

Lithium is an effective and frequently prescribed drug for the treatment of bipolar affective disorders. Unfortunately, lithium has a number of important effects on renal function. These include nephrogenic diabetes insipidus, renal tubular acidosis, and chronic interstitial nephritis.[39] Demonstrable defects in the renal concentrating ability occur in more than half of patients taking lithium, with clinically significant polyuria occurring in approximately 20%. Lithium induces nephrogenic diabetes insipidus through several cellular effects. The most important effect of lithium is to impair generation of cyclic adenosine-3′,5′,-monophospate in the collecting

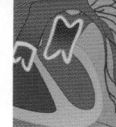

tubule of the distal nephron in response to antidiuretic hormone. This defect results in a failure to reabsorb filtered water adequately, and the result is water wasting, hyperosmolality, and secondary polydipsia. Although this defect usually responds to discontinuation of lithium therapy, some patients clearly have persistent nephrogenic diabetes insipidus for months or even years after cessation.[40]

Despite the clinical concern and evidence that long-term administration of lithium leads to interstitial nephritis and decreased GFR, this has been a very difficult subject to rigorously investigate. Early data were retrospective and biased toward patients who came to medical attention because of renal functional abnormalities. Renal biopsies of a number of these patients showed tubular atrophy and interstitial fibrosis.[41] However, the attribution of these lesions to lithium was questioned because similar renal histologic changes have been observed in patients who have never received lithium.[42] At least one prospective study has demonstrated no difference in renal interstitial fibrosis between psychiatric patients taking lithium for more than 5 years and those who had never received the drug. Nevertheless, prospective studies have suggested an increased incidence of impaired GFR in lithium-treated patients, and a number of well-documented case reports describe patients who had normal baseline renal function yet progressed to end-stage renal disease after long-term therapy with lithium.[3,11,43,44] The incidence of severely impaired renal function in patients receiving lithium is probably low, and it is reasonable to assume that maintenance of serum lithium levels in the therapeutic range would minimize the risk for progressive renal damage. Patients who demonstrate progressive renal insufficiency while receiving lithium should discontinue the drug.

CHEMOTHERAPEUTIC AGENTS

Chloroethylnitrosoureas

The nitrosoureas, including carmustine and streptozocin, are used against a number of malignancies. Long-term administration of these agents frequently produces renal dysfunction.[4,9] The risk for renal injury correlates strongly with the cumulative dose. Common signs of nitrosourea-associated nephrotoxicity include increased serum creatinine concentration and proteinuria. Renal dysfunction can progress despite discontinuation of the drug. In addition to causing intrinsic renal injury, some nitrosoureas (e.g., carmustine) can produce (pre)renal injury as a result of systemic hypotension.

Cisplatin

Cisplatin (cis-diamminedichloroplatinum) has activity against various solid tumors and is frequently used in combination chemotherapy. Its toxicities include myelosuppression and renal dysfunction. Cisplatin can produce both acute renal failure and chronic interstitial nephritis; Fanconi-type tubular dysfunction may also occur, producing salt and magnesium wasting.[4,9,11]

Cisplatin is largely protein bound and is actively taken up by renal cells; it remains in the kidneys for weeks after intravenous administration. Both antitumor and nephrotoxic properties are dependent on the stereoisomer, because trans-dichlorodiammineplatinum has no toxicity. Cisplatin produces focal acute tubular necrosis with tubular dilatation and interstitial edema, but spares the glomerulus. Although doses in excess of 100 mg/m² have caused acute renal failure, a more typical presentation with cumulative administration is the slow progressive rise in creatinine levels. Magnesium wasting, a consequence of impaired tubular reabsorption, may be severe, resulting in hypomagnesemia as well as hypokalemia and hypocalcemia.[4]

Vigorous hydration is important in reducing acute and probably chronic nephrotoxicity. Carboplatin has similar nephrotoxicity; however, nephrotoxicity appears less frequently with this drug.

Methotrexate

Methotrexate is a widely used chemotherapeutic agent. Among its adverse effects is renal injury.[9] Both acute renal failure and chronic insufficiency are associated with methotrexate. Acute renal failure is often the result of tubular necrosis secondary to crystallization of drug and metabolite in the renal tubules (although other mechanisms are suspected).[4] Because methotrexate solubility in renal tubules is pH dependent, with greater solubility in alkaline urine, urine alkalinization is commonly provided before high-dose methotrexate administration.

ENVIRONMENTAL AND OCCUPATIONAL TOXINS

Lead

Adults may be continually exposed to lead through a number of routes. For example, exposure may occur occupationally, for example, in smelting and refining, casting of battery plates, welding, or petroleum distillation. Painters and plumbers are at particular risk for lead exposure. Although now relatively rare, consumption of moonshine made in improper containers or the use of pottery glazed with lead-containing glazes is another source of lead poisoning.

Acute lead poisoning results in proximal tubular dysfunction or Fanconi's syndrome. Long-term exposure leads to hyperuricemia (saturnine gout), hypertension, and chronic renal failure. The pathologic lesion of lead nephropathy is chronic interstitial nephritis.[9,45-47] End-stage renal disease may not develop until 20 or 30 years after exposure, and thus it has been difficult to implicate lead in specific cases of renal failure of unclear etiology.[48] About 5% of patients undergoing hemodialysis have elevated bone lead concentrations.[49] In a cross-sectional study in Belgium, an inverse correlation was found

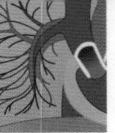

between blood lead concentrations and creatinine clearance.[50]

Severe chronic lead intoxication can often be treated by long-term chelation therapy with EDTA. Improvement in GFR has been reported in patients who have minimal reductions in GFR. However, patients with advanced chronic renal failure do not usually demonstrate improvement after chelation.

Lead-poisoned children develop subclinical but important renal disease; they are at six to seven times greater risk for developing hypertension as adults than less exposed children.[51]

Cadmium

Cadmium is a potent nephrotoxin. Industrial workers may develop chronic renal disease by inhalation exposure to cadmium. The general population may be exposed to cadmium from prevalent sources such as environmental tobacco smoke. Much like lead, cadmium intoxication results in Fanconi's syndrome and chronic interstitial nephritis.[9,52] Workers with high-level industrial exposure develop reductions in GFR and increased urinary excretion of various enzymes such as β_2-microglobulin and N-acetyl-β-glucosaminidase.[9,53] Normally, β_2-microglobulin undergoes glomerular filtration and is then reabsorbed by proximal tubule epithelial cells. Increased excretion of this protein generally suggests impaired proximal tubule function. N-acetyl-β-glucosaminidase is a lysosomal enzyme; increased urinary excretion of this protein suggests chronic cellular injury. Another hallmark of cadmium-induced renal toxicity is the appearance of metallothionein in urine.[54] Metallothionein is closely linked with cadmium nephrotoxicity; synthesized by the liver in response to cadmium exposure, metallothionein, often referred to as an endogenous chelator, binds to cadmium delivering the heavy metal to the proximal renal tubules. The cadmium-metallothionein complex is nephrotoxic, presumably via deposition in the lysosomes of the proximal renal tubules.[9]

Treatment of cadmium nephropathy consists of elimination of exposure. As is true of all forms of chronic renal disease, however, if renal function is already moderately impaired, progressive dysfunction may continue even when the initiating factor is withdrawn.

Mercury

Mercury is toxic to the proximal tubule. Severe exposure can produce acute, severe tubular necrosis. However, low-dose exposures can also result in injury to the proximal tubules.

ACKNOWLEDGMENT

Mark Paller, MD, contributed to a previous version of this chapter.

REFERENCES

1. Parmer MS: Chronic renal disease. BMJ 2002;325:85–90.
2. Yu HT: Progression of chronic renal failure. Arch Intern Med 2003;163:1417–1429.
3. Rahman M, Smith M: Chronic renal insufficiency: a diagnostic and therapeutic approach. Arch Intern Med 1998;158:1743–1752.
4. Kintzel PE: Anticancer drug-induced kidney disorders—incidence, prevention and management. Drug Saf 2001;24:19–38.
5. Blijenberg BG, Brouwer HJ: The accuracy of creatinine methods based on the Jaffe reaction: a questionable matter. Eur J Clin Chem Clin Biochem 1994;32:909–913.
6. Fuhrman SA: General clinical tests, renal function. In Tietz NW (ed): Clinical Guide to Laboratory Tests, 3rd ed. Philadelphia, WB Saunders, 1995, pp 65–86.
7. Andreev E, Koopman M, Arisz L: A rise in plasma creatinine that is not a sign of renal failure. Which drugs can be responsible? J Intern Med 1999;246:247–252.
8. Cockcroft DW, Gault MH: Prediction of creatinine clearance from serum creatinine. Nephron 1976;16:31.
9. Palmer BF, Henrich WL: Toxic nephropathy. In Brenner BM, Rector FC (eds): The Kidney, 7th ed. Philadelphia, WB Saunders/Elsevier, 2004, pp 237–254.
10. Kincaid-Smith P: Analgesic abuse and the kidney. Kidney Int 1980;17:250.
11. Perazella MA: Drug-induced renal failure: update on new medications and unique mechanisms of nephrotoxicity. Am J Med Sci 2003;325:349–362.
12. Noroian G, Clive D: Cyclo-oxygenase-2 inhibitors and the kidney. Drug Saf 2002;25:165–172.
13. Dubach UC, Rosner B, Stürmer T: An epidemiologic study of abuse of analgesic drugs. Effects of phenacetin and salicylate on mortality and cardiovascular morbidity. N Engl J Med 1991;324:155.
14. Sandler DP, Smith JC, Weinberg CR, et al: Analgesic use and chronic renal disease. N Engl J Med 1989;320:1238.
15. Perneger TV, Whelton PK, Klag MJ: Risk of kidney failure associated with the use of acetaminophen, aspirin, and nonsteroidal antiinflammatory drugs. N Engl J Med 1994;331:1675.
16. Weber M, Braun B, Kohler H: Ultrasonic findings in analgesic nephropathy. Nephron 1985;39:216.
17. Elseviers MM, De Schepper A, Corthouts R, et al: High diagnostic performance of CT scan for analgesic nephropathy in patients with incipient to severe renal failure. Kidney Int 1995;48:1316.
18. Gonwa TA, Corbett WT, Schey HM, et al: Analgesic-associated nephropathy and transitional cell carcinoma of the urinary tract. Ann Intern Med 1980;93:249.
19. McCredie M, Stewart JH, Carter JJ, et al: Phenacetin and papillary necrosis: independent risk factors for renal pelvic cancer. Kidney Int 1986;30:81.
20. Myers BD: Cyclosporine nephrotoxicity. Kidney Int 1986;30:964.
21. Remuzzi G, Bertani T: Renal vascular and thrombotic effects of cyclosporine. Am J Kidney Dis 1989;13:261.
22. Garr MD, Paller MS: Cyclosporine augments renal but not systemic vascular reactivity. Am J Physiol 1990;258:F211–F217.
23. Myers BD, Ross J, Newton L, et al: Cyclosporine-associated chronic nephropathy. N Engl J Med 1984;311:699.
24. Young BA, Burdmann, EA Johnson RJ, et al: Cyclosporine A induced arteriolopathy in a rat model of chronic cyclosporine nephropathy. Kidney Int 1995;48:431.
25. Young BA, Burdmann, EA, Johnson RJ, et al: Cellular proliferation and macrophage influx precede interstitial fibrosis in cyclosporine nephrotoxicity. Kidney Int 1995;48:439.
26. Kahan BD: Cyclosporine. N Engl J Med 1989;321:1725.
27. Feutren G, Mihatsch MJ: Risk factors for cyclosporine-induced nephropathy in patients with autoimmune diseases. N Engl J Med 1992;326:1654.
28. Pei Y, Scholey JW, Katz A, et al: Chronic nephrotoxicity in psoriatic patients treated with low-dose cyclosporine. Am J Kidney Dis 1994;23:528.
29. Ludwin D, Alexopoulou I, Esdaile JM, et al: Renal biopsy specimens from patients with rheumatoid arthritis and apparently normal renal function after therapy with cyclosporine. Am J Kidney Dis 1994;23:260.

30. Bertani T, Ferrazzi P, Schieppati A, et al: Nature and extent of glomerular injury induced by cyclosporine in heart transplant patients. Kidney Int 1991;40:243.

31. Bantle JP, Paller MS, Boudreau RJ, et al: Long-term effects of cyclosporine on renal function in organ transplant recipients. J Lab Clin Med 1990;115:233.

32. Ruggenenti P, Perico N, Amuchastegui S, et al: Following an initial decline, glomerular filtration rate stabilizes in heart transplant patients on chronic cyclosporine. Am J Kidney Dis 1994;24:549.

33. Morozumi K, Thiel G, Albert FW, et al: Studies on morphological outcome of cyclosporine-associated arteriolopathy after discontinuation of cyclosporine in renal allografts. Clin Nephrol 1992;38:1.

34. Hauser AC, Derfler K, Stockenhuber F, et al. Effect of calcium-channel blockers on renal function in renal-graft recipients treated with cyclosporine. N Engl J Med 1991;324:1517.

35. Palmer BF, Dawidson I, Sagalowsky A, et al: Improved outcome of cadaveric renal transplantation due to calcium channel blockers. Transplantation 1991;52:640–645.

36. Pirsh JD, D'Allessandro AM, Roecker EB, et al: A controlled, double-blind, randomized trial of verapamil and cyclosporine in cadaver renal transplant patients. Am J Kidney Dis 1993;21: 189–195.

37. Jorkasky DK, Audet P, Shusterman N, et al: Fenoldopam reverses cyclosporine-induced renal vasoconstriction in kidney transplant recipients. Am J Kidney Dis 1992;19:567.

38. Ruggenenti P, Perico N, Mosconi L, et al: Calcium channel blockers protect transplant patients from cyclosporine-induced daily renal hypoperfusion. Kidney Int 1993;43:706.

39. Boton R, Gaviria M, Batlle DC: Prevalence, pathogenesis, and treatment of renal dysfunction associated with chronic lithium therapy. Am J Kidney Dis 1987;10:329.

40. Batlle DC, von Riotte AB, Gaviria M, et al: Amelioration of polyuria by amiloride in patients receiving long-term lithium therapy. N Engl J Med 1985;312:408.

41. Hestbech J, Hansen HE, Amdisen A, et al: Chronic renal lesions following long-term treatment with lithium. Kidney Int 1977; 12:205.

42. Walker RG, Bennett WM, Davies BM, et al: Structural and functional effects of long-term lithium therapy. Kidney Int 1982;21:513.

43. Jorkasky DK, Amsterdam JD, Oler J, et al: Lithium-induced renal disease: a prospective study. Clin Nephrol 1988;30:293.

44. Gitlin MJ: Lithium-induced renal insufficiency. J Clin Psychopharmacol 1993;13:276.

45. Chia KS, Jeyaratnam J, Lee J, et al: Lead-induced nephropathy: relationship between various biological exposure indices and early manifestations of nephrotoxicity. Am J Ind Med 1995;27:883–895.

46. Vyskocil A, Semecky V, Fiala Z, et al: Renal alterations in female rats following subchronic lead exposure. J Appl Toxicol 1995; 15:257–262.

47. Nuyts GD, Daelemans RA, Jorens G, et al: Does lead play a role in the development of chronic renal disease? Nephrol Dial Transplant 1991;6:307–315.

48. Batuman V, Landy E, Maesaka JK, et al: Contribution of lead to hypertension with renal failure. N Engl J Med 1983;309:17.

49. Van De Vyver FL, D'Haese PC, Visser WJ, et al: Bone lead in dialysis patients. Kidney Int 1988;33:601.

50. Staessen JA, Lauwerys RR, Buchet JP, et al: Impairment of renal function with increasing blood lead concentrations in the general population. N Engl J Med 1992;327:151.

51. Hu H: A 50-year follow-up of childhood plumbism. Am J Dis Child 1991;145:681–687.

52. Wedeen RP: Environmental renal disease: lead, cadmium and Balkan endemic nephropathy. Kidney Int 1991;40(Suppl 4):5–20.

53. Smith TJ, Anderson RJ, Reading JC: Chronic cadmium exposure associated with kidney function effects. Am J Industr Med 1980;1:319.

54. Meyer BR, Fischbein A, Rosenman K, et al: Increased urinary enzyme excretion in workers exposed to nephrotoxic chemicals. Am J Med 1984;76:989.

13 *Gastrointestinal Toxicology*

SUZANNE R. WHITE, MD ■ MATTHEW W. HEDGE, MD

INTRODUCTION AND IMPORTANCE

The gastrointestinal (GI) tract provides a key interface between the body and the environment. Symptoms of GI disturbance such as nausea, vomiting, or a change in bowel habits are common complaints, especially in the acute care setting where the diagnosis of "gastroenteritis" is frequently entertained. Of concern, these seemingly benign complaints could either represent acute exposure to life-threatening intoxicants or herald the onset of a serious adverse drug effect. In fact, most drugs have the potential to cause GI tract disturbances at toxic doses or in susceptible individuals. For that reason, it is important to differentiate common medical or surgical conditions from serious intoxicant-induced gastro-intestinal disease. In certain ways, the GI tract is uniquely resistant, but in other ways it is extremely vulnerable to certain poisons. A discussion of certain structural and functional aspects of the GI tract will provide a basis for understanding the effects of a wide range of intoxicants on this system and its subsequent response to exposure.

GI TRACT STRUCTURE, FUNCTION, AND REGULATION

The GI tract comprises the mouth, salivary glands, esoph-agus, stomach, small and large intestines, pancreas, liver, and gallbladder. Functionally, it is characterized by the highly specialized performance and regulation of several critical processes, such as water absorption, nutrient digestion and extraction, and immune surveillance. The GI tract also plays a role in metabolizing and eliminating some xenobiotics through cytochrome P-450, glucuronyl transferases, and sulfotransferases located within small and large intestinal cells.[1] These metabolic processes are discussed in greater detail in Chapter 5. As the largest neuroendocrine organ, the GI tract is directly connected to the vascular and lymphatic systems and indirectly linked with many other systems.

Functional Regulation

PEPTIDES

Gastrointestinal functions are regulated through a complex interplay of neural, hormonal, and paracrine mediators. Five key peptide hormones are responsible for much of this regulatory effect.[2] They are secretin, gastrin, cholecystokinin (CCK), gastric inhibitory peptide (GIP), and motilin. Secretin stimulates biliary and pancreatic aqueous and bicarbonate secretion. Gastrin stimulates secretion of gastric acid, whereas GIP inhibits gastric acid secretion and stimulates insulin release. Motilin stimulates motility of the upper GI tract. CCK stimulates pancreatic aqueous, bicarbonate, and enzyme secretion and gallbladder contraction, in addition to inhibiting gastric emptying and signaling the termi-nation of eating.[3] These five key hormones are located in endocrine cells scattered throughout the GI tract mucosa and are released into the general circulation in response to chemical triggers in food, neural activity, or physical distention. Somatostatin and histamine have important roles as paracrine agents, that is, once released from endocrine cells they locally diffuse to their target tissue. The former inhibits gastrin release and the latter potentiates parietal cell secretion of gastric acid.

NERVES

Autonomic innervations both intrinsic and extrinsic to the GI tract regulate its functional responses. Input from these systems is further modulated by the central nervous system (CNS). Extrinsic nerves are distributed through both parasympathetic and sympathetic auto-nomic pathways. The sympathetic nervous system provides for the stimulation (contraction) of sphincteric muscle and relaxation of nonsphincteric muscle. Parasympathetic innervation via the vagus, splanchnic, and pelvic nerves stimulates (contracts) nonsphincteric muscle.[4] Intrinsic neural pathways comprise the "enteric nervous system" and are grouped into plexuses along the entire length of the GI tract. The myenteric Auerbach's plexus is located between the longitudinal and circular smooth muscle layers and controls peristalsis. The submucosal plexuses predominantly control secretion and absorption. Within these intrinsic pathways, acetylcholine is the major excitatory neurotransmitter, acting at the M_2 and M_3 muscarinic receptor subtypes.[5] Other less ubiquitous intrinsic neurotransmitters also mediate important digestive functions. Nitric oxide and vasoactive intestinal peptide (VIP) have major inhibitory roles in this regard.[6] Other agents function as neurocrines (i.e., they are located in intrinsic neurons, released near target tissue, and diffuse a short distance across synaptic gaps to stimulate or inhibit the release of other hormones or paracrines). Such stimulatory neurocrines are serotonin (5-HT) through $5HT_4$ receptors, substance P in the myenteric plexus, and gastrin releasing peptide (GRP), which mediates the vagal release of gastrin. Finally, leu- and met-enkephalins bind to μ opioid receptors on circular smooth muscle and mucosal cells to slow transit and inhibit glandular secretion.[7,8]

Structure

SALIVARY GLANDS

Functionally, saliva initiates digestion, exhibits anti-bacterial action, and provides lubrication for food passage. Saliva is produced in large volumes, is hypotonic, and

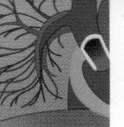

contains high concentrations of potassium. Digestive enzymes present in saliva include α-amylase and lingual lipase. Interestingly, salivation is triggered by both the sympathetic and parasympathetic branches of the autonomic nervous system and can be a manifestation of either cholinergic or sympathomimetic intoxication. Salivation is inhibited by fatigue, fear, sleep, and dehydration and stimulated by conditioning, smell, taste, and nausea.[2]

ESOPHAGUS

The function of the esophagus is strictly one of motility—to propel food from the oropharynx to the stomach. The nonkeratinized stratified squamous epithelial cell lining of the esophagus provides a protective coating of cells for the underlying tissue. Mucus secreted from superficial glands at the levels of the cricoid cartilage and the esophagogastric junction provides a protective and lubricant surface to facilitate the passage of food. No digestion or absorption takes place here, since the process of swallowing takes only seconds. The average volume swallowed by a child is 9.3 mL and by an adult 14 to 21 mL.[9] Swallowing can be initiated voluntarily but proceeds as an involuntary reflex under the control of the brainstem.

STOMACH

The epithelial architecture and cellular makeup of each region of the stomach is distinct. The first portion distal to the gastroesophageal junction, the cardia, is composed of columnar epithelium and mucous cells. The body and fundus have a similar epithelial framework with the addition of parietal cells, chief cells, and endocrine cells. The parietal cells secrete hydrochloric acid and intrinsic factor, necessary for vitamin B_{12} absorption. The chief cells contain pepsinogen granules, precursors of the proteolytic digestive enzyme pepsin. The endocrine argentaffin cells secrete serotonin and histamine. The pyloric antrum occupies a triangular area in the distal fifth of the stomach where gastrin-secreting (G) cells are found. Gastric contractile activity and emptying are highly regulated processes under the influence of the vagus nerve, motilin, and CCK. Gastric emptying also involves feedback inhibition from small intestinal receptor-mediated responses to osmotic pressure, hydrogen ions, and fatty acids. The stomach is capable of directly absorbing un-ionized lipophilic molecules of moderate size.[1]

The H^+ concentration in gastric juice is 3 million times greater than that in blood or tissue. The toxicologic significance of this fact is that agents which disrupt the integrity of the gastric mucosa (ethanol, caustics) allow for back-diffusion of hydrogen ions, potentiating the initial injury. Hydrochloric acid is secreted into the gastric lumen by parietal cells through an adenosine triphosphate (ATP)-dependent process. This process is blocked by omeprazole, a proton pump inhibitor that concentrates selectively in parietal cells and noncompetitively inhibits the H^+/K^+-ATPase. (A related drug, lansoprazole, binds the H^+/K^+-ATPase at the parietal cell surface.[10]) Acid secretion is regulated by three primary endogenous chemicals: acetylcholine, gastrin, and histamine.[10] Acetylcholine released from either vagal efferent or intrinsic nerves at the site of the parietal cell causes direct stimulation of acid secretion, an effect that is potentiated by histamine. Gastrin also causes direct stimulation of acid secretion, and its effects are also potentiated by histamine. Gastrin is most highly concentrated in the antrum, although appreciable amounts are also found in the epithelium of the duodenal bulb. Histamine is abundantly present throughout the gastric mucosa, originating from mast cells and basophils. It is hypothesized that histamine constantly sensitizes the parietal cells to other stimuli. The development of histamine-2 (H_2) receptor antagonists (cimetidine, ranitidine, famotidine, and nizatidine) has clarified this potentiating role of histamine in gastric acid secretion.[10] For example, in the setting of H_2 receptor antagonist use, acid secretion in response to other stimuli, such as gastrin or caffeine, insulin-induced hypoglycemia is inhibited. Of note, proton pump inhibitors are more potent blockers of acid secretion than are H_2 receptor antagonists.

PANCREAS

The exocrine pancreas is a grapelike clustering of acinar glands drained by ductules that ultimately converge to form the pancreatic duct. Through this duct, pancreatic secretions enter the proximal duodenum. Interspersed among the pancreatic acini are islets of Langerhans, or the endocrine pancreas, which produces insulin, glucagon, and somatostatin. Acinar cells manufacture, store (as zymogen granules), and secrete enzymes essential for digestion. These include proteases such as trypsinogen, chymotrypsinogen, proelastase, and carboxypeptidases as well as amylase and lipases. Enzymes are admixed with a large volume of aqueous solution containing sodium and bicarbonate. Pancreatic exocrine secretion is influenced by CCK, secretin, and extrinsic parasympathetic and sympathetic neurons, which are stimulatory and inhibitory, respectively. Specifically, enzymatic secretion from acinar cells is controlled by vagal input and CCK. The primary stimulant of aqueous pancreatic juice secretion is secretin, the effects of which are potentiated by both CCK and acetylcholine. Luminal pH of less than 4.5, dietary fat, and amino acid content are the main triggers of pancreatic exocrine response, stimulating vagal activity, CCK, and secretin release. These triggers potentiate each other through second messengers. Of toxicologic significance, pancreatic injury of sufficient magnitude to decrease enzyme secretion by more than 80% of baseline will result in steatorrhea.

GALLBLADDER

Bile is secreted by the liver as a complex mixture of bile acids, phospholipids, cholesterol, bile pigments, electrolytes, and water. These compounds form mixed micelles that facilitate the digestion of dietary lipids. During fasting, bile is stored and concentrated in the gallbladder. In the fed state, the gallbladder contracts, mostly in response to CCK, expelling bile into the duodenum. Bile acids are then enterohepatically recirculated, with 90% reabsorbed in the small intestine. The remainder reaches the colon, where additional absorption occurs,

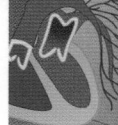

but ultimately 0.3 to 0.6 g is lost in the feces daily. The bile acids, chenodeoxycholic acid and deoxycholic acid, have intrinsic cathartic properties. Diarrhea is therefore a serious consequence of bile salt malabsorption from ileal disease and is a potential side effect during chenodeoxycholic acid therapy for the dissolution of cholesterol gallstones.

SMALL INTESTINE

The small intestine comprises the duodenum, jejunum, and ileum. It is highly proliferative, with an abundance of undifferentiated cells, rendering this portion of the GI tract particularly susceptible to toxic exposure, particularly the effects of mitotic inhibitors or irradiation. Its extensive surface area results from an estimated 25 million finger-like projections called *villi*. The surface lining of these villi, the *brush border*, carries out the major function of the small intestine—digestion and absorption of nutrients. Movement of luminal contents is dependent on segmental (mixing) and peristaltic (aboral transit) contraction, both under the coordination of myenteric nerves, motilin, CCK, and gastrin.

Virtually all food enters the GI tract in polymeric form and requires enzymatic hydrolysis to monomers that can be absorbed by specific transport systems. Some key digestive enzymes originating from the salivary glands, gastric chief cells, and pancreas are discussed above. In the small intestine, luminal degradation of food continues primarily through brush border enzyme activity. In humans, these enzymes are all hydrolases, including disaccharidases, peptidases, phosphatases, and others. Substrate is hydrolyzed outside the cell, so at least some part of the protein faces the external surface of the membrane. The surface exposure of these enzymes renders them susceptible to damage not only by ingested drugs and poisons but also by infectious organisms, foreign antigens, and pancreatic proteases. In fact, the proteolytic digestion of these surface enzymes accounts for their rapid turnover and short half-life, in some cases only 4 to 6 hours. Therefore, the maintenance of activity of some brush border enzymes requires several cycles of protein synthesis during the approximately 5-day life span of small intestinal cells.

Absorption of dietary nutrients follows their digestion from polymers to monomers. Complex starches are digested to hexoses, proteins to dipeptides and amino acids, and vitamin complexes to free vitamins. These monomers are then absorbed by specific carrier-mediated mechanisms. Sodium-dependent active transport systems have been described for glucose and galactose, amino acids and peptides, pteroylglutamate, vitamin C, biotin, bile salts, riboflavin, thiamine, and other water-soluble organic substrates. Most mineral absorption occurs in the small intestine, the best studied being calcium and iron. Calcium is absorbed by both active (duodenum) and passive (jejunum and ileum) processes. Iron is absorbed in the proximal duodenum via a divalent metal transporter. Heme iron is readily absorbed by endocytosis. Other metals may also be absorbed by active transport methods in the intestine. While the exact mechanisms for lead absorption are unknown, it is suspected to follow calcium and iron pathways. Lead absorption is assumed to involve both active and passive transport. Children are known to absorb more lead partly on the basis of their higher calcium absorption efficiency compared with adults, induced by increased calcium demand. Furthermore, iron deficiency will increase lead absorption. It is hypothesized that the sodium gradient across the intestinal absorptive cell membrane is the driving force for active transport. Lithium is a readily absorbed substitute for sodium in the intestinal cells. The carrier systems for these nutrients most likely are integral proteins situated in the lipid membrane of the brush border. As with the surface orientation of brush border digestive enzymes, their external orientation poses susceptibility to toxic injury from ingested poisons.

Lipids do not appear to require a membrane protein for absorption. After dietary neutral fat (triglycerides) is digested to long-chain fatty acids and monoglycerides by pancreatic lipase, the monomers as well as cholesterol are solubilized in bile salts to form micelles. (Orlistat is a synthetic derivative of lipstatin that forms an inactive acyl-enzyme complex with lipase and prevents fat absorption.) Long-chain fatty acids, monoglycerides, and cholesterol are absorbed by diffusion when the molecules by chance collide with the absorptive cell membrane. Fat absorption then is diminished by factors that interrupt the formation of micelles or alter the absorptive membrane.

As described above, the intestinal mucosa is a rapidly proliferating epithelium susceptible to injury by chemicals. Breaks in the mucosal barrier following exposure to intoxicants perturb critical absorptive and secretory transport properties and predispose to infection and systemic illness. Minor mucosal breaches are repaired by "epithelial restitution," a process independent of cell proliferation. Restitution is regulated by a variety of cytokines and growth factors and is modulated by integrin-dependent interactions with the extracellular matrix. Restitution also involves intracellular signaling pathways that remodel the actin cytoskeleton. Deeper injuries require additional reparative mechanisms involving nonepithelial cells, angiogenesis, and scarring.[11]

COLON

The colon comprises several anatomically distinct regions: the cecum, ascending colon, transverse colon, descending colon, sigmoid colon, and rectum. The epithelial lining differs from that of the small bowel in that villi are absent; therefore, the absorptive surface is flat. Like the small intestine, however, the epithelium is highly proliferative, posing susceptibility to toxic insult. Primary colonic functions include (1) absorption of water and electrolytes, (2) secretion of potassium, and (3) storage and discharge of luminal contents. The absorption of metals and toxins from the colon is thought to be minimal.

Each day, the colonic epithelium is confronted by about 1500 mL of water, 200 mEq of sodium, 5 mEq of potassium, 120 mEq of chloride, and 60 mEq of bicarbonate. A normal stool contains about 100 mL water, 5 mEq sodium, 9 to 13 mEq potassium, 2 mEq chloride, and 3 mEq bicarbonate, thus indicating the net

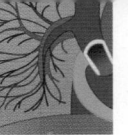

absorption of water, sodium, chloride, and bicarbonate and the net secretion of potassium. Various factors alter colonic fluid and electrolyte movement such as luminal pH, osmolality, and the presence of ions (bile acids, sulfates, hydroxy fatty acids). Additionally, colonic water and electrolyte movement are under the influence of hormones such as aldosterone, 9α-fluorohydrocortisone, and antidiuretic hormone. The storage and discharge functions of the colon depend on its motor activity, which is regulated by intrinsic and extrinsic nerves, gastrin, and CCK. Aboral movement of contents is a slow process usually taking days.

TOXIC EFFECTS ON THE GI TRACT

Diseases of the Mouth

Excessive salivation can be caused by both cholinergic and sympathomimetic agents. It has been reported as an adverse effect of olanzapine, clozapine, and ketamine therapy. Importantly, drooling can signify exposure to phencyclidine, nicotine, thallium, corrosives, or irritants. In children, drooling is a common manifestation of dystonic reaction, since normal swallowing may be impaired. *Decreased salivation* is seen with exposure to anticholinergics, botulism, and hypovolemia. Drug-induced *stomatitis* can occur in isolation or as part of multisystem illness (e.g., Stevens-Johnson syndrome [SJS]). Many drugs cause SJS, most significantly sulfonamides, anticonvulsants, nonsteroidal anti-inflammatory drugs (NSAIDs), and allopurinol. Of note, reports of stomatitis in association with multiple classes of HIV medications are increasing. Cases of isolated recurrent stomatitis related to fluoxetine use are reported.[12] Latent stomatitis can be caused by epithelial cell cycle inhibitors (chemotherapeutics) or irradiation. (With methotrexate, this recurring toxicity is reduced by supplementation with folic acid, 1 mg/day). Glossitis and stomatitis are significant problems in 11% of persons taking the herbal supplement feverfew. *Gingivitis* can be caused by phenytoin and calcium channel blockers and rarely can stem from the chronic inhalation of elemental mercury vapor or from exposure to other metals such as thallium, nickel, or zinc. Oral mucosal ulcerations have been noted following acute exposure to various corrosive or irritant chemicals and also with the chronic misuse of an undiluted mouthwash containing 70% ethanol.[13] The chronic use of hydrogen peroxide as a mouthwash can cause hypertrophy of the tongue papillae. *Dysgeusia* can be related to zinc depletion from excessive metal chelation therapy or from chronic cocaine abuse. Metal toxicity, including metal fume fever, can result in a metallic taste. Oral *discoloration* can signify exposure to substances listed in Table 13-1. Finally, *toxic parotitis* has been associated with L-asparaginase, doxycycline, and general anesthesia.

Diseases of the Esophagus

The most common symptoms that relate to esophageal disease are nonspecific and include retrosternal chest

TABLE 13-1 Causes of Oral Discoloration	
COLOR	**CAUSE**
Tongue	
Brown	Bromine, bismuth, arsenic, phenolphthalein, doxorubicin, quinacrine, tobacco
Green	Vanadium
Black, hairy	Cefoxitin, corticosteroids, lansoprazole, penicillin, sodium perborate, sodium peroxide, tetracyclines
White	Chlorhexidine, phenol, caustic acids, hydrogen peroxide (chronic)
Blue	Methylene blue
Gumline	
Blue-gray	Bigmuth, lead, mercury, copper salts, thallium, zinc

pain and dysphagia. Drug-induced esophageal disorders most commonly derive from either change in motility or disrupted mucosal integrity. Motility disorders include esophageal spasm, which can be caused by β blockers, both therapeutically and in overdose. Reflex esophageal spasm is precipitated by local factors such as corrosive injury or Ewald tube insertion during gastric lavage. Mechanical obstruction of the esophagus has occurred following the ingestion of sucralfate or drug packets, or as a late complication of corrosive-induced stricture. Ethanol, caffeine, opioids, and anticholinergic agents decrease lower esophageal sphincter tone and can cause gastroesophageal reflux.

Esophageal disorders that result from changes in mucosal integrity represent a broad spectrum of disease. Drug-induced esophagitis can vary from diffuse mild inflammation to necrotizing ulceration with hemorrhage. Perforation and stricture have occurred as secondary complications. Drugs implicated in esophagitis include antibiotics (tetracycline, doxycycline, clindamycin, lincomycin), 5-fluorouracil, NSAIDs, oral potassium supplements, emepronium bromide, iron, quinidine, carbachol, ascorbic acid, cromolyn inhalant, cimetidine, and biphosphonates. The mechanism of injury appears to be direct corrosion based on acid or alkaline pH effect. As examples, tetracycline and doxycycline are known to be highly acidic in solution. Although drug-induced esophageal injury is more likely to occur in individuals with underlying mechanical or peristaltic abnormalities, it can occur in the normal esophagus, especially if the agent is taken with insufficient liquid and upright position is not maintained. Caustic alkali and acid chemically induced injuries to the esophagus are discussed in greater detail in Chapter 98.

Diseases of the Stomach

Slowed gastric emptying results from the ingestion of solids, especially high fat substances, and from metabolic disturbances such as hypokalemia. Drugs can increase or decrease gastric emptying time. Those which delay gastric emptying include anticholinergics and opiates. When the stomach fails to empty normally, symptoms

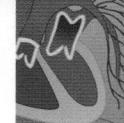

such as satiety, loss of appetite, and nausea are common, and gastric contents are often vomited. Absorption of concurrently administered therapeutic drugs can thus be impaired. Of toxicologic significance is the common example of acetaminophen overdose in combination with opioids or anticholinergics, where peak levels can be delayed well beyond the expected 4-hour time frame.

Drugs that increase gastric emptying can cause symptoms of diarrhea, sweating, palpitations, and abdominal cramps. These prokinetic agents include metoclopramide, domperidone, and cisapride. Domperidone and metoclopramide block the inhibitory effect of dopamine on gut motility. (Metoclopramide also crosses the blood-brain barrier and exerts central antidopaminergic effects, which can trigger extrapyramidal symptoms in 10% to 30% of patients.) Additional prokinetic actions of metoclopramide include agonism of gut 5-HT4 receptors and stimulation of acetylcholine release. Cisapride increases acetylcholine release from the myenteric plexus without antidopaminergic effect. Of toxicologic significance, co-ingestion of prokinetic drugs may cause more rapid absorption of CNS depressants such as antihistamines, benzodiazepines, or ethanol with greater than expected sedation.[10]

A few miscellaneous toxic scenarios with significant gastric implications deserve mention. Gastric bezoars can form after large ingestions of iron, lithium, calcium channel blockers, sustained-release theophylline, and potassium chloride. Gastric outlet obstruction with stricture formation in the pyloric region is a known late complication of iron toxicity. The distal stomach (antrum and pylorus) is the most frequent site of injury following the ingestion of a liquid strong acid owing to a common pathway (magenstrasse) that directs fluid along the lesser curvature to the pylorus.

Intestinal Disorders

Blood flow to the intestines can be compromised in several ways. Oral contraceptives can cause mesenteric venous or arterial thrombosis.[14,15] Through unclear mechanisms, mesenteric ischemia with bowel necrosis in the absence of prolonged hypotension has been noted following acute calcium channel blocker overdose.[16] Various other slow-release formulations, iron products, and osmotic pump delivery systems have caused local lesions, strictures, or perforation. Intestinal vasospasm can be caused by vasopressin, T-2 toxin, and cocaine. Cocaine-induced intestinal ischemia with perforation is described following injection or inhalation or with mechanical bowel obstruction from impacted or ruptured cocaine packets.[17-19] Other unusual but presumptively ischemic complications from "crack" include hemorrhagic diarrhea in a child acutely exposed, pneumoperitoneum, and perforation of gastric ulcers.[20,21] Metformin-associated lactic acidosis can masquerade as mesenteric ischemia.[22] Nausea, bloating, vomiting, and diarrhea, common effects noted with both acute overdose and chronic toxicity, must then be cautiously regarded as potential markers of life-threatening metformin-related lactic acidosis.[23-25] Additional gastrointestinal compli-

cations due to chronic metformin use include GI bleeding and pancreatitis.[23]

Diseases of the Pancreas

Pancreatitis is an acute or chronic inflammatory process characterized by abdominal pain, vomiting, and elevated pancreatic enzymes. The spectrum of severity ranges from mild to rapidly fatal illness. Drug-induced pancreatitis is rare. Most agents, except ethanol, are associated with the acute form of illness with a return to normal pancreatic anatomy and function following withdrawal of the offending agent. Variable mechanisms for drug-induced pancreatitis are proposed, including pancreatic duct constriction, interference with acinar cell protein synthesis/transport/secretion, immunosuppression, direct cytotoxicity from toxic metabolites, elevated triglycerides, arteriolar thrombosis, microcirculatory disruption, and haptene formation. The evidence for a true link between various drugs and human pancreatitis has been evaluated. The strength of association was based on criteria including the absence of other inciting factors, an appropriate temporal sequence, and a positive rechallenge.[26,27] This information is summarized in Box 13-1.

Isolated hyperamylasemia without clinical evidence of pancreatitis has been described with methanol, lithium, organophosphates, T-2 toxin, and opioid intoxication. (Of note, some of these agents can cause true pancreatitis as well.) Beta cell destruction and diabetes mellitus can occur following exposure to alloxan, streptozocin, vacor, and pentamidine.

Diseases of the Gallbladder

A variety of drugs induce a spectrum of gallbladder diseases. An increase in the relative lithogenicity of bile, from bile and cholesterol hypersecretion, is an adverse effect of oral contraceptive use. Whether this in fact

---

BOX 13-1	PROPOSED LINKS BETWEEN INTOXICANTS AND HUMAN PANCREATITIS*

Definite: Aminosalicylate, anticholinesterases, didanosine, ethanol, furosemide, methyldopa, metronidazole, estrogens, scorpion venom, tetracycline, valproic acid
Probable: Hydrochlorothiazide, pentamidine, nitrofurantoin, sulfonamides, olanzapine
Possible: ACE inhibitors, acetaminophen, azathioprine, L-asparaginase, chlorthalidone, cyclosporine, cytosine-ara, corticosteroids, erythromycin, ethacrynic acid, indomethacin, isoniazid, 6-mercaptopurine, metformin, methanol, rifampicin, sulindac, theophylline, vinblastine, zinc chloride
Insufficient evidence: Amphetamines, β blockers, carbamazepine, cimetidine, cholestyramine, clofibrate, clonidine, cyproheptadine, propoxyphene, diazoxide, growth hormone, histamine, isotretinoin, meprobamate, phenformin, procainamide, warfarin

*Modified from Braganza JM, Foster JR: Toxicology of the pancreas. In Ballantyne B, Marro T, Syverson T (eds): General and Applied Toxicology, 4th ed. London, Macmillan Reference, 2004, p 893.

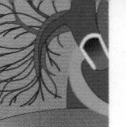

increases the incidence of gallbladder disease is controversial.[28] Clofibrate increases the risk of gallstone formation.[29] Drugs that induce hemolysis such as dapsone can lead to pigment cholelithiasis. Through its precipitation as a calcium salt, ceftriaxone reversibly induces biliary sludge or "pseudolithiasis" in 25% to 45% of patients.[30] Epidemiologic studies conflict regarding the association between acute cholecystitis and thiazide diuretic use. The hepatic artery infusion of chemotherapy agents causes cholecystitis so frequently that prophylactic cholecystectomy is often performed. Finally, hypersensitivity cholecystitis is reported with erythromycin and ampicillin. The role of various opioids in the induction of sphincter of Oddi spasm is controversial.

Malabsorption and Altered GI Tract Flora

Interference with nutrient digestion and absorption results from the toxic effect of a wide variety of exogenous agents. Certain agents can also affect the absorption of therapeutic drugs. The mechanisms leading to maldigestion and malabsorption include (1) alteration of environmental pH (potassium chloride, antacids), (2) chelation (tetracycline, ketoconazole with calcium, cholestyramine with iron), (3) inhibition of digestive enzymes and inhibition of transport processes requiring membrane proteins (drugs that alter mitotic activity such as colchicine and methotrexate), and (4) direct toxic injury to the epithelium (neomycin, mefenamic acid, other caustics). When severe, these toxic effects cause malabsorption of fat, protein, carbohydrate, salt, water, minerals, and water-soluble and fat-soluble vitamins.

Numerous drugs adversely affect the digestion and absorption of nutrients. The absorption of vitamin B_{12} and folic acid is inhibited by anticonvulsants, neomycin, colchicine, metformin, potassium chloride, and cholestyramine. Chronic ethanol abuse alters the absorption of several nutrients, including vitamin B_{12}, folic acid,

thiamine, amino acids, calcium, and magnesium. Drugs that inhibit digestive absorption are listed in Table 13-2.

Alterations in GI tract flora can be associated with consequences; a few of toxicologic significance are mentioned here. Through mechanisms discussed above, H_2 receptor antagonists and proton pump inhibitors effectively raise gastric pH and can increase the risk of foodborne illness and pulmonary infections. In newborns, immature GI tract flora and relative achlorhydria create a milieu that favors botulinum spore germination and growth and predisposes to infantile botulism. Approximately 30% of an oral digoxin dose is metabolized by normal gut flora (*Eubacterium lentum*). A decrease in this bacterial population can result in a relative digoxin dose increase. Digoxin toxicity from this drug-drug interaction is best described with the concurrent use of erythromycin, clarithromycin, and tetracycline. Broad-spectrum antibiotics can decrease GI tract bacterial synthesis of vitamin K. As a result, coagulopathy and bleeding can occur in patients taking warfarin along with these agents. Similarly, antibiotic reduction of normal gut flora can decrease the enterohepatic recirculation of estrogen metabolites, leading to a reduction in the efficacy of certain oral contraceptives, unwanted pregnancy, or menstrual irregularity. Conversion of ingested nitrates to more potent methemoglobin-inducing nitrites can occur in the gut by coliform bacteria. Because infants possess reduced activity of nicotinamide adenine dinucleotide (NADH) methemoglobin reductase, they are most likely to be affected.

Toxic Disorders That Mimic "Gastritis," "Gastroenteritis," or "Enteritis"

Symptoms exhibited during various stages of intoxication caused by myriad drugs or chemicals can mimic those symptoms typical of gastritis, gastroenteritis, or enteritis. Specifically, nausea, vomiting, abdominal cramping, and bloody or nonbloody diarrhea will be

TABLE 13-2 Drugs That Inhibit Digestive-Absorptive Mechanisms

DRUG	NUTRIENT MALABSORBED	PUTATIVE MECHANISMS
Aluminum hydroxide	Phosphate, vitamin A	Intraluminal formation of insoluble complexes
Anion exchange resins (cholestyramine, colestipol)	Water- and fat-soluble vitamins, bile salts, oxalate	Intraluminal binding of nutrient
Biguanides	Glucose, amino acids, folate, B_{12}	Inhibit oxidative phosphorylation
Cimetidine	B_{12} bound to food	Inhibits gastric acid and intrinsic factor
Colchicine	Fat, glucose, B_{12}	Inhibits mitotic spindle
Dilantin	Folate	Inhibits folate conjugase; alkalinizes intestinal contents
Ethanol	Fat, glucose, amino acids, vitamins, minerals	Alters physical properties of the membrane; inhibits Na$^+$/K$^+$-ATPase; stimulates cyclic AMP
Folate antagonists (methotrexate, aminopterin, trimethoprim)	Folate	Inhibit folate transport; inhibit cell proliferation
Neomycin	Fat, cholesterol, fat-soluble vitamins glucose, amino acids, B_{12}, minerals	Precipitates fatty acids and bile acids; causes histologic damage
Oral contraceptives	Folate	Inhibit folate conjugase
p-Aminosalicylic acid	Fat, cholesterol, folate, B_{12}	Unknown
Somatostatin	Fat	Inhibits pancreatic lipase secretion
Sultasalazine	Folate	Inhibits folate transport
Omeprazole	B_{12} bound to protein	Decreases intrinsic factor secretion

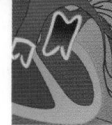

discussed. The most common symptom complex, *nausea and vomiting*, can be attributed to most intoxicants under appropriate conditions, and is also a common psychological or vasovagal response. In some situations (cytotoxic drug use), these symptoms are expected. In other situations, nausea and vomiting can signal the onset of unexpected, severe drug toxicity (theophylline and digoxin). Emesis can result from stimulation of serotonin (5-HT3) receptors, through stimulation of the vomiting center via the chemoreceptor trigger zone (CTZ) or via afferent fibers from the GI tract, the vestibular apparatus, the nucleus of the tractus solitarius, or higher cortical centers. A frequent association is made with drugs that are cholinergic, dopaminergic, or histaminic and with direct GI tract irritation (potassium salts, iron) or pharyngeal irritation (irritant gasses). Drugs such as digoxin, opiates (apomorphine), estrogens, and levodopa have direct action on the CTZ in the floor of the fourth ventricle, outside the blood-brain barrier.[13] While cocaine likewise directly stimulates medullary centers, nausea and vomiting in the setting of abuse can signify the presence of more ominous conditions such as intestinal or myocardial ischemia.[31] In the acute overdose setting, the onset and character or color of emesis can occasionally assist in formulating a differential diagnosis (Table 13-3). Hematemesis may result from the ingestion of caustics, iron, concentrated hydrogen peroxide, or mercury salts. Blue-green emesis can be noted following the ingestion of boric acid, methylene blue, or copper sulfate, and luminescence with yellow phosphorus.

Diarrhea is commonly noted both with acute intoxication and as an adverse therapeutic drug effect. Multiple causal mechanisms include mucosal injury with loss of absorptive or digestive capacity, pancreatic injury, cholinergic excess, or osmotic effect. Some cathartics, for example, increase intestinal motility and decrease transit time based on their osmotic effect. Similarly, antacids such as magnesium hydroxide or aluminum hydroxide can exert osmotic effects within the GI tract that lead to chronic diarrhea and secondary derangements in calcium and phosphorus. Diarrhea caused by antibiotics or high-dose corticosteroids is generally attributed to altered gut flora. An extreme example of this aberration, pseudomembranous colitis, results from antibiotic-related overgrowth of *Clostridium difficile* with toxin elaboration. Erythromycin causes diarrhea through a direct effect on gut motility (through motilin) and has been used in conjunction with metoclopramide to hasten the elimination of ingested drug packets.[32] Drugs or conditions associated with increased serotonin activity (serotonin reuptake inhibitor use, serotonin syndrome), excess acetylcholine (organophosphate poisoning), excess catecholamines (methylxanthine toxicity), or excess histamine (scombroid poisoning) cause diarrhea. Diarrhea in these situations is typically only one of a constellation of dramatic clinical features. Metals such as arsenic and iron cause diarrhea, but this rarely occurs in isolation and typically is accompanied by vomiting and, in severe cases, hypotension. Discolored diarrheal stools can occasionally provide clues to the etiologic agent (Table 13-4). Although it is not feasible to present a comprehensive review of the many drugs and chemicals that adversely affect the GI tract, key agents are discussed below—again, with a focus on those that may mimic "gastroenteritis." Wherever possible, distinguishing features that may point to the diagnosis of poisoning are highlighted.

BIOLOGICALS
Colchicine

Colchicine poisoning can result from pharmaceutical or plant sources (autumn crocus, glory lily). Illness is

TABLE 13-3 Approximate Onset of Gastroenteritis Symptoms by Agent

AGENT	TIME TO ONSET
Arsenic	Early
Caustics	Early
Digoxin (acute)	Early
Iron	Early
Lithium (acute)	Early
Mercury, inorganic	Early
Methylxanthines (acute, non–sustained-release)	Early
Nicotine	Early
Organophosphates	Early
Podophyllum	Early
SSRIs	Early
Abrin/ricin	Delayed 1–3 hours to days
Colchicine	Delayed 2–12 hours
Fluoride	Delayed several hours
Jatropha spp	Delayed 1–2 days
Methotrexate	Delayed 2–4 hours
Methylxanthines (sustained-release)	Delayed for several hours
Opioid withdrawal	Delayed 4–24 hours
Solanum spp	Delayed up to 2 days
Thyroid hormone	Delayed 1–11 days

TABLE 13-4 Agents that Cause Fecal Discoloration

COLOR	AGENT
Black	Acetazolamide, aluminum hydroxide, aminophylline, amphotericin B, barium, benzene, bismuth, bromides, charcoal, chloramphenicol, chlorpropamide, clindamycin, corticosteroids, cyclophosphamide, digitalis, ferrous salts, fluorouracil, formaldehyde, halides (Br, F, I), halothane, heavy metals (Ag, As, Cu, Hg, Mn, Pb, Tl), hydralazine, methotrexate, methylene blue, nitrates, NSAIDs, tetracycline, theophylline, warfarin
Blue	Boric acid, chloramphenicol, manganese dioxide, methylene blue
Yellow-green	Mercurous chloride, yellow phosphorus (stool is luminescent and smoking)
Orange/red	Phenazopyridine, rifampin
Pink	Manganese dioxide, phenolphtalein

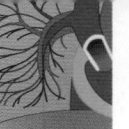

characterized by severe hemorrhagic gastroenteritis beginning 2 to 12 hours postingestion. Along with this GI symptom, dehydration, electrolyte disturbances, shock, dysrhythmias, and marked leukocytosis are found in the early phases of toxicity.[33,34] Later, bone marrow suppression, renal failure, pulmonary edema, alopecia, and neuropathic features develop. Other findings include oral dysesthesias, ileus, colitis, and hepatocellular injury. Colchicine acts through inhibition of the polymerization of tubulin into microtubules, causing mitotic metaphase arrest. As such, gastrointestinal biopsy may be diagnostic, demonstrating numerous metaphases, epithelial pseudo-stratification, loss of epithelial polarity, and frequent apoptosis.[35-37]

Podophyllum

Poisoning from podophyllum resin (made from the roots of mayapple or "wild mandrake") occurs following ingestion or dermal application and manifests with nausea, vomiting, abdominal pain, ileus, and severe diarrhea.[38,39] Symptom onset typically occurs shortly following oral ingestion, although delays of up to 10 hours have been reported.[40] Other clues to the diagnosis include the presence of a sensorimotor neuropathy, bone marrow suppression, CNS depression, and autonomic instability. Illness is similar to that caused by colchicine, as is the pathophysiology—inhibition of microtubular assembly. Additionally, podophyllum is a direct intestinal mucosal irritant, which accounts for the violent peristalsis and catharsis seen in oral poisoning.

Nicotine

Nicotine ingestion most commonly involves tobacco products and can be life threatening. One of the earliest symptoms is a burning sensation in mouth, throat, esophagus, and stomach. This is commonly followed by increased salivation, nausea, vomiting, abdominal pain, and diarrhea. Early emesis, within minutes, occurs in 16% to 63% of pediatric nicotine exposures but does not correlate with the ultimate severity of illness and therefore has limited usefulness in triage.[41] Diarrhea is delayed for 4 to 24 hours in 14% of patients.[37] A diagnostic clue is the constellation of symptoms that includes bronchorrhea, tachycardia, hypertension, pallor, seizures, fasciculations, paralysis, and ultimately hypoventilation, apnea, and cardiovascular collapse. Green tobacco sickness is an occupationally acquired form of nicotine poisoning that typically occurs in teenagers or older males who have been harvesting wet, uncured tobacco leaves. Symptoms begin 3 to 24 hours after a 6-hour exposure period and are mainly gastro-intestinal (nausea, vomiting, abdominal cramping).[42-44] Prevention can be accomplished by use of protective clothing.

Abrin/Ricin

Severe toxic gastroenteritis with hemorrhage is a hallmark of toxicity from toxalbumin-containing seeds such as castor oil plant seeds (*Ricinus communis*), *Jatropha* spp seeds, or rosary peas (*Abrus precatorius*). Abdominal pain, vomiting, and frequent heme-positive stools with tenesmus can occur as early as 1 to 3 hours postingestion or can be delayed for several days.[45-48] To some extent, the onset and severity of symptoms are thought to depend on the extent of seed mastication. Gastro-intestinal symptoms progress over 4 to 36 hours to dehydration and cardiac, renal, and hepatic toxicity in severe poisoning. Pathophysiology involves toxalbumin inhibition of the 60S ribosomal subunit, which arrests protein synthesis and causes cell death. The reticuloendothelial and highly proliferative intestinal cells are particularly vulnerable to the effects of ricin. While one masticated castor bean or rosary pea (containing up to 10 mg ricin) is potentially fatal to a toddler, the frequently cited human fatal oral dose of 1 mg/kg is unconfirmed.[49] In one study of *Jatropha* ingestions, most patients exhibited only vomiting and abdominal pain; 98% were discharged 24 to 48 hours postexposure.[50]

Trichothecene Mycotoxins

This family of dermally active toxins is produced by various molds of the genera *Fusarium*, *Stachybotrys*, and others. Anorexia, vomiting, and diarrhea, possibly hemorrhagic, can occur following either ingestion or dermal exposure to some of the more than 150 toxin derivatives. T-2 toxin gained notoriety as a lethal agent after accidental flour contamination caused a Russian civilian endemic illness termed *alimentary toxic aleukia*. In those who consumed contaminated bread, initial GI symptoms, fever, and chills progressed to a protracted illness characterized by bone marrow suppression and secondary sepsis. In another incident, those who consumed moldy rice contaminated with T-2 toxin experienced chills, dizziness, nausea, vomiting, abdominal distention, abdominal pain, and diarrhea.[51] Pancreatitis due to T-2 toxin has been reported. A clue to the diagnosis of T-2 exposure is intense burning, inflammation, and necrosis of dermally exposed skin, mucous membranes, and the respiratory tract. Pathophysiology of the illness involves the inhibition of protein synthesis and a dose-dependent decrease in gastric and intestinal blood flow.[52] One specific trichothecene mycotoxin—deoxynivalenol, or vomitoxin—consistently causes anorexia and vomiting through unclear mechanisms.[53]

Other Plants and Mycotoxins

A variety of GI syndromes occur following plant ingestion, many through unidentified mechanisms. Immediate mouth irritation can result from chewing plants with insoluble oxalates (e.g., dieffenbachia and philodendron). Emesis with minimal or absent diarrhea can result from the ingestion of certain bulbs (daffodil, jonquil, and narcissus) or wisteria seeds or flowers, owing to their direct action on the gastric mucosa and the CTZ. Irritation of the intestinal mucosa by pokeweed, holly, elderberry, or baneberry can cause rapid onset of emesis, abdominal pain, and diarrhea. Delayed gastroenteritis (up to 2 days) can be seen following the ingestion of solanine-containing plants (potato sprouts, climbing nightshade, Jerusalem cherry), horsenettle, crocus, castor bean, and rosary pea.

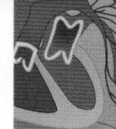

The primary toxic effect of some mushrooms is acute, early-onset gastroenteritis. Members of this "gastrointestinal irritant" class of mushrooms include *Boletus sensibilis, Entoloma lividum, Leucoagaricus putidus, Omphalotus olearius, Pholiota squarrosa,* and *Tricholoma pardinum.* Secondary dehydration or electrolyte abnormalities are described, but hepatic injury, renal failure, and neurologic symptoms are absent. (Paresthesias and tetany, when present, are ascribed to fear or hyperventilation and not to primary neurotoxicity.) The onset of symptoms following mushroom ingestion is a valuable diagnostic clue, with the most toxic species causing delayed GI symptom onset. Notable exceptions to this rule, however, are *Gomphus bonari, G. floccosus,* and *G. kauffmanii,* all associated with delayed-onset diarrhea (8 to 14 hours).

PESTICIDES/HERBICIDES

Nausea, vomiting, abdominal cramps, diarrhea, and fecal incontinence commonly occur following exposure to acetylcholinesterase inhibitors such as organophosphates, carbamates, or nerve agents.[54,55] The pattern of illness varies with route and duration of exposure.[56] In addition, organophosphates cause both pancreatitis and isolated hyperamylasemia, the latter noted in 76% of patients with acute poisoning in one series.[57] In another series, elevated serum amylase levels correlated with respiratory failure necessitating ventilatory support.[58] Puzzling gastrointestinal effects described in organophosphate poisoning include intussusception and acute hemorrhagic panesophagitis.[59,60] A clue to the diagnosis of acetylcholinesterase inhibitor poisoning is the presence of miosis, rhinorrhea, lacrimation, bronchorrhea, bronchoconstriction, CNS depression, seizures, fasciculations, and paralysis. Within the therapeutic arena, the use of reversible cholinesterase inhibitors to treat dementia is consistently associated with nausea, vomiting, and diarrhea in 30% to 50% of patients.[61]

Paraquat is a caustic herbicide and frequent suicidal agent in some countries. Ingestion is often associated with immediate mouth and throat irritation, followed by abdominal pain, nausea, vomiting, and diarrhea.[62,63] Swelling, edema, and ulceration of the mouth, pharynx, esophagus, stomach, and intestines have occurred.[61,62,64] Patients who develop GI tract injury generally have a poor prognosis.[63,65,66] Other clues to this diagnosis are severe pulmonary edema with fibrosis; renal, liver, and myocardial injury; and pancreatitis. The pathophysiology of this poisoning stems from paraquat's potent oxidizing affect and ability to promote free radical formation and redox cycling.

NONSTEROIDAL ANTI-INFLAMMATORY AGENTS/SALICYLATES

An estimated 17,000 deaths per year in the United States are related to nonsteroidal anti-inflammatory medications.[67] Gastric erosion occurs in 30% and 50% of patients taking one or greater than one NSAID respectively for 12 months, with frank ulceration in 10%.[13] These agents, including aspirin, cause extensive damage to the GI tract through both topical irritant effect and inhibition of cyclooxygenase (COX-1) in the gastric mucosa. Injury can occur even at low doses, such as those used for cardioprotection, or with the parenteral route of administration. Gold therapy, used in the treatment of arthritis, can also cause gastric erosions and panenteritis.

ETHANOL AND OTHER ALCOHOLS

Given the per capita annual consumption of 10 L in the United States, it is not surprising that alcohol-induced GI pathology is commonly encountered. Acute ingestions of greater than 8% ethanol or chronic consumption of lower concentrations can result in erosive gastritis, ulceration, and ultimately GI bleeding. (These same complications occur following the acute ingestion of rubbing alcohol, which is typically a concentrated [70%] solution of isopropanol.)[68] Interestingly, low ethanol concentrations (<5%) stimulate gastrin release and increase gastric acid secretion, as do nondistilled beer and wine.[69] While these effects are not noted with higher concentrations of ethanol or distilled products, other physiologic effects such as slowed gastric emptying and decreased lower esophageal sphincter tone and esophageal motility occur. These latter effects predispose chronic alcohol users to reflux esophagitis. Other adverse GI effects of chronic alcohol abuse include increased intestinal mucosal permeability to bacterial pathogens and decreased intestinal motility.[70,71] Despite slowed motility, diarrhea often is seen in persons with alcoholism. Diarrhea stems from alterations in intestinal digestive enzymes, abnormal biliary and pancreatic function, and malabsorption.

The effect of ethanol on the liver and pancreas is even more significant than its effect on the tubular GI tract. Acute and chronic pancreatitis are well-known complications of chronic ethanol abuse.[25] Chronic ethanol consumption has also been associated with acute hepatitis; cirrhosis, with portal hypertension and life-threatening esophageal variceal bleeding; inhibition of glycogen storage; and increased risk of hepatotoxicity following exposure to other chemicals.

METALS AND METALLOIDS
Lead

Lead is a significant environmental hazard to children and occupational hazard to adults. GI effects due to lead intoxication are well described and include abdominal colic, vomiting, constipation, diarrhea, anorexia, a metallic taste in the mouth, and weight loss.[72] Unusual instances of gastrointestinal bleeding following the ingestion of lead bullets, pyloric obstruction following the ingestion of lead glaze frit, and paralytic ileus are reported.[73-75] A clue to the diagnosis is the presence of encephalopathy, anemia, motor neuropathy (adults or children with sickle cell anemia), renal failure, gout, and hypertension. Some of the GI symptoms of lead poisoning may be explained by the ability of lead to induce GI tract smooth muscle spasm.

Iron

Although pediatric mortality due to iron poisoning has declined, accidental ingestion is still a significant

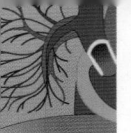

cause of morbidity. Early-onset emesis is common when greater than 20 mg/kg elemental iron is ingested. In fact, protracted vomiting is a useful clinical marker of significant iron toxicity. Gastrointestinal hemorrhage can be seen within the first few hours of severe poisoning. A delayed gastrointestinal effect is pyloric scarring, possibly leading to gastric outlet obstruction 2 to 8 weeks after overdose. Similarly, isolated distal small bowel segmental infarction or stricture following enteric-coated iron tablet ingestion is described.[76] These effects likely result from the direct corrosive effect of iron on the gastrointestinal mucosa. In fact, hemorrhage, ulceration, and necrosis of the esophagus, stomach, and bowel are common autopsy findings in fatal iron overdosing. Clues to the diagnosis of iron poisoning include hypotension (resulting from GI losses, hemorrhage, vasodilatation), hyperlactemia, metabolic acidosis, lethargy, coagulopathy, hepatic or renal dysfunction, and radio-opacities on abdominal x-ray.

Lithium

Acute lithium intoxication frequently manifests with nausea and vomiting.[77] Diarrhea can be noted, particularly after overdose with sustained-release preparations.[78,79] GI effects are reported with chronic therapeutic lithium use in 10% to 20% of patients. As with other metal salts, the mechanism of GI toxicity is one of direct corrosive injury to the intestinal mucosa. Concurrent symptoms that provide diagnostic clues include evidence of dehydration, mental status changes, tremor, neuromuscular hyperexcitability, rigidity, and fever. Hyperamylasemia without clinical evidence of pancreatitis has been reported rarely.[80]

Mercury (Inorganic)

Sources of corrosive inorganic mercury salts include stool fixatives, Chinese herbals, and (historically) disinfectants and teething powders. As with other corrosive metal salts, direct contact between the salt and the gastrointestinal mucosa results in erosion, ulceration, and necrosis. Signs and symptoms include nausea, dysphagia, vomiting, diarrhea, abdominal pain, hematemesis, and hematochezia.[81,82] Diagnostic clues include concurrent hypovolemic shock, acute renal failure, and radio-opacities on abdominal x-ray.

Arsenic

The gastrointestinal effects of arsenic vary with dose and chronicity of exposure. Within minutes to hours following significant acute arsenic ingestion, abdominal pain, vomiting, profuse watery diarrhea (sometimes described as "rice-water-like"), and GI bleeding are present.[83,84] In the absence of a history of ingestion, the diagnosis is difficult. Potential clues include multisystem involvement with cardiovascular collapse, prolonged QT interval, encephalopathy, seizures, pulmonary edema, hepatitis, renal failure, anemia, painful sensorimotor neuropathy, alopecia, hyperpigmentation, a desquamating rash, and Mees' lines. Often, burning and dryness of the mouth is reported. Breath, stool, or emesis may have a garlicky odor.[85]

Thallium

Unlike the other metal salts discussed above, GI symptoms due to thallium are generally less dramatic. In fact, constipation unresponsive to laxatives can be a more common manifestation of poisoning than symptoms of toxic gastroenteritis.[86,87] Nonetheless, nausea, vomiting, paroxysmal abdominal pain, and diarrhea are reported.[88] Gastrointestinal hemorrhage is rare.[86,89] The presence of alopecia and a painful ascending neuropathy point to this diagnosis.

Fluoride

Fluoride is present in dental, industrial, and agricultural products. Once ingested, sodium fluoride reacts with gastric acid to produce highly corrosive hydrofluoric acid, which directly injures the GI tract. In most instances, symptomatology is limited to the GI tract. Epigastric pain, nausea, dysphagia, salivation, hematemesis, and diarrhea occur with acute ingestion of greater than 3 mg/kg or with chronic therapeutic use of greater than 30 mg/day sodium fluoride.[90,91] With acute exposure, symptom onset can be delayed for several hours. The spectrum of GI injury appears to be concentration dependent, with low concentrations of fluoride (1 mg/mL) causing superficial damage to the gastric mucosa, and 13% to 20% bifluoride solutions causing significant burns to the distal esophagus, antrum, and gastric body.[92] With severe poisoning, other clues to the diagnosis include hypocalcemia, hypomagnesemia, hyperkalemia, hypotension, and dysrhythmias.

METHYLXANTHINES

Fortunately, the incidence of theophylline toxicity is declining, and over-the-counter formulations have been removed from the market. The serious nature of theophylline toxicity, however, coupled with the widespread availability of other methylxanthines (such as caffeine found as guarana in dietary supplements) warrant their discussion. GI symptoms due to methylxanthine toxicity include nausea, protracted vomiting, abdominal cramps, diarrhea, and rarely GI bleeding.[93] This symptomatology occurs in more than 80% of patients with acute intoxication compared with only 30% of those with chronic toxicity.[94-96] Emesis can be difficult to control and can interfere with attempts to give multiple-dose activated charcoal, a cornerstone of therapy. With acute overdose, sustained-release formulations can form bezoars in the GI tract.[97] Therapeutic use of theophylline is associated with increased gastric acid secretion and decreased lower esophageal tone due to smooth muscle relaxation. Gastritis or esophagitis can develop as a result. In a retrospective study of low-birth-weight infants, the use of theophylline was associated with feeding intolerance, emesis, GI bleeding, necrotizing enterocolitis, and abdominal radiographic changes (persistently enlarged bowel loops or thickened bowel wall without pneumatosis). These infants also had higher rates of systemic illness, including increased apnea or bradycardia and increased ventilatory support.[98] Clues to the diagnosis of methylxanthine poisoning include

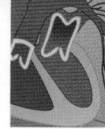

tachycardia, dysrhythmias, agitation, seizures, respiratory alkalosis, lactic acidosis, sweating, tremor, hypokalemia, hypophosphatemia, hyperglycemia, and widened pulse pressure (decreased systemic vascular resistance).

DIGOXIN

As for theophylline, the incidence of digoxin toxicity is becoming less frequent. Nausea, vomiting, and abdominal pain are some of the earliest manifestations of acute overdose. Complaints related to the GI tract are less common with chronic toxicity but are similar to those listed above, including anorexia and weight loss.[99] Diagnostic clues of digoxin toxicity include ventricular ectopy, bradydysrhythmias, syncope, hyperkalemia, lethargy, confusion, and visual disturbances.

SELECTIVE SEROTONIN REUPTAKE INHIBITORS

Because of their improved safety profile relative to cyclic antidepressants, use of selective serotonin reuptake inhibitors (SSRIs) is increasingly widespread. Nausea is a common side effect reported both in the setting of overdose and with therapeutic use.[100] Diarrhea occurred in 38% of patients receiving therapeutic doses of fluoxetine for panic attacks.[101] Fluoxetine has been shown to cause anorexia with resultant weight loss in overweight, nondepressed individuals. These effects are not surprising, given the critical role played by serotonin in the GI tract (see above). Although symptoms of acute SSRI poisoning are relatively nonspecific (dizziness, orthostasis, lethargy, and tachycardia), seizures, QRS prolongation, and QT prolongation are more likely to occur with citalopram overdose.

CORROSIVES

Acid and alkaline corrosive injury to the GI tract is covered in detail in Chapter 98. Commonly available household products that cause direct corrosive injury to the GI tract include sodium hydroxide (lye), toilet cleaners, hydrofluoric acid, ammonia, automatic dishwashing detergents, bleach, and phenols. A few agents with unique features relative to their GI tract toxicity are discussed here.

Hydrogen Peroxide

Ingestion of low concentrations of hydrogen peroxide (3% solutions) typically is not associated with symptoms but on occasion results in mild irritation to mucosal tissue and vomiting.[102] Much higher concentrations are sold as "food grade" health and nutrition products, often without child-resistant closures. Ingestion of these concentrated solutions causes oropharyngeal, esophageal, gastric, and intestinal inflammation that may progress to frank ulceration with hemorrhage. Intestinal gangrene has occurred in extreme cases. Unique among corrosives, hydrogen peroxide ingestion can be associated with the liberation of large volumes of oxygen within the GI tract, causing gastric distention, fatal colonic rupture, or systemic gas embolization.[103-105] Clues to this diagnosis include hematemesis with abdominal distention or the sudden onset of focal neurologic findings.

Boric Acid

Boric acid can be found in homes as an antiseptic, ant killer, roach powder, or homeopathic medication. Most ingestions are typified by early onset of nausea, vomiting, and diarrhea. Hemorrhagic gastroenteritis can occur with the acute ingestion of highly concentrated formulations.[106,107] A clue to the diagnosis of acute boric acid ingestion is blue-green discoloration of the emesis fluid and feces. Chronic boric acid ingestion can be suspected in patients with renal failure, an erythematous desquamating rash, and seizures.

Batteries

Children with esophageal battery lodgment may exhibit irritability, dysphagia, and refusal of oral intake. These symptoms have been mistaken for nonspecific gastritis or viral syndromes, resulting in diagnostic delays. Batteries can become trapped at anatomic narrowings at the level of the cricoid pharynx, aortic knob, gastroesophageal junction, pylorus, ileocecal junction, and Meckel's diverticulum. Esophageal impaction of a disc battery can result in burns, perforation, and mediastinitis. Such injury begins as early as 4 hours after ingestion.[108,109] In the absence of esophageal impaction on chest x-ray, most batteries will pass through the GI tract without complication.[110] Conversely, abdominal pain or other GI complaints indicate the need for urgent evaluation.

OPIOID WITHDRAWAL STATES

Opioid withdrawal is a common occurrence in the adult emergency department and newborn nursery. Symptoms of nausea, vomiting, increased bowel sounds, abdominal cramps, and dehydration are characteristic.[111] The onset, duration and severity of symptoms depend on the pharmacologic properties of the withdrawn opioid and on the pattern of its use. Heroin withdrawal, for example, begins within 4 to 24 hours after the last use and generally peaks at 36 to 48 hours.[112,113] In neonates, failure to thrive, poor suck reflex, and feeding difficulties are noted in about half of those withdrawing from heroin.[114] Similarly, poor feeding is seen in infants and young children withdrawing from chronically administered opioid analgesia. The use of opioid antagonists in those with opioid dependence commonly precipitates vomiting and diarrhea. In the setting of acute oral opioid overdose, some propose that this could theoretically restore peristalsis and further the absorption of ingested drugs, but clinical evidence of this phenomenon is lacking. Clues to the diagnosis of opioid withdrawal include dilated pupils, yawning, lacrimation, rhinorrhea, muscle cramping, myalgias, hyperactive bowel sounds, and piloerection.

THYROID HORMONES

The development of thyrotoxicosis is fairly common after chronic hormone overdose but is unusual after acute ingestion. The development of vomiting and diarrhea relate to the adrenergic effects of triiodothyronine (T_3) or levothyroxine (T_4).[115] Small or modest ingestions of T_3 usually produce few serious symptoms, whereas

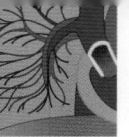
massive overdose can cause symptoms within 12 to 24 hours. Symptoms following T_4 overdose can be delayed up to 11 days as conversion to T_3 takes place. Clinical clues to the diagnosis of thyroid hormone toxicity include palpitations, tachycardia, tremor, anxiety, and behavioral changes.

PROSTAGLANDINS
Misoprostol is a prostaglandin analog used to prevent NSAID-induced GI mucosal toxicity. It is occasionally used as an abortifacient and is contraindicated during pregnancy. In overdose, severe nausea, abdominal cramps, vomiting, induction of labor, and fetal death can result. Other clues to the diagnosis of misoprostol poisoning include hyperthermia, chills, dyspnea, and vaginal bleeding.

METHOTREXATE
Methotrexate is a folate antagonist that is effective in the treatment of various malignancies, ectopic pregnancy, rheumatoid arthritis, psoriasis, inflammatory bowel disease, and other disorders. Intestinal toxicity from methotrexate is a major limitation on its use. Gastrointestinal symptoms of toxicity include nausea, vomiting, abdominal pain, diarrhea, and in severe cases hematemesis and melena with onset 2 to 4 hours postexposure. Mucositis typically begins 7 to 14 days later and persists for 4 to 7 days. It can involve the tongue, buccal mucosa, esophagus, stomach, small intestine, or colon.

Methotrexate is transported into cells by a carrier-mediated system and reaches much higher levels in the intestine than in tumor cells, where it has a substantially longer duration of inhibition of DNA synthesis.[116] Intestinal toxicity is dependent both on duration of exposure and supratherapeutic drug levels and occurs after oral or parenteral routes. Toxic methotrexate doses lead to a sustained reduction in mitoses with loss of intestinal surface absorptive cells. This desquamation of the epithelial cell lining is associated with extensive leukocytic infiltration of the lamina propria. Large areas of ulceration develop, and bleeding eventually occurs. These pathologic features are not specific to methotrexate and can be seen with various poisonous or otherwise noxious agents, a fact that contributes to the intestine's vulnerability based on its limited response to injury. Clues to the diagnosis include bone marrow suppression, hepatotoxicity, renal toxicity, seizures, encephalopathy, and focal neurologic deficits.

LAXATIVES (ACUTE TOXICITY)
Acute laxative poisoning is usually accidental, but laxatives are occasionally used in suicide attempts. Most laxatives have a wide margin of safety, and large doses must be consumed to be fatal. A classification of laxatives and representative examples for each group are presented in Box 13-2.

Acute poisoning can lead to abdominal or rectal pain, vomiting, and watery or bloody diarrhea. In extreme cases, fluid and electrolyte abnormalities and respiratory and circulatory failure can occur. The diagnosis is usually apparent from the history. For laxatives containing magnesium, signs of clinical toxicity are expected at serum magnesium levels of 4 mEq/L and worsen as the concentration rises.

Toxic Disorders Presenting with Constipation

Constipation is commonly associated with drugs that impair GI motility such as opioids and antimuscarinics. An example is severe constipation leading to intestinal perforation in a patient taking amitriptyline therapy.[117] Aluminum hydroxide, calcium carbonate antacids, and iron salts are frequent causes of constipation with therapeutic use. Other constipating agents are discussed in greater detail below.

BOX 13-2	TYPES OF LAXATIVES

Stimulant (or Irritant)
Ricinoleic acid (castor oil)
Dehydrocholic acids (Decholin)
Bisacodyl (Dulcolax)
Phenolphthalein (Ex-Lax, Correctol)*
Oxyphenisatin (Lavema)†
Aloe
Cascara sagrada
Senna (Senokot)
Danthron (Modane)

Stool Softener (Emollient)
Dioctyl sodium sulfosuccinate (DSS)
Dioctyl calcium sulfosuccinate (Surfak)
Mineral oil (Kondremul)

Saline
Magnesium hydroxide (Milk of Magnesia)
Magnesium sulfate
Sodium sulfate
Sodium phosphate (Fleet Phospho-Soda)
Sodium chloride

Osmotic
Polyethylene glycol (GoLYTELY, Colyte)
Lactulose (Chronulac, Duphalac)

Bulk
Psyllium seed derivatives (Konsyl, Metamucil, LA formula, Effer-Syllium, Serutan, Hydrocil)
Methylcellulose (Citrucel)
Bran products

Lubricant

---

*Banned for over-the-counter sale by the FDA in 1998 because of its association with tumors in animals.
†Withdrawn from distribution by the FDA because of its association with chronic active hepatitis.

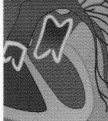

CHARCOAL

Albeit chemically inert, the mechanical effects of charcoal can cause serious complications when used to decontaminate the GI tract following drug overdose. The administration of both single- and multiple-dose activated charcoal with or without cathartic has resulted in GI obstruction or charcoal bezoar formation in patients with carbamazepine, amitriptyline, haloperidol/maprotiline, or theophylline poisoning.[118-121] Intestinal perforation due to a charcoal stercolith was reported in a patient treated with multiple-dose charcoal after an amitriptyline overdose.[122] Intestinal pseudo-obstruction (Olgivie's syndrome) has been reported in association with multidose charcoal treatment of theophylline toxicity.[123] Inadvertent introduction of charcoal into the peritoneum following gastric lavage resulted in significant morbidity.[124]

OPIOIDS

Most members of the opioid group tend to delay gastric emptying, are antisecretory, and slow intestinal motility. Cramping and constipation are therefore common in chronic opioid users. Diphenoxylate is an opioid antidiarrheal agent that exerts its antimotility effect through gastrointestinal μ receptors and is found in combination with atropine. As such, potentially delayed, prolonged anticholinergic and/or opioid toxicity with respiratory depression have occurred in children following ingestion. Loperamide similarly has antisecretory and antimotility effects through μ receptors in the gastrointestinal tract. Although not a true opiate, gastrointestinal effects from this piperidine drug mimic those observed with opioids in overdose. Specifically, constipation, abdominal pain, and ileus are described.[125] Neurologic symptoms including miosis, hypotonia, hypopnea, CNS depression, and fatality are primarily described in infants. Rarely, complications include necrotizing enterocolitis in neonates and elevation of pancreatic enzymes with pancreatitis possibly related to spasm of the sphincter of Oddi, an opioid type effect. Body packing means the ingestion or rectal insertion of multiple packets of illicit drugs for the purpose of smuggling. Complications of heroin body packing include mechanical bowel obstruction and perforation.[126,127]

ANTICHOLINERGICS

Decreased gastric motility and diminished bowel sounds are common with anticholinergic toxicity. Paralytic ileus can occur following oral, intravenous, or nebulized routes of drug administration.[128] Many psychiatric drugs, particularly the phenothiazines, are antimuscarinic and have been associated with intestinal pseudo-obstruction. The antimuscarinic toxidrome is easily recognized and includes mydriasis, xerostomia, hyperthermia, absence of axillary sweating, delirium, tachycardia, seizures, and urinary retention.

CALCIUM CHANNEL BLOCKERS

Nausea, vomiting, and ileus are common findings with calcium channel blocker overdose.[129,130] The formation of large tablet bezoars after the ingestion of sustained-release dose formulations is described. These masses may not be apparent on abdominal films. With therapeutic use, patients taking calcium channel blockers have a twofold increased risk of gastrointestinal bleeding as compared with users of β blockers.[131]

THALLIUM

Constipation in the setting of thallium toxicity is discussed above.

BOTULINUM TOXIN

Multiple forms of botulism exist. Abdominal pain, distention, decreased bowel sounds, and constipation are common features among the various types of illness in both adults and infants.[132-134] Nausea and vomiting are more variable, occurring in only 50% of patients. GI symptom onset can occur before or after the onset of paralysis, and abdominal cramping commonly persists throughout the illness. Some have proposed that GI symptoms are rare in type A botulism, occur variably with type B, and are frequent and severe with type E,[135,136] although reports to the contrary also exist.[137]

CHRONIC LAXATIVE ABUSE

Chronic laxative abuse presents with chronic constipation and occurs in three forms. One is exemplified by constipated patients who therapeutically misuse laxatives, another by bulimic patients who use laxatives for weight loss, and the third by surreptitious laxative abusers.

Cathartic colon is a consequence of prolonged irritant laxative use, typically for 15 or more years. Diarrhea, fever, and blood in the stool are *not* encountered with cathartic colon. The rectal mucosa is not friable, and findings on proctosigmoidoscopy are normal except for the possible presence of melanosis coli, which is discussed below. Clinically, cathartic colon is discovered by barium enema and therefore is primarily a radiologic diagnosis. The earliest radiographic findings are atrophy and shortening of the cecum and ileocecal valve. More extensive changes are a tubular colon with diminished or absent haustrations, which can extend to the distal descending colon. Ulcerations and rigidity are absent. The differential diagnosis of the radiologic findings includes inflammatory bowel disease and amebiasis. Systemic effects of chronic laxative abuse result from the increased fecal loss of sodium and potassium and provide clues to the diagnosis.[138] Specifically, patients can present with potassium depletion, muscle weakness, metabolic alkalosis, hyperaldosteronism, and chronic thirst. Most of the laxatives in the stimulant category are too irritating for continuous use and should be avoided.

The second group of laxative abusers is composed of patients with eating disorders such as bulimia nervosa, estimated to be present in up to 19% of college-aged women. Bulimia is distinct from anorexia and is characterized by secretive binge eating followed by various methods of purging, including cathartics, diuretics, and self-induced vomiting. These patients can develop severe metabolic disturbances and ventricular

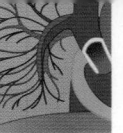

tachydysrhythmias. Sudden death can occur and may be heralded by prolongation of the QT interval.

The third group with chronic laxative abuse includes those who use laxatives surreptitiously and present with diarrhea of unknown cause or with metabolic abnormalities related to long-term laxative misuse. A key feature of the disorder is denial by the patient that he or she takes laxatives. A similar clinical picture may be noted in the setting of Munchausen syndrome by proxy, in which children are given laxatives by adults. Patients often attract at least an initial medical workup designed to rule out infectious, inflammatory, metabolic, and neoplastic diseases before abusive behavior is considered. These studies usually yield normal results. Metabolic abnormalities mentioned above may be present.

A workup for chronic laxative abuse can include blood and urine sampling for laxatives. Clinical laboratories offer a laxative abuse screen of urine for bisacodyl and danthron. Prior to its removal from the market, phenolphthalein abuse was occasionally detected by a pink color change upon alkalinization of stool with sodium hydroxide. Proctosigmoidoscopy itself can be diagnostic by showing the darkened to black mucosa of melanosis coli. Mucosal pigmentation results from melanin accumulation in macrophages in the lamina propria and can begin within 4 months of chronic laxative abuse. Pigmentation is seen most often with use of anthracene derivatives, including cascara, aloes, and senna. When the diagnosis is still suspect in the face of a normal workup, hospital admission is occasionally required, at which point symptoms should improve under direct observation. Meanwhile, stool can be collected while the patient fasts and receives intravenous glucose and fluids. A large stool volume of 500 to 1000 mL or more suggests secretory diarrhea, and the stool is evaluated for sodium, potassium, and osmolality. In secretory diarrhea, the osmolality is accounted for by twice the sodium plus potassium concentration and can be simulated by secretagogue laxatives such as senna, bisacodyl, and phenolphthalein. Osmotic diarrhea is characterized by a wide ion gap that can be caused by magnesium, sulfate, or other laxative ions, and these can be measured in the stool. Since laxatives are not addictive, persons who use them surreptitiously have a serious psychological condition, usually anxiety, depression, or chronic factitious disease with physical symptoms, also known as Munchausen syndrome.

Proctitis

Proctitis can be associated with the local application of nonsteroidal anti-inflammatory agents, ergot suppositories, and lithium, which in addition is associated with painful diarrhea.[139] Severe cases of drug-induced proctitis have been associated with rectovaginal fistulae. Rectal inflammation and hemorrhage can also result from the administration of a 95% ethanol enema.[140] Hydrogen peroxide enemas, as 3% or even more dilute solutions, have caused inflammation and, in some cases, ulceration.[141] Irrigation of endoscopes prior to sigmoidoscopy or colonoscopy with hydrogen peroxide or glutaraldehyde was associated with white rectal plaques, occasional rectal bleeding, tenesmus, and increased stool frequency.[142] Finally, through unclear mechanisms, perineal burning and irritation is well documented after the intravenous administration of dexamethasone.[143]

MECHANICAL INJURY TO THE GI TRACT

Complications occur during gastric decontamination procedures. Orogastric lavage has been associated with esophageal tears, esophageal perforation, and gastric perforation or hemorrhage. Similarly, emesis induced by syrup of ipecac has resulted in esophageal tears and gastric rupture or herniation. Whole-bowel irrigation has been associated with colonic perforation, but this was in the setting of severe underlying diverticulitis.

GASTROINTESTINAL CANCER

Several chemicals have been linked to human gastrointestinal tract malignancy. Gastric cancer can be caused by chronic exposure to asbestos, chromates, coal tar pitch volatiles, nickel compounds, and nitrosamines. Esophageal cancer is associated with asbestos exposure and is also described several years following acid and alkaline corrosive esophageal injury with stricture. Pancreatic cancer has been associated with petroleum refining, coke oven by-products, and rubber and furniture manufacturing. The development of peritoneal mesothelioma has been linked to asbestos exposure.

Ethanol consumption is linked to an increased risk of cancer of the oropharynx, esophagus, stomach, and colon, suggesting possible roles for ethanol (or its metabolites) as either tumor promoters or carcinogens. Other factors associated with chronic alcoholism confound these analyses, however. These include diminished host defenses, hormonal alterations, depletion of vitamin stores, and the occasional presence of nitrosamines, urethanes, microtoxins, inorganic arsenic, pesticides, preservatives, or antifrothing agents in some alcoholic beverages.[68,70]

TREATMENT

Specific treatments, antidotes, and indications for treatment of the many toxicities discussed above are covered in other chapters of this text. Only a few basic management points are discussed here. First, patients with chemical injury of the oropharynx, stomatitis, or angioedema must be monitored for impending airway compromise, systemic allergic reaction, or evidence of Stevens-Johnson syndrome. Those with drug-induced esophagitis generally respond to cessation of the offending drug and management of the complications. Further episodes may be prevented by ensuring that the drug is taken with sufficient liquid and upright position is maintained. Recognition of this disorder is critical

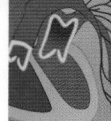

because the disease is usually reversible if discovered early. Malabsorption is usually sufficiently treated by removal of the drug from a patient's regimen and restoration of nutrient deficiencies. Cessation of excessive laxative use and correction of fluid and electrolyte disturbances is usually satisfactory treatment for cathartic colon. Bulimia nervosa and Munchausen syndrome require long-term therapy with medical, psychological, and nutritional professionals. Several investigational therapeutic strategies may someday enhance GI tract wound healing following toxic insult. These include trefoil factors, transforming growth factor β, and the manipulation of the luminal environment with supplemental polyamines or lipid mediators to accelerate mucosal repair.[10] Novel therapeutic neuronal options (e.g., substance P receptor antagonists, somatostatin analogs, and enkephalinase inhibitors) for the treatment of secretory diarrhea are under investigation.[7]

ACKNOWLEDGMENTS

The authors wish to acknowledge the contributions of William B. Strum, MD, who wrote this chapter for a previous edition, and Deborah Mouzon for her technical assistance.

REFERENCES

1. DeSesso JM, Jacobson CF: Anatomical and physiological parameters affecting gastrointestinal absorption in humans and rats. Food Chem Toxicol 2001;39:209.
2. Johnson LR: Gastrointestinal Physiology, 5th ed. St. Louis, Mosby, 1997.
3. Schneeman BO: Gastrointestinal physiology and functions. Br J Nutr 2002;88:S2–S159.
4. Camilleri M: Dyspepsia, irritable bowel syndrome, and constipation: review and what's new. Rev Gastroenterol Disord 2001;1(1):2.
5. Eglen R: Muscarinic receptors and gastrointestinal tract smooth muscle function. Life Sci 2001;68:2573.
6. Takahashi T: Pathophysiological significance of neuronal nitric oxide synthetase in the gastrointestinal tract. J Gastroenterol 2003;38:421.
7. Hansen M: The enteric nervous system. 2. Gastrointestinal functions. Pharmacol Toxicol 2003;92:240.
8. Kurz A, Sessler D: Opioid-induced bowel dysfunction. Drugs 2003;63:649.
9. Ratnapalan S, Potylitsina Y, Tan H, et al: Measuring a toddler's mouthful: toxicologic considerations. J Pediatr 2003;142:729.
10. Mammen JMV, Matthews JB: Mucosal repair in the gastrointestinal tract. Crit Care Med 2003;31:S532.
11. Palop V, Sancho A, Morales-Olivas FJ, et al: Fluoxetine-associated stomatitis. Ann Pharmacother 1997;31:1478.
12. Moghadam BKH, Gier R, Thurlow T: Extensive oral mucosal ulcerations caused by misuse of a commercial mouthwash. Cutis 1999;64:131.
13. Bateman DN: Gastrointestinal disorders. In Davies DM (ed): Textbook of Adverse Drug Reactions, 4th ed. Oxford, Oxford University Press, 1991, pp 230–244.
14. Greig JD: Oral contraceptives and intestinal ischaemia. J R Coll Gen Pract 1989;39:76.
15. Nothmann BJ, Chittinanad S, Schuster MM: Reversible mesenteric vascular occlusion associated with oral contraceptives. Am J Dig Dis 1973;18:361.
16. Donovan JW, O'Donnell S, Burkhart K, et al: Calcium channel blocker overdose causing mesenteric ischemia (abstract). J Toxicol Clin Toxicol 1999;37:628.
17. Brown DN, Rosenholtz MJ, Marshall JB: Ischemic colitis related to cocaine abuse. Am J Gastroenterol 1994;89:1558.
18. Muniz AE, Evans T: Acute gastrointestinal manifestations associated with use of crack. Am J Emerg Med 2001;19:61.
19. Mustard R, Gray R, Maziak D, et al: Visceral infarction caused by cocaine abuse: a case report. Surgery 1992;112:951.
20. Uva JL: Spontaneous pneumothoraces, pneumomediastinum, and pneumoperitoneum: consequences of smoking crack cocaine. Pediatr Emerg Care 1997;13:24.
21. Riggs D, Weibley RE: Acute hemorrhagic diarrhea and cardiovascular collapse in a young child owing to environmentally acquired cocaine. Pediatr Emerg Care 1991;7:154.
22. Chu J, Hoffman RS, Nelson LS: Metformin-associated lactic acidosis versus mesenteric ischemia. J Toxicol Clin Toxicol 2001;39:511.
23. Gan SC, Barr J, Arieff AI, et al: Biguanide-associated lactic acidosis: case report and review of the literature. Arch Intern Med 1992;152:2333.
24. Ben MH, Thabet H, Zaghdoudi I, et al: Metformin associated acute pancreatitis. Vet Hum Toxicol 2002;44:47.
25. Hermann LS, Schersten B, Bitzen PO, et al: Therapeutic comparison of metformin and sulfonylurea, alone and in various combinations: a double-blind controlled study. Diabetes Care 1994;17:1100.
26. Braganza JM, Foster JR: Toxicology of the pancreas. In Ballantyne B, Marro T, Syverson T (eds): General and Applied Toxicology, 2nd ed. London, Macmillan Reference, 2004, p 893.
27. Wilmink T, Frick TW: Drug-induced pancreatitis. Drug Safety 1996;14:406.
28. Michielsen P, Fierens H, Van Maercke Y: Drug-induced gallbladder disease. Drug Safety 1992;7:32.
29. Palmer RH: Prevalence of gallstones in hyperlipidemics and incidence during treatment with clofibrate and/or cholestyramine. Trans Assoc Am Physicians 1978;91:424.
30. Schaud UB, Suter S, Gianelli-Borradori A, et al: A comparison of ceftriaxone and cefuroxime for the treatment of bacterial meningitis in children. N Engl J Med 1990;322:141.
31. Pearman K: Cocaine: a review. J Laryngol Otol 1979;93:1191.
32. Traub SJ, Su M, Hoffman RS, et al: Use of pharmaceutical promotility agents in the treatment of body packers. Am J Emerg Med 2003;21(6):511.
33. Harris RD, Gillett MJ: Colchicine poisoning—overview and new directions. Emerg Med 1998;10:161.
34. Kubler PA: Fatal colchicine toxicity. Med J Aust 2000;172:498.
35. Weakley-Jones B, Gerber JE, Biggs G: Colchicine poisoning. Case report of two homicides. Am J Forensic Med Pathol 2001;22:203.
36. Gilbert JD, Byard RW: Epithelial cell mitotic arrest—a useful postmortem histologic marker in cases of possible colchicine toxicity. Forensic Sci Int 2002;126:150.
37. Iacobuzio-Donahue CA, Lee EL, Abraham SC, et al: Colchicine toxicity:distinct morphologic findings in gastrointestinal biopsies. Am J Surg Pathol 2001;25:1067.
38. Conard PF, Hanna N, Rosenblum M, et al: Delayed recognition of podophyllum toxicity in a patient receiving epidural morphine. Anesth Analg 1990;71:191.
39. Juurlink DN, Sellens C, Tompson M, et al: Danger in the doctor's office: two cases of severe neurologic sequelae after ingestion of podophyllin (abstract). J Toxicol Clin Toxicol 1999;37:620.
40. O'Mahony S, Keohane C, Jacobs J, et al: Neuropathy due to podophyllin intoxication. J Neurol 1990;237:110.
41. Smolinske SC, Spoerke DG, Spiller SK, et al: Cigarette and nicotine chewing gum toxicity in children. Hum Toxicol 1988;7:27.
42. Ross MP, Revolinski D, Taurman L, et al: Detection of a pediatric occupational poisoning in Kentucky (abstract). Vet Hum Toxicol 1994;36:360.
43. McKnight RH, Levine EJ, Rodgers GC: Detection of green tobacco sickness by a regional poison center. Vet Hum Toxicol 1994;36:505.
44. Hipke ME: Green tobacco sickness. South Med J 1993;86:989.
45. Kopferschmitt J, Flesch F, Lugnier A, et al: Acute voluntary intoxication by ricin. Hum Toxicol 1983;2:239.
46. Aplin PJ, Eliseo T: Ingestion of castor oil plant seeds. Med J Aust 1997;167:260.
47. Palatnick W, Tenenbein M: Hepatotoxicity from castor bean ingestion in a child. Clin Toxicol 2000;38:67.
48. Brugsch HG: Toxic hazards: the castor bean. N Engl J Med 1960;262:1039.

49. Bradberry SM, Dickers KJ, Rice P, et al: Ricin poisoning. Toxicol Rev 2003;22(1):65.

50. Makalinao IR: A descriptive study on the clinical profile of Jatropa seed poisoning. Vet Hum Toxicol 1993;35:330.

51. Wang ZG, Fen JN, Tong Z: Human toxicosis caused by moldy rice contaminated with fusarium and T-2 toxin. Biomed Environ Sci 1993;6:65.

52. Beasley VR, Lundeen GR, Poppenga RH, et al: Distribution of blood flow to the gastrointestinal tract of swine during T-2 toxin-induced shock. Fundam Appl Toxicol 1987;9:588.

53. Rotter BA, Prelusky DB, Pestka JJ: Toxicology of deoxynivalenol (vomitoxin). J Toxicol Environ Health 1996;48:1.

54. Wang CL, Chuang HY, Chang CY, et al: An unusual case of organophosphate intoxication of a worker in a plastic bottle recycling plant: an important reminder. Environ Health Perspect 2000;108:1103.

55. Wu ML, Deng JF, Tsai WJ, et al: Food poisoning due to methamidophos-contaminated vegetables. Clin Toxicol 2001;39(4):333.

56. Bjornsdottir US, Smith D: Case report—South African religious leader with hyperventilation, hypophosphataemia, and respiratory arrest. Lancet 1999;354:2130.

57. Lee WC, Yang CC, Deng JF, et al: The clinical significance of hyperamylasemia in organophosphate poisoning. J Toxicol Clin Toxicol 1998;37:673.

58. Matsumiya N, Tanaka M, Iwai M, et al: Elevated amylase is related to the development of respiratory failure in organophosphate poisoning. Hum Exp Toxicol 1996;15:250.

59. Koga H, Yoshinaga M, Aoyagi K, et al: Hemorrhagic panesophagitis after acute organophosphorus poisoning. Gastrointest Endosc 1999;49:642.

60. Crispen C, Kempf J, Greydanus DE, et al: Intussusception as a possible complication of organophosphate overdose and/or treatment. Clin Pediatr 1985;24:140.

61. Williams BR, Nazarians A, Gill MA: A review of rivastigmine: a reversible cholinesterase inhibitor. Clin Ther 2003;25(6):1634.

62. Bismuth C, Garnier R, Baud FJ, et al: Paraquat poisoning: an overview of the current status. Drug Safety 1990;5:243.

63. Pond SM: Manifestations and management of paraquat poisoning. Med J Aust 1990;152:256.

64. Singh S, Bambery P, Chaudhry D, et al: Fatal paraquat poisoning: report of two cases. J Assoc Physicians India 1999;47:831.

65. Honore P, Hantson PH, Fauville JPH, et al: Paraquat poisoning. Acta Clin Belg 1994;49:220.

66. Kalabalikis P, Hatzis T, Papadatos J, et al: Paraquat poisoning in a family. Vet Hum Toxicol 2001;43:31.

67. Whittle BJR: Gastrointestinal effects of nonsteroidal anti-inflammatory drugs. Fundam Clin Pharmacol 2003;17:301.

68. Zaman F, Pervez A, Abreo K: Isopropyl alcohol intoxication: a diagnostic challenge. Am J Kidney Dis 2002;40:E12.

69. Stermer E: Alcohol consumption and the gastrointestinal tract. Isr Med Assoc J 2002;4:200.

70. Thomson ABR, Keelan M, Thiesen A, et al: Small bowel review: diseases of the small intestine. Dig Dis Sci 2001;46(12):2555.

71. Bujanda L: The effects of alcohol consumption upon the gastrointestinal tract. Am J Gastroenterol 2000;95(12):3374.

72. Van Vonderen MGA, Klinkenberg-Knol EC, Craanen ME, et al: Severe gastrointestinal symptoms due to lead poisoning from Indian traditional medicine (letter). Am J Gastroenterol 2000;95:1591.

73. McNutt TK, Dethlefsen M, Shah R, et al: Bite the bullet: lead poisoning after ingestion of 206 lead bullets (abstract). J Toxicol Clin Toxicol 2000;38:549.

74. Zwiener RJ, Owensby JE, Belknap WM, et al: Lead poisoning presenting as intestinal ileus in a child (letter). Am J Dis Child 1990;144:524.

75. Snook C, Spadafora M, Tsipis G, et al: Pyloric obstruction from lead glaze ingestion (abstract). Vet Hum Toxicol 1992;34:339.

76. Tenenbein M, Littman C, Stimpson RE: Gastrointestinal pathology in adult iron overdose. Clin Toxicol 1990;28:311.

77. Bailey B, McGuigan M: Lithium poisoning from a poison control center perspective. Ther Drug Monit 2000;22:650.

78. Bosinski T, Bailie GR, Eisele G: Massive and extended rebound of serum lithium concentrations following hemodialysis in two chronic overdose cases (letter). Am J Emerg Med 1998;16:98.

79. Ehrlich BE, Diamond JM: Lithium absorption: implications for sustained-release lithium preparations. Lancet 1983;1:306.

80. Matsis PP, Fisher RA, Tasman-Jones C: Acute lithium toxicit—chorea, hypercalcemia and hyperamylasemia. Aust N Z J Med 1989;19:718.

81. Toet AE, Dijk AV, Savelkoul TJF, et al: Mercury kinetics in a case of severe mercuric chloride poisoning treated with dimercapto-1-propane sulphonate (DMPS). Hum Exp Toxicol 1994;13:11.

82. Wang RY, Henry GC, Fine J, et al: Mercuric chloride poisonings from stool fixative ingestion (abstract). Vet Hum Toxicol 1992;34:341.

83. Quatrehomme G, Ricq O, Lapalus P, et al: Acute arsenic intoxication: forensic and toxicologic aspects (an observation). J Forensic Sci 1992;37:1163.

84. Bartolome B, Cordoba S, Nieto S, et al: Acute arsenic poisoning: clinical and histopathological features. Br J Dermatol 1999;141:1106.

85. Lee DC, Roberts JR, Kelly JJ, et al: Whole-bowel irrigation as an adjunct in the treatment of radiopaque arsenic (letter). Am J Emerg Med 1995;13:244.

86. Malbrain MLNG, Lambrecht GLY, Zandijk E, et al: Treatment of severe thallium intoxication. Clin Toxicol 1997;35(1):97.

87. Saddique A, Peterson CD: Thallium poisoning: a review. Vet Hum Toxicol 1983;25:16.

88. Desenclos JCA, Wilder MH, Coppenger GW, et al: Thallium poisoning: an outbreak in Florida, 1988. South Med J 1992;85:1203.

89. Meggs WJ, Hoffman S, Shih RD, et al: Thallium poisoning from maliciously contaminated food. Clin Toxicol 1994;32:723.

90. Gessner BD, Beller M, Middaugh JP, et al: Acute fluoride poisoning from a public water system. N Engl J Med 1994;330:95–99.

91. Das TK, Susheela AK, Gupta IP, et al: Toxic effects of chronic fluoride ingestion on the upper gastrointestinal tract. J Clin Gastroenterol 1994;18:194.

92. Swanson L, Filandrinos DT, Shevlin JM, et al: Death from accidental ingestion of an ammonium and sodium bifluoride glass etching compound (abstract). Vet Hum Toxicol 1993;35:351.

93. Paloucek FP, Rodvold KA: Evaluation of theophylline overdoses and toxicities. Ann Emerg Med 1988;17:135.

94. Gaudreault P, Wason S, Lovejoy FH: Acute pediatric theophylline overdose: a summary of 28 cases. J Pediatr 1983;102:474.

95. Sessler CN, Glauser FL, Cooper KR: Treatment of theophylline toxicity with oral activated charcoal. Chest 1985;87:325.

96. Shannon M: Predictors of major toxicity after theophylline overdose. Ann Intern Med 1993;119:1161.

97. Bernstein G, Jehle D, Bernaski E, et al: Failure of gastric emptying and charcoal administration in fatal sustained-release theophylline overdose: pharmacobezoar formation. Ann Emerg Med 1992;21:1388.

98. Hufnal-Miller CA, Blackmon L, Baumgart S, et al: Enteral theophylline and necrotizing enterocolitis in the low-birthweight infant. Clin Pediatr (Phila) 1993;32:647.

99. Gittelman MA, Stephan M, Perry H: Acute pediatric digoxin ingestion. Pediatr Emerg Care 1999;15:359.

100. Borys DJ, Setzer SC, Ling LJ, et al: Acute fluoxetine overdose: a report of 234 cases. Am J Emerg Med 1992;10:115.

101. Gorman JM, Liebowitz MR, Fyer AJ, et al: An open trial of fluoxetine in the treatment of panic attacks. J Clin Psychopharmacol 1987;7:329.

102. Mofenson H, Caraccio T, Wheeler J, et al: Toxicity of 3% hydrogen peroxide (H_2O_2) otc. J Tox Clin Tox 1995;33:488.

103. Christensen DW, Faught WE, Black RE, et al: Fatal oxygen embolization after hydrogen peroxide ingestion. Crit Care Med 1992;20:543.

104. Luu TA, Kelley MT, Strauch JA, et al: Portal vein gas embolism from hydrogen peroxide ingestion. Ann Emerg Med 1992;21:1391.

105. Ijichi T, Itoh T, Sakai R, et al: Multiple brain gas embolism after ingestion of concentrated hydrogen peroxide. Neurology 1997;48:277.

106. Restuccio A, Mortensen ME, Kelley M: Fatal ingestion of boric acid in an adult. Am J Emerg Med 1992;10:545.

107. Litovitz TL, Klein-Schwartz W, Oderda GM, et al: Clinical manifestations of toxicity in a series of 784 boric acid ingestions. Am J Emerg Med 1988;6:209.

108. Litovitz TL: Button battery ingestions: a review of 56 cases. JAMA 1983;249:2502.

109. Gossweiler B, Truttmann B, Guirguis M, et al: Ingestion of button batteries—management (abstract). J Toxicol Clin Toxicol 1999;37:386.

110. Litovitz T, Schmitz BF: Ingestion of cylindrical and button batteries: an analysis of 2382 cases. Pediatrics 1992;89:747.

111. O'Connor PG, Fiellin DA: Pharmacologic treatment of heroin-dependent patients. Ann Intern Med 2000;133:40.

112. Farrell M: Opiate withdrawal. Addiction 1994;89:1471.

113. Cowan DT, Allan LG, Libretto SE, et al: Opioid drugs: a comparative survey of therapeutic and "street" use. Pain Med 2001;2:193.

114. Lifshitz M, Gavrilov V, Galil A, et al: A four year survey of neonatal narcotic withdrawal: evaluation and treatment. Isr Med Assoc J 2001;3:17.

115. Sola E, Gomez-Balaguer M, Morillas C, et al: Massive triiodothyronine intoxication: efficacy of hemoperfusion. Thyroid 2002;12:637.

116. Sirotnak FM, Moccio DM: Pharmacokinetic basis of differences in methotrexate sensitivity of normal proliferative tissue in the mouse. Cancer Res 1980;40:1230.

117. Cass AJ. Stercoral perforation: case of drug-induced impaction. BMJ 1978;2(6142):932.

118. Watson WA, Cremer KF, Chapman JA: Gastrointestinal obstruction associated with multiple-dose activated charcoal. J Emerg Med 1986;4:401.

119. Ray MJ, Padin R, Condie JD, et al: Charcoal bezoar: small-bowel obstruction secondary to amitryptyline overdose therapy. Dig Dis Sci 1988;33:106.

120. Flores F, Battle WS: Intestinal obstruction secondary to activated charcoal. Contemp Surg 1987;30:57–59.

121. Goulbourne K, Cisek JE: Small-bowel obstruction secondary to activated charcoal and adhesions. Ann Emerg Med 1994;24:108.

122. Gomez HF, Brent JA, Munoz DC, et al: Charcoal stercolith with intestinal perforation in a patient treated for amitriptyline ingestion. J Emerg Med 1994;12:57.

123. Brubacher JR, Levine B, Hoffman RS: Intestinal pseudo-obstruction (Ogilvie's syndrome) in theophylline overdose. Vet Hum Toxicol 1996;38:368.

124. Mariani PJ, Pook N: Gastrointestinal tract perforation with charcoal peritoneum complicating orogastric intubation and lavage. Ann Emerg Med 1993;22:606.

125. Litovitz T, Clancy C, Korberly B, et al: Surveillance of loperamide ingestions: an analysis of 216 poison center reports. Clin Toxicol 1997;35:11.

126. Hutchins KD, Pierre-Louis PJB, Zaretski L, et al: Heroin body packing: three fatal cases of intestinal perforation. J Forensic Sci 2000;45:42.

127. Utecht MJ, Stone AF, McCarron MM: Heroin body packers. J Emerg Med 1993;11:33.

128. Markus H: Paralytic ileus associated with ipratropium (letter). Lancet 1990;335(8699):1224.

129. Belson MG, Gorman SE, Sullivan K, et al: Calcium channel blocker ingestions in children. Am J Emerg Med 2000;18:581.

130. Morimoto S, Sasaki S, Kiyama M, et al: Sustained-release diltiazem overdose. J Hum Hypertens 1999;13:643.

131. Kaplan RC, Heckbert SR, Koepsell TD, et al: Use of calcium channel blockers and risk of hospitalized gastrointestinal tract bleeding. Arch Intern Med 2000;160:1849.

132. Werner SB, Chin J: Botulism—diagnosis, management and public health considerations. Calif Med 1973;118:84.

133. Schmidt RD, Schmidt TW: Infant botulism: a case series and review of the literature. J Emerg Med 1992;10:713.

134. Type B botulism associated with roasted eggplant in oil—Italy, 1993. MMWR Morb Mortal Wkly Rep 1995 Jan 20;44(2):33–36.

135. Koenig MG, Drutz DJ, Mushlin AI, et al: Type B botulism in man. Am J Med 1967;42:208.

136. Badhey H, Cleri DJ, D'Amato RF, et al: Two fatal cases of type E adult food-borne botulism with early symptoms and terminal neurologic signs. J Clin Microbiol 1986;23:616.

137. Hughes JM, Blumenthal JR, Merson MH, et al: Clinical features of types A and B food-borne botulism. Ann Intern Med 1981;95:442.

138. Gattuso JM, Kamm MA: Adverse effects of drugs used in management of constipation and diarrhea. Drug Safety 1994;10:47.

139. Perrier A, Martin PY, Favre H, et al: Very severe self-poisoning lithium carbonate intoxication causing a myocardial infarction. Chest 1991;100:863.

140. Triantafillidis JK, Vekini J, Nicolakis D, et al: Ethanol-induced proctitis: another kind of chemical proctitis (letter). 1994;89:1270.

141. Meyer CT, Brand M, DeLuca VA, et al: Hydrogen peroxide colitis: a report of three patients. J Clin Gastroenterol 1981;3:31.

142. Jonas G, Mahoney A, Murray J, et al: Chemical colitis due to endoscope cleaning solutions: a mimic of pseudomembranous colitis. Gastroenterology 1988;95:1403.

143. Baharav E, Harpaz D, Mittelman M, et al: Dexamethasone-induced perineal irritation. N Engl J Med 1986;314:515.

14 *Hematologic Consequences of Poisoning*

STEVEN C. CURRY, MD

This chapter provides an overview of hematologic issues confronted by toxicologists caring for patients who are suffering from acute or chronic poisoning. The thousands of pharmaceutical agents that produce adverse hematologic effects when given at therapeutic doses (e.g., agranulocytosis, aplastic anemia, and thrombocytopenia) or at intentionally toxic doses (e.g., chemotherapy) are not the subject of this chapter. Details concerning specific agents are found in other chapters of this text. The reader is also referred to Chapter 66 for a discussion of thrombolytic agents and anticoagulants.

ERYTHROCYTES

Oxidant Stress

Oxidant stress, or the removal of electrons from molecules, results in three major disorders of toxicologic interest. The removal of electrons from the protein portion of hemoglobin produces *Heinz body hemolytic anemia*. The removal of electrons from iron found in hemoglobin produces *methemoglobinemia*. The oxidation of hemoglobin's porphyrin ring by sulfur produces *sulfhemoglobinemia*. These three disorders are intertwined with respect to the pathophysiology, occurrence,[1] diagnosis, and treatment of poisonings with oxidizing agents (Fig. 14-1).

In many instances, the parent drug or toxin producing hemolysis, methemoglobinemia, or sulfhemoglobinemia possesses no significant oxidizing potential in vivo. Oxidant stress in this setting is caused by electrophilic metabolites, which are frequently generated from metabolism by cytochrome P-450 enzymes. For example, dapsone and sulfonamides are metabolized to hydroxylamines that are responsible for the consequences of oxidant stress.

The mature erythrocyte lacks mitochondria and depends on glycolysis and the hexose monophosphate shunt for energy production (Fig. 14-2). Glycolysis fulfills the cell's adenosine triphosphate and NADH (nicotinamide adenine dinucleotide, reduced form) requirements, the latter being essential to the maintenance of low fractions of methemoglobin. In contrast, the hexose monophosphate shunt mainly serves to facilitate the formation of NADPH (reduced NAD phosphate), which protects against oxidant-induced hemolysis.[2]

Hemolysis

The mature erythrocyte continually undergoes oxidant stress from various sources, including food, infection, oxygen, drugs, and chemicals. Oxidation of the protein portion of hemoglobin (i.e., the removal of an electron from globin) results in denaturation of hemoglobin and attachment of damaged protein to the internal cell membrane. This denatured hemoglobin is visible as Heinz bodies on histologic examination of blood smears with special staining. Red cells containing denatured hemoglobin are removed from the circulation primarily by the spleen. The cells are trapped in the spleen's microcirculation, where they are destroyed; this produces

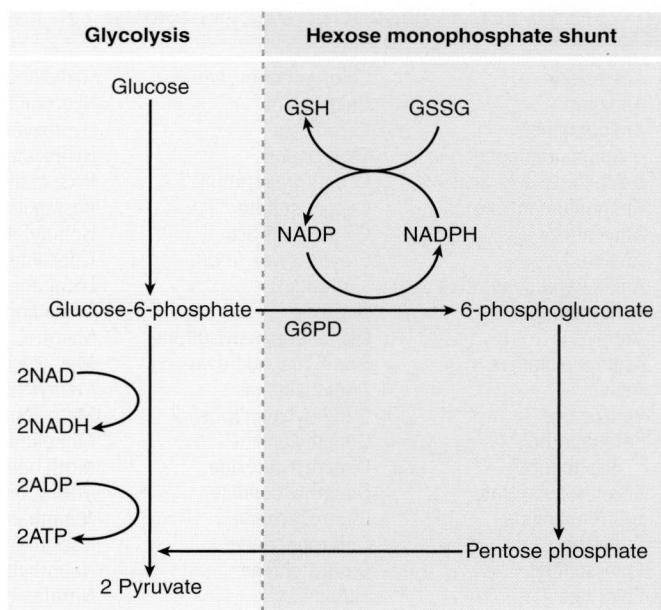

FIGURE 14-2 Metabolism in the erythrocyte. ADP, adenosine diphosphate; ATP, adenosine triphosphate; GSH, reduced glutathione; G6PD, glucose-6-phosphate dehydrogenase; GSSG, oxidized glutathione; NAD, nicotine adenine dinucleotide; NADH, reduced NAD; NADP, nicotine adenine dinucleotide phosphate; NADPH, reduced NADP.

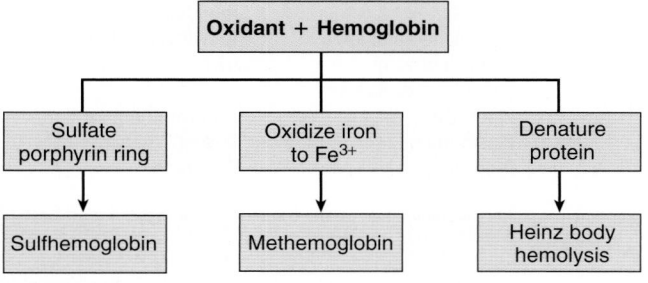

FIGURE 14-1 Results of oxidation of hemoglobin.

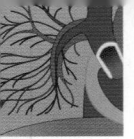

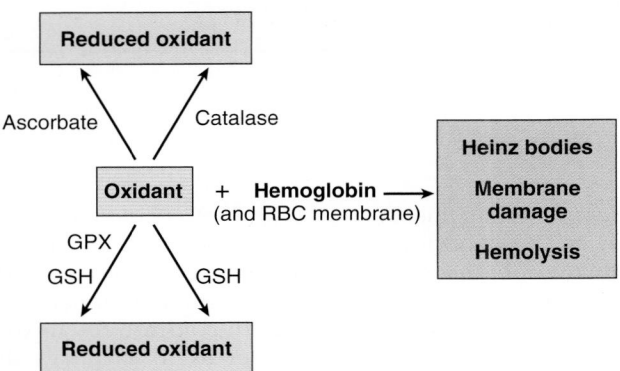

FIGURE 14-3 Inactivation of oxidants to prevent hemolysis. GPX, glutathione peroxidase.

hemoglobin.[2] Reduced glutathione, both nonenzymatically and enzymatically with glutathione peroxidase, is responsible for most reducing capacity in this regard. Catalase reduces hydrogen peroxide, and ascorbate is a mild reducing agent (Fig. 14-3).

Adequate stores of reduced glutathione are maintained within the erythrocyte through conversion of NADPH to NADP (see Fig. 14-2). In turn, NADPH formation requires a properly functioning hexose monophosphate shunt. Patients with the various forms of congenital deficiency of glucose-6-phosphate dehydrogenase (G6PD), the first enzyme in the hexose monophosphate shunt, can be predisposed to hemolysis by sources of oxidant stress that would not affect the ordinary phenotype. The most common sources of oxidant stress in these patients are infection, drugs, and food. However, *Heinz body hemolysis can be produced in anyone* (i.e., normal phenotypes) *if oxidant stress is sufficiently severe* (i.e., after ingestion of dapsone or aniline).

mainly an extravascular hemolysis (nonspherocytic).[3] Oxidant stress may produce hemolysis by several additional mechanisms as well, including the depletion of intracellular glutathione stores with direct damage to the erythrocytic membrane, and the inactivation of several enzymes needed for erythrocyte integrity. In the face of tremendous oxidant stress (e.g., arsine), hemolysis may occur intravascularly as well.

The main mechanism by which the erythrocyte protects itself against oxidant-induced hemolysis is to reduce oxidants before they have a chance to denature

Not surprisingly, substances capable of causing oxidant-induced hemolysis (Box 14-1) share the ability to produce methemoglobinemia and sulfhemoglobinemia. However, some agents are better known for the hemolytic activity they induce than for accompanying dyshemoglobinemias. As examples, arsine and stibine cause massive hemolysis and death following inhalation. Ingestion of naphthalene results in the formation of α-naphthol, a metabolite that is responsible for hemolysis. Patients ingesting, aspirating, or inhaling large amounts of gasoline also can experience significant hemolysis,

BOX 14-1	AGENTS PRODUCING OXIDANT STRESS*			
Acetanilid	Chloronitrobenzene	Hydrazines	p-Nitroaniline	Primaquine
Alloxans	Chloroquine	Hydroquinone	Nitrobenzene and its	Pyridine
Aminophenols	Chromates	Hydroxyacetanilid	derivatives	Pyridium
p-Aminopropiophenone	Clofazimine	Hydroxylamine	Nitroethane	Pyrogallol
p-Aminosalicylic acid	Cobalt preparations	Inks, marking	Nitrofurans	Quinones
Ammonium nitrate	Copper sulfate	Ifosfamide	Nitrogen oxide	Resorcinol
Amyl nitrite	Corning extract	Isobutyl nitrite	Nitroglycerin	Shoe dye or polish
Aniline dyes	Crayons, wax (red/	Lidocaine	Nitrophenol	Spinach
Aniline and derivatives	orange)†	Local anesthetics	Nitrosobenzene	Sulfomethane
Anilinoethanol	Dapsone	Menadione	Pamaquine	Sulfonamides
Antipyrine	Diaminodiphenylsulfone	Menthol	Pentaerythritol	Sulfones
Aromatic amines	Diesel fuel additives	Methylacetanilid	tetranitrate	Tetralin
Arsine	Dimethylamine	Methylene blue	Phenacetin	Tetranitromethane
Benzocaine	Dimethylaminophenol	Metoclopramide	Phenazopyridine	tetronal
Betanaphthol	Dimethylaniline	Monolinuron	Phenetidine	Toluenediamine
disulfonate	Dimethylsulfoxide	Moth balls	Phenols	Toluidine
Bismuth subnitrate	Dimethyltoluidine	Mushrooms	Phenylenediamine	Toluylhydroxylamine
p-Bromoaniline	Dinitrobenzene	Naphthalene	Phenylhydrazine	Trichlorocarbanilide
Cetrimide	Dinitrophenols	Naphthol	Phenylhydroxylamine	(TCC)
Chloranilines	Dinitrotoluene	Naphthylamines	Piperazine	Trinitrotoluene
Chlorates	Flutamide	Nitrates	Plasmoquine	Trional
Chlorobenzene	Food additives	Nitrites	Prilocaine	Valproate

*Poisoning by these agents variously produces Heinz body hemolytic anemia, methemoglobinemia, sulfhemoglobinemia, or any combination of these. Agents best known for causing sulfhemoglobinemia are listed in Box 14-4.
†Children's crayons made in the United States are safe.

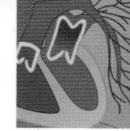

although the exact cause of this outcome is not clear. Perhaps naphthalene, a component of gasoline, is also responsible for hemolysis in gasoline poisoning. Chlorates and chromates produce both severe hemolysis and methemoglobinemia.

The diagnosis of hemolysis is based on the demonstration of a decrease in blood hemoglobin concentration, an increase in plasma free hemoglobin concentration, and a decrease in serum haptoglobin concentration. Other diagnostic clues include hemoglobinuria (after plasma concentrations of hemoglobin have become sufficiently elevated) and the presence of Heinz bodies (confirmed by special staining technique). Heinz bodies are not detectable on a routine Wright stain of blood, but "bite cells" or other abnormally shaped cells may be noted.[4] Spherocytes are typically absent or only mildly increased in number. Reticulocytosis is delayed for several days after onset of hemolysis. Although hemolysis may occur early after poisoning (e.g., with chlorate toxicity), it may not become clinically apparent until several days after ingestion. Other complications of hemolysis include hyperkalemia, pigment nephropathy, and jaundice. In severe cases, impaired oxygen-carrying capacity results in metabolic acidosis, brain failure, and cardiovascular collapse. Methemoglobinemia and, occasionally, sulfhemoglobinemia may accompany Heinz body hemolytic anemia, and evidence of such a combination should be sought.

In general, treatment is supportive and includes giving blood transfusions, ensuring a brisk urine output, and monitoring for hyperkalemia. Specific therapies may be indicated in poisonings with specific toxins (e.g., exchange transfusions for arsine; D-penicillamine therapy for copper). Intravenous administration of N-acetylcysteine prevents severe decreases in whole blood glutathione concentration in cats suffering from acetaminophen-induced methemoglobinemia (this is not a problem in humans).[5] This finding suggests that N-acetylcysteine might be effective in preventing or lessening oxidant-induced hemolysis in humans with acute poisonings, but this conjecture has not been proved.

METHEMOGLOBINEMIA

Pathophysiology

Reduced hemoglobin (deoxyhemoglobin) contains four heme groups, each with a ferrous (Fe^{2+}) ion capable of binding and transporting oxygen. Oxidation (removal of an electron) of iron to the ferric (Fe^{3+}) state produces *methemoglobin*. The fact that oxidant stress produces both denaturation of hemoglobin (Heinz body hemolytic anemia) and methemoglobin explains the common coexistence of hemolysis and methemoglobinemia (see Fig. 14-1).

Methemoglobin continually forms in erythrocytes, to a large extent from the oxidizing power of oxygen. Methemoglobin fractions are most commonly reported in percentages. These values represent the total percentage of hemoglobin pigments present as methemoglobin. Normally, methemoglobin fractions in circulating whole blood are less than 1% to 2%. When fractions exceed this value, methemoglobinemia is said to be present. Although the term *hemoglobinemia* means the presence of excess hemoglobin in plasma, the term *methemoglobinemia* means the presence of elevated circulating fractions of methemoglobin within erythrocytes.

Methemoglobin cannot transport oxygen and thus produces a functional anemia. Furthermore, ferric heme groups impair unloading of oxygen by ferrous heme on the same hemoglobin tetramer, shifting the oxyhemoglobin dissociation curve to the left and thereby further impeding oxygen delivery.[2] Thus, the signs and symptoms of methemoglobinemia result from the impairment of oxygen delivery to tissues.

Unlike hemoglobin, methemoglobin is dark brown. Five grams of normal reduced hemoglobin per deciliter of capillary blood produces visible cyanosis. However, only 1.5 g of methemoglobin per deciliter of blood produces noticeable discoloration. In a patient without anemia, methemoglobin fractions of approximately 10% to 15% produce cyanosis, even before the impairment of oxygen delivery becomes significant. As methemoglobin fractions increase to more than 20% in the nonanemic patient, cardiovascular and central nervous system signs develop and include headache, dyspnea, tachypnea, tachycardia, and mild hypertension. Further increases in methemoglobin fractions into the 40% to 50% range (without anemia) produce confusion, lethargy, and metabolic acidosis. Additional elevation results in coma, seizures, bradyrhythmias, ventricular dysrhythmias, and hypotension; when methemoglobin fractions approach 70%, death ensues. The anemic patient suffers more severe symptoms at given methemoglobin fractions than does the nonanemic patient. In addition, anemic patients exhibit less profound cyanosis at given methemoglobin fractions.

The inactivation of oxidants is relatively unimportant in maintaining methemoglobin fractions within the normal range. For example, patients with congenital glutathione deficiency, G6PD deficiency, catalase deficiency, and scurvy do not have elevated methemoglobin fractions. Rather, methemoglobin fractions are maintained within the normal range by immediate reduction back to ferrous hemoglobin after spontaneous formation.

Cytochrome-b$_5$ reductase is responsible for essentially all methemoglobin reduction in vivo (Fig. 14-4).[6] In the step mediated by this enzyme, electrons are transferred from NADH (from glycolysis) to cytochrome b_5 and then to methemoglobin to form deoxyhemoglobin. Thus, the normal functioning of this enzymatic reduction requires an intact glycolytic pathway, cytochrome b_5, and adequate activity of the reductase enzyme. Usually, the rate of the enzymatic reduction of methemoglobin exceeds the rate of spontaneous background methemoglobin formation by several hundred–fold. Patients who are heterozygous for this enzyme deficiency normally do not have elevated methemoglobin fractions but are

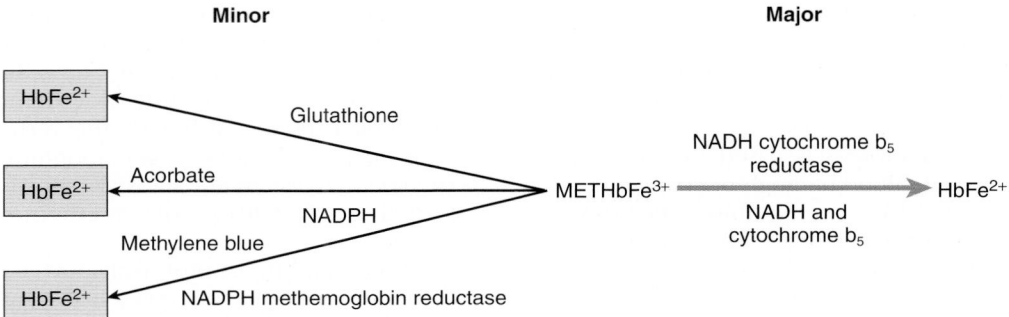

FIGURE 14-4 Reduction of methemoglobin. Essentially all methemoglobin reduction in vivo is catalyzed by cytochrome-b_5 reductase. Methylene blue markedly enhances methemoglobin reduction by acting as a cofactor for NADPH methemoglobin reductase. $HbFe^{2+}$, normal ferrous hemoglobin; NADPH, reduced nicotine adenine dinucleotide phosphate; $METHbFe^{3+}$, methemoglobin.

predisposed to suffering methemoglobinemia in response to oxidant stress that would not affect a patient with a normal phenotype. Patients homozygous for this deficiency have congenital methemoglobinemia.

A second enzyme, *NADPH methemoglobin reductase,* normally remains inactive. However, the addition of a cofactor such as methylene blue markedly accelerates NADPH methemoglobin reductase activity and serves as the basis for treating methemoglobinemia with methylene blue.[2] In this pathway (see Fig. 14-4), electrons are transferred from NADPH (from the hexose monophosphate shunt) to methylene blue and then to methemoglobin to produce deoxyhemoglobin. Thus, reduction of methemoglobin by this pathway requires an intact hexose monophosphate shunt, a cofactor such as methylene blue, and normal activity of the NADPH methemoglobin reductase enzyme. In vitro, some methemoglobin reduction can be demonstrated by glutathione and ascorbate; however, this activity is thought to be insignificant in vivo. Ascorbate generally is not considered an effective agent for the treatment of acute methemoglobinemia because of its slow action.

Infants are predisposed to methemoglobinemia because of their limited cytochrome-b_5 reductase activity and the low cytochrome-b_5 concentrations in their erythrocytes. Oxidant stress resulting from infections such as gastroenteritis or urinary tract infections are by far the most common cause of acquired methemoglobinemia in patients of this age group.[7,8]

Etiology

CONGENITAL CAUSES[3,6]
Homozygous deficiency of cytochrome-b_5 reductase produces congenital methemoglobinemia, which responds to oral methylene blue therapy. Several mutant hemoglobin species collectively termed *hemoglobin M* have been described in which the iron remains in the ferric form. Most patients with hemoglobin M suffer from congenital methemoglobinemia that is unresponsive to methylene blue therapy. Finally, there exist mutant unstable hemoglobins that undergo denaturation to produce congenital Heinz body hemolytic anemias; some of these also oxidize to methemoglobin.

ACQUIRED CAUSES
Most cases of methemoglobinemia are acquired and, except in neonates with infections, result from exposure to drugs or toxic agents (see Box 14-1). Oral overdoses of nitroglycerin and organic nitrates (which are esters of nitrite), as well as therapeutic doses of intravenous nitroglycerin are well known to produce methemoglobinemia.[9] The topical use of benzocaine spray, teething ointments, and hemorrhoidal creams, along with therapeutic doses of most other local anesthetics administered by injection or topical application (e.g., lidocaine spray for bronchoscopy) have produced this disorder. Methemoglobinemia is the rule following overdoses of phenazopyridine (Pyridium) or dapsone, and it occasionally results from the administration of therapeutic doses of the latter. The conversion of nitrates to nitrites by bacteria in the upper gastrointestinal tract has produced fatal methemoglobinemia in infants who ingested well water with high nitrate concentrations.[10] The recreational use of inhalable nitrites such as isobutyl nitrite has resulted in death. Aniline dyes are potent inducers of methemoglobinemia, and topical contact with these agents, which include components of printing ink on diapers, leather dyes in new shoes, and commercial marking crayons, has resulted in significant methemoglobinemia and death.[2] A multitude of prescription drugs have been less frequently associated with methemoglobinemia, including valproic acid, ifosfamide, and flutamide.

As expected, many agents producing methemoglobinemia also produce oxidant-induced hemolysis. For example, profound hemolysis may accompany poisonings with chlorates, arsine, stibine, chromates, and dapsone.

Diagnosis

The diagnosis of methemoglobinemia is confirmed by multiple-wave-length co-oximetry. Other diagnostic clues, however, may be either helpful or misleading. Generalized cyanosis in the presence of a normal arterial oxygen tension almost always represents methemoglobinemia. Failure of cyanosis to resolve with oxygen therapy also is an important diagnostic clue. Many blood gas instruments do not actually measure percent

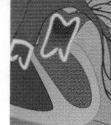

saturation, although they do report a value for saturation. This value is usually calculated from the oxygen tension and pH, and it represents what the saturation should be, assuming a lack of abnormal hemoglobin pigments. Therefore, in methemoglobinemia, the true percent saturation as determined by co-oximetry is much lower than the calculated percent saturation as reported by many blood gas instruments. The difference between these two values, or the *saturation gap,* should be less than 3% to 5% in arterial blood. Large saturation gaps in arterial blood are almost always due to methemoglobinemia or carboxyhemoglobinemia and less commonly to sulfhemoglobinemia.

In the past, most co-oximeters did not differentiate between methemoglobin and sulfhemoglobin and thus reported elevated methemoglobin fractions in the presence of sulfhemoglobinemia. While some of these instruments remain in use, many more recent co-oximeters will not report a falsely elevated methemoglobin fraction in the face of isolated sulfhemoglobinemia (see later section Sulfhemoglobinemia).

Pulse oximetry neither accurately nor reliably measures percent saturation in the presence of methemoglobinemia.[11] Depending on the true oxygen saturation, pulse oximetry may yield falsely low or falsely high values. In an otherwise healthy patient with a normal baseline oxygen saturation, pulse oximetry will read falsely elevated saturations, although they can decline below baseline values. For example, with methemoglobin fractions of 60% and a true oxygen saturation of 40%, a pulse oximeter may report a saturation of 85%. Once the diagnosis of methemoglobinemia has been made, the pulse oximeter should be disconnected from the patient so that medical personnel are not misled by unreliable readings.

Patients with significant methemoglobinemia may be observed to have chocolate-colored blood during blood sampling. A drop of this blood allowed to dry on filter paper appears noticeably brown when compared with venous blood from an asymptomatic patient when methemoglobinemia fractions exceed 10% to 15% in the nonanemic patient.[12] The presence of methemoglobinemia does not alter measurements of total hemoglobin concentration provided by the hematology laboratory. Because co-oximetry determines methemoglobin concentrations by measuring the absorption of light, substances that interfere with light absorption can produce false results on co-oximetry. Hyperlipidemia, such as that seen after the infusion of lipid emulsions or in patients with diabetes mellitus, interferes with the measurement of hemoglobin pigments by some co-oximeters and results in the reporting of a falsely elevated fraction of methemoglobin.[13] Total blood and plasma free hemoglobin concentrations may also be falsely elevated in this situation. Immediately after a dose of methylene blue has been administered, co-oximetry may be unreliable for several minutes.[14] In the foregoing instances, it should be remembered that significant methemoglobinemia is not present in a patient with a normal hemoglobin concentration if he or she does not appear cyanotic.

Methemoglobin fractions increase after death. Therefore, postmortem methemoglobin concentrations are not valid indicators of antemortem methemoglobinemia.[15]

DIFFERENTIAL DIAGNOSIS

Cyanosis caused by methemoglobinemia is most commonly confused with that from hypoxia. However, in cases of isolated methemoglobinemia with or without hemolysis, the arterial oxygen tension remains unchanged from baseline values and, in the absence of other causes, is normal. Furthermore, the cyanosis from methemoglobinemia does not respond to oxygen therapy. An unusual and poorly characterized discoloration of skin and other organs has been reported in patients suffering from hydrogen sulfide poisoning. Rare cases of tellurium exposure are characterized by blue discoloration. Many patients with severe cyanide poisoning experience cyanosis, and many other signs and symptoms of cyanide poisoning are similar to those of methemoglobinemia. Both carbon monoxide poisoning and sulfhemoglobinemia (described later in this chapter) produce saturation gaps in the presence of normal arterial oxygen tensions. Skin contact with new clothing or towels that contain blue dyes may cause discoloration of the skin, but this discoloration is removed by washing or wiping the skin. Excessive administration of methylene blue may also produce cyanosis that can be confused with continuing methemoglobinemia or cyanosis from other causes.

TREATMENT

Patients suffering from methemoglobinemia should receive oxygen to maximize the oxygen-carrying capacity of their remaining normal hemoglobin. Blood should be drawn and analyzed for evidence of hemolysis (hemoglobin measurement, blood smear, Heinz body staining, plasma free hemoglobin determination, and serum haptoglobin measurement). Patients should undergo arterial blood gas analysis and co-oximetry, and routine laboratory studies should be performed. An electrocardiogram should be obtained for ruling out myocardial ischemia.

ASYMPTOMATIC PATIENTS

Many patients suffering from methemoglobinemia exhibit cyanosis but lack signs and symptoms and do not require specific treatment. Once exposure to the offending agent ends, methemoglobin levels usually return to normal within 36 hours. Most of these patients require admission to a hospital for clinical follow-up for worsening of signs and symptoms, monitoring for onset of hemolysis, and serial determination of methemoglobin levels. Assuming normal hemoglobin concentrations, asymptomatic patients usually have methemoglobin fractions between 10% and 15%.

SYMPTOMATIC PATIENTS

Symptomatic patients suffering from methemoglobinemia (e.g., tachycardia, dyspnea, headache) are candidates for antidotal therapy with methylene blue, in the absence of a history of G6PD deficiency. Parenteral

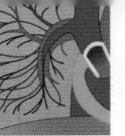

methylene blue is available as a 1% solution (10 mg/mL); it should be administered intravenously over 3 to 5 minutes at an initial dose of 2 mg/kg (0.2 mL/kg of a 1% solution). Resolution of cyanosis usually occurs within 15 to 20 minutes; more time may be required in some instances. If the patient is seriously symptomatic and no response occurs within 15 minutes, or if the patient remains moderately symptomatic without any improvement after 30 minutes, then repeat doses of 1 mg/kg (0.1 mL/kg of a 1% solution) may be given. If methemoglobin levels are readily available, repeat determinations of methemoglobin fractions should be performed before repeat dosing of methylene blue because large doses of methylene blue themselves produce discoloration of the skin. The total dose of methylene blue administered during the first few hours should not exceed 5 to 7 mg/kg.

Some methemoglobin-producing toxins have long half-lives. The classic example is dapsone, which may produce methemoglobinemia and hemolysis that last for days. In this situation, it may be necessary to administer methylene blue as a continuous infusion. Methylene blue may be dissolved in the crystalloid solution of choice and administered, on the basis of case reports in the literature, starting at 0.1 mg/kg per hour (0.01 mL/kg per hour of a 1% solution).[16] However, in the author's experience, higher rates may be required on occasion. Serial methemoglobin fractions are followed to monitor therapy.

Methylene blue largely undergoes renal excretion unchanged (about 75%). Therefore, patients with renal insufficiency do not require changes in initial doses for the treatment of methemoglobinemia but should receive lower continuous infusion doses of the drug determined on the basis of their creatinine clearance.

Adverse effects associated with large or rapidly administered doses of methylene blue in normal volunteers include dysuria, substernal chest pain, nausea, tachycardia, hypertension, and anxiety. Urine initially turns blue and then green as the drug undergoes excretion. Although the literature cautions that methylene blue may produce transient methemoglobinemia when given in large doses (e.g., 5 mg/kg over 35 to 70 minutes),[17] this has not been thought to be a significant problem in humans receiving recommended doses and has been ascribed largely to an in vitro effect occurring in the presence of hypoxic conditions.[18,19] Worsening hemolysis in methemoglobinemia patients has been ascribed to methylene blue therapy, even in those with normal G6PD activity. However, this finding has primarily been noted in case reports of patients in whom hemolysis was not unexpected from the agent producing methemoglobinemia, making causal relationships unclear. Importantly, neonates do seem sensitive to hemolytic actions of methylene blue.[20-22] Regardless of these concerns, the administration of methylene blue to a symptomatic patient with methemoglobinemia (without G6PD deficiency) has never been proved to worsen methemoglobinemia, and so methylene blue continues to be the drug of choice for treating symptomatic patients.

Furthermore, patients with methemoglobinemia should always be closely followed for evidence of hemolysis because hemolysis is common whether or not methylene blue is given.

Methylene blue should never be administered to someone with known G6PD deficiency. Such patients have low red cell NADPH concentrations, which limit augmentation of NADPH methemoglobin reductase by methylene blue. Importantly, methylene blue triggers hemolysis in such patients, which further impairs oxygen delivery to tissues.[2,23] Methylene blue should never be withheld from a symptomatic patient simply because a history concerning the presence or absence of G6PD deficiency cannot be obtained.

Cimetidine has been used to help control methemoglobinemia secondary to dapsone. By inhibiting cytochrome P-450 conversion to the oxidizing metabolite responsible for methemoglobinemia (dapsone hydroxylamine), oral administration of 1200 mg/day cimetidine to patients taking therapeutic doses of dapsone decreased circulating methemoglobin fractions by an average of 25%.[24]

In a manner similar to methylene blue, riboflavin also acts as an electron transfer agent and reduces methemoglobin in the presence of NADPH methemoglobin reductase. While endogenous riboflavin concentrations are not high enough to provide for significant methemoglobin reduction, oral doses of 60 to 100 mg per day have been used with success in patients with congenital methemoglobinemia.[25,26] The safety and efficacy of IV or oral riboflavin for the treatment of acquired, acute methemoglobinemia has not been described.

Incubation of erythrocytes in very high concentrations of N-acetylcysteine appears to enhance methemoglobin reduction in vitro.[27] However, these concentrations of N-acetylcysteine cannot be safely achieved in human beings, and a randomized controlled trial found that conventional doses of IV N-acetylcysteine were ineffective in reducing nitrite-induced methemoglobin fractions in human volunteers.[28]

During the care of patients with methemoglobinemia, care should always be taken to monitor total oxygen-carrying capacity by following both hemoglobin concentrations and methemoglobin fractions. For example, a decrease in the methemoglobin fraction from 30% to 15% will not result in improved oxygen delivery if accompanying hemolysis has resulted in a decrease of hemoglobin concentration from 15 to 5 g/dL. In fact, in this example, oxygen-carrying capacity has worsened. Furthermore, the onset of anemia alone may result in the disappearance of cyanosis if total hemoglobin concentrations decrease to the point where significant amounts of methemoglobinemia do not produce discoloration. For example, a 10% methemoglobin fraction in combination with a hemoglobin concentration of 15 g/dL produces visible cyanosis in most persons. However, a 20% methemoglobin fraction in a patient with a hemoglobin level of 5 g/dL produces no visible discoloration, yet may be lethal. Therefore, caution must be taken in interpreting the disappearance

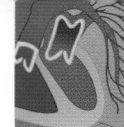

of cyanosis to mean that methemoglobinemia has not worsened or that the patient's status has improved.

After initial signs and symptoms of methemoglobinemia have been addressed, then routine gastrointestinal and skin decontamination should be performed as indicated. If ascorbic acid is used to treat methemoglobinemia, a recommended dose is 0.5 to 1 g intravenously or orally every 6 hours. Again, ascorbic acid works slowly and generally is considered ineffective for the treatment of acute acquired methemoglobinemia.

FAILURE TO RESPOND TO METHYLENE BLUE THERAPY

When patients with methemoglobinemia do not improve with methylene blue therapy, several possibilities should be considered (Box 14-2). They may have been exposed to large amounts of drugs or chemicals that, even with methylene blue therapy, produce methemoglobin at rates greater than the rate of reducing capacity. However, this possibility remains the exception. Although there are certainly times when methemoglobin fractions do not return to normal because of continued methemoglobin formation, methylene blue therapy almost always results in at least a transient decrease in methemoglobin fractions.

The patient who does not respond to methylene blue may also have an unrecognized G6PD deficiency. The rare patient with congenital lack of NADPH methemoglobin reductase also fails to respond to methylene blue treatment. Sulfhemoglobinemia can be mistaken for methemoglobinemia (see later in this chapter). Finally, repeated doses of methylene blue may result in blue discoloration of skin that is mistaken for methemoglobinemia.[29]

Treatment options for the patient who cannot receive or who fails to respond to methylene blue therapy are somewhat limited. Blood transfusions and exchange transfusions may be life saving[30] and are recommended whenever refractory methemoglobin fractions approach 70% in the nonanemic patient. Hyperbaric oxygenation can be a temporizing measure that provides adequate oxygen delivery during preparation for blood transfusion. However, a patient can stay in a hyperbaric chamber only for a relatively limited period of time without suffering from consequences of oxygen toxicity. Although not known to be effective, administration of large doses of ascorbic acid may also be indicated in this situation.

SULFHEMOGLOBINEMIA

Background and Characteristics

Sulfhemoglobin is a green molecule resulting from the incorporation of a sulfur atom into the porphyrin ring of hemoglobin by oxidant stress. Like methemoglobin, sulfhemoglobin cannot transport oxygen (Table 14-1). *Sulfmyoglobin,* a surrogate for one sulfhemoglobin tetramer, has a 2500-fold lower affinity for oxygen than myoglobin does.[31] Although small amounts of methemoglobin normally exist in vivo, no circulating sulfhemoglobin usually occurs. Unlike methemoglobin, sulfhemoglobin persists for the life of the erythrocyte and does not undergo conversion back to hemoglobin. Very little sulfhemoglobin causes typical slate-gray cyanosis. Only 0.5 g/dL of sulfhemoglobin produces noticeable skin discoloration (as compared with 1.5 g/dL of methemoglobin and 5 g/dL of deoxyhemoglobin).

In sulfhemoglobinemia (i.e., in vivo), hemoglobin tetramers usually contain only one or two sulfurated heme isomers. The affected molecules shift unaffected heme moieties toward the unliganded conformation. This reduces the oxygen affinity of the unmodified subunits and shifts the oxyhemoglobin dissociation curve to the right, enhancing oxygen delivery to tissues and partially ameliorating the effects of reduced oxygen-binding capacity.[32] In contrast, methemoglobin and carboxyhemoglobin shift the dissociation curve to the left, worsening the impairment of oxygen delivery to tissues.

Sulfhemoglobin, methemoglobin, and hemoglobin M possess similar light absorption spectra, and many early authors failed to distinguish among these three abnormal pigments. Some multiple-wave-length co-oximeters still in use today report sulfhemoglobin as methemoglobin. Furthermore, early studies of "sulfhemoglobinemia" from hydrogen sulfide mixed with blood

BOX 14-2	POSSIBLE CAUSES OF FAILURE OF METHYLENE BLUE THERAPY IN METHEMOGLOBINEMIA

Profound and overwhelming toxicity from oxidants (e.g., chlorates, aniline)
Glucose-6-phosphate dehydrogenase deficiency
NADPH methemoglobin reductase deficiency
Sulfhemoglobinemia
Discoloration due to large doses of methylene blue

TABLE 14-1   Comparison of Hemoglobin Pigments

Pigment	Deoxyhemoglobin	Methemoglobin	Sulfhemoglobin	Carboxyhemoglobin
Color	Blue	Brown	Green	Bright red
Concentration when cyanosis appears	5 g/dL	1.5 g/dL	0.5 g/dL	—
Oxygen transport?	Yes	No	No	No
Oxyhemoglobin dissociation curve shift	Rightward	Leftward	Rightward	Leftward
Response to methylene blue treatment	None	Decreases	None	None

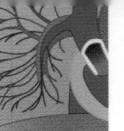

in vitro may have represented nothing more than a mixture of oxidized and denatured hemoglobin pigments that were unrelated to what is termed *sulfhemoglobin* today.[33] Readers interpreting the confusing medical literature on sulfhemoglobinemia must be aware that older literature describing sulfhemoglobin, probably better termed *pseudo-sulfhemoglobin*,[34] might represent true reports of sulfhemoglobinemia, methemoglobinemia, hemoglobin M disease; various species of denatured hemoglobin from hydrogen sulfide mixed with blood in vitro; or perhaps of other chemical compounds.

Etiology

Sulfhemoglobinemia is always acquired (Box 14-3), and chemicals capable of producing sulfhemoglobinemia[35] usually are better known for their ability to produce methemoglobinemia and hemolysis. Thus, methemoglobinemia, sulfhemoglobinemia, and hemolysis may coexist. Why some patients develop sulfhemoglobinemia and others methemoglobinemia after exposure to the same agent remains a mystery.

Sulfhemoglobin forms when sulfur binds to the β-pyrrole ring of the heme moiety (Fig. 14-5A). Based on studies of sulfmyoglobin, it has been suggested that an unstable episulfide bond forms (Fig. 14-5B) that spontaneously converts to the stable conformation (Fig. 14-5C), which persists for the life of the red blood cell.[36] In the past, authors suggested that the source of sulfur responsible for the oxidation of hemoglobin to sulfhemoglobin was the offending chemical producing the oxidant stress. However, many drugs associated with sulfhemoglobinemia do not contain sulfur. Another older belief was that an abnormally functioning gastrointestinal tract alone could produce hemolytic anemia, sulfhemoglobinemia, and methemoglobinemia ("enterogenous cyanosis") from the purported absorption of endogenously produced nitrites and sulfides. However, it appears that such patients were unknowingly ingesting analgesics known to cause such disorders.[37]

In an attempt to identify the source of the sulfur atom when exogenous sulfur was not supplied, Westphal and Azen[38] studied rats with jejunal pouches in which bacterial overgrowth occurred. Rats with jejunal pouches exposed to phenacetin were more likely to develop sulfhemoglobinemia than were the controls. In addition, erythrocytes from both control animals and those with pouches were more likely to become sulfurated when incubated in the urine of pouched rats than when incubated in the urine of controls. Finally, pouched rats were less likely to develop sulfurated hemoglobin when they were treated with neomycin. This suggests that bacterial metabolism in the gastrointestinal tract may

---

BOX 14-3   CLINICAL SUBSTANCES MOST COMMONLY ASSOCIATED WITH "SULFHEMOGLOBINEMIA"*

Acetanilid	Bismuth subnitrite	Hydroxylamine	Nitroglycerin	Sulfathiazole
Aminophenol	Dapsone	Metoclopramide	Phenacetin	Toluenediamine
p-Aminopropiophenone	Dimethylamine	Methylacetylanilide	Phenazopyridine	Tolylhydroxylamine
Ammonium nitrite	Dinitrobenzene	Naphthylamine	Phenylenediamine	Trinitrotoluene
Amyl nitrite	Ethyl nitrite	Nitrites	Phenylhydroxylamine	
Aniline	Flutamide	p-Nitroaniline	Sulfanilamide	
Anilinoethanol	Hydroxyacetylanilide	Nitrobenzene	Sulfapyridine	

*In some instances, it is not known whether older reports of "sulfhemoglobinemia" represented methemoglobinemia, sulfhemoglobinemia, or both.

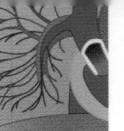

FIGURE 14-5 Proposed formation of sulfhemoglobin as illustrated in a single heme moiety (as in sulfmyoglobin). **A,** Native heme moiety. **B,** Initial episulfide bond across the β–β bond of β-pyrrole. **C,** Terminal sulfhemin in sulfmyoglobin. In sulfmyoglobin, no more than one to two heme moieties of a hemoglobin tetramer are oxidized to the sulfhemin state. (From Chatfield MJ, La Mar GN: 1H nuclear magnetic resonance study of the prosthetic group in sulfhemoglobin. Arch Biochem Biophys 1992;295:290.)

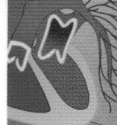

serve as a source for sulfur found in sulfhemoglobin during times of oxidant stress induced by various chemicals. Endogenous sulfhydryl groups may act as sulfur donors during the production of sulfhemoglobin.

Laboratory Diagnosis

In an early attempt to discern what was being measured when "sulfhemoglobin" was reported to be present, Michel and Harris[39] reported that the addition of cyanide or dithionite (hydrosulfite) to blood bound methemoglobin eliminated its spectral absorption immediately, while that of sulfhemoglobin remained. However, this simple test did not exclude hemoglobin M (or perhaps other oxidation products of hemoglobin), which also remains after addition of these compounds. Carrico and colleagues[40] later demonstrated that carbon monoxide bound sulfhemoglobin to produce carbonmonoxy-sulfhemoglobin, a compound with enhanced spectral absorption and a down-field shift, whereas neither methemoglobin nor hemoglobin M bound carbon monoxide. Therefore, light absorption in the presence of cyanide (or dithionite) and carbon monoxide served for several years as laboratory tools to measure "sulfhemoglobin" fractions and concentrations, although it is not known that what we know today as sulfhemoglobin was always the species being measured. Park and Nagel[32] reported that isoelectric focusing (a form of electrophoresis) reliably delineates the three pigments. Although this test is not widely available, it is the most reliable way of distinguishing sulfhemoglobin from methemoglobin and generally serves as the gold standard, although other methods may be used in some reference laboratories.

Various brands and models of co-oximeters detect and report sulfhemoglobin differently. As examples, Instrumentation Laboratory Inc.'s IL282 and IL482 (Lexington, MA) both report sulfhemoglobin as methemoglobin. However, the IL682 by the same manufacturer is reported to indicate the presence of sulfhemoglobin fractions greater than 1.5%.[41] The Radiometer OSM3 (Westlake, OH) has been noted to report falsely elevated oxygen saturations in the presence of sulfhemoglobinemia unless a service program configuration used by factory representatives is used.[42] It is essential that physicians know how the co-oximeter their laboratory uses detects and reports sulfhemoglobinemia. It is wise to remain skeptical about the reliability of some manufacturers' claims and to always use a reference laboratory to quantify sulfhemoglobin if there is any question about the diagnosis.

The exact behavior of pulse oximetry in the face of sulfhemoglobinemia remains unresolved, although reports document that pulse oximeters will not provide reliable estimates of true saturation. This author has seen pulse oximeters read falsely low saturations in the face of sulfhemoglobinemia in two patients. Other authors[43,44] have described falsely elevated saturation reports by pulse oximetry in the face of sulfhemoglobinemia. At present, pulse oximetry should not be used to estimate true saturation when sulfhemoglobinemia is suspected.

Clinical Presentation

Sulfhemoglobinemia enters the differential diagnosis with a cyanotic or gray patient who has a normal oxygen tension, who may or may not have what the laboratory reports to be elevated methemoglobin fractions, and who has failed to respond to methylene blue therapy. Except for cyanosis, most patients with sulfhemoglobinemia are not symptomatic unless other abnormal hemoglobins are present (e.g., methemoglobin) or there is accompanying anemia from hemolysis. The discoloration of skin most often appears slate gray and may persist for weeks or even months owing to the irreversible nature of sulfhemoglobin. Only rarely is sulfhemoglobinemia severe enough to produce tachycardia, tachypnea, dyspnea, and altered level of consciousness due to impairment of oxygen delivery. The coexistence of methemoglobinemia and anemia, of course, may alter the discoloration of cyanosis and clinical symptoms. As with other hemoglobinopathies, arterial oxygen tension is normal unless coexisting disease is present.

Numerous cases of "sulfhemoglobinemia" have been reported in the English literature, and the frequency of reports may be increasing with the use of more modern co-oximeters. However, only rarely has the diagnosis been confirmed with isoelectric focusing. In the past, the drugs most commonly causing sulfhemoglobinemia were acetanilide, phenacetin, and sulfonamides. Use of Bromo-Seltzer was the single most common cause, but acetanilide, the offending ingredient, has since been removed from this product's contents. Over the last several years, reports of sulfhemoglobinemia attributable to flutamide, metoclopramide, phenazopyridine, and dapsone have appeared. Again, these same agents are known to produce methemoglobinemia as well.

Three examples of typical cases follow. Halvorsen[45] reported the case of an 85-year-old woman who received nitrofurantoin and phenazopyridine for a urinary tract infection. She was subsequently hospitalized when she complained of dizziness and was noted to exhibit cyanosis. Co-oximetry reported a methemoglobin fraction of 50.3%. The addition of cyanide to blood produced no change in the methemoglobin fraction. Methylene blue was administered and repeated 1 hour later without effect. On the ninth day of hospitalization, co-oximetry reported a methemoglobin fraction of 26.5%. Her symptoms gradually resolved, but 9 months later she was inadvertently rechallenged with phenazopyridine in combination with cotrimoxazole. She was admitted to the hospital on the seventh day of therapy for cyanosis and what was reported to be a 30% methemoglobin fraction by co-oximetry. Again, methylene blue was given without effect, and cyanosis and reported methemoglobin fractions decreased over several weeks to months.

Basset and associates[46] reported the case of a 37-year-old man who was admitted with chronic anemia and cyanosis. For two weeks he had been taking an average of 100 tablets per week of aspirin, codeine, and phenacetin for headaches. Total hemoglobin concentration was 9 g/dL, the reticulocyte count was 12%, and Heinz body

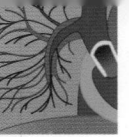

formation was observed. Diagnosis of sulfhemoglo-binemia was made after identification of absorption spectra at 620 nm without change after addition of cyanide. Confirmation was performed with isoelectric focusing.

Chawla and coworkers[47] described a patient who ingested 3 g of dapsone in a suicide attempt and had cyanosis, tachycardia, and tachypnea. Laboratory studies revealed both methemoglobinemia (4.3 g/dL) and sulfhemoglobinemia (0.25 g/dL). Methylene blue therapy produced a resolution in cyanosis and methemoglobinemia and thus was continued for a total of 36 hours. Forty-eight hours later, the patient again became cyanotic, and repeat studies revealed that the methemoglobin concentration had decreased to 0.7 g/dL while the sulfhemoglobin level had risen to 0.39 g/dL.

Treatment

There is no specific antidote for sulfhemoglobinemia. Methylene blue does not confer any beneficial effect. Treatment centers on ensuring adequate oxygen delivery to tissues through the correction of coexistent methemoglobinemia and anemia (frequently from hemolysis) and on promoting maximal oxygen-carrying capacity with administration of oxygen when the patient is symptomatic. In the rare severe case, transfusions have been performed, with a resultant increase in total hemoglobin concentration and a decrease in sulfhemoglobin fraction and concentration.

OTHER ERYTHROCYTE DISORDERS

In addition to oxidant stress, anemia from other or unclear causes may occur in various acute and chronic poisonings (Box 14-4). Hemolysis from damaged red cell membranes may follow some poisonous snake bites or *Loxosceles* envenomation. Impaired heme or erythrocytic synthesis explains at least some of the anemias seen in those with toxicity produced by arsenic, lead, aluminum, colchicine, podophyllum, and nitrous oxide. Acute lead poisoning (from an acute single ingestion of a large amount of lead) may be accompanied by profound hemolysis. The ingestion of zinc supplements prevents

---

BOX 14-4	OTHER CAUSES OF ANEMIA IN ACUTE AND CHRONIC POISONING*

Aluminum
Arsenic
Benzene
Chemotherapeutic
  agents
Colchicine

Ethanol
Lead
Loxosceles spiders
Nitrous oxide
Oxidizing agents
  (see Box 14-1)

Podophyllum
Radiation
Snake
  envenomation
Zinc

*In many cases, the exact mechanism by which anemia occurs remains unknown.

BOX 14-5	AGENTS THAT ELEVATE ERYTHROCYTIC MEAN CELL VOLUME DURING POISONING*

Arsenic
Benzene (myelodysplastic syndrome)
Nitrous oxide

*Excluded are the multitude of agents that elevate erythrocytic mean cell volume when given at therapeutic doses.

---

the absorption of copper and may lead to a sideroblastic anemia.[48]

Elevated values for mean erythrocytic cell volumes suggest the presence of several different toxins (Box 14-5). Refractory anemia seen in benzene-induced myelodysplastic syndromes may also be accompanied by an increased mean cell volume.

Carboxyhemoglobin is covered in Chapter 87. Like other dyshemoglobinemias, carboxyhemoglobin produces a percent saturation gap. Like methemoglobin, carboxyhemoglobin does not carry oxygen and shifts the oxyhemoglobin dissociation curve to the left, further impairing oxygen delivery. Pulse oximetry does not detect low oxygen saturations that result from carboxyhemoglobin. Accurate diagnosis is made with the use of co-oximetry.

Porphyrias are diseases resulting from deficiencies of various enzymes involved in heme synthesis. Although a multitude of agents given at therapeutic doses have exacerbated or triggered crises in patients with porphyrias, the chronic ingestion of grain treated with hexachlorobenzene (a fungicide) serves as the main example of a toxin's being primarily responsible for an outbreak of porphyria (porphyria cutanea tarda).[49] It is now recognized that most patients with idiopathic porphyria cutanea suffer from hepatitis C, and it is unclear whether hepatitis C played an important predisposing role in hexachlorobenzene-induced porphyria.

Leukocytes

Although hundreds of pharmaceutical agents given at therapeutic doses produce leukopenia as an adverse effect, the presence of leukopenia in acute or chronic poisoning suggests only a few causes (Box 14-6). Leukopenia following acute overdoses of chemotherapeutic drugs may not appear for several days and commonly reaches a nadir in 1 to 3 weeks. In contrast, the leukopenia following colchicine poisoning is frequently severe and of rapid onset, appearing within 48 hours after an initial leukocytosis.[50] Leukopenia commonly accompanies the sideroblastic anemia seen in copper deficiency from the ingestion of excessive zinc supplements.[48] Some types of nonlymphocytic leukemias might result as part of a benzene-induced myelodysplastic syndrome after chronic exposure.

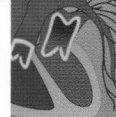

BOX 14-6	TOXINS PRODUCING LEUKOPENIA DURING POISONING

Benzene (myelodysplastic syndrome)
Chemotherapeutic agents
Colchicine
Metals
Podophyllum
Irradiation
Valproic acid

Platelets

Thrombocytopenia may result from bone marrow suppression (e.g., by chemotherapeutic drugs, colchicine, or arsenic), increased destruction by enzymes (e.g., after snake bite), or an intoxication complicated by disseminated intravascular coagulation. Severe acetaminophen toxicity (with hepatic failure) may be accompanied by profound thrombocytopenia.[51] Thrombocytopenia has been reported on several occasions complicating valproic acid overdoses.[52] Most thrombocytopenia seen in patients who have received therapeutic doses of drugs is immune mediated.

Numerous pharmaceutical agents impair platelet function at therapeutic doses and, of course, at toxic doses. Examples include aspirin, nonsteroidal anti-inflammatory drugs, ticlopidine, dipyridamole, and nitroglycerin. Despite inhibition of platelet function, bleeding is a rare cause of serious morbidity or mortality after acute poisonings by these agents.

REFERENCES

1. Evans AS, Enzer N, Eder HA, et al: Hemolytic anemia with paroxysmal methemoglobinemia and sulfhemoglobinemia. Arch Intern Med 1950;86:22.
2. Curry SC: Methemoglobinemia. Ann Emerg Med 1982;11:214.
3. Weatherall DJ, Clegg JB, Higgs DR, et al: The hemoglobinopathies. In Scriver CR, Beaudet AL, Sly WS, et al (eds): The Metabolic and Molecular Bases of Inherited Disease, 7th ed. New York, McGraw-Hill, 1995, pp 4571–4636.
4. Yoo D, Lessin LS: Drug-associated "bite cell" hemolytic anemia. Am J Med 1992;92:243.
5. Savides MC, Oehme FW, Leipold HW: Effects of various antidotal treatments on acetaminophen toxicosis and biotransformation in cats. Am J Vet Res 1985;46:1485.
6. Jaffe ER, Hultquist DE: Cytochrome b_5 reductase deficiency and enzymopenic hereditary methemoglobinemia. In Scriver CR, Beaudet AL, Sly WS, et al (eds): The Metabolic and Molecular Bases of Inherited Disease, 7th ed. New York, McGraw-Hill, 1995, pp 4555–4570.
7. Yano SS, Danish EH, Hsia YE: Transient methemoglobinemia with acidosis in infants. J Pediatr 1982;100:415.
8. Luk G, Riggs D, Luque M: Severe methemoglobinemia in a 3-week-old infant with urinary tract infection. Crit Care Med 1991;19:1325.
9. Curry SC, Arnold-Capell P: Toxic effects of drugs used in the ICU: nitroprusside, nitroglycerin, and angiotensin-converting enzyme inhibitors. Crit Care Clin 1991;7:555.
10. Lukens JN: The legacy of well-water methemoglobinemia. JAMA 1987;257:2793.
11. Ralston AC, Webb RK, Runciman WB: Potential errors in pulse oximetry. 3. Effects of interference, dyes, dyshaemoglobins and other pigments. Anaesthesia 1991;46:291.
12. Henretig FM, Gribetz B, Kearney T, et al: Interpretation of color change in blood with varying degree of methemoglobinemia. Clin Toxicol 1988;26:293.
13. Spurzem JR, Bonekat HW, Shigeoka JW: Factitious methemoglobinemia caused by hyperlipemia. Chest 1984;86:84.
14. Kirlangitis JJ, Middaugh RE, Zablocki A, et al: False indication of arterial oxygen desaturation and methemoglobinemia following injection of methylene blue in urological surgery. Mil Med 1990;155:260.
15. Reay DT, Insalaco SJ, Eisele JW: Postmortem methemoglobin concentrations and their significance. J Forensic Sci 1984;29:1160.
16. Berlin G, Brodin B, Hilden J-O: Acute dapsone intoxication: a case treated with continuous infusion of methylene blue, forced diuresis, and plasma exchange. J Toxicol Clin Toxicol 1985;22:537.
17. Lamont ASM, Roberts MS, Holdsworth G, et al: Relationship between methaemoglobin production and methylene blue plasma concentrations under general anaesthesia. Anaesth Intensive Care 1986;14:360.
18. Way JL, Leung P, Sylvester DM, et al: Methaemoglobin formation in the treatment of acute cyanide intoxication. In Ballantyne B, Marrs TC (eds): Clinical and Experimental Toxicology of Cyanides. Bristol, England, IOP Publishing, 1987, pp 402–412.
19. Stossel TP, Jennings RB: Failure of methylene blue to produce methemoglobinemia in vivo. Am J Clin Pathol 1966;45:600.
20. Kirsch IR, Cohen HJ: Heinz body hemolytic anemia from the use of methylene blue in neonates. J Pediatr 1980;96:276.
21. Crooks J: Haemolytic jaundice in a neonate after intra-amniotic injection of methylene blue. Arch Dis Child 1982;57:872.
22. McEnerney JK, McEnerney LN: Unfavorable neonatal outcome after intraamniotic injection of methylene blue. Obstet Gynecol 1983;61(Suppl):35S.
23. Rosen PH, Johnson C, McGehee WG, et al: Failure of methylene blue treatment in toxic methemoglobinemia: association with glucose-6-phosphate dehydrogenase deficiency. Ann Intern Med 1971;75:83.
24. Coleman MD, Rhodes LE, Scott AK, et al: The use of cimetidine to reduce dapsone-dependent methaemoglobinaemia in dermatitis herpetiformis patients. Br J Clin Pharmacol 1992;34:244.
25. Hirano M, Matsuki T, Tanishima K, et al: Congenital methaemoglobinaemia due to NADH methaemoglobin reductase deficiency: successful treatment with oral riboflavin. Br J Haematol 1981;47:353.
26. Kaplan JC, Chirouze M: Therapy of recessive congenital methaemoglobinaemia by oral riboflavine. Lancet 1978;2:1043.
27. Wright RO, Woolf AD, Shannon MW, et al: N-acetylcysteine reduces methemoglobin in an in-vitro model of glucose-6-phosphate dehydrogenase deficiency. Acad Emerg Med 1998;5:225.
28. Tanen DA, LoVecchio F, Curry SC: Failure of intravenous N-acetylcysteine to reduce methemoglobin produced by sodium nitrite in human volunteers: a randomized controlled trial. Ann Emerg Med 2000;35:369.
29. Goluboff N, Wheaton R: Methylene blue–induced cyanosis and acute hemolytic anemia complicating the treatment of methemoglobinemia. J Pediatr 1961;58:86.
30. Harrison MR: Toxic methaemoglobinaemia: a case of acute nitrobenzene and aniline poisoning treated by exchange transfusion. Anaesthesia 1977;32:270.
31. Berzofsky JA, Peisach J, Blumberg WE: Sulfheme proteins. 2. The reversible oxygenation of ferrous sulfmyoglobin. J Biol Chem 1971;246:7366.
32. Park CM, Nagel RL: Sulfhemoglobinemia: clinical and molecular aspects. N Engl J Med 1984;310:1579.
33. Curry SC, Gerkin RD: A patient with sulfhemoglobin? Ann Emerg Med 1987;16:828.
34. Smith RP, Gosselin RE: Hydrogen sulfide poisoning. J Occup Med 1979;21:93.
35. Finch CA: Methemoglobinemia and sulfhemoglobinemia. N Engl J Med 1948;239:470.
36. Chatfield MJ, La Mar GN: 1H nuclear magnetic resonance study of the prosthetic group in sulfhemoglobin. Arch Biochem Biophys 1992;295:289.
37. Azen EA, Bryan GT, Shahidi NT, et al: Obscure hemolytic anemia due to analgesic abuse: does enterogenous cyanosis exist? Am J Med 1970;48:724.

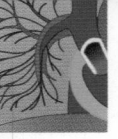
38. Westphal RG, Azen EA: Experimental enterogenous cyanosis and anaemia. Br J Haematol 1972;22:609.

39. Michel HO, Harris JS: The blood pigments: properties and quantitative determination with special reference to spectrophotometric methods. J Lab Clin Med 1940;25:445.

40. Carrico RJ, Peisach RJ, Peisach J, et al: The preparation and some physical properties of sulfhemoglobin. J Biol Chem 1978;253:2386.

41. Demedts P, Wauters A, Watelle M, et al: Pitfalls in discriminating sulfhemoglobin from methemoglobin. Clin Chem 1977;43:1098.

42. Wu C, Kenny MA: A case of sulfhemoglobinemia and emergency measurement of sulfhemoglobin with an OSM3 CO-oximeter. Clin Chem 1997;43:162.

43. Aravindhan N, Chisholm DG: Sulfhemoglobinemia presenting as pulse oximetry desaturation. Anesthesiol 2000;93:833.

44. Langford SL, Sheikh S: An adolescent case of sulfhemoglobinemia associated with high-dose metoclopramide and N-acetylcysteine. Ann Emerg Med 1999;34:538.

45. Halvorsen SM: Phenazopyridine-induced sulfhemoglobinemia: inadvertent rechallenge. Am J Med 1991;91:315.

46. Basset P, Bergerat JP, Lang JM, et al: Hemolytic anemia and sulfhemoglobinemia due to phenacetin abuse: a case with multivisceral adverse effects. Clin Toxicol 1981;18:493.

47. Chawla R, Gurnani A, Bhattacharya A: Acute dapsone poisoning. Anaesth Intensive Care 1993;21:349.

48. Fiske DN, McCoy HE III, Kitchens CS: Zinc-induced sideroblastic anemia: report of a case, review of the literature, and description of the hematologic syndrome. Am J Hematol 1994;46:147.

49. Peters HA: Hexachlorobenzene poisoning in Turkey. Fed Proc 1976;35:2400.

50. Folpini A, Furfori P: Colchicine toxicity—clinical features and treatment: massive overdose case report. J Toxicol Clin Toxicol 1995;33:71.

51. Fischereder M, Jaffe JP: Thrombocytopenia following acute acetaminophen overdose. Am J Hematol 1994;45:258.

52. Anderson GO, Ritland S: Life threatening intoxication with sodium valproate. J Toxicol Clin Toxicol 1995;33:279.

15 *Ocular Toxicology*

ANGELA C. ANDERSON, MD

At a Glance...

- All chemical exposures to the eye require immediate decontamination by copious irrigation with an aqueous solution.
- Rapid irrigation optimizes the chances for full recovery after chemical eye injuries; conversely, a delay in decontamination can negatively affect outcome.
- Tap water is readily available, safe, and effective and, thus, the preferred irrigation fluid.
- Lactated Ringer's solution is theoretically preferable to normal saline as an ocular irrigant because it has a more physiologic pH and osmolarity.
- Newer, specialized irrigation solutions (e.g., hexafluorine or Diphoterine, Prevor Laboratories, France) may become the ideal methods of ocular decontamination, particularly following exposure to chemical warfare agents.
- Some ocular toxins have delayed effects (e.g., mustard agents and hydrofluoric acid).
- Immediate ophthalmologic referral is recommended for all but the most trivial chemical burns to the eye.

In 2005, 133,270 ocular toxic exposures were reported to national poison centers.[1] These exposures accounted for 5.2% of all poison center calls. Toxic injuries to the eye result predominantly from direct, local contact with caustic substances. Some toxins, however, may produce ocular toxicity following systemic absorption, and certain toxins may produce systemic effects following ocular exposure. This chapter reviews the more common and devastating caustic eye injuries and potential abnormalities caused by toxins absorbed systemically.

Consequences of toxic eye injuries may range from minor eye irritation to total loss of vision. Understanding the mechanisms of ocular injury produced by toxic substances requires an understanding of the anatomy, physiology, and repair mechanisms of the eye.

Anatomy of the Eye

The anatomy of the eye is illustrated in Figures 15-1 and 15-2.[2,3] The conjunctiva is the outermost layer of the globe. The portion that overlies the globe itself is called the bulbar conjunctiva, while that which lines the inner surfaces of the eyelids is the palpebral conjunctiva. The next layer is the cornea, which overlies the iris and the anterior chamber of the eye. It is continuous with the sclera, the white part of the eye. The bulbar conjunctiva covers both the cornea and the sclera. The cornea and sclera meet at the limbus (see Figs. 15-1 and 15-2). This area is also the location of the canal of Schlemm, which is the drainage system for aqueous fluid. The space posterior to the cornea and anterior to the iris is the anterior chamber. Behind the iris are the posterior chamber and the lens. Aqueous humor is secreted by the ciliary process into the posterior chamber, travels through the pupil into the anterior chamber, and drains into the canal of Schlemm. The vitreous and the retina are posterior to the lens.

Eye Physiology and Toxin-Induced Physiologic Disturbances

The cornea is normally transparent because it is avascular. It derives nutrition from the aqueous humor and oxygen from that which is dissolved in tears. The cornea comprises five layers. The outermost layer is the epithelium, which has three major purposes: (1) it provides a barrier to microbial pathogens, (2) it produces cytokines that inhibit collagenase production from fibroblasts, and (3) it produces superoxide dismutase, which scavenges free radicals.[4,5] Alkali, acids, and other eye toxins can damage the epithelium and impair these functions.

The next layer is Bowman's membrane. It is not capable of regeneration if damaged. Injuries that extend through this layer always result in scar formation.[6]

The stroma is the third layer and makes up 90% of the cornea. It consists mostly of collagen. Binding of alkali cations to collagen causes stromal hydration; thickening and shortening of collagen meshwork occurs as well. Stromal hydration results in loss of corneal clarity, and contracted meshwork results in an increase in intraocular pressure (glaucoma).[4] The cellular components of the stroma are keratocytes, which are responsible for remodeling damaged stroma. Sensory nerve endings are located in the stroma as well. Consequently, damage to the stromal layer may result in anesthesia of the eye.

The fourth layer of the cornea is Descemet's membrane. Injury to this layer produces corneal hydrops, a condition in which aqueous leaks from the anterior chamber into the stroma and causes corneal clouding.

The endothelium is the innermost layer of the cornea. It is responsible for transporting aqueous back and forth between the anterior chamber and the cornea. Damage to this layer may result in permanent corneal edema.

Damage to the iris and ciliary body may cause either increased intraocular pressure secondary to impaired outflow of aqueous, or hypotony from decreased aqueous production or aqueous leakage. Lens injuries may result in cataract formation.

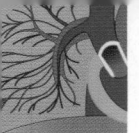

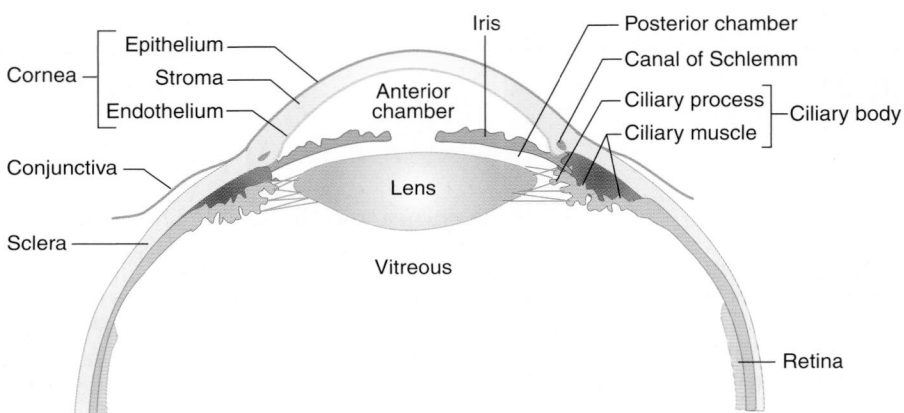

FIGURE 15-1 Anatomy of the anterior eye: transverse section. (From Sullivan J, Krieger G [eds]: Acute Ocular Injury from Hazardous Materials. Baltimore, Williams & Wilkins, 1992.)

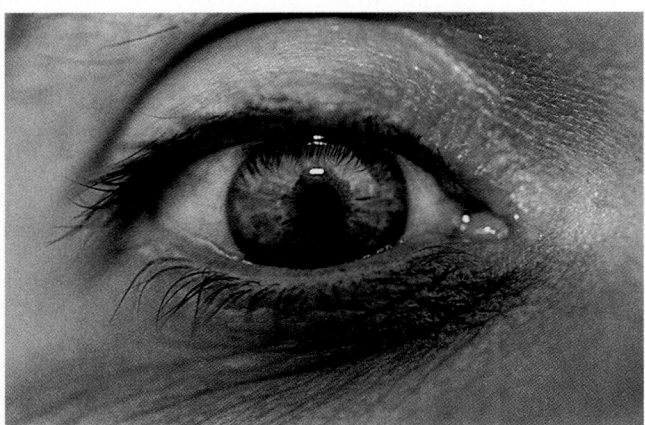

FIGURE 15-2 Anatomy of the anterior eye: surface view.

Mechanisms of Repair

EPITHELIUM

Repair of the epithelium is a two-step process. Reepithelialization is the first step: it involves replacement of lost or damaged epithelium. This is followed by differentiation, in which the newly formed epithelium undergoes further morphologic development. Small defects in the epithelium will be repaired in 1 to 3 days; large defects may take up to 2 weeks.[6] The rate of this process, and the ultimate morphology and physiology of the new epithelial layer, depends on the source of the migrating epithelium.[4] If portions of the corneal or limbal epithelium have remained intact after chemical injury, reepithelialization is rapid and differentiation results in a normal, clear, and stable corneal epithelium. If the corneal and limbal epithelia have both been destroyed, resurfacing must depend on the conjunctival epithelium as a source for the new layer. This is a slower process, which may result in a normal epithelium if the injury was not severe. However, if damage was extensive, the new corneal surface will retain the characteristics of conjunctival epithelium, which will result in vascularization, fibrovascular pannus formation, and loss of clarity. This may cause significant vision loss. Additionally, severe damage to goblet cells may cause abnormal tear film production, leading to chronic ocular surface irritation. This may result in the formation of a symblepharon, an adhesion between the palpebral and bulbar conjunctiva.

STROMA

Stromal keratocytes secrete collagen, collagenase, and matrix mucopolysaccharides. If these cells are injured, balanced regulation of the healing cornea may be disturbed and collagen breakdown may exceed collagen synthesis. This causes sterile ulcerations of the cornea, which may progress to perforation.

SPECIFIC AGENTS AND THEIR MECHANISM OF TOXICITY

Caustic (Corrosive) Chemicals

CHEMICAL IDENTIFICATION AND STRUCTURE OF ALKALIS

The most common and severely damaging alkalis are ammonium hydroxide (NH_4OH), sodium hydroxide ($NaOH$), potassium hydroxide (KOH), and calcium hydroxide ($Ca(OH)_2$) (see Table 15-1 and Chapter 98).

PHARMACODYNAMICS/MECHANISM OF ACTION AND TOXICITY

Alkali burns commonly cause the most severe chemical injuries. The severity of tissue injury is proportional to the degree of increase in tissue pH. The hydroxyl ion saponifies fatty acids (lipids) in cell membranes (Fig. 15-3). This causes cell destruction and allows for further penetration of the substance into the deeper structures of the eye. The depth of destruction influences the potential complications caused by the exposure. Alkali cations react with and hydrate tissue stromal contents (e.g., collagen), which leads to loss of ocular tissue clarity.

In animal studies in which rabbit corneas are removed, the degree of damage caused by various alkalis is directly correlated to the magnitude of the solution's pH, with irreversible damage occurring at a pH greater than 11.0.[7] However, when the corneal epithelium is intact, the extent of damage becomes dependent on the

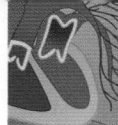

TABLE 15-1 Alkalis: Characteristics, Uses, and Ocular Toxic Effects

ALKALI	CHEMICAL COMPOSITION	DOMESTIC AND INDUSTRIAL USES	COMMENTS	POTENTIAL COMPLICATIONS
Ammonium hydroxide	NH_4OH	Fertilizer, refrigerant, cleaning agents	Highly soluble Extremely rapid penetration	Corneal anesthesia Cataract formation Glaucoma Permanent blindness
Sodium hydroxide	$NaOH$	Drain and oven cleaner Car airbags Acid neutralization Petroleum refining Treatment of cellulose, plastics, and rubber	Second to NH_4OH in rate of penetration	Same as those of NH_4OH
Potassium hydroxide	KOH	Common laboratory reagent	Third highest rate of penetration of the alkalis	Similar to those of $NaOH$
Calcium hydroxide	$CaOH$	Mortar, plaster, cement, whitewash	Calcium soaps cause slower penetration than other alkali Particulate matter may provide reservoir for continued exposure	Superficial ground glass opacification

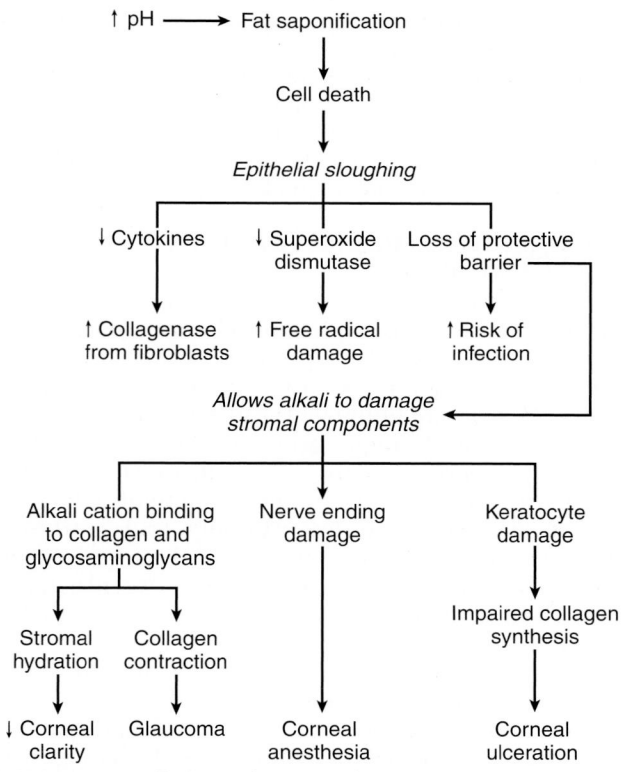

FIGURE 15-3 Alkali: mechanisms of action and toxicity.

rate and manner of penetration through the epithelial barrier. The rate of epithelial penetration is highest for substances with the greatest fat solubility. Penetration rates of various alkalis (controlled for pH), listed from slowest to fastest, are as follows: calcium hydroxide, potassium hydroxide, sodium hydroxide, and ammonium hydroxide.[8]

Other factors important to the injury process include the concentration and amount of the chemical, duration of exposure, and binding of alkali cations (e.g., sodium, calcium) to corneal membranes.[8]

CLINICAL PRESENTATION

Pain is the most common symptom associated with ocular injuries. Ironically, the absence of pain experienced in some exposures may be indicative of a greater severity of injury and poorer prognosis since some injuries destroy sensory nerves of the cornea, causing anesthesia. Injuries in which ocular sensation remains intact are more superficial and more painful. The patient may also complain of decreased visual acuity.

SPECIFIC ALKALIS

Ammonia

Ammonia (NH_3) is a colorless gas used as a fertilizer, a refrigerant, and in the production of other chemicals. It is found most commonly in the household as a 7% solution used for cleaning. Available industrial solutions contain concentrations of ammonia as high as 29% (see Chapter 97).

Fumes of ammonia gas stimulate tearing, which dilutes the chemical and decreases its potential for injury. Consequently, ammonia gas is irritating to the eye, but rarely causes significant damage without prolonged contact.

Ammonia liquefies under pressure to form ammonium hydroxide (NH_4OH). Aqueous ammonium hydroxide and liquid ammonia cause the most devastating eye injuries. These solutions are highly soluble in tissue water. High lipid solubility allows rapid penetration of ammonia into the deeper structures of the eye. The pH of the aqueous humor rises within seconds of exposure to ammonia, while similar increases from sodium hydroxide take 3 to 5 minutes.[4,9] Aqueous pH returns to normal in 30 minutes to 3 hours, with or without irrigation.[10]

Because of its extremely rapid penetration, ammonia exposures are very difficult to ameliorate by rapid

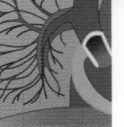

irrigation. As a result, ammonia exposures to the eye may produce serious complications, such as corneal opacification, corneal anesthesia, stromal edema, atrophy of the iris, dense cataract formation, persistent and recurrent glaucoma, and permanent blindness.[8]

Sodium Hydroxide

Sodium hydroxide (also termed *lye, caustic soda,* and *sodium hydrate*) is a white solid that dissolves in water to produce a strongly alkaline solution. Both the solid and liquid forms can cause severe injury to all tissues. It is most commonly found in the home as drain and oven cleaners in concentrations between 0.5% and 54%. Industrial uses include acid neutralization, petroleum refining, and treatment of cellulose, plastics, and rubber. Another potential source of exposure is associated with automobile airbag deployment.[11] Sodium hydroxide and talc powder liberated during airbag deployment have resulted in corneal keratitis, abrasions, and chemical burns.[11]

The penetration rate of sodium hydroxide is second only to that of ammonium hydroxide; consequently, eye damage can be similarly devastating (see discussion of ammonium hydroxide in the earlier section on Ammonia). Studies performed on rabbit eyes demonstrated severe injury and perforation following a 30-second exposure to a drop of 1-N (4%) sodium hydroxide; both mild and severe injury following 15 to 20 seconds of exposure to a 2-N solution; and mild burns from a 0.5-N solution for 30 seconds.[8]

Potassium Hydroxide

Potassium hydroxide (caustic potash) causes the same degree of injury as sodium hydroxide.[8]

Calcium Hydroxide

Calcium hydroxide, or lime, is a common cause of alkali injury in the construction workplace. It is a white powdered or granular solid that is used to make plaster, cement, mortar, and whitewash. Since calcium hydroxide exists in a particulate form, it is commonly retained in the eye (particularly beneath the upper eyelid) and provides a continuous source of exposure. Fortunately, it penetrates the eye much more slowly than ammonium hydroxide or sodium hydroxide, forming insoluble calcium soaps during saponification of cell membrane fatty acids. The calcium soaps precipitate and make penetration of the cornea more difficult. Consequently, lime causes many of the superficial complications seen following other strong alkali injuries, but deeper structures, such as the iris and lens, are routinely spared.[8]

Although calcium hydroxide causes eye injuries that tend to be less severe than those of ammonium or sodium hydroxide, it promotes corneal opacification more quickly than other alkalis.[7] Mild lime burns typically cause a frosted or ground-glass opacity superficially at the level of Bowman's membrane. They usually result in a significant loss of epithelium, but rarely affect the underlying stroma. The opacification of Bowman's membrane observed in mild exposures is secondary to precipitations of calcific material. Therefore, part of the

management of these injuries involves the use of disodium edetate (EDTA) to extract the entrapped calcium (see section on Special Management Considerations).[12] More severe injuries occur when the pH is 12 or higher and are often associated with stromal opacification and corneal anesthesia.[8] Stromal opacification is a result of damage to stromal components and is not responsive to EDTA treatment.

CHEMICAL IDENTIFICATION AND STRUCTURE OF ACIDS

Acids can be classified as inorganic or organic. Inorganic or mineral acids, unlike their organic counterparts, lack carbon atoms (see Table 15-2 and Chapter 98). Strong inorganic acids include sulfuric, hydrochloric, hydrofluoric, and nitric acids, and liquid sulfur dioxide.[3,13] These acids can cause significant ocular damage similar to that of alkalis. Common organic acids include acetic acid, formic acid, and phenol. Acids may also exist as an anhydride, which is the oxide of a metalloid or metal. When combined with water, the anhydride forms its acid. Common organic anhydrides include acetic anhydride and maleic anhydride. Typically, organic acids destroy the conjunctiva and cause little damage to the cornea. Corneal opacification and complete vision loss, however, have been occasionally described with these compounds.[14] Acid anhydrides usually cause more severe damage than their corresponding acids, because of their ability to penetrate the cornea more quickly.[14]

PHARMACODYNAMICS/MECHANISM OF ACTION AND TOXICITY

In acid burns to the eye, the hydrogen ion causes tissue damage by lowering pH, whereas the anion component precipitates and coagulates proteins of the corneal epithelium, forming a relative barrier to further penetration of the acid. Consequently, acids cause fewer stromal and intraocular complications and have a reputation for causing less severe eye injuries than alkalis. However, this is primarily true of weak or dilute mineral acids with concentrations of 10% or less. Although acids tend to be less penetrating and may require a few hours of contact to cause ocular injury, the surface injuries (vascularization and corneal scarring) can be as severe as those of alkali exposures.

Various factors enhance the severity of acid burns. Significant ocular injury does not occur unless the pH of the solution is 2.5 or less. If the protective epithelium of the cornea is removed or compromised, damage can occur with weaker or higher pH substances. Some acids react with water to produce an exothermic reaction. The heat liberated from this reaction damages the corneal epithelium and allows increased tissue penetration. Acids with strong solvent or lipophilic properties destroy cell membranes and penetrate the eye rapidly. Finally, prolonged contact with any acid increases the likelihood of significant ocular injury.

CLINICAL PRESENTATION

As with most chemical eye injuries, pain and irritation are the most common presenting symptoms. Initial

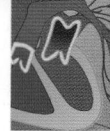

TABLE 15-2 Acids: Characteristics, Uses, and Ocular Toxic Effects

ACID	CHEMICAL COMPOSITION	DOMESTIC AND INDUSTRIAL USES	COMMENTS	POTENTIAL COMPLICATIONS
Inorganic Acids				
Sulfuric acid	H_2SO_4	Automobile batteries Metal, chemical, fertilizer	Causes thermal and chemical injury	Globe perforation Corneal opacification
Hydrochloric acid	HCl	Metal refining, bleach, plumbing	Strong solvent properties promote cell membrane destruction	Corneal opacification
Hydrofluoric acid	HF	See Table 15-3	Free fluoride ion binds Ca^+ and Mg^+ to cause liquefaction necrosis Possible delayed toxicity	Globe perforation Total globe destruction
Nitric acid	HNO_3	Soda, engraving, metal, fertilizer	Causes yellow opacification of the cornea	Corneal opacification Symblepharon formation
Sulfur dioxide	SO_2	Refrigerant, bleach, fruit and vegetable preservative	Causes eye anesthesia Possible delayed toxicity	Symblepharon formation Conjunctival overgrowth of cornea
Organic Acids				
Acetic acid	CH_3OOH	Vinegar (10%) Essence of vinegar (80%) Glacial acetic acid (90%)	>10% needed to cause damage if exposure brief Severity of damage may be delayed	Minor injury unless concentrated solution or prolonged exposure
Formic acid	HCOOH	Airplane glue Cellulose, tanning, formate	Rapidly penetrating	Minor to severe damage
Phenol	C_6H_5O	Antiseptic, disinfectant, barn deodorant	Caustic to skin and eyes	Corneal hypesthesia and opacification Complete vision loss
Organic Anhydrides				
Acetic anhydride	CH_3COOH	Manufacture of acetyl compounds, cellulose acetates, glycerol Dehydrating agent	Severity of damage may be delayed More damaging than dilute acetic acid	Permanent opacification if delayed decontamination
Maleic anhydride	$C_4H_2O_3$	Manufacture of alkyd resins, pharmaceuticals Dye intermediate Agricultural chemicals	More damaging than maleic acid	Produces damage similar to that of alkali

examination of patients with severe damage may reveal iritis, corneal opacification, or corneal anesthesia. Evidence of these abnormalities usually occurs within hours of acid contact, but they may be delayed, particularly following sulfuric acid and hydrogen fluoride exposures.

SPECIFIC ACIDS
Inorganic Acids
SULFURIC ACID
Sulfuric acid is used in fertilizing, metal, and chemical industries. It can be found in household drain cleaners in concentrations as high as 99.5%. However, most sulfuric acid burns to the eye result from exploding automobile batteries. The most common causes of battery explosions include improper use of battery cables, using a match to read the directions on the battery, smoking while working, and improperly connecting battery chargers.[14] When concentrated sulfuric acid reacts with water in the tear film of the cornea, heat is released, causing both thermal and chemical burns to the eye. Very severe burns may cause complete opacification of the cornea or perforation of the globe with loss of significant ocular

fluid.[8] Complications include glaucoma and cataract formation.

Although the ocular damage caused by concentrated sulfuric acid may be devastating, diluted sulfuric acid causes much less damage because the oxygen and hydrogen molecules in the water that dilute the acid partially satiate the acid's avidity for the same molecules in the eye. Consequently, diluted sulfuric acid produces less of an exothermic reaction on contact with the eye and behaves more like simpler acids, such as hydrochloric acid.[8]

SULFUR DIOXIDE
Sulfur dioxide exists in both gas and liquid forms. Sulfur dioxide gas is a common component of smog, but in concentrations likely too low to cause significant eye irritation.[8] Sulfur dioxide gas has a pungent smell and is irritating to the respiratory tract at concentrations lower than those that cause eye irritation. Exposure to sulfur dioxide gas does not cause significant eye injury because of the body's protective mechanisms.

The most damaging form of sulfur dioxide is sulfurous acid, which is formed when sulfur dioxide is combined with water. Sulfurous acid is considered more

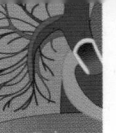

toxic than sulfuric, hydrochloric, or phosphoric acids, because it is highly lipid soluble and, therefore, penetrates the corneal epithelium quickly.[8,15]

Liquid sulfur dioxide is responsible for all significant eye burns. It is used in fruit and vegetable preservatives, bleach, and domestic refrigerators. Eye damage from the refrigerant is attributable to the direct action of the acid itself and not to freezing.[15] The solution is often combined with oil, which facilitates prolonged contact with the eye.

Although damage occurs rapidly, symptoms may be minimal following liquid sulfur dioxide exposure since the acid damages corneal nerves with resultant anesthesia of the eye.[15] The patient may not become aware of eye injury until vision becomes impaired hours to days after the initial contact. Following sulfur dioxide exposure, the corneal epithelium initially becomes opacified but remains adherent to the stroma, similar to acid burns. Later, the opaque corneal epithelium sloughs, which may transiently afford the patient improved vision and allows for a better examination of deeper injury. Slit-lamp evaluation may then reveal stromal edema, corneal opacity, interstitial vascularization, and damage to the endothelium. This deeper damage is similar to that encountered in alkali burns. Vascularization and opacification may continue for months, causing severe vision impairment. Frequent complications include symblepharon formation and conjunctival overgrowth of the cornea.

HYDROCHLORIC ACID (MURIATIC ACID)

Hydrochloric acid is a weak acid but it has strong solvent properties that promote cell membrane destruction. Concentrated solutions of hydrochloric acid (36%) are used primarily in the metal refining, chemical manufacturing, and plumbing industries. More dilute concentrations (8.5% to 15%) are found in bleaching agents and toilet bowl cleaners.

Exposure to hydrochloric acid vapors in concentrations greater than 10 ppm causes immediate eye and mucous membrane irritation.[16] A concentration of 1350 ppm for 1.5 hours causes corneal clouding in animals.[8] Strong protective responses in humans usually limit the degree of exposure so that serious injury from hydrochloric acid gas is rare.

Damage to the eye from hydrochloric acid solutions only occurs when the pH is below 3.[8] The severity of the injury can range from conjunctival irritation to total opacification of the cornea. A 2% solution of hydrochloric acid applied to human eyes for a few seconds does not produce significant injury.[8] Application of a 10% solution to rabbit corneas results in corneal scarring 2 weeks following exposure.[8]

NITRIC ACID

Nitric acid is one of the most commonly used industrial chemicals. It is found in the soda making, engraving, metal refining, electroplating, and fertilizer manufacturing industries. It is also a common laboratory reagent. Nitric acid exists as a colorless liquid that can cause yellow opacification of the corneal epithelium. It causes tissue damage by binding to complex proteins to form a yellow substance called xanthoproteic acid.[17]

Accidental applications of nitric acid to the eyes of newborn babies, given in lieu of dilute silver nitrate, has caused corneal opacification, symblepharon formation, and globe shrinkage.[8] In less severe cases, the opacified corneal epithelium may slough off in 1 or 2 days, and the eye returns to normal as the epithelium regenerates. Nitric acid causes eye injuries similar to those caused by hydrochloric acid burns and is less corrosive than sulfuric acid.

HYDROFLUORIC ACID

Hydrofluoric acid (HF) is formed when hydrogen fluoride is combined with water. Hydrogen fluoride can be a devastating eye, skin, and systemic toxin in both gaseous and liquid states (see Chapter 90). It has multiple industrial and household uses (Box 15-1).

The damage caused by HF is concentration dependent and largely related to the fluoride component rather than its corrosive hydrogen ion. Because HF is a relatively weak acid (pKa 3.8), it is largely nonionized and can penetrate cell membranes easily. During deep tissue penetration, the fluoride ion is released, and subsequently binds avidly to divalent cations to form insoluble salts (predominantly calcium and magnesium fluoride). This results in liquefaction necrosis and significantly decreased tissue concentrations of ionized calcium and magnesium concentrations. Alterations in calcium and magnesium concentrations result in an increase in cellular potassium permeability, which causes spontaneous neuronal depolarization and pain. The onset of pain is immediate following exposure to high-concentration liquids but may be delayed for several hours to days for less concentrated solutions.[18] Despite its deep tissue penetration, systemic fluoride toxicity is highly unlikely following ocular exposure to HF-containing products.

BOX 15-1   USES OF HYDROFLUORIC ACID

Industrial Uses

Semiconductor production
Aluminum manufacturing
Glass polishing and etching
Electropolishing of metals
Ceramic glazing and etching
High-test gasoline production
Manufacture of refrigerants
Fertilizer production
Leather tanning
Control of fermentation in breweries
Plastic production
Germicide production
Rust removal in commercial laundries
Photographic etching
Dispensing agents for insecticides
Dispensing agents for aerosol propellants

Household Uses

Rust remover
Wire cleaner

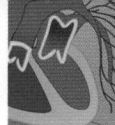

Local ocular penetration of the fluoride ion may continue for 24 hours, causing progressive damage to the corneal epithelium and underlying structures.[19] Reported ocular complications include tearing, conjunctival irritation and scarring, corneal opacification, uveitis, glaucoma, lid deformities, keratitis sicca, blindness, and globe perforation.[20] Anhydrous hydrogen fluoride has caused total eye destruction that necessitated enucleation.[8]

Animal studies have demonstrated complete recovery 10 days after ocular exposure to 0.5% HF solutions, and mild persistent stromal edema and vascularization 40 days following exposure to 2% HF solutions.[21] Instillation of 20% HF caused total corneal opacification, conjunctival ischemia, corneal stroma edema, and necrosis of anterior ocular structures.[8]

Organic Acids
FORMIC ACID
Formic acid is found in the airplane glue, cellulose formate, and tanning industries in concentrations of about 60%. It is one of the most rapidly penetrating acids; consequently, immediate and thorough irrigation is tremendously important. In one case of eye exposure to 90% formic acid, immediate irrigation was associated with complete recovery in 36 to 60 hours (initial examination had revealed loss of epithelium and cells in the anterior chamber).[22] In addition, copious irrigation was associated with complete recovery (initial examination revealed chemosis and epithelial damage) following eye exposure to a solution of 80% formic acid and 2% orthophosphoric acid. Conversely, ocular exposure to the same concentrated formic acid solution resulted in eye perforation and necessitated enucleation in a patient whose eye was less well irrigated.[23,24]

PHENOL
Phenol, also known as carbolic acid, is used primarily as an antiseptic, disinfectant, or barn deodorant. It is available as a pure crystal and in liquid forms in concentrations that range from 1% to 88%.[25] Ocular exposure to 12.5% phenol in 25% glycerol has been reported to cause minor corneal opacification and a temporary decrease in visual acuity; these effects fully resolved in 4 days.[8] Exposure to concentrated phenol, however, can cause conjunctival chemosis, corneal hypesthesia and opacification, and complete vision loss. Phenol is also very caustic to the skin and has damaged eyelids so severely that plastic surgery was required.[8]

ACETIC ACIDS
Acetic acid (CH_3COOH) is an organic acid that is found in the household as common vinegar. Other names include ethanoic acid, ethylic acid, methane carboxylic acid, and glacial acetic acid. Vinegar and most other commercial products contain 4% to 10% acetic acid. "Essence of vinegar" is 80% acetic acid; glacial acetic acid contains 90% acetic acid.

Vinegar routinely produces only minor ocular damage unless contact is prolonged. Consequences of typical exposures include immediate pain, conjunctival hyperemia, and mild, reversible injury to the cornea. Acetic acid typically requires concentrations greater than 10% to cause severe injury.[26] More dilute acetic acid concentrations, however, may produce significant ocular injury after very prolonged contact. Permanent corneal opacification was described in a woman who fainted after having vinegar thrown in her face.[8] Severe, irreversible damage may result from essence of vinegar and glacial acetic acid.[8]

Trichloroacetic acid causes injury similar to that of low-concentration acetic acid.[3,8]

Organic Anhydrides
ACETIC ANHYDRIDE
Acetic anhydride, in both liquid and gaseous forms, is necrotizing to tissues and is more damaging than dilute acetic acid. In its liquid form, acetic anhydride causes immediate burning of the eye, followed hours or days later by increasing corneal and conjunctival edema.[8] Permanent opacification can occur if decontamination is delayed. Acetic anhydride reacts with water to form acetic acid. The severity of injury of both acetic anhydride and acetic acid may not be evident until a few days after exposure.

MALEIC ANHYDRIDE
Maleic acid is a crystalline substance that has the potential to cause severe ocular damage similar to that caused by alkalis. It has a very reactive double bond and may cause protein denaturation.[8]

Solvents

Organic solvents are routinely found in laboratories and in industry. Common solvents include ethyl alcohol, methyl alcohol, toluene, acetone, and butanol. Fortunately, they have no strong alkaline or acidic properties and cause almost no reaction with tissues; therefore, they rarely cause significant eye injury.[8] On contact, solvents cause immediate pain from nonspecific dissolution of superficial lipid membranes; exposure may result in partial or complete loss of the corneal epithelium. Fortunately, these substances do not penetrate deeply and cause little or no damage to the underlying stroma.[26] The epithelium commonly regenerates in a few days without permanent sequelae.

Detergents and Surfactants

Detergents and surfactants cause injury that ranges from minor irritation to extensive injury. Detergents are divided into four categories: inorganic, organic, combination, and oil-soluble agents (see Chapter 102).

Inorganic detergents (sodium carbonate, sodium silicates, sodium metasilicate, and sodium phosphates) are used for laundering and dishwashing. Liquid and granular automatic dishwashing detergents contain combinations of these agents and have pH values that range from 9.7 to 12.7.[27,28] The phosphate detergents (e.g., sodium tripolyphosphate) routinely cause only transient irritation. The non–phosphate-containing detergents (sodium carbonate, sodium silicate, sodium metasilicate) are much more alkaline than phosphate-containing agents. Consequently, sodium carbonate, sodium silicates, and sodium metasilicate have caused significantly more

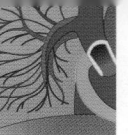

corrosive damage, including total and permanent opacity and corrosion to the cornea.[29] In general, liquid dishwashing and laundry detergents are less corrosive than automatic, granular dishwashing detergents.[30]

Organic detergents are composed of soaps and surfactants. Soaps cause tearing and pain, but they very rarely cause significant eye injury. The exception is commercial laundry soap that contains free alkali and has a pH of 12 or higher. These agents have caused permanent corneal opacification.[8]

Combination detergents are compounds that contain both organic and inorganic detergents. They include sodium dodecylbenzene sulfonate, sodium tripolyphosphate, sodium silicate, and sodium sulfate. These agents have caused corneal opacification in animals that have taken weeks or months to resolve.[8]

Oil-soluble detergents are additives to lubricating oils and produce no known eye hazard.

Surfactants are synthetic organic compounds that have hydrophilic properties at one end and lipophilic properties at the other end. They are used industrially for cleaning and are found in household cosmetics, ophthalmic solutions, shampoos, and detergents.

Surfactants can be classified as cationic, anionic, and nonionic. Cationic surfactants are usually quaternary ammonium compounds (e.g., benzalkonium chloride and benzethonium chloride). They precipitate proteins and routinely cause more damage than either anionic or nonionic agents. Anionic surfactants cause cell lysis. Soaps are included in this category. They tend to cause less damage but produce more pain and irritation than cationic agents. However, irreversible damage has occurred from 10% docusate and 40% dodecyl sodium sulfate.[8] Nonionic surfactants usually cause little or no damage other than local anesthesia of the cornea. However, full-strength tetradecylheptaethoxylate and tridecylhexaethoxylate caused permanent damage in rabbits, and G1690 in concentrations of less than 10% has caused severe irritation and corneal opacity.[8]

Cyanoacrylates

Cyanoacrylate adhesives are the components of common household glues (e.g., Krazy Glue [Elmers Products, Inc., Columbus, OH] and Super Glue [Super Glue, Inc., Rancho Cucamonga, CA]) and commercially available tissue adhesives for laceration repair (e.g., Dermabond [Ethicon, Inc., Somerville, NJ]). A number of accidental applications to the eye have occurred because the bottle was mistaken for an ophthalmic solution.[31,32] Childhood curiosity and ingenuity have resulted in a number of pediatric exposures. Applications to the eye have resulted in focal destruction of the epithelium and mild superficial stromal edema that resolved without sequelae.[31] Use of octylcyanoacrylate for facial laceration repair could also result in inadvertent adhesive application to the eye.

Mustard

Mustard agents are potent alkylating liquid substances that cause severe vesication (blistering) of the mucous membranes and skin (see Chapter 105B). There are two forms of mustard: (1) sulfur mustard (2,2-dichlorethyl sulfide, HD), used as a chemical warfare agent, and (2) nitrogen mustard (usually N-methyl-2,2-dichlorodiethylamine HN₂), a chemotherapeutic agent. Although routinely termed a *gas*, mustard exists as a straw-colored aerosol of oily droplets.[33]

The eye is the organ most susceptible to injury upon exposure to mustard agents delivered via aerosol. In fact, 75% to 90% of mustard casualties in World War I experienced some degree of eye pathology.[34] Ninety percent of those with ocular injury were visually incapacitated for approximately 10 days.[35] In the Iran-Iraq War, the majority of sulfur mustard casualties experienced some degree of ocular injury and 10% developed severe damage with corneal ulceration; 2% of these patients had anterior chamber scarring and neovascularization that caused prolonged disability.

Mustard's lipophilic nature causes it to concentrate in the oily milieu of tears. As an alkylator, mustard interferes with nucleic acid function and protein synthesis. Mustard affects rapidly dividing cells most readily, making the rapidly dividing corneal epithelium a prime target. Mustard agent–induced tissue injury necessitates extensive DNA repair, which leads to depletion of cellular NAD+, which is required for glycolysis. Impaired glycolysis promotes release of tissue proteases, which, in turn, cause cellular necrosis.[33] Oxidative stress also results in free radical formation. Rabbit studies demonstrate that glutathione and ascorbic acid concentrations in the aqueous humor decline 4 hours following sulfur mustard exposure.[36]

Sulfur mustard also has direct effects on cells to induce an inflammatory response that is active even before cell death has occurred; it stimulates the release of cytokines (interleukin-6 [IL-6], IL-8, IL-1β, and tumor necrosis factor-α).[37] This observation has stimulated study of anti-inflammatory agents to treat mustard exposures (see section on Special Management Considerations).

Mustard agents are highly reactive and bind to cellular components within minutes of exposure. Clinical evidence of ocular injury develops gradually over 4 to 12 hours in humans.[33] Symptoms range from mild stinging and dryness, to severe pain, photophobia, blurred vision, and temporary or permanent blindness. Physical findings include blepharospasm, conjunctival injection and edema, chemosis, anterior chamber cellular infiltrates, and decreased visual acuity. Corneal edema begins within 1 hour after exposure, and the corneal epithelium vesicates and sloughs within 4 to 36 hours. The extent of ocular damage is dependent on the concentration and duration of mustard exposure. Resolution of ocular injury occurs over 1 to 2 weeks.

A small percentage (0.5%) of severely injured victims will develop delayed ulcerative keratitis as late as 40 years after the original exposure. These patients undergo a long asymptomatic period followed by recurrent keratitis and areas of porcelain white episcleral tissue that later cause opacification, recurrent ulceration, pain and blindness.[33] Corneal opacification primarily occurs in the lower and central portions of the cornea; the upper

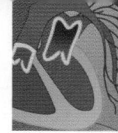

aspect of the cornea is protected during the exposure by the upper eyelid.[38]

Systemic Eye Toxins

Multiple agents taken systemically cause a variety of eye and vision abnormalities. A detailed description of these substances is beyond the scope of this chapter. A partial list of various agents and their effects (noted in humans) is depicted in Box 15-2. Methanol and quinine are two substances whose importance in toxicology requires special mention.

Systemic methanol toxicity is heralded by metabolic acidosis and visual disturbances (see Chapter 32A). Both formaldehyde and formic acid, the metabolites of methanol, are capable of causing ocular injury. However, the metabolite primarily responsible for the ocular damage that occurs following methanol ingestions has

been the subject of controversy. Rabbit studies suggest that direct instillation of formaldehyde into the eye causes injury to the retina and optic nerve, while direct instillation of formate causes little or no damage.[39] The potential reasons for this observation are twofold: (1) formaldehyde is rapidly converted in vivo to formic acid (within 1 to 2 minutes),[40] thereby providing little time to cause significant damage, and (2) in order for formic acid to cause damage, it must be metabolized from methanol within the retina itself.[41] Most investigators believe that formic acid is primarily responsible for methanol-associated blindness.

Formic acid inhibits cytochrome oxidase c in the mitochondria of optic nerve and retinal cells.[42] The resultant disruption of oxidative phosphorylation impairs the ability of the retina and optic nerve to produce adenosine triphosphate (ATP) and inhibits local aerobic metabolism. This inhibition of the electron transport

---

BOX 15-2	EYE AND VISION ABNORMALITIES FROM SYSTEMIC AGENTS

Substances Reported to Cause Papilledema When Taken Systemically

Aspirin	Dynamite	Lead	DL-Penicillamine
Bee sting (venom)	Ergotamine	Levothyroxine	Penicillin
Chloramphenicol	Ethylene glycol	Minocycline	Phosphorus
Chloedecone	Isoniazid	Minoxidil	Sulfonamides
Cisplatin	Isotretinoin	Nalidixic acid	Tetracycline
Contraceptive hormones	Ketoprofen	Nitrofurantoin	Vitamin A
Corticosteroids			

Substances Reported to Cause Nysagmus When Taken Systemically

Barbiturates	Ergot	Methocarbamol	Phenytoin
Carbamazepine	Ethchlorvynol	Methyl bromide	Primidone
Carbon disulfide	Ethyl alcohol	Methyl chloride	Streptomycin
Diazepam	Glutethimide	Methyl iodide	Toluene
Dieldrin			

Substances Reported to Cause Central Scotomas When Taken Systemically

Carbon disulfide*	Digoxin	Ethchlorvynol	Minoxidil
Cassava*	Dinitrochlorobenzene*	Ethyl alcohol	Streptomycin
Chloramphenicol*	Dinitrotoluene*	Ethylene glycol	Sulfonamides
Chloroquine	Disulfiram*	Ibuprofen	Tetraethyl lead*
Chlorpropramide*	Ergotamine	Isoniazid*	Thallium*
Digitalis*	Emetine	Lead*	Wasp sting* (venom)
Digitoxin*	Ethambutol*	Methanol	

Substances Reported to Cause Peripheral Visual Field Constriction When Taken Systemically

Bee sting (venom)	Carbon tetrachloride	Ethambutol	Oxygen
Botulism toxin	Castor beans	Methylmercury compounds	Pheniprazine
Carbon dioxide	Chloramphenicol	Methanol	Quinine
Carbon monoxide	Emitine	Naphthalene	

Substances Reported to Cause Cataracts When Taken Systemically

Acetaminophen†	Busulfan	Deferoxamine	Lead
Allopurinol	Corticosteroids	Ergot	Trinitrotoluene

Substances Reported to Cause Alopecia of the Eyebrows and Eyelids

Dactinomycin	Thallium	Triparanol	Vitamin A

---

*Also reported to cause bulbar neuritis.
†Has been described in animals, not humans.

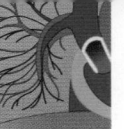

chain promotes the formation of oxidative radicals such as superoxide and hydrogen peroxide. Antioxidant protection is particularly important for the retina because of its frequent exposure to radiation and high metabolic rate. Additional insult to the retina may be caused by a reduction in retinal glutathione concentrations, which has been observed in methanol poisoned rats.[42]

Visual disturbances from methanol intoxication typically occur between 12 and 48 hours postingestion and range from reversible blurred vision and scotomas to permanent blindness. Fundoscopic examination reveals optic disc hyperemia, as well as retinal and disc edema. Macular edema is rare but has been described.[43]

Systemic quinine poisoning may result in significant ocular pathology as well (see Chapter 54). The mechanism by which quinine causes ocular damage remains controversial. Two plausible theories have been promulgated and include: (1) quinine causes vasoconstriction of the retinal artery, leading to retinal ischemic damage or (2) quinine is directly toxic to the retina, which leads to subsequent attenuation of the retinal vessels. Electroretinographic studies indicate that retinal damage precedes vessel narrowing,[44] supporting the later theory. Quinine may additionally exert its retinotoxic effects by blocking acetylcholine neurotransmission in the inner synaptic layer of the retina.[45]

Signs of quinine toxicity usually develop within 1 to 7 hours of an acute ingestion, but can be delayed more than 24 hours. Visual symptoms range from mild deficits in visual acuity to visual field cuts, disturbances in color and light perception, and complete blindness. Most patients recover at least some vision from several days to weeks after acute poisoning, although permanent visual defects may remain.

Fundoscopic evaluation is usually normal early in the course of quinine poisoning. Interestingly, abnormalities are often absent until symptoms begin to improve.[45,46] Findings may include dilated pupils (possibly secondary to the anticholinergic effects of quinine), loss of papillary light reflexes, retinal arteriolar vasoconstriction, a cherry red spot, and macular edema. Optic atrophy may appear days to weeks following exposure.[46]

Patient Examination

A detailed eye examination should not occur until copious irrigation has been performed. Ocular examination should include an assessment of visual acuity, intraocular pressure, tear pH, and corneal debris. The lids should be everted and examined for the presence of debris, particularly in the fornices. Irrigation should be resumed for persistent abnormalities in tear pH (i.e., pH less than 5 or greater than 8). A sterile fluorescein examination (using sterile, single-use strips) should be performed since it will allow evaluation of corneal epithelial defects; however, fluorescein examination alone will not provide adequate information about deeper damage. A slit-lamp examination is essential to assess the depth of the burn, degree of anterior chamber involvement, and potential presence of corneal edema.

Prognosis

The severity of injury at initial presentation correlates with long-term prognosis, such that preserved early vision predicts a preserved long-term visual acuity.[4,47] The most widely used grading system for ocular alkali injuries is the Hughes classification.[4,48] It is based on the degree of corneal epithelial damage and the extent of limbal ischemia. Damage to conjunctival and episcleral blood vessels will cause ischemia and pallor in the area of the limbus.[8,13,49] The degree of ischemia in this area is the most important prognostic sign following alkali injury. The Hughes classification divides injuries into four groups as listed in Table 15-3.

TREATMENT PRINCIPLES

Immediate Management

The initial management of all chemical ocular injuries requires immediate decontamination by irrigation. Early application of a topical anesthetic (e.g., 0.5% to 1.0% proparacaine or tetracaine) is recommended to facilitate irrigation and enhance patient comfort. Occasionally, a lid block may be necessary to relieve severe orbicularis spasm and allow irrigation to proceed.[50] The upper and lower eyelids should be retracted, inspected for retained solid material and injury, and irrigated. Immediate referral to an ophthalmologist is necessary for all significant burns.

TYPE OF IRRIGATION SOLUTION

Any, readily available, sterile, nonirritating solution is appropriate for irrigation. The choice of irrigant is not likely to affect outcome, whereas a delay of seconds to minutes to initiate irrigation could greatly affect outcome. Thus, the most readily available irrigant is what should be used. The most commonly available solutions include sterile water, normal saline, balanced saline solution, and lactated Ringer's. Diphoterine is a newer decontamination solution that may be available at some institutions.

Ordinary tap water is readily available, safe, and effective, and is thus often the initial irrigation fluid

TABLE 15-3 The Hughes Classification System		
GRADE	**DESCRIPTION**	**PROGNOSIS**
I	Corneal epithelial damage	Good
II	Cornea hazy	Good
	Iris details seen	
	Less than a third of limbus ischemic	
III	Total loss of corneal epithelium	Guarded
	Stromal haze blurring iris details	
	A third to half of limbus ischemic	
IV	Cornea opaque, obscures iris or pupil	Poor
	More than half of limbus ischemic	

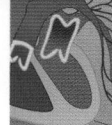

used, particularly in the prehospital environment. Although effective, tap water is hypotonic relative to the cornea. The osmolarity of the corneal stroma is 420 mOsm/L.[51] On theoretical grounds, the osmolarity gradient will promote water flow into the cornea, which will facilitate corneal swelling and toxin entry into ocular tissue. These theoretic concerns should not preclude the use of tap water if it is the most readily available solution.

Normal saline (pH 4.5 to 6.0) has a higher osmolarity than water but is still hypotonic with respect to the cornea. In addition, normal saline is slightly acidic and will not normalize the pH of the anterior chamber even following prolonged irrigation.[51,52]

Balanced saline solution plus (BSS Plus, Alcon Laboratories, Fort Worth, TX) is a pH-neutral solution (pH 7.2) with an osmolarity similar to aqueous humor. In theory, BSS does not cause corneal swelling and has enhanced buffering capabilities.[53] BSS Plus, however, costs more than $100 per bottle, and must be reconstituted prior to use, which will delay initial treatment.

Normal saline buffered with sodium bicarbonate to achieve a pH near 7.4 is attractive because it is inexpensive and causes less discomfort than nonbuffered solutions.[50] It can be made by adding 0.2 mL of bicarbonate (1 mEq/mL) to 500 mL of normal saline.[54] However, initiating immediate irrigation is again paramount; therefore, the use of special solutions is not appropriate unless they are readily available.

Lactated Ringer's solution (pH 6 to 7.5) is a buffered, inexpensive solution available in the hospital setting, and is potentially more effective and better tolerated than nonbuffered normal saline. Warmed solutions and the application of topical anesthesia prior to irrigation may also obviate the need for special formulations.

Diphoterine or hexafluorine is an amphoteric, hypertonic, polyvalent, chelating solution that is currently available in the United States (JR Enterprises, Goldendale, WA). Diphoterine's amphoteric properties allow it to bind and neutralize both acidic and basic compounds; it corrects corneal and aqueous humor pH.[55] Its hypertonicity (820 mOsm/L) attracts substances that have already penetrated tissues. In addition to binding acids and bases, Diphoterine is capable of binding oxidizing, reducing, and alkylating agents, solvents, irritants, and radionuclides.[56] These characteristics make it an appealing choice for decontamination of most ocular toxins, particularly chemical warfare agents (e.g., lacrimating agents and vesicants). Diphoterine is nontoxic (median lethal dose in rats greater than 2000 mg/kg orally and dermally) and nonirritating. The preparation available in the United States is an aerosol that is contained inside a plastic bag and housed within a pressurized can; as a result, no propellant comes in contact with the eye.

DURATION OF IRRIGATION

Prolonged irrigation appears to improve outcome. Thus, irrigation should be performed for at least 30 minutes, 2 L per eye, or until the pH of the eye returns to normal (7.3 to 7.7).[23,53] Severe acid and alkali burns require at least 1 to 2 hours of irrigation regardless of normal ocular pH.[57] A brief irrigation period (1 to 2 minutes) is

needed for most solvent injuries.[8] An irrigation device may facilitate irrigation but is not required.[58]

Special Management Considerations

A few substances deserve special management considerations. Table 15-4 includes a summary of the potential treatments for these compounds.

OCULAR CALCIUM HYDROXIDE BURNS

Irrigation should begin promptly. Following irrigation, a careful search for particulate matter should be performed; attention must be directed to identification and removal of solid material, because particulate matter usually accompanies calcium hydroxide ocular burns. It may be necessary to double-evert the upper eyelid and swab or brush away lodged material, looking especially in the fornices, where particles are frequently hidden. Application of a topical anesthetic followed by a 15-minute irrigation with a 0.01 to 0.05 mol/L (0.3% to 1.86%) solution of EDTA (at a pH between 4.6 and 7.0) may help loosen and dissolve solid matter.[8] A cotton-tipped applicator soaked in EDTA may also facilitate particle removal. To prepare a 0.05 mol/L neutral

TABLE 15-4 Special Management Considerations		
CHEMICAL	**CONCERNS**	**MANAGEMENT**
Calcium hydroxide	Embedded particulate matter Opacification secondary to calcium binding to Bowman's membrane	Swab soaked in 0.3%–1.86% disodium edetate *or* 15-minute irrigation with 0.3%–1.86% disodium edetate
Hydrofluoric acid	Binding of free fluoride ions Do not irrigate with benzethonium chloride or benzalkonium chloride Do not use subconjunctival injections of $CaCl_2$, $MgCl_2$, or calcium gluconate	Irrigate with water, normal saline, lactated Ringer's solution, or isotonic magnesium chloride Consider 1% calcium gluconate drops
Phenol	Decontamination may be difficult	Consider irrigation with 1% diethylenetriamine or 30%–50% polyethylene glycol
Cyanoacrylates	Eyelid adhesions	Consider mineral oil or wet compress applied overnight Antibiotic ointment applied overnight may be somewhat helpful Acetone is effective but may cause transient corneal abrasions

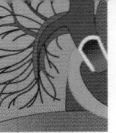

solution of EDTA, dilute 20 mL of Endrate disodium (150 mg/mL) (Abbott Laboratories, North Chicago, IL) with 180 mL of sterile 0.9% sodium chloride.[8] Disodium edetate may also clear the corneal opacification caused by the binding of calcium to Bowman's membrane (see earlier section on Calcium Hydroxide).[12]

OCULAR HYDROFLUORIC ACID BURNS

Management of ocular HF burns deserves special attention for two reasons. First, in addition to simple decontamination measures, treatment of HF burns is targeted at prevention of further penetration of the fluoride ion. Second, application of substances used to treat cutaneous hydrochloric acid burns may cause damage to the eye.

Because the onset of severe symptoms may be delayed, patients with even minor symptoms following hydrogen fluoride exposure may develop significant pain and damage later. Immediate and copious irrigation is imperative, as with all chemical injuries to the eye. Irrigation with benzethonium chloride solutions (0.2% or 0.5%) or benzalkonium chloride solution (0.05%) has been recommended for treatment of HF skin burns, because these compounds deactivate the free fluoride ion. However, these solutions are potentially damaging to the corneal epithelium of the normal eye and provide no benefit for patients with ocular HF burns.[8,20] Multiple irrigations also appear to be deleterious. For ocular HF burns, a single, thorough irrigation with 2 L of sterile lactated Ringer's, saline, water, or isotonic magnesium chloride is recommended.[21] The use of isotonic magnesium chloride solutions have been effective and not irritating.[59]

Injection of divalent cations (e.g., calcium or magnesium salts) binds free fluoride and is also commonly recommended for HF skin burns. Subconjunctival injections with $CaCl_2$, $MgCl_2$, and 10% calcium gluconate can induce significant eye damage and are contraindicated for the treatment of ocular hydrogen fluoride injuries.[20]

The instillation of two to three drops of 1% calcium gluconate solution every 3 hours may be effective in ocular HF burns. This solution, when used with topical cycloplegia and antimicrobial agents, provided complete resolution of signs and symptoms in a patient with ocular burns from 49% HF seen at a 3-month follow-up visit.[20] Further controlled study is necessary prior to formal recommendation of calcium gluconate drops.

Hexafluorine is an amphoteric hypertonic polyvalent compound designed specifically to decontaminate HF eye and skin exposures. It has been shown to prevent chemical burns in workers exposed to 40% HF.[60] However, one study suggests that animals decontaminated with Hexafluorine had a worse outcome than those treated with topical calcium or water irrigation.[61] Further study is warranted.

OCULAR PHENOL BURNS

Although isopropyl alcohol is commonly recommended for skin decontamination of phenol, water remains the solution of choice for eye irrigation. The use of 1% diethylenetriamine or 30% to 50% polyethylene glycol (e.g., PEG 400) has been recommended for eye irrigation, but further investigation is necessary.[8,62]

OCULAR CYANOACRYLATE EXPOSURE

When faced with the task of managing ocular cyanoacrylate exposure, eyelid adhesions are usually the greatest source of aggravation for both the patient and the health care provider. The initial management should include warm fluid irrigation through any available eye opening, as this may decrease the likelihood of corneal abrasions (especially if performed within 15 minutes of exposure).[63]

Acetone has been successfully utilized to loosen glue from the lashes as well as the cornea itself.[64] However, acetone is irritating to the eye and may cause temporary loss of corneal epithelium.[8]

The application of mineral oil has resulted in immediate softening of adhesions.[63,65] Application of a mineral oil compress applied overnight may be necessary to separate eyelids.

OCULAR MUSTARD EXPOSURE

Initial management of mustard eye exposures begins, as always, with irrigation for 10 to 15 minutes; although damage may have already occurred, irrigation may remove potential foreign bodies and debris. Systemic analgesics are usually required. Following irrigation, one should perform a fluorescein examination to initially assess corneal involvement. In mass casualty situations, patients may be divided into two groups: (1) those with conjunctival involvement only; and (2) those with corneal injury evidenced by areas of fluorescein uptake.[33] If injury is confined to the conjunctiva, patients may be discharged with symptomatic therapy, reassurance that vision will return to normal in a few days, and psychological support. Patients with corneal involvement should be referred to an ophthalmologist immediately for further evaluation and care.

A number of therapies specific to management of ocular mustard injuries have been evaluated. Anti-inflammatory agents appear to be promising: dexamethasone eye drops (one drop [50 µL] 4 times daily applied 1 hour postexposure) attenuated the inflammatory response in sulfur mustard exposed rabbits.[66] Diclofenac, a nonsteroidal anti-inflammatory agent, applied in the same manner, gave similar but less notable results.[66]

Topical diltiazem (30 µL of a 10 mmol/L solution) applied prior to nitrogen mustard application, reduced eye irritation and attenuated intraocular pressure elevation in rabbits.[67] Zinc-desferrioxamine or gallium-desferrioxamine (two drops each hour for 12 hours instilled immediately after nitrogen mustard application) significantly reduced conjunctival, corneal, iris, and anterior chamber injury by inhibiting free radical formation.[68] Finally, lowering the incubation temperature of sulfur mustard–exposed cells from 37° C to 31° C transiently decreased apoptotic cell death.[69]

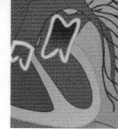

SYSTEMIC METHANOL-INDUCED RETINAL INJURY

Eels and colleagues described the successful use of photobiomodulation to promote recovery of retinal function following methanol-derived formate exposure.[70] Photobiomodulation is a process that uses low-energy lasers or light-emitting diode (LED) rays to accelerate wound healing. LEDs work by up-regulating cytochrome oxidase activity and mitochondrial ATP synthesis. Unlike most lasers, negligible amounts of heat are generated; therefore, thermal damage to biologic tissues does not occur. The Food and Drug Administration has deemed LED technology safe in human trials.[70] Further investigation for the use of LEDs in methanol-poisoned humans is required. See Chapter 32A for a more detailed description of the management of methanol poisoning.

SYSTEMIC QUININE-INDUCED RETINAL INJURY

Specific therapies for quinine-induced ocular injury are limited to isolated case reports and include therapies such as hyperbaric oxygen[71] and intravenous nimodipine.[72] To date, there have been no significant clinical trials in humans or animals. Refer to Chapter 54 for a more detailed description of the management of quinine poisoning.

Special Agents

Many other agents have been found to aid in the healing process following chemical injuries. These therapies are geared toward correcting impediments to reepithelialization and improving transdifferentiation (see earlier section on Mechanisms of Repair). Factors that impair reepithelialization include damage to the basement membrane, abnormal tear production, and infiltration by polymorphonuclear neutrophils.

Toxin-induced damage to the epithelial basement membrane may cause a decrease in fibronectin, which is needed to help the adherence of the advancing epithelium. If fibronectin is decreased, recurrent epithelial erosions can occur. Unfortunately, clinical trials evaluating the efficacy of fibronectin have failed to reveal a benefit.[73,74] Abnormal tear film production may lead to chronic ocular surface irritation, making reepithelialization difficult. Finally, polymorphonuclear neutrophil infiltration will slow the epithelial migration process. Polymorphonuclear neutrophils also produce collagenase and other enzymes that interfere with corneal differentiation. Substances known or currently used to improve corneal healing are listed in Table 15-5.

Final Considerations

After irrigation, the eye should be reinspected for particulate matter and other injuries. The ocular pH should be checked intermittently over the following hour to ensure that the pH remains neutral. An ophthalmic antimicrobial agent should be applied to prevent secondary infection, and a cycloplegic drug may be added to prevent painful ciliary spasms and the development of posterior synechiae. Application of a pressure patch may improve patient comfort. Systemic analgesics rather than topical anesthetics should be administered for additional pain control. Immediate consultation with an ophthalmologist is required for all but the most trivial burns; formal ophthalmologic evaluation is recommended for most patients within 24 hours of exposure. Finally, tetanus prophylaxis should be administered as necessary.

TABLE 15-5   Medical Therapy for Chemical Injuries to the Eye

AGENT	MECHANISM OF ACTION	COMMENTS
Tear substitutes and lubricating ointments	Lubricant Minimizes trauma of eyelid movement	Use only nonpreserved medications
Topical corticosteroids	Reduces inflammation Anticollagenolytic effects	Impairs the stromal repair process that occurs ~14 days after alkali injuries; should not be continued beyond 10–14 days
Medroxyprogesterone (Provera 1%)	Reduces inflammation without affecting corneal wound repair	Can be used after 10–14 days
Ascorbate (topical and systemic)	Necessary for collagen synthesis Replaces ascorbate depletion that accompanies keratocyte damage	Reduces incidence of ulcer formation following alkali injury
Citrate	Decreases polymorphonuclear neutrophils infiltration	
Retinoic acid (vitamin A analog)	Promotes corneal epithelial differentiation	Requires further investigation
Fibronectin	Facilitates adhesion of migrating epithelium	Not currently available for clinical use
Epidermal growth factor	Promotes epithelial mitosis	Not currently available for clinical use

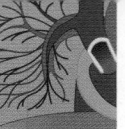

REFERENCES

1. Lai MW, Klein-Schwartz W, Rodgers GC, et al: 2005 annual report of the American Association of Poison Control Centers National Poisoning and Exposure Database. Clin Toxicol 2006;44:803–932.
2. Stein H, Slatt B, Stein R: Ophthalmic Terminology, 3rd ed. St. Louis, MO, Mosby Year Book, 1992.
3. Chernow S: Acute ocular injury from hazardous materials. In Sullivan J, Krieger G (eds): Hazardous Materials Toxicology. Baltimore, Williams & Wilkins, 1992, pp 433–440.
4. Wagoner M, Kenyon K: Chemical injuries. In Singleton B, Hersh P, Kenyon K (eds): Eye Trauma. St. Louis, MO, Mosby Year Book, 1991, pp 79–94.
5. Johnson-Wint B, Gross J: Regulation of connective tissue collagenase production: stimulators from adult and fetal epidermal cells. J Cell Biol 1984;98(1):90–96.
6. Onofrey BE: Management of corneal burns. Optom Clin 1995:4(3):31–40.
7. Grant WM, Kern HL: Action of alkalis on the corneal stroma. Am Arch Ophthalmol 1955;54(6):931–939.
8. Grant W: Toxicology of the Eye, 4th ed. Springfield, IL, Charles C Thomas, 1995.
9. Millea TP, Kucan JO, Smoot EC 3rd: Anhydrous ammonia injuries. J Burn Care Rehabil 1989;10(5):448–453.
10. Paterson CA, Pfister RR, Levinson RA: Aqueous humor pH changes after experimental alkali burns. Am J Ophthalmol 1975;79(3):414–419.
11. Smally AJ, et al: Alkaline chemical keratitis: eye injury from airbags. Ann Emerg Med 1992;21(11):1400–1402.
12. Oosterhuis JA: Treatment of calcium deposits in the cornea by irrigation and by application of EDTA. Ophthalmologica 1963; 145:161–174.
13. Stern AL, Pamel GJ, Benedetto LG: Physical and chemical injuries of the eyes and eyelids. Dermatol Clin 1992;10(4):785–791.
14. Sullivan J, Krieger G: Hazardous Materials Toxicology. Baltimore, Williams & Wilkins, 1992.
15. Minatoya HK: Eye injuries from exploding car batteries. Arch Ophthalmol 1978;96(3):477–481.
16. Grant W: Ocular injury due to sulfur dioxide. Arch Ophthalmol 1947;38:755.
17. Finkel A, Hamilton A, Hardy H: Hamilton and Hardy's Industrial Toxicology. Boston, John Wright & Sons, 1983.
18. Patnaik P: A comprehensive guide to the hazardous properties of chemical substances. New York, Van Nostrand Reinhold, 1992.
19. Hatai J, Weber J, Doizakai K: Hydrofluoric acid burns of the eye: report of possible delayed toxicity. J Toxicol Cutan Ocular Toxicol 1986;5(3):179–184.
20. Ellenhorn M, Barceloux D: Medical Toxicology, 1st ed. New York, Elsevier, 1988.
21. Bentur Y, Tannenbaum S, Yaffe Y, et al: The role of calcium gluconate in the treatment of hydrofluoric acid eye burn. Ann Emerg Med 1993;22(9):1488–1490.
22. McCulley JP, Whiting DM, Petitt MG, et al: Hydrofluoric acid burns of the eye. J Occup Med 1983;25(6):447–450.
23. Sudarsky D: Ocular injury due to formic acid. Arch Ophthalmol 1965;74(805).
24. Martin-Amat G, Tephly T, McMartine K: Methyl alcohol poisoning: II. Development of a model for ocular toxicity in methyl alcohol poisoning using the Rhesus monkey. Arch Ophthalmol 1977;95: 1847–1850.
25. Fink W: The ocular pathology of methyl alcohol poisoning. Am J Ophthalmol 1943;26(694).
26. McCulley J: Chemical agents. In Smolin G, Thoft A (eds): The Cornea. Boston, Little, Brown, 1994, pp 617–633.
27. Teir H: Toxicologic effects on the eyes at work. Acta Ophthalmol Suppl 1984;161:60–65.
28. Krenzelok EP: Liquid automatic dishwashing detergents: a profile of toxicity. Ann Emerg Med 1989;18(1):60–63.
29. Winter ML, Ellis MD: Automatic dishwashing detergents: their pH, ingredients, and a retrospective look. Vet Hum Toxicol 1986; 28(6):536–538.
30. Muhlendahl K, Oberdisse U, Krienke E: Local injuries caused by accidental ingestion of corrosive substances by children. Arch Toxicol 1978;39:299–314.
31. Scharpf LG Jr, Hill ID, Kelly RE: Relative eye-injury potential of heavy-duty phosphate and non-phosphate laundry detergents. Food Cosmet Toxicol 1972;10(6):829–837.

32. Margo CE, Trobe JD: Tarsorrhaphy from accidental instillation of cyanoacrylate adhesive in the eye. JAMA 1982;247(5):660–661.
33. Solberg Y, Alcalay M, Belkin M: Ocular injury by mustard gas. Surv Ophthalmol 1997;41(6):461–466.
34. Hughes W: Mustard gas injuries to the eyes. Arch Ophthalmol 1942;27:582–589.
35. Safarinejad MR, Moosavi SA, Montazeri B: Ocular injuries caused by mustard gas: diagnosis, treatment, and medical defense. Milit Med 2001;166(1):67–70.
36. Kadar T, Turetz J, Fishbine F, et al: Characterization of acute and delayed ocular lesions induced by sulfur mustard in rabbits. Curr Eye Res 2001;22(1):42–53.
37. Arroyo CM, Schafer RJ, Kurt EM, et al: Response of normal human keratinocytes to sulfur mustard (HD): cytokine release using a non-enzymatic detachment procedure. Hum Exp Toxicol 1999; 18(1):1–11.
38. Pleyer U, Sherif Z, Baatz H, et al: Delayed mustard gas keratopathy: clinical findings and confocal microscopy. Am J Ophthalmol 1999;128(4):506–507.
39. Hayasaka Y, Hayasaka S, Nagaki Y: Ocular changes after intravitreal injection of methanol, formaldehyde, or formate in rabbits. Pharmacol Toxicol 2001;89:74–78.
40. McMartin K, Ambre J, Tephly T: Methanol poisoning in human subjects. Am J Med 1980;68:414–418.
41. Garner C: Role of retinal metabolism in methanol-induced retinal toxicity. J Toxicol Environ Health 1995;44:43–56.
42. Seme M, Summerfelt P, Neitz J, et al: Differential recovery of retinal function after mitochondrial inhibition by methanol intoxication. Invest Ophthalmol Vis Sci 2001;42(3):834–841.
43. McKellar M, Hidajat R, Elder M: Acute ocular methanol toxicity: clinical and electrophysiological features. Aust N Z J Ophthalmol 1997;25(3):225–230.
44. Brinton G, Norton EW, Zahn JR, et al: Ocular quinine toxicity. Am J Ophthalmol 1980;90:403–410.
45. Canning C, Hague S: Ocular quinine toxicity. Br J Ophthalmol 1988;72:23–26.
46. Bateman D, Dyson E: Quinine toxicity. Adv Drug React Acute Poison Rev 1896;4:215–233.
47. Morgan SJ, Astbury NJ: Inadvertent self administration of superglue: a consumer hazard. BMJ 1984;289(6439):226–227.
48. Saini JS, Sharma A: Ocular chemical burns—clinical and demographic profile. Burns 1993;19(1):67–69.
49. Hughes W: Alkali burns of the cornea: II. Clinical and pathologic course. Arch Ophthalmol 1946;36:189–194.
50. Reim M: The results of ischaemia in chemical injuries. Eye 1992;6(Pt 4):376–380.
51. Kuckelkorn R, et al: Emergency treatment of chemical and thermal eye burns. Acta Ophthalmol Scand 2002;80(1):4–10.
52. Langefeld S, Press UP, Frentz M, et al: Use of lavage fluid containing diphoterine for irrigation of eyes in first aid emergency treatment. Ophthalmologe 2003;100(9):727–731.
53. Herr RD, White GL, Bernhisel K, et al: Clinical comparison of ocular irrigation fluids following chemical injury. Am J Emerg Med 1991;9(3):228–231.
54. Belin M, Catalano R, Scott J: Burns of the eye. In Ocular Emergencies. Philadelphia, WB Saunders, 1992, pp 179–197.
55. Schrage NF, Kompa S, Haller W, et al: Use of an amphoteric lavage solution for emergency treatment of eye burns. First animal type experimental clinical considerations. Burns 2002;28(8):782–786.
56. Hall AH, Blomet J, Mathieu L: Diphoterine for emergent eye/skin chemical splash decontamination: a review. Vet Hum Toxicol 2002;44(4):228–231.
57. Saari KM, Leinonen J, Aine E: Management of chemical eye injuries with prolonged irrigation. Acta Ophthalmol Suppl 1984;161:52–59.
58. Fernandes CM: Eye irrigating lenses. Arch Emerg Med 1991; 8(4):274–276.
59. McCulley J: Ocular hydrofluoric acid burns: animal model, mechanism of injury and therapy. Trans Am Ophthalmol Soc 1990;88:649–684.
60. Mathieu L, Nehles J, Blomet J, et al: Efficacy of Hexafluorine for emergent decontamination of hydrofluoric acid eye and skin splashes. Vet Hum Toxicol 2001;43(5):263–265.
61. Hojer J, Personne M, Hulten P, et al: Topical treatments for hydrofluoric acid burns: a blind controlled experimental study. J Toxicol Clin Toxicol 2002;40(7):861–866.

62. Brown VK, Box VL, Simpson BJ: Decontamination procedures for skin exposed to phenolic substances. Arch Environ Health 1975;30(1):1–6.

63. Dean BS, Krenzelok EP: Cyanoacrylates and corneal abrasion. J Toxicol Clin Toxicol 1989;27(3):169–172.

64. Turss U, Turss R, Refojo MF: Removal of isobutyl cyanoacrylate adhesive from the cornea with acetone. Am J Ophthalmol 1970;70(5):725–728.

65. Bock G: Skin exposure to cyanoacrylate adhesive. Ann Emerg Med 1984;13(6):486.

66. Amir A, Turetz J, Chapman S, et al: Beneficial effects of topical anti-inflammatory drugs against sulfur mustard-induced ocular lesions in rabbits. J Appl Toxicol 2000;20(Suppl 1):109–114.

67. Gonzalez GG, Gallar J, Belmonte C: Influence of diltiazem on the ocular irritative response to nitrogen mustard. Exp Eye Res 1995; 61(2):205–212.

68. Banin E, Morad Y, Berenshtein E, et al: Injury induced by chemical warfare agents: characterization and treatment of ocular tissues exposed to nitrogen mustard. Invest Ophthalmol Vis Sci 2003; 44(7):2966–2972.

69. Mi L, Gong W, Nelson P, et al: Hypothermia reduces sulphur mustard toxicity. Toxicol Appl Pharmacol 2003;193(1):73–83.

70. Eells J, Henry MM, Summerfelt P, et al: Therapeutic photo-biomodulation for methanol-induced retinal toxicity. Proc Natl Acad Sci U S A 2003;100(6):3439–3444.

71. Wolfe R, Wirtschafter D, Adkinson C: Ocular quinine toxicity treated with hyperbaric oxygen. Undersea and hyperbaric medicine. J Undersea Hyperbaric Med Soc 1997;24(2):131–134.

72. Barrett N, Solano T: Quinine ocular toxicity: treatment of blindness using therapy for vasospasm. Anaesth Intens Care 2002;30:234–235.

73. Gordon JF, Johnson P, Musch DC: Topical fibronectin ophthalmic solution in the treatment of persistent defects of the corneal epithelium. Chiron Vision Fibronectin Study Group. Am J Ophthalmol 1995;119(3):281–287.

74. Boisjoly HM, Beaulieu A: Topical autologous fibronectin in patients with recurrent corneal epithelial defects. Cornea 1991;10(6):483–488.

16 Endocrine Toxicology

HEIKKI ERIK NIKKANEN, MD ■ MICHAEL W. SHANNON, MD, MPH

GLUCOREGULATORY SYSTEM

Glucose is an important source of energy for cellular function. This is especially true of the brain, which is incapable of using free fatty acids. The regulation of blood sugar is accomplished by a complex interplay of systems. Alterations in glucose level can be caused by a variety of agents with endocrine system actions. Hypoglycemia is the most common endocrine emergency, and can be life threatening in certain cases.[1] According to the National Institutes of Health, 6.3% of the U.S. population was afflicted with diabetes in 2002. A correspondingly large number of prescriptions for antidiabetic agents were written as a consequence.

GLUCOSE METABOLISM

Glucose enters the body through the intestinal wall, in some cases after its production in a catabolic reaction involving amylase or a glucosidase. It is then taken up by body tissues with the help of insulin. This hormone, secreted by the β islet cells of the pancreas, facilitates glucose uptake across cell membranes. In adipose tissues, insulin promotes glycogen formation and fatty acid synthesis. Insulin is degraded by insulinase, with a half-life of 5 minutes. In response to hypoglycemia, epinephrine release, or norepinephrine release, glucagon is secreted by the α cells of the pancreas. This hormone, a 29-unit polypeptide, works in the liver through a cyclic adenosine monophosphate pathway to activate phosphorylase. As its name suggests, this enzyme dephosphorylates glucose-1-phosphate to glucose. This reaction is the rate-limiting step in conversion of glycogen to glucose. Glucagon also induces gluconeogenesis. Both of these effects serve to increase glucose levels in the blood. A number of xenobiotics cause hypoglycemia or hyperglycemia through effects on this system.

SPECIFIC AGENTS AND THEIR MECHANISMS OF TOXICITY

Hypoglycemic and Antihyperglycemic Agents

Insulin of various types can be injected intravenously or subcutaneously. Depending on the formulation, dose, and route of administration, the level of hypoglycemia and duration of action are quite variable (Table 16-1). Excess insulin can be the result of greater than necessary insulin administration, decreased caloric intake, or an insulinoma. Once in the bloodstream, exogenous insulin has effects identical to those of the endogenously produced substance. As the kidneys metabolize insulin, patients in renal failure will require decreased doses to avoid hypoglycemic events. Orally, insulin is not bioavailable at all and therefore represents no risk for hypoglycemia when taken in this manner.

Oral antihyperglycemic agents have a variety of mechanisms of action. The α-glucosidase inhibitors prevent the breakdown of oligosaccharides and polysaccharides into simple sugars. Hyperglycemia after meals is prevented, and the delivery of glucose into the bloodstream is delayed. There are few reports of overdose of α-glucosidase inhibitors. Their mechanism of action and the existing animal studies would suggest there are no significant effects in overdose.[2,3] Among the oral antihyperglycemic agents, the sulfonylureas stand out as being able to produce a significant hypoglycemia.[4] They accomplish this by acting on the pancreatic β islet cell to cause it to secrete insulin. Additionally, these drugs increase insulin sensitivity in peripheral tissues. In overdose, approximately one third of children ingesting a sulfonylurea became hypoglycemic; in a case series largely of adults, three fourths developed hypoglycemia.[5,6] Sulfonylureas may result in hypoglycemia many hours after ingestion. Although approximately 90% of patients in several pediatric studies developed hypoglycemia within 8 hours of ingestion, there has been at least one case report of 24 hours' delay in developing significant hypoglycemia following chlorpropamide ingestion.[5,7,8] Between one third and three fourths of pediatric patients had blood glucose measurements below 60 mg/dL.[5,8] There is also a significant risk for prolonged or recurrent hypoglycemic episodes.[9,10]

The thiazolidinedione class exerts its effect by decreasing insulin resistance at peripheral and hepatic sites. These drugs bind selectively to the peroxisome proliferator-activated receptor-γ (PPAR-γ), which is found in fat, liver tissue, and skeletal muscle.[11] Little is known about adverse effects in overdose. In therapeutic doses, hypoglycemia has occurred in conjunction with insulin use, and liver abnormalities have also been noted.[2]

TABLE 16-1 Insulins

INSULIN	ONSET	PEAK	DURATION
Humalog	15–20 min	30–90 min	3–4 hr
Novolog	15–20 min	40–50 min	3–4 hr
Regular	30–60 min	80–120 min	4–6 hr
NPH	2–4 hr	6–10 hr	14–16 hr
Lente	3–4 hr	6–12 hr	16–18 hr
Ultralente	4–6 hr	10–16 hr	18–20 hr
Lantus	2–3 hr	None	18–26 hr

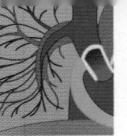

Biguanide oral diabetic agents work by three mechanisms: (1) reduction in intestinal glucose absorption, (2) reduction in hepatic glucose production, and (3) increase in peripheral insulin sensitivity. In overdose, nausea, vomiting, and diarrhea are common. Metabolic acidosis, tachypnea, hypotension, hypoglycemia, and pancreatitis have also been reported. In therapeutic administration, lactic acidosis is the most worrisome adverse effect, but this is relatively rare. In one study, the incidence was only nine cases per 100,000 patient years.[12] Additionally, patients found to be at greater risk are those with underlying chronic or acute renal insufficiency, those with hepatic dysfunction, or those who have a concurrent severe illness.[13-20] There does not seem to be a relationship between serum lactic acid level and outcome.[21] This suggests that biguanide-induced lactic acidosis is of the type B variety.

Meglitinides are among the newest agents available. They stimulate insulin secretion by closing adenosine triphosphate (ATP)-sensitive potassium channels in β cells, with a resultant rise in intracellular calcium and secretion of insulin.[22-27] According to one study, the duration of effect is similar to glyburide.[23] Although data on adverse effects following overdose are scarce, the mechanism of action suggests that hypoglycemia is likely (Table 16-2).

Ethanol can also cause significant hypoglycemia, notably during binge drinking. This generally occurs to those who do not consume enough calories during the event, those with poor glycogen stores, and those in whom nicotinamide adenine dinucleotide (NAD) has been depleted by the metabolism of ethanol. Chronic alcoholics, those who are malnourished, and children are particularly at risk.[28,29]

Vacor, a rodenticide, has particular toxicity to the β islet cells of the pancreas. A massive release of insulin ensues, with resulting hypoglycemia. After the destruction of the β islet cells is complete, type 1 diabetes ensues. Pentamidine poisoning has the same pathophysiology.

Ackee is the national fruit of Jamaica. It is the product of the *Blighia sapida* tree, indigenous to West Africa but carried to Jamaica in the latter part of the 18th century. Two compounds have been isolated in the flesh and seeds. Hypoglycin, also known as hypoglycin A, is the more toxic of the two and is present in much higher concentration in the unripe fruit. When hypoglycin is ingested, it is transaminated and decarboxylated to methylene cyclopropyl acetic acid (MCPA). This metabolite interferes with the process of gluconeogenesis.

Other xenobiotics such as salicylates, β-adrenergic blockers, disopyramide, ritodrine, haloperidol, and quinine have been associated with hypoglycemia. In renal failure, trimethoprim-sulfamethoxazole and propoxyphene have been noted to cause hypoglycemia.[1,4]

Hyperglycemic Agents

Glucagon is used as a hyperglycemic agent in insulin-treated patients who become hypoglycemic and are too obtunded to take oral carbohydrates; nonendocrine uses have included therapy of β-blocker overdose, cardiovascular emergencies, and relaxation of the gastrointestinal (GI) tract for diagnostic procedures. Its toxicity is limited; nausea and vomiting are frequent consequences of its use. The expected increase in glucose does not occur in patients who are depleted of glycogen stores; for example, patients with alcohol-related hypoglycemia show no response, and delaying more effective therapy (such as glucose administration) poses a risk in such a setting. In a patient with an insulinoma, the initial beneficial increase in glucose levels may be followed by a subsequent precipitous glucose drop due to stimulation of further insulin production by the glucagon.

Diazoxide, used infrequently as a parenteral agent in hypertensive crisis, is an inhibitor of insulin secretion and can be used as an oral agent in the therapy of patients with insulinomas. It causes sodium and fluid retention, with associated edema, and simultaneous use of a loop diuretic is a frequent need. In addition to being monitored for development of hyperglycemia related to excessive insulin suppression, patients should be monitored for complications that include GI distress, pancreatitis, thrombocytopenia or leukopenia, impairment of renal function, and proteinuria.

TREATMENT PRINCIPLES

Hypoglycemic Agents

Glucose can be used to rapidly increase blood glucose for use by the target tissues. In most circumstances, it should be the first agent used to counter hypoglycemia. Glucagon can be used to stimulate glycogenolysis and

TABLE 16-2 Oral Antihyperglycemic Agents

CLASS	GENERIC NAME	DURATION OF ACTION (hr)
First-generation sulfonylurea	Chlorpropamide	24–72
First-generation sulfonylurea	Tolazamide	
First-generation sulfonylurea	Tolbutamide	6–10
First-generation sulfonylurea	Glucotrol	12
Second-generation sulfonylurea	Glucotrol XL	24
Second-generation sulfonylurea	Glyburide	18–24
Second-generation sulfonylurea	Glyburide micronized	24
Third-generation sulfonylurea	Glimepiride	24
Biguanide	Metformin	8–12
Biguanide	Metformin XR	24
Meglitinide	Repaglinide	3
Meglitinide	Nateglinide	3
α-Glucosidase inhibitor	Acarbose	4
α-Glucosidase inhibitor	Miglitol	4
Thiazolidinedione	Rosiglitazone	
Thiazolidinedione	Pioglitazone	

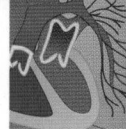

gluconeogenesis, thereby increasing available glucose. One advantage is that it can be administered subcutaneously or intramuscularly. Another advantage is its longer duration of effect. However, patients with poor glycogen stores will not develop an adequate response. Patients with insulinoma should not receive glucagon due to the risk for insulin release and resultant hypoglycemia. Patients with pheochromocytoma should not receive glucagon because it may trigger catecholamine release from the tumor and subsequent hypertension.

Octreotide is a long-acting synthetic somatostatin analog. It acts at somatostatin receptors and inhibits release of a number of pituitary and GI hormones, including insulin and glucagon. It can be used to provide protection against hypoglycemic events due to xenobiotic agents which promote release of insulin by the pancreas. Hypoglycemia caused by sulfonylureas, meglitinides, and perhaps by Ackee fruit, can be treated by its use.

The decision to admit a patient should be based on the nature of the poisoning as well as the clinical picture. It is worth noting that sulfonylurea overdoses in particular benefit from long-term glucose monitoring. Although one study suggests that 8 hours may be sufficient for most cases, many clinicians prefer a period of 24 hours.[8,30]

Hyperglycemic Agents

The hyperglycemia from glucagon is generally transient and does not require any treatment other than stopping the drug. If the patient develops hypertension requiring control, phentolamine mesylate 5 to 10 mg intravenously may be used. Treatment of adverse effects from diazoxide must be tailored to the particular pathology (Table 16-3).

HYPOTHALAMIC AGENTS

Introduction and Importance

The hypothalamus-pituitary axis is the primary interface between the brain and the endocrine system. The circumventricular organs of the hypothalamus play a key role, because their endothelium lacks tight junctions. They are therefore effectively on the outside of the blood-brain barrier, and able to sense levels of various factors and release others.

A number of hormones are secreted by the hypothalamus, with varied target organs. Some of these have been purified or synthesized for medical use. Two hormones secreted by the hypothalamic neurohypophyseal tract have important clinical uses. Oxytocin has a number of functions, but is primarily administered to induce labor and cause postpartum uterine contraction. Vasopressin and its analogs (desmopressin, lypressin) are used primarily for hormone replacement therapy in patients with central diabetes insipidus. Two of the hypothalamic agents, growth hormone-releasing hormone (GHRH) and gonadotropin-releasing hormone (GnRH) are used therapeutically as well.

Specific Agents and Their Mechanisms of Toxicity

Oxytocin is an octapeptide produced in the hypothalamus and stored in the posterior pituitary. It has uterine-stimulatory action, a vasopressive effect, and an antidiuretic effect. It also stimulates the milk letdown reflex. Adverse actions from oxytocin use include overstimulation of the uterus, with potential for fetal distress or uterine rupture, hypertension, or water intoxication. Hyponatremia, resulting from the intrinsic antidiuretic action of the molecule, can lead to various neurologic consequences, including convulsions.

Toxic effects of vasopressin are uncommon if the agent is used in appropriate dosage, and the major adverse effects are related to the expected physiologic action of the molecule in question. Desmopressin (DDAVP) has emerged as the most commonly used vasopressin analog for several reasons, including its convenient forms of administration and its prolonged half-life with enhanced antidiuretic and decreased vasopressor effects compared with the parent arginine vasopressin molecule.[31] Because of the drug's physiologic action, hypertension might also be anticipated as a possible adverse effect of vasopressin administration, but this is also very uncommon, particularly with desmopressin. Hyponatremia is the most likely adverse result of vasopressin administration but is a relatively uncommon problem, because hyponatremia cannot develop unless the vasopressin-stimulated decrease in renal tubular free water clearance is combined with an increase in free water intake.

The hypothalamic-releasing hormones include thyrotropin-releasing hormone (TRH, or protirelin), GnRH (or gonadorelin), GHRH, and corticotropin-releasing hormone. For the most part, these drugs are used as investigative or diagnostic agents, and toxic effects are limited and transient, including flushing, nausea, vomiting, brief abdominal discomfort, and hypotension. In addition to their diagnostic use, two of the releasing hormones, GHRH and GnRH, have potential therapeutic uses.

TABLE 16-3 Treatment of Hypoglycemia		
AGENT	**ADULT DOSE**	**PEDIATRIC DOSE**
Glucose (bolus)	50 mL of 50% dextrose IV	0.5–1 g/kg of 25% dextrose IV
Glucose (infusion)	10%–20% dextrose in water IV	10%–20% dextrose in 0.2% normal saline
Glucagon	1–2 mg IV/IM/SC	0.03–0.1 mg/kg IV/IM/SC
Octreotide	50–100 µg SC/IV q 6–12 hr	4–5 µg/kg/day SC/IV divided into q 6 hr doses

IM, intramuscularly; IV, intravenously; SC, subcutaneously.

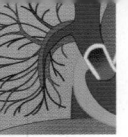

GnRH is used for treatment of infertility in women who have hypothalamic disease with intact pituitary function, enabling them to respond to the hypothalamic agent. Treatment involves episodic pulsatile delivery of the peptide by an infusion pump.[32] Side effects include a potential for ovarian hyperstimulation; because of this potential, this agent should be used only by reproductive endocrinologists who are well trained in its application. Sustained delivery of GnRH analogs suppresses gonadotropin production through down-regulation of the GnRH receptor. These agents are used when inhibition of gonadal function is desired, such as in patients with precocious puberty or carcinoma of the prostate or endometrium. Side effects are minor, with the major effects due to the expected suppression of gonadal function.

GHRH is an investigational agent that may eventually have utility in therapy of individuals who have growth failure due to hypothalamic dysfunction but who maintain normal pituitary function. No significant toxicity has been described.

Treatment Principles

Management of oxytocin toxicity is the same as that for vasopressin toxicity. Careful monitoring during intravenous infusion is essential for prevention of these problems, and the infusion must be discontinued immediately at the first evidence of adverse effect on the mother or her fetus.

Hyponatremia caused by vasopressin or DDAVP is effectively treated by restriction of free water intake and a decrease in, or discontinuation of, vasopressin administration. As with any state of severe hyponatremia or hypo-osmolality, the use of hypertonic saline may be a consideration if the decrease in sodium concentration has been abrupt, is associated with neurologic abnormalities, and has not responded promptly to removal of the precipitating causes.

No therapy is usually required to treat adverse effects of hypothalamic-releasing hormone in view of their brief duration. If hypotension persists, administration of intravenous fluids usually corrects the problem.

PITUITARY AGENTS

Introduction and Importance

Growth hormone (GH) is administered to children who are of short stature due to its deficiency. Gonadotropins are used mostly to treat infertility due to secondary gonadal dysfunction. Adrenocorticotropic hormone (ACTH) stimulates the adrenal cortex and is therefore sometimes used in disorders that respond to glucocorticoid (GC) therapy.

Octreotide is used to treat acromegaly by lowering GH levels, and may be helpful in shrinking pituitary adenomas. Because it has a suppressive effect on many other hormone systems, it can be used in the treatment of other hormone-producing tumors. As has been discussed in the section on glucose metabolism, it can prevent the release of insulin from the pancreas due to sulfonylurea ingestion. Octreotide has a role in the treatment of upper GI hemorrhage due to its inhibition of hormones, which cause vasodilation. Bromocriptine is an ergot alkaloid that has dopaminergic properties useful in treating hyperprolactinemic states, acromegaly, and some nonendocrine disorders.

Specific Agents and Their Mechanisms of Toxicity

The toxicity of GH can be related to two different factors: (1) contaminants that might be inadvertently administered with the hormone, and (2) the metabolic and physiologic effects of the hormone per se. With recombinant DNA-produced GH, the former consideration is not a current concern. However, before the advent of the technology that led to biosynthetic GH production, the only available GH into the mid-1980s was derived from human cadavers, and cases of transmission of the devastating Creutzfeldt-Jakob infection have been described.[33] Because of the long incubation period for this slow virus, it is possible that more cases will develop in the future in patients who previously received virus-contaminated hormone preparations. Patients who have received these human cadaver–based GH injections are at continued risk and should be monitored for neurologic problems; unfortunately, no effective treatment is currently available.

Otherwise, problems with GH occur predominantly in situations in which the agent is used in excessive doses, thereby causing medical problems that are similar to the problems encountered in acromegaly.[34] Long-term administration can cause edema, hypertension, carpal tunnel syndrome, and arthralgias. Insulin resistance and impaired glucose tolerance are also metabolic consequences of GH administration, especially when the drug is used at supraphysiologic doses. Whether GH administration to adults might increase the risk for cardiovascular disease is a concern, based on the observation that acromegalic patients are at increased risk for hypertension and cardiomyopathy. It is not totally clear whether the cardiomyopathy reflects the cardiac response to acromegaly-associated hypertension or is instead evidence of an anabolic effect of GH on cardiac tissue. Whether GH might be a promoter of tumor growth is also speculated, because GH has been shown to exert mitogenic effects in some animal systems, and acromegaly has been associated with an increased risk for premalignant colonic polyps and colon cancer. It has also been suggested that GH therapy in children may be associated with increased risk for leukemia. Despite this speculation, GH therapy has no established association with any malignancy at this time.

Gonadotropin therapy is used in individuals with secondary gonadal dysfunction, primarily as treatment for infertility. Human chorionic gonadotropin (HCG)

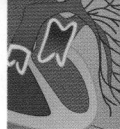

binds to luteinizing hormone receptors and thereby stimulates gonadal function. HCG promotes gonadal steroidogenesis and stimulates the aromatase enzyme that converts testosterone to estradiol; as a result, males have a disproportionate increase in estradiol compared with the increase in testosterone, and gynecomastia may develop. Acne, weight gain, and fluid retention can also occur. In order to achieve fertility in males with secondary hypogonadism, simply stimulating testosterone production with HCG is not sufficient; stimulation of spermatogenesis is also needed, and this requires the use of an agent with follicle-stimulating hormone effect; human menopausal gonadotropin (HMG) is used for this purpose. Because this product contains both follicle-stimulating hormone and luteinizing hormone, the same side effects of weight gain, edema, acne, and gynecomastia are noted.[32] Women who are treated with gonadotropins for infertility can also develop weight gain, edema, and acne. However, a greater clinical concern is the risk for developing ovarian hyperstimulation. This syndrome, which can occur in as many as 15% of HMG-treated patients, consists of cystic ovarian enlargement and fluid shifts (including ascites and pleural effusions), with more severe cases characterized by severe hemoconcentration, electrolyte imbalance, thromboembolism, and even death. The basis of the disorder appears to be increased capillary permeability with major fluid shifts that lead to hemoconcentration, prerenal azotemia, and development of a hypercoagulable state. The likelihood of hyperstimulation syndrome can be minimized by careful monitoring of serum estradiol levels; if the estradiol level becomes excessively elevated during HMG stimulation, subsequent HCG administration should be postponed for that cycle.[35]

ACTH is used for its action of stimulating the adrenal cortex. It is used in disorders that respond to GC treatment. ACTH is used infrequently because of its undesirable properties, which include the need for parenteral administration and an inability to titrate dosage to a specific GC level. The unwanted simultaneous stimulation of mineralocorticoid and androgen activity also complicates its use. In patients with disorders that respond to GC effect, it is preferable to administer a known amount of GC directly rather than to stimulate uncertain GC levels through ACTH administration. Furthermore, the ACTH used for therapeutic purposes is derived from bovine pituitary glands and can produce allergic reactions. ACTH is also used for diagnostic evaluation of adrenal gland function; for this short-term purpose, a synthetic but fully bioactive analog, composed of the first 24 amino acids of the 39–amino acid human ACTH molecule (cosyntropin), is commonly used; this analog is devoid of adverse effects.

Treatment Principles

Mild or moderate ovarian hyperstimulation can be monitored conservatively, with discontinuation of gonadotropin therapy. More severe cases require hospitalization with monitoring of fluid and electrolyte status, weight, fluid intake and output, hematocrit, and renal function. Sodium restriction may also be required, as well as cautious use of plasma expanders or albumin to maintain urine output.

Treatment of other conditions caused by pituitary agents is supportive and should be tailored to the particular pathology encountered.

THYROID

Introduction and Importance

The thyroid is principally responsible for the regulation of the basal metabolic rate. Thyroid hormones act within cells to regulate gene transcription and protein synthesis. Increase in consumption of ATP results in an increase in metabolism of carbohydrates, proteins, and lipids. Thyroid dysfunction falls into two categories. Decreased function of the thyroid gland, or hypothyroidism, is a fairly common disease. Estimates of its prevalence in the United States range from 2% to 10%, and thyroid hormone is therefore one of the most commonly prescribed medications. Thyrotoxicosis, a surfeit of active thyroid hormone, occurs most often as the result of Graves' disease, an autoimmune disease that increases the mass of the gland. This endogenous overproduction of thyroid hormone can be termed *hyperthyroidism*. Alternatively, an excess of thyroid hormone can result from ingestion of xenobiotics. Thyroid tissue is sometimes present in meat from animals' necks, and can be inadvertently consumed. Some people abuse thyroid medications, usually in an attempt to lose weight, but also in intentional overdoses.

Secretion of thyroid hormone results from a complex interplay among the hypothalamus, anterior pituitary, and thyroid. Circulating levels of thyroxine (T_4) and triiodothyronine (T_3) are sensed by the hypothalamus, which secretes TRH or somatostatin (SRIH). TRH has a releasing effect on the anterior pituitary, and SRIH has an inhibiting effect. These signals cause the anterior pituitary to release thyroid-stimulating hormone (TSH, or thyrotropin), which stimulates the thyroid to release both T_3 and T_4. Iodide and, to a much lesser extent, lithium ion have a suppressive effect on the thyroid[36] (Fig. 16-1).

T_4, which has a half-life of about a week, is slowly converted to T_3 in various body tissues. Two enzymes catalyze this process: D1, present in the thyroid, liver, and kidney; and D2, present in the thyroid, smooth muscle, and cardiac muscle. Of the total T_3 in circulation, 80% is formed from T_4 in the periphery, and 20% is released directly from the thyroid.

Toxin-Induced Physiologic Disturbances

NATURAL AND SYNTHETIC T_3 AND T_4/T_3 PRODUCTS

Because of its short half-life, considerable elevation and fluctuation in T_3 levels can occur in patients who

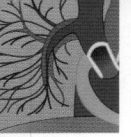

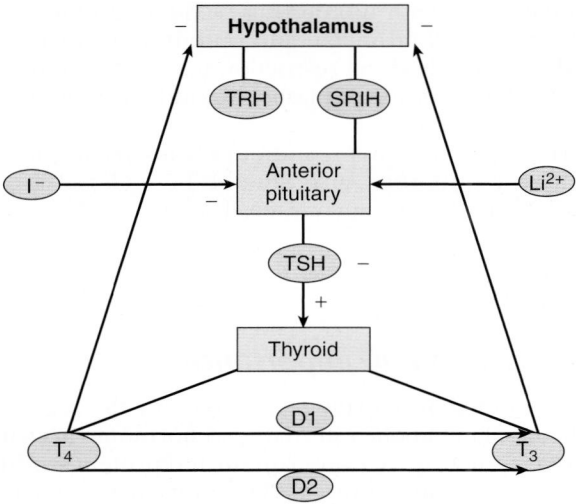

FIGURE 16-1 Hypothalamus-pituitary-thyroid axis.

TABLE 16-4 Signs and Symptoms of Acute Thyroid Hormone Overdose	
SYSTEM	**FINDING**
Cardiovascular	Tachycardia, hypertension, dysrhythmia
Neurologic	Mydriasis, tremor, hyperreflexia, agitation, seizure, coma, psychosis
Skin	Flushing, diaphoresis, dermatitis, rash
Gastrointestinal	Nausea, vomiting, diarrhea
Metabolic	Fever, weight loss

illness. The spectrum of signs and symptoms of acute overdose encompass many organ systems (Table 16-4).

Specific Agents and Their Mechanisms of Toxicity

For a discussion of thyroid hormone–induced physiologic disturbances, see Natural and Synthetic T_3 and T_3/T_4 Products. It is important to note that some xenobiotics have significant effects on the hypothalamus-pituitary-thyroid axis. Thyrotoxicosis due to amiodarone is divided into two varieties. Type 1 occurs mostly in patients with underlying thyroid disease and is characterized by excessive thyroid hormone synthesis due to iodine present in the compound. Type 2 is a destructive thyroiditis that can affect previously euthyroid patients. Differentiation of these two types can be made on the basis of a fine-needle aspiration, which will show evidence of thyroiditis in type 2 disease. Conversely, amiodarone can also cause hypothyroidism via blockade of peripheral conversion of thyroxin to triiodothyronine. Chronic lithium therapy can cause hypothyroidism and goiter. GCs cause a decrease in T_3 production by inhibiting D1 and D2 enzymes. TSH secretion is suppressed by a number of compounds (Table 16-5). A few agents can also cause thyroid storm (Box 16-1).

Radioactive iodine is a frequently used first-line agent in the treatment of Graves' disease and toxic nodular

are treated with pure T_3 or combined T_4/T_3 products. Intermittent peaking to supraphysiologic levels can have adverse effects, especially in older patients with cardiovascular disease. As a result, a number of combined T_4/T_3 preparations have been taken off the market in recent years. Nonetheless, the traditional but outdated standard of an earlier era, desiccated thyroid hormone, is still available and used with surprising frequency. Problems with this preparation include inconsistent absorption and bioavailability, as well as its content of potentially cardiotoxic T_3.[37] Liothyronine (synthetic T_3) has problems similar to those of the animal-derived T_3 and is not in common use.

LEVOTHYROXINE

Levothyroxine is synthetic T_4, which is converted to T_3 by the same enzymatic systems that handle endogenous T_4. Long-term physiologic effects of excessive levothyroxine administration include cardiac changes (shortening of systolic time intervals and increased nocturnal heart rate), elevated levels of liver enzymes, and increased bone resorption; the last is of particular concern in postmenopausal women who already have a high risk for osteoporosis.[36,38] The hypermetabolic consequences of thyrotoxicosis can include weight loss, tremor, heat intolerance, loss of muscle mass and muscle strength, palpitation, and cardiac rhythm disorders, especially supraventricular dysrhythmias. Cases of true thyrotoxicosis are usually encountered in paramedical personnel, although anyone who has access to thyroid medications can potentially be at risk.

Acute overdose of thyroid hormone may cause symptoms in as few as 12 hours in the case of products containing T_3. If levothyroxine is ingested without T_3, a period of 5 to 11 days without symptoms may be followed by the development of illness. Thyrotoxicosis is much more common in chronic overdose than in acute overdose. However, massive acute ingestions may cause profound

TABLE 16-5 Thyrotropin Suppressors	
AGENT	**COMMENT**
Thyroid hormones and analogs	
Dopamine and dopamine agonists	
Somatostatin and its analogs	Effect noted in vitro, not in vivo
Dobutamine	
Glucocorticoids	Effect is transient
IL-1β, IL-6	
Tumor necrosis factor-α	
Phenytoin	
Bexarotene	
IL, interleukin.	

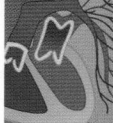

BOX 16-1	AGENTS CAUSING THYROID STORM

Iodine
Thyroid hormone
Radiographic contrast
Thioridazine
Lothiouracil
Premature withdrawal of antithyroid agents

thyroid disease.[39] There has been long experience with this agent, which is extremely safe. The eventual development of hypothyroidism is an expected outcome of the agent, although not universal. Whether radioactive iodine can provoke or worsen the ophthalmopathy of Graves' disease is debated. Radioactive iodine has not been associated with increased risk for malignancy, nor is there evidence for any teratogenic effect in offspring of mothers who were previously treated with radioactive iodine. Pregnancy is an absolute contraindication to the use of radioactive iodine because of the risk for ablation of the fetal thyroid and subsequent congenital hypothyroidism. Because thyroid destruction becomes a risk only after the fetal thyroid has developed, which occurs at 10 weeks of gestation, radioactive iodine is safe and appropriate therapy for women of childbearing age after a negative pregnancy test result has been documented; advice to avoid pregnancy for the following 4 to 6 months is typically given.

Thyroiditis can occur within the first 2 weeks of radiation treatment for hyperthyroidism, with neck pain, swelling, and transient worsening of the hyperthyroidism.

The thionamide derivatives propylthiouracil (PTU) and methimazole are commonly used to treat hyperthyroidism, and they have a generally good track record of limited toxicity.[39] These agents are thought to work by inhibiting human thyroid peroxidase, which catalyzes both incorporation of iodide into tyrosyl residues and the subsequent coupling of iodotyrosyl into T_4 and T_3. Propylthiouracil also inhibits the peripheral deiodination of T_4 to T_3. PTU crosses the placenta to a lesser degree than methimazole and can be used safely during pregnancy and by breast-feeding patients. In pregnancy, fetal exposure should be limited by using the lowest necessary dose to keep the free T_4 index in the high-normal range, and monitoring of thyroid hormone levels in the infant of a breast-feeding woman is advocated to ensure that no effect of drug exposure occurs through the mother's milk.[40]

By far the most serious side effect of these drugs is agranulocytosis, which occurs in about 3 of every 1000 treated patients. This is an idiosyncratic reaction that is more common in patients older than 40 years but can occur regardless of a patient's age, the duration of therapy, or the drug dose.[41] The fall in granulocyte count is abrupt and precipitous, and thus no benefit is derived from periodic monitoring of blood counts. Most patients with drug-induced agranulocytosis present with fever, sore throat, or other features of infection.

Liver disease is also a major potential toxic effect of the thionamides.[41] Drug-related hepatotoxicity seems to be a problem predominantly with PTU, whereas cholestatic jaundice has been associated with methimazole.[42] PTU-related hepatic injury has been fatal in some cases.[43] The presentation is similar to that of viral hepatitis. Mild abnormalities in liver function tests are common in patients who are treated with PTU,[44] and mild abnormalities on liver biopsy have also been demonstrated.

Acute overdoses of methimazole and PTU are rare. Because the duration of effect of these medications is fairly short, the decrease in T_3 levels can be expected to have few significant effects. In one case, between 5 and 13 g of PTU was ingested. An increase in alkaline phosphatase and decrease in T_3 were noted, and the patient recovered fully.[45]

Treatment Principles

THYROID HORMONES AND OTHER MEDICATIONS CAUSING THYROTOXICOSIS

Activated charcoal absorbs thyroid medications and should be given to patients with a recent acute overdose. The onset of any thyrotoxicosis will likely be delayed for hours to days. Sodium ipodate or iopanoic acid has been used in ingestions of levothyroxine and amiodarone thyrotoxicosis to inhibit conversion of T_4 to T_3. In the few patients in whom its use has been documented in case reports, significant improvement has been noted.[46-50] The dose to be used in treatment should likely be determined in consultation with an endocrinologist, because dosing information is limited. Cholestyramine has been used in numerous cases and recommended in a review article for its ability to interrupt enterohepatic recirculation of iodothyronines.[51] In the short term, its only significant side effect is constipation. It is worth consideration in this case.

Adrenergic effects can be rapidly treated by an agent with β_1- and β_2-adrenergic antagonism. The typical agent is propranolol, although labetalol or sotalol might also be used. Fever should be treated aggressively with acetaminophen and external cooling; aspirin should not be used because it displaces T_3 from thyroglobulin, which may worsen the condition. Benzodiazepines are the first-line agents of choice for treatment of agitation and seizure. Congestive heart failure should be managed with diuretics and digoxin, and may not resolve rapidly. There are no data on which antiemetic is best for treating the nausea and vomiting. Supportive care, including airway protection, ventilatory support, and hydration, is also important. Cardiac and hemodynamic monitoring is necessary. Laboratory analysis should include a basic metabolic panel. There is no role for the measurement of T_3 and T_4 levels unless the diagnosis is in doubt.

THIONAMIDES

Patients taking thionamides should be advised to discontinue their medication immediately and arrange for blood count measurements at the first evidence of an infectious process. The hematologic abnormalities

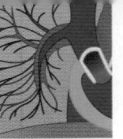

usually resolve within 7 to 10 days; in the meantime, in-patient hospitalization with intravenous antibiotics is usually recommended.[40] The simultaneous use of corticosteroids or granulocyte-stimulating factors has been suggested, but these are not proven interventions and thus are not recommended at this time.[40] Further thionamide therapy should be avoided in patients who have experienced agranulocytosis from one of these drugs. Hepatotoxicity due to PTU generally resolves on withdrawal of the drug. Mild elevations of the transaminases are considered to be transient and asymptomatic. It has been suggested that therapy can be cautiously continued in patients who are symptom free and not jaundiced.[44] Acute overdoses of these medications can generally be managed with supportive care.

OTHER TREATMENTS AFFECTING THE THYROID

Radiation thyroiditis can be effectively treated with analgesic agents and β-adrenergic blockers, as would be used in other types of painful thyroiditis.

Type 2 amiodarone thyrotoxicosis can be treated with steroids, nonsteroidal anti-inflammatories, and antithyroid medications.

PARATHYROID SYSTEM

Introduction and Importance

Calcium plays a number of critical roles in the body. It is essential in the functioning of skeletal, smooth, and cardiac muscle. Its flux through nerve cells results in transmission of neural impulses. Calcium mediates changes in vascular tone. Its presence is essential for the functioning of numerous protein and enzyme systems, including the vitamin K–dependent factors in the clotting cascade. Calcium helps to modulate neurotransmitter release and affects many endocrine and exocrine systems.

Ninety-nine percent of the body's stores of calcium reside in bone, in its mineralized phase. The remaining 1% moves between bone and the intra- and extracellular compartments. In the vascular compartment, 50% is protein bound. In the intracellular compartment, only 1% is free. The rest is bound to the cell membrane or the endoplasmic reticulum, or is within the mitochrondrion.

The parathyroid glands are dedicated to the homeostasis of this mobile 1% of body calcium mentioned above. In response to a decrease of the ionized calcium level in the vascular compartment, chief cells of the parathyroids increase their secretion of parathyroid hormone (PTH). This hormone triggers responses in bone and kidney that increase the blood calcium level. In bone, the effects of PTH are complex, but the net effect is to increase bone resorption and thus increase the amount of available calcium. PTH increases reabsorption of calcium at the renal distal tubule by increasing the opening of calcium channels in the membrane. In addition, the kidney secretes 1,25-dihydroxyvitamin D, which stimulates the intestine to increase absorption of dietary calcium (Fig. 16-2).

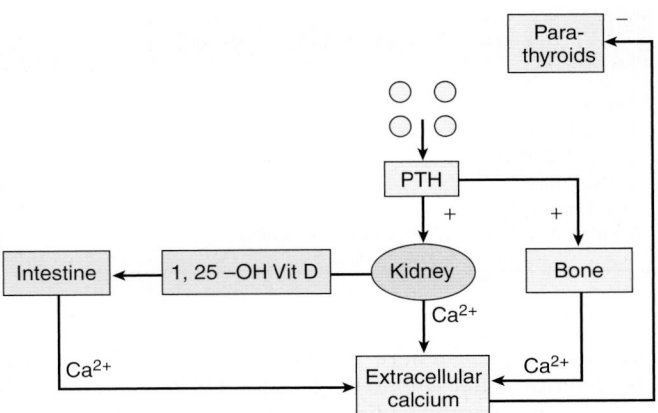

FIGURE 16-2 Parathyroid system.

Disequilibrium of normal calcium homeostasis is a feature of many diseases, including Paget's disease, multiple myeloma, primary hyperparathyroidism, osteoporosis, and hypercalcemia of malignancy. Medications that are intended to treat alterations in calcium metabolism can have significant undesired effects.

Toxin-Induced Physiologic Disturbances

Vitamin D, its metabolites, and its analogs are used to treat osteoporosis (Box 16-2). These medications have a number of effects, because vitamin D receptors exist throughout the body. The receptor then up-regulates transcription of DNA into RNA, bringing about the desired biologic effect. Some actions of vitamin D are thought to occur independently of gene transcription, such as intracellular hypercalcemia, activation of phospholipase C, and opening of calcium channels. The most significant effect, however, is to increase the proportion of dietary calcium that is absorbed. In overdose, nausea, vomiting, diarrhea, and GI bleeding may be seen. The effects of the provoked hypercalcemia include headache, itching, weakness, neuropathy, stupor, and coma; cardiac arrhythmias and hypertension; renal calcium deposits and nephritis; and depression and apathy in chronic overdose.[2,52-54]

Bisphosphonates are synthetic pyrophosphate analogs that inhibit osteoclast-mediated bone resorption (Table 16-6). They are used to treat primary hyperparathyroidism, hypercalcemia, osteoporosis, Paget's disease, and multiple

BOX 16-2	VITAMIN D AND ANALOGS

Calcitriol
Doxercalciferol
Ergocalciferol
Paricalcitol

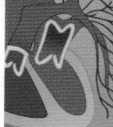

TABLE 16-6 Common Bisphosphonates	
GENERIC NAME	**GENERATION**
Etidronate	First
Clodronate	First
Alendronate	Second
Ibandronate	Second
Pamidronate	Second
Risedronate	Second
Tiludronate	Third
Zoledronate	Third

myeloma. Three generations of these medications have been developed, with the newer compounds having significantly more potency. Adverse effect data are limited, but hypocalcemia is both a theoretical and practical concern. Additional effects include nausea, diarrhea, and GI bleeding; fluid retention, hypokalemia, hypomagnesemia, and hypophosphatemia; nephrotoxicity; muscle and bone pain; avascular necrosis of the jaw; and headaches, paresthesias, malaise, dizziness, and seizure. Other uncommon reactions include a self-limited acute-phase response with fever and myalgia, inflammatory eye reactions or scleritis, skin lesions, erythroderma, and bronchospasm.[2,55-66]

Specific Agents and Their Mechanisms of Toxicity

Calcitonin, an inhibitor of bone resorption, is used in the treatment of Paget's disease, osteoporosis, and hypercalcemia. Both salmon calcitonin and human calcitonin are available, and administration is by injection or nasal spray. Local effects are common, including itching and irritation at the injection site. Systemic symptoms are also frequent, including flushing, nausea, vomiting, and anorexia. Hyperglycemia, hypokalemia, and renal lesions or insufficiency have been reported. There is a case report of anaphylactic shock in response to intramuscular calcitonin injection.[67-81] A slight but asymptomatic decrease in serum calcium levels may occur after injection of calcitonin in patients with Paget's disease. Loss of efficacy is common; this may be related to down-regulation of calcitonin receptors or perhaps development of neutralizing antibodies to the salmon form of this peptide. The use of calcitonin has been limited by the availability of the bisphosphonates, which have similar actions with fewer undesirable effects.

In addition to inhibition of bone resorption, etidronate (but not the other bisphosphonates) can impair bone mineralization, and patients are at risk for developing osteomalacia with chronic etidronate use. As a result, the agent is usually prescribed in a cyclic regimen.[82-86]

Although not approved for use in treatment of metabolic bone disease, sodium fluoride is undergoing investigation as a therapeutic agent for osteoporosis because of its ability to stimulate osteoblast activity and promote new bone formation.[41,87-91] Concerns about its use have centered around the potential for abnormal bone formation with increased fracture risk, as well as other adverse effects such as gastric irritation. In massive overdose, with ingestions of greater than 5 mg/kg of fluoride, adverse effects can occur. These include nausea, vomiting, GI hemorrhage, hypocalcemia, hyperkalemia, hypomagnesemia, and cardiac dysrhythmias.[2,92-94]

Treatment Principles: Vitamin D Agents

Activated charcoal is only needed in massive ingestions, where greater than 100 times the U.S. recommended daily allowance has been ingested.[2] Multiple-dose activated charcoal and dialysis are not helpful in removing vitamin D from the body. Potassium, calcium, magnesium, and phosphate, as well as renal function, should be checked. The patient should have an electrocardiogram and be put on a cardiac monitor. Hypercalcemia above 14 mg/dL or with significant symptoms should be treated initially with normal saline diuresis. This may be followed by furosemide, especially in patients likely to develop fluid overload. Calcitonin can be given in a dose of 4 to 8 IU/kg intramuscularly. Critical hypercalcemia should be treated with hemodialysis. Since the advent of bisphosphonates, mithramycin has fallen out of favor as a treatment. With parent vitamin D (ergocalciferol, or vitamin D_2), the hypercalcemia may persist for many weeks owing to the accumulation of this fat-soluble substance in adipose stores. Additional therapy might include reduction of dietary calcium intake and prescription of a bisphosphonate. Prednisone also may be helpful, because it decreases absorption of dietary calcium; oral hydration and oral phosphate therapy will also decrease the serum calcium level.[2,95]

Bisphosphonate toxicity should be managed mainly with supportive care. Activated charcoal can be given in acute overdoses. Methods of enhanced elimination such as multiple-dose activated charcoal or hemodialysis are not effective. A serum ionized calcium level, as well as potassium, magnesium, and phosphate levels, should be obtained. Renal function tests should be performed. An electrocardiogram and cardiac monitoring are important, because QT prolongation and dysrhythmias can result from hypocalcemia. Severe or symptomatic hypocalcemia can be managed with an intravenous infusion of 10 to 30 mL of 10% calcium gluconate solution. Pediatric dosing of calcium gluconate is 200 to 500 mg/kg/24 hours, divided in every-6-hour doses.[2]

Calcitonin and sodium fluoride toxicities can be managed supportively. Withdrawal of the agent will aid in resolution of the symptoms and signs.

ADRENAL CORTEX

Introduction and Importance

Essential for life, the adrenal gland was first described by Eustachius in 1563. This highly vascular endocrine organ is divided into the medulla, which is a neurosecretory

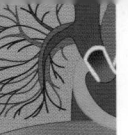

organ dispensing catecholamines; and the cortex, which secretes derivatives of cholesterol. The adrenal cortex is critical to the body's function. Steroids secreted by the adrenal cortex fall into three categories: GCs, which have effects on carbohydrate and protein metabolism; mineralocorticoids, which regulate sodium and extracellular fluid balance; and androgens, which have effects on reproductive function. The latter will be discussed later in this chapter, in the section on gonadal agents.

GC medications (Table 16-7) are commonly used in the treatment of various medical disorders associated with an immunologic or inflammatory component. GC antagonists (Table 16-8) are used in the therapy of Cushing's syndrome and adrenocortical carcinoma. These are not definitive treatments but are instead used for reversal of some of the severe consequences of Cushing's syndrome in preparation for surgery, while awaiting the effects of radiation therapy, or in ameliorating the more devastating effects of Cushing's syndrome in patients with malignancy. Mineralocorticoids are typically used for patients with aldosterone deficiency, such as Addison's disease or other hypoaldosterone states, or for situations in which volume expansion may be desirable, as in patients with idiopathic orthostatic hypotension. Mineralocorticoid antagonists are very useful endocrine agents. Classically used for their action as a competitive inhibitor at the aldosterone receptor, they are also fairly potent antiandrogens. They also possess progestin action.

Toxin-Induced Physiologic Disturbances

GLUCOCORTICOIDS

GCs bind to both the glucocorticoid receptor (GR) and the mineralocorticoid receptor (MR), although more recently synthesized agents have selectivity for the GR alone. Use of GCs causes an increase in expression of anti-inflammatory proteins and a decrease in expression of proinflammatory proteins. This occurs through GR-DNA interactions, which activate certain gene transcriptions and repress others. There may also be direct GR-protein interactions.[96] The resulting suppression of the inflammatory and immune systems represents both the desired clinical effect and a prime adverse effect. A meta-analysis of a number of studies concluded that a relative risk of 1.6 exists for infectious events in patients on moderate chronic doses of systemic corticosteroids.[97] While this may not appear consequential, many of these infections are complicated or opportunistic.

One of the most worrisome consequences of long-term use of GCs is their effect on the musculoskeletal system. Significant bone loss can occur in weeks to months, even with low-dose therapy. Risk factors include age, female gender, body mass, and level and length of steroid therapy.[98] This process occurs through a number of mechanisms, including suppression of osteoblasts; decrease in calcium absorption with an increase in calcium excretion; and suppression of factors important for bone homeostasis, including GH. The effects are most pronounced on cancellous bone: over one third of patients on GCs have evidence of vertebral fractures after 5 years of treatment. In muscle, catabolic effects may lead to myopathy and atrophy. GCs inhibit the uptake of glucose into myocytes, which encourages muscle breakdown. They also up-regulate protein degradation and down-regulate protein synthesis through effects on gene transcription.[97] Muscle enzyme levels will be normal. A biopsy will show type II muscle fiber damage. Longer-acting or halogenated compounds may be more likely to produce this effect. An association between muscle injury and GC therapy with concurrent use of nondepolarizing paralytics has been reported frequently.[99]

In the skin, atrophy of the epidermis and dermis can lead to thinning of the skin as well as the permanent and disfiguring striae rubrae distensae. This results from a decrease in the proliferation of cutaneous cells and protein synthesis, probably from a direct down-regulation of gene expression.[100] These effects can be seen both with

TABLE 16-7 Adrenal Agents

AGENT	CLASS
Betamethasone	Glucocorticoid
Dexamethasone	Glucocorticoid
Methylprednisolone	Glucocorticoid
Prednisone	Glucocorticoid
Triamcinolone	Glucocorticoid
Desoxycorticosterone	Mineralocorticoid
Fludrocortisone	Mineralocorticoid
Aminoglutethimide	Glucocorticoid antagonist
Ketoconazole	Glucocorticoid antagonist
Metyrapone	Glucocorticoid antagonist
Mitotane	Glucocorticoid antagonist
Trilostane	Glucocorticoid antagonist
Mifepristone	Glucocorticoid antagonist
Spironolactone	Mineralocorticoid antagonist
Eplerenone	Mineralocorticoid antagonist

TABLE 16-8 Lipid-Lowering Agents

AGENT	CLASS
Cholestyramine	Bile acid sequestrant
Colesevelam	Bile acid sequestrant
Colestipol	Bile acid sequestrant
Bezafibrate	Fibric acid derivative
Ciprofibrate	Fibric acid derivative
Clofibrate	Fibric acid derivative
Fenofibrate	Fibric acid derivative
Gemfibrozil	Fibric acid derivative
Atorvastatin	HMG-CoA reductase inhibitor
Fluvastatin	HMG-CoA reductase inhibitor
Lovastatin	HMG-CoA reductase inhibitor
Pitavastatin	HMG-CoA reductase inhibitor
Pravastatin	HMG-CoA reductase inhibitor
Rosuvastatin	HMG-CoA reductase inhibitor
Simvastatin	HMG-CoA reductase inhibitor
Niacin	Nicotinic acid
Ezetimibe	Selective cholesterol absorption inhibitor

HMG-CoA, 3-hydroxy-3-methylglutaryl coenzyme A.

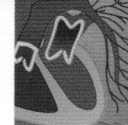

systemic and inhaled GC use. Poor wound healing also represents a significant pathologic effect. It results from suppression of the early inflammatory response and the inhibition of gene expression, which synthesizes matrix protein and collagen.[101,102] Reversible side effects such as hypertrichosis and steroid acne can also be seen.[97]

Effects on the eye from chronic systemic or inhaled GC use include cataract formation and development of glaucoma. These conditions are more likely in middle-aged or elderly patients.[103] One in three patients is susceptible to steroid-induced elevations in intraocular pressure. This risk rises with a personal or family history of primary open-angle glaucoma.[104] Mechanisms for the formation of cataracts include elevation of glucose levels, inhibition of RNA synthesis, and formation of covalent bonds between GC and lysine amino acids present in lens proteins. In the case of glaucoma, increased ocular pressures are commonly seen, the result of GC-induced changes in the trabecular meshwork.[97] Rare complications include retinal emboli and ocular infection.[105]

Central nervous system (CNS) effects of GC range from euphoria to mood swings to suicidal depression and psychosis.[106] The aggregate incidence of these findings, in a meta-analysis of data from several decades, is 5.7%. At least 2 weeks of treatment is usually required before these psychopathologies are manifested. They may be more likely to occur in a patient with a previously existing psychiatric condition, although this point is debated.[107] Some patients suffer depression after the withdrawal of GC. Although it is incompletely understood, repression of the 5-HT$_{1A}$ receptor plays a key role in the pathophysiology of GC induced psychiatric disorders.[108] Memory and cognitive function mediated by the hippocampus can also be affected.[109] This organ appears to be directly injured by GCs. In addition, decreased dendritic branching, loss of neurons, inhibition of neuronal regeneration, and other effects have been noted in the brain.[97] Cases of elevated intracranial pressure (ICP) have been reported, the majority of which occur in boys. The typical case is that of a patient whose long-term GC was stopped, tapered, or changed to another agent. The pathophysiology of this increase in ICP is not clear.[110-113]

Alterations in metabolism and effects on many endocrine organs occur with high frequency in the patient receiving chronic GC therapy. In response to corticosteroids, the pancreas secretes less insulin, and insulin resistance rises.[114] GR-mediated transcription up-regulation increases glucose production. There is evidence to suggest that patients who develop steroid-induced diabetes have a preexisting decrease in insulin secretory reserve. Risk factors include a personal or family history of diabetes. A few patients who develop frank type 2 diabetes may remain diabetic after GC therapy ceases.[115] Most cases of simple hyperglycemia resolve a few days after GC therapy ends. Some of the most common effects of chronic GC therapy result from their influence on the hypothalamic-pituitary-adrenal axis. These include Cushing's syndrome of moon face, buffalo hump, and central obesity; growth inhibition; and adrenal insufficiency.[97] Activation of GRs in the hypothalamus causes a decrease in the secretion of ACTH and corticotropin-releasing hormone, with subsequent downstream effects. There is no clear consensus on how long GC therapy must continue in order to reliably provoke adrenal insufficiency, but even periods of 1 week may be sufficient.[116]

Hypertension, hyperlipidemia, and reduced fibrinolytic potential are the main adverse cardiovascular effects.[117] Although elevated blood pressure is more common in the elderly and those with preexisting hypertension, this adverse event also commonly occurs in children, both with oral and inhaled GC use. This hypertension is the result of increases in systemic vascular resistance, extracellular volume, and cardiac contractility. These effects are mediated by activation of the GR and MR.[97]

In the GI system, the chronic use of GC can lead to peptic ulcers. The relative risk associated with GC use alone ranges from 1.1 to 2.7, but increased to 14.6 when nonsteroidal anti-inflammatory drugs (NSAIDs) are used concurrently.[118] In experimental animals, GCs increase gastric acid secretion, thin gastric mucus, cause gastrin and parietal cell hyperplasia, and slow ulcer healing.[119] It is thought that these effects lead to peptic ulcer disease in humans. Upper GI bleeding and pancreatitis are known adverse effects, as is oral candidiasis with inhaled corticosteroids.[97,120]

MINERALOCORTICOIDS

At therapeutic doses, the toxic effects of these agents are the same as the expected physiologic effects of a mineralocorticoid and tend to be dose related. Mineralocorticoids act at the distal tubule of the kidney to promote the excretion of potassium and reabsorption of sodium. Thus, intravascular volume expansion, hypertension, and hypokalemia are the most likely problems. In supratherapeutic doses, they can inhibit the adrenal cortex and the thymus, and act on the pituitary to decrease corticotropin excretion. They may also stimulate an inappropriate wound healing response in uninjured vascular tissues.[2,121-124]

MINERALOCORTICOID ANTAGONISTS

Toxicity of these agents can be divided into three categories. Classic effects occur at the distal convoluted tubule of the kidney. Because of poor specificity to the MR, antiandrogenic and progestational effects can also be seen. Lastly, pathologic cardiovascular remodeling can also occur. Thus, hyperkalemia is a risk in predisposed patients, such as those with renal insufficiency or long-standing diabetic patients who may have hypoaldosteronism; men can experience impaired libido, impotence, and gynecomastia due to the antiandrogen effects; and women frequently experience menometrorrhagia and mastodynia.[125-127]

Specific Agents and Their Mechanisms of Toxicity

GLUCOCORTICOIDS

In rare cases, methylprednisolone administration has been associated with seizures. Intrathecal infusions of methylprednisolone acetate have caused aseptic meningitis, thought to be due to the polyethylene glycol excipient.[2]

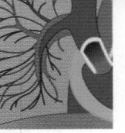

GLUCOCORTICOID ANTAGONISTS

Aminoglutethimide inhibits the conversion of cholesterol to pregnenolone, the first step in steroid synthesis. Thus, in addition to lowering cortisol levels, it also inhibits production of other steroids, including aldosterone and estrogen. Iodine-concentrating abilities of the thyroid are also impaired. Adverse effects can therefore include hypoaldosteronism and hypothyroidism in addition to cortisol deficiency. Common nonendocrine toxic effects include lethargy, somnolence, and a fairly common maculopapular rash. The latter is often associated with fever, occurring within 2 weeks of initiation of therapy, and frequently self-resolving. Patients develop neutropenia, pancytopenia, leukopenia, or agranulocytosis; the incidence of each of these conditions is an estimated 4%.[2]

Ketoconazole is an imidazole antifungal agent. Used primarily as an antimycotic agent, it is a potent inhibitor of enzymes involved in the synthesis of steroids. It is thought to inhibit C-17, 29-desmolase, the enzyme responsible for androstenedione biosynthesis.[128] Ketoconazole has therefore been used effectively to normalize cortisol production in patients with Cushing's syndrome, as well as to treat prostate cancer. Adrenal insufficiency has been reported with its use.[129] It also lowers testosterone production, potentially leading to gynecomastia and reversible loss of libido and impotence in men, as well as a teratogenic effect in male fetuses.[130] Hepatotoxicity is the most significant toxic action of ketoconazole. The injury pattern is usually hepatocellular, although it may be cholestatic.[131-133] Reversible transient abnormalities in liver function seem to occur in about 5% of patients.[134] However, a prospective trial showed some degree of transaminase elevation in 17.5% of patients taking ketoconazole.[135] In a large cohort study, a relative risk of 228, with confidence intervals from 34 to 933, was calculated for development of acute liver injury when taking ketoconazole.[136] Occasional fatal hepatotoxicity is reported.[132,137-140] A case of massive enlargement of the liver, with fatty infiltrate, has been reported.[141] The most common side effect is nausea and vomiting. Fatigue is also a frequent complaint.[134] Skin eruptions are seen in some patients.[142] In the eye, ketoconazole has been associated with papilledema.[143,144] Other rare side effects include weakness and tremor, psychiatric disturbances, and aplastic anemia.[145-148] Ketoconazole strongly inhibits CYP3A4, so potential interactions exist with medications metabolized by this enzyme.[149,150] A disulfiram-like reaction with ethanol ingestion has also been reported.[2] Limited data exist for acute overdose, but headache, fatigue, and tinnitus have been reported.[2]

Metyrapone reduces cortisol and corticosterone production by blocking 11β-hydroxylation of precursor molecules in the adrenal cortex. To a lesser extent, it inhibits 18-hydroxylation and side chain cleavage. In addition to lowering cortisol levels, metyrapone also causes steroidogenesis to be shifted toward increased androgen production. It may also reduce production of aldosterone.[2] Adrenal insufficiency is the most serious adverse effect of metyrapone. It occurs predominantly in patients with diminished adrenal secretory capacity. Monitoring is problematic and potentially misleading because the immediate precursor to cortisol, 11-deoxycortisol, accumulates to high levels with the use of metyrapone. This precursor also cross-reacts to various extents with most cortisol assays, which can give a false sense of security about the appropriateness of cortisol levels. Chronic metyrapone use can cause hirsutism and mild acne in women, although long-term use has also been associated with alopecia.[151,152] Hypertension is a side effect seen in patients as well as in animal studies.[153,154] Metabolic derangements consistent with alteration in mineralocorticoid production occur. Rarely, bone marrow depression or leukopenia have been noted. GI symptoms occur with use of the drug but predominantly when adrenal insufficiency occurs as a result of overtreatment.[2] Rare instances of dissociative psychiatric disturbances have been observed.[155] In overdose, patients may have hypotension and dysrhythmias; nausea, vomiting, diarrhea, and abdominal pain; electrolyte derangements; and adrenal insufficiency.[2]

Mitotane, also known as o,p'-DDD, is a congener of the notorious insecticide DDT (dichlorodiphenyltrichloroethane) and an isomer of another insecticide, p,p'-DDD. Its primary effect is to produce selective atrophic damage to the adrenal cortex. It also reduces the excretion of 17-hydroxycorticosteroids without altering plasma cortisol levels. The mechanisms of action of these effects are not known. Mitotane is used to treat inoperable adrenocortical carcinoma.[156] CNS adverse effects occur in up to 40% of patients, and include depression, lethargy, and vertigo. Long-term use may cause permanent brain damage. GI side effects are frequent and include anorexia, nausea, and vomiting.[157] Elevations of hepatic transaminases are common, and elevated lipid levels have also been seen.[158,159] In one study, all patients developed low serum T_4 levels while being treated with mitotane for Cushing's syndrome.[157] Up to 15% of patients developed skin toxicity. Renal insufficiency and hemorrhagic cystitis, as well as retinopathy and opacification of the lens, have been reported.[2,160-162] Acute overdose information is limited, but effects similar to the above are hypothesized.

Trilostane is a competitive inhibitor of 3-β-hydroxysteroid dehydrogenase. This action slows conversion of biologically inactive δ-5 steroids to their δ-4 derivatives.[163] Trilostane also inhibits testicular 3-β-hydroxysteroid dehydrogenase, resulting in a fall in testosterone levels and elevation of luteinizing hormone levels.[164] Adverse effects in therapeutic doses include hypotension; low testosterone levels; adrenal insufficiency; nausea, vomiting, and diarrhea; palatal edema; rhinorrhea; and flushing.[2,165,166]

Mifepristone (RU 486) is the first synthetic GC and progesterone receptor antagonist.[167] Its only Food and Drug Administration (FDA)-approved use is for the termination of early pregnancy, but it has been used to treat a number of diseases, including Cushing's syndrome. Not surprisingly, uterine pain, cramping, and

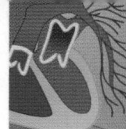

vaginal bleeding are common adverse effects. Headaches, nausea, vomiting, and diarrhea are also seen with regularity. Rash, adrenal insufficiency, elevation of liver transaminases, uterine rupture, hypotension, and myocardial infarction have also been reported.[2,168-176]

MINERALOCORTICOIDS

Fludrocortisone is a halogenated hydrocortisone derivative with a high degree of GC and mineralocorticoid activity. Its action in the distal tubule of the kidney to increase sodium resorption and the subsequent fluid retention make it a useful agent for treatment of orthostatic hypotension. Potassium and hydrogen ions are excreted via the same mechanism. Fludrocortisone is also used for adrenocortical insufficiency as well as adrenogenital syndrome. As expected, common adverse effects include hypertension, peripheral edema, and hypokalemia.[177,178] Adrenal suppression and severe metabolic alkalosis have also been reported.[179-181] Cardiac hypertrophy and heart failure have been described after long-term therapy.[182-184] Topical and inhaled nasal forms of this medication exist, and excess mineralocorticoid activity as well as hypertension have been described with their use.[185,186]

Desoxycorticosterone toxicity is not well described in the literature. In the United States, it is available for veterinary use only. Animal studies have demonstrated hypertension as well as hypernatremia and hypokalemia as adverse effects associated with its use.[187-189] Hypertension has also been documented in humans, in some cases lasting long after the cessation of treatment.[190]

MINERALOCORTICOID ANTAGONISTS

Spironolactone is a competitive inhibitor of aldosterone at the MR. Renally mediated hyponatremia and hyperkalemia are the expected primary effects.[191] It also appears to have effects on the systemic vascular resistance and the cardiac response to adrenergic signaling, which are independent of its mineralocorticoid antagonism.[192] Spironolactone also decreases 17-hydroxylase activity, which explains its effectiveness in the treatment of hirsutism.[193] It has been used to treat a wide array of diseases, with the most common being hyperaldosteronism, hypertension, hypernatremia, and hypokalemia.

Eplerenone is an aldosterone receptor antagonist with high specificity for the MR. This leads to fewer cardiovascular and nonmineralocorticoid effects, although it has less affinity for the MR than does spironolactone. It is used after myocardial infarction to prevent pathologic cardiac remodeling and for the treatment of some types of hypertension.[2,125] The most common and serious effect is hyperkalemia.[194] The manufacturer's experience suggests that gynecomastia and vaginal bleeding are infrequent, and placebo-controlled trials show no difference in incidence. Some patients were noted to have elevations of TSH.[195] Dose-related elevations in transaminases, as well as elevated lipid levels, occurred. No cases of hepatotoxicity were described.[2] There are currently no data on toxicity after acute overdose.

Treatment Principles

For many of the steroid-related complications, there are no specific antidotes. The general recommendation of limiting steroid use to the lowest possible effective dose for the shortest possible interval is a logical maneuver to prevent complications. Withdrawal of the offending agent is suggested as a first step in reversing toxicity. However, this advice may not be practical in the management of a specific patient who has a clearcut need for long-term steroid therapy at high doses. In some situations, other options are available to limit or treat adverse effects. Consultation with a specialist may be helpful.

GLUCOCORTICOIDS

Suppression of the hypothalamic-pituitary-adrenal axis as a result of high-dose GC treatment for greater than 1 month requires that doses be tapered. One recommendation for a prednisone taper is to decrease the dose by 1.0 to 2.5 mg per week, and to assess the adrenal reserve with a cortisol stimulation test when a daily dose of 5 mg has been reached.[115] Stress level steroid coverage is mandatory in acutely ill patients if there is any question of possible adrenal suppression.[196] With severe stress, it is estimated that approximately 200 to 300 mg of hydrocortisone daily, in divided doses, reasonably mimics the response of normally functioning adrenals to a major illness. This stands in contrast to the basal physiologic production of no more than 12 to 15 mg/m² per day for nonstressed individuals.

It is best to prevent development of steroid-induced osteoporosis rather than to treat its sequelae. The 2001 American College of Rheumatology guidelines recommend calcium and vitamin D supplementation as well as the use of bisphosphonates in all men and postmenopausal women.[197,198] Bisphosphonates are well tolerated, and robust data exist to demonstrate their effectiveness.[198-200] It is reasonable to use these agents for all patients who are going to be treated with GC for an extended interval.[201] A cyclic regimen of etidronate, 400 mg per day for 2 weeks every 3 months, has been effective and well tolerated.[202] Loading of the skeleton through exercise is also recommended. Monitoring of bone mineral density on a regular basis is a reasonable way of assessing the effectiveness of prophylaxis. Dual-energy x-ray absorptiometry is a sensitive method of accurately assessing skeletal status. The spine and proximal femur, with a high percentage of trabecular bone, are particularly affected by steroids.[197]

Treatment of steroid myopathy consists of tapering and discontinuing the steroid. In cases where a nondepolarizing paralytic has been used, that agent should be stopped if possible. Clinical recovery may take many weeks. Physical therapy is helpful in prevention as well as recovery.[99]

Diabetes as a complication of GC therapy generally requires administration of insulin at mealtimes to achieve adequate glucose control.[203] Diet control and oral medications have been attempted with some success.[204]

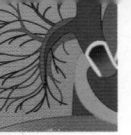

Blood glucose levels only rise significantly after eating. For this reason, regular checks of postprandial glucose are important for the patient receiving long-term corticosteroids.[115]

Increases in intraocular pressure as a result of GC treatment are generally reversible if the treatment duration is under 1 year.[205] Treatment includes stopping the corticosteroid and administration of topical agents for open-angle glaucoma.[206] If cataracts develop, they must be treated in the standard fashion.[207] Regular ophthalmologic examinations, including tonometry, are essential in early detection of ocular side effects.[208]

Standard treatment of corticosteroid-induced psychosis consists of tapering the steroids and treatment with a neuroleptic. Lithium has been used prophylactically with success, but has not been reported as a treatment. Atypical antipsychotics are recommended as treatment for subacute cases.[107] The treatment for elevated ICP is as unclear as its etiology. Changing the corticosteroid, or increasing or decreasing the dose, have been attempted. Therapeutic lumbar puncture has also improved the clinical picture in some patients.[209]

Elevation of low-density lipoprotein (LDL) cholesterol due to GC can be effectively treated with a statin. To lower triglycerides, omega-3 fatty acids or fibrates may be used. Omega-3 agents appear to have fewer interactions with statins than do fibrates. Nicotinic acid may potentiate glucose intolerance and thus may not be ideal for the patient already taking GC.[210]

Treatment of GC-induced hypertension includes stopping the agent, lowering the dose, or moving to an every-other-day dosing regimen.[211,212] Sodium restriction or initiation of a thiazide diuretic may be necessary.[213]

Peptic ulcers seen in association with steroid use are better prevented than treated. Elimination of risks such as NSAID use, smoking, and alcohol may help.[118] Although no data exist on their efficacy, it would be reasonable to treat GC-related ulcers with antacids, H_2 blockers, or proton pump inhibitors, or to initiate this treatment prophylactically.[213]

Acute overdose of GCs generally does not produce significant toxicity. However, in one case Cushing's syndrome was caused in a patient who received a large inadvertent overdose of triamcinolone. Experimentally, a GC antagonist was given and clinical improvement was noted. The dosing regimen was as follows: mifepristone 200 mg daily for 11 days, followed by 600 mg on days 12 and 13, and 200 mg daily for 5 more days.[214] On a theoretical and clinical basis, this therapy is logical and appears to work. However, this is a single experience and cannot be unreservedly recommended.

GLUCOCORTICOID ANTAGONISTS

All GC antagonists may produce adrenocortical insufficiency, which can be treated with exogenous corticosteroids such as hydrocortisone or dexamethasone. Hyperkalemia and hyponatremia should be identified and treated if necessary. In acute ketoconazole overdose, administration of an oral antacid may prevent the absorption of ketoconazole by preventing the tablets from dissolving.[215] Adrenal insufficiency caused by

metyrapone overdose can be treated by administering stress dose GCs. Cardiac monitoring should be implemented, and patients should have fluid and electrolyte replacement. Vasopressor agents may be necessary to reverse hypotension.[2,3] Patients on mitotane treatment should receive GC and mineralocorticoid replacement if necessary.[216] Thyroid function should be tested and levothyroxine administered if necessary. Because of the bleeding complications associated with mifepristone, a complete blood count should be checked and blood products transfused if necessary.

MINERALOCORTICOIDS

Hypertension can be treated by stopping the drug. If this is not possible, sodium restriction to less than 2 g per day may be helpful. Pharmacologic treatment may include amiloride, which blocks the sodium channel in the distal renal tubule. Spironolactone or eplerenone may be used, but these agents will counter the desired effect of the mineralocorticoid. Hypokalemia should be identified and treated by potassium replacement, if necessary.[217]

MINERALOCORTICOID ANTAGONISTS

The serum potassium level should be monitored, and an electrocardiogram obtained. Treatment of hyperkalemia caused by mineralocorticoid antagonists is the same as that caused by other factors. Sodium bicarbonate, sodium polystyrene sulfonate, and insulin/glucose will be effective. Intravenous calcium should be used in severe cases as the first agent. Hypotension can be treated with intravenous crystalloid volume replacement. Vasopressors should be used if the patient remains hypotensive despite adequate fluid resuscitation.[3]

GONADAL

Introduction and Importance

Androgens are endocrine agents commonly used for legitimate purposes such as the treatment of male hypogonadism but are also used illegally in attempts to improve sex drive and athletic performance.[218,219] Androgen replacement for elderly men and postmenopausal women is advocated, although controversial.[220,221] Antiandrogens are primarily used to treat prostate cancer.[31]

Clinical indications for use of estrogen as medical treatment can be divided into at least three categories. Estrogen finds use as a physiologic hormone replacement therapy in estrogen-deficient women. It is also used in premenopausal women for contraceptive purposes. Controversial situations occur when it is used for other purposes, for example, the use of diethylstilbestrol (DES) in years past, for the purposes of improving pregnancy outcome.

Antiestrogens are used for therapy of reproductive disorders and for treatment of estrogen-dependent malignancies. These agents are not pure antagonists but have both estrogen antagonist and estrogen agonist effects, a situation that complicates understanding of

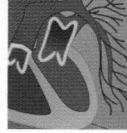

their action and controversy about their toxicity. Tamoxifen's estrogen antagonist action is reflected by improved survival of tamoxifen-treated patients with breast cancer and lowered risk for contralateral breast cancer.

Progestins are at times used as single agents for contraceptive purposes, although they are generally used in conjunction with an estrogen. Megestrol is a progestational agent that suppresses gonadotropin production, lowers testosterone levels, and thus functions as an antiandrogen. It has been used in the treatment of prostate carcinoma, and its antigonadotropic activity has also led to its use in the treatment of breast carcinoma and endometrial carcinoma. It has been observed that cancer victims who are treated with megestrol acetate tend to gain weight, leading to its use for the cachexia associated with malignancy and acquired immunodeficiency syndrome (AIDS).

Toxin-Induced Physiologic Disturbances

ANDROGENS

Many of the androgens that are clinically available are chemically altered versions of the testosterone molecule; without these modifications, effective androgen replacement would be difficult. Unmodified testosterone is quickly absorbed and very quickly metabolized by the liver; oral administration of testosterone is therefore not a useful therapeutic approach. It is now possible to administer unmodified testosterone transdermally. Outside the United States, testosterone implants are also available as a method for delivery of unmodified testosterone. Otherwise, the androgens that are available for administration can be divided into two major categories, based on the way in which the testosterone molecule has been modified for clinical use. Esterification of the 17α-hydroxyl group decreases the molecule's polarity and increases fat solubility. These testosterone esters, testosterone enanthate and testosterone cypionate, are administered in oily injection vehicles and function as depot agents with long half-lives; once absorbed, the esters are hydrolyzed to free testosterone, with subsequent physiologic actions that are no different from those of endogenously produced testosterone.

Acute overdose of androgens is not particularly toxic. Chronic misuse, however, results in significant pathology. The adverse effects of androgens tend to be related to the physiologic effects that result from the interaction of the hormone molecule with the hormone receptor. In the case of the androgens, the prostate gland is a major target organ for androgen action, with prostate cancer and benign prostatic hyperplasia being disorders of particular concern in patients who are treated with androgens.[222] Neither prostate cancer nor benign prostatic hyperplasia develops in the absence of testosterone exposure.[223] Prostatic cancer arises by a two-step process. The first component is the development of microscopic disease, and animal studies suggest that androgens are promoters of this step. The second step is the progression to clinical cancer, and it is not known whether androgens promote this phase of the disease.[224] The androgenic effect on benign prostatic hyperplasia is clearly demonstrated by the finding that prostate size can be reduced, and urinary obstructive symptoms improved, by agents that decrease androgen levels or androgen effect. Testosterone replacement in elderly men is associated with an increase in prostate-specific antigen.[223]

The effects of androgens on classic androgen-sensitive tissues are particularly of concern in athletes who take large and supraphysiologic doses of androgens. In male athletes, suppression of spermatogenesis, subsequent infertility, and testicular atrophy can occur.[225] Female athletes can become virilized, and some of these changes, such as effects on deepening of the voice caused by androgen action on the larynx, can be irreversible. Children and adolescents can experience accelerated skeletal maturation and early epiphyseal closure, which ultimately inhibits their final height.[226] Testosterone administration does not cause excessive stimulation of libido or potency, except in prepubertal boys and young men with long-standing androgen deficiency; in such patients, the possibility of severe and prolonged episodes of priapism dictates that very small initial doses of testosterone be used.

In what may seem to be a paradoxical side effect, administration of testosterone can at times cause gynecomastia. This is related to the conversion of testosterone to estradiol in peripheral tissues by aromatase enzymes and appears to be more common in young boys who are treated with testosterone for induction of puberty and in men with underlying disorders such as hepatic cirrhosis; in these situations, an elevation of the ratio of estradiol to testosterone is the likely mechanism. Testicular shrinkage is noted by chronic users and has been seen at autopsy of such patients.[227]

Androgen effects on nonreproductive tissues include androgen-dependent changes in serum lipoproteins. Men have lower levels than women of the protective high-density lipoprotein (HDL) cholesterol, with the disparity in HDL cholesterol level developing at the time of puberty. A 10% to 15% drop in HDL cholesterol level occurs during testosterone therapy. This androgen-driven decrement in HDL cholesterol may be a major contributor to the increased male risk for cardiovascular disease, although other factors such as a direct protective effect of estrogen on vascular tissue may also be important. Anabolic steroid use has been associated with myocardial infarction in otherwise healthy young athletes with normal coronary anatomy.[228] The cardiovascular risk of androgens may depend on the particular type of androgen used. Orally administered 17α-alkylated steroids cause a much more pronounced lowering of HDL cholesterol level than the testosterone esters, as well as an elevation of LDL cholesterol level that is not noted with the parenteral testosterone products.[222,229] The oral agents may have a greater effect on lipids because of the first-pass effect through the liver; furthermore, the effect of testosterone may be attenuated by its conversion to estrogen, which cannot occur with the 17α-alkylated agents. Although previous work showed an adverse effect of androgens on the cardiovascular system,

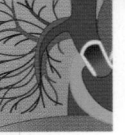

more recent studies suggest that testosterone may protect the arterial vascular system.[230] The musculoskeletal system is also at risk: one study reported unusual cases of tendon rupture among steroid-using bodybuilders. Dysplasia of collagen fibrils was the postulated mechanism.[231]

The initiation of androgen therapy can be associated with modest weight gain, which reflects the anabolic effects of testosterone and a component of sodium retention. Patients with disorders such as congestive heart failure and cirrhosis can have worsening of their edema with testosterone treatment. In combination with other risk factors such as obesity, chronic obstructive lung disease, and advancing age, testosterone administration to hypogonadal men appears to increase the incidence of sleep-related breathing disorders.[32]

Androgens have a number of effects on the body's hematopoietic system. Erythropoiesis increases, especially in the elderly. Cases of thrombosis in the extremities and in the CNS have been described, and it has been suggested that increased platelet aggregation may be the cause.[232-235] Conversely, androgens potentiate the effect of warfarin; a dose reduction up to 25% of this anticoagulant may be necessary.[236,237]

An ongoing controversy is whether or not androgens, when used in high doses, can induce pathologically aggressive and violent behavior or even psychotic symptoms. It is difficult to separate fact from conjecture, because most reports are anecdotal and do not take into account the pretreatment characteristics of the androgen user or consider possible concurrent use of other substances of abuse.[238] However, psychologic effects are suggested by the findings of a full affective disorder in more than 20% of athletes who used 10 to 100 times the usual therapeutic doses of these drugs, with psychotic symptoms appearing in 12%. This is consistent with the concept of androgen-related fluctuations in mood and increased levels of aggressiveness, which have been termed 'roid rage.[227,239] At testosterone doses double the physiologic replacement dose, little change in sexual and aggressive behaviors occurs, and the suggested concerns of adverse effects of exogenous testosterone on male sexual and aggressive behavior thus may be overstated.[240]

The question has also arisen about whether androgens can produce a psychological dependence syndrome. Evidence shows that in some individuals, androgen abuse can develop into a psychoactive substance dependence disorder with features that are similar to those seen with cocaine, alcohol, or opioid abuse. The features of psychological dependence include a preoccupation with the use of androgens, drug craving, and difficulty in discontinuing the agent despite psychological side effects; withdrawal effects are said to include mood swings, violent behavior, and profound depression.[241] In an effort to produce an androgen that can be given by the oral route, testosterone derivatives have been developed in which the molecule has been alkylated at the 17α position, sometimes in association with modification of the ring structure. These changes lead to a slowing of hepatic metabolism, which results in effective drug levels after oral administration. These 17α-alkylated androgens have been associated with severe hepatic toxicity, including cholestasis, liver tumors, and peliosis hepatis.[242-244] Because of these problems, it is generally recommended that these oral androgens should not be used for therapy of male hypogonadism; nonetheless, they can still be prescribed, and their illicit use continues.

Oxymetholone has been associated with development of leukemia in patients being treated for aplastic anemia and Fanconi's anemia. There is no clear causative relationship.[245]

Diabetic patients taking stanozolol may have decreases in glucose tolerance requiring a change in their diabetic medication.[2]

ANTIANDROGENS

Antiandrogens, used for therapy of benign prostatic hyperplasia, inhibit the 5α-reductase enzyme that converts testosterone into the active metabolite dihydrotestosterone. Although testosterone has a direct action in some tissues, it must be converted to dihydrotestosterone to exert an effect on the prostate and skin. No data on acute overdose are available, and adverse effects are rare. The most clinically important chronic toxicity is hepatic, and this effect is noted principally with the agents cyproterone and flutamide. Jaundice and hepatitis occur in 1% to 5% of patients taking these agents, and a few deaths due to liver failure have occurred.[2] Fluid retention, congestive heart failure, and hypertension have been noted.[246] Gynecomastia has been observed.[247] The drug is not approved for use in treatment of hirsutism, because its use in women would be associated with a theoretic risk of impaired virilization of the genitalia of male offspring.

In acute overdose, flutamide can cause CNS depression and decreased respirations.[2] Some cases of methemoglobinemia have been reported following chronic administration of flutamide, both in animals and humans. Methemoglobin levels as high as 32% were measured in one case.[248-250]

Nilutamide has been strongly associated with development of interstitial pneumonitis, with incidence ranging from less than 1% in the general population to 17% in Asians. Oxidative stress resulting from the redox cycling of the drug has been proposed as a mechanism.[251]

ESTROGENS

Acute overdose of oral contraceptive pills is considered a low-toxicity ingestion. GI upset the following day is common, and vaginal bleeding in girls or women in the few days following ingestion may occur.[252]

The use of estrogen replacement in postmenopausal women has risks. An increased risk for endometrial cancer was one of the first described complications of long-term estrogen therapy, with a 2- to 10-fold increase in disease among untreated women. This risk is present only in women who are treated without concurrent use of a progestational agent. The question of whether postmenopausal estrogen therapy leads to an increased risk for breast carcinoma continues to be one of the most

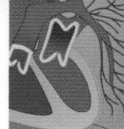

controversial concerns with estrogen treatment. Some studies have not shown any increase in risk, others have demonstrated some risk increase, and some have shown even a decreased risk.[253] When increased risk has been demonstrated, it appears that survival from breast cancer in estrogen-treated patients may be better than that in non-estrogen-treated women; whether this is related to closer medical supervision and monitoring in estrogen-treated women, biologic differences in the cancers, or other unidentified factors is uncertain. The risk question is further complicated by a large number of other variables, including the variety of estrogen products that have been used and the possibility of bias in the selection of patients who take estrogen. Even though at least one meta-analysis has concluded that postmenopausal estrogen therapy does not increase the risk for breast cancer, it is premature to conclude that this issue is settled. In particular, the contemporary tendency to combine estrogen and progestin may negate strict interpretation of earlier studies that evaluated estrogen-only therapy. Further studies will undoubtedly continue to provide more data on this topic; in light of the many conflicting results that have been reported thus far, no conclusive or final answer can be given to the breast cancer question at this time, and this will continue to be a topic of concern.[254]

The risk for gallbladder disease, however, is approximately doubled with estrogen treatment related to changes in the composition of bile.[255] In addition, estrogen can trigger migraine headaches in susceptible women.[253]

Postmenopausal estrogen replacement is usually administered as oral conjugated equine estrogens, oral estradiol, or transdermal estradiol. Transdermal therapy results in direct absorption of the estrogen into the systemic circulation and avoids the first pass effect of estrogen on the liver. The physiologic relevance of this is uncertain; however, in some cases, such as patients with a prior history of thromboembolic disease, the use of transdermal estrogen should minimize risks related to stimulation of clotting cascade protein production. Otherwise, the choice between oral and transdermal estrogen is an issue of individual patient preference.

The current oral contraceptive agents used in the United States are combination pills that contain ethinyl estradiol and one of five possible progestational agents, all of which are 19-nortestosterone derivatives.[256] The risks of estrogen use in these products are a complex issue because of the varying doses of estrogen and the combinations with various progestational agents. All of the data on oral contraceptive risks should be considered to be a moving target, because the earlier agents were relatively rich in estrogen content compared with contemporary agents. Although increased cardiovascular risk was a concern with the initial oral contraceptives, the risk for death due to coronary artery disease does not appear to be increased in present or past birth control pill users in the absence of other cardiovascular risk factors. However, additional risk factors such as hypertension, diabetes, and hypercholesterolemia are synergistic with birth control pills as risk factors for myocardial

infarction, and cigarette smoking in particular is the greatest single factor.

Birth control pills might influence cardiovascular risk factors in a number of ways. All estrogen-containing pills increase fasting triglyceride levels, and patients with underlying hypertriglyceridemia have an increased risk for pancreatitis if the triglyceride level exceeds the 800 to 1000 mg/dL range. Various effects on cholesterol metabolism are noted, depending on the dose of the estrogen and the particular progestin that is used. The addition of progestin may tend to attenuate mildly the generally favorable effects of estrogen on lipoprotein levels. In the various formulations of triphasic pills, changes in total cholesterol, LDL, and HDL are generally very slight. Pills containing only progestin seem to have the least effect on lipids, and it has been suggested that progestin-only pills, implantable levonorgestrel, or pills containing newer progestins such as desogestrel may be the best choice for patients who have a higher than usual risk for coronary artery disease but who would benefit from an effective contraceptive agent.[256]

Before the 1990s, virtually all oral contraceptive pills caused some degree of insulin resistance, with some increase in serum glucose and insulin levels. Both the estrogenic and progestational agents are responsible for the insulin resistance in a dose-dependent manner, and the same effects are less apparent with current oral contraceptives. In a practical sense, the changes in insulin and glucose metabolism are so small that they have no significance for normal women.[256]

Of all the metabolic changes that are related to oral contraceptive use, the changes in liver protein metabolism are the most important, particularly the hepatic proteins associated with coagulation, which increase in proportion to the estrogen content of the oral contraceptive. Oral contraceptive or postmenopausal combination estrogen-progestin therapy is associated with increased risk of thrombosis. This is not the case for low-dose estrogen-only therapy.[257,258]

Venous thromboembolism is the most serious complication related to the use of birth control pills. Its occurrence does not seem to be related to age, parity, obesity, smoking, or other apparent factors. Levels of these serum proteins return to normal within 2 months or so of discontinuation of the pills; the increased risk for thrombophlebitis decreases sooner. A case report describes an ischemic stroke in a young female smoker shortly after inadvertently taking a fourfold overdose of emergency contraception.[259]

Postmenopausal estrogen therapy usually does not affect blood pressure. If it has any effect, it may cause somewhat of a reduction in blood pressure in both normotensive and hypertensive women, with blood pressure elevation being an unusual finding.[254] Blood pressure elevation has been linked to oral contraceptive use, however. Combined oral contraceptives cause hypertension in 4% to 5% of women with normal blood pressure and an increase in blood pressure in 9% to 16% of women with previously established hypertension.[260] An estrogen-related effect on hepatic production of angiotensinogen has been invoked as a possible

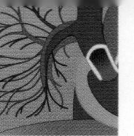

mechanism. In most patients, a compensatory decrease in renin levels seems to prevent the development of hypertension. Ethinyl estrogen at the typical doses of 30 or 35 μg has minimal effects on blood pressure, even in those individuals who may be predisposed to hypertension. Blood pressure is not influenced by progestin-only preparations, and some of the new third-generation progestins may even have an antimineralocorticoid effect that lowers the risk for hypertension.[261] With the triphasic pills, mean blood pressure in groups of patients does not change, although individual patients may have some increase.

DES is a synthesized stilbene with the estrogenic properties of naturally occurring estrogens. It was used for many years because of its effectiveness with oral administration and its low cost of production. DES was eventually banned from use in pregnancy in 1971 because of associated adverse medical effects.[261] The drug was commonly used in pregnancy because of its purported effectiveness in preventing miscarriages and premature births. In the early 1970s, a clear association with clear cell vaginal carcinoma was observed in young women who had been exposed to DES in utero. These women also seem to be at greater risk for anatomic anomalies of the reproductive tract. It is not clear whether males exposed in utero have any increased risk for comparable problems. Men being treated with DES for prostatic cancer have an increased risk for arterial thrombosis.[262] It has also been associated with a case of fatal hemolytic anemia as well as with a number of cases of fluid overload.[263,264] A number of cases of porphyria cutanea tarda have been reported in the literature after DES administration over a period of 1 to 3 years.[265-269]

An industrial exposure to norethindrone and mestranol caused a prolactinoma in a 61-year-old man, with gynecomastia, galactorrhea, and impotence.[270]

ANTIESTROGENS

Although little data exist on acute toxicity, sixfold over-doses in humans have been shown to cause neurotoxicity, including dizziness, ataxia, tremor, hyperreflexia, and seizure, as well as QT prolongation. In animals, respiratory distress and seizures have been generated.[3]

In chronic use, adverse effects include reversible hepatitis, which is thought to be a hypersensitivity reaction, and fatigue, headache, depression, and dizziness.[271,272] The expected estrogen deficiency symptoms of vasomotor instability and vaginal dryness are common. Clomiphene has traditionally been used to induce ovulation in anovulatory women; by masking the estrogen receptor at the hypothalamic-pituitary level, gonadotropin secretion is augmented, with subsequent stimulation of ovarian function. Side effects are infrequent and fairly mild and include occasional pelvic cramping, hot flashes, nausea, and breast tenderness, as well as some visual symptoms. The most significant side effect is ovarian hyperstimulation, with formation of luteinized ovarian cysts.

The estrogen agonist effects of tamoxifen seem to predominate over antagonistic action at the skeleton, where the drug increases bone density; in the metab-

olism of lipoproteins, where it has an estrogen-like action in increasing triglycerides and lowering LDL cholesterol; and at the endometrium, where an increased incidence of endometrial carcinoma has been noted.

PROGESTINS

Many of the effects of progestin therapy were reviewed in the earlier section on oral contraceptives under Estrogens. Because progestins are commonly used in conjunction with estrogens, distinguishing the effects of progestins from those of estrogen has been difficult. It is clear that more information is needed about the consequences, positive and negative, of combining estrogen with progesterone.

Implantable levonorgestrel may not completely suppress gonadotropins, and the subsequent irregularity of estrogen secretion can result in irregular bleeding, which may necessitate removal. No consistent effects on blood pressure, lipoproteins, or coagulation have been noted with this agent. Injectable depot medroxyprogesterone acetate has also been associated with irregular bleeding. Infertility may persist for months after its use. Despite gonadotropin suppression, bone density does not seem to be affected. Decreases in triglycerides and HDL cholesterol may occur without a change in total cholesterol or LDL cholesterol.

At high doses, progestins appear to cross-react with receptors for other steroids, and thus these agents may also have a GC effect. Cushingoid features and hypoadrenalism have been noted in patients taking medroxyprogesterone.[273] Five cases of Cushing's syndrome associated with megestrol therapy have been identified.[274] In one study, 16% of patients receiving high-dose progestins for breast cancer developed hyperglycemia.[275] Adrenal suppression due to ACTH inhibition after abrupt discontinuation of megestrol in a patient with AIDS has been described.[276]

Specific progestin side effects, which are dose dependent, can include breast tenderness, bloating, irritability, and depression.[277] However, a double-blind, placebo-controlled, crossover trial found no significant mood change.[278] Common skin side effects include acne, dermatitis, darkened skin, and hirsutism.[279] There have been 56 cases of intracranial hypertension associated with levonorgestrel use worldwide. Signs and symptoms included headache, nausea, and papilledema.[280] Intrathecal administration of medroxyprogesterone has been linked with the development of arachnoiditis in 17 cases. The mechanism is unclear.[281] However, the agents are generally considered so safe in terms of acute overdose that they have been exempted from poison prevention packaging requirements.[282]

ANTIPROGESTIN

Mifepristone is discussed in this chapter, in the section on the adrenal system.

Treatment Principles

Generally, withdrawal of the agent and supportive care are the mainstays of treatment. Most gonadal agents,

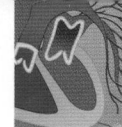

with a few exceptions, are fairly benign in acute overdose (Table 16-9). Laboratory studies should include complete blood count, basic metabolic panel, liver function tests, and coagulation tests.

ANTIANDROGENS

If there is clinical concern, chest radiography should be done to look for pneumonitis. Methemoglobin and sulfhemoglobin levels should be obtained. Methemoglobinemia caused by antiandrogens can be treated with methylene blue, although treatment failures have been described.

ESTROGENS

It is generally recommended that all women who are taking estrogen and who have not had a hysterectomy should also be treated with a progestational agent. Options include the use of medroxyprogesterone acetate, 10 mg for 12 to 14 days monthly, in addition to daily estrogen, with resultant withdrawal bleeding from endometrial sloughing and complete abrogation of the

risk from estrogen treatment. An alternate approach, which avoids menstrual bleeding, is to add medroxyprogesterone, 2.5 mg daily, to the daily estrogen therapy. The progestin reduces the nuclear concentration of estrogen receptors, causing involution of the endometrium; breakthrough bleeding may occur in the first several months.

In women with latent diabetes, such as normoglycemic patients with a history of gestational diabetes, periodic glucose monitoring is reasonable.

Daughters exposed to DES in utero should have careful cervical and vaginal examinations, using half-strength Lugol's solution to stain the entire vaginal wall. If annual Papanicolaou's test results are suspicious, vaginal cytologic tests and colposcopy are recommended. When pregnant, these DES-exposed daughters should be followed as high-risk obstetric patients because of their increased risk for spontaneous abortions, ectopic pregnancies, and premature labor. Although no clear association with testicular cancer has been noted, routine genital examination is also suggested for DES-exposed sons. This is especially true for those with the risk factor of cryptorchidism, which appears to be more prevalent with a DES exposure history.[261]

ANTIESTROGENS

Patients with severe periovulatory or postovulatory pain should undergo pelvic examination or ultrasound evaluation to confirm that the ovaries are of normal size before proceeding with further therapy.

An electrocardiogram should be obtained to evaluate the QT interval. Standard therapy should be used for treatment of seizures or torsades de pointes.

LIPID METABOLISM

Introduction and Importance

Lipids are essential for multiple body functions. Triglycerides are used as fuel stores for the body; cholesterol is a precursor for steroids and bile acids; and other lipids function as cellular signalers. One source of cholesterol is ingestion of cholesterol-containing foods, which are exclusively animal derived. The other source is synthesis of cholesterol within the body. Three molecules of acetate link to form 3-hydroxy-3-methylglutaryl coenzyme A (HMG-CoA). This compound is metabolized to mevalonic acid via the enzyme HMG-CoA reductase. Cholesterol is either excreted unchanged in the stool or converted to bile acids. Half of the cholesterol and almost all of the bile acids are excreted and then reabsorbed in the small bowel.

Control of plasma lipid levels has been proven in multiple large clinical trials to reduce the incidence of symptomatic coronary artery disease in at-risk patients. Prescription of lipid-lowering agents has therefore become ubiquitous, with global sales reaching 15.5 billion dollars in the year 2001.[283] Although many of these agents have excellent safety records, they are not without toxicity and adverse effects.

TABLE 16-9 Gonadal Agents	
AGENT	**CLASS**
Calusterone	Androgen
Danazol	Androgen
Fluoxymesterone	Androgen, 17α-alkylated
Methandrostenolone	Androgen
Methenolone	Androgen
Methyltestosterone	Androgen, 17α-alkylated
Nandrolone	Androgen
Oxandrolone	Androgen, 17α-alkylated
Oxymetholone	Androgen, 17α-alkylated
Stanozolol	Androgen, 17α-alkylated
Testosterone	Androgen
Chlorotrianisine	Estrogen
Dienestrol	Estrogen
Diethylstilbestrol	Estrogen
Estrogen	Estrogen
Promestriene	Estrogen
Quinestrol	Estrogen
Tibolone	Estrogen
Hydroxyprogesterone	Progestin
Levonorgestrel	Progestin
Medroxyprogesterone	Progestin
Megestrol	Progestin
Nomegestrol	Progestin
Norethindrone	Progestin
Progesterone	Progestin
Bicalutamide	Antiandrogen
Cyproterone	Antiandrogen
Dutasteride	Antiandrogen
Finasteride	Antiandrogen
Flutamide	Antiandrogen
Nilutamide	Antiandrogen
Cyclofenil	Antiestrogen
Droloxifene	Antiestrogen
Fulvestrant	Antiestrogen
Levormeloxifene	Antiestrogen
Reloxifene	Antiestrogen
Tamoxifen	Antiestrogen
Testolactone	Antiestrogen
Toremifene	Antiestrogen
Aglepristone	Antiprogestin (not available in USA)
Mifepristone	Antiprogestin

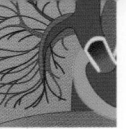
Toxin-Induced Physiologic Disturbances

Bile acid sequestrants lower cholesterol by binding bile acids in the stool and preventing their reabsorption. Subsequently, more bile acid is synthesized through cholesterol-7-α-hydroxylase, decreasing cholesterol stores.[284] This results in an increase in the number of hepatic LDL cholesterol receptors, which remove cholesterol from the circulation.[285] Fat-soluble vitamins A, D, E, and K, as well as vitamin B$_{12}$ and folic acid can be trapped with the bile acids and excreted as well. Depletion of vitamin K–dependent clotting factors and bleeding can occur, as can other conditions related to low levels of these vitamins.[286-290] Patients taking cholestyramine and colestipol at high doses can develop severe hyperchloremic acidosis. This occurs because the chloride ion in the resin is exchanged for HCO$_3$, depleting the body of this buffer.[291] In some cases this has been related to a predisposition to renal tubular acidosis, such as dehydration, renal insufficiency, or concomitant spironolactone administration.[292-297] Bile acid sequestrants also commonly cause constipation; they have been associated with vomiting or diarrhea to a lesser degree. Although no data exist about acute overdose of bile acid sequestrants, it is thought that bowel obstruction from inspissation would be a likely result.[2]

The same binding that seizes bile acids results in another of the adverse effects of this class of lipid-lowering agent. Taking a bile acid sequestrant at the same time as another drug may result in binding of the other medication and a decrease in its absorption.[298] In one study, a group of hypothyroid patients receiving cholestyramine and levothyroxine had a decrease in free T$_4$ levels.[2] It has also been documented that bile acid sequestrants bind endogenous iodothyronines and increase their fecal excretion.[299] This property may be useful in GI decontamination and enhanced elimination of other xenobiotics after toxic ingestions. Reports in the literature abound of cholestyramine being used to enhance elimination of levothyroxine, amiodarone, ochratoxin A, cardiac glycosides, methotrexate, chlordane, and chlordecone.[51,300-310] It is logical that lipid-soluble compounds, especially those that undergo enterohepatic recirculation, could be removed in this way. In one study, cholestyramine was found to be more effective than activated charcoal in absorbing lindane.[311]

Fibric acid derivatives reduce triglycerides and LDL cholesterol, and increase HDL cholesterol. They do this via activation of PPAR-γ. This nuclear hormone receptor exists in peripheral tissues as well as in the liver. Downstream effects include oxidation of fatty acids, increased synthesis of lipoprotein lipase, and reduced expression of apo-CIII.[312]

Gemfibrozil, and potentially other fibric acid derivatives, are likely metabolized by CYP3A4.[313] At least one, gemfibrozil, inhibits CYP2C8. This property has been experimentally shown to significantly raise the concentration of rosiglitazone when the two are administered together.[314] This inhibition may be the mechanism of other interactions between fibrates and oral hypoglycemic agents. In addition, a known interaction between fibric acid derivatives and warfarin results in increased International Normalized Ratio. This may be the result of enzyme inhibition as well as displacement of warfarin from protein binding sites. An interaction with furosemide is also postulated.[315]

A particularly feared complication of fibrate and statin-fibrate combination therapy is the possibility of rhabdomyolysis. Myopathy, which is much more common than frank rhabdomyolysis, has an incidence of 0.1% to 0.5% with monotherapy and 0.5% to 2.5% with combination therapy. Endocrine, metabolic, or genetic factors may play a role.[316] Reports have been published of autoimmune diseases potentiated by statin or fibrate therapy. It has been suggested that myositis is a manifestation of this synergy.[317] Some research suggests that rhabdomyolysis in this case is caused by two elements. First, fibrates strongly induce pyruvate dehydrogenase kinase 4 (PDK4) messenger RNA in muscle. Second, there is a reduction in serum triglyceride and fatty acid levels, which myocytes rely on for energy.[318] Another theory relates the adverse myotonic effects to inhibition of chloride ion channels in muscle.[319] Rhabdomyolysis has been seen to occur in acute overdose as well as chronic therapeutic dosing.[320]

Elevations in liver function tests have been seen in patients on fibrate therapy. Clofibrate has been found to induce peroxisomal enzymes and glutathione peroxidase activity. Reactive oxygen species are thus generated. It is unclear whether this is the pathophysiology which causes liver function test elevation.[321]

Mild creatinine elevations occur in about 10% of patients on fibrates.[322] This increase is on the order of 40%.[323] One study suggests that this is the result of increased creatinine production rather than development of renal insufficiency.[324]

Elevated homocysteine levels are well known to be caused by statin therapy, with the possible exception of gemfibrozil. Hyperhomocysteinemia is an independent risk factor for cardiovascular disease.[325] Elevations range from 20% to 50%.[326] The mechanism by which this occurs is not known.

White blood cell counts may drop in patients on fibric acid derivative medications. Using a chemoluminescence assay, one group of researchers determined that a single therapeutic dose of gemfibrozil strongly increases the production of reactive oxygen species in blood phagocytes. This may explain the leukopenia phenomenon.[327]

Other adverse effects common to the fibric acid derivatives include fatigue, dizziness, headache, nausea, vomiting, diarrhea, and constipation.

HMG-CoA reductase inhibitors, as their name implies, impede the enzyme involved in the rate-limiting step in cholesterol synthesis. Differences in the side chains of these otherwise similar molecules affects their lipophilicity. They are metabolized by CYP3A4, and primarily excreted in the bile. Total serum cholesterol and LDL cholesterol are both reduced. In some studies, but not in others, serum ubiquinone levels have been shown to decrease significantly.[328,329] Ubiquinone, also known as coenzyme Q10, is an antioxidant and membrane stabilizer necessary for mitochondrial respiration. Mevalonic acid

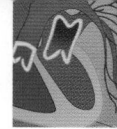

is a precursor for ubiquinone as well as for cholesterol.[330] Treatment with an HMG-CoA reductase inhibitor would therefore theoretically inhibit the production of ubiquinone as well as cholesterol. Its deficiency has been proposed as a cause for the adverse effects of the statins.[331] However, muscle ubiquinone levels were actually elevated.[332] Another proposed mechanism for the adverse effects of the statins is the reduction in cholesterol, which is itself necessary for many biochemical functions.[333]

Myalgias, myopathy, and rhabdomyolysis, with the possibility of renal failure and hyperkalemia, are the most significant adverse effects. The risk for this occurring is greater if the patient is taking a fibric acid derivative or nicotinic acid, which can also have this effect. One medication in this class, cerivastatin, was withdrawn from the market due to concerns about a high incidence of rhabdomyolysis. However, the overall incidence of myopathy is only 1.2 per 10,000 patient-years.[334] Elevations in liver function tests occur in a minority of patients. The incidence is approximately 2% to 3%, and may be dose dependent. Hepatotoxicity is extremely rare.[335] Nervous system changes, including stocking-glove neuropathy, confusion, memory impairment, and headache, have been reported.[336] The relative risk for definite cases of polyneuropathy has been estimated at 14.2 in a case control study. For patients on a statin for more than 2 years, the relative risk rises to 26.2.[337] The cause of these effects has not been elucidated, although some in vitro research suggests that simvastatin is neurotoxic.[338] Colitis has been associated with HMG-CoA reductase inhibitors in extremely rare cases. It is thought that up-regulation of nitric oxide synthase and cytokine production may be the cause, but further study is necessary to establish a causal link.[339] In acute overdose, up to 6 g has been taken without adverse effect.[3] No toxic overdoses have been reported in the literature.

Nicotinic acid therapy lowers the level of triglycerides, LDL and total cholesterol, and increases the HDL cholesterol level. The mechanism of action has not been completely elucidated. Proposed modes of action include inhibition of synthesis of apolipoprotein B-100,[340] up-regulation of lipoprotein lipase activity,[341] and reduction of free fatty acid release.[342] Niacin is a component of coenzymes NAD and nicotinamide-adenine dinucleotide phosphate (NADP) which are essential for redox reactions in numerous tissues.[343]

Adverse effects include atrial arrhythmia, with an incidence of 4.7%, compared with 2.9% in a group receiving placebo.[2,344] Glucose control becomes more difficult in diabetics.[345] Niacin also causes flushing of the skin through vasodilation (niacin flush), especially when the patient is exposed to large initial doses, until plateau serum levels are reached.[346] Nausea, vomiting, diarrhea, and peptic ulcer disease are fairly common. Pruritus can be disabling. Elevations of liver function tests, including some cases of fulminant hepatic necrosis, have been documented.[347] Three preparations are currently available: immediate release (IR), extended release (ER), and sustained release (SR). Hepatotoxicity is more common with the SR preparation, while flushing symptoms and GI distress are less frequent.[348] ER preparations offer less flushing than the IR and fewer hepatic complications than the SR preparations.[349] The differences in adverse effects among the preparations are a function of the drug metabolism. The IR preparation is primarily conjugated; the SR is mostly metabolized through the nicotinamide pathway; the ER is a balance between the two.[350] The presentation of hepatotoxicity is one of hepatocellular death, and can even mimic hepatobiliary neoplasia.[351] Dose-related and reversible visual changes, such as decreased vision or paracentral scotoma, have been noted in a few cases. Cystoid macular edema can be seen on examination.[352,353] In the SR formulation, niacin administration has been associated with a small decrease in platelet count and increase in prothrombin time.[2]

Acute overdose data are limited, but toxicity includes flushing, rash, pruritus, hepatotoxicity, and lactic and anion-gap acidoses.[3,354,355]

Ezetimibe is a novel lipid-lowering agent known as a selective cholesterol absorption inhibitor. It impedes the absorption of dietary and biliary cholesterol across the brush border of the intestine.[356] It appears to have no significant effect on the absorption of nutrients or vitamins. It is glucuronidated in the intestinal wall, and the parent and metabolite undergo enterohepatic recirculation.[357] Varied adverse effects, such as fatigue, headache, sinusitis, diarrhea, viral infections, variations in taste, and elevations in transaminases have been reported in clinical trials. However, the frequency of these effects in the placebo group was almost identical.[358] No data on acute overdose are available. The expected toxicity is low, based on the mechanism of action and metabolism.

Specific Agents and Their Mechanisms of Toxicity

Cholestyramine is a quaternary ammonium anion exchange resin with a high molecular weight. In case reports, it has been associated with platelet gigantism in a 9-year-old boy with hypercholesterolemia. The drug was given on three separate occasions, with recurrence of the finding each time.[359]

Colesevelam is a cross-linked hydrogel polymer bile acid sequestrant. It has been associated with asthenia and myalgias in small numbers of patients.[2] Incidence of adverse GI side effects appears lower. Serum levels of fat soluble vitamins were unaffected by colesevelam administration, and coadministration with a variety of other medications showed no significant impairment of absorption.[360-362]

Colestipol is a basic anion exchange resin, which is composed of amine groups. Occasional reports of chest pain and shortness of breath have been made by patients taking this medication.[2] Reversible elevations in liver function tests have been seen.[363] Some patients reported a decrease in visual acuity, but ocular examination of 10 patients who had been taking colestipol for 1 year showed no changes.[364,365]

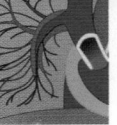

Fenofibrate has been associated with one case report of allergic reaction characterized by asthemia, hyperthermia, and muscular pain. Laboratory abnormalities included pancytopenia and elevated creatine kinase. The patient survived.[366]

Treatment Principles

GENERAL PRINCIPLES

Activated charcoal will bind these agents if administered promptly. Either because of large volume of distribution or high protein binding, hemodialysis is not thought to be helpful in enhancing elimination. Laboratory studies should include a metabolic panel, liver and renal function tests, urinalysis, and creatine kinase or myoglobin to assess for rhabdomyolysis. Care should be supportive and tailored to the toxic manifestations.

BILE ACID SEQUESTRANTS

An agent should be given to prevent constipation. Psyllium has been studied and found to provide significant relief.[367] Fat-soluble vitamins should be replenished. If hyperchloremic acidosis occurs, treatment should include intravenous sodium bicarbonate and replenishment of potassium, if it is low.[291]

FIBRIC ACID DERIVATIVES

Treatment with folic acid and vitamins B_6 and B_{12} significantly limit the hyperhomocysteinemia seen with fibrate therapy.[325,326] Care should be taken to identify drug interactions as described above. Fibric acid–statin combination therapy should be avoided if possible.

HMG-CoA REDUCTASE INHIBITORS

Most of these medications are extensively metabolized by CYP3A4. Xenobiotics that inhibit this liver enzyme should therefore not be used in patients on a statin.

NICOTINIC ACID

Administration of 325 mg of aspirin 1 hour prior to the dose of niacin may help lessen the degree of skin flushing. In cases of acute overdose, the same treatment may be given postingestion.

SELECTIVE CHOLESTEROL ABSORPTION INHIBITOR

Provide supportive care.

REFERENCES

1. Service FJ: Hypoglycemia. Med Clin North Am 1995;79:1–8.
2. Micromedex Healthcare Series: Thomson MICROMEDEX, Greenwood Village, CO (edition 119 expired March 2004).
3. Klasco RK (ed): POISINDEX System. Thomson MICROMEDEX, Greenwood Village, CO (edition 119 expired March 2004).
4. Seltzer HS: Drug-induced hypoglycemia. Endocrine Metab Clin North Am 1989;18:131–163.
5. Spiller HA, Villalobos D, Krenzelok EP: Prospective multicenter study of sulfonylurea ingestion in children. J Toxicol Clin Toxicol 1995;33:509.
6. Palatnick W, Meatherall RC, Tenenbein M: Clinical spectrum of sulfonylurea overdose and experience with diazoxide therapy. Arch Intern Med 1991;151:1859–1862.
7. Greenberg B, Wiehl C, Hug G: Chlorpropamide poisoning. Pediatrics 1968;41:145.
8. Spiller HA, Villalobos D, Krenzelok EP: Prospective multicenter study of sulfonylurea ingestion in children. J Pediatr 1997;131:141–146.
9. Asplund K, Wilholm BE, Lithner F: Glibenclamide-associated hypoglycaemia: a report on 57 cases. Diabetologia 1983;24:412–417.
10. Sonnenblick M, Shilo S: Glibenclamide induced prolonged hypoglycaemia. Age Ageing 1986;15:185–189.
11. Imano E, Kanda T, Kawamori R, et al: Pioglitazone-reduced insulin resistance in patient with Werner syndrome. Lancet 1997;350(9088):1365.
12. Stang MR, Wysowski DK, Butler-Jones D: Incidence of lactic acidosis in metformin users. Diabetes Care 1999;22:925–927.
13. Jurovich MR, Wooldridge JD, Force RW: Metformin-associated nonketotic metabolic acidosis. Ann Pharmacother 1997;31:53–55.
14. Luft D, Schmulling RM, Eggstein M: Lactic acidosis in biguanide-treated diabetics. Diabetologia 1978;14:75–87.
15. Chalopin JM, Tanter Y, Besancenot JF: Treatment of metformin-associated lactic acidosis with closed recirculation bicarbonate-buffered hemodialysis. Arch Intern Med 1984;144:203–205.
16. Gan SC, Barr J, Arieff AI: Biguanide-associated lactic acidosis: case report and review of the literature. Arch Intern Med 1992;152:2333–2336.
17. Schmidt R, Horn E, Richards J: Survival after metformin-associated lactic acidosis in peritoneal dialysis-dependent renal failure. Am J Med 1997;102:486–488.
18. Ryder REJ: Lactic acidotic coma with multiple medication including metformin in a patient with normal renal function. Br J Clin Pract 1984;38:229–230, 232.
19. Hutchison SMW, Catterall JR: Metformin and lactic acidosis—a reminder. Br J Clin Pract 1987;41:673–674.
20. Lalau JD, Westeel PF, Debussche X: Bicarbonate haemodialysis: an adequate treatment for lactic acidosis in diabetics treated by metformin. Intensive Care Med 1987;13:383–387.
21. Lalau JD, Race JM: Lactic acidosis in metformin therapy. Drugs 1999;58:55–60.
22. Kikuchi M: Modulation of insulin secretion in non-insulin dependent diabetes mellitus by two novel oral hypoglycaemic agents, NN623 and A4166. Diabetic Med 1996;13(Suppl):151–155.
23. Ampudia-Blasco FJ, Heinemann L, Bender R: Comparative dose-related time-action profiles of glibenclamide and a new non-sulphonylurea drug, AG-EE 623 ZW, during euglycaemic clamp in healthy subjects. Diabetologia 1994;37:703–707.
24. Gromada J, Dissing S, Kofod H: Effects of the hypoglycaemic drugs repaglinide and glibenclamide on ATP-sensitive potassium channels and cytosolic calcium channels in beta TC3 cells and rat pancreatic beta islet cells [Abstract]. Diabetologia 1995;38:1025–1032.
25. Malaisse WJ: Insulinotropic action of meglitinide analogues: modulation by an activator of ATP-sensitive K+ channels and high extracellular K+ concentrations [Abstract]. Pharmacol Res 1995;32:111–114.
26. Robling MR, Dolben J, Luzio SD: Single dose-response study of a new oral hypoglycaemic agent in diet-treated patients with non-insulin dependent diabetes mellitus [Abstract]. Br J Clin Pharmacol 1992;34:173P.
27. Vinambres C, Villanueva-Penacarillo ML, Valverde I: Repaglinide preserves nutrient-stimulated biosynthetic activity in rat pancreatic islets [Abstract]. Pharmacol Res 1996;34(1–2):83–85.
28. Service FJ: Hypoglycemic disorders. N Engl J Med 1995;332:1144–1152.
29. Service FJ: Factitial hypoglycemia. Endocrinologist 1992;2:173–176.
30. Bosse GM: Antidiabetic and hypoglycemic agents. In Lewin NA (ed): Goldfrank's Toxicologic Emergencies. New York, McGraw-Hill, 2002, pp 593–613.
31. Richardson DW, Robinson AG: Desmopressin. Ann Intern Med 1985;103:228–239.
32. Matsumoto AM: Hormonal therapy of male hypogonadism. Endocrinol Metab Clin North Am 1994;23:857–875.
33. Hintz RL: The prismatic case of Creutzfeldt-Jakob disease associated with pituitary growth hormone treatment. J Clin Endocrinol Metab 1995;80:2298–2301.

34. Corpas E, Harman SM, Blackman MR: Human growth hormone and human aging. Endocr Rev 1993;14:20–39.

35. Miller MM, Hoffman DI: Ovulation induction. In Becker KL (ed): Principles and Practice of Endocrinology and Metabolism. Philadelphia, JB Lippincott, 1995, pp 900–906.

36. Mandel SJ, Brent GA, Larsen PR: Levothyroxine therapy in patients with thyroid disease. Ann Intern Med 1993;119:494–502.

37. Jackson IMD, Cobb WE: Why does anyone still use dessicated thyroid USP? Am J Med 1978;64:284–288.

38. Roti E, Minelli R, Gardini E, Braverman LE: The use and misuse of thyroid hormone. Endocr Rev 1993;14:401–423.

39. Franklyn JA: The management of hyperthyroidism. N Engl J Med 1994;330:1731–1738.

40. Klein I, Becker DV, Levey GS: Treatment of hyperthyroid disease. Ann Intern Med 1994;121:281–288.

41. Pak CYC, Sakhaee K, Adams-Huet B: Treatment of postmenopausal osteoporosis with slow-release sodium fluoride. Final report of a randomized controlled trial. Ann Intern Med 1995;123:401–408.

42. Arab DM, Malatjalian DA, Rittmaster RS: Severe cholestatic jaundice in uncomplicated hyperthyroidism treated with methimazole. J Clin Endocrinol Metab 1995;80:1083–1085.

43. Hanson JS: Propylthiouracil and hepatitis. Two cases and a review of the literature. Arch Intern Med 1984;144:994–996.

44. Liaw Y-F, Huang M-J, Fan K-D: Hepatic injury during propylthiouracil therapy in patients with hyperthyroidism. Ann Intern Med 1993;118:424–428.

45. Jackson GL, Flickinger FW, Wells LW: Massive overdosage of propylthiouracil. Ann Intern Med 1979;91:418–419.

46. Garcia H, Michaud P, Rojas M, Tellez R: Acute poisoning with thyroxine in children [Spanish]. Rev Chil Pediatr 1990;61(6):334–336.

47. Brown RS, Cohen JH III, Braverman LE: Successful treatment of massive acute thyroid hormone poisoning with iopanoic acid. J Pediatr 1998;132(5):903–905.

48. Braga M, Cooper DS: Clinical review 129: oral cholecystographic agents and the thyroid. J Clin Endocrinol Metab 2001;86(5):1853–1860.

49. Bogazzi F, Aghini-Lombardi A, Cosci C, et al: Lopanoic acid rapidly controls type I amiodarone-induced thyrotoxicosis prior to thyroidectomy. J Endocrinol Invest 2002;25:176–180.

50. Bogazzi F, Bartalena L, Cosci C, et al: Treatment of type II amiodarone-induced thyrotoxicosis by either iopanoic acid or glucocorticoids: a prospective, randomized study. J Clin Endocrinol Metab 2003;88(5):1999–2002.

51. Lehrner LM, Weir MR: Acute ingestions of thyroid hormones. Pediatrics 1984;73(3):313–317.

52. Parfitt AM: Renal function in treated hypoparathyroidism. A possible direct nephrotoxic effect of vitamin D. Adv Exp Med Biol 1977;81:455–464.

53. Arya SN, Das GC: Nephropathy after acute hypervitaminosis-D (an experimental study). J Indian Med Assoc 1973;61(12):503–506.

54. Irnell L: Metastatic calcification of soft tissue on overdosage of vitamin D. Acta Med Scand 1969;185(3):147–152.

55. Pfister T, Atzpodien E, Bauss F: The renal effects of minimally nephrotoxic doses of ibandronate and zoledronate following single and intermittent intravenous administration in rats [see comment]. Toxicology 2003;191(2–3):159–167.

56. Marx RE: Pamidronate (Aredia) and zoledronate (Zometa) induced avascular necrosis of the jaws: a growing epidemic [see comment]. J Oral Maxillofac Surg 2003;61(9):1115–1117.

57. Hirschberg R: Nephrotoxicity of third-generation, intravenous bisphosphonates [see comment]. Toxicology 2004;196(1–2):165–170.

58. Fraunfelder FW: Ocular side effects associated with bisphosphonates. Drugs Today 2003;39(11):829–835.

59. Peter R, Mishra V, Fraser WD: Severe hypocalcaemia after being given intravenous bisphosphonate. BMJ 2004;328(7435):335–336.

60. Carter GD, Goss AN: Bisphosphonates and avascular necrosis of the jaws. Aust Dent J 2003;48(4):268.

61. Migliorati CA: Bisphosphonates and oral cavity avascular bone necrosis. J Clin Oncol 2003;21(22):4253–4254.

62. Chang JT, Green L, Beitz J: Renal failure with the use of zoledronic acid. N Engl J Med 2003;349(17):1676–1679.

63. Body JJ: Dosing regimens and main adverse events of bisphosphonates. Semin Oncol 2001;28(4 Suppl 11):49–53.

64. Blank MA, et al: Bisphosphonates and gastrointestinal damage [see comment]. Dig Dis Sci 1999;44(4):728.

65. Wallace JL, Dicay M, McKnight W, et al: N-bisphosphonates cause gastric epithelial injury independent of effects on the microcirculation. Aliment Pharmacol Ther 1999;13(12):1675–1682.

66. Adami S, Zamberlan N: Adverse effects of bisphosphonates. A comparative review. Drug Saf 1996;14(3):158–170.

67. Buemi M, Allegra A, Morabito N, et al: [Flushing due to calcitonin and the opioid system.] [Italian.] Recenti Prog Med 1990;81(12):819.

68. Reginster JY, Almer S, Gaspar S, et al: [Hypocalcemia induced in patients with Paget's disease by nasal salmon calcitonin. Effects of anti-calcitonin salmine antibodies.] Rev Rhum Malad Osteo-Articulaires 1989;56(7):563–567.

69. Conget JI, Vendrell J, Halperin I, Esmatjes E: Widespread tremor after injection of sodium calcitonin. BMJ 1989;298(6667):189.

70. Yamaguchi H, Sakaguchi H, Morisada M: Renal lesions following administration of calcitonin. A consideration on the morphological similarities to IgA nephropathy. Exp Pathol 1987;31(1):17–24.

71. Benito P, Blanch J, Duro JC, Faus S: [Severe hypocalcemia induced by calcitonin.] [Spanish.] Med Clin 1985;85(13):559–560.

72. Anonymous: Side-effects of calcitonins. Lancet 1983;1(8330):926–967.

73. Grunstein HS, Clifton-Bligh P, Posen S: Side effects of calcitonin therapy: a sex-related difference? N Engl J Med 1981;305(5):286.

74. Thomas DW, Frewin DB, Jolley PT: Deterioration in diabetic control during calcitonin therapy. Med J Aust 1979;2(13):699–670.

75. Evans IM, Joplin GF, MacIntyre I: Hyperglycaemic effect of synthetic salmon calcitonin. Lancet 1978;1(8058):280.

76. Gattereau A, et al: Hyperglycaemic effect of synthetic salmon calcitonin. Lancet 1977;2(8047):1076–1077.

77. Staehelin A: [Observations concerning the tolerability and dosage of calcitonin and its effect on disorders of the arterial circulation (author's translation).] Schweiz Rund Med Praxis 1977;66(19):580–584.

78. Cavatorta F, Queirolo C: [Acute renal insufficiency caused by probable allergic nephropathy caused by calcitonin treatment.] Arch Maragliano Patol Clin 1974;30(1):69–74.

79. Caniggia A, Gennari C: [Metabolic effects of calcitonin in man.] Minerva Med 1973;64(43):2249–2258.

80. Hantman DA, Donaldson CL, Hulley SB: Abnormal urinary sediment during therapy with synthetic salmon calcitonin. J Clin Endocrinol Metab 1971;33(3):564–566.

81. Piccone U, Pala M, Caprari M: [Calcitonin-induced anaphylactic shock. Case report and review of the literature.] Minerva Cardioangiol 1994;42(9):435–441.

82. MacGowan JR, Pringle J, Morris VH, Stamp TC: Gross vertebral collapse associated with long-term disodium etidronate treatment for pelvic Paget's disease. Skel Radiol 2000;29(5):279–282.

83. van Staa TP, Leufkens H, Abenhaim L, Cooper C: Postmarketing surveillance of the safety of cyclic etidronate. Pharmacotherapy 1998;18(5):1121–1128.

84. Thomas T, Lafage MH, Alexandre C: Atypical osteomalacia after 2 year etidronate intermittent cyclic administration in osteoporosis. J Rheumatol 1995;22(11):2183–2185.

85. Eyres KS, Marshall P, McCloskey E, Douglas DL, Kanis JA: Spontaneous fractures in a patient treated with low doses of etidronic acid (disodium etidronate). Drug Saf 1992;7(2):162–165.

86. Gibbs CJ, Aaron JE, Peacock M: Osteomalacia in Paget's disease treated with short term, high dose sodium etidronate. BMJ 1986;292(6530):1227–1229.

87. Morabito N, Gaudio A, Lasco A, et al: Three-year effectiveness of intravenous pamidronate versus pamidronate plus slow-release sodium fluoride for postmenopausal osteoporosis. Osteoporosis Int 2003;14(6):500–506.

88. von Tirpitz C, Klaus J, Steinkamp M, et al: Therapy of osteoporosis in patients with Crohn's disease: a randomized study comparing sodium fluoride and ibandronate. Aliment Pharmacol Ther 2003;17(6):807–816.

89. Rubin CD, Pak CY, Adams-Huet B, et al: Sustained-release sodium fluoride in the treatment of the elderly with established osteoporosis. Arch Intern Med 2001;161(19):2325–2333.

90. Pak CY, Sakhaee K, Rubin CD, Zerwekh JE: Sustained-release sodium fluoride in the management of established post-menopausal osteoporosis. Am J Med Sci 1997;313(1):23–32.

91. Pak CY, Sakhaee K, Adams-Huet B, et al: Treatment of postmenopausal osteoporosis with slow-release sodium fluoride. Final report of a randomized controlled trial [see comment]. Ann Intern Med 1995;123(6):401–408.

92. Shulman JD, Wells LM: Acute fluoride toxicity from ingesting home-use dental products in children, birth to 6 years of age. J Pub Health Dent 1997;57(3):150–158.

93. Li Y: Fluoride: safety issues. J Indiana Dent Assoc 1993;72(3):22–26.

94. Cummings CC, McIvor ME: Fluoride-induced hyperkalemia: the role of Ca2+-dependent K+ channels. Am J Emerg Med 1988;6(1):1–3.

95. Schamban N, Borenstein M: Selected oncologic emergencies. In Marx JA, Hockberger RS, Walls RM (eds): Rosen's Emergency Medicine. St. Louis, MO, Mosby, 2002, pp 1707–1708.

96. Reichardt HM, Schutz G: Glucocorticoid signalling—multiple variations of a common theme. Mol Cell Endocrinol 1998;146(1–2):1–6.

97. Schacke H, Docke WD, Asadullah K: Mechanisms involved in the side effects of glucocorticoids. Pharmacol Ther 2002;96(1):23–43.

98. Reid IR: Glucocorticoid-induced osteoporosis. Best Pract Res Clin Endocrinol Metab 2000;14(2):279–298.

99. Sergent JS: Arthritis accompanying endocrine and metabolic disorders. In Ruddy S, Harris ED, Sledge CB (eds): Kelley's Textbook of Rheumatology. Philadelphia, WB Saunders, 2001, p 1584.

100. Perez P, Page A, Bravo A, et al: Altered skin development and impaired proliferative and inflammatory responses in transgenic mice overexpressing the glucocorticoid receptor. FASEB J 2001;15(11):2030–2032.

101. Gras MP, Verrecchia F, Uitto J, Mauviel A: Downregulation of human type VII collagen (COL7A1) promoter activity by dexamethasone. Identification of a glucocorticoid receptor binding region. Exp Dermatol 2001;10(1):28–34.

102. Leibovich SJ, Ross R: The role of the macrophage in wound repair. A study with hydrocortisone and antimacrophage serum. Am J Pathol 1975;78(1):71–100.

103. Jick SS, Vasilakis-Scaramozza C, Maier WC: The risk of cataract among users of inhaled steroids. Epidemiology 2001;12(2):229–234.

104. Tripathi RC, Parapuram SK, Tripathi BJ, et al: Corticosteroids and glaucoma risk. Drugs Aging 1999;15(6):439–450.

105. Carnahan MC, Goldstein DA: Ocular complications of topical, peri-ocular, and systemic corticosteroids. Curr Opin Ophthalmol 2000;11(6):478–483.

106. Carpenter WT Jr, Gruen PH: Cortisol's effects on human mental functioning. J Clin Psychopharmacol 1982;2(2):91–101.

107. Sirois F: Steroid psychosis: a review. Gen Hosp Psych 2003;25(1):27–33.

108. Wissink S, Meijer O, Pearce D, et al: Regulation of the rat serotonin-1A receptor gene by corticosteroids. J Biol Chem 2000;275(2):1321–1326.

109. Wolkowitz OM, Reus VI, Canick J, et al: Glucocorticoid medication, memory and steroid psychosis in medical illness. Ann N Y Acad Sci 1997;823:81–96.

110. Newton M, Cooper BT: Benign intracranial hypertension during prednisolone treatment for inflammatory bowel disease [see comment]. Gut 1994;35(3):423–425.

111. Zadik Z, Barak Y, Stager D, et al: Pseudotumor cerebri in a boy with 11-beta-hydroxylase deficiency—a possible relation to rapid steroid withdrawal. Child Nerv Syst 1985;1(3):179–181.

112. Vyas CK, Talwar KK, Bhatnagar V, Sharma BK: Steroid-induced benign intracranial hypertension. Postgrad Med J 1981;57(665):181–182.

113. Chandra RK: Steroid-induced intracranial hypertension. Indian J Pediatr 1965;32(208):178.

114. Andrews RC, Walker BR: Glucocorticoids and insulin resistance: old hormones, new targets. Clin Sci 1999;96(5):513–523.

115. Trence DL: Management of patients on chronic glucocorticoid therapy: an endocrine perspective. Primary Care Clin Office Pract 2003;30(3):593–605.

116. Henzen C, Suter A, Lerch E, et al: Suppression and recovery of adrenal response after short-term, high-dose glucocorticoid treatment [see comment]. Lancet 2000;355(9203):542–545.

117. Sholter DE, Armstrong PW: Adverse effects of corticosteroids on the cardiovascular system. Can J Cardiol 2000;16(4):505–511.

118. Piper JM, Ray WA, Daugherty JR, Griffin MR: Corticosteroid use and peptic ulcer disease: role of nonsteroidal anti-inflammatory drugs. Ann Intern Med 1991;114(9):735–740.

119. Richardson CT: Pathogenetic factors in peptic ulcer disease. Am J Med 1985;79(2C):1–7.

120. Trainer PJ, Besser M: Cushing's syndrome. Therapy directed at the adrenal glands. Endocrinol Metab Clin North Am 1994;23(3):571–584.

121. Weber KT: Vascular remodeling and mineralocorticoids. J Endocrinol Invest 1995;18(7):533–539.

122. Krishna GG, Kapoor SC: Potassium supplementation ameliorates mineralocorticoid-induced sodium retention. Kidney Int 1993;43(5):1097–1103.

123. Campbell SE, Janicki JS, Matsubara BB, Weber KT: Myocardial fibrosis in the rat with mineralocorticoid excess. Prevention of scarring by amiloride. Am J Hypertension 1993;6(6 Pt 1):487–495.

124. Thommesen N: [Myocardial infarct during mineralocorticoid therapy. A case occurring in a 33-year-old man with Buerger's disease.] Ugeskrift Laeger 1969;131(38):1603–1604.

125. Liew D, Krum H: Aldosterone receptor antagonists for hypertension: what do they offer? Drugs 2003;63(19):1963–1972.

126. Brown NJ: Eplerenone: cardiovascular protection. Circulation 2003;107(19):2512–2518.

127. Rittmaster RS: Clinical review 73: medical treatment of androgen-dependent hirsutism. J Clin Endocrinol Metab 1995;80(9):2559–2563.

128. Weber MM, Lang J, Abedinpour F, et al: Different inhibitory effect of etomidate and ketoconazole on the human adrenal steroid biosynthesis. Clin Invest 1993;71(11):933–938.

129. Tucker WS Jr, Snell BB, Island DP, et al: Reversible adrenal insufficiency induced by ketoconazole. JAMA 1985;253(16):2413–2414.

130. Pont A, Williams PL, Loose DS, et al: Ketoconazole blocks testosterone synthesis. Arch Intern Med 1982;142(12):2137–2140.

131. Findor JA, Sorda JA, Igartua EB, Avagnina A: Ketoconazole-induced liver damage. Medicina 1998;58(3):277–281.

132. Gasior-Chrzan B, Stenvold SE, Falk ES: Juvenile tinea capitis caused by Trichophyton violaceum. Hepatic reactions during ketoconazole treatment. Acta Dermatovenereol 1991;71(1):57–58.

133. Bensaude RJ, Furet Y, Autret E, et al: [Cholestatic hepatitis caused by ketoconazole.] [French]. Ann Gastroenterol Hepatol 1988;24(2):55–57.

134. Sugar AM, Alsip SG, Galgiani JN, et al: Pharmacology and toxicity of high-dose ketoconazole. Antimicrob Agents Chemother 1987;31(12):1874–1878.

135. Chien RN, Yang LJ, Lin PY, Liaw YF: Hepatic injury during ketoconazole therapy in patients with onychomycosis: a controlled cohort study [see comment]. Hepatology 1997;25(1):103–107.

136. Garcia Rodriguez LA, Duque A, Castellsague J, et al: A cohort study on the risk of acute liver injury among users of ketoconazole and other antifungal drugs. Br J Clin Pharmacol 1999;48(6):847–852.

137. Knight TE, Shikuma CY, Knight J: Ketoconazole-induced fulminant hepatitis necessitating liver transplantation [see comment]. J Am Acad Dermatol 1991;25(2 Pt 2):398–400.

138. Bercoff E, Bernuau J, Degott C, et al: Ketoconazole-induced fulminant hepatitis. Gut 1985;26(6):636–638.

139. Zollner E, Delport S, Bonnici F: Fatal liver failure due to ketoconazole treatment of a girl with Cushing's syndrome. J Pediatr Endocrinol Metab 2001;14(3):335–338.

140. Duarte PA, Chow CC, Simmons F, et al: Fatal hepatitis associated with ketoconazole therapy. Arch Intern Med 1984;144(5):1069–1070.

141. Gradon JD, Sepkowitz DV: Massive hepatic enlargement with fatty change associated with ketoconazole [see comment]. DICP 1990;24(12):1175–1176.

142. Graybill JR, Drutz DJ, Murphy AL: Ketoconazole: a major innovation for treatment of fungal disease. Ann Intern Med 1980; 93(6):921–923.

143. Novack GD: Ocular toxicology. Curr Opin Ophthalmol 1994; 5(6):110–114.

144. Or M, Akbatur H, Hasanerisoglu B, Bilgihan K, et al: Ketoconazole induced papilledema. Acta Ophthalmol 1993;71(2):270–272.

145. Bulkowstein M, Mordish Y, Zimmerman DR, Sherman E, et al: Ketoconazole-induced neurologic sequelae. Vet Hum Toxicol 2003;45(5):239–240.

146. Duman D, Turhal NS, Duman DG: Fatal aplastic anemia during treatment with ketoconazole. Am J Med 2001;111(9):737.

147. Finkelstein E, Amichai B, Halevy S: Paranoid delusions caused by ketoconazole. Int J Dermatol 1996;35(1):75.

148. Hanash KA: Neurologic complications of ketoconazole therapy for advanced prostatic cancer. Urology 1989;33(6):466–467.

149. Herman BD, Fleishaker JC, Brown MT: Ketoconazole inhibits the clearance of the enantiomers of the antidepressant reboxetine in humans. Clin Pharmacol Ther 1999;66(4):374–379.

150. Mignat C: Clinically significant drug interactions with new immunosuppressive agents. Drug Saf 1997;16(4):267–278.

151. Tosi A, Misciali C, Piraccini BM, et al: Drug-induced hair loss and hair growth. Incidence, management and avoidance. Drug Saf 1994;10(4):310–317.

152. Harris PL: Alopecia associated with long-term metyrapone use. Clin Pharm 1986;5(1):66–68.

153. Wexler BC, Greenberg BP: Metyrapone-induced cardiovascular degenerative changes in non-arteriosclerotic and arteriosclerotic rats. Br J Exp Pathol 1978;59(1):52–63.

154. Connell JM, Cordiner J, Davies DL, et al: Pregnancy complicated by Cushing's syndrome: potential hazard of metyrapone therapy. Case report. Br J Obstet Gynaecol 1985;92(11):1192–1195.

155. Kellner M, Schick M, Wiedemann K: Prodissociative effects of metyrapone. Am J Psychiatry 2001;158(7):1159.

156. Hutter AM Jr, Kayhoe DE: Adrenal cortical carcinoma. Results of treatment with o,p'DDD in 138 patients. Am J Med 1966; 41(4):581–592.

157. Schteingart DE, Tsao HS, Taylor CI, et al: Sustained remission of Cushing's disease with mitotane and pituitary irradiation. Ann Intern Med 1980;92(5):613–619.

158. Neuman O, Bruckert E, Chadarevian R, Jacob N, et al: [Hepatotoxicity of a synthetic cortisol antagonist: OP'DDD (mitotane).] [French.] Therapie 2001;56(6):793–797.

159. Heilmann P, Wagner P, Nawroth PP, Ziegler R: [Therapy of the adrenocortical carcinoma with Lysodren (o,p'-DDD). Therapeutic management by monitoring o,p'-DDD blood levels.] Med Klin 2001;96(7):371–377.

160. Ng WT, Toohey MG, Mulhall L, Mackey DA: Pigmentary retinopathy, macular oedema, and abnormal ERG with mitotane treatment. Br J Ophthalmol 2003;87(4):500–501.

161. Fraunfelder FT, Meyer SM: Ocular toxicity of antineoplastic agents. Ophthalmology 1983;90(1):1–3.

162. Vizel M, Oster MW: Ocular side effects of cancer chemotherapy. Cancer 1982;49(10):1999–2002.

163. Potts GO, Creange JE, Hardomg HR, Schane HP: Trilostane, an orally active inhibitor of steroid biosynthesis. Steroids 1978;32(2):257–267.

164. Semple CG, Thomson JA, Stark AN, et al: Trilostane and the normal hypothalamic-pituitary-adrenocortical axis. Clin Endocrinol 1982;17(6):569–575.

165. Winterberg B, Vetter H: [Therapy of primary aldosteronism with trilostane.] Schweiz Med Wochenschr 1983;113(46):1735–1738.

166. Beardwell CG, Hindley AC, Wilkinson PM, et al: Trilostane in the treatment of advanced breast cancer. Cancer Chemother Pharmacol 1983;10(3):158–160.

167. Spitz IM, Bardin CW: Clinical pharmacology of RU 486—an antiprogestin and antiglucocorticoid. Contraception 1993;48(5):403–444.

168. Laue L, Lotze MT, Chrousos GP, et al: Effect of chronic treatment with the glucocorticoid antagonist RU 486 in man: toxicity, immunological, and hormonal aspects. J Clin Endocrinol Metab 1990;71(6):1474–1480.

169. Grimes DA, Mishell DR Jr, Shoupe D, Lacarra M: Early abortion with a single dose of the antiprogestin RU-486. Am J Obstet Gynecol 1988;158(6 Pt 1):1307–1312.

170. Hausknecht R: Mifepristone and misoprostol for early medical abortion: 18 months experience in the United States. Contraception 2003;67(6):463–465.

171. Newfield RS, Spitz IM, Isacson C, New MI: Long-term mifepristone (RU486) therapy resulting in massive benign endometrial hyperplasia. Clin Endocrinol 2001;54(3):399–404.

172. Lecorvaisier-Pieto C, Joly P, Thomine E, et al: Toxic epidermal necrolysis after mifepristone/gemeprost-induced abortion. J Am Acad Dermatol 1996;35(1):112.

173. Phillips K, Berry C, Mathers AM: Uterine rupture during second trimester termination of pregnancy using mifepristone and a prostaglandin. Eur J Obstet Gynecol Reprod Biol 1996;65(2):175–176.

174. Thong KJ, Lynch P, Baird DT: Uterine rupture during therapeutic abortion in the second trimester using mifepristone and prostaglandin [see comment]. Br J Obstet Gynaecol 1995; 102(10):844–845.

175. Delay M, Genestal M, Carrie D, et al: [Cardiocirculatory arrest after administration of combined mifepristone (Mifegyne) and sulprostone (Nalador) for induced abortion. Possible role of coronary vasospasm.] [French.] Arch Malad Coeur Vaisseaux 1992;85(1):105–107.

176. Sorbette F, Delay M, Genestal M, et al: [Cardio-circulatory arrest with mifepristone sulprostone combination for pregnancy interruption.] [French.] Therapie 1991;46(5):387–389.

177. Kochar MS, Itskovitz HD: Treatment of idiopathic orthostatic hypotension (Shy-Drager syndrome) with indomethacin. Lancet 1978;1(8072):1011–1014.

178. Holler W, Knorr D: [Hypertension as a complication treatment of adrenogenital syndrome.] Monatsschr Kinderheilk 1982;130(9):734–735.

179. Burns A, Brown TM, Semple P: Extreme metabolic alkalosis with fludrocortisone therapy. Postgrad Med J 1983;59(694):506–507.

180. Husmann F: [Effect of 9-alpha-fluorocortisol on adrenocortical function.] Klin Wochenschr 1971;49(10):607–609.

181. Anonymous: Severe metabolic alkalosis. BMJ 1981;283(6306):1607–8.

182. Chobanian AV, Volicer L, Tifft CP, et al: Mineralocorticoid-induced hypertension in patients with orthostatic hypotension. N Engl J Med 1979;301(2):68–73.

183. Bhattacharyya A, Tymms DJ: Heart failure with fludrocortisone in Addison's disease. J R Soc Med 1998;91(8):433–434.

184. Willis FR, Byrne GC, Jones TW: Fludrocortisone induced heart failure in Addison's disease. J Paediatr Child Health 1994;30(3):280–281.

185. Casellato F, Prina L, Tremolada F, Scolari F, et al: [Arterial hypertension with excessive mineraloactive hormone activity caused by overuse of a nasal spray containing fluorohydrocortisone.] [Italian.] G Ital Cardiol 1981;11(7):1014–1018.

186. Sanchez M, Perez-Garcia R, Lazaro P, et al: Hypermineralocorticoidism due to topical application of 9 alpha-fluoroprednisolone. Clin Nephrol 1984;22(5):267–268.

187. Chow E, Campbell WR, Turnier JC, et al: Toxicity of desoxycorticosterone pivalate given at high dosages to clinically normal beagles for six months. Am J Vet Res 1993;54(11):1954–1961.

188. Terris JM, Berecek KH, Cohen EL, et al: Deoxycorticosterone hypertension in the pig. Clin Sci Mol Med 1976;3(Suppl):303–305.

189. Wisenbaugh PE, Bogaty GV, Hill RW: Deoxycorticosterone acetate hypertension in dogs. Lab Invest 1965;14(12):2140–2149.

190. Marks JF, Fink CW: Prolonged hypertension following cessation of desoxycorticosterone therapy in congenital adrenal hyperplasia. Pediatrics 1967;40(2):184–187.

191. Horisberger JD, Giebisch G: Potassium-sparing diuretics. Renal Physiol 1987;10(3–4):198–220.

192. Schohn DC, Jahn HA, Pelletier BC: Dose-related cardiovascular effects of spironolactone. Am J Cardiol 1993;71(3):40A–45A.

193. Boisselle A, Tremblay RR: New therapeutic approach to the hirsute patient. Fertil Steril 1979;32(3):276–279.

194. White WB, et al: Effects of the selective aldosterone blocker eplerenone versus the calcium antagonist amlodipine in systolic hypertension [see comment]. Hypertension 2003;41(5):1021–1026 [erratum appears in Hypertension 2003;42(6):e20].

195. Weinberger MH, Roniker B, Krause SL, Weiss RJ: Eplerenone, a selective aldosterone blocker, in mild-to-moderate hypertension. Am J Hypertension 2002;15(8):709–716.

196. Dellinger RP, Carlet JM, Masur H, et al: Surviving Sepsis campaign guidelines for management of severe sepsis and septic shock. Crit Care Med 2004;32(3):858–873.

197. Jehle PM: Steroid-induced osteoporosis: how can it be avoided? Nephrol Dial Transplant 2003;18(5):861–864.

198. Anonymous: Recommendations for the prevention and treatment of glucocorticoid-induced osteoporosis: 2001 update. American College of Rheumatology Ad Hoc Committee on Glucocorticoid-Induced Osteoporosis. Arthritis Rheumatism 2001;44(7):1496–1503.

199. Sambrook PN: Glucocorticoid osteoporosis. Curr Pharm Design 2002;8(21):1877–1883.

200. Anonymous: Fractures in adults on systemic steroid therapy: which prophylaxis? Prescrire Int 1999;8(43):153–156.

201. European best practice guidelines for renal transplantation. Section IV: Long-term management of the transplant recipient. IV.8. Bone disease. Nephrol Dial Transplant 2002;17(Suppl 4):43–48.

202. Adachi JD, Bensen WG, Brown J, et al: Intermittent etidronate therapy to prevent corticosteroid-induced osteoporosis [see comment]. N Engl J Med 1997;337(6):382–387.

203. Pagano G, Cavallo-Perin P, Cassader M, et al: An in vivo and in vitro study of the mechanism of prednisone-induced insulin resistance in healthy subjects. J Clin Invest 1983;72(5):1814–1820.

204. Willi SM, Kennedy A, Brant BP, et al: Effective use of thiazolidinediones for the treatment of glucocorticoid-induced diabetes. Diabetes Res Clin Pract 2002;58(2):87–96.

205. Sapir-Pichhadze R, Blumenthal EZ: [Steroid induced glaucoma.] Harefuah 2003;142(2):137–140, 157.

206. Kong L, Zhang C, Chen M, Xue G: Clinical analysis of steroid glaucoma. Yen Ko Hsueh Pao [Eye Science] 1995;11(1):53–56.

207. Jobling AI, Augusteyn RC: What causes steroid cataracts? A review of steroid-induced posterior subcapsular cataracts. Clin Exp Optometry 2002;85(2):61–75.

208. Garbe E, LeLorier J, Boivin JF, Suissa S: Inhaled and nasal glucocorticoids and the risks of ocular hypertension or open-angle glaucoma [see comment]. JAMA 1997;277(9):722–727.

209. Lacomis D, Samuels MA: Adverse neurologic effects of glucocorticoids. J Gen Intern Med 1991;6(4):367–377.

210. Kobashigawa JA, Kasiske BL: Hyperlipidemia in solid organ transplantation. Transplantation 1997;63(3):331–338.

211. Whitworth JA: Mechanisms of glucocorticoid-induced hypertension. Kidney Int 1987;31(5):1213–1224.

212. Truhan AP, Ahmed AR: Corticosteroids: a review with emphasis on complications of prolonged systemic therapy. Ann Allergy 1989;62(5):375–391.

213. Nesbitt LT Jr: Minimizing complications from systemic glucocorticosteroid use. Dermatol Clin 1995;13(4):925–939.

214. Schweitzer DH, et al: Clinical and pharmacological aspects of accidental triamcinolone acetonide overdosage: a case study. Neth J Med 2000;56(1):12–16.

215. Van Der Meer JW, Keuning JJ, Scheijgrond HW, et al: The influence of gastric acidity on the bio-availability of ketoconazole. J Antimicrob Chemother 1980;6:552–554.

216. Hogan TF, Citrin DL, Johnson BM, et al: o,p'-DDD (mitotane) therapy of adrenal cortical carcinoma: observations on drug dosage, toxicity, and steroid replacement. Cancer 1978;42(5):2177–2181.

217. Dluhy RG, Lawrence JE, Williams GH: Endocrine hypertension. In Larsen PR (ed): Williams Textbook of Endocrinology. Philadelphia, WB Saunders, 2003, p 573.

218. Evans NA: Current concepts in anabolic-androgenic steroids. Am J Sports Med 2004;32(2):534–542.

219. Franke WW, Berendonk B: Hormonal doping and androgenization of athletes: a secret program of the German Democratic Republic government. Clin Chem 1997;43(7):1262–1279.

220. Practice Committee of the American Society for Reproductive Medicine: Treatment of androgen deficiency in the aging male. Fertil Steril 2004;81(5):1437–1440.

221. Basaria S, Dobs AS: Safety and adverse effects of androgens: how to counsel patients. Mayo Clin Proc 2004;79(4 Suppl):25–32.

222. Bardin CW, Swerdloff RS, Santen RJ: Androgens: risks and benefits. J Clin Endocrinol Metab 1991;73(1):4–7.

223. Tenover JS: Effects of testosterone supplementation in the aging male. J Clin Endocrinol Metab 1992;75(4):1092–1098.

224. Rolf C, Nieschlag E: Potential adverse effects of long-term testosterone therapy. Baillieres Clin Endocrinol Metab 1998;12(3):521–534.

225. Boyadjiev NP, et al: Reversible hypogonadism and azoospermia as a result of anabolic-androgenic steroid use in a bodybuilder with personality disorder. A case report. J Sports Med Phys Fitness 2000;40(3):271–274.

226. Strauss RH, Liggett MT, Lanese RR: Anabolic steroid use and perceived effects in ten weight-trained women athletes. JAMA 1985;253(19):2871–2873.

227. Thiblin I, Lindquist O, Rajs J: Cause and manner of death among users of anabolic androgenic steroids. J Forensic Sci 2000;45(1):16–23.

228. Varriale P, Mirzai-Tehrane M, Sedighi A: Acute myocardial infarction associated with anabolic steroids in a young HIV-infected patient. Pharmacotherapy 1999;19(7):881–884.

229. Matsumoto AM: Hormonal therapy of male hypogonadism. Endocrinol Metab Clin North Am 1994;23(4):857–875.

230. Weidemann W, Hanke H: Cardiovascular effects of androgens. Cardiovasc Drug Rev 2002;20(3):175–198.

231. Laseter JT, Russell JA: Anabolic steroid-induced tendon pathology: a review of the literature. Med Sci Sports Exerc 1991;23(1):1–3.

232. Ferenchick G, Schwartz D, Ball M, Schwartz K: Androgenic-anabolic steroid abuse and platelet aggregation: a pilot study in weight lifters. Am J Med Sci 1992;303(2):78–82.

233. Alvarado RG, Liu JY, Zwolak RM: Danazol and limb-threatening arterial thrombosis: two case reports. J Vasc Surg 2001;34(6):1123–1126.

234. Akhter J, Hyder S, Ahmed M: Cerebrovascular accident associated with anabolic steroid use in a young man. Neurology 1994;44(12):2405–2406.

235. Nagelberg SB, Laue L, Loriaux DL, Liu L: Cerebrovascular accident associated with testosterone therapy in a 21-year-old hypogonadal man. N Engl J Med 1986;314(10):649–650.

236. Edwards MS, Curtis JR: Decreased anticoagulant tolerance with oxymetholone. Lancet 1971;2(7717):221.

237. Lorentz SM, Weibert RT: Potentiation of warfarin anticoagulation by topical testosterone ointment. Clin Pharm 1985;4(3):332–334.

238. Fudala PJ, Weinrieb RM, Calarco JS, et al: An evaluation of anabolic-androgenic steroid abusers over a period of 1 year: seven case studies. Ann Clin Psychiatry 2003;15(2):121–130.

239. Pope HG Jr, Katz DL: Homicide and near-homicide by anabolic steroid users [see comment]. J Clin Psychiatry 1990;51(1):28–31.

240. Bagatell CJ, et al: Metabolic and behavioral effects of high-dose, exogenous testosterone in healthy men. J Clin Endocrinol Metab 1994;79(2):561–567.

241. Hallagan JB, Hallagan LF, Snyder MB: Anabolic-androgenic steroid use by athletes [see comment]. N Engl J Med 1989;321(15):1042–1045.

242. Hayashi T, Takahashi T, Minami T, et al: Fatal acute hepatic failure induced by danazol in a patient with endometriosis and aplastic anemia. J Gastroenterol 2001;36(11):783–786.

243. Confavreux C, Seve P, Broussolle C, Renaudier P, et al: Danazol-induced hepatocellular carcinoma. QJM 2003;96(4):317–318.

244. Bork K, Pitton M, Harten P, Koch P: Hepatocellular adenomas in patients taking danazol for hereditary angio-oedema [see comment]. Lancet 1999;353(9158):1066–1067.

245. Hirota Y: Effects of androstanes on aplastic anemia—a prospective study. Acta Haematol Jpn 1981;44(7):1341–1359.

246. Goldenberg SL, Bruchovsky N: Use of cyproterone acetate in prostate cancer. Urol Clin North Am 1991;18(1):111–122.

247. Ferrando J, et al: Unilateral gynecomastia induced by treatment with 1 mg of oral finasteride. Arch Dermatol 2002;138(4):543–544.

248. Kouides PA, Abboud CN, Fairbanks VF: Flutamide-induced cyanosis refractory to methylene blue therapy. Br J Haematol 1996;94(1):73–75.

249. Khan AM, Singh NT, Bilgrami S: Flutamide induced methemoglobinemia. J Urol 1997;157(4):1363.

250. Schott AM, Vial T, Gozzo I, Chareyre S, Delmas PD, et al: Flutamide-induced methemoglobinemia. DICP 1991;25(6):600–601.

251. Berger V, Berson A, Wolf C, et al: Generation of free radicals during the reductive metabolism of nilutamide by lung microsomes: possible role in the development of lung lesions in patients treated with this anti-androgen. Biochem Pharmacol 1992;43(3):654–657.

252. Riordan M, Rylance G, Berry K: Poisoning in children 3: common medicines. Arch Dis Child 2002;87(5):400–402.

253. Belchetz PE: Hormonal treatment of postmenopausal women [see comment]. N Engl J Med 1994;330(15):1062–1071.

254. Spitz IM, Bardin CW: Mifepristone (RU 486)—a modulator of progestin and glucocorticoid action. N Engl J Med 1993;329(6):404–412.

255. Kreek MJ: Female sex steroids and cholestasis. Semin Liver Dis 1987;7(1):8–23.

256. Sondheimer SJ: Update on the metabolic effects of steroidal contraceptives. Endocrinol Metab Clin North Am 1991;20(4):911–923.

257. Grodstein F, Stampfer MJ, Goldhaber SZ, et al: Prospective study of exogenous hormones and risk of pulmonary embolism in women [see comment]. Lancet 1996;348(9033):983–987.

258. Rossouw JE, Anderson GL, Prentice RL, et al: Risks and benefits of estrogen plus progestin in healthy postmenopausal women: principal results From the Women's Health Initiative randomized controlled trial [see comment]. JAMA 2002;288(3):321–333.

259. Sanchez-Ojanguren J, Escudero D, Zapata A: [Occlusion of the right common carotid artery due to oral estrogen overdose.] Rev Neurol 1998;27(158):604–606.

260. Baird DT, Glasier AF: Hormonal contraception [see comment]. N Engl J Med 1993;328(21):1543–1549.

261. Giusti RM, Iwamoto K, Hatch EE: Diethylstilbestrol revisited: a review of the long-term health effects. Ann Intern Med 1995;122(10):778–788.

262. Beaumont V, Lemort N, Abbou CC, Beaumont J : Ethinylestradiol and diethylstilbestrol induced antibodies and vascular thrombosis. Biomedicine 1980;32(1):26–31.

263. Rosenfeld DL, Bronson RA: Reproductive problems in the DES-exposed female. Obstet Gynecol 1980;55(4):453–456.

264. Konitturi MJ, Sotaniemi EA, Larmi TK: Body fluid and electrolyte balance during estrogen therapy of prostatic cancer. J Urol 1974;111(5):652–655.

265. Weimar VM, Weimar GW, Ceilley RI: Estrogen-induced porphyria cutanea tarda complicating treatment of prostatic carcinoma. J Urol 1978;120(5):643–644.

266. Reginster JP: [Case of porphyria cutanea tarda appearing during treatment with estrogens.] Arch Belg Dermatol Syphiligr 1972;28(2):179–180.

267. Roenigk HH Jr, Gottlob ME: Estrogen-induced porphyria cutanea tarda. Report of three cases. Arch Dermatol 1970;102(3):260–266.

268. Vail JT Jr: Porphyria cutanea tarda and estrogens. JAMA 1967;201(9):671–674.

269. Becker FT: Porphyria cutanea tarda induced by estrogens. Arch Dermatol 1965;92(3):252–256.

270. Baron SH, Sowers JR, Feinberg M: Prolactinoma in a man following industrial exposure to estrogens. West J Med 1983;138(5):720–722.

271. Rossi G, Gabbi E, Serra L: Acute hepatitis induced by cyclofenil: a case report. Ital J Gastroenterol 1992;24(2):77–78.

272. Bellmunt J, Sole L: European early phase II dose-finding study of droloxifene in advanced breast cancer. Am J Clin Oncol 1991;14(Suppl 2):36–39.

273. Dux S: Medroxyprogesterone acetate-induced secondary adrenal insufficiency. Ann Pharmacother 1998;32(1):134.

274. Mann M, Koller E, Murgo S, et al: Glucocorticoidlike activity of megestrol. A summary of Food and Drug Administration experience and a review of the literature. Arch Intern Med 1997;157(15):1651–1656.

275. Abrams JS, Parnes H, Aisner J: Current status of high-dose progestins in breast cancer. Semin Oncol 1990;17(6 Suppl 9):68–72.

276. Leinung MC, Liporace R, Miller CH: Induction of adrenal suppression by megestrol acetate in patients with AIDS [see comment]. Ann Intern Med 1995;122(11):843–845.

277. Grady D, Rubin SM, Petitti DB, et al: Hormone therapy to prevent disease and prolong life in postmenopausal women [see comment]. Ann Intern Med 1992;117(12):1016–1037.

278. Kirkham C, Hahn PM, Van Vugt DA, et al: A randomized, double-blind, placebo-controlled, cross-over trial to assess the side effects of medroxyprogesterone acetate in hormone replacement therapy. Obstet Gynecol 1991;78(1):93–97.

279. Sivin I, Stern J: Health during prolonged use of levonorgestrel 20 micrograms/d and the copper TCu 380Ag intrauterine contraceptive devices: a multicenter study. International Committee for Contraception Research (ICCR). Fertil Steril 1994;61(1):70–77.

280. Alder JB, Fraunfelder FT, Edwards R: Levonorgestrel implants and intracranial hypertension. N Engl J Med 1995;332(25):1720–1721.

281. Roche J: Steroid-induced arachnoiditis. Med J Aust 1984;140(5):281–284.

282. Consumer Product Safety Commission: Poison prevention packaging requirements; exemption of hormone replacement therapy products. Final rule. Fed Reg 2002;67(212):66550–66552.

283. Anonymous: Cardiovascular drugs: products, applications, and new developments. In RB-151. Norwalk, CT, Business Communications Company, 2001.

284. Lees RS, Wilson DE: The treatment of hyperlipidemia. N Engl J Med 1971;284(4):186–195.

285. Shepherd J: Mechanism of action of bile acid sequestrants and other lipid-lowering drugs. Cardiology 1989;76(Suppl 1):65–74.

286. Gross L, Brotman M: Hypoprothrombinemia and hemorrhage associated with cholestyramine therapy. Ann Intern Med 1970;72(1):95–96.

287. Vroonhof K, van Rijn HJ, van Hattum J: Vitamin K deficiency and bleeding after long-term use of cholestyramine. Neth J Med 2003;61(1):19–21.

288. Shojania AM, Grewar D: Hypoprothrombinemic hemorrhage due to cholestyramine therapy. CMAJ 1986;134(6):609–610.

289. Saraux H, Offret H, Levy VG: [Severe amblyopia caused by vitamin A deficiency induced by prolonged cholestyramine treatment.] Bull Soc Ophtalmol France 1980;80(4–5):367–368.

290. Acuna R, Gonzalez Ceron M: [Hypoprothrombinemia and bleeding associated to treatment with cholestyramine (author's translation).] Rev Med Chile 1977;105(1):27–28.

291. Effros RM, Widell JM: Acid-base balance. In Murray JF, Nadel JA (eds): Textbook of Respiratory Medicine. Philadelphia, WB Saunders, 2000, pp 169–170.

292. Kleinman PK: Cholestyramine and metabolic acidosis [Letter]. N Engl J Med 1974;290(15):861.

293. Clouston WM, Lloyd HM: Cholestyramine induced hyperchloremic metabolic acidosis. Aust N Z J Med 1985;15(2):271.

294. Zapater P, Alba D: Acidosis and extreme hyperkalemia associated with cholestyramine and spironolactone. Ann Pharmacother 1995;29(2):199–200.

295. Scheel PJ Jr, Whelton A, Rossiter K, Watson A: Cholestyramine-induced hyperchloremic metabolic acidosis. J Clin Pharmacol 1992;32(6):536–538.

296. Eaves ER, Korman MG: Cholestyramine induced hyperchloremic metabolic acidosis. Aust N Z J Med 1984;14(5):670–672.

297. Blom HJ, Monasch E: [Metabolic acidosis in a patient with kidney dysfunction following administration of cholestyramine. Ned Tijdschr Geneeskd 1983;127(32):1446–1447.

298. Rosenberg R: Malabsorption of thyroid hormone with cholestyramine administration. Conn Med 1994;58(2):109.

299. Hagag P, Nissenbaum H, Weiss M: Role of colestipol in the treatment of hyperthyroidism. J Endocrinol Invest 1998;21(11):725–731.

300. de Luis DA, Duenas A, Martin J, Abad L, et al: Light symptoms following a high-dose intentional ʟ-thyroxine ingestion treated with cholestyramine. Horm Res 2002;57(1–2):61–63.

301. Kerkadi A, et al: Cholestyramine protection against ochratoxin A toxicity: role of ochratoxin A sorption by the resin and bile acid enterohepatic circulation. J Food Protect 1999;62(12):1461–1465.

302. Krivoy N, Eisenman A: [Cholestyramine for digoxin intoxication.] Harefuah 1995;128(3):145–147, 199.

303. Goddard CJ, Whorwell PJ: Amiodarone overdose and its management. Br J Clin Pract 1989;43(5):184–186.

304. McAnena OJ, Ridge JA, Daly JM: Alteration of methotrexate metabolism in rats by administration of an elemental liquid diet. II. Reduced toxicity and improved survival using cholestyramine. Cancer 1987;59(6):1091–1097.

305. Garrettson LK, Guzelian PS, Blanke RV: Subacute chlordane poisoning. J Toxicol Clin Toxicol 1984;22(6):565–571.

306. Guzelian PS: New approaches for treatment of humans exposed to a slowly excreted environmental chemical (chlordecone). Zeitschr Gastroenterol 1984;22(1):16–20.

307. Guzelian PS: Therapeutic approaches for chlordecone poisoning in humans. J Toxicol Environ Health 1981;8(5–6):757–766.

308. Fresard F, Balant L, Noble J, Garcia B, et al: [Cholestyramine and digoxin intoxication: therapeutic efficacy?] Schweiz Med Wochenschr 1979;109(12):431–436.

309. Cady WJ, Rehder TL, Campbell J: Use of cholestyramine resin in the treatment of digitoxin toxicity. Am J Hosp Pharm 1979;36(1):92–94.

310. Cohn WJ, Boylan JJ, Blanke RV, et al: Treatment of chlordecone (Kepone) toxicity with cholestyramine. Results of a controlled clinical trial. N Engl J Med 1978;298(5):243–248.

311. Kassner JT, Maher TJ, Hull KM, Woolf AD, et al: Cholestyramine as an adsorbent in acute lindane poisoning: a murine model. Ann Emerg Med 1993;22(9):1392–1397.

312. Kersten S, Desvergne B, Wahli W: Roles of PPARs in health and disease. Nature 2000;405(6785):421–424.

313. Miller DB, Spence JD: Clinical pharmacokinetics of fibric acid derivatives (fibrates). Clin Pharmacokinet 1998;34(2):155–162.

314. Niemi M, Backman JT, Granfors M, et al: Gemfibrozil considerably increases the plasma concentrations of rosiglitazone. Diabetologia 2003;46(10):1319–1323.

315. Bays HE, Dujovne CA: Drug interactions of lipid-altering drugs. Drug Saf 1998;19(5):355–371.

316. Hodel C: Myopathy and rhabdomyolysis with lipid-lowering drugs. Toxicol Lett 2002;128(1–3):159–168.

317. Fauchais AL, et al: [Polymyositis induced or associated with lipid-lowering drugs: five cases.] Rev Med Interne 2004;25(4):294–298.

318. Motojima K, Seto K: Fibrates and statins rapidly and synergistically induce pyruvate dehydrogenase kinase 4 mRNA in the liver and muscles of mice. Biol Pharm Bull 2003;26(7):954–958.

319. Feller DR, Kamanna VS, Newman HA, et al: Dissociation of hypolipidemic and antiplatelet actions from adverse myotonic effects of clofibric acid related enantiomers. J Med Chem 1987;30(8):1265–1267.

320. Giraud O, Chanu B, Farge D, et al: [Acute rhabdomyolysis associated with digestive disorders during a voluntary overdose of ciprofibrate.] Gastroenterol Clin Biol 1995;19(2):231–232.

321. Takemura K, Aoyagi K, Nagase S, et al: Biosynthesis of methylguanidine in the hepatic peroxisomes and the effect of the induction of peroxisomal enzymes by clofibrate. Nephron 1998;78(1):82–87.

322. Branco MC, de Moura JP, Pereira M, et al: [Safety of ciprofibrate. Open study in a Portuguese population.] [Portuguese.] Rev Port Cardiol 1995;14(5):395–399, 360.

323. Broeders N, Knoop C, Antoine M, Tielemans C, et al: Fibrate-induced increase in blood urea and creatinine: is gemfibrozil the only innocuous agent? [see comment]. Nephrol Dial Transplant 2000;15(12):1993–1999.

324. Hottelart C, El Esper N, Rose F, Achard JM, et al: Fenofibrate increases creatininemia by increasing metabolic production of creatinine. Nephron 2002;92(3):536–541.

325. Dierkes J, Westphal S, Luley C: The effect of fibrates and other lipid-lowering drugs on plasma homocysteine levels. Exp Opin Drug Saf 2004;3(2):101–111.

326. Melenovsky V, Stulc T, Kozich V, et al: Effect of folic acid on fenofibrate-induced elevation of homocysteine and cysteine. Am Heart J 2003;146(1):110.

327. Scatena R, Nocca G, De Sole P, et al: The priming effect of gemfibrozil on reactive oxygen metabolism of phagocytic leucocytes. An intriguing side effect. Clin Chim Acta 1997;266(2):173–183.

328. Watts GF, Castelluccio C, Rice-Evans C, et al: Plasma coenzyme Q (ubiquinone) concentrations in patients treated with simvastatin. J Clin Pathol 1993;46(11):1055–1057.

329. Bargossi AM, Battino M, Gaddi A, et al: Exogenous CoQ10 preserves plasma ubiquinone levels in patients treated with 3-hydroxy-3-methylglutaryl coenzyme A reductase inhibitors. Int J Clin Lab Res 1994;24(3):171–176.

330. Rosenson RS: Current overview of statin-induced myopathy. Am J Med 2004;116(6):408–416.

331. Bliznakov EG: Lipid-lowering drugs (statins), cholesterol, and coenzyme Q10. The Baycol case—a modern Pandora's box. Biomed Pharmacother 2002;56(1):56–59.

332. Laaksonen R, Jokelainen K, Sahi T, Tikkanen MJ, et al: Decreases in serum ubiquinone concentrations do not result in reduced levels in muscle tissue during short-term simvastatin treatment in humans. Clin Pharmacol Ther 1995;57(1):62–66.

333. Morita I, Sato I, Ma L, Murota S: Enhancement of membrane fluidity in cholesterol-poor endothelial cells pre-treated with simvastatin. Endothelium 1997;5(2):107–113.

334. Gaist D, Rodriguez LA, Huerta C, et al: Lipid-lowering drugs and risk of myopathy: a population-based follow-up study. Epidemiology 2001;12(5):565–569.

335. Bradford RH, Shear CL, Chremos AN, et al: Expanded clinical evaluation of lovastatin (EXCEL) study results: III. Efficacy in modifying lipoproteins and implications for managing patients with moderate hypercholesterolemia. AJM 1991;91(Suppl 1B):18–24.

336. Bakker-Arkema RG, Nawrocki JW, Black DM: Safety profile of atorvastatin-treated patients with low LDL-cholesterol levels. Atherosclerosis 2000;149(1):123–129.

337. Gaist D, Jeppesen U, Andersen M, et al: Statins and risk of polyneuropathy: a case-control study [see comment]. Neurology 2002;58(9):1333–1337.

338. Kumano T, Mutoh T, Nakagawa H, Kuriyama M: HMG-CoA reductase inhibitor induces a transient activation of high affinity nerve growth factor receptor, trk, and morphological differentiation with fatal outcome in PC12 cells. Brain Res 2000; 859(1):169–172.

339. Rea WE, Durrant DC, Boldy DA: Ulcerative colitis after statin treatment. Postgrad Med J 2002;78(919):286–287.

340. Grundy SM: Drug therapy in dyslipidemia. Scand J Clin Lab Invest Suppl 1990;199:63–72.

341. Odetti P, Cheli V, Carta G, et al: Effect of nicotinic acid associated with retinol and tocopherols on plasma lipids in hyperlipoproteinaemic patients. Pharmatherapeutica 1984;4(1):21–24.

342. Nash DT: Gemfibrozil in combination with other drugs for severe hyperlipidemia. Preliminary study comprising four cases. Postgrad Med 1983;73(4):75–82.

343. DiPalma JR, McMichael R: Assessing the value of meganutrients in disease. Bull N Y Acad Med 1982;58(3):254–262.

344. Anonymous: Clofibrate and niacin in coronary heart disease. JAMA 1975;231(4):360–381.

345. Garg A, Grundy SM: Nicotinic acid as therapy for dyslipidemia in non-insulin-dependent diabetes mellitus [see comment]. JAMA 1990;264(6):723–726.

346. Hulshof JH, Vermeij P: The effect of nicotinamide on tinnitus: a double-blind controlled study. Clin Otolaryngol Allied Sci 1987;12(3):211–214.

347. Crouse JR 3rd: New developments in the use of niacin for treatment of hyperlipidemia: new considerations in the use of an old drug. Coron Artery Dis 1996;7(4):321–326.

348. McKenney J: New perspectives on the use of niacin in the treatment of lipid disorders. Arch Intern Med 2004;164(7):697–705.

349. Pieper JA: Overview of niacin formulations: differences in pharmacokinetics, efficacy, and safety. Am J Health Syst Pharm 2003;60(13 Suppl 2):9–14; quiz 25.

350. McKenney J: Niacin for dyslipidemia: considerations in product selection. Am J Health Syst Pharm 2003;60(10):995–1005.

351. Parra JL, Reddy KR: Hepatotoxicity of hypolipidemic drugs. Clin Liver Dis 2003;7(2):415–433.

352. Fraunfelder FW, Fraunfelder FT, Illingworth DR: Adverse ocular effects associated with niacin therapy. Br J Ophthalmol 1995;79(1):54–56.

353. Schwartz SG, Mieler WF: Medications and retinal toxicity. Ophthalmol Clin North Am 2002;15(4):517–528.

354. Paopairochanakorn C, White S, Baltarowich L: Hepatotoxicity in acute sustained-release niacin overdose. Clin Toxicol 2001;39:516.

355. Menna VJ: Index of suspicion. Case 2. Diagnosis: niacin overdose. Pediatr Rev 1993;14(11):433–435.

356. Miettinen TA: Cholesterol absorption inhibition: a strategy for cholesterol-lowering therapy. Int J Clin Pract 2001;55(10):710–716.

357. Bays HE, Moore PB, Drehobl MA, et al: Effectiveness and tolerability of ezetimibe in patients with primary hypercholesterolemia: pooled analysis of two phase II studies. Clin Ther 2001;23(8):1209–1230 [erratum appears in Clin Ther 2001; 23(9):1601].

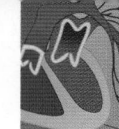

358. Knopp RH, Dujovne CA, Le Beaut A, et al: Evaluation of the efficacy, safety, and tolerability of ezetimibe in primary hypercholesterolaemia: a pooled analysis from two controlled phase III clinical studies. Int J Clin Pract 2003;57(5):363–368.

359. Latger-Cannard V, Sommelet D, Guerci B, et al: Platelet gigantism associated with cholestyramine therapy. Arch Int Med 2001;161(21):2619–2620.

360. Melian EB, Plosker GL: Colesevelam. Am J Cardiovasc Drugs 2001;1(2):141–148.

361. Steinmetz KL: Colesevelam hydrochloride. Am J Health Syst Pharm 2002;59(10):932–939.

362. Donovan JM, Stypinski D, Stiles MR, et al: Drug interactions with colesevelam hydrochloride, a novel, potent lipid-lowering agent. Cardiovasc Drugs Ther 2000;14(6):681–690.

363. Sirmans SM, Beck JK, Banh HL, Freeman DA: Colestipol-induced hepatotoxicity. Pharmacotherapy 2001;21(4):513–516.

364. Fellin R, Briani G, Balestrieri P, et al: Long-term effects of colestipol (U-26,597 A) on plasma lipids in familial type II hyperbetalipoproteinaemia. Atherosclerosis 1975;22(3):431–445.

365. Gross L, Figueredo R: Long-term cholesterol-lowering effect of colestipol resin in humans. J Am Geriatr Soc 1973;21(12):552–556.

366. Rabasa-Lhoret R, Rasamisoa M, Avignon A, Monnier L: Rare side-effects of fenofibrate. Diabetes Metabolism 2001;27(1):66–68.

367. Maciejko JJ, Brazg R, Shah A, et al: Psyllium for the reduction of cholestyramine-associated gastrointestinal symptoms in the treatment of primary hypercholesterolemia. Arch Fam Med 1994;3(11):955–960.

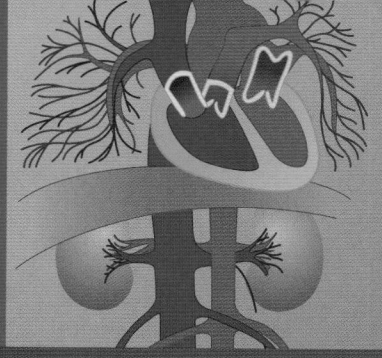

17 *Management Principles of Overdose in Pregnancy*

TIMOTHY B. ERICKSON, MD ■ KIRK CUMPSTON, DO ■ VALERIE A. DOBIESZ, MD

INTRODUCTION AND EPIDEMIOLOGY

The obstetric patient can suffer from various toxicities presenting as acute intentional drug overdose, recreational drug abuse, unintentional exposure from industrial or environmental toxins, and, finally, through iatrogenic causes. Suicide attempts during pregnancy frequently present as intentional drug overdoses, representing a more common means than self-mutilation, gunshot wounds, or jumping from high places.[1] Although an uncommon cause of maternal mortality as a whole (1% to 5%), suicide attempts and gestures can account for significant obstetric morbidity. According to one study, the incidence of attempted suicide for pregnant women ranged from 1% to 22%. Of women who actually committed suicide, 2% to 12% were pregnant.[2] The suicide rate was reported as 1 for every 88,000 to 400,000 live births before abortion became legalized, and is now felt to be much less common.[1] Suicidal gestures are typically impulsive, as a result of untimely pregnancies, interpersonal conflicts, or broken homes. In addition, pregnant women may take overdoses of an abortifacient with no intent of self-harm. Attempts are most common during the early stages of pregnancy and during the early third trimester, and half are by primigravid mothers. Personality disorders are often present, but true mental illness is infrequent, with neurotic depression being the most common psychiatric disorder diagnosed.[1]

Unless routinely screened or tested, early stages of pregnancy can go unrecognized in the overdose patient.[3] Pregnant women also have significant access to multiple medications. According to one study of prescription use in a Medicaid population, pregnant women received an average of 3.1 prescriptions, excluding vitamins.[4] Another study of drug utilization found a median of 4.7 drugs taken by pregnant females, most commonly vitamins, iron preparations, analgesics, antipyretics, anti-inflammatory agents, antiemetics, antacids, and antibiotics.[5]

Illicit drug use is also reported to have an incidence from 10% to 25% among pregnant patients. The rate of herbals/alternative remedy use among pregnant women is unestablished. It is the opinion of some that substance abuse during pregnancy is the most frequently missed diagnosis in perinatal medicine.[6]

The obstetric patient risks toxic exposure from an unprecedented number of chemicals and drugs. The Food and Drug Administration has assigned a risk classification (A, B, C, D, X) for all drugs based on the level of potential risk to the fetus (Table 17-1). These classifications must be interpreted with caution. Category A simply means that controlled studies in women fail to demonstrate a risk to the fetus. Category B means either animal studies have or have not demon-

TABLE 17-1 FDA Fetal Risk Classification

CATEGORIES

A	Controlled studies in pregnant women fail to demonstrate a risk to the fetus in the first trimester with no evidence of risk in later trimesters. The possibility of fetal harm appears remote.
B	Either animal reproduction studies have not demonstrated a fetal risk but there are no controlled studies in pregnant women, or animal reproduction studies have shown an adverse effect (other than a decrease in fertility) that was not confirmed in controlled studies in women in the first trimester and there is no evidence of a risk in later trimesters.
C	Either studies in animals have revealed adverse effects on the fetus (teratogenic or embryocidal effects or other) and only if the potential benefits justify the potential risk to the fetus.
D	There is positive evidence of human fetal risk, but the benefits from use in pregnant women may be acceptable despite the potential risk to the patient.
X	Studies in animals or human beings have demonstrated fetal abnormalities, or there is evidence of fetal risk.

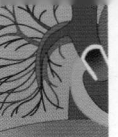

strated a risk to the fetus, and there are no controlled studies in women. Category C means either adverse effects have been discovered in animals and there are no controlled studies in humans, or there are no studies in women or animals. A majority of pharmaceuticals fall into this classification. The "safety" of category C may be based more on the absence of data, rather than the absence of proven teratogenic effects. Category D states there is a risk for teratogenicity to the human fetus, but if the therapeutic benefits of the drug to the pregnant woman outweigh the risks for teratogenicity to the fetus, its use is acceptable. Category X clearly states these drugs are contraindicated in pregnancy due to demonstrated fetal abnormalities in humans.

The potential for teratogenicity is often a concern even in a one-time exposure to a drug. When 1400 acute overdoses in pregnant women were followed over 30 years, there was no increase in congenital abnormalities when compared with women who did not overdose. If the fetus is exposed at 18 to 60 days of gestation, it will either spontaneously abort or survive without abnormalities.[7-10] Therefore, an acute insult by a toxin to the fetus will most likely result in demise of the fetus or survival without congenital malformations.

It is beyond the scope of this text to cover all poisonings and their teratogenicity. Instead, this chapter will focus on the more common toxins pregnant patients may be exposed to and those that have special considerations in the obstetric setting. Additionally, altered physiology, pharmacokinetics, and general management issues regarding poisoning in pregnancy will be discussed.

As with obstetric care in general, the same holds true for the poisoned patient: if you optimally treat the mother, you will also be treating the fetus. Conversely, if treatment is delayed or withheld over concern of inducing fetal harm, and the mother's care is compromised, both maternal and fetal outcome can be jeopardized. Therefore, the well-being of the mother should be of foremost concern in the treatment of a toxic exposure in a pregnant patient.

RELEVANT ANATOMY, PHYSIOLOGY, AND PHARMACOLOGY OF PREGNANCY

There are many physical and physiologic changes that occur during pregnancy that alter the pharmacokinetics of drugs and therefore affect the maternal exposure and toxic response.[11,12] These physiologic changes of pregnancy are summarized by organ system in Box 17-1.

Absorption

Gastrointestinal (GI) absorption is altered secondary to delayed gastric emptying, decreased GI motility, and prolonged transit time through the GI tract. During pregnancy, there is delayed but more complete GI absorption of drugs. Pulmonary changes may increase absorption of inhaled substances because of increased minute ventilation, increased tidal volume, and decreased residual lung volume. Dermal absorption may be enhanced because of increased total surface area and increased blood flow to the skin.

Distribution

The apparent volume of distribution (Vd) of drugs may be increased because of increases in mean plasma volume, extracellular fluid volume, and body fat stores. This Vd is variable in pregnancy because these physiologic changes are dynamic throughout the gestational period. An increase in serum concentrations of many drugs has been documented. Decreases in plasma albumin, protein binding, increased binding competition, and decreased hepatic biotransformation may all increase free drug concentration. This increased unbound or free drug results in larger volumes of distribution as the unbound drug is free to move into tissues. Free fractions of drug may also account for increased clearance rates as it is available for metabolism or elimination.

Metabolism

Hepatic alterations during pregnancy may include hepatic blood flow, bile excretion, and enzyme induction. There appears to be no clinically significant change in hepatic blood flow or bile excretion. Enzyme induction can be variable. Overall hepatic elimination patterns are inconsistent and difficult to predict in the pregnant woman.

Renal Excretion

Increased renal blood flow and glomerular filtration may result in increased renal elimination. Drugs excreted by the kidney are more rapidly excreted during pregnancy.

Placental-Fetal Blood Flow

The maternal-fetal unit is complex in terms of drug disposition and pharmacokinetics.

Increased lipid solubility and low molecular weight promote the transplacental passage of specific compounds. Additionally, drugs that are highly ionized tend to be more protein bound, limiting their transport across the placenta. As a result, with certain drugs, the placenta can act as a barrier protecting the fetus from a toxic insult. Conversely, it may prevent the passage of a beneficial antidote in an overdose setting. For certain toxins (e.g., lead), the placenta seems to provide no barrier to its free transmission to the fetus.

TREATMENT PRINCIPLES

Supportive Measures

The general management principles for a poisoned pregnant patient are the same as for a nonpregnant patient, with the exception of concern for fetal well-being. As with all overdose patients, initial stabilization measures should be addressed regarding ventilatory and hemodynamic status. If the patient is hypotensive, as with

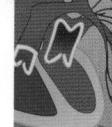

BOX 17-1	**Physiologic Changes of Pregnancy by Organ System (Time of Detected Change)**

Overall Physiologic Changes

↑ body mass 25% by term
↑ body water 7–8 L
↑ body fat 3–4 kg; 21%
↑ body temperature 0.5°C

Specific Organ Physiologic Changes

Renal
↓ Urine concentration (5 days)
  Ureteral dilation due to
  hormonal relaxation,
  mechanical compression
↑ Aldosterone secretion
↑ Antidiuretic hormone secretion
↑ Plasma volume 45%–50% with
  70% increase in volume of extracellular
  fluid space
↑ Renal plasma flow 25%–85%
↓ Serum creatinine; blood urea
  nitrogen

Cardiovascular
↑ Cardiac output (6 wk)
  35% by 10 wk
  48% by 25 wk

↑ Heart rate 20% or 15 bpm
↑ Stroke volume 10%–32% or 17 mL
↓ Peripheral vascular resistance
  due to low resistance
  placental circulatory shunt
↑ Peripheral blood flow
↑ Perfusion of skin, mucosa,
  epidural space

↓ Oxygen extraction
↑ Oxygen consumption 15%–20%

Pulmonary
↑ Ventilatory response to CO_2
↑ Arterial Po_2 10 mm Hg
↓ Arterial Pco_2 10 mm Hg
↑ Minute ventilation 40%–50%
↑ Alveolar ventilation
↓ Vital capacity
↑ Respiratory rate 0–15%
↑ Tidal volume 40%
↓ Functional residual
  capacity 20%
↓ Expiratory reserve
  volume 20%
↓ Residual volume 20%
↓ Subjective dyspnea
↓ Airway resistance 36%
  Pulmonary blood flow

Gastrointestinal
↑ Nausea and vomiting
  Relaxed cardiac sphincter
↑ Gastrointestinal reflux
↓ Gastric acidity 30%–50% (0–4 mo)
↓ Mucus secretion
↓ Gastric motility
↓ Small bowel motility
↑ Stomach emptying time 0–160%
  Hepatic metabolism ↑ or ↓

Urogenital
↑ Weight of uterus
  400% by 10 wk
  2000% by term

Blood
↑ Blood volume 35%–40%
↑ Plasma volume 50%
↑ Red blood cell volume
  18%–20% 300–400 mL
↓ Hematocrit 15%
↓ Serum hemoglobin
↓ Serum iron
↑ White blood count 66%
↓ Total serum proteins
  18% (3rd trimester)

↓ Serum albumin 14%–30%
↑ α_1 α_2 globulins 0–20%
↑ Serum fibrinogen 40%–200%
↑ Phospholipids
↑ Cholesterol
↑ Free fatty acids

Neurologic
↓ Plasma cholinesterases 20%

↑, increase; ↓, decrease.

---

traumatic injury, the patient should be placed in the left lateral decubitus position with aggressive intravenous fluid administration. A thorough history and physical examination should be performed addressing the time of and reason for exposure, type and quantity of the toxin, stage of pregnancy, and symptomatology. The physical examination should include fetal monitoring if gestation is at an appropriate level of development. If the mother is experiencing altered mental status, assessment of her glucose status is indicated, and if hypoglycemic, 50% dextrose solution should be administrated. In the setting of coma, the benefit of giving naloxone to a suspected opioid-intoxicated mother with respiratory compromise outweighs the potential risks of inducing narcotic withdrawal in mother and fetus.[13]

Decontamination Principles

Decontamination principles in the pregnant patient should be practiced in a similar fashion to those used in general overdosed patients, with a few caveats. The emetic agent syrup of ipecac is strongly discouraged from use in pregnancy, keeping with the most recent trends in the poison decontamination literature.[14-17] Syrup of ipecac can induce protracted emesis, resulting in increased abdominal and thoracic pressure. This agent is absolutely contraindicated if the patient has altered mental status, seizures, and toxin-induced vomiting. Additionally, there are potential teratogenic concerns over the chronic use of ipecac.[18] Although there are currently no studies addressing the utility and

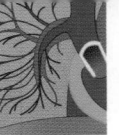
safety of gastric lavage in the pregnant patient, it may be indicated following a very recent ingestion of a potentially life-threatening or fetal toxic drug.[14] Additionally, since the pregnant patient has physiologic delayed gastric emptying and decreased gut motility, delayed lavage may be considered following massive ingestions. The literature is unclear as to the timing and indications for evacuation of drugs that slow gut motility (anticholinergics and opioids), or those toxins that are known to form concretions (salicylates and iron). Activated charcoal, the most efficacious and safe gastric decontamination modality, is not systemically absorbed from the GI tract and is considered safe (low risk of adverse side effects) in the pregnant patient, with no reports of fetal toxicity.

The usefulness of cathartics for GI decontamination has never been well documented; therefore, their addition to general decontamination measures in the pregnant patient is not mandatory. The general use of cathartic agents such as magnesium citrate or sorbitol in the pregnant patient should be used with extreme caution, particularly in later stages of pregnancy. Overzealous use of these agents may stimulate preterm labor, cause dehydration, or produce electrolyte imbalance.[19] Whole bowel irrigation is an osmotically safe, high-molecular-weight, polyethylene glycol solution. This decontamination modality has been shown to be efficacious and safely administered in iron, cocaine packet, lead, and sustained-released product ingestions.[20] Although reported cases are anecdotal, it has been safely used in overdosed pregnant patients.[21,22]

Multiple-dose activated charcoal is indicated for the same toxic overdoses as in the nonpregnant patient: theophylline, phenobarbital, carbamazepine, dapsone, and quinine. Enhanced elimination of these drugs occurs because their physical properties or enterohepatic circulation allow for gut dialysis of the drug from the circulatory system into the GI tract, where it is adsorbed to the charcoal.

Antidotes

Literature on the use of antidotes in the pregnant overdosed patient is limited largely to animal studies and isolated case reports or retrospective case series. There have been no adequate or well-controlled clinical trials. Thus, definitive conclusions regarding their use with obstetric patients are inconclusive.[11] In general, the use of antidote therapy in pregnancy is indicated if needed to reverse the toxic manifestations in the mother. Several cases in the literature have reported both maternal and fetal death when a potentially life-saving antidote was withheld because of fear of harming the fetus.[23,24] As with general poison management, if you appropriately treat the mother, you will be treating the fetus (Table 17-2).

Enhanced Elimination

Literature regarding the use of hemodialysis and hemoperfusion in poisoned pregnant patients is limited. However, if indicated, their implementation is recom-

TABLE 17-2 Placental Permeability of Toxins and Antidotes

	PLACENTAL PERMEABILITY	
	YES	**NO**
Acetaminophen	X	
N-acetylcysteine	X	
Iron	X (receptor-mediated endocytosis)	
Deferoxamine		X
Lead	X	
Carbon monoxide	X	
Oxygen	X	
Organophosphate	X	
Atropine	X	
Cyanide	X	
Sodium thiosulfate		X

mended as there have been few adverse effects reported in women who required these treatments in the acute overdose setting.[25,26] In addition, routine use of hemodialysis in pregnant patients with chronic renal failure is reported as relatively safe. However, premature labor and growth retardation have been described but have been attributed to the chronic disease state and not a consequence of dialysis.[27,28]

Disposition

Specific disposition of the poisoned pregnant patient depends on the type of toxin, symptomatology, stage of pregnancy, and intent of exposure. Unstable overdosed patients should be closely monitored in an intensive care setting. There are reports of complete maternal and fetal recovery after maternal cardiac arrest justifying aggressive, prolonged resuscitation attempts.[29] Under certain circumstances, emergent delivery of a mature or full-term fetus may prove beneficial for the specific treatment of both mother and newborn. When the toxic mother is deemed stable, admission to a general obstetric, labor and delivery, or medical ward is appropriate with close fetal monitoring. If the toxic exposure is intentional, once medically stabilized, a psychiatric consultation should be obtained. If the patient is medically stable and not psychiatrically impaired, she may be discharged home with close outpatient prenatal care.

ABORTIFACIENTS

An abortifacient is any substance that is used to terminate a pregnancy (Box 17-2). Historically, lead and quinine have been used as abortifacients, but now over-the-counter preparations such as acetaminophen, aspirin, iron, and herbal preparations are more commonly used to induce abortion. The greatest dangers of abortifacients are the effect of the toxin on the mother and the potential teratogenic effect on the fetus. Most attempts to chemically abort a fetus are made in the first trimester. Acetaminophen and multidrug ingestions

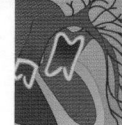

BOX 17-2	**ABORTIFACIENTS**

Angelica root (*Angelica archangelica*)
Black cohosh (*Cimicifuga racemosa*)
Blue cohosh (*Caulophyllum thalictroides*)
Buckthorn bark (*Rhamnus cathartica, frangula, alnifolia*)
Diethylcarbamazine
Ergotamine
Mandrake (*Podophyllum peltatum*)
Mifepristone (approved in France as an abortifacient in 1988)
Misopristol
Mistletoe (*Phoradendron falvescens, macrophyllum rubrum, serotinum, tomentosum; Viscum album*)
Pennyroyal (*Mentha pulegium/Hedeoma pulegioides*)
Poison hemlock (*Conium maculatum*)
Quinine
Rue (*Ruta graveolens*)
Savun/juniper (*Juniperus sabina*)
Sodium chloride 20% by transabdominal intra-amniotic injection
Tansy (*Tanacetum/Chrysanthenum vulgare*)
Windflower (*Anemone pulsatilla*)

are the most common exposures, with minor maternal toxicity reported in most cases.

As a result of the serious nature of an abortion attempt and the often nonspecific clinical manifestation of the ingestion, a high index of suspicion is required to discover if this has occurred in gravid patients. Therefore, every female overdose patient of childbearing age should have a pregnancy test performed. In addition, women who present with significant vaginal bleeding should be questioned about possible abortifacient use.[30,31]

ACETAMINOPHEN

Acetaminophen or paracetamol is readily available to pregnant patients since numerous over-the-counter preparations such as cold remedies, antipyretics, and analgesics contain this compound. It has been cited as the drug most frequently taken in an acute overdose by pregnant patients.[1]

In an acute overdose, sulfonation and glucuronidation metabolic pathways become saturated, causing an increased shift to the cytochrome P-450 pathway. As a result, glutathione stores are depleted, leading to hepatotoxicity via central lobular necrosis. Since acetaminophen crosses the placental barrier, the fetus is at risk for poisoning.[32,33] Evidence of placental transfer has been documented in both animals[34] and humans.[33] The cytochrome P-450 system is present in the fetus by 14 weeks' gestation.[35] Early in fetal development, the cytochrome P-450 activity is only 10% of adult activity and develops in a linear fashion throughout gestation.[18] As a result, in later stages of pregnancy, the fetus is more susceptible to toxicity since it is able to form the toxic metabolite of acetaminophen, *N*-acetyl-*p*-benzoquinone imine. This finding has been observed clinically in selected studies in which the fetal outcome was worse if the overdose occurred during the third trimester,

particularly if the mother demonstrated concomitant signs of hepatotoxicity.[18,35-38]

In an acute ingestion, an acetaminophen level should be drawn and plotted on the Rumack-Matthew nomogram to assess the risk for hepatotoxicity. Peak serum levels and pharmacokinetics of acetaminophen in the pregnant patient are unchanged in standard doses but are as yet undetermined in the overdose setting.[39] In addition, baseline liver function tests and coagulation profiles should be drawn and followed in a serial manner as indicated.

If the time of ingestion is unknown, or is chronic in nature, a serum level is still recommended in order to document the exposure. Subsequent levels should be followed as hepatic damage will prolong the half-life of the drug. The mean half-life of acetaminophen during pregnancy in therapeutic doses has been shown to be 3.7 hours versus 3.1 hours in the nonpregnant patient.[39]

In the acute acetaminophen overdose, general stabilization and decontamination measures should be implemented. If the acetaminophen level is hepatotoxic on the nomogram or if over 140 mg/kg is acutely ingested, administration of the antidote *N*-acetylcysteine is indicated. *N*-acetylcysteine (NAC) acts by replenishing hepatic glutathione stores and is most effective if given within 8 hours postingestion.[40]

Whether NAC administration is protective or toxic to the fetus is unknown. However, Riggs and colleagues, in a study of 60 pregnant patients, demonstrated a significant positive correlation between the time to initial administration of NAC and pregnancy outcome. There was an increase in the incidence of spontaneous abortion or fetal demise when the treatment was delayed.[35] In a large series describing 48 cases, the researchers observed no birth defects associated with first-trimester NAC therapy.[41]

There has been controversy over the ability of NAC to cross the placenta in humans. One ovine study examining whether NAC crossed the placenta documented negligible transfer.[42] Another study in a rodent model clearly demonstrated placental transfer of NAC.[43] NAC has been measured in fetal cord blood from human neonates born to mothers who received NAC as treatment for acetaminophen overdose. The level found in the cord blood was in the therapeutic range.[44] A possible explanation for the discrepancy between animal species could be the number of layers present in the different placentas. The human and rat placenta are composed of three layers while the ewe placenta is made up of five layers.

If deemed hepatotoxic by history, the nomogram, or liver function tests, the standard oral loading dose of 140 mg/kg followed by 70 mg/kg every 4 hours for 17 doses should be administered. Some sources advocate the recently approved intravenous form of NAC in pregnant patients since the oral form produces lower plasma levels, may induce vomiting, and undergoes maternal first-pass hepatic metabolism, lessening its availability to the fetus.[15,18,42,44] The latest literature also supports treatment with NAC in chronic or delayed acetaminophen-induced hepatotoxicity because it may

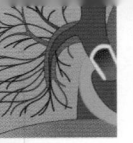

rescue the hepatocytes by acting as a free radical scavenger or through other hepatoprotective mechanisms.[45,46]

Any pregnant patient presenting with a potentially hepatotoxic ingestion of acetaminophen should be admitted for both maternal observation and fetal monitoring. In general, the maternal-fetal outcome is good following an acetaminophen overdose.[35,41,47-49] Thus, acetaminophen poisoning in and of itself should not be an indication for termination of a pregnancy.[50,51] In third-trimester acetaminophen toxicity, a greater risk for infratentorial hemorrhage, fetal demise, and maternal death has been reported when compared with other stages of pregnancy. For this reason, emergent delivery of the fetus by vaginal or cesarean section for extrauterine NAC therapy has been advocated in the third trimester in mothers suffering from fulminant hepatic failure secondary to acetaminophen overdose.[18] If the mother demonstrates signs of hepatic failure or hepatic encephalopathy, she should be admitted to an intensive care unit. In this setting, consultation with a gastroenterologist or hepatologist is recommended for potential maternal liver transplantation.

IRON

As a result of their widely prescribed use in prenatal care, iron preparations are readily available to the obstetric patient and are documented as the second most common drug overdose during pregnancy.[1] Iron normally does not diffuse through the placenta but is actively transported against a gradient into the fetal circulation.[18,51] Iron apparently crosses the placenta by receptor-mediated endocytosis. However, these receptors can become saturated, limiting the rate of transport. As a result, the placenta acts as a barrier to protect the fetus from iron toxicity. Animal studies have demonstrated that acutely elevated maternal serum iron concentrations are not accompanied by significant elevations in fetal serum iron levels.[51] In general, the mother suffers more from the insult of iron than does the fetus. Fetal compromise probably results from maternal instability rather than the direct toxic effects of iron. Although elevated iron levels in the fetus may be detrimental, there are no known reports of anomalies or adverse outcomes in the neonate in cases of maternal toxicity if the mother survives the overdose.[52] However, an increased risk for neonatal infection by bacteria from the *Yersinia* or *Listeria* species (both of which have fastidious iron requirements) has been reported.

In pregnancy, peak serum iron levels have been reported to appear within 2 to 4 hours after ingestion, similar to nonpregnant patients.[53] Historically, the laboratory hallmark of toxicity was when the serum iron levels exceeded the measured total iron-binding capacity (TIBC) of serum. However, these laboratory findings have been inconsistently observed in the poisoned pregnant patient. In one reported case, iron levels in a toxic third-trimester patient did not exceed the TIBC, nor did they correlate with the severity of the poisoning.[15,54] As a result, TIBC measurement should not be used to assess iron toxicity in the pregnant patient.

Therapeutic interventions in iron toxicity begin with general decontamination principles. Specifically, gastric decontamination with lavage may be indicated in any potentially toxic overdose presenting with a very recent ingestion. Syrup of ipecac use is discouraged and absolutely contraindicated if the patient has already vomited or has altered mental status. Activated charcoal, although considered safe in the pregnant patient, is not efficacious in iron poisoning due to the drug's small ionic size.[15] However, charcoal may be administered if multiple drugs were ingested or the history is unclear. Whole bowel irrigation may be indicated in the setting of an iron overdose, particularly if multiple radio-dense pills are noted on an abdominal flat plate radiograph[22] (Fig. 17-1). The amount of radiation risk the fetus is exposed to from a single radiograph to document the presence of iron tablets is minimal compared with the potential toxicity of a maternal iron overdose. Alternatively, ultrasonography can be utilized to detect the presence of pill fragments in the GI tract while additionally assessing the status of the fetus.[55]

Deferoxamine (DFO) is the specific chelating antidote for iron poisoning, capable of binding the free circulating iron. Unlike elemental iron, the DFO-iron complex can be excreted through the kidneys. Hypotension, metabolic acidosis, GI bleeding, shock, and an iron level of more than 500 μg/dL are all signs of severe iron poisoning and are indications for DFO administration. Some believe that the threshold for treatment with DFO in the pregnant patient should be lowered to an iron level of 350 μg/dL or with ingestions greater than 30 mg/kg of elemental iron.[52] As with the

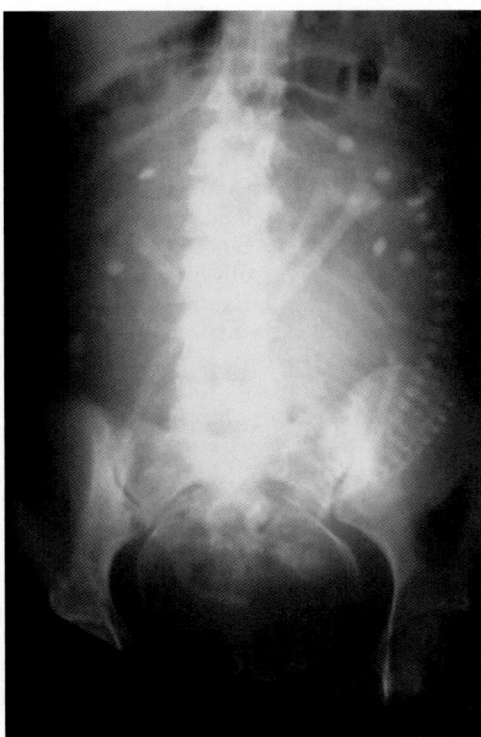

FIGURE 17-1 Radiograph demonstrating radiopaque iron tablets following an overdose in a third-trimester pregnant patient.

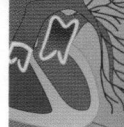

nonpregnant patient, the traditional dose of DFO is 15 mg/kg/hr intravenously, not to exceed a daily dose of 6 g.[52,56] Although some sources have historically recommended chelation therapy until after the urine clears of its "vin rosé" color, more recent literature suggests continued therapy until the acidosis and symptoms resolve. At present, a specific end point of therapy remains controversial.

Chelation is critical in significant maternal iron toxicity and should always override theoretical concerns of fetal teratogenicity.[23,57-59] Cases of maternal death have been reported when DFO was withheld over this concern.[23,24] Two animal studies documented skeletal abnormalities during exposure to high-dose DFO during early gestation.[56,57] However, limited case reports suggest that DFO can be administered to a pregnant patient suffering from iron toxicity without concern for producing adverse fetal effects.[52,54,60] A more recent animal study in an ovine model demonstrated that maternal infusion of DFO resulted in a rapid decrease in maternal serum iron concentrations but had minimal effect on fetal serum iron levels, supporting the theory that DFO does not cross the placenta.[51] To date, infants delivered after DFO therapy appear to have tolerated this antidote well.[54,57] Therefore, pregnancy should not be considered a contraindication to the use of DFO if its administration is indicated in the mother.[24,60-62]

The largest known study to address the effect on the outcome of pregnancy in iron overdose was a retrospective investigation involving 49 pregnant patients with mild to moderate iron overdoses.[63] Twenty-five of these patients (51%) were treated with DFO. Of these, 21 had normal outcomes, and the investigators found no evidence to suggest that DFO given for iron overdose caused toxicity in either the mother or the baby. Any malformations were not considered by the researchers to be directly related to the DFO administration since all were treated after their first trimester.

Any pregnant patient who presents following a serious acute iron ingestion should be aggressively treated, chelated with DFO, and admitted to the intensive care unit for both maternal and fetal monitoring. If the patient is medically stable and only has a potentially toxic ingestion, admission to a general medical or obstetric ward is appropriate with close observation of serial iron levels and possible chelation. If the mother receives chelation therapy with DFO, particularly in later stages of pregnancy, pediatric postpartum monitoring of the infant's serum iron levels is recommended.[52,56,57] Finally, when the mother recovers from a significant iron ingestion, gastroenterology consultation is recommended to diagnose any subsequent GI scarring weeks after ingestion.

SALICYLATES

Salicylate usage is extremely common in pregnancy due to the ubiquitous nature of the drug in over-the-counter preparations. It has been reported in numerous studies as one of the most common drugs taken during pregnancy.[2,5,64] Many of the mothers took these medications both with and without medical supervision.[65] In therapeutic doses, salicylates appear to be safe in early pregnancy but should be avoided in the third trimester because they may affect neonatal coagulation and cause premature closure of the ductus arteriosus.[11]

Maternally ingested salicylates freely cross the placenta and can be detected in fetal serum. The toxicity of salicylates stems from the parent compound and not its toxic metabolites, unlike acetaminophen.[18] Particularly in later stages of pregnancy, the fetus appears to be at greater risk of toxicity than the mother for several reasons. Salicylate concentrations at a given maternal level are higher in the fetus.[66] There is a greater proportion of salicylates that enters the fetal central nervous system (CNS). The fetus has less buffering capacity for the ensuing acidosis. Finally, the fetus has reduced metabolism and excretion as compared with the mother.[18,67] Several studies have documented the characteristic platelet abnormality caused by salicylates, namely, a loss of the secondary phase of platelet aggregation in babies born to mothers ingesting salicylates just prior to delivery.[68] There have been several reports of petechiae, purpura, cephalhematoma, and severe GI and intracranial bleeding in infants whose mothers had taken salicylates late in the third trimester.[68,69] Salicylates also have been found to displace bilirubin from albumin-binding sites and may lead to hyperbilirubinemia in the neonatal period. One study of 144 infants chronically exposed to salicylates in utero found significantly lower birth weights and increased perinatal mortality but no significant difference in rate of congenital anomalies.[70] These infants were found to have elevated cord-blood salicylate levels, but they had no clinical evidence of bleeding or hypoglycemia. In comparison with children, neonatal hypoglycemia has not been commonly observed.[66,71] Pregnant women who ingest salicylates on a frequent basis are reported to have longer gestational periods, prolonged labor, more hemorrhage, and a higher frequency of cesarean section.[66] All of these are believed to be attributed to the antiprostaglandin properties of salicylates.[71]

Treatment guidelines for salicylate poisoning in the pregnant mother are deficient in the literature. Current recommendations are to treat the mother in the same fashion as the nonpregnant patient. Initial stabilization, supportive care, fluid management, and electrolyte and glucose monitoring are essential. Gastric lavage and activated charcoal should be administered when indicated. Although unproven, since salicylates may form gastric concretions, late GI decontamination may prove beneficial. Additionally, because of delayed absorption, serial serum salicylate levels are essential until peak and declining levels have been documented. Enhanced elimination with sodium bicarbonate alkalinization appears to be safe and efficacious in the pregnant patient, particularly if the mother is acidotic. As with any salicylate overdose, the effectiveness of alkalinization is dependent on an adequate potassium supplementation. Hemodialysis is indicated in the toxic mother using the same inclusion criteria as in the nonpregnant patient. However, these treatment methods may not be as effective in the fetus as the mother. As a result, prompt

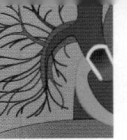

delivery of a mature fetus should be considered for its optimal treatment.[18]

The obstetric patient manifesting signs of severe salicylism (metabolic acidosis, altered mental status, pulmonary edema, or seizures) should be admitted to the intensive care unit with close maternal and fetal monitoring. In this setting, the nephrologist should be consulted for emergent hemodialysis. In the stable maternal patient with a potentially toxic ingestion, admission to an obstetric or medical ward is recommended for serial salicylate levels. If the overdose occurs in later stages of gestation, the pediatrician should be alerted regarding potential bleeding complications in the newborn.

COCAINE

Cocaine use is reported to be increasing in women of all socioeconomic levels in the United States. Cocaine abuse by women is most widespread during the childbearing years, and this age group has shown the greatest increase in recreational use over the past decade.[11,72] In fact, 20% of all women between the ages of 26 and 34 have used cocaine at least once.[73] Additionally, cocaine use is on the increase among pregnant women. In one study, 17% of urban women enrolled in prenatal care were found to have used cocaine at least once during pregnancy.[74] It is estimated that as many as 1 fetus out of every 10 is exposed to cocaine via maternal use.[75] Smoking of crack cocaine has become the predominant route of exposure in pregnant women.[76] Unfortunately, an estimated 60% of pregnant women who use crack cocaine receive no prenatal care.[77] Many addicted women do not discover they are pregnant until well into gestation. Although some seek treatment, others assume that the fetus has already been harmed and therefore continue to abuse.[78] There also exists a false perception in the lay population that cocaine speeds up the labor and delivery process, when in fact it may actually intensify the awareness of pain and prolong delivery time.[79] Finally, one recent study showed that infants of 66 mothers who reported heavy cocaine use during pregnancy already had evidence of delays in auditory comprehension and language development by 1 year of age.[80]

Symptoms and adverse effects of cocaine toxicity in the mother can include agitation, tachycardia, hyperthermia, hypertension, seizures, myocardial ischemia, cerebral vascular accidents, and intracranial bleeds resulting in significant morbidity and mortality.[76] Maternal concentrations of serum cholinesterases are diminished during pregnancy, resulting in more sustained cocaine blood levels than in nonpregnant users.[63] Fetal cholinesterase is relatively deficient compared with adult levels. Cocaine readily crosses the placental barrier, placing the fetus at risk following maternal use of cocaine by any route. Cocaine is biotransformed by the human placenta, presumably by cholinesterase activity. Therefore, the placenta may provide a moderate degree of protection from cocaine-induced morbidity by converting the cocaine into less active metabolites.[75] Cocaine administration in a pregnant ovine model

increased uterine vascular resistance, decreased uterine blood flow, increased fetal heart rate and arterial blood pressure, and decreased fetal oxygen content.[81-83] This animal study also showed that pregnancy in and of itself increased the cardiovascular toxicity to cocaine, thought to be mediated by progesterone.[83] Maternal exposure can cause preterm labor, placenta abruptio, decreased fetal growth, prematurity, urinary congenital anomalies, neonatal neurobehavioral deficits, and fetal death.[84-86] However, assessing maternal and fetal risks of cocaine use is difficult because this patient population may abuse other illicit drugs, alcohol, and cigarettes. In addition, these studies are limited by inconsistent cocaine detection methods, confounding socioeconomic factors, and reporting bias.[85]

Any pregnant patient with suspicion for cocaine toxicity should have a toxicology screen sent for confirmation. Urinary toxicology screens detect cocaine metabolites for only 48 to 72 hours; therefore, an accurate prenatal history may prove more reliable. However, in one urban-based study, 24% of pregnant women denied use of cocaine at the time of their interview but were identified as positive by urinary screens.[74] More recent studies have advocated the use of neonatal hair[87] or meconium tests to measure cumulative intrauterine exposure.[88]

Numerous studies exist in the medical literature addressing the epidemiology, maternal-neonatal outcome, and detoxification efforts of the cocaine-abusing pregnant patient. However, specific treatment recommendations in the acutely intoxicated pregnant patient are lacking. As with other poisonings, optimal treatment of the mother will ultimately benefit the fetus. Agitation, hypertension, tachycardia, and myocardial ischemia experienced by the acutely cocaine-intoxicated mother can often be controlled by the administration of benzodiazepines alone. Clinical experience supports their use as a first-line treatment for cocaine-intoxicated patients. Benzodiazepines have effective anxiolytic properties; they also reduce blood pressure, heart rate, and myocardial oxygen demand in the face of myocardial ischemia.[73] Although controversial, according to one authority, no specific fetal malformations have been attributed to benzodiazepines administered during pregnancy.[11] However, late in gestation or soon after delivery, the newborn can have transient CNS and respiratory sedation. In this setting, the benefit of giving benzodiazepines to a pregnant patient with acute cocaine toxicity may outweigh the potential fetal risks. When presenting with chest pain, the mother should have a baseline electrocardiogram with continuous maternal and fetal monitoring. Cardiac ischemia may also require the administration of nitroglycerin.[73] Cocaine-induced seizures should be treated with intravenous benzodiazepines. If seizure activity is refractory, phenobarbital loading may be an alternative therapy.[11] Phenytoin should be avoided due to its well-documented fetal neurotoxicity.[11] With seizures occurring during the third trimester of pregnancy, the diagnosis of eclampsia should also be entertained and traditional doses of intravenous magnesium administered as indicated. One of the most critical treatment interventions is the rapid

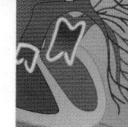

cooling of the acutely hyperthermic patient, because temperature duration and level can have a negative effect on both maternal and fetal mortality.[89] Finally, in a patient presenting with ingestion of cocaine packets (i.e., body packers and stuffers), activated charcoal administration and whole bowel irrigation are recommended. In general, both modalities have been shown to be safe and efficacious in the pregnant patient.

Any pregnant patient presenting with severe cocaine toxicity should be monitored in the intensive care setting. If manifesting cardiotoxicity, a cardiologist should be consulted. If the mother and fetus survive the acute intoxication, prenatal care should be focused on drug rehabilitation and education. If the cocaine exposure occurred throughout the prenatal period, the pediatrician should be aware that the newborn may manifest signs of cocaine withdrawal.

HEROIN

Heroin overdose presents with the triad of respiratory depression, CNS depression, and miosis.[90] Neonates can experience lethargy at birth if there was recent maternal opioid use, or if large doses of an opioid agent were therapeutically administered to the mother during labor. The specific antidote naloxone can be administered to the pregnant patient with an opioid overdose in standard 2-mg doses.[91] Concern over the possibility of fetal and neonatal withdrawal syndrome in heroin-dependent mothers given naloxone is outweighed by the benefit from reversing maternal and fetal hypoxia. The neonate is prone to withdrawal symptoms if the mother had chronic dependency during her later prenatal stages. If acute maternal withdrawal is a concern, smaller doses of naloxone can be administered to lessen the severity of maternal and fetal withdrawal. Withdrawal seizures have been documented in neonates born to opioid-dependent mothers.[92,93]

CARBON MONOXIDE

Carbon monoxide (CO) is a leading cause of poison-induced deaths in the United States.[94] The clinical presentation of CO poisoning can be subtle in pregnant patients, resulting in misdiagnosis and significant maternal-fetal morbidity if not approached with a high index of suspicion. During pregnancy, endogenous CO levels increase about 20% above normal nonpregnant values secondary to increased fetal production and an increase in maternal red cell mass, and from the action of progesterone on hepatic microsomal enzymes.[95] In addition, at a given CO exposure, pregnant patients are more susceptible to toxicity because of her increased minute ventilation. Cigarette smoking also results in higher than normal maternal and fetal CO levels.

In the mother, CO possesses 240 times the binding affinity to hemoglobin than oxygen, resulting in cellular hypoxia. CO decreases the capacity of blood to transport oxygen. CO shifts the oxyhemoglobin saturation curve to the left and alters the shape of the curve to a more hyperbolic form (Fig. 17-2).[95] Fetal carboxyhemoglobin (COHb) is associated with an exaggerated shift to the left, impairing the release of oxygen to the tissues. Under normal circumstances, the fetal COHb is approximately 10% to 15% greater than that of the mother.[95] With maternal exposure, the fetal COHb level rises more slowly than the maternal COHb level but will continue to rise for several hours after acute exposure until it reaches an equilibrium.[94] Fetal hemoglobin appears to falsely elevate COHb concentration.[96]

CO readily crosses the placenta by simple diffusion, and fetal hemoglobin has a higher affinity for CO than adult hemoglobin.[97] As a result, unlike the majority of poisonings, the fetus is at greater risk for toxicity and mortality than the mother.[98] This has been documented in several case reports where the mother has survived a significant CO exposure but fetal demise ensued.[94,99,100] As with the general population, maternal blood CO levels often do not correlate with the severity of symptoms. Maternal symptoms at the scene of exposure are a better predictor of fetal toxicity than CO levels.[94,97,101] These symptoms may include altered mental status, neurologic deficits, seizures, and coma.

The result of fetal CO exposure can lead to different effects on the fetus depending on the stage at which it is exposed. In the embryonic stage, neurologic, skeletal, and cleft palate deformities can be seen. In the fetal stage, anoxic encephalopathy and growth restriction may result. In the third trimester, premature delivery, decreased immunity, right-sided cardiomegaly, sodium channel, and myelin defects have been reported.[102]

Apart from removing the patient from the site of exposure, oxygen therapy is paramount. Oxygen acts by competing with the CO for hemoglobin binding sites.

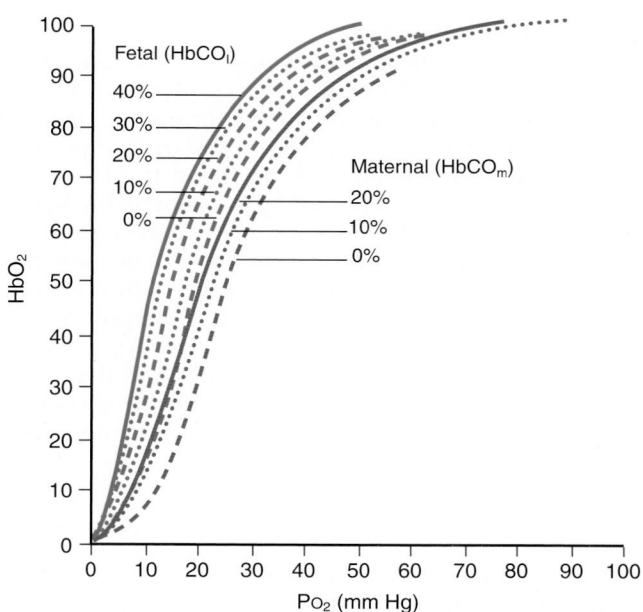

FIGURE 17-2 Oxygen dissociation curve of maternal and fetal hemoglobin demonstrating effects of carbon monoxide exposure.

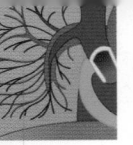

On room air, the half-life of CO is 5 to 6 hours; on 100% oxygen, the half-life is 90 minutes; and with hyperbaric oxygenation (HBO), the half-life falls to 20 minutes. Because the fetal hemoglobin binds CO much more readily than maternal hemoglobin, it is recommended that pregnant patients receive 100% oxygen five times longer than do normal adults to ensure adequate reduction of CO in the fetus.[94,97,101] In the past, controversy existed in treating the pregnant patient with HBO because of adverse effects of high partial pressures of oxygen on the fetus observed in animal investigations.[103] However, several human studies, the majority of which are case reports,[96,101,103,104] advocate the use of HBO in pregnant patients exposed to CO.[15,103,105,106] Although no definitive guidelines have been established, it has been recommended that more liberal HBO treatment be initiated in pregnant patients because of the enhanced vulnerability of the fetus to CO, hypoxia, and permanent brain damage. Additional HBO therapy may also be needed if fetal signs of distress are demonstrated after initial HBO therapy. One source suggests that if cesarean delivery of the fetus is being considered, delivery of the fetus before HBO therapy can lead to a greater probability of fetal death. This opinion is not a result of clinical trials. Despite studies in animals linking HBO therapy with retinopathy, cardiovascular defects, and premature closure of the ductus arteriosus, human case reports and a prospective study have not shown morbidity or mortality in the mother or the fetus after HBO therapy.

The safety of HBO was documented in a prospective study where 44 pregnant patients with CO poisoning tolerated HBO without any fetal or obstetric morbidity.[107] Human clinical experience indicates that the short duration of high-dose oxygen attained during HBO therapy can be tolerated by the fetus in all stages of pregnancy and can reduce the risk for death or deformity to the mother and fetus.[103] Indications for HBO in pregnancy are indicated in (Box 17-2).

All pregnant patients with suspected CO poisoning should be removed from the source of exposure and transported to an emergency facility for evaluation, fetal monitoring, CO level measurement, and oxygen therapy. If symptoms or levels indicate the need for HBO, the patient should be transported to a facility with hyperbaric capabilities.[109] With exposures occurring in early stages of pregnancy, consultation should be obtained regarding potential fetal neurotoxicity. However, one case showed significant first-trimester CO exposure with subsequent normal outcome in the newborn.[110] If the mother presents in late stage pregnancy and delivery is eminent, the pediatric intensivist should be advised of the need for aggressive oxygen delivery to the neonate.

LEAD

Lead poisoning is a major public health problem and a significant paradigm of maternal-fetal toxicity. It is well documented that the fetus is at risk from maternal lead exposure. In fact, lead has been used historically as an

---

BOX 17-2	INDICATIONS FOR HYPERBARIC OXYGEN THERAPY IN THE PREGNANT PATIENT

COHb level ≥ 20%
Mental status depression
Seizures
Metabolic acidosis
Fetal distress
Cardiotoxicity
Any neurologic findings in the mother

---

abortifacient.[111] Pregnant women can suffer from environmental[112] or occupational lead exposure.[113,114]

Removal of lead from gasoline has caused a dramatic reduction in the average blood lead level of children in the United States, from 15 μg/dL in 1978 to 2 μg/dL in 2004. Despite this advancement, lead poisoning is still a major health concern for children. The mother also may unknowingly ingest lead from containers coated with lead glaze[115] or herbal products,[116] or may demonstrate increased pica behavior during the prenatal period.[117-120]

There are limited case reports that describe lead poisoning in the pregnant patient. Most involve the mother exhibiting pica behavior.[119,120] A study of lead exposure of pregnant women in their first trimester in New York City found that blood lead levels were inversely related to maternal age and length of time in the United States, and directly related to gestational age and pica behavior.[121] Another study found that endogenous lead sources in bone continues to influence blood lead levels of immigrants in the United States during and after pregnancy. Due to hormonal changes during pregnancy, chronic maternal lead stores may be mobilized from the bone and transferred to the fetus.[122-124]

Placental transfer of lead has been demonstrated in the human fetus at 12 to 14 weeks' gestation along with increasing fetal tissue lead stores with advancing gestational age.[112] This heavy metal has been shown to induce spontaneous abortion, teratogenesis, and neurodevelopmental delays in the newborn.[25,125] One study measured umbilical cord blood lead levels in over 5000 consecutive deliveries of over 20 weeks' gestation. Lead was found to be associated in a dose-related fashion with an increased risk for minor congenital anomalies such as hemangiomas, lymphangiomas, hydrocele, skin tags, and undescended testicles. This study controlled for other covariables and found no characteristic anatomic defect.[126] An epidemiologic study performed in Turkey found that umbilical cord lead levels that correlated significantly with maternal levels were approximately 70% of the latter.[127] A case report describing the radiographic findings seen in congenital lead poisoning described a dense cranial vault, lead lines in the distal ends of long bones, and delayed emergence of dentition. The investigators recommend using these findings as a screen for subtle presentations of congenital lead poisoning.[128]

Although currently under debate, the highest acceptable lead level in young children is 10 μg/dL.[129] How-

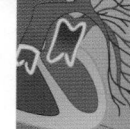

ever, according to one investigation, the fetus appears to be adversely affected at low blood lead concentrations, cautioning against the application of this level toward the fetus.[130] The primary treatment of maternal and congenital lead poisoning is discovery and removal of the mother from the source of exposure.

Data on chelating obstetric patients with elevated blood lead levels are limited. As a result of their nonspecific action on metal binding and subsequent excretion, prior concern existed that chelating agents may be teratogenic or toxic to the fetus.[92] According to one leading authority, maternal toxicity should be the primary reason for initiating lead chelation during pregnancy.[18] Calcium ethylenediaminetetraacetic acid (EDTA) has been used with some success in the later stages of third-trimester pregnancy.[114,117] In one case, a maternal blood level of 86 μg/dL was documented and the mother was given a 3-day chelation course of calcium EDTA. Eight days later, at delivery, her level had fallen to 26 μg/dL, but the cord blood level remained elevated at 79 μg/dL.[117] Based on this and other studies, it is unlikely that EDTA crosses the placenta and would therefore be an ineffective fetal chelator.[18] EDTA chelates calcium and zinc and is a known teratogenic agent when administered in pregnant rats. In two case reports, pregnant women received EDTA, 2 g/day intravenously and 75 mg/kg/day intravenously, respectively. Both mothers delivered a normal fetus post-therapy.[131]

Since intramuscular dimercaprol or bronchoalveolar lavage (BAL) penetrates into the central nervous system tissues, it theoretically should cross into fetal tissues, although little data exist describing its use in pregnant humans with lead poisoning. However, this drug may be of limited value in the pregnant patient due to its known adverse side effects such as hypertension, febrile reactions, tachycardia, and nephrotoxicity. BAL is known to cause skeletal abnormalities in mice at doses greater than 125 mg/kg/day when given subcutaneously. Newborn infants have required continued chelation therapy with calcium EDTA or dimercaprol weeks after delivery since lead levels have been noted to rebound.[115,117] This demonstrates that a short intrauterine course of chelation therapy with these agents may not be adequate to fully treat congenital lead toxicity.

The newer oral lead chelator, dimercaptosuccinic acid (DMSA, succimer), is structurally related to BAL with less severe side effects and may be the treatment of choice for maternal lead toxicity.[18] Animal studies have documented that DMSA is not toxic to fetal development.[132] In one investigation, DMSA was administered to pregnant rodents. On day 20 of gestation, no gross external abnormalities, visceral/skeletal abnormalities, or teratogenicity at any dosage level was noted in the fetal rats.[133]

DMSA has been shown to cause prenatal deaths, reduction in body weight, soft tissue abnormalities, and skeletal anomalies in mice when administered subcutaneously at dosages greater than 410 mg/kg/day. The no observed effect level of fetal-maternal toxicity after oral DMSA is less than 100 mg/kg/day, and no teratogenicity has been seen at levels greater than 1000 mg/kg/day.[134] Because DMSA has not been studied

in humans in controlled trials, it is category C in pregnancy. It has been used during pregnancy at the maximum human dose of 30 mg/kg/day without fetal abnormalities. Nevertheless, in one case report the blood lead level remained essentially unchanged from 44.0 μg/dL to 43.9 μg/dL after 18 days of chelation.[134]

Penicillamine has been found to be a teratogen in both humans and animals. It has been implicated as the cause of congenital connective tissue and other abnormalities in neonates born from women chelated during pregnancy for cystinuria, rheumatoid arthritis, and Wilson's disease. The dosage used in pregnant women is 0.25 to 0.50 g/day. Because safer chelators such as DMSA are available, penicillamine should be avoided when chelating the pregnant patient.[135]

It is unknown if chelation during pregnancy is effective at decreasing the fetal or maternal body lead burden, or improving the outcome of the fetus exposed to lead. The small amount of data on the risk of chelators to the fetus and the mother is provided in animal studies and human case reports.[136] In the literature, a few case reports have documented maternal chelation therapy for lead poisoning during pregnancy. The chelators used were EDTA, BAL, and DMSA. After birth, the blood lead levels were consistently higher in the neonate than the mother. None of these children were born with birth defects.[120] At this time, nutritional supplementation along with analysis of the risk versus benefit of a chelation agent appears to be a sound approach for treatment of gestational lead poisoning.

Nutritional supplementation is a safe adjunct for treatment of lead toxicity. Many lead-toxic patients are deficient in iron, zinc, and calcium. Women taking iron and folic acid have been found to have lower lead levels than matched cohorts.[136] Alcohol and tobacco use have been found to correlate with higher lead levels, so abstinence from their use has multiple benefits.

In a pregnant patient exhibiting signs of acute lead intoxication with encephalopathy, admission is recommended with institution of chelation therapy and close fetal monitoring. When the blood lead levels are elevated yet the mother is asymptomatic, removal from the source is essential with monitoring of serial levels and possible institution of outpatient chelation therapy. If maternal toxicity is documented at any time during the prenatal period, the newborn should be monitored for initial and rebounding lead levels.

ORGANOPHOSPHATES

Insecticide ingestions are uncommon in pregnancy per se, but these chemicals are widely available to an expectant mother with suicidal intentions. Pregnant women may also be occupationally or environmentally exposed to pesticides (organophosphate, carbamates, and pyrethrins). A study of an Ontario farm population[137] exposed to a variety of pesticides found that the timing of the exposure during gestation could predict the toxicity of a pesticide, including organophosphates. There is a significant risk for morbidity and mortality in

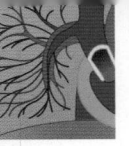

the mother and the fetus exposed to organophosphates, but the relationship between chronic exposure and risk for effects is still uncertain.

A case report documented the use of an organophosphate in conjunction with substance abuse. Because of "street knowledge" that lowering one's cholinesterase activity may prolong the euphoric effects of cocaine, a nearly full-term pregnant woman took an organophosphate with her cocaine and presented in both cholinergic and sympathomimetic crisis.[138] In general, acute organophosphate poisoning can present with maternal cholinergic crisis (diarrhea, urination, miosis, bradycardia, bronchosecretions, emesis, lacrimation, and salivation) along with nicotinic symptoms of central nervous system depression and muscle fasciculations.[139]

Access of terrorists to chemical weapons opens the possibility of pregnant women being exposed to "nerve gas" agents like sarin, soman, tabun, and VX. All of these agents inhibit acetylcholinesterase, causing cholinergic signs of toxicity such as bronchospasm, bradycardia, bronchorrhea, salivation, lacrimation, urinary and fecal incontinence, abdominal pain, and miosis. They may also cause nicotinic signs because of inhibition of the metabolism of acetylcholine at these receptors. Nicotinic symptoms include tachycardia, hypertension, muscle fasciculations, weakness, and mydriasis. In 1995 a Japanese terrorist group released sarin gas into a subway system. Five toxic pregnant women were treated with atropine only. No fetal malformations were reported 1 month and 1 year after the attack.[140,141]

There exist little data accounting for the transplacental passage of specific organophosphate compounds.[18,142] Fetal organophosphate levels have been detected on autopsy of fatalities from organophosphate poisoning.[140] In a case report describing both maternal and fetal fatalities from an organophosphate ingestion, the investigators documented fetal levels of the insecticide on autopsy, indicating that these agents cross the placental barrier.[143] Regarding cholinesterase enzyme levels, studies have noted 50% to 70% decreases in activity of red blood cell cholinesterase in normal neonatal plasma.[144,145] This would intuitively make the fetus more susceptible to the effects of anticholinesterase insecticides.[18]

As with any organophosphate poisoning, the mother should be managed with gastric and skin decontamination when indicated, along with aggressive airway control to maintain adequate maternal and fetal oxygenation. There have been cases where organophosphate poisonings in second- and third-trimester pregnancy have been successfully treated with appropriate doses of atropine for the cholinergic effects and pralidoxime (2-PAM) for the nicotinic manifestations.[146] In two of the cases, both women delivered normal, full-term infants. In one investigation using a chick embryo model, supplemental use of oxime cholinesterase reactivators such as 2-PAM reduced the incidence and severity of developmental defects to specific organophosphate teratogens such as parathion and dicrotophos (bidrin). The protective effect noted was dose related.[147]

Another case report described a woman at 35 weeks' gestation who presented with an unknown overdose in cholinergic crisis.[148] Organophosphate toxicity was presumed and confirmed by markedly depressed serum and erythrocyte cholinesterase levels. Moderate doses of atropine in the mother demonstrated maternal improvement, but profound fetal tachycardia forced the treating physicians to stop the infusion, resulting in worsening of the mother's condition. An emergent cesarean section was performed, with the delivery of a hypotonic infant with low Apgar scores. The mother went on to require 8 days of assisted ventilation and 11 days of atropine infusion. The newborn required mechanical ventilation for 2 days and atropine therapy for 8 days. Neither patient received 2-PAM. Compared with the baby, it took longer for the mother's cholinesterase activity to recover to normal. Interestingly, the mother presented with more serious symptoms of poisoning requiring doses of atropine that proved toxic or intolerable to the fetus. However, it is difficult to ascribe the cause of the fetal distress based on this one case. Several factors may have contributed to both maternal and fetal distress, such as fetal hypoxia secondary to maternal respiratory distress or the direct transplacental fetal action of the atropine. The atropine serum level in the fetus is half the maternal level in 20 minutes in early pregnancy. In late pregnancy, fetal serum atropine reaches 93% of the maternal level in 5 minutes.[140]

Any pregnant patient with an organophosphate poisoning manifesting acute cholinergic or nicotinic manifestations should be managed in an intensive care setting with close maternal-fetal monitoring and appropriate doses of atropine and 2-PAM.[139] Additionally, it may prove efficacious to deliver a mature or full-term fetus in distress for initiation of extrauterine therapy.[18]

CONCLUSION

Pregnant women have significant risk for toxic exposures and may present as a diagnostic and therapeutic dilemma. Unfortunately, few adequate or well-controlled studies are available in the medical literature regarding treatment guidelines for the poisoned obstetric patient. The most critical issue in managing the pregnant patient suffering from any toxin is the stabilization and treatment of the mother, since this will have a beneficial effect on maternal and fetal outcome. If questions arise concerning potential toxins and exposure to the pregnant patient, regional poison control centers and teratogen resources are available.

REFERENCES

1. Rayburn W, Aronow R, DeLancey B, et al: Drug overdose during pregnancy: an overview from a metropolitan poison control center. Obstet Gynecol 1984;64:611–614.
2. Kleiner GJ, Gretson WM: Suicide during pregnancy. In Cherry SH, Merkatz IR (eds): Complications of Pregnancy: Medical, Surgical, Gynecologic, Pyschosocial, and Perinatal, 4th ed. Baltimore, Williams & Wilkins, 1991, pp 269–289.
3. Jones JS, Dickson K, Carlson S: Unrecognized pregnancy in the overdosed or poisoned patient. Am J Emerg Med 1997;15: 538–541.

4. Piper JM, Baum C, Kennedy DL: Prescription drug use before and during pregnancy in a Medicaid population. Am J Obstet Gynecol 1987;157:148–156.

5. Bonasi S, Magnani M, Calvi A, et al: Factors related to drug consumption during pregnancy. Acta Obstet Gynecol Scand 1994;73:535–540.

6. Chasnoff IJ: Drug use and women: establishing a standard of care. Ann N Y Acad Sci 1989;562:208–210.

7. Czeizel A, Szentesi I, Molnar G: Lack of effect of self-poisoning on subsequent reproductive outcome. Mutat Res 1984;127:175–182.

8. Czeizel AE, Tomcsik M, Timar L: Teratologic evaluation of 178 infants born to mothers who attempted suicide by drugs during pregnancy. Obstet Gynecol 1997;90:195–201.

9. Houston H, Jacobson L: Overdose and termination of pregnancy: an important association? Br J Gen Pract 1996;46:737–738.

10. Gbolade BA: Overdose and termination of pregnancy. Br J Gen Pract 1997;47:184.

11. Koren G: Maternal-Fetal Toxicology: A Clinician's Guide, 2nd ed. New York, Marcel Dekker, 1994.

12. Ellenhorn MH, Barceloux DG: Toxic exposure during pregnancy. In Ellenhorn MJ, Barceloux DG (eds): Medical Toxicology: Diagnosis and Treatment of Human Poisoning, 1st ed. New York, Elsevier, 1988, pp 131–152.

13. Fine JS: Reproductive and perinatal principles. In Goldfrank LF, Flomenbaum NE, Lewin NA, et al (eds): Toxicologic Emergencies, 7th ed. Norwalk, CT, McGraw-Hill, 2002, pp 1606–1628.

14. Graves HB, Smith EE, Braen CR, et al: Clinical policy for the initial approach to patients presenting with acute toxic ingestion or dermal or inhalation exposure. Ann Emerg Med 1995;25(4): 570–585.

15. Ford MD, Olshaker JS: Concepts and controversies in toxicology. Emerg Med Clin North Am 1994;12(2).

16. Shannon M: The demise of ipecac? Pediatrics 2003;112(5): 1180–1181.

17. Bond GR: Home syrup of ipecac use does not reduce emergency department use or improve outcome. Pediatrics 2003;112(5): 1061–1064.

18. Tenenbein M: Poisoning in pregnancy. In Koren G (ed): Maternal-Fetal Toxicology: A Clinician's Guide, 2nd ed. New York, Dekker, 1994, pp 223–252.

19. D'Ascoli P, Gall SA: Common poisons. In Gleicher N (ed): Principles of Medical Therapy in Pregnancy. New York, Plenum Press, 1985.

20. Howland MA: Whole bowel irrigation. In Goldfrank LR, Flomenbaum NE, Lewin NA, et al (eds): Toxicologic Emergencies, 5th ed. Norwalk, CT, Appleton & Lange, 1994, pp 74–75.

21. Turk J, Aks SE, Ampuero F, et al: Successful therapy of iron intoxication in pregnancy with intravenous deferoxamine and whole bowel irrigation. Vet Hum Toxicol 1993;35(6):441–444.

22. Van Ameyde KJ, Tenenbein M: Whole bowel irrigation during pregnancy. Am J Obstet Gynecol 1989;160:646–664.

23. Strom RL, Schiller P, Seeds AT, et al: Fatal iron poisoning in a pregnant female. Minn Med 1976;59:483–489.

24. Manoguerra AS: Iron poisoning: report of a fatal case in an adult. Am J Hosp Pharm 1976;59:1088–1090.

25. Kurtz GG, Michael UF, Morosi HJ, et al: Hemodialysis during pregnancy. Report of a case of glutethamide poisoning complicated by acute renal failure. Arch Intern Med 1966;118:30–32.

26. Vaziri ND, Kumar KP, Mirahmadi K, et al: Hemodialysis in the treatment of acute chloral hydrate poisoning. South Med J 1977;70:377–378.

27. Trebbin WM: Hemodialysis in pregnancy. JAMA 1979;441: 1811–1812.

28. Hou S: Pregnancy in women requiring dialysis for renal failure. Am J Kidney Dis 1987;9:368–373.

29. Selden BS, Burke TJ: Complete maternal and fetal recovery after prolonged cardiac arrest. Ann Emerg Med 1988;17:346–349.

30. Perrone J, Hoffman RS: Toxic ingestions in pregnancy: abortifacient use in a case series of pregnant overdose patients. Acad Emerg Med 1997;4:206–209.

31. Netland KE, Martinez J: Abortifacients: toxidromes, ancient to modern—a case series and review of the literature. Acad Emerg Med 2000;7:824–829.

32. Ley G, Garrettson LK, Soda DM: Evidence of placental transfer of acetaminophen. Pediatrics 1975;55:895.

33. Roberts I, Robinson MZ, Mughal JG, et al: Paracetamol metabolites in the neonate following maternal overdose. Br J Pharmacol 1984;18:201–206.

34. Wang LH, Rudolph AM, Benet LZ: Pharmacokinetic studies of the disposition of acetaminophen in the sheep maternal-placental unit. J Pharmacol Exp Ther 1986;238:198–205.

35. Riggs BS, Bronsteine AC, Kulig K, et al: Acute acetaminophen overdose during pregnancy. Obstet Gynecol 1989;74:247–253.

36. Haibach H, Akhter JE, Muscato MS, et al: Acetaminophen overdose with fetal demise. Am J Clin Pathol 1984;82:240–242.

37. Kurzel RB: Can acetaminophen excess result in maternal and fetal toxicity. South Med J 1990;83(8):953–954.

38. Wang PH, Yang MJ, Lee WL, et al: Acetaminophen poisoning in late pregnancy. J Reprod Med 1997;42:367–371.

39. Rayburn W, Skukla U, Stetson P, et al: Acetaminophen pharmacokinetics: comparison between pregnant and nonpregnant women. Am J Obstet Gynecol 1986;155:1353–1356.

40. Smilkstein MJ, Knapp GL, Kulig KW, et al: Efficacy of oral N-acetylcysteine in the treatment of acetaminophen overdose. N Eng J Med 1988;319(24):1557–1562.

41. McElhatton PR, Sullivan FM, Volans GN, et al: Paracetamol poisoning in pregnancy: an analysis of the outcomes of cases referred to the teratology information service of the national poisons information service. Hum Exp Toxicol 1990;9:147–153.

42. Seldon BS, Curry SC, Clark RF, et al: Transplacental transport of N-acetylcysteine in an ovine model. Ann Emerg Med 1991;20: 1069–1072.

43. Ansai N, Kimura T, Chida S, et al: Studies on the metabolic fate of N-acetylcysteine in rats and dogs. Pharmacometrics 1983;26: 249–260.

44. Horowitz RS, Dart RC, Jarvie DR, et al: Placental transfer of N-acetylcysteine following human maternal acetaminophen toxicity. J Toxicol Clin Toxicol 1997;35(5):447–451.

45. Kozer E, Koren G: Management of paracetamol overdose: current controversies. Drug Saf 2001;24(7):503–512.

46. Harrison PM, Keays R, Bray GP, et al: Improved outcome of paracetamol-induced fulminant hepatic failure by late administration of acetylcysteine. Lancet 1990;335:1572–1573.

47. Stokes IM: Paracetamol overdose in the second trimester of pregnancy. Case report. Br J Obstet Gynecol 1984;91:286–288.

48. Ludmir J, Main DM, Landon MB, et al: Maternal acetaminophen overdose at 15 weeks of gestation. Obstet Gynecol 1986;67: 750–751.

49. McElhatton PR, Sullivan FM, Volans GN: Paracetamol overdose in pregnancy: analysis of the outcomes of 300 cases referred to the teratology information service. Reprod Toxicol 1997;11(1): 85–94.

50. Janes J, Routledge PA: Recent developments in the management of paracetamol (acetaminophen) poisoning. Drug Saf 1992;7(3): 170–177.

51. Curry SC, Bond GR, Raschke R, et al: An ovine model of maternal iron poisoning in pregnancy. Ann Emerg Med 1990;19:632–38.

52. Lacoste H, Goyert GL, Goldman LS, et al: Acute iron intoxication in pregnancy: case report and review of the literature. Obstet Gynecol 1992;80:500–501.

53. Rotham JL, Lietman PS: Acute iron poisoning. a review. Am J Dis Child 1980;134:875–879.

54. Olenmark M, Biber B, Dottori O, et al: Fatal iron intoxication in late pregnancy. Clin Toxicol 1987;25(4):347–359.

55. Anderson AC, Share JC, Woolf AD: The use of ultrasound in the diagnosis of toxic ingestions. Vet Hum Toxicol 1990;32(4):355.

56. Blanc P, Hryhorczuk DO, Danel I: Deferoxamine treatment of acute iron intoxication in pregnancy. Obstet Gynecol 1984; 64(Suppl):12–14.

57. Rayburn WF, Donn SM, Wulf ME: Iron overdose during pregnancy: successful therapy with deferoxamine therapy. Am J Obstet Gynecol 1983;147:717–718.

58. Tran T, Wax JR, Philput C, et al: Intentional iron overdose in pregnancy—management and outcome. J Emerg Med 2000; 18(2):225–228.

59. Tran T, Wax JR, Steinfeld JD, et al: Acute intentional iron overdose in pregnancy. Obstet Gynecol 1998;92(4 Pt 2):678–679.

60. Singer ST, Vichinsky EP: Deferoxamine treatment during pregnancy: Is it harmful? Am J Hematol 1999;60:24–26.
61. Czeizel A, Szentesi I, Szekeres I, et al: Pregnancy outcome and health conditions of offspring of self-poisoned women. Acta Pediatr Hung 1984;25:209–236.
62. Perucca E: Drug metabolism in pregnancy, infancy and childhood. Pharmacol Ther 1987;34:129–143.
63. McElhatton PR, Roberts JC, Sullivan FM: The consequences of iron overdose and its treatment with deferroxamine in pregnancy. Hum Exp Toxicol 1991;10:251–259.
64. Corby DG: Aspirin in pregnancy: maternal and fetal effects. Pediatrics 1978;62(Suppl):930–937.
65. Palmisano PA, Cassady G: Salicylate exposure in the perinate. JAMA 1969;209(4):556–558.
66. Levy G, Procnal JA, Garrettson LK: Distribution of salicylate between neonatal and maternal serum at diffusion equilibrium. Clin Pharmacol Ther 1975;18:210–214.
67. Levy G, Garrettson LK: Kinetics of salicylate elimination by newborn infants of mothers who ingested aspirin before delivery. Pediatrics 1974;53(2):201–210.
68. Haslam RH, Ekert H, Gillam GL: Hemorrhage in a neonate possibly due to maternal ingestion of salicylate. J Pediatr 1974;84:556.
69. Karlwicz MG, White LE: Severe intracranial hemorrhage in a term neonate associated with maternal acetylsalicylic acid ingestion. Clin Pediatr 1993;32:740–743.
70. Turner G, Collins E: Fetal effects of regular salicylate ingestion in pregnancy. Lancet 1975;2(7930):338–339.
71. Collins E: Maternal and fetal effects of actaminophen and salicylates in pregnancy. Obstet Gynecol 1981;58(5 Suppl):57–62.
72. Richardson GA, Day NL: Maternal and neonatal effects of moderate cocaine use during pregnancy. Neurotoxicol Teratol 1991;13(4):455–460.
73. Hollander JE: The management of cocaine-associated myocardial ischemia. N Engl J Med 1995;333(19):1267–1272.
74. Frank DA, Amaro H, Bauchner H, et al: Cocaine use during pregnancy: prevalence and correlates. Pediatrics 1988;82:888–895.
75. Roe DA, Little BB, Bawdon RE, et al: Metabolism of cocaine by human placentas: implications for fetal exposure. Am J Obstet Gynecol 1990;163:715–718.
76. Bandstra ES, Burkett G: Maternal-fetal and neonatal effects of in utero cocaine exposure. Semin Perinatol 1991;15(4):288–301.
77. Cherukui R, Minkoff H, Feldman J, et al: A cohort study of alkaloidal cocaine "crack" in pregnancy. Obstet Gynecol 1988;72(2):147–151.
78. Little DR: Cocaine addiction and pregnancy: education in primary prevention. Resd Staff Phys 1993;April:79–81.
79. Dombrowski MP, Wolfe HM, Welch RA, et al: Cocaine abuse is associated with abruptio placentae and decreased birth weight, but not shorter labor. Obstet Gynecol 1991;77:139–141.
80. Singer LT, Arendt R, Minnes S, et al: Developing language skills of cocaine-exposed infants. Pediatrics 2001;107:1057–1064.
81. Hoyme HE, Jones KL, Dixon SD, et al: Prenatal cocaine exposure and fetal vascular disruption. Pediatrics 1990;85(5):743–747.
82. Moore TR, Sorg J, Miller L, et al: Hemodynamic effects of intravenous cocaine on the pregnant ewe and fetus. Am J Obstet Gynecol 1986;155:883–888.
83. Woods JR, Plessinger MA, Clark KE: Effect of cocaine on uterine blood flow and fetal oxygenation. JAMA 1987;257(7):957–961.
84. Meeker JE, Reynolds PC: Fetal and newborn death associated with maternal cocaine use. J Anal Toxicol 1990;14:379–382.
85. Slutsker L: Risks associated with cocaine use during pregnancy. Obstet Gynecol 1992;79:778–789.
86. MacGregor SN, Keith LG, Chasnoff IJ, et al: Cocaine use during pregnancy: adverse prenatal outcome. Am J Obstet Gynecol 1987;157:686–690.
87. Graham K, Koren G, Klein J, et al: Determination of gestational cocaine exposure by hair analysis. JAMA 1989;262:3328–3330.
88. Ostrea E, Brady M, Parks P, et al: Drug screening of meconium in infants of drug dependent mothers: an alternative to urine testing. J Pediatr 1989;115:474–483.
89. Brent RL: Relationship between uterine vascular disruption syndrome, and cocaine teratogenicity. Teratology 1990;41:757–760.
90. Sporer KA: Acute heroin overdose. Ann Intern Med 1999;130:584–590.
91. Chamberlain JM, Klein BL: A comprehensive review of naloxone for the emergency physician. Am J Emerg Med 1994;12:650–660.
92. Thorp JM: Management of drug dependency, overdose, and withdrawal in the obstetric patient. Obstet Gynecol Clin North Am 1995;22(1):131–142.
93. Committee on Drugs: Neonatal drug withdrawal. Pediatrics 1998;101:1079–1088.
94. Farrow JR, Davis GJ, Roy TM, et al: Fetal death due to nonlethal carbon monoxide poisoning. J Forensic Sci 1990;35(6):1448–1452.
95. Longo LD: The biological effects of carbon monoxide on the pregnant women, fetus, and newborn infant. Am J Obstet Gynecol 1977;129:69–103.
96. Perrone J, Hoffman RS: Falsely elevated carboxyhemoglobin levels secondary to fetal hemoglobin. Acad Emerg Med 1996;3(3):287–289.
97. Koren GK, Sharav T, Garrettson LK, et al: A multicenter prospective study of fetal outcome following accidental carbon monoxide poisoning in pregnancy. Reprod Toxicol 1991;5:397–403.
98. Kopelman AE, Plaut TA: Fetal compromise caused by maternal carbon monoxide poisoning. J Perinatol 1998;18(1):74–77.
99. Cramer CR: Fetal death due to accidental maternal carbon monoxide poisoning. J Toxicol Clin Toxicol 1982;19(3):297–301.
100. Muller GH, Graham S: Intrauterine death of the fetus due to accidental carbon monoxide poisoning. N Engl J Med 1955;252(25):1075–1078.
101. Caravati EM, Adams CJ, Joyce SM, et al: Fetal toxicity associated with maternal carbon monoxide poisoning. Ann Emerg Med 1988;17:714–717.
102. Aubard Y, Magne I: Carbon monoxide poisoning in pregnancy. Br J Obstet Gynecol 2000;107:833–838.
103. Van Hoesen KB, Camporesi EM, Moon RE, et al: Should hyperbaric oxygen be used to treat the pregnant patient for acute carbon monoxide poisoning? A case report and review of the literature. JAMA 1989;261(7):1039–1043.
104. Brown DB, Mueller GL, Golich FC: Hyperbaric oxygen treatment for carbon monoxide poisoning in pregnancy: a case report. Aviat Space Environ Med 1992;63(11):1011–1014.
105. Hollander DI, Nagey DA, Welch R, et al: Hyperbaric oxygen therapy for the treatment of acute carbon monoxide poisoning in pregnancy: a case report. J Reprod Med 1987;32(8):615–617.
106. Silverman RK, Montano J: Hyperbaric oxygen treatment during pregnancy in acute carbon monoxide poisoning. J Reprod Med 1997;42:309–311.
107. Elkharrat D, Raphael JC, Jars-Guincestre MC, et al: Acute carbon monoxide intoxication and hyperbaric oxygen in pregnancy. Intens Care Med 1991;17:289–292.
108. Roy B, Crawford R: Pitfalls in the diagnosis and management of carbon monoxide poisoning. J Acad Emerg Med 1996;13(1):62–63.
109. Weaver LK, Hopkins RO, Chan KJ, et al: Hyperbaric oxygen for acute carbon monoxide poisoning. N Engl J Med 2002;347:1057–1067.
110. Copel JA, Bowen F, Bolognese RJ: Carbon monoxide intoxication in early pregnancy. Obstet Gynecol 1982;59(Suppl):26–28.
111. Satin KP, Neutra RR, Guirguis G, et al: Umbilical cord blood lead levels in California. Arch Environ Health 1991;46(3):167–173.
112. Singh N, Donovan CM, Hanshaw JB: Neonatal lead intoxication in a prenatally exposed infant. J Pediatr 1978;93:1019–1021.
113. Ryu JE, Ziegler EE, Fomon SJ: Maternal lead exposure and blood concentration in infancy. J Pediatr 1978;93:476–478.
114. Angle CR, McIntire MS: Lead poisoning during pregnancy. Am J Dis Child 1964;108:436–439.
115. Ghafour SY, Khuffash FA, Ibrahim HS, et al: Congenital lead intoxication with seizures due to prenatal exposure. Clin Pediatr 1984;23(5):282–283.
116. Tait PA, Vora A, James S, et al: Severe congenital lead poisoning in a preterm infant due to a herbal remedy. Med J Aust 2002;177:193–195.
117. Timpo AE, Amin JS, Casalino MB, et al: Congenital lead intoxication. J Pediatr 1979;94:765–767.
118. Horner RD, Lackey CJ, Kolasa K: Pica practices of pregnant women. J Am Diet Assoc 1991;91:34–38.
119. Hamilton S, Rothenberg SJ, Khan FA, et al: Neonatal lead poisoning from maternal pica behavior during pregnancy. J Natl Med Assoc 2001;93:317–319.
120. Shannon M: Severe lead poisoning in pregnancy. Ambul Pediatr 2003;3(1):37–39.

121. Klitzman S, Sharma A, Nicaj L, et al: Lead poisoning among pregnant women in New York City: risk factors and screening practices. J Urban Health 2002;79:225–237.

122. Gomaa A, Hu H, Bellinger D, et al: Maternal bone lead as an independent risk factor for fetal neurotoxicity: a prospective study. Pediatrics 2002;110:110–118.

123. Rothenberg SJ, Khan F, Manalo M, et al: Maternal bone lead contribution to blood lead during and after pregnancy. Environ Res 2000;82:81–90.

124. Rothenberg SJ, Kondrashov V, Manalo M, et al: Increases in hypertension and blood pressure during pregnancy with increased bone lead levels. Am J Epidemiol 2002;156:1079–1087.

125. Hertz-Picciotto I: The evidence that lead increases the risk for spontaneous abortion. Am J Ind Med 2000;38:300–309.

126. Needleman HL, Rabinowitz M, Leviton A, et al: The relationship between prenatal exposure to lead and congenital anomalies. JAMA 1984;251:2956–2959.

127. Furman A: Maternal and umbilical cord blood lead levels: an Instanbul study. Arch Environ Health 2001;56(1):26–28.

128. Pearl M, Boxt LM: Radiographic findings in congenital lead poisoning. Radiology 1980;136:83–84.

129. Canfield RL, Henderson CR, Cory-Slechta DA, et al: Intellectual impairment in children with blood lead concentrations below 10 μg per deciliter. N Engl J Med 2003;348(16):1517–1526.

130. Bellinger D, Leviton A, Waternaux C, et al: Longitudinal analyses of prenatal lead exposure and early cognitive development. N Engl J Med 1987;316(17):1037–1043.

131. O'Hara TM, Bennett L, McCoy CP: Lead poisoning and toxicokinetics in a human fetus treated with CaNA2EDTA and thiamine. Vet Diagn Invest 1995;7(4):531–537.

132. Bosque MA, Domingo JL, Corbella J, et al: Developmental toxicity evaluation of monoisoamyl meso-2,3 dimercaptosuccinate in mice. J Toxicol Environ Heath 1994;42(4):443–450.

133. Domingo JL, Ortega A, Paternain JL, et al: Meso-2,3 dimercaptosuccinic acid in pregnant Sprague-Dawley rats: teratogenicity and alterations in mineral metabolism. J Toxicol Environ Health 1990;30(3):181–190.

134. Horowitz RS, Mirkin DB: Lead poisoning and chelation in a mother-neonate pair. J Toxicol Clin Toxicol 2001;39(7):727–731.

135. Martinez-Frias ML, Rodriguez-Pinilla E, Bermejo E: Prenatal exposure of penicillamine and oral clefts. Am J Med Genet 1998;76(3):274–275.

136. Domingo JL: Developmental toxicity of metal chelating agents. Reprod Toxicol 1998;12(5):499–510.

137. Arbuckle TE, Lin Z, Mery LS: An exploratory analysis of the effect of pesticide exposure on the risk of spontaneous abortion in an Ontario farm population. Environ Health Perspect 2001;109:851–857.

138. Aaron CK, Hirschman Z, Smilkstein M: Street pharmacology: a dangerous new way to prolong the high. Vet Hum Toxicol 1989;31(4):375.

139. Tafuri J, Roberts J: Organophosphate poisoning. Ann Emerg Med 1987;16:193–202.

140. Bailey B: Organophosphate poisoning in pregnancy. Ann Emerg Med 1997;29(2):299.

141. Okumara T, Takasun I, Ishimitus S, et al: Report on 640 victims of the Tokyo subway sarin attack. Ann Emerg Med 1996;28(2):129–135.

142. Astroff BA, Young AD: The relationship between maternal and fetal effects following maternal organophosphate exposure during gestation in the rat. Toxicol Ind Health 1998;14(6):869–889.

143. Padadopoulou-Tsoukali H, Njau S: Mother-fetus postmortem toxicologic analysis in a fatal overdose with mecarbam. Forensic Sci Int 1987;35:249–252.

144. Zsigmond EK, Downs JR: Plasma cholinesterase activity in newborns and infants. Can Anesth Soc J 1971;18:278–285.

145. Karlsen RL, Sterri S, Lyngaas S, et al: Reference values for erythrocyte acetylcholinesterase and plasma cholinesterase activities in children, implications for organophosphate intoxication. Scand J Clin Lab Invest 1981;41:301–302.

146. Karalliedde L, Senanayaka N, Ariaratam A: Acute organophosphate insecticide poisoning during pregnancy. Hum Toxicol 1988;7:363–364.

147. Landauder W: Cholinomimetic teratogens: the effect of oximes and related cholinesterase reactivators. Teratology 1977;15:33.

148. Weis OF, Muller FO, Lyel H, et al: Maternal-fetal cholinesterase inhibitor poisoning. Anesth Analg 1983;62:233–235.

18 *Toxicologic Issues in the Neonate*

JAMES G. LINAKIS, PHD, MD ■ SARA SKARBEK-BOROWSKA, MD

INTRODUCTION AND EPIDEMIOLOGY

In the past few decades, technology has advanced to such a degree that premature and critically ill neonates, who would have previously had no hope for survival, can be saved, often with remarkably good outcomes. With the advent of neonatal intensive care facilities, aggressive pharmacologic intervention has become the norm. Not surprisingly, the increasing use of potent pharmaceuticals in neonates has increased the likelihood of adverse drug reactions occurring in this age group. During the past 50 years, this has been demonstrated on several occasions. In 1956, an increased incidence of kernicterus and associated mortality were reported in premature infants receiving a sulfonamide antibiotic.[1] In 1959, high-dose chloramphenicol was implicated in the cardiovascular collapse of three neonates.[2] Similar outbreaks have been associated with the use of benzyl alcohol as a preservative in bacteriostatic saline[3] and intravenous α-tocopherol[4,5] in newborns. In addition, the escalating ubiquity of toxins in everyday life has also placed the neonate at risk for inadvertent exposure to environmental toxins.

This chapter reviews the current understanding of the pathophysiology of certain toxic reactions in the neonate and discusses those toxins that are most commonly responsible for neonatal toxic emergencies. It is not a comprehensive summary of all the toxic drug reactions reported in neonates. A more complete listing of neonatal drug toxicity is shown in Table 18-1.

Neonatal toxicology is not a simple extension of the established knowledge of clinical toxicology as it pertains to other patient groups. The physiology of the newborn is unique, and organs that play an important role in susceptibility to and moderation of toxic reactions, such as the liver and kidney, are immature in their function. As a result, the manner in which the neonate handles a toxic exposure is frequently quite different from the response of an older child or adult. A working knowledge of neonatal physiology and pharmacokinetic differences from older children and adults is essential for understanding neonatal drug toxicity.

RELEVANT ANATOMY, PHYSIOLOGY, AND PHARMACOLOGY

Neonatal Pharmacokinetics

Pharmacokinetics describes the various processes through which drugs are absorbed, distributed, metabolized, and/or excreted. Several of these processes are markedly different in the neonate than in the adult or even the older child (Table 18-2). In many cases, the peculiarity of

these processes in the neonate predisposes to the development of toxicity. This, combined with the fact that many infants in the neonatal intensive care unit suffer from diseases that may also alter the disposition of medications, places these infants at high risk for drug toxicity.[6]

ABSORPTION

Drug absorption differences in the neonate enhance neonates' susceptibility to toxicity. The neonate has a higher gastric pH due to decreased gastric acid secretion. Since gastrointestinal absorption of many drugs is pH dependent, the continuous changes that occur in gastric pH from birth through the second year of life complicate predictions of drug absorption.[7,8] In addition, the more alkaline gastric environment of infants coupled with their lack of mature mucosal immunologic defenses allows growth of *Clostridium botulinum* and makes them susceptible to botulism (see Chapter 26). As compared with older patient groups, gastric emptying is slower in the neonate and infant. Thus, absorption of drugs may be delayed considerably, leading to a delay in the time to peak serum concentration and a decrease in peak serum concentration. If these factors are not taken into account when initially dosing medications in the neonate, supplemental dosing may be necessary with the consequent increase in potential toxicity.

Absorption of drugs administered by the intramuscular route is also altered in the neonate. Since the relative blood flow of the various muscle groups changes dramatically, particularly in the first 2 weeks of postnatal life, and muscle activity may also undergo alterations, intramuscular administration of medications may produce inconsistent and unreliable absorption in both premature and full-term infants.[7-9]

Transdermal absorption of drugs may also lead to toxicity in the neonate. The comparatively reduced thickness of the stratum corneum, particularly in the premature infant, permits more effective absorption by the cutaneous route.[8,9] Indeed, the literature contains several reports of toxicity in neonates resulting from percutaneous absorption (see Dermatologic Exposures below).[10-13]

DISTRIBUTION

Drug distribution varies considerably in the neonatal period from that which occurs in later life. The differences are due largely to age-related variations in protein binding, body fat, and total body water.[8,9] Overall, protein binding of drugs is reduced and body fat and total body water are increased in the neonate. This may result in an increase in the apparent volume of distribution of drug and consequent increase in the elimination half-life of the drug. Furthermore, the

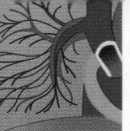

TABLE 18-1 Commonly Used Drugs and Their Potential Toxicity in Neonates

DRUG	TOXICITY
Amikacin	Nephrotoxicity, ototoxicity
Aminophylline	Tachycardia, abdominal distention, GI hemorrhage, jitteriness, or seizures
Amoxicillin	Nephrotoxicity, vitamin K depletion, distal renal tubular acidosis
Ampicillin	Rare; increased, transaminase; eosinophilia; irritability
Atropine sulfate	Tachycardia, urine retention, hyperthermia
Belladonna, tincture of	Hyperthermia, dry secretions, flushing
Bicarbonate	Transient hyperosmolarity, alkalosis, hypernatremia
Caffeine citrate	Tachycardia, seizures, abdominal distention
Calcium gluconate	Bradycardia, sloughing and calcification with IV infiltration; potentiates digitalis effect
Carbenicillin	Hypernatremia, sloughing with IV infiltration; transaminase elevation, platelet dysfunction
Cephalothin	Nephrotoxicity, neutropenia, false-positive Coombs' test results, allergic rash, poor passage through blood-brain barrier
Cefazolin	Neutropenia, thrombocytopenia, false-positive Coombs' test results, transient transaminase elevation
Chloral hydrate	Gastric irritation, paradoxic excitement
Chloramphenicol	May cause "gray baby syndrome" with toxic level; potentiates phenytoin effect, reversible bone marrow depression
Chlorothiazide	Hyperglycemia, hypokalemia, hyponatremia, alkalosis
Cholestyramine	Steatorrhea, GI dysfunction, malabsorption of fat-soluble vitamins; metabolic acidosis
Diazepam	Sodium benzoate diluent, competes with bilirubin for albumin binding sites; respiratory depression, hypotension
Diazoxide	Hypotension, hyperglycemia, sodium and water retention
Digoxin	Bradycardia, vomiting, arrhythmias, poor feeding
Epinephrine	Tachycardia, arrhythmia
Furosemide	Hypokalemia, hyponatremia, hypochloremia, alkalosis, dehydration, ototoxicity with aminoglycosides, renal calcifications; enhances nephrotoxicity of cephaloridine
Gentamicin	Nephrotoxicity, ototoxicity
Glucagon	Rebound hyperglycemia
Hydralazine HCl	May cause hypotension or tachycardia
Indomethacin	Transient renal and liver dysfunction, decreased platelet aggregation, hyponatremia, hypoglycemia
Isoproterenol	Marked inotropic effect, hypotension, arrhythmia
Kanamycin	Nephrotoxicity, ototoxicity
Lidocaine HCl	Hypotension, seizures, respiratory arrest, asystole
Magnesium sulfate	Hypotension, CNS depression
Mannitol	Rebound edema and/or circulatory overload
Moxalactam	Thrombocytopenia, platelet dysfunction, hypothrombinemia
Naloxone HCl	Tachycardia, hypertension, tremors, seizures
Nitroprusside	Hypotension, tachyphylaxis, thiocyanate toxicity with long-term use
Oxacillin	Penicillin sensitivity, nephrotoxicity
Paraldehyde	Cardiopulmonary depression, CNS depression, pulmonary edema
Phenobarbital	CNS depression with respiratory arrest with overdose
Phenytoin	Bone marrow depression, nystagmus
Prostigmine	Respiratory failure, cardiovascular collapse
Streptomycin sulfate	Nephrotoxicity, ototoxicity, cardiovascular collapse
Thorazine	Hypotension, hypothermia rare, liver disease and bone marrow depression
Ticarcillin	Bleeding problems, hypernatremia
Tobramycin sulfate	Nephrotoxicity, ototoxicity
Vancomycin	Nephrotoxicity, ototoxicity, histamine-like response

GI, gastrointestinal; IV, intravenous; CNS, central nervous system.
Modified from Harper RG, Jing JY: Handbook of Neonatology, 2nd ed. Chicago, Year Book Medical Publishers, 1987.

reduction in protein binding may result in an increased concentration of free (unbound, and therefore, active) drug with a potentially augmented pharmacologic response for a given drug concentration in the plasma. For a premature infant, the body fat may be much lower, complicating the pharmacokinetic estimates further.

METABOLISM

Neonates have a decreased capacity to metabolize drugs in the liver. The activity of the enzymes that catalyze the nonsynthetic, phase I metabolic functions of the liver (e.g., cytochrome P-450–dependent mixed-function oxidases) is markedly lower than that of adults. Postnatally, these systems appear to mature at varying rates, and several may increase to levels greater than those observed in adults by a few months of age. The synthetic, phase II reactions are also thought to be reduced at birth and to evolve more slowly (often over several years) postnatally.

Renal clearance of drugs is also reduced in the neonate. Consequently, renally excreted drugs such as the aminoglycoside antibiotics will have significantly

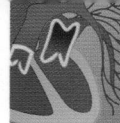

TABLE 18-2 Differences in Specific Pharmacokinetic Processes Between the Neonate and Adult		
VARIABLE	**NEONATE**	**ADULT**
Absorption		
Stomach acidity	Premature: pH, 4.7; Full-term: pH, 2.3–3.6	pH, 1.4–2.0
Gastric emptying time	Prolonged; depends on maturity and gestational age	Adult levels at about 6 mo
Gastrointestinal motility	Irregular and unpredictable	
Percutaneous absorption	Increased in neonate	
Distribution		
Fat content	Premature: 3%–12%; Full-term: 12%	18%
Skeletal muscle content	25%	43%
Extracellular water	60%	20%
Total body water	75%	50%
Plasma protein binding	Decreased binding due to decreased plasma proteins	Adult levels at about 1 yr
Metabolism		
Microsomal tissue	26 mg/g of liver	35 mg/g of liver
NADPH–cytochrome *c* reductase	49% of adult activity	
Cytochrome P-450	25%–50% of adult activity	
Glucuronidation	Low at birth	Adult level at 3 yr
Excretion		
Glomerular filtration rate	Premature: 0.7–2 mL/min Full-term: 2–4 mL/min	130 mL/min
Tubular secretion	20%–30% of adult function	Adult level at 5–7 mo

From Warner A: Drug use in the neonate: interrelationships of pharmacokinetics, toxicity, and biochemical maturity. Clin Chem 1986;32:722.

prolonged elimination and greater potential for producing toxicity. Furthermore, the various renal functions (e.g., glomerular filtration, tubular secretion, etc.) appear to develop at different rates.[9,14]

TREATMENT PRINCIPLES

Toxic Exposures through Breast Milk

Although breast milk offers a nearly ideal source of nutrients for the newborn, there is now considerable evidence that, under certain circumstances, human milk may also become a route of exposure to potentially toxic substances.[15] Neubert has listed three circumstances by which "undesired chemicals" might be transferred to a neonate via the mother's milk: (1) when the nursing mother uses particular medications, (2) when the nursing mother uses "recreational" drugs or drugs of abuse, and (3) when certain environmental toxins have been stored within maternal adipose tissue.[16]

There are a number of routes by which toxins might be transported into breast milk from maternal tissues. According to Berlin, the most probable of these are transcellular diffusion, intercellular diffusion, passive diffusion, and ionophore diffusion.[17] Because diffusion represents the primary mechanism by which drugs enter breast milk, factors such as pH, pK$_a$, protein binding, and lipid solubility of the substance will play an important role in the final concentration of the drug or toxin in breast milk.

For most substances, the concentration of the drug or toxin in breast milk is considerably lower than in the maternal serum[18] (Table 18-3). However, some medications have been shown to be concentrated in breast milk above the concentration in maternal serum. These include iodine 131, propylthiouracil, erythromycin, and gentamicin.[16]

In addition to medications, several environmental substances have been found to accumulate in breast milk. Indeed, there has been increasing concern that for lipophilic toxins such as the organochlorine insecticides, polychlorinated biphenyls, and polybrominated biphenyls, milk may be the only significant path of elimination from the human body.[17] Due to significant exposure variability and uncertainty about the the degree of toxicity produced by these substances, it has been suggested that breast milk should be tested prior to the initiation of breast-feeding for women exposed to these substances.[19]

Box 18-1 lists a number of maternal drug and environmental agent exposures that are thought to be contraindications to breast-feeding.

Toxic Effects of Maternal Drug Dependence

The maternal use and abuse of drugs during pregnancy may have lasting implications for the neonate. For instance, the fetal alcohol syndrome that results from maternal prenatal alcohol abuse has been well documented.[20] The fetal alcohol syndrome is characterized by growth retardation, mental retardation, and facial dysmorphogenesis (i.e., microcephaly, short palpebral fissures, epicanthal folds, maxillary hypoplasia, cleft palate, hypoplastic philtrum, and micrognathia). In addition to teratogenic effects, the maternal use of

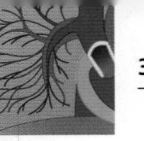

TABLE 18-3 Excretion of Drugs in Human Milk

DRUG	MATERNAL DOSE	PEAK CONCENTRATION IN MILK	MILK/PLASMA RATIO AT PEAK	TIME OF PEAK CONCENTRATION IN MILK	HALF-LIFE IN MILK*	AMOUNT SECRETED IN MILK 24 HR AFTER SINGLE DOSE†	MATERNAL DOSE (%)‡
Acetaminophen	650 mg PO	10–15 µg/mL	0.8	1–2 hr	2.3 hr	0.88 mg	0.14
Antipyrine	18 mg/kg PO	20–30 µg/mL	1.0	10 min	6–22 hr	7–25 mg	0.5–2.4
Caffeine	35–336 mg PO as beverage	2–7 µg/mL	0.6–0.8	½–1 hr	6.1 hr	0.57 mg	0.53
Cefazolin	2 g IV	1.51µg/mL	0.023	3 hr		1.5 mg	0.075
	500 mg IM tid	0		Not detected in milk		0	
Chlorothiazide	500 mg PO	0		Not detected in milk		<1 mg/day	
Diazepam	Not stated	0.27 µg/mL	0.68	3 day	3 day	0.27 mg (peak) on day 3	0.07–0.14
Digoxin	0.25 mg PO	0.6–1.0 ng/mL	0.8–0.9	4 hr	12 hr	0.18–0.36 µg/day	
Ethanol	0.6 g/kg PO	777 µg/mL	0.93	90 min	2.9 hr	300 mg	1
Isoniazid	300 mg PO	16.6 µg/mL	1.6	3 hr	5.9 hr	7 mg	2.3
Lithium	Chronic: dose not specified PO	0.1–0.6 mmol/L	0.5	Levels fairly constant			
Methadone	70 mg/day PO	0.36 µg/mL	0.83			300 µg	0.4
		0.51 µg/mL	1.89		9 hr		
Metronidazole	2.0 g PO	50–57 µg/mL		2–4 hr		21.8 mg	1.1
Nicotine	1 pack/day (400 mg)	91 ng/mL		No correlation		0.68 mg	0.17
		Range: 20–512 ng/mL					
Prednisolone	5 mg PO	26 ng/mL		1 hr	8.2 hr	6 µg	0.12
Prednisone	120 mg PO	154 ng/mL (prednisone)		2 hr	1.8 hr	47 µg (as both prednisone and prednisolone)	0.04
		473 ng/mL (prednisolone)		2 hr	1.1 hr		
Propranolol	20 mg	10 ng/mL	0.56	3 hr		0.6 µg	0.03
	160 mg	150 ng/mL	0.65	3 hr		90 µg	0.05
Salicylate	20 mg/kg						0.18–0.36
Sulfasalazine	2 g/day PO	9–15 mg/mL	0.6	Constant		1.4–2.1 mg	0.16
Sulphone	5 g IM sulphetrone or 500 mg PO dapsone	14 µg/mL	0.16	4–6 hr		10 mg	2
Theophylline	4.25 mg/kg	4 µg/mL	0.7	2 hr	4.0 hr	8 mg	4
Verapamil	80 mg PO tid		0.6	1–2 hr	4.3 hr	31 µg	0.01

IM, intramuscularly; IV, intravenously; PO, orally.
*Half-life is calculated from the elimination (β) phase
†Amount excreted in 24 hr is estimated by assuming that the infant ingests 90 mL of milk every 4 hr.
‡The percentage of maternal dose is calculated by dividing the amount secreted in 24 hr by the maternal dose (single dose or 24-hr total maternal dose).
From Berlin CM Jr: The excretion of drugs and chemicals in human milk. In Yaffe SJ, Aranda JV (eds): Pediatric Pharmacology: Therapeutic Principles in Practice. Philadelphia, WB Saunders, 1992, p 208.

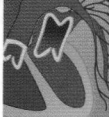

BOX 18-1	**EXPOSURES CONSIDERED TO CONTRAINDICATE BREAST-FEEDING**

Antimetabolites (cancer chemotherapy drugs, including amethopterin, cyclophosphamide, doxorubicin, and methotrexate)
Androgens (e.g., testosterone)
Bromides (high dose)*
Bromocriptine†
Chloramphenicol
Cimetidine*
Clemastine*
Cocaine
Ergot alkaloid (high dose)
Gold salt
Heroin
Indomethacin*
Iodides
Lead (if mother intoxicated)
Lithium

Marijuana†
Mercury, methylmercury§
Methimazole*
Metronidazole
Nalidixic acid
Nitrofurantoin
Phencyclidine (PCP)‡
Phenelzine†
Phenindione*
Pesticides§
Polybrominated biphenyls§
Polychlorinated biphenyls§
Polychlorinated terphenyls§
Radiopharmaceuticals
Strontium 89, strontium 90§
Sulfonamides (for neonates)
Tetrachloroethylene§
Thiouracil*

*Although use of these agents during nursing should not result in excessive infant exposure (at usual doses), alternative therapeutic agents exist that do not share the same risk of serious adverse effects or case reports of adverse occurrences.
†May suppress lactation.
‡Use of these substances as drugs of abuse results in uncontrolled infant exposure because of unknown quality and purity of street drugs. Abstinence should be encouraged.
§Testing of milk indicated if mother is known to be exposed in excess to environmental chemicals for which infant sensitivity is not defined.

numerous drugs during pregnancy has been found to result in neonatal abstinence syndromes, and, occasionally, to long-term neurodevelopmental effects. Opiates, cocaine, barbiturates, benzodiazepines, phencyclidine, and selective serotonin reuptake inhibitors (SSRIs) have all been associated with neonatal withdrawal symptoms. Because of the large number of users, opiates and cocaine represent the largest contributors to neonatal toxicity resulting from in utero exposure.

OPIOIDS

An estimated 10,000 women who are addicted to opioids give birth each year.[21] Of these neonates, as many as 90% may show evidence of opioid withdrawal. Methadone and heroin represent the most commonly implicated opiates, although chronic use of virtually all opioids risks perinatal addiction, including codeine-containing cough preparations.

The time of abstinence syndrome onset is related to the half-life of the narcotic, such that drugs with shorter elimination half-lives will have more rapid onset of symptoms. Withdrawal symptoms are commonly first noted between 24 and 72 hours after delivery in heroin-addicted neonates, dissipating within about 2 weeks. For methadone-addicted infants, withdrawal symptoms typically begin between 3 and 7 days after birth, but delay

of symptoms for as long as 32 days postpartum has been reported.[22] Signs of neonatal opioid withdrawal include irritability, hypertonia, tremors, tachypnea, tachycardia, high-pitched cry, diarrhea, yawning, sneezing, nasal congestion, poor feeding, and occasionally low-grade fever and vomiting. In rare instances, seizures have been reported. Jitteriness and hypertonicity may persist for several months postpartum.

Early diagnosis of neonatal abstinence syndromes is important not only for determining the need for pharmacologic intervention, but also so that appropriate steps can be taken to institute proper monitoring and social services. Opiate-addicted neonates are more commonly born prematurely and are small for gestational age. Monitoring and supportive care must be directed at the provision of ample fluid and calories as well as at the correction of possible hypoglycemia, polycythemia, and other problems ensuing from prematurity.

Determination of the need for pharmacologic intervention in the neonate undergoing opiate withdrawal is frequently a difficult process. Many nurseries use scoring systems similar to those suggested by Kahn and colleagues[23] to dictate therapeutic interventions. In that system, newborns with grade I (symptoms that are mild but obviously abnormal) and grade II (the neonate is symptomatic only when disturbed) effects are treated nonpharmacologically with environmental interventions such as gentle handling, demand feeding, and swaddling. The newborn who is symptomatic even when undisturbed (grade III) is eligible for pharmacologic intervention. These infants typically manifest constant crying, significant diarrhea or tremors, and poor feeding.

There are presently several pharmacologic agents used for the management of opioid withdrawal in neonates.[24] The more common regimens are listed in Table 18-5. When pharmacologic intervention is required, medication is started at the smallest recommended dose and titrated upward as required to achieve the desired level of well-being in the neonate. Once the infant has been asymptomatic for 2 to 3 days, the drug dose is tapered, first by lowering the dose, and subsequently by increasing the dosing interval. This process is continued every 2 to 3 days until symptoms of withdrawal have been completely ameliorated. The total duration of treatment is dependent on a number of factors, including the specific opioid to which the mother is addicted, the severity of maternal addiction, and the medication used for treating withdrawal in the neonate.

COCAINE

Cocaine readily crosses the placenta and the blood-brain barrier. Its use prenatally has been associated with preterm labor and delivery, strokes, abruptio placentae, and poor fetal growth.[22] Intrauterine cocaine exposure has been associated with several postnatal neurobehavioral abnormalities as measured by the Neonatal Behavioral Assessment Scale.[25] These abnormalities include altered interactive behavior in the cocaine-exposed neonate and an abnormal response to environmental stimuli.[26] Hypertonia and coarse tremor have been described

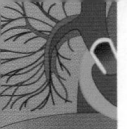

TABLE 18-4 Medications Used to Treat Neonatal Opiate Withdrawal

DRUG	DOSE	DOSING INTERVAL	COMMENTS
Paregoric	0.05–0.1 mL/kg per dose, PO	q4h	Constituents can cause local mucosal irritation and CNS stimulation
Tincture of opium, USP (diluted 25–fold)	0.05–0.1 mL/kg per dose, PO	q4th	No irritating CNS stimulating constituents
Phenobarbital	1–2 mg/kg per dose, PO or IM	q6h	Dose not control diarrhea, may result in poor suck
Chlorpromazine	0.4–0.7 mg/kg per dose, IM or PO	q6h	May cause extrapyramidal symptoms
Clonidine	0.5–1.0 µg/kg per dose, PO	q6h	Experience is limited in neonates

CNS, central nervous system; IM, intramuscularly; PO, orally.

postnatally.[27] In addition, these infants may manifest a syndrome composed of jitteriness, sleep difficulties, poor suck, and behavioral lability. There is disagreement as to the extent that these abnormal behaviors represent an abstinence syndrome versus a direct effect of cocaine.[28-30] Lester and colleagues have suggested that many of the observed cocaine effects can be categorized into two neurobehavioral syndromes, excitable and depressed.[31] They suggest that these two syndromes are the result of direct neurotoxic (excitable) effects of cocaine and indirect or consequent (depressed) effects, such as poor fetal growth. Evidence exists that cocaine metabolites, which can continue to be eliminated for more than a week in the neonate, may additionally contribute to the neonatal cocaine withdrawal syndrome.[32] Fortunately, postnatal effects of intrauterine cocaine exposure infrequently require pharmacologic intervention.

Cocaine also readily passes into breast milk, and maternal use of cocaine in the breast-fed infant has been reported to result in signs and symptoms of cocaine intoxication, including tachycardia, hypertension, irritability, and tremulousness.[28]

SELECTIVE SEROTONIN REUPTAKE INHIBITORS

SSRIs are commonly used in the treatment of depression, panic disorder, and obsessive-compulsive disorder. While in utero exposure to SSRIs does not appear to increase the risk for major fetal malformations,[33,34] exposure to these agents in the third trimester of pregnancy has been associated with a higher rate of neonatal complications, including a neonatal withdrawal syndrome.[33,35-37]

Toxic Environmental Exposures in the Neonate

HEAVY METALS

Although acute neonatal exposure to heavy metals is rare, such exposures have been reported for both lead and mercury. A more common mechanism for heavy metal intoxication in the neonate is from prenatal placental transfer of the metal. This has been reported for a number of heavy metals including lead, mercury, and cadmium.[38-40] Mercury and lead are also secreted into the breast milk of exposed mothers.[15]

Until recently, it was believed that the consequences of prenatal exposure to lead were primarily limited to an increased risk for minor anomalies.[6,41] Cases have now been reported of serious neurodevelopmental injury postnatally in infants whose mothers had high blood lead levels during pregnancy (see Chapter 73).[42,43] Furthermore, there is also significant evidence that low-level fetal lead exposure (maternal levels less than or equal to 25 µg/dL) may lead to mild developmental delay for at least the first few years of life.[44] Although this delay appears to be reversible for many by school age, it is not yet clear whether this is universally true. It is known that infants of mothers with the potential for high-level exposures are at greatest risk. These include pregnant women residing near industrial point sources of lead (e.g., smelters), women with lead-related hobbies (e.g., manufacture of jewelry, stained glass, fishing sinkers), and those involved in construction, particularly the rehabilitation of older, lead-based paint–containing dwellings. Chelation therapy for maternal lead poisoning during pregnancy is controversial partly because of the apparent teratogenic potential of such therapy.[45] Similarly, the blood lead level at which a newborn should be chelated is also undecided, although most authorities agree that chelation is appropriate for levels greater than 40 to 45 µg/dL, with some recommending chelation at even lower levels.[46,47] Further discussion of the treatment of lead poisoning can be found in Chapter 73.

Mercury also readily crosses the placental barrier, particularly organic mercury compounds, such as methylmercury. There have been numerous reported cases of fetal toxicity secondary to maternal exposure to methylmercury (see Chapter 71).[48] It is believed that all forms of mercury are capable of producing fetal toxicity, but that methylmercury is the most toxic. Of the reported cases of fetal mercury poisoning, most have been the result of maternal occupational exposure to mercury compounds or substantial ingestion of contaminated fish.[49] Two epidemics of methylmercury poisoning due to consumption of seafood contaminated by industrial waste occurred in Japan (Minamata Bay in 1956 and Niigata in 1965).[50] Approximately 64 cases of infants with intrauterine methylmercury poisoning, 13 of which resulted in death, have been identified.[51] Clinical manifestations of methylmercury poisoning in these

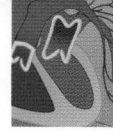

infants included mental retardation, ataxia, dysarthria, abnormalities of posture, chorea, and other nonspecific neurologic findings.[50]

Postnatal exposure to toxic doses of mercury is much less common, although reports of acrodynia in neonates occurred as early as the 1920s.[52] In 1981, several hundred infants in Argentina were poisoned when their commercially laundered diapers were contaminated with mercury.[53] Mercury thermometers in infant incubators have been shown to liberate unacceptably high levels of mercury vapor,[54,55] although few, if any, cases of serious toxicity from this source have been reported. The topical application of merbromin (mercurochrome [no longer manufactured in the United States]) to omphaloceles in neonates has resulted in mercury toxicity,[56,57] including several fatalities.[58-61] Toxic exposure to mercury from breast-feeding has also been well documented, being responsible for an epidemic of methylmercury poisoning in Iraq in 1971 and 1972. In this incident, grain contaminated with methylmercury was used to make bread, and resulted in more than 6500 hospitalizations and over 450 deaths due to mercury poisoning. Numerous infants developed severe toxicity from breast milk exposure alone.[62] Toxic manifestations included mental retardation; impaired motor, sensory, and autonomic function; delayed motor development; and progressively worsening hyperreflexia in several infants.[63,64] Other sources of mercury poisoning in infants have been reported[65,66] but generally represent rare occurrences.

In 1999, an initiative to remove thimerosal, a mercury-containing preservative, from all childhood vaccines was launched following the recognition that the exposure to ethylmercury from a single vaccination could exceed the Environmental Protection Agency's guideline for maximum mercury exposure of 0.1 μg/kg/day.[67]

Results of the Tagum studies conducted in the Philippines suggest that fetal trapping of mercury occurs during pregnancy[68] and that prenatal mercury exposure may result in lower scores on neurodevelopmental screening tests at 2 years of age.[69]

Treatment of mercury poisoning depends on a number of factors, such as the duration of exposure and the form of mercury responsible for the poisoning (metallic, organic, inorganic). Management of mercury poisoning, particularly chelation therapy, is discussed in Chapter 71.

HALOGENATED HYDROCARBONS

Polychlorinated biphenyls (PCBs), dioxins, and furans have been postulated to produce a wide range of toxic effects (see Chapter 93). Due to their persistence in the environment and secretion in breast milk, these compounds have raised concerns as potential toxins to the neonate.[70-73] To date, however, there have been few, if any, reports of acute toxicity due to these substances in newborns. Toxic effects from these compounds are likely to occur only after chronic exposure. Studies are currently being conducted to determine whether such toxicity does occur in infancy.[74-76]

Concern has also been expressed about the potential toxicity of chlorinated hydrocarbon pesticides to neonates.

These compounds, which include dichlorodiphenyl-tricholoroethane (DDT), have well-described toxicities, persist indefinitely in human tissues, and are secreted in the milk of exposed mothers. As with PCBs and dioxin, it is clear that neonates are being exposed to chlorinated hydrocarbon pesticides.[77] The consequences of such exposures, however, are presently unknown. Carbamate pesticides have also been shown to be transmitted transplacentally[78] and could prove toxic to the fetus.

Iatrogenic Poisoning In the Neonate

DERMATOLOGIC EXPOSURES

The newborn infant may be exposed to a large number of chemicals and drugs through topical exposure.[13] Low-molecular-weight substances are particularly well absorbed, and the skin of the premature infant is especially vulnerable.[79] Over the past 100 years, there have been abundant accounts of toxicity caused by transcutaneous absorption of drugs and chemicals in the neonate. Exposure through contamination of diapers has led to outbreaks of methemoglobinemia due to the aniline dyes previously used to mark new cloth diapers.[80,81]

Hexachlorophene is a trichlorophenol antiseptic that was formerly used in nurseries to prevent *Staphylococcus* infections. Frequently, it was used for total-body bathing of newborns. However, after having been considered safe for nearly 20 years, hexachlorophene was implicated as the cause of central nervous system (CNS) depression, seizures, and death in several infants in France. A distinct histologic brain lesion was subsequently found to be present in both animal models of hexachlorophene poisoning and at autopsy in preterm infants regularly bathed in hexachlorophene solutions.[12] Iodine has also been shown to be absorbed systemically when repeatedly administered topically in neonates, with reports of associated goiter and hypothyroidism.[82]

Alcohols are also frequently used topically in newborns, primarily as antiseptic agents. Hemorrhagic necrosis of the skin in preterm infants who have been lying in alcohol-soaked bedding is well described.[12] In addition, isopropyl alcohol has been reported to have systemic effects when used topically as part of umbilical cord care.[83] Similarly, methanol poisoning leading to metabolic acidosis and visual changes has been reported after the use of topical methanol.[84] A cluster of six infant deaths that occurred in Egypt in 1999 was attributed to prolonged exposure to methanol ("red alcohol") compresses at vaccination injection sites.[85] It is also believed that isopropyl alcohol can cause systemic toxicity when used for sponging for fever reduction, although toxicity is thought to occur from inhalation of the isopropyl vapor.[86] A case of fatal inhalational isopropyl alcohol poisoning in a newborn infant following the accidental placement of 70% isopropyl alcohol in the humidifier of a ventilator has also been described.[87]

Adhesive tape remover pads, which often contain solvents such as methylchloroform, have been used in numerous intensive care nurseries. Although systemic toxicity has been rare, cases of toxic epidermal necrosis associated with their use has occurred more frequently.[88]

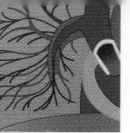

One study has shown that use of these pads produces detectable levels of methylchloroform in incubator air.[89]

Topical corticosteroids have been associated with the development of Cushing's syndrome in the neonate.[90] In addition, there is concern that extended administration may lead to depression of the hypothalamic-pituitary-adrenal axis. Under such circumstances, withdrawal of the topical steroid should occur slowly, by gradually tapering the dosage.

Topical application of over-the-counter products containing camphor has resulted in seizures in a neonate[91] and hepatotoxicity in a 2-month-old infant.[92] While ingestion is the most common route of toxic exposure, toxicity via percutaneous absorption and inhalation has been described.[92] Camphor, which is used in a multitude of cold remedies (e.g., Vicks VapoRub, Vicks VapoSteam, Procter & Gamble, Cincinnati, OH) and in topical anesthetic preparations (e.g., Camphophenique, Bayer Consumer Care, Morristown, NJ), may produce gastrointestinal and CNS toxicity as well as hepatotoxicity in overdose (see Chapter 99).[93]

METHEMOGLOBINEMIA

Neonates are susceptible to the same methemoglobin-producing toxins as older children and adults (see Chapter 14). The risk of methemoglobinemia, however, is increased in neonates due to the immaturity of the methemoglobin reductase pathway in this population.[94] There is additional evidence that neonates may be more sensitive to the oxidizing effects of toxins than older age groups. The problem is further complicated by the high concentration of fetal hemoglobin in the neonate, which further restricts oxygen delivery to tissues. Toxin-induced methemoglobinemia has been reported after inhalational exposures to aniline vapors[95] and nitric oxide,[94,96-98] as well as after administration of local anesthetic agents.[99-110] Since local anesthetics are known to cross the placenta, their use in the mother during labor and delivery may result in methemoglobinemia in the newborn infant.[99-102] Methemoglobinemia secondary to injection of local anesthetic agents in neonates has also been reported.[102-105] Cases of methemoglobinemia related to the use of topical anesthetics, including EMLA (AstraZeneca LP, Wilmington, DE)[94,106-109] and benzocaine,[110] have also been described. EMLA cream is a eutectic mixture of 2.5% lidocaine and 2.5% prilocaine. In its product insert, the manufacturer of EMLA recommends that it not be used in neonates younger than 37 weeks' gestational age, in infants younger than 12 months of age who are receiving treatment with methemoglobin-inducing agents, or in patients with congenital or idiopathic methemoglobinemia. In addition to methemoglobinemia, intoxication with local anesthetics may result in hypotonia, bradycardia, apnea, and seizures (see Chapter 63).[6]

Neonatal methemoglobinemia is relatively uncommon, but when it occurs its treatment must be undertaken with caution. It has been shown that the antidote, methylene blue, is toxic to the neonate at doses only slightly higher than those recommended to treat methemoglobinemia.[111]

ALCOHOLS

In addition to the transcutaneous and inhalational exposures discussed above, ethyl alcohol exposures occasionally occur in infants by accidental or intentional means and may result in severe intoxication (see Chapter 31). Associated hypoglycemia may be particularly problematic in this age group. Similarly, accidental administration of methanol in infant formula has resulted in systemic toxicity.[112] In the early 1980s, administration of intravascular flush solutions containing the preservative benzyl alcohol was noted to produce metabolic acidosis, gasping respirations, CNS depression, seizures, hypotension, renal failure, and occasionally death. This "gasping-baby syndrome" was attributed to large blood concentrations of benzyl alcohol and its metabolite, benzoic acid. In the neonate, immature hepatic metabolism of benzoic acid leads to its bioaccumulation. Benzoic acid was also used as a preservative in a number of parenteral medications frequently administered in neonatal intensive care units.[6] Subsequently, use of intravascular fluids containing benzyl alcohol was discontinued in this setting.

ANTIBIOTICS

Antimicrobials are among the most commonly used medications in neonates and are frequently associated with adverse effects in this age group. Perhaps the best described of the antibiotic-induced toxicities is that produced by chloramphenicol. During the first 2 weeks of life, hepatic glucuronidation of chloramphenicol is significantly less than in later life. Consequently, chloramphenicol may bioaccumulate and lead to the "gray baby syndrome." This syndrome is manifested by lethargy, abdominal distention, hypotension, hypoxemia, and acidosis.[2] Careful attention to dosing and monitoring of chloramphenicol drug levels will minimize this complication. When it occurs, exchange transfusion appears to be the treatment of choice.[113]

Several other antibiotics pose a potential threat to the newborn, particularly the premature infant. As noted earlier, sulfonamide therapy has been associated with an increased incidence of kernicterus[1] and tetracycline treatment with calcification disturbances. In addition, aminoglycoside antibiotics are associated with an augmented risk for nephrotoxicity and ototoxicity to the neonate. Although not unique to infants, neonates are at greater risk for these adverse events since they have impaired renal clearance of aminoglycosides, which results in a prolonged elimination half-life and increased risk for drug accumulation during treatment. Vancomycin administration has also been associated with adverse effects in neonates. Rash and shock occur most commonly,[114] but cardiac arrest has also occurred in a neonate following rapid intravenous injection of vancomycin.[115] As with chloramphenicol, it appears that mindful attention to dose considerations and drug levels will generally prevent these toxic effects.

ANTIFUNGALS

Amphotericin B is frequently used for the treatment of systemic fungal infections in infants. Adverse effects

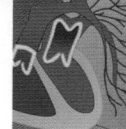

associated with its use include nephrotoxicity, hepatotoxicity, leukopenia, thrombocytopenia, chills, and death.[116] Cardiac toxicity, manifested as frequent premature ventricular contractions (PVCs), was reported in a 6-week-old full-term infant after receiving a cumulative dose of 8.5 mg/kg of amphotericin B. The PVCs ceased on discontinuation of therapy.[117] Two premature infants, who received a 50-fold overdose of amphotericin B, suffered cardiopulmonary collapse and death.[118] Another very-low-birth-weight infant, who received 50-fold overdosing for 3 days, survived.[116] The only adverse effect noted in this neonate was hypokalemia.

ANTIRETROVIRALS

Administering zidovudine (ZDV) antepartum and intrapartum to pregnant women with HIV disease and to the neonate for the first 6 weeks of life reduced the risk for maternal-infant HIV transmission by approximately two thirds in the Pediatric AIDS Clinical Trials Group 076 study.[119] The only toxic effect noted among infants in the ZDV group was a significantly higher incidence of anemia. Hemoglobin values of neonates in the ZDV group and the placebo group were similar by 12 weeks of age. While the HIV transmission rate in the Agence Nationale de Recherches sur le SIDA 075 study was only 1.6%, infants exposed to perinatal lamivudine-ZDV in this study had more adverse effects, including neutropenia, anemia, abnormal liver function tests, elevated lipase, and death in two children from neurologic complications related to mitochondrial dysfunction.[120] Additional cases of mitochondrial dysfunction associated with ZDV alone or in combination with lamivudine in the perinatal period have been reported.[121,122] Severe lactic acidosis in an uninfected neonate who received prophylactic ZDV therapy has also been described.[123]

METHYLXANTHINES

The methylxanthines (e.g., theophylline and caffeine) are commonly used for the treatment of apnea of prematurity. While theophylline is still extensively used, caffeine may emerge as the preferred pharmacologic agent due to its comparable therapeutic efficacy, longer half-life, fewer side effects, and wide therapeutic index.[124] Disadvantages of theophylline administration include fluctuating plasma concentrations that require frequent monitoring and a low therapeutic index for the drug.[124] In addition, theophylline is metabolized to caffeine by methylation, which may result in accumulation of caffeine in the neonate. Manifestations of methylxanthine toxicity generally include agitation, tachycardia, tachypnea, diuresis, hyponatremia, hypokalemia, metabolic acidosis, hyperglycemia, and seizures (see Chapter 65).[125] Other reported manifestations include jitteriness, vomiting, feeding intolerance, hypertonia, diaphoresis, opisthotonus, and tremors.[124,126,127] Numerous cases of neonatal theophylline toxicity[128-135] and caffeine toxicity[125-127,136-138] have been reported in the literature. Management of infants with methylxanthine intoxication

should include fluid and electrolyte replacement as necessary and close monitoring of blood glucose. Dysrhythmias and seizures should be managed in the standard fashion. While most infants with methylxanthine toxicity are managed with supportive care alone, selected cases of severe intoxication may require more invasive therapy. Although charcoal hemoperfusion is the recommended therapy for older children and adults, it has not been tested in infants for this indication. Hemodialysis is an effective and safer alternative to hemoperfusion but may be technically difficult to implement due to the small size and blood volume of certain neonates. Exchange transfusion has been utilized in the setting of both caffeine toxicity[126] and theophylline intoxication.[132] The successful treatment of severe theophylline toxicity in a preterm neonate with hemodialysis[134] and peritoneal dialysis[133] has also been described. In addition, three reports have suggested a role for the administration of activated charcoal.[130,131,139]

SEDATIVE-HYPNOTICS

Chloral hydrate is a sedative-hypnotic agent that has been widely used in the past for conscious sedation of children and for maintenance sedation of ventilated infants. Use of this medication has decreased in recent years due to numerous reports of toxicity and death, including cases involving both preterm[140] and full-term infants.[141-143] Manifestations of toxicity in the neonate include CNS depression, paradoxical excitation, dysrhythmias, hypotension, hyperbilirubinemia, renal failure, and apnea (see Chapter 34).[144]

Fentanyl is a potent opioid that is commonly used for sedation and analgesia in neonates. One well-described adverse effect is generalized muscle and/or chest wall rigidity. A number of cases of chest wall rigidity have been reported following low to moderate dose infusions of fentanyl in infants.[145-147] Chest wall rigidity has also occurred in neonates following maternal fentanyl administration during cesarean section.[148,149] Chest wall rigidity is treated with either an opiate antagonist (e.g., naloxone) or neuromuscular blockade.[147]

OPHTHALMIC DROPS

Because of the risk for retinopathy of prematurity in low-birth-weight infants who have required oxygen therapy, frequent funduscopic examinations are often necessary. To facilitate these examinations, mydriatic and cycloplegic agents must be instilled into the infants' eyes. The potential toxicities of these agents include hypertension, tachycardia, ventricular dysrhythmias, and subarachnoid hemorrhage.[150] Premature infants are especially sensitive to these side effects, and a fatal outcome has been reported.[150] Consequently, current recommendations are to dilate the eyes of infants with a single drop of 0.5% cyclopentolate, one drop of 2.5% phenylephrine, and one drop of 1% tropicamide. Further dilution to 1% phenylephrine and 0.2% cyclopentolate is recommended for premature infants.

In addition to the commonly used mydriatic and cycloplegic agents, toxicity following topical adminis-

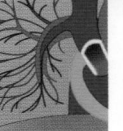

tration of an α_2 agonist for the treatment of glaucoma in infants has also been described.[151] Cases of CNS depression ranging from lethargy to coma in infants following a single drop of brimonidine tartrate 0.2% ophthalmic solution have been reported.[151,152] Infants receiving brimonidine have also been noted to develop hypotonia, hypothermia, apnea, bradycardia, and hypotension.[151] The manufacturer currently recommends that this medication not be given to children younger than 2 years.

Therapy for Neonatal Poisonings

The priorities for management of the poisoned neonate are similar to those for patients of any age with a suspected poisoning: supportive care, decontamination, enhancement of elimination, and administration of any available antidote.[14] Not surprisingly, little research has been conducted to examine the latter three issues in the newborn population. Supportive care is the first priority, and cardiorespiratory status of the infant should be considered particularly fragile in the face of a toxic insult. Once airway, breathing, and circulation have been stabilized, decontamination should be performed whenever acute exposures have occurred. The route of exposure determines the type of decontamination. Bathing may be the only decontamination required when topical exposure has occurred. After gastrointestinal exposure to toxins, decontamination must be carried out carefully due to the frailty of the neonate. Little data exist on the safety of syrup of ipecac in this age group; thus, its routine use cannot be advocated. Nasogastric tubes can be inserted in even the premature neonate with relative ease, although lavage should be conducted with normal saline rather than water, and in aliquots of approximately 15 to 25 mL to avoid fluid and electrolyte shifts. Furthermore, cathartics may represent a risk to the neonate's osmotic balance and therefore should be avoided. The use of activated charcoal is somewhat controversial in the newborn because of the vulnerability of the infant's gastrointestinal tract. Nevertheless, it has been used successfully in this age group.[139] Consequently, the use of activated charcoal may represent a viable treatment option under certain conditions.

Enhancement of the elimination of toxins in neonates is also relatively untested. The use of forced diuresis, a technique more commonly used in older children and adults, may represent a serious risk to even the healthy neonate, since renal function is immature. Furthermore, when the infant has pulmonary or cardiac disease, the risks of this technique are obvious, and thus it is not commonly used. Similarly, hemodialysis and hemoperfusion are technically complex in even full-term infants and can be carried out only in a few specialized centers. Exchange transfusion may be used for eliminating certain toxins in the neonate; it can be performed with relative ease. Its use is restricted to instances in which the toxin is primarily confined to the vascular space (low volume of distribution). This method of treatment is particularly attractive for severe cases of methemoglobinemia and methylxanthine toxicity.

CONCLUSION

The physiologic and pharmacokinetic characteristics of neonates make them particularly vulnerable to poisoning. Toxic exposures in the neonate may be particularly difficult to diagnose, particularly since the signs and symptoms are frequently similar to those that occur with other neonatal ailments, such as sepsis or cardiac disease. While the incidence of toxic exposures is presumably low, it is imperative that all of those caring for newborns maintain a high index of suspicion for poisoning.[112] Due to the possibility of accidental iatrogenic poisoning, a thorough review of administered medications should occur during the initial evaluation of all sick neonates. In instances when a toxic exposure is suspected, the clinical toxicologist must work in concert with the neonatologist or pediatrician, using his or her knowledge of the unique aspects of neonatal physiology to obtain a diagnosis and institute the appropriate therapy.

REFERENCES

1. Andersen DH, Blanc WA, Crozier DN, Silverman WA: A difference in mortality rate and incidence of kernicterus among premature infants allotted to two prophylactic antibacterial regimens. Pediatrics 1956;18(4):614–625.
2. Sutherland JM: Fatal cardiovascular collapse of infants receiving large amounts of chloramphenicol. Am J Dis Child 1959; 97(6):761–767.
3. Menon PA, Thach BT, Smith CH, et al: Benzyl alcohol toxicity in a neonatal intensive care unit. Incidence, symptomatology, and mortality. Am J Perinatol 1984;1(4):288–292.
4. Bodenstein CJ: Intravenous vitamin E and deaths in the intensive care unit. Pediatrics 1984;73(5):733.
5. Lorch V, Murphy D, Hoersten LR, et al: Unusual syndrome among premature infants: association with a new intravenous vitamin E product. Pediatrics 1985;75(3):598–602.
6. Elhassani SB: Neonatal poisoning: causes, manifestations, prevention, and management. South Med J 1986;79(12):1535–1543.
7. Morselli PL: Clinical pharmacokinetics in neonates. Clin Pharmacokinet 1976;1(2):81–98.
8. Routledge PA: Pharmacokinetics in children. J Antimicrob Chemother 1994;34(Suppl A):19–24.
9. Blumer J, Reed M: Principles of neonatal pharmacology. In Yaffe SJ, Aranda JV (eds): Neonatal and Pediatric Pharmacology: Therapeutic Principles in Practice, 3rd ed. Baltimore, Lippincott Williams & Wilkins, 2004.
10. Pyati SP, Ramamurthy RS, Krauss MT, Pildes RS: Absorption of iodine in the neonate following topical use of povidone iodine. J Pediatr 1977;91(5):825–828.
11. Tyrala EE, Hillman LS, Hillman RE, Dodson WE: Clinical pharmacology of hexachlorophene in newborn infants. J Pediatr 1977;91(3):481–486.
12. Rutter N: Percutaneous drug absorption in the newborn: hazards and uses. Clin Perinatol 1987;14(4):911–930.
13. Cetta F, Lambert GH, Ros SP: Newborn chemical exposure from over-the-counter skin care products. Clin Pediatr (Phila) 1991;30(5):286–289.
14. Banner W Jr: Clinical toxicology in the neonatal intensive care unit. Med Toxicol 1986;1(3):225–235.
15. Oskarsson A, Palminger Hallen I, Sundberg J: Exposure to toxic elements via breast milk. Analyst 1995;120(3):765–770.
16. Neubert D: Significance of pharmacokinetic variables in reproductive and developmental toxicity. Xenobiotica 1988;18(Suppl 1):45–58.
17. Berlin C Jr: The excretion of drugs and chemicals in human milk. In Yaffe SJ (ed): Pediatric Pharmacology: Therapeutic Principles in Practice, 2nd ed. Philadelphia, WB Saunders, 1992, pp 205–211.
18. Kunka RL, Venkataramanan R, Stern RM, Ladik CF: Excretion

of propoxyphene and norpropoxyphene in breast milk. Clin Pharmacol Ther 1984;35(5):675–680.

19. Marx C, Pope J, Blumer J: Developmental toxicology. In Haddad LM, Winchester JF (eds): Clinical Management of Poisoning and Drug Overdose, 2nd ed. Philadelphia, WB Saunders, 1990, pp 388–436.

20. Jones KL, Smith DW, Ulleland CN, Streissguth P: Pattern of malformation in offspring of chronic alcoholic mothers. Lancet 1973;1(7815):1267–1271.

21. Hans SL: Developmental consequences of prenatal exposure to methadone. Ann N Y Acad Sci 1989;562:195–207.

22. Mast J: Toxic encephalopathy in the newborn. Semin Neurol 1993;13(1):66–72.

23. Kahn EJ, Neumann LL, Polk GA: The course of the heroin withdrawal syndrome in newborn infants treated with phenobarbital or chlorpromazine. J Pediatr 1969;75(3):495–500.

24. Suresh S, Anand KJ: Opioid tolerance in neonates: mechanisms, diagnosis, assessment, and management. Semin Perinatol 1998; 22(5):425–433.

25. Zuckerman B, Bresnahan K: Developmental and behavioral consequences of prenatal drug and alcohol exposure. Pediatr Clin North Am 1991;38(6):1387–1406.

26. Chasnoff IJ, Burns WJ, Schnoll SH, Burns KA: Cocaine use in pregnancy. N Engl J Med 1985;313(11):666–669.

27. Chiriboga CA, Brust JC, Bateman D, Hauser WA: Dose-response effect of fetal cocaine exposure on newborn neurologic function. Pediatrics 1999;103(1):79–85.

28. Srinivasan G: Infants of drug-dependent mothers. In Yeh TF (ed): Neonatal Therapeutics, 2nd ed. St. Louis: Mosby Year Book, 1991, pp 32–39.

29. King TA, Perlman JM, Laptook AR, et al: Neurologic manifestations of in utero cocaine exposure in near-term and term infants. Pediatrics 1995;96(2 Pt 1):259–264.

30. Frank DA, Augustyn M, Zuckerman BS: Neonatal neurobehavioral and neuroanatomic correlates of prenatal cocaine exposure. Problems of dose and confounding. Ann N Y Acad Sci 1998;846:40–50.

31. Lester BM, Corwin MJ, Sepkoski C, et al: Neurobehavioral syndromes in cocaine-exposed newborn infants. Child Dev 1991;62(4):694–705.

32. Konkol RJ, Murphey LJ, Ferriero DM, et al: Cocaine metabolites in the neonate: potential for toxicity. J Child Neurol 1994;9(3):242–248.

33. Chambers CD, Johnson KA, Dick LM, et al: Birth outcomes in pregnant women taking fluoxetine. N Engl J Med 1996;335(14):1010–1015.

34. Kulin NA, Pastuszak A, Sage SR, et al: Pregnancy outcome following maternal use of the new selective serotonin reuptake inhibitors: a prospective controlled multicenter study. JAMA 1998;279(8):609–610.

35. Nordeng H, Lindemann R, Perminov KV, Reikvam A: Neonatal withdrawal syndrome after in utero exposure to selective serotonin reuptake inhibitors. Acta Paediatr 2001;90(3):288–291.

36. Stiskal JA, Kulin N, Koren G, et al: Neonatal paroxetine withdrawal syndrome. Arch Dis Child Fetal Neonatal Ed 2001;84(2):F134–F135.

37. Costei AM, Kozer E, Ho T, et al: Perinatal outcome following third trimester exposure to paroxetine. Arch Pediatr Adolesc Med 2002;156(11):1129–1132.

38. Alessio L, Dell'Orto A, Calzaferri G, et al: Cadmium concentrations in blood and urine of pregnant women at delivery and their offspring. Sci Total Environ 1984;34(3):261–266.

39. Sikorski R, Paszkowski T, Slawinski P, et al: The intrapartum content of toxic metals in maternal blood and umbilical cord blood. Ginekol Pol 1989;60(3):151–155.

40. Plockinger B, Dadak C, Meisinger V. [Lead, mercury and cadmium in newborn infants and their mothers]. Z Geburtshilfe Perinatol 1993;197(2):104–107.

41. Needleman HL, Rabinowitz M, Leviton A, et al: The relationship between prenatal exposure to lead and congenital anomalies. JAMA 1984;251(22):2956–2959.

42. Sensirivatana R, Supachadhiwong O, Phancharoen S, Mitrakul C: Neonatal lead poisoning. An unusual clinical manifestation. Clin Pediatr (Phila) 1983;22(8):582–584.

43. Ghafour SY, Khuffash FA, Ibrahim HS, Reavey PC: Congenital lead intoxication with seizures due to prenatal exposure. Clin Pediatr (Phila) 1984;23(5):282–283.

44. Dietrich K: Low-level lead exposure during pregnancy and its consequences for fetal and child development. In Pueschel S, Linakis J, Anderson A (eds): Lead Poisoning in Childhood. Baltimore, Paul H. Brookes Publishing, 1996, pp 117–139.

45. Liebelt EL, Shannon MW: Oral chelators for childhood lead poisoning. Pediatr Ann 1994;23(11):616–619, 623–626.

46. Linakis JG: Childhood lead poisoning. RI Med 1995;78(1):22–26.

47. Chisolm J Jr: Medical management. In Pueschel S, Linakis J, Anderson A (eds): Lead Poisoning in Childhood. Baltimore, Paul H. Brookes Publishing, 1996, pp 141–162.

48. Grandjean P, Weihe P, Nielsen JB: Methylmercury: significance of intrauterine and postnatal exposures. Clin Chem 1994;40(7 Pt 2):1395–1400.

49. Koos BJ, Longo LD: Mercury toxicity in the pregnant woman, fetus, and newborn infant. A review. Am J Obstet Gynecol 1976;126(3):390–409.

50. Kondo K: Congenital Minamata disease: warnings from Japan's experience. J Child Neurol 2000;15(7):458–464.

51. Eto K: Minamata disease. Neuropathology 2000;20(Suppl):14–19.

52. Bilderback J: Group of cases of unknown etiology and diagnosis. Northwest Med 1920;19:263.

53. Schumacher E: Outbreak of mercury poisoning in Argentine babies is linked to diapers. New York Times, January 20, 1981, section A, p 18.

54. Waffarn F, Hodgman JE: Mercury vapor contamination of infant incubators: a potential hazard. Pediatrics 1979;64(5):640–642.

55. McLaughlin JF, Telzrow RW, Scott CM: Neonatal mercury vapor exposure in an infant incubator. Pediatrics 1980;66(6):988–990.

56. Schroder CH, Severijnen RS, Monnens LA: [Poisoning by disinfectants in the conservative treatment of 2 patients with omphalocele]. Tijdschr Kindergeneeskd 1985;53(2):76–79.

57. Mullins ME, Horowitz BZ: Iatrogenic neonatal mercury poisoning from Mercurochrome treatment of a large omphalocele. Clin Pediatr (Phila) 1999;38(2):111–112.

58. Stanley-Brown EG, Frank JE: Mercury poisoning from application to omphalocele. JAMA 1971;216(13):2144–2145.

59. Yeh TF, Pildes RS, Firor HV: Mercury poisoning from Mercurochrome therapy of an infected omphalocele. Clin Toxicol 1978;13(4):463–467.

60. Clark JA, Kasselberg AG, Glick AD, O'Neill JA Jr: Mercury poisoning from merbromin (Mercurochrome) therapy of omphalocele: correlation of toxicologic, histologic, and electron microscopic findings. Clin Pediatr (Phila) 1982;21(7):445–447.

61. Festen C, Severijnen RS, vd Staak FH: Nonsurgical (conservative) treatment of giant omphalocele. A report of 10 cases. Clin Pediatr (Phila) 1987;26(1):35–39.

62. Amin-Zaki L, Elhassani S, Majeed MA, et al: Perinatal methylmercury poisoning in Iraq. Am J Dis Child 1976;130(10):1070–1076.

63. Amin-Zaki L, Majeed MA, Greenwood MR, et al: Methylmercury poisoning in the Iraqi suckling infant: a longitudinal study over five years. J Appl Toxicol 1981;1(4):210–214.

64. Bakir F, Rustam H, Tikriti S, et al: Clinical and epidemiological aspects of methylmercury poisoning. Postgrad Med J 1980;56(651):1–10.

65. Meme JS, Brown JD, Kagia J, et al: Mercury poisoning as a cause of acrodynia in Kenya children—a preliminary report. East Afr Med J 1981;58(9):641–649.

66. Moutinho ME, Tompkins AL, Rowland TW, et al: Acute mercury vapor poisoning. Fatality in an infant. Am J Dis Child 1981;135(1):42–44.

67. Goldman LR, Shannon MW: Technical report: mercury in the environment: implications for pediatricians. Pediatrics 2001;108(1):197–205.

68. Ramirez GB, Cruz MC, Pagulayan O, et al: The Tagum study I: analysis and clinical correlates of mercury in maternal and cord blood, breast milk, meconium, and infants' hair. Pediatrics 2000;106(4):774–781.

69. Ramirez GB, Pagulayan O, Akagi H, et al: Tagum study II: follow-up study at two years of age after prenatal exposure to mercury. Pediatrics 2003;111(3):e289–e295.

70. Koppe JG: Dioxins and furans in the mother and possible effects on the fetus and newborn breast-fed baby. Acta Paediatr Scand Suppl 1989;360:146–153.

71. Koppe JG, Pluim HJ, Olie K, van Wijnen J: Breast milk, dioxins and the possible effects on the health of newborn infants. Sci Total Environ 1991;106(1–2):33–41.

72. Koopman-Esseboom C, Huisman M, Weisglas-Kuperus N, et al: Dioxin and PCB levels in blood and human milk in relation to living areas in The Netherlands. Chemosphere 1994;29(9–11): 2327–2338.

73. Sauer PJ, Huisman M, Koopman-Esseboom C, et al: Effects of polychlorinated biphenyls (PCBs) and dioxins on growth and development. Hum Exp Toxicol 1994;13(12):900–906.

74. Lanting CI, Patandin S, Fidler V, et al: Neurological condition in 42-month-old children in relation to pre- and postnatal exposure to polychlorinated biphenyls and dioxins. Early Hum Dev 1998; 50(3):283–292.

75. Patandin S, Koopman-Esseboom C, de Ridder MA, et al: Effects of environmental exposure to polychlorinated biphenyls and dioxins on birth size and growth in Dutch children. Pediatr Res 1998;44(4):538–545.

76. Patandin S, Lanting CI, Mulder PG, et al: Effects of environmental exposure to polychlorinated biphenyls and dioxins on cognitive abilities in Dutch children at 42 months of age. J Pediatr 1999;134(1):33–41.

77. Siddiqui MK, Saxena MC, Bhargava AK, et al: Chlorinated hydrocarbon pesticides in blood of newborn babies in India. Pestic Monit J 1981;15(2):77–79.

78. Sarkar S, Narang A, Singh S: Transplacentally acquired carbamate insecticide (Baygon) poisoning in a neonate. Indian Pediatr 1994;31(3):343–346.

79. Rutter N. Clinical consequences of an immature barrier. Semin Neonatol 2000;5(4):281–287.

80. Scott E, Prince G, Rotondo C: Dye poisoning in infancy. J Pediatr 1946;28:713.

81. Howarth B: Spidemic of methaemoglobinaemia in newborn infants. Lancet 1951;1:934.

82. Chabrolle JP, Rossier A: Goitre and hypothyroidism in the newborn after cutaneous absorption of iodine. Arch Dis Child 1978;53(6):495–498.

83. Vivier PM, Lewander WJ, Martin HF, Linakis JG: Isopropyl alcohol intoxication in a neonate through chronic dermal exposure: a complication of a culturally-based umbilical care practice. Pediatr Emerg Care 1994;10(2):91–93.

84. Kahn A, Blum D: Methyl alcohol poisoning in an 8-month-old boy: an unusual route of intoxication. J Pediatr 1979;94(5):841–843.

85. Darwish A, Roth CE, Duclos P, et al: Investigation into a cluster of infant deaths following immunization: evidence for methanol intoxication. Vaccine 2002;20(29–30):3585–3589.

86. Lacouture PG, Wason S, Abrams A, Lovejoy FH Jr: Acute isopropyl alcohol intoxication. Diagnosis and management. Am J Med 1983;75(4):680–686.

87. Vicas IM, Beck R: Fatal inhalational isopropyl alcohol poisoning in a neonate. J Toxicol Clin Toxicol 1993;31(3):473–481.

88. Ittmann PI, Bozynski ME: Toxic epidermal necrolysis in a newborn infant after exposure to adhesive remover. J Perinatol 1993;13(6):476–477.

89. Gallagher JS, Kurt TL: Neonatal exposure to methyl chloroform in tape remover. Vet Hum Toxicol 1990;32(1):43–45.

90. Gemme G, Ruffa G, Bonioli E, et al: Picture of the month. Cushing's syndrome due to topical corticosteroids. Am J Dis Child 1984;138(10):987–988.

91. Piyaraly S, Boumahni B, Raudrant-Sigogne N, et al: [Percutaneous camphor and convulsions in a neonate]. Arch Pediatr 1998; 5(2):205–206.

92. Uc A, Bishop WP, Sanders KD: Camphor hepatotoxicity. South Med J 2000;93(6):596–598.

93. Siegel E, Wason S: Camphor toxicity. Pediatr Clin North Am 1986;33(2):375–379.

94. Sinisterra S, Miravet E, Alfonso I, et al: Methemoglobinemia in an infant receiving nitric oxide after the use of eutectic mixture of local anesthetic. J Pediatr 2002;141(2):285–286.

95. Montoya Cabrea MA, Hernandez Zamora A, Palacios Trevino JL: [Methemoglobinemia caused by inhalation of aniline vapors by a newborn]. Bol Med Hosp Infant Mex 1980;37(5):1021–1025.

96. Heal CA, Spencer SA: Methaemoglobinaemia with high-dose nitric oxide administration. Acta Paediatr 1995;84(11):1318–1319.

97. Nakajima W, Ishida A, Arai H, Takada G: Methaemoglobinaemia after inhalation of nitric oxide in infant with pulmonary hypertension. Lancet 1997;350(9083):1002–1003.

98. Lopez A, Bernardo B, Lopez-Herce J, et al: Methaemo-globinaemia secondary to treatment with trimethoprim and sulphamethoxazole associated with inhaled nitric oxide. Acta Paediatr 1999;88(8):915–916.

99. Heber G, Hasenburg A, Jaspers V, Spatling L: [Methemo-globinemia in the newborn infant—caused by prilocaine? A case report]. Zentralbl Gynakol 1995;117(2):105–107.

100. Dudley AG, Conrad LL, Martin DM: Newborn methemo-globinemia following propitocaine intrapartum epidural block. First case report. Obstet Gynecol 1970;35(1):75–77.

101. Hrgovic Z: [Methemoglobinemia in a newborn infant following pudendal anesthesia in labor with prilocaine. A case report]. Anasth Intensivther Notfallmed 1990;25(2):172–174.

102. Lloyd CJ: Chemically induced methaemoglobinaemia in a neonate. Br J Oral Maxillofac Surg 1992;30(1):63–65.

103. Duncan PG, Kobrinsky N: Prilocaine-induced methemoglo-binemia in a newborn infant. Anesthesiology 1983;59(1):75–76.

104. Kara A, Yigit S, Aygun C, Oran O: Toxic methemoglobinemia after injection of prilocaine in a newborn. A case report. Turk J Pediatr 1998;40(4):589–592.

105. Ergenekon E, Atalay Y, Koc E, Turkyilmaz C: Methaemo-globinaemia in a premature infant secondary to prilocaine. Acta Paediatr 1999;88(2):236.

106. Jakobson B, Nilsson A: Methemoglobinemia associated with a prilocaine-lidocaine cream and trimethoprim-sulphamethoxazole. A case report. Acta Anaesthesiol Scand 1985;29(4):453–455.

107. Nioloux C, Floch-Tudal C, Jaby-Sergent MP, Lejeune C: [Local anesthesia with Emla cream and risk of methemoglobinaemia in a premature infant]. Arch Pediatr 1995;2(3):291–292.

108. Elsner P, Dummer R: Signs of methaemoglobinaemia after topical application of EMLA cream in an infant with haemangioma. Dermatology 1997;195(2):153–154.

109. Couper RT: Methaemoglobinaemia secondary to topical lignocaine/prilocaine in a circumcised neonate. J Paediatr Child Health 2000;36(4):406–407.

110. Thomas SG, Philips JB 3rd: Methemoglobinemia in a neonate due to topical benzocaine cream. J Perinatol 1989;9(3):361–362.

111. Sills MR, Zinkham WH: Methylene blue-induced Heinz body hemolytic anemia. Arch Pediatr Adolesc Med 1994;148(3): 306–310.

112. Weinstock M, Hartnett L: Toxic emergencies in the neonate. In Haddad LM, Winchester JF (eds): Clinical Management of Poisoning and Drug Overdose, 2nd ed. Philadelphia, WB Saunders, 1990, pp 436–444.

113. Smith A: Chloramphenicol. In Yaffe S, Aranda J (eds): Pediatric Pharmacology: Therapeutic Principles in Practice. Philadelphia, WB Saunders, 1992, pp 276–286.

114. Lacouture PG, Epstein MF, Mitchell AA: Vancomycin-associated shock and rash in newborn infants. J Pediatr 1987;111(4):615–616.

115. Boussemart T, Cardona J, Berthier M, et al: Cardiac arrest associated with vancomycin in a neonate. Arch Dis Child Fetal Neonatal Ed 1995;73(2):F123.

116. Koren G, Lau A, Kenyon CF, et al: Clinical course and pharmacokinetics following a massive overdose of amphotericin B in a neonate. J Toxicol Clin Toxicol 1990;28(3):371–378.

117. Googe JH, Walterspiel JN: Arrhythmia caused by amphotericin B in a neonate. Pediatr Infect Dis J 1988;7(1):73.

118. Perlman JM, Acarregui M, Gard JW: Fatal overdose of amphotericin B in two preterm infants. Dev Pharmacol Ther 1991;17(3–4):187–190.

119. Connor EM, Sperling RS, Gelber R, et al: Reduction of maternal-infant transmission of human immunodeficiency virus type 1 with zidovudine treatment. Pediatric AIDS Clinical Trials Group Protocol 076 Study Group. N Engl J Med 1994;331(18):1173–1180.

120. Mandelbrot L, Landreau-Mascaro A, Rekacewicz C, et al: Lamivudine-zidovudine combination for prevention of maternal-infant transmission of HIV-1. JAMA 2001;285(16):2083–2093.

121. Blanche S, Tardieu M, Rustin P, et al: Persistent mitochondrial dysfunction and perinatal exposure to antiretroviral nucleoside analogues. Lancet 1999;354(9184):1084–1089.

122. Barret B, Tardieu M, Rustin P, et al: Persistent mitochondrial dysfunction in HIV-1-exposed but uninfected infants: clinical screening in a large prospective cohort. AIDS 2003;17(12):1769–1785.

123. Scalfaro P, Chesaux JJ, Buchwalder PA, et al: Severe transient neonatal lactic acidosis during prophylactic zidovudine treatment. Intensive Care Med 1998;24(3):247–250.

124. Bhatia J: Current options in the management of apnea of prematurity. Clin Pediatr (Phila) 2000;39(6):327–336.

125. Ergenekon E, Dalgic N, Aksoy E, et al: Caffeine intoxication in a premature neonate. Paediatr Anaesth 2001;11(6):737–739.

126. Perrin C, Debruyne D, Lacotte J, et al: Treatment of caffeine intoxication by exchange transfusion in a newborn. Acta Paediatr Scand 1987;76(4):679–681.

127. Anderson BJ, Gunn TR, Holford NH, Johnson R: Caffeine overdose in a premature infant: clinical course and pharmacokinetics. Anaesth Intensive Care 1999;27(3):307–311.

128. Larcher VF, Gamsu HR, Sanderson MC, et al: Theophylline toxicity in a neonate. Arch Dis Child 1978;53(9):757–759.

129. Wells DH, Ferlauto JJ: Survival after massive aminophylline overdose in a premature infant. Pediatrics 1979;64(2):252–253.

130. Strauss AA, Modanlou HD, Komatsu G: Theophylline toxicity in a preterm infant: selected clinical aspects. Pediatr Pharmacol (New York) 1985;5(3):209–212.

131. Jain R, Tholl DA: Activated charcoal for theophylline toxicity in a premature infant on the second day of life. Dev Pharmacol Ther 1992;19(2–3):106–110.

132. Osborn HH, Henry G, Wax P, et al: Theophylline toxicity in a premature neonate—elimination kinetics of exchange transfusion. J Toxicol Clin Toxicol 1993;31(4):639–644.

133. Colonna F, Trappan A, de Vonderweid U, Nisi G: Peritoneal dialysis in a 6-weeks old preterm infant with severe theophylline intoxication. Minerva Pediatr 1996;48(9):383–385.

134. Gitomer JJ, Khan AM, Ferris ME: Treatment of severe theophylline toxicity with hemodialysis in a preterm neonate. Pediatr Nephrol 2001;16(10):784–786.

135. Lowry JA, Jarrett RV, Wasserman G, et al: Theophylline toxicokinetics in premature newborns. Arch Pediatr Adolesc Med 2001;155(8):934–939.

136. Sullivan JL: Caffeine poisoning in an infant. J Pediatr 1977;90(6):1022–1023.

137. Banner W Jr, Czajka PA: Acute caffeine overdose in the neonate. Am J Dis Child 1980;134(5):495–498.

138. van den Anker JN, Jongejan HT, Sauer PJ: Severe caffeine intoxication in a preterm neonate. Eur J Pediatr 1992;151(6):466–467.

139. Shannon M, Amitai Y, Lovejoy FH Jr: Multiple dose activated charcoal for theophylline poisoning in young infants. Pediatrics 1987;80(3):368–370.

140. Laptook AR, Rosenfeld CR: Chloral hydrate toxicity in a preterm infant. Pediatr Pharmacol (New York) 1984;4(3):161–165.

141. Anyebuno MA, Rosenfeld CR: Chloral hydrate toxicity in a term infant. Dev Pharmacol Ther 1991;17(1–2):116–120.

142. Kirimi E, Caksen H, Cesur Y, et al: Chloral hydrate intoxication in a newborn infant. J Emerg Med 2002;22(1):104–105.

143. Caksen H, Odabas D, Uner A, et al: Respiratory arrest due to chloral hydrate in an infant. J Emerg Med 2003;24(3):342–343.

144. Goldsmith JP: Ventilatory management casebook. Chloral hydrate intoxication. J Perinatol 1994;14(1):74–76.

145. Wells S, Williamson M, Hooker D: Fentanyl-induced chest wall rigidity in a neonate: a case report. Heart Lung 1994;23(3):196–198.

146. Lemmen RJ, Semmekrot BA: Muscle rigidity causing life-threatening hypercapnia following fentanyl administration in a premature infant. Eur J Pediatr 1996;155(12):1067.

147. MacGregor DA, Bauman LA: Chest wall rigidity during infusion of fentanyl in a two-month-old infant after heart surgery. J Clin Anesth 1996;8(3):251–254.

148. Lindemann R: Respiratory muscle rigidity in a preterm infant after use of fentanyl during Caesarean section. Eur J Pediatr 1998;157(12):1012–1013.

149. Bolisetty S, Kitchanan S, Whitehall J: Generalized muscle rigidity in a neonate following intrathecal fentanyl during caesarean delivery. Intensive Care Med 1999;25(11):1337.

150. Bauer CR, Trottier MC, Stern L: Systemic cyclopentolate (Cyclogyl) toxicity in the newborn infant. J Pediatr 1973;82(3):501–505.

151. Carlsen JO, Zabriskie NA, Kwon YH, et al: Apparent central nervous system depression in infants after the use of topical brimonidine. Am J Ophthalmol 1999;128(2):255–256.

152. Berlin RJ, Lee UT, Samples JR, et al. Ophthalmic drops causing coma in an infant. J Pediatr 2001;138(3):441–443.

19 Toxicologic Issues in the Geriatric Patient

WENDY KLEIN-SCHWARTZ, PHARMD, MPH

INTRODUCTION AND EPIDEMIOLOGY

The elderly are the fastest growing segment of the population of the United States. Twelve percent of the population is 65 years of age or older, and this figure is projected to almost double by the year 2040.[1] Older adults are a heterogeneous group, with marked differences in physiologic aging and disease states. With advancing age, pharmacodynamic and pharmacokinetic responses to drugs and toxins are altered, usually increasing susceptibility to toxicity.[2] Physiologic changes as well as concurrent diseases and medications have an impact on the ability of older adults to compensate for the physiologic stress of an overdose.

Of 2,438,644 human exposure cases reported to the American Association of Poison Control Centers Toxic Exposure Surveillance System in 2004, only 115,232 (4.7%) cases occurred in persons 60 years of age and older.[3] Fatalities occur at a disproportionately high rate, with 157 of the 1183 fatalities (13.3%) occurring in persons 60 years of age and older. Suicide and therapeutic error/unintentional misuse were responsible for 943 and 27 deaths, respectively. Drugs were the primary substance in 73% of deaths. Higher death rates have been reported from poisonings for men 70 years of age and older and for women 60 years of age and older than for younger people.[4]

Unintentional Poisoning

Poison centers report that the majority of potentially toxic exposures in older adults are unintentional.[5-7] Of 237 older patients prospectively evaluated by a poison center, 66% were women; reasons were 83.1% unintentional, 14.9% suicide or attempted suicide, and 1.7% drug abuse.[5] Older patients who require emergency department management are more likely to be admitted than are younger patients.[5,7] The geriatric patient may be less able to cope with acute injury and, therefore, be less likely to improve rapidly while being evaluated and treated in the emergency department. Possible reasons include increased sensitivity to drugs, exaggerated or unusual responses to drugs, and impaired elimination of drugs resulting in prolonged symptomatology.

Adverse Drug Events

As a group, older adults consume more drugs than any other age segment of the population, taking on average 2 to 6 prescription drugs and 1 to 3.4 nonprescription drugs.[8] Older adults account for 25% of total drug expenditures, which is projected to be 40% in 2030.[9] A consequence of age and disease-related effects on drug action and disposition as well as polypharmacy is a high incidence of adverse drug events (ADEs). Of 1523 ADEs during 1 year in ambulatory older adults, 578 (38.0%) were considered serious, life threatening, or fatal, and 244 of these were considered preventable.[10] Most common preventable ADEs were electrolyte/renal, gastrointestinal, hemorrhagic, metabolic/endocrine, and neuropsychiatric. Most commonly implicated drug categories associated with preventable ADEs were cardiovascular drugs, diuretics, nonopioid analgesics, hypoglycemics, and anticoagulants. The severity of ADEs increases with age, and older patients are at higher risk for ADE-related admissions. ADEs are responsible for approximately 10% of hospital admissions in older patients.[11]

Older adults are vulnerable to drug-drug interactions, with important risk factors including number of drugs prescribed and number of physicians treating the patient.[12] Serious interactions most frequently involve drugs commonly used in older adults that have narrow therapeutic indices such as digoxin, calcium channel blockers, antiarrhythmics, oral hypoglycemics, cyclic antidepressants, warfarin, salicylates, centrally acting analgesics, phenytoin, and theophylline. Risk increases when older patients take combinations of drugs that interact to cause additive hypotension, sedation, or anticholinergic effects.

Alcohol, drug misuse, and drug abuse are common, yet frequently underdiagnosed.[13,14] Abuse of legal substances such as sedative-hypnotics, antipsychotics, antidepressants, antianxiety agents, stimulants, and analgesics is more common in older adults than abuse of illicit substances. The incidence of alcohol abuse is 2% to 10%. Psychosocial factors such as inability to deal with loss as well as perceived loss of independence or control of one's life contribute to drug and alcohol abuse.

Suicide

Depression is common among older persons, and suicide rates are higher for older adults than for other age groups.[15,16] Possible explanations for the higher rate of completed suicides in older adults include greater intention to die, social isolation (which decreases chance of early discovery), use of more lethal means, and poorer recuperative powers (e.g., due to chronic disease or impaired drug elimination).[17] Although firearms are most often used in completing suicides, overdose is common in attempting suicide.[18] In women, drug overdose is responsible for suicides almost as frequently as firearms.[19] Drugs commonly used in suicides in older patients include acetaminophen, benzodiazepines, antidepressants, and opiates.[20]

Although suicide attempts by acute overdoses are easy to recognize, purposeful mixing of drugs or failure to

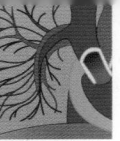

take life-sustaining drugs with the intention of ending one's life may be much less obvious. Underdetection of poisoning is an issue in determining the magnitude of the problem in the older patient. A study of the fatal overdose rates for cyclic antidepressants concluded that lower apparent fatality rates with age were most likely an artifact of underreporting of deaths in older patients. Deaths from poisoning cannot always be easily identified and may be attributed to natural causes in the elderly.[21]

RELEVANT ANATOMY, PHYSIOLOGY, AND PHARMACOLOGY

Table 19-1 summarizes age-related physiologic changes that alter the pharmacodynamics and pharmacokinetics of drugs and toxins.[11] These factors, coupled with pre-existing diseases and poor nutritional status, can increase the likelihood of toxicity, alter toxic manifestations and time course, and affect the geriatric patient's ability to cope with a toxic exposure.

Physiologic and Pharmacodynamic Features

Although deterioration of physiologic functions of all organs occurs with age, there is wide interindividual variability in the extent. Older adults experience changes in neurologic, cardiovascular, pulmonary, hepatic, renal, immunologic, and endocrine function.[11] Older persons have a reduced physiologic reserve, increasing the possibility of decompensation under stress. Older patients are less able to regulate body temperature, blood pH, blood glucose, blood pressure, heart rate, and oxygen consumption. Age-related changes in receptor density and sensitivity have been documented for drugs (e.g., opioids, benzodiazepines), hormones (e.g., androgens, estrogens, gonadotropin, thyroid), and neurotransmitters (e.g., cholinergic, dopaminergic, β-adrenergic, serotonergic receptors, γ-aminobutyric acid [GABA]).[11,22,23]

Geriatric patients are more sensitive to centrally acting drugs such as benzodiazepines, β blockers, central

TABLE 19-1 Age-related Physiologic Changes		
SYSTEM	**AGE-RELATED CHANGE**	**EXAMPLES OF DRUG-RELATED EFFECTS**
Neurologic	Reduced brain weight Loss of neurons Increased conduction time Decreased cerebral blood flow Altered permeability of blood-brain barrier	Enhanced sensitivity to drugs Decreased coordination and prolonged reaction time leading to increased risk of falls
Cardiovascular	Hypertrophy Decreased cardiac output Prolonged contraction Decreased resting heart rate Increased systolic blood pressure Increased vessel thickness Increased total vascular resistance Decreased baroreceptor sensitivity	Decreased response to stress, including overdose Decreased perfusion of organs Increased symptomatic orthostasis
Liver	Decreased mass Decreased blood flow Decreased number of hepatocytes Reduced phase I drug metabolism	Increased bioavailability of drugs with first pass metabolism Altered drug metabolism (usually diminished)
GI tract	Decreased gastric acid secretion Decreased intestinal epithelium surface Decreased splanchnic blood flow Decreased gut motility	Minimal effects on drug absorption
Kidneys	Decreased mass Decreased blood flow Decreased glomerular filtration rate Decreased creatinine clearance Decreased tubular secretion	Decreased drug excretion
Body composition	Decreased total body water Decreased lean body mass Increased adipose tissue Decreased plasma albumin Increased α_1-acid glycoprotein	Decreased volume of distribution and increased plasma concentration of hydrophilic drugs Decreased clearance of lipophilic basic drugs
Endocrine	Decreased estrogens Impaired insulin release Decreased number of insulin receptors Decreased thyroid hormone Decreased response of hypothalamic-pituitary axis to glucocorticoids	Increased susceptibility to drug-induced hypoglycemia Increased risk of drug-induced hypothermia Increased sensitivity to drug effects (e.g., digoxin)
Receptors	Altered density and/or sensitivity of drug, hormone, and neurotransmitter receptors	Altered drug response (usually increased sensitivity to drugs)

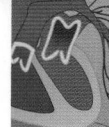

α-agonists, cyclic antidepressants, barbiturates, and opiates than are younger adults.[22,24] Altered thermoregulation can be exacerbated by phenothiazines. Postural hypotension is more likely in older patients taking nitroglycerin, phenothiazines, diuretics, nifedipine, methyldopa, and prazosin because of diminished baroreceptor sensitivity and responsiveness.[22] As a result of reduced postural stability, older adults are more prone to falls and fractures, especially when taking central nervous system (CNS) active drugs.

Geriatric patients are vulnerable to peptic ulcer disease and congestive heart failure associated with nonsteroidal anti-inflammatory drug (NSAID) therapy.[25,26] Salicylates can exacerbate gastritis, resulting in grastrointestinal (GI) bleeding. Older patients with alcoholism, preexisting liver disease, or poor nutritional status are at risk for chronic acetaminophen toxicity. Preexisting alteration in grastrointestinal motility predisposes elderly patients to constipation with therapeutic use of opioids and drugs with anticholinergic properties.

Interplay between organs with diminished function is evident in older persons and may affect drug pharmacokinetics or response. For example, the responsiveness of the cardiovascular system decreases with age. Changes in cardiac output, contractility, total vascular resistance, heart rate, and blood pressure may lead to decreased perfusion of the kidneys and liver, which in turn decreases drug metabolism and excretion. Delivery of drugs to other tissues, such as the CNS, may be reduced. Alternatively, drug-induced changes in blood flow may have adverse consequences in an older person because perfusion of vital organs already is diminished.

Pharmacokinetics

ABSORPTION

Although aging is associated with altered physiology and function of the GI tract, drug absorption is generally unchanged.[11,22] Some drugs (e.g., antihistamines, cyclic antidepressants, opioids) may slow drug absorption by inhibiting GI motility. Reduced first pass metabolism in older adults may increase bioavailability of drugs such as propranolol, verapamil, nifedipine, and nefazodone.[11]

DISTRIBUTION

With aging, intracellular and extracellular water and lean body mass decrease while adipose tissue increases.[22] The increased ratio of fat to lean body mass results in reduced volumes of distribution and increased plasma concentrations for hydrophilic drugs and the reverse for lipophilic drugs. Examples of drugs with reduced volume of distribution in older adults include cimetidine, acebutolol, digoxin, levodopa, lithium, and morphine.[11] Reduced plasma protein binding associated with a decline in plasma albumin may be important for drugs with low volumes of distribution such as oral anticoagulants and sulfonylureas. α_1-Acid glycoprotein, which binds to lipophilic basic drugs such as lidocaine, propranolol, imipramine, and morphine, increases with age, which decreases drug clearance.

METABOLISM

With age, changes in liver mass, blood flow, and hepatocytes alter phase I metabolism (oxidation and reduction) while having little effect on phase II metabolism (conjugation).[11,27] Despite declines in hepatic function, drug metabolism is not significantly diminished, possibly because interindividual variation in metabolism exceeds the effect of age.[11,24]

RENAL EXCRETION

Decrease in drug elimination due to decreased renal function is the most important pharmacokinetic change with age. Serum creatinine does not predictably increase with reduced creatinine clearance, owing to diminished muscle mass, so it is an unreliable guide to renal excretory capacity. Chronic therapeutic intoxications resulting from decreased renal clearance have been reported with drugs such as lithium, digoxin, and salicylates. Impaired renal function may also prolong the course of an overdose for drugs primarily excreted by the kidneys.

High-risk Drugs

Box 19-1 lists drugs with high risk of toxicity as a result of high prevalence of use in older adults and low therapeutic index. Additional detail on drugs of particular concern follows.

SALICYLATES

Older adults have a higher mortality rate following acute salicylate overdoses.[28] Patients with chronic salicylate

---

BOX 19-1   DRUGS WITH HIGH RISK OF TOXICITY IN THE GERIATRIC PATIENT

Analgesic
Acetaminophen
NSAIDs
Opioids
Salicylates

Anticoagulant
Warfarin

Cardiovascular
Antiarrhythmics
β-Adrenergic blockers
Calcium channel blockers
Digoxin

Psychotherapeutic
Cyclic antidepressants
Lithium
Neuroleptics (e.g., phenothiazines)
Sedative-hypnotics (e.g., benzodiazepines)

Theophylline

Anticholinergic
Antihistamines
Cyclic antidepressants
Neuroleptics

Oral Hypoglycemic
Metformin
Oral sulfonylureas

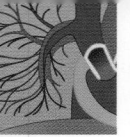

intoxications are older, have associated medical problems, and experience more serious symptomatology, especially CNS effects and pulmonary edema.[29,30] Factors that predispose older patients to salicylate intoxication include impaired renal function and dehydration. Salicylate poisoning can mimic other illnesses, such as diabetic ketoacidosis, cerebrovascular accidents, cardiopulmonary disease, encephalopathy, and alcohol withdrawal, and should be considered whenever an older patient presents with recent deterioration in activities of daily living with no known cause, with delirium or dementia, or with unexplained acid–base disorders.[29,30]

ANTICHOLINERGICS

Diminished cholinergic transmission may increase sensitivity of geriatric patients to drugs having anticholinergic effects (e.g., antihistamines, cyclic antidepressants, phenothiazines).[31] Polypharmacy with more than one drug with anticholinergic properties is contributory. These drugs may worsen medical conditions such as angina, constipation, glaucoma, and urinary dysfunction.[31] Control of bladder function is lessened with advancing age and may be further reduced by anticholinergic drugs with sedating properties.[31] Older patients are more susceptible to anticholinergic-induced cognitive impairment, including disorientation, confusion, delirium, memory impairment, and obtundation.[32] Pupillary dilatation and inability to accommodate may increase the risk of falls.

PSYCHOTHERAPEUTIC DRUGS

Plasma concentrations of *cyclic antidepressants* and long-acting *benzodiazepines* (e.g., diazepam, flurazepam, chlordiazepoxide) are higher because of reduced hepatic clearance with aging.[33,34] ADEs include confusion, delirium, memory impairment, daytime sedation, and ataxia as well as increased risk for falls.[32,35] Older adults with preexisting ischemic heart disease or conduction disturbances may be at greater risk for myocardial infarction, cerebrovascular accident, or congestive heart failure (CHF) following a cyclic antidepressant overdose. *Lithium*'s volume of distribution and renal clearance are reduced with age.[36] Other drugs (e.g., thiazide, angiotensin-converting enzyme [ACE] inhibitors, NSAIDs) and medical conditions (e.g., CHF, renal failure) can also decrease lithium clearance and increase the risk of toxicity in the geriatric patient.

CARDIOVASCULAR DRUGS

Older adults are more likely to experience digoxin toxicity because of high prevalence of use, decreased renal function, lower volume of distribution, increased number of comorbid conditions and concurrent interacting medications, and more frequent occurrence of electrolyte abnormalities (usually related to diuretic therapy).[37] *Calcium channel blockers* and *β blockers* are available at high doses as extended-release products and so only a few extra tablets can cause prolonged toxicity. For some drugs, higher blood concentrations result from either increased bioavailability (e.g., propranolol, verapamil, nifedipine) or decreased clearance (e.g.,

verapamil, nifedipine). Older patients with nodal disease may be at increased risk for bradycardia with therapeutic doses. Older adults are more sensitive to confusion and cognitive impairment associated with β blockers as well as bronchospasm in those with chronic obstructive pulmonary disease (COPD). Hypotension is a potential adverse effect in older patients taking a calcium channel blocker or β blocker while concurrently receiving a drug that lowers blood pressure (e.g., cyclic antidepressant, phenothiazine, nitrate, ACE inhibitor).[12]

ORAL HYPOGLYCEMICS

Oral sulfonylureas, including acetohexamide, tolbutamide, glipizide, and glyburide, can cause hypoglycemia from therapeutic use with inadequate food intake or following an overdose. Risk of hypoglycemia is increased in patients with liver or renal impairment; poor nutrition and living alone compound the potential for severe hypoglycemic episodes in older patients. Prolonged hypoglycemia after small doses of glyburide have been reported in older adults.[38,39] The risk of lactic acidosis from metformin increases with impaired renal function, advancing age, or concomitant use of drugs that affect creatinine clearance or renal tubular secretion of metformin.

TREATMENT PRINCIPLES

Patient Evaluation

History includes information regarding the toxin, patient's condition, and circumstances of the exposure as well as past medical history, including preexisting medical conditions and medications. For older patients with cognitive impairment querying family members or caregivers is necessary.

Older patients treated for toxic exposures in the emergency department are more likely to be admitted.[5] Because of greater susceptibility to toxicity, aggressive initial treatment of acute overdose or chronic intoxication may be required. Recognition of poisoning may be problematic because of atypical manifestations of toxic ingestions in older adults, further compounded by the fact that many diseases present with similar features. Toxicologic syndromes must be diagnosed with caution in the geriatric patient, because normal aging, chronic disease, and polypharmacy may obscure expected findings and lead to misdiagnosis. Toxicity may occur at blood concentrations considered therapeutic in younger adults, further confusing the diagnosis.

Treatment

The principles of management in older patients are similar to those for younger ones (see Chapter 2). Treatment of the ingestion should not exacerbate concomitant disease. Preexisting medical conditions may alter the older patient's response to the overdose and can necessitate additional treatment considerations. Another potential factor complicating management is

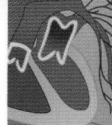

ASSESSMENT/TREATMENT	MANAGEMENT CONSIDERATIONS
TABLE 19-2 Considerations in Managing Poisoning in Geriatric Patients	
History	Need detailed past medical history and medication history
	Query relatives if patient is confused or demented
Seizure management	Greater sensitivity to benzodiazepines and barbiturates may increase need for subsequent intubation and respiratory support
GI decontamination	
Ipecac syrup	Avoid
Activated charcoal	If aspirated, preexisting pulmonary disease may lead to more significant deterioration
Cathartic	Greater susceptibility to fluid and electrolyte problems
Whole-bowel irrigation	Greater susceptibility to fluid and electrolyte problems
Elimination Enhancement	
Multiple-dose activated charcoal	Use cautiously in patients with poor GI motility
Hemodialysis/hemoperfusion	Consider at lower blood concentrations (e.g., salicylates, theophylline, lithium)
Antidote	Adverse effects more likely (e.g., precipitation of heart failure by digoxin-immune Fab in patients who require digoxin's intropic effect to maintain cardiac output; hypernatremia with hyperosmolarity from administration of sodium bicarbonate to alkalinize the blood for cardiotoxic drugs affecting the sodium channel or for salicylate overdose can lead to fluid overload and pulmonary edema, especially in patients with diminished cardiac or renal function)
	Need for dose modifications (e.g., additional Fab dosing if impaired renal function leads to rebound in free digoxin)

the effect of concurrent medications as well as the increased risk of ADEs and drug-drug interactions that the superimposed acute overdose poses during treatment of the overdose. Table 19-2 describes special considerations for managing overdoses in older adults.

PREVENTION

Psychiatric evaluation is imperative in cases of intentional ingestion. In addition to referral for psychiatric care, prevention strategies in older suicidal patients include recognizing and managing depression, treating alcohol abuse, limiting the number of doses dispensed per prescription, and decreasing social isolation.[40]

ADEs can be minimized by evaluating the need for drug therapy and by using the safest drug, starting with low doses and adjusting doses by small increments over long intervals.[32] Drug–drug interactions can be prevented by avoiding or limiting polypharmacy, adjusting drug dosages when interacting drugs are prescribed, and regularly monitoring drug regimens for continued benefit (and possibly eliminating drugs) as well as evidence of toxicity.[12]

Many unintentional poison exposures are preventable. Physiologic changes in older adults (e.g., decreased vision, hearing, memory) contribute to therapeutic errors and unintentional misuse of household products. Examination of unintentional exposures in older adults discloses four types of contributing factors[5]: (1) dementia and confusion (e.g., eating substance for no reason; repeating doses after forgetting earlier dosing), (2) improper use of the product (e.g., topical or inhalation exposures during product use), (3) improper storage of the product (e.g., consuming nonfood products stored in food containers), (4) mistaken identities (e.g., cleaning product mistaken for mouthwash). Using

medication calendars or compliance packaging for ambulatory older patients can reduce confusion regarding dosing schedule. Providing written information for the hearing impaired and larger type size on labels for the visually impaired older adult can aid in proper use of medications and household products. For older adults who are unable to care for themselves or are confused about their medication regimen, help from family members or caregivers is essential. For demented patients, prevention strategies include limiting access to drugs, personal care products, and cleaning products by storing these products so that they are inaccessible.[41]

REFERENCES

1. Chutka DS, Evans JM, Fleming KD, et al: Drug prescribing for elderly patients. Mayo Clin Proc 1995;70:685.
2. Tumer N, Scarpace PJ, Lowenthal DT: Geriatric pharmacology: basic and clinical considerations. Ann Rev Pharmacol Toxicol 1992;32:271.
3. Watson WA, Litovitz TL, Rodgers GC II, et al: 2004 annual report of the American Association of Poison Control Centers Toxic Exposure Surveillance System. Am J Emerg Med 2005;23:589.
4. Woolf A, Fish S, Azzara C, et al: Serious poisonings among older adults: a study of hospitalization and mortality rates in Massachusetts 1983–85. Am J Public Health 1990;80:867.
5. Klein-Schwartz W, Oderda GM, Booze L: Poisoning in the elderly. J Am Geriatr Soc 1983;31:195.
6. Dean BS, Krenzelok EP: Poisoning in the elderly: an increasing problem for health care providers. J Toxicol Clin Toxicol 1987;25:411.
7. Kroner BA, Scott RB, Waring ER, et al: Poisoning in the elderly: characterization of exposures reported to a poison control center. J Am Geriatr Soc 1993;41:842.
8. Stewart RB, Cooper JW: Polypharmacy in the aged: practical solutions. Drugs Aging 1994;4:449.
9. Williams L, Lowenthal DT: Drug therapy in the elderly. South Med J 1992;85:127.
10. Gurwitz JH, Field TS, Rothschild HLR, et al: Incidence and preventability of adverse drug events among older persons in the ambulatory setting. JAMA 2003;289:1107.

11. Turnheim K: Drug dosage in the elderly: is it rational? Drugs Aging 1998;3:357.

12. Seymour RM, Routledge PA: Important drug-drug interactions in the elderly. Drugs Aging 1998;12:485.

13. Barone JA, Holland M: Drug use and abuse in the elderly. U.S. Pharmacist 1987;12:82.

14. King CJ, Van Hasselt VB, Segal DL, et al: Diagnosis and assessment of substance abuse in older adults: current strategies and issues. Addict Behav 1994;19:41.

15. Stevens JA, Hasbrouck LM, Durant TM, et al: Surveillance for injuries and violence among older adults. MMWR CDC Surveill Summ 1999;48:27.

16. Spicer RS, Miller TR: Suicide acts in 8 states: incidence and case fatality rates by demographics and method. Am J Public Health 2000;90:1885.

17. Svenson J: Obtundation in the elderly patient: presentation of a drug overdose. Am J Emerg Med 1987;5:524.

18. Bennett AT, Collins KA: Elderly suicide: a 10-year retrospective study. Am J Forensic Med Pathol 2001;22:169.

19. Meehan PJ, Saltzman LE, Sattin RW: Suicides among older United States residents: epidemiologic characteristics and trends. Am J Public Health 1991;81:1198.

20. Shah R, Uren Z, Baker A, et al: Trends in suicide from drug overdose in the elderly in England and Wales, 1993–1999. Int J Geriatr Psychiatry 2002;17:416.

21. Farmer RD, Pinder RM: Why do fatal overdose rates vary between antidepressants? Acta Psychiatr Scand Suppl 1989;354:25.

22. Hammerlein A, Derendorf H, Lowenthal DT: Pharmacokinetic and pharmacodynamic changes in the elderly: clinical implications. Clin Pharmacokinet 1998;35:49.

23. Severson JA: Neurotransmitter receptors and aging. J Am Geriatr Soc 1984;32:24.

24. Schmucker DL: Aging and drug disposition: an update. Pharmacol Rev 1985;37:133.

25. Solomon DH, Gurwitz JH: Toxicity of nonsteroidal anti-inflammatory drugs in the elderly: is advanced age a risk factor? Am J Med 1997;102:208.

25. Page J, Henry D: Consumption of NSAIDs and the development of congestive heart failure in elderly patients: an underrecognized public health problem. Arch Intern Med 2000;160:777.

27. Wynne HA, Cope LH, Mutch E, et al: The effect of age upon liver volume and apparent liver blood flow in healthy man. Hepatology 1989;9:927.

28. Chapman BJ, Proudfoot AT: Adult salicylate poisoning: deaths and outcome in patients with high plasma salicylate concentrations. Q J Med 1989;72:699.

29. Bailey RB, Jones SR: Chronic salicylate intoxications: a common cause of morbidity in the elderly. J Am Geriatr Soc 1989;37:556.

30. Durnas C, Cusack BJ: Salicylate intoxication in the elderly: recognition and recommendations on how to prevent it. Drugs Aging 1992;2:20.

31. Mintzer J, Burns A: Anticholinergic side-effects of drugs in elderly patients. J R Soc Med 2000;93:457.

32. Moore AR, O'Keefe ST: Drug-induced cognitive impairment in the elderly. Drugs Aging 1999;15:15.

33. Tamayo M, Fernandez de Gatta MM, Gutierrez JR, et al: High levels of tricyclic antidepressants in conventional therapy: determinant factors. Int J Clin Pharmacol Ther Toxicol 1988;26:495.

34. Everitt DE, Avorn J: Drug prescribing for the elderly. Arch Intern Med 1986;146:2393.

35. Ray WA, Griffin MR, Schaffner W, et al: Psychotropic drug use and the risk of hip fracture. N Engl J Med 1987;316:363.

36. Sproule BA, Hardy BG, Shulman KI: Differential pharmacokinetics of lithium in elderly patients. Drugs Aging 2000;16:165.

37. Wofford JL, Ettinger WH: Risk factors and manifestations of digoxin toxicity in the elderly. Am J Emerg Med 1991;9:11.

38. Edwards T, Braunstein G, Davidson M: Glyburide-induced hypoglycemia in an elderly patient: similarity of first generation and second generation sulfonylurea agents. Mt Sinai J Med 1985;32:644.

39. Sketris I, Wheeler D, York S: Hypoglycemic coma induced by inadvertent administration of glyburide. Drug Intell Clin Pharm 1984;18:142.

40. Frierson RL: Suicide attempts by the old and the very old. Arch Intern Med 1991;151:141.

41. Oderda GM, Klein-Schwartz W: Poison prevention in the elderly. Drug Intell Clin Pharm 1984;18:183.

20 *Childhood Poisonings*

A Prevention of Childhood Poisonings

ALAN DAVID WOOLF, MD, MPH

During the past 30 years, childhood morbidity and mortality due to poisoning have decreased as a result of new prevention strategies, along with improved triage and management techniques. Poisoning nevertheless remains a threat to the health of young children. More than 1.2 million poison exposures in children age 5 years and younger were reported by 62 reporting poison centers in the United States in 2004.[1] Although the prevention of poisonings might be broadly defined to include the prevention of excessive morbidity and mortality due to the injury once a poison exposure has taken place, in this chapter the definition is restricted to those measures that attempt to avert the poisoning exposure itself. Indeed, targeted education, improved technology, and more effective government regulations in the interest of poisoning prevention have served as models for efforts to prevent other types of injuries.

PASSIVE VERSUS ACTIVE STRATEGIES

Poisoning prevention strategies can be divided conceptually into passive and active interventions. Passive interventions are those measures that do not depend on behavioral changes by the public for their success. Examples include federal regulations prohibiting the retail sale of caustic agents in household products in concentrations higher than those regarded as safe for home use. Since highly concentrated corrosives have become less accessible to the public, the probability that they will cause poisoning is automatically reduced.

Another example of a passive safety strategy is packaging potentially dangerous medications in child-resistant containers. Such packaging limits a young child's chance of exposure to a toxic dose of a drug before being discovered by a supervising adult. Because the child-resistant cap is automatically part of the packaging, a parent does not need to make an active decision to implement this safety measure.

Active poisoning prevention strategies, on the other hand, are those that require sustained behavioral change in the target population if they are to be effective. For example, counseling parents to poison-proof their household requires continued vigilance to ensure proper handling of potential toxins entering the household and a sustained and repeated effort to ensure that those household products that might be poisonous to toddlers are stored safely.

THE ETIOLOGY OF POISONING

Motor and cognitive developmental milestones achieved by the infant and toddler increase the risk for a poisoning. Children start to walk at about 1 year of age, and thereafter they can explore a much expanded environment. With well-honed gross motor skills, they can climb onto countertops and open cabinets. Fine motor skills, including a newly developed pincer grasp, allow them to undo the lids of containers and place small objects in their mouths. Their oral exploratory behaviors, matched with a lack of discriminatory abilities for potable versus nonpotable objects, put them at high risk for ingesting poisons.[2]

Children living in families whose system of supervision has broken down are vulnerable to poisoning incidents. Some particular stress such as a recent move, family loss, or financial hardship can cause parents to relax their vigilance. Poisonings often occur when a parent is distracted—for example, around mealtime or when entertaining guests. Many poisonings occur when the parent-child interaction is not in the "business-as-usual" routine of everyday life. For example, at holiday time, the parents may be distracted from their usual supervisory activities by parties and family social gatherings. A pregnant woman who already has a toddler at home may inadvertently put him at risk for a poisoning by leaving an open container of prenatal iron pills on the counter. Grandparents may overlook the chore of poison-proofing their home before their grandchildren visit, leaving potent medications in easy reach on a nightstand. Previous studies have suggested that many childhood poisonings occur when a product is in use,[3,4] and the occurrences reinforce the idea that lack of supervision is what places a child at high risk. Another common etiology for childhood poisoning is the circumstance of medication giving; the child has access to an open medicine container, or the parent gives the child the wrong dose or the wrong medicine.[4]

Considerable evidence shows that complex family dynamics sometimes underlie poisoning incidents. Families of childhood poisoning repeaters are charac-

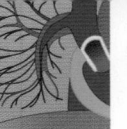

terized as disorganized, socially isolated, and operating under the stress of poor housing, frequent moves, or the psychiatric or physical illness of family members.[5-7] Sobel and Margolis have suggested that children who repeatedly poison themselves use such incidents as tactics in an ongoing power struggle with their parents.[8] They found that the mothers of such poisoning repeaters often came from disorganized households and had poor parental role models. The children were often products of an unwanted pregnancy and tended to be hyperactive and negativistic. The importance of such disordered family relationships in poisoning causation is reinforced by Baltimore and Meyer's findings that the poisoning recognition and storage habits of parents of 52 poisoned children were no different from those of parents of 52 control children.[9] Thus, the environmental hazards present seemed to be the same; what differed between families that had experienced childhood poisoning events and those that had not seemed to involve psychosocial and behavioral factors.

Poisoning prevention strategies that fail to address important moderators such as the behavior of the child, the organization and structure of the family, and the nature of the child-parent interaction have little chance for success. Although child-proofing changes in the house may remain static, the circumstances in which the threshold to a poisoning injury is breached are dynamic (e.g., opened household products or medications, poor supervision, altered family routines). Modification of these circumstances requires patience, counseling, increased social supports, and behavioral adaptations by both children and parents. These goals are somewhat elusive and are part of the challenge in the development of new poisoning prevention strategies.

GENERAL POISONING PREVENTION STRATEGIES

Model poisoning prevention strategies have sought to combine improved technologic advances with enlightened government regulations and effective public education to reduce the risk for a poisoning injury. Baker and colleagues[10] enumerated such general injury prevention strategies, when applied to poisonings, as follows:

1. Banning or reducing the manufacture or sale of an injurious toxin
2. Decreasing the concentration of a poison or the total amount available to the individual to sub-injurious levels
3. Preventing access to the substance
4. Creating barriers between the host and agent during the use of a potentially hazardous product
5. Substituting products with less inherent toxicity but equal efficacy for more dangerous products
6. Changing the formulation of a product to make it less injurious
7. Introduction of an aversive (bittering or pungency) agent to a household product to discourage ingestion

Each of these various principles has been successfully applied to various causes of poisoning among adults as well as children. The banning of dichlorodiphenyl-trichloroethane (DDT) exemplifies legislation targeted at preventing environmental toxic exposures. Limiting the number of baby aspirin to 36 tablets per bottle reduces the likelihood that toddlers can ingest an injurious dose. Child-resistant containers, blister packs for medication, and safe storage of hazardous products prevent access or create a barrier between the child and an injurious dose of the drug or household product. The substitution of acetaminophen for propoxyphene gives equal analgesia while avoiding propoxyphene's considerable toxicity in the event of overdose. The reformulation of children's cough and cold preparations and mouthwashes to exclude alcohol removes a potential source of toxicity to young children and infants. Model legislation in Oregon has required that bittering agents such as denatonium benzoate be added to automotive products such as ethylene glycol–based antifreeze and methanol-based windshield wiper fluid.[11] Whether such measures can decrease the volume of the products swallowed by young children in unintentional exposures and thereby reduce the severity of subsequent injury remains unclear.[11]

Although a number of excellent poisoning prevention strategies have been implemented to reduce adult injuries due to exposure to occupational or environmental poisons, strategies to prevent injuries to children due to environmental toxins are equally compelling if not more so. Such measures include regulations on the amount of pesticide residues allowed in foods or the amounts of contaminants in drinking water. However, this chapter addresses only those specific prevention strategies effective in reducing home poisoning among young children. The following strategies to prevent home poisonings are discussed:

1. Product packaging changes
2. Sticker trials
3. Community-wide programs
4. Clinic-based counseling
5. Growth of poison control centers

SPECIFIC POISONING PREVENTION STRATEGIES

Product Packaging Changes

As early as 1960, the federal government began to take regulatory steps to reduce the incidence of poisoning in the United States by passing the Federal Hazardous Substance Labeling Act. This consumer-oriented legislation required proper labeling of products but did not attempt to regulate their packaging, sale, or use.[12] During the next 15 years, better designs of child-resistant containers were developed and field tested. The rationale for such technology was developmental—that children at highest risk for accidental poisoning (i.e., those 18 to 36 months old) lacked the ability to combine

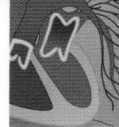

gross motor skills (the palmar exertion of a sufficient straight vector force) simultaneously with fine motor skills (the finger-exerted twisting of sufficient torque) to easily open products secured by child-resistant containers.

The technologic advances in the engineering of child-resistant containers, combined with enough education of the public to convince them of the potential worth of such packaging changes, culminated in passage of the Poison Prevention Packaging Act in 1970.[13] This legislation established standards for special packaging of household products and pharmaceuticals, defined appropriate testing procedures and those products that were subject to the regulation, and set a timetable for gradually phasing in the regulations during an 8-year period. The first products to be regulated were those containing aspirin. The products covered and the dates of implementation are listed in Table 20A-1. This regulation provides that if a consumer product presents a serious danger to children and special packaging is both technically feasible and practical, then a safety closure design must be submitted before the product is approved for marketing. Premarketing tests must demonstrate that 85% of a panel of 200 children younger than 5 years failed to open the package in a 5-minute period. A panel of adults is also allowed a single 5-minute period in which 90% must be able to open the safety closure after reading the opening instructions on the package. The regulations were recently extended to require child-resistant packaging for prescription drugs that are switched to over-the-counter status.[14]

The purpose of child-resistant containers is to separate the child physically from the potential poison by providing a barrier between the two. The intent of the regulation was not to poison-proof the container but simply to delay children long enough in their attempts to get at a poison for an adult to discover and correct the hazardous situation. Follow-up studies suggest that the effectiveness of child-resistant containers has been dramatic.[15-21] As a result of child-resistant packaging, an estimated 86,000 poisoning injuries were averted between the years 1974 and 1981.[15] Walton's study during a 6-year period (1972 to 1978) demonstrated a decline from 7500 to 2300 ingestions during the first 6-year period after the regulations took effect, whereas ingestions of various unregulated products either increased or stayed the same.[16] A recent modeling study estimated a 34% reduction in aspirin-related child mortality rates (preventing about 90 deaths) during 1973 through 1990, attributable to child-resistant packaging.[20]

In one public survey, more than 98% of parents could describe safety packaging.[22] An overwhelming 85% of the 636 families surveyed approved of the idea of safety packaging, and 89% had safety packages in the home. Only 3% of respondents had discontinued use of a product because of difficulty with the package. Vigilance concerning enforcement of the law is important. One study suggested that only 75% of medications dispensed by pharmacists were in compliant child-resistant containers.[23] However, overall the Poison Prevention Packaging Act is a model of well-crafted legislation brought about by successful combination of physician advocacy, improved technology, and effective public education.

The fact that many childhood poisonings occur with open products already in use[2,24] tempers the gains

TABLE 20A-1 Products Covered by the Poison Prevention Packaging Act (PPPA)

PPPA REGULATION	EFFECTIVE DATE	CHARACTERISTICS OF PRODUCTS REGULATED
Aspirin	8/14/72	Products for oral human use
Furniture polish	9/13/72	Nonemulsion liquid form, low viscosity, containing ≥ 10% mineral seal oil or petroleum distillates
Methylsalicylate	9/21/72	Liquid products containing ≥ 5% by weight
Controlled drugs	10/24/72	For oral human use
Sodium and/or potassium hydroxide	4/11/73	Dry form ≥ 10% by weight; other forms ≥ 2% by weight
Turpentin	7/1/73	Liquid from ≥ 10% by weight
Kindling and/or illuminating preparations	10/29/73	Prepackaged liquid, low viscosity, containing ≥ 10% petroleum distillates
Methyl alcohol	7/1/73	Liquids cotaining ≥ 4% by weight
Sulfuric acid	8/14/73	Substances containing ≥ 10% by weight
Prescription drugs	4/16/74	For oral human use
Ethylene glycol	6/1/74	Liquids containing ≥ 10% by weight
Paint solvents	4/23/77	Solvents for paints that contain ≥ 10% by weight of benzene, toluene, xylene
Iron-containing drugs	10/17/78	Noninjectable animal and human drugs containing 250 mg or more elemental iron (total package)
Dietary supplements	10/17/78	Dietary supplements containing 250 mg or more elemental iron (total package)
Acetaminophen	2/27/80	Preparations for oral human use with 1 g or more acetaminophen (total package)

From Walton W: An evaluation of the Poison Prevention Packaging Act. Pediatrics 1982;69:364.

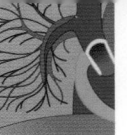

realized by the implementation of child-resistant packaging. Reducing the total number of pills per container sold and reducing the concentration of the drug in each pill are effective strategies for lowering the severity of a poisoning by lowering the attainable total dose.[25] More recent product changes have included the use of unit dosing with blister packs. Such dispensers are expensive but accomplish the dual purposes of lowering the risk for unintentional drug overdoses because of misinterpretation of dosing instruction and decreasing the risk for an overdose by children, who must spend more time unwrapping each individual pill and, thus, it is hoped, cannot ingest a harmful quantity before being discovered. The advent of tamper-resistant containers with protective plastic-wrapped seals has also decreased the risk that a product might be intentionally altered without being noticed by an unwary consumer. Such an outer wrap theoretically imposes yet another barrier to children. The success of such tamper-proof packaging in preventing poisonings has yet to be fully evaluated.

Sticker Trials

Older children can be educated to recognize hazardous agents and to avoid them. Such education usually includes the use of warning stickers that parents affix to hazardous household products to alert children to the danger. These stickers, picturing a skull and crossbones, angry serpent, or frowning face (Mr. Yuk), are meant to evoke psychologically unpleasant or fearsome images in a child's mind so that she or he will be deterred from sampling the poisonous contents. Braden found that such a method of discriminating hazardous agents was necessary; preschool children incorrectly identified 40% of poisonous products with which they were confronted.[26] When children were exposed to an educational program on products labeled with warning stickers, their accuracy of recognition improved to 86%. Krenzelok and Garber introduced poison recognition teaching aids into a daycare center program serving 3285 children 30 to 60 months old and tested 195 randomly selected children 6 weeks later.[27] The children showed improvements in their recognition of the warning symbol, Mr. Yuk, and in their understanding of which products were poisonous. However, no decrease in the incidence of poisonings has been associated with exposure to such a program. When Fergusson's group performed a controlled field trial that distributed labels to 583 families with 543 matched controls, no significant differences in poisoning rates could be appreciated.[28] More than 40% of the parents thought Mr. Yuk labels were not useful, had misgivings about the program, or did not use the warning labels to cover all the poisons in the home. Other concerns have been expressed about the use of warning stickers on household products. Some researchers and parents fear that young children may be attracted instead of repulsed by the warning stickers or may not be able to understand what a poison means.[29] Furthermore, many poisons (e.g., plants) cannot be labeled with a warning. Finally, those poisoning incidents occurring outside the household, which may represent

as many as 13% of all poisonings in children younger than 5 years,[30] cannot be effectively forestalled by a home-centered program.

While well-intentioned home-based educational programs and the teaching of poisoning prevention to children continue to be espoused as important poison prevention measures,[31-33] there is no good evidence that such strategies can effectively reduce the incidence of early childhood poisoning.

Community-Wide Educational Efforts

Relatively few programs have attempted to implement poisoning prevention on a community-wide basis. The health department or a poison control center has usually spearheaded such projects with the cooperation of local government officials, health professionals, community action groups, and even businesses and merchandisers. Fisher and colleagues[34] introduced one such intervention, which included community outreach seminars, school curriculum changes, point-of-purchase education efforts by retailers, and mass media and educational material distribution activities in Monroe County, New York. As a result, the number of poisonings requiring emergency department treatment in area hospitals declined 66%, and poisoning admissions diminished 71%, whereas hospitalization rates in comparable control communities remained stable. Maisel and associates[35] organized a poisoning prevention project in Charleston County, South Carolina, involving education of the public about the recognition of potential poisons and techniques for their safe storage. Activities such as programs for community groups, poster contests, mass media presentations, and group discussions were used. Results of preintervention versus postintervention surveys suggested that 88% of parents had been reached by the educational campaign and had implemented the recommendations. Researchers noted that the number of children hospitalized in Charleston County for poisoning declined. Sumner and associates[36] implemented a similar mass media campaign in North Carolina and demonstrated that it significantly increased the public's knowledge of the poison control center's availability and telephone number. Such model programs have demonstrated that community awareness about poisoning prevention can be increased and can perhaps even lower transiently the rate of poisoning. How long such educational efforts can be sustained remains unclear; whether a more modest but self-perpetuating program of education can be a truly effective long-term deterrent needs to be tested.

Clinic-Based Educational Programs

One strategy for promoting the prevention of poisonings among young children is clinic-based education for their parents. Such education invariably includes information about the recognition of hazardous chemicals in the home environment; elimination of the hazard by not purchasing the poison, safely storing it in the home, and disposing of partially used products; and readiness for a

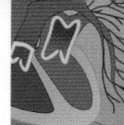

poisoning event by the use of telephone stickers with emergency telephone numbers and knowledge of the appropriate first response (first aid) if a toxic exposure occurs in the home. The Injury Prevention Program (TIPP), an American Academy of Pediatrics–sponsored schedule of safety counseling of families by health care practitioners during a child's primary health care visits, includes such poison prevention advice.[37]

The success of such programs has been found to depend on a number of factors (see Box 20A-1):

1. *Content:* The educational message must be clear, readable at the fifth grade level, succinct, and targeted at the intended audience in terms of sophistication.
2. *Timeliness:* Education is most effective when the audience is addressed during a window of receptivity to such a message, that is, when they recognize its importance, are not distracted, and are personally motivated enough to take action.
3. *Relevance:* The message must be important to the audience and perceived as crucial to their well-being. They must be motivated by its relevance to their own health or that of their family in order to take action.
4. *Lack of barriers:* The education must give information that is practical and for which compliance is not too difficult or beset with barriers (interposed tasks the parent must complete to make the effort effective).
5. *Repetitiveness:* The most effective educational modules are repeated to reinforce the message, if it is intended for the parent to carry out active safety behaviors routinely (e.g., checking labels for toxic ingredients and containers for child-resistant caps).
6. *Educator:* The professional stature of the educator has been found to relate to the success of the compliance with educational recommendations. Parents are much more likely to value their physician's personal suggestions than they are a written summary or slide show, for example. Other cultural, ethnic, and social forces may also enhance or detract from the educator's effectiveness in delivering the message.
7. *Attention span:* The educational program cannot be so abbreviated that the parent does not recognize its importance. Conversely, the education should not be preachy and should not tax the attention or time constraints of the audience. A program that engages parents in an active and collaborative learning experience is more effective.

BOX 20A-1	ATTRIBUTES OF IDEAL POISONING PREVENTION EDUCATION

Clear content
Timeliness
Relevance
Recommendations easy to implement
Repetitive intervention
Effective educator
Brief format

Previous investigations of clinic-based educational programs have been limited by structural or research design problems. Dershewitz and Williamson failed to show an effect when a safety counseling program to child-proof a home was instituted in the clinic setting.[38] Several studies have shown that a more focused message directed at a specific population might be more effective.

Ipecac is no longer routinely recommended as a method of oral decontamination for the poisoned child,[39] so that its universal home storage seems unnecessary. While the storage of activated charcoal in the home has been recommended by some,[40] others are skeptical of its value in home-based poisoning emergencies.[41] However, families can adopt a variety of other prevention strategies applicable to home settings, such as informed choices of nontoxic household products, safe storage of drugs and toxic products, and ready access to the emergency number for poison control (1-800-222-1222). Physicians and other health care providers routinely provide such counseling to families with young children,[42] and medical residents are routinely taught during their training to give such advice.[43] Poisoning prevention advice given in health care settings can substantially improve family safety practices and readiness in the event of an emergency.[44,45] A meta-analysis of 20 studies of injury prevention counseling in primary care settings showed positive effects in the majority.[46]

Poison Control Centers

Regionalization of poison control centers across the United States has contributed to the remarkable progress in poisoning prevention and improvements in poisoning management.[47] This success is derived from the leadership that poison control centers have provided in four different areas:

1. Accuracy of toxicologic information and advice for the management of human poisonings
2. Advocacy as a lead agency in poisoning prevention outreach programs
3. Training for health professionals
4. Research into the etiology, management, and prevention of poisonings

Access to a regional poison control center undoubtedly improves the medical triage and management of a toxic exposure, thus preventing excessive morbidity and mortality. Studies of the use of health services in states with and without poison control centers demonstrate remarkable improvements in telephone triage patterns, avoidance of excess emergency department visits, and improved quality and quantity of pertinent information given for those poisonings in states with regional poison control centers.

It is perhaps underappreciated that poison control centers also serve a focusing role as the lead agency in the community for poisoning prevention programs. They serve as valuable resources for providing public and professional information about the identification of toxic compounds,

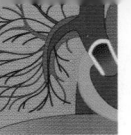

acceptable exposure levels, and safe storage and use. Poison control centers have expanded their roles to include calls requesting information about occupational or environmental exposures, and they serve as a highly visible networking resource, making referrals to other community facilities with more specialized knowledge about teratogenicity, public health implications of specific exposures, and plant or animal identifications.

Poison control centers also serve in poisoning prevention by improving the toxicology training of health professionals through tutorials, staff lectures, in-service programs, and regional workshops and symposia. In addition, poison control centers can alert health professionals, through surveillance of adverse drug reactions, of changes in prescribing style or precautions that must be taken. By pursuing active public education goals via newsletters, public service announcements, health fairs, and media campaigns (e.g., National Poison Prevention Week), poison control centers help to keep the public alert to the principles of poisoning prevention.

Finally, poison control centers often serve as the stimulus to develop new techniques in poisoning prevention. The centers accumulate a dynamic clinical poisoning experience from which epidemiologic trends in poisoning types and circumstances can be identified. Table 20-2 shows the comparative hazard of common drugs and household products as measured by the frequency and extent of injury associated with the poisonings reported to poison control centers nationally.[48] Ideally, such an early warning surveillance system regarding a community's specific toxic exposure problems can lead to directed programs aimed at averting microepidemics of poisoning injuries. Because poison control centers are respected by the public and by health professionals for possessing a particular type of expertise, they can stimulate interest in new research and regulations for poisoning prevention.

THE PHYSICIAN'S RESPONSIBILITY

Physicians have a dual role in the prevention of poisonings, as advocates for their patients' families and as influential and respected community leaders. Physicians must recognize those circumstances that pose a higher than usual potential risk for a poisoning and must take corrective action. This action may include diverse recommendations, such as changing or simplifying a prescribed drug or recommending or advocating daycare, nursing home care, other social supports, psychiatric evaluation, or family counseling. Physicians must give adequate attention to poisoning prevention topics that they discuss with patients as part of their routine health care.

Physicians, in their capacity as community leaders, have an obligation to advocate changes necessary to decrease the risk for poisoning and to alert the community to new or previously unrecognized toxic hazards. Such advocacy includes support for the local or regional poison control service serving the community and for its programs in poisoning prevention. Physicians

TABLE 20A-2 Agents with High Hazard Factors Associated with Poisonings of United States Children Younger than 6 Years (1985–1989)

SUBSTANCE*	TOTAL PEDIATRIC EXPOSURES†	HAZARD FACTOR‡
Pharmaceuticals		
Amphetamines	6409	4.5
Acetaminophen and propoxyphene	2171	4.5
Aspirin	10,002	3.1
Amitriptyline	2897	22.8
Antiarrhythmics	1203	4.0
Anticholinergics	6516	3.2
Antihypertensives	8099	27.6
Barbiturates (long acting)	4475	13.3
Barbiturates (short acting)	1051	6.1
Carbamazepine	4113	32.5
Cardiac glycosides	3846	10.9
Cocaine	546	59.0
Cyclic antidepressant and phenothiazine	832	19.4
Desipramine	935	27.6
Diphenoxylate and atropine	2500	12.2
Doxepin	887	14.5
Imipramine	2503	20.0
Iron	11,234	8.5
Lithium	1054	10.7
Marijuana	694	7.0
Oral hypoglycemics	2609	6.8
Phenothiazines	7451	12.8
Phenytoin	3619	9.3
Propoxyphene	514	6.3
Theophylline	8622	7.7
Valproic acid	1197	6.7
Nonpharmaceuticals		
Alkali	10,267	3.8
Alkali drain cleaners	1474	21.9
Alkali industrial cleaners	938	29.2
Alkali oven cleaners	4619	3.5
Carbon monoxide	3103	31.1
Chlorinated hydrocarbons	9694	4.8
Chlorine gas	2208	4.4
Ethanol	2622	8.0
Ethylene glycol	2321	3.5
Hydrochloric acid	784	6.2
Kerosene	10,751	7.9
Lighter fluid	8865	4.4
Methane, natural gas	700	9.2
Methanol	1883	5.1
Mineral seal oil	6564	3.2
Organophosphate alone	16,560	5.6
Organophosphate and other pesticides	1806	3.6

*Specific substances only—broader categories are not all included; bites and envenomations are not included.
†Only substances with more than 500 exposures included.
‡Only hazard factors > 3.0 included.
Adapted from Litovitz T, Manoguerra A: Comparison of pediatric poisoning hazards: an analysis of 3.8 million exposure incidents. A report from the American Association of Poison Control Centers. Pediatrics 1992;89:1002–1004.

might also make use of public forums to change the public perceptions of poisoning prevention strategies (e.g., the need for child-resistant containers, the importance of following directions for the use of medications, and the dangers of drug abuse). Physicians

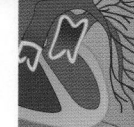

can also be influential consultants to legislative bodies considering new initiatives restricting or regulating the use and disposal of drugs and toxins. Internet websites with educational content on poisoning prevention (see Box 20A-2) can provide physicians with additional resources to assist them in their community advocacy efforts.

Dedicated health professionals must make a concerted effort to continue the momentum and consolidate the gains that have been made in poisoning prevention and to advance new aspects of the field.

POISONING PREVENTION RESOURCES

See Box 20A-2 for online poisoning prevention resources.

BOX 20A-2   SELECT INTERNET WEBSITES: POISONING PREVENTION RESOURCES

American Association of Poison Control Centers (AAPCC): *www.aapcc.org*

This is the official website of the AAPCC, which inventories contact information for all of the poison control centers in the United States. It also includes poisoning fact sheets, a downloadable poison prevention brochure, prevention tips, a list of educators at poison control centers, and information about Poisoning Prevention Week.

American Association of Poison Control Centers' Toll-Free Emergency Number Website: *www.1-800-222-1222.info/poisonhelp.asp*

This website contains information about the AAPCC's toll-free telephone number for poisoning emergencies. It also contains public education information about poisoning prevention and a module targeted to preschool children.

American Academy of Pediatrics: *www.aap.org*

This is the official website of the American Academy of Pediatrics. Under the button "You and Your Family," information is available about the Bright Futures project, which includes injury prevention objectives. The "You and Your Family" section also includes The Injury Prevention Program (TIPP) age-related injury prevention fact sheets, which include poisoning prevention information.

U.S. National Library of Medicine (NLM) and National Institutes of Health (NIH): *www.nlm.nih.gov/medlineplus/poisoningtoxicologyenvironmentalhealth.html*

This website is cosponsored by the NLM and NIH and it includes a variety of poisoning, toxicology, and environmental health topics, from anthrax and air pollution, to water and *Yersinia*.

REFERENCES

1. Watson WA, Litovitz TL, Rodgers GC, et al: 2004 annual report of the American Association of Poison Control Centers toxic exposure surveillance system. Am J Emerg Med 2005;23:589–666.
2. Chatsantiprapa K, Chokkanapitak J, Pinpradit N: Host and environment factors for exposure to poisons: a case-control study of preschool children in Thailand. Injury Prev 2001;7:214–217.
3. Jensen G, Wilson W: Preventive implications of a study of 100 poisonings in children. Pediatrics 1960;65:490–496.
4. Ozanne-Smith J, Day L, Parsons B, et al: Childhood poisoning: access and prevention. J Paediatr Child Health 2001;37:262–265.
5. Sibert R: Stress in families who have ingested poisons. BMJ 1975;3:87–89.
6. Beautrais A, Fergusson D, Shannon T: Accidental poisoning in the first three years of life. Aust Paediatr J 1981;17:104–109.
7. Bithoney B, Snyder J, Michalek J, Newberger E: Childhood ingestions as symptoms of family distress. Am J Dis Child 1985;139:456–459.
8. Sobel R, Margolis J: Repetitive poisoning in children: a psychosocial study. Pediatrics 1985;35:641–651.
9. Baltimore C, Meyer R: A study of storage, child behavioral traits, and mother's knowledge of toxicology in 52 poisoned families and 52 comparison families. Pediatrics 1969;44:816–820.
10. Baker S, O'Neill B, Karpf R: Poisonings. In The Injury Fact Book. Lexington, MA, Lexington Books, 1984.
11. Neumann CM, Giffin S, Hall R, et al: Oregon's toxic household products law. J Public Health Policy 2000;21:342–359.
12. McIntire M: Safety packaging: a model for successful accident prevention. Pediatr Ann 1977;6:706–708.
13. Title 16-commercial practices. Consumer Product Safety Commission, Subchapter E—Poison Prevention Packaging Act of 1970 Regulations (1973). August 7, 1973;38:21247–21250.
14. Consumer Product Safety Commission. Child-resistant packaging for certain over-the-counter drug products. Fed Reg 2001;66(149):40111–40116.
15. Centers for Disease Control: Update: childhood poisonings—United States. MMWR Morb Mortal Wkly Rep 1985;34:117–118.
16. Walton W: An evaluation of the poison prevention packaging act. Pediatrics 1982;69:363–370.
17. Clarke A, Walton WW: Effect of safety packaging on aspirin ingestion by children. Pediatric 1979;63:687–693.
18. Sibert JR, Craft AW, Jackson RH: Child-resistant packaging and accidental child poisoning. Lancet 1977;2:289–290.
19. Rodgers GB: The safety effects of child-resistant packaging for oral prescription drugs: two decades of experience JAMA 1996;275:1661–1665.
20. Rodgers GB: The effectiveness of child-resistant packaging for aspirin. Arch Pediatr Adolesc Med 2002;156:929–933.
21. Assargaard U, Sjoberg G: The successful introduction of child resistant closures for liquid paracetamol. Saf Sci 1995;21:87–91.
22. McIntire M, Angle C, Sathees K, Lee P: Safety packaging—what does the public think? Am J Public Health 1977;67:169–171.
23. Dole EJ, Czaika PA, Rivara FP: Evaluation of pharmacists' compliance with the Poison Prevention Packaging Act. Am J Public Health 1986;76:1335–1336.
24. Jackson R, Walker J, Wynne N: Circumstance of accidental poisoning in childhood. BMJ 1968;4:245–248.
25. Hawton K, Townsend E, Deeks J, et al: Effects of legislation restricting pack sizes of paracetamol and salicylate on self-poisoning in the UK, before and after study. BMJ 2001;322:1203–1207.
26. Braden B: Validation of a poison prevention program. Am J Public Health 1979;69:942–944.
27. Krenzelok E, Garber R: Teaching poison prevention to preschool children, their parents, and professional educators through child care centers. Am J Public Health 1981;71:750–752.
28. Fergusson D, Horwood L, Beautrais A, Shannon F: A controlled field trial of a poisoning prevention method. Pediatrics 1982;69:515–520.
29. Vernberg K, Culver-Dickson P, Spyker D: The deterrent effect of poison-warning stickers. Am J Dis Child 1984;138:1018–1020.
30. Polakoff J, Lacouture P, Lovejoy F: The environment away from home as a source of potential poisoning. Am J Dis Child 1984;138:1014–1017.
31. Phillips W, Little T: Continuity of care and poisoning prevention education. Patient Counsel Health Educ 1980;2:170–173.
32. Broderick M, Dodd-Butera T, Wahl P: A program to prevent iron poisoning using public health nurses in a county health department. Public Health Nursing 2002;19:179–183.
33. Liller KD, Craig J, Crane N, McDermott RJ: Evaluation of a poison prevention lesson for kindergarten and third grade students. Injury Prev 1998;4:218–221.
34. Fisher L, Van Buren J, Nitzkin J, et al: Highlight results of the Monroe County poison prevention demonstration project. Vet Hum Toxicol 1980;22(Suppl 2):15–17.
35. Maisel G, Langdoe B, Jenkins M, Aycock E: Analysis of two surveys evaluating a project to reduce accidental poisoning among children. Public Health Rep 1967;82:555–560.

36. Sumner S, Barkin S, Hudak C, et al: A project to reduce accidental pediatric poisonings in North Carolina. Vet Hum Toxicol 2003;45:266–269.

37. American Academy of Pediatrics: TIPP: The Injury Prevention Program. Elk Grove Village, IL, American Academy of Pediatrics, 2004.

38. Dershewitz R, Williamson J: Prevention of childhood household injuries: a controlled clinical trial. Am J Public Health 1977;67:1148–1153.

39. Committee on Injury, Violence, and Poison Prevention, American Academy of Pediatrics: Policy statement: poison treatment in the home. Pediatrics 2003;112:1182–1185.

40. Spiller HA, Rodgers GC Jr: Evaluation of administration of activated charcoal in the home. Pediatrics 2001;108:e100.

41. Bond GR: Activated charcoal in the home: helpful and important or simply a distraction? Pediatrics 2002;109:145–146.

42. Gerard JM, Klasner AE, Madhok M, et al: Poison prevention counseling—a comparison between family practitioners and pediatricians. Arch Pediatr Adolesc Med 2000;154:65–70.

43. Wright MS. Pediatric injury prevention—preparing residents for patient counseling. Arch Pediatr Adolesc Med 1997;151:1039–1043.

44. Woolf A, Lewander W, Filippone G, Lovejoy F: Prevention of childhood poisoning: efficacy of an educational program carried out in an emergency clinic. Pediatrics 1987;80:359–363.

45. Woolf AD, Saperstein A, Forjuoh S: Poisoning prevention knowledge and practices of parents after a childhood poisoning incident. Pediatrics 1992;90:867–870.

46. Bass JL, Christoffel KK, Widome M, et al: Childhood injury prevention counseling in primary care settings: a critical review of the literature. Pediatrics 1993;92:544–551.

47. Lovejoy FH, Robertson WO, Woolf AD: Poison centers, poison prevention, and the pediatrician. Pediatrics 1994;94:220–224.

48. Litovitz T, Manoguerra A: Comparison of pediatric poisoning hazards: an analysis of 3.8 million exposure incidents—a report from the American Association of Poison Control Centers. Pediatrics 1992;89:999–1006.

B | Poisonings in Children with Unique Metabolism

REBEKAH C. MANNIX, MD ■ MICHAEL W. SHANNON, MD, MPH

At a Glance...

■ Each year, newborn screening identifies approximately 3000 new cases of potentially fatal metabolic disorders, hematologic disorders, and endocrinopathies.

■ These patients with unique metabolism are prone to unique drug responses.

■ Clinicians should review basic metabolic pathways and recognize adverse drug reactions when caring for these patients.

According to the Center for Disease Control and Prevention, approximately 4 million babies in the United States have dried blood spots analyzed through newborn screening programs.[1] These screens, which can detect metabolic disorders, hematologic disorders, and endocrinopathies, identify an estimated 3000 new cases of potentially fatal or debilitating disease each year for which outcomes are improved with early identification and treatment.[1]

Long-term survival of these children poses new challenges for clinicians. Previously well-delineated drug response in the general population may not apply to this subpopulation. Indeed, the toxic effects of drugs in these patients are not merely an extension of current clinical toxicology. The basis for understanding the idiosyncratic drug response of children with unique metabolism requires careful attention to the basics of biochemistry and physiology.

This chapter reviews some of the best characterized adverse drug reactions in children with unique metabolism. It is by no means a complete summary since there is a paucity of information available on drug physiology in these special circumstances. The chapter is intended to act as a guide to clinicians faced with adverse drug reactions in children with unique metabolism and to assist efforts at preventing these adverse drug reactions.

VALPROATE TOXICITY IN PATIENTS WITH DISORDERS OF FATTY ACID METABOLISM

The toxicity of valproic acid (VPA) has been attributed in part to its effects on multiple metabolic pathways, most notably fatty acid synthesis and degradation. It is therefore logical to presume that patients with disorders of fatty acid metabolism are at increased risk for VPA toxicity. An overview of the pharmacokinetics, drug interactions, and manifestations of VPA overdose in the general population may be found in Chapter 40, while the special considerations in patients with defects in fatty acid metabolism are described below.

VPA (2-propylpentanoic acid) is a simple branched-chain carboxylic acid used therapeutically as an anticonvulsant, primarily in pediatric populations.[2] Like other fatty acids, VPA undergoes β-oxidation (incomplete) and competes for the physiologic substrates coenzyme A (CoA) and L-carnitine. This competition does not produce clinically significant derangements in healthy subjects with therapeutic dosing of VPA. However, patients with underlying defects in fatty acid oxidation may develop significant toxicity from "therapeutic" doses of VPA. A review of fatty acid oxidation is necessary to better understand the basis of that toxicity (Fig. 20B-1).

The metabolism of free fatty acids begins with the formation of fatty acid conjugates with CoA to form acyl-CoA esters of varying chain lengths. These are trans-esterified to acylcarnitines at the mitochondrial membrane and shuttled across the mitochondrial matrix

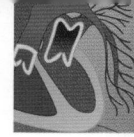

VPA Metabolism

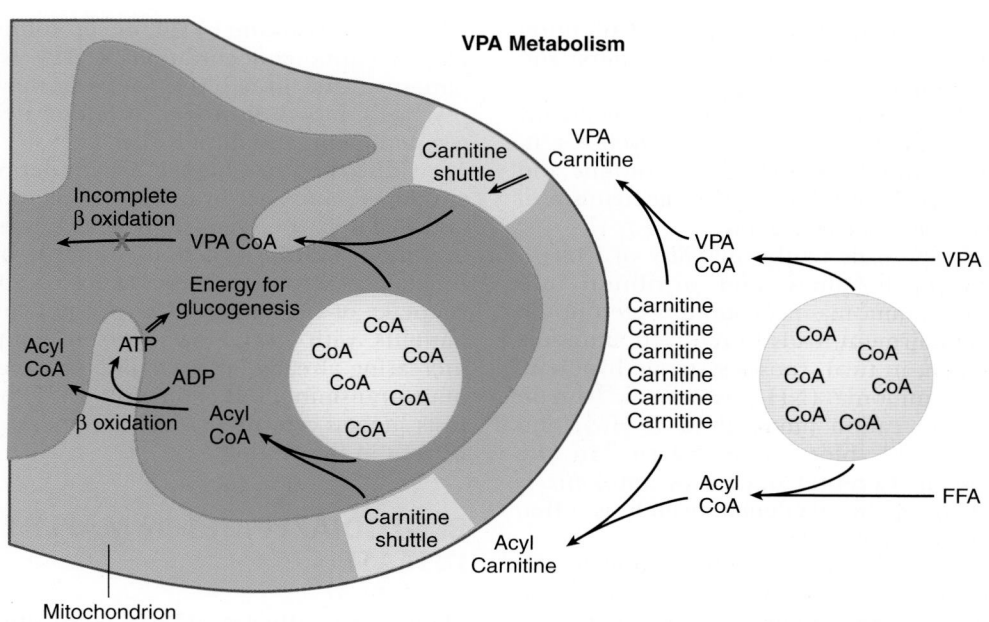

FIGURE 20B-1. Fatty acid metabolism begins with the formation of fatty acid–CoA conjugates to form acyl CoAs. These acyl CoAs are then transesterified to acylcarnitines at the mitochondrial membrane and shuttled across the mitochondrial matrix. Once inside the mitochondrion, acyl CoAs are regenerated and ultimately oxidized the acetyl CoA, which generates ATP via the citric acid cycle. Valproic acid (VPA) competes for the physiologic substrates CoA and carnitine without producing significant amounts of ATP.

where the acyl CoAs are regenerated. The fatty acyl CoAs undergo β-oxidation, forming acetyl CoA, which either enters the citric acid cycle to generate adenosine triphosphate (ATP; fatty acid oxidation being the major source of the ATP required for gluconeogenesis in times of fasting) or becomes the substrate for ketogenesis, lipogenesis, or steroidogenesis.

Regulation of the free and esterified CoA pool of the cell is therefore important in a large number of catabolic and anabolic biochemical reactions. The total cellular CoA pool is small and cannot be increased quickly and the cell is dependent on continued turnover of acyl CoAs to make CoA available.

VPA can be activated to the corresponding acyl CoA (valproyl CoA or VPA CoA), which can be metabolized by mammalian tissues to a variety of energy-poor metabolites.[3-5] The overproduction of poorly metabolized VPA-CoA thioesters jeopardizes multiple biochemical pathways by impeding flux through this entire energy-harvesting pathway, particularly in patients in whom fatty acid metabolism and synthesis are impaired.

Valproylcarnitine (VPA-carnitine) can be generated from VPA CoA, although this is a quantitatively minor pathway of VPA elimination in normal subjects.[6,7] Most studies demonstrate that VPA therapy is associated with a mild decrease in plasma carnitine concentrations, likely through renal excretion of VPA-carnitine esters.[8,9] Data on tissue carnitine contents during VPA therapy are not available.

Recent data suggest that other conjugation pathways, most significantly glutathione, may also play a role in VPA toxicity in both children with fatty acid oxidation defects and healthy, normal children.[10,11] Indeed, it is this depletion of glutathione that may produce the hepatotoxicity associated with VPA overdose.

Although not clinically significant in most therapeutic situations, the depletion of CoA, carnitine, and reduced glutathione by VPA becomes relevant in patients with underlying metabolic disorders as well as those who take a VPA overdose.[12,13] Patients with disorders of fatty acid oxidation such as very long chain acyl-CoA dehydrogenase deficiency, medium chain acyl-CoA dehydrogenase deficiency, long-chain L-3-hydroxyacyl-CoA dehydrogenase deficiency, trifunctional protein deficiency, and medium and short-chain L-3-hydroxyacyl-CoA dehydrogenase deficiency have limited ability to metabolize fatty acids. This deficiency results in a restricted ability to harvest the requisite energy (stored in fatty acids) for gluconeogenesis. Further restriction of the metabolism of free fatty acids (as in the case of the sequestration of CoA by VPA) or increased energy demands (fever, fasting) shifts the relative deficiency to an absolute deficiency. Similarly, patients with relative carnitine deficiency (e.g., in familial epilepsies) may be thrown into metabolic crisis by the VPA-induced depletion of carnitine. Repletion of carnitine and glutathione (in the form of N-acetylcysteine) may ameliorate the toxicity associated with valproate in patients with fatty acid oxidation defects and hereditary carnitine deficiency.

ANTIDEPRESSANTS IN PATIENTS WITH ORNITHINE TRANSCARBAMYLASE DEFICIENCY

Ornithine transcarbamyl transferase (OTC) deficiency is the most common of the urea cycle disorders. OTC deficiency is an X-linked disorder that occurs primarily in males, although it can also manifest itself in females. Clinical presentation of OTC can vary from fulminant

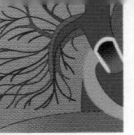
cerebral edema in the neonate, impulsivity and attention deficit in older children, and mood disorders and psychosis in adults; mental status changes are a frequent presentation in adults. Many clinicians have anecdotally noted severe worsening of mood and psychosis in patients with OTC who begin to take serotonin and norepinephrine reuptake inhibitors. The mechanism of this adverse reaction is discussed below.

Deficiency of OTC leads to the inability of liver to condense carbamyl phosphate and ornithine into citrulline, the initial ammonia-incorporating step in the urea cycle. This impairment leads to reduced ammonia incorporation, which, in turn, causes systemic hyperammonemia. Plasma ammonia (NH_3) is a weak base in equilibrium with the cation ammonium (NH_4^+), and only freely crosses the blood-brain barrier in the unionized NH_3 form. Cerebral uptake of ammonia is thus greatly enhanced by alkalemia, which is often present in ammonemic patients.

Elevated levels of NH_3 in the brain stimulate the astrocyte-restricted enzyme glutamine synthetase.[14] The accumulation of astrocyte glutamine drives heteroexchange (the exchange of one amino acid for a different one) of neutral (zwitterionic) amino acids across the LAT1 transporter, leading to accumulation of brain tyrosine, tryptophan, and other essential amino acids.[15-17] The accumulation of tyrosine promotes the formation of norepinephrine (NE) and dopamine (DA), while the build-up of tryptophan produces increased

5-hydroxytryptamine (5-HT, or serotonin) (Fig. 20B-2).[18] High synaptic concentrations of DA, NE, and 5-HT in patients with urea cycle defects may contribute to psychosis, mood disorders, attention deficits, combative temperament, and impulsivity.

As discussed in Chapter 27, antidepressants (tricyclic antidepressants) act by inhibiting the uptake of NE, DA, and 5-HT in the synapse. Selective serotonin reuptake inhibitors (SSRIs) function primarily by inhibiting the reuptake of serotonin; they also possess an ability to inhibit reuptake of DA and NE. Use of these antidepressants in patients with OTC may worsen symptomatology by increasing already high synaptic concentrations of these neurotransmitters. It is uncertain whether 5-HT antagonists such as cyproheptadine and methysergide have any benefit in this setting.

BENZODIAZEPINES IN MAPLE SYRUP DISEASE

Maple syrup disease (MSD) is an autosomal-recessive disorder caused by decreased activity of branched-chain α-ketoacid dehydrogenase, an enzyme in the degradative pathway of the branched-chain amino acids leucine, isoleucine, and valine.[19] The consequence of this deficiency is toxic accumulation of these amino acids in tissues and plasma. The accumulation of leucine further leads to a proportional accumulation of α-ketoisocaproic

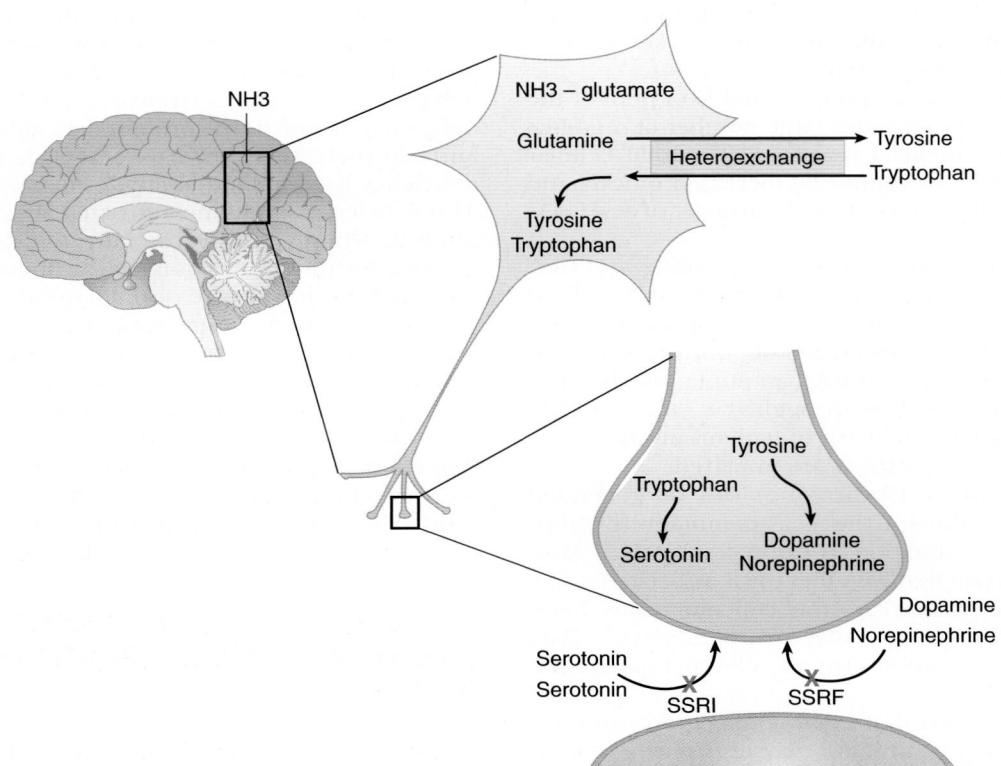

FIGURE 20B-2. Elevated ammonia in the brain of patients with OTC leads to increased formation of glutamine. Increased tissue glutamine drives heteroexchange of glutamine for tryptophan, tyrosine, and other essential amino acids. The accumulation of tyrosine promotes the formation of norepinephrine (NE) and dopamine (DA) while the buildup of tryptophan produces increased serotonin (5-HT).

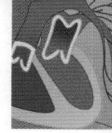

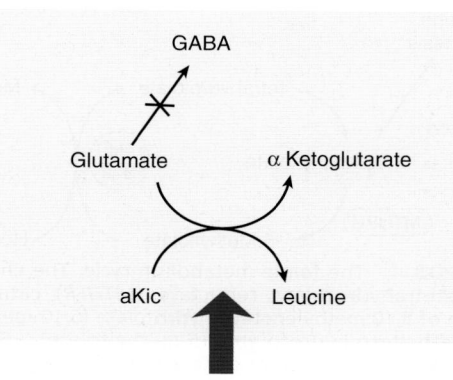

↑ Leucine ⟶ ↑ α Keto isocaproate (aKic)

FIGURE 20B-3. Decreased activity of branched-chain α-ketoacid dehydrogenase (BCKAD) causes buildup of leucine, isoleucine, and valine. The accumulation of leucine further leads to a proportional accumulation of α-ketoisocaproic acid, its ketoacid analog. Excessive intracerebral levels of α-ketoisocaproic acid drive a transamination reaction which depletes glutamate and in turn GABA. (Adapted from Strauss KA, Morton DH: Branched-chain ketoacyl dehydrogenase deficiency: Maple syrup disease. Curr Treat Options Neurol 2003;5:329–341.)

acid, its ketoacid analog. Excessive intracerebral levels of this ketoacid drive a transamination reaction that depletes glutamate and in turn γ-aminobutyric acid (GABA) (Fig. 20B-3).[20-22]

This relative GABA deficiency may lead to chronic up-regulation of GABA receptors and increased sensitivity to the effects of benzodiazepenes at this receptor. Clinicians should be aware that patients with MSD may display toxic effects at doses used therapeutically in the normal population. Reversal with flumazenil should be approached warily by the clinician because increased receptor sensitivity may lower seizure threshold with flumazenil-induced receptor blockade.

GLUCOSE-6-PHOSPHATE DEHYDROGENASE DEFICIENCY AND OXIDANTS

Glucose-6-phosphate dehydrogenase (G6PD) deficiency is the most common human enzyme deficiency, with an estimated 400 million people worldwide affected by this enzymopathy.[23,24] G6PD is the most common hereditary cause of "idiopathic" hyperbilirubinemia in newborns, and can be associated with significant nonhemolytic jaundice in this age group. G6PD catalyzes the first reaction in the hexose monophosphate shunt, an oxidation/reduction reaction that oxidizes glucose-6-phosphate while concomitantly reducing nicotinamide-adenine dinucleotide phosphate (NADP). G6PD is responsible for maintaining adequate cellular levels of reduced NADP (NADPH). NADPH functions as a cofactor in many biosynthetic reactions, including maintenance of glutathione in its reduced form. Reduced glutathione acts as a scavenger for dangerous oxidative metabolites in the cell. While other cells in the body have diverse mechanisms for generating NADPH,

the red cell is fully dependent on G6PD to generate this important molecule.[19] Having only one NADPH-producing enzyme to remove oxidants, red blood cells are therefore especially sensitive to oxidative stresses. Oxidant stress can be precipitated by infection, food, and drugs (Chapter 14). As a result of oxidant stress, these red cells undergo massive hemolysis, leading to hyperbilirubinemia. Removing the cause of oxidative stress is first-line treatment for G6PD hemolysis. Vitamin E and folic acid have both been suggested for treatment of G6PD hemolysis.[25] Treatment for severe cases may include exchange transfusion.

CRIGLER-NAJJAR DISEASE AND CEFTRIAXONE

Crigler-Najjar disease is an autosomal-recessive disorder in which bilirubin metabolism is impaired. Patients with Crigler-Najjar disease are subject to markedly elevated levels of bilirubin that can manifest by icterus, kernicterus, and encephalopathy. Drugs that exacerbate hyperbilirubinemia (either through displacement of bilirubin from albumin or from cholestasis) must be avoided in patients with Crigler-Najjar disease.

Bilirubin is a lipophilic molecule that requires conversion to a polar derivative in order to be eliminated. This conversion of bilirubin occurs in the liver, where the molecule glucuronic acid attaches to bilirubin in a process called glucuronidation. Glucuronidation is carried out by the enzyme uridine diphosphate glucuronyl transferase (UDPGT). Patients with Crigler-Najjar disease have either an absolute lack of this enzyme (type 1) or markedly decrease activity of this enzyme (type 2), resulting in very high levels of unconjugated bilirubin. Importantly, treatment with phenobarbital, which can induce the expression of UDPGT, is not effective in the setting of absolute lack of the enzyme (type 1) but may be effective in ameliorating type 2 disease.

The lipophilic unconjugated bilirubin must be bound to carrier protein to be transported in the aqueous environment of the serum. Albumin has one primary high-affinity binding site for bilirubin and two lower-affinity sites. Albumin bound bilirubin cannot pass through the blood-brain barrier to exert its toxic effect. At physiologic pH, the amount of free bilirubin is very low (less than 0.1% of total) and the brain is protected from the neurotoxic effects of bilirubin. Decreased albumin-binding capacity and/or decreased albumin-binding affinity can increase the amount of free serum bilirubin.

The risk of kernicterus in any jaundiced patient increases as the serum bilirubin-albumin molar ratio exceeds 0.7. Brain injury is imminent when this ratio exceeds 1.0. The quantitative effect of any displacing drug on the toxic level of free bilirubin depends on four major variables: (1) the prevailing bilirubin-albumin molar ratio, (2) peak molar concentration of the drug after administration, (3) fractional protein binding by the drug, and its specific binding affinity for the bilirubin binding pocket, and (4) drug half-life. The latter three

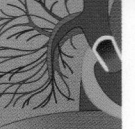

BOX 20B-1	DRUGS TO AVOID IN PATIENTS WITH CRIGLER-NAJJAR DISEASE	
Afelimomab	Edatrexate	Micafungin
Alprostadil	Erlotinib	Molgramostim
Atazanavir	Etoposide	Montelukast
Azacitidine	Flavopiridol	Novobiocin
Busulfan	Ganciclovir	Oxytocin
Capecitabine	Hemoglobin	Pancuronium
Carmustine	Indinavir	Quinupristin/dalfopristin
Ceftazidime	Lamivudine/zidovudine	Ribavirin
Ceftriaxone	Lithium	Tacrine
Clozapine	Menadiol sodium	Tasosartan
Crosfumaril	diphosphate	Temozolomide
Cyclosporine	Methenolone	Trazodone
Cytarabine	Methylene blue	Valspodar
Dapsone	Mezlocillin	

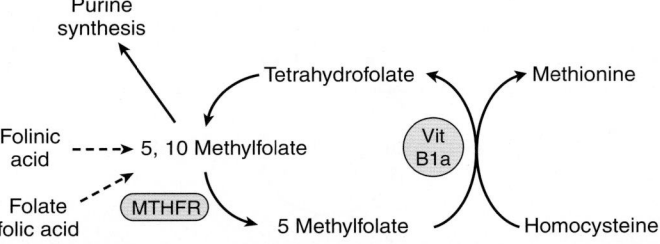

FIGURE 20B-4. The folate metabolism cycle. The enzyme 5,10 methylenetetrahydrofolate reductase (*MTHFR*) catalyzes the conversion of 5,10 methylenetetrahydrofolate (5,10-methylfolate) into 5-methyltetrahydrofolate (5-methylfolate), the major circulating and bioactive form of folate. Abnormally low MTFHR activity leads to lower circulating levels of the bioavailable forms of folate, lower availability of methionine, and higher levels of homocysteine.

variables can be obtained from standard pharmacology texts, while the serum bilirubin-albumin ratio can be calculated as:

$$\text{Bilirubin in mg/dL} \times 17 = \text{Bilirubin in μmol/L}$$
$$\text{Albumin in g/dL} \times 152 = \text{Albumin in μmol/L}$$

Drugs that raise bilirubin either through cholestasis or displacement of bilirubin from albumin should be assiduously avoided in patients with Crigler-Najjar (Box 20B-1).[26-28]

METHOTREXATE AND DISORDERS OF FOLATE AND VITAMIN B₁₂ METABOLISM

The enzyme 5,10-methylenetetrahydrofolate reductase (MTHFR) catalyzes the conversion of 5,10-methylenetetrahydrofolate (5,10-methylfolate) into 5-methyltetrahydrofolate (5-methylfolate), the major circulating and bioactive form of folate. It is important to note that total circulating folate levels (as measured by standard laboratory assays) are normal in these patients, while the fraction of 5-methylfolate in the total folate pool is low (normally more than 50% of total, typically less than 5% of total in patients with severe MTHFR deficiency). Folate is used in many vital biochemical pathways, including the conversion of homocysteine to methionine and the synthesis of nucleotides, and in numerous methylation reactions (Fig. 20B-4).

The effects of abnormal folate metabolism are still incompletely understood, although there is ample evidence that abnormally low MTHFR activity leads to lower circulating levels of the bioavailable forms of folate, lower availability of methionine, and higher levels of homocysteine. Folic acid and folinic acid supplementation do not help these patients; both drugs require activity of MTHFR to be converted to the bioactive 5-methyl-THF.

Similarly, patients with hereditary cobalamin (vitamin B₁₂) disorders are unable to convert homocysteine to methionine. As in the case of MTHFR deficiency, those with elevated levels of homocysteine are at risk for a wide array of metabolic derangements, including neurotoxicity, vasculopathy, and thrombosis.

Dihydrofolate reductase (DHFR) inhibitors, most notably methotrexate, decrease cellular 5-methyltetrahydrofolate. Use of DHFR inhibitors in patients with MTHFR deficiency can lead to a metabolic crisis and significantly increased risk for methotrexate-induced neurotoxicity, vasculopathy, and thrombotic events.[29] Notably, folinic acid ("leucovorin rescue") is ineffective in these patients because folinic acid is not bioavailable due to the underlying enzymatic defect. The best treatment for patients with MTHFR deficiency is to avoid exposure to drugs that disrupt folate metabolism.

Inhaled nitrous oxide anesthesia should also be avoided in patients with disorders of folate and vitamin B₁₂ metabolism because nitrous oxide functions as an irreversible inhibitor of cerebral methionine synthase. Use of nitrous oxide in these patients can produce a sudden and lethal neurologic deterioration due to rapid intracerebral accumulation of *S*-adenosylhomocysteine, adenosine, homocysteine, and excitatory homocysteine metabolites.[30,31]

INHALED ANESTHETICS AND MALIGNANT HYPERTHERMIA

Malignant hyperthermia (MH) is an autosomal-dominant pharmacogenetic disorder triggered by exposure of susceptible individuals to commonly used inhaled anesthetics and depolarizing muscle relaxants.[32] Most patients are asymptomatic prior to the exposure, although MH is associated with central core disease (a rare neuromuscular disorder that is most often characterized by weakness in the legs), other myopathies, and dystonias. Patients with malignant hyperthermia are thought to have abnormal regulation of calcium through the calcium release channel, known as the ryanodine receptor (RYR1), in the sarcoplasmic reticulum of skeletal muscle.[33] About 50% of familial MH is linked to the chromosome 19q13 region, where the RYR1 gene is

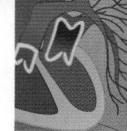

located.[34] To date, more than 30 different mutations in the RYR1 gene have been associated with MH susceptibility.[35]

Administration of an inhaled anesthetic or depolarizing muscle relaxant in patients with a predisposition to MH triggers calcium dysregulation within the muscle cell. Excessive intracellular calcium, or interference with return to storage of calcium, creates a high intracellular calcium level that leads to continuous contractures of skeletal muscles, which manifests clinically as muscle rigidity and spasm. This hyperaction of skeletal muscles increases myocite oxygen consumption, heat production, and use of ATP; these produce the signs of lactic acidosis and hyperthermia. The mortality rate of malignant hyperthermia is as high as 5% to 10%.

Inhalational anesthetics and depolarizing muscle relaxants should be avoided in patients with a known prior history of malignant hyperthermia or strong family history of malignant hyperthermia. The treatment of choice is intravenous dantrolene 2.5 mg/kg per dose to a maximum total dosing of 10 mg/kg, which blocks calcium release. Adjunctive therapy includes cooling, control of acidosis, and 100% O$_2$.[36]

In addition to malignant hyperthermia in patients with congenital myopathies, the use of depolarizing muscle relaxants can produce severe hyperkalemia, rhabdomyolysis, and renal failure. The mechanism of this response is likely due to an adaptive increase in acetylcholine receptors on denervated muscle, leading to massive depolarization.

ACUTE INTERMITTENT PORPHYRIA

Acute intermittent porphyria (AIP) is an autosomal-dominant disorder resulting from an error in pyrrole metabolism due to deficiency of uroporphyrinogen I synthetase (Fig. 20B-5).

AIP is characterized by recurrent attacks of abdominal pain, gastrointestinal dysfunction, neurologic disturbances, and large amounts of aminolevulinic acid and porphobilinogen in the urine. Paresthesias and paralysis

BOX 20B-2	DRUG SAFETY IN ACUTE INTERMITTENT PORPHYRIA

Unsafe (Strong Evidence)	Possibly Unsafe	
Androgens	Alkylkating agents	Methyldopa
Barbiturates	Aminophylline	Metroniazole
Estrogens	Bemegride	Metyrapone
Ethanol	Benzodiazepines	Miconazole
Griseofulvin	Bromobenzine	Nalidixic acid
Hydantoins	Carbamazepine	Nifedipine
Progesterones	Chloramphenicol	Nikethamide
Sulfonamides	Chlorpropamide	Nitrazepam
	Clonidine	Nortriptyline
	Chloroquine	Pentazocine
	Danazol	Phenazone
	Dapsone	Phenoxybenzamine
	Disopyramide	Phensuxamine
	Enflurane	Phenylbutazone
	Ergotamine	Primidone
	Etomidate	Pyrazinamide
	Eucalyptol	Rifampin
	Glutethimide	Spironolactone
	Halothane	Succinimides
	Hyralazine	Theophylline
	Imipramine	Tolazemide
	Ketamine	Tolbutamide
	Ketoconazole	Trimethadone
	Mepivacaine	Troxidone
	Meprobamate	Valproate
	Methsuximide	Verapamil

can also occur, with death resulting from respiratory paralysis.[37]

Multiple drugs have been shown to trigger a porphyric crisis (Box 20B-2). Treatment for acute attacks is mostly supportive with dextrose infusions.[38] Successful treatment of acute attacks with hematin, a specific feedback inhibitor of heme synthesis, has been repeatedly reported, although this is not a viable strategy at most centers due to the unavailability of hematin.[39]

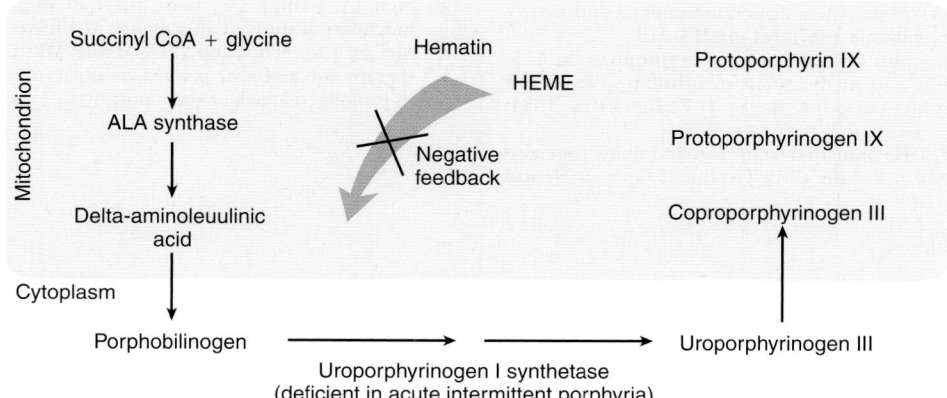

FIGURE 20B-5. Heme synthesis pathway. A defect in the enzyme uroporphyrinogen synthetase causes acute intermittent porphyria. Hematin, a feedback inhibitor of heme synthesis, may be useful in treating acute attacks.

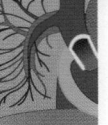

REFERENCES

1. Centers for Disease Control and Prevention: Using tandem mass spectrometry for metabolic disease screening among newborns: a report of a working group. MMWR Morb Mortal Wkly Rep 2001;50(RR-3):1–22.
2. Wallace SJ: Myoclonus and epilepsy in childhood: a review of treatment with valproate, ethosuximide, lamatrigine and zonisamide. Epilepsy Res 1988;29:147–154
3. Bjorge SM, Baillie TA: Studies on the β-oxidation of valproic acid in rat liver mitochondrial preparations. Drug Metab Dispos 1991;19:823–829
4. Li J, Norwood DL, Mao L-F, Schulz H: Mitochondrial metabolism of valproic acid. Biochemistry 1991;30:388–394.
5. Sugimoto T, Muro H, Woo M, et al: Valproate metabolites in high-dose valproate plus phenytoin therapy. Epilepsia 1996;37:1200–1203.
6. Millington DS, Bohan TP, Roe CR, et al: Valproylcarnitine a novel drug metabolite identified by fast atom bombardment and thermospray liquid chromatographymass spectrometry. Clin Chem Acta 1985;145:69–76.
7. Melegh B, Kerner J, Jaszai V, Bieber LL: Differential excretion of xenobiotic acyl-esters of carnitine due to administration of pivampicillin and valproate. Biochem Med Metab Biol 1990; 43:30–38.
8. Ohtani YU, Endo F, Mastsuda I: Carnitine deficiency and hyperammonemia associated with valproic acid therapy. J Pediatr 1982;101:782–785.
9. Castro-Gago M, Eiris-Punal J, Novo-Rodriquez MI, et al: Serum carnitine levels in epileptic children before and during treatment with valproic acid, carbamazepine and phenobarbital. J Child Neurol 1998;13:546–549.
10. Klee S, Johanssen S, Ungemach FR: Evidence for a trigger function of valproic acid in xenobiotic-induced hepatotoxicity. Pharmacol Toxicol 2000;87(2):89–95.
11. Tang W, Abbott FS: Characterization of thiol-conjugated metabolites of 2-propylpent-4-enoic acid (4-ene VPA), a toxic metabolite of valproic acid, by electrospray tandem mass spectrometry. J Mass Spectrom 1996;31(8):926–936.
12. Ponchaut S, van Hoof F, Veitch K: In vitro effects of valproate and valproate metabolites on mitochondrial oxidations. Relevance of CoA sequestration to the observed inhibitions. Biochem Pharmacol 1992;43:2435–2442.
13. Krahenbuhl S, Mang G, Kupferschmidt H, et al: Plasma and hepatic carnitine and coenzyme A pools in a patient with fatal, valproate hepatotoxicity. Gut 1995;37:140–143.
14. Inoue I, Gushiken T, Kobayashi K, Saheki T: Accumulation of large neutral amino acids in the brain of sparse-fur mice at hyperammonemic state. Biochem Med Metab Biol 1987;38(3):378–386.
15. Meier C, Ristic Z, Klauser S, Verrey F: Activation of system L heterodimeric amino acid exchangers by intracellular substrates. EMBO J 2002;21:580–589.
16. Smith QR, Stoll J: Blood-brain barrier amino acid transport. In Pardridge WM (ed): Introduction to the Blood-brain Barrier: Methodology, Biology, and Pathology. Cambridge, UK, Cambridge University Press, 1998, pp 188–197.
17. Colombo JP: Urea cycle disorders, hyperammonemia and neurotransmitter changes. Enzyme 1987;38(1–4):214–219.
18. Bachmann C, Colombo JP: Increase of tryptophan and 5-hydroxyindole acetic acid in the brain of ornithine carbamoyltransferase deficient sparse-fur mice. J Pediatr Res 1984; 18(4):372–375.
19. Strauss KA, Morton DH: Branched-chain ketoacyl dehydrogenase deficiency: maple syrup disease. Curr Treatment Options Neurol 2003;5:329–341.
20. Yudkoff M, Daikhin Y, Nissim I, et al: Inhibition of astrocyte glutamine production by alpha-ketoisocaproic acid. J Neurochem 1994;63:1508–1515.
21. Zielke HR, Huang Y, Baab PJ, et al: Effect of alphaketoisocaproate and leucine on the in vivo oxidation of glutamate and glutamine in the rat brain. Neurochem Res 1997;22:1159–1166.
22. Dwivedi C, James EC, Parmar SS: Effects of abnormal metabolites of maple syrup urine disease on neurotransmitter receptor binding. Biochem Med Metabol Biol 1986;35:275–278.
23. Luzzatto L, Mehta A: Glucose-6-phosphate dehydrogenase deficiency. In Scriver CR (ed): The Metabolic and Molecular Bases of Inherited Disease, 7th ed. New York, McGraw-Hill, 1995, pp 3367–3398.
24. Yoshida A, Beutler E: Glucose-6-Phosphate Dehydrogenase. San Diego, CA, Academic Press, 1986.
25. Corash L, Spielberg S, Bartsocas C, et al: Reduced chronic hemolysis during high-dose vitamin E administration in Mediterranean-type glucose-6-phosphate dehydrogenase deficiency. N Engl J Med 1980;303(8):416–420.
26. Roche Laboratories: Rocephin. Product information. Nutley, NJ, Roche Laboratories, January 1996.
27. Cephalosporins. In Olin BR (ed): Drug Facts and Comparisons. St. Louis, MO, Facts and Comparisons, 1997, pp 335g–336e, 338f–338h.
28. Johnson LH, Bhutani VK, Brown AK: System-based approach to management of neonatal jaundice and prevention of kernicterus. J Pediatr 2002;140(4):396–403.
29. Ullrich CM, Yasui Y, Potter JD, et al: Pharmacogenetics of methotrexate: toxicity among marrow transplantation patients varies with the methylenetetrahydrofolate reductase C677T polymorphism. Blood 2001;98:231–234.
30. Selzer RR, Rosenblatt DS, Laxova R, Hogan K: Adverse effect of nitrous oxide in a child with 5,10-methylenetetrahydrofolate reductase deficiency. N Engl J Med 2003;349(1):45–50.
31. Erbe RW, Salis RJ: Severe methylenetetrahydrofolate reductase deficiency, methionine synthase, and nitrous oxide—a cautionary tale. N Engl J Med 2003;349(1):5–6.
32. Nelson TE, Flewellen EH: The malignant hyperthermia syndrome. N Engl J Med 1983;309:416–418.
33. Jurkat-Rott K, McCarthy TV, Lehmann-Horn F: Genetics and pathogenesis of malignant hyperthermia. Muscle Nerve 2000; 23:4–17.
34. Robinson R, Curran JL, Hall WJ, et al: Genetic heterogeneity and HOMOG analysis in British malignant hypethremia families. J Med Genet 1998;35:196–201.
35. McCarthy TV, Quane KA, Lynch PJ: Ryanodine receptor mutations in malignant hyperthermia and central core disease. Hum Mutat 2000;15:410–417.
36. Taylor P: Agents acting at the neuromuscular junction and autonomic ganglia. In Hardman JG, Limbird LE (eds): Goodman and Gilman's The Pharmacologic Basis of Therapeutics. New York, McGraw-Hill, 2001, pp 193–214.
37. Becker DM, Kramer S: The neurological manifestations of porphyria: a review. Medicine 1977;56:411–423.
38. Stein JA, Tschudy DP: Acute intermittent porphyria: a clinical and biochemical study of 46 patients. Medicine 1970;49:1–16.
39. McColl KEL, Thompson GT, Moore MR, Goldberg A: Haematin therapy and leucocyte gamma-aminolaevulinic-acid-synthase activity in prolonged attack of acute porphyria. Lancet 1978;1:133–134.

PART II

Specific Poisons

II

Specific Poisons

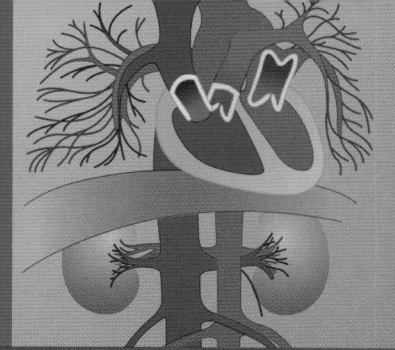

21 *Venomous Snakes*

A   North American Crotalinae Envenomation

FRANK G. WALTER, MD ■ PETER B. CHASE, MD, PHD ■ MIGUEL C. FERNÁNDEZ, MD ■ JUDE MCNALLY, BSPHARM, RPH

At a Glance...

■ North American vipers belong to the subfamily Crotalinae and include rattlesnakes (*Crotalus* and *Sistrurus* spp), copperheads, and water moccasins (both belonging to the genus *Agkistrodon*).

■ Snakebites by North American pit vipers are common, and most victims are seen in health care facilities. Morbidity is usual and may be significant and persistent. Death is rare.

■ Young males are the most frequent victims; ethanol use preceding the bite is not uncommon.

■ Venoms are composed of multiple polypeptides, designed to immobilize, kill, and digest.

■ Coagulopathy, rhabdomyolysis, and hypovolemia dominate the clinical picture of envenomation, with potentially limb-threatening edema of bitten extremities.

■ Treatment is based primarily on the history and physical examination. A simple scoring system of mild, moderate, and severe envenomation is presented.

■ First aid measures include immobilization of the injured part and prompt transport to an appropriate emergency department for evaluation. The practices of packing the wound in ice, applying tourniquets, and "cut and suck" techniques have been abandoned due to lack of efficacy and potential for harm.

■ Crotalidae Polyvalent Immune Fab (CroFab) has largely replaced the use of Wyeth-Ayerst Antivenin (Crotalidae) Polyvalent (ACP) (equine). Antivenoms and their indications, contraindications, and relative efficacies are discussed.

■ Fasciotomy is rarely indicated in snakebites and should be entertained only in the presence of sustained, elevated compartment pressures after the failure of adequate doses of antivenom and limb elevation.

■ Prophylactic antibiotics are not indicated.

ETIOLOGY

North America has two snake families with venomous members, the Viperidae (subfamily Crotalinae) and Elapidae (subfamily Elapinae).[1,2] North America has three genera of Crotalinae (previously known as Crotalidae): *Crotalus*, *Sistrurus*, and *Agkistrodon* (Table 21A-1).[2,3] Rattlesnakes are members of the genera *Crotalus* and *Sistrurus*.[2-4] Members of the genus *Agkistrodon* lack rattles. North America has 18 species of Crotalinae and numerous subspecies (see Table 21A-1).[3,5]

EPIDEMIOLOGY

The 2002 report of the American Association of Poison Control Centers documented 2325 indigenous venomous snakebites (Table 21A-2) from North American snakes.[6] Of these, 50% were by rattlesnakes, 38% by copperheads, 7% by cottonmouths, 4% by coral snakes, and 1% by unspecified crotalines (see Table 21A-2). In this case series, 87% of victims were treated in health care facilities (see Table 21A-2) and 2 patients died (0.1%); 2271 patients suffered morbidity (98%); and 54 patients had no significant health effects (2%). The latter could be considered to have had "dry bites" (i.e., bites from venomous snakes that do not result in signs or symptoms of envenomation) (see Table 21A-2).[4] This 2% dry bite incidence is in contradistinction to the 20% to 25% dry bite incidence quoted by many investigators.[7] Russell estimated that 20% of crotaline bites were dry bites, while Parrish found 27% dry bites; however, Wingert and Chan found a low incidence of dry bites (1%).[4,8,9]

Snakebite is most common in school-aged children, adolescents, and young adults, with the highest snakebite

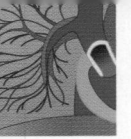

TABLE 21A-1 Some Crotalinae of North America

GENUS	SPECIES	SUBSPECIES	COMMON NAME	U.S. LOCATION
Crotalus	adamanteus		Eastern diamondback rattlesnake	Southeast U.S.
	atrox		Western diamondback rattlesnake	Southwest U.S.
	cerastes		Sidewinder	Southwest U.S.
	helleri		Southern Pacific rattlesnake	California
	horridus		Timber rattlesnake	North and eastern U.S.
	lepidus		Rock rattlesnake	Southwest U.S.
	mitchelli		Speckled rattlesnake	Southwest U.S.
	molossus		Black-tailed rattlesnake	Southwest U.S.
	pricei		Twin-spotted rattlesnake	Southwest U.S.
	ruber		Red diamond rattlesnake	California
	scutulatus	scutulatus	Mojave rattlesnake	Southwest U.S.
	tigris		Tiger rattlesnake	Arizona
	viridis	abyssus	Grand Canyon rattlesnake	Grand Canyon
		cerberus	Arizona black rattlesnake	Arizona
		concolor	Midget faded rattlesnake	Colorado, Utah
		lutosus	Great Basin rattlesnake	Western U.S.
		nuntius	Hopi rattlesnake	Arizona
		oreganus	Northern Pacific rattlesnake	Northwest U.S.
		viridis	Prairie rattlesnake	Rocky Mountains
	willardi		Ridge-nosed rattlesnake	Arizona, New Mexico
Sistrurus	catenatus		Massasauga	Midwest to Southwest
	miliarius		Pigmy rattlesnake	Southeast U.S.
Agkistrodon	contortrix		Copperhead	Massachusetts to Texas
	piscivorus		Cottonmouth	Virginia to Texas

TABLE 21A-2 Epidemiology of Bites from Venomous North American Snakes

TYPE OF SNAKE	NO. (%) OF PATIENTS	NO. (%) OF PATIENTS TREATED IN HEALTH CARE FACILITY	NO. (%) WITH NO MORBIDITY	NO. (%) WITH LIFE-THREATENING MORBIDITY	NO. (%) OF DEATHS
Rattlesnake	1150 (50)	1014 (88)	28 (2)	94 (8)	2 (0.2)
Copperhead	889 (38)	784 (88)	13 (2)	30 (3)	0 (0)
Cottonmouth	173 (7)	138 (80)	4 (2)	8 (5)	0 (0)
Coral	88 (4)	75 (85)	5 (6)	1 (1)	0 (0)
Unspecified crotaline	25 (1)	19 (76)	4 (16)	1 (4)	0 (0)
Total	2325 (100)	2030 (87)	54 (2)	134 (6)	2 (0.1)

From Watson WA, Litovitz TL, Rodgers GC, et al: 2002 annual report of the American Association of Poison Control Centers toxic surveillance system. Am J Emerg Med 2003; 21:394.

rates in 5- to 19-year-olds in two studies.[8,10] Another study found that 55% of victims were 17 to 27 years old, with a mean age of 24 years and a median age of 22 years.[9] Tokish and colleagues found a mean age of 29 years for snakebite victims.[11]

Most snakebite victims are male. Two studies reported 2:1 male-to-female ratios.[8,10] One study reported a 9:1 male-to-female ratio.[9] One study reported 55% males and 45% females.[12]

At least one species of indigenous snake is found in every state of the United States except Alaska, Hawaii, and Maine.[8] Snakebites occur most frequently in the Southeastern, South Central, and Southwestern United States. The 10 states with the highest incidence of snakebite are detailed in Table 21A-3.[8]

Snakebite varies not only by geographic region, but also by anatomic region. In one study, 58% of victims were bitten in a lower extremity; 38% in an upper extremity; 0.7% in the torso; 0.5% in the head, face, or neck; and in 2.8% of bites, the site was not clearly specified. This same study also found more victims were bitten on the right side of their bodies (55%) than the left.[8] In a second study, 55% of snakebites were to upper extremities and 51% were to the right side of the victims' bodies.[11] In a third study, 87% of victims were bitten in an upper extremity, 12% in a lower extremity, and 1% in the torso.[9] In a fourth study, snakebite anatomic region was classified as proximal or distal. Distal was defined as distal to the proximal interphalangeal joint of a finger or toe, or distal to the interphalangeal joint of the thumb or great toe. Distal snakebites occurred in 35% of patients and proximal snakebites occurred in 65%. Distal snakebites produced less severe clinical manifestations than proximal snakebites.[13]

The bite site is related to the victim's activity at the time of the bite. In one study, victims were engaged in

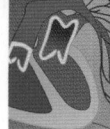

TABLE 21A-3 Geographic Distribution of Snakebite in the United States	
STATE	**INCIDENCE PER 100,000 PEOPLE/YR**
North Carolina	18.79
Arkansas	17.19
Texas	14.70
Georgia	13.44
West Virginia	11.29
Mississippi	10.83
Louisiana	10.25
Oklahoma	8.85
Arizona	7.83
South Carolina	7.72

From Parrish HM: Incidence of treated snakebites in the United States. Pub Health Rep 1966;81:269.

the following activities when they were bitten, in descending order of frequency: playing, working, or walking in their own yards; working on a farm or ranch; playing outside of their own yards; hunting or fishing; pursuing other outdoor recreational activities; handling a venomous snake; walking on or near a highway; working or playing inside a barn or henhouse; picking up logs or lumber; picking berries; reaching into obscure places; and engaging in military maneuvers. Only 4% of patients were handling a venomous snake. This correlates with more numerous lower extremity bites (63%) and fewer upper extremity bites (34%) in this study.[10] This is in contradistinction to another study in which 57% of victims were handling a venomous snake, 28% were clinically intoxicated with ethanol, and 87% were bitten in an upper extremity.[9]

Snakebites occur most commonly during the warmest months of the year, when snakes are most active and people are more frequently outdoors. In one study, 94% of snakebites occurred from April through October.[8] In a second study, 88% of snakebites occurred from April through October.[11] In a third study, 73% of snakebites occurred from April through September.[9] Snakebites occur most commonly during the morning, afternoon, and evening hours when people are most active outdoors. The vast majority of victims are bitten between 9 AM and 10 PM.[8,9]

CROTALINAE SNAKEBITE

Clinical Presentation

PATHOPHYSIOLOGY

Crotaline venom has multitudinous chemical constituents that act in concert to produce snake venom poisoning in a specific victim.[4] The clinician must always remember to treat the patient, not the snake, the venom, or the known or suspected venom constituents.

Venom is 70% water by weight. Lyophilized or desiccated venom is 90% protein and polypeptides by dry weight.[14,15]

The main functions of crotaline venom are immobilization, death, and digestion of prey. Not only do crotalines use venom offensively to obtain food, but also defensively to protect against predators and aggressors. Most crotaline venoms do not produce immobilization through neuromuscular blockade.

Immobilization is usually due to polypeptide, lethal venom components that produce hypovolemic shock so prey cannot escape. These polypeptide, lethal venom components ultimately kill prey due to hypovolemic shock.[4] Digestion is mediated via numerous proteolytic and other enzymes.[1,4] This digestive function is critical to snakes because they swallow prey whole and do not masticate their food. The digestive ability of crotaline venom is facilitated by injection into live prey while some perfusion continues to distribute venom. The venom's polypeptide, lethal components damage endothelial cells and allow plasma to exude and blood to extravasate into surrounding tissues, producing hypovolemic shock due to third spacing. Leaky capillaries also allow delivery of digestive components of snake venom to tissues; this speeds digestion. When live prey was fed to the crotaline *Bothrops jararacussu*, digestion time was 4 to 5 days versus 12 to 14 days for dead prey.[4]

The Mojave rattlesnake *Crotalus scutulatus scutulatus*, with venom A, is the classic exception to the fact that most crotalines immobilize prey with polypeptide, lethal venom components that produce hypovolemic shock.[16-23] Mojave rattlesnakes with venom A have Mojave toxin that immobilizes prey by neuromuscular blockade.[16-24] Mojave toxin is an acidic protein that consists of a basic phospholipase A_2 subunit and an acidic peptide subunit.[16-20] Some other North American crotaline species (e.g., *Crotalus tigris*, *C. viridis concolor*, *C. horridus*, *C. atrox*) have been shown to have some amounts of Mojave toxin in their venoms; however, Mojave rattlesnake venom A has the most Mojave toxin and the lowest median lethal dose (LD_{50}) values of any North American crotaline venom.[12,16-27] Other populations of Mojave rattlesnakes with venom B lack Mojave toxin and immobilize prey by producing hypovolemic shock from third spacing similar to other crotalines.[21-23,25-29] Mojave rattlesnakes with venom B are located predominantly in areas surrounding and between Phoenix and Tucson, Arizona.[21-23]

CLINICAL MANIFESTATIONS

Pathophysiologic, clinical manifestations of crotaline envenomation can be thought of in a familiar "A,B,C,D,E" paradigm.[30] The cardiovascular and neuromuscular systems are primarily at risk because these primary targets of toxicity are fundamentally affected by venom (Table 21A-4).[4,31,32]

The primary target of toxicity for most crotaline venoms is the cardiovascular system, especially vascular endothelial cells.[4,31,33] Crotaline venom produces capillary endothelial cell damage, resulting in endothelial cell swelling and rupture, which leaves large gaps in the microvasculature that allow third spacing of plasma and extravasation of erythrocytes.[33] Endothelial cell damage is caused by relatively low-molecular-weight polypeptides.[1,34] These polypeptides have molecular weights between

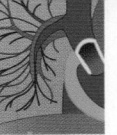

TABLE 21A-4 Targets of Crotaline Venom's Toxic Effects	
BODY COMPONENTS AT RISK	**PRIMARY TARGETS**
Airway	
Breathing	
Cardiovascular system	X
Disability (neuromuscular system)	X
Elimination (kidneys and liver)	

about 4500 and 6000 daltons. They produce shock with intravascular hemoconcentration and hypoproteinemia due to exudation of plasma through the damaged capillary endothelium.[4] This correlates clinically with profound edema that does not necessarily involve extravasation of large numbers of erythrocytes; therefore, hypovolemia can result from third spacing of plasma.[2,4]

While endothelial cells are damaged by lower-molecular-weight nonenzymatic polypeptides, vascular basement membranes and perivascular extracellular matrices are destroyed by hemorrhagic metalloproteinases (zinc-containing enzymes with molecular weights between 20,000 and 100,000 daltons) that allow extravasation of erythrocytes.[35] This correlates clinically with hemorrhage into envenomated parts of the body.[1,35] This extravasation of plasma and erythrocytes leads to shock and death in prey animals and can lead to shock and death in severely envenomated humans.

Other significant cardiovascular effects of venom are its direct actions on the clotting ability of blood.[1,4] Crotaline venom characteristically causes a disseminated intravascular coagulation (DIC)-like syndrome through fibrinogenolysis by thrombin-like, enzymatic venom glycoproteins with molecular weights between 29,000 and 35,000 daltons. These thrombin-like glycoproteins produce fibrin monomers, either fibrinopeptide A, most commonly, or fibrinopeptide B, rarely, depending on the specific venom, without utilizing the victim's own thrombin.[1,4,36-41]

These thrombin-like venom glycoproteins do not activate factor XIII, which rapidly and efficiently produces cross-linked fibrin, whereas thrombin does activate factor XIII in true DIC to rapidly and efficiently produce cross-linked fibrin that yields D-dimer on fibrinolysis. Non-cross-linked fibrin formed from thrombin-like crotaline enzymes is rapidly lysed to fibrin degradation (split) products, but not D-dimer, and the intravascular thrombosis with microangiopathic hemolytic anemia and intravascular consumption of platelets that is typical of true DIC does not occur. Exsanguination is rare from crotaline envenomations because the victim's ability to form thrombin, and thereby cross-linked fibrin, remains intact, and hemostasis can occur.[1,4,36-41]

The fundamental difference between true DIC and DIC-like syndromes from crotaline venoms is that true DIC always involves pathologic generation and activity of the victim's endogenous thrombin, whereas DIC-like syndromes do not. Other differences between true DIC

and DIC-like syndromes from crotaline venoms are outlined in Table 21A-5. The pathophysiologic differences between true DIC and DIC-like syndromes from crotaline venoms have important therapeutic implications. Crotaline antivenom is effective for crotaline, venom-induced coagulopathies, but heparin and blood products are not. Heparin is ineffective for crotaline, venom-induced coagulopathies because crotaline, thrombin-like enzymes are not inhibited by antithrombin III (heparin cofactor).[1,4,36-41] Transfused blood product coagulation factors and platelets are ineffective for crotaline, venom-induced coagulopathies because they are destroyed by circulating venom.[1,4,36-40] Therefore, administration of blood products to patients with crotaline, venom-induced coagulopathies exposes patients to the risks of blood product therapy without the benefits, unless they are actively and significantly bleeding despite copious antivenom administration and intensive supportive care.[1,4,31,36-40,42,43]

Although a characteristic DIC-like syndrome from crotaline venoms is described, crotaline venom–induced coagulopathies often vary markedly from case to case.[4,36] Many crotaline envenomations are accompanied by no significant laboratory abnormalities.[4] Others demonstrate isolated hypofibrinogenemia, isolated thrombocytopenia, or some combination of these, with or without prolongation of the prothrombin time, partial thromboplastin time, or elevated fibrin degradation (split) products.[4,36,38] In general, certain species of crotaline may produce characteristic coagulopathies in their victims.[36] For example, the Southern Pacific rattlesnake (*Crotalus helleri*) characteristically produces severe thrombocytopenia without significant hypofibrinogenemia.[36,43] Timber rattlesnake (*Crotalus horridus*) envenomations characteristically produce severe thrombocytopenia, with or without prothrombin time prolongation.[43,44] Despite generalizations, exceptions always exist; although 90% of victims of pigmy rattlesnake (*Sistrurus miliarius*) bites had no defibrination, 10% did.[36] One pigmy rattlesnake envenomation even resulted in true DIC, a rare and reportable event.[36,45] Not only do venom constituents vary within and between crotaline species, but they also vary in the same snake, depending on its age and the season of the year.[46,47]

Fibrinolysis due to DIC-like syndromes from crotaline venom is caused by indirect activation of plasminogen by release of tissue plasminogen activator from damaged vascular endothelial cells.[39]

Crotaline envenomation can cause thrombocytopenia by multiple mechanisms.[1,4,31,36-40,42,43] Thrombocytopenia is predominantly caused by consumption of platelets at the envenomation site, where disrupted microvasculature exposes platelets to collagen in basement membranes, producing local platelet deposition and aggregation.[33,35,40] Crotaline venom can also cause platelet aggregation without serotonin release.[38,39] Investigators isolated a timber rattlesnake (*Crotalus horridus*) toxin, a serine protease called crotalocytin, that aggregates platelets.[48,49]

The major clinical problems encountered in caring for victims of crotaline envenomations are local tissue

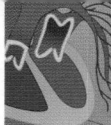

TABLE 21A-5 Comparison of True Disseminated Intravascular Coagulation (DIC) with DIC-like Syndromes from Crotaline Venoms

MANIFESTATION AND THERAPY	DIC	DIC-LIKE SYNDROMES
Pathologic thrombin production and activity	Yes	No
Pathologic activation of factor XIII by thrombin	Yes	No
Thrombin production of both fibrinopeptides A and B	Yes	No
Production of either fibrinopeptide A or B, but not usually both	No	Yes
Production of cross-linked fibrin	Yes	Less common
Production of fibrin degradation (split) products	Yes	Yes
Production of D-dimer	Yes	Less common
Antithrombin III depletion	Yes	No
Thrombocytopenia	Almost always	Sometimes
Active bleeding	Commonly	Rarely
Intravascular thrombosis	Commonly	Rarely
Heparin therapy helpful	Possibly	No
Crotaline antivenin therapy helpful	No	Yes

destruction due to digestive enzymes, edema due to exudation of plasma, hemorrhage due to destruction of the microvasculature, shock due to hypovolemia, and neuromuscular blockade in some victims (see Table 21A-4). Although the cardiovascular and neuromuscular systems are primarily at risk in snake venom poisoning, airway and breathing can be at risk due to massive orofacial or neck edema when the victim is envenomated in the mouth, face, or neck.[50-52] Airway and breathing can also be at risk because of neuromuscular blockade due to Mojave toxin's effect on muscles involved in airway patency and ventilation.[27] Airway and breathing can also be compromised as a result of coma from intravenous or perivenous envenomations, or coma from shock with a decreased ability to maintain airway patency and ventilation.[53,54] Airway and breathing can also be compromised by venom-induced anaphylaxis.[52] Elimination via the kidneys can be disrupted because of acute tubular necrosis due to shock or myoglobinuric renal failure due to rhabdomyolysis.[27,53,55] Canebrake rattlesnake (*Crotalus horridus atricaudatus*) envenomations characteristically produce rhabdomyolysis.[55] The most common clinical manifestations from crotaline bites in one case series are reported in Table 21A-6.[4]

Diagnosis

DIFFERENTIAL DIAGNOSIS

The differential diagnosis of snakebite includes puncture wounds and abrasions from other causes, wound infections, cellulitis, deep venous thrombosis, DIC, thrombocytopenia from other causes, inherited bleeding disorders, septicemia, hypovolemic shock from other causes, weakness as a result of neuromuscular blockade from other causes, and rhabdomyolysis from other causes.

The diagnosis of snake venom poisoning is usually simple because the patient, family, or friends tell the clinician that the patient has been bitten by a snake. However, it is important to consider snake venom poisoning in the differential diagnosis of preschool children, developmentally delayed patients, patients with ethanol or drug intoxication, or unconscious patients who present

TABLE 21A-6 Clinical Manifestations of Crotaline Bites

SIGNS OR SYMPTOMS	% OF PATIENTS
Fang marks (punctures or abrasions)	100
Edema	74
Weakness	72
Pain	65
Diaphoresis	64
Oral, perioral, scalp, or foot paresthesias	63
Abnormal pulse rates	60
Light-headedness, faintness, dizziness	57
Ecchymoses	51
Nausea, vomiting, or both	48
Abnormal blood pressures	46
Paresthesias near the envenomation site	42
Fasciculations	41
Regional lymphadenopathy	40
Abnormal respiratory rates	40
Bullae	40
Thirst	34
Abnormal body temperatures	31
Local tissue necrosis at bite site	27
Cyanosis	16
Hematemesis, melena, or hematuria	15
Unconsciousness	12
Seizures	1

From Russell FE: Snake Venom Poisoning, 2nd ed. Great Neck, NY, Scholium International, 1983, p 281.

with puncture wounds, abrasions, edema, or ecchymoses, with or without coagulopathies, shock, rhabdomyolysis, fasciculations, or neuromuscular blockade. Snake envenomation must be considered in the patient with an unknown bite. This is especially true in areas in which a high incidence of snakebites occurs (see Table 21A-3).[8] Numerous cases of snakebites have been noted in small children who came in crying after playing in the yard.[10]

It is essential to completely undress and examine all nonspeaking patients and patients with altered sensoria to search for snakebite punctures or abrasions, and to search for other local, regional, or systemic signs of envenomation.[54] We have cared for diabetic patients with poor vision due to diabetic retinopathy and poor lower

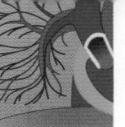

BOX 21A-1   CROTALINE ENVENOMATION: MINIMAL-MODERATE-SEVERE SCORING METHOD

Minimal Envenomation	**Moderate Envenomation**	**Severe Envenomation**
Local swelling	Swelling beyond bite site	Marked local response
Other local changes	Systemic signs and/or symptoms	Severe systemic signs and symptoms
No systemic signs or symptoms	Abnormal laboratory values	Markedly abnormal laboratory values
Normal laboratory values		

From Dart RC, Hurlbut KM, Garcia R, et al: Validation of a severity score for the assessment of crotalid snakebite. Ann Emerg Med 1996;27:321.

---

extremity sensation due to diabetic neuropathy who were unaware of a snakebite but presented with wounds in edematous, ecchymotic legs and had crotaline venom–induced coagulopathies.

CLINICAL DIAGNOSIS

Diagnosis of envenomation from a snakebite is a clinical diagnosis. A history of snakebite is the most helpful diagnostic tool. This history can be obtained from the patient, family, friends, or prehospital health care professionals. Signs and symptoms of crotaline envenomation are detailed in Box 21A-1 and Tables 21A-7 to 21A-9.[4,32,36] The most important aspects of clinical diagnosis of crotaline envenomation are determining the degree of envenomation on presentation (see Box 21A-1 and Tables 21A-7 to 21A-9) and determining whether progression of the envenomation syndrome (i.e., worsening of clinical signs and symptoms) is occurring over time. Three common systems are used to determine the degree of envenomation on presentation: (1) the minimal-moderate-severe scoring method, (2) the

grade 0 through IV scoring method, and (3) the snakebite severity score (see Box 21A-1 and Tables 21A-7 to 21A-9).[56] The snakebite severity score (see Table 21A-8) is a research tool and was not intended for general clinical use. We use a modified minimal-moderate-severe scoring method that integrates portions of all three systems; this is detailed in Table 21A-9.[32]

Serial physical examinations and assessment of vital signs and clinical status, searching for tissue edema, induration and tenderness, progression of swelling, and development of systemic signs and symptoms, are essential to proper diagnosis and management of the snakebite victim.

LABORATORY DIAGNOSIS

Laboratory diagnosis of snake venom poisoning focuses predominantly on detection of the following: coagulopathies; hemoconcentration due to third spacing of plasma; anemia due to extravasation of erythrocytes or other sources of bleeding; rhabdomyolysis as indicated by elevated creatine phosphokinase values, elevated creatinine levels not attributable to renal failure, and myoglobinuria; and hematuria or hemoglobinuria on urinalysis. Laboratory tests to detect these potential abnormalities should be obtained on presentation and periodically thereafter. We recommend obtaining a complete blood count with platelets, prothrombin time, partial thromboplastin time, fibrinogen, and fibrin degradation (split) products on presentation and every 4 hours thereafter for at least the first 12 hours of hospitalization. This is recommended because laboratory evidence of coagulopathy may not be evident initially or can worsen after initial presentation. Frequency of obtaining these laboratory data should be determined by the clinician, depending on the patient's clinical course, the results of the laboratory tests, and whether and when the patient receives antivenom. After administering antivenom, we prefer to obtain these laboratory data every 4 hours until values have returned to normal or to stable near-normal levels.

We often screen for laboratory abnormalities caused by concurrent illnesses that can confound the care of envenomated patients. This also helps to determine whether coagulopathies are the result of an envenomation or of underlying severe liver disease.

Chest radiography and electrocardiograms should be obtained for patients with preexisting cardiopulmonary diseases and for patients with cardiopulmonary signs or symptoms. We do not routinely obtain these for all

---

TABLE 21A-7 Crotaline Envenomation: Grade 0-IV Scoring Method

GRADE	CHARACTERISTICS
0	No envenomation: fang marks and minimal pain
I	Minimal envenomation: fang marks, pain, 1–5 in. of edema and erythema during the first 12 hr; no systemic symptoms
II	Moderate envenomation: fang marks, pain, 6–12 in. of edema and erythema in the first 12 hr; systemic symptoms may be present along with rapid progression of signs from grade I; may be bloody ooze at bite site
III	Severe envenomation: fang marks, pain, edema > 12 in. in first 12 hr; systemic symptoms, including coagulation defects after crotaline bites; signs of grades I and II appear in rapid progression, with immediate systemic signs and symptoms
IV	Very severe envenomation; local reaction develops rapidly; edema may involve ipsilateral trunk; ecchymoses, necrosis, blebs, and blisters develop; at tightly restrictive fascial planes, tension may become great enough to obstruct venous or even arterial flow

From Dart RC, Hurlbut KM, Garcia R, et al: Validation of a severity score for the assessment of crotalid snakebite. Ann Emerg Med 1996; 27:321.

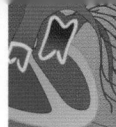

TABLE 21A-8 Crotaline Envenomation: The Snakebite Severity Score

CRITERIA	POINTS*
Pulmonary System	
No symptoms/signs	0
Dyspnea, minimal chest tightness, mild or vague discomfort, or respirations of 20–25/min	1
Moderate respiratory distress (tachypnea, 26–40 breaths/min; accessory muscle use)	2
Cyanosis, air hunger, extreme tachypnea, or respiratory insufficiency/failure	3
Cardiovascular System	
No symptoms/signs	0
Tachycardia (100–25 beats/min), palpitations, generalized weakness, benign dysrhythmia, or hypertension	1
Tachycardia (126–75 beats/min) or hypotension, with systolic blood pressure >100 mm Hg	2
Extreme tachycardia (>175 breaths/min), hypotension with systolic blood pressure <100 mm Hg, malignant dysrhythmia, or cardiac arrest	3
Local Wound	
No symptoms/signs	0
Pain, swelling, or ecchymosis within 5–7.5 cm of bite site	1
Pain, swelling, or ecchymosis involving less than half of the extremity (7.5–50 cm from bite site)	2
Pain, swelling, or ecchymosis involving half to all of the extremity (50–100 cm from bite site)	3
Pain, swelling, or ecchymosis extending beyond affected extremity (>100 cm from bite site)	4
Gastrointestinal System	
No symptoms/signs	0
Pain, tenesmus, or nausea	1
Vomiting or diarrhea	2
Repeated vomiting, diarrhea, hematemesis, or hematochezia	3
Hematologic System	
No symptoms/signs	0
Coagulation parameters slightly abnormal: PT, <20 sec; PTT, <50 sec; platelets, 100,000–150,000/mL; or fibrinogen, 100–150 µg/mL	1
Coagulation parameters abnormal: PT, 20–50 sec; PTT, 50–75 sec; platelets, 50,000–100,000/mL; or fibrinogen, 50–100 µg/mL	2
Coagulation parameters abnormal: PT, 50–100 sec; PTT, 75–100 sec; platelets, 20,000–50,000/mL; or fibrinogen, <50 µg/mL	3
Coagulation parameters markedly abnormal, with serious bleeding or the threat of spontaneous bleeding: unmeasurable PT or PTT; platelets, <20,000/mL; or undetectable fibrinogen; severe abnormalities of other laboratory values also fall into this category	4
Central Nervous System	
No symptoms/signs	0
Minimal apprehension, headache, weakness, dizziness, chills, or paresthesia	1
Moderate apprehension, headache, weakness, dizziness, chills, paresthesia, confusion, or fasciculation in area of bite site	2
Severe confusion, lethargy, seizures, coma, psychosis, or generalized fasciculation	3

PT, prothrombin time; PTT, partial thromboplastin time.
*Points are assessed on the basis of manifestations caused by the venom itself (antivenom reactions not included). Ranges given are for adults; appropriate compensation should be made for age.
From Dart RC, Hurlbut KM, Garcia R, et al: Validation of a severity score for the assessment of crotalid snakebite. Ann Emerg Med 1996;27:321.

patients with crotaline envenomations. All snakebitten patients should receive an intravenous lifeline, continuous cardiac monitoring, frequent automated blood pressure measurements, and pulse oximetry.

Treatment

POISONING TREATMENT PARADIGM
Care of envenomated patients can be thought of in a familiar "A,B,C,D,E" paradigm.[30] Basic resuscitation is similar for all envenomated patients. This includes a primary survey and resuscitation consisting of management of airway and breathing; cardiovascular resuscitation, including administration of intravenous fluids; treatment of any disability (i.e., preserving neuromuscular function); and complete exposure of the patient with environmental control.[30] In addition to the primary survey and resuscitation, the "A,B,C,D,E" mnemonic can be modified to organize care of envenomated patients by utilizing the poisoning treatment paradigm (Box 21A-2).[32] The poisoning treatment paradigm organizes therapy of poisoned patients by considering whether kinetic aspects of a toxin can be modified, by determining whether the effects of the toxin can be modified pharmacodynamically with an antidote, and by reemphasizing basic care of the patient (i.e., the primary survey and resuscitation).

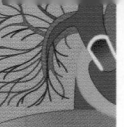

TABLE 21A-9 Crotaline Envenomation: Determining the Degree of Envenomation

DEGREE OF ENVENOMATION	CONTIGUOUS MANIFESTATIONS	SYSTEMIC MANIFESTATIONS	LABORATORY ABNORMALITIES
None or trivial ("dry bite")	Punctures or abrasions; pain and tenderness at bite	None	None
Mild or minimal	Punctures or abrasions; pain, tenderness, edema, and erythema at and adjacent to bite	Perioral paresthesias	None
Moderate	Punctures or abrasions; pain, tenderness, edema, and erythema beyond area adjacent to bite	Perioral paresthesias; peripheral paresthesias; gustatory changes; nausea; emesis; diarrhea; weakness; light-headedness; diaphoresis; chills	↑ PT; ↑ PTT; ↓ platelets; ↓ fibrinogen; ↑ hemoglobin
Severe	Punctures or abrasions; pain, tenderness, edema, and erythema of entire extremity	Ventilatory insufficiency; hypotension; shock; bleeding; altered mental status; fasciculations; seizures	↑↑ PT; ↑↑ PTT; ↓↓ platelets; ↓↓ fibrinogen; ↑↑ hemoglobin

PT, prothrombin time; PTT, partial thromboplastin time.

BOX 21A-2   POISONING TREATMENT PARADIGM

General Paradigm	Specific Therapy for Crotaline Envenomation
Alter absorption	Call 911 with a cell phone and remain still. Apply sling.
Administer antidote	Crotalidae Polyvalent Immune Fab (ovine) or Wyeth-Ayerst Antivenin (Crotalidae) Polyvalent (equine origin)
Basics: Primary survey & resuscitation	Resuscitation basics (A, B, C, D, E) Intravenous isotonic crystalloid Cleanse and dress wounds Tetanus immunization No antibiotics
Change catabolism	None
Distribute differently	None
Enhance elimination	None

IMMEDIATE MEASURES: FIRST AID AND PREHOSPITAL CARE

All patients who may have been bitten by a venomous snake should be taken to a health care facility as soon as possible. The most important principle of first aid for snakebite victims is, "*Primum non nocere,*" that is, "First, do no harm." First-aid measures have never been proven to decrease morbidity or mortality from crotaline envenomations. One study found no differences in clinical courses between those patients who did and those who did not receive first aid.[9] In fact, more recent research found nearly a threefold increase in necrotic and infectious complications that required surgery in patients who received first-aid treatments, such as cryotherapy (ice), cut and suck, tourniquets, or superficial constriction bands.[11]

Pros and cons of first-aid measures have been discussed in detail elsewhere, and first-aid recommendations are summarized in Table 21A-10.[12,57,58] First aid should never be considered a substitute for definitive medical care and should never delay in-hospital admin-

istration of antivenom, if indicated. Any delay can be fraught with danger. The most helpful first-aid tool is a cellular phone. This allows rapid summoning of emergency medical services (EMS) without moving the victim. Walking decreased transit time of ersatz venom in a human study.[59] All patients who may have been bitten by a venomous snake should be taken to an appropriate health care facility as soon as possible. Rapid EMS transport is the safest form of first aid and prehospital care for snakebite.

First aid and prehospital measures for snakebite can be considered to fall into three categories: (1) those that may be helpful and are unlikely to be harmful, (2) those that are controversial and may become harmful, and (3) those that are unhelpful or harmful.

First aid and/or prehospital care that is likely to be helpful, or at least not harmful, includes applying a sling to bitten upper extremities and keeping the bite site in a neutral position (i.e., at heart level). Another reasonable prehospital EMS intervention is to start a large-bore intravenous line in a nonbitten extremity to infuse

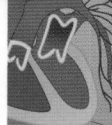

TABLE 21A-10 Immediate Crotaline Snakebite Treatment			
FIRST AID AND PREHOSPITAL CARE	**NO**	**YES**	**CONTROVERSIAL**
Capture snake	X		
Incise fang marks	X		
Oral suction	X		
Electric shock to denature venom	X		
Ice	X		
Tourniquet	X		
Constriction bands	X		X
Splint	X		X
Extraction devices	X		
Sling		X	
Isotonic IV in other extremity		X	
EMS activation with a cellular phone		X	
Rapid transport		X	

EMS, emergency medical services; IV, intravenous line

isotonic crystalloid. This serves as an intravenous lifeline to allow administration of isotonic crystalloids if noticeable swelling begins.

Although snake identification may be helpful, it is unnecessary to capture or kill the snake for identification. Attempts to capture or kill the snake could result in more bites to the victim and bites that could turn potential rescuers into victims.[57,58] Administration of either Crotalidae Polyvalent Immune Fab (ovine) antivenom (Protherics, Nashville, TN) or Antivenin (Crotalidae) Polyvalent (equine origin) (Wyeth-Ayerst, Philadelphia, PA) is effective for all crotaline envenomations and does not require definitive identification of the envenomating crotaline.[31,57,58]

Controversial crotaline bite first aid and prehospital measures that may become harmful include use of constriction bands, and splints involving constriction bands. Most researchers use the term *constriction band* to describe a device that impairs efflux of superficial venous and lymphatic flow from bitten extremities (see Table 21A-10).[42,57-62] Although some studies with envenomated animals and one human study with ersatz venom indicated decreased efflux from extremities with constriction bands, no human clinical studies have proven the safety or efficacy of this practice.[59-62] An animal study showed that systemic absorption of crotaline venom was decreased with constriction band therapy using a sphygmomanometer cuff with the pressure maintained at 45 mm Hg. Continual adjustments, allowing air to escape from the cuff, were necessary to avoid limb-threatening constriction as the envenomated animal's leg swelled.[60] Continual cuff adjustments would be difficult in first aid and prehospital care. In addition, the 45 mm Hg cuff pressure exceeds the normal capillary perfusion pressure of about 30 mm Hg. Another animal study found that elastic wrapping of an envenomated

extremity at 55 mm Hg and splinting decreased systemic absorption of Australian elapid venom; however, Australian elapid venom causes minimal tissue edema.[61] This study also showed that splinting alone or pressure wrapping alone did not limit systemic venom absorption. Both techniques had to be used simultaneously to limit venom absorption.[61] Another study used similar elastic wrapping and splinting and showed decreased systemic absorption of Eastern diamondback rattlesnake venom; however, the high pressure (initially 55 mm Hg) could cause extreme pain in a swollen envenomated extremity and could cause limb-threatening ischemia as swelling increased.[62] Splinting the envenomated limb is also controversial because splinting involves circumferential elastic wrapping that could also compromise limb perfusion as swelling increases because of crotaline envenomation. In summary, constriction bands have not been studied clinically in North American patients with crotaline envenomations; therefore, their safety and efficacy are unproven and we do not recommend them. A constriction band could turn what is uncommonly a life-threatening event (0.1%) into a limb-threatening event (see Table 21A-2).[6]

The remaining first aid and prehospital measures are mentioned only to condemn them, because they are either ineffective or dangerous[31,42,57,58]:

1. Do not incise fang marks.[1,57,58] Incision by persons without training or experience can result in damage to deep structures and can introduce infection and exacerbate tissue necrosis.[31,57,58]

2. Do not use oral suction. Oral suction can introduce human oral flora and carries the theoretical possibility of causing a human bite infection.[31,57,58] Oral suction can also result in envenomation of the lips and/or mouth if the lips are cracked or have lesions or if there is a break in the oral mucosa.

3. Do not apply ice or immerse the envenomated extremity in ice, ice water, or snow.[4,31,57,58,63] So-called cryotherapy can result in profound tissue necrosis due to further vasoconstriction and ischemia in marginally perfused tissues.[4,31,57,58]

4. Do not apply a tourniquet that would result in obstruction of deep venous or arterial flow. This will exacerbate ischemia, infarction, and necrosis in a limb that already may have marginal perfusion due to envenomation. A tourniquet also endangers a limb in which a patient has received a dry bite, without any envenomation or risk of morbidity.[4,31,57,58,63]

5. Do not use electric shock to treat snakebites.[53,57,58,64-68] Studies have shown that electric shocks are ineffective, and clinical experience has shown that they can be dangerous.

Newly published data on extraction devices do not support their use.[69-72] In a study from the 1980s, radiolabeled crotaline venom was injected into rabbits and an extraction device was applied 3 minutes after injection. After 3 minutes of suction (i.e., 6 minutes after venom injection), 23% of the injected venom was removed by the extraction device. Thirty-four percent of radiolabeled

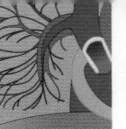

venom was removed after suction for 30 minutes (i.e., 33 minutes after injection).[73] The same group published data on use of extraction devices in patients in an abstract describing three people bitten by rattlesnakes.[74] Two of the three patients exhibited clinical signs of envenomation, and venom was recovered from the wounds of these two patients with an extraction device. The device was left in place until its cup filled with serosanguineous fluid; this was repeated five times in each patient. The largest portion of venom was recovered during the initial application of the extraction device. The clinician should be aware that both of these references are abstracts and include small numbers of subjects. These abstracts raised questions regarding use of extraction devices: Does removal of some portion of injected venom improve the patient's clinical course? Do such devices concentrate venom at the bite site and result in more bite site necrosis? Use of these devices remained unproven and controversial until recently.[69-72] The weight of evidence now does not support the use of extraction devices.[69-72] Bush and colleagues found that an extraction device did not reduce swelling in a randomized, controlled trial injecting rattlesnake venom into study pigs. In fact, some pigs developed circular lesions at the site of application of the extraction device, and these lesions subsequently necrosed and sloughed, with prolonged healing.[71] Similar local lesions have been described in humans after use of these devices.[70,72] Alberts and colleagues found that an extraction device removed virtually no mock venom (radiolabeled albumin) in a simulated snakebite model in human volunteers.[69]

Hospital Care

When a snakebitten patient arrives at the hospital, the clinician should perform a standard primary survey and resuscitation ("A,B,C,D,E").[30] Most patients will not require airway or breathing interventions such as oxygen administration or endotracheal intubation, because most crotaline envenomations are not life threatening.[6] However, patients with signs or symptoms of dyspnea or hypoxia should receive oxygen and assisted ventilation, if necessary. Endotracheal intubation should be performed for the usual indications.[30] Prompt endotracheal intubation is necessary for any patient with any signs of envenomation to the lips, tongue, head, or neck.[46,51,52] Endotracheal intubation must be done as soon as possible, before massive swelling of the airway occurs, which would make endotracheal intubation difficult or impossible, and because cricothyroidotomy would be extremely difficult in the presence of a swollen neck and venom-induced coagulopathy. Not only are airway patency and breathing in danger of being compromised as a result of head and neck envenomations, but also because of rare occurrences of anaphylactoid, angioedematous reactions involving the upper airway caused by intravenous or perivenous envenomations and also because of rare envenomations being associated with acute adult respiratory distress syndrome (ARDS).[29,53,54,75]

Cardiovascular resuscitation is critical in moderate and severe crotaline envenomations with marked third

spacing of plasma into subcutaneous tissue and extravasation of erythrocytes through damaged microvasculature. Intravascular volume resuscitation should be guided by the usual clinical parameters (e.g., administering enough intravenous isotonic crystalloids to relieve the patient's thirst and to produce urine output of at least 1 mL/kg/hr).[29,53,75,76]

Basic neuromuscular resuscitation involves endotracheal intubation with mechanical ventilation for those uncommon patients with moderate to severe Mojave toxin envenomations that produce neuromuscular blockade and ventilatory insufficiency.[16-23,25,27] Ventilatory insufficiency can also develop because of a decreased level of consciousness due to shock and hypoperfusion of the brain,[53] in rare cases of snakebite complicated by seizures,[4] and in rare cases of intravenous or perivenous envenomations associated with coma.[54]

Basic resuscitation to preserve the organs of elimination (i.e., the liver and kidneys) is directed primarily at preserving renal perfusion and urine output. The liver is rarely damaged by crotaline venom poisoning. Occasionally, the kidneys are damaged by acute tubular necrosis from hypoperfusion and hypovolemia or by myoglobinuric renal failure from rhabdomyolysis.[9,27,29,45,55,76-78]

Other basic supportive care for crotaline snakebites includes cleansing the wound and keeping it clean and dry. We usually recommend application of a dry 4 × 4 gauze pad to the wound itself, without tape. Taping the dressing in place can result in vesiculation and formation of bullae caused by shearing forces from the tape on the skin as the affected extremity swells. Tetanus immunization should be given if needed.

Prophylactic antibiotics are not necessary for snakebite because there is no evidence that they are effective.[79,80] Routine use of prophylactic antibiotics is no longer recommended. Broad-spectrum antibiotics are indicated only if signs of wound infection are present.[7,79,80] Older recommendations to prophylactically administer antibiotics to patients with snakebite were based on studies of the oral flora of snakes and not on the incidence of wound infection after North American snakebites.[81]

ADMINISTRATION OF THE ANTIDOTES

Wyeth-Ayerst ACP has been commercially available in the United States since 1954 (Table 21A-11).[82] This antivenom, manufactured by immunizing horses with venom from four crotaline species, *Crotalus adamanteus* (Eastern diamondback rattlesnake), *C. atrox* (Western diamondback rattlesnake), *C. durissus terrificus* (South American or tropical rattlesnake), and *Bothrops atrox* (fer-de-lance),[83] is capable of neutralizing venom from all North, Central, and South American crotalines (see Table 21A-11).[82,83] Because it is of equine origin, it can cause true anaphylactic reactions (type I hypersensitivity), anaphylactoid reactions, and serum sickness (i.e., immune-complex disease [type III hypersensitivity]).[7,31,42,82,83]

A polyvalent, crotaline, ovine-derived, fragment antibody (Fab) antivenom has been developed (initially [premarketing], CroTab, Therapeutic Antibodies, Inc., Nashville, TN; however, now [postmarketing], CroFab, Protherics, Nashville, TN). This new polyvalent

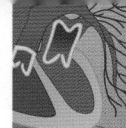

TABLE 21A-11 United States Crotaline Antivenoms

CHARACTERISTICS	ANTIVENIN (CROTALIDAE) POLYVALENT	CROTALIDAE POLYVALENT IMMUNE FAB (OVINE)
FDA approved (year)	1954	2000
Manufacturer	Wyeth-Ayerst Labs	Protherics, Inc.
Distributor	Wyeth-Ayerst Labs	Savage Labs of Altana, Inc.
Immunized animals	Horses (equine)	Sheep (ovine)
Venoms used to immunize animals	*Crotalus adamanteus* (Eastern diamondback)	*C. adamanteus*
	Crotalus atrox (Western diamondback)	*C. atrox*
	Crotalus durissus terrificus (Tropical rattlesnake)	*Crotalus scutulatus* (Mojave rattlesnake with venom type A)
	Bothrops atrox (Fer-de-lance)	*Agkistrodon piscivorus* (cottonmouth)
Immunoglobin	Whole IgG	Fab of IgG
Immunoglobin molecular weight (Daltons)	150,000	50,000
Vial contents	2.1 g lyophilized protein whole 18.9% IgG (wt/wt) 6% albumin (wt/wt)	<1.5 g lyophilized protein >85% Fab (wt/wt) <3% Fc (wt/wt) <0.5% albumin (wt/wt)

antivenom was developed by immunizing sheep with the venom from four North American crotalines: *Crotalus atrox* (Western diamondback rattlesnake), *C. adamanteus* (Eastern diamondback rattlesnake), *C. scutulatus scutulatus* (Mojave rattlesnake with venom A), and *Agkistrodon piscivorus piscivorus* (Eastern cottonmouth) (see Table 21A-11). These venoms were chosen on the basis of their clinical importance in snakebites occurring in the United States and northern Mexico, the geographic ranges of the snakes, genetic dissimilarities of the four immunizing venoms, and cross-antigenicity with venoms from other clinically important crotalines. An animal study showed that CroTab was very effective.[84] Human studies also demonstrated CroTab's and now CroFab's efficacy.[5,85-90] Premarketing CroFab is somewhat different than premarketing CroTab (Table 21A-12).[91]

Prior to administration of any medication, the clinician must ask a five-part question: What are the indications, contraindications, complications, dosage, and route of administration for the medication?[32] Answers to the five elements of this general question are summarized for Wyeth-Ayerst ACP and CroFab in Table 21A-13.

Table 21A-11 compares and contrasts Wyeth-Ayerst ACP with CroFab.[5]

Wyeth-Ayerst ACP (Equine Origin)

Wyeth-Ayerst ACP is indicated in moderate and severe cases of crotaline envenomation and in mild crotaline envenomations with progression (worsening) of clinical signs and symptoms. Progression is defined as worsening of the local injury, laboratory abnormalities, or systemic manifestations.[4]

The clinician should never be lulled into a false sense of security just because the patient and/or clinician knows the envenomation is from a copperhead bite because fatal copperhead bites have been reported.[87,92-95] We have consulted on an intravenous or perivenous copperhead bite to a patient's medial malleolus that

TABLE 21A-12 Minimum Mouse Median Lethal Dose (LD$_{50}$) Neutralizing Units per Vial

VENOM	PREMARKETING CROTAB	POSTMARKETING CROFAB
Crotalus adamanteous	1805	800
Crotalus atrox	985	1350
Crotalus scutulatus	11,630	5210
Agkistrodon piscivorus	755	460

resulted in shock, ventilatory failure, seizure, and coma and required immediate endotracheal intubation, mechanical ventilation, massive intravenous fluid administration, and antivenom therapy. Ultimately, the patient recovered without permanent sequelae.

Relative contraindications to Wyeth-Ayerst ACP include a history of horse product allergy, a history of previous allergic reaction to Wyeth-Ayerst ACP, and inability of the clinician to manage an anaphylactic or anaphylactoid reaction in a patient with a life-threatening envenomation (see Table 21A-11).[32] Absolute contraindications to Wyeth-Ayerst ACP include lack of informed consent and inability of the clinician to manage an anaphylactic and/or anaphylactoid reaction in a patient without a life-threatening envenomation.

The main complications of Wyeth-Ayerst ACP are anaphylactic reactions (type I hypersensitivity), anaphylactoid reactions, and serum sickness (type III hypersensitivity).[7,31,42] Anaphylactic or anaphylactoid reactions are immediate complications of antivenom therapy that occur during antivenom administration. Serum sickness, an immune-complex disease, is a delayed complication of antivenom administration.

Anaphylactic and anaphylactoid reactions are indistinguishable clinically, but differ on the basis of pathogenesis.[96-98] An anaphylactic reaction is a type I

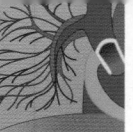
TABLE 21A-13 Guidelines for Use of Crotaline Antivenoms

5 GENERAL QUESTIONS	ANSWERS FOR CROTALINE ANTIVENOMS
Indications	Mild crotaline envenomations with progression
	Moderate and severe crotalid envenomations
Contraindications	Relative contraindications
	Horse product allergy (Wyeth-Ayerst)
	Sheep product allergy (CroFab)
	Papaya or papain allergy (CroFab)
	Inability to manage anaphylactic and anaphylactoid reactions with life-threatening envenomations
	Absolute contraindications
	Refusal after informed consent
	Inability to manage anaphylactic and anaphylactoid reactions with non-life-threatening envenomations
Complications	Immediate
	Anaphylactoid reactions
	Anaphylactic reactions (type I hypersensitivity, IgE mediated)
	More common with Wyeth-Ayerst
	Less common with CroFab
	Delayed
	Serum sickness (type III hypersensitivity; antigen-antibody, immune complex mediated)
	Virtually inevitable with Wyeth-Ayerst
	Uncommon with CroFab
	Recurrent coagulopathy
	Less common with Wyeth-Ayerst
	More common with CroFab

Dosage	DEGREE OF ENVENOMATION	INITIAL NO. OF VIALS	
		WYETH-AYERST	CROFAB
	Dry bite (no envenomation	0	0
	Mild with progression	10	4–6
	Moderate	10–20	6
	Severe	20	6–12
Route	Intravenous in an intensive care setting in the emergency department or intensive care unit		

hypersensitivity reaction, an anamnestic reaction, that requires initial exposure to an antigen that resulted in production of immunoglobulin E (IgE) antibody that attaches to mast cells via its Fc portion. After this initial sensitization step, reexposure to even the smallest concentration of the inciting antigen elicits an anaphylactic reaction due to the antigen binding to preformed IgE attached to mast cells, resulting in degranulation of mast cells with release of histamine and other mediators. Anaphylactoid reactions also result in release of histamine and other mediators from mast cells, but this release is not dependent on IgE. Another important distinction between anaphylactic and anaphylactoid reactions is that the smallest concentrations of the antigen will elicit an IgE-dependent anamnestic response in true anaphylactic reactions; however, substances that elicit anaphylactoid reactions are not acting as antigens for preformed IgE, and therefore the smallest concentrations of these substances will not necessarily elicit an anaphylactoid reaction.[96-98] In other words, anaphylactoid reactions are elicited in a fashion that is dependent on concentration, rate, route, and dose.

This has important therapeutic implications, especially when administering heterologous proteins such as Wyeth-Ayerst ACP. By maximally diluting the Wyeth-Ayerst ACP and administering it slowly, anaphylactoid reactions can be modulated or prevented. True IgE-mediated anaphylactic reactions cannot be prevented with dilution or slower administration. One study showed a 23% incidence of anaphylactic or anaphylactoid reactions in patients treated with Wyeth-Ayerst ACP. Half of these patients manifested only cutaneous signs and symptoms, whereas half of the affected patients manifested systemic signs and symptoms. Treatment of these antivenom reactions was uniformly effective, with no mortality, minimal morbidity, and no permanent sequelae.[99] Another study found that 14% of antivenom-treated patients developed urticaria, 10% developed pruritus, 6% suffered hypotension, 1% suffered bradycardia, and 1% suffered apnea that investigators thought was related to antivenom administration.[9] No patient in this study suffered permanent sequelae from any of these complications. A third study found that 14% of antivenom-treated patients developed a rash, 4% developed a rash and fever, and 14% suffered hypotension and/or respiratory distress.[100]

Serum sickness, a subtype of type III hypersensitivity, is an immune-complex disease due to antigen-antibody complexes.[101] Clinically, serum sickness can manifest the following signs and symptoms: fever, malaise, urticaria, lymphadenopathy, myalgias, arthralgias, and, rarely, vasculitis, glomerulonephritis, or neuritis.[82,101] Onset of

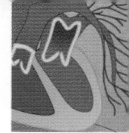

serum sickness after Wyeth-Ayerst ACP administration usually occurs 3 days to 3 weeks after administration, with an average onset of about 1 week.

The incidence of serum sickness seems dose related. One study found an 83% incidence of serum sickness in patients who received more than eight vials of Wyeth-Ayerst ACP versus a 38% incidence in patients who received less than eight vials; however, due to the small sample size, this difference was not statistically significant.[99]

Dosage of Wyeth-Ayerst ACP is determined by the victim's degree of envenomation and has nothing to do with the victim's age or weight.[4,32,56] This is because antivenom neutralizes a specific amount of venom. Clinically, the amount of venom is estimated by the effect that the venom has on the patient. This can be estimated by various grading systems (see Box 21A-1 and Tables 21A-7 to 21A-9).[32,56]

When the decision for antivenom therapy has been made, it is important to note that the recommended dose of antivenom has increased over the years.[4] Although regional differences have been noted, 10 vials (given intravenously) of Wyeth-Ayerst ACP is the initial dose in all treated rattlesnake envenomations.[32,42] In rapidly progressive envenomations or in those with hemodynamic instability, up to 20 vials of Wyeth-Ayerst ACP may be required initially, in addition to aggressive resuscitation.[7,32,42] After the initial antivenom administration, serial laboratory data should be obtained every 4 hours and serial physical examinations at least hourly for evidence of continuing progression (i.e., worsening of clinical signs and/or laboratory data). Repeat antivenom therapy, usually in the range of 10 to 20 vials of Wyeth-Ayerst ACP at a time, may be necessary, until the patient's condition becomes stable.[7,42]

The route of antivenom administration is always intravenous.[7,32,42] Intravenous administration allows systemic antivenom distribution to counteract systemic venom effects and allows precise titration of antivenom to help prevent or modulate anaphylactoid reactions that are dependent on concentration, rate, and dose. Antivenom should not be administered intramuscularly or into the wound area.

Prior to intravenous administration of Wyeth-Ayerst ACP, a skin test can be administered.[7,31,32,42,83,100] The skin test should only be given after the physician has decided to administer antivenom, based on progression of signs or symptoms in mild to moderate crotaline envenomations or based on a severe envenomation at presentation (see Box 21A-1 and Tables 21A-7 to 21A-9. This should be done after the patient has given informed consent, if possible, and before any antihistamines are given. Skin testing can sensitize patients to horse antigens and has resulted in life-threatening anaphylactic and anaphylactoid reactions. Antihistamines can mask the signs of a positive skin test, which can include a wheal and/or flare response larger than 10 mm in diameter, urticaria, and systemic anaphylactic or anaphylactoid reactions. A wheal and/or flare reaction larger than 10 mm in diameter is all that is necessary to declare a skin test result positive.[7,31,32,42,83] Prior to the administration of

the skin test, the clinician should read the package insert and call a consultant in medical toxicology or a regional poison center, unless he or she has sufficient experience in administering the skin test and treating crotaline-envenomated patients. A clinician and all equipment and drugs necessary to manage anaphylactic and anaphylactoid reactions should be at the bedside. Two intravenous lines with isotonic crystalloid should be in place. The patient should be attached to a cardiac monitor, a pulse oximeter, and a blood pressure monitor.[32] After these precautions are taken, 0.02 mL of a 1:10 dilution of normal horse serum is injected intradermally into one shoulder and 0.02 mL of normal saline control is injected into the other shoulder. The 1:10 diluted normal horse serum is already packaged, premixed, and ready for injection.[83] The control and horse serum sites should be observed for 30 minutes to see if wheal, flare, urticaria, or systemic anaphylactic or anaphylactoid reactions develop.[7,31,32,42,83]

If the skin test result is positive, the clinician should reconsider using antivenom in mild and moderate envenomations and discuss the therapeutic pros and cons with the patient in light of the positive result.[32,100] If antivenom will be given, we suggest pretreating the patient with diphenhydramine 1 mg/kg intravenously (50 mg in the average adult) and ranitidine 3 mg/kg intravenously* (150 mg in the average adult).[32] Steroids are not necessarily indicated. Steroids have not been proven safe or effective in treatment of crotaline envenomation.[4,63]

Concurrent with the skin test, the lyophilized Wyeth-Ayerst ACP should be mixed. The antivenom is diluted with enough bacteriostatic water or normal saline to fill the vial. Filling the vial completely helps prevent foaming.[83] Solubilization of the lyophilized antivenom may be facilitated with an automated blood vial rocker. Vigorous shaking of the antivenom denatures it. Foaming may indicate that some denaturation has occurred.[83]

After solubilizing the lyophilized antivenom, we prefer to dilute the antivenom approximately 10:1 (i.e., dilute 10 vials of antivenom in 1 L of normal saline).[32,83] Although this differs from more concentrated solutions recommended by some experts, it is the most dilute solution suggested in the *Physicians' Desk Reference*, and this more dilute solution may help prevent anaphylactoid reactions that are dependent on concentration, rate, and dose.[31,42,83] For children, we dilute the initial dose of antivenom in enough normal saline so the patient will receive an antivenom infusion that does not exceed 20 mL/kg, the usual resuscitation bolus dose for crystalloid infusions in pediatric resuscitation.[30,32] The dilute antivenom infusion should be started slowly and gradually increased over time to help prevent anaphylactoid reactions. We use the antivenom infusion guidelines detailed in Box 21A-3. The guidelines are based on an integration of product information from the

---

*Use of H_2 histamine blockers for prophylaxis and treatment of allergic reactions is a common, but off-label, prescribing practice.

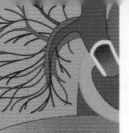

> **BOX 21A-3** **ANTIVENOM INFUSION GUIDELINE FOR 10 VIALS OF WYETH-AYERST ANTIVENIN (CROTALIDAE) POLYVALENT DILUTED IN 1 LITER OF NORMAL SALINE**
>
> Start the antivenom infusion at no more than 60 mL/hr (1 mL/min)
> If no adverse reactions occur in 3 min, increase the drip rate to 120–125 mL/hr
> If no adverse reactions occur in 3 min, increase the drip rate to 240–250 mL/hr
> If no adverse reactions occur in 3 min, increase the drip rate to 480–500 mL/hr
> If no adverse reactions occur in 3 min, increase the drip rate to 960–1000 mL/hr

Physicians' Desk Reference, our own clinical experience, and guidelines from other experts.[7,31,32,42,83] We believe these to be reasonable guidelines, although they have never been validated by a clinical trial. Although life-threatening anaphylactic or anaphylactoid reactions can occur at any time during antivenom infusion, they usually occur while the infusion rate is gradually increased to the maximum of 960 to 1000 mL/hr. It is prudent to have a clinician able to manage all aspects of anaphylaxis at the bedside, until the maximum infusion rate of 960 to 1000 mL/hr has been achieved without complications.

If signs or symptoms of an anaphylactic or anaphylactoid reaction occur during antivenom infusion, one should immediately stop the infusion and treat the patient with intravenous diphenhydramine and ranitidine, or other H_1 and H_2 antagonists. If these steps do not achieve the desired result, epinephrine and steroids (considering glucagon in patients on β-blocker therapy), should be administered, as in any anaphylactic or anaphylactoid reaction. If the clinician has not yet consulted with a regional poison control center or medical toxicologist, he or she should do so at this time.

Life-threatening crotaline envenomations complicated by anaphylactic and/or anaphylactoid reactions to antivenom have been treated with concomitant antivenom and intravenous epinephrine infusions.[7,31,32,42,99,102] Intravenous epinephrine is titrated to effect during antivenom infusions in which the risk-benefit ratio seems to favor administration of antivenom. We are involved in a handful of such cases each snakebite season. To date, the authors' patients have suffered no permanent sequelae from this treatment.

Surgery is rarely necessary for crotaline envenomation. Almost 30 years ago, surgery was recommended by some as the primary treatment for crotaline envenomations with early excisional débridement or fasciotomy[103,104]; however, animal and human studies do not support this position.[105-110]

Fasciotomy should only be performed when clinical signs and symptoms of compartment syndrome are present and hourly, serially measured compartment pressures remain greater than 30 mm Hg despite elevation of the affected limb and administration of 20 vials of Wyeth-Ayerst ACP or 6 to 12 vials of CroFab.[7,31,32,42] This 30 mm Hg pressure limit is based on the fact that capillary perfusion pressure is usually about 30 mm Hg.[111-113]

Compartment perfusion pressure is also dependent on the patient's blood pressure.[112,114-116] Significant decreases in compartmental perfusion occur when compartment pressures rise to within 30 mm Hg of the diastolic blood pressure.[114] An experimental study found that CroFab limited the decrease in perfusion pressure in the anterior leg compartment in a porcine, crotaline envenomation model.[117] Another study found compartment muscle hypoperfusion and anaerobic metabolism when compartment pressures were within 30 mm Hg of the mean arterial pressure (MAP) in nontraumatized muscles.[116] In traumatized muscles, compartment hypoperfusion and anaerobic metabolism occurred when compartment pressures were within 40 mm Hg of the MAP.[116]

The duration of clinical signs and symptoms of compartment syndrome also relates to prognosis. If compartment syndrome signs or symptoms are allowed to persist for 12 hours or more, residual functional deficits almost always occur. Series of patients who undergo fasciotomy within 12 hours of onset of signs or symptoms of compartment syndrome have from 0% to 17% incidence of residual functional deficits.[112,118]

To allow for maximum antivenom dosing and effect, it is reasonable to obtain a few hourly serial compartment pressures if the patient has signs or symptoms of compartment syndrome and the initial pressure was elevated.[7,31,32,42] Consider fasciotomy if the compartment pressure stays pathologically elevated after infusion of at least 20 vials of Wyeth-Ayerst ACP or 6 to 12 vials of CroFab, with elevation of the affected extremity, and well before the patient has had symptoms or signs of compartment syndrome for 12 hours.[7,31,32,42,112,118] Guidelines for management of potential compartment syndromes from crotaline envenomations have been published.[42]

Some experts advocate intravenous mannitol to decrease compartment pressures.[7,31,42] We are unaware of any published experimental or clinical data on mannitol therapy for suspected compartment syndrome from crotaline envenomations and have not used this therapy to date. When considering whether to administer mannitol, the clinician must realize that an antivenom infusion is hyperosmolar and a large volume load. If mannitol, 1 to 2 g/kg, were administered in addition to this, the patient would receive a significant osmotic and volume challenge that could compromise patients with tenuous cardiopulmonary or kidney function. If using CroFab and mannitol, the clinician should be aware of possible increased renal clearance of the antivenom, thereby altering its half-life. In addition, both crotaline antivenoms and mannitol have been associated with anaphylactoid reactions, believed to be related in part to their hyperosmolarity. This is similar to anaphylactoid reactions that occur with hyperosmolar radiographic contrast media.

Surgical débridement of frankly necrotic tissue is reasonable. However, it is difficult to determine which tissue is frankly necrotic and which tissue may still be viable early in the course of snake venom poisoning. In

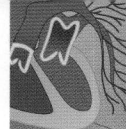

addition, necrosis occurs in a minority of patients with snake venom poisoning.[4] In Russell's series of 100 snakebitten patients in Southern California, 27% developed some necrosis of local tissue.[4] Bullae are usually left intact unless they are on digits and are circumferential or are becoming circumferential and appear to compromise digital perfusion as evidenced by lower skin temperatures measured with a thermistor, by narrower pulse volume amplitude measurements from a Doppler flowmeter, or by lower oxygen content on pulse oximetry distal to a proximal blister.[32,109] Pulse oximetry through a hemorrhagic blister itself is not necessarily accurate, due to the presence of deoxyhemoglobin in blood of the blister. Digital dermotomy has been recommended by some.[119] Potential complications of any surgical procedure include infection, scarring, and anesthetic complications.

Patients who may have had a snakebite from a North American Crotalinae require medical observation for at least 12 hours because development of signs and symptoms of envenomation may be insidious.[7,120,121] During this observation period, hemoglobin, hematocrit, prothrombin time, partial thromboplastin time, fibrinogen, fibrin split products, and platelets should be assayed on presentation and every 4 hours thereafter to assess for development of venom-induced coagulopathies. Every 15 to 60 minutes, the patient's affected extremity should be palpated on both the medial and lateral aspects, starting proximally at the torso and gently moving distally until the leading edge of induration, edema, and tenderness is felt.[7,31,42] This leading edge of induration, edema, and tenderness should be marked on the skin with the corresponding time of observation. If proximal progression of the leading edge of induration, edema, and tenderness occurs, the patient should be admitted and treated with antivenom after his or her informed consent is obtained.[7,31,32,42] Antivenom administration requires an intensive care setting within the emergency department or intensive care unit. If the patient has a coagulopathy on initial presentation or develops one during observation, he or she should be admitted and receive antivenom after informed consent has been given.[7,31,42] If after 12 hours of close clinical observation and serial laboratory tests the clinician is certain that the snakebite was of Crotalinae origin, and the patient has no sign of snakebite other than punctures or abrasions (i.e., no signs of envenomation and no coagulopathy), a reliable patient can be sent home with instructions to return immediately if he or she notes any of the following: increase in pain; onset of redness, swelling, fever, or pus formation; bruising; bloody nose; red or dark urine; weakness; nausea or vomiting; faintness; dyspnea; diaphoresis; or any sign or symptom other than the mildest pain at the bite site.[7,31,42,120,121]

CroFab: Crotalidae Polyvalent Immune Fab (Ovine)

CroFab was approved by the U.S. Food and Drug Administration (FDA) on October 2, 2000. FDA labeling states that CroFab is indicated for the management of patients with minimal or moderate North American crotaline envenomations (see Table 21A-9).[91] In practice, the indications for CroFab are moderate or severe cases of crotaline envenomation and mild crotaline envenomation with progression (worsening) of clinical signs and symptoms (see Table 21A-9).

Relative contraindications for CroFab include a history of allergic reactions to sheep products, papaya, papain, chymopapain, and other papaya extracts; the pineapple enzyme bromelain; dust mites, and latex. CroFab is obtained from sheep immunized with North American crotaline venoms, and papain, a papaya derivative, is used to separate the Fab fragments from the Fc fragments of the immunoglobulins. Bromelain, some dust mite allergens, and some latex allergens share antigenic structures with papain. Obviously, when a relative contraindication is present, the treating clinician must carefully weigh the risks and benefits of CroFab versus the risks of the envenomation. The decision to administer CroFab in a patient with a known relative contraindication is a decision that the treating clinician must make in consultation with the patient. In addition, we recommend that the clinician remain at the bedside for the first administration of CroFab with all critical care equipment and resuscitative medicines at hand.

Absolute contraindications to CroFab are a patient's refusal after informed consent, requiring the patient to be awake, alert, fully oriented, with a clear sensorium, or the inability of the clinician to manage an anaphylactic and/or anaphylactoid reaction in a patient without a life-threatening envenomation.

The main complications of CroFab include anaphylactic and anaphylactoid reactions and serum sickness as well as failure to achieve initial control of local effects; recurrence of local effects, low platelets, elevated protime, high partial thromboplastin time (PTT), low fibrinogen, and hospital readmission; late onset of low platelets, high protime, high PTT, and low fibrinogen; persistent low fibrinogen; and clinical bleeding with recurrent low fibrinogen or late onset of low platelets.

The evidence base for Crotalidae polyvalent immune Fab (ovine) includes two premarketing CroTab studies (Box 21A-4) and four postmarketing CroFab studies, to date. These six studies are summarized in Table 21A-14, with more detailed information from these studies in Tables 21A-15, 21A-16, 21A-17, and 21A-18.

Immediate hypersensitivity (i.e., anaphylactic reactions and anaphylactoid reactions) occurred in 6% of patients (i.e., 8 of 129 patients) in the two premarketing CroTab and four postmarketing CroFab case series published to date (see Table 21A-18).[5,85-90] This incidence of immediate hypersensitivity reactions with CroFab is less than the reported incidence of immediate hypersensitivity reactions to Wyeth-Ayerst antivenom. No hypersensitivity reactions were reported in the first premarketing and the first two postmarketing studies.[85,86,90] In the second premarketing study, 6 of 31 patients (20%) had immediate hypersensitivity reactions to CroFab. On further analysis, 3 of 31 patients (10%) had CroFab that had been incompletely purified of the Fc fragment, which is more allergenic; however, 3 of 31 patients (10%) received normal CroTab. In other

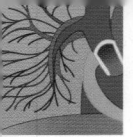

words, immediate hypersensitivity was equally frequent in patients who received standard CroTab and in those who received a batch of CroTab with excess Fc. Therefore, standard CroTab can cause immediate

hypersensitivity.[88] In the two most recent postmarketing case series of CroFab published to date, one patient in each series had an immediate hypersensitivity reaction: 7% in Bush and colleagues' case series and 3% in Lavonas and colleagues' case series.[5,87] In summary, although immediate hypersensitivity reactions to CroFab are uncommon, varying from 0% to 20% in published case series, with an average incidence of 6%, we recommend that the patient give informed consent and that all equipment and drugs necessary to manage immediate hypersensitivity reactions be at the bedside.[7,31,32,42] A clinician capable of managing immediate hypersensitivity reactions should also be at the bedside. Two intravenous lines with isotonic crystalloid should be in place. The patient should be attached to a cardiac monitor, a pulse oximeter, and a blood pressure monitor. These precautions generally require that the patient be managed in an intensive care setting in the emergency department or intensive care unit.

Overall, delayed hypersensitivity reactions were reported in 8% of patients (i.e., 11 of 129 patients) in the two CroTab premarketing and four CroFab postmarketing published studies (see Table 21A-18).[5,85-90] No patients who received only CroTab had delayed hypersensitivity reactions reported in the first CroTab premarketing study; however, only 8 of 11 had follow-up for 14 days to assess for delayed hypersensitivity.[86] In the second premarketing study of CroTab, 6 of 31 patients (19%) developed delayed hypersensitivity reactions to CroTab; however, 5 of the 6 had received a batch of CroTab that had incomplete removal of Fc fragments, predisposing them to greater allergenicity (see Table 21A-18).[88] This predominance of delayed hypersensitivity in patients who received the batch of CroTab that

---

BOX 21A-4   CROTAB PREMARKETING CLINICAL TRIALS

Study Design

Prospective
Multicenter
Open-label (unblinded)
No control group

Inclusion Criteria

Age: ≥10 years
Mild to moderate North American crotaline envenomation
   With progression: worsening clinical signs or lab values
    < 6 hr since snakebite

Exclusion Criteria

Copperhead (*Agkistrodon contortrix*) bite
Dry bite: no venom effects
Lack of progression (worsening) of clinical signs or lab values
Severe crotaline envenomation on presentation
>1 vial of Wyeth-Ayerst antivenom
Significant preexisting comorbidity
Sheep allergy
Systemic steroids within 4 wk
Experimental medications within 4 wk
Pregnancy
Lactation
Inability to give informed consent
Previous entry in this study

TABLE 21A-14 Crotalidae Polyvalent Immune Fab (Ovine) Studies: CroTab and CroFab Studies

REFERENCE	PATIENTS (*N*)	YEAR PUBLISHED	PRE- VS. POSTMARKETING	DESIGN	CROTALINAE	ANTIVENOM
Reference 86 with supplementary data from reference 89	11	1997	Premarketing	Prospective multicenter	Varied	CroTab
Reference 88 with supplementary data from reference 89	31	2001	Premarketing	Prospective multicenter	Varied	CroTab
Reference 85	28	2002	Postmarketing	Retrospective 1 center	Varied	CroFab
Reference 90	12 (9 prospective and 3 retrospective)	2002	Postmarketing	Prospective first center / Retrospective second center	Varied	CroFab
Reference 5	15	2002	Postmaketing	Prospective 1 center	Varied predominantly *Crotalus helleri*	CroFab
Reference 87	32	2004	Postmarketing	Retrospective 1 center	*Agkistrodon contortrix*	CroFab
Total	129	7-year span	2 Premarketing / 4 Postmarketing	3 multicenter / 3 single center	5 Varied / 1 Copperhead	2 CroTab / 4 CroFab

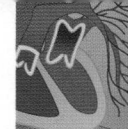

TABLE 21A-15 Evidence-Based Crotalidae Polyvalent Immune Fab (Ovine) Dosing

REFERENCE	PATIENTS (N)	MEAN DOSE TO ACHIEVE INITIAL CONTROL (NO. OF VIALS)	DOSE RANGE TO ACHIEVE INITIAL CONTROL (NO. OF VIALS)	FAILURE TO ACHIEVE INITIAL CONTROL OF LOCAL EFFECTS (PATIENTS)	MEAN TOTAL DOSE (NO. OF VIALS)	TOTAL DOSE RANGE (NO. OF VIALS)
Reference 86 with supplementary data from reference 89	11	6	4–8	1 (9%) required 10 vials of Wyeth-Ayerst in addition to 8 of CroTab for initial control of local effects	6	4–8
Reference 88 with supplementary data from reference 89	31	8	3–12	0 (0%)	12	3–18
Reference 85	28	NR	NR	0 (0%)	16 on initial admission	10–47
Reference 90	12 (9 prospective and 3 retrospective)	8	4–16	0 (0%)	13	4–22
Reference 5	15	7	1–2	0 (0%)	12	1–18
Reference 87	32	4	4–8	2 (6%)	NR	NR
Total	129	6 (weighted average for 101 patients)	1–16	3/129 (2%)	13 (weighted average for 97 patients	1–47

NR, Not reported.

TABLE 21A-16 Evidence-Based Recurrent Complications with Crotalidae Polyvalent Immune Fab (Ovine)

REFERENCE	PATIENTS (N)	LOCAL EFFECTS (%)	LOW PLATELETS (%)	HIGH PROTIME (%)	HIGH PTT (%)	LOW FIBRINOGEN (%)	HOSPITAL ADMISSION (%)
Reference 86 with supplementary data from reference 89	11	0 (0%)	1 (9%)	1 (9%)	NR	1 (9%)	1 (9%)
Reference 88 with supplementary data from reference 89	31	0/15 (0%) with scheduled dosing 8/16 (50%) with prn dosing	6/31 (19%)	4/31 (13%)	2/31 (6%)	6/31 (19%)	0 (0%)
Reference 85	28	2 (7%)	1 (4%)	3 (11%)	NR	3 (11%)	4 (14%)
Reference 90	12 (9 prospective and 3 retrospective	1 (8%)	NR	NR	NR	NR	0 (0%)
Reference 5	15	3 (20%)	NR	NR	NR	NR	0 (0%)
Reference 87	32	6 (19%)	NR	NR	NR	NR	0 (0%)
Total	129	20/129 (16%)	8/70 (11%)	8/70 (11%)	2/31 (6%)	10/70 (14%)	5/129 (4%)

NR, not reported; prn, as needed.

had excess Fc fragments is in contradistinction to the equal incidence of immediate hypersensitivity reactions between those patients who did and those who did not receive batches of CroFab with excess Fc fragments in the second premarketing study (see Table 21A-18).[86,88] Only 26 of 31 patients had 14-day follow-up to assess for delayed hypersensitivity in the second CroTab premarketing study.[88] In the first postmarketing study of CroFab, 2 of 28 patients (7%) had delayed hypersensitivity (see

Table 21A-18).[85] All patients in this study had 14 days of follow-up by phone to assess for delayed hypersensitivity. The second published postmarketing study of CroFab had no patients with delayed hypersensitivity (see Table 21A-18).[90] All patients in this study had clinic or phone follow-up for at least 1 month. In the third postmarketing CroFab study, 1 of 15 patients (7%) had delayed hypersensitivity (see Table 21A-18).[5] All patients in this study had follow-up for at least 21 days. In the fourth

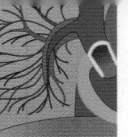

TABLE 21A-17 Evidence-Based Late-Onset and Persistent Coagulopathies with Crotalidae Polyvalent Immune Fab (Ovine)

| | | LATE-ONSET | | | | PERSISTENT | | | |
REFERENCE	PATIENTS (*N*)	LOW PLATELETS (%)	HIGH PROTIME (%)	HIGH PTT (%)	LOW FIBRINOGEN (%)	LOW PLATELETS (%)	HIGH PROTIME (%)	HIGH PTT (%)	LOW FIBRINOGEN (%)
Reference 86 with supplementary data from reference 89	11	2 (18%)	0 (0%)	NR	1 (9%)	0 (0%)	0 (0%)	NR	1 (9%)
Reference 88 with supplementary data from reference 89	31	0 (0%)	2/31 (6%)	3/31 (10%)	4/31 (13%)	0 (0%)	0 (0%)	0 (0%)	2/31 (6%)
Reference 85	28	2 (7%)	0 (0%)	NR	0 (0%)	0 (0%)	0 (0%)	0 (0%)	0 (0%)
Reference 90	12 (9 prospective and 3 retrospective	1 (8%)	NR	NR	NR	0 (0%)	0 (0%)	0 (0%)	0 (0%)
Reference 5	15	NR	NR	NR	NR	0 (0%)	0 (0%)	0 (0%)	0 (0%)
Reference 87	32	0 (0%)	1 (3%)	NR	1 (3%)	NR	NR	NR	NR
Total	129	5/114 (4%)	3/102 (3%)	3/31 (10%)	6/102 (6%)	0/97 (0%)	0/97 (0%)	0/86 (0%)	3/97 (3%)

NR, Not reported.

TABLE 21A-18 Evidence-Based Bleeding and Hypersensitivity Reactions with Crotalidae Polyvalent Immune Fab (Ovine)

REFERENCE	PATIENTS (*N*)	CLINICAL BLEEDING (%)	IMMEDIATE HYPERSENSITIVITY %	DELAYED HYPERSENSITIVITY %
Reference 86 with supplementary data from reference 89	11	1 (9%) had recurrent low fibrinogen bled 2 g/dL of hemoglobin, after hemorrhoidectomy, 12 days after bite	0 (0%)	0 (0%) attributed to CroTab 1 (9%) who received 10 vials of Wyeth-Ayerst
Reference 88 with supplementary data from reference 89	31	0 (0%)	3/31 (10%) had Fc contaminated CroTab batch 3/31 (10%) had standard CroTab	5/31 (16%) had Fc contaminated CroTab batch 1/31 (3%) had standard CroTab
Reference 85	28	1 (4%) had late-onset low platelets and bled 2 g/dL of hemoglobin spontaneously, rectally, 9–10 days after	0 (0%)	2 (7%)
Reference 90	12 (9 prospective and 3 retrospective)	0 (0%)	0 (0%)	0 (0%)
Reference 5	15	0 (0%)	1 (7%)	1 (7%)
Reference 87	32	0 (0%)	1 (3%)	1 (3%)
Total	129	2/129 (2%)	8/129 (6%)	11/129 (8%) 5/123 (4%) excluding 1 patient who received Wyeth-Ayerst and 5 who received Fc contaminated CroTab batch

extant case series with CroFab, 1 of 32 patients (3%) had delayed hypersensitivity (see Table 21A-18).[87] However, only 6 of 32 patients had follow-up for at least 21 days. In summary, in the two premarketing CroTab studies and the four postmarketing CroFab studies, 95 patients had follow-up for at least 2 weeks to assess for delayed hypersensitivity. Overall, 5 of 95 patients (5%) had delayed hypersensitivity reactions to CroTab or CroFab, with no confounding variables such as excess Fc or concurrent Wyeth-Ayerst antivenom.[5,85-90] Confounding variables existed for 6 of 95 (7%) patients with delayed hypersensitivity reactions who had follow-up for at least

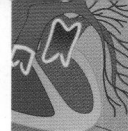

14 days.[86,88] One patient with delayed hypersensitivity in the first CroTab premarketing study also received 10 vials of Wyeth-Ayerst antivenom because 8 vials of CroTab had failed to control the local effects.[86] Delayed hypersensitivity reactions occur in almost all patients receiving 10 vials of Wyeth-Ayerst antivenom. When all patients with and without confounding variables are included for the analysis of the overall incidence of delayed hypersensitivity reactions, 11 of 95 patients (12%) had delayed hypersensitivity (see Table 21A-18).[5,85-90]

Failure to achieve initial control of local effects within 12 hours occurred in 3 of 129 patients (2%) and involved the first premarketing CroTab study and the fourth postmarketing CroFab study (see Table 21A-15).[5,85-90]

Failure to achieve initial control of local effects within 12 hours of envenomation first occurred in one patient in the first CroTab premarketing study, in which the maximal dose of CroTab was only 8 vials.[86] This patient received an additional 10 vials of Wyeth-Ayerst antivenom to control spread of local effects, spreading from his entire right upper extremity onto his chest. Local effects were halted with the additional 10 vials of Wyeth-Ayerst antivenom. The remaining two patients with failure to achieve initial control of local effects within 12 hours occurred in the most recent CroFab postmarketing case series of patients envenomated by the copperhead (*Agkistrodon contortrix*).[87] In one patient, local effects continued after receiving four vials of CroFab but stopped when an additional four vials were given 17 hours later. In the other patient, local effects continued to progress for 31 hours in spite of 24 vials of CroFab. The first two patients with failure to achieve initial control of local effects within 12 hours might be attributable to underdosing of CroTab or CroFab; however, the third patients received 24 vials of CroFab within 31 hours and local effects continued to progress.[87] These data highlight the fact that treatment with antivenom involves empiric titration of dose to achieve initial control.

Overall, local effects recurred in 20 of 129 patients (16%) in the six published CroFab studies (see Table 21A-16).[5,85-90] The incidence of recurrent local effects in individual studies varied between 0% and 25%. Recurrence of local effects were prevented in the second premarketing CroTab study with scheduled administration of two vials of CroFab, repeatedly, 6, 12, and 18 hours after achievement of initial control.[88,89] In contrast, patients who received nonscheduled dosing of CroFab after initial control (i.e., repeat CroTab dosing on an as-needed basis) had a 50% incidence of recurrent local effects in 8 of 16 patients.[88,89] This study finding is the basis for the recommended scheduled dosing with two vials of CroTab, repeatedly, 6, 12, and 18 hours after achievement of initial control.[88,89] Recurrent local effects occurred in some patients in all four postmarketing CroFab studies, in spite of receiving scheduled dosing of two vials of CroFab, repeatedly, 6, 12, and 18 hours after achieving initial control.[5,85,87,90] This highlights the fact that treatment with antivenom is an empiric titration, not only to achieve initial control, but to treat recurrent local effects.

Recurrent coagulopathies, including low platelets and low fibrinogen, as well as high protime and PTT, occurred frequently in premarketing CroTab studies and postmarketing CroFab studies (see Table 21A-16).[5,85-90] In premarketing CroTab studies, 38 of 42 patients had complete laboratory data for 14 days. Among these 38 patients, 28 (74%) had a coagulopathy before or within the first hour of treatment. Of these 38 patients, 14 (37%) developed thrombocytopenia, 22 (58%) developed hypofibrinogenemia, and 17 (45%) developed prolonged protime or PTT. Among the 38 patients, 20 (53%) developed multicomponent coagulopathies involving combinations of the preceding individual component coagulopathies. Coagulopathic abnormalities resolved in all patients with CroTab treatment; however, coagulopathies recurred in 20 (53%) patients (69% of the 28 patients with initial coagulopathy), within 2 to 14 days after envenomation. In other words, recurrent coagulopathies occurred in about half of all treated patients and in about two thirds of those patients with initial coagulopathies studies.[89,122] The only CroFab postmarketing study that documented whether recurrent coagulopathies found them (see Table 21A-16).[85]

Recurrent hospital admissions (readmissions) occurred in the first premarketing CroTab study and the first postmarketing CroFab study.[85] One of 11 patients (9%) in the first premarketing CroTab study developed recurrent hypofibrinogenemia, which was discovered when he had incision and drainage of thrombosed external hemorrhoids 12 days after envenomation. At the time, his fibrinogen was undetectable.[89] His hematocrit had been 36% on the second day after envenomation, and this decreased to 36% on his readmission, 12 days after envenomation. His local bleeding was controlled with pressure, and no blood products were administered. No CroFab was readministered.[89] In the first postmarketing CroFab study, 4 of 28 patients (14%) had recurrent hospital admissions for recurrent coagulopathies.[85] Three of these had no clinical bleeding. The fourth patient had spontaneous rectal bleeding for 2 days prior to readmission on the 10th day after his envenomation, with a platelet count of 15,000/mm^3 at that time. This was a late-onset thrombocytopenia. His hemoglobin had also decreased from 36% at discharge from his previous admission to 30% on readmission for spontaneous rectal bleeding. He was retreated with a total of 18 vials of CroFab, which was temporally associated with a slow, gradual rise in his platelet count. Blood products were not administered and the patient had no further bleeding.[85]

Late-onset coagulopathy manifested by low platelets, high protime, high PTT, or low fibrinogen occurred in 0% to 18% of patients in the two premarketing CroTab studies and four postmarketing CroFab studies. Pooled data for all pre- and postmarketing studies, in patients who had laboratory follow-up for individual coagulopathies for at least 2 weeks, indicated an overall incidence of late-onset thrombocytopenia of 4%, late-onset high protime of 3%, late-onset high PTT of 10%, and late-onset of hypofibrinogenemia 6% (see Table 21A-17).[5,85-90]

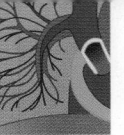

Persistent coagulopathy with low fibrinogen was documented only in the two premarketing CroTab studies occurring in 1 of 11 patients (9%) in the first CroTab study and in 2 of 31 patients (6%) in the second CroTab study (see Table 21A-17).[86,88,89] No persistent coagulopathies were documented in any postmarketing CroFab studies.[5,85,87,90] Pooled data for premarketing CroTab and postmarketing CroFab studies indicate that 3 of 97 patients (3%) had persistent hypofibrinogenemia for up to 14 days of follow-up after envenomation.[5,85-90]

Dosage of CroFab, like other antivenoms, is determined by the victim's degree of envenomation and has nothing to with the victim's age or weight.[4,32,56] This is because antivenom neutralizes a specific amount of venom. Clinically, the amount of venom is estimated by the effect that the venom has on the patient. This can be estimated by various grading systems (see Box 21A-1 and Tables 21A-7 to 21A-9).

According to the FDA-approved labeling, "administration of antivenom should be initiated as soon as possible after crotalid snakebite in patients who develop signs of progressive envenomation (e.g., worsening local injury, coagulation abnormality, or systemic signs of envenomation)." In other words, "time is tissue," analogous to reperfusion in acute myocardial infarction. CroFab was shown to be effective in the premarketing CroTab studies when given within 6 hours of snakebite.

Initial dosing of CroFab is empirically titrated to achieve what is called "initial control," defined as complete arrest of progression of local manifestations and return of coagulation tests and systemic signs to normal.[91] If this initial control is not achieved with the first dose of CroFab, additional CroFab should be repeated until initial control of the envenomation syndrome has been achieved. After initial control has been established, additional two-vial doses of CroFab, every 6 hours for up to 18 hours (six additional vials) is recommended.[91] In the studies reported to date, six vials of CroFab is the overall mean number of vials necessary to achieve initial control in a weighted average of 101 patients for whom these data were available (see Table 21A-15).[5,85-90] The mean number of vials of CroFab needed to achieve initial control in the individual studies varied between 4 and 8 vials, with a dose range of 1 to 16 vials. The overall mean total dose of CroFab vials on the first admission for patients in pre- and postmarketing studies was 13 vials of CroFab, which is a weighted average for 97 patients for whom these data were available. The total dose range of CroFab vials in these studies varied between 1 and 47 vials.[5,85-90]

It is important to remember that the FDA-approved package insert for CroFab, which recommends an initial dose of four to six vials, is based only on two premarketing CroTab studies with a total of 42 patients, all of whom had mild or moderate crotaline envenomations at the time of enrollment in the study (see Table 21A-14).[86,88,89] Data in the second premarketing CroTab study and the third postmarketing CroFab study clearly indicate that up to 12 vials of CroFab may be necessary to achieve initial control (see Table 21A-15).[86,89,90] In fact, the second postmarketing CroFab study had one patient

in whom 16 vials of CroFab were necessary to achieve initial control.[90]

In summary, reasonable dosing guidelines for the initial number of CroFab vials are contained in Table 21A-13, with dose ranges for mild crotaline envenomations with progression (4 to 6 vials) and for severe envenomations (6 to 12 vials). For clinicians desiring an even simpler initial dosing regimen without ranges, a reasonable recommendation is an initial dose of 4 vials of CroFab for mild envenomations with progression, 6 vials of CroFab for moderate envenomations, and 12 vials of CroFab for severe envenomations. These initial dosing guidelines have not been validated by prospective randomized studies, but are reasonable recommendations based on the authors' experiences and review of dosing data in the six extant published studies regarding CroTab and CroFab.[5,85-90]

Each vial of CroFab should be reconstituted with 10 mL of sterile water for injection and mixed by continuous gentle swirling.[91] Studies have shown that CroFab reconstitutes more rapidly than the Wyeth-Ayerst antivenom.[123] The contents of the reconstituted vials should be further diluted in 250 mL of 0.9% sodium chloride and mixed by gentle swirling. The reconstituted and diluted products should be used within 4 hours. The antivenom infusion should be begun at no more than 50 mL/hr. If no adverse reactions occur in 3 minutes, then increase the drip rate to 125 mL/hr. If no adverse reactions occur in another 3 minutes, then increase the drip rate to 250 mL/hr. This dosing guideline will allow the entire 250 mL of reconstituted antivenom to be infused in slightly more than 1 hour. No skin test is recommended nor given prior to administration of CroFab.[91]

After achievement of initial control of the envenomation with CroFab and then scheduled dosing with two vials of CroFab, 6, 12, and 18 hours after achievement of initial control, further CroFab dosing is unnecessary unless or until recurrent local effects, or recurrent or late-onset coagulopathy, occurs. The optimal dosing for recurrent coagulopathy is unclear. Recurrent coagulopathies are difficult to treat and may not respond to copious amounts of repeated CroFab as evinced by dosing up to 47 vials of CroFab in one patient with late-onset thrombocytopenia.[85] Although 127 of 129 patients (98%) in the extant CroTab and CroFab studies had no clinical bleeding, 2 of 129 patients (2%) did have clinical bleeding. Based on these concerns, the most conservative recommendation is that all patients restrict their physical activity and avoid all contact sports and unnecessary driving or other activities that could be dangerous with resultant trauma for at least 2 weeks after any crotaline envenomation. Based on these data, it is also recommended that patients receive follow-up complete blood counts with platelets, as well as a protime, PTT, and fibrinogen, every 2 to 3 days for 2 weeks after discharge for crotaline envenomation.

When coagulopathies recur or have late onset in these patients, it is critical that the patient be informed of this and that they are at greater risk for bleeding with any trauma or surgical procedure. Surgical procedures should be deferred for at least 2 weeks after enven-

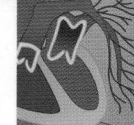

omation and until coagulation studies return to normal, if at all possible. In addition, patients should understand that they should return for clinical evaluation immediately if there are any signs of bleeding.

Redosing of CroFab in patients with recurrent coagulopathy is dependent on the individual clinician's and patient's degree of comfort or discomfort with the possibility of either spontaneous bleeding or bleeding with trauma or a surgical procedure. Researchers have promulgated guidelines for thresholds beyond which CroFab would be administered. Yip recommends giving CroFab in any patient with clinically significant bleeding and any abnormal coagulation parameter or when a symptomatic patient has developed multicomponent coagulopathy with an International Normalized Ratio (INR) of more than 3.0, a PTT of more than 50 seconds, a fibrinogen concentration of less than 75 mg/dL, and a platelet count of less than 50,000/mm³. He further recommends that the treatment should be continued until coagulation parameters are stabilized above what he calls critical values (i.e., INR more than 3.0, PTT more than 50 seconds, fibrinogen concentration less than 75 mg/dL and platelet count less than 50,000/mm³).[124] Boyer and colleagues recommend retreatment of recurrent crotaline coagulopathy with CroFab for the following indications: fibrinogen less than 50 µg/mL, platelet count less than 25,000/mm³, INR more than 3.0, PTT more than 50 seconds, any multicomponent coagulopathy, a worsening trend in the patient with prior severe coagulopathy, patients with high-risk behavior for trauma, and patients with comorbid conditions that increase hemorrhagic risk.[122] Regardless of these published guidelines, each individual clinician and patient must be aware of the risks involved, and the patient must give informed consent to be treated with additional CroFab in the face of recurrent or late-onset coagulopathy. Optimal dosing with CroFab may also be limited by the fact that supplies of CroFab have been extremely limited since it was approved by the FDA. De facto rationing of CroFab has occurred in some regions due to shortages, with clinicians trying to do the greatest good for the greatest number of crotaline-envenomated patients when supplies of CroFab are limited.[92,125]

New Crotaline Antivenoms of the Future

A new antivenom, Antivipmyn (Fab)², is currently being studied and shows great promise.[126]

Prognosis

Although any significant snakebite is potentially lethal, death is unusual (0.1%) after North American Crotalinae bites in cases reported to the American Association of Poison Control Centers (see Table 21A-2).[6] The Western Envenomation Database, a consecutive case series of crotaline bites in which the Arizona Poison Control Center was consulted by clinicians from throughout the United States, reported a mortality rate of 1.4%.[127] This mortality rate may be artifactually high because the Arizona Poison Control Center commonly receives calls from throughout the United States for consultation on severe or unusual crotaline envenomations, resulting in potential selection bias. Selected details from the three fatal cases are provided in Table 21A-19. Common characteristics of these fatal cases include more proximal bite sites, bites due to *Crotalus* species, little or no intravenous fluid infusion in two patients, minimal or no antivenom administration, and nonaccidental upper extremity envenomations in two patients. One treating physician thought that one patient's bite was from a nonvenomous snake prior to the patient's fatal cardiorespiratory arrest 5 hours after the bite.[127]

The Western Envenomation Database has also tabulated nonfatal sequelae from crotaline envenomations. Long-term morbidity (i.e., permanent sequelae) are more common in upper extremity and face bites. This may be caused by the circumstances of these bites. Most patients with upper extremity or facial bites were handling the snake at the time of the bite. Snakes that feel threatened from handling may inject larger amounts of venom. The

TABLE 21A-19 Fatal Crotaline Envenomations			
STUDY PARAMETERS	**PATIENT 1**	**PATIENT 2**	**PATIENT 3**
Age (yr)	2	7	32
Sex	F	M	M
Bite site	Shoulder	Knee	Forearm
Snake	*Crotalus viridis*	*Crotalus*, unknown species	*Crotalus atrox*
Time to hospital	30 min	30 min	40 min
IV fluids	Very slow rate	No	Several liters
Antivenom	1 vial	No	4 vials, hours after shock ensued
Other therapy	No	No	Fasciotomy, steroids
Initial assessment by physician	Severe envenomation	Nonvenomous bite	Severe envenomation
Course	Cardiorespiratory arrest at 3 hr	Cardiorespiratory arrest at 5 hr	Prolonged hypotension and death at 16 hr
Circumstances	Nonaccidental; adult placed snake around child	Accidental, while playing	Nonaccidental; rattlesnake roundup

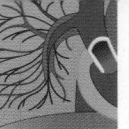

complexity of fine motor functions and sensation in the face and upper extremities may also be more easily impaired by venom effects, and disability would be more apparent. Most long-term morbidity involved weakness, pain, decreased range of motion, hypesthesia, paresthesia, anesthesia, or skin discoloration. The most common long-term morbidity was decreased range of motion. Only one amputation was necessary. This was an amputation of an envenomated finger.[127] These data suggest that a patient's physical therapy should begin as soon as possible after antivenom administration has halted progression of signs of envenomation and no further antivenom therapy is needed.[42,127]

REFERENCES

1. Russell FE: Toxic effects of terrestrial animal venoms and poisons. In Klaassen CD (ed): Casarett and Doull's Toxicology: The Basic Science of Poisons. New York, McGraw-Hill, 2001, pp 945-964.
2. Dart RC, McNally J: Efficacy, safety, and use of snake antivenoms in the United States. Ann Emerg Med 2001;37(2):181–188.
3. Behler J, King F: National Audubon Society Field Guide to North American Reptiles and Amphibians, 2nd ed. New York, Alfred A. Knopf, 1995.
4. Russell FE: Snake Venom Poisoning, 2nd ed. Great Neck, NY, Scholium International, 1983.
5. Bush SP, Green SM, Moynihan JA, et al: Crotalidae polyvalent immune Fab (ovine) antivenom is efficacious for envenomations by Southern Pacific rattlesnakes (Crotalus helleri). Ann Emerg Med 2002;40(6):619–624.
6. Watson WA, Litovitz TL, Rodgers GC Jr, et al: 2002 Annual report of the American Association of Poison Control Centers Toxic Exposure Surveillance System. Am J Emerg Med 2003;21(5):353–421.
7. Warrell DA: Animal toxins. In Cook CG (ed): Manson's Tropical Diseases, 20th ed. Philadelphia, WB Saunders, 1996, pp 468–515.
8. Parrish HM: Incidence of treated snakebites in the United States. Public Health Rep 1966;81(3):269–276.
9. Wingert WA, Chan L: Rattlesnake bites in southern California and rationale for recommended treatment. West J Med 1988;148(1):37–44.
10. Parrish HM, Goldner JC, Silberg SL: Comparison between snakebites in children and adults. Pediatrics 1965;36:251–256.
11. Tokish JT, Benjamin J, Walter F: Crotalid envenomation: the southern Arizona experience. J Orthop Trauma 2001;15(1):5–9.
12. McKinney PE: Out-of-hospital and interhospital management of crotaline snakebite. Ann Emerg Med 2001;37(2):168–174.
13. Moss ST, Bogdan G, Dart RC, et al: Association of rattlesnake bite location with severity of clinical manifestations. Ann Emerg Med 1997;30(1):58–61.
14. Iyaniwura TT: Snake venom constituents: biochemistry and toxicology (Part 1). Vet Hum Toxicol 1991;33(5):468–474.
15. Iyaniwura TT: Snake venom constituents: biochemistry and toxicology (Part 2). Vet Hum Toxicol 1991;33(5):475–480.
16. Cate RL, Bieber AL: Purification and characterization of Mojave (Crotalus scutulatus scutulatus) toxin and its subunits. Arch Biochem Biophys 1978;189(2):397–408.
17. Castilonia RR, Pattabhiraman TR, Russell FE: Neuromuscular blocking effects of Mojave rattlesnake (Crotalus scutulatus scutulatus) venom. Proc West Pharmacol Soc 1980;23:103–106.
18. Gopalakrishnakone P, Hawgood BJ, Holbrooke SE, et al: Sites of action of Mojave toxin isolated from the venom of the Mojave rattlesnake. Br J Pharmacol 1980;69(3):421–431.
19. Ho CL, Lee CY: Presynaptic actions of Mojave toxin isolated from Mojave rattlesnake (Crotalus scutulatus) venom. Toxicon 1981;19(6):889–892.
20. Valdes JJ, Thompson RG, Wolff VL, et al: Inhibition of calcium channel dihydropyridine receptor binding by purified Mojave toxin. Neurotoxicol Teratol 1989;11(2):129–133.
21. Glenn JL, Straight R: Mojave rattlesnake Crotalus scutulatus scutulatus venom: variation in toxicity with geographical origin. Toxicon 1978;16(1):81–84.
22. Glenn JL, Straight RC, Wolfe MC, Hardy DL: Geographical variation in Crotalus scutulatus scutulatus (Mojave rattlesnake) venom properties. Toxicon 1983;21(1):119–130.
23. Glenn JL, Straight RC: Intergradation of two different venom populations of the Mojave rattlesnake (Crotalus scutulatus scutulatus) in Arizona. Toxicon 1989;27(4):411–418.
24. Clark RF, Williams SR, Nordt SP, Boyer-Hassen LV: Successful treatment of crotalid-induced neurotoxicity with a new polyspecific crotalid Fab antivenom. Ann Emerg Med 1997;30(1):54–57.
25. Weinstein SA, Minton SA, Wilde CE: The distribution among ophidian venoms of a toxin isolated from the venom of the Mojave rattlesnake (Crotalus scutulatus scutulatus). Toxicon 1985;23(5):825–844.
26. Huang SY, Perez JC, Rael ED, et al: Variation in the antigenic characteristics of venom from the Mojave rattlesnake (Crotalus scutulatus scutulatus). Toxicon 1992;30(4):387–396.
27. Jansen PW, Perkin RM, Van Stralen D: Mojave rattlesnake envenomation: prolonged neurotoxicity and rhabdomyolysis. Ann Emerg Med 1992;21(3):322–325.
28. Hardy DL: Envenomation by the Mojave rattlesnake (Crotalus scutulatus scutulatus) in southern Arizona, U.S.A. Toxicon 1983;21(1):111–118.
29. Hardy DL: Fatal rattlesnake envenomation in Arizona: 1969–1984. J Toxicol Clin Toxicol 1986;24(1):1–10.
30. American College of Surgeons Committee on Trauma: Initial assessment and management. In Advanced Trauma Life Support Instructor Manual, 5th ed. Chicago, American College of Surgeons, 1993, pp 17–37.
31. Norris RL, Bush SP: North American venomous reptile bites. In Auerbach PS (ed): Wilderness Medicine, 4th ed. St. Louis, MO, Mosby, 2001, pp 896–926.
32. Walter FG: Envenomations. Dallas, TX, American College of Emergency Physicians, 1995.
33. Ownby CL, Kainer RA, Tu AT: Pathogenesis of hemorrhage induced by rattlesnake venom: an electron microscopic study. Am J Pathol 1974;76(2):401–414.
34. Dubnoff JW, Russell FE: Isolation of lethal protein and peptide from Crotalus viridis helleri venom. Proc West Pharmacol Soc 1970;13:98.
35. Bjarnason JB, Fox JW: Hemorrhagic metalloproteinases from snake venoms. Pharmacol Ther 1994;62(3):325–372.
36. Kitchens CS: Hemostatic aspects of envenomation by North American snakes. Hematol Oncol Clin North Am 1992;6(5):1189–1195.
37. Kitchens CS, Van Mierop LH: Mechanism of defibrination in humans after envenomation by the Eastern diamondback rattlesnake. Am J Hematol 1983;14(4):345–353.
38. Hasiba U, Rosenbach LM, Rockwell D, Lewis JH: DIC-like syndrome after envenomation by the snake, Crotalus horridus horridus. N Engl J Med 1975;292(10):505–507.
39. Budzynski AZ, Pandya BV, Rubin RN, et al: Fibrinogenolytic afibrinogenemia after envenomation by western diamondback rattlesnake (Crotalus atrox). Blood 1984;63(1):1–14.
40. Simon TL, Grace TG: Envenomation coagulopathy in wounds from pit vipers. N Engl J Med 1981;305(8):443–447.
41. Mosher DF: Disorders of blood coagulation. In Bennett JC, Plum F (eds): Cecil Textbook of Medicine, 20th ed. Philadelphia, WB Saunders, 1996, pp 987–1003.
42. Dart RC: Reptile bites. In Tintinalli JE, Kelen GD, Stapczynski JS (eds): Emergency Medicine: A Comprehensive Study Guide, 6th ed. New York, McGraw-Hill, 2003, pp 1200–1206.
43. Burgess JL, Dart RC: Snake venom coagulopathy: use and abuse of blood products in the treatment of pit viper envenomation. Ann Emerg Med 1991;20(7):795–801.
44. Bond RG, Burkhart KK: Thrombocytopenia following timber rattlesnake envenomation. Ann Emerg Med 1997;30(1):40–44.
45. Ahlstrom NG, Luginbuhl W, Tisher CC: Acute anuric renal failure after pigmy rattlesnake bite. South Med J 1991;84(6):783–785.
46. Reid HA, Theakston RD: Changes in coagulation effects by venoms of Crotalus atrox as snakes age. Am J Trop Med Hyg 1978;27(5):1053–1057.
47. Gregory VM, Russell FE, Brewer JR, Zawadski LR: Seasonal variations in rattlesnake venom proteins. Proc West Pharmacol Soc 1984;27:233–236.
48. Bond GR: Controversies in the treatment of pediatric victims of Crotalinae snakebite. Clin Pediatr Emerg Med 2001;2:192–202.

49. Schmaier AH, Colman RW: Crotalocytin: characterization of the timber rattlesnake platelet activating protein. Blood 1980;56(6):1020–1028.

50. Gerkin R, Sergent KC, Curry SC, et al: Life-threatening airway obstruction from rattlesnake bite to the tongue. Ann Emerg Med 1987;16(7):813–816.

51. Lewis JV, Portera CA Jr: Rattlesnake bite of the face: case report and review of the literature. Am Surg 1994;60(9):681–682.

52. Brooks DE, Graeme KA, Ruha AM, Tanen DA: Respiratory compromise in patients with rattlesnake envenomation. J Emerg Med 2002;23(4):329–332.

53. Curry SC, Kunkel DB: Toxicology rounds. Death from a rattlesnake bite. Am J Emerg Med 1985;3(3):227–235.

54. Banner W, Russell FE, Barton B: Fatal rattlesnake bite in a child [Abstract]. Vet Hum Toxicol 1984;26:400.

55. Carroll RR, Hall EL, Kitchens CS: Canebrake rattlesnake envenomation. Ann Emerg Med 1997;30(1):45–48.

56. Dart RC, Hurlbut KM, Garcia R, Boren J: Validation of a severity score for the assessment of crotalid snakebite. Ann Emerg Med 1996;27(3):321–326.

57. Forgey W, Norris RL, Blackman J, et al: Rattlesnake bite. J Wilderness Med 1994;5:216–221.

58. Walter FG, Olson KR: First aid for snakebite. Am Acad Clin Toxicol Update 1995;8(2):1.

59. Howarth DM, Southee AE, Whyte IM: Lymphatic flow rates and first-aid in simulated peripheral snake or spider envenomation. Med J Aust 1994;161(11–12):695–700.

60. Burgess JL, Dart RC, Egen NB, Mayersohn M: Effects of constriction bands on rattlesnake venom absorption: a pharmacokinetic study. Ann Emerg Med 1992;21(9):1086–1093.

61. Sutherland SK, Coulter AR, Harris RD: Rationalisation of first-aid measures for elapid snakebite. Lancet 1979;1(8109):183–185.

62. Sutherland SK, Coulter AR: Early management of bites by the eastern diamondback rattlesnake (Crotalus adamanteus): studies in monkeys (Macaca fascicularis). Am J Trop Med Hyg 1981;30(2):497–500.

63. Clark RW: Cryotherapy and corticosteroids in the treatment of rattlesnake bite. Milit Med 1971;136(1):42–44.

64. Dart RC, Lindsey D, Schulman A: Snakebite and shocks [Letter]. Ann Emerg Med 1988;17:1262.

65. Russell FE: A letter on electroshock for snakebite. Vet Hum Toxicol 1987;29(4):320–321.

66. Johnson EK, Kardong KV, Mackessy SP: Electric shocks are ineffective in treatment of lethal effects of rattlesnake envenomation in mice. Toxicon 1987;25(12):1347–1349.

67. Howe NR, Meisenheimer JL Jr: Electric shock does not save snakebitten rats. Ann Emerg Med 1988;17(3):254–256.

68. Dart RC, Gustafson RA: Failure of electric shock treatment for rattlesnake envenomation. Ann Emerg Med 1991;20(6):659–661.

69. Alberts MB, Shalit M, LoGalbo F: Suction for venomous snakebite: a study of "mock venom" extraction in a human model. Ann Emerg Med 2004;43(2):181–186.

70. Bush SP: Snakebite suction devices don't remove venom: they just suck. Ann Emerg Med 2004;43(2):187–188.

71. Bush SP, Hegewald KG, Green SM, et al: Effects of a negative pressure venom extraction device (Extractor) on local tissue injury after artificial rattlesnake envenomation in a porcine model. Wilderness Environ Med 2000;11(3):180–188.

72. Bush SP, Hardy DL Sr: Immediate removal of extractor is recommended. Ann Emerg Med 2001;38(5):607–608.

73. Bronstein AC, Russell FE, Sullivan JB, et al: Negative pressure suction in field treatment of rattlesnake bite. [Abstract]. Vet Hum Toxicol 1985;27:297.

74. Bronstein AC, Russell FE, Sullivan JB, et al: Negative pressure suction in the field treatment of rattlesnake bite victims. Vet Hum Toxicol 1986;28:485.

75. Davidson TM: Intravenous rattlesnake envenomation. West J Med 1988;148(1):45–47.

76. Kitchens CS, Hunter S, Van Mierop LH: Severe myonecrosis in a fatal case of envenomation by the canebrake rattlesnake (Crotalus horridus atricaudatus). Toxicon 1987;25(4):455–458.

77. Bush SP, Jansen PW: Severe rattlesnake envenomation with anaphylaxis and rhabdomyolysis. Ann Emerg Med 1995;25(6):845–848.

78. Cruz NS, Alvarez RG: Rattlesnake bite complications in 19 children. Pediatr Emerg Care 1994;10(1):30–33.

79. Weed HG: Nonvenomous snakebite in Massachusetts: prophylactic antibiotics are unnecessary. Ann Emerg Med 1993;22(2):220–224.

80. Clark RF, Selden BS, Furbee B: The incidence of wound infection following crotalid envenomation. J Emerg Med 1993;11(5):583–586.

81. Goldstein EJ, Citron DM, Gonzalez H, et al: Bacteriology of rattlesnake venom and implications for therapy. J Infect Dis 1979;140(5):818–821.

82. Horowitz RS, Dart RC: Antivenins and immunobiologicals: immunotherapeutics of envenomation. In Auerbach PS (ed): Wilderness Medicine: Management of Wilderness and Environmental Emergencies, 4th ed. St. Louis, MO, Mosby, 2001, pp 952–960.

83. Antivenin (Crotalinae) polyvalent (equine origin). In: Physician's Desk Reference, 49th ed. Montvale, NJ, Medical Economics Data Production Co., 1995, pp 2643–2644.

84. Consroe P, Egen NB, Russell FE, et al: Comparison of a new ovine antigen binding fragment (Fab) antivenin for United States Crotalidae with the commercial antivenin for protection against venom-induced lethality in mice. Am J Trop Med Hyg 1995;53(5):507–510.

85. Ruha AM, Curry SC, Beuhler M, et al. Initial postmarketing experience with crotalidae polyvalent immune Fab for treatment of rattlesnake envenomation. Ann Emerg Med 2002;39(6):609–615.

86. Dart RC, Seifert SA, Carroll L, et al: Affinity-purified, mixed monospecific crotalid antivenom ovine Fab for the treatment of crotalid venom poisoning. Ann Emerg Med 1997;30(1):33–39.

87. Lavonas EJ, Gerardo CJ, O'Malley G, et al: Initial experience with Crotalidae polyvalent immune Fab (ovine) antivenom in the treatment of copperhead snakebite. Ann Emerg Med 2004;43(2):200–206.

88. Dart RC, Seifert SA, Boyer LV, et al: A randomized multicenter trial of Crotalinae polyvalent immune Fab (ovine) antivenom for the treatment for crotaline snakebite in the United States. Arch Intern Med 2001;161(16):2030–2036.

89. Boyer LV, Seifert SA, Clark RF, et al: Recurrent and persistent coagulopathy following pit viper envenomation. Arch Intern Med 1999;159(7):706–710.

90. Offerman SR, Bush SP, Moynihan JA, Clark RF: Crotaline Fab antivenom for the treatment of children with rattlesnake envenomation. Pediatrics 2002;110(5):968–971.

91. Protherics, Inc.: CroFab, Crotalidae polyvalent immune Fab (Ovine) [Package insert]. Nashville, TN, Protherics, Inc., 2000.

92. Caravati EM: Copperhead bites and Crotalidae polyvalent immune Fab (ovine): routine use requires evidence of improved outcomes. Ann Emerg Med 2004;43(2):207–208.

93. Scharman EJ, Noffsinger VD: Copperhead snakebites: clinical severity of local effects. Ann Emerg Med 2001;38(1):55–61.

94. Parrish HM, Carr CA: Bites by copperheads (Agkistrodon contortrix) in the United States. JAMA 1967;201(12):927–932.

95. Litovitz TL, Klein-Schwartz W, Rodgers GC Jr, et al: 2001 Annual report of the American Association of Poison Control Centers Toxic Exposure Surveillance System. Am J Emerg Med 2002;20(5):391–452.

96. Schwartz LB: Systemic anaphylaxis. In Goldman L, Ausiello D (eds): Cecil Textbook of Medicine, 22nd ed. Philadelphia, WB Saunders, 2004, pp 1614–1617.

97. Zull DN: Anaphylaxis. In Harwood-Nuss AL, Wolfson AB, Linden CH, Shepherd SM, eds. The Clinical Practice of Emergency Medicine, 3rd ed. Philadelphia, Lippincott Williams & Wilkins, 2000, pp 1053–1057.

98. Brostoff J, Hall T: Hypersensitivity-type I. In Roitt I, Brostoff J, Male D (eds): Immunology, 6th ed. Edinburgh, Scotland, Mosby, 2001, pp 323–343.

99. Jurkovich GJ, Luterman A, McCullar K, et al: Complications of Crotalidae antivenin therapy. J Trauma 1988;28(7):1032–1037.

100. Spaite D, Dart R, Sullivan JB: Skin testing in cases of possible crotalid envenomation. Ann Emerg Med 1988;17(1):105–106.

101. Hay F, Westwood OMR: Hypersensitivity-type III. In Roitt I, Brostoff J, Male D (eds): Immunology, 6th ed. Edinburgh, Scotland, Mosby, 2001, pp 357–369.

102. Loprinzi CL, Hennessee J, Tamsky L, Johnson TE: Snake antivenin administration in a patient allergic to horse serum. South Med J 1983;76(4):501–502.

103. Huang TT, Lynch JB, Larson DL, Lewis SR: The use of excisional therapy in the management of snakebite. Ann Surg 1974;179(5):598–607.

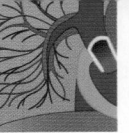

104. Glass TG Jr: Early debridement in pit viper bites. JAMA 1976;235(23):2513–2516.
105. Garfin SR, Castilonia RR, Mubarak SJ, et al: Rattlesnake bites and surgical decompression: results using a laboratory model. Toxicon 1984;22(2):177–182.
106. Stewart RM, Page CP, Schwesinger WH, et al: Antivenin and fasciotomy/debridement in the treatment of the severe rattlesnake bite. Am J Surg 1989;158(6):543–547.
107. Garfin SR, Castilonia RR, Mubarak SJ, et al: The effect of antivenin on intramuscular pressure elevations induced by rattlesnake venom. Toxicon 1985;23(4):677–680.
108. Garfin SR, Castilonia RR, Mubarak SJ, et al: Role of surgical decompression in treatment of rattlesnake bites. Surg Forum 1979;30:502–504.
109. Curry SC, Kraner JC, Kunkel DB, et al: Noninvasive vascular studies in management of rattlesnake envenomations to extremities. Ann Emerg Med 1985;14(11):1081–1084.
110. Hall EL: Role of surgical intervention in the management of crotaline snake envenomation. Ann Emerg Med 2001;37(2):175–180.
111. Ganong WF: Review of Medical Physiology, 21st ed. New York, McGraw-Hill, 2003.
112. Frankel NR, Villarin A: Compartment syndrome evaluation. In Roberts JR, Hedges JR (eds): Clinical Procedures in Emergency Medicine, 4th ed. Philadelphia, WB Saunders, 2004, pp 1058–1072.
113. Hargens AR, Akeson WH, Mubarak SJ, et al: Fluid balance within the canine anterolateral compartment and its relationship to compartment syndromes. J Bone Joint Surg Am 1978;60(4):499–505.
114. Whitesides TE, Haney TC, Morimoto K, Harada H: Tissue pressure measurements as a determinant for the need of fasciotomy. Clin Orthop Rel Res 1975(113):43–51.
115. Zweifach SS, Hargens AR, Evans KL, et al: Skeletal muscle necrosis in pressurized compartments associated with hemorrhagic hypotension. J Trauma 1980;20(11):941–947.
116. Heppenstall RB, Sapega AA, Scott R, et al: The compartment syndrome. An experimental and clinical study of muscular energy metabolism using phosphorus nuclear magnetic resonance spectroscopy. Clin Orthop Rel Res 1988(226):138–155.
117. Tanen DA, Danish DC, Clark RF. Crotalidae polyvalent immune Fab antivenom limits the decrease in perfusion pressure of the anterior leg compartment in a porcine crotaline envenomation model. Ann Emerg Med 2003;41(3):384–390.
118. Matsen FA: Compartmental Syndromes. New York, WB Saunders, 1980.
119. Watt CH Jr: Treatment of poisonous snakebite with emphasis on digit dermotomy. South Med J 1985;78(6):694–699.
120. Guisto JA: Severe toxicity from crotalid envenomation after early resolution of symptoms. Ann Emerg Med 1995;26(3):387–389.
121. Hurlbut KM, Dart RC, Spaite DW: Reliability of clinical presentation for predicting significant pit viper envenomation [Abstract]. Ann Emerg Med 1988;17:438.
122. Boyer LV, Seifert SA, Cain JS: Recurrence phenomena after immunoglobulin therapy for snake envenomations: Part 2. Guidelines for clinical management with crotaline Fab antivenom. Ann Emerg Med 2001;37(2):196–201.
123. Hill RE, Bogdan GM, Dart RC: Time to reconstitution: purified Fab antivenom vs. unpurified IgG antivenom. Toxicon 2001;39(5):729–731.
124. Yip L: Rational use of crotalidae polyvalent immune Fab (ovine) in the management of crotaline bite. Ann Emerg Med 2002;39(6):648–650.
125. Tyler LS, Fox ER, Caravati EM: The challenge of drug shortages for emergency medicine. Ann Emerg Med 2002;40(6):598–602.
126. Sanchez EE, Galan JA, Perez JC, et al: The efficacy of two antivenoms against the venom of North American snakes. Toxicon 2003;41(3):357–365.
127. Dart RC, McNally JT, Spaite DW, Gustafson R: The sequelae of pitviper poisoning in the United States. In Campbell JA, Brody ED (eds): Biology of the Pitvipers. Tyler, TX, Selva Press, 1992, pp 395–404.

B Elapidae: North American and Selected Non-native Species

STEPHEN W. BORRON, MD, MS ■ PETER B. CHASE, MD, PHD ■ FRANK G. WALTER, MD

At a Glance...

■ The Elapidae family is a large group of snakes, characterized by short, anterior, fixed, grooved, venom-conducting fangs.

■ The only native representatives of this family in the United States are the coral snakes, of the subfamily Elapinae.

■ Non-native Elapidae are responsible for bites in the United States, both in zoos and in homes of keepers of pet snakes.

■ Other important Elapidae discussed here include the cobras, kraits, Australian brown snakes, mambas, tiger snakes, and death adders.

■ The primary toxic mechanism for many Elapidae, including the corals, is neurotoxicity, with respiratory failure posing the greatest life threat. However, some species cause significant tissue necrosis and cardiotoxicity as well.

■ Antivenoms are available for many of the Elapidae. While effective against the neural components of toxicity, they are generally derived from horse serum and can cause serious allergic reactions, thus requiring careful administration and consideration of prophylactic measures to reduce anaphylaxis.

■ Anticholinesterases, such as edrophonium and neostigmine have been used successfully in reversing neurotoxicity as well, but are not universally effective.

■ As always, intensive supportive care is paramount to success in treating snakebite victims.

■ It cannot be emphasized too strongly that potentially fatal respiratory failure may occur precipitously more than 12 hours after a bite, so that even well-appearing bite victims should be observed closely for a minimum of 24 hours.

■ It is not uncommon for fang marks to be absent, and local tissue injury is often minimal or absent. Thus, the history of a bite should be considered sufficient evidence for observation and absence of local effect not equated with absence of envenomation.

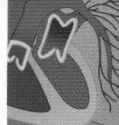

Mortality from snakebite worldwide is an enormous problem, estimated by some at up to 100,000 deaths per year.[1] Even this substantial figure is probably an underestimate of the real incidence, given the number of poor rural victims who do not seek care in hospitals, or simply die at home. Many of these bites are inflicted by members of the Elapidae family, which are found throughout Asia, Africa, Australia, and the Americas, but not in Europe. Worldwide, most bites occur in agricultural workers, fishermen, and hunters,[2] but in the United States a substantial number of bites occurs in handlers of "pet snakes."[3-6] The importance of this problem can be appreciated by examining the cases consulted upon personally by Minton between 1977 and 1995 (Table 21B-1).[5] Clearly, many more bites occurred during this period, suggesting a much higher overall incidence.

Dry bites (nonvenomous bites) are said to occur, on average, in about 50% of cases, with high variability among species.[2] In bites where venom is injected, the case fatality rate remains extremely high in some regions (upwards of 50%), but with antivenom and modern medical care, the mortality rate approaches that of other poisonings (i.e., less than 5%).[7]

The Elapidae family, defined in part by the presence of a pair of short, anterior, fixed, venom-conducting fangs, is composed of five subfamilies (although there is some disagreement as to classification): the Elapinae (coral snakes), Bungarinae (cobras, mambas, kraits) Oxyuraninae (Australian elapids), and Hydrophiinae and Laticaudinae (Sea snakes, which will not be described here). In North America, elapids account for relatively few snakebites and low mortality, compared with the more common bites of the Crotalinae (see Chapter 21A). However, elapids endemic to Asia (cobras) and Australia (taipan, death adder, brown snake, tiger snake, and others) account for significant morbidity and mortality. This chapter will focus primarily on Elapinae (coral snakes), but we will briefly discuss other terrestrial Elapidae of global importance.

U.S. CORAL SNAKES

North America has two genera of Elapidae, *Micruroides* and *Micrurus*.[8] *Micrurus* is represented by two subspecies in the United States: *Micrurus fulvius fulvius*, which is the Eastern coral snake, and *Micrurus fulvius tenere*, which is the Texas coral snake. *Micruroides* consists of one subspecies, *Micruroides euryxanthus euryxanthus*, the Sonoran or Arizona coral snake.[8]

Coral snakes are Elapidae and differ from the Crotalinae in that coral snakes have a pair of short, fixed, grooved, but not hollow, anterior fangs that carry venom along open, unsealed grooves from the ducts located at the base of the fangs.[8-11] This inefficient venom delivery apparatus (proterogliphous) is but one reason why coral snake envenomations are relatively uncommon in the United States, when compared with the more efficient venom delivery system of pit vipers (solenogliphous).[12] Other reasons include the coral snake's small mouth, which is unable to achieve a large jaw aperture to bite a human, the fact that coral snakes are not aggressive, and the fact that they live mostly underground. For an effective envenomation to occur, a coral snake usually must gnaw or hang onto its victim for at least several seconds because its venom is not injected directly through hollow fangs as in crotalids.[10,11,13]

In the United States, only a small percentage of snakebites are caused by coral snakes, usually *M. fulvius fulvius* and *M. fulvius tenere*.[13] The only other U.S. coral snake, *M. euryxanthus euryxanthus* is located in the Sonoran Desert of Arizona, New Mexico, and Mexico. A bite from *M. euryxanthus euryxanthus* may have the distinction of being the only coral snakebite that does not deliver enough venom to kill an adult human.[11,13] The average and maximum extracted venom yields of 0.12 mg and 6 mg, respectively, obtained from *M. euryxanthus euryxanthus*, is significantly below that obtained from the *Micrurus* species. The estimated lethal dose of *M. euryxanthus euryxanthus* venom for an adult human is 6 to 8 mg. This is in contradistinction to bites from *M. fulvius fulvius* in Florida and Alabama, and *M. fulvius tenere* in Texas, where bites by both species have produced adult human fatalities.[14]

Pathophysiology

Elapinae snake venoms contain a complex mixture of polypeptides. Whereas pit viper venom contains protein that causes coagulopathies, thrombocytopenia, and tissue necrosis, coral snake venom contains α neurotoxins and phospholipase A_2 (PLA_2), which cause paralysis and myonecrosis, respectively.[15] The neurotoxic components are polypeptides devoid of enzymatic activity and act primarily by binding postsynaptically at the nicotinic

SPECIES	BITES
Eastern green mamba (*Dendroaspis angusticeps*)	1
Balsan coral snake (*Micrurus laticollaris*)	1
Chinese cobra (*Naja atra*)	1
African ringed cobra (*Naja haje annulifera*)	3
Monocellate cobra (*Naja kaouthia*)	7
Oxus cobra (*Naja oxiana*)	1
Cape cobra (*Naja nivea*)	1
King cobra (*Ophiophagus hannah*)	1
Cobra, species uncertain	9
Collett's snake (*Pseudechis colletti*)	1
Elapidae (total)	26
Viperidae (total)	22
Atractaspididae (total)	2
Colubridae (total)	4
Total of 4 families of snakes	54

TABLE 21B-1 Relative Incidence of Venomous Bites by Non-native Elapid Snakes 1977–1995 in Comparison with Other Families

Only one bite (from an Asian or Indian cobra) resulted in death.
Adapted from Minton SA: Bites by non-native venomous snakes in the United States. Wilderness Environ Med 1996;7(4):297–303.

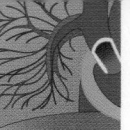

acetylcholine receptors of the neuromuscular junction, causing flaccid paralysis of striated muscles.[13,16-18] This competitive, nondepolarizing blockade of nicotinic acetylcholine receptors differs from the action of curare in that its onset is slower, its duration of action is much longer, and it is not necessarily reversed by anticholinesterases.[9,18-21] In addition, it should be noted that infusion of lethal doses of *M. fulvius fulvius* venom in dogs (0.3 mg/kg) or cats (2 mg/kg) produced profound hemodynamic changes (shock) primarily due to decreases in cardiac output despite ventilatory support.[22,23] The target of myotoxic PLA_2 is the plasmalemma, similar to pit viper PLA_2; however, evidence suggests these phospholipases evolved independently from each other.[21]

Clinical Manifestations

Coral snake envenomations differ clinically from crotaline envenomations in three major ways: Coral snake envenomations primarily produce neurotoxicity with comparatively little local tissue toxicity, although there can be myonecrosis, indicated by serum creatine kinase elevations.[10,11,20,24-27] Coral snake envenomations also differ from crotaline envenomations in that the onset of signs and symptoms can be delayed for more than 13 hours and then occur precipitously.[11,18,26-29] Venom effects can occur earlier; in fact, death due to ventilatory failure has occurred within 4 hours of envenomation.[29] Finally, unlike crotaline envenomation, the signs of coral snake envenomation are difficult to reverse or may even progress after administration of antivenom. Therefore, early coral snake antivenom administration is advisable.[11] Without infusion of antivenom, the neurologic complications of a coral snake bite may last 3 weeks to a month.

Victims of Arizona (Sonoran) coral snakebites (*M. euryxanthus euryxanthus*) have reported local paresthesias, weakness, hand incoordination, drowsiness, nausea, and abdominal pain.[24] Envenomation by Eastern and Texas coral snakes (*M. fulvius*) can produce severe neurotoxic effects. Detailed signs and symptoms of Eastern coral snake envenomations in a 20-patient subset of a 39-patient case series included fang marks (85%), a small amount of local swelling (40%), paresthesias (35%), vomiting (25%), euphoria (15%), weakness (15%), dizziness (10%), dyspnea (10%), diaphoresis (10%), muscle tenderness (10%), fasciculations (5%), and confusion (5%). Six of 39 patients in this case series (15%) were endotracheally intubated. Three of these patients received elective intubation before frank ventilatory failure and none developed aspiration pneumonia; however, three other patients who were intubated immediately before frank ventilatory failure developed aspiration pneumonia.[11] Seizures have also been reported after *M. fulvius* envenomation, particularly in children; it is unclear whether these were caused by hypoxia.[28] Ventilatory failure is the ultimate cause of death and is usually, but not always, preceded by signs of cranial nerve dysfunction, including ptosis, dysarthria, dysphagia, and/or hypersalivation.[28,29]

Diagnosis

Clinical diagnosis of coral snake envenomation can be difficult. Coral snake envenomations can occur with or without visible fang marks.[11,20,25] The patient and clinician may not realize a coral snake envenomation has occurred without positively identifying the snake and realizing that onset of signs and symptoms is often delayed. Although several U.S. snakes resemble the bright red-, yellow-, and black-banded coloration of coral snakes, the mnemonic, "Red on yellow, kill a fellow; red on black, venom lack," identifies the color pattern of coral snakes in the United States, but not elsewhere.[8,10,13] No significant laboratory abnormalities occur, other than hypercarbia or hypoxia in patients who have ventilatory insufficiency.[24]

Treatment

PREHOSPITAL TREATMENT

No first aid should delay rapid transport to a medical facility. Vigorous washing with copious amounts of water and detergent should be done as soon as possible to remove venom that can remain on the skin's surface and could enter through punctures or abrasions. Emergency medical service notification and transportation to a medical facility are the most effective prehospital treatments. During the time of transportation to a medical facility, it is possible to provide a pressure wrap to the victim's extremity similar to what has been recommended for envenomation by the Australian Elapidae species.[30,31] It should be emphasized that the pressure immobilization technique has never been demonstrated clinically to be effective in treatment of *M. fulvius* envenomations. Nonetheless, German and colleagues recently demonstrated marked reduction in mortality in a porcine model of *M. fulvius fulvius* envenomation using this technique.[32] Briefly, the technique involves wrapping a long, wide swath or bandage around the bitten area in a firm but not occlusive manner. The bandage should be extended to cover as much of the bitten extremity as possible and then the limb immobilized to limit activity.

HOSPITAL TREATMENT

Antivenin (*Micrurus fulvius*) (equine origin) (Wyeth-Ayerst Laboratories, Philadelphia, PA) is available for Eastern and Texas coral snake (*M. fulvius*) envenomations, but not for Arizona coral snake (*M. euryxanthus euryxanthus*) envenomations (F.E. Russell, personal communication, 1996).[24-26] However, Wyeth-Ayerst production of *M. fulvius* antivenom was discontinued in 2001. There is evidence that other antivenoms from Mexico, Australia, and Costa Rica may have potential for use in the treatment of coral snake (*M. fulvius fulvius*) envenomations.[12,33,34]

Although it is generally not advisable to capture a venomous snake because of the risk for further envenomations, positive field identification is helpful in determining the duration of patient observation for a potential coral snakebite. If the patient has been bitten and if a reliable, positive, field identification has been

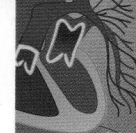

made, or if there are signs or symptoms of *M. fulvius* coral snake envenomation, then *M. fulvius* coral snake antivenom treatment is indicated.[11,24,25]

Before intravenous administration of antivenom, a skin test can be performed. Wyeth-Ayerst *M. fulvius* antivenom skin testing and intravenous administration involve similar risks and require similar precautions as with the Wyeth-Ayerst polyvalent crotalid antivenom, because both are of equine origin. Life-threatening anaphylactic and anaphylactoid reactions can occur.[11]

The recommended initial dose of Wyeth-Ayerst *M. fulvius* antivenom varies among researchers (F.E. Russell, personal communication, 1996).[11,24,35] Investigators agree with the recommendation of a recognized authority who suggested an initial dose of at least 5 vials of Wyeth-Ayerst *M. fulvius* antivenom (F.E. Russell, personal communication, 1996). An initial dose of 10 vials of Wyeth-Ayerst *M. fulvius* antivenom may be necessary with bites caused by large coral snakes, bites involving long exposures with difficulty disengaging the biting snake, and in bites of small children (F.E. Russell, personal communication, 1996).[11,24,35] A subsequent dose of 5 vials of Wyeth-Ayerst *M. fulvius* antivenom is indicated if the patient has worsening of signs or symptoms after the initial dose of antivenom.[11,25,26,35]

Once a patient has developed neurotoxic signs or symptoms, these signs or symptoms may progress in spite of antivenom therapy.[11] Good supportive care is paramount with early endotracheal intubation, before frank ventilatory failure and respiratory arrest.[11,24]

As with other bites, administer tetanus prophylaxis, if indicated. Prophylactic antibiotics are not recommended.

Other Antivenoms to Consider

Presently there are equine immunoglobulin $F(ab)_2$ fragments available from Mexico (Coralmyn, Instituto Bioclon, Mexico) that have good neutralizing capacity for venom of *M. fulvius* from the United States.[12,34] In addition, another nondomestic antivenom from Australia for use against the tiger snake (*Notechis scutatus*, CSL Limited, Parkville, Victoria, Australia) has also been shown to be effective in preventing lethality due to *M. fulvius fulvius* envenomation in an animal model.[34] Niether Coralmyn nor the Australian tiger snake antivenom is FDA approved, but both may become available from U.S. zoos that house Central and South American coral snakes or Australian snakes.[36]

Disposition

Patients should be admitted, observed, and monitored for at least 24 hours, even if bite marks or other signs or symptoms are lacking. Patients may be discharged after at least 24 hours if no signs of toxicity develop.[25,26]

Prognosis

Prognosis is excellent in most cases; however, some patients have required endotracheal intubation and mechanical ventilation for paralysis that has lasted as long as 1 week.[11] Death is caused by ventilatory failure and is unusual.[28,29] Death occurs early in most fatal cases. Approximately 10% of patients treated with antivenom in one case series developed serum sickness[11] (Fig. 21B-1).

NON-NATIVE (NON-ELAPINAE) ELAPIDAE
Epidemiology

Elapid envenomation is rare in the United States, but it is a major cause of morbidity and mortality in other parts of the world. According to Bawaskar,[37] there are 52 known poisonous snake species in India; the major families are of the Elapidae family and including common cobras (*Naja naja*), the king cobra (*Ophiophagus hannah*) and the common krait (*Bungarus caeruleus*). There are an estimated 200,000 snake bites reported annually in India, with an estimated 35,000 to 50,000 deaths.[38] Snakebites are also extremely common in Papua New Guinea, where up to 36% of patients presenting to the major treating hospital will require ventilation. Unfortunately, both ventilators and antivenom are in scarce supply.[39] Fernando, in a report on the first 10 years of the existence of the Sri Lankan National Poisons Information Centre, pointed out that snakebites are responsible for only 6% of enquiries, but for 42% of poisoning hospitalizations. The case fatality rate was, compared with neighboring India, surprisingly low, at 0.5%. Fernando attributes some of this success to a massive information campaign regarding the benefits of antivenom over traditional Ayurvedic therapy. This information resulted in a fivefold increase in hospital admissions over a 10-year period ending in 1996.[40] This case fatality rate compares with that of Australia, where hospitalization is rapid and antivenom widely available. Currie recently catalogued the incidence of snakebite in a hospital in the Northern Territory of Australia. An estimated 23 bites per 100,000 population occur annually. The bite victim is typically male (2:1 predominance), older than 15 years, and Aboriginal (61 bites per 100,000 population versus 20 in others). The most commonly involved elapids were the Western brown snake (*Pseudonaja nuchalis*), Mulga snake (*Pseudechis australis*), and death adder (*Acanthophis* species), all viewed as extremely toxic. The majority of bite victims of these species received antivenom (81%, 75%, and 29%, respectively). In spite of early collapse with unconsciousness occurring in 15% of patients, there were no deaths.[7] In fact, there are only about two fatalities from snakebite in Australia each year, in spite of many incidents. In summary, it appears that the availability of antivenoms and adequate systems for life support have a profound impact on elapid bite mortality. A brief review of some of the specifics regarding the various genera of non-Elapinae elapids is followed by a general overview of treatment.

Pathophysiology and Clinical Manifestations

As is the case for coral venoms, the venoms of non-native Elapidae are complex mixtures, containing neurotoxins,

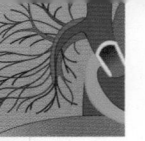

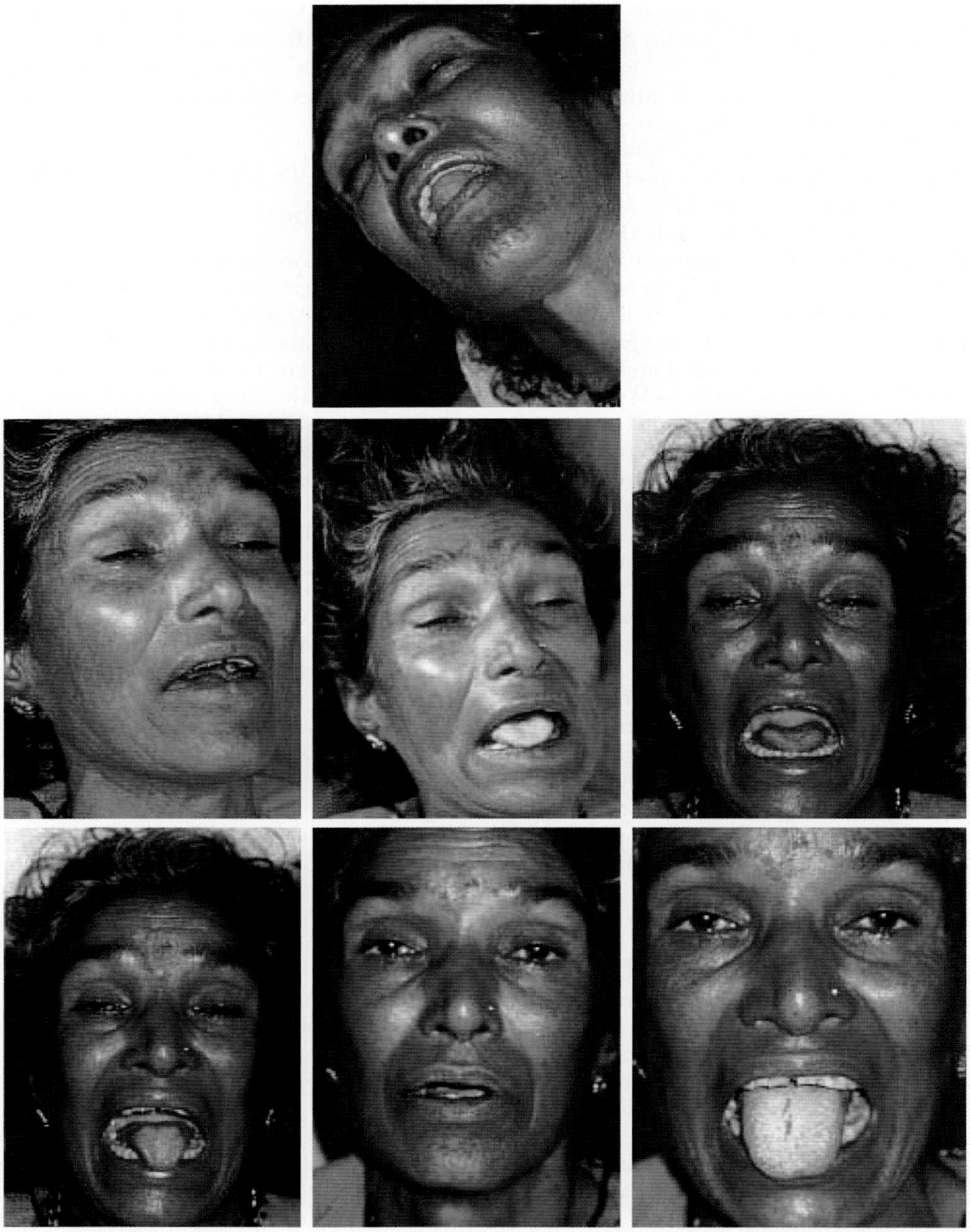

FIGURE 21B-1 Response to antivenom and neostigmine in a patient with decreased mental status and cranial nerve deficits. (From Bawaskar HS, Bawaskar PH: Envenoming by the common krait (*Bungarus caeruleus*) and Asian cobra (*Naja naja*): clinical manifestations and their management in a rural setting. Wilderness Environ Med 2004;15(4):257–266. Used with permission.)

myotoxins, cardiotoxins, and other components. Neurotoxins may act at presynaptic or postsynaptic sites (Table 21B-2), which may affect their onset and, in part, their response to anticholinesterase drugs.

COBRAS (*NAJA* SPECIES, *OPHIOPHAGUS HANNAH,* AND OTHERS)

Cobras produce a venom that is neurotoxic, cardiotoxic, and hemotoxic (Fig. 21B-2). The neurotoxic component is most often cited as predominating, but the venoms vary from one subspecies to another: Some cause more

tissue necrosis than neurotoxicity.[41] Conversely, the Philippine cobra (*Naja naja philippinensis*) has a neurotoxicity:tissue necrosis ratio of 14:1, inducing neurotoxic symptoms in as many as 97% of bite victims in the study by Watt.[42] One of the principal neurotoxic components of the venom is α-bungarotoxin, which reversibly blocks postsynaptic acetylcholine receptors. Neostigmine may reverse these effects.[43] As mentioned, *Naja* species may produce severe local tissue necrosis, which is not prevented by administration of antivenom. The venom contains hyaluronidase[44] and phospholipases,

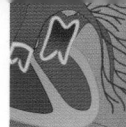

TABLE 21B-2 Representative Neurotoxins and Active Sites of Various Elapid Venoms

GENUS	TOXIN	ACTIVE SITE
Acanthophis species (death adder)	*Acanthophis antiarcticus* b and others	Postsynaptic
Micrurus species (corals)	α neurotoxin	Postsynaptic
Naja species (cobras)	α bungarotoxin	Postsynaptic
Bungarus species (kraits)	β bungarotoxin	Presynaptic
Dendroaspis species (mambas)	Dendrotoxins	Presynaptic
Notechis species (tiger snakes)	Notexin	Presynaptic
Oxyuranus species (taipan)	Taipoxin	Presynaptic

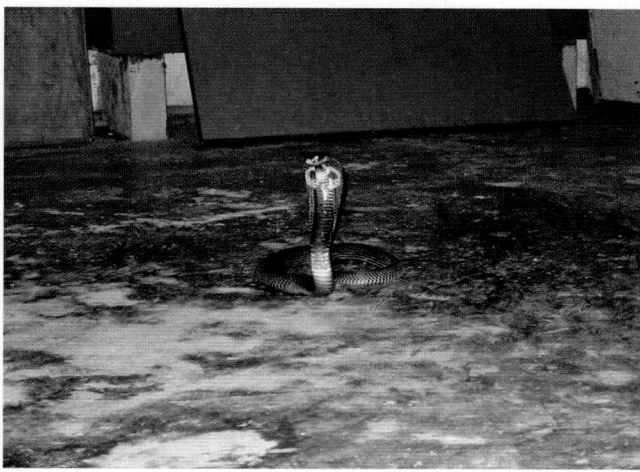

A

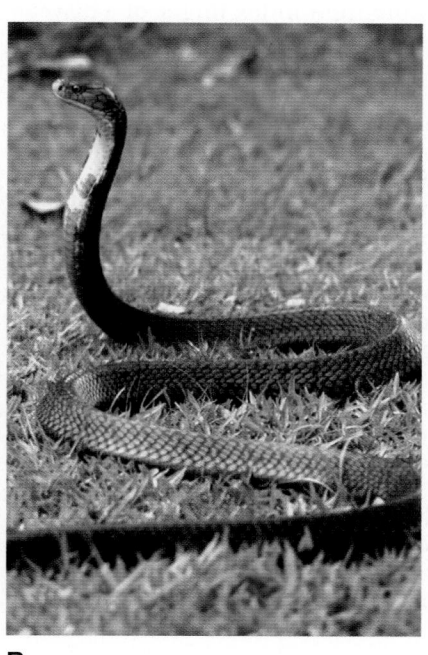

B

FIGURE 21B-2 A, *Naja sumatrana* (spitting cobra). **B,** *Ophiophagus hannah* (king cobra). (Courtesy of Francis Lim, Curator, Singapore National Zoo.)

resulting in anticoagulant effects.[45] A hemolysin, phosphatidase, produces enzymatic destruction of the endothelium and red blood cells. This may lead to hemolysis and acute renal failure. Other components include proteases, cholinesterases, and erepsin.[3] Cardiotoxicity appears to be rare,[3] although some of the venom peptides appear to affect calcium transport. Cobra venom administration results in significant conduction disturbances in rats.[46]

Bawaskar and Bawaskar reported on a series of cobra and krait bites in rural India. Among the seven cobra bites, two were dead on arrival, one died upon seeing the cobra (without apparent bite), for a bite mortality rate of 29%. Four subjects recovered with a combined therapy of antivenom, anticholinesterase drugs, and/or artificial ventilation. According to Bawaskar and Bawaskar, the cobra, unlike the krait, deposits its venom deeply. This, in combination with hyaluronidase, allows spreading of the venom to occur rapidly and symptoms to arise abruptly. Interestingly, this rapidity of onset prompts rural victims in India to seek care quickly after a cobra bite, while the more insidious onset of symptoms induced by the bite of the krait more often results in a visit to the local traditional healer (mantrik or tantrik) for natural curatives. A number of social issues likewise enter into the difficult decision to seek hospital care.[43]

A number of cobra bites have been reported in the United States as well. Britt and Burkhart reported on a bite by *N. naja* (described in this case as a black Pakistani cobra) maintained as a pet. A 26-year-old man with a collection of about 65 snakes was bitten on the right index finger by the snake and suffered severe pain within minutes. He was tachycardic and tachypneic on hospital arrival, was observed on a cardiac monitor for a few hours, and was then discharged. He returned within 8 hours complaining of chest pain, abdominal pain, and nausea. The right arm had swollen considerably since his first admission. The patient was started on five vials of polyvalent cobra antivenom but had received only about one fifth of the infusion when he developed generalized urticaria. He was given diphenhydramine and methyl prednisolone, with resolution of the rash. The remainder

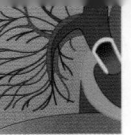

of the antivenom was withheld. The patient was discharged after 3 days with complaints of persistent occasional swelling of the affected finger.[3] This case nicely illustrates several of the typical characteristics of elapid snake bites in the United States: the patient is often a man in his twenties or thirties who keeps the snake for a pet. Symptoms may be delayed for many hours after a bite, and administration of antivenom often results in allergic (anaphylactic or anaphylactoid) phenomena. Although not specifically mentioned in this case, it is not uncommon that consumption of alcohol precedes the bite. Ronan-Bentle and colleagues recently reported on a bite to the right index finger of a 30-year-old man who was feeding his pet Asiatic Suphan cobra (*Naja kaouthia*). The patient presented to an emergency department, was given neostigmine and atropine, and was transferred to a tertiary care center. On arrival there, he complained of paresthesias, muscle cramps, inability to keep his eyes open, and diplopia on lateral gaze. The patient was found to have ptosis, ophthalmoplegia, and tongue fasciculations. He was pretreated with subcutaneous epinephrine and given five vials of South African polyvalent antivenom. Nevertheless, his bulbar palsy worsened and he became cyanotic, requiring intubation. He was given an additional five vials of Thai Red Cross purified antivenom. He was admitted to the intensive care unit and ventilated for 12 hours before successful extubation. He was discharged in good condition but subsequently required amputation of the finger.[6]

Davidson and colleagues have published a nice review of cobras and a (now somewhat dated) list of available antivenoms and sources.[41] The Antivenom Index can provide updated availability information of these vital resources.[36]

KRAITS (*BUNGARUS* SPECIES)

The krait produces β-bungarotoxin, which has a high affinity for, and irreversibly blocks, presynaptic neuromuscular receptors. The krait has the most lethal venom (by weight), but the effects are delayed due to slow absorption from subcutaneous or skin deep bites because of the snake's short sharp fangs. Kraits in India often enter the dwellings of rural families in search of prey, such as rats and mice. Because many rural Indians sleep on the floor, it is common to be bitten at night. In spite of the slow onset of toxic symptoms, the common krait is considered the most dangerous species on the Indian subcontinent, with a 35% to 50% case mortality rate.[43] In a series of 30 elapid bites that occurred in rural India, 23 krait bites were recorded, with 2 patients dead on arrival, 7 deaths in the hospital, and 14 recoveries (mortality rate 39%). Four patients required artificial respiration, antivenom, and anticholinesterases. One had a dry bite and the remaining nine survived with supportive care.[43] The investigators reported success with anticholinesterase treatment (see Fig. 21B-1). While signs and symptoms are similar to those of cobra bites, there are important differences, as illustrated in Table 21B-3.

TIGER SNAKE (*NOTECHIS* SPECIES)

Tiger snakes have venom that is neurotoxic, myotoxic, and procoagulant. Notexin is the major neurotoxin, acting, like β-bungarotoxin, on presynaptic neuromuscular junctions. It is described as resistant to treatment with antivenom. Notexin is also responsible for muscle damage and myoglobinuria. A procoagulant component has been identified, which acts by cleaving peptide bonds of prothrombin, resulting in conversion to thrombin. The procoagulant action is rapid, preceding the onset of neuromuscular paralysis.[47] The tiger snake is the second most common cause of death from snakebite in Australia, following the brown snake (*Pseudonaja* species). It was responsible for 8 of 30 deaths reported on that continent between 1981 and 1994. Ferguson and colleagues studied complete coagulation parameters in 3 patients bitten by *Notechis ater occidentalis*. All three cases had markedly prolonged International Normalized Ratio and activated partial thromboplastin time values and diminished fibrinogen. D-dimers were elevated, indicative of fibrinolysis. Factor V was also markedly diminished, while factor VIII was moderately diminished. Interestingly, platelet counts remained normal in all three. Two of three patients survived their coagulopathy and snakebite after receiving fresh frozen plasma (FFP) and tiger snake antivenom. Two patients, including a 14-year-old boy, received cryoprecipitate as well. The child suffered cardiac arrest approximately 30 minutes after the bite, was resuscitated, but developed ischemic brain damage and died about 30 hours after envenomation.[47] The researchers signaled the importance of giving both FFP and cryoprecipitate to replace the factor V and fibrinogen.

DEATH ADDER (*ACANTHOPHIS* SPECIES)

The death adder is the most common poisonous snake in Papua New Guinea and is likewise found in Irian Jaya, Australia, and parts of eastern Indonesia.[48] The venom of the death adder contains at least four distinct neurotoxins that cause postsynaptic blockade. Like the krait, the death adder is a nocturnal hunter; however, bites do occur during the day as well. According to Lalloo, the death adder causes less severe envenomation than the taipan. The researchers reported signs of neurotoxicity in 15 of their 16 envenomated patients, but intubation was required in only 5 (27.1%).[48]

MAMBAS (*DENDROASPIS* SPECIES)

The venom of mambas contains dendrotoxins, small proteins that enhance acetylcholine release at the neuromuscular junction (thus, presynaptically, like kraits and tiger snakes). The toxins of the green mamba (*Dendroaspis angusticeps*) have been shown to block particular subtypes (Kv1.1, Kv1.2, and Kv1.6) of potassium channels, serving as probes for the study of potassium channels in physiology and pathophysiology.[49] The toxin is likewise used to study subtypes of muscarinic receptors.[50,51]

Munday and colleagues recently reported on a healthy 40-year-old female neurobiochemist who presented with

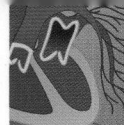

TABLE 21B-3 Representative Symptoms and Signs of Non-native Elapid Envenomations

CLINICAL EFFECT	COBRA (*NAJA SPECIES, N* = 7)	KRAIT (*BUNGARUS CAERULUS, N* = 23)	DEATH ADDER (*ACANTHOPHIS SPECIES, N* = 18)
Reference	43	43	48*
Fang marks	7 (100%)	ND	ND
Swelling and/or ecchymosis at bite site	7 (100%)	2	0
Mild swelling and tenderness	ND	2	ND
Tender adenopathy	ND	ND	11
Abdominal pain or tenderness	ND	17	8
Vomiting	ND	11	5
Bleeding	ND	ND	1
Level of consciousness			
Conscious	1	6	ND
Semiconscious	3	7	ND
Comatose	3	8	ND
Sweating	ND	11	ND
Paresthesias/dysesthesias	ND	18	ND
Ptosis (partial or complete)	ND	19	17
Ophthalmoplegia	1	20	10
Blurred or double vision	1	1	3
Decreased hand grip strength	ND	ND	5
Slurred speech	ND	ND	4†
Dysphagia	ND	ND	5
Jaw restriction	ND	ND	2†
Diminished reflexes	ND	ND	2
Bradycardia	ND	1	ND
Hypotension	ND	2	ND
Hypertension	ND	4	ND
Requirement for intubation	4	11	5
Requirement for mechanical ventilation	4	11	5

ND, no data provided.
*Where numbers of symptoms versus signs differ, the higher number is displayed.
†Not assessed in all patients.

progressive numbness of the left malar region and lateral orbit that progressed to include the medial orbit and tongue. One hour prior to presentation she used her bare hands to remove residual petroleum jelly from a dish that had previously contained 500 nanoliters of 500 nanomolar dendrotoxin. She recalled rubbing her left eye prior to the onset of symptoms. She had previously washed the dish with 70% ethanol while using latex gloves. Physical examination was remarkable only for weakness to superior gaze and some mild tongue fasciculations. The symptoms resolved within 12 hours of exposure.[52]

TAIPANS

The taipan (*Oxyuranus scutellatus*) is one of the deadliest snakes in the world, with the third most lethal venom of all snakes and the second largest average venom yield (120 mg) of Australasian snakes. The rare inland taipan (*Oxyuranus microlepidotus*) has the most potent venom of all Australasian snakes. The principal neurotoxin of the taipan is taipoxin, which acts presynaptically. The taipan has extremely long fangs (8 to 12 mm) and an efficient venom delivery system on biting, with a "snap-release" action. Survival from an effective taipan bite was very rare before antivenom and ventilation were available.[53]

Diagnosis

Diagnosis for non-native elapid bites is largely clinical, based on the history and identification of the snake, when available. Because bite marks are not always visible (apparently a particular problem with kraits) and swelling and ecchymosis are quite variable (see Table 21B-3), the diagnosis may be elusive. The history may sometimes be misleading, as in the case of one man who was about to be whisked off to the operating room for exploratory laparotomy due to abdominal pain, who finally admitted that the scratches on his hand were actually the bite of his pet cobra.[54] Sudden onset of ptosis or other cranial neuropathies and/or respiratory muscle failure should prompt the suspicion of an elapid bite under appropriate circumstances. A micro-ELISA (enzyme-linked immunosorbent assay) kit for the detection of snake venom and venom antibody exists,[37]

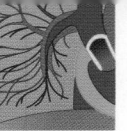

but is unlikely to be found in most hospitals. Hung and colleagues reported good correlation of their ELISA for the Taiwan cobra (*Naja atra*) with the severity of local tissue destruction.[55]

Treatment

SUPPORTIVE CARE

As in all envenomations, the primary treatment for non-native elapid poisonings is careful observation and intensive supportive care. Due to the neurotoxic effects of the venoms, respiratory depression is common and often requires intubation (see Table 21B-3). Given that the median time to requirement for intubation and ventilation in a series of death adder envenomations was 13 hours (range 2 to 23.5 hours), it seems prudent to recommend that patients who suffer bites by non-native elapids be observed for at least 24 hours in the hospital.

ANTIBIOTICS

While prophylactic antibiotics are often recommended in elapid bites, very few studies of their actual need have been undertaken. Blaylock, in a prospective study of snake bites in South Africa, looked at antibiotic use in 310 patients (data were missing for 53 additional bites). The protocol called for antibiotics not to be used unless the bite was necrotic or "necrosis was anticipated." Infected wounds were cultured. A number of protocol violations occurred, but there were no infections in patients who did not receive antibiotics. Where positive cultures occurred, the most frequent organisms were gram-negative enterobacteriaceae. No anaerobes were cultured. The researcher concluded that antibiotics should be reserved for those snakebite patients with necrosis and should cover gram-negative aerobic bacilli and gram-positive aerobic cocci.[56] Studies of antibiotic use in pit viper envenomations[57,58] and nontoxic snake bites[59,60] have strongly suggested that routine antibiotics are not necessary in these cases. While it is thorny to generalize across families and species of snakes, there currently appears to be insufficient evidence to support the use of antibiotic prophylaxis in elapid bites.

SURGICAL INTERVENTIONS

A recent retrospective analysis of snakebites in pediatric patients presenting to a hospital in India over 6 years was conducted by Chattopadhyay and colleagues. Records were reviewed for the type of surgical lesions seen and the treatment offered and their results. Fifty-five percent of bites were from unidentified poisonous snakes, followed by cobras, then nonpoisonous snakes. Forty-four of the 58 children required some form of local, and in most cases, conservative therapy. Twenty-eight percent required débridement for local necrosis, and only five needed a skin graft, with good functional results over a period of 1 to 45 days. One child underwent an above-knee amputation. Patients who required surgical intervention received significantly more vials of antivenom. The investigators concluded that complications of snakebite are frequent, but can be managed conservatively, that delayed excision of the resultant local necrosis is associated with good outcomes, and that the need for fasciotomy is rare.[61]

ANTIVENOMS

Antivenoms for non-native snakes are manufactured around the world, are maintained in a number of zoos across the United States, and can usually be located with the assistance of the regional poison control center. It is advisable to contact the poison center in your area immediately upon presentation of a patient with a bite to see what antivenom may be available for the species involved. Because of the relative rarity of these products, it is not uncommon to use expired antivenom,[3] but as adverse reactions to all horse-derived antivenoms are common, it is probably wise to obtain specific informed consent for their administration, particularly if the product is outdated. Unlike crotaline antivenoms, elapid antivenoms appear to have little effect on the myotoxic properties of the venoms. The antivenom is administered primarily to combat the respiratory effects of the venom. According to Bawaskar and Bawaskar, citing Ponchanugool, antivenom does not prevent local tissue necrosis.[43,62] Accordingly, local swelling should not be used as a guide to the administration of antivenom.[3]

In India[63] and Sri Lanka, it is common to precede antivenom treatment with prophylactic epinephrine, given subcutaneously. Premawardherna and colleagues[64] performed a prospective, double-blind, randomized, placebo-controlled trial in 105 patients with signs of envenomation after snakebite. Fifty-six patients from 14 to 65 years of age received epinephrine (0.25 mL 1:1000 subcutaneously) and 49 controls (ages 17 to 65 years) received placebo as pretreatment. Six patients (11%) receiving epinephrine and 21 control patients (43%) developed acute adverse reactions to antivenom serum ($P = .0002$). Significant reductions in acute adverse reactions to serum were also seen in the epinephrine group of patients for each category of mild, moderate, and severe reactions. There were no significant adverse effects attributable to epinephrine.

Other investigators have recommended corticosteroids and/or antihistamines as prophylaxis. Gawarammana and colleagues performed a double-blind, randomized, placebo-controlled trial of a parallel infusion of hydrocortisone with or without a bolus injection of chlorpheniramine to attempt to reduce acute adverse reactions to antivenom. The group that received both hydrocortisone and chlorpheniramine had significantly fewer reactions (52%) to a polyvalent antivenom (Vins Bioproduct Limited, Mumbai, India) than those who received hydrocortisone alone (80%) or placebo (81%).[65]

ANTICHOLINESTERASES

Edrophonium was shown in a small, double-blind, placebo-controlled study to temporarily reverse the neurotoxic symptoms of bites of the Philippine cobra.[66] A subsequent study by the same group, comparing edrophonium and antivenom, revealed better response to the anticholinesterase.[67] Bawaskar has reported improvement after administration of neostigmine, with some decrease in ptosis within 20 minutes. Gold likewise

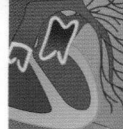

reported dramatic improvement in symptoms using neostigmine after the bite of an Asiatic cobra.[54] The efficacy of neostigmine could not be demonstrated by Tin-Myint and colleagues,[68] however, in a king cobra (*O. hannah*) bite (cited in Gold[4]).

ANTICOAGULANTS

Heparin has been shown in rats to ameliorate the cardiotoxicity associated with cobra venom.[69] Interestingly, heparin and tetracycline can also prevent the corneal opacification induced by the venom of the spitting cobra, *Hemachatus haemachatus*.[70] Tibballs found no benefit of post-exposure heparin treatment in experimental therapy of brown snake (*Pseudonaja textilis*) envenomation in dogs[71] and recommended against its use in humans, but found that preadministration of heparin prevented both cardiovascular and hematologic effects of venoms from the brown snake and the tiger snake.[72,73] While employed in some centers, heparin administration cannot be recommended at present based on lack of published clinical evidence of efficacy.

OBSERVATION

Once again, it must be strongly emphasized that the neurotoxic effects of elapid bites may be delayed by many hours and that envenomation is not disproved by lack of bite wounds or early clinical signs. Observation in an intensive care unit for 24 hours is prudent and justified when the history suggests a bite may have occurred.

SUMMARY

Elapid bites are uncommon in the United States but are quite common throughout Australia, Asia, and Africa. Elapids represent some of the most poisonous snakes, with thousands of deaths reported each year, particularly in developing countries without access to adequate transportation, health centers capable of advanced life support, and antivenoms. Intensive care of victims, concentrating on respiratory support and attention to hemodynamics and hematologic disorders, can be life saving. Antivenoms, when available, may reduce the neurotoxic symptoms. Allergic reactions are common, but may be diminished by prophylactic administration of subcutaneous epinephrine, corticosteroids, and antihistamines. Anticholinesterases may also benefit patients suffering from neurotoxic effects.

REFERENCES

1. Chippaux JP: Snake-bites: appraisal of the global situation. Bull WHO 1998;76(5):515–524.
2. Theakston RD, Warrell DA, Griffiths E: Report of a WHO workshop on the standardization and control of antivenoms. Toxicon 2003;41(5):541–557.
3. Britt A, Burkhart K: Naja naja cobra bite. Am J Emerg Med 1997;15(5):529–531.
4. Gold BS, Pyle P: Successful treatment of neurotoxic king cobra envenomation in Myrtle Beach, South Carolina. Ann Emerg Med 1998;32(6):736–738.
5. Minton SA: Bites by non-native venomous snakes in the United States. Wilderness Environ Med 1996;7(4):297–303.
6. Ronan-Bentle SE, Bryant SM, Williams JB: Naja Kaouthia envenomation in the midwest. Vet Hum Toxicol 2004;46(4):181–182.
7. Currie BJ: Snakebite in tropical Australia: a prospective study in the "Top End" of the Northern Territory. Med J Aust 2004;181(11–12):693–697.
8. Behler J, King F: National Audubon Society Field Guide to North American Reptiles and Amphibians, 2nd ed. New York, Alfred A. Knopf, 1995.
9. Coelho LK, Silva E, Espositto C, Zanin M: Clinical features and treatment of Elapidae bites: report of three cases. Hum Exp Toxicol 1992;11(2):135–137.
10. Dart RC, Sullivan JB: Elapid snake envenomation. In Harwood-Nuss AL (ed): The Clinical Practice of Emergency Medicine. Philadelphia, Lippincott-Raven, 1996, p 1453.
11. Kitchens CS, Van Mierop LH: Envenomation by the Eastern coral snake (Micrurus fulvius fulvius). A study of 39 victims. JAMA 1987;258(12):1615–1618.
12. de Roodt AR, Paniagua-Solis JF, Dolab JA, et al: Effectiveness of two common antivenoms for North, Central, and South American Micrurus envenomations. J Toxicol Clin Toxicol 2004;42:171.
13. Roze JA: Coral Snakes of the Americas: Biology, Identification, and Venoms. Malabar, FL, Krieger, 1996.
14. Parrish HM, Donovan LP: Facts about snakebites in Alabama. J Med Assoc State Ala 1964;33:297–305.
15. Alape-Giron A, Stiles B, Schmidt J, et al: Characterization of multiple nicotinic acetylcholine receptor-binding proteins and phospholipases A2 from the venom of the coral snake Micrurus nigrocinctus. FEBS Lett 1996;380(1–2):29–32.
16. Iyaniwura TT: Snake venom constituents: biochemistry and toxicology (Part 1). Vet Hum Toxicol 1991;33(5):468–474.
17. Iyaniwura TT: Snake venom constituents: biochemistry and toxicology (Part 2). Vet Hum Toxicol 1991;33(5):475–480.
18. Pettigrew LC, Glass JP: Neurologic complications of a coral snake bite. Neurology 1985;35(4):589–592.
19. Lee CY: Elapid neurotoxins and their mode of action. Clin Toxicol 1970;3(3):457–472.
20. Norman S: Poisindex: Coral Snake. Denver, CO, Micromedex, 1998.
21. Rosso JP, Vargas-Rosso O, Gutierrez JM, et al: Characterization of alpha-neurotoxin and phospholipase A2 activities from Micrurus venoms. Determination of the amino acid sequence and receptor-binding ability of the major alpha-neurotoxin from Micrurus nigrocinctus nigrocinctus. Eur J Biochem 1996;238(1):231–239.
22. Weis R, McIsaac RJ: Cardiovascular and muscular effects of venom from coral snake, Micrurus fulvius. Toxicon 1971;9(3):219–228.
23. Ramsey HW, Taylor WJ, Boruchow IB, Snyder GK: Mechanism of shock produced by an elapid snake (Micrurus f. fulvius) venom in dogs. Am J Physiol 1972;222(3):782–786.
24. Russell FE: Snake venom poisoning, 2nd ed. Great Neck, NY: Scholium International, 1983.
25. Norris RL, Dart RC: Apparent coral snake envenomation in a patient without visible fang marks. Am J Emerg Med 1989;7(4):402–405.
26. Moseley T: Coral snake bite: recovery following symptoms of respiratory paralysis. Ann Surg 1966;163(6):943–948.
27. Gaar GG: Assessment and management of coral and other exotic snake envenomations. J Fla Med Assoc 1996;83(3):178–182.
28. McCollough N, Gennaro JF Jr: Coral snake bites in the United States. J Fla Med Assoc 1963;49:968–972.
29. Parrish HM, Khan MS: Bites by coral snakes: report of 11 representative cases. Am J Med Sci 1967;253(5):561–568.
30. Sutherland SK, Coulter AR, Harris RD: Rationalisation of first-aid measures for elapid snakebite. Lancet 1979;1(8109):183–185.
31. McKinney PE: Out-of-hospital and interhospital management of crotaline snakebite. Ann Emerg Med 2001;37(2):168–174.
32. German BT, Hack JB, Brewer K, Meggs WJ: Pressure-immobilization bandages delay toxicity in a porcine model of eastern coral snake (Micrurus fulvius fulvius) envenomation. Ann Emerg Med 2005;45(6):603–608.
33. Arce V, Rojas E, Ownby CL, et al: Preclinical assessment of the ability of polyvalent (Crotalinae) and anticoral (Elapidae) antivenoms produced in Costa Rica to neutralize the venoms of North American snakes. Toxicon 2003;41(7):851–860.
34. Wisniewski MS, Hill RE, Havey JM, et al: Australian tiger snake (Notechis scutatus) and Mexican coral snake (Micrurus species)

antivenoms prevent death from United States coral snake (Micrurus fulvius fulvius) venom in a mouse model. J Toxicol Clin Toxicol 2003;41(1):7–10.

35. Soskis JE: Snakebite Assessment and Treatment in the Eastern United States. Midway, FL, Snakebite Publishing, 1994.

36. American Zoo and Aquarium Association: The Antivenom Index. Baltimore, MD, American Zoo and Aquarium Association, 1999.

37. Bawaskar HS: Snake venoms and antivenoms: critical supply issues. J Assoc Physicians India 2004;52:11–13.

38. McNamee D: Tackling venomous snake bites worldwide. Lancet 2001;357(9269):1680.

39. Cheng AC, Winkel K: Call for global snake-bite control and procurement funding. Lancet 2001;357(9262):1132.

40. Fernando R: The National Poisons Information Centre in Sri Lanka: the first ten years. J Toxicol Clin Toxicol 2002;40(5):551–555.

41. Davidson TM, Schafer S, Killfoil J: Cobras. Wilderness Environ Med 1995;6(2):203–219.

42. Watt G, Padre L, Tuazon L, et al: Bites by the Philippine cobra (Naja naja philippinensis): prominent neurotoxicity with minimal local signs. Am J Trop Med Hyg 1988;39(3):306–311.

43. Bawaskar HS, Bawaskar PH: Envenoming by the common krait (Bungarus caeruleus) and Asian cobra (Naja naja): clinical manifestations and their management in a rural setting. Wilderness Environ Med 2004;15(4):257–266.

44. Tan NH, Tan CS: A comparative study of cobra (Naja) venom enzymes. Comp Biochem Physiol B 1988;90(4):745–750.

45. Doley R, Mukherjee AK: Purification and characterization of an anticoagulant phospholipase A(2) from Indian monocled cobra (Naja kaouthia) venom. Toxicon 2003;41(1):81–91.

46. Omran MA, Abdel-Nabi IM: Changes in the arterial blood pressure, heart rate and normal ECG parameters of rat after envenomation with Egyptian cobra (Naja haje) venom. Hum Exp Toxicol 1997;16(6):327–333.

47. Ferguson LA, Morling A, Moraes C, Baker R: Investigation of coagulopathy in three cases of tiger snake (Notechis ater occidentalis) envenomation. Pathology 2002;34(2):157–161.

48. Lalloo DG, Trevett AJ, Black J, et al: Neurotoxicity, anticoagulant activity and evidence of rhabdomyolysis in patients bitten by death adders (Acanthophis sp.) in southern Papua New Guinea. QJM 1996;89(1):25–35.

49. Harvey AL: Twenty years of dendrotoxins. Toxicon 2001;39(1):15–26.

50. Potter LT: Snake toxins that bind specifically to individual subtypes of muscarinic receptors. Life Sci 2001;68(22–23):2541–2547.

51. Bradley KN: Muscarinic toxins from the green mamba. Pharmacol Ther 2000;85(2):87–109.

52. Munday SW, Williams SR, Clark RF: Dendrotoxin poisoning in a neurobiochemist. J Toxicol Clin Toxicol 2003;41(2):163–165.

53. Currie BJ: Clinical toxicology: a tropical Australian perspective. Ther Drug Monit 2000;22(1):73–78.

54. Gold BS: Neostigmine for the treatment of neurotoxicity following envenomation by the Asiatic cobra. Ann Emerg Med 1996;28(1):87–89.

55. Hung DZ, Liau MY, Lin-Shiau SY: The clinical significance of venom detection in patients of cobra snakebite. Toxicon 2003;41(4):409–415.

56. Blaylock RS: Antibiotic use and infection in snakebite victims. S Afr Med J 1999;89(8):874–876.

57. Kerrigan KR, Mertz BL, Nelson SJ, Dye JD: Antibiotic prophylaxis for pit viper envenomation: prospective, controlled trial. World J Surg 1997;21(4):369–373.

58. LoVecchio F, Klemens J, Welch S, Rodriguez R: Antibiotics after rattlesnake envenomation. J Emerg Med 2002;23(4):327–328.

59. Weed HG: Nonvenomous snakebite in Massachusetts: prophylactic antibiotics are unnecessary. Ann Emerg Med 1993;22(2):220–224.

60. Terry P, Mackway-Jones K: Towards evidence based emergency medicine: best BETs from the Manchester Royal Infirmary. Antibiotics in non-venomous snakebite. Emerg Med J 2002;19(2):142.

61. Chattopadhyay A, Patra RD, Shenoy V, et al: Surgical implications of snakebites. Indian J Pediatr 2004;71(5):397–399.

62. Pochanugool C, Limthongkull S, Meemano K: Clinical features of 37 non-antivenin treated neurotoxic snake bite patients. In Gopalakrishnakone P, Tan CK (eds): Progress in Venom and Toxin Research. Singapore, Faculty of Medicine, National University of Singapore, 1987, pp 46–51.

63. Bawaskar HS, Bawaskar PH: Aphasia in a farmer after viper bite. Lancet 2002;360(9346):1703.

64. Premawardhena AP, de Silva CE, Fonseka MM, et al: Low dose subcutaneous adrenaline to prevent acute adverse reactions to antivenom serum in people bitten by snakes: randomised, placebo controlled trial. BMJ 1999;318:1041–1043.

65. Gawarammana IB, Kularatne SA, Dissanayake WP, et al: Parallel infusion of hydrocortisone +/– chlorpheniramine bolus injection to prevent acute adverse reactions to antivenom for snakebites. Med J Aust 2004;180(1):20–23.

66. Watt G, Theakston RD, Hayes CG, et al: Positive response to edrophonium in patients with neurotoxic envenoming by cobras (Naja naja philippinensis). A placebo-controlled study. N Engl J Med 1986;315(23):1444–1448.

67. Watt G, Meade BD, Theakston RD, et al: Comparison of Tensilon and antivenom for the treatment of cobra-bite paralysis. Trans R Soc Trop Med Hyg 1989;83(4):570–573.

68. Tin-Myint, Rai-Mra, Maung-Chit, et al: Bites by the king cobra (Ophiophagus hannah) in Myanmar: successful treatment of severe neurotoxic envenoming. QJM 1991;80(293):751–762.

69. Sun JJ, Walker MJ: Actions of cardiotoxins from the southern Chinese cobra (Naja naja atra) on rat cardiac tissue. Toxicon 1986;24(3):233–245.

70. Ismail M, al-Bekairi AM, el-Bedaiwy AM, Abd-el Salam MA: The ocular effects of spitting cobras: I. The ringhals cobra (Hemachatus haemachatus) venom-induced corneal opacification syndrome. J Toxicol Clin Toxicol 1993;31(1):31–41.

71. Tibballs J, Sutherland SK: The efficacy of heparin in the treatment of common brown snake (Pseudonaja textilis) envenomation. Anaesth Intensive Care 1992;20(1):33–37.

72. Tibballs J: The cardiovascular, coagulation and haematological effects of tiger snake (Notechis scutatus) prothrombin activator and investigation of release of vasoactive substances. Anaesth Intensive Care 1998;26(5):536–547.

73. Tibballs J, Sutherland SK, Rivera RA, Masci PP: The cardiovascular and haematological effects of purified prothrombin activator from the common brown snake (Pseudonaja textilis) and their antagonism with heparin. Anaesth Intensive Care 1992;20(1):28–32.

22 *Venomous Arthropods*

A Spiders

ANDIS GRAUDINS, MBBS (HONS), PHD

At a Glance...

■ Although virtually all spiders produce venom, only a small number are potentially venomous to humans.

■ Widow spiders (*Latrodectus* species) are responsible for a significant number of spider envenomations worldwide.

■ Widow spider envenomation is also called latrodectism.

■ The most significant symptom occurring with latrodectism is pain.

■ Treatment with widow spider antivenoms appears to be the most effective and rapid way to reverse the effects of latrodectism.

■ Brown recluse spider (*Loxosceles* species) envenomation may result in the production of necrotic skin lesions.

■ Specific treatments for necrotic arachnidism have included dapsone and hyperbaric oxygen therapy, but there is little controlled evidence suggesting that these are effective therapies.

■ In most cases, standard wound care is all that is required to facilitate healing of skin lesions from necrotizing arachnids.

Spiders can be divided into two major groups: (1) the Mygalomorphae (the primitive spiders), which are large, powerful ground-dwelling spiders with vertically down-facing chelicerae, usually living in burrows with rudimentary web structures; and (2) the Araeneomorphae (true spiders), which include all other web-building spiders with horizontally opposed chelicerae. Examples of the Mygalomorphae include the Australian funnel web and mouse spiders and examples of the Araeneomorphae include the black widow and brown recluse spiders.[1] Almost all spiders are venomous. The venom is used to kill and digest their live prey. Of the 20,000 or more species found in the United States, only about 50 of these have fangs that can penetrate human skin.[2] Fortunately, even fewer cause clinical problems because their venom is too weak. Medically important spiders include the genera *Latrodectus* (widow spiders), *Steatoda* (cupboard spiders), *Loxosceles* (recluse spiders), and *Atrax* and *Hadronyche* (Australian funnel web spiders). The true incidence of spider bite is probably underestimated. This is primarily due to the voluntary nature of most reporting processes.

BLACK WIDOW SPIDERS (GENUS *LATRODECTUS*)

Black widow spiders are found on all continents excluding Antarctica. They are, arguably, responsible for the largest number of medically important spider bites around the world. In 2003, there were 2739 black widow spider exposures reported to U.S. poison centers, of which 30% were treated in a health care facility. No deaths were reported, but 12.7% had "moderate" to "major" outcome.[3] In Australia, an estimate of 2000 to 3000 *L. hasselti* (red back spider) bites per year has been made, with clinically significant envenomation requiring antivenom therapy in about 20% of cases.[4] The female is responsible for all significant bites. It is considerably larger than the male, whose chelicerae are not large enough to penetrate human skin. The female is commonly 1 to 1.5 cm in length with a large bulbous black abdomen exhibiting a distinctive red hourglass mark ventrally. Some species, such as the Australian red back spider (*L. hasselti*) also exhibit a dorsal abdominal red/pink stripe of varying length.

Five species have been found in the United States, and *Latrodectus mactans* is the most common. Other species include *L. hesperus* (found more commonly in the west), *L. variolus*, and *L. bishopi*. One notable variant is the brown widow spider of Florida, *L. geometricus*, also found along equatorial regions of many other continents. Widow spiders are known to have been transported large distances, most likely in shipping containers. Colonies of *L. hasselti* (Australian red back spider) have been found in port areas of Osaka, Japan, and in Belgium.

The female black widow spider creates webs near the ground in secluded dark areas such as barns, garages, abandoned burrows, sheds, under unused chairs and benches, and even in outdoor lavatories.[5,6] All *Latrodectus* species produce a similar envenomation syndrome regardless of geographic location.[6-9] However, the potency of venom may vary across species and even within species based on geographic location, seasonality, and size of the spider.[10]

Steatoda spp. (cupboard spiders) are commonly found in houses, in cupboards, and under furniture. They have a similar body shape to widow spiders but are either black or brown and without abdominal coloring and are often misidentified as widow spiders. The bite usually causes local irritation only but can uncommonly produce a systemic envenomation syndrome resembling latrodectism.[11-13]

Pathophysiology

The best characterized widow spider venom is that of the European widow spider, *L. tredecimguttatus*. It contains a

433

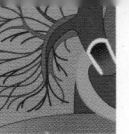

120-kD vertebrate-specific toxin, α-latrotoxin, and a number of insect-specific latroinsectotoxins of similar molecular weight.[14-17] It had long been presumed that similar toxins were also present in other *Latrodectus* spp. This presumption was based on the similar clinical envenomation syndromes produced by all *Latrodectus* spp., similar in vitro effects observed with whole venom extracts, and that antivenoms prepared from one widow spider species reversed the envenomation effects of other *Latrodectus* spp. Recently, this presumption has been proven correct; partial amino acid sequences for α-latrotoxin and α- and δ-latroinsectotoxins have been derived for both *L. mactans* and *L. hasselti*.[18] Venoms from these two *Latrodectus* spp. have high sequence homology and similar toxins to the venom of *L. tredecimguttatus*.[18]

Alpha-latrotoxin binds to synaptic membranes and leads to release of massive amounts of norepinephrine and acetylcholine from nerve terminals. Specifically, α-latrotoxin binds to the calcium-dependent receptor neurexin-1α and calcium-independent receptor latrophilin, found on presynaptic nerve terminal membranes. Subsequent to receptor binding, there is in an influx of calcium from cation channels, exocytosis of the synaptic vesicles, and release of neurotransmitter into the synaptic cleft.[19-21] α-Latrotoxin is also assimilated into the presynaptic membrane directly and produces membrane pores, which result in an influx of calcium into the synaptic nerve terminal. This is partly responsible for the uncontrolled release of neurotransmitters such as acetylcholine and norepinephrine.[21] The toxin is also internalized into the synaptic terminal and exhibits other less defined effects that increase synaptic vesicle degranulation and neurotransmitter release.[22] Amplifying these effects is the fact that the venom also reduces presynaptic neuronal reuptake of acetylcholine and amines.[23] The end result is the stimulation of the autonomic nervous system through the release and depletion of catecholamines at adrenergic nerve endings. *Steatoda* spp. (cupboard spiders) venom is likely to contain latrotoxin-like toxins that may produce an envenomation syndrome similar to latrodectism.[24]

Clinical Presentation

The envenomation syndrome from the bite of a widow spider is known as latrodectism. The initial bite of the widow spider is often described as a mild pinprick sensation or similar to a bee sting. This is followed by a dull ache 20 to 30 minutes later. All that may be visible is one or two puncture wounds 1 to 2 mm apart. Local erythema and, in some cases, a diffuse, erythematous, maculopapular rash extending beyond the bite site may occasionally be noted.[6]

The most significant symptom of latrodectism is pain.[6,8,9,25,26] This may be local to the bite site, regional, or generalized. Mild to moderate envenomation results in localized symptoms at the bite site. Signs and symptoms include increasing pain, sweating, and muscle fasciculation, which develop in the 30 minutes to few hours following the bite. In more severe cases, signs and symptoms may become regional; severe pain, sweating,

and muscle fasciculation may progress to the entire limb over several hours. In cases of generalized envenomation, patients often present with severe systemic pain, sweating, muscle fasciculation, anxiety, moderate hypertension, and insomnia.[6] Abdominal and back pain are common complaints with systemic illness.[25] Abdominal pain may be so severe as to mimic an acute abdomen, particularly in children where a history of spider bite may not be elicited.[27] Other, less common, signs and symptoms seen in severe envenomation include chest pain, priapism, parvor mortis (fear of death), facies latrodectismica (facial grimacing due to pain), flushing, periorbital edema, conjunctivitis, and tachycardia.[6,8,9,25] Death from envenomation is rare and has not been reported since the 1950s.[28,29] Left untreated, systemic signs and symptoms may last for 24 to 48 hours, and occasionally for days to weeks.

Diagnosis

The diagnosis of latrodectism is clinical and based on a positive history of spider exposure (if available) and suggestive signs and symptoms. No laboratory tests will substantiate the diagnosis, although a marked response to antivenom strongly supports the correct diagnosis.

Treatment

Treatment recommendations of latrodectism vary from continent to continent. The bite of *Latrodectus* species may result in a distressing and incapacitating syndrome of envenomation that has a relatively slow onset as compared with snake envenomation. It is extremely painful but unlikely to be fatal. Current recommendations for first aid or prehospital care are to avoid the application of pressure immobilization bandages and tourniquets; these may increase local pain due to pressure on the bite site.[30] Local application of ice to the bite site has been suggested as a temporizing measure, but there are no clinical trials to prove the efficacy of such treatment. Application of heat to the bite site may actually result in worsening of pain.[31] The use of opioids may afford some relief to patients with distressing symptoms until more definitive therapy can be instituted.

Antivenom therapy has been shown to be the most effective treatment in alleviating the symptoms and signs of latrodectism.[5,8,25,32-35] Clark and colleagues reported that patients receiving antivenom therapy (Black widow antivenom from Merck & Company, Inc., West Point, PA) in the United States were more likely to be discharged home from the emergency department and have a much shorter hospital stay than those receiving supportive measures alone. Additionally, patients receiving antivenom had a significant decrease in the signs and symptoms of envenomation, with a mean time of 31 minutes from administration of antivenom until clinical improvement. In this series, the mean duration of symptoms (from time of the bite) was 9 hours for the antivenom-treated patients as compared with 25 hours for patients treated with analgesics alone.[25] Rapid relief of symptoms, usually within 1 to 2 hours, has also been reported with other

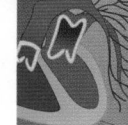

antivenom formulations around the world.[6,8,9] Mild to moderate cases of local envenomation may respond to analgesic therapy alone. In patients with regional or systemic symptoms, treatment with antivenom should be strongly considered because it is likely to significantly reduce the severity and duration of symptoms.

All *Latrodectus* spp. antivenoms appear capable of reversing the effects of envenomation from any widow spider.[36,37] This may have implications for regions of the world where no local antivenom is available. A list of available antivenoms is shown in Table 22A-1.

The threshold for use of antivenom appears to vary from region to region. In the United States, there appears to be the greatest reluctance to use specific immunotherapy in cases of envenomation. This may be due to isolated case reports of death following administration of widow spider antivenom[25] and/or a presumed risk for anaphylaxis extrapolated from the use of crotalid polyvalent snake antivenom. Spaite and colleagues showed that the risk for anaphylaxis to crotalid polyvalent antivenom was as high as 86% in patients who tested positive to skin testing with horse serum and 9% in those who tested negative.[38] These anaphylactic risk estimates were determined for patients that subsequently received large volumes of horse protein intravenously (e.g., as required for most crotalid snake envenomations). It is unlikely that the risk is as large for patients who receive equine-derived widow spider antivenom since the amount of protein administered is significantly lower than for the treatment of crotalid envenomation. In large series of *Latrodectus* spp. envenomations, symptom relief commonly occurs after the administration of one vial of antivenom.[8,25] Occasionally, two or more vials may be necessary. Manufacturer recommendations for the use of widow spider antivenom in the United States suggest that it should be reserved for "severe cases" of envenomation or those occurring at the extremes of age. Little data exist on the true incidence of allergic reactions following the use of widow spider envenomation in

the United States. Clark and colleagues observed an 8% incidence of allergic reactions (urticaria and bronchospasm) with widow spider antivenom use.[25] In general, antivenoms contain a significant amount of protein with anticomplement activity, which may result in anaphylactoid reactions when infused rapidly.[39] This activity is reported to be reduced in trypsin-digested antivenoms, which contain only Fab-IgG fragments, such as Australian red back spider (*L. hasselti*) antivenom, which has a reported incidence of mild allergic reactions of 0.54%.[8] The incidence may be greater in antivenoms produced as crude hyperimmune IgG equine sera, such as Merck & Company's, U.S. widow spider antivenom.[39] Consequently, when given intravenously, antivenom should always be diluted in 100 to 200 mL normal saline or 5% glucose first and then infused slowly (over 30 to 60 minutes). Infusions should occur in a monitored environment with immediate access to resuscitation facilities capable of treating untoward allergic reactions.

Late presentation or pregnancy is not a contraindication to antivenom administration. Antivenom was used successfully in a woman who was 20 weeks pregnant and manifested signs of systemic latrodectism. She subsequently had a normal full-term delivery.[33] Antivenom has been reported to be effective at reversing the effects of latrodectism presenting 1 to 2 days postbite.[21,33-35] Antivenom therapy has been effective up to 2 weeks after bites of *L. hasselti*, the Australian red back spider.[40,41]

Other therapies recommended for the relief of pain and muscle spasms have included intravenous calcium infusions and muscle relaxants such as methocarbamol and diazepam. Controlled trials are lacking, but these therapies have not proven more effective than opioid analgesia or antivenom therapy and do not provide effective or lasting relief of symptoms of latrodectism.[25,42,43] Calcium salts are not recommended based on their lack of efficacy.[25] For patients with mild to moderate latrodectism, when antivenom administration may not be necessary, the administration of opioid analgesics and benzodiazepines are recommended for controlling pain and muscle spasm, respectively.

Red back spider antivenom has also been used successfully to reverse systemic envenomation that followed the bite of *Steatoda grossahas*. Red back spider antivenom has been shown to experimentally reverse and inhibit in vitro toxicity of the venom of this species.[11,12]

BROWN RECLUSE SPIDER (GENUS *LOXOSCELES*)

The genus *Loxosceles* is notorious for producing local wound necrosis (dermonecrotic arachnidism) and, in rare cases, systemic illness. These brown spiders are small (6 to 22 mm) and have a distinctive violin-shaped marking on the dorsum of their cephalothorax (fiddleback spiders). These spiders are found in several areas of the world, such as Africa, Australia, southern Europe, the Mediterranean, the Pacific Islands, South and Central America, and the United States.[44] In the United States, *Loxosceles* spp. are found throughout the South but are

TABLE 22A-1 Currently Available Widow Spider Antivenoms Worldwide

VENOM USED TO RAISE ANTIVENOM	SOURCE	COMPOSITION
	Merck & Co., Inc., West Point, PA	Equine IgG
L. mactans	Instituto Nacional de Microbiologia, Buenos Aires, Argentina	Equine IgG
	Instituto Bioclon, Calzada de Telalpan, Mexico	Polyvalent equine F(ab)₂ IgG
L. indistinctus	South African Institute for Medical Research, Rietfontein, Edenvale, Transvaal, South Africa	Equine IgG
L. hasselti	Commonwealth Serum Laboratories, Melbourne, Australia	Equine F(ab)₂ IgG fragment

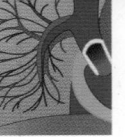
rarely seen because of their shy, reclusive nature. These spiders form small, inconsequential webs and are often encountered in home storage areas or outdoors, typically in woodpiles.

Loxosceles reclusa (the brown recluse spider) is found predominantly in south central and southeastern states (except Florida), whereas *Loxosceles apachea, arizonica,* and *destera* are found in the southwestern states.[44] Two additional species have been discovered in the United States, *Loxosceles laeta* in California and *Loxosceles rufescens* in Hawaii.[44] *Loxosceles laeta* is typically endemic to South America whereas *Loxosceles rufescens* is endemic to Africa. Loxoscelism, the envenomation syndrome seen after a *Loxosceles* spp. bite, is seen most commonly after a bite from *Loxosceles reclusa* or *Loxosceles laeta*.[31]

In a survey of South Carolina physicians, patients seeking medical treatment for presumed brown recluse (*Loxosceles reclusa*) spider bites outnumbered those seeking treatment for black widow spider bites, 478 to 143 for the year 1990.[45] In 2003, there were 2843 brown recluse spider exposures reported to United States poison centers, of which 40% were treated in a health care facility. Of all exposures, 23.3% had a "moderate" to "major" outcome, and one death occurred.[3] Dermonecrotic arachnidism in the United States occurs predominantly from the brown recluse spider. Bites by other genera of spiders, however, can also produce necrotic wounds. These other spiders include *Chiracanthium* species (the clubionid spiders), *Phidippus* (the jumping spider), *Argiope,* and *Tegenaria agrestis* (the hobo spider) and are sometimes the actual culprits when the brown recluse is mistakenly blamed.

Pathophysiology

The venom of the brown recluse spider contains various cytotoxic enzymes, which include sphingomyelinase D, ribonuclease, hyaluronidase, deoxyribonuclease, lipase, phosphohydrolase, and alkaline phosphatase. Sphingomyelinase D, the primary dermonecrotic factor, disrupts cellular membranes.[46,47] Sphingomyelinase D also causes serotonin release, which is associated with platelet aggregation and thus thrombosis of small capillaries.[48-51] Hyaluronidase facilitates the ability of the venom to spread locally in the tissue, thus indirectly enhancing tissue destruction. All the cytotoxic elements of the venom produce local endothelial cell damage, which attracts neutrophils, which subsequently release more destructive enzymes and promote further platelet aggregation and thrombosis.[52,53] Polymorphonuclear leukocyte migration into cutaneous lesions appears to be a significant event in the development of dermonecrosis. The venom can also cause erythrocyte hemolysis, which contributes to systemic effects.[54] The systemic effects of the venom occur largely from the release of cytokines by leukocytes and activation of complement.

Clinical Presentation

A brown recluse spider bite is usually mild and often not noted by those afflicted. Within 24 hours, the patient presents for treatment of a painful purple papule. This central violaceous lesion is often surrounded by a blanched ischemic zone and a rim of indurated erythema. The central papule or vesicle can coagulate and become thrombosed. A necrotic, ulcerating wound results and may progress for as long as a week after the initial bite.[55] The eschar may slough, and the lesion may extend into subcutaneous fat and create a disfiguring ulcer that can take weeks to heal and occasionally requires surgical grafting.[56] Patients may occasionally present with systemic loxoscelism, which can include fever, chills, nausea, arthralgias, a morbilliform rash, and hemolysis.[55] In rare cases, patients can develop disseminated intravascular coagulation, renal failure, and even seizures.[57] Systemic loxoscelism typically develops 24 to 72 hours after the bite and is not correlated with the size or severity of the necrotic skin reaction.

Very young and immunocompromised patients have a greater susceptibility to morbidity and mortality from brown recluse spider envenomations.

Diagnosis

The diagnosis of a brown recluse spider bite is often presumptive and based on suggestive physical findings in an endemic area. A positive history of spider bite is not usually evident since the bite is not very painful and the spider is shy. Patients usually present after several days, when the lesion has become necrotic. Numerous techniques have been developed to facilitate the diagnosis of brown recluse spider bite. They include a serologic assay (i.e., detecting the presence of IgG antibodies to venom components), a passive hemagglutination inhibition assay (i.e., testing for the presence of venom components by inhibition of antiserum-induced agglutination of venom-coated red blood cells), an enzyme-linked immunoabsorbent assay (i.e., detection of specific venom antigens from the wound), and tissue biopsy (i.e., detect the presence of typical histopathologic changes in the wound).[58-61] However, these tests are not routinely or readily available and are not 100% sensitive at the time of patient presentation. Routine laboratory work is indicated in severe envenomations. Blood cell count, urinalysis, renal function tests, and a disseminated intravascular coagulation screen may be indicated in patients with systemic symptoms of loxoscelism. In most cases, however, patients show only a local lesion without any significant systemic effects.

Treatment

Generally, all that is required for most presumed brown recluse spider bites is routine wound care, including tetanus prophylaxis. This can include débridement of necrotic tissue as well as watching for late infection. Routine prophylactic antibiotics are not indicated. If a patient appears ill, blood and urine tests can be performed to preclude systemic hemolysis. Treatment for hemolytic anemia would be supportive, with red blood cell replacement provided as needed. Since serious complications are rare, supportive care is the best approach.[62]

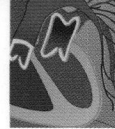

Several experimental therapies have been advocated for patients with brown recluse spider bites, especially for those with the threat of a disfiguring scar. The most popular has been the use of dapsone. The theoretic basis of this agent lies in inhibiting the polymorphonuclear leukocytes from aggregating at the wound site and causing tissue necrosis. In a poorly described study of dermal envenomation, pretreatment of guinea pigs with oral dapsone resulted in skin lesions less than 50% the size of those seen in control animals.[63] In a similar model, initiation of dapsone treatment after envenomation also resulted in smaller necrotic lesions as compared with animals not treated with dapsone.[64] However, two recent studies were unable to reproduce these favorable results.[65,66] Clinical experience has been limited and uncontrolled. In a small, observational study, Rees and colleagues reported that scars were smaller and healing appeared improved in patients administered dapsone.[67]

Dapsone should still be considered an experimental treatment for presumed brown recluse spider bites pending controlled study of its efficacy. If it is to be used, the potential adverse effects of this drug must be acknowledged. The most serious are hemolysis and methemoglobinemia, occurring most commonly in patients with glucose-6-phosphate dehydrogenase deficiency.[67] Short-term therapy can result in dizziness, fatigue, dyspnea, and anxiety. Longer treatment courses have caused agranulocytosis, erythema nodosum, toxic epidermal necrolysis, nephrotoxicity and hepatotoxicity. Adverse effects have been reported with use of dapsone for brown recluse spider bites, including hypersensitivity reactions, methemoglobinemia, and hemolysis.[68] Because of the lack of proven clinical efficacy for dapsone, it should probably only be considered for bites in cosmetically sensitive areas. The recommended dapsone dosing regimen is to begin with 25 mg two to three times a day, increasing the dose gradually to 50 to 100 mg twice a day for 1 to 2 weeks.[69]

Hyperbaric oxygen has been used in brown recluse bites with purported successes in observational studies.[70] More recent controlled studies utilizing animal models have yielded equivocal results. Maynor and colleagues reported that a single hyperbaric oxygen treatment as long as 48 hours postenvenomation caused a 50% reduction in lesion size after experimental envenomation in rabbits.[71] However, two other studies failed to show any beneficial effects of hyperbaric therapy on gross lesion appearance in similar animal models.[66,72] Risks to patients include barotrauma and the expense of an unproven therapy. Potential beneficial effects of hyperbaric oxygen in recluse bites are multifaceted but not specific for this envenomation and are similar to those for patients suffering from chronic skin ulceration from other causes. These include reoxygenation of the wound and sequestration of polymorphonuclear leukocytes away from the wound.[73] Although it has also been purported that hyperbaric therapy inactivates venom toxicity, Merchant and colleagues have reported that activity of sphingomyelinase D in *Loxosceles reclusa* venom is not reduced by exposure to hyperbaric oxygen.[74] The U.S. Undersea and Hyperbaric Medical Society has yet to approve routine hyperbaric treatment for brown recluse spider bites. Hyperbaric therapy could be considered in cases of severe necrotic ulceration that has not responded to routine wound care.

Other recommended treatments, such as antivenom, steroids, electric shock, cyproheptadine, colchicine, and nitroglycerin, either have been disappointing in controlled trials or have not been studied adequately. Intralesional injection of experimental antivenin (Fab fragments) in patients and animals results in attenuated dermonecrosis with little or no scarring.[55,75] The effect of the antivenin becomes minimal when delayed by several hours after envenomation; the venom rapidly spreads away from the bite site. Electric shock was shown to be of no value in a guinea pig envenomation model.[64] Cyproheptadine, an antihistamine with serotonin antagonist properties, was of no benefit in a rabbit model.[66] Surgical excision guarantees a scar at a site that could potentially heal without any disfigurement.[67] Surgical débridement and skin grafting (if necessary) should be reserved for days to weeks later, when the inflammatory effects of the venom have subsided and revascularization of the wound edges have occurred.

OTHER SPIDERS

Although the black widow and brown recluse are the most important spiders clinically, occasional bites by other species are notable. Necrotic arachnidism cannot always be assumed to be due to *Loxosceles*. Several other U.S. spiders have been implicated in the production of direct tissue damage. These include *Chiracanthium* spp. (the clubionid spider),[76] *Phidippus* species (the jumping spider),[77] and *Tegenaria* spp. (the hobo spider).[78,79] The hobo spider, imported to the Pacific Northwest, can cause identical local and systemic symptoms and signs as seen with *Loxosceles*. The majority of cases of necrotic arachnidism in the Pacific Northwest are due to hobo spiders; these cases are often mistaken for brown recluse spider envenomation. Furthermore, clinicians should be wary of making the diagnosis of necrotic arachnidism in cases where there is no objective evidence of spider bite. Many case reports are based on retrospective data with little or no evidence of the spider involved.[80] The best example of this is the *Lampona cylindrata* (Australian white tailed spider), frequently implicated in cases of unexplained dermonecrosis. Following a prospective collection of 130 white tail spider bites with positive identification of the spiders in all cases, it was found that no cases of dermonecrosis were seen.[81] Similar scientific rigor needs to be pursued when necrotic arachnidism is suspected in the differential diagnosis of unexplained skin ulceration. All efforts should be made to identify the spider when possible.

Specific mention should be made of the Australian funnel web spiders (*Atrax* and *Hadronyche* spp.) found along the eastern seaboard of Australia. These large, aggressive, mygalomorphic spiders produce, arguably, the most toxic spider venom to humans and other primates. The venom of the *A. robustus* (Sydney funnel web spider)

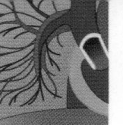

contains a primate-specific δ-atracotoxin-Ar1, which acts by inhibiting the conversion of axon sodium channels from the active to the inactive state. This results in massive neurotransmitter release from all nerve endings.[82] The envenomation syndrome is characterized by marked pain at the bite site, rapid development of muscle fasciculation, diaphoresis, salivation, tachycardia, hypertension, respiratory paralysis, pulmonary edema, and death.[83,84] A specific funnel web antivenom produced from the venom of *A. robustus* is available; it is life saving and also neutralizes the venom of various other Australian funnel web species.[84,85]

Other spiders usually cause only local painful reactions and swelling, most notably *Argiope* (golden orb weaver) and *Lycosa* (wolf spider).[26] Tarantulas, members of the primitive mygalomorph suborder of spiders, can inflict a histamine-like reaction either by a painful bite or by brushing hairs toward their prey. Treatment for all of these envenomations is supportive, with the possible exception of tarantula encounters, which can be treated with oral antihistamines and topical steroids as needed.

ACKNOWLEDGMENT

Christian Tomaszewski, MD, authored the previous edition of this chapter.

REFERENCES

1. York Main B: Spiders, 2nd ed. Sydney, Australia, Collins, 1984, p 296.
2. Horen WP: Arachnidism in the United States. JAMA 1983;185:839–843.
3. Watson SA, Litovitz, TL, Klein-Schwartz W, et al: 2003 Annual report of the American Association of Poison Control Centers toxic exposure surveillance system. Am J Emerg Med 2004;22:443–497.
4. Jelinek GA, Banham ND, Dunjey SJ: Red-back spider-bites at Fremantle Hospital, 1982–1987. Med J Aust 1989;150:693–695.
5. Wiener S: Red-back spider bite in Australia: an analysis of 167 cases. Med J Aust 1961;2:44–49.
6. Maretic Z: Latrodectism: variations in clinical manifestations provoked by *Latrodectus* species of spiders. Toxicon 1983;21:457–466.
7. McCrone JD, Netzloff ML: An immunological and electrophoretical comparison of the venoms of the North American *Latrodectus* spiders. Toxicon 1965;3:107–110.
8. Sutherland SK, Trinca JC: Survey of 2144 cases of red-back spider bites. Med J Aust 1978;2:620–623.
9. Muller G: Black and brown widow spider bites in South Africa. A series of 45 cases. South Afr Med J 1993;83:399–405.
10. McCrone JD: Comparative lethality of several *Latrodectus* venoms. Toxicon 1964;2:201–203.
11. South M, Wirth P, Winkel KD: Redback spider antivenom used to treat envenomation by a juvenile *Steatoda* spider [letter]. Med J Aust 1998;169:642.
12. Graudins A, Gunja N, Broady KW, Nicholson GM : Clinical and in vitro evidence for the efficacy of Australian red-back spider (*Latrodectus hasselti*) antivenom in the treatment of envenomation by a cupboard spider (*Steatoda grossa*). Toxicon 2002;40:767–775.
13. Warrell DA, Shaheen J, Hillyard PD, Jones D: Neurotoxic envenoming by an immigrant spider (*Steatoda nobilis*) in southern England. Toxicon 1991;29:1263–1265.
14. Grasso A: Preparation and properties of a neurotoxin purified from the venom of black widow spider (*Latrodectus mactans tredecimguttatus*). Biochim Biophys Acta 1976;439:406–412.
15. Grishin EV, Himmelreich NH, Pluzhnikov KA, Pozdnyakova NG et al: Modulation of functional activities of the neurotoxin from black widow spider venom. Fed Eur Biol Soc Lett 1993;336:205–207.
16. Kiyatkin NI, Dulubova IE, Chekhovskaya IA, Grishin EV: Cloning and structure of cDNA encoding alpha-latrotoxin from black widow spider venom. Fed Eur Biol Soc Lett 1990;270:127–131.
17. Volkova TM, Galkina TG, Kudelin AB, Grishin EV: [Structure of tryptic fragments of a neurotoxin from black widow spider venom]. Bioorganicheskaia Khimia 1991;17:437–441.
18. Graudins A: Spiders of medical importance in the Asia-Pacific: neurotoxin characterization and antivenom efficacy. PhD thesis, Department of Health Sciences, University of Technology, Sydney, Australia, 2003, p 205.
19. Geppert M, Khvotchev M, Krasnoperov V, et al: Neurexin I alpha is a major alpha-latrotoxin receptor that cooperates in alpha-latrotoxin action. J Biol Chem 1998;273:1705–1710.
20. Sugita S, Ichtchenko K, Khvotchev M, Sudhof TC: α-Latrotoxin receptor CIRL/latrophilin 1 (CL1) defines an unusual family of ubiquitous G-protein-linked receptors. G-protein coupling not required for triggering exocytosis. J Biol Chem 1998;273:32715–32724.
21. Van Renterghem C, Iborra C, Martin-Moutot N, et al: α-Latrotoxin forms calcium-permeable membrane pores via interactions with latrophilin or neurexin. Eur J Neurosci 2000;12:3953–3962.
22. Ichtchenko K, Khvotchev M, Kiyatkin N, et al: Alpha-latrotoxin action probed with recombinant toxin: receptors recruit alpha-latrotoxin but do not transduce an exocytotic signal. Eur Mol Biol Org J 1998;17:6188–6199.
23. Rothlin RP, Pardal JF, Pardal MMF: Supersensitivity to norepinephrine induced in vitro by crude *Latrodectus mactans* venom in the rabbit ear artery. Toxicon 1977;15:71–74.
24. Usmanov PB, Kazakov I, Kalikulov D, et al: The channel-forming component of the Theridiidae spider venom neurotoxins. Gen Physiol Biophys 1985;4:185–193.
25. Clark RF, Wethern-Kestner S, Vance MV, Gerkin R: Clinical presentation and treatment of black widow spider envenomation: a review of 163 cases. Ann Emerg Med 1992;21:782–787.
26. Isbister GK, Gray MR: A prospective study of 750 definite spider bites, with expert spider identification. QJM 2002;95:723–731.
27. White J: *Latrodectism* as a mimic [letter]. Med J Aust 1985;142:75.
28. Parrish HM: Analysis of 460 fatalities from the venomous animals in the United States. Am J Med Sci 1963;24:35–47.
29. White J: Envenoming and antivenom use in Australia. Toxicon 1998;36:1483–1492.
30. Sutherland SK, Duncan AW: New first-aid measures for envenomation: with special reference to bites by the Sydney funnel-web spider (*Atrax robustus*). Med J Aust 1980;1:378–379.
31. White J, Cardoso JL, Fan HW: Clinical toxicology of spider bites. In Meier J, White J (eds): Handbook of Clinical Toxicology of Animal Venoms and Poisons. Boca Raton, FL, CRC Press, 1995, pp 259–329.
32. Bogen E: Arachnism. Arch Intern Med 1926;38:623–632.
33. Russell FE, Marcus P, Streng JA: Black widow spider envenomation during pregnancy. Report of a case. Toxicon 1979;17:188–189.
34. Wiener S: Red back spider bite treated with antivenene. Med J Aust 1956;1:858.
35. Wiener S: The Australian red back spider (*Latrodectus hasselti*): I. Preparation of antiserum by the use of venom adsorbed on aluminium phosphate. Med J Aust 1956;1:739–742.
36. Graudins A, Padula M, Broady K, Nicholson GM: Red-back spider (*Latrodectus hasselti*) antivenom prevents the toxicity of widow spider venoms. Ann Emerg Med 2001;37:154–160.
37. Daly FF, Hill RE, Bogdan GM, Dart RC: Neutralization of *Latrodectus mactans* and *L. hesperus* venom by redback spider (*L. hasselti*) antivenom. J Toxicol Clin Toxicol 2001;39:119–123.
38. Spaite DW, Dart R, Sullivan JB: Skin testing: implications in the management of pit viper envenomation [abstract]. Ann Emerg Med 1988;17:152.
39. Sutherland S: Serum reactions: an analysis of commercial antivenoms and the possible role of anticomplementary activity in de-novo reactions to antivenoms and antitoxins. Med J Aust 1977;1:613–615.
40. Pincus DR: Response to antivenom 14 days after red back spider bite [letter]. Med J Aust 1994;161:226.
41. Banham ND, Jelinek GA, Finch PM: Late treatment with antivenom in prolonged red-back spider envenomation. Med J Aust 1994;161:379–381.

42. Key GF: A comparison of calcium gluconate and methocarbamol (Robaxin) in the treatment of latrodectism (black widow spider envenomation). Am J Trop Med Hyg 1981;30:273–277.

43. Russell FE, Madon NB: New names for the brown recluse and the black widow. Postgrad Med 1981;70:31.

44. Gertsch WJ, Ennik F: The spider genus Loxosceles in North America, Central America, and West Indies (Araneae, Loxscelidae). Bull Am Mus Nat Hist 1983;175:265–360.

45. Schuman SH, Caldwell ST: 1990 South Carolina Physician Survey of tick, spider and fire ant morbidity. J SC Med Assoc 1991;87:429–432.

46. Geren CR, Chan TK, Howell DE, Odell GV: Partial characterization of the low molecular weight fractions of the extract of the venom apparatus of the brown recluse spider and of its hemolymph. Toxicon 1975;13:233–238.

47. Rees RS, Nanney LB, Yates RA, King LE Jr: Interaction of brown recluse spider venom on cell membranes: the inciting mechanism? J Invest Dermatol 1984;83:270–275.

48. Gates CA, Rees RS: Serum amyloid P component: its role in platelet activation stimulated by sphingomyelinase D purified from the venom of the brown recluse spider (Loxosceles reclusa). Toxicon 1990;28:1303–1315.

49. Rees RS: Platelet activation stimulated by the toxin of the brown recluse spider requires serum amyloid P component, not C-reactive protein. Toxicon 1989;27:953–954.

50. Kurpiewski G, Campbell BJ, Forrester LJ, Barrett JT: Alternate complement pathway activation by recluse spider venom. Int J Tissue React 1981;3:39–45.

51. Rees RS, Gates C, Timmons S, et al: Plasma components are required for platelet activation by the toxin of Loxosceles reclusa. Toxicon 1988;26:1035–1045.

52. Patel KD, Modur V, Zimmerman GA, et al: The necrotic venom of the brown recluse spider induces dysregulated endothelial cell-dependent neutrophil activation. Differential induction of GM-CSF, IL-8, and E-selectin expression. J Clin Invest 1994;94:631–642.

53. Futrell JM: Loxoscelism. Am J Med Sci 1992;304:261–267.

54. Hufford DC, Morgan PN: C-reactive protein as a mediator in the lysis of human erythrocytes sensitized by brown recluse spider venom. Proc Soc Exp Biol Med 1981;167:493–497.

55. Rees R, Campbell D, Rieger E, King LE: The diagnosis and treatment of brown recluse spider bites. Ann Emerg Med 1987;16:945–949.

56. Gendron BP: Loxosceles reclusa envenomation. Am J Emerg Med 1990;8:51–54.

57. Vorse H, Seccareccio P, Woodruff K, Humphrey GB: Disseminated intravascular coagulopathy following fatal brown spider bite (necrotic arachnidism). J Pediatr 1972;80:1035–1037.

58. Barbaro KC, Cardoso JL, Eickstedt VR, Mota I: IgG antibodies to Loxosceles sp. spider venom in human envenoming. Toxicon 1992;30:1117–1121.

59. Cardoso JL, Wen FH, Franca FO, et al: Detection by enzyme immunoassay of Loxosceles gaucho venom in necrotic skin lesions caused by spider bites in Brazil. Trans R Soc Trop Med Hyg 1990;84:608–609.

60. Barrett SM, Romine-Jenkins M, Blick KE: Passive hemagglutination inhibition test for diagnosis of brown recluse spider bite envenomation. Clin Chem 1993;39:2104–2107.

61. Chavez-Olortegui C, Zanetti VC, Ferreira AP, et al: Elisa for the detection of venom antigens in experimental and clinical envenoming by Loxosceles intermedia spiders. Toxicon 1998;36:563–569.

62. Wright SW, Wrenn KD, Murray L, Seger D: Clinical presentation and outcome of brown recluse spider bite. Ann Emerg Med 1997;30:28–32.

63. King LE Jr, Rees RS: Dapsone treatment of a brown recluse bite. JAMA 1983;250:648.

64. Barrett SM, Romine-Jenkins M, Fisher DE: Dapsone or electric shock therapy of brown recluse spider envenomation? Ann Emerg Med 1994;24:21–25.

65. Hobbs GD, Anderson AR, Greene TJ, Yealy DM: Comparison of hyperbaric oxygen and dapsone therapy for loxosceles envenomation. Acad Emerg Med 1996;3:758–761.

66. Phillips S, Kohn M, Baker D, et al: Therapy of brown spider envenomation: a controlled trial of hyperbaric oxygen, dapsone, and cyproheptadine. Ann Emerg Med 1995;25:363–368.

67. Rees RS, Altenbern DP, Lynch JB, King LE Jr: Brown recluse spider bites. A comparison of early surgical excision versus dapsone and delayed surgical excision. Ann Surg 1985;202:659–663.

68. Wille RC, Morrow JD: Case report: dapsone hypersensitivity syndrome associated with treatment of the bite of a brown recluse spider. Am J Med Sci 1988;296:270–271.

69. Wasserman GS: Wound care of spider and snake envenomations. Ann Emerg Med 1988;17:1331–1335.

70. Svendsen FJ: Treatment of clinically diagnosed brown recluse spider bites with hyperbaric oxygen: a clinical observation. J Ark Med Soc 1986;83:199–204.

71. Maynor ML, Moon RE, Klitzman B, et al: Brown recluse spider envenomation: a prospective trial of hyperbaric oxygen therapy. Acad Emerg Med 1997;4:184–192.

72. Hobbs GD: Brown recluse spider envenomation: is hyperbaric oxygen the answer? Acad Emerg Med 1997;4:165–166.

73. Tomaszewski CA, Thom SR: Use of hyperbaric oxygen in toxicology. Emerg Med Clin North Am 1994;12:437–459.

74. Merchant ML, Hinton JF, Geren CR: Effect of hyperbaric oxygen on sphingomyelinase D activity of brown recluse spider (Loxosceles reclusa) venom as studied by 31P nuclear magnetic resonance spectroscopy. Am J Trop Med Hyg 1997;56:335–338.

75. Gomez HF, Miller MJ, Trachy JW, et al: Intradermal anti-loxosceles Fab fragments attenuates dermonecrotic arachnidism. Acad Emerg Med 1999;6:1195–1202.

76. Spielman A, Levi HW: Probable envenomation by Chiracanthium mildei; a spider found in houses. Am J Trop Med Hyg 1970;19:729–732.

77. Russell FE: Bite by the spider Phidippus formosus: case history. Toxicon 1970;8:193–194.

78. Vest DK: Envenomation by Tegenaria agrestis (Walckenaer) spiders in rabbits. Toxicon 1987;25:221–224.

79. Vest DK: Necrotic arachnidism in the northwest United States and its probable relationship to Tegenaria agrestis (Walckenaer) spiders. Toxicon 1987;25:175–184.

80. Isbister GK: Data collection in clinical toxinology: debunking myths and developing diagnostic algorithms. J Toxicol Clin Toxicol 2002;40:231–237.

81. Isbister GK, Gray MR: White-tail spider bite: a prospective study of 130 definite bites by Lampona species. Med J Aust 2003;179:199–202.

82. Nicholson GM, Walsh R, Little MJ, Tyler MI: Characterisation of the effects of robustoxin, the lethal neurotoxin from the Sydney funnel-web spider Atrax robustus, on sodium channel activation and inactivation. Pflug Arch Eur J Physiol 1998;436:117–126.

83. Torda TA, Loong E, Greaves I: Severe lung oedema and fatal consumption coagulopathy after funnel-web spider bite. Med J Aust 1980;2:442–444.

84. Miller MK, Whyte IM, White J, Keir PM: Clinical features and management of Hadronyche envenomation in man. Toxicon 2000;38:409–427.

85. Graudins A, Wilson D, Alewood PF, et al: Cross-reactivity of Sydney funnel-web spider antivenom: neutralization of the in vitro toxicity of other Australian funnel-web (Atrax and Hadronyche) spider venoms. Toxicon 2002;40:259–266.

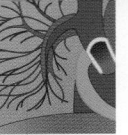

B   Scorpions and Stinging Insects

JERRY D. THOMAS, MD ■ KAREN E. THOMAS, MPH ■ ZIAD N. KAZZI, MD

At a Glance...

■ Scorpion envenomation cause significant morbidity and mortality worldwide.

■ Most envenomations require only supportive treatment.

■ Antivenom use remains controversial. Currently there is no commercially available antivenom in the United States.

■ Hymenoptera and other stinging insects are a frequent cause of human injury.

■ Anaphylaxis from stings is the major cause of morbidity associated with hymenoptera envenomations.

■ For patients with significant sensitivity reactions, education on avoidance, epinephrine auto-injector prescription, and referral to an allergist may be life saving.

SCORPIONS

Introduction and Relevant History

Scorpions are invertebrate arthropods that have existed for longer than 400 million years.[1] They belong to the phylum Arthropoda, the class Arachnida, and the order Scorpiones. Taxonomic classification is evolving and consists of anywhere from 9 to 20 living families. Of the over 1400 species of scorpions worldwide, less than 50 are considered dangerous to humans.[2,3] All potentially lethal scorpions belong to the family Buthidae with the exception of one genus, *Hemiscorpius,* which belongs to the family Scorpionidae.

Scorpions are found on all continents except Antarctica and live in tropical and temperate regions within 50 degrees north and south of the equator.[2,4] The only medically important species in the United States is *Centruroides sculpturatus,* also known as *Centruroides exilicauda* or the bark scorpion (Fig. 22B-1). Recent research may suggest that *C. sculpturatus* and *C. exilicauda* are in fact two distinct species.[5] *C. sculpturatus* is found in the Southwestern United States, primarily in Arizona, but also in parts of California, New Mexico, Texas, and on the shores of Lake Mead, Nevada.[1] Other medically important species and their distribution are shown in Table 22B-1. Scorpions can be transported to other nonendemic locations, either unintentionally as stowaways in shipped goods or intentionally as exotic pets.

The body of the scorpion consists of two major segments: the anterior prosoma and the posterior opisthosoma. The opisthosoma contains seven mesosomal segments, five metasomal segments, and the venom apparatus known as the *telson* (Fig. 22B-2). The scorpion also possesses a pair of claw-like pedipalps used for grabbing prey, a pair of pincher-like chelicerae near the mouth used for feeding, and four pairs of legs. Scorpions range in color from light yellow to black.[6] A unique feature of scorpions is that all are thought to fluoresce under ultraviolet light. Although not well understood, this is thought to be secondary to one or more substances located in the cuticle of their exoskeletons. This phenomenon is used to harvest, study, and protect against them. Freshly molted scorpions, however, do not fluoresce.

There are no hard and fast rules to determine which scorpions are dangerous based on appearance. The size of the scorpion does not correlate to its aggressiveness or venom potency.[7] Commonly, however, scorpions with slender pedipalps are more toxic than those with thicker ones.[6,8] Additionally, one structural difference that helps distinguish Buthidae scorpions from other families is a triangular sternal plate as opposed to a more pentagonal plate seen in the other families.

Scorpions are primarily nocturnal creatures that prey on insects, arachnids, and small lizards. They grab their prey with pedipalps, inject the venom from their telson by arching their tails over the back, and then tear their prey apart with their chelicerae. They are often found around dwellings, hiding in woodpiles and other concealed locations. *C. sculpturatus* does not burrow like some scorpions but prefers to be in or around trees, particularly sycamore, mesquite, and cottonwood trees.[1] The life span of scorpions varies by species but generally ranges from several months to several years.[2]

Epidemiology

Worldwide, scorpions are the most important cause of arachnid morbidity and mortality.[9] In Mexico, Tunisia, Algeria, Morocco, and Libya, scorpions are the most important venomous animal, and in many other tropical areas, they are second only to snakes.[6] There are an estimated 5000 deaths from scorpion stings worldwide each year.[7] In Tunisia, each year an estimated 40,000 people are stung by scorpions, of whom 1000 require

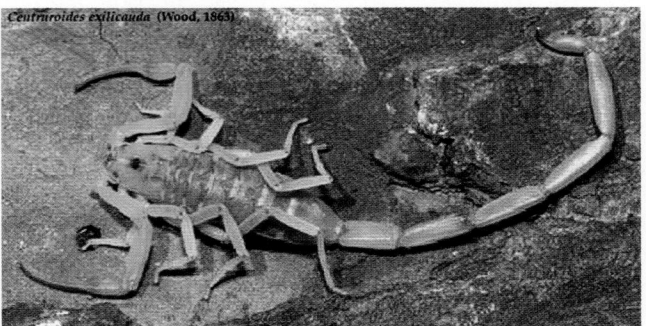

FIGURE 22B-1 *Centruroides sculpturatus* or *exilicauda.* (Courtesy of Scott Stockwell, PhD.)

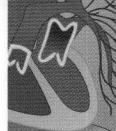

TABLE 22B-1 Medically Important Scorpion Species

NAME	LOCATION	APPROXIMATE SIZE	COLOR
Androctonus australis (Yellow fat tail scorpion, yellow desert scorpion, Sahara scorpion)	North Africa (Tunisia, Algeria), Israel	Up to 10 cm	Brownish yellow
Androctonus crassicauda (Black fat tail scorpion, black scorpion)	North Africa (Egypt), Saudi Arabia, Persian Gulf	Up to 8.5 cm	Black or dark brown
Buthus occitanus (Common European scorpion, Tunisian scorpion, Moroccan scorpion)	North Africa (Tunisia, Algeria), Spain	4–7.5 cm	Yellow
Centruroides sculpturatus (Bark scorpion)	Southwestern United States, Northern Mexico	6.5 cm	Yellow, tan, or brown without stripes
Centruroides suffusus (Mexican scorpion)	Mexico	5–8 cm	Yellow, tan, or brown
Hemiscorpius lepturus	Middle East (Iran, Iraq, Pakistan, Yemen)	Females 5 cm Males 8.5 cm	Yellow to yellow brown
Leiurus quinquestriatus (Yellow scorpion, death stalker, five-keeled gold scorpion, Egyptian scorpion)	Saudi Arabia, Middle East, Egypt	Females 8 cm Males 7 cm	Yellow
Mesobuthus tamulus (Red scorpion, Indian red scorpion, Eastern Indian scorpion)	India	Up to 10 cm	Yellow to black
Parabuthus species	Southern Africa	Up to 10–14 cm, depending on species	Brownish
Tityus serrulatus (Brazilian scorpion, yellow scorpion)	Brazil	6–7 cm	Yellowish brown

Adapted from references 1, 2, 4, 6, 7, 8, and 28.

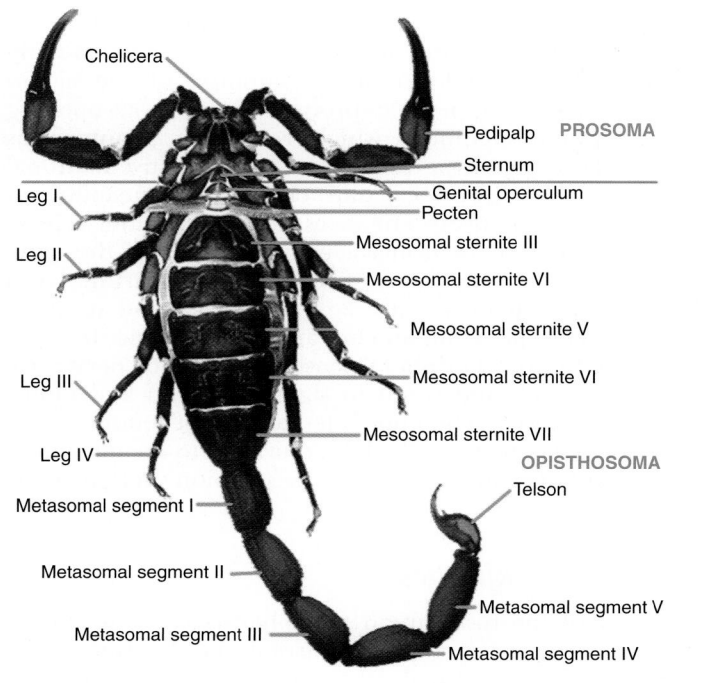

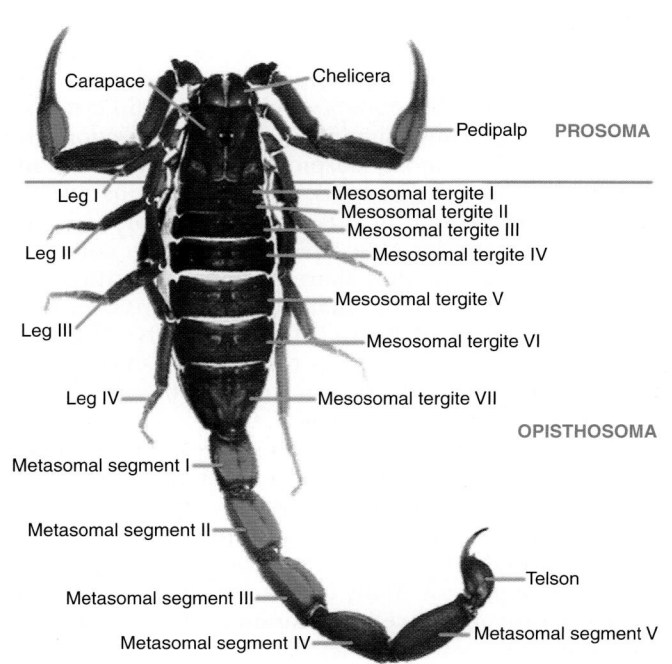

FIGURE 22B-2 Scorpion morphology. **A**, Ventral view. **B**, Dorsal view. (Courtesy of Scott Stockwell, PhD.)

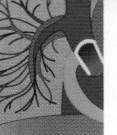

hospitalization and 100 die.[10] In Algeria, 50,000 people are stung and 150 die.[11] Mexico records about 100,000 cases each year, with 800 dying, and North Africa reports about 30 fatalities a year.[6]

In the United States in 2003, the Toxic Exposure Surveillance System reported 14,417 exposures to scorpions, 908 (6.3%) of which were treated in medical facilities. The majority of exposures were in adults 20 years and older (71.7%). Of the 3245 persons in whom follow-up was conducted, most (88%) had no or minor effects from the sting, 11.7% had moderate effects, and 10 people (0.3%) had life-threatening effects.[12] No deaths from scorpions were reported by U.S. poison centers in 2003. In 2002, however, two deaths were reported: one from a *Centruroides* sting and one resulting from the antivenom.[13] In 2000, there was one death due to anaphylaxis from a scorpion sting.[14] The National Vital Statistics System also reported one death in 2001 from a scorpion sting.[15]

Scorpion stings to humans are usually accidental. Scorpions are not aggressive and would rather escape from humans. Stings most commonly occur when a human unintentionally steps on or squeezes a scorpion or reaches under a stone or piece of wood. Children are often stung when playing with scorpions.[6] Since scorpions are nocturnal, envenomations occur more commonly at night. In areas where scorpions are endemic, care should be taken to prevent scorpion envenomations (Box 22B-1).

Pharmacology and Pathophysiology

Scorpion venom has evolved primarily to aid in the immobilization of prey.[7] Scorpion venom in general contains a complex mixture of mucopolysaccharides, hyaluronidase, phospholipase, acetylcholinesterase, serotonin, histamine, protease inhibitors, histamine releasers, and neurotoxins.[4] Serotonin is thought to mediate most of the immediate pain experienced after an envenomation. *Hemiscorpius* venoms contain cytotoxic substances that cause significant tissue destruction; this is not typical of most scorpion venoms, which cause systemic toxicity. In humans, the neurotoxins are the most clinically significant component of scorpion venom. Each species of scorpion has its own collection of neurotoxins, but they share a similar structure. The neurotoxins are low-molecular-weight proteins composed of a single chain of 60 to 70 amino acids. The composition of the venom and its toxicity varies not only by species but also with the season, and with the age and the nutritional status of the scorpion.[16]

Of more than 14,000 scorpion species, the venoms of only 30 or so have been thoroughly characterized.[17] Scorpion venom composition varies by species, and this variation may aid in taxonomy disputes.[5] Only 0.02% of the estimated 100,000 unique peptides have been identified at present. Many of these peptides bind to and alter the function of cell membrane, voltage-dependent ion channels, specifically Na^+, Cl^-, K^+, and Ca^{2+} channels.[3,17] The affinity and effect of these ion channel effectors vary by species. Although not completely understood, action potentials are thought to be affected

---

BOX 22B-1   PREVENTION OF SCORPION STINGS

There are a number of precautions that you can take if you live in or are traveling in an area where scorpions are endemic:

Reduce the amount of garbage and keep it covered. Insects are attracted to garbage and scorpions to insects.

Avoid the accumulation of wood and other building materials near the house; such piles are good homes for scorpions.

Before putting on clothes and shoes, check for the presence of scorpions.

Check the covers and around the room before going to sleep.

Do not walk barefoot at night.

Wear gloves, closed-toe shoes, and other protective clothing when working in areas where scorpions may live (piles of wood, stones, etc.).

Monitor children when they may be playing near areas where scorpions may hide.

Keep beds and other furniture away from walls.

Ensure windows have screens.

In Mexico and other endemic areas, a row of glazed tiles around the walls and steps are recommended because scorpions cannot climb smooth surfaces.

To attract scorpions, lay a piece of damp burlap on the floor before going to sleep. Scorpions will move under the burlap during the night where they can be killed the following morning.

Chickens are natural enemies of scorpions, as are birds, bats, ducks, and monkeys.

If chemical control is employed, it should be understood that scorpions can hide for extended periods of times. Insecticide effect should be long lasting or applied frequently.

If you do feel something crawling on you, removed it with the palm of your hand instead of slapping it.

Data from references 2, 3, 4, 6, 7, and 35.

---

by several mechanisms. Certain peptides produce incomplete inactivation of sodium channels, thus resulting in a slowing and prolonged duration of the action potential. Other peptides produce spontaneous opening of sodium channels, which results in spontaneous depolarization, hyperexcitability, and repetitive neuronal firing.[17] Increased calcium channel permeability of presynaptic neurons enhances neurotransmitter release and enhanced neuronal activity. Neurons of the autonomic nervous system (nicotinic, muscarinic, and adrenergic neurons) are largely affected and result in enhanced parasympathetic and sympathetic nervous system activity. Peripheral sensory and motor nerves are also affected and result in significant pain and motor hyperactivity.[1,4] The human lethal dose of venom ranges from 100 to 600 µg, which is equivalent to the maximum amount of venom present in the scorpion's telson at any one time.[3]

Pharmacokinetics

Many of the distribution and pharmacokinetic studies on scorpion venom were carried out by Ismail and colleagues in animals.[18] Scorpion venom is injected subcutaneously and rapidly absorbed into tissues.[3] Using radiolabeled venom from *Leiurus quinquestriatus*, *Buthus*

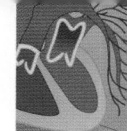

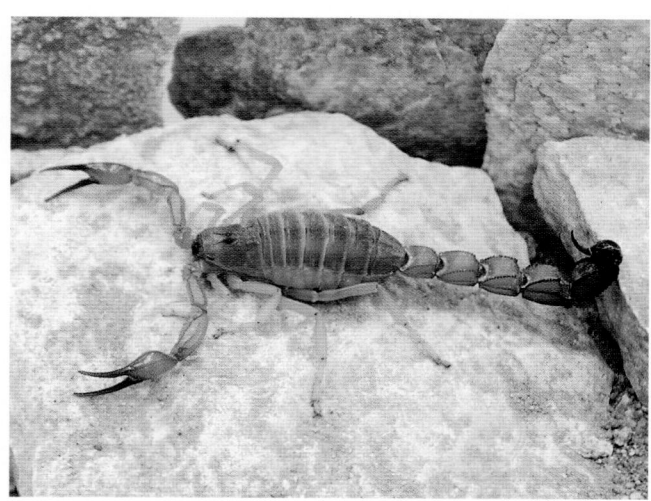

FIGURE 22B-3 *Androctonus australis.* (Courtesy of Scott Stockwell, PhD.)

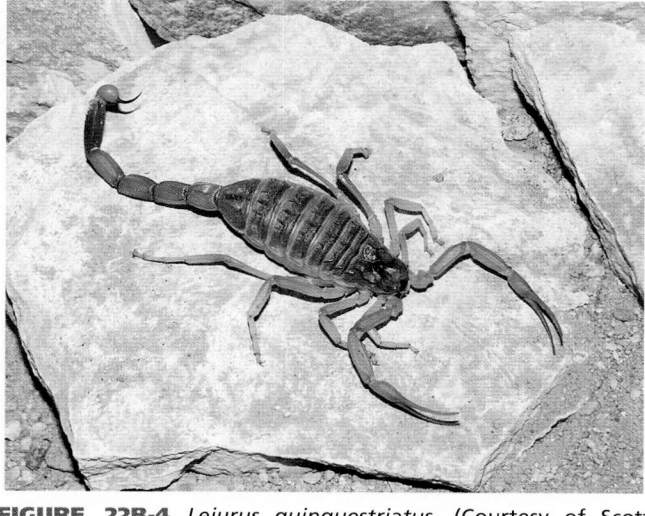

FIGURE 22B-4 *Leiurus quinquestriatus.* (Courtesy of Scott Stockwell, PhD.)

judaicus, and *Androctonus amoreuxi,* they demonstrated that the venoms appeared to demonstrate a two-compartment pharmacokinetic model. Following intravenous administration, there is rapid tissue redistribution (alpha phase) over 4 to 7 minutes followed by an overall elimination (beta phase) half-life of 4.2 to 13.4 hours.[3,18] An Algerian study using an enzyme-linked immunosorbent assay (ELISA) in 182 cases of *Androctonus australis* envenomations showed a correlation between the clinical severity of envenomation on presentation and blood venom concentrations (Fig. 22B-3). They showed an elimination half life of 2 hours, and antivenom administration did not effectively neutralize the scorpion venom.[11] In another study, which used a sandwich ELISA method in three victims of *Centruroides* envenomation, the elimination of venom was consistent with a two-compartment model, with half-lives ranging from 313 to 515 minutes.[19]

Special Populations

The severity of envenomation will depend on both scorpion and host factors. The species and size of the scorpion, number of stings, and amount of venom delivered will affect illness severity.[3] Host factors that are important include age, weight, and health of the victim.[3] Because the severity of symptoms is age and weight dependent, children usually sustain more severe scorpion envenomations than adults.[16] The mortality rate in children is also higher. Children younger than 5 years stung by *Centruroides sculpturatus* are more likely to develop severe neuromuscular hyperactivity and respiratory effects.[20] Elderly patients with preexisting cardiac problems are also considered to be at a greater risk for severe effects and mortality from scorpion envenomation.[3,6]

Little is known about the effect of scorpion envenomation in pregnant women.[21] Animal studies have shown that the uterus of pregnant rats may be more sensitive to scorpion venom early in pregnancy.[22] In humans, there

are some anecdotal reports of first-trimester spontaneous abortion in pregnant women stung by *L. quinquestriatus* (Fig. 22B-4).[21]

Clinical Manifestations

Most scorpion stings are characterized by severe localized pain with little visible evidence of envenomation. There may be slight edema, pruritus, numbness, and occasionally small blisters at the bite site.[6] Paresthesias and hyperesthesias travel up the extremity and may become generalized.[1] Performing a tap test may be helpful to distinguish a *C. sculpturatus* from other envenomations in the United States. Tapping gently on the site of the sting will substantially worsen the pain if the sting is from a *C. sculpturatus* scorpion.[4]

Local tissue effects vary among species. The *Hemiscorpius lepturus* can cause significant dermal lesions. However, the presence of significant local effects practically rules out *C. sculpturatus* envenomation.[23]

There have been several grading systems developed for use in scorpion envenomations. One has been developed for *C. sculpturatus* envenomations commonly seen in the United States (Table 22B-2).[1] Grade I consists of pain and paresthesias at the site of envenomation only. In grade II, the pain and paresthesias have progressed to other areas distant from the envenomation site and the patient may also experience perioral numbness. Patients with a grade III envenomation exhibit either cranial nerve or skeletal neuromuscular dysfunctions. Grade IV consists of both cranial nerve and skeletal neuromuscular dysfunction.

In Algeria, a three-grade system is used to classify scorpion envenomations.[24] Grade I envenomations are considered mild; patients manifest local pain and burning only. Grade II envenomations include systemic signs and symptoms (e.g., shivering, restlessness, faintness, or vomiting and other gastrointestinal signs). Grade III envenomations are characterized by serious systemic

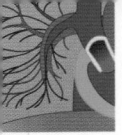

TABLE 22B-2 Grades of *Centruroides sculpturatus* Envenomation

Grade I	Local pain and/or paresthesias at the site of envenomation
Grade II	Pain and/or paresthesias remote from the site of envenomation, in addition to local findings
Grade III	*Either* cranial nerve *or* somatic skeletal neuromuscular dysfunction: 1. Cranial nerve dysfunction: blurred vision, wandering eye movements, hypersalivation, trouble swallowing, tongue fasciculations, problems with upper airway, slurred speech 2. Somatic skeletal neuromuscular dysfunction: jerking of extremities, restlessness, severe involuntary shaking and jerking, which may be mistaken for seizure activity (but are not)
Grade IV	*Both* cranial nerve *and* somatic skeletal neuromuscular dysfunction

Adapted from reference 1.

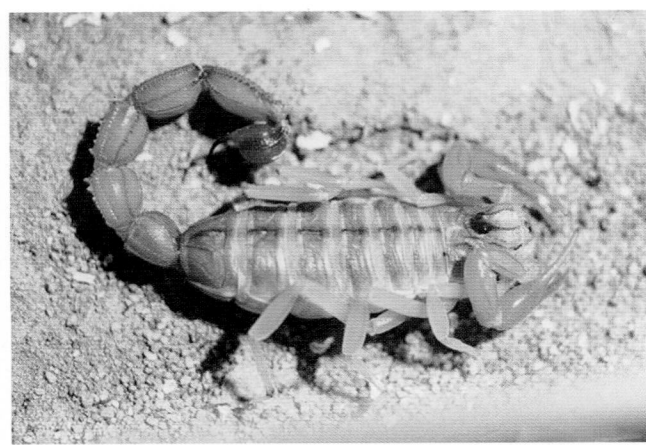

FIGURE 22B-5 *Buthus occitanus.* (Courtesy of R. David Gaban.)

complications such as neurologic findings, hyperthermia, priapism, respiratory failure, pulmonary edema, or shock.

A study of calls to the Arizona Poison Center,[1] where a majority of envenomations would be expected to involve *C. sculpturatus,* showed that evidence of grade I envenomations such as pain and paresthesia was immediate in all cases. Progression to higher grades was variable but always happened in less than 5 hours. Infants sometimes progressed to grade IV in 15 to 30 minutes. A more rapid onset of signs and symptoms in young children is felt to reflect quicker absorption from their thinner dermis.[8,25] In general, clinical effects occur immediately after envenomation (local pain initially), progress to peak effects by 5 hours, and may last for over 24 hours.[4]

Autonomic nervous system effects are prominent in higher-grade scorpion envenomations. Sympathetic or adrenergic signs include extreme agitation, hyperthermia, hypertension, tachycardia, mydriasis, piloerection, and diaphoresis. These effects may culminate in hypotension

and cardiovascular collapse. Priapism has been noted in males. Scorpion envenomations often associated with autonomic storm include the *Tityus* species of the Caribbean and South America, *Androctonus* and *Buthus occitanus* of North Africa, and the *Mesobuthus tamulus* (also known as *Buthus tamulus*) of India (see Figs. 22B-3 and 22B-5). Parasympathetic or cholinergic effects include bradycardia, salivation, bronchorrhea, nausea, vomiting, diarrhea, lacrimation, and urination. Without the history of a sting, these symptoms may be confused with exposure to an anticholinesterase pesticide, especially if such agents are being used for scorpion control.[25] Scorpions often associated with cholinergic excess include the *Centruroides* of the United States and Mexico and *Parabuthus* species of southern Africa (Fig. 22B-6).

Neurologic signs (peripheral and central effects) may include "roving eyes," anisocoria, opsoclonus, disconjugate gaze, pharyngeal muscle dysfunction, and muscle and tongue fasciculations. Extreme muscle rigidity, twitching,

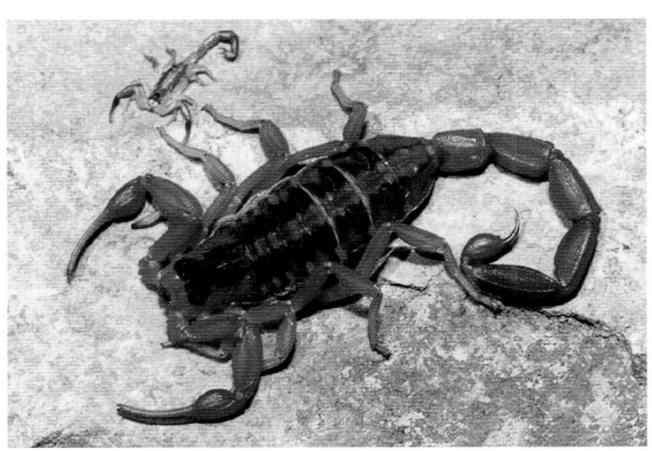

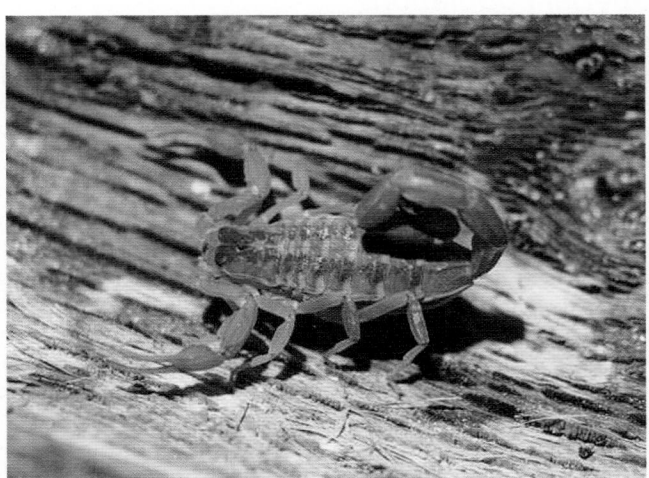

A   B

FIGURE 22B-6 Color variations of *Centruroides vitatus.* (Courtesy of Scott Stockwell, PhD.)

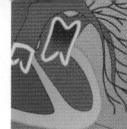

and jerking have also been described. Choreiform and ballistic motor activity is not uncommon. Seizures have been described with some scorpion envenomations but there is significant controversy among experts as to whether those envenomated by *C. sculpturatus* have true seizures. Most patients with motor hyperactivity are conscious. Cerebral infarction, cerebral thrombosis, and acute hypertensive encephalopathy have been described with *Buthidae* envenomations.

Gastrointestinal symptoms may be a reflection of cholinergic excess and profuse nausea, vomiting, and abdominal pain. Envenomation by *Tityus* species are well known to cause pancreatitis and are a major cause in endemic areas.

Severely symptomatic patients should be monitored for cardiac effects. Sequelae have included bradycardia, tachycardia, ventricular dysrhythmias, and cardiovascular collapse. Myocardial infarction has been documented with elevations of creatine kinase. This may be due to a direct myotoxic effect, although it is not well understood. Transient myocardial "stunning" or reversible mechanical dysfunction without tissue necrosis has also been documented with echocardiography.[6] Respiratory function may be compromised by increased secretions and loss of protective reflexes. Pulmonary edema and cardio-respiratory collapse have also been noted. Anaphylactic reactions to scorpion stings, while rare, should be considered in people who have been previously exposed.[7]

Severe dermatologic changes, hemolysis, and central nervous system (CNS) changes are a prominent feature of the *H. lepturus*. In Southwestern Iraq, this scorpion is thought to account for only 10% to 15% of enveno-mations but for the majority of fatalities. Severe skin sloughing and disfiguring wounds have been described.[23]

Diagnosis

The diagnosis of scorpion envenomation is made primarily from the patient's history and physical examination.

LABORATORY TESTING

The extent of laboratory evaluation will depend on the severity of the patient's clinical presentation. Even though venom assays have been used in studies, there are no routinely available tests for the detection of scorpion venom. Laboratory evaluation is used to rule out other medical illnesses and to facilitate the provision of sup-portive care (i.e., evaluate for complications of enven-omation). A complete blood count with platelet count and coagulation studies may be warranted since defibrination syndrome has been reported after *M. tamulus* envenomation,[26,27] and massive hemolysis may occur after *H. lepturus* envenomation.[23] Renal failure has occurred secondary to hemolysis or rhabdomyolysis and may merit monitoring of electrolytes, blood urea nitrogen, creatinine and creatine kinase, and urinary output. Because *T. trinitatus* envenomation has been associated with pancreatitis, amylase and lipase levels may be helpful. In addition, arterial blood gases may be necessary to guide therapy in patients with severe respiratory distress.

OTHER DIAGNOSTIC TESTING

An electrocardiogram (ECG) may be helpful because some scorpions such as *L. quinquestriatus* have caused arrhythmias (e.g., atrioventricular block and bradycardia). Other ECG changes such as ST-T wave abnormalities and QTc segment prolongation have also been reported. Echocardiography of patients with shock typically demonstrates global hypokinesia.[28] Chest radiography may be helpful in patients with respiratory symptoms to assess for pulmonary edema.

DIFFERENTIAL DIAGNOSIS

If the scorpion is not seen at the time of the bite, the differential is wide. It includes spider bites, insect bites, and abrasions. The differential diagnosis for patients presenting with neurologic signs and symptoms includes acute dystonic reactions; seizures; poisoning with CNS stimulants, cholinergic agents, and strychnine; acute cerebrovascular accident; CNS infections; botulism; and tetanus.

Occasionally, the similarity in presentations between *Centruroides* stings and CNS stimulant ingestion is used by parents to conceal the cause of their children's illness. In a case series of 18 cases of methamphetamine ingestion, two children were misdiagnosed as victims of scorpion envenomation. The two children were treated with anti-venom, and one of the patients developed anaphylaxis.[29]

Management

SUPPORTIVE CARE

Most envenomations are minor and can be treated symp-tomatically with analgesics, local wound care, tetanus prophylaxis, and a period of observation to determine whether the envenomation will progress. In healthy adults, many envenomations can be managed at home. Judicious application of ice, light compression wrapping, and immobilization of the effected area often offer some relief.[7] Oral analgesics are helpful, but parenteral therapy may be required. Some recommend local anesthesia with lidocaine, bupivicaine, or dehydroemetine by infiltration or a nerve block.[4] Prophylactic antibiotics are not indi-cated and should be withheld until evidence of infection occurs. The use of steroids has not proven beneficial.[10] If the scorpion has been killed and brought with the patient, it may be helpful to have it identified by an entomologist.

For patients exhibiting systemic envenomation, advanced life support measures (including endotracheal intubation) should be instituted as necessary to treat respiratory compromise. Continuous cardiovascular and respiratory monitoring should be employed. Hyper-thermia and hypothermia should be addressed. Fluid resuscitation should be administered as necessary along with careful observation for pulmonary edema. Excessive secretions may require frequent suctioning.

When envenomation is complicated by hyperthermia, acetaminophen and external cooling methods have been recommended.[18] Dipyrone intravenously has been advo-cated in *Tityus serrulatus* envenomation. Vomiting should be treated with antiemetic therapy (e.g., metoclopramide) and aggressive rehydration with intravenous crystalloid.

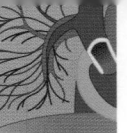

Seizures or neuromuscular hyperactivity should be treated initially with benzodiazepines and/or barbiturates.

Routine administration of atropine or neostigmine for their parasympatholytic effect is controversial. These agents have been used successfully to decrease secretions associated with *Centruroides* and *Tityus* envenomations.[3,30] These agents may also exacerbate sympathetic effects and result in hypertension and pulmonary edema.[3] Thus, anticholinergics should probably be reserved for cases of severe bradycardia.

Hypertension is a hallmark of most severe envenomations and should be treated aggressively. Nitroprusside is the agent of choice for severe hypertension and can be more easily titrated to effect.[7] Prazosin is a selective α_1-adrenergic receptor blocker that has been recommended for scorpion envenomation, particularly from *M. tamulus* envenomation. Case series in India have shown beneficial effect, and Bawaskar strongly recommends early administration.[30] The use of nifedipine for hypertension is discouraged because it may cause reflex stimulation of the sympathetic nervous system and lead to cardiac stimulation and dysrhythmia. Angiotensin converting enzyme inhibitors are discouraged because they may exacerbate venom toxicity by increasing bradykinin levels.[18] Hydralazine has been used extensively for the treatment of hypertension but has been associated with unpredictable hypotension.

When it occurs subsequent to envenomation, pulmonary edema should be treated with oxygen and positive pressure mechanical ventilation as necessary. Loop diuretics should be used with caution due to volume depletion in many patients.

Historically, initial treatment recommendations included heavy sedation with so-called "lytic cocktails." Heavy sedation with benzodiazepines and aggressive opioid analgesic therapy is now sometimes discouraged due to the associated risk for respiratory compromise. When used, these therapies should be used judiciously.

Hemiscorpius stings in Iraq have exhibited local tissue destruction and hemolysis. Local authorities have advocated early local excision, alkalinization of urine to prevent renal failure, and steroids. Randomized trials to support these recommendations have not been conducted.[23]

ANTIDOTES

The use of antivenom for envenomations is controversial. Since the risk for death with scorpion envenomation is so small and the risk for allergic reaction from antivenom administration is high, the benefit of antivenom administration is unclear. Thus, supportive care is probably similar in efficacy and safer than the use of antivenom.[7] Many complex antivenom regimens have been promulgated for symptomatic scorpion envenomations without clear evidence of efficacy. Rigorous testing of these regimens is difficult due to the wide variety of scorpions and the limited resources where most envenomations occur (i.e., limited availability of specific medications, critical care support, or antivenom). Perhaps not surprisingly, the extant regional literature seems to support regimens commonly used in each region.

Antivenom recommendations are not clearly defined, and antivenom is not readily available in many areas or for many specific species. For areas that have antivenoms, there has been little control over their manufacture and quality, yet most are used in the belief that they represent the standard of care. Antivenom use has been predicated on the premise that any venom should respond to antivenom. Trials to prove efficacy have been rare, and future trials are questionable ethically in areas where administration has become the standard of care. In general, use of antivenom should be reserved for patients with severe signs and symptoms of envenomation (grades III and IV), particularly young children.

To date, the greatest use of scorpion antivenoms has occurred in regions of frequent envenomations, such as Northern Africa, the Middle East, Mexico, and Brazil. Large series of patients treated with antivenom have been reported supporting the use of antivenom. In one series of patients, antivenom administration was reported for over 20,000 cases of *Centruroides* scorpions in Mexico.[31] No patient developed immediate hypersensitivity from antivenom, and no deaths were recorded. In another large series of patients from Brazil, antivenom use was reported in 3860 patients stung by *T. serrulatus*.[32] The mortality rate was 0.28%. All deaths occurred in children treated 3 or more hours after envenomation. In the few controlled clinical trials that have been conducted evaluating antivenom therapy, however, a benefit from antidotal therapy has not been shown.[9,10] Proponents of antivenom use argue that antivenom is the only specific treatment to directly counteract the primary physiologic effects of the venom, and its administration significantly improve outcomes. The disappointing results seen from the controlled trials probably result from inadequate dosing.[4] Opponents to antivenom therapy believe that since the major effects of envenomation result not from the toxin, but from the release of endogenous neurotransmitters, antivenom will have minimal effect at reducing morbidity and mortality.[4] However, until more controlled trials are conducted, antivenom use appears to be justified in cases of severe systemic envenomation, particularly in high-risk groups such as children.[6,9,33] In some areas where there is limited access to clinical care (e.g., rural Mexico), early antivenom use has become the standard of care.

Until recently, a goat serum antivenom for *Centruroides sculpturatus* envenomation had been available in the United States from the University of Arizona. This antivenom was not approved by the Food and Drug Administration (FDA), however, and could not be used outside the state of Arizona. In small, uncontrolled studies, this antivenom appeared to be effective but was also associated with a significant incidence of hypersensitivity reactions.[9,34] Its intravenous administration produced rapid resolution of the respiratory, cardiovascular, and neurologic toxicity associated with the sting of *C. sculpturatus*.[4] Symptoms resolved within 3 hours for patients who received antivenom, whereas symptoms lasted 15 to 24 hours for those not treated with antivenom.[34] Of those receiving the antivenom, however, 3% to 8% experienced an immediate hypersensitivity reaction and 58% to 61% developed delayed serum sickness.[25,34] The production of this antivenom has recently ceased, and the remaining supply is becoming depleted. The FDA

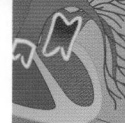

has approved clinical testing of an antivenom, Alacramyn Fab2 fragment, produced by the Mexican Ministry of Health. This product is polyvalent and equine derived and has been used extensively for the Mexican *Centruroides*.[3]

If antivenoms are used, they should be administered as soon as possible after envenomation to contain the release of endogenous reactive substances.[4,6] In addition, the tissue distribution of the antivenom immunoglobulins is much slower than that of the venom, with redistribution half-lives 11 to 102 times longer than that of venom.[10] The antivenom should be administered intravenously because intramuscular administration further slows tissue distribution.[6,35,36] The Mexican antivenom is administered with an H_1-antihistamine (e.g., chlorpheniramine).[3] During administration of antivenom, patients should be observed closely for any signs and symptoms of type I immediate hypersensitivity reactions. Patients should also be monitored for serum sickness (typically occurs 7 to 21 days after antivenom), which can be treated with oral antihistamines and corticosteroids.

Patients with grade III or IV *Centruroides* stings and other severe Buthidae envenomations should be admitted to an intensive care unit (ICU) and/or treated with antivenom. Occasionally, patients with grade III envenomation are discharged home after resolution of their symptoms with antivenom. In general, young children are more likely to require inpatient observation.

Disposition

The disposition of the patient depends primarily on the severity of illness at presentation. Those who exhibit significant symptomatology will require intensive care monitoring and support. Observational monitoring should continue until patients are hemodynamically stable and no longer at risk for rhabdomyolysis. For *C. sculpturatus* envenomations, the rapidity of sign and symptom resolution is dependent on the patient's age and severity of envenomation. Improvement usually occurs by 10 hours for those not treated with antivenom.[4] However, the pain and paresthesias from the scorpion sting may persist for 1 to 2 weeks.

Those treated with antivenom should be followed closely after hospital discharge due to the significant risk for serum sickness. These patients should be educated as to the signs and symptoms of serum sickness (e.g., arthralgias) and appropriate initial treatment (e.g., nonsteroidal anti-inflammatory drugs [NSAIDs]).

STINGING INSECTS AND OTHER VENOMOUS ARTHROPODS

Hymenoptera

INTRODUCTION AND RELEVANT HISTORY
Hymenoptera is a very large order of the phylum Arthropoda and the class Insecta. Species of medical importance belong to the following families: Vespidae (wasps, yellow jackets, and hornets), Apidae (honeybees and bumblebees), and Formicidae (fire ants, Australian

jumper ant, and others). In general, hymenoptera are not aggressive toward humans.[6] The greatest risk to humans is not the toxicity of their venom, but rather the risk of type I allergic reactions. The earliest depiction of such a reaction is in the tomb of the Egyptian pharaoh Menes, who died in 2621 BC following an insect sting.[37]

The family Apidae contains a number of types of bees. Honeybees (*Apis mellifera*) are social creatures that live in colonies of 30,000 to 50,000 workers. These creatures most frequently sting to protect their colony from honey-loving predators.[6] "Killer" bees (*Apis mellifera scutellata*) are African honeybees that were introduced to Brazil because they were thought to be more efficient at producing honey in tropical climates. They first escaped from hives in Brazil in 1957 and have since spread widely, reaching the southern United States in 1990. There are now populations in Texas, Arizona, New Mexico, and California.[38] Killer bees are of concern because they are more aggressive than typical hymenoptera, attack in swarms, and chase victims for greater distances from their hive than other species.[38] Bumblebees (*Bombus* and related genera) are generally mild mannered and live in smaller colonies of around 1,000 individual insects in underground nests or in hollow trees.[6,38] Sweat bees (family Halictidae) are small insects attracted to sweaty skin. Their sting is not very painful but can cause anaphylaxis, and their venom is not immunologically related to that of other bees and wasps.[38]

The family Vespidae mainly contains social wasps; a small number of solitary species are also included. Social wasps are found throughout the world but are predominantly a medical problem in the United States and Europe (Fig. 22B-7).[38] They live in colonies of 30 to several thousand individuals.[39] While some species may use their stinger to capture prey, the stinger is primarily used to defend the colony.[6] Wasps seldom sting away from the nest unless trapped or disturbed.[40]

Ants are social insects whose venom is used primarily for defense and, occasionally, for capturing prey.[6,38] The most medically important ant in the United States is the fire ant. Fire ants (*Solenopsis invicta*) were initially

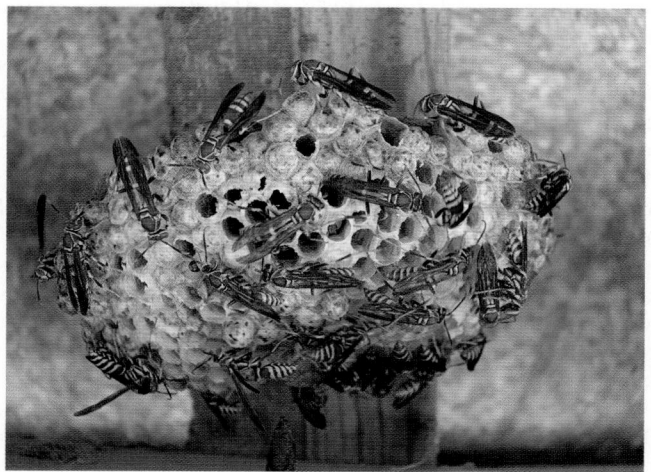

FIGURE 22B-7 Paper wasps. (Courtesy of Nancy Hinkle, PhD, University of Georgia.)

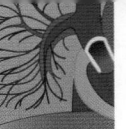

introduced to Mobile, Alabama, in 1939 as a stowaway in a shipment of nursery products and sod.[38,41] Currently, fire ants infest Alabama, Arkansas, Florida, Georgia, Louisiana, Mississippi, North Carolina, Oklahoma, South Carolina, Tennessee, Texas, Virginia, Puerto Rico, Arizona, New Mexico, and California.[42] Harvester ants (*Pogonomyrmex*), which are found in the Southwestern United States and Mexico, also have some medical importance. They can produce a painful sting, which may result in systemic symptoms and anaphylaxis.[38]

The venom apparatus of hymenoptera is located at the end of the abdomen and consists of venom glands, a reservoir for the venom, and a hollow structure for piercing the integument and injecting the venom.[38] The stingers are actually modified ovipositors, and therefore, only the females can sting.[6] When honeybees sting, they leave the entire venom apparatus in their target and eventually die.[6] Because bumblebees and wasps do not have barbed stingers, they can remove their stinger and sting repeatedly.[6,41] In some species of ants, the stinger is absent and the ant sprays venom into a wound created by its bite.[39]

EPIDEMIOLOGY

In 2003, the American Association of Poison Control Centers reported 12,516 exposures to bees, wasps, yellow jackets, and hornets and 2480 exposures to ants.[12] There was one reported death in a 3-month-old from fire ant stings and one death from multiple yellow jackets stings to a 2-year-old.[12] Between 40 and 55 deaths a year in the United States are attributed to insect stings, primarily from anaphylaxis.[6,15] Current numbers may underestimate the problem because many unexplained sudden deaths in outdoor workers and others may be undiagnosed anaphylactic reactions to hymenoptera.[43,44] In the United States and Europe, the majority of deaths due to venomous animals are caused by hymenoptera.[39]

Hymenoptera stings more frequently occur to the head or neck, followed by the lower and upper extremities. Stings in the mouth, pharynx, and esophagus can occur when an insect is accidentally ingested.[38] In temperate areas, stings occur more frequently in the summer and early fall because hymenoptera are more active in higher temperatures and humidity.[38,39] About twice as many men experience severe reactions to stings than females, but this may likely be a difference in exposure rates rather than a physiologic difference.[41] Adults are more likely to experience severe reactions than children[38]; most deaths are in people over 40 years of age.[39] In the United States, 0.4% of the population exhibits some type of allergic reaction to insect venom.[38] Large local reactions to hymenoptera stings occur in 2% to 19% of patients. Systemic reactions are seen in 1% to 3% of adults and less than 1% of children.[37] Of those individuals who exhibit a systemic reaction, 27% to 57% will react systemically to a future envenomation by the same type of insect.[37]

Multiple stings often occur when a nest is disturbed. Either the venom or an alarm pheromone released by the first insects threatened stimulates the other members of the colony to attack.[38,39] Another dangerous situation

BOX 22B-2	PREVENTION OF HYMENOPTERA STINGS

Precautions that can reduce the risk of sustaining a hymenoptera sting:

Bees and wasps are attracted to sweet things and wasps are also attracted to meat, so keep food covered when eating outdoors.

Frequently clean garbage cans and recycling bins and dispose of decaying fruit to make the area less attractive to bees and wasps.

Do not walk around barefoot outside.

Wear gloves, shoes, and other protective clothing when gardening.

Do not wear strong-smelling perfumes and lotions when spending significant time outdoors.

Dark-colored clothing and that with colorful patterns are attractive to bees and wasps; white and light khaki clothing is less attractive.

Exercise caution around fallen tree trunks because wasps may build nests inside.

Avoid fast movements around bees and wasps.

If you disturb a nest, stay still as opposed to running away. Fast movements will attract the attention of the insects and make multiple stings more likely.

Insect repellents used with mosquitoes are not effective with hymenoptera.

Hymenoptera are susceptible to many insecticides. It is safer to spray nests at night.

Antihistamines taken prophylactically before high-risk activities (e.g., beekeeping) can prevent large local reactions but are not protective against more severe reactions.

Allergic individuals should carry an emergency kit with epinephrine and wear a medical identification tag indicating the allergy.

Kits should be available in work and recreation areas where the possibility of stings is high.

Data from references 6, 37 through 40, and 47.

exists when wasps or bees are accidentally trapped in motor vehicles. Not only are the occupants at risk for stings, but they are also at risk for crashes as they attempt to kill or remove the insect from the car.[38] General measures that can be taken to prevent hymenoptera envenomation are listed in Box 22B-2.

Fire ant stings usually occur in children and to the lower extremities. Stings most often occur in the summer, although there may be a seasonal difference in the venom protein concentrations.[42] It is estimated that 30% to 60% of people in endemic areas are stung each year.[42] There have also been reports of massive sting attacks in residents of nursing homes.[42] Approximately 0.6% to 16% of people stung will exhibit an anaphylactic reaction. Most of these individuals have received previous stings, but some will develop a reaction after their first sting. However, most of these people appear to be sensitized to yellow jackets and research suggests that these two venoms cross-react.[42]

PHARMACOLOGY AND PATHOPHYSIOLOGY

The venoms of hymenoptera varies by family and species, but in general, most contain a mixture of low-molecular-weight substances (i.e., peptides) and high-molecular-weight substances (i.e., enzymes). During one single bee

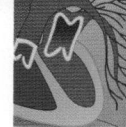

or wasp sting, a volume of only 0.5 to 2 µL of venom is injected.[38,39] Most venoms cause predominantly local pain and discomfort. More severe sequelae can be caused by their respective allergenicity.

The low-molecular-weight substances include histamine, tyramine, dopamine, serotonin, epinephrine, and norepinephrine. These agents predominantly cause pain, mast cell degranulation, and further catecholamine release. Ant venoms contain formic acid, and fire ant venom contains dialkylpiperidines.[39]

Peptides present in hymenoptera venom are responsible for further mast cell degranulation. These include a number of wasp kinins, mastoparans, and chemotactic peptides. About 50% of dry bee venom is melittin, a peptide consisting of 26 amino acids. It acts as a detergent in cell membranes and is responsible for pain. Other peptides found in bee venom are Oa-Adolapsin, apamin, and mast cell degranulating peptide. Apamin blocks calcium-dependent potassium channels.[39]

Enzymes or high-molecular-weight substances include hydrolytic enzymes that have a digestive effect on tissues. These high-molecular-weight substances include phospholipase A2, phospholipase B, hyaluronidase, acidic phosphatase, alkaline phosphatase, cholinesterase, histidincarboxylase, saccharidase, DNAse, and protease. These high-molecular-weight compounds are potential allergens and may precipitate severe allergic reactions in sensitive people.[39]

Allergic manifestations are the result of an immunoglobulin E (IgE)-mediated (type I) hypersensitivity reaction. The initial contact with the allergenic venom components, usually phospholipase A2, hyaluronidase, or melittin, stimulates the body to produce IgE antibodies. Upon subsequent contact with the sensitizing allergen, there is aggregation of the IgE antibodies by mast cells, which leads to degranulation and histamine release.[6]

There is little cross-sensitization between bees and wasps. There is, however, almost 100% cross-sensitivity between yellow jacket and hornet venom. Cross-sensitivity is also seen between fire ants and bees or wasps. Of people allergic to bees or wasps but without exposure to fire ants, 51% of patients had a positive radioallergeosorbent test reaction to fire ant venom.[38]

PHARMACOKINETICS

In general, the venom is injected 2 to 3 mm into the subcutaneous tissue.[6] In the case of intravenous injection or a sting in a highly vascular area, systemic reactions may be more likely.[37]

Toxic reactions are produced by venom in a dose-dependent manner.[37] The amount of venom injected per sting varies by species. Bees usually inject 50 to 100 µg of venom per sting, while wasps and hornets inject 2 to 10 µg per sting.[6] The number of stings necessary to produce a life-threatening reaction vary from 40 to 50 for a large species like the white-faced hornet to 500 to 1400 stings for a honeybee.[38] For Africanized "killer" honeybees, 50 stings can cause systemic toxicity and an estimated 500 are necessary to cause death due to toxicity. The intravenous median lethal dose in mice for honeybees

in 6 mg/kg and for different hornet venoms is 1.6 to 4.1 mg/kg.[38]

SPECIAL POPULATIONS

Due to the dose-dependent toxicity from hymenoptera venom, those with smaller body mass are more susceptible to the toxic effects produced by multiple stings. Thus, fewer stings are needed to become life-threatening in children. Glucose-6-phosphate dehydrogenase deficiency may predispose some populations to greater hemolytic toxicity from envenomation.[40]

CLINICAL MANIFESTATIONS

Most patients will present with instant pain and a wheal and flare reaction at the site of envenomation.[38] Stings in the mouth, throat, or larynx can cause swelling of mucous membranes and laryngeal edema.[6] Local erythema and swelling may also occur.

Large local reactions spreading more than 15 cm and persisting more than 24 hours are thought to represent cell-mediated (type IV) hypersensitivity. Half of the patients with large local reactions, however, will also have elevated serum IgE (indicative of type I reaction) or a positive skin test result. Subsequent stings in these victims usually result in another large local reaction as opposed to a more severe systemic reaction.[44]

Fire ant stings start with the typical wheal and flare reaction that occurs within 20 minutes of the sting. Sterile pustules or necrotic lesions develop within 24 hours, and may last for several days and are pathognomonic for fire ant stings. Pustules are often observed in a ring pattern because the ant bites the skin and then stings as it pivots around the bite site.[41]

The most serious complication of hymenoptera envenomation is an allergic reaction. Severe allergic reactions and anaphylaxis are common. Allergic symptoms may include skin rash, edema, bronchial constriction, cardiovascular failure, difficulties swallowing and speaking, labored breathing, burning sensation in the pharyngeal cavity, itching of palms and soles, hot flashes, hypotension, and general weakness.[6] Over 50% of severe reactions occur within 10 minutes, and almost all in the first 5 hours. Most deaths occur within 1 hour.[38]

Massive hymenoptera envenomations, as occur from multiple stings (i.e., 20 to 50), may also cause systemic effects. These effects include vomiting, diarrhea, generalized edema, dyspnea, hypotension, tachycardia, and cardiovascular collapse. Widespread necrosis of skeletal muscle (rhabdomyolysis) may occur and result in hyperkalemia, acute renal failure from acute tubular necrosis, and hepatorenal syndrome. In addition, hemolysis, hemoglobinuria, acute pancreatitis, disseminated intravascular coagulation, acute respiratory distress syndrome, myocardial infarction, atrial fibrillation, optic neuropathies, and cerebral infarction have been reported after multiple stings.[38]

Atypical reactions can include serum sickness, Arthus reaction, nephritic syndrome, thrombocytopenic purpura, grand mal or focal motor seizures, transient ischemic attacks, Guillain-Barré syndrome, and progressive demyelinating neurologic disease.[38]

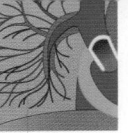
DIAGNOSIS

Diagnosis is usually made by history and suggestive physical findings. If the patient has not seen a hymenoptera insect or is unable to give a history, the diagnosis may be more difficult. It is often difficult to distinguish between symptoms of an immediate allergic reaction and a systemic, dose-related, toxic reaction to multiple stings.[37]

Laboratory Testing

Laboratory evaluation should be based on clinical presentation. Most uncomplicated envenomations will require observation only. For severe allergic reactions and patients with multiple stings, urinalysis, complete blood count, and serum measurements of electrolytes, renal function, creatine phosphokinase, and lactate dehydrogenase should be obtained.[38]

Serum IgE levels and tryptase levels may be elevated following allergic reactions to hymenoptera stings, although this is rarely readily available or helpful in acute management of patients. In a study of sera collected in 142 cases of sudden unexpected death, 23% contained elevated IgE to at least one insect venom as compared with 6% of sera from 92 living blood donors.[43] In an additional study of 68 of the previous samples, 9% were found to have elevated tryptase levels in addition to the elevated IgE levels.[45] Similarly, anti–fire ant IgE and an elevated tryptase level were observed in a fatal fire ant envenomation.[46] Patients with significant reactions should be referred for evaluation by an allergist for more specific testing and consideration of immunotherapy.

Differential Diagnosis

Hymenoptera envenomations can be confused with stings from other insects and spiders. Similar signs and symptoms may also occur with allergic reactions of unknown etiology.

MANAGEMENT

Decontamination

Many authorities recommend immediate removal of retained stingers with the thought that the retained venom apparatus continues to pump venom.[37,47] The time until stinger removal is correlated with severity of reaction.[47] Although many procedures are advocated, the stinger can be removed by gentle scraping of a straight edge such as a credit card. For most cases, washing the area with soap and water is the only decontamination necessary. If the person is sprayed with ant venom, water should be used to rinse the formic acid from the eyes and mucous membranes.[6]

Supportive Care

For most envenomations, all that is necessary is local wound care, analgesia, tetanus prophylaxis, and a brief period of observation to make sure hypersensitivity does not occur. Secondary infections are likely greater with vespid envenomations as compared with honey bees since vespids reuse their stinger and sometimes break the skin with their mandible.[40] Regardless, the risk for infection is small, and prophylactic antibiotics are not recommended. Ice packs, antihistamine lotion/cream, and topical antimicrobials may be helpful. Oral antihistamines are often used but are of questionable effectiveness except with more severe local reactions or generalized urticaria.[37,38] Oral corticosteroids may be effective in extensive local reactions.[38] Immobilization and elevation of the stung extremity will help reduce swelling.[37]

There are no uniformly effective treatments for fire ant envenomation.[48] Cold compresses, oral antihistamine, and corticosteroids may be helpful for symptoms.[42] Reactions are thought to be primarily immunogenic, and prophylactic antibiotics are not routinely recommended. Proactive breaking of blisters is discouraged.[38] Massive fire ant stings in the absence of allergic reactions can usually be managed with topical corticosteroids and oral antihistamines.[42]

Treatment of severe signs and symptoms of anaphylaxis is beyond the scope of this chapter. Multiple stings that produce systemic toxicity or severe hypersensitivity reactions (e.g., anaphylaxis) require aggressive therapy and ICU observation. Those patients with greater than 50 to 100 bee stings should be hospitalized and observed for signs of systemic toxicity.[39] The treatment of all severe reactions includes the administration of intravenous crystalloid, parenteral corticosteroids, H_1- and H_2-receptor antagonists (antihistamines), epinephrine (subcutaneous or intravenous), and inhaled β_2-adrenergic receptor agonists. Close cardiac, hemodynamic, and urine output monitoring is warranted in such patients. All patients with systemic symptoms or that require epinephrine should have a 12-lead electrocardiogram performed.[6,37,38] These patients should be admitted and monitored for 12 to 24 hours for coagulopathy and evidence of renal compromise.[38] Massive envenomations may be at risk for subsequent delayed type III serum sickness reactions that can typically be treated with NSAIDs and corticosteroids.

Antidote

A group in the United Kingdom has developed an antivenom for use in patients with multiple bee stings. While it has been effective in animal models, there has been no documented use in humans.[38]

DISPOSITION

Patients presenting immediately after envenomation should be monitored for an appropriate period of time, usually 1 to 2 hours, for signs and symptoms of hypersensitivity progression and anaphylaxis. Patients who are asymptomatic or have minimal local reactions without progression may then be safely discharged. They should be instructed to return immediately for recrudescent or delayed-onset allergic signs and symptoms (e.g., urticaria, difficulty breathing). For mildly symptomatic patients with appropriate access to health care or asymptomatic patients with a documented prior sensitivity, many advocate a short 3-day course of oral antihistamines and corticosteroids. Moderate hypersensitivity reactions, such as isolated urticaria without hypotension or respiratory difficulty, may be treated with a short

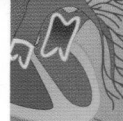

observation period until their signs and symptoms improve or resolve. They should also receive a 3-day course of antihistamines and corticosteroids. If a patient has been treated with epinephrine prior to arrival or during observation, they should be observed for at least 2 hours after the administration of epinephrine to ensure that they exhibit no hypersensitivity recrudescence; significant symptom recurrence is uncommon. Severe symptomatology requires observation for 24 hours or longer if persistently symptomatic. Fifty stings in a child or 100 stings in an adult may also be life threatening,[39] so patients who are victims of severe attacks with multiple stings merit 24-hour observation.

Patients that develop moderate to severe hypersensitivity reactions should always be discharged with a prescription for an epinephrine auto-injector and education regarding the use of the auto-injector and prevention of further hymenoptera stings (see Box 22B-2). In addition, they should schedule outpatient follow-up with an allergist for more specific testing and consideration for immunotherapy.

OTHER VENOMOUS ARTHROPODS

Lepidoptera

Lepidoptera is the order of the class Insecta that includes butterflies and moths. Sixteen families have venomous species, which are largely caterpillars with venomous spines. One such stinging caterpillar is the saddleback caterpillar (*Sibine stimulea*) in the family Limacodidae (Fig. 22B-8). Envenomation generally occurs accidentally when brushing against one of these caterpillars or attempting to remove it by hand from clothing or on the body. These sharp hairs or spines are either hollow, connected to poison glands (venom flows on contact), or similar to glass fibers (hairs break off in skin easily) sometimes causing pain like a needle prick. The venom of stinging caterpillars is poorly characterized and typically produces an urticarial rash and minimal local discomfort after contact.[38] This rash may develop over a few hours and last for a week. In addition, detached spines can lodge in the eye and cause conjunctivitis or keratitis.[38] The recommended treatment is to remove the spines with an adhesive tape while trying to avoid rubbing the area of contact. Analgesics, including anti-inflammatory drugs (e.g., NSAIDs), antihistamines, and topical corticosteroids are also recommended. Patients with a spine lodged in their eye need to be referred to an ophthalmologist for microscope-assisted removal. Lepidoptera envenomations can be prevented by not handling caterpillars, wearing protective clothing when participating in activities that put one in contact with the caterpillar habitat, spraying trees with appropriate pesticides, and using window screens.[6,38]

The puss caterpillar or woolly caterpillar (*Megalopyge opercularis*) is the most medically significant species in the southern United States (Fig. 22B-9); its habitat extends between Texas and Missouri. Puss caterpillar stings can cause dyspnea, seizures, abdominal pain, hypotension, and characteristic hemorrhagic pinpoint papular lesions (Fig. 22B-10).[38]

In South America, *Lonomia achelous* and *Lonomia oblique* are caterpillars that can cause severe envenomations and have a mortality rate three to six times higher than envenomations from snakebites.[6] The venom contains a component (Lonomine V) believed to be responsible for coagulopathy by inactivating factor XIII.[6] Contact with *Lonomia* spines causes immediate pain followed by headache a few hours later. The contact site develops ecchymosis that may spread to the rest of the body. Brain hemorrhages secondary to coagulopathy can develop.[6] Patients with coagulopathy may benefit from administration of *L. oblique* antivenom.[49]

Hemiptera (Sucking Bugs)

These bugs include the traitomines (kissing bugs, vinchuca bugs), assassin bugs (family Reduviidae), and

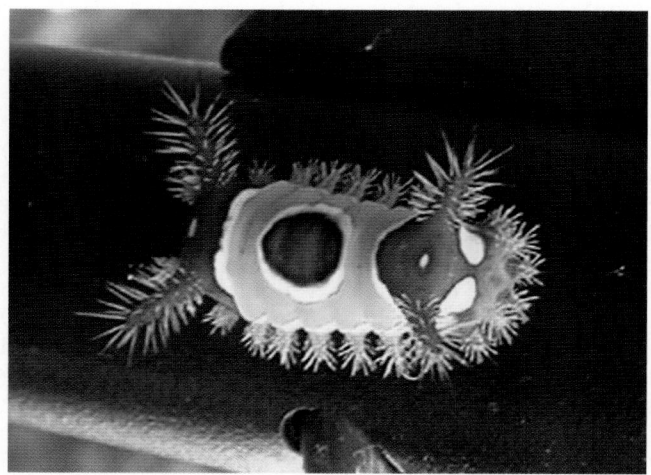

FIGURE 22B-8 Saddleback caterpillar (*Sibine stimulea*). (Courtesy of J.D. Hinkle.)

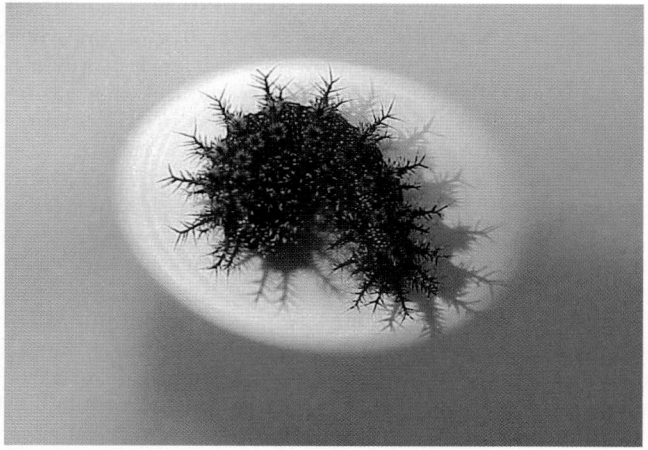

FIGURE 22B-9 Puss caterpillar (*Megalopyge opercularis*). (Courtesy of Christopher Holstege, MD, University of Virginia.)

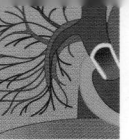

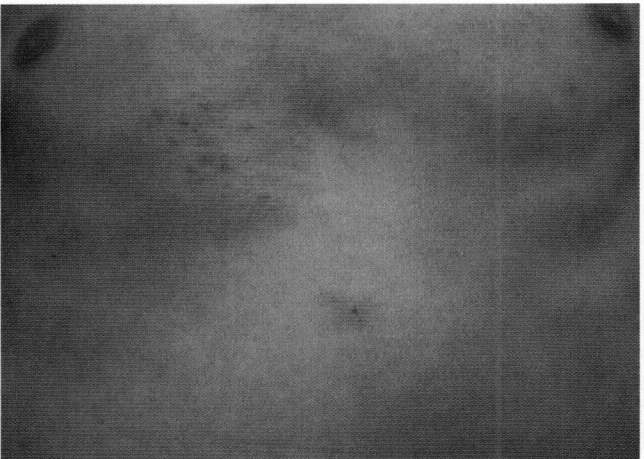

FIGURE 22B-10 Papular lesions from contact with the pus caterpillar. (Courtesy of Alexander Baer, MD, University of Virginia.)

bed bugs (family Cinicidae). They are 2 to 4 cm in length and have a proboscis that allows them to suck blood from their prey. The venom is used to subjugate prey and may aid with their digestion. The bites are painless but cause pruritic papules that form a line or a cluster. Patients may develop fever, lymphadenopathy, hemorrhagic bullae, urticarial wheals, and even anaphylactic reactions. Treatment is supportive and symptomatic. Preventive actions include using insecticides and wearing protective garments.

Beetles

Blister beetles (family Meloidae) and rove beetles (genus *Paederus* from family Staphylinidae) are found in the Eastern United States, Europe, Africa, and Asia. These beetles produce harm to humans primarily when they are crushed against the skin, releasing secretions that contain cantharidin (blister beetles) and pederin (rove beetles), respectively. Skin contact with cantharidin causes noninflammatory vesicles or bullae that are painless unless they are ruptured.[38] Ingestion of Spanish fly, an aphrodisiac composed of dried blister beetles, may lead to burning sensation in the pharynx and esophagus, hematemesis, flank and suprapubic pain, and occasionally nephritis. Eye contact with cantharidin causes severe edema and conjunctivitis.[6] Skin contact with pederin causes vesicular lesions that appear 12 to 36 hours after the exposure. The lesions follow the shape of the area of contact with the crushed beetle. They last up to 2 weeks and are followed by a postinflammatory hyperpigmentation. Other parts of the body such as the eyes may become affected secondary to autoinoculation.[50] The skin should be washed promptly with water after contact with the beetle's secretions. General chemical burn care should be followed; treatment with antihistamines and steroids is not helpful. Preventive actions include turning off lamps at dusk in endemic areas and avoiding crushing the beetles on the skin.[50]

Ticks

Ticks belong to either one of two families: Ixodidae (hard body) or Argasidae (soft body). They are ovoid in shape and reach a maximal size of 1.5 cm when engorged with blood. They are known for their ability to stick to their prey using their teeth and secretions. Ticks are better known as vectors for infectious diseases such as Rocky Mountain spotted fever, typhus, tularemia, and Lyme disease, among others. However, tick paralysis is a toxin-mediated syndrome. Tick paralysis is caused by 43 species of ticks, only 4 of which are medically important. These are *Dermacentor andersoni* and *Dermacentor variabilis* in North America and *Ixodes holocyclus* and *Ixodes cornuatus* in Australia. Ticks produce a neurotoxin in their salivary glands that inhibits the release of acetylcholine at the neuromuscular junction, thus leading to flaccid paralysis. The toxin that is injected along with their saliva has local anesthetic and anticoagulant properties.[6]

Clinically, the symptoms of tick paralysis appear within 4 to 7 days after the bite. It is an acute, ascending, flaccid motor paralysis that can be confused with Guillain-Barré syndrome, botulism, and myasthenia gravis. Prodromal symptoms are seen with *Dermacentor* bites, which include facial and limb paresthesias. Children bit by *Ixodes* ticks may present with ataxia. Symptoms progress further to generalized weakness, flaccid paralysis, and respiratory and bulbar paralysis. Treatment of tick paralysis is tick removal and supportive care. The signs and symptoms typically improve with time after removal of the tick but may initially progress for 48 hours prior to clinical improvement. Australian antivenom is occasionally used in cases of severe muscle paralysis.[6] Its efficacy, however, is unproven.[49] Preventive measures include wearing long-sleeved garments when present in a forest, use of insect repellants, checking for ticks on a regular basis, and avoiding squeezing the tick if attached to the skin. Medium-tipped, blunt forceps may be used, if available, to remove the ticks.[51] When using insect repellants, permethrin applied to garments, and *N,N*-diethyltoluamide applied to exposed skin are effective agents.

Centipedes

Centipedes are arthropods that belong to the Chilopoda family. They comprise more than 3000 species within four orders, only two of which, Scolopendromorpha and Scutigeromorpha, are of medical importance.[52] They have an elongated segmented body with a pair of legs in each segment. The first pair of legs is modified into a biting structure that injects venom stored in a sack to paralyze the prey. Centipedes range in size from 1 to 30 cm and are distributed widely in warm, temperate, and tropical regions.[53] Their venom contains proteins like serotonin, histamine, and various enzymes.[54]

A bite from a centipede consists of two puncture wounds with localized pain, edema, and regional lymphadenopathy (Fig. 22B-11). In a prospective study that examined the clinical course of 44 centipede bites,

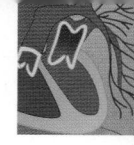

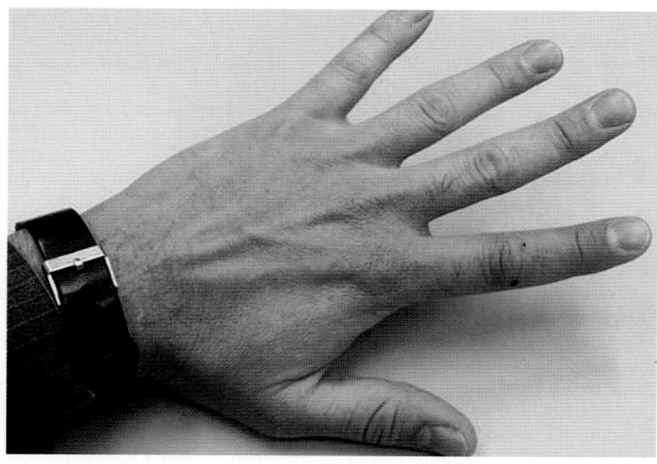

FIGURE 22B-11 Centipede bite. (Courtesy of Scott Stockwell, PhD.)

it was found that systemic symptoms were absent and the clinical course was usually short (less than 2 days).[52] Occasionally, the wound is complicated by necrosis and gangrene, possibly from secondary infections.[6]

Certain tropical centipedes may cause systemic findings such as nausea, headache, restlessness, tachycardia, and fever.[6] Myocardial ischemia has been reported after centipede envenomation.[54,55] Eosinophilic cellulitis or Wells' syndrome has also been associated with a centipede sting.[56] Treatment for centipede envenomation includes local wound care, analgesics, and tetanus prophylaxis. Antibiotics should be reserved for infected wounds.[53,57]

Millipedes

Millipedes are arthropods that belong to the Diplopoda family. They have elongated segmental bodies with one pair of legs per segment. They do not bite, but can secrete and spray a noxious substance that causes a mahogany-colored skin lesion. This skin discoloration has been confused with child abuse, thermal burns, and gangrene. It may persist for months.[58] Some can spray secretions up to 25 cm, which can affect the eyes, leading to periorbital edema, chemical keratoconjunctivitis, corneal ulcers, and even blindness, in rare cases.[59] Management is symptomatic and supportive. Eye exposures require irrigation with normal saline followed by examination with fluorescein dye to look for corneal abrasions. Antibiotic, corticosteroid, and cycloplegic (for ciliary spasm) eyedrops are recommended.[59]

REFERENCES

1. Curry SC, Vance MV, Ryan PJ, et al: Envenomation by the scorpion Centruroides sculpturatus. J Toxicol Clin Toxicol 1983–1984;21: 417–449.
2. Lucas SM, Meier J: Biology and distribution of scorpions of medical importance. In Meier J, White J (eds): Handbook of Clinical Toxicology of Animal Venoms and Poisons. Boca Raton, FL, CRC Press, 1995, pp 205–219.
3. Dehesa-Davila M, Alagon AC, Possani LD: Clinical toxicology of scorpion stings. In Meier J, White J (eds): Handbook of Clinical Toxicology of Animal Venoms and Poisons. Boca Raton, FL, CRC Press, 1995, pp 221–237.
4. Suchard JR, Connor DA: Scorpion envenomation. In Auerbach PS (ed): Wilderness Medicine, 4th ed. St. Louis, MO, Mosby, 2001, pp 839–862.
5. Valdez-Cruz NA, Davila S, Licea A, et al: Biochemical, genetic and physiological characterization of venom components from two species of scorpions: Centruroides exilicauda Wood and Centruroides sculpturatus Ewing. Biochimie 2004;86:387–396.
6. Mebs D: Venomous and Poisonous Animals. Boca Raton, FL, CRC Press, 2002.
7. Saucier JR: Arachnid envenomation. Emerg Med Clin North Am 2004;22:405–422.
8. Amitai Y: Clinical manifestations and management of scorpion envenomation. Public Health Rep 1998;26:257–263.
9. Isbister GK, Volschenk ES, Seymour JE: Scorpion stings in Australia: five definite stings and a review. Intern Med J 2004;34:427–430.
10. Abroug F, ElAtrous S, Nouira S, et al: Serotherapy in scorpion envenomation: a randomised controlled trail. Lancet 1999;354: 906–909.
11. Hammoudi-Triki D, Ferquel E, Robbe-Vincent A, et al: Epidemiological data, clinical admission gradation and biological quantification by ELISA of scorpion envenomations in Algeria: effect of immunotherapy. Trans R Soc Trop Med Hyg 2004;98:240–250.
12. Watson WA, Litovitz TL, Klein-Schwartz W, et al: 2003 annual report of the American Association of Poison Control Centers Toxic Exposure Surveillance System. Am J Emerg Med 2004; 22:335–404.
13. Watson WA, Litovitz TL, Rodgers GC Jr, et al: 2002 annual report of the American Association of Poison Control Centers Toxic Exposure Surveillance System. Am J Emerg Med 2003;21:353–421.
14. Litovitz TL, Klein-Schwartz W, White S, et al: 2000 Annual report of the American Association of Poison Control Centers Toxic Exposure Surveillance System. Am J Emerg Med 2001;19:337–395.
15. Centers for Disease Control and Prevention: Wide-ranging online data for epidemiologic research (WONDER): compressed mortality file. Accessed February 7, 2005, at http://wonder.cdc.gov/mort SQL.html.
16. Ben-Abraham R, Eshel G, Winkler E, et al: Triage for Leiurus quinquestriatus scorpion envenomation in children—is routine ICU hospitalization necessary? Hum Exp Toxicol 2000;19:663–666.
17. Zhijian C, Yingliang W, Jiqun S, et al: Evidence of the existence of a common ancestor of scorpion toxins affecting ion channels. J Biochem Mol Toxicol 2003;17:235–238.
18. Ismail M: The scorpion envenoming syndrome. Toxicon 1995; 33:825–858.
19. Chase PB, Vazquez HL, Boyer L, et al: Serum levels and urine detection of Centruroides sculpturatus venom in significantly envenomated patients. J Toxicol Clin Toxicol 2002;40:650.
20. Gibly R, Williams M, Walter FG, et al: Continuous intravenous midazolam infusion for Centruroides exilicauda scorpion envenomation. Ann Emerg Med 1999;34:620–635.
21. Langley RL: A review of venomous animal bites and stings in pregnant patients. Wilderness Environ Med 2004;15:207–215.
22. Marei ZA, Ibrahim SA: Stimulation of rat uterus by venom from the scorpion L. quinquestriatus. Toxicon 1979;17:251–258.
23. Radmanesh M: Clinical study of Hemiscorpion lepturus in Iran. J Trop Med Hyg 1990;93:327–332.
24. Krifi MN, Kharrat H, Zghal K, et al: Development of an ELISA for the detection of scorpion venoms in sera of humans envenomed by Androctonus australis garzoni (Aag) and Buthus occitanus tunetanus (Bot): correlation with clinical severity of envenoming in Tunisia. Toxicon 1998;36:887–900.
25. Walter FG, Bilden EF, Gibly RL: Envenomations. Crit Care Clin 1999;15:353–386.
26. Murthy K, Zolfagharian H, et al: Disseminated intravascular coagulation & disturbances in carbohydrate & fat metabolism in acute myocarditis produced by scorpion (Buthus tamulus) venom. Indian J Med Res 1988;87:318–325.
27. Devi CS, Reddy CN, Devi SL, et al: Defibrination syndrome due to scorpion venom poisoning. BMJ 1970;1:345-7, 1970.
28. Gueron M, Ilia R, Margulis G: Arthropod poisons and the cardiovascular system. Am J Emerg Med 2000;18:708–714.
29. Kolecki P: Inadvertent methamphetamine poisoning in pediatric patients. Pediatr Emerg Care 1998;14:385.

30. Bawaskar HS, Bawaskar PH: Clinical profile of severe scorpion envenomation in children at rural setting. Indian Pediatr 2003;40:1072–1081.

31. Dehesa-Davila M: Epidemiological characteristics of scorpion sting in Leon, Guanajuato, Mexico. Toxicon 1989;27:281–286.

32. Freire-Maia L, Campos JA: Pathophysiology and treatment of scorpion poisoning. In Ownby CL, Odell GV (eds): Natural Toxins. Characterization, Pharmacology and Therapeutics. New York, Pergamon, 1989, pp 139–159.

33. Bond GR: Antivenom administration for Centruroides scorpion sting: risks and benefits. Ann Emerg Med 1992;21:788–791.

34. LoVecchio F, Welch S, Klemens J, et al: Incidence of immediate and delayed hypersensitivity to Centruroides antivenom. Ann Emerg Med 1999;34:615–619.

35. Hamed MI: Treatment of the scorpion envenoming syndrome: 12-years experience with serotherapy. Int J Antimicrob Agents 2003;21:170–174.

36. Belghith M, Boussarsar M, Haguig H, et al: Efficacy of serotherapy in scorpion sting: a matched pair study. Clin Toxicol 1999; 37:51–57.

37. Mosbech H: Clinical toxicology of hymenopteran stings. In Meier J, White J (eds): Handbook of Clinical Toxicology of Animal Venoms and Poisons. Boca Raton, FL, CRC Press, 1995, pp 349–359.

38. Minton SA, Bechtel HB, Erikson TB: North American arthropod envenomation and parasitism. In Auerbach PS (ed): Wilderness Medicine, 4th ed. St. Louis, Mosby, 2001, pp 863–887.

39. Meier J: Biology and distribution of hymenopterans of medical importance, their venom apparatus and venom composition. In Meier J, White J (eds): Handbook of Clinical Toxicology of Animal Venoms and Poisons. Boca Raton, FL, CRC Press, 1995, pp 331–348.

40. Barss P: Renal failure and death after multiple stings in Papua New Guinea. Med J Aust 1989;151:659–663.

41. Steen CJ, Carbonaro PA, Schwartz RA: Arthropods in dermatology. J Am Acad Dermatol 2004;50:819–842.

42. Kemp SF, deShazo RD, Moffitt JE, et al: Expanding habitat of the imported fire ant (Solenopsis invicta): a public health concern. J Allergy Clin Immunol 2000;105:683–691.

43. Schwartz HJ, Sutheimer C, Gauerke MB, Yuninger JW: Hymenoptera venom-specific IgE antibodies in post-mortem serum from victims of sudden, unexpected death. Clin Allergy 1988;18:461–468.

44. Wright D, Lockey R: Local reactions to stinging insects (Hymenoptera). Allergy Proc 1990;11:23.

45. Schwartz H, Yuninger J, Schwartz L: Is unrecognized anaphylaxis a cause of sudden unexpected death? Clin Exp Allergy 1995; 25:866–870.

46. Prahlow J, Barnard J: Fatal anaphylaxis due to fire ant stings. Am J Forensic Med Pathol 1998;19:137–142.

47. Visscher PK, Vetter RS, Camazine S: Removing bee stings. Lancet 1996;348:301–302.

48. Hile DC, Coon TP, Skinner CG, et al: Treatment of imported fire ant stings with Mitigator Sting and Bile Treatment—a randomized control study. Wilderness Environ Med 2006;17:21–25.

49. Isbister GK, Graudins A, White J, Warrell D: Antivenom treatment in arachnidism. J Toxicol Clin Toxicol 2003;41:291–300.

50. Zargari O, Kimyai-Asadi A, Fathalikhani F, Panahi M: Paederus dermatitis in northern Iran: a report of 156 cases. Int J Dermatol 2003;42:608–612.

51. Gammons M, Salam G: Tick removal. Am Fam Physician 2002; 66:643–645.

52. Balit CR, Harvey MS, Waldock JM, Isbister GK: Prospective study of centipede bites in Australia. J Toxicol Clin Toxicol 2004;42:41–48.

53. Bush SP, King BO, Norris RL, Stockwell SA: Centipede envenomation. Wilderness Environ Med 2001;12:93–99.

54. Yildiz A, Biçeroglu S, Yakut N, et al: Acute myocardial infarction in a young man caused by centipede sting. Emerg Med J 2006;23:e30.

55. Ozsarac M, Karcioglu O, Ayrik C, et al: Acute coronary ischemia following centipede envenomation: case report and review of the literature. Wilderness Environ Med 2004;15:109–112.

56. Friedman IS, Phelps RG, Baral J, Sapadin AN: Wells' syndrome triggered by centipede bite. Int J Dermatol 1998;37:602–605.

57. McFee RB, Caraccio TR, Mofenson HC, McGuigan MA: Envenomation by the Vietnamese centipede in a Long Island pet store [Letter]. Clin Toxicol 2002;40:573–574.

58. Elston DM: What's eating you? Millipedes (Diplopoda). Cutis 2001;67:452.

59. Hudson BJ, Parsons GA: Giant millipede "burns" and the eye. Trans R Soc Trop Med Hyg 1997;91:183–185.

23 *Mushrooms*

JEFFREY BRENT, MD, PHD ■ ROBERT B. PALMER, PHD

At a Glance...

- Life-threatening or major organ–threatening mushroom syndromes typically present with symptoms starting greater than 6 hours following ingestion.
- Gastrointestinal symptoms that occur within a few hours of ingestion do not rule out poisoning by the more dangerous mushrooms.
- As with most poisonings, supportive care is of primary importance in toxic mushroom ingestions.
- The mushrooms of greatest concern are the hepatotoxic species of *Amanita*.
- Although several antidotes have been proposed and are used for the treatment of hepatotoxic *Amanita* poisoning, none have been proven to be efficacious.
- Mushrooms containing orellanine may cause renal failure, which may not become evident for days to weeks postingestion.
- Poisonings by mushrooms containing gyromitrin, such as the *Gyromitra* spp. (false morels), may benefit from treatment with pyridoxine.
- Poisonings by mushrooms containing muscarine, such as some *Inocybe* and *Clitocybe* spp., may benefit from treatment with atropine if there are excessive muscarinic cholinergic effects.

INTRODUCTION AND RELEVANT HISTORY

Mushrooms are the sexual organs, or fruiting bodies, of fungi. The word *mushroom* is derived from an early Greek term which roughly translates to "mucus"—the stuff the ancients thought to be the substance of origin of both mushrooms and frogs.[1] Of the possibly 10,000 species of mushrooms worldwide, only 50 to 100 are known to be toxic. Little is known about the toxic effects of ingestion of most mushrooms, although fatalities do occur. However, toxins derived from mushrooms cannot be universally condemned because many such compounds have been used as leads for antimicrobial and antineoplastic agents. Mushroom poisonings most frequently result from the growing trend worldwide of foraging for edible fungi. They are used for food, in religious ceremonies, and even as medication by herbal healers. Typically, mushrooms are identified by experience, through guidebooks, or simply by feeding them to domestic animals as a bioassay of toxicity. Of the earliest reports of mushroom poisoning, the most notable was the tragic account of the Greek poet Euripides, who described the death of his wife and three children due to the ingestion of poisonous mushrooms.[2]

It is probably easiest to understand mushroom toxicology by categorizing mushrooms into groups based on the toxins they contain and the symptoms and signs they may cause. For a patient with a history of toxic mushroom ingestion, the clinical picture may help determine to which group the mushroom belonged, pending definitive identification. In the majority of cases, the true identity of the offending mushroom is unknown. Analysis of exposures reported to poison control centers in the United States indicates that the precise species of mushroom is identified in only 3.4% of all exposures.[3] However, even in the absence of positive identification, the clinical syndrome being treated may be identified and appropriate therapeutic measures undertaken. In the majority of cases, no illness results from mushroom ingestion.[3] The possible mushroom-associated syndromes and the typical causative species are listed in Table 23-1. Determining the type of mushroom ingested based on the presenting syndrome is analogous to what is encountered daily in the clinical practice of clinical toxicology with patients who overdose on unknown medications.

GENERAL MANAGEMENT

Current concepts of the management of mushroom poisoning are evolutionary and dynamic, and, thus, fraught with debate and controversy. As with all poisonings, supportive care is of primary importance in toxic mushroom ingestions. Airway management and cardiopulmonary resuscitation, along with maintenance of vital signs, should take priority over positively identifying the toxin or searching for specific antidotes.

Guidelines for initial management of toxic mushroom poisoning are listed in Box 23-1. Most patients with symptoms after mushroom ingestion have prominent gastrointestinal (GI) complaints: vomiting, diarrhea (possibly bloody), and abdominal pain. If vomiting and diarrhea are severe enough to result in significant hypovolemia, intravenous fluid and electrolyte repletion with a glucose-containing solution should be initiated. It is critical to determine the time course of the development of symptoms after ingestion. Symptoms developing more than 6 hours after ingestion can be assumed to be due to mushrooms belonging to the cyclopeptide (commonly the deadly *Amanita*), gyromitrin, or orellanine groups. With mushrooms from the orellanine group, symptoms may develop more than 24 hours after ingestion. It is emphasized, however, that GI symptoms occurring within a few hours of ingestion do not rule out poisoning by the more dangerous mushrooms. It is common for people to ingest a number of different mushrooms simultaneously, including those that cause early symptoms. In addition, ingestion of cytotoxic mushrooms may rarely produce symptom onset within 6 hours of ingestion.

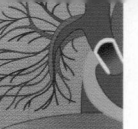

TABLE 23-1 Summary of Common Mushroom-Associated Syndromes*

SYNDROME	CLINICAL COURSE	TOXIN(S)	TYPICAL CAUSATIVE MUSHROOM(S)
Delayed gastroenteritis followed by hepatorenal syndrome	Stage 1: 24 hr after ingestion: onset of nausea, vomiting, profuse cholera-like diarrhea, abdominal pain, hematuria Stage 2: 12–48 hr after ingestion: apparent recovery; levels of hepatic enzymes are rising during this stage Stage 3: 24–72 hr after ingestion: progressive hepatic and renal failure, coagulopathy, cardiomyopathy, encephalopathy, convulsions, coma, death	Cyclopeptides, principally amatoxins	"Deadly *Amanitas*," *Galerina* species
Hyperactivity, delirium, coma	30 min–2 hr after ingestion: delirium, hallucinations, and coma	Muscimol, ibotenic acid	*Amanita muscaria, Amanita pantherina*
Delayed gastroenteritis with central nervous system abnormalities	6–24 hr after ingestion: nausea, vomiting, diarrhea, abdominal pain muscle cramps, delirium, convulsions, coma; hemolysis and methemoglobinemia may occur	Gyromitrin	*Gyromitra esculenta* ("false morel")
Cholinergic syndrome	30 min–2 hr after ingestion: bradycardia, bronchorrhea, bronchospasm, salivation, perspiration, lacrimation, convulsions, coma	Muscarine	*Boletus* species, *Clitocybe* species, *Inocybe* species, *Amanita* species
Disulfiram-like reaction with ethanol	30 min after drinking ethanol (may occur up to 1 wk after eating coprine-containing mushrooms): flushing of skin of face and trunk, hypotension, tachycardia, chest pain, dyspnea, nausea, vomiting, extreme apprehension	Coprine	*Coprinus atramentarius*
Hallucinations	30 min–3 hr after ingestion: hallucinations, euphoria, drowsiness, compulsive behavior, agitation	Psilocybin and psilocyn	*Psilocybe* species
Delayed gastritis and renal failure	Abdominal pain, anorexia, vomiting starting over 30 hr after ingestion, followed by progressive renal failure 3 to 14 days later	Orelline, orellanine	*Cortinarius* species
Immune-mediated hemolytic anemia	Syncope, gastroenteritis, oliguria, hemoglobinuria, back pain, hemolysis	Immunoglobulin mediated	*Paxillus involutus*
General gastrointestinal irritants	30 min–2 hr after ingestion: nausea, vomiting, abdominal cramping, diarrhea; may recover without treatment	Unidentified, probably multiple	*Chlorophyllum molybdites*, backyard mushrooms ("little brown mushrooms"), many others

*See Box 23-2 for an extensive list of mushrooms causing these syndromes.

Activated charcoal, if administered in the first hour or two postinjection, may be of benefit in adsorbing any toxin remaining in the gut. Any gastric contents obtained by spontaneous emesis should be saved and examined for spores. To examine for spores, the gastric aspirate or emesis sample should be filtered through cheesecloth and centrifuged for 10 minutes. The heavier layer at the bottom of the test tube contains the spores, and a sample is carefully removed with a pipette. A drop of water is then added, a coverslip placed, and the slide examined under oil immersion. Generally, mushroom spores are similar in size to red blood cells (8 to 20 μm). Spores found in either the gastric contents or the lamellae of the mushroom should be examined under the microscope for (1) general appearance, (2) shape,

(3) color, (4) thick or thin walls, and (5) the presence of pores.[4]

Identification of suspected toxic mushrooms can be difficult. In fact, because even veteran mushroom hunters occasionally make an error, many have adopted the practice of eating only one kind of mushroom at a time and saving a sample in case unanticipated effects occur. A spore print can be helpful in identifying the mushroom in question. This is formed by placing the cap of the mushroom on a white piece of paper (Fig. 23-1) and allowing the spores to fall on the paper, imparting a characteristic color. An example of a spore print is shown in Figure 23-2. Because an adequate spore print generally takes several hours to develop, one should be started as soon as possible. It is usually helpful to cover the cap with

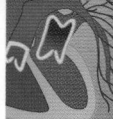

| BOX 23-1 | **GENERAL MANAGEMENT OF MUSHROOM INGESTION** |

1. Determine history of ingestion: how many types of mushrooms ingested, what time, if anyone else ate them, and what symptoms are present.
2. Attempt to determine which of the possible syndromes (see Table 23-1) the patient may have. For example, gastrointestinal symptoms occurring more than 6 hr after ingestion strongly suggest cyclopeptide, gyromitrin, or *Cortinarius* poisoning.
3. Administer activated charcoal. If the patient has diarrhea, do not give a cathartic. If a cathartic is used, give it only with the first dose of activated charcoal. Use repeated doses of activated charcoal for suspected amatoxin poisonings.
4. If feasible and when indicated, send gastric aspirate or emesis, along with any remaining mushrooms, to a mycologist for identification.
5. Try to perform a preliminary identification of mushroom and spores. Start to develop a spore print as soon as possible.
6. Maintain supportive measures, including airway support, intravenous fluids, and vasopressors (if needed). Monitor volume status.
7. Avoid antispasmodics for gastrointestinal symptoms.
8. Anticipate the clinical course (see Table 23-1).

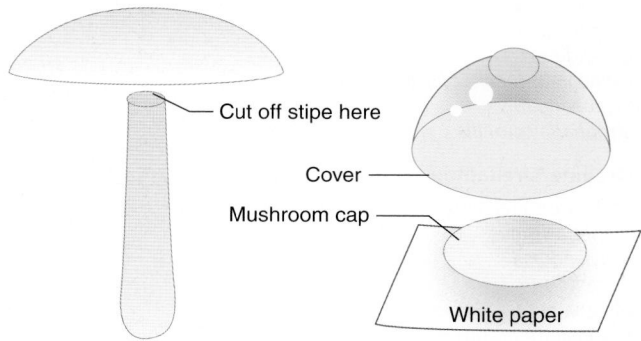

Cut off stipe here

Cover

Mushroom cap

White paper

FIGURE 23-1 Technique of drawing a spore print. (From Rumack BH, Salzman E [eds]: Mushroom Poisoning: Diagnosis and Treatment. West Palm Beach, FL, CRC Press, 1978. Copyright the Chemical Rubber Company, CRC Press, Inc.)

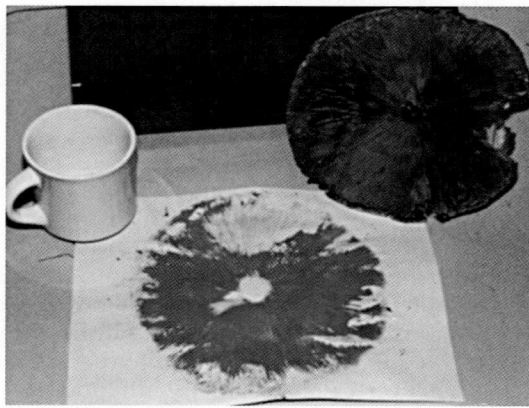

FIGURE 23-2 Spore print of *Chlorophyllum molybdites*. (Courtesy of Lynn Augenstein, MD, and the Rocky Mountain Poison Center, Denver, CO.)

a glass or bowl while the spore print is being formed to prevent the dispersion of spores by drafts. Other techniques, such as digital imaging, may also assist in mushroom identification.[5]

A professional mycologist should be able to describe the principal types of mushrooms in a given region and may also assist in mushroom identification. Local or regional poison centers should know how to reach mycologists in their region. When a patient is seen after a mushroom ingestion, family members or friends should be asked to bring in a similar mushroom (if possible) for identification purposes. The specimen should be refrigerated, wrapped in wax paper, and stored in a paper bag (a thorough discussion of mushroom identification may be found in appropriate references).[6] It should also be kept in mind that, with the Internet and the associated increase in international commerce, even professional mycologists may have difficulty identifying foreign mushroom species.

Of greatest concern in mushroom poisoning is the ingestion of the potentially deadly *Amanita* species. Although many antidotes and treatments have been suggested for *Amanita* poisoning, most of them are unproven. By consulting Table 23-1, the group to which the ingested mushrooms may belong should be apparent. For ease of discussion, further management recommendations are described under the specific toxins. Common mushroom species containing the toxins discussed are listed in Box 23-2.

CYCLOPEPTIDE POISONING

Overview

The cyclopeptide-containing mushrooms are responsible for more than 90% of all deaths due to mushroom poisonings in the Western world. These mushrooms are found predominantly throughout Europe and North America. The cyclopeptides are found mainly in species from three genera: *Amanita*, *Galerina*, and *Lepiota* (see Box 23-2 and Figs. 23-3 to 23-5). The vast majority of serious poisonings and fatalities in this group of mushrooms, however, result from *Amanita*, particularly *Amanita phalloides* (see Fig. 23-3). Ingestion of deadly *Amanita* most commonly occurs after misidentification of the mushroom by foragers, although the possibility of criminal or terrorist use of toxins isolated from *Amanita* species has also been suggested.[7] These mushrooms are most commonly found during the late summer or autumn in well-forested areas. The cyclopeptide toxins consist primarily of amatoxins, which contain eight amino acids, and the seven residue phallotoxins and virotoxins. More than 15 cyclopeptides have been isolated from the genus *Amanita*. Note, however, that not all mushrooms of the *Amanita* species contain significant quantities of amatoxin. *Amanita muscaria* and *Amanita pantherina*, for example, contain no amatoxin, and ingestion of these mushrooms is not associated with development of hepatotoxicity.

The phallotoxins are extremely potent hepatotoxins but are not well absorbed from the GI tract and therefore

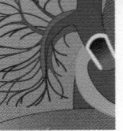

BOX 23-2   SOME MUSHROOM SPECIES, BY CLINICAL GROUPING OF TOXINS

Cyclopeptides (Amatoxins, Phallotoxins)

Amanita phalloides ("death cap" or "green death cap")
A. verna ("death angel")
A. virosa ("destroying angel" or "white destroying angel")
A. bisporigera ("white destroying angel")
A. ocreata
A. suballiacea
A. tenuifolia
Galerina autumnalis
G. marginata
G. venenata
Lepiota helveola
L. brunneoincarnata
L. chlorophyllum
L. vosserandii
Conocybe filaris

Muscimol, Ibotenic Acid

Amanita muscaria ("fly agaric")
A. pantherina
A. gemmata
A. cokeri
A. cothurnata
A. regalis

Monomethylhydrazine

Gyromitra esculenta ("false morel")
G. gigas
G. amabigua
G. infula
G. caroliniana
G. brunnea
G. fastigiata
Paxina spp.
Sarcosphaera coronaria
Cyathipodia macropus

Muscarine

Boletus calopus
B. luridus
B. pulcherrimus
B. satanas
Clitocybe cerrusata
C. dealbata
C. illudens

C. rivulosa
Inocybe fastigiata
I. geophylla
I. lilacina
I. patuoillardi
I. purica
I. rimosus
*Amanita muscaria**
*A. pantherina**

Coprine

Coprinus atramentarious ("inky cap")
Clitocybe clavipes

Indoles

Psilocybe cubensis
P. caerulescens
P. cyanescens
P. baeocystis
P. fimentaria
P. mexicana
P. pelluculosa
P. semilanceata
P. silvatica
Conocybe cyanopus
Gymnopilus aeruginosa
G. spectabilis
G. validipes
Panaeolous foenisecii ("mower's mushroom")
P. subbalteatus
Stropharia coronilla

Orelline/Orellanine

Cortinarius orellanus
C. speciosissinus
C. splendoma
C. gentilis
Mycena pura
Omphalatus orarius

General Gastrointestinal Irritants

Many species from diverse genera
"Little brown mushrooms" (backyard mushrooms)
Chlorophyllum molybdites
Omphalates illudens ("jack-o-lantern")

*Typically contain only trace amounts of muscarine.

---

contribute little to *Amanita* toxicity following ingestion. They may contribute to the initial gastroenteritis-like picture, although this has also been questioned.[8] Laboratory animals cannot be poisoned by oral administration of the phallotoxin phalloidin, whereas they die within hours after intravenous injection of the same compound.

Pathophysiology

Amatoxins are not only extremely potent hepatotoxins but are also actively absorbed from the GI tract.

Although α-amanitine is the principal toxin in this group, nine cyclic octapeptide amatoxins with molecular weights of approximately 900 Daltons, have been identified. Nucleoli of liver cells disintegrate soon after exposure to α-amanitine, resulting in interference with transcription of DNA by inhibiting RNA polymerase II. α-Amanitine accomplishes this by binding to the 140,000-Dalton subunit of RNA polymerase II. Because the primary action of amatoxins is inhibition of DNA transcription, tissues that are highly dependent on protein synthesis (namely, the GI tract and liver) are most sensitive to this poisoning. Once absorbed through

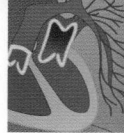

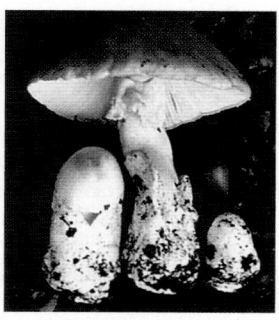

FIGURE 23-3 The death cap, *Amanita phalloides* (cyclopeptide). (Courtesy of Marilyn Shaw, Denver, CO.)

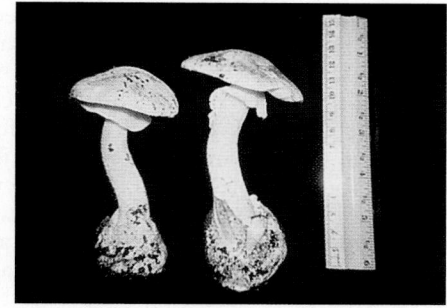

FIGURE 23-4 The destroying angel, *Amanita virosa* (cyclopeptide). (Courtesy of D.H. Mitchel and the Denver Botanic Gardens–Herbarium of Denver, CO.)

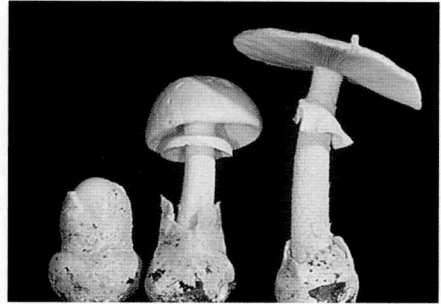

FIGURE 23-5 Fool's mushroom, *Amanita verna* (cyclopeptide). (Courtesy of Donald Simon, Wilmington, DE.)

the gut, amatoxins are transported into hepatocytes by a nonspecific transport system. Circulating amatoxin is not metabolized but excreted by the biliary system and the kidneys. Enterohepatic recirculation and biliary excretion of amatoxins are significant. The cyclopeptides are not denatured by boiling, and hence cooking deadly *Amanita* mushrooms does not render them nontoxic. It is estimated that approximately 0.1 mg/kg of oral amatoxin or the amount contained in one *A. phalloides* mushroom may be lethal to an adult.[6]

Clinical Presentation

The classic clinical presentation of *Amanita* poisoning can be divided into three stages (see Table 23-1). Patients do not have GI symptoms for at least 6 hours after ingestion,

and then they develop colicky abdominal pain, vomiting, and severe diarrhea (stage 1). The onset of symptoms may occur from 6 to 24 hours after ingestion. The diarrhea may contain blood and mucus and may be so severe that it has been termed *cholera-like*.

Even without treatment, patients may apparently recover (stage 2), although their hepatic enzyme levels may be rising. Two to 4 days after ingestion, patients may suffer fulminant hepatic, cardiac, and renal failure (stage 3). Pancreatitis, disseminated intravascular coagulation, convulsions, and death may then occur in the subsequent 2 to 4 days. The pathologic picture of hepatic necrosis tends to be most marked in the centrilobular (zone III) areas. In series of treated patients, the death rate due to *A. phalloides* poisoning ranges from 10% to 30%. Although many patients with cyclopeptide-induced hepatotoxicity recover fully, approximately 20% develop immune complex–mediated chronic active hepatitis with anti–smooth muscle antibodies. It is important to understand that not every patient will develop fulminant hepatic failure but may develop mild gastrointestinal and hepatoxic effects.

Diagnosis

The diagnosis of cyclopeptide mushroom poisoning is made largely from a positive history of ingestion coupled with suggestive physical findings (e.g., acute gastroenteritis, toxic hepatitis). Any patient with gastroenteritis should be specifically questioned about recent wild mushroom foraging and ingestion. Optimally, the mushroom (obtained from meal leftovers or from visiting the site of foraging) could be identified by an experienced mycologist, but this is rarely possible.

Several analytical techniques may be employed to assist diagnosis, which include detection of amatoxins from body fluids or utilization of bedside tests. Circulating amatoxins can be detected for hours after ingestion.[9] Most of the ingested α-amanitine is excreted renally, and urine levels tend to be higher than serum levels. Although amatoxins can be detected by very sensitive radioimmunoassay or high-pressure liquid chromatographic methods, these assays are not usually clinically available. The Meixner test is a bedside assay that can detect substituted indoles such as amatoxins. In this test, gastric material or pulverized mushroom juice is spotted on pulp paper and allowed to dry. Although newspaper is generally recommended in most references, it may be too thin to give a clear reaction and the ink may bleed, further obscuring the result. Telephone book paper gives a more satisfactory result.[10] Several drops of concentrated (10 to 12N) hydrochloric acid are added to the spot. A blue response developing within 30 minutes of acid treatment constitutes a positive test result. If the mushroom has been dried, it should be extracted with methanol and the methanol washings tested as described above. Because some types of paper can actually produce a false-positive result, a section of paper on which no mushroom material has been applied should also be tested as a control. Other substituted indoles such as serotonin or indoles in other mushroom genera may also

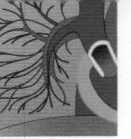
give a positive Meixner test result.[4,10] Thus, the Meixner test is not specific. Although the amount of amatoxin present in deadly amanitas theoretically should give a positive reaction, the sensitivity of the Meixner test in clinical practice has not been determined.

Identifying deadly *Amanita* mushrooms in the field should not be difficult, but for various reasons even those who have picked and consumed mushrooms with impunity for many years are not immune to making that fatal mistake. Figure 23-6 demonstrates the maturation course of a typical *Amanita* mushroom and how the classic annulus and "death cup" develop. These structures are not always obvious, however, and may be obliterated in the act of picking the mushrooms out of the ground. The immature "buttons" in many ways resemble edible puffballs. It is useful to remember that all species of deadly *Amanita* have white gills and spore prints.

Management

The basic facets of treatment of known or suspected cyclopeptide mushroom poisoning includes the provision of supportive care (e.g., fluid and electrolyte repletion and antiemetic therapy), gastrointestinal decontamination (e.g., administration of activated charcoal), enhanced elimination techniques (e.g., multiple-dose activated charcoal and/or charcoal hemoperfusion), antidotal therapy (e.g., penicillin G and silibinin administration), and treatment of secondary complications (e.g., coagulopathy, and liver and renal failure) as necessary. All patients with suspected or confirmed cytotoxic mushroom ingestion should be admitted to the hospital for close observation.

A wide variety of antidotes to *Amanita* poisoning have been touted to be beneficial, but clinical assessments of these therapies have for the most part been anecdotal. The use of thioctic acid has been lauded in the literature on the basis of anecdotal reports. Being a dithiol compound, it has been postulated to function as a free radical scavenger. However, there is no convincing human evidence of its efficacy in *A. phalloides* poisoning.

Intravenous penicillin has also been recommended on the theory that it inhibits the uptake of amatoxins by hepatocytes. Various other protective mechanisms for penicillin have also been proposed. Animal data and retrospective human data suggest that benzylpenicillin (penicillin G) in a dose range of 300,000 to 1,000,000 units/kg per day is hepatoprotective; however, this could not be demonstrated in a prospective study.

Silibinin, a water-soluble preparation of silymarin, which is composed of a group of falvenoligants isolated from milk thistle (*Silybum marianum*), has been shown to be effective in animals in reducing hepatotoxicity by inhibiting amatoxin uptake by hepatocytes and interfering with enterohepatic recirculation of amatoxin.[11,12] It has also been postulated to act as a free radical scavenger. Intravenous silibinin (20–30 mg/kg/day in three or four divided doses or as a continuous infusion) is routinely administered in Europe when amatoxin-containing mushroom ingestion is suspected.[13] The oral preparation of silymarin is the only preparation available for use in the United States. Oral silymarin is available in health food stores as a food supplement and can be dosed at 140 mg two to three times daily. Definitive studies for silibinin and silymarin as treatments in human amatoxin poisoning have not been conducted. Anecdotal reports of efficacy coupled with the lack of adverse effects of this therapy render it a potentially beneficial but still unvalidated therapy for human amatoxin poisoning.[6,13]

A report of 11 patients with apparent poisonous *A. phalloides* poisoning treated with infusion of *N*-acetylcysteine (NAC) reported survival in all, with only one patient requiring liver transplantation.[14] However, these patients were also treated with an intensive regimen of venovenous hemodiafiltration with activated charcoal and high-dose penicillin G; thus, the contribution of the NAC could not be assessed.

Anecdotal reports and preliminary animal data suggest a number of additional antidotes, including hyperbaric oxygen, plasmapheresis, cimetidine, ascorbic acid, cephalosporins, corticosteroids, cytochrome C, bile salts, heavy metal salts, D-penicillamine, and diethyldithiocar-

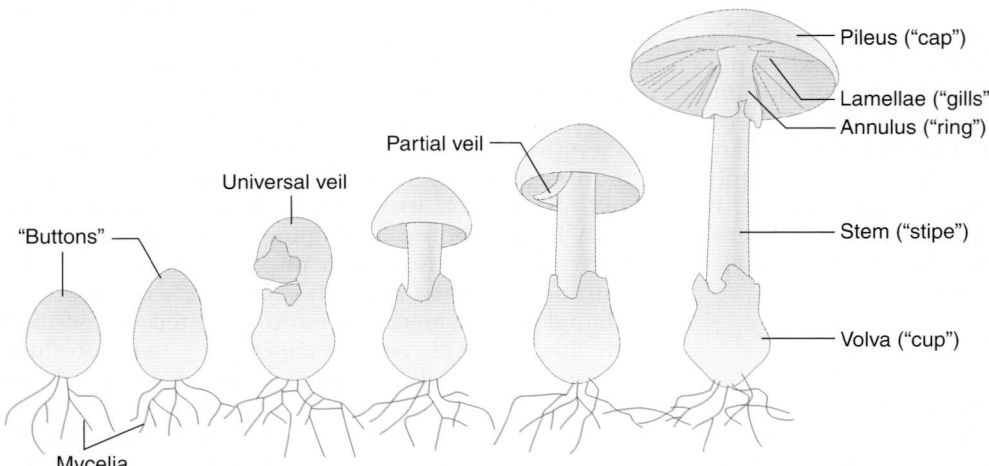

FIGURE 23-6 Maturation of *Amanita* species. The early stages ("buttons") may resemble nontoxic puffballs. The lamellae and spores are white in all *Amanita* species, whereas the pileus may be white, as in *Amanita phalloides, Amanita verna,* or *Amanita virosa,* or bright orange-red, as in *Amanita muscaria.* The distinguishing features of all amanitas include the annulus and volva ("death cup"); however, these are frequently destroyed in the process of picking and preparing the mushroom. Poisonous *Amanita* mushrooms are toxic during all stages of development. (Adapted from Litten W: The most poisonous mushrooms. Sci Am 1975;232;90.)

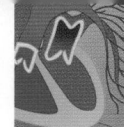

bamate. However, no firm clinical data indicate that any of these are useful.

Although it is unclear if any of these specific antidotes are of value in the management of amatoxin poisoning, there is little doubt that optimization of a patient's fluid status is of great importance.

Hemoperfusion, hemodialysis, or plasma exchange[15] may be theoretically useful in enhancing elimination early after ingestion. However, these have never been proved to be beneficial and may be impractical because most patients present late.

Of these, plasmapheresis appears to be the technique of choice. A recent uncontrolled series of six children poisoned with hepatotoxic mushrooms reported dramatic improvement in multiple biochemical and clinical parameters in four after use of a molecular absorbent regenerating system (MARS) using albumin as the absorbent.[16] One of the two nonresponders had been in cardiac arrest and remained in deep coma postresuscitation. A second series[17] reported using the MARS system on six *A. phalloides*–poisoned patients (mean age 46 years). Although the treatment was started an average of 76 hours postingestion, there was substantial improvement in metabolic parameters, and five of these six survived. Because of the late use of MARS in these patients, it is likely that the survival advantage conferred by MARS was from correction of the effects of hepatic dysfunction rather than the removal of amatoxins. Since both of these series were uncontrolled, it is impossible to conclude definitively that the MARS treatments were beneficial.

Antiamatoxin Fab fragments have been studied in animal models, but these strongly enhance the observed toxicity.

Liver transplantation has been successfully performed on patients with severe cyclopeptide-induced hepatotoxicity. Because most patients with amatoxin poisoning recover with aggressive supportive care, partial or total transplantation should not be considered to be standard treatment for hepatotoxicity. However, if a patient shows signs of severe hepatotoxicity, transfer to a transplantation center may be beneficial to facilitate the procedure should it become necessary. Although no universally agreed on criteria exist for transplantation, high-grade encephalopathy is generally considered such a poor prognostic sign that liver transplantation should be considered.

Because amatoxins have been reported to undergo enterohepatic recirculation, it may be useful to administer multiple doses of activated charcoal for at least 48 hours after ingestion. Duodenal suction is also of theoretic benefit during this period. However, neither of these therapeutic approaches has been proven helpful.

Amanita (see Figs. 23-3 to 23-5) is by far the most commonly ingested genus that results in significant clinical toxicity. As mentioned previously and noted in Box 23-2, several species of *Galerina* and *Lepiota* contain cyclopeptides and are therefore capable of causing similar toxicity to *Amanita* spp.[18-20] *Galerina* spp. (see Fig. 23-7) are common, indiscreet, small brown mushrooms; approximately 15 to 20 *Galerina* mushrooms contain the same

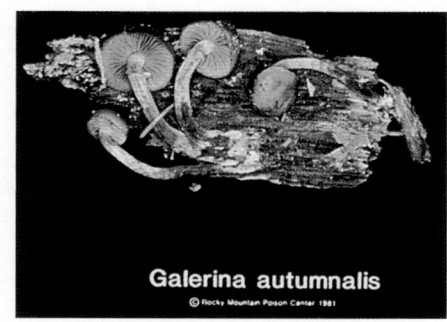

FIGURE 23-7 *Galerina autumnalis* (cyclopeptide). (Courtesy of Linnea Gilman, Denver, CO.)

amount of toxin as one mature *A. phalloides*. They may be ingested by crawling children or by those seeking psychoactive mushrooms. *Galerina* tends to contain small amounts of amatoxins, and it is commonly believed, although not empirically verified, that ingestion of at least one to two dozen mushrooms is required for toxicity. Several species of *Lepiota* contain amatoxin. Ingestion of these mushrooms has been associated with human fatalities from fulminant hepatic failure in France and Germany.[6,21]

One of the common errors made in identification of mushrooms of the *Amanita* and *Lepiota* species is confusing them with *Chlorophyllum molybdites* mushrooms, which also possess an annulus and a swelling at the base resembling a cup. Persons ingesting *C. molybdites* mushrooms, however, usually develop severe vomiting and diarrhea within 2 hours, although many are able to consume these mushrooms without becoming symptomatic. Differentiating between *C. molybdites* and *Amanita* and *Lepiota* spp. should not be difficult. *Chlorophyllum* spp. are the only mushrooms with greenish gills and spores (create greenish spore print), and the spores are thick walled and contain pores. The mushroom itself stains reddish orange where it is injured, and the annulus is movable; in *Amanita* and *Lepiota*, the annulus is fixed.

MUSCIMOL AND IBOTENIC ACID POISONING

Overview

Certain *Amanita* species contain the closely related isoxazoles muscimol (a hallucinogen) and ibotenic acid (a potent insecticide) (see Box 23-2 and Fig. 23-8). Ingestion of these mushrooms often produces the rapid onset of altered sensorium and mentation. *A. muscaria* and *A. pantherina* (Figs. 23-9 and 23-10) are responsible for most cases of isoxazole mushroom poisoning.[6,22] These two mushroom species are very common and have a wide geographic distribution. *A. muscaria* is found in conifer or deciduous forests and *A. pantherina* is usually found under Douglas fir trees.[6] *A. muscaria* is commonly known as the "fly agaric" because it attracts and kills flies that land on it. These mushrooms have been used for their psychoactive effects for at least 3000 years in the

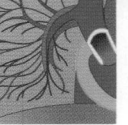

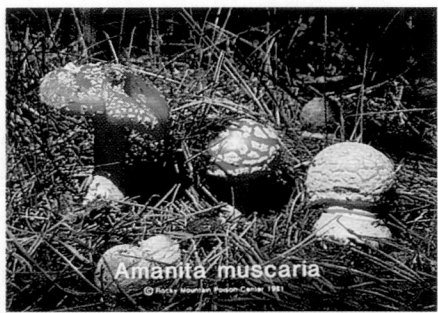

FIGURE 23-8 Chemical structures of ibotenic acid and muscimol and the analogy with the conversion of glutamic acid to γ-aminobutyric acid.

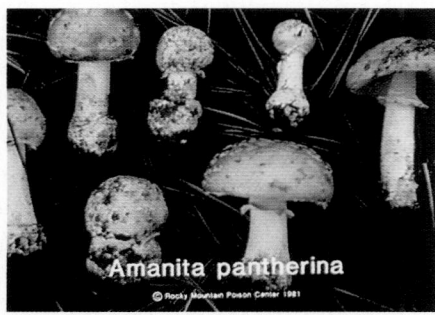

FIGURE 23-9 The fly agaric, *Amanita muscaria* (muscimol, ibotenic acid). (Courtesy of Linnea Gilman, Denver, CO.)

FIGURE 23-10 *Amanita pantherina* (muscimol, ibotenic acid). (Courtesy of Linnea Gilman, Denver, CO.)

rituals of many Asian and Indian tribes. Purposeful ingestion of urine from people who have eaten these mushrooms has been reported as a way to elicit the psychoactive effects of the excreted muscimol.[6] Many cases of *A. muscaria* poisoning still occur in individuals who deliberately seek and ingest the mushroom for its hallucinogenic properties. Exposure history (e.g., patient intent) is, thus, very important in patient evaluation.

A. pantherina ("panther caps") may be confused with edible agarics ("meadow mushrooms") by inexperienced collectors. Despite its toxic effects, *A. pantherina* is used as a food, mostly in the Pacific Northwest. This requires peeling off the skin of the cap, which contains the highest concentration of isoxazoles, and parboiling the

remaining parts. Because the isoxazoles are water soluble, they are extracted by this process. Needless to say, the water should be discarded.

Pathophysiology

The pharmacologically active toxins in these mushrooms include the isoxazoles ibotenic acid, muscimol, and muscazone.[6,23] Additional compounds have been isolated from these mushrooms but are present in insufficient quantity to be physiologically active. These inactive compounds include muscarine, muscaridine, pilzatropin (leveohyoscyamine or "mushroom atropine"), indole derivatives, stizolobic acid, and amino acids.[6]

Although the pathophysiology of muscimol poisoning is imperfectly understood, its central nervous system (CNS) effects seem to be the result of its action as a γ-aminobutyric acid (GABA) agonist. Conversely, ibotenic acid acts as an agonist at excitatory glutamic acid receptors (e.g., N-methyl-D-aspartate receptor).[24] In addition, both toxins have produced increased brain levels of serotonin, decreased levels of brain dopamine, CNS sympathetic effects, and impaired CNS control of motor activity.[6] The resultant picture can be one of alternating CNS depression and stimulation with varied motor effects. Both toxins readily cross the blood-brain barrier. Ibotenic acid is spontaneously decarboxylated to muscimol. Muscimol is approximately five times more potent than ibotenic acid. These compounds are excreted in the urine and detected within 1 hour of mushroom ingestion.

Although toxic doses of both ibotenic acid and muscimol can be found in a single mushroom, large numbers of these mushrooms typically must be ingested before a toxic effect is manifested.[25] Typically, 2 to 4 *A. muscaria* mushrooms must be ingested to produce psychoactive effects and more than 10 mushrooms must be ingested to produce death.[6] Fatalities, however, are rare.

Clinical Presentation

Toxic effects typically occur within 30 minutes of ingestion but may be delayed for up to 3 hours. Signs and symptoms include nausea, vomiting, abdominal cramps, diarrhea, CNS depression alternating with CNS agitation and excitation, ataxia, incoordination, dizziness, euphoria, visual perceptual changes, vivid dreams, hallucinations, frank psychosis, irregular pulse and respirations, hypotension, mydriasis or miosis, diaphoresis, pale or flushed skin, myoclonic jerking, muscle fasciculations, seizures, coma, and death. It appears that seizures are more common in pediatric patients.[23] Death as a result of poisoning from these mushrooms is rare.[6] Waxing and waning mental status and bizarre behavior are common. The clinical duration of toxicity may last from 4 to 24 hours.[6]

Muscarine was first extracted from *A. muscaria* in 1869, and its use as a pharmacologic research tool has enhanced our knowledge of the muscarinic receptors of the parasympathetic nervous system. Paradoxically, most patients poisoned by *A. muscaria* do not have cholinergic findings. In fact, poisoning by this group of mushrooms has been described as causing anticholinergic manifes-

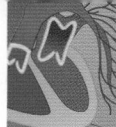

tations. However, despite some similarities to a classic anticholinergic syndrome, neither the pathophysiology nor clinical manifestations of poisoning by this group of mushrooms are truly anticholinergic.

Diagnosis

The diagnosis of isoxazole-containing mushroom poisoning is made from a positive history of mushroom ingestion coupled with the rapid onset of symptoms and the presence of suggestive physical findings (e.g., altered sensorium, alternating agitation and obtundation, myoclonic jerking). Diagnosis is greatly facilitated by either a description of the mushroom or uneaten specimens brought to the health care facility. Identification of *A. muscaria* and *A. pantherina* mushrooms should be relatively easy. The *A. muscaria* cap is 8 to 24 cm in diameter, bright orange or red in color, and covered with small white plaques, which are remnants of the universal veil (see Fig. 23-9). The *A. pantherina* cap is 5 to 12 cm in diameter, yellowish brown in color, with similar small white warts or plaques spread across its surface (see Fig. 23-10). As in all *Amanita* species, the annulus and volva for these mushrooms are prominent, and the spores are hyaline, thin walled, and without pores. The spore prints are white.[6]

Management

Treatment of this group of poisonings consists of appropriate supportive care and GI decontamination (see Box 23-1). There is little to suggest, based on either pathophysiology or published clinical experience, that the once touted antidote physostigmine is effective in controlling any toxic manifestation of ibotenic acid or muscimol poisoning. Patients with unstable vital signs or significant alterations in their mental status should be admitted to an intensive care unit until their toxic effects resolve.

GYROMITRIN

Overview

The *Gyromitra* spp., or false morels, are an extremely interesting genus toxicologically. Many species of *Gyromitra* contain the hydrazone gyromitrin (acetaldehyde methylformylhydrazone) and small amounts of other hydrazones. Gyromitrin is metabolized to monomethylhydrazine (Fig. 23-11). The common toxic species in this genus are listed in Box 23-2.

Gyromitra spp. are found in Asia, Europe, and North America. The *Gyromitra* species are nongilled fungi, the spores of which develop is asci, or microscopic sacs, on the surfaces of the fruiting bodies. The caps of *Gyromitra* are orange-brown to brown in color and highly convoluted, hence the nickname "brain fungi" (Figs. 23-12 and 23-13). Toxicity is variable and unpredictable but typically occurs only after intentional ingestion of *Gyromitra* spp. Many species of *Gyromitra* are edible, but

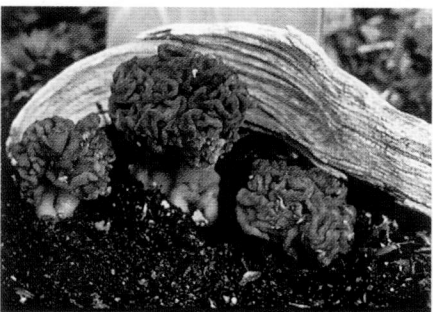

FIGURE 23-11 Chemical structures showing the conversion of gyromitrin to monomethylhydrazine.

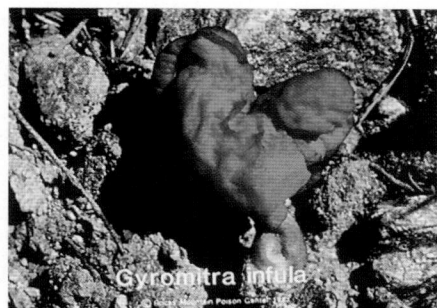

FIGURE 23-12 *Gyromitra esculenta* (monomethylhydrazine). (Courtesy of Joy Spurr, Issaquah, WA.)

FIGURE 23-13 *Gyromitra infula* (monomethylhydrazine). (Courtesy of the late George Grimes.)

determining which ones may be safely ingested is best left to experts. Despite their name, false morel, these mushrooms do not resemble members of the genus *Morchella* or true morels.

In post–World War II Poland, death due to ingestion of *Gyromitra esculenta* exceeded that caused by *A. phalloides*.[26] Poisoning by this mushroom occurs in the spring, in contrast to poisoning by *A. phalloides*, which tends to be common in the autumn.

Poisoning can occur after ingestion of either raw or cooked mushrooms. The hydrazones in these mushrooms may be destroyed and volatilized by cooking; however, this should not be considered a foolproof strategy for rendering them edible. In addition, toxicity has occurred from inhaling the steam during the cooking process.[6,27]

Pathophysiology

The toxin gyromitrin (acetaldehyde *N*-methyl-noformylhydrazone) and its breakdown product, monomethylhydrazine, produce toxic effects similar to those of

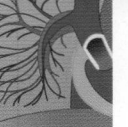

isoniazid overdose. These toxins inhibit the formation of GABA in the brain by inducing a state of pyridoxine (vitamin B_6) deficiency. Specifically, these toxins inhibit the enzyme pyridoxine phosphokinase, thus preventing activation of pyridoxine to pyridoxal phosphate (active form of vitamin B_6). These toxins also bind and inhibit pyridoxal phosphate directly and inhibit glutamic acid decarboxylase, the enzyme that catalyzes the formation of GABA from glutamate. CNS depletion of GABA results in seizures associated with *Gyromitra* spp. poisoning.

Clinical Presentation

Six to 48 hours after ingestion of mushrooms from the *Gyromitra* spp., patients develop nausea, vomiting, abdominal pain and bloating, diarrhea, dizziness, fatigue, and muscle cramps.[28] These symptoms are usually mild and limited largely to gastrointestinal effects. Toxicity, however, may progress to neurologic, hematologic, and hepatorenal dysfunction. Serious neurologic effects include delirium, coma, and convulsions. Hematologic effects include methemoglobinemia and hemolysis. Hepatic failure usually occurs by 48 hours and is heralded by right upper quadrant tenderness, hepatic transaminitis, jaundice, coagulopathy, and hypoglycemia. Renal dysfunction may result from rhabdomyolysis or prolonged hypotension or as part of the hepatorenal syndrome. In parts of Eastern Europe, fatalities due to *G. esculenta* are common; mortality rates as great as 10% have been reported.[29]

Diagnosis

The diagnosis of gyromitrin-containing mushroom poisoning is made from a positive history of mushroom ingestion, positive identification of uneaten specimens, and the presence of suggestive physical findings (e.g., seizures, hepatorenal syndrome). The presence of a latency between mushroom ingestion and the onset of clinical effects may assist diagnosis. Gas chromatography, gas chromatography-mass spectrometry, and thin-layer chromatography may be used to identify hydrazone and hydrazine compounds in mushrooms. Laboratory testing for gyromitrin is not likely to be readily available.

Management

Treatment consists of supportive care, administration of methylene blue for significant methemoglobinemia, blood transfusions if required, and intravenous pyridoxine for monomethylhydrazine-induced seizures. Replacement of ongoing fluid and electrolyte losses is an important aspect of early treatment. Gastrointestinal decontamination is unlikely to be useful due to the long latency between ingestion and patient presentation. Pyridoxine, which is depleted in poisoning by hydrazines, is a necessary cofactor for the synthesis of GABA. Pyridoxine also forms a chemical complex with hydrazines, and this may have a role in its antidotal effect in treating monomethylhydrazine poisoning. Hydrazines also inhibit the metabolic conversion of folic acid to its

active form, tetrahydrofolate, and supplementation with folinic acid has been suggested on theoretical grounds.

High doses of pyridoxine are known to cause peripheral neuropathy, and thus excessive use should be avoided. An empiric initial dose of 5 g administered intravenously (or 25 to 50 mg/kg) is generally regarded as appropriate for the initial management of seizures in an adult suffering from *Gyromitra* poisoning. This should be repeated only for recurrent seizures or coma. Pyridoxine does not reverse the other aspects of poisoning by these mushrooms.[30] Benzodiazepines and/or barbiturates may be useful adjunctive treatments for seizures associated with *Gyromitra* poisoning.

MUSCARINE

Overview

More than 30 species of *Inocybe* and 6 species of *Clitocybe* contain muscarine (see Box 23-2 and Figs. 23-14 and 23-15). These inconspicuous mushrooms are found worldwide but commonly grow in lawns and public parks. *A. pantherina* and *A. muscaria* contain muscarine (hence the name) but usually in quantities that are insufficient to cause a cholinergic syndrome. Muscarine was initially isolated from *A. muscaria*.[31]

Pathophysiology

Mushrooms in this group predictably cause symptoms and signs of poisoning by the cholinergic alkaloid mus-

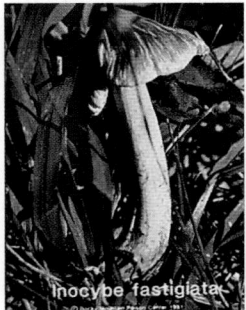

FIGURE 23-14 *Inocybe fastigiata* (muscarine). (Courtesy of the late George Grimes.)

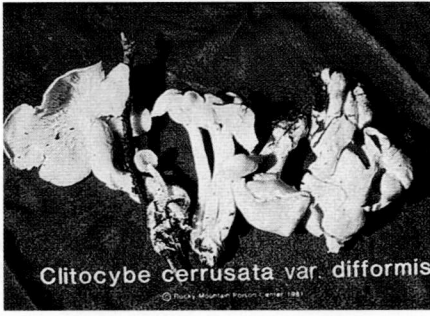

FIGURE 23-15 *Clitocybe cerrusata* (muscarine). (Courtesy of Linnea Gilman, Denver, CO.)

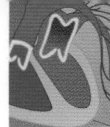

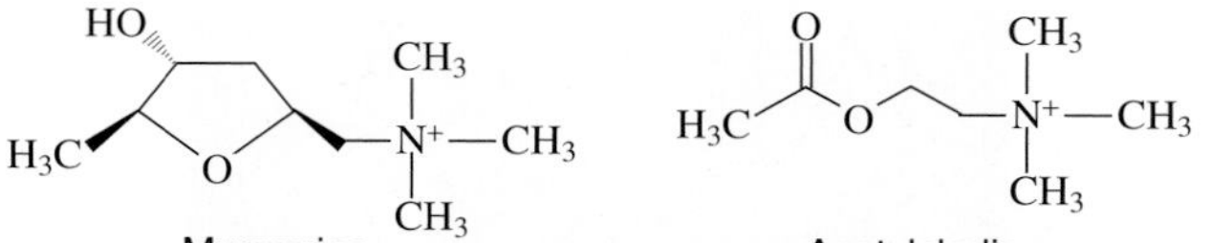

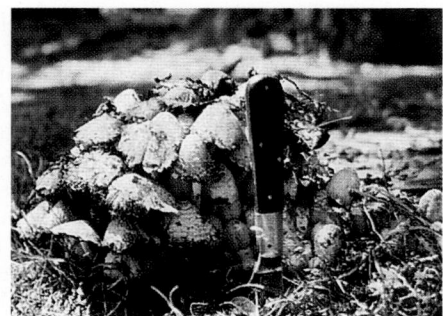

FIGURE 23-16 Chemical structures of muscarine and acetylcholine.

carine. Muscarine is a quaternary ammonium compound structurally similar to acetylcholine and causes depolarization of neurons by binding to the acetylcholine receptor at postganglionic cholinergic neurons (Fig. 23-16). Because muscarine does not possess an ester bond,[32] it is not hydrolyzed by cholinesterases. Thus, the cholinergic or parasympathomimetic effects of muscarine are prolonged. As a quaternary compound that carries a charge, muscarine is not well absorbed from the gastrointestinal tract and does not readily cross the blood-brain barrier. Thus, CNS toxic effects do not readily occur.

Clinical Presentation

Minutes to an hour after ingestion, patients may develop the classic cholinergic syndrome consisting of diaphoresis, bradycardia, bronchospasm, profuse bronchorrhea, miosis, seizures, salivation, lacrimation, involuntary loss of urine and stool, and vomiting. Unlike the cholinergic crisis occurring after poisoning by organophosphate insecticides, the syndrome in these cases, although highly uncomfortable, is usually mild compared with organophosphate poisoning and seldom life threatening. This may be at least partially due to the poor GI absorption of muscarine. Unlike organophosphates, muscarine does not stimulate nicotinic receptors. Muscarine is heat labile, so vigorous cooking of these mushrooms may prevent their cholinergic effects. Clinical effects are usually self-limited and last approximately 2 hours but may persist for 6 to 24 hours if large amounts of muscarine have been consumed.[6]

Diagnosis

The diagnosis of muscarine-containing mushroom poisoning is made from a positive history of mushroom ingestion coupled with the rapid onset of parasympathomimetic clinical effects. The best analytical method for detecting muscarine in mushrooms is high-performance thin-layer chromatography.[33] Although of theoretic utility, this analytical technique has not been applied to body fluids.

Management

Treatment consists of GI decontamination, supportive care, and administration of atropine. Although activated charcoal is theoretically beneficial in preventing absorption of muscarine, it is important to emphasize that cathartics should not be administered to patients with diarrhea syndromes. Atropine has been recognized as a treatment for this poisoning since the mid-1800s.[31] Atropine may

be given in sequential doses until pulmonary secretions are dried. The recommended intravenous starting dose of atropine is 0.1 to 0.5 mg in adults and 0.02 mg/kg in children. Glycopyrrolate is an alternative anticholinergic agent that may be preferable to atropine since it does not cross the blood-brain barrier. Like atropine, it is dosed sequentially with recommended intravenous doses of 0.05 to 0.1 mg in adults and 0.005 to 0.01 mg/kg in children. The use of inhaled ipratropium bromide may be beneficial for patients with significant bronchospasm.

COPRINE

Overview

Coprine poisoning is most commonly associated with ingestion of *Coprinus atramentarius,* or the "inky cap" (Fig. 23-17). It is so called because the mature specimens have lamellae that deliquesce or autodigest into an inky black fluid that is obvious on examination of the mushroom. The mushrooms themselves are edible, but disulfiram-like toxicity occurs when these mushrooms are ingested concurrently with or shortly before alcohol.

Pathophysiology

These mushrooms contain coprine, which is a glutamic acid derivative that induces hyperacetaldehydemia in the presence of ethanol by inhibiting acetaldehyde dehydrogenase. Coprine itself is not an inhibitor of this enzyme.[34,35] However, it has been speculated that a metabolite of coprine, 1-aminocyclopropanol, functions like disulfiram and inhibits the metabolism of ethanol at the acetaldehyde dehydrogenase step, resulting in clinical symptoms (Fig. 23-18).[36] Coprine is not a heat-labile toxin and, thus, toxicity will still occur if these

FIGURE 23-17 *Coprinus atramentarius* (coprine). (Courtesy of Joe H. Restivo, Savannah, GA.)

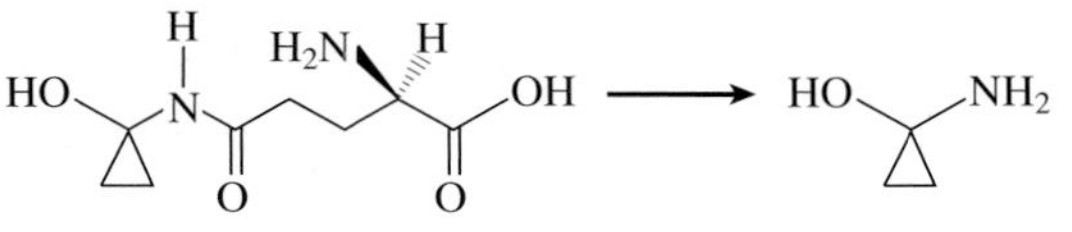

FIGURE 23-18 Chemical structure of coprine and its proposed active metabolite, 1-aminocyclopropanol.

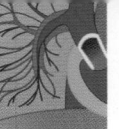

mushrooms are cooked and consumed with alcohol. The active toxin, 1-aminocyclopropanol, irreversibly inactivates aldehyde dehydrogenase by forming a covalent bond with the enzyme. Thus, a disulfiram-like reaction may occur even if alcohol is consumed up to 5 days after coprine-containing mushroom ingestion.[6] The symptom complex engendered by this interaction has been referred to as "Clayton's hangover."[37]

Clinical Presentation

Signs and symptoms usually occur within 20 to 30 minutes of ethanol ingestion and spontaneously resolve after 3 to 6 hours.[6] Symptoms, however, may persist for 24 hours. Sensitivity to alcohol usually occurs within 2 hours of eating coprine-containing mushrooms. Effects will be less prominent when ethanol is consumed concurrently with inky caps than when consumed after the mushrooms since coprine must be bioactivated to 1-aminocyclopropanol to create the disulfiram effect. Clinical effects include flushing of the face, neck, and trunk; headache; a metallic taste; nausea; vomiting; palpitations; dyspnea; chest pain; tachycardia; and diaphoresis. Hypotension may occur secondary to peripheral vasodilatation.[36,38-40] Other effects include cardiac arrhythmias, confusion, coma, and patient apprehension.

Diagnosis

Diagnosis is made by history and clinical effects suggestive of a disulfiram-like reaction. A positive history of mushroom ingestion and the rapid onset of clinical effects after consumption of ethanol is highly suggestive. Coprine may be detected by thin-layer chromatography. Because coprine is an amino acid, a coprine-containing spot stains when sprayed by ninhydrin.[34,40,41]

Management

Treatment of the coprine syndrome is supportive. Patient reassurance and rehydration are often the only necessary treatments. Gastrointestinal decontamination is not likely to be beneficial and is unnecessary. Although antihistamines and propranolol have been suggested as specific treatments, these agents have not been proven useful and are not recommended.[36] The coprine syndrome is self-limited and usually abates within several hours.

Because of its disulfiram-like effect, coprine has been suggested as a potential agent for chemoprevention of alcohol abuse. However, the mutagenic, carcinogenic, and male gonadotoxic effects render it inappropriate for this use.[36]

INDOLES

Overview

The psilocin-psilocybin-containing mushrooms have been used by Aztec and American Indians in religious ceremonies for thousands of years[42] and are frequently

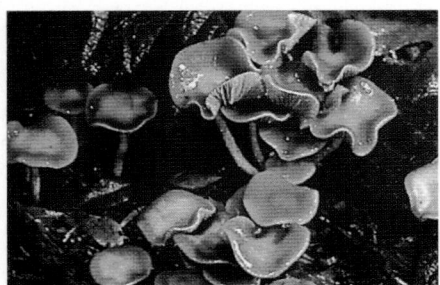

FIGURE 23-19 *Psilocybe cyanescens* (indole). (Courtesy of Kit Scates, Post Falls, ID.)

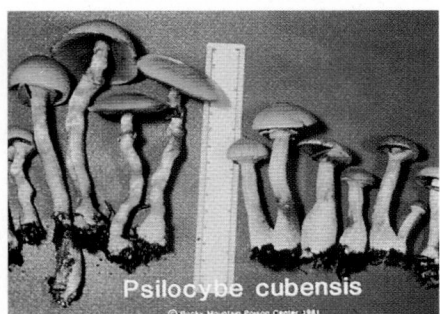

FIGURE 23-20 *Psilocybe cubensis* (indole). (Courtesy of the Rocky Mountain Poison Center, Denver, CO.)

referred to as "magic mushrooms." Psilocybin is found largely in four genera of mushrooms that include *Conocybe, Gynmopilus, Panaeolus,* and *Psilocybe* (see Box 23-2 and Figs. 23-19 and 23-20). These mushrooms are found throughout the United States but are more commonly found in warm climates. The *Psilocybe* genus contains more than 100 species of small brown, slender-stalked mushrooms. They are commonly, but not exclusively, found growing in piles of horse and cow dung and fertilized grasses, especially after a spring rain. Also growing in a similar environment and with a similar appearance is the cyclopeptide-containing mushroom *Conocybe filaris*. Indole-containing mushrooms are found in moist areas all over the United States, most commonly in the South. The spores are smooth purple and contain pores. A classic feature of the *Psilocybe* mushrooms is the blue-green areas where it has been injured or handled. Although this color is usually the result of the oxidation of psilocin,[37] this color change is not specific for hallucinogenic mushrooms.

Pathophysiology

The clinical effects from ingestion of these mushrooms are caused by the psychoactive indole tryptamine derivatives, psilocybin and psilocin, which are chemically related to both lysergic acid and serotonin (Fig. 23-21). The psychedelic effects of these compounds are mediated largely by agonist activity at CNS serotonin 5-HT$_{2A}$ receptors (see Chapter 45). Psilocybin was first isolated in 1958 by Albert Hoffman, the discoverer of lysergic acid diethylamide (LSD). Intravenous use of

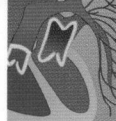

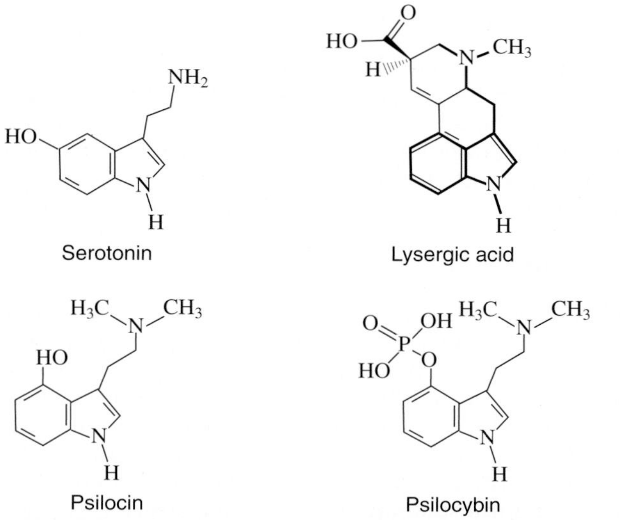

FIGURE 23-21 Chemical structures demonstrating the structural relationships between lysergic acid, serotonin, psilocin and psilocybin. For clarity the structural comparison area in lysergic acid is shown in boldface.

these mushrooms has also been reported.[43,44] Psilocybin is quite stable; both dried mushrooms and boiled extract retain their hallucinogenic potency. Although use of this mushroom is generally limited by its supply, these mushrooms tend not to be expensive.[45]

Concentrations of psilocybin vary greatly from mushroom to mushroom, by season, and location.[6,13] The initial hallucinogenic effects of psilocybin are evident with as little as 4 mg of toxin, while a dose of 12 mg or more produces vivid hallucinations.[6,13] Because of the small amounts of psychoactive indoles in these mushrooms, ingestion of several caps is usually required to elicit a hallucinogenic effect. It may take the ingestion of 3 to 60 mushrooms to achieve the desired effect. In general, 4 to 8 mg of psilocybin is present in 20 g of fresh and 2 g of dried mushroom.

Clinical Presentation

Thirty to 60 minutes after the psychotropic *Psilocybe* is ingested, a feeling of euphoria develops, followed by perceptual distortions and hallucinations that are usually, but not always, considered pleasant.[46] Sensory and perceptual distortions and illusions occur more commonly than true hallucinations. Tachycardia, mydriasis, and paresthesias are common effects. Hyperadrenergic effects may occur. Seizures have been reported.[47] The experience generally lasts 4 to 6 hours. Flashbacks may occur.[45] Among connoisseurs of the psychoactive effects of indoles, these mushrooms are often preferred over LSD.[14,45] Mortality is extremely rare following recreational use of psilocybin-containing mushrooms.

Diagnosis

Diagnosis is based on a positive history of mushroom ingestion and the presence of corroborating clinical effects

(e.g., sensory or perceptual distortions, hallucinosis, sympathomimetic effects). As with any illicitly purchased substance, the actual material used may not be what is suspected by history. In a study of 886 samples sold as psilocybin mushrooms, only 28% contained psilocybin. An additional 31% contained LSD or phencyclidine, and in 37%, no psychoactive substances could be identified.[48]

Many analytic techniques have been described for the identification of psilocybin and other psychoactive indoles.[23] However, it is unlikely that most hospital clinical laboratories will be equipped to perform these assays and the results will generally not affect the treatment or disposition of the patient.

Management

Most patients who ingest psilocybin-containing mushrooms have no serious adverse effects and do not require hospital treatment. Patients who require medical care usually need little more than reassurance,[49] but sedation may be required. Benzodiazepines are generally considered the drugs of choice in this case. Gastrointestinal decontamination is not necessary.

ORELLANINE
Overview

Some mushrooms of the genus *Cortinarius* contain the bipyridyl toxin orellanine (Fig. 23-22).[50] The syndrome of poisoning by these mushrooms was first described after a large outbreak of cases in Poland in 1952. Ingestion of these mushrooms may result in the development of gastroenteritis, thirst, polyuria, chills, headaches, and myalgias, after a hiatus of several days. A small percentage of these cases progress to renal failure, evident days to weeks later.[50-53] Few cases of *Cortinarius* poisoning have been reported in the United States and Australia, but many occurrences have been documented in Europe and Japan. Some species of *Cortinarius* are edible, creating a dangerous temptation to seasoned yet adventurous mushroom hunters. Mushrooms of this genus are distinguished by their medium-sized orange-brown caps (2 to 5 cm) and rusty brown spores (Figs. 23-23 and 23-24). *Cortinarius* is the largest genus of mushrooms, containing more than 800 species, making the differentiation between the edible and poisonous varieties extremely difficult. Although orellanine is the primary nephrotoxin in these fungi, some species appear to contain other related nephrotoxins known as cortinarins (cortinarin A and B).[54,55] These nephrotoxins appear to require activation by cytochrome P-450.[56]

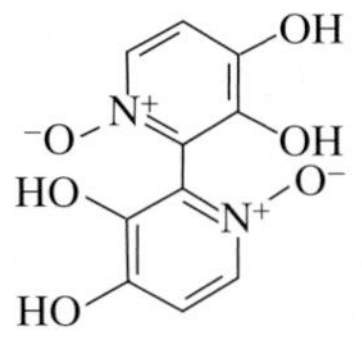

FIGURE 23-22 Chemical structure of orellanine.

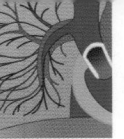

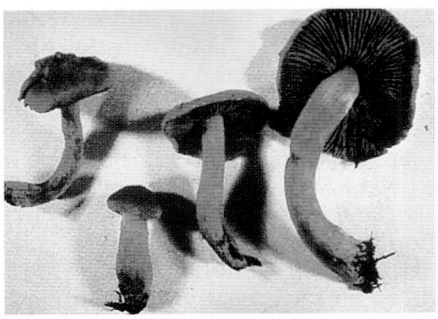

FIGURE 23-23 *Cortinarius speciosissimus* (orellanine). (Reprinted from Lampe KF [ed]: AMA Handbook of Poisonous and Injurious Plants. Chicago, American Medical Association, 1985.)

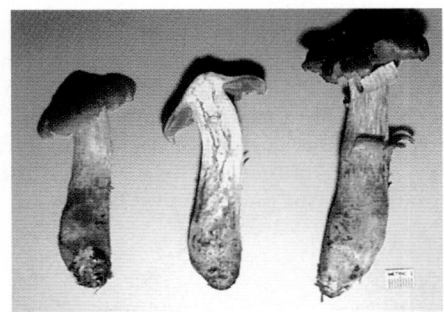

FIGURE 23-24 *Cortinarius orellanoides* (orellanine). (Courtesy of Joseph Ammirati, PhD, University of Washington, Seattle.)

Pathophysiology

Orellanine is a heat-stable toxin that is chemically closely related to the herbicides paraquat and diquat. Orellanine is not deactivated by cooking, parboiling, drying, or freezing the mushrooms. The mechanism of cytotoxicity of orellanine is not well known, but it appears to involve disruption of the actin cytoskeleton and protein synthesis in renal tubular cells.[57,58] Poisoning by these compounds results in tubulointerstitial nephritis and fibrosis.[52] Despite the structural similarity between orellanine and herbicides like paraquat and diquat, no cases of pulmonary damage as a result of *Cortinarius* poisoning have been reported.

Clinical Presentation

The onset of symptoms occurs after a latent period of 36 hours to 17 days following mushroom ingestion.[6] Over a period of days, patients develop headache, thirst, chills, dizziness, malaise, nausea, vomiting, abdominal and back pain, myalgias, and polydipsia. Progressive renal insufficiency develops over 1 to 3 weeks and is manifested by polyuria, oliguria, microscopic hematuria, leukocyturia, proteinuria, and anuria. The severity of poisoning is inversely correlated with the length of the latent period, such that the shorter the latent period, the greater the severity of poisoning.[6] Renal insufficiency occurs in approximately one third (30% to 46%) of patients and becomes chronic in about half of patients.[6] Recovery is gradual and takes several weeks.

Diagnosis

Diagnosis is based on a positive history of mushroom ingestion, a long latency between the ingestion and the onset of clinical effects, and the presence of acute renal failure. Diagnosis is not commonly made prior to the onset of renal insufficiency.[6] Orellanine may be detected by thin-layer or high-performance liquid chromatography.[23]

Management

There are no antidotes for poisoning by these mushrooms. Because patients tend to become symptomatic more than 24 hours after ingestion, activated charcoal is unlikely to be helpful. Treatment therefore consists of aggressive fluid management and close monitoring of renal function. In the majority of cases (50% to 70%), renal failure improves over time.[52] Chronic hemodialysis and renal transplantation may be necessary.

AMANITA SMITHIANA

A syndrome of delayed renal failure similar to orellanine-containing mushrooms has also been more recently attributed to the mushroom *Amanita smithiana*.[59] *A. smithiana* is found in the Pacific Northwest of the United States. These mushrooms contain alienic norleucine, and pentanoic and aminoheadienoic acids, which are believed to produce renal toxicity.[59,60] Unlike *Cortinarius* spp., these mushrooms produce gastrointestinal effects within 2 to 12 hours of ingestion. Renal failure occurs 2 to 5 days after mushroom ingestion. The treatment of *A. smithiana* mushroom toxicity is supportive. Most patients recover renal function within several weeks; hemodialysis may be required temporarily.

TRICHOLOMA EQUESTRE

In 2001, 12 cases of rhabdomyolysis were associated with the ingestion of *Tricholomas equestre* in France (Fig. 23-25). Initial symptoms developed 24 to 72 hours after eating the last of several large consecutive meals of the mushroom.[61] Symptoms included fatigue, myalgias, weakness, nausea, and diaphoresis. Rhabdomyolysis was diagnosed by significant elevations of serum creatinine phosphokinase. Three cases resulted in fatality. In a subsequently performed animal study, extracts from *Tricholomas equestre* have been shown to produce rhabdomyolysis in rats.[61] The myotoxin contained in the mushroom is still unknown.

Tricholomas equestre (also known as *Tricholomas flavovirens* or "Man on Horseback") is found in coniferous forests throughout North America in the late summer and fall. The mushroom has a smooth, yellowish-brown or greenish-brown cap (3 to 5 cm) with yellow gills. Subsequent cases of rhabdomyolysis resulting from repeated ingestion of large amounts of this mushroom have been reported.[62] If this mushroom is to be eaten, small, nonconsecutive meals (less than 100 grams) are recommended so as to avoid human toxicity.[62]

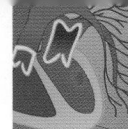

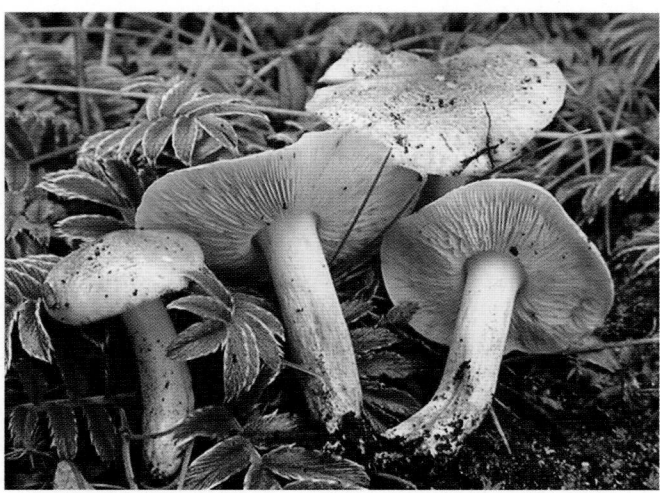

FIGURE 23-25 *Tricholoma equestre* (L.:Fr.) Kummer. (Photograph by R. E. Halling. Copyright 2003.)

PAXILLUS SYNDROME

Overview

Paxillus involutus ("brown rim-roll" mushroom; Fig. 23-26) is, for most people who ingest it, a simple GI irritant.[52,63] However, a small proportion of those eating this mushroom develop immune-mediated hemolytic anemia, referred to as the *Paxillus* syndrome.[64,65] This syndrome typically follows long periods of ingestion of these mushrooms and manifests, once started, as progressively worsening reactions.[64,65] This reaction is not a true mushroom poisoning but rather a food allergy. Given these characteristics, it is of little surprise that the *Paxillus* syndrome is rarely encountered clinically.

Although the *Paxillus* syndrome is generally described as occurring after repeated ingestion of the brown roll-rim mushroom, one case was reported after ingestion of *Suillus luteus* ("slippery Jack"),[66-68] a bolete generally regarded as edible, although this has been questioned.[69,70] The clubfoot mushroom, *Clitocybe clavipes,* has also been suggested as a possible cause of the *Paxillus* syndrome,[54] but it is more likely that any observed reactions to this mushroom are simply the result of its disulfiram-like effect.[71]

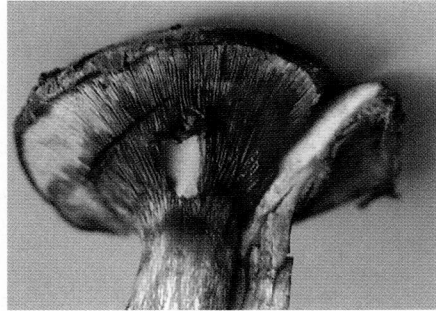

FIGURE 23-26 *Paxillus involutus* (hypersensitivity). (Courtesy of Marilyn Shaw, Denver, CO.)

Pathophysiology

The precise mechanism defining the pathophysiology of the *Paxillus* syndrome is unknown. It appears to be an immunoglobulin-mediated hemolysis provoked by exposure to a yet unidentified antigen.

Clinical Presentation

The *Paxillus* syndrome typically manifests 1 to 2 hours after ingesting the fungi. Clinical features generally reported are syncope, gastroenteritis, decreased urine output, hemoglobinuria, decreased haptoglobins, and low back pain.

Diagnosis

The diagnosis is suggested by the presence of anemia, hemolysis on peripheral blood smear, a decrease in serum haptoglobin, and hemoglobinuria. A hemagglutination test in which a mushroom extract, the patient's serum, and erythrocytes are incubated together has been described to assist diagnosis.[64,72-74] Agglutination that occurs within 30 minutes of incubation is a positive test result and confirms diagnosis.[6]

Management

Treatment consists primarily of aggressive fluid management and, if the mushroom was recently ingested, oral activated charcoal. Plasmapheresis has been used in severe cases,[72] but no convincing evidence shows that this technique provides any therapeutic benefit.

GASTROINTESTINAL IRRITANTS

This group has traditionally been a catch-all category for mushrooms that (1) usually produce nausea, vomiting, and diarrhea shortly (within 2 to 3 hours) after ingestion and (2) do not produce other significant systemic symptoms or signs. The number of species considered in this classification is so great that to list them would be unproductive. Not all species of this group of mushrooms cause symptoms in all people. The same species may cause symptoms in one person at one time and not at another time. The toxins responsible for the GI symptoms are, for the most part, unidentified.

Among the most common species causing acute gastroenteritis is *C. molybdites*.[75] In its juvenile form, it resembles the "shaggy mane," and it is quite often mistaken for this edible mushroom. It is, however, easily distinguished from virtually all other mushrooms by its green gills and spore print (see Fig. 23-2). However, sterile forms of this mushroom, which produce no spores, are known to exist.[75] Another common GI irritant mushroom is *Omphalotus olearius* or *illudens* ("Jack O'Lantern"). This mushroom has a bright orange stalk and large cap (7 to 11 cm) that may glow in the dark. Although formerly classified in the genus *Clitocybe*, more recent study confirms that this mushroom does not

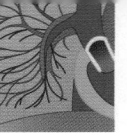

contain muscarine but other GI irritants.[6] This mushroom is commonly found in Europe and North America. The European variety is associated with more severe illness and hepatotoxicity.

Many common backyard mushrooms or "little brown mushrooms" can be considered to be in this group. When these mushrooms are ingested by children or in large quantities by adults, it is still safest to presume them to be toxic and to have them identified.

Generally, no therapy is required for ingestion of gastrointestinal irritant mushrooms. If symptoms are significant or if signs of volume depletion are evident, it is advisable to provide hydration and GI decontamination with activated charcoal. However, it must be emphasized that administration of cathartics with activated charcoal is very likely to exacerbate the condition being treated and thus should be avoided.

ENVIRONMENTAL AND MUSHROOM FARMING ISSUES

Mushrooms are occasionally used as environmental sentinal species for toxins including pesticides[76] and radionuclides.[77,78] This is especially true with respect to monitoring heavy metals such as cadmium, lead, and mercury and radionuclides including potassium 40, cesium 137, cesium 134, and radon 222. These elements may not only be detected on the surface of the mushrooms as a result of atmospheric deposition, but may also be incorporated into the flesh of the mushroom. Mushrooms also appear to be good accumulators of elements such as rubidium, copper, cesium, and selenium.[79] In most cases, the cap accumulates heavy metals to a greater extent than the stipe or stalk of the same mushroom. Furthermore, the species of mushroom may also influence the extent of metal accumulation. For example, fly agaric (*A. muscaria*) demonstrates a preferential uptake of mercury relative to other mushroom species.[78] Despite the accumulation of these potentially toxic elements in mushrooms, the total exposure through ingestion of mushrooms is usually well below any level of concern. No cases of ill health effects as a result of exposure to toxic elements through mushroom ingestion were found. However, mushrooms should be considered as potential contributors to total body burden of metals such as mercury.

Although the majority of mushroom-related toxicity is the result of ingestion, some additional maladies attributable to mushroom exposure in the absence of ingestion have been described. Most often, these noningestion toxicities are the result of hypersensitivity reactions and can be broadly categorized as either dermatologic or pulmonary. The primary dermatologic effect is allergic contact dermatitis, which frequently clears with removal from the source.[80] This is commonly seen in persons working on mushroom farms or mushroom packing facilities.

A syndrome of hypersensitivity pneumonitis termed *mushroom worker's lung* has been described in mushroom farm workers in Japan and numerous American states, including Florida, Pennsylvania, and Washington.[80-83] Patients often present with episodic shortness of breath, persistent cough, fever, chills, and malaise. In some instances, the cough may improve or disappear during weekends and holidays. Pulmonary function testing typically reveals restrictive ventilatory impairment with diffuse interstitial pulmonary infiltrates, while chest radiography shows diffuse infiltrates. Histologic examination of mushroom-related pneumonitis may reveal granulomatous alveolitis. Some cases of mushroom workers lung have been severe enough to cause sufferers to seek alternative employment. One case report exists in which the researchers suggest that chronic hypersensitivity pneumonitis from Shiitake mushroom spores was a causative agent for adenosquamous carcinoma of the lung,[84] although this has not been a commonly reported complication.

The causative agents appear to be constituents of the organic dusts, which are ubiquitous to nearly all areas of the mushroom farms. Spores of a variety of mushroom species as well as elevated airborne endotoxin concentrations are reported causes of chronic cough and pneumonitis in mushroom workers. This has led at least one investigator to ask if mushroom workers' chronic cough is actually the same as byssinosis and what the occupational exposure limits should be for endotoxin.[85] However, it is often not possible to isolate a specific antigen responsible for the condition, and the results of serologic assessments in many asymptomatic workers may demonstrate exposure to antigenic substances.

The medical management of mushroom workers lung is symptomatic and supportive. Removal from the source of the antigenic substances is the first order. β-Adrenergic agonists and steroids may be warranted in cases with acute effects. Follow-up provocation testing may or may not be able to isolate a specific cause.

CONCLUSION

The management of mushroom poisoning is best thought of by dividing mushrooms into clinical syndromes based

---

BOX 23-3 POSSIBLE PITFALLS IN THE TREATMENT OF MUSHROOM POISONING

Forgetting that "mushroom poisoning" may actually be an allergic reaction or food poisoning secondary to bacteria

Forgetting that "mushroom poisoning" may actually be secondary to pesticides sprayed on the mushroom or edible mushrooms laced with drugs (e.g., phencyclidine) or from a concomitant medical or surgical disease

Assuming that all persons ingesting the same mushroom must become ill

Assuming that if symptoms occur before 6 hr after ingestion, deadly *Amanita* species could not have been eaten

Discharging patients when they appear to have recovered from their gastrointestinal symptoms when those symptoms developed more than 6 hr after ingestion and therefore may have been due to a potentially very toxic mushroom

Forgetting the principles of supportive care while concentrating on toxin identification and antidotes on the toxins they contain. The treatment of mushroom poisoning is not significantly different from that for drug overdose; supportive care must take highest priority pending identification of the toxin.

Common pitfalls in the management of mushrooms poisoning are listed in Box 23-3. By avoiding these common errors and emphasizing supportive care and continued monitoring, the outcome in most cases of mushroom poisoning should be favorable.

REFERENCES

1. Baker T: Origins of the word *mushroom*. Mycologist 1990;3:88–90.
2. Klein AS, Hart J, Brems JJ, et al: *Amanita* poisoning: treatment and the role of liver transplantation. Am J Med 1989;86:187–193.
3. Trestrail JH: Mushroom poisoning in the United States—an analysis of 1989 United States Poison Center data. Clin Toxicol 1991;29:459–465.
4. Lampe KF, McCann MA: Differential diagnosis of poisoning by North American mushrooms, with particular emphasis on *Amanita phalloides*–like intoxication. Ann Emerg Med 1987;16:956–963.
5. Fischbein CB, Mueller GM, Leacock PR, et al: Digital imaging: a promising tool for mushroom identification. Acad Emerg Med 2003;10:808–811.
6. Spoerke DG, Rumack BH (eds): Handbook of Mushroom Poisoning: Diagnosis and Treatment. Boca Raton, FL, CRC Press, 1994.
7. Burda A, Sigg T, Fischbein C, et al: *Amanita virosa* poisoning: agent of terrorists or criminal activity? Vet Hum Toxicol 2003;45:226.
8. Duffy TJ, Vergeer PP: *Amanita* poisoning: treatment and role of liver transplantation [Letter]. Am J Med 1989;87:244.
9. Jaeger A, Jehl F, Flesch F, et al: Kinetics of amatoxins in human poisoning: therapeutic implications. Clin Toxicol 1993;31:63–80.
10. Beuhler M, Lee DC, Gerkin R: The Meixner test in the detection of α-amanitine and false-positive reactions caused by psilocin and 5-substituted tryptamines. Ann Emerg Med 2004;44:114–120.
11. Vogel G, Tuchweber V, Trost W, Mengs U: Protection by silibinin against *Amanita phalloides* intoxication in beagles. Toxicol Appl Pharmacol 1984;73:355–362.
12. Vogel G, Braatz R, Mengs U: On the nephrotoxicity of α-amanitin and the antagonistic effects of silymarin in rats. Agents Actions 1979;9:221–226.
13. Benjamin DR: Mushrooms: poisons and panaceas. New York, WH Freeman, 1995.
14. Montanini S, Sinardi D, Pratico C, et al: Use of acetylcysteine as the life-saving antidote in *Amanita phalloides* (death cap) poisoning. Arzneimittelforschung 1999;49:1044–1047.
15. Ponikvar R, Drinovec J, Kandus A, et al: Plasma exchange in management of severe acute poisoning with *Amanita phalloides*. Prog Clin Biol Res 1990;337:327–329.
16. Covic A, Goldsmith DJA, Gusbeth-Tatomir P, et al: Successful use of molecular absorbent regenerating system (MARS) dialysis for the treatment of fulminant hepatic failure in children accidentally poisoned by toxic mushroom ingestion. Liver Int 2003;23:21–27.
17. Faybik P, Hetz H, Baker A, et al: Extracorporeal albumin dialysis in patients with *Amanita phalloides* poisoning. Liver Int 2003;23:28–33.
18. Meunier BC, Camus CM, Houssin DP, et al: Liver transplantation after severe poisoning due to amatoxin-containing *Lepiota*—report of three cases. Clin Toxicol 1995;33:165–171.
19. Paydas S, Kocak R, Erturk F, et al: Poisoning due to amatoxin-containing *Lepiota* species. Br J Clin Pharmacol 1990;44:450–453.
20. Ramirez P, Parrilla P, Bueno FS, et al: Fulminant hepatic failure after *Lepiota* mushroom poisoning. J Hepatol 1993;19:51–54.
21. Schulz-Weddigen I: Beitrage zur kenntnis der gattung Lepiota: I. Eine intoxication mit Lepiota brunneo-incarnata in Nordwest-deutschland. Z Mykol 1986;52:91–100.
22. Benjamin DR: Mushroom poisoning in infants and children: the *Amanita pantherina/muscaria* group. Clin Toxicol 1992;30:13–22.
23. Bresinsky A, Besl H: Giftpilze. Stuttgart, Germany, Wissenschaftliche Verlagsgesellschat, 1985.
24. DeFeudis FV: Binding studies with muscimol: relation to synaptic γ-aminobutyrate receptors. Neuroscience 1980;5:675–688.
25. Hatfield GM, Brady LR: Toxin of higher fungi. Lloydia 1975;38:36–55.
26. Grymala S: Les recherches sur la frequence des intoxications par les champignons. Bull Med Leg Toxicol Med 1965;2:200–210.
27. Pyaysalo H, Niskanen A: On the occurrence of N-methyl-N-formylhydrazones in fresh and processed false morel, Gyromitra esculenta. J Agric Food Chem 1977;25:644–647.
28. Hanrahan J, Gordon M: Mushroom poisoning: case reports and review of therapy. JAMA 1984;251:1057–1061.
29. Gerault A, Girre L: Mise au point sur les intoxications par les champignons superieurs. Bull Soc Mycol Fr 1977;93:373–405.
30. Braun R, Greeff U, Netter KJ: Liver injury by the false morel poison gyromitrin. Toxicology 1979;12:155–163.
31. Schmiedeberg O, Koppe R: Das Muskarin, das giftige Alkaloid des Fliegenpilzes (*Agaricus muscarius* L.). Leipzig, Germany, Vogel, 1869.
32. Kogl F, Salemink CA, Schouten H, et al: Uber Muscarin III. Rec Trav Chim Pays-Bas 1957;76:109–127.
33. Stijve T: High performance thin layer chromatographic determination of the toxic principles of some poisonous mushrooms. Mitt Geb Lebensmittelunters Hyg 1981;72:44–54.
34. Hatfield GM, Schaumberg JP: Isolation and structural studies of coprine, the disulfiram-like constituent of *Coprinus atramentarius*. Lloydia 1975;38:489–496.
35. Herrmann M: Der Rettichhelmling-Mycena pura (Pers. Ex Fr.) Kum.—ist giftig! Mykol Mitt Bl 1973;17:17–18.
36. Michelot D, Toth B: Poisoning by *Gyromitra esculenta*—a review. J App Toxicol 1991;11:235–243.
37. Barbato MP: Poisoning from accidental ingestion of mushrooms. Med J Aust 1993;158:842–847.
38. Hatfield GM, Schaumberg JP: The disulfiram-like effects of *Coprinus atramentarius* and related mushrooms. In Rumack BH, Salzman C (eds): Mushrooms. New York, CRC Press, 1978, pp 181–186.
39. Iten PX: Antialkohol-Wirkstoff des Faltentintlings (*Coprinus atramentarius*) Aufgeklart, Schweiz. Z Pilzkd 1977;55:1–9.
40. Lindberg P: Coprine, a Cyclopropanone-Related Disulphiram-like Constituent of *Coprinus atramentarius* [Thesis]. University of Lund, Lund, Sweden, 1977, p 109.
41. Levine W: Formation of blue oxidation product from psilocybin. Nature 1967;215:1292–1293.
42. Ott J: A brief history of hallucinogenic mushrooms. In Ott J, Bigwood J (eds): Teononacatl: Hallucinogenic Mushrooms of North America. Seattle, WA, Madrona Press, 1978, pp 5–22.
43. Curry SC, Rose MC: Intravenous mushroom poisoning. Ann Emerg Med 1985;14:900–902.
44. Sivyer G, Dorrington L: Intravenous injection of mushroom [Letter]. Med J Aust 1984;140:182.
45. Schwartz RH, Smith DE: Hallucinogenic mushrooms. Clin Pediatr 1988;27:70–73.
46. Peden NR, Bissett AF, Macaulay KEC, et al: Clinical toxicology of "magic mushroom" ingestion. Postgrad Med J 1981;57:543–545.
47. McCrawley EL, Brummett RE, Dana GW: Convulsions from *Psilocybe* mushroom poisoning. Proc West Pharmacol Soc 1962;5:27–33.
48. Renfroe C, Messinger TA: Street drug analysis: an eleven-year perspective on illicit drug alteration. Semin Adolesc Med 1985;1:247–258.
49. Peden NR, Pringle SD, Crooks J: The problem of psilocybin mushroom abuse. Hum Toxicol 1982;1:417–424.
50. Schumacher T, Hoiland K: Mushroom poisoning caused by species of the genus *Cortinarius fries*. Arch Toxicol 1983;53:87–106.
51. Marichal JF, Triby F, Wiederkehr JL, et al: Insuffisance renale chronique apres intoxication par champignons de type *Cortinarius orellanus* Fries. Nouv. Presse Med 1977;6:2973–2975.
52. Bouget J, Bousser J, Pats B, et al: Acute renal failure following collective intoxication by *Cortinarius orellanus*. Intensive Care Med 1990;16:506–510.
53. Delpech N, Rapior S, Cozette AP, et al: Evolution d'une insufficiance renale aigue par ingestion volontaire de *Cortinarius orellanus*. Presse Med 1990;19:122–124.
54. Koppel C: Clinical symptomatology and management of mushroom poisoning. Toxicon 1993;31:1513–1540.
55. Tebbett IR, Caddy B: Mushroom toxins of the genus *Cortinarius*. Experientia 1984;40:441–446.

56. Nieminen L: Effects of drugs on mushroom poisoning induced in the rat by *Cortinarius speciosissimus*. Arch Toxicol 1976;35:235–238.

57. Richard JM, Louis J, Cantin D, et al: Nephrotoxicity of orellanine, a toxin from the mushroom *Cortinarius orelaanus*. Arch Toxicol 1988;62:242–245.

58. Richard JM, Creppy EE, Benoit-Guyod JL, et al: Orellanine inhibits protein synthesis in Madrin-Darby canine kidney cells, in rat liver mitochondria, and in vitro: indication for its activation prior to in vitro inhibition. Toxicology 1991;67:53–62.

59. Warden CR, Benjamin DR: Acute renal failure associated with suspected Amanita smithiana mushroom ingestions: a case series. Acad Emerg Med 1998;5:808–812.

60. Pelizarri CV, Feifal E, Rohrmoser MM, et al: Partial purification and characterization of a toxic component of *Amanita smithiana*. Mycologia 1994;86:555–560.

61. Bedry R, Baudrimont I, Deffieux G, et al: Wild-mushroom intoxication as a cause of rhabdomyolysis. New Engl J Med 2001;345:798–802.

62. Chodorowski Z, Waldman W, Sein Anand J: Acute poisoning with Tricholoma equestre. Prezegl Lek 2002;59:386–387.

63. Flammer R: Hamolyse bei Pilzvergiftungen: Fakten und Hypothesen. Schweiz Med Wochenschr 1983;113:1555–1561.

64. Schmidt J, Hartmann W, Wurstlin A, et al: Akutes Nierenversagen durch immunhamolytische Anamie nach Genuss des Kahlen Kremplings (*Paxillus involutus*). Dtsch Med Wochenschr 1971;96:1188–1191.

65. Deicher H, Stangel W: Akute immunhamolytische Anamie nach Genuss des Kahlen Kremplings. Verh Dtsch Ges Inn Med 1977;83:1606–1609.

66. Bobrowski H: Ostra niewydolnosc nerek w przebiegu ostrego nabytego zespolu hemolitycznego u osoby uczulonej na grzyb maslak (*Boletus luteus*) [Acute renal failure in the course of an acute haemolytic reaction in a subject sensitive to *Boletus luteus*.] Pol Tyg Lek 1966;21:1864–1865.

67. Albrecht W: Gibt es enzymabhangige und blutgruppenspezifische Pilzvergiftnungen. Sudwestdeutsche Pilzrundschau 1983;19:11–14.

68. Hausen BM: Unerwunschte Nebenwirkungen beim Genuss essbarer Pilze. Mat Med Nordm 1977;29:230–253.

69. Lincoff GH: The Audubon Society Field Guide to North American Mushrooms. New York, Knopf, 1981, p 926.

70. Prager MH, Goos RD: A case of mushroom poisoning from *Suillus luteus*. Mycopathologia 1984;85:175–176.

71. Christiansen AL, Rasmussen KE, Tonnesen F: Determination of psilocybin in *Psilocybe semilanceata* using high-performance liquid chromatography on a silica column. J Chromatogr 1981;210:163–167.

72. Winkelmann M, Stangel W, Schedel I, et al: Severe hemolysis caused by antibodies against the mushroom *Paxillus involutus* and its therapy by plasma exchange. Klin Wochenschr 1986;64:935–938.

73. Lefevre H: Immunhamolytische Anamie nach Genuss des Kahlen Krempling (*Paxillus involutus*). Dtsch Med Wochenschr 1982;107:1374.

74. Winkelmann M, Borchard F, Stangel W, et al: Todlich verlaufene immunhamolytische Anamie nach Genuss des Kahlen Kremplings (*Paxillus involutus*). Dtsch Med Wochenschr 1982;107:1190–1194.

75. Lehmann PF, Khazan U: Mushroom poisoning by *Chlorophyllum molybdites* in the midwest United States. Mycopathologia 1992;118:3–12.

76. Mitchell SH, Kilpatrick M: Occurrence of pesticide residues in mushrooms in Northern Ireland. Food Addit Contam 2003;20:716–719.

77. Marzano FN, Bracchi PG, Pizzetti P: Radioactive and conventional pollutants accumulated by edible mushrooms (*Boletus* sp.) are useful indicators of species origin. Environ Res 2001;85:260–264.

78. Falandysc J, Jedrusiak A, Lipka K, et al: Mercury in wild mushrooms and underlying soil substrate from Koszalin, North-Central Poland. Chemosphere 2004;54L:461–466.

79. Gas MI, Segovia N, Morton O, et al: 137Cs and relationships with major and trace elements in edible mushrooms from Mexico. Sci Total Environ 2000;262:73–89.

80. Curnow P, Tam M: Contact dermatitis to Shiitake mushrooms. Aust J Dermatol 2003;44:155–177.

81. Johnson WM, Kleyn JG: Respiratory disease in a mushroom workers. J Occup Med 1981;23:49–51.

82. Sanderson W, Kullman G, Sastre J: Outbreak of hypersensitivity pneumonitis among mushroom farm workers. Am J Ind Med 1992;22:859–872.

83. Tanaka H, Saikai T, Sugawara H, et al: Three-year follow-up study of allergy in workers in a mushroom factory. Resp Med 2001;95:943–948.

84. Suzuki K, Tanaka H, Sugawara H, et al: Chronic hypersensitivity pneumonitis induced by Shiitake mushroom spores associated with lung cancer. Intern Med 2001;40:1132–1135.

85. Lange JH, Fedeli U, Mastrangelo G: Is mushroom workers' chronic cough the same as byssinosis and what should the occupational exposure limit be for endotoxin? Chest 2003;123:2160–2162.

24 Poisonous Plants

SUSAN C. SMOLINSKE, PHARMD ■ G. PATRICK DAUBERT, MD ■ DAVID G. SPOERKE, MS, RPH

At a Glance...

- Most pediatric unintentional ingestions of plants and berries can be safely managed at home.
- A few plants can cause serious toxicity with one bite of berry/leaf/root:
  - Autumn crocus
  - Castor bean
  - Common oleander
  - Glory lily
  - Jequirity bean
  - Lily of the valley
  - Monkshood
  - Poison hemlock
  - Water hemlock, water hemlock dropwort
  - Yellow oleander
- Gastric decontamination is generally not indicated.
- Few specific antidotes are available.
- Physostigmine can be considered for serious *Datura* exposures.
- Digoxin Fab fragments can be considered for cardiac glycoside poisoning.
- Photographs of many toxic plants can be found on pages 14 to 21.

INTRODUCTION AND RELEVANT HISTORY

Plants are one of the most common sources of accidental poisoning in children. In 2003, there were 57,778 plant exposures in children under the age of 6 years reported to the Toxic Exposure Surveillance System (TESS), 4.6% of total poisonings in that age group. In contrast, adult plant poisoning is much less common. In the same year, there were only 10,048 plant poisonings in patients older than 19 years.[1] Fatalities are rare in developed countries. Between 1983 and 2000 in the United States, there were 30 fatal plant exposures; 7 were related to *Cicuta* species, 5 to *Datura* species, 1 to *Conium maculatum*, 1 to oleander extract, and 1 to *Gloriosa superba*.[2] In 2003, there were three plant-related fatalities: a 34-year-old man who drank absinthe liquor and died of complications from aspiration pneumonitis, a 61-year-old man who injected crushed castor beans intravenously, and a 50-year-old patient who ingested yew. A series of five plant-related deaths were reported in Switzerland between 1966 and 1994. Species involved were *Colchicum* (two cases), *Oenanthe crocata*, *Taxus baccata*, and *Narcissus* (daffodil).[3]

These facts are in contrast with international experiences with more widespread plant poisonings, particularly in developing countries, due to unsafe food-handling practices or cultural choice of plants as a common mode of suicide. For example, intentional ingestion of yellow oleander is a major clinical problem in Sri Lanka, with a fatality rate of up to 9%. In two studies, involving 631 patients hospitalized for plant poisoning over 2 years, 12% to 17% were related to *Thevetia*, with 6% to 7% fatal outcomes. A follow-up study in 1996 showed 4361 patients over 3 years, with 32% to 36% related to *Thevetia* and 3% to 4% fatal.[4] In the Indian state of Kerala, plants are responsible for 10% of all poisonings, with *Cerbera odollam* (the suicide tree) accounting for half of the plant exposures, most involving suicide or homicide. *Atractylis* poisoning in Maghreb populations of Morocco, Algeria, and Tunisia carries a 65% case fatality rate. Ingestion of unripe ackee fruit is estimated to cause thousands of deaths annually in the Caribbean. Epidemics of ascending peripheral neuropathy are common in Mexico and Central America due to ingestion of buckthorn fruit. These examples serve as reminders that serious toxicity can occur from plant poisoning, particularly with intentional exposures.

The antimuscarinic symptoms of various plants have been recorded throughout history. Henbane, deadly nightshade, and thorn apple (*Datura* species) are mentioned among favorite poisonings in ancient Rome.[5] The wives of the Roman emperors Augustus and Claudius are reputed to have used deadly nightshade to murder large numbers of Romans. The more famous history of intoxication from *Datura* species came in 1676, when British soldiers were sent to Virginia near Jamestown to stop the Rebellion of Bacon. As part of a final meal before entering the rebellion, several soldiers were offered a salad which included a local weed (Jamestown weed, today known as Jimson weed). The ensuing toxicity rendered the soldiers incapable of fighting for several days.[6,7]

Another historical example is provided by a paper presented by Dr. Barton to the American Philosophical Society in 1794. It described with great detail epidemics of poisoned honey made from toxic plants, including rhododendron, yew, oleander, water hemlock, and others, particularly in colonial America. In one European case cited, he described an account by Xenophon in the *Anabasis* that reported the poisoning of his troops by the honey of *Rhododendron ponticum* flowers.[8]

Table 24-1 lists toxic plants found in the United States and their characteristics.

STRUCTURE-ACTIVITY RELATIONSHIPS

Alkaloids

Webster's online dictionary traces the origin of the term *alkaloid* to popular literature sometime before 1887. At the time it was applied to any organic base, for example, a nitrogenous substance that forms salts with acids. In

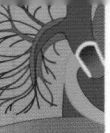

TABLE 24-1 Some Toxic Plants Found in the United States

COMMON NAME	SCIENTIFIC NAME	TOXIC PART	TOXIC AGENT
Akee	*Blighia sapida*	Fruit except aril	Hypoglycin A and B
*Allamanda	*Allamanda cathartica*	All except root	Unknown cathartic
*Alocasia	*Alocasia* species	Leaves, stems	Oxalates
Aloe	*Aloe* species	Latex	Barbaloin
Anthurium	*Anthurium* species	Foliage, fruit	Oxalates
Ape	*Alocasia* species	Leaves, stems	Oxalates
Apple	*Malus* species	Seed	Cyanide glycosides
Apricot	*Prunus* species	Seed kernel	Cyanide glycosides
Autumn crocus	*Colchicum autumnale*	All	Colchicine alkaloids
Azalea	*Rhododendron* species	All	Andromedotoxin
*Baneberry	*Actaea* species	Berries, roots	Protoanemonin
Belladonna	*Atropa belladonna*	All	Atropine, scopolamine
Bethlehem star	*Ornithogalum umbellatum*	All	Colchicine alkaloids
Bird of paradise	*Casesalpinia gilliesii*	Pods	Unknown
Bittersweet	*Solanum dulcamara*	Variable, foliage	Solanine, tropane alkaloids
*Black locust	*Robinia pseudoacacia*	Seeds, young leaves	Robin, robitin, phasin
Bleeding heart	*Dicentra formosa*	Foliage, root	Isoquinolines
*Blue flag	*Iris* species	Leaves, root stalks	Irisin, iridin, irigenin
*Buckeye	*Aesculus glabra*	Foliage, seed, flower	Esculin
Burn bean	*Sophora secundiflora*	All	Cytisine
*Buttercups	*Ranunculus* species	All	Protoanemonin
Daffodil	*Narcissus* species	Bulb	Lycorine, narcissine
*Caladium	*Caladium bicolor*	All	Oxalates
Candlenut	*Aleurites molluccana*	All, seeds	Phorbol
Carolina jasmine	*Gelsemium sempervirens*	All, berries	Gelsemine
*Castor bean	*Ricinus communis*	All (seeds mainly)	Ricin
Celandine	*Chelidonium majus*	Roots	Isoquinoline alkaloids
*Century plant	*Agave americana*	Sap	Unknown
Chinaberry	*Melia azedarach*	Fruit	Possible resinoid
*Christmas rose	*Helleborus niger*	Foliage, root	Helleborin
Corn cockle	*Agrostemma githago*	Seeds	Githagin
*Cowbane	*Cicuta* species	All	Cicutoxin
Crab's eye	*Abrus precatorius*	Seeds	Abrin, abric acid
Daffodil	*Narcissus* species	Bulb	Lycorine and others
Daphne	*Daphne* species	All	Mezereinic anhydride
Deadly nightshade	*Atropa belladonna*	All	Atropine, scopolamine
Delphinium	*Delphinium* species	All	Delphinine, ajacine
Desert potato	*Jatropha macrorhiza*	Root	Phytotoxins
Desert rose	*Adenium* species	All	Cardiac glycosides
Dieffenbachia	*Dieffenbachia* species	All	Oxalates, proteins
*Dogbane	*Apocynum* species	Rhizome	Apocynamarin
Dog's parley	*Aethusa cynapium*	All	Aethusanol A, coniine
Doll's eyes	*Actaea* species	Berries, roots	Protoanemonin
Donkeytail	*Euphorbia myrsinites*	Foliage, sap	Diterpenes, phorbols
Dumbcane	*Dieffenbachia* species	All	Oxalates, proteins
Dutchman's breeches	*Dicentra cucullaria*	Folliage, root	Isoquinlines
Elephant's ear	*Alocasia, Colocasia*	All	Oxalates
Fava beans	*Vicia faba*	Seed, pollen	Enzyme dificiency
Fool's parsley	*Aethusa cynapium*	All	Aethusanol A coniine
Four o'clock	*Mirabilis jalapa*	Root, seed	Trigonelline
*Foxglove	*Digitalis purpurea*	Leaves, seeds	Digitalis glycosides
Golden chain	*Laburnum anagyroides*	Seed capsules	Cytisine
Gordolobo	*Senecio longilobus*	All	Pyrrolizidines
Groundsel	*Senecio longilobus*	All	Pyrrolizidines
Heavenly blue	*Ipomoea violacea*	Seeds	Ergine, isoergine
Holly	*Ilex* species	Berries	Ilicin
Honeysuckle	*Lonicera* species	Berries	Unknown gastrointestinal irritant
Horse chestnut	*Aesculus hippocastanum*	Foliage, seed, flower	Esculin
Hyacinth	*Hyacinthus orientalis*	Bulb	Narcissine
Hydrangea	*Hydrangea* species	All	Cyanide glycosides
*Indian licorice	*Abrus precatorius*	Seeds	Abrin, abric acid
*Indian tobacco	*Lobelia inflata*	All	Lobeline
Indian turnip	*Arisaema triphyllum*	Rhizome	Oxalates
*Inkberry	*Phylolacca americana/decandra*	All parts, fruit least	Saponin, glycoprotein, and phytolaccotoxin
*Iris	*Iris* species	Leaves, root stalks	Irisin, iridin, irigenin
Jack-in-the-pulpit	*Arisaema triphyllum*	Rhizome	Oxalates
Japan oil tree	*Aleurites cordata*	All, seeds	Phorbol

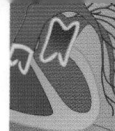

TABLE 24-1   Some Toxic Plants Found in the United States (Cont'd)

COMMON NAME	SCIENTIFIC NAME	TOXIC PART	TOXIC AGENT
Jasmine, yellow	*Gelsemium sempervirens*	All, berries	Gelsemine
*Jequirity bean	*Abrus precatorius*	Seeds	Abrin, abric acid
Jerusalem cherry	*Solanum pseudocapsicum*	Berries	Solanine, tropane alkaloids
Jimsonweed	*Solanum stramonium*	All	Solanine and tropane alkaloids
Narcissus	*Narcissus* species	Bulb	Lycorine, narcissine
Nightshades	*Solanum* species	Variable, foliage	Solanine and tropane alkaloids
Laburnum	*Laburnum anagyroides*	Seed capsules	Cytisine
*Lantana	*Lantana camara*	Berries (unripe)	Lantadene A
Larkspur	*Delphinium* species	Seeds, young foliage	Delphinine
Lesser hemlock	*Aethusa cynapium*	All	Aethusanol A, coniine
Lily of the valley	*Convallaria majalis*	All	Digitalis-like alkaloids
*Marsh marigolds	*Caltha palustris, Caltha leptocephala*	All	Protoanemonin
Mescal	*Lophophora williamsii*	All (button)	Mescaline and others
Mistletoe	*Phoradendron* species	Berries	Phenylethylamine, tyramine, choline
*Monkshood	*Aconitum* species	Roots, seeds, leaves	Aconitine
Moonseed	*Menispermum canadense*	All	Dauricine
Morning glory	*Ipomoea violacea*	Seeds	Ergine, isoergine
Mountain laurel	*Sophora secundiflora*	All	Cytosine
	Kalmia latifolia	All	Andromedotoxin
Narcissus	*Narcissus* species	Bulb	Lycorine and others
Nightshades	*Solanum* species	Variable, foliage	Solanine alkaloids
*Oleanders	*Nerium oleander*	All	Oleandrin, nerioside
Pasque flower	*Anemone patens*	All	Protoanemonin
Peach	*Prunus* species	Seed kernel	Cyanide glycosides
Pearly gates	*Ipomoea violacea*	Seeds	Ergine, isoergine
Pencil tree	*Euphorbia tirucalli*	Foliage, sap	Phorbols
Peyote	*Lophophora williamsii*	All	Mescaline, others
*Philodendron	*Philodendron* species	All	Oxalates
*Pigeon berry	*Phytolacca americana/decandra*	All parts, fruit least	Saponin, glycoprotein, and phytolaccotoxin
Poinciana	*Casesalpinia gilliesii*	Pods	Unknown
*Poison hemlock	*Conium maculatum*	All	Coniine
*Poison ivy	*Toxicodendron radicans*	All	Urushiol
*Pokeweed	*Phytolacca americana/decandra*	All parts, fruit least	Saponin, glycoprotein, and phytolaccotoxin
*Precatory bean	*Abrus precatorius*	Seeds	Abrin, abric acid
Privet	*Ligustrum japonicum*	All	Andromedotoxin
Red squill	*Urginea maritime*	Bulb	Cardiac glycosides
Rhododendron	*Rhododendron* species	All	Andromedotoxin
Rhubarb	*Rheum rhaponticum*	Leave blade	Oxalates, anthraquinones
*Rosary pea	*Abrus precatorius*	Seeds	Abrin, abric acid
Snowdrop	*Ornithogalum umbellatum*	All	Alkaloids (colchicine)
Skunk cabbage	*Symplocarpus foetidus*	All	Oxalates
Sweet pea	*Lathyrus odoratus*	Seeds	Aminopropionitrile
Texas mountain laurel	*Sophora secundiflora*	All	Cytosine
Thornapple	*Solanum stramonium*	All	Solanine and tropane alkaloids
Threadleaf groundsel	*Senecio longilobus*	All	Pyrrolizidines
Tree tobacco	*Nicotiana* species	All	Nicotine alkaloids
Tung nut	*Aleurites fordii*	All, seeds	Phorbols
*Water hemlock	*Cicuta* species	All	Cicutoxin
White snakeroot	*Eupatorium rugosum*	Above ground parts	Tremetone
Wild tobacco	*Nicotiana* species	All	Nicotine alkaloids
Wisteria	*Wisteria floribunda Wisteria sinensis*	Seeds	Gelsemine and gelseminine
*Wolfsbane	*Aconitum* species	Roots, seeds, leaves	Aconitine
Yellow jasmine	*Gelsemium sempervirens*	All, berries	Gelsemine
Yellow oleander	*Thevetia peruviana*	All parts	Thevetin A and B
Yew	*Taxus* species	All part, aril least	Taxine

the updated 1911 version, the definition changed to restrict the term to bases of vegetable origin and characterized by remarkable toxicologic or pharmacologic effects. Treating the plant with a dilute acid and precipitating the bases with potash, soda, lime, or magnesia can chemically extract the base. The separation of the mixed bases obtained occurs through repeated fractional crystallization, or by taking advantage of certain properties

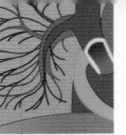

of the constituents. Structure-activity relationships of selected plant toxins are discussed in the ensuing paragraphs.

Pyrrolizidine alkaloids, such as sececionine and symphytine, have three structural requirements for toxicity. They must contain an unsaturated (double bond at the 1:2 position) heterocyclic ring, the ring nucleus must have an esterified hydroxyl group, and the ester side chains must contain at least one branched carbon chain. The parent compounds are converted by CYP1A2 and 2E1 to pyrrolic esters and then further to pyrrolic alcohols. The acute toxicity is most likely related to the more reactive esters, which can alkylate DNA.

Colchicine is an alkaloidal amine without a heterocyclic nitrogen atom. It contains four methyl groups. When hydrolyzed to trimethylcolchicinic acid, with loss of a methyl group, activity is lost.

Grayanotoxins are diterpenoid alkaloids, also known as andromedotoxins. To produce toxicity, a hydroxyl group at R1 is essential. An ester group at R3 decreases toxicity, but larger ester groups have greater toxicity. The interaction of grayanotoxin with the sodium channel involves contact by hydrogen binding with the 3-β-OH, 5-β-OH and 6-β-OH sites and by hydrophobic bonds in binding to the sodium channel. Grayanotoxins, and perhaps aconitine and vertradine as well, appear to contain four hydroxyl groups essential for optimal hydrophobicity and biologic activity. Altering the number of hydroxyl groups reduces the toxin's biologic activity.[9]

Diterpene Ester Alkaloids

Three groups of compounds are considered to be diterpene esters. Phorbol esters are most commonly associated with irritant properties in Euphorbia species. Ingenol esters and daphnane esters are also irritants. Structural requirements for irritancy include an ester group at carbon 13, a rigid tetracyclic structure, a C ring in a cis transfiguration, AB rings in the trans transfiguration, and a four-β function. Irritancy is enhanced when R1 becomes unsaturated and with increasing chain length at R1.

Another diterpene compound, salvinorin A, from Salvia divinorum, is a potent and selective κ opioid receptor agonist, resulting in hallucinations. Screening of salvinorins and derivatives for binding affinity and functional activity at opioid receptors have suggested that the methyl ester and furan ring are required for activity but that the lactone and ketone functionalities are not.[10]

Aconitine alkaloids with diester bonds appear to have the most toxicity compared with those alkaloids with no ester side chain, which have few clinical effects.[11]

Glycosides

Glycosides are defined as any compound that contains a carbohydrate molecule that is convertible by hydrolytic cleavage into a sugar (glycone) and a nonsugar component (aglycone or genin). Examples include the cardenolides, bufadienolides, amygdalin, anthraquinones, and salicin. Saponins consist of an aglycone with a triterpenoid or steroid backbone linked to a carbohydrate molecule. This confers their ability to form soap-like foams in aqueous solutions.

Cardenolides are 23-carbon steroids with an α,β-unsaturated five-membered lactone ring on carbon 17. These include digitoxin, convallatoxin, and evonoside. Bufadienolides are 24-carbon steroids with a double unsaturated six-membered lactone ring on carbon 17. Examples include convallamarin, scillaren, and hellebrin. The lactone ring was initially considered to be responsible for the inotropic activity of the cardiotonic steroids. However, research conducted with digitalis and differing lactone rings demonstrated little cardiotonic activity among the lactone rings.[12] The five- and six-membered lactone rings more likely contribute energy to the cardiac steroid/adenosine triphosphatase (ATPase) bond through a conformational change promoted by the steroidal binding.[13]

Three positions of the steroid nucleus appear to be essential for the activity of the cardiac glycosides. These are the carbons at the 3-, 14-, and 17-positions. The 17-carbon position links the steroid nucleus to the lactone ring. The hydroxyl group at the C14 position is not an essential feature for inotropic activity, although when it is replaced by hydrogen, potency decreases considerably.[14] To retain cardiac toxicity, the hydroxyl group at C14 confers added potency, and the configuration of the C/D ring must be in cis configuration. Additional hydroxyl groups confer more rapid onset and shorter duration of activity. Its larger role probably resides in its ability to modify the spatial disposition of ring D enabling an interaction of the lactone with ATPase.[15] Otherwise, the D ring does not appear to be essential for cardiotonic activity.[16]

The wide range of toxicity among the cardiac glycosides resides in the complex interaction of the steroid nucleus, sugar moiety, and the lactone ring with ATPase. The steroid nucleus is key to the cardiac glycoside interacting with ATPase. Plant cardiotoxin sterols differ from mammalian sterols in the ring orientation. The difference is mostly in the orientation of the A ring to the B ring. In mammalian steroids, the A/B ring juncture is in a trans configuration. However, plant cardiac glycosides have an A/B ring juncture that is cis, and the two hydrogens are on the same side of the rings.[17] The change of the A/B junction does not necessarily imply a decrease of activity of the steroid, although it does for the corresponding glycosides, indicating that the main influence of A/B junction arises from its ability to place the sugar into a suitable position.

Although the fundamental pharmacologic activity of these plant toxins resides in the steroid nucleus, the sugar residues play an integral role in their activity. The sugar residue increases the water solubility of the steroid nucleus, making it more available for translocation into the myocardium. The lipophilic steroid nucleus is important in the compound's onset and duration of action. The presence of an acetyl group on the sugar moiety also affects the lipophilic character and the kinetics of the entire glycoside. In general, cardiac glycosides with more lipophilic character are absorbed faster and exhibit longer duration of actions as a result of slower urinary excretion rate. Lipophilicity is markedly

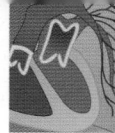

influenced by the number of sugar residues and the number of hydroxyl groups on the aglycone part of the glycoside. As the steroidal rings are substituted with polar hydroxy substitutes, the onset of action becomes faster and the duration decreases.[18] Cardiac glycosides with monosaccharide sugar residues appear to have great potency, suggesting that only the first sugar molecule is involved in receptor binding.[19-21]

Polyacetylenes

Cicutoxin is a noncompetitive γ-aminobutyric acid (GABA)-mediated chloride channel antagonist. The compound is a long π-bond conjugated polyacetylene system, with a terminal hydroxyl, and an allylic hydroxyl group. The length and geometry of the π-bond and O-functional groups correlated with neurotoxicity and with potency in inhibition of the GABA channel. Other polyacetylene compounds, such as falcarinol, which have a carbonyl group conjugated with both double and triple bonds, have been associated with phototoxicity, but not neurotoxicity. Plants containing falcarinol include *Hedera helix*, *Panax pseudoginseng*, *Schefflera arboricola*, *Tagetes patula*, and *Daucus carota*.

PHARMACOLOGY

Pharmacokinetics

Pharmacokinetic data are available for only a few plant-derived constituents. Examples of onset and duration of effect from plant poisonings are given in Box 24-1.

PATHOPHYSIOLOGY

Due to the multiple constituents of many plants, the mechanism by which a plant causes toxicity can be complex. Many plants may also possess features that cause toxicity in more than one organ system. The most common type of plant intoxication is gastrointestinal (GI) irritation.

Gastrointestinal Irritation: Amaryllidaceae Alkaloids

Plants from the Amaryllidaceae family contain several alkaloids that have been linked to GI distress in humans.[22] Most of these alkaloids are derived from phenanthridine, and are typically in highest concentration in the outer layers of the bulbs.[23] Daffodil bulbs may be mistaken for onions by the unwary consumer. Some plants containing Amaryllidaceae alkaloids include *Narcissus* spp. (daffodils and jonquils), Liliaceae spp. (spider lily), *Momordica charantia* (balsam pear), *Hippeastrum equestre* (amaryllis), *Hyacinthus orientalis* (hyacinth), *Amaryllis belladonna* (March lily), *Ammocharis coranica* (ground lily), *Boophone disticha* (fan-leaved boophone, poison bulb, sore-eye flower, tumblehead), *Brunsvigia* spp. (candelabra flowers), *Clivia miniatah* (St. John's lily), *Crinum* spp., *Cyrtanthus* spp., *Galanthus nivalis* (snowdrop), *Haemanthus coccineus* (April

fool), *Nerine* spp., *Scadoxus* spp., and *Zephyranthes* spp. (zephyr lilies). The Amaryllidaceae alkaloids most well described include galanthamine, narciclasine, and lycorine. These alkaloids are specific protein inhibitors and have strong emetic properties. Galanthamine possesses anticholinesterase actions similar to physostigmine and has been evaluated in the treatment of Alzheimer's disease.[24] It also has antimuscarinic and analgesic effects. Narciclasine acts as a microtubule inhibitor similar to colchicine, particularly at concentrations above 0.5 mg/kg.[25]

Gastrointestinal Irritation: Triterpene Saponin

Another group of plant components that cause more specific intestinal mucosa irritation rather than gastric irritation is the triterpene alkaloids. Plants with triterpene alkaloids include *Aesculus hippocastanum* (horse chestnut), *Hedera helix* (English ivy), *Phytolacca americana* (pokeweed), *Actaea* spp. (baneberry), and *Medicago truncatula* (barrel medic). Triterpenes are related to steroids and cholesterol and are broadly described as saponins because of their ability to form a soapy consistency when concentrated. Pokeweed is the most well-described plant in this group. It has been commonly used in cooking, salads, and herbal remedies. Teas from pokeweed are reputed to treat rheumatism, helminth infections, and constipation. The pokeweed root may also be mistaken for horseradish.[26] The triterpene alkaloids are heat labile, but the process of parboiling is recommended if the leaves or berries are to be used. The toxic triterpene saponins of Pokeweed include phytolaccatoxin and phytolaccagenin. *P. americana* also contains proteins exhibiting mitogenic[27,28] and antiviral[29] properties. The mitogenic activity is attributed to pokeweed lectin, specific for *N*-acetylglucosamine-containing saccharides, which stimulates peripheral lymphocytes to undergo mitosis by binding to their cell surfaces.

Irritation from Plants that Contain Calcium Oxalate

Plants may contain several types of oxalates, commonly separated into soluble and insoluble oxalates. Insoluble oxalates produce localized tissue injury. Plants with insoluble oxalates are found in a variety of common houseplants and ornamental plants. The most common include *Philodendron*, *Dieffenbachia*, *Caladium*, *Axisaema triphyllum* (Jack-in-the-pulpit), *Colocasia* (elephant ear), *Rheum raponticum* (rhubarb), *Scindapsus aureus* (pothos), *Calla palustris* (wild calla), and *Symplocarpus foetidus* (skunk cabbage). Oxalic acid is a by-product of a plant's cellular metabolism and often takes the form of a crystal when it combines with calcium.[30] The crystalline structure varies among calcium oxalate crystals, and the shape may dictate the extent of local injury. Parallel needle-shaped crystals arranged in bundles are known as raphides and are a common source of intoxication. Raphides are commonly contained within a cellular structure called an idioblast. Calcium oxalate crystals not contained within idioblasts (*Inpatiens* spp.) have not been shown to produce significant toxicity.[31] When stimulated (chewing

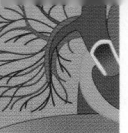

BOX 24-1	TOXIC PRINCIPLES

Aconitine-like Alkaloids

Symptoms: Numbness, tingling of lips and tongue, bradycardia or irregular pulse, gastroenteritis, respiratory failure, vagal nerve stimulation.

Pharmacokinetics: three active metabolites, excreted in urine up to 6 days, not dialyzable due to high molecular weight (645 kD) and lipophilicity; onset 3 minutes to 2 hours, usually 10–20 minutes; dermally absorbed.

Source: monkshood

Agave americana Irritant

Symptoms: Sap contains an unknown dermal irritant that may produce rash (sometimes hemorrhagic). Systemic signs may be fever and leucocytosis.

Source: *Agave americana*

Aminopropionitrile

Symptoms: Skeletal abnormalities, growth suppression, muscle paralysis with chronic ingestion.

Pharmacokinetics: Onset 4–8 weeks; duration 1 month or more after removal from diet.

Source: sweet pea (*Lathyrus*)

Andromedotixin (Synonym: Grayanotoxin)

Symptoms: Gastroenteritis, muscle paralysis, CNS depression, respiratory failure, heart muscle inhibition, cardiac poison, paralyzes vagus and motor nerve ends in striated muscle.

Pharmacokinetics: Onset 30–120 minutes; duration less than 24 hours.

Sources: mountain laurel, buttercups, *Andromeda* species, *Rhododendron* species

Anthraquinone Glycosides

Symptoms: Purgative, irritant, nephritis with large doses.
Pharmacokinetics: Onset 6–8 hours.
Sources: Many Aloe species
Example: barbaloin

Casesalpinia Toxin

Symptoms: Exact toxin unknown, usually produces severe vomiting and diarrhea that may lead to dehydration.

Pharmacokinetics: Symptoms may persist for 24 hours.

Source: *Casesalpinia gilliesii*

Cicutoxin

Symptoms: Abdominal pain, salivation, vomiting, mydriasis, delirium, severe seizures.

Pharmacokinetics: Onset 5 minutes to 1–2 hours; may be dialyzable.

Source: water hemlock

Colchicine-like Alkaloids

Symptoms: Symptoms include oral irritation and pain, vomiting, violent diarrhea, renal failure, and shock.

Pharmacokinetics: Peak plasma levels in 30 minutes to 2 hours. Serious symptom onset may be delayed for 2–6 hours. Lethal cases have occurred after a quiescent period. High enterohepatic circulation; high volume of distribution (10–12 L/kg); elimination half-life 1.7–32 hours.

Sources: autumn crocus, meadow saffron, star of Bethlehem

Coniine

Symptoms: Vomiting, initial CNS stimulation followed by CNS depression, muscle paralysis, respiratory failure.

Pharmacokinetics: Onset within 30 minutes.
Source: poison hemlock

Cyanogenic Glycosides

Symptoms: Cyanide-like, hyperpnea, shock, coma, marked metabolic acidosis. Lethal ingestions recorded, usually of large quantities of kernels or seeds.

Pharmacokinetics: Onset 90 minutes to 2 hours or longer.

Sources: Seed kernels of peach, pear, apricot, apple seeds, purified glycosides used medically, *Hydrangea* species

Examples: amygdalin, prunisin, hydrangin, githagin, linimarin

Cytisine

Symptoms: Nicotine-like in effects; dysphagia, vomiting, headache, incoordination, vertigo, possible confusion, excitement, respiratory stimulation, renal failure, convulsions, mydriasis, death via asphyxiation possible.

Pharmacokinetics: Onset 15–60 minutes; peak plasma level 2 hours in mice; elimination half-life 200 minutes in mice.

Sources: Golden chain tree, *Laburnum* species, Texas mountain laurel

Daphnin

Symptoms: Skin vesicant; ingestion may lead to vomiting, diarrhea, renal failure, convulsions and death.

Source: daphne

Delphinine Alkaloid

Symptoms: Gastroenteritis, respiratory depression, hypotension, paresthesias, salivation, headache, heart arrhythmias.

Sources: larkspur, delphiniums

Digitalis-like Glycosides

Symptoms: Possible dizziness and vomiting; these are cardiac glycosides that may produce arrhythmias. Atrioventricular block may occur.

Pharmacokinetics: Peak effect 4–12 hours; volume of distribution of digitoxin is 0.6 L/kg; digitoxin is metabolized to digoxin; half-life of digitoxin 4–6 days.

Sources: Foxglove, lily of the valley

Examples: digitoxin, digitalin, digitonin, convallarin, convallamarin, convallatoxin, apocynamarin, gitoxin, gitalin, hellebrin, evonoside

Diterpene Irritants

Symptoms: Irritation of skin, eyes, mucous membranes; vomiting, diarrhea.

Pharmacokinetics: Form acyl groups upon hydrolysis, which are cocarcinogenic; onset 2–8 hours; peak skin irritation and vesicle formation 4–24 hours; duration 3–4 days.

Sources: *Euphoria* species like donkey tail, pencil tree, crown of thorns

Examples: phorbols, tigliane

Esculin

Symptoms: Vomiting, diarrhea, muscle twitching, ataxia, paralysis, mydriasis, CNS depression, death.

Sources: horse chestnut, buckeye seeds

Gelsemine

Symptoms: Motor neuron depression and paralysis may lead to respiratory failure.

Sources: yellow or Carolina jasmine

Examples: gelsemine, gelseminine

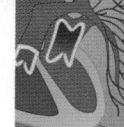

BOX 24-1	TOXIC PRINCIPLES (Cont'd)

Helleborin/Helleborein

Symptoms: If ingested, oral inflammation and numbness leading to vomiting, diarrhea, and convulsions in severe cases. May affect the CNS and has a strong action on the heart, resembling digitalin.
Sources: Christmas rose roots and leaves

Hypoglycin A and B

Symptoms: Vomiting, may progress to severe hypoglycemia convulsions or coma. Lethal ingestions are recorded.
Pharmacokinetics: Hypoglycin is metabolized to a toxic metabolite, methylenecyclopropylacetic acid; onset 2–6 hours.
Source: *Blighia sapida* "ackee" fruit, except edible ripe aril

Ilicin

Symptoms: Vomiting, abdominal pain, diarrhea.
Sources: Primarily berries from various *Ilex* (holly) species
Example: other saponins

Irisin

Symptoms: A resinous agent that may produce dermatitis. Ingestion may cause oral irritation, vomiting, diarrhea, possible pancreas and liver damage.
Sources: *Iris* species, commercial and wild
Examples: Similar resinous agents are irigenin and iridin.

Isoquinoline-type Alkaloids

Symptoms: Dyspnea, excessive salivation, labored breathing, tremors, unusual gait, convulsions, death by paralysis. An uncommon human poisoning, since roots and foliage are most toxic.
Sources: Bleeding heart, Dutchman's breeches, other *Dicentra* species
Examples: apomorphine, dauricine, protoberberine, protopine

Lantadene A

Symptoms: Somewhat similar to anticholinergic poisoning; gastroenteritis, cyanosis, circulatory collapse, muscle weakness. Cholestatic hepatitis, jaundice, photosensitization from ingestion of leaves.
Pharmacokinetics: Onset 2–6 hours.
Source: lantana
Examples: Lantadene is a polycyclic triterpenoid.

Lobeline

Symptoms: An alkaloid with nicotine-like symptoms. May cause vomiting, tremors, convulsions, weakness, coma, or death.
Source: Indian tobacco (*Lobelia species*)
Examples: lobelamine, lobeline

Lycorine-like Alkaloids

Symptoms: Gastroenteritis, possible liver toxicity, convulsions, hypotension. Most human cases result in mild gastroenteritis.
Pharmacokinetics: Peak galantamine level in 2 hours, several active metabolites, duration of effect 3 hours; elimination complete in 72 hours; half-life 5.7 hours.
Sources: daffodils, narcissus, hyacinth (similar)
Examples: lycorine, narcissine, galantamine, others

Melia Resinoid

Symptoms: Dyspnea, slowed movement, tachycardia, vomiting.
Pharmacokinetics: Onset one to several hours: death can occur in 12–24 hours; hepatorenal syndrome can develop after several days in survivors.

Sources: Chinaberry (*Melia azedarach*). Most often a poisoning in animals but gastrointestinal symptoms have been reported after 6 to 8 berries in a child.

Mescaline

Symptoms: Visual hallucinations, altered sensorium.
Pharmacokinetics: Onset 30 minutes to 2 hours; duration 6–12 hours.
Source: peyote

Mezerenic Acid Anhydride

Symptoms: Skin vesicant, oral irritant, produces bloody vomiting and diarrhea. May lead to renal failure, conculsions and death.
Source: daphne

Nicotine

Symptoms: vomiting, muscle tremors, initial CNS stimulation followed by CNS depression, muscle paralysis, and respiratory failure.
Pharmacokinetics: Onset 15 minutes to 1 hour; duration 3–12 hours; inactive metabolite continine is measured in the urine as a marker of exposure; nicotine half-life 0.5 hours in smokers, 1.3 hours in nonsmokers; cotinine half-life 10–20 hours.
Sources: tobacco, tree tobacco

Olavine Alkaloids

Symptoms: Psychotomimetic effects, nausea, euphoria, uterine stimulation.
Pharmacokinetics: One morning glory seed is equivalent to about 1 μg of LSD (effective dose 20–50 seeds); *Agryreia* is more potent (effective dose 4–12 seeds); onset 4–6 hours; duration 12–24 hours.
Sources: Morning glory, Hawaiian baby woodrose (*Agryreia nervosa*)
Examples: ergine, isoergine, elymoclavine

Oleander-type Glycosides

Symptoms: Irritations of mouth and stomach, vomiting, diarrhea, irregular pulse, possible ventricular fibrillation.
Pharmacokinetics: More rapid onset than digoxin; extensive enterophepatic circulation; oleander toxins cross-react with digoxin and digitoxin immunoassays.
Sources: Oleander, red squill, yellow oleander
Examples: oleandroside, oleandrin, nerioside, thevetin A and B, thevetoxin

Oxalates

Symptoms: Symptoms vary greatly. Initial oral pain may lead to swelling of the lips and tongue, dysphagia, and sometimes vomiting. Serious poisonings may lead to renal failure and dyspnea. Ocular exposure may produce corneal opacity.
Sources: Philodendrons, caladiums, dumbcanes, calocasias, alocasias, Virginia creeper, rhubarb leaf, jack-in-the-pulpit, and many others
Examples: Usually calcium oxalates in needle-like structures. Many of these plants also contains additional chemical irritants.

Phytolaccine

Symptoms: Gastroenteritis (characteristic foamy diarrhea), tremors, amblyopia followed by salivation, diaphoresis, weakness, prostration, respiratory depression, leukocytosis, heart block.
Pharmacokinetics: Onset 2–3 hours, duration 48 hours.
Source: pokeberry
Examples: phytolaccine, phytolaccotoxin

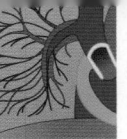
BOX 24-1	TOXIC PRINCIPLES (Cont'd)

Protoanemonin

Symptoms: burning sensation of the mouth and throat, gastroenteritis
Sources: clematis, anemones, buttercups
Examples: anemonin, ranunculin (glycoside containing protoanemonin)

Pyrrolizidine Alkaloids

Symptoms: Hepatotoxicity (veno-occlusive disease), abdominal pain, vomiting, diarrhea, apathy, emaciation.
Pharmacokinetics: Onset days to weeks, metabolized by CYP1A and 2E to toxic pyrrolic esters and alcohols; eliminated within 24 hours.
Sources: Senecio species such as threadleaf groundsel

Saponins

Symptoms: Emetic, mucous membrane irritant, gastroenteritis, growth suppression or bloat in some animals, increase cell membrane permeability, diuretic.
Sources: common in plants
Examples: A diverse group of glycosides; mainly of the triterpenoidal type (e.g., oleanolic acid and hedagenin). Coffee weed, purple sesban, yucca, rattlebox, and soapwort.

Solanine

Symptoms: Intact glycoalkaloid is an irritant. Vomiting, diarrhea, abdominal pain, may lead to respiratory depression, CNS depression, convulsions, circulatory collapse.
Pharmacokinetics: Onset 1–25 hours after eating potatoes; peak levels 4–8 hours; half-life of α-solanine 11 hours; half-life of α-chaconine 19 hours; duration of gastroenteritis 3–6 days.
Sources: potato leaves, tomato leaves, nightshades, eggplant, Jerusalem cherry, ground cherry, horse nettle, and bittersweets
Examples: α-solanine, α-chaconine

Taxine

Symptoms: Gastroenteritis, dyspnea, circulatory failure, heart function depression, prolonged QRS. Possible dermatitis after skin exposure.

Pharmacokinetics: Onset 30 minutes to 3 hours; duration up to 24 hours.
Source: yew

Toxalbumins (RIPs)

Symptoms: Initial symptoms are oral burning, violent vomiting and diarrhea, which may progress to shock, hemolysis, renal failure, CNS depression and death. Many sources have attractive seeds.
Pharmacokinetics: half-life 2 days
Sources: include black locust, castor bean, desert potato, and rosary pea
Examples: abrin (rosary pea), robin, robitin, phasin (black locust), ricin, ricinine (castor bean)

Trigonelline

Symptoms: May cause skin irritation, eye irritation, vomiting, and diarrhea.
Sources: four o'clocks, green coffee beans

Tropane Alkaloids

Symptoms: Antimuscarinic in nature, dry mouth, thirst, irritability, flushing, delirium, tachycardia, mydriasis, fever, convulsion, coma.
Pharmacokinetics: Onset 2–6 hours; duration up to 72 hours.
Sources: *Datura* (one seed equivalent to 0.1 mg atropine), *Hyoscyamus, Atropa* species
Examples: hyoscyamine (atropine), scopolamine (hyoscine)

Urushiol

Symptoms: Allergic dermatitis, inflammation, blistering, vesicles
Pharmacokinetics: Onset hours to 5 days; duration 1–3 weeks.
Source: poison ivy
Example: 3-*N*-pentadecylcatechol

Wisterin

Symptoms: gastroenteritis, dizziness, confusion
Pharmacokinetics: Duration 5–7 days.

---

or biting a leaf or stem), the idioblast releases the raphides with some force for a distance of two to three cell lengths.[32] Raphide microstructure and size both contribute to irritation. In addition, many calcium oxalate crystals contain barbs and grooves that may contribute to local tissue injury. However, tissue irritation is not consistent among crystals and the presence of an additional chemical toxin has been proposed as a second mechanism of toxicity.[33]

Delayed Gastroenteritis from Plants That Contain Ribosome-Inactivating Proteins

A vast amount of research has been conducted into the pathophysiology of plants containing toxins that inhibit ribosomes. Ribosome-inactivating proteins (RIPs) are found in a number of toxic and nontoxic plants. RIPs are divided into two main groups: type 1 RIPs, consisting of a single polypeptide chain, and type 2 RIPs, consisting of an A (active) chain and a B (binding) chain with lectin properties. The type 2 RIPs have also been referred to as toxalbumins or as lectins based on properties of the B chain. The type 1 RIPs are considered nontoxic because they lack the ability to enter the cell membrane. For instance, pokeweed contains a type 1 RIP termed PAP that does not contribute to its cellular toxicity.

The type 2 RIPs have been found in a number of plant species, including *Ricinus communis* (castor bean), *Abrus precatorius* (rosary pea), *Robinia pseudoacacia* (black locust), *Hura crepitans* (sandbox tree), *Jatropha multifida* (coral bush), and *Phoradendron* spp., and in small quantities of *Viscum album* (mistletoe). The most common type 2 RIPs described are ricin from the castor bean and the toxin abrin from the rosary pea. A wide range of toxicity is induced by type 2 RIPs. The mechanism of toxicity of the type 2 RIPs begins with the binding of the B chain to the cell surface. The cytotoxicity of type 2 RIPs

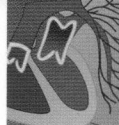

is (partly) determined by the binding of the B chain to a sugar-containing receptor on the cell surface. The B chain (lectin) first binds to glycolipids and/or glyoproteins containing β-1,4-linked galactose residues on the cell surface, inducing endocytosis of the A and B chains. The toxin is transported to the Golgi apparatus and endoplasmic reticulum (ER), with subsequent release into the cytosol.[34] A partial unfolding of the A chain enables it to translocate across the ER membrane via a translocon using the pathway normally followed by misfolded ER proteins targeted for ER-associated degradation. Refolding of the A chain in the cytosol into a protease-resistant, enzymatically active structure enables its interaction with the sarcin-ricin domain of the large ribosome subunit RNA.[35] The A chain acts as an *N*-glycosidase by hydrolyzing a single *N*-glycosidic bond between adenine and ribose within a highly conserved sequence on the large recombinant RNA of animal ribosomes.[36] This interrupts translation at the step of guanosine triphosphate (GTP)-dependent binding of the elongation factor 1 and/or 2 to ribosomes.[37] There is recent evidence that the A chain is also capable of inactivating many nonribosomal nucleic acid substrates,[38] and hence can be considered a polynucleotide: adenosine glycosidase.

Delayed Gastroenteritis from Plants That Contain Glycoalkaloids

Plants containing glycoalkaloids, such as solanine, are a common cause of gastric irritation. This is due in part to the common variety of plants containing such glycoalkaloids, including *Solanum tuberosum* (potato), *Solanum nigrum* (black nightshade), *Lycopersicon esculentum* (tomato), *Solanum pseudocapsicum* (Jerusalem cherry), and *Physalis heterophylla* (ground cherry). Young plants/roots and unripe fruit tend to have a much higher concentration of toxin. Glycoalkaloids have been shown to destabilize membranes and inhibit serum acetylcholinesterase,[39] which may partially explain the GI toxicity. The glycoalkaloids are able to interact strongly with sterol-containing membranes, thereby causing membrane disruption specific for the type of glycoalkaloid and sterol.[40] Several of the glycoalkaloids have also demonstrated inotropic activity, which may be partly explained by the structural resemblance to the cardiac glycosides.[41] Most relevant, the clearance of glycoalkaloids usually takes more than 24 hours, which suggests that the toxicants may accumulate after daily consumption.[42]

Cytotoxic Plants That Produce Multiorgan Failure

This diverse group of plants is commonly involved in research on cancer and cellular function. They contain alkaloids with the common characteristic of binding to microtubules. Microtubules are involved in a wide variety of cellular function, including cell division and axonal transport. Microtubules are required for the transport of various metabolites and the movement of organelles, including mitochondria and secretory granules, along neuronal processes. Microtubules are composed of the protein tubulin, which consists of α and β subunits. The α subunit binds GTP, retaining it within its structure. The β subunit hydrolyzes GTP to guanosine diphospate (GDP) during protofilament formation. The tubulin-binding alkaloids interfere with protofilament formation by binding to various sites along the tubulin molecule. Cell division is arrested during metaphase at the G_2/M phases of the cell cycle.

Colchicine, found in the autumn crocus (*Colchicum autumnale*) and glory lily (*Gloriosa superba*), binds to the β subunit at the colchicine-binding site, inhibiting polymerization of tubulin polymers.[43] Podophyllotoxin from the mayapple plant (*Podophyllum peltatum*) inhibits GTP hydrolysis at the β subunit, thereby preventing β- and α-subunit polymerization during protofilament formation.[44] The vinca alkaloids derived from *Catharamus* spp. (formally *Vinca rosea*) include the toxins vincristine and vinblastine. The vinca alkaloids also bind to the β subunit at the vinca-binding site, inhibiting the hydrolysis of GTP to GDP and inhibiting the binding of GDP to its nucleotide site.[45]

Another antineoplastic drug with plant derivation is *Taxus brevifolia*, containing the alkaloid taxol. Taxol differs in its mechanism of microtubule inactivation by promoting assembly of microtubules. Early assembly of microtubules reduces the critical concentration of tubulin required for assembly. Other intracellular processes affected by microtubule inhibition include inhibition of synthesis of proteins and nucleic acids, elevation of oxidized glutathione, alteration of lipid metabolism and the lipid content of membranes, elevation of cyclic adenosine monophosphate (cAMP), platelet membrane integrity, and inhibition of calcium-calmodulin-regulated cAMP phosphodiesterase.[46]

Plants That Produce Cardiovascular Disturbances

Plants containing cardiac glycosides (steroids) are well known because of their long history in the treatment of heart failure. Plants that have been known to contain cardiac glycosides include foxglove (*Digitalis purpurea*), lily of the valley (*Convallaria majalis*), oleander (*Nerium oleander*), squill (Liliaceae family), yellow oleander (*Thevetia peruviana*), dogbane (*Apocynum cannabimum*), wallflower (*Cheiranthus cheiri*), milkweed (Asclepiadaceae family), *Strophanthus* (*Strophanthus kombe/hispidus*), suicide tree (*Cerbera odollam*), hellebores (*Helleborus* spp.), star of Bethlehem (*Ornithogalum* spp.), spindle tree (Euonymus family), Crassulaceae family, crownvetch (*Coronilla* spp.), witstorm, *Thesium lineatum*, Iridaceae family, Melianthaceae family (*Bersama* and *Melianthus* spp.), Natal plum (*Carissa* spp.), and the frangipani tree (*Plumeria rubra*).

Although a wide variety of plants contain cardiac glycoside toxins, their mechanisms of action are quite similar. The myocardial effects of these compounds are attributable to increased intracellular concentrations of calcium and sodium, resulting from inhibition of the transmembrane Na^+/K^+-ATPase pump. The cardiac glycosides consist of a C_{23} (cardenolide) or C_{24} (bufadienolide) steroid with one or more sugar moieties

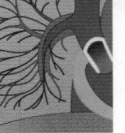

attached to the C_3 carbon of the steroid nucleus.[13] The majority of plant cardiac glycosides are cardenolides. The exceptions are the *Urginea* spp., *Hellebore* spp., several toxins within *Convallaria* spp., several toxins within the Crassulaceae family, *Thesium lineatum*, Iridaceae family, and the Melianthaceae family (*Bersama* and *Melianthus* spp.).

Plants with Sodium Channel–Binding Properties

Plants and their associated toxins with sodium channel–binding properties include aconitine, from monkshood (*Aconitum napellus*); veratridine, from false or green hellebore (Veratrum family); grayanotoxins, from azalea and rhododendron (*Rhododendron* spp.), death camas (*Zigadenus*), mountain laurel (*Kalmia latifolia*), and taxine from *Taxus brevifolia*. The sodium channel–binding characteristics of this group of plants have been known for some time. Aconitine has been found in a number of Chinese herbals, including both *chuanwu* (*A. carmichaeli*) and *caowu* (*A. kusnezoffii*). These herbs are believed to possess anti-inflammatory, analgesic, and cardiotonic effects and have been used in Chinese traditional medicine mainly for the treatment of musculoskeletal disorders.[47] Roots of monkshood have also been mistaken for horseradish (*Armoracia rusticana*).

Grayanotoxins have largely been reported to cause intoxication in regions where honey is produced from *Rhododendron* spp. Approximately 18 different types of grayanotoxins have been isolated, but grayanotoxin I appears to be responsible for the majority of poisonings.[48]

Veratridine has historically been used in both insecticides and medicinals. Major toxicity from veratridine came from the use of sneezing powders in Europe that contained the ground root of white hellebore (*Veratrum album*). *Veratrum* species have also been ingested intentionally after being mistaken for leeks, skunk cabbage, ramps (*Allium tricoccum*), and plants from the Gentian family.[49]

All of the toxins from these plants are large, complex diterpenoid alkaloids. The diterpenoid alkaloids are lipid soluble, allowing them to access the sodium channel–binding site embedded within the plasma membrane.[50] Aconitine, veratridine, and grayanotoxins reversibly bind to site 2 along the inner membrane of the channel. Site 2 is an intracellular region expanding between domains I and IV. This site overlaps the known binding site of local anesthetics, and is shared by the *Phylloides*-derived toxin batrachotoxin. All the diterpenoid alkaloids preferentially bind to the open state of the voltage-gated sodium channel (VGSC.)[51] They exert their action on nerve and muscle membranes by persistent activation of VGSC at the resting membrane potential.[52] Veratridine's persistent opening of the VGSC may reduce single-channel conductance by 75%.[53]

The activation of VGSC is explained by two effects: first, a shift of the voltage dependence of activation of VGSC toward more negative effects, and second, a block of the fast inactivation of these channels.[50] Therefore, their binding is enhanced by other toxins or drugs that enhance prolonged opening of sodium channels.

Prolongation of sodium channels with a subsequent increase in intracellular sodium causes an increase in intracellular calcium due to inhibition of the sodium-calcium pump. This increase in intracellular calcium has a similar effect as that seen with the cardiac glycosides, with increased ionotropicity. However, since Na^+/K^+-ATPase is not inhibited, hyperkalemia is notably absent. The negative ionotropic effects and cardiodepressant effects (particularly aconitine) are most likely due to vagal stimulation, since they are reversed with atropine.[54] Aconitine also has a propensity to cause early and delayed after-depolarizations in ventricular myocytes that may be due to increased intracellular calcium and sodium. This may explain the reports of biventricular tachycardia and torsades de pointes in patients with aconitine intoxication.[55,56] Other effects of these alkaloids include antinociceptive and antiepileptiform properties, and reuptake inhibition of norepinephrine and serotonin.[57] The *Aconitum* species also contain a compound called songorine that has demonstrated noncompetitive antagonism at $GABA_A$ and agonistic action at dopamine receptors in the rat cerebral cortex.[58]

The toxins produced by *Taxus brevifoli* (yew) include both taxol and taxine. In Caesar's time, the yew plant was known as the tree of death. American species, like *Taxus cuspidaande* (Japanese yew) and *Taxus canadensis* may be found as ornamental shrubs or Christmas decorations. All parts of the plant except the fleshy fruit contain taxane alkaloids. Taxine is a mixture of more than seven alkaloids, with taxine A and taxine B as its main constituents. Taxine B is the most potent cardiotoxin of this group. The taxines have been known since the 1940s, but with the discovery of taxol (leading to paclitaxel) the taxines have since been overshadowed. In contrast to aconitine, grayanotoxin, and veratridine, taxine B reduces cardiac contractility and the maximum rate of depolarization of the action potential similar to class I antiarrhythmic drugs.[59,60] Taxine B and paclitaxel share the same skeletal structure and differ only in their side chains. The taxines do not demonstrate antitumor activity, and the cardiotoxicity of taxol is lower than that of taxines.

Plants That Act Primarily on the Nervous System

PLANTS THAT HAVE A NICOTINE-LIKE ACTION

Nicotine alkaloids have been in use for many centuries, and the presence and addictive potential of nicotine in tobacco is well known. The nicotine plant alkaloids are highly toxic. They are widely used as insecticides, which is most likely an extension of their natural role in the plant kingdom. Plants and plant alkaloids with nicotine or nicotine-like mechanisms of action include γ-coniceine and coniine from poison hemlock (*Conium maculatum*), *Aethusa cynaprium* (fool's parsley), nicotine from wild tobacco (*Nicotiana tabacum*; 0.5% to 9% nicotine), *Nicotiana rustica* (18% nicotine), lobeline (*Lobelia* spp.), anabasine (*Anabasis aphylla*), sparteine (*Cytisus scoparius*), N-methylcytisine from blue cohosh (*Caulophyllum thalictroides*), and cytisine from *Sophora* spp., golden chain

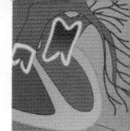

(*Laburnum spp.*), and *Gymnocladus dioicus* (Kentucky coffee bean). Nicotinic pyridine and piperidine alkaloids share common receptor agonism for nicotinic acetylcholine receptors (nAChRs). Nicotine and nicotine-like alkaloids interact with presynaptic nAChRs to facilitate the release of a variety of neurotransmitters, including acetylcholine, dopamine, norepinephrine, serotonin, GABA, and glutamate. Some nicotinic alkaloids also inhibit aromatase, preventing androstenedione conversion to estrogen.[61] However, at high concentrations of nicotine, nAChRs become desensitized due to increasing affinity for substrate at the receptor. With this, initial central nervous system (CNS) and muscle stimulation is typically followed by paralysis of motor nerve endings and CNS depression.

Poison hemlock (*Conium maculatum*) belongs to the Umbelliferae family and is closely related to carrots, parsnips, cow parsley, parsley, and caraway. Death from poison hemlock has often occurred from mistaken identity.[62] Three main alkaloids are responsible for the toxicity of poison hemlock. The most toxic chemical, γ γ-coniceine, is an unsaturated piperidine alkaloid and is abundant in the leaves and flowers but less common in the fruits, where it is quickly converted to coniine and *N*-methylconiine. Gamma-coniceine is considered to be seven or eight times more toxic than coniine.[63] The actions of coniine are similar to nicotine, but produce greater CNS and skeletal muscle nerve ending paralysis. The actions of coniine have been said to resemble that of strychnine.

TROPANE ALKALOIDS: ANTIMUSCARINIC PLANTS

The tropane alkaloids are found in a number of plant families, including Solanaceae, Erythroxylaceae (e.g., *Erythroxylum coca;* cocaine), and Convolvulaceae (morning glory family). Tropane alkaloids possessing antimuscarinic properties are primarily from the Solanaceae family. Common alkaloids in this family include atropine, scopolamine, hyoscyamine, and hyoscine. These plants include *Atropa belladonna* (belladonna; deadly nightshade), *Solandra* spp. (trumpet flower), *Datura stramonium* (jimson weed), *Mandragon officinarum* (mandrake; not to be confused with *Podophyllum peltatum,* also referred to as Mandrake), *Brugmansia* (angel's trumpet), *Cestrum diurnum* (day jessamine), *Lantana camara* (lantana, shrub verbena), and henbane (*Hyoscyamus niger*).

The tropane alkaloids from these plants are all structurally similar. Atropine and hyoscyamine are racemic isomers, as are hyoscine and scopolamine. Atropine consists of a mixture of equal parts of D- and L-hyoscyamine and does not exist as a single alkaloid in plant species. Both hyoscyamine isomers may bind to muscarinic receptors, although the pharmacologic activity is thought to be due almost entirely to L-hyoscyamine.[64,65] Scopolamine and L-hyoscyamine are most likely the primary compounds responsible for the toxic effects of these plants. The toxicity of these compounds results from competitive blockade of acetylcholine at peripheral and central muscarinic receptors. The most commonly affected organ systems include the

CNS, cardiac myocytes and conduction system, exocrine glands, and smooth muscle cells.

NEUROLOGIC INJURY

Plants that cause neurologic injury are some of the most well-known and toxic species. Several of these plants contain specific toxic alkaloids producing seizures upon ingestion. The water hemlock species *Cicuta virosa* and *Cicuta maculata* that belong to the Umbelliferae family have been responsible for a number of reported deaths. The Umbelliferae family also contains several edible plants such as celery, water parsley, parsnip, and wild carrot. Severe poisonings have occurred while foraging for these edible relatives.[66] There are also reported cases of people mistaking wild ginseng for water hemlock.[67] The early practice of making toy whistles from the water hemlock stem has been been associated with several deaths in children.[68] Cicutoxin is a noncompetitive GABA_A receptor antagonist acting at both the GABA agonist site and on the chloride channel of the GABA_A receptor-channel complex.[69,70] This mechanism explains the high rate of seizures reported with cicutoxin exposure.

The ginkgo tree (*Ginkgo biloba*) is the oldest tree living tree species. It has been employed in medicinal treatments for centuries and recently promoted for treatment of memory impairment, commonly as standardized extracts of *G. biloba* leaves. Ginkgo is primarily composed of two constituents: terpenoids and flavonoids. The terpenoids include ginkgolides A, B, C, J, and bilobalide. Flavonoids found in *Ginkgo* include a wide variety of compounds, but the best described is quercetin. Ginkgolides are moderate potent antagonists at GABA_A receptor.[71] They also have been shown to cause vasodilation by inhibiting calcium influx through calcium channels and simulate the activation of nitric oxide release in the endothelium.[72] Ginkgolide B is a potent platelet-activating factor antagonist[73] and ginkgolide C has demonstrated potent and selective antagonism at inhibitory glycine receptors.[74] Ginkgo-induced seizures are probably multifactorial. The flavonoid quercetin is an antagonist at both GABA_A and GABA_C receptors, and probably modulates other ligand-gated ion channels.[75] In a recent case, a ginkgo seed constituent, 4-methoxypyridoxine, was thought to be responsible for seizure activity. The concentration of 4-methoxypyridoxine was elevated in this case and linked to decreased GABA synthesis.[76]

Another hemlock species linked to seizure activity after ingestion is the *Oenanthe* species, hemlock water dropwort. The roots of water dropwort are yellow and typically composed of five or more tubers. This characteristic appearance has earned it the name "dead man's fingers." Water dropwort has produced significant toxicity from concentrated teas made from the plant or in its confusion with edible plants (i.e., water parsnips).[77] The water dropwort produces oenanthotoxin, which is the *cis*-isomer of cicutoxin. Oenanthotoxin is thought to inhibit neuronal sodium and calcium channels, resulting in potential seizure activity.[78] Its effect on GABA receptors has not been demonstrated.

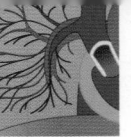

The use and known toxicity of *Anamirta* species of plants also has existed for many centuries. *Anamirta paniculata* produces the toxin picrotoxin. The plant originates from the coast of Malabar and the islands around India. The common names for *Anamirta paniculata* (fishberries or Indian berries) derived from native fishermen using the crushed seeds to stupefy fish. It was also once employed in India and Great Britain as an antidote in morphine overdose.[79] Picrotoxin is an allosteric, noncompetitive inhibitor of both $GABA_A$ and $GABA_C$[80] receptors. The mechanism of picrotoxin is believed to involve binding to residues that line the pore in the second transmembrane domain (M2) of the α subunit. The M2 domain is a common feature of many transmembrane receptors, including GABA, glycine, and acetylcholine receptors. The common binding site is the probable mechanism for picrotoxin's additional antagonism noted at nAChRs and glycine receptors.[81]

The *Coriaria* species of plants are most well known in Great Britain and New Zealand. *Coriaria* grows wild in southern Europe and may be cultivated in gardens because of its rich foliage. The leaves have been found as adulterants in senna and sweet marjoram. In the early 1900s, a reported Mexican drug called *Tlolocopetale* was said to be the product of *C. myrtifolia* and was acutely poisonous.[82] The active toxin in *Coriaria* species is coriamyrtin. The New Zealand species of coriaria (New Zealand toot-plant; *Coriaria ruscifolia, Coriaria sarmentosa*) contains a glucoside similar to coriamyrtin, called tutin. Coriamyrtin and tutin are structurally similar to picrotoxin and appear be antagonists at GABA receptors.[83] However, the extent of their receptor binding and inhibition has not been revealed.

The strychnos plant (*Strychnos nux-vomica*) is associated with violent seizures, paralysis, and death. Strychnos is a native plant of India and Southeast Asia. The strychnine alkaloid is a reversible and competitive inhibitor of glycine receptors in the spinal cord and cerebral cortex.

The indolizidine alkaloid swainsonine isolated from the plants *Swainsona canescens, Astragalus mollissimus* (locoweed), and *Oxytropis* species (also locoweed) causes a debilitating chronic neurologic disease often leading to death. Swainsonine is a potent inhibitor of α-mannosidase II, resulting in a lysosomal storage disease termed mannosidosis.[84] It is currently being investigated in the treatment of advanced neoplasms.[85]

Lathyrism, a disease caused by the grass pea (*Lathyrus sativus*), is mediated by a stereospecific plant amino acid (β-N-oxalylamino-L-alanine) that serves as a potent agonist at the (RS)-α-amino-3-hydroxy-5-methyl-isoxazole-4-propionic acid (AMPA) subclass of neuronal glutamate receptors.[86]

HALLUCINATIONS

The use of hallucinogenic drugs dates back many centuries. The vast majority of early plant use for hallucinogenic effects was through psychoactive snuffs. Recent literature supports the theory that hallucinogenic drugs produce their effects through partial agonist action at serotonin 5-HT_2 receptors.[87] One of the most commonly known hallucinogens found in plant species is lysergic acid amide (LAA). It is structurally similar to lysergic acid (LSD). Lysergic acid amide is found primarily in *Ipomoea violacea* (morning glory) and *Turbina corymbosa* (ololiuqui). The content of LAA varies by plant but is most abundant in the *Ipomoea* varieties pearly gates, wedding bells, and Scarlet O-hara.[88] In addition, *Ipomoea* seeds contain other alkaloids such as isolysergic acid amide 0.005%, chanoclavine 0.005%, elymoclavine 0.005%, and ergometrine 0.005%.[89,90] However, chanoclavine and ergometrine both possess open indole rings and lack hallucinogenic properties.[91] Several species of plants and cacti produce their hallucinogenic effects from phenethylamine derivatives. Mescaline is a phenethylamine (3,4,5-trimethoxy-β-phenethylamine) found in cactus species of *Lophophora williamsii* (peyote), *Trichocereus pachanoi* (San Pedro cactus), and *Trichocereus peruvianus* (Peruvian torch). Its crown, or "button," is used as the source of mescaline. It is cut from the cactus and dried into a hard brown disc.[92]

Nutmeg contains myrisiticin, which is metabolized to a methylenedioxymethamphetamine (MDMA) analog in animals; this pathway has not been demonstrated in humans. Myristicin is also a serotonin 5-HT_2 agonist. It contains elemicin, which is metabolized to 3,4,5-trimethoxy amphetamine.[15]

The leaves of the tropical plant *Mitragyna speciosa* (ithang, korth, kratom) have been traditionally used as a substitute for opium. It has also been used in the Middle East as a traditional medicine for treating stomach and intestinal disorders (diarrhea). *M. speciosa* contains several alkaloids that possess opioid agonistic activities. It has been recently discovered that the 7-hydroxymitragynine metabolite of the parent alkaloid mitragynine (9-methoxy-corynantheidine) has the highest opioid activity of this plant.[93]

DEMYELINATION

An illness associated with peripheral neuropathy has been associated with the plant *Karwinskia humboldtiana* (buckthorn, coyotillo). This plant is a large tree or bush that is commonly seen in northern Mexico and the southern United States. Intoxication typically results from the ingestion of the plant's fruit. Only recently has the toxin been completely identified. The toxin from *K. humboldtiana* is called peroxisomicine. It is also known as T-514 or tullidol. Peroxisomicine destroys peroxisomes and generates free radicals, resulting in lipoperoxidation of cell membranes and leading to cell death.[94] Peroxisomicine has been shown to specifically target thick, distal nerve segments causing demyelination.[95] Histologically, there is widening of the periaxonal space and a redistribution of axonal organelles to a marginal position. Ultimately, axons undergo wallerian degeneration.[96]

CYANOGENIC PLANTS: AMYGDALIN, CYANOGENIC GLYCOSIDES

Approximately 2500 different plant species have the ability to produce cyanogenic glycosides.[97] The compounds all

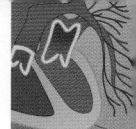

share the common feature of yielding hydrogen cyanide on complete hydrolysis. Considering the vast of amount of plant taxa producing cyanogenic glycosides, the majority of exposures occur with cassava (*Manihot esculenta*) and seeds from the *Prunus* species (apple, peach, apricot, plum, etc.). Cassava contains the cyanogenic glycoside linamarin, which has been responsible for significant acute and chronic toxicity.[98,99] Toxicity typically occurs from improperly cooked cassava. The pathogenesis of the chronic diseases associated with cassava (e.g., epidemic spastic paraparesis or konzo) is probably multifactorial. The neurologic symptoms of konzo resemble that seen with neurolathyrism acquired from the grass pea. The principal metabolite of cyanide, thiocyanate, has been shown to be a potent agonist at AMPA receptors, similar to lectins from the grass pea. The metabolism of cyanide, however, is dependent on the sulfur-dependent enzyme rhodanese. In protein-deficient people where sulfur amino acids are low, cyanide may conceivably be converted to cyanate.[100] Cyanate has been shown to cause neurodegenerative disease in humans and animals.[101] It has been assumed that linamarin is enzymatically converted to cyanide by bacteria in the intestine. However, unmetabolized linamarin has been found in the urine after ingestion of cassava. Linamarin may be neurotoxic by entering cells via a glucose transporter and competing with cytochalasin B and glucose for those transporters.

The principal cyanogenic glycoside found in the *Prunus* species is amygdalin. Amygdalin was first isolated from bitter almonds in 1830. It is metabolized to cyanide by the intestinal enzyme complex emulsin (glucosidase, benzocyanase, nitrilase). Amygdalin is the active ingredient in the apricot extract Laetrile (derived from laevorotatory mandelonitrile) that was promoted as an antineoplastic agent. It continues to be marketed primarily in Mexico as an anticancer drug.

Metabolic Effects

SAPONIN GLYCOSIDES

The licorice root (*Glycyrrhiza gabra*) is one of the oldest known plant-derived medicines, having been used by Egyptians, Romans, and Greeks. It is one of the most frequently used traditional Chinese medicines[102] and has become one of the leading natural compounds for clinical trials of chronic active viral hepatitis or human immunodeficiency virus infections. Glycyrrhizic acid is the major bioactive triterpene glycoside of licorice root. It has demonstrated a wide range of pharmacologic properties, including anti-inflammatory, antiulcer, anti-allergic, and antiviral effects.[103] The content of glycyrrhizic acid in licorice root is 2% to 24% of the dry weight. Upon ingestion, glycyrrhizic acid is hydrolyzed in the intestine to the pharmacologically active compound glycyrrhetic acid, which inhibits the enzyme 11-β-hydroxysteroid dehydrogenase. 11-β-hydroxysteroid is responsible for the interconversion of cortisol to cortisone and confers ligand specificity to the mineralocorticoid receptor.[104] Inhibition of 11-β-hydroxysteroid dehydro-genase leads to increased serum cortisol levels. This promotes a hypermineralocorticoid state since cortisol binds with the same affinity as aldosterone at the mineralocorticoid receptor.[105] The ensuing pseudo-primary hyperaldosteronism is reversible, but may take several months to resolve. The protective function of glycyrrhizic acid on the liver has recently been explained as an inhibitory effect on nuclear factor κ B, which is known to activate genes encoding inflammatory cytokines within the liver.[106]

NEPHROTOXIC PLANTS

Toxicity from *Aristolochia* species has most commonly been seen with Chinese herbal medications.[107,108] An epidemic occurred in Belgium when the Chinese herbal *Stephania tetranda* was substituted by *Aristolochia fangchi*. However, endemic nephropathy in Croatia has recently been linked to wheat grain flour, likely contaminated with seeds of *Aristolochia clematitis* during harvesting.[109] Aristolochic acids present in *Aristolochia* species undergo reduction of the nitro group by CYP1A1 and CYP1A2 peroxidases in extrahepatic tissues to reactive cyclic nitrenium ions.[110] Reaction with intracellular proteins leads to a specific pattern of tubulointerstitial fibrosis[111] and Fanconi syndrome,[112] and may lead to urothelial carcinoma.[113]

HEPATOTOXIC PLANTS

Hypoglycin

The ackee tree (*Blighia sapida*) originates from West Africa and was introduced into Jamaica around 1778. Its scientific name derives from the British explorer Captain William Bligh, who apparently introduced the tree to Jamaica in 1793 as a food source for West African slaves.[114] In West Africa, the green fruits are used for laundering and the crushed fruits are employed as a fish poison. When burned, the ashes from the seeds and jackets may be used as soap due to their oil and potash contents. Various parts of the Ackee tree are still used medicinally in South America for fever, headache, dysentery, and as an antihelminthic. Jamaican vomiting sickness (JVS) has been a well-described illness resulting from eating the fruit from the ackee tree. For many years the source of the toxin was thought to come from the overripe or decomposing arils. It is now known that the toxin in ackee fruit is found in the unripe arils and seeds. The ackee fruit contains two primary toxins, hypoglycin A and B.[115] Hypoglycin A [α-amino-β-(2-methylenecyclo-propyl) propionic acid] is found primarily in the aril of the ackee fruit, but is degraded as the aril opens and ripens.[116] The ripe fruit may still contain a small portion of toxin, however. The seeds contain hypoglycin B [γ-L-glutamyl α-amino-β-(2-methylene cyclopropyl) propionic acid], the γ-glutamyl derivative of hypoglycin A. The seeds are always poisonous, but hypoglycin B is reported to be less toxic than hypoglycin A.

Hypoglycin undergoes transamination and oxidative decarboxylation to form methylene cyclopropyl acetic acid (MCPA), which then combines with coenzyme A (MCPA-CoA). MCPA-CoA is a suicide inhibitor of several

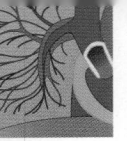

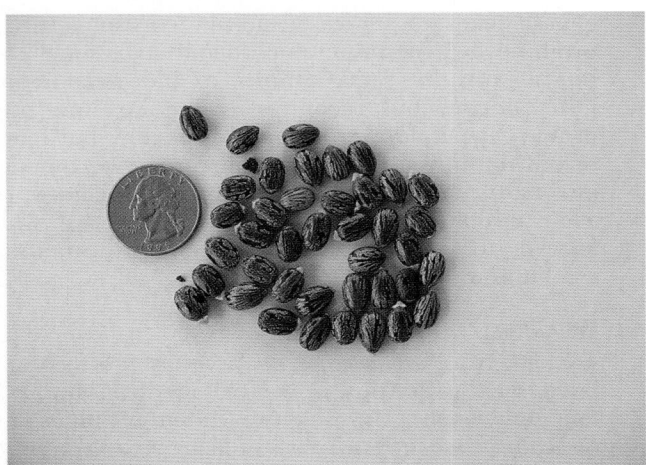

FIGURE 24-1 Castor beans.

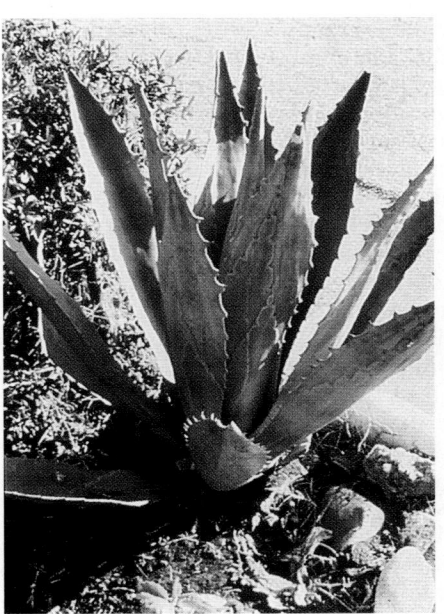

FIGURE 24-2 Century plant. (Courtesy of Donald B. Kunkel, MD.)

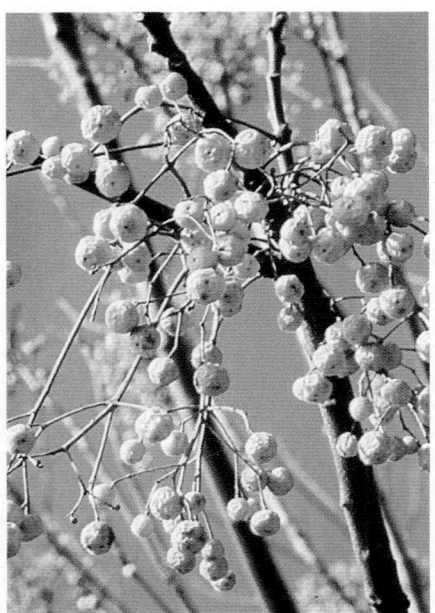

FIGURE 24-3 Chinaberry. (Courtesy of Donald B. Kunkel, MD.)

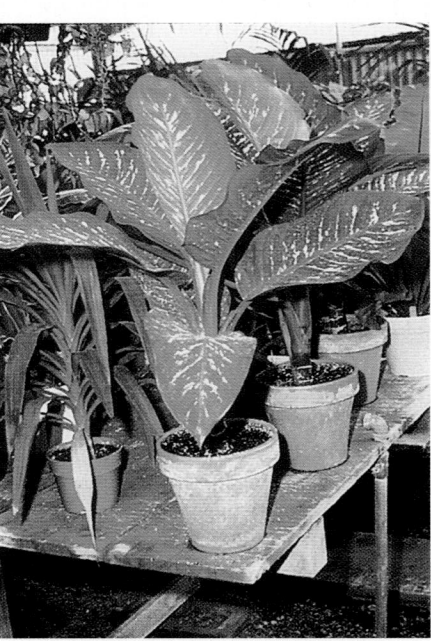

FIGURE 24-4 Dieffenbachia. (Courtesy of Donald B. Kunkel, MD.)

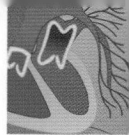

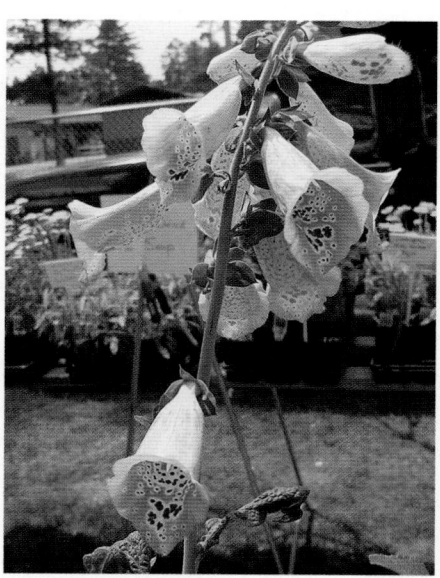

FIGURE 24-5 Foxglove.

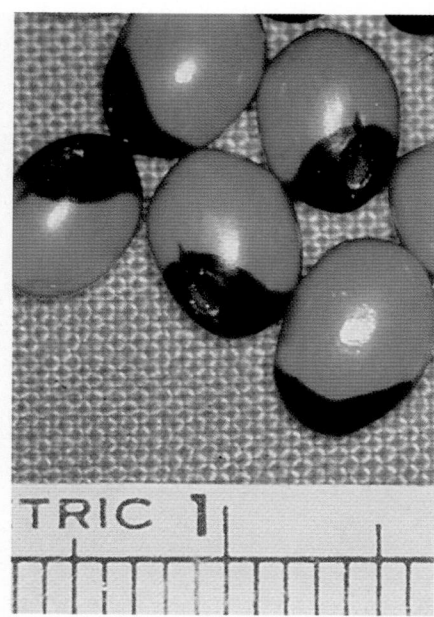

FIGURE 24-6 Jequirity beans. (Courtesy of Donald B. Kunkel, MD.)

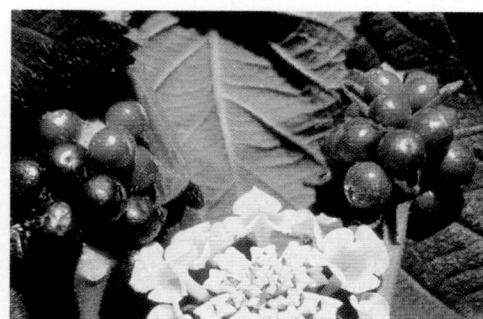

FIGURE 24-8 Lantana. (Courtesy of Donald B. Kunkel, MD.)

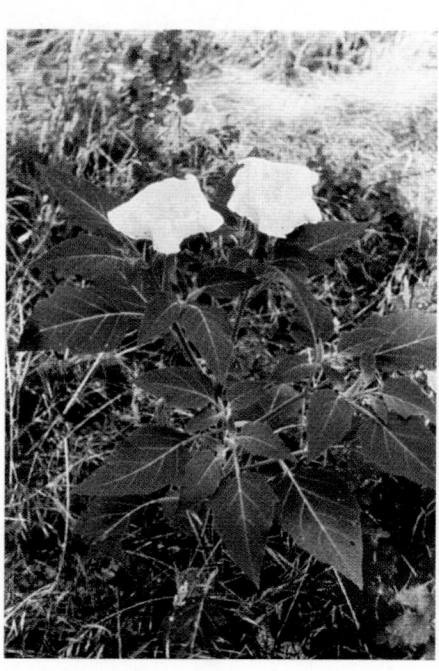

FIGURE 24-7 Jimson weed. (Courtesy of Donald B. Kunkel, MD.)

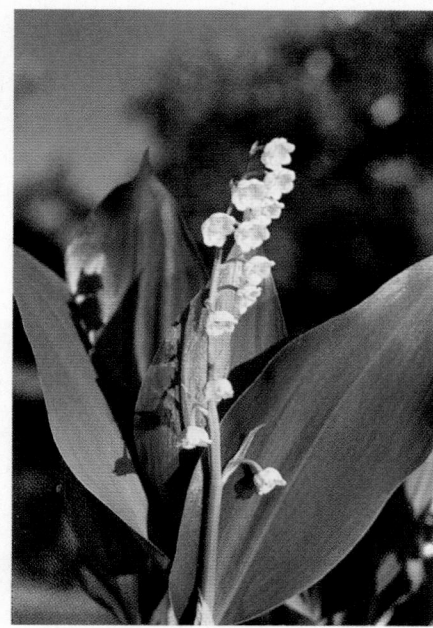

FIGURE 24-9 Lily of the valley. (Courtesy of Donald B. Kunkel, MD.)

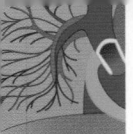

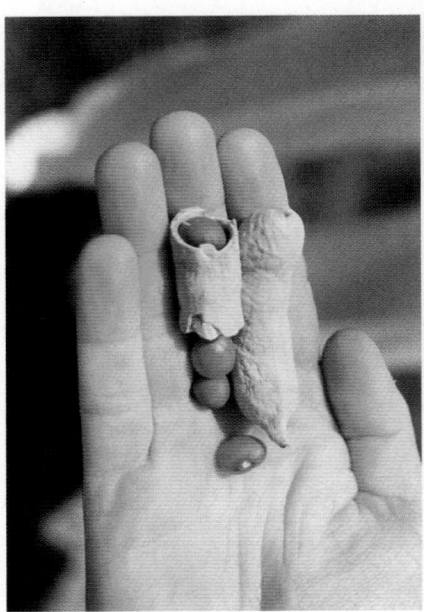

FIGURE 24-10 Mescal beans. (Courtesy of Donald B. Kunkel, MD.)

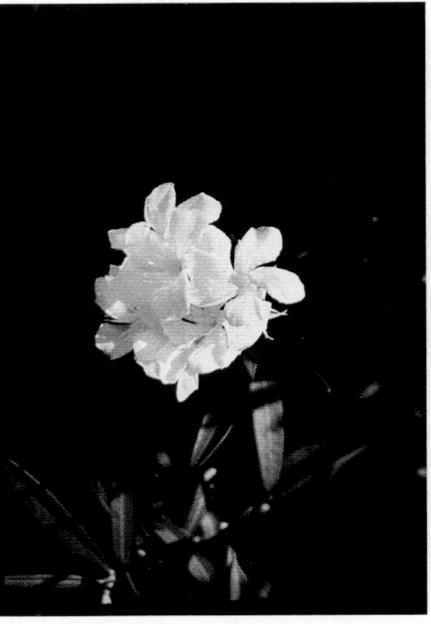

FIGURE 24-11 Yellow oleander. (Courtesy of Donald B. Kunkel, MD.)

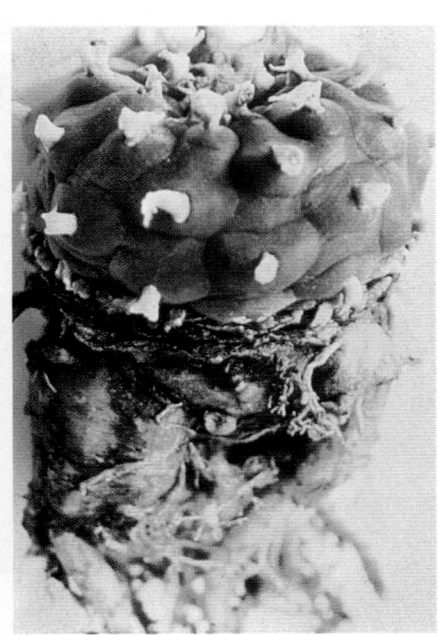

FIGURE 24-12 Peyote. (Courtesy of Donald B. Kunkel, MD.)

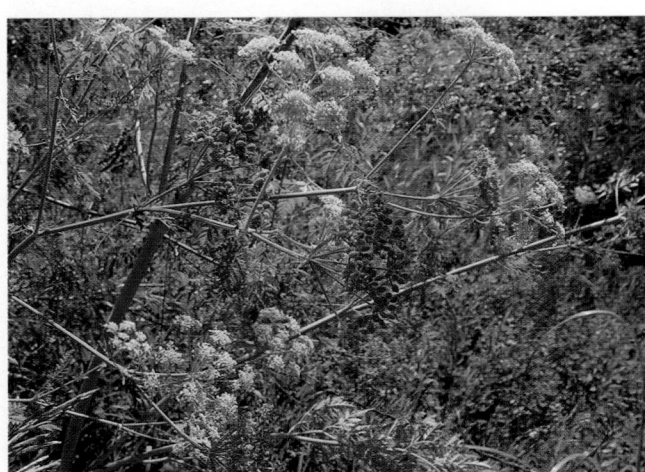

FIGURE 24-13 Poison hemlock. (Courtesy of Donald B. Kunkel, MD.)

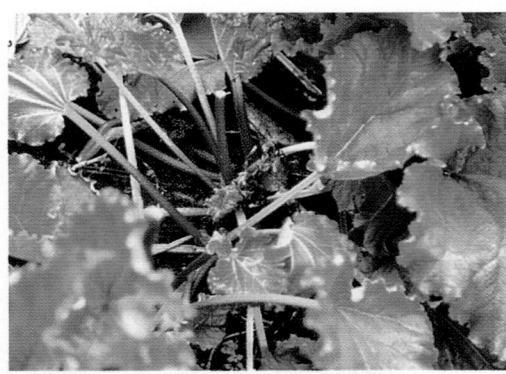

FIGURE 24-14 Rhubarb. (Courtesy of Donald B. Kunkel, MD.)

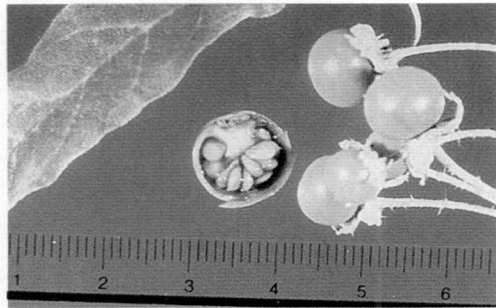

FIGURE 24-15 Silverleaf nightshade. (Courtesy of Donald B. Kunkel, MD.)

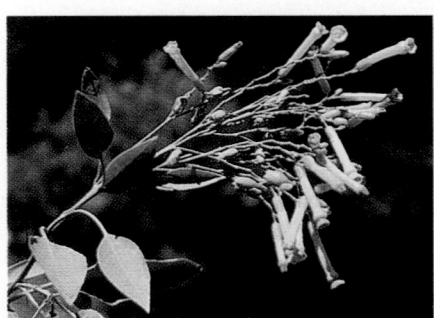

FIGURE 24-16 Tree tobacco. (Courtesy of Donald B. Kunkel, MD.)

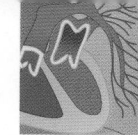

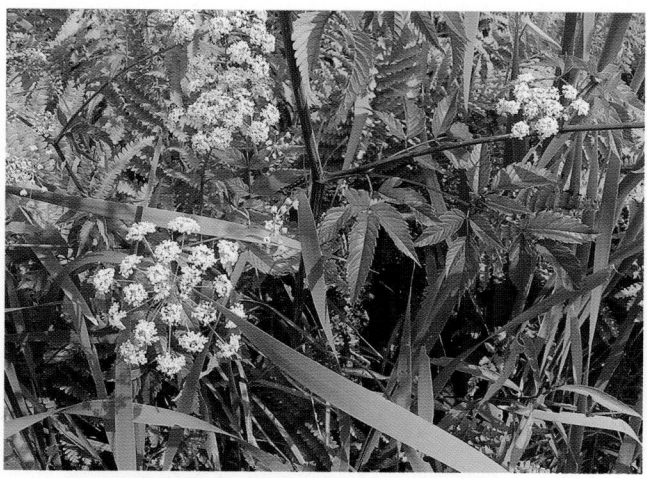

FIGURE 24-17 Water hemlock.

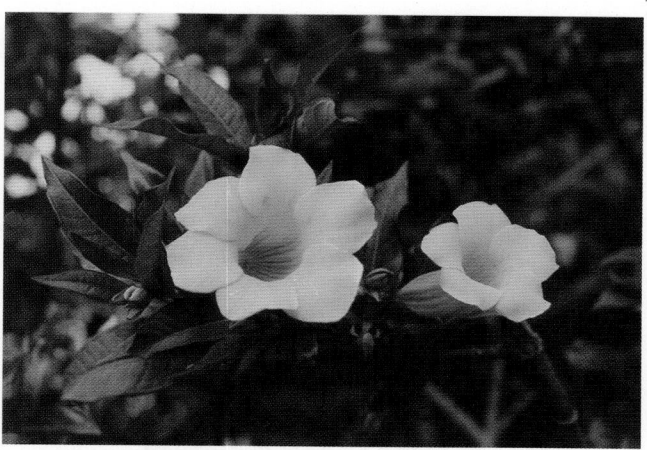

FIGURE 24-18 Allamanda.

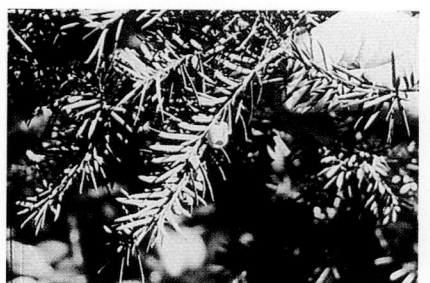

FIGURE 24-19 Yew. (Courtesy of Donald B. Kunkel, MD.)

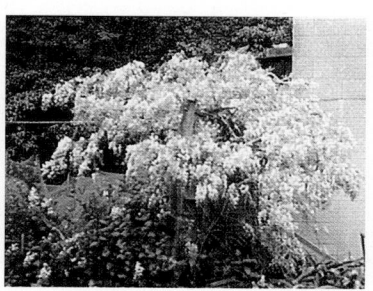

FIGURE 24-20 Wisteria. (Courtesy of Donald B. Kunkel, MD.)

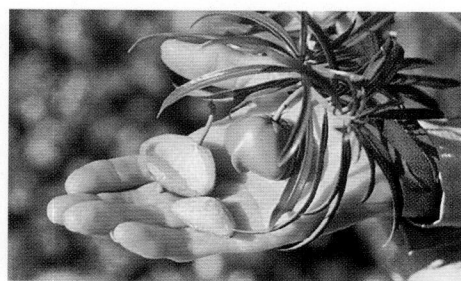

FIGURE 24-21 Yellow oleander, fruit with "lucky nut." (Courtesy of Donald B. Kunkel, MD.)

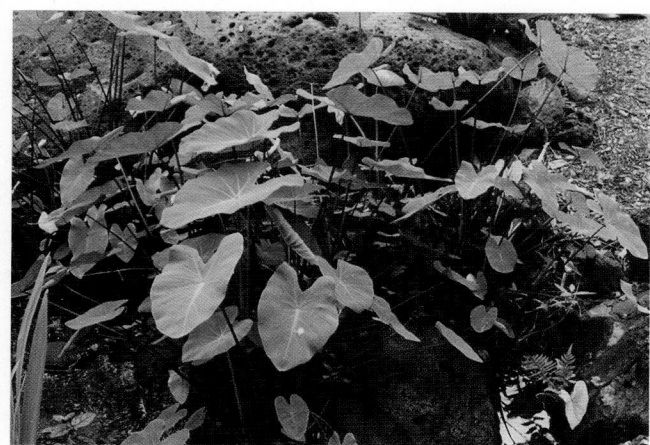

FIGURE 24-22 Alocasia.

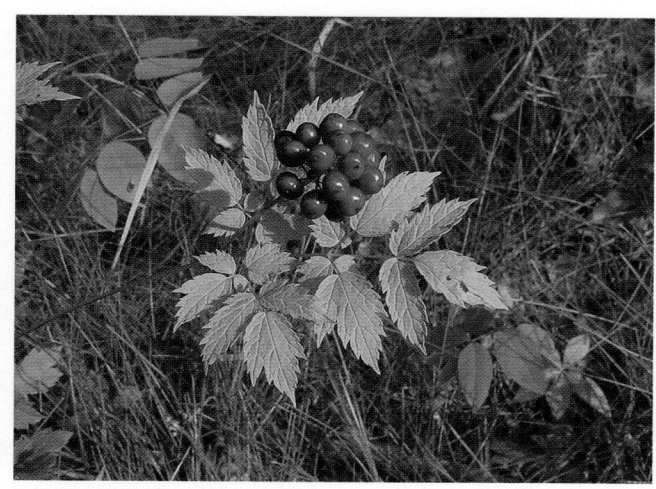

FIGURE 24-23 Red baneberry.

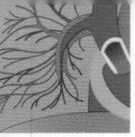

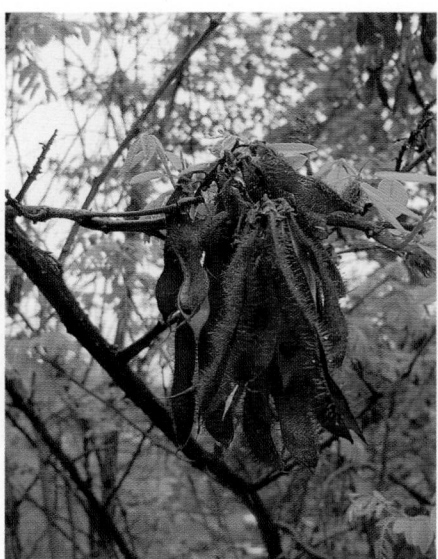

FIGURE 24-24 Black locust pods.

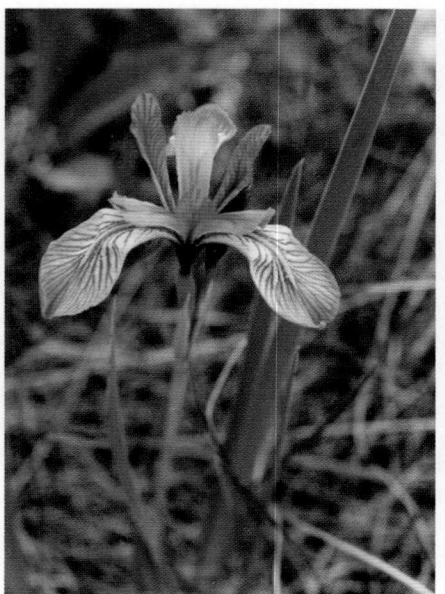

FIGURE 24-25 Iris.

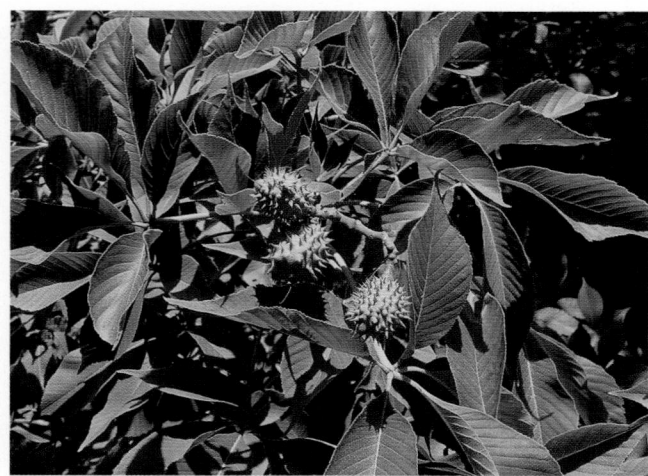

FIGURE 24-26 Buckeye.

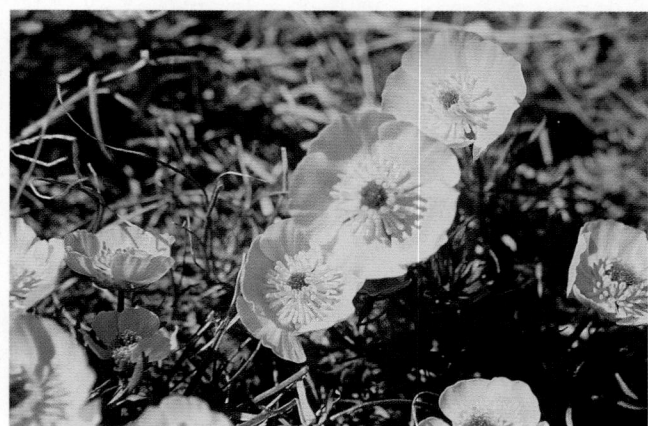

FIGURE 24-27 Buttercup (Courtesy of David G. Spoerke, MS, RPH.)

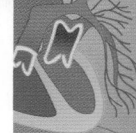

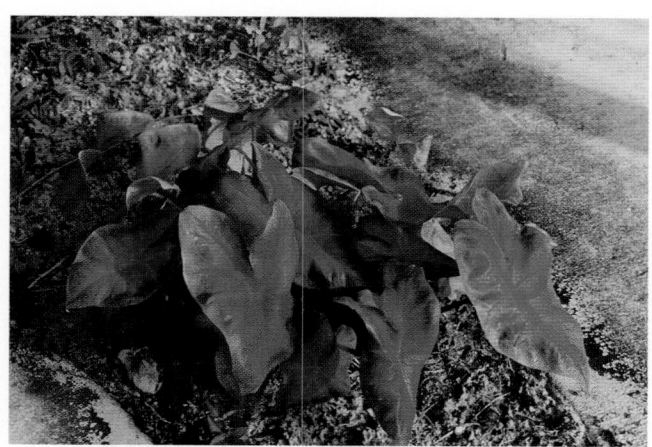

FIGURE 24-28 Caladium.

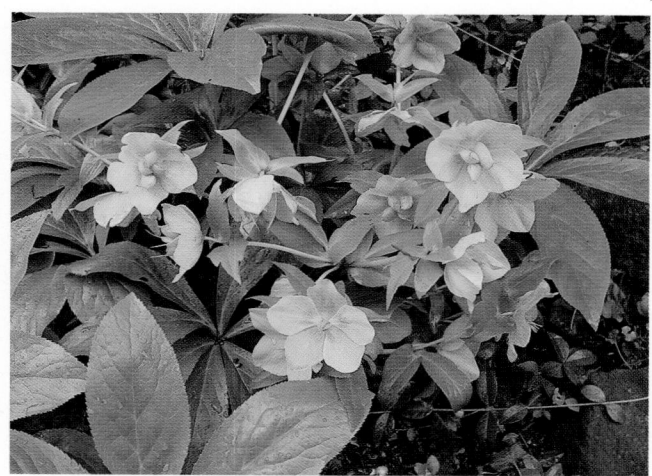

FIGURE 24-29 Lenten rose. (Courtesy of David G. Spoerke, MS, RPH.)

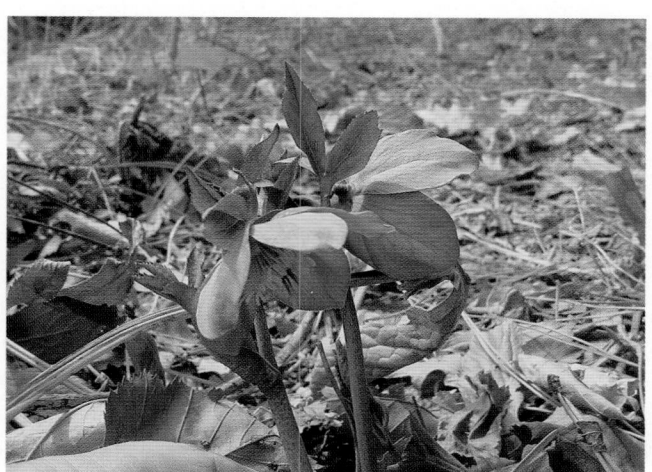

FIGURE 24-30 Dogbane.

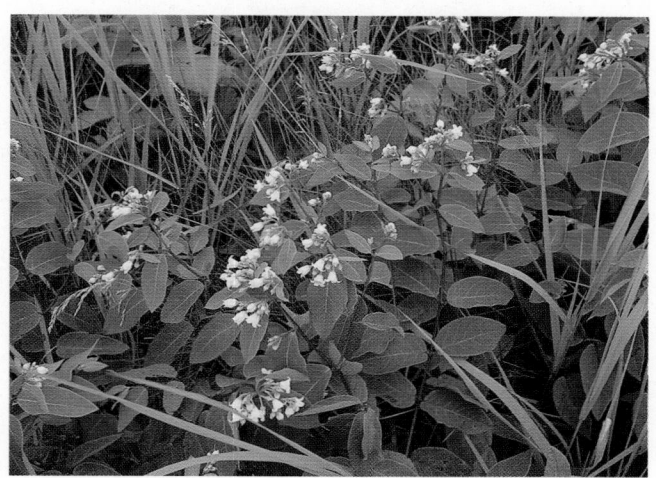

FIGURE 24-31 Four o'clocks.

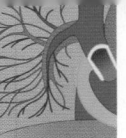

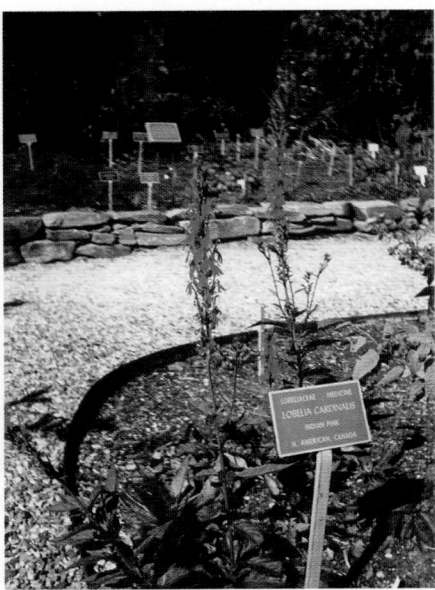

FIGURE 24-32   Lobelia.

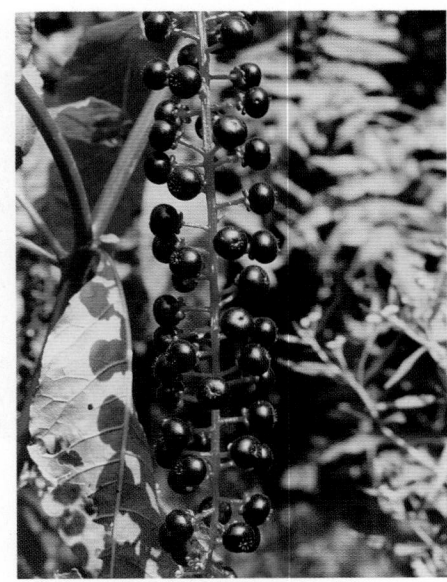

FIGURE 24-33   Pokeweed.

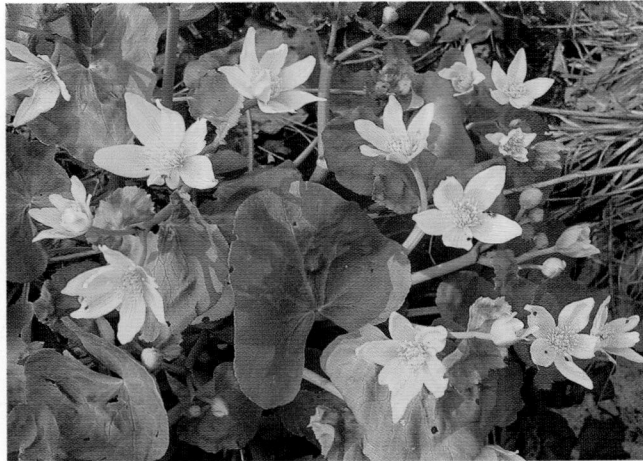

FIGURE 24-34   Marsh marigold.

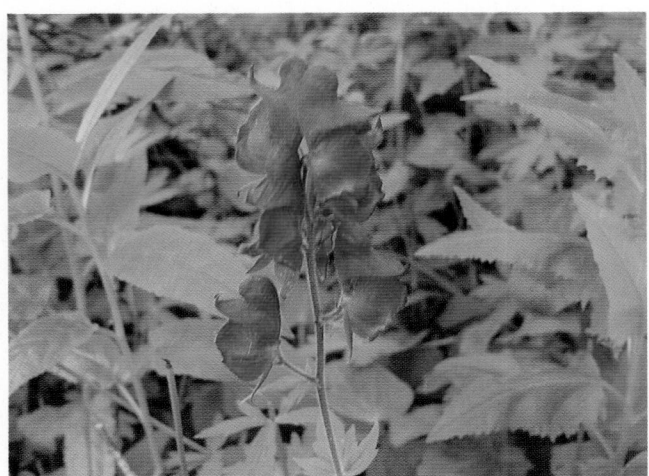

FIGURE 24-35   Monkshood.

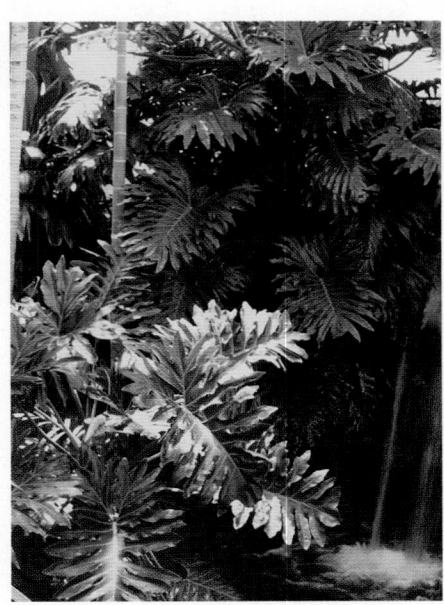

FIGURE 24-36   Lacy tree philodendron.

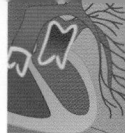

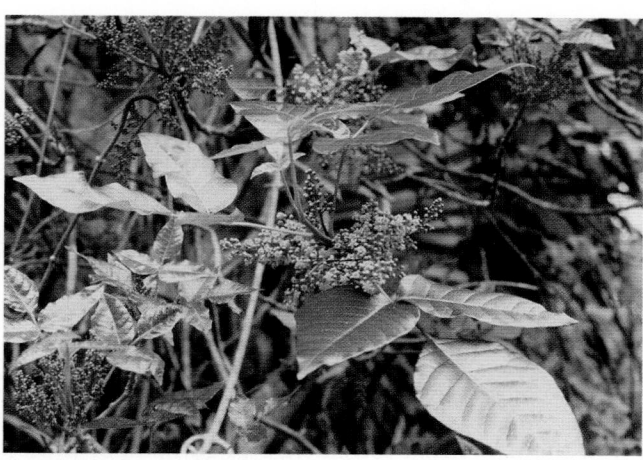

FIGURE 24-37 Poison ivy.

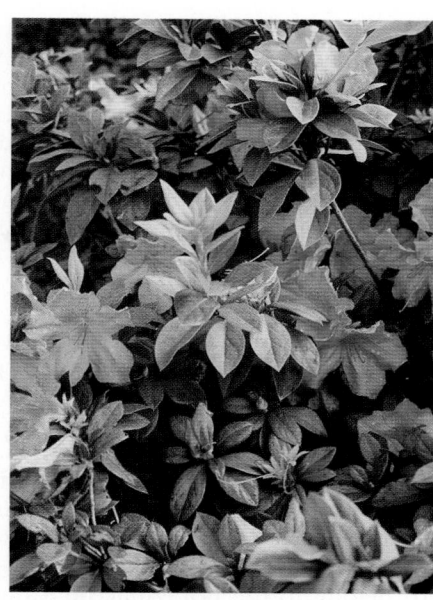

FIGURE 24-38 Balsam azalea.

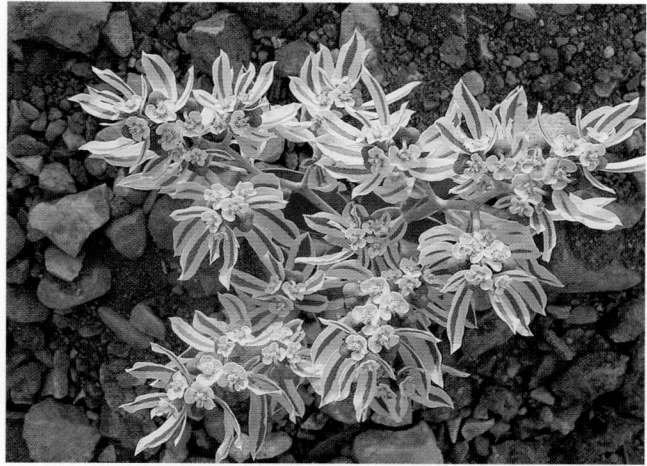

FIGURE 24-39 Snow on the mountain. (Courtesy of David G. Spoerke, MS, RPH.)

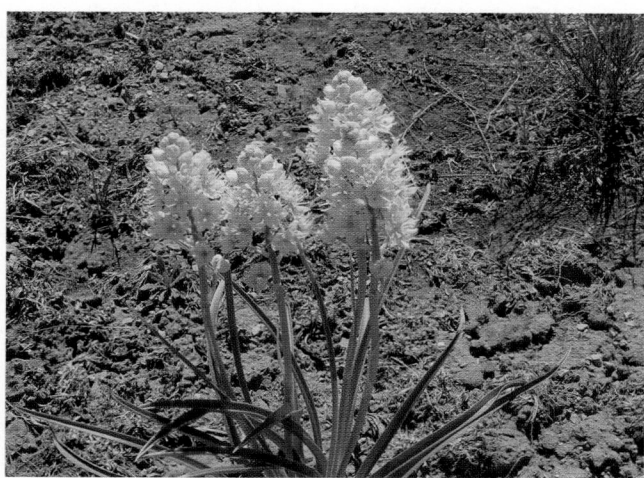

FIGURE 24-40 Sand corn (Zigadenus).

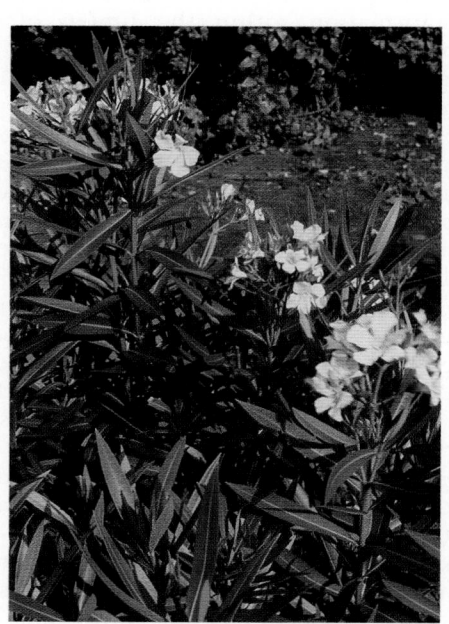

FIGURE 24-41 Common oleander.

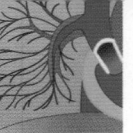

distinct acyl-CoA dehydrogenases: short-chain acyl-CoA, medium-chain acyl-CoA, and isovaleryl-CoA dehydrogenases.[117,118] Long-chain acyl-CoA dehydrogenase does not appear to be significantly inactivated. Inhibition of acyl-CoA dehydrogenase prevents the β-oxidation of fatty acids, leading to a decrease in the substrates needed for gluconeogenesis and oxidative phosphorylation. The release of insulin is not affected by MCPA, MCPA-CoA, or hypoglycin.[119]

Pyrrilizidine Alkaloids

More than 350 pyrrolizidine alkaloids have been identified in over 6000 plants.[120] Not all pyrrolizidine alkaloids are known to be toxic. In those that are known to cause toxicity, a number have been discovered to be carcinogenic in rodents. Due to the vast number of plants containing pyrrolizidine alkaloids and their worldwide distribution, they probably are the most common poisonous plants affecting livestock, wildlife, and humans.[121] Plants containing toxic pyrrolizidine alkaloids belong to the Boraginaceae, Compositae, and Leguminosae families. The most commonly encountered plants containing these alkaloids are *Amsinckia* spp. (fiddle neck, tarweed), *Crotalaria* spp. (rattle box), *Cynoglossum officinale* (hound's tongue), *Echium vulgare* (blue weed), *Heliotropium* species (giant hog weed), *Hypericum perforatum* (heliotrope), *Senecio* spp. (groundsels, *Senecio*), and *Symphytum officinale* (comfrey).

The mechanism of hepatoxicity is thought to be the formation of toxic metabolites by cytochrome P-450.[122] Pyrrolizidine alkaloids are metabolized by CYP450 to highly reactive pyrroles such as dehydroretronecine. The toxicity of the necine alkaloids is inherent upon their ability to bind and alkylate various intracellular constituents. Intracellular toxicity leads to defects of sinusoidal endothelia, with increased permeability and red blood cell extravasation into the space of Disse. Obstruction of vessels is subsequently caused by reticulin fiber formation within the lumen of central and sublobular veins. The thickening of hepatic veins leads to a functional outflow obstruction and massive organ congestion. The end result is necrosis of hepatocytes and mesenchymal cells.[123] Signs of inflammation are usually lacking.[124] Although the liver is the most commonly reported effect, other organ systems may also be affected. Endothelial defects may occur within the lung similar to those seen within the liver parenchyma, leading to the development of pulmonary hypertension.[125]

In Western Europe, comfrey has been applied for inflammatory disorders such as arthritis, thrombophlebitis, and gout and as a treatment for diarrhea. Toxicity is most likely due to various hepatotoxic pyrrolizidine alkaloids such as lasiocarpine, symphytine, and symphytoxide A.[126,127] The main liver injury caused by comfrey (*Symphytum officinale*) is veno-occlusive disease. Symphytoxide A has also exhibited hypotensive effects in anesthetized rats.

In the rat model the alkaloids have been found to be tumorogenic. Hepatocellular adenomas have been induced in rats fed a diet of comfrey roots and leaves.[128] There have been no definitive reports of human cancers in those exposed to pyrrolizidine alkaloids. Maté tea (*Ilex paraguensis*) contains pyrrolizidine alkaloids as well as tannins, and has been associated with increased risk for esophageal cancer, which is related to both amount and temperature of the ingested beverage.[129]

OTHER HEPATIC PLANT TOXINS

Germander has been used in herbal remedies for 2000 years.[130] Alcoholic extracts may use germander as a flavor ingredient, providing a bitter aromatic taste to the beverage. In 1992, several cases of hepatitis surfaced in France due to germander. At that time, germander (*Teucrium chamaedrys*) was being used for supportive treatment of obesity and diarrhea. An interesting feature in the original cases in France was that in approximately half of the patients, a rechallenge of germander caused early recurrence, suggesting an immunoallergic type of hepatitis.[131-133] The furan ring of the diterpenoids in germander has been shown to be oxidized by CYP3A4 to a reactive epoxide neoclerodane.[134,135] Neoclerodane depletes cellular thiols, decreases cell glutathione, increases intracellular calcium, and causes DNA fragmentation, resulting in apoptosis.[136] Research conducted on the mechanism of abrupt disease recurrence with reintroduction of germander demonstrated that epoxide hydrolase was the target of germander-induced autoantibodies on the surface of human hepatocytes. Epoxide hydrolase may in turn act as a target for reactive metabolites from the neoclerodane diterpenoids. *Teucrium polium* (felty germander) has also been used as an herbal medication primarily in Iran as a hypoglycaemic adjunct. The *Teucrium* species contain saponins, glycosides, flavonoids, and a number of furan-containing neoclerodane diterpenoids (teucrolivin, teucrin A). *Teucrium polium* has been shown to reduce high blood glucose levels by enhancing insulin secretion in the β islet cell.[137]

Sassafras (*Sassafras albidum*) contains the toxin safrole that is a potent inhibitor of human CYP1A2, CYP2A6, and CYP2E1.[138] Safrole has been used recently in the manufacturing of MDMA by way of an aminomercuration process. Safrole has been linked, however, to the development of cancer. The carcinogenicity of safrole is mediated through 1'-hydroxysafrole formation, followed by sulfonation to an unstable sulfate that reacts to form DNA adducts.[139]

The primary toxin in pennyroyal is the terpene pulegone. Pulegone may have toxic properties but it is likely its proximate metabolite methofuran that is responsible for significant hepatoxicity. Menthofuran is formed by oxidation of the allylic methyl groups of pulegone by CYP3A4.[140,141] Menthofuran reacts with nucleophilic groups on proteins to form covalent adducts[142] and extensively depletes glutathione.[143] Histologically, dilatation of the central veins and distention of sinusoidal spaces occurs within 6 hours of exposure. Centrilobular necrosis is evident within 12 hours of exposure.[144]

Both *Atractylis gummifera* (Mediterranean thistle) and *Callilepsis laureoa* (impila) have been shown to be considerably toxic, with a high rate of mortality. *C. laureoa*

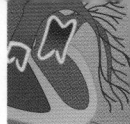

thrives in the KwaZulu-Natal region of South Africa and has been used as a traditional herbal medicine by the Zulu. It is estimated that up to 1500 deaths occur annually in this region due to ingestion of *C. laureoa*.[145] Ingestions of *A. gummifera* continue to occur in the Middle East and southern Europe because of its use as an herbal medicine. Children have been poisoned by this plant, mistaking the root for wild artichoke.[146] The toxicity of *A. gummifera* resides in its three diterpenoid glucosides: atractyloside, carboxyatractyloside, and apo-carboxyatractyloside. The atractylosides are capable of inhibiting mitochondrial oxidative phosphorylation as specific inhibitors of the mitochondrial ADP/ATP translocase.[147] Human poisoning may present with either acute hepatic or renal pathology. At varying concentrations of atractyloside, cells may exhibit frank necrosis or apoptosis.[148] Because of the varying pathology between the liver and renal tissue histologically, it is possible that there is a second, different mechanism of toxicity in hepatocytes.[145]

Plant Dermatitis

CHEMICAL IRRITANT DERMATITIS

The spurge family (Euphorbiaceae) is notorious for its highly irritant latex. The classic plants in this family associated with dermatitis include *Euphorbia myrsinites* (creeping spurge), *Euphorbia tirucalli* (pencil cactus), *Euphorbia lactea* (candelabra cactus), *Euphorbia pulcherrima* (poinsettia), and *Euphorbia milii* (crown of thorns). The latex has been used medicinally for centuries. In AD 50, a Greek physician named Pedanius Dioscorides mentioned several species of *Euphorbia* in the treatment of warts, calluses, and torpid ulcers of the scalp.[149,150] The active toxins in the latex are phorbol (tigliane polyol) and diterpenoid esters.[151,152]

Perhaps the most notorious plant known to cause an irritant dermatitis is the chili pepper. Members of the genus *Capsicum* have been used in recipes longer than any other spice, dating back to 7000 BC.[153] Upon contact with the skin, capsaicin binds to C-polymodal nociceptors, causing depolarization and leading to vasodilation, smooth muscle stimulation, glandular secretions, and sensory nerve activation.[154] Since only C-afferent nerve fibers are affected, and not the skin, no blistering is seen.

Members of the buttercup family (*Ranunculaceae*) have also caused significant skin irritation. Buttercup leaves have long been used in Europe and elsewhere as vesicants.[155] Buttercups contain an unsaturated lactone called protoanemonin, which is formed after injury to the plant by the breakdown of the glycoside ranunculin.[156,157] Local tissue injury may be due to inhibition of DNA polymerase and increase of oxygen free radicals by protoanemonin. Protoanemonin rapidly metabolizes to anemonin, which is nontoxic. Therefore, only freshly damaged plants typically cause a skin reaction.

ALLERGIC CONTACT DERMATITIS

Allergic contact dermatitis is the result of a type IV hypersensitivity reaction that requires a previous exposure before symptoms develop. The most common substances known to elicit such a reaction are the urushiol oleoresins. Urushiol contains a mixture of catechols (1,2-dihydroxybenzenes) and resorcinols (1,3-dihydroxybenzenes) and is found in *Toxicodendron* (poison tree) species, including poison ivy (*Toxicodendron radicans*), poison oak (Eastern, *Toxicodendron toxicarium*; Western, *Toxicodendron diversilobum*), and poison sumac (*Toxicodendron vernix*). It also includes fruit and nut trees such as gingko (*G. biloba*), cashew (*Anacardium occidentale*), and mango (*Mangifera indica*). Cashew nut shell oil contains cardol, a resorcinol with a similar side chain to poison oak and poison ivy allergens. Members of Ginkgoaceae and Proteaceae contain sensitizing resorcinols.[158] In severe cases, type I hypersensitivity reactions may develop.

Occupational exposures to plants represent another common source of toxicity. People working in the tulip industry have known for years of the condition termed "tulip fingers." This painful hyperkeratosis of the fingertips is caused by exposure to the toxin tuliposide A.[159] People working with lilies of the *Alstroemeria* family have developed a similar condition due to the tuliposide found in *Alstroemeria*. Tuliposide is hydrolyzed to a butyrolactone, which probably acts as the true allergen in these cases. Cross-reactivity may occur among workers already sensitized to tulips or *Alstroemeria* species. Occupational exposure to primroses is another cause of allergic dermatitis due to the toxin primin (2-methoxy-6-pentyl-1,4-benzoquinone).[160]

CONTACT URTICARIA

Toxin-mediated contact urticaria occurs without prior sensitization and does not involve a hypersensitivity mechanism. Members of the family Urticaceae, including stinging nettle (*Urtica dioica*), account for the majority of contact urticaria throughout the world.[161] Plant species known to cause contact urticaria contain small outgrowths of epidermal cells known as trichomes. A trichome is composed of two components: a proximal silicaceous hair and a distal calcified bulb. When traumatized, the bulb is dislodged from the end of the hair, revealing a beveled, hypodermic needle–like, silicaceous hollow.[162] Glandular trichomes linked to urticaria most often contain histamine, choline, and serotonin as active toxic components.[163,164] Cowitch (*Mucuna pruriens*) also produces a "sea bean," which contains 6% levodopa and tryptamines.

PHYTOPHOTODERMATITIS

Recognition of plants associated with phytodermatitis developed through treatment of preexisting skin conditions such as vitiligo. Four plant families have been primarily implicated in causing phytophotodermatitis and include Umbelliferae (Apiaceae), Leguminosae (Fabaceae), Moraceae, and Rutaceae. Throughout the late 1800s and early 1900s, the dermatitis of a number of plants was recognized, although the necessity of concomitant ultraviolet radiation (UVR) exposure was not identified until the 1940s. Photochemotherapy (e.g., pulsed ultraviolet actinotherapy) continues to be an avid treatment for skin conditions such as vitiligo, psoriasis, atopic dermatitis, and many others.[165]

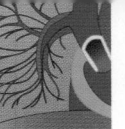

The compounds responsible for phytodermatitis are furocoumarins, which are tricyclic compounds with both linear (psoralens) and angular structures. The two most clinically relevant photosensitizing psoralens are 8-methoxypsoralen (8-MOP, or xanthotoxin) and 5-methoxypsoralen (5-MOP, or bergapten). The photo-toxic effect of furocoumarins is related to their ability to absorb photon energy. In particular, psoralen molecules exposed to UVR are elevated into an excitable state that causes covalent bonding between the psoralen molecule and the cell's DNA. The alteration of DNA structures stimulates mitosis in epidermal skin cells, particularly keratinocytes and melanocytes.[166] Melanocytes have been observed to have enhanced tyrosinase activity as well as larger, dispersed melanosomes contributing to enhance pigmentation. In general, the psoralens are more phototoxic than the angular furocoumarins, with the exception of angular furocoumarin (known as pimpinellin) found in members of the genus *Heracleum* (Umbelliferae). The most severe reactions occur with bergapten isolated from *Citrus bergamia* (Rutaceae), the bergamot orange, and xanthotoxin isolated from *Fagara xanthoxyloides* (Rutaceae). The majority of toxicity develops from common fruits and plants in these families such as *Citrus aurantifolia* (lime), *Apium graveolens* (celery), *Heracleum sphondylium* (cow parsley), *Ruta graveolens* (garden rue), *Ficus carica* (fig tree), and *Psoralea corylifolia* (scurf-pea).

TOXICOLOGY

Clinical Manifestations (Acute and Chronic)

GASTROINTESTINAL IRRITATION

The majority of plant exposures result in mild toxicity, typically in form of GI distress. However, a number of animal cases have demonstrated more a significant level of toxicity, including hypotension, sedation, seizures, and hepatic degeneration with *Narcissus*.[167]

Calcium oxalate crystals are found in a wide variety of common houseplants and are frequently involved in pediatric poisonings. *Dieffenbachia* species are the most potent mucosal irritants. Mechanical stimulation is needed for forced extrusion of the crystals and other bradykinin-like substances, resulting in mucosal injury, salivation, and swelling of the lips, tongue, and mouth. Due to immediate tissue irritation, large amounts of the plant are seldom ingested, reducing the likelihood of systemic oxalate intoxication. In grazing animals, how-ever, oxalic acid poisoning has occurred due to larger ingestions. Swelling rarely causes obstruction, but loss of voice can last for several days. Plant juice exposures to the eye can also produce significant eye irritation, with calcium oxalate crystals detected up to 8 weeks after exposure.[168]

Plants containing RIPs [jequirity bean, castor bean, black locust, Barbados nut (*Jatropha*)] are only toxic if masticated or injected. One masticated seed is potentially lethal to a child, and 8 to 10 seeds to an adult.[169] Clinical effects include severe hemorrhagic gastroenteritis with a delay of 2 to 6 hours, followed by complications of fluid-electrolyte loss (hypotension, tachycardia, prerenal impairment). Transient liver damage occurs in most cases. Metabolic effects include metabolic acidosis, leukocytosis, hyperglycemia or hypoglycemia, and increased creatine kinase. QT prolongation was observed in 5 of 10 serious pediatric cases. Fever is an important initial finding. If death occurs, it is usually related to multiorgan failure after the third day.[170]

Pokeweed contains phytolaccine, a saponin that produces a severe hemorrhagic gastroenteritis within 2 to 4 hours of ingestion, consisting of hematemesis, abdominal cramps, foamy diarrhea, and melena. There is typically initial burning in the mouth and throat. Unripe berries are more toxic, but serious toxicity has occurred with as few as 10 ripe berries in a child. Toxicity can generally be avoided by parboiling the shoots. Mitogens accompany the GI irritants and commonly result in the presence of immature plasma cells on peripheral smears; plasmacytosis may last 2 months or more. A tea made from leaves is more toxic and causes rapid onset of hypotension, respiratory depression, cholinergic symptoms, and seizures.[171]

Solanine is a bitter-tasting alkaloid found in *Solanum* species such as climbing nightshade, horse nettle, potato eyes, eggplant, tomato, and Jerusalem cherry. It is removed by boiling but not baking. Ingestion results in both GI and neurologic symptoms. Unripe berries are more toxic, and it is estimated that up to 10 berries of *Solanum dulcamara* or up to three berries of *Solanum nigrum* or *Solanum pseudocapsicum* can be ingested with-out toxicity. Vomiting, diarrhea, headache, and flushing are the most common symptoms, with the potential for altered mental status, hallucinations, and delirium resembling the antimuscarinic toxidrome.[172]

Holly berries and leaves contain saponins, which may cause gastroenteritis. However, most casual ingestions result in no toxicity. Vomiting generally occurs within 6 hours, and diarrhea follows within 20 hours. It is estimated that ingestion of 20 to 30 berries could be fatal to a child; however, this is poorly documented.[173]

The American variety of mistletoe contains phora-toxin, which is 10 times less toxic than the viscotoxin found in European varieties. Nevertheless, the berries from both remain a common source of GI poisoning, with all parts of the plant being potentially toxic. Up to 20 berries or five leaves have been ingested without toxicity[174]; 90% of exposures reported to poison centers remained asymptomatic in a large series.[175] The ingestion of mistletoe tea is potentially fatal, as concentrated forms of the toxins are cardiotoxic. Mistletoe hepatitis has also been reported.[176]

It is estimated that 15% of the world's total population chews betel nut on a daily basis. The fruit of the areca palm tree (*Areca catechu*) is chewed alone or mixed with other components to form a quid, usually containing catechu gum from the Malaysian acacia tree, and calcium hydroxide. The chief ingredients are arecoline and arecatcine, which act as acetylcholine agonists at central and peripheral sites. Acute effects are similar to nicotine, with dizziness, nausea, diaphoresis, and vomiting.

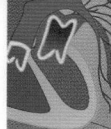

Cholinergic toxicity with classic SLUDGE (salivation, lacrimation, urination, defecation, gastric distress, emesis) syndrome occurs with initial or heavy use. Tachycardia is typically observed. A dose-related bronchospasm occurs in asthmatic subjects. Long-term effects include betel chewer's perleche (fissures at the angles of the mouth), red staining of the oral mucosa, gingival leukoplakia that can progress to squamous cell carcinoma, brown staining of teeth, and milk-alkali syndrome related to the oyster shell lime paste component of the quid.[177]

HEPATOTOXIC PLANTS

JVS remains prevalent in the Caribbean. The Centers for Disease Control and Prevention reviewed reported cases of JVS from 1989 to 1991 and found 38 cases and 6 deaths, with 76% of cases occurring between January and March.[178] Hypoglycin toxin is similar in structure to a valproic acid metabolite and causes hypoglycemia, hyperammonemia, lethargy, vomiting, coma, and cerebral edema resembling Reye's syndrome. The ackee fruit is still available for sale in some European countries, but the U.S. Food and Drug Administration has banned its importation due to the potential risk for toxicity.

Reports of hepatic disease surfaced in South Africa in 1920 after ingestion of *Senecio longilobus* (threadleaf, groundsel) led to the development of liver cirrhosis in several people.[179] Another outbreak of severe liver toxicity occurred in Jamaica in the 1950s when several children developed ascites, hepatomegaly, jaundice, and eventually cirrhosis after the ingestion of "bush tea." The tea consumed contained the leaves from *Crotalaria* species, now known to contain toxic pyrrolizidine alkaloids. More recent cases in both adults and infants have occurred in India, Afghanistan, and the United States.[180,181] Reports to the French Regional Centers of Pharmacovigilance revealed an association of germander ingestion and hepatitis. The severity of the illness ranged from mild hepatitis to cirrhosis to fulminant hepatic failure.[182-185] More recently, the ingestion of *Teucrium polium* was implicated in acute cholestatic hepatitis in Greece.[186] The liver disease that has now been well described for the pyrrolizidine alkaloids resembles that of Budd-Chiari syndrome, with thrombotic and nonthrombotic occlusion of terminal centrilobular hepatic veins.[187,188]

Pennyroyal has long been used as an abortifacient, particularly in areas of central and South America.[189] The oil is also used in cosmetic formulations as a fragrance component. Pennyroyal oil has been an adulterant in mint teas used as home remedies to treat minor ailments and colic, resulting in at least one infant death.[190] Severe toxic effects may develop after ingesting as little as 10 mL, and fulminant hepatic failure may be observed after ingesting as little as 15 mL.[191]

Cardiovascular Toxicity

CARDIAC GLYCOSIDES

Cardiac glycoside poisonings are characterized by initial GI symptoms of nausea and vomiting, followed by bradycardia, dysrhythmias, hypotension, hyperkalemia, and altered mental status. Dysrhythmias generally include various degrees of heart block and bradycardia, with subsequent ventricular ectopy. However, a wide range of toxicity exists among plants containing cardiac glycoside toxins. For example, although poisoning from yellow oleander,[192-194] lily of the valley,[195] and squill[196] are remarkably similar, significant intoxication leading to mortality is rarely reported with lily of the valley ingestions.

A 10-year analysis of TESS exposures to lily of the valley found only three patients with serious outcomes among 2639 cases. The great majority of these exposures occurred in children younger than 6 years (93%), and there is no documentation of amount of exposure in the report.[197]

SODIUM CHANNEL TOXINS

In a series of 356 ingestions of *Taxus baccata* (English yew tree), only 4% of patients had minor symptoms. In more severe cases, systemic toxicity evolves within a few hours and consists of vomiting, abdominal cramps, syncope, bradycardia, hypotension, and cardiovascular collapse. Fatal cases have involved a toddler who chewed berries, a 20-year-old woman who ingested yew to commit suicide, a man who developed ventricular arrhythmias after drinking a tea made from boiled leaves, a 28-year-old woman who ingested yew leaves, three prisoners who ingested a boiled extract of leaves, and ingestion of 150 leaves by a psychotic woman. Preterminal arrhythmias reported in these cases included ventricular flutter, ventricular fibrillation, and idioventricular rhythms. In a previous report of the cardiac toxicity of *Taxus brevifoli*, the cardiac toxicity was partially attributed to cardiac glycoside activity.[198] However, the cardiac toxicity in this case is most likely due to the plant's taxine alkaloids and not a cardiac glycoside, since the plant does not appear to possess any cardenolide and bufadienolide compounds.

Cardiovascular toxins such as hellebore, death camas, rhododendron, azalea, and monkshood share a mechanism of maintaining sodium channels in the open position, resulting in a combination of cardiovascular and neurologic toxicity. Initial symptoms may include sneezing, diaphoresis, chills, and paresthesias, followed by vomiting, diarrhea, bradycardia, dysrhythmias (including torsades de pointes), hypotension, CNS and respiratory depression, and seizures. The amount and composition of *Aconitum* alkaloids are the main factors determining the severity of intoxication and vary greatly with different species, time of harvesting, and the method of processing.[199,200]

NEUROTOXINS

Nicotine is an alkaloid that is well absorbed from the skin, lungs, and GI tract. Initially, it is a potent emetic, which somewhat limits its toxicity in small ingestions. Serious intoxication, however, is well reported. Early symptoms are those of both parasympathetic and sympathetic stimulation (GI distress, miosis, lacrimation, bronchorrhea, transient hypertension, and tachycardia followed by cardiovascular collapse). Neuromuscular

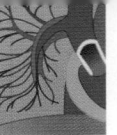

symptoms include fasciculations, weakness, paralysis, coma, and seizures. Several distinct illnesses have been described among the nicotine alkaloids. Green tobacco sickness is an illness associated with nicotine exposures among tobacco harvesters. This illness develops through transdermal absorption of nicotine through contact with the green tobacco plant. Symptoms include weakness, headache, nausea, vomiting, dizziness, abdominal cramps, diarrhea, chills, fluctuations in blood pressure or heart rate, and increased perspiration and salivation. The onset of the illness is 3 to 17 hours after exposure and the duration of illness is 1 to 3 days.[201]

Coniine and its metabolites, found in poison hemlock, act similarly to nicotine and characteristically cause an ascending paralysis with terminal asphyxia. Ataxia, salivation, and coma have been described. Seizures are usually absent. In humans, 3 mg of coniine is said to have produced symptoms, but 150 mg have been tolerated without discomfort. It has been reported that a lethal dose may be six to eight fresh leaves or approximately 100 to 300 mg.[202] The infamous death of Socrates in 399 BC is attributed to the ingestion of a beverage that contained poison hemlock (*Conium maculatum*). After Socrates drank the poison, "he walked about and, when he said his legs were heavy, lay down on his back, for such was the advice of the attendant." The jailor then began to examine Socrates, much in the way a modern physician might do.[62]

> The man . . . laid his hands on him and after a while examined his feet and legs, then pinched his foot hard and asked if he felt it. He said "No"; then after that, his thighs; and passing upwards in this way he showed us that he was growing cold and rigid. And then again he touched him and said that when it reached his heart, he would be gone.[203]

Anticholinergic toxins include scopolamine, atropine, and hyoscyamine and are found in a variety of plants, such as jimson weed (*Datura stramonium*), henbane, deadly nightshade (*Atropa belladonna*), night-blooming jessamine, and mandrake (*Madragora officinarum*). The typical toxidrome involves dry mouth, mydriasis, fever, flushing, blurred vision, hallucinations, urinary retention, ileus, seizures, tachycardia, hypertension, and coma. Symptoms may be recurrent and prolonged. There are also reports of antimuscarinic symptoms developing following the use of Chinese herbal products. The Chinese herb yangjinhua contains dried flowers from *Datura metel* and has been used in treatment of bronchial asthma and chronic bronchitis.[204] Other herbal products linked to antimuscarinic toxicity include Panax ginseng and naoyangua. These products were most likely contaminated with *Mandragon officinarum* or other Solanaceae species and not part of the original Chinese material medica. There is also a case reporting the unintentional poisoning by deadly nightshade in a patient mistaking the plant for burdock (*Arctium lappa*) leaves while foraging.[205] *Datura* has been used as a hallucinogen in the United States, resulting in sporadic cases of antimuscarinic poisoning and death.[206-209]

Cicutoxin, from water hemlock, is the most lethal indigenous North American poison. Most human exposures occur in patients who mistake *Cicuta* for wild edible species, such as wild carrot. The root contains the highest concentration of the toxic alkaloid cicutoxin. Ingestion of a 2- to 3-cm portion of the root can be fatal in adults.[210] Toxicity begins with severe GI symptoms within 15 to 90 minutes of ingestion. Seizures rapidly develop, with status epilepticus and respiratory arrest contributing to the 30% mortality rate. Other movement disorders and spasticity may occur. Complications include rhabdomyolysis and renal failure.

HALLUCINOGENIC PLANTS

Hallucinogenic plants include marijuana, nutmeg, peyote, morning glory seeds, Hawaiian baby woodrose, Scotch broom, ibogaine, khat, *Salvia*, *Mitragyna*, and yohimbine.

Marijuana ingestion in children, with as little as 1 g of hashish or a few "cigarette" butts, causes rapid onset of drowsiness, conjunctival redness, mydriasis, ataxia, pallor, nystagmus, marked hypotonia, and eyelid lag. Rarely, coma, hypothermia, and respiratory obstruction can occur. Recovery typically occurs in 6 to 12 hours. Acute marijuana inhalation or ingestion can induce transient brief episodes of visual hallucinations, illusion, and auditory distortions, particularly with oral ingestion.[211-213]

Morning glory and Hawaiian baby woodrose seeds contain D-lysergic acids and produce a toxidrome similar to LSD. Altered sensorium and sympathomimetic toxidrome occurs with 20 to 50 morning glory seeds (equivalent to 20 to 50 µg of LSD) and 4 to 12 Hawaiian baby woodrose seeds. Very high doses (200 to 300 seeds) have resulted in lethargy, numbness, cool extremities, diarrhea, and dysuria. Onset is typically within 4 to 6 hours and resolves in 12 to 24 hours.[214]

Peyote cactus tops are ingested for the mescaline hallucinogenic effect, which is achieved with seven to eight dried cactus tops. An early phase of mild GI distress occurs, followed by a sympathomimetic phase, with the sensory phase peaking at 4 to 6 hours and lasting 6 to 12 hours.[215]

Nutmeg use continues to be reported among youths. The usual recreational dose is 1 to 3 tablespoons of ground nutmeg (approximately equivalent to one to three whole nutmeg kernels). Initially, nausea, vomiting, diarrhea, abdominal pain, and agitation occur. Later a hallucinogenic/delirium phase may ensue, but is inconsistently present. Onset is 3 to 8 hours, with a duration of up to 24 hours.[15]

Ibogaine, from *Tabernanthe iboga*, is an N-methyl-D-aspartate (NMDA) antagonist and opiate κ agonist that is being used as a treatment for drug withdrawal. The typical experience is a dreamy state lasting 4 to 6 hours. Two fatalities have been reported, from ingestion of 29 and 85 mg/kg. Vomiting, hypotension, and tremor preceded sudden collapse 2 hours and 24 hours after ingestion, respectively.

Scotch broom (*Cytisus scoparius*) is touted as a legal high, containing hydroxytryptamine and sparteine. Blossoms are aged in a sealed jar for 10 days, then rolled into a cigarette and smoked. Deep relaxation, followed

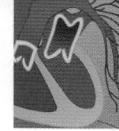

by enhanced color perception, without true hallucinations, is reported by users. Large doses can cause hypotension and tachycardia.[216]

Ayahuasca (also known as daime, yaje, natema, vegetal) is ritually used by shamans in the Amazon. The preparation consists of two herbs prepared as a mixture. All contain a source of harmaline, *Banisteriopsis caapi* The second component is one of two plants that contain *N,N*-dimethyltryptamine (also known as DMT), either *Psychotria viridis* or *Diplopterys cabrerana*. The harmaline alkaloids are monoamine oxidase inhibitors, and prevent presystemic metabolism of DMT, enhancing its psychotomimetic effects. In addition to hallucinations, mild sympathomimetic effects, such as hypertension, tachycardia, and fever, occur.[217]

Salvia divinorum is a hallucinogenic plant in the mint family that contains a diterpene compound called salvinorin A, the most potent known plant-derived hallucinogenic compound, with an effective dose of 200 to 1000 µg when smoked. The plant's leaves are dried and smoked, or chewed, to produce a rapid onset of hallucinations, within a minute, that last about 30 to 60 minutes.[218]

The Rhamnaceae family (buckthorn, wild cherry, coyotillo) consists of small woody shrubs and trees, the seeds of which are potent peripheral neurotoxins, causing a segmental demyelination, presenting as a neurologic syndrome similar to that for Guillain-Barré syndrome or other polyradiculoneuropathies.[219] GI symptoms may also occur. Onset is after a latency of 4 to 7 weeks, with progression over months. The peripheral neuropathy classically starts in the lower extremities and may progress to respiratory compromise and death.[220] Most patients recover after several months with supportive care.

Multisystem Organ Failure

There are several plants with cytotoxic mechanisms of action that produce multisystem organ failure. The most common are the colchicine-containing plants of autumn crocus and glory lily, and *Podophyllum* resin from mayapple.

Colchicine plant poisoning often results from mistaken identity for edible foods such as autumn crocus leaves for salad greens, bulbs for onions, and glory lily tubers for sweet potato. Children have been poisoned from use of the dried seed parts of autumn crocus as rattles. Each seed contains approximately 3.5 mg of colchicine. Ingestion of 10 to 12 flowers has been fatal in adults.[221] *Gloriosa superba* tubers contain 6 mg per 10 g. Colchicine toxicity is characterized by oral paresthesias and hemorrhagic gastroenteritis within 2 to 12 hours, followed by progression in 24 to 72 hours to multisystem organ failure. Symptoms include fever, confusion, coma, ascending polyneuropathy, progressive respiratory distress, renal failure, hepatic failure, leukocytosis followed by disseminated intravascular coagulation and bone marrow suppression, and cardiovascular shock or sudden cardiac arrest. Death is generally related to respiratory failure, cardiovascular collapse, sudden asystole, or sepsis

related to bone marrow suppression. Ingestion of more than 0.8 mg/kg is universally fatal.[222]

Podophyllum toxicity is similar to that of colchicine, with a delay in onset of up to several hours after ingestion, and up to 13 hours, following dermal application. However, neurologic toxicity is more predominant, with sensory motor peripheral neuropathy, paralysis, and encephalopathy reported after as little as 8 to 25 mL of the 25% resin ingested, with progression over months.[223,224]

CYANOGENIC GLYCOSIDES

There are at least 150 plants that contain cyanogenic glycosides. Amygdalin is found in the kernels of plants in the *Prunus* species. The intact seed is not harmful. When the seed is crushed, the release of an enzyme, emulsin, catalyzes the hydrolysis of amygdalin to cyanide. Some gut bacteria also contain glucosidases. The clinical picture is like that of cyanide poisoning. Within 30 minutes of ingestion, dyspnea, cyanosis, vomiting, diaphoresis, weakness, seizures, coma, and cardiovascular collapse occur. Apricot kernels contain the highest concentration of amygdalin (8%), followed by peach pits (6%) and plum pits (2.5%). One gram of amygdalin releases 60 mg of hydrogen cyanide. Ingestion of 20 to 40 apricot kernels has resulted in serious toxicity.[225,226] Apple seeds also contain amygdalin, and ingestion of 50 seeds in one case and a cup of seeds in another case was fatal.[172] Hydrangea contains hydrangin, another cyanide-releasing glycoside, in the leaves and buds; however, there have been no reported cases of cyanide toxicity from hydrangea.

DERMATOLOGIC TOXINS

The most notorious member of the Euphorbiaceae family is the manchineel tree. This tree once grew along beaches throughout the Caribbean, but is now mostly seen in areas of the Virgin Islands and Everglades National Park.[151] The manchineel tree was once planted on graves to deter grave robbers, and the latex has been used to brand horses.[161] The toxic effects from spurges vary by species, but many are capable of producing erythema, blistering, and desquamation. Contact with the latex from the spurge plants produces both local and mild systemic symptoms. Spontaneous, self-limited vomiting may occur in a small percentage of patients. Initial symptoms of skin reddening and swelling occur in 2 to 8 hours, with formation of vesicles and blisters within 4 to 12 hours. Eye contact often causes corneal abrasions, with effects lasting up to 3 weeks. Although poinsettia is in the same family, few cases of toxicity have been reported.[227] Contact with sap caused caustic burns in an adult who was bundling plants in a greenhouse, with a latency of 24 hours. Poinsettia obtained an unwarranted reputation for significant toxicity after a poorly documented case report in Hawaii in 1918. In general, poinsettia latex induces little local skin toxicity in humans and animals.[228] An analysis of TESS data showed oral irritation in 28%, vomiting in 24%, and throat irritation in 15% of poinsettia exposures.[229]

One of the most common plant exposures reported to poison centers is related to *Capsicum* peppers, producing

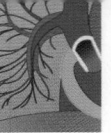

mucosal irritation and increased pain sensitivity, also known as hunan hand syndrome. Erythema and an intense burning sensation occur, generally without vesiculation. Massive ingestions can cause diarrhea or "jaloproctitis." The New Mexico Poison and Drug Information Center receives up to 90 calls per year for "chili burns" of the hands. Their study showed that the best home remedy for chili burns was hand washing with soap and water followed immediately by 1 hour of immersion in vegetable oil.[230]

Dermatitis following exposure to trichomes of such plants as stinging nettle usually lasts about 12 hours. The most impressive skin reactions result from contact with plants and trees from the genus *Dendrocnide*. This tree is primarily found in eastern Australia and has been linked to severe dermatitis lasting up to 3 weeks.[155] This reaction is exacerbated by water and has been attributed to one death.[150]

Delayed contact dermatitis is associated with plants containing urushiol, such as poison ivy, poison oak, and poison sumac. Lacquer also contains urushiol. Cross-reacting compounds are present in mango, cashew, and ginkgo. Onset of rash is typically delayed for 24 to 48 hours. Eruptions are classically linear streaks of erythema, followed by clusters of fluid-filled lesions that are intensely pruritic. The fluid contains no antigen and is not contagious, but patients often spread lesions by scratching areas contaminated with the oleoresin. Resolution typically occurs after 3 weeks or longer. Delayed contact dermatitis has also been reported from contact with ragweed, castor beans, and western red cedar. *Urtica urens* has also been reported to cause allergic contact dermatitis.[231]

Photodermatitis due to furocoumarins and psoralens has been reported following exposures to lime, bergamot, bitter orange (*Citrus aurantium*), dill, celery, carrot, fennel, parsnip, mustard, fig, buttercup, and common rue. Bartenders have developed vesicles on their fingers from squeezing limes into cocktails. Phytophotodermatitis is an oxygen-independent, nonimmunologic reaction that may occur with only 15 to 30 minutes of exposure. The resulting hyperpigmentation may last for several months.

DIAGNOSIS

Laboratory Testing

Osterloh and colleagues[232] described cross-reactivity of oleander glycosides on radioimmunoassay for digoxin. Clinical symptoms, however, are more indicative of toxicity. Postmortem serum concentrations of cardiac glycosides are known to increase and do not predict the premortem levels.[233] The majority of polyclonal assays designed to detect digoxin or digitoxin will probably cross-react sufficiently to detect plant cardiac glycosides. If results are in question, a separate assay may provide additional confirmation. Other diagnostic testing used to detect plant toxins includes ultraviolet absorption, thin layer chromatography, high-performance liquid chromatography and mass spectrometry. There are

sufficient case reports that chromatography can be a used to confirm plant exposure. Similar to the cardiac glycosides, however, clinical symptoms will be more indicative of toxicity.

Differential Diagnosis

The most common diagnostic dilemma is the presentation of an asymptomatic child to an emergency department or a poison center with a history of ingesting an unknown berry. Although crude berry identification keys are available, these are not routinely useful.[234] Identification of the plant through faxed copies of the material and/or having a family member bring the plant to a plant nursery has been successful. In patients presenting with suspected plant-related delirium in the presence of antimuscarinic findings, a diagnostic challenge with physostigmine can often provide the answer. The section on Pathophysiology contains a list of plants contained within each defined presenting toxidrome and can be used as a differential diagnostic tool when plant poisoning is suspected in a symptomatic patient.

MANAGEMENT

Supportive Measures

As with other poisonings, support of airway, breathing, and circulation should be provided when necessary.

Decontamination

Gastric decontamination is not well studied for treatment of plant-related poisonings. The use of syrup of ipecac has declined in the United States to negligible amounts, but plant poisoning remain an indication for some poison centers, despite no evidence to document efficacy. A prospective randomized clinical trial of syrup of ipecac in 103 children who ingested less than six toxic berries showed no benefit from decontamination.[235] It is reasonable to assume that gastric emptying could benefit patients who present early and have ingested a potentially serious plant (see At a Glance section). In theory, large plant parts would be more completely retrieved by ipecac-induced emesis than by gastric lavage, particularly in children, in whom large-bore tubes are not practical. This same group of patients with very toxic plant ingestions may warrant more aggressive decontamination with whole bowel irrigation and activated charcoal. Given the benign nature of most plant ingestions in children, this should be a rare occurrence in the pediatric population.

Nasogastric lavage performed 3 to 9 hours after ingestion of jimson weed seeds did not improve outcomes of length of stay or intensive care unit (ICU) admission, despite recovery of some seeds in 57% of patients where this was attempted. In cases where small seeds of plants with serious toxicity are ingested, it may considered when orogastric lavage cannot be performed.[236]

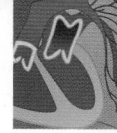

Skin decontamination is indicated for plants causing dermatologic toxicity. Plant trichomes from *Mucuna* or stinging nettle have been removed using such methods as adhesive tape, nontoxic glue dried and peeled, and facial masks. Skin areas in contact with poison ivy can be decontaminated with several washings of soap and water to remove the resinous material and prevent further areas of skin contamination.

Eye decontamination is similar to that with other ocular exposures. It is particularly important following ocular exposures to plant saps known to cause eye irritation or injury, such as insoluble oxalates, Euphorbiaceae family, and trichome-containing plants.

Laboratory Monitoring

Laboratory studies will be dictated by the type of plant poisoning involved. Routine laboratory studies are seldom indicated for accidental plant exposures.

Antidotes

CARDIOVASCULAR PLANT POISONING

Large doses of Fab-anti-digoxin antibodies (60 mg/kg) corrected both rhythm and hyperkalemia in dogs poisoned by oleander.[237] Lower doses might have been effective, but were not tested. Shumaik and colleagues[238] reported the use of digoxin-specific Fab fragments in the treatment of a 37-year-old man who had ingested *Nerium oleander* leaves, and other reports suggest efficacy of Fab fragments in this setting.[239] Indications for Fab fragments include:

1. Hyperkalemia (K$^+$ > 5 to 5.5 mEq/L)
2. Life-threatening supraventricular and ventricular dysrhythmias
3. Hemodynamically significant bradycardia unresponsive to atropine

The treatment of aconitine and other sodium channel–opening plant toxins is therapeutically challenging and based primarily on case report data. Bradycardia may respond to atropine. Amiodarone is a reasonable first-line agent for ventricular tachycardia, and was effective in five of nine patients in one series. Cardioversion was uniformly unsuccessful.[240]

It is reasonable to suppose that plants with sodium channel blocking activity may respond to intravenous sodium bicarbonate infusion. This was ineffective in a swine model of yew (*Taxus*) poisoning with widened QRS. Treated animals had lower blood pressures and wider QRS over time than controls. This treatment was effective in a case report of a patient with suicidal ingestion of yew cookies, however. Other anecdotal treatments have included vasopressors, transvenous pacing, cardioversion, atropine, magnesium sulfate, and lidocaine. Digoxin Fab fragments are ineffective, since the plant alkaloids have no cardiac glycoside structure. Taxine B also displays calcium channel blockade; therefore, intravenous calcium infusion may theoretically be beneficial.[60]

HEPATOTOXICITY

Pulegone is metabolized in a manner analogous to acetaminophen. *N*-acetylcysteine was administered in a patient who did not develop hepatotoxicity in one case, and should be considered in any patient with significant ingestion of the pennyroyal plant,[241] despite lack of efficacy shown in an animal model.[242]

There is no specific antidote or treatment of hepatic veno-occlusive disease caused by plants containing pyrrolizidine alkaloids

MULTIORGAN FAILURE

Anticochicine Fab fragments have been developed in France, with evidence of efficacy in one human poisoning case and favorable animal research. However, these are not in commercial production and are currently not available.[243]

The U.S. army has recently developed an experimental vaccine against ricin. It has shown efficacy in mice.

NEUROLOGIC PLANT TOXICITY

Physostigmine has been compared with benzodiazepine therapy in the treatment of jimson weed–induced delirium in two studies. Burn and colleagues found that only physostigmine reversed delirium, and was associated with decreased agitation, less complications, and shorter recovery time compared with benzodiazepines in a retrospective study of 52 patients with anticholinergic poisoning. *Datura* was the substance in 4 patients in each treatment group.[244] In the second study, the combination of benzodiazepines with physostigmine did not reduce length of stay or ICU admission in 3 patients compared with benzodiazepines alone in 14 patients.[245] Repeated doses of physostigmine are often necessary due to prolonged absorption of the plant toxins.

Benzodiazepines remain part of the supportive care for other plant-related hallucinations and agitation syndromes, as well as initial therapy for plant-related seizures. Pyridoxine should be tried in cases of seizures suspected to be related to *Ginkgo biloba*, particularly with ingestion of the seeds, known to contain a pyridoxine antagonist.

ELIMINATION

There is no evidence for plant toxins to benefit from hemodialysis or hemoperfusion. Digitoxin, derived from *Digitalis lanata*, may benefit from enhanced elimination with multiple-dose activated charcoal. However, given the marked efficacy of the digoxin-specific Fab fragments, the utility of this modality will be low.

DISPOSITION

Patients who have ingested plants with a predilection for delayed onset of toxicity should be admitted, even if initially asymptomatic. This includes pennyroyal, RIPs (ricin, abrin), podophyllum, and colchicine-containing plants. Disposition for other toxic plants will be determined by their exhibiting signs and symptoms.

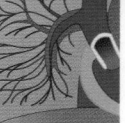
REFERENCES

1. Watson WA, Litovitz TL, Klein-Schwartz W, et al: 2003 Annual Report of the American Association of Poison Control Centers Toxic Exposure Surveillance System. Am J Emerg Med 2004; 22:335–404.
2. Krenzelok EP: Lethal plant exposures reported to poison centers: prevalence, characterization and mechanisms of toxicity. J Toxicol Clin Toxicol 2002;40:303–304.
3. Jaspersno-Schib R, Theus J, Guirguis-Oeschager M, et al: Serious plant poisonings in Switzerland 1966–1994. Case analysis from the Swiss Toxicology Information Centre. Schweiz Med Wochenschr 1996;126:1085–1098.
4. Eddleston M, Persson H: Acute plant poisoning and antitoxin antibodies. J Toxicol Clin Toxicol 2003;41:309–315.
5. Cilliers LR, Retief FP: Poisons, poisoning and the drug trade in ancient Rome. Akroterion 2000;45:88–100.
6. Beverley R: The History and Present State of Virginia. Chapel Hill, NC, University of North Carolina Press, 1947.
7. Thabet H, Brahmi N, Amamour M, et al: Datura stramonium poisoning in humans. Vet Hum Toxicol 1999;41:320.
8. Barton BS: Some account of the poisonous and injurious honey of North America. Trans Am Phil Soc 1802;5:51–70.
9. Masutani T, Seyama I, Narahashi T: Structure-activity relationship for grayanotoxin derivatives in frog skeletal muscle. J Pharmacol Exp Ther 1981;217:812.
10. Munro TA, Rizzacasa MA, Roth BL, et al: Studies toward the pharmacophore of salvinorin A, a potent kappa opioid receptor agonist. J Med Chem 2005;48:345–348.
11. Ameri A: The effects of Aconitum alkaloids on the central nervous system. Prog Neurobiol 1998;56:211–235.
12. Medarde MC, Caballero E, Tomé F, et al: Synthesis and evaluation of cardiotonic activity of simple butenolides, II. Eur J Med Chem 1993;28:887–892.
13. Melero CP, Medarde M, San Feliciano A: A short review on cardiotonic steroids and their aminoguanidine analogues. Molecules 2000;5:51–81.
14. Shigei TT, Tsuru H, Saito Y, Okada M: Structure-activity relationship of the cardenolide, with special reference to the substituents and configurations at C-14 and C-15. Experientia 1973;29:449–450.
15. Sangalli BC, Chiang W: Toxicology of nutmeg abuse. J Toxicol Clin Toxicol 2000;38:671–678.
16. Gobbini M, Benicchio A, Marazzi G, et al: Digitalis-like compounds: synthesis and biological evaluation of seco-D and D-homo derivatives. Steroids 1996;61:572–582.
17. Foye WO, Lemke TL, Williams DA, Mehanna AS: Principles of Medicinal Chemistry, 4th ed. Baltimore, MD, Williams & Wilkins, 1995.
18. Chen JJ, Henderson FG: Pharmacology of sixty-four cardiac glycosides and aglycones. J Pharmacol Exp Ther 1954;111:365–583.
19. Chiu FC, Watson TR: Conformational factors in cardiac glycoside activity. J Med Chem 1985;28:509–515.
20. Brown L, Thomas RE: Arzneimittelforschung 1983;33:814–817.
21. Fullerton DS, Kihara M, Deffo T, et al: Cardiac glycosides. 1. A systematic study of digitoxigenin D-glycosides. J Med Chem 1984;27:256–261.
22. Litovitz TL, Fahey BA: Please don't eat the daffodils. N Engl J Med 1982;306:547.
23. Lopez S, Bastida J, Viladomat F, Codina C: Galanthamine pattern in Narcissus confusus plants. Planta Med 2003;69:1166–1168.
24. Nesterenko L: Influence of the galanthamine on the activity of the acetylcholinesterase in different regions of the brain. Farmakol Toksikol (Moscow) 1965;28:413–414.
25. Ceriotti G: Narciclasine: an antimitotic substance from narcissus bulbs. Nature 1967;213:595–596.
26. Harding A: Ginseng and Other Medicinal Plants: A Book of Valuable Information for Growers as Well as Collectors of Medicinal Roots, Barks, Leaves, Etc. Columbus, OH, AR Harding, 1936.
27. Barker BE, Farnes P, LaMarche PH: Haematological effects of pokeweed [Letter]. Lancet 1967;1:437.
28. Barker BE, Farnes P, LaMarche PH: Peripheral blood plasmacytosis following systemic exposure to Phytolacca americana (Pokeweed). Pediatrics 1966;38:490.
29. Picard D, Kao CC, Hudak KA: Pokeweed antiviral protein inhibits brome mosaic virus replication in plant cells. J Biol Chem 2005; 280:20069–20075.
30. Li X, Zhang D, Lynch-Holm VJ, et al: Isolation of a crystal matrix protein associated with calcium oxalate precipitation in vacuoles of specialized cells. Plant Physiol 2003;133:549–559.
31. Rauber A: Observations on the idioblasts of Dieffenbachia. J Toxicol Clin Toxicol 1985;23:79–90.
32. Gardner DG: Injury to the oral mucous membranes caused by the common houseplant, dieffenbachia. A review. Oral Surg Oral Med Oral Pathol 1994;78:631–633.
33. Sakai WS, Shiroma SS, Nagao MA: A study of raphide microstructure in relation to irritation. Scan Electron Microsc 1984; (Pt 2):979–986.
34. Sandvig K, van Deurs B: Entry of ricin and shiga toxin into cells: molecular mechanisms and medical perspectives. EMBO J 2000;19:5943–5950, 2000.
35. Hartley MR, Lord JM: Cytotoxic ribosome-inactivating lectins from plants. Biochim Biophys Acta 2004;1701:1–14.
36. Endo Y, Tsurugi K: RNA N-glycosidase activity of ricin A-chain. J Biol Chem 1987;262:8128–8130.
37. Nilsson L, Asano K, Svensson B, Poulsen FM, et al: Reduced turnover of the elongation factor EF-1 X ribosome complex after treatment with the protein synthesis inhibitor II from barley seeds. Biochem Biophys Acta 1986;868:62–70.
38. Barbieri L, Valbonesi P, Bonora E, et al: Polynucleotide:adenosine glycosidase activity of ribosome-inactivating proteins: effect on DNA, RNA and poly(A). Nucleic Acids Res 1997;25:518–522.
39. Fletcher SP, Geyer BC, Smith A, et al: Tissue distribution of cholinesterases and anticholinesterases in native and transgenic tomato plants. Plant Mol Biol 2004;55:33–43.
40. Keukens EA, de Vrije T, Fabrie CH, et al: Dual specificity of sterol-mediated glycoalkaloid induced membrane disruption. Biochim Biophys Acta 1992;1110:127–136.
41. Nishie K, Norred WP, Swain AP: Pharmacology and toxicology of chaconine and tomatine. Res Commun Chem Pathol Pharmacol 1975;12:657.
42. Mensinga T, Sips A, Rompelberg CJ, et al: Potato glycoalkaloids and adverse effects in humans: an ascending dose study. Regul Toxicol Pharmacol 2005;41:66–72.
43. Hastie SB: Interactions of colchicine with tubulin. Pharmacol Ther 1991;51:377–401.
44. Sackett DL: Podophyllotoxin, steganacin and combretastatin: natural products that bind at the colchicine site of tubulin. Pharmacol Ther 1993;59:163–228.
45. Himes RH: Interactions of the catharanthus (Vinca) alkaloids with tubulin and microtubules. Pharmacol Ther 1991;51:257–267.
46. Iwasaki S: Natural organic compounds that affect to microtubule functions. Yakugaku Zasshi 1998;118:112–126.
47. Chan TY, Critchley JA: Usage and adverse effects of Chinese herbal medicines. Hum Exp Toxicol 1996;15:5–12.
48. Sutlupinar N, Mat A, Satganoglu Y: Poisoning by toxic honey in Turkey. Arch Toxicol 1993;67:148–150.
49. Prince LA, Stork CM: Prolonged cardiotoxicity from poison lily (Veratrum viride). Vet Hum Toxicol 2000;42:282–285.
50. Denac H, Mevissen M, Scholtysik G: Structure, function and pharmacology of voltage-gates sodium channels. Naunyn Schmiedebergs Arch Pharmacol 2000;362:453–479.
51. Hills B, Barnes S: Veratridine modifies open sodium channel. J Gen Physiol 1988;91:421–443.
52. Lazdunski M, Renaud J-F: The action of cardiotoxins on cardiac plasma membranes. Annu Rev Physiol 1982;44:463–473.
53. Wang GK, Wang SY: Veratridine block of rat skeletal muscle sodium channels in the inner vestibule. J Physiol 2003;548:667–675.
54. Honerjager P, Meissner A: The positive ionotropic effects of aconitine. Naunyn Schmiedebergs Arch Pharmacol 1983;322:49–58.
55. Adaniya H, Hayami H, Hiraoka M, Sawanobori T: Effects of magnesium on polymorphic ventricular tachycardias induced by aconitine. J Cardiovasc Pharmacol 1994;24:721–729.
56. Tai Y, But P: Bidirectional tachycardia induced by herbal aconite poisoning. Pacing Clin Electrophysiol 1992;15:831.
57. Nagata R, Izumi K: Veratramine-induced behavior associated with serotonergic hyperfunction in mice. Jpn J Pharmacol 1991;55: 129–137.

58. Zhao XY, Wang Y, Li Y, et al: Songorine, a diterpenoid alkaloid of the genus Aconitum, is a novel GABA(A) receptor antagonist in rat brain. Neurosci Lett 2003;337:33–36.

59. Alloatti G, Penna C, Levi RC, et al: Effects of yew alkaloids and related compounds on guinea-pig isolated perfused heart and papillary muscle. Life Sci 1996;58:845–854.

60. Ruha AM, Tanen DA, Graeme KA, et al: Hypertonic sodium bicarbonate for Taxus media-induced cardiac toxicity in swine. Acad Emerg Med 2002;9:179–185.

61. Barbieri R, Gochberg J, Ryan K: Nicotine, cotinine, and anabasine inhibit aromatase in human trophoblast in vitro. J Clin Invest 1986;77:1727–1733.

62. Bloch E: Hemlock Poisoning and the Death of Socrates: Did Plato Tell the Truth? Buffalo, NY, Oxford University Press, 2001.

63. Lopez TA, Cid MS, Bianchini ML: Biochemistry of hemlock (Conium maculatum L.) alkaloids and their acute and chronic toxicity in livestock. A review. Toxicon 1999;37:841–865.

64. Palmer L, Lundgren G, Karlen B: A method using L-hyoscyamine for the study of muscarinic acetylcholine receptor binding in vivo. Pharmacol Toxicol 1987;60:54–57.

65. McEvoy G: Anticholinergic Agents. AHFS Drug Information. Bethesda, MD, American Hospital Formulary Service, 2002, pp 1222–1228.

66. Heath KBH: A fatal case of apparent water hemlock poisoning. Vet Hum Toxicol 2001;43:35–36.

67. Sweeney K: Water hemlock poisoning—Maine, 1992. MMWR 1994;43:229–231.

68. Miller M: Water hemlock poisoning. JAMA 1933;101:852–853.

69. Uwai K, Ohashi K, Takaya Y, Virol A: A toxic trans-polyacetylenic alcohol of Cicuta virosa, selectively inhibits the GABA-induced Cl(-) current in acutely dissociated rat hippocampal CA1 neurons. Brain Res 2001;889:174–180.

70. Uwai K, Ohashi K, Takaya Y: Exploring the structural basis of neurotoxicity in C(17)-polyacetylenes isolated from water hemlock. J Med Chem 2000;43:4508–4515.

71. Huang S, Duke R, Chebib M, et al: Ginkgolides, diterpene trilactones of Ginkgo biloba, as antagonists at recombinant alpha1beta2-gamma2L GABAA receptors. Eur J Pharmacol 2004;494:131–138.

72. Satoh H, Nishida S: Electropharmacological actions of Ginkgo biloba extract on vascular smooth and heart muscles. Clin Chim Acta 2004;342:13–22.

73. Negro Alvarez J, Miralles Lopez J, Ortiz Martinez J, et al: Platelet-activating factor antagonists. Allergol Immunopathol (Madr) 1997;25:249–258.

74. Jaracz S, Nakanishi K, Jensen A, et al: Ginkgolides and glycine receptors: a structure-activity relationship study. Chemistry 2004;10:1507–1518.

75. Goutman J, Calvo D: Studies on the mechanisms of action of picrotoxin, quercetin and pregnanolone at the GABAq1 receptor. Br J Pharmacol 2004;141:717–727.

76. Kajiyama Y, Fujii K, Takeuchi H, et al: Ginkgo seed poisoning. Pediatrics 2002;109:325–327.

77. Downs C, Phillips J, Ranger A, et al: A hemlock water dropwort curry: a case of multiple poisoning. Emerg Med J 2002;19:472–473.

78. Dubois JM, Schneider MF: Block of ionic and gating currents in node of Ranvier with oenanthotoxin. Toxicon 1982;20:49–55.

79. Anonymous: Cocculi Fructus. Cocculus Indicis. London, The British Pharmaceutical Codex: Council of the Pharmaceutical Society of Great Britain, 1911.

80. Qian H, Pan Y, Zhu Y, et al: Picrotoxin accelerates relaxation of GABAC receptors. Mol Pharmacol 2005;67:470–479.

81. Erkkila BE, Weiss DS, Wotring VE: Picrotoxin-mediated antagonism of α3β4 and α7 acetylcholine receptors. Neuroreport 2004;15:1969–1673.

82. Remington J, Wood H: The Dispensatory of the United States of America. Philadelphia, JB Lippincott, 1918 (last updated January 19, 2005).

83. Kudo Y, Niwa H, Tanaka A, et al: Actions of picrotoxinin and related compounds on the frog spinal cord: the role of a hydroxyl-group at the 6-position in antagonizing the actions of amino acids and presynaptic inhibition. Br J Pharmacol 1984;81:373–380.

84. Dorling P, Huxtable C, Colegate S: Inhibition of lysosomal alpha-mannosidase by swainsonine, an indolizidine alkaloid isolated from Swainsona canescens. Biochem J 1980;191:649–651.

85. Goss P, Baker M, Carver J, et al: Inhibitors of carbohydrate processing: a new class of anticancer agents. Clin Cancer Res 1995;1:935–944.

86. Spencer P: Food toxins, ampa receptors, and motor neuron diseases. Drug Metab Rev 1999;31:561–587.

87. Aghajanian G: Serotonin and hallucinogens. Neuropsychopharmacology 1999;21(Suppl):16–23.

88. Rice W, Genest K: Acute toxicity of extracts of morning glory seeds in mice. Nature 1965;207:302.

89. Miller M: Isolation and identification of lysergic acid amide and isolysergic acid amide as the principal ergoline alkaloids in Argyreia nervosa, a tropical wood rose. J AOAC Int 1970;53:123–127.

90. Hoffmann A, Tscherter H: Isolierung van lysergsaure Aekaloi den aus der Mexicanischen zauberdroge Oloiqui (Rivea corymbosa). Experientia 1960;16:414.

91. Anonymous: Hallucinogens of morning glory. BMJ 1966;1:814.

92. Halpern J: Hallucinogens and dissociative agents naturally growing in the United States. Pharmacol Ther 2004;102:131–138.

93. Horie S, Koyama F, Takayama H: Indole alkaloids of a Thai medicinal herb, Mitragyna speciosa, that has opioid agonistic effect in guinea-pig ileum. Planta Med 2005;71:231–236.

94. Paunovic K: Morphological changes in the renal tissue of the rat (Abstract 53). In: International Scientific Conference, 1999. Belgrade, Yugoslavia, Medical School of Belgrade University, 1999.

95. Hernandez-Cruz A, Munoz-Martinez E: Distal reduction of the conduction velocity of alpha-axons in tullidora (buckthorn) neuropathy. Exp Neurol 1983;82:335–343.

96. Heath J, Ueda S, Bornstein M, et al: Buckthorn neuropathy in vitro: evidence for a primary neuronal effect. J Neuropathol Exp Neurol 1982;41:204–220.

97. Vetter J: Plant cyanogenic glycosides. Toxicon 2000;38:11–36.

98. Akintonwa A, Tunwashe O: Fatal cyanide poisoning from cassava-based meal. Hum Exp Toxicol 1992;11:47–49.

99. Sreeja VG, Nagahara Li Q, Minami M: New aspects in pathogenesis of konzo: neural cell damage directly caused by linamarin contained in cassava (Manihot esculenta Crantz). Br J Nutr 2003;90:467–472.

100. Tor-Agbidye J, Palmer V, Lasarev M, et al: Bioactivation of cyanide to cyanate in sulfur amino acid deficiency: relevance to neurological disease in humans subsisting on cassava. Toxicol Sci 1999;50:228–235.

101. Tor-Agbidye J, Palmer V, Spencer P: Sodium cyanate alters glutathione homeostasis in rodent brain: relationship to neurodegenerative diseases in protein-deficient malnourished populations in Africa. Brain Res 1999;820:9–12.

102. Shibata S: A drug over the millennia: pharmacognosy, chemistry, and pharmacology of licorice. Yakugaku Zasshi 2000;120:849–862.

103. Baltina L: Chemical modification of glycyrrhizic acid as a route to new bioactive compounds for medicine. Curr Med Chem 2003;10:155–171.

104. Whorwood C, Sheppard M, Stewart P: Licorice inhibits 11 beta-hydroxysteroid dehydrogenase messenger ribonucleic acid levels and potentiates glucocorticoid hormone action. Endocrinology 1993;132:2287–2292.

105. Stormer F, Reistad R, Alexander J: Glycyrrhizic acid in liquorice—evaluation of health hazard. Food Chem Toxicol 1993;31:303–312.

106. Bean P: The use of alternative medicine in the treatment of hepatitis C. Am Clin Lab 2002;21:19–21.

107. Vanhaelen M, Vanhaelen-Fastre R, But P, et al: Identification of aristolochic acid in Chinese herbs. Lancet 1994;343:174.

108. Wooltorton E: Several Chinese herbal products may contain toxic aristolochic acid. CMAJ 2004;171:449.

109. Hranjec T, Kovac A, Kos J, et al: Endemic nephropathy: the case for chronic poisoning by aristolochia. Croat Med J 2005;46:116–125.

110. Zhou S, Koh H, Gao Y, et al: Herbal bioactivation: the good, the bad and the ugly. Life Sci 2004;74:935–968.

111. Nortier J, Vanherweghem J: Renal interstitial fibrosis and urothelial carcinoma associated with the use of a Chinese herb (Aristolochia fangchi). Toxicology 2002;181:577–580.

112. Krumme B, Endmeir R, Vanhaelen M, et al: Reversible Fanconi syndrome after ingestion of a Chinese herbal "remedy" containing aristolochic acid. Nephrol Dial Transplant 2001;16:400–402.

113. Nortier J, Martinez M, Schmeiser H, et al: Urothelial carcinoma associated with the use of a Chinese herb (Aristolochia fangchi). N Engl J Med 2000;342:1686–1692.

114. Morton J: Plants Poisonous to People. Miami, FL, Hurricane House, 1971.

115. Tanaka K, Kean E, Johnson B: Jamaican vomiting sickness. Biochemical investigation of two cases. N Engl J Med 1976;295:461–467.

116. Bressler R, Corredor C, Brendel K: Hypoglycin and hypoglycin-like compounds. Pharmacol Rev 1969;21:105–130.

117. Ikeda Y, Tanaka K: Selective inactivation of various acyl-CoA dehydrogenases by (methylenecyclopropyl)acetyl-CoA. Biochim Biophys Acta 1990;1038:216–221.

118. Addae JI, Melville GN: A re-examination of the mechanism of ackee-induced vomiting sickness. West Indian Med J 1988;37:6–8.

119. Mills J, Melville G, Bennett C, et al: Effect of hypoglycin A on insulin release. Biochem Pharmacol 1987;36:495–497.

120. Stegelmeier B, Edgar JA, Colegate S, et al: Pyrrolizidine alkaloid plants, metabolism and toxicity. J Nat Toxins 1999;8:95–116.

121. Smith L, Culvenor C: Plant sources of hepatotoxic pyrrolizidine alkaloids. J Nat Prod 1981;44:129–152.

122. Huxtable R: New aspects of the toxicology and pharmacology of pyrrolizidine alkaloids. Gen Pharmacol 1979;10:159–167.

123. Yeong M, Wakefield SJ, Ford H: Hepatocyte membrane injury and bleb formation following low dose comfrey toxicity in rats. Int J Exp Pathol 1993;74:211–217.

124. Ridker P, Ohkuma S, McDermott W, et al: Hepatic venoocclusive disease associated with the consumption of pyrrolizidine-containing dietary supplements. Gastroenterology 1985;88:1050–1054.

125. Shubat P, Banner W, Huxtable R: Pulmonary vascular response induced by the pyrrolizidine alkaloid monocrotalinein rats. Toxicon 1987;25:995–1002.

126. Ahmad V, Noorwala M, Mohammad F, et al: Symphytoxide A, a triterpenoid saponin from the roots of Symphytum officinale. Phytochemistry 1993;32:1003–1006.

127. Stickel F, Seitz H: The efficacy and safety of comfrey. Public Health Nutr 2000;3:501–508.

128. Hirono I, Mori H, Haga M: Carcinogenic activity of Symphytum officinale. J Natl Cancer Inst 1978;61:865–869.

129. Sewram V, De Stefani E, Brennan P, Boffeta P: Mate consumption and the risk of squamous cell esophageal cancer in Uruguay. Cancer Epidemiol Biomark Prev 2003;12:508–513.

130. Stickel F, Egerer G, Seitz H: Hepatotoxicity of botanicals. Public Health Nutr 2000;3:113–124.

131. Castot A, Larrey D: Hepatitis observed during a treatment with a drug or tea containing Wild Germander. Evaluation of 26 cases reported to the Regional Centers of Pharmacovigilance [French]. Gastroenterol Clin Biol 1992;16:916–922.

132. Legoux J, Maitre F, Labarriere D, et al: Cytolytic hepatitis and wild Germander: a new case with reintroduction [French]. Gastroenterol Clin Biol 1992;16:813–815.

133. De Berardinis V, Moulis C, Maurice M, et al: Human microsomal epoxide hydrolase is the target of germander-induced autoantibodies on the surface of human hepatocytes. Mol Pharmacol 2000;58:542–551.

134. Kouzi S, McMurtry R, Nelson S: Hepatotoxicity of germander (Teucrium chamaedrys L.) and one of its constituent neoclerodane diterpenes teucrin A in the mouse. Chem Res Toxicol 1994;7:850–856.

135. Lekehal M, Pessayre D, Lereau J, et al: Hepatotoxicity of the herbal medicine germander: metabolic activation of its furano diterpenoids by cytochrome P450 3A depletes cytoskeleton-associated protein thiols and forms plasma membrane blebs in rat hepatocytes. Hepatology 1996;24:212–218.

136. Fau D, Lekehal M, Farrell G: Diterpenoids from germander, an herbal medicine, induce apoptosis in isolated rat hepatocytes. Gastroenterology 1997;113:1334–1346.

137. Esmaeili M, Yazdanparast R: Hypoglycaemic effect of Teucrium polium: studies with rat pancreatic islets. J Ethnopharmacol 2004;95:27–30.

138. Ueng Y, Hsieh C, Don M: Inhibition of human cytochrome P450 enzymes by the natural hepatotoxin safrole. Food Chem Toxicol 2005;43:707–712.

139. Ueng Y, Hsieh C, Don M, et al: Identification of the main human cytochrome P450 enzymes involved in safrole 1'-hydroxylation. Chem Res Toxicol 2004;17:1151–1156.

140. Gordon W, Huitric A, Seth C, et al: The metabolism of the abortifacient terpene, (R)-(+)-pulegone, to a proximate toxin, menthofuran. Drug Metab Dispos 1987;15:589–594.

141. Carmichael P: Pennyroyal metabolites in human poisoning. Ann Intern Med 1997;124:250–251.

142. Nelson S, McClanahan R, Thomassen D, et al: Investigations of mechanisms of reactive metabolite formation from (R)-(+)-pulegone. Xenobiotica 1992;22:1157–1164.

143. Thomassen D, Slattery J, Nelson S: Menthofuran-dependent and independent aspects of pulegone hepatotoxicity: roles of glutathione. J Pharmacol Exp Ther 1990;253:567–572.

144. Moorthy B, Madyastha P, Madyastha K: Metabolism of a monoterpene ketone, R-(+)-pulegone a hepatotoxin in rat. Xenobiotica 1989;19:217–224.

145. Popata A, Sheara N, Malkiewicza I: The toxicity of Callilepis laureola, a South African traditional herbal medicine. Clin Biochem 2001;34:229–236.

146. Skalli S, Alaoui I, Pineau A, et al: Atractylis gummifera L. poisoning: a case report [French]. Bull Soc Pathol Exot 2002;95:284–286.

147. Smith V, Fearnley I, Walker J: Altered chromatographic behaviour of mitochondrial ADP/ATP translocase induced by stabilization of the protein by binding of 6′-O-fluorescein-atractyloside. Biochem J 2003;376:757–763.

148. Stewart M, Steenkamp V: The biochemistry and toxicity of atractyloside: a review. Ther Drug Monit 2000;22:641–649.

149. Gunther P: The Greek herbal of Dioscorides. New York, Hafner, 1909.

150. Lovell C: Plants and the Skin, 1st ed. Oxford, UK: Blackwell Scientific, 1993.

151. Webster G: Irritant plants in the spurge family (Euphorbiaceae). Clin Dermatol 1986;4:36–45.

152. Furstenberger GH, Hecker E: On the active principles of the spurge family (Euphorbiaceae). XI. The skin irritant and tumor promoting diterpene esters of Euphorbia tirucalli L. originating from South Africa. Z Naturforsch 1985;40:631–646.

153. Williams S, Clark R, Dunford J: Contact dermatitis associated with capsaicin: Hunan hand syndrome. Ann Emerg Med 1995;25:713–715.

154. Szolcsanyi J: Forty years in capsaicin research for sensory pharmacology and physiology. Neuropeptides 2004;38:377–384.

155. Southcott RH, Haegi LAR. Plant hair dermatitis. Med J Aust 1992;156:623–632.

156. Shearer G: Some observations on the poisonous properties of buttercups. Vet J 1938;94:22–32.

157. Zadina R: Determination of protoanemonin. Cas Cesk Lek 1950;63:333–335.

158. Baer H: Chemistry and immunochemistry of poisonous Anacardiaceae. Clin Dermatol 1986;4:152–159.

159. Gette MM, Marks JE Jr: Tulip fingers. Arch Dermatol 1990;126:203–205.

160. Connolly M, McCune J, Dauncey E, et al: Primula obconica—is contact allergy on the decline? Contact Dermatitis 2004;51:167–171.

161. Stoner JE Jr: Plant dermatitis. J Am Acad Dermatol 1983;9:1–15.

162. Drugge R, Dunn H, Sheard C, et al: Botanical Dermatology: Chemical Irritant Dermatitis. The Internet Dermatology Society, 2000–2005. www.telemedicine.org/botanica/bot4.htm, accessed April 5, 2005.

163. Kulze AG, Greaves M: Contact urticaria caused by stinging nettles. Br J Dermatol 1988;119:269–270.

164. Oliver F, Amon E, Breathnach A, et al: Contact urticaria due to the common stinging nettle (Urtica dioica)—histological, ultrastructural and pharmacological studies. Clin Exp Dermatol 1991;16:1–7.

165. Pathak M: Phytophotodermatitis. Clin Dermatol 1986;4:102–121.

166. Kavli GV, Volden G: Phytophotodermatitis. Photodermatology 1984;1:65–75.

167. Wilson T: Common daffodil (Narcissus pseudo-narcissus) as a poison. Pharmaceut J Pharmacist 1924;112:141–142.

168. Hsueh KF, Lin PY, Lee SM, et al: Ocular injuries from plant sap of genera Euphorbia and Dieffenbachia. Chin Med Assoc 2004;67:93–98.

169. Balint GA: Ricin: the toxic protein of castor oil seeds. Toxicology 1974;2:77–102.

170. Bradberry SM, Dickers KJ, Rice P, et al: Ricin poisoning. Toxicol Rev 2003;22:65–70.

171. Roberge R, Brader E, Martin ML, et al: The root of evil—pokeweed intoxication. Ann Emerg Med 1986;15:470–473.

172. Frohne D, Pfander HJ: A Colour Atlas of Poisonous Plants. London, Wolfe Publishing, 1984.

173. DerMarderosian A: Topic: Holly—The Review of Natural Products. St. Louis, Facts and Comparisons, 1996.

174. Spiller HA, Willias DB, Gorman SE: Retrospective study of mistletoe ingestion. Clin Toxicol 1996;34:405–408.

175. Krenzelok EP, Jacobsen TD, Aronis J: American mistletoe exposures. Am J Emerg Med 1997;15:516–520.

176. Harvey J, Colin-Jones DG: Mistletoe hepatitis. BMJ 1981;282:186–187.

177. Nelson BS, Heischober B: Betel nut: a common drug used by naturalized citizens from India, Far East Asia, and the South Pacific Islands. Ann Emerg Med 1999;34:238–243.

178. Anonymous: toxic hypoglycemic syndrome—Jamaica, 1989–1991. MMWR 1992;41:53–55.

179. Wilmot F, Robertson G: Senecio disease or cirrhosis of the liver due to senecio poisoning. Lancet 1920;2:828.

180. Mohabat O, Srivastava R, Younos M: An outbreak of hepatic veno-occlusive disease in north-western Afghanistan. Lancet 1976;2:269–271.

181. Stillman A, Huxtable R, Consroe P, et al: Hepatic veno-occlusive disease due to pyrrolizidine (Senecio) poisoning in Arizona. Gastroenterology 1977;73:349–352.

182. Mattei A, Bizollon T, Charles J, et al: Liver damage induced by the ingestion of a product of phytotherapy containing wild germander. Four cases [French]. Gastroenterol Clin Biol 1992;16:798–800.

183. Laliberte L, Villeneuve J: Hepatitis after the use of germander, a herbal remedy. CMAJ 1996;154:1689–1692.

184. Perez Alvarez J, Saez-Royuela F, Gento Pena E, et al: Acute hepatitis due to ingestion of Teucrium chamaedrys infusions [Spanish]. Gastroenterol Hepatol 2001;24:240–243.

185. Diaz D, Ferroudji S, Heran B, et al: Fulminant hepatitis caused by wild germander [French]. Gastroenterol Clin Biol 1992;16:1006–1007.

186. Mazokopakis E, Lazaridou S, Tzardi M, et al: Acute cholestatic hepatitis caused by Teucrium polium L. Phytomedicine 2004;11:83–84.

187. Selzer G, Parker R: Senecio poisoning exhibiting as Chiari's syndrome. Am J Pathol 1951;27:885–907.

188. Sherlock S: Noncirrhotic extrahepatic and intrahepatic portal hypertension. Semin Liver Dis 1982;2:202–210.

189. Ciganda C, Laborde A: Herbal infusions used for induced abortion. J Toxicol Clin Toxicol 2003;41:235–239.

190. Bakerink J, Gospe SJ, Dimand R, et al: Multiple organ failure after ingestion of pennyroyal oil from herbal tea in two infants. Pediatrics 1996;98:944–947.

191. Anderson IB, Mullen WH, Meeker JE, et al: Pennyroyal toxicity: measurement of toxic metabolite levels in two cases and review of the literature. Ann Intern Med 1996;124:725–734.

192. Fonseka MM, Seneviratne SL, de Silva CE, Gunatilake SB, de Silva HJ: Yellow oleander poisoning in Sri Lanka: outcome in a secondary care hospital. Hum Exp Toxicol 2002;21:293–295.

193. Eddleston M, Ariaratnam CA, Sjostrom L, et al: Acute yellow oleander (Thevetia peruviana) poisoning: cardiac arrhythmias, electrolyte disturbances, and serum cardiac glycoside concentrations on presentation to hospital. Heart 2000;83:301–306.

194. Bose TK, Basu RK, Biswas B, et al: Cardiovascular effects of yellow oleander ingestion. J Indian Med Assoc 1999;97:407–410.

195. Edgerton PH: Symptoms of digitalis-like toxicity in a family after accidental ingestion of lily of the valley plant. J Emerg Nurs 1989;15:220–223.

196. Tuncok Y: Urginea maritima (squill) toxicity. J Toxicol Clin Toxicol 1995;33:83–86.

197. Krenzelok EP, Jacobsen TD, Aronis JM: Lily-of-the-valley (Convallaria majalis) exposures: are the outcomes consistent with the reputation? J Toxicol Clin Toxicol 1996;34:601.

198. Cummins R, Haulman J, Quan L, et al: Near-fatal yew berry intoxication treated with external cardiac pacing and digoxin-specific FAB antibody fragments. Ann Emerg Med 1990;19:38–43.

199. Chan TY, Tomlinson B, Tse LK, et al: Aconitine poisoning due to Chinese herbal medicines: a review. Vet Hum Toxicol 1994;35:452–455.

200. Chan T: Aconitine poisoning: a global perspective. Vet Hum Toxicol 1994;36:326.

201. McBride JS, Altman DG, Klein M, White W: Green tobacco sickness. Tob Control 1998;7:294–298.

202. Rizzi D, Basile C, DiMaggio A: Rhabdomyolysis and acute tubular necrosis in coniine (Hemlock) poisoning. Lancet 1989;2:1461–1462.

203. Plato: Phaedo. Loeb Classical Library. Cambridge, MA, Harvard University Press, 1990.

204. Chan T: Anticholinergic poisoning due to Chinese herbal medications. Vet Hum Toxicol 1995;37:156–157.

205. Wood BH, Haq EU: An unusual case of atropine poisoning. Br J Clin Pract 1971;25:469–470.

206. Goetz RS, Siegel E, Scaglione J: Suspected moonflower intoxication—Ohio, 2002. MMWR 2003;52:788–791.

207. Birmes P, Chounet V, Mazerolles M, et al: [Self-poisoning with Datura stramonium. 3 case reports.] Presse Med 2002;31:69–72.

208. Tiongson J, Salen P: Mass ingestion of Jimson Weed by eleven teenagers. Del Med J 1998;70:471–476.

209. Dewitt MS, Swain R, Gibson LB Jr: The dangers of jimson weed and its abuse by teenagers in the Kanawha Valley of West Virginia. WV Med J 1997;93:182–185.

210. Dreisbach R: Handbook of Poisoning, 8th ed. Los Altos, CA, Lange Medical, 1974.

211. Macnab A, Anderson E, Susak L: Ingestion of cannabis: a cause of coma in children. Pediatr Emerg Care 1989;5:238–239.

212. Weinberg D, Lande A, Hilton N: Intoxication from accidental marijuana ingestion. Pediatrics 1983;71:848–850.

213. Pettinger G, Duggan MB, Forrest ARW: Black stuff and babies: accidental ingestion of cannabis resin. Med Sci Law 1988;28:310–311.

214. Whelan FJ, Bennett FW, Moeller WS: Morning glory seed intoxication: a case report. J Iowa Med Soc 1968;58:946–948.

215. Jacobsen E: The clinical pharmacology of hallucinogens. Clin Pharmacol Ther 1963;4:480–503.

216. Duke JA: CRC Handbook of Medicinal Herbs. Boca Raton, FL, CRC Press, 1985.

217. Riba J, Valle M, Urbano G, et al: Human pharmacology of ayahuasca: subjective and cardiovascular effects, monoamine metabolite excretion, and pharmacokinetics. J Pharmacol Exp Ther 2003;306:73–83.

218. Bücheler R, Gleiter CH, Schwoerer P, et al: Use of nonprohibited hallucinogenic plants: increasing relevance for public health? A case report and literature review on the consumption of Salvia divinorum (diviner's sage). Pharmacopsychiatry 2005;38:1–5.

219. Martinez H, Bermudez M, Rangel-Guerra R, et al: Clinical diagnosis in Karwinskia humboldtiana polyneuropathy. J Neurol Sci 1998;154:49–54.

220. Bermudez de Rocha M, Lozano Melendez F, Salazar Leal M, et al: Familial poisoning with Karwinskia humboldtiana [Spanish]. Gac Med Mex 1995;131:100–106.

221. Ellwood MG, Robb HG: Self-poisoning with colchicine. Postgrad Med J 1971;47:129–138.

222. Bismuth C, Gaultier M, Conso F: Aplasie medullaire après intoxicationaigne à la colchicine. Nouv Presse Med 1977;6:1625–1629.

223. Juurlink DN, Sellens C, Tompson M: Danger in the doctor's office: two cases of severe neurologic sequelae after ingestion of podophyllin [Abstract]. J Toxicol Clin Toxicol 1999;37:620.

224. O'Mahony S, Keohane C, Jacobs J: Neuropathy due to podophyllin intoxication. J Neurol 1990;237:110–112.

225. Rubino MJ, Davidoff F: Cyanide poisoning from apricot seeds. JAMA 1979;241:359.

226. Suchard JR, Wallace KL, Gerkin RD: Acute cyanide toxicity caused by apricot kernel ingestion. Ann Emerg Med 1998;32:742–744.

227. Edwards N: Local toxicity from a poinsettia plant: a case report. J Pediatr 1983;102:404–405.

228. Winek C, Butala J, Shanor S, et al: Toxicology of poinsettia. Clin Toxicol 1978;13:27–45.

229. Krenzelok E, Jacobsen T, Aronis J: Poinsettia exposures have good outcomes . . . just as we thought. Am J Emerg Med 1996;14:671–674.

230. Jones LA, Tanberg D, Troutman WG: Household treatment for "chile burns" of the hands. J Toxicol Clin Toxicol 1987;25:483–491.

231. Edwards E Jr, Edwards EK Sr: Immediate and delayed hypersensitivity to the nettle plant. Contact Dermatitis 1992;27:264–265.

232. Osterloh J, Herold S, Pond S: Oleander interference in the digoxin radioimmunoassay in a fatal ingestion. JAMA 1982;247:1596–1597.

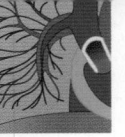

233. Haynes BE, Bessen HA, Wightman WD: Oleander tea: herbal draught of death. Ann Emerg Med 1985;14:350.

234. Spoerke DG, Spoerke SE, Rumack BH: Berry identification using a modified botanic key. Vet Hum Toxicol 1988;30:260–264.

235. Wax PM, Cobaugh DJ, Lawrence RA: Should home ipecac-induced emesis be routinely recommended in the management of toxic berry ingestions? Vet Hum Toxicol 1999;41:394–397.

236. Salen P, Shih R, Sierzenski P, Reed J: Effect of physostigmine and gastric lavage in a Datura stramonium-induced anticholinergic poisoning epidemic. Am J Emerg Med 2003;21:316–317.

237. Clark RF, Selden BS, Curry SC: Digoxin-specific Fab fragments in the treatment of oleander toxicity in a canine model. Ann Emerg Med 1991;20:1073–1077.

238. Shumaik HM, Wu AW, Ping AC: Oleander poisoning treatment with digoxin-specific Fab antibody fragments. Ann Emerg Med 1988;17:732–735.

239. Safadi R, Levy I, Amitai Y, et al: Beneficial effect of digoxin-specific Fab antibody fragments in oleander intoxication. Arch Intern Med 1995;155:2121–2125.

240. Tai Y-T, But PP-H, Young K, Lau C-P: Cardiotoxicity after accidental herb-induced aconite poisoning. Lancet 1992;340:1254–1256.

241. Mullen W, Anderson I, Oishii S: Accidental pennyroyal oil ingestion in a toddler with the first human serum metabolite detection [Abstract]. Vet Hum Toxicol 1994;36:342.

242. Giorgi DF, Lobel D, Morasco R: N-acetylcysteine for pennyroyal oil toxicity [Abstract]. Vet Hum Toxicol 1994;36:358.

243. Baud FJ, Sabourand A, Vicant E, et al: Brief report: treatment of severe colchicine overdose with colchicine-specific Fab fragments. N Engl J Med 1995;332:642–645.

244. Burns MJ, Linden CH, Graudins A, et al: A comparison of physostigmine and benzodiazepines for the treatment of anticholinergic poisoning. Ann Emerg Med 2000;35:374–381.

245. Salen P, Shih R, Sierzenski P, et al: Effect of physostigmine and gastric lavage in a Datura stramonium-induced anticholinergic poisoning epidemic. Am J Emerg Med 2003;21:316–317.

Toxic Marine Life

ROBERT P. DOWSETT, BM, BS

At a Glance...

- Marine life is toxic to humans through envenomation by:
- Stinging: jellyfish, corals, and sea anemones.
- Spinous puncture injury: stingray, catfish, scorpion fish, weever fish, starfish, and sea urchins.
- Bites: sea snake, cone shell, and the blue-ringed octopus.
- Poisoning by ingestion: paralytic shellfish poisoning, scombroid fish poisoning, puffer fish poisoning, and ciguatera.
- Toxins injected by an animal into its prey are usually high-molecular-weight proteinaceous substances, and those that produce symptoms after consumption are generally low-molecular-weight molecules.
- Management of marine toxins is largely supportive.
- Specific first aid is required for jellyfish stings, spinous puncture injury, and envenomation by the blue-ringed octopus, cone shells, and sea snakes.
- Careful débridement and cleaning of marine wounds is important.
- Antivenom is available for the treatment of envenomation by the box jellyfish, stonefish, and sea snake but is only readily accessible in Australia.
- A number of specific therapies have been suggested for the management of ciguatera poisoning, but the use of mannitol is no longer recommended.

MARINE ENVENOMATION

Introduction and Relevant History

Some of the substances known to be most toxic to human beings are found in marine organisms (Table 25-1 and Box 25-1). Important species causing marine envenomation are contained in the phylum Cnidaria, Mollusca, and Echinodermata (all invertebrates) and Chordata, Subphylum, and Vertebrata (vertebrates). The phylum Cnidaria (formerly Coelenterata) is composed of four classes of invertebrates that have the dominant characteristic of tentacles equipped with nematocysts that discharge toxins on contact. Three classes in the phylum are species commonly known as jellyfish; the fourth consists of the corals and anemones. The phylum Mollusca contains the blue-ringed octopus and cone shells. The phylum Echinodermata contains starfish and sea urchins. The phylum Chordata contains venomous fish, stingrays, and sea snakes.[1]

Documented deaths from jellyfish worldwide probably only run into the hundreds, and *Chironex fleckeri* (the Australian box jellyfish) has only been associated with 72 confirmed deaths despite its reputation as being nearly universally fatal. There are only 10 well-recorded deaths from cone shell envenomation, but sea snakes are estimated to cause 150 deaths a year. Deaths from marine spines are rare and, with the exception of the stonefish, appear to result from complications of infection.[1] The three most common marine organisms causing emergency department visits in the mainland United States are stingrays, catfish, and jellyfish.

Epidemiology

The four Cnidaria classes are as follows:

1. Hydrozoa: This group of jelly-fish like animals includes *Physalia physalis* (the Atlantic Portuguese man-of-war and the Pacific man-of-war or blue bottle); *Physalia utriculus*, found off Hawaii and in the Indo-Pacific; and the hydroid corals, which are commonly found growing in tufts on rocks, seaweed, and dock pilings. Examples include *Millepora alcicornis*, the stinging fire coral; *Gonionemus vertens*, the orange-striped jellyfish; and *Lytocarpus philippinus*, the feather hydroid.
2. Cubozoa: This group includes the "box" jellyfish (with tentacles at the corners of a square body), such as the Australian box jellyfish, *Chironex fleckeri*; the sea wasp of Indo-Pacific waters, *Chiropsalmus quadrigatus*; and *Carukia barnesi*, the cause of Irukandji stings to swimmers around Queensland, Australia.
3. Scyphozoa: This group of "true" jellyfish (with tentacles at regular intervals around their bell) includes *Chrysaora quinquecirrha*, the sea nettle of the Atlantic coast, Philippines, and Japan, and the thimble jellyfish, *Linche unguiculata*.
4. Anthozoa: Only some species of coral have stinging nematocysts that harm humans. More dangerous are the cuts and lacerations one can suffer from handling coral or brushing against it. The class also includes the sea anemones, tube anemones, and zoanthids.

Most jellyfish are pelagic (inhabiting the surface of the sea). They may vary in size from a few millimeters to more than 2 m across the bell, with tentacles up to 36 m in length. Because the tentacles in some species are long, it is possible to encounter them without seeing the bell. After a storm during which jellyfish have been broken up and washed ashore, one can be stung while walking along a beach. Even when dry, the nematocysts retain the capacity to discharge and produce typical symptoms.

Nematocysts are cell organelles in specialized epithelial cells. They consist of a capsule wall enclosing a tightly coiled hollow tube that bursts forth like a dart on contact with a human being or animal (Fig. 25-1). During discharge, the coiled internal tubule everts progressively, bringing spines to the external surface. The venom in the capsule is conveyed to the victim through the now

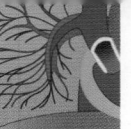

TABLE 25-1 Relative Toxicities of a Selected Group of Toxic Substances

TOXIN	MINIMUM LETHAL DOSE (μg/kg)*	SOURCE
Botulinum toxin A	0.00003	Bacterium: *Clostridium botulinum*
Tetanus toxin	0.00010	Bacterium: *Clostridium tetani*
Ricin	0.02000	Plant: castor bean, *Ricinus communis*
Palytoxin	0.15000	Zoanthid: *Palythoa* species
Crotalus toxin	0.20000	Snake: The rattlesnake, *Crotalus atrox*
Diphtheria toxin	0.30000	Bacterium: *Corynebacterium diphtheriae*
Cobra neurotoxin	0.30000	Snake: *Naja naja*
Kokoi venom	2.7	Frog: *Phyllobates bicolor*
Tarichatoxin	8	Newt: *Taricha torosa*
Tetrodotoxin	8	Fish: *Sphoeroides rubripes*
Saxitoxin	3.4–9	Produced by the dinoflagellate *Gonyaulax catenella* transvected by shellfish
Bufotoxin	390	Toad: *Bufo vulgaris*
Curare	500	Plant: *Chondodendron tomentosum*
Strychnine	500	Plant: *Strychnos nux-vomica*
Muscarin	1100	Mushroom: *Amanita muscaria*
Samandarin	1500	Salamander: *Salamandra maculosa*
Diisopropyl fluorophosphate	3000	Synthetic nerve gas
Sodium cyanide	10,000	Inorganic poison

*Minimal lethal dose refers to mouse, except for ricin, in which it refers to guinea pig, and for bufotoxin and muscarin, in which it refers to cat.
From Mosher HS, Fuhrman FA, Buckwald HD, Fisher HG: Tarichatoxin-tetrodotoxin: A potent neurotoxin. Science 1964;144:1103. Copyright 1964 by The American Association for the Advancement of Science.

BOX 25-1 REPRESENTATIVE TOXIC MARINE LIFE

Envenomation
Jellyfish and the coelenterates
  Hydrozoa
    Portuguese man-of-war (*Physalia physalis*)
    Stinging fire coral (*Millepora alcicornus*)
  Scophozoa
    Jellyfish
    Sea wasp (*Chironex fleckeri, Chiropsalmus quadrigatus, Carukia barnesi*)
  Anthozoa
    Sea anemones (*Actinodendron plumosum*)
    Corals
Stingrays
Catfish
Sea urchins
Weever fish
Scorpion fish and stonefish
The blue-ringed octopus and cone shells
Sea snakes

Infection
Vibrio vulnificus

Poisoning
Paralytic shellfish poisoning
Amnesic shellfish poisoning
Scombroid fish poisoning
Puffer fish poisoning
Ciguatera

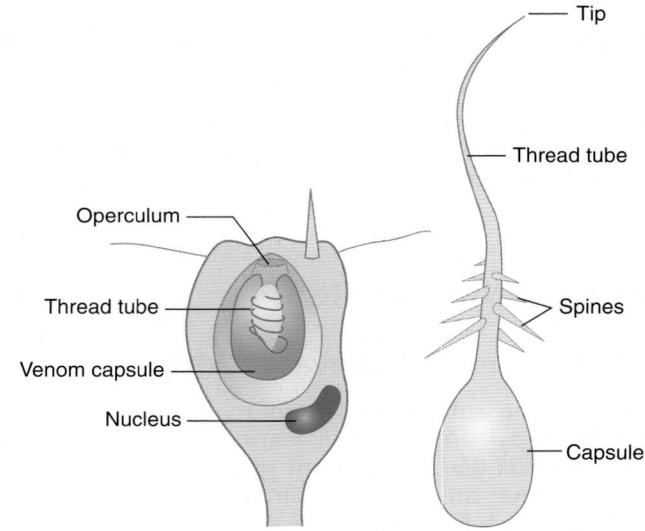

FIGURE 25-1 Generalized coelenterate nematocyst. I, Undischarged. II, Discharged. (Modified from Halstead BW: Poisonous and Venomous Marine Animals of the World, revised ed. Princeton, NJ, Darwin Press, 1980.)

uncoiled tube. Although all coelenterates have nematocysts, most are not injurious to humans.

The Portuguese man-of-war (Fig. 25-2) is characterized by a floating stem with several tentacles dangling from the underside of the float. One or more of the tentacles are markedly elongated and are called fishing tentacles. *Physalia* is found worldwide in warmer waters. One fishing tentacle may contain almost a million nematocysts. Sea wasps (Fig. 25-3) are the potentially lethal cubomedusans, *Chironex fleckeri* of Australia and *Chiropsalmus quadrigatus* of the Philippines. Death in less than 3 minutes has been caused by stings of *C. fleckeri*.

Hydroid corals are upright, clavate, bladelike, or branching calcareous growths that are important in the development of reefs. The stinging coral is not a true coral but a hydroid with an exoskeleton of calcium

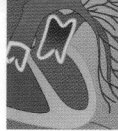

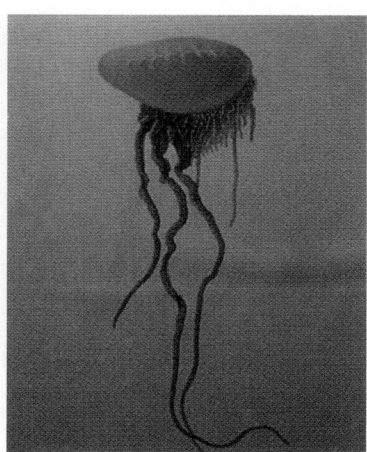

FIGURE 25-2 Portuguese man-of-war, *Physalia physalis.* (Courtesy of Bruce W. Halstead and the World Life Research Institute, Colton, CA.)

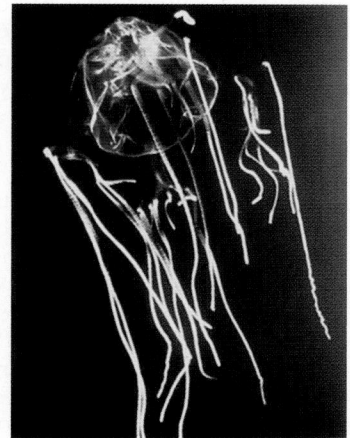

FIGURE 25-3 The sea wasp, *Chironex fleckeri.* (Courtesy of Bruce W. Halstead and the World Life Research Institute, Colton, CA.)

genus can be venomous. The crown-of-thorns starfish inhabit coral reefs in the Indian and Pacific oceans from east Africa to central America. Divers and trawl fishermen are the main victims. Sea urchins (Fig. 25-4) also have spines, some of which may contain toxins. Surfers, fishermen, and divers are those typically stung.

Venomous molluscs include the Australian blue-ringed octopus, *Hapalochlaena maculosa* (Fig. 25-5) and cone shells. The Australian blue-ringed octopus rarely exceeds 8 inches in full extension and can fit in the palm of the hand. The octopus is brown with yellow bands and blue rings; when it becomes excited, the blue rings take on an iridescent glow.[2] Normally reclusive creatures, human bites have occurred mainly when they are captured or provoked. The octopus bites with its beak and secretes tetrodotoxin from its posterior salivary gland. Tetrodotoxin has an unusual distribution in nature; found in such diverse life as puffer fish, the California newt *Taricha,* and the central American frog *Atelopus.*[2] Cone shells are carnivorous snails that have a harpoon-like venom apparatus. They can fire a

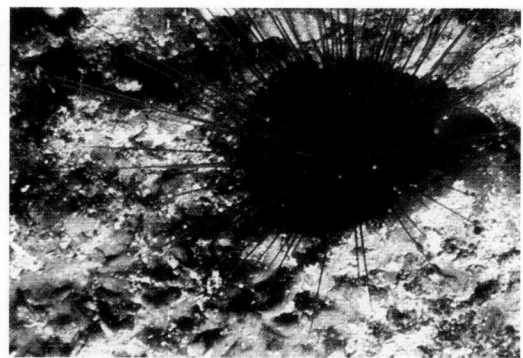

FIGURE 25-4 The sea urchin, *Diadema setosum,* from the Pacific Ocean near the Fiji islands. (Courtesy of Leonard S. Wojnowich, MD, Savannah, GA.)

carbonate, the surface of which is covered with numerous minute pores. Hydroid corals are widely distributed throughout tropical seas in shallow water. *Millepora* is the best-known genus, and includes the fire coral, *Millepora alcicornis,* a nuisance to divers off the Florida Keys and in the Caribbean.

Sea anemones are some of the most abundant seashore animals, especially in tropical and warm temperate waters. Commonly known is the hell's fire sea anemone, *Actinodendron plumosum.* Anemones have a flower-like appearance under water when their tentacles are extended. In addition to having stinging nematocysts, some sea anemones are poisonous if eaten.

Corals, the major constituent of living reefs, are composed of an external calcium carbonate skeleton that houses small anemone-like polyps. Corals of the genera *Goniopora, Plerogyra,* and *Physogyra* contain stinging nematocysts, and *Acropora* species injure by direct mechanical abrasion.

The crown-of-thorns starfish, *Acanthaster planci,* is the main venomous starfish, although other species of the

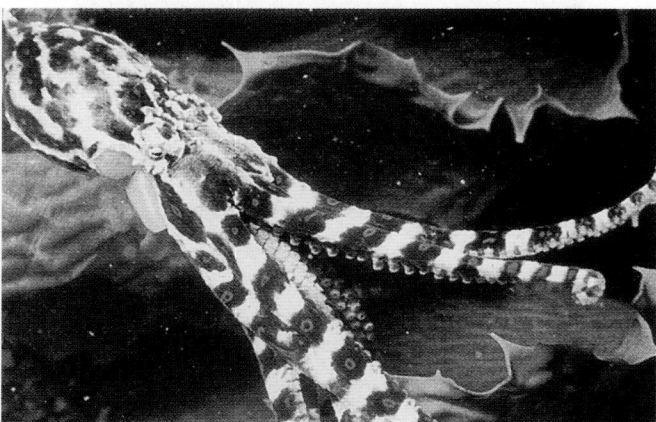

FIGURE 25-5 The Australian blue-ringed octopus, *Hapalochlaena maculosa.* (Copyright David Parer and E. Parer Cook, Auscape International, in VanDenbeld J: Nature and Australia: A Portrait of the Island Continent. New York, Facts on File [in cooperation with the Australian Broadcasting Corporation], 1988.)

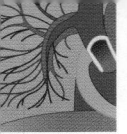

detachable radular tooth into their prey, and this paralyzes the victim.[3,4] Envenomation is uncommon in humans and only occurs when the shells are handled outside of water. *Conus geographus* is the only species known to cause human fatalities.

Marine catfish are abundant silvery fish with smooth, scaleless skin. They have four to five barbels or "whiskers" around the mouth, giving them their name. The dorsal and pectoral spines of many species, especially juvenile catfish, are venomous and capable of inflicting painful wounds. Stinging usually results from handling the fish, such as when removing the fish from the net or taking a hook out of its mouth. There are unsubstantiated claims that the stripped catfish (*Plotosus lineatus*) of the Indian and western Pacific oceans has caused deaths.[1]

Scorpion fish belong to the family Scorpaenidae.[3] Examples of venomous fish in this family include the butterfly fish (*Pterois lunulata*), the zebra fish (*Dendrochirus zebra*; Fig. 25-6), the lionfish (*Pterois volitans*; Fig. 25-7), sculpin (*Scorpaena* species), and rockfish (*Sebastes* species). Most venomous Scorpaenidae are found in tropical water, but a somewhat less venomous species of scorpion fish lives along the coast of California and the southeastern coast of the United States. Most scorpion fish stings occur when handling the fish in home aquariums. The stonefishes (genus *Synanceja*), of which *Synanceja horrida* is the most venomous (Fig. 25-8), are

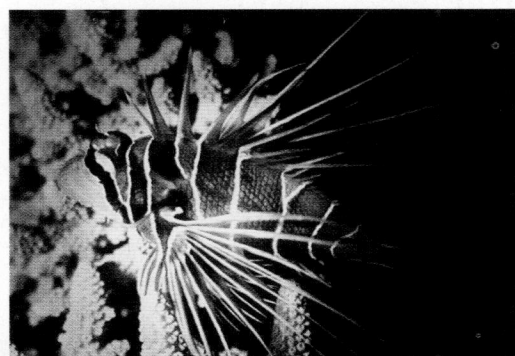

FIGURE 25-6 The zebrafish, *Dendrochirus zebra*. (Courtesy of Sea World, Orlando, FL.)

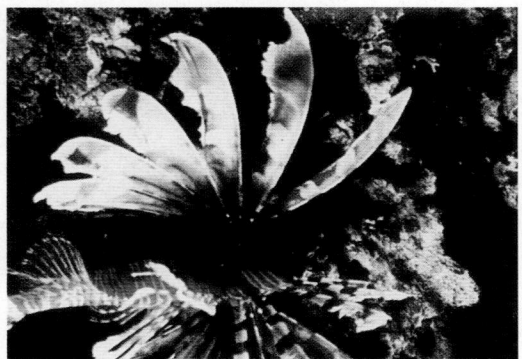

FIGURE 25-7 The lionfish, *Pterois volitans*, near the Fiji islands. (Courtesy of Leonard S. Wojnowich, MD, Savannah, GA.)

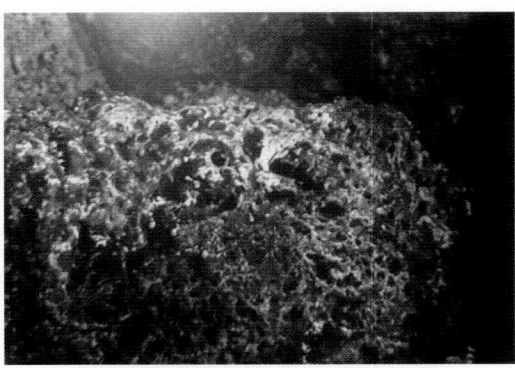

FIGURE 25-8 The stonefish, *Synanceja verrucosa*. (Courtesy of Sea World, Orlando, FL.)

bottom-dwelling fish that are difficult to see and easily trodden on.

The weever fish, of the family Trachinidae, is found in the Mediterranean Sea, along the Atlantic coast of Europe and North Africa, and up to the North Sea. *Trachinus draco*, or dragon fish, has five dorsal and two opercular spines that can inflict on unwary fishermen a painful venom.[3] Weever fish often hide in mud or sand with only the head exposed, only to dart out to attack their prey.[5]

Three common stingrays are the round stingray, *Urolophus halleri*, found along the Pacific coast from California to Panama; the blunt-nosed stingray, *Dasyatis sayi*, found along the eastern Atlantic coast; and the spotted eagle ray, *Aetobatus narinari*, found throughout tropical waters from the Atlantic to the Pacific (Table 25-2). The *Dasyatis* stingrays (Fig. 25-9) are difficult to detect because of their habit of lying buried in the mud or sand with only a portion of the body exposed. Accidents usually occur when bathers step on a buried ray. The ray then whips its tail up and forward, driving the stinger into the foot or leg. Commercial fisherman are sometimes stung on the hand or arms when emptying nets. Divers may be stung on the chest or abdomen.

Sea snakes belong to the family Hydrophiidae and have evolved from the Elapid family of snakes (Table 25-3). Their anatomy has been highly adapted for marine life. The body and particularly the tail are vertically compressed to provide swimming ability, the nostrils are located on top of the head rather than on the side, and specialized glands secrete salt in order to permit life in a saline environment.[3,6] Sea snakes inhabit the Indian and Pacific oceans from the Arabian Sea to Malaysia in the north to Australia and New Zealand in the south. A common sea snake is *Pelamis platurus*, or the yellow-bellied sea snake. This snake has the widest distribution and has been found from the Indian Ocean all the way to the Pacific coast of Central America. It is the only sea snake found to inhabit deep ocean waters; the other species inhabit reefs or coastal waters. No venomous sea snake has ever been found in the Atlantic Ocean or Caribbean Sea. The most highly toxic sea snake is the beaked sea snake, *Enhydrina schistosa*,

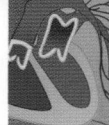

TABLE 25-2 Some Important Venomous Stingrays

FAMILY AND COMMON NAME	PROPER NAME	GEOGRAPHIC DISTRIBUTION
Dasyatidae		
Blunt-nosed stingray	*Dasyatis sayi*	Atlantic coast of the Americas
Southern stingray	*Dasyatis americanus*	Cayman Islands, U.S. Atlantic coast to Brazil
Caribbean stingray	*Himantura scmarde*	Cabribbean
Atlantic stingray	*Dasyatis sabina*	Chesapeake Bay to Gulf of Mexico
Diamond stingray	*Dasyatis brevis*	California to Peru and Galapagos Islands
Red stingray	*Dasyatis akajei*	China, Japan, Korea
Common stingray	*Dasyatis pastinaca*	Mediterranean Sea
Porcupine ray	*Urogymosus africanus*	Indian Ocean from Africa to Australia
Feathertail stingray	*Hypolophus sephen*	Indian and Pacific oceans
Ribbontail ray	*Taeniura lymna*	Indian Ocean, Red Sea to Australia
Thorntail stingray	*Dasyatis thetidis*	New Zealand and Australia
Tahitian stringray	*Himantura fai*	Tahiti, Polynesia, to Thailand
Urolophidae		
Round stingray	*Urolophus halleri*	U.S. Pacific coast to Panama
Yellow stingray	*Urolophus jamaicensis*	U.S. Atlantic, Gulf of Mexico and Caribbean
Crossback stingaree	*Urolophus cruciatus*	Australia, Tasmania
Common stingaree	*Trygonoptera testaceus*	Australia
Myliobatidae		
Spotted eagle ray	*Aetobatus narinari*	Tropical oceans from Atlantic to Indo-Pacific
Bat stingray	*Myliobatis californicus*	U.S. Pacific coast, California to Sea of Cortez
Bull ray	*Myliobatis aquila*	Mediterranean Sea
Southern bat ray	*Myliobatis tentuicaudatus*	Australia and New Zealand
Rhinopteridae		
Cownose ray	*Rhinoptera bonasus*	U.S. Atlantic coast to Brazil
Flapnose ray	*Rhinoptera javanica*	Pacific, Indonesia to Japan

Adapted from Halstead BW: Poisonous and Venomous Marine Animals of the World, revised ed. Princeton, NJ, Darwin Press, 1978; and Michael SW: Reef Sharks and Rays of the World. Monterey, CA, Sea Challengers Publications, 1993.

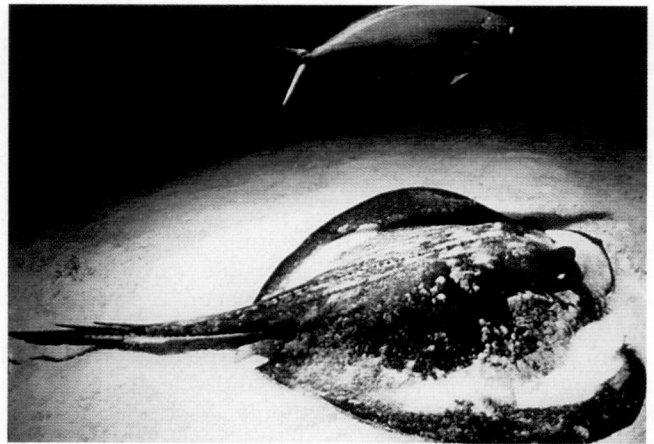

FIGURE 25-9 The blunt-nosed stingray, *Dasyatis sayi*. (Courtesy of Bruce W. Halstead and the World Life Research Institute, Colton, CA.)

responsible for the largest number of envenomations (Fig. 25-10). Divers and fishermen are the usual victims.

Pharmacology

Jellyfish venoms are poorly understood. Potential toxins isolated include vasoactive amines (histamine, serotonin, and dopamine), elastase, hemagglutinin, protease, collagenase, and palytoxins. The venom of *Chironex fleckeri*, the Australian box jellyfish, has been shown to cause skin necrosis, cardiac depression, respiratory depression, and anaphylaxis, but the pharmacologic basis of these effects is uncertain. Some effects may be mediated by interaction with calcium channels. Irukandji venom causes a release of catecholamines that is partly responsible for some of the symptoms of envenomation.[7] Anemone venoms contain neurotoxins, cardiotoxins, hemolysins, and protease inhibitors.[8]

The crown-of-thorns starfish venom contains saponins and possibly hemorrhagic toxins. Sea urchin venom is thought to contain proteins, steroid glycosides, and inflammatory mediators.[1]

Tetrodotoxin blocks the movement of sodium ions by inhibiting the sodium channel, thus causing failure of nerve conduction and subsequent paralysis. Different conopeptides, peptide toxins of cone shells, have been shown to block sodium, potassium, and calcium channels, delay inactivation of sodium channels, and inhibit nicotinic and *N*-methyl-D-aspartate (NMDA)-glutamate receptors.

Catfish venom contains vasoconstrictors. Stonefish venom contain heat-labile proteins that have myotoxic, neurotoxic, and myocardial effects in animals. Stingray venom is primarily protein: extracts contain serotonin and enzymes such as 5-nucleotidase and phosphodiesterase.[9–12] Stingray venom is one of the most powerful

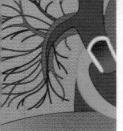

TABLE 25-3 Important Venomous Sea Snakes (Family Hydrophiidae)

COMMON NAME	SCIENTIFIC NAME	GEOGRAPHIC DISTRIBUTION
Beaked sea snake	*Enhydrina schistosa*	Australia, Southeast Asia, India
Stoke's sea snake	*Astrotia stokesi*	Australia, Southeast Asia, India
Annulated sea snake	*Hydrophis cyanocinctus*	Southeast Asia, India
Yellow sea snake	*Hydrophis spiralis*	Southeast Asia, India
	Hydrophis klossi	India
	Hydrophis elegans	Australia
Jerdon's snake	*Kerilia jerdoni*	Southeast Asia, India
Hardwick's (narrow-banded) sea snake	*Lapemis hardwickii*	Australia, Southeast Asia, India
Graceful small-headed sea snake	*Hydrophis gracilis (Disteira gracilis)*	Australia, Southeast Asia, India
Yellow-bellied sea snake	*Pelamis platurus*	All of Pacific and Indian oceans
	Hydrophis obscurus	Australia, India
Reef sea snake	*Hydophis ornatus*	Australia, Southeast Asia, India
	Hydrophis nigra (Thalassophina viperina)	Southeast Asia, India
	Thalassophina anomalus	Southeast Asia

Adapted from Meier J, White J: Handbook of Clinical Toxicology of Animal Venoms and Poisons. Boca Raton, FL, CRC Press, 1995; and Williamson JA, Fenner PJ, Burnett JW: Venomous & Poisonous Marine Animals. Sydney, Australia, University of New South Wales Press, 1996.

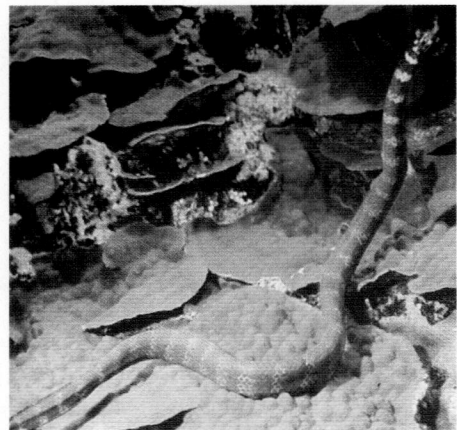

FIGURE 25-10 The sea snake, *Enhydrina schistosa*. (Courtesy of S. Kesier, the Sea Library, and Time-Life, Alexandria, VA.)

vasoconstrictors found among natural toxins. The venom is highly unstable and is markedly heat labile. The venom of scorpion fish, weever fish, and other fish spines are high-molecular-weight proteins that are poorly characterized. Sea snake venom contains postsynaptic neurotoxins and myotoxins.[8,10,11]

Toxicology: Clinical Manifestations

The severity of jellyfish stings in humans depends on the type of nematocysts, their penetrating power, the area of the victim's skin exposed, and the sensitivity of the victim to the venom. Injurious effects resulting from an encounter with coelenterate nematocysts range from mild dermatitis to rapid death.[13] Severe stings can occur with the man-of-war and blue bottle jellyfish; only the former has resulted in fatalities. The sting of a Portuguese man-of-war is far more severe than that of the common jellyfish and produces intense local pain extending up the extremity. Generalized symptoms such as headache, urticaria, muscle cramps, nausea, and vomiting may occur. Two confirmed deaths due to *Physalia* have been reported.[14,15]

Stings by *Chironex fleckeri* and *Chiropsalmus quadrigatus* are potentially dangerous. The effects usually consist of extremely painful localized areas of wheal, edema, and vesiculation, which later result in necrosis involving the full thickness of the skin. The initial lesions, caused by the structural pattern of the tentacles, are multiple linear wheals with transverse barring. The purple or brown tentacle marks form a whip-like skin lesion. Painful muscle spasms, shock, and pulmonary edema can occur rapidly. Death may occur in the water or shortly after leaving it. The prognosis for victims who arrive alive at the hospital is good.

Carukia barnesi is probably not the only species that causes the Irukandji syndrome; similar presentations have occurred in Western Australia and Hawaii, where *C. barnesi* has not been identified. The syndrome typically begins with minor pain at the sting site, low back pain, generalized muscle cramps, sweating, nausea, vomiting, headache, and anxiety.[1] A reversible cardiomyopathy and acute pulmonary edema has been reported. Two deaths have occurred following *C. barnesi* stings.

Stings from anemone contact typically produce a burning pain. The skin blanches and wheals form, with surrounding edema and erythema. Vesicle formation, ulceration, and necrosis may occur.

Coral stings produce initial pain, followed by weeping of the lesion, wheal formation, and itching. If coral cuts or stings are left untreated, a superficial scratch may within a few days become an ulcer, with a septic sloughing base surrounded by a painful zone of erythema. Cellulitis, lymphangitis, enlargement of the local lymph glands, fever, and malaise may ensue. The ulcer may be quite disabling, and the pain is usually out of proportion to the physical signs. If the ulcer occurs in a lower extremity, the patient may be unable to walk for weeks or months after the injury. Relapses, which occur without warning, are common.

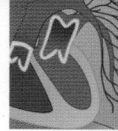

Stings from the crown-of-thorns starfish cause severe pain and the wounds become inflamed and may bleed excessively. The affected limb may become swollen, and infection is common. Sea urchin stings are extremely painful, and the spines often become embedded in the patient. The sea urchin spines of *Diadema setosum* contain purplish dye, which may temporarily stain the skin and give the false impression of a retained foreign body.[16] Multiple stings by the black sea urchin *D. setosum* has been followed by a delayed severe bulbar polyneuritis.[16]

Envenomation by the blue-ringed octopus is described as painless, but the patient rapidly succumbs, becoming weak and unconscious, and develops respiratory arrest, often within 15 minutes. Cardiac arrest and death follow. Because the toxin has a short duration of action, patients may survive with prompt resuscitation.[17,18] Pain following cone shell envenomation is variable, and the skin blanches or has a bluish discoloration. This is followed by numbness and swelling. In severe poisoning nausea, pruritus and muscle weakness occur; vision and hearing may be affected. Death results from respiratory paralysis.[1]

Catfish stings are common, painful, and often become secondarily infected. A patient often has a painful, swollen, and infected wound days after the initial result. A puncture wound by a weever fish produces instantaneous, often crippling pain. Local ischemia, secondary infection at the wound site, and systemic involvement may occur.[10] Intense pain results from stings by stonefish. Systemic symptoms, including headache, seizures, paralysis, abdominal pain, and hypotension, generally result only from envenomation by fish of the Synanceiidae family (stonefishes).[1,3]

The stingray spine has a sharp, arrow-like tip and backward-pointing serrations along the sides so that after penetration the barb is difficult to remove and lacerates the tissues as it is withdrawn. The venom apparatus consists of a spine, integumentary sheath, and associated venom glands. When this is torn, the venom is released. Parts of the spine are typically left behind in the wound. Most stings occur on the ankle or foot. The stingray spine is very sharp, and by virtue of the mechanism of injury, it is common for a patient to receive a laceration rather than a puncture wound. Patients who present to the emergency department may describe walking in the ocean and feeling a fluttering under their foot and then a sudden stabbing pain. The usual presenting symptom is severe shooting pain that increases in intensity during the first hour. Systemic symptoms, such as chest pain, syncope, and other neurologic sequelae, have been described. Death has been reported but is uncommon and is usually related to chest or abdominal injuries. One highly unusual fatality occurred in a 12-year-old boy who was riding in a boat when a manta ray leaped out of the water and impaled him in the chest.[8]

Sea snake bites are often painless. The fangs are often small, frequently only 2 to 3 mm in length; thus, bites are often difficult to detect.[2,8] One third to one half of bites do not result in envenomation.[1] Symptoms occur within 3.5 hours of the bite. The first symptoms are usually muscle pain; this may be preceded by headache and vomiting. After some hours, a flaccid paralysis may develop and can progress to respiratory paralysis.[8,19] Rhabdomyolysis, myoglobinuria, and subsequent renal failure may occur.

Diagnosis

A jellyfish sting can be identified by the patient or a companion. When a patient experiences an unknown sting, the diagnosis is usually made by observing a row of urticarial lesions or the presence of a tentacle adherent to the patient's skin. Stingrays leave a penetrating wound, and snakes leave fang marks. Catfish leave a barb, and this occurs only on handling the catfish.

A differential diagnosis with respect to the type of coelenterate is not so important in the United States, but where lethal coelenterates exist, as in Australia, identification of nematocysts—if time permits—on the patient by examining the skin wheals on the victim may be important. Halstead suggests that the wheal should be scraped with the edge of a microscope slide or scalpel and the material examined microscopically for the presence of nematocysts.[1] Nematocysts may also be obtained by microscopic examination of a strip of transparent tape that has been pressed against the surface of the wheal. The nematocysts adhere to the sticky side of the tape. Identification of nematocysts from the skin of the victim yields positive identification of coelenterate sting, but it requires an expert to identify the species.

LABORATORY TESTING
Biochemistry and hematology analyses should be undertaken in patients with systemic envenomation from jellyfish, blue-ringed octopus, cone shell, and stonefishes. Muscle enzymes should be tested following envenomation by a sea snake.

OTHER DIAGNOSTIC TESTING
X-ray films are indicated in marine spine stings. If the foreign body is seen on the radiograph, the wound should be opened and explored and the spine removed. Patients with chest pain, irregular pulse, or hypotension should have an electrocardiogram and should be placed on a cardiac monitor.

DIFFERENTIAL DIAGNOSIS
The presentation of Irukandji syndrome may be misdiagnosed as a myocardial infarction. When occurring in divers it may be difficult to distinguish from decompression illness. The differential diagnosis of an ascending paralysis, in addition to tetrodotoxin and paralytic shellfish poisoning, include rapidly progressive Guillian-Barré syndrome or a spinal cord hemorrhage.

Management

Treatment of coelenterate stings is symptomatic and supportive. Advanced cardiac life support may be necessary for patients who sustain cardiac arrest, either from toxic effects of the venom (e.g., *C. fleckeri*) or from anaphylaxis. Considerable success has been achieved in

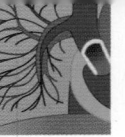

management of jellyfish and Portuguese man-of-war stings in the United States by applying a slurry of paste of sodium bicarbonate (baking soda) to the wound. After an hour the baking soda should be moistened with water and scraped off with a dull object, such as a spoon, to remove any remaining nematocysts.[4] The application of baking soda is not recommended for box jellyfish, which should be scraped off the skin after pouring 5% acetic acid (vinegar) for a minimum of 30 seconds.

Jellyfish can cause allergic reactions, but anaphylaxis is uncommon.[1] For anaphylactic shock, intravenous (IV) epinephrine, oxygen, IV fluids, dopamine, diphenhydramine, and a glucocorticoid may be indicated. Some jellyfish stings may cause severe pain requiring narcotics; morphine or fentanyl is recommended. Generalized symptoms, including hypotension, may be present, and IV fluid therapy with normal saline and general supportive measures may be indicated. For as long as 1 to 4 weeks after the initial sting, it is not uncommon for patients to return with recurrence of urticarial lesions at the site of the sting. These should be treated symptomatically with antihistamines. For this reason, follow-up is recommended for all patients with jellyfish stings.

Symptoms of Irukandji syndrome have responded to the administration of intravenous magnesium.[20] The mechanism may be by antagonism of epinephrine. A loading dose of 20 mEq or 0.2 mEq/kg (10 mmol or 0.1 mmol/kg) over 15 minutes followed by an infusion of 10 mEq/h or 0.02 mEq/kg/h (5 mmol/h or 0.01 mmol/kg/h) is recommended for patients who do not respond to initial opiates. Cardiogenic shock responds to positive pressure ventilation and epinephrine.

Coral cuts or abrasions should be scrubbed using fresh (not salt) water and a soft brush. Large or deep wounds should be surgically débrided, preferably within 3 hours.[1]

There are no clear first aid recommendations for treatment of sea anemone stings; one suggestion is to remove adherent tentacles with forceps or gloved fingers, blot dry, and apply cold packs.[1] Simple analgesia may be effective. Systemic antihistamines and steroids may be needed to treat local allergic reactions. Topical agents are ineffective.

Sea urchin (and starfish) toxin is remarkably heat labile, and hot water immersion therapy is indicated for pain relief and deactivation of the venom.[1] Surgical removal, especially of the thick calcium-containing spines, is indicated.

The immediate treatment for cone shell and blue-ringed octopus envenomation is the application of pressure immobilization by wrapping the limb in a crepe bandage using the same tension as if bandaging a sprained ankle—not sufficient to obstruct blood flow.[8] The limb is then splinted. The bandage can be left on until the patient stabilizes. Treatment is otherwise supportive. Assisted ventilation, if required, may only be necessary for a few hours.

Most cases of marine stings and spine envenomation can be treated in a standard fashion. The key to therapy involves care of the wound, relief of pain, hot water immersion, observation, and hospitalization in severe cases. The affected part should then be immersed continuously in confortably hot water for at least 60 minutes; this deactivates the heat-labile venom and relieves the pain. Patients should not be asked to test the water; they may be too distraught to judge effectively. In the emergency department, hot water immersion should be continued. Hot water immersion alone often provides pain relief, and pain medication may not be necessary. After an hour of continuous hot water immersion, the patient should take the affected part out of the water. If he or she suffers no pain, hot water treatment may stop. Wounds should then be irrigated, cleansed, débrided, and explored if necessary to remove any foreign body. Lacerations may then be surgically closed, although leaving the wound open with follow-up may be preferable, depending on the clinical situation.

Patients who suffer a wound on the chest or abdomen may require surgical exploration. In the case of stingray injuries, all wounds must be surgically explored to exclude injury to deeper tissues and to remove foreign material that is usually left behind when the barb breaks off.

Hot water immersion is effective early in treatment for pain relief and deactivation of weever fish venom; intravenous calcium is useful for pain relief.[5,16] Exploration of the wound is often necessary. Supportive therapy and long-term wound care are generally indicated. Treatment of scorpion fish injury is similar to that for stingray injury. Hot water immersion, wound débridement, and supportive care are indicated.[19]

Tetanus prophylaxis should be given if indicated. Despite the potential for marine wounds to become infected, prophylactic antibiotics are not recommended for healthy people, but a course of doxycycline should be considered for patients who are immunosuppressed, have chronic renal or liver illness, or are diabetic. Empiric therapy for seawater wound infections is doxycycline.

LABORATORY MONITORING

Repeat measurement of creatine kinase (CK), potassium, and renal function is required for patients envenomated by sea snakes.

ANTIDOTES

Box jellyfish antivenom (Commonwealth Serum Laboratories, Melbourne, Australia) is a sheep-derived *Chironex fleckeri* antivenom. It should be administered as soon as possible in settings of collapse, cardiac arrest, or hypotension. Ideally three vials should be given IV, although it can be effective given intramuscularly. In persistent severe toxicity, a further three vials can be given. It is also indicated for severe pain.[17,19] The antivenom may be effective against other chirodropid stings in the Indian and Pacific oceans.[1]

Commonwealth Serum Laboratories (CSL) produces an Australian stonefish antivenom made from horse immunoglobulin. It should be given only intramuscularly, not IV. It is indicated for severe pain: For one to two spine puncture wounds, one vial may be

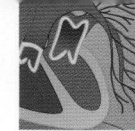

administered; for three to four wounds, two vials; if more than four wounds, three vials. There is limited evidence that it may be effective in stings from the bullrout fish (*Notesthes robusta*), but it is not recommended for use in other species of scorpion fish.[19]

Sea snake antivenom is also produced by CSL and contains horse antiserum against *E. schistosa* (sea snake) and *Notechis scutatus* (terrestrial tiger snake) venoms and is effective for most sea snake envenomations.[17,19] Monovalent sea snake antivenom for *E. schistosa* is also produced by the Halfkine Institute of Bombay, India, and is also effective for most sea snake envenomations in that region.[6] If these are unavailable, CSL monovalent tiger snake *(N. scutatus)* antivenom may be used in a ratio of three vials of tiger snake antivenom to each vial of sea snake antivenom.[17] Sea snake antivenom should be given to any patient with signs of rhabdomyolysis or neuropathy. One vial should be given intravenously, up to three if severely poisoned, and can be repeated, up to a totally of 10 vials if signs are progressing.

Intravenous antivenom should be diluted to a 10% solution and each vial run over 15 to 30 minutes. The preadministration of epinephrine is not currently recommended before administering CSL antivenom, but facilities for the management of anaphylaxis should be immediately available.

ELIMINATION

There are no known effective measures to increase the clearance of marine venoms.

DISPOSITION

Most cases of marine stings and spine envenomation respond to treatment and 4 hours of observation in the emergency department. Serious wounds require outpatient follow-up. Hospitalization may be necessary for surgical débridement of marine wounds or patients who have systemic envenomation. Even with potentially lethal envenomations such as those of the box jellyfish, blue-ringed octopus, or cone shell, signs of systemic poisoning will be evident within 4 hours.

SEAFOOD POISONING

An enormous variety of marine life is toxic to humans because of poisons that are ingested. Common poisonings are paralytic shellfish poisoning (PSP), scombroid fish poisoning, tetrodotoxin poisoning, and ciguatera. Less common are neurotoxic shellfish, clupeotoxic fish, and amnestic shellfish poisoning. With the exception of tetrodotoxin and scombroid poisoning, the causative toxins originate in dinoflagellates; these are unicellular ekaryotic marine algae that are consumed by marine organisms and passed up the food chain, to either shellfish or fish, and ultimately are consumed by humans. Scombroid poisoning and possibly tetrodotoxin have a bacterial origin. The affected fish and shellfish are usually unaffected by the toxins. Scombroid-affected fish are often reported to taste metallic or peppery, but other toxins are tasteless. All toxins are heat stable.

Epidemiology

The dinoflagellates primarily responsible for outbreaks of PSP include *Gonyaulax catenella*, which is found along the Pacific Coast from Alaska and California to Venezuela and west to Japan; *Gonyaulax tamarensis* var. *excavata*, which is found on the Atlantic Coast from Massachusetts and Nova Scotia to the North Sea; and *Pyrodinium bahamense* var. *compressa*, which is found from Central America to the Philippines.[21] Outbreaks of PSP occur worldwide and result from the consumption of shellfish such as mussels, clams, oysters, cockles, and scallops that have fed on toxic dinoflagellates. The shellfish are not adversely affected by the algal toxins, which are known as saxitoxins.[21-26] Less commonly, PSP has resulted from the ingestion of starfish, crabs, and pufferfish.[27]

Red tides result from excessive growth of algae species, including those that cause PSP. Pigments contained within the algae give the water a red-brown appearance. Red tides are a coastal phenomenon that occur sporadically. Poisonings related to red tides of oceans have been described for thousands of years. Because of a red tide in 208 BC, the name Red Sea was given to all the coasts of Arabia by the ancient Greeks. The first large epidemic recorded in the United States was in San Francisco in 1927; 102 persons became ill, and 6 died.[28] The toxin of *Ptychodiscus brevis,* which causes red tides off the Florida coast, can act as an upper respiratory tract irritant. The death of large numbers of fish, seabirds, and shellfish became associated with blooms of this microorganism.[29] Blooms of toxic algae associated with paralytic shellfish poisoning appear to be increasing worldwide.[30]

Greater than 80 µg of saxitoxin per 100 g of raw shellfish meat is considered toxic. The best prevention of paralytic shellfish poisoning in humans is strict adherence to public health agency guidelines on harvesting, processing, and consumption of shellfish.

Scombroid fish poisoning is a clinical syndrome produced by histamine release from spoiled fish of the family Scombroidae, which include tuna and mackerel, skipjack, albacore, and bonito.[31-34] Other fish implicated include mahi-mahi, herring, sardine, anchovy, bluefish, amberjack, and the Japanese saury.[32,33] Proper refrigeration and handling of raw seafood will prevent scombroid poisoning.

Puffer fish (Fig. 25-11) are named for their ability to inflate themselves to a nearly spheric shape when disturbed. Puffer fish poisoning is a highly lethal form of fish poisoning.[35] Fugu in Japan and the tambor puffer in Cuba are species of pufferfish eaten as a delicacy. In Japan, a 59% mortality rate was reported in 6386 cases of puffer fish poisoning during a 78-year period.[3] At least three deaths due to eating puffer fish have been reported in Florida. Some common tetrodotoxic puffers in various areas of the world are blowfish (United States), akeke (Hawaii), tambores (Cuba), fugu (Japan), West Indian swellfish, tinga tinga (Philippines), mamaiacu (Brazil), qarrad (Red Sea), kend (India), buntal pisang (Malaysia), tetraodon, porcupine fish, globefish, tiger

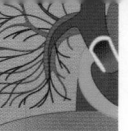

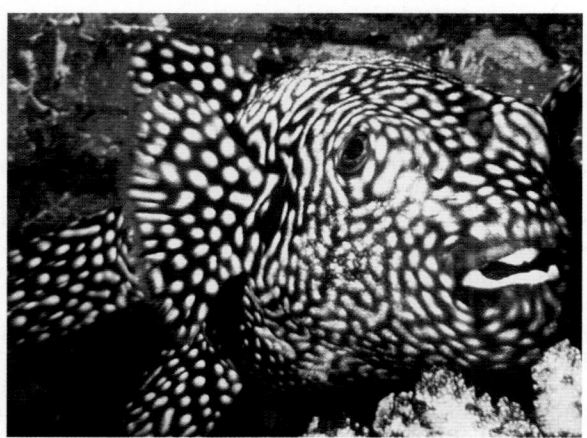

FIGURE 25-11 The puffer fish, *Arophron meleagris*. (Courtesy of Sea World, Orlando, FL.)

puffer, rabbit fish, and botete.[3] Even with extensive regulations, fugu is still a major cause of death due to food poisoning in Japan. Outside of these countries, poisoning occurs when people from other countries misidentify local toxic pufferfish as an edible species.

Numerous species of tropical and subtropical coral reef fish have been linked to ciguatera.[36-40] Toxins from the photosynthetic dinoflagellate *Gambierdiscus toxicus* pass up the food chain when herbivorous fishes consume them.[36-41] These are, in turn, eaten by carnivorous fishes, which are then consumed by humans. Barracuda, amberjack, dolphin fish, the moray eel, surgeonfish, grouper, red snapper, sea bass, and Spanish mackerel are the more common of the 400 species that have been implicated in causing ciguatera.[36-41] Sixty percent of the cases reported in the area around Miami, Florida, followed ingestion of grouper.[39] So many reports of ciguatera followed the ingestion of barracuda that its sale is prohibited in southern Florida.[39] Common causes of ciguatera in Hawaii include the kingfish ulua (*Caranx ignobilis*), the jack papio (*Caranx sexfasciatus*), and the amberjack kahala (*Seriola dumerili*).[36-42] A common cause of ciguatera in the Indo-Pacific, including Hawaii, is the surgeonfish *Ctenochaetus strigosus*, also known as maito in Tahiti.[42]

Neurotoxic shellfish poisoning results from algae blooms of *Ptychodiscus brevis*, a dinoflagellate in the coastal waters of southeastern North America and western Europe. The toxins are accumulated by clams and oysters. The resultant toxins, brevetoxins, can be carried inland, affecting people several miles from the coast.

Clupeotoxin poisoning is caused by herrings, anchovies, and sardines caught offshore of tropical islands after heavy rains or floods. The identity and origin of the toxin is unknown, although a phytoplankton origin is suggested.[43]

A unique illness occurred in Canada in November and December of 1987. It was characterized by gastrointestinal and neurologic symptoms.[44] In a month, more than 250 cases were reported to the Health Department in Canada. The outbreak was tracked to mussel cultivation beds primarily from the Cardigan River estuary of Prince Edward Island.[44-46] Domoic acid, an amino acid neuroexcitatory transmitter, was identified as the causative toxin, the source of which was *Nitzschia pungens,* a form of marine vegetation.[44-47] The poisoning has been termed amnestic shellfish poisoning. No other outbreaks of amnestic shellfish poisoning have been reported, although domoic acid–producing dinoflagellates have been isolated in other parts of the world. Domoic acid produced by the diatom *Pseudo-nitzschia australis* was responsible for the deaths of over 400 California sea lions in the Monterey Bay region in 1998.[48]

Structure and Structure-Activity Relationships

Paralytic shellfish poisoning is caused by saxitoxin and a number of related compounds, sometimes termed gonyautoxins. These compounds are among some of the more potent toxins known. They attach to fast sodium channels in nerve and muscle, blocking the initial influx of sodium during depolarization, resulting in a conduction block.[49,50]

Scombroid fish poisoning results from the activity of bacteria, such as *Proteus morganii*, utilizing the enzyme histidine decarboxylase to metabolize histidine to histamine.[11,51]

Puffer fish poisoning is caused by tetrodotoxin, which, like saxitoxin, inhibits fast sodium channels during depolarization, but at a separate site. Conduction of peripheral motor, sensory, and autonomic nerves is reduced.

Ciguatoxin, the cause of ciguatera, also attaches to fast sodium channels but increases sodium permeability. After an initial stimulation, prolonged refractoriness and decreased conduction velocity occurs.[52]

Neurotoxic shellfish poisoning results from the effects of brevetoxins A, B, and C. These polycyclic ethers bind to fast sodium channels near the binding site for ciguatoxin. Their main effect is on the peripheral cholinergic nerves, increasing the release of acetylcholine.[53]

Amnestic shellfish poisoning is caused by domoic acid, an amino acid neuroexcitatory transmitter.[44,45] It has been suggested that the neurotoxic effect is secondary to through activation of glutamate receptors in the amygdala and hippocampus, resulting in neural necrosis.[45] The exact mechanism is uncertain.

Pharmacology

Paralytic shellfish poisoning results in progressive neurologic impairment that initially affects sensory fibers, bulbar nerves, peripheral motor neurons, and the central nervous system. Scombroid fish poisoning resembles immunoglobulin E–mediated food allergies, replicating the typical features of endogenous histamine production. In addition to inhibiting conduction in peripheral nerves, tetrodotoxin also activates the chemoreceptor trigger zone and may depress the respiratory and vasomotor centers. Effects on cardiac, vascular smooth muscle, and skeletal muscle may occur in high doses. Puffer fish poisoning has a predictable progression of neurologic impairment affecting peripheral sensory nerves, peripheral motor nerves, bulbar

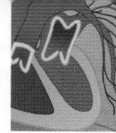

nerves, the central nervous system and respiratory muscles. Ciguatera produces a complex presentation with multiple symptoms affecting many systems; the mechanisms responsible are unclear. Neurotoxic shellfish poisoning, when caused by ingestion of seafood has a similar picture to ciguatera, but when inhaled it can trigger asthma via the stimulation of cholinergic nerve fibers, resulting in bronchospasm. Amnestic (domoic acid) shellfish poisoning results from the destruction of neurones in the amygdala and hippocampus, leading to permanent neurologic deficits.

Pharmacokinetics

Saxitoxin and related toxins associated with paralytic shellfish poisoning are heat stable and water soluble. Histamine is not normally absorbed across the gastrointestinal mucosa but metabolized by diamine oxidase. In scombroid poisoning it may be assisted by the presence of other toxins: putrescine and cadaverine. Tetrodotoxin is heat stable and water soluble. Ciguatoxin is heat stable and can be transferred across the placenta and by semen or breast milk. The pharmacokinetics of these toxins are poorly understood.

Pharmocologic Agents

Taking monoamine oxidase inhibitors, which may also inhibit diamine oxidase, may make patients more sensitive to scombroid.[32] Medications containing cyclic ethers (opiates, barbiturates) may exacerbate the symptoms of ciguatera.

Toxicology: Clinical Manifestations

Patients with paralytic shellfish poisoning may develop neurologic symptoms and, in severe cases, motor paralysis and respiratory failure. Affected shellfish can not be distinguished by odor or taste. A case review reported that in 113 of 117 patients, the initial manifestation of poisoning consisted of paresthesia around the lips, mouth, upper airway, and fingers, which may become apparent within a few minutes after eating poisonous shellfish.[54] Nausea, vomiting, and diarrhea can occur. As the illness progresses, respiratory distress and muscle paralysis become more severe. Death results from respiratory paralysis within 2 to 12 hours. Children appear to be more susceptible.[55] If a patient survives for 24 hours, the prognosis is favorable, and there appears to be no lasting effect.[56]

Patients who have eaten scombroid-affected fish often report a peppery or metallic taste and then present with signs and symptoms of histamine intoxication, often within 30 minutes.[32-34] Flushing of the upper body, urticaria, headache, chills, vomiting, diarrhea, and abdominal cramps are common. Conjunctival erythema may occur.[32] Severe cases that include bronchospasm and hypotension have been reported.[32]

The clinical manifestations of puffer poisoning begin within 45 minutes of ingestion, initially including paresthesia about the lips, then affecting the peripheries.

Diaphoresis, hyperemesis, and salivation occur. Ascending peripheral and bulbar muscle paralysis occurs, ultimately resulting in respiratory failure. In some cases patients may be completely paralyzed, with loss of all brainstem reflex but retain consciousness.[3,35,57]

Features of ciguatera poisoning usually occur within 6 hours of ingestion but may be delayed up to 72 hours. Typically, vomiting and diarrhea are followed by perioral and peripheral paresthesias and ataxia.[36-42,58-63] Reference is often made of a cold-to-hot sensory reversal dysesthesia, with patients usually describing a burning sensation on exposure to cold water, for example. This is not a true sensory reversal, but is probably an exaggerated pain response to minor temperature extremes; patients can accurately detect temperature.[64]

Headache, arthralgias, abdominal pain, tremors, pruritus, and weakness are common complaints. Another unusual feature is that patients may complain that their teeth feel loose and may fall out of their sockets or are painful. Hypotension and bradycardia (including heart blocks) can develop. Paresthesia, pruritus, and prolonged weakness after the acute phase may persist for several weeks to months.[36-41] It has also been noted that repeated episodes of ciguatera may be more severe in character. Ingestion of nonaffected seafood, grains, and alcohol, as well as exercise, may exacerbate symptoms.

Neurotoxic shellfish poisoning produces a similar clinical picture to ciguatera poisoning, but generally less severe. Inhalation of brevetoxins can produce upper and lower airway irritation and bronchospasm. Clupeotoxin poisoning results in a metallic taste, followed by vomiting, diarrhea, and cardiovascular collapse. Headaches, muscle cramps, paresthesia, and progressive muscular paralysis may occur. Seizures and coma resulting in death have occurred.[19] Amnestic (domoic acid) shellfish poisoning was characterized by acute onset of gastrointestinal symptoms within 24 hours of eating mussels, followed by rapid onset of confusion, disorientation, and memory loss within 48 hours.[44] Serious neurologic impairment such as seizures, coma, and mutism have occurred.[45] Deaths have occurred and chronic residual memory deficits may result.[44-46]

Diagnosis

A diagnosis of seafood poisoning is made on the history of seafood ingested and the clinical presentation. Analyses of toxic shellfish and toxic dinoflagellate algal organisms for toxins have helped establish a diagnosis in patients involved in certain outbreaks of shellfish poisonings. A presumptive diagnosis of paralytic shellfish poisoning should be made in a patient who develops neurologic symptoms after ingestion of mussels during seasons of risk in areas where paralytic shellfish poisoning occurs. Other causes of neurologic illness may appropriately have to be ruled out. Patients presenting with allergic symptoms and signs should be asked if they have eaten any of the potentially causative fish and if they noted a peppery taste.

Tetrodotoxin causes an ascending paralysis and the fish ingested are usually distinctive.

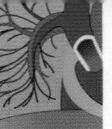
The diagnosis of ciguatera is made on clinical grounds. The history of consumption of fish such as grouper, barracuda, or amberjack with subsequent gastrointestinal symptoms and unusual neurologic symptoms will suggest the clinical diagnosis. Neurotoxic shellfish poisoning can be differentiated from ciguatera by the history of shellfish poisoning.

LABORATORY TESTING

Hospital laboratories generally do not have the capability to detect seafood poisoning toxins, but the appropriate food or health regulatory body may have access to laboratories to detect toxins in any uneaten samples.

DIFFERENTIAL DIAGNOSIS

The clinical presentation of ciguatera and neurotoxic shellfish poisoning may be similar, as may tetrodotoxin and paralytic shellfish; the principal symptoms and the seafood eaten can usually be used to determine the specific etiology.

Infectious gastroenteritis is the main differential diagnosis to consider. The lack of neurologic features should differentiate these diseases.

The history of fish ingested should differentiate scombroid poisoning from true anaphylactic reactions. Other toxic causes of erythema to consider are niacin, vancomycin, rifampicin, monosodium glutamate, and ethanol-disulfiram reactions.

Management

SUPPORTIVE MEASURES

The treatment of seafood poisoning is largely supportive. Careful assessment of airway control and ventilatory function should be undertaken because patients may require intubation and mechanical ventilation. Intravenous saline should be used to replace fluid losses. Ionotropes may be required for paralytic shellfish poisoning or severe ciguatera poisoning. Intravenous calcium gluconate (1 g over 30 minutes, followed by 2 to 4 g/day IV) has been used to treat hypotension secondary to ciguatera.

Seafood toxins are absorbed by activated charcoal and should be given to patients who present within 1 hour of ingestion. Control of vomiting may be required first.

Administration of antihistamines such as the H_2 blocker ranitidine and the H_1 blocker diphenhydramine is key to treatment of scombroid poisoning, as are intravenous fluids, steroids, and general supportive care. Epinephrine may be indicated in the presence of bronchospasm, angioedema, or hypotension. The syndrome is usually self-limited, resolving within a few hours.

Intravenous mannitol has been promoted as a treatment of acute ciguatera poisoning.[65] However, a randomized controlled trial failed to demonstrate that it was superior to normal saline in reducing symptoms by 24 hours, and its use can no longer be recommended.[66] Chronic ciguatera may be bothersome, because symptoms may wax and wane.[60-63] The most success in treatment has been with the use of amitriptyline, possibly

by an affect on sodium channels.[67,68] Treatment is generally begun with amitriptyline 25 mg twice a day. Remissions and exacerbations may occur. Alternatively, gabapentin has provided symptomatic improvement for persistent neurologic sequelae of ciguatera poisoning.[69]

DISPOSITION

Patients poisoned by tetrodotoxin, paralytic shellfish, or clupeotoxin require monitoring of ventilatory function in an appropriate setting. Most other patients can be discharged after treatment in the emergency department. Patients should be admitted if they have severe dehydration, persistent abnormal vital signs, systemic anaphylactoid reactions, or neurologic symptoms. The level of care required depends on clinical severity. Local departments of health should be informed of suspected cases of seafood poisoning.

REFERENCES

1. Williamson JA, Fenner PJ, Burnett JW: Venomous & Poisonous Marine Animals. Sydney, Australia, University of New South Wales Press, 1996.
2. Williamson JAH: The blue-ringed octopus bite and envenomation syndrome. Clin Dermatol 1987;5:127–133.
3. Halstead BW: Poisonous and Venomous Marine Animals of the World, revised ed. Princeton, NJ, Darwin Press, 1978.
4. Gurry D: Marine stings. Aust Fam Physician 1992;21:26–34.
5. Cain D: Weever fish sting: An unusual problem. BMJ 1983;287:406–407.
6. Reid HA: Diagnosis, prognosis, and treatment of sea-snake bite. Lancet 1961;1:399–402.
7. Tiballs J, Hawdon G, Winkel K: Mechanism of cardiac failure in Irukandji syndrome and first aid treatment for stings. Anaesth Intens Care 2001;29:552.
8. Sutherland SK, Tiballs J: Australian Animal Toxins, 2nd ed. Melbourne, Australia, Oxford University Press, 2001.
9. Michael SW: Reef Sharks and Rays of the World. Monterey, CA, Sea Challengers Publications, 1993.
10. McGoldrick J, Marx JA: Marine envenomations. J Emerg Med 1991;9:497–502.
11. Auerbach PS: Marine envenomations. N Engl J Med 1991; 325:486–493.
12. Fenner PJ, Williamson JA, Skinner RA: Fatal and non-fatal stingray envenomation. Med J Aust 1989;151:621–625.
13. Lane CE: Nematocyst toxins of Coelenterates. In Humm HJ, Lane CE (eds): Bioactive Compounds from the Sea. New York, Marcel Dekker, 1974, pp 139–141.
14. Ellis MD: Dangerous Plants, Snakes, Arthropods, and Marine Life. Hamilton, IL, Drug Intelligence Publications, 1978.
15. Burnett JW, Gable WD: A fatal jellyfish envenomation by the Portuguese man-o'-war. Toxicon 1989;27:823–824.
16. Auerbach PS: Wilderness Medicine, 3rd ed. St. Louis, CV Mosby, 1995, pp 1327–1374.
17. White J: Antivenom Handbook. Melbourne, Australia, CLS, 2001.
18. Walker DG: Survival after severe envenomation by the blue-ringed octopus (Hapalochlaena maculosa). Med J Aust 1983;2:663–665.
19. Meier J, White J: Handbook of clinical toxicology of animal venoms and poisons. Boca Raton, FL, CRC Press, 1995.
20. Corkeron M: Magnesium infusion to treat Irukandji syndrome. Med J Aust 2003;178:41.
21. Halstead BW, Walter B: Paralytic Shellfish Poisoning. World Health Organization, 1984, pp 1–59.
22. Ahles MD: Red tide: a recurrent health hazard. Am J Public Health 1974;64:807.
23. Todd E, Avery G, Grant GA: An outbreak of severe paralytic shellfish poisoning in British Columbia. Can Commun Dis Rep 1993;19:99–102.
24. Bond RM, Medcof JC: Epidemic shellfish poisoning in New Brunswick, 1957. Can Med Assoc J 1978;19:19.

25. Collins M: Algal toxins. Microbiol Rev 1978;42:725.
26. Meyer KF: Food poisoning (in 3 parts). N Engl J Med 1953;249:765 (I), 804 (II), 843 (III).
27. Hughes JM, Merson MH: Fish and shellfish poisoning. N Engl J Med 1976;295:1117–1120.
28. Sommer H, Meyer KF: Paralytic shellfish poisoning. Arch Pathol 1937;24:560.
29. Pierce RH: Red tide (Ptychodiscus brevis) toxin aerosols: a review. Toxicon 1986;24:955–965.
30. Anderson DM: Red tides. Sci Am 1994;271:62–68.
31. McInerney J, Sahgal P, Vogel M, et al: Scombroid poisoning. Ann Emerg Med 1996;28:235–238.
32. Sanders WE: Intoxications from the seas: Ciguatera, scombroid, and paralytic shellfish poisoning. Infect Dis Clin North Am 1987;1:665–676.
33. Morrow JD, Margolies GR, Rowland J, Roberts LJ: Evidence that histamine is the causative toxin in scombroid fish poisoning. N Engl J Med 1991;324:716–720.
34. Muller GJ, Lamprecht JH, Barnes JM, et al: Scombroid poisoning. S Afr Med J 1992;81:427–430.
35. Torda TA, Sinclair E, Ulyatt DB: Pufferfish (tetrodotoxin) poisoning. Med J Aust 1973;1:599–602.
36. Gollop JH, Pon EW: Ciguatera: a review. Hawaii Med J 1992;51:91–99.
37. Bagnis R, Kuberski T, Laugier S: Clinical observations on 3009 cases of ciguatera in the South Pacific. Am J Trop Med Hyg 1979;28:1067–1073.
38. Lewis ND: Disease and development: ciguatera fish poisoning. Soc Sci Med 1986;23:983–993.
39. Lawrence DN, Enriquez MB, Lumish RM, Maceo A: Ciguatera fish poisoning in Miami. JAMA 1980;244:254.
40. Gillespie NC, Lewis RJ, Pearn JH, et al: Ciguatera in Australia—occurrence, clinical features, pathophysiology and management. Med J Aust 1986;145:584.
41. Lange WR, Snyder FR, Fudala PJ: Travel and ciguatera fish poisoning. Arch Intern Med 1992;152:2049–2053.
42. Katz AR, Terrell-Perica S, Sasaki DM:. Ciguatera on Kauai. Am J Trop Med Hyg 1993;49:448–454.
43. Halstead BW: Miscellaneous seafood toxicants. In Ragelis EP (ed): Seafood Toxins. Washington, DC, American Chemical Society, 1984, pp 227–238.
44. Perl TM, Bedard L, Kosatsky T, et al: An outbreak of toxic encephalopathy caused by eating mussels contaminated with domoic acid. N Engl J Med 1990;322:1775–1780.
45. Teitelbaum JS, Zatorre RJ, Carpenter S, et al: Neurologic sequelae of domoic acid intoxication due to the ingestion of contaminated mussels. N Engl J Med 1990;322:1761–1767.
46. Kosatsky T: Improving epidemic control: lessons from the 1987 toxic mussels affair. Can Med Assoc J 1992;147:1769–1772.
47. Cendes F, Andermann F, Carpenter S, et al: Temporal lobe epilepsy caused by domoic acid intoxication. Ann Neurol 1995;37:123–126.
48. Scholin CA, Gulland F, Doucette GJ, et al: Mortality of sea lions along the central California coast linked to a toxic diatom bloom. Nature 2000;403:80.
49. Gallagher JP, Shinnick-Gallagher P: Effect of Gynodinium breve toxin in the rate phrenic diaphragm preparation. Br J Pharmacol 1980;69:367.
50. Shinnick-Gallagher P: Possible mechanism of action of Gynodinium breve toxin in the mammalian neuromuscular junction. Br J Pharmacol 1980;69:373.
51. Becker K, Southwick K, Readon J, et al: Histamine poisoning associated with eating tuna burgers. JAMA 2001;285:1327.
52. Cameron J, Flowers AE, Capra MF: Electrophysiological studies on ciguatera in man (part II). J Neurol Sci 1991;101:93.
53. Shimoda T, Krzanowski J, Nelson R: In vitro red tide toxin effect on human bronchial smooth muscle. J Allergy Clin Immunol 1988;81:1187.
54. Gessner BD, Middaugh JP: Paralytic shellfish poisoning in Alaska: a 20 year retrospective analysis. Am J Epidemiol 1995;141:766–770.
55. Rodrigue DC, Etzel RA, Hall S, et al: Lethal paralytic shellfish poisoning in Guatemala. Am J Trop Med Hyg 1990;42:267–271.
56. Centers for Disease Control and Prevention: Paralytic shellfish poisoning—Massachusetts and Alaska, 1990. MMWR Morb Mortal Wkly Rep 1991;40:157–161.
57. Sims JK, Ostman DC: Pufferfish poisoning: emergency diagnosis and management. Ann Emerg Med 1986;15:1094–1098.
58. Losacker W: Ciguatera fish poisoning in the Cook Islands. Bull Soc Pathol Exot 1992;85:447–448.
59. Lewis RJ, Holmes MJ: Origin and transfer of toxins involved in ciguatera. Comp Biochem Physiol 1993;106C:615–628.
60. Chretien JH, Fermaglich J, Garagusi VF: Ciguatera poisoning—presentation as a neurologic disorder. Arch Neurol 1981;38:783.
61. Lange WR: Ciguatera fish poisoning. Am Fam Physician 1994;50:579–584.
62. Engleberg NC, Morris JG, Lewis J, et al: Ciguatera fish poisoning: a major common source outbreak in the U.S. Virgin Islands. Ann Intern Med 1983;98:336.
63. Morris JG, Lewin P, Hargrett N, et al: Clinical features of ciguatera fish poisoning. A study of the disease in the U. S. Virgin Islands. Arch Intern Med 1982;142:1090.
64. Cameron J, Capra MF: The basis of the paradoxical disturbance of temperature perception in ciguatera poisoning. J Toxicol Clin Toxicol 1993;31:571.
65. Palafox NA, Jain LG, Pinano AZ, et al: Successful treatment of ciguatera fish poisoning with intravenous mannitol. JAMA 1988;259:2740.
66. Schnorf H, Taurarii M, Cundy T: Ciguatera fish poisoning. A double-blind randomized trial of mannitol therapy. Neurology 2002;58:873.
67. Bowman PB: Amitriptyline and ciguatera. Med J Aust 1984;140:802.
68. Davis RT, Villar LA: Symptomatic improvement with amitriptyline in ciguatera fish poisoning [Letter]. N Engl J Med 1986;315:65.
69. Perez CM, Vasquez PA, Perret CF: Treatment of ciguatera poisoning with gabapentin. N Engl J Med 2001;344:692–693.

26 Botulism and Other Food-borne Toxins

MICHAEL D. SCHWARTZ, MD ■ BRENT W. MORGAN, MD

At a Glance...

- The clinician must make the initial diagnosis of botulism on clinical grounds.
- Visual disturbances, dysarthria, dysphagia, and dry mouth are the four most specific neurologic symptoms of botulism.
- The treatment of botulism requires meticulous attention to airway and ventilatory status and the early administration of botulism equine trivalent antitoxin.
- Careful history (timing and duration of symptom onset) and physical examination will help narrow the broad differential of food-borne illness.
- Fever, blood in the stool, and a longer incubation period are clues to an enteroinvasive (salmonellosis, shigellosis, campylobacteriosis) food-borne illness.

Many different organisms and toxins are capable of causing food poisoning. This chapter primarily discusses botulism, the most deadly food-related toxicologic disease known. In addition, the food-borne toxicologic syndromes of *Staphylococcus aureus*, *Clostridium perfringens*, cholera and noncholera vibrios, *Bacillus cereus*, *Salmonella*, *Shigella*, and *Campylobacter* are reviewed.

BOTULISM

Introduction

Botulinum toxin is produced by the anaerobic, spore-forming, gram-positive bacillus *Clostridium botulinum*. Botulinum toxin is the most potent toxin known, with as little as 100 ng being lethal to humans.[1] Botulism is the clinical syndrome characterized by neuroparalytic signs and symptoms that result from the actions of the botulinum toxin. Ironically, despite the potency and inherent danger of botulinum toxin, its paralytic actions have made it useful as a therapeutic and cosmetic remedy.

There are three forms of naturally occurring human botulism: food-borne botulism, wound botulism, and intestinal botulism. *Iatrogenic botulism* is a term used to describe patients who develop some symptoms compatible with systemic botulism after receiving botulinum toxin A for therapeutic purposes.[2] Food-borne botulism is the best-known form of botulism. Fortunately, food-borne botulism is rare in the United States, with an average of less than 25 cases a year reported in the past few decades.[3] It occurs when an individual consumes food contaminated with preformed toxin. Historically, wound botulism was extremely rare. Since the 1990s, however, there has been an increased incidence of wound botulism, which has been most commonly associated with the subcutaneous injection of black tar

heroin.[4] Wound botulism occurs when wounds become contaminated with spores of *C. botulinum* that germinate and produce toxin that is absorbed systemically. Intestinal botulism occurs when the gastrointestinal (GI) tract because colonized with *C. botulinum*. This most commonly happens in infants and is frequently termed *infant botulism*. Infant botulism, which is the most common type of botulism in the United States, occurs when an infant consumes foods contaminated with spores of *C. botulinum*. Disease occurs when the spores germinate and proliferate in the GI tract and produce toxin.[5,6] Although uncommon, adults can also develop intestinal botulism.[7] These patients typically have an abnormality of the GI tract that can make them susceptible to intestinal colonization.

Bacteriology/Structure

Botulism spores are ubiquitous; they are found in the soil and in marine sediments worldwide. The species is subdivided into seven antigenically distinct serologic types (A to G), which produce disease in either humans or animals.[8,9] The botulinum toxin is produced after the botulinum spore germinates and begins cell growth. Toxin is released when the mature cell wall lyses.[9] The spores of *C. botulinum* are surrounded by an inner and outer coat of keratin-like structure rich in disulfide bonds that makes them highly resistant to heating, freezing, aerobic and anaerobic conditions, ionizing radiation, and exposure to various chemical agents.[10] Moist heat at temperatures greater than 120° C for at least 30 minutes is required to destroy them.[8,11] Environmental factors that favor spore germination include low acidity, a temperature between 4° C and 70° C, low oxygen, and high water content.[9,12] However, growth of E-type organisms has been reported at temperatures as low as 3° C and in nonanaerobic environments.[8]

Epidemiology and Types of Botulism

Toxin types A, B, and E account for almost all cases of human botulism.[8,13] Types F and G are very rare in humans. Toxin types C and D are associated with botulism in mammalian animals and birds.[13] Between 1973 and 1996, approximately half of the cases of food-borne botulism were caused by type A. In that same period, the remaining cases were almost equally divided between types B and E.[3] Geographic distribution of spore types parallels the toxin type identified in outbreaks. In the western United States, type A spores predominate in the soil, and the majority of disease is due to type A toxin.[8,14] Type B spores predominate in the central and eastern United States, and the majority of cases in these areas are due to type B toxin.[8,14] Type E spores are less

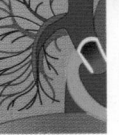

ubiquitous but are most commonly found in damp locations, including sediments around the Great Lakes and the coasts of Washington and Alaska. These coastal areas are the same locations where type E botulism occurs.

The name *botulism* originally comes from the Latin word *botulus*, meaning "sausage." Improperly prepared blood sausage was first implicated in causing the disease in the late 18th century. The organism was first reported to be associated with the disease in 1897 after it was isolated from uncooked ham after an outbreak of 23 cases at a music club in Belgium.[15] Although poorly preserved meat was the cause of most cases of botulism in the past, most present-day cases of types A and B botulism in the United States result from improper home canning of vegetables.

While restaurant-acquired botulism accounts for only 4% of the total number of outbreaks, restaurant-associated outbreaks account for 40% of the total number of cases of botulism.[16] Several large outbreaks have been caused by onions and potatoes that were left at warm temperatures for more than 12 hours in incubator-like conditions.[16-18] Either insufficient heating to kill the spores or introduction of spores to the food after cooking led to proliferation of the organism with subsequent toxin production. Anaerobic conditions may exist, especially if the food is immersed in a liquid or is covered. The onions, which were immersed in butter, were used in patty melt sandwiches and resulted in 28 cases.[16,17] The potatoes were wrapped in aluminum foil and later used in potato salad and caused 34 cases.[18] A similar incubation process has been implicated in other outbreaks involving beef and chicken pot pies, turkey loaf, and beef stew, all of which were kept warm and left to stand for longer than 12 hours without reheating.[16,19,20]

Cases of type E botulinum food poisoning result from either poor vacuum packing or improper home preparation or preservation techniques.[21] Common foods in the Inuit Eskimo communities are urraq (uncooked seal flipper in seal oil), muktuk (chunks of white whale skin, blubber, and meat), and fermented salmon eggs; these foods allow growth of the botulinum organism when left to ferment at room temperature because the foods are low in carbohydrates and thus do not become acidic.[21] The largest outbreak of type E botulism to date recently occurred in Egypt and involved at least 91 people. It resulted from the consumption of faseikh, which is a traditional ungutted, salted fish that was placed in a barrel and kept in a warm environment.[22] Conditions present in the fish intestines during preservation allowed for type E spores to proliferate.[23]

Pathophysiology

The botulinum toxin is the most lethal human toxin known; it has an estimated oral lethal dose of 70 μg in a 70-kg human.[24] Despite its potency, botulinum toxin is easily denatured.[8] Sunlight, chlorine, and heating at 80° C for 30 minutes or 100° C for 10 minutes denatures the active toxin.[13,16] Boiling under pressure is required at

higher altitudes. Botulinum toxins form complexes with other proteins that prevent destruction by proteolytic activity in the stomach after ingestion. The toxins are absorbed in the small intestine. The botulinum toxin is composed of a heavy and light chain held together by a disulfide bond. Once the toxin has been absorbed, it spreads via blood and the lymphatic system to peripheral acetylcholine synapses. Botulinum toxin cannot cross the blood-brain barrier. The heavy chain binds to specific receptors on the presynaptic nerve terminal and the toxin crosses the cell membrane via endocytosis. The heavy chain undergoes a reconfiguration that is triggered by the more acidic pH within the vesicle. The reconfiguration allows the heavy chain to penetrate the vesicle and results in release of the light chain into the cytoplasm. The light chain is a zinc-dependent endopeptidase enzyme that is highly specific for one of three synaptic proteins (SNAP-25, syntaxin, or synaptobrevin) essential for docking and fusion of vesicles.[25,26] Without these synaptic proteins, acetylcholine-containing vesicles cannot fuse with the presynaptic membrane or release the neurotransmitter into the synaptic cleft.

The toxin's blockade of acetylcholine occurs at four separate sites: (1) the neuromuscular junction, (2) ganglionic nerve endings, (3) postganglionic parasympathetic nerve endings, and (4) postganglionic sympathetic nerve endings that use acetylcholine.[9] At high toxin concentrations, adrenergic systems may also be affected.[14] The toxin affects only the release of acetylcholine and does not affect acetylcholine's synthesis, storage, or metabolism.[9] Botulinum toxin does not affect impulse conduction down nerves or impulse conduction at nerve terminals.[11,27]

Food-borne Botulism

CLINICAL MANIFESTATIONS

The first symptoms of botulism usually occur within 12 to 48 hours of ingestion of contaminated foods.[12,28-30] The onset of symptoms, however, may be delayed for as long as 14 days after ingestion. The latent period is inversely proportional to dose of toxin ingested, such that the more toxin consumed, the more rapid the onset of symptoms. The initial signs and symptoms of botulism may be gastrointestinal and can include abdominal pain, nausea, vomiting, and diarrhea. Constipation is the most common GI symptom.

Patients may also present initially with only neurologic signs and symptoms due to cholinergic blockade. Visual disturbances, dysarthria, dysphagia, and dry mouth are the four most specific neurologic symptoms.[8,17,29,31] Additional nonspecific neurologic symptoms associated with botulism include malaise, generalized weakness, headache, dizziness, and paresthesias.[8,17,29,31] As the disease progresses, oculobulbar signs, descending paralysis, and progressive respiratory weakness occurs, which often leads to respiratory failure.

Oculobulbar symptoms are exceedingly common findings in botulism.[8,32,33] Blurring of vision, lateral rectus palsy, ptosis, dilated pupils, and external ophthalmoplegia occur in most patients who develop neurologic

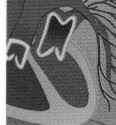

symptoms.[17,29,31] Fixed or dilated pupils are seen in almost half the patients who present in botulism epidemics. Sixth nerve palsy and accommodative paresis are frequent, early ophthalmic signs of botulism.[31,33] Third nerve palsy, if seen, may indicate a higher likelihood of respiratory failure and the need for mechanical ventilation.[31,33] Because botulism is so rare and is associated with nonspecific symptoms, the Centers for Disease Control and Prevention (CDC)[8] and others[17] have suggested various constellations of signs and symptoms to help clinicians consider the diagnosis of botulism early in its presentation (Table 26-1).

Table 26-2 lists the differential diagnoses of botulism.[8,12,34] The disease is most commonly confused with Guillain-Barré syndrome. Approximately 10.5% of persons reported to the CDC with suspected botulism are ultimately diagnosed as having Guillain-Barré syndrome. Other diseases commonly confused with botulism include carbon monoxide poisoning (3.4% of reported cases of botulism), food poisoning of unknown etiology (3.2%), and food poisoning due to staphylococcal organisms (3.0%).[8] Physicians should suspect botulism whenever a patient presents with generalized weakness, particularly if there is ocular or oropharyngeal involvement.

DIAGNOSIS

Because rapid treatment is critically important and results of diagnostic testing take time, the clinician must make the initial diagnosis of botulism on clinical grounds. When botulism is clinically suspected, samples of serum, stool, and stomach contents should be cultured and assayed for botulinum toxin. Epidemiologically suspected foods should also be assayed for the neurotoxin. The mouse neutralization bioassay is the most reliable method for detecting the toxin. Laboratory confirmation cannot be relied on to make treatment decisions because the mouse bioassay requires 4 days to complete. Since *C. botulinum* is ubiquitous, cultures of the suspected food are not usually helpful and can result in false-positive results. Postmortem diagnosis may be aided by detecting toxin or organisms in autopsy specimens of the small intestines, large intestines, or liver.[14]

An electromyogram (EMG) can be useful by correctly differentiating botulism from myasthenia gravis,

Guillain-Barré syndrome, and Eaton-Lambert syndrome. The EMG of a patient suffering from botulism demonstrates a decrease in the evoked action potential at slow-frequency stimulation (2 Hz/s) and incremental increase in amplitude at rapid stimulation (50 Hz/s).[35] The EMG findings in myasthenia gravis show decreased evoked muscle responses at both slow and fast stimulation, and these EMG findings improve with the use of edrophonium chloride.[35] A decrease in evoked potential is usually noted as the muscle is repetitively stimulated, the opposite of what is found in botulism.[35] The EMG findings of a patient with Eaton-Lambert syndrome are very similar to those of a patient suffering from botulism.[35,36] EMG findings for botulism, however, are very dissimilar between different muscle groups and evolve over time, whereas EMG findings between different muscles for Eaton-Lambert syndrome are very similar and stay relatively stable over time. EMG findings for Guillain-Barré usually show patchy slowing, which is indicative of demyelination.

The diagnosis of botulism may be difficult to make on initial patient presentation. The clinician should be familiar with the common presenting signs and symptoms (see Table 26-1) and the clinical features that differentiate it from other illnesses with similar findings (see Table 26-2). The findings on EMG can be helpful to solidify the diagnosis. The physician should consider botulism in the differential diagnosis of any patient who presents with a neurologic or neuromuscular complaint.

MANAGEMENT

The treatment of botulism requires meticulous attention to airway and ventilatory status. Most early deaths result from respiratory failure and occur before a patient has presented for health care or from the failure of health care workers to recognize early signs of respiratory impairment once a patient has presented.[17,37] Patients should be placed in a well-observed treatment area on an electrocardiogram monitor and should have continuous pulse oximetry monitoring. An intravenous line should be established, and equipment necessary for intubation should be readily available. Patients should be asked if any of their family or friends have similar symptoms or whether they have eaten in a restaurant, any home-canned foods, or any unusually prepared meats. Although any food ingested during the prior 8 days could possibly cause botulism, food consumption during the past 2 to 3 days is the more likely source of illness.

Pulmonary function tests are required for all patients with suspected botulism.[38] Although arterial blood gas measurements are helpful in the complete assessment of any patient, they do not accurately predict a declining respiratory reserve.[37,39] Hypercarbia due to respiratory muscle weakness usually develops very late in the course of botulism, just before respiratory arrest.[37] In an effort to predict those patients who will experience a declining ventilatory status, vital capacity and forced inspiratory volume should be measured regularly at 2- to 4-hour intervals. In one study, all adult patients with a vital capacity less than one third that predicted eventually required mechanical ventilation.[37] Elective intubation

TABLE 26-1 Most Common Presentations of Food-borne Botulism	
Presenting complaints	Dry mouth and/or dysphagia
	Abdominal symptoms
Initial appearance	Anxious
	Normal mental status
	Weak
Medical history	Previously well
Vital signs	Afebrile
	Slow or normal pulse
Physical examination	Dysphonia
	Dysarthria
	Symmetric ocular weakness
	Symmetric neurologic abnormalities

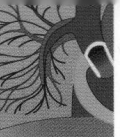

TABLE 26-2 Differential Diagnosis in Botulism

DISEASE OR CONDITION	DIFFERENTIAL MANIFESTATIONS	DISEASE OR CONDITION	DIFFERENTIAL MANIFESTATIONS
Neurologic Diseases			
Guillain-Barré syndrome	Usually ascending paralysis Elevated CSF protein Paresthesias Preceding viral illness common Absent deep tendon reflexes	Eaton-Lambert syndrome	Underlying malignancy, especially oat cell carcinoma Progression much slower Predominant thigh and pelvic muscle involvement
Myasthenia gravis	Lack of autonomic findings Increased fatigability Improvement with edrophonium EMG findings		Extraocular muscle involvement rare Pupillary findings almost never present EMG findings
		Cerebrovascular accident	Asymmetric Unilateral Vascular distribution Asymmetric deep tendon reflexes
Biologic Infections and Toxins			
Bacterial food poisons (staphylococcal, clostridial, and so forth)	Rapid onset Gastrointestinal complaints predominate No paralysis No cranial nerve involvement	Encephalitis	Altered mental status Fever Meningeal signs Abnormal CSF
Diphtheria	Pseudomembrane Pharyngitis Schick's test Limb paralysis occurs weeks after cranial nerve involvement	Saxitoxin Trichinosis	Symptoms within 1 hr of fish ingestion Paresthesias of face predominate Tachycardia Vertigo Fever
Poliomyelitis	Fever Meningeal signs Crampy muscle pain Asymmetric distribution CSF may show encephalitis pattern	*Amanita* Tetanus	Myositis Periorbital edema Eosinophilia Coma Violent vomiting
Tick paralysis	More common in children Tick(s) found on physical examination Paralysis usually ascending Deep tendon reflexes may be absent		Hepatic failure Trismus Risus' sardonicus Neck and jaw stiffness Muscle spasms
Poisoning and Overdose			
Phenothiazine reaction	Spastic muscle contractures Resolution with antihistamines	Aminoglycoside-induced paralysis	Postanesthesia History of renal impairment Serum levels
Carbon monoxide poisoning	Headache Altered mental status Elevated carbon monoxide level	Heavy metal exposure	Exposure history Rapidity of onset Serum or urine levels
Organophosphate overdose	Fasciculations Cholinergic symptoms Resolution with atropine	Hypermagnesemia	Medication history Renal impairment Serum magnesium level
Anticholinergic poisoning	Fever Altered mental status Tachycardia and vasodilation No cranial nerve involvement Medication history		
Medical Conditions and Emergencies			
Acute myocardial infarction Appendicitis Bowel obstruction Bowel infarction	Classic signs and symptoms should evolve over time	Carcinomatous invasion of the base of the skull Hysteria	Cranial nerves V and VIII involvement only Meningeal signs and symptoms Variable, inconsistent findings No objective findings
Acute intermittent porphyria	History or family history Cranial nerve involvement rare Prior psychiatric or CNS complaints Urinary test abnormalities	Sepsis	Fever Leukocytosis Localized sites of infection Abnormal CSF findings Positive blood cultures

CNS, central nervous system; CSF, cerebrospinal fluid; EMG, electromyography.

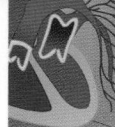

before respiratory arrest decreases mortality from botulism.[29]

The state health department should be contacted in all suspected cases of botulism. The CDC maintains a 24-hour telephone number to provide callers with their state's on-call consultant (404-639-2888). This telephone number provides 24-hour access to consultation regarding suspected cases of botulism. Information is also provided about the nearest location for obtaining the antitoxin. The state health department can assist in the epidemiologic and public health aspects of the outbreak. Samples should be obtained for testing by the CDC.[38] These samples should be kept refrigerated but not frozen.[8]

At the time of diagnosis, unabsorbed toxin-containing food may still be present in a patient's GI tract. While the efficacy of gastric decontamination in suspected cases of botulism is yet to be evaluated, it is recommended. Activated charcoal adsorbs *C. botulinum* type A in vitro and, thus, is recommended for cases of suspected food-borne botulism.[40] The utility of gastric lavage is unknown and should be reserved for patients who ingested known contaminated food within 1 to 2 hours of presentation. Non-magnesium-containing cathartics, enemas, and whole bowel irrigation are other options, but their efficacy is unknown.

Botulism equine trivalent (A, B, E) antitoxin should be administered as soon as possible in all cases of suspected botulism except infantile botulism. The antitoxin binds circulating toxin and is effective in preventing progression of illness but does not reverse neurologic effects that are already present. In a retrospective analysis of 134 cases of type A food-borne botulism, patients who received trivalent antitoxin within 24 hours of symptom onset had a lower mortality rate and a shorter hospital stay than patients who received delayed antitoxin (greater than 24 hours after symptom onset) or no antitoxin at all.[41] Since 1996, the CDC has recommended the administration of only one vial intravenously per patient.[3] Each vial contains 100 times that amount of antitoxin required to neutralize the largest amount of circulating toxin ever measured at the CDC.[42] Pregnancy is not a contraindication to antitoxin administration. It is unknown if asymptomatic individuals that have likely consumed food contaminated with botulinum toxin should be treated empirically with antitoxin. The benefits of early administration must be weighed against the risk for anaphylaxis from the equine-derived antitoxin.

In one investigation, hypersensitivity reactions were noted in 9% of patients treated with the horse serum–prepared antitoxin.[43] Patients in this study were treated with less than one to greater than four vials. More than half of the reactions were nonfatal acute hypersensitivity reactions that ranged from urticaria to true anaphylaxis; the remainder were delayed serum sickness–type hypersensitivity reactions.[43] The incidence of delayed serum sickness–type hypersensitivity reactions was significantly more common in those administered more than four vials. The incidence of hypersensitivity reactions may be lower following administration of one vial, as is currently recommended. Nevertheless, epinephrine should be readily available to treat serious reactions. Skin testing before treatment does not reliably distinguish those patients who will or will not have hypersensitivity reactions.[44]

The incidence of mortality for botulism has declined dramatically during the past 40 years, from more than 60% to between 5% and 15%.[8,16,29,37] There are many reasons for this, which include more widespread media coverage and heightened awareness, more aggressive early care, increased availability of antitoxin, and accumulated intensive care expertise by physicians. Cases of suspected botulism should be cared for by intensivists that are experts in ventilator management. In recent reports, almost all in-hospital deaths have been due to pulmonary and ventilator-related complications.[29,37,45]

Severity of disease appears to be related to the type of toxin. Cases of type A botulism have had a significantly higher incidence of respiratory failure requiring intubation and mechanical ventilation than have cases of types B and E botulism.[16,29,46] Type E botulism has the lowest incidence of intubation but has a shorter incubation period; almost all individuals have symptoms within 24 hours of ingestion.[46] Type B is intermediate in severity between types A and E and has the longest incubation period.

Recovery from botulism may be delayed for months.[35] Patients are often weak and tire easily for as long as a year after the acute phase of their disease. A vaccine developed from a recombinant fragment of *C. botulinum* neurotoxin serotype A has protected mice against intraperitoneal doses of toxin 10 million times the normal lethal dose.[44]

Infant Botulism

Infant botulism, first reported in 1976, is now by far the most common form of botulism in the United States. In one 12-year period, 57 cases were reported at the Children's Hospital of Philadelphia alone.[6] Infant botulism has also been implicated as a possible occult cause of the sudden infant death syndrome. Two non-botulinum *Clostridium* organisms, *Clostridium butyricum* and *Clostridium barati*, have been shown to cause infant botulism by elaboration of botulism toxins type E and F, respectively.[45,47] As of 1996, more than 1400 cases of infant botulism have been reported to the CDC.[3]

Unlike classic adult botulism, which results from ingestion of preformed toxin, infant botulism is due to in vivo germination of botulism spores with concomitant toxin production. The human colon is believed to be the site of bacterial colonization, and symptoms occur when released toxin is absorbed from the gut.[5] Botulism spores do not germinate in the presence of high acidity, a complex mix of aerobic and anaerobic bacteria, or a mature GI immune system.[48] Infants are at risk until about 4 to 6 months of age because of the unique characteristics of their GI tract, including a more alkaline gastric environment, a paucity of normal flora, and a lack of mature mucosal immunologic defenses, including lysozyme, complement, and secretory IgA.[48-50]

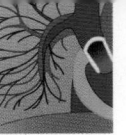

In infants, the median age at presentation is 2 to 4 months; cases of infant botulism after 6 months of age are very uncommon.

Breast-feeding remains a controversial risk factor for the development of infant botulism. A study has shown that before 2 months of age, there is no significant difference between the number of breast-fed and formula-fed infants diagnosed with the disease.[51] The severity of disease in formula-fed infants younger than 2 months appears to be greater, however, and more formula-fed infants require intubation. In infants older than 2 months, those who have been breast-fed have a significantly higher chance of being diagnosed with infant botulism. Other risk factors for infant botulism include residing in regions that have a high soil load of botulism spores. The high spore load in local soils of California, Utah, and Pennsylvania parallels the frequency of disease, and more than half of the reported cases of infant botulism come from these regions.[5] Additional risk factors for infant botulism include alkaline soil, nearby construction, high dust counts, and ingestion of corn syrup or honey.[50,51] Natural honey is one of the causes of infant botulism. As many as 25% of samples have botulism spores. The CDC recommends that natural honey not be given to children younger than 12 months.[51]

Treatment of infant botulism involves aggressive supportive care. Use of equine antitoxin is to be avoided due to the risks associated with use of equine-derived product and the possibility of early sensitization to equine serum.[1] Current evaluation of a human volunteer-derived immune globulin preparation is ongoing and may offer an alternative antibody-based therapy.[1]

Wound Botulism

Wound botulism occurs when *Clostridium botulinum* grows in localized wounds and elaborates sufficient neurotoxin for the systemic signs and symptoms of botulism to develop. First described in 1943, wound botulism has been frequently associated with infected abscesses from injection drug use. In 1982, a case of wound botulism resulted from the intravenous injection of cocaine.[52] More recently cases of wound botulism associated with the intramuscular or subcutaneous ("skin popping") administration of black tar heroin.[53,54] In cases of wound botulism secondary to infected abscesses in which toxin typing is performed, botulinum toxin type A or B is most frequently identified.[53]

Any wound in which *C. botulinum* germinate and elaborate toxin may be associated with clinical botulism. In 1991, botulinum toxin type A was isolated from a case of wound botulism secondary to an odontogenic abscess in a 5-year-old boy.[55]

Treatment of wound botulism includes aggressive supportive care, early surgical débridement of wounds, and the administration of antitoxin.

Iatrogenic Botulism

Subsequent to the use of intradermal botulinum toxin (Botox, Allergan, Inc., Irvine, CA) in cosmetic dermatology, rare cases of systemic botulism have been reported.[56-58] These cases have all involved multiple subcutaneous or intramuscular injections for focal hyperhidrosis, spasticity secondary to multiple sclerosis, spasticity associated with multisystem atrophy, and cervical dystonia.[56-58] Both pharmaceutical formulations, BoTox and Dysport (Ipsen, Ltd., Slough, UK), have been associated with iatrogenic botulism. Patients diagnosed with iatrogenic botulism have all developed generalized muscle weakness and have had EMG evidence of denervation.[56-58] None of these patients received antitoxin treatment or required mechanical ventilation.

OTHER FOOD-BORNE TOXINS

Introduction

Illness caused by food consumption may be due to the direct action of an infecting organism, elaboration of a toxin by an infecting organism, or the presence of a preformed toxin in the ingested food (even in the absence of viable organisms). Food-borne illnesses are vastly underreported in the United States, with most estimates suggesting that about 1% to 5% of cases reach public health awareness.[59] In the past, food-borne illness outbreaks occurred on a small geographic scale with high attack rates and were more easily detected by public health authorities. The changing paradigm of this disease entity is one of broad geographic reach and is characterized by increased numbers of victims and less readily identifiable sources.[60] In a telling example from Minnesota in 1994, 593 cases of *Salmonella enteriditis* were linked to consumption of pasteurized ice cream transported in a tanker truck that had previously carried unpasteurized liquid egg. The inoculum of *Salmonella* found in the contaminated ice cream, if evenly distributed throughout the tanker, was estimated to have been enough to cause 224,000 cases of illness.[61] The underreporting of food-borne illness, compounded by the unavoidable laboratory delay in detecting an event, could have a considerable public health impact if timely intervention to stop an outbreak is not taken.

In the current political climate, the possibility of malicious contamination leading to an outbreak must raise our awareness even more. Determination that the 1984 *Salmonella* outbreak in Oregon was biological terrorism came more than 2 years after the initial public health investigation.[62] Today, the onus is on the frontline physician to report suspected food-borne illnesses, with the intent of identifying an outbreak early enough to intervene, rather than merely retrospectively arriving at a satisfying clinical diagnosis. The following section provides the clinical characteristics associated with the more common toxin-mediated, food-borne syndromes.

Bacterial food toxins may be heat stable or heat labile. Heat-stable enterotoxins are typically smaller proteins that primarily intoxicate intestinal lining cells.[63] The most common heat-stable toxins are those associated with *Staphylococcus aureus*, enterotoxigenic *Escherichia coli*, and *Yersinia enterocolitica*. The most common heat-labile toxins are associated with *Bacillus cereus*, *Clostridium perfringens*, and *Vibrio cholerae*.

Staphylococcal Food Poisoning

INTRODUCTION, EPIDEMIOLOGY, AND BACTERIOLOGY

Staphylococcal food poisoning is the second most common cause of reported food-borne illness in the United States.[64] The self-limited nature of this illness results in a low (10%) rate of presentation to health care facilities and, thus, a vast underreporting of the estimated 6 to 80 million cases that occur each year in the United States.[65]

Approximately 2% to 5% of *S. aureus* isolates produce one of the seven identified heat-stable enterotoxins responsible for human disease.[66] One study of a large outbreak in California and Nevada has also identified and implicated an enterotoxin-producing strain of *Staphylococcus intermedius*.[67] Coagulase-negative staphylococci do not produce enterotoxins and have not been implicated in human food-borne illness.[68] Humans are the natural reservoir for *S. aureus*, although unpasteurized dairy products from cows with mastitis can also be a source of *S. aureus*.[68] Studies show that between 20% and 50% of healthy individuals are asymptomatic carriers of *S. aureus*.[69]

S. aureus contamination occurs when a food handler, who is either a carrier of the organism or has an incidental infection (i.e., impetigo, cellulitis, or an open wound) inoculates the source food with bacteria. The food must maintain a permissive temperature for bacterial growth to allow elaboration of the toxin. For example, centralization of school lunch preparation—where lunches are prepared in one location and then distributed to satellite schools—was felt to contribute to a 1990 outbreak of staphylococcal enterotoxin A illness in two elementary schools in Rhode Island. Ham rolls in 662 lunches, inoculated by a contaminated food handler, were maintained at permissive temperatures for several hours while they were transported to the outlying facilities.[70]

Optimum temperature for bacterial growth is 35° C to 40° C, but the organism can grow and produce toxin at temperatures between 3° C and 60° C.[71] Thorough reheating before serving may kill the bacteria, but the heat-stable toxin will remain active. In a recent, large outbreak in the Kansai district in Japan linked to powdered skim milk produced at a factory in Hokkaido, staphylococci were killed by pasteurization at 130° C, but enterotoxin A remained in concentrations of 3.7 ng/g.[72] Intake among cases was estimated to be 10 to 100 ng.

Foods rich in protein and sugars (e.g., poultry and ham), dairy products (e.g., milk, mayonnaise, cheese), or foods containing dairy products (e.g., sauces, desserts, dressings, and condiments) are most often implicated in *S. aureus* food poisoning.[70] However, any food may be implicated. For example, in a large European outbreak in 1984 that involved Great Britain, France, and Italy, packages of dried lasagna produced at a processing plant in Parma, Italy, were responsible for multiple mini-clusters of staphylococcal food poisoning.[73] This outbreak was a rare event both because of the implicated food item (dried pasta) as well as the point of contamination (during manufacture).

PATHOPHYSIOLOGY

It is well known that staphylococcal enterotoxins A through E and G through J, as well as toxic shock syndrome toxin (TSST, formerly staphylococcal enterotoxin F) act as superantigens and cause toxic shock by means of widespread T-cell activation and resultant cytokine elaboration. Superantigens bind nonspecifically to the T-cell receptor (TCR) of many T cells, resulting in unregulated activation of the inflammatory cascade. However, a different mechanism is implicated in the pathogenesis of staphylococcal food-borne illness, and is only now being intensively investigated. In vitro work has shown that enterotoxin B and TSST will undergo facilitated transport by intestinal lining cells (which lack both TCRs, as well as major histocompatibility complex class II molecules).[74] Mice fed staphylococcal enterotoxin B will demonstrate the presence of the toxin in the blood much more readily than will those fed staphylococcal enterotoxin A.[65] Staphylococcal enterotoxins are not cytotoxic to intestinal lining cells, nor do they stimulate fluid secretion in the gut by uncontrolled cycling of G proteins. Thus, the exact mechanism by which this family of toxins causes emesis and diarrhea remains elusive.

CLINICAL MANIFESTATIONS

The symptoms associated with staphylococcal food poisoning are the classic triad of abdominal pain and nausea, followed by vomiting and often diarrhea. Symptoms usually present between 2 and 6 hours after ingestion and are self-limited to 24 hours. Persistent symptoms should prompt a search for another cause. Significant morbidity is possible, especially in high-risk populations at greatest risk for dehydration, such as the very old and young and those with numerous comorbid conditions. About 9000 deaths a year occur as a result of staphylococcal food poisoning in the United States.

MANAGEMENT

Treatment is symptomatic and supportive.

Clostridium perfringens

INTRODUCTION, EPIDEMIOLOGY, AND BACTERIOLOGY

Clostridium perfringens food poisoning is another common, underreported cause of enterotoxin-mediated food poisoning. Data from 1988 through 1992 indicate that it was the second leading cause of food-borne disease.[75]

C. perfringens is an anaerobic, gram-positive, spore-forming rod that is ubiquitous in the environment and is part of the normal intestinal flora of humans and many other organisms. In this respect, *C. perfringens* differs from *C. botulinum*, which is not considered normal gut flora. The bacterium is known to produce at least 13 different toxins that have been implicated in a number of human disease processes, including gas gangrene.[68] *C. perfringens* is subtyped into strains A through E, and an individual strain may only elaborate a limited repertoire of the 13 recognized toxins.[68] *C. perfringens* type A is the strain most often associated with production of the *C. perfringens* enterotoxin (CPE) implicated as the cause

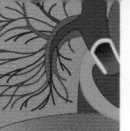

of food poisoning.[68] While 90% of food poisoning isolates are type A, surveys of all *C. perfringens* cultures found the incidence of plasmids containing the *cpe* gene to be fewer than 5%.[76]

Elaboration of enterotoxin occurs during spore formation, and sporulation is required for toxin release from the bacterial cell. The enterotoxin is thought to be a component of the spore coat. When heavily contaminated foodstuffs are ingested, the acidic environment of the stomach probably kills off large numbers of vegetative clostridial cells. However, if sufficient cells reach the small intestine, the bacteria may sporulate, and this leads to elaboration of the enterotoxin.[77] This second sporulation after ingestion suggests that CPE is not exactly a preformed toxin, but exerts its enterotoxigenic effect in such a fashion as to be indistinguishable clinically from ingestion of true preformed toxins associated with other infecting organisms.[68]

C. perfringens tends to contaminate high-protein foods such as meats, poultry, stews, and gravies, because the spores tend to survive the kinds of temperatures associated with roasting. If the food is then left at room temperature, the spores will germinate and proliferate.[68] CPE is heat labile and is inactivated at temperatures greater than 75° C. The toxin has also been shown to be inactivated by freeze-thawing. However, these practices are unlikely to alter or prevent food-borne illness since secondary sporulation in the small intestine is the major source of synthesis and amplification of CPE production.

Improper food handling is the usual source for many food poisoning outbreaks. One of the first and best reported instances occurred in January 1964 at a college in Spokane, Washington.[78] Forty-seven students became ill with diarrhea (81.8%), abdominal pain (75.5%), and headache (40.0%) after eating lamb stew for lunch.

Roast pork was implicated as the source in a diarrheal illness that affected 17 patients in two orthopedic wards at a hospital in England in December 1989.[79] After isolating *C. perfringens* type A from the pork, an inspection of the processing plant showed that a quick-freezing "blast chiller" had been replaced by a slower "shower" that gradually lowered the cooked meats' temperature to 2° C for packaging. Minced beef stew was implicated in a second large hospital outbreak in London in June 1989.[80] Sadly, 2 of the 58 ill patients died.

PATHOPHYSIOLOGY
The molecular mechanism by which CPE causes disease is not fully known. The toxin preferentially binds to intestinal lining cells of the ileum.[77] This results in the formation of a membrane complex that allows leakage of small molecules such as amino acids and ions.[77] In vitro work indicates that CPE does not affect fluid or electrolyte active transport,[77] nor does CPE act via cyclic adenosine monophosphate (cAMP) or cyclic guanosine monophosphate (cGMP).[68] Fluids and electrolytes may passively follow the gradient set up by the membrane complex–mediated loss of small molecules, or the loss of brush border cells and compromised gut integrity may lead to passive fluid losses. The effect of CPE on the brush border ultimately leads to death and sloughing of the intestinal epithelium.[77]

CLINICAL MANIFESTATIONS
Symptoms of *C. perfringens* food poisoning usually develop within 12 to 24 hours of ingestion. In vitro, however, CPE effects are seen in 15 to 30 minutes when applied to rabbit colon.[77] Diarrhea and abdominal cramps occur commonly, whereas nausea occurs only occasionally. Rarely, fever, chills, and vomiting may be present. In a November 1990 outbreak among conventioneers in Michigan linked to minestrone soup, 32 of 42 attendees experienced diarrhea (94%) and abdominal pain (91%) a median 6.5 hours after the meal.[81] Illness is generally self-limited and usually resolves within 24 hours. For instance, among 112 cases of clostridial-associated food poisoning after a firehouse luncheon in Maryland in 1984, illness lasted a mean of 21.2 hours after a median incubation period of 13.4 hours.[82] Death is rare and more often occurs in elderly debilitated patients.[80]

Serious hemorrhagic enteritis associated with toxins other than CPE has been associated with *C. perfringens* type C in both Germany and New Guinea.[83]

MANAGEMENT
Care is generally supportive, with appropriate volume and electrolyte replacement.

Vibrionaceae

INTRODUCTION, EPIDEMIOLOGY, AND BACTERIOLOGY
Vibrios are halophilic (characterized by their salt requirement), motile, gram-negative rods endemic in many coastal areas worldwide, including coastal areas of the western and, more commonly, the southern United States. The family Vibrionaceae includes the genera *Vibrio*, *Aeromonas*, and *Plesiomonas*. Thirteen species of *Vibrio* have the potential to cause human disease: 10 species cause food-borne gastroenteritis or septicemia, while *Vibrio metschnikovii* and *Vibrio damsela* cause wound infections and otitis externa associated with exposure to contaminated water.[84] Vibrios are routine pathogens of seafood worldwide since they reside in the intestinal tracts of fish, in shellfish, and in plankton.

Between 1983 and 1992, seafood (including shellfish) was the third most common vehicle implicated in food-borne illness cases (see Chapter 25).[85] While the most frequently isolated pathogen in shellfish-implicated illness was a virus, 20% of shellfish-related infections were caused by naturally occurring bacteria and only 4% from fecal contaminating bacteria.[85] Reliance on levels of fecal coliform contamination in coastal and estuarine waters is not an accurate indicator of the risk of shellfish-associated illness because fecal contaminating organisms make up such a small percentage of pathogens.

Vibrio cholerae is still associated with large-scale morbidity and mortality in several parts of the world. Cholera is the exception to the fecal contamination rule of shellfish-related illness since the last seven worldwide cholera outbreaks have been related to sewage contamination. The main vehicle in cholera illness associated with the toxigenic 01 (epidemic biotype) strain is raw oysters.[85] The more common strains associated with GI illness in the Unites States include non-01 biotype

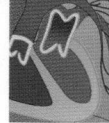

V. cholerae, Vibrio parahaemolyticus, Vibrio mimicus, Vibrio fluvialis, and *Vibrio hollisae.*[86]

V. parahaemolyticus has been isolated from seafood all over the world. It is the leading cause of seafood-borne disease in Japan, and the leading cause of *Vibrio*-associated illness in the United States, followed closely by non-01 *V. cholerae.*[84] *V. parahaemolyticus* survives in slightly colder temperatures than other vibrios and has been isolated from northern U.S. coastal waters. While the organism will not multiply at temperatures below 10° C, intact organisms have been recovered from frozen shrimp.[85] In 1998 in New York, there was a summer outbreak of 23 laboratory-confirmed cases of *V. parahaemolyticus* infection. Harvested shellfish from Long Island Sound and particularly Oyster Bay were implicated in 22 of the 23 cases. A similar outbreak occurred in British Columbia and Washington State in August 1997, when 51 persons became ill from raw oysters harvested on the British Columbia coast.[87]

PATHOPHYSIOLOGY

The mechanism by which *V. cholerae* 01 causes illness is well understood. Ingested organisms adhere to the intestinal lining epithelium and secrete a heterodimeric enterotoxin known as the cholera enterotoxin. One subunit of the cholera enterotoxin binds to ganglioside GM1 and facilitates entry of the active chain into the cell.[84] The active chain up-regulates adenylate cyclase, raising cAMP levels, which leads to uncontrolled chloride secretion into the lumen. Sodium absorption is coupled to chloride secretion, and its uptake into the cell is similarly impaired. Excess water follows the solute into the lumen. Ironically, it is absence or truncation of this chloride and water transmembrane transporter (cystic fibrosis transmembrane rectifier, or CFTR) that leads to lack of sufficient hydration of the mucus in the airways that characterizes classic cystic fibrosis. (The human impact of epidemic cholera in our past, and the high gene frequency of CFTR still maintained today, has led some anthropologists to hypothesize that while two copies of the defective gene confer the lethal recessive phenotype, carrier status for a defective CFTR may have conferred an evolutionary survival advantage against dehydration from cholera to past human populations.[88])

Much less is known about the toxin-mediated mechanisms of disease in non-01 *V. cholerae, Vibrio vulnificus,* and the minor *Vibrio* species. Polysaccharide encapsulation allows some pathogenic strains to evade the host defenses more effectively, and a capsule is associated with septicemia and extraintestinal manifestations.[84] *V. parahaemolyticus* causes diarrhea and gastroenteritis via a thermostable direct hemolysin enterotoxin, and this toxin is isolated from 96% of clinical isolates related to human illness, but only isolated from 1% of isolates in the environment.[84]

CLINICAL MANIFESTATIONS

Symptoms of cholera usually occur within 24 hours of ingestion of all *Vibrio* organisms. With cholera, patients develop an intense watery diarrhea with profuse fluid losses that may be as great as 1 L/hr. Severe cases (cholera gravis) often result in profound dehydration and death within 6 hours if not aggressively treated.

The signs and symptoms of noncholera, *Vibrio*-associated gastroenteritis almost always include diarrhea; vomiting, abdominal cramps, and fever are also common.[86] Bloody stool can also occur; as many as 86% of patients with *V. fluvialis* and 35% with *V. parahaemolyticus*–associated gastroenteritis develop bloody stool.[86] In the *V. parahaemolyticus* outbreak in New York in 1998, 17 of 23 patients (74%) with confirmed cases developed gastroenteritis a median of 19 hours after consumption of tainted shellfish; there were 2 patients (9%) with septicemia who had lower extremity edema and bullae.[89]

MANAGEMENT

Treatment of gastroenteritis due to both cholera and noncholera *Vibrio* infections is generally supportive. Aggressive oral rehydration or intravenous fluids with isotonic saline, glucose, and electrolyte replacement are required. Administration of drugs that interfere with adenylate cyclase or electrolyte fluxes across gut epithelial cells may significantly decrease volume losses. Chlorpromazine, aspirin, indomethacin, and nicotinic acid all have been shown to be effective in treating cholera.[90] Epidemic cholera toxin-mediated diarrhea must be monitored for volume status since assumptions about the adequacy of rehydration efforts are always underestimated. Tetracycline will shorten the course of the diarrheal illness. The widespread use of tetracycline, however, has led to broad resistance patterns.[84]

In non-01 *Vibrio*-associated gastroenteritis, supportive therapy is usually adequate. Special attention, however, must be given to patients at high risk for septicemia and shock (e.g., alcoholics, a history of liver disease, immunosuppression, and extremes of age). If a patient with a history of seafood consumption presents with GI signs or symptoms (particularly bloody diarrhea) and is at higher risk for severe illness, empiric treatment with tetracycline and an aminoglycoside is recommended. If systemic signs or symptoms of illness are present (e.g., shock, edema, and/or bullae), antibiotic treatment is clearly indicated.

Bacillus cereus

INTRODUCTION, EPIDEMIOLOGY, AND BACTERIOLOGY

Bacillus cereus is an aerobic, gram-positive, spore-forming rod that is ubiquitous in the environment and causes two distinct food-borne illness syndromes. These clinically and epidemiologically different illnesses are also associated with different foodstuffs. The rapid onset of emetic illness resembles staphylococcal food poisoning, while the delayed diarrheal disease mimics *C. perfringens* food poisoning. For this reason, *B. cereus* is an infrequently reported cause of food-borne illness outbreaks.[91]

In 1993, 14 of 67 children and daycare workers who ate a catered lunch with fried rice at two centers in Fairfax, Virginia, became ill with vomiting a median 2 hours after the meal and had resolution of symptoms a

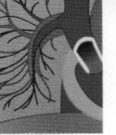

median of 4 hours after onset.[92] Fried rice is the foodstuff usually associated with the emetic form of *B. cereus* infection.[75] Rice that is cooked (boiled or steamed) and then cooled allows the spores of *B. cereus* to multiply and elaborate enterotoxins, including the emetic toxin cereulide. Subsequent reheating, such as pan frying, may not be enough to inactivate the toxins. Chinese food was implicated in 24 of 58 separate outbreaks in the United States between 1973 and 1987.[93] Measures of toxin production in foods implicated in 14 food-borne outbreaks have documented levels ranging from 10 to 1280 ng/g, and toxin titer correlates with the viable colony count of *B. cereus*.[76] Fried rice, boiled rice, dumplings, pasta, bread, noodles, tempura, and soba appear to yield the highest toxin production. Bacterial growth and toxin production are relatively inhibited on meat and eggs, milk products, and vinegar-, mayonnaise-, and tomato-based dishes.[76]

In a food-borne outbreak in Quebec in 1999, 25 of 37 diners at a catered banquet became ill with diarrhea (100%), abdominal pain (100%), and nausea (20%) within 24 hours.[94] Mayonnaise used in potato salad grew *B. cereus*. Another caterer was implicated as the source of a hospital cafeteria outbreak in October 1985 in Memphis, Tennessee. One hundred sixty of 249 hospital employees who ate an ethnic meal on either the day shift (lunch) or evening shift (dinner) suffered diarrhea and abdominal pain within 24 hours of their individual meal.[95] Food items maintained at moderate heat during delivery were implicated in an unusual outbreak associated with Meals-on-Wheels in England in November 1976.[96] Forty-nine of 160 elderly people developed diarrhea and abdominal pain a mean 7 hours after eating; 1 woman was found dead. *B. cereus* was isolated from several patients and the leftovers of one refrigerated meal.[83]

PATHOPHYSIOLOGY

Illness due to *B. cereus* is via the elaboration of two distinct enterotoxins. The emetic toxin cereulide is a 12–amino acid, hydrophobic, highly heat-stable toxin that causes a self-limited vomiting-type illness.[97] In vitro research suggests that cereulide may act as a potential potassium ionophore,[76] and may be a mitochondrial poison that uncouples oxidative phosphorylation.[98]

In contrast to the emetic form of *B. cereus* food poisoning, the diarrheal syndrome of *B. cereus* may be caused by one or more heat-labile enterotoxins. Research has found two similar polypeptide toxins, a hemolytic enterotoxin (HBL) and a nonhemolytic enterotoxin (NHE), to be implicated in *B. cereus* diarrheal food poisoning. The mechanism by which this family of enterotoxins causes diarrheal disease is not well known; however, both HBL and NHE are heterotrimers, and all three peptide chains are required for toxin activity.[68] Similarities to other biologic protein toxins suggests that one peptide chain is responsible for translocation into the cell while another or both exert the cytotoxic effect.

CLINICAL MANIFESTATIONS

The emetic form of *B. cereus* food poisoning has a more rapid onset and shorter clinical course than the diarrheal form. Patients usually become ill within 1 to 5 hours of tainted food ingestion and recover within 24 hours. Diarrhea and abdominal cramps may occur but are not a prominent feature of the emetic form. Despite the apparent innocuous nature of the emetic form of *B. cereus* food poisoning, serious illness is reported. For instance, death from liver failure occurred in a 17-year-old after infection.[99]

The diarrheal form of disease is associated with a broader array of foodstuffs: meat, poultry, eggs, casserole, puddings, and dairy products. After an incubation period of 8 to 24 hours, the symptoms of diarrhea and crampy abdominal pain predominate, with nausea present in a minority of patients.

As with the emetic form of the illness, recovery is usually complete within 24 hours of symptom onset.

DIAGNOSIS

B. cereus food poisoning may be diagnosed by isolation of greater than or equal to 105 organisms per gram of food. The diagnosis in outbreaks of the emetic form, however, may prove difficult if sufficient reheating has killed the organisms but has not inactivated the heat-stable toxin, cereulide. In these instances, testing for the toxin by means of the HEp-2 vacuolation assay may be diagnostic. In suspected outbreaks of the diarrheal form of *B. cereus* food poisoning, stool culture may be more reliable. Commercial assays for the detection of the hemolytic enterotoxin (latex agglutination) and the nonhemolytic enterotoxin (enzyme-linked immunosorbent assay) are available as a public health laboratory tool.[68]

MANAGEMENT

Most cases of *B. cereus* food poisoning are mild and self-limited; treatment is supportive.

Salmonella, Shigella, *and* Campylobacter

Salmonella, *Shigella*, and *Campylobacter* are the most common forms of acute infective bacterial GI illness in the United States.[100] The three genera are remarkably similar in many ways, including source of infection, symptoms of illness, localized invasion of the bowel epithelium, and duration of disease. The clinical syndromes associated with these enteroinvasive pathogens are similar. Toxin-mediated pathophysiology can play a minor role in food-borne illness (*Salmonella* species), or it may lead to serious sequelae, as in the case of Shiga toxin and Shiga-like verocytotoxins.[63] The three infective bacterial food-borne pathogens are presented here with an emphasis on their toxin-mediated effects.

SALMONELLA

Introduction, Epidemiology, and Bacteriology

Salmonellae are motile, gram-negative rods that are ubiquitous in nature and are known to colonize the intestinal tracts of a wide variety of organisms, including mammals, reptiles, and even insects.[101] The bacterium is resistant to freezing and drying but is rapidly killed by high temperatures. More than 2000 serovars of *Salmonella*

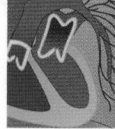

have been identified; the most common associated with food-borne illness are caused by *Salmonella enteridis*, *Salmonella typhimurium*, and *Salmonella paratyphi*.[86]

Salmonella species were the most frequently isolated food-borne pathogen in the United States between 1988 and 1992.[59] From 1992 to 1995, the incidence of both *Salmonella* and *Shigella* infections (both notifiable illnesses) increased in the United States.[102] The Foodborne Diseases Active Surveillance Network (FoodNet) 1996 data indicate that salmonellosis had the second highest incidence rate (16 per 100,000 population) among the top seven pathogens isolated at monitored sites.[103]

In 1984, in Oregon, *Salmonella* was used as a biologic weapon; it was released on the population of several towns in an attempt to influence voter turnout in favor of candidates from a particular religious commune in the county.[62] The disparate sources of infection at several nonchain restaurants, and the panantibiotic sensitivity of the *Salmonella* strain involved raised suspicion among public health authorities. Two years later, during a raid on the groups' compound, the offending strain of *Salmonella* was found in their infirmary freezer. The cult's chief scientist and a clinician were convicted of orchestrating the attack.[104]

The two most common sources of salmonellosis are food or water contaminated with the organism. Transmission normally occurs via the fecal-oral route. Food sources commonly associated with outbreaks include raw or undercooked eggs, unpasteurized milk and dairy products, and various meats, especially poultry.[86] A study conducted in homes in four U.S. cities demonstrated significant levels of *Salmonella* (4.5×10^2 colony-forming units per mL) in the dishwater wrung from used sponges and cotton dishtowels in 15.4% of the samples taken.[105]

Sources implicated in the fecal-oral route include household dogs and cats and occasionally uninfected carriers, particularly children in daycare settings.[85] In the past, a number of infections were associated with pet turtles, which led to a prohibition of their sale in the United States.[85]

Pathophysiology

Once ingested, the *Salmonella* bacterium must survive the host defenses, including gastric acidity and competition with normal flora. Medications that raise gastric pH may reduce the inoculum required.[106] Once past the gastric barrier, the organisms multiply in the small intestine and penetrate the intestinal mucosa, where they proliferate within mesenteric lymphoid tissue.[107] The majority of infections do not spread beyond the local lymphoid tissue. The actual mechanism by which *Salmonella* causes diarrhea is not well understood but may involve local infiltration of polymorphonuclear leukocytes and release of prostaglandins, which increase intestinal fluid secretion.[92] It has been demonstrated that *S. typhimurium* produces a cholera-like enterotoxin, but its role in vivo is not clear.[92]

Clinical Manifestations

Salmonella gastroenteritis has an incubation period of 5 to 72 hours. Symptoms of disease generally last from 2 to 5 days, but in certain cases, an asymptomatic carrier state may persist for as long as a year.[86] Nausea and vomiting are the most common symptoms and are usually followed by low-grade fever, chills, abdominal pain, and diarrhea.[86] In the largest single outbreak of food-borne illness aboard commercial airliners, 186 passengers on 29 transatlantic flights developed diarrhea (99%), abdominal pain (98%), fever (90%), and vomiting (58%) a median 2 to 72 hours after the planes landed.[108] The planes all originated in London and disembarked at 11 U.S. cities. The first-class meal was associated with illness, presumably due to its maintenance at a permissive temperature, and *Salmonella* was isolated from 56 (30%) cases.[108] In the same researchers' subsequent literature review, in 23 reported aircraft-involved food-borne outbreaks, *Salmonella* was the most frequently isolated pathogen (n = 7), followed by staphylococci (n = 5) and *Vibrio* species (n = 5).

Enteric (typhoid) fever, commonly associated with *Salmonella typhi* infection and popularized by the asymptomatic carrier Typhoid Mary, is a more severe form of salmonellosis associated with a longer incubation period (1 to 2 weeks), sustained fever, malaise, weakness, bacteremia, and occasionally shock and multiple organ dysfunction.[85] The largest U.S. outbreak of typhoid fever occurred at a New York hotel during a convention on July 13, 1989.[109] The incubation period was up to 3 weeks in conventioneers who had consumed the contaminated orange juice at a breakfast.[109] While typhoid fever outbreaks do occur, the incidence of typhoid among returning travelers from endemic areas is in decline; an oral vaccine (TY21a, or Vivotif [Berna Biotech, Berne, Switzerland]) with 70% efficacy for a period of 3 to 5 months may account for the decrease.[110]

The course of the disease is more severe and protracted in the very young, the elderly, and immunocompromised patients. Patients with acquired immunodeficiency syndrome and patients with certain hemolytic anemias such as sickle cell anemia are at a much higher risk for developing *Salmonella* bacteremia owing to decreased clearance by the autolyzed spleen.[111] *Salmonella* is the most frequently isolated pathogen from patients with sickle cell disease who develop osteomyelitis.[112]

Diagnosis

The diagnosis of *Salmonella* gastroenteritis is based on a patient's history, and confirmation of diagnosis requires stool culture. Microscopic examination of the stool usually reveals fecal leukocytes, and the stool may contain occult blood.

Management

In most cases, the treatment of salmonellosis is supportive, with fluid and electrolyte replacement as needed. Antibiotics are not recommended in uncomplicated cases because they do not alter the severity of disease and may prolong the carrier state. Antibiotics are reserved for more serious cases such as those associated with significant colitis, or cases in high-risk patients.[86] First-line therapy in typhoid fever is a third-generation cephalosporin. Antimotility agents, which slow intestinal transport times, may lead to intestinal perforation and

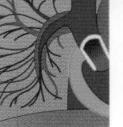
are not recommended in cases of invasive diarrheas such as salmonellosis.

SHIGELLA

Introduction, Epidemiology, and Bacteriology

Members of the genus *Shigella* are small, nonmotile, gram-negative rods that are very similar morphologically and biochemically to *E. coli*. Four different species are associated with human infection: *Shigella dysenteriae*, *Shigella flexneri*, *Shigella sonnei*, and *Shigella boydii*. *S. sonnei* and *S. flexneri* are responsible for the majority of cases in the United States.[113] FoodNet data from 1996 and 1997 showed shigellosis to have the third highest incidence (7.8 per 100,000 population) among the seven pathogens tracked at surveillance sites.[114] A more severe form of infection, bacillary dysentery, is often associated with *S. dysenteriae* infection. The organism has a very low infectious dose, and disease developed in some volunteers fed as few as 100 organisms.[93]

The fecal-oral route is the primary mode of transmitting *Shigella* infection. The majority of infections are spread by consumption of food or water contaminated with fecal material from an infected individual. *Shigella* outbreaks commonly occur in daycare centers, mental health institutions, prisons, and nursing homes, where overcrowding, poor hygiene, and unsanitary conditions may exist.[93]

Outbreaks have been associated with various contaminated foods, and reports indicate that *Shigella* can live for many days on certain foods outside of its normal human host.

Pathophysiology

Shigella organisms possess a high degree of acid resistance and as such are able to survive passage through the acidic gastric barrier quite well. Once ingested, the organisms invade the epithelial lining cells of the intestine, multiply intracellularly, and spread to surrounding cells. Local damage to intestinal epithelium and superficial erosion of the intestinal mucosa are responsible for the presence of blood and fecal leukocytes in the stool.

S. dysenteriae produces the potent cytotoxin Shiga toxin. Shiga toxin is one of a number of naturally occurring cytotoxins that inhibit protein synthesis by inactivating the ribosome (ribosomal inhibitory protein II, or RIP II).[115] This family of heteromeric polypeptides includes various plant-derived RIP IIs such as the toxalbumins (*Abrus precatorius, Viscum album*), of which ricin (*Ricinus communis*) is the most common.

Heterodimeric toxins in this family enter the cell (after binding of the B chain) via endocytosis, and are actively transported in retrograde fashion by carriers through the Golgi apparatus to the endoplasmic reticulum (ER).[63] Once the toxin reaches the ER, the A chain binds to the 60S subunit of the ribosome. The active site of the toxic A chain removes an adenine from the nascent 28S RNA, which prevents the attachment of elongation factor 2 (EF-2).[100] Left unprotected by EF-2, the RNA is rapidly degraded and protein synthesis halted. In the intestinal lining cells of the gut, Shiga toxin's B chain binds to the neutral glycosphingolipid Gb3 to facilitate entry, and the A chain must be cleaved to an A1 fragment before it can bind to the ribosome.[63]

Shigalike toxins (SLTs), also known as verocytotoxins because they act on Vero cells, may be elaborated by certain strains of enterohemorrhagic *E. coli* (EHEC).[63] SLTs are cytotoxic to a range of endothelial cells, whereby they cause end-organ injury. The two best studied of these SLTs (SLT-I and SLT-II) are associated with EHEC strain 0157:H7.[63] These toxins damage endothelial cells in the kidney, leading to renal failure, and vascular endothelial cells, causing microangiopathic anemia and thrombocytopenia: the hemolytic uremic syndrome. Another porcine strain of EHEC produces a variant SLT-IIv, which causes massive edema.[63]

Clinical Manifestations

The incubation period in shigellosis is usually 24 to 48 hours. The clinical presentation has a wide spectrum; some individuals have nonspecific symptoms and a short course of watery diarrhea only.[113] More severe forms of the disease may progress to true dysentery, including high fever, tenesmus, nausea, abdominal pain, and profuse watery diarrhea that evolves over hours to a few days to mucoid, bloody stools.[113] Untreated shigellosis is usually self-limited, and the illness usually persists for 1 week. An individual may continue to shed organisms in the stool for several weeks after clinical infection subsides. Laboratory findings may include leukocytosis and the presence of fecal leukocytes in addition to occult or grossly bloody stool. Complications include seizures (especially in children), dehydration, and death in the very elderly or in children younger than 1 year.[116]

Diagnosis

Shigellosis is the principal bacterial cause of dysentery and should be suspected whenever a patient presents with bloody diarrhea. The diagnosis is based on culture of *Shigella* from stool. Diagnosis may also be suspected when polymerase chain reaction or commercial enzyme immunoassay techniques detect Shiga family toxins in stool.

Management

Treatment for shigellosis is initially supportive, with attention to correcting fluid and electrolyte abnormalities. Antibiotic therapy has been shown to improve the clinical course of the disease, but patients are often already improving when culture results become available. Antibiotics are therefore reserved for patients who are not showing signs of improvement or who have more severe forms of infection. All individuals who have culture-proven *S. dysenteriae* or those with other *Shigella* species who are at high risk for infecting others should receive antibiotics. Specific antibiotics recommended include fluoroquinolones (i.e., ciprofloxacin, 500 mg/day for 5 days in adults), ampicillin (50 to 100 mg/kg/day in children or 2 g/day in adults for 5 days), or trimethoprim-sulfamethoxazole (5/25 mg/kg po bid in children or 160 mg TMP/800 mg 5MX po bid in adults

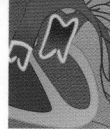

for 5 days). Shigella infection is an invasive enterocolitis and, as such, antimotility agents are not recommended. Recommendations for children in daycare centers with culture-proven *Shigella* require antibiotic therapy and repeat negative follow-up cultures before returning to daycare.[113]

CAMPYLOBACTER

Introduction, Epidemiology, and Bacteriology

Campylobacter species are small, motile, curved or S-shaped, gram-negative bacteria. *Campylobacter* enteritis is today one of the most commonly identified bacterial causes of diarrhea. Human disease is most commonly caused by *Campylobacter jejuni,* which is a part of the normal flora of a wide variety of animals including cattle, sheep, pigs, and poultry.[117] *Campylobacter* may also be found in unpurified drinking water such as that in rural areas or in contaminated springs, and unpasteurized dairy products from infected animals.[96] The primary mode of transmission of *Campylobacter* is fecal-oral.

In addition to infection from contaminated drinking water, various foods are associated with infection. Food may become contaminated with organisms at slaughterhouses whenever improper handling occurs or when intestinal spillage comes into contact with animal carcasses. Contaminated meat and poultry products are commonly associated with infection. *Campylobacter* does not proliferate on foods that it has contaminated as do other enteric organisms such as *Salmonella* species, *Bacillus* species, and *S. aureus*. The organism may actually survive longer if refrigerated and can survive in water or unpasteurized milk for weeks.[116]

Campylobacteriosis was the most frequently isolated food-borne pathogen (incidence 24.7 per 100,000 population) by the FoodNet sites in 1996 and 1997.[103]

Clinical Manifestations

Fever, headache, malaise, myalgias, and cramping abdominal pain usually occur in the first 48 hours after ingestion of an infectious dose of organisms.[118] Diarrhea usually presents within 24 hours after the onset of abdominal pain and may be described as watery, bile stained, mucoid, or grossly bloody.[118]

Clinical disease usually does not persist for more than a week. Relapse is not uncommon, and the organism may be shed for several weeks in the stools of asymptomatic individuals.

Diagnosis

The definitive diagnosis of *Campylobacter* enteritis is based on identification of the organism on stool culture.

Management

Treatment is primarily supportive; fluid and electrolyte repletion should be provided as necessary. The clinical benefit of antibiotic therapy for *Campylobacter* enteritis is not fully known; it is recommended for patients with significant local (e.g., bloody diarrhea) or systemic illness (e.g., high fever, toxic appearance) and protracted symptoms (e.g., beyond 7 days). First-line

therapy is erythromycin (adult, 500 mg erythromycin stearate, base or salt orally every 8 hours for 5 to 7 days; child, 30 to 50 mg/kg/day base orally divided every 6 to 8 hours for 5 to 7 days not to exceed 1 g/day). Alternative therapies include other macrolides (e.g., clarithromycin or azithromycin) or fluoroquinolones (e.g., ciprofloxacin). Full recovery is expected for nearly all patients, regardless of treatment with antimicrobial therapy.

REFERENCES

1. Hatheway CL: Botulism: the present status of the disease. Curr Top Microbiol Immunol 1995;195:55–75.
2. Bakheit AM, Ward CD, McLellan DL: Generalised botulism-like syndrome after intramuscular injections of botulinum toxin type A: a report of two cases. J Neurol Neurosurg Psychiatry 1997;62(2):198.
3. Shapiro RL, Hatheway C, Swerdlow DL: Botulism in the United States: a clinical and epidemiologic review. Ann Intern Med 1998;129(3):221–228.
4. Passaro DJ, Werner WS, McGee J, et al: Wound botulism associated with black tar heroin among injecting drug users. JAMA 1998;279(11):859–863.
5. Wiggington JM, Thill P: Infant botulism: a review of the literature. Clin Pediatr 1993;32:669–674.
6. Shreiner MS, Field E, Ruddy R: Infant botulism: a review of 12 years experience at The Children's Hospital of Philadelphia. Pediatrics 1991;87:159–165.
7. Li LYJ, Kelkar P, Exconde RE, et al: Adult-onset botulism: an unusual cause of weakness in the intensive care unit. Neurology 1999;53(4):891.
8. Centers for Disease Control and Prevention (CDC): Botulism in the United States, 1899–1977: Handbook for Epidemiologists, Clinicians, and Laboratory Workers. Washington, DC, CDC, 1979, pp 1–49.
9. Simpson LL: The origin, structure, and pharmacological activity of botulinum toxin. Pharmacol Rev 1981;33:155–188.
10. Durban EE, Durban M, Grecz N: Production of spore spheroplasts of Clostridium botulinum and DNA extraction for density gradient centrifugation. Can J Microbiol 1974;20:353–358.
11. Simpson LL: The action of botulinal toxin. Rev Infect Dis 1979;1:656–662.
12. Hambleton P: Clostridium botulinum toxins: a general review of involvement disease, structure, mode of action, and preparation for clinical use. J Neurol 1992;239:16–20.
13. Dowell VR Jr: Botulism and tetanus: selected epidemiologic and microbiologic aspects. Rev Infect Dis 1984;6(Suppl 1):202–207.
14. Dodds KL: Clostridium botulinum. In Hui YH, Gorham JR, Murrell KD, Oliver DO (eds): Foodborne Disease Handbook. New York, Marcel Dekker, 1994, pp 97–132.
15. Van Ermengem EP: Über einen neuen anaeroben Bacillus und seine Beziehung zum Botulismus. Z Hyg Infektionskrankh 1897;26:1–56. [English translation: Classics in infectious diseases: a new anaerobic bacillus and its relation to botulism. Rev Infect Dis 1979;4:701–719.]
16. Macdonald KL, Cohen ML, Blake PA: The changing epidemiology of adult botulism in the United States. Am J Epidemiol 1986;124:794–799.
17. MacDonald KL, Spengler RF, Hathaway CL, et al: Type A botulism from sauteed onions: clinical and epidemiologic observations. JAMA 1985;253:1275–1278.
18. Mann JM, Martin S, Hoffman R, et al: Patient recovery from type A botulism: morbidity assessment following a large outbreak. Am J Public Health 1981;71:266–269.
19. Centers for Disease Control and Prevention: Foodborne botulism—Oklahoma, 1994. MMWR Morb Mortal Wkly Rep 1995;44:200–202.
20. Centers for Disease Control and Prevention: Botulism and commercial pot pie—California. MMWR Morb Mortal Wkly Rep 1983;32:39–40, 45.
21. Hauschild AHW, Gavreau L: Food-borne botulism in Canada, 1971–84. CMAJ 1985;133:1141–1146.

22. Webber JT, Tauxe RV, Weber JT, et al: A massive outbreak of type E botulism associated with traditional salted fish in Cairo. J Infect Dis 1993;167:451–454.

23. Centers for Disease Control and Prevention: Fish botulism—Hawaii, 1990. JAMA 1991;266:324, 327.

24. Jaeger A: Botulism as warfare agent: features, management and treatment. J Toxicol Clin Toxicol 2002;40:246–248.

25. Schiavo G, Benefenati F, Poulain B, et al: Tetanus and botulinum-B neurotoxins block neurotransmitter release by a proteolytic cleavage of synaptobrevin. Nature 1992;359:832–835.

26. Blasi J, Chapman ER, Link E, et al: Botulinum neurotoxin A selectively cleaves the synaptic protein SNAP-25. Nature 1993;365:160–163.

27. Sellin LC, Thesleff S, Dasgupta BR: Different affects of types A and B botulinum toxin on transmitter release at the rat neuromuscular junction. Acta Physiol Scand 1983;119:127–133.

28. St. Louis ME, Peck SH, Bowering D, et al: Botulism from chopped garlic: delayed recognition of a major outbreak. Ann Intern Med 1988;108:363–368.

29. Hughes JM, Blumenthal JR, Mersom MH, et al: Clinical features of types A and B food-borne botulism. Ann Intern Med 1981;95:442–445.

30. Ruthman JC, Hendricksen DK, Bonefield R: Emergency department presentation of type A botulism. Am J Emerg Med 1985;3:203–205.

31. Terranova W, Bremen JG, Palumbo JN: Ocular findings in botulism type B. JAMA 1979;241:475–477.

32. Terranova W, Bremen JC, Locey RP, Speck S: Botulism type B: epidemiologic aspects of an extensive outbreak. Am J Epidemiol 1978;108:150–156.

33. Simcock PR, Kelleher S, Dunne JA: Neuro-ophthalmic findings in botulism type B. Eye 1994;8:646–648.

34. Sellin LC: Botulism—an update. Milit Med 1984;149:12–16.

35. Cherington M: Botulism: ten-year experience. Arch Neurol 1974;30:432–437.

36. Sanders AB, Seifert S, Kobernick M: Botulism: clinical review. J Fam Pract 1983;16:987–1000.

37. Schmidt-Nowara WW, Samet JM, Rosario PA: Early and late pulmonary complications of botulism. Arch Intern Med 1983;143:451–456.

38. Centers for Disease Control and Prevention: Release of botulism antitoxin. MMWR Morb Mortal Wkly Rep 1986;35:490–491.

39. Hughes JM, Tacket CO: Sausage poisoning revisited [Editorial]. Arch Intern Med 1983;143:425–427.

40. Gomez HF, Johnson R, Guven H, et al: Adsorption of botulinum toxin to activated charcoal with a mouse bioassay. Ann Emerg Med 1995;25:818–822.

41. Tacket CO, Shandera WX, Mann JM, et al: Equine antitoxin use and other factors that predict outcome in type A foodborne botulism. Am J Med 1984;76:794–798.

42. Hatheway CL, Snyder JD, Seals JE, et al: Antitoxin levels in botulism patients treated with trivalent equine botulism antitoxin to toxin types A, B, and E. J Infect Dis 1984;150:407–412.

43. Black RE, Gunn RA: Hypersensitivity reactions associated with botulinal antitoxin. Am J Med 1980;69:567–570.

44. Clayton MA, Clayton JM, Brown DR, Middlebrook JL: Protective vaccination with a recombinant fragment of Clostridium botulinum neurotoxin serotype A expressed from a synthetic gene in Escherichia coli. Infect Immun 1995;63:2738–2742.

45. Aureli P, Fencia L, Pasolini B, et al: Two cases of type E infant botulism caused by neurotoxigenic Clostridium butyricum in Italy. J Infect Dis 1986;154:207–211.

46. Woodruff BA, Hatheway CL, Griffin PM, et al: Clinical and laboratory comparison of botulism from toxin types A, B, and E in the United States, 1975–1988. J Infect Dis 1992;166:1281–1286.

47. Arnon SS: Infant botulism: anticipating the second decade. J Infect Dis 1986;154:201–206.

48. Arnon SS: Breast feeding and toxigenic intestinal infections: missing links in crib death? Rev Infect Dis 1984;6(Suppl 1):193–201.

49. Long SS, Gajewski JL, Brown LW, Gilligan PH: Clinical, laboratory, and environmental features of infant botulism in southeastern Pennsylvania. Pediatrics 1985;75:935–941.

50. Istre GR, Compton R, Novotny T, et al: Infant botulism: three cases in a small town. Am J Dis Child 1986;140:1013–1014.

51. Schmidt RD, Schmidt TW: Infant botulism: a case series and review of the literature. J Emerg Med 1992;10:713–718.

52. Centers for Disease Control and Prevention: Wound botulism associated with parenteral cocaine abuse—New York City. MMWR Morb Mortal Wkly Rep 1982;37(7):87–88.

53. Passaro DJ, Werner SB, McGee J, et al: Wound botulism associated with black tar heroin among injecting drug users. JAMA 1998;279(11):859–863.

54. Centers for Disease Control and Prevention: Wound botulism among black tar heroin users—Washington, 2003. MMWR Morb Mortal Wkly Rep 2003;52(37):885–886.

55. Weber JT, Goodpasture HC, Alexander H, et al: Wound botulism in a patient with a tooth abscess: case report and review. Clin Infect Dis 1993;16:635–639.

56. Tugnoli V, Eleopra R, Quatrale R, et al: Botulism-like syndrome after botulinum toxin type A injections for focal hyperhidrosis. Br J Dermatol 2002;147:808.

57. Bakheit AMO, Ward CD, McLellan DL: Generalized botulism-like syndrome after intramuscular injections of botulinum toxin type A: a report of two cases. J Neurol Neurosurg Psychiatry 1997;62(2):198.

58. Cobb DB, Watson WA, Fernandez MC: Botulism-like syndrome after injections of botulinum toxin. Vet Hum Toxicol 2000;42(3):163.

59. Todd EC: Epidemiology of foodborne diseases: a worldwide review. World Health Stat Q 1997;50:30–50.

60. Majkowski J: Strategies for rapid response to emerging foodborne microbial hazards. Emerg Infect Dis 1997;3(4):551–554.

61. Hennessey TW, Hedberg CW, Slutsker L, et al: A national outbreak of Salmonella enteriditis infections from ice cream. N Engl J Med 1996;334:1281–1286.

62. Torok TJ, Tauxe RV, Wise RP, et al: A large outbreak of salmonellosis caused by intentional contamination of restaurant salad bars. JAMA 1997;278(5):389–395.

63. Sandvig K, Garred O, van Deurs B: Intracellular transport and processing of protein toxins produced by enteric bacteria. In Paul PS, Francis DH, Benfield DA, et al (eds): Mechanisms in the Pathogenesis of Enteric Diseases. New York, Plenum, 1997.

64. Bunning VK, Lindsay JA, Archer DL: Chronic health effects of microbial foodborne disease. World Health Stat Q 1997;50:51–56.

65. Balaban N, Rasooly A: Staphylococcal enterotoxins. Int J Food Microb 2000;61:1–10.

66. Rosec JP, Guirard JP, Dalet C, et al: Enterotoxin production by staphylococci isolated from food in France. Int J Food Microb 1997;35:213.

67. Kambaty FM, Bennett RW, Shah DB: Application of pulsed field gel electrophoresis to the epidemiological characterization of Staphylococcus intermedius implicated in a food-related outbreak. Epidemiol Infect 1994;113:75–81.

68. Crane JK: Preformed bacterial toxins. Clin Lab Med 1999;19(3):583–599.

69. Martin SE, Myers ER: Staphylococcus aureus. In Hui YH, Gorham JR, Murrell KD, Oliver DO (eds): Foodborne Diseases Handbook. New York, Marcel Dekker, 1994, pp 345–394.

70. Richards MS, Rittman M, Gilbert TT, et al: Investigation of a staphylococcal food poisoning in a centralized school lunch program. Pub Health Rep 1993;108(6):765–771.

71. Holmberg SD, Blake PA: Staphylococcal food poisoning in the United States: new facts and old misconceptions. JAMA 1984;251:487–489.

72. Asao T, Kumeda Y, Kawai T, et al: An extensive outbreak of staphylococcal food poisoning due to low-fat milk in Japan: estimation of enterotoxin A in the incriminated milk and skim milk. Epidemiol Infect 2003;130(1):33–40.

73. Woolaway MC, Bartlett CLR, Wieneke AA, et al: International outbreak of staphylococcal food poisoning caused by contaminated lasagna. J Hygiene 1986;96:67–73.

74. Hamad AR, Marrack P, Kappler JW: Transcytosis of staphylococcal superantigen toxins. J Exp Med 1997;185:1447–1454.

75. Centers for Disease Control and Prevention: Foodborne disease outbreaks, 5 year summary, 1988–1992. MMWR Morb Mortal Wkly Rep 1996;45:1.

76. Ridell J, Bjorkroth J, Eisgruber H, et al: Prevalence of the enterotoxin gene and clonality of Clostridium perfringens strains associated with food-poisoning outbreaks. J Food Protect 1998;61:240.

77. McClane BA: An overview of *Clostridium perfringens* enterotoxin. Toxicon 1996;34:1335–1343.

78. Nelson KE, Ager EA, Marks JA, Emanuel I: *Clostridium perfringens* food poisoning: report of an outbreak. Am J Epidemiol 1966;83(1):86–95.

79. Regan CM, Syed Q, Tunstall PJ: A hospital outbreak of *Clostridium perfringens* food poisoning—implications for food hygiene review in hospitals. J Hosp Infect 1995;29:69–73.

80. Pollock AM, Whitty PM: Outbreak of *Clostridium perfringens* food poisoning. J Hosp Infect 1991;17:179–186.

81. Roach RL, Sienko DG: *Clostridium perfringens* outbreak associated with minestrone soup. Am J Epidemiol 1992;136(10):1288–1291.

82. Gross TP, Kamara LB, Hatheway CL, et al: *Clostridium perfringens* food poisoning: use of serotyping in an outbreak setting. J Clin Microbiol 1989;27(4):660–663.

83. Shandera WX, Tacket CO, Blacke PA: Food poisoning due to *Clostridium perfringens* in the United States. J Infect Dis 1983;147:167–170.

84. Powell JL: *Vibrio* species. Clin Lab Med 1999;19(3):537–552.

85. Lipp EK, Rose JB: The role of seafood in foodborne diseases in the United States of America. Rev Sci Tech 1997;16(2):620–640.

86. Levine WC, Griffin PM: *Vibrio* infections on the Gulf coast: results of first year of regional surveillance. J Infect Dis 1993;167:479–483.

87. Centers for Disease Control and Prevention: Outbreak of *Vibrio parahaemolyticus* infections associated with eating raw oysters—Pacific Northwest, 1997. MMWR Morb Mortal Wkly Rep 1998;47(22):457–462.

88. Cuthbert AW, Halstead J, Ratcliff R, et al: The genetic advantage hypothesis in cystic fibrosis heterozygotes: a murine study. J Physiol 1995;482(Pt 2):449–454.

89. Centers for Disease Control and Prevention: Outbreak of *Vibrio parahaemolyticus* infection associated with eating raw oysters and clams harvested from Long Island Sound—Connecticut, New Jersey, and New York, 1998. MMWR Morb Mortal Wkly Rep 1999;48(3):48–51.

90. Morris JG, Black RE: Cholera and other vibrioses in the United States. N Engl J Med 1985;312:343–350.

91. Bean NH, Griffin PM: Foodborne outbreaks in the United States, 1973–1987: pathogens, vehicles, and trends. J Food Protect 1990;53:804–817.

92. Centers for Disease Control and Prevention: Epidemiologic notes and reports *Bacillus cereus* food poisoning associated with fried rice at two day care centers—Virginia, 1993. MMWR Morb Mortal Wkly Rep 1994;43(10):177–178.

93. Schultz FJ, Smith J: Bacillus: recent advances in *Bacillus cereus* food poisoning research. In Hui YH, Gorham JR, Murrell KD, Oliver DO (eds): Foodborne Disease Handbook. New York, Marcel Dekker, 1994, pp 29–62.

94. Gaulin C, Viger YB, Fillion L: An outbreak of *Bacillus cereus* implicating a part-time banquet caterer. Can J Pub Health 2002;93(5):353–355.

95. Baddour LM, Gaia SM, Griffin R, Hudson R: A hospital cafeteria-related foodborne outbreak due to *Bacillus cereus*: unique features. Infect Contr 1986;7(9):462–465.

96. Jephcott AE, Barton BW, Gilbert RJ, Shearer CW: An unusual outbreak of food-poisoning associated with meals-on-wheels. Lancet 1977;2:129–130.

97. Agata N, Ohta M, Yokoyama K: Production of *Bacillus cereus* emetic toxin (cereulide) in various foods. Int J Food Microbiol 2002;73:23–27.

98. Shinagawa K, Ueno Y, Hu D, et al: Mouse lethal activity of a HEp-2 vacuolation factor, cereulide, produced by *Bacillus cereus* isolated from vomiting-type food poisoning. J Vet Med Sci 1996;58:1027.

99. Mahler H, Pasi A, Kramer JM, et al: Fulminant liver failure in association with the emetic toxin of *Bacillus cereus*. N Engl J Med 1997;336:1142.

100. Stutman HR: *Salmonella, Shigella,* and *Campylobacter*: common causes of infectious diarrhea. Pediatr Ann 1994;23:538–543.

101. Baird-Parker AC: Foodborne salmonellosis. Lancet 1990;336:1231–1235.

102. Centers for Disease Control and Prevention: Summary of notifiable diseases, United States, 1995. MMWR Morb Mortal Wkly Rep 1996;44(53):1–88.

103. Centers for Disease Control and Prevention: Foodborne diseases active surveillance network, 1996. MMWR Morb Mortal Wkly Rep 1997;46(12):258–261.

104. Tucker JB (ed): Toxic Terror: Assessing Terrorist Use of Chemical and Biological Weapons. Cambridge, MA, MIT Press, 2000.

105. Enriquez CE, Enriquez-Gordillo R, Kennedy DI, et al: Bacteriological survey of used cellulose sponges and cotton dishcloths from domestic kitchens. Dairy Food Environ Sanitat 1997;17:20–24.

106. Gordon J, Small PL: Acid resistance in enteric bacteria. Infect Immun 1993;61:364–367.

107. Finlay BB: Molecular and cellular mechanisms of *Salmonella* pathogenesis. Curr Top Microbiol Immunol 1994;192:163–185.

108. Tauxe RV, Tormey MP, Mascola L, et al: Salmonellosis outbreak on transatlantic flights; foodborne illness on aircraft: 1947–84. Am J Epidemiol 1987;125(1):150–157.

109. Birkhead GS, Morse DL, Levine WC, et al: Typhoid fever at a resort hotel in New York: a large outbreak with an unusual vehicle. J Infect Dis 1993;167:1228–1232.

110. Schwartz MD: Fever in the returning traveler, part II: a methodological approach to initial management. Wild Environ Med 2003;14(2):120–130.

111. Workman MR, Philpott-Howard J, Bellingham AJ: Managing patients with an absent or dysfunctional spleen. Guidelines should highlight risk of *Salmonella* infection in sickle cell disease. BMJ 1996;312(7028):430–434.

112. Chambers JB, Forsythe DA, Bertrand SL, et al: Retrospective review of osteoarticular infections in a pediatric sickle cell age group. J Pediatr Orthop 2000;20(5):682–685.

113. Maurelli AT, Lampell KA: Shigella. In Hui YH, Gorham JR, Murrell KD, Oliver DO (eds): Foodborne Disease Handbook. New York, Marcel Dekker, 1994, pp 319–344.

114. Wallace DJ, van Gilder T, Shallow S, et al: Incidence of foodborne illness reported by the foodborne diseases active surveillance network (FoodNet)—1997. J Food Protect 2000;63(3):807–809.

115. Olsnes S, Kozlov JV: Ricin. Toxicon 2001;39:1723–1728.

116. Bennish ML, Harris JR, Wojtyniak BJ, et al: Death in shigellosis: incidence and risk factors in hospitalized patients. J Infect Dis 1990;161:500–506.

117. Franco DA, Williams CE: *Campylobacter jejuni*. In Hui YH, Gorham JR, Murrell KD, Oliver DO (eds): Foodborne Disease Handbook. New York, Marcel Dekker, 1994, pp 71–96.

118. Blaster MJ, Berkowitz ID, LaForce MF, et al: *Campylobacter enteritis*: clinical and epidemiologic features. Ann Intern Med 1979;91:179–185.

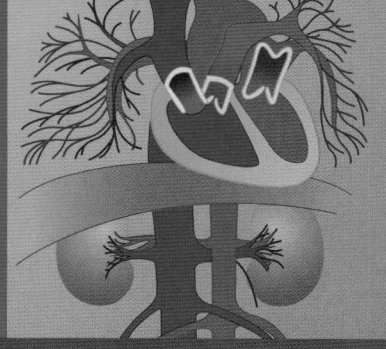

27 *Tricyclic and Other Cyclic Antidepressants*

D. ERIC BRUSH, MD ■ CYNTHIA K. AARON, MD

At a Glance...

■ Primary toxicity related to sodium channel blockade and subsequent effects on cardiac cell depolarization leads to ventricular dysrhythmias. Sodium channel blockade, GABAergic effects, and biogenic amine reuptake effects lead to seizures.

■ Secondary toxicity from inotropic depression and vascular dilation leads to profound hypotension.

■ Hallmark of toxicity seen on electrocardiogram is QRS prolongation and rightward axis deviation of the terminal 40 msec of the QRS complex.

■ Those at highest risk for seizures and ventricular dysrhythmias have a QRS greater than 100 msec or a terminal R wave in aVR greater than 3 mm.

■ Sodium bicarbonate is the primary treatment modality for severe intoxication.

■ Signs of significant toxicity mandate continuous monitoring until symptom free for 24 hours.

Toxicity due to cyclic antidepressant (CA) overdose dates back to 1959, shortly after the introduction of the antidepressant imipramine.[1-3] For several years preceding 1993, antidepressants were deemed responsible for the majority of deaths due to prescription drug overdose in the United States.[4,5] More recently, the number of deaths from antidepressants, including cyclic and noncyclic compounds, has been superseded by analgesic medications, although the number of reported exposures involving antidepressants has not significantly decreased.[6] Evolving epidemiology of antidepressant mortality may be due in part to prescribing practices. Preferential prescription of selective serotonin reuptake inhibitors (SSRIs) for depression, with their improved safety profile compared with cyclic antidepressants, may partly explain this trend. Some data suggest that the death-to-

prescription ratio for CAs exceeds that of other antidepressant classes.[7] Nevertheless, physicians continue to prescribe CAs for depression as well as for neuropathic pain, migraine, obsessive-compulsive disorder, enuresis, and a variety of other maladies. The actual number of prescriptions written for CAs is unknown, which limits interpretation of poison center data regarding exposures and deaths. This fact, coupled with underreporting of exposures and deaths to poison centers, makes conclusions regarding decreased exposure versus improved treatment impossible.[8] Among the antidepressant class of medications, CAs still account for the highest number of deaths. However, according to data from the Toxic Exposure Surveillance System (TESS), the number of deaths caused by SSRIs is gradually approaching that of CAs.[6] Although deaths from CAs have decreased in recent years compared to the 1980s, the number of deaths has remained fairly constant over the last decade, with approximately 100 deaths per year reported by the TESS.[4-6,9-16] These data are based on exposures reported to poison centers and require careful interpretation.

The number of children under 6 years of age exposed to CAs has remained relatively constant over the last few years according to TESS data. The majority of these cases are accidental exposures involving small ingestions or possibly no ingestion. The 2002 TESS data reports 1573 exposures to CAs in children less than 6 years of age.[6] The only deaths occurred from malicious poisonings. A 5-year retrospective study (years 1993 to 1997) of a single poison center's data regarding ingestions of tricyclic antidepressants (excluding monocyclic and tetracyclic drugs) in children less than 6 years of age revealed no deaths.[17] The majority of the children (92%) were asymptomatic, while the remaining patients exhibited mild sedation. Ninety percent of patients in this study ingested less than the age-appropriate dose. Although this study represents a small sample of patients in a retrospective poison center–based review, it identifies the typical features of CA exposure in young children: small

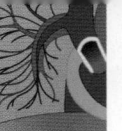

dose and low toxicity. Regardless, exposure histories in young children are difficult to elicit. One or two tablets may be sufficient to cause life-threatening toxicity in small children. Therefore, all exposures in this age group require careful evaluation.

STRUCTURE

Tricyclic antidepressants (TCAs) are a class of drugs that contain a three-ringed nucleus with various side chains and atomic substitutions (Fig. 27-1). The term *cyclic antidepressant* is more encompassing and includes drugs with ring structures beyond the three-ringed TCA nucleus (see Fig. 27-1). These include tetracyclic drugs such as amoxapine, maprotiline, and mirtazapine and bicyclics such as mianserin. The TCAs are broadly classified as secondary or tertiary amines in reference to the number of methyl groups on the propylamine side chain of the structure. The tertiary amines are imipramine, amitriptyline, clomipramine, chloripramine, doxepin, dothiepin, lofepramine, and trimipramine. The secondary amines include desipramine, nortriptyline, and protriptyline. In vivo demethylation of the tertiary amines amitriptyline and imipramine produces the active secondary amines nortriptyline and desipramine, respectively. Metabolism via hydroxylation creates multiple active metabolites (Table 27-1). Intermediate structures display differing degrees of pharmacodynamic actions; the extent of cholinergic receptor blockade in decreasing order of effect is tertiary amine > secondary amine > demethylated metabolites > hydroxylated metabolites.[18-20]

Structural similarities between CAs and phenothiazines as well as other classes of antipsychotic medications yield a likely explanation for shared toxicity as well as cross-reactivity in immunoassays. Anticholinergic, antihistaminic, and some cardiovascular effects such as sodium channel blockade, QT_c prolongation, and peripheral α blockade are shared to various extents by medications from these classes.

PHARMACOLOGY

Pharmacodynamics

Cyclic antidepressants exert their therapeutic action in part by producing varying degrees of reuptake inhibition of norepinephrine, dopamine, and serotonin at nerve terminals in the central nervous system (CNS). While this mechanism of action forms the basis of the monoamine hypothesis of depression, it describes only one of the many effects CAs exert in vivo. Although the monoamine hypothesis remains a likely explanation for much of the therapeutic benefit of antidepressants, alterations in other CNS signaling pathways have recently been discovered and may significantly contribute to drug efficacy in depression. The identification of γ-aminobutyric acid (GABA) and its putative role in depression has recently been elucidated through human brain scans and cerebrospinal fluid analysis as well as in vivo animal and in vitro models.[21] These studies demonstrates that CAs inhibit the influx of chloride through the GABA chloride channel.[22] The extent to which the GABAergic system modulates depression is unclear. This drug effect provides a potential explanation for CA-induced seizures. Additional pharmacologic activity of CAs includes blockade of cholinergic, histaminic, and α_1-adrenergic receptors. Chronic antidepressant dosing alters CNS neurotransmitter receptor expression and sensitivity. Effects on the neurohormonal system have been demonstrated in animal models; CAs have been shown to alter glucocorticoid mRNA receptor expression.[23,24] The significance of this alteration is unknown.

Differences among CAs regarding their effects on neurotransmission are detectable at therapeutic dosing. The nontricyclic antidepressants amoxapine and maprotiline primarily affect norepinephrine while having no effect on serotonin. Amoxapine and its 7-OH-amoxapine metabolite block dopamine receptors to degrees comparable to thioridazine and haloperidol, respectively.[25] All CAs produce some degree of sodium channel blockade in the central and peripheral nervous tissue at

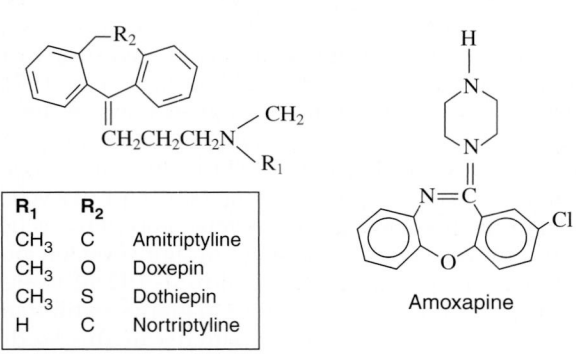

R₁	R₂	
CH₃	C	Amitriptyline
CH₃	O	Doxepin
CH₃	S	Dothiepin
H	C	Nortriptyline

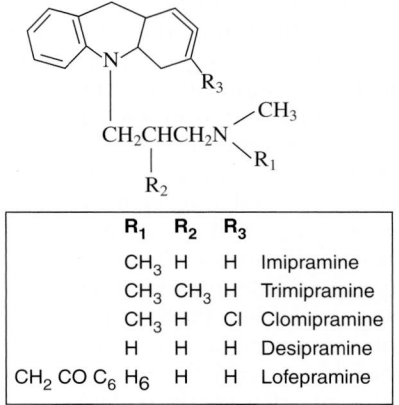

Amoxapine

R₁	R₂	R₃	
CH₃	H	H	Imipramine
CH₃	CH₃	H	Trimipramine
CH₃	H	Cl	Clomipramine
H	H	H	Desipramine
CH₂ CO C₆ H₆	H	H	Lofepramine

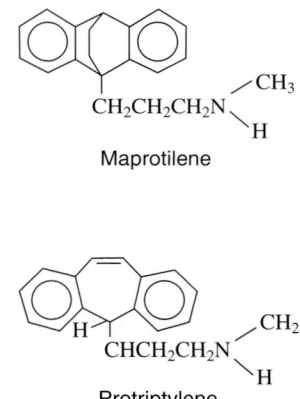

Maprotilene

Protriptylene

FIGURE 27-1 Structures of some cyclic antidepressants.

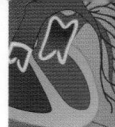

TABLE 27-1 Pharmacokinetic Parameters of Selected Cyclic Antidepressants

DRUG	ELIMINATION HALF-LIFE (hr)*	THERAPEUTIC LEVEL (ng/mL)[†]	CYP METABOLISM[‡]	PRINCIPAL ACTIVE METABOLITES
Amitriptyline	9–25	125–150	1A2, 2C19, 3A4, 2D6, 2C9	Nortriptyline 10-OH amitryptyline 10-OH nortryptiline
Amoxapine	8, (30), (6.5)	160–800	2D6	8-OH amoxapine 7-OH amoxapine
Clomipramine	21, (36)		1A2, 2C19, 3A4, 2D6	Desmethylclomipramine
Desipramine	13–23	50–300	2D6	2-OH despramine
Dothiepin	14–24 (23–46)	50–150		Desmethyldothiepin Dothiepin-S-oxide
Doxepin	8–24	75–200	2D6	Desmethyldoxepin
Imipramine	18–34 (12–30)	150–300	1A2, 2C19, 3A4, 2D6	Desipramine 2-OH imipramine 2-OH desipramine
Lofepramine	1.5–2.5 (12–30)		2D6	Desipramine
Maprotiline	43 (60–90)	50–300		Desmethylmaprotiline
Nortriptyline	16–36	50–150	2D6	10-OH nortriptylline
Protriptyline	55–198	50–150	2D6	
Trimipramine	23	30–170	2D6	Desmethyltrimipramine
Mirtazapine	20–40		2D6, 1A2, 3A4	Dimethylmirtazapine

CYP, cytochrome P-450.
*Numbers in parentheses represent the half-life of the metabolites.
[†]Data are based on small numbers of usual concentrations and may not reflect optimal dosing. Therapeutic concentrations are not well established.
[‡]Metabolic pathways are not fully established for all drugs.

therapeutic dosing. This "membrane stabilizing" or "quinidine-like" effect leads to ventricular dysrhythmias in the setting of overdose. The efficacy of CAs for the treatment of neuropathic pain may stem from this effect.

Pharmacokinetics

Cyclic antidepressants share similar pharmacokinetic parameters. Following oral administration, drug absorption proceeds rapidly,[26] with the exception of the sustained-release (SR) formulation of clomipramine (Anafranil Retard), which has a delayed time to maximum concentration (T_{max}) of 9 hours versus 4.8 hours with the immediate-release (IR) formulation.[27] Currently, clomipramine SR is available only in the United Kingdom. Peak serum concentrations of other CAs are generally achieved within 2 to 6 hours.[26] All drugs in this class are highly lipophilic with a large apparent volume of distribution and rapid tissue redistribution.[26] Typically, CAs exhibit a volume of distribution between 10 and 20 L/kg. Tissue concentrations often exceed serum concentrations by 10- to 100-fold. The fraction of drug in the serum is highly protein bound.[26] Since CAs are weak bases, they are bound to α_1-acid glycoprotein in the intravascular compartment. The fraction of free drug in the serum can be altered with changes in serum pH. Lowering pH creates a higher unbound fraction. Implications of acid–base status for overdose management are discussed in later sections.

Elimination is almost entirely hepatic, with little unchanged drug excreted in the urine. CAs do not undergo biliary excretion in any appreciable amount.[28]

Biotransformation of CAs occurs via the hepatic microoxygenase P-450 enzyme system, and first pass metabolism significantly reduces their oral bioavailability.[29-31] Many CAs form active metabolites following demethylation or hydroxylation (see Table 27-1). Active metabolites may accumulate after a period of 12 to 24 hours and could result in significant toxicity in therapeutic dosing.[32,33] The most common hepatic enzyme isoforms involved in the biotransformation of CAs are CYP2D6 and CYP2C19.[34] Hydroxylation occurs via CYP2D6, whereas the 2C19 isoform is associated with N-demethylation.[26] CAs inhibit CYP2D6 and CYP2C19 activity.[35] Genetic polymorphisms in certain cytochrome P-450 (CYP450) enzymes alter the kinetics of hydroxylation for some CAs.[36] In the United States, 90% to 95% of people are "rapid hydroxylators." In that population, the half-life of desipramine is 13 to 23 hours, whereas the half-life in the subpopulation of "slow hydroxylators" is 81 to 131 hours.[37] Cases of slow recovery from desipramine overdose[38] and toxicity from therapeutic dosing[39] have been reported in slow hydroxylators. Those with genetic defects in CYP2C19 activity have significantly higher plasma concentration curves of amitriptyline compared with normals.[34] Age presents an additional variable that alters serum concentrations of parent drug and metabolites. Across all age groups an increase in serum concentrations of drug and metabolite is seen with increasing age when dosing is weight adjusted. More efficient hepatic biotransformation and renal clearance in children compared with adults likely explains this phenomenon.[40] Half-life of elimination for therapeutic doses of CAs averages 8 to 30 hours with extension to 55 to 127 hours

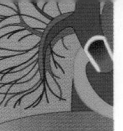
for protriptyline. The same drugs have longer half-lives in the elderly.[41,42] The prolonged elimination half-lives in this population may lead to drug accumulation with daily dosing.[26]

Toxicokinetic parameters for CAs are altered in the setting of overdose. The anticholinergic properties of CAs may lead to delayed gastric emptying, possibly prolonging the absorptive phase, enhancing overall absorption, and delaying time to peak serum concentrations.[26] The onset of toxicity after overdose is typically rapid, and most deaths occur within the first 6 hours postingestion. An increased bioavailability following overdose may result from a decreased first pass metabolism as hepatic enzymes become saturated.[43] Since the unbound fraction of CAs increases with an acid medium, acidemia will enhance overall toxicity.

Kinetics in the postmortem state are dramatically altered. In the steady state, CAs are normally highly tissue bound. Following death, tissues release bound drug, creating a false elevation in serum drug levels. The serum concentrations increase as time proceeds postmortem. This can lead to confusion regarding the manner of death. Strategies for postmortem laboratory analysis are further discussed under Diagnosis.

Drug Interaction

Potential drug-drug interactions may develop through various mechanisms (Table 27-2). Competitive inhibition of CYP isoforms could lead to increased toxicity of CAs or the drugs with which they compete for enzymatic biotransformation. The competitive inhibition of CYP2C19 by imipramine and nortriptyline has resulted in elevated phenytoin concentrations in some patients.[44,45] Induction of CYP isoforms by CAs may, conversely, lead to decreased effectiveness of other medications. Additional drug interactions include medications that may potentiate the serotonergic or sympathomimetic properties of CAs, such as monoamine oxidase inhibitors (MAOIs), SSRIs, amphetamines, and others.

TOXICOLOGY

The most severe toxicities from CA overdose include hypotension, dysrhythmia, coma, seizures, and hyperthermia. Cardiovascular toxicity results primarily from effects on the cardiac cell action potential, negative inotropy, direct effects on vascular tone, and indirect effects mediated by the autonomic nervous system. CNS toxicity is less well understood and is likely a combination of effects on cholinergic and GABA neurotransmission along with sodium channel effects. Deaths are often a result of refractory hypotension.

Cardiovascular System Toxicity

CARDIAC CELL ACTION POTENTIAL

CAs alter the cardiac conduction system in a myriad of ways. The most distinctive toxicity relates to the inhibition of the fast sodium channels in the His-Purkinje tissue, leading to a slowing of phase 0 depolarization.[46,47] This "membrane stabilizing" or "quinidine-like" effect is analogous to that of Vaughn Williams (VW) class I antidysrhythmic drugs.[48] Impaired depolarization of cells within the His-Purkinje system slows the propagation of ventricular depolarization. This appears on the electrocardiogram (ECG) as prolongation of the QRS interval, the hallmark of TCA toxicity. The degree of conduction delay is rate-dependent and worsens with tachycardia.[49] The QRS morphology is generally that of nonspecific intraventricular conduction delay, with discrete bundle branch block being less common. However, the longer refractory period of the right bundle relative to the left leads to the characteristic rightward axis deviation of the terminal 40 msec of the QRS complex seen in many patients with TCA toxicity.[50] On the ECG this appears as an increased R wave amplitude in lead aVR and a deep S wave in leads I and aVL (Fig. 27-2).[51] A less specific finding is prolongation of the corrected QT interval (QT_c). This delay in myocyte repolarization may result from a direct effect of CAs on potassium channels.[52,53] A prolonged QT_c may also be seen in therapeutic dosing.

TABLE 27-2 Cyclic Antidepressant Drug Interactions

DRUG	MECHANISM
Anticoagulants	Inhibition of oral anticoagulant metabolism with subsequent elevated PT
Amphetamines	Enhanced adrenergic stimulation via norepinephrine release
Carbamazepine	TCA metabolism, leading to subtherapeutic levels
Chloroquine	Induction of additive effect of QT prolongation
Cimetidine	Inhibition of TCA metabolism, leading to supratherapeutic levels
Class Ia and Ic antidysrhythmics	Additive effect of QT prolongation via Na channel blockade and QRS prolongation
MAOIs	Enhanced neurotransmitter release, leading to hypertensive crisis or serotonin syndrome
Phenothiazines	Additive effect on QT prolongation
Fluconazole	Inhibition of TCA metabolism, leading to supratherapeutic levels; also increased QT interval
Class III antidysrhythmics	Additive QT prolongation
SSRIs	Risk of serotonin syndrome; competitive inhibition of CYP2D6 and CYP2C19, leading to elevated steady-state TCA levels
Linezolid	Risk of serotonin syndrome
MDMA ("Ecstacy")	Risk of serotonin syndrome

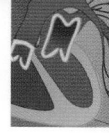

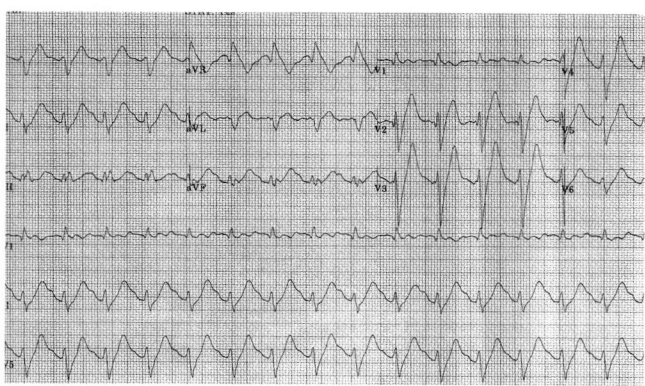

FIGURE 27-2   ECG from a TCA-poisoned patient.

NEGATIVE INOTROPY AND VASCULAR SMOOTH MUSCLE EFFECT

CAs inhibit the influx of calcium into cardiac and neural tissue and interfere with calcium-coupled muscular contraction.[54-56] This may explain the direct depressant effect seen experimentally with isolated human myocardium in response to CAs.[57] Peripheral α-adrenergic blockade may cause postural hypotension at therapeutic doses. At toxic doses, vasodilation contributes to hypotension.[58]

DYSRHYTHMIAS

Sinus tachycardia is the most common rhythm disturbance associated with CA overdose. The etiology is multifactorial and includes anticholinergic effects, increased norepinephrine release, and reflex tachycardia in response to vasodilation. Although the tachycardia does not generally cause morbidity itself, it is clearly a sign of significant toxicity.

Ventricular tachycardia (VT) is the most common ventricular dysrhythmia seen in overdose. However, discriminating this rhythm from the common underlying sinus tachycardia with aberrant conduction (QRS prolongation) may be difficult, since P waves are not always visible. Some cases of VT described in the literature may actually be supraventricular tachycardia (SVT). P waves may be obscured by the preceding T wave owing to the prolonged PR and QT_c intervals along with rapid heart rate. Intraesophageal electrode monitoring may reveal P waves not visible on the standard ECG. An alternative, less sophisticated technique useful in discriminating these rhythms is to follow serial ECGs. A gradual evolution of the QRS prior to loss of the P wave suggests SVT with aberrant conduction. The presence of fusion beats suggests a ventricular origin. Other criteria commonly used to differentiate ventricular and supraventricular rhythms, such as QRS morphology and duration, have not been tested in patients with CA overdose and may not be applicable in this setting.

Torsades de pointes (TdP) has been reported following CA overdose.[59,60] This phenomenon appears to be a more common consequence of therapeutic dosing than of overdose. The increased risk for TdP in conjunction with a slow rhythm likely explains its higher prevalence in therapeutic dosing, since most acutely poisoned patients are tachycardic. Several cases of sudden death in children taking therapeutic doses of CAs have been reported. QT prolongation with resultant TdP is the speculated mechanism for these events.[61] Other less common rhythms seen in overdose are second- or third-degree atrioventricular block[62] and premature ventricular beats. Patients close to death are more likely to develop bradycardia and atrioventricular blocks.

Refractory hypotension is a common cause of death due to CA overdose. Hypotension may occur in the absence of other signs of cardiac toxicity such as QRS prolongation.[63] Hypotension is due in part to vasodilation from α-adrenergic blockade, as well as direct myocardial depression.[57,58,64-66] This inotropic depression is dose-dependent and independent of effects on the cardiac conduction system.[57] Significant sinus tachycardia may contribute to hypotension by decreasing the diastolic period. This effect decreases ventricular filling time and impairs coronary perfusion.

Central Nervous System Toxicity

CNS depression is a common feature of all CAs in overdose. Symptoms range from fatigue to coma. The greatest concern in CNS toxicity in overdose is seizures. Although they most commonly occur in patients who also display signs of cardiac toxicity, seizures may occur in the absence of this finding.[67,68] Maprotiline and amoxapine are more likely than other CAs to cause seizures.[69,70] Seizures due to CAs most often occur within 1 to 2 hours of presentation, are brief in duration, and resolve without the need for anticonvulsant medications.[68] However, seizures may cause a metabolic acidosis that could predispose patients to cardiac dysrhythmias. In some case series, 10% to 20% of patients with seizures abruptly developed cardiovascular deterioration (hypotension, ventricular dysrhythmias) during or within minutes after the seizure.[68,71] Patients with more severe cardiovascular toxicity before the seizure were at highest risk. Therefore, cardiovascular deterioration may have been imminent regardless of the seizure, or potentially worsened by a seizure-induced acidosis. A clear cause and effect has not been identified. Other neurologic symptoms include delirium and myoclonus. Delirium is characterized by agitation, disorientation, and delusions and is most likely attributable to the anticholinergic properties of CAs. Although delirium may appear early in the course of intoxication, it may also manifest several hours later, after the initial period of sedation wanes. It is not uncommon to witness the development of a profound central antimuscarinic syndrome after 24 hours when patients have survived the initial cardiovascular consequences.

Toxicity in Other Systems

Peripheral anticholinergic toxicity may be seen with agents possessing potent anticholinergic properties such as amitriptyline. Signs and symptoms include urinary

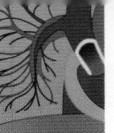

retention, ileus, and dry skin. Pupil size may vary depending on the degree of anticholinergic versus α-adrenergic blockade. Pulmonary complications include aspiration pneumonitis and adult respiratory distress syndrome.[72] These likely represent indirect toxicity secondary to coma, hypotension, excessive fluid administration, or increased capillary permeability from direct endothelial toxicity. Hyperthermia may ensue following excessive heat generation from seizures or myoclonus in the setting of decreased ability to dissipate heat through sweating.

Ultimately, most deaths occur prior to hospital presentation. Of those who survive to the hospital, death occurs within the first few hours of presentation with the majority of deaths occurring in the first 24 hours.[73] It is not uncommon for a patient's clinical condition to deteriorate rapidly with progression from no symptoms to life-threatening cardiotoxicity in less than 1 hour.[74] Late-occurring death results from complications of prolonged hypotension, status epilepticus, or aspiration.

DIAGNOSIS

Electrocardiogram

The ECG is the most rapidly available screening tool for predicting toxicity and guiding the management of CA poisonings. QRS interval prolongation is the most apparent ECG finding in serious CA toxicity and is a marker of the sodium channel blockade resulting from this drug class. The QRS axis is typically shifted to the right, along with the axis of the terminal 40 msec of the QRS complex. An increase in the R wave amplitude in aVR accompanies this finding (see Fig. 27-2).[51,75,76] These parameters are useful in predicting serious adverse outcomes such as seizures and ventricular tachycardia.

In one retrospective study, a maximal limb-lead QRS duration greater than 100 msec identified patients at greatest risk for seizures.[67] However, these and other complications may occur with a lesser degree of QRS prolongation, and patients with any degree of QRS prolongation are considered at risk for developing life-threatening CA toxicity.[77] This was demonstrated in another retrospective study in which a maximal 12-lead ECG QRS duration greater than 100 msec was only 53% sensitive for ventricular dysrhythmias or seizures.[78] The low sensitivity for predicting serious outcomes despite the use of a more sensitive measurement (maximal 12-lead QRS) suggests that life-threatening complications may develop irrespective of narrow QRS duration.

The terminal 40 msec QRS axis deviation greater than 120 degrees has been used to diagnose TCA toxicity, with a range of sensitivities from 29% to 100%.[50,75,77,79] The most common way to detect this measure is to identify a deep S wave in lead I or aVL and a terminal R wave in lead aVR (see Fig. 27-2). The height of the R wave in aVR also provides valuable information when evaluating CA overdoses. A height greater than or equal to 3 mm is 81% sensitive for predicting subsequent seizures or dysrhythmias.[76] This compares with a sensitivity of 82% in

the same study for a QRS duration greater than 100 msec. However, the positive predictive values for the aVR and QRS criteria were 43% and 35%, respectively.

The QT_c interval is mildly prolonged with therapeutic doses of CAs and becomes more prolonged with overdose.[80] A corrected QT_c greater than 480 msec in the setting of CA poisoning has been linked to an increased risk of seizures and dysrhythmias.[51] However, this marker is not useful in the diagnosis of CA toxicity versus non-CA ingestions.[75,79]

Interpretation of ECG criteria should be weighed with the knowledge that the ECG is a dynamic measurement. An initially normal ECG may rapidly evolve to reveal the characteristic changes cited above. At the time of presentation in one study, the maximum recorded QRS interval was present on the ECG in 80% of patients.[81] The remaining patients reached a maximum QRS duration in a median time of 3 hours (range, 1 to 9). The maximum T40 msec axis occurred at the time of presentation in 86% in this same group, with the remaining patients reaching this maximum in a median time of 3 hours (range, 1 to 5). Therefore, frequent ECGs are required during the first few hours following a CA overdose to monitor potential changes.

Laboratory Studies

CAs can be detected qualitatively in urine by thin-layer chromatography or liquid chromatography, or quantitatively in serum by liquid or gas chromatography. Active demethylated metabolites are usually measured via the latter methods. Therapeutic CA concentrations are generally in the range of 50 to 300 ng/mL (see Table 27-1). Bedside immunoassays are available; however, they have not been extensively tested.[82] False-positive results from CA immunoassays are well documented and include cross-reactions with quetiapine, carbamazepine, diphenhydramine, and many others (Table 27-3).[83-86]

The correlation of serum CA concentrations with toxicity is imprecise,[67,73] and their measurement adds little to the management of CA overdose. Life-threatening toxicity is usually accompanied by a serum concentration of greater than 100 ng/mL, while concentrations greater than 300 to 500 ng/mL are often fatal.[47] The serum CA concentration may increase up to fivefold postmortem. When using CA levels to determine cause of death, the measurement of liver drug concentrations rather than blood concentration may avoid the tissue redistribution artifact that leads to dramatic elevations in blood CA content, even with therapeutic dosing.[87-89] Another technique involves examining the ratio of parent drug to metabolite. Typically, the metabolites are found in greater concentration in patients taking therapeutic doses, whereas fatal overdoses lead to a much higher concentration of parent drug compared to metabolites.

Without a clear history of CA ingestion, the diagnosis may be confused with other drugs or disease states. CA toxicity is most likely to resemble other drugs that produce QRS prolongation. Drugs which may induce cardiotoxicity indistinguishable from that of CAs include

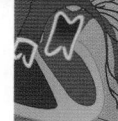

TABLE 27-3 TCA Assays and Drugs Reported to Cause False-Positive Results

ASSAY	FLUID	DRUG CROSS-REACTIVITY
Abbott TDx/TDxFlx TCA immunoassay	Blood	Carbamazepine
Syva EMIT immunoassay	Blood	Thioridazine, chlorpromazine, trimeprazine, cyproheptadine, cyclobenzaprine, norcyclobenzaprine, diphenhydramine, quetiapine
DuPont automatic clinical analyzer	Blood	Thioridazine
Triage plus TCA	Urine	Cyclobenzaprine
Homogenous enzyme immunoassay (Microgenics, Syva)	Urine	Quetiapine
Liquid chromatography	Blood	Diphenhydramine
High-performance liquid chromatography	Blood	Thioridazine, perphenazine, cyclobenzaprine, norcyclobenzaprine
Gas chromatography–mass spectrometry	Blood	No reported drug cross-reactivity

Adapted from Matos ME, Burns MM, Shannon MW: False-positive tricyclic antidepressant drug screen results leading to the diagnosis of carbamazepine intoxication. Pediatrics 2000;105:E66.

VW class IA (quinidine, procainamide) or IC (flecainide, encainide, propafenone) antidysrhythmic agents. Other drugs that may prolong QRS duration in overdose include cocaine, propranolol, quinine, chloroquine, hydroxychloroquine, high-dose antipsychotics (thioridazine, chlorpromazine), propoxyphene, and diphenhydramine. Nondrug causes of QRS prolongation include hyperkalemia, cardiac ischemia, and other conduction system abnormalities.

MANAGEMENT

Supportive Measures

Given the risk of rapid deterioration, patients with known or suspected CA overdose should have an intravenous line started and cardiac rhythm should be monitored continuously. An ECG on arrival can be compared with subsequent ECGs obtained during the monitoring period. Frequent measurement of vital signs including temperature is imperative. Patients with severe toxicity on presentation, including extreme lethargy, agitation, seizures, or dysrhythmias, require early intubation for airway protection. Particular attention to acid–base status is paramount in managing a severe CA overdose. Patients who develop acidosis from increased muscle activity, seizures, or inadequate ventilation may develop an increase in CA-protein dissociation and subsequent clinical deterioration.

Initial measures for blood pressure support include intravenous fluids and vasopressors such as norepinephrine. Because CA toxicity is reversible once the drug is metabolized and excreted, temporary mechanical support of the circulation may prove useful in hypotensive patients who are unresponsive to other measures. Serum CA levels often decline rapidly following overdose owing to distribution of the drug to tissues. A temporary period of mechanically assisted circulation might, therefore, allow time for spontaneous improvement. Isolated reports of a child who survived 2.5 hours of cardiopulmonary resuscitation during nonperfusing ventricular tachycardia and of an adult treated successfully with femoral-femoral extracorporeal circulation for refractory hypotension support this possibility.[90,91] Preliminary data in swine suggest that cardiopulmonary bypass may allow survival after ingestion of an otherwise fatal dose of CA.[92] Augmentation of aortic outflow utilizing a balloon pump device could provide additional perfusion support when myocardial depression is severe.

Decontamination

Prompt administration of activated charcoal is indicated if the ingestion occurs within 1 hour of presentation. Charcoal may be given after this time period; however, its effectiveness diminishes rapidly with time. Patients who appear drowsy and are unable to drink the charcoal without assist should be protected with tracheal intubation prior to charcoal administration to prevent aspiration of charcoal and subsequent serious pulmonary sequelae.

Laboratory Monitoring

As discussed above, measurement of serum CA concentrations provides little information regarding emergent care of poisoned patients. However, qualitative screening immunoassays may occasionally prove useful in the detection of occult ingestion when overt clinical toxicity is not detected. Measurement of serum electrolytes, blood urea nitrogen, creatinine, creatine kinase, hematocrit, and liver function tests provide information regarding co-ingestions and other disease states that may affect drug metabolism and excretion. Arterial blood gas determinations are indicated for intubated patients and for monitoring acid–base status when sodium bicarbonate infusion is employed as a therapy for CA toxicity.

Antidotes

NaHCO₃
When CAs were introduced into clinical practice, the clinical characteristics of overdose were noted as sharing many features of quinidine toxicity, for which hypertonic sodium lactate (which is rapidly metabolized to bicarbonate) resulted in clinical improvement. The proposed

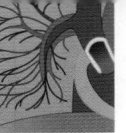

mechanisms for this therapy include increased plasma protein binding of CAs resulting from alkalemia, reduced binding of CAs within the cardiac myocytes, and overcoming the Na channel blockade via sodium loading.[93]

Controlled animal studies clearly established that hypertonic NaHCO₃ is effective in reducing QRS prolongation, increasing blood pressure, and suppressing ventricular ectopy due to CA toxicity.[94-96] This effect is demonstrated experimentally to be independent of and additive to the effect of vasopressors.[97] Some animal data suggest that hypertonic sodium chloride infusions provide additional benefit with respect to treating hypotension and ventricular tachycardia.[98] However, the amount of sodium delivered in these experiments was 15 mEq/kg or 10 mL/kg of 7.5% NaCl, a dose likely to cause severe toxicity in humans. Intracellular pH elevation has been shown to reverse the toxicity of imipramine in cardiac myocytes.[99] This intracellular alkalosis is correlated with a decreased binding of imipramine.[100] In human serum, alkalosis causes a decrease in the free CA concentration.[101]

No randomized controlled human trials are published relating to the efficacy of NaHCO₃ infusion for the treatment of CA poisoning.[93] Retrospective reviews of a few hundred patients in conjunction with case series and case reports provide the basis of confirmation for the effectiveness of NaHCO₃ therapy in the treatment of CA-induced hypotension, cardiac conduction delays, and dysrhythmias in humans.[93,102-105]

Indications for therapy with NaHCO₃ infusion are acidemia (serum pH < 7.35), QRS width greater than or equal to 100 msec, R wave in aVR greater than 3 mm, or wide complex tachydysrhythmias. Optimal serum pH is not well established. The target pH recommended by various clinicians, as determined by survey, vary dramatically and range from a maximum of 7.45 to 7.8.[106] However, the majority of clinicians recommend a maximum serum pH of 7.55.[106] Dosing protocols also vary widely. The most common approach is to administer 1 mEq/kg NaHCO₃ as an intravenous bolus in the setting of a widened QRS or dysrhythmia. This may be increased to achieve resolution of the dysrhythmia or narrowing of the QRS (Fig. 27-3; see also Fig. 27-2). Serum pH should not be permitted to exceed 7.55. Continuous infusion may begin after improved cardiac parameters are achieved with the bicarbonate bolus. Adding 150 mEq of NaHCO₃ to 1 L of D5W yields an isotonic solution that can be infused at a rate 1.5 times maintenance for the patient's weight. The infusion rate may be titrated to hourly serum pH measurements to ensure adequate treatment without overalkalinization. Frequent measurement of serum potassium is critical owing to enhanced renal elimination of potassium in the setting of alkalemia.

PHENYTOIN

Phenytoin was reported to improve QRS duration in an uncontrolled series of patients and one preliminary report that showed more rapid improvement of cardiovascular toxicity in patients randomized to phenytoin.[107,108]

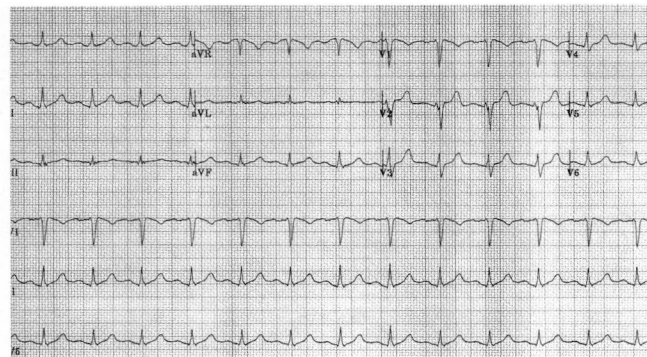

FIGURE 27-3 ECG from a TCA-poisoned patient after NaHCO₃ administration.

Controlled animal studies have not confirmed a benefit, and possible aggravation of ventricular ectopy was noted in one report.[109-111] These data do not support the clinical use of phenytoin for CA cardiotoxicity.

TCA ANTIBODIES

The use of TCA-specific antibody Fab fragments for the treatment of TCA overdose, analogous to those used to treat digoxin overdose, has been studied in rats. Fab doses capable of binding 10% to 30% of the TCA body burden rapidly reverse QRS prolongation and hypotension and prolong survival.[112,113] The toxic dose of TCAs is more than 100 times higher than that of digoxin, however, and the theoretical Fab dose required to reverse toxicity is also much higher (1 to 3 g/kg). One case report details the successful use of experimental ovine Fab in a human amitriptyline overdose.[114] The total dose of Fab administered was only 6% of the molar quantity of TCA ingested. The authors reported a rapid decrease in QRS and QT$_c$ intervals as well as an improvement in mental status. No acute adverse reactions were noted. The ability of the antibodies to bind tetracyclic drugs such as amoxapine and maprotiline is unknown. More extensive experience is required before Fab fragments become part of routine therapy for TCA poisoning.

α₁-ACID GLYCOPROTEIN

α₁-Acid glycoprotein (AAG) has demonstrated some efficacy in the treatment of CA toxicity in animal models. Because CAs are bound to AAG in plasma, the administration of additional AAG would theoretically bind a portion of the free CA fraction, thereby reducing toxicity. Swine and rat studies have shown a trend toward decrease in CA-induced QRS prolongation after the administration of AAG.[115,116] Currently, no evidence suggests that administration of AAG in humans has any role in the treatment of CA toxicity.

PHYSOSTIGMINE

Physostigmine was initially advocated as a treatment for CA poisoning in the 1970s.[117] Indications at the time included seizures, coma, and tachydysrhythmias.[118] The first case reports of asystole following the use of

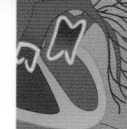

physostigmine were in the context of treating CA-induced seizures.[119] Anecdotal reports of successful treatment of seizures and dysrhythmias are not substantiated by controlled data. Balancing the reported successes are claims that physostigmine induces seizures and asystole when used for CA poisoning. Unfortunately, these are known complications of both CA poisoning as well as physostigmine in isolation. The reported cases linking physostigmine to these complications when used for CA poisonings do not demonstrate a conclusive cause and effect relationship.[120] Thus, seizures may have ceased in response to physostigmine or ceased despite this therapy. Seizures occurring after the administration of physostigmine may have occurred in response to therapy or may have occurred regardless of this drug. Similar logic applies to cases of asystole and bradycardia. Many conclusions may be drawn, and these are based on deductive reasoning rather than scientific evidence.

The pathophysiology of cardiac conduction delays and seizures resulting from CA poisonings is poorly explained by the anticholinergic properties of the drugs. These features are not seen in pure anticholinergic poisonings such as atropine and scopolamine. Rather, the sodium channel effects of CAs provide a more reasonable explanation. Therefore, the use of a purely cholinergic drug for reversal of seizures and dysrhythmias caused by sodium channel blockade lacks a rational basis. In view of the known toxicities including seizures and asystole from physostigmine in the absence of CA poisoning, its use in the context of CA poisoning, where seizures and cardiac dysrhythmias are a known complication, is not recommended. However, patients who survive the acute phase of CA poisoning and have no evidence of cardiac conduction delay may continue to suffer from the anticholinergic drug effects more than 24 hours after the ingestion. Physostigmine could be of benefit for controlling agitated delirium in this subset of patients provided that a patient has demonstrated cardiac stability for a prolonged period of monitoring.

Elimination Enhancement

Enhancing elimination of the CAs is difficult owing to their large volume of distribution. Several uncontrolled case reports note shorter than expected elimination half-lives for CAs with the use of repeated doses of activated charcoal. These data are of limited value because early sampling may have misconstrued the CA distribution phase as evidence of shortened half-life. In controlled studies, repeated oral doses of activated charcoal have been reported either to have no effect on the clearance of subtoxic doses of imipramine[121] or to shorten the elimination half-life of doxepin or amitriptyline by 20%.[122] Most deaths from CA overdose occur within hours of drug ingestion, thereby limiting the utility of a therapy that requires multiple doses over time. It is possible, however, that repeated doses of charcoal might shorten the duration of toxicity in slow hydroxylators who display long CA half-life kinetics. Little active CA is excreted in urine, and measures that enhance urinary CA excretion have a negligible effect on total clearance.[122]

Hemodialysis is ineffective in enhancing the elimination of CAs because of their extensive protein binding and lipid solubility. Hemoperfusion overcomes these limitations but is relatively ineffective because of the drugs' large volume of distribution.[123] One case report noted removal of less than 2% of the ingested dose of imipramine as parent drug or active metabolite during 6 hours of hemoperfusion.[32] Nevertheless, rapid improvement in cardiotoxicity after CA overdose has been anecdotally reported during hemoperfusion.[124-126] However, rapid decline in serum CA levels secondary to drug distribution may explain this observation. In addition, improvements in acid–base status likely contributed to improved cardiovascular status. In the absence of supporting data, there is no role for hemoperfusion in the treatment of CA poisoning.

DISPOSITION

Patients displaying significant signs and symptoms of CA toxicity such as QRS prolongation, lethargy, or hypotension require admission and monitoring until symptom-free for 24 hours.[127,128] QRS duration may be considered normal if it is less than 100 msec or similar to the patient's baseline QRS. When QRS duration is marginally prolonged (100 to 120 msec) and no baseline ECG is available, it may be unclear whether the observed QRS duration is normal for that patient or prolonged from the overdose. In this situation, measurement of the serum CA concentration may be helpful later in hospitalization as grounds for discontinuing therapy and monitoring when drug concentrations are therapeutic or low. A clearly elevated CA concentration would suggest that the QRS prolongation is drug induced, and therefore continued cardiac monitoring is indicated and $NaHCO_3$ therapy should continue. With the exception of overdoses involving a sustained-release drug, patients who are asymptomatic on presentation and do not manifest signs of toxicity after 6 hours require no further medical monitoring other than psychiatric evaluation.

ACKNOWLEDGMENTS

The authors acknowledge Paul R. Pentel, Daniel E. Keyler, and Lester M. Haddad for their contribution to the previous edition of this chapter.

REFERENCES

1. Lancaster NP, Foster AR: Suicidal attempt by imipramine overdosage. BMJ 1959;5164:1458.
2. Azima H, Vispo RH: Imipramine: a potent new anti-depressant compound. Am J Psychiatry 1958;115:245–246.
3. Mann AM, Catterson AG, Macpherson AS: Toxicity of imipramine: report on serious side effects and massive overdosage. Can Med Assoc J 1959;81:23–28.
4. Litovitz TL, Holm KC, Clancy C, et al: 1992 annual report of the American Association of Poison Control Centers Toxic Exposure Surveillance System. Am J Emerg Med 1993;11:494–555.
5. Litovitz TL, Clark LR, Soloway RA: 1993 annual report of the American Association of Poison Control Centers Toxic Exposure Surveillance System. Am J Emerg Med 1994;12:546–584.

6. Watson WA, Litovitz TL, Rodgers GC II, et al: 2002 annual report of the American Association of Poison Control Centers Toxic Exposure Surveillance System. Am J Emerg Med 2003;21:353–421.

7. Henry JA, Alexander CA, Sener EK: Relative mortality from overdose of antidepressants. BMJ 1995;310:221–224.

8. Hoppe-Roberts JM, Lloyd LM, Chyka PA: Poisoning mortality in the United States: comparison of national mortality statistics and poison control center reports. Ann Emerg Med 2000;35:440–448.

9. Litovitz TL, Felberg L, Soloway RA, et al: 1994 annual report of the American Association of Poison Control Centers Toxic Exposure Surveillance System. Am J Emerg Med 1995;13:551–597.

10. Litovitz TL, Felberg L, White S, et al: 1995 annual report of the American Association of Poison Control Centers Toxic Exposure Surveillance System. Am J Emerg Med 1996;14:487–537.

11. Litovitz TL, Klein-Schwartz W, Caravata EM, et al: 1998 annual report of the American Association of Poison Control Centers Toxic Exposure Surveillance System. Am J Emerg Med 1999;17:435–487.

12. Litovitz TL, Klein-Schwartz W, Dyer KS, et al: 1997 annual report of the American Association of Poison Control Centers Toxic Exposure Surveillance System. Am J Emerg Med 1998;16:443–497.

13. Litovitz TL, Klein-Schwartz W, Rodgers GC II, et al: 2001 annual report of the American Association of Poison Control Centers Toxic Exposure Surveillance System. Am J Emerg Med 2002;20:391–452.

14. Litovitz TL, Klein-Schwartz W, White S, et al: 1999 annual report of the American Association of Poison Control Centers Toxic Exposure Surveillance System. Am J Emerg Med 2000;18:517–574.

15. Litovitz TL, Klein-Schwartz W, White S, et al: 2000 annual report of the American Association of Poison Control Centers Toxic Exposure Surveillance System. Am J Emerg Med 2001;19:337–395.

16. Litovitz TL, Smilkstein M, Felberg L, et al: 1996 annual report of the American Association of Poison Control Centers Toxic Exposure Surveillance System. Am J Emerg Med 1997;15:447–500.

17. McFee RB, Caraccio TR, Mofenson HC: Selected tricyclic antidepressant ingestions involving children 6 years old or less. Acad Emerg Med 2001;8:139–144.

18. Snyder SH, Yamamura HI: Antidepressants and the muscarinic acetylcholine receptor. Arch Gen Psychiatry 1977;34:236–239.

19. Richelson E, Nelson A: Antagonism by antidepressants of neurotransmitter receptors of normal human brain in vivo. J Pharmacol Exp Ther 1984;230:94–102.

20. Wagner A, et al: Weak binding of 10-hydroxymetabolites of nortriptyline to rat brain muscarinic acetylcholine receptors. Life Sci 1984;35:1379–1383.

21. Tunnicliff G, Malatynska E: Central GABAergic systems and depressive illness. Neurochem Res 2003;28:965–976.

22. Malatynska E, Crites GJ, Harrawood D, et al: Antidepressant effects on GABA-stimulated 36Cl(-) influx in rat cerebral cortex are altered after treatment with GABA(A) receptor antisense oligodeoxynucleotides. Brain Res 2000;869:78–84.

23. Barden N: Modulation of glucocorticoid receptor gene expression by antidepressant drugs. Pharmacopsychiatry 1996;29:12–22.

24. Barden N: Regulation of corticosteroid receptor gene expression in depression and depressant action. J Psychiatry Neurosci 1999;24:25–39.

25. Calvo B, Garcia MJ, Pedraz JL, et al: Pharmacokinetics of amoxapine and its active metabolites. Int J Clin Pharmacol Ther Toxicol 1985;23:180–185.

26. Rudorfer MV, Potter WZ: Metabolism of tricyclic antidepressants. Cell Mol Neurobiol 1999;19:373–409.

27. Herrera D, Mayet L, Galindo MC, et al: Pharmacokinetics of a sustained-release dosage form of clomipramine. J Clin Pharmacol 2000;40:1488–1493.

28. Breyer-Pfaff U, Prox A, Wachsmuth H, et al: Phenolic metabolites of amitriptyline and nortriptyline in rat bile. Drug Metab Dispos 1987;15:882–889.

29. Greenblatt DJ, von Moltke LL, Shader RI: The importance of presystemic extraction in clinical psychopharmacology. J Clin Psychopharmacol 1996;16:417–419.

30. Alvan G, Borga O, Lind M, et al: First pass hydroxylation of nortriptyline: concentrations of parent drug and major metabolites in plasma. Eur J Clin Pharmacol 1977;11:219–224.

31. Sutfin TA, DeVane CL, Jusko WJ: The analysis and disposition of imipramine and its active metabolites in man. Psychopharmacology (Berl) 1984;82:310–317.

32. Pentel PR, Bullock ML, DeVane CL: Hemoperfusion for imipramine overdose: elimination of active metabolites. J Toxicol Clin Toxicol 1982;19:239–248.

33. Gram LF, Bjerre M, Kragh-Sorensen P, et al: Imipramine metabolites in blood of patients during therapy and after overdose. Clin Pharmacol Ther 1983;33:335–342.

34. Jiang ZP, Shu Y, Chen XP, et al: The role of CYP2C19 in amitriptyline N-demethylation in Chinese subjects. Eur J Clin Pharmacol 2002;58:109–113.

35. Shin JG, Park JY, Kim MJ, et al: Inhibitory effects of tricyclic antidepressants (TCAs) on human cytochrome P450 enzymes in vitro: mechanism of drug interaction between TCAs and phenytoin. Drug Metab Dispos 2002;30:1102–1107.

36. Spina E, Steiner E, Ericsson D, et al: Hydroxylation of desmethylimipramine: dependence on the debrisoquin hydroxylation phenotype. Clin Pharmacol Ther 1987;41:314–319.

37. Brosen K, Otton SV, Gram LF: Imipramine demethylation and hydroxylation: impact of the sparteine oxidation phenotype. Clin Pharmacol Ther 1986;40:543–549.

38. Spina E, Henthorn TK, Eleborg L, et al: Desmethylimipramine overdose: nonlinear kinetics in a slow hydroxylator. Ther Drug Monit 1985;7:239–241.

39. Bluhm RE, Wilkinson GR, Shelton R, et al: Genetically determined drug-metabolizing activity and desipramine-associated cardiotoxicity: a case report. Clin Pharmacol Ther 1993;53:89–95.

40. Wilens TE, Biederman J, Baldessarini RJ, et al: Developmental changes in serum concentrations of desipramine and 2-hydroxydesipramine during treatment with desipramine. J Am Acad Child Adolesc Psychiatry 1992;31:691–698.

41. Schulz P, Turner-Tamiyasu K, Smith G, et al: Amitriptyline disposition in young and elderly normal men. Clin Pharmacol Ther 1983;33:360–366.

42. Dawling S, Crome P, Braithwaite R: Pharmacokinetics of single oral doses of nortriptyline in depressed elderly hospital patients and young healthy volunteers. Clin Pharmacokinet 1980;5:394–401.

43. Brosen K, Gram LF: First-pass metabolism of imipramine and desipramine: impact of the sparteine oxidation phenotype. Clin Pharmacol Ther 1988;43:400–406.

44. Houghton GW, Richens A: Inhibition of phenytoin metabolism by other drugs used in epilepsy. Int J Clin Pharmacol Biopharm 1975;12:210–216.

45. Perucca E, Richens A: Interaction between phenytoin and imipramine. Br J Clin Pharmacol 1977;4:485–486.

46. Weld FM, Bigger JT II: Electrophysiological effects of imipramine on ovine cardiac Purkinje and ventricular muscle fibers. Circ Res 1980;46:167–175.

47. Biggs JT, Spiker DG, Petit JM, et al: Tricyclic antidepressant overdose: incidence of symptoms. JAMA 1977;238:135–138.

48. Connolly SJ, Mitchell LB, Swerdlow CD, et al: Clinical efficacy and electrophysiology of imipramine for ventricular tachycardia. Am J Cardiol 1984;53:516–521.

49. Nattel S: Frequency-dependent effects of amitriptyline on ventricular conduction and cardiac rhythm in dogs. Circulation 1985;72:898–906.

50. Niemann JT, Bessen HA, Rothstein RJ, et al: Electrocardiographic criteria for tricyclic antidepressant cardiotoxicity. Am J Cardiol 1986;57:1154–1159.

51. Caravati EM, Bossart PJ: Demographic and electrocardiographic factors associated with severe tricyclic antidepressant toxicity. J Toxicol Clin Toxicol 1991;29:31–43.

52. Terstappen GC, Pula G, Carignani C, et al: Pharmacological characterization of the human small conductance calcium-activated potassium channel hSK3 reveals sensitivity to tricyclic antidepressants and antipsychotic phenothiazines. Neuropharmacology 2001;40:772–783.

53. Cuellar-Quintero JL, Garcia DE, Cruzblanca H: The antidepressant imipramine inhibits the M-type K+ current in rat sympathetic neurons. Neuroreport 2001;12:2195–2198.

54. Joshi PG, Singh A, Ravichandra B: High concentrations of tricyclic antidepressants increase intracellular Ca2+ in cultured neural cells. Neurochem Res 1999;24:391–398.

55. Park TJ, Shin SY, Suh BC, et al: Differential inhibition of catecholamine secretion by amitriptyline through blockage of nicotinic receptors, sodium channels, and calcium channels in bovine adrenal chromaffin cells. Synapse 1998;29:248–256.

56. Watts JA, Yates KM, Bader SK, et al: Mechanisms of Ca2+ antagonism in imipramine-induced toxicity of isolated adult rat cardiomyocytes, Toxicol Appl Pharmacol 1998;153:95–101.

57. Heard K, Cain BS, Dart RC, et al: Tricyclic antidepressants directly depress human myocardial mechanical function independent of effects on the conduction system. Acad Emerg Med 2001; 8:1122–1127.

58. Langou RA, Van Dyke C, Tahan SR, et al: Cardiovascular manifestations of tricyclic antidepressant overdose. Am Heart J 1980;100:458–464.

59. Davison ET: Amitriptyline-induced Torsade de Pointes: successful therapy with atrial pacing. J Electrocardiol 1985;18:299–301.

60. Alter P, Tontsch D, Grimm W: Doxepin-induced torsade de pointes tachycardia. Ann Intern Med 2001;135:384–385.

61. Alderton HR: Tricyclic medication in children and the QT interval: case report and discussion. Can J Psychiatry 1995;40:325–329.

62. Thorstrand C: Clinical features in poisonings by tricyclic anti-depressants with special reference to the ECG. Acta Med Scand 1976;199:337–344.

63. Shannon M, Merola J, Lovejoy FH II: Hypotension in severe tricyclic antidepressant overdose. Am J Emerg Med 1988;6:439–432.

64. Langslet A, Johansen WG, Ryg M, et al: Effects of dibenzepine and imipramine on the isolated rat heart. Eur J Pharmacol 1971; 14:333–339.

65. Sigg EB, Osborne M, Korol B: Cardiovascular effects of imipramine. J Pharmacol Exp Ther 1963;141:237–243.

66. Cairncross KD, McCulloch MW, Mitchelson F: The action of protriptyline on peripheral autonomic function. J Pharmacol Exp Ther 1965;149:365–372.

67. Boehnert MT, Lovejoy FH II: Value of the QRS duration versus the serum drug level in predicting seizures and ventricular arrhythmias after an acute overdose of tricyclic antidepressants. N Engl J Med 1985;313:474–479.

68. Ellison DW, Pentel PR: Clinical features and consequences of seizures due to cyclic antidepressant overdose. Am J Emerg Med 1989;7:5–10.

69. Litovitz TL, Troutman WG: Amoxapine overdose: seizures and fatalities. JAMA 1983;250:1069–1071.

70. Rudorfer MV, Potter WZ: Antidepressants: a comparative review of the clinical pharmacology and therapeutic use of the "newer" versus the "older" drugs. Drugs 1989;37:713–738.

71. Taboulet P, Michard F, Muszynski J, et al: Cardiovascular repercussions of seizures during cyclic antidepressant poisoning. J Toxicol Clin Toxicol 1995;33:205–211.

72. Shannon M, Lovejoy FH II: Pulmonary consequences of severe tricyclic antidepressant ingestion. J Toxicol Clin Toxicol 1987; 25:443–461.

73. Hulten BA, Heath A: Clinical aspects of tricyclic antidepressant poisoning. Acta Med Scand 1983;213:275–278.

74. Callaham M, Kassel D: Epidemiology of fatal tricyclic anti-depressant ingestion: implications for management. Ann Emerg Med 1985;14:1–9.

75. Lavoie FW, Gansert GG, Weiss RE: Value of initial ECG findings and plasma drug levels in cyclic antidepressant overdose. Ann Emerg Med 1990;19:696–700.

76. Liebelt EL, Francis PD, Woolf AG: ECG lead aVR versus QRS interval in predicting seizures and arrhythmias in acute tricyclic antidepressant toxicity. Ann Emerg Med 1995;26:195–201.

77. Caravati EM: The electrocardiogram as a diagnostic discriminator for acute tricyclic antidepressant poisoning. J Toxicol Clin Toxicol 1999;37:113–115.

78. Foulke GE, Albertson TE: QRS interval in tricyclic antidepressant overdosage: inaccuracy as a toxicity indicator in emergency settings. Ann Emerg Med 1987;16:160–163.

79. Wolfe TR, Caravati EM, Rollins DE: Terminal 40-ms frontal plane QRS axis as a marker for tricyclic antidepressant overdose. Ann Emerg Med 1989;18:348–351.

80. Pentel P, Sioris L: Incidence of late arrhythmias following tricyclic antidepressant overdose. Clin Toxicol 1981;18:543–548.

81. Liebelt EL, Ulrich A, Francis PD, et al: Serial electrocardiogram changes in acute tricyclic antidepressant overdoses. Crit Care Med 1997;25:1721–1726.

82. Schwartz JG, Hurd IL, Carnahan JJ: Determination of tricyclic antidepressants for ED analysis. Am J Emerg Med 1994;12:513–516.

83. Hendrickson RG, Morocco AP: Quetiapine cross-reactivity among three tricyclic immunoassays. J Toxicol Clin Toxicol 2003;41:105–108.

84. Chattergoon DS, Verjee Z, Anderson M, et al: Carbamazepine interference with an immune assay for tricyclic antidepressants in plasma. J Toxicol Clin Toxicol 1998;36:109–113.

85. Sloan KL, Haver VM, Saxon AJ: Quetiapine and false-positive urine drug testing for tricyclic antidepressants. Am J Psychiatry 2000;157:148–149.

86. Matos ME, Burns MM, Shannon MW: False-positive tricyclic antidepressant drug screen results leading to the diagnosis of carbamazepine intoxication. Pediatrics 2000;105:E66.

87. Apple FS: Postmortem tricyclic antidepressant concentrations: assessing cause of death using parent drug to metabolite ratio. J Anal Toxicol 1989;13:197–198.

88. Apple FS, Bandt CM: Liver and blood postmortem tricyclic antidepressant concentrations. Am J Clin Pathol 1988;89:794–796.

89. Davis G, Park K, Kloss J, et al: Tricyclic antidepressant fatality: postmortem tissue concentrations. J Toxicol Clin Toxicol 2001;39:649–650.

90. Southall DP, Kilpatrick SM: Imipramine poisoning: survival of a child after prolonged cardiac massage. BMJ 1974;4:508.

91. Williams JM, Hollingshed MJ, Vasilakis A, et al: Extracorporeal circulation in the management of severe tricyclic antidepressant overdose. Am J Emerg Med 1994;12:456–458.

92. Larkin GL, Graeber GM, Hollingsed HM: Experimental amitriptyline poisoning: treatment of severe cardiovascular toxicity with cardiopulmonary bypass. Ann Emerg Med 1994;23:480–486.

93. Blackman K, Brown SG, Wilkes GJ: Plasma alkalinization for tricyclic antidepressant toxicity: a systematic review. Emerg Med (Fremantle) 2001;13:204–210.

94. Nattel S, Keable H, Sasyniuk BI: Experimental amitriptyline intoxication: electrophysiologic manifestations and management. J Cardiovasc Pharmacol 1984;6:83–89.

95. Nattel S, Mittleman M: Treatment of ventricular tachyarrhythmias resulting from amitriptyline toxicity in dogs. J Pharmacol Exp Ther 1984;231:430–435.

96. Pentel P, Benowitz N: Efficacy and mechanism of action of sodium bicarbonate in the treatment of desipramine toxicity in rats. J Pharmacol Exp Ther 1984;230:12–19.

97. Knudsen K, Abrahamsson J: Epinephrine and sodium bicarbonate independently and additively increase survival in experimental amitriptyline poisoning. Crit Care Med 1997;25:669–674.

98. McCabe JL, Cobaugh DJ, Menegazzi JJ, et al: Experimental tricyclic antidepressant toxicity: a randomized, controlled comparison of hypertonic saline solution, sodium bicarbonate, and hyperventilation. Ann Emerg Med 1998;32:329–333.

99. Bou-Abboud E, Nattel S: Relative role of alkalosis and sodium ions in reversal of class I antiarrhythmic drug–induced sodium channel blockade by sodium bicarbonate. Circulation 1996;94:1954–1961.

100. Bou-Abboud E, Nattel S: Molecular mechanisms of the reversal of imipramine-induced sodium channel blockade by alkalinization in human cardiac myocytes. Cardiovasc Res 1998;38:395–404.

101. Levitt MA, Sullivan JB II, Owens SM, et al: Amitriptyline plasma protein binding: effect of plasma pH and relevance to clinical overdose. Am J Emerg Med 1986;4:121–125.

102. Hoffman JR, McElroy CR: Bicarbonate therapy for dysrhythmia and hypotension in tricyclic antidepressant overdose. West J Med 1981;134:60–64.

103. Koppel C, Wiegreffe A, Tenczer J: Clinical course, therapy, outcome and analytical data in amitriptyline and combined amitriptyline/chlordiazepoxide overdose. Hum Exp Toxicol 1992;11:458–465.

104. Brown TC: Sodium bicarbonate treatment for tricyclic anti-depressant arrhythmias in children. Med J Aust 1976;2:380–382.

105. Brown TC, Barker GA, Dunlop ME, et al: The use of sodium bicarbonate in the treatment of tricyclic antidepressant–induced arrhythmias. Anaesth Intensive Care 1973;1:203–210.

106. Seger DL, Hantsch C, Zavoral T, et al: Variability of recom-mendations for serum alkalinization in tricyclic antidepressant

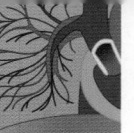
overdose: a survey of U.S. Poison Center medical directors. J Toxicol Clin Toxicol 2003;41:331–338.

107. Hagerman GA, Hanashiro PK: Reversal of tricyclic antidepressant–induced cardiac conduction abnormalities by phenytoin. Ann Emerg Med 1981;10:82–86.

108. Boehnert M, Lovejoy FH II: The effect of phenytoin on cardiac conduction and ventricular arrhythmias in acute tricyclic antidepressant (TCA) overdose. Vet Hum Toxicol 1985;27:297.

109. Callaham M, Schumaker H, Pentel P: Phenytoin prophylaxis of cardiotoxicity in experimental amitriptyline poisoning. J Pharmacol Exp Ther 1988;245:216–220.

110. Kulig K, et al: Phenytoin as treatment for tricyclic antidepressant cardiotoxicity in a canine model. Vet Hum Toxicol 1984;26:399.

111. Mayron R, Ruiz E: Phenytoin: does it reverse tricyclic antidepressant–induced cardiac conduction abnormalities? Ann Emerg Med 1986;15:876–880.

112. Dart RC, Sidki A, Sullivan JB II, et al: Ovine desipramine antibody fragments reverse desipramine cardiovascular toxicity in the rat. Ann Emerg Med 1996;27:309–315.

113. Pentel PR, Scarlett W, Ross CA, et al: Reduction of desipramine cardiotoxicity and prolongation of survival in rats with the use of polyclonal drug-specific antibody Fab fragments. Ann Emerg Med 1995;26:334–341.

114. Heard K, O'Malley GF, Dart RC: Treatment of amitriptyline poisoning with ovine antibody to tricyclic antidepressants. Lancet 1999;354:1614–1615.

115. Pentel PR, Keyler DE: Effects of high dose alpha-1-acid glycoprotein on desipramine toxicity in rats. J Pharmacol Exp Ther 1988;246:1061–1066.

116. Seaberg DC, Weiss LD, Yealy DM, et al: Effects of alpha-1-acid glycoprotein on the cardiovascular toxicity of nortriptyline in a swine model. Vet Hum Toxicol 1991;33:226–230.

117. Manoguerra AS, Ruiz E: Physostigmine treatment of anticholinergic poisoning. JACEP 1976;5:125–127.

118. Slovis TL, Ott JF, Teitebaum DT, et al: Physostigmine therapy in acute tricyclic antidepressant poisoning. Clin Toxicol 1971; 4:451–459.

119. Pentel P, Peterson CD: Asystole complicating physostigmine treatment of tricyclic antidepressant overdose. Ann Emerg Med 1980;9:588–590.

120. Linden C: ACMT net discussion of physostigmine use in the context of TCA poisoning. ACMT.net.

121. Goldberg MJ, Park GD, Spector R, et al: Lack of effect of oral activated charcoal on imipramine clearance. Clin Pharmacol Ther 1985;38:350–353.

122. Karkkainen S, Neuvonen PJ: Pharmacokinetics of amitriptyline influenced by oral charcoal and urine pH. Int J Clin Pharmacol Ther Toxicol 1986;24:326–332.

123. Heath A, Wickstrom I, Martensson E, et al: Treatment of antidepressant poisoning with resin hemoperfusion. Hum Toxicol 1982;1:361–371.

124. Diaz-Buxo JA, Farmer CD, Chandler JT: Hemoperfusion in the treatment of amitriptyline intoxication. Trans Am Soc Artif Intern Organs 1978;24:699–703.

125. Marbury T, Mahoney J, Fuller T, et al: Treatment of amitriptyline overdosage with charcoal hemoperfusion. Kidney Int 1977; 12:485.

126. Pedersen RS, Jorgensen KA, Olesen AS, et al: Charcoal haemoperfusion and antidepressant overdose. Lancet 1978;1:719–720.

127. Frommer DA, Kulig KW, Marx JA, Rumack B: Tricyclic antidepressant overdose: a review. JAMA 1987;257:521–526.

128. Goldberg RJ, Capone RJ, Hunt JD: Cardiac complications following tricyclic antidepressant overdose: issues for monitoring policy. JAMA 1985;254:1772–1775.

28 Serotonin Reuptake Inhibitors and Other Atypical Antidepressants

WESLEY PALATNICK, MD

At a Glance...

- Overdose of selective serotonin reuptake inhibitors is less hazardous than cyclic antidepressants.
- Adverse effects and drug interactions are common during therapy.
- Most overdoses are not life threatening; however, fatalities have been reported.
- Venlafaxine, bupropion, and citalopram have been associated with more toxicity than other selective serotonin reuptake inhibitors.
- Deaths are usually associated with the ingestion of multiple agents.
- Seizures and decreased level of consciousness are the most common manifestations.
- Cardiac effects are usually mild and include prolonged QTc and bradycardia.
- Treatment is supportive.
- The serotonin syndrome may be associated with overdose or during therapy with other serotonergic agents and may be life threatening.
- Asymptomatic patients may be discharged after 6 hours of observation, unless prolonged release products ingested.

Depression is a common problem that results in enormous costs to society. These include the direct costs of treatment, as well as indirect costs due to lost productivity. Pharmacologic therapy is effective, with 65% to 75% of patients showing significant improvement and a complete cure in 40% to 50% of patients. Both the cyclic antidepressants and monoamine oxidase inhibitors (MAOIs) are very effective treatments. However, the cyclic antidepressants have a number of troublesome side effects as well as significant and life-threatening toxicity in overdose. Drug and food interactions with the MAOIs as well as their potential toxicity in overdose limit their acceptability as a treatment option.

The first selective serotonin reuptake inhibitor (SSRI) on the market still in use is fluvoxamine. It was introduced in Europe in 1983. Fluoxetine was introduced in the United States in 1988, followed by sertraline in 1992, paroxetine in 1993, and fluvoxamine in 1995. Bupropion was released in 1989, trazodone in 1992, and venlafaxine in 1994.[1]

SSRI antidepressants are very effective for the management of depression, have a more attractive side effect profile than either the cyclic antidepressants or the MAOIs, and are much less toxic when taken in overdose.[2-8] They are as effective as the cyclic antidepressants in the treatment of depression.[9-11]

Aside from depression, SSRIs are also considered important therapeutic modalities for a number of other common psychiatric disorders such as anxiety, anorexia nervosa, bulimia, and obsessive-compulsive disorder.[10] They are also used in the management of borderline personality disorder, attention-deficit hyperactivity disorder, and fibromyalgia.[12]

EPIDEMIOLOGY

In 2002, the American Association of Poison Control Centers reported 58,817 exposures to SSRIs and trazodone, with 116 deaths. This is in contrast to the 13,198 exposures and 118 deaths associated with cyclic antidepressants.[13] In a review, Barbey reported only six verified overdose deaths involving SSRIs alone from 1985 to 1997. Of these, only two had been reported in the literature.[14]

A comparison of poisoning fatality records for England and Wales from 1993 to 1995 found 1 death per 411,800 3-month treatment episodes for SSRIs as a group compared to 1 death per 8130 3-month treatment episodes for cyclic antidepressants.[15] A comparison of the number of deaths per million prescriptions of antidepressants in England from 1987 to 1992 found a significantly lower number of deaths for the SSRIs compared with both the cyclic antidepressants and MAOIs.[3]

The hospital costs for patients hospitalized for SSRI overdose are significantly lower than those associated with cyclic antidepressant overdose, due to a shorter hospital stay, less need for interventions such as intubation, and less need for admission to the intensive care unit.[16-19]

STRUCTURE

Most of the SSRIs are either aryls or aryl-oxyalkylamines. Citalopram and fluoxetine are racemic mixtures, while sertraline and paroxetine are separate enantiomers. The serotonin uptake blocking of citalopram is primarily due to the (+)-enantiomer with the 1-(S) absolute configuration.[20]

Structure-activity relationships are not well described for the SSRIs. One example is the critical association of the *para*-location of the CF_3 substituent of fluoxetine on serotonin transporter potency.[21]

Bupropion is an aminoketone compound that is unlike most antidepressants. There are four chemical features that contribute to its uniqueness: chloro substituent, ketone function, tertiary alkyl group, and meta orientation of the substituent.[22]

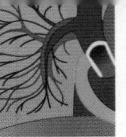

PHARMACOLOGY

The SSRIs all have a similar mechanism of action (Box 28-1). They inhibit the neuronal reuptake of serotonin and thus potentiate the effect of serotonin at the postsynaptic receptors. Most SSRIs have little or no effect on other neuroreceptors such as the histamine, acetylcholine, and adrenergic receptors. However, because the antidepressant effect is often delayed, it is postulated that there also may be a down-regulation of some of the postsynaptic serotonin receptors secondary to the increased serotonin in the synaptic cleft.[23,24] The SSRIs include fluoxetine, paroxetine, sertraline, fluvoxamine, and citalopram.

The atypical antidepressants, including trazodone, nefazodone, venlafaxine, bupropion, and mirtazapine, have distinct pharmacologic properties that differ somewhat from the SSRIs. All are effective antidepressants.

Venlafaxine, a bicyclic phenylethylamine, is a potent inhibitor of serotonin receptors. It has norepinephrine uptake and is a weak inhibitor of dopamine. It has little affinity for muscarinic, histamine, or α-adrenergic receptors.[25]

Trazodone is a triazolopyridine antidepressant that is structurally similar to the tricyclic antidepressants, but has weak inhibition of the reuptake of both norepinephrine and serotonin.[24]

Nefazodone is a 5-HT$_2$ antagonist with limited inhibition of the presynaptic reuptake of both serotonin and norepinephrine with the net effect being enhanced serotonin neurotransmission. It has weak affinity for the 5-HT$_2$, α-adrenergic, and β-adrenergic receptors and does not bind to the histamine, muscarinic, and dopaminergic receptors.[25]

Bupropion is a monocyclic antidepressant structurally related to amphetamine that acts by selectively inhibiting the neuronal reuptake of serotonin as well as dopamine and norepinephrine. It is used as both an antidepressant as well as an aid to smoking cessation.

Mirtazapine has unique pharmacologic effects. It blocks the presynaptic inhibitory α$_2$ autoreceptors, and the presynaptic inhibitory serotonin receptors. Postsynaptically, mirtazapine has little effect of α$_1$ receptors but blocks 5-HT$_2$ and 5-HT$_3$ receptors. The net effect is enhanced release and effects of both norepinephrine and serotonin. Mirtazapine has a high affinity for histamine receptors, but low affinity for cholinergic, muscarinic, and dopaminergic receptors.[1,25,26]

PHARMACOKINETICS

The SSRIs, unlike the cyclic antidepressants, are quite heterogeneous with respect to pharmacokinetic parameters, such as half-life and the presence of active metabolites (Table 28-1).[27] They are well absorbed from the gastrointestinal tract and undergo minimal first pass hepatic metabolism. The effect of food on drug absorption is variable with a decreased absorption for fluoxetine, increased absorption for sertraline, and no effect on paroxetine, fluvoxamine, and citalopram. The time to peak concentration averages 4 to 8 hours. SSRIs are all highly protein bound, varying from a low of 77% for fluvoxamine to over 90% for the remaining agents. The volume of distribution is large for most agents.[28]

The elimination half-life varies considerably among the various agents, ranging from 2 to 4 hours for nefazodone to 48 to 96 hours for fluoxetine. In addition, fluoxetine has an active metabolite, norfluoxetine, that has a half-life of 7 days. Linear pharmacokinetics have been described for sertraline and citalopram, while the other agents undergo nonlinear kinetics.[27-29]

SPECIAL POPULATIONS

The Elderly

SSRIs may be particularly useful in the elderly because of the absence of significant cardiovascular and anticholinergic adverse effects. However, while the pharmacokinetic behavior is similar in all age groups, the drugs may be more slowly metabolized in the elderly and dosage reductions are required. One should start with lower doses and titrate them slowly. In most cases, the final dose in this group of patients should be lower than in the younger population.[30] There are no data supporting one SSRI over another for the elderly, and the choice of drug will be influenced by other factors such as the possibility of drug-drug interactions.[23]

Patients with Renal and Hepatic Disease

Renal and hepatic disease delays the elimination of the SSRIs, and lower dosing or less frequent administration is required to avoid adverse effects. Paroxetine is mainly eliminated by the kidneys, and the dose should be

---

BOX 28-1	**PHARMACOLOGY OF THE NEW ANTIDEPRESSANTS**

Selective Serotonin Reuptake Inhibitors

Fluoxetine
Paroxetine
Sertraline
Fluvoxamine
Citalopram

Atypical Antidepressants

Serotonin Noradrenergic Reuptake Inhibitors (SNaRIs)
Venlafaxine
Nefazodone
Trazodone

Noradrenergic and Specific Serotonergic Antidepressants (NaSSA)
Mirtazapine

Dopamine Reuptake Inhibition
Bupropion

TABLE 28-1 Pharmacokinetics of Selective Serotonin Reuptake Inhibitors and Atypical Antidepressants

DRUG	KINETICS	T_{MAX} (hr)	HALF-LIFE	ACTIVE METABOLITES	PROTEIN BINDING (%)	HEPATIC	RENAL	AGING
Fluoxetine	Nonlinear	6–8	1–9 days	Norfluoxetine (7 days)	94	+	0	0
Sertraline	Linear	6–8	25 hr	No	98	+	0	+
Paroxetine	Nonlinear	5	10–16 hr	No	95	0	0	+
Fluvoxamine	Nonlinear	2–8	8–28 hr	No	77	+	0	+
Citalopram	Linear	2–4	33 hr	Norcitalopram (78 hr)	80	+	+	+
Bupropion	Linear	1–2	10–21 hr	Hydroxy-amfebutamone (15–22 hr) Threo-amfebutamone (9–27 hr)	84	0	?	0
Venlafaxine	Linear	2.1–2.4	2.7–3.8 hr	O-demethyl-venlafaxine (4.0–4.4 hr)	27	+	+	0
Trazodone		1–2	2–4 hr	m-chlorophenylpiperazine	89–95	?	?	+
Nefazodone		1–2			90	90	+	+
Mirtazapine	Linear		20–40 hr	No	85	+	+	+

+, parameter has an effect on pharmacokinetics; 0, parameter has no effect on pharmacokinetics; ?, effect not known; T_{max}, time to peak concentration.
Data derived from references 23, 25, and 28.

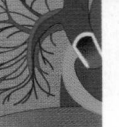

carefully titrated in patients with kidney disease and avoided with renal failure.[23,30,31] Dose reductions in patients with renal or hepatic disease are also required for mirtazapine.[25]

Pregnant and Lactating Patients

Most medications should be avoided in pregnancy if at all possible. Mild depression may be managed with nonpharmacological approaches. However, in severe depression, pharmacologic therapy may be required, and the SSRIs, especially fluoxetine, appear to be relatively safe in pregnancy.[30,32,33] Infant exposure during pregnancy is potentially significant due to placental passage, and therefore the lowest dosage that will provide adequate effects should be prescribed.[34,35] A study of 267 women who took SSRIs (fluoxetine, fluvoxamine, and sertraline) during the first trimester of pregnancy showed no increase in birth defects.[36]

The SSRIs have only been available for a relatively short time, and the potential long-term effects on breast-fed infants are unknown. However, postpartum depression has significant morbidity and mortality, and one needs to weigh the risks and benefits of the treatment of depression in women who are breast-feeding versus the potential risks to the infant. Again, the lowest effective dose of an agent that has minimal secretion in breast milk is recommended.

Paroxetine is secreted in breast milk, but it has no active metabolites, and adverse effects on breast-fed infants have not been reported. The majority of studies describing fluoxetine use in lactating women report no adverse effects on the infant. Sertraline as well as its metabolite desmethylsertraline have been detected in breast milk with low or nondetectable serum concentrations in the infant. Fluvoxamine has also been found in breast milk in very low concentrations, with no reported adverse effect on the infants. Venlafaxine and its metabolites have been found in the sera of breast-fed infants. However, no adverse effects were reported. Limited data exist on the effects of citalopram, trazodone, and nefazodone.[34]

In summary, SSRIs should be avoided in lactating women if possible. A careful weighing of the risk-benefit ratio is required, and if indicated, an agent such as paroxetine, sertraline, or fluoxetine that has minimal secretion in breast milk is suggested.

Children and Adolescents

Although SSRIs are commonly used in the pediatric and adolescent population, its use in this group is controversial.[37-39] Compared with adults, there is a paucity of data from controlled clinical trials in the pediatric population, and the best evidence for efficacy has been for the treatment of depression and obsessive-compulsive disorder. The evidence for other pediatric psychiatric disorders such as autism, social anxiety disorder, and eating disorders is mainly anecdotal.[29,40,41] In addition, there is concern about significant potential adverse effects found in children, such as activation, disinhibition, manic reactions, uncovering of comorbid disorders such as conduct disorders, frontal lobe symptoms (including apathy), and an increase in suicidal ideation.[42,43]

The concern regarding increased suicidal behavior and presumed lack of efficacy has led to a call in the United Kingdom that SSRIs should not be used in children with the possible exception of fluoxetine. Regulatory bodies in the United States and Canada have raised similar concerns.[41] However, this remains controversial.[37]

DRUG INTERACTIONS

Drug interactions may be either pharmacodynamic, where one drug affects the mechanism of action of another drug, or pharmacokinetic, where the drug affects the metabolism of excretion of another drug. Both of these are common with the SSRIs and newer antidepressants[44] (Table 28-2).

The most important pharmacodynamic drug interaction involving the SSRIs is the development of the potentially life-threatening serotonin syndrome. This occurs when an SSRI is combined with another serotonergic agent. The serotonin syndrome is described in Chapter 10A. When SSRIs are combined with a number of agents, the drugs that are of most concern are the MAOIs. A washout period of 2 weeks for most SSRIs and 5 weeks for fluoxetine is mandatory when switching from an SSRI to an MAOI to avoid the development of the serotonin syndrome.[45]

The cytochrome P-450 (CYP450) system metabolizes a number of medications including the SSRIs.[8,46] Drug interactions may result from inhibition of the CYP450 system, thus slowing metabolism of other medications, by acting as a competitive substrate or by the induction of enzymes. A number of enzymes are inhibited by the SSRIs to varying degrees, including CYP2D6, CYP1A2, CYP2C, and CYP3A4. The result is a negative effect on the metabolism of the other drugs and possible elevation in plasma levels. This is especially problematic if the drug in question has a narrow therapeutic window.[12,30]

All of the SSRIs are weak inhibitors of CYP2D6, which is also involved in the metabolism of a number of other common medications, including the cyclic antidepressants, some antipsychotics, β-adrenergic blockers, type Ic antidysrhythmics (encainide, flecainide, mexilitene, and propafenone), codeine, and dextromethorphan. Paroxetine has the greatest effect on CYP2D6 followed by norfluoxetine, fluoxetine, sertraline, fluvoxamine, venlafaxine, nefazodone, and mirtazapine.[44,47]

The SSRIs as well as nefazodone inhibit CYP4A4, which also metabolizes terfenadine and astemizole, as well as the triazolo-benzodiazepines, such as triazalom, alprazalom, and midazolam.[44]

CYP1A2 metabolizes theophylline as well as the tertiary cyclic antidepressants imipramine, clomipramine, and amitryptyline. Fluoxetine, paroxetine, and sertraline are weak inhibitors of this enzyme. Fluvoxamine is a potent inhibitor of this enzyme, and concomitant therapy has

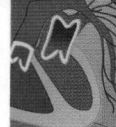

TABLE 28-2 Selected Substrates and Inhibitors of Some Cytochrome P-450 Enzymes*				
CYP ENZYMES			
1A2	**2C19**	**2D6**	**3A4**
Substrates			
TCA†	TCA†	TCA‡	TCA†
Mexiletine	Phenytoin	**Trazodone**	Quinidine
Theophylline	Diazepam	**Fluoxetine**	Terfenadine
Caffeine	Indomethacin	**Paroxetine**	Cyclosporine
Estradiol	S-warfarin	**Venlafaxine**	Tamoxifen
Tacrine	Propranolol	Metoprolol	Lidocaine
R-warfarin	Omeprazole	Timolol	Cisapride
Amiodarone	Phenobarbital	Haloperidol	Rifabutin
	Carbamazepine	Clozapine	Midazolam
		Risperidone	Triazolam
		Thioridazine	Alprazolam
		Perphenazine	Carbamazepine
		Dextromethorphan	Dapsone
		Phenytoin	Lovastatin
Inhibitors			
Fluvoxamine	**Fluoxetine**	**Sertraline**	**Fluoxetine**
Cimetidine	**Fluvoxamine**	Quinidine	**Venlafaxine**
Erythromycin	**Sertraline**	Amiodarone	**Sertraline**
Ciprofloxacin	Citmetidine	Fluphenazine	**Nefazodone**
Enoxacin	Amiodarone	Moclobemide	**Fluvoxamine**
Meclobamine	Ketoconazole		Fluconazole
Disulfiram	Erythromycin		Ketoconazole
	Propoxyphene		Erythromycin
	Felbamate		Clarithromycin
			Amiodarone
			Saquinavir
			Cimetidine

TCA, tricyclic antidepressant.
*Selective serotonin reuptake inhibitors and TCAs are indicated by bold type. Any two drugs that are substrates of the same cytochrome P-450 (CYP) enzyme may potentially compete with each other for that enzyme and thereby inhibit each other's metabolism. Some drugs may also inhibit a CYP enzyme without themselves being a substrate. Note that this table indicates potential interactions; not all have been demonstrated or are necessarily of clinical importance. Some drugs listed as inhibitors may actually be substrates for that particular CYP, but sufficient documentation is not available. Some drugs are substrates or inhibitors of more than one CYP enzyme.
†Demethylation of tertiary amine TCAs; imipramine, amitriptyline, and clomipramine.
‡Hydroxylation of desipramine, imipramine, clomipramine, amitriptyline, and nortriptyline.
Adapted from DeVane CL: Pharmacogenetics and drug metabolism of newer antidepressant agents. J Clin Psychiatry 1994;55(Suppl):38–47.

resulted in elevated plasma theophylline and cyclic antidepressant levels.[44]

Fluvoxamine, fluoxetine, and sertraline are mild to moderate inhibitors of CYP2C9 and -19, and interactions with warfarin and tolbutamide have been reported. Venlafaxine has no effects on CYP2C9 in vitro.[44]

CYP3A4 is the most abundant of the cytochrome enzymes and therefore one of the most important with respect to drug interactions. Nefazodone is the most potent inhibitor of this enzyme, followed by fluvoxamine, norfluoxetine, paroxetine, desmethylsertraline, fluoxetine, sertraline, mirtazapine, and venlafaxine. One should avoid combining these antidepressants with other drugs with potent effects on CYP3A4, such as ketoconazole, terfenadine, and astemizole.[30,44]

In summary, the drugs that are most likely to cause clinically significant pharmacokinetic drug interactions with drugs metabolized by the CYP450 system are fluvoxamine, fluoxetine, paroxetine, and nefazodone. Sertraline has fewer effects, while mirtazapine and ven-lafaxine have the least propensity for such pharmacokinetic interactions.[44]

Starting at lower dosing and careful titration of the medications can minimize drug interactions with the SSRIs and other medications that are oxidized by the P-450 system.[45]

There is no pharmacokinetic interaction or potentiation of psychomotor impairment associated with ethanol.[9]

TOXICOLOGY

The ingestion of 50 to 75 times the therapeutic dose may result in minor symptoms such as drowsiness, tremor, weakness, nausea, and vomiting. Seizures and electrocardiographic (ECG) changes such as widening QRS or QT prolongation and a decreasing level of consciousness occur with larger ingestions. Death has occurred with extremely large overdoses of greater than 150 times the usual therapeutic dose.[14,48]

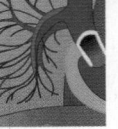
Pure SSRI overdose rarely results in death, and most patients recover without long-term effects. Most of the reported deaths are associated with the ingestion of other drugs or in combination with alcohol.

CLINICAL MANIFESTATIONS

Acute Overdose

The SSRIs and atypical antidepressants are usually benign in overdose and considered much safer than either the cyclic antidepressants or MAOIs. However, each can manifest toxic effects, and there are anecdotal reports of significant toxicity for most of the drugs in this class.[7]

The most common symptoms after acute SSRI overdose include drowsiness, nausea, and vomiting. Other less common effects include dizziness, headache, tremor, and agitation. Serious effects such as dysrhythmias and seizures occur rarely and are much more common with citalopram or venlafaxine overdoses.[49]

The serotonin syndrome has been reported after SSRI overdose, either alone or in combination with other antidepressants.[50] It is a potentially life-threatening syndrome characterized by autonomic dysfunction (hypo- or hypertension, tachycardia, hyperpyrexia, diaphoresis, diarrhea), abnormalities in mental status (disorientation, delirium, confusion, and agitation), and neuromuscular signs and symptoms (myoclonus, especially of the lower extremities, tremor, hyperreflexia, and rigidity). The serotonin syndrome is discussed in Chapter 10A.

Fluoxetine

Fluoxetine overdose is associated with either no or minor effects described in large case series.[51-56] Anecdotally, the most significant toxicities reported are seizures, lethargy, and mild cardiovascular effects such as increased QRS and QT.[57-60]

Sertraline

Sertraline overdose is usually benign.[61-64] Marked diarrhea has been reported with a sertraline overdose,[65] and the serotonin syndrome has been reported with massive overdose.[66-68] Delayed angioedema necessitating tracheal intubation for airway control has been reported after a sertraline and trazodone overdose.[69] Deaths are uncommon, but have been reported associated with asthma[70] and markedly elevated postmortem serum concentrations.[71]

Citalopram

Most citalopram overdoses are associated with little or no clinical effects, although significant toxicity has been reported anecdotally, including seizures, wide complex tachycardia, supraventricular tachycardia, prolonged QTc, and widened QRS.[49,72-75] Severe bradycardia without

QTc prolongation, hypotension, and syncope requiring a temporary pacemaker has also been reported.[76]

Only mild symptoms are associated with ingestions of less than 600 mg, while ECG effects and seizures have been reported after ingestions of greater than 600 mg. All patients will have toxic effects with ingestions of 1900 mg or greater.[77] Cardiovascular effects occur in about 25% of overdoses.[78] Adult respiratory distress syndrome and renal failure, which resolved with supportive care, have been reported after an ingestion of 2400 mg of citalopram.[79] Fatalities with high postmortem blood concentrations have been reported.[80,81] Lower postmortem concentrations may be seen when there are multiple ingestants.[82]

Paroxetine

Paroxetine has a high therapeutic index, and overdose is usually benign in both adults and children. Symptoms are dose related and include minor gastrointestinal complaints, drowsiness, tachycardia, dizziness, and mydriasis.[83,84] Significant hyponatremia occurred 5 days after a paroxetine overdose in an elderly woman.[85] The serotonin syndrome has been reported with combined paroxetine and moclobemide overdose.[86] Deaths have been reported in which there were significant postmortem paroxetine concentrations found in blood. However, there were other drugs involved in all of these cases.[87]

Fluvoxamine

Fluvoxamine overdose is typically not associated with significant toxicity. The most commonly reported effects are drowsiness, tremor, nausea and vomiting, anticholinergic symptoms, and hemodynamically stable bradycardia.[88-90] Nevertheless, a life-threatening intoxication with severe bradycardia, hypotension, seizure activity, and acute respiratory distress syndrome in a 4-year-old child has been reported.[91]

Trazodone

The clinical manifestations of trazodone overdose are generally mild, with drowsiness, nausea, and vomiting being the predominant symptoms, although coma has been reported.[92-96] Because trazodone has little effect on norepinephrine reuptake and does not affect the sodium channels, there is no significant cardiovascular toxicity. A case of severe hyponatremia and late seizure after an overdose of trazodone in an elderly patient has been reported. The hyponatremia was presumed to be due to inappropriate antidiuretic hormone secretion.[97] The terminal half-life of trazodone after overdose was reported to be approximately 8.8 hours in a case report.[98] Deaths are uncommon except when trazodone is ingested with other agents or ethanol.[99]

Nefazodone

Nefazodone has effects on both the serotonin and norepinephrine receptors, and the course after overdose

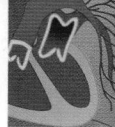

is usually benign, with patients either being asymptomatic or having minor effects such as drowsiness, nausea, vomiting, and dizziness.[99,100] However, more serious effects have also been reported, including hypotension, bradycardia, seizures, and prolongation of the QTc.[101,102]

Bupropion

The majority of cases of bupropion ingestion reported to poison control centers are benign, likely related to minor ingestions. The clinical manifestations seen in minor overdose included nausea and vomiting, tachycardia, hypertension, headache, dizziness, tremor, and mild drowsiness or agitation.[103-105] However, bupropion is potentially more toxic in overdose compared with most of the SSRIs. Significant toxicity has been reported, including seizures and cardiac conduction abnormalities such as widened QRS and prolonged QTc.[106-113] The seizures may occur late in overdose of sustained release preparations.[114] Cardiotoxicity has also been reported in a combined bupropion and ziprasidone overdose.[115] While deaths are uncommon, they have been reported and are usually associated with a massive ingestion[116] or multiple ingestants including alcohol.[117]

Venlafaxine

Venlafaxine is potentially more toxic in overdose than the SSRIs due to its effects on the reuptake of norepinephrine and to a lesser extent dopamine. It is available in both an immediate-release and extended-release formulation.[25] Venlafaxine is considered proconvulsant, and overdose has been associated with seizures.[118-123] Other toxic effects reported include prolonged QRS and QT, ventricular tachycardia, persistent myocardial ischemia, hypertension, and refractory hypotension.[122-127] Serotonin-associated symptoms such as diarrhea, diaphoresis, and rhabdomyolysis, as well as the serotonin syndrome, have also been described.[128-132] Fatalities have been reported,[127,132,133] and its fatality toxicity index is greater than other serotonergic agents and similar to the less toxic cyclic antidepressants.[6]

Mirtazapine

There are only a few reports of mirtazapine overdose in the literature, with only minor effects, including drowsiness, confusion, and tachycardia, described.[134-138] Miosis and coma have also been described with significant overdose.[139]

ADVERSE EFFECTS

Adverse effects associated with SSRI therapy are common and are dose related (Box 28-2).[10,11] SSRI adverse effects, however, are generally mild due to the relative selectivity for serotonin receptors and relative absence of significant interaction with other receptors such as histamine and anticholinergic receptors, and they are better tolerated than the cyclic antidepressants.[4,23,140]

BOX 28-2	ADVERSE EFFECTS OF SELECTIVE SEROTONIN REUPTAKE INHIBITORS

Central Nervous System

Headache
Anxiety
Agitation
Insomnia
Seizures

Gastrointestinal

Nausea
Vomiting
Diarrhea
Anorexia

Other Effects

Hepatotoxicity
Hyponatremia
Discontinuation or withdrawal symptoms

The most common problems encountered include gastrointestinal effects such as nausea and vomiting, anorexia, diarrhea, headache, and stimulant effects such as agitation, anxiety, and insomnia.[9,10,141-143] These are so-called serotonin-type symptoms[4] and are worse at higher doses.[10] Other adverse effects that are less common, but still considered of concern, include weight loss and sexual dysfunction. Trazodone has been associated with priapism.[144]

While the general adverse effects are mild, there are differences between agents. Fluoxetine has been associated with a greater incidence of agitation compared with the other SSRIs, while sertraline appears to cause less agitation. Lethargy and apathy have also been reported.[144] Fluvoxamine has a significant rate of nausea, but this may be less prevalent with paroxetine. Of the SSRIs, sertraline appears to have a lower incidence of side effects.[11]

There is a significant discontinuation rate with SSRI therapy that is directly related to the severity of these adverse effects. Nausea and agitation are the most common reasons for patients stopping therapy.[145]

Cardiovascular side effects are less common with SSRIs. Nevertheless, increased angina, especially in patients with underlying coronary artery disease, has been reported. Dysrhythmias such as atrial fibrillation and bradycardia resulting in syncope, as well as blood pressure changes, have also been reported.[12,144]

Sudden death, syncope, repolarization changes, prolonged QT, and polymorphous ventricular tachycardia (torsades de pointes) in patients taking SSRIs have been reported to regulatory agencies. These effects may be due to the SSRIs themselves or may be a result of increased plasma levels of other medications, due to effects on the CYP450 system.[12]

Severe hyponatremia has been reported in elderly patients taking SSRIs such as fluoxetine and sertraline. The mechanism is unknown, and the hyponatremia

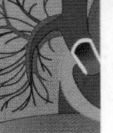

usually responds to withdrawal of the medication.[146] The syndrome of inappropriate antidiuretic hormone (SIADH) has also been reported with SSRIs and may be mediated through serotonin-2A and -2C receptors.[144]

Seizures are uncommon, but have been associated with therapy with a number of the SSRIs.[147] Bupropion has a higher reported incidence of seizures, especially in patients with anorexia. However, the incidence in the general population is comparable with that associated with cyclic antidepressants and is usually associated with higher dosing.[148]

Nefazodone has been associated with hepatic abnormalities and has been removed from the market in Sweden, other parts of Europe, and recently Canada.[149]

Adverse effects reported at therapeutic dosing of mirtazapine include akathisia and hepatotoxicity that resolved with discontinuation of the drug.[150,151] The serotonin syndrome has been described with both monotherapy and in combination with SSRIs therapeutically and in overdose, although the role of mirtazapine in causation of the serotonin syndrome is disputed.[152-157]

Discontinuation reactions or the SSRI withdrawal syndrome have been reported after the abrupt cessation of treatment with all SSRIs as well as venlafaxine and nefazodone. They are most common with paroxetine and fluvoxamine, and much less common with sertraline and fluoxetine. This is most likely related to pharmacologic differences, being much more common with agents with shorter half-lives and can be ameliorated with tapering of the agents when stopping therapy. The symptoms are usually mild and short lived, and common effects include fatigue, headache, nausea, diarrhea, agitation, insomnia, and lethargy. However, more novel discontinuation reactions may also occur with the SSRIs. These can be grouped into three common symptom clusters: effects on balance (vertigo, dizziness, and ataxia), sensory symptoms (numbness, paresthesias, and "shocklike" sensations), and aggressive and impulsive behavior (suicidal and homicidal thoughts). There is often overlap of these symptom clusters.[23,158,159]

DIAGNOSIS

Laboratory Testing

Initial laboratory investigations should include complete blood count and routine biochemistry, including renal function. Specific blood levels of the SSRIs and other atypical antidepressants[160] are rarely available and do not aid management and thus are not routinely indicated.[8] False-positive urine drug screens for amphetamines have been reported with bupropion and trazodone overdose.[112,113,161] A false-positive drug screen for phencyclidine not confirmed by gas chromatography–mass spectrometry has been reported after a massive venlafaxine overdose.[118] If rhabdomyolysis or the serotonin syndrome is suspected, serum creatine kinase and myoglobin should be analyzed.

Other Diagnostic Testing

An electrocardiogram should be obtained because cardiac effects may occur with SSRI and atypical antidepressant overdose. Other investigations may be indicated based on the clinical presentation.

DIFFERENTIAL DIAGNOSIS

There is no specific toxidrome or laboratory test that is diagnostic, and the differential diagnosis will depend on the patient's signs and symptoms. While most overdoses are asymptomatic, patients with an SSRI overdose may present with a decreased level of consciousness, and the differential diagnosis should include the ingestion of any agent or clinical condition that could result in an alteration of the mental status. If the patient has a seizure, then one should consider the differential diagnosis of toxin-induced seizures.

MANAGEMENT

Supportive Measures

Cardiac monitoring and pulse oximetry are indicated in all patients. Venous access is indicated in patients with symptoms or signs of an SSRI overdose. The airway, breathing, and circulation should be evaluated and corrective actions taken if there are any abnormalities. Indications for tracheal intubation include a significant decrease in the patient's level of consciousness or the need to establish or protect their airway. Supplemental oxygen is indicated for hypoxia. Hypotension should be managed initially with intravenous crystalloid solution. Vasopressor therapy is rarely needed, but should be instituted if hypotension persists despite adequate fluid resuscitation.

Patients with an altered mental status should have a bedside glucose determination performed, and hypoglycemia should be treated with hypertonic dextrose.

Decontamination

Activated charcoal is indicated if the patient presents within 2 hours of ingestion of a potentially toxic overdose. However, one must be cautious and protect the airway if the patient has an altered level of consciousness or seizures. Whole bowel irrigation may be considered if a sustained-release preparation is ingested or for late presentation. Gastric lavage or administration of ipecac is not indicated.

Laboratory Monitoring

The indication for serial laboratory testing is initial abnormalities or the development of ongoing toxicity such as the serotonin syndrome or rhabdomyolysis. If

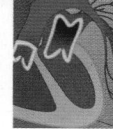

there is QT prolongation on the ECG, then serial ECGs should be obtained until the QT is normalized.

Elimination

Due to the large volume of distribution of the SSRIs and significant protein binding, methods to enhance elimination such as multiple doses of charcoal or hemodialysis are not effective or indicated.

Antidotes

There are no specific antidotes. Anecdotally, sodium bicarbonate has been used to treat presumed sodium channel blockade–induced cardiotoxicity.[60,74] The administration of a sodium bicarbonate bolus followed by an infusion should be considered if there is evidence of QRS prolongation.

Disposition

Patients with significant symptoms will require admission to hospital. Indications for intensive care unit admission include significant decreased level of consciousness, cardiac dysrhythmias, and presence of the serotonin syndrome.

Patients who are asymptomatic with no signs of toxicity may be discharged after 6 hours of observation in the emergency department after appropriate psychiatric consultation.[8]

REFERENCES

1. Sambunaris A, Hesselink JK, Pinder R, et al: Development of new antidepressants. J Clin Psychiatry 1997;58(Suppl 6):40.
2. Henry JA, Alexander CA, Sener EK: Relative mortality from overdose of antidepressants. BMJ 1995;310:221.
3. Henry JA: Epidemiology and relative toxicity of antidepressant drugs in overdose. Drug Saf 1997;16:374.
4. Perreti S, Judge R, Hindmarch I: Safety and tolerability considerations: tricyclic antidepressants vs. selective serotonin reuptake inhibitors. Acta Psychiatr Scand 2000;101(Suppl 403):17.
5. de Jonghe F, Swinkels JA: The safety of antidepressants. Drugs 1992;43(Suppl 2):40.
6. Buckley NA, McManus PR: Fatal toxicity of serotonergic and other antidepressant drugs: analysis of United Kingdom mortality data. BMJ 2002;325:1332.
7. Buckley NA, Faunce TA: Atypical antidepressants in overdose. Clinical considerations with respect to safety. Drug Saf 2003;26:539.
8. Power BM, Hackett LP, Dusci LJ, Ilett KE: Antidepressant toxicity and the need for identification and concentration monitoring in overdose. Clin Pharmacokinet 1995;29:154.
9. Rudorfer MV, Manji HK, Potter WZ: Comparative tolerability profiles of the newer versus older antidepressants. Drug Saf 1994;10:18.
10. Montgomery SA: New antidepressants and 5-HT uptake inhibitors. Acta Psychiatr Scand 1989;80(Suppl 350):107.
11. Rickels K, Schweizer E: Clinical overview of serotonin reuptake inhibitors. J Clin Psychiatry 1990;51(Suppl):9.
12. Dalfen AK, Stewart DE: Who develops severe or fatal adverse drug reactions to selective serotonin reuptake inhibitors? Can J Psychiatry 2001;46:258.
13. Watson WA, Litovitz TL, Rodgers GC, et al: 2002 annual report of the American Association of Poison Control Centers toxic exposure surveillance system. Am J Emerg Med 2003;21:353.
14. Barbey JT, Roose SP: SSRI safety in overdose. J Clin Psychiatry 1998;59(Suppl 15):42.
15. Mason J, Freemantle N, Eccles M: Fatal toxicity associated with antidepressant use in primary care. Br J Gen Pract 2000;50:366
16. Revicki DA, Palmer CS, Phillips SD, et al: Acute medical costs of fluoxetine versus tricyclic antidepressants. A prospective multi-centre study of antidepressant drug overdoses. Pharmacoeconomics 1997;11:48.
17. Kapur N, House A, Creed F, et al: Costs of antidepressant overdose: a preliminary study. Br J Gen Pract 1999;49:733.
18. Ramchandani P, Murray B, Hawton K, et al: Deliberate self poisoning with antidepressant drugs: a comparison of the relative hospital costs of cases of overdose of tricyclics with those of selective-serotonin re-uptake inhibitors. J Affect Disord 2000;60:97.
19. Stoner SC, Marken PA, Watson WA, et al: Antidepressant overdoses and resultant emergency department services: the impact of SSRIs. Psychopharmacol Bull 1997;33:667.
20. Willets J, Lippa A, Beer B: Clinical development of citalopram. J Clin Psychopharmacol 1999;19(Suppl 1):36.
21. Baldessarini RJ, Tarazi FI: Drugs and the treatment of psychiatric disorders. In Hardman JG, Limbird LE (eds): Goodman and Gilman's The Pharmacologic Basis of Therapeutics, 10th ed. 485–529. 2001. New York, McGraw-Hill, 2001, pp 485–529.
22. Mehta NB: The chemistry of bupropion. J Clin Psychiatry 1983;44:56.
23. Vaswani M, Linda FK, Ramesh S: Role of selective serotonin reuptake inhibitors in psychiatric disorders: a comprehensive review. Prog Neuropsychopharmacol Biol Psychiatry 2003;27:85.
24. Frazer A: Pharmacology of antidepressants. J Clin Psychopharmacol 1997;17:(2S Suppl):2S.
25. Kent JM: SNaRIs, NaSSAs and NaRIs: new agents for the treatment of depression. Lancet 2000;355:911.
26. Hartmann PM: Mirtazapine: a newer antidepressant. Am Fam Phys 1999;59:159.
27. Preskorn SH: Pharmacokinetics of antidepressants: why and how they are relevant to treatment. J Clin Psychiatry 1993;54(9 Suppl):14.
28. Goodnick PJ: Pharmacokinetic optimization of therapy with newer antidepressants. Clin Pharmacokinetics 1994;27:307.
29. Ziervogel CE: Selective serotonin re-uptake inhibitors for children and adolescents. Eur Child Adolesc Psychiatry 2000;9:I20.
30. Mourilhe P, Stokes PE: Risks and benefits of selective serotonin reuptake inhibitors in the treatment of depression. Drug Saf 1998;18:57.
31. Mitchell PB: Selective serotonin reuptake inhibitors: adverse effects, toxicity and interactions. Advers Drug React Toxicol Rev 1994;13:121.
32. Gupta S, Masand PS, Rangwani S: Selective serotonin reuptake inhibitors in pregnancy and lactation. Obstet Gynecol Surv 1998;53:733.
33. Wisner KL, Gelenberg AJ, Leonard H, et al: Pharmacological treatment of depression during pregnancy. JAMA 1999;282:1264.
34. Misri S, Kostaras X: Benefits and risks to mother and infant of drug treatment for postnatal depression. Drug Saf 2002;25:903.
35. Misri S, Burgmann A, Kostaras D: Are SSRIs safe for pregnant and breastfeeding women? Can Fam Physician 2000;46:626.
36. Kulin NA, Patuszak A, Sage SR: Pregnancy outcome following maternal use of the new selective serotonin inhibitors. JAMA 1998;279:609.
37. Ramchandani P: Treatment of major depressive disorder in children and adolescents. BMJ 2004;328:3.
38. Varley CK: Psychopharmacological treatment of major depressive disorder in children and adolescents. JAMA 2003;290:1091.
39. Garland EJ: Facing the evidence: antidepressant treatment in children and adolescents. CMAJ 2004;170:489.
40. DeVane CL, Sallee FR: Serotonin selective reuptake inhibitors in child and adolescent psychopharmacology: a review of published experience. J Clin Psychiatry 1996;57:55.
41. Wagner KD, Ambrosini P, Rynn M, et al: Efficacy of sertraline in the treatment of children and adolescents with major depressive disorder. JAMA 2003;290:1033.
42. Walkup J, Labellarte M: Complications of SSRI treatment. J Child Adolesc Psychopharmacol 2001;11:1.

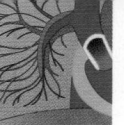

43. Wooltortoon E: Paroxetine (Paxil, Seroxat): increased risk of suicide in pediatric patients. CMAJ 2003;169:446.

44. Richelson E: Pharmacokinetic drug interactions of new antidepressants: a review of the effects on the metabolism of other drugs. Mayo Clin Proc 1997;72:835.

45. Rosenbaum JF: Managing selective serotonin reuptake inhibitor-drug interactions in clinical practice. Clin Pharmacokinetics 1995;29(Suppl 1):53.

46. Greenblatt DJ, von Moltke LL, Harmatz JS, Shader RI: Human cytochromes and some newer antidepressants: kinetics, metabolism, and drug interactions. J Clin Psychopharmacol 1999;(Suppl 1):489–493.

47. Ereshefsky L, Reisenman C, Lam YW: Antidepressant drug interactions and the cytochrome P450 system. The role of cytochrome P450 2D6. Clin Pharmacokinet 1995;29(Suppl 1):10.

48. Glassman AH: Citalopram toxicity. Lancet 1997;350:818.

49. Catalano G, Catalano M, Epstein MA, et al: QTc interval prolongation associated with citalopram overdose. A case report and literature review. Clin Neuropharmacol 2001;24:158.

50. Neuvonen PJ, Pohjola-Sintonen S, Tacke U, et al: Five fatal cases of serotonin syndrome after moclobemide-citalopram or moclobemide-clomipramine overdoses [letter]. Lancet 1993;342:1419.

51. Spiller HA, Morse S: Fluoxetine ingestion: a one year retrospective study. Vet Hum Toxicol 1990;32:153.

52. Borys, DJ, Setzer SC, Ling LJ, et al: The effects of fluoxetine in the overdose patient. Clin Toxicol 1990;28:331.

53. Borys DJ, Setzer SC, Ling LJ, et al: Acute fluoxetine overdose: a report of 234 cases. Am J Emerg Med 1992;10:115.

54. Moore JL, Rodriguez R: Toxicity of fluoxetine in overdose [letter]. Am J Psychiatry 1989;147:1089.

55. Kim SW, Pentel P: Flu-like symptoms associated with fluoxetine overdose: a case study. Clin Toxicol 1989;27:389.

56. Feirabend RH: Benign course in a child with massive fluoxetine overdose. J Fam Pract 1995;41:289.

57. Phillips S, Brent J, Kulig K, et al: Fluoxetine versus tricyclic antidepressants: a prospective multicenter study of antidepressant drug overdoses. J Emerg Med 1997;15:439.

58. Braitberg G, Curry SC: Seizure after isolated fluoxetine overdose. Ann Emerg Med 1995;26:234.

59. Gross R, Dannon PN, Zohar J, et al: Generalized seizures caused by fluoxetine overdose [letter]. Am J Emerg Med 1998;16:328.

60. Graudins A, Vossler C, Wang R: Fluoxetine-induced cardiotoxicity with response to bicarbonate therapy. Am J Emerg Med 1997;15:501.

61. Klein-Schwartz W, Anderson B: Analysis of sertraline-only overdoses. Am J Emerg Med 1996;14:456.

62. Caracci G: Unsuccessful suicide attempt by sertraline overdose [letter]. Am J Psychiatry 1994;151:147.

63. Catalano G, Cooper DS, Catalano MC, et al: Pediatric sertraline overdose. Clin Neuropharmacol 1998;21:59.

64. Lau GT, Horowitz BZ: Sertraline overdose. Acad Emerg Med 1996;3:132.

65. Brown DF, Kerr HD: Sertraline overdose [letter]. Ann Pharmacother 1994;28:1307.

66. Brendel DH, Bodkin JA, Yang JM: Massive sertraline overdose. Ann Emerg Med 2000;36:524.

67. Kaminski CA, Robbins MS, Weibley RE: Sertraline intoxication in a child. Ann Emerg Med 1994;23:1371.

68. Pao M, Tipnis T: Serotonin syndrome after sertraline overdose in a 5-year-old girl [letter]. Arch Pediatr Adolesc Med 1997;151:1064.

69. Adson DE, Erickson-Birkedahl S, Kotlyar M: An unusual presentation of sertraline and trazodone overdose. Ann Pharmacother 2001;35:1375.

70. Carson HJ, Zweigart M, Lueck NE: Death from asthma associated with sertraline overdose. Am J Forensic Med Pathol 2000;21:273.

71. Milner DA, Hall M, Davis GG, et al: Fatal multiple drug intoxication following acute sertraline use. J Anal Toxicol 1998;22:545.

72. Grundemar L, Wohlfart B, Lagerstedt C, et al: Symptoms and signs of severe citalopram overdose. Lancet 1997;349:1602.

73. Bezchlibnyk-Butler K, Aleksic I, Kennedy SH: Citalopram—a review of pharmacological and clinical effects. J Psychiatry Neurosci 2000;25:241.

74. Engebretsen KM, Harris CR, Wood JE: Cardiotoxicity and late onset seizures with citalopram overdose. J Emerg Med 2003;25:163.

75. Cuenca PJ, Holt KR, Hoefle JD: Seizure secondary to citalopram overdose. J Emerg Med 2004;26:177.

76. Rothenhausler H-B, Haberl C, Ehrentraut S, et al: Suicide attempt by pure citalopram overdose causing long-lasting severe sinus bradycardia, hypotension and syncope: successful therapy with a temporary pacemaker. Pharmacopsychiatry 2000;33:150.

77. Personne M, Sjoberg G, Persson H: Citalopram overdose—review of cases treated in Swedish hospitals. Clin Toxicol 1997;35:237.

78. Personne M, Persson H, Sjoberg G: Citalopram toxicity [letter]. Lancet 1997;350:518.

79. Kelly CA, Upex A, Spencer EP, et al: Adult respiratory distress syndrome and renal failure associated with citalopram overdose. Hum Exp Toxicol 2003;22:103.

80. Öström M, Eriksson A, Thorson J, et al: Fatal overdose with citalopram [letter]. Lancet 1996;348:339.

81. Jonasson B, Saldeen T: Citalopram in fatal poisoning cases. Forensic Sci Int 2002;126:1.

82. Fu K, Konrad RJ, Hardy RW, et al: An unusual multiple drug intoxication case involving citalopram. J Anal Toxicol 2000;24:648.

83. Myers LB, Krenzelok EP: Paroxetine (Paxil) overdose: a pediatric focus. Vet Hum Toxicol 1997;39:86.

84. Gorman SE, Rice T, Simmons HF: Paroxetine overdose [letter]. Am J Emerg Med 1993;11:682.

85. Johnsen CR, Hoejlyng N: Hyponatremia following acute overdose with paroxetine. Int J Clin Pharm Ther 1998;36:333.

86. Fitzsimmons CR, Metha S: Serotonin syndrome caused by overdose with paroxetine and moclobemide. J Accid Emerg Med 1999;16:293.

87. Vermeulen T: Distribution of paroxetine in three postmortem cases. J Anal Toxicol 1998;22:541.

88. Garnier R, Azoyan P, Chataigner D, et al: Acute fluvoxamine poisoning. J Int Med Res 1993;21:197.

89. Lebegue B: Survivable fluvoxamine overdose [letter]. Am J Psychiatry 1990;147:1689.

90. Amital D, Amital H, Gross R, et al: Sinus bradycardia due to fluvoxamine overdose. Br J Psychiatry 1994;165:553.

91. Fraser J, South M: Life-threatening fluvoxamine overdose in a 4-year old child. Intensive Care Med 1999;25:548.

92. Ali CJ, Henry JA: Trazodone overdose: experience over 5 years. Neuropsychobiology 1986;15(Suppl 1):44.

93. Henry JA, Ali CJ, Caldwell R, et al: Acute trazodone poisoning: clinical signs and plasma concentrations. Psychopathology 1984;17(Suppl 2):77.

94. Gamble DE, Peterson LG: Trazodone overdose: four years of experience from voluntary reports. J Clin Psychiatry 1986;47:544.

95. Lesar T, Kingston R, Dahms R, et al: Trazodone overdose. Ann Emerg Med 1983;12:221.

96. Flomenbaum N, Price D: Recognition and management of antidepressant overdoses: tricyclics and trazodone. Neuropsychobiology 1986;15(Suppl 1):46.

97. Vanpee D, Laloyaux P, Gillet J-B: Seizure and hyponatremia after overdose of trazodone [letter]. Am J Emerg Med 1999;17:430.

98. Hassan E, Miller DD: Toxicity and elimination of trazodone after overdose. Clin Pharm 1985;4:97.

99. Benson BE, Mathiason M, Dahl D, et al: Toxicities and outcomes associated with nefazodone poisoning: an analysis of 1,338 exposures. Am J Emerg Med 2000;18:587.

100. Gaffney PN, Schuckman HA: Naefazodone overdose [letter]. Ann Pharmacother 1998;32:1249.

101. Isbister GK, Hackett LP: Nefazodone poisoning: toxicokinetics and toxicodynamics using continuous data collection. J Toxicol Clin Toxicol 2003;41:167.

102. Catalano G, Catalano MC, Tumarkin NB: Nefazodone overdose: a case report. Clinical Neuropharmacol 1999;22:63.

103. Spiller HA, Ramoska EA, Krenzelok EP, et al: Bupropion overdose: a 3-year multi-center retrospective analysis. Am J Emerg Med 1994;12:43.

104. Belson MG, Kelley TR: Bupropion exposures: clinical manifestations and medical outcome. J Emerg Med 2002;23:223.

105. Balit CR, Lynch CN, Isbister GK: Bupropion poisoning: a case series. Med J Aust 2003;178:61.

106. Tracey JA, Cassidy C, Casey PB, et al: Bupropion (Zyban) toxicity. Irish Med J 2002;95:23.

107. Paris PA, Saucier JR: ECG conduction delays associated with massive bupropion overdose. Clin Toxicol 1998;36:595.
108. Ayers S, Tobias JD: Bupropion overdose in an adolescent. Pediatr Emerg Care 2001;17:104.
109. Mainie I, McGurk C, McClintock G, et al: Seizures after bupropion overdose [letter]. Lancet 2001;357:1624.
110. Gittelman DK, Kirby MG: A seizure following bupropion overdose [letter]. J Clin Psychiatry 1993;54:162.
111. Storrow A: Bupropion overdose and seizure. Am J Emerg Med 1994;12:183.
112. Paoloni R, Szekely I: Sustained-release bupropion overdose: a new entity for Australian emergency departments. Emerg Med 2002;14:109.
113. Shrier M, Diaz JE, Tsarouhas N: Cardiotoxicity associated with bupropion overdose [letter]. Ann Emerg Med 2000;35:100.
114. Jepsen F, Matthews J, Andrews FJ: Sustained release bupropion overdose: an important cause of prolonged symptoms after overdose. Emerg Med J 2003;20:560.
115. Biswas AK, Zabrocki LA, Mayes KL, et al: Cardiotoxicity associated with intentional ziprasidone and bupropion overdose. J Toxicol Clin Toxicol 2003;41:101.
116. Harris CR, Gualteri, Stark G: Fatal bupropion overdose. Clin Toxicol 1997;35:321.
117. Ramcharitar V, Levine BS, Goldberger BA, et al: Bupropion and alcohol fatal intoxication: case report. Forensic Sci Int 1992;56:151.
118. Bond GR, Steele PE, Uges RA: Massive venlafaxine overdose resulted in a false positive Abbott AxSYM urine immunoassay for phencyclidine. J Toxicol Clin Toxicol 2003;41:999.
119. Whyte IM. Dawson AH, Buckley NA: Relative toxicity of venlafaxine and selective serotonin reuptake inhibitors in overdose compared to tricyclic antidepressants. Q J Med 2003;96:369.
120. White CM, Gailey RA, Levin GM, et al: Seizure resulting from a venlafaxine overdose. Ann Pharmacother 1997;31:178.
121. Zhalkovsky B, Walker D, Bourgeois JA: Seizure activity and enzyme elevations after venlafaxine overdose [letter]. J Clin Psychopharmacol 1997;17:490.
122. Peano C, Leikin JB, Hanashiro PK: Seizures, ventricular tachycardia and rhabdomyolysis as a result of ingestion of venlafaxine and lamotrignine. Ann Emerg Med 1997;30:704.
123. Blythe D, Hackett LP: Cardiovascular and neurological toxicity of venlafaxine. Hum Exp Toxicol 1999;18:309.
124. Coorey AN, Wenck DJ: Venlafaxine overdose [letter]. Med J Aust 1998;168:523.
125. Partridge SJ, MacIver DH, Solanki T: A depressed myocardium. Clin Toxicol 2000;38:453.
126. Fantaskey A, Burkhart KK: A case report of venlafaxine toxicity. Clin Toxicol 1995;33:359.
127. Mazur JE, Doty JD, Krygiel AS: Fatality related to a 30-g venlafaxine overdose. Pharmacotherapy 2003;23:1668.
128. Adesanya A, Varma SL: Overdose of venlafaxine—a new antidepressant [letter]. Med J Aust 1997;167:54.
129. Roxanas MG, Machado JF: Serotonin syndrome in combined moclobemide and venlafaxine ingestion. Med J Aust 1998;168:523.
130. Kolecki P: Isolated venlafaxine-induced serotonin syndrome. J Emerg Med 1997;15:491.
131. Oliver JJ, Kelly C, Jarvie D, et al: Venlafaxine poisoning complicated by a late rise in creatine kinase: two case reports. Hum Exp Toxicol 2002;21:463.
132. Daniels RJ: Serotonin syndrome due to venlafaxine overdose. J Accid Emerg Med 1998;15:333.
133. Banham ND: Fatal venlafaxine overdose [letter]. Med J Aust 1998;169:445.
134. Velasquez C, Carlson A, Stokes KA, et al: Relative safety of mirtazapine overdose. Vet Hum Toxicol 2001;43:342.
135. Holzbach R, Holger J, Pajonk F-G, et al: Suicide attempts after mirtazapine overdose without complications. Biol Psychiatry 1998;44:925.
136. Gerritsen AW: Safety in overdose of mirtazapine: a case report [letter]. J Clin Psychiatry 1997;58:271.
137. Bremner JD, Wingard P, Walshe TA: Safety of mirtazapine in overdose. J Clin Psychiatry 1998;59:233.
138. Raja M, Azzoni A: Mirtazapine overdose with benign outcome [letter]. Eur Psychiatry 2002;17:107.
139. Langford NJ, Ferner RE, Patel H, et al: Mirtazapine overdose and miosis [letter]. J Toxicol Clin Toxicol 2003;41:1037.
140. Nelson JC: Safety and tolerability of the new antidepressants. J Clin Psychiatry 1997;58(Suppl 6):26.
141. Edwards JG, Anderson I: Systemic review and guide to selection of selective serotonin reuptake inhibitors. Drugs 1999;57:507.
142. Leonard BE: Pharmacological differences of serotonin reuptake inhibitors and possible clinical relevance. Drugs 1992;43 (Suppl 2):3.
143. Spigset O: Adverse reactions of selective serotonin reuptake inhibitors: report from a spontaneous reporting system. Drug Saf 1999;20:277.
144. Settle EC: Antidepressant drugs: disturbing and potentially dangerous adverse effects. J Clin Psychiatry 1998;59(Suppl 16):25.
145. Trindale E, Menon D, Topfer L-A, Coloma C: Adverse effects associated with selective serotonin reuptake inhibitors and tricyclic antidepressants: a meta-analysis. CMAJ 1998;159:1245.
146. Taylor IC, McConnell JG: Severe hyponatremia associated with selective serotonin reuptake inhibitors. Scot Med J 1995;40:147.
147. Kim KY, Craig, JM Hawley JM: Seizure possibly associated with fluvoxamine. Ann Pharmacother 2000;34:1276.
148. Peck AW, Stern WC, Watkinson C: Incidence of seizures during treatment with tricyclic antidepressant drugs and bupropion. J Clin Psychiatry 1983;44(Sec 2):197.
149. Choi S: Nefazodone (Serzone) withdrawn because of hepatotoxicity. CMAJ 2003;169:1187.
150. Girischandra BG, Johnson L, Cresp RM, et al: Mirtazapine-induced akathisia [letter]. Med J Aust 2002;176:242.
151. Hui C-K, Yuen M-F, Wong W-M, et al: Mirtazapine-induced hepatotoxicity. J Clin Gastroenterol 2002;35:270.
152. Hernandez JL, Ramos FJ, Infante J, et al: Severe serotonin syndrome induced by mirtazapine monotherapy. Ann Pharmacother 2002;36:641.
153. Ubogu EE, Katirji B: Mirtazapine-induced serotonin syndrome. Clin Neuropharmacol 2003;26:54.
154. Benazzi F: Serotonin syndrome with mirtazapine-fluoxetine combination [letter]. Int J Geriatr Psychiatry 1998;13:495.
155. Demers JC, Malone M: Serotonin syndrome induced by fluvoxamine and mirtazapine. Ann Pharmacother 2001;35:1217.
156. McDaniel WW: Serotonin syndrome: early management with cyproheptadine. Ann Pharmacother 2001;35:870.
157. Isbister GK, Dawson AH, Whyte IM: Comment: serotonin syndrome induced by fluvoxamine and mirtazapine [letter]. Ann Pharmacother 2001;35:1674.
158. Haddad P: Newer antidepressants and the discontinuation syndrome. J Clin Psychiatry 1997;58(Suppl 7):17.
159. Rajagopalan M, Little J: Discontinuation symptoms with nefazodone. Aust N Z J Psychiatry 1999;33:594.
160. Titier K, Castaing N, Scotto-Gomez E, et al: High performance liquid chromatographic method with diode array detection for identification of the eight new antidepressants and five of their active metabolites in plasma after overdose. Ther Drug Monit 2003;25:581.
161. Roberge RJ, Luellen JR, Reed S: False-positive amphetamine screen following a trazodone overdose [letter]. Clin Toxicol 2001;39:181.

29 Monoamine Oxidase Inhibitors and Serotonin Syndrome

JEFFREY BRENT, MD, PHD ■ ROBERT PALMER, PHD

At a Glance...

- Monoamine oxidase types A and B are responsible for the intracellular degradation of biogenic amines.
- Serotonin is metabolized almost exclusively by monoamine oxidase type A.
- Hypertensive reactions can occur if monoamine oxidase is inhibited and indirect-acting amine-releasing substances are ingested (tyramine or cheese reaction).
- In overdose, monoamine oxidase type A inhibition is associated with a severe multisystem syndrome involving neuromuscular and sympathetic hyperactivity and cardiovascular collapse.
- Treatment of monoamine oxidase inhibitor overdoses is mostly supportive.
- Direct-acting vasopressors (e.g., norepinephrine or phenylephrine) should be used for monoamine oxidase inhibitor overdose; indirect agents (e.g., dopamine) should be avoided.
- If monoamine oxidase type A is inhibited and another serotonergic agent is administered, there is a high likelihood of developing a serotonin-excess syndrome.
- Serotonin syndrome is characterized by altered mental status, myoclonus, hyperreflexia, diaphoresis, diarrhea, ataxia, and shivering.
- The treatment of serotonin syndrome is primarily supportive, but preliminary data suggest that cyproheptadine may be effective.

The monoamine oxidase inhibitors (MAOIs) are a structurally diverse group of pharmaceuticals whose place in therapy has been the center of considerable controversy during the past 40 years. This controversial position is largely caused by the many toxic reactions and interactions for which MAOIs are responsible. This chapter reviews the biochemistry of the enzyme MAO, the pharmacology of the MAOIs, and the diagnosis, pathophysiology, and treatment of the various toxic responses associated with these agents.

RELEVANT HISTORY

In 1951, isoniazid and its isopropyl derivative, iproniazid, were introduced for the treatment of tuberculosis. Although the latter antibiotic is no longer marketed, it was quickly noted that patients treated with it experienced elevated mood. This psychotropic effect was attributed to the ability of iproniazid to inhibit MAO. Although severe hepatotoxicity resulted in the removal of iproniazid from the market, the effect on mood prompted the use of other MAOIs for the treatment of depression. These compounds were the first true specific antidepressant agents used. In 1962, enthusiasm for the use of MAOIs as antidepressants was tempered when a fatality associated with Stilton cheese ingestion in a patient taking an MAOI was reported.[1] The realization of the potential severity of adverse MAOI interactions caused considerable retrenchment from their use, a situation that has only recently been reconsidered.

The mood-elevating properties of MAOIs are attributable to the inhibition of an MAO isoenzyme family referred to as MAO type A (MAO-A), which is distinctly different from the MAO type B (MAO-B) isoenzyme. Although less useful as a target of antidepressant therapy, inhibition of the MAO-B isozyme also has therapeutic application. In 1989, several reports[2,3] suggested that a selective MAO-B inhibitor, L-deprenyl (selegiline), had a marked effect in the treatment of Parkinson's disease. Inhibitors of MAO-B, including selegiline and rasagiline mesylate (not available in the United States), appear to slow the progression of Parkinson's disease and extend the time before it is necessary to treat patients with this condition with L-dihydroxyphenylalanine.[4] This observation has sparked numerous investigations into the therapeutic role of MAO-B inhibition.

Currently, MAOIs are used for a variety of psychiatric indications, the most common of which is the treatment of depression refractory to standard antidepressant therapy. MAOIs have assumed this secondary role partly because of the reluctance to use these agents as a first-line drug given the concerns about the danger of major toxic effects. Other therapeutic applications of MAOIs include the treatment of vascular headaches, narcolepsy, panic disorders, phobias, obsessive-compulsive disorder, eating disorders, and post-traumatic stress disorder. For a full description of the numerous medical uses of MAOIs, readers are referred to several of the excellent references on this topic.[5-7]

THE PHYSIOLOGY OF MONOAMINE OXIDASE

Catecholamines are metabolized by MAO and catechol-O-methyl transferase (COMT). COMT is responsible for the degradation of extracellular catecholamines, such as those in the synaptic cleft. In contrast, MAO, a flavin-containing intracellular enzyme tightly bound to the outer mitochondrial membrane, is the major enzyme responsible for the catabolism of intracellular bioactive amines. Because MAO is confined to the intracellular compartment, the physiologic response to the administration of direct-acting pressor amines (e.g., norepinephrine) is unaffected by MAOIs.[8]

The intracellular location of MAO is a critical factor in understanding the pathogenesis of toxic reactions

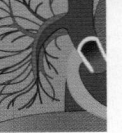

associated with MAOIs. Normally, the presence of functioning MAO keeps the intracellular concentration of free biogenic amines quite low. Because of its location, inhibition of MAO raises concentrations of intracellular biogenic amine substrates. Those amine substrates that are located in storage vesicles, however, are protected from MAO degradation. Similarly, exogenous biogenic amines that act directly at extracellular receptors are relatively unaffected by MAO. Thus, inhibition of MAO does not result in increased concentrations of, and subsequent toxic reactions to, directly acting agents.

MAO catalyzes the oxidative deamination biogenic amines such as epinephrine, norepinephrine, dopamine, 5-hydroxytryptamine (5-HT, serotonin), and tyramine. The generic reaction of MAO on primary biogenic amines is described as follows.[9]

Note that one of the products of the MAO reaction is hydrogen peroxide, which is a generator of highly toxic free radicals.[10] Examples of the specific reactions of MAO with specific biogenic amines are shown in Figure 29-1.

With the exceptions of erythrocytes, blood serum, and skeletal muscle, virtually all tissues contain some small amounts of MAO. This enzyme is found primarily in brain, peripheral noradrenergic neuronal axons, intestine, and liver. First pass catabolism by hepatic and gastrointestinal MAO prevents systemic absorption and significant physiologic effects following the oral ingestion of pressor amines (e.g., tyramine or phenylethanolamine). In general, MAO levels tend to increase with age. The two isoenzymes of MAO are separate gene products, although they share considerable sequence homology. Both genes for MAO are found on the X chromosome.

Monoamine Oxidase Isoenzymes

The two MAO isoenzymes differ in both their anatomic distribution and substrate specificity (Table 29-1). Because of these differences, the roles of the two isozymes in the pathophysiology of toxic syndromes associated with MAOIs must be considered separately.

The highest concentration of MAO is in the liver, which contains a slight predominance of MAO-A. Brain similarly contains both isoenzymes, although type B is found primarily in glial cells and serotonergic neurons. Platelets contain exclusively MAO-B.[11]

Although qualitatively most substrates are oxidized by both isoenzymes, the substrate specificities of the MAOs[12-14] exhibit quantitative differences (see Table 29-1). The Michaelis constant (K_m) and maximal velocity (V_{max}) for epinephrine, norepinephrine, dopamine, and tyramine are similar for both isoenzymes. However, serotonin (5-HT) is almost exclusively metabolized by MAO-A, while 2-phenylethylamine (the parent compound for amphetamine and its derivatives) is primarily metabolized by MAO-B.

The substrate preferences of the MAO isoenzymes are determined by the relative electrostatic, steric, and lipophilic properties of the substrate when compared with the enzyme active site. The three-dimensional structure of both isoenzymes is such that they have two active sites, a larger one for bulky substituents, and a smaller lipophilic one. However, the relative sizes of these sites are different in the two isoenzymes.[15]

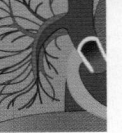

FIGURE 29-1 Representative reactions of monoamine oxidase (MAO).

Tryptamine → MAO → Indoleacetaldehyde

5-hydroxytryptamine (Serotonin; 5-HT) → MAO → 5-hydroxyindole-acetaldehyde

Norepinephrine → COMT → Normetanephrine → MAO →

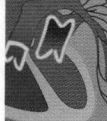

TABLE 29-1 Monoamine Oxidase Isoenzymes

	LOCATIONS	SUBSTRATE SPECIFICITY
MAO-A		
	Intestinal mucosa	Serotonin
	Placenta	Dopamine
	Biogenic amine terminals	Norepinephrine
	Liver	Tyramine
	Brain*	Epinephrine
MAO-B		
	Brain*	Dopamine
	Platelets	Tyramine
	Liver	Phenylethylamine
		Epinephrine
		Norepinephrine

MAO-A, monoamine oxidase type A; MAO-B, monoamine oxidase type B.
*Approximately equal quantities of both isoenzymes exist in the brain, but there are considerable differences in their regional distribution. In addition, monoamine oxidase type B is found primarily in glial tissue.

PHARMACOLOGY AND PHARMACOKINETICS OF MONOAMINE OXIDASE INHIBITORS

The MAOIs are available only as oral preparations. In general, MAOIs are rapidly and completely absorbed from the gastrointestinal tract, with peak plasma concentrations ranging from 1 to 4 hours after ingestion.[16-18] Plasma elimination of these agents occurs largely by hepatic metabolism and is also rapid; half-lives range from 1 to 3 hours. In general, MAOIs are transported into cells by the neurotransmitter amine reuptake system. For irreversible MAOIs, maximal MAO inhibition takes 5 to 10 days after initiation of drug therapy. Thus, plasma drug concentrations do not correlate with the level of MAO inhibition.[16-18] For reversible MAOIs, however, maximal inhibition of MAO occurs within a few hours of the first dose.

As can be seen in Table 29-2, MAOIs are generally classified according to their preferential effect on the isoenzyme they inhibit. For most of these agents, however, the selectivity is not complete and tends to be lost at higher doses and especially in overdose. The selective MAO-B inhibitor selegiline has been reported to lose some of its selectivity at doses as low as 10 mg/day, a dose that is in the therapeutic range.[19]

MAOIs may also be classified as either reversible or irreversible inhibitors of MAO. The classic MAOIs are irreversible inhibitors of the enzyme. Although serum concentrations of the MAOIs decline rapidly after last use, their effects are long-lived. It is generally believed that a period of 2 to 3 weeks is necessary to regain MAO activity after the cessation of the administration of an irreversible inhibitor, because new enzyme must be synthesized.[17]

A new class of reversible inhibitors of MAO,[20-26] the prototype of which is moclobemide, have been devel-

oped (see Table 29-2). Other agents include befloxatone, brofaromine, cimoxatone, and teloxantrone. The reversible inhibitors act primarily on MAO-A and are therefore referred to as reversible inhibitors of MAO-A (RIMAs). The effect of RIMAs is short lived, with MAO activity being reconstituted within hours to days of the last dose. Because of the reversible nature of the binding of RIMAs with MAO, adverse reactions such as the pressor effect with tyramine ingestion ("cheese reaction") are unlikely to occur.[24] Approximately 150 mg of tyramine is needed to cause an increase in blood pressure while taking moclobemide. This is the equivalent of eating approximately 300 g of a tyramine-containing cheese.[27] Thus, although a tyramine reaction is theoretically possible, it is highly unlikely to occur given the doses required. The reason why MAO-A inhibition by moclobemide does not predispose to a tyramine reaction is a result of competitive substrate binding; the tyramine displaces the RIMA from the enzyme active site, allowing normal metabolism of the substrate.

Several of the older MAOIs are substituted hydrazine (NH_2-NH_2) derivatives (see Table 29-2). These MAOIs tend to be metabolized into active products and, like the well-known hydrazine isoniazid, are inactivated by N-acetylation at a genetically determined rate. The human population can be broadly separated into fast and slow acetylators on the basis of the rate of this reaction. For example, approximately equal numbers of American and European whites may be classified as fast versus slow acetylators. The rate of slow acetylators is higher in Asian populations. Slow acetylators may be at greater risk for developing adverse effects (e.g., drug and dietary interactions) with therapeutic doses. Various adverse effects are specifically associated with the hydrazine-derived MAOIs.[28] Most prominent among these are the inhibition of multiple enzyme systems, hepatotoxicity, and the induction of pyridoxine (vitamin B_6) deficiency with the associated problem of seizures. The hepatotoxicity of MAOI hydrazines has been well reviewed.[29-31]

Among the various other enzyme systems inhibited by hydrazine MAOIs, the most important are pyridoxal kinase, L-amino acid decarboxylase, diamine oxidase, and cytochrome P-450.[28] In addition, hydrazines tend to form soluble complexes with pyridoxine, resulting in a deficiency of this vitamin by enhancing its urinary excretion.

In addition to the induction of pyridoxine deficiency, hydrazines prevent the use of pyridoxine for important metabolic reactions. Pyridoxine is not active as an enzyme cofactor until it is phosphorylated to pyridoxal phosphate by the enzyme pyridoxal kinase. Among the reactions for which pyridoxal phosphate is a cofactor is the synthesis of γ-aminobutyric acid (GABA) by the decarboxylation of glutamic acid, catalyzed by L-amino acid decarboxylase. Reduced production of GABA may cause the development of profound seizures as a result of poisoning by hydrazine MAOIs. The specific treatment for these seizures is administration of pyridoxine.

Virtually all MAOIs have a terminal phenyl group attached to a short aliphatic side chain, thus mimicking

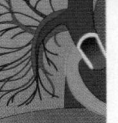
TABLE 29-2 Characteristics of Monoamine Oxidase Inhibitors

GENERIC NAME	TRADE NAME	SELECTIVITY	REVERSIBILITY	HYDRAZINE
Clorgyline		A*	No	No
Isocaboxazid	Marplan	A§	No	Yes
Moclobemide	Aurorix	A*	Yes	No
Pargyline	Eutonyl	B‖	No	No
Phenelzine	Nardil	A§	No	Yes
Selegiline	Deprenyl, Eldepryl	B*	No	No
Tranylcypromine	Parnate	A§	No	No
Brofaromine	Consonar	A*	Yes	No
Iproniazid	Marsilid†	A§	No	Yes
Isoniazid		No‡	No	Yes
MDMA		A§	Yes	No
Fluoxetine	Prozac	B*	Probably	No

MDMA, 3,4-methylenedioxymethamphetamine ("Ecstasy").
*Selectivity is lost at supratherapeutic doses.
†No longer manufactured.
‡Weak monoamine oxidase inhibitor.
§Weak inhibitor of monoamine oxidase type B.
‖Weak inhibitor of monoamine oxidase type A.

the phenethylamine structure of amphetamines (Fig. 29-2). It is thus possible that excessive doses of these agents may cause amphetamine-like reactions. Conversely, amphetamine or its derivatives tend to have some inhibitory effects on MAO.

MAOIs enhance synaptic biogenic amine transmitter concentrations by various mechanisms (Box 29-1). By inhibiting the enzymatic degradation, the cytoplasmic concentrations of these neurotransmitters are increased, resulting in the tendency for release of these biogenic amines by a mass action effect. In addition, the act of transporting the MAOI into the cell by the amine reuptake system causes the ligand-binding site of the membrane-bound transporter molecule to face inward, and it thus becomes available for the transport of neurotransmitter out of the cytoplasm into the synapse or neuroeffector junction. By being transported into the cell by the amine reuptake pump, the MAOIs act as competitive inhibitors of bioactive amine transport out of the synapse by this system. All of these factors tend to increase both intracellular and extracellular amine levels.

FIGURE 29-2 Chemical structures of selected monoamine oxidase inhibitors. The structures of phenethylamine, amphetamine, and methamphetamine are included for comparison.

Iproniazid

Phenelzine

Tranylcypromine

Moclobemide

Isocarboxazid

Selegiline

MDMA

Pargyline

Fluoxetine

Phenthylamine

Amphetamine

Methamphetamine

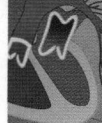

BOX 29-1	FACTORS CONTRIBUTING TO MONOAMINE OXIDASE TYPE A INHIBITOR TOXICITY

Decreased biogenic amine degradation
Amphetamine-like effect and increased catecholamine release from intracellular vesicles
GABA deficiency (hydrazines)
Decreased amine reuptake
Depletion of biogenic amine stores
GABA antagonism (tranylcypromine, isocarboxazid)
Increased amine release
Metabolism to amphetamine (tranylcypromine)

GABA, γ-aminobutyric acid.

Being amphetamine congeners, MAOIs provoke release of stored amines from presynaptic vesicles, and thus the free intracellular concentrations of these molecules are increased. Given the decreased degradation of these amines by virtue of inhibition of MAO, any free bioactive amine molecules resulting from either release from vesicles or from reuptake are relatively protected from catabolism.

As noted in Table 29-2, the MAOIs differ in their characteristics. Several of them, however, merit specific comment.

Although no longer available as a therapeutic agent, clorgyline is the prototypic inhibitor of MAO-A. By virtue of the fact that nanomolar concentrations of this agent irreversibly inhibit MAO-A in a selective manner, this particular isoenzyme was defined.

Moclobemide is the prototype RIMA.[20-26] Although not available in the United States, moclobemide is available in most other parts of the world. In general, it appears that moclobemide and other RIMAs are safer than the traditional MAOIs.

In addition to the MAOIs noted in Table 29-2, various other agents have weak inhibiting properties of this enzyme. For example, procarbazine (Matulane, Sigma-Tau Pharmaceuticals, Gaithersburg, MD), a chemotherapeutic agent used in regimens to combat Hodgkin's disease, is also a weak, nonselective, irreversible MAOI. Linezolid (Zyvox [Pfizer, New York, NY]), a novel antimicrobial, is a reversible, nonselective MAOI. In addition, St. John's wort, an herbal supplement, has been noted to have weak MAOI activity. Fortunately, MAO inhibition by these agents is unlikely to have significant therapeutic implications.

Tranylcypromine is an MAOI with great structural similarity to amphetamine. It may be metabolized to amphetamine, which may have a role in some of the toxicity of this agent. In addition, tranylcypromine can inhibit the action of GABA at the $GABA_A$ receptor by preventing chloride influx. This inhibition of GABA activity by tranylcypromine may be responsible for the seizures observed with therapeutic doses of this agent. A similar effect on GABA channels is possible with isocarboxazid.

Selective MAO-B inhibition with selegiline is utilized in the treatment of Parkinson's disease since it inhibits striatal dopamine degradation. Selegiline is metabolized to *l*-methamphetamine, which is substantially less active than its *d*-isomer. Although the serum half-life of selegiline is short (0.15 hour), it is an irreversible inhibitor of MAO-B and thus its effects are long-lasting. Although relatively safe compared with the nonselective MAOIs, when selegiline and levodopa are concurrently administered, dopaminergic effects (hallucinations and dyskinesia) may occur.

TOXICOLOGY AND CLINICAL MANIFESTATIONS OF OVERDOSE

Overdose with the classic irreversible inhibitors of MAO-A, although infrequent, is associated with extremely high morbidity and mortality. All classic MAO-A inhibitors can cause a similar severe toxic syndrome in overdose. Ingestion of these agents in amounts greater than approximately 2 mg/kg should generally be considered potentially life threatening.[32] Although many factors affect the course of poisoning by these agents, a general chronologic framework may be noted in the construct of MAOI overdose. This syndromic description, promulgated by Linden and coworkers,[32] highlights the following four phases:

1. Asymptomatic (latent)
2. Neuromuscular excitation and sympathetic hyperactivity
3. Central nervous system (CNS) depression with the potential for cardiovascular collapse
4. Secondary complications for survivors of the above

As noted in this scheme, a relatively asymptomatic period may precede the significant clinical manifestations of MAOI poisoning. Although it is unusual for this latent period to last for more than 6 to 12 hours, it is generally believed that patients ingesting these agents should be observed for a full 24 hours to adequately rule out significant toxicity.[32-35]

The clinical effects of MAO-A inhibitor overdose are varied. Early manifestations frequently include headache and mild agitation, which may progress to profound central and peripheral nervous system stimulation associated with increased agitation, hyperthermia, hyperreflexia, diaphoresis, tremor, myoclonus, seizures, rhabdomyolysis, and a general hypersympathetic state. More serious cases may evolve to frank rigidity. The hyperadrenergic state is often followed by obtundation and a sympatholytic syndrome, which may deteriorate to cardiovascular collapse. Common in cases of acute overdose are manifold complications that include adult respiratory distress syndrome, disseminated intravascular coagulation, multiple organ system failure, and rhabdomyolysis.[32,33,35-39]

The pathophysiology of MAO-A inhibitor overdose involves many factors (see Box 29-1). The exact weight of the contribution of each of these factors is variable and

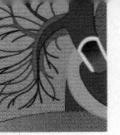

may depend on multiple factors, including exact drug, dose ingested, and the underlying physiology of the patient.

Inhibition of MAO-A is associated with various effects on the degradative metabolism of intracellular catecholamines, indoles, and histamine. Because MAO-A is the major enzyme involved in degradation of these intracellular amines, inhibition results in increased cytoplasmic concentrations of these substances. Normally stored in intracytoplasmic vesicles, these amines are generally inaccessible to MAO. However, any amine that is released from these vesicles, metabolically generated, or free amine resulting from reuptake will not be normally degraded by MAO.

5-HT is the major biologically active indole metabolized by MAO-A (Fig. 29-3). Thus, inhibition of MAO-A results in elevated levels of intracytoplasmic 5-HT.[40] It should be noted, however, that alternative minor pathways for 5-HT metabolism also exist.[40-42] Tryptamine is an eleptogenic indole produced by the metabolic decarboxylation of tryptophan.[43] MAO is the major enzymatic pathway for the catabolism of tryptamine, which is oxidatively deaminated to indoleacetic acid.[40,44] After poisoning by MAO-A inhibitors, urinary excretion of unmetabolized tryptamine increases.[40] This inhibition of tryptamine catabolism may contribute to the CNS excitation and seizures that occur after overdose with these agents.

FIGURE 29-3 Metabolism of tryptophan.

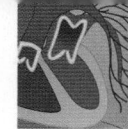

Histamine is metabolized either oxidatively to imidazole acetic acid or by *N*-acetylation to *N*-acetylhistamine.[9] The oxidative metabolism of histamine is accomplished by either MAO or diamine oxidase. As already noted, hydrazine MAOIs inhibit both of these enzymes. Thus, overdoses with hydrazine MAOIs are expected to result in elevated histamine levels,[40] which would contribute to flushing and hypotension.

All of these factors associated with an overdose of an MAO-A inhibitor may be anticipated to increase intracytoplasmic biologically active amine concentrations. However, the exact contribution of the inhibition of MAO to the toxidrome engendered by an acute overdose of these agents is unknown. Some doubt may be raised about the significance of the inhibition of MAO in acute overdose because clinically effective MAO inhibition takes approximately 1 week with therapeutic dosing. It is possible that higher doses may cause faster inhibition of this enzyme.

Although moclobemide is safer than the traditional MAOIs, there are reports of overdose patients sustaining cardiovascular collapse after a delay of many hours. Fatalities have been reported at serum moclobemide concentrations of 55 mg/L and higher (therapeutic 1.5 to 2.5 mg/L).[45]

DIAGNOSIS

The diagnosis of MAOI poisoning is made by a positive history of exposure and corroborating evidence from the physical examination. The presence of an altered mental status coupled with autonomic and neuromuscular dysfunction (e.g., a hyperadrenergic and hyperserotonergic state) suggest MAOI toxicity. In the absence of a positive history of ingestion, however, it is extremely difficult to make a definitive diagnosis of MAOI toxicity. The presence of "ping-pong" gaze (slow, rhythmic, saccadic eye movements or ocular clonus) may suggest MAOI toxicity, but there are no pathognomonic physical findings or laboratory findings commonly associated with MAOI poisoning. Serotonin syndrome and MAOI poisoning have a significant degree of overlap in their pathophysiology and clinical manifestations. Other conditions that could create a similar clinical picture include the neuroleptic malignant syndrome, sepsis, tetanus, meningoencephalitis, intracranial hemorrhage, heatstroke, malignant hyperthermia, sympathomimetic syndrome, central hallucinogen toxicity, lithium toxicity, salicylism, hypoglycemia, thyrotoxicosis, and pheochromocytoma.

Although toxicology screening may be useful to exclude other intoxications, screening methods are unlikely to detect MAOIs. Specific qualitative and quantitative testing for MAOIs are not readily available and do not correlate with the severity of toxicity.

TREATMENT

The treatment of MAO-A inhibitor overdose is primarily supportive. The early sympathomimetic component of MAO-A inhibitor poisoning may have associated hypertension, which can be severe. However, caution must be used in the treatment of this hypertension because this early sympathomimetic state may unpredictably and suddenly be replaced by a sympatholytic syndrome. Thus, the treatment of MAOI-induced hypertension should involve a short-acting titratable agent such as phentolamine or nitroprusside. Standard agents should be used to treat cardiac dysrhythmias. Gastrointestinal decontamination for patients presenting after an MAOI overdose should include administration of activated charcoal if the ingestion occurred within 1 to 2 hours of patient presentation.

Although not systematically studied in a controlled trial, aggressive management of MAOI-induced hyperthermia should be considered to be of paramount importance in favorably altering a patient's prognosis.

The muscular hyperactivity and CNS stimulation in MAOI overdoses contribute to catecholamine release,[46] hyperthermia, and rhabdomyolysis. Thus, sedation of agitated, rigid, or hyperactive patients with benzodiazepines or barbiturates is generally beneficial. Benzodiazepines may be preferable because they are typically associated with fewer hemodynamic side effects. Linden and colleagues suggested that amobarbital would be an appropriate barbiturate to use because of its short duration of effect and rapid onset of action.[32] If rigidity, agitation, or muscular activity cannot be readily and effectively controlled by simple pharmacologic maneuvers, then neuromuscular paralysis should be induced. It must be remembered, however, that neuromuscular blockade obscures the ability to observe seizures, and thus paralyzed patients may be experiencing unappreciated CNS seizure activity. It is therefore important to use a short-acting paralytic agent, induce a state of partial paralysis as measured by twitches, or to perform continuous electroencephalographic monitoring.

Blood pressure support should be accomplished using direct-acting sympathomimetic amines such as epinephrine, norepinephrine, or phenylephrine. The benefits of the direct agonists are that they act directly at smooth muscle receptors on blood vessels and do not require intracellular metabolism to generate an active pressor amine. In addition, direct agonists undergo COMT-mediated catabolism. However, because of decreased reuptake of these amines coupled with diminished degradation of any that is transported to the intracellular compartment, an exaggerated response is a theoretical possibility.[47] Therefore, low and titrated doses should initially be used.

The indirect-acting amines that are used for blood pressure support (e.g., dopamine) are metabolized to active pressors (epinephrine and norepinephrine) intracellularly. MAO normally prevents excessive amounts of these active metabolites from being generated; however, in the setting of MAO inhibition, elevated concentrations of these amines may lead to an exaggerated hemodynamic response. Thus, indirect pressor amines are generally considered to be contraindicated, although this notion is based primarily on theoretical grounds.

As already discussed, a hyperexcitable state or seizures in patients who have overdosed on a hydrazine

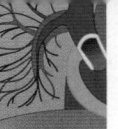

type of MAOI (see Table 29-2) should be treated with pyridoxine. Because one element of the toxidrome observed following MAOI overdose is an excess of 5-HT, it seems reasonable that a serotonin antagonist would be of benefit. However, this treatment approach has not been well studied. The primary sites at which excess serotonin causes significant clinical effects are the 5-HT$_1$ and 5-HT$_2$ receptors. Cyproheptadine is an antagonist at 5-HT$_1$ and 5-HT$_2$ receptors and is relatively devoid of potentially harmful effects; however, it is available only as an oral preparation. Methysergide is a 5-HT$_1$ and 5-HT$_2$ antagonist but is also not available as a parenteral preparation. Ondansetron is a 5-HT$_3$ antagonist, and it is unlikely that this receptor is involved in the pathogenesis of the MAOI toxidrome or serotonin syndrome. Procainamide, propranolol, and trazodone also have 5-HT antagonist properties; however, little is known about the effects of these agents in MAOI overdose, and these drugs may produce undesirable hemodynamic effects. Bromocriptine is an ergot derivative that is a direct partial agonist at the dopamine receptor and blunts the effects of excess dopamine. Its use has not been proven effective for the MAOI toxidrome. Dantrolene sodium is an inhibitor of calcium release from the sarcoplasmic reticulum of skeletal muscle and thereby attenuates excitation-contraction coupling. Theoretically, it may be of use in decreasing the muscle rigidity associated with MAOI poisoning. As noted earlier, hydrazine MAOIs (see Table 29-2) block histamine catabolism, and therefore antihistamines (e.g., diphenhydramine) may be of some benefit in these cases.

The antihypertensives tolazoline, pentolinium, and clonidine have been touted as appropriate agents to treat the hypertension associated with the early stages of MAOI poisoning.[48,49] However, no evidence shows that these agents are preferable to other antihypertensives, and their half-lives may be too long.

Urinary acidification has a minor enhancing effect on the urinary excretion of tranylcypromine.[50] No data suggest that urinary acidification will further the clearance of other MAOIs. Given the almost inevitable rhabdomyolysis associated with the MAOI toxidrome and the lack of proven efficacy of urinary acidification, this treatment should be considered contraindicated.

INTERACTION OF MONOAMINE OXIDASE INHIBITORS WITH DIETARY AMINES

One of the greatest concerns in the therapeutic use of MAOIs is the potential hypertensive reaction associated with the ingestion of dietary amines. The amine most commonly implicated in these reactions is tyramine. Because the vast majority of all reported reactions and deaths have been associated with the ingestion of tyramine-containing cheese,[51,52] the name generally applied to this phenomenon is the cheese reaction. Spontaneous cases in the absence of any apparent

exogenous amine have also been reported in patients taking both classic MAOIs and RIMAs.[53,54]

Tyramine does not cross the blood-brain barrier. Therefore, the manifestations of the cheese reaction are due to its peripheral actions. Tyramine is an indirect-acting agonist that, similar to cocaine, competes for reuptake and thus increases synaptic concentrations of norepinephrine and dopamine.

Dietary tyramine is normally metabolized by gastrointestinal MAO-A,[55-58] and, thus, little of it gains access to the systemic circulation. Approximately 87% of an oral dose of tyramine is metabolized by this pathway to *p*-hydroxyphenylacetic acid.[59] That fraction which is absorbed is further subject to degradation by neuronal MAO-A. Although tyramine is a substrate for both MAO isoenzymes, MAO-A provides protection from the cheese effect. Patients taking MAO-B inhibitors are much less vulnerable to a cheese reaction; they become susceptible only at supratherapeutic doses of the inhibitor when isoenzyme selectivity may be substantially reduced.[60]

The literature contains considerable debate and misunderstanding about the potential dietary sources of tyramine and the resulting restrictions required of patients being treated with MAO-A inhibitors. The list of various foods that have been implicated in hypertensive reactions associated with MAO-A inhibitors is lengthy (Box 29-2). Such an extensive list of dietary restrictions is both impractical and not justified by scientific data. However, certain dietary restrictions do appear to be necessary.

The greatest concern with regard to food interactions with MAO-A inhibitors involves cheeses. On average, European cheeses contain 20 mg tyramine per 100 g of cheese.[59] However, marked differences may exist between individual types of cheese. Many aged cheeses are high in tyramine content and therefore should be restricted, but other aged cheeses such as Brie, Emmenthal, Mozzarella,[61,62] and Gruyère contain little tyramine and can be eaten without concern.[51] Cottage cheese, processed cheese slices, ricotta, cream cheese, Romano,[61] Havarti, Boursin, Parmesan, bleu cheese dressing, Gorgonzola, feta, Muenster, sour cream, and yogurt can likewise be eaten because of their low tyramine content.[51] Thus, it appears that a cheese pizza may be safe to eat when taking an MAO.[61] Alcoholic beverages have been a source of concern, although few contain dangerously high concentrations of tyramine. Beer, even dealcoholized, has been implicated in hypertensive reactors.[63] Chianti wine has traditionally been singled out because of a 1964 report showing dangerously high tyramine levels.[64] However, more recent studies have failed to confirm this.[51]

The original reports of high levels of tyramine in pickled herring[65] have not been replicated by more recent studies.[51,66] It has been suggested that the original report by Nuessle and colleagues in 1965[65] alleging a high concentration of tyramine in this fish was due to either an unreliable assay method or spoilage. Similarly, studies of smoked fish and caviar have also failed to demonstrate any significant tyramine content.[51]

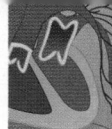

BOX 29-2	**FOODS IMPLICATED IN HYPERTENSIVE REACTIONS WITH MONOAMINE OXIDASE INHIBITORS**				
Cheese	**Alcoholic Beverages**	**Fish**	**Meat**	**Fruit**	**Yeast Extracts**
All cheeses except cottage cheese and yogurt	Red wine (especially Chianti) Sherry Vermouth Cognac Beer Liqueurs	Smoked fish Pickled Herring Caviar	All fermented/aged meat, including: Corned beef, Salami Pepperoni Liver Sausage	Spoiled or overripe fruits Canned or overripe figs Stewed or whole bananas (including peeled)	Vitamin supplements (brewer's yeast)
Sauerkraut	**Bouillon**	**Soy Sauce**	**Beans** Broad bean pods (Italian green beans) Fava beans		

Processed meat such as salami and some sausage have been shown to be high in tyramine.[51,66] However, other meats such as liver, bologna, aged meat, corned beef, and pâtés have failed to demonstrate any significant tyramine content. Fruits and figs, including avocado, have virtually no tyramine content and should not be restricted. The one exception is banana peels, which contain approximately 1.4 mg of tyramine per peel. Therefore, preparations of whole banana should be eaten only in moderation.

Concentrated yeast extracts (Marmite [Unilever Best Foods, UK]) contain a significant amount of tyramine and should be restricted in patients taking MAO-A inhibitors.[51,67] However, various brewer's yeasts have low to nonexistent tyramine content and may be eaten without concern.[51] Sauerkraut contains nearly 14 mg of tyramine per 250-g serving and therefore should be considered contraindicated in patients who are taking MAO-A inhibitors. Bouillon and soy sauce have been found to contain very low amounts of tyramine and therefore can be eaten without any concern.[51] Fava beans contain virtually no tyramine.[51] Italian green broad bean pods are not a concern with regard to their tyramine content, although they do contain the indirect-acting pressor dihydroxyphenylalanine (DOPA) and therefore should not be eaten.[68]

Given these data, it is clear that many of the existing lists of foodstuffs to be avoided by patients taking MAO-A inhibitors are unduly restrictive, and more liberalized and scientifically based suggestions have evolved.[51,69,70] It appears to be safe for patients using MAO-A inhibitors simply to avoid aged cheeses, concentrated yeast extract (Marmite), Italian broad bean pods, sauerkraut, salami, and sausage.

If a patient does have a hypertensive response associated with the ingestion of a dietary amine, treatment is generally considered to consist of pharmacologic control of blood pressure and management of any complications associated with the hypertensive episode. If the ingestion was within the last 1 or 2 hours, administration of activated charcoal may be considered on theoretical grounds. Although no controlled studies have investigated the appropriate management of these hypertensive responses, phentolamine in doses of 5 to 10 mg is generally recommended because it is an α-receptor antagonist and will antagonize the hypertensive effect of norepinephrine. However, no data suggest that other antihypertensive regimens would be any less effective.

It is generally considered that there is a lower risk for a cheese reaction with MAO-B inhibitors,[24,71,72] except if they are taken in high doses, which may cause these agents to lose their isoenzyme selectivity.[27,60] However, hypertensive reactions have been reported in patients taking selegiline.[19] In contrast to case reports, a meta-analysis of clinical trials with selegiline found no difference in the incidence of clinical effects between those taking the drug and placebo.[73] Thus, it appears that these reactions are less likely to occur clinically with these agents than with MAO-A inhibitors, although the possibility cannot be ruled out. Data from human volunteer studies indicate that selegiline does appear to decrease the catabolism of tyramine.[19]

Reversible inhibitors of MAO-A are unlikely to cause a pressor response from ingested cheese because tyramine can displace RIMAs from the MAO-A binding site.[24,25,60] Very large doses of tyramine can cause an elevation in blood pressure in patients taking RIMAs.[27] However, hypertensive responses to dietary amines have not been reported with the use of these agents.

SEROTONIN SYNDROME

Relevant History

In 1955, a "fatal toxic encephalitis" was described in a patient who received meperidine while he was being treated for tuberculosis with iproniazid. Before the patient's death, he exhibited severe muscular hyperactivity, rigidity, and clonus.[74] Shortly thereafter, Oates and Sjoerdsma[75] noted that tryptophan administered to patients who were taking an MAOI caused a phenomenon of unsteady gait, clonus, tremor, incoordination, feeling of lightheadedness, paresthesias, CNS excitation, dilated pupils, and hyperactive reflexes. Noting that

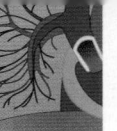

tryptophan is a precursor in the biosynthetic pathway of both 5-HT and the neuroexcitatory transmitter tryptamine (see Fig. 29-3), the researchers concluded that inhibition of MAO caused an increase in levels of these molecules.[75] That these effects were indeed likely due to a derivative of tryptophan was verified by Smith and Prockop,[76] who showed that high doses of this amino acid can cause a similar effect. The following year, similar effects were observed when rhesus monkeys were fed high doses of tryptophan.[77] That these effects were likely not due to the tryptophan itself but to a metabolic derivative was shown in 1964 by Hodge and colleagues,[78] who demonstrated that they can be prevented by the administration of an inhibitor of the enzyme L-amino acid decarboxylase, which prevents the formation of tryptamine and 5-HT from tryptophan (see Fig. 29-3).

In 1971, Grahame-Smith[79] produced a similar phenomenon in rats, thus creating the animal model most commonly used to study serotonin syndrome. That the observed syndrome is due to heightened levels of serotonin and not tryptamine was suggested by the clinical report by Beaumont,[80] which described four cases of a fatal interaction associated with similar symptoms as the prior reports, in patients taking an MAOI and the serotonergic antidepressant clomipramine (Anafranil). Although not specifically discussed in this report, this interaction suggested that 5-HT was responsible for this syndrome. In 1982, Insel and associates[81] described a similar syndrome in patients taking clomipramine plus an MAOI and coined the term *serotonin syndrome*. The reader is referred to Chapter 10A for additional information on serotonin syndrome.

Pathophysiology of Serotonin Syndrome

Since the mid-1930s, it has been known that a substance in intestinal enterochromaffin cells had a stimulating effect on bowel motility.[82] In 1948, a vasoconstrictor material was isolated from serum and named *serotonin*. This material was subsequently chemically characterized as 5-HT.[83] By 1952, it was known that 5-HT was the gut-stimulating material from the enterochromaffin cells.[82]

It is now known that serotonin is synthesized from tryptophan (see Fig. 29-3) intracellularly and stored in vesicles by ion trapping. Any free 5-HT that is not so stored is metabolized by intracellular MAO to 5-hydroxyindoleacetaldehyde.

Serotonin is found in high concentrations in platelets, enterochromaffin cells of the gastrointestinal tract, and the brain. Platelet 5-HT is important in hemostasis. Intestinal enterochromaffin cells contain approximately 90% of the total-body 5-HT. Tumors of these cells produce excess amounts of 5-HT and give rise to the carcinoid syndrome.

Serotonin acts by interaction with a specific family of receptors. The universe of serotonin-binding sites was originally thought to be composed of two separate receptors known as M and D.[84] However, by the early 1970s, studies of lysergic acid diethylamide (LSD)

binding to serotonin receptors indicated that this scheme of two receptor types was too simple. Subsequently, seven families of serotonin receptors were demonstrated. Because there are subtypes within these families, we now know of 13 separate serotonin receptors.[85] All are G-protein coupled except the 5-HT$_3$ receptor, which is a ligand-gated ion channel (see Chapter 10). The 5-HT$_{1A}$ and 5-HT$_{2A}$ receptors appear to be of importance in the pathogenesis of the serotonin syndrome. Agonists at the 5-HT$_{1A}$ receptor, which include LSD and 5-HT, inhibit the firing of raphe neurons. These neurons tend to modulate and attenuate sensory input. 5-HT$_{2A}$ receptors are excitatory and stimulate vascular smooth muscle and the CNS neurons. Serotonin is an indole compound structurally similar to LSD and psilocybin. The effects of these hallucinogens are mediated through interaction with the serotonin receptors (see Chapter 45). Because 5-HT$_{1A}$ and 5-HT$_2$ antagonists block features of the serotonin syndrome, it has been concluded that these receptors are responsible for the various manifestations of 5-HT excess. An alternative explanation for the serotonin syndrome derives from the similarity in clinical features between this condition and the neuroleptic malignant syndrome, which results from blockade of central dopamine effects (see Chapters 10A and 38). An excess of 5-HT inhibits brain dopaminergic neurons by blocking dopamine release or synthesis.[86-88] If this hypothesis is true, then some or all of the clinical features of the serotonin syndrome could potentially be blocked or attenuated by dopamine agonists. This has not been well studied experimentally.

Clinical Manifestations

Serotonin syndrome is commonly identified by the presence of the triad of alteration of mental status, autonomic hyperactivity, and neuromuscular dysfunction. In 1991, Sternbach[89] reviewed 38 reported patients with serotonin syndrome and used the observed clinical features to define his diagnostic criteria (see next section). The most common manifestations were, in decreasing order of frequency, restlessness, confusion, myoclonus, hyperreflexia, diaphoresis, shivering, tremor, hypomania, diarrhea, and incoordination. A later review found that the most common reported manifestations were, in order of decreasing frequency, hyperreflexia, altered mental status, myoclonus, ataxia, diaphoresis, fever, shivering, and diarrhea.[90] Mills conducted the most comprehensive analysis of reported cases and reported the signs and symptoms in 100 previously reported cases, dividing them into cognitive/behavioral, autonomic, and neuromuscular. The results of his analysis are shown in Table 29-3.

Diagnosis of Serotonin Syndrome

Given the clinical presentation of serotonin syndrome, the differential diagnosis to be entertained is broad and includes withdrawal states, tetanus, neuroleptic malignant syndrome, thyrotoxicosis, sepsis, and overdose of

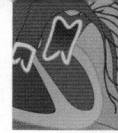

TABLE 29-3 Signs and Symptoms of Serotonin Syndrome (Review of 100 Cases)

SIGN/SYMPTOM	FREQUENCY (%)
Cognitive-Behavioral Symptoms	
Confusion/disorientation	51
Agitation/irritability	34
Coma/unresponsiveness	29
Anxiety	15
Euphoria/hypomania	14
Headache	13
Drowsiness	13
Seizures	12
Insomnia	11
Hallucinations (visual and auditory)	6
Dizziness	5
Autonomic Nervous System	
Hyperthermia	45
Diaphoresis	45
Sinus tachycardia	36
Hypertension	35
Dilated pupils	28
Tachypnea	26
Nausea	23
Unreactive pupils	20
Flushing	16
Hypotension	15
Diarrhea	8
Ventricular tachycardia	6
Cyanosis	5
Abdominal cramps	4
Salivation	2
Neuromuscular	
Myoclonus	58
Hyperreflexia	52
Muscle rigidity	51
Restlessness/hyperactivity	48
Tremor	43
Ataxia/incoordination	40
Clonus	23
Babinski's sign (bilateral)	16
Nystagmus	15
Trismus	7
Teeth chattering	6
Opisthotonos	6
Paresthesias	6

sympathomimetics, strychnine, MAOIs, or lithium. Sternbach[89] proposed the following three diagnostic criteria for the serotonin syndrome:

A. Coincident with the addition of a known serotonergic agent to an established medication regimen or an increase in its dose, at least three of the following clinical features are present:
1. Mental status changes (confusion, hypomania)
2. Agitation
3. Myoclonus
4. Hyperreflexia
5. Diaphoresis
6. Shivering
7. Tremor
8. Diarrhea
9. Incoordination
10. Fever

B. Other causes (e.g., infectious, metabolic, substance abuse or withdrawal) have been ruled out.
C. A neuroleptic had not been started or increased in dose before the onset of the signs and symptoms listed earlier.

Insel[81] and Dursun[91,92] and their colleagues have suggested modifications of Sternbach's criteria by replacing the 10 items under the first diagnostic criterion with the following, of which three were believed to be required:
1. Uncontrollable shivering
2. Incoordination
3. Restlessness in the feet while sitting
4. Initial involuntary contractions followed by myoclonus-like movements in the legs
5. Hyperreflexia
6. Frightened, diaphoretic hyperarousal state
7. Agitation
8. Oculogyric crisis
9. Diarrhea
10. Fear

The diagnosis of serotonin syndrome is clinical. No laboratory tests confirm the diagnosis. It requires the presence of known exposure to serotonin-potentiating agents and the appropriate constellation of physical findings. More recently, an alternative algorithm for diagnosis has been proposed that is considered simpler to use and to have a higher sensitivity and specificity.[93-96] Using this algorithm, the diagnosis of serotonin syndrome is made if a serotonergic agent has been recently introduced and there is the presence of any of the following: (1) tremor and hyperreflexia; (2) spontaneous clonus; (3) muscle rigidity, temperature greater than 38° C, and either ocular clonus or inducible clonus; (4) ocular clonus and either agitation or diaphoresis; or (5) inducible clonus and either agitation or diaphoresis. With this latter clinical algorithm, the presence of clonus is the single most important physical finding that suggests the diagnosis of serotonin syndrome.[93] It is also important to understand that the serotonin syndrome encompasses a broad spectrum of illness severity, from very mild to severe and immediately life-threatening stigmata.[93]

Agents That Cause Serotonin Syndrome

Theoretically, any scenario that produces an increase of 5-HT concentrations can result in serotonin syndrome. However, this syndrome typically results from a combination of serotonergic agents rather than simply an increase in a single medication. This occurs most commonly when two agents that increase serotonin levels by different mechanisms are taken. The various serotonergic agents are listed in Table 29-4. In 1995, Bodner and associates[97] compiled a six-page table documenting the various interactions of serotonergic agents that may cause the serotonin syndrome. A comprehensive list would be much longer now and difficult to commit to memory. It is, thus, best to understand that any two serotonergic agents in combination are at least theoretically capable of causing this

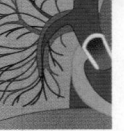

TABLE 29-4 Serotonergic Agents	
AGENT	**MECHANISM**
MAOIs	Inhibit serotonin breakdown
Clomipramine	Inhibits serotonin reuptake
Selective serotonin reuptake inhibitors	Inhibit serotonin reuptake
Tryptophan	Metbolized in serotonin
Lithium	Enhances serotonin release, potentiates effects of 5-HT$_{1A}$ receptor
Amitryptyline/impramine	Inhibits serotonin reuptake
Meperidine	Inhibits serotonin reuptake
Dextromethorphan	Inhibits serotonin reuptake
Levodopa	Causes serotonin release
Trazodone	Inhibits serotonin reuptake
MDMA	MAOI, cause serotonin release
Amphetamines	Cause serotonin release
Cocaine	Causes serotonin release
Lysergic acid diethylamide (LSD)	5-HT$_{1A}$ agonist

MAOI, monoamine oxidase inhibitor; 5-HT, 5-hydroxytryptamine; MDMA, 3,4-methylenedioxymethamphetamine.

syndrome. The most common drug combinations reported to cause serotonin syndrome are MAOIs plus selective serotonin reuptake inhibitors (SSRIs)[89,90,97-100] and MAOIs plus clomipramine.[97,101] Another combination that has been frequently implicated in causing the serotonin syndrome is simultaneous administration of an MAOI and tryptophan.[75,78,81,97,102-110] Overdose of a single serotonin-potentiating agent may also produce the serotonin syndrome. In one study, serotonin syndrome was diagnosed in 14% to 16% of patients that overdosed on SSRIs.[111] The serotonin syndrome may also occur when a drug is administered that interferes with the metabolism of a serotonin-potentiating agent (e.g., SSRI combined with erythromycin).[112]

One particular drug combination that has received considerable attention is the interaction between an MAOI and meperidine. In 1962, a woman who received meperidine in labor was reported to have developed coma and hypotension. It was subsequently noted that she had been self-administering phenelzine, and thus concern was raised about a possible drug interaction.[113] Shortly thereafter, a patient on pargyline therapy was reported to have developed rigidity, coma, and clonus after receiving meperidine.[114] Since then, several other cases of an interaction of a similar nature in patients taking meperidine in MAOIs have been reported.[90,97] There are several unexplained curiosities about the serotonin syndrome generated by the interaction between meperidine and MAOIs. Despite the diverse group of serotonergic drugs in common clinical practice (see Table 29-4) and the frequent use of meperidine, few reports have described a serotonin syndrome with any other agent in combination with meperidine. Similarly, Ebrahim reported a series of 42 patients who were taking isocarboxazid and who were premedicated with meperidine for surgery; none of them had an adverse effect.[115]

An animal model developed for this syndrome almost three decades ago involved the sole administration of high doses of tryptophan to rats, which caused a unique constellation of tremors and movement abnormalities.[79] The same syndrome could be induced by simply administering high doses of an MAOI.[79] This observation provided evidence that some aspects of the clinical syndrome engendered by MAOI overdoses are related to serotonin excess. It is possible that a serotonin excess syndrome could occur after overdoses of SSRIs. However, this appears to occur rarely[116-118] and was not a feature in a series of fluoxetine overdoses (see Chapter 28).[119] A child ingested an excessive amount of sertraline and appeared to develop a serotonin syndrome manifested by tachycardia, hypertension, hallucinations, coma, hyperthermia, tremors, and skin flushing.[120]

A serotonin syndrome–like toxidrome has been reported to follow the ingestion of methylenedioxymethamphetamine (MDMA, or "Ecstasy").[121-129] Being a phenylethylamine type of agent, it is structurally similar to amphetamines and primarily affects serotonergic neurons. In addition, MDMA is frequently ingested in the context of a "rave," a gathering at which so-called *smart drinks*, which are amino acid supplements that possibly contain significant amounts of tryptophan, are also ingested.[123,130] Thus, it is possible that the complex clinical syndrome noted after MDMA ingestion may often be a drug interaction between two serotonergic agents. MDMA, in combination with other serotonergic agents, should be considered to have the potential of causing a serotonin syndrome. A series of deaths have been reported from serotonin syndromes caused by the intentional mixing of MDMA with moclobemide, the latter ingested in an attempt to heighten serotonergic effects.[131]

Although they appear to be safer than classic MAOIs, RIMAs are capable of causing a drug interaction resulting in a serotonin syndrome. Reported cases have involved the interaction of moclobemide and either clomipramine, citalopram, or another serotonin reuptake inhibitor, after both overdose[5,132-134] and therapeutic use.[135] Two of the fatalities involve purposeful taking of the combination to achieve a psychologic "high."[132]

As noted in Table 29-4, lithium has several serotonergic effects, which include stimulation of 5-HT release[136] and enhancement of the response to stimulation of 5-HT$_{1A}$ receptors.[137,138] Several case reports describe a serotonin syndrome caused by the therapeutic combination of lithium with SSRIs.[139-141] Given the frequency with which lithium is prescribed in combination with SSRIs, the relatively few cases of serotonin syndrome induced by these combinations suggest that this is an unusual interaction.

The use of MAOIs with tricyclic antidepressants has been the subject of considerable debate. Combining these two agents has been associated with a serotonin syndrome–like picture.[142,143] However, given the frequency of the use of this combination and the rarity of adverse reports, it appears that the likelihood of an adverse effect from this combination is small.[144] However, particular caution must be exercised when using clomipramine,

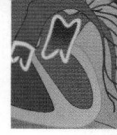

which is a tricyclic antidepressant (3-chloroimipramine) that has a significant effect on inhibiting serotonin reuptake (see Table 29-4). The combination of a TCA with an RIMA appears to be safe, with the exception of agents such as clomipramine, which have a significant effect on serotonin uptake.[145]

A body of literature suggests that the serotonergic effects of dextromethorphan (DM), in consort with other agents, may produce a serotonin syndrome. In 1970, Rivers and Horner described profound hyperthermia in a patient ingesting a DM-containing preparation while taking phenelzine.[146] Several reports have since described similar interactions.[147-149] A similar syndrome has been described in rabbits pretreated with MAOIs.[150] Whether DM can cause a serotonin syndrome in concert with an SSRI has been the subject of controversy. Several cases have been reported.[148,149] It has been proposed that the nature of the interaction in two cases, involving paroxetine and fluoxetine, respectively, is a result of an interaction at the level of the hepatic microsomal P-450 isoenzyme CYP2D6 (debrisoquin hydroxylase).[151-154] DM is metabolized by this enzyme to dextrorphan, in a genetically determined manner by one of two phenotypes, known as extensive and poor metabolizers. Administration of DM to subjects who have had this isoenzyme inhibited by quinidine results in profoundly elevated DM levels and signs and symptoms similar to the serotonin syndrome. Both paroxetine and fluoxetine are inhibitors of this isoenzyme,[153,154] as are sertraline and fluvoxamine.[155,156] However, the significance of this enzymatic inhibition in the generation of a serotonin syndrome associated with the administration of DM has been questioned on the basis of the small amounts of DM requisite to the formation of a manifestation of 5-HT in these combinations.[100]

Sandyk[157] reported an apparent serotonin syndrome in a patient with parkinsonism treated with bromocriptine in whom levodopa was started. The reported syndrome consisted of tremor, mild clonus, hyperreflexia, clonus, hypertension, tachycardia, diaphoresis, and diarrhea. Support that this was due to serotonin excess was suggested by its prompt response to the serotonin antagonist methysergide. Both bromocriptine and levodopa are serotonergic agents. Serotonergic neurons are capable of decarboxylating levodopa to dopamine, during which 5-HT may be released.[158,159] Bromocriptine appears to increase brain levels of serotonin, inhibiting 5-HT catabolism[160,161]; however, only one case of such an interaction has been described.[157]

Trazodone is an antidepressant with complex serotonergic effects. At low doses, it appears to be a serotonin antagonist.[162] At higher doses, however, it appears to be a mixed agonist/antagonist.[162] Low doses appear to be safe when trazodone is taken in combination with an MAOI.[163] Cases of serotonin syndrome have been reported after the combined administration of trazodone and other serotonergic agents.[164]

Selegiline and MAO-B inhibitors have been reported to cause the serotonin syndrome. Although 5-HT is metabolized by MAO-A, selegiline may cause an excess serotonin effect by virtue of its loss of MAO specificity

at higher doses. Cases of the serotonin syndrome, including death, have been reported with the combination of selegiline and SSRIs,[165-167] tricyclic antidepressants,[90,168] and other serotonergic agents.[19]

Buspirone is an anxiolytic agent that is a partial agonist at the 5-HT$_{1A}$ receptor. Its potential role in the generation of the serotonin syndrome is unclear but probably unlikely because animals treated with high doses do not develop a full-blown serotonin syndrome. Several cases of the serotonin syndrome have been reported when buspirone has been used in conjunction with other serotonergic agents.[164]

The "triptans" are serotonergic antimigraine agents that are generally implicated in the etiology of the serotonin syndrome. They act primarily on 5-HT$_{1D}$ receptors. Their antimigraine effect is related to vasoconstriction of cephalic blood vessels. However, most of the triptans are catabolized by MAO and thus their use with an MAOI may cause elevated levels of these agents. A recent report, however, found no evidence of an adverse reaction from the combined use of moclobemide and sumatriptan.[5]

Tramadol is a serotonergic agent that blocks 5-HT reuptake[169,170] and has been implicated in causing a serotonin syndrome.[134] The antibiotic linezolid represents the first of the oxazolidinones class and is a weak, nonspecific reversible inhibitor of MAO. Case reports have suggested the possibility of a serotonin syndrome when linezolid is used with SSRIs.[171] A curious interaction, suggestive of a serotonin syndrome, has been reported in patients taking serotonergic medications and atypical neuroleptics, such as olanzapine.[172] The significance of this is that the atypical agents are 5-HT$_2$ receptor antagonists, and thus would be expected to be protective against serotonin syndrome. However, it has been hypothesized that such blockade of the 5-HT$_2$ receptor may result in overactivation of the 5-HT$_{1A}$ receptor.[172]

St. John's wort (*Hypericum perforatum*), a very popular and widely available herbal agent marketed as an antidepressant, is a weak MAOI that inhibits 5-HT reuptake. It has been reported to cause or contribute to serotonin syndrome[172] probably on the basis of the latter activity.

Treatment of Serotonin Syndrome

No controlled prospective studies have investigated any specific treatment for serotonin syndrome. Virtually all of the data that we have to rely on come from anecdotal case reports and animal studies. From these, it can be gleaned that discontinuation of the provoking agents and supportive care are the cardinal principles in the treatment of this syndrome. Patients with agitation or neuromuscular hyperactivity should be treated initially with benzodiazepines. Benzodiazepines have been shown to improve survival in animal models of serotonin survival.[173,174] Severe cases should be treated in the same manner as an MAOI overdose. Prompt neuromuscular paralysis with nondepolarizing agents is indicated for patients with severe neuromuscular

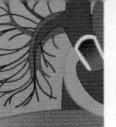

hyperreactivity and hyperthermia.[93,174] The life-threatening complications associated with the serotonin syndrome (e.g., metabolic acidosis, rhabdomyolysis, hepatitis, renal failure, and disseminated intravascular coagulopathy) occur as a result of severe and/or prolonged hyperthermia.

Cyproheptadine, a general 5-HT receptor antagonist that is most potent at the 5-HT$_2$ receptor,[175] is the most commonly touted antidote for the serotonin syndrome. The apparent utility of cyproheptadine is derived from evidence that suggests that the 5-HT$_2$ receptor is important in the pathophysiology of the serotonin syndrome. In addition to being a serotonin antagonist, cyproheptadine is antihistaminic and anticholinergic. Animal studies suggest that cyproheptadine can block serotonin syndrome.[176]

Several anecdotal reports describe treatment of serotonin syndrome with cyproheptadine.[88,141,164,177] Unfortunately, cyproheptadine is available only as an oral preparation. A standard starting dose is 4 to 8 mg, typically followed by doses of 4 mg every 2 to 4 hours. Because of its antimuscarinic properties, anticholinergic side effects may occur; therefore, doses should not exceed more than 0.5 mg/kg per day (typically, 32 mg for an adult).

Methysergide maleate is a nonspecific serotonin antagonist that appears to have some efficacy in animal studies in preventing serotonin syndrome.[178] Clinical data evaluating the efficacy of methysergide in this toxidrome are sparse. In one case report, it appeared to be effective in the treatment of a serotonin syndrome induced by the therapeutic use of the combination of levodopa and bromocriptine.[157] Methysergide is available only as an oral preparation. It is usually given in doses of 2 to 6 mg, the latter being the typical total dose. It is frequently administered in a twice-a-day regimen.

β-Adrenergic receptor antagonists also tend to have some serotonin antagonist qualities. Propranolol is a 5-HT$_{1A}$ blocker[179] that is effective in blocking the serotonin syndrome in animals.[178,180] Responses to propranolol in human cases of serotonin syndrome have been inconsistent.[88,98,108]

Dantrolene has been mentioned as an agent that might inhibit the neuromuscular hyperactivity component of the serotonin syndrome; however, there has been little clinical experience with it in this setting. In addition, dantrolene does not alter survival in animal models of serotonin syndrome.[181,182]

Although certain antipsychotics (e.g., chlorpromazine, ziprasidone, olanzapine, risperidone) are 5-HT$_2$ antagonists and are available for parenteral administration, there has been little experience with them in the treatment of the serotonin syndrome. The few case reports studied have shown mixed results.[145,183-185] Olanzapine (10 mg in a sublingual dose) was used with favorable results in one case of serotonin syndrome.[186]

REFERENCES

1. Hemmeloch JM: Monoamine oxidase inhibitors. In Kaplan HI, Saddock BJ (eds): Comprehensive Textbook of Psychiatry, 6th ed. Baltimore, Williams & Wilkins, 1995, pp 2038–2053.
2. Parkinson Study Group: Effect of deprenyl on the progression of disability in early Parkinson's disease. N Engl J Med 1989; 321:1364–1371.
3. Tetrud JW, Langston JW: The effect of deprenyl on the natural history of Parkinson's disease. Science 1989;245:519–522.
4. Tipton KF: What is it that *l*-deprenyl (selegiline) might do? Clin Pharmacol Ther 1994;56:781–795.
5. Bonnet U: Moclobemide: therapeutic use and clinical studies. Drug Rev 2003;9:97–140.
6. Yamada M, Yasuhara H: Clinical pharmacology of MAO inhibitors: safety and future. Neurotoxicology 2004;25:215–221.
7. Siderowf A, Kurlan R: Monoamine oxidase and catechol-*O*-methyltransferase inhibitors. Med Clin North Am 1999;83: 445–467.
8. Elis J, Laurence DR, Mattie H, Prichard BNC: Modification by monoamine oxidase inhibitors of the effect of some sympathomimetics on blood pressure. BMJ 1967;2:75–78.
9. Davidson AN: Physiological role of monoamine oxidase. Physiol Rev 1958;38:729–747.
10. Brent J, Rumack BH: The role of free radicals in toxic hepatic injury. II. Are free radicals the cause or the consequences of toxin-induced injury? J Toxicol Clin Toxicol 1993;31:173–196.
11. Wells DG, Bjorksten AR: Monoamine oxidase inhibitors revisited. Can J Anaesth 1989;36:64–74.
12. O'Carroll A-M, Fowler CJ, Phillips JP, et al: The deamination of dopamine by human brain monoamine oxidase: specificity of the two forms in seven brain regions. Naunyn Schmiedebergs Arch Pharmacol 1983;323:198–202.
13. O'Carroll A-M, Bardsley ME, Tipton KF: The oxidation of adrenaline and noradrenaline by the two forms of monoamine oxidase from human and rat brain. Neurochem Int 1986;8: 493–500.
14. Kinemuchi H, Fowler CJ, Tipton KF: Substrate specificities of the two forms of monoamine oxidase. In Tipton KF, Dostert P, Strolin Benedetti M (eds): Monoamine Oxidase and Disease: Prospects for Therapy with Reversible Inhibitors. New York, Academic Press, 1984, pp 53–62.
15. Ramsay RR, Hunter DJB: Inhibitors alter the spectrum and redox properties of monoamine oxidase A. Biochim Biophys Acta 2002;1601:178–184.
16. Baker GB, Urichuk LJ, McKenna KF, Kennedy SH: Metabolism of monoamine oxidase inhibitors. Cell Mol Neurobiol 1999;19: 411–426.
17. Baldessarini RJ: Drugs and the treatment of psychiatric disorders. In Hardman JG, Limbird LE, Gilman AG (eds): Goodman & Gilman's the Pharmacological Basis of Therapeutics, 10th ed. New York, McGraw-Hill, 2001, pp 447–483.
18. Mallinger AG, Smith E: Pharmacokinetics of MAO inhibitors. Psychopharmacol Bull 1991;27:493–502.
19. Jacob JE, Wagner ML, Sage JL: Safety of selegiline with cold medications. Ann Pharmacother 2003;37:438–441.
20. Da Prada M, Keller H, Keller R, et al: Ro 11-1163, a specific short acting MAO inhibitor with antidepressant properties. In Kamito K, Usdin E, Nagatsu T (eds): Monoamine Oxidase. Basic and Clinical Frontiers. Amsterdam, Excerpta Medica, 1981, pp 183–196.
21. Youdim MBH, Da Prada M, Amrein R (eds): The cheese effect and new reversibly MAO-A inhibitors. J Neural Transm Suppl 1988;26.
22. Haefely W, Burkard WP, Cesura AM, et al: Biochemistry and pharmacology of moclobemide, a prototypical RIMA. Psychopharmacology 1992;106(Suppl):S6–S14.
23. Haefely W, Burkard WP, Cesura A, et al: Pharmacology of moclobemide. Clin Neuropharmacol 1993;16(Suppl 2):S8–S18.
24. Youdim MBH: The advent of selective monoamine oxidase A inhibitor antidepressants devoid of the cheese reaction. Acta Psychiatr Scand 1995;91(Suppl 386):5–7.
25. Callingham BA: Possible drug interactions with reversible MAO inhibitors. Clin Neuropharmacol 1992;15(Suppl 1):339A–340A.
26. Amrein R, Allen SR, Guentert TW, et al: The pharmacology of reversible monoamine oxidase inhibitors. Br J Psychiatry 1989;155(Suppl 6):66–71.
27. Dallow S: Selective MAOIs. Lancet 1995;345:1055.
28. Tollefson GD: Monoamine oxidase inhibitors: a review. J Clin Psychiatry 1983;44:280–288.

29. Browne B, Linter S: Monoamine oxidase inhibitors and narcotic analgesics. A critical review of the implications for treatment. Br J Psychiatry 1987;151:210–212.
30. Ciraulo DA, Shader RI: Fluoxetine drug-drug interactions: I. antidepressants and antipsychotics. J Clin Psychopharmacol 1990;10:48–50.
31. Dupont H, Davies DS, Strolin Benedetti M: Inhibition of cytochrome P-450-dependent oxidation reactions by MAO inhibitors in rat liver microsomes. Biochem Pharmacol 1987; 36:1651–1657.
32. Linden CH, Rumack BH, Strehlke C: Monoamine oxidase inhibitor overdose. Ann Emerg Med 1984;13:1137–1144.
33. Matell G, Thorstrand C: A case of fatal nialamide poisoning. Acta Med Scand 1967;181:79–82.
34. Reid DD, Kerr WC: Phenelzine poisoning responding to phenothiazine. Med J Aust 1969;2:1214–1215.
35. Mawdsley JA: "Parstelin." A case of fatal overdose. Med J Aust 1968;2:292.
36. Platts MM, Usher A, Stentiford NH: Phenelzine and trifluoperazine poisoning. Lancet 1965;2:738.
37. Robertson JC: Recovery after massive MAOI overdose complicated by malignant hyperpyrexia, treated with chlorpromazine. Postgrad Med J 1972;48:64–65.
38. King J, Barnett PS, Kew MC: Drug-induced hyperpyrexia. A case report. S Afr Med J 1979;567:190–191.
39. Coulter S, Edmunds J, Pyle PO: An overdose of Parstelin. Anaesthesia 1971;26:500–501.
40. Baldridge ET, Miller LV, Haverback BJ, Brunjes S: Amine metabolism after an overdose of a monoamine oxidase inhibitor. N Engl J Med 1962;267:421–426.
41. Melsaac WM, Page IH: New metabolites of serotonin in carcinoid urine. Science 1958;128:537.
42. Davidson J, Sjoerdsma A, Loomis LN, Udenfriend S: Studies with serotonin precursor. 5-hydroxytryptophan in experimental animals and man. J Clin Invest 1957;36:1594–1599.
43. Tedeschi DH, Tedeschi RE, Fellows EJ: Effects of tryptamine on central nervous system including pharmacological procedure for evaluation of iproniazid-like drugs. J Pharmacol Exp Ther 1959;126:223–232.
44. Sjoerdsma A, Oates JA, Zaltzman P, Udenfriend S: Identification and assay of urinary tryptamine: Application as index of monoamine oxidase inhibition in man. J Pharmacol Exp Ther 1959;126:217–222.
45. Bleumink GS, van Vliet ACM, van der Tholen A, Stricker BHC: Fatal combination of moclobemide overdose and whisky. J Med 2003;61:88–90.
46. von Euler US, Hellner S: Excretion of noradrenaline and adrenaline in muscular work. Acta Physiol Scand 1952;26:183–191.
47. Boakes AJ, Laurence DR, Teoh PC, et al: Interactions between sympathomimetic amines and antidepressant agents in man. BMJ 1973;1:311–315.
48. Reynolds JEF: Martindale, the Extra Pharmacopoeia, 28th ed. London, Pharmaceutical Press, 1982, p 28.
49. Cain NN, Cain RM: A compendium of antidepressants. Drug Ther 1978;8:114–150.
50. Turner P, Young JH, Paterson J: Influence of urinary pH on the excretion of tranylcypromine sulphate. Nature 1967;215:881–882.
51. Shulman KI, Walker SE, MacKenzie S, Knowles S: Dietary restriction, tyramine and the use of monoamine oxidase inhibitors. J Clin Psychopharmacol 1989;9:397–402.
52. Livingston MG: Reply to Dallow [letter]. Lancet 1995;345:1056.
53. Fallon B, Foote B, Walsh BT, Roose SP: "Spontaneous" hypertensive episodes with monoamine oxidase inhibitors. J Clin Psychiatry 1988;49:163–165.
54. Lavin MR, Mendelowita A, Kronig MH: Spontaneous hypertensive reactions with monoamine oxidase inhibitors. Biol Psychiatry 1993;34:146–151.
55. Blackwell B, Marley E: Interactions with cheese and its constituents with monoamine oxidase inhibitors. Br J Pharmacol Chemother 1966;26:120–141.
56. Ilett KF, George CF, Davies DS: The effect of monoamine oxidase inhibitors on "first pass" metabolism tyramine in dog intestine. Biochem Pharmacol 1980;29:2551–2556.
57. Davies DS, Yasuhara H, Boobis AR, George CF: The effects of reversible and irreversible inhibitors of monoamine oxidase on

tyramine deamination by the dog intestine. In Tipton KF, Dostert P, Strolin Benedetti M (eds): Monoamine Oxidase and Disease: Prospects for Therapy with Reversible Inhibitors. London, Academic Press, 1984, pp 443–448.
58. Hasan F, McCrodden JM, Kennedy NP, Tipton KF: The involvement of intestinal monoamine oxidase in the transport and metabolism of tyramine. J Neural Transm Suppl 1988;26:1–9.
59. Bieck PR, Antonin KH, Schmidt E: Clinical pharmacology of reversible monoamine oxidase-A inhibitors. Clin Neuropharmacol 1993;16(Suppl):34–41.
60. Callingham BA: Drug interactions with reversible monoamine oxidase-A inhibitors. Clin Neuropharmacol 1993;16(Suppl 2):42–50.
61. Shulman KI, Walker SE: Clarify the safety of the MAOI diet and pizza. J Clin Psychiatry 2000;61:145–146.
62. Shulman KI, Walker SE: Refining the MAOI diet: Tryamine content of pizzas and soy products. J Clin Psychiatry 1999;60: 191–193.
63. Murray J, Walker JF, Doyle JS: Tyramine in alcohol-free beer. Lancet 1988;337:1167–1168.
64. Horowitz D, Lovenberg W, Engelman K, Sjoerdsma A: Monoamine oxidase inhibitors, tyramine, and cheese. JAMA 1964;188:1108–1110.
65. Nuessle WF, Norman FC, Mille HE: Pickled herring and tranylcypromine reaction. JAMA 1965;192:726–727.
66. Da Prada M, Zurcher G, Wuthrich I, Haefely WE: On tyramine food, beverages and the reversible MAO inhibitor moclobemide. J Neural Transm 1988;26:31–56.
67. Blackwell B, Mabbitt LA: Effects of yeast extract after monoamine oxidase inhibition. Lancet 1965;1:940–943.
68. Hodge JV, Nye ER, Emerson GW: Monoamine-oxidase inhibitors, broad beans and hypertension. Lancet 1964;1:1108.
69. Sweet RA, Brown EJ, Hemiberg RG, et al: Monoamine oxidase inhibitor dietary restrictions: what are we asking patients to give up? J Clin Psychiatry 1995;56:196–201.
70. Larsen JK: MAO inhibitors: Pharmacodynamic aspects and clinical implications. Acta Psychiatr Scand 1988;78(Suppl 345):74–80.
71. Kalir A, Sabbagh A, Youdim MBH: Selective acetylenic "suicide" and reversible inhibitors of monoamine oxidase A and B. Br J Pharmacol 1981;73:55–64.
72. Finberg JPM, Tenne M, Youdim MBH: Tyramine antagonistic properties of AGN-1135, an irreversible inhibitor of monoamine oxidase B. Br J Pharmacol 1981;73:65–70.
73. Birks J, Flicker L: Selegiline for Alzheimer's disease (Cochrane Review). Cochrane Database Syst Rev 1999;(1):CD000442.
74. Mitchell RS: Fatal toxic encephalitis occurring during iproniazid therapy in pulmonary tuberculosis. Ann Intern Med 1955;42: 417–424.
75. Oates JA, Sjoerdsma A: Neurologic effects of tryptophan in patients receiving a monoamine oxidase inhibitor. Neurology 1960;10:1076–1078.
76. Smith B, Prockop DJ: Central-nervous system effects of ingestion of L-tryptophan by normal subjects. N Engl J Med 1962;267:1338–1341.
77. Curzon G, Ettlinger G, Cole M, et al: The biochemical, behavioral and neurologic effects of high L-tryptophan intake in the rhesus monkey. Neurology 1963;12:431–438.
78. Hodge JV, Oates JA, Sjoerdsma A: Reduction of the central effects of tryptophan by a decarboxylase inhibitor. Clin Pharmacol Ther 1964;5:149–155.
79. Grahame-Smith DG: Studies in vivo on the relationship between brain tryptophan, brain 5-HT synthesis hyperactivity in rats treated with a monoamine oxidase inhibitor and L-tryptophan. J Neurochem 1984;18:1053–1066.
80. Beaumont G: Drug interactions with clomipramine (Anafranil). J Intern Med Res 1973;1:480–484.
81. Insel R, Roy B, Cohen R, Murphy D: Possible development of the serotonin syndrome in man. Am J Psychiatry 1982;139:954–955.
82. Erspamer V: Occurrence of indolealkylamines in nature. Handb Exp Pharmakol 1966;19:132–181.
83. Rapport MM, Green AA, Page IH: Serum vasoconstrictor (serotonin), IV: isolation and characterization. Biol Chem 1948; 176:1243–1251.
84. Gaddun JH, Hameed KA: Drugs which antagonize 5-hydroxytryptamine. Br J Pharmacol 1957;9:240–248.
85. Saxena PR: Serotonin receptors: subtypes, functional responses, and therapeutic relevance. Pharmacol Ther 1995;66:339–368.

86. Meltzer H, Young M, Metz J, et al: Extrapyramidal side effects and increased serum prolactin following fluoxetine, a new antidepressant. J Neural Transm 1979;45:165–175.

87. Baldessarini RJ, Marsh E: Fluoxetine and side effects [letter]. Arch Gen Psychiatry 1990;47:191.

88. Lappin R, Auchincloss E: Treatment of serotonin syndrome with cyproheptadine. N Engl J Med 1994;331:1021–1022.

89. Sternbach H: The serotonin syndrome. Am J Psychiatry 1991; 148:705–713.

90. Sporer KA: The serotonin syndrome. Drug Saf 1995;13:94–104.

91. Dursun SM, Mathew VM, Reveley MA: Toxic serotonin syndrome after fluoxetine plus carbamazepine. Lancet 1993;342:442.

92. Dursun SM, Burke JG, Reveley MA: Toxic serotonin syndrome or extrapyramidal side-effects? [letter]. Br J Pharmacol 1995;166: 401–402.

93. Boyer EW, Shannon M: The serotonin syndrome. N Engl J Med 2005;352:1112–1120.

94. Dunkley EJ, Isbister GK, Sibbritt D, et al: The Hunter Serotonin Toxicity Criteria: Simple and accurate diagnostic decision rules for serotonin toxicity. Q J Med 2003;96:635–642.

95. Kaneda Y, Ohmori T, Fujii A: The serotonin syndrome: investigation using the Japanese version of the Serotonin Syndrome Scale. Psychiatry Res 2001;105:135–142.

96. Hegerl U, Bottlender R, Gallinat J, et al: The serotonin syndrome scale: first results on validity. Eur Arch Psychiatry Clin Neurosci 1998;248:96–103.

97. Bodner RA, Lynch T, Lewis L, Kahn D: Serotonin syndrome. Neurology 1995;45:219–223.

98. Ruiz F: Fluoxetine and the serotonin syndrome. Ann Emerg Med 1994;24:983–985.

99. Feighner JP, Boyer WF, Tyler DL, Nebrosky RJ: Adverse consequences of fluoxetine-MAOI combination therapy. J Clin Psychiatry 1990;51:222–225.

100. Corkeror MA: Serotonin syndrome—a potentially fatal complication of antidepressant therapy. Med J Aust 1995;163:481–482.

101. Nierenberg DW, Semprebon M: The central nervous system serotonin syndrome. Clin Pharmacol Ther 1993;53:84–87.

102. Price LH, Charney DS, Heninger GR: Serotonin syndrome [letter]. Am J Psychiatry 1992;111:116–117.

103. Pope HG, Jonas JM, Hudson JI, Kafka MP: Toxic reactions to the combination of monoamine oxidase inhibitors and tryptophan. Am J Psychiatry 1985;142:491–492.

104. Baloh RW, Dietz J, Spooner JW: Myoclonus and ocular oscillations induced by L-tryptophan. Ann Neurol 1982;11:95–97.

105. Thomas JM, Rubin EH: Case report of a toxic reaction from a combination of tryptophan and phenelzine. Am J Psychiatry 1984;141:281–283.

106. Glassman AH, Platman SR: Potentiation of a monoamine oxidase inhibitor by tryptophan. J Psychiatr Res 1969;83–88.

107. Levy AB, Bucher P, Votolato N: Myoclonus, hyperreflexia and diaphoresis in patients on phenelzine-tryptophan combination treatment. Can J Psychiatry 1985;30:434–436.

108. Guze BH, Baxter LR Jr: The serotonin syndrome: case responsive to propranolol. J Clin Psychopharmacol 1986;6:119–120.

109. Brennan D, MacManus M, Howe J, McLoughlin J: "Neuroleptic malignant syndrome" without neuroleptics. Br J Psychiatry 1988;152:578–579.

110. Kline SS, Mauro LS, Scala-Barnett DM, Zick D: Serotonin syndrome versus neuroleptic malignant syndrome as a cause of death. Clin Pharmacol 1989;8:510–514.

111. Isbister GK, Bowe SJ, Dawson A, Whyte IM: Relative toxicity of selective serotonin reuptake inhibitors (SSRIs) in overdose. J Toxicol Clin Toxicol 2004;42:277–285.

112. Lee DO, Lee CD: Serotonin syndrome in a child associated with erythromycin and sertraline. Pharmacotherapy 1999;19:894–896.

113. Cocks DP, Passmore-Towe A: Dangers of monoamine oxidase inhibitors. BMJ 1962;1:1545–1546.

114. Vigran IM: Dangerous potentiation of meperidine hydrochloride by pargyline hydrochloride. JAMA 1964;18:163–164.

115. Ebrahim ZY, O'Hara J, Borden L, Tetzlaff J: Monoamine oxidase inhibitors and elective surgery. Cleve Clin J Med 1993;60:129–130.

116. Kelly CA, Dhaun N, Laing WJ, et al: Comparative toxicity of citalopram and the newer antidepressants after overdose. J Toxicol Clin Toxicol 2004;42:67–71.

117. Whyte IM, Dawson AH, Buckley NA: Relative toxicity of venlafaxine and selective serotonin reuptake inhibitors in overdose compared to tricyclic antidepressants. Q J Med 2003;96: 369–74.

118. Graudins A, Dowsett RP, Liddle C: The toxicity of antidepressant poisoning: is it changing? A comparative study of cyclic and newer serotonin-specific antidepressants. Emerg Med 2002; 14:440–446.

119. Phillips SD, Heiligenstein J, Burkett M, et al: Fluoxetine vs tricyclic antidepressants: a prospective multicenter study of antidepressant drug overdoses [abstract]. Vet Hum Toxicol 1994;36:37.

120. Kaminski CA, Robbins MS, Weibley RE: Sertraline intoxication in a child. Ann Emerg Med 1994;23:1371–1374.

121. Parrott AC: Recreational ecstasy/MDMA, the serotonin syndrome, and serotonergic neurotoxicity. Pharmacol Biochem Behav 2002;71:837–844.

122. Demirkiran Y, Jankovic J, Dean JM: Ecstasy intoxication: an overlap between serotonin syndrome and neuroleptic malignant syndrome. Clin Neuropharmacol 1996;19:157–164.

123. Randall T: Ecstasy-fueled "rave" parties become dances of death for English youths. JAMA 1992;268:1505–1506.

124. Iwerson S, Schmoldt A: Two very different fatal cases associated with the use of methylenedioxyethylamphetamine (MDEA): Eve as deadly as Adam [letter]. Clin Toxicol 1996;34:241–244.

125. Brown C, Osterloh J: multiple severe complications from recreational ingestion of MDMA (ecstasy). JAMA 1987;258:780–781.

126. Screaton GR, Singer M, Cairns HS, et al: Hyperpyrexia and rhabdomyolysis after MDMA ("ecstasy") abuse. Lancet 1992;339: 677–678.

127. Singarajah C, Lavies NG: An overdose of ecstasy. Role for dantrolene. Anaesthesia 1992;47:686–687.

128. Chadwick IS, Curry PD, Linsley A, et al: 3,4-Methylenedioxymethamphetamine (MDMA), a fatality associated with coagulopathy and hyperthermia. J R Soc Med 1991;84:371.

129. Tehan B, Hardern R, Bodenham A: Hyperthermia associated with 3,4-methylenedioxyethamphetamine ("Eve"). Anaesthesia 1993; 48:507–510.

130. Friedman R: Ecstasy, the serotonin syndrome, and neuroleptic malignant syndrome—a possible link [letter]. JAMA 1993;269: 869–870.

131. Vuori E, Henry JA, Ojanpera I, et al: Death following ingestion of MDMA (ecstasy) and moclobemide. Addiction 203;98:365–368.

132. Neuvonen PJ, Pohjola-Sintonen S, Tacke U, Vuori E: Five fatal cases of serotonin syndrome after moclobemide-citalopram or moclobemide-clomipramine overdoses. Lancet 1993;342:1419.

133. Kuisma MJ: Fatal serotonin syndrome with trismus [letter]. Ann Emerg Med 1993;26:108.

134. Hernandez AF, Montero MN, Pla A, Villanueva E: Fatal moclobemide overdose or death caused by serotonin syndrome? J Forensic Sci 1995;40:128–130.

135. Spigset O, Mjorndal T, Lovhein O: Serotonin syndrome caused by a moclobemide-clomipramine interaction. BMJ 1993;306:248.

136. Treiser SL, Cascio CS, O'Donohue TL, et al: Lithium increases serotonin release and decreases serotonin receptors in the hippocampus. Science 1981;231:1529–1531.

137. Goodwin GM, De Souza RJ, Green AR, Heal DJ: The enhancement by lithium of the 5-HT$_{1A}$ mediate serotonin syndrome produced by 8-OH-DPAT in the rat: evidence for a post-synaptic mechanism. Psychopharmacology 1986;90:488–493.

138. Price LH, Charney DS, Delgado PL, Heninger GR: Lithium and serotonin function: implications for the serotonin hypothesis of depression. Psychopharmacology 1990;100:2–12.

139. Salama AA, Shafey M: A case of severe lithium toxicity induced by combined fluoxetine and lithium carbonate. Am J Psychiatry 1989;148:705–713.

140. Ohman R, Spigset O: Serotonin syndrome induced by fluvoxamine-lithium interaction. Pharmacopsychiatry 1993;26:263–264.

141. Muly EC, McDonald W, Steffens D, Book S: Serotonin syndrome produced by a combination of fluoxetine and lithium [letter]. Am J Psychiatry 1993;150:1565.

142. McDaniel KD: Clinical pharmacology of monoamine oxidase inhibitors. Clin Neuropharmacol 1986;9:207–234.

143. Brodribb TR, Downey M, Gilbar PJ: Efficacy and adverse effects of moclobemide. Lancet 1994;343:475.

144. Goldberg RS, Thornton WW: Combined tricyclic-MAOI therapy for refractory depression: a review, with guidelines for appropriate use. J Clin Pharmacol 1978;18:143–146.

145. Zimmer R, Gieschke R, Fischbach R, Gasic S: Interaction studies with moclobemide. Acta Psychiatr Scand 1990;360(Suppl):84–86.

146. Rivers N, Horner B: Possible lethal reaction between Nardil and dextromethorphan. Can Med Assoc J 1970;103:85.

147. Sovner R, Wolfe J: Interaction between dextromethorphan and monoamine oxidase inhibitor therapy with isocarboxazid. N Engl J Med 1988;2:850–851.

148. Shamsie SJ, Barriga C: The hazards of use of monoamine oxidase inhibitors in disturbed adolescents. Can Med Assoc J 1971; 104:715.

149. Sauter D, Macneil P, Weinstein E, et al: Phenelzine sulfate dextromethorphan interaction: a case report. Vet Hum Toxicol 1991;33:365.

150. Sinclair JG, Lo GF: The blockade of serotonin uptake and the meperidine-monoamine oxidase inhibitor interaction. Proc West Pharmacol Soc 1977;20:373–374.

151. Skop BP, Finkelstein JA, Mareth TR, et al: The serotonin syndrome associated with paroxetine, an over-the-counter cold remedy, and vascular disease. Am J Emerg Med 1994;12:642–644.

152. Achamallah NS: Visual hallucinations after combining fluoxetine and dextromethorphan. Am J Psychiatry 1992;149:1406.

153. Harvey AT, Burke M: Comment on the serotonin syndrome associated with paroxetine, an over-the-counter cold remedy, and vascular disease [letter]. Am J Emerg Med 1995;13:605–606.

154. Bloomer JC, Woods FR, Haddock RE, et al: The role of cytochrome P-4502D6 in the metabolism of paroxetine by human liver microsomes. Br J Clin Pharmacol 1992;33:521–523.

155. Preskorn SH, Alderman J, Chung M, et al: Pharmacokinetics of desipramine coadministered with sertraline or fluoxetine. J Clin Psychopharmacol 1994;14:90–98.

156. Spina E, Pollicino AM, Avenoso A, et al: Effect of fluvoxamine on the pharmacokinetics of imipramine and desipramine in healthy subjects. Ther Drug Monit 1993;15:243–246.

157. Sandyk R: L-dopa induced "serotonin syndrome" in a parkinsonian patient on bromocriptine [letter]. J Clin Psychopharmacol 1986;6:194.

158. Klawans HL, Goetz C, Bergen D: Levodopa-induced myoclonus. Arch Neurol 1975;32:331–334.

159. Karobath M, Diaz JL, Huttunen M: The effect of L-dopa on the concentration of tryptophan, tyrosine and serotonin in rat brain. Eur J Pharmacol 1971;14:393–396.

160. Hutt CS, Snider SR, Fahn S: Interaction between bromocriptine and levodopa. Neurology 1977;27:505–510.

161. Snider SR, Hutt CS, Stein B, et al: Increase in brain serotonin produced by bromocriptine. Neurosci Lett 1975;1:237–241.

162. Palider Maj J, Rawlow A: Trazodone, a central antagonist and agonist. J Neurol Transm 1979;44:236–248.

163. Jacobsen FM: Low-dose trazodone as a hypnotic in patients treated with MAOI and other psychotropics-pilot study. J Clin Psychiatry 1990;51:298–302.

164. Goldberg RJ, Huk M: Serotonin syndrome from trazodone and buspirone. Psychosomatics 1992;33:235–236.

165. Suchowersky O, deVries JD: Possible interactions between deprenyl and Prozac. Can J Neurol Sci 1990;17:571–572.

166. Suchowersky O, deVries JD: Interaction of fluoxetine and selegiline. Can J Psychiatry 1990;35:571–572.

167. Jermain DM, Hughes PL, Follender AB: Potential fluoxetine-selegiline interaction. Ann Pharmacother 1990;26:1300.

168. U.S. Government Printing Office: Eldepryl and Antidepressant Interaction. FDA Medical Bulletin. Washington, DC, U.S. Food and Drug Administration, 1995, p 6.

169. Driessen B, Reimann W: Interaction of the central analgesic, tramadol, with the uptake and release of 5-hydroxytryptamine in the rat brain in vitro. Br J Pharmacol 1992;105:147–151.

170. Raffa RB, Friderichs E, Reimann W, et al: Opioid and non-opioid components independently contribute to the mechanism of action of tramadol, an atypical opioid analgesic. J Pharmacol Exp Ther 1992;260:275–285.

171. Lavery S, Ravi H, McDaniel WW, et al: Linezolid and serotonin syndrome. Psychomatics 2001;42:432–434.

172. Sternbach H: Serotonin syndrome—how to avoid, identify, and treat dangerous drug interactions. Curr Psychiatry 2003;2:14–24.

173. Nisijima K, Shioda K, Yoshino T, et al: Diazepam and chlormethiazole attenuate the development of hyperthermia in an animal model of the serotonin syndrome. Neurochem Int 2003;43:155–164.

174. Gillman PK: The serotonin syndrome and its treatment. J Psychopharmacol 1999;13:100–109.

175. Peroutka SJ: Serotonin receptors. In Meltzer HY (ed): Psychopharmacology: The Third Generation of Progress. New York, Raven Press, 1987, pp 303–311.

176. Gerson SC, Baldessarini RJ: Motor effects of serotonin in the central nervous system. Life Sci 1980;27:1435–1451.

177. Beasley CM, Masica DN, Heiligenstein JH, et al: Possible monoamine oxidase inhibitor-serotonin uptake inhibitor interaction: Fluoxetine clinical data and preclinical findings. J Clin Psychopharmacol 1993;13:312–320.

178. Heal DJ, Luscombe GP, Martin KF: Pharmacological identification of 5-HT receptor subtypes using behavioral models. In Marsden CA, Heal DJ (eds): Central Serotonin Receptors and Psychotropic Drugs. Boston, Blackwell Scientific, 1992, pp 56–99.

179. Sprouse JS, Aghajanian GK: Propranolol blocks the inhibition of serotonergic dorsal raphe cell firing by HT1A selective agonists. Eur J Pharmacol 1986;128:295–298.

180. Deakin JFW, Green AR: The effects of putative 5-hydroxytryptamine antagonists on the behaviors produced by administration of tranylcypromine and L-tryptophan or tranylcypromine and L-DOPA to rat. Br J Pharmacol 1978;64:201–209.

181. Isbister GH, Whyte IM: Serotonin toxicity and malignant hyperthermia: role of 5-HT2 receptors. Br J Anaesth 2002;88:603–604.

182. Nisijima K, Yoshino T, Yui K, Katoh S: Potent serotonin (5-HT_{2A}) receptor antagonists completely prevent the development of hyperthermia in an animal model of the 5-HT syndrome. Brain Res 2001;890:23–31.

183. Graham PM, Potter JM, Paterson J: Combination monoamine oxidase inhibitor/tricyclic antidepressant interaction. Lancet 1982;2:440.

184. Grantham J, Neel W, Brown W: Reversal of imipramine-monoamine oxidase inhibitor induced toxicity with chlorpromazine. J Kans Med Soc 1964;65:279–280.

185. Tackley RM, Tregaskis B: Fatal disseminated intravascular coagulation following a monoamine oxidase inhibitor/tricyclic interaction. Anaesthesia 1987;42:760–763.

186. Boddy R, Ali R, Dowsett R: Use of sublingual olanzapine in serotonin syndrome [abstract]. J Toxicol Clin Toxicol 2004;42:725.

30 Lithium

JOSEF G. THUNDIYIL, MD, MPH ■ KENT R. OLSON, MD

At a Glance...

■ Lithium is a drug with a narrow therapeutic index.
■ It has a two-compartment volume of distribution moving from extracellular to intracellular compartments.
■ Lithium is eliminated almost entirely by the kidneys.
■ Its toxicity is most commonly manifested by CNS symptoms.
■ Acute lithium overdose differs significantly from chronic lithium intoxication.
■ Serum levels do not correlate with systemic toxicity.
■ Hemodialysis is an ideal treatment modality but should be reserved for patients exhibiting signs of severe intoxication and should be based on clinical and kinetic criteria.

INTRODUCTION

Lithium was discovered in 1818 and initially used for the treatment of gout, rheumatism, and renal calculi.[1,2] In the early 1900s it was used as a salt substitute but was later abandoned because of toxic effects. It was also once present in the soft drink 7-Up.[3] Although Aulde and Lange recognized in the 1880s that lithium could be used to treat depression, it was not until the 1950s that Cade and Schou established its use as a treatment for bipolar disorder.[4] In 1970, the U.S. Food and Drug Administration (FDA) approved its use for the treatment of acute mania. Currently, lithium is used to treat a wide variety of disorders (Box 30-1) from bipolar affective disorder and alcoholism to prophylaxis for cluster

headache. It remains the drug of choice for the treatment of recurrent bipolar illness.[5]

With increasing use of lithium comes an increased risk for toxic effects. It is estimated that up to 90% of patients taking lithium have at some time experienced signs and symptoms of toxicity.[6] In 1991, the American Association of Poison Control Centers reported 4149 cases of lithium exposure, with 622 (15%) resulting in moderate to severe intoxication and 12 in death.[7] In 2002, 4954 cases were reported (one third being unintentional exposures) with 1527 resulting in moderate to severe intoxication and 15 in death. Although death is rare, the risks for morbidity and prolonged hospitalization emphasize the importance of appropriate management.

PHARMACOLOGY

Lithium is the lightest alkali metal and has no known physiologic role. Its mechanism of action is not clearly understood. It inhibits the release of norepinephrine and augments its reuptake.[8] It also depletes brain inositol, which is a precursor in the phosphatidylinositol pathway assisting in signal transduction of hormones and neurotransmitters.[1] This effect may result in reduced responsiveness to α-adrenergic stimulation.[9] Other proposed mechanisms include inhibition of G proteins crucial to ion channel opening,[10] stimulation of release of serotonin from the hippocampus, and inhibition of adenylate cyclase.[8] These inhibitory effects may decrease neuronal responsiveness to neurotransmitters. Additionally, because lithium is a cation, it behaves similarly to potassium and sodium, thereby affecting ion transport and cell membrane potential.

PHARMACOKINETICS

Lithium is dispensed in a variety of formulations (Table 30-1) some of which are sustained-release preparations. Lithium is rapidly absorbed, reaching peak levels in 1 to 3 hours in regular preparations and 4 to 12 hours in sustained-release preparations. The bioavailability for most preparations is nearly 100%. It is neither protein bound nor metabolized. Lithium initially has a volume of distribution approximately 0.4 L/kg. However, as the ion moves from extracellular compartments to intracellular compartments over 6 to 8 hours, the final volume of distribution is between 0.6 and 0.9 L/kg.[11] This process, which takes up to 6 to 10 days to reach final equilibrium, reflects the amount of time required to achieve therapeutic response. Serum lithium levels measure only the extracellular concentration of lithium. Yet, lithium exerts its effects once it has moved to its intracellular

---

BOX 30-1   THERAPEUTIC USES OF LITHIUM

Psychiatric Disorders

Manic-depressive (bipolar) illness*
Unipolar depressive illness
Behavior disorders
Character disorders
Pain
Alcoholism/drug abuse
Premenstrual tension
Organic brain syndrome
Cycloid psychosis
Anorexia nervosa
Schizoaffective disorders
Steroid-induced psychosis

Nonpsychiatric Disorders

? Pain
  Graves' disease
? Premenstrual tension
? Leukopenia/chemotherapy
? Felty's syndrome
? Thyrotoxicosis
? Tardive dyskinesia
? Huntington's chorea
? Pancreatic cholera syndrome
? Syndrome of inappropriate antidiuretic hormone secretion

*Only approved use for lithium in the United States; other uses are experimental.

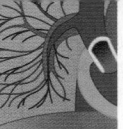

TABLE 30-1 Some Available Lithium (Li) Preparations*		
TRADE NAME	**CHEMICAL FORMULATION**	**DOSE FORMS**
United States		
Lithane (Miles Pharmaceutical)	Lithium carbonate	Tablets, 300 mg
Lithium carbonate USP	Lithium carbonate	Capsules, 150 mg, 300 mg, 600 mg; tablets, 300 mg
Lithium citrate syrup USP (Roxane)	Lithium citrate	Syrup, 8 mEq/5 mL—equivalent to 300 mg of lithium carbonate
Cibalith-S (CIBA)	Lithium citrate	Syrup, 8 mEq/5 mL—equivalent to 300 mg of lithium carbonate
Lithobid (CIBA)	Lithium carbonate	Tablets, 300 mg (sustained release)
Eskalith (SmithKline)	Lithium carbonate	Capsules and tablets, 300 mg
Eskalith CR (SmithKline)	Lithium carbonate	Tablets, 300 mg, 450 mg; capsules, 300 mg (sustained release)
Canada		
Carbolith (ICN)	Lithium carbonate	Capsules and tablets, 300 mg
Lithane (Pfizer)	Lithium carbonate	As above
Lithizine (Maney)	Lithium carbonate	As above
United Kingdom	Lithium carbonate	400 mg tablets also available
Scandinavia		
Litarex	Lithium carbonate	Sustained-release formulation

*Molecular mass = 73.89 daltons; atomic number, 3; atomic weight, 6.94; emission line on flame photometer, 671 nm.

compartment. This two-compartment phenomenon explains why patients can be initially asymptomatic in the setting of significantly elevated serum levels.

Lithium has a predilection for accumulation in liver, bone, muscle, brain, kidney, and thyroid.[12] The highest levels are found in the brain and kidney,[11] and toxicity is most commonly associated with these organs.

Ninety-five percent of lithium is excreted by the kidneys, while the remainder is eliminated via sweat and feces. Lithium is handled similarly to sodium by the kidney, and approximately 75% of the filtered load is reabsorbed in the proximal tubule.[13] The renal clearance is between 10 mL and 40 mL/min.[14] Sodium depletion can increase lithium reabsorption significantly. Consequently, volume depletion from diuretics, dehydration, febrile illness, or gastrointestinal (GI) loss can lead to elevated lithium levels in the serum.

The serum elimination half-life of lithium can vary from 12 to 27 hours. In patients with chronic intoxication the half-life can be prolonged up to 48 hours.[15] The half-life of lithium may vary significantly with duration of therapy.[16] It has been hypothesized that this phenomenon may be due in part to inhibition of lithium efflux from cells by the drug itself during chronic therapy.

The usual renal clearance of lithium is 10 to 40 mL/min. In the elderly, renal clearance may be reduced to 15 mL/min and the elimination half-life can be as long as 58 hours. There is also a propensity toward a smaller final volume of distribution in the elderly.[17] In a study of hospitalized patients with lithium toxicity, age greater than 65 years was associated with a significantly higher likelihood of toxic lithium level.[18]

During the third trimester of pregnancy, lithium clearance will usually increase, thereby creating difficulties with serum monitoring.[17] Lithium freely crosses the placenta and is also excreted in breast milk.[19] It is labeled as pregnancy class D and has been implicated in causing

an increased risk of congenital cardiac defects, particularly Ebstein's anomaly. Breast-feeding infants of mothers taking lithium have been reported to have signs of cyanosis, hypotonia, and lethargy.[20]

Multiple medication interactions are associated with lithium (Table 30-2). It has been reported to cause neuroleptic malignant syndrome in combination therapy with neuroleptic agents or by itself in overdose. Additionally, diuretics that deplete sodium and water will indirectly result in lithium toxicity by enhancing its reabsorption in the proximal tubules. Most notable, however, are the drug interactions that affect lithium clearance. Studies in both healthy patients given lithium and those receiving chronic lithium therapy have shown that nonsteroidal anti-inflammatory drugs (NSAIDs) can decrease lithium clearance and raise plasma lithium levels.[23] This may be secondary to prostaglandin inhibition causing a reduction in glomerular filtration rate (GFR) and subsequent sodium (and lithium) reabsorption in patients with preexisting volume depletion. Angiotensin-converting enzyme (ACE) inhibitors also contribute to lithium toxicity in volume-depleted patients by causing a further decrease in GFR.

TOXICOLOGY

Lithium toxicity can be classified into three major categories. It may occur as the result of an *acute* overdose (in a lithium-naive patient), acute overdose in a patient on chronic therapy (*acute-on-chronic*), or *chronic* overmedication or drug accumulation. Generally, chronic intoxication is associated with the most serious toxicity.

Accumulation of lithium may result from excessive intake or impaired excretion. Excessive intake is seen in the acute and acute-on-chronic overdose settings in which a patient intentionally ingests an excessive amount

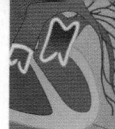

TABLE 30-2   Known Drug Interactions with Lithium

DRUG	EFFECTS OF INTERACTION
Haloperidol	Rigidity, ataxia, oral tardive dyskinesia, ↑ depression, ↑ haloperidol toxicity
Tricyclic antidepressants (TCAs)	Additive antidepressant effect, hypotension, delirium, seizures, increase in blood pressure if hypotension secondary to TCA
Phenothiazines	↑ Lithium and phenothiazine toxicity, ↑ depression along with toxicity
Benzodiazepines	↑ Depression
Neuromuscular blockers	↑ Neuromuscular blockade
Methyldopa	↑ Parkinsonian syndrome
Nonsteroidal anti-inflammatory drugs: indomethacin, piroxicam, mefenamic acid, phenylbutazone	Partial reversal of nephrogenic diabetes insipidus and ↑ serum lithium, ↓ renal lithium clearance
Phenytoin	Polyuria, polydipsia, tremor
Calcium channel blockers: verapamil, nifedipine, diltiazem	Additive or synergistic action with lithium
Angiotensin-converting enzyme inhibitors (e.g., captopril, enalapril)	Reduced glomerular filtration rate, ↓ lithium clearance
Diuretics	
Thiazides	↑ Serum lithium
Osmotics, acetazolamide, sodium bicarbonate	↑ Urinary lithium excretion
Furosemide	No change in serum lithium, unless induces significant sodium loss
Potassium-sparing diuretics and potassium supplements	Abolish distal renal tubular acidosis and may prevent renal lithium toxicity

of lithium tablets in a suicidal or accidental ingestion. Excessive intake also occurs when dose modifications are made for the patient chronically taking lithium.

Impaired excretion of lithium occurs from a variety of factors. Any condition in which sodium and volume depletion occurs may lead to increased reabsorption of the drug in the kidneys. Vomiting, diarrhea, febrile illness, renal insufficiency, excessive exercise, water restriction, excessive sweating, low sodium diet, and congestive heart failure all can increase the risk for lithium toxicity. Concomitant administration of drugs that decrease GFR will also contribute to chronic toxicity. Other factors that play a role in toxicity include duration of therapy[16] and individual tolerance to lithium.[2]

Patients on chronic lithium therapy may develop nephrogenic diabetes insipidus (NDI), which can trigger a cascade of symptoms and signs of lithium toxicity. However, most patients will develop symptoms of polyuria without full-blown NDI. Up to 37% of patients taking therapeutic doses of lithium experience symptoms of polyuria.[24] This is attributable to impaired urinary concentrating ability by the kidneys. This effect coupled with any intercurrent illness can trigger the vicious cycle of lithium toxicity (Fig. 30-1). With sodium and volume depletion, the excretion and clearance of lithium decreases as the kidney increases its reabsorption of the cation. The increased reabsorption leads to elevated levels of serum lithium, which in turn continues to adversely affect the kidneys' ability to concentrate urine. Consequently, patients on chronic lithium therapy who exhibit symptoms of polyuria (or NDI) are at increased risk for developing lithium toxicity.[6]

CLINICAL MANIFESTATIONS

The clinical manifestations of lithium toxicity are primarily related to the central nervous system (CNS)

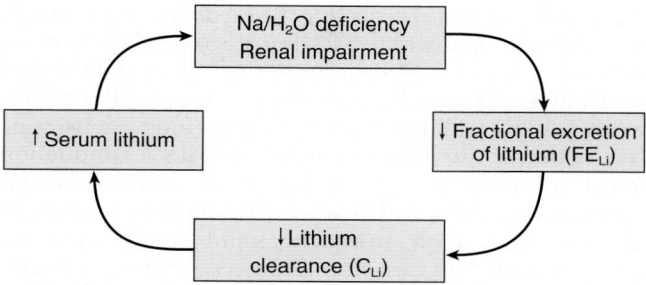

FIGURE 30-1 The vicious cycle of sodium and water depletion and lithium toxicity.

and kidneys. In addition, gastrointestinal, cardiovascular, and endocrine side effects are commonly reported.

Neurologic symptoms of intoxication include coarse tremor, dysarthria, ataxia, nystagmus, slurred speech, hyperreflexia, and myoclonia. Patients often have alterations in level of consciousness ranging from mild confusion to delirium, agitation, seizures, and coma. Some patients on chronic therapy complain of prodromal symptoms of nervousness prior to more objective signs of intoxication.[8] Although most patients recover after lithium intoxication, there are reports of neurologic sequelae including scanning speech, ataxia, memory deficits, and choreoathetoid movements persisting for 12 months or even permanently.[25-28]

Renal toxicity is more common in patients on chronic lithium therapy. Toxicity includes impaired urinary concentrating ability, NDI, and sodium-losing nephritis. Previous studies have suggested the incidence of polyuria to be as high as 37% and worsened by concomitant use of serotoninergic antidepressants.[24] Nephrotic syndrome, acute tubular necrosis, and chronic interstitial nephropathy have also been described in association with lithium therapy.

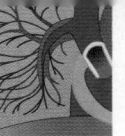

Lithium is the most common cause of drug-induced NDI.[29] The mechanism is not entirely understood. Lithium enters the renal tubules via sodium channels and modulates the function of certain G proteins, thereby lowering the levels of cyclic adenosine monophosphate (cAMP). The lowered intracellular cAMP may contribute to a decrease in transcription and expression of the antidiuretic hormone–sensitive aquaporin-2 water channels[30] responsible for water reabsorption in the kidney. NDI is characterized by polyuria, polydipsia, hypernatremia, and low urine osmolality. Elevated serum osmolality is also expected, but most patients are able to compensate by excessive fluid intake on a daily basis. NDI can significantly predispose patients to lithium toxicity via volume depletion, lithium reabsorption, and the vicious cycle of renal toxicity. Treatment of lithium-induced NDI includes discontinuation of the drug and administration of amiloride,[31] NSAIDS, or thiazide diuretics.[32-34] Cases of persistent NDI after discontinuation of lithium for up to 57 months have been described.[35]

Cardiovascular effects are usually mild and non-specific. Patients may experience mild hypertension, bradycardia, or tachycardia. Electrocardiographic changes can include transient ST depression, flattened or inverted T waves, QRS widening, QT prolongation, or intraventricular conduction delays. Nearly all patients taking lithium will develop T wave flattening. Sinus node dysfunction is the most commonly reported conduction defect followed by QT prolongation, intraventricular conduction defects, and U waves. Although these findings are reversible, their prevalence and significance are undetermined.[36] In rare circumstances, severe ventricular arrhythmias and myocardial infarction have been described in acute overdoses.[37]

Gastrointestinal symptoms are also more common in the acute overdose setting. Symptoms include nausea, vomiting, diarrhea, anorexia, and bloating and typically occur within 1 hour of ingestion.

Endocrine effects from lithium toxicity most commonly include hypothyroidism via inhibition of thyroid hormone synthesis and subsequent release (in 3% to 60% of patients taking lithium).[38] Less commonly seen is hyperthyroidism, which may not only mask symptoms of lithium toxicity but can increase toxicity by inducing cellular unresponsiveness and altered renal tubular handling of lithium.[38] Lithium is also associated with hyperparathyroidism, hypothermia, and less frequently hyperthermia.

DIAGNOSIS

Degree of intoxication is important for understanding the diagnosis and management of lithium toxicity. Severity of lithium toxicity is most frequently arbitrarily divided into three grades: mild, moderate, and severe[6] (Table 30-3). This grading system was first described by Hansen and Amdisen in 1978[4] and has been used with some degree of consistency throughout the literature. *Mild* symptoms include nausea, vomiting, lethargy, tremor, and fatigue. Symptoms of *moderate* intoxication are confusion, agitation, delirium, tachycardia, and hypertonia. Coma, seizures, hyperthermia, and hypotension characterize *severe* intoxication.

Patient History

Diagnosis and classification (acute, acute-on-chronic, or chronic) of lithium intoxication can be difficult. The prevalence of neurologic symptoms should alert the clinician to the possibility of lithium poisoning. Additional history from the patient and outside sources regarding previous level of functioning, other medications, prodromal symptoms, and recent intercurrent illness may be necessary. Other pertinent history should include the type of lithium preparation that was ingested and any underlying illnesses that predispose to toxicity. The diagnosis can be further complicated by the fact that many patients with toxicity on presentation may not have taken an intentional overdose of lithium, but rather may be suffering from chronic toxicity.

Physical Examination

Particular attention should be paid to the vital signs, degree of neurologic involvement, and cardiovascular status. Documentation of a thorough initial neurologic

TABLE 30-3 Serum Lithium and Toxic Manifestations†		
SEVERITY OF SYMPTOMS	**APPROXIMATE SERUM LITHIUM CONCENTRATION (mEq/L)**	**SYMPTOMS**
No toxicity (therapeutic)	0.4–1.3	Usually none
Mild toxicity	1.5–2.5	Nausea, vomiting, lethargy, tremor CNS depression, fatigue, diarrhea
Moderate toxicity	2.5–3.5	Confusion, agitation, delirium, tachycardia, hypertonia
Severe toxicity	>3.5	Coma, seizures, hyperthermia, hypotension

*Lithium toxicity may be manifested even at therapeutic levels, especially in the elderly, when the therapeutic level may be 0.2 mEq/L.
†Classification of Hansen and Amdisen.[4] (Stages I and II: apathy, tremor, weakness, ataxia, motor agitation, rigidity, fascicular twitching, nausea, vomiting and diarrhea. Stage III: Latent convulsive movements, stupor, and coma.)

examination may be helpful in patients who may endure a prolonged hospital course.

Laboratory and Imaging Studies

Initial studies should include cardiac monitoring, electrocardiogram (ECG), assessment of oxygenation and monitoring of urine output, serum electrolytes, calcium, renal function, glucose, serum lithium level, and thyroid-stimulating hormone (TSH). Leukocytosis can be seen with therapeutic lithium use as well as intoxication. A low anion gap can also be present after acute ingestion of lithium carbonate[8] possibly owing to the presence of and interference by the carbonate anion in the calculation of anion gap. In addition, in chronic poisoning, patients are likely to demonstrate evidence of renal insufficiency with elevated blood urea nitrogen and creatinine. In some cases in which the diagnosis is initially unclear, imaging of the brain may be necessary. Although some formulations of lithium may be radiopaque, radiography is not reliable for excluding ingestion.[39]

Many hospitals have readily available serum testing for lithium levels (normal range, ~0.6 to 1.2 mEq/L). Serum levels should ideally be drawn at least 6 to 12 hours after the last therapeutic dose to avoid misinterpretation of predistributional levels. However, these levels can still be misleading because lithium has a low therapeutic index and levels frequently do not correlate with level of toxicity. Levels as high as 10.6 mEq/L (10.6 mmol/L) have been reported without evidence of neurologic toxicity after an acute overdose[40] because of the multicompartment kinetics of the drug. Furthermore, a normal level does not exclude toxicity, because serum levels do not accurately reflect the intracellular concentration or toxicity of the drug.

It is important to note that some specimen tubes contain lithium heparin as an anticoagulant and can falsely elevate serum lithium results. This phenomenon has been demonstrated to factitiously elevate serum lithium levels by as much as 2.0 mEq/L in healthy volunteers.[41] Others have reported these tubes producing falsely elevated levels by as much as 6 to 8 mEq/L.[42]

There is relatively poor correlation between serum levels and systemic toxicity, particularly after an *acute* or *acute-on-chronic* overdose. Hansen and Amdisen described 23 patients with lithium intoxication and concluded that there is *no clear-cut relationship between serum lithium levels and severity of symptoms*. However, 21 of their patients were suffering from chronic lithium intoxication. They suggested that levels of 1.5 to 2.5 mEq/L are associated with mild symptoms of toxicity, 2.5 to 3.5 mEq/L are considered serious, and greater than 3.5 mEq/L are considered life threatening (see Table 30-3). These levels, which were all drawn at approximately 12 hours after the last dose of lithium,[43] hold relevance only for patients with chronic lithium exposure.

Bailey and McGuigan prospectively studied all cases of lithium exposure brought to the attention of a poison control center over a 1-year period, and their study group included patients with acute, acute-on-chronic,

and chronic exposures plus one patient with *severe* lithium intoxication after a chronic exposure and a peak serum level of 1.5 mEq/L.[44] They noted that toxicity occurred at lower levels in patients with chronic exposures compared with those with acute-on-chronic exposures. They concluded that the Hansen and Amdisen classification is not a useful tool for predicting morbidity or mortality and does not correlate well with lithium level.

Oakley and colleagues conducted a retrospective analysis of 97 cases of lithium exposure at a regional center over a 13-year period. They concluded that peak serum levels are significantly higher in patients with severe intoxication and that chronic exposure carries a substantially higher risk of severe neurotoxicity than acute exposure. Furthermore, they identified risk factors contributing independently to the development of chronic intoxication: NDI, age over 50 years, thyroid dysfunction, and baseline endogenous creatinine clearance below normal.[45]

Currently, most authors agree that clinical symptoms are more reliable than serum lithium levels. Additionally, management should be based on these clinical parameters rather than on drug levels.[46] Clinicians are cautioned about reliance on an isolated serum lithium level.

It has been suggested that erythrocyte, urine, or cerebrospinal fluid (CSF) levels of lithium might be useful in the assessment of lithium toxicity. The erythrocyte concentration does not fluctuate as much as plasma lithium levels, perhaps reflecting an intracellular lithium concentration. However, this value has not been shown to have clinical significance. CSF levels are about 40% to 50% of plasma lithium levels, but in animal studies they have demonstrated no advantage over plasma lithium levels in assessing toxicity.[47] In addition to being more invasive, CSF levels do not reflect intracellular levels of lithium. Urine levels do not correlate with clinical toxicity but can be useful in the calculation of renal lithium clearance.

Differential Diagnosis

Differential diagnosis of lithium toxicity includes psychosis, hypoglycemia, meningitis, encephalitis, gastroenteritis, food poisoning, drug withdrawal, intracranial bleeding, trauma, thyrotoxicosis, Parkinson's disease, and neuroleptic malignant syndrome. Intoxication by other psychotropic drugs that may be available to the patient should be considered, such as tricyclic antidepressants, selective serotonin reuptake inhibitors (SSRIs), valproic acid, and antipsychotic drugs.

MANAGEMENT

Supportive Measures

Initial treatment of lithium toxicity includes appropriate airway management, assessment of vital signs, and continuous cardiac monitoring. Peripheral IV lines should be inserted for the administration of fluids as well

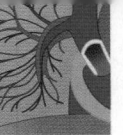

as other general emergency treatment measures including dextrose and naloxone if needed. Hyperthermia or hypothermia should be treated appropriately. If seizures develop, they should be treated with standard measures including benzodiazepines and barbiturates (see Chapter 2A). Electrocardiographic findings such as flattened or inverse T waves and mild QT prolongation do not usually require treatment; however, severe arrhythmias should be treated with usual measures, including magnesium for marked QT prolongation or torsades de pointes.

The goal of fluid therapy is to maintain GFR and urine output in order to reduce the continued reabsorption of lithium. Fluid replacement should begin with isotonic saline. A few reports have suggested marked improvement with forced diuresis using very large volumes of normal saline along with diuretics,[48] achieving lithium clearance values of 39 mL/min (in patients with normal renal function).[49] However, other studies have suggested less than favorable outcomes with forced diuresis, including a reduction in lithium clearance.[43] Because of inconsistent results and the risk of electrolyte imbalances, forced diuresis is not recommended. On the other hand, volume resuscitation to replace fluid losses and to maintain adequate urine output is crucial to the treatment of lithium intoxication.

Decontamination

There is no known antidote for lithium, so particular attention should be paid to gastric decontamination. Although it has been demonstrated in in vitro studies that lithium does not bind well to activated charcoal,[50] charcoal should be given if co-ingestants are suspected. In patients with early presentation, consideration should be given to gastric lavage, especially for regular-release preparations. After ingestion of sustained-release preparations (e.g., Litho-Bid), whole bowel irrigation may be preferable. In a crossover study of healthy volunteers who were given GoLYTELY at 2 L/hr for 5 hours after lithium ingestion, there was a significant reduction in peak lithium concentrations by more than 50% and reduction in lithium absorption by 67%.[51] Whole-bowel irrigation should also be considered after massive ingestion of regular-release products.

Limited evidence supports the use of sodium polystyrene sulfonate (SPS; Kayexalate) to bind lithium in the gut and to enhance elimination. Animal studies have demonstrated that the SPS resin effectively binds lithium and can reduce serum lithium concentrations even after IV lithium dosing.[7] Studies in healthy human volunteers have shown small but statistically significant reductions in lithium absorption after treatment with SPS, without significant changes in serum sodium or potassium levels.[52,53] However, the reductions were not large enough to likely affect the clinical course of an acute overdose.[52] Furthermore, there is no consensus regarding optimal dosing or whether electrolyte alterations in a sick patient population could be more pronounced. At this time, SPS is not recommended for acute lithium ingestion.

Elimination

Besides hemodialysis, a variety of methods have been suggested or reported to enhance the elimination of lithium, including alkaline diuresis, IV theophylline, and dopamine. However, in addition to posing potential adverse effects, these alternative methods are not supported by clinical studies.

Lithium renal clearance can be estimated using the serum and urine lithium levels. Renal lithium clearance = urine flow rate (mL/min) × urine lithium (mEq/L)/ serum lithium (mEq/L). The normal renal lithium clearance is estimated to be between 10 and 40 mL/min. Hansen and Amdisen, however, reported in their study of chronic lithium intoxicated patients that the lithium clearance of this group ranged from 0.9 to 18.4 mL/min.[43] Similar variable clearances for patients on chronic lithium therapy have been found in other studies.[54]

Peritoneal dialysis has been shown to achieve lithium clearance rates of between 9 and 15 mL/min.[23,49] This modality might be considered in patients who have poor renal function if hemodialysis facilities are unavailable (e.g., in remote areas). Otherwise, it should not be substituted for hemodialysis.

Because lithium has a small volume of distribution and minimal protein binding, hemodialysis is an appropriate method for lithium removal. Lithium clearances of 70 to 170 mL/min have been reported with hemodialysis. However, there is controversy about indications for hemodialysis. Removal of lithium from the plasma and extracellular fluid may have little effect on intracellular lithium concentrations, and toxic effects may persist even after serum levels fall. This is consistent with the clinical observation that serum lithium levels correlate poorly with signs and symptoms of toxicity. It could be argued that dialysis is most likely to be effective soon after an acute ingestion while the serum lithium level is markedly elevated and prior to intracellular redistribution. However, these patients generally experience less severe toxic effects,[45] and patients with levels as high as 10.6 or higher[40] may remain asymptomatic and recover with supportive measures alone.

Amdisen recommended that patients with impaired renal function or those who have taken an overdose and have persistent levels greater than 1.4 mEq/L should undergo hemodialysis.[6] Jaeger and coworkers studied the kinetics of lithium in intoxicated patients and concluded that no rigid indication for hemodialysis can be set. They further stated that hemodialysis is not an emergency therapy but one that should be initiated only after observation of the patient as an inpatient and based on a combination of clinical and kinetic criteria.[54] Other authors have suggested that the rapid correction of lithium by hemodialysis might contribute to persistent neurologic toxicity similarly to rapid correction of hyponatremia.[28]

Bailey and McGuigan in a prospective study recommended hemodialysis for patients with any of the following criteria: (1) severe toxicity, (2) alteration in level of consciousness, (3) cardiac toxicity, (4) creatinine greater than 2.3 mg/dL associated with an acute lithium level greater than 2.0 mEq/L or chronic level greater

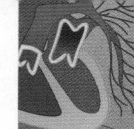

than 1.5, or (5) creatinine greater than 1.7 mg/dL associated with a chronic level of 2.5 mEq/L or acute level of 4.0 mEq/L. Serum creatinine levels were obtained after several hours of hydration. The authors compared the outcomes for patients in whom dialysis was recommended but not performed to those of patients who actually received hemodialysis. Although fewer patients received dialysis than was recommended, there was no outcome difference between the two groups. They concluded that indications for hemodialysis should be based on clinical symptoms and reserved for the more severe cases.[55]

Clearly, there is no consensus on precisely when to dialyze. Most agree that patients exhibiting signs and symptoms of severe lithium poisoning (seizures, coma, cardiac arrhythmias) or who have renal failure should undergo hemodialysis. In addition, dialysis should be considered in acute overdose patients with clinical deterioration and patients with chronic lithium toxicity whose serum levels are greater than 3.5 mEq/L. Patients with acute or acute-on-chronic overdose with elevated levels but who are asymptomatic or minimally symptomatic and have normal renal function should be treated with IV fluids and monitored closely for deterioration. There may be rebound (Fig. 30-2) in serum levels after dialysis, and the procedure should be repeated until the serum level 6 to 8 hours after dialysis is less than 1 mEq/L.

Several case reports have demonstrated success in adults and children[56] for treating lithium intoxication with the use of continuous renal replacement therapy (CRRT). This includes methods such as continuous venovenous hemodialysis (CVVHD), continuous arteriovenous hemodialysis (CAVHD), continuous venovenous hemodiafiltration (CVVHDF), and continuous arteriovenous hemodiafiltration (CAVHDF). The reported lithium clearance rates for CVVHD, CVVHDF, CAVHD, and CAVHDF are given in Table 30-4.[56-60] While these clearances are less than for hemodialysis, the procedures require less specialized staff and facilities and can be done continuously for several hours or days, compared with typical dialysis runs of 2 to 3 hours at a time. In addition, CVVHD is pump-driven and therefore does not rely on the patient's arterial pressure to provide a pressure gradient. One particular case study documented success with CVVHD in a hemodynamically unstable lithium-intoxicated patient in whom hemodialysis had to be discontinued.[58]

CRRT has the added advantage of ease of implementation and avoidance of rebound lithium levels (see Fig. 30-2). One author suggests that the combination of hemodialysis and CVVHD may have the potential to decrease length of hospital stay and health care costs.[56] CRRT procedures have been used for periods of 14 to 72 hours, with an average duration of 34.7 hours in one study.[60] It is not yet clear, however, whether CRRT will shorten the length of hospital stay or change outcome when compared with intermittent hemodialysis. There are no controlled studies to date comparing safety and efficacy of CRRT over other methods of therapy for routine treatment of lithium toxicity. Continuous renal

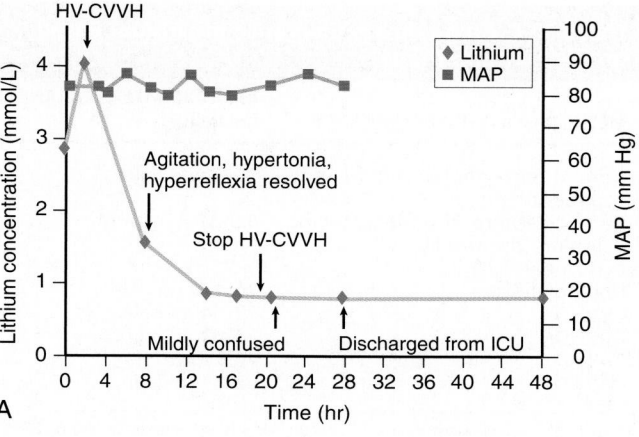

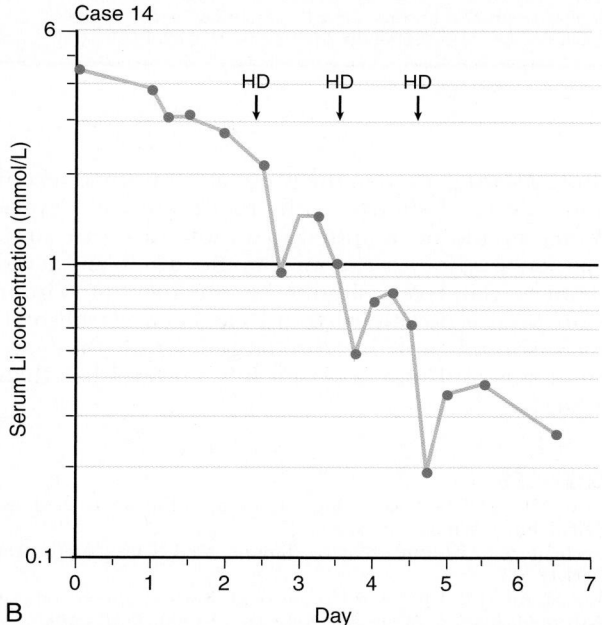

FIGURE 30-2 Serum lithium concentration after **(A)** high-volume continuous venovenous hemofiltration (HV-CVVH) vs. **(B)** intermittent hemodialysis (HD). Note the steady decline in lithium concentration during HV-CVVH in **A** in contrast with the rebound in lithium concentration after each run of hemodialysis in **B**. Although hemodialysis remains the gold standard for lithium elimination, other modes of continuous renal replacement therapy demonstrate promise. (Reproduced from Jaeger A, Sauder P, Kopferschmidt J, et al: When should dialysis be performed in lithium poisoning? A kinetic study in 14 cases of lithium poisoning. J Toxicol Clin Toxicol 1993;31:429–447, and van Bommel EF, Kalmeijer MD, Donssen H: Treatment of life-threatening lithium toxicity with high-volume continuous venovenous hemofiltration. Am J Nephrol 2000;20:408–411.)

replacement therapy may be considered in treating patients in facilities in which dialysis is not readily available or who are considered too unstable for immediate hemodialysis.

Disposition

All patients with symptoms of lithium intoxication should be admitted to the hospital for observation in a

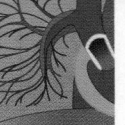

TABLE 30-4 Approximate Clearance of Lithium Based on Different Methods*

METHOD OF LITHIUM CLEARANCE	APPROXIMATE CLEARANCE (mL/min)
Normal renal clearance in healthy patient	10–40 mL/min
Renal clearance of patients taking lithium chronically	0.9–18.4 mL/min
Peritoneal dialysis	9–15 mL/min
Hemodialysis	70–170 mL/min
CVVHD	23–54 mL/min
CVVHDF	28–62 mL/min
CAVHD	20.5 mL/min
CAVHDF	27–55 mL/min

*Approximate clearances are based on data from references 56 to 60. CVVHD, continuous venovenous hemodialysis; CVVHDF, continuous venovenous hemodiafiltration; CAVHD, continuous arteriovenous hemodialysis; CAVHDF, continuous arteriovenous hemodiafiltraton.

monitored setting, even in the presence of normal serum lithium levels. Patients with moderate or severe symptoms should be admitted to an intensive care unit. For patients who are asymptomatic after an acute ingestion, serial levels should be obtained at 6-hour intervals until a downward trend has been established. Patients should not be discharged until they are asymptomatic and have a serum lithium level less than 1.5 mEq/L.

REFERENCES

1. Ford MD, Delaney KA, Ling LJ, et al: Clinical Toxicology. Philadelphia, WB Saunders, 2001.
2. Groleau G: Lithium toxicity. Emerg Med Clin North Am 1994;12:511.
3. Aita JF, Aita JA, Aita VA: 7-Up anti-acid lithiated lemon soda or early medicinal use of lithium. Nebr Med J 1990;75:277–279.
4. Timmer RT, Sands JM: Lithium intoxication. J Am Soc Nephrol 1999;10:666–674.
5. Schou M: Forty years of lithium treatment. Arch Gen Psychiatry 1997;54:9–13.
6. Amdisen A: Clinical features and management of lithium poisoning. Med Toxicol Adverse Drug Exp 1988;3:18.
7. Scharman FJ: Methods used to decrease lithium absorption or enhance elimination. J Toxicol Clin Toxicol 1997;35:601–608.
8. Haddad LM, Shannon MW, Winchester JF (eds): Clinical Management of Poisoning and Drug Overdose, 3rd ed. Philadelphia, WB Saunders, 1998.
9. Baldessarini RJ: Drugs and the treatment of psychiatric disorders. In Goodman LS, Gillman AG (eds): The Pharmacologic Basis of Therapeutics, 8th ed. Singapore, McGraw-Hill, 1991.
10. Waldmeier PC: Mechanisms of action of lithium in affective disorders: a status report. Pharmacol Toxicol 1990;66(Suppl): 121–132.
11. Singer I, Rotenberg D: Mechanism of lithium action. N Engl J Med 1973;289:254–260.
12. Schou M: Lithium studies: distribution between serum and tissue. Acta Pharmacol 1958;15:115–124.
13. Hayslett JP, Kashgarian M: A micropore study of the renal handling of lithium. Pflugers Arch 1979;380:159–163.
14. Amdisen A: Serum level monitoring and clinical pharmacokinetics of lithium. Clin Pharmacokinet 1977;2:73–92.
15. Dyson EH, Simpson D, Prescott LF, et al: Self poisoning and therapeutic intoxication with lithium. Hum Toxicol 1987;6:325.
16. Goodnick PJ, Fieve RR, Meltzer HL, et al: Lithium elimination half-life and duration of therapy. Clin Pharmacol Ther 1981; 29:47–50.
17. Lehmann K, Merten K: Elimination of lithium in correlation with age in normal subjects and in renal insufficiency. Int J Clin Pharmacol Ther Toxicol 1974a; 10:292.
18. Webb AL, Solomon DA, Ryan CE: Lithium levels and toxicity among hospitalized patients. Psychiatr Serv 2001;52:229–231.
19. Iqbal MM, Sohhan T, Mahmud SZ: The effect of lithium, valproic acid, and carbamazepine during pregnancy and lactation. Clin Toxicol 2001;39:381–392.
20. Tunnesen WW II, Hertz CG: Toxic effects of lithium in newborn infants: a commentary. J Pediatr 1972;81:804–807.
21. Berry N, Pradhan S, Sagar R, et al: Neuroleptic malignant syndrome in an adolescent receiving olanzapine-lithium combination therapy. Pharmacotherapy 2003;23:255–259.
22. Gill J, Singh H, Nugent K, et al: Acute lithium intoxication and neuroleptic malignant syndrome. Pharmacotherapy 2003;23: 811–815.
23. Okusa MD, Crystal LJ: Clinical manifestations and management of acute lithium intoxication. Am J Med 1994;97:383–389.
24. Movig KL, Baumgarten R, Leufkens HG, et al: Risk factors for the development of lithium-induced polyuria. Br J Psychiatry 2003; 182:319–323.
25. Von Hartitzsch B, Hoenich NA, Leigh RJ, et al: Permanent neurological sequelae despite haemodialysis for lithium intoxication. BMJ 1972;30:757–759.
26. Schou M: Long-lasting neurological sequelae after lithium intoxication. Acta Psychiat Scand 1984;70:594–602.
27. Apte SN, Langston JW: Permanent neurological deficits due to lithium toxicity. Ann Neurol 1982;13:453–455.
28. Swartz CM, Jones P: Hyperlithemia correction and persistent delirium. J Clin Pharmacol 1994;34:865–870.
29. Bendz H, Aurell M: Drug-induced diabetes insipidus: incidence, prevention and management. Drug Saf 1999;21:449–456.
30. Oksche A, Rosenthal W: The molecular basis of nephrogenic diabetes insipidus. J Mol Med 1998;76:326–337.
31. Battle DC, von Riotte AB, Gaviria M, et al: Amelioration of polyuria by amiloride in patients receiving long-term lithium therapy. N Engl J Med 1985;312:408–414.
32. Eustatia-Rutten CF, Tamsma JT, Meinders AE, et al: Lithium-induced nephrogenic diabetes insipidus. Neth J Med 2001;58: 137–142.
33. Stoff JS, Rosa RM, Silva P, et al: Indomethacin impairs water diuresis in the DI rat: role of prostaglandins independent of ADH. Am J Physiol 1981;241:F231–F237.
34. Allen HM, Jackson RL, Winchester MD, et al: Indomethacin in the treatment of lithium-induced nephrogenic diabetes insipidus. Arch Intern Med 1989;149:1123–1125.
35. Guirguis AF, Taylor HC: Nephrogenic diabetes insipidus persisting 57 months after cessation of lithium carbonate therapy: report of a case and review of the literature. Endocr Pract 2000;6:324–328.
36. Brady HR, Horgan JH: Lithium and the heart: unanswered questions. Chest 1988;93:166–168.
37. Perrier A, Martin PY, Favre H, et al: Very severe self-poisoning lithium carbonate intoxication causing a myocardial infarction. Chest 1991;100:863–865.
38. Oakley PW, Dawson AH, Whyte IM, et al: Lithium: thyroid effects and altered renal handling. J Toxicol Clin Toxicol 2000;38:333–337.
39. Tillman DJ, Ruggles DL, Leikin JB, et al: Radiopacity study of extended-release formulations using digitalized radiography. Am J Emerg Med 1994;12:310–314.
40. Nagappan R, Parkin WG, Holdsworth SR: Acute lithium intoxication. Anaesth Intensive Care 2002;30:90–92.
41. Lee DC, Klachko MN: Falsely elevated lithium levels in plasma samples obtained in lithium containing tubes. J Toxicol Clin Toxicol 1996;34:467–469.
42. Olson KR (ed): Poisoning and Drug Overdose, 4th ed. San Francisco, McGraw-Hill, 2004.
43. Hansen HE, Amdisen A: Lithium intoxication. Q J Med 1978; 47:123–144.
44. Bailey B, McGuigan M: Lithium poisoning from a poison control center perspective. Ther Drug Monit 2000;22:650–655.

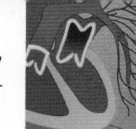

45. Oakley PW, Whyte IM, Carter GL: Lithium toxicity: an iatrogenic problem in susceptible individuals. Aust N Z J Psychiatry 2001;35:833–840.

46. Sadosty AT, Groleau GA, Atcherson MM: The use of lithium levels in the emergency department. J Emerg Med 1999;17:887–891.

47. Cooper JR, Thomas B: Psychopharmacology: The Third Generation of Progress. New York, Raven Press, 1987.

48. Parfrey PS, Ikeman R, Anglin D, et al: Severe lithium intoxication treated by forced diuresis. Can Med Assoc J 1983;129:979–980.

49. O'Connor J, Gleeson J: Acute lithium intoxication: peritoneal dialysis or forced diuresis? NZ Med J 1982;95:790–791.

50. Favin FD, Klein-Schwartz W, Oderda GM, et al: In vitro study of lithium carbonate adsorption by activated charcoal. J Toxicol Clin Toxicol 1988;26:443–450.

51. Smith SW, Ling LJ, Halstenson CE: Whole-bowel irrigation as a treatment for acute lithium overdose. Ann Emerg Med 1991;20:536–539.

52. Belanger DR, Tierney MG, Dickinson G: Effect of sodium polystyrene sulfonate on lithium bioavailability. Ann Emerg Med 1992;21:1312–1315.

53. Tomaszewski C, Musso C, Pearson JR, et al: Lithium absorption prevented by sodium polystyrene sulfonate in volunteers. Ann Emerg Med 1992;21:1308–1311.

54. Jaeger A, Sauder P, Kopferschmitt J, et al: When should dialysis be performed in lithium poisoning? A kinetic study in 14 cases of lithium poisoning. J Toxicol Clin Toxicol 1993;31:429–447.

55. Bailey B, McGuigan M: Comparison of patients hemodialyzed for lithium poisoning and those for whom dialysis was recommended by PCC but not done: what lesson can we learn? Clin Nephrol 2000;54:388–392.

56. Meyer RJ, Flynn JT, Brophy PD, et al: Hemodialysis followed by continuous hemofiltration for treatment of lithium intoxication in children. Am J Kidney Dis 2001;37:1044–1047.

57. Bellomo R, Kearly Y, Parkin G, et al: Treatment of life-threatening lithium toxicity with continuous arterio-venous hemodiafiltration. Crit Care Med 1991;19:836–837.

58. Beckmann U, Oakley PW, Dawson AH, et al: Efficacy of continuous venovenous hemodialysis in the treatment of severe lithium toxicity. J Toxicol Clin Toxicol 2001;39:393–397.

59. van Bommel EF, Kalmeijer MD, Ponssen HH: Treatment of life-threatening lithium toxicity with high-volume continuous venovenous hemofiltration. Am J Nephrol 2000;20:408–411.

60. LeBlanc M, Raymond M, Bonnardeaux A, et al: Lithium poisoning treated by high-performance continuous arteriovenous and venovenous hemodiafiltration. Am J Kidney Dis 1996;27:365–372.

31 *Ethanol*

KURT C. KLEINSCHMIDT, MD

At a Glance...

- Chronic ethanol use is associated with many medical problems including osteoporosis, electrolyte abnormalities, polyneuropathy, endocrine disorders, dementia, alcoholic heart disease, cardiac dysrhythmias, liver dysfunction, and suppression of all hematopoietic elements.

- The elderly and children are more prone to experience ethanol's intoxicating effects.

- Benzodiazepines are the mainstay of therapy of alcohol withdrawal. Very large doses may be needed for severe withdrawal. Sympatholytic agents should not be used alone in severe withdrawal management.

- Delirium tremens is uncommon today. It manifests with significant autonomic hyperactivity and gross disorientation. Hyperthermia or seizures during delirium tremens is particularly associated with poor outcome.

- Wernicke's encephalopathy is difficult to diagnose, so all persons with alcoholism should receive thiamine during an evaluation.

INTRODUCTION

Ethanol is derived from fermentation of sugars in fruits, cereals, and vegetables. Valued for its medicinal and mood altering effects, ethanol has played a significant historical role in the medical, social, and religious rituals of humankind. While modern medical uses of ethanol are limited, it remains a popular social lubricant and is widely used in religious and social ceremonies. Ethanol is commonly abused by humans, resulting in significant medical and social morbidity. Its widespread availability also makes it a common cause of unintentional poisoning in children. In addition to alcoholic beverages, many household products such as food extracts, mouthwashes, and cough preparations contain ethanol, often in large amounts (Table 31-1).[1,2]

Chronic alcohol-related problems are common. Approximately 8.2 million persons in the United States are dependent on alcohol. In a primary care practice, 15% of the patients had an "at-risk" pattern of alcohol use or an alcohol-related health problem.[3] Chronic use of ethanol is associated with many medical problems including physical dependence and withdrawal, neuropsychiatric problems including Wernicke's encephalopathy, and significant effects on many body organs.

PHARMACOKINETICS

Ethanol is a clear, low-molecular-weight hydrocarbon that is highly soluble in water and lipids. Its volume of distribution (0.6 L/kg) is similar to that of water. Ethanol does not bind proteins or tissues and does not affect the binding of other agents.[4] Environmental and genetic factors influence its absorption, bioavailability, metabolism, and elimination.[5] The significance of these factors is difficult to assess owing to great variations among individuals.

Ethanol is rapidly absorbed by passive diffusion across the lipid membranes of the stomach ($\approx$20%) and small intestine ($\approx$80%), reaching peak levels 20 to 60 minutes after ingestion.[4-6] Various factors affect absorption (Table 31-2). Inter- and intraindividual differences in gastric emptying rate affect absorption.[4] The time to maximum concentration can vary by as much as fourfold between subjects, and the maximum concentration itself can vary by twofold.[4] The major factor decreasing the rate of gastric emptying, thus delaying ethanol absorption, is the presence of food.[4] Decreased gastrointestinal motility also delays absorption.[5] Activated charcoal binds ethanol poorly, minimally affecting its absorption.[7]

Ethanol is metabolized in a series of oxidative steps; initially to acetaldehyde and then to acetate. Three hepatic enzyme systems contribute to the initial metabolism to acetaldehyde: the microsomal cytochrome P-450 (CYP) isoenzyme CYP2E1, the cytosol-based enzyme alcohol dehydrogenase (ADH), and the hydrogen peroxide–dependent peroxisome catalase system (Fig. 31-1). The catalase system contributes minimally and is not discussed further.[8]

In the nonalcoholic person, 90% of the oxidation of ethanol to acetaldehyde is done by ADH. Multiple isoenzyme forms of ADH occur with variable frequency in different human populations. These ADH isoenzymes have different affinities for ethanol, resulting in variations in ethanol elimination rates among individuals and racial groups. The activity of ADH does not change with chronic ethanol consumption.[9] However, liver ADH is degraded in the fasting state, which may result in as much as a 40% decrease in ADH activity.[10]

CYP2E1 (CYP2E1 is the specific isoenzyme) contributes less than 10% to the oxidation of ethanol in the

TABLE 31-1 Alcohol Content of Common Products and Medications

PRODUCT	ETHANOL CONTENT (%)
Aftershave lotions	15–80
Cold/allergy medications	5–16
Cough preparations	2–25
Glass cleaners	10
Mouthwashes	15–25
Perfumes/colognes	25–95

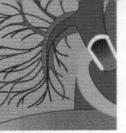

TABLE 31-2 Absorption and Metabolic Factors Affecting Blood Ethanol Concentrations

FACTOR	EFFECT ON BLOOD ETHANOL	REASON
Adiposity	↑	Relative ↓ in Vd
Age	↑ in elderly	↓ Vd secondary to ↑ adipose/lean body mass ratio
	↓ in those < 13 years of age	↑ in metabolic rate
Chronic use	↑	If severe alcoholic liver disease present
	↓	↑ in metabolic rate secondary to ↑ CYP2E1 oxidation
Fasting state	↑	↑ Absorption secondary to faster gastric emptying and temporary ↓ in gastric ADH activity
Delayed gastric emptying	↓	Longer exposure to gastric ADH
Increased lung tidal volume	↓	↑ in elimination from breath
Medications	Variable	Often secondary to change in CYP2E1 activity
Sex	↑ in females	↑ in absorption secondary to ↓ gastric metabolism
		↑ in adipose tissue
		↓ in lean body weight
Cigarette smoking	↓	↑ in metabolic rate
Lean body weight (increased)	↓	Relative ↑ in Vd

↑, increase; ↓, decrease; ADH, alcohol dehydrogenase; Vd, volume of distribution.

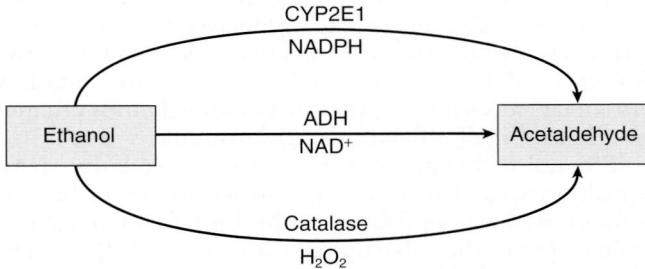

FIGURE 31-1 Pathways for ethanol oxidation to acetaldehyde. ADH, alcohol dehydrogenase; H_2O_2, hydrogen peroxide; NAD^+, nicotinamide adenine dinucleotide, oxidized form; NADPH, nicotinamide adenine dinucleotide phosphate, reduced form.

moderate drinker. The K_m (the concentration of a substrate which yields half-maximal enzyme activity) of ADH for ethanol is much lower than that for CYP2E1. The contribution of CYP2E1 to the oxidation of ethanol increases as the blood ethanol concentration rises. The activity of CYP2E1 is significantly increased in chronic drinkers.[8] Unlike ADH, which requires oxidized nicotinamide adenine dinucleotide (NAD^+) and generates nicotinamide adenine dinucleotide reduced form (NADH), CYP2EI requires the reduced form of nicotinamide adenine dinucleotide phosphate (NADPH) and yields nicotinamide adenine dinucleotide phosphate, oxidized form ($NADP^+$). Oxidation of ethanol by ADH results in an increased $NADH/NAD^+$ ratio, creating an unfavorable "redox" state for oxidative metabolism, decreasing the oxidative capacity of the liver. Interestingly, the "revved up" CYP2E1 in chronic alcoholics creates excess $NADP^+$, which improves the redox state of the liver and enhances ADH activity.[8]

The next step in ethanol metabolism is the oxidation of acetaldehyde to acetate, which also yields more NADH (Fig. 31-2). The reaction is catalyzed by various acetaldehyde dehydrogenase (ALDH) isoenzymes.

These isoenzymes are very efficient, having a K_m approximately 1000 times lower than that of ADH for ethanol.[10] Fifty-percent of Japanese and Chinese persons have isoenzymes with decreased activity, resulting in increased levels of acetaldehyde after ingestion of ethanol.[8,10] This may be the cause of the increased incidence of facial flushing, vasodilation, and tachycardia (acetaldehyde syndrome) noted in some Japanese after drinking.[10] The increased acetaldehyde levels found in chronic alcoholics result from its increased production and are not due to inadequate ALDH activity.[11] Acetaldehyde itself is hepatotoxic by decreasing cellular capacity to repair DNA, increasing free radical–mediated lipid peroxidation, and augmenting hepatic collagen synthesis.[12]

Ethanol's bioavailability, and thus blood ethanol concentration (BEC), is affected by first pass metabolism (FPM). FPM primarily results from liver ADH. However, the mucosa of the intestinal tract, particularly the stomach, also contains ADH. Stomach ADH can contribute up to 20% of the metabolism of ethanol.[13]

Metabolism is affected by other factors. Persons with chronic alcoholism and severe liver disease have decreased rates of ethanol metabolism that correlate with severity of hepatic damage. This mechanism may contribute to the loss of previously attained tolerance in some persons with chronic alcoholism.[11] Abnormalities of liver function tests are not associated with changes in BECs.[14]

Elimination involves multiple processes. Most ethanol is metabolized by the above-noted oxidative processes, resulting in carbon dioxide and water production. A small percentage of ethanol is eliminated unchanged in the breath. For example, lung volume affects levels, since ethanol is excreted unchanged in the breath. The contribution of this mechanism may be significant at high BECs.[9]

The elimination kinetics of ethanol are complex and not clearly defined. It was considered to be linear and to

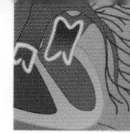

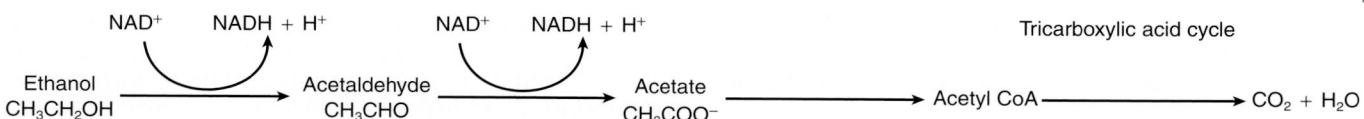

FIGURE 31-2 Ethanol metabolism. CoA, coenzyme A; NAD$^+$, nicotinamide adenine dinucleotide, oxidized form; NADH, nicotinamide-adenine dinucleotide, reduced form.

follow zero order kinetics, that is, an absolute amount is eliminated per unit time. However, more recent work reflects that the kinetics are complicated. Elimination kinetics are difficult to evaluate because many enzyme systems with different K_ms are involved, different BEC ranges have been studied, and individual variability exists in the rates of ethanol elimination. One case report described a patient with a BEC of 1500 mg% whose ethanol elimination followed first order kinetics (an absolute percentage eliminated per unit time) down to 400 mg%.[15] When BECs are high, the initial availability of free enzymes plus activation of CYP2E1 contributes to a rapid decline in ethanol that is most consistent with a first order process. The contribution of CYP2E1 decreases at moderate ethanol concentrations where the more linear decline reflects saturation of alcohol dehydrogenase. Ethanol elimination slows even further at low concentrations, a pattern consistent with the final phase of first order kinetics.

Because of ethanol's complex pharmacokinetics, BECs are variable and difficult to predict (see Table 31-2). Although the absolute dose of ethanol roughly correlates with the resulting BEC, it is not associated with the time to the peak level.[6] The metabolism rate correlates directly with the degree of drinking done by individuals; however, there is much overlap between groups. Metabolism rates for nondrinkers are 12 to 24 mg%/hr and for persons with alcoholism 15 to 49 mg%/hr. Not all studies have demonstrated differences between chronic and intermittent drinkers.[14] The only way to definitely know an individual's elimination rate is to obtain serial BECs. It is reasonable to assume a metabolic rate of 20 mg%/hr for unselected patients in an emergency department setting.[14]

SPECIAL POPULATIONS

The metabolism of ethanol is not significantly different in the elderly. However, age-related increases in adipose tissue and decreases in lean body mass result in decreased total body water. This results in higher BECs than those obtained by younger individuals ingesting equal amounts of ethanol.[16] Cognitive impairment and dementia may also be worsened by chronic ethanol use.[16] In addition, ethanol interacts with many medications commonly used by the elderly, including central nervous system (CNS) depressants, analgesics, anticoagulants, and antidiabetic agents.[16]

Childhood exposure to ethanol is uncommon, representing less than 1% of contacts with poison control centers (PCCs).[17] Reports of pediatric deaths due to ethanol alone are rare. In 2002, exposures in children aged 6 to 19 years were alcoholic beverages in 93%, whereas exposure in those younger than 6 years of age were not beverage related in 77%.[17] Unlike many pediatric exposures, older children were involved with ethanol more than younger ones.[17] Approximately 75% of the exposures reported to PCCs involve perfumes, colognes, and aftershave lotions; alcoholic beverages and mouthwashes make up 15% and 7% of the ingestions, respectively.[2] Most emergency department visits and hospital admissions result from drinking alcoholic beverages rather than nonbeverage items.[17] Intentional exposure must always be considered and the appropriate child protection network initiated if this concern exists. While the pharmacokinetics are similar, children less than 13 years of age appear to metabolize ethanol faster than do adults with alcoholism.[2] Children have more severe effects at lower BECs than do adults, and fatal complications have been reported at less than 50 mg%.[2] Children commonly present with marked sleepiness or coma and may also have vomiting, ataxia, and seizures.[2] Ethanol-induced hypoglycemia occurs more frequently in children than in adults and has occurred with a BEC level as low 20 to 30 mg%.[2] Hypoglycemia is usually associated with ingestion of alcoholic beverages but does not appear to be dose dependent.[2] Seizures may occur and are often associated with hypoglycemia.[2] The etiology of hypoglycemia in children versus adults is not fully understood but may be related to smaller glycogen stores.[2]

An estimate of the potential BEC can be obtained by using the relationship between the volume of distribution (Vd), specific gravity of ethanol (SG), and volume ingested (A):

$$\text{BEC (mg/dL)} = A \text{ (mL)} \times \%\text{EtOH} \times SG \text{ (0.80 g/mL)} \div Vd$$
$$\text{(0.6 L/kg)} \times \text{body weight (kg)}$$

For example, a concerned individual calls because a 20-kg toddler grabbed a half-ounce (15 mL) shot glass of 100-proof (50% ethanol) whiskey and drank it. The numerator determines the absolute amount of ethanol ingested (15 mL × 0.50 × 0.80 g/mL) and is divided by the volume in which it is distributed (0.6 L/kg × 20 kg). After correcting for the units used, the expected BEC is 49 mg%. This is a potentially dangerous level in so young a child, and immediate evaluation in an emergency department would be appropriate. Conversely, the formula can be rearranged to determine the amount ingested once the BEC has been determined. This information may be used to verify the history when considering the possibility of a nonaccidental exposure.

Women attain higher BECs after ingesting equal amounts to men. Women generally have a smaller body mass but more fat, resulting in decreased total body

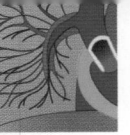

water and a decreased volume of distribution of ethanol.[18] Women have decreased gastric ADH activity compared with men, also contributing to higher BECs.[13]

DRUG INTERACTIONS

Ethanol's complex pharmacology results in many potential drug interactions (Table 31-3). Because of cross-tolerance between ethanol and barbiturates, alcohol-dependent individuals who are abstaining from ethanol require relatively larger doses of barbiturates for induction of anesthesia.[19] Conversely, barbiturate and benzodiazepine metabolism is inhibited in actively drinking individuals, since ethanol already occupies the microsomal CYP oxidizing system. Ethanol-associated CNS sedation is additive to that produced by benzodiazepines and other sedative-hypnotics such as chloral hydrate, ethchlorvynol, meprobamate, methylqualone, and glutethamide.[19] Sedation associated with phenothiazines, antihistamines, and narcotics is also enhanced by ethanol.[20] The use of long-term β-blockers in persons with alcoholism may mask sympathomimetic symptoms associated with hypoglycemia or early withdrawal.[20] The significance of the interaction between the H_2 antagonists and ethanol is debated. All H_2 blockers except famotidine inhibit gastric alcohol dehydrogenase and have been associated with increased BECs.[21]

Disulfiram (Antabuse) irreversibly inhibits acetaldehyde dehydrogenase. If ethanol is ingested after pretreatment with disulfiram, a 5- to 10-fold increase in acetaldehyde develops within 15 minutes. Patients experience flushing and throbbing pains of the head and neck, which are secondary to vasodilation. In addition, abdominal cramps, nausea, vomiting, chest pain, weakness, dizziness, dyspnea, hyperventilation, tachycardia, diaphoresis, and hypotension occur.[19,20,22] Symptoms last 30 minutes to several hours. This reaction develops even up to 2 weeks after disulfiram exposure.[20] Toxicity can be precipitated by as few as 7 mL ethanol.[22] Patients using disulfiram should be made aware of the presence of ethanol in over-the-counter products to prevent unexpected reactions.

Diethyldithiocarbamate, the major metabolite of disulfiram, chelates metals and thus inactivates metalloenzymes including ADH and dopamine β-hydroxylase (DBH). The increased BECs sometimes associated with disulfiram therapy have been attributed to ADH suppression. The sometimes intractable hypotension associated with disulfiram reactions may be secondary to DBH inhibition, which causes decreased nerve terminal norepinephrine production.[22] Long-term users of disulfiram have an increased incidence of depression, which may be secondary to altered dopamine metabolism owing to suppression of central nervous system DBH.[19] Although other medications have been associated with disulfiram-like reactions (see Table 31-3), their effects are generally inconsistent and mild.[19] Management of patients with disulfiram reactions is generally supportive. However, hypotension secondary to vomiting and vasodilation can be severe and aggressive volume resuscitation may be needed. If vasopressor support is indicated, direct α agonists such as nor-epinephrine should be used, since dopamine's effect is blocked by disulfiram's inhibition of DBH. Antiemetics should be considered if vomiting is present.

TABLE 31-3 Medications That Interact with Ethanol		
MEDICATIONS	**MECHANISM OF INTERACTION**	**FINAL EFFECT**

Acetaminophen
Anesthetics (chloroform, halothane)
Barbiturates
Benzodiazepines
Isoniazid
Phenytoin
Warfarin
	Chronic ethanol use enhances CYP2E1 activity if
	  (1) alcoholic is currently abstaining from drinking
	  (2) alcoholic is currently drinking alcohol
		Fulminant hepatic failure
		↓ in medication levels
		↑ in medication levels

Cimetidine Ranitidine	Inhibits gastric ADH, increasing ethanol bioavailability	↑ in blood ethanol concentration
Barbiturates Benzodiazepines Chloral hydrate	Synergistic with effects of ethanol	↑ in sedation ↑ in respiratory depression
Allopurinol	Synergistic with the ↑ in serum uric acid levels secondary to ethanol	↑ in gouty arthritis
Cephalosporins Chloramphenicol Griseofulvin Metronidazole Quinacrine Sulfonylurea oral hypoglycemics	Disulfiram-like reaction with inhibition of acetaldehyde dehydrogenase	Acetaldehyde syndrome

↑ increase; ↓ decrease; ADH, alcohol dehydrogenase.

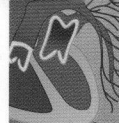

The significance of the interaction between acetaminophen and ethanol in persons with chronic alcoholism is debated. Both acetaminophen and ethanol are metabolized by the CYP isoenzyme CYP2E1. Acetaminophen metabolism results in a small amount of the hepatotoxic metabolite *N*-acetyl-*p*-benzoquinone imine (NAPQI), which is eliminated by conjugation with glutathione. Hepatic injury, however, occurs when NAPQI production overwhelms the detoxification mechanism. Conditions that result in increased NAPQI production or in decreased glutathione detoxification can cause hepatotoxicity; patients with chronic alcoholism have these conditions. Ethanol use induces the CYP2E1 isoenzyme, resulting in increased NAPQI production. Chronic ethanol use and starvation decrease glutathione availability; further contributing to potential toxicity.[23,24] One retrospective series describes patients with chronic alcoholism who have developed hepatotoxicity despite having minor overdoses or even after using less than 4 g/day.[23] Some authors have recommended that acetaminophen be used in decreased doses or not at all in patients with alcoholism.[25] However, a randomized, double-blind, prospective comparison of acetaminophen with placebo in 201 chronic alcoholics did not find increased transaminases with acetaminophen.[26]

TOXICOLOGY

Acute Toxicity (Intoxication)

It is unusual for persons with alcoholism to present for acute care with intoxication as their only medical problem. In one urban emergency department (ED) series, only 26% of patients intoxicated with ethanol had intoxication as their sole problem.[14] A different ED series found that 50% of 289 patients with positive ethanol screens had at least one other drug.[27] Fifty-three percent of 116 consecutive motor vehicle accident admissions to an urban trauma service had BECs greater than 100 mg%.[28]

A toxic dose is considered to be 5 g/kg in an adult or 3 g/kg in a child. The ethanol content of popular beverages ranges from 3% to 6% in beers to as high as 90% in some distilled liquors. One ounce of whiskey (80 proof, or 40%), 12 ounces of beer, or 4 ounces of wine are approximately equipotent and will raise the BEC 25 mg% in the average adult. The majority of states in the United States use 0.08% (80 mg%) as the legal limit for ethanol.

Symptoms of intoxication begin with a perception of stimulation due to the suppression of central inhibitory mechanisms. However, as BEC rises, sedation, incoordination, ataxia, and impaired psychomotor performance appear.[29] Even higher levels can result in coma and death. While BECs typically correlate with symptoms in nondrinkers (Table 31-4),[30-33] chronic drinkers require higher levels to reach similar states of intoxication. The degree of intoxication also correlates with the rate of rise of the BEC. Slower ethanol ingestion results in less intoxication.[30] Acute tolerance has been

TABLE 31-4 Signs and Symptoms of Intoxication and Blood Ethanol Concentrations in a Non-Alcohol-Dependent Population*

ETHANOL CONCENTRATION (MG%)	SIGNS AND SYMPTOMS
<25	Sense of warmth Sense of well-being Talkativeness Mild incoordination
25–50	Euphoria Clumsiness Decreased judgment and control
50–100	Decreased sensorium Worsened coordination, ataxia Decreased reflexes/increased reaction time Emotional lability
100–250	Cerebellar/vestibular dysfunction (ataxia, diplopia, slurred speech, visual impairment, nystagmus) Severe emotional lability, confusion, stupor Nausea, vomiting
250–400	Stupor or coma Little response to stimuli Incontinence Respiratory depression
>400	Respiratory paralysis Loss of protective reflexes Hypothermia Death

*Correlation between signs and symptoms and blood ethanol levels show wide variability among individuals.

demonstrated with a single large ingestion of ethanol. This manifests as a greater degree of intoxication at any BEC when the level is rising compared to when the level is falling.[30] Visual tracking of objects is decreased as much as 25% with a BEC of 80 mg%.[34] Coma is unusual when the BEC is below 200 mg%.[31] The lethal level for 50% of the non-ethanol-dependent population is 450 mg%[31] although individuals have survived BECs as large as 1500 mg%.[15]

DIAGNOSIS OF ACUTE INTOXICATION

The differential diagnosis is vast because it involves altered mentation or coma. Conditions that must routinely be considered include hypoglycemia, hypoxia, intracranial pathology, seizure, encephalopathy, uremia, cerebral infection, and shock. Many medications cause an alteration in mental status including sedative-hypnotics, opioids, antidepressants, and antipsychotics.

The patient's history and physical examination should guide the selection of ancillary laboratory data. The usefulness of routine measurement of the BEC in the emergency department is controversial. Its use is appropriate in a patient with an altered mental status. However, the BEC is less likely to affect management decisions in an intoxicated individual who is awake and alert. The disposition of intoxicated patients is a clinical decision and should not be based on BEC.

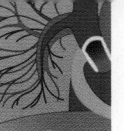

The BEC may be obtained by using various body fluids; however, venous blood and breath samples are most commonly used. BECs are *not* affected by the use of ethanol in the skin preparation, despite theoretical concerns.[35] The accuracy of the breath ethanol analyzer (BEA) depends on the constant equilibrium of ethanol in the blood to alveolar air at a ratio of 2100:1.[4] BEA results are slightly lower than those from venous blood, especially at higher levels of ethanol, and may be affected by the patient's ability to cooperate.[36] BEA results are also consistently less than venous blood estimations in patients with poor pulmonary function, including the elderly.[37] Testing within 15 to 20 minutes of the last drink or if vomitus is in the mouth may cause small false elevations. Conversely, false negatives are rare.[36]

MANAGEMENT OF ACUTE INTOXICATION

Other causes of altered mental status must be assessed depending on the clinical situation. Hypoglycemia should routinely be considered. The threshold to perform a head computed tomographic (CT) scan must be low. Because steady improvement occurs when mental status is depressed by ethanol, a head CT scan is indicated if a patient's sensorium does not improve during a period of observation.

Fluid administration is indicated, since the intoxicated patient is frequently volume depleted secondary to ethanol-induced diuresis, vomiting, and poor oral intake. However, IV fluids do not affect blood ethanol clearance.[38] Patients with alcoholism should also receive multivitamins, thiamine, and folate. The routine administration of glucose to sick alcoholic patients is rational because of the significant incidence of ketoacidosis and glycogen deficiency. Studies have not shown caffeine,[39] naloxone,[40] fructose,[41] or flumazenil[42] to hasten the reversal of intoxication. Gastric emptying is ineffective at decreasing BECs due to ethanol's rapid absorption. Charcoal should be considered in patients who may have ingested other toxins.

The timing of the disposition of an intoxicated patient is controversial. However, most would agree that patients should walk away from an acute care facility only when they actually can walk without difficulty and can demonstrate clear, appropriate thought processes. These points should be documented at the time of disposition.

Chronic Toxicity

NEUROPSYCHIATRIC EFFECTS OF CHRONIC INTOXICATION

In addition to the neuropsychiatric effects of acute intoxication, chronic ethanol use is associated with polyneuropathy, Wernicke's encephalopathy, Korsakoff's psychosis, cerebellar degeneration, dementia, and central pontine myelinolysis. Controversy exists over the etiology and management of these disorders and the relationship between them.

The most common chronic neurologic symptom in alcoholics is polyneuropathy. The axonal degeneration and demyelination likely results from both nutritional deficiencies and direct toxic ethanol effects.[33] Common findings include painful dysesthesia, anesthesia, weakness, decreased pain and temperature sensation, and decreased touch and vibration sense.[32,33] Disease progression is gradual, bilateral, and symmetric. The most common site of involvement is the distal legs.[32,33] If severe, muscle atrophy occurs and the deep tendon reflexes are decreased. Abstinence may result in slow and incomplete recovery.[33]

Wernicke's encephalopathy (WE) results from a deficiency of vitamin B_1 (thiamine) and is characterized by the classic clinical triad of oculomotor abnormalities, ataxia, and global confusion. Thiamine is an enzyme cofactor in various metabolic pathways. Although WE is classically associated with alcoholism, thiamine deficiency may also occur in any nutritionally depleted state.[32,33,43] Indeed, one autopsy series demonstrated that only 18% of cases occurred in persons with alcoholism.[43] Thiamine deficiency occurs in persons with alcoholism because of poor diet, reduced absorption and liver storage, and decreased conversion to its active form.[33,43]

Glucose loading in thiamine-depleted individuals has been proposed to induce WE.[43] It is common for authors to recommend that thiamine be given *prior to* glucose in patients with altered mental status. The usual reference[44] cited in support describes four patients. None of these developed WE after a single, acute administration of glucose; however, all required hours of glucose administration. Thus, the specific order of administration of thiamine and glucose likely does not matter as long as they are given around the same time.[45]

Only a small minority of thiamine-deficient patients develop WE. A low serum thiamine level has poor specificity for the diagnosis. The development of clinical disease in so few thiamine-deficient individuals reflects either a genetic contribution, unknown affecting variables, or underdiagnosis.[46] The diagnosis is usually established by the combination of clinical symptoms and magnetic resonance imaging revealing mammillary body shrinkage. On autopsy, findings include mammillary body shrinkage and petechial hemorrhages.[33,37]

WE is likely more common than generally perceived, since the diagnosis is difficult to establish. Autopsy series have demonstrated cerebral and cerebellar neuropathologic changes specific for WE in 0.8% to 2.8% of the general population and in 12% of persons with alcoholism.[43] Reviews of premorbid patient symptoms from these series found stupor and coma to be the most common presentations, while WE was diagnosed in less than 20% of the patients.[43,47]

Based on pathologic studies and chart reviews, WE presents with the classic triad in only 10% to 33% of the patients and up to 20% have none of the three.[32,43] The onset occurs over several days to many weeks. The hallmark of WE is the extraocular movement abnormalities, with horizontal nystagmus noted in 85%, bilateral lateral rectus paralysis in 54%, and paresis of conjugate gaze in 44%.[48] The equilibrium loss is secondary to vestibular paresis and cerebellar dysfunction and typically produces ataxia of gait but not of the limbs.[48] The global confusional state consists of apathy, poor concentration, spatial and temporal disorientation, and slow and irrational thinking. Most patients have a normal level of consciousness. Impairment of memory and ability to learn is present in a majority but is often difficult to demonstrate because of poor concentration skills.[30] Other manifestations include hypothermia and hypotension secondary to altered temperature regulation and decreased sympathetic outflow.[43] Wernicke's encephalopathy evolves over time, with mild, subclinical episodes progressing until the clinical triad is apparent.[43] The mortality for treated WE is 17% during the initial weeks after diagnosis, most of which is related to associated diseases including infections and cirrhosis.[48]

WE is partially reversible with the administration of thiamine. It should be considered a medical emergency because of the associated morbidity and mortality. Thiamine absorption from the gastrointestinal tract is significantly poorer in thiamine-deficient patients than in healthy controls. In addition, ethanol loading decreases thiamine absorption by 50%.[49] It is recommend that patients with WE be hospitalized and receive 100 mg thiamine intravenously daily for at least 5 days.[32,33] Ocular abnormalities generally reverse completely within hours to days except for a fine horizontal nystagmus on lateral gaze that persists in 60%.[48] Recovery from ataxia usually takes more than a month and is complete in only 33% of patients. Virtually all patients recover from the global confusion within 2 months, although most have persistent memory difficulties.[48]

Abnormal thought processing is common in persons with chronic alcoholism. Neuropsychological impairment is present in 50% to 70% of detoxified persons with alcoholism.[50] Diagnoses that have been applied to these patients include both Korsakoff's psychosis (KP) and alcoholic dementia. Much overlap between dementia and KP exists and differentiation between the two is not clear. KP is classically described as an "abnormal mental state in which memory and learning are affected out of all proportion to other cognitive functions in an otherwise alert and responsive patient."[48] It is characterized by anterograde (events occurring now) and some retrograde (recent events) amnesia. Patients are alert, responsive, and can interact well socially but are apathetic and unaware of their disability.[48] The term *psychosis* is confusing, since patients with KP do not have the gross distortion of mental capacity typically associated with a psychosis.

The classic work of Victor reflected that 80% of those with WE will have KP evident once the global confusion of WE has cleared following thiamine treatment. He suggests that the memory impairment associated with WE is likely the beginning of KP—all primarily related to thiamine deficiency.[48] However, not all patients with KP will have had WE. In particular, patients with non-alcoholic WE uncommonly develop severe permanent memory disorders. This argues against WE and KP being the acute and chronic phases of the same thiamine deficiency.[50] KP may have a multifactorial etiology including a drinking lifestyle, multiple episodes of withdrawal, seizures, and repeated head injury.[50]

Management of KP includes routine nursing care, proper diet, and abstinence from alcohol. The role of thiamine is not clear. Complete recovery from KP occurs over 1 to 3 months in 20% of afflicted patients, while 25% do not recover at all.[48]

Alcoholic dementia has been used to describe cases in which amnesia occurs in conjunction with global intellectual decline.[50] It likely has multiple etiologies including a direct toxic effect of ethanol on the CNS. Cerebral atrophy is common. Some feel the dementia is a manifestation of KP.[33] Central pontine myelinolysis is also associated with alcoholism. It evolves over days to weeks and is associated with hyponatremia.[33] The pontine corticobulbar white fibers undergo demyelination, causing mental confusion, dysarthria, dysphagia, facial and neck weakness, dysfunctional tongue movements, and gaze palsies.[32,33]

Alcoholic cerebellar degeneration affects chronic drinkers and is characterized by a gradual onset of ataxia that affects the trunk more than the limbs and the legs more than the arms.[32,33] The symptoms and cerebellar abnormalities are similar to those found in WE, suggesting that these diseases may actually be parts of the same process.[33] While the gait ataxia is similar to that of WE, patients with cerebellar degeneration have more limb ataxia and dysarthria and much less nystagmus.[32] Various causes have been proposed, including thiamine deficiency, electrolyte abnormalities, and direct toxicity from ethanol.[33] The disease stabilizes or improves with the cessation of drinking.[33]

OTHER EFFECTS OF CHRONIC INTOXICATION

Ethanol alters many aspects of endocrine function including all levels of the hypothalamic-pituitary-adrenal axis, gonadal and carbohydrate activity, and mineral metabolism. Some of these effects may reverse with prolonged abstinence.[51] Ethanol and its metabolites directly decrease testosterone production.[51] Up to 50% of persons with alcoholism and cirrhosis have atrophic testes and many have gynecomastia. Women who drink moderately have more anovulatory cycles, and amenorrhea occurs more often in those with cirrhosis.[51]

Alcoholism is associated with osteoporosis in both men and women. Etiologies include ethanol's direct toxicity to osteoblasts, hypogonadism, decreased calcium intake, malabsorption, increased urinary calcium excretion, minimal exercise, and an altered parathormone response to hypocalcemia.[51]

Acute and chronic ethanol ingestion cause stimulation of the hypothalamic-pituitary-adrenal axis. Elevated adrenocorticotropin hormone and cortisol levels in some persons with alcoholism suggest Cushing's syndrome.[31,51] These individuals have classic clinical stigmata such as central obesity and laboratory abnormalities including altered dexamethasone suppression tests.[51] Glucocorticoid secretion returns to normal within a few weeks of abstinence.[51]

Ethanol alters fat and carbohydrate metabolism. Hepatic lipogenesis, peripheral fat mobilization, and hepatic uptake of circulating lipids are increased while hepatic lipoprotein release is decreased. The

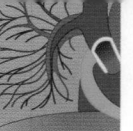

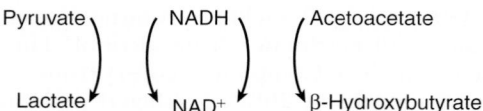

FIGURE 31-3 Some effects of the increased NADH/NAD⁺ ratio.

altered NADH/NAD⁺ ratio impedes the function of the tricarboxylic acid cycle and slows fatty acid oxidation.[12] These actions cause triglycerides to accumulate in hepatocytes (steatosis) and increase serum triglycerides. Hypoglycemia results from nutrition-related glycogen depletion and decreased gluconeogenic activity resulting from the altered redox ratio.[12,51,52]

Malnutrition leads to vitamin deficiency disorders such as pellagra, stomatitis, and scurvy. Thiamine deficiency is particularly common because its total body supply can be depleted within 33 days.[46] Electrolyte disorders include hypokalemia, hypophosphatemia, and hypomagnesemia. Hypokalemia is also caused by gastrointestinal losses and urinary excretion due to altered mineralocorticoid activity.[52,53] Acid–base abnormalities occur in persons with alcoholism; however, ethanol itself does not cause an acidosis. The anion-gap acidosis sometimes seen in alcoholic patients results from a combination of keto acids and lactic acid. The increased NADH/NAD⁺ ratio favors lactate over pyruvate production (Fig. 31-3).[52,54] Metabolic alkalosis secondary to vomiting and volume contraction may occur.[52]

Alcoholic ketoacidosis (AKA) typically begins with abdominal pain (from gastric irritation, pancreatitis, hepatitis, etc.) and vomiting. Volume depletion occurs, and ethanol ingestion decreases as the patient becomes more ill. Comorbid conditions often cloud the typical clinical characteristics (Table 31-5). The stress-related catecholamine increase and resurgent gluconeogenesis (since the patient has stopped drinking) result in normal to mildly elevated serum glucose levels. Ketoacidosis results from acetyl CoA shunting to ketone production, increased lipolysis and free fatty acid (FFA) release, decreased peripheral tissue uptake and metabolism of ketones, and decreased urinary elimination of ketones (Fig. 31-4).[54] The primary keto acids are β-hydroxybutyrate and acetoacetate. In AKA, the increased NADH/NAD⁺ ratio favors β-hydroxybutyrate production (see Fig. 31-3).

The treatment of AKA includes volume resuscitation, thiamine and glucose supplementation, and management of associated disorders. Glucose administration causes endogenous insulin release, which suppresses FFA release and ketogenesis. Treatment of AKA results in a decreased NADH/NAD⁺ ratio, which decreases the β-hydroxybutyrate-to-acetoacetate ratio. Because the nitroprusside test for ketones measures only acetoacetate, this is paradoxically reflected by an increasingly positive nitroprusside test for ketones. Most urine dipsticks and in-laboratory tests for ketones are still based on nitroprusside color changes.

Acute ethanol ingestion causes dose-dependent suppression of pituitary antidiuretic hormone, resulting in its familiar diuretic effect. This causes free water loss

TABLE 31-5 Alcoholic Ketoacidosis Presentation Summary	
SOURCE OF DATA	**FINDINGS**
History taking	Alcoholism
	Cessation or decrease of ethanol intake over prior 24–72 hours
	Fasted state
	Abdominal pain
	Vomiting
Physical examination	Consciousness
	Status consistent with volume depletion
	Tachycardia
	Tachypnea
Laboratory	Anion-gap metabolic acidosis
	pH may be acidemic, normal, or alkalemic
	Acidemia secondary to ketoacidosis
	Alkalosis secondary to tachypnea and vomiting
	Hypokalemia
	Hypophosphatemia
	Glucose level mildly elevated, normal, or low
	Serum and urinary ketones increased (elevation may be underestimated with the nitroprusside test because this test only measures acetoacetate, whereas β-hydroxybutyrate is the primary ketoacid)

without significant urinary electrolyte loss.[53] The effect of chronic ethanol intake on total body water is debatable. Ethanol-induced diuresis and periodic abdominal upset and vomiting may lead to dehydration in persons with chronic alcoholism. However, chronic ethanol use may cause a lowering of the pituitary osmole receptor set-point that increases antidiuretic hormone secretion, resulting in eventual volume overload.[53] Fluid supplementation of the patient with chronic alcoholism should be based on the clinical evaluation.

Cardiac abnormalities associated with ethanol use include alcoholic cardiomyopathy with congestive heart failure, dysrhythmias, hypertension, and coronary artery disease. The term *alcoholic heart disease* is replacing the term *alcoholic cardiomyopathy*, since cardiomyopathy technically is the primary disease of the cardiac muscle of unknown etiology. Alcoholic heart disease is affected by genetic predisposition and the amount and length of ethanol abuse.[55] Once alcoholic heart disease is present, the prognosis is poor unless patients abstain from further ethanol intake.[55] The postulated pathophysiology includes changes in the sarcolemma, the Na⁺/K⁺-activated ATPase pump, calcium homeostasis, and contractile proteins.[55] Changes in cardiac structure and function include four chamber dilatation, reduced left ventricular compliance and ejection fraction, mild endocardial and valve-leaflet scarring, and mural thrombi.[55]

Chronic, heavy ethanol use increases both systolic and diastolic blood pressures.[55,56] Conversely, acute ethanol ingestion causes decreased blood pressure that may be due to a combination of decreased vascular resistance and cardiac function.[57]

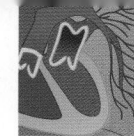

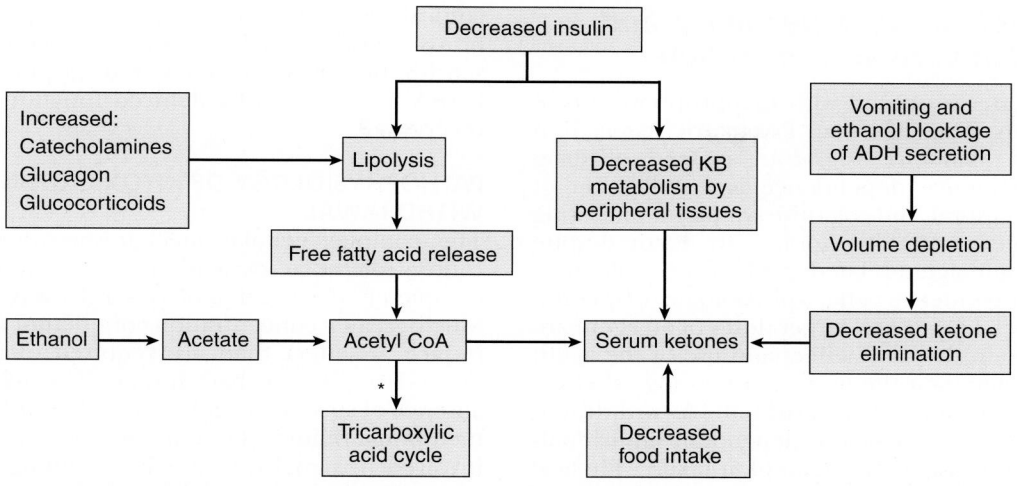

FIGURE 31-4 Factors causing ketonemia in alcoholic ketoacidosis. ADH, antidiuretic hormone. *The tricarboxylic acid cycle is significantly slowed because intermediates are used for gluconeogenesis.

The effect of ethanol on coronary atherosclerotic disease (CAD) and on stroke is biphasic. Regular light-to-moderate alcohol intake appears to provide protection against both CAD and ischemic stroke. This protective effect may be related to an increase in high-density lipoprotein and to a decrease in low-density lipoprotein, platelet aggregation, and fibrinolytic activity.[56-59] Low doses of ethanol increase nitric oxide release, augmenting vasodilation. Conversely, heavy consumption increases the risk of CAD and both hemorrhagic and ischemic stroke.[56,59] Excessive alcohol use increases atherosclerotic disease by increasing blood pressure, triglycerides, and insulin resistance and by altering coagulation.[56,59]

Ethanol is associated with atrial and ventricular dysrhythmias. Ettinger and others described the "holiday heart syndrome" in persons with alcoholism without overt alcoholic heart disease who developed dysrhythmias. Atrial fibrillation and flutter are the most common signs; they clear with abstinence.[60] This relationship was supported by a review that found ethanol caused or contributed to 63% of admissions for atrial fibrillation. Eighty-nine percent of the ethanol-related cases converted to sinus rhythm within 24 hours of admission in contrast to only 42% of those with atrial fibrillation secondary to other etiologies.[61]

The effects of ethanol on the gastrointestinal tract include esophagitis, gastritis, peptic ulcer disease, malabsorption, gastrointestinal bleeding secondary to numerous causes, and liver and pancreatic diseases. Ethanol-associated liver disorders include fatty infiltration, alcoholic hepatitis, and fibrosis (cirrhosis). Fatty infiltration of the liver can start within days of the onset of heavy drinking. It is due primarily to triglyceride deposition, but dietary fat intake also contributes.[18] Inflammation resulting from alcoholic hepatitis hastens the deposition of collagen. Inflammation associated with fatty infiltration results in the deposition of collagen, the primary protein of fibrous tissues, into liver lipocytes. The lipocytes eventually transform into collagen-producing cells. Cirrhosis develops when collagen production outpaces its degradation.[18]

Ethanol's induction of the CYP system increases the conversion of xenobiotic compounds such as anesthetics and industrial solvents to toxic metabolites. The system also activates carcinogens that may contribute to the increased incidence of upper alimentary and respiratory tract cancers in persons with alcoholism. Acetaldehyde accumulation is associated with impaired hepatic oxygen utilization, increased free radical production, lipid peroxidation, and fibrinogenesis.[12]

Ethanol abuse suppresses hematopoietic elements of the bone marrow through malnutrition-related vitamin deficiency and direct ethanol toxicity. Ethanol causes decreased bone marrow cellularity, vacuolization of marrow precursor cells, and a macrocytosis independent of folate deficiency. Chronic ethanol abuse causes thrombocytopenia that resolves with abstinence; however, its effect on platelet function is not clear.[62] Ethanol also causes many types of anemia including iron and folate deficiency, hemolytic, and sideroblastic. Classic folate-dependent megaloblastic anemia occurs in 4% of ambulatory persons with alcoholism and generally affects those who imbibe hard liquor, since beer is actually a good folate source.[62] Folate deficiency in persons with alcoholism is secondary to poor diet, malabsorption, disruption of the enterohepatic circulation, and a direct antifolate effect of ethanol.

Infection in alcoholics is associated with increased morbidity. Immunosuppression occurs with acute and chronic ethanol abuse. Acute ingestion causes decreased neutrophil delivery to infection sites and decreased adherence, whereas chronic abuse results in marrow suppression, decreased chemotaxis, and neutropenia. Neutrophil bactericidal and phagocyte activity are not affected by ethanol.[63] Abstinence results in the reversal of leukopenia within a few days.[62] Ethanol is also associated with decreased pulmonary macrophage mobilization, bactericidal activity, and reticuloendothelial system clearance.[62]

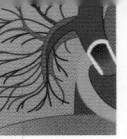

Addiction, Tolerance, Dependency, and Withdrawal in Chronic Intoxication

Various terms are associated with inappropriate use of addicting agents. The American Psychiatric Association uses the term *substance dependence* instead of drug addiction.[29] Substance dependence is a collection of physiologic, behavioral, and cognitive symptoms indicating that a person is continuing to use an agent despite having significant agent-related problems.[29] Tolerance and physical dependence reflect physiologic adaptation at a cellular level. Larger and larger doses of an agent are required to obtain the same effect and use of the agent is necessary to maintain the desired psychological effect or prevent symptoms of withdrawal. A withdrawal syndrome occurs in physically dependent individuals who reduce or cease their ethanol intake.[29] Physical dependence is not required for the diagnosis of substance dependence. Addictive drugs provide a "reward" by acting as positive reinforcers (producing euphoria) or as negative reinforcers (alleviating symptoms of withdrawal or dysphoria).[29] The brain system involved in the reward mechanism becomes hypersensitized to both the direct effects of the drug and associated environmental stimuli (cues) that are not directly attributable to the drug. The hypersensitization results in pathologic wanting, or craving, independent of symptoms of withdrawal. Substance abuse incorporates recurrent and significant adverse effects related to the use of an agent including the use of the agent in dangerous situations, failure to fulfill major role obligations, legal problems, and continued use despite all the attendant problems.[29]

The pathophysiology of addiction is complex but interestingly is shared by different addicting agents. The center is the mesocorticolimbic dopamine systems that originate in the ventral tegmental area (VTA). Projections from the VTA go to limbic structures such as the nucleus accumbens, amygdala, and hippocampus and to the prefrontal cortex and anterior cingulate. These circuits affect reinforcement, memory, craving, and the emotional and motivational changes of the withdrawal syndrome. Addictive drugs provide a "reward" by stimulating release of dopamine from the VTA into the nucleus accumbens, causing euphoria and reinforcement of the behavior. Ethanol increases dopamine by activating the inhibitory neurotransmitter γ-aminobutyric acid (GABA) receptors or by inhibiting the stimulatory *N*-methyl-D-aspartate (NMDA) receptors. Chronic ethanol use enhances the function of NMDA receptors by modifying the subunits.[29] Opioid and serotonin receptors have a role in the reinforcing effects of ethanol.[29] Interestingly, during withdrawal, there is a decrease in dopamine levels in the nucleus accumbens.

The severity of withdrawal syndrome is related to three major factors: the degree of drug exposure, duration of exposure, and (of less clarity) the history of previous withdrawal episodes.[64] Persons with alcoholism with a longer history of recurrent withdrawal experience more severe withdrawal. This phenomenon has been referred to as "kindling."[64,65] "Reinstatement" is another clinical entity that refers to the ever-shortening drinking bouts required before cycles of withdrawal.[65] This sensitization is likely related to hypofunction of the GABA receptors and enhanced function of the NMDA receptors.[64]

PATHOPHYSIOLOGY OF INTOXICATION AND WITHDRAWAL

The complex cellular mechanisms of ethanol intoxication, tolerance, dependence, and withdrawal are not completely clear. Ethanol is a relatively weak sedative. Much greater concentrations of ethanol are required to induce an effect than are required of agents such as benzodiazepines or barbiturates. This likely reflects the absence of specific receptors for ethanol.[32] Ethanol alters membrane fluidity, the function of membrane structures involved in signal transduction, binding of neurotransmitters, and regulation of gene expression.[32,33] Selective sites of toxicity include the receptor complex of GABA, the areas regulating excitatory amino acids, calcium channels, the central adrenergic system, dopamine and adenosine receptors, and the hypothalamic-pituitary-adrenal axis.[32,33]

GABA receptors are part of a large membrane protein complex that includes a GABA-activated chloride channel and closely linked benzodiazepine receptors whose effect is mediated by the same chloride channels.[32,33] Ethanol causes neuronal inhibition by a direct effect on the chloride channel and indirectly by potentiating GABA.[32] The physical proximity of these receptors may explain the cross-tolerance that occurs between ethanol and the benzodiazepines. Chronic ethanol use decreases the magnitude of GABA complex–mediated neuroinhibition, an effect that probably contributes to the development of tolerance.[32] Decreased GABA-activated chloride channel flux during abstinence contributes to the CNS hyperexcitability of ethanol withdrawal.[32] The sedating effect of benzodiazepines on patients with symptoms of ethanol withdrawal is likely due to activation of these same channels.

Calcium channels and their receptors also contribute to the cellular mechanisms of tolerance and withdrawal. A few days of ethanol use causes an increase in both calcium channel flux and binding site availability that persists for several hours after drinking has ceased. Calcium channel blockers decrease tremors, seizures, and death in ethanol-dependent rodents deprived of ethanol. Calcium channel blockers attenuate some of the sympathetic symptoms of withdrawal in humans; however, they do not prevent seizures or delirium tremens.[33]

Ethanol affects the activity of excitatory amino acids, particularly NMDA, in certain areas of the brain.[33] Ethanol decreases NMDA-receptor-associated calcium channel flux and changes the cell's response to its activation. Of particular interest is ethanol's inhibition of NMDA receptors in the hippocampus, an area involved in learning and memory. This is a proposed mechanism of cognitive defects and "blackouts" associated with ethanol use.[32,33]

Adrenergic activity affects withdrawal symptoms. The excitatory neurotransmitter norepinephrine (NE) is released by presynaptic vesicles. It interacts with various receptors and is then resequestered into the presynaptic terminal. Within the hypothalamus, intersynaptic NE is taken up by extraneuronal cells (possibly astrocytes) and converted to epinephrine, which is then released back into the synapse. Phenylethanolamine-N-methyltransferase (PNMT) catalyzes this extraneuronal conversion of NE to epinephrine. Epinephrine activates presynaptic α_2 receptors, which inhibit NE release. Ethanol increases PNMT activity, leading to central adrenergic inhibition. Chronic ethanol ingestion leads to compensatory down-regulation of presynaptic α_2 receptors. Ethanol withdrawal is associated with decreased PNMT activity that results in less epinephrine being available to stimulate the previously down-regulated α_2 receptors. Since the α_2 receptors provide negative feedback to the presynaptic neurons, the resulting loss of negative inhibition yields increased sympathomimetic activity.[65] This pathophysiologic process explains the effect of the central α_2 agonist clonidine in decreasing the sympathomimetic activity associated with withdrawal. The stimulatory central adrenergic β receptors also appear to contribute to the withdrawal syndrome. Ethanol causes uncoupling between the β receptor proteins and their second messengers, which prevents the receptor down-regulation that typically occurs during sympathetic states. Increased adrenergic activity during withdrawal results in hyperstimulation of these receptors.[66] This mechanism may explain the effects of atenolol in management of the withdrawal syndrome. Excess dopaminergic states are associated with psychosis, hallucinosis, cravings, and the mechanisms of reward and reinforcement.[33] However, the roles of serotonin and dopamine in ethanol intoxication and withdrawal are not clearly defined.[33]

Adenosine is also associated with physical dependence and tolerance.[33] While not a neurotransmitter itself, it modulates the effects of neurotransmitters. Acute ethanol ingestion inhibits intracellular transport of adenosine, leading to increased stimulation of extracellular membrane adenosine α_2 receptors. This stimulation of the α_2 receptors causes increased G protein–mediated adenylcyclase activity and increased intracellular adenosine 3',5'-cyclic phosphate (cyclic AMP). Chronic ethanol intake eventually causes an adaptive decrease in cyclic AMP production. Adapted cells require ethanol to maintain adequate cAMP production. The adenosine nucleoside transporter also loses its sensitivity to ethanol inhibition with chronic ethanol use. Protein kinase A activity, which requires cyclic AMP, is responsible for the decreased adenosine nucleoside transporter uptake. The decrease in available cyclic AMP associated with chronic ethanol ingestion eventually results in increased adenosine transporter activity. These membrane changes reflect "tolerance" at the cellular level.[33]

WITHDRAWAL SYNDROMES

Into the 1950s, the cause of the clinical syndrome that we now refer to as "withdrawal" was hotly debated. It was unclear whether the syndrome was due to cessation of drinking, a direct toxic effect of ethanol, or nutritional deficiencies. Isbell and others settled the debate in 1953.[67] In their study, ethanol was given daily to 10 healthy, former opiate addicts in controlled conditions that provided adequate diets and vitamins but prevented the introduction of other agents. Upon cessation of drinking, four subjects who drank for up to 34 days all developed tremor, perspiration, gastrointestinal distress, and anorexia lasting 1 to 3 days. Three of these four drank for no more than 16 days, reflecting the little time needed to develop physical dependence. The six subjects who drank between 48 and 87 days developed vomiting, diarrhea, insomnia, hyperreflexia, and fever in addition to the above symptoms. Five also had hallucinations, two had seizures, and three developed delirium tremens.[67] Ethanol withdrawal developed even if the study participants did not become intoxicated as long as the amount of ethanol ingested remained large over time.[67]

Symptoms of ethanol withdrawal range from mild anxiety and tremors to seizures, delirium tremens (DTs), and death. Symptoms start 6 to 8 hours after a significant drop in ethanol level. Sympathetic symptoms include tremors, tachycardia, hypertension, irritability, and/or hyperreflexia. Neuropsychiatric symptoms include anxiety, agitation, hyperalertness, easy startling, insomnia, craving for rest, self-preoccupation, inattention, and mild disorientation to time with no gross confusion.[30,67] The absence of significant disorientation, confusion, and autonomic instability differentiates minor withdrawal from the more serious DTs. Tremors may be minimally noticeable (shaky inside) but worsen with activity or agitation and can become so coarse that the patient many not be able to talk, walk, or eat.[30] Symptoms often peak and begin to resolve within 24 hours but can last days to more than a week. Without treatment, the hyperalertness, shakiness, and insomnia can last as long as 10 to 14 days.[30] A mild symptom complex occurs in 70% to 80%, while 15% to 20% become moderately ill if treatment is not provided.[68]

Hallucinations can occur in up to 25% of patients. Three quarters begin within 48 hours, but they may not occur until 6 to 8 days after the cessation of drinking.[30] Pure visual hallucinations are five times more frequent than auditory.[30] They may also rarely be tactile or olfactory. Other disorders of perception such as illusions are transient and rarely last longer than 3 days.[30]

An unusual manifestation of ethanol withdrawal is "acute auditory hallucinosis," which occurred in 2% of patients in one series.[30] The patients did not have significant autonomic hyperactivity. The auditory hallucinations affected only chronic alcoholics, were usually threatening in nature, and lasted a few days to 2 weeks. Patients were oriented and appropriate during the hallucinatory events. Upon recovery, patients realized that the voices were imaginary but could vividly recall the events.[30]

Alcoholic withdrawal seizures, or "rum fits," are generalized and tonic–clonic. Unlike idiopathic seizures, this is an adult-onset disease, with 94% beginning after the age of 30 years.[69] Electroencephalograms (EEGs) of patients with ethanol withdrawal seizures demonstrate diffuse

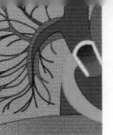
slowing that normalizes after the seizures have ceased. This is different from idiopathic seizure in patients whose baseline EEGs are abnormal.[67,69] The frequency of withdrawal seizures in patients with concomitant idiopathic epilepsy is increased relative to those without epilepsy.[30] Three to 12 percent of untreated withdrawal patients have seizures, with 50% occurring 13 to 24 hours after cessation of drinking and 90% within 48 hours.[30,69] Seizures occurring within 12 hours of the cessation of drinking often have other contributing factors including prior ethanol tapering or head trauma.[30,69] Fifty-four percent of patients with alcohol withdrawal seizures have more than one seizure, all occurring within a few hours of each other.[30,69] One third of patients who have seizures eventually develop DTs if not treated,[30,69] while one third of those who have DTs will have had a seizure during the current withdrawal.[70] Seizures are unusual after the onset of DTs. Patients who have both withdrawal seizures and DTs typically have the seizures first. Delirium tremens begins during the postictal period in 25%, and most episodes begin within 3 days of the seizure.[30]

While ethanol withdrawal can cause seizures, it is proposed that ethanol itself causes seizures. One retrospective series of 308 inner-city patients with new-onset seizures found that only 30% of the alcoholic patients had reduced or stopped their drinking during the 2 weeks prior to their seizures.[71] It has been noted[72] that even patients in the older, classic series[30,69] had seizures outside the typical time frames or while still ingesting ethanol. It has been suggested that seizures in the setting of ethanol use should simply be referred to as "ethanol-related seizures."[71]

Delirium tremens is an infrequent but potentially fatal syndrome. It can occur in individuals who have drunk steadily for as few as 48 days[67] and develops in approximately 5% of patients with untreated ethanol withdrawal.[30,73] It typically begins 3 to 5 days after ethanol intake has decreased but can start within 24 hours or as late as 14 days.[30] Delirium tremens is marked by severe autonomic hyperactivity (hypertension, tachycardia, fever, tremors, diaphoresis, dilated pupils) and significant disorientation. Patients may demonstrate brief moments of insight and reality if their attention can be obtained. While 83% recover within 3 days, 10% can have relapses, with the entire process lasting up to a month.[30] Patients are typically amnestic for events during the delirium.[30]

Prior to the 1950s, the mortality associated with DTs was as high as 50% but averaged 20% to 25%.[73] A 1950s series had a 15% mortality.[30] Mortality today is often quoted to be 5% to 15% in treated patients.[68] However, mortality has not been well studied since the benzodiazepines have become the mainstay of therapy. Mortality likely is relatively low in patients with DTs who have received adequate doses of benzodiazepines and appropriate nursing care. Death during DTs is usually related to patients' underlying medical conditions including pancreatitis, subarachnoid hemorrhage, gastrointestinal hemorrhage, infection, dehydration, seizure disorders, severe electrolyte abnormalities, cardiac rhythm disturbances, and liver disease.[70,73] Hyperthermia or seizures in patients with DTs are particularly associated with a poor outcome. In one series, seizures occurred in 31% of those who died versus 13% of survivors. Even more significant was that 51% of those with temperatures greater than 104° F died, compared with 8% of survivors.[70]

Management of Withdrawal Syndrome

The treatment goals for individuals with the withdrawal syndrome are to prevent the progression of withdrawal to seizures or DTs, allay symptoms, treat underlying disorders, and prepare patients for long-term rehabilitation. Both pharmacologic and nonpharmacologic approaches have been used. Benzodiazepines are the mainstay of pharmacologic therapy. Nonpharmacologic approaches include reassurance, reality orientation, frequent monitoring of signs and symptoms, and general nursing care.[74] Nonpharmacologic therapy has been effective, but it has only been used on patients with mild withdrawal symptoms and without seizures or concomitant medical problems.[74,75]

Patients in withdrawal should receive supplementary multivitamins, thiamine, glucose, and folate. Multivitamins are included because of malnutrition resulting from the "empty" ethanol calories. Thiamine is given by the oral, intramuscular, or intravenous routes. The safety of IV thiamine was demonstrated in a prospective series of 989 patients. Eleven had local irritation and only one developed mild generalized pruritis.[76] Dextrose is given because hypoglycemia is common owing to poor oral intake, glycogen depletion, and decreased carbohydrate production. Potassium, phosphate, and magnesium supplementation may also be beneficial, but there are no data to support this.

Patients with severe symptoms, altered mental status, or significant comorbid conditions should be hospitalized. Hayashida and others demonstrated that outpatient management was effective, safe, and less costly in a population with mild to moderate symptoms, no comorbid disease, and accessibility to daily follow-up.[77] Social issues including homelessness and social support must also be considered when making management decisions.

Benzodiazepines (BDZs) are cross-tolerant with ethanol and are the drugs of choice because of their sedative, anxiolytic, and anticonvulsive properties.[78] Their efficacy was established initially in two classic papers. Sereny and Kalant performed a five-armed, randomized, double-blind comparison of two doses of chlordiazepoxide, two doses of promazine, and placebo. Chlordiazepoxide improved study parameters more consistently than did promazine, and the latter was also associated with an increased progression to DTs.[79] Kaim and others compared chlordiazepoxide, chlorpromazine, hydroxyzine, thiamine, and placebo for the treatment of withdrawal. Chlordiazepoxide was clearly the best at preventing progression of withdrawal.[80] BDZs should be started at the onset of withdrawal symptoms, regardless of the blood ethanol concentration. Problems associated with the use of BDZs include excessive sedation and minor cardiovascular and respiratory depression.[31] However, their safety profile is excellent.

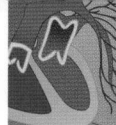

No trials exist that compare oral to parenteral BDZs in patients with severe withdrawal, seizures, or DTs. However, most use intravenous BDZs because they can be better titrated to effect. Intramuscular administration of lorazepam is appropriate if intravenous access cannot initially be obtained.

The optimal choice of BDZ for the treatment of withdrawal is debated, especially with regard to the desirability of drug characteristics such as half-life, lipid solubility, the mechanism of metabolism and the presence of active metabolites, and abuse potential. An extensive meta-analysis found all BDZs to be equally effective in reducing signs and symptoms of withdrawal.[81] However, the longer acting agents, with their active metabolites, may be more effective at preventing seizures during a fixed-dose taper owing to smoother withdrawal with fewer rebound symptoms.[3,81] The potential for abuse is another consideration in BDZ choice. Faster acting agents such as lorazepam, diazepam, and alprazolam have a higher abuse potential than agents with a slower onset of action such as oxazepam or chlordiazepoxide.[82] Oversedation is a concern, particularly with oral dosing. Agents with long half-lives or active metabolites may accumulate and cause extended periods of sedation.[78,81] Interestingly, while oversedation is a concern, this author could not find any cases that reflected this has ever had any clinical significance in the alcohol withdrawal setting. Indeed, as noted above, the long-acting agents likely provide a "smoother" withdrawal with fewer symptom flares. This concept was supported by a comparison of diazepam and lorazepam that found the latter agent to be associated with significantly more anxiety, depression, and poorer performance on cognitive testing.[83] Severe liver dysfunction slows the metabolism of BDZs eliminated by oxidation (diazepam, chlordiazepoxide) more than those eliminated by glucuronidation alone (lorazepam oxazepam).[78,84] It is possible that the metabolism of long-acting agents is decreased in the presence of cirrhosis, chronic active hepatitis, and old age, and half-lives are increased by concomitant administration of disulfiram, cimetidine, or ethanol.[85,86] Such patients may become oversedated, especially with oral regimens, if dosing is not adjusted appropriately.[78,84-86] The significance of lipophilicity is unclear. More lipophilic agents (midazolam > diazepam > lorazepam) penetrate the CNS faster (of unclear clinical significance) but also undergo faster redistribution back out of the CNS (shortening the duration of a single injection).[78] Chlordiazepoxide continues to be one of the most commonly used agents for a fixed-dose taper. It was the first to enter the market (1960); is inexpensive; has long-acting metabolites that accumulate with multiple doses, enabling a smooth taper; and has a relatively low abuse potential. Comparisons among BDZs are shown in Table 31-6.

Few conclusions can be drawn from large reviews or meta-analyses. Three meta-analyses have reached similar conclusions: that BDZs are the agents of choice and the data are not clear as to the optimal BDZ.[81,87,88] Bird and Makela conducted a literature review to determine whether lorazepam should be the agent of choice over the long-acting agents and concluded that no experimental evidence documented the clinical superiority of lorazepam.[78]

Three treatment protocols with BDZs have been used. The most commonly used BDZ dosing method in the United States is a fixed-dose, 3- to 5-day taper of chlordiazepoxide.[89] A slower taper should be considered for the BDZs that only undergo glucuronidation—lorazepam and oxazepam.[31] Tapering should be done by decreasing the dose and not by increasing the interval between doses.[31]

Another approach is the "loading dose technique," which takes advantage of the sustained action of the long-acting agents. A high dose of a long-acting agent is given every 1 to 2 hours until the withdrawal symptoms clear or sedation occurs.[90,91] For example, diazepam 20 mg orally has been used for each dose. Patients averaged four doses over 12 hours and then received no further medications. The long half-lives of diazepam's active metabolites facilitate this approach, since therapeutic levels persist beyond 72 hours.[90] A pharmacokinetic study of the diazepam loading dose technique revealed that some patients did not reach maximum concentration until 90 minutes, reflecting that the dosing intervals should be at least 90 minutes long.[92]

The third protocol is symptom-triggered therapy, in which patients receive medication only when symptoms exceed a threshold of severity, enabling individualized tapering regimens.[89] This approach uses an assessment

TABLE 31-6 Comparison of Benzodiazepines Used for the Treatment of Withdrawal				
CHARACTERISTIC	**CHLORDIAZEPOXIDE**	**DIAZEPAM**	**LORAZEPAM**	**OXAZEPAM**
Routes	IV, IM*, PO	IV, IM*, PO	IV, IM, PO	PO
Initial dosing regimen	15–50 mg tid/qid	5–20 mg tid/qid	1–2 mg bid/qid	15–30 mg tid/qid
Liver metabolism	Oxidation	Oxidation	Glucuronidation	Glucuronidation
Active metabolites	Yes	Yes	No	No
Half-life (hr)†	(Long)	(Long)	(Intermediate)	(Intermediate)
	Range: 6–30	Range: 20–70	Range: 5–25	Range: 5–20
	Average: 10	Average: 33	Average: 15	Average: 8

IM, intramuscular; IV, intravenous; PO, oral; tab, tablet.
*IM absorption is erratic, and thus this route of delivery should be avoided if possible. Inject in the deltoid muscle if administration must be IM.
†Chlordiazepoxide's and diazepam's active metabolites have half-lives from 25 to 100 hr.

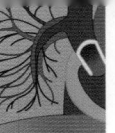

scale to establish severity. The most extensively studied scales are the Clinical Institute Withdrawal Assessment–Alcohol (CIWA-A) and the revised, shortened version of the same. The scales are reliable, reproducible, and valid. High scores predict increased likelihood of seizures or delirium.[3,81] Symptom-triggered therapy decreases the total dose of BDZ and the duration of treatment.[3,81,89] Unfortunately, studies of symptom-triggered therapy have been only in patients with mild to moderate withdrawal.[81,86,89,93] Concerns over the approach include inducing drug-seeking behavior, undertreating patients, and causing "kindling" sensitization because too little treatment has been given.[93]

For patients with severe withdrawal, very large doses of BDZs may be required. Reported doses include 2640 mg of diazepam over 48 hours[94] and 3600 mg of lorazepam over 3 days.[95] A common mistake in the management of patients with severe withdrawal is to not be aggressive enough with the use of BDZs. Use of the "usual" doses may be very inadequate.

Other sedative-hypnotic medications have been assessed. Barbiturates have been used extensively; however, there are few data to support them. They have a narrow safety margin, have abuse potential, and are very sedating. Barbital, a long-acting oral barbiturate, decreases symptoms comparably to BDZs.[81] Phenobarbital is supported by various uncontrolled trials. It has less abuse potential than other barbiturates, can be administered by multiple routes, and is inexpensive.[96] However, it has a greater risk of respiratory depression and a lower safety profile than BDZs.[3,81] γ-Hydroxybutyrate (GHB) compared favorably with diazepam in a prospective series of 60 patients with mild to moderate withdrawal.[97] Propofol is reported to decrease the symptoms of DTs in patients who were refractory to benzodiazepines.[95,98] A problem with these and other sedatives is that they have not clearly been shown to decrease the progression of withdrawal.

Anticonvulsant medications have long been used for ethanol withdrawal, with a main action of cross-tolerance with ethanol at the GABA$_A$ receptors.[3,96] Various open-label trials and anecdotal reports indicate that valproic acid is effective at reducing symptoms.[96] Gabapentin relieved withdrawal symptoms in a four-patient series.[99] Carbamazepine is the best studied of these agents. It is superior to placebo and at least equal to oxazepam, lorazepam, and barbital for the suppression of mild to moderate alcohol withdrawal. Compared with lorazepam, it is associated with fewer protracted symptoms, less relapse during a 3-month follow-up, and fewer adverse events such as dizziness or incoordination.[3,81,96] Like the nonbenzodiazepine sedative-hypnotics, the anticonvulsant medications have not been shown to prevent the progression of withdrawal in humans.

The neuroleptic phenothiazines and butyrophenones have no role in the management of withdrawal despite their ability to attenuate the signs and symptoms of withdrawal. They are less effective than BDZs in preventing delirium and have actually been associated with an increase in seizures compared with placebo.[3,81] Neuroleptics can also modify the body's ability to regulate hyperthermia and can cause hypotension.[31]

The sympatholytic centrally acting α_2 agonists and β blockers are also used. Their primary benefit is attenuation of hyperadrenergic symptoms such as tremor, tachycardia, and hypertension while permitting normal cognitive function.[81,100,101] They usually are used in conjunction with other agents. They have not been shown to prevent seizures or progression to DTs.[81,101] In seriously ill patients, the reduction of sympathetic symptoms masks the progression of DTs and the worsening of associated medical problems.[100,101] β Blockers may be contraindicated for medical reasons including hypoglycemia, cardiomyopathy, and chronic obstructive pulmonary disease.[100]

Alcohol-related seizures should be treated with BDZs. Intravenous lorazepam significantly decreased the frequency of recurrent seizures in one prospective, randomized series of 229 patients who presented following an alcohol withdrawal seizure.[102] Phenytoin, valproic acid, carbamazepine, and primidone are not effective.[101] In addition, except for phenytoin, these agents also cannot be rapidly loaded.

REFERENCES

1. Petroni NC, Cardoni AA: Alcohol content of liquid medicinals. Clin Toxicol 1979;14:407–432.
2. Vogel C, Caraccio T, Mofenson H, et al: Alcohol intoxication in young children. J Toxicol Clin Toxicol 1995;33:25–33.
3. Kosten TR, O'Connor PG: Management of drug and alcohol withdrawal. N Engl J Med 2003;348:1786–1795.
4. Norberg A, Jones AW, Hahn RG, et al: Role of variability in explaining ethanol pharmacokinetics: research and forensic applications. Clin Pharmacokinet 2003;42:1–3.
5. Holt S, Stewart MJ, Adam RD, et al: Alcohol absorption, gastric emptying and a breathalyser. Br J Clin Pharmacol 1980;9:205–208.
6. Jones AW, Jonsson KA, Neri A: Peak blood-ethanol concentration and the time of its occurrence after rapid drinking on an empty stomach. J Forensic Sci 1991;36:376–385.
7. Minocha A, Herold DA, Barth JT, et al: Activated charcoal in oral ethanol absorption: lack of effect in humans. J Toxicol Clin Toxicol 1986;24:225–234.
8. Crabb DW, Bosron WF, Li TK: Ethanol metabolism. Pharmacol Ther 1987;34:59.
9. Bogusz M, Pach J, Stasko W: Comparative studies on the rate of ethanol elimination in acute poisoning and in controlled conditions. J Forensic Sci 1977;22:446–451.
10. Li TK, Bosron WF: Genetic variability of enzymes of alcohol metabolism in human beings. Ann Emerg Med 1986;15:997–1004.
11. Panes J, Caballeria J, Guitart R, et al: Determinants of ethanol and acetaldehyde metabolism in chronic alcoholics. Alcohol Clin Exp Res 1993;17:48–53.
12. Lieber CS: Hepatic and metabolic effects of ethanol: pathogenesis and prevention. Ann Intern Med 1994;26:325–330.
13. Caballeria J: First-pass metabolism of ethanol: its role as a determinant of blood alcohol levels after drinking. Hepato-gastroenterology 1992;39(Suppl 1):62–66.
14. Gershman H, Steeper J: Rate of clearance of ethanol from the blood of intoxicated patients in the emergency department. J Emerg Med 1991;9:307–311.
15. O'Neill S, Tipton KF, Prichard JS, et al: Survival after high blood alcohol levels: association with first-order elimination kinetics. Arch Intern Med 1984;144:641–642.
16. Dufour MC, Archer L, Gordis E: Alcohol and the elderly. Clin Geriatr Med 1992;8:127–141.
17. Watson W, Litovitz T, Rodgers GC II, et al: 2002 annual report of the American Association of Poison Control Centers Toxic Exposure Surveillance System. Am J Emerg Med 2003;21:353–364.
18. Lieber CS: Medical disorders of alcoholism. N Engl J Med 1995;333:1058–1065.
19. Seixas FA: Alcohol and its drug interactions. Ann Intern Med 1975;83:86–91.

20. Interactions of drugs with alcohol. Med Lett Drugs Ther (April 3) 1981;23:33–36.
21. Gugler R: H₂-antagonists and alcohol: do they interact? Drug Saf 1994;10:271–280.
22. Gilman AG, Rall TW, Nies AS, et al: The Pharmacological Basis of Therapeutics, 8th ed. New York, Pergamon, 1990.
23. Schiodt FV, Rochling FA, Casey DL, et al: Acetaminophen toxicity in an urban county hospital. N Engl J Med 1997;337:1112–1117.
24. Lee WM: Drug-induced hepatotoxicity. N Engl J Med 2003; 349:474–485.
25. Zimmerman HJ, Maddrey WC: Acetaminophen (paracetamol) hepatotoxicity with regular intake of alcohol: analysis of instances of therapeutic misadventure. Hepatology 1995;22:767–773.
26. Kuffner EK, Dart RC, Bogdan GM, et al: Effect of maximal daily doses of acetaminophen on the liver of alcoholic patients: a randomized, double-blind, placebo-controlled trial. Arch Intern Med 2001;161:2247–2252.
27. Bailey DN: Comprehensive toxicology screening: the frequency of finding other drugs in addition to ethanol. J Toxicol Clin Toxicol 1984;22:463–471.
28. Fantus RJ, Zautcke JL, Hickey PA, et al: Driving under the influence: a level-I trauma center's experience. J Trauma 1991; 31:1517–1520.
29. Cami J, Farre M: Drug addiction. N Engl J Med 2003;349:975–986.
30. Victor M, Adams RD: The Effect of Alcohol on the Nervous System. Baltimore, Williams & Wilkins, 1953.
31. Adinoff B, Bone GH, Linnoila M: Acute ethanol poisoning and the ethanol withdrawal syndrome. Med Toxicol Adverse Drug Exp 1988;3:172–196.
32. Charness ME, Simon RP, Greenberg DA: Ethanol and the nervous system. N Engl J Med 1989;321:442–454.
33. Diamond I, Messing RO: Neurologic effects of alcoholism. West J Med 1994;161:279–287.
34. Bittencourt P, Wade P, Richens A, et al: Blood alcohol and eye movements. Lancet 1980;2:981.
35. McIvor RA, Cosbey SH: Effect of using alcoholic and non-alcoholic skin cleansing swabs when sampling blood for alcohol estimation using gas chromatography. Br J Clin Pract 1990;44:235–236.
36. Gibb K: Serum alcohol levels, toxicology screens, and use of the breath alcohol analyzer. Ann Emerg Med 1986;15:349–353.
37. Wilson A, Sitar DS, Molloy WD, et al: Effect of age and chronic obstructive pulmonary disease on the breathalyzer estimation of blood alcohol level. Alcohol Clin Exp Res 1987;11:440–443.
38. Li J, Mills T, Erato R: Intravenous saline has no effect on blood ethanol clearance. J Emerg Med 1999;17:1–5.
39. Nuotto E, Mattila MJ, Seppala T, et al: Coffee and caffeine and alcohol effects on psychomotor function. Clin Pharmacol Ther 1982;31:68–76.
40. Nuotto E, Palva ES, Lahdenranta U: Naloxone fails to counteract heavy alcohol intoxication. Lancet 1983;2:167.
41. Brown SS, Forrest JA, Roscoe P: A controlled trial of fructose in the treatment of acute alcoholic intoxication. Lancet 1972;2:898–899.
42. Fluckiger M, Hartmann D, Leishman B, et al: Lack of effect of the benzodiazepine antagonist flumazenil (Ro 15-1788) on the performance of healthy subjects during experimentally induced ethanol intoxication. Eur J Clin Pharmacol 1988;34:273–276.
43. Reuler JB, Girard DE, Cooney TG: Current concepts: Wernicke's encephalopathy. N Engl J Med 1985;312:1035–1039.
44. Watson AJS, Walker JF, Tomkin GH, et al: Acute Wernicke's encephalopathy precipitated by glucose loading. Ir J Med Sci 1981;150:301–303.
45. Hack JB, Hoffman RS: Thiamine before glucose to prevent Wernicke's encephalopathy: examining the conventional wisdom. JAMA 1998;279:583.
46. Wilson JD, Madison LL: Deficiency of thiamine (beriberi), pyridoxine, and riboflavin. In Isselbacher KJ (ed): Harrison's Principles of Internal Medicine, 9th ed. New York, McGraw-Hill, 1980, pp 425–429.
47. Naik P, Lawton J: Pharmacological management of alcohol withdrawal. Br J Hosp Med 1993;50:265–269.
48. Victor M, Adams RD, Collins GH: The Wernicke-Korsakoff Syndrome. Philadelphia, FA Davis, 1971.
49. Thomson AD, Baker H, Leevy CM: Patterns of S-thiamine hydrochloride absorption in the malnourished alcoholic patient. J Lab Clin Med 1970;76:34–45.
50. Homewood J, Bond NW: Thiamin deficiency and Korsakoff's syndrome: failure to find memory impairments following nonalcoholic Wernicke's encephalopathy. Alcohol 1999;19:75–84.
51. Adler RA: Clinically important effects of alcohol on endocrine function. J Clin Endocrinol Metab 1992;74:957–960.
52. Halperin ML, Hammeke M, Josse RG, et al: Metabolic acidosis in the alcoholic: a pathophysiologic approach. Metabolism 1983; 32:308–315.
53. Ragland G: Electrolyte abnormalities in the alcoholic patient. Emerg Med Clin North Am 1990;8:761–773.
54. Duffens K, Marx JA: Alcoholic ketoacidosis: a review. J Emerg Med 1987;5:399–406.
55. Piano MR, Schwertz DW: Alcoholic heart disease: a review. Heart Lung 1994;23:3–17.
56. Puddey IB, Zilkens RR, Croft KD, et al: Alcohol and endothelial function: a brief review. Clin Exp Pharm Physiol 2001;28: 1020–1024.
57. Lang RM, Borow KM, Neumann A, et al: Adverse cardiac effects of acute alcohol ingestion in young adults. Ann Intern Med 1985;102:742–747.
58. Ahlawat SK, Siwach SB: Alcohol and coronary artery disease. Int J Cardiol 1994;44:157–162.
59. Reynolds K, Lewis B, Nolen JD, et al: Alcohol consumption and risk of stroke: a meta-analysis. JAMA 2003;289:579–588.
60. Ettinger PO, Wu CF, De La Cruz C II, et al: Arrhythmias and the "holiday heart": alcohol-associated cardiac rhythm disorders. Am Heart J 1978;95:555–562.
61. Lowenstein SR, Gabow PA, Cramer J, et al: The role of alcohol in new-onset atrial fibrillation. Arch Intern Med 1983;143: 1882–1885.
62. Girard DE, Kumar KL, McAfee JH: Hematologic effects of acute and chronic alcohol abuse. Hematol Oncol Clin North Am 1987;1:321–334.
63. MacGregor RR: Alcohol and immune defense. JAMA 1986; 256:1474–1478.
64. Gonzalez LP, Veatch LM, Ticku MK, et al: Alcohol withdrawal kindling: mechanisms and implications for treatment. Alcohol Clin Exp Res 2001;25:197S–201S.
65. Linnoila M, Mefford I, Nutt D, et al: NIH conference: alcohol withdrawal and noradrenergic function. Ann Intern Med 1987; 107:875–889.
66. Rosenbloom A: Emerging treatment options in the alcohol withdrawal syndrome. J Clin Psychiatry 1988;49:28–31.
67. Isbell H, Fraser HF, Wikler A, et al: An experimental study of the etiology of rum fits and delirium tremens. Q J Stud Alcohol 1955;16:1–33.
68. Lerner WD, Fallon HJ: The alcohol withdrawal syndrome. N Engl J Med 1985;313:951–952.
69. Victor M, Brausch C: The role of abstinence in the genesis of alcoholic epilepsy. Epilepsia 1967;8:1–20.
70. Tavel ME, Davidson W, Batterton TD: A critical analysis of mortality associated with delirium tremens. Am J Med Sci 1961;242:18–29.
71. Ng SK, Hauser WA, Brust JC, et al: Alcohol consumption and withdrawal in new-onset seizures. N Engl J Med 1988;319:666–673.
72. Simon RP: Alcohol and seizures. N Engl J Med 1988;319:715–716.
73. Moore M, Gray MG: Delirium tremens: a study of cases at the Boston City Hospital, 1915–1936. N Engl J Med 1939;220:953–956.
74. Sellers EM, Naranjo CA: New strategies for the treatment of alcohol withdrawal. Psychopharmacol Bull 1986;22:88–92.
75. Sullivan JT, Swift RM, Lewis DC: Benzodiazepine requirements during alcohol withdrawal syndrome: clinical implications of using a standardized withdrawal scale. J Clin Psychopharmacol 1991;11:291–295.
76. Wrenn KD, Murphy F, Slovis CM: A toxicity study of parenteral thiamine hydrochloride. Ann Emerg Med 1989;18:867–870.
77. Hayashida M, Alterman AI, McLellan AT, et al: Comparative effectiveness and costs of inpatient and outpatient detoxification of patients with mild-to-moderate alcohol withdrawal syndrome. N Engl J Med 1989;320:358–365.
78. Bird RD, Makela EH: Alcohol withdrawal: what is the benzodiazepine of choice? Ann Pharmacother 1994;28:67–71.
79. Sereny G, Kalant H: Comparative clinical evaluation of chlordiazepoxide and promazine in treatment of alcohol-withdrawal syndrome. BMJ 1965;1:92–97.

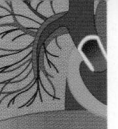
80. Kaim SC, Klett CJ, Rothfeld B: Treatment of the acute alcohol withdrawal state: a comparison of four drugs. Am J Psychiatry 1969;125:1640–1646.

81. Mayo-Smith MF: Pharmocological management of alcohol withdrawal. JAMA 1997;278:144–151.

82. Griffiths RR, Wolf B: Relative abuse liability of different benzodiazepines in drug abusers. J Clin Psychopharmacol 1990;10:237–243.

83. Ritson B, Chick J: Comparison of two benzodiazepines in the treatment of alcohol withdrawal: effects on symptoms and cognitive recovery. Drug Alcohol Depend 1986;18:329–334.

84. Solomon J, Rouck LA, Koepke HH: Double-blind comparison of lorazepam and chlordiazepoxide in the treatment of the acute alcohol abstinence syndrome. Clin Ther 1983;6:52–58.

85. Miller WC II, McCurdy L: A double-blind comparison of the efficacy and safety of lorazepam and diazepam in the treatment of the acute alcohol withdrawal syndrome. Clin Ther 1984; 6:364–371.

86. Massman JE, Tipton DM: Signs and symptoms assessment: a guide for the treatment of the alcohol withdrawal syndrome. J Psychoactive Drugs 1988;20:443–444.

87. Moskowitz G, Chalmers TC, Sacks HS, et al: Deficiencies of clinical trials of alcohol withdrawal. Alcohol Clin Exp Res 1983; 7:42–46.

88. Holbrook AM, Crowther R, Lotter A, et al: Meta-analysis of benzodiazepine use in the treatment of acute alcohol withdrawal. CMAJ 1999;160:649–655.

89. Saitz R, Mayo-Smith MF, Roberts MS, et al: Individualized treatment for alcohol withdrawal: a randomized double-blind controlled trial. JAMA 1994;272:519–523.

90. Sellers EM: Alcohol, barbiturate and benzodiazepine withdrawal syndromes: clinical management. CMAJ 1988;139:113–120.

91. Lejoyeux M, Solomon J, Ades J: Benzodiazepine treatment for alcohol-dependent patients. Alcohol Alcohol 1998;33:563–575.

92. Heinala P, Piepponen T, Heikkinen H: Diazepam loading in alcohol withdrawal: clinical pharmacokinetics. Int J Clin Pharmacol Ther Toxicol 1990;28:211–217.

93. Sullivan JT: Individualized treatment of alcohol withdrawal. JAMA 1995;273:183–184.

94. Nolop KB, Natow A: Unprecedented sedative requirements during delirium tremens. Crit Care Med 1985;13:246–247.

95. McCowan C, Marik P: Refractory delirium tremens treated with propofol: a case series. Crit Care Med 2000;28:1781–1784.

96. Malcolm R, Myrick H, Brady KT, et al: Update on anticonvulsants for the treatment of alcohol withdrawal. Am J Addict 2001; 10(Suppl):16–23.

97. Addolorato G, Balducci G, Capristo E, et al: Gamma-hydroxy-butyric acid (GHB) in the treatment of alcohol withdrawal syndrome: a randomized comparative study versus benzo-diazepine. Alcohol Clin Exp Res 1999;23:1596–1604.

98. Coomes TR, Smith SW: Successful use of propofol in refractory delirium tremens. Ann Emerg Med 1997;30:825–828.

99. Bonnet U, Banger M, Leweke FM, et al: Treatment of alcohol withdrawal syndrome with gabapentin. Pharmacopsychiatry 1999;32:107–109.

100. Baumgartner GR, Rowen RC: Transdermal clonidine versus chlordiazepoxide in alcohol withdrawal: a randomized, controlled clinical trial. South Med J 1991;84:312–321.

101. Liskow BI, Goodwin DW: Pharmacological treatment of alcohol intoxication, withdrawal and dependence: a critical review. J Stud Alcohol 1987;48:356–370.

102. D'Onofrio G, Rathlev NK, Ulrich AS, et al: Lorazepam for the prevention of recurrent seizures related to alcohol. N Engl J Med 1999;340:915–919.

32 *Methanol, Ethylene Glycol, and Other Toxic Alcohols*

A Methanol

DAG JACOBSEN, MD, PHD ■ KNUT ERIK HOVDA, MD, PHD

At a Glance...

- Methanol or methyl alcohol is converted to the toxic metabolite formic acid, which causes acidosis and inhibits cell cytocromes.
- Clinical manifestations vary and are usually delayed for 12 to 24 hours: Visual disturbances, gastrointestinal symptoms, dyspnea, headache, and sometimes chest pain occur. In late stages, coma and respiratory arrest may be observed.
- Diagnosis is based on clinical signs, acid-base status, measurement of serum formate and/or direct serum methanol analyses, or calculation of the anion and osmolal gaps.
- Treatment consists of buffer, an antidote (either ethanol or fomepizole), folinic acid, and often hemodialysis.
- One should always consider multiple victims, especially if the source is contaminated alcohol.
- Permanent sequelae, such as impaired vision and brain damage, may develop if treatment is delayed.

Methanol (HCOOH, methyl alcohol, wood spirits) is a clear, colorless liquid at room temperature. It is a widely used commercial, industrial, and marine solvent and paint remover, as well as a solvent in paints, varnishes, shellacs, and photocopying fluid. It may be used as an antifreeze fluid and is commonly used in windshield-washing fluids. In addition, it can be formulated as a solid canned fuel (4%), along with ethanol and soap, or as a liquid fuel for heating small engines used in various hobbies. In the United Kingdom, methanol is adulterated with a purple dye to distinguish it from ethanol. However, its high industrial production and its use in laboratories, schools, and industrial processes account for the fact that large volumes may be obtained and contribute to epidemic outbreaks of methanol poisoning.

Methanol is also used as an adulterant to make ethyl alcohol unfit to drink when the latter is used for cleaning purposes. Because methanol can be purchased tax free and is considerably less expensive than normal alcoholic beverages, it is not surprising that chronic alcoholics may consume such compounds.[1] Methanol outbreaks are therefore most common in countries with high taxes on alcohol.[2] Methanol has no therapeutic properties and is considered to be only a toxicant.

TOXICOLOGY AND PHARMACOLOGY

The lethal dose of methanol is variably given as 30 to 240 mL, with 1 g/kg (1.2 mL/kg) as the best estimate.[3]

However, with aggressive treatment, survival may be achieved despite much higher intake. Because toxicity in methanol poisoning depends on the degree of metabolic acidosis, there is really no lethal or toxic concentration of methanol if its metabolism to formic acid is blocked. The minimum dose that can cause permanent visual defects is unknown, but most probably ingestion of more than 30 mL (adults) is necessary.

The main route of toxicity is ingestion, but toxicity may also occur after inhalation or skin absorption.[4,5] Methanol is readily absorbed from the gastrointestinal (GI) tract after ingestion and reaches peak blood levels in 30 to 90 minutes. It is widely distributed in body tissues, with a volume of distribution of 0.6 to 0.7 L/kg.[6,7] A small amount of methanol is found in the expired breath of normal persons, presumably due to endogenous metabolic production. The kidneys and lungs in untreated patients excrete less than 5% to 10% of unchanged methanol. The majority of methanol, therefore, is metabolized in the liver, by alcohol dehydrogenase to formaldehyde. Thereafter, formaldehyde is converted by the enzyme aldehyde dehydrogenase to formic acid, which is primarily responsible for the toxicity in methanol poisoning (Fig. 32A-1). This toxicity results from a combination of metabolic acidosis (H+ production) and an intrinsic toxicity of the anion formate.[7] The metabolism and hence elimination of formate depends on the folate pool in the liver.[8] Primates have a small

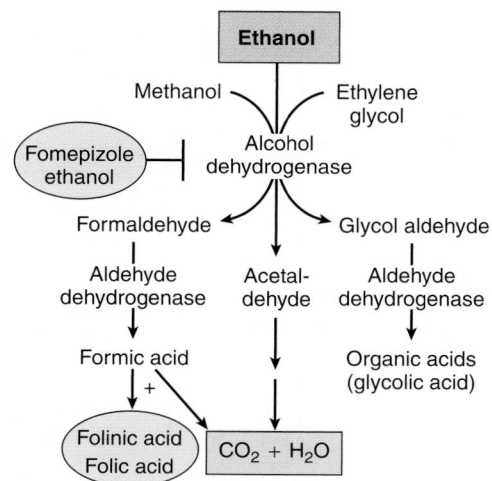

FIGURE 32A-1 The metabolic pathways of methanol, ethylene glycol, and ethanol.

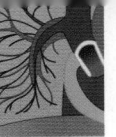

folate reserve and are the only species that accumulate formate and thus suffer from methanol toxicity.[9,10] Other animals only develop acidosis and methanol toxicity if they are made folate deficient.[11] In our latest study,[12] the renal elimination of formate was unexpectedly high in nonacidotic patients. Based on experimental studies demonstrating that this renal elimination depends on pH, we have postulated that increasing acidosis may, by this mechanism, also contribute to the ensuing metabolic acidosis. Thus, metabolic acidosis may itself be a trigger for increasing accumulation of formate. If correct, this adds further importance to the correction of metabolic acidosis in these patients.

The elimination of methanol is usually of zero order because of saturation of alcohol dehydrogenase. Data on this elimination are limited, but elimination rates of 2.7 mmol/L/hr (8.5 mg/dL/hr)[13] and 6.3 mmol/L/hr (20 mg/dL/hr)[12] have been reported. If ethanol metabolism is inhibited by antidote (ethanol or fomepizole) administration, methanol elimination is of first order with a half-life of 22 to 87 hours.[12] For unknown reasons, this half-life seems to increase with increasing serum methanol concentrations.[12,14]

In the early stage of methanol poisoning, the toxic effects are due to the increasing metabolic acidosis caused by the production of formic acid. At this stage, there is a good correlation between the degree of metabolic acidosis reflected by the base deficit or the increase in anion gap, and the formate concentration.[15] In late stages, as formate accumulates, the toxicity is mainly caused by acidosis and the histotoxic effects of formate, which inhibits mitochondrial respiration.[16] The resulting lactate production increases acidosis and thereby

toxicity of formate, as more formate is protonated and thereby able to penetrate the blood-brain barrier.[11] Thus, a vicious hypoxic circle is initiated.[17] In this late stage, the metabolic acidosis reflected by the increased anion gap usually is a combined formate and lactate acidosis.[18]

Why the eye is the primary target organ for methanol's toxic effects is unknown.[19,20] In the late stages, specific lesions of the basal ganglia may develop.[9,21] It is not known why this structure is particularly vulnerable in late stages of methanol toxicity. Although the mechanism of these lesions is not known, it is reasonable to believe that the histotoxic effect of formate in late stages, causing a so-called hypoxic circle, is a contributing factor (Fig. 32A-2).

Formate inhibits the enzyme cytochrome oxidase in the mitochondrial electron transport chain by binding to the ferric iron in the heme moiety of that enzyme. This inhibition occurs in the 5- to 30-millimolar range,[16] which correlates with formate concentrations found in symptomatic patients[17,18] and other primates.[22,23] This inhibition of mitochondrial energy metabolism increases the production of reactive oxidative molecules and thus the likelihood of oxidative injury.[24] Formate also causes depletion of glutathione, which is the major endogenous molecule protecting against oxidative stress in the retina.[25] Because the retina is exposed to several sources of oxidative stress by virtue of its high intrinsic metabolic rate and its exposure to ambient radiation, retinal glutathione concentrations are relatively high compared with other organs.[26] Glutathione synthesis depends on mitochondrial respiration.[27] Experimental studies indicate that cones may be more sensitive than rods to long-term damage from methanol poisoning, possibly because of their greater number of mitochondria.[25]

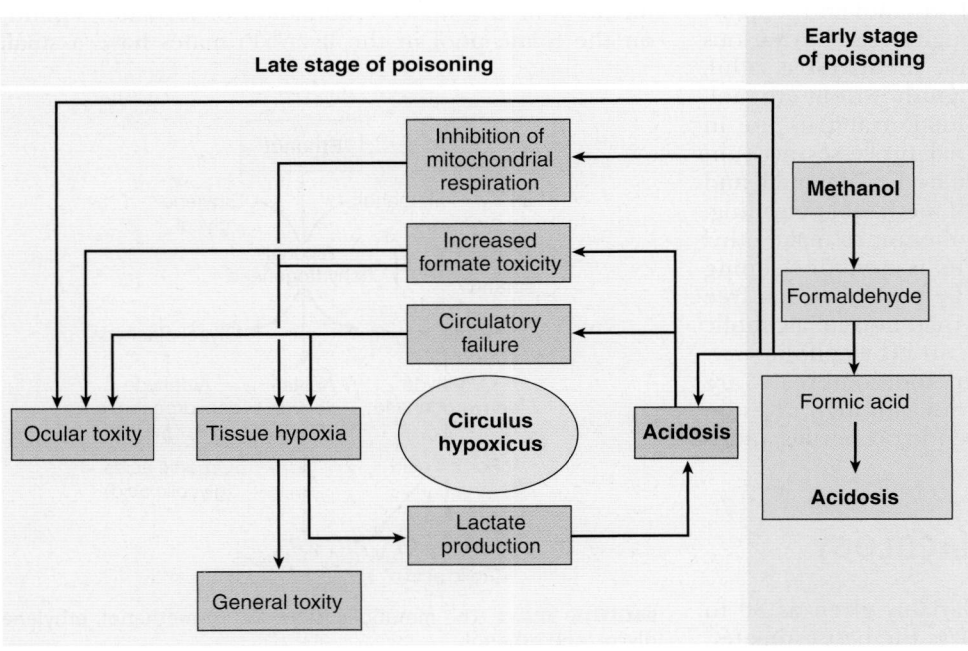

FIGURE 32A-2 Circulus hypoxicus; a proposed description of the toxic effects of methanol in humans. (Modified from Jacobsen D, McMartin KE: Methanol and ethylene glycol poisonings. Mechanism of toxicity, clinical course, diagnosis and treatment. Med Toxicol 1986;1[5]: 309–334.)

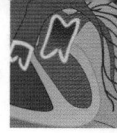

CLINICAL MANIFESTATIONS OF METHANOL INTOXICATION

Symptoms of methanol poisoning may be delayed for 12 to 24 hours, or even longer if ethanol is also ingested before, concomitantly, or just after methanol consumption. This characteristic latent period is thought to result from the slow metabolism of methanol to the principal toxic product, formic acid. In contrast to ethanol (or ethylene glycol), methanol does not cause significant central nervous system (CNS) depression and ethanol-like inebriation. Early clinical features are nausea, vomiting, and abdominal pain, but these are also seen in later stages.[28] A few cases may also present as acute abdomen, probably because of pancreatitis.[9,29]

Clinical features of systemic toxicity are usually anorexia, headache, nausea, accompanied or followed by increasing hyperventilation as metabolic acidosis progresses.[9,28] The first complaint may often be shortness of breath because of hyperventilation. Some patients may also have chest pain and may therefore be admitted acutely with the diagnosis of acute myocardial infarction. Visual symptoms (of all kinds, such as blind spots, blurred vision, or "snow fields") may appear first, or with the symptoms above. Usually ocular symptoms precede objective signs, such as dilated pupils that are partially reactive or nonreactive to light and fundoscopy showing optic disc hyperemia with blurring of the margins (pseudopapillitis).[7]

If treatment is not initiated at this early stage of poisoning, the patient may develop coma and respiratory and circulatory failure. Respiratory arrest is a dramatic complication associated with a mortality rate of 75%.[28] The toxic effect on the basal ganglia may not be evident in the acute stage because it is concealed by pronounced CNS depression. Survivors may later manifest a parkinsonian-like syndrome.[7,9,21]

DIAGNOSIS

In the absence of an exposure history, methanol poisoning is difficult to diagnose, especially if ethanol is co-ingested and the latency period is prolonged. Therefore, methanol poisoning should be considered in every patient presenting with a metabolic acidosis of unknown origin.[18] Methanol is usually determined by gas chromatography or radioimmunoassay techniques. Formate analyses are usually not available in the clinical setting, but a recent simple enzymatic method has proven to be both sensitive and specific and may therefore replace the need for more complicated gas chromatography.[30] Laboratory evaluation of suspected methanol poisoning should always include arterial blood gas analysis in addition to standard blood samples. If ethylene glycol poisoning is considered a differential diagnosis, urinalysis including microscopy should be performed in search of crystalluria (see Chapter 32B). The presence of crystals may suggest ethylene glycol, although their absence has no diagnostic value.

The standard physical examination should focus on vital signs (especially respiratory rate). Visual acuity and fundoscopy examinations should be performed. The objective signs of ocular toxicity of methanol include dilated pupils, which are partially reactive or nonreactive to light, and optic disc hyperemia with blurring of the disc margins (pseudopapillitis). The blurring of the disc margin may look like papillary edema, but there is no diopter difference between the fundus and the disc. Several days after the acute stage, this hyperemia turns into pallor, which is usually associated with blindness. A computed tomography scan or magnetic resonance scan of the brain may show necrosis of the putamenal areas, a finding seen late in the course of methanol poisoning.[9,21]

If the patient presents with a metabolic acidosis of unknown origin, especially if diabetic ketoacidosis and renal failure are ruled out, the anion and osmolal gaps should be calculated as a clue to the diagnosis. The accumulation of formate causes a metabolic acidosis with an increased anion gap.[18] The "normal" range for the anion gap ($[Na^+ + K^+] - [Cl^- + HCO_3^-]$) in unselected acutely hospitalized patients is 12 ± 8 mmol/L (mean $\pm$ 2 SD; reference range is then 4 to 20 mmol/L).[31] In concentrations associated with toxicity, methanol also increases the serum osmolality, as do other alcohols. This effect can be demonstrated by calculating the difference between the measured osmolality (O_m) and the calculated osmolality (O_c):

$$\text{Osmolal gap (OG)} = O_c - O_m$$

The calculated osmolality is determined as follows:

$$\frac{1.86 \times Na + glucose + urea}{0.93}$$

where all concentrations are in mmol/L. To convert from SI units, divide glucose (mg/dL) by 18 and urea (BUN in mg/dL) by 2.8. Correct for co-ingested ethanol (mg/dL/4.6).

The reference range for the osmolal gap in unselected acutely admitted patients is 5 ± 14 mOsm/kg H_2O (mean $\pm$ 2 SD).[31] An osmolal gap above 19 (5 $\pm$ 2 SD) therefore indicates exogenous osmoles of some kind. Although the value of the osmolal gap has been questioned in recent years,[32] as demonstrated by us in a recent epidemic, a decision level or cutoff value for the osmolal gap of 25 mOsm/kg H_2O works very well.[18] Osmometry must be performed by the freezing point depression technique and not by the vapor pressure technique, because the latter does not detect the increased osmolality caused by volatile alcohols. The osmolal contribution from methanol and other alcohols is shown in Table 32A-1.

The relationships between the osmolal gap and methanol and between the anion gap and formate are presented in Figures 32A-3 and 32A-4. Note the good correlation for the patients studied. In the two patients with the highest anion gap (see Fig. 32A-4), there was a significant accumulation of lactate. Therefore, the increase of the anion gaps is slightly higher than the respective serum formate levels.

It must be noted that the magnitude of the increase in the osmolal and anion gap in methanol poisoning varies with time since ingestion, as illustrated in Figure 32A-5. In early stages, or if ethanol is co-ingested, only the osmolal gap is elevated, because the metabolism of methanol to

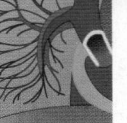

TABLE 32A-1 Molecular Mass of Alcohols and Their Contribution to the Osmolal Gap

ALCOHOL	MOLECULAR WEIGHT (DALTONS)	OSMOLAL CONTRIBUTION (mOsm/kg H₂O) per 100 mg/dL (*)	ANION GAP ELEVATED
Dietylene glycol	106	9	(+)
Ethanol	46	22	−
Ethylene glycol	62	16	+
Isopropyl alcohol	60	17	−
Isobutyl alcohol	74	14	−
Methanol	32	34	+
Propylene glycol	76	13	−

*A methanol concentration of 32 mmol/L (100 mg/dL) increases the osmolal gap by 32/0.93 = 34 mOsm/kg H₂O. Divide by 0.93 because serum consists of 93% water.

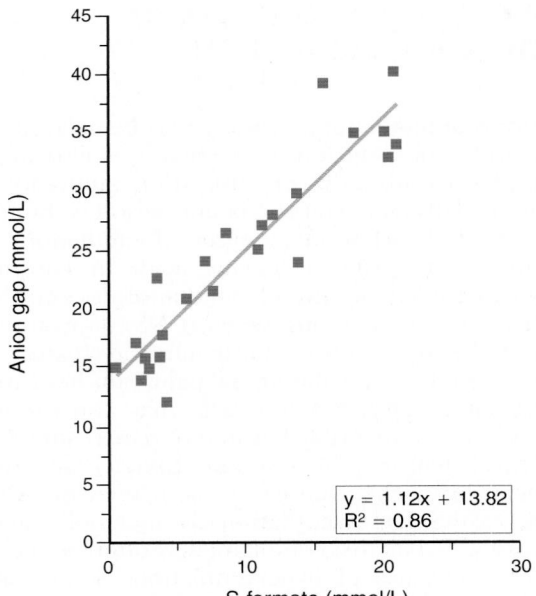

FIGURE 32A-4 S-formate versus anion gap in eight methanol poisoned patients. Equation of correlation: y = 1.12x + 13.82, R² = 0.86. (From Hovda KE, Hunderi OH, Rudberg N, et al: Anion and osmolal gaps in the diagnosis of methanol poisoning: clinical study in 28 patients. Intensive Care Med 2004;30[9]:1842–1846.)

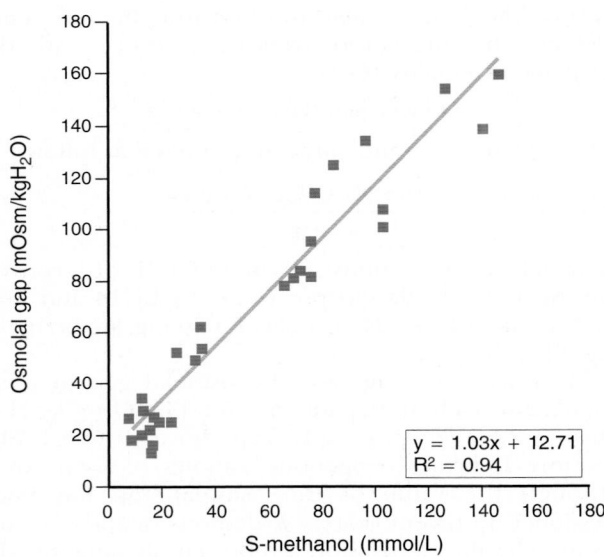

FIGURE 32A-3 S-methanol versus osmolal gap in 28 methanol-poisoned patients. Equation of correlation: y = 1.03x + 12.71, R² = 0.94. (From Hovda KE, Hunderi OH, Rudberg N, et al: Anion and osmolal gaps in the diagnosis of methanol poisoning: clinical study in 28 patients. Intensive Care Med 2004;30[9]:1842–1846.)

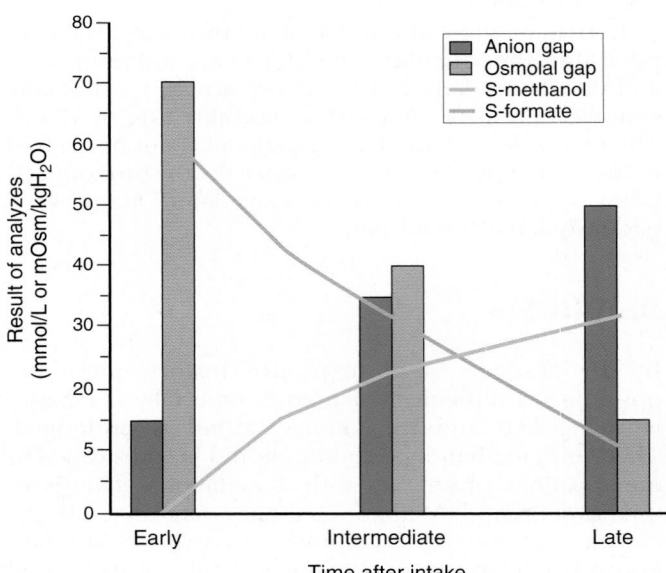

FIGURE 32A-5 Changes in osmolal and anion gaps with time in methanol poisoning. (From Hovda KE, Hunderi OH, Rudberg N, et al: Anion and osmolal gaps in the diagnosis of methanol poisoning: clinical study in 28 patients. Intensive Care Med 2004;30[9]:1842–1846.)

formate has not yet begun. In late stages of methanol poisoning, most of the methanol is metabolized to formate. At this stage the anion gap is elevated but the osmolal gap may be normal; formate detection may then be the only way to confirm the diagnosis.[30]

If the diagnosis is based on the osmolal and anion gaps, it must be noted that elevated gaps also occur in ethylene glycol intoxication. Differentiating the two may be difficult, but the treatment is essentially the same. Hypocalcemia, seizures, and urine oxalate crystals indicate ethylene glycol poisoning; visual symptoms and/or optic

disc hyperemia indicate methanol poisoning.[20] Differential diagnoses when both the gaps are elevated are few (Table 32A-2). A proposed algorithm for diagnosis and triage in suspected methanol poisoning is given in Figure 32A-6.

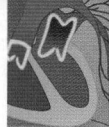

TREATMENT OF METHANOL INTOXICATION

General treatment measures include intensive supportive care and gastric decontamination. If the patient is seen soon (within 1 hour) after ingestion, which is rarely the case, gastric aspiration is recommended. Activated charcoal is probably of limited value because of limited binding.

Specific treatment of methanol poisoning includes intravenous (IV) sodium bicarbonate to combat the metabolic acidosis, antidotal therapy with ethanol or fomepizole to inhibit methanol metabolism to formate, and hemodialysis to remove methanol and formate and correct the metabolic acidosis. Folinic acid, 1 mg/kg IV up to 50 mg every 4 hours, may be of value in increasing the metabolism of formate.[33] If folinic acid is unavailable, folic acid, in the same dose, can be used.

Metabolic acidosis should be immediately and aggressively treated by infusing sodium bicarbonate, aiming for a full correction of acidosis.[3] As much as 400 to 600 mEq may be required during the first few hours. It is important to realize that bicarbonate treatment also decreases the amount of undissociated formic acid, resulting in less access of formate to the CNS, and thereby less toxicity.[11,12,20] Hence, metabolic acidosis resulting from methanol poisoning, in contrast to most other causes of metabolic acidosis, should always be treated with bicarbonate.

Alkali treatment must be accompanied by administration of fomepizole or ethanol; otherwise, the acidosis becomes so-called bicarbonate resistant, because more formic acid will be produced from the metabolism of methanol. If a methanol level cannot readily be obtained and anion and osmolal gaps are difficult to interpret, ethanol or fomepizole therapy should be started in any patient with acidosis, symptoms, or a history of a potentially toxic alcohol ingestion. Antidotal treatment can be discontinued when the methanol level drops below about 6 mmol/L (20 mg/dL), provided that the acid-base status is normal and there are no complications.

The recommended therapeutic blood ethanol level is about 22 mmol/L (100 mg/dL). However, the amount of ethanol necessary to block methanol metabolism depends on the concomitant methanol level, because there is a dynamic competition for the enzyme alcohol dehydrogenase in the liver. If the blood methanol level is known, the molar ethanol concentrations should be at least one fourth of the molar methanol concentration.[7]

A blood ethanol level of 100 mg/dL may be achieved by giving a bolus dose of 600 mg/kg, followed by 66 to 154 mg/kg/hr IV or orally, with the higher maintenance dose for heavy drinkers. Mixing 50 mL of absolute ethanol with 450 mL isotonic glucose yields a 10% solution if a 10% ethanol solution for IV use is unavailable. With this solution, a bolus of 8 mL/kg (over 0.5 hour), followed by 1.5 mL/kg/hr, will produce the desired ethanol

TABLE 32A-2 **Differential Diagnoses with Elevated Osmolal (>25) and/or Anion Gap (>20)**		
DIAGNOSIS	**INCREASED OSMOLAL GAP**	**INCREASED ANION GAP**
Methanol	Yes	Yes
Ethylene glycol	Yes	Yes
Isopropanol	Yes	No
Ethanol	Yes	No
Other alcohols	Yes	Rarely
Lactic acids	No	Yes
Ketoacidosis	Minimally	Yes
Acidosis in alcoholics	Minimally	Yes
Renal failure	No	Yes
Shock following trauma	Minimally	Yes

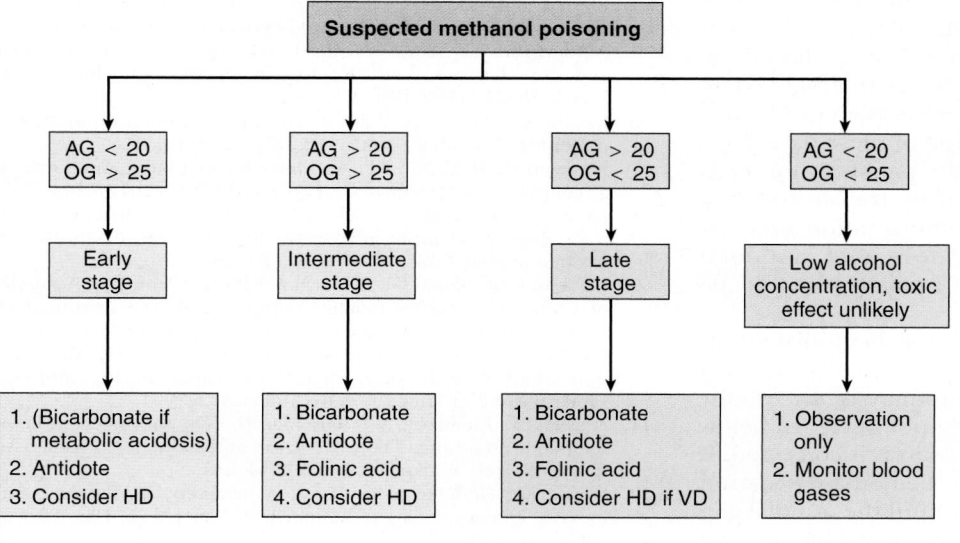

FIGURE 32A-6 "Hovdalgorithm" for diagnosis and triage in suspected methanol poisoning. (From Hovda KE, Hunderi OH, Rudberg N, et al: Anion and osmolal gaps in the diagnosis of methanol poisoning: clinical study in 28 patients. Intensive Care Med 2004;30[9]:1842–1846.)

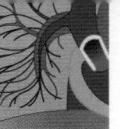

concentration. The maintenance infusion should be increased or decreased according to frequently measured ethanol levels.

Monitoring the blood ethanol level is important, especially during hemodialysis, because this procedure also removes ethanol. As a rule of thumb, the maintenance dose of ethanol should be doubled during hemodialysis. If not, methanol metabolism can resume when the ethanol level drops, resulting in worsening toxicity despite hemodialysis.

Fomepizole (4-methylpyrazole; Antizol [Jazz Pharmaceuticals, Palo Alto, CA]) is commercially available from manufacturers in the United States and in Europe and has been approved for the treatment of methanol poisoning.[9,14,34] While various dosing regimens have been proposed, we recommend a loading dose of fomepizole of 15 mg/kg IV, followed by doses of 10 mg/kg IV every 12 hours four times, thereafter 15 mg/kg every 12 hours. If hemodialysis is begun, fomepizole dosing frequency should be increased to every 4 hours. We generally recommend fomepizole over ethanol, like others.[9] However, if diagnosis is uncertain (no serum methanol level available) and the osmolal gap is only a little elevated (less than 30 to 40 mOsm/kg H$_2$O), then ethanol may be preferable if no visual disturbances are present, because it is inexpensive.

Hemodialysis effectively removes methanol and formate and also counteracts metabolic acidosis.[6,35] The only absolute indication for hemodialysis is visual impairment of any degree in a patient with metabolic acidosis or a detectable methanol level. Other indications usually mentioned are severe metabolic acidosis (particularly if unresponsive to bicarbonate and ethanol therapy), a blood methanol level above 15.6 mmol/L (50 mg/dL) (because of the very slow elimination of methanol during antidotal therapy), and ingestion of more than 1 g/kg of methanol. Following the approval of fomepizole for methanol poisoning, the situation has somewhat evolved. In most patients (i.e., those with no visual disturbances), dialysis is now only indicated to shorten the length of time on fomepizole treatment, since the methanol half-life is then 22 to 87 hours. In severe poisoning, however, with pronounced metabolic acidosis (base deficit greater than 20 mmol/L) and visual disturbances, in our opinion hemodialysis should be performed to remove formate and methanol.[9,36] The role of dialysis in removing formate has been doubted,[37] but others have questioned the value of these data.[38]

If hemodialysis is unavailable, the patient who needs it, or will probably need it, should be transferred to a facility with this capability. Alkali administration aimed at full correction of metabolic acidosis and antidotal therapy (preferably fomepizole, if available) should be given prior to transport.

There is no clear cutoff level for hemodialysis in methanol poisoning, because the presence of acidosis also must be considered. Hemodialysis is usually continued until the blood methanol level is below 6.3 mmol/L (20 mg/dL) and the acidosis is corrected. If methanol analyses are unavailable, hemodialysis should be continued for at least 8 hours or until the osmolal gap is normal in two samples 1 hour apart (possible osmolal contribution from ethanol must be subtracted). This latter approach has been proven to save dialysis time and may be especially valuable in large outbreaks or in other circumstanced where dialysis facilities are limited.[39] Serum formate concentration may also be used as a guide to hemodialysis.[33] Continuous venovenous hemodialysis and peritoneal dialysis may also remove methanol but not as effectively as hemodialysis.[40] Hemoperfusion is ineffective.

ADDENDUM

It should be emphasized that diagnosing and treatment of methanol poisoning is difficult. Because treatment is so effective but often is initiated too late, "time is vision" in this medical emergency. Consultation with a poison center or toxicologist is therefore strongly recommended if the physician is unfamiliar with the management of methanol poisoning. In addition, information on where to obtain methanol or formate levels may be provided.

The possibility of multiple victims should be considered when the source of methanol is unknown or is known to be contaminated ethanol. It should also be remembered that even if some patients are treated at a very late stage and brain circulation has stopped, the damage caused to the rest of the vital organs is often reversible upon standard supportive care. Organ donation has therefore often been performed in such patients.[28,41]

REFERENCES

1. Bennett JL Jr, Cary FH, Mitchell GL Jr, Cooper MN: Acute methyl alcohol poisoning: a review based on experiences in an outbreak of 323 cases. Medicine (Baltimore) 1953;32:431–463.
2. Sejersted OM, Ostborg J, Jansen H: [Methanol poisoning. Emergency measures, diagnostic and therapeutic problems during the Kristiansand outbreak in 1979] [Norwegian]. Tidsskr Nor Laegeforen 1981;12:706.
3. Roe O: The metabolism and toxicity of methanol. Pharmacol Rev 1955;7(3):399–412.
4. Kahn A, Blum D: Methyl alcohol poisoning in an 8-month-old boy: an unusual route of intoxication. J Pediatr 1979;94(5):841–843.
5. Aufderheide TP, White SM, Brady WJ, Stueven HA: Inhalational and percutaneous methanol toxicity in two firefighters. Ann Emerg Med 1993;22(12):1916–1918.
6. Jacobsen D, Jansen H, Wiik-Larsen E, et al: Studies on methanol poisoning. Acta Med Scand 1982;212(1–2):5–10.
7. Jacobsen D, McMartin KE: Antidotes for methanol and ethylene glycol poisoning. J Toxicol Clin Toxicol 1997;35(2):127–143.
8. Jacobsen D, McMartin KE: Methanol and ethylene glycol poisonings. Mechanism of toxicity, clinical course, diagnosis and treatment. Med Toxicol 1986;1(5):309–334.
9. Barceloux DG, Bond GR, Krenzelok EP, et al: American Academy of Clinical Toxicology practice guidelines on the treatment of methanol poisoning. J Toxicol Clin Toxicol 2002;40(4):415–446.
10. McMartin KE, Martin-Amat G, Makar AB, Tephly TR: Methanol poisoning. V. Role of formate metabolism in the monkey. J Pharmacol Exp Ther 1977;201(3):564–572.
11. Herken W, Rietbrock N, Henschler D: [On the mechanism of methanol poisoning. The toxic agent and influence of acid-base balance.] Arch Toxikol 1969;24(2):214–238.
12. Hovda KE, Andersson KS, Urdal P, Jacobsen D: Methanol and formate kinetics during treatment with fomepizole. Clin Toxicol 2005;43(4):221–227.

13. Jacobsen D, Webb R, Collins TD, McMartin KE: Methanol and formate kinetics in late diagnosed methanol intoxication. Med Toxicol Adverse Drug Exp 1988;3(5):418–423.

14. Megarbane B, Borron SW, Trout H, et al: Treatment of acute methanol poisoning with fomepizole. Intensive Care Med 2001; 27(8):1370–1378.

15. Sejersted OM, Jacobsen D, Ovrebo S, Jansen H: Formate concentrations in plasma from patients poisoned with methanol. Acta Med Scand 1983;213(2):105–110.

16. Nicholls P: The effect of formate on cytochrome aa3 and on electron transport in the intact respiratory chain. Biochim Biophys Acta 1976;430(1):13–29.

17. Jacobsen D, McMartin KE: Methanol and ethylene glycol poisonings. Mechanism of toxicity, clinical course, diagnosis and treatment. Med Toxicol 1986;1(5):309–334.

18. Hovda KE, Hunderi OH, Rudberg N, et al: Anion and osmolal gaps in the diagnosis of methanol poisoning: clinical study in 28 patients. Intensive Care Med 2004;30(9):1842–1846.

19. Baumbach GL, Cancilla PA, Martin-Amat G, et al: Methyl alcohol poisoning. IV. Alterations of the morphological findings of the retina and optic nerve. Arch Ophthalmol 1977;95(10):1859–1865.

20. Jacobsen D, McMartin KE: Antidotes for methanol and ethylene glycol poisoning. J Toxicol Clin Toxicol 1997;35(2):127–143.

21. Server A, Hovda KE, Nakstad PH, et al: Conventional and diffusion-weighted MRI in the evaluation of methanol poisoning. Acta Radiol 2003;44(6):691–695.

22. Hayreh MS, Hayreh SS, Baumbach GL, et al: Methyl alcohol poisoning III. Ocular toxicity. Arch Ophthalmol 1977;95(10): 1851–1858.

23. Hayreh MM, Baumbach GL, Cancilla P, et al: In Merigan W, Weiss B (eds): Neurotoxicity of the Visual System. New York, Raven, 1980, pp 35–53.

24. Erecinska M, Wilson DF: Inhibitors of cytochrome c oxidase. Pharmacol Ther 1980;8(1):1–20.

25. Seme MT, Summerfelt P, Neitz J, et al: Differential recovery of retinal function after mitochondrial inhibition by methanol intoxication. Invest Ophthalmol Vis Sci 2001;42(3):834–841.

26. Schutte M, Werner P: Redistribution of glutathione in the ischemic rat retina. Neurosci Lett 1998;246(1):53–56.

27. Meister A: Mitochondrial changes associated with glutathione deficiency. Biochim Biophys Acta 1995;1271(1):35–42.

28. Hovda KE, Hunderi OH, Tafjord AB, et al: Methanol outbreak in Norway 2002–2004. Epidemiology, clinical features, and prognostic signs. J Intern Med 2005;258(2):181–190.

29. Hantson P, Mahieu P: Pancreatic injury following acute methanol poisoning. J Toxicol Clin Toxicol 2000;38(3):297–303.

30. Hovda KE, Urdal P, Jacobsen D: Increased serum formate in the diagnosis of methanol poisoning. J Anal Toxicol 2005;29(6): 586–588.

31. Aabakken L, Johansen KS, Rydningen EB, et al: Osmolal and anion gaps in patients admitted to an emergency medical department. Hum Exp Toxicol 1994;13(2):131–134.

32. Hoffman RS, Smilkstein MJ, Howland MA, Goldfrank LR: Osmol gaps revisited: normal values and limitations. J Toxicol Clin Toxicol 1993;31(1):81–93.

33. Osterloh JD, Pond SM, Grady S, Becker CE: Serum formate concentrations in methanol intoxication as a criterion for hemodialysis. Ann Intern Med 1986;104(2):200–203.

34. Brent J, McMartin K, Phillips S, et al: Fomepizole for the treatment of methanol poisoning. N Engl J Med 2001;344(6):424–429.

35. Jacobsen D, Ovrebo S, Sejersted OM: Toxicokinetics of formate during hemodialysis. Acta Med Scand 1983;214(5):409–412.

36. Hovda KE, Froyshov S, Gudmundsdottir H, et al: Fomepizole may change the indication for HD in methanol poisoning: prospective study in 7 cases. Clin Nephrol 2005; 64(3):190–197.

37. Kerns W, Tomaszewski C, McMartin K, et al: Formate kinetics in methanol poisoning. J Toxicol Clin Toxicol 2002;40(2):137–143.

38. Yip L, Jacobsen D: Endogenous formate elimination and total body clearance during hemodialysis. J Toxicol Clin Toxicol 2003;41(3):257–258.

39. Hunderi OH, Hovda KE, Jacobsen D: Use of the osmolol gap to guide start and duration of dialysis in methanol poisoning. Scand J Urol Nephrol 2006;40(1):70–74.

40. Kan G, Jenkins I, Rangan G, et al: Continuous haemodiafiltration compared with intermittent haemodialysis in the treatment of methanol poisoning. Nephrol Dial Transplant 2003;18(12): 2665–2667.

41. Hantson P, Vanormelingen P, Lecomte C, et al: Fatal methanol poisoning and organ donation: experience with seven cases in a single center. Transplant Proc 2000;32(2):491–492.

B Ethylene Glycol

BRUNO MÉGARBANE, MD, PHD ■ STEPHEN W. BORRON, MD, MS ■ FRÉDÉRIC J. BAUD, MD

At a Glance...

- Ethylene glycol is a readily available and extremely toxic substance by ingestion.
- The hallmarks of intoxication are an increased osmolal gap early in the intoxication that steadily declines and an increased anion gap that increases as ethylene glycol is metabolized.
- When present, an increased osmolal gap should raise suspicion of ethylene glycol poisoning, but a normal osmolal gap does not rule out intoxication. Likewise, a normal anion gap early in the course of the poisoning does not rule out intoxication, as time is required for the formation of toxic acid metabolites.
- Ethylene glycol poisoning should be suspected in any case of altered mental status where the anion gap is increased. Laboratory interference may result in increased glycolic acid being reported as increased lactic acid, thus caution in interpretation is warranted.
- Fomepizole (4-methylpyrazole) is the antidote of choice for ethylene glycol poisoning. It should be administered without waiting for confirmation of poisoning.
- Ethanol can be administered orally or intravenously (IV) if fomepizole is not available, but blood concentrations must be carefully monitored, along with blood glucose and level of consciousness.
- Hemodialysis is often required, particularly in the case of significant acidosis and very high blood concentrations of ethylene glycol, and in the presence of renal insufficiency. Hemodialysis removes not only the toxic metabolites of ethylene glycol, but ethylene glycol itself, as well as the antidotes fomepizole and ethanol. Adjustments in antidotal dosing are required during dialysis.
- Consultation with a medical toxicologist is advised for defining ideal management.

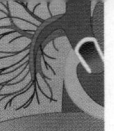

Ethylene glycol poisoning is relatively uncommon, but still represents a significant threat in suicide or accidental poisonings, resulting in numerous deaths and serious sequelae. The American Association of Poison Control Center's Toxic Exposure Surveillance System reported 5081 exposures to ethylene glycol, with 16 deaths and 468 moderate and major outcomes in 2003.[1] Among these exposures, 71% occurred in adults older than 20 years, 16% in individuals 6 to 19 years, and 12% in children younger than 6 years. That 85% of exposures were unintentional (and presumably smaller) may explain the relatively low overall mortality. About 3% experienced life-threatening or significant symptoms or signs resulting in residual disability.

Ethylene glycol poisoning represents the most common poisoning among the toxic alcohols. Ethylene glycol (molecular weight 62.07 Daltons) is an odorless, colorless, volatile, slightly viscous, and sweet-tasting liquid, used in many chemical manufacturing processes (painting, plastics, safety explosives, synthetic fibers) (Table 32B-1). It is present in solvents and added to cosmetics and antifreeze solutions. Examples of uses include automobile antifreeze, hydraulic brake fluid (although diethylene and triethylene glycols are more commonly employed for this use), foam stabilizer, window cleaners, leather dyes, metal cleaners, degreasing agents, cellophane softening agent, printers' inks, stamp pad and ballpoint pen inks, synthetic waxes, and so on. Colorants, often fluorescent, are frequently added to automotive antifreeze products. Ethylene glycol is also used to de-ice airport runways and aircraft. Its evaporation rate is low (2.6 times smaller than ethanol), its boiling point is 197°C, and its pH is neutral. It is not miscible in hydrocarbons, but is easily miscible in water and low-molecular-weight aliphatic alcohols.

TOXICOKINETICS AND TOXICOLOGY

Ethylene glycol itself is nontoxic. Gastrointestinal absorption is rapid, with peak blood levels occurring between 1 and 4 hours after ingestion. Percutaneous and pulmonary absorption is limited. No evidence of toxic accumulation was reported in volunteers, following inhalation exposures to concentrations up to 27 ppm for 4 weeks.[2] However, anecdotal skin irritation and iridocyclitis have been reported after accidental eye contact and cases of chronic poisoning with nystagmus and recurrent attacks of unconsciousness were described after exposure of factory workers to ethylene glycol vapors in 1950.[3]

The accepted lethal dose of ethylene glycol ingestion is 100 mL in a 70-kg adult, although methods used to determine it do not meet the usual scientific criteria. Moreover, death has been reported after ingestion of as little as 30 mL, while recovery with adequate medical intervention has occurred after ingestion of as much as 3000 mL.[4] There are interspecies differences regarding preferential ethylene glycol metabolism to oxalate and relative susceptibility to poisonings. Humans, like monkeys, cats, and dogs, are highly susceptible, while rats, mice, guinea pigs, and rabbits are rather resistant.[5]

Following absorption, ethylene glycol is rapidly distributed throughout the body tissues, with a distribution volume of 0.5 to 0.8 L/kg.[6] Ethylene glycol is successively oxidized by liver alcohol dehydrogenase (ADH) to glycoaldehyde and then by aldehyde dehydrogenase (AldDH) to glycolate (rapid step) and to glyoxylate (rate-limiting step) (Fig. 32B-1).[7] Only a small part of glyoxylate is transformed into oxalate, which precipitates as calcium oxalate crystals in tissues and urine. Possible production of multiple other acids from glyoxalic acid have been described, including oxalomalic acid, γ-hydroxy-α-ketoglutaric acid, formic acid, glycine, benzoic acid, hypuric acid, and α-hydroxy-β-ketoadipic acid; their respective roles in toxicity are controversial. Pyridoxine and thiamine are two cofactors in the metabolic pathways involving glyoxylate. However, they play only a small role in ethylene glycol detoxification. Liver metabolism is responsible for 80% of the absorbed dose of ethylene glycol. The remaining 20% undergoes glomerular filtration, passive tubular reabsorption, and urinary elimination. Ethylene glycol's renal clearance is about 27 mL/min, depending on renal function.[8] There is limited elimination from the lungs due to ethylene glycol's high water solubility and low vapor pressure. The elimination half-life of ethylene glycol is about 3 hours, but markedly prolonged in the presence of an alcohol dehydrogenase competitor: 17 to 18 hours in the case of ethanol[9] and 20 hours in the presence of fomepizole.[10] Only 1% of the ingested dose appears as oxalic acid in urine. Ethylene glycol toxicokinetic parameters are given in the Table 32B-2.[8,11-13]

Toxicity is related to the production of toxic metabolites. Accumulation in the blood of glycolate results in an anion gap metabolic acidosis. Glycolate accumulation correlates well with the anion gap and the decrease in serum bicarbonate concentration.[14] On the other hand, glyoxalate and oxalate's contributions to the anion gap are limited.[15,16] Two other factors, including lactate production and bicarbonate consumption, may

TABLE 32B-1 Ethylene Glycol Physical Properties	
Chemical formula	$C_2H_6O_2$
Molecular weight	62.07 g/mol
Volumetric mass	1 ppm = 2.54 mg/m³
Density	1.113 at 25°C
Vapor pressure	0.06 mmHg at 20°C
Log octanol/water partition coefficient (low Kow)	−1.36
Boiling point	197.5°C
Melting point	−13°C
Flash point	232°F
Properties	Colorless, sweet-tasting, hygroscopic liquid
Solubility	Miscible with water and alcohol
	Slightly soluble in ether
	Insoluble in benzene and its homologs, chlorinated hydrocarbons, and petroleum ethers

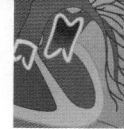

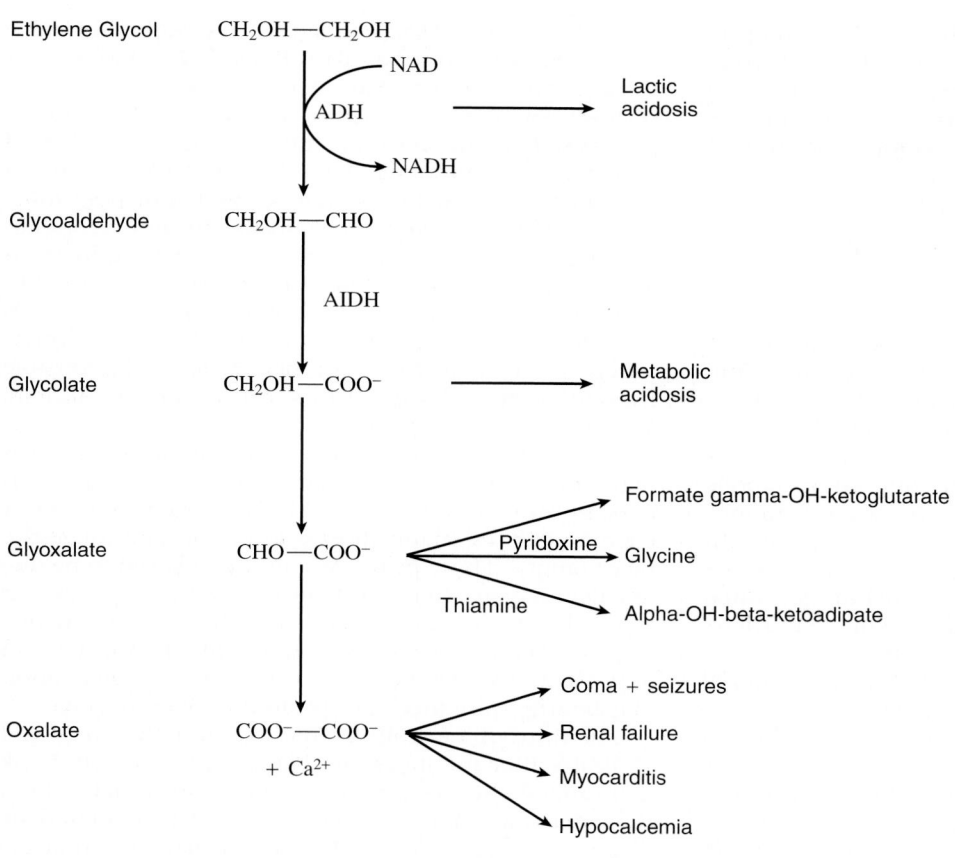

FIGURE 32B-1 Pathogenesis of ethylene glycol poisonings with the main symptoms related to the toxic metabolites resulting from oxidation by alcohol dehydrogenase (ADH) and aldehyde dehydrogenase (AlDH).

TABLE 32B-2 Ethylene Glycol Toxicokinetic Parameters and Their Modifications in Relation to Hemodialysis or Antidotal Treatment	
Lethal dose	1.4–1.6 mL/kg
Distribution volume	0.5–0.8 L/kg
Elimination	0 or 1st order (?)
Total body clearance	70 mL/min
Renal clearance*	17–39 mL/min
Half-life	
+ Ethanol	11–18 hr
+ 4-MP	20 hr
Dialysis half-life	2.5–3.5 hr
Dialyser clearance†	156–210 mL/min
Main metabolite (glycolate) clearance	254 mL/min

*Dependent on renal function
†Dependent on blood flow during hemodialysis.

account for worsening acidosis. Lactic acid is produced in response to nicotinamide-adenine dinucleotide (NAD) trapping that occurs during the breakdown of ethylene glycol and the by-products of glyoxalate metabolism, which inhibit the citric acid cycle and result in the conversion of pyruvate to lactate (see Fig. 32B-1). In addition, acidosis may be worsened by bicarbonate consumption due to glycine production, resulting from

glycolate (and to a lesser extent glyoxalate) recondensing under the activity of pyridoxal phosphate and glyoxalate transaminase enzymes.

Deposition of birefringent calcium oxalate crystals (see Fig. 32B-2) induces tissue destruction. Reversible oliguric or anuric acute renal failure is the primary injury due to oxalate crystal deposition in the proximal renal tubules,[17] with evidence of interstitial nephritis, cortical focal hemorrhagic necrosis, and acute tubular necrosis.[18] Damage is predominant in the proximal tubules, compared with distal ones, while glomeruli and basement membrane remain intact. A direct cytotoxic action of metabolites has also been proposed as a complementary mechanism of toxicity.[19] This hypothesis is reinforced by the absence of correlation in pathologic findings between the extent of renal damage and the number of deposited crystals.[20] Although renal failure is usually reversible, persistent renal insufficiency has been reported. Initial central nervous system (CNS) depression is believed to be related to the glycol itself or the production of glycoaldehyde, whereas later in the course, persistent stupor or coma is probably the consequence of brain edema, hemorrhage, or metabolic encephalopathy.[21] Hypocalcemia, for which the hypothesized mechanism is calcium chelation by oxalate, may contribute to the development of seizures, dysrhythmias, and negative inotropic effects. In fulminant forms, patients experience coma with seizure

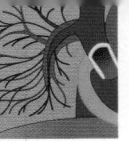
activity, respiratory failure, cardiovascular collapse, pulmonary edema, and adult respiratory distress syndrome. Death may follow multiorgan failure. In these cases, autopsy reveals diffuse hemorrhage, inflammatory infiltration, and edema, in addition to the deposition of calcium oxalate crystals in kidneys, brain, pleura, lungs, pericardium, heart, pancreas, and spleen.[22]

CLINICAL PRESENTATION

Presentation of ethylene glycol–poisoned patients is polymorphous, depending on the delay since ingestion, the ingested dose, the co-ingestion of ethanol, and the timing of medical intervention (Table 32B-3).[23] Early after ingestion, patients are usually asymptomatic or present only with hyperventilation due to metabolic acidosis (Kussmaul's respiration). In these patients, underestimation of poisoning severity may occur. In stark contrast, late presentation is responsible for life-threatening signs and symptoms, including coma, seizures, respiratory distress, and renal failure.[24] Ethylene glycol toxicity occurs in three classical theoretical stages, although the onset and progression of this condition are not always straightforward or predictable.[25,26]

The first phase (called neurologic) occurs within 30 minutes to 12 hours after ingestion. Patients appear inebriated and euphoric, but without the characteristic alcohol smell. Nausea, vomiting, and hematemesis are possible, reflecting ethylene glycol gastrointestinal direct irritation. It is not uncommon, however, to observe an initial latent period, reflecting the time required for the toxic metabolites to accumulate. Rapidly, the most severely intoxicated patients may develop coma, myoclonic seizures, nystagmus, ataxia, ocular external muscle paralysis, CNS depression, and meningismus. Loss of light reflexes and papilledema have been reported but are more frequent in relation to methanol poisoning. Sustained hypocalcemia is responsible for muscle spasms and hyperreflexia. Cranial computed tomography scans are usually normal, despite the neurologic symptoms. However, various radiologic abnormalities have been reported, including diffuse cerebral edema, intra-parenchymal hemorrhage or petechiae, and reversible hypodense areas localized in various brain, brainstem, and cerebellum territories.

The second phase (called cardiopulmonary) starts between 12 and 24 hours after the ingestion. Patients present with tachycardia, mild hypertension, pulmonary edema, adult respiratory distress syndrome, and congestive heart failure. These presentations are believed to be due to calcium oxalate crystal deposition within the vascular tree, the myocardium, and the lung parenchyma. Hypoxia may be related to aspiration pneumonia or CNS depression. Dysrhythmias with QTc interval prolongation may be the consequence of profound hypocalcemia.

The third phase (called renal) begins between 24 and 72 hours after the ingestion. Patients present with flank pain and tenderness, oliguria, and acute renal failure. Bone marrow suppression has been reported, but hepatic damage is usually minimal. Calcium oxalate or hippurate crystals are present in the urine.

Delayed symptoms are possible in the most severe cases: persistent renal insufficiency requiring prolonged hemodialysis, as well as delayed cranial nerve deficits (5 to 20 days after ingestion)[27,28] involving cranial nerves II, V, VII, VIII, IX, X, and XII that are related to calcium oxalate crystal deposition–associated local infiltration, which may be observed on magnetic resonance imaging. All these injuries slowly resolve, but last as long as several months, particularly after severe encephalopathy or profound acidemia with reported arterial pH as low as 6.46.[29,30] Ultimately, recovery of renal function is usually complete. However, exceptional cases requiring chronic hemodialysis or renal transplantation have been reported.

LABORATORY DIAGNOSIS OF ETHYLENE GLYCOL POISONING

Ethylene glycol poisoning should be strongly suspected in patients exposed to presumed ethylene glycol–containing products, patients inebriated without the smell of alcohol, patients presenting with metabolic acidosis and elevated anion gap unexplained by an increased plasma lactate concentration, and finally, patients presenting with acute renal failure or multiorgan failure of unexplained origin.[31] Caution is advised in interpreting plasma lactate values, as glycolate has been shown to cause interference in laboratory analysis of lactate.[32,33] The evolving laboratory profile reflects ethylene glycol metabolism, organic acid

TABLE 32B-3 Ethylene Glycol Poisoning	
MAJOR SYMPTOMS AND SIGNS	**LABORATORY FINDINGS**
Early	
Inebriation, drowsiness	Elevated osmolal gap
Coma, ataxia, CNS depression	Detectable ethylene glycol
Vomiting, nausea	
Delayed	
Dyspnea, hyperventilation, tachypnea	Acidosis with elevated anion gap
Kussmaul's respiration	Detectable ethylene glycol and metabolites
Coma, seizure, cerebral edema	Elevation of serum creatinine
Tetany, muscle paralysis, myoclonus	Elevation of blood urea nitrogen
Tachycardia, hypertension, dysrhythmias, myocarditis	Hypocalcemia
Acute renal failure	Elevation of creatine phosphokinase
Respiratory distress, noncardiogenic pulmonary edema	Hematuria, proteinuria, leukocyturia
Multiorgan failure	Calcium oxalate crystals in urine
Very Delayed (rare)	
Persistent renal insufficiency	
Cranial nerves deficiencies (including bilateral facial paralysis and ophthalmoplegia)	

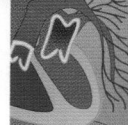

accumulation, and medical intervention timing. The combination of an osmolal gap and an anion gap is strongly suggestive of ethylene glycol poisoning, but is not specific.[7] At a given time after ingestion, the concentrations of remaining ethylene glycol and the accumulated acid metabolites affect the magnitude of the osmolal and anion gap, respectively.

Osmolal gap is the difference between the measured osmolality (by the freezing point depression method) and the calculated one, based on sodium, blood urea nitrogen (BUN), and glucose concentrations: (1.86 [Na^+] + [BUN] + [glucose]) / 0.93, in SI units. If values are reported in mg/dL, the BUN should be divided by 2.8 and the blood glucose by 18. Note that vapor pressure methods may underestimate the contribution of volatile alcohols like ethylene glycol. An elevated osmolal gap (normal values 10 to 15 mOsm/kg H_2O) corresponds to the presence of ethylene glycol in blood, with an increase of 2 mOsm/kg H_2O for every 0.1 g/L (1.6 mmol/L) of ethylene glycol. Other alcohols and ketones may of course contribute to the osmolal gap (Table 32B-4). Normal osmolal gap may be encountered very early (before significant absorption) or very late in the course of poisoning, when ethylene glycol is completely metabolized.[34] Contribution of metabolites to the osmolal gap is reduced, explaining its transient elevation due to ethylene glycol's short half-life. However, persistent high osmolal gap with low ethylene glycol level has been reported and attributed to plasma glycolate.[35] A normal osmolol gap does not rule out poisoning.

Anion gap (normal values 12 to 16 mmol/L) is the difference between measured cations and anions in plasma and is calculated as follows: ([Na^+] + [K^+]) − ([HCO_3^-] + [Cl^-]). Significant acidosis is produced with the production of ethylene glycol metabolites. Glycolic acid, which accounts for approximately 96% of the anion gap, significantly correlates with the decline in serum bicarbonate concentration and the elevation in anion gap.[7,35] Other toxicants, including methanol-derived formate, may be responsible for increased anion gap. Differential diagnoses exist, with endogenous organic acid accounting for the anion gap: diabetic, alcoholic, or starvation-related ketoacidosis (with accumulation of acetone, acetoacetate, and β-hydroxybutyrate), circulatory hepatic failure (with elevation of lactate), renal failure (with accumulation of phosphates, sulfates, and nitrogen acid compounds), and critical illness.[23] Thus, specificity

of the diagnosis value of anion gap is increased in the absence of hypotension, diabetes, seizures, and alcoholism. Consistently, ethanol co-ingestion delays the appearance of anion gap, also reducing the symptoms of intoxication. Simultaneous ingestion of bromide (not distinguished from chloride on electrolyte analysis) may also mask the anion gap.[36]

Other laboratory features of ethylene glycol poisoning include elevation of serum creatinine and BUN concentrations, rhabdomyolysis (elevation of serum creatine phosphokinase concentration), hypocalcemia, hyperkalemia (in the case of acute renal failure), and nonspecific leukocytosis (see Table 32B-3). If lumbar tap is performed, high cerebrospinal fluid protein, neutrophils or monocytes, red blood cells, or xanthochromia may be observed. The presence of either monohydrate (whewellite) or dihydrate (weddellite) calcium oxalate crystals in the urine is characteristic of ethylene glycol renal injury (Fig. 32B-2). These crystals appear 4 to 8 hours after ingestion and may persist for up to 10 days in the presence of renal failure. Identification of the nature of these crystals requires polarized light microscopy and repeated urinalysis. Crystals are birefringent, variegated and pleomorphic, octahedral, or tent shaped for dihydrate forms, and they are prism or needle shaped for monohydrate forms. Other forms of calcium oxalate include dumbbell, ovoid, and elliptical crystals. Other clinical settings may include calcium oxalate crystals, like primary hyperoxaluria, or oxalate-rich dietary excess foods. However, detection of calcium oxalate crystalluria, particularly the monohydrate forms, supports the diagnosis of ethylene glycol poisoning.[31] In addition to crystals, microscopic hematuria, proteinuria, leukocyturia, and urine with low specific gravity may be observed. The absence of crystals does not exclude the diagnosis of ethylene glycol exposure.

Definitive diagnosis is assessed by the measurement of plasma ethylene glycol concentration. Early after ingestion, the plasma ethylene glycol concentration is elevated in relation to the ingested amount. On the other hand, late in the course, low plasma ethylene glycol concentrations are observed, contrasting with the severity of the clinical presentation. In fact, severity of poisoning better correlates with reduced bicarbonate level, elevated anion gap, and elevated glycolic acid than with serum ethylene glycol concentration. The method of choice for measuring ethylene glycol concentration is gas chromatography with flame ionization detection.[31] Commonly, ethylene glycol is analyzed as the boronic ester derivative by using packed or capillary columns. Underivatized ethylene glycol is difficult to analyze due to the poor detection limit of flame ionization detectors. However, direct injection of ethylene glycol on a wide-bore capillary column has been described, with the advantage of eliminating the derivatization step and extending the analytical life of the column. Thus, in practice, separate dedicated columns are preferred, rendering this technique reserved for specialized laboratories of toxicology. Propanediol and butanediol are used as appropriate internal standards. Consequently, some IV medication solvents containing propylene glycol (diazepam, phenytoin) may produce false-positive

TABLE 32B-4   Molecular Weight and Contribution of Various Alcohols and Ketones to the Osmolal Gap

NAME OF THE COMPOUND	MOLECULAR WEIGHT (DALTONS)	OSMOLAL GAP (mOsm/kg H_2O) AT 1 g/L CONCENTRATION
Propylene glycol	90	13
Ethylene glycol	62	16
Isopropanol	60	17
Acetone	64	18
Ethanol	46	22
Methanol	32	34

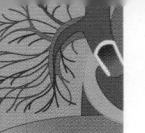

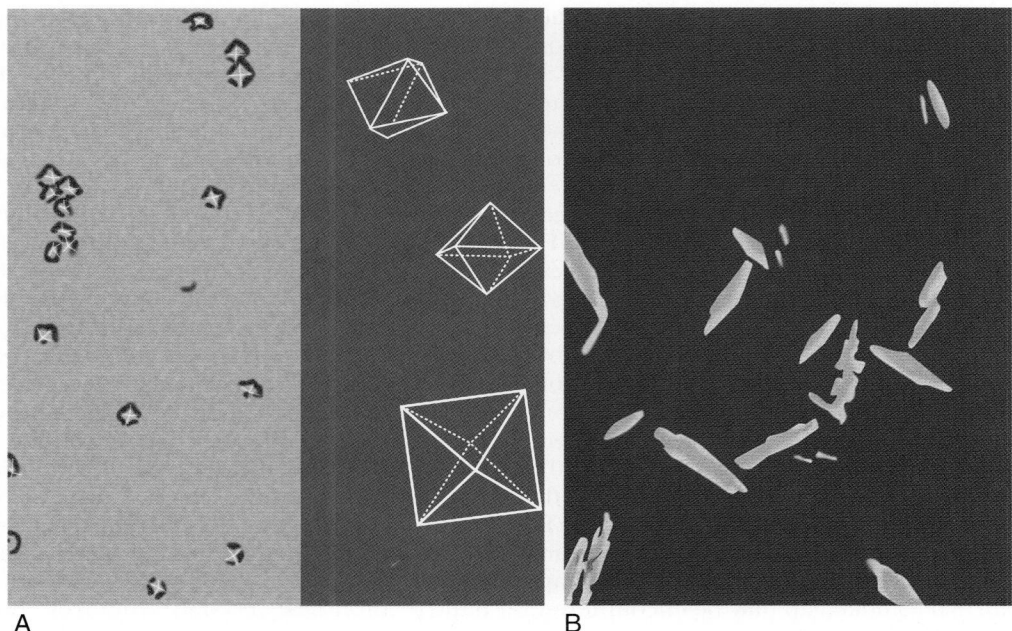

A   B

FIGURE 32B-2 Calcium oxlatae crystalluria in the urine of an ethylene glycol–poisoned patient. **A,** Calcium oxalate dihydrate. (Courtesy of Dr. G.E. Schreiner). **B,** Calcium oxalate monohydrate crystals. (Courtesy of Dr. A. Terlinsky.)

results. Confirmation by mass spectrometry is thus required, especially in ketotic patients.[37] Enzymatic screening assays based on ethylene glycol oxidation using *Enterobacter aerogenes* glycerol dehydrogenase have been described.[38] The produced NADH is measured by spectrophotometer. Cross-reactions are possible with glycerol and glycoaldehyde, the short half-lives of which make them unlikely to interfere with the assay. However, their use in critically ill patients may be limited due to several glycerol-containing IV medications. Consistently reliable screening tests can eliminate ethylene glycol as a cause of increased anion gap metabolic acidosis in a comatose patient, preventing the patient from receiving invasive and inappropriate treatments.

POISONING MANAGEMENT

Recommended management of ethylene glycol poisonings includes (1) supportive care; (2) infusion of sodium bicarbonate to correct metabolic acidosis, to increase renal elimination of glycolate, and to inhibit precipitation of calcium oxalate crystals; (3) antidotes, such as a competitive ADH substrate (ethanol) or inhibitor (fomepizole) to block ADH metabolism of the toxic alcohol; and (4) intermittent dialysis to remove the toxic alcohol and its toxic metabolites.[7,23]

Usual supportive treatments include correction of life-threatening signs, dehydration, acid-base, and fluid imbalances. Particular attention should be directed to adapt fluid load to diuresis in the case of acute renal failure. Treatment of seizures is standard: benzodiazepines (diazepam or lorazepam), phenobarbital, and (perhaps) phenytoin. Gastric lavage is useful only within the first hour after ingestion because of the very rapid

gastrointestinal absorption of ethylene glycol. Activated charcoal is not useful because ethylene glycol is not adsorbed. Hemoperfusion is not recommended because of column saturation and the absence of correction of acid-base disturbances. Hypocalcemia should be corrected with IV calcium only in case of symptoms related to low levels of calcium (tetany, muscle paralysis, or seizures). Two cofactors of ethylene glycol metabolism may be administered: pyridoxine (500 mg IV every 6 hours over 2 days) to stimulate glyoxalate to glycine metabolism and thiamine (100 mg IV every 6 hours over 2 days) to enhance transformation of glyoxalate to α-OH-β-ketoadipate.

ANTIDOTES

Fomepizole

Fomepizole (4-methylpyrazole, 4MP) [Antizol, Orphan Medical, Minnetonka, MN, in the United States, and Fomepizole, Opi & Isotec, France, in Europe) is a potent inhibitor of ADH, with limited toxicity in animals and humans, that prevents the metabolism of ethylene glycol or methanol into their toxic metabolites. Fomepizole was approved by the U.S. Food and Drug Administration in 1997 for the treatment of ethylene glycol poisoning. It has been successfully used in France since 1981 in several cases of ethylene glycol poisoning.[39-41] No lethality or significant morbidity occurred if patients were treated before significant toxic metabolism of ethylene glycol had occurred, and all such patients recovered from their poisoning. A recent multicenter prospective clinical trial performed in the United States confirmed the efficacy of fomepizole in the treatment of ethylene glycol intoxication.[10] There was clinical improvement

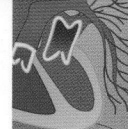

with rapid resolution of acidosis and an absence of any new symptoms of poisoning after the initiation of therapy. Renal injury was prevented if fomepizole was administered early in the course of ethylene glycol intoxication. Treatment with fomepizole resulted in alteration of the toxicokinetics of ethylene glycol, with a prolongation of its first-order elimination (to 19.7 ± 1.3 hours) and a reduction in glycolate formation.[10]

Fomepizole pharmacokinetics have been largely studied. Although mostly used by the IV route, fomepizole is rapidly and almost completely absorbed orally. In fact, the three initial cases of ethylene glycol poisoning were treated with fomepizole by the oral route.[40] Thereafter, 4 of 11 cases of ethylene poisonings in the series reported by Borron and colleagues received this antidote orally.[41] When intravenously administered, fomepizole is typically infused in 100 mL of 0.9% sodium chloride or 5% dextrose over 30 minutes. Fomepizole's volume of distribution has been reported to be in the range of 0.6 to 1.0 L/kg. Its plasma protein binding is low. Fomepizole has three metabolites: 4-hydroxymethylpyrazole, the only active metabolite with approximately one third of the potency of the parent compound, 4-carboxypyrazole, and a glucuronide metabolite.[42] Fomepizole is virtually entirely eliminated by saturable hepatic metabolism, with a Michaelis constant (K_m) of 6 μmol/L, a concentration always markedly exceeded during therapeutic use.[43] Fomepizole is a competitive inhibitor of ADH with an in vitro inhibitory constant for human ADH of 0.2 μmol/L.[44] Its affinity for ADH is 500- to 8000-fold greater than that of ethanol. A plasma concentration of 10 μmol/L was shown in experimental studies to be sufficient to inhibit formate accumulation in the methanol-poisoned monkey.[42] Thus, this plasma concentration of fomepizole was considered to be sufficient in prospective human trials of this antidote. In the Methylpyrazole for Toxic Alcohols (META) studies in the United States, complete inhibition was reached in each reported case.[10] Plasma fomepizole concentrations using the prescribed dosing regimen exceeded the target concentration of 10 μmol/L. At therapeutic concentrations, elimination is characterized by dose-dependent, nonlinear, zero-order kinetics, with a rate of 4 to 15 mmol/L/hr.[43,45]

While fomepizole blocks ADH activity, repeated doses induce cytochrome P-450, and particularly cytochrome P-450 2E1, resulting in an increase in its own elimination rate. Initial studies with human volunteers demonstrated that fomepizole has the ability to induce its own metabolism after 48 hours of treatment.[43] Thus, an increase of up to 15 mg/kg in patients treated over 48 hours is currently recommended by North American authors and was incorporated into practice guidelines developed by the American Academy of Clinical Toxicology to account for its enhanced metabolism.[23] This dosing protocol has been validated in the U.S. META study.[10] However, it is noteworthy that fomepizole is expensive and a dosage regimen using the minimal effective cumulative dose remains to be determined. The French dosing regimen consists of a loading dose of 15 mg/k followed by 10 mg/kg every 12 hours until the

alcohol concentration is <0.2 g/L (3.2 mmol/L) or becomes undetectable. Borron and colleagues reported a series of ethylene glycol poisonings treated with tapering doses of fomepizole.[41] In the French experience, no failure was noted in any patient who was treated without a dose increase, except in one case. In this severely poisoned patient (initial ethylene glycol concentration 4.2 g/L [67.6 mmol/L], peaking at 6.4 g/L [101.9 mmol/L] 4 hours later), anion gap decreased following the administration of a 6.4 mg/kg loading dose of fomepizole.[46] However, the beneficial effect was reported to be transient and dose dependent, requiring further maintenance doses of 11.3, 4.8, and 2.4 mg/kg, and the patient ultimately recovered without sequelae. This early treatment failure was likely due to an inadequate initial dose rather than failure to up-regulate the dose for induced fomepizole metabolism. Based on this clinical experience, a different dosage regimen is recommended in Europe (Table 32B-5).

During concomitant hemodialysis, fomepizole is extracted with a mean extraction coefficient of 49.6 ± 42.5%, a mean hemodialysis clearance of 99 ± 33 mL/min, and a mean hourly extracorporeal extraction of 83 ± 31%.[47,48] Although not systematically validated, two different schemes were proposed to compensate for fomepizole loss in the dialysate. The U.S. manufacturer recommends a reduction in the dosing interval from 12 to 4 hours, while European researchers have proposed a continuous IV infusion of 1 to 1.5 mg/kg/hr for the entire duration of the hemodialysis session following the initial loading dose.[47,48] Since the duration of hemodialysis depends on the initial plasma ethylene glycol concentration to be lowered below the toxic range, the continuous infusion protocol appears better adapted, rather than a shortening of the dosing interval. Moreover, this regimen appears simpler and sufficient to maintain fomepizole at or above the minimally effective concentrations (greater than 10 μmol/L). However, the dosage of fomepizole during continuous venovenous hemodiafiltration or continuous arteriovenous hemodialysis and the pharmacokinetics in patients with liver disease or liver failure are not known.

In patients with normal renal function throughout the course of the poisoning, the renal clearance of ethylene glycol is consistently reported to be about 20 mL/min (see Table 32B-2).[23] In relation to ADH blockade, fomepizole administration results in first-order elimination of ethylene glycol with a prolonged half-life to 20 hours.[10,49] Thus, the antidotal regimen (dose and duration) blocks the metabolism of the toxic alcohol, resulting in its retention in the body for a longer time.

The usual contraindications of fomepizole administration are previously known allergy to pyrazole derivatives (such as phenylbutazone) and pregnancy, due to the lack of data on safety in these cases. The randomized, placebo-controlled, double-blinded studies in human volunteers[48] as well as the various clinical trials in poisoned patients[10] indicated that fomepizole is well tolerated at doses used therapeutically, although headaches (12%), nausea (11%), dizziness (7%), and irritation at the injection site were reported. Other

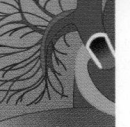

TABLE 32B-5   Dosage Regimen of Fomepizole and Ethylene Glycol Poisoning

ETHYLENE GLYCOL PLASMA CONCENTRATION		FOMEPIZOLE (mg/kg)					
g/L	mmol/L	2ND DOSE LOADING DOSE	3RD DOSE T + 12 hr	4TH DOSE T + 24 hr	5TH DOSE T + 36 hr	6TH DOSE T + 48 hr	T + 60 hr
European Dosing Regimen*							
6	96	15	10	10	10	7.5	5
3	48	15	10	10	10	7.5	
1.5	24	15	10	10	7.5		
0.75	12	15	10	7.5			
0.35	5.6	15	7.5				
0.1–0.3	1.6–5.5	15					
American Dosing Regimen‡							
	Not specified	15	10	10	10	10	15†

*Fomepizole is administered each 12 hours, by oral or intravenous route, in relation to plasma ethylene glycol concentration.
†All subsequent doses are administered as 15 mg/kg until plasma ethylene glycol level is 0.2 g/L (20 mg/dL) and the patient is asymptomatic with normal pH.
‡Data from Brent J, McMartin K, Phillips S, et al: Fomepizole for the treatment of ethylene glycol poisoning. Methylpyrazole for Toxic Alcohols Study Group. N Engl J Med 1999;340:832–838.

adverse reactions included rash, lymphangitis, vomiting, diarrhea, abdominal pain, tachycardia, hypotension, vertigo, slurred speech, inebriation, fever, mild transient eosinophilia, and slight increases in hepatic transaminases. None required the discontinuation of therapy. Drug interactions are possible with the ones modifying cytochrome P-450 activity, such as phenytoin, carbamazepine, cimetidine, or ketoconazole. Reciprocal metabolic interaction also exists between ethanol and fomepizole. In rats, the concurrent administration of ethanol with a 1 mmol/kg dose of fomepizole markedly increased the duration of fomepizole elimination.[51] The concomitant acute administration of ethanol decreased by about 50% the concentration of 4-hydroxymethylpyrazole. Similarly, in rats chronically fed diets containing fomepizole and/or ethanol, plasma fomepizole levels were higher with concomitant ethanol administration, suggesting that ethanol delays fomepizole metabolism. In human volunteers, using double-blind crossover designs, therapeutic doses of fomepizole (10 to 20 mg/kg) caused a 40% reduction in the rate of elimination of ethanol (0.5 to 0.7 g/kg). Ethanol was demonstrated to inhibit fomepizole metabolism, consequently increasing its blood concentrations.[43] Thus, the previous intake or administration of ethanol before fomepizole therapy does not decrease the efficiency of the antidotal therapy. However, the clinical relevance of the effect of fomepizole on ethanol elimination remains to be determined. Although not formally studied in children, there have been several pediatric cases reported where the drug appears to be efficacious and without severe side effects,[52-54] other than nystagmus.[55]

However, unlike ethanol, therapeutic concentrations are reliably achieved with the proposed dosing regimens, and no severe central nervous system or significant liver toxicity or hypoglycemia occurred in fomepizole-treated patients. To reduce ethanol therapy side effects, appropriate monitoring and IV glucose intake in a controlled environment such as an intensive care unit (ICU) are necessary. Monitoring of therapeutic concentrations of fomepizole does not appear to be necessary in patients with normal hepatic function. Therefore, considering its demonstrated clinical efficacy and safety, fomepizole should be recommended as a first-line antidotal treatment in poisoned patients. In the case of exposure to a toxic alcohol or diagnosis of a metabolic acidosis with elevated anion gap unexplained by a concomitant increase in serum lactate concentration, a loading dose of fomepizole should be administered while awaiting measurement of the toxic alcohol concentrations, which will permit a definitive diagnosis. Indications to begin empiric treatment for ethylene glycol poisoning are summarized in Box 32B-1.

Ethanol

Ethyl alcohol is an ADH competitive substrate blocking ethylene glycol liver metabolism when plasma ethanol

---

BOX 32B-1   **INDICATIONS TO START EMPIRIC TREATMENT FOR ETHYLENE GLYCOL POISONING, PREFERRING FOMEPIZOLE ADMINISTRATION (LOADING DOSE: 15 mg/kg) IF AVAILABLE**

History of ethylene glycol ingestion (accidental, suicidal, criminal or as alcohol substitute)
Intoxication associating decreased level of consciousness, ataxia, slurred speech, and/or focal neurologic examination in an inebriated patient without the odor of ethanol or with the absence of ethanol in blood
Unexplained metabolic acidosis, with anion gap (> 16mmol/L) and/or osmolar gap (> 15mOsmol/kg)
Calcium oxalate crystals in urine or urine that fluoresces under the Wood's lamp
Ethylene glycol concentration > 0.2 g/L

From Barceloux DG, Krenzelok EO, Olson K, Watson W: American Academy of Clinical Toxicology practice guidelines on the treatment of ethylene glycol poisoning. J Toxicol Clin Toxicol 1999;37:537–560.

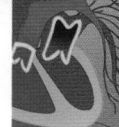

levels of 1 to 1.5 g/L are maintained. ADH is 50% inhibited for an ethanol concentration of 0.02 g/L and more than 90% for 0.5 g/L. However, ethylene glycol concentrations of greater than or equal to 3.26 g/L (5.26 mmol/L) are required to saturate the enzyme by 50%.[56] Ethanol may be administered orally or given as an IV infusion of 10% ethanol diluted in 5% dextrose. The IV route is possible in comatose patients and does not induce gastrointestinal upset. The oral route has the advantage of being simple and rapid, with various forms and concentrations readily available. However, first-pass liver metabolism reduces ethanol bioavailability. Thus, in chronic alcoholics or in case of hepatic enzyme induction, higher doses of ethanol may be required than in abstinent patients.

During ethanol administration, ethylene glycol's elimination half-life is prolonged to 17 hours but is only 2.5 hours in association with hemodialysis. The recommended ethanol regimen in ethylene glycol poisoning management is a loading dose of 0.6 to 0.7 g/kg of 50% ethanol, followed by a maintenance dose of 110 mg/kg/hr of 20% ethanol, or greater, if large amounts of ethylene glycol were ingested. The ethanol should be diluted to 10% if given IV (Table 32B-6). This median dose may vary between 66 mg/kg/hr (for nondrinkers) to 154 mg/kg/hr (for alcoholics). Ethanol therapy should be continued until plasma ethylene glycol concentration is less than 0.2 g/L or undetectable.[23] Plasma ethanol concentrations should be closely monitored, every 1 to 2 hours. During hemodialysis, ethanol should be administered at a rate of 230 mg/kg/hr to maintain blood ethanol levels between 1.0 and 1.5 g/L. Ninety-five percent ethanol can be added to the dialysate bath to reach concentrations of 1.0 g/L, allowing easier ethanol blood level stabilization.[57] Adverse effects are numerous, limiting indications of ethanol to centers where fomepizole is unavailable: inebriation, obtundation, CNS depression (with the risk of need for intubation), pancreatitis, hypoglycemia in children, and local phlebitis requiring infusions by central venous access. That said, a recent study demonstrated a low rate of clinically important adverse effects related to ethanol used as an antidote to treat methanol poisoning in children.[58] Despite wide variation in ethanol levels, but with appropriate monitoring and IV glucose intake in a controlled environment such as a pediatric intensive care unit, ethanol therapy does not carry as many risks as generally believed.

HEMODIALYSIS

Hemodialysis is considered to be an integral part of the treatment of patients receiving ethanol or fomepizole therapy to expedite removal of the alcohol and thus reduce the duration of antidote treatment. Hemodialysis clearance of toxicant depends on molecular size, charge, distribution, and protein- or lipid-binding status. Ethylene glycol is efficiently cleared by dialysis (see Table 32B-2). The traditional end-point of dialysis is a plasma concentration of less than 0.2 g/L or undetectable, with disappearance of acid-base imbalance and correction of the anion and osmolar gap.[23] More recently, a simple method to estimate the required dialysis time was validated in 13 ethylene glycol– and 5 methanol-poisoned patients.[59,60] The required dialysis time (RDT) to reach a 5 mmol/L toxin concentration target was obtained by the following formula: RDT (h) = [-V· Ln (5/A)] / 0.06k, where V (L) is Watson's estimate of total body water, A is the initial toxin concentration in mmol/L, and k (mL/min) is 80% of the manufacturer-specified dialyzer urea clearance. In these studies, there was no difference between the predicted hemodialysis duration and that actually carried out based on hourly concentration sampling.

Hemodialysis has usually been recommended in cases of confirmed ethylene glycol poisoning, severe or refractory metabolic acidosis, and deteriorating vital signs, and in the onset of acute renal failure (Box 32B-2). A serum ethylene glycol concentration above 50 mg/dL was a well-recognized indication, even though not all investigators agree.[61] In the U.S. META study, 17 of 19 ethylene glycol–poisoned patients treated with fomepizole were hemodialyzed.[10] Among them, 18 survived, whereas only 1 died secondary to a myocardial infarction. All the patients in whom renal injury developed (9 of

TABLE 32B-6 Therapeutic Doses of Ethanol in Ethylene Glycol Poisoning, According to the Patient Status and Equivalence Between the Different Ethanol Presentations

	ABSOLUTE ETHANOL	VOLUME (43% ORAL SOLUTION)	VOLUME (10% IV SOLUTION)
Loading dose	600 mg/kg	1.8 mL/kg	7.6 mL/kg
Standard maintenance dose			
Nondrinker	66 mg/kg/hr	0.2 mL/kg/hr	0.83 mL/kg/hr
Chronic alcoholic	154 mg/kg/hr	0.46 mL/kg/hr	1.96 mL/kg/hr
Standard maintenance dose during hemodialysis			
Nondrinker	169 mg/kg/hr	0.5 mL/kg/hr	2.13 mL/kg/hr
Chronic alcoholic	257 mg/kg/hr	0.77 mL/kg/hr	3.26 mL/kg/hr

BOX 32B-2   REVISED RECOMMENDATIONS FOR HEMODIALYSIS IN ETHYLENE GLYCOL

Arterial pH < 7.10
Drop in arterial pH > 0.05 resulting in a pH outside the normal range despite bicarbonate infusion
Inability to maintain arterial pH > 7.3 despite bicarbonate therapy
Decrease in bicarbonate concentration > 5 mmol/L despite bicarbonate therapy
Rise in serum creatinine by > 90 mmol/L
Recently released: Initial plasma ethylene glycol concentration ≥ 50 mg/dL

Data from references 23 and 61.

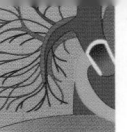

19, 46%), had a plasma glycolate concentration on admission of greater than 98 mg/dL. Renal elimination and hemodialysis are the only significant routes of ethylene glycol elimination, as long as fomepizole concentrations are maintained well above 10 μmol/L.[49] Hemodialysis effectively clears glycolate, with an elimination rate of 170 ± 23 mmol/L/min and a half-time of 155 ± 474 minutes, compared with the spontaneous elimination rate of 1.8 ± 0.67 mL/L/min and half-time of 625 ± 474 min.[16]

In a retrospective study, Borron and colleagues demonstrated the lack of requirement of systematic dialysis in the management of ethylene glycol poisoning treated with fomepizole.[41] Among 38 patients treated for suspicion of ethylene glycol exposure, 11 patients had ethylene glycol concentrations of greater than 0.2 g/L. Among these, 21% presented in coma, 34% in metabolic acidosis, and 11% with an initial plasma creatinine of greater than 110 μmol/L (1.2 mg/dL). Hemodialysis was performed in only 3 of these 11 patients, 2 with renal insufficiency and acidosis and 1 with a very high ethylene glycol concentration (134 mmol/L, or 837.5 mg/dL), but with normal renal function. Among the 7 patients with normal renal function treated with fomepizole, no subsequent deterioration was noted. Among all the 38 patients, only 1 died within a few hours after his admission, with severe multiorgan failure, whose onset started before fomepizole administration. Patients who were dialyzed were significantly more acidotic (arterial pH 7.11 vs. 7.31) than those who were not. Patients treated with fomepizole prior to the onset of significant acidosis did not require hemodialysis. Since this study, new insights have been developed with regard to hemodialysis criteria. An absolute concentration above 0.5 g/dL is no longer considered to be an independent criterion for hemodialysis in patients treated with fomepizole.[49] The use of hemodialysis should be based on the presence of renal insufficiency or severe metabolic acidosis rather than unsupported criteria of serum concentrations greater than 0.5 g/L alone.[62] The recommended criteria are now the existence of a significant metabolic acidosis (pH < 7.25), renal failure, or electrolyte imbalances unresponsive to conventional therapy and deteriorating vital signs despite intensive supportive care.[23] Before fomepizole availability, repeated hemodialysis had been recommended in case of redistribution of ethylene glycol within 12 hours after its cessation.[63] Initial serum glycolic acid concentration appears to be a good indicator for hemodialysis. However, it is not readily available in the majority of hospitals. An initial glycolic acid level higher than 10 mmol/L predicts acute renal failure, with a sensitivity of 100%, a specificity of 94%, and an efficiency of 98%.[64] In a retrospective study including 41 ethylene glycol–poisoned patients, these researchers demonstrated that a glycolic acid concentration higher than 8 mmol/L is a criterion for the initiation of hemodialysis. On the contrary, ethylene glycol concentration was not predictive of acute renal failure or central nervous system toxicity, while an anion gap of greater than 20 mmol/L or pH of less than 7.30 predicts acute renal failure. There was no need to dialyze, regardless of ethylene glycol level, if the glycolic acid level was less than or equal to 8 mmol/L in patients receiving antidotal treatment.[64]

CRITICAL ANALYSIS OF ETHYLENE GLYCOL TREATMENT

Although ethanol and hemodialysis constituted the recommended therapy for many years, it is unlikely that applying principles of evidence-based medicine would justify such recommendations now, given the significant experience with fomepizole and dialysis.[62] While it would have been desirable in the U.S. prospective trial[10] to have a comparison group with the standard of practice (ethanol plus hemodialysis), this was not done for a variety of reasons. Nonetheless, until demonstration that ethanol therapy results in equivalent efficacy and outcomes, it is difficult not to recommend fomepizole. To date, there has been no randomized comparative study regarding efficacy and cost effectiveness among hemodialysis + ethanol versus hemodialysis + fomepizole or fomepizole alone. There are frequent references to the minimal cost of parenteral ethanol in comparison with the relatively high cost of fomepizole. Such comparisons generally ignore the critical issue of laboratory costs for monitoring serum ethanol and blood glucose, the increased nursing care required for patients maintained in a state of ethanol intoxication, and the requirement for intensive care (which may not be necessary in patients receiving fomepizole in the absence of extant toxicity). Considering the high cost of fomepizole (about $1000 per gram), smaller hospital centers that only occasionally see ethylene glycol poisoning might prefer to continue to stock inexpensive and readily available parenteral ethanol rather than fomepizole.[65] However, it should be kept in mind that the suggested shelf life of fomepizole is 3 years and that, in some cases, the manufacturer will replace it at no charge after this period, rendering it economical even for smaller emergency departments to have this antidote in their armamentarium.

Why is it worthwhile to confirm that fomepizole may obviate hemodialysis under certain conditions? First, there is a significant downside to the use of hemodialysis: it is not universally available, rendering it difficult to obtain in case of epidemic poisonings. It represents an invasive technique with risks of adverse effects, such as hemorrhage, catheter infections, and metabolic disorders (hypophosphatemia). Moreover, hemodialysis of poisoned patients often requires hospitalization in an ICU. If significant toxicity and hemodialysis can be avoided by the early administration of fomepizole, ICU admissions may be limited to a relatively brief (24-hour) period of observation (Fig. 32B-3). There are also advantages to the use of fomepizole in comparison with ethanol: fomepizole is a more potent ADH inhibitor (and not a substrate), with a wider therapeutic index, a longer duration of action, easier dosing, and more predictable kinetics. There is no need for blood fomepizole concentration monitoring, treatments are well tolerated, and there are no similar data to prove ethanol efficacy. Use of ethanol, in our estimation, should now be limited to settings where fomepizole is

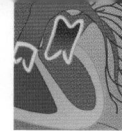

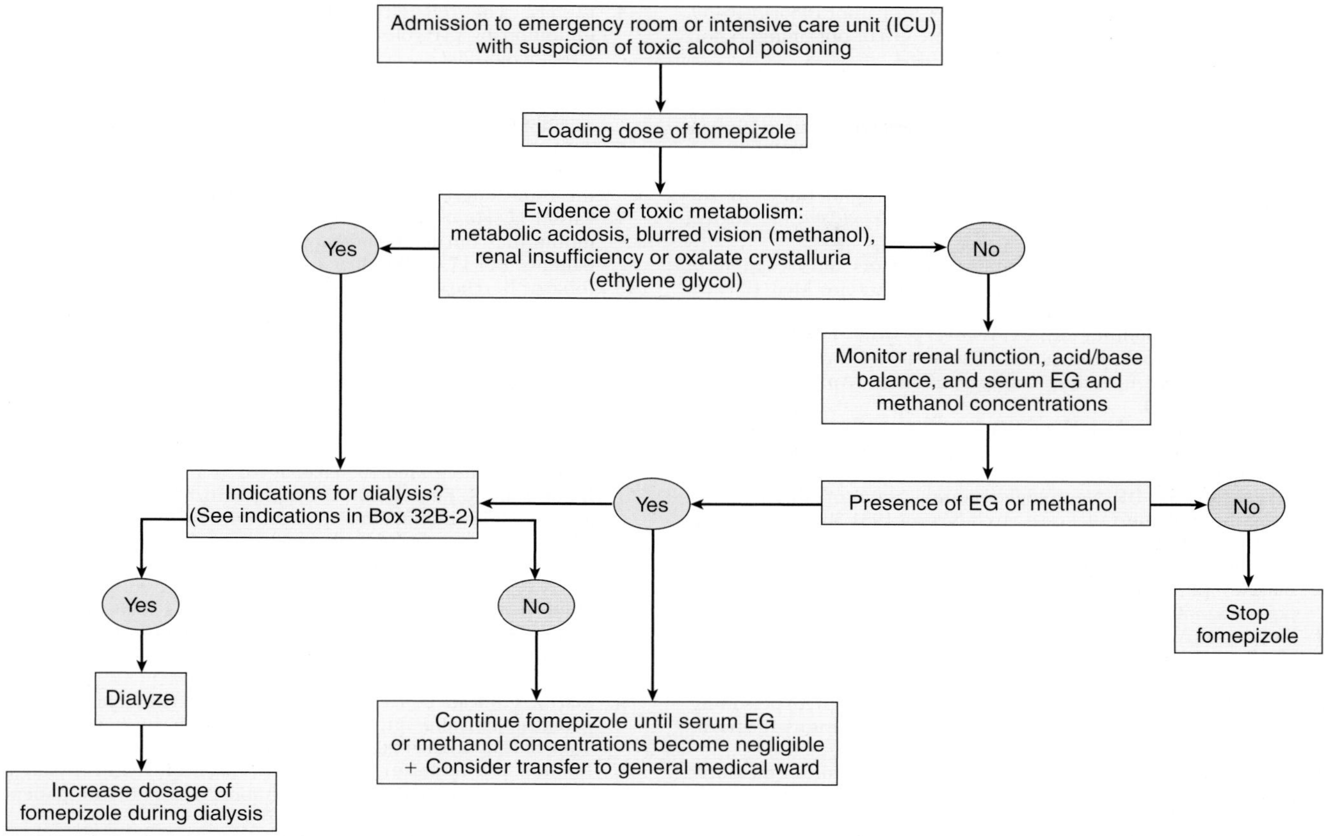

```
┌─────────────────────────────────────────┐
│ Admission to emergency room or intensive │
│ care unit (ICU) with suspicion of toxic  │
│ alcohol poisoning                        │
└─────────────────────────────────────────┘
                    │
                    ▼
        ┌──────────────────────────┐
        │ Loading dose of fomepizole│
        └──────────────────────────┘
                    │
                    ▼
        ┌──────────────────────────────────────┐
  ┌Yes─┤ Evidence of toxic metabolism:          ├─No─┐
  │    │ metabolic acidosis, blurred vision     │    │
  │    │ (methanol), renal insufficiency or     │    │
  │    │ oxalate crystalluria (ethylene glycol) │    │
  │    └──────────────────────────────────────┘    │
  │                                                 ▼
  │                            ┌──────────────────────────┐
  │                            │ Monitor renal function,  │
  │                            │ acid/base balance, and   │
  │                            │ serum EG and methanol    │
  │                            │ concentrations           │
  │                            └──────────────────────────┘
  │                                                 │
  │                                                 ▼
  │  ┌──────────────────────┐        ┌──────────────────────────┐
  └─▶│ Indications for      │◀─Yes───┤ Presence of EG or methanol├─No─┐
     │ dialysis? (See       │        └──────────────────────────┘    │
     │ indications in Box   │                                        ▼
     │ 32B-2)               │                              ┌──────────────┐
     └──────────────────────┘                              │ Stop         │
       │                │                                  │ fomepizole   │
      Yes               No                                 └──────────────┘
       │                │
       ▼                ▼
  ┌─────────┐   ┌──────────────────────────────────┐
  │ Dialyze │   │ Continue fomepizole until serum  │
  └─────────┘   │ EG or methanol concentrations    │
       │        │ become negligible + Consider     │
       ▼        │ transfer to general medical ward │
  ┌──────────┐  └──────────────────────────────────┘
  │ Increase │
  │ dosage of│
  │ fomepizole│
  │ during   │
  │ dialysis │
  └──────────┘
```

FIGURE 32B-3 Proposed algorithm for treatment of ethylene glycol– and methanol-poisoned patients. This algorithm is based on series and case reports and has not been validated prospectively. (Adapted from Megarbane B, Borron SW, Baud FJ: Current recommendations for treatment of severe toxic alcohol poisonings. Intensive Care Med 2005;31:189–195.)

unavailable or in patients for whom fomepizole is contraindicated. Given its safety, especially in patients who may subsequently be found not to be poisoned with toxic alcohols, fomepizole is of value in emergency medicine because it permits a margin of diagnostic error. In selected exposed patients, fomepizole may obviate the need for hemodialysis. However, the risks and benefits of fomepizole must be weighed against those of hemodialysis. Accelerated blood clearance by an adequate single hemodialysis session provides for a shorter hospital stay and fewer required doses of ADH inhibitors.[66]

REFERENCES

1. Watson WA, Litovitz TL, Klein-Schwartz W, et al: 2003 annual report of the American Association of Poison Control Centers Toxic Exposure Surveillance System. Am J Emerg Med 2004;22:325–404.
2. Wills JH, Coulston F, Harris ES, et al: Inhalation of aerosolized ethylene glycol by man. Clin Toxicol 1974;7:463–476.
3. Troisi FM: Chronic intoxication with ethylene glycol vapour. Br J Ind Med 1950;1:65.
4. Johnson B, Meggs WJ, Bentzel CJ: Emergency department hemodialysis in a case of severe ethylene glycol poisoning. Ann Emerg Med 1999;33:108–110.
5. Mundy RL, Hall LM, Teague RS: Pyrazole as an antidote for ethylene glycol poisoning. Toxicol Appl Pharmacol 1974;28:320–322.
6. Gessner PK, Parke DV, Williams RT: Studies in detoxication. 86. The metabolism of 14C-labelled ethylene glycol. Biochem J 1961;79:482–489.

7. Jacobsen D, McMartin KE: Antidotes for methanol and ethylene glycol poisoning. J Toxicol Clin Toxicol 1997;35:127–143.
8. Cheng JT, Beysolow TD, Kaul B, et al: Clearance of ethylene glycol by kidneys and hemodialysis. J Toxicol Clin Toxicol 1987;25:95–108.
9. Weiss B, Coen G: Effect of ethanol on ethylene glycol oxidation by mammalian liver enzymes. Enzymol Biol Clin (Basel) 1966;6:297–304.
10. Brent J, McMartin K, Phillips S, et al: Fomepizole for the treatment of ethylene glycol poisoning. Methylpyrazole for Toxic Alcohols Study Group. N Engl J Med 1999;340:832–838.
11. Jacobsen D, Hewlett TP, Webb R, Brown ST: Ethylene glycol intoxication: evaluation of kinetics and crystalluria. Am J Med 1988;84:145–151.
12. Peterson CD, Collins AJ, Himes JM, Keane WF: Ethylene glycol poisoning: pharmacokinetics during therapy with ethanol and hemodialysis. N Engl J Med 1981;304:21–23.
13. Hoffman RS, Smilkstein MJ, Howland MA, Goldfrank LR: Osmol gaps revisited: normal values and limitations. Clin Toxicol 1993;31:81–93.
14. Clay KL, Murphy RC: On the metabolic acidosis of ethylene glycol intoxication. Toxicol Appl Pharmacol 1977;39:39–49.
15. Jacobsen D, Ovrebo S, Ostborg J, Sejersted OM: Glycolate causes the acidosis in ethylene glycol poisoning and is effectively removed by hemodialysis. Acta Med Scand 1984;216:409–416.
16. Moreau CL, Kerns W II, Tomaszewski CA, et al: Glycolate kinetics and hemodialysis in ethylene glycol poisoining. J Toxicol Clin Toxicol 1998;36:659–666.
17. Berman LB, Schreiner GE, Feys J: The nephrotoxic lesion of ethylene glycol. Ann Intern Med 1957;46:611–619.
18. Pons CA, Custer RP: Acute ethylene glycol poisoning: a clinicopathologic report of eighteen fatal cases. Am J Med Sci 1946;211:544.

19. Bove KE: Ethylene glycol toxicity. Am J Clin Pathol 1966;45:46–50.

20. Munro KMH, Adams JH: Acute ethylene glycol poisoning: report of a fatal case. Med Sci Law 1967;7:181–184.

21. Mair W: Cerebral computed tomography of ethylene glycol intoxication. Neuroradiology 1983;24:175–177.

22. Milles G: Ethylene glycol poisoning with suggestions for its treatment as oxalate poisoning. Arch Pathol 1946;41:631–638.

23. Barceloux DG, Krenzelok EO, Olson K, Watson W: American Academy of Clinical Toxicology practice guidelines on the treatment of ethylene glycol poisoning. J Toxicol Clin Toxicol 1999;37:537–560.

24. Hylander B, Kjellstrand CM: Prognostic factors and treatment of severe ethylene glycol intoxication. Intensive Care Med 1996;22:546–552.

25. Kahn HS, Brotchner RJ: A recovery from ethylene glycol (antifreeze) intoxication: a case of survival and two fatalities from ethylene glycol including autopsy findings. Ann Intern Med 1950;32:284–294.

26. Davies D, Bramwell KJ, Hamilton RS, Williams SR: Ethylene glycol poisoning: case report of a record-high level and a review. J Emerg Med 1997;15:653–667.

27. Berger JR, Ayyar DR: Neurological complications of ethylene glycol intoxication. Report of a case. Arch Neurol 1981;38:724–726.

28. Spillane L, Roberts JR, Meyer AE: Multiple cranial nerve deficits after ethylene glycol poisoning. Ann Emerg Med 1991;20:208–210.

29. Blakeley KR, Rinner SE, Knochel JP: Survival of ethylene glycol poisoning with profound acidemia. N Engl J Med 1993;328:515–516.

30. Steinke W, Arendt G, Mull M, et al: Good recovery after sublethal ethylene glycol intoxication: serial EEG and CT findings. J Neurol 1989;236:170–173.

31. Eder AF, McGrath CM, Dowdy YG, et al: Ethylene glycol poisoning: toxicokinetic and analytical factors affecting laboratory diagnosis. Clin Chem 1998;44:168–177.

32. Morgan TJ, Clark C, Clague A: Artifactual elevation of measured plasma l-lactate concentration in the presence of glycolate. Crit Care Med 1999;27:2177–2179.

33. Porter WH, Crellin M, Rutter PW, Oeltgen P: Interference by glycolic acid in the Beckman Synchron Method for lactate: a useful clue for unsuspected ethylene glycol intoxication. Clin Chem 2000;46:874–875.

34. Steinhart B: Case report: severe ethylene glycol intoxication with normal osmolal gap—"a chilling thought." J Emerg Med 1990;8:583.

35. Hewlett TP, McMartin RE: Ethylene glycol intoxication: the value of glycolic acid determination for diagnosis and treatment. Clin Toxicol 1986;24:389.

36. Heckerling PS: Ethylene glycol poisoning with a normal anion gap due to occult bromide intoxication. Ann Emerg Med 1987;16:1384.

37. Bjellerup P, Kallner A, Kollind M: GLC determination of serum-ethylene glycol, interferences in ketotic patients. J Toxicol Clin Toxicol 1994;32:85–87.

38. Standefer J, Blackwell W: Enzymatic method for measuring ethylene glycol with a centrifugal analyzer. Clin Chem 1991;37:1734–1736.

39. Baud FJ, Galliot M, Astier A, et al: Treatment of ethylene glycol poisoning with intravenous 4-methylpyrazole. N Engl J Med 1988;319:97–100.

40. Baud FJ, Bismuth C, Garnier R, et al: J Toxicol Clin Toxicol 1986;24:463–483.

41. Borron SW, Mégarbane B, Baud FJ: Fomepizole in treatment of uncomplicated ethylene glycol poisoning. Lancet 1999;354:831.

42. McMartin KE, Hedström KG, Tolf BR, et al: Studies on the metabolic interactions between 4-methylpyrazole and methanol using the monkey as an animal model. Arch Biochem Biophys 1980;199:606–614.

43. Jacobsen D, Barron SK, Sebastian CS, et al: Non-linear kinetics of 4-methylpyrazole in healthy human subjects. Eur J Clin Pharmacol 1989;37:599–604.

44. Li TK, Theorell H: Human liver alcohol dehydrogenase: inhibition by pyrazole and pyrazole analogs. Acta Chem Scand 1969;23:892–902.

45. Jacobsen D, Sebastian CS, Dies DF, et al: Kinetic interactions between 4-methylpyrazole and ethanol in healthy humans. Alcohol Clin Exp Res 1996;20:804–809.

46. Tournaud C, Kopferschmidt J, Sauder P, et al: Ethylene glycol poisoning treated with 4-methylpyrazole [abstract]. Presented at the 15th Congress of the EAPCCT, Istanbul, 1992.

47. Faissel H, Houze P, Baud FJ, Scherrmann JM: 4-methylpyrazole monitoring during hemodialysis of ethylene glycol intoxicated patients. Eur J Clin Pharmacol 1995;49:211–213.

48. Jobard E, Harry P, Turcant A, et al: 4-methylpyrazole and hemodialysis in ethylene glycol poisoning. J Toxicol Clin Toxicol 1996;34:379–381.

49. Sivilotti MLA, Burns MJ, McMartin KE, Brent J: Toxicokinetics of ethylene glycol during fomepizole therapy: implications for management. Ann Emerg Med 2000;36:114–125.

50. Jacobsen D, Sebastian CS, Barron SK, et al: Effects of 4-methylpyrazole, methanol/ethylene glycol antidote, in healthy humans. J Emerg Med 1990;8:455–461.

51. Blomstrand R, Ellin A, Löf A, Ostling-Wintzell H: Biological effects and metabolic interactions after chronic and acute administration of 4-methylpyrazole and ethanol to rats. Arch Biochem Biophys 1980;199:591–605.

52. Harry P, Jobard E, Briand M, et al: Ethylene glycol poisoning in a child treated with 4-methylpyrazole. Pediatrics 1998;102:31–33.

53. Baum CR, Langman CB, Oker EE, et al: Fomepizole treatment of ethylene glycol poisoning in an infant. Pediatrics 2000;106:1489–1491.

54. Martin Caravati E, Heileson HL, Jones M: Treatment of severe pediatric ethylene glycol intoxication without hemodialysis. J Toxicol Clin Toxicol 2004;42:255–259.

55. Benitez JG, Swanson-Biearman B, Krenzelok EP: Nystagmus secondary to fomepizole administration in a pediatric patient. J Toxicol Clin Toxicol 2000;38:795–798.

56. Pietruszko R, Voigtlander K, Lester D: Alcohol dehydrogenase from human and horse liver: substrate specificity with diols. Biochem Pharmacol 1978;27:1296.

57. Peterson CD, Collins A, Himes JM, et al: Ethylene glycol poisoning. Pharmacokinetics during therapy with ethanol and hemodialysis. N Engl J Med 1981;304:21.

58. Roy M, Bailey B, Chalut D, et al: What are the adverse effects of ethanol used as an antidote in the treatment of suspected methanol poisoning in children? J Toxicol Clin Toxicol 2003;41:155–161.

59. Hirsch DJ, Jindal KK, Wong P, Fraser AD: A simple method to estimate the required dialysis time for cases of alcohol poisoning. Kidney Int 2001;60:2021–2024.

60. Youssef GM, Hirsch DJ: Validation of a method to predict required dialysis time for cases of methanol and ethylene glycol poisoning. Am J Kidney Dis 2005;46:509–511.

61. Ellenhorn MJ: Alcohols and glycols. In Ellenhorn MJ, Schonwald S, Ordog G, Wasserberger J (eds): Ellenhorn's Medical Toxicology: Diagnosis and Treatment of Human Poisoning, 2nd ed. Baltimore, Williams & Wilkins, 1997, pp 1127–1166.

62. Watson WA: Ethylene glycol toxicity: closing in on rational, evidence-based treatment. Ann Emerg Med 2000;36:114–125.

63. Gabow PA, Clay K, Sullivan JB, Lepoff R: Organic acids in ethylene glycol intoxication. Ann Intern Med 1986;105:16–20.

64. Porter WH, Rutter PW, Bush BA, et al: Ethylene glycol toxicity: the role of serum glycolic acid in hemodialysis. J Toxicol Clin Toxicol 2001;39:607–615.

65. Goldfarb DS: Fomepizole for ethylene glycol poisoning. Lancet 1999;354:1646.

66. Vasavada N, Williams C, Hellman RN: Ethylene glycol intoxication: case report and pharmacokinetic perspectives. Pharmacotherapy 2003;23:1652–1658.

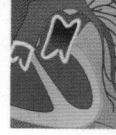

C   Other Toxic Alcohols

MARCO L. SIVILOTTI, MD, MSc

At a Glance...

- These alcohols range considerably in their degree of toxicity.
- Multiple routes of exposure are possible, which in turn affect the degree of toxicity.
- Poisoning with certain alcohols may produce early central nervous system depression and elevation of serum osmolality followed by a delayed-onset metabolic acidosis and renal failure.
- Fomepizole or ethanol are potential antidotes in selected cases.
- Isopropanol poisoning results in ketosis (acetonemia and acetonuria) without significant metabolic acidosis, and can almost always be managed supportively in a manner analogous to ethanol intoxication.

Although ethanol, methanol, and ethylene glycol account for the vast majority of toxicity from alcohols encountered in clinical practice, other members of this chemical class can also be harmful to human health. An alcohol is any compound with a hydroxyl (-OH) group attached to a carbon chain. The chemical structures of commonly encountered alcohols are shown in Table 32C-1. Since their toxicities vary considerably, they will be discussed individually.

ISOPROPANOL

Isopropanol (2-propanol, isopropyl alcohol) is widely used as a solvent, rubefacient, and sterilizing agent and is found in many skin lotions, mouthwashes, rubbing alcohols, and cleaning fluids. Being readily available and less expensive than ethanol, it is often abused as an ethanol substitute. The IDLH (immediate danger to life and health) workplace standard according to the

National Institute of Occupational Safety and Health is 2000 ppm.

Isopropanol is rapidly absorbed after oral ingestion into a volume of distribution of 0.7 L/kg. Peak serum concentrations occur from 30 to 120 minutes after ingestion, whereas peak concentrations of its metabolite, acetone, do not occur until 4 hours after ingestion.[1] Inhalation and dermal application can also result in substantial absorption and subsequent toxicity.[2-5] Isopropanol is metabolized primarily by alcohol dehydrogenase (ADH) in the liver (80%). A smaller fraction is eliminated unchanged by the kidneys. The serum elimination half-life is 2.5 to 16.2 hours, and increases substantially when ethanol or fomepizole are also present.[6-12] Because isopropanol is a secondary alcohol (the hydroxyl group is attached to a carbon atom bonded to two other carbon atoms), oxidation yields a ketone (acetone), which cannot be further oxidized to an organic acid.[13] Acetone is slowly eliminated by the lungs and kidneys with a half-life ranging from 7.6 to 26 hours.[7,14,15] As a result, the biochemical hallmark of isopropanol metabolism is the presence of a substantial ketonemia and ketonuria without acidemia.

Clinically, isopropanol ingestion resembles acute ethanol poisoning. Central nervous system (CNS) depression develops rapidly, and has generally reached its nadir within a few hours of the ingestion. Animal data suggest that the CNS depressant effects of isopropanol are two to three times more potent than ethanol, whereas its metabolite, acetone, has CNS depressant effects equivalent to ethanol.[16] CNS depression can range from mild lethargy with slurred speech and ataxia to deep coma with areflexia. The fruity breath odor of ketones may be appreciated on physical examination. Other clinical findings include hemorrhagic gastritis, vomiting, abdominal pain, hemorrhagic tracheobron-

TABLE 32C-1 Chemical Structure and Molecular Weight of Selected Alcohols

	CHEMICAL STRUCTURE	MOLECULAR WEIGHT (DALTONS)
Methanol	CH_3OH	32
Ethanol	CH_3-CH_2OH	46
Isopropanol	$CH_3-CHOH-CH_3$	60
Benzyl alcohol	$(C_6H_5)-CH_2OH$	108
Ethylene glycol	CH_2OH-CH_2OH	62
Propylene glycol	$CH_2OH-CHOH-CH_3$	76
Polyethylene glycols	$CH_2OH-CH_2-O-(CH_2-CH_2-O)_nH$	
Diethylene glycol	n = 1	106
Triethylene glycol	n = 2	150
PEG-400	n = 8–9	~400
PEG-3350	n = 68–84	~3350
Ethylene glycol ethers (cellosolves)	$CH_3-(CH_2)_n-O-CH_2-CH_2OH$, n = 0	
Ethylene glycol monomethyl ether	n = 0	76
Ethylene glycol monoethyl ether	n = 1	90
Ethylene glycol monobutyl ether	n = 3	118

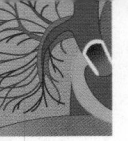

chitis, tachycardia, muscle weakness, and pulmonary aspiration. Rarely, massive ingestion results in hypotension from vasodilatation and negative cardiac inotropic effects, and respiratory arrest. The duration of CNS depression may be prolonged due to the added CNS depressant effects and slower rate of elimination of the acetone metabolite.

Serum isopropanol concentrations can be measured by gas chromatography, and may be reported on an "alcohol screen" in addition to methanol and ethanol (but not necessarily ethylene glycol). Serum concentrations of at least 50 to 100 mg/dL (8 to 17 mmol/L) result in intoxication, and of at least 150 mg/dL (25 mmol/L) result in coma, although tolerance can diminish these effects. Cardiovascular depression is generally seen at concentrations above 450 mg/dL (75 mmol/L). Because treatment is largely supportive and determined by clinical findings, serum isopropanol concentrations usually add little information beyond identifying and quantifying the exposure. Small concentrations of isopropanol may be detectable in the serum of patients with alcoholic, starvation, and diabetic ketoacidosis due to acetone reduction back to isopropanol.[17,18] In one study, 15% of patients with diabetic ketoacidosis had detectable serum concentrations of isopropanol, ranging as high as 30 mg/dL.[17] Breath analysis for ethanol by infrared absorption may detect isopropanol as an interferent.[19] Some enzymatic assays may misrepresent isopropanol as ethanol.

In general, the presence or absence of an osmol gap is neither sensitive nor specific and cannot be used to rule in or out a toxic alcohol ingestion (see Chapter 3). Both isopropanol and acetone will increase serum osmolality. For each 1 mg/dL of either isopropanol (molecular weight 60 daltons) or acetone (58 daltons) in the serum, the serum osmolality will increase by about 0.17 mOsm/kg. Therefore, either isopropanol or acetone contribute approximately 10 mOsm/kg at a combined concentration of 60 mg/dL (10 mmol/L), and the osmolal gap multiplied by 6 approximates the summed serum concentrations of isopropanol and acetone in mg/dL. Thus, when history, physical examination, and initial laboratory data suggest poisoning with isopropanol and conclusive measurement of this alcohol is not immediately available, the osmolal gap can be used to quantify and follow the exposure with good sensitivity, since the metabolite, acetone, is both osmotically active and uncharged.

Acetone is detectable in the serum within 30 minutes, and in the urine within 3 hours after isopropyl alcohol ingestion.[1] Conversely, the absence of serum acetone effectively rules out isopropanol ingestion, unless ethanol is also present. Acetone can interfere with serum creatinine assays,[20-22] and persists after isopropanol is undetectable. Other laboratory findings associated with isopropanol poisoning include rhabdomyolysis, hemolytic anemia, and renal tubular acidosis.

Patient management closely parallels acute ethanol ingestion. Gastrointestinal decontamination is rarely indicated due to the delay that usually occurs between ingestion and hospital presentation. Large doses of activated charcoal have been shown to adsorb both isopropanol and acetone in vitro.[23] Administration of such large doses of activated charcoal, however, is impractical in the care of poisoned patients. Thus, in circumstances where a patient can be treated immediately after a massive ingestion, small nasogastric tube aspiration is the only decontamination necessary. Supportive care must emphasize airway protection and ensure adequate tissue oxygenation. Careful monitoring and frequent reassessment are essential. As with ethanol, the pharmacokinetics are such that peak CNS effects typically occur by the time of hospital presentation. If symptoms have not developed within 2 hours after reported ingestion, they will not develop, and patients can be cleared for discharge.[24] Unlike ethanol, however, the duration of CNS depression may be prolonged. Regardless, serial observation should demonstrate an improving level of consciousness with time. Indeed, a deterioration should lead the clinician to investigate alternate causes of the depressed level of consciousness. Similarly, the presence of a metabolic acidosis demands a careful evaluation of alternate diagnoses, including alcoholic ketoacidosis (see Chapter 6) and inadequate tissue perfusion following massive ingestion.

Inhibition of ADH using either fomepizole or ethanol is not indicated and would only serve to prolong toxic effects.[12,13] Hemodialysis, while effective at removing both isopropanol and acetone, is not necessary for the vast majority of patients. Hemodialysis should be reserved for the rare patient with severe hemodynamic compromise despite fluid resuscitation.[25,26]

THE HIGHER ALCOHOLS

The higher saturated aliphatic alcohols may also have some toxicity. The higher liquid alcohols are butyl, amyl, ethyl, hexyl, and so on, and the solid fatty alcohols include lauryl, myristyl, cetyl, and stearyl. The liquid alcohols are used as solvents, and the solid fatty alcohols are used in cosmetics. The term *fusel alcohol* is used to describe the higher-order alcohols produced by natural fermentation, and are present in beer and other alcoholic beverages at concentrations as high as 2200 ppm.[27] In general, the CNS potency of an alcohol increases with increasing carbon chain length.[16] The order of increasing toxicity by single oral doses is as follows: ethanol, isopropanol, *n*-propanol, *sec*-butyl, *n*-butyl, *tert*-butyl, isobutyl, and amyl alcohol. *n*-Butyl alcohol vapors have produced conjunctivitis and keratitis. Although skin irritation is common with the liquid alcohols, percutaneous absorption does not seem to occur. Vapor inhalation may produce pulmonary injury. The amyl alcohols are more potent, and ingestion or rectal instillation of about 30 mL has proved lethal in human adults. Glycosuria and methemoglobinemia may result from ingestion of isoamyl alcohol.

The primary alcohols, such as ethanol, *n*-propanol, *n*-butyl, and isobutyl alcohol, are oxidized to aldehydes and carboxylic acids. Therefore, significant metabolic acidosis may result from their ingestion. The secondary

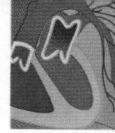

alcohols, such as isopropanol and *sec*-butyl alcohol, are converted to ketones, which may also cause CNS depression. The tertiary alcohols such as *tert*-butyl alcohol are metabolized slowly and incompletely, and excreted in the urine as glucuronides.

Very few cases of human toxicity have been described. In general, the major clinical effects are in the CNS, particularly with vaporizing compounds, and include headache, muscle weakness, giddiness, ataxia, confusion, delirium, and coma. If these agents are ingested, GI effects predominate and consist of vomiting and diarrhea. The odor of the alcohol may be noted. Fusel alcohols may contribute to both the flavor and side effects ("hangover") of certain alcoholic beverages. Death from higher alcohols is mainly due to respiratory failure but may also result from cardiac arrhythmias.

BENZYL ALCOHOL

Benzyl alcohol (α-hydroxytoluene) is an aromatic alcohol used as an antimicrobial preservative at concentrations ranging from 0.9% to 2.0% in many multidose medication vials and parenteral solutions. It is readily oxidized in vivo to benzoic acid, and conjugated with glycine to form hippuric acid. Neonates have reduced capacity to metabolize benzoic acid, and toxicity may result from bioaccumulation of benzyl alcohol and benzoic acid with repetitive dosing. Neonates inadvertently given 100 to 240 mg/kg/day of benzyl alcohol (mostly in bacteriostatic catheter flush solutions) developed a syndrome of CNS depression, severe metabolic acidosis, gasping respiration, thrombocytopenia, hepatorenal failure, seizures, intracranial hemorrhage, bradycardia, skin breakdown, cardiovascular collapse, and death, termed the "gasping baby syndrome."[28] The evidence for causation rests on the original case-control description, elevated concentrations of serum and urine metabolites, and the disappearance of the syndrome with the removal of bacteriostatic solutions from the nursery.[28,29] A reduction in kernicterus, intracranial hemorrhage, neurologic deficit, and perhaps mortality has also been associated with elimination of benzyl alcohol solutions in neonates.[30-32] The daily dose of benzyl alcohol should not exceed 5 mg/kg body weight.[33] Some common parenteral medications formulated with benzyl alcohol include amiodarone, atracurium, atropine sulfate, bacteriostatic water and saline for injection, bumetanide, chlordiazepoxide, diazepam, furosemide, glycopyrrolate, heparin, hydroxyzine, metoclopramide, midazolam, lorazepam, pancuronium, physostigmine, procainamide, prochlorperazine, succinylcholine, and trimethoprim-sulfamethoxazole.

PROPYLENE GLYCOL

Propylene glycol (1,2-propanediol; PG) is a clear, colorless, odorless, sweet-tasting liquid that is widely used as a solvent and antimicrobial preservative. PG is considerably less toxic than ethylene glycol,[34] and thus commonly used as the main ingredient in many "ethylene glycol–free" antifreeze, de-icing and heat-exchanger solutions. Being generally recognized as safe by the U.S. Food and Drug Administration, it is routinely used as a solvent in pharmaceutical preparations, and as a humectant and preservative in food products. Deaths are rare following exposure to PG. Nevertheless, the relatively high concentration of PG in intravenous formulations of phenytoin (40%), diazepam (40%), chlordiazepoxide (20%), etomidate (35%), phenobarbital (70%), pentobarbital (40%), and lorazepam (80%) can result in toxicity during rapid or prolonged infusion of high doses of these medications. PG is also present in parenteral preparations of esmolol, digoxin, multivitamins, nitroglycerin, and trimethoprim-sulfamethoxazole. Toxicity following dermal exposure is possible, particularly in infants and burn patients.[35,36] The use of silver sulfadiazine cream has produced serum hyperosmolality, hypoglycemia, seizures, and CNS depression from transdermal absorption of PG.[36-38] The oral median lethal dose (LD50) is 20 g/kg or greater in rodents.[34] The daily dose should not exceed 25 mg/kg.[39]

Similar to other alcohols and glycols, PG is rapidly absorbed from the gastrointestinal tract with peak serum levels after 1 to 2 hours, and distributes into a volume of 0.6 L/kg. The terminal hydoxyl group of PG is readily oxidized via ADH to form lactic acid (2-hydroxypropanoic acid), which subsequently can be converted to pyruvate and enter the Kreb's cycle. Up to half of the parent glycol is excreted unchanged in the kidneys. The serum elimination half-life in adults is 2.3 ± 0.7 hours, but becomes saturated above 50 mg/dL, and can be up to 17 hours (or zero-order 13.5 mg/dL/hr) in neonates.[36,40,41] With chronic dosing of racemic PG, D-lactate accumulates in cats.[42] The significance of chirality is not known in human exposures. In an adult patient treated with continuous ethanol infusion and ethanol: PG serum concentrations of 1:2 mol/mol, zero-order elimination of 13 mg/dL/hr was observed across PG concentrations ranging from 300 to 500 mg/dL.[43] PG concentrations greater than 17.7 mg/dL are required to increase the lactate concentration and increase the anion gap.[44] PG concentrations of 76 mg/dL will increase the serum osmolality by about 10 mOsm/kg.[45] PG can be detected by gas chromatography. PG is a potential interferent when testing for ethylene glycol, so mass spectrometry should be used to confirm glycol identity.[46-48]

High doses result in abrupt cardiovascular depression, cardiac conduction abnormalities including QRS widening and bradyasystole, lactic acidosis, hyperosmolality, CNS depression and seizures, hypoglycemia, deafness, and thrombophlebitis, as described in various case reports.[49-53] Bradycardia is vagally mediated, as evidenced by pretreatment with atropine or vagotomy in animals.[54] Most toxic effects from PG are attributed to the parent glycol rather than its metabolites, suggesting that ADH inhibitor therapy is of limited benefit.[55] Hemodialysis has been used in critically ill patients.[56,57] The role of fomepizole is unknown.[55] Continuous venovenous hemofiltration with dialysis removes PG more slowly, and one patient receiving up to 9 g PG hourly developed toxicity despite simultaneous venovenous hemofiltration.[58]

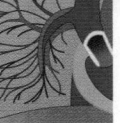

DIETHYLENE GLYCOL

Diethylene glycol (2,2'-dihydroxydiethyl ether, ethylene diglycol, 2,2'-oxydiethanol, 3-oxapentane-1,5-diol) is a viscous, sweet-tasting hydroscopic liquid. It is used as a plasticizer, antifreeze, lubricant, and liquid fuel (e.g., Sterno Wick Chafing Fuel, Des Plaines, IL). Its solubility in both organic and aqueous solutions has resulted in its occasional incorporation into pharmaceutical elixirs, with tragic results. The use of diethylene glycol to dissolve the early sulfa drug sulfanilamide by the Messengill company in 1937 resulted in 105 deaths, and triggered a national outcry.[59] This tragedy led to the federal Food, Drug and Cosmetic Act in 1938, which initiated the close regulation of the safety of medicinals by the Food and Drug Administration. Unfortunately, outbreaks continue to occur in developing countries following the inadvertent substitution of diethylene glycol for PG or glycerin in elixirs usually intended for children, with mortality rates of 40% to 100%.[60-64] (Table 32C-2) The oral LD50 ranges from 4.9 g/kg (rabbits) to 28.2 g/kg (mice), but is only 1.1 to 2.2 g/kg in mice when given intravenously. A human infant fatality has been reported following ingestion of 3.6 g.

After ingestion, diethylene glycol is rapidly absorbed, and 40% to 70% is excreted unchanged in the urine. The remainder is oxidized to 2-hydroxyethoxy acetic acid by ADH and aldehyde dehydrogenase, which may esterify under physiologic conditions to the cyclic lactone *p*-dioxanone, a nonacid.[65,66] The parent ether link is stable in vivo, accounting for the absence of ethylene glycol, glycolate, and glyoxalate in animal toxicity studies, and the inconsistent observation of oxalate in human cases.[65-68] Lactic acid accounts for a substantial portion of the metabolic acidosis.[69] Pyrazole and ethanol both reduce but do not eliminate the toxicity in animal models,[69] suggesting that the parent compound is also toxic.

Nephrotoxicity (tubular necrosis) is the prominent feature in animal poisoning studies. Other findings include CNS depression and hemorrhage, metabolic acidosis, and fatty liver. In poisoned humans, characteristic findings include delayed-onset renal failure with vacuolar nephropathy and acute tubular necrosis, and centrilobular hepatic necrosis following single or subacute ingestion of about 1 g/kg. In the Haiti outbreak, the maximum possible median toxic dose was 1.5 g/kg (95% confidence interval 0.25 to 4.9 g/kg).[62] In serious poisonings, headache, dizziness, CNS depression, anorexia, nausea, vomiting, diarrhea, and abdominal pain are commonly seen within 24 hours after ingestion. Unlike poisoning with ethylene glycol, the metabolic acidosis is not as prominent until renal toxicity is advanced. Laboratory findings include elevated serum osmolality, hypoglycemia, elevated blood urea nitrogen and creatinine, anion gap metabolic acidosis, elevated liver function test results, and an abnormal urinalysis result with cells and casts. In addition to hepatorenal failure, other late findings include cerebral and pulmonary edema, encephalopathy progressing to coma, facial nerve paralysis, demyelinating neuropathy, seizures, hypertension, adrenal cortical hemorrhage, and pancreatitis.

Although there is little reported experience in humans, both early dialysis and the inhibition of ADH is recommended for all symptomatic diethylene glycol exposures, especially patients with acidemia or renal insufficiency.[67,70] Using fomepizole to inhibit ADH is rational,[71] and has been used empirically in human cases.[69,70] The toxicity of the parent compound suggests that fomepizole without hemodialysis is unwise. In addition to dialysis and ADH inhibition, the need for intensive care to multiple patients with multiorgan failure may overwhelm a health care system in the context of an outbreak.[62,64]

POLYETHYLENE GLYCOLS

Triethylene glycol is the next higher molecular weight polymer after diethylene glycol in the series of polyethylene glycols. This series consists of subunits of ethylene glycol joined by an ether link. As the number of subunits increases, the polyethylene glycols are typically a mixture of varying chain lengths and are described by a number (e.g., PEG-3350). This number denotes the average molecular weight of the mixture.

TABLE 32C-2 Diethylene Glycol (DEG) Poisoning Outbreaks

YEAR	COUNTRY	SOURCE (% DEG)	AGES	FATALITIES IDENTIFIED	REFERENCES
1937	USA	Sulfonilamide (72%)	30% children	105 of 353	59
1969	South Africa	Sedatives	Children	7	103
1985	Spain	Topical silver Sulfadiazine		5	104
1985	Netherlands	Wine	Adults		105
1986	India	Glycerin (18.5%)	Adults	14	106
1990	Nigeria	Acetaminophen	Children	47	63
1990–1992	Bangladesh	Acetaminophen	Children	236	60
1992	Argentina	Propolis		7	68
1995/1996	Haiti	Acetaminophen (14%)	Children	101 of 109	61, 62
1998	India	Cough syrup (17.5%)	Children	33 of 36	64

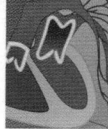

These compounds are liquids at room temperatures until the molecular weight exceeds 1000 daltons, after which they become solids and are termed carbowaxes. The toxicity also decreases substantially with increasing molecular weight. The higher polyethylene glycols are commonly used as excipients in medications and ointments. Intravenous lorazepam contains nearly 20% PEG-400, and burn ointments may contain over 99% PEG-300. PEG-3350 combined with an electrolyte solution (PEG-ELS) is used as a bowel evacuant for whole bowel irrigation (e.g., Go-Lytely [Braintree Laboratories, Braintree, MA] and CoLyte [Schwarz Pharma, Milwaukee, WI]).

Only lower-molecular-weight polyethylene glycols are absorbed in significant quantities after ingestion. These compounds can be metabolized via ADH to mono- and diacid metabolites,[72] but the majority is excreted unchanged in the urine. The ether link appears to be stable in vivo (see earlier section on Diethylene Glycol), and toxic amounts of ethylene glycol are not generated. In animals, 10 g/kg of polyethylene glycols over a wide range of molecular weights are well tolerated after single intravenous administration.

Although uncommon, toxicity associated with polyethylene glycols includes CNS depression, serum hyperosmolality, anion gap metabolic acidosis, and renal failure. Triethylene glycol has been reported to cause acute toxicity after ingestion in humans.[73] In this case report, intentional ingestion of nearly pure triethylene glycol resulted in coma and profound anion gap metabolic acidosis (initial arterial pH 7.03, anion gap 30 mmol/L, lactate 2 mmol/L, osmol gap 7) within 90 minutes of ingestion. In another case report, an intentional ingestion of brake fluid containing both diethylene glycol (10%) and triethylene glycol (55% vol/vol) resulted in coma, clonus, and anion gap acidosis (pH 7.34, anion gap 28 mmol/L, lactate 12 mmol/L, osmol gap 31) at least 2 hours after ingestion.[69] The third report of toxicity following intentional ingestion involved the liquid contents of a lava light (18% PEG-200) by a 65-year-old man who presented with confusion, nystagmus, renal failure, and acidosis (anion gap 15, creatinine 5.7 μg/dL). Burn patients absorb PEG-300 from creams applied topically and eliminate acid metabolites in urine,[72] perhaps resulting in toxicity.[74] For instance, serum hyperosmolality, anion gap metabolic acidosis, and acute tubular necrosis have been described in this patient population and may be attributed to PEG percutaneous absorption.[74] One case of hyperosmolar metabolic acidosis in a patient administered 1.7 g lorazepam intravenously (18% PEG-400, 80% PG) was attributed to the 150 mL of polyethylene glycol excipient,[57] but the coadministered 704 g of PG are a more plausible explanation.[55] The relative safety of PEG-3350 is illustrated by a case report of a 2-year-old child treated with 3 L/kg of whole bowel irrigation over 5 days without adverse effects.[75]

Treatment with ADH blockade using either fomepizole or ethanol appears to be appropriate for symptomatic ingestions of low-molecular-weight polyethylene glycols.[69,73] The role of hemodialysis is not defined, but should be instituted for persistent metabolic acidosis or renal insufficiency. The acute oral toxicity of the higher-molecular-weight polyethylene glycols is minimal.

GLYCOL ETHERS

The glycol ethers, or cellosolves, are a family of organic compounds in which at least one alkyl hydrocarbon is joined by an ether link to a diol such as ethylene glycol. Thus, the basic structure is $R1\text{-}O\text{-}(CH_2)x\text{-}O\text{-}R2$. The most common glycol ether, accounting for about half of the annual production in North America, is ethylene glycol n-butyl ether (EGBE), in which $R1 = CH_3(CH_2)_3$- (i.e., n-butyl), x = 2 (ethylene glycol), and R2 = H. Replacing R1 with methyl results in ethylene glycol methyl ether (EGME). Other commonly encountered glycol ethers are listed in Table 32C-3.

Since the glycol ethers combine the solubility properties of both alcohols and ethers, they are miscible in a wide range of aqueous and organic solutions, and have numerous household and industrial applications. The first reports of human toxicity appeared in the 1930s following the introduction of EGME into the manufacture of stiffened shirt collars. Workers producing "fused collar" shirts developed toxic encephalopathy and bone marrow toxicity following chronic pulmonary and dermal exposure.[76] Today, various glycol ethers are found as the primary component of automotive brake fluids, as well as in fuel injector and carburetor cleaners, degreasing agents, stain removers, carpet and fabric cleaners, inks and ink removers, leather dyes, shoe polish, leather conditioners, and many window and surface cleaning products. Their coating properties lead to their use in lacquers, paints, varnishes, and surface preparation agents. They are used extensively in the semiconductor industry, as well as the plastics, rubber, photography, and printing industries.

Although the first human fatality attributed to intentional ingestion of a glycol ether was reported over 50 years ago,[77] there are very few published case reports of toxicity following acute use. This is in contrast with their prevalence in the household environment. For the years of 1998 to 2000, the American Association of Poison Control Centers Toxic Exposure Surveillance System shows over 26,000 human exposures (54% age younger than 6 years) to products containing any glycol other than ethylene glycol, out of a total of 6.6 million cases reported to U.S. poison control centers. Of these, 64 (0.2%) resulted in major toxicity, and 2 deaths are listed, both in adults, presumably following intentional ingestion with suicidal intent. Indeed, toxicity was not observed in a retrospective poison control center study of 24 young children following accidental ingestion of a mouthful of products containing less than 10% glycol ethers.[78]

Following oral ingestion, absorption of low-molecular-weight glycol ethers such as EGME and EGBE is rapid, and comparable with ethanol.[79] Pulmonary absorption is also possible, particularly of the more volatile agents. Thus, methyl derivatives such as EGME (vapor pressure

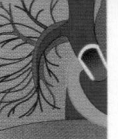

TABLE 32C-3 Glycol Ethers

NAME	ABBREVIATION	CAS NO.	SYNONYMS	STRUCTURE
Ethylene glycol methyl ether	EGME	109-86-4	2-methoxyethanol, Methyl Cellosolve, methyl oxitol	$CH_3O-CH_2CH_2OH$
Ethylene glycol ethyl ether	EGEE	110-80-5	2-ethoxyethanol, Cellosolve, Oxitol	$C_2H_5O-CH_2CH_2OH$
Ethylene glycol n-butyl ether	EGBE	111-76-2	2-butoxyethanol, Butyl Cellosolve, 3-oxa-1-heptanol	$C_4H_9O-CH_2CH_2OH$
Diethylene glycol methyl ether	DEGME	111-77-3	2-(2-methoxy-ethoxy)ethanol, methoxydiglycol, methyl dioxitol, 3,6-dioxa-1-heptanol	$CH_3O-CH_2CH_2O-CH_2CH_2OH$
Diethylene glycol n-butyl ether	DEGBE	112-34-5	2-(2-butoxyethoxy)ethanol, butoxydiglycol, butyl dioxitol, Dowanol DB	$C_4H_9O-CH_2CH_2O-CH_2CH_2OH$
2-Propylene glycol-1-methyl ether	α-PGME	107-98-2	1-methoxy-2-propanol	$CH_3O-CH_2CH(CH_3)OH$
1-Propylene glycol-2-methyl ether	β-PGME	1589-47-5	2-methoxy-1-propanol (4 isomers)	$CH_3O-CH(CH_3)CH_2OH$
Dipropylene glycol methyl ether	DPGME	34590-94-8	1,2-dimethoxyethane, Glyme, Dimethyl Cellosolve	$CH_3O-C_3H_6O-C_3H_6OH$
Ethylene glycol dimethyl ether	EGDME	110-71-4	2,5-dioxahexane	$CH_3O-CH_2CH_2O-CH_3$

9.7 mm Hg at 25° C) are more hazardous than EGBE (vapor pressure 0.9 mm Hg). The diethylene and dipropylene glycol ethers have vapor pressures ranging from about 0.4 to 0.004 mm Hg under ambient conditions, reducing the risk for exposure, and triethylene glycol ethers or higher are essentially nontoxic via the pulmonary route.[80] The glycol ethers readily diffuse across intact skin in inverse proportion to molecular weight. EGME diffuses across human skin more quickly than ethanol, then in decreasing order propylene glycol methyl ether (PGME), ethylene glycol ethyl ether (EGEE), dimethylene glycol methyl ether (DEGME), diethylene glycol ethyl ether, and EGBE.[81] Both the pulmonary and dermal routes of exposure can lead to toxicity in the occupational setting.[82] Once absorbed, the volume of distribution for EGBE has been estimated at 0.7 L/kg.[83]

The monoalkyl ethers are predominantly metabolized to alkoxyacetic acid by hepatic ADH and aldehyde dehydrogenase.[80] For example, EGME is oxidized to methoxyacetic acid and EGBE to butoxyacetic acid (BAA). This metabolism is inhibited in animals by pyrazole (a fomepizole analog) or relatively low concentrations of ethanol. O-dealkylation to ethylene glycol and a mono-alcohol plays a minor role in mammals. The alkoxyacetic acid and its glycine conjugate are the major urinary metabolites recovered.[83] Only trivial amounts of the parent compound are eliminated in feces or breath. Despite reports of moderate increases in oxaluria in two case reports,[84,85] the absence of detectable ethylene glycol, methanol, and tissue calcium oxalate crystals in most other published reports demonstrates that the toxicity of EGME and EGBE is not due to the release of ethylene glycol.[77,79,85,86] Two other case reports may represent ethylene glycol ingestions.[87,88] In contrast to all

the ethylene glycol monoalkyl ethers and β-PGME, ADH oxidizes secondary alcohols such as α-PGME more slowly, and O-dealkylation presumably via CYP450 can produce substantial quantities of PG.[80]

Because of the paucity of published reports of acute toxicity following oral ingestion, careful scrutiny of these case reports is justified, as summarized in Table 32C-4. Analogous to most other toxic alcohols, the acid metabolites appear to be more potent toxins than the parent glycol ether. Rapid onset coma may occur within 1 hour of ingestion,[79] but an anion gap metabolic acidosis follows several hours later if ADH metabolism is not inhibited.[79,84-86] Mild to moderate hemolysis has been observed in humans following large ingestions of EGBE,[79,84,89,90] but not after inhalational exposure or with other glycol ethers. Animal models demonstrate that BAA is the proximate hemolytic agent.[91] Human erythrocytes appear to be resistant to hemolysis in vitro.[92] Other reported toxic effects following glycol ether ingestion are hypotension requiring pressors, mild renal dysfunction with proteinuria, lactic acidosis, and less commonly disseminated intravascular coagulopathy, acute lung injury, hepatic dysfunction, and hypochloremic metabolic acidosis.

Chronic exposure can result in bone marrow suppression, encephalopathy, developmental toxicity, and subfertility. The neurologic effects range from personality changes to amnesia, headache, and lethargy, with tremor, clonus, ataxia, and dysarthria. Both erythroid and myeloid hypoplasia have been described on the bone marrow aspirates of workers exposed to higher concentrations of EGME, but not following low level exposures to EGBE.[93,94] Several epidemiologic studies have reported an association between decreased fertility in female workers and exposure to EGME, EGBE (and

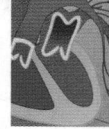

TABLE 32C-4   Human Case Reports of Symptomatic Glycol Ether Ingestion

REFERENCE	AGE (yr)	SEX	INTENTIONAL	INGESTION	TIME POST ARRIVAL	FEATURES	TREATMENT	COMMENTS
77	46	M	Yes	250 mL pure EGME + some ethanol	0	Comatose, RR 28/min		Acute hemorrhagic gastritis, toxic changes renal tubules and pancreas
					5 hr	Dead; no methanol/some ethanol in urine		
85	41	M	Yes	100 mL pure EGME 8 hr PTA	0	Agitated, confused, restless, increased RR		
					12 hr	Restless, AG 24, creat 2.0 mg/dL, pH 7.18, Ca oxalate crystalluria	Ethanol × 3 days	
					5 days	Creat N; no methanol or EGME in urine		Proteinuria × 7 day, alopecia, dermatitis
85	23	M	Yes	100 mL pure EGME 20 hr PTA	-2 hr	Motor weakness		
					0	Confused, increased RR, AG 30, creat 1.5 mg/dL, pH 7.22; no methanol, EGME, or Ca oxalate in urine	Ethanol × 3 days	
					1 day	Creat N		
					5–9 days	27–54 mg/day oxaluria (N)		Proteinuria × 7 day
84	50	F	Yes	250+ mL 12% EGBE 12 hr PTA	0	Coma inc creat, pH 7.23, oxalate crystaluria		
					3–6 days	Hemolysis		
					5 days	Extubated; BAA up to 40 g/g creat, EGBE 2 g/g creat, and oxalate 200 mg/g creat (peaks day 1 and 7) in urine		
79	23	F	Yes	250 mL 12.7% EGBE + 3.2% ethanol 1 hr PTA	0	Coma, AG N, creat N; EGBE 432 mg/L, ethanol 35.6 mg/L in serum		
					2 hr	EGBE 304 mg/L, ethanol 1 mg/L in serum		
					3 hr	Awake		
					6 hr	RR 28/min, AG 28, creat N, lactate 7.1 mM, pH 7.08, OG N		Rapid onset coma, dopamine for hypotension, coingested ethanol appears to have delayed onset of acidosis and serum elimination of EGBE
					22 hr	Creat N, urine oxalate N, mild hemolysis	HD × 6 hr	
86	1.3	F	No	10%–30% EGBE 2 hr PTA	0	GCS 7, AG 19, lactate 1.0 mM		
					2 hr	AG 20, no ethylene glycol in serum	Fomepizole × 1 dose	
					4 hr	AG N		
					26 hr	Awake		Early hypoglycemia, late pancreatitis (mild)
89	19	M	Yes	600 + mL 25%–35% EGBE + 15%–25% propylene glycol 20 min PTA	1 hr	Lethargic, RR 24/min		Hypotension on 3 pressors; DIC; propylene glycol coingestion; peak BAA 170 mg/dL, no increased elimination during hemodialysis; lactate also cleared slowly

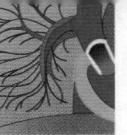

TABLE 32C-4 Human Case Reports of Symptomatic Glycol Ether Ingestion—*Cont'd*

REFERENCE	AGE (yr)	SEX	INTENTIONAL	INGESTION	TIME POST ARRIVAL	FEATURES	TREATMENT	COMMENTS
					3 hr	Coma, AG 10, lactate 5.0 mM, pH 7.36; propylene glycol 43 mg/dL		
					29 hr		HD × 4 hr	
					2 days	Hemolysis		
107	59	F	Yes	20%–30% DPGME	0	Coma, AG increased, OG 12; no methanol or ethylene glycol in serum	Ethanol	Hypotensive eventually needing CPR; skin burns attributed to urine leak
					24 hr	AG N		
101	51	F	Yes	240 mL 10%–30% EGBE + 10%–40% isopropanol 1.5 hr PTA	0	Vomited, RR 24/min, AG 15, creat 0.8 mg/dL, pH 7.31; isopropanol 3 mg/dL, acetone 3 mg/dL		Deteriorated shortly after ethanol begun; hyperchloremic metabolic acidosis resolved when ethanol discontinued; EGBE and BAA levels much lower than expected
					4 hr	Obtunded	Ethanol × 3 days	
					3 days	AG 11–15, creat N, no oxaluria, no hemolysis		
90	18	M	Yes	360 + mL 22% EGBE 3 hr PTA	0	Awake, AG N, creat 1.2 mg/dL, pH 7.34, OG N		
					10 hr	Lethargic, inc RR		
					16 hr	Creat 1.5 mg/dL, lactate 5.9 mM, pH 7.46; no ethylene glycol, peak BAA 4.9 mM, peak EGBE 0.001 mM in serum		
					21 hr	Creat 1.1 mg/dL, no ethylene glycol in serum	HD × 4.5 hr; ethanol × 30 hr	
					30 hr	Awake, mild hemolysis		
					60 hr	AG N, creat N		Mild epigastric discomfort; ketonuria, hematuria, proteinuria
90	18	M	Yes	480 mL 22% EGBE 6 hr PTA	0	Alert, creat 1.3 mg/dL, pH 7.40, no ethylene glycol in serum	Ethanol × 28 hr	
					8 hr	OG 8, peak BAA 2 mM, EGBE 0.1 mM	HD	Time of peak BAA relative to HD not clear

The table summarizes published reports of serious glycol ether ingestion
AG, anion gap (mM); CPR, external chest compressions; creat, serum creatinine; DIC, disseminated intravascular coagulation; HD, hemodialysis; N, normal; OG, osmolal gap; PTA, prior to hospital arrival; RR, respiratory rate.

their acetate derivatives which are deesterified in vivo to the parent glycol ether), and other ethylene and PG ethers used in photolithography during semiconductor fabrication.[95-97] EGME, EGEE, and perhaps higher glycol ethers are teratogenic.[98-100]

The diagnosis of acute exposure to glycol ether depends on a reliable history, since laboratory testing for the parent glycol ether or its acid metabolite is generally not possible within a clinically relevant turnaround time. CNS depression should be present on physical examination following significant poisoning. The presence of an anion gap metabolic acidosis, with or without a concurrent lactic acidosis, is an indirect marker of exposure and metabolism, but is not specific. The osmol gap is usually normal despite severe symptoms.[79,90,101,102] In fact, in one patient with rapid onset coma, the serum

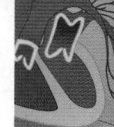

concentration of EGBE was 3 mmol/L, and would therefore not be expected to increase the osmol gap appreciably.

Treatment must therefore be predicated upon clinical effects such as mental status, acid-base status, and other readily apparent end-organ effects. Many of the patients in case reports were treated with ADH blockade or delayed hemodialysis, or both. Fomepizole was used in one instance.[86] There are insufficient data on which to base a firm recommendation at this time. The use of an ADH inhibitor is based on the premise that the acid metabolite is the more toxic species, and is justified only if substantial amounts of the parent glycol ether remain at the time of initiation of therapy. It is difficult to interpret the human toxicokinetics of the parent glycol ether, because the reported methodologies for quantifying EGBE appear to yield inconsistent results. From these imprecise published estimates, it would appear that the glycol ether is absorbed and cleared rapidly from the serum. The available data also suggest that full-dose ethanol therapy can result in hemodynamic compromise and a hyperchloremic metabolic acidosis.[101] The use of hemodialysis is recommended to correct refractory metabolic acidosis and to remove the glycol ether metabolites. Here again, the literature is unsatisfactory. The only report of serial serum BAA levels suggests that hemodialysis does not increase BAA elimination substantively.[89] This observation is at odds with the low molecular weight and volume of distribution of BAA, and should be confirmed prior to reconsidering the role of hemodialysis.

Pending better information, it seems prudent to recommend fomepizole or low-dose ethanol for symptomatic patients who present shortly after an intentional ingestion of a product known to contain nontrivial concentrations of glycol ethers. Hemodialysis should be offered to patients with a metabolic acidosis not responsive to fluids and sodium bicarbonate. Accidental sips of solutions with less than 10% glycol ether can be managed with home observation if the patient remains asymptomatic.[78]

REFERENCES

1. Lacouture PG, Heldreth DD, Shannon M, Lovejoy FH Jr: The generation of acetonemia/acetonuria following ingestion of a subtoxic dose of isopropyl alcohol. Am J Emerg Med 1989; 7(1):38–40.
2. Leeper SC, Almatari AL, Ingram JD, Ferslew KE: Topical absorption of isopropyl alcohol induced cardiac and neurologic deficits in an adult female with intact skin. Vet Hum Toxicol 2000;42(1):15–17.
3. Lewin GA, Oppenheimer PR, Wingert WA: Coma from alcohol sponging. JACEP 1977;6:165–167.
4. Martinez TT, Jaeger RW, deCastro FJ, et al: A comparison of the absorption and metabolism of isopropyl alcohol by oral, dermal and inhalation routes. Vet Hum Toxicol 1986;28(3):233–236.
5. Vivier PM, Lewander WJ, Martin HF, Linakis JG: Isopropyl alcohol intoxication in a neonate through chronic dermal exposure: a complication of a culturally-based umbilical care practice. Pediatr Emerg Care 1994;10(2):91–93.
6. Monaghan MS, Ackerman BH, Olsen KM, et al: The use of delta osmolality to predict serum isopropanol and acetone concentrations. Pharmacotherapy 1993;13(1):60–63.
7. Pappas AA, Ackerman BH, Olsen KM, Taylor EH: Isopropanol ingestion: a report of six episodes with isopropanol and acetone serum concentration time data. J Toxicol Clin Toxicol 1991; 29(1):11–21.
8. Parker KM, Lera TA Jr: Acute isopropanol ingestion: pharmacokinetic parameters in the infant. Am J Emerg Med 1992; 10(6):542–544.
9. Daniel DR, McAnalley BH, Garriott JC: Isopropyl alcohol metabolism after acute intoxication in humans. J Anal Toxicol 1981;5(3):110–112.
10. Gaudet MP, Fraser GL: Isopropanol ingestion: case report with pharmacokinetic analysis. Am J Emerg Med 1989;7(3):297–299.
11. Natowicz M, Donahue J, Gorman L, et al: Pharmacokinetic analysis of a case of isopropanol intoxication. Clin Chem 1985;31(2):326–328.
12. Bekka R, Borron SW, Astier A, et al: Treatment of methanol and isopropanol poisoning with intravenous fomepizole. J Toxicol Clin Toxicol 2001;39(1):59–67.
13. Su M, Hoffman RS, Nelson LS: Error in an emergency medicine textbook: isopropyl alcohol toxicity. Acad Emerg Med 2002;9(2):175.
14. Jones AW: Elimination half-life of acetone in humans: case reports and review of the literature [Review]. J Anal Toxicol 2000; 24(1):8–10.
15. Vicas IM, Beck R: Fatal inhalational isopropyl alcohol poisoning in a neonate. J Toxicol Clin Toxicol 1993;31(3):473–481.
16. Wallgren H: Relative intoxicating effects on rats of ethyl, propyl and butyl alcohols. Acta Pharmacol Toxicol 1960;16:217–222.
17. Bailey DN: Detection of isopropanol in acetonemic patients not exposed to isopropanol. J Toxicol Clin Toxicol 1990;28(4):459–466.
18. Jones AE, Summers RL: Detection of isopropyl alcohol in a patient with diabetic ketoacidosis. J Emerg Med 2000;19(2): 165–168.
19. Logan BK, Gullberg RG, Elenbaas JK: Isopropanol interference with breath alcohol analysis: a case report. J Forensic Sci 1994; 39(4):1107–1111.
20. Linden CH: Unknown alcohol [Letter; Comment]. Ann Emerg Med 1996;28(3):371.
21. Blijenberg BG, Brouwer HJ: The accuracy of creatinine methods based on the Jaffe reaction: a questionable matter. Eur J Clin Chem Clin Biochem 1994;32(12):909–913.
22. Rich J, Scheife RT, Katz N, Caplan LR: Isopropyl alcohol intoxication [Review; see comments]. Arch Neurol 1990;47(3):322–324.
23. Burkhart KK, Martinez MA: The adsorption of isopropanol and acetone by activated charcoal. J Toxicol Clin Toxicol 1992;30(3): 371–375.
24. Stremski E, Hennes H: Accidental isopropanol ingestion in children. Pediatr Emerg Care 2000;16(4):238–240.
25. Rosansky SJ: Isopropyl alcohol poisoning treated with hemodialysis: kinetics of isopropyl alcohol and acetone removal. J Toxicol Clin Toxicol 1982;19(3):265–271.
26. King LH Jr, Bradley KP, Shires DL Jr: Hemodialysis for isopropyl alcohol poisoning. JAMA 1970;211(11):1855.
27. Chen EC, David JJ: Quantitative determination of fusel alcohols in beer and fermenting wort. J Sci Food Agric 1974;25(11): 1381–1387.
28. Gershanik J, Boecler B, Ensley H, et al: The gasping syndrome and benzyl alcohol poisoning. N Engl J Med 1982;307(22):1384–1388.
29. Brown WJ, Buist NR, Gipson HT, et al: Fatal benzyl alcohol poisoning in a neonatal intensive care unit. Lancet 1982;1(8283):1250.
30. Jardine DS, Rogers K: Relationship of benzyl alcohol to kernicterus, intraventricular hemorrhage, and mortality in preterm infants. Pediatrics 1989;83(2):153–160.
31. Benda GI, Hiller JL, Reynolds JW: Benzyl alcohol toxicity: impact on neurologic handicaps among surviving very low birth weight infants. Pediatrics 1986;77(4):507–512.
32. Hiller JL, Benda GI, Rahatzad M, et al: Benzyl alcohol toxicity: impact on mortality and intraventricular hemorrhage among very low birth weight infants. Pediatrics 1986;77(4):500–506.
33. Brunson EL: Benzyl alcohol. In Kibbe AH (ed): Handbook of Pharmaceutical Excipients. Washington, DC, American Pharmaceutical Association, 2000, pp 41–43.
34. LaKind JS, McKenna EA, Hubner RP, Tardiff RG: A review of the comparative mammalian toxicity of ethylene glycol and propylene glycol [Review]. Crit Rev Toxicol 1999;29(4):331–365.

35. Peleg O, Bar-Oz B, Arad I: Coma in a premature infant associated with the transdermal absorption of propylene glycol. Acta Paediatr 1998;87(11):1195–1196.

36. Fligner CL, Jack R, Twiggs GA, Raisys VA: Hyperosmolality induced by propylene glycol. A complication of silver sulfadiazine therapy. JAMA 1985;253(11):1606–1609.

37. Kulick MI, Wong R, Okarma TB, et al: Prospective study of side effects associated with the use of silver sulfadiazine in severely burned patients. Ann Plast Surg 1985;14(5):407–419.

38. Kulick MI, Lewis NS, Bansal V, Warpeha R: Hyperosmolality in the burn patient: analysis of an osmolal discrepancy. J Trauma 1980;(3):223–228.

39. Dandiker Y: Propylene glycol. In Kibbe AH (ed): Handbook of Pharmaceutical Excipients. Washington, DC, American Pharmaceutical Association, 2000; pp 442–444.

40. Speth PA, Vree TB, Neilen NF, et al: Propylene glycol pharmacokinetics and effects after intravenous infusion in humans. Ther Drug Monit 1987;9(3):255–258.

41. Ruddick JA: Toxicology, metabolism, and biochemistry of 1,2-propanediol [Review]. Toxicol Appl Pharmacol 1972;21(1):102–111.

42. Christopher MM, Eckfeldt JH, Eaton JW: Propylene glycol ingestion causes D-lactic acidosis. Lab Invest 1990;62(1):114–118.

43. Brooks DE, Wallace KL: Acute propylene glycol ingestion. J Toxicol Clin Toxicol 2002;40(4):513–516.

44. Kelner MJ, Bailey DN: Propylene glycol as a cause of lactic acidosis. J Anal Toxicol 1985;9(1):40–42.

45. Hall AH, Bronstein AC, Smolinske SC, et al: Propylene glycol plasma level. Pediatrics 1985;76(4):654.

46. Tuohy KA, Nicholson WJ, Schiffman F: Agitation by sedation. Lancet 2003;361(9354):308.

47. Robinson CA Jr, Scott JW, Ketchum C: Propylene glycol interference with ethylene glycol procedures. Clin Chem 1983;29(4):727.

48. DeWitt C, Palmer R, Phillips S, Dart RC: False positive ethylene glycol level [Abstract]. J Toxicol Clin Toxicol 2003;41(5):736.

49. Bedichek E, Kirschbaum B: A case of propylene glycol toxic reaction associated with etomidate infusion. Arch Intern Med 1991;151(11):2297–2298.

50. Arbour RB: Propylene glycol toxicity related to high-dose lorazepam infusion: case report and discussion. Am J Crit Care 1999;8(1):499–506.

51. Guillot M, Bocquet G, Eckart P, et al: [Home environment and acute propylene glycol intoxication in a two-year old. An unusual case report] [French]. Arch Pediatr 2002;9(4):382–384.

52. Wilson KC, Reardon C, Farber HW: Propylene glycol toxicity in a patient receiving intravenous diazepam. N Engl J Med 2000;343(11):815.

53. Reynolds HN, Teiken P, Regan ME, et al: Hyperlactatemia, increased osmolar gap, and renal dysfunction during continuous lorazepam infusion. Crit Care Med 2000;28(5):1631–1634.

54. Louis S, Kutt H, McDowell F: The cardiocirculatory changes caused by intravenous dilantin and its solvent. Am Heart J 1967;74(4):523–529.

55. Mullins ME, Barnes BJ: Hyperosmolar metabolic acidosis and intravenous Lorazepam [see comment]. N Engl J Med 2002;347(11):857–858.

56. Parker MG, Fraser GL, Watson DM, Riker RR: Removal of propylene glycol and correction of increased osmolar gap by hemodialysis in a patient on high dose lorazepam infusion therapy. Intens Care Med 2002;28(1):81–84.

57. Tayar J, Jabbour G, Saggi SJ: Severe hyperosmolar metabolic acidosis due to a large dose of intravenous lorazepam [see comment]. N Engl J Med 2002;346(16):1253–1254.

58. Al Khafaji AH, Dewhirst WE, Manning HL: Propylene glycol toxicity associated with lorazepam infusion in a patient receiving continuous veno-venous hemofiltration with dialysis. Anesth Analg 2002;94(6):1583–1585.

59. Wax PM: Elixirs, diluents, and the passage of the 1938 Federal Food, Drug and Cosmetic Act. Ann Intern Med 1995;122(6):456–461.

60. Hanif M, Mobarak MR, Ronan A, et al: Fatal renal failure caused by diethylene glycol in paracetamol elixir: the Bangladesh epidemic [see comment]. BMJ 1995;311(6997):88–91.

61. Junod SW: Diethylene glycol deaths in Haiti. Public Health Rep 2000;115(1):78–86.

62. O'Brien KL, Selanikio JD, Hecdivert C, et al: Epidemic of pediatric deaths from acute renal failure caused by diethylene glycol poisoning. Acute Renal Failure Investigation Team [see comment]. JAMA 1998;279(15):1175–1180.

63. Okuonghae HO, Ighogboja IS, Lawson JO, Nwana EJ: Diethylene glycol poisoning in Nigerian children [see comment]. Ann Trop Paediatr 1992;12(3):235–238.

64. Singh J, Dutta AK, Khare S, et al: Diethylene glycol poisoning in Gurgaon, India, 1998 [see comment]. Bull WHO 2001;79(2):88–95.

65. Mathews JM, Parker MK, Matthews HB: Metabolism and disposition of diethylene glycol in rat and dog. Drug Metab Dispos 1991;19(6):1066–1070.

66. Lenk W, Lohr D, Sonnenbichler J: Pharmacokinetics and biotransformation of diethylene glycol and ethylene glycol in the rat. Xenobiotica 1989;19(9):961–979.

67. Rollins YD, Filley CM, McNutt JT, et al: Fulminant ascending paralysis as a delayed sequela of diethylene glycol (Sterno) ingestion. Neurology 2002;59(9):1460–1463.

68. Drut R, Quijano G, Jones MC, Scanferla P: [Pathologic findings in diethylene glycol poisoning.] Medicina 1994;54(1):1–5.

69. Borron SW, Baud FJ, Garnier R: Intravenous 4-methylpyrazole as an antidote for diethylene glycol and triethylene glycol poisoning: a case report. Hum Exp Toxicol 1997;39(1):26–28.

70. Brophy PD, Tenenbein M, Gardner J, et al: Childhood diethylene glycol poisoning treated with alcohol dehydrogenase inhibitor fomepizole and hemodialysis. Am J Kidney Dis 2000;35(5):958–962.

71. Wiener HL, Richardson KE. Metabolism of diethylene glycol in male rats. Biochem Pharmacol 1989;38(3):539–541.

72. Herold DA, Keil K, Bruns DE: Oxidation of polyethylene glycols by alcohol dehydrogenase. Biochem Pharmacol 1989;38(1):73–76.

73. Vassiliadis J, Graudins A, Dowsett RP: Triethylene glycol poisoning treated with intravenous ethanol infusion. J Toxicol Clin Toxicol 1999;37(6):773–776.

74. Bruns DE, Herold DA, Rodeheaver GT, Edlich RF: Polyethylene glycol intoxication in burn patients. Burns 1982;9(1):49–52.

75. Kaczorowski JM, Wax PM: Five days of whole-bowel irrigation in a case of pediatric iron ingestion. Ann Emerg Med 1996;27(2):258–263.

76. Browning RG, Curry SC: Clinical toxicology of ethylene glycol monoalkyl ethers [Review]. Hum Exp Toxicol 1994;13(5):325–335.

77. Young EG, Woolner LB: A case of fatal poisoning from 2-methoxyethanol. J Ind Hyg Toxicol 1946;28:267–268.

78. Dean BS, Krenzelok EP: Clinical evaluation of pediatric ethylene glycol monobutyl ether poisonings [see comment]. J Toxicol Clin Toxicol 1992;30(4):557–563.

79. Gijsenbergh FP, Jenco M, Veulemans H, et al: Acute butylglycol intoxication: a case report. Hum Toxicol 1989;8(3):243–245.

80. Miller RR: Metabolism and disposition of glycol ethers [Review]. Drug Metab Rev 1987;18(1):1–22.

81. Dugard PH, Walker M, Mawdsley SJ, Scott RC: Absorption of some glycol ethers through human skin in vitro. Environ Health Perspect 1984;57:193–197.

82. Ohi G, Wegman DH: Transcutaneous ethylene glycol monomethyl ether poisoning in the work setting. J Occup Med 1978;20(10):675–676.

83. Johanson G, Kronborg H, Naslund PH, Byfalt NM: Toxicokinetics of inhaled 2-butoxyethanol (ethylene glycol monobutyl ether) in man. Scand J Work Environ Health 1986;12(6):594–602.

84. Rambourg-Schepens MO, Buffet M, Bertault R, et al: Severe ethylene glycol butyl ether poisoning. Kinetics and metabolic pattern. Hum Toxicol 1988;7(2):187–189.

85. Nitter-Hauge S: Poisoning with ethylene glycol monomethyl ether. Report of two cases. Acta Med Scand 1970;188(4):277–280.

86. Osterhoudt KC: Fomepizole therapy for pediatric butoxyethanol intoxication. J Toxicol Clin Toxicol 2002;40(7):929–930.

87. Nisse P, Coquelle-Couplet V, Forceville X, Mathieu-Nolf M: Renal failure after suicidal ingestion of window cleaner: a case report. Vet Hum Toxicol 1998;40:173.

88. Litovitz TL, Bailey KM, Schmitz BF, et al: 1990 annual report of the American Association of Poison Control Centers National Data Collection System. Am J Emerg Med 1991;9(5):461–509.

89. Burkhart KK, Donovan JW: Hemodialysis following butoxyethanol ingestion. J Toxicol Clin Toxicol 1998;36(7):723–725.

90. Gualtieri JF, DeBoer L, Harris CR, Corley R: Repeated ingestion of 2-butoxyethanol: case report and literature review. J Toxicol Clin Toxicol 2003;41(1):57–62.

91. Ghanayem BI, Burka LT, Matthews HB: Metabolic basis of ethylene glycol monobutyl ether (2-butoxyethanol) toxicity: role of alcohol and aldehyde dehydrogenases. J Pharmacol Exp Ther 1987;242(1):222–231.

92. Bartnik FG, Reddy AK, Klecak G, et al: Percutaneous absorption, metabolism, and hemolytic activity of n-butoxyethanol. Fundam Appl Toxicol 1987;8(1):59–70.

93. Cullen MR, Solomon LR, Pace PE, et al: Morphologic, biochemical, and cytogenetic studies of bone marrow and circulating blood cells in painters exposed to ethylene glycol ethers. Environ Res 1992;59(1):250–264.

94. Johanson G: Toxicity review of ethylene glycol monomethyl ether and its acetate ester [Review]. Crit Rev Toxicol 2000;30(3):307–345.

95. Correa A, Gray RH, Cohen R, et al: Ethylene glycol ethers and risks of spontaneous abortion and subfertility. Am J Epidemiol 1996;143(7):707–717.

96. Swan SH, Beaumont JJ, Hammond SK, et al: Historical cohort study of spontaneous abortion among fabrication workers in the Semiconductor Health Study: agent-level analysis. Am J Ind Med 1995;28(6):751–769.

97. Chen PC, Hsieh GY, Wang JD, Cheng TJ: Prolonged time to pregnancy in female workers exposed to ethylene glycol ethers in semiconductor manufacturing. Epidemiology 2002;13(2):191–196.

98. Saavedra D, Arteaga M, Tena M: Industrial contamination with glycol ethers resulting in teratogenic damage. Ann NY Acad Sci 1997;837:126–137.

99. Cordier S, Szabova E, Fevotte J, et al: Congenital malformations and maternal exposure to glycol ethers in the Slovak Republic [see comment]. Epidemiology 2001;12(5):592–593.

100. Cordier S, Bergeret A, Goujard J, et al: Congenital malformation and maternal occupational exposure to glycol ethers. Occupational Exposure and Congenital Malformations Working Group [see comment]. Epidemiology 1997;8(4):355–363.

101. McKinney PE, Palmer RB, Blackwell W, Benson BE: Butoxyethanol ingestion with prolonged hyperchloremic metabolic acidosis treated with ethanol therapy. J Toxicol Clin Toxicol 2000;38(7):787–793.

102. Browning RG, Curry SC: Effect of glycol ethers on plasma osmolality. Hum Exp Toxicol 1992;11(6):488–490.

103. Bowie MD, McKenzie D: Diethylene glycol poisoning in children. South Afr Med J 1972;46(27):931–934.

104. Cantarell MC, Fort J, Camps J, et al: Acute intoxication due to topical application of diethylene glycol. Ann Intern Med 1987;106(3):478–479.

105. van der Linden-Cremers PM, Sangster B: [Medical sequelae of the contamination of wine with diethylene glycol] [Dutch]. Nederlands Tijdschrift voor Geneeskunde 1985;129(39):1890–1891.

106. Pandya SK: Letter from Bombay. An unmitigated tragedy. BMJ 1988;297(6641):117–119.

33 *Opioids*

LUKE YIP, MD ■ BRUNO MÉGARBANE, MD, PHD ■ STEPHEN W. BORRON, MD, MS

At a Glance...

- Opioids elicit the same overall physiologic effects as morphine but may demonstrate conspicuous differences following an overdose.
- The classic "opioid toxidrome" (mental status depression, respiratory depression, miosis, and decreased bowel motility) may not be apparent following a mixed overdose.
- Purity and adulterants play a considerable role in the outcome and complications of heroin use.
- Inhalation of heated heroin vapors may result in a progressive spongiform leukoencephalopathy.
- Acute lung injury may occur following opioid overdose or naloxone therapy.
- Higher doses of naloxone may be required to antagonize the effects of high-potency opioids (e.g., fentanyl and its analogs, methadone, pentazocine, propoxyphene, and diphenoxylate).
- Naloxone has a short half-life, and the effects of most opioids will significantly outlast several doses of naloxone.
- Judicious use of naloxone infusion may obviate the need for endotracheal intubation.

HISTORY AND INTRODUCTION

Opium, one of the oldest known pharmacologic agents, is derived from the poppy *Papaver somniferum*. The Sumerians first reported the psychotherapeutic benefits of juice from immature poppy heads about 4000 BC. Opium solutions contained morphine, codeine, and numerous other related alkaloids. In 1806, morphine was isolated from opium by Sertürner. Other alkaloids were later isolated, including codeine in 1832 by Robiquet and papaverine in 1848 by Merck. Morphine was soon recognized to be as addictive as opium. Attempts were made to increase morphine's antinociceptive and antidiarrheal properties while decreasing tolerance and dependence. The result was Dreser's synthesis of diacetylmorphine (heroin) in 1898.

The existence of specific opioid receptors was definitively established in 1973 by Snyder and colleagues in the United States and Terenius and colleagues in Sweden. In 1975, Kosterlitz and Hughes identified two endogenous pentapeptides with morphine-like activity—the leu-enkephalin and the met-enkephalin—opening the door to the characterization of additional endogenous ligands. Work continues on opioid receptors with the aim of improving our understanding of their biopharmacology and manipulating the beneficial effects of opioids, while reducing their undesirable consequences.

The term *opiate* specifically refers to all naturally occurring alkaloids derived from opium, including morphine, 6-mono-acetyl-morphine, codeine, codethyline, and pholcodine. In contrast, the term *opioid* refers to all drugs, natural or synthetic, with morphine-like actions or actions mediated through binding to opioid receptors. This chapter focuses on the clinical issues concerning the acute and chronic toxicology of opioids and appropriate treatment relevant to current clinical practice.

EPIDEMIOLOGY

The dangers of opioid overdose have been recognized for as long as the use of opium itself. Overdose from illicit opioid use has increased in many countries over the past decade,[1] as has the illicit production, transportation, and consumption of opioids, especially heroin. Higher production, increasing purity, and lower prices have considerably contributed to the worldwide expansion of opioid use. Higher heroin purity enables users to smoke or snort rather than inject it, contributing to widespread popularity, illustrated by a recently reported epidemic of heroin use.[2] Changes in the route of opioid administration over time may occur in relation to opioid tolerance or drug purity increase. Heroin vapor inhalation produced by heating heroin on aluminum foil is increasingly common. The majority of drug users currently entering treatment programs are noninjectors. There is a trend toward multidrug use, with attendant drug-drug interactions and the risk of polyintoxication.

In 2004, the Substance Abuse and Mental Health Services Administration (SAMHSA) and the Drug Abuse Warning Network (DAWN) estimated that 19.1 million Americans ages 12 or older (about 7.9% of the population) were current illicit drug users.[3] However, the prevalence of heroin use remains low in the general population when compared with alcohol, tobacco, or cannabis. Typically, less than 2% of the adult population has ever used heroin, and less than 1% is dependent on heroin. An estimated 300,000 persons in the United States suffer from heroin dependence or abuse (Fig. 33-1), and 118,000 persons have used heroin for the first time within the past 12 months with an average age of initiation at 24 years. The number of injectors has been estimated to be about 5.3 million worldwide, which appears to be constant. For 2003, the American Association of Poison Control Centers (AAPCC) reported 22,600 opioid overdoses among the 270,000 exposures to analgesics (around 8%), which resulted in 213 of 656 deaths (around 35%) attributed to this pharmacological class.[4]

The SAMHSA reported 709,000 hospital facility visits in 2004 related to illicit drug use, versus 638,484 in 2001

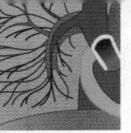

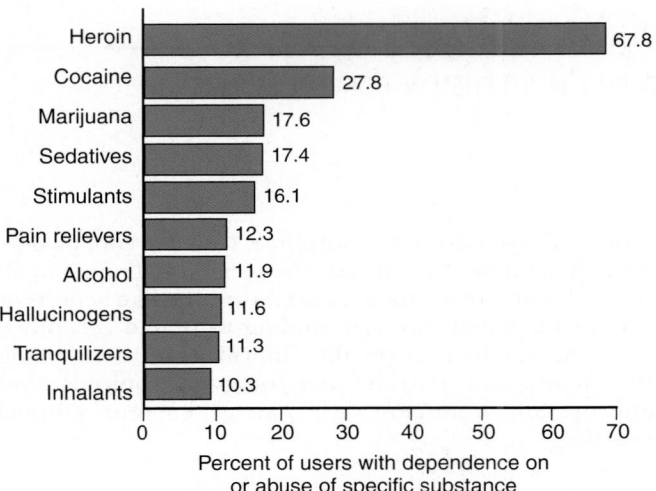

FIGURE 33-1 Comparative incidence of dependence or abuse of specific substances among past users of substances in the United States in 2004. (Courtesy of the Substance Abuse and Mental Health Services Administration, http://www.icpsr.umich.edu/SAMHDA.)

and 323,100 in 1978.[3] This increase does not necessarily reflect an elevation in the number of heroin users, but rather a greater number of individuals seeking help. Emergency department admissions for opioid overdose were estimated in the United States at 93,000 per year in 2002 versus 72,000 in 1995. In contrast, heroin use is decreasing in western Europe, with a rise in the mean age, presumably in relation to the widespread introduction of opioid maintenance treatment programs and to the development of dependence on other illicit drugs (cannabis, cocaine, and amphetamines). In France, for example, traditional opiate use has decreased since 1996, when both prescribed and diverted buprenorphine appeared on the scene.[5] In other countries, various locally produced opioids are used, including "home-back" in Australia and New Zealand, prepared with codeine and other opiates; "kompot" in Poland, made from poppy straw; and "black water opium" in Vietnam.

Opioids represent the most lethal illicit drug, with most of the fatalities occurring in young males, resulting in 33,662 potential years of life lost and 42 years of life lost per death.[6] A dependent heroin injector has a 20 to 30 times greater estimated risk for premature death than a similar-aged non–drug-using person. In 1995, opioid overdose deaths accounted for 76% of all deaths due to illicit drug use and 9% of deaths among young adults 15 to 44 years of age in Australia.[2] In Glasgow, nearly a third of all deaths among young adults 15 to 35 years of age were related to opioids.[7] However, after a rise in the second half of the 1980s, the number of overdose deaths has generally stabilized or declined in the majority of Western countries.[1,5] Nearly two thirds of all long-term heroin users have self-overdosed on heroin at least once.[8]

Mortality for opioid users in maintenance treatment is reduced (about four times), in comparison to opioid users involved in opioid-related emergencies.[9] Substi-

tution therapy with methadone, levomethadyl acetate, or buprenorphine may result in a substantial reduction in consumption of illicit opiate and psychoactive substances.[10-12] However, deaths have been attributed to maintenance treatment as well, in relation to their overdose or misuse. Deaths have been reported in relation to buprenorphine "overdose."[13-16] Forensic studies concluded that these deaths were due to asphyxia, with the underlying cause attributed to misuse and/or coadministration of psychotropic substances. Buprenorphine is injected by some users, despite the labeling for sublingual use.[17-19] However, despite an estimated 90,000 patients treated with high-dose buprenorphine (8 to 16 mg/day) in France since 1996, the number of significant reported side effects has been limited.[5,20] Interestingly, it appears that a strict limitation on the number of patients per prescribing physician for buprenorphine substitution programs has been associated with very limited abuse of the product since its launch in the United States in 2002.[21] Similarly, most lethal methadone intoxications are due to diverted or illegal methadone, in association with medications or other illicit drugs.[22,23] Recent increases in methadone prescription under strict medical control have not increased the number of lethal methadone intoxications but may have contributed to a large decrease in overall drug intoxication deaths.[24]

PHARMACOLOGY

The Various Opioid Molecules

Morphine is still obtained from opium or extracted from poppy straw. A number of natural alkaloids are derived from *Papaver somniferum,* including phenanthrenes (morphine, codeine, and thebaine) and benzylisoquinolines (papaverine, noscapine). Codeine is methylmorphine. Thebaine, the precursor of several compounds such as oxycodone and naloxone, differs from morphine in the methylation of its two hydroxyl groups and the presence of double bonds in the ring. Heroin is a diacetylmorphine, in the 3 and 6 positions. Hydromorphone, oxymorphone, hydrocodone, and oxycodone are also made by modifying the morphine molecule. Synthetic opioids can be structurally divided into five classes: morphinans, phenylpiperidines, benzomorphans, methadones, and propionanilides. Levorphanol is the only commercially available opioid agonist from the morphinan series. The phenylpiperidine family includes meperidine, diphenoxylate, loperamide, fentanyl, sufentanil, alfentanil, and remifentanil. Methadone and propoxyphene are structurally related opioids. Some partial opioid antagonists are clinically used, including pentazocine (a benzomorphan derivative), nalbuphine (structurally related to naloxone and oxymorphone), buprenorphine (a semisynthetic opioid derived from thebaine), and meptazinol. Minor changes in the chemical structure may convert an agonist into an antagonist opioid, like nalorphine (derived from morphine) or naloxone and naltrexone (both derived

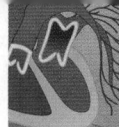

from oxymorphone). These substitutions are critical in determining agonist or antagonist properties, as well as their interactions with the various opioid receptors.

A simple classification scheme including all opioids, whether clinically used or not, distinguishes natural exogenous opioids, synthetic opioids, and endogenous opioids.

THE EXOGENOUS NATURAL OPIOIDS

This class includes opiates derived from *Papaver somniferum*, like morphine, as well as other animal-derived peptides, like deltorphines, extracted from the skin of South American frogs belonging to the *Phyllomedusa* genus and characterized by a high affinity to δ receptors.

THE SYNTHETIC OPIOIDS

This group may be subdivided into nonpeptide and peptide-like molecules. The first subgroup includes morphine derivatives, like heroin, buprenorphine, methadone, and etorphine (Fig. 33-2), as well as some δ selective agonists.

THE ENDOGENOUS OPIOIDS

Endogenous opioids are naturally occurring peptides with various types of opioid activity. They are produced after the cleavage of high-molecular-weight precursors. This group includes endorphins, enkephalins, and dynorphins or neoendorphins. They are found at various sites and in differing quantities throughout the central and peripheral nervous system. Complex interactions with multiple opioid receptors result in modulation of the response to painful stimuli. More recently, two tetrapeptides have been described and dubbed "endomorphins" due to their high affinity to μ opioid receptors, making them good candidates as endogenous ligands of these receptors.[25]

FIGURE 33-2 Chemical structures of the main opiate/opioid molecules.

Etorphin

Heroin

Buprenorphine

Methadone

PHARMACODYNAMICS

The clinically used opioids exert a common activity profile, mainly through μ opioid receptors. The central analgesic action of opioids is the most important property used in therapeutics.[26] These antinociceptive effects are mediated through spinal and supraspinal opioid receptors. Analgesia occurs without loss of consciousness. Given to patients in pain, opioids reduce the pain, while drowsiness commonly occurs and euphoria may be experienced. Given to normal pain-free subjects, opioids may induce nausea, vomiting, drowsiness, apathy, or lessened physical activity.

Mood alterations including euphoria, tranquility, and rewarding properties may follow opioid administration. Their mechanism is still not clearly understood but seems mediated by dopaminergic pathways, independently from those involved in physical dependence and analgesia. Pinpoint miosis is a near pathognomonic consequence of opioids on the parasympathetic innervation of pupils. The cough reflex is depressed through a direct action on the cough center in the medulla. This antitussive action represents the target effect of some opioid agents. Nausea and vomiting are caused by direct stimulation of the chemoreceptor trigger zone for emesis in the area postrema of the medulla.

Opioids may be responsible for respiratory depression, mainly by a direct effect on the brainstem respiratory centers. Opioids may also depress the pontine and medullary centers involved in regulation of respiratory rhythmicity. With usual opioid doses, in the absence of underlying pulmonary or neurologic diseases, clinically significant respiratory depression is rare, unless other psychotropic or sedative medications are concomitantly used. Respiratory depression increases with the dose and is the incriminated mechanism of death following opioid overdose. All phases of respiration may be depressed, including respiratory rate and tidal and minute volumes. Following an intravenous (IV) injection of morphine, maximal respiratory depression is obtained within 5 to 10 minutes. High doses of certain opioids (fentanyl, alfentanil, remifentanil, and sufentanil) may produce acute muscular rigidity, involving the trunk and the chest wall, sometimes compromising respiration. The mechanism for this is still debated and may involve basal ganglia dopamine receptor blockade, α_2-adrenergic or δ opioid receptor stimulation. In patients undergoing anesthesia, muscle rigidity may necessitate the administration of neuromuscular blocking agents to facilitate mechanical ventilation.

Endocrine effects have also been reported, including the inhibition of gonadotropin-releasing hormone and corticotropin-releasing factor production, inducing a diminution in concentrations of luteinizing hormone, follicle-stimulating hormone, adrenocorticotropic hormone, and β-endorphin circulating. Antidiuretic hormone release is also reduced. Opioids increase the muscular tonus of the gastrointestinal (GI) tract and diminish peristaltic contractions. They also diminish biliary, pancreatic, and intestinal secretions, but increase anal sphincter tone. Intestinal resting tone is increased and

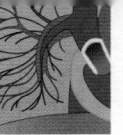

spasms may result. All these effects induce desiccation of the feces, leading to constipation and the therapeutic use of some opioid compounds as antidiarrheic substances. Opioids also increase bladder external sphincter tone, resulting in urinary retention, sometimes requiring bladder catheterization.

Opioid-related cardiovascular side effects are well known: mild reduction in blood pressure, risk for orthostatic hypotension, or, uncommonly, bradycardia. Only propoxyphene is associated with significant cardiovascular toxicity due to sodium channel blockade. Opioids also induce peripheral vasodilatation at therapeutic doses. The skin of the face, neck, and upper thorax may flush due to histamine liberation. The immune system also may be considered a potential therapeutic target of opioids, including central immunomodulatory activity or direct effects on immune cells. This latter effect is related to an activation of δ opioid receptors expressed on peripheral blood cells. Met-enkephalin and β-endorphin may stimulate the chemotactic properties of neutrophils, monocytes, or lymphocytes. In contrast, morphine reduces the activity of natural killer lymphocytes and neutrophil activity. The latter immunosuppressive effects appear to be mediated through μ receptors.[27]

Prolonged treatment with opioids may induce a tolerance to their effect, characterized by the loss of their effectiveness and the necessity to increase doses to obtain the same effects. Dependence on opioids is responsible for the appearance of withdrawal when the opioid therapy is abruptly stopped. Addiction results from an altered behavior with the compulsive use of opioids and an overwhelming need for their procurement and use. The molecular mechanisms of dependence and tolerance appear very complex, involving opioid and *N*-methyl-D-aspartate receptors. These pathways are physiologic responses to opioid treatments and may be distinct from those involved in addiction.

Morphine, tramadol, meperidine, fentanyl, and related opioids are used primarily for their analgesic properties. Codeine is used widely for its antitussive action. Given their dynamic and kinetic properties, methadone (with a long half-life) and buprenorphine (with partial μ agonist activity) are used as maintenance therapies in heroin abusers. Naloxone, the therapeutic antagonist of reference, is used to reverse neurologic and respiratory depression induced by acute opioid poisoning.

OPIOID RECEPTORS

The International Union on Receptor Nomenclature has recently recommended a nomenclature change from the historical Greek alphabet to one similar to other neurotransmitter systems, the receptors δ, κ, and μ, becoming OP_1, OP_2, and OP_3, respectively.[28]

1. *The μ opioid receptors (OP_3).* The μ receptors were the first opioid binding sites described, in relation to morphine agonist activity and high affinity.[29] Morphine has a 50-times higher affinity for μ receptors in comparison with other opioids. Fentanyl and other piperidyl agonists also have good affinity and selectivity for μ receptors (Table 33-1).

Naloxone is the only clinically used opioid receptor antagonist, with a higher affinity for the μ than for the other receptors.[30] Other antagonists also have good selectivity for μ receptors (Fig. 33-3).

μ Receptors are further classified into μ_1 and μ_2 subclasses (Table 33-2). The μ_1 receptors found in the periaqueductal gray matter, the nucleus raphe magnus, and the locus caeruleus are postulated to have supraspinal analgesic properties. The μ_1 receptors are responsible for almost all opioid analgesic properties, and to some extent, their side effects. The μ_2 receptors, characterized by a lower affinity for opioids than μ_1, are responsible for the untoward side effects of opioids, including respiratory depression, delayed GI motility (nausea, vomiting, and constipation), urinary retention, bradycardia, miosis, euphoria, and physical dependence.

2. *The κ receptors (OP_2).* The κ agonists produce analgesia that is unaffected by tolerance or antagonists to μ receptors (see Table 33-2). The κ_1 receptors appear to be concentrated in the spinal cord, whereas κ_2 and κ_3 receptors appear to predominate in the supraspinal region. They may even outnumber μ receptors in that region. Untoward effects of κ stimulation include respiratory depression (less than μ), miosis, dysphoria, and psychotomimetic effects.

3. The δ receptors (OP_1). The δ receptors mediate spinal analgesia, specifically via thermal nociception. Both enkephalins and β-dynorphin bind to this class. The δ receptors also have a cortical distribution and may have a role interacting with centrally located μ receptors. Untoward side effects include respiratory depression via decreased respiratory rate.[29]

All these opioid receptors have now been cloned and sequenced. They each consist of seven transmembrane segments (Fig. 33-4). The molecular conformations of the opioid receptors play an important role in their activity.[31,32] All the opioid receptors belong to the G-protein–binding superfamily, with significant sequence homology between their transmembrane regions. However, important differences exist within their intracellular and extracellular segments, determining the differences in their binding properties (Table 33-3). Different mechanisms of cellular transduction are now described, depending not on the receptor type but on its localization. The G-protein structure contains three subunits (α, β, γ), from which the βγ subunit is liberated on the binding of the α subunit to guanosine triphosphate. The βγ is then able to activate various effector systems, including phospholipase C, adenylate cyclase, other channels, or transport proteins (Fig. 33-5). The main postsynaptic signal trasduction mechanism is based on the inhibition of the adenylate cyclase, mediated by inhibitory G proteins (Gi), associated with μ, κ, and δ opioid receptors.[33,34] Opening of potassium channels may result from opioid receptor stimulation, yielding membrane hyperpolarization and neuronal excitability reduction.[35,36] On the presynaptic membrane, the opioid receptor activation is associated with a closure

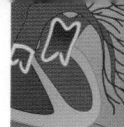

TABLE 33-1 Opioid Pharmacological Properties

	α RECEPTOR, [³H]HU-69,593	δ RECEPTOR, [³H]NALTRINDOL	μ RECEPTOR, [³H]DAMGO
Nonselective Compounds			
Dynorphin A	0.5	>1000	32
Leu-enkephalin	>1000	4.0	3.4
Met-enkephalin	>1000	1.7	0.65
β-Endorphin	52	1.0	1.0
Des-Tyr¹-β-endorphin	>1000	>1000	>1000
(−)-Naloxone	2.3	17	0.93
(+)-Naloxone	>1000	>1000	>1000
Levorphanol	6.5	5.0	0.086
Dextrorphan	>1000	>1000	>1000
(±)-Bremazocine	0.089	2.3	0.75
Ethylketocyclazocine	0.40	101	3.1
Etorphine	0.13	1.4	0.23
Pentazocine	7.2	31	5.7
Diprenorphine	0.017	0.23	0.072
β-CNA	0.083	115	0.90
β-FNA	2.8	48	0.33
Naltrexone	3.9	149	1.0
Nalbuphine	3.9	>1000	11
Nalorphine	1.1	148	0.97
μ-Selective Compounds			
CTOP	>1000	>1000	0.18
Dermorphin	>1000	>1000	0.33
Methadone	>1000	>1000	0.72
DAMGO	>1000	>1000	2.0
PLO17	>1000	>1000	30
Morphiceptin	>1000	>1000	56
Codeine	>1000	>1000	79
Fentanyl	255	>1000	0.39
Sufentanil	75	50	0.15
Lofentanil	5.9	5.5	0.68
Naloxonazine	11	8.6	0.054
Morphine	538	>1000	14
κ-Selective Compounds			
Norbinaltorphimine	0.027	65	2.2
Spiradoline	0.036	>1000	21
U-50,488	0.12	>1000	>1000
U-69,593	0.59	>1000	>1000
ICI 204,488	0.71	>1000	>1000
δ-Selective Compounds			
DPDPE	>1000	14	>1000
D-Ala²-deltorphin II	>1000	3.3	>1000
DSLET	>1000	4.8	39
BW 3734	17	0.013	26
DADL	>1000	0.74	16
SIOM	>1000	1.7	33
Naltrindole	66	0.02	64
NTB	13	0.013	12
BNTX	55	0.66	18

Receptor affinity (Kᵢ) were obtained using competition with [³H]naltrindol (δ), [³H]U69,593 (κ), and [³H]DAMGO (μ) in the presence of the indicated molecules.
β-CNA, β-chlornaltrexamine; β-FNA, β-funaltrexamine; CTOP, D-Phe-Cys-Tyr-D-Trp-Orn-Thr-Pen-Thr-NH₂; SIOM, 7-spiroindinooxymorphone.
Data from Raynor K, Kong H, Chen Y, et al: Pharmacological characterization of the cloned kappa-, delta-, and mu-opioid receptors. Mol Pharmacol 1994;45(2):330–334.

of N-type calcium channels, resulting in a reduction of intracellular calcium concentration at the end of the synapse and leading to the blockage of presynaptic vesicle fusion with the terminal membrane and the reduction in neurotransmitter release.[37]

PHARMACOKINETICS

Opioids are available in numerous formulations, allowing various routes of administration, including oral, parenteral, transdermal (fentanyl), transmucosal (morphine

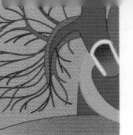

FIGURE 33-3 Selective μ opioid receptor agonists and antagonists.

DAMGO

Tyr—D—Ala—Gly—N(Me)Phe—Gly—oI

Morphine

PLO17

Tyr—Pro—τ—MePhe—D—Pro—NH₂

Fentanyl

Naloxone

Naloxonazin

Naltrexone

β-FNA

TABLE 33-2 The Different Opioid Receptor Type and Subtypes

RECEPTORS	AGONISTS*	ANTAGONISTS	SPECIFIC REPORTED EFFECTS OF EACH RECEPTOR SUBTYPE
μ	Morphine, methadone, DAMGO	CTOP	Sedation, euphoria
μ₁	Meptazinol	Naloxonazin	Supraspinal analgesia, peripheral analgesia, euphoria, prolactin release
μ₂	Metkephamid		Spinal analgesia, respiratory depression, physical dependence, gastrointestinal effects, bradycardia, puritis, dopamine, and growth hormone release
δ	DSLET	Naltrindol, NTB, BNTX	Modulation of μ receptor function and dopaminergic neurons
δ₁	DPDPE		Spinal and supraspinal analgesia
δ₂	Deltorphin		Supraspinal analgesia
κ	Dynorphin A, ethylketocyclazocine	Nor-binaltorphimin (nor-BNI)	Sedation, gastrointestinal effects
κ₁	U50,488H, spiradolin		Spinal analgesia, diuresis, miosis
κ₂	Bremazocin		Psychotomimesis, dysphoria
κ₃	Nalorphin		Supraspinal analgesia

*Leverphanol and etorphin are nonspecific agonists of the three opioid receptor types, whereas naloxone and naltrexone are nonselective antagonists of these three receptor types.

and hydromorphone), epidural, intrathecal, intranasal, and even intrapulmonary (by smoking) administration. In opioid overdoses, dosage, duration, and route of administration may influence symptoms and their duration. Thus, considering opioid pharmacokinetic properties is useful in understanding their toxicologic consequences and choosing the best methods of treatment.

Variable reduction in bioavailability results from first pass metabolism when absorbed through the GI tract. Morphine bioavailability by the oral route is only 25%, in contrast to codeine at 60%. Buprenorphine undergoes

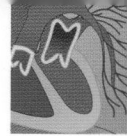

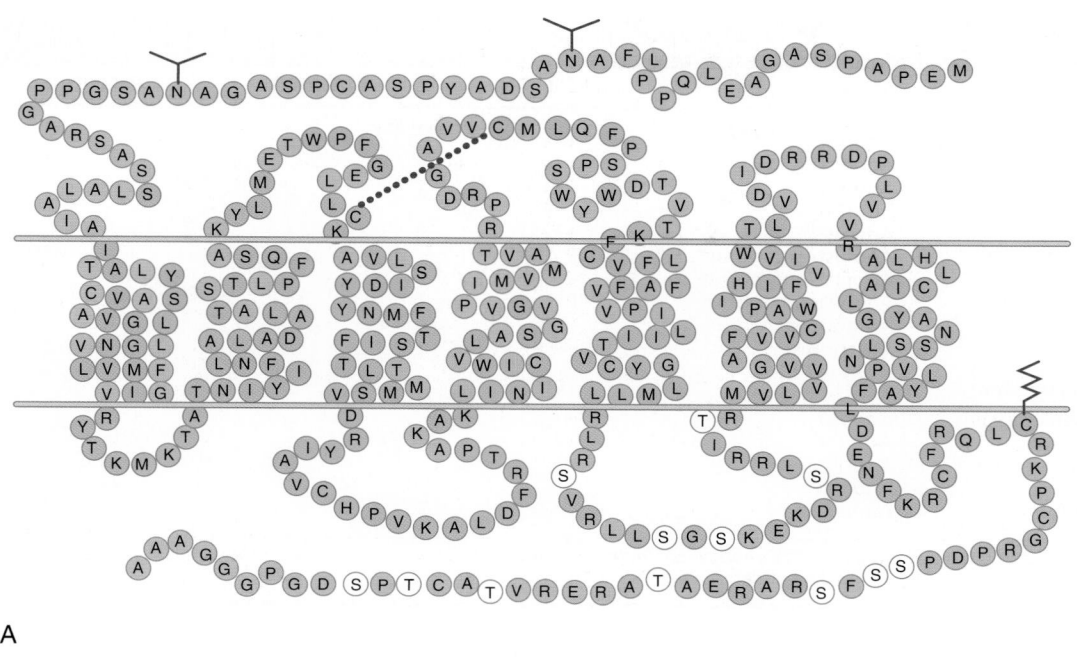

A

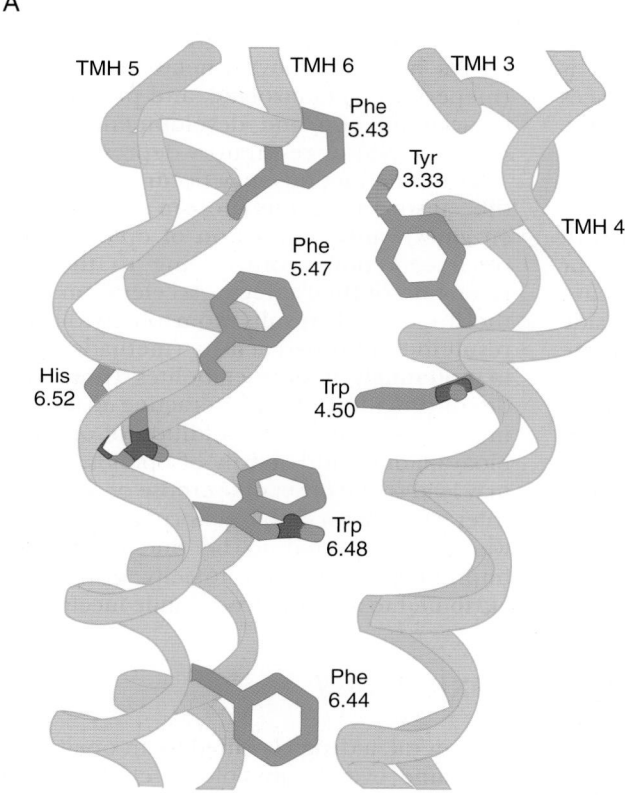

B

FIGURE 33-4 **A,** Molecular representation of opioid receptors. All receptors exhibit seven transmembrane segments with differences determining specific binding properties. **B,** As an example, we represented the aromatic and polar residues of the δ receptors, which are specific for its binding sites.

extensive first pass metabolism after oral administration, making the sublingual route mandatory for a bio-availability of 50%.[38]

Protein binding and any interaction that alters it also play a vital role in pharmacodynamics. The range of protein-bound opioid varies from a low of 7% for codeine to greater than 90% for methadone and buprenorphine. Depression in albumin and other serum proteins (α- or β-globulin) resulting in decreased binding may produce higher levels of free opioid with possible opioid toxicity. Changes in serum pH may also alter protein binding of opiates. Transport system

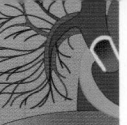

TABLE 33-3 Selective Activity of the Main Opiate/Opioid on the Different Opioid Receptors

MOLECULES	ACTIVITY	μ RECEPTOR	δ RECEPTOR	κ RECEPTOR
Morphine	Agonist	+++		+
Methadone	Agonist	+++		
Etorphin	Agonist	+++	+++	+++
Fentanyl	Agonist	+++		
Sufentanyl	Agonist	+++	+	+
Buprenorphine	Agonist–antagonist	P	?	– –
Nalorphin	Agonist–antagonist	– – –		+
Pentazocin	Agonist–antagonist	P		++
Naloxone	Antagonist	– – –	–	– –
Naltrexone	Antagonist	– – –	–	– – –
Endogenous Peptides*				
Met- et Leu-enkephalins	Agonist	++	+++	
β-endorphin	Agonist	+++	+++	
Dynorphin A	Agonist	++		+++
Dynorphin B	Agonist	+	+	+++
α-neoendorphin	Agonist	+	+	+++

*Enkephalins and endorphins are considered the endogenous ligands of μ and δ receptors; dynorphin A activity is related to κ receptors.
+, agonist; –, antagonist; P, partial agonist; ?, not determined.

proteins, such as P-glycoproteins, may also influence tissue distribution. Crossing the blood-brain barrier is dependent on lipid solubility and polarity and influences clinical effects. Heroin (diacetylmorphine) enters the brain more readily than both of its metabolites, 6-monoacetylmorphine (6-MAM) and morphine, explaining its greater addictive potential.

Opioids generally undergo hepatic metabolism with some form of conjugation, hydrolysis, oxidation, or dealkylation. Some of the resulting metabolites have been implicated in the activity or recognized toxic side effects of various opioids. Examples of this include the metabolism of codeine to morphine, morphine to the more active morphine-6-glucuronide, buprenorphine to norbuprenorphine, meperidine to the potentially neurotoxic normeperidine, and propoxyphene to the potentially cardiotoxic norpropoxyphene. Figure 33-6 illustrates the metabolism of buprenorphine, which undergoes extensive cytochrome P-450 3A4-mediated N-dealkylation to norbuprenorphine and then glucuronidation.[39] Cytochrome genotype appears to be an important parameter in opioid efficacy or toxicity. Small doses of codeine, which is bioactivated into morphine by cytochrome P-450 2D6, may be responsible for life-threatening intoxication in patients with allele patterns inducing ultrarapid metabolism, in combination with inhibition of cytochrome P-450 3A4 activity and a transient reduction in renal function.[40]

Excretion of opiates occurs primarily via the renal route, with about 90% of the opioid metabolites eventually being excreted in the urine, usually via glomerular filtration. A small amount may end up in the GI tract via enterohepatic circulation. The urinary detection of opioids or metabolites is a routinely used diagnostic test. The presence of 6-MAM in the urine is a reliable marker of recent heroin consumption, because humans cannot acetylate morphine but only deacetylate heroin. Renal failure leads to toxic effects via accumulated drug or active metabolites (morphine-6-

glucuronide or normeperidine). Hepatic dysfunction results in delayed liver metabolism of certain opioids (meperidine, pentazocine, and propoxyphene), leading to accumulation and development of central nervous system (CNS) or respiratory depression.

Drug interactions may occur at various sites affecting the absorption, metabolism (induction of hepatic enzymes), and elimination of opioids (competition for renal excretion) contributing to the potentiation or reduction of their effects. Acceleration of metabolism in the liver, which results from phenytoin induction, may result in diminished activity (methadone) or an increase in potentially toxic metabolites (normeperidine). The discontinuation of an interacting drug may play just as important a role as the addition of one in changing the bioavailability and activity of opioids. These interactions may lead to the onset of overdose or withdrawal symptoms. Interaction between buprenorphine and benzodiazepines, which is suspected to be one of the mechanisms of buprenorphine-related toxicity or fatality,[41] has been attributed to a pharmacodynamic mechanism.[42]

TOXICOLOGY

In general, a drug classified as an opiate or opioid elicits the same overall physiologic effects as morphine, the prototype of this group. However, there are conspicuous differences among these agents, which will be specifically addressed. Varying degrees of the classic "opiate toxidrome" (i.e., mental status depression, respiratory depression, miosis, and decreased bowel motility) may manifest in patients administered opioids.

Central Nervous System Effects

A dose of 5 to 10 mg of morphine usually produces analgesia without altering mood or mental status in a patient. Sometimes dysphoria rather than euphoria may

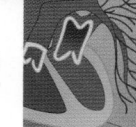

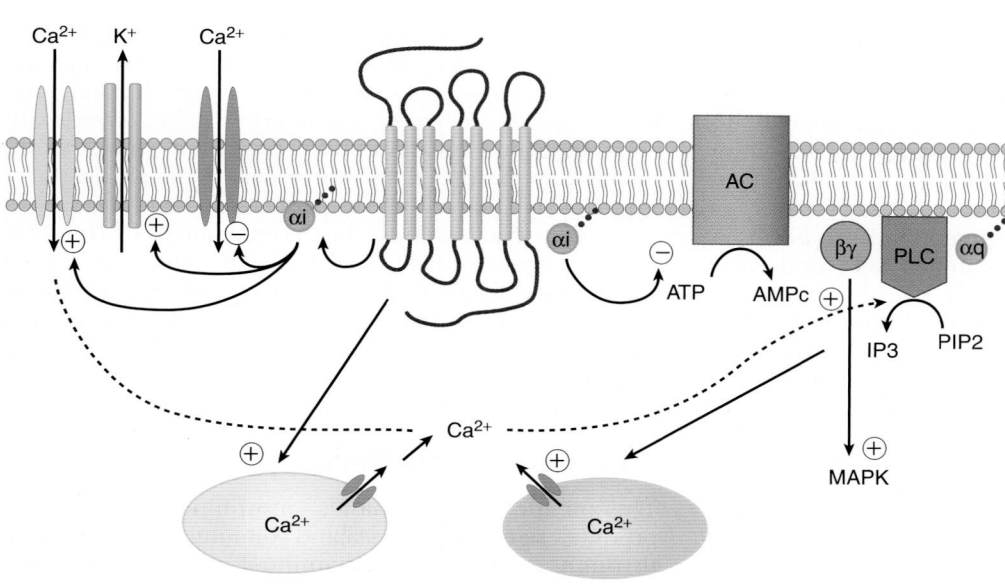

FIGURE 33-5 Regulation of the different cellular effectors by the opioid receptors MAPK (mitogen-activated protein kinases), AC (adenylate cyclase), PLC (phospholipase C), IP3 (inositol 1,4,5 triphosphate), and PIP2 (phosphatidylinositol 4,5 biphosphate).

FIGURE 33-6 Liver metabolism of buprenorphine (Bup), as demonstrated in vitro, using liver microsomes. Various cytochromes P-450 (CYP) are involved, resulting in the production of a predominant active metabolite, the norbuprenorphine (Norbup). Other metabolites (M1 to M5) are also produced, but their role and importance in vivo are unknown. (From Chang Y, Moody DE, McCance-Katz EF: Novel metabolites of buprenorphine detected in human liver microsomes and human urine. Drug Metab Dispos 2006;34(3):440–448.

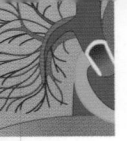

manifest, resulting in mild anxiety or a fear reaction. Nausea is frequently reported, whereas vomiting is occasionally observed. The clinical effects of morphine are accentuated with increasing doses (e.g., analgesia is stronger, lethargy and drowsiness progress to sleepiness and coma). Slurred speech and significant motor incoordination are usually absent.

Morphine and most of its congeners cause pupillary constriction. This effect is predominantly a central effect and is accentuated following an overdose. Not all patients taking opioids present with miosis. Patients taking meperidine or propoxyphene regularly maintain normal pupillary size, and patients taking pentazocine may not develop miosis.[43] Mydriasis may occur in severely poisoned patients secondary to hypoxic or anoxic brain injury. Combination drug use such as cocaine and heroin ("speedball"), scopolamine-adulterated heroin, and Lomotil (diphenoxylate hydrochloride and atropine sulfate; Pfizer, New York, NY) or the presence of adulterants may produce variable pupil size depending on the relative contribution by each agent.

Cerebral circulation does not appear to be altered by therapeutic doses of morphine, unless respiratory depression and carbon dioxide retention result in cerebral vasodilation.[44] Seizures are rare adverse drug events associated with most therapeutic opioid dosing. In an acute opioid overdose, seizures are most likely to be caused by hypoxia. Morphine-induced seizures have only been reported in neonates,[45] and seizures should be anticipated in patients with meperidine, propoxyphene, or tramadol toxicity.

Respiratory Effects

Respiratory failure is the most serious consequence from opioid overdose. Opioids reduce ventilation by diminishing the sensitivity of the medullary chemoreceptors in the respiratory centers to an increase in carbon dioxide tension ($PaCO_2$) and depress the ventilatory response to hypoxia.[46] The combined diminution in hypercapnic and hypoxic drive leaves virtually no stimulus to breathe, and apnea ensues. Even small doses of morphine depress respiration by directly affecting the brainstem respiratory centers. Morphine-induced respiratory depression initially relates more closely to changes in tidal volume and a reduction of respiratory rate with escalating doses.[30,44] The peak respiratory depressant effect is usually noted within 7 minutes of IV morphine administration, and may be delayed for up to 30 minutes if the drug is administered intramuscularly. Normal carbon dioxide sensitivity usually returns within 2 to 3 hours, while minute volume may remain below normal for up to 5 hours following a therapeutic dose.[47]

Cardiovascular Effects

Therapeutic opioid doses cause arteriolar and venous dilation and may result in a mild decrease in blood pressure.[48] This change in blood pressure is clinically insignificant while the patient is supine, but significant orthostatic changes are common.[49] Hypotension appears to be mediated by histamine release[50] and may be related to the nonspecific ability of certain opioids to activate mast cell

G protein,[51] which induces degranulation of histamine-containing vesicles. The combination of H_1 and H_2 antagonists appears to be effective in ameliorating the hemodynamic effects of opioids.[52] Not all opioids are equivalent in their ability to release histamine. In one study, meperidine produced the most, and fentanyl the least, hypotension and elevation of plasma histamine levels.[53]

Bradycardia is unusual, but a reduction in heart rate is common as a result of the associated reduction in CNS stimulation. Myocardial damage (necrotizing angiitis) in opiate overdose associated with prolonged hypoxic coma may be mediated by cellular components released during rhabdomyolysis, direct toxic effects, or hypersensitivity to the opioids or adulterants.[54]

Gastrointestinal Effects

Therapeutic use of opioids, morphine in particular, produces significant nausea and vomiting.[55] It is mediated through agonism at dopamine-2 receptor subtypes within the chemoreceptor trigger zone of the medulla. Opioid-induced constipation is an adverse drug event of both the therapeutic and recreational use of opioids. It is mediated by μ_2 receptors within the smooth muscle of the intestinal wall. Morphine and related drugs may cause a delay in the passage of gastric contents through the pylorus up to 12 hours and marked decrease in intestinal peristalsis.

SPECIFIC OPIOIDS

Heroin

Heroin has two to five times the analgesic potency of morphine, with similar effects on the CNS.[56] Virtually all street heroin in the United States is produced in clandestine laboratories and is adulterated prior to distribution. The purity of street heroin is between 5% and 90%, and is usually less than 50%.[57] Adulterants may include noscapine, caffeine, procaine, various sugars, phenobarbital, methaqualone, quinine, and acetaminophen in combination with caffeine.[58,59] Heroin is generally bought by the "bag" (25 mg) or quarter gram and may also be mixed with other drugs of abuse (e.g., "speed ball"). Purity and adulterants may play a considerable role in the outcome and complications of heroin use. Interindividual variation in sensitivity and tolerance makes correlation of serum heroin levels with clinical symptoms difficult.

Heroin is available as either a hydrochloride salt or a base, with the base being the prevalent form in most regions of the world. The hydrochloride salt form is typically a white or beige powder and is highly water soluble, which allows simple IV administration. Heroin base is often brown or black in color, and "black tar heroin" is one designation referring to an impure form available in the United States. Heroin base is virtually insoluble in water, and requires heating until it liquefies prior to IV administration. This process involves heating the powder in a spoon or bottle cap until it is dissolved, passing the heroin through cotton or a cigarette filter

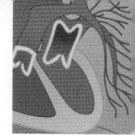

into a syringe, and boiling the cotton or filters to extract additional drug. The filtered heroin and the extract are injected IV or subcutaneously ("skin popping"). Some drug users may become acutely ill with a benign febrile, leukocytic syndrome following an IV injection. This condition is known as "cotton fever," and its etiology has been attributed to bacteremia following injection of *Enterobacter agglomerans* that has colonized in the cotton or cigarette filters.[60]

Heroin may also be taken intranasally (snorted) and by inhalation of heated vapors. Inhalation of heated vapors is known as "chasing the dragon," "Chinesing," or "Chinese blowing," and involves placing heroin base on aluminum foil, heating it from below with a flame, and inhaling the thick white pyrolysate through a straw. The bioavailability of heroin administered by this route is comparable with that of heroin administered by other routes, and the clinical and toxicological effects are dose dependent.[61,62]

Physiologically, the effects of heroin are identical to those described for morphine.[63,64] The plasma half-life of heroin is 5 to 15 minutes. Heroin is initially deacetylated in the liver and plasma and then is renally excreted as a conjugate, with small amounts of morphine, diacetyl-morphine, and 6-MAM.[65] The initial heroin rush is probably due to its high lipid solubility and rapid penetration into the CNS.[56] The majority of its lasting effects are attributable to its metabolites 6-MAM and morphine.[49] Fatal overdoses with heroin have been reported with serum morphine concentrations of 0.1 to 1.8 µg/mL.[66]

Acute lung injury (noncardiogenic pulmonary edema) as a complication of heroin overdose was first described by William Osler during an autopsy.[67] Its presentation and clinical course following nonfatal heroin overdoses were first described in 1953,[68] and later in case series and reports.[69] Patients with acute lung injury may present early on in their course; within 2 hours of parenteral heroin use and up to 4 hours following intranasal heroin use.[66,69,70] Typically, the patient awakens from an opioid coma, either spontaneously or following an opioid antagonist, and over the subsequent several minutes to hours develops hypoxemia and pulmonary rales. Classic frothy, pink sputum is occasionally observed in the patient's airway. Acute lung injury was reported in 48% of hospitalized heroin overdose patients[71] and was noted in 50% to 90% of heroin overdose patients at postmortem examinations, many of whom died in a prehospital setting.[72,73] Postmortem studies of patients who succumbed to heroin-induced acute lung injury showed no gross cardiac pathology.[74] The mechanism for acute lung injury may be multifactorial and includes profound hypoxemia, hypersensitivity reactions, immune complex deposition in the alveolar capillary membrane, histamine-induced capillary leakage, neurogenic sympathetic discharge, and transient lymphatic pumping irregularities.[70-72,75-79]

A consequence of "chasing the dragon" is a progressive spongiform leukoencephalopathy and was first reported from the Netherlands.[80] The initial symptoms include pronounced motor restlessness (e.g., compulsion to move), apathy, bradyphrenia, soft (pseudobulbar) speech, disturbed cerebellar speech, and ataxia. After 2 to 4 weeks some patients developed rapid worsening of the cerebellar symptoms (e.g., gait disturbance). Hyperactive deep tendon reflexes and pathologic reflexes with hypertonic hemiplegia or tetraplegia developed. Some patients developed tremor of the head and shoulders, and others developed myoclonic jerks or choreoathetoid movements. In most cases palmomental, snout, and oculomandibular reflexes became evident. Patients who did not deteriorate remained stable with subsequent partial improvement. Within the next 2 to 4 weeks some patients further progressed in their clinical course and developed stretching spasms, profuse perspiration, central pyrexia, and blindness. The spastic paresis became hypotonic and resulted in areflexia. Some patients developed akinetic mutism. All patients who had progress to this stage died, most because of respiratory difficulties. The mortality rate was 25%. Survivors have stabilized with severe deficits or shown modest degrees of improvement.[81,82]

Heroin toxicity may be associated with cardiac conduction abnormalities and dysrhythmias,[83-85] which may be the result of metabolic derangements associated with hypoxia, a direct effect of heroin or its metabolites or of adulterants.[54,86,87] Quinine-adulterated heroin has been associated with dysrhythmias,[88,89] amblyopia,[90] and thrombocytopenia.[91] Patients exposed to heroin that has been adulterated with scopolamine may present in acute anticholinergic crisis.[92] Surreptitious addition of cocaine to heroin may cause significant myocardial ischemia or infarction.[93] Other reported adulterants include thallium,[94] lead,[95] amphetamines,[96] chloroquine,[97] and strychnine.[98]

Codeine

Codeine (methylmorphine) is available as a sole ingredient and in combination with aspirin or acetaminophen. Codeine is rapidly absorbed by the oral route, producing a peak plasma level within 1 hour of a therapeutic dose.[99] Ten percent of codeine is metabolized to morphine.[100] Both codeine and morphine appear in the urine within 24 to 72 hours, with only morphine being detected in the urine at 96 hours.[99] The effect of codeine on the CNS is comparable but less pronounced than that of morphine. An IV codeine phosphate dose of 750 to 900 mg produces symptoms similar to those seen with acute heroin overdose.[101] Fatal ingestions with codeine alone are rare. The estimated lethal dose in a nonabuser is 800 mg, with a serum codeine concentration of 0.14 to 4.8 mg/dL.[102,103]

Fentanyl

Fentanyl is a synthetic opioid with rapid onset of action and short duration of action, and has a potency 100 times that of morphine. It is highly lipid soluble and has a volume of distribution of 60 to 300 L.[104] Legitimate fentanyl use is limited to anesthesia and conscious sedation, and it has been abused mostly by medical and paramedical personnel because of limited access since it was first introduced. Numerous fentanyl analogs (e.g., α-

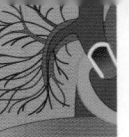

methylfentanyl ["China White"], 3-methylfentanyl, α-methyl-acetyl-fentanyl, α-methyl-fentanyl acrylate, and benzyl fentanyl) have been illicitly synthesized and distributed on the street as heroin substitutes.[105-109] They can be 200 to 6000 times more potent than morphine. Toxic effects may be experienced with very small amounts. Typically, the patients present comatose and apneic. In such cases, unsuspecting users administer their usual "dose" of heroin, which surreptitiously contains variable amounts of an illicit fentanyl analog. A number of "heroin-related" deaths have been attributed to these agents secondary to marked increased potency compared with heroin.[106-108]

Rapid IV injection of certain high-potency opioids (e.g., fentanyl) may result in acute muscular rigidity primarily involving the trunk, and may impair chest wall movement and exacerbate hypoventilation. Similar effects contribute to lethality during epidemics of fentanyl-adulterated heroin.[107] Although motor activity resembling seizures has been associated with fentanyl use,[110-112] simultaneous electroencephalogram recording during fentanyl induction of general anesthesia did not show epileptiform activity.[113-116] This suggests a myoclonic rather than epileptic nature of the observed muscle activity.[115]

Fentanyl is available as a patch; a transdermal delivery system establishes a depot of drug in the upper skin layers, where it is available for systemic absorption. After removal of the patch, drug absorption from the dermal reservoir continues and the effective fentanyl half-life is 17 hours, versus 2 to 4 hours associated with the IV route (Duragesic [fentanyl], Janssen Pharmaceutica, Piscataway, NJ). The availability of a transdermal fentanyl delivery system provides a widening pool of individuals with access. Prescribed transdermal fentanyl patches can be sold or stolen. Disabling myoclonus has been reported after several days of fentanyl therapy by the transdermal delivery system.[117] Misuse and abuse of the fentanyl patch has been reported in the form of simultaneous application of multiple patches, ingestion, inhalation, and IV injection of the transdermal fentanyl patch contents, which has resulted in respiratory arrest and death.[118-124]

Meperidine

Meperidine is a synthetic opioid and is chemically different from the traditional opiates. Although considered to possess strong analgesic properties when given by the parenteral route, it is less than half as effective if given by the oral route.[125] It appears to be a common drug of abuse among medical personnel, with few reports of meperidine poisoning or fatalities.[126-128] Meperidine is metabolized in the liver primarily by N-demethylation to normeperidine, an active metabolite with half the analgesic and euphoric potency of meperidine, and twice the neurotoxic properties.[129,130] Excretion is primarily through the kidneys as conjugated metabolites.[131] Meperidine and normeperidine may be detected in either urine or serum.[131] Meperidine toxicity

has been attributed to the accumulation of normeperidine in patients with renal impairment, which has an elimination half-life of 14 to 24 hours.[132-134] However, when meperidine is used in large doses and at frequent dosing intervals, seizures may occur in patients with normal renal function.[135-138]

Meperidine also interacts with serotonin receptors by blocking presynaptic reuptake of serotonin. A potentially fatal form of serotonin syndrome may occur in patients on monoamine oxidase inhibitors (MAOIs) and is treated with meperidine.[139]

Meperidine is the prototype for a series of homologs that are used as heroin substitutes. In a process to synthesize a meperidine analog, 1-methyl-4-phenyl-propionoxypiperidine (MPPP), as a heroin substitute, a clandestine drug laboratory inadvertently introduced 1-methyl-4-phenyl-1,2,3,6-tetrahydropyridine (MPTP) by incorrect heating of the synthetic mixture. When MPTP is introduced into the body, monoamine oxidase-B in glial cells metabolizes MPTP to MPP^+, which selectively destroys dopamine-containing cells in the substantia nigra by inhibiting mitochondrial oxidative phosphorylation.[140,141] MPTP contaminant led to an epidemic of severe parkinsonism among IV drug abusers ("frozen addicts") within days of repeated injections.[142-144]

Diphenoxylate and Loperamide

Diphenoxylate is structurally similar to meperidine, with limited absorption from the GI tract that contributes to its strong local constipating effects, and is used in the management of diarrhea. Diphenoxylate (2.5 mg) is formulated with 0.025 mg of atropine sulfate (Lomotil). In therapeutic doses, the drug has no significant CNS effects. However, the standard adult formulation may result in significant systemic absorption and toxicity in children. One half tablet of Lomotil has been reported to cause serious toxicity in children.[145-147] Signs and symptoms arising from a toxic ingestion may be delayed, prolonged, or recurrent.[147] This is related to the delayed gastric emptying effects inherent to both opioids and anticholinergics, and more important, the accumulation of the hepatic metabolite difenoxin, which is a significantly more potent opioid than diphenoxylate and possesses a longer serum half-life.[148,149]

Loperamide, an over-the-counter antidiarrheal agent, is another meperidine analog with limited absorption from the GI tract, and appears to have a high safety profile.[150]

Methadone

Methadone is a synthetic opioid commonly used in the treatment of chronic pain or detoxification, or as a maintenance substitute for opioid addiction, and is also sold on the streets.[151,152] Methadone is well absorbed from the GI tract, resulting in a peak plasma level within 2 to 4 hours, with peak effect occurring within 2 hours.[153] It has an average half-life of 25 hours and may be

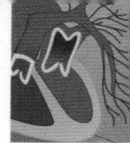

as long as 52 hours during long-term maintenance therapy.[154] Methadone and its inactive metabolite, an *N*-demethylated pyrolidine, may be detected in either urine or plasma.[155] Its analgesic, sedative, euphoric, and respiratory depressive effects are comparable with those seen with analogous doses of morphine.[156,157] In a nontolerant person, a 40- to 50-mg dose may produce coma and respiratory depression.[155,158] Rapid escalation of methadone doses have been associated with choreoathetoid movements and may be due to enhanced striatal dopamine release.[159] Unintentional pediatric poisoning with fatal consequences has occurred in situations in which parents on methadone maintenance treatment had improperly stored their methadone at home.[160] A protracted clinical course is expected following an overdose. There is a possible association between patients on very high doses of methadone and having torsades de pointes, particularly in a setting of additional dysrhythmia risk factors (e.g., hypokalemia).[161] In these patients the mean daily methadone dose was 397 ± 283 mg and their mean QTc interval was 615 ± 77 msec.

Buprenorphine

Buprenorphine is a semisynthetic, highly lipophilic opioid, with 25 to 50 times more potent analgesic activity than morphine.[162] Sublingual buprenorphine is well absorbed, with 60% to 70% of the bioavailability of the IV route. Buprenorphine is mainly metabolized in the liver by CYP3A4 to an active dealkylated metabolite, norbuprenorphine. There is no direct relation of buprenorphine's clinical effects with plasma concentrations.

Buprenorphine is a partial μ receptor agonist and a weak κ receptor antagonist, with ceiling effects. Dose-effect relationships, both in animals and humans, suggest a plateau of respiratory effects.[163] Buprenorphine shows a very slow dissociation from opioid receptors, and consequently, has a long duration of action. These pharmacologic properties appear to be of utmost importance regarding its safety for use in substitution treatment. They confer a low level of physical dependence and mild withdrawal symptoms on cessation after prolonged administration. Although respiratory depression can be prevented by prior administration of naloxone, buprenorphine is weakly antagonized by naloxone given after buprenorphine.[164]

Buprenorphine 8 to 16 mg/day has been used in France as a maintenance treatment for opioid-dependent patients since 1996. In 2002, buprenorphine was approved by the Food and Drug Administration for the treatment of opioid addiction in certified physicians' offices. A mixture of buprenorphine and naloxone named Suboxone (Reckitt Benckiser Healthcare, Ltd., Hull, UK) is also available, designed to discourage IV use. Since the advent of office-based availability, buprenorphine has been successfully used for opioid detoxification, with a good safety profile.[10,11] In France, the introduction of high-dose buprenorphine coincided with a decrease in opiate/opioid poisoning mortality rates.[5] In the United States, restricted conditions for drug prescription (no more than 30 patients per qualifying certified physician) have resulted in little abuse since its launch.[21]

As with other opioids, buprenorphine intoxication includes coma, respiratory depression, and pinpoint pupils. Several deaths have been associated with buprenorphine misuse or psychotropic drug coingestion, including benzodiazepines.[14] However, forensic determination of the exact role of buprenorphine in the death process appears difficult, because other factors may be involved (and potentially unknown), including substitution modality and concomitant intake of other drugs.[20] Moreover, the exact mechanism of interaction between buprenorphine and benzodiazepines (often implicated in buprenorphine deaths) is unknown.[165] The clinical role of drugs that interact with CYP3A4 and that may modify production of norbuprenorphine (an active metabolite with more potent respiratory depressant effects) is unknown.

Propoxyphene

Propoxyphene is structurally related to methadone, and toxicity has resulted in significant morbidity and mortality.[166-168] It is available alone or in combination with aspirin or acetaminophen. Oral administration is followed by rapid absorption, with peak serum levels occurring within 1 hour.[169] The plasma half-lives of propoxyphene and its main active hepatic metabolite norpropoxyphene are 6 to 12 hours and 37 hours, respectively. Norpropoxyphene is also the primary metabolite excreted in the urine and is believe to play a role in the prolonged clinical course following an overdose.[170,171] Prominent cardiovascular effects may occur with propoxyphene toxicity and manifest by wide-complex dysrhythmias and negative contractility through sodium channel antagonism similar to that of type IA antidysrhythmic agents. Propoxyphene appears to be responsible for both CNS (e.g., respiratory depression and seizures) and cardiac toxicity (e.g., QRS prolongation, negative inotropy, and dysrhythmias), whereas norpropoxyphene contributed only to the cardiotoxicity.[172]

The clinical course following an overdose may be severe and rapidly progressive, with cardiac dysrhythmias, circulatory collapse, seizures, and respiratory arrest developing within 1 hour.[173-178] Propoxyphene toxicity may result in focal and generalized seizures.[176,178] The minimum toxic dose reported is 10 mg/kg, and 20 mg/kg is considered potentially fatal,[179] but tolerance develops with chronic use. Doses of 1000 to 2000 mg may be ingested or injected with minimal signs of intoxication in chronic propoxyphene abusers and heroin addicts.[178,180-182] Blood levels in fatal overdose cases range from 0.1 to 2.5 mg/dL.[167,168]

Pentazocine

Pentazocine is a synthetic analgesic class with both agonist and weak antagonist activity at the opioid

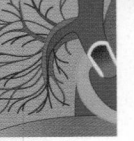

receptors.[183] The physiologic effects of pentazocine are similar to morphine, and with one third of its analgesic potency.[183] When administered by the oral route, peak plasma pentazocine levels occur within 1 hour.[184] Pentazocine is extensively metabolized in the liver,[183,184] with the parent compound and metabolites detectable in either urine or plasma.[183] Anxiety, dysphoria, and hallucinations may be more common with pentazocine than with other opiate derivatives.[183]

Pentazocine (Talwin, Sandoz, Princeton, NJ) is associated with a fairly specific scenario of parenteral abuse when used in combination with the antihistamine tripelennamine (Pyribenzamine, Novartis, Basel, Switzerland), a blue capsule. This combination forms a street product known as "T's and blues" and, once solubilized and injected, was used as a heroin substitute that was previously popular among addicts because of its heroin-like "rush" and lower cost.[185-187] Newer combination street products, such as pentazocine with methylphenidate, have been reported.[188] Acute toxicity results in the typical opiate intoxication syndrome, as well as dyspnea, hyperirritability, hypertension, and seizures. It is believed that these effects may be directly related to the tripelennamine dose.[186,189,190]

In an effort to curtail IV pentazocine abuse, the oral preparation was reformulated to contain 0.5 mg of naloxone (Talwin-NX, Sandoz, Princeton, NJ).[191] The naloxone component is inactivated when taken orally, and avoids withdrawal symptoms. However, when Talwin-NX is parenterally administered, pentazocine's effects are antagonized by naloxone, which causes withdrawal in opiate-dependent individuals. Because pentazocine's duration of action exceeds that of naloxone, delayed respiratory depression may occur.

Dextromethorphan

Dextromethorphan, an analog of codeine and the optical isomer of levorphanol (a potent opioid analgesic), is found in a large number of nonprescription cough and cold remedies. Within the therapeutic dose, dextromethorphan lacks analgesic, euphoriant, and physical dependence properties.[192] Dextromethorphan is formulated as the hydrobromide salt. It is available as a single ingredient or in combination with decongestants (sympathomimetics) and antihistamines. Dextromethorphan is well absorbed from the GI tract, with peak plasma levels occurring 2.5 and 6 hours after ingestion of regular and sustained-release preparations, respectively. The therapeutic effect lasts 3 to 6 hours, with a corresponding plasma half-life of 2 to 4 hours. The predominant antitussive effect is attributed to the active metabolite dextrorphan.[193]

Over-the-counter access appears to be the primary reason for its popularity in abuse, although its abuse pattern seems to be self-limiting due to adverse drug events, such as lethargy, somnambulism, and ataxia, after a few weeks of abuse.[194] Dextromethorphan abuse appears to be associated with a psychological rather than a physiologic dependence syndrome.[192] Recreation dextromethorphan abusers report increased perceptual awareness, altered time perception, euphoria, and visual hallucinations.[194-196] Long-term dextromethorphan use may result in bromide toxicity.[197] Since dextromethorphan frequently appears in combination products, the contribution of these co-ingestants should be considered in assessing overdose or abuse cases.

Dextromethorphan blocks presynaptic serotonin reuptake and may elicit the serotonin syndrome in patients on MAOI therapy.[198,199] Interaction between dextrorphan and the "σ receptor" produces a phencyclidine-like dysphoria.[200] The metabolism of dextromethorphan to dextrorphan is dependent on CYP2D6 activity, an enzyme with a significant genetic polymorphism. Patients who express extensive metabolizer polymorphism appear to experience more drug-related psychoactive effects, whereas patients with poor metabolizers experience more adverse effects related to the parent compound.[201] Occasionally, a patient may experience choreoathetoid or dystonia-like movements while on dextromethorphan.[202]

Tramadol

Tramadol is structurally similar to morphine and has both opioid and nonopioid mechanisms responsible for its clinical effects. It is a centrally acting analgesic with moderate affinity for μ opioid receptors. However, the metabolite O-demethyl tramadol appears to have a higher affinity than the parent compound for the same receptors. In therapeutic doses, tramadol does not appear to produce significant respiratory depression or have significant cardiovascular effects. Most of the analgesic effects are attributed to the nonopioid properties of the drug. Tramadol may exert its analgesic effect by blocking the reuptake of biogenic amines (e.g., norepinephrine and serotonin) at synapses in the descending neural pathways, which inhibits pain responses in the spinal cord.[203] Serotonin syndrome may develop in patients concurrently taking tramadol and serotonin reuptake inhibitor medication.[204,205] Seizures may occur during therapeutic dosing.[206]

BODY PACKERS

The transportation of illicit drugs by internal concealment is an important means of international smuggling, with accounts of body packing worldwide. Body packers are sometimes called "mules," "swallowers," "internal carriers," or "couriers." These are people who transport large numbers of meticulously prepared illicit drug packets in their GI tracts across borders with the intent to sell or receive compensation for transporting the drug. Typically, the packets contain either concentrated cocaine or heroin. If one of these packets ruptures, the amount of drug released may cause life-threatening toxicity.[207,208]

CLINICAL MANIFESTATIONS

Mental status depression, respiratory depression, miosis, and decreased bowel motility are the hallmarks of opiate intoxication, with the magnitude and duration of toxicity dependent on the dose and individual degree of tolerance. The clinical effects of an overdose with any one of the agents in this class are similar. However, as discussed, there are important differences between certain drugs. Overdoses resulting in toxicity often have a prolonged clinical course, partially due to an opioid-induced decrease in GI motility and prolonged half-life of the drug or its active metabolites.

Miosis is considered a consistent finding in opioid poisoning, with the exception of meperidine, propoxyphene, petazocin, dextromethorphan use, in case of a mixed overdose with an anticholinergic or sympathomimetic drug, or when severe acidemia, hypoxemia, hypotension, or a CNS structural disorder is present.

Patients presenting with CNS depression following an opioid overdose represent the most seriously intoxicated patients. However, codeine, meperidine, and dextromethorphan intoxications are remarkable for CNS hyperirritability, resulting in a mixed syndrome of stupor and delirium. In addition, patients with meperidine toxicity may also have tachypnea, dysphoric and hallucinogenic episodes, tremors, muscular twitching, and spasticity,[126,132,133,135] whereas patients with dextromethorphan toxicity may also manifest restlessness and clonus.[196,209-212]

Acute lung injury after heroin overdose may not be unique. It has been reported with overdoses of opioids that include methadone, propoxyphene, codeine, buprenorphine, and nalbuphine.[76,102,103,189,213-222] Acute lung injury may not develop until 24 hours following methadone overdose.[70,71,223,224]

Patients with heroin-induced acute lung injury typically have normal capillary wedge pressures and elevated pulmonary arterial pressures.[224,225] In contrast, elevated systemic, pulmonary arterial, and pulmonary capillary wedge pressures and total systemic vascular resistance are seen with pentazocine intoxication.[226] These effects are believed to result from transient endogenous catecholamine release.[227] Signs and symptoms of heroin-induced acute lung injury usually resolve within 24 to 36 hours.[69,228,229] Persistent pulmonary symptoms beyond 24 to 48 hours may indicate aspiration or bacterial pneumonitis, with atelectasis, fibrosis, bronchiectasis, granulomatous disease, or pneumomediastinum.[230]

Adulterants in street drugs are potential pulmonary toxicants.[231] The injection of adulterants such as talc (magnesium trisilicate) has produced granulomatosis in small pulmonary arteries, resulting in pulmonary thrombosis, pulmonary hypertension, and acute cor pulmonale.[189,190,230,232] Other potential pulmonary complications associated with IV opioid use include pulmonary arteritis, septic emboli, lung abscess, bacterial pneumonia, aspiration pneumonitis, pulmonary edema, and respiratory arrest.

Seizures and focal neurologic signs are usually absent following opiate intoxication[233] unless precipitated by severe hypoxia, dysrhythmia and hypotension, an intracranial process (e.g., brain abscess and subarachnoid hemorrhage), hypersensitive immune vascular injury or vasculitis, proconvulsive adulterants, meperidine, propoxyphene, pentazocine (T's and blues), or tramadol use.[176,178,186,234-242] Normeperidine neurotoxicity may manifest as delirium, tremor, myoclonus, or seizures.

Meperidine- and propoxyphene-related seizures may be more frequent in chronic drug abusers with renal dysfunction.

Hypotension may occur following opiate overdose, although pentazocine intoxication may result in hypertension.[186] Heroin and propoxyphene toxicity may be associated with nonspecific ST-segment and T-wave changes, first-degree atrioventricular block, atrial fibrillation, prolonged QTc intervals, and ventricular dysrhythmias.[83-85,173-175] Cardiovascular findings may be exacerbated by electrolyte abnormalities, metabolic derangements associated with hypoxia, or adulterants (e.g., quinine) in street drugs.

The anticholinergic and opioid effects may be significantly delayed, prolonged, or recurrent following a Lomotil overdose.[147,243] The relevance of delayed toxicity is highlighted by a patient with an asymptomatic presentation 8 hours postingestion who was observed for several hours and discharged. This patient returned to the emergency department 18 hours postingestion with severe atropinism.[243] Toxicity may manifest as a biphasic clinical syndrome, and patients may manifest anticholinergic toxicity (CNS excitement, hypertension, fever, flushed dry skin) before, during, or after opioid effects. However, opioid effects (CNS and respiratory depression with miosis) may predominate or occur without any signs of atropinism. Cardiopulmonary arrest has been reported to occur 12 hours after Lomotil ingestion.[244]

Patients presenting after a tramadol overdose may exhibit lethargy, nausea, tachycardia, agitation, seizures, coma, hypertension, and respiratory depression.[240] Tramadol-associated seizures are brief, and significant respiratory depression is uncommon.

Interaction between meperidine and MAOIs, dextromethorphan and MAOIs, and tramadol and selective serotonin reuptake inhibitors may result in the serotonin syndrome.[245-246] Patients with severe serotonin syndrome exhibit rapid onset of altered mental status, muscle rigidity, hyperthermia, autonomic dysfunction, coma, seizures, and death.

Rhabdomyolysis, hyperkalemia, myoglobinuria, and renal failure may complicate the clinical course of an acute opioid overdose or opioid dependence.[86,247,248] Rhabdomyolysis has been reported following IV, inhalational, and intranasal heroin abuse.[249] Acute renal failure may be due to direct insult by the abused substance, adulterants in the street drugs, and prolonged coma.[86,247,248] Chronic parental drug use may result in glomerulonephritis and renal amyloidosis and has been associated with concurrent bacterial infections.[250-253]

Body packers are typically asymptomatic, but are at risk for delayed and prolonged toxicity from packet rupture.[254] Symptomatic patients will exhibit the typical signs and symptoms of opiate intoxication. Body packers may also present with or develop signs and symptoms of intestinal obstruction, and occasionally intestinal perforation and peritonitis.[255]

Clandestine laboratories have produced exceedingly potent and toxic drugs as new manufacturing methods have been developed to circumvent the use of controlled or unavailable precursor compounds. As government

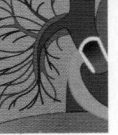

authorities stringently regulate these products and their precursors, new drugs and methods are designed to take their place.[105] Since these drugs may contain a wide variety of active ingredients, adulterants, and contaminants, the clinical syndromes seen in the abuser may be only partly related to the opioid component.

DIAGNOSIS

Laboratory Studies

Laboratory studies such as complete blood count, serum electrolytes, blood urea nitrogen, creatinine, creatine phosphokinase, urinalysis, arterial blood gas, electrocardiography, imaging studies, and lumbar puncture should be obtained as clinically indicated. Laboratory investigations should also include infections associated with IV drug abuse (e.g., endocarditis, aspergillosis, bacterial meningitis, cutaneous abscess, mycotic aneurism, intracranial abscess, epidural abscess, transverse myelitis, viral hepatitis, wound botulism, tetanus, osteomyelitis, and acquired immunodeficiency syndrome).

MANAGEMENT

Opioid toxicity should be part of the differential diagnosis in all comatose patients. However, the classic "opioid toxidrome" may not be apparent following a mixed overdose. Respiratory support is paramount in the management of patients with opioid toxicity; and the patient should be managed according to current advanced cardiac life support guidelines. Priorities include assessment and establishment of effective ventilation and oxygenation, followed by ensuring adequate hemodynamic support. Initial support with a bag-valve-mask (BVM) device is appropriate, along with 100% oxygen supplementation. Oral or nasal airway placement may be helpful, and caution is advised with their use given the potential for vomiting and/or aspiration. A suction apparatus should be available for immediate use at the patient's bedside. Ventilatory support can usually be safely provided with a BVM device while awaiting the reversal of respiratory depression by an opioid antagonist. Endotracheal intubation is indicated in severely compromised patients in whom there is a real risk for aspiration or in patients who do not satisfactorily respond to opioid antagonists.

GI decontamination should be considered after vital signs have been stabilized. Opioids may cause decreased GI motility, and this suggests there may be some benefit to GI decontamination several hours postingestion. Gastric lavage may be of benefit in patients who are critically ill, do not respond to naloxone, are suspect of polypharmacy overdose, or have overdosed on Lomotil; retrieval of Lomotil pills as late as 27 hours postingestion has been reported.[147] In the obtunded patient, endotracheal intubation should be performed prior to the placement of the orogastric tube to minimize the risk of aspiration. Early administration of activated charcoal has been advocated as the sole GI decontamination procedure. Although the clinical benefits of multiple oral doses of activated charcoal remain to be established, it has potential benefit because of the prolonged absorption phase typically encountered with opioid overdoses. Patients should be closely monitored for the presence of bowel sounds and passing of charcoal-laden stool. Repeat charcoal doses should not be used in the absence of active bowel sounds or in the presence of an ileus. Ipecac-induced emesis in patients with opioid overdose is not recommended given the potential for rapid deterioration and the risk for aspiration.

Naloxone is a pure competitive opioid antagonist at the μ, κ, and δ receptors, and has a greater affinity for the μ receptor than for the κ or δ receptors. It can reverse the analgesia, respiratory depression, miosis, hyporeflexia, and cardiovascular effects of opiate toxicity[256,257] and is effective in terminating opioid-induced vomiting. The goal of naloxone therapy is to reestablish adequate spontaneous ventilation and maintain adequate airway reflexes without precipitating an acute withdrawal syndrome.[258] Naloxone is relatively contraindicated in the pregnant patient, in whom precipitation of acute narcotic withdrawal may induce premature labor or miscarriage. However, this does not preclude judicious naloxone use in pregnant patients with severe respiratory depression. A judicious starting dose for IV naloxone may be 0.05 to 0.1 mg if the patient is possibly opioid dependent. Otherwise, an initial 2-mg dose can be administered. The recommended pediatric naloxone dose is 0.1 mg/kg, up to 2 mg. For high-potency opioids (e.g., fentanyl and its analogs) or opioids with a greater affinity for the κ or δ receptor (e.g., pentazocine, propoxyphene) a larger than usual dose of naloxone may be needed to successfully antagonize the opioid effects.[259] Repeat IV naloxone boluses up to 10 to 20 mg should be considered if there is a history of opioid exposure, a strong clinical suspicion based on presenting signs and symptoms, or a partial response to the initial naloxone dose. Submental, intranasal, intralingual, endotracheal, intraosseous, intramuscular, and subcutaneous routes of naloxone administration are acceptable alternatives when vascular access is not readily available.[260-264] However, intramuscular and subcutaneous injections are less desirable in the emergent situation. Repeat naloxone boluses may be required every 20 to 60 minutes because of its short elimination half-life (60 to 90 minutes) compared with that of most opioids.[265] A continuous naloxone infusion may be considered in patients who have a positive response and require repeated bolus doses because of recurrent respiratory depression.[266-268] A therapeutic naloxone infusion may be made up by multiplying the effective naloxone bolus dose by 6.6, adding that quantity to 1000 mL normal saline, and infusing the solution at 100 mL/hr. The infusion is titrated to maintain adequate spontaneous ventilation without precipitating acute opioid withdrawal and is empirically continued for 12 to 24 hours. The patient should be admitted to an intensive care setting where the patient will be frequently assessed during this time. After discontinuing the naloxone therapy, the patient should be carefully observed for 2 to 4 hours for recurrent respiratory depression. In the event of acute iatrogenic opioid withdrawal, allow the

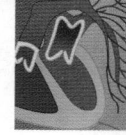

effect of naloxone to abate and avoid administering additional opioids.

Clinical experience has demonstrated naloxone to be an extremely safe drug. It has been administered at a bolus dose of 5.4 mg/kg followed by infusion at 4 mg/kg/hr for 23 hours in the treatment of acute spinal cord injury.[269] Although naloxone is ordinarily a safe drug, there have been reports ascribing acute lung injury,[222,270-275] hypertension, cardiac dysrhythmias, and death to naloxone therapy.[276-279] Typically, the patient has a depressed consciousness and respiration. After naloxone administration, the patient awakens and over minutes to hours is noted to become hypoxic with an adequate respiratory rate and to develop pulmonary edema. Pink, frothy sputum may be evident in the nasopharyngeal area. Acute naloxone-induced withdrawal has been associated with massive CNS sympathetic discharge, which may be a precipitating factor in the development of "neurogenic" pulmonary edema.[280-282] It appears that the pulmonary injury is at the alveolar-capillary membrane, resulting in manifestations consistent with acute respiratory distress syndrome.[77,218] Abrupt heroin withdrawal precipitated by naloxone may contribute to the development of acute lung injury. However, it cannot be the only effect. Naloxone does not appear to directly alter the vascular permeability of the lung.[283] Pulmonary edema was reported in 50% to 90% of the autopsies performed on heroin overdose patients, many of whom were declared dead in the prehospital setting and never received naloxone.[72,73] In addition, opioid antagonist was unavailable when the initial cases of pulmonary edema were reported. A mechanical effect in which negative intrathoracic pressure generated by attempted inspiration against a closed glottis creates a large pressure gradient across the alveolar membrane and draws fluid into the alveolar space may be responsible for the observed association between naloxone administration and acute lung injury, similar to ventilator-associated pulmonary edema (Müller maneuver) prior to the advent of demand ventilators and neuromuscular blockers.[284] Opioid poisoning may result in glottic laxity, prevent adequate air entry during inspiration, and may be especially prominent at the time of naloxone administration. This may result in breathing being reinstituted prior to the return of adequate upper airway function.

Naloxone is effective in reversing diphenoxylate (Lomotil)-induced opioid toxicity, but recurrence of respiratory and CNS depression is common.[243] All patients with significant diphenoxylate overdose should be admitted for monitored observation in the hospital for at least 24 hours.[147] Naloxone has been reported to reverse, though inconsistently, the CNS effects of ethanol, benzodiazepines, clonidine, chlorpromazine, and valproic acid following an overdose.[285-288]

Naloxone administration may "unmask" cocaine toxicity in patients using "speedballs"[289] or anticholinergic toxicity in patients using heroin and scopolamine.[290]

Hypotension may respond to naloxone therapy, but may require fluid resuscitation and vasopressors. Overzealous fluid resuscitation should be avoided because of the risk for pulmonary edema. Cardiac dysrhythmias should be managed according to current advance cardiac life support guidelines. Sodium bicarbonate may be useful in treating cardiotoxicity from drugs with "quinidine-like effects" (type IA antidysrhythmics) that impair sodium channel functioning, manifested by widened QRS complexes, dysrhythmias, and hypotension. Sodium bicarbonate has been reported to be effective in narrowing the QRS complex in the setting of propoxyphene-induced wide complex dysrhythmias.[291] Sodium bicarbonate (1 to 2 mEq/kg) may be administered as an IV bolus over a period of 1 to 2 minutes. Greater amounts may be required to treat unstable ventricular dysrhythmias. Sodium bicarbonate boluses can then be repeated as needed with the end point of stabilizing or narrowing the QRS interval. Excessive alkalemia (pH greater than 7.55) and hypernatremia should be avoided.

Management of seizures should follow current treatment guidelines and should include benzodiazepines or barbiturates. Adjunct naloxone therapy may be effective in propoxyphene-[292] but not meperidine- or tramadol-related seizures. Experimental evidence suggests naloxone may potentiate normeperidine-induced seizures by inhibiting an anticonvulsant effect of meperidine.[293] Naloxone appears to potentiate the anticonvulsant effects of benzodiazepines and barbiturates, and may antagonize the effects of phenytoin.[294] Seizure has been reported immediately following naloxone administration for tramadol overdose.[240,295] The tramadol package insert cautions against naloxone use in overdose situations.

The management of serotonin syndrome is primarily supportive. Sedation, paralysis, intubation and ventilation, anticonvulsants, antihypertensives, and aggressive rapid cooling may all be necessary. There has been some success with nonspecific serotonin antagonist cyproheptadine (4 to 8 mg every 8 hours orally).[296]

The occurrence of acute lung injury appears to be clinically unpredictable,[70,71,76,297] and it has been suggested that a man in his late thirties who is a relatively inexperienced heroin user and has a Glasgow Coma Scale score of 4 to 5, has a respiratory rate of 6, and requires naloxone to maintain his respiratory drive in the prehospital setting would have a high likelihood of developing acute lung injury.[298] It has been recommended to observe all patients for at least 24 hours following emergence from an opioid overdose. However, some clinicians suggest that 4 hours patient observation may be sufficient following a pure IV heroin or short-acting opioid overdose.[69,299] An even shorter observation of at least 1 hour in an emergency department has been investigated and may be acceptable, and remains to be validated.[300] This study suggests that patients with presumed opioid overdose can be safely discharged 1 hour after naloxone administration if they (1) can mobilize as usual, (2) have oxygen saturation on room air greater than 92%, (3) have a respiratory rate between 10 and 20 breaths per minute, (4) have a temperature between 35.0° C and 37.5° C, (5) have a heart rate between 50 and 100 beats per minute, and (6) have a Glasgow Coma Scale score of 15.

The management of acute lung injury should include adequate ventilation, oxygenation, and positive-pressure

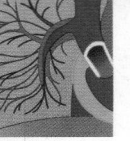

ventilation as needed. Inotropic and chronotorpic agents and preload- and afterload-reducing agents appear to be of little value. In one case series, the majority of patients only required supplemental oxygen, and 33% of patients required mechanical ventilation.[69]

Asymptomatic body packers may be managed conservatively by the prograde route provided the condition of packaging does not appear to be compromised. Some clinicians suggest whole bowel irrigation with polyethylene glycol electrolyte lavage solution based on retrospective case series and case reports.[207,301-303] A proposed method, based on more than 100 cases of cocaine body packers, together with more than 10 years' experience, suggests a safe and efficient method for the medical management of asymptomatic body packers. This same method may be applied to heroin body packers and involves the oral administration of a water-soluble contrast solution followed by serial abdominal radiographs (Box 33-1).[304,305]

Body packers who develop opiate toxicity can often be managed with continuous naloxone infusion, activated charcoal, and whole bowel irrigation. Surgical intervention is indicated for patients with intestinal obstruction or perforation, and may be indicated when packets fail to progress through the GI tract after conservative management. Endoscopic retrieval of a few packets that are retained in the stomach may be considered, and should be performed by an experienced endoscopist.

Pruritis is a common opioid adverse drug event. It may be localized or general and range from mild to severe. Antihistamines are usually ineffective, but naloxone has frequently been found to offer relief. Ondansetron has been reported to provide relief in refractory cases.[307]

Treatment of spongiform leukoencephalopathy is supportive, and antioxidant therapy with coenzyme Q (30 mg four times daily), vitamin E (2000 mg daily), and vitamin C (2000 mg daily) has been advocated.[310]

Constipation may be ameliorated by oral naloxone. Enteral naloxone is poorly absorbed, and opioid withdrawal symptoms are usually not evident when the oral dose of naloxone does not exceed hepatic glucuronidase capacity.[308] Methylnal-trexone is a quaternary ammonium molecule and is unable to cross the blood-brain barrier. It antagonizes the effects of opioids on the GI tract without precipitating opioid withdrawal.[309]

Forced diuresis and manipulation of urine pH have not been demonstrated to be of clinical benefit in opioid overdose. Hemodialysis may be indicated in patients with compromised renal function and are toxic from opioids or its metabolites (e.g., normeperidine) that depend on renal elimination.[310]

OTHER OPIOID ANTAGONISTS

Nalmefene is effective for the reversal of opioid-induced CNS effects and may be administered orally or intravenously. Its half-life and dose-dependent duration of action are 4 to 8 hours following IV administration.[311,312] The initial adult dose is 0.5 mg for those who are not opioid dependent and 0.1 mg for those suspected of having opioid dependency. If there is an incomplete response or no response, additional doses can be given at 2- to 5-minutes intervals. A total dose of 1.5 mg may be necessary to exclude the possibility of opioid poisoning. Nalmefene has proven safety and efficacy in the management of meperidine-induced sedation and opiate overdose in the emergency department.[313-315] The principal advantage over naloxone is its considerably longer duration of antagonistic action, which translates into fewer complications arising from fluctuations in the level of consciousness, reduced incidence of resedation, better long-term control of longer-acting opiate ingestions, and fewer indications for naloxone infusions. Withdrawal syndrome precipitated by the use of nalmefene would also be prolonged.

Naltrexone is a potent, long-acting, pure opiate antagonist that is effective orally. Its use is primarily limited as adjunctive therapy for opioid detoxification. Naltrexone may induce a withdrawal syndrome lasting up to 72 hours.

DISPOSITION

The minimum observation period following a patient's emergence from an opioid overdose remains to be determined. Data seem to suggest that observation for 1 to 4 hours may be sufficient following a pure IV heroin or short-acting opioid overdose.[69,299,300] Factors that favor extended observation or hospital admission include exposure to agents with long half-lives (e.g., methadone, L-α-acetylmethadol, propoxyphene, diphenoxylate, and buprenorphine); agents whose toxicity may be delayed, prolonged, or recurrent (e.g., diphenoxylate); large amounts of ingestant or co-ingestant; low tolerance to opioids (as compared to that of the chronic abuser); respiratory or cardiovascular instability; and comorbid conditions. Although administering an opioid antagonist can have a temporizing effect, overdose on an opioid with a long half-life (e.g., methadone) will significantly

---

BOX 33-1	**MANAGEMENT OF ASYMPTOMATIC BODY PACKERS**

Abdominal radiographs with oral contrast:
1. Administer an oral dose of water-soluble contrast (e.g., Gastrografin): 1 mL/kg.
2. Perform abdominal radiographs (supine and upright) at least 5 hours after oral contrast administration.
3. If radiographs are positive, administer an oral dose of 100 mL mineral oil twice daily.
4. Perform daily abdominal radiographs and after a spontaneous bowel movement.
5. All bowel movements are checked for drug packets.
6. The patient may be discharged after passage of two packet-free bowel movements and negative abdominal radiographs.

Patients are permitted to feed normally and vascular access should be maintained.

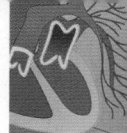

outlast several doses of naloxone and may require a continuous naloxone infusion or the use of nalmefene. Because of the potential for delayed onset and recurrent respiratory and CNS depression following naloxone therapy, it is recommended to observe patients for at least 24 hours. Patients who are on high-dose methadone therapy and have a prolonged QTc interval on ECG should be admitted to an intensive care unit because of its association with torsades de pointes and risk for sudden death.[161]

ACKNOWLEDGMENT

Michael Schwartz, MD, contributed to this chapter in a previous edition.

REFERENCES

1. World Health Organization: Opioid overdose. Trends, risk factors, interventions and priorities for action. In Social Change and Mental Health. Geneva, Switzerland, World Health Organization, 1998.
2. Hall W, Darke S: Trends in opiate overdose deaths in Australia 1979–1995. Drug Alcohol Depend 1998;52(1):71–77.
3. Substance Abuse and Mental Health Services Administration: Results from the 2004 National Survey on Drug Use and Health: national findings. Rochville, MD, Substance Abuse and Mental Health Services Administration, 2005.
4. Watson WA, Litovitz TL, Klein-Schwartz W, et al: 2003 annual report of the American Association of Poison Control Centers Toxic Exposure Surveillance System. Am J Emerg Med 2004;22(5):335–404.
5. Gueye PN, Megarbane B, Borron SW, et al: Trends in opiate and opioid poisonings in addicts in north-east Paris and suburbs, 1995–99. Addiction 2002;97(10):1295–1304.
6. Single E, Rehm J, Robson L, Truong MV: The relative risks and etiologic fractions of different causes of death and disease attributable to alcohol, tobacco and illicit drug use in Canada. CMAJ 2000;162(12):1669–1675.
7. Frischer M, Goldberg D, Rahman M, Berney L: Mortality and survival among a cohort of drug injectors in Glasgow, 1982–1994. Addiction 1997;92(4):419–427.
8. White JM, Irvine RJ: Mechanisms of fatal opioid overdose. Addiction 1999;94(7):961–972.
9. Risser D, Honigschnabl S, Stichenwirth M, et al: Mortality of opiate users in Vienna, Austria. Drug Alcohol Depend 2001;64(3):251–256.
10. Gowing L, Ali R, White J: Buprenorphine for the management of opioid withdrawal. Cochrane Database Syst Rev 2004(4):CD002025.
11. Johnson RE, Chutuape MA, Strain EC, et al: A comparison of levomethadyl acetate, buprenorphine, and methadone for opioid dependence. N Engl J Med 2000;343(18):1290–1297.
12. Mattick RP, Kimber J, Breen C, Davoli M: Buprenorphine maintenance versus placebo or methadone maintenance for opioid dependence. Cochrane Database Syst Rev 2003(2):CD002207.
13. Gaulier JM, Marquet P, Lacassie E, et al: Fatal intoxication following self-administration of a massive dose of buprenorphine. J Forensic Sci 2000;45(1):226–228.
14. Kintz P: Deaths involving buprenorphine: a compendium of French cases. Forensic Sci Int 2001;121(1–2):65–69.
15. Kintz P: A new series of 13 buprenorphine-related deaths. Clin Biochem 2002;35(7):513–516.
16. Tracqui A, Kintz P, Ludes B: Buprenorphine-related deaths among drug addicts in France: a report on 20 fatalities. J Anal Toxicol 1998;22(6):430–434.
17. Comer SD, Collins ED, Fischman MW: Intravenous buprenorphine self-administration by detoxified heroin abusers. J Pharmacol Exp Ther 2002;301(1):266–276.
18. Obadia Y, Perrin V, Feroni I, et al: Injecting misuse of buprenorphine among French drug users. Addiction 2001;96(2):267–272.
19. Thirion X, Lapierre V, Micallef J, et al: Buprenorphine prescription by general practitioners in a French region. Drug Alcohol Depend 2002;65(2):197–204.
20. Pirnay S, Borron SW, Giudicelli CP, et al: A critical review of the causes of death among post-mortem toxicological investigations: analysis of 34 buprenorphine-associated and 35 methadone-associated deaths. Addiction 2004;99(8):978–988.
21. Cicero TJ, Inciardi JA: Potential for abuse of buprenorphine in office-based treatment of opioid dependence. N Engl J Med 2005;353(17):1863–1865.
22. Bryant WK, Galea S, Tracy M, et al: Overdose deaths attributed to methadone and heroin in New York City, 1990–1998. Addiction 2004;99(7):846–854.
23. Perret G, Deglon JJ, Kreek MJ, et al: Lethal methadone intoxications in Geneva, Switzerland, from 1994 to 1998. Addiction 2000;95(11):1647–1653.
24. Seymour A, Black M, Jay J, et al: The role of methadone in drug related deaths in the west of Scotland. Addiction 2003;98(7):995–1002.
25. Zadina JE, Hackler L, Ge LJ, Kastin AJ: A potent and selective endogenous agonist for the mu-opiate receptor. Nature 1997;386(6624):499–502.
26. Reisine T, Pasternak G: Opioid analgesics and antagonists. In Hardman J, Limbird LE, Gilman AG, et al (eds): Goodman & Gilman's The Pharmacological Basis of Therapeutics. New York, McGraw-Hill, 1996, pp 521–555.
27. Gaveriaux-Ruff C, Matthes HW, Peluso J, Kieffer BL: Abolition of morphine-immunosuppresion in mice lacking the mu-opioid receptor gene. Proc Natl Acad Sci U S A 1998;95(11):6326–6230.
28. Dhawan BN, Cesselin F, Raghubir R, et al: International Union of Pharmacology. XII. Classification of opioid receptors. Pharmacol Rev 1996;48(4):567–592.
29. Shook JE, Watkins WD, Camporesi EM: Differential roles of opioid receptors in respiration, respiratory disease, and opiate-induced respiratory depression. Am Rev Respir Dis 1990;142(4):895–909.
30. Emmerson PJ, Liu MR, Woods JH, Medzihradsky F: Binding affinity and selectivity of opioids at mu, delta and kappa receptors in monkey brain membranes. J Pharmacol Exp Ther 1994;271(3):1630–1637.
31. Janecka A, Fichna J, Janecki T: Opioid receptors and their ligands. Curr Top Med Chem 2004;4(1):1–17.
32. Salvadori S, Temussi PA: Antagonism in opioid peptides: the role of conformation. Curr Top Med Chem 2004;4(1):145–157.
33. Ueda H, Harada H, Nozaki M, et al: Reconstitution of rat brain mu opioid receptors with purified guanine nucleotide-binding regulatory proteins, Gi and Go. Proc Natl Acad Sci U S A 1988;85(18):7013–7017.
34. Yasuda K, Raynor K, Kong H, et al: Cloning and functional comparison of kappa and delta opioid receptors from mouse brain. Proc Natl Acad Sci U S A 1993;90(14):6736–6740.
35. Grudt TJ, Williams JT: Kappa-opioid receptors also increase potassium conductance. Proc Natl Acad Sci U S A 1993;90(23):11429–11432.
36. North RA, Williams JT, Surprenant A, Christie MJ: Mu and delta receptors belong to a family of receptors that are coupled to potassium channels. Proc Natl Acad Sci U S A 1987;84(15):5487–5491.
37. Schoffelmeer AN, Van Vliet BJ, De Vries TJ, et al: Regulation of brain neurotransmitter release and of adenylate cyclase activity by opioid receptors. Biochem Soc Trans 1992;20(2):449–453.
38. Elkader A, Sproule B: Buprenorphine: clinical pharmacokinetics in the treatment of opioid dependence. Clin Pharmacokinet 2005;44(7):661–680.
39. Chang Y, Moody DF, McCance-Kate EF: Novel metabolites of buprenorphine detected in human liver microsomes and human urine. Drug Metab Dispos 2006;34(3):440–448.
40. Gasche Y, Daali Y, Fathi M, et al: Codeine intoxication associated with ultrarapid CYP2D6 metabolism. N Engl J Med 2004;351(27):2827–2831.
41. Borron SW, Monier C, Risede P, Baud FJ: Flunitrazepam variably alters morphine, buprenorphine, and methadone lethality in the rat. Hum Exp Toxicol 2002;21(11):599–605.

42. Kilicarslan T, Sellers EM: Lack of interaction of buprenorphine with flunitrazepam metabolism. Am J Psychiatry 2000;157(7):1164–1166.

43. Ghoneim MM, Dhanaraj J, Choi WW: Comparison of four opioid analgesics as supplements to nitrous oxide anesthesia. Anesth Analg 1984;63(4):405–412.

44. Eckenhoff JE, Oech SR: The effects of narcotics and antagonists upon respiration and circulation in man. A review. Clin Pharmacol Ther 1960;1:483–524.

45. Koren G, Butt W, Pape K, Chinyanga H: Morphine-induced seizures in newborn infants. Vet Hum Toxicol 1985;27(6):519–520.

46. Weil JV, McCullough RE, Kline JS, Sodal IE: Diminished ventilatory response to hypoxia and hypercapnia after morphine in normal man. N Engl J Med 1975;292(21):1103–1106.

47. Eckenhoff JE, Helrich M, Hege MJ, Jones RE: Respiratory hazards of opiates and other narcotic analgesics. Surg Gynecol Obstet 1955;101(6):701–708.

48. Ward JM, McGrath RL, Weil JV: Effects of morphine on the peripheral vascular response to sympathetic stimulation. Am J Cardiol 1972;29(5):659–666.

49. Zelis R, Mansour EJ, Capone RJ, Mason DT: The cardiovascular effects of morphine. The peripheral capacitance and resistance vessels in human subjects. J Clin Invest 1974;54(6):1247–1258.

50. Fahmy NR, Sunder N, Soter NA: Role of histamine in the hemodynamic and plasma catecholamine responses to morphine. Clin Pharmacol Ther 1983;33(5):615–620.

51. Barke KE, Hough LB: Opiates, mast cells and histamine release. Life Sci 1993;53(18):1391–1399.

52. Philbin DM, Moss J, Akins CW, et al: The use of H1 and H2 histamine antagonists with morphine anesthesia: a double-blind study. Anesthesiology 1981;55(3):292–296.

53. Flacke JW, Flacke WE, Bloor BC, et al: Histamine release by four narcotics: a double-blind study in humans. Anesth Analg 1987;66(8):723–730.

54. Melandri R, Re G, Lanzarini C, et al: Myocardial damage and rhabdomyolysis associated with prolonged hypoxic coma following opiate overdose. J Toxicol Clin Toxicol 1996;34(2):199–203.

55. Cepeda MS, Gonzalez F, Granados V, et al: Incidence of nausea and vomiting in outpatients undergoing general anesthesia in relation to selection of intraoperative opioid. J Clin Anesth 1996;8(4):324–328.

56. Lasagna L: The clinical evaluation of morphine and its substitutes as analgesics. Pharmacol Rev 1964;16:47–83.

57. Darke S, Hall W, Weatherburn D, Lind B: Fluctuations in heroin purity and the incidence of fatal heroin overdose. Drug Alcohol Depend 1999;54(2):155–161.

58. Griffiths P, Gossop M, Powis B, Strang J: Transitions in patterns of heroin administration: a study of heroin chasers and heroin injectors. Addiction 1994;89(3):301–309.

59. Kaa E: Impurities, adulterants and diluents of illicit heroin. Changes during a 12-year period. Forensic Sci Int 1994;64(2–3):171–179.

60. Ferguson R, Feeney C, Chirurgi VA: Enterobacter agglomerans–associated cotton fever. Arch Intern Med 1993;153(20):2381–2382.

61. Hendriks VM, van den Brink W, Blanken P, et al: Heroin self-administration by means of "chasing the dragon": pharmaco-dynamics and bioavailability of inhaled heroin. Eur Neuro-psychopharmacol 2001;11(3):241–252.

62. Jenkins AJ, Keenan RM, Henningfield JE, Cone EJ: Phar-macokinetics and pharmacodynamics of smoked heroin. J Anal Toxicol 1994;18(6):317–330.

63. Elliott HW, Parker KD, Wright JA, Nomof N: Actions and metabolism of heroin administered by continuous intravenous infusion to man. Clin Pharmacol Ther 1971;12(5):806–814.

64. Tress KH, El-Sobky AA: Cardiovascular, respiratory and tempera-ture responses to intravenous heroin (diamorphine) in depen-dent and non-dependent humans. Br J Clin Pharmacol 1980;10(5):477–485.

65. Boerner U: The metabolism of morphine and heroin in man. Drug Metab Rev 1975;4(1):39–73.

66. Nakamura GR: Toxicologic assessments in acute heroin fatalities. Clin Toxicol 1978;13(1):75–87.

67. Osler W: Oedema of left lung—Morphia poisoning. Montreal Gen Hosp Rep 1880;1:291–293.

68. Troen P: Pulmonary edema in acute opium intoxication. N Engl J Med 1953;248:364–366.

69. Sporer KA, Dorn E: Heroin-related noncardiogenic pulmonary edema: a case series. Chest 2001;120(5):1628–1632.

70. Steinberg AD, Karliner JS: The clinical spectrum of heroin pulmonary edema. Arch Intern Med 1968;122(2):122–127.

71. Duberstein JL, Kaufman DM: A clinical study of an epidemic of heroin intoxication and heroin-induced pulmonary edema. Am J Med 1971;51(6):704–714.

72. Helpern M, Rho YM: Deaths from narcotism in New York City. Incidence, circumstances, and postmortem findings. NY State J Med 1966;66(18):2391–2408.

73. Hine CH, Wright JA, Allison DJ, et al: Analysis of fatalities from acute narcotism in a major urban area. J Forensic Sci 1982;27(2):372–384.

74. Levine SB, Grimes ET: Pulmonary edema and heroin overdose in Vietnam. Arch Pathol 1973;95(5):330–332.

75. Dettmeyer R, Schmidt P, Musshoff F, et al: Pulmonary edema in fatal heroin overdose: immunohistological investigations with IgE, collagen IV and laminin–no increase of defects of alveolar-capillary membranes. Forensic Sci Int 2000;110(2):87–96.

76. Frand UI, Shim CS, Williams MH Jr: Heroin-induced pulmonary edema. Sequential studies of pulmonary function. Ann Intern Med 1972;77(1):29–35.

77. Katz S, Aberman A, Frand UI, et al: Heroin pulmonary edema. Evidence for increased pulmonary capillary permeability. Am Rev Respir Dis 1972;106(3):472–474.

78. Paranthaman SK, Khan F: Acute cardiomyopathy with recurrent pulmonary edema and hypotension following heroin overdosage. Chest 1976;69(1):117–119.

79. Smith WR, Glauser FL, Dearden LC, et al: Deposits of immunoglobulin and complement in the pulmonary tissue of patients with "heroin lung." Chest 1978;73(4):471–476.

80. Wolters EC, van Wijngaarden GK, Stam FC, et al: Leuco-encephalopathy after inhaling "heroin" pyrolysate. Lancet 1982;2(8310):1233–1237.

81. Tan TP, Algra PR, Valk J, Wolters EC: Toxic leukoencephalopathy after inhalation of poisoned heroin: MR findings. Am J Neuroradiol 1994;15(1):175–178.

82. Weber W, Henkes H, Moller P, et al: Toxic spongiform leuco-encephalopathy after inhaling heroin vapour. Eur Radiol 1998;8(5):749–755.

83. Glauser FL, Downie RL, Smith WR: Electrocardiographic abnor-malities in acute heroin overdosage. Bull Narc 1977;29(1):85–89.

84. Labi M: Paroxysmal atrial fibrillation in heroin intoxication. Ann Intern Med 1969;71(5):951–959.

85. Lipski J, Stimmel B, Donoso D: The effect of heroin and multiple drug abuse on the electrocardiogram. Am Heart J 1973;86(5):663–668.

86. Pearce CJ, Cox JG: Heroin and hyperkalaemia. Lancet 1980;2(8200):923.

87. Perry DC: Editorial. Heroin and cocaine adulteration. Clin Toxicol 1975;8(2):239–243.

88. Lupovich P, Pilewski R, Sapira JD, Juselius R: Cardiotoxicity of quinine as adulterant in drugs. JAMA 1970;212(7):1216.

89. Shesser R, Jotte R, Olshaker J: The contribution of impurities to the acute morbidity of illegal drug use. Am J Emerg Med 1991;9(4):336–342.

90. Brust JC, Richter RW: Quinine amblyopia related to heroin addiction. Ann Intern Med 1971;74(1):84–86.

91. Christie DJ, Walker RH, Kolins MD, et al: Quinine-induced thrombocytopenia following intravenous use of heroin. Arch Intern Med 1983;143(6):1174–1175.

92. Scopolamine poisoning among heroin users—New York City, Newark, Philadelphia, and Baltimore, 1995 and 1996. Morb Mortal Wkly Rep MMWR 1996;45(22):457–460.

93. Hollander JE, Lozano M Jr: Cocaine-associated myocardial infarction secondary to a contaminant. Am J Emerg Med 1993;11(6):681–682.

94. Questel F, Dugarin J, Dally S: Thallium-contaminated heroin. Ann Intern Med 1996;124(6):616.

95. Parras F, Patier JL, Ezpeleta C: Lead-contaminated heroin as a source of inorganic-lead intoxication. N Engl J Med 1987;316(12):755.

96. Choudry N, Doe J: Inadvertent abuse of amphetamines in street heroin. Lancet 1986;2(8510):817.

97. O'Gorman P, Patel S, Notcutt S, Wicking J: Adulteration of "street" heroin with chloroquine. Lancet 1987;1(8535):746.

98. Hoffman R: The toxic emergency: strychnine. Emerg Med 1994;26:111–112.

99. Solomon MD: A study of codeine metabolism. Clin Toxicol 1974;7(3):255–257.

100. Adler TK, Fujimoto JM, Way EL, Baker EM: The metabolic fate of codeine in man. J Pharmacol Exp Ther 1955;114(3):251–262.

101. Huffman DH, Ferguson RL: Acute codeine overdose: correspondence between clinical course and codeine metabolism. Johns Hopkins Med J 1975;136(4):183–186.

102. Peat MA, Sengupta A: Toxicological investigations of cases of death involving codeine and dihydrocodeine. Forensic Sci 1977;9(1):21–32.

103. Wright JA, Baselt RC, Hine CH: Blood codeine concentrations in fatalities associated with codeine. Clin Toxicol 1975;8(4):457–463.

104. Fung DL, Eisele JH: Fentanyl pharmacokinetics in awake volunteers. J Clin Pharmacol 1980;20(11–12):652–658.

105. Buchanan JF, Brown CR: "Designer drugs." A problem in clinical toxicology. Med Toxicol Adverse Drug Exp 1988;3(1):1–17.

106. Hibbs J, Perper J, Winek CL: An outbreak of designer drug–related deaths in Pennsylvania. JAMA 1991;265(8):1011–1013.

107. Kram TC, Cooper DA, Allen AC: Behind the identification of China White. Anal Chem 1981;53(12):1379A–1386A.

108. Martin M, Hecker J, Clark R, et al: China White epidemic: an eastern United States emergency department experience. Ann Emerg Med 1991;20(2):158–164.

109. Ziporyn T: A growing industry and menace: makeshift laboratory's designer drugs. JAMA 1986;256(22):3061–3063.

110. Rao TL, Mummaneni N, El-Etr AA: Convulsions: an unusual response to intravenous fentanyl administration. Anesth Analg 1982;61(12):1020–1021.

111. Safwat AM, Daniel D: Grand mal seizure after fentanyl administration. Anesthesiology 1983;59(1):78.

112. Sebel PS, Bovill JG: Fentanyl and convulsions. Anesth Analg 1983;62(9):858–859.

113. Murkin JM, Moldenhauer CC, Hug CC Jr, Epstein CM: Absence of seizures during induction of anesthesia with high-dose fentanyl. Anesth Analg 1984;63(5):489–494.

114. Scott JC, Sarnquist FH: Seizure-like movements during a fentanyl infusion with absence of seizure activity in a simultaneous EEG recording. Anesthesiology 1985;62(6):812–814.

115. Smith NT, Benthuysen JL, Bickford RG, et al: Seizures during opioid anesthetic induction—are they opioid-induced rigidity? Anesthesiology 1989;71(6):852–862.

116. Sprung J, Schedewie HK: Apparent focal motor seizure with a jacksonian march induced by fentanyl: a case report and review of the literature. J Clin Anesth 1992;4(2):139–143.

117. Adair JC, el-Nachef A, Cutler P: Fentanyl neurotoxicity. Ann Emerg Med 1996;27(6):791–792.

118. Arvanitis ML, Satonik RC: Transdermal fentanyl abuse and misuse. Am J Emerg Med 2002;20(1):58–59.

119. DeSio JM, Bacon DR, Peer G, Lema MJ: Intravenous abuse of transdermal fentanyl therapy in a chronic pain patient. Anesthesiology 1993;79(5):1139–1141.

120. Edinboro LE, Poklis A, Trautman D, et al: Fatal fentanyl intoxication following excessive transdermal application. J Forensic Sci 1997;42(4):741–743.

121. Kramer C, Tawney M: A fatal overdose of transdermally administered fentanyl. J Am Osteopath Assoc 1998;98(7):385–386.

122. Marquardt KA, Tharratt RS: Inhalation abuse of fentanyl patch. J Toxicol Clin Toxicol 1994;32(1):75–78.

123. Reeves MD, Ginifer CJ: Fatal intravenous misuse of transdermal fentanyl. Med J Aust 2002;177(10):552–553.

124. Tharp AM, Winecker RE, Winston DC: Fatal intravenous fentanyl abuse: four cases involving extraction of fentanyl from transdermal patches. Am J Forensic Med Pathol 2004;25(2):178–181.

125. Stambaugh JE, Wainer IW, Sanstead JK, Hemphill DM: The clinical pharmacology of meperidine—comparison of routes of administration. J Clin Pharmacol 1976;16(5–6):245–256.

126. Green RC Jr, Carroll GJ, Buxton WD: Drug addiction among physicians. The Virginia experience. JAMA 1976;236(12):1372–1375.

127. Putnam PL, Ellinwood EH Jr: Narcotic addiction among physicians: a ten-year follow-up. Am J Psychiatry 1966:122(7):745–748.

128. Ward CF, Ward GC, Saidman LJ: Drug abuse in anesthesia training programs. A survey: 1970 through 1980. JAMA 1983;250(7):922–925.

129. Hershey LA: Meperidine and central neurotoxicity. Ann Intern Med 1983;98(4):548–549.

130. Miller JW, Anderson HH: The effect of N-demethylation on certain pharmacologic actions of morphine, codeine, and meperidine in the mouse. J Pharmacol Exp Ther 1954;112(2):191–196.

131. Mather LE, Tucker GT, Pflug AE, et al: Meperidine kinetics in man. Intravenous injection in surgical patients and volunteers. Clin Pharmacol Ther 1975;17(1):21–30.

132. Kaiko RF, Foley KM, Grabinski PY, et al: Central nervous system excitatory effects of meperidine in cancer patients. Ann Neurol 1983;13(2):180–185.

133. Morisy L, Platt D: Hazards of high-dose meperidine. JAMA 1986;255(4):467–468.

134. Szeto HH, Inturrisi CE, Houde R, et al: Accumulation of normeperidine, an active metabolite of meperidine, in patients with renal failure of cancer. Ann Intern Med 1977;86(6):738–741.

135. Goetting MG, Thirman MJ: Neurotoxicity of meperidine. Ann Emerg Med 1985;14(10):1007–1009.

136. Marinella MA: Meperidine-induced generalized seizures with normal renal function. South Med J 1997;90(5):556–558.

137. Mauro VF, Bonfiglio MF, Spunt AL: Meperidine-induced seizure in a patient without renal dysfunction or sickle cell anemia. Clin Pharm 1986;5(10):837–839.

138. McHugh GJ: Norpethidine accumulation and generalized seizure during pethidine patient-controlled analgesia. Anaesth Intensive Care 1999;27(3):289–291.

139. Browne B, Linter S: Monoamine oxidase inhibitors and narcotic analgesics. A critical review of the implications for treatment. Br J Psychiatry 1987;151:210–212.

140. Nicklas WJ, Youngster SK, Kindt MV, Heikkila RE: MPTP, MPP+ and mitochondrial function. Life Sci 1987;40(8):721–729.

141. Uhl GR, Javitch JA, Snyder SH: Normal MPTP binding in parkinsonian substantia nigra: evidence for extraneuronal toxin conversion in human brain. Lancet 1985;1(8435):956–957.

142. Ballard PA, Tetrud JW, Langston JW: Permanent human parkinsonism due to 1-methyl-4-phenyl-1,2,3,6-tetrahydropyridine (MPTP): seven cases. Neurology 1985;35(7):949–956.

143. Burns RS, LeWitt PA, Ebert MH, et al: The clinical syndrome of striatal dopamine deficiency. Parkinsonism induced by 1-methyl-4-phenyl-1,2,3,6-tetrahydropyridine (MPTP). N Engl J Med 1985;312(22):1418–1421.

144. Langston JW, Ballard P, Tetrud JW, Irwin I: Chronic parkinsonism in humans due to a product of meperidine-analog synthesis. Science 1983;219(4587):979–980.

145. Henderson W, Psaila A: Lomotil poisoning. Lancet 1969;1(7589):307–308.

146. Penfold D, Volans GN: Overdose from Lomotil. BMJ 1977;2(6099):1401–1402.

147. Rumack BH, Temple AR: Lomotil poisoning. Pediatrics 1974;53(4):495–500.

148. Karim A, Ranney RE, Evensen KL, Clark ML: Pharmacokinetics and metabolism of diphenoxylate in man. Clin Pharmacol Ther 1972;13(3):407–419.

149. Rubens R, Verhaegen H, Brugmans J, Schuermans V: Difenoxine (R 15403), the active metabolite of diphenoxylate (R 1132). 5. Clinical comparison of difenoxine and diphenoxylate in volunteers and in patients with chronic diarrhea. Double-blind cross-over assessments. Arzneimittelforschung 1972;22(3):526–529.

150. Litovitz T, Clancy C, Korberly B, et al: Surveillance of loperamide ingestions: an analysis of 216 poison center reports. J Toxicol Clin Toxicol 1997;35(1):11–19.

151. Aronow R, Brenner SL, Woolley PV Jr: An apparent epidemic: methadone poisoning in children. Clin Toxicol 1973;6(2):175–181.

152. Persky VW, Goldfrank LR: Methadone overdoses in a New York City hospital. JACEP 1976;5(2):111–113.

153. Berkowitz BA: The relationship of pharmacokinetics to pharmacological activity: morphine, methadone and naloxone. Clin Pharmacokinet 1976;1(3):219–230.

154. Anggard E, Nilsson MI, Holmstrend J, Gunne LM: Pharmacokinetics of methadone during maintenance therapy: pulse labeling with deuterated methadone in the steady state. Eur J Clin Pharmacol 1979;16(1):53–57.

155. Garriott JC, Sturner WQ, Mason MF: Toxicologic findings in six fatalities involving methadone. Clin Toxicol 1973;6(2):163–173.

156. Kreek MJ: Medical complications in methadone patients. Ann N Y Acad Sci 1978;311:110–134.

157. Norris JV, Don HF: Prolonged depression of respiratory rate following methadone analgesia. Anesthesiology 1976;45(3): 361–362.

158. Gordon E: Treatment of methadone poisoning. JAMA 1972;220(5):728–731.

159. Bonnet U, Banger M, Wolstein J, Gastpar M: Choreoathetoid movements associated with rapid adjustment to methadone. Pharmacopsychiatry 1998;31(4):143–145.

160. Binchy JM, Molyneux EM, Manning J: Accidental ingestion of methadone by children in Merseyside. BMJ 1994;308(6940): 1335–1336.

161. Krantz MJ, Lewkowiez L, Hays H, et al: Torsade de pointes associated with very-high-dose methadone. Ann Intern Med 2002;137(6):501–504.

162. Cowan A, Doxey JC, Harry EJ: The animal pharmacology of buprenorphine, an oripavine analgesic agent. Br J Pharmacol 1977;60(4):547–554.

163. Walsh SL, Preston KL, Stitzer ML, et al: Clinical pharmacology of buprenorphine: ceiling effects at high doses. Clin Pharmacol Ther 1994;55(5):569–580.

164. Gal TJ: Naloxone reversal of buprenorphine-induced respiratory depression. Clin Pharmacol Ther 1989;45(1):66–71.

165. Megarbane B, Pirnay S, Borron SW, et al: Flunitrazepam does not alter cerebral distribution of buprenorphine in the rat. Toxicol Lett 2005;157(3):211–219.

166. Carson DJ: Fatal dextropropoxyphene poisoning in Northern Ireland. Review of 30 cases. Lancet 1977;1(8017):894–897.

167. Hudson P, Barringer M, McBay AJ: Fatal poisoning with propoxyphene: report from 100 consecutive cases. South Med J 1977;70(8):938–942.

168. Sturner WQ, Garriott JC: Deaths involving propoxyphene. A study of 41 cases over a two-year period. JAMA 1973;223(10): 1125–1130.

169. Wolen RL, Gruber CM Jr, Kiplinger GF, Scholz NE: Concentration of propoxyphene in human plasma following oral, intramuscular, and intravenous administration. Toxicol Appl Pharmacol 1971;19(3):480–492.

170. Bellville JW, Seed JC: A comparison of the respiratory depressant effects of dextropropoxyphene and codeine in man. Clin Pharmacol Ther 1968;9(4):428–434.

171. Verebely K, Inturrisi CE: Disposition of propoxyphene and norpropoxyphene in man after a single oral dose. Clin Pharmacol Ther 1974;15(3):302–309.

172. Lund-Jacobsen H: Cardio-respiratory toxicity of propoxyphene and norpropoxyphene in conscious rabbits. Acta Pharmacol Toxicol (Copenh) 1978;42(3):171–178.

173. Bogartz LJ, Miller WC: Pulmonary edema associated with propoxyphene intoxication. JAMA 1971;215(2):259–262.

174. Gary NE, Maher JF, DeMyttenaere MH, et al: Acute propoxyphene hydrochloride intoxication. Arch Intern Med 1968;121(5):453–457.

175. Gustafson A, Gustafsson B: Acute poisoning with dextropropoxyphene. Clinical symptoms and plasma concentrations. Acta Med Scand 1976;200(4):241–248.

176. McCarthy WH, Keenan RL: Propoxyphene hydrochloride poisoning. Report of the first fatality. JAMA 1964;187:460–461.

177. Sloth Madsen P, Strom J, Reiz S, Bredgaard Sorensen M: Acute propoxyphene self-poisoning in 222 consecutive patients. Acta Anaesthesiol Scand 1984;28(6):661–665.

178. Tennant FS Jr: Complications of propoxyphene abuse. Arch Intern Med 1973;132(2):191–194.

179. Strom J: Acute propoxyphene self-poisoning—with special reference to propoxyphene cardiotoxicity and treatment. Dan Med Bull 1989;36(4):316–336.

180. D'Abadie NB, Lenton JD: Propoxyphene dependence: problems in management. South Med J 1984;77(3):299–301.

181. Miller RR, Feingold A, Paxinos J: Propoxyphene hydrochloride. A critical review. JAMA 1970;213(6):996–1006.

182. Woody GE, Tennant FS, McLellan AT, et al: Lack of toxicity of high dose propoxyphene napsylate when used for maintenance treatment of addiction. NIDA Res Monogr 1979;27:435–440.

183. Brogden RN, Speight TM, Avery GS: Pentazocine: a review of its pharmacological properties, therapeutic efficacy and dependence liability. Drugs 1973;5(1):6–91.

184. Ehrnebo M, Boreus LO, Lonroth U: Bioavailability and first-pass metabolism of oral pentazocine in man. Clin Pharmacol Ther 1977;22(6):888–892.

185. Challoner KR, McCarron MM, Newton EJ: Pentazocine (Talwin) intoxication: report of 57 cases. J Emerg Med 1990;8(1):67–74.

186. De Bard ML, Jagger JA: "T's and B's"—Midwestern heroin substitute. Clin Toxicol 1981;18(9):1117–1123.

187. Stahl SM, Kasser IS: Pentazocine overdose. Ann Emerg Med 1983;12(1):28–31.

188. Carter HS, Watson WA: IV pentazocine/methylphenidate abuse—the clinical toxicity of another Ts and blues combination. J Toxicol Clin Toxicol 1994;32(5):541–547.

189. Bhargava HN: Mechanism of toxicity and rationale for use of the combination of pentazocine and pyribenzamine in morphine-dependent subjects. Clin Toxicol 1981;18(2):175–188.

190. Farber HW, Falls R, Glauser FL: Transient pulmonary hypertension from the intravenous injection of crushed, suspended pentazocine tablets. Chest 1981;80(2):178–182.

191. Poklis A: Decline in abuse of pentazocine/tripelennamine (T's and Blues) associated with the addition of naloxone to pentazocine tablets. Drug Alcohol Depend 1984;14(2): 135–140.

192. Bem JL, Peck R: Dextromethorphan. An overview of safety issues. Drug Saf 1992;7(3):190–199.

193. Silvasti M, Karttunen P, Tukiainen H, et al: Pharmacokinetics of dextromethorphan and dextrorphan: a single dose comparison of three preparations in human volunteers. Int J Clin Pharmacol Ther Toxicol 1987;25(9):493–497.

194. McCarthy JP: Some less familiar drugs of abuse. Med J Aust 1971;2(21):1078–1081.

195. Murray S, Brewerton T: Abuse of over-the-counter dextromethorphan by teenagers. South Med J 1993;86(10):1151–1153.

196. Wolfe TR, Caravati EM: Massive dextromethorphan ingestion and abuse. Am J Emerg Med 1995;13(2):174–176.

197. Ng YY, Lin WL, Chen TW, et al: Spurious hyperchloremia and decreased anion gap in a patient with dextromethorphan bromide. Am J Nephrol 1992;12(4):268–270.

198. Rivers N: Possible lethal reaction between Nardil and dextromethorphan. Can Med Assoc J 1970;103:85.

199. Sovner R, Wolfe J: Interaction between dextromethorphan and monoamine oxidase inhibitor therapy with isocarboxazid. N Engl J Med 1988;319(25):1671.

200. Szekely JI, Sharpe LG, Jaffe JH: Induction of phencyclidine-like behavior in rats by dextrorphan but not dextromethorphan. Pharmacol Biochem Behav 1991;40(2):381–386.

201. Zawertailo LA, Kaplan HL, Busto UE, et al: Psychotropic effects of dextromethorphan are altered by the CYP2D6 polymorphism: a pilot study. J Clin Psychopharmacol 1998;18(4):332–337.

202. Graudins A, Fern RP: Acute dystonia in a child associated with therapeutic ingestion of a dextromethorphan containing cough and cold syrup. J Toxicol Clin Toxicol 1996;34(3):351–352.

203. Raffa RB, Friderichs E, Reimann W, et al: Opioid and nonopioid components independently contribute to the mechanism of action of tramadol, an "atypical" opioid analgesic. J Pharmacol Exp Ther 1992;260(1):275–285.

204. Kesavan S, Sobala GM: Serotonin syndrome with fluoxetine plus tramadol. J R Soc Med 1999;92(9):474–475.

205. Lantz MS, Buchalter EN, Giambanco V: Serotonin syndrome following the administration of tramadol with paroxetine. Int J Geriatr Psychiatry 1998;13(5):343–345.

206. Nightingale SL: From the Food and Drug Administration. JAMA 1996;275(16):1224.

207. Traub SJ, Hoffman RS, Nelson LS: Body packing—the internal concealment of illicit drugs. N Engl J Med 2003;349(26): 2519–2526.

208. Wetli CV, Rao A, Rao VJ: Fatal heroin body packing. Am J Forensic Med Pathol 1997;18(3):312–318.

209. Katona B, Wason S: Dextromethorphan danger. N Engl J Med 1986;314(15):993.

210. Pender ES, Parks BR: Toxicity with dextromethorphan-containing preparations: a literature review and report of two additional cases. Pediatr Emerg Care 1991;7(3):163–165.

211. Schneider SM, Michelson EA, Boucek CD, Ilkhanipour K: Dextromethorphan poisoning reversed by naloxone. Am J Emerg Med 1991;9(3):237–238.

212. Shaul WL, Wandell M, Robertson WO: Dextromethorphan toxicity: reversal by naloxone. Pediatrics 1977;59(1):117–118.

213. Gould DB: Buprenorphine causes pulmonary edema just like all other mu-opioid narcotics. Upper airway obstruction, negative alveolar pressure. Chest 1995;107(5):1478–1479.

214. Jaffe RB, Koschmann EB: Intravenous drug abuse. Pulmonary, cardiac, and vascular complications. Am J Roentgenol Radium Ther Nucl Med 1970;109(1):107–120.

215. Kjeldgaard JM, Hahn GW, Heckenlively JR, Genton E: Methadone-induced pulmonary edema. JAMA 1971;218(6):882–883.

216. Pearson MA, Poklis A, Morrison RR: A fatality due to the ingestion of (methyl morphine) codeine. Clin Toxicol 1979;15(3):267–271.

217. Schaaf JT, Spivack ML, Rath GS, Snider GL: Pulmonary edema and adult respiratory distress syndrome following methadone abuse. Am Rev Respir Dis 1973;107(6):1047–1051.

218. Sklar J, Timms RM: Codeine-induced pulmonary edema. Chest 1977;72(2):230–231.

219. Stadnyk A, Grossman RF: Nalbuphine-induced pulmonary edema. Chest 1986;90(5):773–774.

220. Thammakumpee G, Sumpatanukule P: Noncardiogenic pulmonary edema induced by sublingual buprenorphine. Chest 1994;106(1):306–308.

221. Winek CL, Collom WD, Wecht CH: Codeine fatality from cough syrup. Clin Toxicol 1970;3(1):97–100.

222. Zyroff J, Slovis TL, Nagler J: Pulmonary edema induced by oral methadone. Radiology 1974;112(3):567–568.

223. Presant S, Knight L, Klassen G: Methadone-induced pulmonary edema. Can Med Assoc J 1975;113(10):966–967.

224. Wilen SB, Ulreich S, Rabinowitz JG: Roentgenographic manifestations of methadone-induced pulmonary edema. Radiology 1975;114(1):51–55.

225. Gopinathan K, Saroja J, Spears R: Hemodynamic studies in heroin induced acute pulmonary edema. Circulation 1970;42:44.

226. Lee G, DeMaria AN, Amsterdam EA, et al: Comparative effects of morphine, meperidine and pentazocine on cardiocirculatory dynamics in patients with acute myocardial infarction. Am J Med 1976;60(7):949–955.

227. Tammisto T, Jaattela A, Nikki P, Takki S, et al: Effect of pentazocine and pethidine on plasma catecholamine levels. Ann Clin Res 1971;3(1):22–29.

228. Addington W: The pulmonary edema of heroin toxicity—an example of stiff lung syndrome. Clinical Conference in Pulmonary Disease. Chest 1972;62:199–205.

229. Morrison WJ, Wetherill W, Zyroff J: The acute pulmonary edema of heroin intoxication. Radiology 1970;97(2):347–351.

230. Pare JA, Fraser RG, Hogg JC, et al: Pulmonary "mainline" granulomatosis: talcosis of intravenous methadone abuse. Medicine (Baltimore) 1979;58(3):229–239.

231. Glassroth J, Adams GD, Schnoll S: The impact of substance abuse on the respiratory system. Chest 1987;91(4):596–602.

232. Sieniewicz DJ, Nidecker AC: Conglomerate pulmonary disease: a form of talcosis in intravenous methadone abusers. Am J Roentgenol 1980;135(4):697–702.

233. Sternbach G, Moran J, Eliastam M: Heroin addiction: acute presentation of medical complications. Ann Emerg Med 1980; 9(3):161–169.

234. Angiitis in drug abusers. N Engl J Med 1971;284(2):111–113.

235. Amine AR: Neurosurgical complications of heroin addiction: brain abscess and mycotic aneurysm. Surg Neurol 1977;7(6):385–386.

236. Brust JC, Richter RW: Stroke associated with addiction to heroin. J Neurol Neurosurg Psychiatry 1976;39(2):194–199.

237. Jensen R, Olsen TS, Winther BB: Severe non-occlusive ischemic stroke in young heroin addicts. Acta Neurol Scand 1990;81(4): 354–357.

238. King J, Richards M, Tress B: Cerebral arteritis associated with heroin abuse. Med J Aust 1978;2(9):444–449.

239. Niehaus L, Meyer BU: Bilateral borderzone brain infarctions in association with heroin abuse. J Neurol Sci 1998;160(2):180–182.

240. Spiller HA, Gorman SE, Villalobos D, et al: Prospective multicenter evaluation of tramadol exposure. J Toxicol Clin Toxicol 1997;35(4):361–364.

241. Vila N, Chamorro A: Ballistic movements due to ischemic infarcts after intravenous heroin overdose: report of two cases. Clin Neurol Neurosurg 1997;99(4):259–262.

242. Woods BT, Strewler GJ: Hemiparesis occurring six hours after intravenous heroin injection. Neurology 1972;22(8):863–866.

243. McCarron MM, Challoner KR, Thompson GA: Diphenoxylate-atropine (Lomotil) overdose in children: an update (report of eight cases and review of the literature). Pediatrics 1991;87(5): 694–700.

244. Cutler EA, Barrett GA, Craven PW, Cramblett HG: Delayed cardiopulmonary arrest after Lomotil ingestion. Pediatrics 1980; 65(1):157–158.

245. Dunkley EJ, Isbister GK, Sibbritt D, et al: The Hunter Serotonin Toxicity Criteria: simple and accurate diagnostic decision rules for serotonin toxicity. QJM 2003;96(9):635–642.

246. Sternbach H: The serotonin syndrome. Am J Psychiatry 1991; 148(6):705–713.

247. Richter RW, Challenor YB, Pearson J, et al: Acute myoglobinuria associated with heroin addiction. JAMA 1971;216(7):1172–1176.

248. Schwartzfarb L, Singh G, Marcus D: Heroin-associated rhabdomyolysis with cardiac involvement. Arch Intern Med 1977;137(9): 1255–1257.

249. D'Agostino RS, Arnett EN: Acute myoglobinuria and heroin snorting. JAMA 1979;241(3):277.

250. Cunningham EE, Brentjens JR, Zielezny MA, et al: Heroin nephropathy. A clinicopathologic and epidemiologic study. Am J Med 1980;68(1):47–53.

251. Cunningham EE, Venuto RC, Zielezny MA: Adulterants in heroin/cocaine: implications concerning heroin-associated nephropathy. Drug Alcohol Depend 1984;14(1):19–22.

252. Cunningham EE, Zielezny MA, Venuto RC: Heroin-associated nephropathy. A nationwide problem. JAMA 1983;250(21):2935–2936.

253. Dubrow A, Mittman N, Ghali V, Flamenbaum W: The changing spectrum of heroin-associated nephropathy. Am J Kidney Dis 1985;5(1):36–41.

254. Utecht MJ, Stone AF, McCarron MM: Heroin body packers. J Emerg Med 1993;11(1):33–40.

255. Hutchins KD, Pierre-Louis PJ, Zaretski L, et al: Heroin body packing: three fatal cases of intestinal perforation. J Forensic Sci 2000;45(1):42–47.

256. Handal KA, Schauben JL, Salamone FR: Naloxone. Ann Emerg Med 1983;12(7):438–445.

257. Hantson P, Evenepoel M, Ziade D, et al: Adverse cardiac manifestations following dextropropoxyphene overdose: can naloxone be helpful? Ann Emerg Med 1995;25(2):263–266.

258. American Heart Association in collaboration with the International Liaison Committee on Resuscitation: Guidelines 2000 for Cardiopulmonary Resuscitation and Emergency Cardiovascular Care. Part 8: advanced challenges in resuscitation: section 2: toxicology in ECC. Circulation 2000;102(8 Suppl):I223–I228.

259. Moore RA, Rumack BH, Conner CS, Peterson RG: Naloxone: underdosage after narcotic poisoning. Am J Dis Child 1980; 134(2):156–158.

260. Barton ED, Ramos J, Colwell C, et al: Intranasal administration of naloxone by paramedics. Prehosp Emerg Care 2002;6(1):54–58.

261. Maio RF, Gaukel B, Freeman B: Intralingual naloxone injection for narcotic-induced respiratory depression. Ann Emerg Med 1987;16(5):572–573.

262. Salvucci AA Jr, Eckstein M, Iscovich AL: Submental injection of naloxone. Ann Emerg Med 1995;25(5):719–720.

263. Tandberg D, Abercrombie D: Treatment of heroin overdose with endotracheal naloxone. Ann Emerg Med 1982;11(8):443–445.

264. Wanger K, Brough L, Macmillan I, et al: Intravenous vs subcutaneous naloxone for out-of-hospital management of presumed opioid overdose. Acad Emerg Med 1998;5(4):293–299.

265. Longnecker DE, Grazis PA, Eggers GW Jr: Naloxone for antagonism of morphine-induced respiratory depression. Anesth Analg 1973;52(3):447–453.

266. Goldfrank L, Weisman RS, Errick JK, Lo MW: A dosing nomogram for continuous infusion intravenous naloxone. Ann Emerg Med 1986;15(5):566–570.

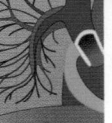

267. Lewis JM, Klein-Schwartz W, Benson BE, et al: Continuous naloxone infusion in pediatric narcotic overdose. Am J Dis Child 1984;138(10):944–946.

268. Romac DR: Safety of prolonged, high-dose infusion of naloxone hydrochloride for severe methadone overdose. Clin Pharm 1986;5(3):251–254.

269. Bracken MB, Shepard MJ, Collins WF, et al: A randomized, controlled trial of methylprednisolone or naloxone in the treatment of acute spinal-cord injury. Results of the Second National Acute Spinal Cord Injury Study. N Engl J Med 1990;322(20):1405–1411.

270. Brimacombe J, Archdeacon J, Newell S, Martin J: Two cases of naloxone-induced pulmonary oedema—the possible use of phentolamine in management. Anaesth Intensive Care 1991; 19(4):578–580.

271. Flacke JW, Flacke WE, Williams GD: Acute pulmonary edema following naloxone reversal of high-dose morphine anesthesia. Anesthesiology 1977;47(4):376–378.

272. Olsen KS: Naloxone administration and laryngospasm followed by pulmonary edema. Intensive Care Med 1990;16(5):340–341.

273. Prough DS, Roy R, Bumgarner J, Shannon G: Acute pulmonary edema in healthy teenagers following conservative doses of intravenous naloxone. Anesthesiology 1984;60(5):485–486.

274. Schwartz JA, Koenigsberg MD: Naloxone-induced pulmonary edema. Ann Emerg Med 1987;16(11):1294–1296.

275. Taff RH: Pulmonary edema following naloxone administration in a patient without heart disease. Anesthesiology 1983;59(6): 576–577.

276. Andree RA: Sudden death following naloxone administration. Anesth Analg 1980;59(10):782–784.

277. Cuss FM, Colaco CB, Baron JH: Cardiac arrest after reversal of effects of opiates with naloxone. BMJ 1984;288(6414):363–364.

278. Michaelis LL, Hickey PR, Clark TA, Dixon WM: Ventricular irritability associated with the use of naloxone hydrochloride. Two case reports and laboratory assessment of the effect of the drug on cardiac excitability. Ann Thorac Surg 1974;18(6):608–614.

279. Tanaka GY: Hypertensive reaction to naloxone [Letter]. JAMA 1974;228(1):25–26.

280. Mills CA, Flacke JW, Flacke WE, et al: Narcotic reversal in hypercapnic dogs: comparison of naloxone and nalbuphine. Can J Anaesth 1990;37(2):238–244.

281. Mills CA, Flacke JW, Miller JD, et al: Cardiovascular effects of fentanyl reversal by naloxone at varying arterial carbon dioxide tensions in dogs. Anesth Analg 1988;67(8):730–736.

282. Pallasch TJ, Gill CJ: Naloxone-associated morbidity and mortality. Oral Surg Oral Med Oral Pathol 1981;52(6):602–603.

283. Silverstein JH, Gintautas J, Tadoori P, Abadir AR: Effects of naloxone on pulmonary capillary permeability. Prog Clin Biol Res 1990;328:389–392.

284. Kollef MH, Pluss J: Noncardiogenic pulmonary edema following upper airway obstruction. 7 cases and a review of the literature. Medicine (Baltimore) 1991;70(2):91–98.

285. Chandavasu O, Chatkupt S: Central nervous system depression from chlorpromazine poisoning: successful treatment with naloxone. J Pediatr 1985;106(3):515–516.

286. Jefferys DB, Flanagan RJ, Volans GN: Reversal of ethanol-induced coma with naloxone. Lancet 1980;1(8163):308–309.

287. Kulig K, Duffy J, Rumack BH, et al: Naloxone for treatment of clonidine overdose. JAMA 1982;247(12):1697.

288. Montero FJ: Naloxone in the reversal of coma induced by sodium valproate. Ann Emerg Med 1999;33(3):357–358.

289. Merigian KS: Cocaine-induced ventricular arrhythmias and rapid atrial fibrillation temporally related to naloxone administration. Am J Emerg Med 1993;11(1):96–97.

290. Hamilton RJ, Perrone J, Hoffman R, et al: A descriptive study of an epidemic of poisoning caused by heroin adulterated with scopolamine. J Toxicol Clin Toxicol 2000;38(6):597–608.

291. Stork CM, Redd JT, Fine K, Hoffman RS: Propoxyphene-induced wide QRS complex dysrhythmia responsive to sodium bicarbonate—a case report. J Toxicol Clin Toxicol 1995;33(2): 179–183.

292. Gilbert PE, Martin WR: Antagonism of the convulsant effects of heroin, d-propoxyphene, meperidine, normeperidine and thebaine by naloxone in mice. J Pharmacol Exp Ther 1975; 192(3):538–541.

293. Cowan A, Geller EB, Adler MW: Classification of opioids on the basis of change in seizure threshold in rats. Science 1979;206(4417):465–467.

294. Jackson HC, Nutt DJ: Investigation of the involvement of opioid receptors in the action of anticonvulsants. Psychopharmacology (Berl) 1993;111(4):486–490.

295. Van Derburgh K, Hantsch C, Meredith T: Is naloxone contraindicated in tramadol overdose? [Abstract]. J Toxicol Clin Toxicol 1998;36:435.

296. Graudins A, Stearman A, Chan B: Treatment of the serotonin syndrome with cyproheptadine. J Emerg Med 1998;16(4):615–619.

297. Frand UI, Shim CS, Williams MH Jr: Methadone-induced pulmonary edema. Ann Intern Med 1972;76(6):975–979.

298. Sterrett C, Brownfield J, Korn CS, et al: Patterns of presentation in heroin overdose resulting in pulmonary edema. Am J Emerg Med 2003;21(1):32–34.

299. Smith DA, Leake L, Loflin JR, Yealy DM: Is admission after intravenous heroin overdose necessary? Ann Emerg Med 1992; 21(11):1326–1330.

300. Christenson J, Etherington J, Grafstein E, et al: Early discharge of patients with presumed opioid overdose: development of a clinical prediction rule. Acad Emerg Med 2000;7(10): 1110–1118.

301. Farmer JW, Chan SB: Whole body irrigation for contraband bodypackers. J Clin Gastroenterol 2003;37(2):147–150.

302. Hoffman RS, Smilkstein MJ, Goldfrank LR: Whole bowel irrigation and the cocaine body-packer: a new approach to a common problem. Am J Emerg Med 1990;8(6):523–527.

303. Traub SJ, Kohn GL, Hoffman RS, Nelson LS: Pediatric "body packing." Arch Pediatr Adolesc Med 2003;157(2):174–177.

304. Marc B, Baud FJ, Aelion MJ, et al: The cocaine body-packer syndrome: evaluation of a method of contrast study of the bowel. J Forensic Sci 1990;35(2):345–355.

305. Marc B, Baud F: Paraffin and body-packers. Lancet 1999; 353(9148):238–239.

306. Larijani GE, Goldberg ME, Rogers KH: Treatment of opioid-induced pruritus with ondansetron: report of four patients. Pharmacotherapy 1996;16(5):958–960.

307. Kriegstein AR, Shungu DC, Millar WS, et al: Leukoencephalopathy and raised brain lactate from heroin vapor inhalation ("chasing the dragon"). Neurology 1999;53(8):1765–1773.

308. Meissner W, Schmidt U, Hartmann M, et al: Oral naloxone reverses opioid-associated constipation. Pain 2000;84(1):105–109.

309. Yuan CS, Foss JF, O'Connor M, et al: Methylnaltrexone for reversal of constipation due to chronic methadone use: a randomized controlled trial. JAMA 2000;283(3):367–372.

310. Hassan H, Bastani B, Gellens M: Successful treatment of normeperidine neurotoxicity by hemodialysis. Am J Kidney Dis 2000;35(1):146–149.

311. Dixon R, Howes J, Gentile J, et al: Nalmefene: intravenous safety and kinetics of a new opioid antagonist. Clin Pharmacol Ther 1986;39(1):49–53.

312. Gal TJ, DiFazio CA: Prolonged antagonism of opioid action with intravenous nalmefene in man. Anesthesiology 1986;64(2): 175–180.

313. Barsan WG, Seger D, Danzl DF, et al: Duration of antagonistic effects of nalmefene and naloxone in opiate-induced sedation for emergency department procedures. Am J Emerg Med 1989;7(2):155–161.

314. Kaplan JL, Marx JA: Effectiveness and safety of intravenous nalmefene for emergency department patients with suspected narcotic overdose: a pilot study. Ann Emerg Med 1993;22(2): 187–190.

315. Kaplan JL, Marx JA, Calabro JJ, et al: Double-blind, randomized study of nalmefene and naloxone in emergency department patients with suspected narcotic overdose. Ann Emerg Med 1999;34(1):42–50.

34

Sedative-Hypnotics

JOHN G. BENITEZ, MD, MPH, FACMT, FACPM ■ LINDA G. ALLISON, MD, MPH
■ SHARON TERNULLO, BS, PHARMD, CSPI

At a Glance...

- All sedative-hypnotics are not the same.
- Central nervous system depression is their main effect.
- Additive CNS effects occur with other CNS depressants.
- There is no specific antidote for any of the sedative-hypnotics.
- Plasma concentrations of these agents do not assist in management.
- Hemodialysis does not help in clinical management.

INTRODUCTION AND HISTORY

Sedative-hypnotic is a term that describes different medications that sedate or calm a person or induce drowsiness and sleep. The substances covered in this chapter are all chemically different from benzodiazepines and barbiturates (see Chapters 35 and 36). This chapter will focus on the multiple, diverse sedative-hypnotic drugs that are not structurally similar (Fig. 34-1).

Sedatives and hypnotics were among the earliest medications to be introduced into medical practice. Chloral hydrate was synthesized in 1832 and first used clinically starting in 1869. Deaths from this agent were reported as early as 1890.[1] Chloral hydrate, urethane, and paraldehyde were used prior to the introduction of barbital in 1903 and phenobarbital in 1912. As the physical dependence, withdrawal, and abuse potential of these agents began to be appreciated, a search was made for sedative-hypnotics that minimized these risks. Chlorpromazine, the first phenothiazine, was introduced in the early 1950s, and meprobamate, a bis-carbamate ester, was introduced in 1955. Other sedative-hypnotics were introduced during this time period that were presumed to have more selectivity and less abuse potential, including glutethimide, methyprylon (piperidine-diones), chlormezanone, ethinamate (urethane derivative), ethchlorvynol, and methaqualone (quinazolines and their derivatives).[2-5]

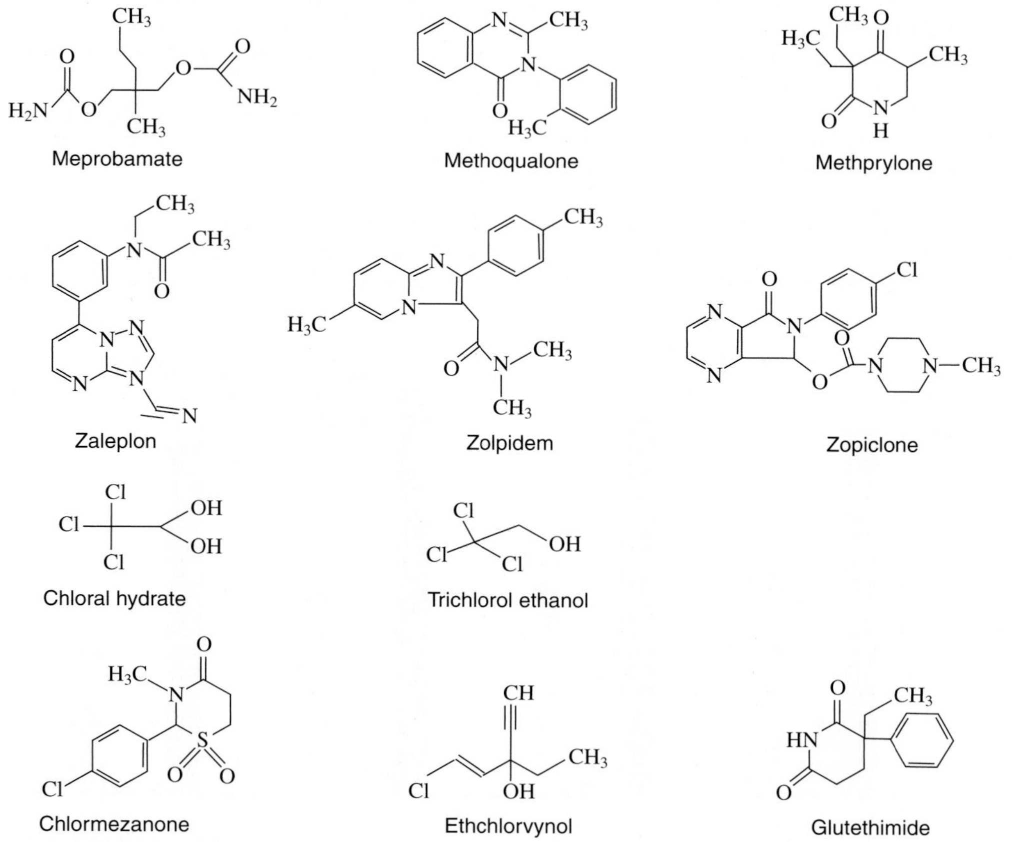

FIGURE 34-1 Chemical structures of sedative-hypnotics described in this chapter. (All structures drawn and identified using ChemIDplus, accessed at http://chem.sis.nlm.nih.gov/chemidplus/.)

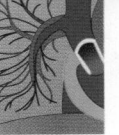

Because of the high abuse potential, tolerance, and acute toxicity of the early sedatives and hypnotics, their use was eventually discontinued. Ethinamate, chlormezanone, methyprylon, paraldehyde, and methaqualone were withdrawn in the 1980s and 1990s. These agents had dependence and abstinence syndromes at least equal to those of the barbiturates, and intoxication was more difficult to manage. During the 1980s to 1990s, selective benzodiazepine receptor agonists were identified and synthesized, including zolpidem, zaleplon, zopiclone (not available in the United States), and alpidem. Zopiclone was first introduced in France in 1987. It was the first cyclopyrrolone hypnotic and was chemically unrelated to other existing sedatives. Ultimately, zolpidem and zaleplon were marketed in the United States. Alpidem was not marketed in the United States due to inconsistent results during clinical trials and was withdrawn from the French market in 1993 due to reports of hepatic toxicity.[6,7]

Sedative-hypnotics are used worldwide, but overall use has steadily decreased since the 1980s. Over the years, barbiturate and benzodiazepine use has increased, replacing the older sedative-hypnotics. In the United States, American Association of Poison Control Centers (AAPCC) data show that exposures to sedative-hypnotics (nonbarbiturates and nonbenzodiazepines) decreased from 2000 to 2003 (Fig. 34-2). Exposures to chloral hydrate, however, remain steady, with approximately 220 toxic exposures reported per year. Fewer than five deaths per year from these agents were reported to U.S. poison centers from 2000 to 2003 (Fig. 34-3).[8]

In Australia, the ratio of female-to-male overdoses was 1.5 to 1. Most overdoses were from the barbiturate or benzodiazepine class, with a small percentage in the "other" class, but specific agents were not described.[9] Chloral hydrate was noted in 0.3% of admissions and 3.5% of deaths from self-poisoning between 1987 and 1992.[10] Chloral hydrate was 4.5 times as likely (odds ratio [OR] 4.5, confidence interval 2–10, 95%) to be used for self-poisoning and had a high likelihood of death (OR

58.1) between 1989 and 1992. In London, 3.1% of overdoses were with sedative-hypnotics, excluding benzodiazepines and barbiturates, during 1984 to 1988. The female-to-male ratio was 1.3:1 for all overdoses.[11,12]

Chlormethiazole was the most popular medication for ethanol withdrawal in Great Britain during the mid-1980s, but its use was discontinued secondary to drug interactions. The drug exhibits cross-tolerance with ethanol, and with long-term use alcoholics readily transferred dependence and often used it while continuing to drink, resulting in a significantly increased mortality rate. There were 95.7 deaths per million prescriptions for this drug, which was twice that of chloral hydrate. By comparison, the newer less toxic alternatives zolpidem and zopiclone resulted in approximately 2 deaths per million prescriptions each.[4,5]

During the late 1960s and early 1970s, 22% of overdose fatalities were due to glutethimide. Mortality approaches 20% after glutethimide-only overdoses and 17% in mixed ingestions, and is greater than any other drug in the sedative-hypnotic group.[13]

Meprobamate was the second most commonly prescribed sedative in the United States after barbiturates during this same time period, and was available in combination dosage forms containing anticholinergics, conjugated estrogens, antianginal agents, and antidepressants.[14,15] In France, mortality from meprobamate overdose was approximately 2.6%.[16] Until 1992, the drug was sold over the counter in some European countries, including Belgium. Moving it to prescription status decreased the number of meprobamate poisoning cases requiring admission from 120 to 18 per year.[17]

STRUCTURE AND STRUCTURE-ACTIVITY RELATIONSHIPS

The exact mechanism of action is unknown or unclear for many sedative-hypnotics. Some affect the γ-aminobutyric acid (GABA) chloride channel but differently from

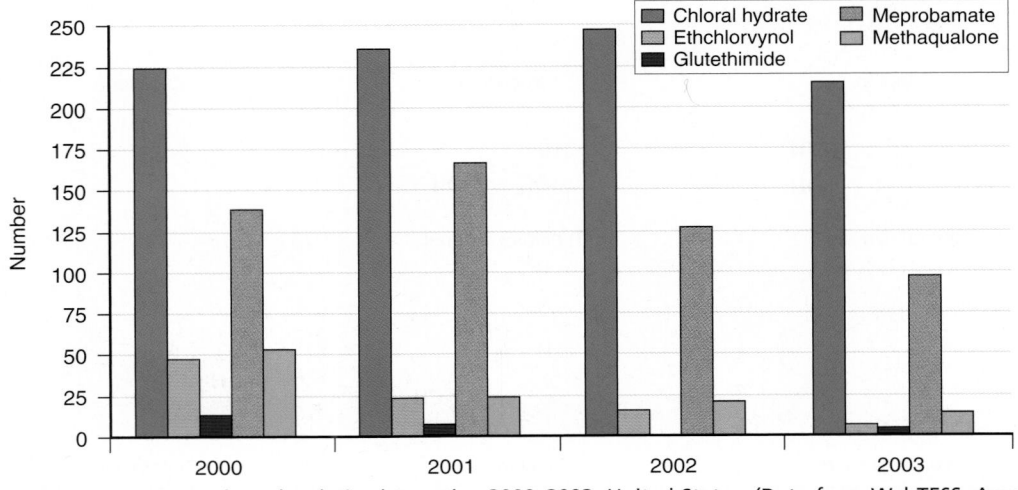

FIGURE 34-2 Human exposures to selected sedative-hypnotics, 2000–2003, United States. (Data from WebTESS, American Association of Poison Control Centers, http://webtess.aapcc.org, accessed June 2004.)

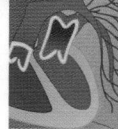

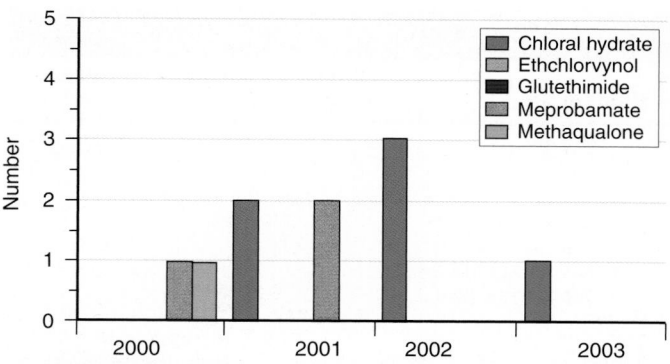

FIGURE 34-3 Human deaths attributed to selected sedative-hypnotics, 2000–2003, United States. (Data from WebTESS, American Association of Poison Control Centers, http://webtess., aapcc.org, accessed June 2004.)

benzodiazepines and barbiturates. The primary metabolite of chloral hydrate is trichloroethanol (TCE), which seems to produce the main sedative-hypnotic effect. TCE affects the $GABA_A$ receptor–ion channel complex similar to other sedative-hypnotic agents by altering chloride currents and decreasing excitability of neurons, but only when GABA is present. In addition, TCE inhibits ion currents activated by excitatory amino acids. This combined effect leads to central nervous system (CNS) sedation.[18] TCE also sensitizes the myocardium to endogenous catecholamines and may induce arrhythmias, similar to other halogenated hydrocarbons.[19-21]

Chlormethiazole similarly affects $GABA_A$-evoked currents in a dose-dependent fashion. It modulates the GABA receptor via a site separate from that of the benzodiazepines. At low doses it potentiates GABA-evoked responses; at high doses it directly activates the GABA receptor. Chlormethiazole prolongs the GABA channel burst duration similar to that of the barbiturates. In addition, chlormethiazole potentiates glycine-evoked currents. This potentially explains its efficacy in treating status epilepticus resistant to therapy with benzodiazepines or barbiturates.[22] It does not seem to have any direct interaction with the N-methyl-D-aspartate receptor.[4]

Meprobamate potentiates GABA at the $GABA_A$ receptors and also activates the chloride channel in the absence of GABA.[23]

Zaleplon, zolpidem, and zopiclone are selective $GABA_A$ benzodiazepine receptor agonists (type 1 omega-1).[7,24] It is unknown at this time how this receptor site mediates pharmacologic activities.[25-27]

The mechanisms of action for ethchlorvynol, glutethimide, and methyprylon are unknown. Glutethimide has an active metabolite, 4-hydroxy-2-ethyl-2-phenyl-glutarimide.

SPECIFIC DRUGS

The pharmacology and toxicology of the different sedative-hypnotics will be considered individually for similar agents. The diagnosis and treatment sections consider all drugs together due to the similar diagnostic approach and management of all of these agents.

General Comments on Pharmacology and Pharmacokinetics

Absorption varies greatly between the sedative-hypnotic agents; some have significant first pass clearance. Due to their high lipid solubility, many of these agents can be described by a two- or even three-compartment model of distribution and eventual elimination. The initial plasma elimination reflects partitioning into fat stores, and the later slow elimination reflects gradual release from fat stores back into the plasma. All are extensively metabolized in the liver along complex multiple pathways and all are enzyme inducers. Specific pathways of metabolism have not been fully elucidated. Many agents have at least one active metabolite.[1,7,14,15,24,28,29]

The pharmacokinetic parameters of selected agents are summarized in Table 34-1. It is noteworthy that with the exception of the newer agents, zaleplon and zolpidem, data from various studies with the older agents are inconsistent. See Table 34-2 for a summary of important drug interactions.

General Comments on Toxicology

The sedative-hypnotics generally produce drowsiness and sedation, hence their classification. Overdose of these agents is associated with sedation, dizziness, hypothermia, and hypotension that can progress to coma and respiratory depression. Patients may vomit and aspirate, leading to pneumonia or even death. In all of these patients, respiratory depression may lead to hypoxia, which could result in devastating neurologic injury if not recognized and treated. There are a few exceptions to this general picture, and there are a few additional findings with specific agents, which are described under the individual agents.

Adverse Effects

Physical dependence and cross-tolerance exists between many of these agents, and withdrawal symptoms have been reported after chronic use and abuse. Maternal administration has resulted in respiratory depression or withdrawal in neonates exposed for many of these agents, including chlormethiazole and ethchlorvynol.[30,31]

Chloral Hydrate/Trichloroethanol

PHARMACOLOGY AND PHARMACOKINETICS
See Table 34-1.

SPECIAL POPULATIONS
For chloral hydrate, toxicity has been particularly pronounced in neonates due to accumulation and persistence of TCE for several days after chloral hydrate has been discontinued. Because TCE competes with bilirubin for protein binding sites and metabolic (glucuronidation)

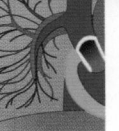

TABLE 34-1 Pharmacokinetic Parameters of Selected Agents

	HALF-LIFE (hr)	Vd	RENAL EXCRETION	METABOLISM	PROTEIN BINDING %	BIOAVAIL-ABILITY	PEAK (hr)
Chloral hydrate (*Noctec*)	Rapid reduction to TCE TCE 7–11, Avg 8		Less than 10% parent compound	Liver extensive Metabolized to trichloroethanol active metabolite and trichloroacetic acid	70%–80%		0.3–1
Chlormethiazole (investigational in USA)	2.6–8.9	0.28 L/kg	0.1–5%	Hepatic 70%–80% 2 inactive metabolites	56%–64%	10%–15% increase in liver disease	0.5
Chlormezanone (*Trancopal*) (TEN reactions led to discontinuation in 1996)	19–24	1.2 L/kg	40% less than 3% unchanged	Stomach-hydrolyzed Liver: hydrolysis and oxidation with nonglucuronide conjugation	48%–64%		1–2
Ethchlorvynol (*Placidyl*)	10–25	4 L/kg	Less than 10%				
Ethinamate (discontinued 1990 in USA)	1.9–2.5		36%	Extensive hydroxylation and glucuronidation			0.5–1.0
Glutethimide (*Doriden*)	Parent 11.6–13.5	1.6 L/kg	Less than 2% unchanged	2–3 active metabolites	47%–59%		1–6
Meprobamate (*Equanil, Miltown*)	9–11	0.5–0.8 L/kg	10%–20%	90% liver to inactive metabolites	0–30%		2–3
Methaqualone (*Mandrax*) (discontinued in 1983 in USA)	10–43 Avg 16		Feces 1%–4%	Site of metabolism to phenolic derivatives unknown	Parent highly protein bound	67%–99%	1–2
Methyprylon (*Noludar*) (discontinued by Roche in 1988)	9.2	0.97 L/kg	3% unchanged 60% metabolites	2 identified P-450 enzyme system, some dose dependency	38%	Assumed at least 90%	2
Paraldehyde (removed from U.S. market)	7.4	1.73 L/kg	0% unchanged	Liver: 70%–80% to acetaldehyde 30% exhaled via lungs		Well absorbed IM PO:93% PR:80%	
Zaleplon (*Sonata*)	1	1.4 L/kg	Less than 1% active, 71% inactive	CYP3A4 4 inactive metabolites	60%	30% first pass effect	1.1
Zopiclone	3.5–6	1.5 L/kg	4–5% parent Extensive metabolites	Extensive:1 active (*N*-oxide) 1: *N*-desmethyl (inactive)	45%	80%	1–1.5
Zolpidem (*Ambien*)	1.2–4	0.54 L/kg	Less than 1% active, 79%–96% inactive	Extensive No active metabolites	89%–92%	70%	1.6–2

IM, intramuscularly; PO, orally; PR, rectally; TCE, trichloroethanol; TEN, toxic epidermal necrolysis; Vd, volume of distribution.

systems, resulting in both impaired transport and elimination, it should be used with caution in neonates. There have been reports of indirect hyperbilirubinemia, apnea, and difficulty in weaning neonates from mechanical ventilation after chloral hydrate therapy.[32]

DRUG INTERACTIONS

The prototypical drug interaction for this class of medications has been the interaction between chloral hydrate and ethanol. Chloral hydrate is rapidly converted to TCE.[21] TCE successfully competes with ethanol for the dehydrogenase enzymes that metabolize ethanol, thereby decreasing elimination of ethanol. Ethanol stimulates NADH production and therefore increases the rate of chloral hydrate reduction to TCE by liver alcohol dehydrogenase. This dual mechanism results in an increased production of TCE and decreased elimination of ethanol that is the basis for the toxicity of the "Mickey Finn."[33] Other interactions with chloral hydrate are based on its ability to induce microsomal enzymes and displace other agents such as furosemide and warfarin from plasma protein binding sites.[1,20] Chloral hydrate increases myocardial sensitivity to catecholamines, with the potential for inducing recalcitrant and fatal dysrhythmias when these agents are used. See section on Management below.[21]

TOXICOLOGY: MANIFESTATIONS

For chloral hydrate, cardiac toxicity is a hallmark of severe overdose, manifested by atrial and ventricular

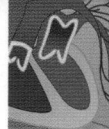

TABLE 34-2 Summary of Important Drug Interactions

SEDATIVE	INTERACTING MEDICATION	MECHANISM	RESULT
Chloral hydrate	Ethanol	Competition for alcohol dehydrogenase system	Accumulation of trichloroethanol and elevated ethanol levels
	Furosemide	Displacement of furesemide from protein binding sites	Cardiovascular toxicity
	Warfarin	Displacement of warfarin from protein binding sites	Increased risk of bleeding
Chlromethiazole	Cimetidine	Decreased metabolism	50% increase in half-life
Ethchlorvynol	Warfarin	Microsomal enzyme induction	Decreased prothrombin time
Glutethimide	Warfarin	Microsomal enzyme induction	Decreased prothrombin time
Meprobamate	Ethanol	Microsomal enzyme induction	Variable; increased sedation
Zaleplon	Cimetidine	Enzyme inhibition	Increased plasma concentration of zaleplon by 85%
	Rifampin	Enzyme induction	Decreased Cpmax and AUC by 80% and increased clearance fivefold
Zolpidem	Ritonavir	Decreased metabolism	Increased serum concentrations
	Rifampin (*both phenytoin and carbamazepine could potentially interact as well)	Induction of CYP3A4	Decreased serum concentrations
	Ketoconazole	Inhibition of metabolism	Decreased clearance by 40%–65%
	Sertraline, venlafaxine, bupropion, desipramine, fluoxetine	Unknown	Hallucinations
	Oral contraceptives	Increased clearance	Decreased half-life of zolpidem
	Cigarette smoking	Increased clearance	Decreased half-life
Zopiclone	Erythromycin	Decreased plasma clearance or increased oral bioavailability	Increased plasma concentrations and AUC
	Rifampin (*both phenytoin and carbamazepine could potentially interact as well)	Induction of CYP3A4	Decreased plasma concentrations of zopiclone

AUC, area under the curve; Cpmax, maximum plasma concentration of the drug.

dysrhythmias, including unifocal and multifocal ventricular premature contractions, bigeminy, torsades de pointes, ventricular fibrillation, and asystole.[1,19-21] When ethanol and chloral hydrate are ingested together (a Mickey Finn), the CNS depressant actions of both are enhanced, leading to the so-called "knock-out drop" effect, or rapid, decreased level of consciousness; some persons also experience vasodilation, tachycardia, facial flushing, headache, and hypotension.[33]

Chlormethiazole

PHARMACOLOGY AND PHARMACOKINETICS
Chlormethiazole exhibits a 10-fold increase in bioavailability if co-ingested with alcohol and in patients with cirrhosis, presumably from an impaired first pass effect. Low serum albumin in alcoholics leads to decreased protein binding, allowing for an increased free drug serum concentration. This may account for the high death rate in alcoholics who continue to drink while taking chlormethiazole.[12]

DRUG INTERACTIONS
Ethanol and imipramine produce additive clinical effects.[25]

TOXICOLOGY: MANIFESTATIONS
The coma associated with chlormethiazole overdose may be prolonged and has been reported to last from 40 to 92 hours. Victims also have increased salivation and bronchial secretions.[34] A direct effect on thermoregulatory centers contributes to significant hypothermia. The addition of alcohol to chlormethiazole leads to a deep coma, severe respiratory depression, and increased mortality.[5]

Chlormezanone

PHARMACOLOGY AND PHARMACOKINETICS
Chlormezanone is rapidly absorbed and metabolized into at least six compounds, which are excreted in the urine. In one series of eight elderly patients, oral absorption of chlormezanone was delayed but not reduced, and the half-life was prolonged to 54 hours. The volume of distribution calculated from these data was approximately 85 L, which is consistent with other agents of this class. The half-life following an overdose without evidence of shock has been estimated at 29 to 35 hours.[35] Chlormezanone is similar to baclofen in chemical structure, and its metabolite exerts a similar muscle relaxant effect.[36]

DRUG INTERACTIONS
Ethanol and imipramine produce additive clinical effects.[25]

TOXICOLOGY: MANIFESTATIONS
Chlormezanone overdose signs and symptoms are similar to those of other sedatives; metabolic acidosis has also been noted. In addition, drug-induced hepatitis may

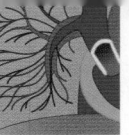
occur, with abrupt elevation of liver enzymes, prolonged prothrombin time, elevated bilirubin, and hypoglycemia. Diffuse hydropic degeneration and necrosis of hepatocytes with pericentral vein congestion are noted on liver biopsy.[37-39] Central anticholinergic syndrome has been reported in chlormezanone overdose both as a result of single agent ingestion and in combination with ofloxacin and diphenhydramine.[40]

ADVERSE EFFECTS

Even with the recommended dose of chlormezanone, a hypersensitivity reaction can result in a transient hepatitis, which is associated with eosinophilia, cholestasis, and mild periportal infiltration. A fixed skin eruption may also occur at normal doses.[37-39]

Ethchlorvynol

PHARMACOLOGY AND PHARMACOKINETICS

Ethchlorvynol is rapidly absorbed after oral administration. It is highly lipophilic, and concentrates in adipose tissue and the CNS.[41] Because of this high lipid solubility, it exhibits a biphasic elimination, with a secondary plasma peak occurring between 7 and 14 hours postingestion, reflecting gradual elimination from extensive body stores. This may explain the large variation in the duration of coma reported after large ingestions (50 to 300 hours). Ethchlorvynol is metabolized by hepatic glucuronidation and/or hydroxylation. Some of the volatile oil is eliminated via the lung. It is unknown whether the parent compound or the metabolite of the drug is responsible for the pungent breath odor that is noticed in intoxicated patients. Ethchlorvynol may accumulate in circulating and developing blood cells; severe pancytopenia has been reported.[42]

DRUG INTERACTIONS

Ethanol and imipramine produce additive clinical effects.[25] Ethchlorvynol is a microsomal enzyme inducer that enhances the metabolism of warfarin, decreasing its effectiveness.[43]

TOXICOLOGY: MANIFESTATIONS

Ethchlorvynol overdose presents with the typical symptoms, but bradycardia rather than tachycardia may be present. A distinctive pungent aromatic odor may be noted on the breath. There is a direct relationship between the dose and the duration and level of coma, but no such relationship exists between dose and the occurrence or level of hypothermia. Interestingly, however, the level of coma does not change appreciably after hemodialysis and a reduction in the ethchlorvynol level. Deep prolonged coma may last from 10 to 288 hours, with a mean of 119 hours. Deep tendon reflexes are usually absent, and there may be loss of the corneal and pupillary light reflexes. The prolonged coma places victims at risk for complications such as gram-negative pneumonia, pressure ischemia and neuropathy, thrombophlebitis, and thromboembolism. Pressure necrosis similar to that reported for barbiturates,

glutethimide, opiates, and carbon monoxide has been noted.[44] An autopsy performed on one patient who had severe multisystem disease revealed bilateral bronchopneumonia, pulmonary embolism, thrombophlebitis of the ovarian vein, renal infarct, focal hepatic necrosis, acute cystitis, marked cerebral edema, and passive congestion of viscera.[45] Intravenous injection, and possibly oral ingestion, of ethchlorvynol may lead to noncardiogenic pulmonary edema. Noncardiogenic pulmonary edema appears to be mediated by cyclooxygenase products since it can be blunted by the prior administration of nonsteroidal anti-inflammatory agents.[46,47] After intravenous injection, patients experience a mintlike taste, marked shortness of breath, and nonproductive cough; physical findings include diffuse end-inspiratory rales and a normal cardiac examination. Other findings include hypoxemia, respiratory acidosis, bilateral alveolar infiltrates on chest x-ray without cardiomegaly, and a normal electrocardiogram.[48,49]

Glutethimide

PHARMACOLOGY AND PHARMACOKINETICS

Absorption of glutethimide is slow and erratic due to its poor solubility. The absorption is hastened and increased with concurrent ethanol ingestion.[13] The apparent volume of distribution for glutethimide is greater than that of body water.[28] Due to its high lipid solubility, 80% of the parenterally administered drug appears to be sequestered in the gastrointestinal tract, adipose tissue, and the central nervous system. Less than 2% is found in the blood.[50] The majority of the metabolites undergo enterohepatic circulation in animals, with slow urinary excretion. At least one metabolite, 4-hydroxy-2-ethyl-2-phenylglutarimide (4-HG), contributes to toxicity.[51] In mice, 4-HG is approximately twice as potent as the parent compound in producing death.[41,52] The drug is 90% conjugated in the liver as two glucoronides with delayed excretion. As with other highly lipophilic agents, it is eliminated following a biphasic elimination curve. Further complicating elimination is the racemic nature of the drug, with each enantiomer being metabolized differently.[41]

DRUG INTERACTIONS

Ethanol and imipramine produce additive clinical effects.[25] Glutethimide is a microsomal enzyme inducer that enhances the metabolism of warfarin, decreasing its effectiveness.[43] Glutethimide potentiates codeine's sedative effect, with increased risk for death when both are taken together.[53]

TOXICOLOGY: MANIFESTATIONS

Intoxication with glutethimide results in a prolonged coma with variations in coma depth and sudden apnea, but little correlation between blood levels and the patient's clinical condition.[53] Cerebral edema and seizures appear to be more common than with other sedative-hypnotics. Acute renal failure is rare but has been reported.[13] Anticholinergic activity of glutethimide

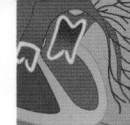

probably contributes to reduced gastric motility and delayed gastrointestinal transit, urinary retention, mydriasis, and some of the hallucinations and delusions reported in acute ingestions of the drug.[54] In the 1970s, there were reports of neonatal withdrawal from glutethimide. Infants born to mothers addicted to glutethimide responded well initially, then had recurrence of symptoms about 5 days later, including overactivity, restlessness, tremors, hyper-reflexia, hypotonus, vasomotor instability, incessant crying, and general irritability. The infants usually responded to treatment with benzodiazepines, phenobarbital, and morphine/methadone/paregoric over 6 to 7 weeks.[55]

Meprobamate

PHARMACOLOGY AND PHARMACOKINETICS

Meprobamate has a low solubility in water, is resistant to gastric and intestinal juices, and decreases gastric motility; bezoar formation is more likely than with other sedative-hypnotics. The metabolism of meprobamate is induced by ethanol.[15] Meprobamate has characteristics of a drug whose elimination might be increased by hemoperfusion, including a low intrinsic clearance, a relatively low volume of distribution, and charcoal adsorption.[56] Carisoprodol is a muscle relaxant (half-life of 100 minutes) that is converted to meprobamate (half-life of 11.3 hours).[57,58]

DRUG INTERACTIONS

Ethanol and imipramine produce additive clinical effects.[25]

TOXICOLOGY: MANIFESTATIONS

Meprobamate intoxication may be difficult to distinguish from other sedatives, but some differences may be noted. Fluctuating coma and seizures may occur, although the drug has been reported to have anticonvulsant activities. Cardiac dysrhythmias include both tachycardia and bradycardia; hypotension can be profound and protracted, and is attributed to direct action on the CNS vasomotor center. Pulmonary edema has been reported, as has bullous skin lesions. Meprobamate deaths have been attributable to shock, pulmonary edema, or complications such as pneumonia or sepsis. Carisoprodol overdose presents with the same clinical picture.[16,57,58]

Methaqualone

PHARMACOLOGY AND PHARMACOKINETICS
See Table 34-1.

TOXICOLOGY: MANIFESTATIONS

Methaqualone is no longer available either as a single drug or in combination with diphenhydramine (Mandrax) in the United States or United Kingdom; however, some is available on the black market and is used to adulterate heroin. Patients presenting with a methaqualone overdose exhibit a range of neurologic symptoms, including lethargy to coma, slurred speech, and gait disturbance. Sensorimotor abnormalities include hyperacusis, blurred vision, ophthalmoplegia, hallucinations, and paresthesias. Increased muscular tone and rigidity, hyper-reflexia, clonus, myoclonus, and seizures may occur, leading to rhabdomyolysis and hyperthermia. In general, hypotension and respiratory depression occur less frequently with methaqualone than with other drugs in this class, but can be exacerbated by co-ingestion of additional depressants or ethanol. Markedly increased tracheobronchial secretions and salivation are also seen in intoxication. One case of unilateral pulmonary edema has been reported. Retinal hemorrhages, purpura, and gastrointestinal hemorrhages can occur. Studies in animal models noted that the drug inhibits adenosine diphosphate (ADP) and decreases both collagen- and ADP-induced platelet aggregation.[59] Many of these findings may be related to or exacerbated by diphenhydramine combined with methaqualone in a preparation available earlier.[59-62]

Methyprylon

PHARMACOLOGY AND PHARMACOKINETICS

Methyprylon is structurally and pharmacologically related to glutethimide, but is more water soluble and therefore has nearly complete gastrointestinal absorption. Its distribution and elimination are generally described as a two-compartment model. Hepatic metabolism is via the P-450 dehydrogenase system, with production of at least four metabolites. A second oxidative pathway has also been identified with multiple metabolites. The elimination half-lives of methyprylon reported in the literature vary greatly (4 to 50 hours).[63]

DRUG INTERACTIONS

Ethanol and imipramine produce additive clinical effects.[25]

TOXICOLOGY: MANIFESTATIONS

Patients with methyprylon overdose may demonstrate inconsistent findings. Various studies have reported cases with no hypotension, moderate to severe hypotension that was recurrent, no decrease in peripheral reflexes except in mixed ingestions, hyperreflexia and seizure activity, hyperreflexia and areflexia, pinpoint, sluggish pupils, or fixed and dilated pupils. The one fatal case in the literature was deeply comatose, cyanotic, and hypotensive, and presented approximately 18 hours postingestion. Other cases that presented earlier, but with equally severe initial findings recovered with supportive treatment or supportive treatment plus hemodialysis.[63-70]

Zaleplon, Zolpidem, and Zopiclone

PHARMACOLOGY AND PHARMACOKINETICS

The kinetics of zaleplon, zolpidem, and zopiclone have been characterized to a greater extent than the preceding agents. Neither zaleplon nor zolpidem appear to exhibit dose-dependent kinetics within the therapeutic range. Zaleplon has a more rapid elimination than zolpidem.[7] Zolpidem has a rapid absorption, rapid distribution into the CNS, and rapid onset of activity.[71]

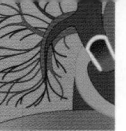

Zolpidem is metabolized in the liver by four different P-450 pathways. Sixty-one percent of the drug is metabolized through the 3A4 enzyme system, 22% through 2C9, 14% through 1A2, and less than 3% through the combined 2D6 and 2C19 pathways.[72] Because it is less lipophilic than other similar agents, it is cleared from the CNS more rapidly.[6]

Zopiclone has a high bioavailability, which suggests absence of a significant first pass effect. Thirteen metabolites through seven pathways have been identified. A low volume of distribution, confirmed by autopsy results, indicates that the agent has no particular preferential distribution into solid organs.[73] The drug's elimination follows a two-compartment model.[74] The half-life of its primary active metabolite is approximately equal to the half-life of the parent drug. The half-life of zopiclone is longer in patients with cirrhosis and in elderly patients, so the dosage should be reduced by half in these patients. The half-life of the drug is also prolonged in patients with renal disease, but the changes are slight and probably not clinically significant.[25,75,76]

SPECIAL POPULATIONS

Zopiclone dosage should be reduced by half in elderly patients and those with severe liver insufficiency.[75]

DRUG INTERACTIONS

Ethanol and imipramine appear to have no effect on the kinetics or pharmacodynamics of zopiclone.[25] Rifampin has been shown to enhance the metabolism of zaleplon, zolpidem, and zopiclone due to its potent induction of cytochrome P-450, resulting in decreased maximum peak concentration, reduction of the area under the curve (AUC), and increased total clearance. This potential effect also exists for other inducers of the cytochrome isoenzymes, such as phenytoin and carbamazepine.[77-79] Zaleplon appears to have no significant pharmacokinetic drug interactions with digoxin, ibuprofen, warfarin, imipramine, or paroxetine; however, additive psychomotor effects have been reported when it is combined with imipramine, paroxetine, or thioridazine. Cimetidine increases the plasma concentration of zaleplon by 85%.[77,80-83] Erythromycin has been shown to increase the AUC and peak concentrations of zopiclone, but the differences are not likely to be of clinical significance.[84] Ranitidine did not increase drowsiness when used in patients receiving a single dose of zopiclone as a preoperative medication.[85] No pharmacokinetic interactions have been observed between digoxin, warfarin, or ranitidine and zolpidem.[86,87] The half-life of zolpidem is reduced by smoking and oral contraceptive use; this is not likely to be clinically significant.[88] There is an increase in peak serum concentration and a decrease in time to peak concentration of zolpidem in patients who also take sertraline, but this is also unlikely to be of routine clinical significance.[89] Ketoconazole decreases the clearance of zolpidem by approximately 40%; itraconazole and fluconazole produce only small changes in the drug's elimination kinetics. Ritonavir also reduces the clearance of zolpidem.[72,90] Decreased psychomotor performance has been observed with the combination of chlorpromazine and zolpidem, but no pharmacokinetic interaction was found with single-dose administration.[87] There is an increased risk for hallucinations with concurrent use of zolpidem and select antidepressants, including bupropion, fluoxetine, sertraline, venlafaxine, and desipramine. The mechanism of this interaction has not been established.[91]

TOXICOLOGY: MANIFESTATIONS

Two cases of zaleplon overdose have been reported, and both patients recovered uneventfully. Zolpidem overdose usually presents with a mild clinical picture, including drowsiness and vomiting. Some patients experience gait abnormalities, blurred vision, mydriasis, visual hallucinations, and memory impairment. More severe symptoms are consistent with multiple-drug overdose, including respiratory depression or failure and hypotension.[92-97] Fatalities have occurred with zolpidem taken with co-ingestants such as morphine, hydrocodone, meprobamate, lidocaine, and carisoprodol.[93,97,98]

ADVERSE EFFECTS

Withdrawal symptoms after chronic use have been reported with zopiclone and zolpidem but are not generally life threatening. Hallucinations and sensory distortion may occur with therapeutic doses of zolpidem. Amnesic psychotic reactions and agitation with disorganization of thoughts may occur.[6,97,99-101]

DIAGNOSIS

Laboratory Testing

A toxicology screen may confirm the presence of these agents, but will generally not be helpful in establishing the level of toxicity and planning treatment; severity of toxicity is generally a clinical diagnosis. General laboratory testing should include a complete blood count, serum electrolytes, blood urea nitrogen (BUN), creatinine, liver enzymes, and arterial blood gas. Pulse oximetry should be monitored.

Therapeutic serum chlormezanone levels are normally 4 to 6 mg/L, with levels greater than 50 mg/L considered toxic. Ethchlorvynol levels are directly proportional to the amount ingested, but they do not correlate with clinical symptoms.[45]

Meprobamate levels of 3 to 10 mg/dL are associated with mild to moderate signs of toxicity, 10 to 20 mg/dL with deeper coma, and greater than 20 mg/dL with severe toxicity and increased fatality rate. Rising levels may indicate continued absorption, which would suggest the formation of concretions in the gastrointestinal tract.

Methaqualone levels of 2 to 5 μg/dL are generally considered to be in the toxic range.[62] Multiple complications have been associated with methaqualone, and therefore baseline laboratory evaluation should include a complete blood count, liver enzymes, coagulation studies, platelet count, serum creatine phosphokinase (CPK), BUN, creatinine, and electrolytes. Coagulation abnormalities, with prolonged prothrombin and partial

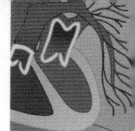

thromboplastin times, inhibition of platelet aggregation, and decreases in factors V and VII may lead to bleeding problems. Rhabdomyolysis and hyperthermia may affect renal function.[59,62] Methyprylon levels of greater than 3.0 mg/dL are associated with coma, and levels less than 3.0 mg/dL are generally associated with somnolence. Other symptoms do not demonstrate a correlation between dose and severity.[63,70] Most laboratory values are not affected in methyprylon overdose, although slight transient elevations of liver enzymes have been noted.[65,68]

Other Diagnostic Testing

Additional testing, such as electrocardiography (ECG) and chest radiography should be performed as indicated in specific clinical situations. Chloral hydrate is radio-paque and may be seen on radiography.[102] Metha-qualone ECG abnormalities are reversible and include right bundle branch block and nonspecific T wave abnormalities.[59,62]

On examination, a pear-like odor to the breath may be noted in chloral hydrate overdose, and a pungent, vinyl-like odor may be associated with ethchlorvynol overdose.

Differential Diagnosis

The differential diagnosis of these agents typically includes other CNS depressant drugs, CNS lesions, other endocrine or infectious processes, and fluid and electrolyte abnormalities. Organophosphate poisoning is included in the differential diagnosis of methaqualone overdose because of the copious secretions associated with this agent.

MANAGEMENT

Supportive Measures

The standard "ABCs" approach is appropriate in cases of sedative-hypnotic overdose. For comatose patients, the main goal is supporting the airway, ventilation, and cardiovascular system. Vital signs must be monitored frequently, including respirations, pulse, blood pressure, and temperature. Unresponsive patients should be intubated to protect the airway and to ensure adequate respirations and ventilation. Ventilation/oxygenation should be monitored with pulse oximetry and arterial blood gas, making adjustments in fraction of inspired oxygen (FIO_2) or rate of ventilation as indicated. Aggressive management of the respiratory status decreases the risk factors for cardiac arrest. Hypotension may be treated with isotonic fluid boluses; vasopressors and inotropes should be used as indicated. Cardiac dysrhythmias should be treated according to advanced cardiac life support (ACLS) protocols with the exception of chloral hydrate (see Specific Treatment). Seizures may be treated with benzodiazepines. Normal body temperature should be maintained; warming blankets

may be sufficient, but use of warmed IV fluids, radiant warming, and other methods may also be required. This is especially important if the patient is hypothermic and develops cardiac dysrhythmias; patients may not respond to usual ACLS protocols during hypothermia. One must anticipate the sequelae of coma and immobilization. The overall incidence and severity of pneumonia is directly proportional to the duration of coma; gram-negative organisms are frequently the cause of pneumonia in these patients. Patients may develop pressure ischemia and neuropathy from prolonged immobilization; such patients should be repositioned frequently. Victims are also at risk for thrombophlebitis and thromboembolism.

Decontamination

Gastric lavage should be considered in patients presenting with mixed ingestions or a potentially lethal ingestion of a single drug if they present within 1 to 2 hours of ingestion. Activated charcoal 1 g/kg may decrease absorption and should be administered. Multiple-dose activated charcoal has been advocated for meprobamate and glutethimide ingestions to prevent ongoing absorption from concretions and delayed motility and to interrupt enterohepatic circulation; however, its efficacy in these ingestions is unproved. Gastric lavage, multiple-dose activated charcoal, and whole bowel irrigation should be considered with meprobamate because of the tendency toward bezoar formation. Recovery of a bezoar weighing only 25 g could be clinically significant because the minimum lethal dose is approximately 20 g. However, it is important to evaluate whether ileus is present before instituting these measures.[56,103-105]

Laboratory Monitoring

Arterial blood gases and pH provide information about ventilation and acid–base status. Mixed respiratory and metabolic acidosis may be seen due to hypoventilation, immobilization, hypotension, and hypothermia.

Monitoring for complications related to prolonged coma and immobilization should be considered.[45] One should monitor for rhabdomyolysis and hyperthermia in cases of myoclonus and seizures, including serum CPK, creatinine, BUN, and electrolytes. Special attention should be focused on maintaining renal function. One should monitor liver enzymes, platelet count, and coagulation times after methaqualone ingestion.[62]

Antidote

There are no specific antidotes currently available for sedative-hypnotic overdoses. Flumazenil has been reported to reverse the effects of chloral hydrate, but there are concerns that it may also precipitate seizures in chloral hydrate overdose, so it should be used with caution, if at all.[105] Flumazenil may reverse CNS depression from severe zolpidem toxicity and zaleplon overdose.[106]

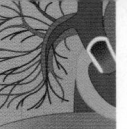

Specific Treatment

Chloral hydrate and trichloroethanol sensitize the myocardium to endogenous catecholamines. Naloxone and flumazenil may precipitate ventricular dysrhythmias. Ventricular dysrhythmias associated with chloral hydrate overdose may be treated with β blockers: propranolol (adults 1.0 to 2.0 mg IV bolus followed by 1.0 to 2.0 mg/hr infusion, children 0.01 to 0.1 mg/kg, maximum 1 mg) or esmolol (adults 500 µg/kg IV slow bolus over 2 minutes followed by 25 to 100 µg/kg/min, children 100 to 500 µg/kg given over 1 minute, followed by infusion of 25 to 100 µg/kg/min, titrated to dysrhythmias cessation). Torsades de points may be treated with IV magnesium or overdrive pacing.

Platelets, fresh frozen plasma, and vitamin K should be administered for uncontrolled bleeding after methaqualone ingestion.[62]

Elimination Enhancement

In general, there is no convincing evidence to support the use of hemodialysis or hemoperfusion in the treatment of sedative-hypnotic overdose. Historically, these methods have been attempted for severe chloral hydrate (TCE) poisoning or inadequate response to supportive care, but clinical improvement has not correlated with reduced levels of drug.[107] There is no evidence to support the use of hemodialysis or hemoperfusion in treating chlormethiazole, glutethimide, or chlormezanone overdoses.[108,109] The use of forced diuresis, hemodialysis, peritoneal dialysis, and hemoperfusion in accelerating the removal of ethchlorvynol remains somewhat controversial. Although these modalities have been shown to reduce the half-life of ethchlorvynol, they have not been shown to shorten the duration of coma, or to reduce morbidity or mortality.[45,110] Hemodialysis and hemoperfusion can enhance the elimination of meprobamate, but these invasive methods are rarely indicated when aggressive decontamination and supportive measures are used.[103] Hemodialysis and hemoperfusion do not alter the clinical outcome of methaqualone overdose, but do increase clearance.[111] Although dialysis has been used in cases of severe methyprylon overdoses, reports of clinical improvement and elimination of the active drug have been inconsistent. Most cases can be managed with supportive care. Osmotic diuresis has also been used, but there is little evidence that this is helpful.[63,65,68,70] There is no experience with hemodialysis for zaleplon or zopiclone overdose. Zolpidem is not dialyzable.[76]

Disposition

Symptomatic patients should be admitted and monitored for 24 hours, or until symptoms resolve; asymptomatic patients for 2 to 6 hours. Patients who are comatose, hypotensive, hypothermic, or show signs of cardiac instability should be admitted to the intensive care unit for supportive care and close monitoring. It may take a day or up to a week to stabilize the patient, depending on level of coma, respiratory compromise, and development of complications. The patient may be discharged to home or psychiatric care when he or she is stable.

The prolonged deep coma and severe respiratory depression associated with ethchlorvynol overdose may last up to 17 days. Patients who improve initially should be observed for at least 24 hours due to the biphasic distribution of ethchlorvynol.[45]

Patients who have ingested significant amounts of chloral hydrate should be admitted for observation and their cardiac status monitored for at least 24 hours. Asymptomatic patients with suspected ingestions should be monitored for 6 to 8 hours. Because of the gastric irritation and vomiting associated with chloral hydrate overdose, the patient should be followed for later development of esophageal stricture.[20]

Asymptomatic patients should be monitored for 6 to 8 hours after meprobamate or glutethimide ingestion. Patients with mild symptoms should be observed for 12 to 24 hours; those with more severe symptoms require longer observation and support due to the biphasic recurrence of toxic symptoms after an initial resolution.[51,109]

Infants born to mothers who have received chlormethiazole should be monitored for 36 to 48 hours for development of respiratory depression or apnea.[30] Neonatal withdrawal symptoms may persist for up to 45 days in infants born to mothers addicted to glutethimide.[67]

REFERENCES

1. Graham SR, Day RO, Lee R, Fulde GWO: Overdose with chloral hydrate: a pharmacological and therapeutic review. Med J Aust 1988;149:686–688.
2. Charney DS, Mihic SJ, Harris RA: Hypnotics and sedatives. In Hardman JG, Limbird LC (eds): Goodman & Gilman: The Pharmacologic Basis of Therapeutics, 10th ed. New York, McGraw-Hill, 2001, pp 399–427.
3. Bailey D, Shaw R: Interpretation of blood glutethimide, meprobamate, and methyprylon concentrations in nonfatal and fatal intoxications involving a single drug. J Toxicol Clin Toxicol 1983;20(2):113–145.
4. Green AR, Cross AJ: The neuroprotective actions of chlormethiazole. Prog Neurobiol 1994;44:463–484.
5. McInnes GT: Chlormethiazole and alcohol: a lethal cocktail. BMJ 1987;294(6572):592.
6. Durand A, Thenot JP, Bianchetti B, et al: Comparative pharmacokinetic profile of two imidazopyridine drugs: zolpidem and alpidem. Drug Metab Rev 1992;24(2):239–266.
7. Greenblatt DJ, Harmatz JS, von Moltke LL, et al: Comparative kinetics and dynamics of zaleplon, zolpidem, and placebo. Clin Pharmacol Ther 1998;64(5):553–561.
8. WebTESS, American Association of Poison Control Centers: http://webtess.aapcc.org, accessed June 2004.
9. McGrath J: A survey of deliberate self-poisoning. Med J Aust 1989;150:317–324.
10. Buckley NA, Whyte IM, Dawson AH, et al: Self-poisoning in Newcastle, 1987–1992. Med J Aust 1995;162:190–193.
11. Buckley NA, Whyte IM, Dawson AH, et al: Correlations between prescriptions and drugs taken in self-poisoning. Implications for prescribers and drug regulation. Med J Aust 1995;162:194–197.
12. Fuller GN, Rea AJ, Payne JF, Lant AF: Parasuicide in central London 1984–1988. J R Soc Med 1989;82:653–656.
13. Arieff A, Friedman E: Coma following non-narcotic drug overdosage: management of 208 adult patients. Am J Med Sci 1973;266(6):405–426.
14. Breimer DD: Clinical pharmacokinetics of hypnotics. Clin Pharmacokinet 1977;2:93–109.
15. Gomolin I: Meprobamate. Clin Toxicol 1981;18(6):757–760.

16. Kintz P, Tracqui A, Mangin P, et al: Meprobamate self-poisoning. Am J Forensic Med Pathol 1988;9(2):139–140.

17. Lambert WE, De Leenheer AP, Van Bocxlaer JF, et al: Meprobamate intoxication: rare and difficult to find. Clin Toxicol 1992; 30(4):683–684.

18. Peoples RW, Weight FF: Trichloroethanol potentiation of γ-aminobutyric acid-activated chloride current in mouse hippocampal neurones. Br J Pharmacol 1994;113:555–563.

19. Brown AM, Cade JF: Cardiac arrhythmias after chloral hydrate overdose. Med J Aust 1980;1:28–29.

20. Bowyer K, Glasser SP: Chloral hydrate overdose and cardiac arrhythmias. Chest 1980;77:232–235.

21. Sing K, Erickson T, Amitai Y, Hryhorczuk D: Chloral hydrate toxicity from oral and intravenous administration. Clin Toxicol 1996;34(1):101–106.

22. Hales TG, Lambert JJ: Modulation of GABA$_A$ and glycine receptors by chlormethiazole. Eur J Pharmacol 1992;210:239–246

23. Rho JM, Donevan SD, Rogawski MA: Barbiturate-like actions of the propanediol dicarbamates felbamate and meprobamate. J Pharmacol Exp Ther 1997;280(3):1383–1391.

24. Sanger DJ, Morel E, Perrault G: Comparison of the pharmacological profiles of the hypnotic drugs, zaleplon and zolpidem. Eur J Pharmacol 1996;313(1–2):35–42.

25. Goa KL, Heel RC: Zopiclone: a review of its pharmacodynamic and pharmacokinetic properties and therapeutic efficacy as an hypnotic. Drugs 1986;32:48–65.

26. Trifiletti RR, Snyder SH: Anxiolytic cyclopyrrolones zopiclone and suriclone bind to a novel sited linked allosterically to benzodiazepines receptors. Mol Pharmacol 1984;26:458–469.

27. Depoortere M, Zivkovic B, Lloyd KG, et al: Zolpidem, a novel nonbenzodiazepine hypnotic. I. Neuropharmacological and behavioral effects. J Pharmacol Exp Ther 1986;237(2):649–658.

28. Curry SH, Riddall JS, Gordon MB, et al: Disposition of glutethimide in man. Clin Pharmacol Ther 1971;12(5):849–856.

29. Gwilt PR, Pankaskie MC, Thornburg JE, et al: Pharmacokinetics of methyprylon following a single oral dose. J Pharm Sci 1985; 74(9):1001–1003.

30. Johnson RA: Adverse neonatal reaction to maternal administration of intravenous chlormethiazole and diazoxide. BMJ 1976;1(6015):943.

31. Rumack BH, Walravens PA: Neonatal withdrawal following maternal ingestion of ethchlorvynol (Placidyl). Pediatrics 1973;52(5):714–716.

32. Birner G, Rutkowska A, Dekant W: N-acetyl-S (1,2,2-trichlorovinyl)-L-cysteine and 2,2,2-trichloroethanol; two novel metabolites of tetrachloroethene in humans after occupational exposure. Drug Metab Dispos 1996;24:41–48.

33. Sellers EM, Lang B, Koch-Weser J, et al: Interaction of chloral hydrate and ethanol in man. Clin Pharmacol Ther 1971;13:37–49.

34. Illingworth RN, Stewart MJ, Jarvie DR: Severe poisoning with chlormethiazole. BMJ 1979;2(6195):902–903.

35. Bernard N, Fauvel JP, Pozet N, et al: Pharmacokinetics of chlormezanone in elderly patients. Eur J Clin Pharmacol 1991;40:603-607.

36. Bor-Shyang S, Ching-Yih L, Kuan-Wen, C, et al: Severe hepatocellular damage induced by chlormezanone overdose. Am J Gastroenterol 1995;90:833–835.

37. Sheu BS, Lin CY, Chen KW, et al: Severe hepatocellular damage induced by chlormezanone overdose. Am J Gastroenterol 1995;90:833–835.

38. Armstrong D, Braithwaite RA, Vale JA: Chlormezanone poisoning. BMJ (Clin Res Ed) 1983;286:845–846.

39. Ohsawa T, Konishi K: Hepatitis associated with chlormezanone. Drug Intell Clin Pharm 1986;20:506.

40. Koppel C, Hopfe T, Menzel J: Central anticholinergic syndrome after ofloxacin overdose and therapeutic doses of diphenhydramine and chlormezanone. Clin Toxicol 1990;28(2):249–253.

41. Bertino J, Reed M: Barbiturate and nonbarbiturate sedative hypnotic intoxication in children. Pediatr Clin North Am 1986;33(3):703–723.

42. Klock J: Hemolysis and pancytopenia in ethchlorvynol overdose. Ann Intern Med 1974;81(1):131–132.

43. Yell RP: Ethchlorvynol overdose. Am J Emerg Med 1990;8(5):246–250.

44. Chamberlain JM, Klein-Schwartz W, Gorman R: Pressure necrosis following ethchlorvynol overdose. Am J Emerg Med 1990;8(5):467–468.

45. Teehan BP, Maher JF, Carey JJ, et al: Acute ethchlorvynol (Placidyl) intoxication. Ann Intern Med 1970;72:875–882.

46. Yagi K, Baudendistel LJ, Dahms TE: Ibuprofen reduces ethchlorvynol lung injury: possible role of blood flow distribution. J Appl Phys 1992;72(3):1156–1165.

47. Zanaboni PB, Bradley JD, Webster RO, Dahms TE: Cyclo-oxygenase inhibitors prevent ethchlorvynol-induced injury in rat and rabbit lungs. J Appl Phys 1991;71(1):43–49.

48. Reed CR, Glauser FL: Drug-induced noncardiogenic pulmonary edema. Chest 1991;100:1120–1124.

49. Glauser, FL, Smith WR, Caldwell A, et al: Ethchlorvynol (Placidyl®)-induced pulmonary edema. Ann Intern Med 1976;34:46–48.

50. Keberle H, Hoffmann K, Bernhard K: The metabolism of glutethimide (Doriden). Experientia 1962;18:105–111.

51. Decker WJ, Thompson HL, Arneson LA: Glutethimide rebound. Lancet 1970;1(7650):778–779.

52. Jones AH, Mayberry JF: Chronic glutethimide abuse. Br J Clin Pract 1986;40:213.

53. Bailey D, Shaw R: Blood concentrations and clinical findings in nonfatal and fatal intoxications involving glutethimide and codeine. Clin Toxicol 1985–1986;23(7,8):557–570.

54. Campbell R, Schaffer CB, Tupin J: Catatonia associated with glutethimide withdrawal. J Clin Psychiatry 1983;44(1):32–33.

55. Reveri M, Pyati SP, Pildes RS: Neonatal withdrawal symptoms associated with glutethimide (Doriden) addiction in the mother during pregnancy. Clin Pediatr 1977;16(5):424–425.

56. Jacobsen D, Wiik-Larson E, Saltvedt E, et al: Meprobamate kinetics during and after terminated hemoperfusion in acute intoxications. Clin Toxicol 1987;25(4):317–331.

57. Lin JL, Lim PS, Lai BC, Lin WL: Continuous arteriovenous hemoperfusion in meprobamate poisoning. Clin Toxicol 1993;31(4):645–652.

58. Hassan E: Treatment of meprobamate overdose with repeated oral doses of activated charcoal. Ann Emerg Med 1986;15(1):73–76.

59. Mills DG: Effects of methaqualone on blood platelet function. Clin Pharmacol Ther 1978;23(6):685–691.

60. Trese M: Retinal hemorrhage caused by overdose of methaqualone. Am J Ophthalmol 1981;91(2):201–203.

61. Oh TE, Gordon TP, Burden PW: Unilateral pulmonary oedema and "Mandrax" poisoning. Anaesthesia 1978;33(8):719–721.

62. Matthew H, Proudfoot AT, Brown SS, Smith ACA: Mandrax poisoning: conservative management of 116 patients. BMJ 1968;2:101–102.

63. Contos DA, Dixon KF, Guthrie RM, et al: Nonlinear elimination of methylprylon (Noludar) in an overdosed patient: correlation of clinical effects with plasma concentration. J Pharm Sci 1991; 80(8):768–771.

64. Pancorbo AS, Palagi PA, Piecoro JJ, Wilson HD: Hemodialysis in methyprylon overdose: some pharmacokinetic considerations. JAMA 1977;237:470–471.

65. Mandelbaum JM, Simon NM: Severe methyprylon intoxication treated by hemodialysis. JAMA 1971;216:139–140.

66. Xanthaky G, Freireich AW, Matusiak W, Lukash L: Hemodialysis in methyprylon poisoning. JAMA 1966;198(11):190–191.

67. Yudis M, Swartz C, Onesti G, et al: Hemodialysis for methyprylon (Noludar) poisoning. Ann Intern Med 1968;68(6):1301–1304.

68. Burnstein N, Stauss HK: Attempted suicide with methyprylon. JAMA 1965;194(10):1139–1140.

69. Reidt WU: Fatal poisoning with methyprylon (Noludar), a nonbarbiturate sedative. N Engl J Med 1956;255(5):231–232.

70. Bailey DN, Jatlow PI: Methyprylon overdose: interpretation of serum drug concentrations. Clin Toxicol 1973;6(4):563–569.

71. Kurta DL, Myers LB, Krenzelok EP: Zolpidem (Ambien) a pediatric case series. Clin Toxicol 1997;35(5):453–457.

72. von Moltke LL, Greenblatt DJ, Granda BW, et al: Zolpidem metabolism in vitro: responsible cytochromes, chemical inhibitors, and in vivo correlations. Br J Clin Pharmacol 1999;48:89–97.

73. Pounder DJ, Davies JI: Zopiclone poisoning: tissue distribution and potential for postmortem diffusion. Forensic Sci Int 1994;65:177–183.

74. Gaillot J, Heusse D, Houghton GW, et al: Pharmacokinetics and metabolism of zopiclone. Pharmacology 1983;27(Suppl 2):76–91.

75. Gaillot H, Le Roux Y, Houghton GW, et al: Critical factors for pharmacokinetics of zopiclone in the elderly and in patients with liver and renal insufficiency. Sleep 1987;10(Suppl 1):7–21.

76. Marc-Aurele J, Caille G, Bourgoin J: Comparison of zopiclone pharmacokinetics in patients with impaired renal function and normal subjects. Effect of hemodialysis. Sleep 1987;10(Suppl 1): 22–26.

77. Dooley M, Plosker GL: Zaleplon: a review of its use in the treatment of insomnia. Drugs 2000;60(2):413–445.

78. Villikka K, Kivisto KT, Lamberg TS, et al: Concentrations and effects of zopiclone are greatly reduced by rifampicin. Br J Clin Pharmacol 1997;43:471–474.

79. Villikka K, Kivisto KT, Luurila H, et al: Rifampin reduces plasma concentrations and effects of zolpidem. Clin Pharm Ther 1997;62(6):629–634.

80. Garcia PS, Carcas A, Zapater P, et al: Absence of an interaction between ibuprofen and zaleplon. Am J Health Syst Pharm 2000;57:1137–1141.

81. Garcia PS, Paty I, Leister CA, et al: Effect of zaleplon on digoxin pharmacokinetics and pharmacodynamics. Am J Health Syst Pharm 2000;57:2267–2270.

82. Hetta J, Broman JE, Darwish M, et al: Psychomotor effects of zaleplon and thioridazine coadministration. Eur J Clin Pharmacol 2000;56:211–217.

83. Sonata Product Information Sheet. Philadelphia, Wyeth-Ayerst Phamaceuticals Inc., 2003.

84. Aranko K, Luurila H, Backman JT, et al: The effect of erythromycin on the pharmacokinetics and pharmacodynamics of zopiclone. Br J Clin Pharmacol 1994;38:363–367.

85. Wilson CM, Robinson FP, Thompson EM, et al: Effect of pretreatment with ranitidine on the hypnotic action of single doses of midazolam, temazepam and zopiclone: a clinical study. Br J Anaesth 1986;58:483–486.

86. Hullhoven R, Desager JP, Harvengt C, et al: Lack of interaction between zolpidem and H2 antagonists, cimetidine and ranitidine. Int J Clin Pharmacol Res 1988;8:471–476.

87. Ambien Product Information Sheet. New York, Sanofi-Synthelabo, Inc., 2004.

88. Olubodun JO, Ochs HR, Truten V, et al: Zolpidem pharmaco-kinetic properties in young females: influence of smoking and oral contraceptive use. J Clin Pharmacol 2002;42:1142–1146.

89. Allard S, Sainati SM, Roth-Schecter BF: Coadministration of short-term zolpidem with sertraline in healthy women. J Clin Pharmacol 1999;39:184–191.

90. Greenblatt DJ, von Moltke LL, Harmatz JS, et al: Kinetic and dynamic interactions study of zolpidem with ketoconazole, itraconazole, and fluconazole. Clin Pharmacol Ther 1998;64: 661–671.

91. Elko CJ, Burgess JL, Robertson WO: Zolpidem-associated hallucinations and serotonin reuptake inhibition: a possible interaction. Clin Toxicol 1998;36:195–203.

92. Gock SB, Wong SH, Nuwayhid N, et al: Acute zolpidem overdose — report of two cases. J Anal Toxicol 1999;23(6):559–562.

93. Winek CL, Wahba WW, Janssen JK, et al: Acute overdose of zolpidem. Forensic Sci Int 1996;78(3):165–168.

94. Hamad A, Sharma N: Acute zolpidem overdose leading to coma and respiratory failure. Intensive Care Med 2001;27(7):1239.

95. Tracqui A, Knitz P, Mangin P: A fatality involving two unusual compounds—zolpidem and acepromazine. Am J Forensic Med Pathol 1993;14(4):309–312.

96. Lichtenwalner M, Tully R: A fatality involving zolpidem. J Anal Toxicol 1997;21(7):567–569.

97. Garnier R, Guerault E, Muzard D, et al: Acute zolpidem poisoning—analysis of 344 cases. J Toxicol Clin Toxicol 1994; 32(4):391–404.

98. Meeker JE, Som CW, Macapagal EC: Zolpidem tissue concentrations in a multiple drug related death involving Ambien. J Anal Toxicol 1995;19:531–534.

99. Iruela LM, Ibanez-Roho V, Baca E: Zolpidem-induced macropsia in anorexic woman. Lancet 1993;342:443–444.

100. Pitner JK, Gardner M, Neville M, et al: Zolpidem-induced psychosis in an older woman. J Am Geriatr Soc 1997;45(4):533–534.

101. Hoyler CL, Tekell JL, Silva JA: Zolpidem-induced agitation and disorganization. Gen Hosp Psychiatry 1996;18:452–453.

102. Maes V, Huyghens L, Dekeyser J, et al: Acute and chronic intoxication with carbromal preparations. Clin Toxicol 1985;23:341.

103. Hassan E: Treatment of meprobamate overdose with repeated oral doses of activated charcoal. Ann Emerg Med 1986;15(1): 73–76.

104. Felby S: Concentrations of meprobamate in the blood and liver following fatal meprobamate poisoning. Acta Pharmacol Toxicol 1970;28:334–337.

105. Donovan KL, Fisher DJ: Reversal of chloral hydrate overdose with flumazenil. BMJ 1989;298(6682):1253.

106. Lheureux P, Debailleul G, De Witt O, Askensasi R: Zolpidem intoxication mimicking narcotic overdose: response to flumazenil. Hum Exp Toxicol 1990;9(2):105–107.

107. Stalker NE, Gambertoglio JG, Fukumitsu CJ, et al: Acute massive chloral hydrate intoxication treated with hemodialysis: a clinical pharmacokinetic analysis. J Clin Pharmacol 1978;18(2–3): 136–142.

108. Chazan JA, Cohen JJ: Clinical spectrum of glutethimide intoxication: hemodialysis reevaluated. JAMA 1969;208(5): 837–839.

109. Chazan JA, Garella S: Glutethimide intoxication: a prospective study of 70 patients treated conservatively without hemodialysis. Arch Intern Med 1971;128:215–218.

110. Benowitz N, Abloin C, Tozer T, et al: Resin hemoperfusion in ethchlorvynol overdose. Clin Pharmacol Ther 1980;27(2):346–242.

111. Baggish D, Gra S, Jatlow P, Bia MJ: Treatment of methaqualone overdose with resin perfusion. Yale J Biol Med 1981;54(2): 147–150.

35 *Benzodiazepines*

SUSAN E. FARRELL, MD ■ TANIA M. FATOVICH, MD

At a Glance...

- Benzodiazepines are widely prescribed and used for sedative, hypnotic, amnestic, anxiolytic, anticonvulsant, and muscle relaxant properties.
- Benzodiazepines are relatively safe in isolated overdose but may be dangerous when co-ingested with other agents.
- Laboratory testing is of limited value in overdose.
- Treatment of overdose is primarily supportive.
- Flumazenil, a competitive antagonist at the γ-aminobutyric acid A receptor, will reverse the toxic effects of benzodiazepines but should be used with caution in benzodiazepine poisoning.
- Patients with benzodiazepine overdose that remain asymptomatic after 4 to 6 hours of observation are medically safe for psychiatric evaluation and disposition.

INTRODUCTION AND RELEVANT HISTORY

The first commercially marketed benzodiazepine, chlordiazepoxide, was accidentally synthesized in 1955 by Roche Laboratories in Nutley, New Jersey. The scope of its pharmacologic properties and clinical applications, however, were not appreciated until 1957, when it was noted to possess effective sedative, hypnotic, and anticonvulsant properties.[1] Subsequent to its clinical release as Librium (Roche Pharmaceuticals of Hoffman-La Roche, Inc., Nutley, NJ) in 1960, chlordiazepoxide spawned an era of widespread benzodiazepine use that still persists today. Diazepam, perhaps the best known and most commercially successful of all the benzodiazepines, was synthesized in 1959 and marketed as Valium (Roche Pharmaceuticals of Hoffman-La Roche, Inc. Nutley, NJ) in 1963. Since the early 1960s, more than 3000 benzodiazepines have been developed, more than 120 have been tested for biologic activity, and approximately 50 different benzodiazepines are currently marketed worldwide. Fourteen benzodiazepines are currently available for clinical use in the United States. They are classified as schedule IV drugs by the Food and Drug Administration (FDA). These agents and a few related compounds available outside the United States are listed in Table 35-1.

Benzodiazepines have various sedative, hypnotic, amnestic, anxiolytic, anticonvulsant, and muscle relaxant properties. All benzodiazepines are effective in the treatment of anxiety and insomnia. However, individual drugs are approved by the FDA and marketed for specific indications on the basis of their clinical and pharmacologic characteristics. For example, alprazolam may have significant antidepressant activity in addition to its sedative properties. Benzodiazepines such as alprazolam and clonazepam have gained use in the treatment of social phobias and panic disorders,[2,3] and clonazepam and lorazepam may be effective in place of, or in combination with, a neuroleptic and lithium for the treatment of acute mania in bipolar disorder.[4] Reports also describe the efficacy of benzodiazepines for the initial treatment of catatonia[5-8] and neuroleptic-induced akathisia and dystonias.[9] In addition, short-acting benzodiazepines such as temazepam and triazolam have found new uses in the prevention and treatment of jet lag.[10,11] Their action is presumed to be through the readjustment of sleep patterns and body temperature, and they shorten the time to resynchronize activity rhythms when used in conjunction with regular exercise. In the past several years, certain benzodiazepines have also been reported to be of benefit in the treatment of pain syndromes,[12] by both decreasing situational anxiety in the setting of acute pain and relieving muscle tension related to some chronic musculoskeletal pain syndromes. Finally, benzodiazepines are also increasingly used in the treatment of cancer patients for the relief of anticipatory anxiety and nausea, insomnia, chemotherapy-induced emesis, neuralgias, and psychiatric disorders secondary to high-dose steroids.[13]

Since their introduction, the benzodiazepines have enjoyed a meteoric rise in popularity and have largely replaced other sedative-hypnotics. Their extraordinary acceptance in clinical medicine has been based on their safety, efficacy, minimal side effects, relatively low addiction potential, and the medical and public demand for sedative and anxiolytic agents. In 1979, the U.S. National Household survey reported that 11% of the adult population in the United States had taken an anxiolytic on one or more occasions in the previous year.[14] Benzodiazepine use peaked in the late 1970s and mid-1980s. Since that time, the annual prevalence of benzodiazepine use in the United States has declined, from a prevalence of 13% in 1981 to 8.3% in 1990.[15] Similar declining rates in benzodiazepine prescriptions have been reported in Australia, Great Britain, and Canada. This decline has largely been attributed to widespread negative publicity and concern about potential misuse, abuse, and long-term side effects, particularly dependence and withdrawal.

Benzodiazepine prescriptions vary by age. In a recent nationwide U.S. survey, 5% of children were prescribed benzodiazepines, a rate that has remained stable from 1987 to 1996.[16] Data from a Canadian study of benzodiazepine prescriptions dispensed for the elderly demonstrated rates that decreased from 25.1% in 1993 to 22.5% in 1998. Prescription rates, however, were still significantly higher for older patients: approximately 20% for those 65 to 69 years of age, and approximately 30% for those at least 85 years of age.[17]

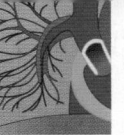
TABLE 35-1 Benzodiazepines Available in the United States

GENERIC NAME	TRADE NAME	YEAR OF INTRODUCTION	RECOMMENDED ADULT DOSE*	AVAILABLE DOSAGE FORMS	FDA-APPROVED INDICATIONS	RATE OF ORAL ABSORPTION
Alprazolam	Xanax	1981	Oral: 0.75–4 mg/day divided tid	0.25-, 0.5-, 1-mg tablets	Anxiety Anxious depression	Intermediate
Chlordiazepoxide	Librium	1960	Oral: 15–100 mg/day divided tid to qid	5-, 10-, 25-mg tablets or capsules	Alcohol withdrawal Anxiety Preoperative sedation	Intermediate
Clonazepam	Klonopin	1974	Oral:7.5–20 mg/day divided tid	0.5-, 1-, 2-mg tablets	Seizure disorder	Intermediate
Clorazepate	Tranxene	1972	Oral: 7.5–60 mg/day divided qd to qid	2.75-, 7.5-, 15-mg capsules	Anxiety Alcohol withdrawal	Rapid
Diazepam	Valium	1963	Oral: 6–40 mg/day divided qd to qid IV: 0.1 mg/kg per dose	2-, 5-, 10-mg tablets	Anxiety/insomnia Alcohol withdrawal Muscle spasm/ seizures Preoperative sedation	Rapid
Flurazepam	Dalmane	1970	Oral: 15–30 mg/day hs	15-, 30-mg capsules	Insomnia	Rapid
Halazepam	Paxipam	1981	Oral: 80–160 mg/day divided tid to qid	20-, 40-mg capsules	Anxiety	Intermediate to slow
Lorazepam	Ativan	1977	Oral: 1–10 mg/day divided bid to tid IM: 0.5 mg/kg IV: 0.05 mg/kg	0.5-, 1-, 2-mg tablets	Anxiety/insomnia Anxious depression Preoperative sedation	Intermediate
Midazolam	Versed	1986	Oral: not available IM: 0.07–0.08 mg/kg IV: Begin 1–2.5 mg, titrate to effect; 0.05 mg/kg total		Preoperative sedation Anesthesia induction Conscious sedation	Rapid†
Oxazepam	Serax	1963	Oral: 30–120 mg/day divided tid to qid	10-, 15-, 30-mg capsules 15-mg tablets	Anxiety Alcohol withdrawal Anxious depression	Slow
Prazepam	Centrax	1977	Oral: 20–60 mg/day divided bid	5-, 10-mg capsules 10-mg tablets	Anxiety	Ultraslow
Temazepam	Restoril	1981	Oral: 15–30 mg qhs	15-, 30-mg capsules	Insomnia	Slow
Triazolam	Halcion	1983	Oral: 0.125–0.5 mg qhs	0.125-, 0.25-, 0.5-mg capsules	Insomnia	Intermediate

IM, intramuscularly; IV, intravenously.
*Maximum dose not established.
†Oral form of midazolam is not yet commercially available, but may administer parenteral formulation orally at 0.3 to 0.7 mg/kg (typically in children).

Because of their widespread availability, benzodiazepines are also among the most frequently misused drugs. Dependence and abuse by the general population, however, are minor when compared to those of alcohol, cocaine, or opiates. As a class, benzodiazepines are not powerful euphoriants and are therefore not frequently abused as a primary agent. Secondary drug abuse is common, however, usually in the form of self-medication, to decrease the adverse side effects of stimulants or hallucinogens, to ameliorate the unpleasant symptoms of withdrawal from more highly addictive substances, or to substitute for the drug of primary dependence when it is not available.

Benzodiazepines are often used by intravenous drug abusers. This combination of intravenous drug use and benzodiazepine abuse has been correlated with increased incidence of needle sharing, polydrug use, psychosocial dysfunction, depression, anxiety, and poor health.[18] The U.S. Treatment Outcome prospective study reported that 73% of heroin abusers also used benzodi-

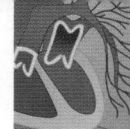

azepines on their entry into treatment.[18] A 1999 study found a similarly high prevalence of benzodiazepine abuse among patients entering a methadone treatment clinic, with lifetime and current prevalences of 66.3% and 50.8%, respectively.[19]

In an attempt to limit such widespread availability and the incidence of misuse and abuse, various laws regulating the prescribing of benzodiazepines have been enacted, with mixed results.[20] For example, in 1989, the State of New York enacted a regulation that required prescriptions for benzodiazepines to be written in triplicate, with mandatory reporting of prescriptions to the New York State Department of Health. The purpose of the regulation was to decrease improper prescribing practices, to restrict overall use of benzodiazepines, and to help eliminate fraud and illegal misdirection of the drugs. As a result of this regulation, benzodiazepine prescriptions decreased by 2 million, but were accompanied by a concurrent increase in the use of other anxiolytics.[21,22] The number of elderly patients using benzodiazepines was reduced by 33%, and the number of prescriptions written was reduced by 45%.[23] Weintraub compared the use of benzodiazepine alternatives in New York to prescribing practices in other unlegislated areas, and concluded that "an undesirable increase has occurred in the prescribing of less acceptable medications."[24] Other unintended consequences of this legislation included an increase in patient visits to an urban psychiatric emergency department for a recurrence of previously controlled psychiatric symptoms or acute benzodiazepine withdrawal. Sales of distilled spirits also increased during the first 4 months after the law was implemented. Similar findings have been reported in European studies.[25]

A more recent study reported another unintended effect of the New York ruling. A marked decrease in new benzodiazepine prescriptions was found among patients discharged from the hospital after cardiac- or cancer-related admissions, 72.5% and 69.4%, respectively.[20] Over the past decade, six states have enacted legislation to restrict benzodiazepine prescribing.

Although benzodiazepines have a low likelihood for producing fatal central nervous system (CNS) depression and are, thus, remarkably safe as compared with older sedative-hypnotics, their potential for addiction and abuse is still well-recognized and a matter of medical and legal controversy.

STRUCTURE AND STRUCTURE-ACTIVITY RELATIONSHIPS

All benzodiazepines are organic bases composed of a benzene ring fused to a seven-membered diazepine ring[26] (Figs. 35-1 and 35-2) All of the important benzodiazepines have a 5-aryl substituent and various substitutions at the R1 and R4 positions of the diazepine ring. The aryl ring at position R5 confers greater potency of the molecule. Specific benzodiazepine agonists vary in the substitutions at the R1, R2, R3, R4, R7, and R2′ positions. Substitution of a keto group at R5 and a methyl group at R4 creates the benzodiazepine antagonist flumazenil. Despite the myriad benzodiazepine

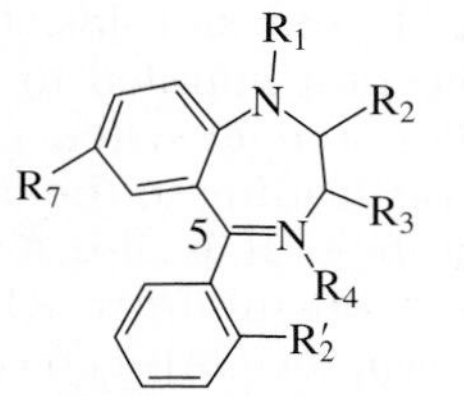

FIGURE 35-1 The general chemical structure of benzodiazepines.

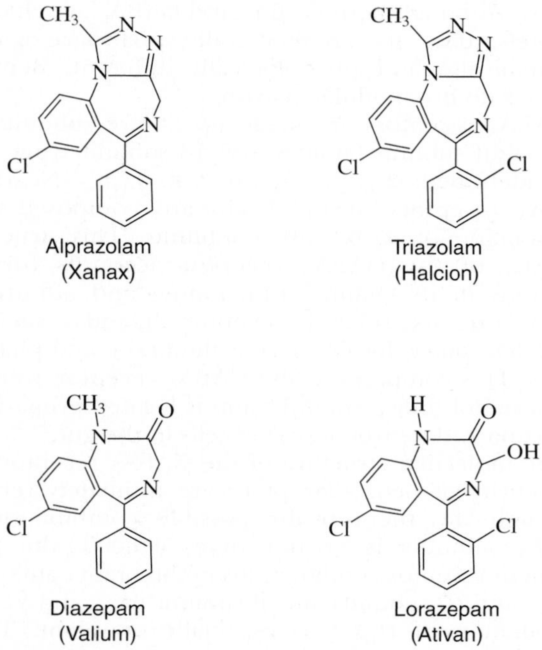

Alprazolam
(Xanax)

Triazolam
(Halcion)

Diazepam
(Valium)

Lorazepam
(Ativan)

FIGURE 35-2 The four most prescribed benzodiazepines in the United States.

compounds available, all derivatives can be expected to have similar qualitative pharmacologic and clinical effects when adjusted for differences in potency. Variations in the pharmacokinetics of an individual drug's onset, duration of action, and metabolism make it more suitable for certain indications.

PHARMACOLOGY

Benzodiazepines produce their sedative, hypnotic, anxiolytic, and anticonvulsant effects through their ability to potentiate the activity of γ-aminobutyric acid (GABA), the major inhibitory neurotransmitter in the CNS. GABA is involved in sleep induction, control of neuronal excitation and epileptic potentials, anxiety, memory, hypnosis, and modulation of the hypothalamic-pituitary axis. GABA is found in high concentrations in the basal ganglia, hippocampus, cerebellum, hypothalamus, and substantia gelatinosa of the dorsal horn of the spinal cord.[27]

Three types of GABA receptors have been defined. $GABA_A$ is a hetero-oligomeric chloride channel composed of five subunits of various types, which is modulated by chemicals such as benzodiazepines,

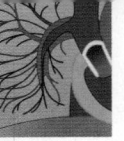
barbiturates, ethanol, and steroids. $GABA_B$ is a seven trans-membrane receptor coupled to G proteins, which activate the second messenger system of phospholipase C and adenylate cyclase, leading to the opening of calcium and potassium channels. It is also a hetero-oligomeric receptor, composed of subunits R1a, R1b, and R2. Baclofen is an agonist at the $GABA_B$ receptor. $GABA_C$ is an ionotropic chloride channel, similar to $GABA_A$. In fact, $GABA_C$ receptors may actually be homomeric $GABA_A$ receptors, composed entirely of one subunit type, unlike $GABA_A$. Although both $GABA_A$ and $GABA_C$ are chloride channels, they are architecturally, pharmacologically, biochemically, and physiologically different. Benzodiazepines do not modulate $GABA_C$.[28]

$GABA_A$ receptors are made up of five subunits. To date, eight subunit families and 18 subunit types have been identified: α_{1-6}, β_{1-3}, γ_{1-3}, δ, ε, π, θ, ρ_{1-3}. Nearly all $GABA_A$ receptors in the brain are composed of a combination of α, β, and γ subunits. This structural diversity of the $GABA_A$ receptor accounts for the variations in its channel functioning and affinity for GABA and its related receptor ligands, such as benzodiazepines, localization in the brain, and pharmacology. This compares to the $GABA_C$ receptor, which is composed of only ρ subunits and is located primarily in the retina and neuroendocrine cells in the gut.[29,30]

The molecular structure of the $GABA_A$ receptor and the activity of benzodiazepines are intimately related. Although the theoretically possible combination of $GABA_A$ subunits is greater than 500,000, the most prevalent receptor combinations in the brain contain α_1, α_2, α_3, and α_5 subunits, any β subunit type, and γ_2. The combination of $\alpha_1\beta_2\gamma_2$ is especially prevalent. These subunits are encoded as a cluster on chromosome 5 of the genome, such that their expression is regulated in a coherent manner.[31]

Benzodiazepine recognition sites, termed *benzodiazepine receptor (BZ) types I and II*, are located on the $GABA_A$ receptor. Because these sites are also binding sites for nonbenzodiazepine ligands, they have been termed w_1 and w_2 *receptors*. A "peripheral type" benzodiazepine receptor, or "P" site, has also been identified in most peripheral tissues and glial cells in the brain. It is unrelated to central benzodiazepine receptors, but may be involved in the modulation of central benzodiazepine effects, the synthesis of neurosteroids, and steroid hormones in peripheral glands.[32-34] Benzodiazepine receptor ligands can act as agonists, antagonists, or inverse agonists at the $GABA_A$ receptor. In other words, binding of these ligands may increase, decrease, or block the effects of GABA at $GABA_A$ receptors, respectively.

Recent studies now show that the ω_1 and ω_2 receptors actually correspond to the interface of the α subunits and the γ_2 subunit on the $GABA_A$ receptor complex.[35] Specifically, ω_1 receptors correspond to the interface at the α_1 subunit, and ω_2 receptors correspond to the interface at the α_2, α_3, or α_5 subunit on $GABA_A$.[36] This interface is the active binding site for benzodiazepines, which bind at the α subunit. After benzodiazepine binding, a conformational change, mediated through the γ_2 subunit, occurs at the β subunit, enhancing the

binding of GABA at the β subunit. The chloride ion channel opens, hyperpolarizing the cell, and limiting excitatory impulses. Benzodiazepines potentiate GABA effects by increasing the frequency of channel opening (Fig. 35-3). They are positive modulators of the GABA receptor. In the absence of GABA, however, benzodiazepines have no direct effect on $GABA_A$ receptor function; benzodiazepine effects depend on the presynaptic release of GABA.

Although classic benzodiazepines act at all $\alpha\gamma_2$ interfaces of the $GABA_A$ receptor complex, animal studies, which target individual subunit formation through genetic single point mutations and knockouts, have elucidated the important relationship between the phamacologic effects of benzodiazepine agonists and the subunit composition of individual $GABA_A$ receptors.[29,37] For example, $GABA_A$ receptors, which contain α_1 subunits, mediate the sedative and amnestic effects produced by benzodiazepines. The anticonvulsant effects of these drugs are also partially mediated by α_1-containing receptors. Anxiolysis and muscle tone are mediated through α_2-containing $GABA_A$ receptors, which comprise only 15% of all $GABA_A$ receptors, but are particularly dense in the amygdala and the dorsal horn cells of the spinal cord.

$GABA_A$ receptors, which are the active binding sites of benzodiazepines, are extremely heterogeneous receptor complexes. It is this complexity that accounts for the variety of effects of $GABA_A$-related modulators. Classic benzodiazepines act at all $GABA_A$ receptors, accounting for their many side effects. The creation of drugs that act at specific receptor subunits will allow for selective therapeutic effects devoid of the side effects, which are common to the benzodiazepines. For example, zopiclone, zolpidem, alpidem, and zaleplon, nonbenzodiazepine sedatives, preferentially bind to α_1 $GABA_A$ receptors, accounting for their therapeutic efficacy as hypnotics.[29,37] Future research into the development of subtype-selective drugs with specific activity mediated at specific $GABA_A$ receptor subunits is certain to enhance the therapy of many neuropsychiatric disorders, which involve GABA regulation.

Endogenous benzodiazepine-like substances, diazepam-binding inhibitors, have been recently isolated. Although the actual source of diazepam-binding inhibitors is controversial, research into their role in neuroendocrine function,[34] panic disorder,[38] anxiety,[39] memory and learning,[40] and hepatic encephalopathy,[41,42] may further elucidate the normal regulatory functions of GABA.

PHARMACOKINETICS

Although some benzodiazepines form water-soluble salts at acidic pH, at physiologic pH all are moderately to highly lipid-soluble molecules that are rapidly and completely absorbed from the proximal small bowel (see Tables 35-1 and 35-2). Significant differences in lipid solubility affect the rate of gastrointestinal absorption and subsequent distribution. Highly lipophilic benzodiazepines, such as diazepam and flurazepam, are rapidly

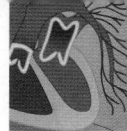

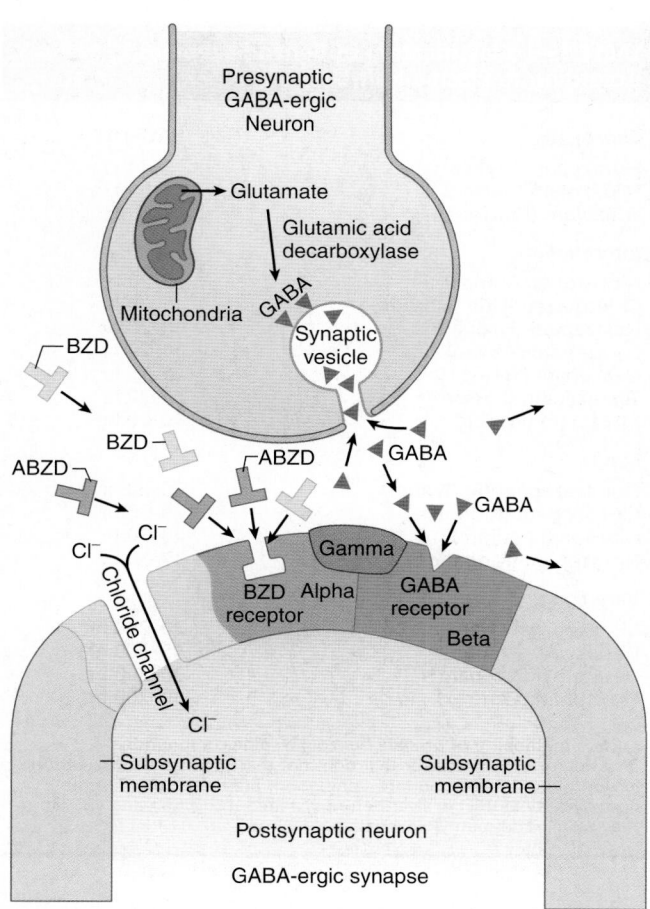

FIGURE 35-3 Benzodiazepine receptors and the GABAergic synapse. Central nervous system neurotransmission occurs via a complex circuitry consisting of multiple connections, pathways, feedback mechanisms, and inhibitory/disinhibitory neurons, all under the control of neurotransmitters and neuroinhibitors. The body's most important neuroinhibitor, γ-aminobutyric acid (GABA), is synthesized in nerve endings of presynaptic GABAergic neurons from glutamate, under the influence of the enzyme glutamic acid decarboxylase. GABA is stored in synaptic vesicles located in presynaptic nerve endings and is released into the synapse to function as a neuroinhibitor. GABA activity is terminated by diffusion out of the synapse or reuptake into presynaptic nerve endings. Specific GABA receptors have been identified on the subsynaptic membrane of postsynaptic neurons. GABA receptors are adjacent to and coupled with chloride ion channels in such a way that activation of a GABA receptor "opens" the associated channel, increasing chloride ion influx. The end result is hyperpolarization of the cell membrane and decreased neuronal excitability. The activity of GABA or its functional relationship to GABA receptors may be related to GABA modulin, an endogenous peptide located in synaptic membranes. The benzodiazepine receptor is located on a subunit of the benzodiazepine-GABA pharmacophore, spatially adjacent to the GABA receptor. Binding of benzodiazepines to the benzodiazepine receptor subunit induces a change in the receptor complex, which facilitates GABA binding to the GABA receptor subunit, increasing the frequency of chloride ion channel opening. Benzodiazepine antagonists competitively block specific benzodiazepine receptor sites and either block the benzodiazepine binding or displace already bound drug, thereby offsetting any benzodiazepine-enhanced GABAergic transmission. GABA, γ-aminobutyric acid; BZD, benzodiazepine; ABZD, benzodiazepine antagonist.

TABLE 35-2 Absorption Rates of Orally Administered Benzodiazepines

	TIME OF PEAK PLASMA CONCENTRATION
Rapid	<1.2 hr
Desmethyldiazepam (from clorazepate [Tranxene])	
Diazepam (Valium)	
Flurazepam (Dalmane)	
Midazolam* (Versed)	
Intermediate	1.2–2.0 hr
Alprazolam (Xanax)	
Chlordiazepoxide (Librium)	
Clonazepam (Klonopin)	
Flunitrazepam (Rohypnol)	
Halazepam (Paxipam)	
Lorazepam (Ativan)	
Triazolam (Halcion)	
Slow	2.0–3.0 hr
Oxazepam (Serax)	
Temazepam (Restoril)	
Ultraslow	>3.0 hr
Desmethyldiazepam (from prazepam [Centrax])	
Diazepam CR (slow release)	

*Oral form midazolam not yet commercially available.

absorbed, and less lipophilic compounds, such as oxazepam and temazepam, are more slowly absorbed.[26,43]

The rate of oral absorption is influenced by other factors, such as the co-ingestion of ethanol[44] (enhanced absorption), or co-ingestion of food or antacids[45] (slowed). Depending on the drug preparation and the presence of co-ingestants, the time from ingestion to appearance of the drug in the systemic circulation is approximately 10 to 20 minutes. In general, the time to maximal serum concentration (T_{max}) is inversely related to the maximal serum concentration (C_{max}) and may be influenced by the aforementioned factors.[46]

Certain benzodiazepines, such as clorazepate, flurazepam, and prazepam, do not reach the systemic circulation in clinically significant amounts. Clorazepate is rapidly decarboxylated in the acidic environment of the stomach to its active metabolite, N-desmethyldiazepam (nordiazepam), which is then absorbed completely. Flurazepam and prazepam undergo first pass metabolism in the liver and reach the systemic circulation only as metabolites.

Benzodiazepine absorption from intramuscular injection is variable. Lorazepam and midazolam are the only benzodiazepines rapidly and completely absorbed after intramuscular administration. Chlordiazepoxide absorption is particularly slow and erratic; plasma concentration may not peak for 6 to 12 hours. Diazepam is inconsistently absorbed after intramuscular administration. Serum levels of diazepam and chlordiazepoxide are more rapidly achieved by the oral route than by intramuscular administration.

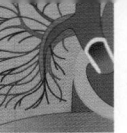

After absorption, benzodiazepines are highly protein bound, ranging from 70% to 99%. Protein binding is greatest with highly lipid-soluble drugs (e.g., diazepam 99% bound) and least with more water-soluble agents (e.g., alprazolam 70% bound). Only unbound drug is available to cross the blood-brain barrier and interact with CNS receptors. Drug concentrations in the cerebrospinal fluid are generally 2% to 4% of plasma levels, roughly equivalent to the concentration of free drug in the plasma. Alterations in protein binding affect the amount of free drug available to the CNS at sites of action, and the subsequent clinical effects.

All benzodiazepines distribute widely and rapidly to highly perfused organs. Their volume of distribution ranges from 0.3 to 5.5 L/kg, and tissue concentrations within the brain, liver, and spleen typically exceed that of the serum. Because penetration into the CNS is rapid, the onset of clinical effects is limited more by the rate of systemic absorption of individual compounds than by their rate of distribution.

After initial distribution within the central compartment, benzodiazepines slowly redistribute to less perfused tissues, such as adipose and muscle. The rate of initial distribution and redistribution, and thus onset and offset of clinical effect, correlates with the individual drug lipophilicity.

Benzodiazepine activity is terminated by at least three mechanisms. Two of these are pharmacokinetic, and the third is a function of alterations of the GABA(A)/benzodiazepine recognition site. The rate of redistribution of drug from the central compartment to the peripheral compartment is the most important determinant of the duration of clinical effect. The second mechanism responsible for the duration of action is hepatic metabolism and renal excretion. The third mechanism is acute tolerance that occurs at the level of the receptor.

The duration of action of benzodiazepines is a function of the CNS elimination half-life, which correlates with drug lipophilicity. During single-dose administration, the most lipophilic benzodiazepines have the shortest duration of action due to their rapid and extensive redistribution. They have the longest calculated plasma half-lives after redistribution because they remain in clinically inactive peripheral storage compartments (fat, muscle) for prolonged periods. In contrast, drugs that are less lipophilic have a longer duration of action, but a shorter plasma half-life due to slower redistribution from the CNS. This is illustrated by comparing the clinical anticonvulsant activity of lorazepam and diazepam. Lorazepam, a drug of relatively low lipophilicity, has more prolonged anticonvulsant activity than the highly lipophilic diazepam. The benzodiazepine midazolam is extremely lipophilic and rapidly metabolized in the liver. It has an extremely rapid onset but short duration of action due to both rapid redistribution and hepatic metabolism. Benzodiazepines may be classified into four different groups based on plasma elimination half-lives of the parent in combination with its active metabolites (see Tables 35-1 and 35-3).

TABLE 35-3 Classification of Benzodiazepines According to Plasma Half-Life

Short	HALF-LIFE
Flurazepam (Dalmane)	1–4 hr
Midazolam (Versed)	2–5 hr
Triazolam (Halcion)	2–6 hr
Intermediate	
Alprazolam (Xanax)	6–20 hr
Chlordiazepoxide (Librium)	5–20 hr
Halazepam (Paxipam)	10–20 hr
Lorazepam (Ativan)	10–20 hr
Oxazepam (Serax)	5–15 hr
Temazepam (Restoril)	5–20 hr
Estazulam (Prosem)	10–20 hr
Long	
Flunitrazepam (Rohypnol)	20–50 hr
Clonazepam (Klonopin)	20–30 hr
Diazepam (Valium)	20–70 hr
Nitrazepam (Mogadon)	17–50 hr
Very Long	
Clorazepate[†] (Tranxene)	30–200 hr
Desalkylflurazepam*	45–300 hr
Desmethyldiazepam*	30–200 hr
Prazepam[†] (Centrax)	30–200 hr

*Active metabolite of primary benzodiazepine compounds.
[†]Prodrug or drug precursor that does not reach the system circulation in clinical significant amounts. Compounds are metabolized in the gastrointestinal tract or liver before systemic absorption and appear in the serum as desmethyldiazepam.

During prolonged administration, the plasma half-life is a more reliable predictor of clinical response (intensity and duration) to the highly lipophilic agents. Repeated doses of lipid-soluble benzodiazepines cause the eventual saturation of peripheral fat stores during redistribution. As they become saturated, the concentration gradient from plasma to peripheral lipid compartment decreases, increasing the drug concentration and duration of action at CNS receptor sites. In addition, the lipid stores act as a depot for the drug and its active metabolites, resulting in prolonged release of drug and persistence of drug effects.[45] Benzodiazepines with longer elimination half-lives have a greater potential for accumulation after multiple doses and are more likely to exhibit prolonged "washout" periods after termination of multiple-dose therapy. In contrast, these agents are less likely to be associated with rebound side effects upon termination of treatment.[46]

Hepatic biotransformation via phase I oxidation or phase II conjugation accounts for virtually all benzodiazepine metabolism and clearance in humans. Oxidative metabolism occurs primarily at the cytochrome families CYP3A, CYP2D, and CYP2C.[47] These drugs undergo aliphatic hydroxylation or N-demethylation to pharmacologically active intermediates, and/or conjugation to inactive glucuronides, sulfates, and acetylated compounds; these inactive compounds are subsequently renally excreted (Fig. 35-4).

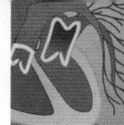

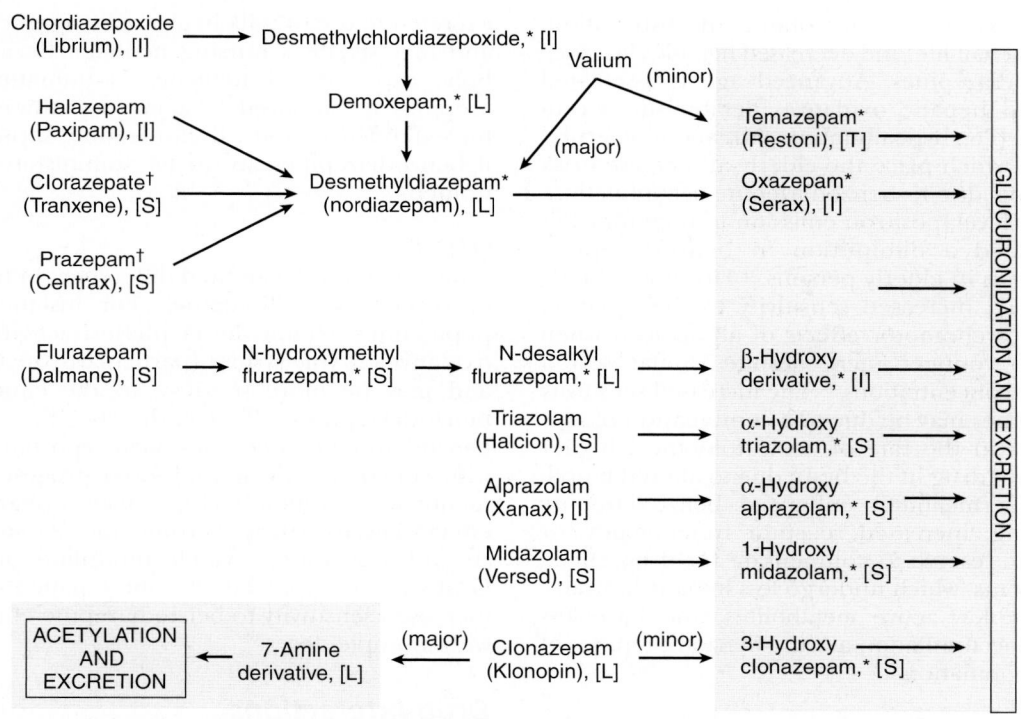

FIGURE 35-4 Major metabolic pathways of benzodiazepines approved for use in the United States. [S], conversion half-life of less than 6 hours; [I], conversion half-life of 6 to 20 hours; [L], conversion half-life of greater than 20 hours; *, active metabolite; †, prodrug or drug precursor, which does not reach the systemic circulation in clinically significant amounts. Shaded areas denote processes that proceed via phase II metabolism.

Several benzodiazepines are biotransformed to active metabolites, which possess half-lives that far exceed those of the parent compound. In such instances, persistent clinical effects are a consequence of the metabolite, its blood concentration, lipophilicity, and affinity for the GABA$_A$/benzodiazepine receptor complex. For example, flurazepam has a plasma half-life of 1 to 4 hours, but its pharmacologically active metabolite, desalkylflurazepam, has a serum half-life of 45 to 300 hours. Due to biotransformation to active metabolites with slow elimination, the duration of action of most benzodiazepines often bears little resemblance to the elimination half-life of the administered (parent) drug. For those agents that are biotransformed to inactive metabolites (e.g., lorazepam and oxazepam) or active metabolites that are subsequently rapidly eliminated (e.g., temazepam and triazolam), the duration of action will be more closely correlated with their clinical duration of action. Elimination of benzodiazepine metabolites usually occurs via renal clearance.

Tolerance can develop rapidly to nearly all of the clinical effects of benzodiazepines, although the effect on anxiolytic properties is limited. Several studies have been performed to evaluate the mechanism of tolerance. Mice made tolerant to lorazepam exhibited decreased benzodiazepine-receptor binding and GABA$_A$ function, consistent with down-regulation of the receptor. Subsequent discontinuation of lorazepam was accompanied by increased motor activity, receptor binding, and function, consistent with up-regulation. Lorazepam-tolerant mice

also had markedly reduced levels of messenger RNA for some subunits of the GABA$_A$/benzodiazepine receptor.[48] Tolerance to chronic lorazepam was attenuated in mice, and the down-regulation of the GABA$_A$ receptor reversed when the benzodiazepine antagonist flumazenil was administered concomitantly with lorazepam.[49] Tolerance is likely due to acute uncoupling of the benzodiazepine effect at the GABA receptor, as well as changes in gene expression for certain subunits of the GABA receptor, particularly the α_1 and γ_2 subunits, in conjunction with up-regulation of genes encoding less common subunits, such as α_4 and α_5.[31,33]

The incidence of tolerance is unclear. In one retrospective study of 191 patients that received long-term benzodiazepine therapy, 92% had not needed to increase their dose of benzodiazepine, despite drug treatment for a mean of 5.6 years.[50] Conversely, the development of tolerance to these medications has limited their long-term utility as sedatives and anticonvulsants. Interventions to prevent or reduce tolerance are under study and consist of intermittent dosing, tapering schedules, use of benzodiazepine antagonists, or coadministration of anticonvulsants.[49]

Special Populations

GERIATRICS

The clinical responses of elderly patients to benzodiazepines are altered as a result of age-related changes in both pharmacokinetics and pharmacodynamics. Aging is

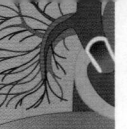

associated with an increased volume of distribution, increased plasma half-life, and decreased hepatic clearance of some benzodiazepines. Advanced age is associated with diminished hepatic oxidative metabolism, serum protein-binding (i.e., hypoalbuminemia), and glomerular filtration, all of which place the elderly at increased risk for complications due to benzodiazepine accumulation. At the receptor level, positron emission tomography has not demonstrated a diminution in benzodiazepine-binding potentials in elderly persons.[51] However, elderly men experienced increased sensitivity to the sedative, hypnotic, and psychomotor effects of alprazolam when compared with younger men, despite similar serum benzodiazepine concentrations.[52] The increased sensitivity to benzodiazepines may be due to a combination of age-related changes in the rate of acute tolerance, higher concentrations of drug in the brain due to altered blood-brain barrier permeability, enhanced benzodiazepine receptor binding, increased receptor functionality, or less homeostatic reserve to compensate for drug effect. Short-acting agents, which undergo less hepatic biotransformation, have few active metabolites, and have less capacity for bioaccumulation are the benzodiazepines of choice in this population.

HEPATIC AND RENAL IMPAIRMENT

Because benzodiazepines are primarily metabolized by the liver, their pharmacokinetics may be altered in patients with cirrhosis.[45,46,53] In general, agents that undergo phase I biotransformation may accumulate in cirrhotic patients due to increased volumes of distribution, decreased protein binding, prolonged half-life, and decreased oxidative clearance.[45] Dose adjustment is usually unnecessary for agents, which are biotransformed by phase II glucuronidation alone. Elimination of benzodiazepine metabolites occurs via renal clearance. Patients with renal insufficiency may be at risk for the accumulation of active metabolites.

PREGNANCY

Benzodiazepines readily cross the placenta and may accumulate in the fetus, with serum concentrations that exceed those achieved in the mother. High doses of benzodiazepines administered during the immediate prepartum period may produce a floppy baby syndrome in newborn infants. This syndrome may be attributed to the persistence of long-acting benzodiazepine metabolites in neonatal serum.[54,55] The incidence may decrease when benzodiazepines, which undergo only phase II metabolism, are administered.[56]

Most benzodiazepines are categorized as class D in pregnancy by the FDA, indicating that these drugs have caused or are expected to cause an increased incidence of human fetal malformations with maternal use. The teratogenic potential of benzodiazepines is unknown, and categorization comes from early human data that are inconsistent.

Fetal benzodiazepine dependence occurs, and subsequent withdrawal may be delayed up to 10 days postpartum due to diminished neonatal benzodiazepine clearance.[57] Benzodiazepines and their metabolites are excreted in breast milk in clinically significant amounts[58] and may sedate a nursing neonate. Because the metabolic capability of neonates is immature,[59] benzodiazepines metabolized by phase I pathways may persist for extended periods. Breast-feeding should be avoided if benzodiazepines are to be administered to lactating women.

OTHER

There are ethnic-associated differences in the metabolism of certain benzodiazepines. For instance, East Asian populations exhibit slower phase I activity of the P-450 oxidative enzyme system (particularly the CYP2C family) and may be more sensitive to the clinical effects of benzodiazepines.[47,60] Gender-specific sensitivity to benzodiazepine effects has been reported in association with concomitantly administered progesterone in post-menopausal women.[61] This is likely a pharmacodynamic effect, because progesterone and its metabolites are steroid hormones, which modulate activity at the GABA(A) receptor. Finally, obese patients may have an increased sensitivity to benzodiazepine effects associated with multiple doses.[62]

Drug Interactions

Benzodiazepine drug interactions can be pharmacodynamic or pharmacokinetic; they may be associated with effects at the $GABA_A$/benzodiazepine recognition site or associated with benzodiazepine absorption and hepatic metabolism.

Benzodiazepines potentiate the CNS-depressant effects of ethanol and numerous other drugs. Many of these interactions occur at the $GABA_A$ receptor, where ethanol, barbiturates, propofol, some general anesthetics, and other sedative-hypnotics (e.g., meprobamate, zaleplon, zolpidem, and zopiclone) also have binding sites and act as positive GABA modulators. Methylxanthines and some antibiotics diminish benzodiazepine-induced sedation.

Since phase I biotransformation is a primary metabolic pathway for many benzodiazepines (e.g., diazepam, alprazolam, and temazepam), drugs that induce or inhibit the function of the P-450 CYP3A4 and CYP2D or 2C enzyme families can enhance or diminish the normal metabolism of benzodiazepines. The result may be shortened elimination half-life and reduced efficacy, or prolonged duration of action and oversedation.[47,63] Phase II conjugation reactions are effected to a lesser degree, inhibited by probenecid and induced by oral contraceptive agents.[47] These alterations in conjugative enzyme function will not produce significant clinical effects as related to benzodiazepines.

Certain drugs also inhibit renal tubular secretion of benzodiazepine metabolites. Probenecid inhibits the tubular secretion of organic bases, and has been shown to decrease the renal clearance of N-desmethyladinazolam, the active metabolite of adinazolam.[64] The coadministration of probenecid with adinazolam was associated with a decrease in psychomotor skill performance in healthy volunteers, and was presumed to be secondary to N-desmethyladinazolam accumulation.

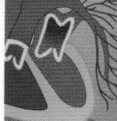

TOXICOLOGY

Clinical Manifestations

ACUTE

The acute clinical manifestations of benzodiazepines are mainly those of CNS depression. Patients with a pure benzodiazepine overdose display mild to moderate sedation, often with dysarthria and ataxia, without serious neurologic, cardiovascular, or respiratory impairment.

CHRONIC

The long-term effects of benzodiazepines on the $GABA_A$ receptor and GABA physiology are not known. Research into the neurochemical effects of chronic benzodiazepine use indicates the possibility of subtle and delayed effects on cognitive function and memory acquisition. The reversibility of these effects is unclear. In one study of long-term benzodiazepine users who were detoxified from benzodiazepines, some cognitive defects persisted for up to 6 months.

Adverse Effects

Therapeutic doses of benzodiazepines cause various degrees of sedation, drowsiness, lightheadedness, lethargy, and lassitude in virtually all patients, especially when therapy is initiated. Dysarthria, ataxia, motor incoordination, impairment of cognition, and amnesia may also occur. Uncommonly, fatigue, headache, blurred vision, vertigo, nausea and vomiting, diarrhea, arthralgias, chest pain, and incontinence have been reported. The frequency and severity of side effects increase with age.

Uncommon side effects of rapid intravenous benzodiazepine administration include respiratory arrest, cardiac arrest, hypotension, and phlebitis at the site of injection. Severe adverse reactions are more common in the elderly, patients with severe cardiopulmonary disease, and those taking cardiorespiratory depressant medications. Other extremely rare side effects reported after benzodiazepine overdose include neuromuscular blockade; hematologic, renal, and hepatic toxicity; acute rhabdomyolysis; anaphylaxis; dermatitis; and acute respiratory distress syndrome. Postoperative exposure to benzodiazepines may increase the risk for delirium in recovering surgical patients.

Long- and short-acting benzodiazepines have different side effect profiles.[65] Long-acting benzodiazepines are associated with residual sedation and daytime drowsiness and may cause greater respiratory depression in patients with pulmonary disease. In addition, long- and intermediate-acting benzodiazepines are considered to have reinforcing properties that may lead to their persistent use and potential for abuse.[65] In comparison, short-acting benzodiazepines (those used as hypnotics) are more commonly associated with daytime anxiety and rebound insomnia upon discontinuation.

The anxiolytic benzodiazepines have been reported to unmask bizarre, uninhibited behavior in some patients, as well as hostility, rage, paranoia, and depression. These reactions occur more frequently in elderly patients or those with overt or latent psychoses and organic brain syndrome. Such disinhibition or dyscontrol reactions are quite rare and usually are related to the patient's preexisting expectations and pretreatment level of aggression and hostility.[66]

Rates of benzodiazepine usage increase with age, and elderly patients thus account for a disproportionately large percentage of benzodiazepine prescriptions. In addition, the elderly are more likely to be long-term users of these drugs. These facts, in combination with age-related differences in benzodiazepine pharmacokinetics and pharmacodynamics, place this population at greater risk for adverse side effects, namely, excess sedation, falls, and cognitive impairment.

Multiple studies demonstrate adverse effects suffered by elderly benzodiazepine users.[67-69] Chronic use and higher-than-recommended dosages are associated with an increased risk for accelerated decline in physical performance in community-dwelling elderly women.[70] In one review of 11 epidemiologic studies, at least a 50% increase in the risk for hip fracture secondary to falls was associated with benzodiazepine use, especially during the initiation of therapy and at higher doses.[71] After adjustment for covariates, the risk for hip fracture was also increased with benzodiazepine dosage regimens greater than or equal to 3 mg/day of diazepam equivalents, during initiation (first 2 weeks) of benzodiazepine therapy, and continuous benzodiazepine use for greater than 1 month.[72] Short-acting benzodiazepines were not found to be safer than long-acting agents in these studies.

Benzodiazepines, particularly long-acting agents, are the drug class most commonly associated with cognitive impairment in elderly people, often producing confusion, forgetfulness, slowing of thought processes, and loss of the ability to care for oneself.[73] In a 4-year longitudinal study, chronic elderly benzodiazepine users had a greater risk for cognitive decline, independent of age, sex, education, ethanol, and other psychotropic drug use.[74] A subgroup of elderly patients with neurodegenerative processes, such as dementia, may be at greater risk for cognitive impairment.[69,75] Although a recent study notes the difficulty of quantifying benzodiazepine exposure in relation to adverse events,[76] and outcomes of cognitive studies depend on the battery of tests applied to the study patients, it is still prudent to be cautious when using benzodiazepines in the elderly. Low doses should be administered for brief periods, and patients should be closely monitored for the development of side effects. If excess sedation, confusion, agitation, or other signs of cognitive impairment develop in an elderly patient taking benzodiazepines, the drug should be discontinued immediately pending further clinical investigation. The benzodiazepine effect may be overlooked by family and physicians and wrongly attributed to senility or a worsening of an underlying disease process.

Benzodiazepine use in pregnancy may be associated with teratogenic effects and fetal loss. A syndrome of benzodiazepine embryopathy was reported in the 1980s, consisting of growth retardation, dysmorphic features, and CNS dysfunction, after oxazepam exposure.[45] These

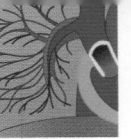

findings may be linked to potential benzodiazepine-induced regulation of GABA$_A$ subunit expression in the embryo. For example, mice, which lack β_3 subunits, have an associated cleft palate. A recent review of the teratogenicity of benzodiazepines concluded that current data are insufficient to make informed decisions regarding benzodiazepine use in pregnancy, but suggest that diazepam and chlordiazepoxide, but not alprazolam, are safe.[77] These drugs, however, are still categorized as pregnancy class D by the FDA.

In an animal model, fetal exposure to benzodiazepines alters function and stressor-induced responsiveness of the GABA$_A$ receptor in the brains of the exposed adult animals. It is hypothesized that the GABA receptor has a developmental role in integrated stress responses, in addition to developmental changes in non-neural systems. Research is ongoing into the effect of prenatal exposure to benzodiazepines on the development of both the neurologic and immunologic systems. Central GABA$_A$ receptors and "peripheral" benzodiazepine receptors may interact with exogenous benzodiazepines in a way that adversely affects fetal development of these systems.

Fetal benzodiazepine dependence and subsequent neonatal withdrawal can occur. The syndrome resembles neonatal narcotic withdrawal; symptoms include hypertonicity, irritability, tremors, hyperreflexia, tachypnea, and weight loss.[57] Benzodiazepine administration to ill neonates may be associated with an increased risk for respiratory depression and hypotension.[78]

Early animal data suggested that benzodiazepine use may influence the risk for selected cancers. However, no association between the use of these drugs and the incidence of cancers, including breast, large bowel, malignant melanoma, lung, endometrium, or ovarian, has been proven.[79,80]

Acute Overdose

Numerous clinical reports support the relatively benign nature and uncomplicated course of benzodiazepine overdose.[44,81,82] In contrast to older sedative-hypnotic drugs, benzodiazepines have a high therapeutic index. Deaths attributable to benzodiazepines taken alone are extremely rare,[1,81,82] and often involve short-acting benzodiazepines.[83] For instance, death has been associated with isolated ingestions of flunitrazepam, flurazepam, nitrazepam, and triazolam.

CNS depression is the hallmark of benzodiazepine overdose. Patients become acutely drowsy, stuporous, and ataxic, or may present in low-grade coma without focal neurologic abnormalities. These patients can generally be aroused from this state with verbal or painful stimulation. In one series of 38 patients with pure benzodiazepine overdose, 16 were awake and none were more symptomatic than grade 0 coma (asleep but arousable).[84] In a series of 93 cases of diazepam overdose, patients required only supportive therapy, and no patient who ingested benzodiazepines alone required hospital admission.[84] Occasionally, patients may manifest mild hypothermia, bradycardia, and hypotension.

Profound and significant coma, hypotension, respiratory depression, or hypothermia is extremely uncommon in oral overdose, unless other drugs have also been ingested. Although prolonged deep coma, cyclic coma, and focal neurologic signs[85] have been reported with benzodiazepine overdose, such clinical scenarios are distinctly unusual. Most acutely poisoned patients become easily arousable or awaken within 12 to 36 hours. The duration of coma, however, may be prolonged in elderly and nonhabituated patients. After recovery of consciousness, it is typical for overdosed patients to feel dizzy, depressed, and apathetic for an extended period of time. Recovery may also be prolonged for those who develop complications (e.g., aspiration pneumonia).

When they do occur, deaths are almost always due to benzodiazepines taken in combination with other drugs. The risk for toxicity is substantially increased when co-ingested with other CNS depressants.[82] In this series, the combination of benzodiazepines and barbiturates was noted to be particularly dangerous, and 50% of these overdose patients required mechanical ventilation. Ethanol, identified as a co-ingestant in 38% of benzodiazepine overdoses,[44] also enhances the CNS toxicity of benzodiazepines.[86] These clinical outcomes are predictable, based on the synergistic effects of these drugs at the GABA$_A$/benzodiazepine receptor complex.

DIAGNOSIS

Laboratory Testing

Qualitative urine screening for the presence of parent benzodiazepines or their metabolites provides rapid, useful information in the evaluation of patients with an unknown cause of CNS depression. Qualitative screening techniques, however, are fallible and should not be used in isolation to make clinical treatment decisions. Most laboratories perform initial screens for benzodiazepines with diagnostic immunoassays, the results of which are confirmed by gas or high-pressure liquid chromatography and/or mass spectrometry. Quantitative plasma measurements are not available in most hospitals, and provide no significant therapeutic direction to the treating physician.[81,84,87,88] Plasma concentrations of benzodiazepines correlate very poorly with the severity of toxic effects (e.g., degree of CNS depression) or mortality.

Various urine immunoassay screens are available and are standardized against the detection of a single benzodiazepine compound, usually oxazepam. Other structurally similar benzodiazepines are subsequently detected through immunologic cross-reactivity with the compound that is used as the standard. The concentration of benzodiazepine metabolites in urine can vary by several orders of magnitude, depending on the ingested drug, drug dose, and time of sample collection relative to dosing. Therefore, the sensitivity for detecting any individual benzodiazepine may vary significantly.

Laboratory detection of benzodiazepines depends on the particular toxicologic screen used. For example, the

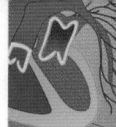

enzyme-multiplied immunoassay technique (EMIT) screen cross-reacts with chlordiazepoxide, clonazepam, demoxepam, desalkylflurazepam, desmethyldiazepam, flurazepam, lorazepam, oxazepam, prazepam, and temazepam.[89] However, several of these compounds are inconsistently detected unless they are present in extremely high concentrations. Enzymatic hydrolysis may improve the yield of EMIT screens.[90] Triazolobenzodiazepine derivatives, such as alprazolam or triazolam,[91] may be particularly difficult to detect in small but clinically significant ingestions because they possess poor immunologic cross-reactivity with oxazepam. The radioimmunoassay screening test, Abuscreen (Roche Diagnostic Systems, Inc., Somerville, NJ), identifies alprazolam, chlordiazepoxide, demoxepam, clorazepate, diazepam, temazepam, desmethyldiazepam, desalkylflurazepam, halazepam, lorazepam, midazolam, and prazepam but does not detect clonazepam or flurazepam.[92]

Various urine screens have been compared in their ability to accurately detect benzodiazepines.[93,94] The metabolites that most commonly produce false-negative results were lorazepam and 7-aminoclonazepam. None of the screens were able to detect α-hydroxytriazolam or α-hydroxyalprazolam. Although some urine screens have sensitivities of 90% to 98%, as compared with gas chromatography/mass spectrophotometry, the range in sensitivities is 80% to 100%.[95] In summary, the cross-reactivity lists quoted by screen manufacturers may be incomplete, and it is important to realize that some commonly used screens may produce negative results despite a clinically significant benzodiazepine ingestion. In addition, positive screens for benzodiazepines may not correlate with clinical toxicity and may reflect the presence of an inactive metabolite (e.g., N-desmethyldiazepam) that cross-reacts with the screen.

False-positive benzodiazepine screens have been reported in the urine of patients using the nonsteroidal anti-inflammatory agent oxaprozin.[96,97] Its urinary metabolite is probably responsible for these results. Similar false-positive results have been reported for etodolac, naproxen sodium, fenoprofen calcium, and tolmetin sodium.[94] False-positive screens have also been reported in the presence of sertraline.[98,99] In this era of drug screening for legal and management decisions in the workplace, it is important to be aware of the limitations of some screening technologies.

Although some research toxicology laboratories have the capacity to measure quantitative benzodiazepine levels, their measurement is not useful in the management of acute overdose. Therapeutic diazepam levels range between 0.5 and 2.0 μg/mL, while levels of 5 to 20 μg/mL are generally regarded as toxic. Yet, many patients with "toxic" levels may exhibit no or only mild clinical toxicity. Quantitative measurement of serum benzodiazepines and their metabolites may be useful for differentiating acute from chronic ingestions or for medicolegal or forensic cases.

Other sources of tissue used for benzodiazepine detection include hair[100,101] and oral fluids.[95] Both sources may yield false-negative results and lack the sensitivity to be used as screening tests. Forensic studies have also examined benzodiazepine detection in postmortem samples of bile and bone, with fairly good yield.[102,103]

Other Diagnostic Testing

Other diagnostic testing should be performed as necessary to identify or exclude coexisting conditions, which may also require treatment. Such testing often includes, but is not limited to, computed tomography of the head, laboratory testing for ethanol and other toxicants for which qualitative or quantitative testing may be beneficial, measurements of serum electrolytes and glucose, as well as electroencephalography for subclinical status epilepticus. Arterial blood gas analysis and capnography may be performed to assess the adequacy of respiration in those patients with CNS depression.

Differential Diagnosis

Patients with a pure benzodiazepine overdose display mild to moderate sedation, often with dysarthria and ataxia, without serious focal neurologic, cardiovascular, or respiratory derangement. There are no specific diagnostic clinical features unique to benzodiazepine overdose. Toxicity from benzodiazepines produces signs and symptoms that are similar to many toxicologic and nontoxicologic entities. The CNS depressant effects may be similar to effects produced by alcohols, antiepileptics, antipsychotics, barbiturates, carbon monoxide and other gases, lithium, opiates, other sedative-hypnotics, and skeletal muscle relaxants. CNS infection, traumatic head injury, cerebrovascular accidents, and metabolic disturbances should be considered and ruled out with appropriate testing.

MANAGEMENT

Supportive Measures and Laboratory Testing

Treatment for benzodiazepine overdose is primarily supportive. Patients with significant CNS or respiratory depression should have their airways protected, breathing assisted, and cardiovascular support provided supportive as necessary. All patients should have continuous cardiac monitoring, an intravenous line established, and electrocardiography performed. Supplemental oxygen, continuous pulse oximetry, and parenteral thiamine, dextrose (or rapid fingerstick glucose determination), and naloxone should be considered for patients with altered mental status or seizures. Semi-comatose patients should be placed in the left lateral, head-down position to minimize the risk for aspiration. Frequent vital sign and neurologic evaluations are necessary. Routine laboratory analysis should include a complete blood count and measurement of electrolytes, blood urea nitrogen, creatinine, glucose concentrations, and pregnancy testing for women of childbearing age. Serum acetaminophen and

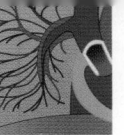
salicylate concentrations should be performed for all intentional overdose patients. Co-ingestion of other toxic substances, concurrent trauma, or other underlying medical conditions significantly alter the diagnostic and therapeutic approach. Urine screening may confirm the presence of benzodiazepines or their metabolites. Negative screening does not rule out the presence of certain benzodiazepines, as mentioned above.

Decontamination and Enhanced Elimination Techniques

Single-dose administration of activated charcoal (1 g/kg orally or by nasogastric tube) is the preferred method of gastrointestinal decontamination and may be beneficial if administered within 1 hour of drug ingestion. Orogastric lavage is not recommended for isolated benzodiazepine overdose since the risk for death is very low in this patient population. The clinical benefit of activated charcoal administration beyond 1 hour following benzodiazepine ingestion is likely low.

Antidotes

Flumazenil (Romazicon [Roche Pharmaceuticals of Hoffman-La Roche, Inc., Nutley, NJ]) was synthesized in 1979 and is the benzodiazepine antagonist available in the United States. It is a 1,4-imidazobenzodiazepine, a derivative of the antibiotic anthramycin,[104] which contains a diazepine ring that binds at the benzodiazepine receptor complex (Fig. 35-5).

Flumazenil is administered intravenously. It has also been studied as a potential reversal agent after subcutaneous,[105] sublingual, intramuscular, rectal,[106] submucosal,[107] intranasal,[108] and endotracheal administration.[109] Orally administered flumazenil has been studied in the treatment of epilepsy[110-112] and hepatic encephalopathy.[113]

Flumazenil has a volume of distribution of 1.1 L/kg, is 40% to 50% protein bound, and is highly lipid soluble.[104] It has a distribution half-life of 5 minutes and rapidly crosses the blood-brain barrier to reverse benzodiazepine-induced sedation within 1 to 2 minutes after intravenous administration. The mean half-life of flumazenil is 57 minutes; therefore, resedation may occur within 1 to 2 hours after administration, requiring subsequent doses. Flumazenil is hepatically metabolized by conjugation, and the metabolite is renally excreted. In oral dosage form, flumazenil is rapidly absorbed but has low bioavailability secondary to significant first pass metabolism in the liver.

The dose of flumazenil is 0.2 IV per dose, to a total of 3 mg, in adults and 0.01 mg/kg IV per dose, to a total of

0.05 mg/kg or 1 mg, in children. A continuous infusion of flumasenil has been used in both children[114] and adults.[115] The adult dose of flumazenil is 0.2 mg intravenously over 30 seconds, followed by 0.3 and 0.5 mg at 1-minute intervals to a maximum dose of 3 mg. Alternatively, flumazenil may be administered in 0.2-mg aliquots intravenously every 30 to 60 seconds until a dose of 3 mg is reached. Flumazenil rapidly reverses the sedative, anxiolytic, anticonvulsant, ataxic, anesthetic, and muscle relaxant effects of benzodiazepines in animals and humans.[116] It restores an electroencephalogram to the baseline waking state in patients who have been administered benzodiazepines,[117,118] and is an effective antidote for benzodiazepine overdose.[119]

Patients with benzodiazepine-induced coma respond dramatically within 1 to 5 minutes after flumazenil administration.[120,121] A number of benzodiazepine effects have been reversed by flumazenil, which include respiratory depression,[122] midazolam-induced laryngospasm,[123] first-degree atrioventricular block in alprazolam overdose,[124] lorazepam-induced acute delirium,[125] and midazolam-associated myoclonic movements in full-term newborns.[126]

Incomplete or partial antagonism of benzodiazepine-induced sedation has been reported[121] but may be secondary to co-ingestion of other sedative-hypnotics or concomitant medical causes of depressed consciousness. In addition, residual memory deficits may persist. Finally, orally administered flumazenil may only partially reverse the effects of benzodiazepines.[127]

Flumazenil acts as an antagonist, competitively removing both positive and negative GABA modulators from the benzodiazepine recognition site. It binds at the same $\alpha\gamma_2$ interface on the GABA(A) complex where benzodiazepines bind and interacts with amino acid residues that are not associated with benzodiazepine binding. At high doses, it is reported to have agonist-like anticonvulsant activity. However, it is also reported to have weak inverse agonist properties.[128] Based on its mechanism of action, flumazenil has been used to reverse sedation in cases of hepatic encephalopathy.[129] Anecdotal reports also describe partial reversal of ethanol- and carbamazepine-induced CNS depression.

When administered to normal volunteers, flumazenil has produced dizziness, facial erythema, anxiety, and headache. Symptoms are often mild and disappear within several minutes. Flumazenil has been shown to further increase intracranial pressure when administered to head-injured patients with elevated intracranial pressure. Reports of ventricular dysrhythmias have been associated with its administration.[114] Additionally, flumazenil has been noted to precipitate seizures in epileptic patients who take benzodiazepines for seizure control and in patients who have co-ingested drugs that lower the seizure threshold.[130,131] Older case series demonstrated an increased risk for seizures after flumazenil administration to patients who had ingested cyclic antidepressants. A more recent study, however, did not show such serious complications occurring in this setting. The lack of seizure precipitation in this latter study may have been due to slow incremental flumazenil dosing or smaller total doses of the antagonist.[132] Flumazenil has

FIGURE 35-5 The chemical structure of flumazenil (Ro 15-1788), a specific benzodiazepine antagonist.

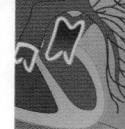

also precipitated acute benzodiazepine withdrawal and seizures in dependent persons. For these reasons, the role of flumazenil in patients who present with suspected benzodiazepine overdose and CNS depression or undifferentiated drug coma is controversial.

Flumazenil has been used in the pediatric population for both reversal of sedation and for empiric treatment in the unconscious patient. Pediatric case reports of flumazenil-associated seizures have also been reported,[133] one in the setting of iatrogenic apnea induced by diazepam and treated with flumazenil after an infant presented with febrile seizures.[134] The Flumazenil Pediatric Study Group suggests flumazenil dosing of 0.01 mg/kg infusion (max 0.2 mg) each minute to a maximum of 0.05 mg/kg (or 1 mg) for reversal of sedation.[135]

As mentioned, flumazenil has the potential to precipitate withdrawal symptoms in benzodiazepine-dependent individuals.[136] In animal studies, the severity of withdrawal depends on the specific benzodiazepine used, the dose and duration of treatment, and the dose of flumazenil administered.[137] Abrupt withdrawal symptoms are usually more severe when induced by flumazenil administration.

Although the potential toxicity of benzodiazepines is relatively low and aggressive therapy for pure overdose is rarely required, flumazenil offers several important potential uses in clinical medicine. Its use can help to confirm a suspected diagnosis of benzodiazepine overdose and obviate the need for other diagnostic testing (e.g., cranial computed tomography and lumbar puncture). Flumazenil may reverse overdose of zolpidem and zopiclone, and may be indicated for benzodiazepine-associated respiratory depression, particularly if intubation and mechanical ventilation would otherwise be indicated. Flumazenil may be useful postoperatively to reverse the effects of preoperative sedation or to reverse iatrogenic overdose when benzodiazepines are used for conscious sedation. Flumazenil may be used in select circumstances with experienced practitioners in these settings. The use of flumazenil for undifferentiated coma, even when administered slowly, is dangerous and not recommended. Despite its potential usefulness, flumazenil should not become "routine" antidote in the treatment of coma secondary to overdose.

Elimination

There are no practical ways to significantly enhance the elimination of benzodiazepines. Forced diuresis is of no value. Extracorporeal removal techniques are not recommended as part of treatment for benzodiazepine poisoning since these agents have large volumes of distribution and high plasma protein binding.

Disposition

Most patients with isolated benzodiazepine overdose develop minimal to mild toxicity and are medically safe after an observation period of 4 to 6 hours in the emergency department. Patients who are able to safely ambulate after observation may be discharged after appropriate psychiatric consultation. Patients who develop more significant CNS depression or have continued evidence of mild toxicity at 6 hours should be admitted to a monitored bed for continued observation.

REFERENCES

1. Greenblatt DJ, Shader RI: Drug therapy. Benzodiazepines. N Engl J Med 1974;291:1011–1015.
2. Johnson MR, Lydiard RB, Ballenger JC: Panic disorder. Pathophysiology and drug treatment. Drugs 1995;49:328–344.
3. Blanco C, Schneier FR, Schmidt A, et al: Pharmacological treatment of social anxiety disorder: a meta-analysis. Depress Anxiety 2003;18:29–40.
4. Practice guidelines for the treatment of patients with bipolar disorder. Am J Psychiatry 1994;151:1–36.
5. Ungvari GS, Leung CM, Wong MK, Lau J: Benzodiazepines in the treatment of catatonic syndrome. Acta Psychiatr Scand 1994;89:285–288.
6. Rosenfeld MJ, Friedman JH: Catatonia responsive to lorazepam: a case report. Mov Disord 1999;14:161–162.
7. Ungvari GS, Kau LS, Wai-Kwong T, Shing NF: The pharmacological treatment of catatonia: an overview. Eur Arch Psychiatry Clin Neurosci 2001;251(Suppl 1):31–34.
8. Pommepuy N, Januel D: Catatonia: resurgence of a concept. A review of the international literature. Encephale 2002;28(6 Pt 1):481–492.
9. Rosebush PI, Mazurek MF: Do benzodiazepines modify the incidence of neuroleptic-induced dystonia? [Letter]. Am J Psychiatry 1993;150:528.
10. Redfern P, Minors D, Waterhouse J: Circadian rhythms, jet lag, and chronobiotics: an overview. Chronobiol Int 1994;11:253–265.
11. Buxton OM, Copinschi G, Van Onderbergen A, et al: A benzodiazepine hypnotic facilitates adaptation of circadian rhythms and sleep-wake homeostasis to an eight hour delay shift simulating westward jet lag. Sleep 2000;23:915–927.
12. Dellemijn PLI, Fields HL: Do benzodiazepines have a role in chronic pain management? Pain 1994;57:137–152.
13. Greenberg DB: Strategic use of benzodiazepines in cancer patients. Oncology 1991;5:83–88.
14. Livingston MG: Benzodiazepine dependence. Br J Hosp Med 1994;51:281–286.
15. Woods JH, Winger G: Current benzodiazepine issues. Psychopharmacology 1995;118:107–115.
16. Olfson M, Marcus SC, Weissman MM, Jensen P: National trends in the use of psychotropic medications by children. J Am Acad Child Adolesc Psychiatry 2002;41:514–521.
17. Tu K, Mamdani MM, Hux JE, Tu J: Progressive trends in the prevalence of benzodiazepine prescribing in older people in Ontario, Canada. J Am Geriatr Soc 2001;49:1341–1345.
18. Darke S: Benzodiazepine use among injecting drug users: problems and implications. Addiction 1994;89:379–382.
19. Gelkopf M, Bleich A, Hayward R, et al: Characteristics of benzodiazepine abuse in methadone maintenance treatment patients: a 1-year prospective study in an Israeli clinic. Drug Alcohol Depend 1999;55:6368.
20. Wagner AK, Soumerai SB, Zhang F, et al: Effects of state surveillance on new post-hospitalization benzodiazepine use. Int J Qual Health Care 2003;15:423–431.
21. Schwartz HI, Blank K: Regulation of benzodiazepine prescribing practices: clinical implications. Gen Hosp Psychiatry 1991;13:219–224.
22. Schwartz HI: Negative clinical consequences of triplicate prescription regulation of benzodiazepines. NY State J Med 1991;91(Suppl 11):9–12.
23. McNutt LA, Coles FB, McAuliffe T, et al: Impact of regulation on benzodiazepine prescribing to a low income elderly population, New York State. J Clin Epidemiol 1994;47:613–625.
24. Weintraub M, Singh S, Byrne L, et al: Consequences of the 1989 New York State triplicate benzodiazepine prescription regulations. JAMA 1991;266:2392–2397.

25. Linden M, Gothe H: Benzodiazepine substitution in medical practice. Analysis of pharmacoepidemiologic data based on expert interviews. Pharmacopsychiatry 1993;26:107–113.

26. Charney DS, Mihic SJ, Harris RA: Hypnotics and sedatives. In Hardman JG, Limbrid LE, Gilman AG (eds): Goodman & Gilman's the Pharmacological Basis of Therapeutics, 10th ed. New York, McGraw-Hill, 2001, pp 399–427.

27. Goodchild CS: GABA receptors and benzodiazepines. Br J Anaesth 1993;71:127–133.

28. Chebib M: The "ABC" of GABA receptors: a brief review. Clin Exp Pharm Phys 1999;26:937–940.

29. Enz R: GABAC receptors: a molecular view. Biol Chem 2001;382:1111–1122.

30. Möhler H, Fritshy JM, Rudolph U: A new benzodiazepine pharmacology. Pharm Exp Ther 2002;300:2–8.

31. Doble A: New insights into the mechanism of action of hypnotics. J Psychopharm 1999;13(Suppl 1):11–20.

32. Whitehouse BJ: Benzodiazepines and steroidogenesis. J Endocrinol 1992;134:1–3.

33. Sanger DJ, Benavides J, Perrault G, et al: BZ-omega receptor subtypes—activity of various benzodiazepines may be due to different activity at various subtypes. Neurosci Biobehav Rev 1994;18:355–372.

34. Arvat E, Giordano R, Grottoli S, Ghigo E: Benzodiazepines and anterior pituitary function. J Endocrinol Invest 2002; 25:735–747.

35. Griebel G, Perrault G, Letang V, et al: New evidence that the pharmacological effects of benzodiazepine receptor ligands can be associated with activities at different BZ(?) receptor subtypes. Psychopharmacology 1999;146:205–213.

36. Sanger DJ, Griebel G, Perrault G, et al: Discriminative stimulus effects of drugs acting at GABAA receptors; differential profiles and receptor selectivity. Pharm Biochem Behav 1999; 64:269–273.

37. Rudolph U, Crestani F, Möhler H: GABAA receptor subtypes: dissecting their pharmacological functions. Trends Pharm Sci 2001;22:188–194.

38. Nutt DJ, Smith CF, Bennett R, Jackson HC: Investigations on the "set-point" theory of benzodiazepine receptor function. Adv Biochem Psychopharmacol 1992;47:419–429.

39. Malizia AL, Coupland NJ, Nutt DJ: Benzodiazepine receptor function in anxiety disorders. Adv Biochem Psychopharmacol 1995;48:115–133.

40. Izquierdo I, Medina JH: GABAa receptor modulation of memory: the role of endogenous benzodiazepines. Trends Pharmacol Sci 1991;12:260–265.

41. Rothstein JD: Benzodiazepine-receptor ligands and hepatic encephalopathy: a causal relationship? Hepatology 1994;19:248–250.

42. Mullen KD: Benzodiazepine compounds and hepatic encephalopathy. N Engl J Med 1991;325:509–511.

43. Baselt RC: Disposition of Toxic Drugs and Chemicals in Man, 7th ed. Foster City, CA, Biomedical Publications, 2004.

44. Finkle BS, McCloskey KL, Goodman LS: Diazepam and drug-associated deaths: a survey in the United States and Canada. JAMA 1979;242:429–434.

45. Bailey L, Ward M, Musa MN: Clinical pharmacokinetics of benzodiazepines. J Clin Pharmacol 1994;34:804–811.

46. Greenblatt DJ: Benzodiazepine hypnotics: sorting the pharmacokinetic facts. J Clin Psychiatry 1991;52(Suppl 9):4–10.

47. Obach RS: Drug-drug interactions: an important negative attribute in drugs. Drugs Today 2003;39:301–338.

48. Miller LG: Chronic benzodiazepine administration: from the patient to the gene. J Clin Pharmacol 1991;31:492–495.

49. Miller LG, Koff JM: Interaction of central and peripheral benzodiazepine sites in benzodiazepine tolerance and discontinuation. Prog Neuropsychopharmacol Biol Psychiatry 1994;18:847–857.

50. Logan KE, Lawrie SM: Long term use of hypnotics and anxiolytics [Letter]. BMJ 1994;309:27–28.

51. Suhara T, Inoue O, Kobayashi K, et al: No age-related changes in human benzodiazepine receptor binding measured by PET with [11C]Ro 15-4513. Neurosci Lett 1993;159:207–210.

52. Bertz RJ, Kroboth PD, Kroboth FJ, et al: Alprazolam in young and elderly men: sensitivity and tolerance to psychomotor,

53. Kroboth PD, Maxwell RA, Fleishaker JC, et al: Comparison of adinazolam pharmacokinetics and effects in healthy and cirrhotic subjects. J Clin Pharmacol 1991;31:580–586.

54. Spreight ANP: Floppy-infant syndrome and maternal diazepam and/or nitrazepam. Lancet 1977;2:878.

55. Whitelaw AGL, Cummings AJ, McFadyen IR: Effect of maternal lorazepam on the neonate. BMJ 1981;282:1106–1108.

56. Drury KAD: Floppy-infant syndrome: is oxazepam the answer? Lancet 1977;2:1126.

57. Smith DE, Wesson DR: Benzodiazepine dependency syndromes. In Smith DE, Wesson DR (eds): The Benzodiazepines: Current Standards for Medical Practice. Lancaster, UK, MTP Press, 1985.

58. Cole AP, Hailey DM: Diazepam and active metabolites in breast milk and their transfer to the neonate. Arch Dis Child 1975;50:741–742.

59. Kaplan SA: Pharmacokinetics of the benzodiazepines. In Priest RG, Vianna Filho U, Amrein R, Skreta M (eds): Benzodiazepines Today and Tomorrow. Lancaster, UK, MTP Press, 1980.

60. Ajir K, Smith M, Keh-Ming L, et al: The pharmacokinetics and pharmacodynamics of adinazolam: multi-ethnic comparisons. Psychopharmacology 1997;129:265–270.

61. McAuley JW, Reynolds IJ, Kroboth FJ, et al: Orally administered progesterone enhances sensitivity to triazolam in postmenopausal women. J Clin Psychopharmacol 1995;15:3–11.

62. Derry CL, Kroboth PD, Pittenger AL, et al: Pharmacokinetics and pharmacodynamics of triazolam after two intermittent doses in obese and normal-weight men. J Clin Psychopharmacol 1995;15:197–205.

63. Dresser GK, Bailey DG: A basic conceptual and practical overview of interactions with highly prescribed drugs. Can J Clin Pharmacol 2002;9:191–198.

64. Golden PL, Warner PE, Fleishaker JC, et al: Effects of probenecid on the pharmacokinetics and pharmacodynamics of adinazolam in humans. Clin Pharmacol Ther 1994;56:133–141.

65. Mendelson WB: Clinical distinctions between long-acting and short-acting benzodiazepines. J Clin Psychiatry 1992;53(Suppl): 4–7.

66. Rothschild AJ: Disinhibition, amnestic reactions, and other adverse reactions secondary to triazolam: a review of the literature. J Clin Psychiatry 1992;53(Suppl):69–79.

67. Dealberto MJ, Mcavay GJ, Seenan T, Berkman L: Psychotropic drug use and cognitive decline among older men and women. Int J Geriatr Psychiatry 1997;12:567–574.

68. Paterniti S, Dufouil C, Bisserbe JC, Alperovitch A: Anxiety, depression, psychotropic drug use and cognitive impairment. Psychol Med 1999;29:421–428.

69. Pat McAndrews M, Weiss RT, Sandor P, et al: Cognitive effects of long-term benzodiazepine use in older adults. Hum Psychopharmacol 2003;18:51–57.

70. Gray SL, Penninx BW, Blough DK, et al: Benzodiazepine use and physical performance in community-dwelling older women. J Am Geriatr Soc 2003;51:1563–1570.

71. Cumming RG, LeCouteur DG: Benzodiazepines and risk of hip fractures in older people: a review of the evidence. CNS Drugs 2003;17:825–837.

72. Wang PS, Bohn RL, Glynn RJ, et al: Hazardous benzodiazepine regimens in the elderly: effects of half-life, dosage, and duration on risk of hip fracture. Am J Psychiatry 2001;158:892–898.

73. Larson EB, Kukill WA, Buchner D, Reifler BV: Adverse drug reactions associated with cognitive impairment in elderly persons. Ann Intern Med 1987;107:169–173.

74. Paterniti S, Dufouil C, Alperovitch A: Long-term benzodiazepine use and cognitive decline in the elderly: the Epidemiology of Vascular Aging Study. J Clin Psychopharmacol 2002;22:285–293.

75. Allard J, Artero S, Ritchie K: Consumption of psychotropic medication in the elderly: a re-evaluation of its effect on cognitive performance. Int J Geriatr Psychiatry 2003;18:874–878.

76. Ray WA, Thapa PB, Gideon P: Misclassification of current benzodiazepine exposure by use of a single baseline measurement and its effects upon studies of injuries. Pharmacoepidemiol Drug Saf 2002;11:663–669.

77. Iqbal MM, Sobhan T, Ryals T: Effects of commonly used benzodiazepines on the fetus, the neonate, and the nursing infant. Psychiatr Serv 2002;53:39–49.

78. Ng E, Klinger G, Shah V, Taddio A: Safety of benzodiazepines in newborns. Ann Pharmacother 2002;36:1150–1155.

79. Rosenberg L, Palmer JR, Zauber AG, et al: Relation of benzodiazepine use to the risk of selected cancers: breast, large bowel, malignant melanoma, lung, endometrium, ovary, non-Hodgkin's lymphoma, testis, Hodgkin's disease, thyroid, and liver. Am J Epidemiol 1995;141:1153–1160.

80. Dublin S, Rossing MA, Heckbert SR, et al: Risk of epithelial ovarian cancer in relation to use of antidepressants, benzodiazepines, and other centrally acting medications. Cancer Causes Control 2002;13:35–45.

81. Busto U, Kaplan HL, Sellers EM: Benzodiazepine-associated emergencies in Toronto. Am J Psychiatry 1980;137:224–227.

82. Greenblatt DJ, Allen MD, Noel BJ, et al: Acute overdosage with benzodiazepine derivatives. Clin Pharmacol Ther 1977;21:497–514.

83. Martin CD, Chan SC: Distribution of temazepam in body fluids and tissues in lethal overdose. J Anal Toxicol 1986;10:77–78.

84. Jatlow P, Dobular K, Bailey D: Serum diazepam concentrations in overdose: their significance. Am J Clin Pathol 1979;72:571–579.

85. Deleu D, Keyser J: Flunitrazepam intoxication simulating a structural brainstem lesion. J Neurol Neurosurg Psychiatry 1987;50:236–237.

86. Sellers EM, Busto U: Benzodiazepines and ethanol: assessment of the effects and consequences of psychotropic drug interactions. J Clin Pharmacol 1982;22:249–262.

87. Allen-Divoll M, Greenblatt DJ, Lacasse Y: Pharmacokinetic study of lorazepam overdosage. Am J Psychiatry 1980;137:1414–1415.

88. Bailey DN: Blood concentrations and clinical findings following overdose of chlordiazepoxide alone and chlordiazepoxide plus ethanol. Clin Toxicol 1984;22:433–446.

89. Package insert, EMIT. Urine immunoassay. Sylva Company, Palo Alto, CA, August 1985.

90. Borrey D, Meyer E, Duchateau L, et al: Enzymatic hydrolysis improves the sensitivity of emit screening for urinary benzodiazepines. Clin Chem 2002;48:2047–2049.

91. Fraser AD: Urinary screening for alprazolam, triazolam and their metabolites with the EMIT®d.a.u.TM benzodiazepine metabolite assay. J Anal Toxicol 1987;11:263–266.

92. Package insert, Abuscreen-Radioimmunoassay for benzodiazepines. Roche Diagnostic Systems, Nutley, NJ, July 1987.

93. Fitzgerald RL, Rexin DA, Herold DA: Detecting benzodiazepines: immunoassays compared with negative chemical ionization gas chromatography/mass spectrometry. Clin Chem 1994;40:373–380.

94. Peace MR, Poklis JL, Tarnai LD, Poklis A: An evaluation of the OnTrak Testcup-er® on-site urine drug-testing device for drugs commonly encountered from emergency departments. J Anal Toxicol 2002;26:500–503.

95. Gronholm M, Lillsunde P: A comparison between on-site immunoassay drug-testing devices and laboratory results. Forensic Sci Int 2002;121:37–46.

96. Pulini M: False-positive benzodiazepine urine test due to oxaprozin [Letter]. JAMA 1995;273:1905–1906.

97. Fraser AD, Howell P: Oxaprozin cross-reactivity in three commercial immunoassays for benzodiazepines in urine. J Anal Toxicol 1998;22:50–54.

98. Gear JL: False-positive toxicology screens. J Am Acad Child Adolesc Psychiatry 1996;35:1571–1572.

99. Fitzgerald RL, Herold DA: Improved CEDIA benzodiazepine assay eliminates sertraline crossreactivity. J Anal Toxicol 1997;21:32–35.

100. Sramek JJ, Baumgartner WA, Ahrens TN, et al: Detection of benzodiazepines in human hair by radioimmunoassay. Ann Pharmacother 1992;26:469–472.

101. Yegles M, Mersch F, Wennig R: Detection of benzodiazepines and other psychotropic drugs in human hair by GC/MS. Forensic Sci Int 1997;84:211–218.

102. Gorczynski LY, Melbye FJ: Detection of benzodiazepines in different tissue, including bone, using a quantitative ELISA assay. J Forensic Sci 2001;46:916–918.

103. Vanbinst R, Koenig J, Di Fazio V, Hassoun A: Bile analysis of drugs in postmortem cases. Forensic Sci Int 2002;128:35–40.

104. Longmire AW, Seger DL: Topics in clinical pharmacology: flumazenil, a benzodiazepine antagonist. Am J Med Sci 1993;306:49–52.

105. Luger TJ, Morawetz RF, Mitterschiffthaler G: Additional subcutaneous administration of flumazenil does not shorten recovery time after midazolam. Br J Anaesth 1990;64:53–58.

106. Heniff MS, Moore GP, Trout A, et al: Comparison of routes of flumazenil administration to reverse midazolam-induced respiratory depression in a canine model. Acad Emerg Med 1997;4:1115–1118.

107. Oliver FM, Sweatdown TW, Unkel JH, et al: Comparative pharmacokinetics of submucosal vs. intravenous flumazenil (Romazicon) in an animal model. Pediatr Dent 2000;22:489–493.

108. Scheepers LD, Montgomery CJ, Kinaham AM, et al: Plasma concentration of flumazenil following intranasal administration in children. Can J Anaesth 2000;47:120–124.

109. Weiner AL, McKay CA Jr: Endotracheal administration of flumazenil. Am J Emerg Med 1998;16:436–437.

110. Scollo-Lavizzari G: The clinical anti-convulsant effects of flumazenil, a benzodiazepine antagonist. Eur J Anaesthesiol Suppl 1988;2:129–138.

111. Sharief MK, Sander JW, Shorvon SD: The effect of oral flumazenil on interictal epileptic activity: results of a double-blind, placebo-controlled study. Epilepsy Res 1993;15:53–60.

112. Reisner-Keller LA, Pham Z: Oral flumazenil in the treatment of epilepsy. Ann Pharmacother 1995;29:530–531.

113. Blei AT: Diagnosis and treatment of hepatic encephalopathy. Baillieres Clin Gastroenterol 2000;14:959–974.

114. Sugarman JM, Paul RI: Flumazenil: a review. Pediatr Emerg Care 1994;10:37–43.

115. Guglielminotti J, Maury E, Alzieu M, et al: Prolonged sedation requiring mechanical ventilation and continuous flumazenil infusion after routine doses of clonazepam for alcohol withdrawal syndrome. Intensive Care Med 1999;25:1435–1436.

116. Darragh A, Lambe R, Scully M, et al: Investigation in man of the efficacy of a benzodiazepine antagonist, Ro15-1788. Lancet 1981;2:8–10.

117. Laurian S, Gailard M, Le PK, et al: Effects of a benzodiazepine antagonist on the diazepam-induced electrical brain activity modifications. Neuropsychobiology 1984;11:55–58.

118. Wojna V, Guerrero L, Guzman J, Cotto M: Effect of flumazenil on electroencephalographic patterns induced by midazolam. P R Health Sci J 2000;19:353–356.

119. Hofer P, Scollo-Lavizzari G: Benzodiazepine antagonist Ro 15-1788 in self-poisoning: diagnostic and therapeutic use. Arch Intern Med 1985;145:663–664.

120. Scollo-Lavizzari G: First clinical investigation of the benzodiazepine antagonist Ro 15-1788 in comatose patients. Eur Neurol 1983;22:7–11.

121. Chern CH, Chern TL, Hu SC, et al: Complete and partial response to flumazenil in patients with suspected benzodiazepine overdose [Letter]. Am J Emerg Med 1995;13:372–375.

122. Gross JB, Blouin RT, Zandsberg S, et al: Effect of flumazenil on ventilatory drive during sedation with midazolam and alfentanil. Anesthesiology 1996;85:713–720.

123. Davis DP, Hamilton RS, Webster TH: Reversal of midazolam-induced laryngospasm with flumazenil. Ann Emerg Med 1998;32:263–265.

124. Mullins ME: First degree atrio-ventricular block in alprazolam overdose reversed by flumazenil. J Pharm Pharmacol 1999;51:367–370.

125. Olshaker JS, Flanigan J: Flumazenil reversal of lorazepam-induced acute delirium. J Emerg Med 2003;24:181–183.

126. Zaw W, Knoppert DC, da Silva O: Flumazenil's reversal of myoclonic-like movements associated with midazolam in term newborns. Pharmacotherapy 2001;21:642–646.

127. Girdler NM, Lyne JP, Wallace R, et al: A randomised, controlled trial of cognitive and psychomotor recovery from midazolam sedation following reversal with oral flumazenil. Anaesthesia 2002;57:868–876.

128. Philip BK: Drug reversal: benzodiazepine receptors and antagonists. J Clin Anesth 1993;5(Suppl 1):46–51.

129. Hoffman EJ, Warren EW: Flumazenil: a benzodiazepine antagonist. Clin Pharm 1993;12:641–656.

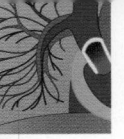

130. Haverkos GP, DiSalvo RP, Imhoff TE: Fatal seizures after flumazenil administration in a patient with mixed overdose. Ann Pharmacother 1994;28:1347–1349.

131. Spivey WH: Flumazenil and seizures: analysis of 43 cases. Clin Ther 1992;14:292–305.

132. Weinbroum A, Rudick V, Sorkine P, et al: Use of flumazenil in the treatment of drug overdose: a double-blind and open clinical study in 110 patients. Crit Care Med 1995;24:199–206.

133. McDuffee AT, Tobias JD: Seizure after flumazenil administration in a pediatric patient. Pediatr Emerg Care 1995;11:186–187.

134. Davis CO, Wax PM: Flumazenil associated seizure in an 11-month-old child. J Emerg Med 1996;14:331–333.

135. Shannon M, Albers G, Burkhart K, et al: Safety and efficacy of flumazenil in the reversal of benzodiazepine-induced conscious sedation. The Flumazenil Pediatric Study Group. Curr Opin Pediatr 1996;8:243–247.

136. Cumin R, Bonetti EP, Scherchlicht R, et al: Use of the specific benzodiazepine antagonist, Ro 15-1788, in studies of physiological dependence on benzodiazepines. Experientia 1982;38:833–834.

137. Investigational drug brochure, intravenous flumazenil (Ro 15-1788). Hoffmann-La Roche, Nutley, NJ, March 1987.

36 *Barbiturates*

RICHARD LYNTON, MD

At a Glance...

- The barbiturates are a family of sedative-hypnotics. Their clinical use has fallen dramatically over the past 3 decades as benzodiazepines and other safer sedative-hypnotics have been created.

- Barbiturates are associated with significant morbidity and mortality, the result of their ability to produce profound central nervous system and myocardial depression.

- There are nine barbiturates in clinical use, each having a unique pharmacokinetic profile.

- Barbiturate use is associated with a number of significant drug interactions.

- Tolerance and dependence with barbiturates can lead to significant addiction as well as an abstinence syndrome (withdrawal) with acute discontinuation.

- Barbiturate overdose produces a syndrome of central nervous system depression; severe intoxication may lead to hemodynamic instability. Other manifestations, for example, skin changes ("barb blisters"), are less common.

- Treatment of barbiturate overdose begins with supportive care that includes airway and blood pressure support

- The elimination of phenobarbital can be enhanced through three measures: multiple-dose activated charcoal, urine alkalinization, and hemodialysis. Hemodialysis and other extracorporeal drug removal techniques are generally reserved for patients with severe phenobarbital toxicity (serum concentration > 100 µg/L). These elimination techniques are not effective with other barbiturates.

Over the past 30 years, barbiturates as a class have slowly been replaced by safer sedative-hypnotics such as benzodiazepines. Their role to toxicologists as drugs in overdose settings are therefore significantly less, as shown in cumulative data from poison centers in North America (Fig. 36-1). Barbiturate overdose now results in less morbidity and mortality when compared with more commonly used benzodiazepines. However, barbiturates continue to be important in sedation, anesthesia, and seizure control, and as an adjunct in headache treatment. With such widespread use, the barbiturates continue to have overdose potential.

HISTORY

In 1864, research assistant Adolph von Baeyer in Ghent, Belgium, produced barbituric acid, a cyclic diureide, from the condensation of malonic acid and urea.[1] Barbituric acid itself does not possess any central nervous system (CNS) properties. The hypnotic and CNS-depressant effects of its congeners were discovered after various substitutions were made to it.

In 1903, Fisher and von Mehring introduced diethylbarbituric acid or barbital as the first barbiturate to enter medicine, under the trade name Veronal. In 1912, phenobarbital, under the trade name Luminal, was independently and simultaneously brought to medicine by Loewe, Juliusburger, and Impens.[1-3]

In the mid-20th century, barbiturates became the most popular class of sedative-hypnotics. During this time they also became popular substances of abuse, along with other sedative-hypnotics of that era; collectively these agents were known as "downers." Sold on the street with such names as "red devils," barbiturates were taken either alone or with ethanol to produce a pleasurable feeling of intoxication. The death of actress Marilyn Monroe was attributed to barbiturates; an empty bottle of Nembutal was found at her side. As safer sedative-hypnotics for those with insomnia or other sleep disturbances were created, use of barbiturates declined quickly; they are rarely used for these purposes any longer. Finally, among advocates of euthanasia and suicide, barbiturates remain one of the most commonly recommended drugs.

PHARMACOLOGY AND PHARMACOKINETICS

Table 36-1 shows the general formula of barbituric acid and where the substitutions occur that give each chemical its characteristics. Most barbiturates carry oxygen at carbon position 2 on the ring and hence are called oxybarbiturates. Barbiturates where sulfur replaces oxygen are called thiobarbiturates; of these, only thiopental is currently in use in the United States.

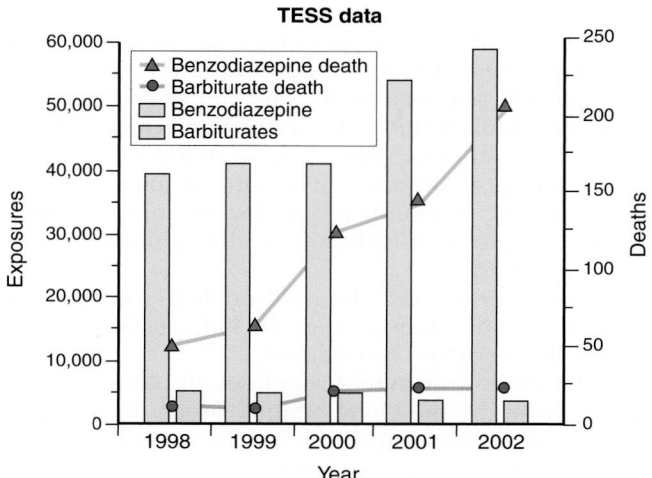

FIGURE 36-1 Toxic Exposure Surveillance System (TESS) Data. (Data from references 65 through 69.)

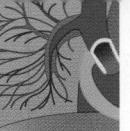
TABLE 36-1 Barbiturate Classification

GENERAL FORMULA AND SUBSTITUTED DERIVATIVES

BARBITURATE	TRADE NAME	pKa	DURATION OF ACTION (hr)	PLASMA HALF-LIFE (hr)	R_{5a}	R_{5b}	R_3
Short-Acting Barbiturates							
ULTRASHORT							
Thiopental	Pentothal	7.6	0.3	6–46	Ethyl	1-Methylbutyl	H
Methohexital	Brevital	7.9	0.3		Allyl	1-Methyl-2-pentynyl	CH_3
SHORT							
Pentobarbital	Nembutal	7.96	3.0	21–42	Ethyl	1-Methylbutyl	H
Secobarbital	Seconal	7.90	3.0	20–28	Allyl	1-Methylbutyl	H
INTERMEDIATE							
Amobarbital	Amytal	7.75	3–6	15–40	Ethyl	Isopentyl	H
Butabarbital	Butisol	7.74	3–6	34–42	Ethyl	sec-Butyl	H
Long-Acting Barbiturates							
Barbital	Veronal	7.74	6–12	48	Ethyl	Ethyl	H
Mephobarbital	Mebaral	8.5	6–12	48–52	Ethyl	Phenyl	CH_3
Phenobarbital	Luminal	7.24	6–12	48–144	Ethyl	Phenyl	H
Primidone	Mysoline	—	6–12	6–22	Ethyl	Phenyl	H

*S= Substitution for O= in thiopental, H_2 substitution for O= in primidone.

Lipid solubility is important in barbiturate pharmacokinetics. In general, increased lipid solubility decreases drug latency of onset and duration of action, and increases metabolic degradation rate and hypnotic potency. Methylation of one or both of the nitrogens increases drug affinity for lipids and hence decreases duration of action; methohexital is an example of such a drug. Other methylated barbiturates are demethylated in the body, producing long-acting compounds; mephobarbital conversion to phenobarbital is such an example. Sulfur in general makes thiobarbiturates more lipid soluble than oxybarbiturates; this explains thiopental's rapid onset and short duration. The anticonvulsant activity of barbiturates is produced by discrete moieties such as a phenyl group at carbon 5 or alkyl groups on both nitrogen atoms.[1,4]

Barbiturates are well absorbed orally as sodium salts. Other routes of administration include rectal (particularly in children) and intravenous.

Barbiturates distribute throughout all body compartments, including the blood-brain barrier, and can cross the placenta, depending on their lipid solubility, protein binding, and extent of ionization.

Barbiturates are metabolized by either oxidation at carbon 5, n-dealkylation, cleavage of the barbituric acid ring, or desulfuration as in the case of thiobarbiturates. Of these, oxidation is the most important, yielding polar compounds that appear in urine as free compounds or glucoronide conjugates. Barbital, because of its low lipid solubility, is one of the few barbiturates that rely almost exclusively on renal elimination for removal of drug from the body.[1]

Primidone is unique in that it is oxidized to phenobarbital and phenylethylmalonamide, the latter having no anticonvulsant activity.[5] In neonates the half-life of phenobarbital is very long (45 to 409 hours) but decreases with age. Primidone conversion to its active metabolites generally does not occurs with neonates.[6]

THERAPEUTIC USES OF BARBITURATES

Table 36-2 displays some of the currently used barbiturates and their indications. Barbiturates continue to play an important role in seizure treatment. Phenobarbital is used as maintenance therapy for patients with seizure disorders. It is useful for both generalized tonic-clonic seizures and simple partial seizures. Several, including phenobarbital and pentobarbital, are useful for treating status epilepticus in the intensive care unit

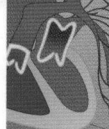

TABLE 36-2 Common Barbiturates and Their Uses

BARBITURATE	SCHEDULE	INDICATION	PREPARATIONS
Thiopental	III	Anesthetic Pediatric sedation ICP management Status epilepticus	250, 400, and 500 mg intectable 1, 2.5, 5 g injectable
Methohexital	IV	Anesthetic	500 mg, 2.5 g, 5 g injectable
Secobarbital	II	Insomnia Status epilepticus	100 mg capsule
Amobarbital	II	Insomnia Narcoanalysis Schizophrenia aid	500 mg injectable 50 mg capsules
Butabarbital	II (secobarbital/phenobarbital combination) III	Sedation, anxiety	30 mg/5 mL elixir 30 and 50 mg tablets
Mephobarbital	IV	Sedation Seizure prophylaxis	32, 50 and 100 mg tablets
Pentobarbital	II III (suppositories)	Insomnia Status epilepticus Barbiturate withdrawal Coma induction	18.2 mg/5 mL elixir 50, 100 mg capsules 50 mg/mL injectable 30, 60, 120, 200 mg suppositories
Phenobarbital	IV	Seizure prophylaxis Barbiturate withdrawal Sedation, anxiety	20 mg/5 mL elixir 15, 16, 30, 32, 60 65, and 100 mg tablets 30, 60, 65, and 130 mg/mL
Primidone		Psychomotor seizure prophylaxis Refractory tonic-clonic seizures	

ICP, intracranial pressure.
Adapted from McEvoy G (ed): AHFS Drug Information 2004. Bethesda, MD, American Society of Health-System Pharmacists, 2004.

where a "barbiturate coma" can be employed in attempts to treat refractory seizures. Pentobarbital as a second-tier agent for the treatment of refractory intracranial hypertension is also commonly used.[7,8] However, a recent Cochrane review found no evidence of improved outcome when barbiturates were used to treat increased intracranial pressure in severely head-injured patients.[9]

Several over-the-counter (OTC) and prescription medications contain barbiturates (e.g., butalbital in combination with acetaminophen, codeine, aspirin, or caffeine) that are used to treat migraine headaches. Barbiturates are also used to treat insomnia and anxiety states; as hypnotics, they are also used to provide general anesthesia as in the case of thiopental and methohexital.

Less well known uses for barbiturates include primidone for the treatment of essential hand tremor[10] and phenobarbital for cyclic vomiting,[11] to prevent and treat hyperbilirubinemia in neonates,[12] or as an intervention for chronic anovulation.[13] There is anecdotal evidence that pentobarbital may be useful for treating γ-hydroxybutyrate (GHB) and γ-butyrolactone withdrawal.[14,15]

Phenobarbital, thiopental, and methohexital have all been useful for sedation and immobilization in young children and can be given by different routes. Barbiturate use is contraindicated in patients with porphyrias.[16]

TOLERANCE, ABUSE, AND DEPENDENCE

The abuse potential of barbiturates results from pharmacologic characteristics such as rapid onset and lipid solubility that facilitates entry across the blood-brain barrier. Barbiturates bind to γ-aminobutyric acid A [GABA$_A$] through an ionotropic or ligand gated mechanism that mediates fast synaptic transmission, causing a conformational change in the GABA$_A$ channel and an influx of chloride that goes on to activate proteins essential in producing CNS-depressant effects.[17] In the presence of a depressant such as a barbiturate, stimulatory effects will increase neurologically to keep the body in homeostasis. Over time, if that drug becomes unavailable due to abrupt cessation in use, unfavorable neuroexcitation symptoms predominate, such as tremors, anxiety, insomnia, tachycardia, hypertension, and even seizures. These symptoms usually resolve once the drug is reintroduced, creating an environment for dependence potential.

Tolerance also manifests because of pharmacokinetic and pharmocodynamic properties of barbiturates. Because they are microsomal inducers, enhanced metabolism and resulting decreased drug at the site of action can produce tolerance within days. A reduced response in the face of unchanged or higher drug concentration through cellular adaptive changes can develop over weeks to months.[18]

Patients who use medications with butalbital for treatment of migraines are particularly at risk for abuse. Care should be taken when treating these patients and in consideration of withdrawal from the medication. There is anecdotal evidence that withdrawal seizures, personality changes, and psychotic behavior can occur.[19] A syndrome of a rebound headache commonly occurs in these patients, which worsens as the dose of butalbital is increased to prevent headache induction. This syndrome has been treated with a long-acting barbiturate such

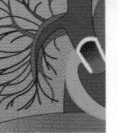

as phenobarbital. Patients generally require inpatient monitoring until they are symptom free.[20,21] There is an ongoing debate whether butalbital should be removed from the U.S. formulary, given its relative lack of therapeutic value.[22,23]

DRUG INTERACTIONS AND ADVERSE DRUG REACTIONS

One of the potential common drug interactions with barbiturates occurs when they are given in conjunction with other sedative-hypnotics. Benzodiazepines, alcohol, anesthetics such as propofol and etomidate, glutethimide, and zolpidem, to name a few, all can have a synergistic effect with serious consequences if dosage adjustments are not made.

Certain herbs used in conjunction with phenobarbital appear to lower seizure threshold. These include thujone-containing herbs such as wormwood and sage, and gamolenic acid–containing herbs such as evening primrose oil and borage.[24] Table 36-3 lists some important drug-herb interactions.

Anticonvulsant hypersensitivity syndrome (AHS) is a rare life-threatening adverse drug reaction seen with phenobarbital and primidone use. The syndrome usually occurs 1 to 8 weeks after initiation of the drug and may present with fever, cervical adenopathy, pharyngitis, skin findings ranging from skin eruption to Stevens-Johnson syndrome, and systemic injury. There is anecdotal evidence suggesting that severe cases of AHS may respond to steroids and immunoglobulin therapy.[25,26] Other findings seen with barbiturate hypersensitivity include urticaria, erythema multiforme, leukocytoclastic vasculitis, bullous eruption, and fixed drug eruptions.[27] At therapeutic doses, barbiturates have also been implicated in toxic epidermal necrolysis, and when abused by injection through skin-popping, tender erythematous plaques can lead to deep ulcers caused by the alkalinity of barbiturates.[28]

Tubular interstitial nephritis has been seen with phenobarbital therapy.[29] Barbiturates are known to cause the syndrome of inappropriate antidiuretic hormone as well.[30]

Barbiturates have been implicated in cytochrome P-450 interactions. Phenobarbital is known to be a potent inducer of CYP1A2, 2A6, 2C8, 2C9, 2C19, and 3A4. Phenobarbital is also a known substrate for CYP2E1; it may be a substrate for CYP2C9 and 2C19 as well. Vulnerable populations such as children, pregnant women, the elderly, and patients with genetic polymorphisms can be adversely affected. Care must also be taken when using phenobarbital as an anticonvulsant in combination with other anticonvulsants.[31] Phenobarbital increases oral contraceptive, warfarin, theophylline, and corticosteroid metabolism. Valproate is known to increase serum phenobarbital concentrations by inhibiting p-hydroxylation and n-glucosidation, significantly reducing its clearance.[32]

Primidone and phenobarbital are known to cause hypocalcemia; however, primidone has been shown to shorten the QT interval.[33] Thiopental has been implicated in treatment-resistant hypokalemia, with severe rebound hyperkalemia occurring in patients treated with barbiturate coma for traumatic brain injury and subarachnoid hemorrhage.[34]

There are also data implicating them in gingival hyperplasia[35] and various embryonic malformations in mothers receiving long-standing therapy for epilepsy[36]; this may result from folate antagonism.[37] Adverse drug reactions can occur in infants whose mothers are breast-feeding while taking phenobarbital or primidone. Although no clear consensus exists for recommendations to this specific subpopulation of anticonvulsant users, lactation should be regarded as potentially unsafe, and such mothers should observe infants for sedation or poor suckling.[38] To those who must be maintained on antiseizure medication such as phenobarbital, monthly levels are recommended.[39]

Primidone has been implicated in the development of rare cases of hyperammonemia.[40] Another rare reported effect includes shoulder-hand syndrome.[41,42]

Phenobarbital and primidone have also been implicated in the development of bone disorders. Patients

TABLE 36-3 Common Herbs and Their Potential Barbiturate Interactions		
HERB	**USE**	**EFFECT ON BARBITURATE**
Kava	Relaxation beverage Uterine relaxation	Synergistic CNS depression in animal studies
Valerian	Anxiety, insomnia	Increased CNS depression
St. John's Wort	Depression	Decreased efficacy of barbiturates
Cayenne	Food additive Local irritant (mace)	Increased or decreased effect of barbiturates
Passion flower	Nervous restlessness, insomnia	Increased CNS depression
Tylophora indica	Treat asthma	Increased sedation
Eucalyptus	Rubefacient URI treatment	Decreased sedative and depressant effects
Catnip	Treat muscle spasms, asthma, newborn colic, sedative	Increased CNS depression and psychomotor retardation
Calamus	Sedative, pain relief, vasodilator	Increased sedation, potentiates the hypnotic effect of barbiturates

CNS, central nervous system; URI, upper respiratory infection.
Adapted from Thomson MICROMEDEX: MICROMEDEX Healthcare Series, I. Greenwood Village, CO, Thomson MICROMEDEX, 2007.

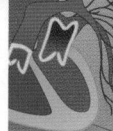

taking these medications chronically demonstrate a drop in bone mineral density. Although low 25-hydroxyvitamin levels have been noted, the exact etiology of osteopenia is unclear. At-risk patients include postmenopausal women, older men, children, and institutionalized patients.[43,44]

CLINICAL PRESENTATION OF BARBITURATE OVERDOSE

Barbiturates are sedatives and as such their physiologic effects are depressive. The differential diagnosis of barbiturate overdose includes other drugs and toxins that produce CNS and cardiovascular depression, such as other sedative-hypnotics, toxic alcohols, cellular asphyxiants, and other psychotropic agents. Medical conditions such as hypoglycemia must always be ruled out in any patient presenting with an altered level of consciousness.

Manifestations of acute barbiturate toxicity can be divided into (1) mild intoxication (victims are somnolent but arousable with slurred speech, unsteady gait, and nystagmus); (2) moderate intoxication (victims have depressed level of consciousness, decreased deep tendon reflexes, and slowed respirations), and (3) severe intoxication (victims are unresponsive to painful stimuli; respiratory, cardiovascular, and neurologic collapse occur).[45]

Four grades of coma from barbiturate overdose are shown in Table 36-4.[46]

Cardiovascular effects most commonly include hypotension, but cardiovascular collapse and cardiac arrest are also possible. In severe overdoses, respiratory depression and apnea may occur. Hypothermia is commonly seen after barbiturate overdose.[47-49] Along with clonidine, guanfacine, GHB and its congenors, and narcotics, barbiturates are among the few drugs associated with significant hypothermia. Barbiturate overdose victims can also present with renal failure due to acute tubular necrosis. Several case reports describe massive crystalluria from primidone overdose[50,51]; however, this has also been seen during maintenance therapy.[52]

TABLE 36-4	Stages of Coma in Barbiturate Overdose
GRADE	**FEATURES**
I	Patient is comatose, the patient withdraws from painful stimuli, and the reflexes are intact.
II	Patient is comatose and fails to respond to painful stimuli, but the reflexes are intact and the vital signs are stable.
III	Patient is comatose and fails to respond to painful stimuli, deep tendon reflexes are absent, but vital signs are stable.
IV	Patient is comatose and fails to respond to painful stimuli, deep tendon reflexes are absent, and vital signs are unstable, with respiratory and cardiovascular depression.

Muscle necrosis and calcification associated with acute renal failure have also been described.[53]

Barbiturate blisters, also known as coma blisters, although not specific for barbiturate overdose, have been seen. They are noted in patients profoundly poisoned with associated neurologic sequale such as loss of consciousness, hence the latter name. They typically appear as blanchable erythematous patches at pressure points of normal skin within 24 hours of coma. A biopsy of the lesion shows intraepidermal or subepidermal blisters with characteristic necrosis of sweat glands. Over the next 2 to 3 days these patches become blisters or erosions, but they usually heal spontaneously over 1 to 2 weeks[28] (Fig. 36-2).

EVALUATION AND MANAGEMENT

As with most drug overdoses, the mainstay of treatment and good outcome is attention to supportive care principles. Since respiratory and CNS depression are the most common findings, attention to the airway and prevention of hypoxia are of the utmost importance.

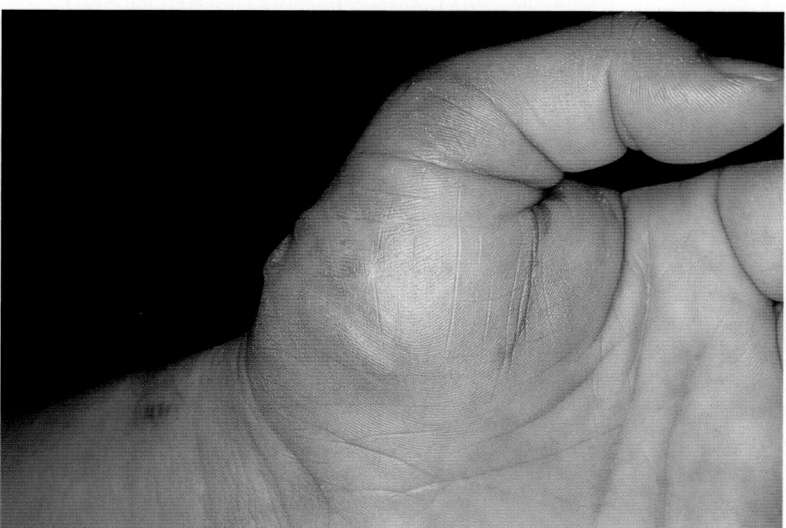

FIGURE 36-2 Coma blisters. (From Bolognia J, Jorizzo JL, Rapini RP [eds]: Dermatology, Vol 1. St. Louis, Mosby, 2003.)

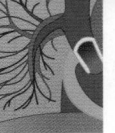

Given the risk for cardiovascular compromise and hypothermia, attention should be directed to vital signs as soon as possible. Also, ruling out hypoglycemia is essential; missing this diagnosis can have grave consequences.

Activated charcoal should be given in a dose of 50 to 60 g (1 g/kg in children). For patients who have a compromised airway, endotracheal intubation is advised prior to giving charcoal. With very large overdoses, antecedent gastric lavage may be considered; however, it should be performed cautiously, given the morbidity associated with this procedure.

Laboratory evaluation should include basic electrolytes and glucose. Screening assays employing semi-quantitative immunoassays of serum and urine are readily available. Serum barbiturate levels can be useful in gauging the clinical course or therapy. In patients who have taken primidone, it is important to measure serum concentrations of phenobarbital, its active metabolite.

The therapeutic range for phenobarbital is generally considered 15 to 40 µg/mL. Toxic effects from phenobarbital can be seen at 50 µg/mL.[54] Parenthetically, cross-reaction among various barbiturates and nonbarbiturates have been reported, requiring special consideration of a false-positive result.[55,56]

Urine alkalinization is of theoretical value in the treatment of phenobarbital overdose but not overdose of other barbiturates. According to the theory of ion trapping, phenobarbital, as a weak acid, will be poorly reabsorbed by the renal tubules if it can be ionized in the milieu of an alkaline urine. The administration of sodium bicarbonate is therefore typically recommended to produce such an alkaline environment. However, having a pKa of 7.4, phenobarbital is difficult to ionize without producing profound changes in urine pH; such alkalinization is rarely achieved in clinical practice without the unwanted effects of metabolic alkalosis or hypernatremia. Given the risks versus benefits, routine urinary alkalinization in barbiturate overdose is no longer recommended.[57]

Multiple-dose activated charcoal (MDAC) has been shown to be more effective in decreasing phenobarbital half-life, increasing its total body clearance in adults and neonates.[57-60] Working by the principle of "gastrointestinal dialysis," MDAC reduces the elimination half-life of phenobarbital by more than 50%; this effect occurs even when the drug has been administered intravenously. However, while MDAC greatly accelerates phenobarbital elimination, its clinical value in the treatment of phenobarbital overdose has been questioned. In a seminal study by Pond and colleagues, MDAC, while greatly reducing the elimination half-life of phenobarbital in a cohort of severely poisoned patients, was ineffective in reducing length of intensive care unit stay and other measures of therapeutic benefit.[61] In a more recent study of 30 patients equally divided into three groups who received MDAC only, urine alkalinization alone, or both, clinical parameters, including the duration of assisted ventilation, intubation, and coma, were all appreciably reduced the greatest in the group that only received MDAC.[62]

Extracorporeal removal by hemodialysis or hemoperfusion is also effective in removing the barbiturates, although they are reserved for the most severe cases. Hemoperfusion is thought to be more effective in barbiturate clearance; however, it has a high rate of adverse effects, is less available than hemodialysis, and, in the era of the high-flux hemodialysis apparatus, does not produce substantially greater clearance rates.[63] As a result, hemodialysis has become the extracorporeal treatment of choice for severe phenobarbital overdose. It is important to note that while phenobarbital is readily removed by hemodialysis, other barbiturates are not. Exchange transfusion has been reported to be useful in an underweight newborn with phenobarbital intoxication.[64]

Indications for hemodialysis after phenobarbital have not been clearly established. Prevailing recommendations call for the procedure in all patients with serum phenobarbital concentrations of 100 µg/mL or greater. This recommendation is based on the clinical observation that as serum phenobarbital concentrations reach and exceed this range, victims are more likely to develop signs of life-threatening intoxication, including severe hypotension and, in the face of fluid support, pulmonary edema. Unfortunately, victims with serum phenobarbital concentrations in this range are often too hypotensive to become ideal hemodialysis candidates. Given the ease and efficacy of hemodialysis in patients with severe barbiturate overdose, its early use should always be considered.

All patients with a barbiturate overdose will need to be admitted. Disposition will depend on clinical affects. Patients with severe mental status depression will need intensive care unit admission, possible intubation with mechanical ventilation, and close monitoring. Less poisoned patients must also be watched closely, in an inpatient setting. In all intentional overdose patients, disposition should include a psychiatric evaluation.

REFERENCES

1. Goodman L, Gilman AG (eds): The Pharmacological Basis of Therapeutics, 5th ed. New York, Macmillan, 1975.
2. Ball C, Westhorpe R: The history of intravenous anaesthesia: the barbiturates. Part 1. Anaesth Intensive Care 2001;29(2):97.
3. Ball C, Westhorpe R: The history of intravenous anaesthesia: the barbiturates. Part 2. Anaesth Intensive Care 2001;29(3):219.
4. Hardman J, Limbird LE (eds): Goodman & Gilman's The Pharmacological Basis of Therapeutics, 10th ed. New York, McGraw-Hill, 2001.
5. Baselt R: Disposition of Toxic Drugs and Chemicals in Man, 6th ed. Foster City, CA, Biomedical Publications, 2002.
6. Battino D, Estienne M, Avanzini G: Clinical pharmacokinetics of antiepileptic drugs in paediatric patients. Part I: Phenobarbital, primidone, valproic acid, ethosuximide and mesuximide. Clin Pharmacokinet 1995;29(4):257–286.
7. Censullo JL, Sebastian S: Pentobarbital sodium coma for refractory intracranial hypertension. J Neurosci Nurs 2003;35(5):252–262.
8. Claassen J: Treatment of refractory status epilepticus with pentobarbital, propofol or midazolam: a systematic review. Epilepsia 2002;43(2):146–153.
9. Roberts I: Barbiturates for acute traumatic brain injury. Cochrane Database Syst Rev 2000(2):CD000033.
10. Chen JJ, Swope DM: Essential tremor: diagnosis and treatment. Pharmacotherapy 2003;23(9):1105–1122.

11. Gokhale R, Huttenlocher PR, Brady L, Kirschner BS: Use of barbiturates in the treatment of cyclic vomiting during childhood. J Pediatr Gastroenterol Nutr 1997;25(1):64–67.

12. Dennery PA: Pharmacological interventions for the treatment of neonatal jaundice. Semin Neonatol 2002;7(2):111–119.

13. Gocze PM, Szabo I, Porpaczy Z, Freeman DA: Barbiturates inhibit progesterone synthesis in cultured Leydig tumor cells and human granulosa cells. Gynecol Endocrinol 1999;13(5):305–310.

14. Sivilotti ML, Burns MJ, Aaron CK, Greenberg MJ: Pentobarbital for severe gamma-butyrolactone withdrawal. Ann Emerg Med 2001;38(6):660–665.

15. Rosenberg MH, Deerfield LJ, Baruch EM: Two cases of severe gamma-hydroxybutyrate withdrawal delirium on a psychiatric unit: recommendations for management. Am J Drug Alcohol Abuse 2003;29(2):487–496.

16. Krauss B, Green SM: Sedation and analgesia for procedures in children. N Engl J Med 2000;342(13):938–945.

17. Cami J, Farre M: Drug addiction. N Engl J Med 2003;349(10): 975–986.

18. Silberstein SD, McCrory DC: Butalbital in the treatment of headache: history, pharmacology, and efficacy. Headache 2001;41(10):953–967.

19. Raja M, Altavista MC, Azzoni A, Albanese A: Severe barbiturate withdrawal syndrome in migrainous patients. Headache 1996; 36(2):119–121.

20. Loder E, Biondi D: Oral phenobarbital loading: a safe and effective method of withdrawing patients with headache from butalbital compounds. Headache 2003;43(8):904–909.

21. Sands GH: A protocol for butalbital, aspirin and caffeine (BAC) detoxification in headache patients. Headache 1990;30(8): 491–496.

22. Young WB, Siow HC: Should butalbital-containing analgesics be banned? Yes. Curr Pain Headache Rep 2002;6(2):151–155.

23. Solomon S: Butalbital-containing agents: should they be banned? No. Curr Pain Headache Rep 2002;6(2):147–150.

24. Miller LG: Herbal medicinals: selected clinical considerations focusing on known or potential drug-herb interactions. Arch Intern Med 1998;158(20):2200–2211.

25. Mostella J, Pieroni R, Jones R, Finch CK: Anticonvulsant hypersensitivity syndrome: treatment with corticosteroids and intravenous immunoglobulin. South Med J 2004;97(3):319–321.

26. Bessmertny O, Pham T: Antiepileptic hypersensitivity syndrome: clinicians beware and be aware. Curr Allergy Asthma Rep 2002;2(1):34–39.

27. McKenna JK, Leiferman KM: Dermatologic drug reactions. Immunol Allergy Clin North Am 2004;24:399–423.

28. Bolognia J, Jorizzo JL, Rapini RP (eds): Dermatology, 1st ed, Vol 1. St. Louis, CV Mosby, 2003.

29. Sawaishi Y, Komatsu K, Takeda O, et al: A case of tubulo-interstitial nephritis with exfoliative dermatitis and hepatitis due to phenobarbital hypersensitivity. Eur J Pediatr 1992;151(1):69–72.

30. Asconape JJ: Some common issues in the use of antiepileptic drugs. Semin Neurol 2002;22(1):27–39.

31. Patsalos PN, Froscher W, Pisani F, van Rijn CM : The importance of drug interactions in epilepsy therapy. Epilepsia 2002;43(4): 365–385.

32. Yukawa E: Investigation of phenobarbital-carbamazepine-valproic acid interactions using population pharmacokinetic analysis for optimisation of antiepileptic drug therapy: an overview. Drug Metab Drug Interact 2000;16(2):86–98.

33. Loukeris K, Mauri D, Pazarlis P: QT length and heart function in primidone hypocalcaemia. Acta Cardiol 2002;57(5):367–369.

34. Cairns CJ, Thomas B, Fletcher S, et al: Life-threatening hyper-kalaemia following therapeutic barbiturate coma. Intensive Care Med 2002;28(9):1357–1360.

35. Sinha S, Kamath V, Arunodaya GR, Taly AB: Phenobarbitone induced gingival hyperplasia. J Neurol Neurosurg Psychiatry 2002;73(5):601.

36. Holmes LB, Harvey EA, Coull BA, et al: The teratogenicity of anticonvulsant drugs. N Engl J Med 2001;344(15):1132–1138.

37. Hernandez-Diaz S, Werler MM, Walker AM, Mitchell AA: Folic acid antagonists during pregnancy and the risk of birth defects. N Engl J Med 2000;343(22):1608–1614.

38. Hagg S, Spigset O: Anticonvulsant use during lactation. Drug Saf 2000;22(6):425–440.

39. Pennell PB: Antiepileptic drug pharmacokinetics during pregnancy and lactation. Neurology 2003;61(6 Suppl 2):35–42.

40. Katano H, Fukushima T, Karasawa K, et al: Primidone-induced hyperammonemic encephalopathy in a patient with cerebral astrocytoma. J Clin Neurosci 2002;9(1):79–81.

41. Rovetta G, Baratto L, Farinelli G, Monteforte P: Three-month follow-up of shoulder-hand syndrome induced by phenobarbital and treated with gabapentin. Int J Tissue React 2001;23(1):39–43.

42. De Santis A, Ceccarelli G, Cesana BM, et al: Shoulder-hand syndrome in neurosurgical patients treated with barbiturates: a long term evaluation. J Neurosurg Sci 2000;44(2):69–76.

43. Pack AM, Morrell MJ: Adverse effects of antiepileptic drugs on bone structure: epidemiology, mechanisms and therapeutic implications. CNS Drugs 2001;15(8):633–642.

44. Farhat G, Yamout B, Mikati MA, et al: Effect of antiepileptic drugs on bone density in ambulatory patients. Neurology 2002;58(9): 1348–1353.

45. Lindberg MC, Cunningham A, Lindberg NH: Acute pheno-barbital intoxication. South Med J 1992;85(8):803–807.

46. Arieff AI, Friedman EA: Coma following nonnarcotic drug over-dosage: management of 208 adult patients. Am J Med Sci 1973; 266(6):405–426.

47. Fell RH, Gunning AJ, Bardhan KD, Triger DR: Severe hypothermia as a result of barbiturate overdose complicated by cardiac arrest. Lancet 1968;1(7539):392–394.

48. Rosenberg J, Benowitz NL, Pond S: Pharmacokinetics of drug overdose. Clin Pharmacokinet 1981;6(3):161–192.

49. Hernandez E, Praga M, Alcazar JM, et al: Hemodialysis for treatment of accidental hypothermia. Nephron 1993;63(2):214–216.

50. van Heijst AN, de Jong W, Seldenrijk R, van Dijk A: Coma and crystalluria: a massive primidone intoxication treated with haemoperfusion. J Toxicol Clin Toxicol 1983;20(4):307–318.

51. Lehmann DF: Primidone crystalluria following overdose: a report of a case and an analysis of the literature. Med Toxicol Adverse Drug Exp 1987;2(5):383–387.

52. Sigg T, Leikin JB: Massive crystalluria in a patient taking primidone. Ann Emerg Med 1999;33(6):726–727.

53. Clark JG, Sumerling MD: Muscle necrosis and calcification in acute renal failure due to barbiturate intoxication. BMJ 1966;5507:214–215.

54. Warner A, Privitera M, Bates D: Standards of laboratory practice: antiepileptic drug monitoring. National Academy of Clinical Biochemistry. Clin Chem 1998;44(5):1085–1095.

55. Drost RH, Plomp TA, Maes RA: EMIT-st drug detection system for screening of barbiturates and benzodiazepines in serum. J Toxicol Clin Toxicol 1982;19(3):303–312.

56. Nordt SP: Butalbital cross-reactivity to an Emit assay for phenobarbital. Ann Pharmacother 1997;31(2):254–255.

57. Proudfoot AT, Krenzelok EP, Vale JA: Position paper on urine alkalinization. J Toxicol Clin Toxicol 2004;42(1):1–26.

58. Frenia ML, Schauben JL, Wears RL, et al: Multiple-dose activated charcoal compared to urinary alkalinization for the enhancement of phenobarbital elimination. J Toxicol Clin Toxicol 1996;34(2): 169–175.

59. Veerman M, Espejo MG, Christopher MA, Knight M: Use of activated charcoal to reduce elevated serum phenobarbital concentration in a neonate. J Toxicol Clin Toxicol 1991;29(1):53–58.

60. Bradberry SM, Vale JA: Multiple-dose activated charcoal: a review of relevant clinical studies. J Toxicol Clin Toxicol 1995;33(5):407–416.

61. Pond SM, Olson KR, Osterloh JD, Tong TG: Randomized study of the treatment of phenobarbital overdose with repeated doses of activated charcoal. JAMA 1984;251(23):3104–3108.

62. Mohammed Ebid AH, Abdel-Rahman HM: Pharmacokinetics of phenobarbital during certain enhanced elimination modalities to evaluate their clinical efficacy in management of drug overdose. Ther Drug Monit 2001;23(3):209–216.

63. Palmer BF: Effectiveness of hemodialysis in the extracorporeal therapy of phenobarbital overdose. Am J Kidney Dis 2000;36(3): 640–643.

64. Sancak R, Kucukoduk S, Tasdemir HA, Belet N: Exchange trans-fusion treatment in a newborn with phenobarbital intoxication. Pediatr Emerg Care 1999;15(4):268–270.

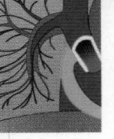

65. Watson WA, Litovitz TL, Rodgers GC Jr, et al: 2002 annual report of the American Association of Poison Control Centers Toxic Exposure Surveillance System. Am J Emerg Med 2003;21(5): 353–421.

66. Litovitz TL, Klein-Schwartz W, Rodgers GC Jr, et al: 2001 annual report of the American Association of Poison Control Centers Toxic Exposure Surveillance System. Am J Emerg Med 2002;20(5): 391–452.

67. Litovitz TL, Klein-Schwartz W, White S, et al: 2000 annual report of the American Association of Poison Control Centers Toxic Exposure Surveillance System. Am J Emerg Med 2001;19(5): 337–395.

68. Litovitz TL, Klein-Schwartz W, White S, et al: 1999 annual report of the American Association of Poison Control Centers Toxic Exposure Surveillance System. Am J Emerg Med 2000;18(5): 517–574.

69. Litovitz TL, Klein-Schwartz W, Caravati EM, et al: 1998 annual report of the American Association of Poison Control Centers Toxic Exposure Surveillance System. Am J Emerg Med 1999;17(5): 435–487.

37 Muscle Relaxants

MATTHEW D. SZTAJNKRYCER, MD, PHD

At a Glance...

- The skeletal muscle relaxants comprise a structurally and pharmacologically heterogeneous group of compounds, all of which are purported to decrease skeletal muscle tone.
- Central nervous system depression is the predominant finding in acute toxicity.
- Cardiac conduction abnormalities and dysrhythmias are rare, with the exception of orphenadrine.
- Management is primarily supportive, focusing on central nervous system and cardiopulmonary support.

Muscle tone reflects a complex interplay among the central nervous system, spinal cord, and musculoskeletal system. Skeletal muscle relaxants comprise a structurally and pharmacologically heterogeneous group of compounds, all of which are purported to decrease skeletal muscle tone. Mechanistically, this may occur at the level of the central nervous system, spinal cord, or musculoskeletal system. These agents are prescribed for acute post-traumatic muscle spasm (e.g., acute lumbar strain) or the management of spasticity associated with chronic neuropathologic processes (e.g., multiple sclerosis, cerebral palsy, spinal cord injury). Dantrolene is also used in the treatment of severe muscle hypertonia due to malignant hyperthermia, neuroleptic malignant syndrome (NMS), and tetanus.

Significant abuse potential exists for several of these agents.[1,2] Carisoprodol has additionally been used to modify the effects of other abused drugs, including benzodiazepines, alcohol, and cocaine.[3]

In addition to the benzodiazepines (see Chapter 35), 10 skeletal muscle relaxants have clinical and toxicologic significance (Table 37-1). An 11th agent, chlormezanone, was voluntarily recalled from worldwide markets in 1996 due to severe hypersensitivity reactions.

According to the American Association of Poison Control Centers, 21,793 exposures were reported in 2003. Of these, 4084 resulted in moderate toxicity, 1024 resulted in major toxicity, and 59 resulted in death. A total of 2490 exposures occurred in children 5 years old or younger, and 14,019 occurred in patients over the age of 19.

STRUCTURE

Baclofen (Lioresal, para-chlorophenyl-γ-aminobutyric acid; Novartis, East Hanover, NJ) differs from GABA (γ-aminobutyric acid) solely due to the presence of an additional phenylchloride group. Carisoprodol (Rela [Schering-Plough, Kenilworth, NJ], Soma [Wallace, Somerset, NJ], n-isopropyl-meprobamate) is structurally similar to the sedative-hypnotic agent meprobamate (see Chapter 34). Cyclobenzaprine (Flexeril, McNeil, Chattanooga, TN) is a tricyclic amine, structurally related to amitriptyline (see Chapter 27), while orphenadrine (Norflex, 3M Pharmaceuticals, St. Paul, MN) is structurally related to diphenhydramine (see Chapter 39). Dantrolene (Dantrium, Procter & Gamble, Cincinnati, OH) and metaxalone (Skelaxin, Mallinckrodt, Hazelwood, MO) are structurally related to phenytoin (see Chapter 40), while tizanidine (Zanaflex, Acorda Therapeutics, Hawthorn, NY) is an imidazoline derivative similar to clonidine (see Chapter 62). Chlorzoxazone (Parafon Forte, Ortho-McNeil Pharmaceutical, Raritan, NJ), methocarbamol (Robaxin, Wyeth-Ayerst, Collegeville, PA), and the chemically related chlorphenesin (Maolate, Upjohn, Pfizer, Inc., New York, NY) are unrelated to other agents.

PHARMACOLOGY

With the exception of dantrolene, the skeletal muscle relaxants act centrally, in part through central nervous system (CNS) modulation of interneurons, modifying pain perception without affecting pain threshold.[4]

Baclofen, a $GABA_B$ agonist, acts predominantly at presynaptic sites, as well as by decreasing spinal γ motor neuron activity.[5] Carisoprodol acts pharmacologically through its primary metabolite meprobamate, increasing chloride ion flux through the $GABA_A$ receptor complex. At high concentrations, meprobamate is capable of blocking N-methyl-D-aspartate (NMDA)–receptor mediated calcium currents.[6] Cyclobenzaprine possesses antimuscarinic, antihistaminic, and sedative properties with (in contrast to the tricyclic antidepressants) only weak inhibition of presynaptic norepinephrine and serotonin reuptake. Skeletal muscle activity is attributed to brainstem-mediated inhibition of α and γ motor neurons.[7] Although orphenadrine demonstrates peripheral antimuscarinic properties, NMDA receptor blockade, and sodium channel blockade, its skeletal muscle relaxant properties appear to be centrally mediated.[8] Orphenadrine-mediated dopamine release may be partly responsible for its abuse potential.[9] Tizanidine, a centrally acting $α_2$ agonist, is believed to reduce spasticity by increasing presynaptic inhibition of motor neurons.[10] Dantrolene is unique among the muscle relaxants, acting directly on skeletal muscle. It functions by inhibiting calcium release from the sarcoplasmic reticulum, decreasing the force of skeletal muscle contraction without affecting cardiac or smooth muscle.[11]

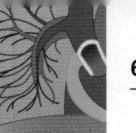

TABLE 37-1 Selected Pharmacologic Properties of Muscle Relaxants

AGENT	Vd (L/kg)	TIME TO PEAK LEVEL (hr)	ELIMINATION	METABOLITES	SPECIAL POPULATIONS	DRUG INTERACTIONS
Baclofen	1.3	2	2–6	Deaminated metabolites	Renal insufficiency	NSAIDs Levodopa
Carisoprodol	1	1–4	1.5–6	Meprobamate, hydroxycarisoprodol Hydroxymeprobamate	Renal insufficiency, hepatic insufficiency	
Chlorphenesin	1.27	1.9	3–4		Renal insufficiency, hepatic insufficiency, Asthamtics (secondary to tartrazine)	
Chlorzoxazone	Small	3–4	1.1	6-hydroxy-chlorzoxazone	Porphyria	Isoniazid Disulfiram Guanethidine Tramadol
Cyclobenzaprine	6	4–6	24–72	Glucuronide conjugate Cyclobenzaprine-N-oxide Norcyclobenzaprine, bis-10, 11-dihydroxy-nortriptyline 3-hydroxy-cyclobenzaprine		
Dantrolene	0.54 (pediatric)	4–8	8–10	5-hydroxy-dantrolene	Liver insufficiency Women Age > 35 years Amyotrophic lateral sclerosis	Calcium channel antagonists Vecuronium Theophyllline
Metaxalone Methocarbamol	1–2	3.3–4.3 1	2.4–9.2 1.2–2.2	3-(2-hydroxyphenoxy)-1, 2-propanediol-1-carbamate 3-(4-hydroxy-2 methoxyphenoxy)-1,2 propanediol-1-carbamate		
Orphenadrine	Large	2–4	14	N-monodemethyl orphenadrine Orphenadrine-N-oxide O-methylbenzhydrol conjugate O-methylbenzhydroxyacetic acid conjugate	Porphyria	
Tizanidine	2.4	1.5	2.1–4.1	Metabolite 3 (DS-200-717) Metabolite 4 (DS-201-341)	Renal insufficiency, hepatic insufficiency	Oral contraceptives, phenytoin

Vd, volume of distribution.

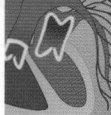

PHARMACOKINETICS

The heterogeneous nature of the muscle relaxants results in a wide range of pharmacokinetic properties (see Table 37-1). Baclofen is rapidly and completely absorbed from the gastrointestinal tract with therapeutic dosing. Absorption is both decreased and prolonged as ingested dose increases. Although penetration of the blood-brain barrier is limited at therapeutic doses, baclofen demonstrates central effects at higher doses.[12] Carisoprodol is rapidly absorbed after ingestion.[13] Cyclobenzaprine is slowly but completely absorbed after ingestion, while 70% of an ingested dantrolene dose is absorbed. Orphenadrine is readily absorbed after ingestion, demonstrating 100% bioavailability. Peak orphenadrine plasma levels may be delayed in overdose.[14]

Metabolism of the muscle relaxants is primarily hepatic, and elimination is primarily renal. Less than 1% of ingested carisoprodol and chlorzoxazone are eliminated unchanged in the urine, while 85% of baclofen is excreted unchanged. After extensive first pass hepatic metabolism, 50% of an ingested cyclobenzaprine dose is excreted in the urine. Substantial enterohepatic recirculation occurs, with 15% excreted in the bile unchanged.[15] Orphenadrine and tizanidine also demonstrate significant enterohepatic recirculation. The elimination half-life of cyclobenzaprine is 1 to 3 days, substantially longer than that of the other muscle relaxants. Approximately 60% of an ingested orphenadrine dose is excreted in the urine, with up to 30% excreted unchanged in the setting of urinary acidification.

Selected At-Risk Patient Populations

With the exception of cyclobenzaprine, safety in pregnancy is uncertain (category C). Cyclobenzaprine is presumed safe in pregnancy (category B). Carisoprodol is concentrated in breast milk and is considered unsafe in lactation. Methocarbamol is considered safe in lactation, and the safety of the remaining agents is unknown. Baclofen and tizanidine should be used cautiously in patients with renal insufficiency.[16] Tizanidine and dantrolene are contraindicated in the setting of liver disease. Dantrolene should also be used cautiously in women and individuals over the age of 35 due to an increased risk for idiosyncratic hepatotoxicity (see Adverse Effects with Therapeutic Use), and in patients with amyotrophic lateral sclerosis due to potential worsening of neuromuscular weakness.[17] Orphenadrine and carisoprodol are associated with acute porphyria and are contraindicated in patients with porphyria.

Adverse Drug Interactions

All skeletal muscle relaxants have the potential for adverse drug interactions with other CNS depressants. Concomitant baclofen and levodopa administration has resulted in hallucinations and worsening of parkinsonian symptoms.[18] Chlorzoxazone metabolism is decreased with concomitant disulfiram administration and in slow acetylators on isoniazid.[19,20] Due to structural similarities with the tricyclic antidepressants, potential adverse interactions have been suggested for cyclobenzaprine and guanethidine or tramadol. Animal studies have demonstrated potentially lethal interactions between dantrolene and verapamil or theophylline.[21,22] In the former, dantrolene administration to verapamil-pretreated swine resulted in profound myocardial depression, hyperkalemia (8.0 ± 0.7 mEq/L), and cardiac arrest preceded by complete heart block in 50% of the experimental group. In the latter, rat studies demonstrated increased theophylline mortality from concomitant therapeutic dantrolene doses in the absence of increased seizure frequency. Dantrolene prolonged neuromuscular blockade in a patient receiving vecuronium.[23] Oral contraceptive use has been associated with decreased tizanidine clearance, while tizanidine use is associated with decreased phenytoin clearance.[24]

TOXICOLOGY

Adverse Effects with Therapeutic Use

Numerous adverse effects have been associated with therapeutic use of the muscle relaxants (Table 37-2). CNS depression has been noted with all the agents, although it is less commonly associated with dantrolene. Additional CNS findings associated with baclofen therapy include movement disorders, memory impairment, muscle weakness, flapping tremor, nystagmus, diplopia, and dysarthria. Increased seizure activity, including status epilepticus, has been observed in patients with preexisting seizure disorders. Chlorzoxazone use is associated with opisthotonus and torticollis, while visual blurring and sensorineural hearing loss have been described with therapeutic use of intravenous and oral dantrolene, respectively. Neuropsychiatric effects, including mania, depression, psychosis, confusion, and amnesia, have been described with all skeletal muscle relaxants.

Cardiovascular complaints associated with baclofen administration include palpitations, flushing, bradycardia, hypotension, and hypertension. Facial flushing and orthostatic hypotension have been reported with carisoprodol use. Cyclobenzaprine, methocarbamol, and chlorphenesin are associated with hypotension, palpitations, and syncope. Although possessing only 2% to 10% of clonidine's antihypertensive potency, mild hypotension, symptomatic orthostatic hypotension, and syncope have been described with tizanidine use. Pericarditis, pleural effusions, and pleural fibrosis have been described with chronic therapeutic dantrolene use.[25]

Gastrointestinal complaints typically include nausea, vomiting, abdominal pain, and diarrhea or constipation. Idiosyncratic, potentially fatal hepatotoxicity is associated with chronic chlorzoxazone and dantrolene use. Onset of chlorzoxazone-associated hepatotoxicity is variable, typically occurring within weeks of initiation of therapy, but occasionally occurring after 5 or more months. Although reversible, centrilobular hepatotoxi-

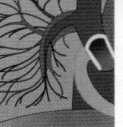
TABLE 37-2 Clinical Toxicity of the Muscle Relaxants

AGENT	CHRONIC EXPOSURE	ACUTE INTOXICATION
Baclofen	Neuropsychiatric dysfunction, GI upset, uinary retention, morbilliform rash, palpitations, physical dependence	Coma, respiratory depression, seizures, hypothermia
Carisoprodol	Sedation, nausea, vomiting, orthostatic hypotension, allergic reactions, physical dependence	Coma, nystagmus, seizures, cardiovascular instability
Chlorphenesin	CNS depression, neuropsychiatric dysfunction, allergic reactions	CNS depression
Chlorzoxazone	CNS depression, amnesia, parasthesias, opisthotonis, torticollis, urticaria, nausea/vomiting, idiosyncratic hepatitis	Coma, GI distress, hypotonia, hypotension
Cyclobenzaprine	CNS depression, antimuscarinic syndrome, hypotension, palpitations, syncope	Antimuscarinic syndrome, coma
Dantrolene	CNS depression, neuropsychiatric dysfunction, idiosyncratic heptotoxicity, pericarditis, pleural effusions, muscle weakness	Severe muscle weakness, CNS depression, hypotension
Metaxalone	CNS depression, neuropsychiatric dysfunction, syncope	CNS depression, nephrotoxicity, seizures, muscular rigidity
Methocarbamol	CNS depression, neuropsychiatric dysfunction, syncope, hypotension, hypersensitivity reactions	CNS depression, seizures
Orphenadrine	Antimuscarinic syndrome	Antimuscarinic syndrome, coma, seizures, cardiac conduction abnormalities, ventricular dysrhythmias, hypoglycemia, pulmonary hemorrhage
Tizanidine	CNS depression, syncope, urinary retention, orthostatic hypotension	Coma, hypotonia, miosis, bradycardia, apnea, hypothermia

CNS, central nervous system; GI, gastrointestinal.

city has recurred upon rechallenge to chlorzoxazone.[26] Risk factors for fatal hepatic necrosis after dantrolene use include age greater than 30 years, chronic use greater than 2 months, female gender, doses greater than 300 mg/day, high bilirubin levels, and concomitant illness.[27,28]

Urinary retention has been associated with baclofen, cyclobenzaprine, orphenadrine, and tizanidine. Dantrolene and baclofen use is associated with acneiform and morbilliform rashes, respectively. Cyclobenzaprine and orphenadrine are associated with central and peripheral antimuscarinic symptoms. Profound muscle weakness can occur with dantrolene use, resulting in diminished protective airway reflexes.[29] Severe allergic reactions have been reported with carisoprodol and chlorphenesin, associated with the additives sodium metabisulfite and tartrazine, respectively.

Acute Intoxication

Severe baclofen poisoning is characterized by coma, respiratory depression, bradycardia, and hypotension. Other CNS findings include hyporeflexia and encephalopathy.[30,31] Seizure activity has been observed after oral and intrathecal overdose, including generalized tonic–clonic activity, focal motor seizures, and status epilepticus. Two of eight patients in a case series of recreational abuse and 5 patients in a series of 12 overdoses developed seizures.[31,32] Seizure activity is believed secondary to the inhibitory effects of baclofen at presynaptic $GABA_B$ receptors and resultant inhibition of presynaptic GABA release, and may be delayed as long as 12 hours after acute ingestion. Cardiovascular findings are typically limited to bradycardia and hypotension, although cardiac conduction disturbances including first-

and second-degree AV block and QTc prolongation have rarely been reported in overdose. Mechanical ventilation was required in 10 of 12 patients after acute baclofen overdose in one case series.[31] Accidental intrathecal bolus administration of 10 mg resulted in coma and respiratory arrest within 80 minutes.[33] Mild hypothermia is common in overdose. Minimum adult oral lethal doses in case reports range from 1000 to 2500 mg, while acute ingestions of 300 to 970 mg have resulted in severe poisoning. In overdose, elimination half-life increases to 8.6 hours, with one report suggesting an elimination half-life of 34.5 hours.[34]

Acute carisoprodol toxicity presents similarly to meprobamate, with potentially abrupt onset of coma, cardiovascular instability, and death. Coma may persist for several days, and cerebral and pulmonary edema have been noted in severe overdose. Sixteen of 50 patients in a case series of meprobamate intoxications required mechanical ventilation.[35] Hypotension is likely multifactorial, related to CNS depression, direct effects on the CNS vasomotor center, and myocardial depression.[36] Ingestion of 700 mg by a toddler was associated with severe toxicity, and ingestion of 3.5 g by a 5-year-old resulted in death.[37,38]

Antimuscarinic findings predominate in acute cyclobenzaprine poisoning. CNS findings range from agitated delirium to coma. Symptoms typically occur within 4 hours of ingestion, although they may be delayed up to 12 hours. In one case series, sinus tachycardia occurred in one third of patients and CNS depression in 54%.[39] Three percent of patients required mechanical ventilation. Despite chemical similarity to the tricyclic antidepressants, impaired cardiac conduction, ventricular dysrhythmias, and seizures have only rarely been reported. Less than 1% of patients manifested

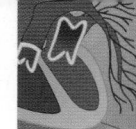

dysrhythmias other than sinus tachycardia, none of which were life threatening. While one case report suggested a minimum lethal adult dose of 100 mg, a case series suggested that adult ingestions of less than 100 mg were asymptomatic, and no deaths were reported after ingestions of up to 1000 mg.[39,40]

Severe orphenadrine intoxication is associated with respiratory and CNS depression, ranging from lethargy to coma. Antimuscarinic findings are noted in overdose, including mydriasis and sinus tachycardia, and may predominate in milder toxicity. Unlike cyclobenzaprine, orphenadrine poisoning is associated with seizures (including status epilepticus), cardiac conduction abnormalities, ventricular dysrhythmias, and cardiac arrest.[41-43] Life-threatening symptoms may appear precipitously, necessitating prompt, aggressive management. Additional manifestations of severe toxicity include hypoglycemia (especially in children), hypokalemia, hypothermia, pulmonary hemorrhage, and disseminated intravascular coagulation (DIC).[44] A 3-year-old child died after ingestion of 400 mg of orphenadrine, and a 23-month-old child developed severe toxicity after ingestion of 300 mg.[42,43]

Acute tizanidine toxicity presents similarly to clonidine, with decreased level of consciousness, hypotonia, hyporeflexia, hypotension, bradycardia, miosis, respiratory depression, apnea, and hypothermia (see Chapter 62). A 3-year retrospective review of 45 cases demonstrated lethargy in 38 patients (84%), bradycardia in 14 (31%), hypotension in 8 (18%), agitation in 7 (16%), and coma in 2 (4%).[45] The minimum adult ingested doses associated with hypotension and coma were 28 and 120 mg, respectively.

In acute overdose, chlorzoxazone toxicity presents as varying degrees of CNS depression, gastrointestinal distress, and hypotonia. Coma, flacidity, hyporeflexia, and subsequent secondary respiratory failure have been described. With the exception of hypotension, cardiovascular toxicity has not been described. Acute dantrolene overdose is not well described in the literature.[46,47] Severe muscle weakness may occur, with CNS depression occurring less frequently. Hypotension has been reported. Metaxalone overdose manifests predominantly as CNS depression, ranging from sedation to coma. Seizures may rarely occur, as may nephrotoxicity, and elevated hepatic transaminases. In one case report, severe muscular rigidity with subsequent prolonged weakness required placement in an extended care facility.[48] Findings in acute methocarbamol and chlorphenesin overdose are similar to metaxalone, with CNS depression and rare seizures noted. Cardiotoxicity is extremely rare in isolated ingestions.

Withdrawal

Chronic carisoprodol use is associated with tolerance, dependence, and a withdrawal syndrome, attributed to the metabolite meprobamate.[49] Symptoms are analogous to those seen with withdrawal from other sedative-hypnotic agents, with death reported after sudden withdrawal.[50] After long-term baclofen use, a withdrawal syndrome has been described, manifesting as hallucinations, agitated delirium, and seizures, typically within 12 to 96 hours of discontinuation.[51,52] Withdrawal may last as long as 8 days. This syndrome is particularly severe after abrupt discontinuation of intrathecal infusion, manifesting as an NMS-like syndrome. Severe dysautonomia, spasticity and rigidity, marked hyperthermia (43°C), tachycardia, rhabdomyolysis, agitated delirium, seizures, and DIC have been reported. In one case, an infant born to a paraplegic mother receiving chronic baclofen therapy developed status epilepticus resistant to multiple antiepileptic agents 7 days postdelivery. The seizures abated within 30 minutes of receiving baclofen.[53]

DIAGNOSIS

Diagnosis of skeletal muscle relaxant poisoning is based on history and clinical examination. Although analytic laboratory monitoring methods exist to confirm exposure to these agents, they are not routinely available, nor do specific levels correlate with outcome. Baclofen may be detected in serum using either high-performance liquid chromatography or gas chromatography/mass spectrometry technology. Therapeutic serum concentrations range from 80 to 395 ng/mL. Postmortem levels of 17 µg/mL have been reported 12 hours after ingestion.[54] Cyclobenzaprine has been reported to cross-react with the Syva EMIT (Dade-Behring, Deerfield, IL) technique and Abbott Adx tricyclic antidepressant (TCA) immunoassay (Abbott Laboratories, North Chicago, IL), and migrates similarly to amitriptyline on the Toxilab thin layer chromatography (TLC) system (Varian, Inc., Palo Alto, CA).[55] Therapeutic blood concentrations range from 10 to 40 ng/mL, with postmortem levels of 260 to 300 ng/mL reported.[55,56] Therapeutic blood levels of orphenadrine are less than 0.2 µg/mL, while moderate effects have been described at levels of 5.1 µg/mL and severe effects at 12.3 µg/mL. Postmortem levels have ranged from 7 to 33 µg/mL.[42,57] Therapeutic serum levels for carisoprodol range from 4 to 7 mg/L, while coma has been reported with a serum level of 13.4 mg/L 19 hours after ingestion, and death has been reported with a level of 36 mg/L 4.5 hours after ingestion.[58]

No specific laboratory analyses are routinely indicated, and clinical investigations are directed toward identification of end-organ toxicity. Creatine phosphokinase, electrolytes, and urine output should be monitored in patients with prolonged seizures or coma. Serum glucose should be rapidly determined in patients presenting with altered mental status. Coagulation studies and hepatic transaminase levels are indicated in orphenadrine intoxication, while hepatic and renal studies are indicated in metaxalone toxicity. Acetaminophen levels may be indicated in patients presenting after acute intentional ingestion. Electrocardiographic monitoring should be considered to detect the presence of conduction abnormalities and dysrhythmias. Computed tomography of the head and electroencephalographic assessment may be indicated to evaluate altered mental status, prolonged coma, and status epilepticus.

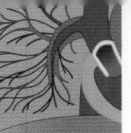

BOX 37-1	DIFFERENTIAL DIAGNOSIS OF MUSCLE RELAXANT INTOXICATION

Antidepressants
Antihistamines
Antiepileptic agents
Barbiturates
Benzodiazepines
Buspirone
Carbon monoxide
Cyanide
Ethanol
Ethylene glycol
γ-hydroxybutyrate (GHB)
Ketamine
Lithium
Hydrogen sulfide
Imidazolines
Isoniazid
Isopropanol
Organophosphate and carbamate pesticides
Phencyclidine
Sedative-hypnotic agents
Solvents
Zolpidem

Differential Diagnosis

Signs and symptoms of skeletal muscle relaxant poisoning are nonspecific, reflecting the CNS depressant effects of the agents (Box 37-1). The differential diagnosis for cyclobenzaprine and orphenadrine also includes sympathomimetic agents, antihistamines, antipsychotic agents, antispasmodic agents, cyclic antidepressants, and antimuscarinic plants and preparations. Toxicologic causes of altered mental status and seizures include cyanide, carbon monoxide, organophosphates and carbamates, buproprion, camphor, isoniazid, lithium, meperidine, propoxyphene, phencyclidine, oral hypoglycemics, phenothiazines, venlafaxine, and cyclic antidepressants. Toxicologic causes of cardiac conduction abnormalities include antidysrhythmics, antidepressants, antihistamines, antimuscarinic agents, β-adrenergic antagonists, propoxyphene, phenothiazines, and cocaine. The differential diagnosis for tizanidine intoxication includes opiates and opioids, clonidine and imidazolines, organophosphates and carbamates, and olanzapine.

MANAGEMENT

Management of skeletal muscle relaxant toxicity is primarily supportive, focusing on respiratory, CNS, and cardiovascular monitoring and support.

Given the potential for profound CNS and respiratory depression, early aggressive airway management is paramount in patient management. Cardiovascular toxicity predominantly presents as hypotension, bradycardia, or tachycardia. Hypotension should initially be treated with intravenous crystalloid boluses, provided no contraindication exists. Inotropic support is indicated for patients failing to respond to fluid boluses. Atropine is the first-line agent for symptomatic bradycardia. Cardiac dysrhythmias are treated according to standard guidelines, except as noted below. Benzodiazepines are first-line agents for patients with psychomotor agitation or seizures. Benzodiazepine-resistant seizures may be treated with barbiturates. Administration of oral or intrathecal baclofen may be required for seizures associated with baclofen withdrawal.[53] Core body temperature should be monitored due to the potential for hypothermia (baclofen) or hyperthermia (agitation, seizures, antimuscarinic syndrome, or sedative-hypnotic withdrawal syndrome).

Activated charcoal administration may be considered for patients presenting within 1 hour from time of ingestion, in accordance with the published guidelines of the American Academy of Clinical Toxicology and European Association of Poisons Centres and Clinical Toxicologists. Agents with delayed gastric emptying secondary to anticholinergic properties may benefit from activated charcoal beyond this time frame, although data are sparse. Whole bowel irrigation may be considered after ingestion of sustained-release preparations. Hemodialysis is not beneficial in the management of skeletal muscle relaxant toxicity.

Agent-Specific Management Strategies

Physostigmine has reversed baclofen-induced coma and orphenadrine-associated CNS toxicity, but is not universally effective, and has been associated with cardiac arrest[59-62] (Table 37-3). As a result, physostigmine use is limited to severe toxicity unresponsive to meticulous supportive care. Although flumazenil has successfully reversed coma and stupor in chlorzoxazone and carisoprodol intoxications, respectively, routine use cannot be recommended due to concern of flumazenil-induced seizures.[63,64] Given similarities to clonidine, naloxone may have a role in the management of tizanidine-associated CNS depression, bradycardia, and hypotension.[65] Cyproheptadine has been used in the management of intrathecal baclofen withdrawal.[66]

Atropine appears beneficial in the management of baclofen-associated bradycardia and hypotension.[67] QRS prolongation associated with orphenadrine and cyclobenzaprine toxicity is initially managed with sodium bicarbonate, analogous to tricyclic antidepressant toxicity (see Chapter 27). Ventricular dysrhythmias unresponsive to sodium bicarbonate therapy are treated with lidocaine. Physostigmine has reversed orphenadrine-associated ventricular tachycardia.[68] Quinidine, disopyramide, and procainamide are contraindicated due to their effects on sodium channels.

Multidose activated charcoal may be beneficial in the management of cyclobenzaprine and orphenadrine, which demonstrate enterohepatic recirculation, although outcome data are lacking. Hemoperfusion may be of benefit in carisoprodol toxicity, due to its

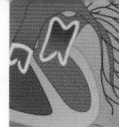

TABLE 37-3 Specialized Treatment Recommendation for Muscle Relaxant Toxicity

ANTIDOTAL AGENT	MUSCLE RELAXANT	INDICATION	DOSE
Atropine	Baclofen Tizanidine	Bradycardia and hypotension	Adult: 0.5–1 mg IV every 5 min (maximum dose 3 mg) Pediatrics: 0.02 mg/kg every 5 min minimum 0.1 mg, maximum dose 1 mg in children, 2 mg in adolescents)
Physostigmine	Baclofen Cyclobenzaprine Orphenadrine	Severe antimuscarinic syndrome	Adult: 1–2 mg IV over 5 min (may repeat once) Pediatrics: 0.02 mg/kg IV (maximum dose 0.5 mg)
Flumazenil	Carisoprodol Chlorzoxazone	CNS depression	Adult: 0.2 mg IV over 30 s every 1 min (maximum dose 5 mg) Pediatrics: 0.01 mg/kg IV over 30 s every 1 min (maximum dose 1 mg)
Naloxone	Tizanidine	CNS depression	Adult: 0.4–2 mg IV (maximum dose 10 mg) Pediatrics ≤ 20 kg: 0.01 mg/kg, then 0.1 mg/kg if needed Pediatrics > 20 kg: 0.4–2 mg IV (maximum dose 10 mg)
Cyprohepatidine	Baclofen	Withdrawal	Adult: 4–8 mg PO every 1–4 hr until therapeutic response (maximum dose 32 mg/day) Pediatrics: 0.25 mg/kg/day PO divided every 6 hr (maximum dose 12 mg/day)

CNS, central nervous system; IV, intravenously; PO, orally.

ability to effectively remove the primary metabolite, meprobamate.[69] Brisk diuresis may increase the elimination of baclofen, which is predominantly excreted in an unchanged form.

Patient Disposition

Asymptomatic or mildly symptomatic patients presenting after ingestion of a non-sustained-release preparation may be medically cleared after a 6-hour observation period. In the case of cyclobenzaprine and orphenadrine, an observation period of 6 to 12 hours has been suggested. Due to the potential for CNS and respiratory depression, significantly intoxicated patients should be admitted to a monitored setting. Hemodynamically unstable patients require continuous cardiopulmonary monitoring in an intensive care setting. Patients may be medically cleared for hospital discharge after signs and symptoms of toxicity have resolved.

REFERENCES

1. Schifano F, Marra R, Magni G: Orphenadrine abuse. South Med J 1988;8:546–547.
2. Bailey DN, Briggs JR: Carisoprodol: an unrecognized drug of abuse. Am J Clin Pathol 2002;117:396–400.
3. Reeves RR, Carter OS, Pinkofsky HB: Use of carisoprodol by substance abusers to modify the effects of illicit drugs. South Med J 1999;92:441.
4. De Lee JC, Rockwood CA: Skeletal muscle spasm and a review of muscle relaxants. Curr Ther Res 1980;27:64–74.
5. Gerkin R, Curry SC, Vance MV, et al: First-order elimination kinetics following baclofen overdose. Ann Emerg Med 1986;15:843–846.
6. Rho JM, Donevan SD, Rogawski MA: Barbiturate-like actions of the propanediol dicarbamates felbamate and meprobamate. J Pharmacol Exp Ther 1997;280:1383–1391.
7. Share NN, McFarlane CS: Cyclobenzaprine: a novel centrally acting skeletal muscle relaxant. Neuropharmacology 1975;12:675–684.
8. Product information: Norflex®, orphenadrine. 3M Pharmaceuticals, Northridge CA, 1998.
9. Cami J, Farre M: Mechanisms of disease: drug addiction. N Engl J Med 2003;349:975–986.
10. Coward DM: Tizanidine: neuropharmacology and mechanism of action. Neurology 1994;44(Suppl 9):6–10.
11. Ward A, Chaffman MO, Sorkin EM: Dantrolene. A review of its pharmacodynamic and pharmacokinetic properties and therapeutic use in malignant hyperthermia, the neuroleptic malignant syndrome and an update of its use in muscle spasticity. Drugs 1986;32:130–168.
12. Nugent S, Katz MD, Little TE: Baclofen overdose with cardiac conduction abnormalities: care report and review of the literature. J Toxicol Clin Toxicol 1986;24:321–328.
13. Hurlbut KM: Skeletal muscle relaxants—central acting. Micromedex Healthcare Series, Vol 117. Greenwood Village, CO, Thomson Healthcare Inc., September 2003.
14. Ellison T, Snyder A, Bolger J, et al: Metabolism of orphenadrine citrate in man. J Pharmacol Exp Ther 1971;176:284–295.
15. Hucker HB, Stauffer SC, Balletto AJ, et al: Physiological disposition and metabolism of cyclobenzaprine in the rat, dog, rhesus monkey, and man. Drug Metab Dispos 1978;6:659–672.
16. Skausig OB, Korsgaard S: Hallucinations and baclofen. Lancet 1977;1(8024):1258.
17. Rivera VM, Breitbach WB, Swanke L: Dantrolene in amyotrophic lateral sclerosis. JAMA 1975;233:863–864.
18. Lees AJ, Shaw KM, Stern GM: Baclofen in Parkinson's disease. J Neurol Neurosurg Psychiatry 1978;41:707–708.
19. Kharasch ED, Thummel KE, Mhyre J, et al: Single-dose disulfiram inhibition of chlorzoxazone metabolism: a clinical probe for P450 2E1. Clin Pharmacol Ther 1993;53:643–650.
20. Zand R, Nelson SD, Slattery JT, et al: Inhibition and induction of cytochrome P4502E1-catalyzed oxidation by isoniazid in humans. Clin Pharmacol Ther 1993;54:142–149.
21. Tayeb OS: A serious interaction of dantrolene and theophylline. Vet Hum Toxicol 1990;32:442–443.
22. Saltzman LS, Kates RA, Corke BC, et al: Hyperkalemia and cardiovascular collapse after verapamil and dantrolene administration in swine. Anesth Analg 1984;63:473–478.

23. Driessen JJ, Wuis EW, Gielen MJ: Prolonged vecuronium neuromuscular blockade in a patient receiving orally administered dantrolene. Anesthesiology 1985;62:523–524.

24. Ueno K, Miyai K, Mitsuzane K: Phenytoin-tizanidine interaction. Ann Pharmacother 1991;25:1273.

25. Mahoney JM, Bachtel MD: Pleural effusion associated with chronic dantrolene administration. Ann Pharmacother 1994;28:587–589.

26. Powers BJ, Cattau EL Jr, Zimmerman HJ: Chlorzoxazone hepatotoxic reactions. Arch Intern Med 1986;146:1183–1186.

27. Chan CH: Dantrolene sodium and hepatic injury. Neurology 1990;40:1427–1432.

28. Utili R, Boitnott JK, Zimmerman HJ: Dantrolene-associated hepatic injury: incidence and character. Gastroenterology 1977;72:610–616.

29. Watson CB, Reierson N, Norfleet EA: Clinically significant muscle weakness induced by oral dantrolene sodium prophylaxis for malignant hyperthermia. Anesthesiology 1986;65:312–314.

30. Lee TH, Chen SS, Su SL: Baclofen intoxication: report of four cases and review of literature. Clin Neuropharmacol 1992;15:56–62.

31. Nugent S, Katz MD, Little TE: Baclofen overdose with cardiac conduction abnormalities: case report and review of the literature. Clin Toxicol 1986;2:321–328.

32. Perry HE, Wright RO, Shannon MW, et al: Baclofen overdose: drug experimentation in a group of adolescents. Pediatrics 1998;101:1045–1048.

33. Saltuari L, Baumgartner H, Kofler M, et al: Failure of physostigmine in treatment of acute severe intrathecal baclofen intoxication. N Engl J Med 1990;322:1533.

34. Ghose K, Holmes K: Complications of baclofen overdosage. Postgrad Med J 1980;56:865–867.

35. Allen MD, Greenblatt DJ, Noel BJ: Meprobamate overdosage: a continuing problem. Clin Toxicol 1977;11:501–515.

36. Blumberg AG, Rosett HL, Dobrow A: Severe hypotensive reactions following meprobamate overdosage. Ann Intern Med 1959;51:607–612.

37. Green DI, Caravati EM: Coma in a toddler from low-dose carisoprodol. J Toxicol Clin Toxicol 2001;39:503.

38. Adams HR, Kerzee T, Morehead CD: Carisoprodol-related death in a child. J Forensic Sci 1975;20:200–202.

39. Spiller HA, Winter ML, Mann KV, et al: Five year multicenter retrospective review of cyclobenzaprine toxicity. J Emerg Med 1995;13:781–785.

40. Hurlbut KM, Rumack BH: Cyclobenzaprine. Micromedex Healthcare Series Vol 117. Greenwood Village, CO, Thomson Micromedex, September 2003.

41. Garza MB, Osterhoudt KC, Rutstein R: Central anticholinergic syndrome from orphenadrine in a 3 year old. Pediatr Emerg Care 2000;16:97–98.

42. Gill DG, Sowerby HA: Orphenadrine poisoning in childhood. Practitioner 1975;214:542–544.

43. Sangster B, van Heijst A, Zimmerman A: Intoxication by orphenadrine HCl: mechanism and therapy. Acta Pharmacol Toxicol 1977;41(Suppl 2):129–136.

44. Bozza-Marrubini M, Frigerio A, Ghezzi R, et al: Two cases of severe orphenadrine poisoning with atypical features. Acta Pharmacol Toxicol 1977;41(Suppl 2):137–152.

45. Adamson LA, Spiller HA, Bosse GM: Tizanidine (Zanaflex®) exposure. J Toxicol Clin Toxicol 2003;41:664.

46. Paloucek FP, Erickson TE, Lundquist S, et al: Oral dantrolene ingestion: a case series. Vet Hum Toxicol 1991;33:362.

47. Robillart A, Bopp P, Vailly B, et al: Cardiac failure caused by an overdose of dantrolene [French]. Ann Fr Anesth Reanim 1986;5:617–619.

48. Snyder LK, Sint T, Kirk MA: Metaxalone induced muscular rigidity. J Toxicol Clin Toxicol 2001;39:503.

49. Littrell RA, Sage T, Miller W: Meprobamate dependence secondary to carisoprodol (Soma) use. Am J Drug Alcohol Abuse 1993;19:133–134.

50. Swanson LA, Okada T: Death after withdrawal of meprobamate. JAMA 1963;184:780–781.

51. Kao LW, Amin Y, Kirk MA, et al: Intrathecal baclofen withdrawal mimicking sepsis. J Emerg Med 2003;24:423–427.

52. Alden TD, Lytle RA, Park TS, et al: Intrathecal baclofen withdrawal: a case report and review of the literature. Childs Nerv Syst 2002;18:522–525.

53. Ratnayaka BDM, Dhaliwal H, Watkin S: Neonatal convulsions after withdrawal of baclofen. BMJ 2001;323:85.

54. Fraser AD, MacNeil W, Isner F: Toxicological analysis of a fatal baclofen (Lioresal) ingestion. J Forensic Sci 1991;36:1596–1602.

55. Hucker HB, Stauffer SC, Albert KS, et al: Plasma levels and bioavailability of cyclobenzaprine in human subjects. J Clin Pharmacol 1977;17:719–727.

56. Levine B, Jones R, Smith ML, et al: A multiple drug intoxication involving cyclobenzaprine and ibuprofen. Am J Forensic Med Pathol 1993;14:246–248.

57. Clarke B, Mair J, Rudolf M: Acute poisoning with orphenadrine. Lancet 1985;1:1386.

58. Adams H, Kerzee T, Morehead C: Carisoprodol-related death in a child. J Forensic Sci 1975;20:200–202.

59. Rushman S, McLaren I: Management of intra-thecal baclofen overdose. Intensive Care Med 1999;25:239.

60. Saltuari L, Baumgartner H, Kofler M, et al: Failure of physostigmine in treatment of acute severe intrathecal baclofen intoxication. N Engl J Med 1990;322:1533–1534.

61. Delhass EM, Brouwers JR: Intrathecal baclofen overdose: report of 7 events in 5 patients and review of the literature. Int J Clin Pharmacol Ther Toxicol 1991;29:274–280.

62. Snyder BD, Kane M, Plocher D: Orphenadrine overdose treated with physostigmine. N Engl J Med 1976;295:1435.

63. Roberge RJ, Atchley B, Ryan K, et al: Two chlorzoxazone (Parafon Forte) overdoses and coma in one patient: reversal with flumazenil. Am J Emerg Med 1998;16:393–395.

64. Roberge RJ, Lin E, Krenzelok EP: Flumazenil reversal of carisoprodol (soma) intoxication. J Emerg Med 2000;18:61–64.

65. Seger DL: Clonidine toxicity revisited. J Toxicol Clin Toxicol 2002;40:145–155.

66. Meythaler JM, Roper JF, Brunner RC: Cyproheptadine for intrathecal baclofen withdrawal. Arch Phys Med Rehabil 2003;84:638–642.

67. Cohen MB, Gailey R, McCoy GC: Atropine in the treatment of baclofen overdose. Am J Emerg Med 1986;4:552–553.

68. Danze LK, Langdorf MI: Reversal of orphenadrine-induced ventricular tachycardia with physostigmine. J Emerg Med 1991;9:453–457.

69. Lin JL, Lim PS, Lain PC, et al: Continuous arteriovenous hemoperfusion in meprobamate poisoning. J Toxicol Clin Toxicol 1993;31:645–652.

38 *Antipsychotic Agents*

MICHAEL LEVINE, MD ■ MICHAEL J. BURNS, MD

At a Glance...

■ The toxic effects of antipsychotic agents are often an amplification of their pharmacologic effects; overdose findings can be predicted by knowledge of relative receptor binding affinities.

■ The presence of central nervous system or respiratory depression, miosis, sinus tachycardia, anticholinergic findings, and extrapyramidal signs should suggest antipsychotic agent poisoning.

■ Clinical effects occur within 1 to 4 hours following antipsychotic agent overdose.

■ Timely supportive care should ensure a good outcome for the vast majority of patients with antipsychotic poisoning.

■ The optimal treatment of neuroleptic malignant syndrome requires prompt recognition, immediate withdrawal of antipsychotic agents, and the provision of good supportive care.

INTRODUCTION AND RELEVANT HISTORY

Prior to 1952, drug therapy for schizophrenia was ineffective and often involved the nonspecific use of sedative-hypnotics (e.g., barbiturates) to calm patients during periods of agitation. The discovery of the traditional antipsychotics (e.g., chlorpromazine and haloperidol) in the early 1950s revolutionized the treatment of schizophrenia. These agents provided specific and effective therapy for the positive signs and symptoms (e.g., delusions, disorganized behavior, hallucinations) of psychosis. Subsequent to their introduction, however, it was realized that traditional agents were associated with disabling extrapyramidal motor and neuroendocrine (e.g., hyperprolactinemia) side effects, and were dangerous in overdose (significant cardiac and neurotoxicity). In addition, it became apparent that these agents were not effective for the negative signs and symptoms (e.g., alogia, avolition, and social withdrawal) and neurocognitive deficits of schizophrenia. This led to the development of second-generation or atypical antipsychotic agents in the 1990s. Atypical agents produce minimal extrapyramidal side effects (EPS) at clinically effective antipsychotic doses and are effective for the negative signs and symptoms and neurocognitive deficits of schizophrenia. Atypical agents, however, are also associated with a variety of adverse effects (e.g., glucose intolerance, weight gain, prolonged QTc interval) that limit efficacy and patient compliance. In 2002, further advance in drug therapy for schizophrenia was marked by the release of the third-generation antipsychotic aripiprazole. It is anticipated that this novel antipsychotic and the class it represents will provide equal or greater antipsychotic efficacy combined with a lower incidence and severity of side effects.

Terminology

The term *antipsychotic* is somewhat of a misnomer because these agents are often used for purposes other than treating psychoses: They are also used as pre-anesthetics and for the treatment of the manic phase of bipolar disorder, agitated behavior, drug-induced hallucinations, nausea and vomiting, migraine and tension headaches, hiccups, pruritus, Tourette's syndrome, and various extrapyramidal movement disorders (e.g., tics, chorea, and hemiballismus).[1] Historically, this class of agents was termed *major tranquilizer*s due to their ability to calm agitated patients. To think of these agents as simple sedatives, however, is overly simplistic. Until recently, the term *neuroleptic* was synonymous with and preferred to antipsychotic, because all traditional antipsychotics produce EPS at therapeutic doses. The introduction of agents that produce minimal EPS, or atypical antipsychotics, has allowed separation of antipsychotic from neuroleptic effects, and prevents the ready interchange of terms. Consequently, the term *antipsychotic* is more commonly used.

Epidemiology

Toxicity from the antipsychotic drugs may be dose related and occur following unintentional or intentional overdose, or may be idiosyncratic and occur as unanticipated adverse effects during therapeutic administration. Dose-related toxicity will vary according to agent, patient age and habituation, and comorbid conditions. Toxic effects are often an overextension of an agent's pharmacologic effects.[1] Because of a large toxic-to-therapeutic ratio, fatalities rarely occur. Death, when it occurs, is usually a consequence of polysubstance overdose. The agents with the greatest individual toxicity or highest fatal toxicity index (most deaths caused per prescription written) are the low-potency traditional agents, such as chlorpromazine, loxapine, mesoridazine, and thioridazine.[2-4] These agents, however, are now implicated in fewer deaths from antipsychotic agents in the United States due to their lower frequency of usage. In 2004, there were 42,833 antipsychotic agent exposures reported to U.S. poison centers, of which 38,315 (89%) were due to atypical antipsychotics and 4518 (11%) were due to phenothiazines.[5] Major toxicity and death occurred in 5.5% and 0.2% of atypical agent exposures and 4.1% and 0.4% of phenothiazine exposures, respectively.[5] While antipsychotic drugs often have a wide margin of safety, these drugs are commonly used, have a

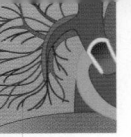

large number of adverse effects, and can produce significant toxicity in the nonhabituated host or those at the extremes of age.

CLASSIFICATION AND STRUCTURE-ACTIVITY RELATIONSHIPS

Antipsychotics can be classified by structure, pharmacologic profile, and whether they are typical (traditional or conventional) or atypical (novel, second and third generation). Classification by structure is challenging since antipsychotics are a structurally diverse group of heterocyclic compounds. Currently more than 50 neuroleptics are available worldwide, with numerous others in various stages of development.[1] Chemical classes include benzamide, benzepine, butyrophenone (phenylbutylpiperidine), diphenylbutylpiperidine, indole, phenothiazine, quinolinone, rauwolfia alkaloid, and thioxanthene derivatives (Table 38-1).[1] The phenothiazines and thioxanthenes are traditional tricyclic antipsychotic agents for which structure predicts function. These agents have two benzene rings linked by a sulfur atom and either a nitrogen (phenothiazines) or carbon (thioxanthenes) atom double bonded to the side chain at position 10 of the central ring (Fig. 38-1).[1] The presence of an electron-withdrawing group at position 2 increases antipsychotic efficacy and potency. Phenothiazines and thioxanthenes are subdivided into three groups (aliphatic, piperidine, and piperazine), based on the side chain substitution at position 10 on the central ring (see Fig. 38-1). The nature of the substitution influences pharmacologic activity. The aliphatic and piperidine subclasses have a higher antipsychotic potency and incidence of EPS, but a lower incidence of sedation, hypotension, and anticholinergic effects than do the piperazine class.[1] In general, the antihistaminergic and anticholinergic properties of the phenothiazines and thioxanthenes are derived from the presence of a tertiary amino group in the side chain connected by two or three carbons to position 10 of the central ring (see Fig. 38-1 and Chapter 39).[1] Aside from the phenothiazine and thioxanthene classes, structure-activity relationships have not been well characterized for most antipsychotics. Therefore, classification based on chemical structure has limited clinical utility for most agents.

A more clinically useful method of antipsychotic agent classification is to identify agents by their relative receptor-binding profiles (Table 38-2). Because clinical toxicity of antipsychotics results from exaggerated pharmacologic activity, knowledge of the agent's binding affinity at various receptors allows one to predict adverse effects in both therapeutic and overdose situations.[6-8]

The most commonly used method of classifying antipsychotics is to identify them as typical or atypical. This classification is clinically based. Agents are considered atypical if they (1) produce minimal EPS at clinically effective antipsychotic doses; (2) have a low propensity to cause tardive dyskinesia (TD) with long-term treatment; and (3) are effective for treating both the positive and negative signs and symptoms of schizophrenia.[6-10] Interestingly, this clinically determined classification

system is rooted in receptor binding. Drug atypia is defined by unique, relative receptor-binding profiles (see Pharmacology section). In the preclinical area, knowledge of an agent's relative receptor-binding affinities can be used to predict whether it will be atypical or typical.

PHARMACOLOGY

All antipsychotic agents bind and block presynaptic (autoreceptors) and postsynaptic D_2 receptors in the central nervous system (CNS).[1] Initially, this receptor antagonism stimulates increased presynaptic production and release of dopamine. With continued antipsychotic treatment, however, depolarization inactivation occurs at the synapse, and decreased production and release occurs simultaneous with continued postsynaptic receptor blockade. Partial receptor agonists and agents with lower receptor affinity (e.g., atypical agents) are less likely to lead to depolarization inactivation at the synapse.

Antipsychotic agents block D_2-subtype receptors in nigrostriatal (basal ganglia), tuberoinfundibular (hypothalamus to pituitary), mesocortical, and mesolimbic pathways of the brain.[1,6,8,9] These agents also antagonize D_2 receptors in the medulla oblongata and the anterior hypothalamus. Blockade of the D_2 receptors in the area postrema (chemotactic trigger zone) is responsible for the antiemetic activity of antipsychotics. Antipsychotic efficacy is mediated by a drug's ability to block mesocortical and mesolimbic D_2 receptors; all antipsychotics share this property.[1,6,8,9] For most neuroleptics, there is a strong correlation between the affinity (potency) at D_2 receptors and daily dose necessary to treat the positive symptoms of schizophrenia (see Tables 38-1 and 38-2).[1,8,11] Based on in vivo studies utilizing positron emission tomography, the therapeutic effects of neuroleptics correlate with 70% or greater D_2 receptor occupancy in the mesolimbic pathway.[12]

Antagonism of the D_2 receptors in other brain regions, however, accounts for many of the undesired side effects of antipsychotics. For example, antagonism of the D_2 receptors in the tuberoinfundibular pathway in the pituitary gland causes hyperprolactinemia, which can result in galactorrhea, gynecomastia, menstrual changes, and sexual dysfunction.[1,6] Antagonism of the nigrostriatal D_2 receptors produces EPS (e.g., acute dystonia, parkinsonism, akathisia). Agents with higher D_2 receptor affinity (e.g., fluphenazine, haloperidol, and thiothixene) have a high likelihood for producing EPS.[6] In contrast, agents with minimal D_2 receptor affinity (i.e., clozapine, quetiapine) or those that selectively inhibit the limbic D_2 receptors over the nigrostriatal D_2 receptors (e.g., sulpiride, remoxipride) are less likely to produce EPS.[6,7,10] Unfortunately, for most traditional antipsychotics, basal ganglia D_2 receptor blockade occurs in the same dose range necessary for limbic D_2 blockage.[12] This produces a high incidence of EPS at therapeutic doses for traditional antipsychotics.[1,6]

Regulation of core body temperature involves dopamine. D_2 receptor blockade by antipsychotics in the anterior hypothalamus (preoptic area) can alter the core temperature set point, block thermosensitive neuronal

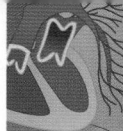

TABLE 38-1 Classification and Dosing of Antipsychotic Agents

STRUCTURAL CLASS	GENERIC NAME (TRADE NAME)	DAILY DOSE RANGE (mg)
Typical Agents		
Butyrophenone (phenylbutylpiperidine)	Droperidol (Inapsine)	1.25–30
	Haloperidol (Haldol)	1–30
	Other: benperidol, bromperidol, melperone, pipamperone, trifluperidol	
Diphenylbutylpiperidine	Pimozide (Orap)	1–20
	Other: fluspirilene, penfluridol	
Indole	Molindone (Moban)	15–225
	Other: oxypertine	
Phenothiazine		
Aliphatic	Chlorpromazine (Thorazine)	25–2000
	Promazine (Sparine)	50–1000
	Promethazine (Phenergan)	25–150
	Triflupromazine (Vesprin)	5–90
Piperazine	Acetophenazine (Tindal)	40–400
	Fluphenazine (Prolixin)	0.5–30
	Perphenazine (Trilafon)	4–64
	Prochlorperazine (Compazine)	10–150
	Trifluoperazine (Stelazine)	2–40
	Thiethylperazine (Torecan)	10–30
Piperidine	Mesoridazine (Serentil)	30–400
	Thioridazine (Mellaril, Millazine)	20–800
	Other: diethazine, ethopropazine, levomepromazine, perazine, pipotiazine thiopropazate, thioproperazine, pericyazine	
Thioxanthene	Chlorprothixene (Taractan)	30–600
	Clopenthixol	—
	Flupenthixol	4
	Thiothixene (Navane)	6–60
	Zuclopenthixol (Cisordinal, Clopixol)	10–50
Atypical Agents		
Benzamides	Amisulpiride	100–1200
	Raclopride	5–8
	Remoxipride	150–600
	Sulpiride	100–1600
	Sultopride	100–1200
	Other: epidepride, eticlopride levosulpiride, nemonapride, tiapride	
Benzepine		
Dibenzodiazepine	Clozapine (Clozaril, Leponex)	150–900
Dibenzooxazepine	Loxapine (Loxitane)	20–250
Thienobenzodiazepine	Olanzapine (Zyprexa)	5–20
Dibenzothiazepine	Quetiapine (Seroquel)	300–600
Dibenzothiazepine	Zotepine	100–300
	Other: butaclamol, fluperlapine, clothiapine, metiapine, savoxepine	
Indole		
Benzisoxazole	Risperidone (Risperdal)	2–16
Imidazolidinone	Sertindole (Serlect)	12–24
Benzisothiazole	Ziprasidone (Zeldox)	40–160
	Other: iloperidone	
Quinolinone	Aripiprazole (Abilify, Abitat)	10–30

inputs, and inhibit centrally mediated thermoregulatory responses.[1] Thus, either hypothermia or hyperthermia can occur from antipsychotic therapy. D_2 receptor antagonism in the hypothalamus and the nigrostriatum mediates the neuroleptic malignant syndrome (NMS), a fulminant hyperthermic adverse reaction associated with antipsychotic therapy. Decreased tolerance to heat and fatal heat stroke have been described in patients who take phenothiazines.[9] Antipsychotics have also been used successfully to treat hyperthermia associated with cocaine and amphetamines.[10-12]

In addition to their D_2 receptor antagonism, most antipsychotics are competitive antagonists at a wide variety of other neuroreceptors. Since the D_2 receptor binding affinity determines the daily (therapeutic) dose, the relative binding affinity at other neuroreceptor

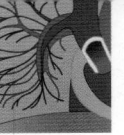

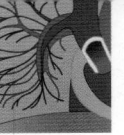

FIGURE 38-1 Phenothiazine structure.

sites compared with that at D_2 receptors predicts the likelihood of producing clinical effects from other neuroreceptors (see Table 38-2).[6,13] Knowledge of relative binding affinities can be used to predict clinical effects at both therapeutic doses and overdoses.[6,13] For instance, high relative antagonism at the H_1-histamine receptor (e.g., aliphatic and piperidine phenothiazines, clozapine, loxapine, olanzapine, and quetiapine) results in sedation, hypotension, and appetite stimulation.[1,6,13,14] Significant blockade of the M_1-muscarinic receptor (e.g., aliphatic and piperidine phenothiazines, clozapine, and olanzapine) produces anticholinergic effects (e.g., agitation, hallucinations, delirium, blurred vision, dry skin and mucous membranes, hyperpyrexia, ileus, mydriasis, tachycardia, and urinary retention). Sialorrhea, a feature unique to clozapine, is likely mediated by its partial agonism at M_1 and M_4 receptors.[6] Significant antagonism of the α_1-adrenergic receptor (e.g., aliphatic and piperidine phenothiazines, clozapine, risperidone, ziprasidone, olanzapine, and sertindole) results in orthostatic hypotension, reflex tachycardia, nasal congestion, and miosis.[1] Blockade of the α_2-adrenergic receptor by certain agents (e.g., clozapine and risperidone) may produce sympathomimetic effects (e.g., tachycardia). The ability of certain agents (e.g., loxapine, clozapine) to block neuronal reuptake of norepinephrine and antagonize $GABA_A$ receptors partly accounts for the high prevalence of seizures with these drugs. High relative binding affinities at M_1 and $5\text{-}HT_{1A}$- and $5\text{-}HT_{2A}$-serotonin receptors are inversely related to the likelihood of producing EPS.[1,13,15,16]

Although drug atypia is defined clinically, it also appears to be determined by one or more of several different pharmacologic mechanisms. Atypical agents belong to one of four distinct receptor-binding groups: (1) D_2 and D_3 receptor antagonists (e.g., amisulpiride, remoxipride, raclopride, sulpiride); (2) D_2, α_1, and 5-

TABLE 38-2 Relative Neuroreceptor Affinities for Antipsychotics*

NEUROLEPTIC AGENT	D_2†	H_1	α_1	α_2	M_1	$5\text{-}HT_{2A}$	OTHER RECEPTOR BINDING
Typical Agents							
Chlorpromazine	2+	2+	3+	0	1+	3+	$D_{1,3,4}$
Fluphenazine	3+	0	0	0	0	0	
Haloperidol	2+	0	1+	0	0	1+	$D_{1,4}$, σ
Loxapine	1+	3+	3+	0	2+	3+	D_4, blocks NE reuptake
Mesoridazine	2+	3+	3+		1+		
Molindone	1+	0	0	1+	0	0	
Perphenazine	3+	1+	1+		0		
Pimozide	2+	0	1+		0	1+	
Prochlorperazine	2+	1+	1+		0	0	
Thioridazine	2+	2+	3+	0	3+	2+	
Thiothixene	3+	0	0	0	0	0	
Trifluoperazine	3+	0	1+		0	1+	
Atypical Agents							
(Ami)sulpiride	2+	0	0	0	0	0	D_3
Aripiprazole	3+‡	2+	2+	0	0	3+	$D_{3,4}$, $5\text{-}HT_{1A,2C,7}$, blocks 5-HT reuptake
Clozapine	1+	3+	3+	3+	3+	3+	$D_{1,4}$, M_{2-5}, $5HT_{2C,2D,3,6,7}$, blocks NE reuptake
Olanzapine	2+	2+	2+	0	3+	3+	$D_{1,3,4}$, M_{2-5}, $5HT_{1C,3,6}$
Quetiapine	1+	3+	3+	0	3+	1+	$5\text{-}HT_{1A}$, D_1
Remoxipride	1+	0	0		0	0	σ
Risperidone	3+	0	2+	1+	0	3+	$D_{1,4}$
Sertindole	3+	0	1+	0	0	3+	$5HT_{1C,2C}$
Ziprasidone	3+	0	3+	0	0	3+	$5HT_{1A,1C,1D,2C}$, D_1 blocks NE, 5-HT reuptake
Zotepine	2+	2+	0	2+	0	3+	$D_{1,3,4}$, $5\text{-}HT_{2C}$, blocks NE reuptake

*Relative neuroreceptor affinity is the neuroreceptor affinity at receptor X/dopamine D_2 receptor affinity.
†Binding affinity (potency) at D_2 receptor correlates inversely with the daily dose of antipsychotic agent.
‡High binding affinity but partial agonist at receptor.
0, minimal to none; 1+, low; 2+, moderate; 3+, high; 4+, very high. NE, norepinephrine.
Data from references 1, 6–8, 57, 58, and 181.

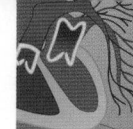

HT$_{2A}$ receptor antagonists (e.g., ziprasidone, sertindole, risperidone), also known as the serotonin-dopamine antagonists; (3) broad-spectrum, multireceptor antagonists (e.g., clozapine, olanzapine, quetiapine); and (4) D$_2$ and 5-HT$_{1A}$ receptor partial agonists (e.g., aripiprazole), also known as dopamine and serotonin system stabilizers.[7] Characteristics associated with drug atypia include low D$_2$ receptor potency (high milligram drug dosing); low D$_2$ receptor occupancy (less than 70%) in the mesolimbic and nigrostriatal areas at therapeutic doses; partial agonist activity at D$_2$ receptors; high affinities for M$_1$, D$_1$, D$_3$, α$_2$, 5-HT$_{1A}$, and 5-HT$_{2A}$ receptors relative to the D$_2$ receptor; multiple neuroreceptor antagonism; and a low likelihood of raising serum prolactin concentrations.[6-8,10,12,14,16]

CNS serotonin antagonism is now recognized as an important mechanism of antipsychotic action and minimizing the likelihood of EPS.[1,14-18] Normally, serotonergic fibers inhibit dopamine release in the nigrostriatum and prefrontal cortex. Thus, blockade of the 5-HT$_{2A}$ receptors in the CNS increases dopamine release in the striatum and prefrontal cortex. Antipsychotics that have high relative 5-HT$_{2A}$ receptor antagonism (5-HT$_{2A}$/D$_2$ binding ratio greater than 1) (e.g., amperozide, clozapine, risperidone, sertindole, ziprasidone) have enhanced efficacy for treating the negative signs and symptoms of schizophrenia and provide a lower EPS liability.[16-18] Agents with partial agonist activity at 5-HT$_{1A}$ autoreceptors (e.g., ziprasidone, aripiprazole) have similar beneficial effects.

Pathophysiology

CARDIAC EFFECTS

The aliphatic and piperidine phenothiazines (e.g., chlorpromazine, thioridazine, and mesoridazine) have direct negative inotropic and quinidine-like (type IA) antiarrhythmic effects on cardiac myocytes.[1] These agents block voltage-gated fast sodium channels; blockade is enhanced at less negative membrane potentials and faster heart rates.[1,19] Thus, conduction disturbances will be augmented for drugs that also produce tachycardia (e.g., those with anticholinergic properties) or tissue acidemia (e.g., as a result of drug-associated seizure or shock). In addition, certain antipsychotic agents antagonize delayed-rectifier, voltage-gated potassium channels (encoded by the HERG gene) responsible for membrane repolarization during phase 3 of the action potential.[1,20,21] Potassium channel antagonism is concentration, voltage, and reverse frequency dependent; block is augmented at higher drug tissue concentrations, less negative membrane potentials, and slower heart rates.[20,21] Potassium channel blockade may induce early after depolarization and triggered ventricular activity (e.g., torsades de pointes [TdP]). Some neuroleptics, (e.g., haloperidol, mesoridazine, pimozide, and thioridazine) are also calcium channel antagonists.[22] The cardiac channel effects of antipsychotics produce a depressed rate of phase 0 depolarization, decreased amplitude and duration of phase 2, and prolongation of phase 3. In addition, early after-depolarizations that result from the blockade of the rectifying potassium channels can trigger ventricular arrhythmias (e.g., TdP).

CARDIOVASCULAR

Hypotension results from α$_1$-adrenergic antagonism and loss of peripheral vasomotor tone, α$_2$-adrenergic antagonism and loss of central vasomotor tone, and direct membrane-depressant cardiac effects. Membrane-depressant effects result in impaired cardiac conduction and contractility.[1] Cardiovascular effects are dose related. Tachycardia occurs as a vasomotor reflex to hypotension or from anticholinergic drug effects.

SEIZURES

All antipsychotic agents appear to lower the seizure threshold and produce dose-related electroencephalographic (EEG) abnormalities that are similar to discharge patterns observed in epileptic patients.[1,23-27] The degree of EEG changes and incidence of seizures are greatest with certain agents (e.g., clozapine, loxapine, and aliphatic and piperidine phenothiazines).[1,23-29] The mechanisms of seizure production are not well elucidated but appear to involve GABA$_A$ receptor antagonism, norepinephrine reuptake inhibition, and disrupted ionic flow through neuronal membrane channels.

EXTRAPYRAMIDAL SIDE EFFECTS

All EPS result from D$_2$ receptor blockade by antipsychotics in basal ganglia nuclei.[1,6,14,30,31] This leads to a disruption of neurotransmission in numerous basal ganglia and thalamocortical pathways critical for coordinated movement. These pathways utilize acetylcholine, serotonin, glutamate, γ-aminobutyric acid (GABA), and various neuropeptides for communication.[16,17,32] Drug-induced parkinsonism is a result of decreased nigrostriatal dopaminergic activity with resultant striatal cholinergic excess.[1,6,30,31] Akathisia is likely produced by D$_2$ receptor blockade in mesocortical pathways.[1,6,30,31] The pathophysiology of acute dystonic reactions (ADRs) is still unknown. One attractive theory posits that dystonia is the manifestation of an acute compensatory response to nigrostriatal D$_2$ receptor blockade produced by antipsychotics. The acute administration of antipsychotics provokes increased dopamine synthesis and release from nigrostriatal neurons and postsynaptic receptor up-regulation.[30,31,33,34] As brain concentrations of the neuroleptic decline hours to days after a dose, a state of dopamine excess develops and hyperkinesis or dystonia results. TD is likely secondary to an increased number and up-regulated dopamine receptor as a compensatory response to chronic D$_2$ receptor blockade by antipsychotics in the nigrostriatum.[1,6,30,31,33,34] TD signifies a state of dopaminergic supersensitivity and cholinergic underactivity in the basal ganglia.

NMS appears to involve dopaminergic hypoactivity in the CNS. Blockade of D$_2$ receptors in the striatum and hypothalamus results in muscular rigidity (similar to parkinsonism) and altered thermoregulation, respectively.[35-37] Fever occurs largely from increased heat production from muscular rigidity but is also due to impaired heat dissipation and an altered set point of

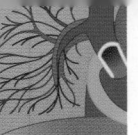

core temperature in the hypothalamus.[1,35-37] Blockade of D_2 receptors in the mesolimbic and mesocortical regions produces altered mentation. Blockade of D_2 receptors in peripheral sympathetic nerve terminals and the vasculature may cause autonomic disturbances.[38,39] The pathophysiology of NMS may involve iron. Iron is a positive modulator of dopamine receptor activity, and low serum iron levels often displayed in those with NMS may lead to a decreased number of dopamine receptors in the brain.[40,41]

PHARMACOKINETICS

Although most classes of antipsychotics have similar pharmacokinetics, there is substantial interindividual variability. Following oral administration, absorption is generally rapid and nearly complete. Because of extensive first-pass hepatic and intestinal metabolism, however, bioavailability is erratic and unpredictable (range 10% to 70%).[1,42,43] Peak plasma concentrations occur within 1 to 6 hours after oral administration. Intramuscular (IM) administration increases bioavailability by a factor of 4 to 10.[1] Peak plasma concentrations occur within 30 to 60 minutes after IM administration of immediate-release preparations but are delayed up to 24 hours following IM administration of depot preparations.[1,42,43] Following an oral overdose, absorption occurs more rapidly but peak plasma concentrations are delayed; clinical effects may occur earlier and last longer. The depot (sustained-release) injectable preparations are created by esterifying the hydroxyl group of the antipsychotic with a long-chain fatty acid (e.g., enanthate or decanoate) and dissolving it in a sesame oil vehicle.[1]

Most antipsychotics are highly protein bound (75% to 99%) and lipophilic. These drugs have large volumes of distribution (usual range 10 to 40 L/kg) and tend to accumulate in brain and other tissues.[1,42,43] Removal of these agents by hemodialysis or hemoperfusion is impossible.

Antipsychotic agents are largely and extensively eliminated by hepatic metabolism. Less than 1% of an ingested dose is excreted unchanged by the kidney. Hepatic metabolism occurs via flavin-containing monooxygenase or cytochrome P-450 mixed-function oxidase systems or by hydroxylation, sulfoxidation, N-dealkylation, and conjugation.[42,43] Hepatic metabolites are not easily measured but often remain pharmacologically active and will extend the parent drug's effects after therapeutic doses or overdose. Thus, there is often a poor correlation between serum concentration and clinical effects.[42-44] Metabolites are variably excreted in the urine and stool after conjugation and enterohepatic circulation, respectively. Elimination half-lives of most antipsychotic agents range from 20 to 40 hours after oral dosing. Depot IM preparations have elimination half-lives of 7 to 21 days.[1,42] With newer sustained-release preparations (e.g., Risperdal Consta, Janssen, LP, Titusville, NJ), steady-state plasma concentrations are maintained for 4 to 6 weeks after the last IM injection.[45]

Risperdal Contra contains an aqueous suspension of risperidone mixed with a biodegradable copolymer. The pharmacokinetic profile of common neuroleptic drugs is presented in Table 38-3.

Special Populations

PREGNANCY AND BREAST-FEEDING
Due to their high lipophilicity, most antipsychotics readily enter the fetal circulation across the placenta and are readily secreted into breast milk.[1] Data that establish the safety of antipsychotics during pregnancy are lacking, and these drugs are thus considered pregnancy class C; their use in pregnant women is warranted only if the benefits to the mother justify the potential risks to the fetus. While most manufacturers recommend against the use of antipsychotics during breast feeding, toxic effects and impaired development have not been demonstrated to date in infants who have been breast-fed by women regularly taking antipsychotics.[46]

RENAL IMPAIRMENT
Most of the antipsychotics are metabolized almost exclusively in the liver before excretion and are not significantly affected by alterations in renal function. Risperidone and the benzamide derivatives (e.g., sulpiride and remoxipride), however, require dosage alterations for patients in renal failure because large amounts of these drugs are excreted unchanged by the kidneys.[43]

HEPATIC IMPAIRMENT
Patients with advanced hepatic disease (e.g., cirrhosis) and conditions that impair hepatic blood flow (e.g., congestive heart failure) have diminished clearance of antipsychotic agents. Thus, dose reduction is recommended for this group of patients during chronic therapy.[43] The presence of hepatic disease, however, is unlikely to affect clinical outcome following acute overdose in this group of patients.

AGE
Infants and geriatric patients have reduced capacity to metabolize and eliminate antipsychotic agents, whereas children tend to metabolize these drugs more rapidly than adults.[1] In general, however, elderly and pediatric patients are more sensitive to the effects of neuroleptics than are young adults. Thus, patients at the extremes of age have a greater tendency to develop anticholinergic stigmata, EPS, sedation, confusion, and postural hypotension. The safety and efficacy of many antipsychotics have not been adequately studied in pediatric patients.

GENETIC POLYMORPHISMS
There is large interindividual variation in the hepatic biotransformation of antipsychotic agents, which largely reflects CYP enzyme polymorphisms. For instance, 5% to 10% of white individuals are CYP2D6 "poor metabolizers," which may result in certain antipsychotic drug concentrations (e.g., risperidone, haloperidol, thioridazine) that are up to 10-fold higher than those in

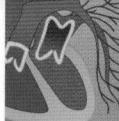

TABLE 38-3 Pharmacokinetics of Various Antipsychotics

ANTIPSYCHOTIC AGENT	TIME TO PEAK AFTER ORAL DOSING (hr)	ELIMINATION HALF-LIFE (hr)	PROTEIN BINDING (%)	Vd (L/KG)	ROUTE OF METABOLISM	ACTIVE METABOLITE
Typical Agents						
Chlorpromazine	2–4	8–35	90–95	7–20	CYP2D6	Yes
Haloperidol	1–6	17–36	92	10–35	CYP2D6 CYP3A4	Yes
Fluphenazine	2–5	5–27	90–95	220	Hepatic	Yes
Loxapine	1–6	2–8	91–99	NA	CYP1A2 CYP2D6 CYP3A4	Yes
Perphenazine	2–6	8–21	90–95	10–35	CYP2D6	No
Prochlorperazine	1.5–5	17–27	>90	13–32	Hepatic	No
Promethazine	3.3	9–16	93	9–19	Hepatic	Yes
Pimozide	6–8	28–214	99	11–62	CYP3A4 CYP1A2	Yes
Thioridazine	2–4	9–36	99	18	CYP2D6	Yes
Thiothixene	1–3	12–36	90–95	NA	Hepatic	No
Atypical Agents						
Aripiprazole	3–5	75	99	4.9	CYP3A4 CYP2D6	Yes
Clozapine	1–4	10–105	92–96	2–5	CYP1A2 CYP3A4	Yes
Iloperidone	2–3.5	5–14	93	NA	Hepatic	
Olanzapine	5–6	20–70	93	10–20	CYP1A2 CYP2D6	No
Quetiapine	1–2	4–10	83	10	CYP3A4	Yes
Remoxipride	1–2	4–7	80	0.7	Hepatic, renal	No
Risperidone	1–1.5	3–24	90	1–1.5	CYP2D6	Yes
Sertindole	10	24–200	>99	20–40	CYP3A4 CYP2D6	Yes
Sulpiride	3–6	5–14	40	2.7	Hepatic, renal	No
Ziprasidone	5	4–10	>99	2	CYP3A4	No

NA, data not available.
Pharmacokinetic data obtained from references 1, 8, 10, 42–44, and 182.

"normal" CYP2D6 individuals.[47,48] Dose adjustment for these patients is unknown. Theoretically, these patients are at greater risk for adverse drug interactions.

Drug Interactions

The coadministration of antipsychotics with other drugs has the potential for numerous clinically significant pharmacodynamic and pharmacokinetic interactions.[49] The CNS and respiratory depressant effects of neuroleptics are potentiated when co-ingested with alcohols, antihistamines, opiates, other psychotropics, and sedative-hypnotics. Fatal cardiopulmonary arrest has occurred when therapeutic doses of clozapine have been taken with lorazepam.[50] Exaggerated anticholinergic effects could occur when certain antipsychotics are coadministered with tricyclic antidepressants, antihistamines, antiparkinson agents, and some skeletal muscle relaxants (e.g., cyclobenzaprine). Hypotension could occur when antipsychotics with α_1-adrenergic antagonistic effects are co-ingested with antihypertensives with similar properties (e.g., prazosin, hydralazine). QT prolongation may occur when cardioactive agents are coadministered with certain antipsychotics (e.g., droperidol,

haloperidol, thioridazine). The combination of lithium and neuroleptic agents can produce a syndrome similar to NMS.[51,52]

Since many neuroleptics are metabolized by the CYP2D6, CYP1A2, and CYP3A4 enzymes, their clearance can be significantly altered when coadministered with inhibitors or inducers of these enzymes (see Table 38-3). A thorough knowledge of the neuroleptic's unique receptor-binding profile and hepatic metabolism will facilitate recognition and treatment of clinically significant drug interactions.

TOXICOLOGY

Clinical Manifestations Following Overdose

Isolated antipsychotic agent overdose is rarely fatal; most patients who overdose on these agents will remain asymptomatic or develop only mild toxicity.[5] Ingested doses that produce acute toxicity and lethality are highly variable; many patients have survived ingestions reported to be lethal in others.[53] Toxicity largely depends on age,

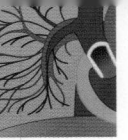

habituation, and comorbid illness of the patient, agent identity, and time to treatment. Tolerance develops to the sedative effects of antipsychotics over a period of days to weeks.[1] Thus, nonhabituated adults and young children (rarely prescribed these agents) are more sensitive to the toxic effects of antipsychotics than those who have ingested the drug chronically. The ingestion of a single tablet of chlorpromazine, clozapine, loxapine, mesoridazine, olanzapine, quetiapine, or thioridazine may cause CNS and respiratory depression in young children.[53–58] Multireceptor, low-potency agents (e.g., clozapine, loxapine, chlorpromazine, thioridazine, and mesidorazine) are more toxic than more selective, high-potency agents (e.g., fluphenazine, haloperidol).[1-5] When death occurs, it usually results from respiratory arrest (prior to medical intervention), arrhythmias, or aspiration-induced respiratory failure.[2]

Clinical effects begin within 30 to 90 minutes and peak within 2 to 6 hours of ingestion. Delayed onset and peak toxicity are possible after ingestion of drugs that slow gastrointestinal motility (e.g., anticholinergic drugs). Resolution of serious toxicity usually occurs by 24 to 48 hours. The toxic effects are similar in adults and children.

CNS depression is the most common finding following overdose.[3,54-64] CNS effects range from lethargy, slurred speech, ataxia, and confusion in mild intoxication, to mild coma with respiratory depression in moderate intoxication, to deep coma with apnea and loss of brainstem and deep tendon reflexes in severe intoxication. Paradoxical agitation and delirium may occur with mixed overdoses and those involving antipsychotic agents with anticholinergic properties (e.g., chlorpromazine, clozapine, mesidorazine, olanzapine, and thioridazine). Respiratory depression that necessitates endotracheal intubation is uncommon but occurs with greater frequency in children, polydrug overdoses, and sedating, multireceptor, low-potency antipsychotics (e.g., aliphatic and piperidine phenothiazines, clozapine, olanzapine, and quetiapine). Apnea and sudden infant death syndrome have been associated with the use of antipsychotic agents.[65] Pulmonary edema can rarely occur.[66]

Seizures are uncommon in overdose, reported in about 1% of patients in large series.[3,57] Seizures, however, appear to occur with greater frequency after ingestion of chlorpromazine, clozapine, loxapine, mesoridazine, and thioridazine. A seizure incidence of 60% and 10% have been reported following loxapine and clozapine overdose, respectively.[28,57,60] Loxapine-induced seizures can be recurrent and severe, resulting in rhabdomyolysis, myoglobinuria, and acute renal failure.[28]

Anticholinergic manifestations (peripheral and central) are frequent following overdoses of thioridazine, mesoridazine, chlorpromazine, clozapine, and olanzapine. These effects include dry, flushed skin; dry mucous membranes; mydriasis; sinus tachycardia; decreased bowel sounds; urinary retention; myoclonic jerking and tremulousness; hyperthermia; agitation; delirium; and coma. Both hyperthermia and hypothermia have been described following antipsychotic overdose. Neuro-

muscular hyperactivity, seizures, the inability to sweat, and cutaneous vasodilation at high ambient temperature increase the likelihood of drug-associated hyperthermia. Coma, hypotension, suppressed shivering capability, and cutaneous vasodilation at low ambient temperatures increase the likelihood of drug-associated hypothermia. Miosis or mydriasis may occur with antipsychotic overdose. Miosis is more likely to occur in seriously poisoned patients with both atypical and typical agents; it has been described in 75% of adults and 72% of children after phenothiazine overdose.[57,60,61,63,67]

The most common cardiovascular manifestations of antipsychotic overdose are sinus tachycardia and orthostatic hypotension.[57,59,60,63] Other cardiovascular effects occur uncommonly and include hypertension, sinus bradycardia, conduction abnormalities, and supraventricular and ventricular tachyarrhythmias. Electrocardiographic (ECG) abnormalities include prolongation of the PR, QRS, and QT intervals, nonspecific ST-T wave changes, depressed ST segments, T wave abnormalities (widening, flattening, notching, and inversion), increased U wave amplitude, rightward shift of the terminal 40 milliseconds of the QRS (i.e., the presence of R in aVR), atrioventricular, bundle branch, fascicular, and intraventricular blocks, and supraventricular and ventricular arrhythmias.[3,68-72] Other than sinus tachycardia, repolarization abnormalities are the earliest and most common ECG abnormalities.[68-72] Serious cardiotoxicity is more common with the aliphatic and piperidine phenothiazines and less common with atypical agents.[3,57] TdP ventricular tachycardia has been reported after overdose of droperidol, haloperidol, mesoridazine, pimozide, and thioridazine.[72-77] Cardiovascular and ECG abnormalities should be apparent within several hours of an acute overdose.

Although EPS are often idiosyncratic reactions that follow therapeutic neuroleptic doses, these effects may also be dose related, and have occurred following overdose with many neuroleptics.[54,59,64] EPS can be the presenting manifestation in a child following accidental neuroleptic poisoning.[54,64,78]

Adverse Effects

All antipsychotics, typical or atypical, are associated with numerous adverse effects. Adverse effects may be idiosyncratic or dose related, can occur early or late in the course of therapy, and are often the result of receptor antagonism.[1] Neurologic and cardiovascular side effects occur most commonly.

EXTRAPYRAMIDAL SIDE EFFECTS

EPS are a group of sustained movement disorders that can occur in approximately 30% of patients treated with antipsychotic agents and often lead to medication noncompliance in those with psychosis.[1,79] All antipsychotics can produce EPS, but the incidence is significantly reduced for newer generation, atypical agents. The incidence of EPS is similar to that with placebo during chronic therapy with clozapine, olanzapine, quetiapine, ziprasidone, and aripiprazole.[14,34,79-81] There are six EPS

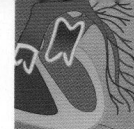

syndromes. They can be divided into the reversible syndromes that occur within hours to days (e.g., acute dystonia, akathisia) or days to weeks (e.g., parkinsonism, NMS) and the potentially irreversible syndromes that occur after months to years of therapy (e.g., TD, focal perioral tremor).[1]

Acute dystonia is a hyperkinetic movement disorder characterized by intermittent, uncoordinated, spasmodic, or sustained involuntary contractions of muscles of the face, tongue, neck, trunk, and extremities. Clinical manifestations include facial grimacing, trismus, blepharospasm, oculogyric crisis, tongue protrusion, buccolingual crisis, retrocollis, torticollis, opisthotonus, abnormal postures and gait, tortipelvis, and respiratory difficulty. ADRs, although distressing to patients, are rarely life threatening. Pharyngeal and laryngeal muscle spasm has produced respiratory distress and asphyxia.[82]

ADRs usually occur soon after initiation of antipsychotic therapy or after an increase in dose. Fifty percent occur within 48 hours and 90% within the first 5 days of treatment.[83,84] The peak incidence occurs when antipsychotic concentrations are declining in the serum. In one study of pediatric patients, ADRs occurred 5 to 50 hours (mean 23 hours) after the first therapeutic dose and 1 to 20 hours (mean 5 hours) after single accidental ingestion of phenothiazines.[85] The incidence of ADRs varies according to the agent's identity, dose, route of administration, and duration of therapy, and the presence of individual risk factors. The incidence is lowest with agents that have low D_2 receptor potency and/or high relative potency at $5\text{-}HT_2$, $5\text{-}HT_{1A}$, M_1, α_2, or D_4 receptors (atypical agents). Incidence rates of 25%, 16%, 8.3%, 3.5%, and less than 1% have been described for IM fluphenazine decanoate, haloperidol, thiothixene, chlorpromazine, and atypical agents, respectively.[33,83,84] Individual risk factors include male gender, young age (peak range 5 to 45 years), a family history or personal history of ADRs, or a recent history of cocaine or alcohol use.[33,83,84,86,87]

Akathisia is a condition of subjective unease and motor restlessness that occurs within minutes to days of initiation or increase of antipsychotic drug dosing.[14,81] It is usually observed within the first 3 months of treatment.[1] Akathisia may be misinterpreted as anxiety or agitation related to an underlying psychiatric condition. Akathisia is characterized by the inability to sit still and the overwhelming need to continuously move the legs or get up and walk or pace. Patients are frequently anxious, agitated, or unable to concentrate. About 30% of patients ingesting traditional agents develop akathisia.[1,8,10,14,81] The incidence is less with atypical agents, with an incidence range of 5% to 15%.[88,89] Akathisia is more likely to occur with the use of higher-potency D_2 antagonists, larger doses, rapid dose escalation, and parenteral antipsychotic administration.[14,81,88]

Parkinsonism is a reversible, intermediate-stage EPS that typically occurs gradually over days to weeks and is evident by 2 to 3 months of therapy.[1] Parkinsonism is characterized by muscle rigidity (cogwheel type), bradykinesia or akinesia, mask facies, shuffling gait, tremor (e.g., pill rolling), and cognitive impairment.

Antipsychotic-induced parkinsonism occurs in 13% of patients who take antipsychotic agents chronically.[6,14] Antipsychotic-induced parkinsonism occurs in all age groups but occurs with greater frequency in the elderly. Other risk factors for its occurrence include female sex, the presence of organic brain injury, use of high-potency agents, and long duration of therapy.[1,6,14,81] The rabbit syndrome is an uncommon reversible late-onset EPS characterized by perioral lip tremor. It usually occurs after months or years of antipsychotic treatment and is considered a variant of parkinsonism.[1]

TD is a hyperkinetic, late-onset EPS that typically occurs after 2 years of antipsychotic therapy and only rarely before 6 months.[1,14,81] It is characterized by involuntary, painless, stereotyped, repetitive movements of orofacial structures and, occasionally, the trunk and arms. These movements include chewing; tongue protrusion; lip smacking, sucking, and pursing; facial grimacing; grunting; rapid eye blinking; and occasionally choreoathetosis of the trunk and limbs. TD is associated with all antipsychotic agents, but the incidence is significantly lower with atypical agents, particularly clozapine. TD develops in 15% to 25% of patients on long-term antipsychotic therapy. An annual incidence of 3% to 5% is described with traditional antipsychotics, whereas atypical agents have an annual incidence of less than 2%.[90] TD occurs in patients of all ages (including children) but occurs more commonly in women older than 50 years.[91] TD is frequently elicited in patients who have their drug discontinued or dose lowered after years of therapy.[1,91]

NMS is an uncommon but potentially fatal idiosyncratic complication of antipsychotic drug therapy. NMS is often considered an extreme, severe form of EPS[92-95] (see also Chapter 10A). NMS usually occurs early in the course of treatment or soon after a change in dose but may appear at any time during therapy. It is estimated that NMS occurs in 2 out of every 1000 patients treated with neuroleptics.[95] While NMS has been associated with all antipsychotic agents, most cases have been secondary to the high-potency agents haloperidol and fluphenazine, particularly their depot formulations. NMS is not a result of overdose and usually occurs with antipsychotic serum concentrations in the therapeutic range. Potential risk factors for development of NMS include rapid initiation of antipsychotic therapy; use of high-potency agents and depot preparations; dehydration; severe patient agitation or catatonia; requirement of restraints or patient seclusion; preexisting organic brain disease, mental retardation, or affective disorder; a history of NMS or electroconvulsive therapy (ECT); poorly controlled EPS; and concomitant use of predisposing drugs, namely lithium, anticholinergic agents, and antiparkinson agents.[92-98] NMS occurs more commonly in men (2:1 male:female ratio), with a mean age of 40 years.[92-98]

NMS typically develops over a period of 24 to 72 hours and is commonly characterized by the tetrad of altered consciousness, fever (temperature greater than 38° C), muscular rigidity, and autonomic dysfunction.[92-98] Altered mental status includes lethargy, agitation, mutism,

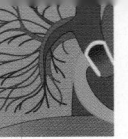

stupor, and coma. Muscular rigidity is lead pipe and cogwheel type, similar to parkinsonism.[1] Autonomic dysfunction includes fever, tachycardia, tachypnea, hypertension or hypotension, diaphoresis, sialorrhea, pallor, flushing, urinary incontinence, and cardiac arrhythmias. Other common findings include EPS (e.g., tremor, bradykinesia, akinesia, festinating gait, chorea, dystonia, dysphagia, dysarthria, aphonia), mutism, seizures, abnormal reflexes, dyspnea, and hypoxemia. Laboratory abnormalities include elevated serum creatine phosphokinase (greater than three times normal) in up to 97% of cases, leukocytosis, elevated levels of hepatic transaminases, hyper- or hyponatremia, metabolic acidosis, myoglobinuria, elevated serum blood urea nitrogen and creatinine, and decreased serum iron levels.[40,41,92-99] Medical complications of NMS include rhabdomyolysis, myoglobinuric renal failure, aspiration pneumonitis, pulmonary edema, pulmonary embolism, respiratory failure, sepsis, coagulopathy, disseminated intravascular coagulation, seizures, myocardial infarction, cardiac arrhythmias, peripheral neuropathy, necrotizing enterocolitis, and periarticular ossification.[92-99]

The presence of fever and muscle rigidity is usually required for diagnosis, but their absence has been associated with certain NMS variants. NMS is best considered a heterogeneous syndrome with variable signs, symptoms, and severity.[93-95] Most cases of NMS seem to follow a sequence of development. Mental status changes and muscular rigidity precede autonomic dysfunction and fever in over 80% of cases.[100] Early recognition of confusion, catatonia, or worsening EPS may facilitate timely treatment and halt progression to the fulminant syndrome.[100]

Once antipsychotics are discontinued, the signs and symptoms of NMS resolve over a period of 1 to 61 days, with a mean duration of approximately 10 days.[94-97] The clinical course is nearly twice as long in patients who have received IM depot preparations.[94-97] NMS was initially characterized as malignant due to its frequent fatal outcome. Mortality rate, once estimated to range from 17% to 28%, now ranges from 0 to 11.6%.[92-102]

SEIZURES

Seizures are usually generalized and major motor type. Risk factors for seizures include a history of organic brain disease, epilepsy, drug-associated seizures, or ECT, an abnormal baseline EEG, polypharmacy, initiation of antipsychotic therapy, rapid dose titration and/or use of large antipsychotic doses, and the use of certain antipsychotic agents.[23-29] Seizures occur most commonly with chlorpromazine, clozapine, and loxapine; the risk is dose dependent with these agents.[25,28,29,57] A 0.5% incidence of seizures has been reported with low to moderate doses of chlorpromazine (30 to 900 mg/day) and 9% incidence with daily doses greater than 1 g.[23] A seizure incidence of 1.8% has been reported with moderate doses of clozapine (300 to 600 mg/day), whereas those taking greater than 600 mg/day have an incidence of 4.4%.[24,27,29] Seizures are unlikely to occur during therapeutic dosing with other antipsychotics;

the incidence is comparable with that of placebo (less than 1%).[24]

CARDIOVASCULAR

Although repolarization abnormalities (e.g., prolongation of the QT interval) and arrhythmias are dose dependent and have been reported most frequently with antipsychotic overdose, these findings can also occur with therapeutic doses of these agents. QT prolongation has been associated with therapeutic dosing and overdose of aliphatic and piperidine phenothiazines, droperidol, haloperidol, loxapine, pimozide, quetiapine, risperidone, sertindole, and ziprasidone.[3,28,68-77,103-117] The U.S. manufacturer of sertindole (Abbott Laboratories, North Chicago, IL) withdrew its new drug application for consideration by the Food and Drug Administration (FDA) due to concern that therapeutic dosing would be associated with TdP and sudden death. The rare association of ventricular arrhythmia (e.g., TdP) with therapeutic doses of droperidol (typically large doses) caused the FDA to issue a "black box" warning to U.S. health care practitioners in December 2001.[115] Sudden unexplained death has been described in otherwise healthy patients taking therapeutic doses of many antipsychotic drugs.[104,115-117] These deaths are presumed to be the result of malignant ventricular arrhythmias (e.g., TdP).[116,117] In one series of sudden death from antipsychotics, more than half were associated with thioridazine.[104]

Myocarditis and cardiomyopathy have rarely been associated with the therapeutic use of antipsychotic agents. Ten cases of myocarditis, some with eosinophilic cellular infiltrates, have been described in association with clozapine; this adverse effect is rare, idiosyncratic, often occurs within 1 to 2 weeks of starting therapy, is likely the result of acute hypersensitivity, and may be fatal.[118,119]

METABOLIC

Recently, the therapeutic use of the benzepines (e.g., clozapine, olanzapine, and quetiapine) and aripiprazole has been associated with an increased risk for developing type 2 diabetes mellitus or diabetic ketoacidosis (DKA).[120-124] Numerous cases of fatal DKA or hyperglycemic hyperosmolar nonketotic coma have been reported in patients taking either clozapine or olanzapine.[125-129] African Americans appear to be affected disproportionately as compared with other races.[130] Hypertriglyceridemia has also been reported in patients taking olanzapine, clozapine, and quetiapine.[131-134] Nonalcoholic steatohepatitis has been associated with the therapeutic use of olanzapine and risperidone, and pancreatitis has been associated with the use of clozapine.[135,136] Asymptomatic elevations of hepatic transaminases (both cholestatic and hepatitic pattern) have been reported with most neuroleptics.[137-139] These elevations are usually idiosyncratic, self-limiting, and typically occur during the first 3 months of therapy. Most atypical antipsychotics produce increased appetite and weight gain; these side effects occur most commonly

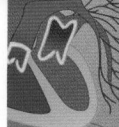

with benzepine agents and are likely associated with the increased risk for acquired diabetes mellitus.[1,14,57] Priapism, allergic dermatitis, photosensitivity, cholestatic jaundice, and pigmentation of the skin, cornea, lens, and retina have been associated with therapeutic phenothiazine use.[1]

HEMATOLOGIC TOXICITY

Agranulocytosis (absolute neutrophil count of less than 500 per cubic millimeter) is a life-threatening idiosyncratic reaction that can rarely occur with phenothiazine and clozapine therapy. Agranulocytosis occurs in approximately 1 in 10,000 patients taking chlorpromazine and 1 in 100 patients taking clozapine.[140-143] Early recognition (by regular white blood cell monitoring) and treatment (use of granulocyte colony-stimulating factor [G-CSF]) of clozapine-associated agranulocytosis has reduced its mortality to 3% to 4%.[130] Prompt treatment with the use of G-CSF and granulocyte-macrophage colony-stimulating factor (GM-CSF) has reduced the duration of granulocytopenia from a mean of 16 days to 8 days.[144] Agranulocytosis has also been reported with the use of olanzapine, quetiapine, and risperidone.[145-147] Clozapine has been associated with an increased risk for thromboembolic disease.[148]

DIAGNOSIS

The diagnosis of antipsychotic poisoning is based on a positive history of ingestion, suggestive physical findings, and supporting evidence from the ECG, laboratory, and other adjunctive tests. Physical findings that suggest antipsychotic agent toxicity include CNS and/or respiratory depression, anticholinergic stigmata, miosis, hypotension, and EPS. The presence of sinus tachycardia and/or repolarization abnormalities on ECG supports a history of antipsychotic agent poisoning. Phenothiazines and butyrophenones are radiopaque and often visible on abdominal radiographs. The use of abdominal radiography as a diagnostic aid is not recommended, however, since a normal radiograph does not rule out significant ingestion of these or other antipsychotic agents. Similarly, although the Forrest, ferric chloride, and Phenistix colorimetric urine tests can be positive in the setting of phenothiazine ingestion, the tests are both insensitive and nonspecific.[149] Thus, they should not be used to confirm or rule out ingestion of either phenothiazine or nonphenothiazine antipsychotics.

Comprehensive screening of urine (using gas chromatography and mass spectrometry) may be used to qualitatively confirm the presence of most antipsychotics. Comprehensive testing, however, is not routinely available at most hospitals, and results are often delayed beyond 4 to 6 hours. In addition, comprehensive tests have other limitations. False-negative results may occur with newer atypical agents or if testing is performed too early or late following exposure. For instance, a false-negative screen is likely to occur for a patient who presents with EPS more than 24 hours after ingestion of a single antipsychotic tablet. Quantitative drug concentrations can also be performed for most antipsychotic agents (usually from the drug manufacturer). Serum drug concentrations, however, will not guide therapy; they do not correlate well with clinical toxicity and are not readily available. It should be recognized that certain antipsychotics (e.g., chlorpromazine, mesoridazine, quetiapine, and thioridazine) will often produce false-positive results for tricyclic antidepressants on many commercial immunoassay screens for drugs of abuse.[150]

The diagnosis of NMS is clinical and based on a positive history of antipsychotic exposure and suggestive physical findings. The adoption and use of standardized criteria to make the diagnosis is recommended (Box 38-1).[35,95,151,152] Fever and muscular rigidity should be present to make the diagnosis of NMS, and the diagnosis should not be made before other medical illnesses (e.g., CNS infection) have been excluded.

Differential Diagnosis

Toxicity from antipsychotic agents produces signs and symptoms that are similar to many toxicologic and nontoxicologic entities. The CNS and cardiovascular manifestations of antipsychotic overdose may be similar to effects produced by alcohols, antiarrhythmics, anticholinergics, antiepileptics, antihistamines, barbiturates, cyclic antidepressants, lithium, opiates, sedative-hypnotics, and skeletal muscle relaxants. Toxicity from chlorpromazine, loxapine, mesoridazine and thioridazine can be clinically indistinguishable from that of cyclic antidepressants. CNS infection, traumatic head injury, cerebrovascular accidents, and metabolic disturbances should be considered and ruled out with appropriate testing. ADRs must be differentiated from anticholinergic, antiepileptic, and strychnine poisoning, CNS or oropharyngeal infections, hypocalcemia, hypomagnesemia, temporomandibular joint dislocations, cerebrovascular accidents, and conversion disorders. Akathisia may be mistaken for acute anxiety or agitation associated with underlying psychosis.[1] NMS must be differentiated from the anticholinergic, serotonin, and sedative-hypnotic withdrawal syndromes; poisoning by hallucinogens, lithium, monoamine oxidase inhibitors, strychnine, and sympathomimetics; and intracranial hemorrhage, thyrotoxicosis, heat stroke, pheochromocytoma, malignant hyperthermia, and lethal catatonia.

Malignant hyperthermia should not be confused with NMS. Malignant hyperthermia is a rare, inherited disorder of skeletal muscle calcium metabolism. Exposure to certain anesthetic agents (e.g., succinylcholine, halothane) or stress precipitates enhanced release and impaired reuptake of calcium from the sarcoplasmic reticulum in skeletal muscle cells. The result is excessive excitation-contraction coupling and a syndrome of muscle rigidity and fever that may appear clinically similar to NMS. Unlike NMS, malignant hyperthermia is associated with general anesthesia and not antipsychotics.

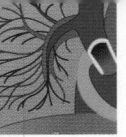

| BOX 38-1 | USEFUL DIAGNOSTIC CRITERIA FOR NEUROLEPTIC MALIGNANT SYNDROME (NMS) |

Criterion 1*

A. Treatment with neuroleptic agents within 7 days of symptom onset (2–4 weeks for depot agents)

B. Fever > 38° C

C. Muscle rigidity

D. Five of the following:
1. Change in mental status
2. Tachycardia
3. Hypertension or hypotension
4. Tachypnea or hypoxia
5. Diaphoresis or sialorrhea
6. Tremor
7. Incontinence
8. Increased CPK or myoglobinuria
9. Leukocytosis
10. Metabolic acidosis

Criterion 2†

A. Major:
1. Fever
2. Rigidity
3. Elevated CPK concentration

B. Minor:
1. Tachycardia
2. Abnormal arterial blood pressure
3. Tachypnea
4. Altered mental status
5. Diaphoresis
6. Leukocytosis

C. The presence of all three major criteria, or two major and three minor criteria indicate a high likelihood of NMS

D. Symptoms are supported by an appropriate clinical history

Criterion 3‡

A. Development of muscle rigidity and fever associated with the use of neuroleptics

B. At least two of the following:
Change in level of consciousness
Mutism
Tachycardia
Hypertension or labile blood pressure
Diaphoresis
Dysphagia
Tremor
Incontinence
Leukocytosis
Laboratory evidence of muscle injury (e.g., elevated CPK)

C. Symptoms in A and B are not due to another substance or to a neurologic or general medical condition

D. Symptoms in A and B are not better accounted for by a mental disorder

CPK, creatine phosphokinase.
*Data from reference 95.
† Data from reference 152.
‡ Data from reference 151.

MANAGEMENT

Overdose

OVERVIEW

Treatment for antipsychotic agent poisoning is mainly supportive.[58] Patients with significant CNS or respiratory depression should have their airway protected, breathing assisted, and cardiovascular support provided as necessary. All patients should have continuous cardiac monitoring, an intravenous (IV) line established, and an ECG performed. Supplemental oxygen, continuous pulse oximetry, and parenteral thiamine, dextrose (or rapid fingerstick glucose determination), and naloxone should be considered for patients with altered mental status or seizures. Semicomatose patients should be placed in the left lateral, head-down position to minimize the risk for aspiration. Frequent vital sign and neurologic evaluations are necessary. Routine laboratory analysis should include a complete blood count and measure-

ment of electrolytes, blood urea nitrogen, creatinine, glucose concentrations, and pregnancy testing for women of childbearing age. Serum acetaminophen and salicylate concentrations should be performed for all intentional overdose patients. For patients with seizures or hyperthermia, laboratory evaluation should also include an arterial blood gas, urinalysis, and measurement of serum creatine phosphokinase, calcium, and magnesium concentrations. A complete blood count should also be obtained on any patient who presents with a fever while taking clozapine or chlorpromazine.

SEIZURES

Seizures are often self-limited and may not require specific treatment. If prolonged or recurrent, seizures should be treated with benzodiazepines (e.g., lorazepam 0.05 to 0.1 mg/kg IV). Barbiturates (e.g., phenobarbital 10 to 20 mg/kg IV) are reserved for seizures refractory to benzodiazepine therapy. Pentobarbital coma may rarely be necessary for patients with status epilepticus

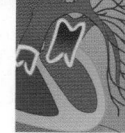

associated with certain antipsychotics (e.g., loxapine). The efficacy and safety of phenytoin treatment for antipsychotic-associated seizures is unknown. Measurements of blood glucose concentration and core temperature are imperative for those with seizures.

CARDIOVASCULAR

Hypotension is treated initially by placing the patient in the Trendelenberg position and administering IV crystalloid boluses (10 to 40 mL/kg). α-Adrenergic agonists (e.g., norepinephrine, phenylephrine) are the preferred vasopressors for treatment of refractory hypotension. Dopamine, an indirect-acting vasopressor, may be ineffective and is not recommended as a first-line agent for hypotension. Central venous, peripheral arterial, or pulmonary arterial catheter monitoring is recommended for patients requiring prolonged vasopressor therapy. Intraventricular conduction delay (e.g., prolonged QRS on ECG) and ventricular arrhythmias should be treated with sodium bicarbonate (1 to 2 mEq/kg IV bolus followed by intermittent boluses or continuous infusion).[153] Lidocaine (1 to 1.5 mg/kg IV) is an acceptable alternative or second-line agent for ventricular arrhythmias.[154] Types Ia (e.g., quinidine, procainamide), Ic (e.g., propafenone), II, III (e.g., amiodarone), and IV antiarrhythmic agents should be avoided in patients with cardiac conduction disturbances and/or ventricular arrhythmias. Their use may potentiate such cardiotoxicity.[154] TdP ventricular tachycardia should be treated in the standard fashion (e.g., IV magnesium and/or lidocaine, overdrive pacing with isoproterenol or electrical pacing, correction of electrolyte disturbances).[155-158] Sinus tachycardia associated with antipsychotic poisoning does not require specific treatment.

ANTICHOLINERGIC SYNDROME

Physostigmine may be used to control agitation and reverse delirium in patients with the anticholinergic syndrome (ACS) from certain antipsychotics (see Chapter 39). It has been used successfully for patients with ACS associated with chlorpromazine, clozapine, olanzapine, and thioridazine.[57,60,159,160] Physostigmine is safe provided that the ECG does not demonstrate cardiac conduction disturbances (e.g., prolonged PR or QRS intervals).[159] Physostigmine should be given slowly IV (0.02 mg/kg in children, or 2 mg in adults) over 3 minutes. Because the clinical duration of action of physostigmine is short (20 to 90 minutes) compared with that of antipsychotic agents, resolution of the anticholinergic stigmata after physostigmine administration should not alter patient disposition. Agitation associated with the ACS from antipsychotics may also be treated with benzodiazepines.

DECONTAMINATION AND ENHANCED ELIMINATION

Gastrointestinal decontamination should be initiated rapidly after patient stabilization. Single-dose administration of activated charcoal (1 g/kg orally or by nasogastric tube) is the preferred method of gastrointestinal

decontamination. Orogastric lavage is not routinely recommended since the risk for death following acute neuroleptic overdose is very low. If performed, gastric lavage should be followed by the administration of activated charcoal. Due to slowed gut motility and delayed drug absorption produced by the anticholinergic effects of many antipsychotics, activated charcoal administration is still recommended when patients present several hours after an overdose. The clinical benefit of this recommendation, however, is likely minimal. Forced emesis, use of cathartics, whole bowel irrigation, and multiple-dose activated charcoal are not recommended for antipsychotic poisoning due to their low likelihood to provide clinical benefit. Extracorporeal removal techniques are not recommended as part of treatment for antipsychotic poisoning since these agents have large volumes of distribution and high plasma protein binding.

Extrapyramidal Side Effects

ADRS

Treatment of ADRs may rarely require supplemental oxygen and assisted ventilation for patients with respiratory difficulty from laryngeal and pharyngeal dystonia. The usual treatment is parenteral administration of either diphenhydramine (1 mg/kg IV or IM) or benztropine (1 to 2 mg IV or IM in adults, or 0.02 to 0.05 mg/kg in pediatric patients). ADRs typically respond within 5 to 10 minutes of IV anticholinergic administration, but repeat dosing may be necessary for its complete resolution. If dystonia does not respond to anticholinergic therapy, diazepam (0.1 mg/kg IV) or lorazepam (0.05 to 1.0 mg/kg IV) may be effective. Following parenteral therapy, an oral anticholinergic agent should be administered for the next 48 to 72 hours to prevent dystonia recurrence.[161]

AKATHISIA

No treatment for akathisia is uniformly effective.[88] Anticholinergic drugs significantly reduce the incidence of akathisia when administered prior to or concomitant with antipsychotic agents.[162] Although recommended as first-line treatment for established akathisia, anticholinergic therapy often fails to provide consistent and adequate symptom relief.[81,163] Alternatively, benzodiazepines may provide effective symptom relief.[88] Patients who develop akathisia but require chronic antipsychotic treatment may benefit from reduction of the antipsychotic dose, substitution with another atypical agent, administration of propranolol (10 mg orally three times per day), clonidine (0.1 mg orally three times per day), cyproheptadine (16 mg/day), anticholinergic agents (e.g., benztropine or diphenhydramine), or benzodiazepines (e.g., diazepam).[88,164-167]

PARKINSONISM

Drug-induced parkinsonism may be minimized by using low doses of traditional antipsychotics, changing to an atypical agent, or adding either an anticholinergic agent (e.g., benztropine or diphenhydramine) or one that enhances dopaminergic activity (e.g., amantadine).[81]

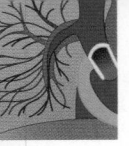

TARDIVE DYSKINESIA

Once tardive dyskinesia (TD) develops, it is difficult to treat and may be irreversible. The best treatment is to minimize its risk for occurrence.[168] Antipsychotic drugs should be administered at the lowest possible effective doses, and periodic reevaluation should be performed to determine the continued need for antipsychotic therapy and evaluate for the earliest signs of TD.[81,168] Because TD is a progressively irreversible disorder, early detection and prompt antipsychotic withdrawal will increase the likelihood of complete recovery. Atypical agents should preferentially be used for long-term therapy since they have a lower propensity for producing TD. Anticholinergic agents will exacerbate TD and should not be used.[1] While higher doses of antipsychotic agents will temporarily relieve the symptoms of TD, this treatment is discouraged because it will further enhance dopamine receptor dysfunction and lead to worsening dyskinesia.[1,81,168]

NEUROLEPTIC MALIGNANT SYNDROME

Successful treatment of neuroleptic malignant syndrome (NMS) requires prompt recognition, immediate withdrawal of antipsychotic and NMS-potentiating drugs (e.g., lithium or anticholinergics), exclusion of other medical conditions that could simulate or complicate NMS, and the provision of good supportive care. Good supportive care necessitates the provision of adequate ventilation and oxygenation, rehydration, aggressive temperature reduction, nutritional support, low-dose heparin to prevent thromboembolic disease, antibiotics to treat concurrent infection, and treatment of cardiopulmonary, metabolic, and renal complications.[99] Gastrointestinal decontamination is not necessary since NMS is associated with therapeutic dosing of antipsychotic agents. Empirical antibiotic administration is prudent due to the difficulty in differentiating NMS from a systemic infectious process and the high incidence of concurrent infection. Prophylactic intubation should be strongly considered for patients with excessive sialorrhea, swallowing dysfunction, coma, hypoxia, acidosis, or muscular rigidity associated with their hyperthermia.

The role of specific pharmacotherapies for NMS is controversial since most data on individual agent efficacy comes from retrospective studies and case reports. Although each therapy has been reported effective anecdotally in the management of NMS, none has been consistently beneficial or clearly superior to supportive care alone.[94,95,99,169] Specific treatment measures include dantrolene, nondepolarizing neuromuscular paralysis, benzodiazepines, bromocriptine, amantadine, levodopa/carbidopa, nifedipine, nitroprusside, and ECT.

Anticholinergic agents are not recommended for treatment of NMS; they are considered ineffective and may worsen hyperthermia.[37,94,95] One retrospective study in children and adolescents with NMS, however, noted a reduction in the duration of illness associated with the use of anticholinergic agents.[97]

Dantrolene is a hydantoin derivative that inhibits the release of ionized calcium from the sarcoplasmic reticulum. It causes direct muscle relaxation by uncoupling excitation-contraction in the skeletal muscle. It is used to control NMS-associated rigidity and hyperthermia. It can be administered orally or intravenously. While the initial dosing is 1 to 2.5 mg/kg every 6 hours, doses up to 10 mg/kg/day are considered safe.[94,95,170,171] Dantrolene should be continued until the signs and symptoms of NMS resolve.

Bromocriptine, a dopamine receptor agonist, is given orally three times daily (2.5 to 10 mg/dose).[94,95,99] Amantadine, which enhances presynaptic dopamine release, is given orally two times per day (100 to 200 mg per dose).[94,95,99] Levodopa/carbidopa, which increases presynaptic dopamine stores, is given orally three to four times daily (25/250 mg per dose). Dopamine agonists are given alone or in conjunction with dantrolene or other muscle relaxants. For both dantrolene and dopamine agonist therapy, it is recommended that treatment be tapered over a period of days.[92,172] Signs of NMS have returned when pharmacotherapies have been abruptly discontinued.[173]

In one retrospective analysis of 67 cases of NMS, dantrolene or bromocriptine reduced mean times to improvement and complete resolution of toxicity as compared with supportive care alone.[174] Mean response time to clinical improvement was 1.0 day for bromocriptine, 1.7 days for dantrolene, and 6.8 days for supportive care alone. Mean time to complete resolution was 9.0 days for dantrolene, 9.8 days for bromocriptine, and 15.8 days for supportive care alone. A prospective nonrandomized study of 20 patients with NMS, however, demonstrated a more prolonged illness and greater complication rates with bromocriptine or dantrolene treatment as compared with supportive care alone.[175] The mean duration of illness was 9.9 days for patients receiving bromocriptine/dantrolene versus 6.8 days for patients receiving supportive care. In retrospective analyses, dopamine agonists have been reported to reduce NMS mortality rates significantly, from 21% to 9.2%.[176,177] The addition of dantrolene to bromocriptine treatment does not offer additional survival advantage.

ECT has been employed successfully for NMS. In one review of 29 patients, a positive response occurred in 83% of patients.[178] Some suggest that the mortality rate of NMS patients treated with ECT is lower than that of patients treated supportively.[178] ECT should be reserved for severely affected patients since this therapy has been associated with cardiac arrhythmias, cerebral edema, and death.[95]

Prompt reduction of NMS-associated muscle rigidity and hyperthermia can be expected to minimize the risk for rhabdomyolysis, renal failure, pneumonia, respiratory failure, disseminated intravascular coagulation, and cardiovascular collapse. These complications are responsible for most NMS-associated deaths, and, thus, their prevention is paramount. Since NMS-associated hyperthermia occurs primarily from muscular rigidity, rapid peripheral muscle relaxation is imperative. Dantrolene and bromocriptine take a day or more to achieve fever reduction. Nondepolarizing neuromuscular paralysis will provide rapid, predictable, and effective resolution of rigidity and fever and should be the first-

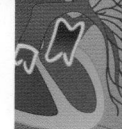

line treatment for patients who have severe hyperthermia (e.g., core temperature greater than or equal to 40° C). Pancuronium administration has been effective for the rapid control of fever and rigidity in patients with severe NMS.[179]

For patients with less severe NMS, a logical first approach to the management of fever and rigidity is the administration of benzodiazepines (e.g., diazepam 0.1 to 0.4 mg/kg or lorazepam 0.05 to 0.1 mg/kg IV) coupled with antipyretics, evaporative cooling, ice packs, and cooled IV fluids.[180] The addition of dopamine agonist therapy and dantrolene may be helpful. If muscle rigidity persists and core temperature reaches 40° C despite these therapies, neuromuscular paralysis with a nondepolarizing paralytic agent is recommended. The level of intervention depends on the severity of illness.

Disposition

Most patients with pure neuroleptic overdose develop only mild toxicity and are medically safe for psychiatric evaluation and disposition after an observation period of 4 to 6 hours in the emergency department. Patients who have continued evidence of mild toxicity (e.g., sinus tachycardia, mild CNS depression, QTc prolongation) at 6 hours should be admitted to a monitored bed for continued observation. Patients with evidence of moderate or severe toxicity at any time (e.g., significant CNS and/or respiratory depression, cardiac arrhythmias or conduction disturbances, acidosis, prolonged hypotension, seizures, ACS) should be admitted to the intensive care unit for supportive care. Due to its significant associated morbidity, all patients suspected of having NMS should be admitted initially to the intensive care unit.

REFERENCES

1. Baldessarini RJ, Tarazi FI: Drugs and the treatment of psychiatric disorders: psychosis and mania. In Hardman JG, Limbrid LE, Gilman AG (eds): Goodman & Gilman's The Pharmacological Basis of Therapeutics, 10th ed. New York, McGraw-Hill, 2001, pp 485–520.
2. Buckley N, McManus P: Fatal toxicity of drugs used in the treatment of psychotic illnesses. Br J Psychiatry 1998;172:461–464.
3. Buckley NA, Whyte IM, Dawson AH: Thioridazine has greater cardiotoxicity in overdose than other neuroleptics, J Toxicol Clin Toxicol 1995;33:199–204.
4. Schreinzer D, Frey R, Stimpfl T, et al: Different fatal toxicity of neuroleptics identified by autopsy. Eur Neuropsychopharmacol 2001;11:117–124.
5. Watson WA, Litovitz TL, Rodger GC, et al: 2004 annual report of the American Association of Poison Control Centers Toxic Exposure Surveillance System. Am J Emerg Med 2005;23:589–666.
6. Richelson E: Receptor pharmacology of neuroleptics: relation to clinical effects. J Clin Psychiatry 1999;60(Suppl 10):5–14.
7. Blin O: A comparative review of new antipsychotics. Can J Psychiatry 1999;44:235–244.
8. Jibson MD, Tandon R: New atypical antipsychotic medications. J Psychiatr Res 1998;32:215–218.
9. Tandon R, Milner K, Jibson MD: Antipsychotics from theory to practice: integrating clinical and basic data. J Clin Psychiatry 1999;60(Suppl 8):21–28.
10. Borison RL: Recent advances in the pharmacotherapy of schizophrenia. Harvard Rev Psychiatry 1997;4:255–271.
11. Seeman P, Lee T, Chau-Wong M, Wong K: Antipsychotic drug doses and neuroleptic dopamine receptors. Nature 1976;261:717–719.
12. Farde L, Nordstrom AL, Wiesel FA, et al: Positron emission tomographic analysis of central D1 and D2 dopamine receptor occupancy in patients treated with classical neuroleptics and clozapine. Relation to extrapyramidal side effects. Arch Gen Psychiatry 1992;49:538–544.
13. Black JL, Richelson E: Antipsychotic drugs: prediction of side effect profiles based on neuroreceptor data derived from human brain tissue. Mayo Clin Proc 1987;62:369–372.
14. Casey DE: The relationship of pharmacology to side effects. J Clin Psychiatry 1997;58(Suppl 10):55–62.
15. Meltzer HY, Li Z, Kaneda Y, et al: Serotonin receptors: their key role in drugs to treat schizophrenia. Prog Neuropsychopharmacol Biol Psychiatry 2003;27:1159–1172.
16. Kapur S, Remington G: Serotonin-dopamine interaction and its relevance to schizophrenia. Am J Psychiatry 1996;153:466–476.
17. Kinon BJ, Lieberman JA: Mechanisms of action of atypical antipsychotic drugs: a critical analysis. Psychopharmacology 1996;124:2–34.
18. Risch SC: Pathophysiology of schizophrenia and the role of newer antipsychotics. Pharmacotherapy 1996;16(Suppl):11–14.
19. Ogata N, Narahashi T: Block of sodium channels by psychotropic drugs in single guinea-pig cardiac myocytes. Br J Pharmacol 1989;97:905–913.
20. Drolet B, Cincet F, Rail J, et al: Thioridazine lengthens repolarization of cardiac ventricular myocytes by blocking the delayed rectifier potassium current. J Pharmacol Exp Ther 1999;288:1261–1268.
21. Rampe D, Murawsky K, Grau J, Lewis EW: The antipsychotic agent sertindole is a high affinity antagonist of the human cardiac potassium channel HERG. J Pharmacol Exp Ther 1998;286:788–793.
22. Gould RJ, Murphy KMM, Reynolds IJ, et al: Antischizophrenic drugs of the diphenylbutylpiperidine type act as calcium channel antagonists. Proc Natl Acad Sci U S A 1983;86:5122–5125.
23. Logothetis J: Spontaneous epileptic seizures and electroencephalographic changes in the course of phenothiazine therapy. Neurology 1967;17:869.
24. Cold JA, Wills BG, Froemming JH: Seizure activity associated with antipsychotic therapy. DICP 1990;24:601–606.
25. Hedges D, Jeppson K, Whitehead P: Antipsychotic medication and seizures: a review. Drugs Today (Barc) 2003;39:551–557.
26. Pisani F, Oteri G, Costa C, et al: Effects of psychotropic drugs on seizure threshold. Drug Saf 2002;25:91–110.
27. Alldredge BK: Seizure risk associated with psychotropic drugs: clinical and pharmacokinetic considerations. Neurology 1999;53(Suppl 2):68–75.
28. Peterson C: Seizures induced by acute loxapine overdose. Am J Psychiatry 1981;138:1089–1091.
29. Devinsky D, Honigfeld G, Patin J: Clozapine-related seizures. Neurology 1991;41:369–371.
30. Marsden CD, Jenner P: The pathophysiology of extrapyramidal side-effects of neuroleptic drugs. Psychol Med 1980;10:55–72.
31. Baldessarini RJ, Tarsy D: Dopamine and the pathophysiology of dyskinesia induced by antipsychotic drugs. Ann Rev Neurosci 1980;3:23–41.
32. Carlsson A, Walters N, Carlsson ML: Neurotransmitter interactions in schizophrenia—therapeutic implications. Biol Psychiatry 1999;46:1388–1395.
33. Rupniak NMJ, Jenner P, Marsden CD: Acute dystonia induced by neuroleptic drugs. Psychopharmacology 1986;88:403–419.
34. Kolbe H, Clow A, Jenner P, et al: Neuroleptic-induced acute dystonic reactions may be due to enhanced dopamine release or to supersensitive postsynaptic receptors. Neurology 1981;31:434–439.
35. Mann SC, Caroff SN, Lazarus A: Pathogenesis of neuroleptic malignant syndrome. Psychiatr Ann 1991;21:175–180.
36. Henderson VW, Wooten GF: Neuroleptic malignant syndrome: a pathophysiologic role for the dopamine receptor blockade? Neurology 1981;1331:132–137.
37. Ebadi M, Pfeiffer RF, Murrin LC: Pathogenesis and treatment of neuroleptic malignant syndrome. Gen Pharmacol 1990;21:367–386.

38. Lindvall O, Bjorklung A, Skagerberg G: Dopamine-containing neurons in the spinal cord: anatomy of some functional aspects. Ann Neurol 1983;14:255–260.

39. Stoof JC, Kebabian JW: Two dopamine receptors: biochemistry, physiology and pharmacology. Life Sci 1984;34:2281–2286.

40. Rosebush PI, Mazurak MF: Serum iron and neuroleptic malignant syndrome. Lancet 1991;338:149–151.

41. Garcia FM, Duarte J, Perez A, et al: Low serum iron and neuroleptic malignant syndrome. Ann Pharmacother 1993;27:101–102.

42. Javid JI: Clinical pharmacokinetics of antipsychotics. J Pharmacol 1994;34:286–295.

43. Ereshefsky L: Pharmacokinetics and drug interactions: update for new antipsychotics. J Clin Psychiatry 1996;57(Suppl 11):12–25.

44. Fang J, Gorrod JW: Metabolism, pharmacogenetics, and metabolic drug-drug interactions of antipsychotic drugs. Cell Mol Neurobiol 1999;19:491–510.

45. Micromedex Healthcare Series, Vol. 123. DRUGDEX drug evaluations, Risperdal Consta. Greenwood Village, CO, Thomson MICROMEDEX, 2004. Accessed December 29, 2004.

46. Howard L, Webb R, Abel K: Safety of antipsychotic drugs for pregnant and breastfeeding women with non-affective psychosis [Editorial]. BMJ 2004;329:933–934.

47. Dahl ML: Cytochrome p450 phenotyping/genotyping in patients receiving antipsychotics: useful aid to prescribing? Clin Pharmacokinet 2002;41:453–470.

48. Ozaki N: Pharmacogenetics of antipsychotics. Nagoya J Med Sci 2004;67:1–7.

49. Goff DC, Baldessarini RJ: Drug interactions with antipsychotic agents. J Clin Psychopharmacol 1993;13:57–67.

50. Klimke A, Klieser E: Sudden death after intravenous application of lorazepam in a patient treated with clozapine. Am J Psychiatry 1994;151:780.

51. Berry N, Pradhan S, Sagar R, et al: Neuroleptic malignant syndrome in an adolescent receiving olanzapine-lithium combination therapy. Pharmacotherapy 2003;23:255–259.

52. Joseph JK, Thomas K: Lithium toxicity—a risk factor for neuroleptic malignant syndrome. J Assoc Physicians India 1991;39:572–573.

53. Trenton A, Currier G, Zwemer F: Fatalities associated with therapeutic use and overdose of atypical antipsychotics. CNS Drugs 2003;17:307–324.

54. Mady S, Wax P, Wang D, et al: Pediatric clozapine intoxication. Am J Emerg Med 1996;14:462–463.

55. Yip L, Dart RC, Graham K: Olanzapine toxicity in a toddler [Letter]. Pediatrics 1998;102:1494.

56. Bond GR, Thompson JD: Olanzapine pediatric overdose [Letter]. Ann Emerg Med 1999;34:292–293.

57. Burns MJ: The pharmacology and toxicology of atypical antipsychotic agents. J Toxicol Clin Toxicol 2001;39:1–14.

58. Parsons M, Buckley NA: Antipsychotic drugs in overdose: practical management guidelines. CNS Drugs 1997;6:427–441.

59. Acri AA, Henretig FM: Effects of risperidone in overdose. Am J Emerg Med 1998;16:498–501.

60. LeBlaye I, Donatini B, Hall M, et al: Acute overdosage with clozapine: a review of the available clinical experience. Pharm Med 1992;6:169–178.

61. O'Malley GCF, Seifert S, Heard K, et al: Olanzapine overdose mimicking opioid intoxication. Ann Emerg Med 1999;34:279–281.

62. Harmon TJ, Benitez JG, Krenzelok EP, et al: Loss of consciousness from acute quetiapine overdosage. J Toxicol Clin Toxicol 1998;36:599–602.

63. Barry D, Meyskens FL, Becker CE: Phenothiazine poisoning: a review of 48 cases. Calif Med 1973;118:1–5.

64. Bonin MM, Burkhart KK: Olanzapine overdose in a 1-year old male. Pediatr Emerg Care 1999;15:266–267.

65. Dyer KS, Woolf AD: Use of phenothiazines as sedatives in children: what are the risks? Drug Saf 1999;21:81–90.

66. Li C, Gefter WB: Acute pulmonary edema induced by overdosage of phenothiazines. Chest 1992;101:102–104.

67. Mitchell AA, Lovejoy FH, Goldman P: Drug ingestions associated with miosis in comatose children. J Pediatr 1976;89:303.

68. Elkayam U, Frishman W: Cardiovascular effects of phenothiazines. Am Heart J 1980;100:397–401.

69. Fowler ND, McCall D, Chou T, et al: Electrocardiographic changes and cardiac arrhythmias in patients receiving psychotropic drugs. Am J Cardiol 1981;37:223–230.

70. Fletcher GF, Kazamias TM, Wenger NK: Cardiotoxic effects of Mellaril: conduction disturbances and supraventricular arrhythmias. Am Heart J 1961;78:135–138.

71. Thornton CC, Wendkos MH: EKG T-wave distortions among thioridazine-treated psychiatric inpatients. Dis Nerv Syst 1971;32:320–323.

72. Frye MA, Coudreaut MF, Hakeman SM, et al: Continuous droperidol infusion for management of agitated delirium in an intensive care unit. Psychosomatics 1995;36:301–305.

73. Riker RR, Fraser GL, Cox PM: Continuous infusion of haloperidol controls agitation in critically ill patients. Crit Care Med 1994;22:433–440.

74. Krahenbuhl SI, Sauter B, Kupferschmidt H, et al: Reversible QT prolongation with torsades de pointes in a patient with pimozide intoxication. Am J Med Sci 1995;309:315–316.

75. Hulisz DT, Dasa SL, Black LD, et al: Complete heart block and torsade de pointes associated with thioridazine poisoning. Pharmacotherapy 1994;14:239–245.

76. Wilt JL, Minnema AM, Johnson RF, et al: Torsade de pointes associated with the use of intravenous haloperidol. Ann Intern Med 1993;119:391–394.

77. Sharma ND, Rosman HS, Padhi D, Tisdale JE: Torsades de pointes associated with intravenous haloperidol in critically ill patients. Am J Cardiol 1998;81:238–240.

78. Cheslik TA, Erramouspe J: Extrapyramidal symptoms following accidental ingestion of risperidone in a child. Ann Pharmacother 1996;30:360–363.

79. Muscettola G, Barbato G, Pampallona S, et al: Extrapyramidal syndromes in neuroleptic-treated patients: prevalence, risk factors, and association with tardive dyskinesia. J Clin Psychopharmacol 1999;19:203–208.

80. Balestrieri M, Vampini C, Bellantuono C: Efficacy and safety of novel antipsychotics: a critical review. Hum Psychopharmacol Clin Exp 2000;15:499–512.

81. Cortese L, Pourcher-Bouchard E, Williams R: Assessment and management of antipsychotic-induced adverse events. Can J Psychiatry 1998;43(Suppl 1):15–20.

82. Koek RJ, Edmond HP: Acute laryngeal dystonic reactions to neuroleptics. Psychosomatics 1989;30:359–364.

83. Swett C: Drug-induced dystonia. Am J Psychiatry 1982;132:532–534.

84. Ayd FJ: A survey of drug-induced extrapyramidal reactions. JAMA 1961;175:1054–1060.

85. Gupta JM, Lovejoy FH: Acute phenothiazine toxicity in childhood: a five-year survey. Pediatrics 1967;39:771.

86. Hegarty AM, Lipton RB, Merriam AE, et al: Cocaine as a risk factor for acute dystonic reactions. Neurology 1991;41:1670–1672.

87. Freed E: Alcohol-triggered neuroleptic-induced tremor, rigidity and dystonia. Med J Aust 1981;2:44–45.

88. Nelson DE: Akathisia—a brief review. Scott Med J 2001;46:133–134.

89. Kurz M, Hummer M, Oberbauer H, Fleischhacker WW: Extrapyramidal side effects of clozapine and haloperidol. Psychopharmacology 1995;118:52–56.

90. Kobayashi RM: Drug therapy of tardive dyskinesia. N Engl J Med 1977;296:257.

91. Yassa R, Ananth J, Cordozo S, et al: Tardive dyskinesia in an outpatient population: prevalence and predisposing factors. Can J Psychiatry 1983;28:391–394.

92. Nierenberg D, Disch M, Manheimer E, et al: Facilitating prompt diagnosis and treatment of the neuroleptic malignant syndrome. Clin Pharmacol Ther 1991;50:580–586.

93. Levinson DF, Simpson GM: Neuroleptic-induced extrapyramidal symptoms with fever: heterogeneity of the "neuroleptic malignant syndrome." Arch Gen Psychiatry 1986;43:839–848.

94. Addonizio G, Susman VL, Roth SD: Neuroleptic malignant syndrome: review and analysis of 115 cases. Biol Psychiatry 1987;22:1004–1020.

95. Caroff SN, Mann SC: Neuroleptic malignant syndrome. Med Clin North Am 1993;77:185–202.

96. Shalev A, Munitz H: The neuroleptic malignant syndrome: agent and host interaction. Acta Psychiatr Scand 1986;73:337–347.

97. Silva RR, Munoz DM, Alpert M, et al: Neuroleptic malignant syndrome in children and adolescents. J Am Acad Adolesc Psychiatry 1999;38:187–194.

98. Pearlman CA: Neuroleptic malignant syndrome: a review of the literature. J Clin Psychopharmacol 1986;6:257–273.

99. Pelonero AL, Levenson JL, Pandurangi AK: Neuroleptic malignant syndrome: a review. Psychiatr Serv 1998;49:1163–1172.

101. Velamoor VR, Norman RMG, Caroff SN, et al: Progression of symptoms in neuroleptic malignant syndrome. J Nerv Ment Dis 1994;182:168–173.

102. Keck PE, Pope HG, McElroy SL: Declining frequency of neuroleptic malignant syndrome in a hospital population. Am J Psychiatry 1991;148:880–882.

103. Kellam AMP: The (frequently) neuroleptic (potentially) malignant syndrome. Br J Psychiatry 1990;157:169–173.

104. Ravin DS, Levenson JW: Fatal cardiac event following initiation of risperidone therapy. Ann Pharmacother 1997;31(7–8):867–870.

105. Mehtonen OP, Aranko K, Malkonen L, et al: A survey of sudden death associated with the use of antipsychotic or antidepressant drugs: 49 cases in Finland. Acta Psychiatr Scand 1991;84:58–64.

106. Hollister LE, Kosek JV: Sudden death during treatment with phenothiazine derivatives. JAMA 1965;192:1035–1038.

107. Lee AM, Knoll JL, Suppes R: The atypical antipsychotic sertindole: a case series. J Clin Psychiatry 1997;58:410–416.

108. Brown K, Levy H, Brenner C, et al: Overdose of risperidone. Ann Emerg Med 1993;22:1908–1910.

109. Lynch S, Fill S, Hoffman RS: Intentional quetiapine (Seroquel) overdose [Abstract]. J Toxicol Clin Toxicol 1999;37:631.

110. Hustey FM: Acute quetiapine poisoning. J Emerg Med 1999;17:995–997.

111. Kopala LC, Day C, Dillman B, Gardner D: A case of risperidone overdose in early schizophrenia: a review of potential complications. J Psychiatry Neurosci 1998;23:305–308.

112. Flugelman MY, Tal A, Pollack S, et al: Psychotropic drugs and long QT syndromes: case reports. J Clin Psychiatry 1985;46:290–291.

113. Aunsholt NA: Prolonged QT interval and hypokalemia caused by haloperidol. Acta Psychiatr Scand 1989;79:411–412.

114. Lawrence KR, Nasraway SA: Conduction disturbances associated with administration of butyrophenone antipsychotics in the critically ill: a review of the literature. Pharmacotherapy 1997;17:531–537.

115. Lischke V, Behne M, Doelken P, et al: Droperidol causes a dose-dependent prolongation of the QT interval. Anesth Analg 1994;79:983–986.

116. MedWatch 2001 Safety Information Summaries: Inapsine (Droperidol). Accessed January 16, 2005, from http://www.fda.gov/medwatch/safety/2001/safety01.htm#inapsi.

117. Glassman AH, Bigger JT Jr: Antipsychotic drugs: prolonged QT interval, torsades de pointes, and sudden death. Am J Psychiatry 2001;158:1774–1782.

118. Haddad PM, Anderson IM: Antipsychotic-related QTc prolongation, torsades de pointes and sudden death. Drugs 2002;62:1649–1671.

119. Anonymous: Clozapine and myocarditis. WHO Drug Information 1994;8:212–213.

120. Merrill DB, Dec GW, Goff DC: Adverse cardiac effects associated with clozapine. J Clin Psychopharmacol 2005;25:32–41.

121. Lebovitz HE: Metabolic consequences of atypical antipsychotic drugs. Psychiatr Q 2003;74:277–290.

122. Liebzeit KA: New onset diabetes and atypical antipsychotics. Eur Neuropsychopharmacol 2001;11:25–32.

123. Gianfrancesco F, White R, Ruey-hua W, et al: Antipsychotic-induced type 2 diabetes: evidence from a large health plan database. J Clin Psychopharmacol 2003;23:328–335.

124. Citrone LL, Jaffe AB: Relationship of atypical antipsychotics with development of diabetes mellitus. Ann Pharmacother 2003;37:1849–1857.

125. Torrey EF, Swalwell CI: Fatal olanzapine-induced ketoacidosis. Am J Psychiatry 2003;160:2241.

126. Koller EA, Doraiswamy PM: Olanzapine-associated diabetes mellitus. Pharmacotherapy 2002;22:841–852.

127. Avella J, Wetli CV, Wilson JC, et al: Fatal olanzapine-induced hyperglycemia. Am J Forensic Med Pathol 2004;25:172–175.

128. Meatherall R, Younes J: Fatality from olanzapine-induced hyperglycemia. J Forensic Sci 2002;47:893–896.

129. Wehring HJ, Kelly DL, Love RC, et al: Deaths from diabetic ketoacidosis after long-term clozapine treatment. Am J Psychiatry 2003;160:2241–2242.

130. Koller E, Schneider B, Bennett K, et al: Clozapine-associated diabetes. Am J Med 2001;15:716–723.

131. Iqbal MM, Rahman A, Husain K, et al: Clozapine: a clinical review of adverse effects and management. Ann Clin Psychiatry 2003;15:33–48.

132. Haupt DW, Newcomer JW: Hyperglycemia and antipsychotic medications. J Clin Psychiatry 2001;62(Suppl 27):15–26.

133. Meyer JM: Novel antipsychotics and severe hyperlipidemia. J Clin Psychopharmacol 2001;21:369–374.

134. Domon SE, Webber JC: Hyperglycemia and hypertriglyceridemia secondary to olanzapine. J Clin Adolesc Psychopharmacol 2001;11:285–288.

135. Kingsbury SJ, Fayek M, Trufasiu D: The apparent effects of ziprasidone on plasma lipids and glucose. J Clin Psychiatry 2001;62:347–349.

136. Haberfellner EM, Honsig T: Nonalcoholic steatohepatitis: a possible side effect of atypical antipsychotics. J Clin Psychiatry 2003;64:851.

137. Koller EA, Cross JT, Doraiswamy PM: Pancreatitis associated with atypical antipsychotics: from the Food and Drug Administration's Med Watch surveillance system and published reports. Pharmacotherapy 2003;23:1123–1130.

138. Selem K, Kaplowitz N: Hepatotoxicity of psychotropic drugs. Hepatology 1999;29:1347–1351.

139. Hummer M, Kurz M, Kurzthalaer I, et al: Hepatotoxicity of clozapine. J Clin Psychopharmacol 1997;17:314–317.

140. Whitworth AB, Liensberger D, Fleischhacker WW: Transient increase of liver enzymes induced by risperidone: two case reports [Letter]. J Clin Psychopharmacol 1999;19:475–476.

141. Trayle WH: Phenothiazine-induced agranulocytosis [Letter]. JAMA 1986;256:1957.

142. Wren P, Frizzell LA, Keltner NL, et al: Three potentially fatal adverse effects of psychotropic medications. Perspect Psychiatr Care 2003;39:75–81.

143. Litvak R, Kaelbling R: Agranulocytosis, leukopenia and psychotropic drugs. Arch Gen Psychiatry 1971;24:265–267.

144. Alvir J, Lieberman J, Safferman A, et al: Clozapine-induced agranulocytosis; incidence and risk factors in the United States. N Engl J Med 1993;329:162–167.

145. Gerson SL: G-CSF and the management of clozapine-induced agranulocytosis. J Clin Psychiatry 1994;55(Suppl B):139–142.

146. Steinwachs A, Grohmann R, Pedrosa F, et al: Two cases of olanzapine-induced reversible neutropenia. Pharmacopsychiatry 1999;32:154–156.

147. Ruhe HG, Becker HE, Jessurun P: Agranulocytosis and granulocytopenia associated with quetiapine. Acta Psychiatr Scand 2001;104:311–313.

148. Dernovsek Z, Tavcar P: Risperidone-induced leucopenia and neutropenia. Br J Psychiatry 1997;171:393–394.

149. Hagg S, Spigset O, Soderstrom TG: Association of venous thromboembolism and clozapine. Lancet 2000;355:1155–1156.

150. Forrest FM, Forrest IS, Mason AS: Review of rapid urine tests for phenothiazine and related drugs. Am J Psychiatry 1961;118:300–307.

151. Sloan KL, Haver VM, Saxon AJ: Quetiapine and false-positive urine drug testing for tricyclic antidepressants [Letter]. Am J Psychiatry 2000;157:148–149.

152. American Psychiatric Association: Diagnostic and Statistical Manual of Mental Disorders, 4th ed. Washington, DC, American Psychiatric Association, 1994, pp 739–742.

153. Adnet P, Lestavel P, Krivosic-Horber R: Neuroleptic malignant syndrome. Br J Anaesth 2000;85:129–135.

154. Albertson TE, Dawson A, de Latorre FJ, et al: TOX-ACLS: toxicologic-oriented advanced cardiac life support. Ann Emerg Med 2001;37(Suppl 4):78–90.

155. Kawamura T, Kodama I, Toyama J, et al: Combined application of class I antiarrhythmic drugs causes "additive," "reductive," or "synergistic" sodium channel block in cardiac muscles. Cardiovasc Res 1990;24:925–931.

156. Tranum BL, Murphy ML: Successful treatment of ventricular tachycardia associated with thioridazine (Mellaril). South Med J 1969;62:357–358.

157. Lumpkin J, Watanabe AS, Rumack BH, et al: Phenothiazine-induced ventricular tachycardia following acute overdose. JACEP 1979;8:476–478.

158. Pietro DA: Thioridazine-associated ventricular tachycardia and isoproterenol [Letter]. Ann Intern Med 1981;94:411.

159. Kemper A, Dunlop R, Pietro D: Thioridazine-induced torsades de pointes successful therapy with isoproterenol. JAMA 1983;249:2931–2934.

160. Burns MJ, Linden CH, Graudins A, et al: A comparison of physostigmine and benzodiazepines for the treatment of anticholinergic poisoning. Ann Emerg Med 2000;35:374–381.

161. Schuster P, Gabriel E, Luefferie B, et al: Reversal by physostigmine of clozapine-induced delirium. Clin Toxicol 1977;10:437–441.

162. Corre K, Neimann J, Bessen H: Extended therapy for acute dystonic reactions. Ann Emerg Med 1984;13:194–197.

163. Vinson DR, Drotts DL: Diphenhydramine for the prevention of akathisia induced by prochlorperazine: a randomized, controlled trial. Ann Emerg Med 2001;37:125–131.

164. Lima AR, Weiser KV, Bacaltchuk J, Barnes TR: Anticholinergics for neuroleptic-induced akathisia. Cochrane Database Syst Rev 2004;1:CD003727.

165. Adler L, Angrist B, Peselow E, et al: A controlled assessment of propranolol in the treatment of neuroleptic-induced akathisia. Br J Psychiatry 1983;149:42–45.

166. Zubenko GS, Cohen BM, Lipinski JF, et al: Use of clonidine in treating neuroleptic-induced akathisia [Letter]. Psychiatry Res 1985;13:253.

167. Fischel T, Hermesh H, Aizenberg D, et al: Cyproheptadine versus propranolol for the treatment of acute neuroleptic-induced akathisia: a comparative double-blind study. J Clin Psychopharmacol 2001;21:612–615.

168. Miller CH, Fleischhacker WW: Managing antipsychotic-induced acute and chronic akathisia. Drug Saf 2000;22:73–81.

169. Sachdev PS: The current status of tardive dyskinesia. Aust N Z J Psychiatry 2000;34:355–369.

170. Susman VL: Clinical management of neuroleptic malignant syndrome. Psychiatr Q 2001;72:325–336.

171. Guze BH, Baxter LR: Neuroleptic malignant syndrome. N Engl J Med 1985;313:163–166.

172. Krause T, Gerbershagen MU, Fiege M, et al: Dantrolene—a review of its pharmacology, therapeutic use and new developments. Anaesthesia 2004;59:364–373.

173. Velamoor VR, Swamy GN, Parmar Late-RS, et al: Management of suspected neuroleptic malignant syndrome. Can J Psychiatry 1995;40:545–550.

174. Dhib-Jalbut S, Hesselbrock R, Mouradian MM, et al: Bromocriptine treatment of neuroleptic malignant syndrome. J Clin Psychiatry 1987;48:69–73.

175. Rosenberg MR, Green M: Neuroleptic malignant syndrome: review of response to therapy. Arch Intern Med 1989;149:1927–1931.

176. Rosebush PI, Stewart TD, Marzurek MF: The treatment of neuroleptic malignant syndrome: are dantrolene and bromocriptine useful adjuncts to supportive care? Br J Psychiatry 1991;159:709–712.

177. Sakkas P, Davis JM, Hua J, et al: Pharmacotherapy of neuroleptic malignant syndrome. Psychiatr Ann 1991;21:157–164.

178. Sakkas P, Davis JM, Janicak PG, et al: Drug treatment of the neuroleptic malignant syndrome. Psychopharmacol Bull 1991;27:381–384.

179. Davis JM, Janicak PG, Sakkas P, et al: Electroconvulsive therapy in the treatment of the neuroleptic malignant syndrome. Convuls Ther 1991;7:111–120.

180. Sangai R, Dimitrijevic R: Neuroleptic malignant syndrome: successful treatment with pancuronium. JAMA 1985;254:2795–2796.

181. Khaldarov V: Benzodiazepines for treatment of neuroleptic malignant syndrome. Hosp Physician 2000;36:51–55.

182. Burris KD, Molski FR, Xu C, et al: Aripiprazole, a novel antipsychotic, is a high-affinity partial agonist at human dopamine D2 receptors. J Pharmacol Exp Ther 2002;302:381–389.

183. Baselt RC: Disposition of Toxic Drugs and Chemicals in Man, 7th ed. Foster City, CA, Biomedical Publications, 2004.

39 *Anticholinergics and Antihistamines*

MARK A. KIRK, MD ■ ALEXANDER B. BAER, MD

At a Glance...

- Anticholinergic and sedating antihistamine agent poisoning is common and should be included in the differential diagnosis of any patient with an altered mental status and sinus tachycardia, particularly those with agitated delirium.
- The diagnosis of the anticholinergic syndrome is based on the clinical examination; the absence of patient sweating is a key physical finding.
- The majority of patients with anticholinergic poisoning have a good outcome with supportive care.
- Treatment with physostigmine is indicated for select patients with agitated delirium and the absence of conduction disturbances on the electrocardiogram.

INTRODUCTION AND RELEVANT HISTORY

Anticholinergic drugs and plants have a distinct place in world history. Marc Anthony's military troops were neutralized and defeated after ingesting hallucinogenic anticholinergic plants. In 1676, a witness wrote of British soldiers' antics after they had consumed salad containing *Datura stramonium*. His account is a vivid description of anticholinergic poisoning[1]:

> . . . some of them eat plentiful of it [James-town weed], the Effect of which was a very pleasant Comedy; for they turn'd natural Fools upon it for several Days: One would blow up a Feather in the Air; another wou'd dart Straws at it with much Fury; and another stark naked was sitting up in a Corner, like a Monkey, grinning and making Mows at them; a Fourth would fondly kiss, and paw his Companions, and snear in their faces . . . and after Eleven Days return'd to themselves again, not remembring any thing that had pass'd.

In the world of crime, scopolamine has been "truth serum," "date-rape drug," and "knockout drops" for great detective novels. In the real world, it has produced temporary psychosis so that victims could be robbed. Analgesia for broken bones and cure for the common cold are only a few of the historical uses of anticholinergic drugs. These drugs continue to contribute to modern medicine.

Today, many classes of prescription and over-the-counter medications have anticholinergic properties. Anticholinergic effects are the desired therapeutic actions for some medications but may occur as unintended or exaggerated adverse drug effects for others. In addition to medications, a number of plants and mushrooms contain anticholinergic alkaloids. Some may be ingested deliberately for their mind-altering effects. Others may be added to illicit drugs to enhance the drug experience but produce inadvertent effects. For instance, scopolamine-tainted heroin[2,3] and atropine-adulterated cocaine[4] has led to hospitalizations for anticholinergic poisoning. Anticholinergic toxicity has also been associated with the use of herbal supplements.[5] Antihistamines are a diverse group of medications, most with potent anticholinergic effects and numerous other pharmacologic activities.

The clinical syndrome of anticholinergic poisoning is one of the most common and readily recognized toxidromes. The ability to identify the signs and symptoms of this syndrome and differentiate it from other drug intoxications and medical illnesses is a basic skill that is necessary for all health care practitioners that care for poisoned patients.

CLASSIFICATION AND STRUCTURE

Anticholinergics

Anticholinergic (antimuscarinic) agents may be classified by their source (natural, semisynthetic, or synthetic) or structure (tertiary amine or quaternary ammonium compounds). The naturally occurring agents, atropine (*d,l*-hyoscyamine) and scopolamine (*l*-hyoscine), are tropane alkaloids of the belladonna (family Solanaceae) plants.[6] Specifically, atropine and scopolamine are esters of tropic acid (aromatic acid) and tropine and scopine (organic bases), respectively (Fig. 39-1). Semisynthetic derivatives are created by the addition of a different organic base to tropic acid or a methyl group to the base's nitrogen. Synthetic derivatives have a wide variety of structures but maintain the ester bond in close proximity to a nitrogen to preserve anticholinergic activity. In general, anticholinergic activity requires the presence of a tertiary or quaternary amino group linked by two or three carbons to an ester, ether, or nitrogen and one or more aromatic rings (see Fig. 39-1). Embedded in each anticholinergic compound is a portion that resembles the structure of acetylcholine, which allows for competitive binding at muscarinic receptors. The most potent antimuscarinic agents have an ester and -OH group in close proximity to the amino group.

Antimuscarinic compounds contain a tertiary amine or quaternary ammonium structure. The tertiary amines are readily absorbed from the gastrointestinal (GI) tract and freely cross the blood-brain barrier (BBB). Quaternary ammonium compounds, however, have a charge on their nitrogen and are, thus, not well absorbed from the GI tract and penetrate the BBB poorly. Quaternary deriv-

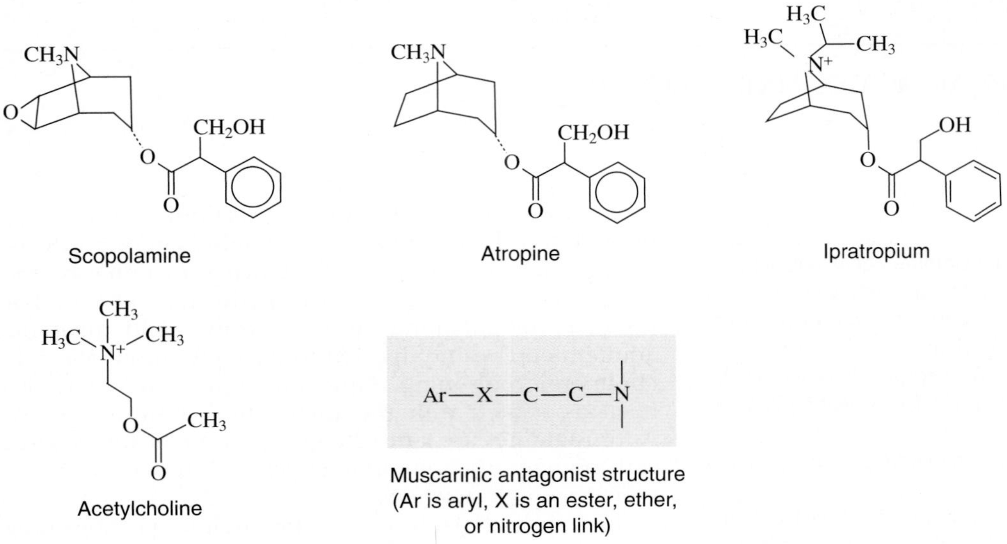

FIGURE 39-1 Structures of some anticholinergic agents.

Scopolamine

Atropine

Ipratropium

Acetylcholine

Muscarinic antagonist structure
(Ar is aryl, X is an ester, ether,
or nitrogen link)

atives, however, have more potency at both muscarinic and nicotinic receptors. The charge, like that of acetylcholine, enables greater attraction to the anionic active site of target receptors.

Antihistamines

H_1-receptor antagonists are typically divided into six structural classes. They include ethanolamines (diphenhydramine), ethylenediamines (pyrilamine), alkylamines (chlorpheniramine), piperazines (hydroxyzine), phenothiazines (promethazine), and piperidines (loratadine, acrivastine, cetirizine, and fexofenadine). Although potent antihistamines, doxepin (a dibenzoxepine) and other tricyclic antidepressants (TCAs) are classified by their other drug effects and considered separately (see Chapter 27). Except for the novel class of piperidines, all first-generation agents readily cross the BBB and are often referred to as *sedating antihistamines*.

First-generation H_1-receptor antagonists have a tertiary amino group connected by two or three carbons to a nitrogen or ether link and then two to three aromatic rings (Fig. 39-2).[7] Like histamine, antihistamines have a β-aminoethyl side chain. Unlike histamine, antihistamines have substitutions on their amino group and more than a single aromatic ring. As shown in Figures 39-1 and 39-2, sedating antihistamines possess the structural characteristics necessary to bind and competitively antagonize muscarinic receptors (tertiary amine linked by an ethyl group to an aromatic ring). This large overlap of structure accounts for a large overlap in pharmacologic and toxic effects and is why these agents are considered together.

Agents That Produce the Anticholinergic Syndrome

Both pharmaceutical agents and plants may cause significant anticholinergic toxicity (Box 39-1). For many medications, such as the GI antispasmodics or the local mydriatics, the anticholinergic properties produce the desired therapeutic effect for the drug. Hence, many of the primary pharmacologic effects are not considered toxic. The desired therapeutic effects of other medications (e.g., antipsychotics and antiparkinsonian drugs), however, are not the anticholinergic manifestations. Thus, mydriasis, constipation, tachycardia, and dry mouth are frequently considered adverse effects. The more potent the anticholinergic binding relative to other drug effects, the more likely the antimuscarinic side effects will occur with therapeutic drug dosing.

Combining medications with anticholinergic properties produces synergistic effects.[8-10] For example, when antiparkinsonian medications are administered in combination with phenothiazines to prevent the occurrence of undesirable extrapyramidal reactions, this greatly increases the incidence of toxic confusional states.[11] Small changes in the dose of either drug may precipitate the central anticholinergic syndrome in a previously unaffected individual.[12] Many over-the-counter medications have anticholinergic properties and can precipitate the anticholinergic syndrome when ingested by an unknowing layperson who is already prescribed an agent with antimuscarinic activity. For example, the combined use of oral diphenhydramine with topical application of Caladryl lotion (calamine lotion and diphenhydramine [Parke-Davis, Morris Plains, NJ]) has produced central anticholinergic toxicity in children.[13-15]

An unusual form of toxicity involves the use of transdermal scopolamine patches.[16] Several cases of the central anticholinergic syndrome have been reported in adults and children using the patches for treatment of motion sickness. Accidental instillation of the drug into the eyes has occurred after manipulation of the patch. This has resulted in a unilateral fixed dilated pupil or bilateral fixed dilated pupils without focal neurologic changes.[17,18] This finding is also known as the "cornpicker's pupil" and has been described in cornfield workers who have unintentionally rubbed pulverized jimsonweed in their eyes during harvesting.[19] An additional

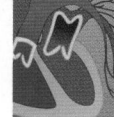

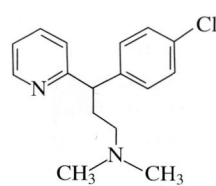

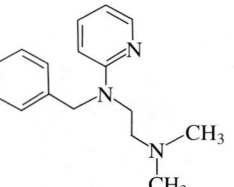

Diphenhydramine   Promethazine   Chlorpheniramine   Tripelenamine

Histamine

H₁-antagonist structure
(Ar is aryl, X is a nitrogen, carbon,
or ether link)

FIGURE 39-2 Structures of some H₁-histamine antagonists.

BOX 39-1   EXAMPLES OF AGENTS WITH ANTICHOLINERGIC PROPERTIES

Plants and Mushrooms

Atropa belladonna (Deadly nightshade)
Datura stramomium (Jimsonweed)
Mandrigora officinarum (Mandrake)
Hyoscyamine niger (Henbane)
Amanita muscaria (Fly agaric)
Amanita pantherina (Panther)

Belladonna Alkaloids and Related Synthetic Compounds

Atropine
Scopolamine
Glycopyrrolate (Robinul)

Antispasmodics

Clidinium bromide (Librax)
Dicyclomine (Bentyl)
Propantheline bromide (Pro-Banthíne)
Methantheline bromide (Banthíne)
Flavoxate (Urispas)
Oxybutynin (Ditropan)

Antiparkinsonism Medications

Benztropine mesylate (Cogentin)
Biperiden (Akineton)
Trihexyphenidyl (Artane)

Local Mydriatics

Cyclopentolate (Cyclogyl)
Homatropine (Isopto Homatropine)
Tropicamide (Mydriacyl)

Muscle Relaxants

Cyclobenzaprine (Flexeril)
Orphenadrine (Norflex)

Antihistamines

Brompheniramine (Dimetane)
Chlorpheniramine (Ornade, Chlor-Trimeton)
Cyclizine (Marezine)
Dimenhydrinate (Dramamine)
Diphenhydramine (Benadryl, Caladryl)
Hydroxyzine (Atarax)
Meclizine (Antivert)

Antipsychotics

Chlorpromazine (Thorazine)
Clozapine (Clozaril)
Loxapine (Loxitane)
Mesoridazine (Serentil)
Olanzapine (Zyprexa)
Thioridazine (Mallaril)

Over-the-Counter Sleep Aids

Diphenhyramine (Benadryl)
Doxylamine (Unisom)

Cyclic Antidepressants

Amitriptyline (Elavil)
Clomipramine (Anafranil)
Doxepin (Sinequan)
Imipramine (Tofranil)

Others

Amantadine (Symmetrel)
Carbamazepine (Tegretol)
Cyproheptadine (Periactin)
Ipratropium (Atrovent)

---

method of systemic anticholinergic toxicity involves the absorption of ophthalmologic agents or nasal decongestants through the conjunctiva, nasal mucosa, or GI tract.[20,21]

Scopolamine eyedrops have allegedly been used deliberately to disorient subsequent victims of theft.[22] The victim is often found naked, disoriented, hallucinating, and amnestic to the events before hospital-

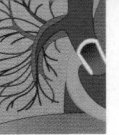

ization. Scopolamine was believed to have been placed in a beverage ingested by the victim.[23] Many toxicologic laboratories do not routinely screen for scopolamine; therefore, these patients had negative results on toxicologic screens.

Both anticholinergic pharmaceuticals and plants may be abused. Central anticholinergic effects of intentional ingestion may produce euphoria and hallucinogenic effects.[24] It has been proposed that a physiologic dependence and the development of withdrawal symptoms exist when the agent is withheld.[24] Among the most frequently reported anticholinergic drugs abused are the antiparkinsonian agents trihexyphenidyl and benztropine mesylate.[25] These drugs have potent dopamine reuptake inhibition. The resulting dopamine excess is a proposed mechanism for craving of many abused drugs.[25,26] Drug seekers may feign extrapyramidal symptoms to receive additional anticholinergic agents.[24,27-30]

Many types of plants contain alkaloids that produce anticholinergic stigmata in humans. Most of these are found in the family Solanaceae, which include the genera *Atropa, Datura, Hyoscyamus, Lycium,* and *Solanum.* The principal alkaloids found in these plants include solanine, atropine (a racemic mixture of *d-* and *l-*hyoscyamine, of which only the levorotatory isomer is pharmacologically active), and scopolamine (*l-*hyoscine). The mushrooms *Amanita muscaria* and *Amanita pantherina* have rarely been reported to cause anticholinergic or cholinergic toxicity. Anticholinergic effects can be severe but are rarely the prominent finding with poisoning by these mushrooms (see Chapter 23).[31] The alkaloid content of each species and each plant varies greatly and depends on many parameters such as the time of year, the available moisture, and the temperature. For this reason, it is very difficult to determine predicted toxicity in relation to the amount and the origin of the plant material. Recreational abusers of anticholinergic mushrooms and *D. stramonium* (jimsonweed) are unable to titrate the dose of ingested substance because of this tremendous biologic variability and, therefore, are prone to severe anticholinergic poisoning.

PHARMACOLOGY

Anticholinergics

Acetylcholine is an endogenous neurotransmitter found in various synaptic sites and neuroeffector junctions (e.g., secretory glands and smooth and cardiac muscle) in the central and peripheral nervous systems.[6] The actions of acetylcholine are mediated by muscarinic and nicotinic cholinergic receptors. Muscarinic receptor sites are in the brain (e.g., cerebral cortex, thalamus, hippocampus, reticular activating system), postganglionic parasympathetic nervous system, and select postganglionic sympathetic nervous system sites (e.g., sweat glands). Nicotinic receptors are located at the skeletal muscle motor end plate and spinal cord and autonomic ganglia.[32] There are five subtypes of muscarinic receptors (M_{1-5}) and all are transmembrane proteins that interact with G proteins.[32] Acetylcholine binds to and activates muscarinic receptors, and the result is stimulation or inhibition of cellular function. Nicotinic receptors are ligand-gated cation channels in autonomic ganglia and postsynaptic membranes. Their activation results in increased permeability to sodium and calcium ions, depolarization, and excitation. Nicotinic receptor activation is responsible for enhanced autonomic neurotransmission and skeletal muscle contraction. Acetylcholine is inactivated when metabolized at the synaptic cleft by the enzyme acetylcholinesterase.

Anticholinergic drugs block acetylcholine's action by competitively binding to and blocking muscarinic receptors. Receptor blockade and clinical effects are dose dependent. Clinical effects, however, are nonuniform since there is variable sensitivity of the neuroeffector organ sites to blockade by muscarinic receptor antagonists.[6] Differential sensitivity is largely from the variable parasympathetic tone of each organ system but is also influenced by the effects of other neuronal inputs and the ability of the drug to reach the end organ. In general, small doses of anticholinergic drugs decrease secretions of the sweat, bronchial, and salivary glands. Larger doses produce mydriasis, cycloplegia, and increased heart rate from blockade of the sphincter muscle of the iris, ciliary muscle of the lens, and vagus nerve innervation to the heart, respectively. Even larger doses cause urinary retention and ileus from depressed bladder tone and GI motility, respectively. These classic peripheral anticholinergic effects are caused by blocking postganglionic cholinergic nerves and predominate in most cases of acute poisoning.[33] Cholinergic neurons are spread widely through the cerebral cortex and subcortical areas.[32] Because of this ubiquitous distribution, they likely have a role in regulation and modulation of other neurotransmitters.[34] Central cholinergic pathways are important to memory, wake-sleep cycle, alertness, and orientation and for fine-tuning motor movements. *Central anticholinergic syndrome* refers to an acute psychosis or delirium resulting from inhibition of central cholinergic transmission. The degree of central anticholinergic activity is related to a medication's ability to cross the BBB.

Muscarinic antagonists are highly selective for muscarinic over nicotinic sites. Thus, the nicotinic receptors at autonomic ganglia and the motor end plates are unaffected by drugs that block muscarinic receptors.

Antihistamines

Histamine is a mediator of the allergic response, a regulator of gastric acid secretion, and a central nervous system (CNS) neurotransmitter.[35] Four distinct receptors have been identified (H_1, H_2, H_3, H_4). Stimulation of H_1 receptors constricts bronchioles, dilates peripheral vasculature, increases vascular permeability, and triggers proinflammatory effects through B cells, T cells, monocytes, and lymphocytes.[36] H_1 receptors have also been detected in the brain, GI tract, and genitourinary tract. H_2 receptors are primarily regulators of gastric acid secretion but are also present in the brain, lymphoid

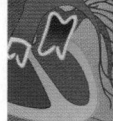

cells, and uterus. In the CNS, histamine (H_1 and H_2) modulates activities such as arousal, thermoregulation, and neuroendocrine and vegetative functions that are controlled by the neocortex, hypothalamus, and hippocampus.[35] H_3 receptors are expressed in the brain and the bronchial smooth muscle and are presynaptic regulators of synthesis and release of histamine into the synapse. The recently characterized H_4 receptor is expressed on mononuclear cells, neutrophils, eosinophils, mast cells, and resting cluster of differentiation CD_4 T lymphocytes.

The antihistamines are reversible competitive inhibitors of H_1-histamine receptors.[35] Except for the newer, second-generation piperidines, all first-generation agents readily cross the BBB and produce both CNS excitation and depression. All H_1 antagonists inhibit both the early vasodilatory effects and later vasoconstrictive effects of histamine. In addition, these agents block histamine-mediated increases in capillary permeability, pruritus, and salivary, lacrimal, and other exocrine secretions. First-generation antihistamines (but not second-generation agents) are also competitive antagonists at both central and peripheral muscarinic receptors and produce clinical effects that are often clinically indistinguishable from those of other anticholinergic drugs. Therapeutic antimuscarinic effects are likely responsible for the prevention of motion sickness with these agents. In addition, antihistamines alter cortical neurons and block fast-sodium channels. These effects cause CNS symptoms, local anesthetic effects, and cardiac conduction abnormalities.[37,38] Diphenhydramine and orphenadrine have been associated with QRS prolongation following overdose.[38] Promethazine and other phenothiazines have α_1-adrenergic blocking effects, which may result in hypotension. The piperidines block the outward potassium rectifier current of cardiac cells, and may result in QTc prolongation and torsades de pointes–type cardiac dysrhythmias. Some H_1 antagonists affect serotonin receptors. Specifically, cyproheptadine is a competitive antagonist at $5\text{-}HT_1$- and $5\text{-}HT_2$-serotonin receptors.[39]

PHARMACOKINETICS

Relevant pharmacokinetic parameters for the anticholinergic and antihistaminergic agents are listed in Table 39-1. Clinical toxicity is usually evident within 1 to 4 hours after ingestion of these agents, but the severity and duration of toxic effects are highly variable. The pharmacokinetic parameters of these agents may change significantly after overdose. Anticholinergic agents decrease gut motility and may produce delayed, erratic, and prolonged absorption with excessive doses.

TABLE 39-1 Pharmacokinetic Parameters of Common Anticholinergic and Antihistaminergic Compounds*

GENERIC NAME (TRADE NAME)	ROUTES OF ADMINISTRATION AND THERAPEUTIC DOSING FOR ADULTS	TIME TO PEAK AFTER ORAL DOSING (hr)	ELIMINATION HALF-LIFE (hr)	PROTEIN BINDING (%)	Vd (L/kg)	ROUTE OF METABOLISM	ACTIVE METABOLITE
Anticholinergic Agents							
dl-Hyoscyamine (Atropine)	Oral: 0.3–1.2 mg q 4–6 hr ETT: 0.6–2 mg Ophtho: 1 drop of 1%–2% solution up to tid IM/IV 0.04 mg/kg (0.5–1 mg, up to 3 mg)	1–2	3–4	4.9–23	2.3–3.9	Hepatic	Yes
Benztropine (Cogentin)	Oral/IV/IM: 1–2 mg bid to tid	—	—	—	—	—	—
Biperiden (Akineton)	Oral/IV/IM: 2–16 mg/day	1.5	18–24	—	20–28	Hepatic	—
Cyclobenzaprine (Flexeril, Lisseril)	Oral: 10–20 mg bid to tid	3.8	24	97	—	Hepatic	Yes
Dicyclomine (Bentyl)	Oral/IM: 10–40 mg tid to qid	1.5–2	5	—	—	Renal	—
Orphenadrine (Disipal, Norflex, Norgesic)	Oral/IM/IV: 25–100 mg bid to tid	3	13–20	20	4.3–7.8	Hepatic; renal (8%)	Yes
Oxybutynin (Cystrin, Ditropan, Tropax)	Oral: 5–20 mg/day divided qd to qid	1–2	2–5	—	1.3–2.8	Hepatic	Yes
Scopolamine (Hyoscine, Transderm Scop, Donnatol)	Oral/IM: 0.01–0.5 mg single dose; Transdermal patch: 1.5 mg q 3 days	1	2–6	10	1.4–2.0	Hepatic	No
Trihexylphenidyl (Artane, Bentex, Broflex, Parkinane)	Oral: 2–15 mg/day, divided qd to bid	1–2	24–41	—	—	Hepatic	—

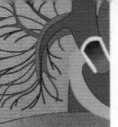

TABLE 39-1 Pharmacokinetic Parameters of Common Anticholinergic and Antihistaminergic Compounds* (Cont'd)

GENERIC NAME (TRADE NAME)	ROUTES OF ADMINISTRATION AND THERAPEUTIC DOSING FOR ADULTS	TIME TO PEAK AFTER ORAL DOSING (hr)	ELIMINATION HALF-LIFE (hr)	PROTEIN BINDING (%)	Vd (L/kg)	ROUTE OF METABOLISM	ACTIVE METABOLITE
Sedating H1 Antihistamines							
Brompheniramine (Dimetane, Puretane)	Oral/IM/IV 4 mg 4–6 hr	3–5	25	—	9–15	Hepatic (90%); renal (10%)	Yes
Chlorpheniramine	Oral/IM: 0.5–8 mg qd to tid	2–3	12–43	72	5.9	Hepatic	Yes
Clemastine (Tavist)	Oral:1–2 mg qd to tid	2–3	21	—	7–16	Hepatic	Yes
Cyclizine (Marezine)	Oral/IM: 50 mg q 4–6 hr	2	7–24	75	13–21	Hepatic	Yes
Cyproheptadine (Periactin)	Oral: 4 mg tid	—	—	—	—	Hepatic	—
Diphenhydramine (Benadryl)	Oral/IM/IV: 25–50 mg tid to qid; 1 mg/kg/dose	1–4	3–14	78–98	3–4	Hepatic	Yes
Doxylamine (Bendectin, Diclectin, Unisom, Nyquil)	Oral: 12.5–25 mg q 4–6 hr	1–4	10	—	2.7	Hepatic; renal	—
Hydroxyzine (Atarax, Vistaril)	Oral/IM: 25–100 mg tid to qid	2	13–27	—	13–31	Hepatic	Yes
Meclizine (Antivert, Bonamine, Bonine, Dramamine)	Oral: 12.5–50 mg/day, divided bid to tid	4	—	—	—	Hepatic	No
Promethazine (Phenergan, Remsed, Zipan)	Oral/IM/IV rectal: 12.5–25 mg tid	2–3	9–19	93	7–19	Hepatic	Yes
Pyrilamine (Midol-PMS, Robitussin Night Relief)	Oral: 25 mg tid to qid	—	—	—	—	Hepatic	—
Tripelennamine (Pyribenzamine)	Oral: 25–50 mg bid to qid	2–3	2.9–5.3	—	9–12	Hepatic	—
Triprolidine (Actifed)	Oral: 1.25–2.5 mg q 4–6 hr	2	1.2–3.3	—	6–9	Hepatic	—
Nonsedating H1 Antihistamines							
Acrivastine (Duact, Semprex-D)	Oral: 4–12 mg qd to qid	1–2	1.7–3.5	50	0.6	Renal (67%); hepatic; fecal	Yes
Cetirizine (Zyrtec)	Oral: 5–10 mg qd	1	6.5–10	93–98	0.58	Renal (70%); hepatic; fecal (10%)	No
Desloratadine (Clarinex)	Oral: 5 mg qd	3–6	21–27	82–87	10–30	Hepatic	Yes
Loratadine (Alavert, Claritin)	Oral: 10 mg qd	2	3–20	97	32–261	Hepatic	Yes
Fexofenadine (Allegra)	Oral: 60 mg bid	2–4	9–20	60–70	12	Fecal (80%); renal (10%)	No
H2 Antihistamines							
Cimetidine (Tagamet)	Oral/IM/IV: 1200–2400 mg/day, divided bid to tid	0.5–3	1–4	18–26	1.4	Renal (35%–60%); hepatic (30%)	No
Famotidine (Pepcid)	Oral: 20–40 mg qd to bid	1–2	2–4	15–22	1–1.3	Renal (25%–70%); hepatic (30%–35%)	—
Nizatidine (Axid)	Oral: 150–300 qd to bid	0.5–3	1.3–1.7	30	1.2–1.8	Renal (70%); renal (10%)	No
Ranitidine (Zantac)	Oral: 150–300 mg qd to bid	0.5–2.0	2.1	15	1.5	Renal (60%); hepatic (30%)	No

*Pharmacokinetic data may be inaccurate when applied to overdose situation. Anticholinergic agent–induced decreased gut motility may create delayed and prolonged absorption following oral ingestion.
—,data not available; bid, twice daily; ETT, endotracheal tube; IM, intramuscularly; IV, intravenously; Ophtho, ophthalmic.
Pharmacokinetic data obtained from references 94 and 95.

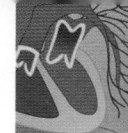

SPECIAL POPULATIONS: PREGNANCY AND LACTATION

Most anticholinergic and antihistaminergic drugs are categorized as Class B or C by the U.S. Food and Drug Administration. Although largely unknown, most agents are likely secreted into breast milk as suggested by their large volumes of distribution.

DIPHENHYDRAMINE

There is one case-control study in which there was a slight statistical association between cleft palate and diphenhydramine exposure in the first trimester. Other than this single study, the vast majority of animal and human data support the safe usage of diphenhydramine in pregnancy. Diphenhydramine is excreted into human breast milk, and the manufacturer concludes that the drug is contraindicated in nursing mothers.[40]

CIMETIDINE

Although the use of cimetidine in pregnancy has not been associated with congenital malformations, multiple animal studies and one human study of nonpregnant patients suggest an antiandrogen effect in the form of decreased prostate, seminal vesicle, and testes size and decreased human libido. Cimetidine is excreted into breast milk, but the effect on the infant is unknown.[40]

ATROPINE

Atropine readily crosses the placenta. No fetal or neonatal adverse effects were noted in two human studies in which atropine was used to reduce gastric secretions before cesarean section. The largest study of fetal exposure to atropine demonstrated no associated congenital anomalies. Another smaller study, however, demonstrated a possible association of atropine exposure to neonatal limb reduction, but other factors could have contributed as well.[40]

TOXICOLOGY

Clinical Manifestations

Although anticholinergic agents often have activity at sites other than muscarinic receptors, the major clinical toxicity from these agents is the anticholinergic syndrome. Manifestations are divided into peripheral and central antimuscarinic effects (Box 39-2). Peripheral manifestations include (1) thirst, dry mucous membranes and hot, dry skin from inhibition of secretions from salivary glands, bronchioles, and sweat glands; (2) skin flushing from dilation of cutaneous blood vessels, especially those of the face; (3) hyperpyrexia from the inability to sweat and neuromuscular hyper-reactivity; (4) mydriasis, poor pupillary light response, and blurred vision from pupillary sphincter and ciliary muscle paralysis; (5) tachycardia from vagolytic effects; (6) urinary retention from inhibition of ureter and bladder contraction; and (7) decreased bowel sounds from inhibition of gastric emptying and GI motility. Sinus

---

BOX 39-2	SYMPTOMS/SIGNS OF ANTICHOLINERGIC TOXICITY

Peripheral (Muscarinic Blockade)

Tachycardia
Dry, flushed skin
Dry mucous membranes
Dilated pupils
Hyperpyrexia
Urinary retention
Decreased bowel sounds
Hypertension
Hypotension (late finding)

Central Anticholinergic Syndrome

Confusion
Disorientation
Loss of short-term memory
Ataxia
Psychomotor agitation
Picking and grasping movements
Extrapyramidal reactions
Visual/auditory hallucinations
Frank psychosis
Coma
Seizures
Respiratory failure
Cardiovascular collapse

---

tachycardia is one of the earliest and most reliable signs of muscarinic receptor blockade.[41] Thus, the absence of tachycardia early after anticholinergic poisoning suggests inaccurate history or co-ingestion of a cardiotoxic agent. The urinary bladder may be palpable from bladder atony, and impaired bowel motility may produce an ileus and delayed and prolonged drug absorption. This latter effect may result in prolonged symptoms secondary to protracted drug absorption.

Anticholinergic delirium, or the central anticholinergic syndrome, is characterized by patient hyperactivity; tremulousness; disorientation; short-term memory impairment; agitation; delirium; visual and auditory hallucinosis; slurred, nonsensical, or incoherent speech; meaningless motor activity such as repetitive picking at bed clothes or grabbing at nonexistent objects; removal of clothing; seizures; and coma.[8-10,42-44]

In overdose, both central and peripheral anticholinergic signs are commonly present. Indeed, the famous mnemonic, "Mad as a hatter, red as a beet, dry as a bone, blind as a bat, and hot as a hare" describes the syndrome well. The central anticholinergic syndrome may occasionally occur without evidence of peripheral signs.[45-48] Although one study reported that "isolated" central anticholinergic signs and symptoms were present in 17% of their patients with the anticholinergic syndrome, dry skin was preserved in those with central sign predominance.[49] Thus, "isolated" central anticholinergic syndrome will likely have at least some peripheral signs of poisoning present and should be more appropriately termed *central predominance* anticholinergic syndrome.

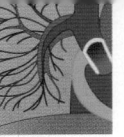

Central predominance anticholinergic syndrome seems more likely to occur in the very young and old, those with underlying organic brain syndrome, those with exaggerated antimuscarinic responses to therapeutic doses, and late following an acute overdose (when peripheral effects have decreased in intensity).[10]

Anticholinergic agents may produce seizures following both therapeutic and excessive doses. Seizures are more commonly dose related and, thus, occur more frequently in overdose. Anticholinergic-induced seizures are usually short lived and require no specific therapy. However, large overdoses of diphenhydramine, pyrilamine, hydroxyzine, orphenadrine, cyclic antidepressants, and carbamazepine have caused prolonged or repeated seizures.

The mechanism of anticholinergic-induced seizures remains unclear. The majority of seizures related to anticholinergic toxicity seem to be associated with medications having other toxic manifestations rather than purely anticholinergic drugs. Seizures have been reported with antihistamine, cyclic antidepressant, phenothiazine, and carbamazepine poisonings but are infrequently reported in jimsonweed abusers and atropine-poisoned infants. Interestingly, researchers have suggested that histamine may have a role as a natural anticonvulsant. Positron emission tomography has demonstrated possible H_1 receptors' coalescence around epileptogenic foci in brain, and this may inhibit generalization of epileptic discharges in the brain.[50] Histamine and its precursor, histidine, seem to act as anticonvulsants in the mammalian brain by their actions on presynaptic H_3 receptors and postsynaptic H_1 receptors.[51-54] H_1 antagonists have been shown to decrease the seizure threshold in rats and mice by heat and electrical stimuli to the brain, respectively.[52,53] Similarly, antihistamines increase electroencephalographic abnormalities and are suspected of producing seizures in epileptic patients. Retrospective data have suggested that phenothiazines, a class of antihistamine, decrease the seizure threshold.[55,56] Doxepin and other cyclic antidepressants are potent histamine blockers that frequently cause seizures when taken in serious overdoses. In addition, seizure activity from some medications with anticholinergic activity is due to interactions at γ-aminobutyric acid (GABA) receptors (cyclic antidepressants) or adenosine receptors (carbamazepine).

Sinus tachycardia is the most common arrhythmia in anticholinergic poisoning and occurs by blocking vagal effects on M_2-muscarinic receptors on the sinoatrial node pacemaker.[6] Sinus tachycardia is most prevalent in young, healthy adults who normally have high resting vagal tone.[6] Tachycardia may not be as evident in the very young and old. Some anticholinergic agents cause life-threatening cardiac arrhythmias by mechanisms other than muscarinic blockade. Medications with anticholinergic effects and the potential to cause quinidine-like conduction abnormalities include cyclic antidepressants, phenothiazines, diphenhydramine, chlorpheniramine, orphenadrine, pyrilamine, and class IA antiarrhythmics.[38] These drugs have sodium channel–blocking properties that not only slow conduction but also

decrease myocardial contractility. Phenothiazines also block rectifying potassium channels and may prolong the QT interval and cause torsades de pointes or other ventricular dysrhythmias.

Rhabdomyolysis is an occasional complication of anticholinergic poisoning, particularly for patients that have psychomotor agitation.[57] Drug-induced rhabdomyolysis from anticholinergic poisoning is due to excess energy use or inadequate oxygen and nutrient delivery to the muscle, which causes myocyte breakdown. Patients at greatest risk are those who have repetitive or prolonged seizures, coma, compartment syndrome, hyperthermia, or severe agitation requiring restraint.

Death from anticholinergic or antihistamine poisoning is most often from cardiac arrhythmia and is frequently associated with seizures. Death is not likely to occur from antimuscarinic receptor antagonism but rather the sodium and potassium channel–blocking effects of these drugs.[58]

Diagnosis

The diagnosis of anticholinergic or sedating antihistamine poisoning is based on a positive history of ingestion and physical findings consistent with the anticholinergic syndrome. When a history of ingestion is not available from the patient due to delirium or obtundation, patient belongings and the exposure environment should be searched for clues to diagnosis. Any knowledge of a patient's past medical history, particularly a list of medications, may greatly assist diagnosis. Any history obtainable from friends or relatives about abuse of drugs or hallucinogenic plants (particularly jimsonweed and mushrooms) may be of value. A history of recent travel and the use of scopolamine patches should be sought.

In a mixed ingestion, the physical findings may be variable and make the diagnosis more challenging. Electrocardiographic (ECG), laboratory, and other adjunctive tests are not often helpful to confirm or refute the diagnosis of anticholinergic poisoning. An ECG often demonstrates sinus tachycardia alone. The presence of repolarization abnormalities (e.g., nonspecific ST-T changes, QT prolongation) is consistent with certain agents (e.g., diphenhydramine). As with many poisonings, a toxicology screen has limited value. Agents that produce anticholinergic toxicity are not often part of a routine immunoassay screen.[23] Comprehensive qualitative screening techniques (e.g., gas chromatography/mass spectrometry) and quantitative assays are not readily available and do not routinely guide treatment. These tests may be useful for confirmation of the presence of a drug after treatment has been initiated. Toxicology screens are more useful to identify other causes of altered mental status or to identify unsuspected co-ingestions (e.g., acetaminophen).

As stated, the diagnosis and treatment of the anticholinergic syndrome is guided by the clinical examination. This cause of delirium can be missed if the physician fails to recognize associated peripheral signs or inappropriately dismisses the diagnosis because common

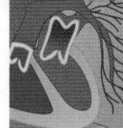

peripheral anticholinergic signs (e.g,, sinus tachycardia and mydriasis) are absent. Anticholinergic delirium has been misdiagnosed as dementia or psychotic depression in elderly patients and varicella encephalitis in children.[45,47]

DIFFERENTIAL DIAGNOSIS OF ANTICHOLINERGIC POISONING

The constellation of symptoms that identify the anticholinergic syndrome can be mimicked, in part, by many other toxins and medical conditions (Box 39-3). Distinguishing it from adrenergic excess (sympathomimetic poisoning, thyrotoxicosis, or pheochromocytoma) can be difficult. The pupillary, cardiovascular, and CNS effects of sympathomimetic poisons are similar to those produced by anticholinergic poisoning. Sweating frequently accompanies adrenergic stimulation, whereas dry skin and mucous membranes are characteristic of anticholinergic poisoning. Paranoid hallucinations and violent behavior often accompany adrenergic-induced hallucinations, whereas anticholinergic poisoning causes mumbling speech, picking at sheets, and disorientation. Urinary retention may also be helpful in distinguishing anticholinergic from sympathomimetic poisoning. The anticholinergic syndrome has similarities to the autonomic dysfunction and altered mental status that occurs with ethanol or sedative-hypnotic withdrawal, serotonin syndrome, neuroleptic malignant syndrome, or a disulfiram reaction. The absence of sweat with the anticholinergic syndrome is a key differentiating feature from these other drug-associated syndromes. Chronic salicylate poisoning can appear similar to anticholinergic poisoning because patients often present with altered mental status, tachycardia, and fever. Medical conditions can also mimic the anticholinergic syndrome. Hypoxia or hypoglycemia causes delirium, agitation, or CNS depression. Dry, hot skin and altered sensorium due to heat stroke, dehydration, or sepsis can be mistaken for anticholinergic toxicity. Central anticholinergic effects in the absence of peripheral signs can be similar to those caused by some hallucinogenic substances, steroid-induced psychosis, vascular or infectious CNS disease, sepsis, or psychiatric illnesses.

BOX 39-3	**TOXINS AND MEDICAL CONDITIONS EASILY CONFUSED WITH THE ANTICHOLINERGIC SYNDROME**

Toxins

Adrenergic poisons
  Amphetamines
  Caffeine
  Cocaine
  Methylphenidate
  Pseudoephedrine
  Theophylline
Autonomic dysfunction
  Disulfiram reactions
  Neuroleptic malignant syndrome
  Serotonin syndrome
  Withdrawal from ethanol or benzodiazepines
Central hallucinogen poisoning
  Lysergic acid diethylamide
  Mescaline
  Phencyclidine
  Psilocybin mushrooms
Lithium poisoning
Salicylate poisoning
Steroid-induced psychosis

Medical Conditions

Adrenergic excess
  Pheochromocytoma
  Thyrotoxicosis
Central nervous system infection
Cerebral vasculitis
Dehydration
Heat stroke
Hypoglycemia
Hypoxia
Psychiatric illnesses
Sepsis

TREATMENT OF ANTICHOLINERGIC TOXICITY

General Management

The majority of patients poisoned by anticholinergic agents are adequately treated with supportive care and observation.

Anticholinergics inhibit GI motility and can cause prolonged, erratic, or delayed drug absorption. After a large overdose of benztropine, a patient demonstrated erratic absorption and repeated worsening of anticholinergic symptoms over 9 days.[59] Because of slowed GI absorption, gastric emptying procedures may be useful even when patients present many hours after toxicant ingestion. Administration of charcoal is effective for preventing further drug absorption. Repeated doses of activated charcoal may play a role in preventing continued absorption, although the development of ileus limits its use. There is no role for enhanced elimination techniques (e.g., hemodialysis or hemoperfusion) with anticholinergic agents and antihistamines due to their large volumes of distribution and high protein binding (see Table 39-1).

A search for and removal of a transdermal patch should be initiated in all patients with altered mental status that could be attributed to the anticholinergic syndrome.

Treatment of Agitation

Anticholinergic-induced delirium ranges from mild confusion to severe agitation and possibly violence. Controlling agitation is necessary for adequate patient assessment and to prevent rhabdomyolysis, hyperthermia, and physical injury. Physical and chemical re-

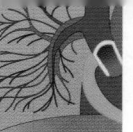

straints are indicated for the treatment of severe agitation. Benzodiazepines may be tried initially to control patient agitation, but they are often ineffective when anticholinergic-associated agitation is severe.[60] Adjunctive therapy with haloperidol or other neuroleptics is not recommended to control agitation since these agents can impair thermoregulation. Provided no contraindications for its use exist (see Antidote Theraphy), physostigmine has been shown to be both safe and effective for the treatment of agitated delirium in the setting of known or suspected anticholinergic syndrome.[49] As compared with benzodiazepine therapy, physostigmine treats patient delirium better, controls patient agitation more effectively, may decrease the need for mechanical ventilation, and shortens the course of neurologic morbidity.[49] When the diagnosis is initially suspected but uncertain, physostigmine may obviate the need for further testing (e.g., head computed tomography and lumbar puncture) upon resolution of delirium.[49]

Treatment of Seizures

Although the mechanism of seizures is not well understood for this class of agents, drug-associated seizures are generally best treated with benzodiazepines (e.g., diazepam or lorazepam) followed by barbiturates (e.g., phenobarbital) when necessary. Data from case reports suggest that physostigmine may be effective for seizure termination, but clinical experience is limited and efficacy not well established.[61,62] The administration of physostigmine for seizures from this class of agents is not recommended, particularly since seizures are a known major adverse effect from physostigmine.

Treatment of Rhabdomyolysis

Agitation and excessive neuronal stimulation increase the risk of rhabdomyolysis. Controlling agitation and seizures is important to prevent rhabdomyolysis. Serial measurements of creatine phosphokinase in blood and determination of occult blood positivity in the urine will help identify those at risk for developing acute renal failure from rhabdomyolysis. Ensuring adequate urine output with intravenous (IV) fluids is the mainstay of treatment for preventing acute tubular necrosis.[57] The efficacy of mannitol and urine alkalinization has not been established for the routine treatment of rhabdomyolysis.[63]

Treatment of Cardiovascular Toxicity

Sinus tachycardia is the most common toxic cardiovascular effect from anticholinergic poisoning but rarely requires intervention. A large number of drugs with anticholinergic effects cause QRS prolongation and dysrhythmias by blocking fast-sodium channels (type 1a activity).[64-66] IV sodium bicarbonate improves impaired conduction from fast-sodium channel blockers such as cyclic antidepressants, diphenhydramine, and orphenadrine.[38,67] Rarely, myocardial pump failure occurs with large overdoses. Case reports have demonstrated that

refractory shock can occur despite aggressive medical intervention. Patients with such profound cardiovascular toxicity have been successfully resuscitated after cardiac bypass or intra-aortic balloon pump procedures.[68]

Antidote Therapy

Although its use is controversial, physostigmine is a well-recognized antidote that can be used to treat the anticholinergic syndrome. Physostigmine, a naturally occurring alkaloid obtained from the West African vine *Physostigma venosum*, is a reversible, carbamate cholinesterase inhibitor.[6] After a single dose of physostigmine, the action of acetylcholine is potentiated at postganglionic parasympathetic and central cholinergic neuroreceptors, and the competitive blockade by anticholinergic agents is reversed by mass action. As a tertiary amine, physostigmine readily crosses the BBB and is capable of reversing central anticholinergic effects (e.g., agitation, hallucinations, delirium, and coma).[69-73] Peripherally, physostigmine may reverse the tachycardia, mydriasis, ileus, and urinary retention that occur secondary to muscarinic blockade.

Physostigmine is a nonspecific analeptic. Its administration results in cholinergic modulation of other CNS neurotransmitter pathways by poorly understood mechanisms. The sedating effects of drugs without anticholinergic activity have responded to physostigmine administration through nonspecific arousal.[73] Because of this, physostigmine was employed as part of a "coma cocktail" in the 1970s and often administered to patients with undifferentiated drug-induced coma. When used for this indication, physostigmine was neither consistently effective nor safe. Physostigmine resulted in an unacceptable high incidence of side effects (e.g., seizures, cholinergic crisis, bradyarrhythmias, and asystole), particularly when used for TCA poisoning.[60]

In one clinical series, 2 of 21 patients who received physostigmine had seizures after its administration, and 2 developed cholinergic symptoms (hypersalivation in 1 patient, bradycardia and hypotension in the other). The author of this series concluded that physostigmine has "little part to play in routine management" because patients with anticholinergic symptoms usually fare well with supportive therapy alone.[74] In another clinical series of 26 patients (of which 17 had ingested a TCA), seizures occurred in 3 (12%) patients and bradycardia in 1 patient given physostigmine.[75] In a recent retrospective chart review of 39 adults who were administered physostigmine for the anticholinergic syndrome, 1 (2.6%) developed a brief seizure. However, this individual had presented after a 1- to 2-minute seizure, so it is impossible to say that physostigmine caused the seizure.[76] In a retrospective study that compared treatment of physostigmine with benzodiazepines in a group of 52 patients with anticholinergic delirium, physostigmine was more effective for the control of agitation and reversing delirium.[49] One case report described a patient poisoned by *D. stramonium* (jimsonweed), who developed atrial fibrillation and a short run of ventricular tachycardia 45 minutes after administration of physostigmine.[77] In an additional case report, an 85-year-old man developed ventricular ectopy 30 minutes after receiving 1 mg of physostigmine.[78]

Physostigmine is no longer indicated in the treatment of cyclic antidepressant poisoning, and evidence strongly suggests that it is dangerous for use.[74,75,79,80] A series of 41 patients taking intentional overdoses of maprotiline showed that 6 of 7 patients treated with physostigmine developed seizures.[74] The investigators concluded that the use of physostigmine should be abandoned in overdoses of maprotiline and other cyclic antidepressants. The danger of physostigmine administration is further illustrated in another cases series of two patients with acute severe TCA poisoning. The administration of physostigmine was temporally associated with the occurrence of bradyasystole.[80] The potential risks associated with physostigmine are greater than the benefits gained from its use in cyclic antidepressant toxicity.

There is a long history of clinical use of physostigmine as an antidote. It is apparent that when used inappropriately (e.g., nondifferentiated drug-induced coma, known or suspected TCA poisoning, rapid IV administration), it is associated with an unacceptably high incidence of side effects. Conversely, when used appropriately, it is both safe and effective and the preferred treatment for the anticholinergic syndrome. The use of physostigmine is indicated for the treatment of patient agitation and delirium in known or suspected anticholinergic syndrome, particularly when patients are dangerous to themselves or others. Although efficacy is not well-established, physostigmine may also be appropriate for narrow complex supraventricular arrhythmias in the setting of the anticholinergic syndrome that result in hemodynamic instability (hypotension, myocardial ischemia, or congestive heart failure) when other attempts to control heart rate have failed or are believed to be too risky in a particular patient. Neostigmine, a quaternary cholinesterase inhibitor that does not cross the BBB, may play a selective role for severe ileus or intestinal pseudo-obstruction associated with anticholinergic drugs.[81] Absolute contraindications for the use of physostigmine include any evidence of cardiac conduction disturbances on ECG (e.g., prolonged PR or QRS intervals) or known or suspected acute cyclic antidepressant poisoning. Although physostigmine has been previously recommended for the treatment of ventricular tachyarrhythmias and seizures associated with the anticholinergic syndrome, these should be considered relative, if not absolute, contraindications for use of this antidote. Conversely, although contraindications for the use of physostigmine have historically included the presence of patient asthma, ischemic heart disease, peripheral vascular disease, and mechanical obstruction of the GI or urogenital tract, these contraindications are theoretical, unsubstantiated, and no longer considered true.[6,82]

The suggested doses of physostigmine are as follows:

For children: a dose of 0.02 mg/kg slowly IV over 3 to 5 minutes.

For adults: 1 to 2 mg slowly IV; may be repeated every 10 minutes until cessation of the life-threatening condition. Schneck has recommended an IV infusion of 2 mg in 100 mL of normal saline infused over 10 minutes to avoid adverse effects from too rapid administration.[34]

In one study of adults, the mean initial dose necessary to treat agitated delirium associated with the anticholinergic syndrome was 2.2 mg (range, 0.5 to 6 mg) with a mean initial response time of approximately 11 minutes.[49] The duration of action is usually 20 to 60 minutes, and recurrence of anticholinergic symptoms may require repeated doses. In this same study, relapse of symptoms occurred in 78% of patients with a mean relapse time of 100 minutes.[49] Adverse effects are more likely after repeated doses. Cholinergic excess due to physostigmine use is not often life threatening. It has been suggested that atropine should be available and given in half the dose of physostigmine should severe cholinergic toxicity develop.[70] The use of glycopyrrolate, a pure peripheral anticholinergic agent, has been proposed as an alternative to atropine to treat the cholinergic toxicity of physostigmine.

Whenever physostigmine is used, it should (1) be given very slowly (over 3 to 10 minutes) IV; (2) not be given merely to "wake the patient up"; (3) be used only in a setting where advanced life support is available; (4) be used only when central and peripheral anticholinergic findings are present; (5) be used only in the absence of cardiac conduction abnormalities suggesting sodium channel blockade; and (6) always be preceded and followed by proper supportive care.

SPECIAL CONSIDERATIONS FOR ANTIHISTAMINE AND ANTICHOLINERGIC TOXICITY

Nonsedating Piperidine Antihistamines

Acrivastine, cetirizine, fexofenadine, desloratadine, and loratadine are currently marketed in the United States as nonsedating piperidine antihistamines. In therapeutic doses, their lack of CNS effects is secondary to an inability to cross the BBB.[39] Acrivastine, the active metabolite of triprolidine, was given to humans for 1 week at 100 times the recommended dose without cardiovascular effects.[83] Cetirizine, the carboxylated metabolite of hydroxyzine, lacked cardiovascular toxicity and sedation in overdose.[84] Fexofenadine, the metabolite of terfenadine, has a safety profile similar to placebo with no significant drug interactions, cardiotoxicity, or sedation.[85] In vitro, loratadine significantly inhibited the potassium rectifier current.[86] Loratadine, when given with nefazodone, resulted in significantly increased QT interval in humans.[87] Desloratadine, the active metabolite of loratadine, does not seem to effect the potassium rectifier current.[88,89] This finding was likely from the inhibition of the CYP3A4-mediated metabolism of loratadine, leading to increased concentrations.

From a historical perspective, terfenadine and astemizole were withdrawn from the market in the late 1990s because of the high incidence of ventricular dys-

U: Unclear what you mean by 'dangerous for use'. Do you mean for any use?

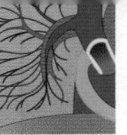

rhythmias. Terfenadine and astemizole inhibit the delayed potassium rectifier current and thus slow repolarization.[90] Accumulation of these drugs in the serum as occurred with overdose or impaired metabolism from coadministration of CYP3A4 inhibitors, was manifested clinically as prolongation of the QT interval and torsades de pointes. Agents that inhibit CYP3A4 metabolism of terfenadine include erythromycin, clarithromycin, ketoconazole, fluconazole, itraconazole, and grapefruit juice. Underlying liver disease in the absence of P-450 inhibitors can also cause cardiac toxic effects.

H_2 Receptor Blockers

The H_2 blockers are competitive antagonists at H_2 receptors and block gastric acid secretion. These agents are used to treat peptic acid diseases and include cimetidine, ranitidine, famotidine, and nizatidine. They are highly selective receptor antagonists and do not block H_1 receptors or have antimuscarinic activity. Blocking central H_2 receptors alters neurotransmitter function and causes delirium, confusion, agitation, and seizures. Confusion is more likely to occur in elderly patients and those who have elevated blood concentrations of these agents after acute deterioration of renal and hepatic function.[91] Only cimetidine causes significant inhibition of hepatic microsomal mixed-function oxidases that may impair metabolism of other drugs.

Acute overdose of the specific H_2 receptor antagonists typically causes only minor toxic effects such as drowsiness and mild bradycardia.[92] More serious effects such as hypotension or bradycardia are likely to occur with IV overdoses and not with ingestion of the drug. Other effects rarely reported include hypersensitivity hepatitis, bone marrow suppression, and renal failure with long-term therapeutic doses.

Chemical Weapons

Anticholinergic chemicals have been used both as an agent and an antidote in chemical warfare. 3-Quinuclidinyl benzylate (QNB) was first developed for the treatment of GI illness but later turned over to the U.S. Army because of the multiple cases of delirium at very low doses. QNB is a competitive antagonist at the muscarinic receptors in the central and peripheral nervous systems. The reader is referred to Chapter 105E for a detailed discussion of this agent

Atropine is a component, along with pralidoxime, of the Mark I kits developed as an antidote for nerve agent poisoning. There are multiple cases of anticholinergic poisoning from unjustified injections in the Scud missile attacks on Israel in 1991. There were 208 unjustified injections of atropine accounting for 47% of all the injuries during this 8-day barrage of surface-to-surface missiles[93] (see Chapter 105A).

DISPOSITION

Clinical toxicity is usually evident within 1 to 4 hours after ingestion, but the severity and duration of toxic effects are highly variable. The potential for prolonged toxin absorption and, thus, prolonged toxicity from anticholinergic agents must be considered when determining patient disposition. Patient discharge or medical clearance is reserved for patients who do not develop toxic effects or who develop mild toxic effects initially that resolve during a 6-hour period of observation (provided that GI ileus and significant co-ingestants with delayed toxicity are not present). No patient should be discharged without suicide assessment, substance abuse counseling, or poison prevention counseling.

Those patients who manifest mild toxicity (e.g., ataxia, lethargy, mild agitation, sinus tachycardia, repolarization abnormalities on ECG) should be admitted to a monitored bed for continued observation. Patients with moderate to severe toxicity (e.g., significant CNS depression or agitation, respiratory depression, hypotension, seizures, acid–base disturbances, nonsinus arrhythmias, and cardiac conduction disturbances) should be admitted to an intensive care unit for aggressive supportive care. In addition, patients who are given large doses of benzodiazepines for the control of agitation require intensive care unit observation. Patients whose agitation and delirium resolve following the administration of physostigmine still require hospital admission due to the short duration of antidotal activity and, consequently, high incidence of recrudescent toxicity. When the appropriate disposition of a patient is in question, consultation with a medical toxicologist or poison control center is recommended.

REFERENCES

1. Labianca DA, Reeves WJ: Scopolamine: a potent chemical weapon. J Chem Educ 1984;61:678–680.
2. Beaver K, Gavin T: Treatment of acute anticholinergic poisoning with physostigmine. Am J Emerg Med 1998;16(5):505–507.
3. Centers for Disease Control and Prevention: Scopolamine poisoning among heroin users—New York City, Newark, Philadelphia, and Baltimore, 1995 and 1996. MMWR Morb Mortal Wkly Rep 1996; 45:457–460.
4. Weiner A, Bayer M, McKay C, et al: Anticholinergic poisoning with adulterated intranasal cocaine. Am J Emerg Med 1998;16(5): 517–520.
5. Chan T: Anticholinergic poisoning due to Chinese herbal medicines. Vet Hum Toxicol 1995;37(2):156–157.
6. Brown JH, Taylor P: Muscarinic receptor agonists and antagonists. In Hardman JG, Limbird LE (eds): Goodman and Gilman's The Pharmacological Basis of Therapeutics. New York, McGraw-Hill, 1996, pp 141–160.
7. Brown N, Roberts L: Histamine, bradykinin, and their antagonists. In Hardman JG, Limbird LE (eds): Goodman and Gilman's The Pharmacological Basis of Therapeutics. New York, McGraw-Hill, 2001, pp 645–667.
8. Hall RC, Fox J, Stickney SK, Gardner ER: Anticholinergic delirium: etiology, presentation, diagnosis and management. J Psychedelic Drugs 1978;10:237–241.
9. Hall RC, Feinsilver DL, Holt RE: Anticholinergic psychosis: differential diagnosis and management. Psychosomatics 1981; 22:581–587.
10. Hvizdos AJ, Bennet JA, Wells BG, et al: Anticholinergic psychosis in a patient receiving usual doses of haloperidol, desipramine, and benztropine. Clin Pharm 1983;2:174–178.
11. Cole J: Atropine-like delirium and anticholinergic substances. Am J Psychiatry 1972;128:898–899.
12. Forrester PA: An anticholinergic effect of general anaesthetics on cerebrocortical neurones. Br J Pharmacol 1975;55:275–278.

13. Woodward GA, Baldassano RN: Topical diphenhydramine toxicity in a five year old with varicella. Pediatric Emerg Care 1988; 4:18–20.

14. Reilly JF, Weisse ME: Topically induced diphenhydramine toxicity. J Emerg Med 1990;8:59–61.

15. Filloux F: Toxic encephalopathy caused by topically applied diphenhydramine. J Pediatr 1986;108:1018–1020.

16. Wilkinson JA: Side effects of transdermal scopolamine. J Emerg Med 1987;5:389–392.

17. Price BH: Anisocoria from scopolamine patches. JAMA 1985; 253:1561.

18. Patterson JH, Ives T, Greganti MA: Transient bilateral pupillary dilation from scopolamine discs. Drug Intell Clin Pharm 1986;20:986–987.

19. Thompson H: Cornpicker's pupil: Jimson weed mydriasis. J Iowa Med Soc 1971;61(8):475–477.

20. Reid D, Fulton JD: Tachycardia precipitated by topical homatropine. BMJ 1989;299:795–796.

21. Fitzgerald DA, Hanson RM, West C: Seizures associated with 1% cyclopentolate eyedrops. J Paediatr Child Health 1990;26:106–107.

22. Brizer DA, Manning DW: Delirium induced by poisoning with anticholinergic agents. Am J Psychiatry 1982;139:1343–1344.

23. Goldfrank L, Flomenbaum N, Lewin N, et al: Anticholinergic poisoning. Clin Toxicol 1982;19:17–25.

24. Dilsalver SC: Antimuscarinic agents as substance of abuse: a review. J Clin Psychopharmacol 1988;8:14–22.

25. Smith JM: Abuse of the antiparkinson drugs: a review of the literature. J Clin Psychiatry 1980;41:351–354.

26. Modell JG, Tandon R, Beresford TP: Dopaminergic activity of the antimuscarinic antiparkinsonian agents. J Clin Psychopharmacol 1989;9:347–351.

27. Land W, Pinsky D, Salzman C: Abuse and misuse of anticholinergic medications. Hosp Commun Psychiatry 1991;42:580–581.

28. MacVicar K: Abuse of antiparkinsonian drugs by psychiatric patients. Am J Psychiatry 1977;134:809–811.

29. Pullen GP, Best NR, Maguire J: Anticholinergic drug abuse: a common problem. BMJ 1984;289:612–613.

30. Crawshaw JA, Mullen PA: A study of benzhexol abuse. Br J Psychiatry 1984;145:300–303.

31. Benjamin MB: Mushroom poisoning in infants and children: the Amanita Pantherina/Muscaria Group. Clin Toxicol 1992;30:13–22.

32. Taylor P, Brown JH: Acetylcholine. In Siegel GJ (ed): Basic Neurochemistry: Molecular, Cellular, and Medical Aspects. New York, Raven, 1989, pp 203–231.

33. Cuello AC, Sofroniew MV: The anatomy of the CNS cholinergic neurons. Trends Neurosci 1984;7:74–78.

34. Schneck HJ, Rupreht J: Central anticholinergic syndrome in anesthesia and intensive care. Acta Anaesthesiol Belg 1989;40:219–228.

35. Green JP: Histamine. In Siegel GJ (ed): Basic Neurochemistry: Molecular, Cellular, and Medical Aspects. New York, Raven, 1994, pp 309–318.

36. Gefland EW: Role of histamine in the pathophysiology of asthma: immunomodulatory and anti-inflammatory activities of the H1-receptor antagonists. Am J Med 2002;113(9A):2s–7s.

37. Sastry BS, Phillis JW: Depression of rat cerebral cortical neurons by H1 and H2 histamine receptor agonists. Eur J Pharmacol 1976;38:269–273.

38. Clark RF, Vance MV: Massive diphenhydramine poisoning resulting in a wide-complex tachycardia: successful treatment with sodium bicarbonate. Ann Emerg Med 1992;21:318–321.

39. Simons FE, Simons KJ: The pharmacology and use of H1-receptor-antagonist drugs. N Engl J Med 1994;330:1663–1670.

40. Briggs G, Freeman R, Yaffe S: Drugs in Pregnancy and Lactation, 6th ed. Philadelphia, Lippincott Williams & Wilkins, 2002.

41. Greenblatt DJ, Shader RI: Anticholinergics. N Engl J Med 1973;288:1215–1217.

42. Gowdy JM: Stramonium intoxication: review of symptomatology in 212 cases. JAMA 1972;221:585–587.

43. Perry PJ, Wilding DC, Juhl RP: Anticholinergic psychosis. Am J Hosp Pharm 1978;35:725–727.

44. Fisher CM: Visual hallucinations on eye closure associated with atropine toxicity. A neurological analysis and comparison with other visual hallucinations. Can J Neurol Sci 1991;18:18–27.

45. Johnson AL, Hollister LE, Berger PA: The anticholinergic intoxication syndrome: diagnosis and treatment. J Clin Psychiatry 1981;42:313–316.

46. Klein-Schwartz W, Oderda GM: Jimson weed intoxication in adolescents and young adults. Am J Dis Child 1984;138:737–739.

47. Moreau A, Jones BD, Banno V: Chronic central anticholinergic toxicity in manic depressive illness mimicking dementia. Can J Psychiatry 1986;31:339–340.

48. Richmond M, Seger D: Central anticholinergic syndrome in a child: a case report. J Emerg Med 1985;3:453–456.

49. Burns M, Linden C, Graudins A, et al: A comparison of physostigmine and benzodiazepines for the treatment of anticholinergic poisoning. Ann Emerg Med 1999;35(4):374–381.

50. Tuomisto L, Tacke U: Is histamine an anticonvulsive inhibitory transmitter? Neuropharmacology 1986;25:955–958.

51. Chen Z, Li W-D, Zhu L-J, et al: Effects of histidine, a precursor of histamine, on phenylenetetrazole-induced seizures in rats. Acta Pharmacol Sin 2002;23(4):361–366.

52. Yokoyama H, Sato M, Iinuma K, et al: Centrally acting histamine H1 antagonists promote the development of amygdala kindling in rats. Neurosci Lett 1996;217:194–196.

53. Yokoyama H, Onodera K, Iinuma K, Watanabe T: 2-Thiazolylethylamine, a selective histamine H1 agonist, decreases seizure susceptibility in mice. Pharmacol Biochem Behav 1994;47:503–507.

54. Scherkl R, Hashem A, Frey H: Histamine in brain—its role in regulation of seizure susceptibility. Epilepsy Res 1991;10:111–118.

55. Markowitz J, Brown R: Seizures with neuroleptics and antidepressants. Gen Hosp Psychiatry 1987;9:135–141.

56. Donlon P, Tupin J: Successful suicides with thioridazine and mesoridazine. Ach Gen Psychiatry 1977;34:955–957.

57. Curry SC, Chang D, Conner D: Drug- and toxin-induced rhabdomyolysis. Ann Emerg Med 1989;18:1068–1084.

58. Glauser J: Tricyclic antidepressant poisoning. Cleve Clin J Med 2000;67(10):709–713.

59. Fahy P, Arnold P, Curry SC, Bond R: Serial serum drug concentrations and prolonged anticholinergic toxicity after benztropine (Cogentin) overdose. Am J Emerg Med 1989;7:199–202.

60. Manoguerra AS, Ruiz E: Physostigmine treatment of anticholinergic poisoning. J Am Coll Emerg Physicians 1976;5:125–127.

61. Magera BE, Betlach CJ, Sweatt AP, Derrick CW: Hydroxyzine intoxication in a 13-month-old child. Pediatrics 1981;67:280–283.

62. Gillick JS: Atropine toxicity in a neonate. Br J Anaesth 1974; 46:793–794.

63. Homsi E, Barreiro M, Orlando J, Higra E: Prophylaxis of acute renal failure in patients with rhabdomyolysis. Ren Fail 1997; 19(2):283–288.

64. Lindsay CA, Williams GD, Levin DL: Fatal adult respiratory distress syndrome after diphenhydramine toxicity in a child: a case report. Crit Care Med 1995;23:777–781.

65. Danze LK, Langdorf MI: Reversal of orphenadrine-induced ventricular tachycardia with physostigmine. J Emerg Med 1991; 9:453–457.

66. Farrell M, Heinrichs M, Tilelli JA: Response of life threatening dimenhydrinate intoxication to sodium bicarbonate administration. Clin Toxicol 1991;29:527–535.

67. Sharma A, Hexdall A, Chang E, et al: Diphenhydramine-induced wide complex dysrhythmia responds to treatment with sodium bicarbonate. Am J Emerg Med 2003;21(3):212–215.

68. Freedberg RS, Friedman GR, Palu RN, Feit F: Cardiogenic shock due to antihistamine overdose: reversal with intra-aortic balloon counterpulsation. JAMA 1987;257:660–661.

69. Granacher RP, Baldessarini RJ, Messner E: Physostigmine treatment of delirium induced by anticholinergics. Am Fam Physician 1976;13:99.

70. Rumack BH: Anticholinergic poisoning: Treatment with physostigmine. Pediatrics 1973;52:449–451.

71. Burks JS, Walker JE, Rumack BH, Oh JE: Tricyclic antidepressant poisoning. Reversal of coma, choreoathetosis, and myoclonus by physostigmine. JAMA 1974;230:1405–1407.

72. Duvoisin RC, Katz R: Reversal of central anticholinergic syndrome in man by physostigmine. JAMA 1968;206:1963.

73. Nattel S, Bayne L, Ruedy J: Physostigmine in coma due to drug overdose. Clin Pharmacol Ther 1979;25:96.

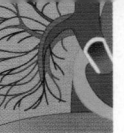

74. Knudsen K, Heath A: Effects of self poisoning with maprotiline. BMJ 1984;288:601–603.

75. Walker WE, Levy RC, Henenson IB: Physostigmine—its use and abuse. J Am Coll Emerg Physicians 1976;5:335.

76. Schneir A, Offerman S, Ly B, et al: Complications of diagnostic physostigmine administration to emergency department patients. Ann Emerg Med 2003;42(1):14–19.

77. Levy R: Arrhythmias following physostigmine administration in Jimson weed poisoning. J Am Coll Emerg Physicians 1977;6:107.

78. Dysken MW, Janowsky DS: Dose-related physostigmine induced ventricular arrhythmia: case report. J Clin Psychiatry 1985;46:446–447.

79. Munoz RA, Kuplic JB: Large overdoses of tricyclic antidepressants treated with physostigmine salicylate. Psychosomatics 1975;16:77–78.

80. Pentel P, Peterson CD: Asytole complicating physostigmine treatment of tricyclic antidepressant overdose. Ann Emerg Med 1980;9:588–590.

81. Isbister G, Oakley P, Whyte I, Dawson A: Treatment of anti-cholinergic-induced ileus with neostigmine. Ann Emerg Med 2001;38(6):689–693.

82. Nilsson E, Meretoja OA, Neuvonen P: Hemodynamic responses to physostigmine in patients with a drug overdose. Anesth Analg 1983;62:885–888.

83. Berlin J, King A, Tutsch K, et al: A phase II study of vinblastine in combination with acrivastine in patients with advanced renal cell carcinoma. Invest New Drugs 1994;12:137–141.

84. Spiller H, Villalobos D, Benson B, et al: Retrospective evaluation of cetirizine (Zyrtec) ingestion [Letter]. Clin Toxicol 2002;40(4):525–526.

85. Mason J, Reynolds R, Rao N: The systemic safety of fexofenadine HCl. Clin Exp Allergy 1999;29(Suppl 3):163–170.

86. Crumb W: Loratadine blockage of K (+) channels in human hear, comparison with terfenadine under physiological conditions. J Pharmacol Exp Ther 2000;292:261–264.

87. Abernathy D, Barbey J, Franc J, et al: Loratadine and terfenadine interaction with nefazodone, both antihistamines are associated with QTc prolongation. Clin Pharmacol Ther 2001;69:96–103.

88. Kreutner W, Chiu J, Barnett A: Preclinical pharmacology of desloratadine, a selective and nonsedating histamine H1 receptor antagonist. Second communication, lack of central nervous system and cardiovascular effects. Arzneimittelforschung 2000;50:441–448.

89. Paakkari I: Cardiotoxicity of new antihistamines and cisapride [Review]. Toxicol Lett 2002;127:279–284.

90. Berul CI, Morad M: Regulation of potassium channels by nonsedating antihistamines. Circulation 1995;91:2220–2225.

91. Schentag JJ: Cimetidine-associated mental confusion: further studies in 36 severely ill patients. Ther Drug Monit 1980;2:133–142.

92. Krenzelok EP, Litovitz T, Lippold KP: Cimetidine toxicity: an assessment of 881 cases. Ann Emerg Med 1987;16:1217–1221.

93. Bleich A, Dycian A, Koslowsky M, et al: Psychiatric implications of missile attacks on a civilian population. JAMA 1992;268(5):613–615.

94. Baselt RC: Disposition of Toxic Drugs and Chemicals in Man, 7th ed. Foster City, CA, Biomedical Publications, 2004.

95. Thummal KE, Shen DD: Design and optimization of dosage regimens. In Hardman JG, Limbird LE, Gilman AG (eds): Goodman & Gilman's The Pharmacological Basis of Therapeutics, 10th ed. New York, McGraw-Hill, 2001, pp 1924–2023.

40 *Anticonvulsants*

DONNA SEGER, MD

At a Glance...

- Many anticonvulsants are used to treat nonconvulsive disorders such as mood disorders.
- Drugs that are hepatically metabolized via the cytochrome system interact with other drugs metabolized via the same system.
- Data on overdose is minimal for most newer anticonvulsants. Unless otherwise stated, treatment is supportive.
- Gastrointestinal decontamination recommendations supported by the American Academy of Clinical Toxicology/European Association of Poison Control Centres and Clinical Toxicologists are as follows:
  - Gastric lavage may be considered if the patient is obtunded within an hour of ingestion.
  - Whole-bowel irrigation may be considered when tablets are sustained release or enteric coated.

Prior to 1993, the only drugs available to treat epilepsy—phenobarbital, primidone, phenytoin, carbamazepine, and valproate—caused significant side effects. Many patients taking these drugs still had refractory seizures. Since 1993, eight new anticonvulsants with better side effect profiles and less hepatic enzyme induction have been approved. However, they are more expensive than the traditional drugs and may not be more cost effective.[1]

EPILEPSY AND DRUG DEVELOPMENT

Epilepsy is a chronic neurologic condition in which the patient suffers recurrent, unprovoked seizures.[2] Seizures, a paroxysmal transient disturbance of brain function, affect 1% of the world's population. Side effects of anticonvulsants (ACs) and the 25% of the epileptic population who are not seizure-free have driven the development of new ACs that are less toxic and more efficacious.[3]

Choice of Drug

The ideal AC has the following pharmacokinetic characteristics: rapid absorption after oral ingestion, high bioavailability, rapid achievement of steady-state concentrations, minimal protein binding, linear kinetics, long elimination half-life that allows twice a day dosing, minimal hepatic metabolism, primary renal excretion, and constant interpatient pharmacokinetics. The ideal drug is also effective for a wide range of seizure types, causes few adverse effects, and interacts with few drugs.[4]

Sudden Unexpected Death

Sudden unexpected death (SUD) is increased in patients with epilepsy and reflects population rates, not drug effect. Mechanism and role of AC in SUD are unknown and may depend on the unique circumstances.[5]

Teratogenicity

Major malformation, growth retardation, and hypoplasia of the midface and fingers is called anticonvulsant embryopathy. The incidence of embryopathy correlates with exposure to the anticonvulsant drug.[6] Its incidence is not increased in infants whose mother had epilepsy but did not take anticonvulsant drugs during pregnancy.

Anticonvulsant Hypersensitivity Syndrome

Anticonvulsant hypersensitivity syndrome (AHS), a rare, life-threatening syndrome consisting of rash and internal organ (most frequently liver) involvement, occurs within 8 weeks of initiation of an AC and is not related to dose or serum concentration of the drug. AHS occurs in one in 1000 to 10,000 exposures and is most frequently caused by the aromatic AC (phenobarbital, phenytoin, carbamazepine). Its cause is unknown. Treatment is discontinuation of the anticonvulsant and aggressive supportive care. The syndrome is associated with substantial morbidity and mortality, including fulminant hepatic failure and death.[7]

PHENOBARBITAL

Pharmacology

Phenobarbital (PB) inhibits seizures by potentiating synaptic inhibition through two separate actions on the γ-aminobutyric acid ($GABA_A$) receptor—that is, enhanced effects of GABA-evoked chloride currents, and direct activation of the receptor at supratherapeutic concentrations.[8]

Pharmacokinetics

PB is slowly absorbed, with peak concentrations occurring several hours after a single dose. It is 40% to 60% bound to plasma proteins. Up to 23% of the dose is eliminated unchanged by pH-dependent renal excretion. The remainder of the drug is metabolized primarily by hepatic CYP2C9.[8]

735

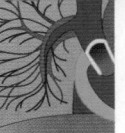

Toxicology

ACUTE TOXICITY (OVERDOSE)

Central nervous system (CNS) depression is caused by the effects of the drug on the reticular activating system and the cerebellum. Vasodilation, decreased sympathetic output, and negative inotropic cardiac effects cause hypotension. Decreased consciousness, respiratory depression, hypotension, and hypothermia follow overdose. Less severe toxicity is manifest by slurred speech, ataxia, nystagmus, and confusion. The patient may appear intoxicated. Pupils may be constricted or dilated. Brainstem and deep tendon reflexes are usually depressed or absent. Bullous skin lesions may also be seen.[9] Owing to PBs rapid CNS redistribution, patients may become more alert despite persistently elevated serum drug concentrations. Fatalities result from cardiorespiratory arrest or (direct) myocardial depression.

CHRONIC TOXICITY

Sedation and impaired cognition occurs in both children and adults.[9]

ADVERSE EFFECTS

Children manifest altered sleep, fussiness, irritability, and hyperactivity.

Diagnosis

The relationship between plasma concentration and adverse effects depends on the development of tolerance. Side effects usually disappear with continued use even when serum concentrations are supratherapeutic. The usual therapeutic serum concentration is 15 to 40 µg/mL. Concentrations greater than 60 µg/mL are associated with significant toxicity in the nontolerant individual.[9]

Management

Administration of multiple-dose activated charcoal (MDAC) and urinary alkalinization to a pH of 7.5 to 8.0 increases elimination of the parent compound. Although both MDAC and urinary alkalinization decrease elimination half-life, treatment with these modalities may neither shorten the clinical course nor change outcome. Hemoperfusion and hemodialysis increase clearance of the drug, although they are rarely needed for this overdose.[10,11] A serum PB concentration of greater than 100 to 125 µg/mL is an indication for extracorporeal drug removal.

PHENYTOIN

Pharmacology

Phenytoin (PHT) causes voltage-frequency and use-dependent block of sodium channels, inhibits calcium channels, and stimulates the Na^+/K^+-ATPase pump.[12]

Pharmacokinetics

Limited phenytoin solubility (i.e., dissolution rate decreases with increasing dose) causes prolonged absorption and delays peak serum concentrations, which have been reported to occur days after ingestion of a large dose. After a 400-mg dose, peak serum concentrations occur in 8 hours. The drug is 90% protein bound with a volume of distribution of 0.6 to 0.7 L/kg. Half-life is 20 to 30 hours. Metabolism is hepatic. Inactive metabolites and 5% of the parent drug are renally excreted.[13,14]

Metabolism is dose dependent. At therapeutic serum concentrations, elimination is first order (i.e., rate of drug metabolism increases as the concentration of the drug increases). In the upper therapeutic and toxic serum concentrations, the hydroxylation reaction reaches maximum velocity and elimination is zero order (i.e., rate of metabolism is constant).[13-15]

Absorption from bone is rapid following intraosseous administration. Pharmacokinetics approximate those following intravenous administration.[16]

Toxicology

ACUTE TOXICITY (OVERDOSE)

Initial cerebellar symptoms (nystagmus, ataxia, and drowsiness) are followed by basal ganglia signs (movement disorders) as serum concentrations exceed 20 mg/L. At higher concentrations, the CNS becomes depressed, ultimately producing coma. PHT overdose does not cause cardiac toxicity. The occurrence of paradoxical seizures following overdose has not been confirmed. Treatment is supportive.[17]

CHRONIC TOXICITY

Chronic PHT toxicity may occur during therapeutic ingestion owing to (1) small increases in maintenance doses that saturate enzyme systems, leading to zero order kinetics; (2) decrease in protein binding of the drug (e.g., addition of another drug); or (3) drug-induced alteration in hepatic metabolism.

Although head computed tomography (CT) may demonstrate cerebellar atrophy and cerebellar tissue loss in patients chronically receiving phenytoin, seizures can cause the same changes.[18]

ADVERSE EFFECTS

Adverse effects of PHT usually occur when serum concentrations are greater than 15 mg/L. Gingival hyperplasia and folic acid deficiency are among the most common and are dose related. Rash, acne, lupus-like syndrome, Stevens-Johnson syndrome, thyroid function inhibition, hirsutism, hypertrichosis, benign intracranial hypertension (pseudotumor cerebri), carbohydrate intolerance, peripheral neuropathy, osteomalacia, and altered vitamin D metabolism (increased alkaline phosphatase) may occur. The most serious adverse effect is a hypersensitivity syndrome manifested by fever, rash, lymphadenopathy, hepatitis, and eosinophilia. Death

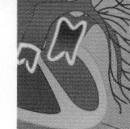

typically occurs from fulminant hepatic failure. Elevated liver enzymes should be monitored closely to distinguish transient enzyme elevation from progression to hepatic failure.[19]

Diagnosis

Symptoms correlate with free rather than total phenytoin concentrations; free concentrations are usually not available. Therapeutic serum concentrations (10 to 20 mg/L) equate with a free PHT concentration of 1.0 to 2.0 mg/L. Symptoms of toxicity occur when free PHT concentrations are greater than 5 mg/L.[20]

Management

Treatment of acute overdose and chronic PHT toxicity is supportive. The drug's prolonged elimination half-life may cause prolonged symptoms. The main concern in patients with PHT toxicity is ataxia causing a fall and resultant injury. The patient must be in the appropriate setting for observation.[17]

Intravenous Phenytoin

PHT is administered intravenously when a therapeutic concentration is needed as rapidly as possible (e.g., subtherapeutic concentrations following a seizure). Propylene glycol is necessary to maintain solubility and stability of parenteral PHT, but it can cause hypotension and bradycardia if administered too rapidly. In concentrations of 6 to 10 mg/L of normal saline (NS), PHT maintains solubility for about 1 hour. Oral loading results in delayed therapeutic concentrations, since limited PHT absorption (with a large dose) prolongs the time needed to reach therapeutic concentration.[21]

An IV dose of 15 to 18 mg/kg produces therapeutic serum concentrations lasting 12 to 24 hours. Distribution to the brain is rapid, and anticonvulsant activity begins within 3 to 5 minutes after IV infusion. If serum concentration of phenytoin is known, each 100 mg of IV phenytoin will increase serum concentration approximating 1.2 mg/L.[21]

Rapid IV administration of the drug (because of propylene glycol) and high PHT solution concentrations can cause cardiovascular toxicity. A PHT concentration of 4 to 10 mg/mL NS can be safely administered at a rate of 50 mg/min in patients younger than 50 years of age, and a concentration of 4 mg/mL NS (1 g phenytoin in 250 mL NS) at a rate of 25 mg/min in patients less than 50 years of age. Patients should be on a cardiac monitor. A constant infusion pump should monitor intravenous piggyback delivery. PHT should not be administered to patients with marked bradycardia, second- or third-degree heart block, active severe arteriosclerotic heart disease (ASHD), or hypotension. Fatalities have occurred in elderly patients with ASHD and in younger patients when the IV delivery rate or phenytoin concentration was greater than recommended.[23,24]

If the total dose administered is greater than 1 g, ataxia, dizziness, and confusion may occur despite appropriate administration rate and concentration. The infusion should be stopped if systemic side effects occur.[23]

Solvent alkalinity may cause burning and aching of the arm if infused into a small vein and buffering capacity of the blood is exceeded. Decreasing the rate or concentration may alleviate the symptoms. Soft tissue and vascular injury have occurred in elderly women with cardiovascular disease. A 20-gauge IV catheter and administration rate less than 25 mg/min may decrease the risk of injuries.[25]

FOSPHENYTOIN

Pharmacology

Fosphenytoin (FOS) is a disodium phosphate ester prodrug of PHT that is water-soluble and therefore does not require propylene glycol. Phosphatases present in the liver, red blood cells, and other tissues remove the phosphate molecule and convert FOS to active PHT in 8.4 minutes following intravenous administration.[26]

Pharmacokinetics

Maximal serum concentration is reached within 10 to 20 minutes of starting the infusion. Therapeutic PHT concentrations (10 to 20 mg/mL) occur within 10 minutes of infusions administered at a rate of 100 mg/min and within 30 minutes of infusions administered at less than 100 mg/min.[27]

ADVERSE EFFECTS

Nystagmus, headache, ataxia, and somnolence are the most frequent symptoms. Paresthesias and perineal and generalized pruritus have been reported in 30% to 60% of patients.

Diagnosis

Determination of FOS concentrations is of no value, since the drug is not clinically active. However, serum PHT levels are useful in guiding therapy.

Intravenous PHT vs. Intravenous FOS

FOS may be administered more rapidly than PHT. However, owing to the need for observation and other medical issues in patients who have just had a seizure, emergency department (ED) time is not decreased by administration of FOS. The adverse effect profile of FOS is different from that of PHT but not necessarily better. A significant number of people suffer perineal pruritus. FOS is more expensive than PHT. Cost analysis does not justify administration of FOS over PHT.[28,29]

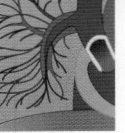

CARBAMAZEPINE

Pharmacology

Carbamazepine (CBMZ) inhibits sodium channels, interferes with release of glutamate (and possibly other neurotransmitters), and inhibits muscarinic and nicotinic acetylcholine receptors, N-methyl-D-aspartate (NMDA) receptors, and CNS adenosine receptors.[30]

Pharmacokinetics

CBMZ is an iminostilbene derivative that is chemically and structurally similar to imipramine, yet shares few of its pharmacologic properties. Absorption is slow, and peak serum concentrations usually occur within 4 to 8 hours but may be as late as 12 hours after ingestion.[31,32] A serum therapeutic concentration is 4 to 12 µg/mL.

The drug is 75% protein bound and has a volume of distribution of 0.79 to 1.19 L/kg. It is metabolized by liver cytochrome P4503A4 to an active metabolite (10,11-epoxide) with a half-life of 10 to 20 hours. The epoxide concentration is 10% to 15% of the parent compound in adults and 20% in children. The epoxide may be responsible for the neurotoxicity of the drug. Because CMBZ induces its own metabolism, its half-life after an isolated single dose (35 hours) is much longer than the half-life of the drug at steady state (10 to 20 hours). Autoinduction takes about a month. Elimination of the parent compound follows zero order kinetics, and 3% of the parent compound is excreted unchanged in the urine. The epoxide is metabolized to inactive compounds, which are excreted in the urine.[32,33]

Toxicology

ACUTE TOXICITY (OVERDOSE)

Delayed and erratic absorption due to CMBZ's anticholinergic properties and low water solubility can cause delayed clinical deterioration and a cyclic clinical course. Peak serum concentrations may occur 72 hours after ingestion of immediate-release (IR) and 96 hours after ingestion of controlled-release (CR) formulations. Half-life may be prolonged (39 hours) after an isolated ingestion or shorter when chronic therapeutic ingestion has induced metabolism.[31,32]

Symptoms of toxicity include coma, respiratory failure, ataxia, nystagmus, mydriasis, ileus, hypertonicity, increased deep tendon reflexes, movement disorders, and anticholinergic toxidrome. Seizures are more likely to occur in patients with high serum drug concentrations and an underlying seizure disorder. Left ventricular dysfunction with heart failure has been reported. Complete heart block (without hemodynamic compromise) has been reported in children. Cardiac arrhythmias are rarely seen. Laboratory abnormalities include hyponatremia, hyperglycemia, and transient elevation of serum liver enzymes.[34-38]

CHRONIC TOXICITY

CBMZ-induced bradycardia (including complete heart block) may occur in elderly patients with a defective conduction system or sick sinus syndrome. Benign cardiac conduction disturbances have been found in up to 57% of patients with CBMZ toxicity. Patients over 50 years of age should have an electrocardiogram (ECG) performed prior to initiation of CBMZ therapy.[37,38]

ADVERSE EFFECTS

Adverse effects occur in 25% of patients ingesting CBMZ. A mild transient leukopenia that may occur during the first month of treatment is unrelated to aplastic anemia, which occurs in 1 in 575,000 patients taking CBMZ. Hematologic monitoring is recommended. Discontinuation of the drug is not required for the mild liver enzyme elevation that occurs in up to 10% of patients taking CBMZ.

Diagnosis

Although serum CBMZ concentrations do not accurately correlate with the clinical severity of the poisoning, serum concentrations greater than 40 mg/L are associated with an increased risk of serious complications such as coma, seizures, respiratory failure, and cardiac conduction defects. Serum concentrations greater than 60 to 80 mg/mL may be associated with a fatal outcome. The seriousness of toxicity should be judged by the clinical status of the patient, not by the serum CBMZ concentration.[37,38]

Because of its ringed structure, CBMZ can cause a false-positive tricyclic antidepressant (TCA) result on the urine drug screen (UDS). Both CBMZ and carbamazepine 10,11-epoxide are measured by the standard enzyme multiplied immunoassay test (EMIT). A ratio of parent compound to epoxide greater than 2.5 is suggestive of continuing gastrointestinal (GI) absorption.[39]

Management

Gastric lavage may be considered if the patient is obtunded within 1 hour of ingestion of CBMZ. Prolonged absorption is possible. MDAC may decrease half-life but may not decrease time to recovery or change outcome. The benefit:risk ratio of MDAC administration in a sleepy patient or a patient who may require intubation must be assessed in each case. Similarly, although charcoal hemoperfusion (CHP) decreases the half-life of both CBMZ and the epoxide, the efficacy of charcoal hemoperfusion has not been compared with administration of multiple doses of activated charcoal or supportive care. If extracorporeal removal is considered in a life-threatening overdose, hemodialysis usually is the treatment of choice, since CHP cartridges are not readily available.[40-42]

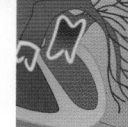

VALPROATE

Pharmacology

Valproate (VPA) has a number of indirect actions on the GABAergic system, causing increased GABA concentration. VPA reduces release of γ-hydroxybutyrate (an eliptogenic amino acid) and blocks cell firing induced by NMDA glutamate receptors. In rat brain sections, VPA increases brain endogenous opioid. Active metabolites may add to the drug's antiepileptic actions.[43-46]

Pharmacokinetics

VPA is a simple eight-carbon, branch-chained fatty acid. It is rapidly and completely absorbed, with peak serum concentrations occurring 1 to 4 hours after ingestion. The drug is extensively metabolized in the liver by glucuronic acid conjugation and mitochondrial β-oxidation, which may be inhibited by long-term or high-dose VPA therapy. VPA enters the mitochondria by a transport system that uses L-carnitine as a cofactor. Cytosolic ω-oxidation plays a smaller role in metabolism. Protein binding is determined by serum concentration with 90% of the drug protein bound at concentrations of 40 μg/mL. Concentrations greater than 150 μg/mL saturate protein binding sites, and less than 70% of the drug is protein bound. VPA has a small volume of distribution (0.13 to 0.23 L/kg) The half-life of VPA is 8 to 21 hours but may be up to 42 hours after overdose. In therapeutic concentrations and following overdose, elimination kinetics of the parent compound appear to be first order. Less than 3% of the drug is excreted unchanged in urine and feces.[47,48]

Toxicology

ACUTE TOXICITY (OVERDOSE)

If the enteric-coated or CR formulation has been ingested, peak serum concentration may be delayed for 12 to 16 hours. Patients who have ingested these formulations cannot be medically cleared until the clinical picture and serum concentration are assessed at the end of this time period.[49]

CNS depression, ranging from drowsiness to coma, is the most frequent sign following overdose. Serum concentrations greater than 850 μg/mL uniformly cause coma. Respiratory depression, hypotension, hypoglycemia, hypocalcemia, hypernatremia, hypophosphatemia, and anion-gap metabolic acidosis may persist for days. Serum aminotransferases, ammonia, amylase, and lactate may be elevated. Pancreatitis may occur. Thrombocytopenia, the most common hematologic toxicity, may be clinically significant and severe.[49]

VPA increases renal ammonia production and blocks hepatic ammonia metabolism. Resultant hyperammonemia may increase intracellular osmolarity, which promotes influx of water into the cell and causes cerebral edema. Hyperammonemia (in the absence of liver failure) and cerebral edema have been reported following VPA overdose. Whether increased ammonia is the cause of cerebral edema and the resultant increased intracranial pressure is unknown.[50]

CHRONIC TOXICITY

Increased serum liver enzymes and bilirubin occur in up to 60% of patients with therapeutic VPA serum concentrations. Liver enzymes normalize with dose reduction or discontinuation of the drug.

Hepatic failure, histologically evident as microvesicular steatosis, occurs in 1 in 20,000 patients. VPA-induced hepatotoxicity may be either intrinsic (reversible, reproducible, and dose dependent) and benign, occurring in 44% or patients, or idiosyncratic (unpredictable, not dose dependent, long latent period) and fatal. Children less than 3 years of age who are receiving multiple antiepileptic agents and have additional medical problems are at highest risk for fatal hepatotoxicity (incidence of 1 in 500). Liver enzymes and ammonia should be checked in children therapeutically ingesting VPA who demonstrate somnolence, lethargy, or even coma.[51]

Asymptomatic hyperammonemia without hepatic damage occurs in 20% of patients taking this drug. The origin of the ammonia is hepatic, a result of impaired urea cycle function and inability to metabolize nitrogen loads. The mechanism of this impairment is unknown. Carnitine deficiency may play a role in impaired urea production.[50]

Thirty-six cases of VPA-associated pancreatitis, including nine deaths, have been reported. Patients receiving multiple anticonvulsants may be at highest risk for developing pancreatitis. The cause of the pancreatitis is unknown. Abdominal pain, lethargy, or coma may be the presenting symptoms. Thrombocytopenia, usually transient despite continuing the drug, has rarely induced bone marrow toxicity.[52]

ADVERSE EFFECTS

Fifteen percent of patients experience GI side effects such as anorexia, nausea, and diarrhea. CNS effects of sedation, ataxia, and tremor also occur.

Diagnosis

Serum concentration does not correlate well with either seizure control or toxicity. Therapeutic concentrations are 50 to 100 μg/mL. The incidence of adverse side effects increases at concentrations greater than 120 μg/mL.

EMIT will yield higher values of serum VPA than will the gas-liquid chromatographic assay, requiring consistent analytic methodology. VPA is eliminated partly as ketone bodies and may cause a false-positive test result for ketones in the urine.

Management

Administration of high-dose naloxone has been reported to reverse VPA-induced CNS depression, possibly by reversal of VPA-induced release of endogenous opioids or reversal of VPA blockade of GABA uptake.[53]

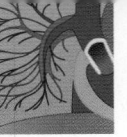

Because of delayed peak serum concentrations, serial concentrations should be obtained. Whole-bowel irrigation may be considered if the patient ingests Depakote or an extended-release preparation and presents within 5 hours of ingestion. Serum ammonia concentrations should be obtained in all patients with an altered level of consciousness. Serum glucose, calcium, phosphate, and platelets must be monitored.[54]

β-Oxidation, the primary metabolic pathway, may be decreased following overdose. Hypocarnitinemia, which inhibits β-oxidation, may occur following long-term VPA therapy. The clinical relevance of hypocarnitinemia in patients with seizures on chronic VPA therapy or in overdose patients is unknown. L-Carnitine has been administered to overdose patients in an attempt to increase VPA metabolism via β-oxidation. L-Carnitine causes few adverse side effects. However, its administration is experimental.[55]

Hemoperfusion (HP) and hemodiafiltration without HP have been performed to treat severe VPA overdose. Although the significant protein binding should not make it amenable to dialysis, the hypothesis is that unbound (free) drug is markedly increased in overdose. None of the extracorporeal means of detoxification have been compared with supportive care to determine whether these measures improve outcome.[56]

FELBAMATE

Introduction

Shortly after U.S. Food and Drug Administration (FDA) approval, it became apparent that felbamate was not well tolerated owing to GI complaints, insomnia, weight loss, dizziness, fatigue, ataxia, and lethargy. Felbamate-induced aplastic anemia (with an incidence 100 times higher than in the general population) and hepatic failure caused many physicians to discontinue the drug. Unfortunately, acute withdrawal of felbamate precipitated status epilepticus in some patients, causing some fatalities.[57,58]

Currently, felbamate is recommended only when other treatment regimens have failed. It remains on the market with a black box warning for aplastic anemia and hepatic failure and is not considered a first-line anticonvulsant.[1]

Pharmacology

Felbamate decreases the sodium current, enhances inhibitory actions of GABA, and blocks NMDA and α-amino-3-hydroxy-5-methyl-4-isoxazole propionic acid (AMPA) receptors. There is no effect on benzodiazepine receptors or GABA receptor binding.[1,59]

Pharmacokinetics

Felbamate is a dicarbamate derivative structurally related to meprobamate. The drug is 90% bioavailable after ingestion. Time to peak plasma level is 1 to 4 hours.

Volume of distribution is 0.75 L/kg. It is 25% bound to plasma protein, and elimination half-life is 20 hours. Forty to fifty percent is excreted unchanged in the urine.[59]

Toxicology

ACUTE TOXICITY (OVERDOSE)

Somnolence and GI symptoms may occur. Following overdose of felbamate and VPA, massive felbamate crystalluria and acute renal failure occurred. Crystalluria may have been caused by felbamate alone or in combination with VPA.[60]

CHRONIC TOXICITY

Fatal hepatitis and aplastic anemia are potential life-threatening effects.

ADVERSE EFFECTS

Weight gain, weakness, malaise, influenza-like symptoms, palpitations, tachycardia, agitation, psychological disturbance, aggressive reaction, pruritus, and Stevens-Johnson syndrome have been reported.

Diagnosis

Liver enzymes and white blood counts must be monitored when felbamate is taken. Although there is no recommended therapeutic range for felbamate, plasma concentrations as high as 140 μg/mL have been tolerated without significant adverse effects.[61] Acute overdose is treated with supportive care; there is no means of enhancing the drug's removal.

GABAPENTIN

Pharmacology

Structurally related to GABA, gabapentin does not bind to GABA receptors but is thought to enhance the release or actions of GABA. Unlike GABA, gabapentin readily crosses the blood-brain barrier. Gabapentin inhibits voltage-dependent sodium currents.[12]

Pharmacokinetics

Bioavailability is dose-dependent owing to facilitated transport during absorption by the L-amino acid transporter. The transport system becomes saturated at higher doses, limiting absorption. (The drug is presumed to be transported across the blood-brain barrier in the same way.) Oral bioavailability is 60% after a 300 mg dose and decreases to 35% when the dosage is 1600 mg three times a day. It is neither metabolized (and therefore does not induce hepatic enzymes) nor bound to plasma proteins. Gabapentin half-life is 5 to 7 hours. Kinetics are linear. Since gabapentin is eliminated by the kidneys, its renal clearance is dependent on creatinine clearance; the dose should be adjusted in patients with renal impairment.[62]

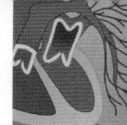

Toxicology

ACUTE TOXICITY (OVERDOSE)

Serious toxicity has not been reported after gabapentin overdose, probably because of its limited bioavailability.[63]

ADVERSE REACTIONS

Side effects of dizziness, somnolence, fatigue, ataxia, headache, tremor, diplopia, nausea and vomiting, and rhinitis are usually transient and disappear with prolonged therapy.[64]

CARCINOGENICITY

While the drug was being developed, preclinical studies temporarily ended owing to increased incidence of pancreatic acinar cell tumors in male Wistar rats fed high doses of gabapentin. The tumors did not occur in female rats, mice, or monkeys. Human pancreatic cancer tends to be ductal. The relevance of the tumors in animals to human carcinogenesis is unknown.[64]

Diagnosis

In adults receiving 900 to 1800 mg/day, plasma concentrations range from 2.7 to 4.1 µg/mL following a single dose and from 4.0 to 8.5 µg/mL following multiple doses.

Management

The treatment of gabapentin overdose is supportive. There is no established role for forced diuresis to enhance its urinary elimination.

LAMOTRIGINE

Pharmacology

Lamotrigine (LTG) stabilizes presynaptic neuronal membranes by blocking voltage-dependent sodium channels and thereby preventing the release of excitatory amino acids, especially glutamate and aspartate. Although LTG is a weak inhibitor of dihydrofolate reductase, antifolate drugs have not been shown to possess anticonvulsant activity.[65]

Pharmacokinetics

The drug is well absorbed; bioavailability is 98%. Its half-life is 22 to 36 hours. Being 55% protein bound, LTG is metabolized by hepatic glucuronidation, which is a target for enzyme inducers and inhibitors. Not surprisingly, metabolism of LTG is markedly increased by inducing drugs. Less than 10% is excreted unchanged.[65]

DRUG INTERACTIONS

Hepatic drug enzyme inducers such as carbamazepine, phenytoin, and phenobarbital reduce the half-life of LTG by 15 hours. Sodium valproate reduces the clearance of LTG by 21% and increases its half-life to 59 hours. LTG does not induce or inhibit hepatic enzymes. LTG increases symptoms when added to carbamazepine through pharmacodynamic rather than pharmacokinetic interactions.[66]

Toxicology

ACUTE TOXICITY (OVERDOSE)

Serious toxicity has not been reported in adults. In a single case report, ataxia and rotational nystagmus were described. An analysis of serum concentrations suggests the elimination pharmacokinetics are first order. Seizures and coma have been reported in children ingesting LTG; all recovered without sequelae.[67,68]

ADVERSE REACTIONS

Hypersensitivity reactions evidenced by multiorgan dysfunction and hepatic abnormalities, with and without the presence of a rash, have been reported. All patients who developed LTG-associated hypersensitivity syndrome were concomitantly taking ACs. Supratherapeutic dosing of LTG has also been associated with hypersensitivity reaction.[68]

Rashes, including Stevens-Johnson syndrome, toxic epidermal necrolysis, and hypersensitivity reaction occur in up to 25% of children less than 16 years of age and 0.3% (3/1000) of adults. Rarely, death has occurred. Rash usually occurs within 2 to 8 weeks of initiation of the drug, but isolated cases occurring after prolonged treatment (6 months) have been reported. Risk factors include coadministering VPA and exceeding the recommended initial doses of LTG or escalating the dose. LTG should be discontinued at the first sign of a rash. Other reported side effects are headache, nausea, vomiting, dizziness, diplopia, ataxia, and tremor.[69]

Diagnosis

At therapeutic doses, trough plasma concentrations are 2 to 4 mg/L. Maximum reported concentration following overdose is 35.8 mg/L. Serum concentrations are of no clinical value following overdose.[67]

Treatment of overdose is supportive.

TOPIRAMATE

Pharmacology

Topiramate, a sulfamate-substituted monosaccharide, is structurally distinct from other ACs. Topiramate causes a state-dependent blockade of sodium channels and potentiates GABA-mediated neuroinhibition by acting at a unique modulatory site. It enhances GABA-mediated chloride influx into neurons (similarly to diazepam), increasing the frequency at which GABA activates $GABA_A$ receptors. The drug itself does not interact with GABA binding sites or BZDP binding sites on $GABA_A$. Topiramate also causes blockade of glutamate-mediated neuroexcitation. It is a weak carbonic anhydrase inhibitor.[70]

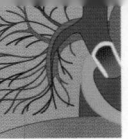

Pharmacokinetics

Topiramate is rapidly and completely absorbed from the GI tract and is minimally protein bound (9% to 17%) but extensively bound to erythrocytes until the binding sites are saturated. The drug's half-life is 19 to 23 hours. Hepatic metabolism is minimal, and there are no active metabolites. The drug is primarily (70%) excreted in the urine.[70]

Toxicology

ACUTE TOXICITY (OVERDOSE)

Coma, status epilepticus, and hyperchloremic metabolic acidosis have been reported following acute overdose.[71]

ADVERSE EFFECTS

CNS side effects (sedation) and cognitive side effects (trouble concentrating and finding words, decreased attention span) are worse with rapid titration of topiramate. Weight loss, ataxia, dizziness, nystagmus, tremor, and fatigue may occur. Since the drug is a carbonic anhydrase inhibitor, exchange of hydrogen ion for sodium ion and reabsorption of bicarbonate is decreased at the proximal renal tubule. Metabolic acidosis can therefore develop. Carbonic anhydrase inhibitors also decrease urinary citrate. Both decreased urinary citrate and acidosis increase the chance of calcium phosphate stones.[72,73]

Treatment of topiramate overdose is supportive; there are no antidotes.

TIAGABINE

Pharmacology

Tiagabine (TGB) prolongs the action of GABA by selectively inhibiting GABA transporters in the glia and neurons. TGB does not affect voltage-gated sodium or calcium channels.[74]

Pharmacokinetics

TGB is oxidized via the cytochrome P-450 system but does not affect hepatic enzyme function and therefore does not affect other drug metabolism. Its half-life is 5 to 8 hours although it may be decreased to 3 hours by inducing drugs.[1,75]

Toxicology

ACUTE TOXICITY (OVERDOSE)

TGB overdose may precipitate seizures and non-convulsive status.[76]

ADVERSE REACTIONS

Side effects associated with therapeutic use include dizziness, headache, asthenia, and tremor. Visual field defects (VFDs) have been reported. Whether VFDs are completely reversible when the drug is discontinued is unclear.[77]

Diagnosis

Therapeutic monitoring of plasma concentration is not recommended, since there is no clinical correlation between plasma concentrations and clinical course. Treatment of TGB overdose is supportive.

VIGABATRIN (VGB)

Introduction

Early experiments revealed that brain microvacuoles developed in some animal species taking vigabatrin (VGB). An extensive clinical monitoring program since 1982 throughout the United States and Europe has not revealed evidence of VGB-related CNS vacuolation in humans.[78]

Pharmacology

VGB is a structural analog of GABA and an irreversible inhibitor of GABA transaminase, the enzyme primarily responsible for GABA catabolism. VGB also reduces GABA reuptake activity. Both mechanisms increase brain GABA concentrations.

Pharmacokinetics

The bioavailability of VGB is 90%, and volume of distribution is 0.8L/kg. The drug is not protein bound, has negligible hepatic metabolism, and is primarily cleared by the kidneys. Its half-life is 5 to 7 hours. The pharmacologic half-life is much longer than the elimination half-life, with the duration of action being 5 to 7 days.[79]

Toxicology

ACUTE TOXICITY (OVERDOSE)

Symptoms following overdose include drowsiness, decreased level of consciousness, and coma. Respiratory depression, bradycardia, hypotension, agitation, irritability, confusion, and abnormal behavior have also been reported.[80]

ADVERSE REACTIONS

Mood and behavior changes such as depression, psychosis, and acute encephalopathy may occur. Sedation, fatigue, headache, and weight gain are usually mild and short lasting.

Diagnosis

There is no correlation between plasma concentration and seizure control or adverse effects. Treatment of overdose is supportive.

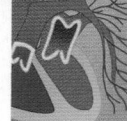

LEVETIRACETAM

Pharmacology

Levetiracetam is structurally unrelated to other antiepileptic drugs. It does not affect the GABA system, nor does it block sodium or calcium channels. In vitro, the drug binds to brain cell membranes in reversible, saturable, and stereoselective fashion.[81]

Pharmacokinetics

Levetiracetam is rapidly and completely absorbed, and peak plasma concentrations occur in an hour. Minimal protein binding and lack of hepatic metabolism prevent drug interactions. Sixty-six percent is excreted unchanged in the urine, of which 27% is excreted as inactive metabolites. The drug's volume of distribution is 0.5 to 0.7 L/kg. Its half-life in adults is 6 to 8 hours; in the elderly, 10 to 12 hours; and in children, 6 hours. Because it is primarily renally excreted, dosage adjustments are necessary for patients with renal impairment.[81,82]

Toxicology

ACUTE TOXICITY (OVERDOSE)
Levetiracetam may cause CNS and respiratory depression. Recovery is rapid with supportive care. Elimination kinetics are first order following overdose. Treatment of overdose is supportive.[83]

ZONISAMIDE

Pharmacology

Zonisamide (ZNS) is a sulfonamide. The drug blocks sodium channels and T-type calcium channels and is a weak carbonic anhydrase inhibitor.[82,84]

Pharmacokinetics

Peak plasma concentrations are achieved in 2.4 to 3.6 hours after ingestion. Japanese studies have reported linear pharmacokinetics, whereas U.S. studies have reported nonlinear pharmacokinetics with first order clearance. CYP3A4 is the isoenzyme that metabolizes the drug. The drug's elimination half-life is 63 hours. The drug is excreted in the urine as unchanged drug, as an acetylation product, and as the glucuronide of a metabolite.[84]

Toxicology

CHRONIC TOXICITY
Carbonic anhydrase inhibitors decrease urinary citrate, an inhibitor of stone formation. Whether ZNS increases the risk of nephrolithiasis is unknown.

In 2001, oligohidrosis and hyperthermia were reported in 38 patients in Japan and 2 patients in the United States. Pediatric patients may be at increased risk for this dangerous adverse effect.[85]

ZNS may contribute to psychosis during polytherapy. The incidence of psychotic episodes in epileptic patients taking ZNS is higher than the prevalence of epileptic psychosis in those not receiving the drug.[86]

SIDE EFFECTS
Drowsiness (24%), ataxia (13%), anorexia, dizziness, forgetfulness, slowness of thought, and irritability are usually mild and transient.

OXCARBAZEPINE

Pharmacology

Oxcarbazepine (OXZ) is the 10-keto analog of carbamazepine. Similarly to CBMZ, oxcarbazepine blocks voltage-sensitive sodium channels, causing stabilization of hyperexcited neural membranes, inhibition of repetitive neuronal firing, and inhibition of the spread of discharges. The drug also increases potassium conductance, decreases glutaminergic transmission, and modulates the calcium channel.[87]

Pharmacokinetics

OXZ is well absorbed; its absorption is not affected by food. Peak serum concentrations occur 4 to 6 hours after ingestion. It is rapidly metabolized in the liver to an active, nontoxic metabolite, which is widely distributed in the brain and lipophilic tissues and is responsible for the pharmacologic action of the drug. Metabolite half-life is 8 to 10 hours and is not affected by other ACs. Compared with CBMZ, OXZ has fewer side effects owing to lack of toxicity of the metabolite. OXZ is 38% bound to plasma protein. Since the active drug is excreted by the kidneys, the dose may need to be reduced in patients with renal impairment.[88]

Toxicology

ADVERSE EFFECTS
Duration and frequency of side effects are less than for CBMZ. Side effects include fatigue, headache, dizziness, ataxia, and nausea. Skin rash occurs in up to 10% of patients and is the main reason for discontinuation of the drug. OXZ may be administered to patients who have developed a rash while taking carbamazepine. Cross-reactivity is about 25%. Clinically insignificant hyponatremia occurs in 20% of patients.[89]

DRUG INTERACTIONS
An advantage of OXZ is that it causes few drug interactions. If OXZ is substituted for carbamazepine, deinduction can occur.

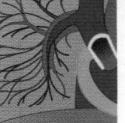

REFERENCES

1. LaRoche SM, Helmers SL: The new antiepileptic drugs: clinical applications. JAMA 2004;291:605–614.
2. Kwan P, Brodie MJ: Early identification of refractory epilepsy. N Engl J Med 2000;342:314–319.
3. Diaz-Arrastia R, Agostini MA, Van Ness PC: Evolving treatment strategies for epilepsy. JAMA 2002;287:2917–2920.
4. Perucca E: Marketed new antiepileptic drugs: are they better than old-generation agents? Ther Drug Monit 2002;24:74–80.
5. Lathers CM, Schraeder PL: Clinical pharmacology: drugs as a benefit and/or risk in sudden unexpected death in epilepsy? J Clin Pharmacol 2002;42:123–136.
6. Holmes LB, Harvey EA, Coull BA, et al: The teratogenicity of anticonvulsant drugs. N Engl J Med 2001;344:1132–1138.
7. Knowles SR, Shapiro LE, Shear NH: Anticonvulsant hypersensitivity syndrome: incidence, prevention and management. Drug Saf 1999;21:489–501.
8. Rho JM, Donevan SD, Rogawski MA: Direct activation of GABAA receptors by barbiturates in cultured rat hippocampal neurons. J Physiol 1996;497:509–522.
9. Shubin H, Weil MH: The mechanism of shock following suicidal doses of barbiturates, narcotics and tranquilizer drugs, with observations on the effects of treatment. Am J Med 1965;38:853–863.
10. Pond SM, Olson KR, Osterloh JD, et al: Randomized study of the treatment of phenobarbital overdose with repeated doses of activated charcoal. JAMA 1984;251:3104–3108.
11. Frenia ML, Schauben JL, Wears RL, et al: Multiple-dose activated charcoal compared to urinary alkalinization for the enhancement of phenobarbital elimination. J Toxicol Clin Toxicol 1996;34:169–175.
12. Russell RJ, Parks B: Anticonvulsant medications. Pediatr Ann 1999;28:238–245.
13. McNamara J: Drugs effective in the therapy of the epilepsies. In Hardman J, Limbird L (eds): Goodman and Gilman's The Pharmacological Basis of Therapeutics, 10th ed. New York, McGraw-Hill, 2001, pp 436–444.
14. Jung D, Powell JR, Walson P, et al: Effect of dose on phenytoin absorption. Clin Pharmacol Ther 1980;28:479–485.
15. Dichter MA: Old and new mechanisms of antiepileptic drug actions. Epilepsy Res Suppl 1993;10:9–17.
16. Walsh-Kelly CM, Berens RJ, Glaeser PW, et al: Intraosseous infusion of phenytoin. Am J Emerg Med 1986;4:523–524.
17. Wyte CD, Berk WA: Severe oral phenytoin overdose does not cause cardiovascular morbidity. Ann Emerg Med 1991;20:508–512.
18. Masur H, Elger CE, Ludolph AC, et al: Cerebellar atrophy following acute intoxication with phenytoin. Neurology 1989;39:432–423.
19. Flowers FP, Araujo OE, Hamm KA: Phenytoin hypersensitivity syndrome. J Emerg Med 1987;5:103–108.
20. Gordon MF, Gerstenblitt D: The use of free phenytoin levels in averting phenytoin toxicity. N Y State J Med 1990;90:469.
21. Donovan PJ, Cline D: Phenytoin administration by constant intravenous infusion: selective rates of administration. Ann Emerg Med 1991;20:139–142.
22. Carducci B, Hedges JR, Beal JC, et al: Emergency phenytoin loading by constant intravenous infusion. Ann Emerg Med 1984;13:1027–1031.
23. Earnest MP, Marx JA, Drury LR: Complications of intravenous phenytoin for acute treatment of seizures: recommendations for usage. JAMA 1983;249:762–765.
24. York R, Coleridge ST: Cardiopulmonary arrest following intravenous phenytoin loading. Am J Emerg Med 1988;6:255–259.
25. Spengler RF, Arrowsmith JB, Kilarski DJ, et al: Severe soft-tissue injury following intravenous infusion of phenytoin. Arch Intern Med 1988;148:1329–1333.
26. DeToledo JC, Ramsay RE: Fosphenytoin and phenytoin in patients with status epilepticus. Drug Saf 2000;22:459–466.
27. Browne TR, Kugler AR, Eldon MA: Pharmacology and pharmacokinetics of fosphenytoin. Neurology 1996;46(6 Suppl 1):S3–S7.
28. Rudis MI, Touchette DR, Swadron SP, et al: Cost-effectiveness of oral phenytoin, intravenous phenytoin, and intravenous fosphenytoin in the emergency department. Ann Emerg Med 2004;43:386–397.

29. Swadron SP, Rudis MI, Azimian K, et al: A comparison of phenytoin-loading techniques in the emergency department. Acad Emerg Med 2004;11:244–252.
30. Yoshimura R, Yanagihara N, Terao T, et al: Inhibition by carbamazepine of various ion channels: mediated catecholamine secretion in cultured bovine adrenal medullary cells. Naunyn Schmiedebergs Arch Pharmacol 1995;352:297–303.
31. Graudins A, Peden G, Dowsett RP: Massive overdose with controlled-release carbamazepine resulting in delayed peak serum concentrations and life-threatening toxicity. Emerg Med (Fremantle) 2002;14:89–94.
32. Winnicka RI, Topacinski B, Szymczak WM, et al: Carbamazepine poisoning: elimination kinetics and quantitative relationship with carbamazepine 10,11-epoxide. J Toxicol Clin Toxicol 2002;40:759–765.
33. Graves NM, Brundage RC, Wen Y, et al: Population pharmacokinetics of carbamazepine in adults with epilepsy. Pharmacotherapy 1998;18:273–281.
34. Seymour JF: Carbamazepine overdose. Drug Saf 1993;8:81–88.
35. Apfelbaum JD, Cavarati EM, Kerns WP II, et al: Cardiovascular effects of carbamazepine toxicity. Ann Emerg Med 1995;25:631–635.
36. Lifshitz M, Gavrilov V, Sofer S: Signs and symptoms of carbamazepine overdose in young children. Pediatr Emerg Care 2000;16:26–27.
37. Stremski ES, Brady WB, Prasad K, et al: Pediatric carbamazepine intoxication. Ann Emerg Med 1995;25:624–630.
38. Hojer J, Malmlund HO, Berg A: Clinical features in 28 consecutive cases of laboratory confirmed massive poisoning with carbamazepine alone. J Toxicol Clin Toxicol 1993;31:449–458.
39. Matos ME, Burns MM, Shannon MW: False-positive tricyclic antidepressant drug screen results leading to the diagnosis of carbamazepine intoxication. Pediatrics 2000;105:E66.
40. Boldy DA, Heath A, Ruddock S, et al: Activated charcoal for carbamazepine poisoning. Lancet 1987;1:1027.
41. Wason S, Baker RC, Carolan P, et al: Carbamazepine overdose: the effects of multiple-dose activated charcoal. J Toxicol Clin Toxicol 1992;30:39–48.
42. Tapolyai M, Campbell M, Dailey K, et al: Hemodialysis is as effective as hemoperfusion for drug removal in carbamazepine poisoning. Nephron 2002;90:213–215.
43. Andersen GO, Ritland S: Life threatening intoxication with sodium valproate. J Toxicol Clin Toxicol 1995;33:279–284.
44. Albus H, Williamson R: Electrophysiologic analysis of the actions of valproate on pyramidal neurons in the rat hippocampal slice. Epilepsia 1998;39:124–129.
45. Loscher W: Effects of the antiepileptic drug valproate on metabolism and function of inhibitory and excitatory amino acids in the brain. Neurochem Res 1993;18:485–502.
46. Asai M, Talavera E, Massarini A, et al: Valproic acid–induced rapid changes of met-enkephalin levels in rat brain. Neuropeptides 1994;27:203–210.
47. Dupuis RE, Lichtman SN, Pollack GM: Acute valproic acid overdose: clinical course and pharmacokinetic disposition of valproic acid and metabolites. Drug Saf 1990;5:65–70.
48. Rho JM, Sankar R: The pharmacologic basis of antiepileptic drug action. Epilepsia 1999;40:1471–1483.
49. Spiller HA, Krenzelok EP, Klein-Schwartz W, et al: Multicenter case series of valproic acid ingestion: serum concentrations and toxicity. J Toxicol Clin Toxicol 2000;38:755–760.
50. Patsalos PN, Wilson SJ, Popovik M, et al: The prevalence of valproic acid–associated hyperammonaemia in patients with intractable epilepsy. J Epilepsy 1993;6:228–232.
51. Bryant AE III, Dreifuss FE: Valproic acid hepatic fatalities. 3. U.S. experience since 1986. Neurology 1996;46:465–469.
52. Yazdani K, Lippmann M, Gala I: Fatal pancreatitis associated with valproic acid. Medicine 2002;81:305–310.
53. Alberto G, Erickson T, Popiel R, et al: Central nervous system manifestations of a valproic acid overdose responsive to naloxone. Ann Emerg Med 1989;18:889–891.
54. Ingels M, Beauchamp J, Clark RF, et al: Delayed valproic acid toxicity: a retrospective case series. Ann Emerg Med 2002;39:616–621.
55. Ishikura H, Matsuo N, Matsubara M, et al: Valproic acid overdose and L-carnitine therapy. J Anal Toxicol 1996;20:55–58.

56. Kane SL, Constantiner M, Staubus AE, et al: High-flux hemodialysis without hemoperfusion is effective in acute valproic acid overdose. Ann Pharmacother 2000;34:1146–1151.

57. Leppik IE: Felbamate. Epilepsia 1995;36(Suppl 2):S66–S72.

58. Welty TE, Privitera M, Shukla R: Increased seizure frequency associated with felbamate withdrawal in adults. Arch Neurol 1998;55:641–645.

59. Hachad H, Ragueneau-Majlessi I, Levy RH: New antiepileptic drugs: review on drug interactions. Ther Drug Monit 2002; 24:91–103.

60. Rengstorff DS, Milstone AP, Seger DL, et al: Felbamate overdose complicated by massive crystalluria and acute renal failure. J Toxicol Clin Toxicol 2000;38:667–669.

61. Harden CL, Trifiletti R, Kutt H: Felbamate levels in patients with epilepsy. Epilepsia 1996;37:280–283.

62. Fisher JH, Andrews CO, Taber JE, et al: Multidose evaluation of gabapentin pharmacokinetics in patients with epilepsy. Epilepsia 1995;36(Suppl 4):121.

63. Fischer JH, Barr AN, Rogers SL, et al: Lack of serious toxicity following gabapentin overdose. Neurology 1994;44:982–983.

64. U.S. Gabapentin Study Group No. 5: Gabapentin as add-on therapy in refractory partial epilepsy: a double-blind, placebo-controlled, parallel-group study. Neurology 1993;43:2292–2298.

65. Goa KL, Ross SR, Chrisp P: Lamotrigine: a review of its pharmacological properties and clinical efficacy in epilepsy. Drugs 1993;46:152–176.

66. Yuen AW, Land G, Weatherby BC, et al: Sodium valproate acutely inhibits lamotrigine metabolism. Br J Clin Pharmacol 1992; 33:511–513.

67. O'Donnell J, Bateman DN: Lamotrigine overdose in an adult. J Toxicol Clin Toxicol 2000;38:659–660.

68. Briassoulis G, Kalabalikis P, Tomiolaki M, et al: Lamotrigine childhood overdose. Pediatr Neurol 1998;19:239–242.

69. Schlumberger E, Chavez F, Palacios L, et al: Lamotrigine in treatment of 120 children with epilepsy. Epilepsia 1994;35:359–367.

70. Garnett WR: Clinical pharmacology of topiramate: a review. Epilepsia 2000;41(Suppl 1):S61–S65.

71. Fakhoury T, Murray L, Seger D, et al: Topiramate overdose: clinical and laboratory features. Epilepsy Behav 2002;3:185–189.

72. Stowe CD, Bollinger T, James LP, et al: Acute mental status changes and hyperchloremic metabolic acidosis with long-term topiramate therapy. Pharmacotherapy 2000;20:105.

73. Wasserstein AG, Rak I, Reife RA: Nephrolithiasis during treatment with topiramate. Epilepsia 1995;36(Suppl 3):S153.

74. Suzdak PD, Jansen JA: A review of the preclinical pharmacology of tiagabine: a potent and selective anticonvulsant GABA uptake inhibitor. Epilepsia 1995;36:612–626.

75. Leach JP, Brodie MJ: Tiagabine. Lancet 1998;351:203–207.

76. Ostrovskiy D, Spanaki MV, Morris GL II: Tiagabine overdose can induce convulsive status epilepticus. Epilepsia 2002;43:773–774.

77. Kaufman KR, Lepore FE, Keyser BJ: Visual fields and tiagabine: a quandary. Seizure 2001;10:525–529.

78. Gidal BE, Privitera MD, Sheth RD, et al: Vigabatrin: a novel therapy for seizure disorders. Ann Pharmacother 1999;33:1277–1286.

79. Hoke JF, Yuh L, Antony KK, et al: Pharmacokinetics of vigabatrin following single and multiple oral doses in normal volunteers. J Clin Pharmacol 1993;33:458–462.

80. Davie MB, Cook MJ, Ng C: Vigabatrin overdose. Med J Aust 1996;165:403.

81. Patsalos PN: Pharmacokinetic profile of levetiracetam: toward ideal characteristics. Pharmacol Ther 2000;85:77.

82. Perucca E, Bialer M: The clinical pharmacokinetics of the newer antiepileptic drugs: focus on topiramate, zonisamide and tiagabine. Clin Pharmacokinet 1996;31:29–46.

83. Barrueto F II, Williams K, Howland MA, et al: A case of levetiracetam poisoning with clinical and toxicokinetic data. J Toxicol Clin Toxicol 2002;40:881–884.

84. Mimaki T: Clinical pharmacology and therapeutic drug monitoring of zonisamide. Ther Drug Monit 1998;20:593–597.

85. Oommen KJ, Mathews S: Zonisamide: a new antiepileptic drug. Clin Neuropharmacol 1999;22:192.

86. Miyamoto T, Kohsaka M, Koyama T: Psychotic episodes during zonisamide treatment. Seizure 2000;9:65–70.

87. Shorvon S: Oxcarbazepine: a review. Seizure 2000;9:75–79.

88. Tecoma ES: Oxcarbazepine. Epilepsia 1994;40(Suppl 5):S37–S46.

89. Rouan MC, Lecaillon JB, Godbillon J, et al: The effect of renal impairment on the pharmacokinetics of oxcarbazepine and its metabolites. Eur J Clin Pharmacol 1994;47:161–167.

41 *Marijuana*

JOÃO DELGADO, MD

At a Glance...

- Marijuana is the most commonly used illicit drug in the United States.
- Marijuana intoxication is self-limited and typically produces mild symptoms.
- There is no specific antidote—treatment of intoxication is supportive.

INTRODUCTION AND RELEVANT HISTORY

Marijuana is by far the most extensively used illicit drug in the United States. The hemp plant, *Cannabis sativa*, from which it is prepared, has been used for centuries not only for its psychoactive resin but also for hemp fiber and rope. The cannabinoid Δ^9-tetrahydrocannabinol (THC) is the principal psychoactive constituent and is found in highest concentration in the leaves and the flowering tops of the plant. In addition, the plant contains hundreds of other chemicals, including several cannabinoids. Marijuana and its synthetic analogs (e.g., dronabinol) have also been used medicinally to treat a variety of chronic conditions.

The term *marijuana* refers to dried, tobacco-like preparations of the leaves, stems, and flowers. The THC content of marijuana is variable and may range from 0.4% to 20%, depending on cultivation techniques. The average THC content of confiscated marijuana has increased over the past two decades from under 2% in the late 1970s to 7.79% in 2005.[1] A typical marijuana cigarette contains 500 to 1000 mg of plant material, which is equivalent to approximately 25 to 50 mg of THC. Hashish is the resin extracted from the tops of the flowering plants and has a THC concentration that may exceed 10%. Hash oil is an organic solvent extract of cannabis that may have a THC concentration of 20% or higher.

The modern phase of therapeutic cannabis use began in 1842, when O'Shaughnessy reported on its effectiveness as an analgesic and anticonvulsant.[2] Cannabis was subsequently touted as a treatment for psychiatric illnesses, insomnia, poor appetite, opium addiction, chronic alcoholism, delirium tremens, and a wide variety of painful disorders. However, as synthetic analgesics and sedatives became available, the medical use of cannabis faded. The Marijuana Tax Act of 1937 officially eliminated it from medical practice in the United States.

Current therapeutic uses of cannabinoids include alleviating chemotherapy-induced nausea and vomiting and attenuation of anorexia and nausea associated with AIDS. In general, enthusiasm for the medicinal use of marijuana has been tempered by inconsistent clinical trial results, modest therapeutic effectiveness, the adverse health consequences of delivery by smoking, undesirable side effects, and the superiority of already marketed drugs. Those advocating the use of marijuana for medicinal purposes argue that THC is delivered more effectively in smoke than in oral preparations, that marijuana is less expensive than synthetic THC, and that marijuana produces few if any harmful side effects.

The most common form of marijuana use in the United States is in cigarettes. Generally, smoke is inhaled deeply and held in the lungs for 15 to 30 seconds, which results in rapid intoxication or "high." Other psychoactive substances, such as phencyclidine or cocaine, may be mixed with marijuana and then smoked. Ingestion is the second most common means of intoxication and is typically accomplished by baking marijuana inside cookies or brownies. In contrast to inhalation, the effects after ingestion occur more gradually and the level of intoxication is not as readily controlled as with inhalation. Illicit intravenous injection of crude marijuana plant extracts remains an unusual practice. The gummy consistency of the plant resin and its poor water solubility limit its use via this route.

EPIDEMIOLOGY

The National Institute on Drug Abuse (NIDA) funds an ongoing national research and reporting program called the Monitoring the Future Study, in which secondary school students, college students, and young adults are surveyed annually about drug use.[3] This study has consistently shown that alcohol is the most frequently used substance in all subgroups, and marijuana is the most frequently used illicit substance. The most recent data show that nearly one half of 12th graders have used marijuana at least once and that 22% are current users.[4] Another large national survey indicates that 37% of the U.S. population (83 million people) has used marijuana at least once and 14.6 million are currently using marijuana.[5] Such widespread use has significant public health implications. For example, workers who smoke marijuana frequently have higher rates of absenteeism and miss more days of work due to illness than nonsmokers.[6] Perhaps more concerning is marijuana's role as a "gateway" drug, meaning that marijuana users are more likely to move on to other more harmful drugs, such as cocaine, heroin, and amphetamines.[7]

STRUCTURE

Cannabinoids are aryl-substituted monoterpenes unique to the genus *Cannabis*. *C. sativa* contains over 60 cannabi-

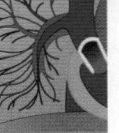

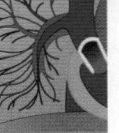

FIGURE 41-1 Chemical structure of 1-*trans*-Δ9-tetrahydro-cannabinol.

noids, the most pharmacologically potent of which is THC (Fig. 41-1).

PHARMACOLOGY AND PATHOPHYSIOLOGY

THC produces numerous pharmacologic and behavioral effects through its action on the CB_1 cannabinoid receptor. This receptor is a member of a large family of receptors that are coupled to G proteins and modulate adenylate cyclase.[8] CB_1 receptors are distributed primarily in axons and nerve terminals. Their presynaptic localization suggests a modulatory role on neurotransmitter release. In fact, THC is known to inhibit the release of a variety of neurotransmitters, including acetylcholine, dopamine, γ-aminobutyric acid, L-glutamate, serotonin, and norepinephrine.[9] A number of arachidonic acid derivatives have been shown to serve as endogenous CB_1 ligands. These derivatives include arachidonolyl-glycerol (Ara-G1) and anandamide.[10,11] The establishment of a cannabinoid receptor and several endogenous ligands with biosynthetic and degradative pathways suggests the possible presence of a distinct neurochemical system. A peripheral cannabinoid receptor, designated CB_2, has been identified in macrophages but its role remains unknown.[12]

The highest density of cannabinoid receptors is found in the cerebral cortex, particularly the frontal areas, cerebellum, basal ganglia, hypothalamus, and hippocampus.[9] This distribution explains the prominent effects of THC on memory, cognition, and motor function. Scarce levels of CB_1 receptors in the brainstem regions are thought to account for the low lethality of cannabinoids. Binding has also been found in the B-lymphocyte-rich areas, including the marginal zone of the spleen, the nodular corona of Peyer's patches, and the cortex of lymph nodes.[13]

Pharmacologic effects begin rapidly and generally peak within 30 minutes of smoking a marijuana cigarette. Behavioral and physiologic effects generally return to baseline levels 4 to 6 hours after smoking. However, impairment of various performance measures related to complex tasks, such as driving a car or flying an airplane, has been demonstrated immediately after marijuana use and persisting for as long as 24 hours.[14,15] Marijuana is classified as a schedule I controlled substance ("no currently accepted medical use") by the U.S. Drug Enforcement Administration, whereas pharmaceutical THC is classified as a schedule III controlled substance.

The THC analogs dronabinol, levonantradol, nabilone, and nabitan have been used to treat chemotherapy-induced nausea and vomiting.[16] A systematic review of the medical literature determined that cannabinoids appear to be more effective than conventional antiemetics in treating mild to moderate nausea but were associated with significant side effects that limited their usefulness.[17] The development of 5-HT$_3$ receptor antagonists, such granisetron and ondasetron, has further limited the use of THC for this indication. Dronabinol is approved by the Food and Drug Administration for chemotherapy-associated nausea and vomiting refractory to conventional antiemetics. The recommended dose is 5 to 15 mg/m². Dronabinol is also approved for appetite stimulation in patients with AIDS wasting syndrome.[18] The typical starting dose for appetite stimulation is 2.5 mg twice a day. Dronabinol is marketed under the trade name Marinol (Solvay Pharmaceuticals, Inc., Marietta, GA)

Although THC has analgesic properties, it is no more effective than codeine and produces considerable side effects in the effective analgesic dose range.[19] Marijuana, THC, and several synthetic derivatives have been shown to lower intraocular pressure in patients with glaucoma but are not widely used for this indication.[20] A topical preparation of marijuana intended for the treatment of glaucoma is marketed as Canasol in Jamaica (Medi-Grace Ltd., Kingston, Jamaica).[21] Extensive animal studies have shown that THC is capable of producing both proconvulsant and anticonvulsant effects. Cannabidiol, in particular, showed some promise as an anticonvulsant in animal studies.[22] However, its efficacy was not sufficient to warrant clinical use in humans. Recently, there has been an interest in using *Cannabis* for tremor and spasticity associated with multiple sclerosis. Clinical trials have not shown improvement in objective measures of tremor or spasticity despite the perception by participants of an improvement of their symptoms.[23,24]

PHARMACOKINETICS

THC is readily absorbed when marijuana is smoked, with peak serum concentrations obtained within 10 to 20 minutes. Peak clinical effects occur within 30 minutes of smoking.[25] Heavy marijuana smokers absorb THC more efficiently (23% to 27% bioavailability) than light smokers (10% to 14% bioavailability).[26] Although oral ingestion of marijuana produces similar pharmacologic effects, THC is absorbed more slowly and erratically than when smoked. Oral bioavailability is only 6% to 10% because of extensive first pass metabolism. Peak plasma THC concentrations occur 1 to 3 hours after ingestion and are much lower than those achieved by smoking.

THC is highly protein bound (97% to 99%) and lipophilic, with an apparent volume of distribution of 4 to 14 L/kg.[25] THC is metabolized first to hydroxylated metabolites, followed by conversion to carboxylic acids. The metabolites are subsequently excreted as conjugates. The initial hydroxylated metabolites of THC (i.e., 11-hydroxy-THC and 8-β-hydroxy-THC) are active but do not achieve appreciable plasma concentrations and are not likely to contribute to the acute behavioral

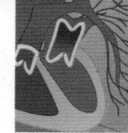

effects of marijuana.[25] Approximately 15% and 50% of THC is excreted in urine and feces, respectively, over several days.[27] The urinary elimination half-life of THC averages 5 days in heavy users of marijuana as compared with 20 to 57 hours for infrequent users.[25,28] The primary urinary metabolite is conjugated 11-*nor*-9-carboxy-Δ^9–THC, which has a urinary elimination half-life of 3 days in heavy users.[29] Only trace amounts of THC are excreted in urine unchanged.

Blood concentrations of THC peak before behavioral effects and do not correlate well with pharmacologic effects.[30] Peak behavioral effects lag behind the time of peak plasma THC levels by 10 to 30 minutes for smoking and 1 to 3 hours for ingestion; significant effects may last for 4 to 8 hours.[25,31,32] In clinical settings, blood and urine levels of THC and metabolites are only useful for determining whether or not an individual has used marijuana and not in determining degree of resulting impairment.

TOXICOLOGY

Overall, toxicity arising from cannabinoid use is mild. Even when large doses are used, the effects are not usually prolonged or life threatening. Exceptions to this rule are ingestions involving small children, who may become severely obtunded after ingesting hashish or marijuana, and individuals who experience severe allergic reactions to *Cannabis,* both of which are rare occurrences.[33,34]

Psychological and Neurologic Effects

Marijuana's effects on central nervous system functions such as behavior, cognition, perception, and performance are its most important physiologic effects. Individuals who consume low to moderate quantities generally report a feeling of well-being and pleasant relaxation, euphoria, a dreamlike state, alteration of time and space perception, and a heightening of their senses. Smoking a large quantity of marijuana can produce a range of effects including mild anxiety, paranoid behavior, acute psychosis, problems in dealing with reality, and obsessional thought content characterized by delusions, hallucinations, illusions, and bizarre behavior. These adverse effects sometimes occur in inexperienced users even after low doses.

Cognitive functioning, such as speaking, problem solving, and memory recall, are affected by marijuana use.[35] Marijuana's interference with short-term memory is thought to be a major cause of poor cognitive performance during marijuana intoxication. Information learned while intoxicated is less well recalled than in a sober state.

Impairment of complex motor functions also occurs in intoxicated individuals.[35] Some parameters that affect driving performance continue to be impaired even several hours after a marijuana user no longer feels high. Epidemiologic data suggest that drivers who recently used *Cannabis* are approximately three to seven times more likely to have caused a crash than sober drivers.[36] This impairment is exacerbated by the common combination of marijuana with alcohol.

Adverse psychological reactions to marijuana use occur relatively frequently.[37] The exaggeration of the more usual marijuana response, in which an individual loses perspective (i.e., the realization that what he or she is experiencing is a transient drug-induced distortion of reality), may produce anxiety. This reaction appears to occur primarily in inexperienced users, although unexpectedly higher doses of the drug can cause such a response even in experienced users. Symptoms usually resolve in a few hours as the immediate effects of acute intoxication recede. Typically, only authoritative assurance and limiting sensory input are required.

Uncommon cannabinoid-induced symptoms may include severe panic and anxiety states, paranoia, depression, personality changes, confusional states, and psychoses, which are indistinguishable from primary psychiatric syndromes unless the drug-induced etiology is known. Whether marijuana use can precipitate permanent psychiatric illness in individuals who have no underlying predisposition remains controversial. Marijuana has also been linked to transient ischemic attacks and strokes, but definitive evidence of a causative role is lacking.[38,39] There is no convincing evidence that cannabinoids are neurotoxic to humans.[40]

Respiratory Effects

Inhalation of marijuana smoke is associated with rhinitis, pharyngitis, laryngitis, cough, hoarseness, and bronchitis, which are symptoms commonly reported by tobacco smokers as well. Interestingly, marijuana smoke also produces bronchodilatation in both normal and asthmatic patients. Prolonged marijuana use is associated with chronic bronchitis and changes in respiratory tract cells.[41] In contrast to tobacco smoke, which affects primarily the smaller airways and the alveoli, marijuana smoke is associated with large airways disease.[42,43] Longitudinal data suggest an additive effect of marijuana plus tobacco with respect to symptom prevalence. Uncommon adverse effects include pneumothorax and pneumomediastinum from the Valsalva maneuver that marijuana users frequently employ in an attempt to increase THC absorption by the lung; partial upper airway obstruction from marijuana smoke–induced uvulitis; and pulmonary aspergillosis.[44-46]

As with tobacco smoke, marijuana smoke has a high content of particulate matter, or tar. Compared to tobacco smoke, marijuana smoke contains threefold more tar and results in fivefold higher carbon monoxide concentrations.[47] No large-scale epidemiologic studies have been carried out to determine if there is a relationship between smoking marijuana and the incidence of lung cancer. Nevertheless, there is good reason for concern about the possibility that lung cancer might result from prolonged use. Several reports have noted a higher-than-expected incidence of head and neck squamous cell carcinoma.[48] Like tobacco smoke residuals, so-called tar *Cannabis* residuals, when applied to the skin

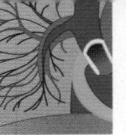

of experimental animals, produce tumors. Analysis of marijuana smoke has also revealed high concentrations of carcinogenic hydrocarbons.

Cardiovascular Effects

Dose-related sinus tachycardia is the most common cardiovascular effect observed after the administration of THC, regardless of route.[49] Orthostatic hypotension may occur with higher doses. Electrocardiographic changes in intoxicated individuals include nonspecific ST-T changes as well as occasional premature ventricular contractions. One report implicated marijuana use in causing atrial fibrillation.[50] The cardiovascular effects are caused primarily by stimulation of the autonomic nervous system with involvement of both the parasympathetic and sympathetic pathways. These effects are not likely to have serious consequences in young, healthy adults but may be significant in patients with preexisting cardiovascular disease. For example, one study found that the risk of having a myocardial infarction increases fourfold in the hour following marijuana use.[51] No long-term cardiovascular effects have been described to date.

Reproductive Effects

No definitive evidence shows that marijuana use alters reproductive function in either gender to such an extent that reproduction is compromised. Changes in sex hormone levels after heavy marijuana use have been described, but these effects have not been consistently demonstrated. For example, one study found depressed testosterone levels in heavy marijuana users but another found no difference in levels of testosterone, luteinizing hormone, follicle-stimulating hormone, prolactin, or cortisol.[52,53] Even when lower testosterone levels have been noted, the levels have been within normal limits. Whether long-term use of marijuana might result in persistently depressed levels of serum testosterone is unknown.

An increased incidence of gynecomastia and elevated estrogen levels have been noted in some men who use marijuana chronically. Studies of the semen of male long-term users found abnormalities in count, motility, and structural characteristics of the sperm examined.[54,55] In men with already marginal fertility, decreased fertility might well result, although definitive evidence of this has not emerged. Marijuana use does not appear to affect the ovulatory cycle in women.[56]

Pregnancy and Fetal Development

In laboratory animals, exposure to high doses of THC results in an increased number of stillbirths and decreased litter size.[57] Malformations in offspring have also been described, but these occur only when dams received very high doses of THC during the initial stages of organogenesis. Many of these studies conducted with high doses of THC more likely reflect maternal toxicity rather than direct effects on embryonic and fetal development.[58]

The effects of maternal marijuana use on fetal development and the outcome of pregnancy are difficult to study in humans because these effects are confounded by alcohol and drug use, smoking, nutritional status, and socioeconomic status. A reduction in birth weight of infants born to women who used marijuana during pregnancy has been noted in some studies but not in others.[59] In general, marijuana users are more likely than nonusers to have had an unplanned pregnancy, premature labor, and abruptio placentae, and their children are more likely to have lower birth weight and congenital features compatible with fetal alcohol syndrome or other major malformations.[60-62] Because women who smoke marijuana frequently smoke tobacco, drink alcohol, and abuse other drugs, it is difficult to isolate a marijuana effect. The long-term consequences of prenatal marijuana exposure are not clear. Some alterations in language skills are observed at 2 years of age, and verbal ability and memory were different between marijuana-exposed and nonexposed 4-year-olds.[63,64] However, these differences were not observed in 5- and 6-year-olds.

Immune System

The presence of a unique subpopulation of cannabinoid receptors in macrophages suggests that cannabinoids are capable of affecting the immune system. Although there has been concern that cannabinoids could contribute to immunosuppression, particularly in already compromised individuals, convincing evidence is lacking in humans.[65,66] Marijuana smoke has been shown to alter numerous immune parameters in vitro. Described changes in macrophages include suppression of superoxide production, altered morphology, diminished phagocytic and spreading ability, increased interleukin-1 production, suppression of extrinsic antivirus activity, and alteration of tumor necrosis factor levels.[67-73] Studies examining cellular and humoral responses have produced inconsistent results, with some showing differences in immunoglobulin production and alteration in CD4 to CD8 ratios, while others have not been able to demonstrate differences.[74,75] Perhaps most concerning is the observation that cannabinoids may decrease host resistance to infection. While these effects are unlikely to affect normal hosts, they may be significant in compromised hosts.

Tolerance and Dependence

The development of tolerance to the effects of marijuana is well established.[76] Marijuana dependence, defined as experiencing physical symptoms (such as irritability, restlessness, sleep disturbance, nausea, and diarrhea) on cessation of use may occur in settings of heavy use.[77] It is estimated that more than 200,000 individuals in the United States seek treatment for marijuana dependence each year.[78] The gradual release of accumulated THC from fat stores creates a "tapered dose" effect and is thought to account for the relatively mild manifestations of marijuana withdrawal.

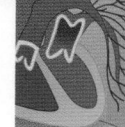

EFFECTS OF MARIJUANA IN COMBINATION WITH ALCOHOL AND OTHER DRUGS

Marijuana is most commonly used along with ethanol. Several studies have reported that concomitant marijuana and ethanol use produces either additive or supra-additive effects on psychomotor performance.[79,80] One study, however, reported that marijuana attenuates plasma ethanol levels, with a resultant decrease in the duration of subjective effects for both agents.[81] Concomitant use of intranasal cocaine and marijuana smoke enhances the tachycardia observed with marijuana alone. The duration of the effects of marijuana and cocaine are unaltered when both drugs were given together; however, marijuana pretreatment reduces the time required for the onset of cocaine effects and decreases the duration of negative cocaine effects. Moreover, marijuana pretreatment increases cocaine levels almost twofold.[82] These observations are thought to occur because marijuana-induced dilation attenuates the vasoconstrictive properties of cocaine, enhancing the absorption of the latter. Simultaneous use of marijuana and amphetamines increases the intensity and duration of a subjective high.

DIAGNOSIS

The clinical features of acute marijuana intoxication are nondescript. Conjunctival hyperemia, nasopharyngeal irritation, tachycardia, and difficulty with short-term memory with its attendant effects on fluency of speech and performance of complex tasks, may be noted. Acute anxiety reactions as well as an acute toxic psychosis with hallucinations, delusions, illusions, and agitation are primarily observed in inexperienced individuals or in those who take large doses. Symptoms, even when severe, generally subside within 4 to 6 hours. In individuals with underlying schizophrenia, marijuana may exacerbate existing symptoms or precipitate a relapse.[37] Urine immunoassay is the easiest way to confirm marijuana use. Although a marijuana-induced toxic psychosis that lasted days has been described, symptoms that persist beyond a few hours after marijuana use are more likely to indicate the presence of a cointoxicant or an underlying psychiatric disorder.

Laboratory Testing

The typical means of detecting marijuana use is through measurement of the THC metabolite 11-*nor*-Δ^9-THC carboxylic acid in urine using an immunoassay screen. Common cutoff limits for commercially available kits are 20, 50, and 100 ng/mL. When the results from the initial screen are confirmed by gas chromatography/mass spectrometry, the results are extremely reliable, with sensitivity and specificity approaching 100%. Therapeutic use of synthetic THC may result in a positive urine screen.

The length of time that marijuana metabolites can be detected in urine depends on the cutoff limit, the amount absorbed, and the frequency of use. Using a urine screen with a 50 ng/mL cutoff, THC may be detected for 1 to 3 days after acute marijuana use. Lower detection cutoffs permit detection for as long as a week or more.[83] Heavy users may have detectable cannabinoids in urine for weeks following last use. The reason for this is that THC accumulates in fat stores and upon cessation gradually redistributes back to blood and is then eliminated. Obese individuals who have large lipid stores of THC and lose weight rapidly may have detectable THC in their urine despite a prolonged period of abstinence.

A number of purported methods to defeat urinary assays have been described. These include dilution, bleach, lemon juice, potassium nitrite, niacin, salt, tetrahydrozoline, and vinegar. Marijuana use may be distinguished from dronabinol use by measuring urinary Δ^9-tetrahydrocannabivirin, which is a THC analog found only in plant material.[84]

Passive inhalation of marijuana smoke may lead to low concentrations of THC and the 11-carboxy metabolite in both serum (up to 20 ng/mL) and urine (up to 40 ng/mL).[85] However, this requires such an intense exposure to ambient marijuana smoke that it would be unlikely to occur outside research settings. Passive exposure to marijuana smoke ordinarily does not trigger a positive immunoassay nor does it produce psychotomimetic effects.[25,86] A group of rock concert attendees who were in an area where marijuana was smoked did not have detectable THC metabolites using a radioimmunoassay with a detection limit of 50 ng/mL.[87] Ingestion of hemp seed oil and other hemp seed food products has resulted in positive urine screens.[88]

Antenatal exposure to cannabinoids may be documented by testing urine as soon as possible after birth. When routine urine testing is negative but clinical suspicion remains high, meconium may be tested for *Cannabis* and other illicit substances. In fact, meconium is more sensitive than urine or hair testing in determining antenatal exposure to cannabinoids and may indicate exposure as remote as the second trimester.[89] Methods for meconium analysis for the presence of THC have been described.[90]

Federal regulations require that workers employed in certain transportation-related occupations, such as aviation, mass transit, railroads, and trucking, undergo drug and alcohol testing. The Department of Transportation develops and publishes the rules that govern the testing of these transportation workers. The Department of Transportation cutoff concentration for THC is 50 ng/mL for initial screening and 15 ng/mL for confirmatory testing.

MANAGEMENT

Treatment of marijuana intoxication is supportive. Anxiety associated with inexperience or excessive dosescan generally be managed with a quiet, protective environment, reassurance, and mild sedation with

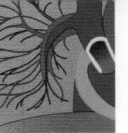

benzodiazepines, if needed. Patients who experience psychotic symptoms should be treated with antipsychotic medications. Activated charcoal may help prevent the absorption of THC after ingestion but data are not available on its effectiveness. Because THC toxicity is rarely life threatening, gastric emptying is not recommended. Patients who present with anxiety or a toxic psychosis may be discharged when their symptoms have abated. Admission is almost never required.

Elimination

THC is not amenable to enhanced elimination techniques due to high protein binding and a large volume of distribution.

Prevention and Addiction Treatment

No prevention model has been successful on a broad scale. Although recent data suggest that the prevalence of marijuana use in school-aged children may be declining, it is unknown which public health measures or policies, if any, are responsible for this decline.[4] The standard treatment modality for marijuana use has been psychotherapy similar to that of a 12-step Alcoholics Anonymous model. This approach, coupled with urine monitoring, can be effective in terminating marijuana use. However, as with most other drugs of abuse, relapse is common.

REFERENCES

1. The University of Mississippi Potency Monitoring Project, 2002. http://www.dea.gov/concern/18862/marijuan.htm.
2. O'Shaughnessy WB: On the preparation of Indian hemp and gunjah. Trans Med Phys Soc Bombay 1842;8:421–461.
3. Johnston LD, O'Malley PM, Bachman JG: National survey results on drug use from the Monitoring the Future Study, 1975–1995. Washington, DC, US Department of Health and Human Services, 1995.
4. Johnston LD, O'Malley PM, Bachman JG, Schulenberg JE: Monitoring the Future National Survey results on drug use, 1975–2003. Volume I: Secondary school students (National Institutes of Health Publication No. 04-5507). Bethesda, MD, National Institute on Drug Abuse, 2004.
5. Substance Abuse and Mental Health Services Administration: Results from the 2002 National Survey on Drug Use and Health: national findings (Department of Health and Human Services Publication No. SMA 03-3836). Rockville, MD, Department of Health and Human Services, 2003.
6. Polen MR, Sidney S, Tekawa IS, et al: Health care use by frequent marijuana smokers who do not smoke tobacco. West J Med 1993;158:596–601.
7. Ferguson DM, Horwood LJ: Does cannabis use encourage other forms of illicit drug use? Addiction 2000;95:505–520.
8. Matsuda LA, Lolait SJ, Brownstein MJ, et al: Structure of a cannabinoid receptor and functional expression of the cloned cDNA. Nature 1990;346:561–564.
9. Iversen L: Cannabis and the brain. Brain 2003;126:1252–1270.
10. Axelrod J, Felder CC: Cannabinoid receptors and their endogenous agonist anandamide. Neurochem Res 1998;23:575–581.
11. Calignano A, La Rana G, Giuffrida A, Piomelli D: Control of pain initiation by endogenous cannabinoids. Nature 1998;394:277–281.
12. Munro S, Thomas KL, Abu-Shaar M: Molecular characterization of a peripheral receptor for cannabinoids. Nature 1993;365:61–64.
13. Lynn A, Herkenham M: Localization of cannabinoid receptors and nonsaturable high-density cannabinoid binding sites in peripheral tissues of the rat: Implications for receptor-mediated immune modulation by cannabinoids. J Pharmacol Exp Ther 1994;268:1612–1623.
14. Leirer VO Yesavage JA, Morrow DG: Marijuana, aging and task difficulty effects on pilot performance. Aviat Space Environ Med 1989;60:1145–1152.
15. Kurzthaler I, Hummer M, Miller C, et al: Effects of cannabis on cognitive functions and driving ability. J Clin Psychiatry 1999; 60:395–399.
16. Joy JE, Watson SJ, Benson JA: The Medical Value of Marijuana and Related Substances in Marijuana and Medicine: Assessing the Science Base. Washington, DC, National Academy Press, 1999.
17. Tramèr MR, Carroll D, Campbell FA, et al: Cannabinoids for control of chemotherapy induced nausea and vomiting: quantitative systematic review. BMJ 2001;323:16–21.
18. Regelson W, Butler JR, Schulz J, et al: Δ^9-Tetrahydrocannabinol as an effective antidepressant and appetite-stimulating agent in advanced cancer patients. In Braude MC, Szara S (eds): The Pharmacology of Marihuana. New York, Raven, 1976.
19. Campbell FA, Tramèr MR, Carroll D, et al: Are cannabinoids an effective and safe treatment option in the management of pain? A qualitative systematic review. BMJ 2001;323:1–6.
20. Adler MW, Geller EB: Ocular effects of cannabinoids. In Mechoulam R (ed): Cannabinoids as Therapeutic Agents. Boca Raton, FL, CRC Press, 1986.
21. West ME, Homi J: Cannabis as a medicine. Br J Anaesth 1996; 76:167.
22. Karler R, Turkanis SA: The cannabinoids as potential antiepileptics. J Clin Pharmacol 1981;21(Suppl):417–448.
23. Fox P, Bain PG, Glickman S, et al: The effect of cannabis on tremor in patients with multiple sclerosis. Neurology 2004;62:1105–1109.
24. Zajicek J, Fox P, Sanders H, et al: Cannabinoids for treatment of spasticity and other symptoms related to multiple sclerosis (CAMS Study): multicentre randomized placebo-controlled trial. Lancet 2003;362:1517–1526.
25. Baselt RC: Disposition of toxic drugs and chemicals in man, 7th ed. Foster City, CA, Biomedical Publications, 2004, pp 1083–1088.
26. Ohlsson A, Agurell S, Londgren J, et al: Pharmacokinetics studies of delta-1-tetrahydrocannabinol in man. In Barnett G, Chiang C (eds): Pharmacokinetics and Pharmacodynamics of Psychoactive Drugs. Foster City, CA, Biomedical Publications,1985.
27. Wall ME, Sadler BM, Brine D, et al: Metabolism, disposition, and kinetics of Δ^9-tetrahydrocannabinol in men and women. Clin Pharmacol Ther 1983;34:352–363.
28. Johansson E, Halldin MM, Agurell S, et al: Terminal elimination plasma half-life of delta^9-tetrahydrocannabinol (delta^9-THC) in heavy users of marijuana. Eur J Clin Pharmacol 1989;37:273–277.
29. Johansson E, Halldin MM: Urinary excretion half-life of delta L-tetrahydrocannabinol-7-oic acid in heavy marijuana users after smoking. J Anal Toxicol 1989;13:218–223.
30. Huestis MA, Sampson AH, Holicky BJ, et al: Characterization of the absorption phase of marijuana smoking. Clin Pharmacol Ther 1992;52:31–41.
31. Hollister LE, Gillespie HK, Ohlsson A, et al: Do plasma concentrations of delta-9-tetrahydrocannabinol reflect the degree of intoxication? J Clin Pharm 1981;21(Suppl):171–177.
32. Chiang CN, Barnett G: Marijuana effect and delta-9-tetrahydrocannabinol plasma level. Clin Pharm Ther 1984;36:234–238.
33. MacNab A, Anderson E, Susak L: Ingestion of cannabis: a cause of coma in children. Pediatr Emerg Care 1989;5:238–239.
34. Stadtmauer G, Beyer K, Bardina L, Sicherer SH: Anaphylaxis to ingestion of hempseed (Cannabis sativa). J All Clin Immunol 2003;112:216–217.
35. Chait LD, Pierri J: Effects of smoked marijuana on human performance: a critical review. In Murphy L, Bartke A (eds): Marijuana/Cannabinoids: Neurobiology and Neurophysiology. Boca Raton, FL, CRC Press, 1992.
36. Ramaekers JG, Berghaus G, van Laar M, Drummer OH: Dose related risk of motor vehicle crashes after cannabis use. Drug Alcohol Depend 2004;73:109–119.
37. Johns A: Psychiatric effects of cannabis. Br J Psychiatry 2001;179: 116–122.
38. Mouzak A, Agathos P, Kerezoudi E, et al: Transient ischemic attack in heavy cannabis smokers: how safe is it? Eur Neurol 2000;44:44–44.

39. Russmann S, Winkler A, Lovblad KO, et al: Lethal ischemic stroke after cisplatin-based chemotherapy for testicular carcinoma and cannabis. Eur Neurol 2002;48:178–180.

40. Zimmer L, Morgan JP: Marijuana Myths, Marijuana Facts. New York, Lindemith Center, 1997.

41. Gong H, Fligiel S, Tashkin DP, Barbers RG: Tracheobronchial changes in habitual, heavy smokers of marijuana with and without tobacco. Am Rev Respir Dis 1987;136:142–149.

42. Tashkin DP, Calvarese BM, Simmons MS, Shapiro BJ: Respiratory status of seventy-four habitual marijuana smokers. Chest 1980;78:699–706.

43. Tashkin DP, Coulson AH, Clark VA, et al: Respiratory symptoms and lung function in habitual heavy smokers of marijuana alone, smokers of marijuana and tobacco, smokers of tobacco alone, and nonsmokers. Am Rev Respir Dis 1987;135:209–216.

44. Birrer RB, Calderon J: Pneumothorax, pneumomediastinum and pneumopericardium following Valsalva's maneuver during marijuana smoking. NY State J Med 1984;84:619–620.

45. Boyce SH, Quigley MA: Uvulitis and partial upper airway obstruction following cannabis inhalation. Emerg Med 2002;14:106–108.

46. Levitz SM, Diamond RD: Aspergillosis and marijuana. Ann Intern Med 1991;115:578–579.

47. Wu TC, Tashkin DP, Djahed B, Rose JE: Pulmonary hazards of smoking marijuana as compared with tobacco. N Engl J Med 1988;318:347–351.

48. Zhang ZF, Morgenstern H, Spitz MR, et al: Marijuana use and increased risk of squamous cell carcinoma of the head and neck. Cancer Epidemiol Biomarkers Prev 1999;6:1071–1078.

49. Jones RT: Cardiovascular system effects of marijuana. J Clin Pharmacol 2002;42(11 Suppl):58–63.

50. Kosior DA, Filipiak KJ, Stolarz P, Opolski G: Paroxysmal atrial fibrillation following marijuana intoxication: a two-case report of possible association. Int J Cardiol 2001;78:183–184.

51. Mittleman MA, Lewis RA, Maclure M, et al: Triggering myocardial infarction by marijuana. Circulation 2001;103:2805–2809.

52. Kolodny R, Leasin P, Tora G, et al: Depression of plasma testosterone with acute marihuana administration. In Braude MC, Szara S (eds): The Pharmacology of Marihuana. New York, Raven, 1976.

53. Block R, Farinpour R, Schlechte J: Effects of chronic marijuana use on testosterone, luteinizing hormone, follicle stimulating hormone, prolactin and cortisol in men and women. Drug Alcohol Depend 1991;28:121–128.

54. Hembree W, Nahas GG, Zeidenberg P, Huang HFS: Changes in human spermatozoa associated with high dose marihuana smoking. In Nahas GG, Paton WDM (eds): Marihuana: Biological Effects. New York, Pergamon, 1979.

55. Issidorides MR: Observations on chronic hashish users: nuclear aberrations in blood and sperm and abnormal acrosomes in spermatozoa. In Nahas GG, Paton WDM (eds): Marihuana: Biological Effects. New York, Pergamon, 1979.

56. Mendelson JH, Mello NK: Effects of marijuana on neuroendocrine hormones in human males and females. In Braude MC, Ludford JP (eds): Marijuana Effects on the Endocrine and Reproductive Systems. Washington, DC, US Government Printing Office, 1984.

57. Wenger T, Croix D, Tramu G, Leonardelli J: Effects of Δ⁹-tetrahydrocannabinol on pregnancy, puberty, and the neuroendocrine system. In Murphy L, Bartke A (eds): Marijuana/Cannabinoids: Neurobiology and Neurophysiology. Boca Raton, FL, CRC Press, 1992.

58. Abel EL: Effects of prenatal exposure to cannabinoids. In Pinkert TM (ed): Current Research on the Consequences of Maternal Drug Abuse. Washington, DC, U.S. Government Printing Office, 1985.

59. Fried PA, O'Connell CM: A comparison of the effects of prenatal exposure to tobacco, alcohol, cannabis and caffeine on birth size and subsequent growth. Neurotoxicol Teratol 1987;9:79–85.

60. Hingston R, Zuckerman B, Frank DS, et al: Effects on fetal development of maternal marijuana use during pregnancy. In Harvey DJ (ed): Marijuana '84: Proceedings of the Oxford Symposium on Marijuana. Oxford, IRL Press, 1984.

61. Gibson GT, Baghurst PA, Colley DP: Maternal alcohol, tobacco and cannabis consumption and the outcome of pregnancy. Aust N Z J Obstet Gynaecol 1983;23:15–19.

62. Linn S, Schoenbaum SC, Monson RR, et al: The association of marijuana use with outcome of pregnancy. Am J Public Health 1983;73:1161–1164.

63. Fried PA, O'Connell CM, Watkinson B: 60- and 72-month follow-up of children prenatally exposed to marijuana, cigarettes, and alcohol: cognitive and language assessment. J Dev Behav Pediatr 1992;13:383–391.

64. Day N, Richardson G, Goldschmidt L, et al: Effect of prenatal marijuana exposure on the cognitive development of offspring at age three. Neurotoxicol Teratol 1994;16:169–175.

65. Morahan PS, Klykken PC, Smith SH, et al: Effects of cannabinoids on host resistance to Listeria monocytogenes and herpes simplex virus. Infect Immun 1979;23:670–674.

66. Ashfaq MK, Watson ES, ElSohly HN: The effect of subacute marijuana smoke inhalation on experimentally induced dermonecrosis by *S. aureus* infection. Immunopharmacol Immunotoxicol 1987;9:319–331.

67. Davies P, Somberger GC, Huber GL: Effects of experimental marijuana and tobacco smoke inhalation on alveolar macrophages. Lab Invest 1979;41:220–223.

68. Cabral GA, Stinnett AL, Bailey J, et al: Chronic marijuana smoke alters alveolar macrophage morphology and protein expression. Pharmacol Biochem Behav 1991;40:643–649.

69. Lopez-Cepero M, Friedman M, Klein T, Friedman H: Tetrahydrocannabinol induced suppression of macrophages spreading and phagocytic activity in vivo. J Leukoc Biol 1986;39:679–686.

70. Spector S, Lancz G: Suppression of human macrophage function in vitro by Δ⁹-tetrahydrocannabinol. J Leukoc Biol 1991;50:423–426.

71. Shivers SC, Newton C, Friedman H, Klein TW: Δ⁹-Tetrahydrocannabinol (THC) modulates IL-1 bioactivity in human monocyte/macrophage cell lines. Life Sci 1994;54:1281–1289.

72. Cabral GA, Vasquez R: Δ⁹-Tetrahydrocannabinol suppresses macrophage extrinsic antiherpes virus activity. Proc Soc Exp Biol Med 1992;199:255–263.

73. Fischer-Stenger K, Pettit DAD, Cabral GA: Δ⁹-Tetrahydrocannabinol inhibition of tumor necrosis factor-α: suppression of post-translational events. J Pharmacol Exp Ther 1993;267:1558–1565.

74. Wallace JM, Tashkin DP, Oishi JS, Barbers RG: Peripheral blood lymphocyte subpopulations and mitogen responsiveness in tobacco and marijuana smokers. J Psychoactive Drugs 1988;20:9–14.

75. Nahas GG, Ossweman EF: Altered serum immunoglobulin concentration in chronic marijuana smokers. In Friedman H, Spector S, Klein TW (eds): Drug of Abuse, Immunity, and Immunodeficiency. New York, Plenum, 1991.

76. Tennant FS: The clinical syndrome of marijuana dependence. Psychiatr Ann 1986;16:225–234.

77. Weller RA, Halikas JA: Objective criteria for the diagnosis of marijuana abuse. J Nerv Ment Dis 1980;168:98–103.

78. Office of Applied Studies: Results from the 2001 National Household Survey on Drug Abuse: Volume II. Technical Appendices and Selected Data Tables (Department of Health and Human Services Publication No. SMA 02-3759). Rockville, MD, Substance Abuse and Mental Health Services Administration, 2002.

79. Bird KD, Boleyn T, Chesher GB, et al: Intercannabinoid and cannabinoid-ethanol interactions and their effects on human performance. Psychopharmacology 1980;71:181–188.

80. Sutton L: The effects of alcohol, marijuana and their combination on driving ability. J Stud Alcohol 1983;44:438–445.

81. Lukas SE, Benedikt R, Mendelson JH, et al: Marihuana attenuates the rise in plasma ethanol levels in human subjects. Neuropsychopharmacology 1992;7:77–81.

82. Lukas S, Sholar M, Kouri E, et al: Marihuana smoking increases plasma cocaine levels and subjective reports of euphoria in male volunteers. Pharmacol Biochem Behav 1994;48:715–721.

83. Huestis MA, Mitchell JM, Cone EJ: Detection times of marijuana metabolites in urine by immunoassay and GC/MS. J Anal Toxicol 1995;19:443–449.

84. ElSohly MA, DeWit H, Wachtel SR, et al: Δ⁹-Tetrahydrocannabivarin as a marker for the ingestion of marijuana versus Marinol: results of a clinical study. J Anal Toxicol 2001;25:565–571.

85. Stein IN: Marijuana testing. West J Med 1988;148:78.

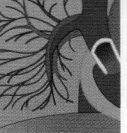

86. Morland J, Bugge A. Shuterud B, et al: Cannabinoids in blood and urine after passive inhalation of cannabis smoke. J Forensic Sci 1985;30:997–1002.
87. Toussi A: Side-stream inhalation of marijuana: the Grateful Dead experience. Ann Emerg Med 1996;27:816–817.
88. Alt A, Reinhartdt G: Positive cannabis results in urine and blood samples after consumption of hemp food products. J Anal Toxicol 1998;22:80–81.
89. Bar-Oz B, Klein J, Karaskov T, Koren G: Comparison of meconium and neonatal hair analysis for detection of gestational exposure to drugs of abuse. Arch Dis Childhood 2003;88:F98–F100.
90. Moore C, Negrusz A, Lewis D: Determination of drugs of abuse in meconium. J Chromatogr B Biomed Sci Appl 1998;713:137–146.

42 Cocaine

TIMOTHY E. ALBERTSON, MD, MPH, PhD ■ ANDREW CHAN, MD ■
R. STEVEN THARRATT, MD, MPVM

At a Glance...

- Cocaine is the most frequent cause of emergency department visits and death associated with illicit drug use in the United States.
- The major routes of administration of cocaine are sniffing, injecting, and smoking (free-base or "crack" cocaine).
- Local anesthetic effects and the blockade of catecholamine and serotonin uptake define cocaine's principal mechanisms of action.
- Toxicity is manifested primarily by behavioral alterations, hyperthermia, seizures, and cardiac abnormalities. Less commonly, gastrointestinal, liver, kidney, muscle, renal, and pulmonary damage have been reported.
- Treatment is primarily supportive in nature.

INTRODUCTION AND RELEVANT HISTORY

Cocaine continues to be a significant drug of abuse in the United States, as well as in many other parts of the world. It is often associated with drug-related emergency department (ED) visits, intensive care unit (ICU) admissions, and death.[1-3] Cocaine is frequently detected on drug screens performed on reckless or impaired drivers[4] and trauma patients that present to EDs.[5,6] Although the central nervous and cardiovascular systems are most commonly affected by cocaine, the drug can have toxic manifestations in nearly every organ system. Due to the prevalence and medical significance of cocaine toxicity, health care providers must be knowledgeable of and alert for cocaine toxicity.

Cocaine, an alkaloid that is derived from the leaves of *Erythroxylum coca,* has an interesting history that interfaces with the history of medicine and drug abuse. The first recorded medicinal uses were reported by Spanish physicians in 1596.[7] Cocaine was first isolated from coca leaves in 1859 by Albert Nieman, a graduate student at the University of Göttingen.[8] By 1863, Angelo Mariani was marketing a wine in France that was fortified with about 6 mg per ounce of the cocaine alkaloid extract.[8] In the United States, the Parke-Davis Company was selling a fluid extract containing 0.5 mg/mL of a crude cocaine by 1880.[8] By 1884, Sigmund Freud had proposed that cocaine be used for the treatment of depression, cachexia, and asthma and also as a local anesthetic.[9] That same year, cocaine was also first used in eye surgery, a field that was revolutionized by the discovery of this drug. William Steward Halsted, the father of modern American surgery, first used cocaine in regional nerve blocks also in 1884. Unfortunately, Halsted, like Freud, became heavily dependent on cocaine.[9] In 1885, the Georgia pharmacist John Styth Pemberton registered the cocaine-containing "French Wine Cola" in the United States; later, he renamed the product Coca-Cola.[3,8] Coca-Cola was initially a mixture of extracts from the cocaine-containing coca leaf and the caffeine-containing African kola nut. The soft drink was first introduced in 1892 as a brain tonic for elderly people who were easily tired; it was also marketed as a cure for all nervous afflictions.[3]

By 1893, fatalities from the use of cocaine had been reported. In 1895, a series of six fatalities was reported in the *Lancet*.[6,10] In 1909, more than 10 tons of cocaine was imported into the United States without legal restraint. Multiple over-the-counter medical products and elixirs containing various amounts of cocaine were created. A product for nasal application called Dr. Tucker's Asthma Specific contained 420 mg of cocaine per ounce.[8] The passage of the Harrison Narcotics Act of 1914 finally banned nonprescription use of cocaine-containing products. Subsequently, a significant reduction in the use of cocaine occurred in the United States. Although amphetamines surpassed cocaine as the most prevalent stimulant of abuse in the 1950s, the use of cocaine surged again in the 1970s. Cocaine currently remains the most commonly abused stimulant and illicit drug of abuse.[1,9,11] The Controlled Substances Act of 1970 prohibited the manufacture, distribution, and possession of cocaine in the United States, except for increasingly limited medical uses.[9] It has since been designated as a schedule II drug by the U.S. Drug Enforcement Agency (DEA). By the 1980s, chunks of an alkaloidal cocaine called "crack" had become widely available. Cocaine is still used medicinally as a local anesthetic. Topical application of the hydrochloride (1%, 4%, or 10% solution) to the eyes or upper respiratory tract mucosa provides local anesthesia and vasoconstriction with a single agent.[12]

EPIDEMIOLOGY

Cocaine use and dependence remains an epidemic in the United States. The widespread availability of a highly pure, relatively inexpensive, easy-to-use, and highly addictive formulation crack cocaine has ensured the continued American addiction to this illicit drug.[13,14] In 1999, it was estimated that 25 million Americans had used cocaine at least once, 3.7 million used it within the past year, and 1.5 million were current regular users.[1,14] Each year, the number of new users steadily increases, with 900,000 new users estimated in 2000.[15] The prevalence of cocaine use is greatest in Americans 18

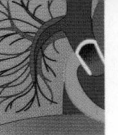

to 25 years of age. Approximately 11% of Americans older than 12 years have used cocaine, with 7% of adults between 18 and 34 years of age having used it within the previous year.[3] According to the Drug Abuse Warning Network, cocaine continues to be the most frequent cause of ED visits associated with illicit drug use in the United States; it accounted for 30% of all such ED visits in 2002 (approximately 200,000 ED visits).[1] In addition, from 1995 to 2002, cocaine-related ED visits have increased by 33%.[1]

Death after cocaine use is one of the five leading causes of death in the 15- to 44-year-old age group.[16] Between 1990 and 1992, as many as 26.7% of all deaths in New York City were associated with the presence of cocaine or a cocaine metabolite in the blood or urine.[16] More than 30% of these deaths were attributed to cocaine directly, and 65% involved traumatic injuries associated with cocaine.[16] Cocaine overdose appears from surveys of users to be less associated with crack cocaine smoking than with intravenous use.[17] Accidental overdose deaths have slightly decreased from its peak between 1993 and 1995 in New York.[18] Regardless, cocaine alone or in combination with alcohol and or an opiate was determined to be the cause of death in 69.5% of these cases.[18] In a study of intravenous drug users in San Francisco, the use of heroin and cocaine together ("speedballs") was frequently associated with overdose.[19] A survey of cocaine users in Brazil noted that 20% had experienced one or more episodes of overdose.[20] In Tennessee in 1993, more than 25% of reckless drivers who did not smell of alcohol were found to be intoxicated with cocaine alone or in combination with marijuana.[4] Again, both the direct effects of cocaine and related trauma contribute to the high rate of cocaine-associated deaths.[3,6,16] In 2001, cocaine was the most frequent cause of drug-related deaths reported to medical examiners in the United States.[2,14]

Cocaine remains a major drug of abuse, with the majority coming into the United States from South and Central America.[21] The DEA noted that in 2002, federal drug seizures of cocaine in Florida alone amounted to 26,258 kg.[21] Acute and chronic cocaine toxicity represents a major challenge to the clinician. Cocaine's ability to cause significant multiorgan system dysfunction contributes to this challenge. Preventive care and new carefully tested approaches to therapy can help reduce the incidence and improve the outcome of patients with this modern affliction.

STRUCTURE/STRUCTURE-ACTIVITY RELATIONSHIPS

Cocaine is a naturally occurring drug; it is the principal active alkaloid that is derived from the leaves of the shrub *Erythroxylum coca*, found in South and Central America, India, and Java, and also from *Erythroxylum novogranatense*, found in South America. Coca leaves may be chewed or ingested as a tea (*mate de coca*).[3] This is how the ancient Incas used and native South Americans still

currently use cocaine. Each coca leaf contains 0.1% to 0.9% cocaine by weight.[3,22] A partly purified product, cocaine sulfate (also known as *pasta, basuco, basa, pitillo,* and *paste*) is made when coca leaves are mixed with water and dilute sulfuric acid. Coca paste is commonly mixed with tobacco and smoked in South America.[3,22] Coca paste is often further refined to cocaine hydrochloride (an odorless, white, crystalline powder) by repetitive mixings with various solvents (e.g., kerosene, methyl alcohol, and sulfuric acid). Refined cocaine hydrochloride powder is 30% to 40% pure.[3,22]

Cocaine hydrochloride is freely soluble in water and can be injected intravenously or readily absorbed across all mucous membranes. Alternatively, the free base of cocaine can be made by dissolving the hydrochloride salt in a solvent and separating and drying the precipitate. Cocaine free base is not water soluble and, thus, cannot be injected intravenously or readily absorbed across mucosal surfaces.[3,13,22] Cocaine base, however, is lipophilic and rapidly absorbed across the alveolar-capillary and blood-brain barrier.

Free-basing is a process of converting cocaine hydrochloride back to cocaine base for smoking. Traditionally, free base was made by dissolving the hydrochloride salt in water, adding ammonia to remove the hydrochloride, adding ether to solubilize the base, and then letting the ether evaporate from the base.[3,13] An alternative form of cocaine free base, crack is made by dissolving the hydrochloride salt in water, adding sodium bicarbonate (baking soda) to remove the hydrochloride, heating the mixture until the water evaporates, and cooling the free base into a soft mass that subsequently dries into a hard rock.[3,13] Cocaine free base has a relatively low melting point as compared with the hydrochloride form (98° C versus 197° C) and is stable to pyrrolysis.[3,14] Thus, the free base can be heated, vaporized, and inhaled (smoked). The base is commonly smoked in a glass or regular pipe or mixed with tobacco or marijuana in cigarette form. If the ether is not fully evaporated from the free base prior to smoking, airway burns are a possibility.[13] The hydrochloride form of cocaine breaks down with pyrrolysis.[9] The term *crack* comes from the popping sound that occurs when the rock is smoked.[3,13,14] Due to ease of production, relative inexpense, ease of use, and rapid onset of effects after use, crack has become a very popular means of cocaine abuse.[13,19] It also appears to be the most potent and addictive form of cocaine.[13,14] Crack and free-base cocaine are 85% to 90% pure, whereas cocaine hydrochloride preparations are often adulterated with one or more of several compounds (e.g., sucrose, mannitol, lactose, quinine, caffeine, amphetamine, phencyclidine, talc, procaine, lidocaine, or strychnine).[23]

The stimulant cocaine (benzoylmethylecgonine, $C_{17}H_{21}NO_4$) is an ester of benzoic acid and the amino alcohol base methylecgonine (Fig. 42-1).[12] Its molecular weight is 303.4. In its natural form, cocaine is a weak base with a pKa of 8.6.[24] The ester structure of cocaine predicts rapid hydrolysis by esterases and a short duration of action. Its structure is similar to other ester-type local anesthetics.[12]

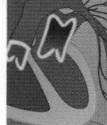

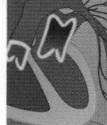

FIGURE 42-1 The chemical structure of the alkaloid cocaine hydrochloride.

PHARMACOLOGY

Cocaine produces its clinical effects predominantly from reuptake blockade and enhanced presynaptic release of catecholamines (e.g., norepinephrine and dopamine) and serotonin from central and peripheral nerve terminals.[3,24] Reuptake blockade of norepinephrine in the sympathetic nervous system innervation to the adrenal gland results in postsynaptic medullary release of catecholamines (predominantly epinephrine) and systemic sympathetic effects.[25] Reuptake inhibition of dopamine in the central nervous system (CNS) produces stimulation of both D_1- and D_2-dopamine receptors in mesocortical, mesolimbic (e.g., nucleus accumbens), and basal ganglia areas of the brain; this accounts for the euphoric, psychostimulatory, and motor effects from cocaine.[12,26] Cocaine also enhances release of the excitatory amino acids glutamate and aspartate in the limbic system, which adds to its psychostimulatory effects.[27,28] Reuptake inhibition with repetitive cocaine use leads to accelerated catabolism and depletion of presynaptic catecholamines and serotonin. In addition, compensatory processes work to down-regulate the overstimulated neuronal pathways. Cocaine craving and movement disorders (e.g., parkinsonism) likely occur from depletion of dopaminergic stores or a down-regulated dopamine pathway.[12]

Cocaine also causes marked local anesthetic effects from the blockade of membrane sodium channels (see Chapter 63).[11,12,24] Sodium channel blockade is concentration, frequency, pH, and voltage dependent; block is greater at higher frequencies of stimulation, lower pH, and more positive membrane potentials.[12] Vasoconstrictive effects of cocaine will increase local drug concentration and membrane effects.[12] Cocaine may also inhibit potassium channels and sodium-calcium exchange mechanisms in some cellular membranes.[29]

PHARMACOKINETICS

Cocaine is readily absorbed across all mucous membranes.[3,12,14] The onset of action and peak effects depend on the dose and route of absorption. Mucosal and oral administration of cocaine result in a slower absorption, slower onset of action, later peak effect, and longer duration of action than the inhalation and intravenous routes.[14] Although absorption is rapid after ingestion, the oral bioavailability of both the hydrochloride and free-base forms are only 30% to 40%.[3] After nasal insufflations of cocaine, the onset of effects occurs within 1 to 5 minutes.[3,14] Constriction of nasal vessels inhibits and prolongs drug absorption, such that the duration of effects are extended, peak levels are blunted, and dose-dependent toxicity is reduced.[13,30] When cocaine is snorted, chewed, or ingested, peak levels and effects occur within 30 to 120 minutes.[3,24,30] The inhalation route produces a more rapid increase in plasma and brain cocaine levels and more intense euphoria than the nasal and oral routes; the cardiovascular effects are similar to those produced by an equivalent intravenous dose of cocaine.[22] When inhaled and injected intravenously, the onset of action occurs within seconds, and peak effects occur within 3 to 5 minutes. The duration of effects typically lasts 5 to 15 minutes after inhalation and 20 to 60 minutes after intravenous use of cocaine.[12,14,30] The rapid decrease in plasma and brain cocaine concentrations that follow an initial surge (i.e., brief duration of euphoria) probably accounts for the desire to reuse within 10 to 30 minutes of inhalant (crack) use.[12]

Although dependent on dose and route of administration, peak cocaine blood concentrations of 200 to 600 mg/mL are seen with typical doses (0.2 to 2 mg/kg or 10 to 140 mg).[24,30] Peak blood concentrations of several thousand milligrams per milliliter have been reported in intoxicated patients.[24,30] Blood cocaine concentrations averaged 4600 mg/mL in one study of 37 cocaine-related fatalities.[31]

Cocaine has a volume of distribution of 2 to 3 L/kg.[24,30] About 35% to 45% of cocaine is rapidly metabolized by nonenzymatic hydrolysis to benzoylecgonine. Another 32% to 49% of cocaine is metabolized to ecgonine methyl ester by enzymatic hydrolysis with hepatic and plasma esterases (e.g., pseudocholinesterase). A small amount of the benzoylecgonine is metabolized on to ecgonine in a 24-hour period. Although these metabolites tend not to be very active, a small percentage of cocaine, particularly after toxic exposure, undergoes hepatic microsomal oxidative metabolism (N-demethylation) to norcocaine, a potentially active metabolite, and then to N-hydroxynorcocaine, a metabolite potentially toxic to the liver.[24,30] Endogenous (genetic) loss or induced (e.g., by organophosphate pesticide exposure) loss of cholinesterase activity in a patient may result in a delay in metabolism of cocaine and may increase the toxic risk of a given exposure. Blood or plasma samples must be frozen, or fluoride or cholinesterase inhibitors must be added to samples, to prevent cocaine from being hydrolyzed to ecgonine methyl ester by serum cholinesterases.

The serum half-life of cocaine is approximately 30 to 90 minutes. The fact that only 1% to 9% of cocaine appears in the urine unchanged (dependent on urine pH) makes the analysis of the major cocaine metabolites benzoylecgonine and ecgonine more useful for diagnostic and forensic purposes. Benzoylecgonine and ecgonine have serum half-lives of approximately 4 to 6 hours and 3 to 4 hours, respectively.[12,24,30]

Intravenous use of cocaine alone or in combination with heroin, benzodiazepines, or other sedative-hypnotics

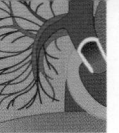

is commonly seen. As previously noted, the intravenous use of heroin in combination with cocaine is called "speedballing" and is thought to be responsible for 12% to 15% of toxic cocaine episodes managed in EDs in the United States.[1] The combined use of ethanol and cocaine facilitates the formation of cocaethylene.[32] This potent cocaine metabolite has a half-life of approximately 2 hours. Animal studies and human epidemiologic studies suggest that cocaethylene is more toxic to the brain and heart than cocaine or its usual metabolites.[33] The risk of sudden death is 21.5-fold greater with the combined use of ethanol and cocaine than with cocaine use alone.[33] The exact contribution of cocaethylene to this increased toxicity in humans is controversial.[34] In a randomized, double-blind trial, daily oral cocaine treatment at doses without subjective effects or signs of toxicity significantly decreased physiologic responses to intravenous cocaine.[35] Whether this is a form of tachyphylaxis is not clear.

TOXICOLOGY

The toxicity of cocaine comes from the extension of its pharmacology and mechanisms of action. Acute toxicity is frequently noted from CNS and sympathetic nervous system overstimulation. Toxic cardiac manifestations are likely from cocaine's effect on sodium and potassium exchange channels along with its catecholaminergic effects.

In addition to acute toxic effects, binge use depletes central and peripheral nervous system catecholamines and serotonin, resulting in depression and potential reduced vascular tone. Cocaine withdrawal may represent an extension of this type of depleted state. The toxicity associated with cocaine abuse often results in ED and ICU admissions.

CLINICAL MANIFESTATIONS

Cocaine is capable of inducing toxicities in many organ systems. Both acute and chronic abnormalities have been reported with cocaine exposures. Studies have not established the exact prevalence or incidence of the toxicities, which are summarized in Table 42-1.

Cardiovascular

Cocaine use and abuse is frequently associated with a wide array of cardiovascular complications.[14,36,37] Acute and chronic cardiovascular toxicity results from an exaggeration of both β- and α-adrenergic receptor stimulation, augmented myocardial cellular calcium influx and elevation of cytosolic free calcium concentrations, and increased secondary messenger (e.g., phospholipase C, inositol triphosphate) activation.[37]

Chest pain is the most frequent presenting complaint of patients who have used cocaine and is responsible for approximately 16% of cocaine admissions to EDs.[5,14,38-41] Although most of cocaine-associated chest pain is

noncardiac in origin, ruling out myocardial ischemia is the principal concern when such patients present to the ED.[14,41] This is because acute myocardial infarction (MI) is the most frequently reported cardiac consequence of cocaine abuse.[41,42] Prospective studies have shown that approximately 6% of patients with cocaine-associated chest pain that present to the ED have an MI by enzyme analysis.[41,43] The risk for MI is increased 24-fold in the hour following use of cocaine.[14,44] Cocaine-associated MI is not route, dose, or duration dependent; it occurs following all routes of administration, with a wide range of doses, and occurs in both first-time and long-term users.[14,41] Cocaine-associated MI cannot be distinguished from noncardiac chest pain on the basis of chest pain location, quality, duration, associated symptoms, or the presence of traditional risk factors for atherosclerosis.[14,41,43] A recent retrospective study of patients with cocaine-associated chest pain found that a 9- to 12-hour period of ED observation without evidence of ischemic or cardiac complications predicted a very low risk for death or MI for a 30-day period after ED discharge.[45]

Several mechanisms may lead to cocaine-induced MI.[46] These include increased myocardial oxygen demand in the setting of limited myocardial oxygen supply, coronary artery vasoconstriction, enhanced platelet aggregation, in situ coronary artery thrombosis formation, left ventricular hypertrophy, and accelerated atherosclerosis.[14,37,41,46] Increased oxygen demand is created by cocaine-induced tachycardia, enhanced contractility, and increased blood pressure (enhanced afterload). Decreased oxygen supply is the result of coronary vasoconstriction, which is greatest in diseased coronary artery segments.[47] Cocaine-induced coronary artery vasoconstriction is mediated by α-adrenergic stimulation, as evidenced by its reversal after administration of the α-adrenergic receptor antagonist phentolamine and exacerbation with β-adrenergic antagonist therapy.[48,49] Cocaine potentiates vasoconstriction by stimulating release of endothelin and thromboxane (vasoconstrictors) and impairing release of nitric oxide and prostacyclin (vasodilators) from endothelial cells.[50,51] Coronary artery spasm leading to MI has been widely reported in cocaine users.[38] Both epicardial and microvascular cardiac flow is impaired by cocaine.[52] Enhanced platelet activity occurs from α-adrenergic-mediated increases in platelet aggregation and increased releases of thromboxane and adenosine diphosphate.[53,54] In situ thrombosis formation may occur from cocaine-induced vasoconstriction and resultant disruption in the endothelial surface (i.e., plaque rupture).[55] In addition, concentrations of antithrombin III and protein C are decreased and concentrations of tissue plasminogen activator inhibitor are increased after cocaine use.[3,56] Cocaine may promote atherosclerosis by enhancing endothelial cell permeability to low-density lipoprotein and enhancing endothelial cell expression of adhesion molecules and leukocyte migration to their surface.[14,57,58]

Most patients with cocaine-associated MI are young (mean age 38 years), nonwhite (72%) tobacco smokers (91%). They have a history of cocaine use within the past

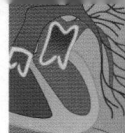

TABLE 42-1 Major Noninfectious Medical Complications Associated with Cocaine Use

COMPLICATION	FREQUENCY AND MAGNITUDE OF EVENTS*	COMPLICATION	FREQUENCY AND MAGNITUDE OF EVENTS*
Respiratory		**Cardiac**	
BAROTRAUMA	++	Chest pain	+++
Pneumothorax		Myocardial infarction	+++
Pneumopericardium		Arrhythmias	++
Pneumomediastinum		Cardiomyopathy	++
Subcutaneous emphysema		Myocarditis	+
Pulmonary hemorrhage/infarct	+	Hypertension	+++
Diffuse alveolar hemorrhage	+	Sudden death	++
Pulmonary edema	+++		
Exacerbation of asthma	++	**Psychiatric**	
Eosinophilic lung disease	+	Anxiety	++
Recurrent transient pulmonary infiltrates with peripheral eosinophilia	+	Depression	++
		Paranoia	++
		Delirium	++
Chronic diffuse interstitial pneumonia with mild fibrosis	+	Psychosis	++
		Suicide	+++
Sudden infant death syndrome (SIDS)	+	**Obstetric**	
Pulmonary hypertension	+	Low birth weight	+
"Crack lung" with transient pulmonary infiltrates	++	Placental abruption	+
Nasal septum perforation/aspiration	+	**Neurologic**	
Bronchiolitis obliterans organizing pneumonia	+	Headaches	++
		Strokes	++
Airway burns/tracheal stenosis	+	Seizures	+++
Sinusitis	+	Cerebral infarcts	++
Epiglottitis	+	Cerebral hemorrhage	++
Bronchitis	++	Cerebral vasculitis	+
Pulmonary cellulose granulomas in lung	+	**Gastrointestinal, Renal, and Other**	
Panlobar emphysema	+	Renal failure	+
Foreign body aspiration/needle	+	Rhabdomyolysis	++
Alveolar accumulation of carbonaceous material	++	Hyperthermia	+
		Disseminated vasculitis	+
Central nervous system respiratory stimulant effect	++	Bowel ischemia/colitis	++
		Thrombocytopenia/platelet aggregation	+
NEUROGENIC PULMONARY EDEMA	+++	Hepatitis	+
Respiratory depression—overdose/postictal	+++		
Abnormal hypoxic response in infants of cocaine-abusing mother	+		

*Estimated.
+, rarely reported; ++, commonly reported; +++, frequently seen with chronic use or overdose.

24 hours (88%), have a history of repeated use of cocaine (mean duration of use of 5 years), and do not have other traditional risk factors for atherosclerosis.[37,14,41,43,44] Q-wave and non-Q-wave infarctions are seen with equal frequency.[14] Although most patients have the onset of pain within an hour of cocaine use, MI has been reported several days after use.[42-44] MI has also been associated with therapeutic doses and use of cocaine and in the setting of cocaine withdrawal.[41,42] Angiographic studies of these patients have demonstrated both atherosclerotic and normal coronary arteries with about equal frequency.[13,14,59] Left ventricular hypertrophy, hypertension, and coronary atherosclerosis are thought to occur as a result of chronic cocaine use. Accelerated atherosclerosis is found in animals that are administered cocaine chronically and in 40% of autopsies of young patients who used cocaine regularly.[3,60]

Early cardiovascular complications occur in up to 36% of patients with cocaine-associated MI.[14,41,60] Ventricular arrhythmias occur in 4% to 17%, congestive heart failure in 5% to 7%, and death in less than 2%.[14,60] Most complications (90%) occur within 12 hours of hospital arrival, and death is extremely unlikely for those patients who are alive on hospital arrival.[41,60]

The cardiovascular toxicity of cocaine is potentiated by concomitant cigarette smoking or use of alcohol. Similar to cocaine, cigarette smoking produces coronary vasoconstriction by an α-adrenergic mechanism.[61] Simultaneous use of cocaine and cigarettes produces synergistic increases in blood pressure, heart rate, and coronary vasoconstriction.[41,61] When cocaine is used concomitantly with alcohol, the heart rate increase is greater than when each drug is used alone.[62] Patients who die of a combined overdose of cocaine and ethanol

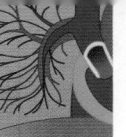

have lower blood cocaine concentrations than those who die from cocaine alone.[14,63] The hepatic transesterification product cocaethylene is considered to be largely responsible for the synergistic toxicity that occurs when cocaine and ethanol are used in close proximity.[64] Animal models have demonstrated that cocaethylene is more lethal than cocaine.[14,65] Cocaethylene increases myocardial oxygen demand by producing hypertension and increased vascular resistance; it does not have direct effects on coronary blood flow.[66]

A number of clinical reports have described left ventricular hypertrophy, systolic dysfunction, dilated cardiomyopathy and myocarditis from long-term use of cocaine. Myocardial hypertrophy is frequently discovered at autopsy in patients who die from cocaine toxicity.[67] Seven percent of long-term abusers of cocaine demonstrate left ventricular systolic dysfunction by radionuclide ventriculography.[14,68] Numerous mechanisms may explain cocaine-associated cardiomyopathy. Repetitive elevations of plasma catecholamines as occur with repetitive cocaine use may produce subendocardial contraction band necrosis, mononuclear cell myocardial infiltration, myocytolysis, myocarditis, and resultant fibrosis.[69] These effects may be reversible with discontinuation of cocaine use. Alternatively, cocaine-induced cardiomyopathy may be the result of repetitive episodes of ischemia or infarction, long-standing hypertension, an immune-mediated or hypersensitivity reaction to cocaine, altered myocyte collagen production, or from the toxic effects of cocaine adulterants or contaminants, including heavy metals such as manganese.[14,37]

Because of cocaine's local anesthetic properties and its effects on catecholamines, it is not surprising that both cardiac conduction disturbances and arrhythmias are common in patients who abuse cocaine. Although sinus bradycardia, complete heart block, and bundle branch block have been described, supraventricular and ventricular tachyarrhythmias occur most commonly.[14,37] At low doses, sinus bradycardia and ectopic rhythms may occur.[70] At high doses, cocaine produces direct sodium and potassium channel blockade, prolonged QRS and QTc intervals and ST-T wave changes on electrocardiograms (ECGs), and resultant intraventricular conduction delays and reentrant ventricular dysrhythmias (e.g., ventricular tachycardia and torsades de pointes).[14,29,37,70] Enhanced sympathetic stimulation will increase myocardial intracellular calcium concentrations, enhance automaticity, produce afterdepolarizations, and possibly lead to ectopic rhythms (e.g., tachyarrhythmias).[14,37] Cardiac conduction abnormalities and arrhythmias occur most commonly in the context of myocardial ischemia, profound metabolic acidosis, seizures, hypoxia, or hypotension.[14,37,71] These latter effects minimally play a potentiating role and may often be the primary cause of cardiac toxicity from cocaine.

Acute aortic dissection and rupture and papillary muscle rupture have been associated with cocaine use in otherwise healthy patients.[72] Endocarditis is a frequent complication of intravenous drug use, and thus is seen in the patient abusing intravenous cocaine.[73]

Central Nervous System

Neurologic complaints occur in 17% to 42% of patients with cocaine-related medical problems necessitating ED treatment in the United States.[3,5,39,40] Altered mental status, anxiety, paranoid behavior, dizziness, headaches, paresthesias, tremors, seizures, strokes, transient ischemic attacks, and coma represent the majority of these neurologic complaints.[74] Cocaine-associated strokes may be ischemic or hemorrhagic. The mechanisms of cerebrovascular accidents are multifactorial and include cerebral vasoconstriction, thrombosis, vasculitis, and loss of vasomotor autoregulation in the setting of acute hypertension, and embolism of particulate matter.[3,74-77] Increased activity of platelets and other mediators of thrombosis potentiate the likelihood of an ischemic stroke. Cocaine-induced agitated delirium may result from disrupted dopaminergic function and is often associated with fulminant hyperthermia, rhabdomyolysis, and sudden death.[78]

Seizures are a very common manifestation of cocaine toxicity and have been reported in up to 9% of ED patients with cocaine toxicity.[39] Drug-induced seizures are frequently caused by stimulants. Cocaine-induced seizures accounted for the increase in all drug-induced seizure cases from 4% in 1981 to 23% in 1988.[79] Although not fully elucidated, the mechanism of cocaine-induced seizures involves interaction of the drug with voltage-dependent sodium channels and numerous neurotransmitter systems. It appears that 5-HT_2-serotonergic, D_1-dopaminergic, α_1- and α_2-adrenergic, GABA_A, and glutamatergic receptors are all involved in cocaine-induced seizures.[80] Human and animal data suggest that cocaine-induced seizures are usually generalized, single seizures without long-lasting neurologic consequences.[81,82] The majority of cocaine-related seizures are associated with intravenous injection or inhalation of cocaine. In one study, Pascual-Leone and colleagues found that when habitual cocaine abuse was associated with seizures, computed tomography and electroencephalography frequently showed diffuse brain atrophy and diffuse slowing, respectively.[81] Multiple or focal seizures are often seen with acute intracerebral complications (e.g., hemorrhage) or with the toxic manifestations of other medications.[81] Recurrent generalized seizures have been reported in children after mucosal application of the topical anesthetic tetracaine-adrenaline-cocaine. Seizures may be a major determinant of cocaine lethality.[83] This justifies aggressive immediate treatment of sustained cocaine-induced seizures with the correction of seizure-associated metabolic acidosis and hypoxemia. Repetitive or prolonged seizures attributed to the use of cocaine indicate the need for further diagnostic workup that includes computed tomography of the brain and, possibly, lumbar puncture.

Cerebral vasculitis, headaches, toxic encephalopathies, transient ischemic events, migraine-like events, and a wide array of extrapyramidal side effects (e.g., acute dystonic reactions, Tourette's syndrome, akathisia, choreoathetosis, tardive dyskinesia) have been reported

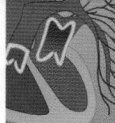

with both acute and chronic use of cocaine.[3,13,84,85] Choreoathetoid movements associated with crack use have been termed "crack dancing."[85] Extrapyramidal movement disorders occur from dopamine disturbances in the basal ganglia; choreoathetosis is from an overabundance of dopamine, and acute dystonia from dopamine deficiency. As expected, cerebral hemorrhage, cerebral infarction, and cerebral vasculitis are associated with significant morbidity and mortality among cocaine users. Kaku and Lowenstein reported that 34% of patients between the ages of 15 and 44 years with a diagnosis of ischemic or hemorrhagic stroke had associated drug abuse. Cocaine and amphetamines accounted for the largest percentage of cases.[86] Psychological dependence and a cocaine withdrawal or abstinence syndrome have been reported.[12,24] The cocaine abstinence syndrome has been described as having three phases.[24] The first phase is a "crash" that lasts up to 4 days and is characterized by dysphoria, depression, irritability, anxiety, and insomnia followed by hypersomnolence, exhaustion, and drug craving. The second phase lasts from 1 to 10 weeks and is characterized by anergia, anxiety, listlessness, and drug craving. The third phase, which has been called the "extinction phase," may last indefinitely and is associated with normalization of mood and actions but also episodic drug craving that is often triggered by environmental cues.[24] Acute psychiatric disturbances, including agitation, anxiety, depression, psychosis, paranoia, and suicidal ideation have been widely reported in cocaine users.[87] The cocaine "washed out" syndrome is similar to the "crash" associated with the abstinence syndrome and occurs soon after a several day binge of cocaine.[12] Patients are lethargic with normal vital signs and sleep deeply for a period of 24 to 48 hours. The syndrome is considered to result from an acute depletion of catecholamines that follows a several day binge of cocaine.

Pulmonary

Cocaine can produce a wide range of pulmonary complications (see Table 42-1).[88,89] Cocaine-induced pulmonary disturbances occur in up to 25% of users and often result in ED and ICU admissions.[3,90] Primary respiratory depression or reduced respiratory drive has been associated with toxic cocaine exposures. This has occurred both in conjunction with and independent of cardiac arrhythmias and seizure-induced cardiovascular collapse.

Cocaine smoking is associated with significant barotrauma and may result in pneumothorax, pneumomediastinum, pneumopericardium, and subcutaneous air.[3,89] The self-application of a Valsalva maneuver (to increase positive airway or intrapleural pressures) by cocaine smokers seeking enhancement of its euphoric effects may precipitate barotraumatic complications. High positive airway pressures can also be generated by an "assistant" who blows back into the cocaine pipe being used. Thermal injury from smoking cocaine may also contribute to the development of barotrauma.

Noncardiogenic pulmonary edema is associated with cocaine use.[88,89,91] Although pulmonary edema may be cardiogenic and occur secondary to acute or chronic left ventricular failure from increased vascular resistance, the majority of cases appear to be caused by a noncardiogenic "capillary leak" syndrome.[92] Both neurogenic and non-neurogenic mechanisms for cocaine-induced noncardiogenic pulmonary edema can be postulated. Cocaine may directly injure pulmonary endothelium and increase local capillary permeability.[91]

Exacerbation of reversible airway diseases, including asthma, has been reported in association with the use of cocaine. These exacerbations may be the consequences of heat or of exposure to the impurities in cocaine, since its catecholamine effects would not be expected to produce airway bronchospasm.[23,88,89] An increase in bronchial hyperactivity has been seen in patients who inhaled "rebujo" (vaporized heroin and cocaine on aluminum foil compound) compared with controls using lung function tests before and after methacholine challenge.[93]

Dyspnea is a frequent presenting complaint of patients with cocaine-induced toxicity, occurring in 3% to 22% of cases in various series.[3,5,39,40] Hemoptysis, bronchitis, and expectoration of carbonaceous sputum are frequent complaints of cocaine users in the ED. An increased incidence of pulmonary hypertension, pulmonary infarction, pulmonary hemorrhage, and pulmonary foreign body granulomas have been reported in cocaine users.[3,89] Bronchiolitis obliterans and organizing pneumonia (BOOP) associated with fever and dyspnea may also occur.[88,89,94] Loss of a functional alveolocapillary interface as measured by a reduction in carbon monoxide diffusion capacity has been observed in studies of frequent cocaine users.[88] The interpretation of this finding is complicated by other pulmonary exposures to tobacco and marijuana in the population studied. Other studies have suggested that the reduction can be attributed to tobacco use alone.[95]

A specific syndrome known as "crack lung" is a hypersensitivity pneumonitis associated with the smoking of cocaine; it is characterized by fever, chest pain, dyspnea, wheezing, hemoptysis, productive cough, and diffuse interstitial and alveolar infiltrates.[3,89,96] Clinically inapparent alveolar hemorrhage has been demonstrated to occur frequently in crack cocaine users.[97] Again, whether these manifestations of pulmonary toxicities are related to cocaine exposure itself, to the inhalation of superheated adulterants, or to exposure to combustion products is unknown.

Hyperthermia

The majority of cocaine deaths are associated with drug-induced hyperthermia.[98-100] Cocaine may produce hyperthermia from increased heat production (e.g., psychomotor agitation, neuromuscular hyperactivity, seizures), impaired heat dissipation (e.g., cutaneous vasoconstriction), and altered thermoregulation (e.g., hypothalamic dysfunction). Although psychomotor

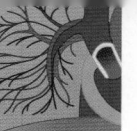

agitation and seizures are the principal etiologies of hyperthermia, temperature elevations from cocaine have been reported in their absence.[59,60,101,102] Altered thermoregulation may be the result of an altered core temperature set point from D_2-dopamine or 5-HT$_2$-serotonin receptor agonism effects in the hypothalamus.[60,102] In general, the duration and severity of hyperthermia from drug-associated heatstroke are correlated closely with mortality.[98] Patient dehydration and high ambient temperature will increase the lethal effects of cocaine and other drugs. Interestingly, in one study, it was shown that mortality from cocaine in New York City increased at higher ambient temperatures.[103] Like exertional heatstroke, hyperthermia from cocaine toxicity may precipitate a cascade of complications that includes agitated delirium, coma, seizures, cerebral edema, rhabdomyolysis, acute renal failure, hepatocellular necrosis, disseminated intravascular coagulation, metabolic acidosis, and cardiovascular collapse.[98,101,102,104] Rectal temperatures as high as 45.6° C (104° F to 114.1° F) have been reported.[102]

Rhabdomyolysis and Renal Failure

Similar to the vascular beds of other organ systems, cocaine produces vasoconstriction as well as thrombosis of both large and small skeletal muscle and renal vessels; ischemia and cell death may ensue with the amount of tissue injury dependent on the size of the occluded vessel.[3,105] Cocaine-associated rhabdomyolysis may result from ischemia, seizures, and trauma.[101,104] Approximately one third of patients with cocaine-associated rhabdomyolysis develop acute renal failure.[101] Renal failure usually occurs from acute tubular necrosis, either from direct cocaine-induced renal cortical vasoconstriction or from rhabdomyolysis with myoglobinuria and renal tubular obstruction. The presence of profound hypotension, hyperpyrexia, and marked elevations of serum creatine kinase levels at admission are useful for predicting renal failure.[101] Cocaine-induced rhabdomyolysis is often associated with seizures, coma, hypotension, arrhythmia, or cardiac arrest. In one series, six of seven patients who developed cocaine-induced rhabdomyolysis, disseminated intravascular coagulation, and renal failure died.[101] The systemic release of tissue thromboplastin from local ischemic injury may partly precipitate disseminated intravascular coagulation.[3,101] Chest wall, skeletal muscle rhabdomyolysis is felt to account for the majority of cocaine-associated chest pain and is often mistaken for myocardial ischemia.[3,14,41]

Head and Neck

Although rarely life-threatening, head and neck complications of cocaine toxicity are not uncommon. An ophthalmologic condition called "crack eye" has been described; it is characterized by pain, photophobia, lacrimation, chemosis, and hyperemia in association with corneal epithelial defects. In addition, microbial keratitis may complicate the syndrome of crack eye, leading to potential long-term corneal alterations.[106] Central retinal artery occlusion and blindness have been associated with cocaine use.[107]

Chronic sinusitis as a result of cocaine abuse, including osteolytic sinusitis and secondary bilateral optic nerve involvement, has been described.[108] Midline granulomas and loss of olfaction have also been reported with cocaine use. Acute epiglottitis has followed crack cocaine inhalation. It is not known whether epiglottitis is a direct effect of cocaine or is induced by the inhalation of hot gases. Cocaine-induced dental erosions and gingival necrosis have been reported.[109] A perforated nasal septum is commonly noted with chronic nasal inhalation of cocaine. At least one case of the pulmonary aspiration of a fragment of nasal septum has been described.[88]

Gastrointestinal

Gastrointestinal (GI) tract ischemic injury may occur when cocaine is used by all routes of administration.[3] The fear of GI tract injury is heightened when "body stuffers" (people who ingest a relatively small amount of loosely wrapped drugs to avoid arrest) or "body packers" or "mules" (people who ingest large amounts of well-wrapped drugs to smuggle them across borders) ingest the drug. Cocaine ingestion has been associated with bowel obstruction, ischemia, necrosis, and perforation.[110-112] Although it commonly occurs in the small bowel, obstruction and perforation may occur in the esophagus.[113] Ischemia and perforation occur in the small or large bowel and are usually focal and segmental.[3] Patients with cocaine-induced bowel ischemia will often manifest constant pain in the midabdomen and may have associated low-grade fever and leukocytosis.[3,114] Symptomatic body stuffers or body packers may present with a seizure, vomiting, abdominal pain, an adrenergic crisis, or cardiac arrest.[115,116] Acute pyloric and GI perforations have been reported after prolonged crack cocaine smoking.[111] The intense vasoconstriction from stimulation of α-adrenergic receptors in the mesenteric vasculature is believed to contribute to focal tissue ischemia and perforation. Thermal injury of the esophagus has been reported after smoking free-base cocaine.[112] Nontraumatic splenic infarction, hemorrhage, and hematomas have been reported from cocaine use.[3,117]

Pregnancy

Significant alteration in menstrual cycle function, including amenorrhea and infertility, have been noted with cocaine abuse.[118] If the female cocaine user becomes pregnant, increased risk for placental abruption exists.[119] Cocaine causes uterine contractions, decreased uterine blood flow, and constriction of placental blood flow.[3,120] As a result, premature rupture of membranes, spontaneous abortion, pregnancy-induced hypertension, intrauterine growth retardation, precipitous delivery, and fetal death have been associated with cocaine use.[119] A meta-analysis suggests that increased congenital malformations of the limbs, the GI tract, and the cardiovascular and neurologic systems occur in children of cocaine users.[121] Congenital urinary tract anomalies

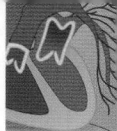

and bilateral cleft lip may be associated with maternal cocaine use.[119,121,122] Abnormal ventilatory patterns and increased incidence of sudden infant death syndrome have been reported with maternal cocaine use.[123,124]

Other neurobehavioral abnormalities in the neonate, including tremulousness and an increased startle reflex ("crack baby" behavior), have been noted after maternal cocaine use.[119,124] Infants born to women who were heavy cocaine users during pregnancy demonstrate altered "executive" functioning at 9.5 to 12.5 months of age.[124] Brain dopamine and serotonin concentrations and pathways are abnormal at birth in rats that have significant prenatal exposure to cocaine. These neurotransmitter concentrations return to normal as the rat ages.[125] The duration and long-term implications of these neurobehavioral abnormalities are unknown. Both cocaine and cocaethylene are found in breast milk and may be transferred to breast-fed infants.[126]

Urologic Effects

Several cases of impotence and priapism from acute cocaine use have been reported. Intranasal, intraurethral, and topical application (to the glans penis) of cocaine have all been reported to cause priapism.[127] The risk for priapism is greater when cocaine is used in combination with trazodone.[128]

Hepatic

Oxidative processes centered around the tropane nitrogen are responsible for about 10% of cocaine metabolism, using the cytochrome P-450 enzyme system within the liver.[30,129] This minor pathway appears to be responsible for hepatic toxicity. It produces norcocaine, norcocaine nitroxide, hydrogen peroxide, and superoxide radicals.[129,130] These products are thought to reduce hepatocyte nicotinamide-adenine dinucleotide phosphate (NADPH) and glutathione levels.[129]

The formation of lipid peroxidation and the resultant superoxide or hydroxyl radical injury are believed to lead to the intrinsic hepatotoxicity seen with cocaine abuse.[129] A case of fulminant liver failure that recovered after snorting large doses of cocaine has been reported with centrilobular necrosis.[131] Agents that deplete NADPH and intracellular glutathione (e.g., acetaminophen) can enhance the risk for cocaine hepatotoxicity. Human cocaine hepatotoxicity is seen most frequently as necrosis in zone 3 of the liver that corresponds to the cytochrome P-450 distribution.[129,130] Although many case reports of cocaine-induced hepatotoxicity exist and hepatocyte tissue cultures confirm intrinsic toxicity, the clinical incidence of cocaine hepatotoxicity is unknown, but is probably low. The explanation for the low frequency of hepatitis secondary to cocaine toxicity is as yet unknown, and the determination of its exact incidence is complicated by the high prevalence of viral and alcohol-induced liver disease in this patient population. Most instances of toxic hepatitis (manifested as hepatic transaminitis) attributed to cocaine will occur in the setting of fulminant hyperthermia and multiorgan dysfunction.

Hematologic

The association of disseminated intravascular coagulation, rhabdomyolysis, and renal failure has been discussed.[101] Severe destructive thrombocytopenia unrelated to retroviral infection has been reported in a small series of both intravenous and inhalation cocaine users.[132] Cocaine-associated thrombocytopenia has been described and has a clinical course similar to that of immunopathic thrombocytopenic purpura. In one series, five of six patients with thrombocytopenia responded favorably to corticosteroids. The sixth patient had a partial response to corticosteroids and a complete response to splenectomy.[132] Whether this thrombocytopenia reflects a direct or an indirect immunologic stimulus from cocaine or a contaminant is not known. In addition, increased platelet aggregation is believed to contribute to thrombocytopenia in some cocaine users.

In a study of 19 patients presenting to an ED with acute cocaine use, hemoglobin and hematocrit levels were significantly elevated, but no evidence of erythrocytosis was seen. Male patients presenting with chest pain were more likely than females to demonstrate these effects.[133]

Endocrine

Thyroid function tests are not significantly different from normal values in heavy users of cocaine. Hyperprolactinemia with resultant galactorrhea has been described in chronic cocaine abusers. Higher peak and trough levels of prolactin-releasing factor have also been reported in male cocaine users with hyperprolactinemia.[118] In one study, prolactin levels remained elevated for 4 weeks in men and women during hospitalization for cocaine withdrawal.[69] The persistent elevation of prolactin was attributed to cocaine-induced derangement in the dopaminergic neural regulatory systems. In this same study, levels of plasma luteinizing hormone, testosterone, and cortisol were found to be within the normal range. Chronic cocaine use also alters plasma growth hormone levels, dexamethasone suppression of cortisol, and thyroid-stimulating hormone response to thyroid-releasing hormone.[134] Many of these neuroendocrine abnormalities are augmented when cocaine abuse is combined with ethyl alcohol.[135] The clinical importance of these findings is unclear, but they may account for the impotence and gynecomastia reported in men who chronically abuse cocaine.

DIAGNOSIS

The diagnosis of cocaine toxicity is based on a suggestive history, physical findings consistent with the known toxicity of cocaine (e.g., sympathomimetic effects), and laboratory testing that confirms the presence of cocaine. The physical examination may need to include a thorough cavity search (e.g., vaginal and rectal examinations) when body packing or body stuffing is suspected.

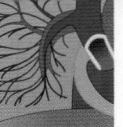
Laboratory Testing

If the history of use is clear and symptoms or signs of intoxication are mild, laboratory testing is often unnecessary. If patients have moderate to severe toxic effects, routine laboratory investigations should include a complete blood count; measurements of electrolytes, blood urea nitrogen, creatinine, glucose, creatine phosphokinase (CPK), or troponin T or I; and a urinalysis. The diagnosis of acute MI in the setting of cocaine-associated chest pain is most accurately made with serial measurements of troponin T or I.[41] Troponin measurements are more specific than CPK-MB measurements; the latter can be falsely elevated with concomitant cocaine-associated rhabdomyolysis.[14,41,136] Patients with agitated delirium, seizures, hyperthermia, or severe rhabdomyolysis should have liver function tests, calcium, phosphate, and coagulation (e.g., prothrombin time, international normalized ratio, disseminated intravascular coagulation [DIC] screen) parameters measured. Arterial blood gas analysis and lactate concentrations may be helpful for patients with significant toxicity.

Analysis of both blood and urine for cocaine and its metabolites can be readily and routinely performed at most hospitals. Testing of saliva, hair, meconium, gastric aspirates, and breast milk can also be performed, if necessary. An enzyme-linked immunoassay directed against benzoylecgonine is useful for the rapid, qualitative screening of samples for cocaine and its metabolites. This method usually detects benzoylecgonine in body fluids at or above a concentration of 300 ng/mL.[30] False-positive results are rare. Other screening tests include thin-layer and high-pressure liquid chromatography. Gas chromatography followed by mass spectrometry (GC-MS) of urine or blood represents one of the most sensitive and specific assays available for identifying cocaine and its metabolites and can be used to confirm the presence of cocaine in a body fluid specimen. Quantification of cocaine and its major metabolites in saliva using GC-MS have been reported.[137] Typically, cocaine metabolites will be detected in the urine for 48 to 72 hours after cocaine use. Rarely, heavy use may allow metabolite detection for up to 22 days.[138,139] Quantification of cocaine and its metabolites from body fluids is generally not recommended because no correlation has been found between cocaine or metabolite levels and the severity of clinical effects and mortality.[85,140] Cocaine concentrations in tissues of patients who die from cocaine intoxication vary greatly, depending on the dose, route of administration, period of survival, and manner of storage of specimens prior to analysis.[30]

Other Laboratory Testing

A chest radiograph and ECG should be performed on all patients with chest pain, cardiopulmonary complaints, or moderate to severe toxicity from cocaine. Arrhythmias, conduction disturbances, and repolarization abnormalities (e.g., prolonged QRS and QTc intervals) can be readily identified on the ECG. The ability to detect acute MI on the ECG, however, is significantly more limited.

The ECG is abnormal in 56% to 84% of patients with cocaine-associated chest pain, yet its sensitivity and positive predictive value for detecting acute MI are only 36% and 18%, respectively.[41,43,141,142] Up to 43% of patients with cocaine-associated chest pain that are determined subsequently not to have an MI meet ECG criteria for thrombolytic therapy.[41,43,141]

A normal ECG has greater diagnostic utility for those with cocaine-associated chest pain. The specificity and negative predictive value of the ECG for ruling out acute MI are 90% and 96%, respectively.[141] A normal ECG in a patient with cocaine-associated chest pain, however, cannot be used to rule out MI.[43]

Chest radiography is used to facilitate diagnosis of pneumothorax, pneumopericardium, pneumomediastinum, pneumonia, "crack lung," pulmonary edema, or pulmonary hemorrhage or infarct. Abdominal plain films may be useful as a screening tool to detect the presence of foreign bodies in a suspected body packer. Plain abdominal radiography has a sensitivity of 85% to 90%.[115,143] In contrast, plain abdominal radiography is not useful or recommended to detect the presence of drug packets in a "body stuffer."[144] Contrast-enhanced computed tomography (CT) or barium-enhanced radiography are recommended when plain radiography is negative and clinical suspicion for ingested or retained packets is high.[115] The incidence of false-positive and -negative results with contrast-enhanced radiography has been reported to be 4%.[145] Head CT imaging should be performed for patients with recurrent seizures, headache, or altered mental status associated with cocaine to rule out intracerebral hemorrhage. Lumbar puncture may be necessary to rule out subarachnoid hemorrhage. Chest and abdominal CT imaging with oral and intravenous contrast may be necessary for patients with significant chest, back, and abdominal pain to evaluate for the presence of a vascular catastrophe (e.g., aortic dissection) or pulmonary, renal, or GI tract hemorrhage, ischemia, or infarct.

Differential Diagnosis

Cocaine may produce effects similar to those of other toxicants, such as sympathomimetic drugs (e.g., amphetamines, methylxanthines, nicotine, ephedrine, β- and α-adrenergic agonists, monoamine oxidase inhibitors), central hallucinogens (e.g., tryptamine derivatives, phencyclidine, lysergic acid diethylamide, hallucinogenic amphetamines), drug withdrawal states (e.g., alcohol and sedative-hypnotic withdrawal), metabolic poisons (e.g., salicylates, dinitrophenol), psychotropics (e.g., cyclic antidepressants, lithium, antipsychotics, amantadine), membrane-active drugs (e.g., local anesthetics and antiarrhythmics), and certain drug-associated syndromes (e.g., malignant hyperthermia, serotonin syndrome, and neuroleptic malignant syndrome). Certain medical emergencies may present in a similar manner, such as endocrinologic disorders (e.g., pheochromocytoma, thyrotoxicosis, hypoglycemia), infections (e.g., meningoencephalitis, sepsis, tetanus), neuropsychiatric disorders (e.g., paranoid schizophrenia, bipolar disorder, intra-

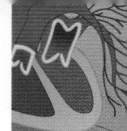

cerebral hemorrhage, head trauma, status epilepticus), and environmental disorders (e.g., exertional and non-exertional heatstroke).

MANAGEMENT

Table 42-2 outlines an algorithm for the general approach to patients with suspected cocaine toxicity. Prospective human studies evaluating different treatment options for such patients are lacking. Thus, recommendations are based on the findings from animal studies and small series of human poisonings with cocaine. The initial management strategy is to institute airway, breathing, and circulatory support as necessary. Supplemental oxygen, vascular access, and continuous cardiac and respiratory monitoring should be provided rapidly. All patients with altered mental status and seizures should have their serum glucose checked or be given dextrose infusion for possible neuroglycopenia. A critical component to successful management is to obtain a core (i.e., rectal) temperature early and treat hyperthermia promptly. Aggressive control of seizures and psychomotor agitation are equally important, particularly since these manifestations often precipitate cocaine-associated hyperthermia. After initial supportive care has been provided, subsequent treatment will depend on the signs, symptoms, and organ system(s) affected. Early GI decontamination should be strongly considered for patients who have ingested cocaine. Activated charcoal with or without a cathartic is administered (1 g/kg body weight) initially; other GI decontamination modalities (e.g., whole bowel irrigation) are also recommended for body stuffers and packers.[115,146] Specific measures for each complication are discussed below. Even patients with cocaine-induced brain death have been successfully stabilized so that organs can be harvested for transplantation.[147]

Given the relatively large volume of distribution and short elimination half-life, enhanced elimination techniques (e.g., urine acidification, hemodialysis) are unlikely to improve the clearance of cocaine and are also not necessary. These approaches have not been formally studied in humans. No specific antidotes exist. However, efforts to develop immunologic ways to bind or neutralize cocaine with antibodies, FAB fragments, vaccines, and specific dopamine receptor antagonists are ongoing and would have potential utility in treating both acute toxicity and drug addiction.[148,149]

Cardiovascular Toxicity

As a result of the relatively short half-life of cocaine and its metabolites, supportive care with minimal pharmacologic intervention is usually adequate for most patients with acute cocaine-related cardiovascular toxicity.

Hypertension and sinus tachycardia usually respond to sedation alone. Nonspecific sympatholysis with benzodiazepines is recommended as first-line treatment.[14,41,150-152] When hypertension and tachycardia do not respond to sedation and are associated with end-organ dysfunction

(e.g., myocardial ischemia, confusion, headache, congestive heart failure), treatment with nitroprusside, calcium channel blockers (e.g., verapamil), or nonselective α-adrenergic agents (e.g., phentolamine) are recommended.[14,41,48,151,152] The use of a β-adrenergic antagonist therapy alone is generally contraindicated for treatment of cocaine toxicity. These agents may result in unopposed α-adrenergic stimulation and worsened end-organ toxicity (e.g., increased coronary vasospasm, worsening hypertension).[14,41,49,151,152]

Patients with cocaine toxicity may present with palpitations and supraventricular tachycardia. Treatment of the patient with no evidence of coronary artery disease includes observation, sedation with benzodiazepines, and the occasional judicious use of calcium channel blockers (e.g., verapamil or diltiazem) for heart rate control.[153] Adenosine may be used but its efficacy is questionable due the transient nature of its effects as compared with the sympathomimetic effects of cocaine. Synchronized cardioversion may be necessary for unstable patients with arrhythmias. The use of β-adrenergic antagonists is contraindicated in these patients for the reasons stated above. Although the data are controversial, the use of labetalol is usually not recommended since it is largely a β-adrenergic antagonist (β- to α-effect of 6 to 1).[14,41,151,152,154,155]

Ventricular arrhythmias are best treated with lidocaine, sodium bicarbonate, and nonspecific sedation with benzodiazepines.[14,41,151,152] The correction of hypoxia and metabolic and electrolyte abnormalities are critically important. Sodium bicarbonate (1-2 mEq/kg intravenous boluses) administration is recommended as a first-line treatment for ventricular or wide-complex arrhythmias immediately after cocaine use, when the fast sodium-channel (type I) blocking effects of cocaine are most likely to be operative.[14,41,151,152] Sodium bicarbonate has been shown to reverse cocaine-induced QRS complex prolongation in animal studies and human case reports.[71,156,157] Lidocaine is recommended as first-line treatment when ventricular arrhythmias are attributed to cocaine-induced myocardial ischemia.[14,41,151,157,158] Although lidocaine itself is a fast-sodium channel blocker, lidocaine competitively antagonizes the sodium channel-blocking activity of cocaine.[157] Unlike cocaine, which has slow on-off sodium channel-binding kinetics, lidocaine has rapid on-off binding kinetics at the sodium channel.[157] Lidocaine does not prolong action potential duration or the QRS interval, and its presence could partly reverse the prolongation that occurs in the presence of toxic concentrations of cocaine. Based on most animal and human clinical data, lidocaine is likely safe and effective for use in cocaine poisoning.[157,158]

Intravascular volume replacement, diuretics, cardiotonic and inotropic agents, and careful vasopressor support have all been utilized in cocaine-induced cardiomyopathy with congestive heart failure.[14] Monitoring of central venous or pulmonary artery wedge pressure may be necessary for titration of these agents. Short-term use of intra-aortic balloon pumps also has been reported to augment cardiac function during transient myocardial dysfunction. General supportive care is important in

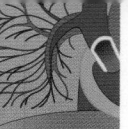
TABLE 42-2 Cocaine Toxicity and Treatment Decision Algorithm

SUSPECTED COCAINE TOXICITY

MILD COCAINE TOXICITY	SEVERE COCAINE TOXICITY	EVALUATE FOR OTHER AGENTS

Psychologic support
Decontamination of oral ingestions/
   administration of activated charcoal
Observe
	Immediate Supportive Care
	Airway control
	Oxygenation
	Vascular access
		Initiate specific treatment for
		   additional agents
		Consider interactions with cocaine
		Monitor for early and late
		   toxicities of other agents

Decontaminate/Antagonists

In oral exposures, administer
  activated charcoal
Consider whole-bowel lavage
  with polyethylene glycol
  solutions for "body packers"
Consider empiric dextrose, thiamine,
  and naloxone
Avoid using benzodiazepine
  antagonists (e.g., flumazenil)

Terminate Seizures

Benzodiazepines (e.g., diazepam,
  lorazepam)
Barbiturates (e.g., pentobarbital,
  phenobarbital)

Correct Immediate Metabolic,
Oxygenation, and Electrolyte
Abnormalities

Correct Local Tissue Ischemia,
Improve Perfusion

Local α-Adrenergic Blockers for
Cocaine (e.g., phenoxybenzamine,
phentolamine)

Treat Hyperthermia

Second-Level Evaluations to Check
for Persistent Abnormalities

PERSISTENT HYPOTENSION	CNS ABNORMALITIES	SUPPORTIVE CARE

Intravascular volume resuscitation
Acute cardiopulmonary support
Central hemodynamic monitoring
	Seizures
	Strokes
	Bleeds
	Terminate seizures
		Psychologic and pharmacologic
		  support for cocaine abstinence
		  and long-term recovery

VENTRICULAR ARRHYTHMIA Antiarrhythmics (e.g., lidocaine) Electrolyte correction Acid-base correction	**PULMONARY EDEMA/RESPIRATORY** **FAILURE** Ventilator Oxygen PEEP	

RENAL FAILURE
Hemodialysis
Intravascular volume
HYPERTENSION
Sedation (e.g., diazepam)
Calcium channel blockers
  (e.g., nifedipine, nicardipine)
Nitroprusside
CORONARY ARTERY ISCHEMIA
Antiplatelet agents (e.g., aspirin)
Calcium channel blockers (e.g., nifedipine,
  diltiazem, nicardipine)
α-Adrenergic blockers (e.g., phentolamine)
	Electrolyte Abnormalities
	Correct hypokalemia (e.g.,
	  potassium chloride)
	Correct hypocalcemia
	  (e.g., calcium gluconate)
	RHABDOMYOLYSIS
	Alkalinize urine (e.g., IV bicarbonate)
	Calcium replacement (e.g., calcium
	  gluconate)
	Intravascular volume	

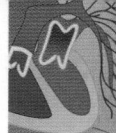

TABLE 42-2 Cocaine Toxicity and Treatment Decision Algorithm (*Con't*)		
SUSPECTED COCAINE TOXICITY		
▼	▼	▼
MILD COCAINE TOXICITY	**SEVERE COCAINE TOXICITY**	**EVALUATE FOR OTHER AGENTS**
▼		
β-Adrenergic blockers (e.g., esmolol, metoprolol) may be contraindicated (see text) Nitrates (e.g., nitroglycerin) Sedation (e.g., diazepam)		

CNS, central nervous system; PEEP, positive end-expiratory pressure; IV, intravenous.

maintaining cardiovascular function during cocaine-induced cardiac toxicities. Discontinuation of cocaine use appears to be the most prudent way of reversing or limiting the progression of cocaine-induced chronic cardiomyopathy.

Myocardial Ischemia

Recommendations are based on two recent reviews of cocaine-induced myocardial ischemia and the recently revised consensus guidelines on emergency cardiovascular care from the American Heart Association in collaboration with the International Liaison Committee on Resuscitation.[14,41,151,152] Patients with suspected cocaine-induced myocardial ischemia or MI should be treated initially with oxygen, parenteral benzodiazepines, aspirin, and nitrates. Both benzodiazepines and nitroglycerin have been shown to improve hemodynamics (reduce rate-pressure product) and resolve chest pain in patients with cocaine-associated chest pain and suspected myocardial ischemia.[41,150,159] As previously noted, use of β-adrenergic antagonists is contraindicated because they may result in unopposed α-adrenergic effects and exacerbate coronary vasoconstriction associated with cocaine.[14,41,49,151,152,154] The specific use of labetalol, although not recommended, cannot be considered an absolute contraindication based on the scientific data available to date.[151,152] In humans undergoing cardiac catheterization and given intranasal cocaine, labetalol reversed cocaine-induced increases in mean arterial pressure but had no effect on cocaine-induced vasoconstriction of coronary arteries.[155] The use of calcium channel blockers (specifically, verapamil), the α-blocker phentolamine, and heparin therapy are considered second-line therapies for cocaine-induced coronary ischemia.[41,151-153] Both verapamil and phentolamine have been shown to reverse coronary artery vasoconstriction in human volunteers given intranasal cocaine immediately prior to cardiac catheterization.[48,153]

If medical management does not eliminate cocaine-induced myocardial ischemia, primary percutaneous intervention (diagnostic and therapeutic cardiac catheterization) is recommended over rapid reperfusion with thrombolytic therapy.[14,41] The increased risk for cerebrovascular hemorrhage with cocaine-induced toxicity requires that the use of thrombolytics in this patient population be carried out with extreme care.[14,41] Thrombolytic therapy has not been proven safe or effective in patients with cocaine-associated MI.[160] In addition, it is usually difficult to base treatment decisions in this patient population on ECG criteria for an MI, which are both insensitive and nonspecific. In general, the mortality of cocaine-induced MI patients that make it to the hospital alive is less than 2%.[14,41] The morbidity and mortality are likely to be increased with the use of thrombolytic therapy. Major intracerebral hemorrhage has been reported in more than 5% of published cases of cocaine-induced MI treated with thrombolytic therapy. Thrombolysis should only be considered when the diagnosis of cocaine-induced MI is firm and cardiac catheterization is not available. As mentioned, the use of lidocaine is recommended for ventricular arrhythmias felt secondary to myocardial ischemia. In review of the use of lidocaine in 29 patients with cocaine-associated MIs, no enhanced cocaine toxicity was seen.[158]

Central Nervous System Toxicity

Sedation with benzodiazepines (e.g., diazepam) is the first-line treatment for CNS agitation associated with cocaine; large doses may be necessary.[99,100,161] Although controversial, the adjunctive use of neuroleptics (e.g., droperidol, haloperidol, or ziprasidone) may be effective for the control CNS agitation produced by cocaine.

Successful treatment of cocaine-induced hyperthermia requires early recognition, rapid cooling, and aggressive supportive care.[98-100,102] Cooling methods include rehydration with cooled intravenous fluids; cool water mist and fans (evaporative and convective cooling); ice packs; ice water baths; and ice water, gastric, peritoneal, rectal, or bladder lavage. Since cocaine-induced hyperthermia is predominantly secondary to increased muscle activity, prompt peripheral muscle relaxation is essential to minimize morbidity and mortality. Sedation with benzodiazepines may be tried initially for mild cases of hyperthermia. Nondepolarizing neuromuscular paralysis (e.g., pancuronium), however, which provides rapid, predictable, and effective termination of motor hyperactivity, should be instituted for severe or refractory hyperthermia.[98,100,102] When canines given intravenous

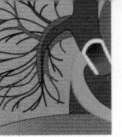

lethal doses of cocaine are ventilated and pretreated with pancuronium, hyperthermia, metabolic acidosis, and mortality can be prevented.[99]

Seizures associated with cocaine are generally best treated with benzodiazepines (e.g., lorazepam) followed by barbiturates (e.g., phenobarbital, pentobarbital), if necessary. The efficacy and safety of phenytoin has not been established. Animal studies suggest that other antiepileptics (e.g., felbamate and gabapentin) may also be effective for cocaine-induced seizures.[162]

Treatment for other neurologic complications of cocaine abuse is supportive. Subarachnoid hemorrhage and intracerebral bleeding may be associated with an underlying cerebral saccular aneurysm or vascular malformation and may require neurosurgical intervention. Transient ischemic attacks and ischemic cerebrovascular accidents are treated symptomatically and may require empiric therapy with aspirin and heparin. The use of thrombolytic therapy for acute ischemic strokes associated with cocaine has not been studied and is theoretically dangerous. Migraine-like headaches produced by cocaine have been reported to improve with ergotamine treatment. However, there is theoretical concern about the use of another vasospastic agent such as ergotamine in view of the vasospastic side effects of cocaine itself. The use of serotonergic agonists (e.g., triptans) for cocaine-induced migraine headaches has not been reported.

Pulmonary Complications

The management of pulmonary complications associated with cocaine use is supportive.[89] Supplemental oxygen, bronchodilator therapy, steroids, and mechanical support may be necessary for cocaine-induced bronchospasm. Oxygen, diuretics, and intubation with or without positive end-expiratory pressure (PEEP) have been used successfully and may be necessary for patients with cocaine-induced pulmonary edema.[89] In addition to PEEP, the lengthening of inspiratory time intervals can also to increase the functional residual capacity and may also enhance oxygenation. Empiric treatment with corticosteroids for BOOP and eosinophilic pulmonary syndromes is recommended, but efficacy has been variable.[88,89] Patients with pneumomediastinum or pneumopericardium should be admitted and observed for the subsequent development of a pneumothorax.[89] Chest tube placement is necessary for patients with large pneumothoraces or those who do not resolve or worsen with high-flow oxygen. It is important to inform patients that barotraumatic complications may recur with repeated use of crack cocaine.[89]

Rhabdomyolysis and Renal Failure

Treatment of cocaine-induced rhabdomyolysis and renal failure is supportive. Aggressive rehydration is recommended to correct hypovolemia and prevent myoglobin precipitation in the renal tubules. Isotonic normal saline is recommended initially to establish and maintain a urine flow of at least 2 mL/kg/hr. Careful monitoring of electrolytes (e.g., phosphate, calcium, potassium) is necessary. Although not proven effective, most experts recommend the administration of bicarbonate-rich fluids to alkalinize the urine (urine pH > 7) and prevent myoglobin precipitation in the renal tubules. Hemodialysis may be necessary for acute renal failure.

Body Stuffers and Packers

Whole bowel irrigation, endoscopy, surgery, cathartics, and repeat doses of activated charcoal have been used to treat patients who have ingested packets of cocaine.[115,143,145,146,163-165] In a series of 34 body stuffers in Chicago, 74% remained asymptomatic, 18% had mild symptoms, 4% had moderate symptoms, and 4% had severe symptoms leading to death. Abdominal radiography, decontamination, and benzodiazepines appeared to be useful.[166] In another series of patients, approximately 3% of patients that ingested cocaine packets required surgical removal for obstruction or toxic effects.[167]

Asymptomatic body packers and stuffers may be treated conservatively with simple observation in an ICU until spontaneous passage of the packets has occurred.[115,116,167] Alternatively, GI tract decontamination with activated charcoal (to bind any cocaine that may leak out of the packets) coupled with whole bowel irrigation may be performed to enhance passage of the packets (see Chapter 2B). Whole bowel irrigation should be continued until complete clearance of the drug packets has occurred from the GI tract. Abdominal imaging with contrast and the passage of several packet-free stools is used to confirm passage of all cocaine packets.[115,145] Symptomatic body stuffers should be treated similarly to other symptomatic cocaine-intoxicated patients. In addition, GI tract decontamination with activated charcoal is important for these patients to limit further cocaine absorption.[115,146] Symptomatic body packers, either from mechanical bowel obstruction or perforation or from cocaine poisoning, require immediate surgical removal of drug packets.[115,116] Although endoscopy has been used to remove cocaine packets from the stomach or proximal small bowel, operative removal is still recommended due to the risk for packet rupture during endoscopic removal.[115]

DISPOSITION

The level (intensive care or floor) and duration of medical care are dependent on the severity and duration of toxicity. If signs and symptoms of toxicity are mild to moderate and resolve after a 4- to 6-hour observation period in the ED, patients may be medically discharged. Patients with altered mental status, persistent abnormal vital signs, nonsinus rhythms, or significant end-organ toxicity (e.g., rhabdomyolysis) should be admitted for further care and observation. Patients with cocaine-associated chest pain who are not at high risk for acute coronary syndrome may be admitted to a 9- to 12-hour chest pain observation unit.[45] These patients may

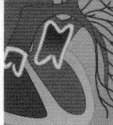

subsequently be discharged with close follow-up if they "rule out" for MI by troponin testing and cardiovascular complications do not occur during their 12-hour observation.[45] Body packers and stuffers usually require ICU admission for observation and treatment.[115] After clinical toxicity has resolved, referral for psychiatric follow-up care may be needed, as may serologic testing for viral hepatitis and human immunodeficiency virus. Evaluation for complications attendant to intravenous drug abuse (e.g., endocarditis, sexually transmitted diseases, etc.) should also be considered.[168]

REFERENCES

1. Substance Abuse and Mental Health Services Administration, Office of Applied Studies: Emergency department trends from the Drug Abuse Warning Network: final estimates 1995–2002, DAWN series: D-24. DHHS publication no. (SMA) 03-3780. Rockville, MD, Department of Health and Human Services, 2003.
2. Substance Abuse and Mental Health Services Administration, Office of Applied Studies: Mortality data from the Drug Abuse Warning Network, 2002. DAWN Series D-25, DHHS publication no. (SMA) 04-3875. Rockville, MD, Department of Health and Human Services, 2004.
3. Shanti CM, Lucas CE: Cocaine and the critical care challenge. Crit Care Med 2003;31:1851–1859.
4. Brookoff D, Cook CS, Williams C, et al: Testing reckless drivers for cocaine and marijuana. N Engl J Med 1994;331:518–522.
5. Rich JA, Singer DE: Cocaine-related symptoms in patients presenting to an urban emergency department. Ann Emerg Med 1991;20:616–621.
6. Loiselle JM, Baker MD, Templeton JM Jr, et al: Substance abuse in adolescent trauma. Ann Emerg Med 1993;22:1530–1534.
7. Cregler LL, Mark H: Medical complications of cocaine abuse. N Engl J Med 1986;315:1495–1500.
8. Karch SB: The history of cocaine toxicity. Hum Pathol 1989;20:1037–1039.
9. Warner EA: Cocaine abuse. Ann Intern Med 1993;119:226–235.
10. Garland O: Fatal acute poisoning by cocaine. Lancet 1895;2:1104–1105.
11. Gawin FH, Ellinwood EH Jr: Cocaine and other stimulants. Actions, abuse, and treatment. N Engl J Med 1988;318:1173–1182.
12. Catterall W, Mackie K: Local anesthetics. In Hardman JG, Limbird LE, Gilman AG (eds): Goodman & Gilman's The Pharmacologic Basis of Therapeutics, 10th edition. New York, McGraw-Hill, 2001, pp 367–384, 634–638.
13. Boghdadi MS, Henning RJ: Cocaine: pathophysiology and clinical toxicology. Heart Lung 1997;26:466–481.
14. Lange RA, Hillis LD: Cardiovascular complications of cocaine use. N Engl J Med 2001;345:351–358.
15. Office of Applied Studies: 2002 National Survey on Drug Use & Health, trends in initiation of substance abuse. Accessed April 2004 from http://oas.samhsa.gov/nhsda/2k2nsduh/Results/2k2results.htm#chap6.
16. Marzuk PM, Tardiff K, Leon AC, et al: Fatal injuries after cocaine use as a leading cause of death among young adults in New York City. N Engl J Med 1995;332:1753–1757.
17. Pottieger AE, Tressell PA, Inciardi JA, et al: Cocaine use patterns and overdose. J Psychoactive Drugs 1992;24:399–410.
18. Coffin PO, Galea S, Ahern J, et al: Opiates, cocaine and alcohol combinations in accidental drug overdose deaths in New York City, 1990–98. Addiction 2003;98:739–747.
19. Ochoa KC, Hahn JA, Seal KH, et al: Overdosing among young injection drug users in San Francisco. Addict Behav 2001;26:453–460.
20. Mesquita F, Kral A, Reingold A, et al: Overdoses among cocaine users in Brazil. Addiction 2001;96:1809–1813.
21. Drug Enforcement Agency: Florida: Drug Situation: Cocaine Statistics. Accessed December 2003 from http://www.dea.gov/pubs/states/florida.html.
22. Gay GR, Inaba DS, Sheppard CW, et al: Cocaine: history, epidemiology, human pharmacology, and treatment. Clin Toxicol 1975;8:149–178.
23. Shannon M: Clinical toxicity of cocaine adulterants. Ann Emerg Med 1988;17:1243–1247.
24. Benowitz NL: Clinical pharmacology and toxicology of cocaine. Pharmacol Toxicol 1993;72:3–12.
25. Tella SR, Schindler CW, Goldberg SR: Cocaine: cardiovascular effects in relation to inhibition of peripheral neuronal monoamine uptake and central stimulation of the sympathoadrenal system. J Pharmacol Exp Ther 1993;267:153–162.
26. Leshner AI: Molecular mechanisms of cocaine addiction. N Engl J Med 1996;335:128–129.
27. Reid MS, Hsu K, Berger SP: Cocaine and amphetamine preferentially stimulate glutamate release in the limbic system: studies on the involvement of dopamine. Synapse 1997;27:95–105.
28. Smith JA, Mo Q, Guo H, et al: Cocaine increases extraneuronal levels of aspartate and glutamate in the nucleus accumbens. Brain Res 1995;683:264–269.
29. Perera R, Kraebber A, Schwartz MJ: Prolonged QT interval and cocaine use. J Electrocardiol 1997;30:337–339.
30. Baselt RC: Disposition of Toxic Drugs and Chemicals in Man, 5th ed. Foster City, CA, Chemical Toxicology Institute, 2000, pp 205–210.
31. Spiehler VR, Reed D: Brain concentrations of cocaine and benzoylecgonine in fatal cases. J Forensic Sci 1985;30:1003–1011.
32. Rose JS: Cocaethylene: a current understanding of the active metabolite of cocaine and ethanol. Am J Emerg Med 1994;12:489–490.
33. Henning RJ, Wilson LD, Glauser JM: Cocaine plus ethanol is more cardiotoxic than cocaine or ethanol alone. Crit Care Med 1994;22:1896–1906.
34. Cami J, Farre M, Gonzalez ML, et al: Cocaine metabolism in humans after use of alcohol. Clinical and research implications. Recent Dev Alcohol 1998;14:437–455.
35. Walsh SL, Haberny KA, Bigelow GE: Modulation of intravenous cocaine effects by chronic oral cocaine in humans. Psychopharmacology (Berl) 2000;150:361–373.
36. Knuepfer MM: Cardiovascular disorders associated with cocaine use: myths and truths. Pharmacol Ther 2003;97:181–222.
37. Mouhaffel AH, Madu EC, Satmary WA, et al: Cardiovascular complications of cocaine. Chest 1995;107:1426–1434.
38. Hollander JE, Hoffman RS, Burstein JL, et al: Cocaine-associated myocardial infarction. Mortality and complications. Cocaine-Associated Myocardial Infarction Study Group. Arch Intern Med 1995;155:1081–1086.
39. Derlet RW, Albertson TE: Emergency department presentation of cocaine intoxication. Ann Emerg Med 1989;18:182–186.
40. Brody SL, Slovis CM, Wrenn KD: Cocaine-related medical problems: consecutive series of 233 patients. Am J Med 1990;88:325–331.
41. Hollander JE: The management of cocaine-associated myocardial ischemia. N Engl J Med 1995;333:1267–1272.
42. Osula S, Stockton P, Abdelaziz MM, et al: Intratracheal cocaine induced myocardial infarction: an unusual complication of fibreoptic bronchoscopy. Thorax 2003;58:733–734.
43. Hollander JE, Hoffman RS, Gennis P, et al: Prospective multicenter evaluation of cocaine associated chest pain. Acad Emerg Med 1994;1:330–339.
44. Mittleman MA, Mintzer D, Maclure M, et al: Triggering of myocardial infarction by cocaine. Circulation 1999;99:2737–2741.
45. Weber JE, Shofer FS, Larkin GL, et al: Validation of a brief observation period for patients with cocaine-associated chest pain. N Engl J Med 2003;348:510–517.
46. Kloner RA, Rezkalla SH: Cocaine and the heart. N Engl J Med 2003;348:487–488.
47. Flores ED, Lange TA, Cigarroa RG, Hillis LD: Effect of cocaine on coronary artery dimensions in atherosclerotic coronary artery disease: enhanced vasoconstriction at sites of significant stenoses. J Am Coll Cardiol 1990;16:74–79.
48. Lange RA, Cigarroa RG, Yancy CW Jr, et al: Cocaine-induced coronary-artery vasoconstriction. N Engl J Med 1989;321:1557–1562.
49. Lange RA, Cigarroa RG, Flores ED, et al: Potentiation of cocaine-induced coronary vasoconstriction by beta-adrenergic blockade. Ann Intern Med 1990;112:897–903.
50. Wilbert-Lampen U, Seliger C, Zilker T, Arendt RM: Cocaine increases the endothelial release of immunoreactive endothelin

and its concentrations in human plasma and urine: reversal by coincubation with sigma-receptors antagonists. Circulation 1998;98:385–390.

51. Mo W, Singh AK, Arruda JA, Dunea TG: Role of nitric oxide in cocaine-induced acute hypertension. Am J Hypertens 1998;11:708–714.

52. Weber JE, Hollander JE, Murphy SA, et al: Quantitative comparison of coronary artery flow and myocardial perfusion in patients with acute myocardial infarction in the presence and absence of recent cocaine use. J Thromb Thrombolysis 2002;14:239–245.

53. Rezkalla SH, Mazza JJ, Kloner RA, et al: The effects of cocaine on human platelets in healthy subjects. Am J Cardiol 1993;72:243–246.

54. Togna G, Tempesta E, Togna AR, et al: Platelet responsiveness and biosynthesis of thromboxane and prostacyclin in response to in vitro cocaine treatment. Haemostasis 1985;15:100–107.

55. Stenberg RG, Winniford MD, Hillis LD, et al: Simultaneous acute thrombosis of two major coronary arteries following intravenous cocaine use. Arch Pathol Lab Med 1989;113:521–524.

56. Moliterno DJ, Lange RA, Gerard RD, et al: Influence of intranasal cocaine on plasma constituents associated with endogenous thrombosis and thrombolysis. Am J Med 1994;96:492–496.

57. Kolodgie FD, Wilson PS, Mergner WJ, Virmani R: Cocaine-induced increase in the permeability function of human vascular endothelial cell monolayers. Exp Mol Pathol 1999;66:109–122.

58. Gan X, Zhang L, Berger O, et al: Cocaine enhances brain endothelial adhesion molecules and leukocyte migration. Clin Immunol 1999;91:68–76.

59. Minor RL Jr, Scott BD, Brown DD, Winniford MD: Cocaine-induced myocardial infarction in patients with normal coronary arteries. Ann Intern Med 1991;115:797–806.

60. Hollander JE, Hoffman RS, Burstein JL, et al: Cocaine-associated myocardial infarction: mortality and complications. Arch Intern Med 1995;155:1081–1086.

61. Winniford MD, Wheelan KR, Kremers MS, et al: Smoking-induced coronary vasoconstriction in patients with atherosclerotic coronary artery disease: evidence for adrenergically mediated alterations in coronary artery tone. Circulation 1986;73:662–667.

62. Foltin RW, Fischman MW, Levin FR: Cardiovascular effects of cocaine in humans: laboratory studies. Drug Alcohol Depend 1995;37:193–210.

63. Escobedo LG, Ruttenber AJ, Agocs MM, et al: Emerging patterns of cocaine use and the epidemic of cocaine overdose deaths in Dade Country, Florida. Arch Pathol Lab Med 1991;115:9800–9805.

64. Hearn WL, Flynn DD, Hime GW, et al: Cocaethylene: a unique cocaine metabolite displays high affinity for the dopamine transporter. J Neurochem 1991;56:698–701.

65. Hearn WL, Rose S, Wagner J, et al: Cocaethylene is more potent than cocaine in mediating lethality. Pharmacol Biochem Behav 1991;39:531–533.

66. Wilson LD, French S: Cocaethylene's effects on coronary artery blood flow and cardiac function in a canine model. J Toxicol Clin Toxicol 2002;40:535–546.

67. Karch SB, Green GS, Young S: Myocardial hypertrophy and coronary artery disease in male cocaine users. J Forensic Sci 1995;40:591–595.

68. Bertolet BD, Freund G, Martin CA, Perchalski EL, et al: Unrecognized left ventricular dysfunction in an apparently healthy cocaine abuse population. Clin Cardiol 1990;13:323–328.

69. Tazelaar HD, Karch SB, Stephens BE, Billingham ME: Cocaine and the heart. Hum Pathol 1987;18:195–199.

70. Mehta A, Jain AC, Mehta MC: Electrocardiographic effects of intravenous cocaine: an experimental study in a canine model. J Cardiovasc Pharmacol 2003;41:25–30.

71. Wang RY: pH-dependent cocaine-induced cardiotoxicity. Am J Emerg Med 1999;17:364–369.

72. Perron AD, Gibbs M: Thoracic aortic dissection secondary to crack cocaine ingestion. Am J Emerg Med 1997;15:507–509.

73. Chambers HF, Morris DL, Tauber MG, Modin G: Cocaine use and the risk for endocarditis in intravenous drug users. Ann Intern Med 1987;106:833–836.

74. Spivey WH, Euerle B: Neurologic complications of cocaine abuse. Ann Emerg Med 1990;19:1422–1428.

75. Qureschi AI, Akbar MS, Czander E, et al: Crack cocaine use and stroke in young patients. Neurology 1997;48:341–345.

76. Kaufman MJ, Levin JM, Ross MH, et al: Cocaine-induced cerebral vasoconstriction detected in humans with magnetic resonance angiography. JAMA 1998;279:376–380.

77. Merkel PA, Koroshetz WJ, Irizarry MC, et al: Cocaine-associated cerebral vasculitis. Semin Arthritis Rheum 1995;25:172–183.

78. Ruttenber AJ, Lawler-Heavner J, Yin M, et al: Fatal excited delirium following cocaine use: epidemiologic findings provide new evidence for mechanisms of cocaine toxicity. J Forensic Sci 1997;42:25–31.

79. Olson KR, Kearney TE, Dyer JE, et al: Seizures associated with poisoning and drug overdose. Am J Emerg Med 1993;11:565–568.

80. Lason W: Neurochemical and pharmacological aspects of cocaine-induced seizures. Pol J Pharmacol 2001;53:57–60.

81. Pascual-Leone A, Dhuna A, Altafullah I, et al: Cocaine-induced seizures. Neurology 1990;40:404–407.

82. Dhuna A, Pascual-Leone A, Langendorf F, et al: Epileptogenic properties of cocaine in humans. Neurotoxicology 1991;12:621–626.

83. Jonsson S, O'Meara M, Young JB: Acute cocaine poisoning. Importance of treating seizures and acidosis. Am J Med 1983;75:1061–1064.

84. Kaye BR, Fainstat M: Cerebral vasculitis associated with cocaine abuse. JAMA 1987;258:2104–2106.

85. Daras M, Koppel BS, Atos-Radzion E: Cocaine-induced choreo-athetoid movements ("crack dancing"). Neurology 1994;44:751–752.

86. Kaku DA, Lowenstein DH: Emergence of recreational drug abuse as a major risk factor for stroke in young adults. Ann Intern Med 1990;113:821–827.

87. Lowenstein DH, Massa SM, Rowbotham MC, et al: Acute neurologic and psychiatric complications associated with cocaine abuse. Am J Med 1987;83:841–846.

88. Albertson TE, Walby WF, Derlet RW: Stimulant-induced pulmonary toxicity. Chest 1995;108:1140–1149.

89. Haim DY, Lippmann ML, Goldberg SK, Walkenstein MD: The pulmonary complications of crack cocaine. Chest 1995;107:233–240.

90. Cruz R, Davis M, O'Neil H, et al: Pulmonary manifestations of inhaled street drugs. Heart Lung 1998;27:297–305.

91. Cucco RA, Yoo OH, Gregler L, et al: Non-fatal pulmonary edema after "freebase" cocaine smoking. Am Rev Respir Dis 1987;136:174–181.

92. Lang SA, Maron MD: Hemodynamic basis for cocaine-induced pulmonary edema in dogs. J Appl Physiol 1991;71:1166–1170.

93. Boto de los Bueis A, Pereira Vega A, Sanchez Ramos JL, et al: Bronchial hyperreactivity in patients who inhale heroin mixed with cocaine vaporized on aluminum foil. Chest 2002;121:1223–1230.

94. Patel RC, Dutta D, Schonfeld SA: Free-base cocaine use associated with bronchiolitis obliterans organizing pneumonia. Ann Intern Med 1987;107:186–187.

95. Kleerup EC, Koyal SN, Marques-Magallanes JA, et al: Chronic and acute effects of "crack" cocaine on diffusing capacity, membrane diffusion, and pulmonary capillary blood volume in the lung. Chest 2002;122:629–638.

96. Forrester JM, Steele AW, Waldron JA, et al: Crack lung: an acute pulmonary syndrome with a spectrum of clinical and histopathologic findings. Am Rev Respir Dis 1990;142:462–467.

97. Baldwin GC, Choi R, Roth MD, et al: Evidence of chronic damage to the pulmonary microcirculation in habitual users of alkaloidal ("crack") cocaine. Chest 2002;121:1231–1238.

98. Rosenberg J, Pentel P, Pond S, et al: Hyperthermia associated with drug intoxication. Crit Care Med 1986;14:964–969.

99. Catravas JD, Waters IW: Acute cocaine intoxication in the conscious dog: studies on the mechanism of lethality. J Pharmacol Exp Ther 1981;217:350–356.

100. Guinn MM, Bedford JA, Wilson MC: Antagonism of intravenous cocaine lethality in nonhuman primates. Clin Toxicol 1980;16:499–508.

101. Roth D, Alarcon FJ, Fernandez JA, et al: Acute rhabdomyolysis associated with cocaine intoxication. N Engl J Med 1988;319:673–677.

102. Callaway CW, Clark RF: Hyperthermia in psychostimulant overdose. Ann Emerg Med 1994;24:68–76.

103. Marzuk PM, Tardiff K, Leon AC, et al: Ambient temperature and mortality from unintentional cocaine overdose. JAMA 1998;279: 1795–1800.

104. Merigian KS, Roberts JR: Cocaine intoxication: hyperpyrexia, rhabdomyolysis and acute renal failure. J Toxicol Clin Toxicol 1987;25:135–148.

105. Kramer RK, Turner RC: Renal infarction associated with cocaine use and latent protein C deficiency. South Med J 1993;86: 1436–1438.

106. Strominger MB, Sachs R, Hersh PS: Microbial keratitis with crack cocaine. Arch Ophthalmol 1990;108:1672.

107. Devenyi P, Schneiderman JF, Devenyi RG, Lawby L: Cocaine-induced central retinal artery occlusion. Can Med Assoc J 1988;138:129–130.

108. Newman NM, DiLoreto DA, Ho JT, et al: Bilateral optic neuropathy and osteolytic sinusitis. Complications of cocaine abuse. JAMA 1988;259:72–74.

109. Quart AM, Small CB, Klein RS: The cocaine connection. Users imperil their gingiva. J Am Dent Assoc 1991;122:85–87.

110. Yang RD, Han MW, McCarthy JH: Ischemic colitis in a crack abuser. Dig Dis Sci 1991;36:238–240.

111. Cheng CL, Svesko V: Acute pyloric perforation after prolonged crack smoking. Ann Emerg Med 1994;23:126–128.

112. Lee HS, LaMaute HR, Pizzi WF, et al: Acute gastrointestinal perforations associated with use of crack. Ann Surg 1990;211:15–17.

113. Cohen ME, Kegel JG: Candy cocaine esophagus. Chest 2002;121:1701–1703.

114. Herrine SK, Park PK, Wechsler RJ: Acute mesenteric ischemia following intranasal cocaine use. Dig Dis Sci 1998;43:586–589.

115. Traub SJ, Hoffman RS, Nelson LS: Body packing of illicit drugs. N Engl J Med 2003;349:2519–2526.

116. Caruana DS, Weinbach B, Goerg D, et al.: Cocaine-packet ingestion. Diagnosis, management, and natural history. Ann Intern Med 1984;100:73–74.

117. Homler HJ: Nontraumatic splenic hematoma related to cocaine abuse. West J Med 1995;163:160–161.

118. Mendelson JH, Mello NK, Teoh SK, et al: Cocaine effects on pulsatile secretion of anterior pituitary, gonadal, and adrenal hormones. J Clin Endocrinol Metab 1989;69:1256–1260.

119. Slutsker L: Risks associated with cocaine use during pregnancy. Obstet Gynecol 1992;79:778–789.

120. Hurd WW, Betz AL, Dombrowski MP, et al: Cocaine augments contractility of the pregnant human uterus by both adrenergic and nonadrenergic mechanisms. Am J Obstet Gynecol 1998;178: 1077–1081.

121. Kain ZN, Kain TS, Scarpelli EM: Cocaine exposure in utero: perinatal development and neonatal manifestations—review. J Toxicol Clin Toxicol 1992;30:607–636.

122. Markov D, Jacquemyn Y, Leroy Y: Bilateral cleft lip and palate associated with increased nuchal translucency and maternal cocaine abuse at 14 weeks of gestation. Clin Exp Obstet Gynecol 2003;30:109–110.

123. Durand DJ, Espinoza AM, Nickerson BG: Association between prenatal cocaine exposure and sudden infant death syndrome. J Pediatr 1990;117:909–911.

124. Noland JS, Singer LT, Mehta SK, et al: Prenatal cocaine/polydrug exposure and infant performance on an executive functioning task. Dev Neuropsychol 2003;24:499–517.

125. Keller RW Jr, Snyder-Keller A: Prenatal cocaine exposure. Ann NY Acad Sci 2000;909:217–232.

126. Bailey DN: Cocaine and cocaethylene binding to human milk. Am J Clin Pathol 1998;110:491–494.

127. Fiorelli RL, Manfrey SJ, Belkoff LH, et al: Priapism associated with intranasal cocaine abuse. J Urol 1990;143:584–585.

128. Myrick H, Markowitz JS, Henderson S: Priapism following trazodone overdose with cocaine use. Ann Clin Psychiatry 1998;10:81–83.

129. Kloss MW, Rosen GM, Rauckman EJ: Cocaine-mediated hepatotoxicity. A critical review. Biochem Pharmacol 1984;33:169–173.

130. Wanless IR, Dore S, Gopinath N, et al: Histopathology of cocaine hepatotoxicity. Report of four patients. Gastroenterology 1990;98:497–501.

131. Campos Franco J, Martinez Rey C, Perez Becerra E, et al: [Cocaine related fulminant liver failure.] Ann Med Interna 2002;19: 365–367.

132. Leissinger CA: Severe thrombocytopenia associated with cocaine use. Ann Intern Med 1990;112:708–710.

133. Weber JE, Larkin GL, Boe CT, et al: Effect of cocaine use on bone marrow-mediated erythropoiesis. Acad Emerg Med 2003;10: 705–708.

134. Di Paolo T, Rouillard C, Morissette M, et al: Endocrine and neurochemical actions of cocaine. Can J Physiol Pharmacol 1989;67:1177–1181.

135. Farre M, de la Torre R, Gonzalez ML, et al: Cocaine and alcohol interactions in humans: neuroendocrine effects and cocaethylene metabolism. J Pharmacol Exp Ther 1997;283:164–176.

136. Hollander JE, Levitt MA, Young GP, et al: The effect of cocaine on the specificity of cardiac markers. Am Heart J 1998;135:245–252.

137. Ambre J: The urinary excretion of cocaine and metabolites in humans: a kinetic analysis of published data. J Anal Toxicol 1985;9:241–245.

138. Weiss RD: Protracted elimination of cocaine metabolites in long-term high-dose cocaine abuse. Am J Med 1988;85:879–880.

139. Campora P, Bermejo AM, Tabernero MJ, et al: Quantitation of cocaine and its major metabolites in human saliva using gas chromatography-positive chemical ionization-mass spectrometry (GC-PCI-MS). J Anal Toxicol 2003;27:270–274.

140. Blaho K, Logan B, Winbery S, et al: Blood cocaine and metabolite concentrations, clinical findings, and outcome of patients presenting to an ED. Am J Emerg Med 2000;18:593–598.

141. Gitter MJ, Goldsmith SR, Dunbar DN, Sharkey SW: Cocaine and chest pain: clinical features and outcome of patients hospitalized to rule out myocardial infarction. Ann Intern Med 1991;115: 277–282.

142. Zimmerman JK, Dellinger RP, Majid PA: Cocaine-associated chest pain. Ann Emerg Med 1991;20:611–615.

143. McCarron MM, Wood JD: The cocaine "body-packer" syndrome: diagnosis and treatment. JAMA 1983;250:1417–1420.

144. Hoffman RS, Chiang WK, Weisman RS, et al: Prospective evaluation of "crack-vial" ingestions. Vet Hum Toxicol 1990;32: 164–166.

145. Marc B, Baud FJ, Aelion MJ, et al: The cocaine body-packer syndrome: evaluation of a method of contrast study of the bowel. J Forensic Sci 1990;35:345–355.

146. Tomaszewski C, McKinney P, Phillips S: Prevention of toxicity from oral cocaine by activated charcoal in mice. Ann Emerg Med 1993;22:1804–1806.

147. Caballero F, Lopez-Navidad A, Gomez M, et al: Successful transplantation of organs from a donor who died from acute cocaine intoxication. Clin Transplant 2003;17:89–92.

148. Kantak KM: Vaccines against drugs of abuse: a viable treatment option? Drugs 2003;63:341–352.

149. Deng SX, de Prada P, Landry DW: Anticocaine catalytic antibodies. J Immunol Methods 2002;269:299–310.

150. Baumann BM, Perrone J, Hornig SE, et al: Randomized, double-blind, placebo-controlled trial of diazepam, nitroglycerin, or both for treatment of patients with potential cocaine-associated acute coronary syndrome. Acad Emerg Med 2000;7:878–885.

151. The American Heart Association in collaboration with the International Liaison Committee on Resuscitation: Guidelines 2000 for cardiopulmonary resuscitation and emergency cardiovascular care: toxicology in ECC. Circulation 2000;102(Suppl I): 223–228.

152. Albertson TE, Dawson A, de Latorre F, et al: TOX-ACLS: toxicologic-oriented advanced cardiac life support. Ann Emerg Med 2001;37(Suppl):78–90.

153. Negus BH, Willard JE, Hillis LD, et al: Alleviation of cocaine-induced coronary vasoconstriction with intravenous verapamil. Am J Cardiol 1994;73:510–513.

154. Sand IC, Brody SL, Wrenn KD, et al: Experience with esmolol for the treatment of cocaine associated cardiovascular complications. Am J Emerg Med 1991;9:161–163.

155. Boehrer JE, Moliterno DJ, Willard JE, et al: Influence of labetalol on cocaine-induced coronary vasoconstriction in humans. Am J Med 1993;94:608–610.

156. Beckman KJ, Parker RB, Hariman RJ, et al: Hemodynamic and electrophysiological actions of cocaine: effects of sodium bicarbonate as an antidote in dogs. Circulation 1991;83:1799–1807.

157. Winecoff AP, Hariman RJ, Grawe JJ, et al: Reversal of the electrocardiographic effects of cocaine by lidocaine. Part 1.

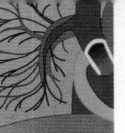
Comparison with sodium bicarbonate and quinidine. Pharmacotherapy 1994;14:698–703.

158. Shih RD, Hollander JE, Burstein JL, et al: Clinical safety of lidocaine in patients with cocaine-associated myocardial infarction. Ann Emerg Med 1995;26:702–706.

159. Brogan WC III, Lange RA, Kim AS, et al: Alleviation of cocaine-induced coronary vasoconstriction by nitroglycerin. J Am Coll Cardiol 1991;18:581–586.

160. Hollander JE, Burstein JL, Hoffman RS, et al: Cocaine-associated myocardial infarction. Clinical safety of thrombolytic therapy. Cocaine Associated Myocardial Infarction (CAMI) Study Group. Chest 1995;107:1237–1241.

161. Derlet RW, Albertson TE: Diazepam in the prevention of seizures and death in cocaine-intoxicated rats. Ann Emerg Med 1989;18:542–546.

162. Gasior M, Ungard JT, Witkin JM: Preclinical evaluation of newly approved and potential antiepileptic drugs against cocaine-induced seizures. J Pharmacol Exp Ther 1999;290:1148–1156.

163. Schaper A, Hofmann R, Ebbecke M, et al: [Cocaine-body-packing. Infrequent indication for laparotomy.] Chirurg 2003;74:626–631.

164. Klein C, Balash Y, Pollak L, et al: Body packer: cocaine intoxication, causing death, masked by concomitant administration of major tranquilizers. Eur J Neurol 2000;7:555–558.

165. Swan MC, Byrom R, Nicolaou M, et al: Cocaine by internal mail: two surgical cases. J R Soc Med 2003;96:188–189.

166. June R, Aks SE, Keys N, et al: Medical outcome of cocaine bodystuffers. J Emerg Med 2000;18:221–224.

167. Aldrighetti L, Paganelli M, Giacomelli M, et al: Conservative management of cocaine-packet ingestion: experience in Milan, the main Italian smuggling center of South American cocaine. Panminerva Med 1996;38:111–116.

168. Feist-Price S, Logan TK, Leukefeld C, et al: Targeting HIV prevention on African American crack and injection drug users. Subst Use Misuse 2003;38:1259–1284.

43 Dissociative Agents: Phencyclidine, Ketamine, and Dextromethorphan

IVAN E. LIANG, MD ■ EDWARD W. BOYER, MD, PHD

At a Glance...

- Phencyclidine, ketamine, and dextromethorphan are structurally related chemicals referred to as dissociative agents.
- The dissociative agents produce their psychotomimetic effects by antagonizing N-methyl-D-aspartate receptors in the central nervous system.
- Clinical effects of overdose include euphoria, a trance-like state, nystagmus, and, occasionally, violent behavior; hyperthermia, rhabdomyolysis, metabolic acidosis, and cardiovascular collapse may ensue. Coma and seizures may occur in severe overdose.
- Patients are often anesthetic and may be unaware of serious injuries.
- All of the dissociative agents may produce a positive urine toxicology screen for phencyclidine.
- Treatment for dissociative agent overdose is supportive. Benzodiazepines or haloperidol are preferred agents for chemical restraint.

Phencyclidine (phenylcyclohexyl piperidine, or PCP), ketamine [2-(O-chlorophenyl)-2-methylamino cyclohexanone], and dextromethorphan [(+)-3-methoxy-17-methyl-9a,13a,14a-morphinan] (Fig. 43-1) are structurally related chemicals that are abused for their dissociative properties. Because these drugs are often used in club settings, the prevalence of their use may have increased dramatically over the past decade. Intoxication with these agents produces a syndrome of sympathetic activation, central nervous system depression, and hallucinations.

EPIDEMIOLOGY

Accurate estimation of the abuse prevalence of phencyclidine, ketamine, and dextromethorphan is difficult. Because these substances are frequently taken in conjunction with other drugs, individuals suffering the effects of multiple drug use may present with a confusing clinical picture that prevents clinicians from accurately identifying the substances used. Nonetheless, the Drug Abuse Warning Network (DAWN) in 2003 identified a dramatic increase in the use of phencyclidine in several metropolitan areas. Data from the American Association of Poison Control Centers' Toxic Exposure Surveillance System (TESS) in 2002 identified 918 phencyclidine exposures with 6 deaths.[1] The DAWN data also observed significant increases in ketamine reports that were likely related to its abuse in party settings such as in raves and circuit parties. In 2002, TESS reported 342 ketamine exposures. Similarly, dextromethorphan was identified by DAWN as having a significantly increased prevalence of abuse. Data from TESS suggest that abuse or misuse of the drug by adolescents between ages 13 and 19 has increased more than 300% over a 3-year period.[2] Dextromethorphan abuse has been observed in children as young as 11.[3]

Dissociative agents are widely available in pill, powder, and injectable form. Phencyclidine is more commonly sold as a powder, but has been recently reported as an additive to marijuana cigarettes in metropolitan areas. Ketamine is difficult to synthesize; therefore, it is diverted from pharmaceutical or veterinary sources in injectable or powdered formulations.[4] Abused dextromethorphan is commonly diverted from over-the-counter cough and cold products that are widely available in stores.[4] Even individuals not intending to take dissociative agents may inadvertently receive them since ketamine and dextromethorphan are commonly used as adulterants in tablets purportedly containing methylenedioxymethamphetamine (MDMA, or "Ecstasy").[5-7]

NEUROPHARMACOLOGY

Phencyclidine, ketamine, and dextromethorphan exert their psychotomimetic effects by antagonizing with high affinity the N-methyl-D-aspartate (NMDA) receptors in limbic and cortical structures, inhibiting the release of excitatory amino acid neurotransmitters.[8,9] Dissociative drugs bind to the Ca^{2+} cation channel of the NMDA receptor to modulate glutamate neurotransmission, the end result of which is the production of specific neurobehavioral findings such as dissociative, "out-of-body" experiences.[7,9] When used for licit purposes such as procedural sedation, these experiences are known as "emergence reactions." NMDA receptor antagonism may selectively interrupt association pathways of the brain before producing somesthetic sensory blockade, and may also selectively depress the thalamoneocortical system before depressing the reticular activating and limbic systems. Dissociative agents also produce dose-dependent reuptake blockade of norepinephrine, dopamine, and serotonin, which contributes to the psychomotor, sympathomimetic, and psychotomimetic effects associated with these agents.[9] In recreational doses, PCP,

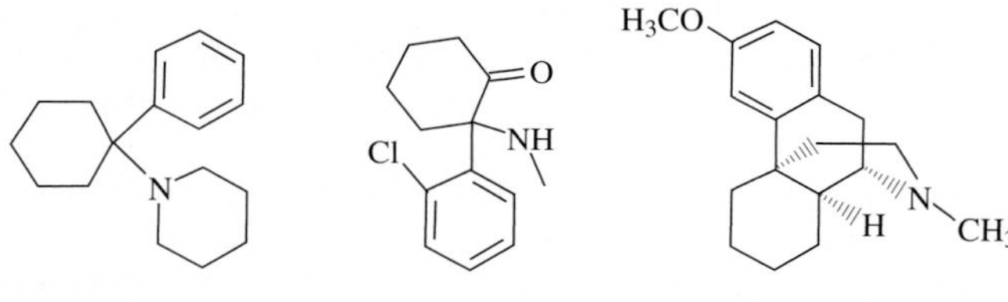

Phencyclidine (PCP)　　Ketamine　　Dextromethorphan
FIGURE 43-1 Chemical structure of dissociative agents.

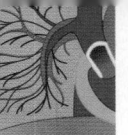

ketamine, and dextromethorphan (large via its active metabolite, dextrorphan) bind with high affinity to nonopiate σ receptors, which may contribute to their antinociceptive and sedative activities. As a nonanalgesic opiate, dextromethorphan produces antitussive activity by selectively binding to δ receptors without exhibiting classic opiate effects that occur from binding to μ and κ opiate receptors. In high doses, PCP and ketamine also bind to opioid and nicotine and muscarinic acetylcholine receptors.

PHENCYCLIDINE

Phencyclidine (PCP, "angel dust," "PeaCe Pill") was originally marketed in 1957 as a preinduction anesthetic agent that was not associated with cardiorespiratory depression.[10] Many patients in their postoperative course, however, developed extreme agitation and dysphoria.[10] Phencyclidine therefore was removed from the marketplace, although it was reintroduced as the veterinary product Senylan (Parke-Davis, Detroit, MI). Phencyclidine emerged as a hallucinogen in the 1960s but did not reach full popularity until the 1970s.[11,12] It was classified as a schedule I substance in 1978, and its use declined during the 1980s.[13] Over the past 5 years, however, increasing numbers of PCP abusers appear to smoke the drug with another substance such as marijuana.[14-17]

Pharmacology

Phencyclidine is a highly lipophilic, water-soluble weak base. It is rapidly absorbed following oral, intranasal, intramuscular, intravenous, pulmonary, or rectal administration. Absorption is minimal in the stomach, but occurs rapidly in the duodenum and jejunum.[15,16] Onset of effects occurs within 30 to 60 minutes when ingested, but may be as rapid as 2 minutes after smoking.[15] Acute toxicity often persists for 4 to 6 hours, and generally resolves within 48 hours.[16] At oral doses of between 5 and 10 mg, toxic psychoses and violent behavior are described.[18] Oral doses greater than 10 mg are associated with schizophreniform reactions, although the dose-response relationship is incompletely defined.[18]

Phencyclidine distributes widely in tissues.[16,18] It possesses an unusual enterogastric circulation in which significant amounts of the drug are actively secreted into the stomach and then reabsorbed in the small intestine.[15] The concentration of PCP in gastric fluid may be 50 times higher than in the serum.[15] The concentration in the brain may be up to nine times that of the serum.[15,16] The slightly acidic milieu of the cerebrospinal fluid (CSF) induces ion trapping of the compound, an effect that explains the prolonged neurologic effects of the drug.[16]

The apparent volume of distribution of phencyclidine is 6.3 L/kg, and the drug is 78% protein bound.[15] The large volume of distribution and lipophilicity contribute to PCP's persistence in the body and its long duration of action. Phencyclidine is hepatically metabolized in a stepwise manner, first by oxidative hydroxylation to an inactive metabolite that undergoes glucuronidation. This water-soluble derivative is the major metabolite that is renally eliminated. Significant first pass metabolism occurs after ingestion, an effect that is not observed following pulmonary or parenteral administration.[15] More than 90% of users excrete metabolites in the urine for up to 7 days after exposure, while chronic abusers do so for up to 4 weeks after last use.[19] Ten percent of an ingested dose is excreted unchanged in the urine.

Clinical Effects

No therapeutic indications are described for PCP, although NMDA antagonists may have theoretical utility in preventing neuronal injury following cerebral hypoxic/ischemic insult.[20,21]

Phencyclidine exhibits a broad variety of clinical effects, some of which are unpredictable but which are generally dose related.[21] Violent behavior, rotatory nystagmus, hypertension, anesthesia, and analgesia are the most characteristic signs of intoxication.[21,22] At elevated doses, PCP will produce a dissociative condition characterized by a catatonic, trancelike state but may include a sense of euphoria, omnipotence, tremendous strength, and sexual prowess.[23] Seizures are described at high doses, and coma may occur, persisting for up to 10 days.[22] Lower doses of phencyclidine will produce ataxia, slurred speech, profuse diaphoresis, and neuromuscular rigidity.[21] The most common causes of death from PCP overdose involve trauma or occur as the sequela of physical restraint of severely agitated patients, with attendant hypothermia, rhabdomyolysis, metabolic acidosis, and cardiovascular collapse.[24]

The neurologic examination may reveal horizontal, vertical, or rotatory nystagmus, a prominent finding that occurs in over half of all intoxicated patients.[21,22] Pupils may be miotic and reactive, and reflexes are briskly hyperactive. Increased muscle strength is commonplace, and several attendants may be required to restrain agitated patients. Patients are anesthetic and are often unaware of injuries, a quality that results from the dissociative effects of the drug.[22]

Prominent psychiatric effects of phencyclidine include violent, aggressive behavior that, when combined with a sense of tremendous strength, is troublesome for caretakers.[21] Patients may also demonstrate mania, but catatonia and visual hallucinations are common.[25] Physiologic dependence on PCP in the absence of clear physiologic symptoms is described, as is an abstinence syndrome characterized by depression, anxiety, and irritability.[26] Long-term PCP abuse is associated with diminished abstract thought and incidental memory.[26]

A temperature greater than 38.8°C (101.8°F) was identified in 2.6% of patient in one series of PCP intoxications.[22] Hyperthermia in PCP overdose may arise from isometric muscle contraction and may portend significant morbidity.[27] Elevations in serum transmamines, rhabdomyolysis, clotting abnormalities, hepatic injury, and renal failure probably arise as a consequence of poorly treated hyperthermia and muscle trauma.

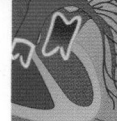

Diagnosis

The diagnosis of phencyclidine poisoning can be inferred from history and physical examination findings, and is confirmed by laboratory testing. Rotatory nystagmus is an important clinical clue to establishing the diagnosis.[21,22] Because PCP is lipophilic and may be detected in the urine for up to 4 weeks, urine is the preferred specimen for detection.[19] If present, PCP should elicit a positive result on qualitative urine toxicologic screen. Quantitative measurement of phencyclidine in plasma is not recommended because clinical signs and symptoms do not correlate well with plasma concentrations.

Patients in whom phencyclidine intoxication is suspected should have electrolytes, blood urea nitrogen, creatinine, transaminases, coagulation times, glucose, and serum creatine phosphokinase concentrations measured. Hyperthermic patients deserve measurement of arterial pH. Clinicians should remain vigilant for electrolyte disturbances, metabolic acidosis, and renal failure.

KETAMINE

Initially developed as a veterinary anesthetic, ketamine is structurally similar to PCP (see Fig. 43-1). Ketamine is often diverted from veterinary or pharmaceutical sources and is sold either in powdered or liquid form or as an adulterant in club drug ("Ecstasy") pills.

Pharmacology

The pharmacology of ketamine is similar to that of phencyclidine. Ketamine can be administered via oral, intranasal, intramuscular, intravenous, and rectal routes.[28] Ketamine is a weakly basic amino compound (pKa of 7.5) with close structural similarity to phencyclidine.[28] It is commercially available as 1:1 racemic mixtures of the S(+) and R(-) enantiomers of the hydrochloride salt. Ketamine undergoes rapid absorption via all routes and distributes within 7 to 10 minutes of intravenous administration into highly perfused tissues such as the brain, heart, and lungs. Concentrations in these organs may be four to five times greater than corresponding plasma levels. Ketamine then undergoes a second redistribution into muscle and, eventually, adipose with a distribution half-life of approximately 10 to 15 minutes.[8,28-30] Ketamine and its metabolites are moderately protein bound in the serum 60%, 50%, and 69% for ketamine, norketamine, and dehydronorketamine, respectively, in human serum.[31] Volumes of distribution of ketamine have been reported ranging from 2 to 5 L/kg.[29]

Ketamine undergoes significant first-pass metabolism via hepatic *N*-demethylation by CYP2D6 to produce norketamine, a compound with one third the activity of the parent compound.[28,32,33] This metabolite is subsequently hydroxylated and conjugated to water-soluble compounds that undergo renal elimination. Approximately 90% of an administered ketamine dose is eliminated as the conjugated hydroxyl metabolite; about

4% is excreted unchanged. Interestingly, the elimination half-life is approximately 2.5 to 3 hours in adults, but only 1 to 2 hours in children.[29,33]

The onset of effects depends on the method of administration. In general, anesthetic or therapeutic doses of ketamine are between 1 and 2 mg/kg (approximately 1 mg for a 70-kg patient) for intravenous administration; the dose of ketamine used for recreational purposes is somewhat lower.[29] Recreational doses begin at approximately 25 mg and are titrated upward to clinical effect. One method of titration, for example, involves insufflating approximately 25-mg "bumps" of ketamine until the user can no longer feel his or her legs. Clinical effects often resolve within 10 minutes of intraparenteral dosing, but may persist for up to 90 minutes after oral administration.[32]

Clinical Effects

Recommended doses of 1 to 2 mg/kg intravenously, up to 4 mg/kg intramuscularly, and 7 mg/kg orally will produce anesthesia and analgesia accompanied by catalepsy with minimal purposeful response to noxious stimuli. The eyes often remain open, with a slow nystagmic gaze; corneal and light responses often remain normal.[34] Hypertonic and occasionally purposeful movements may be intermittently noted.[34] Subanesthetic doses will produce a spectrum of symptoms, but will often interfere with normal cognition and appropriate responses to environment.[34]

Ketamine evokes a number of physiologic responses besides anesthesia.[28,30] The drug increases sympathetic outflow and effect that can be blunted by sedation with benzodiazepines.[28,30] Ketamine produces elevated cerebrospinal fluid and intraocular pressures, although this effect may be abolished by maintenance of normocapnia and/or benzodiazepine administration.[28] The salivary and tracheal-bronchial secretions that accompany ketamine administration are due to the drug's cholinergic characteristics.[28] Despite these secretions, ketamine has been associated with decreases in airway resistance and bronchospasm.[28] Respiratory failure from massive doses of ketamine has been described, although this finding occurred in multiple drug use.[28]

Hallucinations that occur as ketamine anesthesia decreases are described as "emergence reactions" and are the reason for which the drug is diverted to illicit use.[7,35] Drug users frequently describe cosmic, religious, or near death experiences, visualization of psychedelic colors, and out-of-body experiences that can be characterized as ranging from pleasurable to nightmarish.[7] During the episode, patients may be mildly agitated, sympathomimetic, or frankly psychotic and delirious. Incidence of emergence reactions is low among children, but has been reported to be as high as 30% in adults.[35]

Diagnosis

Establishing the diagnosis of ketamine intoxication requires the recognition of subtle physical examination findings. When used illicitly, ketamine does not, in general,

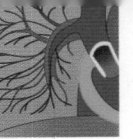

produce the extreme agitation of phencyclidine.[35] Instead, intoxicated patients may demonstrate a distinctive, plodding gait as the legs dissociate from the remainder of the body.[7] Patients may lose fine motor control and experience nausea and vomiting with movement. They may deliver pronouncements that are confusing to sober observers.[7] In addition to the acute dissociative effects, ketamine is associated with dystonia, paranoia, and rhabdomyolysis.[35] This latter finding occurs almost exclusively in patients who receive physical restraints without chemical sedation.

Dependence on ketamine has been described. The chronic effects of ketamine abuse include poor concentration, inhibited learning capabilities, and decreased memory. Ketamine users have described "flashbacks" up to several months after use of the drug.[7] In addition, habitual users describe tolerance to established doses of ketamine, which can be explained by the ability of ketamine to induce the expression of cytochrome P-450 enzyme subtypes.[28]

The diagnosis of ketamine intoxication may be confused by the observation that ketamine produces a false-positive result on qualitative urine assays for phencyclidine.[36]

DEXTROMETHORPHAN

The easy availability of dextromethorphan in over-the-counter preparations contributes to its increasing abuse by younger adults. Data from the TESS database suggest that abuse or misuse of the drug has increased more than 300% over a 3-year period in adolescents between the ages of 13 and 19.[2] Abused dextromethorphan products are sometimes known by users as "Triple C" from the three Cs whose imprint is used to identify some products that are preferred for abuse, but gelcap formulations of dextromethorphan are also called "Skittles" or "Red Hots" because of the similarity in appearance between the drug and the popular candies.[37,38] Unwitting users may not recognize that some over-the-counter dextromethorphan formulations may contain acetaminophen or anticholinergic agents, which cause their own toxicity.

Pharmacology

Dextromethorphan is available in oral formulation; it is well absorbed following ingestion with maximum serum concentrations at 2.5 hours.[39] The major metabolite of dextromethorphan, dextrorphan, achieves peak plasma concentrations at 1.6 to 1.7 hours following ingestion.[40] The volume of distribution of dextromethorphan in humans is not firmly established, but is thought to be large (5.0 to 6.7 L/kg).[29] Dextromethorphan and its metabolites undergo renal elimination, with less than 0.1% of the drug being eliminated in the feces.[29] The half-life of the parent compound is approximately 2 to 4 hours in individuals with normal metabolism.

Dextromethorphan is metabolized by cytochrome CYP2D6. In humans, CYP2D6 is a genetically polymorphic enzyme responsible for metabolizing numerous substances.[41] Rapid metabolizers—those individuals with extensive CYP2D6 activity and, hence, increased rates of dextromethorphan metabolism—constitute about 85% of the U.S. population. Dextromethorphan undergoes 3-demethylation to dextrorphan and, to a lesser extent, N-demethylation to 3-methoxymorphinan.[40,41] Both of these metabolites are further demethylated to 3-hydroxymorphinan. Dextrorphan is the active metabolite that produces neurobehavioral effects, while dextromethorphan does not exhibit the same actions. Dextromethorphan is therefore a prodrug, and the metabolic conversion of dextromethorphan to dextrorphan is an important determinant of the abuse potential of dextromethorphan in an individual. Experienced dextromethorphan users describe tachyphylaxis to the drug, but whether this effect is from alterations in cytochrome function or other effects is not known.

Clinical Effects

The dose of ingested dextromethorphan determines the neurobehavioral outcome. Recreational users of dextromethorphan describe several intensities of effect from the drug, known as "plateaus."[42] The first plateau is a mild stimulant effect similar to that of methylenedioxyamphetamine. The second plateau is described as similar to a combination of concurrent ethanol and marijuana intoxication, although some users describe hallucinations as occurring at this stage.[43] The third level is a dissociative, "out-of-body" state like that produced by a low recreational dose of ketamine, and the fourth plateau is a fully dissociative condition similar to that produced by ketamine intoxication.[42] Neurobehavioral effects begin within 30 to 60 minutes of ingestion and persist for approximately 6 hours.

To produce nominal effects from dextromethorphan—the first plateau—online drug encyclopedias such as Erowid (www.erowid.org) describe a dose of between 100 and 200 mg (1.5–2.5 mg/kg). The second plateau may be achieved with 200 to 400 mg (2.5–7.5 mg/kg), and the third plateau can be achieved with 300 to 600 mg (7.5–15 mg/kg) of the drug. An ingested dose of 600 to 1500 (>15 mg/kg) mg of dextromethorphan may produce a full-blown dissociative state. These doses depend on several factors, such as an individual's CYP2D6 subtype and body weight as well as the degree of tolerance to dextromethorphan.

The clinical presentation of dextromethorphan intoxication therefore depends on the ingested dose. Minimally intoxicated persons may develop tachycardia, hypertension, vomiting, mydriasis, diaphoresis, nystagmus, euphoria, loss of motor coordination, and giggling or laughing.[42] In addition to the above findings, persons with moderate intoxication may demonstrate hallucinations and a distinctive, plodding ataxic gait that has been compared to "zombie-like" walking.[43] Severely intoxicated individuals in a dissociated state may be agitated or somnolent.[38,42,44,45] Extremely agitated patients may develop hyperthermia and metabolic acidosis.

Experienced dextromethorphan users describe a rapidly developing and persistent tolerance to the drug.[42] Dependence on dextromethorphan is rarely described.[46-48]

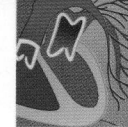

Although dextromethorphan is not thought to have addictive properties, susceptible individuals may develop craving and habitual use of the drug.[44,49] An abstinence syndrome may be associated with cessation of dextromethorphan abuse that is characterized by dysphoria and intense cravings.[46,48,50,51] Toxic psychosis and cognitive deterioration may arise from chronic use of the drug.[46,50,51]

Toxicity in the setting of dextromethorphan abuse can arise from additional sources. Over-the-counter cough formulations frequently contain, in addition to dextromethorphan, other pharmaceutical agents such as chlorpheniramine, acetaminophen, or pseudoephedrine.[52] Chlorpheniramine is an H_1 receptor antagonist. Consequently, individuals who have abused chlorpheniramine-containing dextromethorphan formulations may also exhibit anticholinergic signs and symptoms, such as tachycardia; warm, dry, flushed skin; dry mucosa; mydriasis; agitated delirium; urinary retention; and gastrointestinal dysmotility (see Chapter 39). Severe chlorpheniramine intoxication has also been associated with seizure activity, rhabdomyolysis, and hyperthermia.[38] Pseudoephedrine intoxication may mimic that of chlorpheniramine except that patients may exhibit diaphoresis. In contrast, overdose of acetaminophen, an antipyretic and analgesic that is a component of over 100 cough and cold preparations, produces delayed hepatic injury and, potentially, death. Lastly, because dextromethorphan is produced as the crystalline hydrobromide salt, bromism is a rare consequence that has been identified in heavy chronic abusers of dextromethorphan.[53]

Drug interactions exist between dextromethorphan and other substances, the best characterized of which is serotonin syndrome. Dextromethorphan and its active metabolite, dextrorphan, block reuptake of serotonin in central nerve terminals. This condition typically occurs from the interaction between dextromethorphan and selective serotonin reuptake inhibitors or monoamine oxidase inhibitors, but concurrent administration of antibiotics (e.g., linezolide), opiate analgesics (e.g., meperidine and tramadol), or drugs of abuse (e.g., Syrian rue) could precipitate the condition.[54] Patients with serotonin syndrome may demonstrate the clinical triad of mental status changes, autonomic instability, and muscular hypertonicity[55] (see Chapters 10A and 29).

Diagnosis

The diagnosis of dextromethorphan intoxication relies on epidemiologic, historical, and physical examination findings. Younger adolescents may be at increased risk for dextromethorphan abuse.[56] In addition, data from the National Institute on Drug Abuse's Community Epidemiology Working Group and other sources suggests that pharmaceutical abuse may be more prevalent among females.[57-59] On history, patients may report the abuse of dextromethorphan-containing products. The diagnosis of dextromethorphan intoxication is otherwise made on clinical grounds, with attention directed to signs and symptoms of dissociative use: tachycardia, hypertension, diaphoresis, ataxia, nystagmus, and, potentially, hallucinations, but clinicians should remain aware that specific findings depend on the degree to which individuals are intoxicated. The differential diagnosis of dextromethorphan intoxication includes other potentially serious toxidromes. Patients with ataxia, nystagmus, and mental status changes may suffer from ketamine or phencyclidine abuse, lithium intoxication, phenytoin or carbamazepine poisoning, serotonin syndrome, Wernicke-Korsakoff syndrome, and sedative-hypnotic, including ethanol, abstinence syndromes.[48]

Although dextromethorphan does not produce true positive results on toxic screens or cross-react with the opiate portion of the screen, the molecule may produce false-positive results on qualitative urine assays for phencyclidine.[60,61]

TREATMENT

Supportive management is often sufficient to care for dissociative agent overdose.[38,45,62] Because airway reflexes are preserved in dissociative agent toxicity, relatively few patients require orotracheal intubation and airway support. Excessive airway secretions can be controlled by atropine or glycopyrrolate; clinicians should be aware that phencyclidine may hyperstimulate oropharyngeal musculature, and care should be taken to prevent laryngospasm during passage of an orotracheal tube.

Basic emergency measures that include measurement of vital signs and intravascular access should be performed immediately. All patients should receive intravenous saline solution; this therapy corrects dehydration and prevents renal failure secondary to rhabdomyolysis from muscle breakdown. Hypertension and tachycardia may respond well to sedating agents such as diazepam, but nitroprusside may be necessary in patients who fail chemical sedation.

Patients should receive sedation if necessary. Auditory, tactile, and visual stimuli should be minimized. The technique of "talking down" a patient, often applied effectively to ketamine and dextromethorphan overdose, is generally ineffective in PCP poisoning; the practice may even provoke hostile behavior in PCP-poisoned patients. Combative or hostile patients should receive chemical sedation with either benzodiazepines or phenothiazines. The preferred agent is intravenous lorazepam (initial dose 0.1 mg/kg, total dose titrated to desired level of sedation). However, intramuscular haloperidol (5 to 10 mg) has been demonstrated to improve schizophreniform symptoms seen in PCP poisoning. Notably, phenothiazines may produce unintended adverse reactions such as anticholinergic reactions, dystonia, or seizure activity. These adverse reactions are, however, rare. Physical restraints are highly undesirable and may contribute to mortality by enforcing isometric muscle contractions that are associated with severe lactic acidosis and hyperthermia.[27] If used, physical restraints must be rapidly replaced with chemical sedation.

Hyperthermia and metabolic acidosis arise from excess muscle activity; treatment of these findings may require neuromuscular blockage and mechanical ventilation. Although benzodiazepines have a beneficial

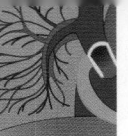
effect in moderate cases, severely ill, hyperthermic patients (T ≥ 40° C) should receive immediate paralysis with nondepolarizing agents such as vecuronium followed by orotracheal intubation and ventilation. Clinicians should avoid succinylcholine because of the risks of arrhythmia from rhabdomyolysis-associated hyperkalemia. There is no role for antipyretics in the management of hyperthermia from dissociative agent overdose; the increase in body temperature is due to muscular activity, not an alteration in the hypothalamic temperature set point.

Activated charcoal is indicated in cases of recent dextromethorphan ingestion (e.g., less than 1 hour after ingestion), but is of unclear benefit in PCP or ketamine toxicity since these agents are infrequently administered via oral routes. Because PCP is actively secreted in the stomach, multiple-dose activated charcoal may offer some benefit, although its efficacy has not been rigorously established. Continuous gastric suctioning has also been recommended for evacuating PCP-laden secretions. Close monitoring of electrolytes is warranted since continuous suctioning may remove potassium, hydrogen, and other essential ions.

There are no antidotes for dissociative agent poisoning. Respiratory depression, rarely described in severe dextromethorphan intoxication, intermittently responds to high-dose intravenous naloxone.[48] Clinicians should consider physostigmine to reverse anticholinergic signs if present.

Laboratory assessment of intoxicated individuals should include measurement of serum electrolytes, hepatic and renal function, acid–base status, serum creatinine phosphokinase, a toxic screen, and urinalysis. In addition, physicians should always measure the serum acetaminophen concentration and treat potentially toxic concentrations or hepatic injury with *N*-acetylcysteine.

REFERENCES

1. Litovitz T, Klein-Schwartz W, Caravati E: 2002 Annual report of the American Association of Poison Control Centers toxic exposure surveillance system. Am J Emerg Med 2003;22:517–575.
2. Watson W: TESS Dextromethorphan Data. Washington, DC, American Association of Poison Control Centers, 2003.
3. Boyer EW: 2003 Poisoning Data. Boston, Massachusetts Poison Control Center, 2003.
4. Anonymous: Trouble in the medicine chest (I): Rx drug abuse growing. Prevention Alert 2003;6.
5. Boyer E, Quang L, Woolf A, Shannon M, Magnani B: Dextromethorphan and ecstasy pills. JAMA 2001;285:409–410.
6. Baggott M, Heifets B, Jones R, Mendelson J, et al: Chemical analysis of ecstasy pills. JAMA 2000;284:2190.
7. Boyer EW, Woolf AW: What's new on the street. Clin Pediatr Emerg Med 2000;1:12–15.
8. Kohrs R, Durieux M: Ketamine: teaching an old drug new tricks. Anesth Analg 1998;87:1186–1193.
9. Lindefors N, Barati S, O'Connor W: Differential effects of single and repeated ketamine administration on dopamine, serotonin, and GABA transmission in rat medial prefrontal cortex. Brain Res 1997;759:205.
10. Pradhan S: Phencyclidine (PCP): some human studies. Neurosci Behav Physiol 1984;8:493–501.
11. Lundberg G, Gupta R, Montgomery M: Phencyclidine (PCP): patterns seen in street drug analysis. J Toxicol Clin Toxicol 1976;9:503–510.
12. Rainey J, Crowder M: Prevalence of phencyclidine in street drug preparations. N Engl J Med 1974;290:466–467.
13. Bailey D: Phencyclidine detection during toxicology testing of a university medical patient population. J Toxicol Clin Toxicol 1987;25:517–526.
14. O'Brien M: Emerging trends in drug use. Presented at the CEWG Annual Conference, Atlanta, GA, December 9–12, 2003. Bethesda, MD, National Institute on Drug Abuse.
15. Showalter C, Thornton W: Clinical pharmacology of phencyclidine toxicity. Am J Psychiatry 1977;134:1234–1238.
16. Misra A, Pontani R, Bartolomeo J: Persistence of phencyclidine and metabolites in brain and adipose tissue and implications for long-lasting behavioral effects. Res Commun Chem Pathol Pharmacol 1979;24:431–435.
17. Holland J, Nelson L, Ravikumar P: Embalming-fluid soaked marijuana: a new high or new guise for PCP? J Psychoactive Drugs 1998;30:215–219.
18. Cook C, Brine D, Quin G: Phencyclidine and phenylcyclohexane disposition after smoking phencyclidine. Clin Pharmacol Ther 1982;31:635–641.
19. Simpson G, Khajawall A: Urinary phencyclidine excretion in chronic abusers. J Toxicol Clin Toxicol 1982;19:1051–1059.
20. Liden C, Lovejoy F: Phencyclidine: nine cases of poisoning. JAMA 1975;234:513–516.
21. McCarron M, Schulze B, Thompson G: Acute phencyclidine intoxication: clinical patterns, complications, and treatment. Ann Emerg Med 1981;10:290–297.
22. McCarron M, Schulze B, Thompson G: Acute phencyclidine intoxication: incidence of clinical findings in 1000 cases. Ann Emerg Med 1981;10:232–242.
23. Burns R, Lerner S: Perspectives: acute phencyclidine intoxication. Clin Toxicol 1976;9:477–501.
24. Heilig S, Diller J, Nelson F: A study of 44 PCP related deaths. Int J Addiction 1982;17:1175–1184.
25. Balster R: Clinical implications of behavioral pharmacol-ogy research on phencyclidine. NIDA Res Monogr 1986;64:148–162.
26. Rawson R, Tennant F, McCann M: Characteristics of 68 chronic phencyclidine users who sought treatment. Drug Alcohol Depend 1981;8:223–227.
27. Hick J, Smith S, Lynch M: Metabolic acidosis in restraint-associated cardiac arrest: a case series. Acad Emerg Med 1999;6:239–245.
28. White P: Ketamine: its pharmacology and therapeutic uses. Anesthesiology 1982;56:119–136.
29. Baselt R, Cravey R: Disposition of Toxic Drugs and Chemicals in Man. Chicago, Yearbook Medical Publishers, 1989.
30. Reich D, Silvay G: Ketamine: an update on the first twenty-five years of clinical experience. Can J Anaesth 1989;36:186–197.
31. Hajazi Y, Boulieu R: Protein binding of ketamine and its active metabolites to human serum. Eur J Clin Pharmacol 2002;58:37–40.
32. Grant I, Nimmo W, Clements J: Pharmacokinetics and analgesic effects of intramuscular and oral ketamine. Br J Anaesth 1981;53:805–810.
33. Grant I, Nimmo W, Clements J: Ketamine disposition in children and adults. Br J Anaesth 1983;55:1107–1111.
34. Weiner A, Vieira L, McKay C, Bayer M: Ketamine abusers presenting to the emergency department: a case series. J Emerg Med 2000;18:447–451.
35. Green S, Li J: Ketamine in adults: what emergency physicians need to know about patient selection and emergence reactions. Acad Emerg Med 2000;7:278–281.
36. Shannon M: Recent ketamine administration can produce urine toxic screen which is falsely positive for phencyclidine. Pediatr Emerg Care 1998;14:180.
37. Boyer EW: Dextromethorphan abuse. Pediatr Emerg Care 2004;20:858–863.
38. Kirages T, Sule H, Mycyk M: Severe manifestations of coricidin intoxication. Am J Emerg Med 2003;21:648–651.
39. Barnhart J, Massad E: Determination of dextromethorphan in serum by gas chromatography. J Chromatogr 1979;163:390–395.
40. Silvasti M, Karttunen P, Tukiannen H: Pharmacokinetics of dextromethorphan and dextrorphan: a single dose comparison of three preparations in human volunteers. Int J Clin Pharmacol Ther 1987;9:493–497.

41. Schadel M, Wu D, Otton S, et al: Pharmacokinetics of dextromethorphan and metabolites in humans: influence of the CYP2D6 phenotype and quinidine inhibition. J Clin Psychopharmacol 1995;15:263–269.

42. White W: DXM FAQ. Vol. 2004: Erowid, www.erowid.org, 1995.

43. Anonymous: RFG's guide to DXM (dextromethorphan). Vol. 2004: DXM Harm Reduction Project, www.dextromethorphan.ws, 2004.

44. Banerji S, Anderson I: Abuse of Coricidin HBP Cough & Cold: episodes recorded by a poison center. Am J Health System Pharmacy 2001;58:1811–1814.

45. Graudins A, Ferm R: Acute dystonia in a child associated with therapeutic ingestion of a dextromethorphan-containing cough and cold syrup. J Toxicol Clin Toxicol 1996;34:351–352.

46. Hinsberger A, Sharma V: Cognitive deterioration from long-term abuse of dextromethorphan: a case report. J Psychiatry Neurosci 1994;19:375–377.

47. Fleming P: Dependence on dextromethorphan. BMJ 1986; 293:597.

48. Wolfe T, Caravati E: Massive dextromethorphan ingestion and abuse. Am J Emerg Med 1995;13:174–176.

49. Nicholson K, Hayes B, Balster R: Evaluation of the reinforcing properties and phencyclidine-like discriminative stimulus effects of dextromethorphan and dextrorphan in rates and rhesus monkeys. Psychopharmacology 1999;146:49–59.

50. Dodds A: Toxic psychosis due to dextromethorphan. Med J Aust 1967;2:231.

51. Schadel M, Sellers E: Psychosis with Vicks Formula 44-D abuse. Can Med Assoc J 1992;147:843–844.

52. Helfer J, Kim O: Psychoactive abuse potential of Robitussin-DM. Am J Psychiatry 1990;147:672–673.

53. Ng Y, Lin W, Chen T, Tsai S: Spurious hyperchloremia and decreased anion gap in a patient with dextromethorphan bromide. Am J Nephrol 1992;12:268–270.

54. Bowdle T: Adverse effects of opioid agonists and agonist-antagonists in anaesthesia. Drug Saf 1998;19:173–189.

55. Shannon M: Methylenedioxymethamphetamine. Pediatr Emerg Care 2000;16:377–380.

56. Baker D, Borys D: Coricidin use and abuse in Texas during 1998 and 1999. J Toxicol Clin Toxicol 2000;38:533.

57. Anonymous: Group discussion: pharmaceutical abuse. Presented at the CEWG Annual Conference, Atlanta, GA, December 9–12, 2003. Bethesda, MD: National Institute on Drug Abuse.

58. Cutler S: Philadelphia report. Presented at the CEWG Annual Conference, Atlanta, GA, December 9–12, 2003. Bethesda, MD: National Institute on Drug Abuse.

59. Dooley D: Boston report. Presented at the CEWG Annual Meeting, Atlanta, GA, December 9–12, 2003. Bethesda, MD: National Institute on Drug Abuse.

60. Darboe M, Keenan G, Richards T: The abuse of dextromethorphan: a pilot study of the community of Waynesboro, PA. Adolescence 1996;31:633–644.

61. Schier J, Diaz J: Avoid unfavorable consequences: dextromethorphan can bring about a false-positive phencyclidine urine drug screen. J Emerg Med 2000;18:379–380.

62. Henretig F, Cugini D, Dubin D: Dextromethorphan overdose in children. Vet Hum Toxicol 1988;3:364.

44 *Amphetamines and Derivatives*

TIMOTHY E. ALBERTSON, MD, MPH, PHD ■ NICHOLAS J. KENYON, MD ■ BRIAN MORRISSEY, MD

At a Glance...

■ Amphetamine abuse and toxicity account for significant morbidity, mortality, and emergency medicine and intensive care unit admissions.

■ The impact of amphetamine toxicity is amplified by its association with violent crime and trauma.

■ The ability of the various amphetamine-related compounds to cause significant behavioral and multiple organ system dysfunction contributes to the clinical challenge.

■ After decontamination, treatment is primarily supportive.

■ Community education and prevention approaches can reduce the incidence of this increasing problem.

INTRODUCTION AND RELEVANT HISTORY

Amphetamines and related stimulant compounds represent an increasingly important class of recreational drugs of abuse in the United States as well as in many other parts of the world. In some locales, they rival cocaine as a cause of drug-related Emergency Department (ED) and intensive care unit (ICU) admissions. Although altered mental status, psychiatric disorders, and cardio-vascular symptoms are most commonly encountered with amphetamine use, toxic manifestations in nearly every organ system have been reported (Box 44-1).

The amphetamine-like compounds have a long medical history. Related phenylisopropylamines including the alkaloids ephedrine, obtained from *Ephedra mahuang,* and norpseudoephedrine, or cathine, obtained from *Catha edulis,* have been used for more than 5000 years in China and 600 years in East Africa, respectively.[1] Ephedrine was classified as a food additive in the United States. Because of this classification, the Food and Drug Administration (FDA) had little regulatory jurisdiction over it. Documentation of increasing cases of toxicity and deaths associated with its use resulted in an FDA ban of ephedrine in April 2004.

Although racemic β-phenylisopropylamine was first synthesized in 1887, initial investigations into the phar-macology of amphetamine derived from the basic phenylethylamine structure (Fig. 44-1) were not reported until 1930 by Piness.[2,3] Early medicinal uses of amphet-amine included the treatment of rhinitis and asthma.[1] The Smith, Kline and French Pharmaceutical Company introduced the Benzedrine Nasal Inhaler in the United States in 1932. Each inhaler contained 250 mg of synthetic racemic amphetamine base with menthol and various other aromatics.[4] Abuse of amphetamines was quickly noted and increased with a 1936 report claiming enhanced intellectual performance with use of the inhaler.[4,5] Because of reports of medical complications, amphetamines became prescription drugs in the United States in 1938; however, inhalers initially remained available without prescription. Limited use and abuse of amphetamine and related compounds continued until World War II, when they were extensively used by the Allies and the Axis powers as stimulants in combat. D-Amphetamine is still used by the U.S. military as a "go pill" for sustained operations and during deployments, and often followed by a benzodiazepine as a "no go pill."

The psychologically addicting characteristics were first realized when amphetamine abuse became epidemic in

---

BOX 44-1	MAJOR SIGNS, SYMPTOMS, AND NONINFECTIOUS MEDICAL COMPLICATIONS ASSOCIATED WITH USE OF AMPHETAMINES AND RELATED COMPOUNDS

Cardiac		Neurologic	
Chest pain	+++	Headaches	+
Myocardial infarction	+	Seizures	++
Palpitations	++	Cerebral infarcts/strokes	++
Arrhythmias	++	Cerebral vasculitis	++
Cardiomyopathy	+	Cerebral edema	+
Myocarditis	+	Mydriasis	++
Hypertension	++	Cerebral hemorrhage	++
Sudden death	+	Subarachnoid	++
		Intraventricular	+++
		Intracerebral	++
Psychiatric		**Respiratory**	
Anxiety	+++	Pulmonary edema	+
Depression	++	Dyspnea	++
Paranoia	++	Bronchitis	+
Delirium/ hallucinations	+++	Pulmonary hypertension	+
		Hemoptysis	+
Psychosis	+++	Pleuritic chest pain	++
Suicide	++	Asthma exacerbations	+
Aggressive behavior	++	Pulmonary granuloma	+
Euphoria/ hyperactivity	++		
Irritability	++	**Other**	
		Hyperpyrexia	++
		Renal failure	+
		Ischemic colitis	+
		Obstetric complications	++
		Anorexia/weight loss	+++
		Rhabdomyolysis	++
		Nausea/vomiting	+
		Disseminated vasculitis	+

Estimated frequency of events: +, reported rare case; ++, commonly reported; +++, frequently seen or reported with chronic use or overdose.

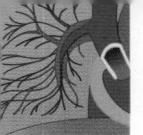

Phenylethylamine	Amphetamine	Methamphetamine
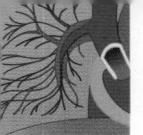		

Ephedrine	3,4-Methylenedioxymethamphetamine (MDMA)

3,4-Methylenedioxy-amphetamine (MDA)	4-Methyl-2,5-Dimethoxyphenylethylamine (DOM/STP)

FIGURE 44-1 Chemical structures of several amphetamine-like compounds. The basic phenylethylamine structure is labeled. Both α and β side chain positions and the phenyl ring itself can be modified to alter the pharmacologic effects of these related compounds.

BOX 44-2   AMPHETAMINES AND RELATED COMPOUNDS

Aminorex fumarate
Amphetamine
Benzphetamine
4-Bromo-2,5-methoxyphenylethylamine (2-CB/MFT)
Cathinone (khat)
Cinnamedrine
Desoxyphedrine
Dextroamphetamine
Diethylpropion
4-Bromo-2,5-dimethoxyamphetamine (DOB)
4-Methyl-2,5-dimethoxyamphetamine (DOM/STP)
Fenfluramine
Mescaline (3,4,5-trimethoxyphenylethylamine)
3,4-Methylenedioxyamphetamine (MDA)
3,4-Methylenedioxyethamphetamine (MDEA)
3,4-Methylenedioxymethamphetamine (MDMA)
Methamphetamine
Methcathinone
Methylphenidate
Methoxyamphetamine (PMA)
Pemoline
Phendimetrazine
Phenmetrazine
Phentermine
Phenylephrine
Phenylethylamine
Phenylpropanolamine
Propylhexadrine
Pseudoephedrine

several countries including Japan and Sweden after World War II.[6] The 1950s and 1960s brought widespread abuse of amphetamines to the United States. Abuse was initially limited to use as an anorectic or as a stimulant in an effort to improve intellectual and physical performance or to combat fatigue.[7] A second pattern of abuse emerged later, with recreational use of amphetamines in an attempt to achieve a euphoric state.[7] In addition to oral use, nasal and intravenous routes were popularized at this time.

Large amounts of amphetamines were legally produced in the United States, peaking in 1965 with more than 10 billion pills (10,000 kg) manufactured.[7] Much of this amphetamine was diverted from legitimate pharmaceutical sales, mainly for the treatment of obesity, to illicit street use. Additional amphetamine-like compounds that have emerged have limited proven medical uses and varying abuse potential (Box 44-2). Compounds such as methamphetamine, propylhexedrine, aminorex fumarate, fenfluramine, and methylphenidate (Ritalin) are a few of these agents. After the passage of the Controlled Substances Act of 1970, manufacture and distribution of amphetamines were better regulated in the United States, and legal production was markedly reduced.[7]

The use of the phenethylamine derivative and amphetamine-like compound methylphenidate (Ritalin) has increased over the last 20 years primarily for the treatment of attention-deficit hyperactivity disorder (ADHD) in children and increasingly in adults. Toxic effects are similar to those of other amphetamines with agitation, tachycardia, and lethargy being the most common symptoms.[8] Exposures in children tend to be due to dosing errors or ingestion of a sibling's drug. Teenage and adult exposures tend to be associated with abuse or suicide attempts.

With reduced amounts of diverted pharmaceutical-grade amphetamines such as D-amphetamine (Dexedrine), large-scale illegal manufacture and illegal importation of amphetamines began. Methamphetamine is synthesized easily in crude street laboratories from readily available precursors such as L-ephedrine.[6] Methamphetamine provides illicit users with equal or longer acting stimulant and euphoric action than that of D-amphetamine. During the past 20 years, "designer" illicit amphetamines have enjoyed popularity on the street (see Box 44-2).

EPIDEMIOLOGY

Colorful names have been used to refer to methamphetamines on the street, including "meth," "speed," "crystal," and "crank." Studies in the late 1980s established the illicit manufacture of methamphetamine to be a 3 billion dollar per year industry in the United States, localized primarily in Hawaii, California, Oregon, and Texas.[1] By the early 1990s, the crude techniques had given way to illicit manufacturers who were able to synthesize very pure methamphetamine. A 99% to 100% pure form of methamphetamine called "ice" (because of

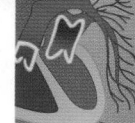

its purity) demonstrates increased volatility when heated. Inhaling these volatile vapors, or "smoking meth," provides the same "rush" as IV use of methamphetamine. Increasing use has been noted in many western states, and nearly epidemic use is reported in some parts of Hawaii and California.

Death associated with amphetamine use has been frequently reported the past 25 years to the present.[9-11] These deaths are often associated with assault, suicide, or homicide.[9,10] Cocaine was involved in one fifth and methamphetamine in about one eighth of all homicides in San Diego County in 1987.[12] By 1989, methamphetamine accounted for 60% of illicit drug seizures by San Diego County law enforcement agencies and 40% of all drug rehabilitation referrals in the area.[13] A large university teaching hospital in San Diego found an increase in the detection of amphetamine compounds on toxicology screens from 3% to 10% of all tests during a 7- to 8-year period.[14] Predominantly men (56%) between the ages of 21 and 30 years (61%) had positive results.[14] Between 1986 and 1988, a 1.7-fold increase in ED visits for methamphetamine abuse was reported nationwide.[13] White males that are unemployed and of low income are most likely to use methamphetamine.[15] Abuse of methcathinone, a cathinone-methamphetamine analog easily made as an oxidative product of ephedrine, has been widely reported in Russia and most recently in the midwestern United States. *p*-Methoxyamphetamine (PMA) is a substituted synthetic amphetamine used in the recreational drug culture including at "raves." A number of fatal overdoses of this drug have been reported in South Australia and the United States.[16-18]

Stimulants are used differently in different regions. In California in 2003, the DEA identified methamphetamine as the primary drug threat, with MDMA ("ecstasy") as the most popular "club" or "rave" drug.[19] The 2002 federal drug seizures in California alone included 9551 kg of cocaine and 311.2 kg of methamphetamine along with the destruction of 1718 clandestine drug laboratories. In contrast, in Florida in 2002, 26,258 kg of cocaine and only 103.1 kg of methamphetamine were seized. A 2000 report noted that more than 35 million individuals abuse amphetamines compared with approximately 15 million who regularly abuse cocaine worldwide.[20]

STRUCTURE AND STRUCTURE-ACTIVITY RELATIONSHIPS

As noted above, the various "designer" illicit amphetamines (see Box 44-2) have additional hallucinogenic properties gained by methoxyl group substitutions on the phenyl ring, especially at the 3,4 position (see Fig. 44-1). These drugs include agents such as 3,4-methylenedioxymethamphetamine (MDMA), 3,4-methylenedioxyamphetamine (MDA), and 2,5-dimethoxy-4-methylamphetamine (DOM). These agents have had intermittent popularity on the streets of various communities. The addition of the methyl group on the nitrogen of D-amphetamine generates methamphetamine, a longer

acting compound with more profound euphoric action. The appetite suppression effect is unchanged.

PHARMACOLOGY AND PATHOPHYSIOLOGY

Amphetamines have complicated and diverse pharmacologic mechanisms. They work primarily (as indirect sympathomimetics) by affecting the release of catecholamines at the neuronal presynaptic terminal.[1-3] Amphetamines and related compounds work indirectly to cause neuronal stimulation by increasing postsynaptic catecholamines. This is accomplished by blocking the presynaptic uptake transport activity from the synaptic cleft, by blocking presynaptic vesicular storage, and by reducing cytoplasmic destruction of catecholamines by inhibiting mitochondrial monoamine oxidase.[1-3] Together these activities increase the rate of postsynaptic receptor stimulation. Both central and peripheral norepinephrine and dopamine neurotransmitters are affected. Some amphetamine-related compounds (e.g., ephedrine) are thought also to have the ability to directly stimulate sympathetic receptors (direct sympathomimetics), but this is probably not a major mechanism of action for most of these compounds.[7] Amphetamines lack the local anesthetic effects of cocaine on cardiac and nervous tissue. The catecholamine toxicity of amphetamines is similar qualitatively to that of cocaine.

Increased norepinephrine postsynaptically causes sympathetic nervous system stimulation. This results in bronchodilation and increased heart rate, cardiac output, pupil size, and blood pressure, all of which are seen in the fight-or-flight response.[1] The central nervous system (CNS) effects of amphetamine appear to be mediated primarily by dopaminergic alterations, which cause changes in mood, excitation, motor movements, and appetite.[1] Some evidence suggests that repeated high-dose amphetamine exposure in both adults and fetuses or neonates results in long-lasting destruction or depletion of central dopamine neurons.[1] Further alteration in mood, psychotic behavior, and aggressiveness may be the result of CNS serotonin release or reuptake blockade.[2] The extent to which serotonin neurotransmission alterations function in the clinical manifestations of amphetamine toxicity is controversial.[1-3]

PHARMACOKINETICS

Amphetamines are weak bases with pK_a values around 8.8 to 10.4. For example, amphetamine has a pK_a of 9.9.[7,21] Amphetamines are easily absorbed across most biologic membranes including gut, airway, nasopharynx, muscle, and vagina. Peak plasma concentrations occur in minutes by the intravenous route, in about 30 minutes by the intramuscular or topical nasal route, and within 2 to 3 hours after ingestion.[7] Tissue redistribution is extensive, and the high lipid solubility of the amphetamines leads to increased concentrations relative to serum in the liver, kidneys, and lungs. This results in

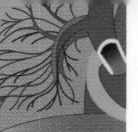

large volumes of distribution ranging from 3 to 6 L/kg for amphetamine, phentermine, and phenylephrine and 12 to 33 L/kg for fenfluramine and methylphenidate.[7]

Cerebrospinal fluid levels are about 80% of plasma levels at steady state. Therapeutic levels of amphetamine itself range between 30 and 40 ng/mL (0.030 to 0.040 mg/L), and death is associated with average levels of 8600 (range, 500 to 44,000) ng/mL in the blood.[7,21] Wide variations in doses and blood levels are reported to cause toxicity. This is in part related to the tolerance to amphetamines that can develop. The serum half-lives of various amphetamine-related compounds are urine pH dependent and range between 7 and 34 hours.[21] The more acidic the urine, the shorter the half-life because of reduced renal reabsorption of ionized urinary amphetamines. This leads to increased renal clearance of the iodized amphetamines.

Both active and inactive metabolites exist. Metabolism that results in aromatic hydroxylation, aliphatic hydroxylation, and *n*-dealkylation of amphetamines can give rise to active metabolites such as the potent hallucinogen *p*-hydroxyamphetamine.[7] Other metabolic pathways, including deamination and subsequent side chain oxidation, produce inactive amphetamine derivatives.[7] Glucuronide and glycine conjugation pathways result in urinary excretion of metabolites.[21] As much as 30% of amphetamine is excreted unchanged in the urine, whereas between 86% and 97% of ephedrine, pseudoephedrine, and phenylpropanolamine is excreted unchanged.[7,21]

Methylphenidate is metabolized by various pathways to ritalinic acid, *p*-hydroxymethylphenidate, or lactam. Increasing evidence suggests that the co-ingestion of ethanol and methylphenidate results in the novel metabolite ethylphenidate that may contribute to its toxicity.[22,23]

Concomitant use of drugs such as the opiates ("speedballing") can increase the overall toxicity of amphetamines. However, major alterations of the metabolic pathways of amphetamine have not been postulated as an explanation for the increased toxicity.[21] Simultaneous use of methamphetamine and ethanol has more psychological and cardiac effects than use of methamphetamine alone. This response also is presumed to be pharmacodynamic in nature rather than a result of any specific pharmacokinetic interaction.[24]

TOXICOLOGY

The amphetamines can cause toxic effects to every organ system. Both acute and chronic and direct and indirect abnormalities have been reported. Figure 44-2 summarizes the clinical presentation of acute amphetamine toxicity. The exact prevalence and incidence of the toxicities summarized in Box 44-1 have not been determined and probably vary with route, dose, and length of exposure to each of the amphetamine-related agents.

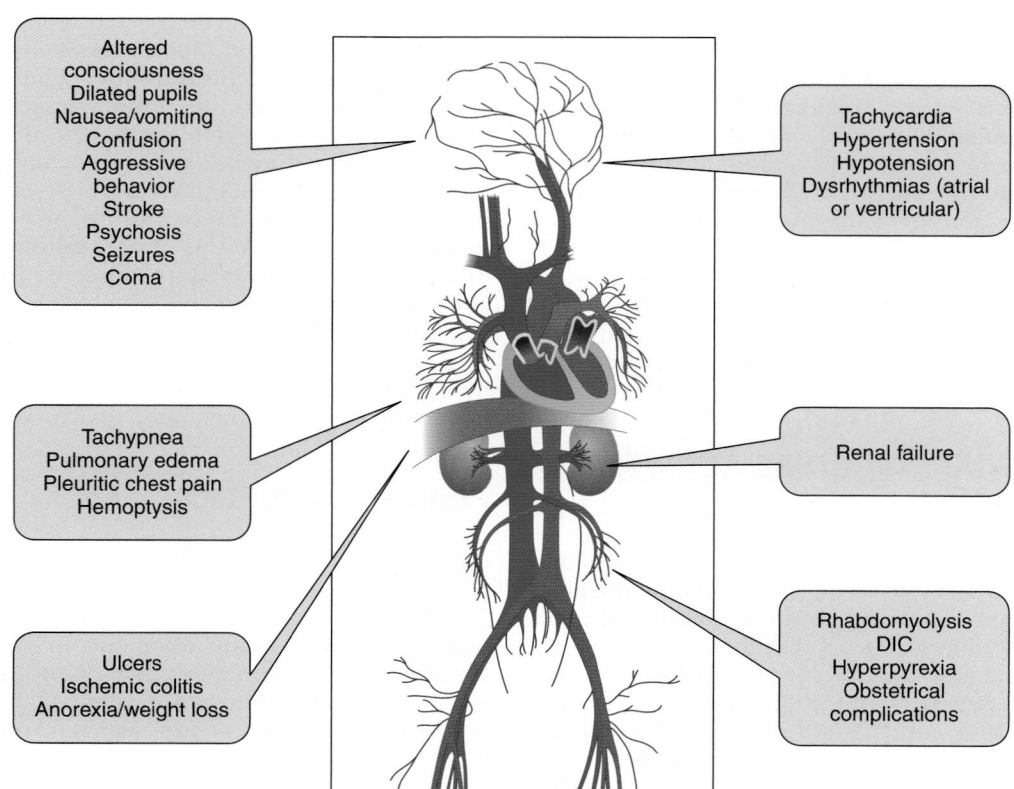

Altered consciousness
Dilated pupils
Nausea/vomiting
Confusion
Aggressive behavior
Stroke
Psychosis
Seizures
Coma

Tachycardia
Hypertension
Hypotension
Dysrhythmias (atrial or ventricular)

Tachypnea
Pulmonary edema
Pleuritic chest pain
Hemoptysis

Renal failure

Ulcers
Ischemic colitis
Anorexia/weight loss

Rhabdomyolysis
DIC
Hyperpyrexia
Obstetrical complications

FIGURE 44-2 Major signs and symptoms associated with acute amphetamine toxicity.

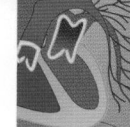

Central Nervous System Toxicity

The CNS is the target organ for the pharmacologic effects of most amphetamine-related compounds. As such, significant CNS toxicity can result from use of amphetamines. With the resurgence of amphetamines as drugs of abuse in the 1960s, it was quickly recognized that the initial sensation of extreme physical and mental powers following amphetamine use could rapidly deteriorate with high doses or chronic moderate doses to recurrent affective lability, confusion, and hallucinations.[25,26] In a series of 127 amphetamine-poisoned patients presenting to an ED, 57% were determined to have altered mental status.[27] Agitation, suicidal ideation, hallucinations, delusions, confusion, and despondent affect were the most common major signs and symptoms noted. The presenting manifestations of headache affected 4%, seizure 3%, and paresthesia 2%.[27] An additional 10% were unresponsive.[27]

Tolerance to the autonomic effects of amphetamine has been reported for body temperature, blood pressure, heart rate, and respirations. The anorectic effects of amphetamines exhibit tolerance as well.[28] In contrast, the motor stimulant and stereotypic behavior effects of amphetamine display progressive enhancement with repeated intermittent administration.[28] This is termed *behavioral sensitization* or *reverse tolerance.*

Researchers have postulated that the acute paranoid delusional psychosis associated with amphetamine use may produce a psychosis similar to schizophrenia that persists through behavioral sensitization long after elimination of the amphetamine.[29] Whether this represents emergence of an underlying psychiatric disorder or simply a lowering of the threshold for drug-induced psychosis is not known.[30,31] When challenged with large doses of IV methamphetamine, patients dependent on amphetamine developed drug-induced psychosis.[31] This same dose of methamphetamine failed to produce drug-induced psychosis in non–amphetamine users.[31] Drug-induced psychotic states have been reported with abuse of most of the stimulant amphetamine-related compounds, including cathinone, pemoline, and phenmetrazine.[32-34] Psychosis is common with derivatives of amphetamine that are hallucinogens, such as mescaline, DOM, MDA, *p*-methoxyamphetamine, and MDMA.[33] Although tolerance to the hallucinogenic properties of these agents has been noted, prolonged psychotic reactions are also well documented.[33] Acute severe hallucinations with bizarre and risky behavior due to the use of agents such as MDA, MDMA, and 3,4-methylenedioxyethamphetamine have resulted in traumatic deaths.[35] Mild to moderate amphetamine-induced agitated behavior and psychosis can be treated with benzodiazepines (e.g., diazepam or lorazepam), but severe symptoms should be treated with high-potency antipsychotic agents (e.g., haloperidol, droperidol, or thiothixene).[7,27,36] Minimizing sensory stimuli with low doses of benzodiazepines in combination with low doses of antipsychotic agents has been a useful approach to amphetamine-induced psychosis.

In addition to behavioral effects including agitation, hallucinations, and psychosis, amphetamine use is associated with several other neurologic toxicities. Amphetamine-induced changes in sexual function and performance including enhancement and inhibition are complicated and have been reviewed.[37]

Cases of juvenile parkinsonism associated with MDMA have been reported.[38] Positron-emission tomography (PET) scans suggest that amphetamine compounds have profiles of binding to the dopamine transporter and changes in synaptic dopamine levels similar to cocaine.[39] The chorea of patients with Huntington's disease is exacerbated by use of amphetamines.[40] The dopaminergic receptor blocker haloperidol was shown to inhibit the amphetamine-induced exacerbation of the choreoathetoid movements.[40] Choreoathetoid movement disorders have also been seen with acute and chronic amphetamine exposures in patients who do not have Huntington's disease.[41,42] Treatment of acute amphetamine-induced choreoathetoid movement disorders includes supportive care, gastrointestinal decontamination with activated charcoal, and administration of haloperidol.[41]

Seizures have been reported with severe intoxications of amphetamine and related compounds.[27,43-45] The seizures have been isolated or associated with hyperpyrexia, coma, metabolic acidosis, and shock. IV benzodiazepines (e.g., diazepam, lorazepam), phenytoin, and barbiturates (e.g., pentobarbital, amobarbital) have been used to terminate amphetamine-induced seizures.[7,44]

Intracerebral hemorrhage is associated with the use of amphetamines and related compounds. Amphetamine-related cerebral hemorrhage has occurred in patients with arteriovenous malformations[46] and drug-induced cerebral vasculitis.[47-50] Both oral and IV amphetamine exposures have resulted in cases of cerebral vasculitis.[47-51] Traditional approaches to intracerebral hemorrhage have focused on supportive care, correction of the hypotension, use of corticosteroids, and employment of antifibrinolytic agents such as ε-aminocaproic acid.[47-50] Treatment directed at the vasculitis in these cases has included use of dexamethasone and cyclophosphamide therapy.[47,48] The efficacy of these agents in the treatment of amphetamine-associated vasculitis is unknown.

Ischemic strokes have been reported with amphetamine compounds taken orally, intravenously, and by inhalation.[52] Supportive care and hypervolemic hemodilution therapy using albumin or 10% dextran 40 has been advocated after angiographic demonstration of cerebral artery spasm and occlusion.[52] Elective extracranial/intracranial bypass was performed in at least one case of amphetamine-associated occlusive stroke, but its efficacy is unproved.[52] A case of transient cortical blindness in an infant exposed to methamphetamine has been reported.[53] The blindness resolved within 12 hours without specific therapy. It was postulated to represent a manifestation of amphetamine-induced cerebral vasospasm.[53]

Methamphetamine neurotoxicity in human abuse is thought to be in part due to necrotic and apoptotic mechanisms.[54] The central nervous system is the main

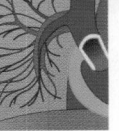

target of the pharmacologic actions of the amphetamines and is also the most frequent organ system to manifest amphetamine-induced toxicity.

Cardiovascular System Toxicity

In a retrospective study of patients with amphetamine toxicity presenting to an ED, hypertension and tachycardia were commonly encountered. The same study found that patients complained of chest pain 9% and palpitations 3% of the time.[27] Direct pharmacologic effects of the amphetamines most likely account for the frequently encountered hypertension and the tachycardia. In a double-blind, placebo-controlled study of eight healthy adults, modest doses of MDMA increased heart rate, blood pressure, and myocardial oxygen consumption in a magnitude similar to that of dobutamine without causing the positive inotropic effects of dobutamine.[55] Hypertension and agitated behavior associated with amphetamine use are initially approached by minimizing stimulus or sensory inputs and by using sedating agents. If more specific treatment is needed, the use of IV nitroprusside or oral or IV calcium channel blockers (e.g., nifedipine or nicardipine) may be indicated. β blockers should not be used in the treatment of amphetamine-induced hypertension without concomitant α blockade, because unopposed α blockade can produce intense vasospasm and paradoxical hypertension.

Appetite suppressants and amphetamine derivatives have been associated with an increased risk of cardiac valvular insufficiency.[56-58] The use of fenfluramine or dexfenfluramine for 4 months or longer was associated with an increased risk of valvular changes.[59] Fenfluramine has been used with the phenylethylamine derivative phentermine (Fen-Phen) extensively to suppress appetite. By 1997, reports of aortic mitral regurgitation associated with the use of these drugs surfaced. The mechanism of this effect is unknown; incidence estimates vary from less than 1% to greater than 20% after exposure to Fen-Phen for more than 4 months.[60,61] Some echocardiographic improvement with cessation of use has been noted. These findings coupled with evidence of associated pulmonary hypertension resulted in the removal of fenfluramine from the market.

Ectopic ventricular beats as well as supraventricular and ventricular tachyarrhythmias have been reported with amphetamine use. Direct catecholamine effects and ischemic effects secondary to coronary vasospasm generated by amphetamine use are probably responsible for the arrhythmias.[62] Although not normally studied, short-acting β-adrenergic receptor blockers (e.g., esmolol), calcium channel blockers (e.g., verapamil, diltiazem), or lidocaine can be used to treat these arrhythmias. Correction of hypoxia and electrolyte abnormalities also is required.

Myocardial infarction associated with amphetamine use is thought to be secondary to direct cardiac toxicity (myocarditis), vasospasm, and thrombus formation.[62,63] Cardiac irritability and myocardial infarction in a 13-year-old has been reported after amphetamine overdose.[64] In addition to treatment with nitrates and analgesics, at least one report describes the use of thrombolytics in treating amphetamine-induced myocardial infarctions.[63] Profound hypotension, bradycardia, and metabolic acidosis have occurred with massive amphetamine overdoses. Treatment includes aggressive hemodynamic support with intravascular volume replacement and vasopressor agents (e.g., norepinephrine or phenylephrine). Direct-acting catecholamines (norepinephrine or phenylephrine rather than dopamine) are preferred because massive overdoses may result in a relative catecholamine-depleted state.

Both acute and chronic cardiomyopathies have been associated with amphetamine use. This effect is thought to be secondary to direct amphetamine toxicity and indirect hypertension.[65] Treatment includes avoidance of amphetamines, use of diuretics and digoxin, and afterload reduction (e.g., nitroprusside acutely and angiotensin-converting enzyme inhibitors such as captopril for long-term use).[66] IV amphetamine use is associated with bacterial endocarditis, which can lead to abnormal cardiac valves, dilated cardiomyopathy, and formation of mycotic aneurysms. Acute aortic dissection, necrotizing angiitis, and both visceral and cerebral aneurysms have also been reported to occur in amphetamine users.[62,67]

Arterial or tissue-extravasated amphetamine quickly leads to tissue ischemia. Immediate intra-arterial or local tissue injection of α-adrenergic blocking agents such as phentolamine or phenoxybenzamine is indicated to reverse the local vasopressor effects of amphetamines. General supportive or symptomatic care is most important to maintain the cardiac system during acute amphetamine toxicity.

Pulmonary System Toxicity

Respiratory symptoms including chest pain and dyspnea have been presenting complaints of patients with amphetamine toxicity presenting to an ED.[27] The actual incidence of respiratory toxicity with amphetamines is not known. The incidence and types of toxicity may vary, depending on the amphetamine compound and the route of exposure. One review examined pulmonary effects of exposure to amphetamine-related compounds.[68] Although amphetamines are often snorted, inhaled, and smoked, the literature does not note an association with barotrauma. On the other hand, a few case reports have associated cocaine, which has similar routes of administration, with barotrauma.[68]

Despite increased use of inhaled or smoked methamphetamine, no extensive reports of exacerbation of reactive airway disease have been noted. In comparison, the association between asthma and cocaine, which has similar pharmacologic properties and patterns of abuse to methamphetamine, is much stronger. One death due to asthma has been reported with the use of the hallucinogenic amphetamine MDMA.[35] In that case, a young man was found dead clutching an inhaler and had pathologic features of asthma at postmortem examination. The contribution of his MDMA use to his

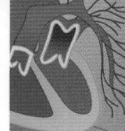

asthma death is speculative. Thirteen patients in two small case series have noted obstructive findings associated with 20% to 60% reductions in carbon monoxide diffusion capacity after IV methylphenidate use.[69,70] These patients showed variable responses to β-adrenergic agonist bronchodilators (e.g., albuterol) and were noted to have panlobular emphysema. Foreign particle embolization from IV dosing of methylphenidate was postulated as the cause rather than a direct drug effect, as similar findings have been found with other IV drugs (e.g., methadone).[68,71]

Case reports describe acute noncardiogenic pulmonary edema associated with amphetamine toxicity.[68] Not only smoking but also ingesting amphetamines has been associated with the development of pulmonary edema.[72] At least one death with pulmonary edema has been related to the use of MDMA.[35] Animal data suggest, at least in part, a direct amphetamine toxicity leading to leaky pulmonary capillaries partly mediated by free-radical and oxidant injury.[73] Alternatively, edema may occur owing to indirect neurogenic (e.g., seizure) or cardiovascular (e.g., shock, hydrostatic leak) consequences. Although noncardiogenic pulmonary edema with cocaine abuse is reported more frequently in the literature than with amphetamine abuse, its mechanism also has not been determined and may be similar.[68]

The literature has for some time described amphetamine use associated with pulmonary hypertension. Users of IV amphetamines obtained from nasal inhalers available until the 1960s were noted to have pulmonary artery foreign body granulomas and muscle hypertrophy.[4,68] Long-term inhalation of methamphetamine and propylhexedrine also has been associated with marked pulmonary hypertension at autopsy in at least one case and in a second case of sudden death.[74,75] Proposed mechanisms include direct toxic endothelial injury caused by the drugs or their contaminants, recurrent hypoxic insults, direct spasm in genetically determined sensitive hosts, vasculitis, and dysregulation of the mediators of vascular tone such as nitric oxide. The amphetamine-like anorectic agents fenfluramine and aminorex fumarate have also been associated with several European reports of pulmonary hypertension.[68] Pulmonary artery vasodilation and remodeling agents have been used for these drug-induced cases of pulmonary hypertension, along with the avoidance of stimulants and supportive care, including supplemental oxygen for hypoxic patients.

With the increased incidence of smoking methamphetamine, the authors have noted pulmonary toxicities similar to those reported with the use of the stimulant crack cocaine. These include hemoptysis, alveolar hemorrhage, and alveolar accumulation of carbonaceous material associated with cough, bronchitis, sinusitis, and thermal epiglottitis.[68] Basic airway management and supportive care are the only approaches to these complications. In severe cases of amphetamine-induced pulmonary edema, aggressive mechanical ventilatory support with the addition of positive end-expiratory pressure and high levels of inspired oxygen flow often are required.

Systemic Toxicity

Severe systemic toxicity has been reported with overdoses of amphetamine-related compounds. A pattern of fulminant hyperthermia, convulsions, disseminated intravascular coagulation (DIC), hepatocellular damage, rhabdomyolysis, acute renal failure, arrhythmias, and refractory hypotension has been seen with use of MDMA.[43]

Hyperthermia, shock, pulmonary edema, rhabdomyolysis, acute renal failure, and DIC have been encountered with use of "designer" amphetamines as well as with phenmetrazine and methamphetamine.[43,45,76-78] In certain parts of the country, trauma may have a high association with methamphetamine. Severe metabolic acidosis associated with methamphetamine use has exaggerated the estimated severity of the injury in trauma patients.[79] Aggressive cooling, cardiopulmonary support, large amounts of intravascular volume replacement, electrolyte replacement, temperature control measures, and early extracorporeal hemodialysis are needed to overcome the amphetamine-induced hyperthermia with severe rhabdomyolysis in these patients.[43,76] If cooling and sedation do not control the hyperthermia, then neuromuscular blockade and mechanical ventilation may be needed.[77] This combination of severe systemic toxicity from amphetamines appears to predict a poor outcome.

Hepatotoxicity with hepatocellular damage has occurred with use of MDMA and other amphetamines.[80-82] Postulated mechanisms for the hepatotoxicity include direct toxic effects, lipid peroxidation, necrotizing angiitis, contaminants, hypotension, and genetic variations in metabolism, which create toxic intermediates. Treatment consists of supportive care and avoidance of amphetamines. At least one liver transplant has been attempted.[43] To further complicate this issue, a case of thrombocytopenic purpura after MDMA-induced acute liver failure has been reported.[83]

In addition to the severe systemic toxicities described above, reversible ischemic colitis induced by methamphetamine abuse has been reported. Abdominal pain was the presenting complaint in 4% of amphetamine-poisoned patients presenting to an ED.[27] The exact incidence of amphetamine-related ischemic bowel and hemorrhagic colitis in abusers of amphetamines is unknown.[84] Diagnostic efforts to rule out necrotic bowel would be prudent in amphetamine-associated cases of persistent abdominal pain, particularly with bloody stools. Giant gastric and duodenal ulcers are strongly associated with methamphetamine use.[85]

Skin changes including lichenoid drug eruptions and burns complicated by "rave" use of amphetamine derivatives have been noted.[86,87]

Obstetric and Prenatal Toxicity

Gestational exposure to amphetamines has been postulated but not proved to have lasting effects on neonates.[88] After illicit amphetamine exposure, infants have had hypoglycemia, sweating, poor feeding, poor visual tracking, and seizures.[88] As with cocaine exposure,

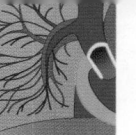

fetal amphetamine exposure was associated with intrauterine growth retardation, decreased head circumference, preterm delivery with fetal distress, anemia, and placental abruption in one study.[88] An amphetamine withdrawal pattern similar to that of cocaine withdrawal was noted in these infants. This pattern consisted of abnormal sleep patterns, tremors, hypertonia, high-pitched cry, poor feeding, vomiting, sneezing, frantic sucking, and tachycardia.[89] Although long-term behavioral and neurologic follow-up of these infants is not yet available, early reports suggest that chaotic lifestyles with minor neurologic abnormalities continue for these infants after discharge from the hospital.[88] Other studies have reported reduced birth weight with methamphetamine exposure relative to normal populations but no increase in other adverse outcomes.[89] In a report of eight cases of fetal and infant deaths, blood levels of methamphetamine averaged 0.36 µg/mL (range, 0.03 to 1.20 µg/mL).[90]

A large retrospective study in the United States and Canada of vasoactive compounds such as pseudoephedrine, phenylpropanolamine, ephedrine, and methylenedioxymethamphetamine exposure during the first 2.5 months of pregnancy resulted in doubling the risk of gastroschisis and small intestinal atresia.[91] Combination exposure to vasoactive drugs and 20 or more cigarettes per day increased the risk with an odds ratio of 3.6 (1.3 to 10.3) for gastroschisis and 4.2 (1.1 to 16.2) for small bowel atresia.[91] One hypothesis is that these small intestine defects are the result of vascular disruption by toxins in early gestation.

Pregnant women exposed to amphetamines are at increased risk of serious obstetric complications, including intracranial hemorrhage, seizures, and amniotic fluid embolism.[89] No specific therapy has been identified for neonates or pregnant women heavily exposed to amphetamines. Identification of at-risk women before pregnancy and during prenatal care would afford an opportunity to educate. Unfortunately, many pregnant women using amphetamines do not seek prenatal care and may be unable or unwilling to reduce their gestational exposures.

DIAGNOSIS

The clinician should consider the diagnosis of toxicity from amphetamine-related compounds in the differential diagnosis when behavioral stimulation is coupled to evidence of catecholamine excess. Inadvertent exposure to amphetamines can occur in pediatric patients, particularly around adults participating in illegal manufacture and distribution.

Urine screening tests primarily utilizing immunoassay techniques exist for amphetamine-related compounds and are often part of "drug abuse" screens.[92] Confirmation of urine and blood samples is made by a gas chromatography coupled with mass spectroscopy (GC-MS) analysis.[93] Urine can remain positive for greater than 48 hours after exposure depending on route, rate of absorption, urine pH, and hydration status.[94] Many

laboratories used to monitor persons in sensitive occupations have thresholds for reporting positive amphetamine results in the urine. Drug detected below these thresholds is not reported. Some laboratories require the D-isomer of methamphetamine to be present along with detectable amphetamine (a metabolite) to report a urine sample positive for methamphetamine. For example, selegiline is metabolized to L-amphetamine and L-methamphetamine (both have minimal toxicity) and will be reported as positive for methamphetamine unless an isomer analysis is performed.[95] Other drugs such as clobenzorex, a Mexican anorectic drug, are metabolized to actual D-amphetamine and will give a positive result on confirmation by GC-MS analysis.[96] Infrared transmission spectroscopy has been used to detect methamphetamines.[97] A rapid-detection, nonaqueous capillary electrophoresis-fluorescence spectroscopy method for MDMA has been reported.[98] The use of hair analysis for amphetamine-related compounds has also been reported but is of little use clinically because of interlaboratory variability.[99-102]

MANAGEMENT

An algorithm for the general approach to a suspected amphetamine-poisoned patient is shown in Table 44-1. No prospective human trials have evaluated different treatment options. Most recommendations are based on animal studies or case reports of humans. For example, the efficacy of activated charcoal in treating oral methamphetamine exposure has been demonstrated in a study in mice but lacks human trials.[103] Early recommendations to acidify the urine in amphetamine overdoses were based on a single case.[104] The risks of systemic acidification and the potential problems for the kidneys when rhabdomyolysis is present have prevented this recommendation from being widely adopted until controlled trials have demonstrated improved patient outcomes. Clinicians must be aware of the problem of contaminants in addition to the direct toxic effects of amphetamines. A cluster of at least 14 cases of acute lead poisoning was found in IV methamphetamine users in Oregon in 1988. Amphetamine products manufactured in clandestine laboratories may be grossly contaminated with toxic heavy metals and chemicals. In addition, the authors have noticed a cluster of 20 cases of acute botulism poisoning associated with illicit drug use.[105,106]

General supportive care; decontamination of the gastrointestinal tract with activated charcoal for ingestions; and control of behavior, seizures, arrhythmias, and temperature remain the mainstay of therapy for amphetamine-poisoned patients. An animal model failed to demonstrate the utility of multiple doses of activated charcoal after IV methamphetamine.[107] In the absence of renal failure, dialysis and hemoperfusion have no role in amphetamine overdose. Specific measures when available for each complication associated with amphetamine use have been mentioned above. Vaccines and antibodies directed against methamphetamine are currently under development to treat overdoses and long-term drug

TABLE 44-1 Amphetamine and Related Compound Toxicity and Treatment and Decision Algorithm

Suspected Amphetamine Toxicity

MILD AMPHETAMINE TOXICITY

Evaluate
Decontamination of oral ingestions/activated
  charcoal
Observe
Psychologic support/environmental control
Health care maintenance
  HIV testing
  Hepatitis screening, etc.

SEVERE AMPHETAMINE TOXICITY

Immediate Supportive Care
Airway control
Oxygenation
Vascular access
Appropriate monitoring

Decontaminate/Antagonists
Oral ingestion/activated charcoal
Consider empirical 50% dextrose, thiamine,
  naloxone
Avoid benzodiazepine antagonists

Terminate Seizures
Benzodiazepines (e.g., diazepam, lorazepam)
Barbiturates (e.g., pentobarbital, phenobarbital)

Control Severe Psychotic Agitation
Minimize sensory stimulation
Benzodiazepines (e.g., diazepam, lorazepam)
Butyrophenones (e.g., droperidol, haloperidol)
Protect from aggressive or self-destructive
  behavior

*Correct Immediate Metabolic, Oxygenation,
  and Electrolyte Abnormalities*
Avoid acidification of the urine

*Local α blockers for Exuded or Intra-Arterial
  Amphetamines (e.g., Phenoxybenzamine,
  Phentolamine)*

Treat Hyperthermia
Passive/active cooling measure

Treat Arrhythmias
Antiarrhythmic (e.g., lidocaine)
Supraventricular arrhythmias (e.g., esmolol)
Electrolyte correction
Acid–base/oxygenation correction

*Second-Level Evaluations to Check for
Persistent Abnormalities*

EVALUATE FOR OTHER AGENTS

Initiate specific treatment
  for additional agents
Consider interactions with
  amphetamine
Monitor for early and late
  toxicities of other agents

Persistent Hypotension

Intravascular volume resuscitation
Acute cardiopulmonary support
Central hemodynamic monitoring

Pulmonary Edema/Respiratory Failure
Ventilator
Oxygen
Positive end-expiratory pressure

Rhabdomyolysis
Alkalize urine (e.g., intravenous bicarbonate)
Calcium replacement (e.g., calcium gluconate)
Intravascular volume

Renal Failure/Rhabdomyolysis/Renal Ischemia
Hemodialysis
Intravascular volume

Supportive Care

Observation/monitoring
Psychologic and pharmacologic support for
  amphetamine abstinence and long-term
  recovery
Health maintenance/education (e.g., HIV and
  hepatitis testing)
Coronary Artery Ishemia
Calcium channel blockers (e.g., nifedipine,
  diltiazem)
β blockers (e.g., esmolol, metoprolol)
Nitrates (e.g., nitroglycerin)
Hypertension
Sedation (e.g., diazepam, haloperidol)
Calcium channel blockers (e.g., nifedipine,
  nicardipine)
β blockers (e.g., esmolol)
Nitroprusside
Electrolyte Abnormalities
Correct hypokalemia (e.g., potassium chloride)
Correct hypocalcemia (e.g., calcium gluconate)
Correct hypoglycemia (e.g., dextrose as D_{50})

*Central Nervous System
Abnormality*
Seizures
Strokes
Bleeds
Vasculitis
Agitation

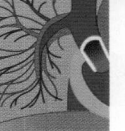

abuse.[108] Infectious diseases should be considered. Patients should be evaluated for complications attendant to IV drug abuse such as bacterial endocarditis, viral hepatitis, and human immunodeficiency virus. Once the acute symptoms of amphetamine poisoning have passed, treating physicians should consider referring patients for rehabilitation or psychiatric care to break up the destructive drug abuse pattern.

REFERENCES

1. Cho AK: Ice: a new dosage form of an old drug. Science 1990;249:631–634.
2. Gawin FH, Ellinwood EH Jr: Cocaine and other stimulants: actions, abuse, and treatment. N Engl J Med 1988;318:1173–1182.
3. Piness G, Miller H, Alles GA: Clinical observations on phenylaminoethanol sulfate. JAMA 1930;94:790–791.
4. Anderson RJ, Reed WG, Hillis LD, et al: History, epidemiology, and medical complications of nasal inhaler abuse. J Toxicol Clin Toxicol 1982;19:95–107.
5. Myerson A: Effect of benzedrine sulphate on mood and fatigue in normal and in neurotic persons. Arch Neurol Psychiatry 1936;36:816–822.
6. Derlet RW, Heischober B: Methamphetamine. Stimulant of the 1990s? West J Med 1990;153:625–628.
7. Linden CH, Kulig KW, Rumack BH: Amphetamines. Top Emerg Med 1985;7:18–32.
8. Klein-Schwartz W: Abuse and toxicity of methylphenidate. Curr Opin Pediatr 2002;14:219–223.
9. Ellinwood EH Jr: Assault and homicide associated with amphetamine abuse. Am J Psychiatry 1971;127:1170–1175.
10. Kalant H, Kalant OJ: Death in amphetamine users: causes and rates. Can Med Assoc J 1975;112:299–304.
11. Katsumata S, Sato K, Kashiwade H, et al: Sudden death due presumably to internal use of methamphetamine. Forensic Sci Int 1993;62:209–215.
12. Bailey DN, Shaw RF: Cocaine- and methamphetamine-related deaths in San Diego County (1987): homicides and accidental overdoses. J Forensic Sci 1989;34:407–422.
13. Beebe DK, Walley E: Smokable methamphetamine ("ice"): an old drug in a different form. Am Fam Physician 1995;51:449–453.
14. Bailey DN: Amphetamine detection during toxicology screening of a university medical center patient population. J Toxicol Clin Toxicol 1987;25:399–409.
15. Wermuth L: Methamphetamine use: hazards and social influences. J Drug Educ 2000;30:423–433.
16. Caldicott DG, Edwards NA, Kruys A, et al: Dancing with "death": p-methoxyamphetamine overdose and its acute management. J Toxicol Clin Toxicol 2003;41:143–154.
17. Kraner JC, McCoy DJ, Evans MA, et al: Fatalities caused by the MDMA-related drug paramethoxyamphetamine (PMA). J Anal Toxicol 2001;25:645–648.
18. Martin TL: Three cases of fatal paramethoxyamphetamine overdose. J Anal Toxicol 2001;25:649–651.
19. U.S. Drug Enforcement Agency: http://www.dea.gov/pubs/states/california.html. Accessed 1/6/05.
20. Rawson RA, Gonzales R, Brethen P: Treatment of methamphetamine use disorders: an update. J Subst Abuse Treat 2002;23:145–150.
21. Baselt RC, Cravey RH: Amphetamine. In Disposition of Toxic Drugs and Chemicals in Man. Foster City, CA, Chemical Toxicology Insitute, 1995, pp 44–47.
22. Markowitz JS, DeVane CL, Boulton DW, et al: Ethylphenidate formation in human subjects after the administration of a single dose of methylphenidate and ethanol. Drug Metab Dispos 2000;28:620–624.
23. Markowitz JS, Logan BK, Diamond F, Patrick KS: Detection of the novel metabolite ethylphenidate after methylphenidate overdose with alcohol coingestion. J Clin Psychopharmacol 1999;19:362–366.
24. Mendelson J, Jones RT, Upton R, Jacob P III: Methamphetamine and ethanol interactions in humans. Clin Pharmacol Ther 1995;57:559–568.
25. Kramer JC, Fischman VS, Littlefield DC: Amphetamine abuse: pattern and effects of high doses taken intravenously. JAMA 1967;201:305–309.
26. Smith DE, Fischer CM: An analysis of 310 cases of acute high-dose methamphetamine toxicity in Haight-Ashbury. Clin Toxicol 1970;3:117–124.
27. Derlet RW, Rice P, Horowitz BZ, Lord RV: Amphetamine toxicity: experience with 127 cases. J Emerg Med 1989;7:157–161.
28. Robinson TE, Becker JB: Enduring changes in brain and behavior produced by chronic amphetamine administration: a review and evaluation of animal models of amphetamine psychosis. Brain Res 1986;396:157–198.
29. Sato M: A lasting vulnerability to psychosis in patients with previous methamphetamine psychosis. Ann N Y Acad Sci 1992;654:160–170.
30. Ellinwood EH: Amphetamine Psychosis. 1. Description of the individuals and process. J Nerv Ment Dis 1967;144:273–283.
31. Bell DS: The experimental reproduction of amphetamine psychosis. Arch Gen Psychiatry 1973;29:35–40.
32. Polchert SE, Morse RM: Pemoline abuse. JAMA 1985;254:946–947.
33. Castellani S, Petrie W, Ellinwood E: Drug-induced psychosis: neurobiological mechanisms. In Alterman A (ed): Substance Abuse and Psychopathology. New York, Plenum Press, 1985, pp 173–210.
34. Schechter MD, Glennon RA: Cathinone, cocaine and meth-amphetamine: similarity of behavioral effects. Pharmacol Biochem Behav 1985;22:913–916.
35. Dowling GP, McDonough ET, Bost RO: "Eve" and "Ecstasy": a report of five deaths associated with the use of MDEA and MDMA. JAMA 1987;257:1615–1617.
36. Dubin WR, Weiss KJ, Dorn JM: Pharmacotherapy of psychiatric emergencies. J Clin Psychopharmacol 1986;6:210–222.
37. Meston CM, Gorzalka BB: Psychoactive drugs and human sexual behavior: the role of serotonergic activity. J Psychoactive Drugs 1992;24:1–40.
38. Kuniyoshi SM, Jankovic J: MDMA and parkinsonism. N Engl J Med 2003;349:96–97.
39. Fowler JS, Volkow ND: PET imaging studies in drug abuse. J Toxicol Clin Toxicol 1998;36:163–174.
40. Klawans HL, Weiner WJ: The pharmacology of choreatic movement disorders. Prog Neurobiol 1976;6:49–80.
41. Rhee KJ, Albertson TE, Douglas JC: Choreoathetoid disorder associated with amphetamine-like drugs. Am J Emerg Med 1988;6:131–133.
42. Lundh H, Tunving K: An extrapyramidal choreiform syndrome caused by amphetamine addiction. J Neurol Neurosurg Psychiatry 1981;44:728–730.
43. Henry JA, Jeffreys KJ, Dawling S: Toxicity and deaths from 3,4-methylenedioxymethamphetamine ("ecstasy"). Lancet 1992;340:384–387.
44. Simpson D, Rumack B: Methylenedioxyamphetamine clinical description of overdose, death, and review of pharmacology. Arch Intern Med 1987;141:1507–1509.
45. Chan P, Chen JH, Lee MH, Deng JF: Fatal and nonfatal methamphetamine intoxication in the intensive care unit. J Toxicol Clin Toxicol 1994;32:147–155.
46. Lukes SA: Intracerebral hemorrhage from an arteriovenous malformation after amphetamine injection. Arch Neurol 1983;40:60–61.
47. Salanova V, Taubner R: Intracerebral haemorrhage and vasculitis secondary to amphetamine use. Postgrad Med J 1984;60:429–430.
48. Matick H, Anderson D, Brumlik J: Cerebral vasculitis associated with oral amphetamine overdose. Arch Neurol 1983;40:253–254.
49. Hughes JC, McCabe M, Evans RJ: Intracranial haemorrhage associated with ingestion of "ecstasy." Arch Emerg Med 1993;10:372–374.
50. Conci F, D'Angelo V, Tampieri D, Vecchi G: Intracerebral hemorrhage and angiographic beading following amphetamine abuse. Ital J Neurol Sci 1988;9:77–81.
51. Brorholt-Petersen JU, Christensen HR: (Fatal intracerebral hemorrhage after amphetamine intake). Ugeskr Laeger 2000;162:4156–4157.
52. Rothrock JF, Rubenstein R, Lyden PD: Ischemic stroke associated with methamphetamine inhalation. Neurology 1988;38:589–592.

53. Gospe SM Jr: Transient cortical blindness in an infant exposed to methamphetamine. Ann Emerg Med 1995;26:380–382.

54. Davidson C, Gow AJ, Lee TH, Ellinwood EH: Methamphetamine neurotoxicity: necrotic and apoptotic mechanisms and relevance to human abuse and treatment. Brain Res Brain Res Rev 2001;36:1–22.

55. Lester SJ, Baggott M, Welm S, et al: Cardiovascular effects of 3,4-methylenedioxymethamphetamine. A double-blind, placebo-controlled trial. Ann Intern Med 2000;133:969–973.

56. Khan MA, Herzog CA, St Peter JV, et al: The prevalence of cardiac valvular insufficiency assessed by transthoracic echocardiography in obese patients treated with appetite-suppressant drugs. N Engl J Med 1998;339:713–718.

57. Weissman NJ, Tighe JF Jr, Gottdiener JS, Gwynne JT: An assessment of heart-valve abnormalities in obese patients taking dexfenfluramine, sustained-release dexfenfluramine, or placebo. Sustained-Release Dexfenfluramine Study Group. N Engl J Med 1998;339:725–732.

58. Devereux RB: Appetite suppressants and valvular heart disease. N Engl J Med 1998;339:765–766.

59. Jick H, Vasilakis C, Weinrauch LA, et al: A population-based study of appetite-suppressant drugs and the risk of cardiac-valve regurgitation. N Engl J Med 1998;339:719–724.

60. Gardin JM, Schumacher D, Constantine G, et al: Valvular abnormalities and cardiovascular status following exposure to dexfenfluramine or phentermine/fenfluramine. JAMA 2000;283:1703–1709.

61. Wee CC, Phillips RS, Aurigemma G, et al: Risk for valvular heart disease among users of fenfluramine and dexfenfluramine who underwent echocardiography before use of medication. Ann Intern Med 1998;129:870–874.

62. Davis GG, Swalwell CI: Acute aortic dissections and ruptured berry aneurysms associated with methamphetamine abuse. J Forensic Sci 1994;39:1481–1485.

63. Furst SR, Fallon SP, Reznik GN, Shah PK: Myocardial infarction after inhalation of methamphetamine (letter). N Engl J Med 1990;323:1147–1148.

64. Sztajnkrycer MD, Hariharan S, Bond GR: Cardiac irritability and myocardial infarction in a 13-year-old girl following recreational amphetamine overdose. Pediatr Emerg Care 2002;18:E11–E15.

65. Frishman WH, Del Vecchio A, Sanal S, Ismail A: Cardiovascular manifestations of substance abuse. 2. Alcohol, amphetamines, heroin, cannabis, and caffeine. Heart Dis 2003;5:253–271.

66. Hong R, Matsuyama E, Nur K: Cardiomyopathy associated with the smoking of crystal methamphetamine. JAMA 1991;265:1152–1154.

67. Swalwell CI, Davis GG: Methamphetamine as a risk factor for acute aortic dissection. J Forensic Sci 1999;44:23–26.

68. Albertson TE, Walby WF, Derlet RW: Stimulant-induced pulmonary toxicity. Chest 1995;108:1140–1149.

69. Schmidt RA, Glenny RW, Godwin JD, et al: Panlobular emphysema in young intravenous Ritalin abusers. Am Rev Respir Dis 1991;143:649–656.

70. Sherman CB, Hudson LD, Pierson DJ: Severe precocious emphysema in intravenous methylphenidate (Ritalin) abusers. Chest 1987;92:1085–1087.

71. Pare JP, Cote G, Fraser RS: Long-term follow-up of drug abusers with intravenous talcosis. Am Rev Respir Dis 1989;139:233–241.

72. Maury E, Darondel JM, Buisinne A, et al: Acute pulmonary edema following amphetamine ingestion. Intensive Care Med 1999;25:332–333.

73. Huang KL, Shaw KP, Wang D, et al: Free radicals mediate amphetamine-induced acute pulmonary edema in isolated rat lung. Life Sci 2002;71:1237–1244.

74. Nishida N, Ikeda N, Kudo K, Esaki R: Sudden unexpected death of a methamphetamine abuser with cardiopulmonary abnormalities: a case report. Med Sci Law 2003;43:267–271.

75. Schaiberger PH, Kennedy TC, Miller FC, et al: Pulmonary hypertension associated with long-term inhalation of "crank" methamphetamine. Chest 1993;104:614–616.

76. Kendrick WC, Hull AR, Knochel JP: Rhabdomyolysis and shock after intravenous amphetamine administration. Ann Intern Med 1977;86:381–387.

77. Callaway CW, Clark RF: Hyperthermia in psychostimulant overdose. Ann Emerg Med 1994;24:68–76.

78. Wallace ME, Squires R: Fatal massive amphetamine ingestion associated with hyperpyrexia. J Am Board Fam Pract 2000;13:302–304.

79. Burchell SA, Ho HC, Yu M, Margulies DR: Effects of methamphetamine on trauma patients: a cause of severe metabolic acidosis? Crit Care Med 2000;28:2112–2115.

80. Jones AL, Jarvie DR, McDermid G, Proudfoot AT: Hepatocellular damage following amphetamine intoxication. J Toxicol Clin Toxicol 1994;32:435–444.

81. Andreu V, Mas A, Bruguera M, et al: Ecstasy: a common cause of severe acute hepatotoxicity. J Hepatol 1998;29:394–397.

82. Shannon M: Methylenedioxymethamphetamine (MDMA, "Ecstasy"). Pediatr Emerg Care 2000;16:377–380.

83. Schirren CA, Berghaus TM, Sackmann M: Thrombotic thrombocytopenic purpura after Ecstasy-induced acute liver failure. Ann Intern Med 1999;130:163.

84. Johnson TD, Berenson MM: Methamphetamine-induced ischemic colitis. J Clin Gastroenterol 1991;13:687–689.

85. Pecha RE, Prindiville T, Pecha BS, et al: Association of cocaine and methamphetamine use with giant gastroduodenal ulcers. Am J Gastroenterol 1996;91:2523–2527.

86. Deloach-Banta LJ: Lichenoid drug eruption: crystal methamphetamine or adulterants? Cutis 1994;53:97–98.

87. Cadier MA, Clarke JA: Ecstasy and Whizz at a rave resulting in a major burn plus complications. Burns 1993;19:239–240.

88. Dixon SD: Effects of transplacental exposure to cocaine and methamphetamine on the neonate. West J Med 1989;150:436–442.

89. Catanzarite VA, Stein DA: "Crystal" and pregnancy—methamphetamine-associated maternal deaths. West J Med 1995;162:454–457.

90. Stewart JL, Meeker JE: Fetal and infant deaths associated with maternal methamphetamine abuse. J Anal Toxicol 1997;21:515–517.

91. Werler MM, Sheehan JE, Mitchell AA: Association of vasoconstrictive exposures with risks of gastroschisis and small intestinal atresia. Epidemiology 2003;14:349–354.

92. Lekskulchai V, Mokkhavesa C: Evaluation of Roche Abuscreen ONLINE amphetamine immunoassay for screening of new amphetamine analogues. J Anal Toxicol 2001;25:471–475.

93. Valentine JL, Middleton R: GC-MS identification of sympathomimetic amine drugs in urine: rapid methodology applicable for emergency clinical toxicology. J Anal Toxicol 2000;24:211–222.

94. Smith-Kielland A, Skuterud B, Morland J: Urinary excretion of amphetamine after termination of drug abuse. J Anal Toxicol 1997;21:325–359.

95. Meeker JE, Reynolds PC: Postmortem tissue methamphetamine concentrations following selegiline administration. J Anal Toxicol 1990;14:330–331.

96. Tarver JA: Amphetamine-positive drug screens from use of clobenzorex hydrochlorate. J Anal Toxicol 1994;18:183.

97. Chappell JS: Infrared discrimination of enantiomerically enriched and racemic samples of methamphetamine salts. Analyst 1997;122:755–760.

98. Fang C, Chung YL, Liu JT, Lin CH: Rapid analysis of 3,4-methylenedioxymethamphetamine: a comparison of nonaqueous capillary electrophoresis/fluorescence detection with GC/MS. Forensic Sci Int 2002;125:142–148.

99. Nakahara Y, Kikura R: Hair analysis for drugs of abuse. 18. 3,4-Methylenedioxymethamphetamine (MDMA) disposition in hair roots and use in identification of acute MDMA poisoning. Biol Pharm Bull 1997;20:969–972.

100. Rohrich J, Kauert G: Determination of amphetamine and methylenedioxy-amphetamine-derivatives in hair. Forensic Sci Int 1997;84:179–188.

101. Kronstrand R, Grundin R, Jonsson J: Incidence of opiates, amphetamines, and cocaine in hair and blood in fatal cases of heroin overdose. Forensic Sci Int 1998;92:29–38.

102. Kintz P, Cirimele V: Interlaboratory comparison of quantitative determination of amphetamine and related compounds in hair samples. Forensic Sci Int 1997;84:151–156.

103. McKinney PE, Tomaszewski C, Phillips S, et al: Methamphetamine toxicity prevented by activated charcoal in a mouse model. Ann Emerg Med 1994;24:220–223.

104. Gary NE, Saidi P: Methamphetamine intoxication: a speedy new treatment. Am J Med 1978;64:537–540.

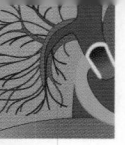

105. Lead poisoning associated with intravenous-methamphetamine use—Oregon, 1988. MMWR Morb Mortal Wkly Rep 1989;38: 830–831.
106. Sandrock CE, Murin S: Clinical predictors of respiratory failure and long-term outcome in black tar heroin-associated wound botulism. Chest 2001;120:562–566.
107. Hutchaleelaha A, Mayersohn M: Influence of activated charcoal on the disposition kinetics of methamphetamine enantiomers in the rat following intravenous dosing. J Pharm Sci 1996;85: 541–545.
108. Kantak KM: Vaccines against drugs of abuse: a viable treatment option? Drugs 2003;63:341–352.

45 *Hallucinogens*

STEPHEN J. TRAUB, MD

At a Glance...

- Most hallucinogens are indoleamine or phenylethylamine derivatives that are structurally similar to the neurotransmitter serotonin.

- Hallucinogens commonly used today include lysergic acid diethylamide, mescaline, 5-methoxy-*N,N*-diisopropyltryptamine ("foxy methoxy"), and psilocybin (in "magic mushrooms").

- Hallucinogens produce disturbances of perception, mood, and thought.

- Occasionally, hallucinogens produce negative experiences, often referred to as a "bad trip."

- Treatment of hallucinogen toxicity is primarily supportive; agitation often necessitates "talking the patient down" and/or treatment with benzodiazepines.

- Hallucinogen persisting perceptual disorder, more commonly known as "flashbacks," is a syndrome whereby previous users of LSD experience perceptual distortions despite abstinence from the drug.

- Hallucinogens rarely cause life-threatening alterations in physiology, but severe impairments in judgment may lead to severe disability or death.

The term *hallucination* is derived from the Latin word *hallucinari*, which means "to wander in mind." Hallucinations are false sensory perceptions that occur in the absence of real external stimuli; hallucinogens are substances that produce these perceptions. Many drugs may produce hallucinations, but those classified as hallucinogens or "psychedelics" produce disturbances of perception, mood, and thought as their primary effect with each use.

HISTORY

Although most commonly associated with the "psychedelic" era of San Francisco's Haight-Ashbury district during the 1960s, hallucinogens have a rich history and have been used by humans for millennia.[1] Hallucinogens have been and still are regularly used as integral parts of religious rituals. The Aztecs consumed psilocybin-containing mushrooms (*teonanacatl,* or "flesh of the gods") during their ceremonies. Mescaline, the major active alkaloid of the peyote cactus (*Lophophora williamsii*), is still used in religious ceremonies by Native American tribes in the Desert Southwest of the United States.

The modern era of hallucinogen use was inadvertently ushered in by Albert Hoffman of Sandoz Laboratories in 1943. Hoffman was working with synthetic ergot derivatives in an attempt to create new vasoactive medications when he inadvertently absorbed one of them, lysergic acid diethylemide (LSD), percutaneously. Soon afterward, he reportedly began to experience sensations we now recognize as characteristic of hallucinogen use:

> The external world became changed as in a dream. Objects appeared to gain in relief; they assumed unusual dimensions; and colors became more glowing. Even self-perception and the sense of time were changed. When the eyes were closed, colored pictures flashed past in a quickly changing kaleidoscope. After a few hours, the not unpleasant inebriation, which had been experienced whilst I was fully conscious, disappeared.[2]

Sandoz later marketed LSD as Delysid. It was touted as a cure for several psychiatric ailments, including alcoholism[3] and, interestingly, schizophrenia.[4] It was also used regularly by psychiatrists for analytical psychotherapy[5,6] and as an adjunct to treat those with terminal illness. LSD, however, was prohibited from use in the United States in 1966, and the drug was classified as a schedule I substance by the Drug Enforcement Agency as part of the Controlled Substances Act of 1970. This dramatically curtailed further human research with hallucinogenic drugs.

The use of hallucinogens as a means to "expand the mind" was popularized in the 1960s. In 1960, Dr. Timothy Leary, a Harvard psychologist, used psilocybin for the first time. His interest in this drug led to the development of the Harvard Psilocybin Project, in which hallucinogens were given to volunteers. Leary first tried LSD in 1962, and shortly thereafter began touting its benefits. He was (not coincidentally) fired from his Harvard position in 1963 but went on to become one of the strongest public advocates of hallucinogen use. The popularity of LSD and other hallucinogens grew during the rest of that decade, until it reached its height of popularity in the late 1960s.

At the same time that Leary was urging people to "tune in, turn on, and drop out," however, more established institutions began paying attention to—and expressing alarm at—the "epidemic" of hallucinogen use. A review of LSD in the *New England Journal of Medicine* in 1968 opened with the statement that "no drug use by man has stimulated greater public debate than lysergic acid diethylamide," and opined that "the widespread use of LSD, or similar drugs waiting in the psychedelic wings, could lead to a whole generation of psychedelic dropouts, incapable of and uninterested in addressing themselves to the important sociologic problems that challenge our times. If this happened, the very structure of this democratic society would be threatened."[7]

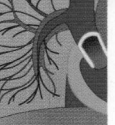
EPIDEMIOLOGY

Although the use of LSD and other hallucinogens has decreased since the 1960s, it has not disappeared. According to a 1999 report by the National Institutes of Health National Institute on Drug Abuse, approximately 10% of the U.S. population aged 12 and older has experimented with hallucinogens.[8] Use generally begins between ages 15 and 19, peaks at age 19, and becomes less common after age 30.[9] Whites are more likely than African Americans or Hispanics to report hallucinogen use[9] and are less likely to perceive that LSD is a dangerous drug.

A recent report from the Drug Abuse Warning Network (DAWN) notes a significant decline in emergency department (ED) visits related to LSD from 1994 to 2001.[10] DAWN estimates that in 2001, LSD was associated with 2821 ED visits in the coterminous United States; this represents a 45% decline from that reported in 1994. In 2001, LSD accounted for only 11% of ED visits associated with club drugs and 0.4% of all drug-related ED visits. Still, adolescents (12 to 17 years of age) and young adults (18 to 25 years) account for 34% and 48% of all ED visits related to LSD, respectively.

Members of previous generations may have relied on friends to tell them about their experiences with hallucinogenic drugs before trying them. Today, however, websites such as Erowid (www.erowid.org) and Lycaeum (www.lycaeum.org) contain information and descriptions (many very positive) of the effects of hallucinogen use. These websites are attractive to adolescents and young adults and may serve to reinforce the use of hallucinogenic drug use in this group of patients.

CLASSIFICATION

There are several classes of hallucinogens that are commonly used today. They include the indoleamines, phenylethylamines, piperazines, arylcyclohexylamines, tetrahydrocannabinoids, anticholinergics, and diterpene alkaloids (Table 45-1). The indoleamines include lysergamides (e.g., LSD) and alkyltryptamines (e.g., *N,N*-dimethyltryptamine [DMT], psilocybin, and bufotenine). The phenylethylamines include mescaline, dimethoxymethylamphetamine, methylenedioxymethamphetamine, and other amphetamine derivatives. Piperazines are structurally similar to phenylalkylamines and include benzylpiperazine and trifluromethylphenylpiperazine. The synthetic amphetamine and piperazine derivatives are discussed in Chapter 44. The arylcyclohexylamines include phencyclidine, ketamine, and dextromethorphan and are discussed in Chapter 43. Tetrahyrocannabinoids include marijuana and hashish and are discussed in Chapter 41. The anticholinergics include belladonna alkaloids and a wide variety of pharmaceutical agents (see Chapter 39). The diterpene alkaloids are found in the plant *Salvia divinorum*. This chapter will largely discuss the two primary hallucinogen classes, indoleamines and phenylalkylamines, as well as diterpene alkaloids.

Lysergamides

The lysergamides or ergolines include the synthetic D-lysergic acid diethylamide and naturally occurring indole alkaloids from the morning glory and Hawaiian baby wood rose plants. LSD is synthesized from lysergic acid and diethylamine; the former is derived from the wheat or rye fungus *Claviceps purpurea*. Seeds from the morning glory plants *Ipomoea violaceae* and *Rivea corymbosa* (Mexican ololiuqui), the Hawaiian baby woodrose (*Argyreia nervosa*), and the Hawaiian woodrose (*Merremia tuberose*) contain D-lysergic acid amide and D-isolysergic acid amide; these indole alkaloids have about one tenth the potency of LSD.[11] LSD is the most potent hallucinogenic drug known, with psychedelic effects occurring with doses as little as 25 to 50 µg.[12] The psychedelic effects from morning glory occur after ingestion of approximately 250 seeds.[11]

Tryptamines

The alkyltryptamines include both synthetic and naturally occurring compounds. These agents include DMT, α-methyl- and α-ethyltryptamine (AMT and AET), 5-methoxy-*N,N*-diisopropyltryptamine (5-MeO-DIPT, "foxy methoxy," or "methoxy"), 5-methoxy-*N,N*-dimethyltryptamine (5-MeO-DMT), psilocin, psilocybin, and bufotenine (5-hydroxydimethyltryptamine [5-OH-DMT]). Both bufotenine and 5-MeO-DMT are present in the secretions and skin of the cane toads, *Bufo* genus. The toad *Bufo alvarius* (Colorado River toad) produces the hallucinogen 5-MeO-DMT.[13] AMT and 5-MeO-DIPT are relatively new, potent, synthetic, hallucinogenic tryptamines popularized by their easy access via the Internet and as club drugs.[14,15] These drugs were recently made schedule I by the Drug Enforcement Administration.[14] DMT is another hallucinogenic tryptamine that is produced synthetically (known as the "businessman's trip") and found naturally in the bark of the yackee plant (*Vivola calophylla*). In Brazil, DMT is known as *yurema* and is basic to the Brazilian Indian Kariri religion.[16] DMT is prepared as snuff from the seeds, leaves, and pods of *Piptadenia peregrina*, *Prestonia amazenicum*, *Anadenanthera peregrina* (yopo tree), and *Mimosa hostilis*. The dose of tryptamines necessary to produce hallucinations varies according to the agent and route of exposure. Hallucinogenic effects have been demonstrated with oral doses of 4 to 10 mg for 5-MeO-DIPT, 100 mg for AMT, and 0.2 to 0.4 mg/kg IV for DMT.[14,15,17] Another naturally occurring, hallucinogenic alkaloid is ibogaine, which is derived from the shrub *Tabernanthe igoba*.

Psilocybin and psilocin are found naturally in mushrooms that belong mainly to the genera *Psilocybe*, *Conocybe*, *Gymnopilus*, *Lycoperdon*, *Pluteus*, *Panaeolus*, and *Stropharia* (see Chapter 23).[16,18,19] Some specific mushrooms containing psilocybin and/or psilocin include *Psilocybe mexicana*, *Psilocybe cubensis*, *Stropharia cubensis*, *Psilocybe semilanceata*, *Psilocybe pelliculosa*, *Panaeolus subbalteatus*, *Psilocybe cyanescens*, *Gymnopilus spectabilis*, and *Psilocybe baeocystis*. Psilocybin mushrooms are usually

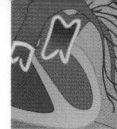

TABLE 45-1 Classes of Hallucinogens

CHEMICAL NAMES	PLANTS OR NATURAL SOURCES; SYNTHETIC AGENTS; "SLANG NAMES"
Indoleamines	
LYSERGAMIDES (ERGOLINES)	
D-Lysergic acid diethylamide	LSD; Delysid; "acid," "blotter," "stamps," "dots," "trips," "paper," "a-bombs," "pyramids"
D-Lysergic acid amide	*Ipomoea violaceae* (morning glory), *Rivea corymbosa* (Mexican ololiuqui), *Argyreia nervosa* (Hawaiian baby woodrose), *Merremia tuberose* (Hawaiian woodrose)
ALKYTRYPTAMINES	
α-methyltryptamine	AMT; "alpha"
N,N-dimethyltryptamine (DMT)	*Piptadenia peregrine, Anadenanthera peregrina, Prestonia amazenicum, Mimosa hostilis, Vivola calophylla*; "businessman's trip"
5-methoxy-*N,N*-dimethyltryptamine (5-MeO-DMT)	*Bufo alvarius*
Psilocybin (4-phophoryloxy-DMT)	*Psilocybe* sp, *Panaeolus* sp, *Conocybe* sp,
Psilocin (4-OH-DMT)	*Inocybe* sp, *Gymnopilus* sp, *Lycoperdon* sp, *Pluteus* genus; "magic mushrooms," "shrooms," "alice"
5-methoxy-*N,N*-diisopropyltryptamine (5-MeO-DIPT)	"Foxy methoxy," "foxy"
Bufotenine (5-OH-DMT)	Ch'an Su
Diethyltryptamine	DET
Ibogaine	*Tabernanthe igoba*
Phenylethylamines	
Mescaline (3,4,5-trimethoxyphenethylamine)	Peyote cactus (*Lophophora williamsii*)
3,4-methylenedioxymethamphetamine (MDMA)	Ecstasy; "XTC," "X," "E," "Adam," "the hug drug"
3,4-methylenedioxyethamphetamine (MDEA)	"Eve"
Methylenedioxyamphetamine (MDA)	
4-bromo-2,5-dimethoxyamphetamine (DOM)	"Serenity, tranquility, and peace" [STP]
Paramethoxyamphetamine (PMA)	
Arylcyclohexylamines (Piperidine Derivatives)	
Phencyclidine (PCP)	Angel dust; "hog," "wacky weed," "T," "killer weed"
Ketamine	Ketalar, ketaject, ketanest, "special K," "K," "K-hole," "vitamin K"
Dextromethorphan	"DXM," "dex," "robotripping," "CCC," "skittles," "red devils"
Piperazines	
Benzylpiperazine (BZP)	"Legal E," "legal X," "A²"
Trifluoromethylphenylpiperazine (TFMPP)	
Methylenedioxybenzylpiperazine (MDBP)	
m-chlorophenylpiperazine (mCPP)	
p-methoxyphenylpiperazine (MeOPP)	
Tetrahydrocannabinoids	
Tetrahydrocannabinol (Δ^9-THC, Δ^1-THC)	Dronabinol (Marinol); *Cannabis sativa* (marijuana, hashish)
Diterpene Alkaloids	
Salvinorin A, C	*Salvia divinorum*; sage
Myrisicin, saffrole	*Myristica fragrans* (nutmeg, mace)
Anticholinergic Agents	
Atropine (D,L-hyoscyamine)	*Atropa belladonna* (deadly nightshade), *Datura stramonium* (jimson weed)
Scopolamine (L-hyoscine)	Transderm Scop; *Datura stramonium* (jimson weed), *Hyoscyamus niger* (henbane)

found in moist warm climates but are widely distributed across the United States. These mushrooms grow overnight in cow pastures after a rainfall. Characteristically, the stalks of some psilocybin mushrooms turn blue with handling secondary to oxidation.[18] Psilocybin is quite stable; both dried mushrooms and boiled extract retain their hallucinogenic potency. Concentrations of psilocybin vary greatly from mushroom to mushroom (both within and between species), by season, and by location.[19] The initial hallucinogenic effects (e.g.,

detachment and relaxation) of psilocybin are evident with as little as 4 mg of toxin.[18,19] There is a dosage effect, with a dose of 12 mg or more producing vivid hallucinations. Due to the varied psilocybin content of each mushroom, it may take the ingestion of from 3 to 60 mushrooms to achieve the desired effect. In general, 4 to 8 mg of psilocybin is present in 20 g of fresh and 2 g of dried mushroom. Psilocybin sold on the street may be nonspecific mushrooms adulterated with LSD or other substances.

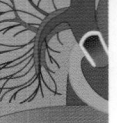

Phenylethylamines

Mescaline is the active phenylethylamine alkaloid from the peyote cactus (*Lophophora williamsii*), which is found in the deserts of the southwestern United States and Mexico. Peyote is a spineless cactus, which forms buttons with seven to ten ribs. The cactus contains about 6% mescaline when dried. Peyote buttons are the round fleshy tubercles from the cactus. One peyote button contains about 40 to 50 mg of mescaline. The average hallucinogenic dose of synthetic mescaline is 5 mg/kg body weight or 4 to 12 peyote buttons.[20] The legal use of peyote and mescaline in the United States is limited to Indian tribes in the Native American Church, who use peyote as part of religious ceremonies.

Nutmeg

Both nutmeg and mace are narcotic hallucinogens derived from a tall evergreen tree, *Myristica fragrans*, native to the Molucca Islands of the South Pacific and now cultivated on Grenada and Trinidad. Nutmeg is the dried seed kernel of the fruit and mace is derived from the fleshy outer covering of the seed.[21,22] Nutmeg and mace are commonly used as spices. The volatile oils present in nutmeg and mace contain the active ingredients, which include myristicin, saffrole, and terpenes. The toxic dose of nutmeg is one to three whole nutmegs, or 5 to 15 g of the ground spice. To produce toxicity from ingestion of nutmeg, the seeds must first be crushed to release the active oils.

Salvinorin A and C

Salvia divinorum is a perennial herb in the mint family native to certain areas of the Sierra Mazateca region of Oaxaca, Mexico.[23-25] *Salvia* is used medicinally and for divination by Mazatec Indians. Numerous species of *Salvia* are found in North and South America. *Salvia* is grown locally as sage or imported from Mexico. The active component of *S. divinorum* is salvinorin A and C, neoclerodane diterpenes (terpenoid essential oils). The hallucinogenic dose of *Salvia* is 10 to 20 fresh leaves chewed or two to five dried leaves smoked or vaporized. This is equivalent to inhaling 200 to 500 µg of salvinorin A.[24,25] Thus, salvinorin A is a very potent hallucinogen, similar to LSD.

STRUCTURE, STRUCTURE-ACTIVITY RELATIONSHIPS, AND PHARMACOLOGY

The neurotransmitter serotonin (5-hydroxytryptamine [5-HT]) is thought to play a major role in the pharmacology of most hallucinogens.[26] The two major classes of hallucinogens, indoleamines and phenylalkylamines, display similar euphoric and psychedelic effects, are cross-tolerant, and are close structural analogs to serotonin (Fig. 45-1).[27,28] These observations suggest that these hallucinogens share a common mechanism of

FIGURE 45-1 Chemical structures of serotonin and select hallucinogens.

action that involves serotonin. Evidence for this is solidified by numerous human studies that demonstrate a strong correlation between the relative affinity that these compounds have for $5\text{-}HT_{2A}$ receptors and their potency as hallucinogens.[29-31] When normal subjects are pretreated with adequate doses of the $5\text{-}HT_{2A}$ antagonists ketanserin or risperidone, the hallucinogenic effects of psilocybin are completely blocked.[32] These findings suggest further that the $5\text{-}HT_{2A}$ receptor mediates the psychedelic effects of indoleamines and phenylethylamines. The importance of receptor subtype selectivity is underscored by the fact that drugs and medications that increase overall serotonergic tone (such as the serotonin selective reuptake inhibitors) do not produce the same clinical effects as hallucinogens. Partial agonist activity at $5\text{-}HT_{2A}$ receptors is central to the hallucinatory effects of these agents, and binding at other serotonin receptor subtypes likely modulates these effects. Both hallucinogen classes are also agonists at $5\text{-}HT_{2C}$ receptors.[26] In addition, the indoleamines are agonists at $5\text{-}HT_{1A}$ and dopamine D_2 receptors.[33] Interestingly, LSD has the structures of both serotonin and dopamine embedded in its nucleus; this latter finding may explain its dopamine receptor agonist properties.

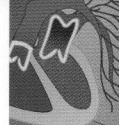

In general, addition of methyl hydroxyl groups to the benzene ring of the tryptamines or phenylethylamines increases lipophilicity, central nervous system (CNS) penetration, and hallucinogenic potency. For instance, addition of a methyl hydroxy group to bufotenine creates 5-MeO-DMT, a hallucinogen with greater CNS potency. Addition of methyl hydroxy groups to the benzene ring of phenylethylamines (e.g., mescaline) markedly increases CNS penetration and effects.

Anatomically, the regions of the brain that appear to be the major targets of hallucinogens are the olfactory bulb, locus ceruleus, dorsal raphe nucleus, nucleus accumbens, and cerebral cortex (in particular, the medial prefrontal cortex).[26,34,35] These brain regions are heavily concentrated with 5-HT$_{2A}$ receptors. These brain areas receive and process a large amount of sensory inputs from the body and environment and transfer this information to the cerebral cortex via extensive cortical projections.[36,37] The cerebral cortex is responsible for final processing and interpretation of neuronal data. Hallucinogens facilitate neuronal activation in the aforementioned brain areas in response to external stimuli. They activate afferent inputs to the cortex while also filtering out tonic inhibitory influences; the end result is asynchronous neuronal activation of numerous cortical regions.

Although serotonin pathways are integral to hallucinogen effects, other neurotransmitters are involved, and include glutamate, norepinephrine, dopamine, and γ-aminobutyric acid (GABA).[26,38] Hallucinogen binding to central 5-HT$_{2A}$ receptors activates release of norepinephrine from the locus ceruleus, serotonin from raphe nuclei, GABA from specific cortical interneurons, and glutamate from multiple cortical areas.[26] Enhanced glutamate activity is diffuse and asynchronous and results in cognitive, perceptual, and affective distortions.

Tolerance to hallucinogens develops rapidly after regular use of these drugs.[39,40] This is likely due, at least in part, to a rapid down-regulation of 5-HT$_{2A}$ receptors.[41,42] Cross-tolerance between hallucinogens is also reported.[27,28] Tolerance occurs to the euphoric and psychedelic effects, but not to autonomic effects.

Although some users elect to use hallucinogens extensively, this class of drugs is not considered physiologically addicting. Tolerance does develop to the psychedelic effects, but no withdrawal syndrome has been observed. A recent review[43] noted that there are no studies in which animals are trained to self-administer hallucinogens; animal self-administration is an important predictor of addiction. In rhesus monkeys, LSD was actually a negative reinforcer.[44]

The hallucinogenic mint S. divinorum contains the psychoactive neoclerodane diterpenes salvinorin A and C. These bioactive compounds are structurally distinct from other naturally occurring hallucinogens (e.g., indoleamines and phenylalkylamines) and do not bind 5-HT$_2$ receptors. Rather, salvinorin A and C are potent, selective, opioid, κ receptor agonists and activate the dynorphin peptide system to induce analgesia, sedation, and perceptual distortion.[23,45-48]

PHARMACOKINETICS

Formulations and Route of Administration

Most hallucinogens are ingested but may also be chewed and absorbed orally, administered sublingually, insufflated, smoked, or injected intramuscularly or intravenously. LSD is a clear or white, odorless, tasteless powder. The powder is formulated as capsules, tiny tablets ("microdots"), and small gelatin squares ("windowpanes") or applied to postage stamp–sized sheets ("blotter acid") or sugar cubes.[49] Each unit dose varies from 50 to 300 µg or more.[12] LSD is typically ingested but may be smoked or injected. Exposure to natural lysergamides (e.g., morning glory) occurs following ingestion of seeds. The hallucinogenic tryptamines are typically ingested with the exception of DMT and 5-methoxy-DMT; these latter compounds are often insufflated, smoked, or injected IV. S. divinorum is administered in many ways; it is smoked (roll dried leaves into a "joint"), ingested ("oral infusion"), or chewed ("the quid") and absorbed sublingually or from the buccal mucosa.

Bufotenine can be isolated from secretions of the parotid and sebaceous glands of Bufo toads. "Toad licking" has been touted by some as a means to intoxication with this hallucinogen. This is misguided for two reasons. First, N,N-hydroxydimethyltryptamine is not well absorbed from the gastrointestinal (GI) tract and does not readily cross the blood-brain barrier; hallucinations will not result from toad licking. Second, several species of toads secrete potent cardioactive steroids or bufadienolides (e.g., bufalin) from their skin glands. Thus, toad licking may result in serious cardiac toxicity without a hallucinogenic effect.[50]

Absorption, Peak Clinical Effects, and Duration of Clinical Effects

Certain pharmacokinetic parameters and clinical characteristics for select hallucinogens are provided in Tables 45-2 and 45-3. The time of onset and duration of clinical effects from hallucinogens vary according to the route of exposure and agent administered. In general, most hallucinogens are rapidly absorbed and distributed to the CNS after ingestion; clinical effects begin within 30 to 60 minutes after ingestion, peak by 2 to 4 hours, and last 4 to 8 hours. Certain agents have a very rapid onset and short duration of effects (e.g., DMT), whereas others may have effects that last 12 to 24 hours or more (e.g., mescaline, nutmeg, and ibogaine).

Metabolism and Excretion

Most agents are extensively metabolized in the liver (by N-demethylation, hydroxylation, and glucuronidation) to inactive metabolites (see Table 45-2). Mescaline is also excreted unchanged in the urine.

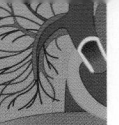

TABLE 45-2 Pharmacokinetics of Select Hallucinogens

HALLUCINOGEN	TIME TO PEAK SERUM CONCENTRATION AFTER ORAL DOSING (hr)	ELIMINATION HALF-LIFE (hr)	PROTEIN BINDING (%)	Vd (L/kg)	ROUTE OF METABOLISM	ACTIVE METABOLITE
LSD	3–5	2–4	80–90	0.27	Hepatic	No
Psilocybin	1–2	1.8–4.5	*	2.5–5	Hepatic	Yes (psilocin)
DMT	1.5	0.5–1.5		38–53	Hepatic	No
Mescaline	2	6			Renal (55%–60%); hepatic	No

*Data not available.
DMT, *N,N*-dimethyltryptamine; LSD, lysergic acid diethylamide; Vd, volume of distribution.
Pharmacokinetic data obtained from references 18 and 55.

TABLE 45-3 Time of Onset and Duration of Effects of Select Hallucinogens

HALLUCINOGEN	HUMAN RECREATIONAL DOSE	TIME OF ONSET OF CLINICAL EFFECTS	DURATION OF CLINICAL EFFECTS (hr)
LSD	Oral: 25–250 µg (3 µg/kg) IV: 140 µg (2 µg/kg)	Oral: 0.5–1 hr	4–12
AMT	Nasal insufflation: 100 mg	Smoke, nasal: 5 min Oral: 15 min	8–16
DMT	Smoke: 30–150 mg IV/IM: 0.2–0.4 mg/kg	IV: 1–5 min IM: 10 min Oral: 30–60 min	0.5–1
5-MeO-DMT	IV or smoked: 5–10 mg	IV: 1–5 min	0.33–0.5
5-MeO-DIPT	Oral: 5–30 mg	Oral: 20 min Smoke: 10 min	3–6
Psilocybin	Oral: 4–12 mg (0.02 mg/kg); 20–30 fresh mushrooms or 1–2 g dried mushroom*	Oral: 20–30 min	4–6
Mescaline	Oral: 200–600 mg (5 mg/kg)	45–60 min	10–12
Nutmeg	Oral: 5–15 g ground spice; 1–3 nutmegs	2–4 hr	24
Salvia divinorum	Oral: 1 mg Smoked: 200–500 µg	15 min	1–3

*The recreational dose of mushroom varies by mushroom genus and species, season, geographic location, and habituation of the user.
AMT, α-methyltryptamine; DMT, *N,N*-dimethyltryptamine; 5-MeO-DIPT, 5-methoxy-*N,N*-diisopropyltryptamine; 5-MeO-DMT, 5-methoxy-*N,N*-dimethyltryptamine; IM, intramuscularly; IV, intravenously; LSD, lysergic acid diethylamide;
Adapted from references 2, 18, 19, 43, and 55, and from Shulgin AT: Profiles of psychedelic drugs. Psilocybin. J Psychedelic Drugs 1980,12:79.

TOXICOLOGY

Physiologic Disturbances

In addition to their CNS effects, most hallucinogens produce a variety of autonomic (parasympathetic and sympathetic) effects that include mydriasis, tachycardia, hypertension, cutaneous flushing, salivation, lacrimation, hyper-reflexia, nausea, vomiting, abdominal cramps, hyperthermia, and tachypnea. These effects may occur directly from the drug or indirectly from the anxiety and CNS stimulation produced by the hallucinogen. The sympathomimetic effects from hallucinogens, for instance, may be mediated by stimulation of noradrenergic neurons in the locus ceruleus. Physiologic effects occur concurrently with the CNS disturbances. Other non-specific effects include dizziness, ataxia, vertigo, weakness, headache, and paresthesias. Seizures have been rarely reported. Nutmeg, mescaline, and psilocybin ingestion have a greater frequency of GI adverse effects (i.e., nausea, vomiting, epigastric cramps) than those associated with other hallucinogens.[18,51] An anticholinergic-type syndrome has been associated with nutmeg intoxication.[52] Although life-threatening physiologic disturbances are unusual, one series of eight patients with massive LSD overdose developed hyperthermia, coma, respiratory arrest, and coagulopathy.[53]

Central Nervous System Psychedelic Effects

Acute perceptual distortions are the common thread that links the hallucinogens. Inanimate objects may begin to pulsate or move. Concrete physical boundaries, such as a wall or a person's face, may appear to waver or even blend in with the surroundings; users frequently perceive that inanimate objects are "melting." Geometric patterns are frequently described, and may be readily

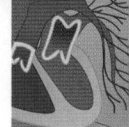

"visible" even when the eyes are closed. An object that moves across the user's visual field may leave a "trail" that persists for several seconds. Synesthesias (the melding of sensory modalities) may occur, in which users may hear colors or see sounds. Sensory inputs such as sights or noises may seem more striking, and ordinary thoughts may seem quite profound. The user's sense of time may be markedly distorted, or completely lost. Time contraction is common such that the user overestimates chronologic time.

Most people who knowingly ingest hallucinogens welcome these perceptual distortions and find the experience quite pleasant. Occasionally, however, users have a profoundly dysphoric experience when using hallucinogens, typically referred to as a "bad trip." The reason why one experience with hallucinogens is good and another bad is not entirely clear. Drug dose, the user's environment, and the user's attitude when taking the drug may all play a role. An interesting but uncontrolled convenience study of LSD users compared a group of 25 users with positive experiences with 25 users with negative experiences. There were no historical or clinical variables that accurately predicted a bad trip. Those with bad trips were not more likely to have a previous psychiatric diagnosis.[54]

Dose-Response Characteristics

The usual recreational doses that produce hallucinogenic effects in humans are listed in Table 45-3. Psychedelic effects are dose related, such that low doses produce mild illusions and perceptual distortions whereas large doses may produce severe neurovegetative disturbances, extreme anxiety or dysphoria, disorientation, or the inability to discriminate between reality and illusion (true hallucinations).[18] In general, hallucinogens have a remarkably low likelihood for producing significant acute morbidity and mortality. For instance, LSD has a therapeutic index of approximately 1000.[55]

"Flashbacks": Hallucinogen Persisting Perception Disorder

Perceptual distortions may recur months or years after hallucinogen abstinence. Commonly referred to as "flashbacks," these perceptual distortions are formally known as hallucinogen persisting perception disorder (HPPD). HPPD is a recognized psychiatric diagnosis in which distressing "geometric hallucinations, false perceptions of movement in the peripheral visual fields, flashes of color, intensified colors, trails of images of moving objects, positive afterimages, halos around objects, macropsia, and micropsia"[56] cannot be ascribed to an acute drug intoxication or another psychiatric illness or condition.

The physiologic basis of HPPD is incompletely understood. Various theories have been proposed, including an LSD-induced decrease in tonic inhibitory tone in visual areas of the brain[57] and/or LSD-induced sensitization of areas of visual processing within the brain.[58] A genetic predisposition has also been postulated.[59]

Although several quantitative studies have addressed HPPD, this literature suffers from methodologic flaws, and firm conclusions are difficult to draw.[60]

Various pharmacologic treatments have been proposed to treat HPPD, which include clonidine[61,62] and clonazepam.[63,64] Interestingly, risperidone (which possesses antagonist activity at the $5-HT_2$ receptor) has been reported to exacerbate this condition,[65] as have the serotonin selective reuptake inhibitors.[66]

Hallucinogen-Induced Psychiatric Disorders

Prolonged perceptual distortions and hallucinosis that last a few days may occasionally occur after hallucinogen use. In addition, hallucinogens may induce acute anxiety, panic disorder, major depression, or schizophrenic episodes in susceptible individuals. There is some evidence that repeated hallucinogen use is a risk factor for the development of chronic or persistent thought disturbances.[67] One case series described four patients diagnosed with schizophrenia within a few years of ingesting LSD between 50 and 300 times.[68] The lack of a control group in this study significantly limits their findings. In addition, all of the patients were in their early 20s and an age at which first psychotic breaks occur in those who subsequently develop chronic schizophrenia. Another paper compared 46 schizophrenics and 46 controls and found no statistical difference in drug use in general, but a trend toward more LSD use among schizophrenics.[69] A poorly chosen control group (all controls were employed, students, or hospital volunteers) significantly limits this study's findings. Subsequent reviews of this subject[70,71] have noted the flawed methodology of these and other similar reports, and concluded that there is no significant association between hallucinogen use and chronic thought disorders.

Chromosomal Abnormalities

Reports suggesting that LSD use led to chromosomal damage both in vitro[72] and in vivo[73] surfaced in the late 1960s and early 1970s and received sensational media attention. Subsequent reports,[74-77] however, disputed the link between LSD use and chromosomal damage. The belief that LSD damages human chromosomes is no longer widely held.

Morbidity and Mortality Due to Impaired Judgment

Hallucinogens are generally thought to be "safe" drugs, in that they do not produce the potentially life-threatening alterations in physiology that one might see with opiates, barbiturates, or cocaine. It should be noted, however, that significant injury or death may result from decisions that are made when hallucinogens have markedly impaired the user's judgment. People under the influence of hallucinogens have mistakenly believed they could fly[78] or have stared directly into the sun[79-81] with disastrous consequences.

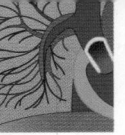

DIAGNOSIS

The diagnosis of hallucinogen intoxication is made clinically and based on a positive history of exposure and suggestive physical findings. Most patients should be able to provide a history of hallucinogen use. Suggestive physical findings include mild to moderate sympathomimetic and GI effects coupled with a patient with ongoing perceptual and sensory illusions (e.g., visual distortions). Hallucinogens do not produce any characteristic abnormalities of the electrolytes or the complete blood count, so these basic ancillary tests are unlikely to aid in the diagnosis. Standard urinary toxicology (immunoassay) screens do not detect LSD or most other hallucinogens; specialized urinary testing kits for LSD are commercially available but not stocked by most hospitals. Even when available, false-positive test results[82-85] limit the utility of such kits (Box 45-1). It should be understood that drugs of abuse screens designed to detect amphetamines and PCP are both insensitive and nonspecific for detection of designer drugs that are frequently abused. Confirmatory testing by gas chromatography/mass spectroscopy or high-pressure liquid chromatography is sensitive and specific, but the results of such testing often take days to return.

In the absence of a clear history of hallucinogen use, patients who have ingested this class of drugs are best approached as an undifferentiated patient with an alteration in mental status. A thorough history and physical examination should be obtained. Comprehensive ancillary testing, both basic (blood glucose level, serum electrolytes, complete blood count) and advanced (computed tomography of the head, lumbar puncture) should be considered.

Differential Diagnosis

The manifestations of hallucinogen intoxication may be similar to intoxication with anticholinergic, sympatho-mimetic (e.g., cocaine, amphetamines, methylxanthines), and other psychotropic (e.g., lithium) agents; withdrawal from alcohol or sedative-hypnotics; functional psychiatric disorders (e.g., acute panic disorder, schizophrenia); CNS or systemic infections; traumatic head injury; cerebrovascular accidents; and several metabolic disturbances (e.g., uremia, hepatic encephalopathy, hyponatremia, or hypoglycemia). In addition, the various hallucinogenic classes may be difficult, if not impossible, to differentiate from each other clinically. Patients may be differentiated from anticholinergic agent toxicity by the absence of delirium, repetitive picking behavior, urinary retention, ileus, or dry skin. Patients may be differentiated from amphetamine poisoning by the absence of stereotypic behavior (e.g., formication, lip smacking, and teeth grinding). Unlike those with hallucinogen intoxication, patients with functional psychoses are alert and oriented, have auditory hallucinations predominantly, lack synesthesias, and cannot differentiate their illusion from reality (true hallucinosis).

MANAGEMENT

Most patients with hallucinogen intoxication have an uncomplicated course and do not require medical treatment. For those patients who require hospital evaluation due to unexpected adverse clinical effects, treatment is largely supportive.

Although uncharacteristic for hallucinogen poisoning, patients with significant CNS or respiratory depression should have their airway protected, breathing assisted, and cardiovascular support provided as necessary. Supplemental oxygen, continuous pulse oximetry, and parenteral thiamine, dextrose (or rapid fingerstick glucose determination), and naloxone should be considered for patients with altered mental status or seizures. Significant CNS or respiratory depression, seizures, and hypotension are unlikely findings after hallucinogen use; their presence should prompt a search for another process. Hypertension, when present, is usually mild and rarely requires treatment. In the event that the clinician is concerned about hypertension in an agitated, hallucinating patient, a benzodiazepine (i.e., lorazepam, 1 to 2 mg IV) is an appropriate first intervention.

GI decontamination is not routinely necessary for hallucinogen poisoning unless there is concern for co-ingestants. Since hallucinogens are rapidly absorbed after ingestion, the effectiveness of GI decontamination is marginal. In addition, since uncomplicated hallucinogen poisoning usually resolves without sequelae, the risks involved in performing decontamination procedures, particularly in the anxious patient, may outweigh any benefits. If GI decontamination is performed, single-dose administration of activated charcoal (1 g/kg orally or by nasogastric tube) is the preferred method. Orogastric lavage is not recommended for this group of patients due to lack of efficacy and associated procedural morbidity. Gastric emptying procedures have not been found to have an effect on the severity and duration of

BOX 45-1	**SUBSTANCES THAT MAY CAUSE FALSE-POSITIVE URINARY LSD TESTING**

Ambroxol (mucolytic)
Amitryptyline
Brompheniramine
Bupivacaine
Diphenhydramine
Doxepin
Doxylamine
Ergonovine
Fentanyl
Imipramine
Lidocaine
Methylphenidate
Metoclopramide
Prilocaine
Ranitidine
Tramadol

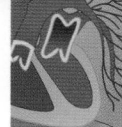

symptoms when performed on series of patients intoxicated with hallucinogenic mushrooms.[86,87]

Patients that are anxious, frightened, or agitated due to negative or punitive distortions (a bad trip) should be provided rest and reassurance in a dark, quiet environment; this approach has been advocated successfully for over 30 years.[88] In the event that concurrent sedation is indicated, benzodiazepines are the preferred pharmacotherapy, providing safe, nonspecific sympatholysis.[89] The use of atypical antipsychotic agents, which specifically antagonize $5-HT_2$ receptors (e.g., ziprasidone, risperidone, clozapine), are theoretically attractive for the treatment of bad trips but have not been adequately studied.

DISPOSITION

Most patients with hallucinogen poisoning develop only mild toxicity and are medically safe for psychiatric evaluation (if necessary) and disposition after an observation period of 4 to 6 hours in the ED. Patients who have continued evidence of agitation, perceptual distortions, and physiologic disturbances at 6 hours should be admitted to a monitored bed for continued observation.

REFERENCES

1. Bruhn JG, De Smet PA, El-Seedi HR, Beck O: Mescaline use for 5700 years. Lancet 2002;359(9320):1866.
2. Erowid website: LSD. Accessed February 28, 2005, at http://www.erowid.org/chemicals/lsd/lsd.shtml
3. Mangini M: Treatment of alcoholism using psychedelic drugs: a review of the program of research. J Psychoactive Drugs 1998;30(4):381–418.
4. Itil TM, Keskiner S, Holden JM: The use of LSD and ditran in the treatment of therapy resistant schizophrenics (symptom provocation approach). Dis Nerv Syst 1969;30(2 Suppl):93–103.
5. Neill JR: "More than medical significance": LSD and American psychiatry 1953 to 1966. J Psychoactive Drugs 1987;19(1):39–45.
6. Novak SJ: LSD before Leary. Sidney Cohen's critique of 1950s psychedelic drug research. Isis 1997;88(1):87–110.
7. Louria DB: Lysergic acid diethylamide. N Engl J Med 1968;278:435–438.
8. National Institutes of Health, National Institute on Drug Abuse: Sixth Triennial Report to Congress. Bethesda, MD, National Institute on Drug Abuse, 1999.
9. Chilcoat HD, Schutz CG: Age-specific patterns of hallucinogen use in the US population: an analysis using generalized additive models. Drug Alcohol Depend 1996;43(3):143–153.
10. Drug Abuse Warning Network: The DAWN Report, Club Drugs, 2001 Update. Rockville, MD, Office of Applied Studies, Substance Abuse and Mental Health Services Administration, Drug Abuse Warning Network, 2001 (March 2002 update). Accessed October 2004 at www.drugabusestatistics.samhsa.gov
11. Ingram AL: Morning glory seed reaction. JAMA 1964;190:107–108.
12. O'Brien CP: Drug addiction and drug abuse. In Hardman JG, Limbird LE, Gilman AG (eds): Goodman & Gilman's the Pharmacological Basis of Therapeutics, 10th ed. New York, McGraw-Hill, 2001, pp 557–577.
13. Weil AT, Davis W: Bufo alvarius: a potent hallucinogen of animal origin. J Ethnopharmacol 1994;41(1–2):1–8.
14. Meatherall R, Sharma P: Foxy, a designer tryptamine hallucinogen. J Anal Toxicol 2003;27(5):313–317.
15. Long H, Nelson LS, Hoffman RS: Alpha-methyltryptamine revisited via easy internet access. Vet Hum Toxicol 2003;45:149.
16. Schultes RE: Hallucinogens of plant origin. Science 1969;163:245–254.
17. Strassman RJ: Human psychopharmacology of N,N-dimethyltryptamine. Behav Brain Res 1996;73:121–124.
18. Spoerke DG, Rumack BH: Handbook of mushroom poisoning: diagnosis and treatment. Boca Raton, FL, CRC Press, 1994.
19. Benjamin DR: Mushrooms: poisons and panaceas. New York, W.H. Freeman & Company, 1995.
20. Schultes RE, Hofmann A: Plants of the Gods. Rochester, VT, Healing Arts Press, 1992.
21. Mack RB: Toxic encounters of the dangerous kind. NC Med J 1982;43:439.
22. Kalbhen DA: Nutmeg as a narcotic. Angew Chem Internat Edit 1971;10:370–374.
23. Giroud C, Felber F, Augsburger M, et al: Salvia divinorum: an hallucinogenic mint which might become a new recreational drug in Switzerland. Forensic Sci Int 2000;112:143–150.
24. Valdes LJ, Chang HM, Visger DC, Koreeda M: Savinorin C, a new neoclerodane diterpene from a bioactive fraction of the hallucinogenic Mexican mint Salvia divinorum. Org Lett 2001;3:3935–3937.
25. Bigham AK, Munro TA, Rizzacasa MA, Robins-Browne RM: Divinatorins A-C, new neoclerodane diterpenoids from the controlled sage Salvia divinorum. J Nat Prod 2003;66:1242–1244.
26. Aghajanian G, Marek G: Serotonin and hallucinogens. Neuropsychopharmacology 1999;21(Suppl 1):16–23.
27. Balestireri A, Fontanari D: Acquired and crossed tolerance to mescaline, LSD-25, and BOL-148. Arch Gen Psychiatry 1959;1:279–282.
28. Isbell H, Wolbach AE, Wikler A, Miner EJ: Cross tolerance between LSD and psilocybin. Psychopharmacology (Berl) 1961;2:147–159.
29. Glennon RA, Titeler M, McKenney JD: Evidence for 5-HT2 involvement in the mechanism of action of hallucinogenic agents. Life Sci 1984;35(25):2505–2511.
30. Sadzot B, Baraban JM, Glennon RA, et al: Hallucinogenic drug interactions at human brain 5-HT2 receptors: implications for treating LSD-induced hallucinogenesis. Psychopharmacology (Berl) 1989;98(4):495–499.
31. Titeler M, Lyon RA, Glennon RA: Radioligand binding evidence implicates the brain 5-HT2 receptor as a site of action for LSD and phenylisopropylamine hallucinogens. Psychopharmacology (Berl) 1988;94(2):213–216.
32. Vollenweider FX, Vollenweider-Scherpenhuyzen MF, Babler A, et al: Psilocybin induces schizophrenia-like psychosis in humans via a serotonin-2 agonist action. Neuroreport 1998;9(17):3897–3902.
33. Winter JC, Filipink RA, Timineri D, et al: The paradox of 5-methoxy-N,N-dimethyltryptamine: an indoleamine hallucinogen that induces stimulus control via 5-HT1A receptors. Pharmacol Biochem Behav 2000;65:75–82.
34. Aghajanian GK: Mescaline and LSD facilitate the activation of locus coeruleus neurons by peripheral stimuli. Brain Res 1980;186(2):492–498.
35. McKenna DJ, Mathis CA, Shulgin AT, et al: Autoradiographic localization of binding sites for 125I-DOI, a new psychotomimetic radioligand, in the rat brain. Eur J Pharmacol 1987;137(2–3):289–290.
36. Aston-Jones G, Bloom FE: Norepinephrine-containing locus coeruleus neurons in behaving rats' exhibit pronounced responses to non-noxious environmental stimuli. J Neurosci 1981;1(8):887–900.
37. Cedarbaum JM, Aghajanian GK: Activation of locus coeruleus neurons by peripheral stimuli: modulation by a collateral inhibitory mechanism. Life Sci 1978;23(1):1383–1392.
38. Winter JC, Eckler JR, Rabin RA: Serotonergic/glutamatergic interactions: the effects of mGlu(2/3) receptor ligands in rats trained with LSD and PCP as discriminative stimuli. Psychopharmacology (Berl) 2004;172(2):233–270.
39. Isbell H, Belleville RE, Fraser HF, et al: Studies on lysergic acid diethylamide (LSD-25): 1. Effects in former morphine addicts and development of tolerance during chronic intoxication. Arch Neurol Psychiatry 1956;76:468–478.
40. Angrist B, Rotrosen J, Gershon S: Assessment of tolerance to the hallucinogenic effects of DOM. Psychopharmacologia 1974;36(3):203–207.
41. Buckholtz NS, Zhou DF, Freedman DX: Serotonin2 agonist administration down-regulates rat brain serotonin2 receptors. Life Sci 1988;42(24):2439–2445.

42. Buckholtz NS, Freedman DX, Middaugh LD: Daily LSD administration selectively decreases serotonin2 receptor binding in rat brain. Eur J Pharmacol 1985;109(3):421–425.

43. Nichols DE: Hallucinogens. Pharmacol Ther 2004;101(2):131–181.

44. Hoffmeister F: Negative reinforcing properties of some psychotropic drugs in drug-naive rhesus monkeys. J Pharmacol Exp Ther 1975;192(2):468–477.

45. Valdes LJ 3rd: Salvia divinorum and the unique diterpene hallucinogen, Salvinorin (divinorin) A. J Psychoactive Drugs 1994;26(3):277–283.

46. Chavkin C, Sud S, Jin W, et al: Salvinorin A, an active component of the hallucinogenic sage Salvia divinorum is a highly efficacious κ-opioid receptor agonist: structural and functional considerations. J Pharmacol Exp Ther 2004;308(3):1197–1203.

47. Butelman ER, Harris TJ, Kreek MJ: The plant-derived hallucinogen, salvinorin A, produces kappa-opioid agonist-like discriminative effects in rhesus monkeys. Psychopharmacology (Berl) 2004;172(2):220–224.

48. Roth BL, Baner K, Westkaemper R, et al: Salvinorin A: a potent naturally occurring nonnitrogenous kappa opioid selective agonist. Proc Natl Acad Sci U S A 2002;99(18):11934–11939.

49. Kilmer SD: The isolation and identification of lysergic acid diethylamide (LSD) from sugar cubes and a liquid substrate. J Forensic Sci 1994;39(3):860–862.

50. Hitt M, Ettinger DD: Toad toxicity. N Engl J Med 1986;314(23):1517–1518.

51. Stein U, Greyer H, Hentschel H: Nutmeg (myristicin) poisoning—report on a fatal case and a series of cases recorded by a poison information centre. Forensic Sci Int 2001;118(1):87–90.

52. Lavy G: Nutmeg intoxication in pregnancy. A case report. J Reprod Med 1987;32(1):63–64.

53. Klock J, Boermer V, Berher C: Coma, hyperthermia and bleeding associated with massive LSD overdose: a report of 8 cases. Clin Toxicol 1975;8:191–203.

54. Ungerleider JT, Fisher DD, Fuller M, et al: The "bad trip"—the etiology of the adverse LSD reaction. Am J Psychiatry 1968;124(11):1483–1490.

55. Baselt RF: Disposition of Toxic Drugs and Chemicals in Man. Foster City, CA, Biomedical Publications, 2004.

56. American Psychological Association: Diagnostic and Statistical Manual of Mental Disorders, 4th ed, text revision. Washington, DC, American Pyschological Association, 2000.

57. Abraham HD, Aldridge AM: Adverse consequences of lysergic acid diethylamide. Addiction 1993;88(10):1327–1334.

58. Phillips TJ: Behavior genetics of drug sensitization. Crit Rev Neurobiol 1997;11:21–31.

59. Abraham HD: Visual phenomenology of the LSD flashback. Arch Gen Psychiatry 1983;40(8):884–889.

60. Halpern JH, Pope HG Jr: Hallucinogen persisting perception disorder: what do we know after 50 years? Drug Alcohol Depend 2003;69(2):109–119.

61. Lerner AG, Finkel B, Oyffe I, et al: Clonidine treatment for hallucinogen persisting perception disorder. Am J Psychiatry 1998;155(10):1460.

62. Lerner AG, Gelkopf M, Oyffe I, et al: LSD-induced hallucinogen persisting perception disorder treatment with clonidine: an open pilot study. Int Clin Psychopharmacol 2000;15(1):35–37.

63. Lerner AG, Skladman I, Kodesh A, et al: LSD-induced hallucinogen persisting perception disorder treated with clonazepam: two case reports. Isr J Psychiatry Relat Sci 2001;38(2):133–136.

64. Lerner AG, Gelkopf M, Skladman I, et al: Clonazepam treatment of lysergic acid diethylamide-induced hallucinogen persisting perception disorder with anxiety features. Int Clin Psychopharmacol 2003;18(2):101–105.

65. Morehead DB: Exacerbation of hallucinogen-persisting perception disorder with risperidone. J Clin Psychopharmacol 1997;17(4):327–328.

66. Markel H, Lee A, Holmes RD, et al: LSD flashback syndrome exacerbated by selective serotonin reuptake inhibitor antidepressants in adolescents. J Pediatr 1994;125:817–819.

67. McLellan AT, Woody GE, O'Brien CP: Development of psychiatric illness in drug abusers: possible role of drug preference. N Engl J Med 1979;301:1310–1314.

68. Glass GS, Bowers MB Jr: Chronic psychosis associated with long-term psychotomimetic drug abuse. Arch Gen Psychiatry 1970;23(2):97–103.

69. Breakey W, Goodell H, Lorenz PC, et al: Hallucinogenic drugs as precipitants of schizophrenia. Psychol Med 1974;4:255–261.

70. Strassman RJ: Adverse reactions to psychedelic drugs. A review of the literature. J Nerv Ment Dis 1984;172(10):577–595.

71. Halpern JH, Pope HG Jr: Do hallucinogens cause residual neuropsychological toxicity? Drug Alcohol Depend 1999;53(3):247–256.

72. Cohen MM, Marinello M, Bark N: Chromosomal damage in human leudocytes induced by lysergic acid diethylamide (LSD-25). Science 1967;155:1417–1419.

73. Corey MJ, Andrews JC, McLeao MJ, et al: Chromosome studies on patients (in vivo) and in cells (in vitro) treated with LSD-25. N Engl J Med 1970;282:939–942.

74. Robinson JT, Chitham RG, Greenwood RM, Taylor JW: Chromosome aberrations and LSD. A controlled study in 50 psychiatric patients. Br J Psychiatry 1974;125(0):238–244.

75. Tjio JH, Pahnke WN, Kurland AA: LSD and chromosomes. A controlled experiment. JAMA 1969;210(5):849–856.

76. Muneer RS: Effects of LSD on human chromosomes. Mutat Res 1978;51(3):403–410.

77. Cohen MM, Shiloh Y: Genetic toxicology of lysergic acid diethylamide (LSD-25). Mutat Res 1977–1978;47(3–4):183–209.

78. Reynolds PC, Jindrich EJ: A mescaline associated fatality. J Anal Toxicol 1985;9(4):183–184.

79. Fuller DG: Severe solar maculopathy associated with the use of lysergic acid diethylamide LSD). Am J Ophthalmol 1976;81(4):413–416.

80. Ewald RA: Sun gazing associated with the use of LSD. Ann Ophthalmol 1971;3(1):15–17.

81. Schatz H, Mendelblatt F: Solar retinopathy from sun-gazing under the influence of LSD. Br J Ophthalmol 1973;57(4):270–273.

82. Rohrich J, Zorntlein S, Lotz J, et al: False-positive LSD testing in urine samples from intensive care patients. J Anal Toxicol 1998;22(5):393–395.

83. Gagajewski A, Davis GK, Kloss J, et al: False-positive lysergic acid diethylamide immunoassay screen associated with fentanyl medication. Clin Chem 2002;48(1):205–206.

84. Grobosch T, Lemm-Ahlers U: Immunoassay screening of lysergic acid diethylamide (LSD) and its confirmation by HPLC and fluorescence detection following LSD ImmunElute extraction. J Anal Toxicol 2002;26(3):181–186.

85. Wiegand RF, Kletter KL, Stout PR, et al: Comparison of EMIT II, CEDIA, and DPC RIA assays for the detection of lysergic acid diethylamide in forensic urine samples. J Anal Toxicol 2002;26(7):519–523.

86. Young RE, Hutchison S, Milroy R, Kesson CM: The rising price of mushrooms. Lancet 1982;1:213.

87. Peden NR, Pringle SD, Crooks J: The problem of psilocybin mushroom abuse. Hum Toxicol 1982;1:417.

88. Martin CM: Caring for the "bad trip." A review of current status of LSD. Hawaii Med J 1970;29(7):555–560.

89. Miller PK, Gay GR, Ferris KC, Anderson S: Treatment of acute adverse psychedelic reactions: "I've tripped and I can't get down." J Psychoactive Drugs 1992;24:277–279.

46 *GHB and Related Compounds*

LAWRENCE S. QUANG, MD

At a Glance...

■ GHB, a schedule I drug, is a potent central nervous system depressant that is abused illicitly for its sedative, euphoric, and hallucinogenic effects.

■ GHB has also been popular as a sports and dietary health supplement for its growth hormone–releasing, anxiolytic, and soporific effects as well as numerous other unproven "natural health benefits."

■ GBL and 1,4-BD are chemical precursors that are converted in vivo to GHB via simple enzymatic biotransformation steps; GVL, GHV, and THF are GHB structural analogs with anecdotal case reports of abuse and overdose.

■ Acute toxicity from GHB and its chemical precursors and analogs consists primarily of central nervous system and respiratory depression; chronic abuse of GHB, GBL, and 1,4-BD has resulted in chemical dependency and a severe withdrawal state upon abrupt cessation.

■ Treatment of acute GHB overdose and its withdrawal state consists of aggressive supportive care.

Despite the known dangers of illicit γ-hydroxybutyric acid (GHB) abuse, greatly publicized by the harmful, illicit, and unlawful use of GHB by high-profile celebrities, such as professional basketball player Tom Gugliotta,[1] Hollywood actor Nick Nolte,[2] and Max Factor heir Andrew Luster,[3,4] GHB has developed into a favorite party drug in popular culture during the past 15 years.[5-8] GHB and its many chemical precursors and structural analogs, most notably γ-butyrolactone (GBL) and 1,4-butanediol (1,4-BD), have become fashionable and trendy recreational drugs during the past decade as reports of its "natural" euphoric and hallucinogenic properties popularized its illicit abuse. GHB, GBL, and 1,4-BD represent an emerging group of drugs among the broad class of recreational drugs known as "club drugs." According to the National Institute on Drug Abuse/ National Institutes of Health, the term *club drugs* derived from the association of these drugs with dance clubs and all-night dance parties called "raves," and include other such drugs as *N*-methyl-3,4-methylenedioxymethamphetamine (see Chapter 44), ketamine (see Chapter 43), flunitrazepam (see Chapter 35), methamphetamine, (see Chapter 44), and lysergic acid diethylamide (see Chapter 45).[9] Like most club drugs, GHB, GBL, and 1,4-BD are physically and psychologically addictive, with acute and chronic toxicity that may be severe or lethal. However, GHB, GBL, and 1,4-BD possess many epidemiologic characteristics and pharmacologic properties that are distinctive from other club drugs. Ironically, before their recent emergence as popular recreational club drugs, GHB, GBL, and 1,4-BD had a relatively quiescent history of medical research and licit therapeutic use spanning more than six decades. This chapter will review the unique history and complex evolution of GHB into a contemporary drug of abuse as well as its pharmacology, toxicology, and clinical diagnosis, management, and disposition.

RELEVANT HISTORY

Of the three principal GHB analogs, GBL was discovered first, in 1947, 13 years before GHB and 19 years before 1,4-BD.[10,11] GHB was subsequently discovered in 1960 by the French scientist Henri Laborit, who synthesized it as a structural analog of the inhibitory neurotransmitter γ-aminobutyric acid (GABA), which was capable of traversing the blood-brain barrier (BBB) after peripheral administration.[12-14] Three years after its laboratory synthesis, GHB was discovered to be a naturally occurring neurochemical in the mammalian brain.[15,16] In 1966, Sprince and colleagues were the first investigators to make the association of 1,4-BD with GHB. Noting the close structural similarity of 1,4-BD with GHB, they demonstrated that 1,4-BD could produce an anesthetic response similar to that of GHB and GBL. In this rodent study, GHB, GBL, and 1,4-BD all produced an anesthetic state that was characterized by the loss of voluntary movement, righting reflex, struggle response, and body and limb tone, as well as myoclonic jerking. They further demonstrated that the electroencephalographic (EEG) tracings of GHB, GBL, and 1,4-BD had very similar wave patterns.[17] As a result of these discoveries, GHB found its first clinical application as an anesthetic agent in the early 1960s.[12-14] Several clinical studies in the 1960s, involving a total of 376 patients, confirmed the potential of GHB to serve as an adjuvant to anesthesia.[18,19] However, those same studies also documented several adverse reactions to GHB anesthesia, including the occurrence of gross muscular movements when rapidly administered, as well as inadequate analgesia (abrupt rise in systolic and diastolic pressure during surgical incision), emergence delirium, and bradycardia. Although GHB continues to be investigated and used as an anesthetic adjuvant abroad,[20-22] it has never gained widespread acceptance in the United States for this clinical application.

In the decades since its initial scientific discovery as a GABA-mimetic neurochemical, GHB has been diverted from an investigational drug with legitimate research applications and licit medical uses to the toxic ingredient in banned nutritional supplements and illicit recreational drugs. An important milestone in this devolution occurred in 1977, when Takahara and colleagues reported that an intravenous dose of 2.5 g of GHB resulted in a

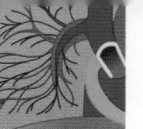

significant increase in plasma growth hormone (GH) and REM sleep in six healthy male subjects.[23] This discovery launched concerted efforts to study and develop GHB as a potential therapeutic agent for sleep disorders such as narcolepsy. However, as an unintended and misappropriated consequence of this and similar other studies, GHB became popular as a sports supplement and "natural" soporific. Subsequently, in the late 1980s, GHB was introduced to the health and dietary supplement market with dubious claims that it could metabolize fat, enhance muscle building, and improve sleep. However, it was quickly associated with severe adverse effects and deaths as overzealous self-administration of GHB-containing nutritional supplements resulted in a well-characterized toxidrome of coma, cardiorespiratory depression, apnea, seizure-like activity, and, in several instances, death.[5,6,7] Accordingly, the U.S. Food and Drug Administration (FDA) intervened in November 1990 to prohibit over-the-counter (OTC) sale of GHB in nutritional supplements.[7] However, GHB purveyors easily circumvented the FDA ban on OTC sale of GHB-containing products by substituting GBL for GHB as the active ingredient. Predictably, toxic effects similar to GHB, including deaths, were reported and confirmed to be attributable to GBL soon after its substitution into dietary health supplements.[8,24-34] Consequently, the FDA issued a recall of GBL-containing health supplements in February 1999, which was easily evaded by the substitution of GBL with 1,4-BD.[35,36] Predictably, the consequences of 1,4-BD misuse and abuse were clinically similar to that of GHB and GBL, including death.[35-42]

In the midst of its emergence as an illicit drug, GHB received both orphan drug and investigational new drug (IND) status from the FDA for clinical trials as a therapeutic agent for narcolepsy. Confounding and nearly preventing its clinical development as a narcolepsy treatment, GHB also developed forensic notoriety as a chemical submission agent used in the commission of drug-facilitated sexual assault, or "date rape." After several highly publicized GHB-related date rape deaths, the Hillory J. Farias and Samantha Reid Date-Rape Prohibition Act (Public Law 106-72) was legislated by Congress and signed into law by President Clinton on March 11, 2000.[43,44] Under this federal statute, GHB received dual scheduling as a schedule III drug for IND use in clinical trials for narcolepsy and as a schedule I drug for illicit purposes. GBL, which has numerous legitimate uses as an industrial solvent, was recognized as a federal list I chemical under this federal statute. Under this law, authority was granted to federal law enforcement agencies to monitor the commercial and industrial sale and distribution of GBL for potential diversionary activity. There was no specific mention of 1,4-BD in this federal law, but 1,4-BD, which also has many legitimate uses as an industrial solvent, was classified by the FDA as a class I health hazard in response to several 1,4-BD-related deaths in 1999.[29,37,38,42] This FDA categorization recognized 1,4-BD to be a potentially life-threatening health hazard but did not impose any regulatory actions on its commercial sale or distribution.

EPIDEMIOLOGY

National statistics from the American Association of Poison Control Centers–Toxic Exposure Surveillance System (AAPCC-TESS), Drug Abuse Warning Network (DAWN), and Monitoring the Future Study (MTFS) have demonstrated a trend of escalating GHB abuse and poisoning throughout the past decade. In 2002, 1386 exposures with GHB and its analogs and precursors were reported to the AAPCC-TESS, representing more than a twofold increase from approximately 600 GHB cases reported in 1996. Among these, 1181 exposures (85%) required treatment in a health care facility and resulted in 272 major outcomes and 3 deaths.[45] Eighty-five percent of these exposures involved individuals over the age of 19. According to DAWN, emergency department (ED) episodes related to GHB increased significantly from 1994 to 1999, and GHB mentions increased dramatically from 1997 to 2000 (Fig. 46-1).[46] Since 2000, trends in ED mentions of GHB appear to have leveled off, with GHB mentions lower in 2002 than in 2000 (Fig. 46-2). ED mentions of GHB appeared to have peaked in 2000, but there was nevertheless a significant long-term increase in ED episodes for GHB from 1995 to 2002 (2197% increase, from 145 to 3330). Almost half (46%) of these ED mentions of GHB were attributed to patients age 20 to 25, nearly 90% were white, and two thirds were male. In 2001, the estimated rate of GHB ED mentions per 100,000 population, by metropolitan area, was highest for San Francisco (9.3%), Dallas (6.7%), New Orleans (5.6%), and Atlanta (4.6%), and GHB abuse increased in 9 of the 21 cities monitored in 2001.[47] Overdose was the predominant reason for ED contact in episodes involving GHB (88%), and the recreational pursuit of its psychic effects was the predominant motive for use among patients with adverse events from GHB (46%).

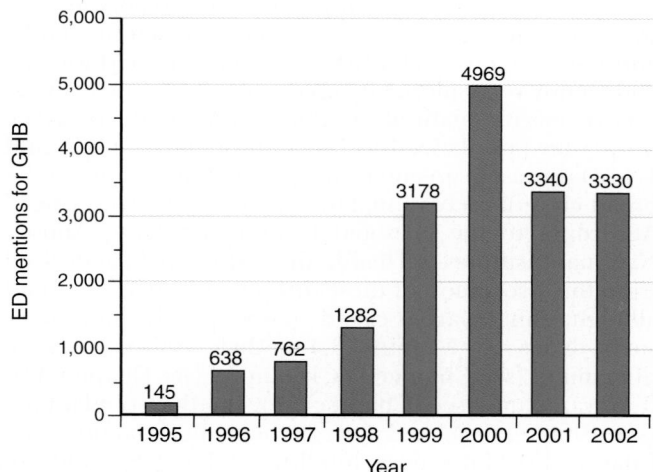

FIGURE 46-1 Emergency department trends for GHB. Final estimates from the Drug Abuse Warning Network (DAWN), 1995–2002. (Compiled from the Substance Abuse and Mental Health Services Administration, Office of Applied Studies: Emergency Department Trends from DAWN, Final Estimates 1995–2002, DAWN Series: D-24. DHHS Publication No. SMA 03-3780. Rockville, MD, Department of Health and Human Services, 2003.)

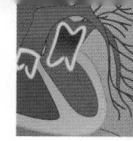

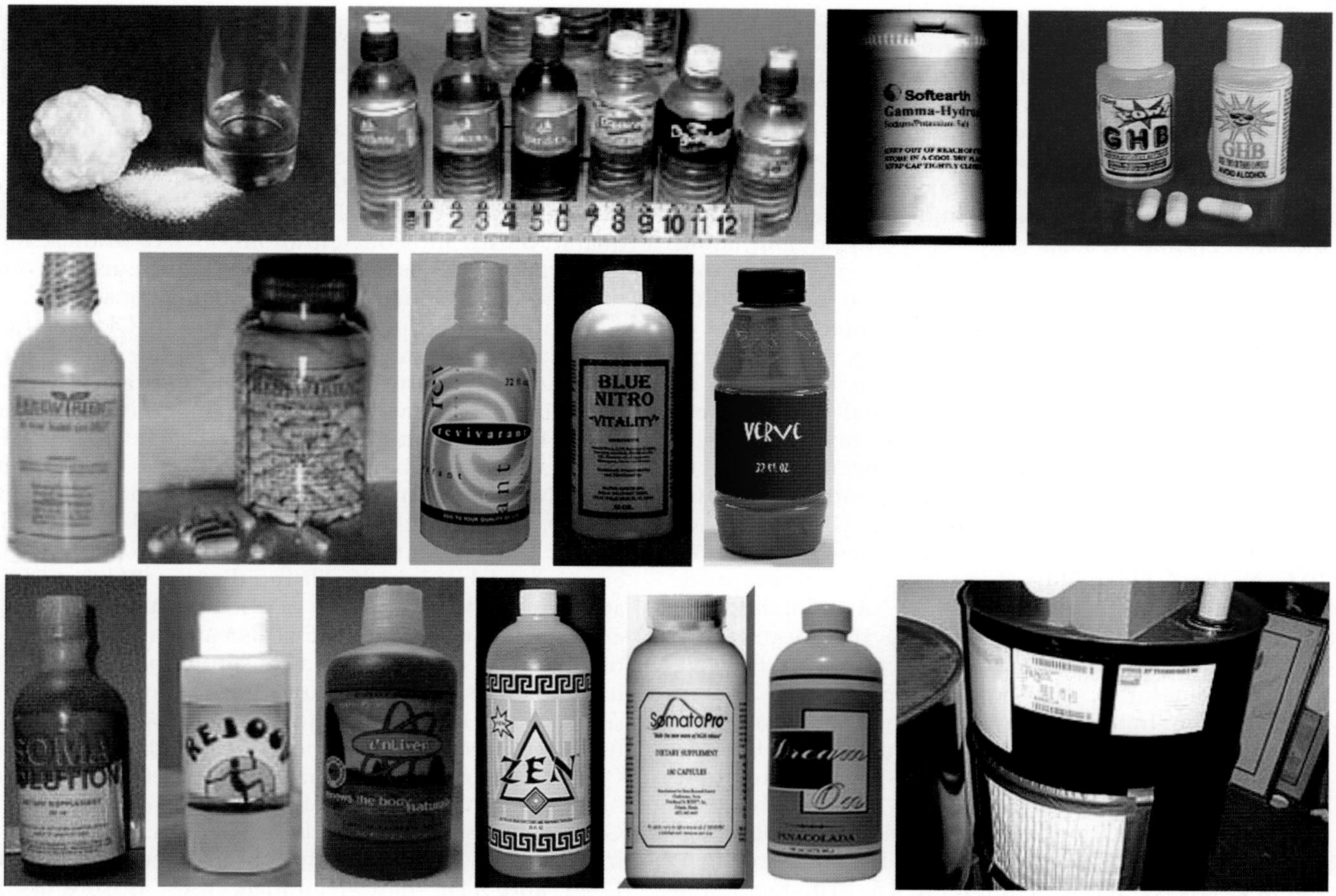

FIGURE 46-2 A, GHB powder, GHB powder dissolved in a water vial and in water bottles, and GHB capsules and drinking solutions. **B,** GBL in various dietary supplements. **C,** 1,4-Butanediol in various dietary supplements and in a 55-gallon drum confiscated by the Drug Enforcement Agency.

Seventy-four percent of ED visits for GHB intoxication involved another club drug. Alcohol was the most frequently mentioned co-ingestant in visits that involved GHB (54%), followed by marijuana (14%) and 3,4-methylenedioxymethamphetamine (MDMA, or "Ecstasy," 12%).[48] While most GHB abusers are young adults, adolescents have also abused GHB, and the 2002 MTFS reported an annual prevalence rate of GHB use of 0.8%, 1.4%, and 1.5% in grades 8, 10, and 12, respectively.[49] These prevalence rates have shown little change since they were first measured for GHB in 2000. Although epidemiologic data are unavailable for each specific GHB analog, the rising abuse of GHB documented by AAPCC-TESS, DAWN, and MTFS likely reflects a parallel increase in GHB analog abuse as well.

The illicit use of GHB and its precursors appears to have plateaued in the United States, but recent international statistics have reported GHB abuse to be on the rise worldwide. The escalating international abuse of GHB has resulted in its scheduling by the United Nations (UN). On March 20, 2001, the UN's Commission on Narcotic Drugs, at the recommendation of the World Health Organization, added GHB to schedule IV of the 1971 Convention on Psychotropic Substances.[50,51] Schedule IV mandates international licensing for manu-

facture, trade, and distribution of GHB and requires all nation signatories of this treaty to comply with prohibition of and restrictions on export and import of GHB, and to "adopt measures for the repression of acts contrary to these laws and regulations." However, since the implementation of this international GHB schedule in 2001, most of the literature reporting toxicity from acute overdoses with GHB has emerged from outside the United States, including the United Kingdom,[52] Spain,[53] Switzerland,[54] the Netherlands,[55] and Australia and New Zealand.[56,57] In Spain, GHB was responsible for 3.1% of all toxicologic emergencies in an urban public hospital ED during a 15-month study period and ranked second in illicit drugs requiring emergency consultation.[53] Conversely, while European and Asian countries have reported recent rises in acute poisonings from GHB and its chemical precursors and structural analogs, virtually all of the reports of GHB dependence and withdrawal have emerged from the United States.

Illicit use of GHB and its analogs have primarily occurred in one of four settings: in the recreational setting of dance raves or night clubs, in the athletic setting of bodybuilding gyms and fitness centers, in the home consumer setting of individuals seeking its "natural health benefits," and in the criminal setting of drug-

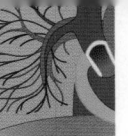

facilitated sexual assault. At raves and nightclubs, GHB is used to achieve effects that have been equated to a combination of alcohol (euphoria, disinhibition, and anxiolysis) and ecstasy (enhanced sensuality, emotional warmth).[51] Current street names for GHB and its precursors and analogs include liquid ecstasy, liquid E, Fantasy, grievous bodily harm, Georgia home boy, great hormones at bedtime, great human benefit, organic quaalude, liquid X, soap, salty water, easy lay, and liquid FX.[42,58-61] In gyms and health food stores, GHB is sold as a performance-enhancing additive in bodybuilding formulas and drinks that are promoted as growth hormone releasers and muscle builders. GHB and its analogs have also been sold to home consumers as "natural" health food and nutritional supplements purporting to enhance weight loss, sexual potency, baldness reversal, and eyesight improvement, and to decrease aging, depres-sion, insomnia, and alcohol, and drug addiction.[62] Products containing GHB, GBL, or 1,4-BD and marketed for these purposes—Somatomax PM, Natural Sleep-500, Renewtrient, Revivarant or Revivarant G, Blue Nitro or Blue Nitro Vitality, GH Revitalizer, Gamma G, Remforce, Invigorate, Jolt, Renewtrient, Verve Revitalize Plus, Serenity, Enliven, GHRE, SomatoPro, NRG3, Thunder Nectar, Weight Belt Cleaner, Inner G, Serenity, Soma Solutions, Blue Nitro, and others—are generally no longer sold because of law enforcement pressure; however, comparable products with similar brand names are available (see Fig. 46-1).[38,42,58-61] Criminally, GHB has been employed in the commission of date rape, and the Drug Enforcement Agency (DEA) has documented 15 drug-facilitated sexual assaults involving 30 victims under the influence of GHB.[58] In the only known published study on the prevalence of drugs used in cases of alleged sexual assault, urine specimens from 1179 cases were submitted to forensic toxicologists nationwide to test specifically for date rape drugs. Approximately 711 samples (60%) tested positive for one or more drugs, and GHB was specifically detected in 48 of these positive samples (6.75%).[63]

Presently, the major distributors of street GHB are clandestine laboratories, both domestic and foreign, that manufacture GHB using a relatively simple synthesis procedure with commercially available, easily accessible, and inexpensive solvents (GBL) and reagents (a base, such as sodium hydroxide). An alternative source for GHB has been home synthesis via recipes and kits that have been available thorough the Internet and mail order.[38,64] Once synthesized, GHB is a clear and odorless liquid that is often distributed in "spring water" bottles and dispensed to the user by the water-bottle cap, with a "capful" being the most common dosage unit.[58,59] GBL and 1,4-BD have been directly substituted for GHB in such packaging. In many instances, these illicit preparations are disguised by adding food coloring and flavoring agents and stored in water or sports drink bottles or in unsuspecting packaging such as eye-dropper bottles, glass vials, and mouthwash bottles. At nightclubs, bars, and "rave" parties, GHB is often sold for $5 to $20 per capful, which is orally consumed in an average dose

of 1 to 5 g.[58-61] When consumed by the capful, one 55-gallon drum of GBL can yield 240,000 capfuls, potentially yielding $1.9 million per 55-gallon drum.[59] While oral ingestion of liquid GHB is the most common route of consumption, capsule and tablet forms are also available, as is powdered GHB, which is snorted or dissolved in a liquid.[61] Because of its salty taste, powdered or liquid GHB is typically mixed into a beverage. The quality, purity, and concentrations of GHB in these illicit preparations are usually so varied that the user is often unaware of the actual dose that is being consumed.

An important epidemiologic trend in GHB abuse is the increased use of analogs. To evade law enforcement detection, GHB distributors have recently developed and distributed new analogs, which are abused in substitution of GHB or used to synthesize GHB. The list of GHB analogs known to be used for these purposes continues to evolve and expand. At present, this list includes GBL, 1,4-BD, GHV, GVL, and THF.[58-61,65] Both GBL and 1,4-BD are well documented to be abused as chemical pre-cursors of GHB, which will rapidly metabolize to GHB after ingestion. Although rarely reported in cases of acute GHB poisoning, THF is also a chemical precursor of GHB. GVL is abused as a substitute for GHB because it metabolizes to GHV, an analog with physiologic effects similar to GHB. Among the GHB analogs, only GBL is used as a precursor ingredient for the illicit synthesis of GHB. GHB analogs are usually distributed as liquids and orally consumed. Despite federal anti-GHB legislation, GHB analogs remain legally available in products not intended for human consumption, since GBL, 1,4-BD, GVL, and THF have legitimate uses as solvents for industrial production of polyurethane, pesticides, elastic fibers, coatings on metals and plastics, and other manufacturing products. Exploiting this legal loophole, GHB purveyors have recently diverted these analogs into thinly veiled household products sold as "fish tank cleaner," "ink stain remover," "ink cartridge cleaner," and "nail enamel remover" for approximately $100 per bottle.

STRUCTURE AND STRUCTURE-ACTIVITY RELATIONSHIPS

GHB has several endogenous structural analogs and chemical precursors as well as several well-characterized synthetic structural analogs and precursors. The chemical structures, structure-activity relationships, and biotrans-formation steps of GHB and its numerous endogenous and synthetic analogs are shown in Figure 46-3. The structure-activity relationships of GHB and these analogs have been methodically examined with the use of [3H]GHB binding studies by Bourguignon and colleagues and are summarized in Table 46-1.[66-68]

PHARMACOLOGY

GHB has a dual pharmacologic profile, with the intrinsic neuropharmacology of endogenous GHB distinct and divergent from that of exogenously administered GHB.

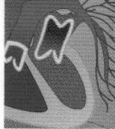

FIGURE 46-3 Chemical structures, biotransformation reactions, and metabolic steps of gamma-hydroxybutyric acid and its chemical precursors and analogues. Numbered enzymes/reactions include *1,* tetrahydrofuran hydroxylase; *2,* 2-hydroxy tetrahydrofuran dehydrogenase; *3,* 2-hydroxy tetrahydrofuran isomerase; *4,* alcohol dehydrogenase; *5,* aldehyde dehydrogenase; *6,* nonezymatic hydrolysis or peripheral tissue and serum lactonases; *7,* GHB dehydrogenase or hydroxyacid-oxoacid transhydrogenase; *8,* succinic semialdehyde reductase; *9,* β-oxidation; *10,* succinic semialdehyde dehydrogenase, *11,* GABA transaminase; and *12,* an uncharacterized reaction (involving 2-carbon condensation?) forming 4,5-dihydroxyhexanoic acid from succinic semialdehyde.

The principal difference between their profiles is that the intrinsic neuropharmacologic activity of endogenous GHB appears to be mediated by the GHB receptor, while the neuropharmacologic activity of exogenously administered GHB is likely mediated by the GABA(B) receptor. Whereas other pharmacologic aspects of endogenous GHB are presently well characterized, research on exogenous GHB neuropharmacology is only in its nascent stages. Therefore, while other pharmacologic differences probably exist between endogenous and exogenous GHB, they are under investigation and have yet to be clarified.

Endogenous GHB

Although the precise physiologic function of endogenous GHB is unknown, GHB is a putative neurotransmitter or neuromodulator because it possesses the requisite pharmacologic properties for recognition as such:

1. It has a discrete regional and subcellular distribution in the central nervous system (CNS).[69-72]

2. It has subcellular systems for synthesis, vesicular uptake, and storage in presynaptic terminals.[71,73-92]

3. It is released in a Ca^{2+}-dependent manner following depolarization of neurons.[71,93-95]

4. Subsequent to neuronal release, GHB binds to GHB-specific receptors and modulates neurotransmitter systems.[71,96-118]

5. Following neuronal release, GHB activity is terminated by active uptake from the synaptic cleft for metabolism by specific cytosolic and mitochondrial enzymes.[71,119-140]

6. Localized application of GHB can produce a response that mimics the action of endogenous GHB released by nerve stimulation (i.e., synaptic mimicry).[141-146]

These pharmacologic properties of GHB are major preconditions if GHB is to play a role in interneuronal signaling or neuromodulation. GHB is heterogeneously distributed throughout the mammalian CNS, with its highest concentrations found in the hippocampus, basal ganglia, hypothalamus, striatum, and substantia nigra.[69-71] GHB is concentrated in the cytosolic and

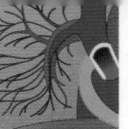

TABLE 46-1 Structure-Activity Relationships of Substituted GHB and Structurally Related Synthetic Compounds

NO. AND NAME OF GHB DERIVATIVE	SUBSTITUTION/MODIFICATION ON GHB MOLECULE	GHB RECEPTOR BINDING (% INHIBITION)		
		AT 10 μmol/L	AT 1 μmol/L	IC$_{50}$, μmol/L
Endogenous Structural Analogs				
1 GABA	γ-NH$_2$	NA		
2 Trans-4-hydroxycrotonic acid (T-HCA)	Unsaturation of GHB by double bond between α and β carbon	64	44	2.9
Endogenous Precursors				
3 γ-butyrolactone (GBL)	Lactone ring of GHB	NA		
4 γ-crotonolactone (GCL)	Unsaturation of GBL by double bond between α and β carbon	NA		
5 1,4-Butanediol (1,4-BD)	Substitution of —C-OH for —C-OOH	NA		
Synthetic Structural Analogs				
6 5-Hydroxyvaleric acid	Lengthening of GHB chain by one carbon	53	22	NR
7 γ-methyl-GHB	γ-CH$_3$	63	12	NR
8 γ-phenyl-GHB	γ—⬡	56	13	6.8
9 γ-(p-chlorophenyl)-GHB	γ—⬡—Cl	NR		
10 γ-(p-methoxyphenyl)-GHB	γ—⬡—OCH$_3$	NR		
11 γ-benzyl-GHB	γ—CH$_3$—⬡	NR	NR	2.3
12 γ-benzyl-GHB (R enantiomer)	γ·····CH$_3$—⬡	NR	NR	1.8
13 γ-benzyl-GHB (S enantiomer)	γ—CH$_3$—⬡	NR	NR	25.0
14 γ-(p-methoxybenzyl)-GHB (NCS 435)	γ—CH$_3$—⬡—OCH$_3$	NR	NR	0.1
Synthetic Structural Precursors				
15 γ-valerolactone (GVL)	Addition of γ-CH$_3$ on GBL; precursor of γ-methyl-GHB	NA		
16 Tetrahydrofuran (THF)	Cyclic ether ring precursor of GBL and GHB	NA		

The names and structures of endogenous and synthetic GHB analogues and precursors are presented with respect to their substitutions and modifications on the GHB molecule:

$$HO-\underset{4}{\overset{\gamma}{C}}-\underset{3}{\overset{\beta}{C}}-\underset{2}{\overset{\alpha}{C}}-\underset{1}{\overset{O}{C}}-OH$$

The structure-activity relationships of these endogenous and synthetic GHB analogs and precursors have been examined by binding studies with [³H]GHB. The GHB analogs and precursors in this table have been tested at concentrations of 1 and 10 μmol/L for their ability to inhibit [³H]GHB (25 μmol/L) binding to GHB receptors on rat brain membrane preparations. The IC$_{50}$ concentrations were available for the most active compounds. Not depicted in the table, GHB itself produced 55% and 35% inhibition of [³H]GHB binding at concentrations of 10 and 1 μmol/L, respectively, and shows an IC$_{50}$ value of 6.6 μmol/L. The GHB derivatives that demonstrated a greater potency than GHB (IC$_{50}$ < 6.6 μmol/L) for inhibiting [³H]GHB binding to GHB receptors were the endogenous structural analog T-HCA (IC$_{50}$ 2.9 μmol/L) and the synthetic structural analogs γ-benzyl-GHB (IC$_{50}$ 2.3 μmol/L), R-γ-benzyl-GHB (IC$_{50}$ 1.8 μmol/L), and γ-(p-methoxybenzyl)-GHB (NCS 435, IC$_{50}$ 0.1 μmol/L). Of note, none of the endogenous or synthetic GHB ring analogs (GBL, GCL, GVL, THF) were recognized by the GHB receptor, evidence that the open form of ring analogs is necessary for GHB receptor binding. Also, the endogenous precursor 1,4-BD and the endogenous structural analog GABA were recognized by the GHB receptor. IC$_{50}$, inhibition concentration of 50%; NA, no affinity; NR, not reported.

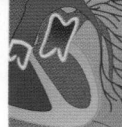

synaptosomal fractions in studies of the subcellular distribution of GHB in rat brain, signifying a mechanism for its presynaptic synthesis and accumulation.[127]

As summarized in Figure 46-3, the subcellular presynaptic synthesis of endogenous GHB involves three precursors (GABA, GBL, and 1,4-BD) and five enzymes (GABA-transaminase [GABA-T], succinic semialdehyde reductase [SSR], alcohol dehydrogenase [ADH], aldehyde dehydrogenase, and serum and peripheral tissue lactonases). The major precursor of endogenous brain GHB is GABA,[71,77,78] which is converted to succinic semialdehyde (SSA) by the brain mitochondrial enzyme, GABA-T. SSA can enter into one of two subsequent biotransformation pathways. In the major pathway, SSA is oxidized by the mitochondrial enzyme succinic semialdehyde dehydrogenase (SSADH) to succinic acid. Production of succinic acid by SSADH allows entry of the GABA carbon skeleton into the tricarboxylic acid cycle for catabolism to H_2O and CO_2.[71-74,77,78] Alternatively, in the minor pathway, SSA is reduced by the neuronal cytosolic enzyme SSR to GHB. The vast majority of GABA enters the mitochondrial oxidative pathway to produce succinic acid by SSADH, because only about 0.05% (in vitro) to 0.16% (in vivo) of the metabolic flux coming from GABA enters the cytosolic reductive pathway to form GHB by SSR.[74,85] Thus, GHB formation is colocalized in GABAergic neurons, or in neurons that can synthesize GABA, which are regionally most prominent in the cerebellum, colliculi, median hypothalamus, and hippocampus.[80,82,84,85]

The second source for subcellular presynaptic synthesis of endogenous GHB is the precursor 1,4-BD, which is present at brain concentrations of about 1/10 of those of GHB.[86] 1,4-BD is the dihydroxy alcohol precursor of GHB, which undergoes in vivo biotransformation by oxidation of one alcohol group on the molecule to γ-hydroxybutyraldehyde by liver ADH followed by the subsequent formation of GHB either by liver aldehyde dehydrogenase or auto-oxidation.[17,73,86-88] The potential sources of the small endogenous concentrations of 1,4-BD found in the mammalian brain are the polyamines ornithine, spermine, spermidine, and putrescine.[89] The third source for subcellular presynaptic synthesis of endogenous GHB is the precursor GBL, which is also present at brain concentrations (200 pmol/g tissue weight) of about 1/10 of those of GHB.[75,90] GBL can undergo rapid in vivo biotransformation to GHB by serum or peripheral tissue lactonases.[91] However, in contrast to ADH and aldehyde dehydrogenase, no lactonase activity has been described in the brain cell.[92] Therefore, the role of GBL as a brain precursor to endogenous GHB is enigmatic. Nevertheless, the equilibrium of GBL and GHB in the mammalian brain might be explained by a chemical nonenzymatic hydrolysis rather than an enzymatic process.[71]

Although the existence of a putative GHB-specific receptor has been speculated[96-98] and disputed for some time, its existence was recently verified by the cloning of a G protein–coupled receptor in the rat that is activated by endogenous GHB.[99] This newly cloned receptor exhibits no binding affinity for GABA, baclofen, or glutamate, which have no capacity to displace radioactive GHB from this binding site, but it does exhibit binding affinity for the GHB structural derivative γ-p-phenyl-hydroxybutyrate (see discussion of GHB analogs earlier under Structure and Structure-Activity Relationships) and the GHB β-oxidation derivative trans-4-hydroxycrotonic acid and its γ-p-chloro-phenyl and γ-p-nitro-phenyl substitute derivatives. Interestingly, however, this receptor exhibited no binding affinity for the GHB receptor-specific antagonist NCS 382. This observation, in combination with the study's additional finding that three distinct bands were present on Northern blot analysis of total RNA extracted from several rat organs (including brain), suggests the existence of a family of GHB receptors in the brain with NCS 382–sensitive and –insensitive subtypes identified.

GHB modulates several neurotransmitter systems. GHB appears to exert a dose-related effect on both the GABAergic and dopaminergic systems. The administration of low-dose GHB inhibits GABA release in the thalamus, thereby implicating a role for GHB in producing absence seizures,[101] and decreases the extracellular GABA concentration in the frontal cortex.[102] However, higher doses of GHB have been shown to enhance GABA concentrations in the frontal cortex.[102] The accentuation of GABA neurotransmission produced by high-dose GHB might underlie the CNS-depressant effect of GHB in experimental animals and overdose patients (see later section on Exogenous GHB). GHB also exerts a prominent modulatory effect on dopamine neurotransmission. Acute administration of GHB inhibits dopamine release and results in the accumulation of dopamine in the presynaptic cells. This effect has been shown to be mediated by GHB inhibition of dopamine neuron firing in the substantia nigra and mesolimbic regions[103-105] and the subsequent autoreceptor-mediated stimulation of tyrosine hydroxylase activity, resulting in increased presynaptic dopamine production.[106,107] The attenuation of dopamine neurotransmission following GHB administration may be the pharmacologic basis for the loss of locomotor activity in experimental animals and overdose patients. Interestingly, it also has been proposed that GHB can produce a biphasic effect on dopamine neurotransmission that is dose and time dependent. While attenuated dopaminergic activity is the primary response after GHB administration, several investigators have demonstrated a second phase of GHB modulation that ensues after the initial decrement in dopamine release, when dopamine neurotransmission is enhanced in the striatum and corticolimbic structures.[71,104,108] Such a biphasic, secondary increase of dopaminergic neurotransmission might represent the pharmacologic basis for its reported euphoric effect and the reward mechanism responsible for its abuse potential.

Other systems modulated by GHB include the serotonin system, cholinergic system, and opioid system. GHB modulates the serotonin system by increasing its turnover rate, without altering total brain serotonin levels, likely by elevating presynaptic tryptophan concentrations.[71,109,110] GBL, but not GHB itself, has been shown to increase total brain acetylcholine concen-

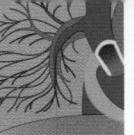

trations by decreasing firing of cholinergic neurons.[111-113] Such an increase in brain acetylcholine might underlie the pharmacologic basis for the reported analeptic effect of GHB in narcolepsy. Despite having no binding affinity for opioid receptors, GHB has been reported to stimulate an increase in release of endogenous opioids in various brain regions.[104,114-116] Furthermore, despite naloxone having no affinity for the GHB receptor, the administration of the opioid antagonists naloxone and naltrexone can attenuate or reverse the electrophysiologic and behavioral actions of GHB on dopamine neuron firing and catalepsy in experimental animals.[117,118]

After its release from GHBergic presynaptic membranes, GHB activity is terminated by an active vesicular uptake system driven by the vesicular inhibitory amino acid transporter (the same transporter that mediates the vesicular uptake of GABA and glycine) or by an active cellular uptake from the synaptic cleft by means of a high affinity Na^+-dependent transport protein specific for GHB and its analogs.[96,119,120] Once within the cell, the degradation of endogenous GHB in the mammalian brain can occur via four pathways leading to (1) succinic acid (which enters the tricarboxylic acid cycle, and represents the most quantitatively significant degradative pathway), (2) GABA, (3) *trans*-4-hydroxycrotonic acid, or (4) 4,5-dihydroxyhexanoic acid (see Fig. 46-3).

Exogenous GHB

Although accumulating evidence favors the role of endogenous GHB as a neuromodulator, because it is synthesized, stored, and released at particular synapses that express GHB-specific receptors, the study of the pharmacologic profile of exogenous GHB is still in its infancy, having only recently been impelled by the increasing problem of GHB abuse. Nevertheless, accumulating data suggest that the $GABA_B$ receptor is a major component of the neural substrate mediating the pharmacologic, behavioral, clinical, and toxicologic actions of exogenous GHB and its precursors, particularly when the brain GHB concentration exceeds its physiologic concentration by two to three orders of magnitude, saturating GHB-specific receptors and producing $GABA_B$ receptor-mediated brain perturbations.[147-153] Thus, data accumulated since 2001 support the role of the $GABA_B$ receptor in mediating acute and chronic toxicity from GHB and its precursor 1,4-BD. Under conditions of excess exogenous administration or endogenous production (see Human Inborn Error of Metabolism, 4-hydroxybutric aciduria/SSADH deficiency),[154] it is theorized that GHB may act both directly as a partial $GABA_B$ receptor agonist and indirectly through a GHB-derived GABA pool. GHB itself is a weak $GABA_B$ receptor agonist with an affinity in the mmol/L range, which far exceeds the 1 to 4 µmol/L physiologic concentrations of GHB in the brain.[147,155,156] Therefore, the supraphysiologic concentration of GHB that could accumulate after its exogenous administration may exert its effects through a weak, direct agonistic effect on $GABA_B$ receptor-mediated mechanisms. Alternatively, GHB could act as an indirect agonist of the $GABA_B$ receptor by its biotrans-

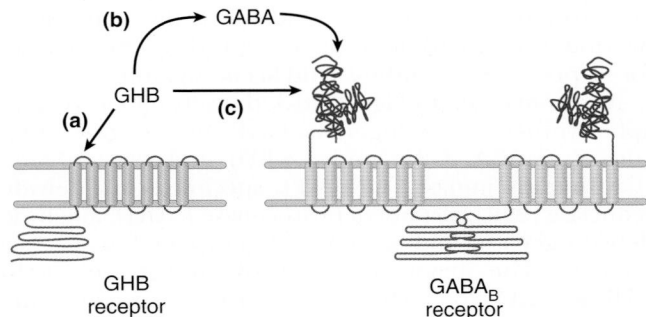

FIGURE 46-4 Schematic model of GHB receptor pharmacology. *a*, Physiologic concentrations of GHB in the human and mammalian brain (nanomolar to micromolar) activate the GHB receptor, which exists as NCS 382–sensitive and –insensitive subtypes. *b*, Supraphysiologic concentrations of GHB (high micromolar to millimolar) might be metabolized to a concentration of GABA sufficient enough to activate the $GABA_B$ receptor. *c*, Supraphysiologic concentrations of GHB may alternatively result in the direct binding of GHB itself to the GABAB receptor. (From Wong CGT, Gibson KM, Snead OC III: From the street to the brain: neurobiology of the recreational drug γ-hydroxybutyric acid. Trends Pharmacol Sci 2004;25[1]:29–34.)

formation to GABA.[71] This hypothesis is supported by the previous observation that inordinately high concentrations of GHB (high µmol/L to low mmol/L) are needed to produce enough GHB-derived GABA to induce displacement and induce $GABA_B$ receptors.[157] In summary, it appears that the pharmacologic and toxicologic effects of supraphysiologic concentrations of GHB, either from exogenous administration (overdose) or endogenous production (inherited SSADH deficiency), are due to saturation of GHB receptors, direct and indirect activation of $GABA_B$ receptors, and/or a combination of these effects (Fig. 46-4).

PHARMACOKINETICS

Human pharmacokinetic data are available only for GHB and are summarized in Table 46-2,[158-161] but such data are lacking for its precursors and analogs, GBL, 1,4-BD, GVL, GHV, and THF. Following oral administration, GHB is rapidly absorbed from the gastrointestinal tract and reaches peak plasma concentrations within 1 hour of dosing. Due to a probable first-pass mechanism, GHB has a low oral bioavailability (less than 30%). GHB does not bind to plasma proteins, readily crosses the placenta and the blood-brain barrier, and has an apparent volume of distribution of 202 to 384 mL/kg. Orally administered GHB exhibits nonlinear elimination pharmacokinetics, with elimination from the human body being dose dependent. As the oral dose is increased, there is a disproportionate increase in systemic exposure, and the elimination half-life is increased. However, plasma GHB was nondetectable or only at negligible concentrations 8 hours after oral administration of 9 g (2.5 times the coma-inducing dose). In general, only 1% to 7% of an oral GHB dose is renally eliminated as parent compound in human urine. Therefore, metabolism is the major elimination pathway for GHB.

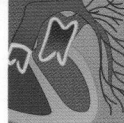

TABLE 46-2 Pharmacokinetic Parameters for GHB (Sodium Oxybate) in Healthy Volunteers after Oral Dosing

STUDY POPULATION	N	ROUTE	DOSE	DURATION	C_{max} (µg/mL)	T_{max} (hr)	$T_{1/2}$ (hr)	AUC_{inf} (mL·min·kg)	CL/F (mL/min·kg)	V_z/F (mL/kg)
			GHB ADMINISTRATION							
Healthy volunteers[1]	8	Oral	12.5 mg/kg	Single	23	0.42	0.45	15.1	14	NR
			25 mg/kg	Single	23	0.5	0.37	21.2	9	NR
			50 mg/kg	Single	23	0.75	0.38	26.1	7	NR
Healthy volunteers[3]	15	Oral	3 g	Single	83.8	0.50	0.74	136	4.3	260
Healthy volunteers[3]	12	Oral	4.5 g	Single	146	0.50	0.76	302	3.1	190
Healthy volunteers (male)[5]	18	Oral	4.5 g	Single	88.3	1.25	0.65	241	3.8	202
Healthy volunteers (female)[5]	18	Oral	4.5 g	Single	83.0	1.14	0.61	233	4.2	218
Healthy volunteers (fed)[5]	36	Oral	4.5 g	Single	60.1	2.00	0.68	188	6.2	384
Healthy volunteers (fasted)[5]	36	Oral	4.5 g	Single	142	0.75	0.57	288	3.7	190
Healthy volunteers[3]	12	Oral	4.5 g (2 × 2.25 g)	Single	64.6	0.50	0.57	178	5.7	248
			4.5 g (2 × 2.25 g)	Single	60.1	0.64	0.59	138	6.6	325
Healthy volunteers[3]	12	Oral	9.0 g (2 × 4.5 g)	Single	142	0.72	0.83	518	3.6	249
Healthy volunteers (fasted)[6]	8	Oral	25 mg/kg	Single	39.4	0.33–0.75	0.5	NR	NR	NR

AUC, area under the curve from time zero to time infinity; CL/F, plasma clearance divided by absolute bioavailability; C_{max}, peak plasma concentration; NR, not reported; $T_{1/2}$, elimination half-life; T_{max}, corresponding peak time; V_z/F, volume of distribution divided by absolute bioavailability.

Special Populations

Human pharmacokinetic data for GHB in special patient populations with narcolepsy, alcoholism, and liver cirrhosis as well as those undergoing general surgery and cesarean section are summarized in Table 46-3.[162-168] There are no significant variations in the kinetics of GHB between males and females (see Table 46-2)[159] or between healthy human volunteers and narcoleptic patients[162,163] and alcohol-dependent patients[165] (see Tables 46-2 and 46-3). However, compared with healthy adult volunteers, the mean oral clearance and elimination half-life were markedly reduced and significantly prolonged, respectively, in patients with biopsy-proven liver cirrhosis[164] (see Tables 46-2 and 46-3).

Pharmacologic Agents

ANESTHESIA

GHB found its first clinical application as an anesthetic agent in the early 1960s. Several clinical studies in the 1960s, involving a total of 376 patients, confirmed the potential of GHB to serve as an adjuvant to anesthesia.[169,170] However, those same studies also documented several adverse reactions to GHB anesthesia, including the occurrence of gross muscular movements when rapidly administered, as well as inadequate analgesia (abrupt rise in systolic and diastolic pressure during surgical incision), emergence delirium, and bradycardia. Although GHB continues to be used and investigated as an anesthetic adjuvant abroad,[171-173] it has never gained widespread acceptance in the United States for this clinical application. At present, GHB use as an anesthetic agent is limited to France, as well as Germany and Austria.[174]

NARCOLEPSY

The clinical development of GHB in the United States began in 1994, when the National Organization of Rare Disorders and the FDA Orphan Products Development Division encouraged the development of GHB as a treatment for narcolepsy based on the promising results of several preliminary clinical studies.[175-179] After the safety and efficacy of GHB as a narcolepsy treatment were established by two randomized, double-blind, placebo-controlled studies,[180-183] the FDA approved GHB (sodium oxybate, Xyrem [Jazz Pharmaceuticals, Palo Alto, CA]) as a treatment for narcolepsy-related cataplexy on July 17, 2002.

ALCOHOL DEPENDENCE AND WITHDRAWAL

GHB has been widely used in Italy to treat alcohol dependence and withdrawal since 1988.[184] The use of a GHB pharmaceutical for this clinical indication was

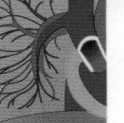

TABLE 46-3 Pharmacokinetic Parameters for GHB (Sodium Oxybate) in Select Patient Populations after Oral or Intravenous Administration

| STUDY POPULATION | N | GHB ADMINISTRATION | | | C_{max} (µg/mL) | T_{max} (hr) | $T_{1/2}$ (hr) | AUC_{inf} (mL/min·kg) | CL/F (mL/min·kg) | V_z/F (mL/kg) |
		ROUTE	DOSE	DURATION						
Narcoleptic patients[9]	13	Oral	4.5 g	Single	90.0	0.75	0.67	226	4.0	226
			4.5 g	8 weeks	104	0.50	0.67	254	3.5	197
Narcoleptic patients[10]	6	Oral	6 g (2 × 3 g)	Single	91.2	0.59	0.88	295	4.2	307
Liver disease (child's class A patients)[11]	8	Oral	25 mg/kg (1.75 g)	Single	68	0.75	0.53	85	4.5	198
Liver disease (child's class C patients)[11]	8	Oral	25 mg/kg (1.75 g)	Single	47	0.75	0.93	94.1	4.1	285
Alcoholic-dependent patients[12]	10	Oral	25 mg/kg (1.75 g)	Single	54	0.5	0.45	52	9.6	NR
			25 mg/kg (1.75 g)	13 doses	55	0.5	0.43	52	9.2	NR
			50 mg/kg (3.5 g)	Single	45	0.75	0.58	90.3	5.3	NR
Surgical patients[13]	3	IV	50 mg/kg (3.5 g)	Single	NR	NR	~0.5	ND	ND	ND
Surgical patients or sedation[14]	6	IV	30–100 mg/kg bolus (2.1–7 g)	Single bolus and infusion	NR	NR	~0.67	ND	ND	ND
Cesarian section patients[15]	14	IV	26.7–50 mg/kg (1.9–3.5 g)	Single infusion	NR	NR	ND	ND	ND	ND

AUC, area under the curve from time zero to time infinity; CL/F, plasma clearance divided by absolute bioavailability; C_{max}, peak plasma concentration; ND, not determined; NR, not reported; $T_{1/2}$, elimination half-life; T_{max}, corresponding peak time; V_z/F, volume of distribution divided by absolute bioavailability.

based on two randomized, double-blind, placebo-controlled clinical trials conducted by Gallimberti and colleagues. In the first trial, 23 patients who met the *Diagnostic and Statistical Manual of Mental Disorders* (DSM-IIIR) criteria for alcohol withdrawal syndrome were recruited for treatment with GHB 50 mg/kg/day (n = 11) or placebo (n = 12).[185] GHB treatment resulted in a significant decrease in the Alcohol Withdrawal Score.[185] This was followed by a second randomized, double-blind clinical trial with 71 alcoholic patients who were randomized to receive GHB 50 mg/kg/day (n = 36) or placebo (n = 35). After the study period and a 3-month follow-up period, GHB-treated patients significantly increased their days of abstinence and reduced the number of drinks they consumed daily. Furthermore, GHB-treated patients reported a significant reduction in Alcohol Craving Scale scores.[186] Similar results were also reported by fellow Italian investigators in clinical studies.[187,188] As a result of these clinical trials, GHB is widely used in Italy today to treat alcohol dependence at the dosage of 50 mg/kg/day in three or more divided doses.[184]

EXPERIMENTAL THERAPIES

Presently, GHB is undergoing clinical and preclinical investigations for diverse indications. Although GHB received FDA approval for treating narcolepsy-related cataplexy, it failed to receive approval for treatment of excessive daytime sleepiness. Therefore, GHB is presently undergoing clinical reevaluation for this narcolepsy indication. Pilot studies have shown promising results, since the nocturnal administration of sodium oxybate in narcoleptic patients recently produced significant improvements in sleep architecture, which coincided with significant improvements in daytime functioning.[189] GHB is also presently being evaluated as a treatment for fibromyalgia, with several recent clinical studies reporting GHB capable of effectively reducing the symptoms of pain, fatigue, and sleep abnormalities characteristic of this disorder.[190,191] Preclinically, interesting and compelling data recently have been generated to demonstrate the potential use of GHB as a neuroprotective agent in stroke[192-195] and traumatic brain[196] and spinal cord injury,[197] as well as an angiogenesis inhibitor in tumors.[198,199]

DRUG INTERACTIONS

The potential for drug interactions by an inhibitory effect of GHB on human hepatic microsomal cytochrome P-450 (CYP) isozymes has been assessed in vitro with pooled human liver microsomal fractions. In these studies, the activities of CYP1A2, CYP2C9, CYP2C19, CYP2D6, CYP2E1, and CYP3A were not inhibited by GHB at concentrations of 3 to 300 µmol/L. Therefore, metabolic interactions of GHB with drugs metabolized through these pathways are not anticipated.[200]

TOXICOLOGY

Clinical Manifestations

Toxicity from GHB and its analogs have occurred in the settings of acute overdose/poisoning, withdrawal after abrupt cessation from chronic misuse, and human inborn error of SSADH expression.

ACUTE OVERDOSE

Clinical experience accumulated during the past 15 years with acute toxicity from GHB overdose has resulted in a fairly homogeneous and easily recognized pattern of symptoms and signs. The hallmark of this "GHB toxidrome" is CNS and respiratory depression of relatively short duration.[5,6,7,8,24-42] There is a dose-response relationship such that the level of CNS and respiratory depression progressively worsens with increasing doses, with doses of greater than 50 mg/kg leading to coma, apnea, and death. These dose-response relationships are summarized in Table 46-4. Respiratory depression is particularly prominent in the published cases of pediatric GHB/GBL poisonings. Among the seven published case reports of pediatric GHB/GBL poisonings, apnea occurred in six patients.[31-33,201] Other adverse clinical effects from acute GHB overdose are summarized by systems in Box 46-1. The occurrence of generalized clonic seizures is controversial because they have been inconsistently reported in acute GHB, GBL, and 1,4-BD overdoses. It is possible that such motor activity may actually represent myoclonic movements mistaken for seizure activity. Such myoclonic activity has been clearly documented during anesthesia induction with GHB and occurs without epileptiform EEG patterns. It is further possible that such seizures may be attributable to hypoxia, co-ingestion with a stimulant drug, or withdrawal. Nevertheless, GHB has been clearly established to produce absence seizures in laboratory animals so that seizures may be a plausible adverse effect from acute GHB overdose. Deaths from GHB ingestion

---

TABLE 46-4 In Vivo and In Vitro Dose-Response Effects of GHB

DOSE OR CONCENTRATION OF GHB	CLINICAL OR PHYSIOLOGIC EFFECT
Oral Dose (Humans)	
10 mg/kg	Short-term amnesia
20–30 mg/kg	Sleep and drowsiness
50–60 mg/kg	Coma, cardiorespiratory depression, seizures
Systemic Dose (Rodents)	
10–50 mg/kg	Memory impairment
75–200 mg/kg	Absence seizures, EEG spike-and-wave discharges
200–300 mg/kg	Stupor, EEG slowing
>300 mg/kg	Coma, EEG burst suppression
1.7 g/kg	LD_{50}
In Vitro Concentration	
Nanomolar to low micromolar	Activation of GHB receptor
Low micromolar	Alter GABA and glutamate release
Millimolar	Activation of GABA(B) receptor, possible conversion to physiologically active concentrations of GABA

EEG, electroencephalographic; GABA, γ-aminobutyric acid.
Adapted from Wong CGT, Gibson KM, Snead OC III: From the street to the brain: neurobiology of the recreational drug γ-hydroxybutyric acid. Trends Pharmacol Sci 2004;25(1):29–34.

BOX 46-1	**CLINICAL EFFECTS OF GHB AND ITS PRODRUGS AND ANALOGS**

Central Nervous System
Euphoria
Hallucinations
Headache
Ataxia
Confusion
Amnesia
Hypotonia
Somnolence
Unconsciousness
Coma
Agitation/combativeness
Delirium
Seizure/myoclonic jerking

Respiratory
Respiratory depression
Apnea
Cheyne-Stokes respirations

Cardiovascular
Bradycardia
Hypotension
Right bundle branch block (pediatric)
ST-segment elevation (pediatric)
P-wave inversion (pediatric)
U waves (adult)

Gastrointestinal
Excessive salivation
Vomiting

Metabolic
Metabolic acidosis
Respiratory acidosis

Other
Miosis
Hypothermia
Diaphoresis
Urinary incontinence
Acute psychosis
Withdrawal syndrome
Wernickle-Korsakoff syndrome

From Shannon M, Quang LS: Gamma-hydroxybutyrate, gamma-butyrolactone, and 1,4-butanediol: a case report and review of the literature. Pediatr Emerg Care 2000;16(6):435–440.

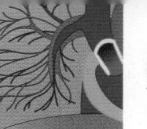

have occurred, with the majority of these incidents involving polysubstance ingestion with either alcohol or a narcotic. Co-ingestion of 1,4-BD with alcohol is particularly dangerous because both substances are competitive substrates for the metabolizing enzyme ADH. Because ADH has a greater substrate affinity for alcohol than 1,4-BD, the adverse effects from ADH-mediated biotransformation of 1,4-BD to GHB will be delayed in this co-ingestion.[40] When co-ingested with GHB or GBL, alcohol has been shown to produce additive or potentiated toxicity as well. Lastly, given the proscriptive status of GHB and its analogs, improperly performed "kitchen synthesis" of GHB has resulted in caustic oral burns and subsequent esophageal strictures when the neutralization process for potassium hydroxide (a key ingredient for home synthesis of GHB from GBL) was inadequately performed.[202]

WITHDRAWAL SYNDROME

The GHB withdrawal syndrome, which occurs after the abrupt cessation of chronic, high-dose abuse, is a rapidly emerging clinical disorder.[42,203-233] As of this writing, there are 87 published case reports of GHB withdrawal in the clinical literature. Eight of these cases predated 2000,[203-211] with the first case report published in 1994.[203] The remaining 79 case reports of GHB withdrawal were published after 2000, which represents nearly a 10-fold increase in incidence during the past 5 years.[42,211-233] The clinical experience derived from the sum of case reports has begun to yield a preliminary characterization of the GHB withdrawal state. Most of the patients experiencing the GHB withdrawal state have been males, with a mean age in the early thirties. Among these 87 case reports of withdrawal, GHB, GBL, and 1,4-BD were responsible for 72 (82.8%), 11 (12.6%), and 4 (4.6%) cases, respectively. While most individuals did not know their exact daily dose, they were estimated to be about 48 g and 27 g for GHB and GBL, respectively, with an average daily dosing interval of 4 to 5 hours. The mean duration of misuse was just over 1 year. The onset of withdrawal symptoms occurred within a mean of 46 hours after the last dose of GHB, and the mean duration of the withdrawal syndrome was 9 days. The clinical features of the GHB withdrawal syndrome were similar to ethanol withdrawal and included, in the relative order of frequency of occurrence, tremor, tachycardia, anxiety, restlessness, hallucinations (primarily visual and auditory), delirium, insomnia, delusions, paranoia, diaphoresis, hypertension, nausea or vomiting, and psychosis. Two seizures have been reported in GHB withdrawal, one of which was associated with death.[223,233]

HUMAN INBORN ERROR OF METABOLISM (4-HYDROXYBUTYRIC ACIDURIA/SUCCINIC SEMIALDEHYDE DEHYDROGENASE DEFICIENCY)

Although acute poisoning from illicit GHB use has been seen by clinicians only in the past 15 years, chronic GHB poisoning from an inherited defect of GABA metabolism has been recognized by molecular biologists and geneticists for nearly 25 years. In 1981, Jakobs and colleagues were the first to describe a 20-month-old boy of related Turkish parents with developmental delay (absent speech), motor retardation, hypotonia, and ataxia, in association with elevated concentrations of GHB in urine, serum, and cerebrospinal fluid.[135] Based on the well-defined metabolic pathway of GABA, Jakobs and colleagues postulated that an enzyme defect of SSADH was responsible. Subsequent investigators verified this theory by demonstrating that the conversion of radiolabeled SSA to CO_2 (via the tricarboxylic acid [TCA] cycle) in intact cultured lymphoblasts of patients was only 2.4% to 6.2% of control values.[234,235] In patients with 4-hydroxybutyric aciduria, SSADH residual activity in these cells was significantly reduced or absent compared with controls.[236-244] Parental and sibling white blood cell extracts demonstrated a "gene-dose effect," with reduction of SSADH activity to approximately 50% of controls. These patterns of patient and parent SSADH activity were consistent with an autosomal-recessive mode of inheritance. As a result of this error of GABA catabolism, Gibson and colleagues reported urine GHB concentrations of 130 to 7600 mmol/mol creatinine (normal less than 2), plasma GHB concentrations of 98 to 1500 µmol/L (normal less than 3), and cerebrospinal fluid GHB concentrations of 263 to 830 µmol/L (normal less than 3) in their large case series. Presently, more than 350 patients have been diagnosed with 4-hydroxybutyric aciduria or SSADH deficiency.[245] Recently, Trettel and colleagues mapped the gene encoding for SSADH to chromosome 6p22.[246] Shortly thereafter, Chambliss and colleagues identified two exon-skipping point mutations in the SSADH genes of four patients. These genetic defects alter highly conserved sequences at intron/exon boundaries, preventing the RNA splicing apparatus from recognizing the normal splice junction. These RNA splicing errors consequently result in SSADH deficiency.[247] Clinical diagnosis can be rather challenging due to some variability of the phenotypic expression of this disease, but in general, clinical findings in patients include psychomotor retardation, absent/delayed speech, mental delay, hypotonia, ataxia, hyporeflexia, seizures/EEG abnormalities, oculomotor apraxia, hyperkinesis, choreoathetosis, aggressive behavior, and somnolence.[248,249]

DIAGNOSIS

Laboratory Testing

GENERAL CONSIDERATIONS

GHB poisoning is generally diagnosed based on clinical history and presentation and confirmed by laboratory testing. Laboratory testing for GHB and its analogs is confounded by several limiting considerations. First, there is a relatively small window of opportunity to recover GHB from biologic fluids. Following oral administration of GHB at toxic doses (12.5 to 50 mg/kg), GHB is almost completely eliminated from blood and urine within 2 to 8 and 8 to 12 hours of administration, respectively.[158-167] Second, immunoassay urine drug screens generally

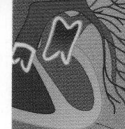

employed by hospitals do not detect GHB and its analogs. Third, while numerous qualitative and quantitative analytical methods have been developed to detect GHB in recent years, they are not routinely available at most hospitals. Fourth, even when theses analytical methods are available to the clinician, they are presently incapable of distinguishing between GHB and its numerous analogs. Fifth, even if a laboratory test is available to confirm and/or quantify the presence of GHB or its analogs, this information is unlikely to alter management or disposition of the GHB-intoxicated patient. Lastly, accurate interpretation of quantitative GHB analysis must also take into consideration complex confounding factors such as specimen collection and storage, spontaneous GHB and GBL chemical interconversion, and endogenous GHB production.

SPECIMEN COLLECTION AND STORAGE

GHB concentrations from collected biologic fluids can be spuriously elevated if improperly collected and stored. Whole blood specimens undergoing laboratory analysis for GHB should be collected and stored in purple-top anticoagulant ethylenediaminetetraacetic acid (EDTA) tubes, avoiding yellow-top anticoagulant-citrate buffer tubes, which artificially generate GHB.[250] Cold storage and use of sodium fluoride or sodium azide preservatives in urine specimens have been shown to minimize spurious GHB concentrations.[251,252]

Spontaneous Chemical Interconversion

The proper identification of GHB versus one of its many analogs, especially GBL, is also complicated by a spontaneous chemical interconversion of GHB and GBL that can occur in aqueous solutions. Generally, this GHB-GBL interconversion is pH dependent, with GHB exhibiting greater stability than GBL in a variety of aqueous solutions. In aqueous solution with water, spontaneous interconversion of GBL to GHB occurs at a ratio of 2:1 within 202 days in pure water, within 9 days in acidic solution (pH 2.0), and within 15 minutes in alkaline solution (pH 12.0). Conversely, spontaneous interconversion of GHB to GBL occurred at a ratio of 1:2 only in acidic solution (pH 2.0) and did not occur at all in pure water or in alkaline solution (pH 12.0).[253] Thus, aqueous solutions of alkaline pH 7.0 favor the spontaneous hydrolysis of GBL to GHB and true equilibrium between GHB and GBL occurring at approximately pH 2.0.

ENDOGENOUS GHB PRODUCTION

In clinical cases that have forensic implications (determination of cause of death) or medicolegal allegations (GHB use for chemical submission/date rape), the endogenous production of GHB must be carefully considered and an analytical chemist/toxicologist consulted. Endogenous production of GHB can occur spontaneously in postmortem biologic specimens and is dependent on both preservative use and storage temperature.[254] Little to no endogenous production of

GHB will occur in postmortem blood preserved with sodium fluoride 10 mg/mL and stored at either room temperature or refrigeration at 4° C. Conversely, 50% higher endogenous GHB formation can occur when postmortem blood was not preserved but stored under refrigeration. Furthermore, when stored at room temperature, endogenous GHB production nearly doubled the value of those unpreserved specimens stored under refrigeration. Therefore, both preservative use and refrigeration of blood specimens will reduce the confounding influence of endogenous GHB production. While virtually all studies do not show elevation of endogenous GHB in postmortem urine, one investigator has reported elevations of endogenous GHB in both postmortem blood and urine specimens.[255]

In clinical cases when there is a medicolegal allegation of sexual assault facilitated by surreptitious placement of GHB into a beverage, it is important to consider that GBL has been discovered to be a natural constituent of a variety of wines. GBL has been detected in extracts from samples of unadulterated red and white wines at concentrations of 5 µg/mL and was easily quantified using a simple chloroform extraction technique followed by gas chromatography/mass spectrometry (GC/MS) analysis.[256] It was additionally demonstrated that grape juice did not contain GBL, suggesting that GBL may be a natural by-product of the wine fermentation process. The observation that many varieties of wine may contain GBL reinforces the need to run proper controls in the forensic analysis of GBL. Hence, during the analysis of allegedly adulterated wine samples, it is important to conduct appropriate comparative quantitative analyses to assess accurately whether the amount of GBL present is at a naturally occurring or elevated level before rendering a decision that the material has been tainted.

QUALITATIVE SCREENING METHODS AND QUANTITATIVE CONFIRMATION METHODS

The dramatic surge in GHB abuse during the 1990s led to rapid advances in the laboratory detection of GHB, which can be useful to the clinician despite the myriad complexities associated with accurate GHB laboratory analysis and interpretation. Presently, at least two rapid colorimetric assays have been commercially developed for rapid screening of the presence of GHB.[257,258] Both rely on the chemical conversion of GHB to GBL and are reported to be capable of producing qualitative results with 0.25 to 1.0 mL of urine within 5 to 10 minutes and with a sensitivity of 0.1 to 0.5 mg/mL. Such qualitative screening methods require confirmation by quantitative methods, which are the most sensitive and reliable methods.

Typically, this quantitative confirmation analysis is performed commercially using a GC/MS technique, for which over two dozen methods have been developed for analysis of GHB.[259] A GC/MS technique was recently used in a clinical study examining the correlation of serum and urine GHB concentrations in 16 patients with a clinical suspicion of GHB-like drug overdose and a Glasgow Coma Scale (GCS) score of 8 or lower.[260] All 16

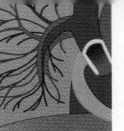

suspected severe GHB overdose patients had significant serum and urine GHB concentrations, which ranged from 45 to 295 mg/L (median 180 mg/L) and 432 to 2407 mg/L (median 1263 mg/L), respectively. Patients who developed a GCS score of 3 had serum concentrations that ranged from 72 to 300 mg/L (median 193 mg/L). Although these GC/MS serum GHB concentrations correlated well with the occurrence of GHB toxicity, they did not correlate with the degree of coma or the time to awakening. Lastly, routine urine organic acid analysis may also accurately detect GHB in the overdose setting when available at a hospital.[261]

Other Diagnostic Testing

Additional diagnostic laboratory testing should be performed as clinically indicated, particularly when the clinician is confronted with a conflicting or complicated clinical picture due to polysubstance ingestion. Because GHB is commonly ingested with ethanol, which exacerbates and/or prolongs the clinical toxicity of GHB, a serum ethanol concentration should be checked in all patients with suspected GHB poisoning. Also, MDMA is a relatively common co-ingestant, which is detectable in routine immunoassay urine drug screens. A 12-lead electrocardiogram is indicated, because GHB may produce cardiac effects (see Table 46-4), but primarily to rule out co-ingestion or intoxication with another potential cardiotoxic agents. A chest x-ray is indicated if there is clinical evidence of aspiration, which the severely GHB-intoxicated patient is at risk for, and which can increase the risk for morbidity and mortality. In cases of prolonged unconsciousness, a serum creatine phosphokinase and basic metabolic panel should be obtained and renal function monitored due to the risk for development of rhabdomyolysis. Other adjunct diagnostic studies for the comatose patient, such as a head computed tomography scan and lumbar puncture, may be deferred if there is a strong clinical index of suspicion for GHB poisoning.

Differential Diagnosis

The differential diagnosis for diminished mental status/coma and respiratory depression, the hallmarks of GHB poisoning, is exhaustive and includes trauma, medical conditions (such as CNS infection or masses, stroke, and hypoglycemia), and other medication overdoses (such as benzodiazepines, barbiturates, opioids, central α_2-adrenergic agonists, anticonvulsants, and ethanol or toxic alcohols). However, while no true pathognomonic sign exists for GHB poisoning, the occurrence of extreme combativeness or agitation during noxious stimuli (such as an attempt on oroendotracheal intubation), followed by relapse into coma, may aid the clinician in differentiating this overdose from other sedative-hypnotic agents. Often, there is a history of GHB ingestion offered by friends, bystanders, or emergency services personnel at the scene, or the patient may be found in possession with containers or products whose label verifies the ingestion of GHB or one of its analogs.

MANAGEMENT

Supportive Measures

The medical management of symptomatic acute overdoses with GHB and its analogs, as well as their withdrawal syndrome, generally only requires vigilant monitoring and anticipatory supportive care. With supportive measures, 54% of patients were treated and released in the majority of episodes involving GHB according to 2002 ED trends reported by DAWN.[48] Recovery with supportive care is often spontaneous and abrupt, since patients have regained consciousness within 1 to 6 hours and without adverse sequelae. At present, there are less data and experience available for the management of the GHB withdrawal syndrome.

ACUTE OVERDOSE

Box 46-2 summarizes the medical management principles for the patient with symptomatic acute overdose with GHB and its analogs. Airway assessment and support is the first priority. A patent airway should be ensured, initially with proper positioning, suctioning of oral secretions, and placement of a temporizing oropharyngeal or nasopharyngeal airway if needed, and supplemental O_2 delivered. Bag-valve mask ventilation followed by endotracheal intubation and mechanical ventilation will be required for patients with loss of airway protective reflexes (coma or severe obtundation), respiratory distress (aspiration pneumonitis), or apnea. When invasive airway management is required, rapid sequence intubation protocols should be applied in order to facilitate a prompt intubation and minimize the occurrence of complications. Intravenous access should be secured and a crystalloid solution administered if hypotensive. Atropine and benzodiazepines are clinically indicated if bradycardia and seizures occur, respectively. As with any patient presenting with coma, dextrose,

---

BOX 46-2	MEDICAL MANAGEMENT AND DISPOSITION OF OVERDOSES FROM GHB AND ITS PRODRUGS AND ANALOGS

Airway support
   Suction airway
   Supplemental oxygen
   Endotracheal intubation
   Mechanical ventilation
Activated charcoal
Intravenous access
Cardiorespiratory monitoring
Atropine for symptomatic bradycardia
Benzodiazepines for seizures
Discharge if clinically stable after 6 hours of observation
Admit if initially presented comatose or if clinically intoxicated after 6 hours of observation

From Shannon M, Quang LS: Gamma-hydroxybutyrate, gamma-butyrolactone, and 1,4-butanediol: a case report and review of the literature. Pediatr Emerg Care 2000;16(6):435–440.

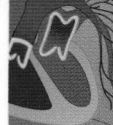

naloxone, and thiamine may be administered as clinically warranted.

WITHDRAWAL SYNDROME

Because the withdrawal syndrome from GHB and its analogs has been reported to be clinically similar to the ethanol withdrawal syndrome, it is managed in much the same manner. In general, high doses of benzodiazepines are used to manage the common withdrawal symptoms of dysautonomia (tachycardia, hypertension), anxiety, agitation, hallucinations, and pyschosis. The limited clinical literature on the GHB withdrawal syndrome also reports cases that are refractory to high-dose benzodiazepines. In such case reports, benzodiazepines have been augmented with and/or substituted by barbiturates (pentobarbital or phenobarbital), anticonvulsants (valproic acid, carbamazepine, gabapentin), chloral hydrate, baclofen, clonidine, β-blockers (propanolol or labetolol), propofol, bromocriptine, trazadone, or antipsychotics.[203–233] At present, no GHB withdrawal treatment regimen has undergone rigorous prospective clinical study.

Decontamination

Induced emesis with syrup of ipecac is contraindicated due to the high likelihood for rapid onset of CNS depression. Although there are no studies demonstrating adsorption of GHB or its analogs to oral activated charcoal (AC), gastrointestinal decontamination with single-dose oral AC may be beneficial if it can be administered in a timely manner. Given the rapid absorption of liquid preparations of GHB and its analogs, decontamination with AC should be initiated within 30 minutes of most ingestions or within 60 minutes of a polydrug ingestion. Accurate assessment for airway integrity and provision of an invasive airway, if clinically indicated, should precede the administration of oral AC.

Laboratory Monitoring

Continuous cardiorespiratory, pulse oximetry, and blood pressure monitoring are required for the patient with a symptomatic acute overdose or the withdrawal syndrome from GHB and its analogs.

Antidotes

Two pharmacologic antidotes, physostigmine and 4-methylpyrazole (4-MP, fomepizole), have been reported to reverse the clinical effects of acute GHB and 1,4-BD overdose, respectively. At present, the administration of these antidotal agents has not been validated with rigorous prospective clinical trials.

PHYSOSTIGMINE

There are several case reports of the successful administration of physostigmine, a carbamate inhibitor of acetylcholinesterase, to reverse GHB-induced sedation in the ED setting. Caldicott and Kuhn reported the reversal of GHB intoxication with physostigmine.[262] Their notion that GHB may be reversed with physostigmine was based on two studies where "GHB reversal" was produced in surgical patients receiving GHB as an anesthestic adjuvant.[263,264] In the two anesthesia case series and in the Caldicott and Kuhn case series, it is likely that investigators may have confused physostigmine "reversal" with the clinical course of GHB, since physotigimine was administered to patients at a time when GHB clinical effects can be expected to wane. Furthermore, pharmacologic studies have found no relationship between GHB and acetylcholine-mediated neurotransmission in the CNS.[265] Therefore, at present, there is a lack of sufficient data to recommend empirical administration of physostigmine as an antidote in the setting of symptomatic acute overdose with GHB or its analogs.

4-METHYLPYRAZOLE

4-Methylpyrazole (4-MP) is a pharmacologically plausible antidotal agent for 1,4-BD overdose. A potent competitive antagonist for ADH, 4-MP would be expected to block the biotransformation of 1,4-BD to GHB, and there are many in vitro and in vivo experimental data to support the use of 4-MP to block 1,4-BD toxicity.[266-271] Furthermore, there is a case report of the successful administration of 4-MP to treat 1,4-BD poisoning.[272] Following a 30-mL ingestion of a homemade 1,4-BD solution, a 43-year-old man developed generalized seizures and coma. This patient awoke shortly after the administration of the initial 4-MP dose of intravenous 10 mg/kg. However, initial GC/MS plasma 1,4-BD and GHB concentrations were 24 and 222 mg/L, respectively. These analytical data are inconsistent with the proposed pharmacologic antidotal mechanism of 4-MP, which is to block 1,4-BD biotransformation to the toxic compound GHB. Although basic investigations support the use of 4-MP in the setting of early 1,4-BD acute overdose,[150,272-274] the empirical administration of 4-MP as an antidote cannot be recommended until more rigorous clinically derived data are available.

Elimination

Given the known pharmacokinetic profile of GHB, it is unlikely that gastric lavage, whole bowel irrigation, or other extracorporeal methods of enhanced elimination will be useful in the management of acute overdoses with GHB or its analogs.

Disposition

Box 46-2 summarizes the disposition of a patient with an acute overdose of GHB or its analogs. Patients should be observed in the ED for 6 hours and may be discharged if they remain asymptomatic. If a patient arrives at the ED with a clinical presentation consistent with an acute overdose of GHB or its analogs, or develops these symptoms during ED observation, inpatient admission is indicated. Disposition of a patient with a GHB polydrug ingestion, particularly when a narcotic or ethanol is involved, requires caution because most GHB-related deaths have been associated with these co-ingestions. In the case of ethanol, animal studies and clinical case

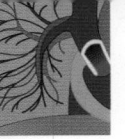
reports have documented potentiated toxicity, prolonged toxicity, and in the case of 1,4-BD, delayed GHB toxicity.

ACKNOWLEDGMENTS

I wish to thank Hai Thong Nguyen, MD, attending physician, Ste. Anne Hospital, Montreal, Quebec (Veterans Affairs, Canada), for his valuable assistance in translating the French-written GHB papers cited in this manuscript (references 12 through 14). Preparation of this chapter was supported in part by National Institutes of Health/National Institute on Drug Abuse Grant 1RO3 DA14951.

REFERENCES

1. Close Call. Retrieved January 2005 from http://espn.go.com/magazine/vol3no7gugliotta.html.
2. CBS News: Nick Nolte cops a plea. Retrieved January 2005 from http://www.cbsnews.com/stories/2002/10/24/entertainment/main526796.shtml.
3. CNN: Max Factor heir returns to face prison term. Retrieved January 2005 from http://www.cnn.com/2003/LAW/06/19/max.factor.heir/.
4. CBS News: Fugitive Max Factor heir caught. Retrieved January 2005 from http://www.cbsnews.com/stories/2003/06/19/national/main559376.shtml.
5. Centers for Disease Control and Prevention: Multistate outbreak of poisonings associated with illicit use of gamma hydroxybutyrate. MMWR 1990;39:861–863.
6. Dyer JE: Gamma-hydroxybutyrate: a health food product producing coma and seizure-like activity. Am J Emerg Med 1991;9:321–324.
7. Food and Drug Administration: Gamma hydroxybutyric acid. Press Release P90-53. Rockville, MD, Food and Drug Administration, November 8, 1990.
8. Higgins TF, Borron SW: Coma and respiratory arrest after exposure to butyrolactone. J Emerg Med 1996;14:435–437.
9. National Institute on Drug Abuse: Club Drugs. Retrieved January 2005 from http://www.drugabuse.gov/drugpages/clubdrugs.html.
10. Giacamino NJ, McCawley EL: On the toxic reactions of unsaturated lactones and their saturated analogs. Fed Proc 1947;6:331–332.
11. Rubin BA, Giarman NJ: The therapy of experimental influenza in mice with antibiotic lactones and related compounds. Yale J Biol Med 1947;19:1017–1024.
12. Laborit H, Jouany JM, Gerard J, et al: Generalities concerning the experimental study and clinical use of gamma hydroxybutyrate of Na [French]. Agressologie 1960;1:397–406.
13. Laborit H, Buchard F, laborit G, et al: Use of sodium 4-hydroxybutyrate in anesthesia and resuscitation [French]. Agressologie 1960;1:549–560.
14. Laborit H, Jouany JM, Gerard J, et al: Summary of an experimental and clinical study on a metabolic substrate with inhibitory central action: sodium 4-hydroxybutyrate [French]. Presse Med 1960;68:1867–1869.
15. Bessman SP, Fishbein WN: Gamma hydroxybutyrate a new metabolite in brain [Letter]. FASEB J 1963;22:334.
16. Bessman SP, Fishbein WN: Gamma-hydroxybutyrate, a normal brain metabolite. Nature 1963;200:1207–1208.
17. Sprince H, Josephs JA, Wilpizeski CR: Neuropharmacological effects of 1,4-butanediol and related congeners compared with those of gamma-hydroxybutyrate and gamma-butyrolactone. Life Sci 1966;5:2041–2052.
18. Blumenfeld M, Suntay RG, Harmel MH: Sodium gamma-hydroxybutyric acid: a new anaesthetic adjuvant. Anesth Analg 1962;41:721–726.
19. Solway J, Sadove MS: 4-Hydroxybutyrate: a clinical study. Anesth Analg 1965;44:532–539, 1965.
20. Kleinschmidt S, Grundmann U, Janneck U, et al: Total intravenous anesthesia using propofol, gamma-hydroxybutyrate or midazolam in combination with sufentanil for patients undergoing coronary artery bypass surgery. Eur J Anaesthesiol 1997;14:590–599.
21. Kleinschmidt S, Grundmann U, Knocke T, et al: Total intravenous anaesthesia with gamma-hydroxybutyrate (GHB) and sufentanil in patients undergoing coronary artery bypass graft surgery: a comparison in patients with unimpaired and impaired left ventricular function. Eur J Anaesthesiol 1998;15:559–564.
22. Kleinschmidt S, Schellhase C, Mertzufft F: Continuous sedation during spinal anaesthesia: gamma-hydroxybutyrate vs propofol. Eur J Anaesthesiol 1999;16:23–30.
23. Takahara J, Yunoki S, Yakushiji W, et al: GHB Stimulatory effects of gamma-hydroxybutyric acid on growth hormone and prolactin release in humans. J Clin Endocrinol Metab 1977;44(5):1014–1017.
24. Rambourg-Schepens MO, Buffet M, Durak C, et al: Gamma butyrolactone poisoning and its similarities to gamma-hydroxybutyric acid: two case reports. Vet Hum Toxicol 1997;39:234–235.
25. LoVecchio F, Curry SC, Bagnasco T: Butyrolactone-induced central nervous system depression after ingestion of Renewtrient, a "dietary supplement." N Engl J Med 1998;339:847–848.
26. Centers for Disease Control and Prevention: Adverse effects associated with ingestion of gamma-butyrolactone. Minnesota, New Mexico, and Texas, 1998–1999. MMWR 1999;48(7):137–140.
27. Hardy CJ, Slifman NR, Klontz KC, et al: Adverse events reported with the use of gamma-butyrolactone products marketed as dietary supplements [Abstract]. J Toxicol Clin Toxicol 1999;37(5):650.
28. Food and Drug Administration: FDA Talk Paper: FDA warns about products containing gamma butyrolactone or GBL and asks companies to issue a recall. Retrieved January 2005 from http://www.fda.gov/bbs/topics/ANSWERS/ANS00937.html.
29. Food and Drug Administration: FDA Talk Paper: FDA warns about GBL-related products. Retrieved January 2005 from http://www.fda.gov/bbs/topics/ANSWERS/ANS00953.html.
30. Kohrs FP, Porter WH: Gamma-hydroxybutyrate intoxication and overdose. Ann Emerg Med 1999;33(4):475–476.
31. Winickoff JP, Houck CS, Rothman EL, et al: Experience and reason: Verve and Jolt: Deadly new internet drugs. Pediatrics 2000;106(4):829–830.
32. Leblanc F, Blais R: Gamma butyrolactone exposure from nail polish remover [Abstract]. J Toxicol Clin Toxicol 2000;38(5):535.
33. Boyer EW, Fearon D, Anderson AC, et al: Child neglect leading to gamma-hydroxybutyrate ingestion [Abstract]. J Toxicol Clin Toxicol 2000;38(5):534–535.
34. Vandevenne L, Beckers J, Van de Velde E, et al: A case of gamma-butyrolactone overdose [Abstract]. J Toxicol Clin Toxicol 2000;38(2):227.
35. Eckstein M, Henderson SO, DelaCruz P, et al: Gamma hydroxybutyrate (GHB): report of a mass intoxication and review of the literature. Prehosp Emerg Care 1999;3(4):357–361.
36. Cisek J, Holstege C, Rose R: Seizure associated with butanediol ingestion [Abstract]. J Toxicol Clin Toxicol 1999;37(5):510.
37. Food and Drug Administration: Medwatch—More on GBL, GHB, BD. Retrieved January 2005 from http://www.fda.gov/medwatch/SAFETY/1999/gblghb.htm.
38. Shannon M, Quang LS: Gamma-hydroxybutyrate, gamma-butyrolactone, and 1,4-butanediol: a case report and review of the literature. Pediatr Emerg Care 2000;16(6):435–440.
39. Ingels M, Rangan C, Bellezzo J, et al: Coma and respiratory depression following the ingestion of GHB and it precursors: three cases. J Emerg Med 2000;19(1):47–50.
40. Schneidereit T, Burkhart K, Donovan JW, et al: Butanediol toxicity delayed by preingestion of ethanol. Int J Med Toxicol 2000;3(1):1–3.
41. Kraner J, Plassard J, McCoy D, et al: Fatal overdose from ingestion of 1,4-butanediol, a GHB precursor [Abstract]. J Toxicol Clin Toxicol 2000;38(5):534.
42. Zvosec DL, Smith SW, McCutcheon JD, et al: Adverse events, including death, associated with the use of 1,4-butanediol. N Engl J Med 2001;344(2):87–94.
43. Drug Enforcement Agency, Department of Justice: Schedules of controlled substances: addition of gamma hydroxybutyric acid to schedule I. Fed Reg 2000;65:13235–13238.

44. Drug Enforcement Administration, Department of Justice: Placement of gamma-butyrolactone in List I of the Controlled Substances Act (21 U.S.C. 802 (34)): final rule. Fed Reg 2000;65(79):21645–21647.

45. Watson WA, Litovitz TL, Klein-Schwartz W, et al: 2003 annual report of the American Association of Poison Control Centers Toxic Exposure Surveillance System. Am J Emerg Med 2004; 22(5):335–404.

46. Substance Abuse and Mental Health Services Administration, Office of Applied Studies: Emergency department trends from the Drug Abuse Warning Network, final estimates 1995–2002, DAWN Series: D-24. DHHS publication no. (SMA) 03-3780. Rockville, MD, Department of Health and Human Services, 2003.

47. Community Epidemiology Work Group, National Institutes of Health, National Institute on Drug Abuse: Epidemiologic trends in drug abuse, advance report, June 2001. Retrieved July 2004 from http://www.nida.nih.gove/CEWG/AdvanceRep/601ADV/601adv.html.

48. Substance Abuse and Mental Health Services Administration, Office of Applied Studies: The DAWN report: club drugs 2001 update. Drug Abuse Warning Network. Rockville, MD, Department of Health and Human Services, March 2002.

49. Johnston LD, O'Malley PM, Bachman JG: Monitoring the future national results on adolescent drug use: overview of key findings, 2002. NIH publication no. 03-5374. Bethesda, MD, National Institute on Drug Abuse, 2003.

50. United Nations Commission on Narcotic Drugs: Implementation of the international drug control treaties: changes in the scope of control of substances. Retrieved December 2004 from http://www.unodc.org/pdf/document_2001-01-29_1.pdf.

51. Galloway GP, Frederick-Osbourne SL, Seymour R, et al: Abuse and therapeutic potential of gamma-hydroxybutyric acid. Alcohol 2000;20:263–269.

52. Elliot SP: Nonfatal instances of intoxication with gamma-hydroxybutyrate in the United Kingdom. Ther Drug Monit 2004;26(4):432–440.

53. Miro O, Nogue S, Espinosa G, et al: Trends in illicit drug emergencies: the emerging role of gamma-hydroxybutyrate. J Toxicol Clin Toxicol 2002;40(2):129–135.

54. Liechti ME, Kupferschmidt H: γ-Hydroxybutyrate (GHB) and γ-butyrolactone (GBL): analysis of overdose cases reported to the Swiss Toxicological Information Centre. Swiss Med Wkly 2004;134:534–537.

55. Bosman IJ, Lusthof KJ: Forensic cases involving the use of GHB in the Netherlands. Forensic Sci Int 2003;133(1–2):17–21.

56. Caldicott DGE, Chow FY, Burns BJ, et al: Fatalities associated with the use of γ-hydroxybutyrate and its analogues in Australasia. Med J Aust 2004;181(6):310–313.

57. Brown TCK: Epidemic of γ-hydroxybutyrate (GHB) ingestion. Med J Aust 2004;181(6):343.

58. Drug Enforcement Administration, Office of Diversion Control, Drug and Chemical Evaluation Section: Fact sheet: gamma hydroxybutyric acid (GHB, liquid X, goop, Georgia home boy). DEA/ODE #(000811). Washington, DC, Drug Enforcement Administration, August 11, 2000.

59. Drug Enforcement Agency, U.S. Department of Justice: GHB/GBL. Retrieved March 2005 from http://www.usdoj.gov/dea/concern/drug_trafficking.html.

60. National Drug Intelligence Center, U.S. Department of Justice: Information bulletin: GHB analogs: GBL, BD, GHV, and GVL. Product no. 2002-L0424-003. Washington, DC, National Drug Intelligence Center, August 2002.

61. National Drug Intelligence Center, U.S. Department of Justice: Intelligence bulletin: GHB trafficking and abuse. Product no. 2004-L0424-015. Washington, DC, National Drug Intelligence Center, September 2004.

62. Zvosec DL, Smith SW: Unsupported "efficacy" claims of gamma hydroxybutyrate (GHB). Acad Emerg Med 2003;10(1):95–96.

63. ElSohly MA, Salamone SJ: Prevalence of drugs used in cases of alleged sexual assault. J Anal Toxicol 1999;23:141–146.

64. Henretig F, Vassalluzo C, Osterhoudt K, et al: "Rave by net": gamma-hydroxybutyrate (GHB) toxicity from kits sold to minors via the internet [Abstract]. J Toxicol Clin Toxicol 1998; 36:503.

65. Cartigny B, Azaroual N, Imbenotte M, et al: 1H NMR spectroscopic investigation of serum and urine in a case of acute tetrahydrofuran poisoning. J Anal Toxicol 2001;25:270–274.

66. Benavides J, Rumigny JF, Bourguignon JJ, et al: A high-affinity, Na⁺-dependent uptake system for gamma-hydroxybutyrate in membrane vesicles prepared from rat brain. J Neurochem 1982;38(6):1570–1575.

67. Bourguignon JJ, Schoenfelder A, Schmitt M, et al: Analogues of γ-hydroxybutyric acid. Synthesis and binding studies. J Med Chem 1988;31(5):893–897.

68. Bourguignon JJ, Schmitt M, Didier B: Design and structure-activity relationship analysis of ligands of gamma-hydroxybutyric acid receptors. Alcohol 2000;20:227–236.

69. Vayer P, Maitre M: Regional differences in depolarization-induced release of γ-hydroxybutyrate from rat brain slices. Neurosci Lett 1988;87:99–103.

70. Mamelak M: Gammahydroxybutyrate: an endogenous regulator of energy metabolism. Neurosci Biobehav Rev 1989;13:187–198.

71. Maitre M: The γ-hydroxybutyrate signaling system in brain: organization and functional implications. Prog Neurobiol 1997; 51:337–361.

72. Snead OC: γ-Hydroxybutyric acid in subcellular fractions of rat brain. J Neurochem 1987;48:196–201.

73. Roth RH, Giarman NJ: Evidence that central nervous system depression by 1,4-butanediol is mediated through a metabolite, gamma-hydroxybutyrate. Biochem Pharmacol 1968;17:735–739.

74. Gold BI, Roth RH: Kinetics of in vivo conversion of γ-[³H]aminobutyric acid to γ-[³H]hydroxybutyric acid by rat brain. J Neurochem 1977;28:1069–1073.

75. Snead OC 3rd, Furner R, Liu CC: In vivo conversion of gamma-aminobutyric acid and 1,4-butanediol to gamma-hydroxybutyric acid in rat brain. Studies using stable isotopes. Biochem Pharmacol 1989;38(24):4375–4380.

76. Eli M, Cattabeni F: Endogenous γ-gammahydroxybutyrate in rat brain areas: postmortem changes and effects of drugs interfering with γ-aminobutyric acid metabolism. J Neurochem 1983;41:524–530.

77. Wong CG, Chan KF, Gibson KM, et al: γ-Hydroxybutyric acid: neurobiology and toxicology of a recreational drug. Toxicol Rev 2004;23(1):3–20.

78. Wong CG, Gibson KM, Snead OC 3rd: From the street to the brain: neurobiology of the recreational drug γ-hydroxybutyric acid. Trends Pharmacol Sci 2004;25(1):29–34.

79. Rumigny JF, Cash C, Mandel P, et al: Evidence that a specific succinic semialdehyde reductase is responsible for γ-hydroxybutyrate synthesis in brain tissue slices. FEBS Lett 1981;134:96–98.

80. Cash CD, Maitre M, Mandel P: Purification from human brain and some properties of two NADPH-linked aldehyde reductases which reduce succinic semialdehyde to 4-hydroxybutyrate. J Neurochem 1979;33:1169–1175.

81. Vayer P, Schmitt M, Bourguignon JJ, et al: Evidence for a role of high K_m aldehyde reductase in the degradation of endogenous γ-hydroxybutyrate from rat brain. FEBS Lett 1985;190:55–60.

82. Weissmann-Nanopoulos D, Belin MF, Mandel P, et al: Immunocytochemical evidence for the presence of enzymes synthesizing GABA and GHB in the same neuron. Neurochem Int 1984;6:333–338.

83. Weissmann-Nanopoulos D, Rumigny JF, Mandel P, et al: Immunocytochemical localization in rat brain of the enzyme that synthesizes γ-hydroxybutyric acid. Neurochem Int 1982;4:523–529.

84. Rumigny JF, Cash C, Mandel P, et al: Ontogeny and distribution of specific succinic semialdehyde reductase apoenzyme in the rat brain. Neurochem Res 1982;7:555–561.

85. Rumigny JF, Maitre M, Cash C, et al: Regional and subcellular localization in rat brain of the enzymes that can synthesize γ-hydroxybutyric acid. J Neurochem 1981;36:1433–1438.

86. Barker SA, Snead OC, Poldrugo F, et al: Identification and quantitation of 1,4-butanediol in mammalian tissues: an alternative biosynthesis pathway for gamma-hydroxybutyric acid. Biochem Pharmacol 1985;34:1849–1852.

87. Pietruszko R, Voigtlander K, Lester D: Alcohol dehydrogenase from human and horse liver-substrate specificity with diols. Biochem Pharmacol 1978;27:1296–1297.

88. Maxwell R, Roth RH: Conversion of 1,4-butanediol to gamma-hydroxybutyric acid in rat brain and in peripheral tissue. Biochem Pharmacol 1972;21:1521–1533.

89. Tillakaratne NJ, Medina-Kauwe L, Gibson KM: Gamma-aminobutyric acid (GABA) metabolism in mammalian neural and nonneural tissues. Comp Biochem Physiol A 1995;112(2):247–263.

90. Doherty JD, Hattox SE, Snead OC, et al: A sensitive method for quantitation of γ-hydroxybutyric acid and γ-butyrolactone in brain by electron capture gas chromatography. Anal Biochem 1975;69:268–277.

91. Roth RH, Delgado JMR, Giarman NJ: Gamma-butyrolactone and gamma-hydroxybutyric acid. II. The pharmacologically active form. Int J Neuropharmacol 1966;5:421–428.

92. Fishbein WN, Bessman SP: Purification and properties of an enzyme in human blood and rat liver microsomes catalyzing the formation and hydrolysis of γ-lactones. J Biol Chem 1966;241:4835–4841.

93. Maitre M, Mandel P: Liberation de γ-hydroxybutyrate calcium-dependente après depolarisation de coupes de cerveau de rat. C R Acad Sci Paris 1982;295:741–743.

94. Maitre M, Cash C, Weissmann-Nanopoulos D, et al: Depolarization-evoked release of γ-hydroxybutyrate from rat brain slices. J Neurochem 1983;41:287–290.

95. Vayer P, Maitre M: Regional differences in depolarization-induced release of γ-hydroxybutyrate from rat brain slices. Neurosci Lett 1988;87:99–103.

96. Benavides J, Rumigny JF, Bourguignon JJ, et al: High affinity binding sites for gamma-hydroxybutyric acid in rat brain. Life Sci 1982;30:953–961.

97. Maitre M, Rumigny JF, Benavides J, et al: High affinity binding site for gamma-hydroxybutyric acid in rat brain. Adv Biochem Psychopharmacol 1983;37:441–453.

98. Snead OC, Liu CC: Gamma-hydroxybutyric acid binding sites in rat and human brain synaptosomal membranes. Biochem Pharmacol 1984;33:2587–2590.

99. Andriamampandry C, Taleb O, Viry S, et al: Cloning and characterization of a rat brain receptor that binds the endogenous neuromodulator γ-hydroxybutyrate (GHB). FASEB J 2003;17:1691–1693.

100. Vayer P, Maitre M: γ-Hydroxybutyrate stimulation of the formation of cyclic GMP and inositol phosphates in rat hippocampal slices. J Neurochem 1989;52:1382–1387.

101. Banerjee PK, Snead OC III: Presynaptic gamma-hydroxybutyric acid (GHB) and gamma-aminobutyric acidB (GABAB) receptor-mediated release of GABA and glutamate (GLU) in rat thalamic ventrobasal nucleus (VB): a possible mechanism for the generation of absence-like seizures induced by GHB. J Pharmacol Exp Ther 1995;273:1534–1543.

102. Gobaille S, Hechler V, Andriamampandry C, et al: γ-Hydroxybutyrate modulates synthesis and and extracellular concentration of γ-aminobutyratic acid in discrete rat brain regions in vivo. J Pharmacol Exp Ther 1999;290:303–309.

103. Roth RH, Doherty JD, Walters JR: Gamma-hydroxybutyrate: a role in the regulation of central dopaminergic neurons? Brain Res 1980;189:556–560.

104. Hechler V, Gobaille S, Bourguignon J, et al : Extracellular events induced by gamma-hydroxybutyrate in striatum: a microdialysis study. J Neurochem 1991;56:938–944.

105. Howard SG, Feigenbaum JJ: Effect of γ-hydroxybutyrate on central dopamine release in vivo. Biochem Pharmacol 1997;53:103–110.

106. Walter JR, Roth RH: Effect of gamma-hydroxybutyrate on dopamine and dopamine metabolites in the rat striatum. Biochem Pharmacol 1972;21:2111–2121.

107. Morgenroth V, Walters JR, Roth R: Dopaminergic neurons—alteration in the kinetic properties of tyrosine hydroxylase after cessation of impulse flow. Biochem Pharmacol 1976;25:655–661.

108. Nissbrandt H, Elverfors A, Enberg G: Pharmacogiclly induced cessation of burst activity in nigral dopamine neurons: significance for the terminal dopamine efflux. Synapse 1994;17:217–224.

109. Waldmeier PC, Fehr B: Effects of baclofen and γ-hydroxybutyrate on rat striatal and mesolimbic 5-HT metabolism. Eur J Pharmacol 1978;49:177–184.

110. Hedner T, Lundborg P: Effect of gammahydroxubutyric acid on serotonin synthesis, concentration and metabolism in the developing rat brain. J Neural Trans 1983;57:39–48.

111. Giarman NJ, Schmidt KF: Some neurochemical aspects of the depressant action of gamma-butyrolactone on the central nervous system 1. Br J Pharmacol 1963;20:563–568.

112. Sethy VH, Roth RH, Walters JR, et al: Effect of anesthetic doses of γ-hydroxybutyrate on the acetylcholine content of rat brain. Naunyn Schmiedebergs Arch Pharmacol 1976;295:9–14.

113. Ladinsky H, Consolo S, Zatta A, et al: Mode of action of gamma-butyrolactone on the central cholinergic system. Naunyn Schmiedebergs Arch Pharmacol 1983;322:42–48.

114. Feigenbaum JJ, Simatov R: Lack of effect of γ-hydroxybutyrate on μ, κ, and δ opioid receptor binding. Neurosci Lett 1996;212:5–8.

115. Larson W, Przewlocka B, Przewlocka R: The effect of gamma-hydroxybutyrate and anticonvulsants on opioid peptide content in the rat brain. Life Sci 1983;33:599–602.

116. Gobaille S, Schmidt C, Cupo A, et al: Characterization of methionine-enkephalin release in the rat striatum by in vivo dialysis: effects of gamma-hydroxy butyrate on cellular and extra-cellular methionine enkephalin levels. Neuroscience 1994;60:637–648.

117. Snead OC III, Bearden LJ: Naloxone overcomes the dopaminergic, EEG, and behavioral effects of γ-hydroxybutyrate. Neurology 1980;30:832–838.

118. Feigenbaum JJ, Howard SG: Naloxone reverses the inhibitory effects of γ-hydroxybutyrate on central DA release in vivo in awake animals: a microdialysis study. Neurosci Lett 1997;224:71–74.

119. Muller C, Viry S, Miehe M, et al: Evidence for a gamma-hydroxybutyrate (GHB) uptake by rat brain synaptic vesicles. J Neurochem 2002;80(5):899–904.

120. Hechler V, Bourguignon JJ, Wermuth CG, et al: γ-Hydroxybutyrate uptake by rat brain striatal slices. Neurochem Res 1985;10:387–396.

121. Chambliss KL, Gibson KM: Succinic semialdehyde dehydrogenase from mammalian brain: subunit analysis using polyclonal antiserum. Int J Biochem 1992;24:1493–1499.

122. Margolis RK: The effect of γ-hydroxybutyric acid on amino-acid levels in brain. Biochem Pharmacol 1969;18:1243–1246.

123. Doherty JD, Stout RW, Roth RH: Metabolism of [1-^{14}C]γ-hydroxybutyric acid by rat brain after intraventricular injection. Biochem Pharmacol 1975;24:469–474.

124. Della Pietra G, Illiano G, Capano V, et al: In vivo conversion of γ-hydroxybutyrate into γ-aminobutyrate. Nature 1966;210:733–734.

125. De Feudis FV, Collier B: Conversion of γ-hydroxybutyrate to γ-aminobutyrate by mouse brain in vivo. Experientia 1970;26:1072–1073.

126. Vayer P, Mandel P, Maitre M: Conversion of γ-hydroxybutyrate to γ-aminobutyrate in vitro. J Neurochem 1985;45:810–814.

127. Snead OC: γ-Hydroxybutyric acid in subcellular fractions of rat brain. J Neurochem 1987;48:196–201.

128. Chan-Palay V, Wu JY, Palay SL: Immunocytochemical localization of γ-aminobutyric acid transaminase at cellular and ultrastructural levels. Proc Natl Acad Sci U S A 1979;76:2067–2071.

129. Walsh JM, Clark JB: Studies on the control of 4-aminobutyrate metabolism in synaptosomal and free rat brain mitochondria. Biochem J 1976;160:147–157.

130. Bloch-Tardy M, Buzenet A, Fages C, et al: Two forms of GABA-T in pig brain. Purification and properties. Neurochem Res 1980;5:1147–1154.

131. Vincent SR, Kimura H, McGreer EG: The histochemical localization of GABA transaminase in the efferents of the striatum. Brain Res 1981;222:198–203.

132. Walkenstein SS, Wiser R, Gudmundsen C, et al: Metabolism of γ-hydroxybutyratic acid. Biochem Biophys Acta 1964;86:640–642.

133. Niwa T, Maeda K, Asada H, et al: Gas chromatographic-mass spectrometric analysis of organic acids in renal tissue biopsy: 4-hydroxybutyric acid and 4-hydroxy-2-butenoic acid. J Chromatogr 1982;230:1–6.

134. Vayer P, Ehrhardt JD, Gobaille S, et al: Gamma hydroxybutyrate distribution and turnover rates in discrete brain regions of the rat. Neurochem Int 1988;12:53–59.

135. Jakobs C, Bojasch M, Monch E, et al: Urinary excretion of gamma-hydroxybutyric acid in a patient with neurologic abnormalities. The probability of a new inborn error of metabolism. Clin Chim Acta 1981;111:169–178.

136. Hechler V, Schmitt M, Bourguignon JJ, et al: Trans-gamma-hydroxycrotonic acid binding sites in brain: evidence for a subpopulation of gamma-hydroxybutyrate sites. Neurosci Lett 1990;110:204–209.

137. Hechler V, Peter P, Gobaille S, et al: Gamma-hydroxybutyrate ligands possess antidopaminergic and neuroleptic-like activities. J Pharmacol Exp Ther 1993;264:1406–1414.

138. Kaufman EE, Nelson T, Fales HM, et al: Isolation and characterization of a hydroxyacid-oxoacid transhydrogenase from rat kidney mitchondria. J Biol Chem 1988;263:16872–16879.

139. Brown GK, Cromby CH, Manning NJ, et al: Urinary organic acids in succinic semialdehyde dehydrogenase deficiency: evidence of alpha-oxidation of 4-hydroxybutyric acid, interaction of succinic semialdehyde with pyruvate dehydrogenase and possible secondary inhibition of mitochondrial beta-oxidation. J Inherit Metab Dis 1987;10:367–375.

140. Gibson KM, Jakobs C: Disorders of beta- and gamma-amino acids in free and peptide-linked forms. In Scriver CR, Beaudet AL, Sly WS, Valle D (eds): The Metabolic and Molecular Bases of Inherited Disease. New York, McGraw-Hill, 2001, pp 2079–2105.

141. Olpe HR, Koella WP: Inhibition of nigral and neocortical cells by γ-hydroxybutyrate: a microiontophoretic investigation. Eur J Pharmacol 1979;53:359–364.

142. Kozhechkin SX: Microiontophoretic study of the mechanism of action of gamma-hydroxybutyric acid. Bull Exp Biol Med 1980;88:1293–1296.

143. Hosli L, Hosli E, Lehmann R, et al: Action of γ-hydroxybutyrate and GABA on neurons of cultured rat central nervous system. Neurosci Lett 1983;37:257–260.

144. Snead OC, Liu CC: GABA$_A$ receptor function in the gamma-hydroxybutyrate model of generalized absence seizures. Neuropharmacology 1993;32:401–409.

145. Williams SR, Turner JP, Crunelli V: Gamma-hydroxybutyrate promotes oscillatory activity of rat and cat thalamocortical neurons by a tonic GABA$_B$ receptor-mediated hyperpolarization. Neuroscience 1995;66:133–141.

146. Xie X, Smart TG: γ-Hydroxybutyrate hyperpolarizes hippocampal neurons by activating GABA$_B$ receptors. Eur J Pharmacol 1992;212:291–294.

147. Lingenhoehl K, Brom R, Heid J, et al: γ-Hydroxybutyrate is a weak agonist at recombinant GABA$_B$ receptors. Neuropharmacology 1999;38:1667–1673.

148. Emri Z, Antal K, Crunelli C, et al: Gamma-hydroxybutyric acid decreases thalamic sensory excitatory postsynaptic potentials by an action on presynaptic GABA$_B$ receptors. Neurosci Lett 1996;216:121–124.

149. Erhardt S, Andersson B, Nissbrandt H, et al: Inhibition of firing rate and changes in the firing pattern of nigral dopamine neurons by γ-hydroxybutyratic acid (GHBA) are specifically induced by activation of GABA$_B$ receptors. Naunyn Schmiedebergs Arch Pharmacol 1998;357:611–619.

150. Quang LS, Desai MC, Kraner JC, et al: Enzyme and receptor antagonists for preventing toxicity from the gamma-hydroxybutyric acid precursor 1,4-butanediol in CD-1 mice. Ann NY Acad Sci 2002;965:461–472.

151. Carai MAM, Colombo G, Reali R, et al: Central effects of 1,4-butanediol are mediated by GABA$_B$ receptors via its conversion into γ-hydroxybutyric acid. Eur J Pharmacol 2002;441:157–163.

152. Carai MAM, Colombo G, Brunetti G, et al: Role of GABAB receptors in the sedative/hypnotic effect of γ-hydroxybutyric acid. Eur J Pharmacol 2001;428:315–321.

153. Carai MAM, Colombo G, Gessa GL: Resuscitative effect of a GABA$_B$ receptor antagonist on γ-hydroxybutyric acid (GHB) mortality in mice. Ann Emerg Med 2005;45:614–619.

154. Hogema BM, Taylor M, Jakobs C, et al: Pharmacologic rescue of lethal seizures in mice deficient in succinic semialdehyde dehydrogenase. Nat Genet 2001;29:212–216.

155. Mathivet P, Bernasconi R, Froestl W, et al: Binding characteristics of gamma-hydroxybutyric acid as a weak but selective GABA$_B$ receptor agonist. Eur J Pharmacol 1997;321:67–75.

156. Doherty JD, Hattox SE, Snead OC: Identification of endogenous γ-hydroxybutyrate in human and bovine brain and its regional distribution in human, guinea pig, and rhesus monkey brain. J Pharmacol Exp Ther 1978;207:130–139.

157. Hechler V, Ratomponirina C, Maitre M: Gamma-hydroxybutyrate conversion into GABA induces displacement of GABAB binding that is blocked by valproate and ethosuxisimide. J Pharmacol Exp Ther 1997;281:753–760.

158. Palatini P, Tedeschi L, Frison G, et al: Dose-dependent absorption and elimination of gamma-hydroxybutyric acid in healthy volunteers. Eur J Clin Pharmacol 1993;45:353–356.

159. Orphan Medical, Inc.: NDA #21-196 Xyrem (sodium oxybate) oral solution. Peripheral and Central Nervous System Drugs Advisory Committee Briefing Booklet for June 6, 2001, presentation. Minnetonka, MN, Orphan Medical, Inc., 2001, pp 201–220.

160. Borgen LA, Okerholm R, Morrison D, et al: The influence of gender and food on the pharmacokinetics of sodium oxybate oral solution in healthy subjects. J Clin Pharmacol 2003;43:59–65.

161. Brenneisen R, ElSohly MA, Murphy TP, et al: Pharmacokinetics and excretion of gamma-hydroxybutyrate (GHB) in healthy subjects. J Anal Toxicol 2004;28(8):625–630.

162. Borgen LA, Okerholm RA, Lai A, et al: The pharmacokinetics of sodium oxybate oral solution following acute and chronic administration to narcoleptic patients. J Clin Pharmacol 2004;44:253–257.

163. Scharf MB, Lai AA, Branigan B, et al: Pharmacokinetics of gammahydroxybutyrate (GHB) in narcoleptic patients. Sleep 1998;21(5):507–514.

164. Ferrara SD, Tedeschi L, Frison G, et al: Effect of moderate or severe liver dysfunction on the pharmacokinetics of γ-hydroxybutyric acid. Eur J Clin Pharmacol 1996;50(4):305–310.

165. Ferrara SD, Zotti S, Tedeschi L, et al: Pharmacokinetics of gamma-hydroxybutyrate in alcohol dependent patients after single and repeated oral doses. Br J Clin Pharmacol 1992;34:231–235.

166. Vree TB, Baars AM, Van Der Kleijn E: Capacity-limited elimination of 4-hydroxybutyrate (Gamma OH®), ethanol and vinylbital (Bykonox®). Pharmaceutisch Weekblad 1975;110(50):1257–1262.

167. Vree TB, Damsma J, Van den Bogert AG, van Der Kleijn E: Pharmocokinetics of 4-hydroxybutyric acid in man, rhesus monkey and dog. Anaesthesiol Intensive Med 1978;110:21–39.

168. van den Bogert AG, Vree TB, van den Kleijn E, et al: Placenta transfer of 4-hydroxybutyric acid in man. Anaesthesiol Intensive Med 1978;110:55–65.

169. Blumenfeld M, Suntay RG, Harmel MH: Sodium gamma-hydroxybutyric acid: a new anaesthetic adjuvant. Anesth Analg 1962;41:721–726.

170. Solway J, Sadove MS: 4-Hydroxybutyrate: a clinical study. Anesth Analg 1965;44:532–539.

171. Kleinschmidt S, Grundmann U, Janneck U, et al: Total intravenous anesthesia using propofol, gamma-hydroxybutyrate or midazolam in combination with sufentanil for patients undergoing coronary artery bypass surgery. Eur J Anaesthesiol 1997;14:590–599.

172. Kleinschmidt S, Grundmann U, Knocke T, et al: Total intravenous anaesthesia with gamma-hydroxybutyrate (GHB) and sufentanil in patients undergoing coronary artery bypass graft surgery: a comparison in patients with unimpaired and impaired left ventricular function. Eur J Anaesthesiol 1998;15:559–564.

173. Kleinschmidt S, Schellhase C, Mertzufft F: Continuous sedation during spinal anaesthesia: gamma-hydroxybutyrate vs propofol. Eur J Anaesthesiol 1999;16:23–30.

174. European Monitoring Centre for Drugs and Drug Addiction: Report on the risk assessment of GHB in the framework of the joint action on new synthetic drugs. Retrieved April 2005 from http://www.emcdda.eu.int/?nnodeid=2821.

175. Broughton R, Mamelak M: The treatment of narcolepsy-cataplexy with nocturnal γ-hydroxybutyrate. Can J Neurol Sci 1979;6:1–6.

176. Scharf M, Brown D, Woods M, et al: The effects and effectiveness of γ-hydroxybutyrate in patients with narcolepsy. J Clin Psychiatry 1985;46:222–225.

177. Bedard MA, Montplaisir J, Godbout R, et al: Nocturnal γ-hydroxybutyrate: effect on periodic leg movements and sleep organization of narcoleptic patients. Clin Neuropharmacol 1989;12:29–36.

178. Scrima L, Hartman PG, Johnson FH, et al: The effects of γ-hydroxybutyrate on the sleep of narcolepsy patients: a double-blind study. Sleep 1990;13:479–490.

179. Lammers GJ, Arends J, Declerck AC, et al: γ-Hydroxybutyrate and narcolepsy: a double-blind placebo-controlled study. Sleep 1993;6:216–220.

180. U.S. Xyrem Multicenter Study Group: A randomized, double-blind, placebo-controlled multicenter trial comparing the effects of three doses of orally administered sodium oxybate with placebo for the treatment of narcolepsy. Sleep 2002;25:42–49.

181. Orphan Medical, Inc.: Xyrem physician's monograph. Minnetonka, MN, Orphan Medical, Inc., 2002.

182. U.S. Xyrem Multicenter Study Group: The abrupt cessation of therapeutically administered sodium oxybate (GHB) does not cause withdrawal symptoms. J Toxicol Clin Toxicol 2003;41:131–135.

183. U.S. Xyrem Multicenter Study Group. A 12-month, open-label, multi-center extension trial of orally administered sodium oxybate for the treatment of narcolepsy. Sleep 2003;26:31–35.

184. Gallimberti L, Spella MR, Soncini CA, et al: Gamma-hydroxybutric acid in the treatment of alcohol and heroine dependence. Alcohol 2000;20:257–262.

185. Gallimberti L, Canton G, Gentile N, et al: Gamma-hydroxybutyric acid for treatment of alcohol withdrawal syndrome. Lancet 1989;2:787–789.

186. Gallimberti L, Ferri M, Ferrara SD, et al: Gamma-hydroxybutyric acid in the treatment of alcohol dependence: a double blind study. Alcohol Clin Exp Res 1992;16:673–676.

187. Addolorato G, Cibin M, Capristo E, et al: Maintaining abstinence from alcohol with gamma-hydroxybutyric acid. Lancet 1999;351(9095):38.

188. Addolorato G, Castelli E, Stefanini GF, et al: An open multicentric study evaluating 4-hydroxybutyric acid sodium salt in the medium-term treatment of 179 alcohol dependent subjects. Alcohol Alcoholism 1996;31:341–345.

189. Mamelak M, Black J, Montplaisir J, et al: A pilot study on the effects of sodium oxybate on sleep architecture and daytime alertness in narcolepsy. Sleep 2004;27(7):1327–1334.

190. Scharf MB, Baumann M, Berkowitz DV: The effects of sodium oxybate on clinical symptoms and sleep patterns in patients with fibromyalgia. J Rheumatol 2003;30:1070–1074.

191. Scharf MB, Hauck M, Stover R, et al: Effect of gamma-hydroxybutyrate on pain, fatigue, and the alpha sleep anomaly in patients with fibromyalgia. Preliminary report. J Rheumatol 1998;25:1986–1990.

192. Ottani A, Saltini S, Bartiromo M, et al: Effect of gamma-hydroxybutyrate in two rat models of focal cerebral damage. Brain Res 2003;986(1–2):181–190.

193. Vergoni AV, Ottani A, Botticelli AR, et al: Neuroprotective effect of gamma-hydroxybutyrate in transient global cerebral ischemia in the rat. Eur J Pharmacol 2000;397(1):75–84.

194. Quang LS, Sadasivan S, Maher TJ, et al: Neuroprotective effect of gamma-hydroxybutyrate and its chemical precursors, gamma-butyrolactone and 1,4-butanediol, in the rodent model of focal cerebral ischemia by permanent middle cerebral artery occlusion [Abstract]. Acad Emerg Med 2003;10(5):438.

195. Quang LS, Sadasivan S, Maher TJ: Neuroprotective effects of gamma-hydroxybutyrate and its precursors 1,4-butanediol and gamma-butyrolactone in MCAo cerebral ischemia [Abstract]. FASEB J 2003;17(4–5):391.12.

196. Yosunkaya A, Ustun ME, Bariskaner H, et al: Effect of gamma-hydroxybutyric acid on tissue Na+, K-ATPase levels after experimental head trauma. Acta Anaesthesiol Scand 2004;48(5):631–636.

197. Guney O, Bengi Celik J, Arazi M et al: Effects of gamma-hydroxybutyrate on cerebrospinal fluid lactate and glucose levels after spinal cord trauma. J Clin Neurosci 2004;11(5):517–520.

198. Yonekura K, Basaki Y, Chikahisa L, et al: UFT and its metabolites inhibit the angiogenesis induced by murine renal cell carcinoma, as determined by a dorsal air sac assay in mice. Clin Cancer Res 1999;5:2185–2191.

199. Basaki Y, Chikahisa L, Aoyagi K, et al. Gamma-hydroxybutyric acid and 5-fluorouracil, metabolites of UFT, inhibit the angiogenesis induced by vascular endothelial growth factor. Angiogenesis 2001;4(3):163–173.

200. Orphan Medical, Inc.: Covance study no. 6627-129, Xyrem (sodium oxybate) oral solution NDA #21-196. Briefing Booklet for the Peripheral and Central Nervous System Drugs Advisory Committee Meeting for June 6, 2001, presentation. Minnetonka, MN, Orphan Medical, Inc., 2001.

201. Suner S, Szlatenyi CS, Wang RY: Pediatric gamma hydroxybutyrate intoxication. Acad Emerg Med 1997;4(11):1041–1045.

202. Dyer JE, Reed JH: Alkali burns from illicit manufacture of GHB [Abstract]. J Toxicol Clin Toxicol 1997;35:553.

203. Galloway GP, Frederick SL, Staggers F Jr: Physical dependence on sodium oxybate [Letter]. Lancet 1994;343:57.

204. Friedman J, Westlake R, Furman M: "Grievous bodily harm": gamma hydroxybutyrate abuse leading to Wernicke-Korsakoff syndrome. Neurology 1996;46:469–471.

205. Addolorato G, Caputo F, Stefanini GF, et al: Gamma-hydroxybutyric acid in the treatment of alcohol dependence: possible craving development for the drug [see comment]. Addiction 1997;92(8):1035–1036.

206. Galloway GP, Frederick-Osborne SL, Seymour R, et al: Gamma-hydroxybutyrate: an emerging drug of abuse that causes physical dependence. Addiction 1997;92:89–96.

207. Dyer JE, Andrews KM: Gamma hydroxybutyrate withdrawal. J Toxicol Clin Toxicol 1997;92:89–96.

208. Galloway GP, Frederick SL, Staggers FE Jr, et al: Gamma-hydroxybutyrate: an emerging drug of abuse that causes physical dependence. Addiction 1997;92:89–96.

209. Hernandez M, McDaniel CH, Costanza CD, et al: GHB-induced delirium: a case report and review of the literature of gamma hydroxybutyric acid. Am J Drug Alcohol Abuse 1998;24:179–183.

210. Addolorato G, Caputo F, Capristo E, et al: A case of gamma-hydroxybutyric acid withdrawal syndrome during alcohol addiction treatment: utility of diazepam administration. Clin Neuropharmacol 1999;22(1):60–62.

211. Price G: In-patient detoxification after GHB dependence. Br J Psychiatry 2000;177:181.

212. Craig K, Gomez HF, McManus JL, et al: Severe gamma-hydroxybutyrate withdrawal: a case report and literature review. J Emerg Med 2000;18(1):64–70.

213. Hutto B, Fairchild A, Bright R: γ-Hydroxybutyrate withdrawal and chloral hydrate. Am J Psychiatry 2000;157:10.

214. Miglani JS, Kim KY, Chahil R: Gamma-hydroxybutyrate withdrawal delirium: a case report. Gen Hosp Psychiatry 2000;22:213–215.

215. Price G: In-patient detoxification after GHB dependence. Br J Psychiatry 2000;177:181.

216. Greene T, Dougherty T: Gamma-butyrolactone withdrawal presenting as acute psychosis. J Toxicol Clin Toxicol 2000;37:651.

217. Sharma AN, Nelson L, Hoffman RS: Severe gamma-butyrolactone withdrawal. J Toxicol Clin Toxicol 2000;38:535.

218. Catalano MC, Glass JM, Catalano G, et al: Gamma butyrolactone (GBL) withdrawal syndromes. Psychosomatics 2001;42(1):83–88.

219. Mullins ME, Fitzmaurice SC: Lack of efficacy of benzodiazepines in treating gamma-hydroxybutyrate withdrawal. J Emerg Med 2001;20(4):418–420.

220. Sharma AN, Lombardi MH: Management of gamma-hydroxybutyrate withdrawal. Ann Emerg Med 2001;38(5):605–607.

221. Su M, Traub SJ, Hussain E, et al: 1,4-Butanediol withdrawal complicated by urinary retention. J Toxicol Clin Toxicol 2001;39:542.

222. Bowles TM, Sommi RW, Amiri M: Successful management of prolonged γ-hydroxybutyrate and alcohol withdrawal. Pharmacotherapy 2001;21(2):254–257.

223. Dyer JE, Roth B, Hyma BA: Gamma-hydroxybutyrate withdrawal syndrome. Ann Emerg Med 2001;37(2):147–153.

224. Mahr G, Bishop CL, Orringer DJ: Prolonged withdrawal from extreme gamma-hydroxybutyrate (GHB) abuse. Psychosomatics 2001;42(5):439–440.

225. McDaniel CH, Miotto KA: Gamma hydroxybutyrate (GHB) and gamma butyrolactone (GBL) withdrawal: five case studies. J Psychoactive Drugs 2001;33(2):143–149.

226. Miotto K, Darakjian J, Basch J, et al: Gamma-hydroxybutyric acid: patterns of use, effects and withdrawal. Am J Addict 2001;10:232–241.

227. Schneir AB, Ly BT, Clark RF: A case of withdrawal from the GHB precursors gamma-butyrolactone and 1,4-butanediol. J Emerg Med 2001;21(1):31–33.

228. Sivilotti ML, Burns MJ, Aaron CK, et al: Pentobarbital for severe gamma-butyrolactone withdrawal. Ann Emerg Med 2001;38(6):660–665.

229. Mycyk MB, Wilemon C, Aks SE: Two cases of withdrawal from 1,4-butanediol use. Ann Emerg Med 2001;38(3):345–346.

230. Chin RL: A case of severe withdrawal from gamma-hydroxy-butyrate. Ann Emerg Med 2001;37(5):551–552.

231. Harold AH, Sneed KB: Treatment of a young adult taking gamma-butyrolactone (GBL) in a primary care clinic. J Am Board Fam Pract 2002;15(2):161–163.

232. Zvosec DL, Smith SW: γ-Hydroxybutyrate addiction and withdrawal: From the γ-hydroxybutyrate addiction study. Ann Emerg Med 2004;44(4):pS91.

233. Chew G, Fernando A 3rd: Epileptic seizure in GHB withdrawal. Aust Psychiatry 2004;12(4):410–411.

234. De Vivo DC, Gibson KM, Resor LD, et al: 4-Hydroxybutyric acidemia: clinical features, pathogenetic mechanisms, and treatment strategies. Ann Neurol 1988;24(2):304.

235. Pattarelli PP, Nyhan WL, Gibson KM: Oxidation of [U-14C] succinic semialdehyde in cultured human lymphoblasts: measurement of residual succinic semialdehyde dehydrogenase activity in 11 patients with 4-hydroxybutyric aciduria. Pediatr Res 1988; 24(4):455–460.

236. Haan EA, Brown GK, Mitchell D, et al: Succinic semialdehyde dehydrogenase deficiency—a further case. J Inherit Metab Dis 1985;8:99.

237. Jakobs C, Smit LM, Kneer J, et al: The first adult case with 4-hydroxybutyric aciduria. J Inherit Metab Dis 1990;13:341–344.

238. Gibson KM, Sweetman L, Nyhan WL, et al: Defective succinic semialdehyde dehydrogenase activity in 4-hydroxybutyric aciduria. Eur J Pediatr 1984;142:257–259.

239. Gibson KM, Lee CF, Chambliss KL, et al: 4-Hydroxybutyric aciduria: application of a fluorometric assay to the determination of succinic semialdehyde dehydrogenase activity in extracts of cultured human lymphoblasts [Letter]. Clin Chim Acta 1991;196: 219–222.

240. Gibson KM, Goodman SI, Frerman FE, et al: Succinic semialdehyde dehydrogenase deficiency associated with combined 4-hydroxbutyric and dicarboxylic acidurias: potential for clinical misdiagnosis based on urinary organic acid profiling. J Pediatr 1989;114(4):607–610.

241. Gibson KM, Doskey AE, Jakobs C, et al: Differing clinical presentation of succinic semialdehyde dehydrogenase deficiency in adolescent siblings from Lifu Island, New Caledonia. J Inherit Metab Dis 1997;20:370–374.

242. Gibson KM, Hoffman G, Nyhan WL, et al: 4-Hydroxybutyric aciduria in a patient without ataxia or convulsions. Eur J Pediatr 1988;147:529–531.

243. Gibson KM, Sweetman L, Nyhan WL, et al: Succinic semialdehyde dehydrogenase deficiency: an inborn error of gamma-aminobutyric acid metabolism. Clin Chim Acta 1983;133:33–42.

244. Gibson KM, Jansen I, Sweetman L, et al: 4-Hydroxybutyric aciduria: a new inborn error of metabolism. III. Enzymology and inheritance. J Inherit Metab Dis 1984;7(Suppl 1):95–96.

245. Gibson KM: 4-Hydroxybutyric aciduria: In Tunnicliff G, Cash CD (eds): Gamma-hydroxybutyrate: Molecular, Functional and Clinical Aspects. New York, Taylor & Francis, 2002, pp 197–217.

246. Trettel F, Malaspina P, Jodice C, et al: Human succinic semialdehyde dehydrogenase: molecular cloning and chromosomal localization. Adv Exp Med Biol 1996;414:253–260.

247. Chambliss KL, Hinson DD, Trettel F, et al: Two exon-skipping mutations as the molecular basis of succinic semialdehyde dehydrogenase deficiency (4-hydroxybutyric aciduria). Am J Hum Genet 1998;63:399–408.

248. Rating D, Hanefeld F, Siemes H, et al: 4-Hydroxybutyric aciduria: a new inborn error of metabolism. I. Clinical review. J Inherit Metab Dis 1984;7(Suppl 1):90–92.

249. Gibson KM, Christensen E, Jakobs C, et al: The clinical phenotype of succinic semialdehyde dehydrogenase deficiency (4-hydroxy-butyric aciduria): case reports of 23 new patients. Pediatrics 1997;99(4):567–574.

250. LeBeau M, Montgomery MA, Jufer RA, et al: Elevated GHB in citrate-buffered blood [Letter]. J Anal Toxicol 2000;24:383–384.

251. LeBeau MA, Miller ML, Levine B: Effect of storage temperature on endogenous GHB levels in urine. Forensic Sci Int 2001; 119(2):161–167.

252. Kerrigan S: In vitro production of gamma-hydroxybutyrate in antemortem urine samples. J Anal Toxicol 2002;26(8):571–574.

253. Ciolino LA, Mesmer MZ, Satzger D, et al: The chemical interconversion of GHB and GBL: forensic issues and implications. J Forensic Sci 2001;46(6):1315–1323.

254. Stephens BG, Coleman DE, Baselt RC, et al: In vitro stability of endogenous gamma-hydroxybutyrate in postmortem blood [Letter]. J Forensic Sci 1999;44(1):231–232.

255. Elliot S: The presence of gamma-hydroxybutyric acid (GHB) in postmortem biological fluids [Letter]. J Anal Toxicol 2001;25:152.

256. Vose J, Tighe T, Schwartz M, et al: Detection of gamma-butyrolactone (GBL) as a natural component in wine. J Forensic Sci 2001;46(5):1164–1167.

257. Baddock N, Zotti R: Rapid screening test for gamma-hydroxybutyric acid (GHB, fantasy) in urine [Letter]. Ther Drug Monit 1999;21(3):376–377.

258. Alston WC II, Ng K: Rapid colorimetric screening test for γ-hydroxybutyric acid (liquid X) in human urine. Forensic Sci Int 2002;126:114–117.

259. Morris-Kukoski CL: γ-Hydroxybutyrate: bridging the clinical-analytical gap. Toxicol Rev 2004;23(1):33–43.

260. Sporer KA, Chin RL, Dyer JE, et al: γ-Hydroxybutyrate serum levels and clinical syndrome after severe overdose. Ann Emerg Med 2003;42:3–8.

261. Quang LS, Levy HM, Law T, et al: Laboratory diagnosis of 1,4-BD and GHB overdose by routine urine organic acid analysis. J Toxicol Clin Toxicol 2005;43(4):1–3.

262. Caldicott DGE, Kuhn M: Gamma-hydroxybutyrate overdose and physostigmine: teaching new tricks to an old drug. Ann Emerg Med 2001;37(1):99–102.

263. Henderson RS, Holmes CM: Reversal of the anesthetic action of sodium gamma-hydroxybutyrate. Anaesth Intensive Care 1976; 4(4):351–354.

264. Holmes CM, Henderson RS: The elimination of pollution by a non inhalational technique. Anaesth Intensive Care 1978;6(2): 120–124.

265. Persson B, Henning M: Central cardiovascular effects of gamma-hydroxybutyric acid; interactions with noradrenaline, serotonin, dopamine and acetylcholine transmission. Acta Pharmacol Toxicol (Copenh) 1980;47:335–346.

266. McCabe ER, Layne EC, Sayler DF, et al: Synergy of ethanol and a natural soporific-gamma hydroxybutyrate. Science 1971; 171(969):404–406.

267. Poldrugo F, Snead OC: 1,4-Butanediol, gamma-hydroxybutyric acid, and ethanol: relationship and interaction. Neuropharmacology 1984;23:109–113.

268. Poldrugo F, Snead OC, Barker S: Chronic alcohol administration produces an increase in liver 1,4-butanediol concentration [Letter]. Alcohol Alcohol 1985;20(2):251–253.

269. Poldrugo F, Snead OC: 1,4-Butanediol and ethanol compete for degradation in rat brain and liver in vitro. Alcohol 1986;3(6): 367–370.

270. Poldrugo F, Snead OC: Ethanol blocks the conversion of 1,4-butanediol to gamma-hydroxybutyric acid in vivo. Neurosci Abstr 1983;9:1234.

271. Poldrugo F, Barker S, Basa M, et al: Ethanol potentiates the toxic effects of 1,4-butanediol. Alcohol Clin Exp Res 1985;9(6): 493–497.

272. Quang LS, Shannon MW, Woolf AD, et al: Pretreatment of CD-1 mice with 4-methylpyrazole blocks toxicity from the gamma-hydroxybutyrate precursor, 1,4-butanediol. Life Sci 2002;71: 771–778.

273. Quang LS, Desai MC, Shannon MW, et al: 4-methylpyrazole decreases 1,4-butanediol toxicity by blocking its in vivo biotransformation to gamma-hydroxybutyric acid. Ann N Y Acad Sci 2004;1025:528–537.

274. Carai MA, Colombo G, Quang LS, et al: Resuscitative treatments on 1,4-butanediol mortality in mice. Ann Emerg Med 2006;47: 184–189.

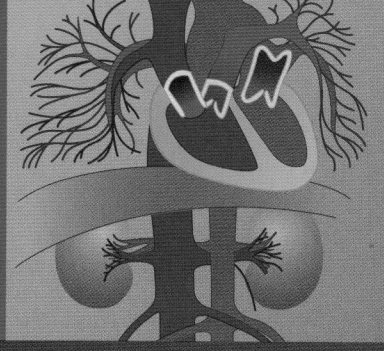

47 Acetaminophen

STEVEN D. SALHANICK, MD ■ MICHAEL W. SHANNON, MD, MPH

At a Glance...

■ Acetaminophen toxicity is a frequent cause of hepatic toxicity and should be considered in the differential diagnosis of any patient presenting with acute hepatic failure.

■ Toxicity is resultant of the metabolism of the drug in overdose.

■ Onset of hepatic toxicity is delayed 12 to 36 hours after acute overdose.

■ Therapy after acute overdose is based on the level of drug if this can be measured 4 to 24 hours after overdose, according to the Rumack-Mathews nomogram.

■ Subacute and late-presenting cases cannot be managed according to the nomogram.

■ Acute overdose that is thought to put the patient at high risk for developing hepatic toxicity is treated with N-acetylcysteine administered as a loading dose of 140 mg/kg followed by 17 maintenance doses at 70 mg/kg. Shorter courses of therapy are routine in Europe, Canada, Australia, and elsewhere, and have been administered in the United States as well.

■ The efficacy of N-acetylcysteine therapy declines beginning 8 hours after acute overdose; therefore, therapy should be started within 8 hours of overdose.

■ Patients with acute ingestion and nontoxic levels do not require therapy. Short courses of therapy in other cases may be required if potential toxicity is unclear.

Acetaminophen (paracetamol, APAP) is a widely used analgesic and antipyretic agent. Use of APAP as an antipyretic was first reported by von Mehring in 1893, in fact preceding the medicinal use of salicylates.[1] Despite its effectiveness, an undesirable side effect profile led to discouragement of its use. It is likely that an impure preparation was used, accounting for the adverse effects.[2] Related compounds including acetanilide (marketed as Antifebrin) were in use since the late 1880s. APAP was subsequently abandoned until the late 1940s, when Brodie and Axelrod published their data indicating that APAP was in fact a metabolite of acetanilide and was responsible for the analgesic and antipyretic effects.[2] Subsequent to these investigations, APAP was substituted for phenacetin in the combination product Trigesic in 1950. Trigesic was withdrawn from the market in 1951 after reports of agranulocytosis associated with its use. APAP was never clearly implicated as causal. APAP use was essentially abandoned in the United States until the advent of Tylenol in 1955. However, aspirin was more widely prescribed until the early 1970s.[2] APAP, marketed as Panadol in the United Kingdom in 1956, increased in popularity throughout the 1960s and 1970s in a fashion parallel to that in the United States.[2]

Currently, APAP poisoning represents the most frequent poisoning reported to U.S. poison centers, is the cause of the majority of poisoning deaths reported to U.S. poison centers, and is the most frequent cause of acute hepatic failure in the United States.[3-5]

PHARMACOLOGY

Despite its widespread use, APAP's mechanism of action remains elusive. Cyclooxygenase inhibition has been long postulated, but APAP has been shown to be a poor inhibitor of COX-1 and COX-2, the two well-described cyclooxygenases involved in the early inflammatory response. Furthermore, unlike nonsteroidal anti-inflammatory drugs, APAP has not shown antiplatelet activity.[6-8] Chandrasekharan and colleagues recently demonstrated the presence of a COX-3 enzyme that is inhibited by APAP. The COX-3 enzyme is primarily expressed in the central nervous system, implying a central location of action for APAP.[6] COX-3 inhibition by APAP is weak, however; therefore, that COX-3 inhibition does not fully explain the analgesic and antipyretic actions of APAP.[8]

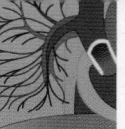

PHARMACOKINETICS

APAP in therapeutic doses is rapidly and nearly completely absorbed. Absorption occurs primarily in the small bowel with the rate of absorption consequently dependent on the rate of gastric emptying. APAP is distributed throughout the body, having a volume of distribution of 0.95 L/kg. Half-life is approximately 1.5 to 2 hours.[9] Hepatic metabolism produces two major metabolites, the sulfate conjugate and the glucuronide conjugate. Approximately 5% of APAP is excreted unchanged, while approximately 4% to 5% undergoes reductive metabolism by the cytochrome P-450 (CYP) system, principally CYP2E1 and CYP1A2 to N-acetyl-parabenzoquinone-imine (NAPQI). NAPQI is subsequently bound to intracellular thiols, principally glutathione, and is excreted as the cysteine and mercapturic acid conjugates in urine[9] (Fig. 47-1). This reductive metabolism and its products are implicated in the toxicity of APAP.

Glucuronide conjugation occurs to a much lesser degree in young children and neonates than in adults, and sulfate conjugation predominates; the plasma half-life may also be prolonged in young children.[10] Patients with severe liver dysfunction may have decreased excretion of APAP as well.[11]

The urinary excretion of APAP is via glomerular filtration with a significant fraction of tubular reabsorption. The glucuronide and sulfate conjugates are actively secreted by the tubules, with renal clearance rates of 130 and 170 mL/min, respectively.[12] Patients with renal failure accumulate metabolites, although the plasma half-life of APAP is unaffected.[11]

APAP readily crosses the placenta and is risk category B in pregnancy, meaning that safety is presumed based on animal studies.[13] Maternal pharmacokinetics are similar to those of humans in the nonpregnant state.[14,15] Several studies have investigated the effects of APAP in therapeutic doses and overdose in all trimesters.[16-22] APAP toxicity appears to occur in utero. One report describes plasma levels in an infant delivered by cesarean section similar to maternal levels following maternal APAP overdose.[23] Therapeutic dosing has not been shown to have any negative effects on pregnancy or the fetus. APAP is excreted in breast milk in milk:plasma ratios reported to range from 1:0.50 to 1:1.42.[24]

Pharmacologic agents that can theoretically affect APAP pharmacokinetics include those that delay gastric emptying, notably the anticholinergic agents. Several case reports describe delay in absorption following APAP overdose with co-ingestants that delay gastric emptying.[25-27] Absorption of liquid preparations is slightly more rapid.[9] No significant drug interactions are known to occur with APAP following therapeutic dosing.

TOXICOLOGY

Death due to hepatic failure following APAP overdose was first reported in 1966.[28,29] Research into the cause of toxicity ensued, and in 1974 Mitchell and Jollow published their work that provided the basis for the widely accepted theory of free radical arylation of hepatic proteins as causative.[30-33] These investigators demonstrated in vivo and in vitro that radiolabeled acetaminophen was recovered bound to proteins in the hepatocyte following administration of high doses of acetaminophen. Furthermore, they found that glutathione depletion preceded other signs of hepatic injury and that glutathione precursors administered prior to experimental poisoning were hepatoprotective. This work formed the basis for N-acetylcysteine (NAC) antidotal therapy. Later studies identified the metabolite responsible for binding to be NAPQI.[34,35] Further work has gone into determining the critical protein or proteins responsible for hepatic failure. At present, approximately 28 proteins subject to arylation have been identified.[36,37] Binding is highly selective, however. Several specific proteins account for the majority of binding, specifically the cytosolic 56- to 58-kD acetaminophen binding protein, the 100-kD N-10-formyl-tetrahydrofolate dehydrogenase, and 50- and 54-kD mitochondrial dehydrogenases.[38] Several investigators have worked extensively to determine the critical protein or proteins that, when arylated, result in cell death. No decrease in protein function has been determined that could likely account for the cell death. Most enzymes show only modest reduction in function postpoisoning, with the most prominent being glutamine synthetase, which has a 50% reduction in activity.[37]

These and other inconsistencies of the NAPQI binding hypothesis have led to consistent challenges to this hypothesis.[37,39] Covalent binding does not always correlate with severity of injury.[37] Inhibition of Kupffer cell activity alters or abolishes toxicity despite a high degree of covalent binding.[40,41] High levels of covalent binding will occur in young female rats with no detectable hepatic injury.[42] 3'-Hydroxyacetanilide, a regioisomer of APAP administered in similar doses, results in a high degree of protein covalent binding without toxicity as well.[43,44] Also, the critical protein or proteins have never been identified in nearly 30 years of investigation. A complete review of the criticism of the NAPQI theory is beyond the scope of this chapter; however, these and other inconsistencies have led to the investigation of several other causes of toxicity.

Wendel and co-workers proposed the hypothesis that reactive oxygen species formed during the CYP metabolism of APAP produce massive lipid peroxidation, and they produced data to strongly support this contention.[45-47] The data were challenged on the basis that due to technical difficulties in the measurement of products of lipid peroxidation, the animal model used by Wendel's group was particularly susceptible to lipid peroxidation and that it was not therefore relevant.[48] Other investigators have not reproduced the work using other models.[37]

Oxidant stress due to the action of reactive oxygen species has been proposed due to the generation of these species from a variety of sources, including injured mitochondria, activated Kupffer cells, infiltrating neutrophils, and xanthine oxidase.[37] Evidence supporting each of these mechanisms exists, but the question

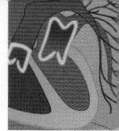

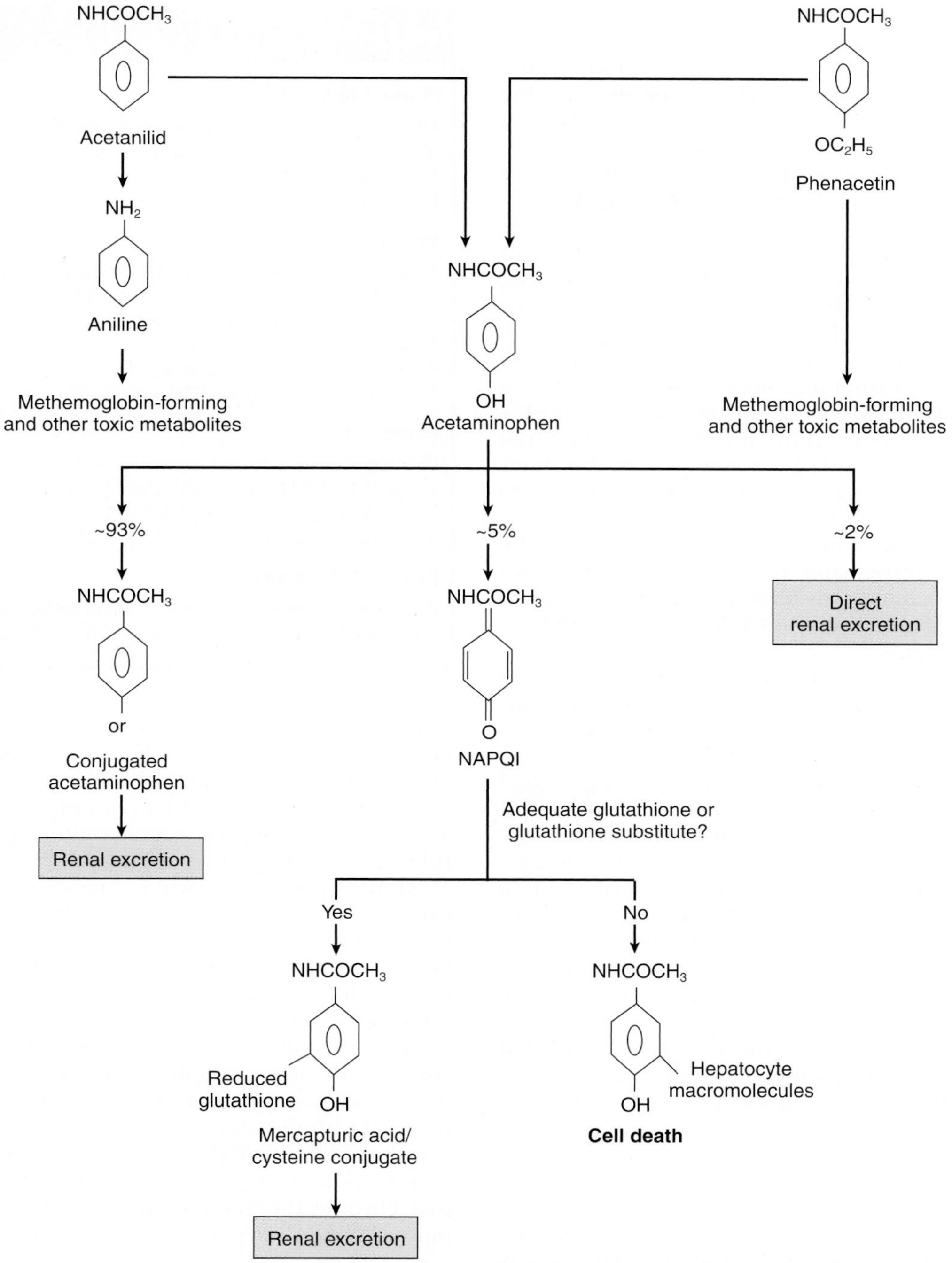

NHCOCH₃

Acetanilid

NH₂

Aniline

Methemoglobin-forming
and other toxic metabolites

NHCOCH₃

OC₂H₅

Phenacetin

NHCOCH₃

OH
Acetaminophen

Methemoglobin-forming
and other toxic metabolites

~93%

NHCOCH₃

or

Conjugated
acetaminophen

Renal excretion

~5%

NHCOCH₃

O
NAPQI

~2%

Direct
renal excretion

Adequate glutathione or
glutathione substitute?

Yes

NHCOCH₃

Reduced
glutathione   OH

Mercapturic acid/
cysteine conjugate

Renal excretion

No

NHCOCH₃

Hepatocyte
macromolecules

OH

Cell death

FIGURE 47-1 Metabolism of acetaminophen and other coal tar analgesics. NAPQI, *N*-acetyl-*p*-benzoquinoneimine; R, glucuronide or sulfate.

remains as to whether oxidant stress is a cause of hepatocyte injury or occurs as a result of hepatocyte injury.

Peroxynitrate formation occurs when nitric oxide is formed in the presence of superoxide anions, a reactive oxygen species.[49] Peroxynitrate is a powerful oxidant and produces nitrotyrosine adducts in tissue, which have been demonstrated by immunohistochemistry in hepatic tissue following experimental APAP overdose. Time course of nitrotyrosine adducts indicates that they bind concurrently or immediately preceding hepatocyte injury. Furthermore, peroxynitrate can deplete cellular glutathione stores.[37]

Finally, early mitochondrial dysfunction is an important early finding in all models of APAP overdose and may occur as soon as 15 minutes after APAP exposure.[50-55] Mitochondrial dysfunction is implicated as playing a role in nearly every aspect of the pathogenesis of APAP toxicity, including failure of energy substrate, increase in reactive oxygen species, and increased cytosolic calcium concentrations. The cause of this early failure is not

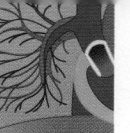

known. Reactive metabolite arylation of mitochondrial proteins has not been demonstrated to have a significant enough effect to be accepted as causal.[37] Early mitochondrial failure remains a crucial missing piece of the puzzle of APAP-induced hepatic injury. One mechanism that has been proposed in the past and is currently undergoing investigation is the concept of hypoxia as causal regarding the early mitochondrial failure.[56,57] Centrilobular hepatocytes are relatively hypoxic at baseline. Mitochondria are susceptible to a lack of available oxygen due to the use of oxygen for drug metabolism. Early work has shown promise but mixed results with regard to APAP poisoning.[57] Hypoxia has been demonstrated in a more convincing fashion in relation to other centrilobular toxins, including ethanol and carbon tetrachloride.[58-62] Another proposed mechanism of mitochondrial failure involves mitochondrial permeability transition (MPT), a state where the inner mitochondrial membrane becomes depolarized due to increased ion permeability. The proposed mechanism involves NAPQI binding to vicinal thiols in the membrane pore responsible for MPT. Other quinones known to bind vicinal thiols have been demonstrated to induce MPT. NAPQI has not been demonstrated to have this effect, however.[63]

Recently, attention has been turned to the delay in fulminant hepatic failure following overdose. Humans and animals typically will have a delay following metabolism of APAP before the rise in transaminases occurs. This phenomenon has been referred to as stage 1 and stage 2 of toxicity.[64] Stage 1 is the metabolism phase of poisoning, where plasma drug level declines and serologic and clinical evidence for hepatotoxicity is absent. Stage 2 refers to the hepatic injury phase that occurs 12 to 36 hours after drug metabolism is complete. Current investigation is focused on the identification of inflammatory mediators that may be responsible for the second stage.[37] It is important to note that the exact cause of the initiating events, while clearly related to metabolism, remains in question. An immune response to arylated proteins has not been demonstrated. Kupffer cell involvement is thought to be imperative in toxicity.

CLINICAL MANIFESTATIONS

Acute human toxicity has traditionally been divided into four clinical phases (Box 47-1). Initially, patients may be asymptomatic or may develop nausea and vomiting. Transaminases may begin to rise by 16 hours after overdose.[65] Between 24 and 72 hours, signs of hepatic insult become prominent. Transaminases begin or continue to rise, the patient may develop right upper quadrant pain, and signs of hepatic synthetic failure (i.e., elevated prothrombin time) may appear, as may evidence of cholestasis with elevated bilirubin. Renal injury will become evident in a small fraction of patients at this point.[66] A few reports of renal injury without hepatic failure exist, but these are exceedingly rare and not well documented.[67] Most cases include some degree of hepatic injury. Between 72 and 96 hours, hepatic and

> ### BOX 47-1   PHASES OF ACETAMINOPHEN POISONING
>
> **Phase 1 (0.5 –24 hr)**
>
> Anorexia, nausea, and vomiting are frequently present.
> Malaise and diaphoresis may be present.
> Transaminases may be elevated.
> Patients may appear normal.
>
> **Phase II (24–72 hr)**
>
> Anorexia, nausea, and vomiting become less pronounced.
> Right upper quadrant pain may be present.
> Transaminase levels continue to increase.
> Bilirubin level may be elevated.
> Prothrombin time may be prolonged.
> Renal function may deteriorate.
>
> **Phase III (72–96 hr)**
>
> Characterized by the sequelae of hepatic necrosis: jaundice, coagulation defects, renal failure, and hepatic encephalopathy.
> Liver biopsy reveals centrilobular necrosis.
> Death due to multiorgan failure may result.
>
> **Phase IV (4–14 days)**
>
> If patients survive, complete resolution of hepatic dysfunction occurs and the liver heals without evidence of fibrosis.

renal failure may worsen. Death occurs due to hepatic failure. Early hepatic transplant may allow survival at this point. Alternatively, hepatic injury may resolve and transaminases may return to normal over the ensuing 4 to 14 days. Complete regeneration of the liver is the rule. Renal insult will resolve as well.[67]

APAP toxicity following supratherapeutic administration, often referred to as chronic toxicity, has been observed in both children and adults. The patients manifest essentially the same course of toxicity. One case of hepatic fibrosis following chronic administration of supratherapeutic doses has been reported.[68]

More recently, chronic administration of therapeutic amounts of acetaminophen has been shown to cause hepatocellular injury. Injury was relatively mild and resolved with discontinuation of the drug.[69] Case reports exist implicating APAP in analgesic nephropathy.[11] However, epidemiologic data do not support the contention that chronic therapeutic administration leads to renal injury.[70-72] APAP hypersensitivity is exceedingly rare.[11]

DIAGNOSIS

The diagnosis of APAP poisoning is based primarily on history and laboratory screening, given the nonspecific nature of the initial presentation and the delay in manifestations of hepatotoxicity. Nausea and vomiting are consistent with early toxicity. A serum APAP concentration should be sent when any patient presents with a history of intentional overdose of any substance due to the wide availability of the drug and the 5% incidence of undeclared ingestion. Because the manifestations of hepatic injury are delayed, the decision to initiate

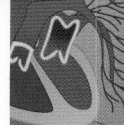

therapy is based on the risk of developing hepatotoxicity. In the setting of the acute ingestion at a single point in time, the decision to treat is relatively straightforward. An accurate time of ingestion must first be established. Establishment of the risk for toxicity is based on the Rumack-Matthews nomogram (Fig. 47-2). The nomogram was developed in 1975 by retrospective review of 64 patients following acute APAP overdose. Patients were found to have a 60% chance of developing severe hepatotoxicity if the plasma level was above the line drawn from the 200 µg/mL level at 4 hours to the 50 µg/mL level at 12 hours. Severe hepatotoxicity was defined as an aspartate aminotransferase (AST) level of greater that 1000 IU/L.[73] It is important to recognize that the nomogram is not applicable to modes of ingestion other than the acute single overdose. Furthermore, the nomogram is not applicable prior to 4 hours or after 24 hours. Levels prior to 4 hours may be markedly elevated because APAP may not have distributed from the vascular compartment to the tissues. It is also important to recognize that the nomogram comprises a series of data points rather than representing the elimination half-life of APAP in overdose.

Rarely, patients following a massive overdose causing levels in the range of 800 to 1000 µg/mL will present with severe acidosis and coma.[74] The mechanism of this presentation is not understood. Animal and in vitro data indicate reversible binding of APAP to mitochondrial proteins inhibiting respiration, and this mechanism has been suggested to be the cause of the acidosis seen in these massive overdoses.[56,75]

Patients presenting late or following ingestion over a prolonged period of time present a more difficult diagnosis because the nomogram cannot be used. A careful history of ingestion should be sought. APAP level should be measured to confirm ingestion, but the level cannot be used to determine risk for resultant hepatotoxicity. Transaminase values should be obtained and elevation should be assumed due to APAP poisoning unless proven otherwise.

The differential diagnosis includes all causes of hepatic centrilobular necrosis. Principal are other toxic causes, including hepatotoxic mushrooms, carbon tetrachloride, halothane and other inhaled anesthetics, brominated and chlorinated benzenes, and dioxane. Shock, vascular obstruction, and other causes of acute hepatic ischemia will also produce a centrilobular necrosis with the resultant clinical picture consistent with acute APAP poisoning. APAP poisoning may be worsened in patients with cardiac insufficiency.[76]

MANAGEMENT

Supportive Measures

Initial supportive measures should be those applicable to any poisoned patient. If the patient presents late in the course of poisoning, then resuscitative measures may be necessary. These should include standard measures to control airway, ventilation, and hemodynamic status. Supportive care for the patient with hepatic failure from APAP poisoning does not differ from that due to any other cause of hepatic failure. Acute renal failure may require dialysis.

Decontamination

Activated charcoal should be given unless the clinician is certain that the time of ingestion is so remote that there is no chance that any APAP remains in the gut. Every patient who presents within 6 hours of ingestion, or for whom the time of ingestion is in question, should therefore be treated with activated charcoal. Multiple-dose charcoal is not indicated following APAP ingestion.

Activated charcoal will bind and reduce the absorption of NAC if given simultaneously; however, no clinical detriment has been shown by this practice.[77-79] NAC should never be delayed beyond 8 hours following ingestion to facilitate decontamination, and concurrent administration of charcoal likely will not be detrimental.

Laboratory Monitoring

Initial management should include obtaining baseline serum transaminase levels, blood urea nitrogen, creatinine, and prothrombin time along with the APAP level. Appropriate screening for co-ingestants should be dictated by the clinical situation. If there is no laboratory evidence of hepatic injury, then daily transaminase levels should suffice for laboratory monitoring. Should any abnormalities in transaminase levels appear at any time, then evidence of synthetic failure should be sought. Serial prothrombin time should be added to the serial transaminases. The frequency of laboratory evaluation

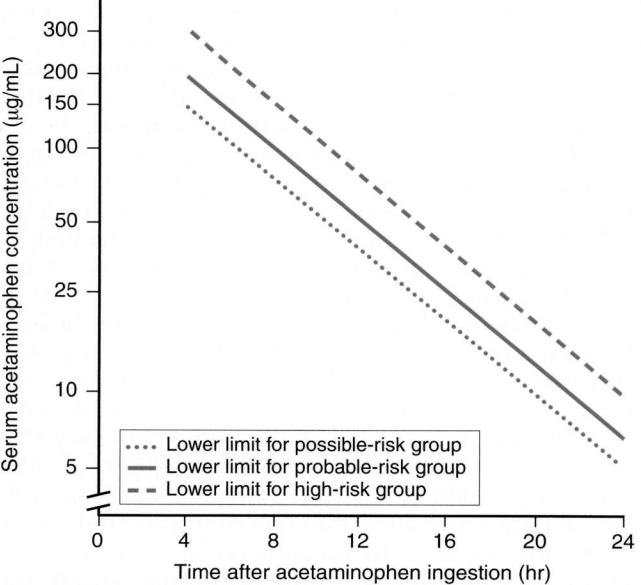

FIGURE 47-2 Acetaminophen (APAP) overdose treatment nomogram. (Adapted from Smilkstein MJ, Knapp GL, Kully KW, et al: Efficacy of oral *N*-acetylcysteine in the treatment of acetaminophen overdose: analysis of the National Multicenter Study [1976 to 1985]. N Engl J Med 1988;319:1557.)

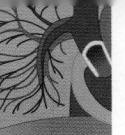
should be dictated by the clinical situation. A modest rise in transaminase levels (less than 500 IU/L) does not warrant more than daily monitoring. As levels approach 1000 IU/L, more frequent (i.e., every 6 to 12 hours) laboratory monitoring should be instituted. With any signs of synthetic failure the evaluation should be expanded to include data with prognostic value. Renal function tests should be followed due to the renal dysfunction that occurs infrequently. Should the patient develop signs of hepatic failure, he or she should be admitted to an intensive care unit and monitored closely for developing acidosis and renal and hepatic failure. This is important because the prognostic factors associated with death include a metabolic acidosis (arterial pH less than 7.3), renal insufficiency (serum creatinine greater than 3.3), or hepatic synthetic failure (International Normalized Ratio [INR] greater than 2 at 24 hours, 4 at 48 hours, or 6 at 72 hours).[80] Recently, attention has been drawn to the use of blood lactate as an early predictor of hepatic failure. Blood lactate greater than 3.5 mmol/L or 3.0 mmol/L after fluid resuscitation was predictive of mortality and has been suggested as criteria to list for transplantation.[81]

Prothrombin time and INR may be elevated following APAP ingestion without evidence of hepatocellular injury. Inhibition of factor VII by high levels of APAP and the anticoagulant effects of NAC have been proposed as mechanisms.[82,83] This early elevation in INR has no prognostic value.

Antidotes

NAC is the current antidote employed worldwide for the treatment of APAP toxicity. The rationale for NAC therapy is based on the theory that glutathione depletion leads to a state where the toxic free radical NAPQI can injure cellular macromolecules. NAC is given as both a glutathione precursor to provide substrate for NAPQI binding as well as a sulfate precursor to help drive the metabolism of APAP down the sulfonation pathway.[73]

Dosing

The standard course of NAC therapy in the United States is to administer a loading dose of 140 mg/kg followed by 17 maintenance doses of 70 mg/kg every 4 hours. This regimen was developed in the 1970s by Rumack and colleagues based on their observations of patients suffering from APAP overdose and applying the theory of NAC as a binding substrate for NAPQI.[73] The amount of NAC administered is based on the theoretical molar amount of NAPQI formation. The duration of therapy is based on the period of time required to metabolize APAP. The duration is purposefully long because some patients display a markedly extended half-life. Standard practice in Europe, Canada, Australia, and other countries is to administer NAC for 20 to 36 hours. Rates of fulminant hepatic failure, death, and transplantation are not significantly different, prompting several investigators in the United States to begin trials of shorter courses of NAC following the acute single overdose.[84,85]

NAC therapy is typically given orally in the United States, while in other countries, intravenous (IV) administration is the preferred route. There are several reasons for this discrepancy. Proponents of oral administration cite the theoretical advantage that oral NAC is presented to the liver in high concentration because it is initially circulated via the portal system. No data exist to support this contention, however. IV NAC can and should be given to patients in the United States, however, if the patient is unable to tolerate the medication orally. The oral preparation sold in the United States is sterile and can be given by the IV route. As with oral administration, NAC should be given as a 5% solution in saline. A 22-μm filter typically used for blood administration should be used. NAC dosing is identical to the oral protocol: 140 mg/kg loading dose followed by 17 maintenance doses of 70 mg/kg. The rate of administration is related to complications. Anaphylactoid reactions are reported in approximately 6% of patients when the loading dose is administered over 15 to 30 minutes.[86,87] Typically, these resolve with cessation of administration.[86] Restarting administration at a lower rate following the administration of diphenhydramine is sufficient treatment. Administration at slower rates reduces the rate of anaphylactoid reaction. Consequently, administering IV NAC over the course of 1 hour is a reasonably conservative practice. More recently, an intravenous form of NAC was approved by the U.S. Food and Drug Administration. The approved dosing protocol applies only to acute ingestion and is given over 21 hours. A loading dose of 150 mg/kg is given over 1 hour, followed by 50 mg/kg over 4 hours, followed by 100 mg/kg over 16 hours.

Patients who ingest APAP over a period greater than several hours due to repeat attempts or therapeutic misadventure and patients who present greater than 24 hours after ingestion present a more difficult decision with regard to initiating treatment. Generally, if the patient gives a history of overdose, has a measurable APAP level, and/or has a rise in AST or alanine transaminase, then NAC should be initiated. If the patient remains without biochemical evidence of toxicity by 24 hours, it is reasonable to discontinue therapy. Therapy should continue if there is evidence of toxicity.

The decision to treat patients who have ingested an overdose at one time point is aided by the use of the Rumack-Matthews nomogram (see Fig. 47-2). It is important to note that this is the only clinical scenario in which the nomogram is applicable. The nomogram was constructed using a series of data points, which represent the presenting plasma level of APAP versus time. A line is drawn through those points representing patients with a greater than 60% likelihood of developing an AST greater than 1000 IU/L. A second line was arbitrarily lowered in order to allow for error in history of the time of ingestion and is the treatment level most commonly in use in the United States. Most physicians outside the United States use the first line as indication for therapy. The lines are drawn from a time point of 4 hours after ingestion. This is because levels during the absorptive phase following ingestion are not reliable in terms of

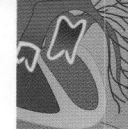

prognosis. APAP levels obtained prior to 4 hours after ingestion should not be used to base treatment decisions. Furthermore, levels obtained after 24 hours similarly have not been determined to have prognostic value. Patients presenting following ingestion should have a level checked as close to 4 hours after the ingestion as possible. Treatment should be based on that level. If the level is above the lowest treatment line, a course of NAC therapy is indicated. If it is below the line, no therapy is needed. A caveat to this rule occurs following co-ingestion of drugs that slow gastric motility, particularly anticholinergics such as diphenhydramine. Case reports indicate that delayed absorption may result in a 4-hour level that is not considered treatable followed by a 6- or 8-hour level that is toxic.[88] In this case a second level should be determined at 6 hours to ensure that the level is trending down and that levels subsequent to the initial 4-hour level will be unlikely to be in the treatable range. If the patient presents 8 or more hours after the ingestion or if a level will not be available before that time, treatment based on history of ingestion alone while awaiting an APAP level is indicated due to the decreasing efficacy of NAC therapy following delay to treatment greater than 8 hours.[89] Patients who present greater than 24 hours after the ingestion pose a more difficult decision to treat because the nomogram is not directly applicable to their treatment. It is reasonable practice to treat patients with persistently elevated APAP levels who present later than 24 hours after ingestion because it is reasonable to assume that the level was in a toxic range at prior to the 24-hour mark. Notably, this is an assumption only, and such levels have no prognostic significance. Patients who present greater than 24 hours after ingestion without an elevated APAP level pose a more difficult treatment decision because it is impossible to know if they had a level placing them at risk for hepatic injury during first 24 hours. Consequently, a reasonable practice is to administer a course of therapy for 24 hours and to follow transaminase levels. Patients will likely begin to display elevated transaminase levels by 36 hours after ingestion.[65,90] If they show no signs of hepatic injury, therapy may be discontinued. Also, any patients with evidence of hepatic injury at the time of presentation warrant therapy. Patients whose evidence of liver injury can clearly be attributed to a cause other than APAP toxicity who do not show progression of liver injury after 24 hours may have NAC therapy discontinued.

It is important to note that NAC therapy is effective at any point after poisoning and that if hepatic injury occurs, therapy is continued until evidence of hepatic dysfunction has resolved and transaminase values are declining and near normal. Therapy should never be stopped following the prescribed 18 doses when evidence of hepatic injury is still present. The reason for this apparent discrepancy is that NAC therapy is proven effective in reducing mortality when started and continued during any point in the course of APAP-induced hepatic injury.[91] Lack of a measurable APAP level is not an indication to withhold NAC therapy because late-presenting patients without measurable APAP levels are clearly benefited by NAC therapy. The

reasons for this are unclear. Several theories have been advanced. "Extrahepatic" effects such as free radical scavenging have been suggested, but experimental evidence is lacking. NAC has been shown to increase hepatic blood flow and oxygen extraction.[92-94] It is following these observations that have led to the advent of NAC therapy for other causes of hepatic failure.

Other suggested antidotes include the CYP inhibitor cimetidine. Cimetidine was recognized early on as an inhibitor of the CYP system, and its use as an antidote for APAP poisoning was considered. Early animal data showed promise.[95] Human experience was less promising and met with little enthusiasm.[96] One argument against cimetidine is that it does not affect the specific CYP isoforms involved in the metabolism of APAP. Specific CYP2E1 inhibitors such as 4-methyl-pyrrizole and disulfiram have been investigated in animals with positive results.[97,98] Human data do not yet exist.

Elimination

Dialysis has been used to enhance elimination following APAP poisoning. Its use has largely been abandoned following the advent of NAC therapy due to the effectiveness of this treatment. However, a role for dialysis has been suggested in cases of massive overdose where the patient presents with coma, acidosis, and levels near 1000 μg/mL, at which point the risk for mortality is very high. There are no data addressing the effectiveness of this intervention. Liver dialysis has been reported to be of benefit in an uncontrolled case series of four patients.[99] More data will be needed to determine benefit of liver dialysis.

DISPOSITION

Patients presenting with a history of APAP ingestion should be screened for co-ingestants in the usual fashion. A careful physical examination aimed at identifying a toxidrome suggestive of co-ingestants should be performed. Serum APAP level should be determined at 4 hours postingestion or as soon as possible after the 4-hour mark. Levels prior to 4 hours are of no prognostic significance. Patients with a single time of ingestion between 4 and 24 hours prior to presentation may be treated according to the Rumack-Matthews nomogram. Patients ingesting APAP at more than one time point warrant an abbreviated course of therapy while monitoring transaminase levels. Any patient with evidence of hepatic injury should have therapy continued until evidence of hepatic injury is resolved. Patients not meeting these criteria do not warrant therapy. As with any ingestion, a careful investigation of the circumstances surrounding the ingestion should be performed. It is important to educate any patient who has overdosed due to misuse of APAP. Intentional overdoses warrant psychiatric evaluation before the patient is discharged from medical care. Patients who suffer hepatic injury and recover may be safely discharged from care because no sequelae will occur once the injury is resolved.

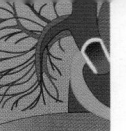
The question of referral to a center capable of transplantation often arises. Given the rapidity of demise in patients who suffer hepatic injury, referral should be discussed with the appropriate personnel at the referral center when the patient begins to display evidence of hepatic functional impairment in order to allow the transplant service adequate time to assess the patient and place him or her on a transplant list. Patients who have only elevation in transaminase levels and a transient, slight elevation in prothrombin time and INR can be managed expectantly with NAC therapy alone. Patients who undergo transplantation will need careful follow-up care as with any transplant patient.

REFERENCES

1. Mehring JV: Beitrage zur Kenntniss der Antipyretica. Ther Monatsschr 1893;7:577.
2. Spooner JB, Harvey JG: The history and usage of paracetamol. J Int Med Res 1976;4(4 Suppl):1–6.
3. Ostapowicz G, Fontana RJ, Schiodt FV, et al: Results of a prospective study of acute liver failure at 17 tertiary care centers in the United States. Ann Intern Med 2002;137(12):947–954. [Summary for patients in Ann Intern Med 2002;137(12):I24; PMID: 12484742.]
4. Litovitz TL, Klein-Schwartz W, Rodgers GC Jr, et al: 2001 annual report of the American Association of Poison Control Centers Toxic Exposure Surveillance System. Am J Emerg Med 2002;20(5):391–452.
5. Larson AM, Polson J, Fontana RJ, et al: Acetaminophen-induced acute liver failure: Results of a United States multicenter prospective study. Hepatology 2005;42(6):1364–1372.
6. Chandrasekharan NV, Dai H, Roos KL, et al: COX-3, a cyclooxygenase-1 variant inhibited by acetaminophen and other analgesic/antipyretic drugs: cloning, structure, and expression [see comment]. Proc Natl Acad Sci U S A 2002;99(21):13926–13931.
7. Botting RM: Mechanism of action of acetaminophen: is there a cyclooxygenase 3? Clin Infect Dis 2000;31(Suppl 5):202–210.
8. Schwab JM, Schluesener HJ, Laufer S: COX-3: just another COX or the solitary elusive target of paracetamol? Lancet 2003;361(9362):981–982.
9. Forrest JA, Clements JA, Prescott LF: Clinical pharmacokinetics of paracetamol. Clin Pharmacokinet 1982;7(2):93–107.
10. Prescott LF: Kinetics and metabolism of paracetamol and phenacetin. Br J Clin Pharmacol 1980;10(Suppl 2):291–298.
11. Clissold SP: Paracetamol and phenacetin. Drugs 1986;32(Suppl 4):46–59.
12. Morris ME, Levy G: Renal clearance and serum protein binding of acetaminophen and its major conjugates in humans. J Pharm Sci 1984;73(8):1038–1041.
13. Levy G, Garrettson LK, Soda DM: Evidence of placental transfer of acetaminophen [Letter]. Pediatrics 1975;55(6):895.
14. Beaulac-Baillargeon L, Rocheleau S: Paracetamol pharmacokinetics during the first trimester of human pregnancy. Eur J Clin Pharmacol 1994;46(5):451–454.
15. Rayburn W, Shukla U, Stetson P, et al: Acetaminophen pharmacokinetics: comparison between pregnant and nonpregnant women. Am J Obstet Gynecol 1986;155(6):1353–1356.
16. Byer AJ, Traylor TR, Semmer JR: Acetaminophen overdose in the third trimester of pregnancy. JAMA 1982;247(22):3114–3115.
17. Friedman S, Gatti M, Baker T: Cesarean section after maternal acetaminophen overdose. Anesth Analg 1993;77(3):632–634.
18. Ludmir J, Main DM, Landon MB, et al: Maternal acetaminophen overdose at 15 weeks of gestation. Obstet Gynecol 1986;67(5):750–751.
19. McElhatton PR, Sullivan FM, Volans GN: Paracetamol overdose in pregnancy: analysis of the outcomes of 300 cases referred to the Teratology Information Service. Reprod Toxicol 1997;11(1):85–94.
20. Riggs BS, Bronstien AC, Kulig K, et al: Acute acetaminophen overdose during pregnancy. Obstet Gynecol 1989;74(2):247–253.
21. Rosevear SK, Hope PL: Favourable neonatal outcome following maternal paracetamol overdose and severe fetal distress. Case report. Br J Obstet Gynaecol 1989;96(4):491–493.
22. Stokes IM: Paracetamol overdose in the second trimester of pregnancy. Case report. Br J Obstet Gynaecol 1984;91(3):286–288.
23. Wang PH, Yang MJ, Lee WL, et al: Acetaminophen poisoning in late pregnancy. A case report. J Reprod Med 1997;42(6):367–371.
24. Findlay JW, DeAngelis RL, Kearney MF, et al: Analgesic drugs in breast milk and plasma. Clin Pharmacol Ther 1981;29(5):625–633.
25. Tighe TV, Walter FG: Delayed toxic acetaminophen level after initial four hour nontoxic level. J Toxicol Clin Toxicol 1994;32(4):431–434.
26. Bartle WR, Paradiso FP, Derry JE, Livingstone DJ: Delayed acetaminophen toxicity despite acetylcysteine use. Drug Intell Clin Pharmacol 1989;23:509.
27. Augenstien WL, Kulig KW, Rumack BH: Delayed rise in serum drug levels in overdose patients despite multiple dose charcoal and after charcoal stools. Vet Hum Toxicol 1987;29:491.
28. Thomson JS, Prescott LF: Liver damage and impaired glucose tolerance after paracetamol overdosage. BMJ 1966;5512:506–507.
29. Davidson DG, Eastham WN: Acute liver necrosis following overdose of paracetamol. BMJ 1966;5512:497–499.
30. Mitchell JR, Jollow DJ, Potter WZ, et al: Acetaminophen-induced hepatic necrosis. I. Role of drug metabolism. J Pharmacol Exp Ther 1973;187(1):185–194.
31. Mitchell JR, et al: Acetaminophen-induced hepatic necrosis. IV. Protective role of glutathione. J Pharmacol Exp Ther 1973;187(1):211–217.
32. Mitchell JR, Thorgiersson SS, Potter WZ, et al: Acetaminophen-induced hepatic injury: protective role of glutathione in man and rationale for therapy. Clin Pharmacol Ther 1974;16(4):676–684.
33. Jollow DJ, Mitchell JR, Potter WZ, et al: Acetaminophen-induced hepatic necrosis. II. Role of covalent binding in vivo. J Pharmacol Exp Ther 1973;187(1):195–202.
34. Dahlin DC, Miwa FT, Lu AY, et al: N-acetyl-p-benzoquinone imine: a cytochrome P-450-mediated oxidation product of acetaminophen. Proc Natl Acad Sci U S A 1984;81(5):1327–1331.
35. Nelson SD: Molecular mechanisms of the hepatotoxicity caused by acetaminophen. Semin Liver Dis 1990;10(4):267–278.
36. Qiu Y, Benet LZ, Burlingame AL: Identification of the hepatic protein targets of reactive metabolites of acetaminophen in vivo in mice using two-dimensional gel electrophoresis and mass spectrometry. J Biol Chem 1998;273(28):17940–17953.
37. Jaeschke H, Knight TR, Bajt ML: The role of oxidant stress and reactive nitrogen species in acetaminophen hepatotoxicity. Toxicol Lett 2003;144(3):279–288.
38. Cohen SD, Khairallah EA: Selective protein arylation and acetaminophen-induced hepatotoxicity. Drug Metab Rev 1997;29(1–2):59–77 [erratum in Drug Metab Rev 1997;29(4):1285].
39. Smith CV, Lauterberg BH, Mitchell JR: Covalent binding and acute lethal injury in vivo: how has the original hypothesis survived a decade of critical examination? In Wilkinson GR, Rawlins MD (eds): Drug Metabolism and Disposition: Considerations in Clinical Pharmacology. Lancaster, UK, MTP Press, 1985, pp 161–181.
40. Michael SL, Rumford NR, Mayeux PR, et al: Pretreatment of mice with macrophage inactivators decreases acetaminophen hepatotoxicity and the formation of reactive oxygen and nitrogen species. Hepatology 1999;30(1):186–195.
41. Laskin DL, Gardiner CR, Price VF, et al: Modulation of macrophage functioning abrogates the acute hepatotoxicity of acetaminophen. Hepatology 1995;21(4):1045–1050.
42. Tarloff JB, Khaifallah EA, Cohen SD, et al: Sex- and age-dependent acetaminophen hepato- and nephrotoxicity in Sprague-Dawley rats: role of tissue accumulation, nonprotein sulfhydryl depletion, and covalent binding. Fund Appl Toxicol 1996;30(1):13–22.
43. Tirmenstein MA, Nelson SD: Subcellular binding and effects on calcium homeostasis produced by acetaminophen and a nonhepatotoxic regioisomer, 3′-hydroxyacetanilide, in mouse liver. J Biol Chem 1989;264(17):9814–9819.
44. Myers TG, Dietz EC, Anderson NL, et al: A comparative study of mouse liver proteins arylated by reactive metabolites of acetaminophen and its nonhepatotoxic regioisomer, 3′-hydroxyacetanilide. Chem Res Toxicol 1995;8(3):403–413.

45. Wendel A, Feuerstein S: Drug-induced lipid peroxidation in mice. I. Modulation by monooxygenase activity, glutathione and selenium status. Biochem Pharmacol 1981;30(18):2513–2520.

46. Wendel A, Jaeschke H, Gloger M: Drug-induced lipid peroxidation in mice. II. Protection against paracetamol-induced liver necrosis by intravenous liposomally entrapped glutathione. Biochem Pharmacol 1982;31(22):3601–3605.

47. Wendel A, Feuerstein S, Konz KH: Acute paracetamol intoxication of starved mice leads to lipid peroxidation in vivo. Biochem Pharmacol 1979;28(13):2051–2055.

48. Mitchell JR, Smith CV, Hughes H, et al: Overview of alkylation and peroxidation mechanisms in acute lethal hepatocellular injury by chemically reactive metabolites. Semin Liver Dis 1981;1(2):143–150.

49. Squadrito GL, Pryor WA: Oxidative chemistry of nitric oxide: the roles of superoxide, peroxynitrite, and carbon dioxide. Free Radic Biol Med 1998;25(4–5):392–403.

50. Burcham PC, Harman AW: Mitochondrial dysfunction in paracetamol hepatotoxicity: in vitro studies in isolated mouse hepatocytes. Toxicol Lett 1990;50(1):37–48.

51. Ruepp SU, Tonge RP, Shaw J, et al: Genomics and proteomics analysis of acetaminophen toxicity in mouse liver. Toxicol Sci 2002;65(1):135–150.

52. Walker RM, Racz WJ, McElligott TF: Scanning electron microscopic examination of acetaminophen-induced hepatotoxicity and congestion in mice. Am J Pathol 1983;113(3):321–330.

53. Donnelly PJ, Walker RM, Racz WJ: Inhibition of mitochondrial respiration in vivo is an early event in acetaminophen-induced hepatotoxicity. Arch Toxicol 1994;68(2):110–118.

54. Katyare SS, Satav JG: Impaired mitochondrial oxidative energy metabolism following paracetamol-induced hepatotoxicity in the rat. Br J Pharmacol 1989;96(1):51–58.

55. Meyers LL, Beierschmidt WP, Khairallah EA, et al: Acetaminophen-induced inhibition of hepatic mitochondrial respiration in mice. Toxicol Appl Pharmacol 1988;93(3):378–387.

56. Marzella L, Muhvich K, Myers RA: Effect of hyperoxia on liver necrosis induced by hepatotoxins. Virchows Arch 1986;51(6):497–507.

57. Salhanick SD, Belikoff B, Orlow D, et al: Hyperbaric oxygen reduces acetaminophen toxicity and increases HIF-1alpha expression. Acad Emerg Med 2006;13(7):707–714.

58. Burkhart KK, Hall AH, Gerace R, Rumack BH: Hyperbaric oxygen treatment for carbon tetrachloride poisoning. Drug Saf 1991;6(5):332–338.

59. Arteel GE, Iimuro Y, Yin M, et al: Chronic enteral ethanol treatment causes hypoxia in rat liver tissue in vivo. Hepatology 1997;25(4):920–926.

60. Arteel GE, Raleigh JA, Bradford BU, et al: Acute alcohol produces hypoxia directly in rat liver tissue in vivo: role of Kupffer cells. Am J Physiol 1996;271(3 Pt 1):G494–G500.

61. Cohen SD, Khairallah EA: Selective protein arylation and acetaminophen-induced hepatotoxicity. Drug Metab Rev 1997;29(1–2):59–77 [erratum in Drug Metab Rev 1997;29(4):1285].

62. Lieber CS: Alcohol and the liver: 1994 update. Gastroenterology 1994;106:1085–1105.

63. James LP, Mayeux PR, Hinson JA: Acetaminophen-induced hepatotoxicity. Drug Metab Dispos 2003;31(12):1499–1506.

64. Bessems JG, Vermeulen NP: Paracetamol (acetaminophen)-induced toxicity: molecular and biochemical mechanisms, analogues and protective approaches. Crit Rev Toxicol 2001;31(1):55–138.

65. Singer AJ, Carracio TR, Mofenson HC: The temporal profile of increased transaminase levels in patients with acetaminophen-induced liver dysfunction. Ann Emerg Med 1995;26(1):49–53.

66. Boutis K, Shannon M: Nephrotoxicity after acute severe acetaminophen poisoning in adolescents. J Toxicol Clin Toxicol 2001;39(5):441–445.

67. Blakely P, McDonald BR: Acute renal failure due to acetaminophen ingestion: a case report and review of the literature. J Am Soc Nephrol 1995;6(1):48–53.

68. O'Dell JR, Zetterman RK, Burnett DA: Centrilobular hepatic fibrosis following acetaminophen-induced hepatic necrosis in an alcoholic. JAMA 1986;255(19):2636–2637.

69. Watkins PB, Kaplowitz N, Slattery JT, et al: Aminotransferase elevations in healthy adults receiving 4 grams of acetaminophen daily: a randomized controlled trial. JAMA 2006;296(1):87–93.

70. Barrett BJ: Acetaminophen and adverse chronic renal outcomes: an appraisal of the epidemiologic evidence. Am J Kidney Dis 1996;28(1 Suppl 1):14–19.

71. Blantz RC: Acetaminophen: acute and chronic effects on renal function. Am J Kidney Dis 1996;28(1 Suppl 1):3–6.

72. Buckalew VM Jr: Habitual use of acetaminophen as a risk factor for chronic renal failure: a comparison with phenacetin. Am J Kidney Dis 1996;28(1 Suppl 1):7–13.

73. Rumack BH: Acetaminophen hepatotoxicity: the first 35 years. J Toxicol Clin Toxicol 2002;40(1):3–20.

74. Flanagan RJ, Mant TG: Coma and metabolic acidosis early in severe acute paracetamol poisoning. Hum Toxicol 1986;5(3):179–182.

75. Esterline RL, Ray SD, Ji S: Reversible and irreversible inhibition of hepatic mitochondrial respiration by acetaminophen and its toxic metabolite, N-acetyl-p-benzoquinoneimine (NAPQI). Biochem Pharmacol 1989;38(14):2387–2390.

76. Bonkovsky HL, et al: Acute hepatic and renal toxicity from low doses of acetaminophen in the absence of alcohol abuse or malnutrition: evidence for increased susceptibility to drug toxicity due to cardiopulmonary and renal insufficiency. Hepatology 1994;19(5):1141–1148.

77. Ekins BR, Ford DC, Thompson MI, et al: The effect of activated charcoal on N-acetylcysteine absorption in normal subjects. Am J Emerg Med 1987;5(6):483–487.

78. Spiller HA, Krenzelok EP, Grande GA, et al: A prospective evaluation of the effect of activated charcoal before oral N-acetylcysteine in acetaminophen overdose [see comment]. Ann Emerg Med 1994;23(3):519–523.

79. Smilkstein MJ: A new loading dose for N-acetylcysteine? The answer is no [see comment]. Ann Emerg Med 1994;24(3):538–539.

80. Makin AJ, Williams R: Acetaminophen-induced hepatotoxicity: predisposing factors and treatments. Adv Intern Med 1997;42:453–483.

81. Bernal W, Donaldson N, Wyncoll D, et al: Blood lactate as an early predictor of outcome in paracetamol-induced acute liver failure: a cohort study [see comment]. Lancet 2002;359(9306):558–563.

82. Whyte IM, Buckley NA, Reith DM, et al: Acetaminophen causes an increased International Normalized Ratio by reducing functional factor VII. Ther Drug Monit 2000;22(6):742–748.

83. Schmidt LE, Knudsen TT, Dalhoff K, et al: Effect of acetylcysteine on prothrombin index in paracetamol poisoning without hepatocellular injury [see comment]. Lancet 2002;360(9340):1151–1152.

84. Yip L, Dart RC: A 20-hour treatment for acute acetaminophen overdose. N Engl J Med 2003;348(24):2471–2472.

85. Woo OF, Mueller RD, Olson KR, et al: Shorter duration of oral N-acetylcysteine therapy for acute acetaminophen overdose. Ann Emerg Med 2000;35(4):363–368.

86. Schmidt LE, Dalhoff K: Risk factors in the development of adverse reactions to N-acetylcysteine in patients with paracetamol poisoning. Br J Clin Pharmacol 2001;51(1):87–91.

87. Appelboam AV, Dargan PI, Knighton J: Fatal anaphylactoid reaction to N-acetylcysteine: caution in patients with asthma. Emerg Med J 2002;19(6):594–595.

88. Ho SY, Arellano M, Zolkowski-Wynne J: Delayed increase in acetaminophen concentration after Tylenol PM overdose. Am J Emerg Med 1999;17(3):315–317.

89. Smilkstein MJ, Knapp GL, Kulig KW, et al: Efficacy of oral N-acetylcysteine in the treatment of acetaminophen overdose. Analysis of the national multicenter study (1976 to 1985) [see comment]. N Engl J Med 1988;319(24):1557–1562.

90. Prescott LF: Paracetamol overdosage. Pharmacological considerations and clinical management. Drugs 1983;25(3):290–314.

91. Keays R, Harrison PM, Wendon JA, et al: Intravenous acetylcysteine in paracetamol induced fulminant hepatic failure: a prospective controlled trial. BMJ 1991;303(6809):1026–1029.

92. Harrison PM, Wendon JA, Gimson AE, et al: Improvement by acetylcysteine of hemodynamics and oxygen transport in fulminant hepatic failure. N Engl J Med 1991;324(26):1852–1857.

93. Devlin J, Ellis AE, McPeake J, et al: N-acetylcysteine improves indocyanine green extraction and oxygen transport during hepatic dysfunction [see comment]. Crit Care Med 1997;25(2):236–242.

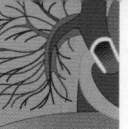

94. Spies CD, Reinhart K, Witt I, et al: Influence of *N*-acetylcysteine on indirect indicators of tissue oxygenation in septic shock patients: results from a prospective, randomized, double-blind study. Crit Care Med 1994;22(11):1738–1746.
95. Speeg KV: Potential use of cimetidine for treatment of acetaminophen overdose. Pharmacotherapy 1987;7(6 Pt 2 Suppl): 125–133.
96. Critchley JA, Dyson EH, Scott AW, et al: Is there a place for cimetidine or ethanol in the treatment of paracetamol poisoning? Lancet 1983;1(8338):1375–1376.
97. Brennan RJ, Mankes RF, Lefevre R, et al: 4-Methylpyrazole blocks acetaminophen hepatotoxicity in the rat. Ann Emerg Med 1994;23(3):487–494.
98. Eszter Hazai LV, Monostory K: Reduction of toxic metabolite formation of acetaminophen. Biochem Biophys Res Commun 2002;291(4):1089–1094.
99. Akdogan M, El-Sahwi K, Ahmed U, et al: Experience with liver dialysis in acetaminophen induced fulminant hepatic failure: a preliminary report. Turk J Gastroenterol 2003;14(3):164–167.

48 *Salicylates*

FERGUS KERR, MBBS, MPH ■ EDWARD P. KRENZELOK, PHARMD

At a Glance...

■ Salicylate poisoning may be a difficult diagnosis to make, particularly in the chronic setting, where salicylism is often unrecognized or mistaken for other illnesses.

■ Serial assessments of a patient's physical examination, acid–base state, and serum salicylate concentrations are essential to guide appropriate treatment.

■ Activated charcoal is the preferred method of gastrointestinal decontamination.

■ Fluid, electrolyte, and metabolic abnormalities occur commonly and should be treated promptly.

■ Urinary alkalinization enhances salicylate elimination and should be instituted in all symptomatic patients and those with serum salicylate concentrations greater than or equal to 30 mg/dL.

■ Hemodialysis is recommended for seriously poisoned patients.

INTRODUCTION AND RELEVANT HISTORY

Salicylates have been used since ancient times. Hippocrates, Galen, and medieval herbalists relied on salicylate-containing plants for their palliative properties. The medicinal properties of willow bark (*Salix alba vulgaris*) have been appreciated by native peoples for centuries. In the mid-19th century, the active ingredient of willow bark, salicylic acid, was isolated and subsequently synthesized from phenol. It gained widespread use in compounded pharmaceuticals as a pain reliever, anti-inflammatory, and antipyretic. In the latter portion of the 19th century, the Bayer company in Germany developed a salicylic acid derivative, aspirin (or acetylsalicylic acid), for commercial use. Aspirin and its chemically related analogs (all known as salicylates) have since been prescribed widely by the medical profession and used extensively in numerous pharmaceuticals for nonprescription use by the public. Since the 1960s, the development of analgesic, antipyretic, and anti-inflammatory alternatives (e.g., acetaminophen, ibuprofen) to salicylates has curtailed their use for these purposes. More recently, aspirin has become widely used as an antiplatelet agent in the treatment of cardio- and cerebrovascular disease. Because of its ubiquitous use and availability, aspirin continues to result in a significant number of acute and chronic poisonings.

EPIDEMIOLOGY

Salicylate poisoning (salicylism) can be accidental or intentional and acute or chronic. Salicylate poisoning occurs largely as an accidental overdose in the pediatric age group or intentional overdose with suicidal intent in the adult and teenage population. Therapeutic misadventure (misuse or error) can result in poisoning at any age. Although acute intoxication is more common, chronic salicylism also occurs with regularity. Untreated, both forms of poisoning can result in significant morbidity and mortality, particularly in the elderly population.

A review of salicylate exposures reported to the American Association of Poison Control Centers Toxic Exposure Surveillance System (AAPCC TESS) for the 10-year period of 1993 through 2002 reveals that 26.3% of all salicylate exposures occurred in children younger than 6 years (Fig. 48-1). Although a significant number of exposures occurred in the pediatric age group (birth–19 years of age), only five fatalities related to accidental overdose were reported—0.003% of all salicylate exposures reported to American poison centers. During this time period, 468 fatalities were attributed to salicylate poisoning. The mean age of those with fatal outcomes was 47.25 years. Most salicylate fatalities occur in older adults who intentionally ingest salicylates acutely in combination with other pharmaceuticals with suicidal intent.

Based on poison center data, the number of salicylate-related poisonings in children younger than 6 years has declined steadily from 1993 through 2002. This is especially noteworthy since the number of pediatric salicylate exposures decreased by nearly 10% since 1993

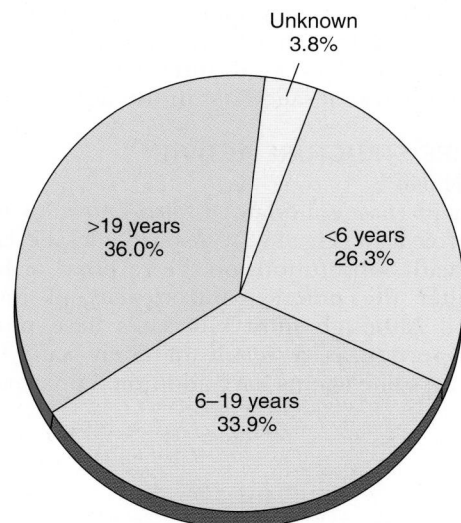

FIGURE 48-1 Age distribution: unintentional salicylate exposures, 1993 through 2002. Mean age, 47.25 years. The data were derived from the American Association of Poison Control Centers Toxic Exposure Surveillance System annual reports, 1993–2002 (retrieved September 16, 2003, from http://www.aapcc.org/annual.htm).

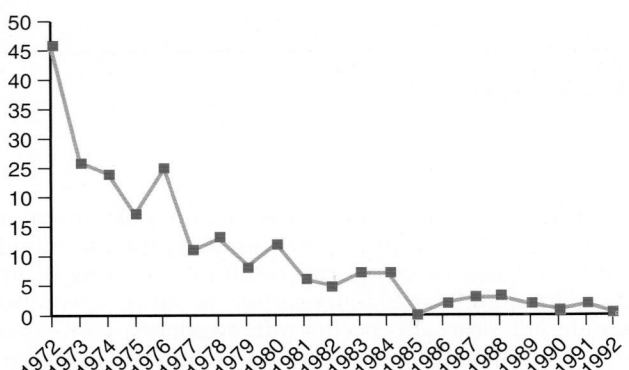

FIGURE 48-2 Aspirin-related fatalities in children younger than 5 years, 1972 through 1992. (From National Center for Health Statistics: Unpublished data.)

(9707 in 1993 versus 8753 in 2002), while the number of exposures reported to poison continued to increase (1,751,476 in 1993 versus 2,380,028 in 2002). Therefore, relative to all poisoning exposures, the incidence of reported pediatric salicylate exposures has dropped dramatically. A number of factors may account for this trend. Most important was the enactment of the 1970 Poison Prevention Packaging Act that mandated the use of child-resistant closures on aspirin-containing products. In addition, the enticingly flavored children's aspirin tablets were restricted to 81 mg per tablet and 36 tablets per bottle, thereby limiting the amount taken by children in accidental ingestions. The possible association between Reye's syndrome and the use of aspirin to treat viral diseases in children has led to a significant decline in the pediatric use of aspirin. As a result, the number of annual fatalities due to aspirin in children younger than 5 years dropped from 46 in 1972 to 0 in 1992 (Fig. 48-2). The introduction of alternatives to aspirin-containing products such as acetaminophen and ibuprofen, which have a considerably higher therapeutic index, have contributed to the decreased number of fatalities by decreasing the use of salicylates in this age group.

STRUCTURE/STRUCTURE-ACTIVITY RELATIONSHIPS

Salicylic acid (base salicylate) is also known as orthohydroxybenzoic acid (Fig. 48-3).[1] Aspirin is a salicylate ester of acetic acid. Substitutions on the carboxyl or hydroxyl groups alter the potency and toxicity of individual salicylates.[1] Although most salicylates have pharmacologic properties as a result of their salicylic acid component, some agents have additional pharmacologic

activity from other substitutions. For instance, the acetyl group substitution of aspirin allows it to acetylate proteins, which is the basis for most of its antiplatelet effects.

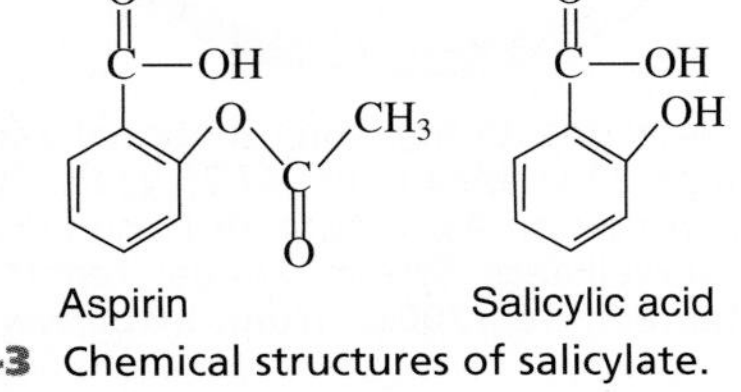

PHARMACOKINETICS

A thorough understanding of salicylate pharmacokinetics and changes that occur with salicylate overdose (toxicokinetics) is essential to understanding the genesis of salicylism and its appropriate management.

Dosing

Salicylates are formulated in oral, rectal, and topical preparations. The therapeutic dose of salicylate depends on the condition being treated. In general, the recommended dose for antipyresis and analgesia is 10 to 20 mg/kg orally every 6 hours for children (up to 75 mg/kg or 3.6 g/day) and 325 to 650 mg every 4 hours for adults (following an initial dose of 1 g). Larger doses of salicylate (4 to 6 g/day) are sometimes recommended for its full anti-inflammatory effects in adults with chronic illnesses (e.g., rheumatoid arthritis).

Absorption

Most cases of salicylate poisoning involve the ingestion of a product that contains aspirin. As a weak acid (pKa 3.5), aspirin is largely nonionized in the stomach and absorbed passively as acetylsalicylic acid.[2] The majority of salicylate absorption, however, occurs as the ionized form in the jejunum due to its greater absorptive surface. In addition, the alkaline jejunum enhances salicylate solubility, and thus tablet dissolution.[3] Absorption is rapid with therapeutic dosing; measurable levels are observed within 30 minutes, and peak serum concentrations of 10 to 20 mg/dL (0.7 to 1.4 mmol/L) usually occur within 1 to 2 hours of a single therapeutic dose. Chronic therapy with anti-inflammatory doses will produce peak serum salicylate concentrations of up to 30 mg/dL (2.2 mmol/L).

Absorption will be significantly influenced by the dose ingested, product formulation (different dissolution characteristics), mucosal pH, and gastric emptying time.[1,2] The presence of food may delay absorption by retarding gastric emptying. Enteric-coated products are resistant to the acid environment of the stomach; tablet dissolution is delayed until the more alkaline medium of the distal intestines is reached. Buffered (alkaline) aspirin tablets have enhanced solubility and more rapid dissolution in the small intestine, which can result in greater bioavailability. Overdose of salicylates can produce pylorospasm, delaying gastric emptying and subsequent absorption. While not a common phenomenon, salicylates have the potential to form gastric concretions or bezoars, which retard the otherwise rapid absorption and result in slow, continuous absorption that simulates a sustained-release pharmaceutical. Salicylate absorption may be slowed when it is co-ingested with other agents that retard gastric emptying and intestinal motility (i.e., anticholinergic drugs, opioids). Peak blood concentrations are often not reached for 4 or more hours in overdose situations. In one reported overdose of enteric-coated aspirin, the peak serum salicylate concentration

FIGURE 48-3 Chemical structures of salicylate.

Aspirin   Salicylic acid

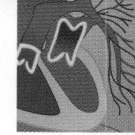

did not occur until 24 hours after ingestion.[4] Coexistent pathophysiology such as hypotension or decreased splanchnic circulation may also impede the absorption of salicylates. Liquid forms of salicylate, such as methyl salicylate, are more bioavailable and not subject to the rate-limiting process of dissolution; therefore, the absorption of liquid products may be more rapid and not retarded by physical or pathophysiologic factors. The route of administration will also affect absorption; rectal administration frequently results in delayed and erratic absorption.

Biliary secretion of salicylate is minimal.[5] Therefore, reabsorption secondary to enterohepatic circulation does not occur.

Dermal absorption of salicylates is a reported but rarely encountered etiology of salicylism.[6,7] Salicylate-containing liniments, keratolytics, and topical rubifacients are unlikely to represent a significant risk due to poor absorption through normal skin and use that is limited to the nonprescription treatment of minor musculoskeletal discomfort. The chronic use of highly concentrated products that are applied to large surface areas of compromised skin, however, may create a condition that allows sufficient salicylate absorption with resultant toxicity.

Chronic excessive use of salicylate suppositories has the potential to produce toxicity. However, it is rarely a cause of acute salicylism. The intentional use of a salicylate enema that contained 700 aspirin tablets produced profound salicylism.[8]

The natural source of salicylates (e.g., willow bark, herbals, etc.) or their pharmaceutical formulation, in conjunction with other variables, will affect salicylate absorption. Once absorption and metabolic conversion to salicylic acid occur, toxicokinetics are unaffected.

Distribution

Salicylates are distributed throughout body fluids and tissues. The low apparent volume of distribution (Vd = 0.16 to 0.35 L/kg) in salicylate overdose victims suggests that salicylate remains largely in the central compartment.[9] The apparent Vd and, thus, tissue distribution increases with supratherapeutic salicylate concentrations (saturation of plasma protein binding sites), lower blood pH, and the presence of drugs that compete with serum protein binding.

Salicylates are amenable to enhanced extracorporeal clearance (e.g., hemodialysis) due to their low molecular weight, small Vd, high water solubility, and increased fraction of free salicylate at supratherapeutic concentrations.

At therapeutic concentrations, salicylates are largely protein bound (50% to 80%), predominantly to serum albumin.[3,10] The degree of protein binding is a function of both the concentration of salicylic acid and the amount of albumin. As protein binding sites become saturated following salicylate overdose or with co-ingestion of other drugs that compete with albumin binding sites (e.g., phenytoin), the amount of free non-protein-bound salicylic acid increases and creates a climate for more significant toxicity. Any condition that depletes albumin or competes with its available binding sites predisposes the patient to a disproportionate risk for severe salicylism at a given plasma concentration.

Under normal physiologic conditions (pH 7.4), salicylates are highly ionized (>99%), which significantly reduces their ability to diffuse across the blood-brain barrier and into the central nervous system (CNS). In advanced salicylate poisoning, the development of metabolic acidosis (acidemia) significantly increases the fraction of nonionized salicylate and results in greater CNS penetration and elevated cerebral spinal fluid (CSF) concentrations. High CSF concentrations are associated with CNS toxicity and greater morbidity.

Salicylates cross the placenta readily and pose a significant risk to the fetus after maternal overdose. Salicylates are also found in breast milk but present a threat to the breast-fed infant only when the mother is taking large daily doses. The infant is prone to toxicity due to immature metabolism and, thus, impaired ability to eliminate salicylates and their metabolites.

Metabolism and Excretion

After gastrointestinal absorption, aspirin is hydrolyzed rapidly by nonspecific plasma esterases to the pharmacologically and toxicologically active chemical salicylic acid. This is a first-order process with a half-life of 15 to 20 minutes.[11] At therapeutic doses, salicylic acid then undergoes hepatic biotransformation and renal elimination via first-order processes[1,12,13]:

1. Glucuronidation → salicyl phenolic (10%) and salicyl acyl (5%) glucuronides
2. Oxidation → gentisic acid (<1%)
3. Microsomal oxidation or glycine conjugation → salicyluric acid (75%)
4. Salicylic acid → elimination via the urine (10%)

The major hepatic metabolic pathways (formation of salicyl phenolic glucuronide and salicyluric acid) become saturated when serum salicylate concentrations exceed 20 to 30 mg/dL.[1,12,13] Biotransformation converts from a dose-dependent first-order process (rate proportional to the dose) to a zero-order process, which means that a fixed amount of salicylic acid is metabolized per unit of time, regardless of the dose. This is referred to as Michaelis-Menten kinetics (see Chapter 4).

Because salicyluric acid and salicyl phenolic glucuronide formation is a saturable process, the biotransformation of salicylic acid proceeds more slowly and creates more opportunity for toxicity to occur.[12,13] The elimination half-life of salicylate is 2 to 3 hours after a single therapeutic dose, 6 to 12 hours with high therapeutic doses (20 to 30 mg/dL), and 20 to 40 hours after overdosage. Importantly, small increases in the dose can result in a significant increase in serum concentration.[1] Awareness of the accumulation kinetics of salicylic acid is essential to understanding the long half-life of salicylates in the overdose situation and the subsequent long duration of toxic manifestations. For the same reasons, the well-intentioned Done nomogram is not applicable in the determination of patient

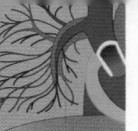

prognosis and the management of either acute or chronic salicylism.[14] Done considered that salicylates followed a first-order elimination process and developed the nomogram accordingly.[15]

SPECIAL POPULATIONS

Kinetics in Children

Neonates absorb salicylate as rapidly as any other age group but metabolize it more slowly than those with mature hepatic function. Renal elimination is slower in children, and they have reduced albumin concentrations that increase plasma salicylate concentrations. The Vd increases proportional to the dose, suggesting that children may have higher tissue concentrations than inferred by their plasma concentration.

Kinetics in the Elderly

Salicylate toxicokinetics in the elderly have not been well defined. However, the same accumulation kinetics apparent in younger adults apply to the elderly. It is likely that elderly patients are more predisposed to salicylate toxicity due to impaired hepatic and renal function that occurs with advanced age.

PHARMACOLOGIC AGENTS

Aspirin is the most common salicylate-containing preparation available. In addition, numerous over-the-counter and prescription products contain aspirin or salicylate analogs (e.g., bismuth subsalicylate, methyl salicylate) in combination with other pharmaceutical agents (Table 48-1). The salicylates are available in many different formulations (i.e., immediate-release, enteric-coated, and effervescent tablets; capsules; suppositories; powder papers; and liquids) for oral and rectal use. In addition, methyl salicylate is found commonly in liniments, lotions, creams, and ointments for the treatment of minor musculoskeletal complaints (concentration of methyl salicylate from 10% to 30%). Methyl salicylate is found in high concentration in oil of wintergreen, a product that is used to flavor confections. One teaspoon of oil of wintergreen contains the equivalent of 5 g of salicylate. Bismuth subsalicylate is used in popular antidiarrheal agents (e.g., Kaopectate [Pfizer, Morris Plains, NJ] and Pepto-Bismol [Proctor & Gamble, Cincinnati, OH]) and often is not recognized as a possible cause of salicylate poisoning (especially when other salicylates are ingested concomitantly). Salicylic acid is present in corn and wart removers. The most common use of salicylates is as an oral analgesic, antipyretic, and anti-inflammatory. For this application, salicylates may be ingested as the sole pharmaceutical (e.g., salicylsalicylic acid in Disalcid [3M Pharmaceuticals, St. Paul, MN]) or in combination with synergistic pain relievers such as opioids (e.g., aspirin with oxycodone in Percodan [Endo Labs, Chadds Ford, PA]). Salicylates may also be found in certain herbal preparations that contain willow bark (*Salix* species) or wintergreen leaf (see Chapter 68).

TOXICOLOGY

Clinical Manifestations

Acute salicylate poisoning produces a diverse array of signs and symptoms. Common clinical findings include tachypnea and hyperpnea, nausea and vomiting, abdominal pain, dehydration, hyperpyrexia, diaphoresis, tachycardia, pallor, and a variety of CNS disturbances (Box 48-1). CNS effects include dizziness, ataxia, tinnitus, deafness, confusion, psychosis, agitation, delirium, stupor, coma, and seizures. More uncommon clinical features may include bleeding, pulmonary edema, acute renal failure, and anaphylaxis. Chronic salicylate poisoning is often misdiagnosed initially due to an insidious onset, lack of history of an overdose, and the presence of nonspecific clinical findings. This category of poisoned patients is discussed in more detail at the end of this chapter.

The mechanisms by which salicylates exert their toxic effects are complex and not completely understood (Table 48-2). However, the pathophysiology includes direct and indirect respiratory center stimulation, uncoupling of oxidative phosphorylation, inhibition of the tricarboxylic acid (TCA) cycle, inhibition of amino acid metabolism, and stimulation of glycolysis, gluconeogenesis, and catabolism of proteins and fats. In addition, there is an interference with hemostatic mechanisms.

TABLE 48-1 Common Salicylate Preparations

COMPOUND	TRADE/COMMON NAME
Acetylsalicylic acid	Aspirin
Bismuth subsalicylate	Pepto-Bismol, Kaopectate
Choline magnesium trisalicylate	Trilisate
Choline salicylate	Arthropan
Magnesium salicylate	Doan's pills, Magan
Homomenthyl salicylate	Sunscreens
Methylsalicylate	Oil of wintergreen
Salicylic acid	Topical ketatolytics
Salicylsalicylic acid	Salsalate, Disalcid, Salsitab
Sodium salicylate	Analgesic
Trolamine salicylate	Aspercreme

BOX 48-1 COMMON CLINICAL FINDINGS IN SALICYLISM

Nausea and vomiting
Dehydration
Tachypnea and hyperpnea
Hyperpyrexia
Confusion
Coma
Tinnitus
Abdominal pain
Diaphoresis

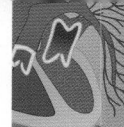

TABLE 48-2 Mechanisms and Manifestations in Salicylate Poisoning

MECHANISM	MANIFESTATION
Respiratory center stimulation	Respiratory alkalosis
	Renal HCO_3 elimination increased osmotic diuresis
	Increased insensible fluid loss
Oxidative-phosphorylation uncoupling	Metabolic acidosis
	Increased heat production and fluid loss
	Hypoglycemia
Inhibition of tricarboxylic acid cycle	Metabolic acidosis
Enhancement of protein metabolism and	Metabolic acidosis
inhibition of amino acid metabolism	Aminoaciduria — osmotic diuresis
Stimulation of gluconeogenesis	Hyperglycemia
	Glycosuria — osmotic diuresis
Stimulation of lipid metabolism	Metabolic acidosis (ketoacidosis)
	Ketonuria — osmotic diuresis
Increased pulmonary capillary permeability	Pulmonary edema

Acid–Base Disturbances

Acid–base disturbances are one of the most common manifestations of salicylate toxicity. Respiratory alkalosis and a high anion gap metabolic acidosis may occur alone or together. Generally, one will observe an initial respiratory alkalosis. However, metabolic acidosis may supervene in sensitive or severely poisoned patients. The coingestion of other drugs may influence acid-base balance. For example, Gabow and colleagues found that 40% of the patients in their series who ingested other drugs had a normal anion gap metabolic acidosis.[16] In children younger than 4 years, the metabolic component is usually more prominent, and these patients invariably demonstrate metabolic acidosis.[17] In contrast, older children and adults tend to have a predominating respiratory component.[18] In a review of 97 adults patients with high salicylate levels, Chapman and Proudfoot recorded patients in four categories of acid–base disturbance, with mixed respiratory alkalosis and metabolic acidosis or respiratory alkalosis alone predominating in 61% and 19% of patients, respectively. The arterial pH, rather than the type of acid-base disturbance, was of greater value in determining clinical severity and mortality.[19] The concomitant ingestion of respiratory depressant drugs may manifest as a mixed or isolated respiratory acidosis.[16]

It is commonly held that in adult salicylate poisoning a dominant metabolic acidosis follows an initial respiratory alkalosis. This latter phase may be very brief.[17] Adults may develop severe acidemia within as little as 3 to 4 hours of a massive aspirin overdose.

The underlying pathophysiology of the acid-base disturbances in salicylate intoxication is complex and not fully elucidated. Salicylates have been shown to stimulate the central respiratory center directly.[20,21] Respiratory alkalosis occurs due to hyperventilation, with an increase in the depth and rate of respirations. As a result there is a low partial pressure of CO_2 in arterial blood ($PaCO_2$), an increased plasma pH, and an elevated serum $[HCO_3^-]$. As a compensatory measure, $[HCO_3^-]$ is then excreted vigorously in the urine. There are animal data that suggest a role for peripheral arterial chemoreceptors in the development of hyperventilation.[22] The respiratory

stimulant effects of salicylates also occur indirectly from an increased production of tissue CO_2. Tissue CO_2 stimulates the respiratory center in the medulla oblongata.

Metabolic acidosis occurs after the inhibition of TCA cycle enzymes and of mitochondrial oxidative phosphorylation.[23,24] The uncoupling of oxidative phosphorylation reduces the production of cellular adenosine triphosphate and hence increases the production of pyruvic and lactic acid. Bartels and Lund-Jacobsen cast doubt on the significance of excessive lactate production due to salicylate-induced uncoupling of oxidative phosphorylation.[25] They postulated that observed elevations in lactate may be due to decreased hepatic elimination of lactate. The inhibition of key TCA cycle enzymes (e.g., α-ketoglutaric dehydrogenase and succinic acid dehydrogenase) further increase pyruvic and lactic acid levels.

The inability to produce cellular energy from oxidative phosphorylation results in enhanced but inefficient cellular metabolism. Gluconeogenesis and glycolysis are stimulated, and protein and lipid catabolism occur. Increased lipid and protein metabolism lead to the production and accumulation of ketone bodies (e.g., β-hydroxybutyric acid, acetoacetic acid, and acetone) and amino acids. Concurrent aminotransferase inhibition by salicylate prevents amino acid (e.g., alanine) metabolism and further augments levels of circulating amino acids.[26] Accumulation of these organic acids leads to the increased anion gap metabolic acidosis associated with salicylate poisoning; only a small contribution occurs from salicylate itself.

Both salicylate in the CSF and acidemia are powerful stimuli to respiration, and the latter facilitates the former.[27] Together they might be expected to enhance hyperventilation in comparison to patients with normal or low arterial $[H^+]$. Chapman and Proudfoot, however, found that the mean $PaCO_2$ was higher in fatal cases (most of whom were acidemic) than in survivors (most of whom had normal or low arterial $[H^+]$). This failure to hyperventilate appropriately in response to an acid stimulus may be a factor in the development of acidemia in these patients.[19]

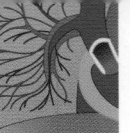

A final contributing factor to the development of acidosis is the depletion of buffering capacity as a result of increased renal loss of [HCO$_3^-$] through the compensatory mechanisms that are a consequence of the initial respiratory alkalosis.[28]

Fluid and Electrolyte Abnormalities

Fluid and electrolyte aberrations are not uncommon in salicylate poisoning and are multifactorial. Fluid and electrolyte losses occur from vomiting, decreased oral intake, diaphoresis, hyperventilation, osmotic diuresis (from bicarbonate, glucose, organic acid loss in urine), and increased metabolism and heat production. Water losses may reach 4 to 6 L/m^2.[29] With increased bicarbonate excretion at the kidney in the early alkalotic stage, there is concomitant loss of sodium and potassium as the body attempts to conserve hydrogen ions. Robin and colleagues reported six severely poisoned patients who presented with hypokalemia manifesting as a low serum potassium concentration, electrocardiographic changes, and neuromuscular abnormalities.[30] All patients demonstrated respiratory alkalosis. It was postulated that the hypokalemia resulted from a subsequent shift of potassium into the cells and excessive renal loss. In a similar way, forced alkaline diuresis may also lead to significant hypokalemia.[31] In both of the above situations, patients responded to potassium supplementation. Hypocalcemia may also complicate attempts to alkalinize the urine.[32] Conversely, transient hypercalcemia has been reported after overdose with soluble aspirin, possibly due to the calcium content of the tablet.[33] Hypernatremia is common, presumably resulting from dehydration. Hyponatremia is less common but does occur, and may be associated with inappropriate fluid retention.[34]

Pulmonary Edema

Pulmonary edema is an uncommon but well-recognized complication of acute salicylate intoxication, first being reported in 1950. More importantly, it is considered to be the most common cause of significant morbidity in chronic salicylate intoxication.[35] In the 1970s, the noncardiogenic origin of the edema was suspected by Zitnik and colleagues after pulmonary artery catheterization revealed a normal pulmonary artery wedge pressure, and by Bowers and colleagues in their studies on sheep.[36,37] Since that time, a number of studies have suggested an increase in pulmonary capillary permeability as the underlying pathologic process. Three prominent theories attempt to explain this.[37] First, aspirin is known to inhibit prostacyclin, a chemical that acts to reduce capillary permeability. Second, mild cerebral edema may result in a catecholamine surge, leading to elevated pulmonary vascular pressures. And third, salicylates' effect on platelet-vessel interaction may result in increased capillary permeability.

Radiologic studies in salicylate intoxication indicate that pulmonary edema occurs in about 35% of patients over the age of 30 years.[37] Chronic ingestion of the drug, smoking, and the presence of metabolic acidosis and/or neurologic features on admission were major risk factors for its development. In the same study, by Walters and colleagues, none of the patients younger than 16 years developed pulmonary edema, whereas Fisher and colleagues demonstrated that 2 out of 20 children developed the complication.[38]

Central Nervous System Abnormalities

CNS toxicity is an important indicator of severe salicylate toxicity. Coma is rare, with patients more often agitated, confused, and restless before unconsciousness occurs. In children younger than 5 years, in whom acidemia is the usual acid–base disturbance, these neurologic features are more common.[17,39]

Adults display CNS toxicity less often, but when they do, it is also associated with acidemia.[16,19] The severity of CNS manifestations and salicylate mortality appears to have a direct relationship to brain salicylate concentrations.[27,40] In a rat model, Hill demonstrated that the presence of acidemia facilitates the shift of salicylate from the extracellular fluid into the intracellular space, especially in the brain.[27,40] With a pKa of 3.0 for salicylic acid, as the pH of the blood falls, a higher percentage of the compound will be found in the nonionized form. This results in enhanced lipid solubility and hence an increased ability to cross cell membranes and the blood-brain barrier. Some patients with significant CNS effects have been alkalemic, but in those cases the plasma salicylate concentrations were very high.

Cerebral edema has been reported, but is uncommon. Hypernatremia and fluid retention or overload may contribute to its development. Seizures may occur in patients with severe toxicity. Some animal studies indicate that they may result from hyperventilation or reduced brain glucose levels, which paradoxically can occur despite normoglycemia.

Concomitant ingestion of CNS depressants, such as alcohol and benzodiazepines, may enhance the toxicity from salicylate independent of the toxic effects that occur directly from these CNS depressants themselves. By reducing the central drive to hyperventilate in response to acidemia, these drugs will enhance the CNS distribution and morbidity from salicylate.[16]

Metabolic Derangement

The principal metabolic derangement in salicylate poisoning is a change in glucose metabolism, which may produce either hypoglycemia or hyperglycemia. In addition, hypoglycorrhachia (low CSF glucose concentrations) may occur despite normal or even high serum glucose concentrations.[41] Increased demand for glucose occurs simultaneously with a decreased ability of certain tissues to utilize the glucose substrate. Increased glucose demand results in glycogenolysis and gluconeogenesis. Initially, patients may present with a short-lived, or in some cases persistent, hyperglycemia, which may be of high enough magnitude to produce glycosuria.[18,29] Sustained and persistent hyperglycemia reflects a failure of the tissues to utilize glucose adequately. Glucose stores

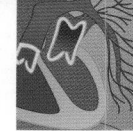

may also become exhausted and result in hypoglycemia. Contributing to the development of hypoglycemia is enhanced insulin secretion, which may result from the inhibition of prostaglandin synthesis.[42]

Hyperpyrexia

Hyperpyrexia is more common in children than adults.[19] It may result from the increased heat production that occurs following the uncoupling of oxidative phosphorylation. Additionally, toxic levels of salicylate impair the efficiency of the body's cooling mechanisms. This is compounded by the presence of dehydration.[29] Hyperpyrexia is uncommon in acute adult salicylate poisoning, and its presence is associated with a poor prognosis.[19] Other causes of an elevated temperature should also be considered, for example, infection or concomitant drug ingestion.

Hematologic Abnormalities

Decreased production of prothrombin and factors V, VII and X, increased capillary fragility, decreased platelet adhesiveness, and thrombocytopenia have all been observed in salicylate intoxication.[43] Rarely do any of these changes become clinically significant. On occasion, transient petechial rashes may be observed over the face and neck. Significant hemorrhagic complications, however, are very uncommon in salicylate poisoning.

Gastrointestinal and Hepatic Abnormalities

As discussed above, gastrointestinal bleeding is rare in salicylate poisoned patients. Gastric perforation has been reported after an acute overdose with enteric-coated aspirin.[41] Nausea, vomiting, and epigastric abdominal pain are the most common and consistent gastrointestinal tract findings in acute salicylate poisoning. Hemorrhagic gastritis, pylorospasm, and decreased gastric motility may also occur.

Direct hepatotoxicity, histologically similar to Reye's syndrome on biopsy, may occur with chronic salicylate use. Differentiating salicylate poisoning from Reye's syndrome is the presence of larger fatty droplets and a lack of mitochondrial changes.[44,45] Salicylate-associated hepatotoxicity is usually mild and resolves with discontinuation of salicylates.

Renal Abnormalities

Kimberly and Plotz have reported a reduced creatinine clearance, an elevated urea, and an increase in celluria as adverse effects of aspirin.[46] This acute renal impairment may possibly be explained by either a reduction in renal blood flow or as a result of direct nephrotoxicity. The renal abnormalities may result from the anti-prostaglandin effects of salicylates. It is thought that salicylates acutely inhibit prostaglandin synthesis, which results in vasoconstriction, reduced renal blood flow, and reduced glomerular filtration.[47] The resultant oliguria is exacerbated by the presence of dehydration. Preexisting renal disease may predispose patients to the development of renal impairment.

Other

Tinnitus is well-described with salicylate intoxication, and frequently precedes the onset of deafness. Both effects are reversible. Mongan and colleagues reported tinnitus beginning at levels from 20 to 45 mg/dL.[48] It has been postulated that salicylates increase intralabyrinthine pressure, but Ramsden and colleagues suggested that salicylates cause their effect by acting at the hair cell–neural interface, causing a transient metabolic blockade.[49] Alternatively, tinnitus and deafness may result from vasoconstriction of the auditory microvasculature (serving cochlea and hair cells).[1]

Ralston and colleagues reported on a 13-month-old boy with mild to moderate salicylate intoxication who experienced bradyarrhythmias and global myocardial dysfunction that they could not attribute to acidosis, hypoxia, ischemia, or metabolic or electrolyte abnormalities.[50] Therapeutic doses of salicylates have no significant cardiovascular effects.

Fatal in utero salicylism has been reported following an aspirin overdose in an 8-month pregnant primigravida.[51] Palatnick and Tenenbein described a 37-week pregnant 17-year-old girl who presented with fetal demise after ingesting 50 aspirin tablets a day for 1 month.[52] A number of factors may explain the apparent increased fetal susceptibility to salicylate poisoning. First, the fetus has immature pathways to metabolize and excrete the drug; second, the fetal concentration of salicylate is higher; and third, the more acidotic fetal blood facilitates the movement of salicylate across the blood-brain barrier.[53,54]

A number of investigators have reported on multiple-system organ failure following salicylate overdose, sometimes associated with rhabdomyolysis.[55,56] Vadas and colleagues demonstrated increased phospholipase A_2 concentrations and postulated that this may result from an aspirin-induced intestinal permeability to endotoxin and that these elevated phospholipase A_2 levels may play a role in the development of multiple-system organ failure.[56]

Hypersensitivity reactions to aspirin and salicylate-containing products have been well documented. Most patients develop a mild urticarial rash, but life-threatening anaphylaxis can occur. Botma and colleagues reported a case of an 18-month-old girl who ingested oil of wintergreen.[57] In addition to the typical features of salicylate poisoning, she also developed local laryngeal edema and stridor that necessitated endotracheal intubation.

DIAGNOSIS

Following an acute overdose of salicylate, the diagnosis is often straightforward. In the pediatric age group, a history of recent ingestion is usually present. The history in the adult population is more circumspect, but these

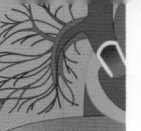

patients are seldom comatose and commonly admit to their actions. Where CNS depressant drugs have also been ingested, the history is more difficult, and a greater reliance should be placed on physical findings. If possible, the history should include the time and intent of ingestion, specific product and amount ingested, and the presence of co-ingestants and pertinent comorbid illnesses.

The severity of an acute salicylate overdose can be determined by history, physical findings, and laboratory data. Although potentially unreliable, the history may be used to predict the clinical severity of illness.[18] Generally, acute ingestions of less than 150 mg/kg follow a benign course, with symptomatic salicylate toxicity unlikely to occur.[58] With ingestions above 150 mg/kg, toxicity is dose dependent and have been traditionally divided into mild (150 to 300 mg/kg), moderate (300 to 500 mg/kg), and severe (>500 mg/kg) poisoning.[18] These categories are not absolute and should be utilized in conjunction with the patient's clinical condition.

Physical findings can also be used to grade the severity of salicylate poisoning.[18] The physical examination should focus on the vital signs, neurologic and cardiovascular examinations, and state of hydration. Early in the course of an acute salicylate overdose, symptoms and signs may be mild and subtle. Hence, it is important to evaluate patients serially, rather than relying on a single initial assessment as an indicator of clinical severity. Traditionally, cases of mild poisoning are said to demonstrate hyperpnea and/or tachypnea, mild lethargy or ataxia, tinnitus, and mild nausea and/or vomiting. Moderate toxicity is characterized by more prominent tachypnea, tachycardia, orthostatic hypotension, and neurologic disturbances (e.g., slurred speech, disorientation, confusion). Severe poisoning is represented by stupor or coma, seizures, respiratory depression, and hyperpyrexia. It is vital to remember, however, that salicylate poisoning is a dynamic process, and regular assessments and management appraisals are required. It is unwise to rigidly categorize such patients.

Finally, the severity of salicylate poisoning can be assessed with various laboratory parameters. Historically, the use of serum salicylate concentrations alone was used by some to assess severity of salicylate poisoning. In 1960, Done studied 38 patients (29 of whom were children), who presented after an acute aspirin overdose.[15] Based on their clinical symptoms and signs and their plasma levels, he created a nomogram that plots salicylate concentrations at differing times in an attempt to estimate the degree of intoxication—asymptomatic, mild, moderate, or severe—and hence predict expected symptoms. Measurements made before 6 hours were considered misleading since the drug may still be in the absorptive phase. In practice, plasma salicylate concentrations do not correlate well with features of acute toxicity, especially in those patients who are assessed as moderately or severely intoxicated.[14] The nomogram has been demonstrated to be unrepresentative of toxicity.[58,59] More specifically, the nomogram is not useful in the following circumstances: salicylate ingestion over a prolonged time (chronic ingestion), a sustained-release preparation or oil

of wintergreen ingestion, the presence of renal insufficiency, an unknown time of ingestion, and an acidemic patient.[60] Furthermore, the nomogram is based on the misconception that salicylates are eliminated via first-order kinetics.[60] Due to these limitations, most toxicologists do not utilize the nomogram to determine severity of salicylate poisoning.

For those with chronic salicylate poisoning, more severe toxicity is typically manifested at lower plasma salicylate concentrations as compared with acute intoxication. For these patients as well, clinical features correlate poorly with concentrations and the Done nomogram is of no use.

Use of laboratory data other than salicylate concentrations will allow a better assessment of the severity of salicylate poisoning. In particular, concurrent measurements of plasma (arterial or venous) and urine pH identify the presence of a systemic acid-base disturbance and allow for estimation of the phase and severity of salicylism.[61] Early or mild poisoning is represented by alkalemia (plasma pH >7.4) and alkaluria (urine pH >6); intermediate or moderate poisoning by alkalemia and paradoxical aciduria (urine pH <6); and late or severe poisoning by acidemia (plasma pH <7.4) and aciduria. Simultaneous measurement of each of these two parameters helps to determine the severity and stage of poisoning and will facilitate treatment. Ultimately, assessment of salicylate severity, whether acute or chronic, is best determined by combining data obtained from history, clinical signs and symptoms, plasma salicylate concentration, and urine and plasma pH together.

Laboratory Testing

When a patient's clinical signs and symptoms suggest salicylism, a plasma salicylate concentration is essential to confirm diagnosis and guide management decisions. A concentration greater than 30 mg/dL is usually associated with toxicity. Chronic therapeutic plasma concentrations in rheumatoid arthritis sufferers range from 10 to 30 mg/dL. A single level drawn too early may not be representative. Therefore, repeated levels at 2- to 3-hourly intervals should be obtained until a downward trend is established. It is important not to rely on a single concentration because of the possibility of prolonged or delayed absorption following the ingestion of sustained-release products, enteric-coated tablets, or the formation of a pharmacologic bezoar. Concentrations should be interpreted in conjunction with the patient's overall clinical and acid-base status. The presence of significant acidemia may imply a more serious intoxication, since higher concentrations of nonionized salicylate can penetrate into the CNS.

Several methods are available through which to determine plasma salicylate concentrations,[59] the most common one being the colorimetric technique, which utilizes the reaction between salicylate and ferric ion, and gives an estimate of the total plasma salicylate concentration. High-performance liquid chromatography and gas chromatography can distinguish acetylsalicylic acid (aspirin) from salicylic acid, something the colori-

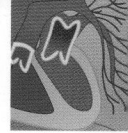

metric test cannot differentiate. Colorimetric testing is, however, easy and fast. So-called "routine" toxicologic screening for salicylate poisoning has a low positive yield.[62] Spot tests performed in the emergency department have little prognostic value and are fraught with problems due to misinterpretation by inexperienced individuals.

In all symptomatic patients and those with intentional salicylate overdose, measurements of serum electrolytes, glucose, BUN, creatinine, and calcium should be obtained and an anion gap calculated. Other tests should include a venous or arterial blood gas, urinalysis (including urine pH), and toxic screening for co-ingestants and qualitative pregnancy testing, as indicated. A complete blood count, coagulation profile, and liver function tests are appropriate in moderate to severe poisonings. A chest x-ray should be performed if pulmonary edema is suggested on examination or if arterial blood gases demonstrate a widened arterial-alveolar gradient.[38]

The concentration of salicylate in the CSF reflects the concentration of unbound drug in the plasma, and studies in children and animals have shown that the severity of intoxication is closely related to the CSF salicylate concentrations. These in turn are related to the total plasma concentration and the $[H^+]$. High $[H^+]$ reduces ionization and thereby facilitates the shift of salicylate into the cells. However, CSF levels are not used routinely to assess the magnitude of salicylism.

Differential Diagnosis

Salicylate toxicity should be considered in patients with unexplained acid–base disturbances, hyperventilation, tinnitus, or CNS disturbances. In severe cases, the presence of an altered mental status may prevent the disclosure of salicylate ingestion and erroneously lead to an involved neuropsychiatric evaluation, delaying the diagnosis and potentially increasing morbidity. Chronic salicylism is insidious and often mistaken for other illnesses, such as diabetic ketoacidosis, alcoholic ketoacidosis, metabolic encephalopathy, systemic infection or sepsis, dementia, organic psychosis, alcohol withdrawal, viral meningitis, Reye's syndrome (in children), delirium, pancreatitis, and other causes of high anion gap acidemia.

MANAGEMENT

Supportive Measures

As with all poisoned patients, initial management should be directed toward establishing and maintaining an adequate airway, and then optimizing respiratory and cardiovascular function. Intravenous access should be established and supplemental oxygen applied when appropriate. Although endotracheal intubation can be life-saving when an airway is compromised, Greenberg and Hendrickson described a 58-year-old man who presented with a mixed metabolic acidosis/respiratory

alkalosis and marked tachypnea following an overdose of aspirin. After intubation, the pH fell and the patient deteriorated and subsequently died. They postulated that mechanical ventilation was an inadequate substitute for manual ventilation and could not provide the rates needed to prevent acid accumulation.[63] If endotracheal intubation becomes clinically necessary, it is critical to maintain or establish patient alkalemia (plasma pH 7.50 to 7.55) to minimize salicylate distribution into the CNS. Patient hyperventilation (to produce hypocarbia) before and after intubation, along with the adjunctive administration of sodium bicarbonate (see Urinary Manipulation) can minimize the entry of salicylates into the CNS.

It is absolutely essential that careful attention be directed to the fluid balance status of the patient. Patients with moderate to severe poisoning should have an indwelling bladder catheter placed to closely monitor urine output. Central venous or pulmonary artery catheter monitoring is recommended for severely poisoned patients. Most patients are dehydrated on presentation. Thus, Temple suggests that the initial amount of fluid given should be in the range of 10 to 15 mL/kg/hr, administered over the first 1 to 2 hours.[18] This may be an important consideration in patients with chronic poisoning or in those who present several hours after the ingestion. Subsequent fluid therapy should be based on the clinical need for rehydration, the renal function, and the risks of inducing or complicating pulmonary edema. Ultimately the aim of fluid replacement is to replace fluid deficits and maintain a urine output of between 100 and 200 mL/hr.

Because hypoglycemia has been implicated in the pathophysiology of CNS injury in salicylate-poisoned patients, glucose should be added (50 to 100 g/L), despite the presence of normoglycemia or even mild hyperglycemia. The potential benefit of giving glucose supplementation is empiric, and there are no clinical data concerning the real glucose requirements.[62]

Patients poisoned seriously by salicylates are at risk for developing pulmonary edema and/or fluid retention through an inappropriate antidiuretic hormone secretion. In these patients, particularly if at the extremes of age, aggressive fluid replacement may be counterproductive. Urine output, renal function, and central venous pressure readings will be helpful in assessing these persons.

Hypernatremia is common; hence, some clinicians recommend hypotonic solutions in the initial management phase. Hypokalemia should also be monitored for and treated. The presence of a significant acidemia may result in a normal serum K^+ level, but mask a true total body potassium deficiency.

As outlined previously, a low serum pH increases the tissue penetration of salicylate, and hence increases CNS concentrations. For this reason, acidemia should be corrected using sodium bicarbonate (see Urinary Manipulation). Hypokalemia should be corrected simultaneously. It should be understood that sodium bicarbonate therapy is often indicated in mild/early and intermediate/moderate poisoning despite the

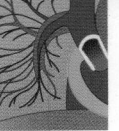

presence of alkalemia. Alkalemia rarely requires specific treatment.

Pulmonary edema in salicylate-poisoned patients is noncardiogenic. Therefore, therapy should begin with oxygen and progress to continuous positive airway pressure ventilation (CPAP), and finally may require intubation with positive end-expiratory pressure ventilation (PEEP). Pulmonary edema will improve as salicylate concentrations fall.[35,62]

All patients with an altered mental status should receive intravenous dextrose (or have a fingerstick blood glucose analysis), naloxone (as indicated), and thiamine. As described above, normoglycemia, or even a slightly elevated blood glucose concentration, may be present in the face of depressed CNS glucose concentrations. The presence of CNS symptoms or signs or hypoglycemia should be treated with an intravenous bolus of 50% glucose, approximately 1 mL/kg.

Seizures are not common in salicylate intoxication. Those that occur should be treated in standard fashion (e.g., dextrose, lorazepam or diazepam, and phenobarbital). Other causes for seizures should also be considered, including electrolyte abnormalities (e.g., hypocalcemia) and hypoglycemia. For those patients with suspected cerebral edema, the head of the bed should be elevated, hyperventilation should be performed, and mannitol administration should be considered.

Hyperpyrexia is more common in children than adults. The possibilities of other causes should be considered, including infection or other drug ingestions. If severe, evaporative cooling (tepid water spray and fans), cooling blankets, and neuromuscular paralysis should be considered (for those with associated neuromuscular agitation).

Decontamination

In recent years the role of syrup of ipecac has been significantly curtailed and most toxicologists do not recommend it in the setting of salicylate poisoning.[64] Gastric lavage has also been the focus of considerable attention. The joint position statement from the American Academy of Clinical Toxicology and the European Association of Poisons Centers and Clinical Toxicologists recommends gastric lavage only for those patients presenting within 1 hour of ingesting a potentially life-threatening amount of poison.[65] Gut decontamination following aspirin ingestion is controversial and can raise considerable debate.[66] Contemporary practices dictate the sole and expeditious use of oral activated charcoal in most acute salicylate overdoses, especially if it can be administered within 1 hour of the ingestion.[67,68] Although uncommon, pharmacologic bezoars may form after very large overdoses. Their presence, as indicated by sustained or rising salicylate concentrations, may necessitate gastric lavage and/or multiple-dose activated charcoal administration or even endoscopic procedures to break up the concretions if there is evidence of continued gut absorption. Comatose patients who undergo gastric lavage should be intubated endotracheally.

Activated charcoal is effective in reducing the gut absorption of salicylates.[12,69] An initial oral bolus of 50 g (adults) or 1 g/kg (children) should be administered as soon as possible, but preferably within 1 hour of ingestion.[70] Charcoal should not be withheld for patients who present late after oral salicylate overdose; pylorospasm and decreased gut motility associated with overdose may provide continued efficacy with late charcoal administration. Subsequent doses should be considered at 2- to 6-hour intervals if there is evidence that continued absorption is occurring. Given that absorption has already occurred in most patients, the use of activated charcoal in those with chronic poisoning is probably of no benefit. Conceptually, as enteric-coated salicylates dissolve in the distal gastrointestinal tract, activated charcoal should be effective. However, whole bowel irrigation (WBI) may be a more effective means of eliminating enteric-coated products. Kirshenbaum and colleagues studied the effectiveness of WBI, compared with single-dose activated charcoal with sorbitol, in preventing salicylate absorption following the ingestion of enteric-coated aspirin in volunteers.[71] They concluded that WBI was more effective in reducing absorption. Generally, the use of WBI in the prevention of salicylate absorption has not been validated, and it cannot be recommended routinely in the management of salicylate overdoses.[72]

Antidotes

There are no specific antidotes for salicylate poisoning.

Elimination

MULTIDOSE ACTIVATED CHARCOAL

The use of multidose activated charcoal (MDAC) to enhance the elimination of salicylates is controversial.[73-75] Hillman and Prescott demonstrated that MDAC was effective for enhancing elimination in patients with mild to moderate toxicity. Most subsequent studies, however, have failed to demonstrate efficacy of MDAC for elimination enhancement. MDAC should not be used as a means of enhancing elimination, bur rather as an intervention to prevent the ongoing absorption of salicylates.[76]

URINARY MANIPULATION

Normally, salicylate undergoes both glomerular filtration and tubular secretion. At high therapeutic doses, the hepatic metabolic pathways for salicylates become saturated. Renal excretion, therefore, becomes very important for the total body elimination of salicylate at high therapeutic and toxic levels. Although only the unbound fraction of salicylate is available for glomerular filtration, this fraction increases with supratherapeutic salicylate concentrations. Salicylate is also reabsorbed at the proximal convoluted tubules (PCTs). This latter process depends on both urine flow rate and urine pH. As explained previously, in an acid environment, salicylate is maximally nonionized, facilitating transfer across cell membranes, and hence PCT reabsorption. During periods of high urine output, the urinary concentration of salicylate falls, which reduces the urine:tubular cell concentration gradient and, thus, PCT

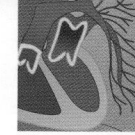

reabsorption. Overall, urinary salicylate clearance is directly proportional to urinary flow rate but logarithmically proportional to urine pH.[77] Forced diuresis, forced alkaline diuresis, and urinary alkalinization are methods that apply these principles to enhance the urinary elimination of salicylates.

Traditionally, to achieve a forced alkaline diuresis, crystalloid fluid with sodium bicarbonate was administered intravenously at a rate of approximately 2 L/hr for 3 hours.[31] Forced diuresis requires the same volume of fluid at the same rate, without the concomitant use of sodium bicarbonate.[78] Urinary alkalinization calls for the administration of sodium bicarbonate alone in an attempt to increase the urine pH above 7.5, while maintaining a normal urine output and avoiding the risks of fluid overload.[79]

In 1982, Prescott and colleagues compared these three methods by studying 44 salicylate-poisoned adults.[78] They concluded that the administration of sodium bicarbonate alone was at least as effective as and, possibly, more effective than either forced diuresis or forced alkaline diuresis. Furthermore, unlike the other two regimens, fluid retention was not a problem with urinary alkalinization alone. The large fluid load produced by regimens designed to force a diuresis are usually well tolerated by young adults with normal renal function; however, even in this age group pulmonary edema and cerebral edema have occurred. The addition of furosemide does reduce the risk of fluid retention, but it may decrease rather than increase renal salicylate elimination.[79] Utilizing urinary alkalinization, the apparent elimination half-life of salicylate poisoning decreased to 6 to 12 hours. In the Prescott and colleagues study, the significant decreases in plasma salicylate seen with forced diuresis and forced alkaline diuresis were greater than expected based on the urinary salicylate excretion. It was felt that this was due in part to hemodilution, and that this phenomenon may give a false impression of efficacy. Patients treated with alkalinization alone in this study, however, received 375 to 500 mL/hr of intravenous fluid during the treatment period, suggesting that fluid resuscitation and the initiation of a diuresis is also important to enhance the renal clearance of salicylate.

The effectiveness of urinary alkalinization to enhance the clearance of salicylate was demonstrated in another human volunteer study. Vree and colleagues conducted a randomized study in six volunteers who received 1.5 g sodium salicylate orally before initiation of urine alkalinization or urine acidification. The mean peak salicylate concentrations were 93.3 mg/L and 109.8 mg/L, respectively. As compared with urinary acidification, the mean elimination half-life was significantly less and the mean total clearance was significantly increased during urine alkalinization.[80]

In the care of poisoned salicylate patients, most patients are dehydrated on presentation, thus necessitating fluid resuscitation simultaneous with urinary alkalinization. While urinary alkalinization is more important to augment renal salicylate clearance than forced diuresis alone, aggressive fluid resuscitation until an adequate flow of urine (>2 mL/kg/hr) is achieved is also

important to competent patient care. The indications for urinary alkalinization include the presence of signs or symptoms of salicylism (symptomatic poisoning), acid-base disturbances, or elevated salicylate levels (>30 mg/dL). The latest recommendations from the American Academy of Clinical Toxicology and the European Association of Poison Control Centres and Clinical Toxicologists Position Statement is that "Based on volunteer and clinical studies, urine alkalinization should be considered as first line treatment for patients with moderately severe salicylate poisoning who do not meet the criteria for hemodialysis."[79]

The procedure for performing urine alkalinization in salicylate poisoning is described in Box 48-2.

Effective alkalinization of the urine may be very difficult to achieve. More recently, the effectiveness of urinary alkalinization has been confirmed by Higgins and colleagues.[81] They reported two separate episodes of salicylate poisoning in the same patient. In the first poisoning episode, hemodialysis was used without alkalinization; in the second, alkalinization was performed without hemodialysis. When urinary alkalinization was performed, the salicylate level fell by 45% 5 hours after admission as compared with a fall of only 4% in the 4 hours prior to hemodialysis where alkalinization had not been attempted.

The use of sodium bicarbonate in salicylate-poisoned patients is associated with certain side effects and has some contraindications. Adverse effects of alkalinization include the creation of severe alkalemia (arterial pH > 7.55) and electrolyte disturbances (e.g., hypocalcemia, hypokalemia, hypernatremia) that may lead to arrhythmia or seizure, and to a lesser extent, fluid overload and congestive heart failure. Theoretical contraindications to the use of sodium bicarbonate include the presence of cerebral or pulmonary edema, oliguric renal failure, and an arterial pH of more than 7.55.

The use of acetazolamide to alkalinize the urine is contraindicated, since it produces metabolic acidosis through renal elimination of bicarbonate, which may worsen salicylism and result in increased tissue penetration of salicylate. Tromethamine is not preferable to the use of bicarbonate when alkalinization is required.

Extracorporeal Techniques

Salicylates are readily removed by extracorporeal means due to a small Vd (approximately 0.2 L/kg) and low molecular weight. At supratherapeutic levels, extracorporeal removal of salicylate is further facilitated by increased concentrations of free drug in the plasma. A number of extracorporeal removal techniques (e.g., exchange transfusion, peritoneal dialysis, hemoperfusion, hemodiafiltration, and hemodialysis) have been utilized in severe poisoning to decrease morbidity and mortality. As compared with hemodialysis, hemoperfusion provides a greater clearance of salicylate from plasma. Hemodialysis, however, is the preferred technique due to its superior safety, familiarity, and ability to correct fluid, electrolyte, and acid-base disturbances (see Chapter 2C).[82] Hemodialysis can reduce the salicylate elimination half-life to 2 to 3 hours.[82] Continuous veno-

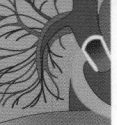

BOX 48-2 | **PROCEDURE FOR PERFORMING URINE ALKALINIZATION IN SALICYLATE POISONING[79]**

Baseline Biochemical Assessment

Measure plasma creatinine and electrolytes.
Measure plasma glucose.
Measure arterial acid-base status.

Clinical Preliminaries

Establish an intravenous line.
Insert a central venous line, if appropriate.
Insert a bladder catheter.
Correct any fluid deficit.
Correct hypokalemia, if indicated.
Measure urine pH using narrow-range indicator paper (use fresh urine because pH will change as carbon dioxide blows off on standing) or pH meter.

Achieving Alkalinization

In an adult, give sodium bicarbonate 225 mmol or mEq (225 mL of an 8.4% [1mEq/mL] solution) intravenously over 1 hour.
In a child, give sodium bicarbonate 25–50 mmol (25 mL of an 8.4% solution) intravenously over 1 hour.
The period of administration of the loading dose of sodium bicarbonate may be shortened and/or the dose increased if there is preexisting acidemia.
The goals of alkalinization are to achieve a blood pH of 7.50 and urine pH of 8.0.

Maintaining Urine Alkalinization

Give additional boluses of intravenous sodium bicarbonate to maintain urine pH in the range 7.5–8.5. This can be achieved by administering a continuous infusion of 100–150 mmol or mEq $NaHCO_3$ mixed in 1 L D5W at 150–200 mL/hr or two times maintenance IV requirements.

Monitor

Urine pH every 15–30 minutes.
Plasma potassium hourly.
Central venous pressure hourly.
Acid-base status hourly (note: arterial pH should not exceed 7.55).
Plasma salicylate concentrations hourly.
Urine output—should not exceed 200 mL/hr.

Discontinue Urine Alkalinization

When plasma salicylate concentrations fall below 30 mg/dL in an adult or 25 mg/dL in a child.

---

venous hemodiafiltration (CVVHDF) is an alternative extracorporeal technique to hemodialysis. CVVHDF may be a more tangible option for patients who are too unstable to undergo hemodialysis or for whom hemodialysis is not available. Although its efficacy is not as well established as for hemodialysis, CVVHDF has provided significant reductions in salicylate levels for poisoned patients.[83] Exchange transfusion has been used successfully for salicylate-poisoned infants, where hemodialysis is not technically feasible in this patient population.[84] Manikian and colleagues described the successful double-volume exchange transfusion in a 4-month-old (5-kg) male infant with severe salicylate poisoning.[85]

The decision to perform hemodialysis is usually made on clinical parameters rather than plasma salicylate concentrations. Clinical indications for hemodialysis include the presence of coma, seizures, cerebral or pulmonary edema, renal failure, refractory acid-base disturbances, or clinical worsening despite treatment. Little information exists on which to base this decision, and in each case an individual assessment is best. The sole reliance on the plasma salicylate concentration is not advised. Serious consideration for hemodialysis, however, should be given to acutely poisoned patients with salicylate concentrations of at least 100 mg/dL or chronic patients with salicylate concentrations of at least 60 mg/dL. Early consultation with a renal medicine specialist is prudent to avoid any possible bureaucratic delays in establishing dialysis. Once initiated, hemodialysis should be continued until clinical improvement, correction of major acid-base disturbances, or a return to nontoxic salicylate levels occurs. Since greater morbidity and mortality are associated with chronic salicylism, hemodialysis is recommended at lower salicylate levels as compared with acutely poisoned patients.

DISPOSITION

Disposition decisions for salicylate-poisoned patients necessitate an assessment of the actual and predicted severity of illness, the initial salicylate concentration, the trend of that concentration, and the patient's clinical

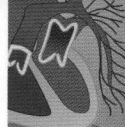

state. Symptomatic patients should be admitted to the hospital, regardless of the amount ingested or of the plasma concentration. Mildly poisoned patients may be managed safely on a regular medical floor or short-stay observation unit, if available. Moderately or severely poisoned patients should be admitted to an intensive care unit. Patients with normal and falling concentrations, who are asymptomatic, and have normal acid-base status, electrolytes, and renal function may be medically discharged, provided there are no psychiatric issues that need to be addressed.

REFERENCES

1. Roberts LJ II, Morrow JD: Analgesic-antipyretic and anti-inflammatory agents and drugs employed in the treatment of gout. In Hardman JG, Limbrid LE, Gilman AG (eds): Goodman & Gilman's The Pharmacological Basis of Therapeutics, 10th ed. New York, McGraw-Hill, 2001, pp 687–731.
2. Rowland M, Riegelman S, Harris PA, et al: Absorption kinetics of aspirin in man following oral administration of an aqueous solution. J Pharm Sci 1972;61:379–385.
3. Needs CJ, Brooks PM: Clinical pharmacokinetics of salicylates. Clin Pharmacokinet 1985;10:164–177.
4. Wortzman DJ, Grunfeld A: Delayed absorption following enteric-coated aspirin overdose. Ann Emerg Med 1987;16:434–436.
5. Brune K, Nuernberg A, Schneider HT: Biliary elimination of aspirin after oral and intravenous administration in patients. In Variability in Response to Anti-Rheumatic Drugs. Basel, Switzerland, Birkhauser Verlag, 1993, pp 51–57.
6. Davies MG, Briffa DV, Greaves MW: Systemic toxicity from topically applied salicylic acid. BMJ 1979;1:661.
7. Brubacher JR, Hoffman RS: Salicylism from topical salicylates: review of the literature. Clin Toxicol 1996;34:431–436.
8. Watson JE, Tagupa ET: Suicide attempt by means of aspirin enema. Ann Pharmacother 1994;28:467–468.
9. Levy G, Yaffe SJ: Relationship between dose and apparent volume of distribution of salicylate in children. Pediatrics 1974;54:713–717.
10. Kwong TC: Salicylate measurement: clinical usefulness and methodology. CRC Crit Rev Clin Lab Sci 1987;25:137–159.
11. Rowland M, Riegelman S: Pharmacokinetics of acetylsalicylic acid and salicylic acid after intravenous administration in man. J Pharm Sci 1968;57:717–720.
12. Levy G, Tsuchiya T: Salicylate accumulation kinetics in man. N Engl J Med 1972;287:430–432.
13. Levy G, Tsuchiya T, Amsel LP: Limited capacity for salicyl phenolic glucuronide formation and its effect on the kinetics of salicylate elimination in man. Clin Pharmacol Ther 1972;13:258–268.
14. Dugandzic RM, Tierney MG, Dickinson GE, et al: Evaluation of the validity of the Done nomogram in the management of acute salicylate intoxication. Ann Emerg Med 1989;18:1186–1190.
15. Done AK: Salicylate intoxication—significance of measurements of salicylate in blood in cases of acute ingestion. Pediatrics 1960;26:800–807.
16. Gabow PA, Anderson RJ, Potts DE, Schrier RW: Acid-base disturbances in the salicylate-intoxicated adult. Arch Intern Med 1978;138:1481–1484.
17. Winters RW, White JS, Hughes MC, Ordway NC: Disturbances of acid-base equilibrium in salicylate intoxication. Pediatrics 1959;23:260–285.
18. Temple AR: Acute and chronic effects of aspirin toxicity and their treatment. Arch Intern Med 1981;141:364–369.
19. Chapman BC, Proudfoot AT: Adult salicylate poisoning: deaths and outcome in patients with high plasma salicylate concentrations. QJM 1989;72:699–707.
20. Tenney SM, Miller RM: The respiratory and circulatory actions of salicylate. Am J Med 1965;19:498–508.
21. Cameron IR, Semple SJR: The central respiratory stimulation action of salicylates. Clin Sci 1968;35:391–401.
22. McQueen DS, Ritchie IM, Birrell GJ: Arterial chemoreceptor involvement in salicylate-induced hyperventilation in rats. Br J Pharmacol 1989;98:413–424.
23. Kaplan EH, Kennedy J, Davis J: Effects of salicylate and other benzoates on oxidative enzymes of the tricarboxylic acid cycle in rat tissue homogenates. Arch Biochem Biophys 1954;51:47–61.
24. Miyahara JT, Karler R: Effect of salicylate on oxidative phosphorylation and respiration of mitochondrial fragment. Biochem J 1965;97:194–198.
25. Bartels PD, Lund-Jacobsen H: Blood lactate and ketone body concentrations in salicylate intoxication. Hum Toxicol 1986;5:363–366.
26. Schwartz R, Landy G, Taller D: Organic acid excretion in salicylate intoxication. J Pediatr 1965;66:658–666.
27. Hill JB: Salicylate intoxication. N Engl J Med 1973;288:1110–1113.
28. Done AK: Treatment of salicylate poisoning: Review of personal and published experiences. Clin Toxicol 1968;1:451–467.
29. Temple AR: Pathophysiology of aspirin overdosage toxicity, with implications for management. Pediatrics 1978;62:873–876.
30. Robin ED, Davis RP, Rees SB: Salicylate intoxication with special reference to the development of hypokalemia. Am J Med 1959;26:869–882.
31. Lawson AAH, Proudfoot AT, Brown SS, et al: Forced diuresis in the treatment of acute salicylate poisoning in adults. QJM 1969;38:31–48.
32. Fox GN: Hypocalcemia complicating bicarbonate therapy for salicylate poisoning. West J Med 1984;141:108–109.
33. Reid IR: Transient hypercalcemia following overdoses of soluble aspirin tablets. Aust N Z J Med 1985;15:364.
34. Temple AR, George DJ, Done AK, Thompson JA: Salicylate poisoning complicated by fluid retention. Clin Toxicol 1976;9:61–68.
35. Anderson RJ, Potts DE, Gabow PA, et al: Unrecognized adult salicylate intoxication. Ann Intern Med 1976;85:745–748.
36. Zitnik RJ, Cooper JA: Pulmonary disease due to antirheumatic agents. Clin Chest Med 1990;11:139–150.
37. Walters JS, Woodring JH, Stelling CB, Rosenbaum HD: Salicylate-induced pulmonary edema. Radiology 1983;146:289–293.
38. Fisher CJ, Albertson TE, Foulke GE: Salicylate-induced pulmonary edema. Clinical characteristics in children. Am J Emerg Med 1985;3:33–37.
39. Gaudreault P, Temple AR, Lovejoy FH: The relative severity of acute versus chronic salicylate poisoning in children: a clinical comparison. Pediatrics 1982;70:566–569.
40. Hill JB: Experimental salicylate poisoning: observations on the effects of altering blood pH on tissue and plasma salicylate concentrations. Pediatrics 1971;47:658–665.
41. Farrand RJ, Green JH, Haworth C: Enteric-coated aspirin overdose and gastric perforation. BMJ 1975;4:85–86.
42. Robertson RP: Eicosanoids as pluripotential modulators of pancreatic islet function. Diabetes 1988;37:367–370.
43. Smith MJH: The metabolic bases of the major symptoms in acute salicylate intoxication. Clin Toxicol 1968;1:387–407.
44. Rich RR, Johnson JS: Salicylate hepatotoxicity in patients with juvenile rheumatoid arthritis. Arthritis Rheum 1973;16:1–9.
45. Wolfe JD, Metzger AL, Goldstein RC: Aspirin hepatitis. Ann Intern Med 1974;80:74–76.
46. Kimberly RP, Plotz PH: Aspirin-induced depression of renal function. N Engl J Med 1977;296:418–424.
47. Rupp DJ, Seaton RD, Weigmann TB: Acute polyuric renal failure after aspirin intoxication. Arch Intern Med 1983;143:1237–1238.
48. Mongan E, Kelly P, Nils K, et al: Tinnitus as an indication of therapeutic serum salicylate levels. JAMA 1973;226:142–145.
49. Ramsden RT, Latif A, O'Malley S: Electrocochleographic changes in acute salicylate overdosage. J Laryngol Otol 1985;99:1269–1273.
50. Ralston ME, Pearigen PD, Ponaman ML, Erickson LC: Transient myocardial dysfunction in a child with salicylate toxicity. J Emerg Med 1995;5:657–659.
51. Rejent TA, Baik S: Fatal in utero salicylism. J Forensic Sci 1985;30:942–944.
52. Palatnick W, Tenenbein M: Aspirin poisoning during pregnancy: increased fetal sensitivity. Am J Perinatol 1998;15:39–41.
53. Levy G, Garrettson LK: Kinetics of salicylate elimination by newborn infants of mothers who ingested aspirin before delivery. Pediatrics 1974;53:201–210.
54. Levy G, Procknal JA, Garrettson LK: Distribution of salicylate between neonatal and maternal serum at diffusion equilibrium. Clin Pharmacol Ther 1975;18:210–214.

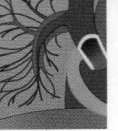

55. Montgomery H, Porter JC, Bradley RD: Salicylate intoxication causing a severe systemic inflammatory response and rhabdomyolysis. Am J Emerg Med 1994;12:531–532.

56. Vadas P, Schouten BD, Stefanski E, et al: Association of hyperphospholipasemia A2 with multiple system organ dysfunction due to salicylate intoxication. Crit Care Med 1993;21:1087–1091.

57. Botma M, Colquhoun-Flannery W, Leighton S: Laryngeal oedema caused by accidental ingestion of oil of wintergreen. Int J Pediatr Otorhinolaryngol 2001;58:229–232.

58. Hurlbut KM, Fish S, Kulig K, et al: Micromedex Healthcare Series Vol. 118. Expires December 2003. Englewood, CO.

59. Kwong TC: Salicylate measurement: clinical usefulness and methodology. CRC Crit Rev Clin Lab Sci 1987;25:137–159.

60. Yip L, Dart RC, Gabow PA: Concepts and controversies in salicylate toxicity. Emerg Med Clin North Am 1994;12:351–364.

61. Linden CH, Rumack GH: The legitimate analgesics: aspirin and acetaminophen. In: Hanson W Jr (ed): Toxic Emergencies. New York, Churchill Livingstone, 1984, p 118.

62. Krenzelok EP, Guharoy SL, Johnson DR: Toxicology screening in the emergency department: ethanol, barbiturates and salicylates. Am J Emerg Med 1984;2:331–332.

63. Greenberg MI, Hendrickson RG: Deleterious effects of endotracheal intubation in salicylate poisoning [Letter]. Ann Emerg Med 2003;41:583–584.

64. Krenzelok EP, McGuigan M, Lheureux P: AACT/EAPCCT position statement: ipecac syrup. J Toxicol Clin Toxicol 1997; 35:699–709.

65. Vale JA: AACT/EAPCCT position statement: gastric lavage. J Toxicol Clin Toxicol 1997;35:711–719.

66. Juurlink DN, McGuigan MA: Gastrointestinal decontamination for enteric-coated aspirin overdose: what to do depends on who you ask. Clin Toxicol 2000;38:465–470.

67. Prescott LF: Clinical features and management of analgesic poisoning. Hum Toxicol 1984;3(Suppl):75–84.

68. Chyka PA, Seger D: AACT/EAPCCT position statement: activated charcoal. J Toxicol Clin Toxicol 1997;35:721–741.

69. Filippone GA, Fish SS, Lacoutre PG, et al: Reversible adsorption (desorption) of aspirin from activated charcoal. Arch Intern Med 1987;147:1390–1392.

70. Dargan PI, Wallace CI, Jones AL: An evidence based flowchart to guide the management of acute salicylate (aspirin) overdose. Emerg Med J 2002;19:206–209.

71. Kirshenbaum LA, Mathews SC, Sitar DS: Whole-bowel irrigation versus activated charcoal in sorbitol for the ingestion of modified-release pharmaceuticals. Clin Pharmacol Ther 1989;46:264–271.

72. Tenenbein M. AACT/EAPCCT position statement: whole bowel irrigation. J Toxicol Clin Toxicol 1997;35:753–762.

73. Kirshenbaum LA, Mathews SC, Sitar DS, Tenenbein M: Does multi-dose charcoal therapy enhance salicylate excretion? Arch Intern Med 1990;150:1281–1283.

74. Johnson D, Eppler J, Giesbrecht E, et al: Effect of multi-dose activated charcoal on the clearance of high-dose intravenous aspirin in a porcine model. Ann Emerg Med 1995;26:569–574.

75. Hillman RJ, Prescott LF: Treatment of salicylate poisoning with repeat oral charcoal. BMJ 1985;291:1472.

76. Vale JA, Krenzelok EP, Barceloux DG: AACT/EAPCCT position statement and practice guidelines on the use of multi-dose activated charcoal in the treatment of acute poisoning. J Toxicol Clin Toxicol 1999;37:731–751.

77. Smith PK, Gleason HL, Stoll CG, et al: Studies on the pharmacology of salicylates. J Pharmacol Exp Ther 1946;87:253.

78. Prescott LF, Balali-Mood M, Critchley JAJH, et al: Diuresis or urinary alkalinisation for salicylate poisoning? BMJ 1982;285: 1383–1386.

79. Proudfoot AT, Krenzelok EP, Vale JA: Position paper on urine alkalization. J Toxicol Clin Toxicol 2004;42:1–26.

80. Vree TB, Van Ewijk-Beneken Kolmer EWJ, Verwey-Van Wissen CPWGM, Hekster YA: Effect of urinary pH on the pharmacokinetics of salicylic acid, with its glycine and glucuronide conjugates in human. Int J Clin Pharmacol Ther 1994;32:550–558.

81. Higgins RM, Connolly JO, Hendry BM: Alkalinization and hemodialysis in severe salicylate poisoning: comparison of elimination techniques in the same patient. Clin Nephrol 1998;50:178–183.

82. Jacobsen D, Wiik-Larsen E, Bredesen JE: Haemodialysis or haemoperfusion in severe salicylate poisoning? Hum Toxicol 1988;7:161–163.

83. Wrathall G, Sinclair R, Moore A, Pogson D: Three case reports of the use of haemodiafiltration in the treatment of salicylate overdose. Hum Exp Toxicol 2001;20:491–495.

84. Leikin SL, Emmanouilides GC: The use of exchange transfusion in salicylate intoxication. J Pediatr 1960;57:715–720.

85. Manikian A, Stone S, Hamilton R, et al: Exchange transfusion in severe infant salicylism. Vet Hum Toxicol 2002;40:224–227.

49 *The Triptans*

ANTHONY J. TOMASSONI, MD, MS ■ CARL A. GERMANN, MD

At a Glance...

■ Triptans have improved safety and side effect profiles in the treatment of migraine relative to older ergot derivatives.

■ Triptans activate the 5-HT_{1B} and 5-HT_{1D} receptors within the trigeminovascular system, including serotonin receptors on cerebral vessels and, to a lesser extent, on coronary arteries.

■ Triptans are contraindicated in patients with ischemic heart disease because of concerns about vasospasm of coronary vessels that could lead to myocardial ischemia.

■ If a patient taking triptans experiences chest pain that may be ischemic in origin, further triptan use should be avoided and appropriate evaluation initiated.

■ Second-generation triptans have improved pharmacokinetics and may reduce the likelihood of chest pain in migraineurs; however, differences between these medications and first-generation triptans are subtle.

■ Risk for precipitating serotonin syndrome may be increased by combining triptan therapy with other serotonergic medications.

The development of the triptans nicely illustrates the process of stepwise drug design. The medicinal properties of serotonin agonists have been recognized for hundreds of years.[1] Long ago, midwives used the vasoconstrictive effects of ergot to accelerate labor or reduce postpartum bleeding. Liquid extracts of ergot have also been used to treat "vascular headaches" in Europe and the United States for more than 100 years. However, the use of early ergot-derived medications frequently resulted in undesirable effects, including severe peripheral vasoconstriction, emesis, paresthesias, and psychosis.

Human experience with related compounds has been well documented since the outbreaks of ergotism in the Middle Ages, then known as St. Anthony's fire. When contaminated rye enters the food supply, generally in the form of bread, epidemic ergotism may result. Vivid descriptions of individuals afflicted with gangrene of the extremities, burning neuropathic pain, and autoamputation survive to document this form of ergotism. An even more dramatic form of ergotism may result in psychosis, seizures, and death. It has been hypothesized that those accused of witchcraft in Salem, Massachusetts, in the late 1600s were stricken with this second form of ergotism. Ironically, it was in that same century that the cause of St. Anthony's fire was traced to ergot (*Claviceps purpurea*), a fungus that grows on the kernels of rye during damp, cold weather.[2]

Before the availability of the triptans, ergotamines were used extensively for relieving migraine pain. Ergotamine was first isolated by Arthur Stoll of Sandoz (Novartis) in 1918. The drug was then found effective in the treatment of migraine headache in the 1930s. Further research at Sandoz resulted in the synthesis of ergonovine, lysergic acid diethylamide, and other serotonin agonist and antagonist drugs.[2,3] Armed with improved understanding of the potential role of serotonin in migraine headache developed during the 1970s, efforts to synthesize a safer, more selective, serotonin agonist were undertaken. This resulted in the introduction of sumatriptan in the early 1990s. Subsequent second-generation triptans seek to improve on the properties of sumatriptan by offering more rapid relief, longer duration of action, improved bioavailability and availability to the central nervous system (CNS), and reduced side effects. Since sumatriptan became available in 1992, six additional triptans have been introduced in the United States (Table 49-1).

Several theories and models have been advanced to explain the pathophysiology of migraine headache, but no unified model explains all the symptoms of a migraine headache. It seems possible that more than one mechanism may be responsible, and this may explain interindividual variations in response to migraine medications. Reductions in serotonin levels have been noted during migraine headaches. Of note, the triptans are structurally similar to serotonin (5-hydroxytryptamine [5-HT]) (Fig. 49-1)

The number of migraineurs in the United States has been estimated as approximately 23 million.[4] GlaxoSmithKline reports that their sumatriptan products have been used to treat more than 646 million migraines over the past decade, approximately equal to treating one migraine headache every second.[5] Of note, there are many similarities, but also significant differences between these selective serotonin agonists. Therefore, patients may be advised that if one of these drugs does not offer sufficient relief from their migraine pain, it is often worthwhile to try another drug from this class with different pharmacologic or pharmacokinetic characteristics. However, the overall efficacy rate for all orally administered triptans is approximately 65%.[6] Little has been reported regarding substantial overdose of these medications; however, adverse effects associated with therapeutic use of the triptans are well described.

STRUCTURE

Sumatriptan is 3-[2-(dimethylamino) ethyl]-*N*-methyl-1H-indole-5-methanesulfonamide. Structures of serotonin and the triptans available in the United States may be compared in Figure 49-1. When compared with sumatriptan, the second-generation agents are characterized by enhanced lipophilicity and greater 5-HT_1 receptor selectivity. These chemical properties are associated with pharmacokinetic and pharmacodynamic improvements such as improved oral bioavailability,

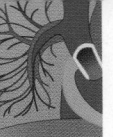

TABLE 49-1 Some Available Triptans and Dates of Approval by the U.S. Food and Drug Administration (FDA)

GENERIC NAME	TRADE NAME	FORMULATION	DATE OF FDA APPROVAL
Sumatriptan	Imitrex Imigran	Injections	December 28, 1992
Sumatriptan	Imitrex Imigran	Tablets	June 1, 1995
Sumatriptan	Imitrex Imigran	Nasal spray	August 26, 1997
Zolmitriptan	Zomig	Tablets	November 25, 1997
Naratriptan	Amerge Naramig	Tablets	February 10, 1998
Rizatriptan	Maxalt Maxalt-MLT	Tablets Orally dissolvable tablets	June 29, 1998
Zolmitriptan	Zomig-ZMT	Orally dissolvable tablets	February 13, 2001
Almotriptan	Axert	Tablets	May 17, 2001
Frovatriptan	Frova	Tablets	November 8, 2001
Eletriptan	Relpax	Tablets	December 26, 2002
Zolmitriptan	Zomig	Nasal spray	September 30, 2003

Some triptans were available in Europe before FDA approval in the United States.[57]
From http://www.fda.gov, Drug Approvals.

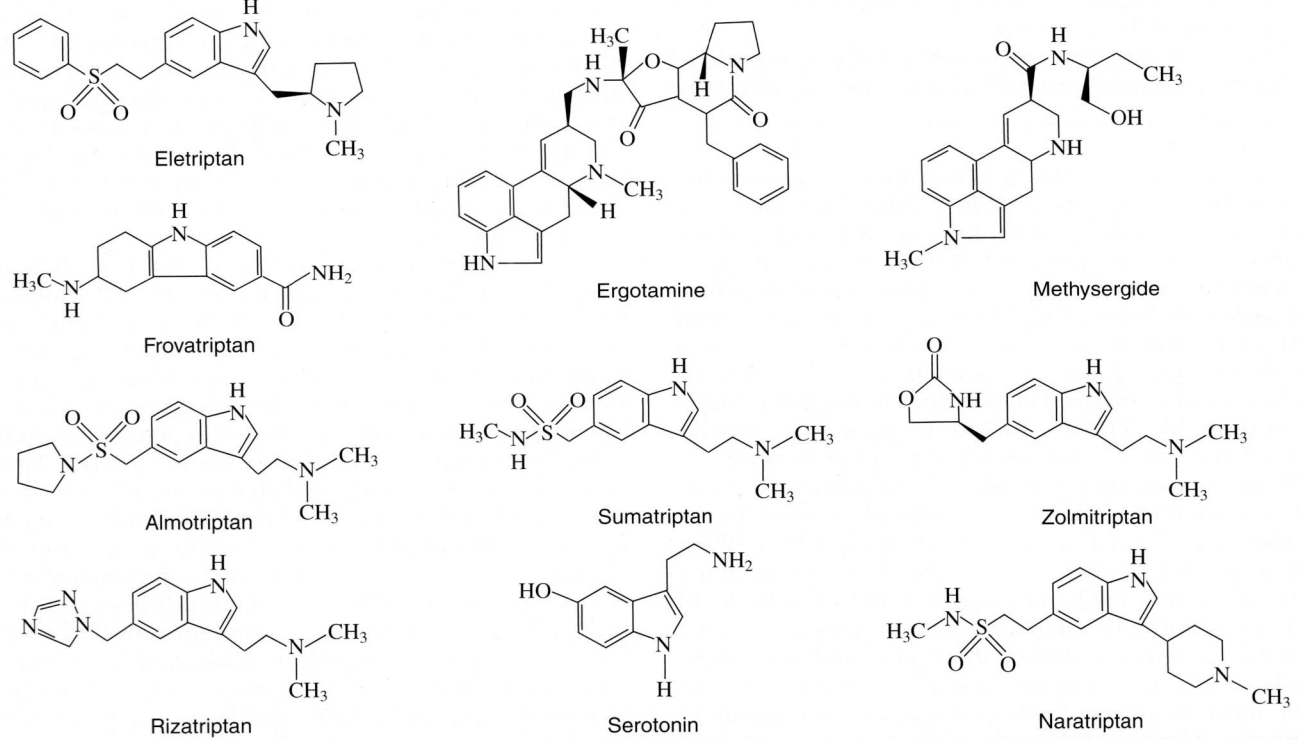

FIGURE 49-1 Comparative structures of serotonin and selected antimigraine drugs. [Modified from Hart C: Forged in St. Anthony's fire: drugs for migraine. Mod Drug Discovery 1999;2(2):20–21, 23–24, 28, 31.]

rapid absorption to achieve maximum plasma levels faster (shorter time to maximum concentration [T_{max}]), longer elimination half-lives ($t_{1/2}$), better CNS penetration, and/or reduced cardiac effects. Improved central penetration and increased receptor affinity and selectivity for the 5-HT$_{1D}$ (neuronal) receptor permit lower total oral dosing and reduced peripheral exposure to the coronary vasoconstrictor 5-HT$_{1B}$ (vascular)

receptor, reducing the incidence and severity of chest pain that occurs with sumatriptan. Frovatriptan has a high affinity for the 5-HT$_{1B}$ receptor when compared with other second-generation triptan agonists.[7,8]

The chemical structure of frovatriptan conforms to structure-activity relationships established for 5-HT$_1$ receptor agonists. These include a nuclear indole heterocycle and a 3-alkylamine structure (incorporated into an

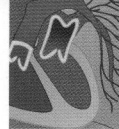

indole-fused cyclohexylamine moiety in frovatriptan). The 3-alkylamine function facilitates formulation of the triptans as water-soluble salts of acids. Of note, the 3-alkylamine feature serves as a substrate for MAO-A catabolism, except in the case of naratriptan.[7] New agents that target the 5-HT$_{1F}$ receptor are under investigation. Such agents may lack the vascular contractile effects of the current triptans that target 5-HT$_{1B/1D}$ receptors.[9]

PHARMACOLOGY

At least seven classes of 5-HT receptors with different biologic effects have been identified. These classes are noted as 5-HT$_1$ through 5-HT$_7$. Except for the 5-HT$_3$ receptor, which is linked to an ion channel, all are G protein linked. The 5-HT$_1$ receptor class differs from the others in that it is inhibitory via adenylate cyclase, while the other receptor classes are excitatory. In general, 5-HT$_1$ receptors are the site of action of the migraine-abortive triptans and dihydroergotamine, which function as agonists at this receptor. In contrast, some migraine-preventative treatments such as amitriptyline and methysergide have 5-HT$_2$ antagonist activity. 5-HT$_2$ receptors are excitatory via phosphatidyl hydrolysis. 5-HT$_3$ antagonists have antiemetic activity.[3]

All triptans activate the 5-HT$_{1B}$ and 5-HT$_{1D}$ receptors and, to a lesser extent, the 5-HT$_{1A}$ and 5-HT$_{1F}$ receptors.[10] Inhibition of vasodilation of meningeal vessels occurs via the 5-HT$_{1B}$ receptor. Triptans are believed to relieve migraine, in part, by stimulating 5-HT$_{1B}$ receptors on meningeal, dural, cerebral, or pial vessels to cause vasoconstriction, which counteracts the pain-inducing vasodilation involved in migraine. Inhibition of trigeminal nuclei cell excitability in the brainstem occurs via 5-HT$_{(1B/1D)}$ receptor agonism; direct inhibition of these receptors is reported to have an antimigraine effect. Additionally, stimulation of presynaptic 5-HT$_{1D}$ receptors inhibits both dural vasodilation and inflammation.[7,8] Triptans have low or no affinity for α- or β-adrenergic, cholinergic, or dopaminergic receptors.[11,12] Anatomic studies using antibodies selective for human 5-HT$_{1B}$ or 5-HT$_{1D}$ receptors found that 5-HT$_{1B}$ receptors are located primarily in the cranial circulation but are also found in the coronary circulation.[13,14] While triptans constrict meningeal arteries more potently than they constrict coronary arteries, there have been concerns regarding potential myocardial ischemia secondary to induced coronary vasoconstriction. A summary of affinities of the triptans for receptor types is provided in Table 49-2.

Of interest, data have demonstrated potent antiinflammatory effects in bacterial meningitis with administration of triptans to rats. Leukocyte influx into the cerebrospinal fluid was reduced, as was intracranial pressure and the formation of brain edema. Survival and clinical score were increased. That these findings may eventually be applicable to humans is suggested by clinically observed activation of the trigeminovascular system.[15]

PHARMACOKINETICS

Since this class of compounds was developed for affinity at specific receptors, there are only minor pharmacodynamic differences between the triptans. Despite significant pharmacokinetic improvements in the newer members of this class, only modest improvements have resulted in their ability to treat migraine. Pharmacokinetic relationships between the triptans are displayed in Table 49-3. Sumatriptan has low oral bioavailability (14%) due to first pass metabolism and incomplete absorption and, relative to newer triptans, a short elimination half-life of approximately 2 hours when administered subcutaneously or intranasally (approximately 2.5 hours when administered orally). Protein binding is approximately 14% to 21%; therefore, the effect of sumatriptan on the protein binding of other

TABLE 49-2 Affinities of Some Ergopeptides and Triptans for Serotonin Receptor Types

DRUG	RECEPTOR TYPE						
	5-HT$_{1A}$	5-HT$_{1B}$	5-HT$_{1D}$	5-HT$_{1E}$	5-HT$_{1F}$	5-HT$_{2A}$	5-HT$_{2B}$
Ergotamine*	+	+	+		+	+	+
Dihydroergotamine	+++	++	+++	++	+	+	+
Sumatriptan	+	++	++	−	+		
Zolmetriptan		+	+		+		
Naratriptan	+	+	+	+	+		
Rizatriptan		+	+				
Eletriptan		++	++	+	++		
Almotriptan	+	++	++				
Frovatriptan	+				+		

Of note, ergotamines also have activity at noradrenergic α and β receptors and on dopamine D$_1$ and D$_2$ receptors.
*The published data for the ergopeptides relate mainly to dihydroergotamine, but the literature infers that the situation for ergotamine is generally similar.
+, degree of agonist activity at the receptor from low (+) to high (+++); −, inactive.
Adapted from references 3 and 58.

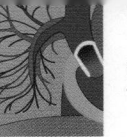

TABLE 49-3 Comparative Pharmacokinetics of Some Triptans

DRUG, FORMULATION, AND DOSE	T_{MAX} (hr) OUTSIDE ATTACK	T_{MAX} (hr) DURING ATTACK	LIPOPHILICITY	$t_{1/2}$ (hr)	BIOAVAILIBILITY (%)	ELIMINATION ROUTE, METABOLISM	PROTEIN BINDING (%)	Vd (L/kg)
Sumatriptan			Low			Hepatic; MAO-A; 60% renal	14–21	2.4
50 mg PO	2.5			2–2.5	14			
20 mg IN	1			2	17			
6 mg SQ	0.2–0.25			2	96–97			
Zolmitriptan			Moderate			Hepatic (1 active and 2 inactive metabolites; CYP1A2; MAO-A)	25	7
2.5 mg PO	2	2.5		2.5–3	40–48			
2.5 mg ZMT	3.3			2.5–3	40–48			
2.5 mg IN	2			2.82	42			
Rizatriptan			Moderate		45–47	Hepatic; MAO-A; 30% renally unchanged	14	110–140
PO tab	1–1.2	1		2–3				
PO melt	1.6–2.5							
Naratriptan			High		63 (m)–74 (f)	50%–70% excreted renally unchanged; CYP	28–31	170
2.5 mg PO	1.5–3	3.5		5.0–6.3				
1 mg SQ	0.2	0.2		5				
Almotriptan	1.4–3.8		Unknown	3.2–3.7	70–80	Hepatic; CYP3A4, 2D6; MAO-A; 15% active metabolite 26%–35% excreted renally unchanged		
Eletriptan	1.0–2.0	2.8	High	3.6–5.5	50	Hepatic CYP3A4, 1A2; 15% active metabolite		
Frovatriptan	2.0–4.0		Low	25	24 (m)–30 (f)	Hepatic; CYP1A2; MAO-A; 26%–35% excreted renally unchanged		

CYP, cytochrome P-450 system; (f), female; IN, intranasal spray; (m), male; MOA, monoamine oxidase; PO, oral; SQ, subcutaneous injection; tab, tablet; $t_{1/2}$, half-life; T_{max}, time to peak plasma concentration.
Adapted from references 58 through 62.

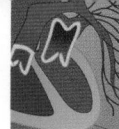

drugs may be minor. The mean volume of distribution of sumatriptan after subcutaneous administration is 2.7 L/kg, and its total plasma clearance is approximately 1200 mL/min. Newer triptans have improved oral bioavailability. The absorption rate of rizatriptan is comparatively fastest when measured by the time to peak plasma concentration, and rizatriptan has been reported to result in more rapid relief of cephalalgia when compared with sumatriptan and zolmitriptan. Eletriptan and naratriptan have somewhat longer half-lives than sumatriptan, while frovatriptan has the longest half-life (up to 25 hours) of the triptans approved in the United States. Plasma levels of frovatriptan may be higher in elderly patients and in females.[8,16]

SPECIAL POPULATIONS

All triptans are 5-HT_{1B} agonists and thus are contraindicated in patients with ischemic heart disease, uncontrolled hypertension, and cerebrovascular disease. Prudence dictates that patients should also be screened for conditions leading to accelerated atherosclerosis and coronary artery spasm. Related conditions may include family history of coronary artery disease or heart attacks, risk factors for coronary artery disease, long-standing or uncontrolled diabetes, hypercholesterolemia and hyperlipidemia, smoking, and physiologic or surgical menopause.

Clinical trials in the pediatric population have yielded positive results that triptans decrease symptoms of migraine, but often in the context of high placebo response rates. Although dosing for sumatriptan in younger patients has been reported, the manufacturer indicates that the use of sumatriptan injection, tablets, and nasal spray in those younger than 18 years is not recommended.[16] In fact, a myocardial infarction has been reported in a 14-year-old boy following the use of oral sumatriptan with clinical signs occurring within 1 day of drug administration.[16] While studies have demonstrated that adolescents may find triptans efficacious and tolerable, clinical data regarding the frequency of events in the pediatric population is still lacking.[17-19]

Since elderly patients may have decreased hepatic or renal function, since they may be more sensitive to drug-induced increases in blood pressure, and since they may be at higher risk for coronary artery disease, the use of triptans in the elderly is not advisable.

Triptans are category C drugs and should not be recommended for use by pregnant women. Review of data available from clinical trials, postmarketing monitoring, and the Sumatriptan Pregnancy Registry suggest no currently measurable increased risk for birth defects after prenatal exposure to sumatriptan. Sample sizes remain too small to draw definitive conclusions. Although use of triptans during pregnancy cannot be encouraged, data are reassuring where inadvertent exposure to sumatriptan has occurred during pregnancy.[20,21]

DRUG INTERACTIONS

Triptans and ergotamines both stimulate serotonergic receptors; therefore, their combined use is not recommended. Monoamine oxidase (MAO) inhibitors, especially MAO-A inhibitors, can slow the metabolism of triptans and are thus contraindicated when using these medications. Also, the vasoconstrictive effects of the triptans may be additive to those of catecholamines. There have also been numerous case reports of suspected serotonin syndrome when MAO inhibitors and triptans are used concurrently.[22-24] Given the fact that little reliable information exists regarding the combination of these two medicines, use of triptans should continue to be avoided in patients taking MAO inhibitors until further data demonstrating safety become available.

It is plausible that the combination of triptans and selective serotonin reuptake inhibitors may precipitate serotonin syndrome. Although serotonin syndrome has been reported with combinations of psychotropic medications, neurologists have considered the potential of triptans combined with selective serotonin reuptake inhibitors (SSRIs) to produce this syndrome as well. In general, clinical experiences and published reports indicate a low risk for serotonin syndrome with the combined use of an SSRI and a triptan.[23] However, considering the large volumes of SSRIs and other serotonergic drugs in use, the paucity of data regarding serotonin syndrome as a consequence of drug interactions with triptans suggests that further study is indicated to ascertain the relative risk of precipitating serotonin syndrome through drug interactions. Some documented and potential (but less likely) drug-drug interactions with triptans are listed in Table 49-4 and Box 49-1.

TOXICOLOGY

Triptans differ from each other in terms of tolerability but not in terms of safety.[10] Animal overdose of sumatriptan has resulted in seizures, tremor, paralysis, behavioral changes, ptosis, erythema of the extremities, abnormal respiration, cyanosis, ataxia, mydriasis, salivation, lacrimation, and death.[16] Clinical manifestations of triptans have been largely compiled from clinical experience, case reports, and systematic retrospective and prospective research. Therefore, the information that follows is derived primarily from observations of patients using an appropriate therapeutic dose.

The most frequent side effects, often called "triptan sensations," are taste disturbances, tingling, paresthesias, and sensations of warmth in the head, neck, chest, and limbs.[10] Other symptoms may include drowsiness, dizziness, flushing, and neck pain or tightness.

The most serious adverse consequences of triptan use involve the cardiovascular system. These insults are presumably due to coronary and cerebral vessels narrowing secondary to 5-HT_{1B} receptor activation. All triptans narrow coronary arteries by about 10% to 20% at

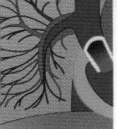

TABLE 49-4 Some Potential Drug Interactions with Triptans

INTERACTION TYPE	AGENT AND MECHANISM	EFFECT
Pharmacokinetic		
	Macrolide antibiotics: inhibition of CYP3A4	Increased almotriptan or eletriptan level
	Monoamine oxidase A inhibitor	Increased 5-HT$_1$ agonism by sumatriptan, zolmitriptan, or rizatriptan
	Propranolol: inhibition of CYP1A2	Increased zolmitriptan level
	Dihydroergotamine	15% reduction in area under the curve for naratriptan
	Acetaminophen	Sumatriptan delays acetaminophen absorption
Pharmacodynamic		
	Ergopeptide	Vasospasm; postpartum cerebral angiopathy
	Methysergide	Myocardial infarction reported with sumatriptan
	Serotonin reuptake inhibitors	Increased serotonin concentration loading to serotonin syndrome (uncommon)
	Loxapine	Dystonia and movement disorder

The magnitude of these effects may be variable ranging from theoretical only or clinically insignificant to potentially life threatening.
Compiled from Eadie MJ: Clinically significant drug interactions with agents specific for migraine attacks. CNS Drugs 2001;15(2):105–118.

BOX 49-1 POTENTIAL INTERACTIONS WITH THE TRIPTANS THAT ARE UNLIKELY TO OCCUR IN PRACTICE*

With Sumatriptan

Butorphanol nasal
Flunarazine
Propranolol
Naproxen
Naratriptan
Pizotifen

With Naratriptan

Ergotamine

With Zolmitriptan

Ergotamine
Pizotifen
Dihydroergotamine
Acetaminophen
Metoclopramide
Fluoxetine
Selegiline

*Given the relative newness of the triptans it is likely that additional drug-drug interactions may come to light.
From Eadie MJ: Clinically significant drug interactions with agents specific for migraine attacks. CNS Drugs 2001;15(2):105–118.

---

conventional doses.[25-27] Numerous studies have established the coronary vasoconstrictive effects of triptans.[25,27-29] This constriction of coronary arteries may cause chest symptoms that closely mimic angina pectoris.[10] However, the chest pain reported by 3% to 5% of patients taking oral triptans has generally not been associated with electrocardiographic changes and is unlikely to be due to cardiac ischemia.[30-32] In fact, in vitro data have shown that at therapeutic concentrations, triptans have little potential to cause clinically significant constriction of nondiseased coronary arteries.[11] Large retrospective studies show no increase in risk for myocardial infarction with triptan use in a general population of migraine sufferers.[33,34] Noncardiac explanations for chest pain associated with the use of triptans include pulmonary vasoconstriction, esophageal spasm, muscle spasm, and anxiety.[30,35,36]

In June 2002, the American Headache Society convened the Triptan Cardiovascular Safety Expert Panel to evaluate the evidence on triptan-associated cardio-

vascular risk and to formulate a consensus regarding the safety of triptans.[37] This consensus stated that chest symptoms occurring during the use of triptans are usually nonserious and usually not attributed to ischemia.[37] Also, while serious cardiovascular adverse events have occurred after the use of triptans, their incidence in both clinical trials and clinical practice appears to be extremely low.[37] Most of these data, however, are derived from clinical trials that typically excluded patients with cardiovascular risk factors or known ischemic heart disease. Therefore, the panel concluded that the cardiovascular risk-benefit profile of triptans favors their use in the absence of contraindications and that in patients at low risk for coronary artery disease, triptans can be safely prescribed without the need for prior cardiac status evaluation.[37]

Triptan effects on diseased coronary arteries have not been well studied. It is plausible that even a small amount of induced vasoconstriction in patients with obstructive coronary artery disease may potentiate myocardial ischemia. Indeed, in rare instances triptan therapy has been associated with severe cardiovascular events.[10,38-42] There have also been published reports of atrial fibrillation, ventricular tachycardia, and ventricular fibrillation following doses of sumatriptan.[40,43-47] A majority of these episodes were reported to occur within 35 minutes of triptan administration. The evidence of increased risk for myocardial ischemia and infarction is largely based on the known pathophysiology of triptans and isolated case reports rather than epidemiologic data.[30]

There is a paucity of data to support a correlative risk of ischemic stroke with triptan use.[33,34,48] A study performed by Hall and colleagues showed no association between triptan prescription and stroke risk in 13,664 patients.[48] In another study of 12,339 patients who used injectable sumatriptan, there was an incidence of 1.08 strokes per 100,000 treated migraine episodes, which correlates with the natural occurrence of migraine and stroke.[34] It is also conceivable that some reports of stroke associated with triptans may have resulted from misiden-

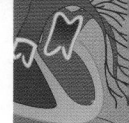

tification of the primary cause of headache (i.e., some patients complaining of headache who received triptans may have had a primary stroke that was only definitively diagnosed after triptan administration).

Triptan-induced vasoconstriction has also been thought to induce ischemic colitis. There have been at least 11 reported cases associating triptan use with ischemic colitis.[49-51] However, no association was found in a large-scale prospective trial of the safety of subcutaneous sumatriptan.[34] Further studies are needed to explore this relationship because there is insufficient evidence thus far associating triptans and ischemic bowel disease.

Serotonin syndrome may result from the combined use of triptans with SSRIs. A handful of case reports describe such events.[22-24] However, in one large prospective study combining SSRIs with triptans, there were no significant adverse neurologic events within 24 hours.[52] Serotonin syndrome consists of a triad of altered mental status, dysautonomia, and neuromuscular changes.

There have been only a handful of case reports describing triptan overdose. Most of these articles report a paucity of adverse events with overuse.[43,53,54] There are no published reports of death secondary to human overdose with triptans to date. However, there is one report of a woman with no underlying cardiovascular disease who presumably died secondary to complications of prolonged cardiac arrest following a single dose of oral sumatriptan.[40]

Ocular toxicity consisting of corneal opacity and defects in the corneal epithelium has been reported in dogs at 30 days after daily administration of oral sumatriptan at three to five times the human daily exposure rate.[16]

Withdrawal of triptans following overuse (approximately 10 days per month for at least several months) may result in rebound (triptan-induced) headache. Triptan use should be limited to 3 days per week. Rebound headache may be characterized by refractoriness to preventive medication, and increasing attack frequency may be the first sign. Withdrawal headaches have also been described. Patients undergoing triptan withdrawal have been reported to request less symptomatic medication than patients undergoing withdrawal from ergot or analgesic medications, suggesting that their headaches were less severe than patients in the other study groups. Substituting medications that do not share cross-tolerance, or discontinuing the medication after the "washout" period is complete, may prove effective. Some patients may require inpatient therapy and/or psychiatric and social assessment and support.[55,56]

DIAGNOSIS

Because adverse effects reported with triptan use are also associated with migraine headaches, effects of the drugs may be difficult to distinguish from those of the disease. Any adverse events, including myocardial ischemia, that occur more than a few hours after triptan use generally do not fit within the period of pharmacokinetic activity of these medications.[30] It may be prudent to exercise

longer periods of observation after potential adverse effects in the case of those triptans that have longer duration of action (i.e., frovatriptan and eletriptan), active metabolites, and elimination times.

MANAGEMENT

Treatment of symptoms following therapeutic doses or potentially toxic doses largely involves supportive measures along with management of any potential cardiovascular or neurologic effects. Benzodiazepines can be useful to control agitation and muscle spasticity associated with serotonin syndrome. Nitroprusside can be used to treat hypertension if end-organ damage is suspected. Labetalol, nitroglycerine, and phentolamine may be used as alternatives with a goal of 20% to 25% reduction in mean arterial pressure.

Decontamination

Activated charcoal is regarded as most effective in absorbing unabsorbed drug from the gastrointestinal tract if given within 1 hour of ingestion after oral overdose. Some absorption of orally administered triptans might also be prevented by early gastric lavage, although the efficacy of this procedure may be no better than oral activated charcoal alone. In the event of massive triptan ingestion, a toxicologist should be consulted regarding decontamination procedures and management. No specific antidote exists.

Laboratory Studies

No specific laboratory work is generally indicated for inadvertent exposure to small amounts of triptans in asymptomatic patients. Specific drug levels are not clinically useful. For patients experiencing chest pain, a 12-lead electrocardiogram and continuous electrical monitoring should be performed if symptoms suggest myocardial ischemia or dysrhythmia. Serial cardiac enzymes may be considered. Since hepatic metabolism and renal excretion are important mechanisms of triptan and triptan metabolite formation and clearance, measures of hepatic and renal function might be useful, especially where presystemic "first pass" clearance of orally administered triptans is concerned. Patients with large exposures may be at risk for sequelae, including seizures and acidosis; laboratory studies should be obtained accordingly.

Disposition

There is a paucity of information regarding risk stratification of patients with triptan overdoses. Should a patient who is exposed to triptans experience chest pain that is believed to be ischemic in origin, further triptan use should be avoided until proper risk stratification can be completed.

A 3-year retrospective study of unintentional pediatric exposures to single-agent triptan acute ingestions has

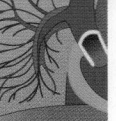
been reported. Exposures to oral formulations of suma-triptan, zolmitriptan, naratriptan, and rizatriptan were documented in children younger than 7 years. Of 32 cases that met inclusion criteria, 26 patients ingested one or two adult doses, three patients ingested three or more doses, and three ingested an unknown amount. Five patients reported at least one effect (vomiting, nausea, abdominal pain, and/or drowsiness). Four of those five patients were treated in the emergency department, and three of the five received activated charcoal. None of the patients required admission or other treatment. Of those five symptomatic patients, one ingested a single tablet, one ingested two tablets, and the others ingested three or four tablets. All of those patients were asymptomatic at the time of follow-up phone call. This limited review suggests that while children who ingest only one to two adult doses of the triptans studied are likely to do well and might be observed at home, more experience and further investigation is needed to establish safe triage and observation guidelines.[63]

Review of limited data available in the literature suggests that some patients who overuse triptans in the setting of acute accidental exposure or overuse do well. However, in the current absence of sufficient data to risk stratify patients with triptan overdose, it is safest to observe or admit patients with large triptan overdoses, comorbid conditions, and abnormal vital signs, as well as symptomatic patients or those with exposure to multiple serotonergic medications, since the consequences of serotonin syndrome or massive triptan overdose may be severe. Those with supratherapeutic exposure to triptans with long half-lives should, at a minimum, be observed for an extended period until such time as further data become available to assist with risk stratification of patients taking excess doses of such triptans.

REFERENCES

1. De Costa C: St Anthony's fire and living ligatures: a short history of ergometrine. Lancet 2002;359:1768–1770.
2. Hart C: Forged in St. Anthony's fire: drugs for migraine. Mod Drug Discovery 1999;2(2):20–21, 23–24, 28, 31.
3. Silberstein SD: The pharmacology of ergotamine and dihydro-ergotamine. Headache 1997;37(Suppl 1):15–25.
4. Stewart WF, Lipton RB, Celentano DD, Reed ML: Prevalence of migraine headache in the United States: relation to age, income, race, and other sociodemographic factors. JAMA 1992;267(1):64–69.
5. GlaxoSmithKline: Press release: Imitrex® (sumatriptan succinate) tablets now available in an innovative formulation for migraine sufferers: new formulation designed to rapidly release in the stomach. Research Triangle Park, NC, GlaxoSmithKline, February 4, 2004.
6. Lipton RB: The triptans and beyond. Addendum to agenda, program for the 1998 American Association for the Study of Headache, Scottsdale Symposium, Scottsdale, AZ, 1998.
7. Deleu D, Hanssens Y: Current and emerging second-generation triptans in acute migraine therapy: a comparative review. J Clin Pharmacol 2000;40:687–700.
8. Tfelt-Hansen P, De Vries P, Saxena PR: Triptans in migraine. Drugs 2000;60:1259–1287.
9. Cohen ML, Schenck K: 5-Hydroxytryptamine1F receptors do not participate in vasoconstriction: lack of vasoconstriction to LY344864, a selective serotonin1F receptor agonist in rabbit saphenous vein. J Pharmacol Exp Ther 1999;290:935–939.
10. Goadsby PJ, Lipton RB, Ferrari MD: Drug therapy: migraine—current understanding and treatment. N Engl J Med 2002;346(4):257–270.
11. Maassen VanDenBrink A, Saxena PR: Coronary vasoconstrictor potential of triptans: a review of in vitro pharmacologic data. Headache 2004;44(Suppl 1):13–19.
12. Hargreaves RJ, Shepheard SL: Pathophysiology of migraine—new insights. Can J Neurol Sci 1999;26(Suppl):12–19.
13. Smith D, Shaw D, Hopkins R, et al: Development and characterizations of human 5-HT1B or 5-HT1D receptor specific antibodies as unique research tools. J Neurosci Methods 1998;80:155–161.
14. Longmore J, Shaw D, Smith D, et al: Differential distribution of 5-HT1D and 5-HT1B immunoreactivity within the human trigemino-cerebrovascular system: implications for the discovery of new antimigraine drugs. Cephalalgia 1997;17:833–842.
15. Hoffmann O, Keilwerth N, Bille MB, et al: Triptans reduce the inflammatory response in bacterial meningitis. J Cereb Blood Flow Metab 2002;22(8):988–996.
16. GlaxoSmithKline: Imitrex®. In Physicians' Desk Reference. Montvale, NJ, Thomson PDR, 2005, pp 1513–1526.
17. Winner P: Triptans for migraine in adolescents. Headache 2002;42:675–679.
18. Rothner AD, Winner P, Nett R, et al: One-year tolerability and efficacy of sumatriptan nasal spray in adolescents with migraine: results of a multicenter, open-label study. Clin Ther 2000; 22(12):1533–1546.
19. Winner P, Rothner AD, Saper J, et al: A randomized, double-blind, placebo-controlled study of sumatriptan nasal spray in the treatment of acute migraine in adolescents. Pediatrics 2000; 106(5):989–997.
20. Loder E: Safety of sumatriptan in pregnancy: a review of the data so far. CNS Drugs 2003;17(1):1–7.
21. Ephross SA, Verp MS: Sumatriptan exposure during pregnancy: what we have learned about the risk of birth defects? Obstet Gynecol 2003;101(4 Suppl):83–84.
22. Bodner RA, Lynch T, Lewis L, et al: Serotonin syndrome. Neurology 1995;45:219–223.
23. Matthew NT, Tietjen Gem Lucker C: Serotonin syndrome complicating migraine pharmacotherapy. Cephalalgia 1999;16:323–327.
24. Gardner DM, Lynd LD: Sumatriptan contraindications and the serotonin syndrome. Ann Pharmacother 1998;32:33–38.
25. Maassen VanDenBrink A, Reekers M, Bax WA, et al: Coronary side-effect potential of current and prospective antimigraine drugs. Circulation 1998;98:25–30.
26. Tepper SJ: Safety and rational use of the triptans. Med Clin North Am 2001;85:959–970.
27. MacIntrye PD, Bhargava B, Hogg KJ, et al: Effect of subcutaneous sumatriptan, a selective 5-HT1 agonist, on the systemic, pulmonary, and coronary circulation. Circulation 1993;87:401–405.
28. Goldstein JA, Massey KD, Kirby S, et al: Effects of high-dose intravenous eletriptan on coronary artery diameter. Cephalalgia 2004;24(7):515–521.
29. Parsons AA, Raval P, Smith S: Effects of the novel high-affinity 5-HT(1B/1D)-receptor ligand frovatriptan in human isolated basilar and coronary arteries. J Cardiovasc Pharmacol 1998;32(2): 220–224.
30. Jamieson DG: The safety of triptans in the treatment of patients with migraine. Am J Med 2002;112:135–140.
31. Visser WH, Jaspers NM, de Vriend RH, et al: Chest symptoms after sumatriptan: a two year clinical practice review in 735 consecutive migraine patients. Cephalalgia 1996;16:554–559.
32. Tfelt-Hansen P: Efficacy and adverse events of subcutaneous, oral and intranasal sumatriptan used for migraine treatment: a systematic review based on number needed to treat. Cephalalgia 1998;18:532–538.
33. Velentgas P, Cole P, Mo J, et al: Severe vascular events in migraine patients. Headache 2004;44:642–651.
34. O'Quinn S, Davis RL, Gutterman DL, et al: Prospective large-scale study of the tolerability of subcutaneous sumatriptan for acute treatment of migraine. Cephalalgia 1999;19:223–231.
35. Cortijo J, Marti-Cabrera M, Bernabeu E, et al: Characteristics of 5-HT receptors on human pulmonary artery, and vein: functional and binding studies. Br J Pharmacol 1997;122:1455–1463.
36. Houghton LA, Foster JM, Whorwell PJ, et al: Is chest pain after sumatriptan oesophageal in origin? Lancet 1994;244:985–986.
37. The Triptan Cardiovascular Safety Expert Panel: Consensus statement: cardiovascular safety profile of triptans (5-HT1B/1D

agonists) in the acute treatment of migraine. Headache 2004;
44:414–425.

38. Humphrey PPA, Feniuk W, Perren MJ, et al: Serotonin and
migraine. Ann N Y Acad Sci 1990;600:587–598.

39. Abbrescia VD, Pearlstein L, Kotler M: Sumatriptan-associated
myocardial infarction: report of a case with attention to potential
risk factors. J Am Osteopath Assoc 1997;97:162–164.

40. Laine K, Raasakka T, Mantynen J, et al: Fatal cardiac arrhythmia
after oral sumatriptan. Headache 1999;39:511–512.

41. Mueller L, Gallagher RM, Ciervo CA: Vasospasm-induced myocardial infarction with sumatriptan. Headache 1996;36:329–331.

42. O'Connor P, Gladstone P: Oral sumatriptan-associated transmural
myocardial infarction. Neurology 1995;45:2274–2276.

43. Centonze V, Bassi A, Causarano V, et al: Sumatriptan overuse in
episodic cluster headache: lack of adverse events, rebound
syndromes, drug dependence and tachyphylaxis. Funct Neurol
2000;15(3):167–170.

44. Main ML, Ramaswamy K, Andrews TC: Cardiac arrest and
myocardial infarction immediately after sumatriptan injection
[letter]. Ann Intern Med 1998;128:874.

45. Kelly KM: Cardiac arrest following use of sumatriptan. Neurology
1995;45:1211–1213.

46. Morgan DR, Trimble M, McVeigh GE: Atrial fibrillation associated
with sumatriptan. BMJ 2000;321:275.

47. Curtain T, Brooks AP, Roberts JA: Cardiorespiratory distress
after sumatriptan given by injection [letter]. BMJ 1992;305:713–714.

48. Hall GC, Brown MM, Jingoing M, et al: Triptans in migraine: the
risks of stroke, cardiovascular disease, and death in practice.
Neurology 2004;62:563–568.

49. Knudsen JF, Friedman B, Chen M, et al: Ischemic colitis and
sumatriptan use. Arch Intern Med 1998;158:1946–1948.

50. Liu JJ, Ardolf JC: Sumatriptan-associated mesenteric ischemia
[letter]. Ann Intern Med 2000;132:597.

51. Naik M, Potluri R, Almasri E, et al: Sumatriptan-associated
ischemic colitis. Dig Dis Sci 2002;47:2015–2016.

52. Putnam GP, O'Quinn S, Bolden-Watson CP, et al: Migraine
polypharmacy and the tolerability of sumatriptan: a large-scale,
prospective study. Cephalalgia 1999;19:668–675.

53. Turhal NS: Sumatriptan overdose in episodic cluster headache: a
case report of overuse without event. Cephalalgia 2001;21:700.

54. Ottervanger JP, Valkenburg HA, Grobbee DE, et al: Pattern of
sumatriptan use and overuse in general practice. Eur J Clin
Pharmacol 1996;50(5):353–355.

55. Silberstein SD, Liu D: Drug overuse and rebound headache. Curr
Pain Headache Rep 2002;6:240–247.

56. Katsarva Z, Fritsche G, Muessig M, et al: Clinical features of
withdrawal headache following overuse of triptans and other
headache drugs. Neurology 2001;57(9):1694–1698.

57. A Catalog of FDA Approved Drug Products. Available at
http://www.fda.gov. Accessed May 10, 2006.

58. Eadie MJ: Clinically significant drug interactions with agents
specific for migraine attacks. CNS Drugs 2001;15(2):105–118.

59. Bigal ME, Bordini CA, Antoniazzi AL, Speciali JG: The triptan
formulations: a critical evaluation. Arq Neuropsiquiatr 2003;
61(2A):313–320.

60. Jhee SS, Shiovitz T, Crawford AW, Cutler NR: Pharmacokinetics
and pharmacodymanics of the triptan antimigraine agents: a
comparative review. Clin Pharmacol 2001;40(3):189–205.

61. Millson DS, Stewart JT, Rapoport AM: Migraine pharmacotherapy
with oral triptans: a rational approach to clinical management.
Exp Opin Pharmacother 2000;1(3):391–404.

62. Armstrong SC, Cozza KL: Med-psych drug-drug interactions
update: triptans. Psychosomatics 2002;43(6):502–504.

63. Borys D, Hill K, Morgan D: Triptans in pediatric overdose: is
medical treatment necessary? [abstract]. J Toxicol Clin Toxicol
2002;40(5):665.

50 *Colchicine*

J. WARD DONOVAN, MD

At a Glance...

- Colchicine has a narrow therapeutic index and serious toxicity; fatalities can occur even with therapeutic doses.
- Colchicine is contraindicated in hepatic disease or renal failure, and should be avoided with macrolide antibiotics.
- The latent period of 4 to 12 hours after an overdose may mislead clinicians into discharging the patient prematurely.
- Toxicity develops in a first phase of severe gastroenteritis with hypovolemia; a second phase of bone marrow depression, cardiac and respiratory failure, hepatorenal syndrome, coagulopathy, and weakness; and a third phase of recovery with alopecia and rebound leukocytosis.
- Initial treatment includes gastric decontamination (even in late presentation), respiratory support, aggressive fluid replacement, and vasopressor use as needed.
- Elimination may be enhanced by multiple dosing of activated charcoal, but hemodialysis has no effect.
- Colchicine-specific Fab fragments show promise for future therapy, but are not currently available.
- Granulocyte colony-stimulating factor may aid in recovery from leukopenia.

INTRODUCTION AND RELEVANT HISTORY

Colchicine is an alkaloid that can be extracted from two plants of the lily family, *Colchicum autumnale* (autumn crocus, meadow saffron) and *Gloriosa superba* (glory lily), and is used as an anti-inflammatory agent in gouty arthritis. Colchicum was first recognized as a poison in the 3rd century BC by the Egyptian Dioscorides.[1] In the 6th century AD, Alexander of Trallis first recommended colchicum as a cathartic in the treatment of joint pain.[2] It was advocated as a diuretic in the New Edinburgh Dispensatory in 1788 and recommended as specific therapy for gout in medical texts of the early 1800s. It was probably introduced into the United States as therapy for gout by Benjamin Franklin.[1] In 1820, colchicine was isolated from the *C. autumnale* tuber and rapidly gained popularity. It is now used to treat acute gouty arthritis, primary biliary cirrhosis, amyloidosis, Behçet's disease, and condyloma acuminata, as prophylaxis for familial Mediterranean fever, and experimentally to study cell division in cytogenetics because of its antimitotic activity.[3]

The infrequency of colchicine toxicity is reflected in the annual report by the American Association of Poison Control Centers (AAPCC). In 2003, there were 213 colchicine exposures reported to the AAPCC, of which only 4 resulted in major toxicity and 4 resulted in death.[4]

Nevertheless, toxic effects may be encountered after accidental, suicidal, or therapeutic use of colchicine tablets. The tubers of the glory lily have also been mistakenly ingested due to their similarity to sweet potatoes. Large volumes of the plants are required to cause toxicity, but the effects are similar to those observed with tablet ingestion.

CLASSIFICATION AND STRUCTURE

The alkaloid colchicine has the chemical formula *N*-(5,6,7,9-tetrahydro-1,2,3,10-tetramethoxy-9-oxobenzo[a]heptalen-7-yl) acetamide. The structure is shown in Figure 50-1.[5] Pharmaceutical colchicine is available as 0.5- and 0.6-mg tablets and as a parenteral solution of 0.5 mg/mL. *Colchicum* species are cultivated and are popular as houseplants. The species *C. autumnale* has long, tubular purple or white flowers with seeds, and plants emerge from an underground corm or bulb (see Chapter 24); colchicine is present at a concentration of approximately 1% in the flowers of this plant.[6]

PHARMACOKINETICS

Colchicine is rapidly absorbed from the gastrointestinal (GI) tract, reaching peak plasma levels within 0.5 to 2 hours.[1] Oral bioavailability has been estimated to be 25% to 44%.[2,6] Because higher doses depress jejunal and ileal function, prolonged absorption may occur in toxic doses.[2] However, this was not observed in one study of human poisoning cases.[7]

Approximately 50% of circulating colchicine is bound to plasma proteins. Initial distribution half-lives range from 45 to 90 minutes, and distribution is complete after 3 to 6 hours.[8] The reported volume of distribution has varied across a wide range; it has been estimated to be 2.2 to 8.5 L/kg with therapeutic doses and 21 L/kg in patients with toxic effects.[6,8] A range of 12% to 44% of colchicine is excreted unchanged in the urine with therapeutic doses, similar to the 30% excretion found in overdose. In patients with liver disease, a larger fraction

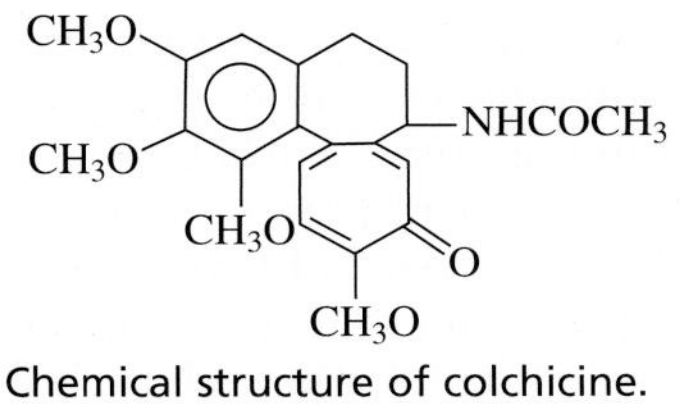

FIGURE 50-1 Chemical structure of colchicine.

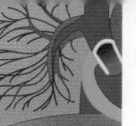

of the drug is excreted unchanged. Metabolism is primarily via deacetylation in the liver mediated by cytochrome P-450 (CYP) 3A4, followed by biliary excretion. Significant enterohepatic recirculation occurs, as demonstrated by the presence of the parent drug and metabolites in large amounts in bile and intestinal secretions.

The terminal plasma elimination half-life in therapeutic doses has ranged from 9.3 to 41 hours.[2,6-8] This is similar to half-lives of 10.6 to 31.7 hours in toxic ingestions. However, serum concentrations were essentially unchanged for 3 days in one case of colchicine co-ingested with drugs that prolonged drug absorption and caused renal and hepatic failure.[8]

DRUG INTERACTIONS

The CYP3A4 inhibitors cimetidine and ketoconazole can cause an increase in colchicine elimination half-life.[2] Likewise, the macrolide antibiotics erythromycin and clarithromycin have the potential for inhibiting the CYP3A4 isoenzyme and, thus, decreasing hepatic metabolism of colchicine. Any known inhibitor of CYP3A4 has the potential for impairing colchicine metabolism and potentiating toxicity from this agent (see Chapter 5). The macrolide antibiotics, including josamycin, also inhibit P-glycoprotein, a transporter involved in cellular efflux and biliary elimination of drugs.[8] Thus, the coadministration of macrolides has been reported to cause serious colchicine toxicity.[8,9] Cyclosporine toxicity has resulted with concomitant use of colchicine.

PATHOPHYSIOLOGY

Colchicine binds to intracellular tubulin, a structural protein necessary for normal cellular motility, shape, endocytosis and exocytosis, axonal transport, and cell division. As a result of tubulin binding, microtubule polymerization is inhibited, spindle formation cannot occur, and cell mitosis is inhibited in metaphase.[10] Those cells with the highest turnover rate, such as intestinal epithelium, bone marrow, and hair follicles, are affected the earliest and to the greatest extent. By inhibiting tubulin polymerization, colchicine affects microtubule function and interferes with the transport of intracellular nutrients and organelles. Failed microtubule function may explain some aspects of the multiorgan failure seen in colchicine toxicity, particularly cardiac failure.[11] There may be a direct toxic effect on the myocardial cells with impairment of impulse generation and cardiac conduction. Alternatively, depressed cardiac conduction and inotropy associated with severe colchicine toxicity may be due to profound acidosis and electrolyte derangements.[3] The action of colchicine in gout is largely due to impaired phagocytosis of urate crystals by leukocytes; these effects probably result from failed microtubule function in leukocytes and their inability to alter cellular shape and engulf crystals.

RANGE OF TOXIC EFFECTS

For acute gouty arthritis, the usual colchicine dose is 0.5 to 1.0 mg every 2 to 3 hours until relief or GI symptoms occur. Because GI warning symptoms do not occur with IV dosing, the recommended IV dose is half of the equivalent oral dose to a maximum of 2 to 4 mg per acute episode.[2] There is a significant risk for death when this cumulative IV dose is exceeded.[12] Maintenance colchicine therapy is usually provided as daily doses of 0.5 to 2 mg for adults and 0.5 mg per day for children. Colchicine is contraindicated in patients with combined hepatorenal disease, creatinine clearances below 10 mL/min, or extrahepatic biliary obstruction.[5] Because of reduced elimination in those with renal impairment, doses should be no larger than 0.6 mg/day if the creatinine clearance is less than 50 mL/min or serum creatinine is greater than 1.6 mg/dL.[13]

Fatalities have occurred with total doses of 8 to 11 mg given therapeutically over several days.[2] Ingestions of 0.5 to 0.8 mg/kg result in severe toxic effects, and doses greater than 0.8 mg/kg or a total of 40 mg are considered to be uniformly fatal.[2,14] However, outcome is dependent on the duration between exposure and treatment, and the use of appropriate aggressive therapy.[15] Severe toxic effects followed by survival have occurred with doses of 50 to 60 mg (greater than 1 mg/kg).[2,10] In children, the fatal dose may be as low as 0.37 mg/kg.[15] Colchicine-containing plants rarely produce severe toxicity due to the low concentrations of toxin, but large ingestions can be fatal.[16] Ten grams of tuber contain about 6 mg of colchicine, and 100 to 125 g of tubers (60 to 95 mg of colchicine) have produced severe toxic effects.[17]

Colchicine plasma levels do not correlate well with the severity of toxicity and are not clinically useful. For instance, in acute ingestions, plasma concentrations that are associated with GI effects alone have ranged from 11 to 63 ng/mL within 4 hours of exposure.[7] In contrast, a level of 24 ng/mL was noted 27 hours after acute colchicine ingestion in a patient with severe hemodynamic instability.[11] In addition, reported colchicine plasma levels have ranged from 11 to 66 ng/mL in fatal cases.[8] Because of enterohepatic recirculation, the drug accumulates in the bile in levels as high as over 5000 ng/mL. Thus, the bile may be the best source for analysis in forensic cases.[18]

CLINICAL MANIFESTATIONS

The clinical manifestations of colchicine overdose involve multiple organ systems, including GI, respiratory, hematologic, cardiovascular, renal, and neurologic. After a latent period of 4 to 12 hours, signs and symptoms of toxicity occur in three phases.[19] The first phase is manifested largely by GI signs and symptoms with fluid losses, electrolyte imbalance, and hypovolemic shock. Life-threatening complications occur during the second stage, or from 24 to 72 hours after exposure. At this

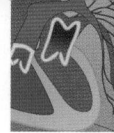

time, cardiac insufficiency, arrhythmias, bone marrow depression, renal failure, hepatic injury, respiratory distress, coagulopathy, and neuromuscular abnormalities are present. This phase can last for 5 to 7 days and is followed by a recovery phase marked by a rebound leukocytosis and alopecia. The duration and features of each phase are outlined in Table 50-1, and details of each involved organ system are discussed separately.

Gastrointestinal

Nausea, vomiting, diarrhea, and burning abdominal pain are the initial symptoms of colchicine toxicity. The presence of GI symptoms can serve a protective effect by warning of the potential for further toxicity with continued use of the drug. In addition, the presence of early GI effects may be the earliest indicator of impending severe toxic effects that will occur after acute overdose. Severe dehydration, hypovolemia, and cardiovascular collapse can result if aggressive treatment is not instituted. GI effects are not prominent after IV use, suggesting a local action of colchicine on gut epithelial cells. Hepatocellular damage (with associated elevations of transaminases and alkaline phosphatase) and hepatomegaly can also occur with colchicine toxicity, but fulminant hepatic failure occurs very rarely.[10] Pancreatitis and a paralytic ileus also frequently occur.

Cardiovascular

Hypotension occurs due to volume losses, extravasation of fluid into extracellular spaces, and myocardial depression. Development of cardiogenic shock due to a postulated direct myocardial injury is a poor prognostic sign.[20] Colchicine is also thought to impair cardiac conduction, leading to arrhythmias and even late asystole.[19] Marked electrocardiographic changes indicative

of myocardial injury can occur, with ST and T wave changes.[17] Elevation of serum troponin I may be indicative of acute myocardial injury and the risk for cardiovascular collapse.[21]

Respiratory

Respiratory distress occurs in about one third of cases and is a result of generalized muscle weakness and acute respiratory distress syndrome (ARDS).[5] Colchicine is also thought to have a direct toxic effect on the lungs, causing capillary leakage. Prolonged hypotension, sepsis, and multiorgan failure probably also play a major role in this syndrome.

Neurologic

Mental status depression may progress to delirium, seizures, and coma. Peripheral neuropathy, loss of deep tendon reflexes, and ascending paralysis can also occur late in the course.[2,19,20] Myelin degeneration is thought to be the cause of these neuropathic effects.[5]

Hematologic

The first phase of acute toxicity includes a peripheral leukocytosis, followed by bone marrow depression in the second phase. Severe leukopenia, thrombocytopenia, and a consumptive coagulopathy peak at 4 to 7 days postingestion.[10] Disseminated intravascular coagulation and sepsis often complicate this phase. Hematologic studies show hypoprothrombinemia, decreased fibrinogen, and increased fibrin split products. At 8 to 10 days postingestion, bone marrow recovery is apparent, and a rebound leukocytosis occurs during the recovery phase. Neutropenia may occur without other toxic effects after several days of therapeutic use.[22]

TABLE 50-1 Phases of Colchicine Toxicity		
PHASE	**COMPLICATION**	**TREATMENT**
I (0–12 hr)	GI symptoms	Gastric lavage to ensure removal of all pills from stomach
	Volume depletion	IV fluid replacement; treatment of shock with use of pressure if needed
	Peripheral leukocytosis	
II (2–7 days)	Respiratory distress, ARDS, hypoxemia	Supplemental oxygen, ET intubation and mechanical ventilation, PEEP
	Cardiovascular shock	Monitor, CVP, Swan-Ganz, fluids, pressors
	Thrombocytopenia, DIC	Replacement therapy with blood products
	Myelosuppression, neutropenia	Blood cultures, treament with antibiotics
	Hyponatremia, hypocalcemia, hypophosphatemia	Electrolyte replacement
	Metabolic acidosis	Maintain volume status; treatment with HCO_3 if necessary
	Rhabdomyolysis, myoglobinuria, oliguric renal failure	Fluids, diuretics to maintain urine output
III (1–2 wk)	Rebound leukocytosis, alopecia	

ARDS, acute respiratory distress syndrome; CVP, central venous pressure; DIC, disseminated intravascular coagulopathy; ET, endotracheal; GI, gastrointestinal; IV, intravenous; PEEP, positive end-expiratory pressure.

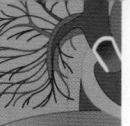

Renal

Renal failure is common in severe colchicine toxicity, probably secondary to hypovolemia, hypoxia, and myoglobinuria.[5] The typical clinical findings are an oliguria responsive to fluids, hematuria, and proteinuria.[17] There is no evidence of direct renal toxicity, although colchicine does concentrate in the kidneys.[7]

Metabolic/Electrolytes

A lactic acid, anion-gap metabolic acidosis is common, again due to hypotension and hypovolemia. This is exacerbated by inhibition of intracellular metabolism and accumulation of organic acids.[19] Hypophosphatemia, hyponatremia, hypocalcemia, and hypomagnesemia occur, primarily due to fluid losses. Hypocalcemia is also thought to be due to direct suppression of bone resorption by colchicine.[2]

Musculoskeletal

A direct myopathic effect of colchicine can lead to muscle weakness, necrosis, and rhabdomyolysis, especially with chronic colchicine use.[10] Reported cases have been associated with preexisting renal failure, and either acute or long-term colchicine in low therapeutic doses.[23,24] Typically, there is rhabdomyolysis with elevated creatine kinase and aminotransferases.[24] The diagnosis is aided by electromyography and muscle biopsy. If respiratory failure occurs, pulmonary function testing is recommended to determine if skeletal muscle weakness is a significant contributing factor. The myopathy is usually rapidly resolved with discontinuation of colchicine.

Dermatologic

Scalp hair loss is common and typically occurs during the recovery phase, but it can occur anytime between 6 and 30 days postingestion.[2,10] Hair growth almost always recovers several weeks after exposure. A vesiculating, erythematous rash resembling toxic epidermal necrolysis has been reported in rare cases, with histopathology showing subepidermal bullae and apoptosis of keratinocytes.[25]

Miscellaneous

Colchicine has been associated with delayed corneal ulcer healing, azoospermia, and oligospermia.[26]

DIAGNOSIS

The diagnosis should be suspected in anyone with access to colchicine and displaying the typical colchicine toxidrome of gastroenteritis, hypotension, lactic acidosis, and prerenal azotemia. In the early phases of colchicine toxicity, the diagnosis could be mistaken for sepsis, nonsteroidal anti-inflammatory drug or iron toxicity, or pancreatitis.[27] Findings associated with the later phase of colchicine toxicity (e.g., peripheral neuropathy and alopecia) could be mistaken for heavy metal poisoning. Differentiation from both is possible by the presence of severe bone marrow suppression in the second phase of colchicine toxicity.

Laboratory monitoring should include frequent measurements of electrolytes (including calcium, magnesium, and phosphate), platelets, and creatine kinase; complete blood count; prothrombin time; serum troponin I; renal and liver function tests; and urinalysis for myoglobinuria. If coagulopathy is suspected, fibrinogen and fibrin split products should be monitored. In severe or persistent hypotension, echocardiography and pulmonary catheter monitoring is warranted.[21] Colchicine measurements are not clinically useful except to establish or confirm the diagnosis.

TREATMENT

Initial Supportive Measures

Treatment for colchicine poisoning is mainly supportive. Patients with significant central nervous system or respiratory depression should have their airway protected, breathing assisted, and cardiovascular support provided as necessary. Initial therapy for hypotension includes aggressive replacement of fluid losses with IV crystalloid (20 to 60 mL/kg of normal saline or lactated Ringer's solution); vasopressors are indicated for hemodynamic instability that is not fluid responsive or severe. If the vasopressor therapy is necessary, it should be guided by Swan-Ganz catheter placement and measurement of hemodynamic parameters. This is important, given the propensity for myocardial depression, hypovolemia, alterations in systemic vascular resistance, and ARDS. Respiratory failure may require mechanical ventilation with positive end-expiratory pressure.

Transfusions of whole blood, fresh frozen plasma, vitamin K, and platelets may be necessary to treat coagulopathies. Because of frequent sepsis complicating neutropenia, the use of broad-spectrum antibiotics should be considered for febrile patients.

Decontamination

Gastric decontamination is warranted if the patient presents during the latent period prior to the onset of gastroenteritis and a potentially toxic amount (greater than 5 to 10 mg in adults) has been ingested. Adsorption of colchicine by activated charcoal has not been studied but is thought to be effective. Even late decontamination should be performed, because large residual amounts of colchicine have been found in the stomach many hours after ingestion. The known enterohepatic recirculation of colchicine also supports late and repeated doses of activated charcoal, but paralytic ileus may complicate this approach.[15] In such cases, duodenal tube suction could be utilized. Cathartics should not be routinely employed due to the expected onset of spontaneous diarrhea, and whole bowel irrigation would also be of limited value for this reason.

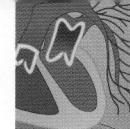

Antidotes

Colchicine-specific Fab fragments have been developed and used with success in studies in laboratory animals.[11] The Fab fragments are prepared from the antiserum of goats immunized with colchicine, and their infusion results in reversal of colchicine binding to tubulin. This investigational agent has been successfully employed in a case of severe toxicity in a human without any adverse effects.[11] Administration of the Fab fragments resulted in a rapid reversal of life-threatening hemodynamic instability, although bone marrow suppression did not significantly improve. The dose given was 480 mg of colchicine-specific Fab fragments, with half given over 1 hour and the remainder over the ensuing 6 hours.[11] However, this agent remains an investigational antidote and is available only in France, in very limited quantities.

Granulocyte colony-stimulating factor (G-CSF) has been used in colchicine toxicity in an attempt to accelerate production of neutrophils within the bone marrow.[10,28] In such cases, an accelerated leukocytosis was observed within 1 to 2 days, but at a time when rebound leukocytosis may naturally occur. Because colchicine-induced bone marrow suppression is short-lived, use of G-CSF should be considered only in life-threatening sepsis during the second phase of toxicity.

Enhanced Elimination

As discussed with decontamination, repeated doses of activated charcoal should theoretically enhance colchicine elimination because of its enterohepatic recirculation, but this has not been tested. This treatment would be problematic in some cases due to the presence of emesis and, possibly, paralytic ileus. With its large volume of distribution, high protein binding, and relatively small fraction of renal excretion, it is unlikely that forced diuresis, hemodialysis, exchange transfusion, or hemoperfusion would be effective for drug removal.[13] Hemodialysis may be necessary to treat the associated renal failure.

Disposition

Because of its narrow therapeutic index and latent phase, any patient should be observed for 8 to 12 hours after acute ingestion of colchicine. The onset of GI symptoms or leukocytosis warrants hospital admission until at least the second phase of toxicity has ended.

REFERENCES

1. Mack RB: Achilles and his evil squeeze: colchicine poisoning. NC Med J 1991;52:581–583.
2. Putterman C, Chetrit EB, Caraco Y, et al: Colchicine intoxication: clinical pharmacology, risk factors, features, and management. Semin Arthritis Rheum 1991;21:143–155.
3. Maxwell MJ, Muthu P, Pritty PE: Accidental colchicine overdose. A case report and literature review. Emerg Med J 2002;19:265–266.
4. Watson WA, Litovitz TL, Klein-Schwartz W, et al: 2003 annual report of the American Association of Poison Control Centers Toxic Exposure Surveillance System. Am J Emerg Med 2004;22:335–404.
5. Hood RL: Colchicine poisoning. J Emerg Med 1992;12:171–177.
6. Baselt RC: Disposition of Toxic Drugs and Chemicals in Man, 7th ed. Foster City, CA, Biomedical Publications, 2004, pp 266–267.
7. Rochdi M, Sabouraud A, Baud FJ: Toxicokinetics of colchicine in humans: analysis of tissue, plasma and urine data in ten cases. Hum Exp Toxicol 1992;11:510–516.
8. Borron SW, Scherrmann JM, Baud FJ: Markedly altered colchicine kinetics in a fatal intoxication: examination of contributing factors. Hum Exp Toxicol 1996;15:885–890.
9. Rollot F, Pajot O, Chauvelot-Moachon L, et al: Acute colchicine intoxication during clarithromycin administration. Ann Pharmacother 2004;38:2074–2077.
10. Folpini A, Furfori P: Colchicine toxicity clinical features and treatment: massive overdose case report. Clin Toxicol 1995;33:71–77.
11. Baud FJ, Sabouraud A, Vicaut E, et al: Brief report: treatment of severe colchicine overdose with colchicine-specific Fab fragments. N Engl J Med 1995;332:642–643.
12. Bonnel RA, Villalba ML, Karwoski CB, Beitz J: Deaths associated with inappropriate intravenous colchicine administration. J Emerg Med 2002;22:385–387.
13. Wallace SL, Singer JZ, Duncan GJ, et al: Renal function predicts colchicine toxicity: guidelines for the prophylactic use of colchicine in gout. J Rheumatol 1999;18:264–269.
14. Bismuth C, Baud F, Dally S, et al: Standardized prognosis evaluation in acute toxicology: its benefit in colchicine, paraquat, and digitalis poisonings. J Toxicol Clin Exp 1986;6:33–38.
15. Atas B, Caksen H, Tuncer O, et al: Four children with colchicine poisoning. Hum Exp Toxicol 2004;23:353–356.
16. Brncic N, Viskovic I, Peric R, et al: Accidental plant poisoning with Colchicum autumnale: report of two cases. Croat Med J 1990;42:673–675.
17. Mendis S: Colchicine cardiotoxicity following ingestion of Gloriosa superba tubers. Postgrad Med J 1989;65:752–755.
18. Devaux M, Hubert N, Demarly C: Colchicine poisoning: case report of two suicides. Forensic Sci Int 2004;143:219–222.
19. Stapczynski JS, Rothstein RJ, Gaye WA, et al: Colchicine overdose: report of two cases and review of the literature. Ann Emerg Med 1981;10:364–369.
20. De Deyn PP, Cauterick C, Saxena V, et al: Chronic colchicine-induced myopathy and neuropathy. Acta Neurol Belg 1995;95:29–32.
21. Mullins ME, Robertson DG, Norton RL: Troponin I as a marker of cardiac toxicity in acute colchicine overdose. Am J Emerg Med 2000;18;743–744.
22. Dixon AJ, Wall GC: Probable colchicine-induced neutropenia not related to intentional overdose. Ann Pharmacother 2001;35:192–195.
23. Tanios MA, Gamal HE, Epstein SK, Hassoun PM: Severe respiratory muscle weakness related to long-term colchicine therapy. Respir Care 2004;49:189–191.
24. Wilbur K, Makowsky M: Colchicine myotoxicity: case reports and literature review. Pharmacotherapy 2004;24:1784–1792.
25. Arroyo MP, Sanders S, Yee H, et al: Toxic epidermal necrolysis-like reaction secondary to colchicines overdose. Br J Dermatol 2004;150:581–588.
26. Alster Y, Varssano D, Loewenstein A, et al: Delay of corneal wound healing in patients treated with colchicine. Ophthalmology 1997;104:118–119.
27. Guven AG, Bahat E, Akman S, et al: Late diagnosis of severe colchicines intoxication. Pediatrics 2002;109:971–973.
28. Harris R, Marx G: Colchicine-induced bone marrow suppression: treatment with granulocyte colony stimulating factor. J Emerg Med 2000;18:435–440.

51

Nonsteroidal Anti-Inflammatory Drugs

J. WARD DONOVAN, MD

At a Glance...

- Acute nonsteroidal anti-inflammatory drug toxicity may produce gastrointestinal (nausea, vomiting), neurologic (lethargy, coma, hallucinations, seizures), and metabolic (acidosis, renal failure) effects.
- Nonsteroidal anti-inflammatory drug toxicity should be included in the differential diagnosis of an anion gap metabolic acidosis, which can be severe (pH < 7.1) in large overdoses.
- Absorption and onset of effects are rapid (1 to 4 hours) following acute overdose.
- Cyclooxygenase-2 nonsteroidal anti-inflammatory drugs have fewer adverse gastrointestinal effects with chronic use, but have similar toxic effects in overdose and have a risk for inducing adverse cardiovascular events in chronic use due to their prothrombic effects.
- Management is supportive and must include rehydration to prevent and reverse the renal and metabolic effects.

INTRODUCTION AND RELEVANT HISTORY

Nonsteroidal anti-inflammatory drugs (NSAIDs) were first developed in the late 19th century; they achieved widespread use even before the marketing of acetylsalicylic acid. The first NSAIDs were the pyrazolones, phenazone and amidopyrine; phenylbutazone, of the same class, was not introduced until after World War II. Other NSAIDs were identified in the late 1950s and the 1960s, and they have undergone an explosive increase in use over the past 30 years. Ibuprofen was first introduced in the United States in 1974 and was approved for over-the-counter use in 1984.

The widespread availability of NSAIDs has naturally resulted in a marked increase in the number of overdoses and reported adverse effects. In the 4-year period 1985 through 1988, 55,800 cases of ibuprofen exposure were reported to the American Association of Poison Control Centers (AAPCC), but 71,043 ibuprofen exposures and a total of 97,123 NSAID exposures were reported in 2003 alone.[1,2] Ibuprofen exposures account for more than 5% of the total cases reported to the London Poisons Information Centre.[3] NSAIDs are now the most commonly utilized class of medications in the world, accounting for more than 4% of all prescriptions, with 73 million prescriptions written per year.[4,5] Piroxicam, with its extended plasma half-life, potency, and safety, has become one of the most widely prescribed NSAIDs in the world.[6]

Despite their extensive use, NSAIDs are among the safest pharmaceuticals in use. Adverse drug reaction frequency is reported as only 24.4 per million prescrip-

tions, with fatal adverse reactions of 1.1 per million prescriptions.[7] Symptoms were absent or minor in 33.6% of cases with known outcomes reported to the AAPCC.[2] However, the potential does exist for serious illness and even death in a few cases, as reflected in the 578 reported serious outcomes and 47 deaths involving NSAIDs in the United States in 2003. NSAIDs are now a common cause of renal failure, and at some regional poison treatment centers, mefenamic acid has accounted for the majority of reported drug-induced seizures.[8,9] Chinese herbal medications have been found to contain NSAIDs, and their use has caused renal failure and aplastic anemia.[10]

STRUCTURE AND STRUCTURAL RELATIONSHIPS

The NSAIDs are a heterogeneous group of chemicals that share similar therapeutic properties. These acids are classified as subgroups of one of two families: the carboxylic or enolic acids. The carboxylic acids are further subdivided into arylacetic (phenylacetic) acids, propionic acids, fenamic acids, isoxazoles, and carbocylic and heterocyclic acetic acids. The enolic acetic acids are subdivided into pyrazolones and oxicams (Box 51-1). Aspirin, a salicylic acid of the carboxylic family, is discussed in Chapter 48. The structures of various NSAIDs are shown in Figure 51-1.[11]

NSAIDs are also classified by their activity as a specific or nonspecific inhibitor of the cyclooxygenase isoenzymes COX-1 and COX-2. Selective inhibition of COX-2, which affects inflammatory responses, is desirable, while inhibition of COX-1, affecting gastric mucosal protection, is not. Selective COX-2 inhibitors celecoxib and rofecoxib have up to a 200 to 300 times greater selectivity for COX-2 than COX-1.[12] The novel coxibs etoricoxib, valdecoxib, parecoxib, and lumiracoxib have even greater COX-2 selectivity, with the possibility of using increased doses to improve efficacy.[13] However, they have renal side effects similar to those of the nonselective NSAIDs, thereby limiting the use of higher doses. Some other NSAIDs also have a modest degree of COX-2 selectivity, particularly etodolac, nabumetone, and meloxicam.[12] A potential disadvantage of the COX-2 inhibitors are that they are prothrombotic, whereas COX-1 inhibition has antithrombotic activity.[14]

PHARMACOLOGY: MECHANISM OF ACTION

The primary mechanism of action of NSAIDs is via inhibition of prostaglandin synthesis. Prostaglandins are derived from phospholipids in cell membranes synthesized

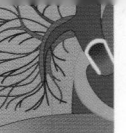

BOX 51-1   CLASSIFICATION OF NSAIDS

Salicylic Acids

Acetylsalicylic acid (aspirin)
Choline salicylate (arthropan)
Diflunisal (Dolobid)
Magnesium salicylate (Doan's, Magan)
Salicylamide
Salsalate (Disalcid)
Sodium salicylate
Sodium thiosalicylate
Trolamine salicylate (Aspercreme, Myoflex Crème)

Phenylacetic Acids

Diclofenac (Voltaren)

Carbocyclic and Heterocyclic Acetic Acids

Aceclofenac
Acemetacin
Bromfenac (Duract)
Diclofenac
Etodolac (Lodine)
Indomethacin (Indocin)
Ketorolac (Toradol)
Nabumetone
Sulindac (Clinoril)
Tolmetin (Tolectin)
Zomepirac

Fenamic Acids

Benzydamine (Tantum, Difflam, Andolex, Opalgyne)
Floctafenine
Flufenamic acid
Mefenamic acid (Ponstel)
Meclofenamate (Meclomen)

Propionic Acids

Carprofen
Ibuprofen (Advil, Nuprin, Motrin)
Naproxen (Naprosyn, Anaprox)
Fenbufen
Flurbiprofen (Ansaid)
Fenoprofen (Nalfon)
Indoprofen
Ketoprofen (Orudis)
Loxoprofen
Oxaprozin (Daypro)
Pirprofen
Suprofen (Suprol)
Tiaprofenic acid

Furanones

Rofecoxib (Vioxx)

Isoxazoles

Valdecoxib (Bextra)

Pyrazoles

Celecoxib (Celebrex)

Pyrazolones

Azapropazone
Fenprazone
Phenylbutazone (Butazolidin)
Oxyphenbutazone (Oxalid)

Oxicams

Isoxacam
Lornoxicam
Piroxicam (Feldene)
Meloxicam (Mobic)
Sudoxicam

---

from arachidonic acid. This synthesis is mediated by the enzyme cyclooxygenase, which is reversibly inhibited by NSAIDs. Thus, NSAIDs block the conversion of arachidonic acid to the various prostaglandins, which are involved in renin release, local vascular tone, regional circulation, water homeostasis, and potassium balance. The prostaglandin pathway and functions are outlined in Figure 51-2.

Prostaglandin E_2 (PGE_2), PGD_2, PGF_2, and prostacyclin (PGI_2) promote salt and water excretion, and the renal vasodilatory action of PGE_2, PGD_2, and prostacyclin enhances this effect. It is thought that PGE_2 and prostacyclin also stimulate renin release.[15] In addition, prostaglandins antagonize the effects of antidiuretic hormone.[16] The net effect of NSAIDs is decreased inhibition of prostaglandins, decreased renal blood flow, and decreased glomerular filtration rate, leading to sodium, potassium, and water retention (Fig. 51-3).

PGE_2 also inhibits lymphocytes and other cells involved in inflammation and allergic response, and this may play a role in the development of interstitial nephritis and hepatotoxic effects in some patients using NSAIDs.[16,17] This has occurred most with fenoprofen and the carbocyclic and heterocyclic acetic acids.

Other actions of NSAIDs are inhibition of platelet activation and mast cell mediation. The former contributes to prolonged bleeding, and the latter may be involved in NSAID-induced anaphylactic reactions and idiosyncratic hypersensitivity reactions. Also, prostaglandins, particularly prostacyclin, are formed in gastric tissue and exert gastric mucosal protective actions. Inhibition of this action by NSAIDs as well as their direct disruption of the gastric mucosal barrier can cause gastritis and gastrointestinal (GI) bleeding. The selective COX-2 inhibitors have less likelihood of adverse GI events, and large clinical trials have validated this theory.[18] However, by decreasing vasodilatory and antiaggregatory prostacyclin production, COX-2 inhibitors may be prothrombotic. This is discussed further under cardiopulmonary effects.

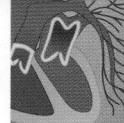

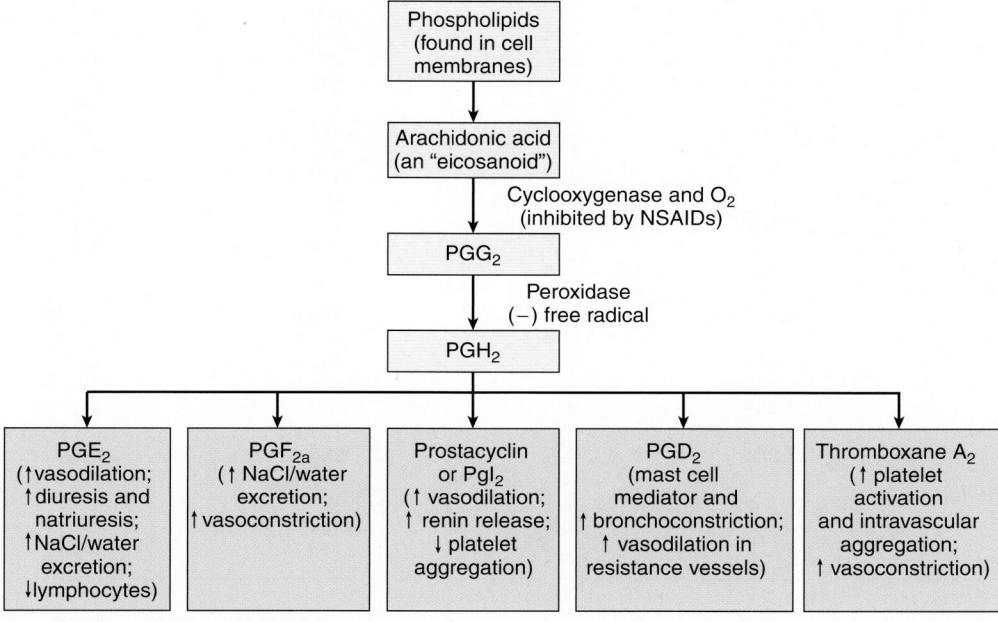

FIGURE 51-1 Chemical structures of various nonsteroidal anti-inflammatory drugs. **A,** Ibuprofen, a propionic acid. **B,** Rofecoxib, a furanone. **C,** Acetylsalicylic acid, an acetylated salicylate. **D,** Meloxicam, an oxicam or enolcarboxamide. **E,** Valdecoxib, an isoxazole. **F,** Indomethacin, an acetic acid. **G,** Salsalate, a nonacetylated salicylate. (From Brent J, Wallace KL, Burkhart KK, et al [eds]: Critical Care Toxicology. Philadelphia, Mosby, 2005.)

FIGURE 51-2 Prostaglandin pathway and function.

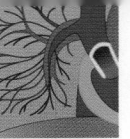

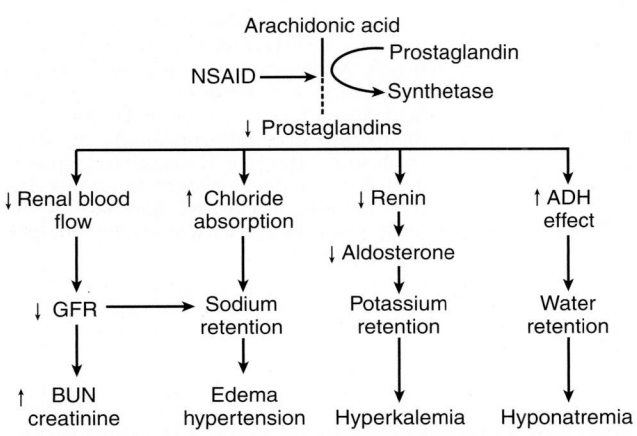

FIGURE 51-3 The net effect of NSAIDs with prostaglandins. ADH, antidiuretic hormone; BUN, blood urea nitrogen; GFR, glomerular filtration rate.

PHARMACOKINETICS

The carboxylic acid and enolic acid NSAIDs share similar pharmacokinetics, pharmacodynamic properties, and metabolic pathways. However, there are some clinically significant differences in rates of absorption and elimination and in drug interactions (Table 51-1).[19,20]

Absorption

Therapeutic oral doses for most NSAIDs are absorbed almost completely, producing peak levels within 1 to 2 hours. Exceptions to this are oxaprozin, mefenamic acid, and diflunisal, which have delays of peak levels of up to 3 to 4 hours. The presence of food can delay the absorption of all NSAIDs.[20] In overdose, some delay may take place in achievement of peak serum levels. Five patients in a series of 29 patients with mefenamic acid overdoses had increasing serum levels after admission, which peaked at 8 to 12 hours postingestion.[8]

Distribution

The NSAIDs are extensively protein bound (98% to 99%), primarily to albumin. Sulindac and indomethacin have slightly lower degrees of binding, in the range of 90% to 93%.[6,20] Principally because of their high protein binding, apparent volumes of distribution are low, ranging from 0.10 to 0.36 L/kg.[6,20] Acute renal insufficiency, liver disease, and hypoalbuminemic states can decrease plasma protein binding and increase volumes of distribution.[20] Plasma protein binding can also decrease when NSAIDs are taken in high doses.

Metabolism

The elimination of NSAIDs is primarily by hepatic biotransformation to metabolites, which are excreted in

TABLE 51-1 Pharmacokinetics of NSAIDs

NSAID	T_{MAX} (hr)	Vd (L/kg)	RENAL EXCRETION OF UNCHANGED DRUG (%)	CLEARANCE (mL/min)	$T_{1/2}$ (hr) (THERAPEUTIC DOSE)	$T_{1/2}$ (hr) (OVERDOSE)
Nonselective COX Inhibitors						
Benzydamine	4–6	1.57	—	160	7.8	>10
Diclofenac	1–3	0.12–0.17	<14	260.4	1–2	41.0
Diflunisal	2–3	0.10	3–5	448.4	48–12	19.4
Etodolac	1.5	0.36	<14	448.4	7.3	—
Fenoprofen	1–2	0.12	2–5	40–90	3.4	
Flurbiprofen	1–2	0.10	20–25	422.4	3–4	
Ibuprofen	0.1–1.5	0.11–0.19	1	470.4	0.42–2.5	1.5–6.4
Indomethacin	1–2	0.12	20	470–140	6.4	3–7
Ketoprofen	0.5–2.4	0.11	<14	487.4	1.5	44.4
Ketorolac	1	0.15–0.33	<58	432.4	4–6	
Meclofenamate	0.5–2.4	—	2–4	190.4	3.4	—
Mefenamic acid	2–3	1.34	<64	—	3–4	2–3
Nabumetone	—	—	<54	—	—	—
Naproxen	2	0.10	<14	445.4	12–15	14.4
Oxaprozin	3–5	0.14–0.18	<14	442.8	21–25	
Phenylbutazone	2	0.24	5	442.5	60–72	
Piroxicam	2	0.12–0.15	10	442.8	38–50	35.4
Sulindac	1	2.44	7	105.4	8.4	—
Tolmetin	0.5–1.4	0.10–1.44	17	125.4	0.41–1.5	
Zomepirac	1	1.84	0–5	180.4	4.4	10.4
Selective COX-2 Inhibitors						
Celecoxib	1.4–2.8	5.7–7.1	2.6	462	11–16	—
Refecoxib	2–3	1.2	<1	119	9–21	—

$t_{1/2}$ elimination half-life; T_{max}, time of maximum concentration; Vd, volume of distribution.
Adapted from Verbeeck RK, Blackburn JL, Loewen GR: Clinical pharmacokinetics of non-steroidal anti-inflammatory drugs. Clin Pharmacokinet 1983;8:302–303.

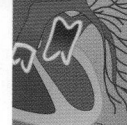

the urine. The major mechanism is conjugation with glucuronic acid, and in some cases this is preceded by oxidation and hydroxylation.[20] Some NSAIDs undergo significant enterohepatic recirculation, including sulindac, indomethacin, diclofenac, flufenamic acid, ibuprofen, phenylbutazone, and piroxicam.[20] Urinary excretion of unchanged drug is less than 5% for most NSAIDs, but larger amounts of indomethacin, flurbiprofen, tolmetin, and piroxicam are eliminated by this route.[20] Sulindac and nabumetone are metabolized to active metabolites.[19]

The elimination half-lives of NSAIDs vary widely and range from as brief as 1 to 1.5 hours for tolmetin, ketoprofen, and diclofenac, 2.5 hours for ibuprofen, and up to 25 to 50 hours for oxaprozin and piroxicam.[20,21] The half-lives of many NSAIDs are also prolonged in neonates and patients in renal failure. In overdose, some NSAIDs follow nonlinear kinetics at high serum levels and have prolonged half-lives, although this did not occur with a massive ingestion of ibuprofen.[21-23] Reported half-lives of NSAIDs in overdose are listed in Table 51-1.[8,20,22-29]

Pregnancy

Most NSAIDs are classified by the U.S. Food and Drug Administration as pregnancy category C or D, indicating that their use in pregnancy is not recommended. Certain propionic derivatives (e.g., ibuprofen, naproxen), however, are classified as pregnancy category B in the first and second trimesters. In the third trimester, all NSAIDs are pregnancy category D due to their ability to produce premature closure of the ductus arteriosus.

DRUG INTERACTIONS

Drug interactions with NSAIDs may be both pharmacokinetic and pharmacodynamic, but the latter is of greatest clinical significance. Significant interactions lead primarily to toxicity from the other agents rather than from the NSAID.

The most serious NSAID interactions are with oral anticoagulants, sulfonylurea agents, and methotrexate.[30] The risk for GI bleeding from NSAIDs is enhanced by coumarin-type anticoagulants. NSAID-induced GI bleeding can also be increased by inhibition of NSAID metabolism by the pyrazolones. Risk for GI bleeding is also increased if NSAIDs are used with alcohol or tobacco, or with other NSAIDs, including COX-2 inhibitors. Methotrexate renal clearance is inhibited by several NSAIDs, and this can result in bone marrow toxic effects and renal or hepatic dysfunction. Lithium clearance may be reduced and lead to increased lithium levels during concurrent use, both by nonselective NSAIDs and COX-2 inhibitors.[31] This is thought to be due to the inhibition of prostaglandins, which are involved in the renal clearance of lithium. NSAIDs may decrease the effect of antihypertensives, including β blockers, angiotensin-converting enzyme inhibitors, central α$_2$-receptor agonists, and angiotensin II blockers.[32] Renal failure may result from concurrent

TABLE 51-2 Drug Interactions with NSAIDs

DRUG	EFFECT
Alcohol	Increased risk for GI bleeding
Antacids	Reduced absorption of NSAIDs
Antihypertensives	Increased risk for NSAID-induced renal failure, reduced antihypertensive effect
Anticoagulants	Increased risk for NSAID-induced GI bleeding; pyrazolones inhibit warfarin metabolism
Aminoglycosides	Decreased renal clearance
Antineoplastic agents	Inreased risk for bleeding due to thrombocytopenia
Cholestyramine	Binds to and interrupts enterohepatic recirculation of NSAIDs, lowers NSAID levels
Cholinesterase inhibitors	Increased risk for GI adverse effects
Corticosteroids	Prolonged concurrent use increases risk for adverse GI effects
Cyclosporine	Increased risk for renal failure; reduced cyclosporine clearance
Sulfinpyrazone	Increased NSAID concentrations; decreased platelet aggregation
Sulfonylureas	Metabolism is inhibited and hypoglycemia enhanced
Methotrexate	Decreased renal clearance
Pemetrexed	Decreased renal clearance
Digoxin	Decreased renal clearance
Lithium	Decreased renal clearance
Ofloxacin/ levofloxacin	Concurrent use may lower seizure threshold
Phenytoin	Displacement of phenytoin from albumin
Diuretics	Effect antagonized by salt and water retention of NSAIDs
SSRIs	Increased risk for GI bleeding due to enhanced antiplatelet activity
Triamterine	Hyperkalemia; indomethacin combination may precipitate renal failure
Valproic acid	Clearance decreased; decreased plasma protein binding

GI, gastrointestinal

diuretic and NSAID use due to inadequate renal blood flow, especially in those who rely upon renal prostaglandins to maintain perfusion. NSAID-drug interactions are summarized in Table 51-2.[30]

TOXICOLOGY

Range of Toxic Effects

Despite their widespread use, reports of serious acute NSAID overdose have been relatively few. They enjoy a wide therapeutic index, and most overdose cases do not result in serious morbidity and mortality. Nevertheless, severe toxic effects and death can occur with large ingestions. Lethal doses have not been firmly established for the various agents.

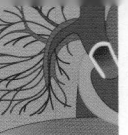

Chronic NSAID use, particularly in the elderly, causes a greater incidence of toxic and adverse effects. The risk for upper GI tract bleeding is 1.5 to 2.7 times higher in those using NSAIDs than in the general population, with an incidence of 1.0 to 3.3 bleeding events per 1000 users.[33]

The enolic acid NSAIDs are thought to be more toxic in overdose than the carboxylic acids.[6,22] However, there are multiple exceptions to this, such as the high incidence of serious neurologic effects with mefenamic acid.[8] In chronic use for rheumatoid arthritis, toxicity was consistently greater for indomethacin, tolmetin, meclofenamate, and ketoprofen, whereas the least toxic were the propionic acids ibuprofen and naproxen.[34] Based on case reports, some ranges of toxic doses and serum levels can be established. However, serum quantification for all NSAIDs is neither generally available nor clinically useful.

Ibuprofen

Because of the frequency of its use, considerable data are available on ibuprofen toxicity. In children, doses of less than 100 mg/kg are very unlikely to induce symptoms. In one study, asymptomatic children had a mean ibuprofen dose of 114 mg/kg, but symptoms occurred in those with a mean ingestion of 440 mg/kg.[25,35] In adults, central nervous system (CNS) symptoms occur only in those who ingest more than 3 g, and renal effects require more than 6 g.[1] Severe symptoms in adults are associated with ingestions of greater than 20 g, although estimated ingestions of up to 60 g have resulted in few or no toxic effects.[1,21,35,36] Complications leading to death have occurred in overdoses of 6.8 g in a child and 24 g in an adult.[25,35]

As with most overdoses, symptoms correlate better with ibuprofen blood levels than with the history of the ingested amount. In one study, all patients with significant symptoms had plasma ibuprofen levels of greater than 50 µg/mL within 10 hours after ingestion.[1] At 1 to 5 hours postingestion, those with symptoms had a significantly greater mean level (294 µg/mL) than those who were asymptomatic (144 µg/mL). Renal impairment is associated with levels greater than 280 µg/mL any time within 10 hours postingestion.[26] Multiple organ failure, including coma, renal failure, GI bleeding, and severe metabolic acidosis, has been reported with levels of greater than 200 to 300 µg/mL at 10 hours postingestion.[21,36] However, levels up to 725 µg/mL have occurred in asymptomatic patients.[36]

A nomogram of ibuprofen plasma levels versus time postingestion has been constructed to predict the likelihood of toxicity (Fig. 51-4).[1] The nomogram plots a semilogarithmic line connecting 100 µg/mL at 1 hour and 25 µg/mL at 12 hours postingestion, below which no significant symptoms are expected to occur. However, most ingestions with levels above the line are characterized by only minor symptoms. Considering that symptoms develop within 4 hours of ingestion in most cases, and that ibuprofen levels are usually not readily available, the utility of the nomogram is minimal.[26,37]

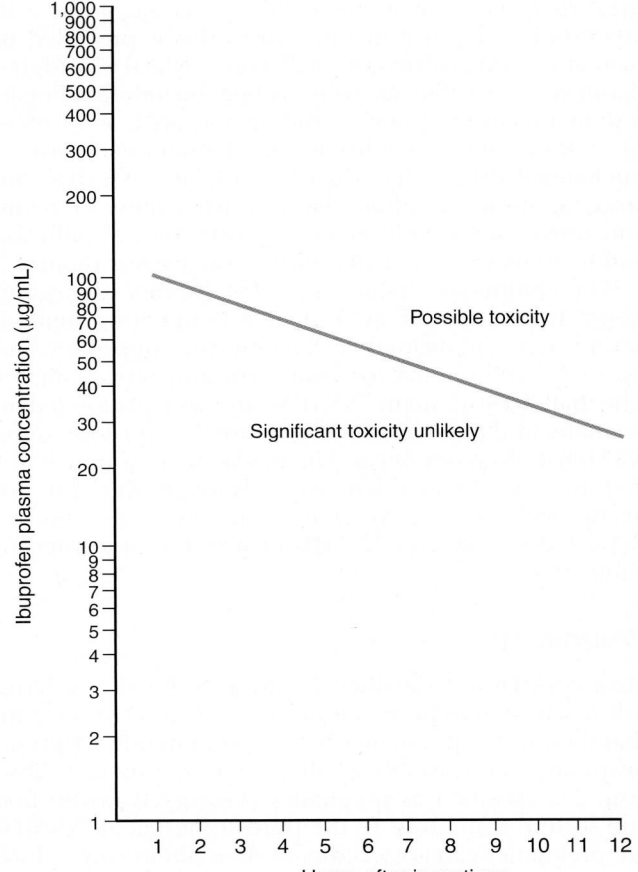

FIGURE 51-4 Nomogram of ibuprofen plasma levels versus time postingestion, used to predict likelihood of toxicity.

Diflunisal

In children, mild GI symptoms and drowsiness can occur with ingestions of 3.5 g. In adults, only mild symptoms are expected with ingestions of less than 7.5 to 10 g.[22] Serious symptoms can occur with as little as 10 g, although usually more than 15 g is required.[22] Death has been reported with an ingestion of 33 g, but a patient who ingested 29 g survived after a deep coma of 10 hours.[38] The plasma diflunisal level was 500 µg/mL at 16 hours postingestion in a patient with severe symptoms.[22] Levels in fatal cases typically exceed 600 µg/mL.[22] Diflunisal is a difluorophenyl derivative of salicylic acid but is not converted to salicylic acid in vivo. Due to its structural similarity to salicylate, diflunisal often produces positive qualitative screens for salicylate and false elevations in serum salicylate concentrations.

Diclofenac

An acute diclofenac overdose of 1500 mg in a 19-year-old man caused confusion and hypotonia.[24] The serum level at 7 hours postingestion during the peak toxic effects was 60.1 µg/mL. A 2-g ingestion resulted in renal injury.[39]

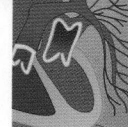

Indomethacin

Doses of 75 to 175 mg in children and 175 to 1500 mg in adults have caused only mild CNS or GI symptoms. In a series of 31 indomethacin overdoses in adults, 61% of patients remained asymptomatic and the rest developed only minor GI toxic effects, drowsiness, headache, and tinnitus.[22] Ingestions of 0.5 and 0.9 g caused mild symptoms and plasma levels of 21 and 84 µg/mL, respectively.[27]

Sulindac

Ingestions of 5 to 8 g of sulindac have resulted in mild GI symptoms and brief courses of hematemesis and renal insufficiency.[39] Ingestions of 10 g or more have caused prolonged courses of renal dysfunction.

Naproxen

Ingestions of 3 to 5 g of naproxen have caused mild GI distress and temporary renal insufficiency.[22,39] Larger overdoses have caused seizures and acidosis.[22,28]

Flurbiprofen

An ingestion of 3 to 6 g in an adult caused coma and respiratory depression, but it was unknown whether other ingestants were involved.[22]

Fenoprofen

Ingestions of 300 to 3000 mg in children and 2 to 15 g in adults have been reported to cause only mild drowsiness, ataxia, tinnitus, and nausea. However, ingestions of as little as 3.75 g in adults have caused hypotension, tachycardia, and tachypnea.[22] Ingestions of greater than 30 g have resulted in hypotension, coma, and renal failure. A postmortem blood level following death from ingestion of an unknown amount was 711 µg/mL.[22]

Ketoprofen

Overdoses of 2 to 5 g in adults have produced only drowsiness, abdominal pain, and vomiting.[22] Ingestion of an unknown amount in an adolescent resulted in seizures, with a serum level of 1128 µg/mL.[23]

Mefenamic Acid

Seizures can occur with acute overdoses only modestly greater than the recommended maximum daily dose of 1.5 g. A 12-year-old had seizures after a 2.5 g ingestion, and adults can suffer convulsions after doses of less than 5 g.[22] Ingestions of 12 to 15 g have produced status epilepticus, coma, and renal failure.[8,22]

Seizures have occurred in patients with mefenamic acid plasma levels at or just above the maximum therapeutic level of 10 µg/mL. In one study, plasma concentrations in patients who had convulsions were significantly higher than in those without (73 versus 38 µg/mL).[8] Most patients with seizures have concentrations above a semilogarithmic line plot connecting 100 µg/mL at 2 hours and 5 µg/mL at 15 hours postingestion.[8] However, seizures can occur with levels well below this line.

Benzydamine

Oral administration of 500 mg of a topical preparation resulted in immediate vomiting, followed 2 hours later by hallucinations lasting 17 hours.[40] No other symptoms or metabolic abnormalities occurred.

Phenylbutazone

Acute phenylbutazone overdoses in children of 1.7 to 3 g result in toxic effects, and death can occur after doses of 2 to 5 g.[22] Severe toxic effects occur in adults after ingestions of 4 to 8 g or more, and death occurs with doses of 14 to 28 g.[9,22]

Piroxicam

Ingestion of 200 to 400 mg appears to cause only mild symptoms, although 100 mg in a child caused severe multisystem toxicity.[22] Doses of 600 mg in adults have the potential for severe toxicity.

CLINICAL EFFECTS

NSAID overdose usually produces minimal or no toxicity. When present, signs and symptoms of toxicity typically include mild GI or neurologic effects such as abdominal pain, nausea, vomiting, lethargy, confusion, headache, or blurred vision.

In studies of acute overdoses of ibuprofen in adults, about 60% remain asymptomatic, 30% to 40% develop mild to moderate symptoms, and fewer than 3% suffer severe symptoms.[1,41] Of the symptomatic group, onset is within 4 hours of ingestion and effects are usually of short duration. Severe and life-threatening toxic effects include metabolic acidosis, GI bleeding, dizziness, seizures, coma, respiratory depression, hypotension, and hepatic and renal injury.

The elderly and those with preexisting renal, cardiovascular, or hepatic disease are at particular risk for development of adverse effects with chronic NSAID use. Most organ systems can be involved, but GI effects are the most common and account for the majority or deaths from chronic use.

Gastrointestinal

GI effects, primarily nausea, vomiting, diarrhea, and abdominal pain, are common in both overdose and chronic use.[22,25,41] The incidence of GI complaints in acute ibuprofen overdose has ranged from 6% to 42%.[35,36,41] The associated fluid losses and resultant dehydration cause hypotension, acidosis, and acute renal failure. Peptic ulceration and GI hemorrhage are rare in acute overdose; the incidence in chronic use is 1.5%.[8,41] Perforation of a duodenal ulcer has been reported

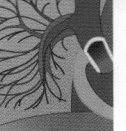

following acute overdose.[42] In another acute overdose, gangrenous ischemic colitis occurred, probably due to inhibition of the cyclooxygenase enzyme, increased vasoconstrictor leukotrienes, and direct injury to GI epithelial cells.[43] Acute mild pancreatitis has also been reported after short courses of NSAIDs.[44]

Neurologic

CNS depression is one of the most common effects of NSAID overdose and chronic use.[4,22,25] In one series of ibuprofen overdose cases, CNS effects occurred in 30% of patients.[36] CNS effects may range from drowsiness to coma. Coma can occur independent of hypotension, respiratory depression, seizures, or acidosis.[45] Decreased memory and ability to concentrate have been reported with chronic NSAID use, particularly in the elderly taking indomethacin, sulindac, and naproxen.[4]

Seizures occur most commonly after mefenamic overdose, but they have also been reported in overdoses of naproxen, phenylbutazone, piroxicam, ibuprofen, and ketoprofen.[8,22,25,28] Acute delirium, psychosis, hallucinations, and myoclonus have been described, particularly with indomethacin, sulindac, diclofenac, benzydamine, and mefenamic acid, but also with ibuprofen.[4,8,40,46,47] The mechanism for these CNS effects is unexplained, but the structural similarities that indomethacin and sulindac have with serotonin suggest a possible causal role from this neurotransmitter.

Aseptic meningitis has occurred rarely with therapeutic NSAID use, usually in patients with systemic lupus erythematosus, but it can occur in otherwise healthy patients.[4] Other neurologic effects include tinnitus, deafness, ataxia, nystagmus, headache, and disorientation.[6,27]

Metabolic

Metabolic acidosis has been described in adults and children, usually in association with coma, seizures, hypotension, or renal failure.[22,28,35,48] However, metabolic acidosis with increased anion gap has also been reported in the absence of these other effects.[1] Acidosis may be remarkably severe, with a serum pH of less than 7.1, and serum bicarbonate of less than 10 mEq/L despite only mild hypotension.[48,49] The weakly acidic nature of NSAIDs and their metabolites may account for some of this acidosis, along with possible uncoupling of oxidative phosphorylation.[41,50]

Hyperkalemia is a reported but unusual complication of NSAIDs after therapeutic use and overdose.[16] Hyperkalemia could be the result of direct NSAID effect on cellular potassium uptake and delivery to distal renal tubules or of transient renal impairment. Hyponatremia and fluid losses result from both NSAID-induced gastroenteritis and inhibition of prostaglandin-mediated diuresis and natriuresis.

Hematologic

Thrombocytopenia, prolonged prothrombin times, agranulocytosis, and pancytopenia have been reported with acute ibuprofen, piroxicam, naproxen, and etodolac overdoses.[27,51] Decrease of platelet aggregation and adhesiveness contribute to bleeding disorders and GI hemorrhage. With therapeutic use, hematologic effects are uncommon, but they cause a disproportionate number of deaths. Aplastic anemia, agranulocytosis, hemolytic anemia, and thrombocytopenia have been associated with therapeutic use of various NSAIDs.[41,44,52]

Hepatic

Hepatotoxicity of both hepatocellular and cholestatic types has occurred with use of all classes of NSAIDs, but it is most common with phenylbutazone and sulindac. The incidence of chronic NSAID-induced hepatic injury is low at 1.1 events per 100,000 prescriptions, and it is seen only rarely in acute overdose.[53] The usual finding is mild elevation of transaminase levels, which resolves after discontinuation of the drug. More severe involvement can occur as part of multiorgan involvement. The at-risk populations appear to be the elderly and patients with autoimmune connective tissue diseases. The mechanism of hepatotoxicity is likely a hypersensitivity reaction. One case report described subfulminant liver failure requiring transplantation, but there was also a history of alcohol abuse and arterial hypertension.[54]

Renal

Problems associated with chronic use of NSAIDs are now among the most common reasons for hospitalization of patients with renal function abnormalities. It has been estimated that about 1% of those taking NSAIDs on a chronic basis will develop some deterioration of renal function.[16] In acute overdose, renal failure has also been well described in case series and in isolated case reports.[25,54-56]

Acute renal insufficiency, as a result of alterations in renal blood flow and glomerular filtration rates, is the most common renal complication. Those dependent on prostaglandin-mediated renal regulation are most at risk, including those with volume depletion, congestive heart failure, cirrhosis, hypoalbuminemia, advanced age, and preexisting renal disease.[54] However, renal failure has also been described after acute overdose in healthy individuals and in brief therapeutic use after binge alcohol drinking.[25,54-56] This may be mediated by increased formation of the leukotrienes, causing renal vasoconstriction and mesangial cell contraction.[55] The renal insufficiency is typically mild; it resolves within 24 to 72 hours and may be oliguric or nonoliguric. The presentation consists of flank pain, elevated blood urea nitrogen (BUN) and creatinine levels, and, in chronic cases, weight gain and hyperkalemia. Urinalysis may show microscopic hematuria and cell casts. In cases associated with other severe manifestations such as coma, acidosis, and hypotension, recovery may be prolonged and require hemodialysis.[48]

Acute interstitial nephritis and the nephrotic syndrome have been reported after short courses of NSAIDs or with chronic use.[10] This syndrome has most often been

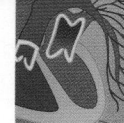

associated with the acetic and propionic acid derivatives and is a hypersensitivity reaction.[15] Proteinuria is usually, but not always, present. Hemodialysis is required in as many as a third of these cases.[10]

Cardiopulmonary

Hypotension and tachycardia, most likely secondary to volume depletion, occur in fewer than 5% of cases.[25,41] Congestive heart failure may result from chronic NSAID-induced fluid and salt retention.[41] Most recently, the COX-2 inhibitors have been found to be associated with an increased risk for cardiovascular adverse effects.[14,57,58] In one study, rofecoxib was associated with a greater than twofold increased risk of a thrombotic cardiovascular event as compared with naproxen; no increased risk for adverse cardiovascular events was associated with the use of celecoxib in two other studies.[18,58] In another trial, however, celecoxib at doses of greater than or equal to 400 mg/day was associated with a 2.5 to 3.4 times greater risk for a cardiovascular event as compared with placebo.[18] As a result of these reports, rofecoxib has been withdrawn from the U.S. market and warnings issued to avoid COX-2 inhibitors as first-line therapy, particularly for those with cardiovascular risk factors.[18]

Respiratory depression and arrest are unusual-but-reported manifestations of NSAID overdose.[25,45] Adult respiratory distress syndrome has occurred in the setting of severe multiorgan toxic effects.[48] This may be due to prostaglandin inhibition causing increased alveolar capillary permeability.[48] Bronchospasm may be precipitated by NSAIDs, especially in persons with drug allergies or asthma.[41]

DIAGNOSIS

NSAID toxicity should be suspected in the case of any overdose that is accompanied by a symptom constellation of gastroenteritis, CNS depression, metabolic acidosis, and renal insufficiency. Ibuprofen (and other NSAIDs) should be included in the differential diagnosis of an increased anion gap acidosis, particularly in large overdoses with very low serum bicarbonate levels and serum pH. The clinical appearance with NSAID toxicity can mimic that with salicylate toxicity (acidosis, tachypnea, altered mental status, gastritis) without tinnitus, and salicylate levels should be measured to exclude this diagnosis. Note that diflunisal cross-reacts with some salicylate assays to produce false-positive results.[59] NSAID toxicity should also be suspected with a history of over-the-counter analgesic ingestion when acetaminophen and salicylates are undetected in the blood.

Laboratory studies for serious overdoses should include assay of electrolytes with anion gap calculation, complete blood count, coagulation studies, and arterial blood gas, BUN, creatinine, and transaminase levels. Renal insufficiency is unlikely to occur if an adult ingests less than 6 g, so renal function tests are not routinely necessary in these cases.[1] In patients at high risk for renal or hepatic complications, baseline renal and liver function tests should be performed prior to initiating NSAID therapy and again in 5 to 7 days.

Routine ibuprofen assays are not particularly useful or predictive of outcomes, and are not routinely available.[41] However, quantification of ibuprofen levels might be useful to determine if an initially asymptomatic patient will remain so. If the ibuprofen level is in the "significant toxicity unlikely" region (see Fig. 51-4), the patient can safely be discharged from medical care without further observation.[1]

MANAGEMENT

Supportive Measures

The therapy of NSAID toxicity is primarily supportive and symptomatic, and there is no antidote. Early correction of any volume depletion is essential to maintain adequate renal blood flow, and 1 to 2 L (15 to 20 mL/kg) normal saline should be given rapidly. Hypotension usually responds to fluid replacement, but a short course of vasopressors may be required. Dopamine may be the best option to maintain renal blood flow in patients at high risk for renal insufficiency.[45] Acidosis should resolve with aggressive hydration, but intravenous (IV) administration of 1 to 2 mEq/kg sodium bicarbonate may be required if the serum pH is less than 7.1.

The coagulopathies of NSAID overdose rarely warrant specific therapy unless active bleeding is occurring. In such cases, fresh frozen plasma and 10 mg phytonadione (vitamin K_1) subcutaneously would be appropriate.

Seizures may require immediate therapy with benzodiazepines, such as 5 to 10 mg IV (0.2 mg/kg in children) diazepam. As with most drug-induced seizures, phenytoin is unlikely to be effective, and long-term treatment is usually unnecessary.

Antacids, H_2-receptor antagonists, and/or sucralfate may be considered for reducing any prolonged GI effects.[6]

Decontamination

Activated charcoal has been shown to reduce absorption of ibuprofen, piroxicam, mefenamic acid, and phenylbutazone, and it is likely to adsorb other NSAIDs as well.[6,60] Single-dose activated charcoal is the GI decontamination procedure of choice. Syrup of ipecac and gastric lavage have also been recommended, but effectiveness of these methods has not been studied in NSAID overdose.

Decontamination has been recommended if the amount ingested is more than 10 times the therapeutic dose for adults or 5 times the dose for children.[6] For ibuprofen, decontamination is thought to be unnecessary in children if less than 100 mg/kg is ingested (10 times the therapeutic dose).[25] Although syrup of ipecac has been suggested for child ingestions of ibuprofen of 100 to 400 mg/kg, the symptoms created by ipecac are indistinguishable from ibuprofen toxicity in this dosage range.[6,25,41] Because of the rapid absorption of NSAIDs, it is unlikely that decontamination will be of benefit more

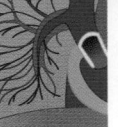
than 2 to 4 hours postingestion.[6,20] Patients who have taken overdoses of NSAIDs that carry a high risk for seizures (e.g., mefenamic acid), CNS depression (e.g., phenylbutazone), or large amounts of other NSAIDs (e.g., more than 400 mg/kg of ibuprofen) should not be given syrup of ipecac.[6,25]

Elimination Enhancement

Because NSAIDs are greater than 90% protein bound, extensively metabolized, and excreted in essentially unchanged form, it is unlikely that elimination would be enhanced by any method.[6,20] This has been supported by a lack of efficacy of hemodialysis and hemoperfusion in limited studies.[6,9] Nevertheless, hemoperfusion has been employed in phenylbutazone overdoses with some limited success.[6] Hemodialysis may be necessary in cases of prolonged or severe renal failure following NSAID overdose.[10,48]

Multiple doses of activated charcoal have been reported to enhance the elimination of phenylbutazone, indomethacin, and piroxicam by interrupting entero-hepatic and/or enteroenteric recirculation.[6,60] This benefit might also be expected in sulindac, diclofenac, flufenamic acid, and ibuprofen, all of which also undergo some enterohepatic recirculation.[25] However, this therapy would be warranted only in the small number of severely symptomatic patients.

DISPOSITION

Ingestions of greater than 10 times the therapeutic dose of NSAIDs other than ibuprofen in adults, or greater than 5 times in children, probably warrant observation in a medical facility for 4 to 6 hours postingestion.[6,25] For ibuprofen, ingestions of more than 300 mg/kg in children and more than 6 to 20 g in adults warrant observation.[25] Mild symptoms usually resolve quickly and may not necessitate hospitalization. The development of CNS depression, acidosis, seizures, or renal insufficiency should mandate admission and careful monitoring.

REFERENCES

1. Hall AH, Smolinske SC, Stover B, et al: Ibuprofen overdose in adults. J Toxicol Clin Toxicol 1992;30:23.
2. Watson WA, Litovitz TL, Klein-Schwartz W, et al: 2003 annual report of the American Association of Poison Control Centers Toxic Exposure Surveillance System. Am J Emerg Med 2004;22:335–404.
3. Volans G, Monaghan J, Colbridge M: Ibuprofen overdose. Int J Clin Pract Suppl 2003;135:54–60.
4. Hoppmann RA, Peden JG, Ober SK: Central nervous system side effects of nonsteroidal anti-inflammatory drugs. Arch Intern Med 1991;151:1309.
5. Simon LS: Actions and toxicity of nonsteroidal anti-inflammatory drugs. Curr Opin Rheumatol 1995;7:159.
6. Vale JA, Meredith TJ: Acute poisoning due to non-steroidal anti-inflammatory drugs. Clinical features and management. Med Toxicol 1986;1:12.
7. Boynton CS, Dick CF, Mayor GH: NSAIDs: an overview. J Clin Pharmacol 1988;28:512.
8. Balali-Mood M, Critchley JA, Proudfoot AT, Prescott LF: Mefenamic acid overdosage. Lancet 1981;1(8234):1354.

9. Prescott LF, Critchley JAJH, Balali-Mood M: Phenylbutazone overdosage: abnormal metabolism associated with hepatic and renal damage. BMJ 1980;281:1106.
10. Abt AB, Oh JY, Huntington RA, et al: Chinese herbal medicine induced acute renal failure. Arch Intern Med 1995;155:211.
11. Graeme KA, Morkunas A: Nonsteroidal antiinflammatory drugs. In Brent J, Wallace KL, Burkhart KK, et al (eds): Critical Care Toxicology. Philadelphia, Elsevier Mosby, 2005, pp 631–640.
12. Oviedo JA, Wolfe M: Clinical potential of cyclo-oxygenase-2 inhibitors. Biodrugs 2001;15:563–572.
13. Tacconelli S, Capone ML, Patrignani P: Clinical pharmacology of novel selective COX-2 inhibitors. Curr Pharm Des 2004;10:589–601.
14. Mukherjee D, Nissen SE, Topol EJ: Risk of cardiovascular events associated with selective COX-2 inhibitors. Can Fam Physician 2002;48:1449–1451.
15. Aronoff GR: Nonsteroidal anti-inflammatory drug induced renal syndromes. J Ky Med Assoc 1992;90:336.
16. Whelton A, Hamilton CW: Non-steroidal anti-inflammatory drugs: effects on kidney function. J Clin Pharmacol 1991;31:588.
17. Boelsterli UA, Zimmerman HJ, Kretz-Rommel A: Idiosyncratic liver toxicity of nonsteroidal antiinflammatory drugs: molecular mechanisms and pathology. Crit Rev Toxicol 1995;25:207.
18. Finckh A, Aronson MD: Cardiovascular risks of cyclooxygenase-2 inhibitors: where we stand now. Ann Intern Med 2005;142:212–213.
19. Murray MD, Brater DC: Renal toxicity of the nonsteroidal anti-inflammatory drugs. Annu Rev Pharmacol Toxicol 1993;33:435.
20. Verbeeck RK, Blackburn JL, Loewen GR: Clinical pharmaco-kinetics of non-steroidal antiinflammatory drugs. Clin Pharmacokinet 1983;8:297.
21. Seifert SA, Bronstein AC, McGuire T: Massive ibuprofen ingestion with survival. Clin Toxicol 2000;38:55–57.
22. Court H, Volans GN: Poisoning after overdose with non-steroidal and anti-inflammatory drugs. Adverse Drug React Toxicol Rev 1984;3:1.
23. Bond GR, Curry SC, Arnold-Capell PA, et al: Generalized seizures and metabolic acidosis after ketoprofen overdose. Vet Hum Toxicol 1989;31:369.
24. Netter P, Lambert H, Larcan A, et al: Diclofenac sodium-chlormezanone poisoning. Eur J Clin Pharmacol 1984;26:535.
25. Hall AH, Smolinske SC, Conrad FL, et al: Ibuprofen overdose: 126 cases. Ann Emerg Med 1986;15:1308.
26. Jenkinson ML, Fitzpatrick R, Streete PJ, et al: The relationship between plasma ibuprofen concentrations and toxicity in acute ibuprofen overdose. Hum Toxicol 1988;7:319.
27. Sheehan TMT, Boldy DAR, Vale JA, et al: Indomethacin poisoning. Clin Toxicol 1986;24:151.
28. Martinez R, Smith DW, Frankel LR: Severe metabolic acidosis after acute naproxen sodium ingestion. Ann Emerg Med 1989;18:129.
29. Backer RC, Kshirsagar VH, Sopher IM: Case report: zomepirac suicide. J Anal Toxicol 1983;7:223.
30. Johnson AG, Seideman P, Day RO: Adverse drug interactions with nonsteroidal anti-inflammatory drugs (NSAIDs): recognition, management and avoidance. Drug Saf 1993;8:99.
31. Phelan KM, Mosholder AD, Lu S: Lithium interaction with the cyclooxygenase 2 inhibitors rofecoxib and celecoxib and other nonsteroidal anti-inflammatory drugs. J Clin Psychiatry 2003;64:1328–1334.
32. Frishman WH: Effects of nonsteroidal anti-inflammatory drug therapy on blood pressure and peripheral edema. Am J Cardiol 2002;89(Suppl):18D–25D.
33. Carson JL, Willett LR: Toxicity of nonsteroidal anti-inflammatory drugs: an overview of the epidemiological evidence. Drugs 1993;46(Suppl 1):243.
34. Fries JF, Williams CA, Bloch DA: The relative toxicity of non-steroidal antiinflammatory drugs. Arthritis Rheum 1991;34:1353.
35. Hall AH, Rumack BH: Treatment of patients with ibuprofen overdose. Ann Emerg Med 1988;17:185.
36. Court H, Streete P, Volans GN: Overdose with ibuprofen causing unconsciousness and hypotension. BMJ 1981;282:1073.
37. McElwee NE, Veltri JC, Bradford DC, et al: A prospective, population-based study of acute ibuprofen overdose: complications are rare and routine serum levels not warranted. Ann Emerg Med 1990;19:657.
38. Upadhyay HP, Gupta SK: Diflunisal (Dolobid) overdose. BMJ 1978;2:640.

39. Kulling PE, Backman EA, Skagius AS: Renal impairment after acute diclofenac, naproxen, and sulindac overdoses. J Toxicol Clin Toxicol 1995;33:173.
40. Gomez-Lopez L, Hernandez-Rodriguez J, Pou J, Nogue S: Acute overdose due to benzydamine. Hum Exp Toxicol 1999;18:471–473.
41. Halpern SM, Fitzpatrick R, Volans GN: Ibuprofen toxicity: a review of adverse reactions and overdose. Adverse Drug React Toxicol Rev 1993;12:107.
42. Clarke SFJ, Arepalli N, Armstrong C, Dargan PI: Duodenal perforation after ibuprofen overdose. J Toxicol Clin Toxicol 2004;42:983–985.
43. Appu S, Thompson G: Gangrenous ischaemic colitis following non-steroidal anti-inflammatory drug overdose. ANZ J Surg 2001;71:694–695.
44. Jick SS, Walker AM, Perera DR, et al: Non-steroidal anti-inflammatory drugs and hospital admission for perforated peptic ulcer. Lancet 1987;2:380.
45. Bright TP, McNulty CJ: Suspected central nervous system toxicity from inadvertent nonsteroidal antiinflammatory drug overdose. DICP 1991;25:1066.
46. Ritter A, Eskin B: Ibuprofen overdose presenting with severe agitation and hypothermia. Am J Emerg Med 1998;16:549–550.
47. Bright TP, McNulty CJ: Suspected central nervous system toxicity from inadvertent nonsteroidal antiinflmmatory drug overdose. DICP 1991;25:1066–1067.
48. Le HT, Bosse GM, Tasi YY: Ibuprofen overdose complicated by renal failure, adult respiratory distress syndrome, and metabolic acidosis. J Toxicol Clin Toxicol 1994;32:315.
49. Wolfe TR: Ibuprofen overdose. Am J Emerg Med 1995;13:375.
50. Masabuchi Y, Yamada S, Horie T: Possible mechanism of hepatocyte injury induced by diphenylamine and its structurally related non-steroidal anti-inflammatory drugs. J Pharmacol Exp Ther 2000;292:982–987.
51. Waugh PK, Keatinge DW: Hypoprothrombinemia in naproxen overdosage. Drug Intell Clin Pharmacol 1983;17:549.
52. Inman WHW: Study of fatal bone marrow depression with special reference to phenylbutazone and oxyphenbutazone. BMJ 1977;1:1500.
53. Rodriguez LAG, Williams R, Derby LE, et al: Acute liver injury associated with nonsteroidal anti-inflammatory drugs and the role of risk factors. Arch Intern Med 1994;154:311.
54. Wen SF, Parthasarathy R, Iliopoulos O, et al: Acute renal failure following binge drinking and nonsteroidal antiinflammatory drugs. Am J Kidney Dis 1992;20:281.
55. Perazella MA, Buller GK: Can ibuprofen cause acute renal failure in a normal individual? A case of acute overdose. Am J Kidney Dis 1991;18:600.
56. Kim J, Gazarian M, Verjee Z, et al: Acute renal insufficiency in ibuprofen overdose. Pediatr Emerg Care 1995;11:107.
57. Kimmel SE, Berlin JA, Reilly M, et al: Patients exposed to rofecoxib and celecoxib have different odds of nonfatal myocardial infarction. Ann Intern Med 2005;142:157–164.
58. Silverstein FE, Faich G, Goldstein JL, et al: Gastrointestinal toxicity with celecoxib vs nonsteriodal anti-inflammatory drugs for osteoarthritis and rheumatoid arthritis: The CLASS study: A randomized controlled trial. JAMA 2000;284:1247–1255.
59. Smolinske SC, Hall AH, Vandenberg SA, et al: Toxic effects of non-steroidal anti-inflammatory drugs in overdose. Drug Saf 1990;5:252–274.
60. Laufen H, Leitold M: The effect of activated charcoal on the bioavailability of piroxicam in man. Int J Clin Pharmacol Ther Toxicol 1986;24:48.

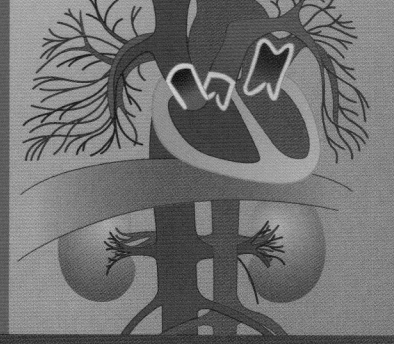

SECTION D
ANTIMICROBIAL, CHEMOTHERAPEUTIC, AND IMMUNOSUPPRESSIVE AGENTS

52 *Antibacterial and Antifungal Agents*

MELISSA L. GIVENS, MD, MPH ■ JAVIER R. CALDERA, MD ■ ROUHOLLAH PRUEITT, MD

At a Glance...

- Antibacterial and antifungal agents include a broad range of chemically and toxicologically diverse substances.
- The major toxicities from antibacterial and antifungal agents result from adverse effects of therapeutic dosing and consist primarily of hypersensitivity reactions.
- In overdose, selected antibacterial and antifungal agents have significant toxicity. These include seizures from penicillins, renal injury from aminoglycosides and amphotericin, cardiovascular collapse from chloramphenicol, and "gasping baby syndrome" from benzyl alcohol.
- The imidazole antifungal agents (e.g., ketoconazole) are potent inhibitors of CYP3A4, producing significant drug-drug interactions.
- Treatment of antibacterial and antifungal overdose is supportive.

Antibiotics are a diverse class of medications used to kill microorganisms. They can cause adverse effects from hypersensitivity reactions, drug-drug interactions, and direct drug toxicity. Many of the complications associated with antibiotic toxicity occur with routine use or as a result of iatrogenic complications; they are less often related to intentional abuse. Antibiotics are well known to be involved in drug-drug interactions, primarily through cytochrome P-450 interactions (Box 52-1), but also through various other mechanisms.

Because antibiotics are commonly prescribed both for use in the hospital and in the home, they are a common source of toxic exposures. There were 65,623 cases of human exposure to antibiotics reported to the American Association of Poison Control Centers (AAPCC) Toxic Exposure Surveillance System (TESS) in 2003, which accounted for 2.7% of all exposures.[1] Fortunately, antibiotic toxicity rarely results in death. In the 2003 TESS data, only three deaths were attributed solely to antimicrobial toxicity. Two deaths were a result of exposure to parenteral tilmicosin, a veterinary-grade macrolide, and one death occurred in a suicidal ingestion of hydroxychloroquine and methotrexate.[1]

HISTORY

The discovery of antibiotics constitutes one of medicine's major breakthroughs. Antimicrobial efficacy predates Alexander Fleming because the use of sulfonamide subcutaneously lowered the mortality from meningococcal meningitis from 70% to 90% to about 10%.[2] Fleming's discovery of the inhibition of staphylococcal growth by the mold *Penicillium notatum* while cleaning his laboratory at Saint Mary's Medical School in London in 1928 was a landmark moment in medicine. Fleming later received the Nobel Prize along with Florey and Chain for the discovery and use of penicillin in infectious disease. Other fortuitous discoveries, such as cephalosporin C–producing organisms found in sewer water, further advanced the science of antimicrobials.[3]

HYPERSENSITIVITY REACTIONS

A history of antibiotic hypersensitivity, or drug allergy, is reported in as many as 25% of hospitalized patients.[4] Hypersensitivity reactions occur as a result of immunologic phenomena, are unpredictable, and are independent

---

BOX 52-1	ANTIBIOTICS WITH IMPORTANT P-450 EFFECTS
Inhibitors	**Inducers**
Azole antifungals (CYP3A4)	Rifampin/rifabutin (CYP1A2,
Ciprofloxacin/enoxacin > norfloxin (CYP1A2)	2C, 3A4)
Clarithromycin/erythromycin (CYP3A4)	
Metronidazole	
Sulfonamides (CYP2C9)	
Trimethoprim	

Data from Gregg CR: Drug interaction and anti-infective therapies. Am J Med 1999;106:227–237.

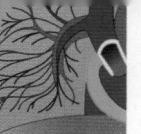

of the expected pharmacology of the drug. Risk factors for hypersensitivity are most closely tied to the chemical properties of the medication, but may also be related to dose, route of administration, duration of treatment, and host factors such as age, gender, atopy, and genetic polymorphisms.[5,6] An allergic response requires previous exposure to the drug or to an immunochemically related substance and usually occurs within the first 2 weeks of administration.[7] There are also pseudo-allergic (anaphylactoid) responses, which are immunoglobulin E (IgE)–independent reactions clinically indistinguishable from an IgE-mediated reaction. The most classic example of an anaphylactoid reaction occurs in response to radiocontrast material, but anaphylactoid reactions have been reported with antibiotics such as ciprofloxacin.[8,9] Vancomycin and polymyxin are also known to cause direct release of mediators from mast cells, which results in urticaria or even anaphylaxis-like symptoms.[10] Other investigators have used the term *pseudo-anaphylactic* for well-described reactions following the administration of procaine penicillin. This response is believed to be related to the procaine and not the β-lactam structure.[11]

True drug allergy requires an antigen-antibody reaction. Most drugs are low-molecular-weight compounds that cannot alone prompt an antibody response. However, when these drugs, or more commonly their metabolites, bind to carrier molecules, antigenic processing can occur. β-Lactam antibiotics are well-known haptens that can bind to carrier molecules both as parent drug and as highly reactive metabolites.[12] Cross-reactivity is often a concern, especially among β-lactam antibiotics such as penicillins and cephalosporins, which share the β-lactam ring structure.[13,14] The true extent of cephalosporin cross-reactivity in penicillin-allergic patients is hard to determine because much variability exists in the literature. The risk for allergic reactions to cephalosporins in penicillin-allergic patients can be from two times to four times the normal population.[15,16] To further confound the issue, many patients who are sensitive to penicillin also have a higher incidence of hypersensitivity reaction to immunologically unrelated compounds.[12,17,18] In addition, immunohematologic reactions must be considered separately because they are usually IgG and IgM mediated in comparison with IgE-mediated

anaphylaxis and urticaria.[15] Skin testing in penicillin-allergic patients reveals a 30% to 50% cephalosporin cross-reactivity of IgE antibodies.[19] However, only about 50% to 70% of those with IgE reactivity to penicillin will develop clinical symptoms, and this reaction rate is expected to be much lower with cephalosporins, especially second- and third-generation drugs.[16,20-22] Many authors recommend avoiding administration of β-lactam antibiotics to penicillin-allergic patients until formal skin testing and desensitization (if indicated) has been performed.[5,7,12,23-26] Unfortunately, the majority of patients who suffer anaphylaxis have no prior history of systemic reaction.[27] Cephalosporins are not the only β lactams with cross-reactivity. Carbapenems show similar cross-reactivity and should be used with discretion in penicillin-allergic patients.[28] The monobactam aztreonam lacks an adjoining ring structure to the β-lactam ring and thus has negligible cross-reactivity and is weakly immunogenic in general.[29-31]

Immunologic reactions can precipitate an array of responses. Table 52-1 is a synopsis of the four types of immunologic response as described by Gell and Coombs. Penicillin alone has been known to cause all four types of immunologic response. Immune responses to drugs can also be classified by clinical presentation and organ system involvement, as described below.

Multisystem Involvement

Because anaphylaxis and anaphylactoid reactions produce similar clinical reactions, they can both be considered multisystem, generalized reactions and will be discussed together.

ANAPHYLAXIS

Portier and Richet were the first to describe anaphylaxis (from Greek *ana*, meaning "backward," and *phylaxis*, meaning "protection") after dogs paradoxically reacted to repeat exposure of a sea anemone–derived toxin intended to produce a protective immunization effect.[32] Richet earned a Nobel Prize in 1913 for his work related to anaphylaxis and is recognized as the founder of the science of allergy.

Antibiotics, especially penicillins, are the leading cause of anaphylaxis in the United States.[33,34] Penicillins

---

TABLE 52-1 Gell and Coombs' Classification of Immune Reactions

CLASSIFICATION	IMMUNOREACTANTS	CLINICAL PRESENTATION	EXAMPLE
Type I	Mast cell mediated IgE dependent IgE independent	Anaphylaxis, urticaria, angioedema, asthma, rhinitis	Penicillin anaphylaxis
Type II	Antibody mediated IgG and IgM	Immune cytopenias Organ inflammation	Amoxicillin: hemolytic anemia Sulfonamide: thrombocytopenia
Type III	Immune complex Complement IgG/IgM immune complexes	Serum sickness, vasculitis	Drug fever Cefaclor serum sickness–like reaction
Type IV	T-lymphocyte mediated Type 1 cytokines	Contact dermatitis	Topical penicillin

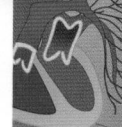

TABLE 52-2 Antibotics Known to Cause Anaphylaxis/Anaphylactoid Reaction

SUBSTANCE	IgE MEDIATED
β lactams	Yes
Tetracyclines	Yes
Sulfonamides	Yes
Nitrofurantoin	Possible
Streptomycin	Possible
Vancomycin	No
Chloramphenicol	No
Ciprofloxacin	No
Amphotericin B	No

are reported to cause fatal anaphylaxis at a rate of 0.002% and nonfatal anaphylaxis at a rate of 0.7% to 10%.[14,35] Penicillins and radiocontrast material may be responsible for 1300 of the predicted 1500 annual deaths from anaphylaxis/anaphylactoid reactions. Although parenteral administration is frequently associated with anaphylaxis, oral administration may also cause anaphylaxis and death.[36] Table 52-2 lists some drugs known to cause anaphylactic and anaphylactoid reactions.[8,9,37]

Pathophysiology

Anaphylaxis is a result of IgE-mediated release of chemical mediators from mast cells and basophils. The reaction is initiated when an allergen combines with an IgE antibody bound to the surface membranes of mast cells and basophils, leading to a signal transduction cascade that results in degranulation and the release of anaphylaxis mediators. Histamine, a preformed mediator stored in mast cell and basophil cytoplasmic granules, can cause bronchoconstriction, vasodilatation, enhanced mucus secretion, and enhanced vascular permeability by acting on histamine (H_1 and H_2 receptors). Other preformed mast cell mediators include neutral proteases such as tryptase, acid hydrolase, oxidative enzymes, chemotactic factors, and proteoglycans. Tryptase is often used as a clinical marker for anaphylaxis because it peaks 60 to 90 minutes after anaphylaxis onset, but its role in the pathophysiology of anaphylaxis is not yet fully understood.[36,38,39]

Leukotrienes B4, C4, and E4; prostaglandin D_2; and platelet-activating factor are membrane-derived mediators formed from arachidonic acid metabolism. Release of these mediators can cause bronchoconstriction, mucus secretion, and alterations in vascular permeability.[35,40] Platelet-activating factor can additionally lower blood pressure and activate clotting.[41] These mediators, in addition to the activation of other proinflammatory pathways and enhanced nitric oxide synthesis, can lead to a severe systemic reaction with the potential for disastrous outcomes.[40]

Clinical Presentation

Clinical features of anaphylaxis include a variety of organ systems. The majority of patients with anaphylaxis manifest symptoms within 1 hour of exposure, but delayed onset has been reported.[35] Cutaneous involvement may present as urticaria, flushing, pruritis, erythema, or even angioedema. Mucous membrane congestion is commonly reported along with edema of the tongue or lips, and even edema of the larynx or epiglottis, which may lead to airway obstruction. Bronchoconstriction, manifested as chest tightness, shortness of breath, or wheezing, can lead to severe hypoxia and hypercapnia. Cardiovascular compromise from distributive shock can be profound. There are also reports of cardiac arrhythmias and evidence of tissue ischemia.[42] Central nervous system hypoperfusion can lead to dizziness, confusion, seizures, and loss of consciousness. Gastrointestinal (GI) disturbances such as nausea, vomiting, abdominal pain, and diarrhea also may occur.[35]

Treatment

Anaphylaxis is a life-threatening reaction that requires immediate medical attention and aggressive supportive care (Fig. 52-1). The first step is to remove the antigenic source as soon as features of anaphylaxis develop. Other treatment modalities are aimed at counteracting mediator release, supporting vital functions, and preventing further mediator release. Special attention should be directed to airway, breathing, and circulation. The patient should have large-bore intravenous access and continuous cardiovascular and pulse oximetry monitoring. Early airway support may be crucial in the setting of laryngeal edema.

Epinephrine is the mainstay of treatment in anaphylaxis.[5] The β1 effects support cardiac output, the β2 stimulation promotes smooth muscle relaxation aiding in bronchial dilation, while the α effects counteract mediator-induced vasodilatation. Epinephrine may also prevent further release of anaphylactic mediators. Epinephrine is administered as a 1:1000 solution, and the standard dose is 0.3 mL intramuscularly in adult patients with urticaria and reactive airways with stable blood pressure. The pediatric dose is 0.01 mL/kg of the 1:1000 solution. In the setting of hypotension or cardiac arrest, 1 mg of epinephrine may be given intravenously as a 1:10,000 solution (0.1 mL/kg in children). Persistent hypotension may require a continuous infusion, and there is much variability in the literature regarding concentrations and dosage.[43] Advanced cardiac life support guidelines recommend diluting 30 mg of 1:1000 epinephrine (30 mL) in 250 mL of normal saline or 5% dextrose, starting the infusion at 100 mL/hr, and then titrating to effect.[44] Patients who receive epinephrine should be closely monitored for side effects, which include cardiac arrhythmias, myocardial ischemia, or severe hypertension. Patients on β-adrenergic blocking agents may have hypotension refractory to epinephrine.[45] These patients may require 1 to 5 mg glucagon given as a bolus followed by a glucagon infusion run at 5 to 15 µg/min.[36,46] Patients should also receive intravenous fluids for vascular support.

Supplemental oxygen may be necessary for patients with cardiac or respiratory symptoms. Clinical signs of airway reactivity, such as wheezing and chest tightness, may require inhaled β agonists in addition to epinephrine. Corticosteroids (hydrocortisone 5 mg/kg or

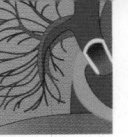

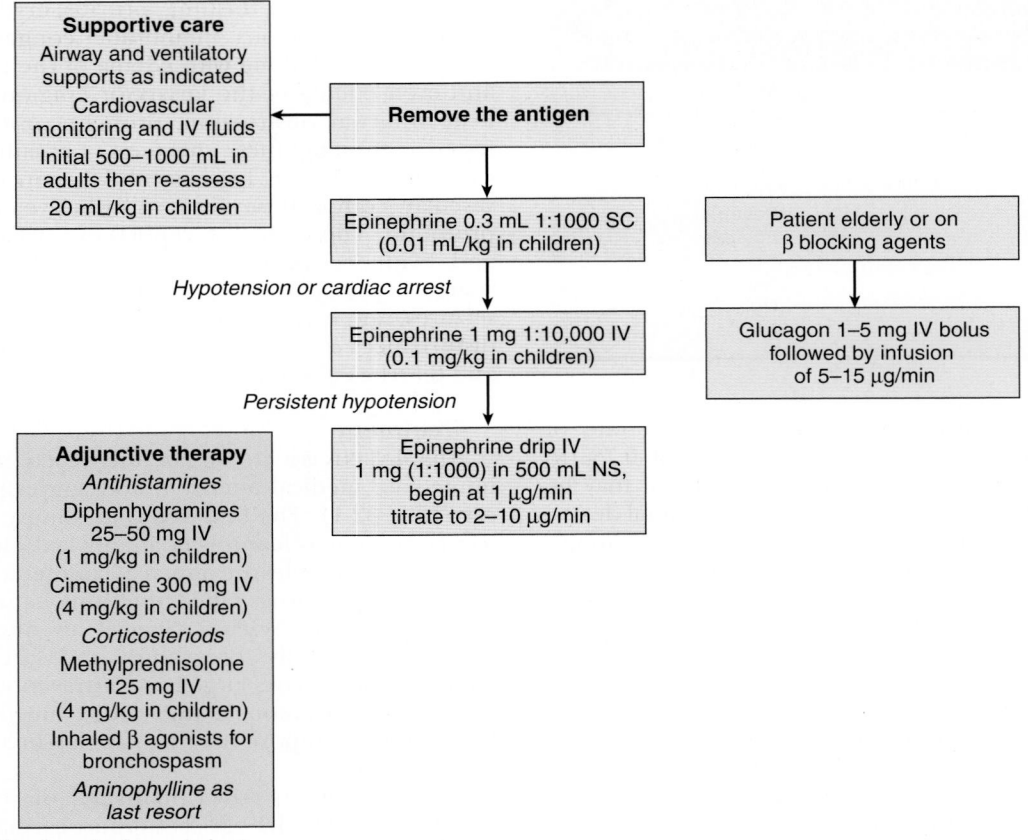

FIGURE 52-1 Treatment of anaphylaxis.

methyprednisolone 125 mg in an adult or 1 mg/kg in children) and antihistamines are unlikely to affect the acute response but may serve a role in reducing prolonged or recurrent symptoms.[47] However, one study by Stark showed little effect of corticosteroids on the occurrence of biphasic or prolonged anaphylaxis.[48] Antihistamines, to include both H_1 (diphenhydramine or hydroxyzine 25 to 50 mg) and H_2 blockers (cimetidine 300 mg) have been widely used both intravenously and orally to reduce pruritis and urticaria associated with the type I immune response. Patients who manifest clinical symptoms of anaphylaxis should be admitted to the hospital as a precaution to avoid premature dismissal of patients at risk for recurrence. Risk factors for recurrent or prolonged symptoms included a delayed onset (greater than 30 minutes) from exposure to manifestation of symptoms and patients who suffered a reaction to oral medications.[48]

SERUM SICKNESS AND SERUM SICKNESS–LIKE REACTIONS

β-Lactam antibiotics are one of the most common causes of nonserum, serum sickness–like reactions. Although this phenomenon is well described in the literature, the reaction is uncommon (estimated at 1.8 per 100,000 prescriptions of cefaclor and 1 per 10 million for cephalexin and amoxicillin).[49-52] Serum sickness–like reactions have also been ascribed to other antibiotics, including sulfonamides, ciprofloxacin, metronidazole, and streptomycin.[53] Serum sickness usually occurs 6 to 21 days after drug exposure. This time course allows for antibody production and the development of IgG and IgM immune complexes. Symptoms include fever, malaise, skin eruptions, joint symptoms, and lymphadenopathy. Treatment is supportive, and antihistamines and/or corticosteroids may provide some benefit.[10]

DRUG-INDUCED AUTOIMMUNITY

Hypersensitivity vasculitis (HSV) is an inflammatory condition of blood vessels and has been associated with antibiotic use, specifically penicillin and sulfonamides. HSV mortality may approach 25%, but if the causative agent is identified and exposure eliminated, the prognosis is very good.[10]

Organ-Specific Reactions

DERMATOLOGIC MANIFESTATIONS

Cutaneous reactions are one of the most common adverse drug events, occurring in 2% to 3% of hospitalized patients, and antibiotics are often the culprit.[54] The most commonly implicated antibiotics include amoxicillin, trimethoprim-sulfamethoxazole, and ampicillin. Exanthematous (or morbilliform) eruptions are the most

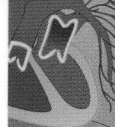

common drug-induced skin eruptions, and the clinical course is usually benign. Urticaria follows morbilliform rashes in frequency and may occur with or without anaphylaxis.[55] The rash may be a result of IgE or pseudo-allergic mechanisms. Onset may be immediate or delayed and will increase with ongoing exposure. Symptoms usually respond to antihistamines, but corticosteroids may be necessary.[7]

Allergic contact dermatitis is a type IV immune response following topical sensitization. Neomycin is a well-known sensitizer, but other implicated antibiotics include other aminoglycosides, penicillin, sulfonamides, chloramphenicol, and antifungal agents.[56] Cross-reactions may occur when these agents are administered systemically.[57]

Erythema multiforme is another cutaneous reaction that has been reported most commonly with the use of sulfonamides but also with aminopenicillins, cephalosporins, fluoroquinolones, tetracyclines, vancomycin, and imidazole antifungals.[58] The reaction can manifest as a spectrum of illness from erythema multiforme minor to major and some even consider toxic epidermal necrolysis (TEN) the extreme of this spectrum (others consider it a separate entity). Symptoms usually begin 1 to 3 weeks after institution of the offending drug. High-dose corticosteroids are indicated early in the course of erythema multiforme. Patients with TEN should be transferred to a burn center, where the risk for mortality may be reduced from 50% to 30%.[59] The safety and efficacy of corticosteroid therapy in TEN patients is controversial.[7,59]

Photosensitivity is another common skin reaction to antibiotic exposure. The reaction may be a nonimmunologic phototoxic reaction seen with tetracycline therapy or the less common photoallergic reaction, which requires sensitization. Photoallergic reactions have been described with the use of sulfonamides and fluoroquinolones.[5]

PULMONARY MANIFESTATIONS

Pulmonary infiltrates with eosinophilia have been associated with penicillins, sulfonamides, and nitrofurantoin. The patient may have nonproductive cough, fever, malaise, and chest discomfort. Treatment is withdrawal of the offending drug and corticosteroids.[60]

HEMATOLOGIC MANIFESTATIONS

Antibiotics may influence hematologic parameters in various ways to include eosinophilia, thrombocytopenia, hemolytic anemia, and agranulocytosis. These reactions are believed to be mediated by immunologic mechanisms; however, agranulocytosis may also occur from direct bone marrow suppression. Eosinophilia in the absence of other clinical manifestations of an immune response may occur with ampicillin, sulfonamides, vancomycin, and streptomycin. Discontinuation of the drug is indicated in the presence of rising eosinophilia.[10] Thrombocytopenia has been described with many pharmaceuticals, but the most commonly implicated antibiotics are the sulfonamides. Recovery usually occurs within 2 weeks of withdrawal of the drug.

Hemolytic anemia may occur through several immune mechanisms, including (1) immune complex, (2) hapten

formation, or (3) autoimmune induction. Nitrofurantoin, rifampin, and streptomycin are all known to cause hemolytic anemia through immune complex formation. The antidrug antibody binds to drug and a specific blood group antigen on the red blood cell membrane, leading to hemolysis, and the direct Coombs' test results are usually positive.[61] Hapten-induced hemolysis results with high-dose penicillin therapy (more than 10 million units daily intravenously) and may also occur with tetracycline and cephalosporins.[61-63] Hemolysis usually occurs after 1 week of therapy and the Coombs' test result is positive.

RENAL MANIFESTATIONS

Drug-induced immunologic nephropathy is known to occur with the use of large doses of benzyl penicillin, methicillin, or sulfonamides. These patients often have fever, rash, and eosinophilia in addition to evidence of renal tubular dysfunction, which reverts to normal after drug discontinuation.[5]

OTHER MANIFESTATIONS OF HYPERSENSITIVITY

Drug-induced vasculitis, as a result of immune complex deposition, has been described with most antibiotic classes. A leukocytoclastic vasculitis is most common, but Henoch-Schönlein purpura and polyarteritis nodosum are known to occur with β lactams and sulfonamides. Affected patients may present with petechiae, purpura, arthralgias, myalgias, or nephritis. Symptoms usually resolve with discontinuation of the drug, but corticosteroids may be necessary.[64]

Drug hypersensitivity due to altered hepatic metabolism that results in reactive metabolites has been commonly associated with the use of sulfamethoxazole in HIV-infected patients who present with fever and rash.[65] This reaction is usually self-limited, and most patients tolerate reexposure.[66] Altered hepatic metabolism has also been implicated in the pathogenesis of the serum sickness–like reaction seen with cefaclor.[52]

In addition to hypersensitivity reactions, antibiotics can cause direct toxicity both at therapeutic doses and in overdose. The following is a discussion of the more significant toxicities associated with antibiotics and antifungals.

ANTIBIOTICS

Penicillins and β Lactams

Penicillins and other β lactams in acute overdose can usually be safely handled by the poison center at home due to their wide margin of safety. However, penicillins can produce toxic effects, especially at high doses. One that is widely known is the central nervous system (CNS) toxicity of penicillins either in large intravenous doses (more than 50 million units) or intraventricular injection.[67-69] Seizures are thought to be related to binding of penicillin near the γ-aminobutyric acid (GABA) binding site, which prevents GABA from binding on its receptor, resulting in lack of inhibition.[70] Other β lactams, such as monobactams and carbepenems, may be

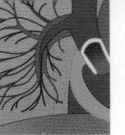

epileptogenic at therapeutic doses; and cephalosporins are known to have epileptogenic effects in acute overdose in patients with acute and chronic renal failure.[71,72] Benzodiazepines or barbiturates can be used for penicillin-induced seizures, and cerebrospinal fluid exchange may be performed in case of intraventricular penicillin injection.[67,68]

Penicillin G may also rarely cause hyperkalemia when given in large doses to patients with renal failure.[73,74] Injection of procaine penicillin has been associated with Hoigne syndrome. This syndrome is characterized by anxiety, psychomotor instability, altered mental status, hallucinations, and paranoid thoughts. Procaine is thought to be the causative agent.[75-77] Other β lactam agents are known to cause adverse events at therapeutic doses. Amoxicillin/clavulanic acid has been associated with intrahepatic cholestatic hepatitis that usually resolves after discontinuing therapy.[78,79] Ampicillin is well known for producing a rash in children with infectious mononucleosis, but the mechanism of this phenomenon is poorly understood.[80] Cephalosporins with the N-methylthiotetrazole (nMTT) side chain, such as cefazolin, cefotetan, and cefoperazone, have the unique toxicity of causing a disulfiram-like reaction due to nMTT inhibition of aldehyde dehydrogenase. nMTT also has been associated with hypothrombinemia by depleting vitamin K–dependent factors.[74,81,82]

Sulfonamides

Sulfonamides in an acute single overdose are usually not life threatening and typically cause only nausea and GI upset. Hemolysis has been described in patients with glucose-6-phosphate deficiency (G6PD) treated with sulfonamides. Newborns given sulfonamides may develop kernicterus due to displacement of bilirubin.[83,84] Sulfonamides have rarely been associated with methemoglobinemia.[85-88]

Fluoroquinolones

Disturbances of the GI tract, CNS symptoms, and photosensitivity are well-known adverse effects of therapy with fluoroquinolones.[89] Fluoroquinolones may also possess epileptogenic effects due to GABA inhibition. Norfloxacin is the most potent GABA inhibitor in the class.[90] Use of fluoroquinolones in young children and pregnant women is generally discouraged due to their known adverse effect on the development of collagen and glucosaminoglycans that results in faulty cartilage formation. However, newer literature suggests that these agents can be safely used in children.[89,91,92] Achilles tendon rupture in adults is another well-known complication of fluoroquinolone treatment.[89,93] Fluoroquinolones, most notably sparfloxacin and grepafloxacin, are known to cause QT interval prolongation by blocking myocardial potassium currents much like class III antiarrhythmics, so caution should be used when prescribing these agents to patients that may be taking other drugs known to prolong the QT interval.[89,94,95]

Aminoglycosides

The aminoglycosides are one of the most commonly used antibiotics due to their efficacy against gram-negative bacteria. They are elaborated from the actinomycetes *Streptomyces* and *Micromonospora*. They have poor GI tract absorption, low protein binding, and small volumes of distribution, making them removable via hemodialysis. Aminoglycosides are only available in parenteral forms; therefore, most of the toxicity is due to dosing errors, which occurs most commonly in neonates. Nephrotoxicity usually presents in patients who receive long courses of the drug and resolves after the drug is retired. Acute single overdoses in persons with normal renal function are unlikely to cause nephrotoxicity.[96,97] Aminoglycoside nephrotoxicity may be diminished by the concomitant use of ticarcillin.[98] Ototoxicity is more common with prolonged use, and the effect is usually permanent. As few as two doses in a dialysis patient have led to ototoxicity.[99] Treatment of aminoglycoside overdose includes removal of the offending agent, hemodialysis, and supportive treatment.

Tetracyclines

Tetracyclines are also broad-spectrum antibiotics. Significant toxicity after acute overdose is unlikely. Side effects are well recognized and include GI irritation and discoloration of the teeth. Tetracycline has been associated with esophagitis, ulcers, pancreatitis, and hepatitis.[100-102] Declomycin has been reported to cause nephrogenic diabetes insipidus.[103]

Macrolides

Macrolides, derived from *Streptomyces*, have poor GI absorption, are known to cross the placenta, and are transmitted into breast milk. Pancreatitis and GI upset are known adverse effects.[104] Erythromycin has been associated with hypoacusis that resolved after stopping the drug.[105]

QT prolongation has been reported on several occasions after therapeutic doses of erythromycin, particularly when it is given intravenously.[106] Daleau, in an animal study in 1994, postulated that erythromycin blocks the rapid component of the delayed rectifier potassium current and lengthens the repolarization phase of cardiac muscle.[107] Stanat and Carlton reported in an in vitro study that clarithromycin and erythromycin inhibit the HERG (the human ether-a-go-go–related gene) potassium current at therapeutic doses, thus increasing repolarization time.[108]

Vancomycin

Vancomycin is produced by the actinomycete *Streptococcus orientalis* and is effective against a number of gram-positive organisms, most notably methicillin-resistant *Staphylococcus aureus*. Acute oral overdose rarely causes significant problems and can be managed with

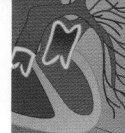

supportive care alone. Multiple-dose activated charcoal decreased the half-life of vancomycin in neonates who received an iatrogenic overdose.[91,109] Vancomycin is known to cause reversible nephrotoxicity and ototoxicity, both of which resolve after stopping the drug.[91] Probably the most well-known toxicity of vancomycin, red man syndrome, is an infusion rate–related reaction that consists of chest pain, dyspnea, pruritus, urticaria, flushing, and angioedema. This is best treated by stopping the drug and supportive measures, such as intravenous fluids and diphenhydramine. Because red man syndrome is not a true allergic reaction, subsequent use of the drug is not prohibited.[110-112]

Nitrofurantoin

Nitrofurantoin is an antibiotic with great specificity for the pathogens of the urinary tract and is commonly used in pregnant patients. Side effects include GI upset and acute pulmonary toxicity that ranges from mild dyspnea to noncardiogenic pulmonary edema. Full recovery can be expected with discontinuation of the drug and use of steroids, bronchodilators, and supportive care.[113]

Chloramphenicol

Chloramphenicol is a nitrobenzene-based antibiotic capable of inhibiting protein synthesis in rapidly proliferating eukaryotic and bacterial cells. In acute overdose it is known to cause nausea and vomiting. It has been shown to cause cardiovascular collapse at levels of 30 to 277 μg/mL and after doubling the dose for 60 hours.[114,115] In early, massive overdoses, orogastric lavage may have a role in decontamination. Extracorporeal removal of the drug by hemodialysis or charcoal hemoperfusion may also be effective in patients with hepatic or renal insufficiency.[116] Chloramphenicol is well known for causing "gray baby syndrome," which was first described in 1959. Infants on chloramphenicol (doses of 100 to 165 mg/kg) for more than 72 hours developed vomiting, refusal to suck, irregular respirations, abdominal distention, diarrhea, acidosis, cyanosis, ashen color, flaccidity, and cardiovascular collapse.[115] Chloramphenicol also can cause dose-dependent bone marrow depression, which most commonly affects erythropoiesis. Resolution occurs with discontinuation of the drug.

Oxazolidinones

Oxazolidinones (linezolid and eperezolid), currently used for multidrug-resistant gram-positive organisms, are the newest antibiotic class; thus, information on human overdose is limited. Common side effects of therapy include GI symptoms, headache, and thrombocytopenia in up to 10% of patients.[117] Linezolid causes a reversible brownish tongue discoloration in up to 33% of patients on therapeutic doses.[118,119] Linezolid is a weak monoamine oxidase inhibitor and concomitant use of selective serotonin reuptake inhibitors has resulted in serotonin syndrome.[120]

Benzyl Alcohol

Historically, benzyl alcohol was used as a bacteriostatic flush for intravenous lines. In 1981 and 1982, several deaths in the neonatal intensive care unit were attributed to the use of benzyl alcohol. These patients presented with neonatal gasping syndrome, characterized gradual neurologic deterioration, severe metabolic acidosis, sudden onset of gasping respirations, skin breakdown, hepatic and renal failure, hypotension, and cardiovascular collapse.[121,122]

Extensive workup in these patients revealed that the illness was the result of repetitive administration of the bacteriostatic solutions containing the benzyl alcohol. Benzoic acid is a by-product of benzyl alcohol, and it is likely that neonates are unable to detoxify the benzoic acid when benzyl alcohol is given repetitively.[122] The syndrome disappeared after use of benzyl alcohol was discontinued in nurseries.

Dapsone

Dapsone (4-4'-diaminodiphenylsulfone [DDS]) is a synthetic sulfone that has been used as a bacteriostatic antimicrobial and as an anti-inflammatory agent in many dermatologic conditions. The first use of oral dapsone was in the treatment of *Mycobacterium leprae* in 1949.[123] Shortly thereafter, several dermatologic uses for sulfones where discovered, including the treatment of acne vulgaris, dermatitis herpetiformis, and subcorneal pustular dermatosis.[124-126] Dapsone, with or without trimethoprim or pyrimethamine, also has strong anti–*Pneumocystis carinii* activity. Oral dapsone is readily absorbed by the GI tract and reaches peak serum concentrations between 0.5 and 4 hours. The volume of distribution is 1.0 to 1.5 L/kg, approximately 70% is protein bound, and the elimination half-life ranges from 12 to 30 hours. Dapsone undergoes enterohepatic circulation, and about 85% is excreted in the urine and 10% in the bile.[127,128] The drug blocks dihydropteroate synthase. This enzyme catalyzes the conversion of para-aminobenzoic acid and pteridine into dihydropteroic acid in the first step of folic acid synthesis. Therefore, dapsone affects bacteria that are dependent on intrinsic folic acid synthesis.[129] The mechanism involved in the anti-inflammatory influence of dapsone has been related to the suppression of leukocyte chemotactic and cytotoxic functions.[130] The most widely known toxicities of dapsone are hemolytic anemia and methemoglobinemia. Other less common effects of dapsone include sulfhemoglobinemia, agranulocytosis, hepatitis, maculopathy, and acute renal failure.[131-134] Dapsone causes an oxidative stress on the hematologic system by dapsone-derived free radicals. These radicals bind erythrocyte membranes and hemoglobin molecules and form precipitates and denatured proteins (Heinz-bodies). These proteins are subsequently sequestered by the reticuloendothelial system and destroyed, causing drug-induced hemolytic anemia.[135] This hemotoxicity is dose dependent, with a few cases reported at 100 mg/day, and

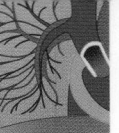

almost all patients involved in one study who were taking 250 mg/day.[136-138] Significant methemoglobinemia has been reported in patients chronically receiving 100 mg/day.[139] Most cases of mild dapsone-induced methemoglobinemia and hemolytic anemia respond to discontinuation of dapsone and observation. Intravenous methylene blue continues to be the mainstay of treatment for severe methemoglobinemia but does not treat sulfhemoglobinemia. Exchange transfusion can be considered for methemoglobinemia or sulfhemoglobinemia unresponsive to supportive care and methylene blue.[140] Studies demonstrate that the use of multidose activated charcoal increases dapsone elimination by interfering with its enterohepatic circulation. In one report, the elimination half-life of dapsone was reduced from 20.5 (±2) to 10.8 (±0.4) hours after multiple doses of charcoal.[141] However, multiple-dose activated charcoal has not been clinically proven to decrease the incidence of methemoglobinemia and hemolytic anemia.[142] Dapsone is poorly dialyzable due to its high protein binding and large volume of distribution.

ANTIFUNGALS

Amphotericin B

Amphotericin B is an intravenous polyene antifungal agent produced by the microorganism *Streptomyces nodosus*. It has been available in the United States since 1956. Amphotericin B lipid complex, amphotericin B cholesteryl sulfate complex, and amphotericin B liposome are alternative formulations that have been developed to reduce nephrotoxicity. Amphotericin B is usually reserved for life-threatening fungal infections due to its high incidence of nephrotoxicity. Amphotericin B causes reduced renal blood flow, decreased glomerular filtration rate, and direct tubular injury, resulting in acute tubular necrosis.[143,144] Approximately 80% to 87% of patients receiving therapeutic doses of amphotericin B experience a decrease in renal function that appears to be dose related and cumulative, and is generally reversible over several months.[144-149] Permanent renal damage may occur in patients receiving 4 g or more. Nausea, anorexia, vomiting, fever, and chills are also seen with therapeutic amphotericin B therapy. The fever and chills have been observed to be independent of the infusion rate and are likely mediated through prostaglandin E_2 synthesis.[145,146,150] Amphotericin-induced electrolyte disturbances include hypokalemia, hypomagnesemia, and, rarely, hyperkalemia.[151-153] Anemia, leukopenia, and thrombocytopenia have also been reported with therapeutic administration.[154-156]

There is no antidote for amphotericin B toxicity. In addition to general supportive care, limiting dosage, and correcting volume deficits, other therapies have also been found to be useful in preventing or treating amphotericin toxicity. Both ibuprofen and meperidine have been advocated to prevent or ameliorate the fever and chills caused by amphotericin B.[157-159] Supplementing dietary sodium chloride intake daily with 150 mEq of sodium chloride intravenously or orally when amphotericin B therapy is initiated may prevent nephrotoxicity.[160]

Triazoles and Imidazoles

Fluconazole, itraconazole, terconazole, and voriconazole are triazole antifungal agents that inhibit ergosterol synthesis in fungal cell membranes. This causes cell leakage and death in the fungal cell. With therapeutic use, the most common adverse effects include nausea, vomiting, and bloating.[161,162] Elevation of transaminase levels has been observed during fluconazole, itraconazole, and voriconazole therapy.[161,163,164]

The imidazoles include clotrimazole, econazole, ketoconazole, and miconazole. Imidazoles also inhibit the biosynthesis of ergosterol or sterols, triglycerides, and phospholipids in fungal cells.[165] Severe toxic effects following oral overdose are expected to be negligible due to minimal oral absorption. Ingestion of even large quantities should produce only minor GI symptoms. At therapeutic doses, adverse effects of ketoconazole include hypertension, nausea, vomiting, gynecomastia, adrenal suppression, suppression of androgen synthesis, and menstrual irregularities. Ketoconazole-induced inhibition of steroid synthesis is a consequence of cytochrome P-450 enzyme inhibition. The competitive inhibition of CYP3A4 makes the triazoles (fluconazole and itraconazole) and the imidazoles (ketoconazole and miconazole) potentiators of other drugs that are more likely to cause serious toxicities such as phenytoin, cyclosporine, and warfarin. Prolonged QT syndrome, torsades de pointes, seizures, and death have been reported in coadministration of ketoconazole with astemizole, cisapride, or terfenadine (all of which are no longer available in the United States). This interaction is less frequently observed with itraconazole and fluconazole.[166-169] Other side effects of ketoconazole include alopecia, drug-induced hepatitis, pruritus, and allergic rash.[168]

REFERENCES

1. Watson WA, Litovitz TL, Klein-Schwartz W, et al: 2003 Annual report of the American Association of Poison Control Centers Toxic Exposure Surveillance System. Am J Emerg Med 2004; 22(5):335–404.
2. Schwentker FF, Gelman S, Long PH: The treatment of meningococcal meningitis. JAMA 1937;108:1407–1408.
3. Powers JH: Antimicrobial drug development. Clin Microbiol Infect 2004;10(Suppl 4):23–31.
4. Lee CE, Zembower TR, Fortis MA, et al: The incidence of antimicrobial allergies in hospitalized patients: implications regarding prescribing patterns and emerging bacterial resistance. Arch Intern Med 2000;160:2819–2822.
5. Executive summary of disease management of drug hypersensitivity: a practice parameter. Joint Task Force on Practice Parameters, the American Academy of Allergy, Asthma and Immunology, and the Joint Council of Allergy, Asthma and Immunology. Disease management of drug hypersensitivity: a practice approach. Ann Allergy Asthma Immunol 1999;83 (6 Suppl):672–700.
6. Adkinson NF Jr: Risk factors for drug allergy. J Allergy Clin Immunol 1984;74:567.

7. Sheperd GM: Hypersensitivity reactions to drugs: evaluation and management. Mt Sinai J Med 2003;70(2):113–125.

8. Assouad M, Willcort RJ, Goodman PH: Anaphylactoid reactions to ciprofloxin. Ann Intern Med 1995;122:396–397.

9. Davis H, McGoodwin E, Reed TG: Anaphylactoid reactions reported after treatment with ciprofloxacin. Ann Intern Med 1989;111:1041.

10. Ditto AM: Drug allergy. In Grammer LC, Greenberger PA (eds): Patterson's Allergic Diseases. Philadelphia, Lippincott, Williams & Wilkins, 2002, pp 295–334.

11. Galpin GE, Chow AW, Yoshikawa TT, et al: "Pseudo-anaphylactic" reactions from inadvertent infusion of procaine penicillin. Ann Intern Med 1974;81:358–359.

12. Weiss ME, Adkinson NF: Immediate hypersensitivity reactions to penicillin and related antibiotics. Clin Allerg 1988;18:515–540.

13. Levine BB: Antigenicity and crossreactivity of penicillin and cephalosporins. J Infect Dis 1973;128:364–366.

14. Idsoe O, Guthe T, Willcox RR, et al: Nature and extent of penicillin side reactions with particular reference to fatalities from anaphylactic shock. Bull WHO 1968;38:159.

15. Petz L: Immunologic cross-reactivity between penicillins and cephalosporins: a review. J Infect Dis 1978;137:574.

16. Anne S, Reisman RE: Risk of administering cephalosporin antibiotics to patients with histories of penicillin allergy. Ann Allergy Asthma Immunol 1995;83:381–385.

17. Smith JW, Johnson JE, Cluff LE: Studies on the epidemiology of adverse drug reactions II. An evaluation of penicillin allergy. N Engl J Med 1966;274:998–1002.

18. Khoury L, Warrington R: The multiple drug allergy syndrome: a matched control-retrospective study in patients allergic to penicillin. J Allergy Clin Immunol 1996;98:462–464.

19. Girard JP: Common antigenic determinants of penicillin G, ampicillin and the cephalosporins demonstrated in men. Int Arch Allergy Appl Immunol 1968;33:428–438.

20. Moskovitz BL: Clinical adverse events during ceftriaxone therapy. Am J Med 1984:84–88.

21. Levine BB, Zolov DM: Prediction of penicillin allergy by immunologic tests. J Allergy 1969;43:231–244.

22. Brown B, Price EV, Moore MB: Penicolloyl-polylysine as an intradermal test of penicillin sensitivity. JAMA 1964;189:599–604.

23. Sullivan TJ, Yecies LD, Shatz GS, et al: Desensitization of patients allergic to penicillin using orally administered beta-lactam antibiotics. J Allergy Clin Immunol 1982;69:275–282.

24. Sheperd GM, Burton DA: Administration of cephalosporins antibiotics to patients with a history of allergy to penicillin [abstract]. J Allergy Clin Immunol 1993;91:262.

25. Blanca M, Fernandez J, Miranda A, et al: Cross-reactivity between penicillins and cephalosporins: clinical and immunological studies. J Allergy Clin Immunol 1989;83:381–385.

26. Sogn DD, Evan R III, Sheperd GM: Results of the National Institute of Allergy and Infectious Disease collaborative clinical trial to test the predictive value of skin testing with major and minor penicillin derivatives in hospitalized adults. Arch Intern Med 1992;152:1025–1032.

27. Kemp SF, Lockey RF, Wolf BL, et al: Anaphylaxis: a review of 266 cases. Arch Intern Med 1995;155:1749–1754.

28. Saxon A, Beall GN, Rohr AS, Adelman DC: Immediate hypersensitivity reactions to beta-lactam antibiotics. Ann Intern Med 1987;107:204–215.

29. Adkinson NF Jr: Immunogenicity and cross-allergenicity of aztreonam. Am J Med 1990;88(Suppl 3C):12–16.

30. Saxon A, Hassner A, Swabb EA, et al: Lack of cross reactivity between aztreonam, a monobactam antibiotic and penicillin in penicillin allergic patients. J Infect Dis 1984;149:16–22.

31. Ennis DM, Cobbs CG: The newer cephalosporins aztreonam and imipenem. Infect Dis Clin North Am 1995;9:687–713.

32. Portier P, Richet C: De l'action anaphylactique de certaines venins. Compt Rend Soc Biol 1902;54:170–172.

33. Matasar MJ, Neugut AI: Epidemiology of anaphylaxis in the United States. Curr Allergy Asthma Rep 2003;3:30–35.

34. Anderson JA: Allergic reaction to drugs and biologic agents. JAMA 1992;268:2845–2857.

35. Bochner BS, Lichtenstein LM: Anaphylaxis. N Engl J Med 1991;324:1785–1790.

36. Atkinson TP, Kaliner MA: Anaphylaxis. Med Clini North Am 1992;76:841–855.

37. Carrington DM, Earl HS, Sullivan TJ: Studies of human IgE to a sulfonamide determinant. J Allergy Clin Immunol 1987;79:442.

38. Tanus T, Mines D, Atkins PC, et al: Serum tryptase in idiopathic anaphylaxis: a case report and review of the literature. Ann Emerg Med 1994;24:104–107.

39. Schwartz LB: Tryptase, a mediator of mast cells. J Allergy Clin Immunol 1990;86:594–598.

40. McGrath KG: Anaphylaxis. In Grammer LC, Greenberger PA (eds): Patterson's Allergic Diseases, 6th ed. Philadelphia, Lippincott, Williams & Wilkins, 2002, pp 415–435.

41. Choi IH, Ha T, Lee D, et al: Occurrence of disseminated intravascular coagulation in active systemic anaphylaxis: role of platelet activating factor. Clin Exp Immunol 1995;100:390–394.

42. Petsas AA, Kotler MN: Electrocardiographic changes associated with penicillin anaphylaxis. Chest 1973;64:66–69.

43. Barach EM, Nowak RM, Lee TG, et al: Epinephrine for the treatment of anaphylactic shock. JAMA 1984;251:2118–2122.

44. AHA Appendix 4: ACLS drugs, cardioversion, defibrillation, and pacing. In Cummins RO (ed): Advanced Cardiac Life Support: Provider Manual. Dallas, TX, American Heart Association, 2003, p 290.

45. Toogood JH: Risk of anaphylaxis in patients receiving beta blocker drugs. J Allergy Clin Immunol 1988;81:1.

46. Zaloga GP, Delacey W, Holmboe E, et al: Glucagon reversal of hypotension in a case of anaphylactoid shock. Ann Intern Med 1986;105:65–66.

47. Lieberman P: The use of antihistamines in the prevention and treatment of anaphylaxis and anaphylactoid reactions. J Allergy Clin Immunol 1990;86:684.

48. Stark BJ, Sullivan TJ: Biphasic and protracted anaphylaxis. J Allergy Clin Immunol 1986;78:76–83.

49. Hebert AA, Sigman ES, Levy ML: Serum sickness like reactions from cefaclor in children. J Am Acad Dermatol 1991;25:805–808.

50. Lowery N, Kearns GL, Young RA, Wheeler G: Serum sickness like reactions with cefprozil. J Pediatr 1994;125:325–328.

51. Platt R, Drewis MW, Kennedy DL, et al: Serum sickness-like reactions to amoxicillin, cefaclor, cephalexin, and trimethoprim-sulfamethoxazole. J Infect Dis 1988;158:474–477.

52. Kearnes GL, Wheeler GJ, Childress SH, et al: Serum sickness reactions to cefaclor: role of hepatic metabolism and individual susceptibility. J Pediatr 1994;125:805–811.

53. Erffmeyer JE: Serum sickness. Ann Allergy 1986;56:105–110.

54. Alanko K, Stubb S, Kauppinen K: Cutaneous drug reactions: clinical types and causative agents. A five year survey of in-patients. Acta Derm Venereol 1989;69:223.

55. Bigby M, Jick S, Jick H, et al: Drug induced cutaneous reactions: a report from the Boston Collaborative Drug Surveillance Program on 15,438 consecutive patients. JAMA 1986;256:3358–3363.

56. Reitschel RL: Dermatologic manifestations of antimicrobial adverse reactions with special emphasis on topical exposure. Infect Dis Clin North Am 1994;8:607–615.

57. Pirila V, Hirvonen ML, Rouhunkoski S: The pattern of cross-sensitivity to neomycin. Dermatologia 1968;136:321.

58. Roujeau JC, Kelly JP, Naldi L, et al: Medication use and the risk of Stevens-Johnson syndrome or toxic epidermal necrolysis. N Engl J Med 1995;333:1600–1607.

59. Heinbach DM, Engrav LH, Martin JA, et al: Toxic epidermal necrolysis: a step forward in treatment. JAMA 1987;257:2171.

60. Pisani RJ, Rosenow EC III: Drug induced pulmonary disease. In Simmons DH, Tierney DF (eds): Current Pulmonology. St Louis, Mosby Year Book, 1992, p 311.

61. Garratty G, Petz LD: Drug-induced immune hemolytic anemia. Am J Med 1975;58:398.

62. Levine BB: Immunologic mechanisms of penicillin allergy: a haptenic model system for the study of allergic diseases in man. N Engl J Med 1966;275:1115.

63. Petz LD, Fudenberg HH: Coombs positive hemolytic anemia caused by penicillin administration. N Engl J Med 1966;274:171–178.

64. Somer T, Finegold SM: Vasculitides associated with infections, immunization and antimicrobial drugs. Clin Infect Dis 1995;20:1010–1036.

65. Reider MJ, Uetrecht J, Shear NH, et al: Diagnosis of hypersensitivity reactions by in-vitro "rechallenge" with hydroxylamine metabolites. Ann Intern Med 1989;110:286–289.

66. Demoly P, Messaad D, Sahla H, et al: Trimethoprim-sulfamethoxazole-graded challenge in HIV infected patients. J Allergy Clin Immunol 2000;102(6 Pt 1):1033–1036.

67. Kristof RA, Clusmann H, Koehler W, et al: Treatment of accidental high dose intraventricular mezlocillin application by cerebrospinal fluid exchange. J Neurol Neurosurg Psychiatry 1998;64(3):379–381.

68. Brozanski BS, Scher MS, Albright AL: Intraventricular nafcillin-induced seizures in a neonate. Pediatr Neurol 1988;4(3):188–190.

69. Seamans KB, Gloor P, Dobell RA, Wyant JD: Penicillin-induced seizures during cardiopulmonary bypass. A clinical and electroencephalographic study. N Engl J Med 1968;278(16):861–868.

70. Baka M, Uyanikgil Y, Yurtseven M, Turgut M: Influence of penicillin-induced epileptic activity during pregnancy on postnatal hippocampal nestin expression in rats: light and electron microscopic observations. Childs Nerv Syst 2004;20(10):726–733.

71. Chatellier D, Jourdain M, Mangalaboyi J, et al: Cefepime-induced neurotoxicity: an underestimated complication of antibiotherapy in patients with acute renal failure. Intensive Care Med 2002;28(2):214–217.

72. Chedrawi AK, Gharaybeh SI, Al-Ghwery SA, et al: Cephalosporin-induced nonconvulsive status epilepticus in a uremic child. Pediatr Neurol 2004;30(2):135–139.

73. Debrand M, Tsueda K: Ventricular tachycardia due to hyperkalemia induced by potassium penicillin G overdose. Acta Anaesthesiol Belg 1980;31(1):35–37.

74. Matsubara T, Otsubo S, Ogawa A, et al: Effects of beta-lactam antibiotics and N-methyltetrazolethiol on the alcohol-metabolizing system in rats. Jpn J Pharmacol 1987;45(3):303–315.

75. Cummings JL, Barritt CF, Horan M: Delusions induced by procaine penicillin: case report and review of the syndrome. Int J Psychiatry Med 1986;16(2):163–168.

76. Robertson CR Jr: Hallucinations after penicillin injection. Am J Dis Child 1985;139(11):1074–1075.

77. Schreiber W, Krieg JC: [Hoigne syndrome. Case report and current literature review]. Nervenarzt 2001;72(7):546–548.

78. Chawla A, Kahn E, Yunis EJ, Daum F: Rapidly progressive cholestasis: an unusual reaction to amoxicillin/clavulanic acid therapy in a child. J Pediatr 2000;136(1):121–123.

79. Nathani MG, Mutchnick MG, Tynes DJ, Ehrinpreis MN: An unusual case of amoxicillin/clavulanic acid-related hepatotoxicity. Am J Gastroenterol 1998;93(8):1363–1365.

80. Kerns DS, Shira JE, Go S: Ampicillin rash in children. Am J Dis Child 1973;125:187–189.

81. Goss TF, Walawander CA, Grasela TH Jr, et al: Prospective evaluation of risk factors for antibiotic-associated bleeding in critically ill patients. Pharmacotherapy 1992;12(4):283–291.

82. Obata H, Iizuka B, Uchida K: Pathogenesis of hypoprothrombinemia induced by antibiotics. J Nutr Sci Vitaminol (Tokyo) 1992;Spec No:421–424.

83. Ali NA, al-Naama LM, Khalid LO: Haemolytic potential of three chemotherapeutic agents and aspirin in glucose-6-phosphate dehydrogenase deficiency. East Mediterr Health J 1999;5(3):457–464.

84. Reinke CM, Thomas JK, Graves AH: Apparent hemolysis in an AIDS patient receiving trimethoprim/sulfamethoxazole: case report and literature review. J Pharm Technol 1996;11(6):256–262; quiz 93–95.

85. Dunn RJ: Massive sulfasalazine and paracetamol ingestion causing acidosis, hyperglycemia, coagulopathy, and methemoglobinemia. J Toxicol Clin Toxicol 1998;36(3):239–242.

86. Heard K, O'Malley G, Dart RC, Smith M: Is sulfasalazine toxic? J Toxicol Clin Toxicol 1998;36(7):757–760.

87. Karpman E, Kurzrock EA: Adverse reactions of nitrofurantoin, trimethoprim and sulfamethoxazole in children. J Urol 2004;172(2):448–453.

88. Lopez A, Bernardo B, Lopez-Herce J, et al: Methaemoglobinaemia secondary to treatment with trimethoprim and sulphamethoxazole associated with inhaled nitric oxide. Acta Paediatr 1999;88(8):915–916.

89. Stahlmann R, Lode H: Toxicity of quinolones. Drugs 1999;58(Suppl 2):37–42.

90. Tsuji A, Sato H, Kume Y, et al: Inhibitory effects of quinolone antibacterial agents on gamma-aminobutyric acid binding to receptor sites in rat brain membranes. Antimicrob Agents Chemother 1988;32(2):190–194.

91. Burkhardt JE, Hill MA, Lamar CH, et al: Effects of difloxacin on the metabolism of glucosaminoglycans and collagen in organ cultures of articular cartilage. Fundam Appl Toxicol 1993;20(2):257–263.

92. Grady R: Safety profile of quinolone antibiotics in the pediatric population. Pediatr Infect Dis J 2003;22(12):1128–1132.

93. Szarfman A, Chen M, Blum MD: More on fluoroquinolone antibiotics and tendon rupture. N Engl J Med 1995;332(3):193.

94. Demolis JL, Charransol A, Funck-Brentano C, Jaillon P: Effects of a single oral dose of sparfloxacin on ventricular repolarization in healthy volunteers. Br J Clin Pharmacol 1996;41(6):499–503.

95. Takahara A, Sugiyama A, Satoh Y, Hashimoto K: Effects of mexiletine on the canine model of sparfloxacin-induced long QT syndrome. Eur J Pharmacol 2003;476(1–2):115–122.

96. Fuquay D, Koup J, Smith AL: Management of neonatal gentamicin overdosage. J Pediatr 1981;99(3):473–476.

97. Ho PW, Pien FD, Kominami N: Massive amikacin "overdose." Ann Intern Med 1979;91(2):227–228.

98. English J, Gilbert DN, Kohlhepp S, et al: Attenuation of experimental tobramycin nephrotoxicity by ticarcillin. Antimicrob Agents Chemother 1985;27(6):897–902.

99. Lu CM, James SH, Lien YH: Acute massive gentamicin intoxication in a patient with end-stage renal disease. Am J Kidney Dis 1996;28(5):767–771.

100. Boyle MP: Minocycline-induced pancreatitis in cystic fibrosis. Chest 2001;119(4):1283–1285.

101. Shiff AD: Doxycycline-induced esophageal ulcers in physicians. JAMA 1986;256(14):1893.

102. Teitelbaum JE, Perez-Atayde AR, Cohen M, et al: Minocycline-related autoimmune hepatitis: case series and literature review. Arch Pediatr Adolesc Med 1998;152(11):1132–1136.

103. Castell D: Nephrogenic diabetes insipidus due to demethychlortetracycline hydrochloride. JAMA 1965;193(3):237–239.

104. Fang C: Erythromycin-induced acute pancreatitis. J Toxicol Clin Toxicol 1996;34(1):93.

105. Sacristan J: Erythromycin-induced hypoacusis: 11 new cases and literature review. Ann Pharmacol 1993;27:950–955.

106. Gitler B. Torsades de pointes induced by erythromycin. Chest 1994;105:168–172.

107. Daleau P: Erythromycin block the rapid component of the delayed rectifier potassium current. Circulation 1995;91:3010–3016.

108. Stanat SJ, Carlton CG, Crumb WJ Jr, et al: Characterization of the inhibitory effects of erythromycin and clarithromycin on the HERG potassium channel. Mol Cell Biochem 2003;254(1–2):1–7.

109. Kucukguclu S: Multiple-dose activated charcoal in an accidental vancomycin overdose. J Toxicol Clin Toxicol 1996;34:83–86.

110. El Harrar E, Miloudi Y, Bensaid A, Alaoui Yazidi A: [An unusual biologic manifestation of the red man syndrome]. Ann Fr Anesth Reanim 2004;23(10):1015–1016.

111. Garrelts JC, Peterie JD: Vancomycin and the "red man's syndrome." N Engl J Med 1985;312:245.

112. Rothenberg H: Anaphylactoid reaction to vancomycin. JAMA 1959;171(4):1101–1102.

113. Chudnofsky C: Acute pulmonary toxicity to nitrofurantoin. J Emerg Med 1989;7:15–19.

114. Phelps S: Chloramphenicol-induced cardiovascular collapse in an anephric patient. Pediatr Infect Dis J 1987;6(3):285–288.

115. Sutherland J: Fatal cardiovascular collapse of infants receiving large amounts of chloramphenicol. AMA J Dis Child 1959;97:761–767.

116. Slaughter R: Effect of hemodialysis on total body clearance of chloramphenicol. Am J Hosp Pharm 1980;37:1983–1986.

117. Pharmacia & Upjohn Company: Product Information: Zyvox, linezolid. Kalamaozoo, MI, Pharmacia & Upjohn Company, 2000.

118. Diekema DJ, Jones RN: Oxazolidinones: a review. Drugs 2000;59:7–16.

119. Dresser LD, Rybak MJ: The pharmacologic and bacteriologic properties of oxazolidinones. Pharmacotherapy 1998;18:456–462.

120. Lavery S, Ravi H, McDaniel WW: Linezolid and serotonin syndrome. Psychosomatics 2001;42:432–434.

121. Brown WJ, Buist NR, Gipson HT: Fatal benzyl alcohol poisoning in a neonatal intensive care unit. Lancet 1982;2(8302):1250.

122. Gershanik J: The gasping syndrome and benzyl alcohol poisoning. N Engl J Med 1982;307:1384–1388.

123. Wozel G: The story of sulfones in tropical medicine and dermatology. Int J Dermatol 1989;28(1):17–21.

124. Sneddon IB, Wilkinson DS: Subcorneal pustular dermatosis. Br J Dermatol 1956;68(12):385–394.

125. Fry L, Seah PP, Hoffbrand AV: Dermatitis herpetiformis. Clin Gastroenterol 1974;3(1):145–157.

126. Barranco VP: Dapsone—other indications. Int J Dermatol 1982; 21(9):513–514.

127. Ellard GA: Absorption, metabolism and excretion of di(rho-aminophenyl) sulphone (dapsone) and di(rho-aminophenyl) sulphoxide in man. Br J Pharmacol 1966;26(1):212–217.

128. Pieters FA, Zuidema J: The pharmacokinetics of dapsone after oral administration to healthy volunteers. Br J Clin Pharmacol 1986;22(4):491–494.

129. Triglia T, Menting JG, Wilson C, Cowman AF: Mutations in dihydropteroate synthase are responsible for sulfone and sulfonamide resistance in Plasmodium falciparum. Proc Natl Acad Sci U S A 1997;94(25):13944–13949.

130. Booth SA, Moody CE, Dahl MV, et al: Dapsone suppresses integrin-mediated neutrophil adherence function. J Invest Dermatol 1992;98(2):135–140.

131. Chugh KS, Singhal PC, Sharma BK, et al: Acute renal failure due to intravascular hemolysis in the North Indian patients. Am J Med Sci 1977;274(2):139–146.

132. Coleman MD, Coleman NA: Drug-induced methaemoglobinaemia. Treatment issues. Drug Saf 1996;14(6):394–405.

133. Kenner DJ, Holt K, Agnello R, Chester GH: Permanent retinal damage following massive dapsone overdose. Br J Ophthalmol 1980;64(10):741–744.

134. Lambert M, Sonnet J, Mahieu P, Hassoun A: Delayed sulfhemoglobinemia after acute dapsone intoxication. J Toxicol Clin Toxicol 1982;19(1):45–50.

135. Goldstein BD: Exacerbation of dapsone-induced Heinz body hemolytic anemia following treatment with methylene blue. Am J Med Sci 1974;267(5):291–297.

136. Degowin RL, Eppes RB, Powell RD, Carson PE: The haemolytic effects of diaphenylsulfone (DDS) in normal subjects and in those with glucose-6-phosphate-dehydrogenase deficiency. Bull WHO 1966;35(2):165–179.

137. Smith WC: Are hypersensitivity reactions to dapsone becoming more frequent? Lepr Rev 1988;59(1):53–58.

138. Weetman RM, Boxer LA, Brown MP, et al: In vitro inhibition of granulopoiesis by 4-amino-4'-hydroxylaminodiphenyl sulfone. Br J Haematol 1980;45(3):361–370.

139. Manfredi G, De Panfilis G, Zampetti M, Allegra F: Studies on dapsone induced haemolytic anaemia. I. Methaemoglobin production and G-6-PD activity in correlation with dapsone dosage. Br J Dermatol 1979;100(4):427–432.

140. Coleman MD: Dapsone-mediated agranulocytosis: risks, possible mechanisms and prevention. Toxicology 2001;162(1):53–60.

141. Neuvonen PJ, Elonen E, Mattila MJ: Oral activated charcoal and dapsone elimination. Clin Pharmacol Ther 1980;27(6):823–827.

142. American Academy of Clinical Toxicology; European Association of Poisons Centres and Clinical Toxicologists: Position statement and practice guidelines on the use of multi-dose activated charcoal in the treatment of acute poisoning. J Toxicol Clin Toxicol 1999;37(6):731–751.

143. Hoitsma AJ, Wetzels JF, Koene RA: Drug-induced nephrotoxicity. Aetiology, clinical features and management. Drug Saf 1991;6(2):131–147.

144. Butler WT, Bennett JE, Alling DW, et al: Nephrotoxicity of amphotericin B; early and late effects in 81 patients. Ann Intern Med 1964;61:175–187.

145. Chabot GG, Pazdur R, Valeriote FA, Baker LH: Pharmacokinetics and toxicity of continuous infusion amphotericin B in cancer patients. J Pharm Sci 1989;78(4):307–310.

146. Garnacho-Montero J, Ortiz-Leyba C, Garcia Garmendia JL, Jimenez Jimenez F: Life-threatening adverse event after amphotericin B lipid complex treatment in a patient treated previously with amphotericin B deoxycholate. Clin Infect Dis 1998;26(4):1016.

147. Johnson JR, Kangas PJ, West M: Serious adverse event after unrecognized substitution of one amphotericin B lipid preparation for another. Clin Infect Dis 1998;27(5):1342–1343.

148. Sabra R, Zeinoun N, Sharaf LH, et al: Role of humoral mediators in, and influence of a liposomal formulation on, acute amphotericin B nephrotoxicity. Pharmacol Toxicol 2001;88(4): 168–175.

149. Zager RA, Bredl CR, Schimpf BA: Direct amphotericin B-mediated tubular toxicity: assessments of selected cytoprotective agents. Kidney Int 1992;41(6):1588–1594.

150. Cleary JD, Weisdorf D, Fletcher CV: Effect of infusion rate on amphotericin B-associated febrile reactions. Drug Intell Clin Pharm 1988;22(10):769–772.

151. McChesney JA, Marquardt JF: Hypokalemic paralysis induced by amphotericin B. JAMA 1964;189:1029–1031.

152. Craven PC, Gremillion DH: Risk factors of ventricular fibrillation during rapid amphotericin B infusion. Antimicrob Agents Chemother 1985;27(5):868–871.

153. Brent J, Hunt M, Kulig K, Rumack B: Amphotericin B overdoses in infants: is there a role for exchange transfusion? Vet Hum Toxicol 1990;32(2):124–125.

154. Goodpasture HC, Voth DW, Romig DA, et al: Clinical correlations during amphotericin B therapy. J Kans Med Soc 1972;78(11): 486–490.

155. Stein JB, Tolle SW: Episodic leukopenia associated with amphotericin B. South Med J 1983;76(3):409–410.

156. Chan CS, Tuazon CU, Lessin LS: Amphotericin-B-induced thrombocytopenia. Ann Intern Med 1982;96(3):332–333.

157. Burks LC, Aisner J, Fortner CL, Wiernik PH: Meperidine for the treatment of shaking chills and fever. Arch Intern Med 1980; 140(4):483–484.

158. Gigliotti F, Shenep JL, Lott L, Thornton D: Induction of prostaglandin synthesis as the mechanism responsible for the chills and fever produced by infusing amphotericin B. J Infect Dis 1987;156(5):784–789.

159. Oldfield EC 3rd: Meperidine for prevention of amphotericin B-induced chills. Clin Pharm 1990;9(4):251–252.

160. Anderson CM: Sodium chloride treatment of amphotericin B nephrotoxicity. Standard of care? West J Med 1995;162(4): 313–317.

161. Sugar AM, Saunders C: Oral fluconazole as suppressive therapy of disseminated cryptococcosis in patients with acquired immunodeficiency syndrome. Am J Med 1988;85:481–489.

162. Group AMS: Treatment of vaginal candidiasis with a single oral dose of fluconazole. Eur J Clin Microbiol Infect Dis 1988;7: 364–367.

163. Stern JJ HB, Sharkey P: Oral fluconazole therapy for patients with acquired immunodeficiency syndrome and cryptococcosis: experience with 22 patients. Am J Med 1988;85:477–480.

164. Tucker RM, Williams PL, Arathoon EG: Pharmacokinetics of fluconazole in cerebrospinal fluid and serum in human coccidioidal meningitis. Antimicrob Agents Chemother 1988;32:369–373.

165. Bennett J: Antimicrobial Agents, 9th ed. New York, McGraw-Hill, 1996.

166. Monahan BP, Ferguson CL, Killeavy ES, et al: Torsade de pointes occurring in association with terfenadine use. JAMA 1990; 264(2):2788–2790.

167. Honig PK, Wortham DC, Zamani K, et al: Terfenadine-ketoconazole interaction—pharmacokinetic and electrocardiographic consequences. JAMA 1993;269:1513–1518.

168. Bennett JE: Antifungal agents. In Hardman JG, Limbird LE, Molinoff PB, et al (eds): Goodman and Gilman's The Pharmacologic Basis of Disease. New York, McGraw-Hill, 1996, pp 1175–1190.

169. Tsai WC, Tsai LM, Chen JH: Combined use of astemizole and ketoconazole resulting in torsades de pointes. J Formos Med Assoc 1997;96(2):144–146.

53

Antiviral Agents

J. MEULENBELT, MD, PHD ■ J.W. FIJEN, MD, PHD

At a Glance...

■ The nucleoside reverse-transcriptase inhibitors, including didanosine, lamivudine, and stavudine, used to treat human immunodeficiency virus infection, is among the largest class of antiviral agents. They also have a broad range of significant adverse effects.

■ Protease inhibitors, another large class of antiviral agents, have important effects on the cytochrome P-450 enzymes, producing important drug interactions.

■ The guanosine analogs, another important class of antiviral agents, include acyclovir and ganciclovir. As prodrugs that require biotransformation to become active, these agents are important in the treatment of herpes simplex and varicella-zoster viruses.

■ M2 protein blockers, which include amantadine, are the third most important class of antiviral agents; they are used commonly in the treatment of influenza.

Ten to 15 years ago only a few drugs were licensed for the treatment of viral infections. Recently, the drive to combat the human immunodeficiency virus (HIV) along with a better understanding of the viral life cycle resulted in the discovery of new antiviral medicines. New antiviral drugs have been developed against HIV, cytomegalovirus, herpes simplex virus, varicella-zoster virus, respiratory syncytial virus, hepatitis C, and the influenza viruses.

Antiviral medicines can be targeted against viral or human cellular proteins. The first approach is more specific against viruses and yields more specific and less toxic drugs; however, the development of drug resistance is more likely. The latter approach yields antiviral drugs with a broader activity and a higher likelihood of toxicity.

It is relevant to understand the viral life cycle in order to develop suitable antiviral medicines that have minimal toxicity to the patient. The viral life cycle encompasses several crucial steps, starting with the attachment of the virus to the cell followed by the replicative cycle and the release of the progeny virions from the cell. In retroviruses, this replicative cycle begins with reverse transcription (RNA→DNA); the proviral DNA then becomes integrated into the cellular genome and follows the classical transcription and translation processes of the human host cell. Cytolytic viruses (e.g., the herpesviruses) replicate their genome and express their genes autonomously, independent of the human host cell.

The following steps can be targeted by antiviral medicines: virus adsorption, virus–host cell fusion, viral RNA or DNA synthesis, and viral enzyme activity, for example, proteases and neurominidases. Two host enzymes, inosine 5'-monophosphate (IMP) dehydrogenase and S-adenosylhomocysteine hydrolase can also be targets for certain classes of antiviral agents.[1,2] Medicines have been developed to interfere with one of the steps in the viral life cycle. However, the emergence of viral resistance to antiviral drugs and the appearance of drug-related side effects are the main reasons that further research and refinement of antiviral medicines are needed.

The most important goals for treating viral infections in immunocompetent patients are to reduce the severity of illness and to decrease the rate of transmission of the virus. Thus, efficacy, safety, and convenience are key factors in antiviral drug development. Treatment efficacy is of primary importance in order to prevent viral damage to vital organs such as the liver, kidneys, lungs, gastrointestinal tract, and nervous system. Antiviral drugs are used for prophylaxis, suppression of viral replication in order to prevent tissue damage, or treatment of overt disease.

In this chapter the potency and ranked value of antiviral agents against particular viruses will not be discussed. The reader is referred to the website http://AIDSinfo.nih.gov and references.[2-6] The main adverse effects that are important from a clinical toxicology point of view are summarized below and in Table 53-1. For an extensive overview of adverse effects of antiviral drugs, the reader is referred to handbooks, review articles, and websites concerning antiviral treatment. The endogenous antiviral agent interferon is also not discussed here. While drug interactions are discussed, in-depth discussion can be found in several of the cited articles.[7,8]

NUCLEOSIDE REVERSE-TRANSCRIPTASE INHIBITORS

Nucleoside reverse-transcriptase inhibitors (NRTIs) are a class of anti-HIV drugs. They include abacavir, didanosine, lamivudine, zalcitabine, stavudine, zidovudine, adefovir, tenovir, and emtricitabine. Structurally, they are analogs of the natural nucleotides that form the building blocks of RNA and DNA in both human cells and viruses. Nucleoside and nucleotide analogs typically require intracellular phosphorylation by human cellular kinases to achieve their triphosphate form. This triphosphate form competes with the natural nucleotide for inclusion in the growing DNA chain. Absence of the hydroxyl group at the 3' position of the ribose ring in the analogs means a new 3',5'-phosphodiester bond cannot be formed with the next nucleotide, and hence the further extension of this DNA strand is prevented. Thus, NRTIs are competitive inhibitors of mitochondrial DNA

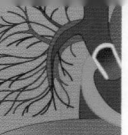

TABLE 53-1 Currently Available Antiretroviral Drugs (See Text for References)

SUBSTANCE NAME	TRADE NAME	RECOMMENDED DAILY DOSE (mg)*	ORAL AVAIL-ABILITY (%)	T_{max} (hr)	Vd (L/kg)	THERA-PEUTIC PLASMA CONCEN-TRATION (mg/L)	PROTEIN BINDING	AVERAGE PLASMA HALF-LIFE (hr)
Nucleoside-Reverse-Transcriptase-Inhibitors (NRTIs)								
NUCLEOSIDE ANALOGS								
Abacavir (guanosine analog)	Ziagen	300 mg po bid, Child: 8mg/kg po bid	83	1.5	0.8–1.9		50	0.8–1.5
Didanosine (adenosine analog)	Videx, ddl	Adult < 60 kg: po 250 mg; Adult > 60 kg: po 400 mg; Child > 6 yr: po 240 mg/m² body surface	30–50	0.7–1	0.8–1.2		<5	1–1.8 (in children 0.8)
Lamivudine (cytidine analog)	Epivir, 3TC	150 mg po bid	86 for adults, 55–65 for children < 12 yr	1	1.3–2			1.2–9
Stavudine (thymidine analog)	Zerit, d4T	> 60 kg: 40 mg po bid Child: 1 mg/kg po bid	86	0.6–1.5	0.5			1–2
Zalcitabine (cytidine analog)	Hivid, ddC	0.75 mg po tid Child: 0.01 mg/kg po tid	85, child: 55	1	0.5–0.6		<5	1.2–2
Zidovudine (thymidine analog)	AZT, Retrovir	300 mg po bid Child: 160 mg/m2 po tid	60	0.5–1	1.5–2.5		20–38	1.1
ACYCLIC NUCLEOTIDE ANALOGS								
Adefovir	Hepsera	10 mg po daily	59	1.75 (0.6–4)	0.3–0.4		4	7.5
Tenofovir	Viriad	300 mg po for adults with CrCl > 60 mL/min; in children unknown	25 in fasting state, 39 with fatty meal	1–2.3	1.3		7	14,417
THICYTIDINE NUCLEOTIDE ANALOG								
Emtricitabine	Emtriva	200 mg po daily; in children unknown	93	1–2			<4	10

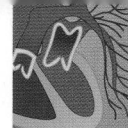

INTRACELLULAR HALF-LIFE TIME (hr)	ADVERSE EFFECTS	TOXIC EFFECT	RELEVANT ISSUES FOR DRUG METABOLISM	REMARKS
3.3	Nausea, vomiting, diarrhea, abdominal pain, headache, fever, lethargia, hypersensivity reaction, bone marrow depression	Lactate acidosis, generally in combination with hepatomegalia	Metabolized by alcohol dehydrogenase and glucoronyl transferase	Contraindications: severe liver and renal failure, metabolites are for 82% excreted with the urine.
25–40	Numbness in extremities caused by periferal neuropathy, nausea,vomiting, diarrhea, headache, fever, lethargia, seizures, bone marrow depression, diabetes mellitus, pancreatitis more common, hyperuricemia	Lactate acidosis, generally in combination with hepa-tomegalia, 1600 mg has been survived by 28 yr-old man without relevant toxicity		Be careful in cases with history of pancreatitis and liver disease. About 50% of the dose is excreted with the urine. Be careful with comedication rifampacine, rifabutin, ribavirin, tenofovir.
16–19	Nausea, vomiting, diarrhea, abdominal pain, fever, pancreatitis	Lactate acidosis, generally in combination with hepatomegalia		Unchanged excreted in the urine. Plasma concentration increases with renal failure.
3.5	Peripheral neuropathy, rare pancreatitis, gastrointestinal complaints, headache	Lactate acidosis, generally in combination with hepatomegalia		About 50% of the dose is excreted with the urine.
3	Peripheral neuropathy, stomatitis, rare pancreatitis	Lactate acidosis, generally in combination with hepatomegalia		About 70% of the dose is excreted with the urine.
3	Gastrointestinal complaints, headache, insomnia, asthenia, bone marrow depression, myopathy	Lactate acidosis, generally in combination with hepatomegalia	Metabolized to AZT, glucuronidated GAZT, renal excretion of GAZT	15%–20% is excreted unchanged with the urine, the rest mainly as zidovudine glucorinide.
	Fever, headache, nausea, vomiting, diarrhea, flatulence, liver failure, weakness, renal failure			Elimination is impaired in renal failure, hemodialysis is useful.
10–50	Asthenia, headache, nausea, vomiting, diarrhea, flatulence		Induces a slight inhibition of CYP1A2	Primarily excreted by glomerular filtration and active tubular excretion; not recommended for patients with creatinine clearance < 60 mL/min.
	Headache, nausea, diarrhea rash	Lactate acidosis, generally in combination with hepatomegalia, 1200 mg was tolerated in 11 patients, without severe adverse reactions		85% is excreted with the urine and 15% in the feces, hemodialysis is useful, adjust dose in renal impairment.

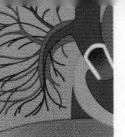

TABLE 53-1 Currently Available Antiretroviral Drugs (See Text for References)—*cont'd*

SUBSTANCE NAME	TRADE NAME	RECOMMENDED DAILY DOSE (mg)*	ORAL AVAIL-ABILITY (%)	T_{max} (hr)	Vd (L/kg)	THERA-PEUTIC PLASMA CONCEN-TRATION (mg/L)	PROTEIN BINDING	AVERAGE PLASMA HALF-LIFE (hr)
Non-NRTIs								
Delaviridine (delavirdine)	Rescriptor	400 mg po tid; in children unknown	85	1.0-4	0.7		97	2–11
Efavirenz	Sustiva, Stocrin	600 mg po daily; children: 12–15 mg/kg once per day	65	3-5		1.8–4.1	99.5	40–55
Nevirapine	Viramune	200 mg po for 14 days, then if no rash 200 mg po bid	> 90 ≈	0.8-2.2	1.2–1.5	3.7–5.9	60	25–30
Protease Inhibitors (PI)								
Amprenavir	Agenerase	1200 po bid; child < 50 kg: 22.5 mg /kg po bid	90 in fasting state (see also tenofovir in this table)	0.5–2	5–6.1 l/kg		90	6–11
Indinavir	Crixivan	800 po tid; child: 500 mg/m² po tid	60–65 in fasting state	0.7–1	0.4–2.25	0.15–8	60–70	1.8–2
Lopinavir	Kaletra (+ combi-nation with ritonavir)	400 (+ 100) mg po bid; child < 40 kg 10–12 mg (+2.5–3 mg) po bid		2–5			98–99	5–6
Nelfinavir	Viracept	750 mg po tid	20–80	2–4	2.0–7.0	1.6–4	>98	3.0–5
Ritonavir	Norvir	600 mg po bid; child: 350–400 mg/m² po bid	66–75	1–1.5	0.4–0.5	3.5–9.6	98–99	3.0–5

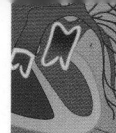

INTRACELLULAR HALF-LIFE TIME (hr)	ADVERSE EFFECTS	TOXIC EFFECT	RELEVANT ISSUES FOR DRUG METABOLISM	REMARKS
	Rash in ≈ 4.3%, increased transaminase levels, headache		Metabolized by cytochrome P450 (CYP3A4 and CYP2D6)	Be carefull with co-medications that interact with P450 metabolism, 50% is excreted with the urine as glucuronidated metabolites, 44% in feces.
	Rash in ≈ 1.7%, increased transaminase levels, dizziness, somnolence, insomnia, abnormal dreams, confusion, impaired concentration, amnesia, agitation, depersonalization, hallucinations, euphoria, retinal toxicity		Metabolized by cytochrome P450 (CYP3A4 and CYP2B6)	Be careful with co-medications that interact with P450 metabolism, 14%–34% exreted with the urine as glucuronidated metabolities, 16%–61% in feces, false positive cannabinoid test.
	Skin rash in ≈ 7%, even in 0.3% a Stevens Johnson's toxic necrotic epidermolysis, nausea, fever, insomnia, increased transaminase levels, hepatitis		Metabolized by cytochrome P450 (CYP3A4 and CYP2B6)	Be careful with co-medications that interact with P450 metabolism, 80% excreted with the urine as glucuronidated metabolites, 10% in feces.
	GI symptoms, transient rash 7–14 d after start, hyper-triglyceridemia, perioral paresthesias, buffalo hump, hyperglycemia, hemolytic anemia		Metabolized by CYP3A4, inhibition of CYP3A4; avoid terfenadine, astemizole, bepridil, ergotamine, potent benzodiazepines such as midazolam and triazolam	Be careful with comedications that interact with P450 metabolism, ≈ 75% is in the feces excreted and 15% with the urine.
	Nausea; diarrhea; nephrolithiasis in days till weeks after start (3%–15%); hyperbiliru-binemia; elevated AST, ALT, and amylase levels; acute hemolytic anemia	6 g in 47 yr-old man transient neurologic and gastrointestinal symptoms; ARF, renal atrophy, interstitial nephritis	Metabolized by CYP3A4, inhibition of CYP3A4; avoid terfenadine, astemizole, ergotamine, potent benzodiazepines like midazolam	Be careful with comedications that interact with P450 metabolism; take care for adequate hydration.
			Standard combination with ritonavir 100 mg bid	Be careful with comedications that inter-act with P450 metabolism.
	Dose-dependent diarrhea		Metabolized by CYP3A4; avoid terfenadine, propafenone, flecainide, astemizole, ergotamine, potent benzodiazepines like midazolam and triazolam	Be careful with comedications that interact with P450 metabolism.
	GI complaints, fatigue, perioral paresthesias, hypertriglyceridemia 5%, elevated AST, ALT, and GGT	3 g results in transient paresthesias	Metabolized by CYP3A4; avoid terfenadine, propafenone, flecainide, astemizole, ergotamine, potent benzodiazepines like midazolam and triazolam	Be careful with comedications that interact with P450 metabolism.

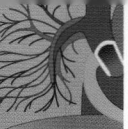

TABLE 53-1 Currently Available Antiretroviral Drugs (See Text for References)—*cont'd*

SUBSTANCE NAME	TRADE NAME	RECOMMENDED DAILY DOSE (mg)*	ORAL AVAIL-ABILITY (%)	T_{max} (hr)	Vd (L/kg)	THERA-PEUTIC PLASMA CONCEN-TRATION (mg/L)	PROTEIN BINDING	AVERAGE PLASMA HALF-LIFE (hr)
Saquinavir	Invirase Fortovase	600 mg po tid 1200 po tid	<4, during high fatty meals up to 30	1–1.2	10–19.7	0.08–0.7	98	9–15
Atazanavir	Reyataz	200 mg po bid. or tid; children not approved	Food enhances absorp-tion	2			86	3–7.9
Fusion Inhibitors								
Enfuvirtide T-20	Fuzeon	90 mg sc bid; child: 2 mg/kg sc bid	84–89	4.0–6.9	5.5	3.4	92	3.8
Guanosine analogs								
Acyclovir	Zovirax	5–20 mg/kg intravenously tid or 5 times po 800 mg; child (3 mo–12 yr) 250 mg/m² body surface intravenously tid	20	1.5–2	48	0.5–3.0		3, in neonates 3–4
Famciclovir	Famvir	500 mg po tid	72–83	0.7–1	1–1.5		20	2–2.5
Ganciclovir	Cymevene, Cytovene	5 mg/kg intravenously bid or 1000 mg orally tid	6–9	2–4				2.5–4
Penciclovir		Topical use			1–1.5		20	2–2.5
Valacyclovir	Zelitrex, Valtrex	1000 tid till 2000 mg po qid; children unknown	60–90	1.5	48	0.8–1.0		2.2–3.1
Valganciclovir	Valcyte	900 mg po bid, after induction period of 21 days, 900 daily	60; with food 75–85	2–2.9				3.5–5
M2 Protein Blocker								
Amantadine	Symmetrel, Amantan, Mantadix	100 mg po bid–tid; child: 4.4 mg/kg po bid (max 150 mg/day)	>90	4	4.4–5.1	< 0.8		9–37
Rimantadine	Flumadine	100 mg po bid–tid	>90	3–6	21			24.9–30
Neurominidase Inhibitors								
Oseltamivir	Tamiflu	75 mg po bid; child (1 to 13 yr-old) 2 mg/kg po bid	75–80	2–3	23–26 L (similar to ECV of body water)		42	6–10.0

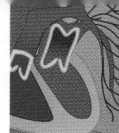

INTRACELLULAR HALF-LIFE TIME (hr)	ADVERSE EFFECTS	TOXIC EFFECT	RELEVANT ISSUES FOR DRUG METABOLISM	REMARKS
	Nausea diarrhea, peripheral neuropathy, headache, hyperbilirubinemia, elevated AST, rash, athralgia, pancreatitis	In adults: safe till single dose 8 g or 7.2 g/day for 25 wk	Metabolized by CYP3A4, all inhibitors P450 (ketoconazole) increase AUC plasmaconc by 300%; avoid terfenadine, astemizole, ergotamine, potent benzodiazepines like midazolam and triazolam	Be careful with comedications that interact with P450 metabolism.
	5% hypertriglyceridemia, elevated AST, ALT, hyperglycemia, first degree AV block (heart)		Metabolized by CYP3A4; avoid terfenadine, propafenone, flecainide, astemizole, ergotamine, potent benzodiazepines like midazolam and triazolam	Be careful with comedications that interact with P450 metabolism; 80% excreted via feces, 7% unchanged with the urine, 6% of the metabolites is excreted with the urine; in liver dysfunction adjust dosages.
	Injection site reactions		No effect on CYP450 enzymes	Unknown in liver dysfunction or severe renal failure. Clearance was not affected in patients with CrCl > 35 mL/min.
	Nausea, vomiting, diarrhea, phlebitis	Nephrotoxic (tubular crystal formation), neurotoxic: tremor, myoclonus, confusion, lethargy, agitation, hallucination, dysarthria, seizures or hemiparesthesia	Be careful in dehydration, previous neurological symptoms.	80% excreted unchanged with the urine, during hemodialysis plasma half-life is reduced to 5.7 L.
	Nausea, diarrhea, vomiting, hepatitis			70% is excreted unchanged with the urine.
	Nausea, diarrhea, vomiting, hepatitis, neurotoxicity, psychosis, nephrotoxic	Granulocytopenia (40%), thrombocytopenia (15%), ventricular ectopia, TTP		70% is excreted unchanged with the urine.
	Nausea, vomiting, diarrhea, headache, phlebitis	Nephrotoxic, neurotoxic	Be careful in dehydration, previous neurological symptoms.	
	Neurotoxicity, nephrotoxic, trombocytopenia, hepatitis	Neutropenia, anemia, diarrhea		80% excreted unchanged with the urine, 50% is removed by hemodialysis.
	Nausea, anorexia, nervousness, difficulty concentrating, fatigue, arrhythmias	Hyperthermia, long QT interval, ARDS, psychosis, coma, ventricular ectopia, torsades de pointes, rhabdomyolysis, anticholinergic syndrome		Elimination by glomerular filtration and tubular secretion of the intact drug; in elderly (>65 yr), in renal or liver dysfunction 50% dose reduction
	Nausea, anorexia	NA	75% metabolized in the liver by hydroxylation	50% dose reduction in elderly (>65 yr), renal or liver dysfunction
	Gastrointestinal symptoms (10%)	None	No effect on CYP450 enzymes	Elimination exclusively by renal excretion

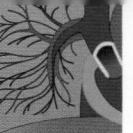

TABLE 53-1 Currently Available Antiretroviral Drugs (See Text for References)—cont'd

SUBSTANCE NAME	TRADE NAME	RECOMMENDED DAILY DOSE (mg)*	ORAL AVAIL-ABILITY (%)	T_{max} (hr)	Vd (L/kg)	THERA-PEUTIC PLASMA CONCEN-TRATION (mg/L)	PROTEIN BINDING	AVERAGE PLASMA HALF-LIFE (hr)
Zanamivir	Relenza	Inhaled 10–20 mg daily for adults and children > 12 yr	10–20	Poorly absorbed following oral admin-istration bioavail-ability about 2%				NA
Pyrofosfate Analogs								
Foscarnet	Foscavir	60 mg/kg intravenously tid, or 90 mg/kg intravenously bid	10–20		0.4–0.7	0.33–0.50 mmol/L	17	first phase, 0.5–1.4 second phase, 3.3–6.8 third phase, up to 18
Others								
Ribavirin	Rebetol, Copegus	>75 kg: 600 mg po bid (generally + interferon); <75 kg: 400 mg in the morning and 600 mg po in the evening	50	1–2	5–29 L/kg		nihil	20–50
Ribavirin	Virazole	20 mg/mL as aerosol 18–20 hr per day and 3–7 days long					nihil	9.5
Cidofovir	Vistide	5 mg/kg IV once weekly for 14 days, thereafter once per 14 days	<5		0.26–0.51		<10	2.2
Palivizumab	Synagis	15 mg/kg in once monthly		0.7	0.07–0.11			18–20 days

(mtDNA) polymerase-γ, which is responsible for mtDNA synthesis, leading to decreased mtDNA. Furthermore, these agents are chain terminators.[9] mtDNA is the only extrachromosomal, extranuclear DNA in humans. The mitochondria perform an essential respiratory role known as oxidative phosphorylation. The mechanism of mitochondrial toxicity by antiviral agents such as NRTIs has been discussed by several investigators.[9-11] Mitochondrial toxicity leads to impairment of normal oxidation of long-chain fatty acids in mitochondria. This causes esterification of triglycerides and an increase in nonesterified fatty acids. These accumulate as intra-cellular vesicles or are released on cell death. Impaired energy production and probably direct toxic effects of nonesterified fatty acids are likely etiologic in cell death.[12] Different human cells carry varying levels of mito-chondria; therefore, impairment of mitochondrial function is likely to become apparent in tissues that are metabolically most active. Common NRTI-associated mito-chondrial dysfunction includes lactic acidosis, hepatic steatosis, peripheral neuropathy, pancreatitis, myopathy, and lipodystrophy.[13-19] Free radicals may also contribute to nucleoside toxicity, potentially playing a role in didanosine-associated pancreatitis.[9,16] The most relevant and regularly occurring adverse effects are summarized below. These effects have been reported in all NRTIs.

Adverse Effects of Nucleoside Reverse-Transcriptase Inhibitors

LACTATE ACIDOSIS
Lactic acidosis most commonly occurs in patients undergoing prolonged therapy with NRTIs. The onset of lactic acidosis can be either abrupt or insidious. Clinical

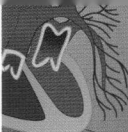

INTRACELLULAR HALF-LIFE TIME (hr)	ADVERSE EFFECTS	TOXIC EFFECT	RELEVANT ISSUES FOR DRUG METABOLISM	REMARKS
	None	None		All absorbed drug is excreted unchanged in urine.
	Renal failure, hypo- and hyperphosphatemia, hypocalcemia, bone marrow depression, headache, paresthesia, dizziness, anorexia, nausea, vomiting, fever skin rash, anemia. Less frequently: several other adverse effects (phlebitis after peripheral intra-venous administration), penile ulceration, nephrogenic diabetes insipidus, thrombocytemia	Acute hypocalciemia, convulsions, renal toxicity. One patient died after 12.5 g for 3 instead of 10.9 mg/day. He suffered a grand mal seizure and became comatose. Of nine patients with 1.14 to 8 times their recommended dose, three suffered seizures, three renal failure, four had paresthesia, and five calcium and phosphate disturbances.	Preverably do not administer in combination with other nefrotoxic drugs	Elimination increased by hemodialysis; Foscarnet is hardly metabolized and the majority of the dose is unchanged excreted with the urine. Be aware for hypo- and hypercalciemia, hypomagnesemia and hyper- and hypophos-phatemia. Hemodialysis and hydration may be of benefit in reducing drug plasma concentrations.
	Nausea, joint and muscle pain, bone marrow depression, tachycardia, pancreatitis, hyperuricemia			Mainly excreted with the urine, for 30% unchanged
		Water intoxication has been reported.		
	Nausea, vomiting, fever, neutropenia, renal toxicity with proteinuria, rare pancreatitis, very rarely ototoxicity	Nephrotoxicity (proximal tubula cell injury)		Co-administration of probenecid may reduce nephrotoxicity, 80%–100% is excreted unchanged with the urine. The compound is hemodialysable.
	Injection site reactions			

symptoms can include abdominal distention and pain, nausea, vomiting, diarrhea, anorexia, tachypnea, weakness, weight loss, and hepatomegaly. Liver and/or renal failure, clotting abnormalities, seizures, and cardiac arrhythmias may be present. In addition to hyperlactatemia, laboratory evaluation may reveal an increased anion gap, elevated aminotransferases, creatine phosphokinase, lactic dehydrogenase, lipase, and amylase.[16,19-23] Echography and computed tomography scans may indicate an enlarged fatty liver; histologic examination of the liver might reveal microvesicular steatosis.[19]

Antiretroviral treatment should be ceased if clinical and laboratory manifestations of the lactic acidosis syndrome occur. For certain patients, this adverse event resolves after discontinuation of NRTIs[19,24] and a revised NRTI-containing regimen can be resumed.[19,25] However, insufficient data exist to recommend this strategy versus treatment with an NRTI-sparing regimen. Intensive therapeutic strategies and intensive care treatment may be necessary. Thiamine[26] and riboflavin[27,28] have been administered on the basis of the pathophysiologic hypothesis that sustained cellular dysfunction of the mitochondrial respiratory chain is responsible for this fulminant clinical syndrome. However, efficacy of these latter interventions requires clinical validation. Although cases of severe lactic acidosis with hepatomegaly and steatosis are rare, when it occurs, this syndrome is associated with a poor prognosis.[14,16,23,29]

PERIPHERAL NEUROPATHY

NRTIs cause a dose-dependent distal, bilateral, symmetrical peripheral neuropathy. This neuropathy typically manifests as pain and have abrupt onset and progression. The main features are pain, numbness, and

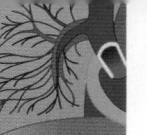

paresthesia. Lower extremities are more involved than upper extremities. Zalcitabine and stavudine are associated with comparable rates of peripheral neuropathy, and didanosine a lower rate. Zidovudine, lamivudine or abacavir are not generally associated with peripheral neuropathy. Acetyl-L-carnitine has analgesic effects in painful neuropathy and may have some benefit in these patients.[30] However, efficacy of this latter intervention requires clinical validation.

MYOPATHY

In the myopathy of NRTI use, skeletal muscles are most commonly affected, leading to proximal weakness, fatigue, muscle pain, and muscular wasting, together with a raised creatine kinase level.[16,31-33] Skeletal myopathy has been reported predominantly with zidovudine and is dose dependent.[33] It is unusual with the other NRTIs.[34] Tissue-specifity studies with zidovudine have demonstrated that the greater impact of muscle cells may involve inhibition of succinate transport systems rather than direct mitochondrial toxicity.[35] In vitro studies have established that L-carnitine may both prevent zidovudine-induced myotoxicity and hasten recovery.[36,37]

FAT MALDISTRIBUTION

Fat maldistribution is often referred to as the lipodystrophy syndrome. Clinical findings include central obesity, lipomas, visceral and dorsocervical ("buffalo") fat accumulation, as well as breast enlargement, peripheral fat wasting, and facial thinning.[38-40] Lipodystrophy may occur in association with insulin resistance and hyperlipidemia.[41] The prevalence of this adverse effect has been reported to increase with long-term NRTI exposure.[39,42,43] Theories on the role of NRTIs in fat redistribution have focused on mitochondrial toxicity and the potential impact on peripheral versus visceral and brown fat cells.[15,17]

No clearly effective therapy for fat accumulation or lipoatrophy has been found. In the majority of victims, discontinuation of antiretroviral medications or class switching has not resulted in substantial benefit; however, among a limited number of persons, improvement in physical appearance has been reported.

Specific Agents

ABACAVIR

Pharmacokinetic information and adverse effects of abacavir (Fig. 53-1) are summarized in Table 53-1.[44-46] Among the NRTIs, skin rash occurs most frequently with abacavir. Skin rash may be a symptom of abacavir-associated systemic hypersensitivity reaction; in that case,

FIGURE 53-1 Abacavir.

therapy should be discontinued without future attempts to resume abacavir therapy. Single doses of up to 1200 mg and daily doses of up to 1800 mg have been administered to patients in clinical studies without adverse effects. Acute overdose with abacavir has not been reported but is presumed to produce minimal toxicity.

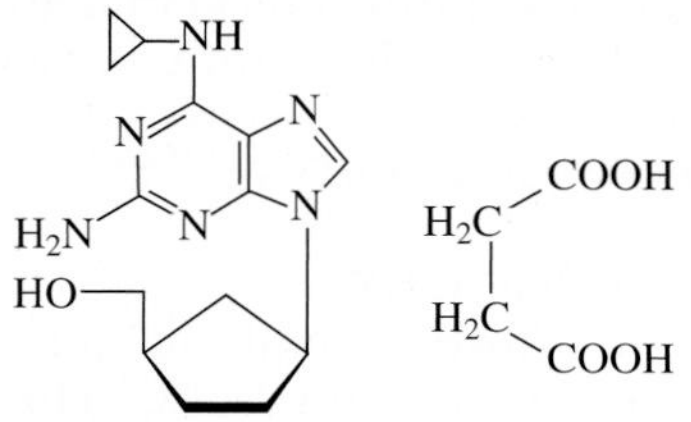

DIDANOSINE

Pharmacokinetic information and adverse effects of didanosine (Fig. 53-2) are summarized in Table 53-1.[46-50] Diarrhea is the most common adverse effect associated with didanosine. Further treatment-limiting toxicities of

FIGURE 53-2 Didanosine.

didanosine are peripheral neuropathy and pancreatitis.[51] Acute overdose with didanosine has not been widely reported. In one case, hemodialysis for 4 hours removed approximately 20% of the amount present in the body at the start of dialysis.[50]

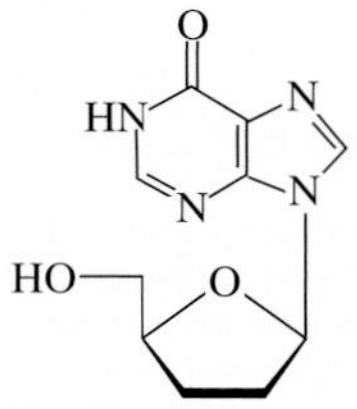

LAMIVUDINE

Pharmacokinetic information and adverse effects of lamivudine (Fig. 53-3) are summarized in Table 53-1.[46,52,53] Adverse effects associated with lamivudine use are primarily gastrointestinal and include nausea, vomiting, abdominal pain or cramps, and diarrhea.

FIGURE 53-3 Lamivudine.

Acute, single overdoses produce minimal toxicity. In one reported case, an adult ingested 6 g of lamivudine. No clinical symptoms were reported. Hematologic indices remained normal.[5]

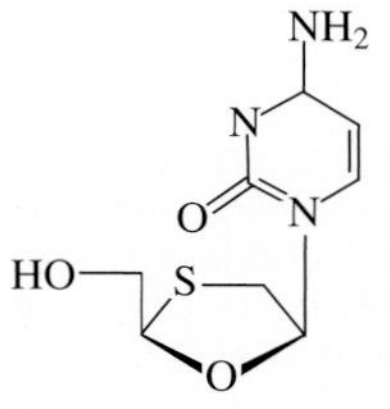

ZALCITABINE

Pharmacokinetic information and adverse effects of zalcitabine (Fig. 53-4) are summarized in Table 53-1.[46,47,54,55]

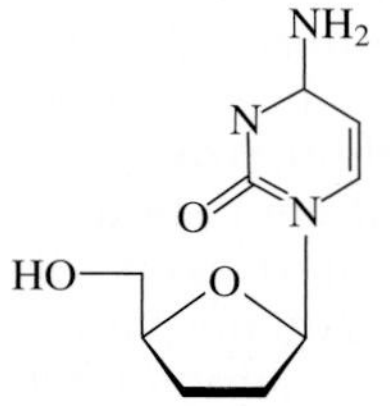

FIGURE 53-4 Zalcitabine.

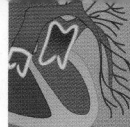

Peripheral neuropathy and oral stomatitis are frequently reported adverse effect with zalcitabine therapy. Acute overdoses with zalcitabine have not been reported.

STAVUDINE
See also Table 53-1.[46,56] The major clinical toxicity with stavudine (Fig. 53-5) is dose-related reversible peripheral

FIGURE 53-5 Stavudine.

neuropathy. Experience with adults exposed to 12 to 24 times the recommended dose has indicated that no significant acute toxicity develops.

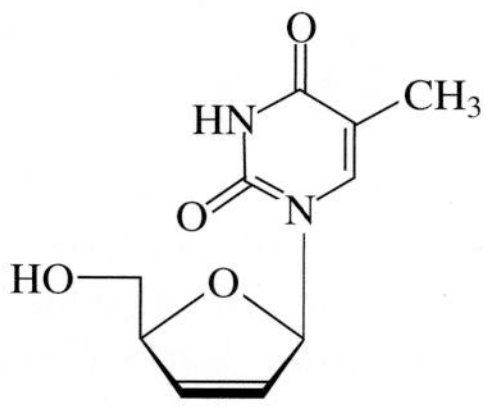

ZIDOVUDINE
See also Table 53-1.[46,47,57,58] Zidovudine (Fig. 53-6) is the most extensively used of the NRTIs. Overdoses have been reported both in pediatric and adult patients. After acute overdose, the only consistent findings have been nausea and vomiting. Headache, dizziness, drowsiness, lethargy, and confusion have also been reported. In one case report, ocular nystagmus and ataxia occurred, resolving

FIGURE 53-6 Zidovudine.

48 hours after ingestion of 10 to 20 g.[59,60] When a 34-year-old man ingested 100 tablets of 200-mg zidovudine, the zidovudine level 12 hours after ingestion was 185 μmol/L (normal range 0.6 to 4.4 μmol/L). He was drowsy but otherwise asymptomatic.[61] In an unusual case, a patient who ingested 36 g zidovudine had a grand mal seizure 3 hours after ingestion.[62]

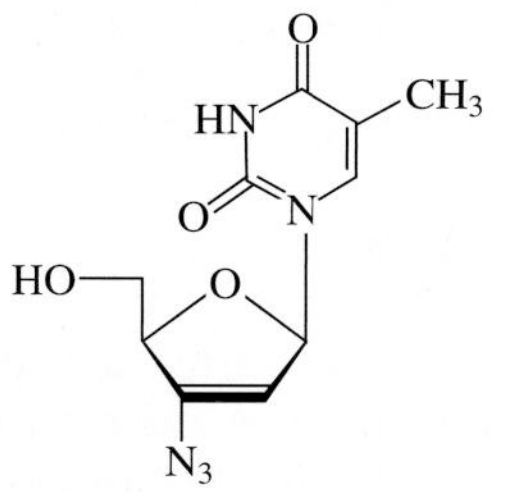

Hematologic variables remain generally normal after acute overdose; in long-term use myelodepression may occur.[59,63,64] Treatment of this overdose is supportive.

ADEFOVIR
For a summary of pharmacokinetic information and adverse effects of adefovir (Fig. 53-7), see Table 53-1.[65] (See also adefovir dipivoxil, FDA Advisory Committee Briefing Document, NDA 21-449, July 5, 2002.) Acute overdoses with adefovir have not been reported; its toxicity profile is therefore largely unknown.

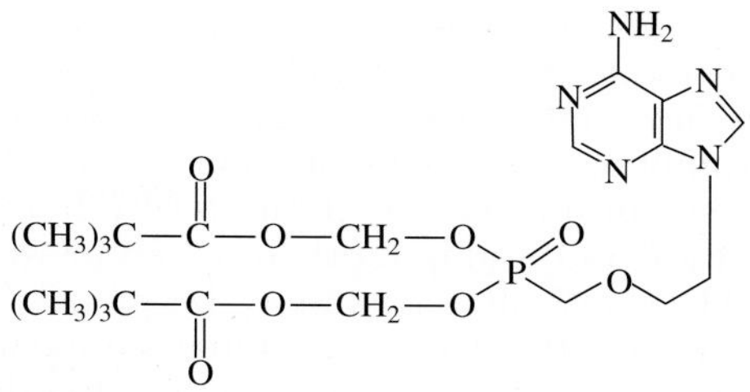

FIGURE 53-7 Adefovir.

TENOFOVIR
See Table 53-1.[66-69] Acute overdoses with tenofovir (Fig. 53-8) have not been reported.

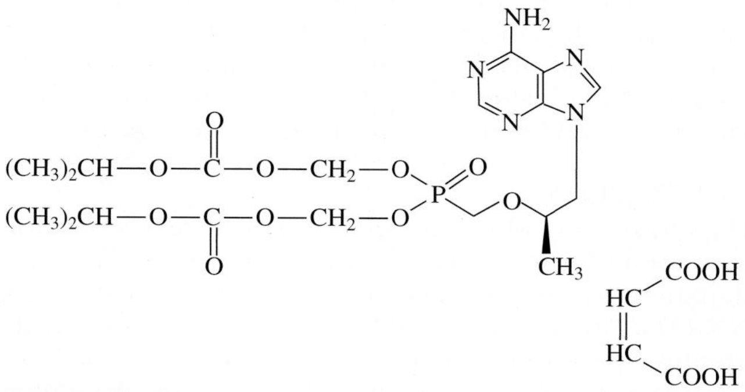

FIGURE 53-8 Tenofovir.

EMTRICITABINE
See Table 53-1.[49,70] Acute overdoses with emtricitabine (Fig. 53-9) have not been reported.

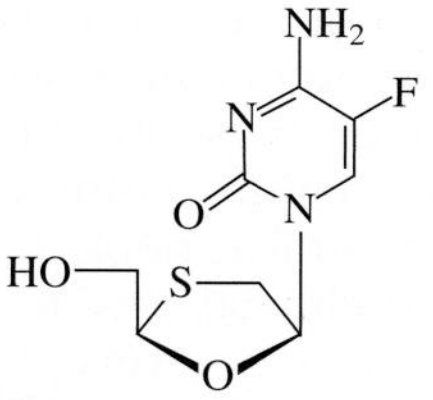

FIGURE 53-9 Emtricitabine.

NON-NUCLEOSIDE REVERSE-TRANSCRIPTASE INHIBITORS

The non-nucleoside reverse-transcriptase inhibitors (NNRTIs) include delavirdine, efavirenz, and nevirapine. These agents interrupt the reverse transcription of viral RNA to DNA, a crucial step for HIV replication, by a mechanism of action different from nucleoside analogs. The NNRTIs bind to reverse transcriptase and block the RNA-dependent and DNA-dependent DNA polymerase activities by causing a disruption of the enzyme catalytic site.

Adverse Effects

SKIN RASH
Skin rash appears to be a class-wide adverse reaction of the NNRTIs. The majority of skin eruptions are mild to moderate, occurring within the first weeks of therapy. A syndrome of drug rash with severe or even life-

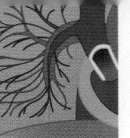
threatening manifestations (e.g., Stevens-Johnson syndrome, toxic epidermal necrosis [TEN], and eosinophilia with systemic symptoms) is frequently described and should prompt permanent discontinuation of NNRTIs.[71,72] Systemic symptoms can include fever, hematologic abnormalities, and multiple organ involvement. Among the NNRTIs, skin rash occurs more frequently and with greater severity with nevirapine. Females appear to have a higher risk for developing severe skin rashes than male patients.[73,74] The prophylactic use of systemic corticosteroid or antihistamine therapy at the time of nevirapine initiation has not proven to be effective.[73]

The incidence of cross-reactivity in the adverse effects among these agents is unknown. In a limited number of reports, patients with nevirapine-associated skin rashes have been able to tolerate efavirenz without increased rates of cutaneous reactions.[75,76] Initiating NNRTI for a patient with a history of mild to moderate skin rash with another NNRTI should be performed with caution.

HEPATOXICITY

Hepatotoxicity, which is defined as a three- to fivefold increase in serum transaminases, with or without clinical hepatitis, has been reported among patients receiving NNRTIs. Among the NNRTIs, nevirapine possesses the greatest potential for producing clinical hepatitis.[77] Nevirapine-associated hepatitis can also be present as part of a hypersensitivity syndrome (e.g., skin rash, fever, and eosinophilia). Approximately two thirds of the cases of nevirapine-associated clinical hepatitis occur within the first 12 weeks of therapy. Fulminant and even fatal cases of hepatic necrosis have been reported. Victims may also experience nonspecific gastrointestinal and flu-like symptoms with or without increased liver enzyme levels. The syndrome can progress rapidly to hepatomegaly, jaundice, and hepatic failure within days. Because of the potential severity of clinical hepatitis, close monitoring of liver enzymes and clinical symptoms after nevirapine initiation is necessary (e.g., every 2 weeks for the first month; then monthly for the first 12 weeks, and every 1 to 3 months thereafter). Patients who experience severe hepatotoxicity while receiving nevirapine should not receive nevirapine therapy again in the future.

Specific Agents

DELAVIRDINE

Pharmacokinetic information and adverse effects of delavirdine (Fig. 53-10) are summarized in Table 53-1.[46,48,78-82] Consequences of acute overdose with delavirdine have not been characterized.

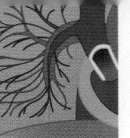

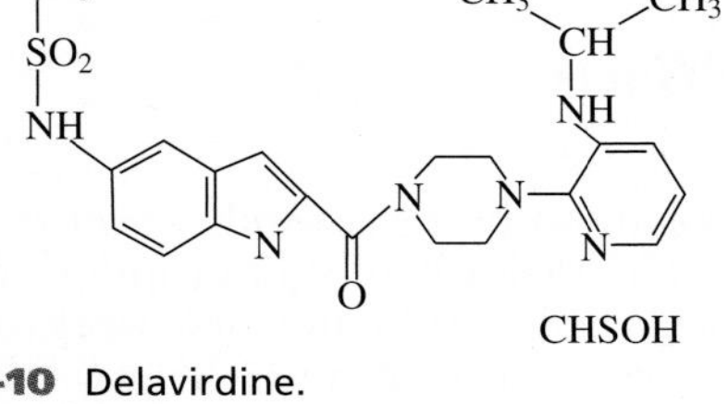

FIGURE 53-10 Delavirdine.

EFAVIRENZ

For pharmacokinetic information and adverse effects of efavirenz (Fig. 53-11) see Table 53-1.[46,49,80,81,83,84] The most significant adverse events observed in patients who take efavirenz chronically are neurotoxicity and rash.

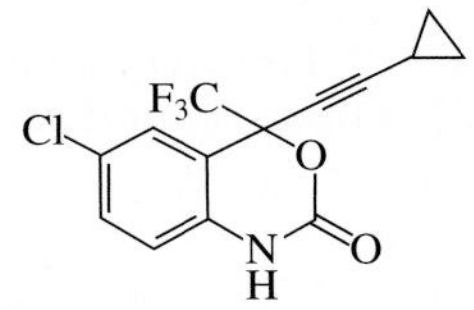

FIGURE 53-11 Efavirenz.

Occasional cases of pancreatitis have also been described; increases in serum amylase levels have been observed in a significantly higher number of patients treated with 600 mg of efavirenz than in control patients. Increases in total cholesterol of 10% to 20% have been observed in clinical trials. Acute overdoses with efavirenz have not been reported.

NEVIRAPINE

For pharmacokinetic information on nevirapine (Fig. 53-12) see Table 53-1.[46,53,80,81,85,86] Rash is the most frequently observed adverse effect with nevirapine, manifesting as a maculopapular eruption with or without fever, edema, myalgia, and arthralgia. This rash is in general mild and transient. However, severe fatal reactions such as Stevens-Johnson syndrome may occur. Nevirapine-associated rashes have been reported to

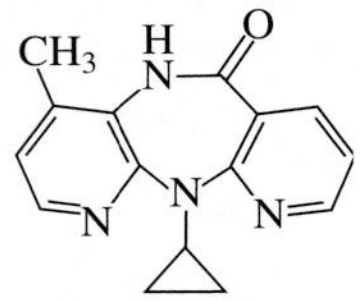

FIGURE 53-12 Nevirapine.

occur in as many as 48% after a starting dose of 400 mg/day. Starting with a lower dose and slowly increasing the dose reduced the occurrence of rashes to 9% to 32%. Hepatotoxicity is frequently observed in patients receiving nevirapine, occurring predominantly in the first 8 weeks of administration. Granulocytopenia has also been observed, particularly in children. Conse-quences of acute overdose with nevirapine have not been characterized.

GUANOSINE ANALOGS

The guanosine analogs include acyclovir, valaciclovir, ganciclovir, penciclovir, famciclovir, and valganciclovir. These agents exert their effect after being metabolized to their triphosphate form. The initial step in this process, the formation of the monophosphate form, is catalyzed by a thymidine kinase induced by herpes simplex virus types 1 and 2 and varicella-zoster virus in the infected cells or by a protein kinase produced by cytomegalovirus.[1,2,87-89] In the triphosphate form, guanosine analogs inhibit the synthesis of viral DNA, either as a competitive inhibitor or as an alternative substrate with respect to the natural substrate (2'-deoxyguanosine triphosphate) for viral DNA poly-

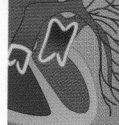

merase. Once the guanine analog is inserted into the replicating viral DNA, synthesis stops. In this process, the triphosphate form of the guanosine analog is a potent inhibitor of herpes simplex type 1 DNA polymerase and of human cellular α-DNA polymerase.[1,90] The limited production of the guanosine analog triphosphate form in uninfected cells and its specificity for viral DNA polymerase result in minimal cellular toxic effects.

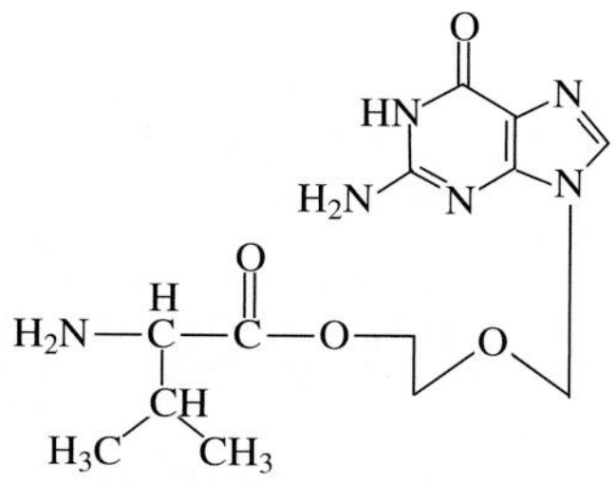

Specific Agents

ACYCLOVIR

Pharmacokinetic information and adverse effects of acyclovir (Fig. 53-13) are summarized in Table 53-1.[91-94] The kidneys account for 75% of the total clearance of acyclovir. Renal clearance of this drug is approximately three times that of creatinine, suggesting that elimination occurs both by glomerular filtration and tubular secretion.[95] Neurotoxicity and nephrotoxicity by tubular crystal formation or by acute interstitial nephritis are potentially serious complications of acyclovir.[93,96-99] The potential for neurotoxicity is increased when renal elimination is impaired.[100] Peak plasma acyclovir levels do not correlate well with symptoms of neurotoxicity.[101-105]

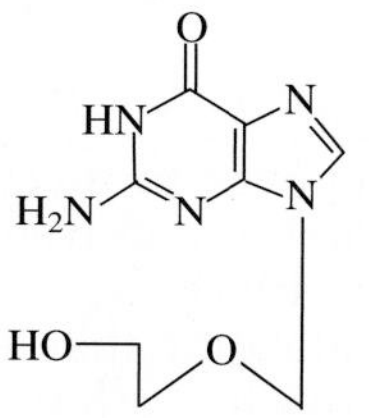

FIGURE 53-13 Acyclovir.

There have been several reports of acyclovir overdose. In one, a neonate received an inadvertent overdose of 750 mg (220 mg/kg) intravenous acyclovir. Treated with saline hydration alone, he had only a transient increase in serum creatinine.[106] Neurotoxicity from acyclovir is more common in the elderly, in patients with renal dysfunction, or in patients taking other neurotoxic drugs.[92,107-110] Acyclovir nephrotoxicity typically resolves after discontinuation of the drug. Extracorporeal clearance of acyclovir with hemodialysis can be of modest benefit.[91,96,111] In serious neurotoxicity, hemodialysis should be considered.[112] Further treatment is supportive.

VALACYCLOVIR

For pharmacokinetic information and adverse effects of valacyclovir (Fig. 53-14) see Table 53-1.[113-115] Valacyclovir, a prodrug, is the L-valyl ester of acyclovir.[116] After ingestion, the drug is rapidly converted to acyclovir by the enzyme valacyclovir hydrolase in the gastrointestinal tract and liver.[117] Its oral bioavailability is three to five times that of acyclovir.[118] In terms of toxicity, a few cases of neurotoxicity in patients with end-stage renal disease are described.[114,115,119] High-dose valacyclovir (8 g/day) has been associated with the development of thrombotic thrombocytopenic purpura, although HIV itself could not be excluded as the etiology in these reported cases.[113,120] Treatment principles follow that of acyclovir.

FIGURE 53-14 Valacyclovir.

GANCICLOVIR

For pharmacokinetic information and adverse effects of ganciclovir (Fig. 53-15) see Table 53-1.[121,122] Ganciclovir differs from acyclovir by the addition of a hydroxymethyl group at the 3′ position of the acyclic side chain.[5] The value of the oral formulation is limited due to its low bioavailability. The metabolism and action of ganciclovir are similar to those of acyclovir, although it is not an absolute DNA chain terminator.[123] Ganciclovir is converted to ganciclovir monophosphate by a viral-encoded phosphotransferase produced in cytomegalovirus-infected

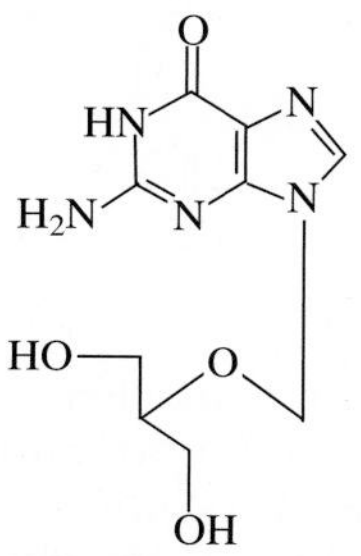

FIGURE 53-15 Ganciclovir.

cells. Gancyclovir's affinity for this phosphotransferase is better than that of acyclovir. The intracellular half-life of ganciclovir triphosphate (12 hours) is significantly longer than that of acyclovir (1 to 2 hours). Hematologic toxicity from ganciclovir is increased by its combination with other myelotoxic drugs.[124] In one reported case, a cardiac transplant recipient received 50 mg/kg ganciclovir for 36 hours without immediate or delayed adverse effects or toxicity. In another series, two patients developed ventricular tachycardia and died after the intravenous administration of 5 mg/kg ganciclovir.[125] Retinal toxicity has been observed after a high intravitreal dose (400 μg/0.1 mL).[126]

PENCICLOVIR

For pharmacokinetic information and adverse effects of penciclovir (Fig. 53-16) see Table 53-1.[5] Penciclovir is similar to the ganciclovir molecule, differing only by the substitution of a methylene bridge for the ether oxygen in the acyclic ribose part of the molecule.[5] The oral bioavailability of penciclovir is poor. The drug is only approved for topical treatment of herpes labialis. Following intravenous administration, the volume of distribution is approximately 1.5 L/kg, with a mean terminal-phase half-life of 2.0 hours. Approximately 70% of drug is excreted unchanged in the urine.[127]

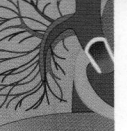

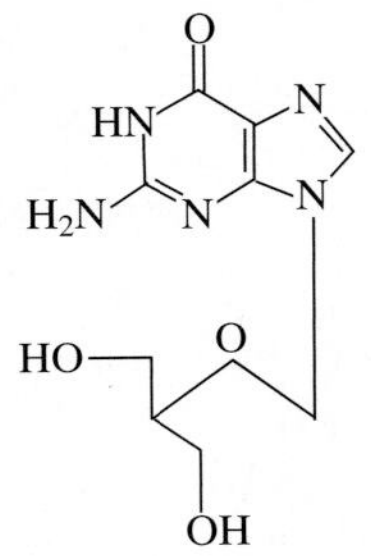

FIGURE 53-16 Penciclovir.

FAMCICLOVIR

For pharmacokinetic information and a summary of adverse of famciclovir (Fig. 53-17) effects see Table 53-1.[117,128,129] Famciclovir is an oral prodrug of penciclovir. It is well absorbed after oral administration and is

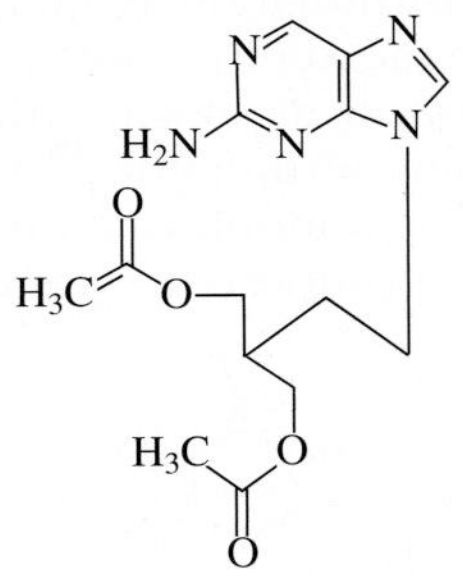

FIGURE 53-17 Famciclovir.

rapidly metabolized to penciclovir by deacetylation in the gastrointestinal tract, blood, and liver, after which it is oxidized by the liver at position 6 of the purine ring. The intracellular half-life of the active drug, penciclovir triphosphate, is long.[117] Experience with acute toxicity is limited. A report of acute overdosage of 10.5 g was notable in the absence of significant symptoms.

VALGANCICLOVIR

For pharmacokinetic information and adverse effects of valganciclovir (Fig. 53-18), see Table 53-1.[130-135]

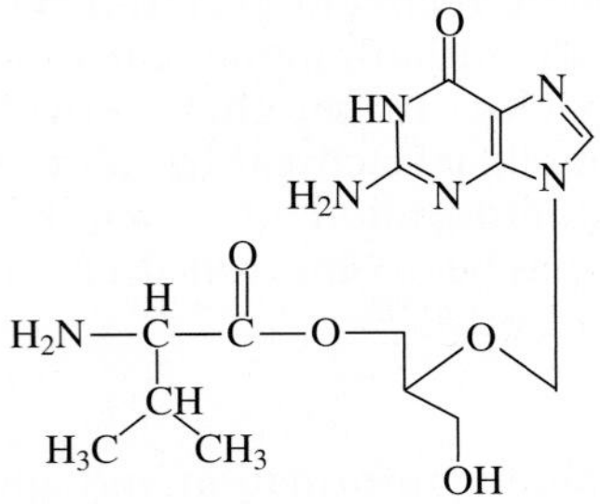

FIGURE 53-18 Valganciclovir.

Valganciclovir, the L-valyl ester of ganciclovir, is an orally administered prodrug of ganciclovir. Its oral bioavailability is good (10 times higher than ganciclovir). Valganciclovir is rapidly converted to ganciclovir. After its absorption the drug has pharmacokinetic properties approaching those of intravenously administered ganciclovir. Adverse effects are similar to those of intravenous ganciclovir and require periodic monitoring of complete blood count and renal function.

PROTEASE INHIBITORS

Most protease inhibitors contain a synthetic analog of the phenylalanine-proline sequence of the GAG-POL polyprotein.[136,137] HIV protease inhibitors prevent cleavage of GAG and GAG-POL protein precursors in all infected cells, arresting maturation and blocking the infectivity of nascent viral particles. In order to achieve maximal drug levels, protease inhibitors often must be administered at high doses, potentially compromising tolerability and adherence.

Protease inhibitor–associated liver enzyme abnormalities can occur any time during the treatment course. In a retrospective review, severe hepatotoxicity (defined as an increase of greater than five times over baseline aspartate aminotransferase or alanine aminotransferase) was observed more often among patients receiving ritonavir or ritonavir/saquinavir-containing regimens than those receiving indinavir, nelfinavir, or saquinavir.[138] Other potential risk factors for hepatotoxicity include hepatitis B or C infection,[139-142] alcohol abuse,[141] baseline elevated liver enzymes,[143] stavudine use,[142] and concomitant use of other hepatotoxic agents.

Adverse Effects

HYPERLIPIDEMIA

Dyslipidemias are known to occur with the use of protease inhibitors; however, its frequency varies from an increased association with ritonavir to limited association with newer agents, indicating that hyperlipidemia might be a drug-specific toxicity rather than a class-specific toxicity.[41] Morevoer, the magnitude of changes varies substantially and occurs inconsistently. Frequently, antiretroviral-associated dyslipidemias are sufficiently severe to require therapeutic intervention.

Indications for monitoring and intervention in HIV therapy–associated dyslipidemias are the same as among uninfected populations. Hypercholesterolemia might respond to 3-hydroxy-3-methylglutaryl-CoA reductase inhibitors (statins). There is an increased risk for fat accumulation with the protease inhibitors, and whether specific drugs are more strongly associated with this toxicity is unclear.[38,41]

HYPERGLYCEMIA

Protease inhibitors are associated with the development of hyperglycemia; the incidence does not vary substantially between the agents within this class.[144] The pathogenesis of these abnormalities has not been fully elucidated; it may result from peripheral and hepatic insulin resistance, relative insulin deficiency, or an impaired ability of the liver to extract insulin.[145,146]

Specific Agents

AMPRENAVIR

Pharmacokinetic information and adverse effects of amprenavir (Fig. 53-19) are summarized in Table 53-1.[81,82,147-150] Amprenavir is well tolerated. Acute overdoses with amprenavir have not been reported, but can be predicted to produce little significant toxicity.

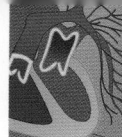

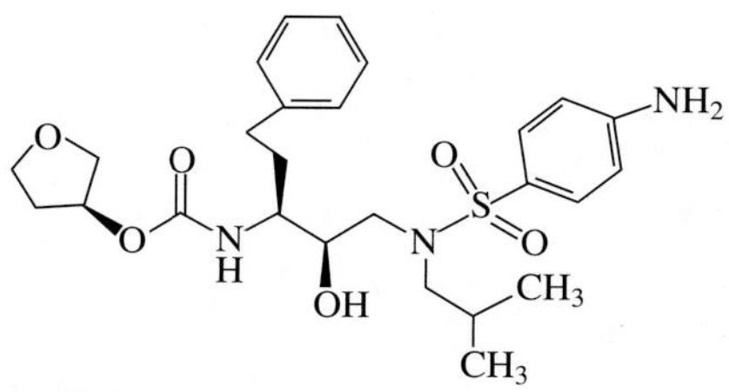

FIGURE 53-19   Amprenavir.

INDINAVIR

See Table 53-1.[81,136,150-152] The most significant adverse effect from indinavir (Fig. 53-20) is nephrolithiasis, which typically resolves after hydration. In one described

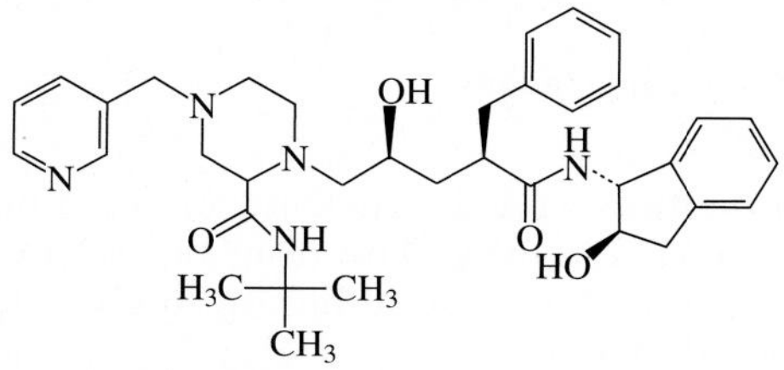

FIGURE 53-20   Indinavir.

case a patient ingested 6 g of indinavir, developing nausea and limb paresthesias. The patient was treated with activated charcoal and hydration. The symptoms resolved within 4 hours, and no nephrolithiasis occurred.[151]

LOPINAVIR

For pharmacokinetic information and adverse effects of lopinavir (Fig. 53-21) see Table 53-1.[81,150] Acute overdoses with lopinavir have not been reported to date.

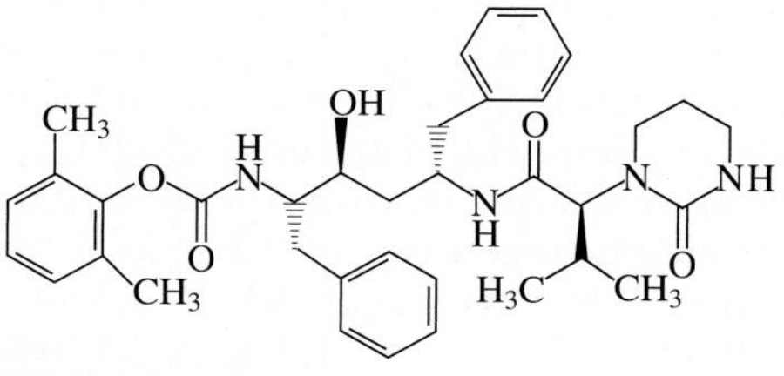

FIGURE 53-21   Lopinavir.

NELFINAVIR

For pharmacokinetic information and adverse effects of nelfinaviar (Fig. 53-22) see Table 53-1.[81,136,150,152,153] Nelfinavir is well tolerated. Other adverse events are rare. Rash (30%) and diarrhea (18%) are common with nelfinavir.[154]

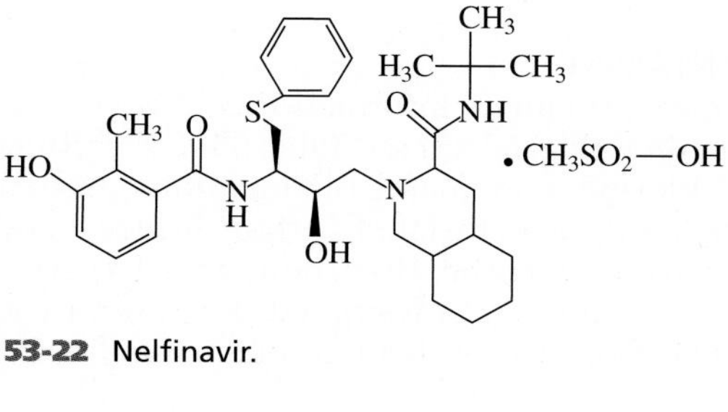

FIGURE 53-22   Nelfinavir.

RITONAVIR

For pharmacokinetic information and adverse effects of ritonavir (Fig. 53-23) see Table 53-1.[81,136,150,152] Diarrhea is the most common adverse effect reported with ritonavir. One death due to pancreatitis was possibly caused by lopinavir/ritonavir, but it could have been related to the thymidine nucleoside analogs as well.[153] In a clinical trial, one patient ingested 1500 mg/day for 2 days. Paresthesias developed, which resolved after the dose was decreased.

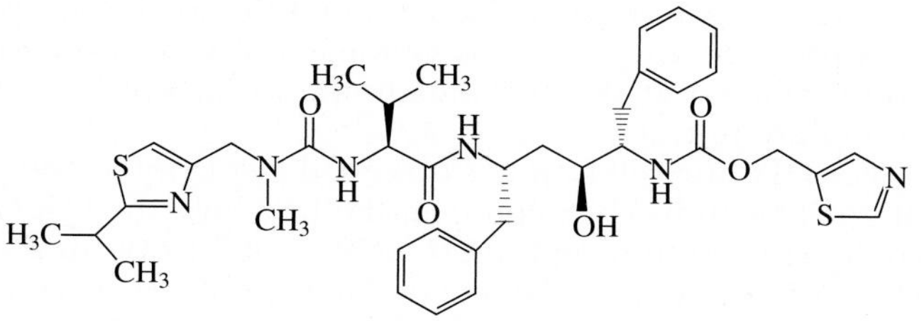

FIGURE 53-23   Ritonavir.

OTHER AGENTS

Pharmacokinetic information and adverse effects for saquinavir (Fig. 53-24) and atazanavir (Fig. 53-25) are summarized in Table 53-1.[81,136,150,152]

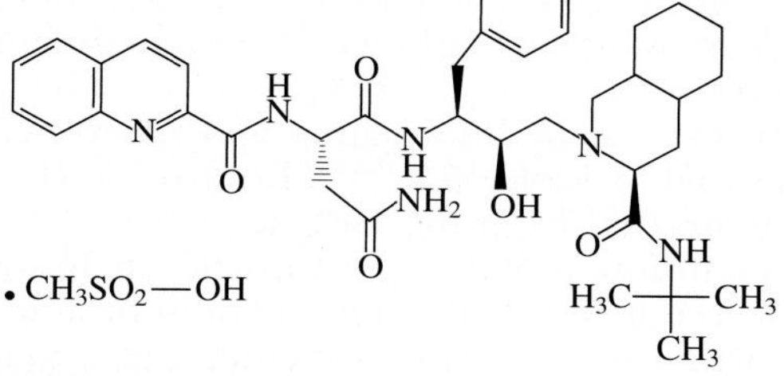

FIGURE 53-24   Saquinavir.

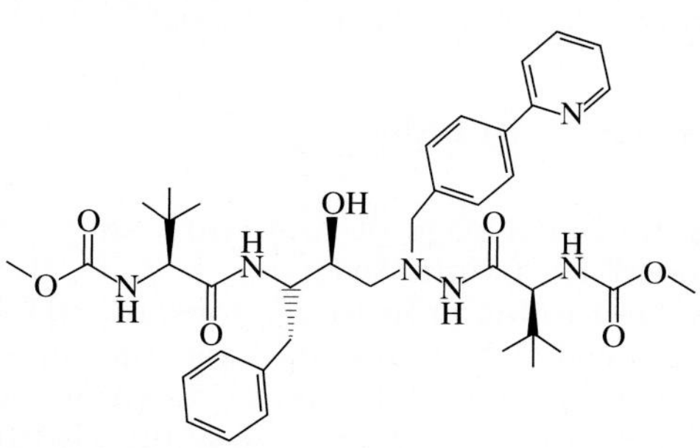

FIGURE 53-25   Atazanavir.

VIRUS CELL FUSION INHIBITORS (ENFUVIRTIDE)

Enveloped viruses undergo a fusion between their envelope and the host cell membrane that is followed by uncoating, after which the virus RNA enters the host cell. Thereafter, the RNA is read by reverse transcription to form DNA. The DNA integrates with the host DNA after which, via transcription replication of the virus genome,

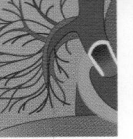

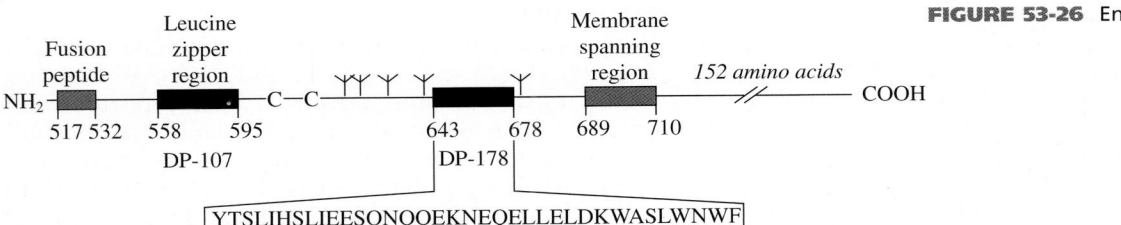

FIGURE 53-26 Enfuvirtide.

YTSLIHSLIEESQNQQEKNEQELLELDKWASLWNWF

the viral RNA is formed. After proteolytic processing by viral protease, the new virus genome and viral proteins are assembled at the cell membrane, from which new virions are released.

For HIV, the cell fusion is preceded by the interaction of gp120 with its coreceptor on the host cell: the C-X-C chemokine motif receptor-4 (CXCR4) for T-tropic or X4 HIV strains, or the C-C chemokine motif receptor 5 (CCR5) for M-tropic or R5 HIV strains. CXCR4 and CCR5 normally act as the receptors for the C-X-C chemokine stromal cell derived factor 1 (SDF1) and the C-C chemokines RANTES (regulated upon activation, normal T-cell expressed and secreted) and macrophage inflammatory protein 1 (MIP1), respectively. The interaction of gp120 with its coreceptor (CCR5 or CXCR4) triggers a series of changes in the gp120-gp41 complex. These changes ultimately lead to fusion of the viral and host cell membranes. Consequently, agents that interfere with the gp120-gp41 complex and its interaction with the cellular membrane might be expected to inhibit this fusion process.[1,155]

Pharmacokinetic information and adverse effects are summarized in Table 53-1.[156,157] Enfuvirtide (Fig. 53-26), or T-20, derived from the HR2 sequence of HIV-1, is a virus cell fusion inhibitor.[158] Enfuvirtide, a 36-amino-acid peptide, is not absorbed orally and must be administered subcutaneously.[159,160] Mild injection site reactions are common with enfuvirtide. Approximately 3% of patients discontinue treatment because of local reactions.

M2 PROTEIN BLOCKERS

During the initial stage of viral entry, after it has been surrounded by a lipid layer, the cell. In the formed vesicles, after influx of hydrogen ions, the pH falls. This acidity is needed to allow the viral uncoating process (decapsidation), so that the ribonucleoprotein can enter the cell nucleus and initiate replication. Hydrogen ions pass through the M2 channel.[2,161] Amantadine and rimantadine exert their function by blocking the viral M2 protein ion channel and its ability to modulate intracellular pH. Consequently, viral replication is hampered.

Specific Agents

AMANTADINE

For pharmacokinetic information and adverse effects of amantadine (Fig. 53-27) see Table 53-1.[162-166] Amantadine hydrochloride is an amine with a unique 10-carbon ring.

FIGURE 53-27 Amantadine.

Besides anti-influenza A virus activity, amantadine is used as an antiparkinson drug. The drug blocks presynaptic reuptake of dopamine, resulting in higher levels of postsynaptic dopamine.

Amantadine is excreted unchanged in the urine; dose adjustments are required for relatively modest decrements in renal function (creatinine clearance less than 60 to 80 mL/min). However, even reduced dosage has been associated with excess rates of adverse effects and has required discontinuation of the drug.

Amantadine has many adverse effects, particularly in those with renal dysfunction and in the elderly, in whom peak concentrations are approximately three times as high as in younger adults given the same dose. The plasma half-life in the elderly is about 12 hours longer. Many cases of amantadine overdose and toxicity are reported in the literature. In general, iatrogenic poisoning occurred in the elderly or was related to renal or liver dysfunction. Hyperthermia, long QT interval, adult respiratory distress syndrome (ARDS), and death, resulting from one overdose of 12 g in a 37-year-old suicidal woman, have been reported.[167] Acute psychosis and hallucinations in adults (1.2 g in 24 hours) and children, coma (after ingestion of 600 mg), and death (after ingestion of 2 g) have all been reported.[163,164,168-171] Furthermore, cardiac ventricular ectopic beats after ingesting 1.4 g (in 17-year-old girl) and torsades de pointes after ingesting 2.5 g (in a 37-year-old woman) have been reported.[165,172] Rhabdomyolysis and an anticholinergic syndrome were seen in a patient with a combined poisoning of phenobarbital and amantadine (0.8 g).[162] Treatment is mainly supportive.[167] Physostigmine may reverse anticholinergic neurologic symptoms in adults and children.[166,171]

RIMANTADINE

For pharmacokinetic information and adverse effects of rimantadine (Fig. 53-28) see Table 53-1.[173-175] Rimantadine hydrochloride is an analog of amantidine, with anamine inserted with a methylated carbon bridge between the amino group and the 10-carbon ring. Experience with overdose by this agent is limited. However, its profile of toxicity is likely to parallel that of amantadine.

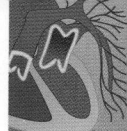

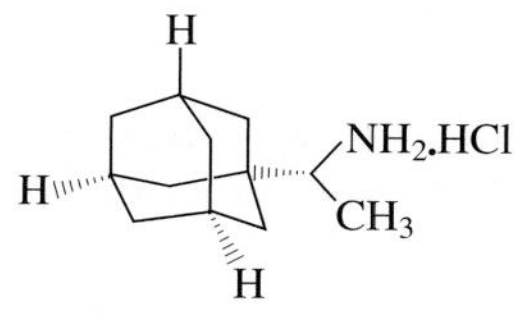

FIGURE 53-28   Rimantadine.

NEURAMINIDASE INHIBITORS

Neuraminidase (sialidase) is a surface glycoprotein with enzymatic activity. Neuraminidase cleaves off the terminal sialic acid of the host cell receptor, allowing virus particles to leave the cell after the viral replicative cycle has been completed. The viral neuromidase is therefore needed for the elution of newly formed particles from the cell. In addition, the viral neuraminidase might promote viral movement through the respiratory tract mucus, thereby enhancing viral infectivity.[1,176]

Zanamivir and oseltamivir are both neuraminidase inhibitors with a similar rate of effectiveness against influenza A and B viruses.[177,178]

Specific Agents

ZANAMIVIR

For pharmacokinetic information and adverse effects of zanamivir (Fig. 53-29) see Table 53-1.[176,179,180] Zanamivir is administered by inhalation.[181] Scintigraphic studies showed 13% of the inhaled 10-mg dose to be deposited

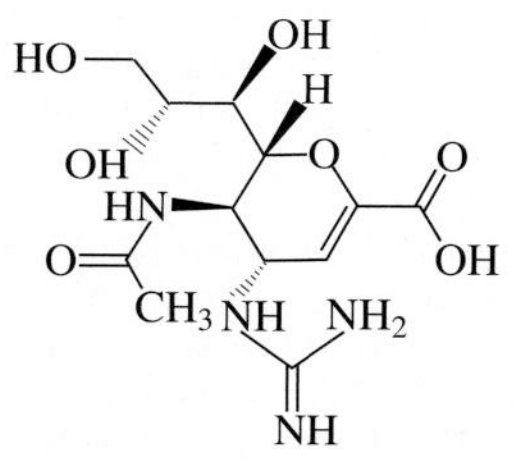

FIGURE 53-29   Zanamivir.

in bronchi and lungs, with 78% being deposited in the oropharynx. High concentrations are retained in tracheal and bronchial epithelium for 24 hours after a single 10-mg dose.[179] Impairment of renal function has no effect on maximal concentration (Cmax) values.[180] Minor adverse effects have been reported in a minority of persons (fewer than 5%), although these effects were similar to those in placebo-control groups.[179] In patients with chronic respiratory disease (e.g., asthama), bronchospasm and ARDS have been reported.

OSELTAMIVIR

For pharmacokinetic information and adverse effects of oseltamivir (Fig. 53-30) see Table 53-1.[179,182] Oseltamivir produces GI symptoms such as nausea and vomiting in about 10% of persons. When the drug is taken with food, the incidence of side effects is reduced, while pharmacokinetics were not altered.

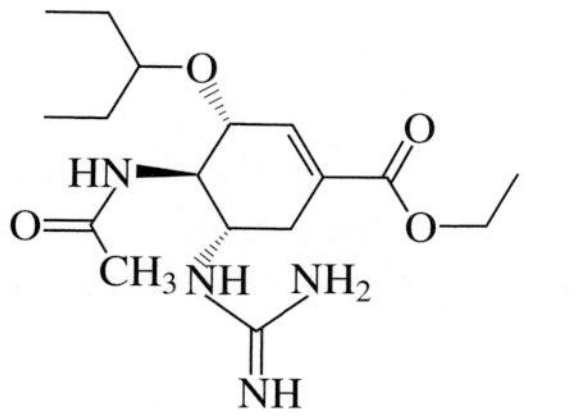

FIGURE 53-30   Oseltamivir.

FOSCARNET

Foscarnet (Fig. 53-31) is a competitive inhibitor of the pyrophosphate binding site on the polymerases. Therefore, it acts by blocking viral DNA polymerase and reverse transcriptase, which are necessary for copying genetic material (from RNA to DNA). This copying process is required for the reproduction of the virus.

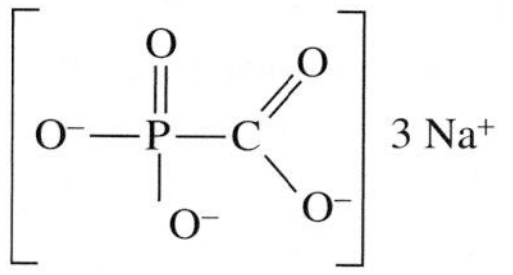

FIGURE 53-31   Foscarnet.

For pharmacokinetic information and adverse effects see Table 53-1.[183-185] The most common adverse effect from foscarnet, nephrotoxicity, seems to be dose dependent.[186] To reduce the risk for nephrotoxicity, creatinine clearance should be calculated even if the serum creatinine is within the normal range. Drug dose should be adjusted accordingly. Adequate hydration reduces the risk for nephrotoxicity. Due to foscarnet's propensity to chelate divalent metal ions, such as calcium, magnesium, iron, and zinc, serum concentrations of these ions should be monitored. Hypocalciemia has been reported after foscarnet is administered in combination with pentamidine or after rapid infusion. Severe hypocalciemia might lead to Trousseau's and Chvostek's signs, seizures, and heart rhythm disturbances.[183,187-190] Other electrolyte changes (e.g., hypokalemia, hypophosphatemia, and hyperphosphatemia) have been reported. Since foscarnet is excreted in high concentrations in the urine, local irritation and ulceration may ensue.[191,192] In patients with severe intoxication, hemodialysis and hydration may be of benefit in reducing drug plasma concentrations, but the effectiveness of these interventions has not been evaluated.

CIDOFOVIR

For pharmacokinetic information and adverse effects of cidofovir (Fig. 53-32) see Table 53-1.[65,193-195] After

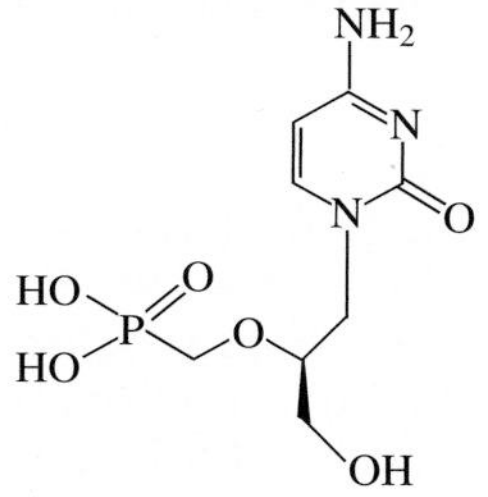

FIGURE 53-32   Cidofovir.

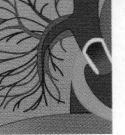

intracellular phosphorylation to the diphosphate form, and incorporation at the 3' end of the viral chain, cidofovir acts as a chain terminator.[2] Nephrotoxicity is common after overdose with this agent. Concomitant oral probenecid decreases both the renal clearance of cidofovir and the incidence of nephrotoxicity.

RIBAVIRIN

For pharmacokinetic information and adverse effects of ribavirin (Fig. 53-33) see Table 53-1.[196-201] Ribavirin interacts (in its 5'-monophosphate form) with inosine monophosphate (IMP) dehydrogenase, which converts (IMP) to xanthosine monophosphate, a key step in the biosynthesis of guanosine triphosphate and deoxyguanosine triphosphate. In its 5'-trophosphate form, ribavirin can also interfere with the viral RNA polymerase and the 5'-capped oligonucleotide primer formation required for transcription of the influenza genome. It is administered in an aerosol and orally.

FIGURE 53-33 Ribavirin.

Adverse effects from ribavirin have been reported. Water intoxication in a 6-week-old girl was observed after a nebulized dose of 6 g in 100 mL distilled water four times daily. On day 2, convulsions occurred and plasma sodium was 108 mmol/L.[202] An 8-week-old girl was treated with 6 g in 300 mL distilled water nebulized for 18 hours when seizures occurred, and plasma sodium was 116 mmol/L.[203] Treatment is supportive.

Ribavirin is administered as an aerosol, with delivery of the drug into a mist tent, hood, or ventilator. In certain small animals dosed systematically with ribavirin, teratogenity and embryopathy have been found. Furthermore, ribavirin can significantly affect sperm morphology in rats; it is a germ cell mutagen in rats. These effects in experimental models have led to concerns abaout exposure to health care personnel administering aerosolized ribavirin and have significantly reduced its use in the health care setting. Though the effect on fetal development in humans is not known, it is recommended that occupational exposure to ribavirin aerosol be minimized as much as possible.

PALIVIZUMAB

For pharmacokinetic information and adverse effects of palivizumab see Table 53-1.[204,205] Palivizumab is a humanized monoclonal immunoglobulin G1 antibody to the fusion protein of the respiratory syncytial virus (RSV) that is highly active against RSV A and B strains. Adverse effects are mild and transient.

ACKNOWLEDGMENT

The molecular figures were taken from a review article by E. de Clercq: Antiviral drugs in current clinical use. J Clin Virol 2004;30(2):115–133.

REFERENCES

1. De Clercq E: Strategies in the design of antiviral drugs. Nat Rev Drug Discov 2002;1(1):13–25.
2. De Clercq E: Antiviral drugs in current clinical use. J Clin Virol 2004;30(2):115–133.
3. National Institutes of Health: Guidelines for the use of antiretroviral agents in HIV-1-infected adults and adolescents. Retrieved October 29, 2004, from http://AIDSinfo.nih.gov.
4. National Institutes of Health: Guidelines for the use of antiretroviral agents in pediatric HIV infection. Retrieved January 20, 2004, from http://AIDSinfo.nih.gov.
5. Balfour HH Jr: Antiviral drugs. N Engl J Med 1999;340(16): 1255–1268.
6. De Clercq E: Antivirals and antiviral strategies. Nat Rev Microbiol 2004;2(9):704–720.
7. Piscitelli SC, Gallicano KD: Interactions among drugs for HIV and opportunistic infections. N Engl J Med 2001;344(13):984–996.
8. Kovacs JA, Masur H: Prophylaxis against opportunistic infections in patients with human immunodeficiency virus infection. N Engl J Med 2000;342(19):1416–1429.
9. Moyle G: Toxicity of antiretroviral nucleoside and nucleotide analogues: is mitochondrial toxicity the only mechanism? Drug Saf 2000;23(6):467–481.
10. Kakuda TN: Pharmacology of nucleoside and nucleotide reverse transcriptase inhibitor-induced mitochondrial toxicity. Clin Ther 2000;22(6):685–708.
11. Lewis W, Day BJ, Copeland WC: Mitochondrial toxicity of NRTI antiviral drugs: an integrated cellular perspective. Nat Rev Drug Discov 2003;2(10):812–822.
12. Fromenty B, Pessayre D: Impaired mitochondrial function in microvesicular steatosis. Effects of drugs, ethanol, hormones and cytokines. J Hepatol 1997;26(Suppl 2):43–53.
13. John M, Moore CB, James IR, et al: Chronic hyperlactatemia in HIV-infected patients taking antiretroviral therapy. AIDS 2001;15(6):717–723.
14. Fortgang IS, Belitsos PC, Chaisson RE, Moore RD: Hepatomegaly and steatosis in HIV-infected patients receiving nucleoside analog antiretroviral therapy. Am J Gastroenterol 1995;90(9):1433–1436.
15. Brinkman K, Smeitink JA, Romijn JA, Reiss P: Mitochondrial toxicity induced by nucleoside-analogue reverse-transcriptase inhibitors is a key factor in the pathogenesis of antiretroviral-therapy-related lipodystrophy. Lancet 1999;354(9184):1112–1115.
16. Moyle G: Clinical manifestations and management of antiretroviral nucleoside analog-related mitochondrial toxicity. Clin Ther 2000;22(8):911–936.
17. Kakuda TN, Brundage RC, Anderson PL, Fletcher CV: Nucleoside reverse transcriptase inhibitor-induced mitochondrial toxicity as an etiology for lipodystrophy. AIDS 1999;13(16):2311–2312.
18. Mallal SA, John M, Moore CB, et al: Contribution of nucleoside analogue reverse transcriptase inhibitors to subcutaneous fat wasting in patients with HIV infection. AIDS 2000;14(10): 1309–1316.
19. Lonergan JT, Behling C, Pfander H, et al: Hyperlactatemia and hepatic abnormalities in 10 human immunodeficiency virus-infected patients receiving nucleoside analogue combination regimens. Clin Infect Dis 2000;31(1):162–166.
20. Scalfaro P, Chesaux JJ, Buchwalder PA, et al: Severe transient neonatal lactic acidosis during prophylactic zidovudine treatment. Intensive Care Med 1998;24(3):247–250.
21. Sundar K, Suarez M, Banogon PE, Shapiro JM: Zidovudine-induced fatal lactic acidosis and hepatic failure in patients with acquired immunodeficiency syndrome: report of two patients and review of the literature. Crit Care Med 1997;25(8):1425–1430.
22. McKenzie R, Fried MW, Sallie R, et al: Hepatic failure and lactic acidosis due to fialuridine (FIAU), an investigational nucleoside

analogue for chronic hepatitis B. N Engl J Med 1995;333(17): 1099–1105.

23. Olano JP, Borucki MJ, Wen JW, Haque AK: Massive hepatic steatosis and lactic acidosis in a patient with AIDS who was receiving zidovudine. Clin Infect Dis 1995;21(4):973–976.

24. Miller KD, Cameron M, Wood LV, et al: Lactic acidosis and hepatic steatosis associated with use of stavudine: report of four cases. Ann Intern Med 2000;133(3):192–196.

25. Mokrzycki MH, Harris C, May H, et al: Lactic acidosis associated with stavudine administration: a report of five cases. Clin Infect Dis 2000;30(1):198–200.

26. Schramm C, Wanitschke R, Galle PR: Thiamine for the treatment of nucleoside analogue-induced severe lactic acidosis. Eur J Anaesthesiol 1999;16(10):733–735.

27. Luzzati R, Del Bravo P, Di Perri G, et al: Riboflavine and severe lactic acidosis. Lancet 1999;353(9156):901–902.

28. Fouty B, Frerman F, Reves R: Riboflavin to treat nucleoside analogue-induced lactic acidosis. Lancet 1998;352(9124):291–292.

29. ter Hofstede HJ, de Marie S, Foudraine NA, et al: Clinical features and risk factors of lactic acidosis following long-term antiretroviral therapy: 4 fatal cases. Int J STD AIDS 2000;11(9):611–616.

30. Moyle GJ, Sadler M: Peripheral neuropathy with nucleoside antiretrovirals: risk factors, incidence and management. Drug Saf 1998;19(6):481–494.

31. Gold R, Meurers B, Reichmann H: Mitochondrial myopathy caused by long-term zidovudine therapy. N Engl J Med 1990;323(14):994.

32. Simpson DM, Citak KA, Godfrey E, et al: Myopathies associated with human immunodeficiency virus and zidovudine: can their effects be distinguished? Neurology 1993;43(5):971–976.

33. Cupler EJ, Danon MJ, Jay C, et al: Early features of zidovudine-associated myopathy: histopathological findings and clinical correlations. Acta Neuropathol (Berl) 1995;90(1):1–6.

34. Pedrol E, Masanes F, Fernandez-Sola J, et al: Lack of muscle toxicity with didanosine (ddI). Clinical and experimental studies. J Neurol Sci 1996;138(1–2):42–48.

35. Pereira LF, Oliveira MB, Carnieri EG: Mitochondrial sensitivity to AZT. Cell Biochem Funct 1998;16(3):173–181.

36. Semino-Mora MC, Leon-Monzon ME, Dalakas MC: Effect of L-carnitine on the zidovudine-induced destruction of human myotubes. Part I: L-carnitine prevents the myotoxicity of AZT in vitro. Lab Invest 1994;71(1):102–112.

37. Semino-Mora MC, Leon-Monzon ME, Dalakas MC: The effect of L-carnitine on the AZT-induced destruction of human myotubes. Part II: Treatment with L-carnitine improves the AZT-induced changes and prevents further destruction. Lab Invest 1994;71(5): 773–781.

38. Miller KD, Jones E, Yanovski JA, Shankar R, Feuerstein I, Falloon J. Visceral abdominal-fat accumulation associated with use of indinavir. Lancet 1998;351(9106):871–875.

39. Lo JC, Mulligan K, Tai VW, et al: "Buffalo hump" in men with HIV-1 infection. Lancet 1998;351(9106):867–870.

40. Herry I, Bernard L, de Truchis P, Perronne C: Hypertrophy of the breasts in a patient treated with indinavir. Clin Infect Dis 1997;25(4):937–938.

41. Carr A, Samaras K, Thorisdottir A, et al: Diagnosis, prediction, and natural course of HIV-1 protease-inhibitor-associated lipodystrophy, hyperlipidaemia, and diabetes mellitus: a cohort study. Lancet 1999;353(9170):2093–2099.

42. Saint-Marc T, Partisani M, Poizot-Martin I, et al: A syndrome of peripheral fat wasting (lipodystrophy) in patients receiving long-term nucleoside analogue therapy. AIDS 1999;13(13):1659–1667.

43. Carr A, Miller J, Law M, Cooper DA: A syndrome of lipoatrophy, lactic acidaemia and liver dysfunction associated with HIV nucleoside analogue therapy: contribution to protease inhibitor-related lipodystrophy syndrome. AIDS 2000;14(3):F25–F32.

44. Kumar PN, Sweet DE, McDowell JA, et al: Safety and pharmacokinetics of abacavir (1592U89) following oral administration of escalating single doses in human immunodeficiency virus type 1-infected adults. Antimicrob Agents Chemother 1999;43(3): 603–608.

45. Hughes W, McDowell JA, Shenep J, et al: Safety and single-dose pharmacokinetics of abacavir (1592U89) in human immunodeficiency virus type 1-infected children. Antimicrob Agents Chemother 1999;43(3):609–615.

46. Barry M, Mulcahy F, Merry C, et al: Pharmacokinetics and potential interactions amongst antiretroviral agents used to treat patients with HIV infection. Clin Pharmacokinet 1999;36(4): 289–304.

47. Burger DM, Meenhorst PL, Beijnen JH: Concise overview of the clinical pharmacokinetics of dideoxynucleoside antiretroviral agents. Pharm World Sci 1995;17(2):25–30.

48. Morse GD, Fischl MA, Shelton MJ, et al: Single-dose pharmacokinetics of delavirdine mesylate and didanosine in patients with human immunodeficiency virus infection. Antimicrob Agents Chemother 1997;41(1):169–174.

49. Molina JM, Peytavin G, Perusat S, et al: Pharmacokinetics of emtricitabine, didanosine and efavirenz administered once-daily for the treatment of HIV-infected adults (pharmacokinetic substudy of the ANRS 091 trial). HIV Med 2004;5(2):99–104.

50. Singlas E, Taburet AM, Borsa LF, et al: Didanosine pharmacokinetics in patients with normal and impaired renal function: influence of hemodialysis. Antimicrob Agents Chemother 1992;36(7):1519–1524.

51. Moyle GJ, Nelson MR, Hawkins D, Gazzard BG: The use and toxicity of didanosine (ddI) in HIV antibody-positive individuals intolerant to zidovudine (AZT). QJM 1993;86(3):155–163.

52. Yuen GJ, Morris DM, Mydlow PK, et al: Pharmacokinetics, absolute bioavailability, and absorption characteristics of lamivudine. J Clin Pharmacol 1995;35(12):1174–1180.

53. Sabo JP, Lamson MJ, Leitz G, Yong CL, MacGregor TR: Pharmacokinetics of nevirapine and lamivudine in patients with HIV-1 infection. AAPS Pharm Sci 2000;2(1):E1.

54. Adkins JC, Peters DH, Faulds D: Zalcitabine. An update of its pharmacodynamic and pharmacokinetic properties and clinical efficacy in the management of HIV infection. Drugs 1997;53(6): 1054–1080.

55. Deviveni D, Gallo JM: Zalcitabine. Clinical pharmacokinetics and efficacy. Clin Pharmacokinet 1995;28(5):351–360.

56. Rana KZ, Dudley MN: Clinical pharmacokinetics of stavudine. Clin Pharmacokinet 1997;33(4):276–284.

57. Acosta EP, Henry K, Page LM, et al: Pharmacokinetics and safety of concentration-controlled oral zidovudine therapy. Pharmacotherapy 1997;17(3):424–430.

58. Rachlis A, Fanning MM: Zidovudine toxicity. Clinical features and management. Drug Saf 1993;8(4):312–320.

59. Spear JB, Kessler HA, Lehrman SN, de Miranda P: Zidovudine overdosage. Ann Intern Med 1988;109(1):76–77.

60. Pickus OB: Overdose of zidovudine. N Engl J Med 1988;318(18): 1206.

61. Hargreaves M, Fuller G, Costello C, Gazzard B: Zidovudine overdose. Lancet 1988;2(8609):509.

62. Routy JP, Prajs E, Blanc AP, et al: Seizure after zidovudine overdose. Lancet 1989;1(8634):384–385.

63. Valentine C, Williams O, Davis A, et al: Case study of zidovudine overdose. AIDS 1993;7(3):436–437.

64. Lafeuillade A, Poizot-Martin I, Dhiver C, et al: Zidovudine overdose: a case with bone-marrow toxicity. AIDS 1991;5(1):116–117.

65. Cundy KC: Clinical pharmacokinetics of the antiviral nucleotide analogues cidofovir and adefovir. Clin Pharmacokinet 1999; 36(2):127–143.

66. Kearney BP, Flaherty JF, Shah J: Tenofovir disoproxil fumarate: clinical pharmacology and pharmacokinetics. Clin Pharmacokinet 2004;43(9):595–612.

67. Hazra R, Balis FM, Tullio AN, et al: Single-dose and steady-state pharmacokinetics of tenofovir disoproxil fumarate in human immunodeficiency virus-infected children. Antimicrob Agents Chemother 2004;48(1):124–129.

68. Fung HB, Stone EA, Piacenti FJ: Tenofovir disoproxil fumarate: a nucleotide reverse transcriptase inhibitor for the treatment of HIV infection. Clin Ther 2002;24(10):1515–1548.

69. Barditch-Crovo P, Deeks SG, Collier A, et al: Phase I/II trial of the pharmacokinetics, safety, and antiretroviral activity of tenofovir disoproxil fumarate in human immunodeficiency virus-infected adults. Antimicrob Agents Chemother 2001;45(10):2733–2739.

70. Gish RG, Leung NW, Wright TL, et al: Dose range study of pharmacokinetics, safety, and preliminary antiviral activity of emtricitabine in adults with hepatitis B virus infection. Antimicrob Agents Chemother 2002;46(6):1734–1740.

71. Bourezane Y, Salard D, Hoen B, et al: DRESS (drug rash with eosinophilia and systemic symptoms) syndrome associated with nevirapine therapy. Clin Infect Dis 1998;27(5):1321–1322.

72. Bossi P, Colin D, Bricaire F, Caumes E: Hypersensitivity syndrome associated with efavirenz therapy. Clin Infect Dis 2000;30(1):227–228.

73. Antinori A, Baldini F, Girardi E, et al: Female sex and the use of anti-allergic agents increase the risk of developing cutaneous rash associated with nevirapine therapy. AIDS 2001;15(12):1579–1581.

74. Bersoff-Matcha SJ, Miller WC, Aberg JA, et al: Sex differences in nevirapine rash. Clin Infect Dis 2001;32(1):124–129.

75. Clarke S, Harrington P, Barry M, Mulcahy F: The tolerability of efavirenz after nevirapine-related adverse events. Clin Infect Dis 2000;31(3):806–807.

76. Soriano V, Dona C, Barreiro P, Gonzalez-Lahoz J: Is there cross-toxicity between nevirapine and efavirenz in subjects developing rash? AIDS 2000;14(11):1672–1673.

77. Martinez E, Blanco JL, Arnaiz JA, et al: Hepatotoxicity in HIV-1-infected patients receiving nevirapine-containing antiretroviral therapy. AIDS 2001;15(10):1261–1268.

78. Borin MT, Cox SR, Herman BD, et al: Effect of fluconazole on the steady-state pharmacokinetics of delavirdine in human immunodeficiency virus-positive patients. Antimicrob Agents Chemother 1997;41(9):1892–1897.

79. Cheng CL, Smith DE, Carver PL, et al: Steady-state pharmacokinetics of delavirdine in HIV-positive patients: effect on erythromycin breath test. Clin Pharmacol Ther 1997;61(5):531–543.

80. Tran JQ, Gerber JG, Kerr BM: Delavirdine: clinical pharmacokinetics and drug interactions. Clin Pharmacokinet 2001;40(3):207–226.

81. Boffito M, Back DJ, Blaschke TF, et al: Protein binding in antiretroviral therapies. AIDS Res Hum Retroviruses 2003;19(9):825–835.

82. Tran JQ, Petersen C, Garrett M, et al: Pharmacokinetic interaction between amprenavir and delavirdine: evidence of induced clearance by amprenavir. Clin Pharmacol Ther 2002;72(6):615–626.

83. Villani P, Regazzi MB, Castelli F, et al: Pharmacokinetics of efavirenz (EFV) alone and in combination therapy with nelfinavir (NFV) in HIV-1 infected patients. Br J Clin Pharmacol 1999;48(5):712–715.

84. Adkins JC, Noble S: Efavirenz. Drugs 1998;56(6):1055–1064.

85. Luzuriaga K, Bryson Y, McSherry G, et al: Pharmacokinetics, safety, and activity of nevirapine in human immunodeficiency virus type 1-infected children. J Infect Dis 1996;174(4):713–721.

86. Cheeseman SH, Hattox SE, McLaughlin MM, et al: Pharmacokinetics of nevirapine: initial single-rising-dose study in humans. Antimicrob Agents Chemother 1993;37(2):178–182.

87. Fyfe JA, Keller PM, Furman PA, et al: Thymidine kinase from herpes simplex virus phosphorylates the new antiviral compound, 9-(2-hydroxyethoxymethyl)guanine. J Biol Chem 1978;253(24):8721–8727.

88. Biron KK, Elion GB: In vitro susceptibility of varicella-zoster virus to acyclovir. Antimicrob Agents Chemother 1980;18(3):443–447.

89. Biron KK, Stanat SC, Sorrell JB, et al: Metabolic activation of the nucleoside analog 9-[(2-hydroxy-1-(hydroxymethyl)ethoxy] methyl)guanine in human diploid fibroblasts infected with human cytomegalovirus. Proc Natl Acad Sci U S A 1985;82(8):2473–2477.

90. de Miranda P, Blum MR: Pharmacokinetics of acyclovir after intravenous and oral administration. J Antimicrob Chemother 1983;12(Suppl B):29–37.

91. Krieble BF, Rudy DW, Glick MR, Clayman MD: Case report: acyclovir neurotoxicity and nephrotoxicity—the role for hemodialysis. Am J Med Sci 1993;305(1):36–39.

92. Feldman S, Rodman J, Gregory B: Excessive serum concentrations of acyclovir and neurotoxicity. J Infect Dis 1988;157(2):385–388.

93. Peterslund NA, Larsen ML, Mygind H: Acyclovir crystalluria. Scand J Infect Dis 1988;20(2):225–228.

94. Brigden D, Whiteman P: The mechanism of action, pharmacokinetics and toxicity of acyclovir—a review. J Infect 1983;6(1 Suppl):3–9.

95. de Miranda P, Whitley RJ, Blum MR, et al: Acyclovir kinetics after intravenous infusion. Clin Pharmacol Ther 1979;26(6):718–728.

96. Spiegal DM, Lau K: Acute renal failure and coma secondary to acyclovir therapy. JAMA 1986;255(14):1882–1883.

97. Hernandez E, Praga M, Moreno F, Montoyo C: Acute renal failure induced by oral acyclovir. Clin Nephrol 1991;36(3):155–156.

98. Johnson GL, Limon L, Trikha G, Wall H: Acute renal failure and neurotoxicity following oral acyclovir. Ann Pharmacother 1994;28(4):460–463.

99. Jones PG, Beier-Hanratty SA: Acyclovir: neurologic and renal toxicity. Ann Intern Med 1986;104(6):892.

100. Revankar SG, Applegate AL, Markovitz DM: Delirium associated with acyclovir treatment in a patient with renal failure. Clin Infect Dis 1995;21(2):435–436.

101. Saral R, Burns WH, Laskin OL, et al: Acyclovir prophylaxis of herpes-simplex-virus infections. N Engl J Med 1981;305(2):63–67.

102. Haefeli WE, Schoenenberger RA, Weiss P, Ritz RF: Acyclovir-induced neurotoxicity: concentration-side effect relationship in acyclovir overdose. Am J Med 1993;94(2):212–215.

103. McDonald LK, Tartaglione TA, Mendelman PM, et al: Lack of toxicity in two cases of neonatal acyclovir overdose. Pediatr Infect Dis J 1989;8(8):529–532.

104. Eck P, Silver SM, Clark EC: Acute renal failure and coma after a high dose of oral acyclovir. N Engl J Med 1991;325(16):1178–1179.

105. Fletcher CV, Chinnock BJ, Chace B, Balfour HH Jr: Pharmacokinetics and safety of high-dose oral acyclovir for suppression of cytomegalovirus disease after renal transplantation. Clin Pharmacol Ther 1988;44(2):158–163.

106. Baker KL, Baker SD, Morgan DL: Largest dose of acyclovir inadvertently administered to a neonate. Pediatr Infect Dis J 2003;22(9):842.

107. Bradley J, Forero N, Pho H, Escobar B, Kasinath BS, Anzueto A: Progressive somnolence leading to coma in a 68-year-old man. Chest 1997;112(2):538–540.

108. Da Conceicao M, Genco G, Favier JC, et al: [Cerebral and renal toxicity of acyclovir in a patient treated for meningoencephalitis.] Ann Fr Anesth Reanim 1999;18(9):996–999.

109. Selby PJ, Powles RL, Janeson B, et al: Parenteral acyclovir therapy for herpesvirus infections in man. Lancet 1979;2(8155):1267–1270.

110. Strong DK, Hebert D: Acute acyclovir neurotoxicity in a hemodialyzed child. Pediatr Nephrol 1997;11(6):741–743.

111. Swan SK, Bennett WM: Oral acyclovir and neurotoxicity. Ann Intern Med 1989;111(2):188.

112. Gomez Campdera FJ, Verde E, Vozmediano MC, Valderrabano F: More about acyclovir neurotoxicity in patients on haemodialysis. Nephron 1998;78(2):228–229.

113. Rivaud E, Massiani MA, Vincent F, et al: Valacyclovir hydrochloride therapy and thrombotic thrombocytopenic purpura in an HIV-infected patient. Arch Intern Med 2000;160(11):1705–1706.

114. Izzedine H, Mercadal L, Aymard G, et al: Neurotoxicity of valacyclovir in peritoneal dialysis: a pharmacokinetic study. Am J Nephrol 2001;21(2):162–164.

115. Linssen-Schuurmans CD, van Kan EJ, Feith GW, Uges DR: Neurotoxicity caused by valacyclovir in a patient on hemodialysis. Ther Drug Monit 1998;20(4):385–386.

116. Soul-Lawton J, Seaber E, On N, et al: Absolute bioavailability and metabolic disposition of valaciclovir, the L-valyl ester of acyclovir, following oral administration to humans. Antimicrob Agents Chemother 1995;39(12):2759–2764.

117. Snoeck R: Antiviral therapy of herpes simplex. Int J Antimicrob Agents 2000;16(2):157–159.

118. Perry CM, Faulds D: Valaciclovir. A review of its antiviral activity, pharmacokinetic properties and therapeutic efficacy in herpesvirus infections. Drugs 1996;52(5):754–772.

119. Izzedine H, Launay-Vacher V, Baumelou A, Deray G: An appraisal of antiretroviral drugs in hemodialysis. Kidney Int 2001;60(3):821–830.

120. Bell WR, Chulay JD, Feinberg JE: Manifestations resembling thrombotic microangiopathy in patients with advanced human immunodeficiency virus (HIV) disease in a cytomegalovirus prophylaxis trial (ACTG 204). Medicine (Baltimore) 1997;76(5):369–380.

121. Crumpacker CS: Ganciclovir. N Engl J Med 1996;335(10):721–729.

122. Buhles WC Jr, Mastre BJ, Tinker AJ, et al: Ganciclovir treatment of life- or sight-threatening cytomegalovirus infection: experience

in 314 immunocompromised patients. Rev Infect Dis 1988;10 (Suppl 3):495–506.

123. Hamzeh FM, Lietman PS: Intranuclear accumulation of sub-genomic noninfectious human cytomegalovirus DNA in infected cells in the presence of ganciclovir. Antimicrob Agents Chemother 1991;35(9):1818–1823.

124. Hochster H, Dieterich D, Bozzette S, et al: Toxicity of combined ganciclovir and zidovudine for cytomegalovirus disease associated with AIDS. An AIDS Clinical Trials Group Study. Ann Intern Med 1990;113(2):111–117.

125. Cohen AJ, Weiser B, Afzal Q, Fuhrer J: Ventricular tachycardia in two patients with AIDS receiving ganciclovir (DHPG). AIDS 1990; 4(8):807–809.

126. Saran BR, Maguire AM: Retinal toxicity of high dose intravitreal ganciclovir. Retina 1994;14(3):248–252.

127. Fowles SE, Pierce DM, Prince WT, Staniforth D: The tolerance to and pharmacokinetics of penciclovir (BRL 39,123A), a novel antiherpes agent, administered by intravenous infusion to healthy subjects. Eur J Clin Pharmacol 1992;43(5):513–516.

128. Rolan P: Pharmacokinetics of new antiherpetic agents. Clin Pharmacokinet 1995;29(5):333–340.

129. Gill KS, Wood MJ: The clinical pharmacokinetics of famciclovir. Clin Pharmacokinet 1996;31(1):1–8.

130. Brown F, Banken L, Saywell K, Arum I: Pharmacokinetics of valganciclovir and ganciclovir following multiple oral dosages of valganciclovir in HIV- and CMV-seropositive volunteers. Clin Pharmacokinet 1999;37(2):167–176.

131. Pescovitz MD, Rabkin J, Merion RM, et al: Valganciclovir results in improved oral absorption of ganciclovir in liver transplant recipients. Antimicrob Agents Chemother 2000;44(10):2811–2815.

132. Czock D, Scholle C, Rasche FM, et al: Pharmacokinetics of valganciclovir and ganciclovir in renal impairment. Clin Pharmacol Ther 2002;72(2):142–150.

133. Martin DF, Sierra-Madero J, Walmsley S, et al: A controlled trial of valganciclovir as induction therapy for cytomegalovirus retinitis. N Engl J Med 2002;346(15):1119–1126.

134. Fortun AJ, Martin-Davila P, Moreno S, et al: Pharmacokinetics of oral valganciclovir and intravenous ganciclovir administered to prevent cytomegalovirus disease in an adult patient receiving small-intestine transplantation. Antimicrob Agents Chemother 2004;48(7):2782–2783.

135. Burri M, Wiltshire H, Kahlert C, et al: Oral valganciclovir in children: single dose pharmacokinetics in a six-year-old girl. Pediatr Infect Dis J 2004;23(3):263–266.

136. Flexner C: HIV-protease inhibitors. N Engl J Med 1998;338(18): 1281–1292.

137. Debouck C: The HIV-1 protease as a therapeutic target for AIDS. AIDS Res Hum Retroviruses 1992;8(2):153–164.

138. Sulkowski MS, Thomas DL, Chaisson RE, Moore RD: Hepatotoxicity associated with antiretroviral therapy in adults infected with human immunodeficiency virus and the role of hepatitis C or B virus infection. JAMA 2000;283(1):74–80.

139. den Brinker M, Wit FW, Wertheim-van Dillen PM, et al: Hepatitis B and C virus co-infection and the risk for hepatotoxicity of highly active antiretroviral therapy in HIV-1 infection. AIDS 2000; 14(18):2895–2902.

140. Saves M, Raffi F, Clevenbergh P, et al: Hepatitis B or hepatitis C virus infection is a risk factor for severe hepatic cytolysis after initiation of a protease inhibitor-containing antiretroviral regimen in human immunodeficiency virus-infected patients. The APROCO Study Group. Antimicrob Agents Chemother 2000; 44(12):3451–3455.

141. Nunez M, Lana R, Mendoza JL, et al: Risk factors for severe hepatic injury after introduction of highly active antiretroviral therapy. J Acquir Immune Defic Syndr 2001;27(5):426–431.

142. Gisolf EH, Dreezen C, Danner SA, et al: Risk factors for hepatotoxicity in HIV-1-infected patients receiving ritonavir and saquinavir with or without stavudine. Prometheus Study Group. Clin Infect Dis 2000;31(5):1234–1239.

143. Bonfanti P, Landonio S, Ricci E, et al: Risk factors for hepatotoxicity in patients treated with highly active antiretroviral therapy. J Acquir Immune Defic Syndr 2001;27(3):316–318.

144. Tsiodras S, Mantzoros C, Hammer S, Samore M: Effects of protease inhibitors on hyperglycemia, hyperlipidemia, and

145. Carr A, Cooper DA: Images in clinical medicine. Lipodystrophy associated with an HIV-protease inhibitor. N Engl J Med 1998;339(18):1296.

146. Carr A, Samaras K, Chisholm DJ, Cooper DA: Pathogenesis of HIV-1-protease inhibitor-associated peripheral lipodystrophy, hyperlipidaemia, and insulin resistance. Lancet 1998;351(9119): 1881–1883.

147. Falloon J, Piscitelli S, Vogel S, et al: Combination therapy with amprenavir, abacavir, and efavirenz in human immunodeficiency virus (HIV)-infected patients failing a protease-inhibitor regimen: pharmacokinetic drug interactions and antiviral activity. Clin Infect Dis 2000;30(2):313–321.

148. Sadler BM, Gillotin C, Lou Y, et al: Pharmacokinetic study of human immunodeficiency virus protease inhibitors used in combination with amprenavir. Antimicrob Agents Chemother 2001;45(12):3663–3668.

149. Polk RE, Brophy DF, Israel DS, et al: Pharmacokinetic Interaction between amprenavir and rifabutin or rifampin in healthy males. Antimicrob Agents Chemother 2001;45(2):502–508.

150. Zeldin RK, Petruschke RA: Pharmacological and therapeutic properties of ritonavir-boosted protease inhibitor therapy in HIV-infected patients. J Antimicrob Chemother 2004;53(1):4–9.

151. Burkhart KK, Kemerer K, Donovan JW: Indinavir overdose. J Toxicol Clin Toxicol 1998;36(7):747.

152. Beach JW: Chemotherapeutic agents for human immunodeficiency virus infection: mechanism of action, pharmacokinetics, metabolism, and adverse reactions. Clin Ther 1998;20(1):2–25.

153. Walmsley S, Bernstein B, King M, et al: Lopinavir-ritonavir versus nelfinavir for the initial treatment of HIV infection. N Engl J Med 2002;346(26):2039–2046.

154. Starr SE, Fletcher CV, Spector SA, et al: Combination therapy with efavirenz, nelfinavir, and nucleoside reverse-transcriptase inhibitors in children infected with human immunodeficiency virus type 1. Pediatric AIDS Clinical Trials Group 382 Team. N Engl J Med 1999;341(25):1874–1881.

155. Root MJ, Kay MS, Kim PS: Protein design of an HIV-1 entry inhibitor. Science 2001;291(5505):884–888.

156. Dando TM, Perry CM. Enfuvirtide. Drugs 2003;63(24):2755–2766.

157. Fung HB, Guo Y: Enfuvirtide: a fusion inhibitor for the treatment of HIV infection. Clin Ther 2004;26(3):352–378.

158. Cooper DA, Lange JM: Peptide inhibitors of virus-cell fusion: enfuvirtide as a case study in clinical discovery and development. Lancet Infect Dis 2004;4(7):426–436.

159. Lalezari JP, Henry K, O'Hearn M, et al: Enfuvirtide, an HIV-1 fusion inhibitor, for drug-resistant HIV infection in North and South America. N Engl J Med 2003;348(22):2175–2185.

160. Lazzarin A, Clotet B, Cooper D, et al: Efficacy of enfuvirtide in patients infected with drug-resistant HIV-1 in Europe and Australia. N Engl J Med 2003;348(22):2186–2195.

161. Bui M, Whittaker G, Helenius A: Effect of M1 protein and low pH on nuclear transport of influenza virus ribonucleoproteins. J Virol 1996;70(12):8391–8401.

162. Yang CC, Deng JF: Anticholinergic syndrome with severe rhabdomyolysis—an unusual feature of amantadine toxicity. Intensive Care Med 1997;23(3):355–356.

163. Snoey ER, Bessen HA: Acute psychosis after amantadine overdose. Ann Emerg Med 1990;19(6):668–670.

164. Macchio GJ, Ito V, Sahgal V: Amantadine-induced coma. Arch Phys Med Rehabil 1993;74(10):1119–1120.

165. Pimentel L, Hughes B: Amantadine toxicity presenting with complex ventricular ectopy and hallucinations. Pediatr Emerg Care 1991;7(2):89–92.

166. Berkowitz CD: Treatment of acute amantadine toxicity with physostigmine. J Pediatr 1979;95(1):144–145.

167. Brown CR, Hernandez S, Kelly MT: Hyperthermia and death from amantadine overdose. Vet Hum Toxicol 1987;29(6):463.

168. Simpson DM, Ramos F, Ramirez LF: Death of a psychiatric patient from amantadine poisoning. Am J Psychiatry 1988;145(2):267–268.

169. Fahn S, Craddock G, Kumin G: Acute toxic psychosis from suicidal overdosage of amantadine. Arch Neurol 1971;25(1):45–48.

170. Cook PE, Dermer SW, McGurk T: Fatal overdose with amantadine. Can J Psychiatry 1986;31(8):757–758.

171. Casey DE: Amantadine intoxication reversed by physostigmine. N Engl J Med 1978;298(9):516.

172. Sartori M, Pratt CM, Young JB: Torsade de pointe. Malignant cardiac arrhythmia induced by amantadine poisoning. Am J Med 1984;77(2):388–391.

173. Hayden FG, Gwaltney JM Jr, Van de Castle RL, et al: Comparative toxicity of amantadine hydrochloride and rimantadine hydrochloride in healthy adults. Antimicrob Agents Chemother 1981;19(2):226–233.

174. Tominack RL, Wills RJ, Gustavson LE, Hayden FG: Multiple-dose pharmacokinetics of rimantadine in elderly adults. Antimicrob Agents Chemother 1988;32(12):1813–1819.

175. Holazo AA, Choma N, Brown SY, et al: Effect of cimetidine on the disposition of rimantadine in healthy subjects. Antimicrob Agents Chemother 1989;33(6):820–823.

176. Dunn CJ, Goa KL: Zanamivir: a review of its use in influenza. Drugs 1999;58(4):761–784.

177. Hayden FG, Atmar RL, Schilling M, et al: Use of the selective oral neuraminidase inhibitor oseltamivir to prevent influenza. N Engl J Med 1999;341(18):1336–1343.

178. Treanor JJ, Hayden FG, Vrooman PS, et al: Efficacy and safety of the oral neuraminidase inhibitor oseltamivir in treating acute influenza: a randomized controlled trial. US Oral Neuraminidase Study Group. JAMA 2000;283(8):1016–1024.

179. Couch RB: Prevention and treatment of influenza. N Engl J Med 2000;343(24):1778–1787.

180. Freund B, Gravenstein S, Elliott M, Miller I: Zanamivir: a review of clinical safety. Drug Saf 1999;21(4):267–281.

181. Hayden FG, Gubareva LV, Monto AS, et al: Inhaled zanamivir for the prevention of influenza in families. Zanamivir Family Study Group. N Engl J Med 2000;343(18):1282–1289.

182. Dutkowski R, Thakrar B, Froehlich E, et al: Safety and pharmacology of oseltamivir in clinical use. Drug Saf 2003;26(11):787–801.

183. Chrisp P, Clissold SP: Foscarnet. A review of its antiviral activity, pharmacokinetic properties and therapeutic use in immunocompromised patients with cytomegalovirus retinitis. Drugs 1991;41(1):104–129.

184. Koks CHW, Beijnen JH: Foscarnet. Pharmaceutisch Weekblad 1989;31:584–586.

185. Noormohamed FH, Youle MS, Tang B, et al: Foscarnet-induced changes in plasma concentrations of total and ionized calcium and magnesium in HIV-positive patients. Antivir Ther 1996;1(3):172–179.

186. Seidel EA, Koenig S, Polis MA: A dose escalation study to determine the toxicity and maximally tolerated dose of foscarnet. AIDS 1993;7(7):941–945.

187. Youle MS, Clarbour J, Gazzard B, Chanas A: Severe hypocalcaemia in AIDS patients treated with foscarnet and pentamidine. Lancet 1988;1(8600):1455–1456.

188. Jacobson MA, Gambertoglio JG, Aweeka FT, et al: Foscarnet-induced hypocalcemia and effects of foscarnet on calcium metabolism. J Clin Endocrinol Metab 1991;72(5):1130–1135.

189. Jacobson MA: Review of the toxicities of foscarnet. J Acquir Immune Defic Syndr 1992;5(Suppl 1):11–17.

190. Jayaweera DT: Minimising the dosage-limiting toxicities of foscarnet induction therapy. Drug Saf 1997;16(4):258–266.

191. Van Der Pijl JW, Frissen PH, Reiss P, et al: Foscarnet and penile ulceration. Lancet 1990;335(8684):286.

192. Moyle G, Nelson M, Barton SE, et al: Penile ulcerations with foscarnet. Lancet 1990;335(8688):547–548.

193. Wachsman M, Petty BG, Cundy KC, et al: Pharmacokinetics, safety and bioavailability of HPMPC (cidofovir) in human immunodeficiency virus-infected subjects. Antiviral Res 1996;29(2–3):153–161.

194. Cundy KC, Petty BG, Flaherty J, et al: Clinical pharmacokinetics of cidofovir in human immunodeficiency virus-infected patients. Antimicrob Agents Chemother 1995;39(6):1247–1252.

195. Brody SR, Humphreys MH, Gambertoglio JG, et al: Pharmacokinetics of cidofovir in renal insufficiency and in continuous ambulatory peritoneal dialysis or high-flux hemodialysis. Clin Pharmacol Ther 1999;65(1):21–28.

196. Preston SL, Drusano GL, Glue P, et al: Pharmacokinetics and absolute bioavailability of ribavirin in healthy volunteers as determined by stable-isotope methodology. Antimicrob Agents Chemother 1999;43(10):2451–2456.

197. Glue P, Schenker S, Gupta S, et al: The single dose pharmacokinetics of ribavirin in subjects with chronic liver disease. Br J Clin Pharmacol 2000;49(5):417–421.

198. Glue P: The clinical pharmacology of ribavirin. Semin Liver Dis 1999;19(Suppl 1):17–24.

199. Connor E, Morrison S, Lane J, et al: Safety, tolerance, and pharmacokinetics of systemic ribavirin in children with human immunodeficiency virus infection. Antimicrob Agents Chemother 1993;37(3):532–539.

200. Lertora JJ, Rege AB, Lacour JT, et al: Pharmacokinetics and long-term tolerance to ribavirin in asymptomatic patients infected with human immunodeficiency virus. Clin Pharmacol Ther 1991;50(4):442–449.

201. Tsubota A, Hirose Y, Izumi N, Kumada H: Pharmacokinetics of ribavirin in combined interferon-alpha 2b and ribavirin therapy for chronic hepatitis C virus infection. Br J Clin Pharmacol 2003;55(4):360–367.

202. Van Bever HP, Desager KS, Van Hoeck K: Water intoxication after nebulised tribavirin. Lancet 1995;345(8947):451.

203. Titus BJ, Perez AF, Arcala Bares LI: Water intoxication after nebulised tribavirin. Lancet 1995;345(8957):1116.

204. Saez-Llorens X, Moreno MT, Ramilo O, et al: Safety and pharmacokinetics of palivizumab therapy in children hospitalized with respiratory syncytial virus infection. Pediatr Infect Dis J 2004;23(8):707–712.

205. Boeckh M, Berrey MM, Bowden RA, et al: Phase 1 evaluation of the respiratory syncytial virus-specific monoclonal antibody palivizumab in recipients of hematopoietic stem cell transplants. J Infect Dis 2001;184(3):350–354.

54 Anthelmintics

MAHESH SHRESTHA, MD ■ DANIEL C. KEYES, MD, MPH

At a Glance...

- The anthelmintics include:
  - Imidazoles (mebendazole, albendazole, thiabendazole, flubendazole, niridazole)
  - Piperazines (diethylcarbamazine)
  - Antischistosomal agents (praziquantel, metrifonate, oxamniquine, hycanthone)
  - Unclassified (ivermectin, niclosamide, suramin, pyrantel pamoate, pyrvinium pamoate, antimony)
- The anthelmintics are a broad range of substances with variable toxicity. Most are designed to be neurotoxic to helminths and other parasites.
- While many of the older anthelmintics contain known toxins (e.g., antimony), newer agents have a significantly better safety profile.
- The major clinical toxicity of these agents is neurologic; many produce seizures.
- Treatment of anthelmintics overdose is supportive; no antidotes are available.

Infections caused by worms, or helminths, may be the most prevalent of all human infections. It has been estimated that there may be as many worms infecting people as there are people.[1] A thorough review of all the helminths, the clinical syndromes caused, and their diagnoses and treatments are beyond the scope of this chapter. The major organisms are briefly examined, followed by a discussion of the individual chemotherapeutic agents used to treat the infections they cause. Although the mechanisms of action of the anthelmintic medications are poorly understood,[2] they are presented whenever available. A discussion of toxicities of individual agents concludes this chapter.

Helminths are divided into three broad categories: nematodes (roundworms), trematodes (flatworms, or flukes), and cestodes (tapeworms).

Nematodes include two general categories, intestinal nematodes and tissue nematodes. Intestinal nematodes include the abundant *Ascaris lumbricoides* (giant roundworm), *Trichuris trichiura* (whipworm), and *Enterobius vermicularis* (pinworm), as well as the hookworms *Ancylostoma duodenale* (European hookworm), *Necatur americanus* (North American hookworm), and *Strongyloides stercoralis*. In the United States, *E. vermicularis*, which causes pruritus ani, is the most common of all helminthic parasites, infecting 42 million people.[3] The prevalence of strongyloidiasis in the southern United States is estimated at 0.4% to 4%. The other helminths are found mainly in tropical areas of the globe, but they are also present in the southeastern United States. It is estimated

that 1 billion of the world's population (4.4 million in the United States) are infected with *A. lumbricoides*, 800 million (2.2 million in the United States) with *T. trichiura*, and one fourth of the world's population with hookworm. Hookworm disease was controlled almost in its entirety in the United States during the early part of this century and is uncommon here. The treatment of choice for all of these intestinal nematode infections, except strongyloidiasis, is mebendazole, an imidazole. Thiabendazole, a related compound, is currently the treatment of choice for strongyloidiasis. Albendazole is the newest of this group of medications. It achieves greater tissue levels and has a broader spectrum of activity. Pyrantel pamoate can also be used.

Tissue nematodes include *Trichinella spiralis* (the causative agent of trichinosis), *Dracunculus medinensis* (causing skin ulcers through which the worm appears), the three causative agents of filariasis (*Wuchereria bancrofti*, *Brugia malayi*, and *Brugia timori*), *Loa loa*, and *Onchocerca volvulus*. No completely effective treatment has been found for trichinosis, but use of thiabendazole is recommended within 24 hours for patients known to have ingested trichinous meat. Thiabendazole or metronidazole is recommended for the inflammation of dracunculiasis so that the worms themselves can be physically removed by rolling them on a stick during the course of a week. Filariasis is characterized by acute and chronic lymphatic inflammation eventually resulting in elephantiasis, hydrocele, and chyluria. There is no satisfactory treatment, but administration of diethylcarbamazine reduces the number of microfilaria. Diethylcarbamazine is also effective against *L. loa* and *O. volvulus*. *L. loa* is characterized by transient subcutaneous swellings (Calabar swellings). *O. volvulus* is the causative agent of river blindness, named for the blackfly that breeds in fast streams, which has caused blindness in whole African villages. The newer drug ivermectin is safer and more effective than diethylcarbamazine for onchocerciasis (but may be contraindicated for *L. loa*, which has been associated with encephalopathy[1]). Albendazole is the newest of this group of medications (imidazoles) and produces greater tissue levels and a broader spectrum of activity.

Trematodes include the blood flukes, or schistosomes (*Schistosoma mansoni*, *Schistosoma japonicum*, *Schistosoma haematobium*, and *Schistosoma mekongi*), which are one of the world's major public health concerns; the liver flukes (*Clonorchis sinensis* and *Fasciola hepatica*); the lung fluke *Paragonimus westermani*; and the intestinal fluke *Fasciolopsis buski*. Praziquantel is the drug of choice for all of these organisms (except *F. hepatica*, for which bithionol is used) and has revolutionized treatment. Metrifonate is effective against *S. haematobium*, and oxamniquine is effective against *S. mansoni*.

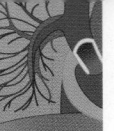

Cestodes, segmented worms or tapeworms, include the beef tapeworm (*Taenia saginata*), the pork tapeworm (*Taenia solium*, whose eggs cause human cysticercosis), the fish tapeworm (*Diphyllobothrium latum*), the dwarf tapeworm (*Hymenolepis nana*), and *Echinococcus granulosus*, the causative agent of echinococcosis, or hydatid disease. Niclosamide is the usual drug given to eradicate the adult tapeworms, but paromomycin and praziquantel are also effective. For human cysticercosis, praziquantel (with corticosteroids) is the drug of choice, and for hydatid cyst disease, albendazole with surgical removal is effective.

Other helminthic infections include visceral larval migrans (toxocariasis), cutaneous larva migrans (creeping eruption, caused by *Ancylostoma braziliense*, the dog or cat hookworm), and dirofilariasis. Most patients recover from visceral larva migrans without specific therapy. Thiabendazole has been used along with other agents for severe cases. Thiabendazole administered either orally or topically has also been used successfully for cutaneous larva migrans. *Dirofilaria immitis* is the causative agent of the dog heartworm. In humans, the immature filariae die, causing a local vasculitis in the pulmonary circulation. This may be seen occasionally as a coin lesion on the chest radiograph.

The drugs mentioned earlier are the most common anthelmintics used. Older drugs such as those in the antimony group—pyrantel pamoate, poquil, bephenium hydroxynaphthoate, and hycanthone—have special applications and may still be in use, especially in less developed countries and in veterinary medicine. Levamisole, related to mebendazole, and suramin, in use since 1920, have found newer uses as chemotherapeutic agents in the treatment of certain cancers.

In general, the older medications are more toxic to humans than the newer ones. The older medications have reported protean side effects, some of which are worse than the disease being treated. On other occasions, the side effects may be mistaken for progression or complications of the disease itself. It is important to remember that many of the side effects of treatment, such as with praziquantel for cysticercosis or with diethylcarbamazine for onchocerciasis (ivermectin is now used), are due to the large antigenic mass of dying worms released into the bloodstream. Similarly, many side effects are really not side effects of the medication because they probably would not occur if uninfected patients were given the same treatment. Pretreatment or concurrent treatment with corticosteroids is used in some cases, and slow progressive therapy is used in others. Medications that are not significantly absorbed (and thus have insignificant systemic toxicity), such as mebendazole, are ideal for susceptible helminths that are limited to the lumen of the gastrointestinal (GI) tract.

In the review that follows, the many agents available are divided into intuitive groups: imidazoles (mebendazole and related compounds), piperazines (diethylcarbamazine and piperazine), drugs identified for schistosomiasis (praziquantel, metrifonate, and others), and other important anthelmintics, such as ivermectin and suramin.

IMIDAZOLES

Mebendazole

Mebendazole is a drug commonly used in the treatment of intestinal nematodal disease, such as ascariasis, trichiuriasis, hookworm (*N. americanus* or *A. duodenale*), and enterobiasis (pinworm). Like the other benzimidazoles, it is thought to selectively and irreversibly block microtubular-dependent glucose uptake by nematodes and cestodes by binding to free β-tubulin and inhibiting tubulin polymerization.[5] Only 5% to 10% of an orally ingested dose is absorbed from the GI tract. Most of what is absorbed is metabolized in the liver (P-450 system) with a significant first pass effect. Thus, adverse reactions attributable to the medication itself are practically nonexistent, although diarrhea and abdominal pain have been reported. The usual dose used is 100 mg twice daily for 3 days. For pinworm infection, one 100-mg tablet given once is sufficient. A repeat dose a week later is recommended to kill nematodes that were protected as eggs at the time of initial mebendazole administration. Treatment of all family members is also recommended.

Mebendazole has also been used to treat hydatid disease (echinococcal cysts); a reduction in cyst size has been demonstrated with prolonged treatment. Albendazole, a related imidazole with better absorption, has now replaced mebendazole for this use. Albendazole is given in 4-week cycles of 400 mg, twice daily, separated by 2-week rest periods. At least three cycles are given. When albendazole is given in these higher doses, pyrexia has been noted; it is thought to be due to tissue necrosis of the hydatid cyst.

Another reported side effect of mebendazole is agranulocytosis. In a Russian study, this complication was found in 2 of 75 patients with hydatid cysts treated with 50 mg/kg per day for 30 days, resulting in the death of one patient.[6] Mebendazole has been shown to be teratogenic and embryotoxic in laboratory animals and so is contraindicated in pregnancy and in those younger than 2 years. Cimetidine, by inhibiting the P-450 system, may increase blood levels. There have been reports of contact urticaria and contact dermatitis from albendazole.[7] An outbreak of Stevens-Johnson syndrome/toxic epidermal necrolysis among those treated with both mebendazole and metronidazole has been reported.[8]

Treatment of poisoning includes decontamination in cases of overdose and is otherwise symptomatic and supportive.

Albendazole

Albendazole is similar to mebendazole but is more completely absorbed from the GI tract. It has a broader spectrum of activity. Its absorption is enhanced by taking it with fatty meals.[9] One of its main uses is in adjunctive treatment with surgery (or single-agent treatment without surgery) in hydatid cyst disease due to echinococci.[10] Mebendazole is probably as effective for most nematodal diseases isolated to the lumen of the

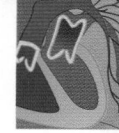

GI tract. Albendazole appears to be more effective for hookworm.[11] It is also effective against intestinal tapeworms and neurocysticercosis, for which it is an alternative to niclosamide and praziquantel, respectively. In one trial, it was more effective than praziquantel in neurocysticercosis.[12]

Albendazole is rapidly metabolized by the liver into an active metabolite that has a terminal half-life of 8.5 hours. It is given in at least three 4-week cycles separated by 2-week rest periods at a dose of 400 mg twice daily (10 to 14 mg/kg/day) when used for hydatid cyst disease. Side effects are similar to those for mebendazole and usually do not require discontinuation. It, too, has been shown to be teratogenic in animals (rats and rabbits) and is not recommended in pregnancy or in infants younger than 2 years. In one review only GI side effects were seen, and only at the low rate of slightly over 1%.[13] Treatment of poisonings is symptomatic and supportive (see also the later discussion of side effects in the section on Thiabendazole).

Thiabendazole

Thiabendazole, like albendazole, is also rapidly absorbed through the GI tract, metabolized by the hepatic P-450 system, and excreted by the kidneys in the first 24 hours. It is also available for topical application for cutaneous larva migrans. In addition to binding free β-tubulin, it inhibits the helminth-specific fumarate reductase enzyme system. It is the treatment of choice for strongyloidiasis, for which the dosage is 25 mg/kg twice daily (maximum, 3 g/day) for 2 days. In immunocompromised hosts (e.g., human immunodeficiency virus–infected patients or those with cancer), a hyperinfection syndrome from *S. stercoralis* can develop. Infective filariform larvae reenter the host via the lower GI tract or perianal regions in massive numbers. For this, thiabendazole is given at 25 mg/kg twice daily for 2 to 3 weeks.[14]

Thiabendazole has also been used for cutaneous larva migrans (creeping eruption, caused by *A. braziliensis*), visceral larva migrans, and trichinosis (*T. spiralis*), all of which have no proven therapy. Thiabendazole may serve only to decrease the load of growing organisms. It has also been used, at a dose of 25 mg/kg twice daily for 2 days, to treat *D. medinensis* infection (dracontiasis), when it helps to decrease inflammation, allowing slow removal of the helminth by winding it on stick during the course of a week.[15] Metronidazole has also been used for this same purpose.

Numerous adverse reactions have been loosely attributed to thiabendazole. Most reactions are transient and not serious. These include GI effects such as anorexia, nausea, epigastric discomfort, and diarrhea; generalized complaints such as dizziness, drowsiness, weakness, and pruritus; and nervous system complaints such as headaches, tinnitus, and blurred vision. Also reported are hypotension, bradycardia, crystalluria, and malodorous urine. Self-limited abnormalities may be cholestasis, leukopenia, elevated liver transaminase levels, jaundice, and hyperglycemia. Nephrotoxicity has been reported, as has inhibition of hepatic metabolism of theophylline, which would be expected because both drugs are metabolized by the hepatic P-450 system. In mice, subchronic exposure caused slight anemia (hemosiderosis and extramedullary hematopoiesis), liver injury (elevated transaminases), and kidney injury (tubular atrophy).[16] Hypersensitivity reactions are also reported and include fever/chills, rashes, angioedema, erythema multiforme, Stevens-Johnson syndrome, and anaphylaxis. Allergy to topically applied medication has also been reported.[17]

Treatment for intoxication with this agent is supportive. Thiabendazole should be avoided by patients with liver and kidney disease. Levels of other hepatic P-450–metabolized medications should be monitored. Because of the possibility of drowsiness due to this drug, heavy machinery should not be operated by patients under treatment. Its safety has not been established in pregnancy or lactation.

Flubendazole

Flubendazole is the parafluoro analog of mebendazole. Interestingly, it is absorbed better from the GI tract when taken with or after a meal. It is also available in a slow-release parenteral preparation given subcutaneously or intramuscularly, which allows sustained release over 5 days. The usual dosage is 750 mg/wk for onchocerciasis. It is used to treat hookworm, *T. trichiura*, and *A. lumbricoides*. Side effects are vague and mostly abdominal, such as nausea, abdominal pain and rumbling, soft/loose stools, and dyspepsia. Also reported are fatigue and breathlessness. Unlike mebendazole, it has not yet been shown to be teratogenic in laboratory animals. Treatment of poisoning is supportive. If side effects are severe, flubendazole may have to be withdrawn.

Levamisole

Levamisole is the more nematocidal L-isomer of tetramisole. Its mechanism of action is thought to be rapid and reversible muscle paralysis of the helminth due to ganglionic stimulation. Like thiabendazole, at high doses, it also inhibits the helminthic fumarate reductase system. It is available as syrup or in a tablet, is rapidly absorbed from the GI tract, and is extensively metabolized. Its use is mainly for nematodal disease such as ascariasis, for which it can be given in a single 120- to 150-mg dose.

Today levamisole is used more in combination chemotherapy for cancer (e.g., with 5-fluorouracil in colon cancer) than as an anthelmintic. The doses when used in this manner are different, and more side effects have become evident. Agranulocytosis develops when levamisole is used for a prolonged period.[18] Thrombocytopenia occurring as late as 2 years after its use has been reported.[19] Many skin reactions have been reported, most recently a fixed toxic erythema with pigmentation.[20] Also reported are cases of multifocal inflammatory leukoencephalopathy when used with 5-fluorouracil.[21] In patients taking warfarin, the international normalization

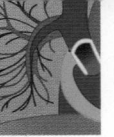

ratio has been reported to increase.[22] This may be because of its competitive inhibition of hepatic P-450 system metabolism of warfarin.

Treatment of poisoning is supportive. Severe effects mandate discontinuation of its use.

Niridazole

Niridazole is also an imidazole (a substituted nitrothiazole), but it does not have the same uses as the others. It also has the distinction of suppressing cellular immunity and possibly being carcinogenic. Fifty percent of oral intake is absorbed. It is excreted in the feces and urine after it has been metabolized in the liver. It has a metabolite with a half-life of 40 hours, and this is responsible for the prolonged immune suppression encountered. It causes the urine to become very dark, and patients should be warned about this.

Its main uses are for *S. japonicum* and *S. mansoni* infections, amebiasis, and dracontiasis, in which it may be used like thiabendazole as an anti-inflammatory. It is not as effective against the other species of schistosomes. In general, its use has become obsolete.

Its toxicity includes nervous system problems such as seizures (usually limited to patients with a seizure disorder), subclinical electroencephalographic changes, headaches, dizziness, agitation, insomnia, and hallucinations (usually only in patients with a history of psychosis). In the treatment of schistosomiasis, it is possible that some of the central nervous system effects are due to high drug levels because of hepatic shunting. Other side effects include GI effects such as nausea, vomiting, and abdominal pain. Also reported are rash, slight electrocardiographic abnormalities, and hemolytic anemia in patients with glucose-6-phosphatase deficiency.

Treatment of the toxicity is supportive. It should not be used by patients with a seizure disorder, liver disease, or psychosis.

PIPERAZINES

Piperazine

Piperazine causes paralysis of the helminth and is thought to precipitate expulsion of the helminth from the GI tract. It is orally absorbed and is excreted unchanged in the urine within 24 hours. Its uses include treatment of enterobiasis (pinworm infection), 65 mg/kg/day (maximum 2.5 g) for 7 days; and ascariasis, 75 mg/kg/day (maximum 3.5 g) for 2 days. In cases of intestinal obstruction due to large worm burdens, it is recommended that piperazine syrup be given via nasogastric tube at a dose of 150 mg/kg then 65 mg/kg every 12 hours for 6 doses. It narcotizes the worm in the intestinal or biliary tract, allowing its passage distally.[23]

Side effects are rare but can affect many organ systems. GI symptoms include nausea and vomiting, diarrhea, and abdominal pain. General symptoms include fever, weakness, and rash. Angioneurotic edema has been reported in sensitive patients.[24] Neurologic abnormalities include visual disturbances, seizures and electroen-cephalographic abnormalities, and cerebellar ataxia, known as "worm wobble."[25] The latter abnormalities are seen mainly in patients with overdoses or with renal failure in which the accumulated levels have become toxic.

Treatment of side effects and toxicities includes discontinuation of treatment and administration of antihistamines if the effects seem to be allergic in nature. Other side effects are treated symptomatically. Piperazine is not recommended for patients with hepatic or renal disturbance or with seizures. Its safety in pregnancy has not been established. There has been a report that it may be linked with cleft hand and foot.[26]

Diethylcarbamazine

Diethylcarbamazine is still in use in many parts of the world. In the United States, it may be found in dog-owning households because it is a treatment for *D. immitis*, the dog heartworm. Ivermectin has become popular for prophylaxis of this condition (discussed later). Diethylcarbamazine is highly soluble in water and is well absorbed through the GI tract. Its renal clearance is reduced in alkaline urine. It is also available as a lotion for onchocerciasis. In addition to its canine use, it can be used to treat filariasis and *O. volvulus*. In filariasis, like thiabendazole, it may do no more than reduce the number of microfilariae of *W. bancrofti* and *B. malayi* (6 mg/kg daily for 2 weeks). Its effect on adult worms is uncertain, although a higher dose repeated monthly or weekly may be effective.[27] In the treatment of *L. loa*, it eliminates the microfilariae and may also kill the adult worms.

In the treatment of onchocerciasis (and also of filariasis to a lesser degree) with diethylcarbamazine, a severe reaction, probably an immune response to the mass of dying antigenic microfilariae, may develop 16 hours after treatment. It consists of severe pruritus, a fine papular rash, skin edema, fever, tachycardia, headache, swollen lymph nodes, and possibly hypotension. This reaction was first described in 1948 and is called the Mazzotti reaction.[28] For this reason, it is recommended that the diethylcarbamazine dose be gradually increased from 50 mg once per day on day 1, to 50 mg three times per day on day 2, to 100 mg three times per day on day 3, to the full 3 mg/kg three times per day on days 4 through 21. Levels of the immune mediator interleukin-6 correlate with the occurrence and severity of clinical symptoms after treatment. Tumor necrosis factors also are elevated in patients with reactions.[29] The Mazzotti reaction can also be used to test whether a rash is caused by *O. volvulus*. This is done by giving a test dose of 50 mg of diethylcarbamazine. If the rash worsens, it probably is due to a reaction against *O. volvulus*. Ivermectin (discussed later) has replaced diethylcarbamazine as the drug of choice in the treatment of onchocerciasis because it is safer and more effective. The Mazzotti reaction has also been seen with ivermectin treatment.[30]

Other side effects include changes in the posterior segment of the eye (transient pigment lesions, optic disc leakage, and visual loss).[31] *L. loa* encephalopathy may be aggravated. Pretreatment or concurrent treatment

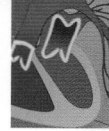

with corticosteroids is helpful. A transient proteinuria, possibly resulting from circulating immune complexes, has also been described in patients.[32]

ANTISCHISTOSOME MEDICATIONS

Praziquantel

The development of praziquantel has been a major advance in the control of schistosomiasis. It also has many other anthelmintic uses. It is readily absorbed through the GI tract and excreted by the kidneys. It can be detected in human breast milk. Its mode of action is not clearly understood. Bioavailability is limited by an extensive first pass effect through liver metabolism. This is exacerbated by dexamethasone and antiepileptic medication (through P-450 induction), often given concomitantly with praziquantel in patients with neurocysticercosis.[33,34] Cimetidine, which inhibits P-450 metabolism, lengthens the drug's elimination half-life.[35]

It is effective against all schistosomes as well as most of the other trematodes (flukes).[36] For *S. haematobium* and *S. mansoni,* it is given as a single 40 mg/kg dose, and for *S. japonicum* it is given as 20 mg/kg three times in 1 day. For *C. sinensis,* it is the treatment of choice. Surgery may be necessary for biliary obstruction. *Clonorchis* and intestinal flukes (*F. buski* and *Heterophyes heterophyes*) are treated with a dose of 25 mg/kg three times per day for 1 day. The lung fluke (*Paragonimus*) is treated with 25 mg/kg three times per day for 2 days. The only fluke not responsive to praziquantel is *F. hepatica,* for which bithionol must be used.

In addition to the trematodes, praziquantel is also effective against the cestodes (tapeworms). *T. saginata* (beef tapeworm), *T. solium* (pork tapeworm), and *Diphyllobothrium nana* (fish tapeworm) are treated with 10 mg/kg as a single dose, and *H. nana* (dwarf tapeworm) is treated with 25 mg/kg as a single dose. For human cysticercosis, infection with *T. solium* eggs, treatment is with 50 mg/kg per day in three divided doses for 2 weeks. This is usually given with corticosteroids to avoid the immunologic reaction common with the large antigenic load that is released. It may also have a role in the treatment of *Echinococcus.*

Side effects and toxicity from praziquantel are usually a result of the treatment of the infection rather than of the medication per se. When all inhabitants in an area of high prevalence of *S. mansoni* (61.8%) were treated, 27.2% had side effects (abdominal discomfort, fever, headache), mostly mild, disappearing in 24 hours, correlating with those that were infected.[37]

Toxicity is rare. Mild toxicity does not require discontinuance of medication. If toxicity is from the rapid killing of worms, corticosteroids may be administered if not already given.

Metrifonate

Metrifonate, also called trichlorfon, is an organophosphorus compound that is selective for treatment of *S. haematobium.* It is nonenzymatically transformed into dichlorvos and inhibits plasma cholinesterase activity. It inhibits erythrocyte cholinesterase to a lesser degree. The dose is 7.5 mg/kg (range, 5 to 15) every 2 weeks for 6 weeks.

Side effects include those of other cholinergic medications if taken in sufficient quantity. Suicide attempts among patients using metrifonate have been reported. Also reported have been cases of polyneuropathy.[38] Management of toxicity is similar to that with other cholinergic medication.

Oxamniquine

Oxamniquine is an antischistosomal quinoline compound selective for *S. mansoni.* Fifty percent of an oral dose is absorbed; most is excreted in the urine. A metabolite turns the urine dark orange or reddish on the second day. The dosage used varies from 60 mg/kg over 3 days in Egypt or East Africa to a low of 12 mg/kg as a single dose.

Side effects are frequent but usually mild and are likely due to immune reactions to the release antigenic load rather than the medication itself. They include dizziness, headache, vague abdominal pain, nausea, vomiting, and transient increases in results of liver function tests, especially in older patients. In one report, 38% had fever of 38° C to 39° C often 24 to 72 hours after completing a 3-day treatment. Six of 40 developed Löffler's syndrome with transient pulmonary infiltrates and eosinophilia.[32,39] Treatment is supportive.

Hycanthone

Hycanthone (Etronol) has an unknown mechanism of action but is effective against *S. haematobium* and *S. mansoni.* It has good GI absorption and can also be given intramuscularly. It is not sold in the United States.

Side effects are frequent but mild and self-limited. The complaints usually are of GI origin (nausea, vomiting, and abdominal pain) or generalized (weakness, dizziness, headache, and myalgias). Very rarely a serious hepatic necrosis can occur. Hycanthone is mutagenic, carcinogenic, and teratogenic in animals and therefore should not be given to pregnant women until 1 month after delivery, nor to children or young adults. It should also be avoided by patients with liver disease. Treatment is symptomatic and supportive.

Niridazole was discussed earlier in the section on imidazoles.

OTHER ANTHELMINTICS

Other anthelmintics, such as ivermectin and niclosamide, are in common use around the world, and others are of primarily historical importance. Some of the latter are still used in developing countries.

Ivermectin

Ivermectin enjoys widespread use around the world. In the United States, it is used primarily for prophylaxis and

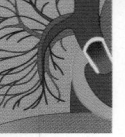

treatment of heartworm in dogs. It is often the object of calls to regional poison control centers.

Ivermectin is from a family of chemicals called avermectins. These are macrocyclic lactones from the fermentation broth of *Streptomyces avermitilis*. It is thought to work by opening chloride-sensitive channels. In the free-living nematode *Aenorhabditis elegans,* it binds to a glutamate-gated chloride channel.[40]

It is active primarily in nematodes and is the drug of choice for the treatment of onchocerciasis. It kills the microfilariae of *O. volvulus* but not the adults. Sumarin (discussed later) is the only agent that kills the adults. It is also used to treat *D. immitis* (heartworm) in dogs. For onchocerciasis, it is given in a dose of 150 μg/kg as a single dose. It has been tried in the treatment of lymphatic filariasis (single dose), clearing microfilariae from the blood, but is not active against adult filarial worms in the lymphatic system.[41] It can also be used as an alternative to mebendazole in the treatment of intestinal nematodes.[42]

Adverse reactions are fairly numerous and may be related to the worm burden rather than the medication itself. Encephalopathy has been temporally related to ivermectin administration, most cases when the patients may have also had *L. loa*.[4] In another report, 97% had side effects when ivermectin was used to treat *W. bancrofti*. These consisted of fever, headache, pruritic rash, weakness, myalgias, lymphatic nodules, cough, and elevated alkaline phosphatase levels, all of which subsided in 12 to 72 hours after treatment. Some patients with very dense infection developed serious pulmonary symptoms consisting of cough with production of blood-tinged sputum, shortness of breath, and patchy pneumonitis.[43] Some patients, however, had heavy worm burdens but did not develop side effects. Other reported side effects include facial edema and bullous skin disease.[44] Treatment is symptomatic.

Niclosamide

Niclosamide (Yomesan) is not absorbed through the GI tract and therefore has almost no side effects. It is used to treat cestodes (tapeworms), which include *T. saginata* (beef tapeworm), *T. solium* (pork tapeworm), *D. latum* (fish tapeworm), and *H. nana* (dwarf tapeworm). It is not effective against cysticercosis (eggs of *T. solium*) or *E. granulosus* (hydatid disease), because these require tissue penetration.

Patients occasionally complain of GI symptoms, such as abdominal cramping and nausea. Treatment is supportive and symptomatic.

Suramin

Suramin is an antiparasitic drug that is now used in cancer chemotherapy. It was introduced in 1920 for the treatment of African trypanosomiasis and began to be used in 1947 for the treatment of onchocerciasis. It is the only medication that kills the adult *O. volvulus*. It is not well absorbed orally, and intramuscular injection causes significant local skin irritation; thus, it is given

intravenously. Its elimination half-life is 36 to 54 hours. Nearly 100% (99.9%) is protein bound.

It is recommended for onchocerciasis only if the patient has recurrent skin disease after treatment with ivermectin and several courses of diethylcarbamazine or for patients with eye disease. A test dose of 100 mg is first given, and if this is tolerated, 1.0 g is given intravenously each week for 6 weeks. Treatment is stopped if proteinuria or casts appear in the urine or if exfoliative dermatitis develops.

Suramin toxicity can result in renal and adrenal insufficiency, coagulation factor abnormalities, immune suppression, and polyneuropathy.

Other side effects include a wide variety of skin eruptions,[45] including a lethal toxic epidermal necrolysis,[46] and weakness due to hypophosphatemia, mitochondrial myopathy,[47] or motor axonal polyneuropathy (some with sensory symptoms).[48] Treatment is supportive and symptomatic. The drug should be withdrawn if side effects occur.

Pyrantel Pamoate

Pyrantel pamoate is a depolarizing neuromuscular blocker. It results in spastic neuromuscular paralysis of the parasite, allowing its expulsion. It is poorly absorbed from the GI tract; 40% is excreted in the feces, and small amounts are detectable in the urine. It is used for enterobiasis (pinworm), ascariasis (giant roundworm), and *N. americanus* (hookworm) infections. The usual dose is 11 mg/kg orally once (maximum 1 g), repeated after 2 weeks.

Because most of an oral ingestion remains in the lumen of the GI tract, the medication itself has very few side effects. Most of the side effects are from the parasitic burden. These include nausea, vomiting, abdominal pain, tenesmus, headache, dizziness, insomnia, drowsiness, fever, rash, and nasal congestion. Liver transaminase levels may become transiently elevated. Use of pyrantel pamoate is contraindicated in pregnancy, in those younger than 1 year, and in patients with liver disease. Treatment is symptomatic and supportive.

Pyrvinium Pamoate

Pyrvinium pamoate, like pyrantel pamoate, is useful to eliminate certain intestinal parasites because of its minimal absorption from the GI tract. Patients should be warned of changes in stool color, which most often becomes red. It has been largely replaced by mebendazole for the treatment of enterobiasis (oxyuriasis).

It produces minimal side effects, with occasional nausea, vomiting, and abdominal pain. A photosensitive skin reaction has also been reported. Treatment is symptomatic.

Poquil

Poquil has been used for the treatment of enterobiasis (oxyuriasis) at a dose of 1.5 mg/kg per day for 8 days. Mebendazole treatment is simpler (one dose) and is the agent of choice. Poquil is well tolerated, although occasional nausea and vomiting are reported. It causes a bitter taste in the mouth. Treatment of intoxication is symptomatic and supportive. If vomiting or other effects are severe, it should be discontinued.

Antimony

The trivalent antimonials act by inhibition of phosphofructokinase. They have to be administered intravenously because oral ingestion leads to significant GI irritation. They bind to erythrocytes and thus have slow renal excretion, on the order of weeks to months.

Trivalent antimony has been replaced by other medications for most helminthiasis, but on occasion they are used, mainly for schistosomiasis. *S. japonicum* responds to antimony potassium tartate and antimony sodium dimercaptosuccinate. *S. haematobium* and *S. mansoni* also respond to antimony sodium dimercaptosuccinate. *S. mansoni* also responds to stibophen.

The antimonials have many toxicities. They are contraindicated in hepatic disease, unless it is due to schistosomiasis, because they can cause worsening of liver function. They can rarely cause hepatitis. A host of immunologic reactions can occur, such as an anaphylactoid reaction and anaphylaxis, arthralgias, arthritis, myalgias, headache, fainting, skin rashes, and facial edema. Pulmonary symptoms include pneumonia (especially with tartrates), coughing, dyspnea, and apnea.

More specific side effects include fever, fainting, rashes, and vomiting with use of dimercaptosuccinate; hemolytic anemia, thrombocytopenia, vomiting, and albuminuria with stibophen; and phlebitis, cough, and death due to rapid injection with tartrates. Dimercaptosuccinate is contraindicated in the presence of bacterial infection or herpes (simplex or zoster) infection.

The medication should be withdrawn if the side effects are severe. Treatment is supportive and symptomatic.

Pentavalent antimony is used in the treatment of protozoan infections such as leishmaniasis.

Bephenium Hydroxynaphthoate

Bephenium hydroxynaphthoate is a quaternary ammonium used for the treatment of hookworm (*N. americanus*, 5 g twice per day for 3 days; and *A. duodenale*, 5 g twice per day for 5 days); and also for giant roundworm (*A. lumbricoides*). It has been replaced for the most part by mebendazole but is more effective than tetrachloroethylene.

Bephenium hydroxynaphthoate has minimal GI absorption. It does have a bitter taste, and this is what usually causes the nausea and vomiting. Treatment is symptomatic.

Bithionol

Bithionol may still be used for human fascioliasis (30 to 50 mg/kg on alternate days for 10 to 15 doses), for which it is the treatment of choice. It may be used for paragonimiasis (30 mg/kg every other day for 20 days),

but for the most part, treatment of this and other trematode infections has been replaced by praziquantel.

Side effects are skin reactions and GI irritation, which are rarely severe enough to discontinue medication. Treatment is symptomatic.

Paromomycin

Paromomycin can be used to eradicate the cestodes (tapeworms) *T. saginata, T. solium, D. latum,* and *H. nana.* It is given in a dosage of 1 g every 4 hours for 4 days. Treatment with paromomycin has largely been replaced by niclosamide.

ACKNOWLEDGMENT

The authors wish to thank Donald G. Barceloux, MD, for his thoughtful review and commentary on this chapter.

REFERENCES

1. Stoll NR: This wormy world. J Parasitol 1947;33:1–18.
2. Liu LX, Weller PF: Antiparasitic drugs. N Engl J Med 1996; 334:1178–1184.
3. Warren KS: Helminthic diseases endemic in the United States. Am J Trop Med Hyg 1974;23:723.
4. Nana AYTD: Loa loa encephalopathy temporally related to ivermectin administration reported from onchocerciasis mass treatment programs from 1989–2001: implications for the future. Filaria J 2003;2(Suppl):7.
5. Lacey E: Mode of action of benzimidazoles. Parasitol Today 1990;6:112–115.
6. Shcherbakov AM, Kozlova TL, Bebris NK: Agranulocytosis—a complication of the chemotherapy of echinococcosis with mebendazole. Med Parazitol (Mosk) 1992;5–6:9–11.
7. Macedo NA, Piseyro MI, Carmona C: Contact urticaria and contact dermatitis from albendazol. Contact Dermatitis 1991;25:73–75.
8. Chen KT, Twu SJ, Chang JH, Lin RS: Outbreak of Stevens-Johnson syndrome/toxic epidermal necrolysis associated with mebendazole and metronidazole use among Filipino laborers in Taiwan. Am J Public Health 2003;93:489–492.
9. Awadzi K, Hero M, Opoku NO, et al: The chemotherapy of onchocerciasis XVII: a clinical evaluation of albendazole in patients with onchocerciasis; effects of food and pretreatment with ivermectin on drug response and pharmokinetics. Trop Med Parasitol 1994;45:203–208.
10. Dickson B: Albendazole for hydatid cysts. Lancet 1984;1:37.
11. Albonico M, Smith PG, Hall A, et al: A randomized controlled trial comparing mebendazole and albendazole against Ascaris, Trichuris and hookwork infections. Trans R Soc Trop Med Hyg 1994;88: 585–589.
12. Takayanagui OM, Jardim E: Therapy for neurocysticercosis: comparison between albendazole and praziquantel. Arch Neurol 1992;49:290–294.
13. Horton J: Albendazole: a review of anthelmintic efficacy and safety in humans. Parasitology 2000;121(Suppl):113–132.
14. Grove DI: Treatment of strongyloidiasis with thiabendazole: an analysis of toxicity and effectiveness. Trans R Soc Trop Med Hyg 1982;76:114–118.
15. Sastry SC, Jayakumar K, Lakshminarayana V: The treatment of dracontiasis with thiabendazole. J Trop Med Hyg 1978;81:32.
16. Tada Y, Funjitani T, Yoneyama M: Subchronic toxicity of thiabendazole (TBZ) in ICR mice. Food Chem Toxicol 1996;34:709–716.
17. Mancuso G: Topical thiabendazole allergy. Contact Dermatitis 1994;31:207.
18. Renoux G: The general immunopharmacology of levamisole. Drugs 1980;19:89–90.
19. Winquist EW, Lassam NJ: Reversible thrombocytopenia with levamisole. Med Pediatr Oncol 1995;24:262–264.

20. Clavere P, Bonnafoux-Clavere A, Delrous JL, et al: Fixed pigmented erythema caused by levamisole administration. Ann Dermatol Venereol 1994;121:238–239.

21. Enterline DS, Davey NC, Tien RD: Multifocal inflammatory leukoencephalopathy due to treatment with 5-fluorouracil and levamisole. AJR Am J Roentgenol 1995;165:214–215.

22. Scarfe MA, Israel MK: Possible drug interaction between warfarin and combination of levamisole and fluorouracil. Ann Pharmacol 1994;28:264–267.

23. Swartwelder JC, Miller JH, Sappenfield RW: The use of piperazine for the treatment of human helminthiases. Gastroenterology 1957;33:87.

24. Eedy DJ: Angioneurotic oedema following piperazine ingestion in an ethylenediamine-sensitive subject. Contact Dermatitis 1993;28:48–49.

25. Conners GP: Piperazine neurotoxicity: worm wobble revisited. J Emerg Med 1995;13:341–343.

26. Meyer HH, Brenner P: Cleft hand and foot deformity as a possible teratogenic side effect of antihelminthic agent piperazine. Internist 1988;29:217–219.

27. Ottesen EA: Efficacy of diethylcarbamazine in eradicating infection with lymphatic-dwelling filariae in humans. Rev Infect Dis 1985;7:341.

28. Mazzotti L: Posibilidad de utilizar como medio diagnóstico en la onchocercosis las reacciones alérgicas consecutivas a la administratión de Heterozan. Rev Inst Salubr Enferm Trop 1948;9:235–237.

29. Turner PF, Rockett KA, Ottesen EA, et al: Interleukin-6 and tumor necrosis factor in the pathogenesis of adverse reactions after treatment of lymphatic filariasis and onchocerciasis. J Infect Dis 1994;169:1071–1075.

30. Mackenzie CD, Geary TG, Gerlach JA: Possible pathogenic pathways in the adverse clinical events seen following Ivermectin administration to onchocerciasis patients. Filaria J 2003;2(Suppl):5.

31. Bird AC, Hall EL, Sheil CH, et al: Changes in visual function and in the posterior segment of the eye during the treatment of onchocerciasis with diethylcarbamazine citrate. Br J Ophthalmol 1980;64:1191.

32. Ngu JL, Mate A: Proteinuria associated with diethylcarbamazine. Lancet 1980;1:710.

33. Vazquez ML, Jung H, Sotelo J: Plasma levels of praziquantel decrease when dexamethasone is given simultaneously. Neurology 1987;37:1561–1562.

34. Bittencourt PR, Garcia CM, Martins R, et al: Phenytoin and carbamazepine decrease and bioavailability of praziquantel. Neurology 1992;42:492–496.

35. Duchman WD, Adubofour KO, Biken DS, et al: Cimetidine-induced rise in praziquantel levels in a patient with neurocysticercosis being treated with anti-c. J Infect Dis 1994;169:689–691.

36. Day TA, Bennett JL, Pax RA: Praziquantel: the enigmatic antiparasitic. Parisitol Today 1992;8:342–344.

37. Boisier P, Ravaoalimalala VA, Serieye J, et al: Schistosoma mansoni infection in a hyperendemic region of midwestern Madagascar: epidemiology, morbidity and secondary effects of praziquantel [French]. Arch Inst Pasteur Madagascar 1994;61:43–48.

38. Akimor GA, Buchko VM, Kremleva RV: Neurological disorders in trichlorfon poisoning. Klin Med (Mosk) 1975;5:65.

39. Higashi GI, Farid Z: Oxamniquine-drug-induced or immune-complex reaction? BMJ 1979;2:830.

40. Cully DF, Vassilatis DK, Liu KK, et al: Cloning of an ivermectin-sensitive glutamate-gated chloride channel from *Caenorhabiditis elegans*. Nature 1994;371:707–711.

41. Ottesen EA, Vijayasekaran V, Kumaraswami V, et al: A controlled trial of ivermectin and diethylcarbamazine in lymphatic filariasis. N Engl J Med 1990;322:1113–1117.

42. Naquira C, Jimenez G, Guerra JG, et al: Ivermectin for human strongyloidiasis and other intestinal helminths. Am J Trop Med Hyg 1989;40:304–309.

43. Kar SK, Patnaik S, Kumaraswami V, Murty RS: Side reactions following ivermectin therapy in high density bancroftian microfilaraemics. Acta Trop 1993;55:21–31.

44. Burnham GM: Adverse reactions to ivermectin treatment for onchocerciasis. Results of a placebo-controlled, double-blind trial in Malawi. Trans R Soc Trop Med Hyg 1993;87:313–317.

45. Lowitt MH, Eisenberg M, Sina B, Kao GF: Cutaneous eruptions from suramin. A clinical and histopathologic study of 60 patients. Arch Dermatol 1995;131:1147–1153.

46. Falkson G, Rapoport BL: Lethal toxic epidermal necrolysis during suramin treatment. Eur J Cancer 1992;28A:1294.

47. Rago RP, Miles JM, Sufit RL, et al: Suramin-induced weakness from hypophosphatemia and mitochondrial myopathy. Cancer 1994;73:1954–1959.

48. Bitton RJ, Figg WD, Venzon DJ, et al: Pharmacologic variables associated with the development of neurologic toxicity in patients treated with suramin. J Clin Oncol 1995;13:2223–2229.

55 *Isoniazid*

ANN-JEANNETTE GEIB, MD ■ MICHAEL W. SHANNON, MD, MPH

At a Glance...

■ Isoniazid, which is structurally related to nicotinic acid, pyridoxine, and other pyridines, remains the most common treatment for tuberculosis.

■ Isoniazid produces a broad range of adverse effects, including drug-drug interactions, hypersensitivity reactions, and hepatotoxicity.

■ In overdose, isoniazid produces the pathognomonic triad of seizures, severe metabolic acidosis, and coma.

■ Treatment of isoniazid overdose begins with supportive care that includes seizure control, which begins with administration of benzodiazepines.

■ The specific antidote and treatment of choice for isoniazid-induced seizures is intravenous vitamin B_6 (pyridoxine), given in a gram-for-gram dose. If the ingested dose of isoniazid is unknown, 5 g (75 mg/kg in children) should be administered intravenously.

Isoniazid (INH) was introduced in 1952 and remains the antibiotic most commonly used in the treatment of tuberculosis. It is first-line treatment for both latent tuberculosis and in combination with other agents for active tuberculosis. Because the incidence of tuberculosis remains high worldwide, INH continues to be more widely prescribed.[1] With this expanded use has come a greater opportunity for INH adverse effects and poisoning. Fortunately, a greater understanding of the biochemical mechanisms underlying its effects has led to the development of effective strategies for the treatment of INH intoxication.[2,3]

PHARMACOLOGY

INH, which contains a pyridine nucleus, is a structural analog of the nutrients nicotinic acid (niacin, vitamin B_3), nicotinamide-adenine dinucleotide (NAD), and pyridoxine (vitamin B_6) (Fig. 55-1). INH is also a congener of the monoamine oxidase inhibitor antidepressant isocarboxazid. Its complete name, isonicotinic acid hydrazide, identifies INH as a congener of nicotinic acid.[3] INH has primary pKa of 1.9.[4]

As monotherapy in latent tuberculosis, INH is given daily in 5 mg/kg (adult) or 10 mg/kg (pediatric) doses.[5] Treatment regimens vary for active tuberculosis.[6] Details about isoniazid pharmacotherapy go beyond the scope of this chapter; the reader is referred to sources specific for the treatment of tuberculosis.[7] Isoniazid also may be given as an intramuscular injection and has been given intravenously in experimental settings.

INH is rapidly absorbed from the gastrointestinal tract (primarily the small intestine), and peak serum concentrations are achieved within 1 to 2 hours.[3,4] Absorption is delayed by concomitant administration of antacids.[3] Once absorbed, INH is distributed throughout body water and has an apparent volume of distribution of 0.6 L/kg.[4,5] INH has negligible binding to plasma proteins.[4,5]

The primary metabolic pathway for INH is acetylation by the enzyme *N*-acetyltransferase (NAT). This enzyme is located in the liver and intestinal mucosa. NAT has been identified as a polymorphic enzyme whose pharmacokinetic activity follows Michaelis-Menten (saturable) kinetics. Additionally, the activity of this enzyme is genetically controlled by autosomal-dominant inheritance.[3,4] Phenotypically, slow and fast acetylators can be identified. The fast acetylation phenotype is found primarily among Eskimos and Japanese, and slow acetylation among Scandinavians, Jews, and North Africans. In the United States, the prevalence of slow acetylation is about 50% of the general population. Acetylation activity is responsible for a number of the clinical differences observed in slow versus fast acetylators: (1) slow acetylators have a smaller degree of hepatic clearance (first pass effect) than fast acetylators, (2) fast acetylators metabolize INH five to six times faster than slow acetylators, and (3) plasma INH concentrations are 30% to 50% lower in fast versus slow acetylators. Daily INH treatment regimens usually do not result in any differences in response rates between slow and fast acetylators. Fast acetylators may have a suboptimal response in once-weekly regimens.[5] It is thought that slow acetylators may be more prone to the hepatotoxic effects of INH.[8]

The elimination half-life of INH in fast acetylators is approximately 70 minutes, compared with a mean of 3 hours in slow acetylators. The primary metabolites after

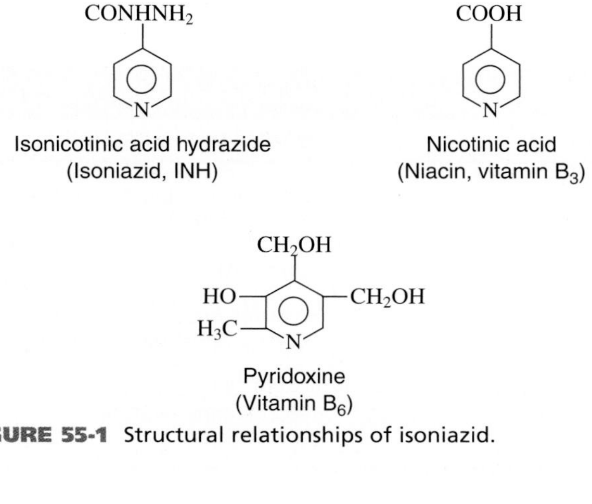

CONHNH$_2$

Isonicotinic acid hydrazide
(Isoniazid, INH)

COOH

Nicotinic acid
(Niacin, vitamin B$_6$)

CH$_2$OH

HO— —CH$_2$OH

H$_3$C—

Pyridoxine
(Vitamin B$_6$)

FIGURE 55-1 Structural relationships of isoniazid.

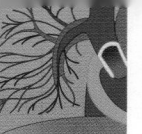

INH biotransformation are acetylisoniazid and isonicotinic acid.[3,4,9] Based on urinary concentrations of these metabolites and the parent compound, it is possible to determine acetylation status with a technique outlined by Kohno and colleagues.[10,11] Both INH and its inactive metabolites are excreted in the urine, and 75% to 95% of a single dose is eliminated within 24 hours. Twenty-seven percent of INH is excreted unchanged in slow acetylators, in contrast to 11% in fast acetylators.[4] The clearance of INH averages 46 mL/min.[4] The half-life is especially prolonged in those with end-stage renal disease (up to 17 hours). Compliance with therapy may be measured using either urine or serum testing (colorimetric urine tests have been developed), but serum concentrations are not routinely monitored.

Hydrazine, a component of rocket fuel that is also touted as an alternative treatment for cancer, and monomethylhydrazine, the toxic component of *Gyromitra* mushrooms, are derivatives of INH. They produce neurotoxicity and hepatotoxicity in a similar manner.[12] Hydrazine is well-known as a human carcinogen. Isoniazid has not been demonstrated to be carcinogenic. INH is an inhibitor of several cytochrome P-450–mediated functions, particularly demethylation, oxidation, and hydroxylation.[13] In vitro, INH has been shown to inhibit CYP2C19 and CPY3A4 isoenzymes at clinically relevant plasma concentrations; coadministration with substrates of these enzymes may result in drug interactions.[14] INH appears to exert a biphasic effect on the CYP2E1 isoenzyme with inhibition followed by induction.[15-17] Significant drug interactions exist with INH.[1,2] Table 55-1 demonstrates the more clinically significant interactions. An effect on the anticonvulsant phenytoin has been well described; altered mental status (occasionally coma) has occurred in patients who were simultaneously prescribed INH and phenytoin, associated with the development of toxic serum phenytoin concentrations. Phenytoin toxicity results from INH inhibition of cytochrome P-450 hydroxylases.[3,5] This decrease in phenytoin clearance tends to occur in the second week of combined treatment.[18] Other drugs whose elimination is reduced by concomitant administration of INH are carbamazepine, valproate,[19] coumarin anticoagulants, and rifampin.[13]

When coadministered with INH, serum theophylline concentrations are increased, resulting from inhibition of its metabolism.[3,5] Case reports have suggested a significant adverse interaction between INH and acetaminophen,[20] the result of CYP2E1 enzyme induction. However, well-controlled clinical studies have failed to demonstrate a greater risk for hepatotoxicity when these two are taken simultaneously.[16] The degree of acetaminophen toxic metabolite formation also may be dependent on the patient's acetylation phenotype.[21]

Certain herbal medications have been associated with fulminant hepatic failure when taken with INH.[5] One case of central nervous system (CNS) depression and hemodynamic instability has been reported when INH was coadministered with meperidine, a serotonergic opioid.[22] No cases of interactions with serotonin reuptake inhibitors have been reported.

INH has a significant effect on several biochemical pathways (Table 55-2). INH also affects the enzymes involved in the metabolism of the CNS neurotransmitter γ-aminobutyric acid (GABA). GABA is the primary neurotransmitter at the motor inhibitory neurons of the CNS. GABA levels are regulated by two enzymes, glutamic acid decarboxylase (GAD) and GABA aminotransferase. GAD catalyzes the synthesis of GABA, whereas GABA aminotransferase promotes GABA breakdown. Both enzymes require pyridoxal phosphate as a cofactor. INH is an inhibitor of both enzymes but has a greater inhibitory effect on GAD, leading to reduced GABA levels.[8,23,24] Reduction in GABA has been directly associated with the development of seizures.[23,24] Monomethylhydrazine has a similar pharmacologic action.

INH's effect on pyridoxine metabolism is pivotal in the drug's toxicity. Pyridoxine activity is markedly reduced by INH, and pyridoxine depletion ultimately results. At least two mechanisms are responsible for this loss of pyridoxine activity: (1) INH inhibition of the enzyme pyridoxine phosphokinase, which converts pyridoxine to its active form, pyridoxal phosphate,[26] and (2) INH binding to pyridoxal phosphate, which forms an inactive hydrazone complex that is excreted in the urine.[4,25] Daily urinary excretion of pyridoxine is doubled with INH doses of 3 to 5 mg/kg and is quadrupled

TABLE 55-1 Drug Interactions with Isoniazid			
DRUG	**NATURE OF INTERACTION**	**CLINICAL EFFECT**	**REFERENCES**
Phenytoin	Inhibition of parahydroxylation	Increased phenytoin level	3, 5, 18
Carbemazepine	P-450 inhibition (3A4)	Increased carbamazepine level	5
Valproic acid	Unknown; possible enzymatic inhibition	Increased valproic acid level	19
Coumarin anticoagulants	Unknown	Increased warfarin levels; increased prothrombin time	5
Rifampin	Possible enzyme induction by rifampin	Isoniazid hepatotoxicity	5, 13
Theophylline	Unclear; possible P-450 inhibition	Increased theophylline levels; tachycardia, neurotoxicity	5
Acetaminophen	P-450 2E1 inhibition	Hepatotoxicity	16, 20, 21
Meperidine	Monoamine oxidase inhibition	Coma, hemodynamic instability, possible serotonin syndrome	22

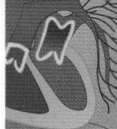

TABLE 55-2 Metabolic Actions of Isoniazid

BIOCHEMICAL EFFECT	CLINICAL EFFECT	REFERENCES
Enzyme inhibition		
P-450	↓ Clearance of other drugs	13, 14
Monoamine oxidase	↑ Sensitivity to tyramine	2
	Mood elevation	
Glutamate decarboxylase	↓ GABA activity	23, 24, 65
GABA aminotransferase	↑ GABA activity	23
Apotryptophanase	Peripheral neuritis	2
Histaminase	↑ Sensitivity to scombroid fish poisoning	13, 55
Pyridoxine phosphokinase	↓ Conversion of pyridoxine to pyridoxal phosphate	23, 70
Transaminases; decarboxylases	↓ Catecholamine synthesis	70
Binding of pyridoxal phosphate	↓ Pyridoxine activity	70
Replacement of nicotinic acid, producing inactive nicotinamide-adenine dinucleotide	Impaired glucose and fatty acid oxidation, metabolic acidosis	26, 66, 70

GABA, γ-aminobutyric acid.

with INH doses of 20 mg/kg.[26] The consequences of pyridoxine depletion include impaired activity of pyridoxine-dependent transaminases and decarboxylases (including GAD). Catecholamine synthesis also is affected by inhibition of these enzymes.

Because of INH's structural similarity to nicotinic acid, it may replace nicotinic acid in the synthesis of NAD, and an inactive compound may form.[4,27]

INH readily crosses the placenta and enters breast milk. No teratogenic or mutagenic effects have been identified with INH use during pregnancy.[4] The American Academy of Pediatrics has determined that it is safe to continue breast-feeding while a woman is taking isoniazid.[28]

CLINICAL TOXICOLOGY

Adverse Events

Because of its many biochemical effects, INH is associated with a myriad of adverse reactions when taken in therapeutic doses. The overall incidence of adverse drug reactions with INH therapy is 5.4%.[3] The most common of these are rash, neuropsychiatric abnormalities, and abnormal liver function with the appearance of jaundice. INH hepatotoxicity may result from the generation of hydrazines.[3,12,29] INH-induced liver enzyme elevation occurs in up to 20% of patients and in most cases is asymptomatic.[5] Approximately 0.6% of patients develop frank jaundice and hyperbilirubinemia, and approximately 0.4% go on to develop ongoing liver disease.[5] Hepatotoxicity appears to occur more often in older patients and in slow acetylators.[8] A study of health care workers found elevation of transaminases to levels requiring discontinuation of the drug in 9.6%.[30] A study of patients in a public health tuberculosis clinic found a hepatotoxicity incidence of 0.1% in those starting a regimen containing INH.[30,31] A British study found mild aminotransferase elevation in 30% of children receiving triple therapy for tuberculosis disease, but treatment was discontinued in only one child.[32] Fulminant hepatitis

occurs in an estimated 20.7 per 1000 persons; approximately 1 to 4.2 cases per 100,000 result in death.[33-35] Liver transplantation may be necessary.[33] It is well established that the risk for hepatotoxicity is increased with multidrug antitubercular regimens. Other risk factors for INH-induced or -associated hepatotoxicity are alcoholism and active hepatitis B infection (as evidenced by positive hepatitis Be antigen).[36,37] Hepatitis C seropositivity was not considered to be a risk factor for INH-induced hepatitis.[36] The Centers for Disease Control and Prevention has recommended discontinuation of isoniazid when transaminases reach elevations greater than three times the upper limit of normal and the patient is symptomatic, or an asymptomatic elevation greater than five times the upper limit of normal. The reader again should refer to these guidelines for more specific details of tuberculosis management.[7]

Acute pancreatitis has also been associated with INH use but is rare.[38,39] Autoimmune phenomena ranging from an asymptomatic ANA seropositivity to frank lupus erythematosus occurs.[40] Approximately 25% of those taking INH develop antinuclear antibodies.[41] The mechanism is unknown, although it may be related to the hydrazine structure of INH; slow acetylators may be at higher risk.[8,40] Symptoms usually consist of fever, rash, arthralgias or frank arthritis, and pleuritis.[8] Life-threatening complications such as pericardial tamponade have been reported.[41] The syndrome usually resolves with discontinuation of the drug; corticosteroids and/or immunosuppressants may be required in some cases.[40,42]

Peripheral or optic neuritis may also occur with INH use. Peripheral neuritis has been observed in up to 20% of those taking INH at doses greater than 6 mg/kg. Those at greater risk include patients with poor nutritional status, alcoholism, pregnancy, or hemodialysis-requiring renal disease. Children appear to be at lesser risk for neuropathy.[3,8] Symptoms of peripheral neuritis include paresthesias in a stocking-glove distribution, which may progress proximally.[2] Although primarily a sensory neuritis, myalgias and weakness may occur.[2] Optic neuritis generally is manifested as decreased visual acuity (often unilateral).[2,3,39,43-45] Less commonly, CNS toxicity

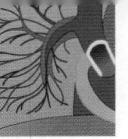

occurs, with manifestations of dysarthria, ataxia, and psychiatric disturbances.[45] Suicidal psychosis has been observed with therapeutic dosing and resolved with discontinuation of the drug.[46,47] Neurologic complications are usually reversible and may be due to INH inhibition of the neuronal enzyme apotryptophanase.[2] Coadministration of pyridoxine with INH prevents their occurrence.[3]

INH may precipitate seizures in those with such a predisposition, even at therapeutic dosing.[3,48] Patients receiving hemodialysis appear to be at greater risk.[8] Pellagra in the setting of INH use has been documented. The result of vitamin B_3 (niacin) depletion, pellagra is characterized by a triad of dermatitis, diarrhea, and dementia or alteration in mental status. INH is thought to act as an analog for niacin in biochemical reactions and may precipitate pellagra in those with niacin depletion. Some investigators have attempted to treat INH-induced pellagra with pyridoxine (vitamin B_6), only to find it ineffective.[49,50] However, when INH was discontinued, and in some cases, niacin supplemented, the pellagra resolved.[49-52] Patients with the slow acetylator phenotype may be at greater risk.[52]

INH use also may have a significant effect on diet. INH is known to be a weak monoamine oxidase inhibitor. In fact, soon after the introduction of INH to the market, tuberculosis patients were noted to have improvement in their mood. One derivative of INH, isocarboxazid, was used as an monoamine oxidase inhibitor antidepressant. This property predisposes the patient to similar interactions with tyramine-containing foods (e.g., cheese, wine, aged sausages). Symptoms of a tyramine reaction include hypertension, flushing, and tachycardia. A syndrome similar to scombroid poisoning may occur after ingestion of certain fish due to INH inhibition of histaminase. Patients should be forewarned about the possibility of these food reactions.[8,14,53-55] Isoniazid also has been linked to hematologic disturbances, including red cell aplasia, agranulocytosis, hemolytic anemia, sideroblastic anemia, thrombocytopenia, eosinophilia, and megaloblastic anemia.[8,56] Skin disorders associated with INH use range from simple rash to exfoliative dermatitis to Stevens-Johnson syndrome.[8,57,58]

Acute Intoxication

Acute ingestion of 2 to 3 g of INH leads to toxicity, whereas ingestion of more than 10 to 15 g or 80 mg/kg is usually fatal without aggressive treatment.[5,59] Severe INH toxicity correlates with serum INH concentrations of greater than 30 mg/L.[60] Clinical manifestations of INH intoxication may appear as early as 30 minutes after ingestion.[60,61-63] Early signs and symptoms include nausea, vomiting, slurred speech, dizziness, mydriasis, and tachycardia. A subsequent cascade of biochemical events soon leads to the striking clinical features that characterize INH intoxication, namely, recurrent seizures, severe metabolic acidosis, and coma. As described earlier, INH prevents pyridoxine-dependent synthesis of GABA, the major inhibitory neurotransmitter. A proposed mechanism for this sequence is shown in Figure 55-2.

Seizures after INH overdose are episodic and tend to occur at regular intervals; either hyperreflexia or areflexia precedes their onset.[2] Improvement in consciousness may occur between seizures.[59] Once they begin, seizures are difficult to control despite the administration of anticonvulsants. *Seizures refractory to conventional anticonvulsant therapy are a hallmark of INH intoxication.*

Severe metabolic acidosis is another prominent feature of INH overdose. Although pH ranges of 6.80 to 7.30 are common, surviving victims may present with a systemic pH as low as 6.49.[64] The etiology of metabolic acidosis appears to be an increase in the generation of lactic acid because of the muscular activity of recurrent seizures. Experimental data have demonstrated that paralyzed animals with INH intoxication do not develop severe metabolic acidosis.[65] Other theories of metabolic acidosis have been proposed, however, including (1) the generation of acidic INH metabolites, (2) an increase in keto acids (specifically, β-hydroxybutyric acid) due to altered fatty acid oxidation, and (3) the formation of inactive NAD, leading to impairment of both glucose and fatty acid metabolism. The last-named theory has led to the suggestion that nicotinic acid be administered in INH overdose, although no clinical studies have been performed to this end.[4,27,66-68]

Coma may be protracted after overdose (lasting more than 24 hours) and may continue after seizures have abated and metabolic acidosis has been corrected. This profound CNS depression has been attributed to CNS catecholamine depletion.[63,69]

Other clinical effects of acute INH intoxication are severe hypotension, hyperglycemia, acetonuria, abnormal results of liver function tests, and renal failure.[2,69,70] INH-induced renal failure is often exacerbated by the myoglobinuria that develops from seizure-induced rhabdomyolysis.[71]

DIAGNOSIS

In the absence of a history of overdose, INH overdose may be suspected in patients who present with the characteristic symptom complex. The differential diagnosis of severe metabolic acidosis includes diabetic ketoacidosis and the ingestion of cyanide, methanol, ethylene glycol, iron, ibuprofen, or salicylates. Of these, only INH overdose has recurrent seizures as its hallmark.

The toxic screen generally does not detect the presence of INH, although serum INH concentrations can be measured if confirmation is required. These results likely will return well after the patient's acute toxicity has resolved. Other important laboratory tests are an arterial blood gas determination, electrocardiogram, electrolyte measurements, liver function tests, creatine phosphokinase determination, and urinalysis.

MANAGEMENT

The initial management of INH intoxication requires stabilization of vital signs with provision of a patent

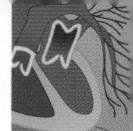

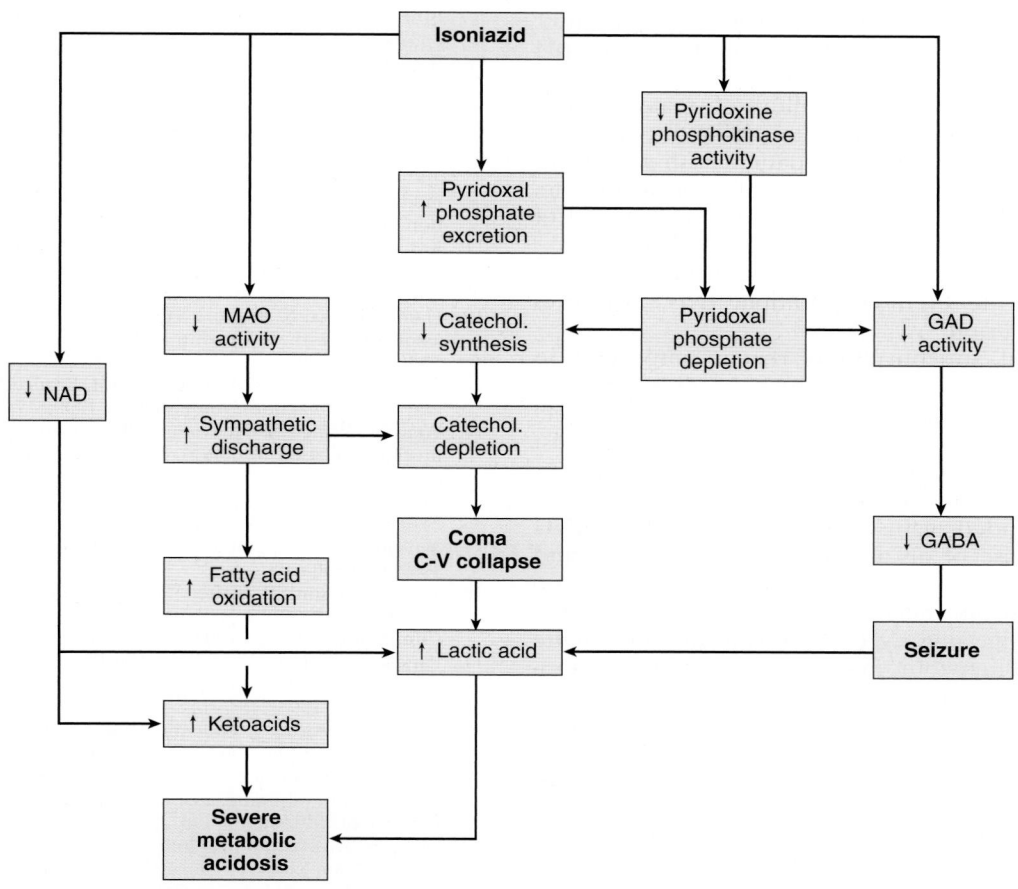

FIGURE 55-2 Proposed mechanisms of isoniazid toxicity.

airway, oxygen, cardiovascular support with intravenous fluids, and administration of sodium bicarbonate to treat metabolic acidosis (Box 55-1).

If emergency department arrival is within 1 hour of ingestion, administration of activated charcoal with a cathartic is indicated. Ipecac-induced emesis is contraindicated owing to the potentially rapid onset of seizures and risk for airway compromise. Delayed absorption of INH after an overdose has not been observed, and it is thus suggested that late gastrointestinal decontamination may be ineffective.

Intravenous pyridoxine has been shown to be highly effective for INH intoxication and should be administered to all symptomatic patients.[60,72] The milligram dose of pyridoxine should equal the ingested dose of INH. Pyridoxine (given as pyridoxine hydrochloride) has been shown to terminate seizures, correct metabolic acidosis, and abbreviate the duration of coma.[2,73] The efficacy of pyridoxine is directly correlated with the administered dose; in one study, recurrent seizures occurred in 60% of patients who received no pyridoxine, 47% of those who received 10% of the ideal pyridoxine dose, and none of the patients who received a full dose of pyridoxine.[73] When the quantity of ingested INH is unknown, a pyridoxine dose of 5 g (75 mg/kg in children) should be administered. Repeated doses of pyridoxine may be required based on the resolution of

signs and symptoms. Pyridoxine is commonly dispensed as 100 mg/mL solution with a pH ranging from 2 to 3.8. A relatively large volume of such an acidic solution may

---

BOX 55-1   SUMMARY OF TREATMENT STRATEGIES FOR ISONIAZID OVERDOSE

Supportive Care

Ventilatory support
Vascular access
Fluids, vasopressors

Gastrointestinal Decontamination

Activated charcoal plus cathartic

Pharmacologic Treatment

Sodium bicarbonate to correct metabolic acidosis
Benzodiazepines and/or barbiturates as anticonvulsants
Pyridoxine: gram for gram per dose ingested, 5 g (75 mg/kg for children) if isoniazid dose is unknown; may be repeated if necessary

Elimination Enhancement

Hemodialysis
? Multiple-dose activated charcoal

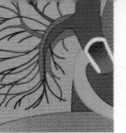

temporarily worsen a metabolic acidosis soon after administration. This transient decline in serum pH should resolve within approximately 30 minutes and should not be interpreted as a failure of treatment, nor should it be a contraindication to pyridoxine administration for INH overdose.[74,75] A patient with significant INH overdose may deplete local supplies of pyridoxine. Santucci and colleagues suggest stocking at least 5 g of pyridoxine in the emergency department at all times.[76] Contingency plans should be created for access to pyridoxine in the event of multiple INH exposures within a brief period.[76,77]

Conventional anticonvulsants remain important in the early treatment of seizures. The benzodiazepines are agents of choice because they have a synergistic effect with pyridoxine as well as inherent GABA agonist activity.[2,73,78,79] Prophylactic administration of benzodiazepines has no proven efficacy. Several investigators have recommended against the use of phenytoin in INH overdose because of an apparent lack of efficacy and the potential for phenytoin intoxication.[2,70] However, impaired phenytoin metabolism has been documented only in those ingesting INH continually, not after acute intoxication. Phenytoin may be an acceptable anticonvulsant, although its efficacy remains in question.[79] Phenobarbital, like the benzodiazepines, is a potent GABA agonist that may be effective in the treatment of seizures. Phenobarbital may worsen CNS depression, especially if administered after a benzodiazepine.

INH has a small volume of distribution and low protein binding, pharmacokinetic features that make it amenable to hemodialysis and peritoneal dialysis. Up to 75% of serum INH may be removed within 5 hours by hemodialysis, with clearance rates as high as 120 mL/min.[4,8] Hemodialysis should be reserved for patients with severe acidosis or who develop renal failure. These same characteristics make isoniazid similar to theophylline and phenobarbital, two drugs whose elimination is enhanced by the "gut dialysis" effect of multiple-dose activated charcoal. While data are lacking, multiple-dose activated charcoal should be considered as a potential means of elimination enhancement in patients with severe intoxication.

REFERENCES

1. Corbett E, Watt CJ, Walker N, et al: The growing burden of tuberculosis. Arch Intern Med 1999;163:1009–1021.
2. Holdiness M: Neurological manifestations and toxicities of the antituberculosis drugs—a review. Med Toxicol 1987;2:33–51.
3. Mandell G, Sande MA: Antimicrobial agents [continued]. In Hardman JL, Limbird LE, Gilman AG (eds): Goodman and Gilman's Pharmacologic Basis of Therapeutics, 10th ed. New York, McGraw-Hill, 2001, pp 1146–1149.
4. Weber W, Hein DW: Clinical pharmacokinetics of isoniazid. Clin Pharmacol 1979;4:401–422.
5. Isoniazid. In DRUGDEX System [Intranet database]. Version 5.1. Greenwood Village, CO: Thomson MICROMEDEX, 2004.
6. Joint Tuberculosis Committee of the British Thoracic Society: Chemotherapy and management of tuberculosis in the United Kingdom: recommendations 1998. Thorax 1998;53:536–548.
7. Anonymous: Treatment of tuberculosis. MMWR Morbid Mortal Weekly Rep 2003;52(RR11):1–77.
8. Huang YS, Chern HD, Su WJ, et al: Polymorphism of the N-acetyltransferase 2 gene as a susceptibility risk factor for anti-tuberculosis drug-induced hepatitis. Hepatology 2002;35(4):883–889.
9. Boxenbaum H, Riegelman S: Pharmacokinetics of isoniazid and some metabolites in man. J Pharmacokinet Biopharm 1976;4(4):287–325.
10. Institute for Algorithmic Medicine: Determining the isoniazid acetylation phenotype based on measurement of urinary isoniazid and acetylisoniazid. Retrieved October 26, 2004, from http://www.medalreg.com/www/sheets/ch32/phenotype%20INH%20acetylation.xls
11. Kohno H, Kubo H, Takada A, et al: Isoniazid acetylation phenotyping in the Japanese: the molar metabolic ratio INH/AcINH. Am J Ther 1996;3:74–78.
12. Hainer M, Tsai N, Komura ST, Chiu CL: Fatal hepatorenal failure associated with hydrazine sulfate. Ann Intern Med 2000;133(1):877–880.
13. Self TH, Chrisman CR, Baciewicz AM, Bronze MS: Isoniazid drug and food interactions. Am J Med Sci 1999;317(5):304–311.
14. Wen X, Wang JS, Neuvonen PJ, Backman JT: Isoniazid is a mechanism-based inhibitor of cytochrome P450 1A2, 2A6, 2C19 and 3A4 isoforms in human liver microsomes. Eur J Clin Pharmacol 2002;57(11):799–804.
15. O'Shea D, Kim RB, Wilkinson GR: Modulation of CYP2E1 activity by isoniazid in rapid and slow N-acetylators. Br J Clin Pharmacol 1997;43(1):99–103.
16. Zand R, Nelson SD, Slattery JT, et al: Inhibition and induction of cytochrome P4502E1-catalyzed oxidation by isoniazid in humans. Clin Pharmacol Ther 1993;54(2):142–149.
17. Park K, Sohn DH, Veech RL, Song BJ: Translational activation of ethanol-inducible cytochrome P450 (CYP2E1) by isoniazid. Eur J Pharmacol 1993;248:7–14.
18. Miller RR, Porter J, Greenblatt DJ: Clinical importance of the interaction of phenytoin and isoniazid. Chest 1979;75:356–358.
19. Jonville AP, Gauchez AS, Autret E, et al: Interaction between isoniazid and valproate: a case of valproate overdosage. Eur J Clin Pharmacol 1991;40:197–198.
20. Crippin JS: Acetaminophen hepatotoxicity: potentiation by isoniazid. Am J Gastroenterol 1993;88(4):590–592.
21. Chien JY, Peter RM, Nolan CM, et al: Influence of polymorphic N-acetyltransferase phenotype on the inhibition and induction of acetaminophen bioactivation with long-term isoniazid. Clin Pharmacol Ther 1997;61(1):24–34.
22. Gannon R, Pearsall W, Rowley R: Isoniazid, meperidine, and hypotension. Ann Intern Med 1983;99(3):415.
23. Wood JD, Peesker SJ: A correlation between changes in GABA metabolism and isonicotinic acid hydrazide-induced seizures. Brain Res 1972;45(2):489–498.
24. Wood JD, Peesker SJ: The effect on GABA metabolism in brain of isonicotinic acid hydrazide and pyridoxine as a function of time after administration. J Neurochem 1972;19(6):527–537.
25. Marcus RCA: Water-soluble vitamins: the vitamin B complex and ascorbic acid. In Hardman JL, Limbird LE, Gilman AG (eds): Goodman and Gilman's Pharmaceutical Basis of Therapeutics, 10th ed. New York, McGraw-Hill, 2001, pp 1753–1771.
26. Biehl JP, Vilter RW: Effects of isoniazid on pyroxidine metabolism. JAMA 1954;156(7):1549–1552.
27. Pahl MV, Vaziri ND, Ness R, et al: Association of beta hydroxy-butyric acidosis with isoniazid intoxication. Clin Toxicol 1984;22(2):167–176.
28. American Academy of Pediatrics Committee on Drugs: The transfer of drugs and other chemicals into human milk. Pediatrics 2001;108(3):776–789.
29. Mitchell JR, Zimmerman HJ, Ishak KG, et al: Isoniazid liver injury: clinical spectrum, pathology and probable pathogenesis. Ann Intern Med 1976;84:181–192.
30. Stuart RL, Wilson J, Grayson ML: Isoniazid toxicity in health care workers. Clin Infect Dis 1999;28(4):895–897.
31. Nolan CM, Goldberg SV, Buskin SE: Hepatotoxicity associated with isoniazid preventive therapy: a 7-year survey from a public health tuberculosis clinic. JAMA 1999;281(11):1014–1018.
32. Corrigan D, Paton J: Hepatic enzyme abnormalities in children on triple therapy for tuberculosis. Pediatr Pulmonol 1999;27(1):37–42.
33. Anonymous: Severe isoniazid-associated hepatitis—New York, 1991–1993. MMWR Morbid Mortal Weekly Rep 1993;42(28):545–547.

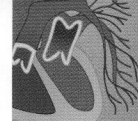

34. Millard PS, Wilcosky TC, Reade-Christopher SJ, Weber DJ: Isoniazid-related fatal hepatitis [see comment]. West J Med 1996;164(6):486–491.

35. Salpeter S: Fatal isoniazid-induced hepatitis. West J Med 1993;159:560–564.

36. Sadaphal P, Astemborski J, Graham NM, et al: Isoniazid preventive therapy, hepatitis C virus infection, and hepatotoxicity among injection drug users infected with *Mycobacterium tuberculosis.* Clin Infect Dis 2001;33(10):1687–1691.

37. Patel PA, Voight MD: Prevalence and interaction of hepatitis B and latent tuberculosis in Vietnamese immigrants to the United States. Am J Gastroenterol 2002;97(5):1198–1203.

38. Izzedine H, Launay-Vacher V, Storme T, Deray G: Acute pancreatitis induced by isoniazid. Am J Gastroenterol 2001; 96(11):3208–3209.

39. Rabassa AA, Trey G, Shukla U, et al: Isoniazid-induced acute pancreatitis. Ann Int Med 1994;121(6):433–434.

40. Drug-induced systemic lupus erythematosus. In DRUGDEX consults [Intranet database]. Version 5.1. Greenwood Village, CO, Thomson MICROMEDEX, 2004.

41. Siddiqui MA, Khan IA: Isoniazid-induced lupus erythematosus presenting with cardiac tamponade. Am J Ther 2002;9(2): 163–165.

42. Price EJ, Venables PJ: Drug-induced lupus. Drug Saf 1995;12(4): 283–290.

43. To TQ, Townsend JC: Ocular toxicity of systemic medications: a case series. Optometry 2000;71(1):29–39.

44. Gonzalez-Gay MA, Sanchez-Andrade A, Aguero JJ, et al: Optic neuritis following treatment with isoniazid in a hemodialyzed patient. Nephron 1993;63(3):360.

45. Siskind MS, Thienemann D, Kirlin L: Isoniazid-induced neurotoxicity in chronic dialysis patients: report of three cases and a review of the literature. Nephron 1993;64:303–306.

46. Iannaccone R, Sue YJ, Avner JR: Suicidal psychosis secondary to isoniazid. Pediatr Emerg Care 2002;18(1):25–27.

47. Alao AO, Yolles JC: Isoniazid-induced psychosis. Ann Pharmacother 1998;32(9):889–891.

48. Martinjak-Dvorsek I, Gorjup V, Horvat M, Noc M: Acute isoniazid neurotoxicity during preventive therapy. Crit Care Med 2000; 28(2):567–568.

49. Bender DA, Russell-Jones R: Isoniazid-induced pellagra despite vitamin-B6 supplementation. Lancet 1979;2(8152):1125–1126.

50. Darvay A, Basarab T, McGregor JM, Russell-Jones R: Isoniazid induced pellagra despite pyridoxine supplementation. Clin Exp Dermatol 1999;24(3):167–169.

51. Ishii N, Nishihara Y: Pellagra encephalopathy among tuberculous patients: its relation to isoniazid therapy. J Neurolog Neurosurg Psychiatry 1985;48(7):628–634.

52. Muratake T, Watanabe H, Hayashi S: Isoniazid-induced pellagra and the N-acetyltransferase gene genotype. Am J Psychiatry 1999;156(4):660.

53. O'Sullivan TL: Drug-food interaction with isoniazid resembling anaphylaxis. Ann Pharmacother 1997;31(7–8):928–929.

54. DiMartini A: Isoniazid, tricyclics and the "cheese reaction." 1995;Sep:197–198.

55. Morinaga S, Kawasaki A, Hirata H, et al: Histamine poisoning after ingestion of spoiled raw tuna in a patient taking isoniazid. Intern Med 1997;36(3):198–200.

56. Marseglia GL, Locatelli F: Isoniazid-induced pure red cell aplasia in two siblings. J Pediatr 1998;132(5):898–900.

57. Lee AY, Jung SY: Two patients with isoniazid-induced photosensitive lichenoid eruptions confirmed by photopatch test. Photodermatol Photoimmunol Photomed 1998;14(2):77–78.

58. Scheid P, Kanny G, Trechot P, et al: Isoniazid-induced bullous skin reaction. Allergy 1999;54(3):294–296.

59. Caksen H, Odabas D, Erol M, et al: Do not overlook acute isoniazid poisoning in children with status epilepticus. J Child Neurol 2003;18(2):142–143.

60. Romero JA, Kuczler FJ Jr: Isoniazid overdose: recognition and management. Am Fam Physician 1998;57(4):749–752.

61. Steinmann RA, Rickel MK: A 23-year-old with refractory seizures following an isoniazid overdose. J Emerg Nurs 2002;28(1):7–10.

62. Knapp JF, Johnson T, Alander S: Seizures in a 13-year-old girl. Pediatr Emerg Care 2003;19(1):38–40.

63. Salkind AR, Hewitt CC: Coma from long-term overingestion of isoniazid. Arch Intern Med 1997;157(21):2518–2520.

64. Hankins D, Saxena K, Faville RJ, et al: Profound acidosis caused by isoniazid ingestion. Am J Emerg Med 1987;5:165–166.

65. Chin L, Sievers ML, Herrier RN, Picchioni AL: Convulsions as the etiology of lactic acidosis in acute isoniazid toxicity in dogs. Toxicol Appl Pharmacol 1979;49(2):377–384.

66. Piliero PJ, Fish DG: Isoniazid-induced beta-hydroxybutyric acidosis. Ann Intern Med 2001;134(9 Pt 1):799.

67. Miller J, Robinson A, Percy AKL: Acute isoniazid poisoning in childhood. Am J Dis Child 1980;134:290–292.

68. Terman DS, Teitelbaum DT: Isoniazid self-poisoning. Neurology 1970;20:299–304.

69. Hankins DG, Saxena K, Faville RJ, et al: Profound acidosis caused by isoniazid ingestion. Am J Emerg Med 1987;5:165–166.

70. Orlowski J, Paganini EP, Pippenger CE: Treatment of a potentially lethal dose isoniazid ingestion. Ann Emerg Med 1988;17(1):73–76.

71. Blowey D, Johnson D, Verjee Z: Isoniazid-associated rhabdomyolysis. Am J Emerg Med 1995;13:543–544.

72. Nelson LS, Rella J, Hoffman RS: Status epilepticus. N Engl J Med 1998;339(6):409–410; author reply 10.

73. Wason S, Lacouture PG, Lovejoy FH: Single high-dose pyridoxine treatment for isoniazid overdose. JAMA 1981;246(10):1102–1104.

74. Lovecchio F, Curry SC, Graeme KA, et al: Intravenous pyridoxine-induced metabolic acidosis. Ann Emerg Med 2001;38(1):62–64.

75. Pyroxidine. In DRUGDEX consults [Intranet database]. Version 5.1. Greenwood Village, CO, Thomson MICROMEDEX, 2004.

76. Santucci KA, Shah BR, Linakis JG: Acute isoniazid exposures and antidote availability. Pediatr Emerg Care 1999;15(2):99–101.

77. Scharman E, Rosencrance JG: Isoniazid toxicity: a survey of pyridoxine availability. Am J Emerg Med 1994;12(3):386–388.

78. Chin L, Sievers ML, Laird HE, et al: Evaluation of diazepam and pyridoxine as antidotes to isoniazid intoxication in rats and dogs. Toxicol Appl Pharmacol 1978;45:713–722.

79. Chin L, Sievers ML, Herrier RN, Picchioni AL: Potentiation of pyridoxine by depressants and anticonvulsants in the treatment of acute isoniazid intoxication in dogs. Toxicol Appl Pharmacol 1981;58:504–509.

56 *Chemotherapeutic Agents and Thalidomide*

A Chemotherapeutic Agents

RICHARD Y. WANG, DO

At a Glance...

- Overdoses from chemotherapeutic agents occur infrequently, but are associated with devastating outcomes.
- The majority of unintentional exposures occur iatrogenically, resulting from errors in either dosage regimen or drug preparation.
- Mucositis, emesis, pancytopenia, and alopecia are common clinical manifestations of toxicity.
- Management includes stabilization of life-threatening disorders, decontamination, prevention of overwhelming sepsis, the timely use of rescue agents, and enhanced elimination in specific instances.

The use of chemotherapeutic agents in the treatment of cancer stems from the discovery that mustard agents used during World Wars I and II caused bone marrow toxicity. Mustard gas (sulfur mustard) was first used in World War I as a chemical warfare agent at Ypres, Belgium, in 1917, and was later found to cause myelosuppression in animals and in sailors unintentionally exposed to this agent while on a U.S. naval vessel.[1] Upon further evaluation of this class of agents, it was demonstrated that they were effective against tumors in animals and the nitrogen mustards were less toxic to the host than sulfur mustard. These findings led to the production of mechlorethamine (Mustargen) for the treatment of lymphoma by Merck & Co, West Point, Pennsylvania, in 1943. The next class of chemotherapeutic agents developed for clinical use was the folate analogs. Pteroyltriglutamic acid was identified in 1946 as the active agent in the fermentation products of *Lactobacillus casei* that caused the remission of breast tumors in mice.[2] Since then, other folate analogs and several other classes of agents have been developed and used successfully in cancer therapy. These agents can be generally classified as antimetabolites, alkylating agents, antibiotics, and antimitotics. Certain tumor cells (e.g., prostate, breast, endometrial) are responsive to hormonal therapy, and these agents comprise another class. Unlike other classes of pharmaceutical agents, the chemotherapeutic agents are more likely to cause toxicity in people with exposures because of the unique mechanism of action and narrow therapeutic window of these agents.

The occurrence of toxicity from chemotherapeutic agents in patients during therapy was characterized in a review of the Surveillance, Epidemiology, and End Results (SEER) tumor registry of the hospitalizations of women with breast cancer from 1991 to 1996.[3] There were 35,060 women diagnosed with breast cancer in this period, and 4134 underwent chemotherapy that included doxorubicin, mitoxantrone, cyclophosphamide, fluorouracil, methotrexate (MTX), and paclitaxel. The observed frequency of hospital admissions for adverse effects attributed to chemotherapy (i.e., neutropenia, thrombocytopenia, fever, and unspecified adverse effects of systemic therapy) was 14%, which was higher than the 0.5% of women admitted for the same diagnoses who did not receive chemotherapy. Neutropenia accounted for about half of the admissions in the treated women, and the rate of hospitalizations for these adverse effects increased by about 2-fold with advancing stages of tumor. Chemotherapy was associated with a 10-fold higher mortality rate and a 6-fold higher likelihood for death in women admitted for health effects associated with treatment. The host factors that were associated with hospital admission for toxicity related to chemotherapy were advanced stage of tumor and type of chemotherapeutic agent. Women treated with anthracycline agents were two to three times more likely to be admitted for toxicity than those who were treated with cyclophosphamide, fluorouracil, MTX, or paclitaxel.

Unintentional exposures to chemotherapeutic agents may occur by confusing the amount to be administered, the route of administration, the dose frequency, or the agent itself. The following discussion is intended to familiarize health care providers with the clinical manifestations of toxicity and management of the commonly observed chemotherapeutic agents in therapy.

MECHANISMS OF ACTION AND TOXICITY

Chemotherapeutic agents cause cell death by primarily disrupting DNA synthesis or function during cell replication. These agents can alter DNA structure, impair DNA synthesis, or inhibit chromosomal separation by a variety of mechanisms. The alkylating agents interact through reactive intermediates with electrophilic DNA side groups to form a covalent bond by nucleophilic substitution. The alkylated DNA can form inter- or intrastrand cross-linkages, which can promote errors in base pairing during DNA replication or transcription and lead to cell death. The 7 nitrogen in the imidazole ring of guanine is a favored substitution site because it can alter the DNA structure by either forming the unfavorable enol tautomer or disrupting the imidazole ring complex. The nitrogen mustard agents are most

927

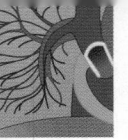

likely to form cross-linkages because each molecule contains two reactive 2-chloroethyl side chains. The reactive intermediates of the alkylating agents can be formed by spontaneous hydrolysis or an enzymatic-dependent process. The anthracycline antibiotics impair DNA structure by causing breaks in the strand, which can result from any one of several mechanisms. The planar structures of these agents allow them to intercalate with DNA to cause single-strand breaks. Similar results can occur from the generation of oxygen free radicals from the formation of a semiquinone intermediate during the hepatic metabolism of these agents. The anthracyclines can bind and inhibit topoisomerase II to cause permanent double-strand breaks in DNA, which are more damaging to the cell than single-strand breaks.

The antimetabolites indirectly disrupt DNA synthesis by serving as inhibitory analogs to either cofactors or nitrogenous bases of nucleic acids. These agents can be categorized as folate analogs (e.g., MTX), pyrimidine analogs (e.g., 5-fluorouracil, 5FU), and purine analogs (e.g., mercaptopurine). The antimitotic agents, such as vinca alkaloids, disrupt chromosomal separation during cell division by impairing microtubule function. These agents bind to tubulin, which is a protein subunit of microtubules, and cause cells to stop at metaphase during mitosis.

In recent years, hormonal active agents have become part of chemotherapy because of their ability to alter gene transcription and to cause cell death. Topotecan and irinotecan belong to a new class of chemotherapeutic agent that inhibits toposisomerase I, which is responsible for reversible DNA breaks and is necessary for DNA replication. These agents are derived from camptothecin, which is isolated from the tree *Camptotheca acuminata*. Bone marrow suppression with resultant overwhelming sepsis and death can occur from an overdose with topotecan.[4]

PHARMACOLOGY

The chemotherapeutic agents can be administered by a variety of routes, including intravenous (IV), intra-arterial, intravesicular, intracavitary (pleural, peritoneal), intralesional, topical, and oral. The majority of chemotherapeutic agents are administered by the IV route, and only a few are given orally. The intrathecal (IT) route of administration is limited to MTX and cytarabine (cytosine arabinoside). These three routes are the common ones associated with overdoses. The selection of the route of administration depends on drug stability and the intended site of action. Some medications poorly penetrate the blood-brain barrier and must be given intrathecally for them to be effective in cases of existing (or the potential for) brain metastasis. The agents available as tablets and associated with overdoses in the literature include MTX, busulfan, and melphalan. MTX is rapidly absorbed from the gut, with peak serum levels achievable within 1 to 2 hours after oral administration. Gut bacteria metabolize about 5% of MTX to 2,4-diamino-*N*(10)-methylpteroic acid (DAMPA), which is

inactive at the dihydrofolate reductase (DHFR) site, but will cross react on the clinical TDx assay (Abbott Laboratories, Abbott Park, IL) to contribute to the overall serum MTX level. In an oral overdose of 4 mg/kg busulfan tablets, the peak plasma busulfan level was observed at 4 hours after ingestion.[5] Typically, busulfan does not distribute well into the cerebrospinal (CS) space, but at doses higher than 16 mg/kg, appreciable CSF levels can be achieved to result in seizures. A similar situation occurs when a high dose of vincristine is administered. Unique to paclitaxel is its 49.7% ethanol diluent, which can cause its own toxicity in the overdose setting.

Many of the chemotherapeutic agents distribute in the body according to a multicompartment model based on the decay of the plasma level. The initial plasma half-life for these agents ranges from minutes to hours and the terminal half-life ranges from hours to days (Table 56A-1). Several agents have high plasma protein or tissue binding capacities and large volumes of distribution, which would limit their ability to be removed by hemodialysis. MTX can distribute into third space fluids (e.g., peritoneal, pleural) to prolong the terminal half-life, which is associated with increased host toxicity. Bowel obstruction can also increase MTX's terminal half-life by allowing for the re-uptake of MTX by entero-hepatic circulation.

The majority of the chemotherapeutic agents are metabolized in the liver and the metabolites are eliminated by the kidneys through either glomerular filtration or active tubular secretion. For some agents, they are eliminated unchanged in the urine and require their dose adjusted in patients with diminished renal function. Biliary elimination accounts for a small amount of total drug elimination for certain agents, such as MTX. Some agents (e.g., mechlorethamine, cisplatin) undergo spontaneous hydrolysis and quickly become reactive intermediates upon the administration of the drug. Cisplatin's chloride molecule is replaced by a hydroxyl molecule to form monohydroxymonochloro *cis*-diammine platinum, which contributes to renal tubular toxicity. This hydrolytic reaction is limited in the presence of a high chloride concentration, which is why sodium chloride diuresis is performed during high-dose cisplatin therapy. For some agents, additional drug metabolism occurs intracellularly. MTX undergoes polyglutamation inside the cell by the enzyme folyl polyglutamate synthetase. This prolongs MTX's duration in the cytosol and activity at the DHFR site.

Some of the metabolites of the chemotherapeutic agents can contribute to host toxicity. For example, cyclophosphamide is metabolized by a series of hepatic and intracellular enzymatic reactions to phosphoramide mustard and acrolein, which are both renally eliminated and biologically active. Phosphoramide mustard is the active alkylating intermediate, and acrolein is a by-product. Acrolein is a highly reactive aldehyde because of the close proximity between the carbonyl and vinyl groups in its structure, and is highly irritating to epithelial cells. The latter effect may result from acrolein's ability to bind to sulfhydryl groups, which can

TABLE 56A-1 Pharmacologic Parameters Pertaining to Selected Chemotherapeutic Agents Discussed in This Chapter.

AGENT	MOLECULAR WEIGHT (Da)	ROUTE OF ADMINISTRATION	VOLUME OF DISTRIBUTION (L/kg)	PLASMA PROTEIN BINDING	METABOLISM (PRIMARY)	METABOLITES	ELIMINATION	TERMINAL PLASMA HALF-LIFE (hr)
Alkylating								
Busulfan	246	PO IV*	0.6–1.0	3%–32%	Hepatic	Methanesulfonic acid	Renal	2–3
Chlorambucil	304	PO	0.14–0.29	99%	Hepatic	Phenylacetic acid mustard (PAM)* Hydroxylated derivatives	Renal	2 (PAM) 1.5 (parent)
Cisplatin	300.1	IV	0.17–1.47	90%	Nonezymatic hydrolysis	Hydrolytic derivatives* (e.g., Monohydroxymonochloro cis-diammine platinum [II])	Renal	58–73
Cyclophosphamide	279.1	PO, IV	0.34–1.2	12%–14%	Hepatic	4-Hydroxycyclophosphamide (HC), Phosphoramide mustard (PM)* 4-Ketocyclophosphamide Carboxyphosphamide Acrolein*	Renal	3–12 (parent) 9 (PM) 7 (HC)
Ifosfamide	261.1	IV	0.34–0.9	Not appreciable	Hepatic	4-Hydroxyifosfamide Ifosphoramide mustard* Dechloroethylifosfamide derivatives 4-Ketoifosfamide 4-Carboxyifosfamide Acrolein*	Renal	4–15
Melphalan	305.2	PO, IV	0.5	90%	Nonezymatic hydrolysis	Hydrolytic derivatives	Biliary > renal (10%–15% unchanged)	2 (parent)
Antibiotic								
Daunorubicin	563.9	IV	20–40	50%–60%	Hepatic	Daunorubicinol (DNL)*	Biliary > renal	55 (parent) 25 (DNL)
Doxorubicin	543.5	IV	25	70%–85%	Hepatic	Doxorubicinol (DXL)*	Biliary	30 (parent) 29 (DXL)
Idarubicin	533.9	IV	25	94%–97%	Hepatic	Idarubicinol (IDL)*	Biliary > renal	15–24 (parent) 45 (IDL)
Mitoxantrone	517.4	IV	1000–2000 L/m²	80%	Hepatic	Mono- and dicarboxylic acid derivatives	Biliary > renal	20–200
Antimetabolite								
5-Fluorouracil	130.1	Topical, IV	0.25	8%–12%	Hepatic	Fluorodeoxyuridine monophosphate* Alpha-fluoro-beta-alanine	Respiratory, renal	16 min (parent)
Methotrexate	454.5	PO,IV,IT	0.4–0.8	50%	Hepatic	Polyglutamated derivatives* 7-hydroxymethotrexate* 2, 4-diamino-N(10)-methylpteroic acid	Renal > biliary	8–15 (parent)
Antimitotic								
Vinblastine	923.1	IV	27	40%–99%	Hepatic	Desacetylvinblastine*	Biliary > renal	23
Vincristine	923	IV	8.4	44%	Hepatic	Uncharacterized	Biliary > renal	20–150
Paclitaxel	853.9	IV	2	90%–98%	Hepatic	6-hydroxypaclitaxel	Biliary > renal	3–20

*Biologically active

IT, intrathecal; IV, intravenous; PO, oral.

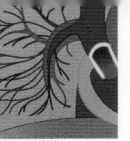
lead to the disruption of cellular protein activity. In the urinary bladder and in high concentration, acrolein can cause a hemorrhagic cystitis. This is prevented by hydrating the patient to promote urinary flow and to lower the urinary acrolein level and by administering the thiol agent sodium 2-mercaptoethane sulfonate (MESNA) during high-dose cyclophosphamide therapy (>120 mg/kg) before bone marrow transplantation. Another example of a toxic metabolite is when MTX is administered at a dose higher than 1 g/m². MTX is metabolized by aldehyde oxidase to 7-hydroxymethotrexate (7OHMTX), which is not active as a folate analog and is eliminated uneventfully in the urine. However, this metabolite is less soluble than MTX and tends to precipitate in acidic pH. During high-dose MTX therapy, appreciable levels of 7OHMTX can be achieved to cause precipitation in the renal tubules with resultant necrosis and renal failure.

TOXICOLOGIC MANIFESTATIONS

The toxicologic effects of the chemotherapeutic agents in the body are most apparent in cells with a high turnover rate, such as those in the epithelium, bone marrow, and hair follicle. This is because these agents were designed to limit cancerous cell growth by exploiting their high rate of mitosis. Thus, patients with toxicity will present with mucositis, alopecia, and leukopenia. The occurrence of these events post-treatment will vary by agent, but can be expected at about 3 to 5 days for mucosal epithelial loss and 7 to 13 days for the nadir effect of leukopenia. The mucosal epithelial loss can lead to gastrointestinal bleeding and serve as a source for sepsis from the entry of gut bacteria into the systemic circulation. MTX, 5FU, bleomycin, and doxorubicin are highly associated with mucosal ulcerations during therapy. The white blood cell count usually returns to baseline at 21 to 24 days. For some agents, the nadir of the leukopenia can be delayed by weeks (e.g., carmustine) or the duration of bone marrow suppression is much more sustained and can last for months to years after the exposure (e.g., busulfan). During this period of myelosuppression, patients may require blood product replacement, use of granulocyte colony-stimulating factors,[6,7] reverse isolation, and antibiotic therapy to protect them from overwhelming sepsis. Granulocyte colony-stimulating factor has been demonstrated to improve neutrophil count response, improve rate of recovery from neutropenia, decrease duration of febrile neutropenia, and decrease hospital length of stay in patients undergoing chemotherapy. Additional findings common to overdoses of chemotherapeutic agents include nausea, vomiting, and hyperuricemia. The onset of nausea and vomiting is within 6 hours of exposure, and the effect can last for as long as 24 hours.

Chemotherapeutic agents are highly emetogenic, especially cisplatin, mechlorethamine, and doxorubicin because of their ability to stimulate the emetic center located in the medulla from various pathways. These include the chemoreceptor trigger zone (CTZ), which can be affected by constituents in the blood or CSF, and the solitary tract nucleus, which receives vagal and sympathetic innervation by the enterochromaffin cells in the intestinal mucosa. The vagal and sympathetic afferents can stimulate the emetic center by way of the CTZ as well. Because serotonin is involved in many of these pathways, ondansetron is an effective antiemetic agent for chemotherapeutic agent–induced vomiting. In order to assist patients with protracted emesis from these agents, the pharmacologic inhibition of the other neurotransmitters involved in these pathways (e.g., dopamine) is often necessary, requiring combination drug therapy. Certain chemotherapeutic agents cause unique toxicologic manifestations and they are further discussed in the advancing sections.

Cardiac

The chemotherapeutic agents causing cardiotoxicity in a dose-dependent fashion are cyclophosphamide and the anthracycline antibiotics. The pyrimidine analog 5FU appears to be associated with manifestations consistent with coronary vasopasm during high-dose continuous infusion therapy.[8] Doxorubicin and daunorubicin are the original anthracycline agents, and their use is limited by their oxidative-induced damage to myocardial tissue, which can lead to irreversible congestive cardiomyopathy. Cardiomyopathy is a significant and consequential effect of anthracycline therapy because it is irreversible, can lead to congestive heart failure, and is associated with a 48% mortality rate.[9] The availability of structural analogs (e.g., epirubicin and idarubicin) and liposomal encapsulated formulations of the original anthracyclines allows for the continued use of this class of agents with less toxicity to the host. For example, the cumulative dose for doxorubicin and epirubicin to cause a 20% incidence of congestive cardiomyopathy is 550 mg/m² and 720 mg/m², respectively.[10,11] Daunorubicin and mitoxantrone are associated with a 2% incidence at the cumulative doses of 600 mg/m² and 140 mg/m², respectively. In addition to cardiomyopathy, which is a delayed effect, the anthracycline agents can cause immediate manifestations of cardiac toxicity. These immediate effects, occurring within 24 hours of administration, include dysrhythmias, ST segment and T wave changes on the electrocardiogram, diminished left ventricular ejection fraction leading to congestive heart failure, pericarditis, myocarditis, and sudden death.[12-15] The repolarization changes on the electrocardiogram are observed in about 40% of patients receiving doxorubicin therapy, and are transient and not associated with either total dose or peak serum levels.[13,16,17] The onset of cardiomyopathy is heralded by manifestations consistent with biventricular heart failure and its timing, since the last course of treatment can be quite variable, ranging from months to years. Although this period is usually 1 to 4 months, it tends be longer for the less toxic anthracycline analogs.[18-20]

Cyclophosphamide's toxic effects on the heart are described in patients receiving high-dose therapy for

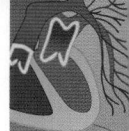

bone marrow transplantation and in the overdose setting.[21] These patients can develop congestive heart failure, hemorrhagic pericarditis, or cardiac tamponade resulting in death within days of exposure.[22,23] Patients receiving a mean cyclophosphamide dose of 174 mg/kg were observed to have greater reductions in QRS voltage and increases in left ventricular mass index compared with patients treated at a lower dose.[24] These findings were attributed to myocardial swelling from either edema or hemorrhage.[25] Patients at increased risk for cardiac effects from cyclophosphamide therapy include those who are older than 50 years, have a history of cardiac dysfunction,[26] or received treatment with anthracycline agents or thoracic radiotherapy.

5FU is associated with myocardial ischemia and cardiogenic shock when administered as a high-dose continuous infusion.[27] The incidence of cardiac symptoms in patients receiving high-dose continuous infusion therapy was observed to be about 10%, which was 10-fold higher than patients receiving bolus therapy.[8] In some of these patients, diminished QRS voltage and ventricular wall motion normalized within 48 hours of discontinuation of 5FU treatment. These manifestations are attributed to increased myocardial oxygen demand[28] and coronary vasospasm,[29] which may be a response to endothelial damage caused by the metabolite fluoroacetate.[30] Patients with coronary artery disease or prior thoracic radiotherapy are at risk for these events during 5FU therapy, and they should be treated by discontinuation of 5FU and with coronary artery vasodilators (e.g., nitrates, calcium channel blockers) for myocardial ischemia.

Neurologic

The chemotherapeutic agents can cause a variety of neurologic effects, including central nervous system (CNS) and peripheral nervous system disorders, from the systemic administration of an excessive dose. Altered mental status and seizures are commonly observed during overdoses from the nitrogen mustards, MTX, and vincristine. The inappropriate IT administration of vincristine or MTX (by dose) can result in seizures as well. The putative neurotoxin from chlorambucil and ifosfamide overdoses is chloroacetaldehyde, which is produced by N-dechloroacetylation in the liver.[31-33] The seizures from chlorambucil overdoses typically present within 6 hours of exposure and are generalized tonic-clonic activity, which can last for 24 hours.[34,35] Vincristine-induced seizures occur much later than those caused by the nitrogen mustards; typically at 1 to 7 days after exposure. Patients with underlying seizure disorders, delayed drug elimination,[36-39] or altered drug pharmacokinetics (e.g., nephrotic syndrome) (salloum) are at risk for seizures during treatment with these agents. Vincristine toxicity can cause hypothalamic stimulation as well as central autonomic instability. The former can lead to fevers and the syndrome of inappropriate secretion of antidiuretic hormone (SIADH).[40] The duration of the fevers can be protracted, lasting for 1 week after the exposure, and serum electrolyte abnormalities may not present until 10 days after drug exposure. The manifestations of central autonomic instability include bowel ileus, constipation, atony of the urinary bladder, hypertension, and hypotension.[38] Other chemotherapeutic agents associated with altered mental status include L-asparaginase, 5FU, and procarbazine.[41] 5FU is associated with cerebellar ataxia in less than 5% of treated patients, and the mechanism remains to be determined.[42]

The neurologic effects from MTX toxicity are variable and depend on the nature of the exposure. Chemical arachnoiditis occurs within hours of IT treatment and manifests as cephalgias, meningismus, pleocytosis, sterile CSF, and increased CSF protein and CSF MTX levels. The early administration of systemic steroids may limit the inflammatory response that is believed to occur during this process. A CSF MTX level higher than 100 μmol/L during IT therapy suggests either an excessive amount of MTX administered or a CSF outflow obstruction.[43] Transverse myelopathy can occur from the lumbar subarachnoid administration of MTX and is typically not a reversible process, which is unlike that of chemical arachnoiditis. Neurobehavioral disorders and depressed mental status presenting months to years after treatment is characteristic of MTX-induced leukoencephalopathy. The overall incidence of this disorder is variable, ranging from 10% to 70%, and patients with increased age, intraventricular or IT administration of MTX, or prior cranial radiation appear to be at risk for developing this finding.[44] Computed tomography scan and magnetic resonance imaging of the brain can demonstrate findings consistent with demyelination and necrosis of the white matter.[45]

IT overdoses with MTX occur infrequently and are associated with devastating outcomes, including permanent neurologic deficits and death. IT therapy is used to prevent CNS spread of cancerous cells in patients with acute lymphoblastic leukemia. The common cause of IT errors is confusing IV for IT medication, which can occur with similarly named drugs, multiple medications at the bedside, or when varying doses by different routes of administration are available for the same medication.[46] This latter reason accounts for some MTX IT overdoses because the higher IV dose was administered as the IT dose. The manifestations of toxicity present within minutes of the drug's administration, and include pain in the lower extremities, cephalgia, meningismus, and depressed level of consciousness. An electroencephalograph can demonstrate diffuse alterations in electrical activity.[47] IT overdoses with vincristine also have occurred, and the clinical outcome is more devastating than other chemotherapeutic agents administered in a similar manner.[48-50] Patients present with findings consistent with an ascending myelopathy, and the outcome is typically fatal or includes permanent neurologic sequelae.

Peripheral neuropathies are observed with cisplatin and vincristine toxicities and occur in a dose-dependent fashion. The neuropathy is classic in its clinical presentation, ascending in nature, and can involve both sensory and motor components. The incidence of paresthesia with vincristine therapy is about 60% at a dose of 12 to 25 μg/kg and increases sixfold at a dose of

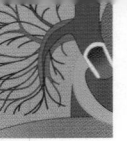

75 µg/kg.[51] The occurrence of neuropathies is higher for vincristine than vinblastine. The onset of symptoms during therapy ranges from 2 to 8 weeks after treatment, and limits the dosing regimen for vincristine.[52] For the vinca alkaloids, the loss of the Achilles tendon reflex is an early finding that can be expected to resolve within 7 weeks upon discontinuation of further therapy.[53] Cranial nerve (III–VII and X) and laryngeal nerve involvement have been described in association with the vinca alkaloids.[41,54] In comparison to vincristine, paclitaxel (taxol)-induced neuropathies have more of a sensory deficit and a shorter recovery period. This may be related to the difference in the mechanism of activity of these two agents on microtubule synthesis. The peripheral neuropathy associated with cisplatin toxicity is primarily a sensory disorder, and it is potentiated by the concomitant use of other neurotoxic agents, such as paclitaxel. The patient will present with paresthesia, and loss of vibratory sense and proprioception. Other clinical findings associated with cisplatin toxicity include tinnitus, high-frequency hearing loss, and retinopathy.[55]

Renal

Chemotherapeutic agents can cause renal toxicity either directly or indirectly, resulting from the accumulation of breakdown products of cell death (i.e., uric acid). Acute uric acid nephropathy is commonly observed during the use of these agents for the treatment of leukemia or lymphoma. MTX is associated with renal insufficiency at doses higher than 500 mg/m² (100 mg/kg). Prior to the institution of prophylactic measures, such as hydration and urinary alkalinization, MTX was associated with renal insufficiency in 30% of the patients receiving therapy, and mortality in patients with severe renal failure.[56] The cause is the precipitation of the 7OHMTX metabolite in the renal tubules to cause acute tubular necrosis. This metabolite is less soluble than MTX and crystallizes in renal tubules in an acidic environment. The solubility of 7OHMTX at pH 5.5 is 2 mmol/L and increases at a higher pH. Cisplatin is another agent that causes renal tubular necrosis in a dose-dependent manner, and when repeat doses are administered in close succession. Protein unbound cisplatin freely enters into renal tubular cells, accumulating in the corticomedullary region of the kidney to cause distal and proximal tubular necrosis. Pretreatment with sodium chloride reduced the level of cisplatin and cisplatin metabolites in the kidney tissue and urine of treated animals.[57] When the cisplatin dose is higher than 50 mg/m², the frequency of renal failure is about 30%. The time of onset for the increase in serum blood urea nitrogen (BUN) and creatinine is about 1 to 2 weeks after treatment, which is slightly delayed compared to MTX. Hypomagnesemia and hypocalcemia are observed during cisplatin toxicity and may be attributed to renal loss from tubular injury.[58] Patients at risk for renal toxicity from these agents include the elderly, those with underlying renal disease, and those receiving concomitant therapy with nephrotoxic agents (e.g., aminoglycosides).

DIAGNOSIS

The diagnosis of a patient with an overdose from a chemotherapeutic agent is based on the presence of clinical manifestations consistent with the toxicity of the agent, historic evidence of the exposure, and laboratory findings supporting the exposure or toxicity. In most instances, the event will be clearly evident based on the history alone because these agents are typically administered in the controlled setting of a hospital. However, for agents associated with delayed onset of clinical toxicity or toxicity from chronic exposure, a heightened level of awareness will be necessary to establish the relationship between exposure and clinical findings.[20]

The mechanisms responsible for the unintentional administration of chemotherapeutic agents involve either errors in dosage regimens or drug preparations, and they should be investigated in situations where the exposure is not apparent but suspected.[59] Some of the reasons for the dosage regimen errors include inappropriate dosage, misinterpretation of the protocol, and incorrect number for current treatment cycle. Such occurrences result from the lack of familiarity with the treatment protocol, errors in prescribing, errors in administration, errors in interpretation of the written order, and lack of familiarity with the patient's medical background. Two common examples of errors in administration include doxorubicin (correct, 100 mg/m² for over 4 days in divided doses; incorrect, 100 mg/m² daily for 4 days) and vincristine (correct, IV dose [0.06 mg/kg]; incorrect, administered IT). A systemic approach to prevent medical errors with chemotherapeutic agents is discussed elsewhere.[60] Patient risk factors for toxicity from these agents need to be considered during the assessment because these may explain the clinical findings. These include inability to eliminate or metabolize the drug (i.e., renal or hepatic insufficiency), pre-existing disorder (e.g., seizures, congestive heart failure, coronary artery disease) of the target organ of toxicity, the presence of third space fluid compartments (e.g., peritoneal, pleural) that can sequester the drug or metabolite, and concomitant treatments (e.g., medications or radiotherapy) that can potentiate the target organ's toxicity.

Drug levels for this class of agents are not routinely available in the clinical setting to assist in confirming the diagnosis of toxicity. However, analytical assays to measure MTX, busulfan,[5] cisplatin (platinum),[58] and vincristine[61] are available, and the levels of these agents can be used to assess for exposure. Some of the chemotherapeutic agents are associated with unique manifestations of toxicity such that when these are present, the agents should be suspected. For example, the anthracyclines are associated with congestive heart failure and cardiomyopathy; cisplatin with renal insufficiency, ototoxicity, and peripheral neuropathy; the vinca alkaloids with peripheral neuropathy, SIADH, and central autonomic instability; and ifosfamide with seizures.

Certain studies can assist the diagnostic process by either confirming the findings on clinical examination

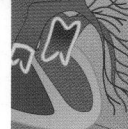

or by evaluating for other disorders that may present with similar findings. For example, myocardial biopsies can evaluate for infectious and ischemic causes of cardiomyopathy when anthracycline toxicity is being considered. Although this procedure is infrequently used for this purpose, it is still used in conjunction with the left ventricular ejection fraction to determine the course of anthracycline treatment in select cases. The electroretinogram can identify retinal disorders of the post-photoreceptor neural function that is described in patients with visual loss and color aberrations from cisplatin toxicity.[55] Other studies include audiometry to evaluate for high-frequency hearing loss from cisplatin toxicity; brain computed axial tomography or magnetic resonance imaging to evaluate for leukoencephalopathy from MTX, hemorrhage, and metastatic lesions; and nerve conduction studies to evaluate for sensorimotor deficits attributed to a peripheral neuropathy. Drug-induced peripheral neuropathies in cancer patients need to be differentiated from paraneoplastic syndromes.[62]

MANAGEMENT

The initial approach toward the patient with a chemotherapeutic agent overdose requires the stabilization of immediate life-threatening findings. These include dysrhythmias, congestive heart failure, seizures, and complications of pancytopenia (e.g., sepsis). Furosemide, inotropic agents, and fluid restriction can be used to treat heart failure. Uncontrolled hypertension can be managed with a peripheral vasodilating agent, such as a calcium channel blocker. This may be necessary because vincristine toxicity central autonomic instability can occur in this setting. Seizures can be treated with benzodiazepines, barbiturates, and phenytoin. For busulfan, phenytoin is used in a prophylactic manner during high-dose therapy (>16 mg/kg). Methylene blue (50 mg IV as a 1% solution) is used to treat encephalopathy from ifosfamide, and it was attributed to an improved patient outcome in a small case series.[63] Blood product replacement may be necessary because of either anemia or thrombocytopenia. In order to protect febrile neutropenic patients from overwhelming sepsis, granulocyte colony-stimulating factor, reverse isolation, and broad-spectrum antibiotics will be necessary.

There are two events when decontamination is important, and they are oral and IT exposures. The application of gut decontamination is limited to only a few chemotherapeutic agents because of their availability as oral formulations. These include MTX, busulfan, melphalan, and chlorambucil. The oral administration of activated charcoal is indicated when patients present in a timely manner following the ingestion. Repeat doses of activated charcoal can be used in the setting of delayed MTX elimination (e.g., renal failure) to limit enterohepatic recirculation of the drug.[64] As for IT overexposures, it is imperative to decontaminate immediately the cerebrospinal space so that the maximal amount of drug can be removed. IT decontamination consists of CSF drainage, lavage of the cerebrospinal

space, and ventriculolumbar perfusion.[47] The volume of CSF that can be safely removed at one time is dependent on the age of the patient. For an adult, up to 75 mL can be removed and replaced with an equal volume of Ringer's lactate. Cerebrospinal space lavage is accomplished by exchanging CSF with isotonic saline or lactated Ringer's mixed with fresh-frozen plasma to minimize protein loss from the CSF.

Patients need to be adequately hydrated to promote renal perfusion because they are at risk for volume depletion from gastrointestinal fluid loss. Specific approaches to limit renal toxicity by stabilizing either parent drug or metabolite are recommended for cisplatin and MTX. Sodium chloride promotes the anionic state of cisplatin and decreases urine platinum concentrations to limit renal toxicity.[65,66] Therapy with 0.9% saline hydration and osmotic diuresis with mannitol to achieve a urinary output of 1 to 3 mL/kg/hr for 6 to 24 hours is recommended. It is important to maintain urinary output because platinum renal elimination is dependent on urine flow and not on creatinine clearance.[67] For MTX, the patient needs to be adequately hydrated and the urine alkalinized to limit renal toxicity from the precipitation of drug metabolite.[68] The urine pH should be maintained at >7.0, which can be accomplished with a sodium bicarbonate infusion.

Baseline studies should be obtained upon initial evaluation of the patient, and they include complete blood count, serum electrolytes, BUN, creatinine, liver function tests (i.e., aspartate transaminase, alanine transaminase, lactate dehydrogenase, alkaline phosphatase, bilirubin), prothrombin time/partial thromboblastin time, urine analysis, and electrocardiogram. If the woman may be pregnant, a pregnancy test is necessary to evaluate the consequences of the exposure to the pregnancy. Trace elements such as magnesium should be monitored in the setting of cisplatin toxicity because renal wasting can lead to hypomagnesemia. In general, hematologic indices should be followed weekly for up to 2 weeks after hospital discharge of the patient because myelosuppression may not present until weeks after the exposure. For many of the chemotherapeutic agents, patients with an excessive exposure will require intensive management for their condition. This will include close and constant monitoring for existing and evolving toxicities (e.g., cardiac, CNS, renal), or treatment with either rescue agents or the use of enhanced elimination therapy. Thus, these patients need to be admitted to the area in the hospital that can provide them with the appropriate level of care.

Drug levels are infrequently monitored during chemotherapy and thus are not available in the routine clinical setting. However, MTX is an exception, and drug levels are monitored to assist patient management in the course of therapy. A serum MTX level should be obtained initially and repeated at 24 and 48 hours to determine the risk for toxicity and the duration of leucovorin treatment. An MTX half-life greater than 3.5 hours within the first 24 hours of exposure or a serum MTX level greater than 5 μmol/L at 28 hours post-exposure is associated with increased risk for toxicity.

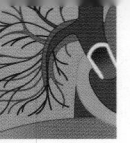

MTX CSF levels can assist in evaluating symptomatic patients at risk for neurotoxicity (e.g., prior meningeal disease) from either an overdose or a CSF outflow obstruction. In both cases, the CSF MTX level would be elevated. The common clinical method for measuring MTX is the fluorescence polarization immunoassay (TDx), which has a level of sensitivity of 0.01 μmol/L and can accept various biologic specimens (e.g., plasma, serum, urine, and CSF). The notable interferents with this method are MTX metabolites, such as 7OHMTX and DAMPA.

Rescue Agents

Rescue agents or chemoprotectants[69] are medications that limit host toxicity from the effects of drugs used in chemotherapy. The role for rescue agents in the management of patients with chemotherapeutic agent toxicity is limited because of the few drugs available and the need to use them in a timely manner. These rescue agents were designed for pretreatment and not post-treatment therapy. Thus, when an exposure is recognized, it is important to administer the rescue agent immediately once the decision is made to use it. Rescue agents are available for MTX (folinic acid, carboxypeptidase), cisplatin (amifostine, thiosulfate), and the anthracycline antibiotics (dexrazoxane). Although glutamic acid is not considered a rescue agent because of its nonspecific activity, it has been used during vincristine therapy to limit peripheral neuropathy based on animal evidence.[70] Patients treated with glutamic acid were observed to have improved deep tendon reflex and sensory responses,[71] and a shorter duration of myelosuppression.[72] The therapy is benign and should be offered to overdosed patients. The dose for glutamic acid is 500 mg every 8 hours, by mouth or IV.

Folinic acid (leucovorin) is used to limit the toxic effects of MTX on host cells by allowing for the continuation of biochemical processes that are dependent on tetrahydrofolate. Tetrahydrofolate is necessary for single carbon transfer reactions that are critical to the formation of certain amino acids, purine nucleotides, and thymidylate. The latter two products are necessary for the synthesis of DNA and RNA. MTX blocks the reduction of dihydrofolate to tetrahydrofolate by inhibiting DHFR. The addition of reduced folate analogs (e.g., folinic acid [5-formyl-5,6,7,8-tetrahydro-folic acid]) allows for continued cell function and survival by bypassing this enzymatic blockade. The beneficial effects of folinic acid have been demonstrated to decrease gastrointestinal mucosal disruption and bone marrow–suppressive effects during high-dose MTX therapy. The use of folinic acid is indicated when the serum MTX level is anticipated to be greater than 0.01 μmol/L, which can occur during high-dose MTX therapy, in the overdosed patient or in a patient with delayed MTX elimination. Although the effective MTX concentration to inhibit DHFR is 0.5 μmol/L, it is generally accepted that a level of 0.01 μmol/L is not likely to have any toxicologic effects, and folinic acid rescue treatment is recommended until this level is achieved. The IV route of administration is preferred for folinic acid in the acute setting or in the patient with toxic manifestations. This is because of the efficiency of drug administration and the limitations associated with the oral route in this setting. These include incomplete gut absorption[73] and lack of compliance, which can result in the patient with mucosal ulcerations. The dose of folinic acid is from 15 to 25 mg orally, and up to 1000 mg/m² IV, and is administered every 6 to 8 hours. When 100 mg/m² folinic acid was administered IV over 4 hours, it achieved a steady-state reduced folate level of 4 μmol/L.[74] Folinic acid should be administered IV during IT MTX overexposures to limit systemic toxicity from the distribution of MTX from the cerebrospinal space to the systemic circulation. Folinic acid is not to be administered intrathecally for IT MTX overdoses because this route of administration was associated with a fatal outcome.[75] Serum MTX levels should be monitored daily to determine adjustments in dose and therapeutic end point during the use of folinic acid. Folinic acid therapy is benign, and treatment should not be delayed in anticipation of a serum MTX level in patients with an MTX overdose.

Carboxypeptidase (NSC-641273) is a bacterial enzyme that effectively deactivates MTX by cleaving the glutamyl residue. This rescue agent is under investigatory use to degrade MTX during situations of host toxicity. Carboxypeptidase has been used systemically (i.e., IV) and in the cerebrospinal space for IT overdoses with success.[43] This agent is made available through the National Institutes of Health, and the indications for use include renal failure and an elevated serum MTX level[76] or IT overdoses (protocol number 92-C-0137). The contact information is as follows: Clinical Studies Support Center/National Cancer Institute, telephone (888) 624-1937, fax (301) 881-8239, website http://ccr.ncifcrf.gov/trials/cssc/patients/search.asp, and e-mail address ncicssc@mail.nih.gov. A limitation to the use of carboxypeptidase is host sensitization, which has not been previously described.

Amifostine (Ethyol, MedImmune Oncology, Inc., Gaithersburg, MD), and sodium thiosulfate are thiol agents that have been clinically used to limit cisplatin-induced nephrotoxicity. Although only amifostine is approved by the Food and Drug Administration to protect against nephrotoxicity, the mechanism by which these thiol agents work to counteract cisplatin are different. Thiol agents have long been studied for their protective effects from cisplatin toxicity. Several mechanisms are proposed by which these agents elicit their protection, and they include binding to reactive cisplatin intermediates, scavenging for free radicals, or regenerating intracellular glutathione.[77] Amifostine is an organic thiol agent and is activated by intracellular alkaline phosphatase. It is most effective when administered prior to cisplatin, and may offer additional beneficial effects by limiting myelosuppression, mucositis, and neuro-toxicity.[78,79] Amifostine administration can cause hypotension; thus, the patient needs adequate hydration and frequent blood pressure monitoring during the use of this drug. Sodium thiosulfate works by binding to extracellular protein unbound platinum species, which limits the metal's

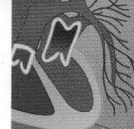

deposition in the renal tubules to cause damage.[58] There is some evidence that thiosulfate may limit neurotoxicity from cisplatin as well.[80,81] Thiosulfate needs to be administered soon after cisplatin exposure to obtain maximal benefit, and as an infusion because of its short plasma half-life (approximately 20 minutes). When thiosulfate was administered as an IV bolus of 4 g/m^2 and continued as an infusion of 12 g/m^2 over 6 hours, it was shown to limit renal toxicity in patients receiving cisplatin at a dose as high as 270 mg/m^2.[82,83] BNP7787 is a disulfide of MESNA and is being investigated as another thiol rescue agent for cisplatin toxicity. In controlled animal trials, BNP7787 was shown to limit cisplatin-induced nephrotoxicity and myelosuppression.[84]

Dexrazoxane is used to limit cardiotoxicity during doxorubicin therapy of women with breast cancer and who are receiving doses higher than 300 mg/m^2. This agent is a cyclic analog of ethylenediaminetetra-acetic acid (EDTA) and forms an intracellular intermediate to chelate iron to interrupt the formation of free radicals responsible for cardiotoxicity. Dexrazoxane treatment is associated with improved left ventricular ejection fraction and decreased incidence of congestive heart failure following doxorubicin therapy.[85] During chemotherapy, dexrazoxane is administered 30 minutes prior to doxorubicin treatment, and in a dose ratio of 10:1. Although further investigations are necessary to define the role of this rescue agent in the overdose setting, its use may benefit patients with doxorubicin overdoses, and the oncologist should be consulted on this topic. Amifostine[86] and monohyroxyethylrutoside[87] are being considered as new rescue agents to protect patients from the cardiotoxic effects of the anthracycline agents.

Enhanced Elimination

The application of enhanced elimination for patients with chemotherapeutic agent overdoses is based on the limited experience and variable success with a few agents. These include busulfan, ifosfamide, cisplatin, doxorubicin, mitoxantrone, MTX, and vincristine. The factors significantly contributing to the effectiveness of these approaches include timeliness of intervention and the extent of either tissue binding or tissue distribution by the chemotherapeutic agent. The protein-binding capacity of the agent is important when hemodialysis is being considered. Hemodialysis has been used to enhance the elimination of busulfan in renal failure patients during therapy[88,89] and in an overdosed patient. This procedure may be effective for ifosfamide exposures[90] as well. In a 4.6-kg infant who received a four-fold overdose of busulfan tablets, hemodialysis was instituted at 9 hours following exposure and continued for 3 hours at a flow rate of 68.3 mL/min.[5] During hemodialysis, the plasma half-life for busulfan was 1 hour and the clearance was 61 mL/min/kg, which were improved from the pretreatment values of 1.6 hours and 41 mL/min/kg, respectively.

Hemoperfusion is the preferred method for the enhanced elimination of MTX because of its greater efficiency compared to hemodialysis.[91] Hemodialysis should be reserved for patients with both an elevated serum MTX level and renal failure because MTX is efficiently eliminated by normal functioning kidneys.[92,93] At 24 hours, about 85% of MTX administered IV is eliminated by the body. Delayed endogenous clearance of MTX occurs when the creatinine clearance is less than 60 mL/m^2/min. Hemoperfusion may be effective in removing doxorubicin because it was shown to increase doxorubicin clearance by 20-fold in animal experiments,[94] and to rapidly decrease serum drug levels in patients with doxorubicin overdoses.[95] However, hemoperfusion was less successful in removing mitoxantrone in an overdosed patient even though it was initiated within hours of the drug's administration.[96] The lack of efficacy in this latter situation may be attributed to this drug's extensive tissue-binding capacity or tissue distribution.

Plasmapheresis is best used to enhance the elimination of chemotherapeutic agents with a high capacity for protein binding. Plasmapheresis is the preferred approach to remove cisplatin because it was shown to be more effective than hemodialysis,[52,97-99] and associated with improved symptoms following a decline in plasma drug level.[52] In an event where a patient received 400 mg/m^2 of cisplatin, plasmapheresis was initiated the day after drug exposure and continued for 12 days for a total of nine sessions. The plasma cisplatin level declined from 2470 ng/mL to 216 ng/mL, and the patient's mental status improved after the fifth session.[52] Plasmapheresis should be initiated soon after the exposure to limit further distribution of cisplatin into the intracellular space, but can still be of benefit when administered days after the initial exposure.[67] For vincristine overdoses, plasmapheresis[100,101] and exchange transfusion[72] have been demonstrated to lower plasma drug levels and, possibly, shorten the duration of toxicity. Plasmapheresis and exchange transfusion were initiated at 6 hours post-exposure, and drug levels decreased from pretreatment levels by 23% and 65%, respectively. It is important to institute these procedures soon after exposure to maximize removal of the drug while it remains in the blood compartment.

SUMMARY

Chemotherapeutic agent overdoses are associated with high morbidity and mortality because of the cell-specific mechanism of action and the narrow therapeutic window of the drugs in this class. The causes of the exposure are typically iatrogenic and involve several mechanisms that can be categorized as errors in either dosage regimen or drug preparation. The manifestations of toxicity common to these agents include pancytopenia, nausea, vomiting, mucositis, and alopecia. The presence of additional clinical findings, such as cardiac dysrhythmias and failure, renal insufficiency, seizures, peripheral neuropathies, and electrolyte abnormalities will vary by the chemotherapeutic agent. The management of these patients includes stabilization of immediate life-threatening disorders, decontamination,

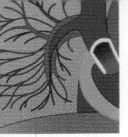

administration of rescue agents, and institution of enhanced elimination. Despite all of these modalities, prevention remains the best treatment for these patients.

This chapter was written by Richard Y. Wang in his private capacity. No official support or endorsement by the CDC is intended or should be inferred.

REFERENCES

1. Einhorn J: Nitrogen mustard: the origin of chemotherapy for cancer. Int J Radiat Oncol Biol Phys 1985;11(7):1375–1378.
2. Angier RB, Boothe JH, Hutching BL, et al: The structure and synthesis of the liver L. casei factor. Science 1946;103:667–669.
3. Du XL, Osborne C, Goodwin JS: Population-based assessment of hospitalizations for toxicity from chemotherapy in older women with breast cancer. J Clin Oncol 2002;20(24):4636–4642.
4. Royal W 3rd, Dupont B, McGuire D, et al: Topotecan in the treatment of acquired immunodeficiency syndrome-related progressive multifocal leukoencephalopathy. J Neurovirol 2003; 9(3):411–419.
5. Stein J, Davidovitz M, Yaniv I, et al: Accidental busulfan overdose: enhanced drug clearance with hemodialysis in a child with Wiskott-Aldrich syndrome. Bone Marrow Transplant 2001;27(5):551–553.
6. Steger GG, Mader RM, Gnant MF, et al: GM-CSF in the treatment of a patient with severe methotrexate intoxication. J Intern Med 1993;233(6):499–502.
7. Jirillo A, Gioga G, Bonciarelli G, Dalla Valle G: Accidental overdose of melphalan per os in a 69-year-old woman treated for advanced endometrial carcinoma. Tumori 1998;84(5):611.
8. de Forni M, Malet-Martino MC, Jaillais P, et al: Cardiotoxicity of high-dose continuous infusion fluorouracil: a prospective clinical study. J Clin Oncol 1992;10(11):1795–1801.
9. Pratt CB, Ransom JL, Evans WE: Age-related adriamycin cardiotoxicity in children. Cancer Treat Rep 1978;62(9):1381–1385.
10. Von Hoff DD, Layard MW, Basa P, et al: Risk factors for doxorubicin-induced congestive heart failure. Ann Intern Med 1979;91(5):710–717.
11. Michelotti A, Venturini M, Tibaldi C, et al: Single agent epirubicin as first line chemotherapy for metastatic breast cancer patients. Breast Cancer Res Treat 2000;59(2):133–139.
12. Bristow MR: Toxic cardiomyopathy due to doxorubicin. Hosp Pract (Off Ed) 1982;17(12):101–108, 110–111.
13. Steinberg JS, Cohen AJ, Wasserman AG, et al: Acute arrhythmogenicity of doxorubicin administration. Cancer 1987;60(6): 1213–1218.
14. Wortman JE, Lucas VS Jr, Schuster E, et al: Sudden death during doxorubicin administration. Cancer 1979;44(5):1588–1591.
15. Schwartz CL, Hobbie WL, Truesdell S, et al: Corrected QT interval prolongation in anthracycline-treated survivors of childhood cancer. J Clin Oncol 1993;11(10):1906–1910.
16. Lefrak EA, Pitha J, Rosenheim S, et al: A clinicopathologic analysis of adriamycin cardiotoxicity. Cancer 1973;32(2):302–314.
17. Von Hoff DD, Rozencweig M, Piccart M: The cardiotoxicity of anticancer agents. Semin Oncol 1982;9(1):23–33.
18. Jensen BV, Skovsgaard T, Nielsen SL: Functional monitoring of anthracycline cardiotoxicity: a prospective, blinded, long-term observational study of outcome in 120 patients. Ann Oncol 2002;13(5):699–709.
19. Siegert W, Hiddemann W, Koppensteiner R, et al: Accidental overdose of mitoxantrone in three patients. Med Oncol Tumor Pharmacother 1989;6(4):275–278.
20. Gbadamosi J, Munchau A, Weiller C, Schafer H: Severe heart failure in a young multiple sclerosis patient. J Neurol 2003; 250(2):241–242.
21. Roush W: Dana-Farber death sends a warning to research hospitals. Science 1995;269(5222):295–296.
22. Mills BA, Roberts RW: Cyclophosphamide-induced cardiomyopathy: a report of two cases and review of the English literature. Cancer 1979;43(6):2223–2226.
23. Appelbaum F, Strauchen JA, Graw RG Jr, et al: Acute lethal carditis caused by high-dose combination chemotherapy. A unique clinical and pathological entity. Lancet 1976;1(7950):58–62.
24. Braverman AC, Antin JH, Plappert MT, et al: Cyclophosphamide cardiotoxicity in bone marrow transplantation: a prospective evaluation of new dosing regimens. J Clin Oncol 1991;9(7): 1215–1223.
25. Kumar S, Gupta RK, Bhake AS, Samal N: Cardiotoxic effects of high doses of cyclophosphamide in albino rats. Arch Int Pharmacodyn Ther 1992;319:58–65.
26. Steinherz LJ, Steinherz PG, Mangiacasale D, et al: Cardiac changes with cyclophosphamide. Med Pediatr Oncol 1981;9(5):417–422.
27. Tsavaris N, Kosmas C, Vadiaka M, et al: Cardiotoxicity following different doses and schedules of 5-fluorouracil administration for malignancy—a survey of 427 patients. Med Sci Monit 2002;8(6): PI51–PI57.
28. Millart H, Brabant L, Lorenzato M, et al: The effects of 5-fluorouracil on contractility and oxygen uptake of the isolated perfused rat heart. Anticancer Res 1992;12(2):571–576.
29. Gorgulu S, Celik S, Tezel T: A case of coronary spasm induced by 5-fluorouracil. Acta Cardiol 2002;57(5):381–383.
30. Arellano M, Malet-Martino M, Martino R, Gires P: The anti-cancer drug 5-fluorouracil is metabolized by the isolated perfused rat liver and in rats into highly toxic fluoroacetate. Br J Cancer 1998;77(1):79–86.
31. Brock N, Stekar J, Pohl J, et al: Acrolein, the causative factor of urotoxic side-effects of cyclophosphamide, ifosfamide, trofosfamide and sufosfamide. Arzneimittelforschung 1979;29(4):659–661.
32. Kupfer A, Aeschlimann C, Wermuth B, Cerny T: Prophylaxis and reversal of ifosfamide encephalopathy with methylene-blue. Lancet 1994;343(8900):763–764.
33. Goren MP, Wright RK, Pratt CB, Pell FE: Dechloroethylation of ifosfamide and neurotoxicity. Lancet 1986;2(8517):1219–1220.
34. Ammenti A, Reitter B, Muller-Wiefel DE: Chlorambucil neurotoxicity: report of two cases. Helv Paediatr Acta 1980;35(3):281–287.
35. Byrne TN Jr, Moseley TA 3rd, Finer MA: Myoclonic seizures following chlorambucil overdose. Ann Neurol 1981;9(2):191–194.
36. Hurwitz RL, Mahoney DH Jr, Armstrong DL, Browder TM: Reversible encephalopathy and seizures as a result of conventional vincristine administration. Med Pediatr Oncol 1988;16(3):216–219.
37. Johnson FL, Bernstein ID, Hartmann JR, Chard RL Jr: Seizures associated with vincristine sulfate therapy. J Pediatr 1973;82(4): 699–702.
38. Kaufman IA, Kung FH, Koenig HM, Giammona ST: Overdosage with vincristine. J Pediatr 1976;89(4):671–674.
39. Stones DK: Vincristine overdosage in paediatric patients. Med Pediatr Oncol 1998;30(3):193.
40. Rosenthal S, Kaufman S: Vincristine neurotoxicity. Ann Intern Med 1974;80(6):733–737.
41. Weiss HD, Walker MD, Wiernik PH: Neurotoxicity of commonly used antineoplastic agents. N Engl J Med 1974;291(2):75–81
42. Pirzada NA, Ali II, Dafer RM: Fluorouracil-induced neurotoxicity. Ann Pharmacother 2000;34(1):35–38.
43. O'Marcaigh AS, Johnson CM, Smithson WA, et al: Successful treatment of intrathecal methotrexate overdose by using ventriculolumbar perfusion and intrathecal instillation of carboxypeptidase G2. Mayo Clin Proc 1996;71(2):161–165.
44. Gowan GM, Herrington JD, Simonetta AB: Methotrexate-induced toxic leukoencephalopathy. Pharmacotherapy 2002;22(9):1183–1187.
45. Allen JC, Rosen G, Mehta BM, Horten B: Leukoencephalopathy following high-dose iv methotrexate chemotherapy with leucovorin rescue. Cancer Treat Rep 1980;64(12):1261–1273.
46. Fernandez CV, Esau R, Hamilton D, et al: Intrathecal vincristine: an analysis of reasons for recurrent fatal chemotherapeutic error with recommendations for prevention. J Pediatr Hematol Oncol 1998;20(6):587–590.
47. Riva L, Conter V, Rizzari C, et al: Successful treatment of intrathecal methotrexate overdose with folinic acid rescue: a case report. Acta Paediatr 1999;88(7):780–782.
48. Alcaraz A, Rey C, Concha A, Medina A: Intrathecal vincristine: fatal myeloencephalopathy despite cerebrospinal fluid perfusion. J Toxicol Clin Toxicol 2002;40(5):557–561.
49. Iqbal Y, Abdullah MF, Turner C, Al-Sudairy R: Intrathecal vincristine: long-term survivor of potentially fatal chemotherapeutic error. Ann Saudi Medicine 2002;22(1):108.
50. Dettmeyer R, Driever F, Becker A, et al: Fatal myeloencephalopathy due to accidental intrathecal vincristin administration: a report of two cases. Forensic Sci Int 2001;122(1):60–64.

51. Holland JF, Scharlau C, Gailani S, et al: Vincristine treatment of advanced cancer: a cooperative study of 392 cases. Cancer Res 1973;33(6):1258–1264.

52. Choi JH, Oh JC, Kim KH, et al: Successful treatment of cisplatin overdose with plasma exchange. Yonsei Med J 2002;43(1):128–132.

53. Legha SS: Vincristine neurotoxicity. Pathophysiology and management. Med Toxicol 1986;1(6):421–427.

54. Sandler SG, Tobin W, Henderson ES: Vincristine-induced neuropathy. A clinical study of fifty leukemic patients. Neurology 1969;19(4):367–374.

55. Katz BJ, Ward JH, Digre KB, et al: Persistent severe visual and electroretinographic abnormalities after intravenous cisplatin therapy. J Neuroophthalmol 2003;23(2):132–135.

56. Bleyer WA: New vistas for leucovorin in cancer chemotherapy. Cancer 1989;63(6 Suppl):995–1007.

57. Choie DD, Longnecker DS, del Campo AA: Acute and chronic cisplatin nephropathy in rats. Lab Invest 1981;44(5):397–402.

58. Erdlenbruch B, Pekrun A, Schiffmann H, et al: Topical topic: accidental cisplatin overdose in a child: reversal of acute renal failure with sodium thiosulfate. Med Pediatr Oncol 2002;38(5):349–352.

59. Favier M, de Cazanove F, Saint-Martin F, Bressolle F: Preventing medication errors in antineoplastic therapy. Am J Hosp Pharm 1994;51(6):832–833.

60. American Society of Health-System Pharmacists (ASHP) Council on Professional Affairs: ASHP guidelines on preventing medication errors with antineoplastic agents. Am J Health Syst Pharm 2002;59(17):1648–1668.

61. Desai ZR, Van den Berg HW, Bridges JM, Shanks RG: Can severe vincristine neurotoxicity be prevented? Cancer Chemother Pharmacol 1982;8(2):211–214.

62. Grisold W, Drlicek M: Paraneoplastic neuropathy. Curr Opin Neurol 1999;12(5):617–625.

63. Pelgrims J, De Vos F, Van den Brande J, et al: Methylene blue in the treatment and prevention of ifosfamide-induced encephalopathy: report of 12 cases and a review of the literature. Br J Cancer 2000;82(2):291–294.

64. Gadgil SD, Damle SR, Advani SH, Vaidya AB: Effect of activated charcoal on the pharmacokinetics of high-dose methotrexate. Cancer Treat Rep 1982;66(5):1169–1171.

65. Al-Sarraf M, Fletcher W, Oishi N, et al: Cisplatin hydration with and without mannitol diuresis in refractory disseminated malignant melanoma: a Southwest Oncology Group study. Cancer Treat Rep 1982;66(1):31–35.

66. Vogl SE, Zaravinos T, Kaplan BH: Toxicity of cis-diamminedichloroplatinum II given in a two-hour outpatient regimen of diuresis and hydration. Cancer 1980;45(1):11–15.

67. Chu G, Mantin R, Shen YM, Baskett G, et al: Massive cisplatin overdose by accidental substitution for carboplatin. Toxicity and management. Cancer 1993;72(12):3707–3714.

68. Christensen ML, Rivera GK, Crom WR, et al: Effect of hydration on methotrexate plasma concentrations in children with acute lymphocytic leukemia. J Clin Oncol 1988;6(5):797–801.

69. Schuchter LM, Hensley ML, Meropol NJ, Winer EP: American Society of Clinical Oncology Chemotherapy and Radiotherapy Expert Panel. 2002 update of recommendations for the use of chemotherapy and radiotherapy protectants: clinical practice guidelines of the American Society of Clinical Oncology. J Clin Oncol 2002;20(12):2895–2903.

70. Boyle FM, Wheeler HR, Shenfield GM: Glutamate ameliorates experimental vincristine neuropathy. J Pharmacol Exp Ther 1996;279(1):410–415.

71. Jackson DV, Wells HB, Atkins JN, et al: Amelioration of vincristine neurotoxicity by glutamic acid. Am J Med 1988;84(6):1016–1022.

72. Kosmidis HV, Bouhoutsou DO, Varvoutsi MC, et al: Vincristine overdose: experience with 3 patients. Pediatr Hematol Oncol 1991;8(2):171–178.

73. Straw JA, Szapary D, Wynn WT: Pharmacokinetics of the diastereoisomers of leucovorin after intravenous and oral administration to normal subjects. Cancer Res 1984;44(7):3114–3119.

74. Mehta BM, Glass JP, Shapir WR: Serum and cerebrospinal fluid distribution of 5-methyltetrahydrofolate after intravenous calcium leucovorin and intra-Ommaya methotrexate administration in patients with meningeal carcinomatosis. Cancer Res 1983;43:435–438.

75. Jardine LF, Ingram LC, Bleyer WA: Intrathecal leucovorin after intrathecal methotrexate overdose. J Pediatr Hematol Oncol 1996;18(3):302–304.

76. Windemann BC, Balis FM, Murphy RF, et al: Carboxypeptidase-G2, thymidine, and leucovorin rescue in cancer patients with methotrexate-induced renal dysfunction. J Clin Oncol 1997;15(5):2125–2134.

77. Korst AE, Eeltink CM, Vermorken JB, van der Vijgh WJ: Pharmacokinetics of amifostine and its metabolites in patients. Eur J Cancer 1997;33(9):1425–1429.

78. Kemp G, Rose P, Lurain J, et al: Amifostine pretreatment for protection against cyclophosphamide-induced and cisplatin-induced toxicities: results of a randomized control trial in patients with advanced ovarian cancer. J Clin Oncol 1996;14(7):2101–2112.

79. Alberts DS, Bleyer WA: Future development of amifostine in cancer treatment. Semin Oncol 1996;23(4 Suppl 8):90–99.

80. Markman M, Cleary S, Pfeifle CE, Howell SB: High-dose intracavitary cisplatin with intravenous thiosulfate. Low incidence of serious neurotoxicity. Cancer 1985;56(10):2364–2368.

81. van Rijswijk RE, Hoekman K, Burger CW, et al: Experience with intraperitoneal cisplatin and etoposide and i.v. sodium thiosulphate protection in ovarian cancer patients with either pathologically complete response or minimal residual disease. Ann Oncol 1997;8(12):1235–1241.

82. Hirosawa A, Niitani H, Hayashibara K, Tsuboi E: Effects of sodium thiosulfate in combination therapy of cis-dichlorodiammine-platinum and vindesine. Cancer Chemother Pharmacol 1989;23(4):255–258.

83. Pfeifle CE, Howell SB, Felthouse RD, et al: High-dose cisplatin with sodium thiosulfate protection. J Clin Oncol 1985;3(2):237–244.

84. Hausheer FH, Kanter P, Cao S, et al: Modulation of platinum-induced toxicities and therapeutic index: mechanistic insights and first- and second-generation protecting agents. Semin Oncol 1998;25(5):584–599.

85. Speyer JL, Green MD, Kramer E, et al: Protective effect of the bispiperazinedione ICRF-187 against doxorubicin-induced cardiac toxicity in women with advanced breast cancer. N Engl J Med 1988;319(12):745–752.

86. Catino A, Crucitta E, Latorre A, et al: Amifostine as chemoprotectant in metastatic breast cancer patients treated with doxorubicin. Oncol Rep 2003;10(1):163–167.

87. van Acker FA, van Acker SA, Kramer K, et al: 7-mono-hydroxyethylrutoside protects against chronic doxorubicin-induced cardiotoxicity when administered only once per week. Clin Cancer Res 2000;6(4):1337–1341.

88. Masauzi N, Higa T, Nakagawa S, et al: Pharmacokinetic study of busulfan in an AML patient treated with regular hemodialysis. Ann Hematol 1998;77(6):293–294.

89. Ullery LL, Gibbs JP, Ames GW, et al: Busulfan clearance in renal failure and hemodialysis. Bone Marrow Transplant 2000;25(2):201–203.

90. Carlson L, Goren MP, Bush DA, et al: Toxicity, pharmacokinetics, and in vitro hemodialysis clearance of ifosfamide and metabolites in an anephric pediatric patient with Wilms' tumor. Cancer Chemother Pharmacol 1998;41(2):140–146.

91. Relling MV, Stapleton FB, Ochs J, et al: Removal of methotrexate, leucovorin, and their metabolites by combined hemodialysis and hemoperfusion. Cancer 1988;62(5):884–888.

92. Saland JM, Leavey PJ, Bash RO, et al: Effective removal of methotrexate by high-flux hemodialysis. Pediatr Nephrol 2002;17(10):825–829.

93. Wall SM, Johansen MJ, Molony DA, et al: Effective clearance of methotrexate using high-flux hemodialysis membranes. Am J Kidney Dis 1996;28(6):846–854.

94. Winchester JF, Rahman A, Tilstone WJ, et al: Will hemoperfusion be useful for cancer chemotherapeutic drug removal? Clin Toxicol 1980;17(4):557–569.

95. Curran CF: Acute doxorubicin overdoses. Ann Intern Med 1991;115(11):913–914.

96. Hachimi-Idrissi S, Schots R, DeWolf D, et al: Reversible cardiopathy after accidental overdose of mitoxantrone. Pediatr Hematol Oncol 1993;10(1):35–40.

97. Brivet F, Pavlovitch JM, Gouyette A, et al: Inefficiency of early prophylactic hemodialysis in cisplatinum overdose. Cancer Chemother Pharmacol 1986;18(2):183–184.
98. Lagrange JL, Cassuto-Viguier E, Barbe V, et al: Cytotoxic effects of long-term circulating ultrafiltrable platinum species and limited efficacy of haemodialysis in clearing them. Eur J Cancer 1994; 30A(14):2057–2060.
99. Pike IM, Arbus MH: Cisplatin overdosage. J Clin Oncol 1992; 10(9):1503–1504.
100. Lotz JP, Chapiro J, Voinea A, et al: Overdosage of vinorelbine in a woman with metastatic non-small-cell lung carcinoma. Ann Oncol 1997;8(7):714–715.
101. Pierga JY, Beuzeboc P, Dorval T, et al: Favourable outcome after plasmapheresis for vincristine overdose. Lancet 1992;340(8812):185.

B Thalidomide

MICHAEL W. SHANNON, MD, MPH

At a Glance...

- Thalidomide has many useful clinical properties, possessing sedative-hypnotic, antibiotic, anti-inflammatory, anti-angiogenesis, and immunomodulatory effects. It consequently has a wide range of potential clinical uses.
- Thalidomide is also a very potent teratogen, capable of producing birth defects after a single dose. The limb deformity phocomelia is the best characterized of thalidomide's effects.
- Adverse effects of thalidomide when taken therapeutically include somnolence, rash (including Stevens-Johnson syndrome), peripheral neuropathy, and hepatotoxicity.

Thalidomide is one of the most notorious drugs ever created. The agent was used around the world for approximately 5 years before its role as a potent teratogen was recognized. Banned after producing a generation of children with severe birth defects, the drug began making a surprise comeback in the 1980s. In 1998, thalidomide was approved by the Food and Drug Administration (FDA) for use in erythema nodosum leprosum. Since that time, the drug's list of clinical indications has proliferated as its broad range of pharmacologic actions are exploited to treat leprosy, multiple myeloma, leprosy, and many other disorders.

HISTORY

Thalidomide was first released in Germany as the drug Contergan in 1956 and in England in 1958 as Distaval. Originally developed to be an antibiotic, it was found to have a useful sedative effect. It was approved as a sedative-hypnotic, safer than barbiturates and other central nervous system (CNS) depressants of its era. Its liquid form was often given to crying children, earning it the title "West Germany's baby sitter."[1] Proving to be effective in hyperemesis gravidarum, it became a popular drug for the nausea of pregnancy, with the added benefit of offering women a full night's sleep. Having an excellent safety profile, its use rapidly grew; it quickly became the third largest selling drug in Europe; at its peak it was sold in 48 countries.[2] In North America, it was used briefly in Canada as the drug Kevadon; for a brief period Kevadon was distributed illegally in the United States. However, when a new drug application to market Kevadon in the United States was filed with the FDA in 1960, the drug's approval was deferred by Dr. Frances O. Kelsey because reports of thalidomide-associated peripheral neuropathy had begun to appear and because animal safety data seemed inadequate. As the FDA continued to seek more data, in November 1961 thalidomide's role in causing phocomelia ("seal limb") in the offspring of women who used the drug during pregnancy was reported almost simultaneously by Drs. Lenz in West Germany and McBride in Australia. The drug was promptly removed from the market. By 1962, phocomelia, amelia, and other birth defects in more than 12,000 children in 46 countries were attributed to thalidomide; at least 17 cases of phocomelia occurred in the United States.[3] While phocomelia, an obvious and debilitating birth defect, became synonymous with thalidomide, cardiac defects and other anomalies were also found in the progeny of pregnant women who used thalidomide.[4] Birth defects were associated with ingestion of as little as a single dose.

After its worldwide withdrawal in 1961, the drug was shunned for only a few years. In 1965 its efficacy in the treatment of erythema nodosum leprosum (ENL) was discovered. After years of growing scientific interest, and drug research and development, in July 1998 the FDA approved thalidomide for the treatment of ENL, a debilitating condition associated with lepromatous leprosy. Soon thereafter it was shown to be valuable as a treatment for aphthous ulcers, leading to its approval for this indication in 2001. Once clinical and experimental data indicated that thalidomide was also a potent angiogenesis inhibitor, its clinical role expanded even

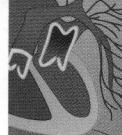

BOX 56-1	**POTENTIAL CLINICAL USES FOR THALIDOMIDE**

Dermatologic
Prurigo nodularis
Pyoderma gangrenosum
Actinic prurigo
Erythema multiforme
Uremic pruritis
Bullous pemphigoid
Cicatricial pemphigoid
Toxic epidermal necrolysis

Autoimmune
Chronic graft-versus-host
  disease
Lupus erythematosus
Rheumatoid arthritis
Cold hemagglutination disease
Ankylosing spondylitis

Neurologic
Postherpetic neuralgia

Other
Sarcoidosis
Behçet's disease

Digestive/Gastrointestinal
Recurrent aphthous ulcers
Ulcerative colitis

Oncologic
Langerhans' cell histiocytosis
Multiple myeloma
Lymphoma
Prostate cancer
Renal cell carcinoma

Infectious
Erythema nodosum leprosum
HIV-associated wasting syndrome
Tuberculosis-associated weight
  loss
HIV–associated proctitis
HIV-associated *Microsporidium*
  diarrhea
Hepatitis

Vascular
Diabetic retinopathy
Macular degeneration

HIV, human immunodeficiency virus

more. Thalidomide is now used for a broad range of conditions (Box 56-1).

PHARMACOLOGY

Thalidomide is a glutamic acid derivative. Its structure is shown in Figure 56-1. The agent is available in 50-, 100-, and 200-mg capsules. For most of its clinical uses, thalidomide is prescribed in a dose of 3 to 6 mg/kg/day, taken in one to four divided doses. Customary doses are 200 to 800 mg daily. Absorption of thalidomide from the gut is slow but extensive; a 200-mg dose produces a peak concentration of 1 to 2 mg/L at 3 to 4 hours.[5] Distribution characteristics include plasma protein binding of approximately 60% and an apparent volume of distribution (Vd) of approximately 1 L/kg.[5,6]

Thalidomide is primarily biotransformed through spontaneous, nonenzymatic hydrolytic cleavage.[5] The drug also undergoes metabolism by the cytochrome P-450 isoenzyme CYP2C19. Multiple metabolites have been identified; certain drug effects (e.g., antiangio-

genesis activity) are attributed to its metabolites rather than to the parent drug. The drug's elimination half-life is approximately 6 hours. Thalidomide metabolites are eliminated in urine and feces within 48 hours of a dose; there is little excretion of unchanged drug. Drug pharmacokinetics are not altered by repeat dosing. Thalidomide possesses no significant drug interactions.

Having a broad range of clinical effects, thalidomide has unclear cellular mechanisms of action. However, on a macroscopic level, the drug appears to have four primary actions: (1) immunomodulatory, (2) anti-inflammatory,[7-9] (3) antiangiogenesis, and (4) hypnosedative. Thalidomide is an immunostimulant, producing an increase in total lymphocyte count and CD8+ T cells. It also increases interferon-γ production[2] while significantly lowering levels of circulating tumor necrosis factor-α (TNF-α, also referred to as cachectin). For many conditions, its efficacy is based on this action. For example, ENL is associated with high circulating levels of TNF-α; thalidomide's efficacy correlates with falling TNF-α concentrations. Recurrent aphthous ulcers and Behçet's disease, other conditions for which thalidomide is useful, are also associated with elevated circulating TNF-α.[10,11] Sedative effects of the drug appear to have a mechanism different from barbiturates; rather than enhancing γ-aminobutyric acid (GABA)-mediated neurotransmission, thalidomide appears to activate sleep centers in the forebrain.[5] Recent data also suggest that thalidomide is an inhibitor of nitric oxide synthase.[12]

Although thalidomide is FDA approved only for the treatment of recurrent aphthous ulcers and erythema nodosum leprosum, the range of disorders for which it has been used, with reported clinical benefit, is extensive (see Fig. 56B-1). It has been used successfully to treat infectious conditions such as HIV-associated wasting syndrome and tuberculosis-associated weight loss. It has also been used to treat chronic graft-versus-host disease. However, its most rapidly expanding use has been as a chemotherapeutic agent for select cancers, including multiple myeloma,[13-16] prostate cancer, myelofibrosis, renal cell carcinoma, lymphoma, Kaposi's sarcoma, and thyroid cancer.[17] It has also been used to treat a number of autoimmune or idiopathic disorders, including ankylosing spondylitis, sarcoidosis,[18] and inflammatory bowel disease.[19,20]

TOXICITY

The mechanisms of thalidomide toxicity are equally unclear. By whatever mechanisms, the drug is associated with a very broad range of adverse effects (Box 56-2). These toxicities are found in those taking the drug chronically; acute single overdose of thalidomide appears to produce only mild sedation; ingestions of as much as 14 g have led to minimal toxicity.[5]

The adverse effects associated with chronic thalidomide use include somnolence, rash, fatigue, constipation, abdominal pain, Stevens-Johnson syndrome, elevated liver enzymes, and peripheral edema.[8] Endocrine effects are also multiple and include hyperprolactinemia (with

FIGURE 56-1 Thalidomide structure.

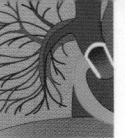

BOX 56-2   ADVERSE CLINICAL EFFECTS ASSOCIATED WITH THALIDOMIDE

Neurobehavioral
Dizziness
Increased appetite
Mood changes
Peripheral neuropathy
Sedation or drowsiness

Digestive/Gastrointestinal
Elevated hepatic transaminases
Constipation
Nausea

Endocrinologic/Reproductive
Antithyroid effect
Decreased libido
Galactorrhea
Hyperprolactinemia
Hypoglycemia
Increased adrenocorticotropic hormone
Menstrual abnormalities

Dermatologic
Brittle fingernails
Exfoliative dermatitis
Face/limb edema
Pruritus
Red palms
Stevens-Johnson syndrome

Hematologic
Neutropenia
Thrombocytopenic purpura

Cardiovascular
Allergic vasculitis
Deep venous thrombosis
Thromboembolism

---

accompanying galactorrhea), an antithyroid effect,[21] and amenorrhea.[22,23]

Peripheral neuropathy has been a recognized adverse effect of thalidomide since it was first released. The neuropathy characteristically affects sensory rather than motor neurons and lower more than upper extremities.[24] Victims often complain of distal lower extremity painful paresthesias. The neuropathy seems to be dose related, although dose-unrelated occurrences have also been reported.[25] At-risk groups are females rather than males and the elderly. The neuropathy is partially reversible and can be either an axonal length–dependent neuropathy or a ganglionopathy.[26]

Other clinical toxicities include sinus bradycardia, particularly in those taking other medications that decrease heart rate,[27] deep venous thrombosis, pulmonary embolus, and other thromboembolic events.[28,29]

As many as 30% of subjects must cease thalidomide use due to unacceptable adverse effects.[30]

TERATOGENICITY

Thalidomide is a powerful teratogen, producing effects when taken during much of pregnancy, particularly days 34 to 50 after the final period. The main categories of thalidomide embryopathy include limb deformity, craniofacial defects (microtia or anotia, eye defects, choanal atresia), cardiac disturbances (ductus arteriosus, conotrocal defects, septal defects), intestinal disorders (duodenal atresia, anal atresia, pyloric stenosis), genitourinary tract abnormalities (ectopic kidney, vaginal duplication, renal/testicular agenesis), and lung abnormalities. Limb deformities such as phocomelia occurred

when women took any amount of thalidomide during the 20th to the 36th day of pregnancy. Most birth defects, including phocomelia, have been attributed to the drug's antiangiogenesis effects. Thalidomide does not produce second-generation birth defects.[31]

When it approved thalidomide, the FDA and drug manufacturer instituted severe controls over the drug. To minimize the risk for birth defects, the FDA has mandated that physicians prescribing thalidomide be registered in the System for Thalidomide Education and Prescribing Safety (STEPS) program. Patients taking the drug must receive drug education and acknowledge that they received this education. Women must agree in writing to have no intercourse or to use two methods of birth control should they engage in intercourse. Women must also undergo periodic pregnancy tests.

MANAGEMENT

Acute overdose of thalidomide should be treated with initial stabilization and supportive care. Sedation can be anticipated. Activated charcoal adsorbs thalidomide and is a potentially valuable intervention, particularly if administered within 1 to 2 hours of ingestion. There are no specific laboratory data that would be useful in the diagnosis and management of thalidomide toxicity. An electrocardiogram and an arterial blood gas or pulse oximetry with end-tidal CO_2 monitoring can be useful adjuncts in management. Other tests (e.g., toxic screen testing) may be useful to rule out coingestions. There is no known method of enhancing the elimination of thalidomide; elimination enhancement should not be necessary since patients quickly recover without sequelae. A pregnancy test should be considered in women of childbearing age since thalidomide ingestion during pregnancy has grave implications that may require pregnancy counseling. Patients with acute overdose who are asymptomatic or who have only transient lethargy can be safely discharged from the emergency department with close follow-up.

REFERENCES

1. McFadyen RE: Thalidomide in America: a brush with tragedy. Clio Med 1976;11:79–93.
2. Bernstein JR: Thalidomide. Clin Toxicol Rev 1999;21(5):1–3.
3. Taussig HB: Thalidomide and phocomelia. Pediatrics 1962; 30:654–659.
4. Taussig HB: The evils of camouflage as illustrated by thalidomide. N Engl J Med 1963;269:92–94.
5. Teo SK, Colburn WA, Tracewell WG, et al: Clinical pharmacokinetics of thalidomide. Clin Pharmacokinet 2004;43:311–327.
6. Eriksson T, Bjorkman S, Hoglund P: Clinical pharmacology of thalidomide. Eur J Clin Pharmacol 2001;57(5):365–376.
7. Nasca MR, Micali G, Cheigh NH, et al: Dermatologic and non-dermatologic uses of thalidomide. Ann Pharmacother 2003;37(9):1307–1320.
8. Laffitte D, Revuz J: Thalidomide, an old drug with new clinical applications. Exp Opin Drug Saf 2004;3:47–56.
9. Matthews SJ, McCoy C: Thalidomide: a review of approved and investigational uses. Clin Ther 2003;25(2):342–395.
10. Jacobson JM, Greenspan JS, Spritzler J, et al: Thalidomide for the treatment of oral aphthous ulcers in patients with human immunodeficiency virus infection. N Engl J Med 1997;336:1487–1493.

11. Sayarlioglu M, Kotan MC, Topcu N, et al: Treatment of recurrent perforating intestinal ulcers with thalidomide in Behcet's disease. Ann Pharmacother 2004;38(5):808–811.

12. Shimazawa R, Sano H, Tanatani A, et al: Thalidomide as a nitric oxide synthase inhibitor and its structural development. Chem Pharm Bull (Tokyo) 2004;52:498–499.

13. Kyle R, Rajkumar S: Multiple myeloma. N Engl J Med 2004;351: 1860–1873.

14. Ghobrial I, Rajkumar S: Management of thalidomide toxicity. J Supportive Oncol 2003;1:194–205.

15. Ribas C, Colleoni G: Advances in the treatment of multiple myeloma: the role of thalidomide. Leuk Lymphoma 2003;44:291–298.

16. Singhal S, Mehta J, Desikan R, et al: Antitumor activity of thalidomide in refractory multiple myeloma. N Engl J Med 1999;341(21):1565–1571.

17. Joglekar S, Levin M: The promise of thalidomide: evolving indications. Drugs Today (Barc), 2004;40(3):197–204.

18. Baughman RP, Judson MA, Teirstein AS, et al: Thalidomide for chronic sarcoidosis. Chest 2002;122(1):227–232.

19. Bariol C, Meagher AP, Vickers CR, et al: Early studies on the safety and efficacy of thalidomide for symptomatic inflammatory bowel disease. J Gastroenterol Hepatol 2002;17(2):135–139.

20. Bousvaros A, Mueller B: Thalidomide in gastrointestinal disorders. Drugs 2001;61(6):777–787.

21. deSavary N, Lee R, Vaidya B: Severe hypothyroidism after thalidomide treatment. J R Soc Med 2004;97:422.

22. Dharia S, Steinkampf M, Cater C: Thalidomide-induced amenorrhea: case report and literature review. Fertil Steril 2004; 82:460–462.

23. Frances C, El Khoury S, Gompel A, et al: Transient secondary amenorrhea in women treated by thalidomide. Eur J Dermatol 2002;12(1):63–65.

24. Jones G: Thalidomide: 35 years on and still deforming. Lancet 1994;343:1041.

25. Chaudhry V, Cornblath DR, Corse A, et al: Thalidomide-induced neuropathy. Neurology 2002;59(12):1872–1875.

26. Isoardo G, Bergui M, Durelli L, et al: Thalidomide neuropathy: clinical, electrophysiological and neuroradiological features. Acta Neurol Scand 2004;109:188–193.

27. Kaur A, Yu SS, Lee AJ, Chiao TB: Thalidomide-induced sinus bradycardia. Ann Pharmacother 2003;37:1040–1043.

28. Bennett CL, Schumock GT, Desai AA, et al: Thalidomide-associated deep vein thrombosis and pulmonary embolism. Am J Med 2002;113(7):603–606.

29. Bowcock SJ, Rassam SM, Ward SM, et al: Thromboembolism in patients on thalidomide for myeloma. Hematology 2002;7(1): 51–53.

30. Gordon JN, Goggin PM: Thalidomide and its derivatives: emerging from the wilderness. Postgrad Med J 2003;79(929): 127–132.

31. Smithells D: Does thalidomide cause second generation birth defects? Drug Saf 1998;19(5):339–341.

57 Transplant Agents and Other Immunosuppressives

SHARITA E. WARFIELD, MD, MS ■ MATTHEW W. HEDGE, MD

At a Glance...

- Transplant agents and other immunosuppressives are being used increasingly as the prevalence of solid organ and cell transplant recipients increases.
- All transplant agents have important drug–drug or drug–food interactions, requiring careful dosing and close monitoring.
- Tacrolimus and cyclosporine, the most common transplant agents, are metabolized by CYP3A3. Their metabolism can be significantly slowed in the presence of CYP3A inhibitors, leading to elevated concentrations and resulting toxicity.
- The major toxicity resulting from tacrolimus and cyclosporine overdose is renal injury.

Transplantation of vital organs such as the kidney, liver, pancreas, heart, and bone marrow is efficiently used as a form of treatment for end-stage organ disease. It is the role of the body's immune system to discriminate between self and nonself cells in the body and destroy the nonself cells. When an organ transplant is introduced to the body, it is recognized as foreign. It is this response that leads to transplants being rejected. Historically, immunosuppressive agents have been used to ensure the success of organ transplantation. However, the use of these agents was not without consequence. Older agents used in single and multiple drug protocols had many undesirable effects. The discovery and refinement of current conventional immunosuppressive agents, which function in a nonspecific manner to suppress the immune system, has helped revolutionize the field of transplantation.

Until recently, these agents provided the mainstay of clinical immunosuppression with antiproliferative activity. They included antimetabolites, alkylating agents, and irradiation. The current belief is that T lymphocytes are primarily responsible for graft rejection. The introduction of agents that specifically act on T lymphocytes (cyclosporine, tacrolimus [FK506], and azathioprine) dramatically changed the outcome after transplantation.

The use of immunosuppressive agents extends beyond organ graft protection. Many newer agents have shown efficacy in the treatment of dermatologic disorders including seborrheic dermatitis, cutaneous lupus erythematous, vulvar lichen sclerosus, and vitiligo.[1-4] Some older agents have shown efficacy in the treatment of the vasculitides, rheumatoid arthritis, and multiple sclerosis.[5,6] In general, overdose of transplant agents is rare. However, increasing indications for the newer agents coupled with the occasional dosing errors with the older agents have sparked an interest in better understanding the toxicity and adverse effects of these drugs.

TACROLIMUS (FK506)

Pharmacology

Tacrolimus (FK506) is a macrolide immunosuppressant derived from *Streptomyces tsukubaensis*. It has been used in liver, heart, kidney, and other experimental forms of transplantation. It is similar to cyclosporine in its mode of action, efficacy, and toxicity profile. The exact mechanism by which tacrolimus produces immunosuppression remains unknown. It is proposed that tacrolimus inhibits T-lymphocyte activation by binding to an intracellular protein, FKBP-12. A complex is formed between tacrolimus and FKBP-12, calcium, calmodulin, and calcineurin. This complex inhibits the phosphatase activity of calcineurin. The inhibition of calcineurin is believed to prevent the dephosphorylation and translocation of nuclear factor of activated T cells (NF-AT), which is the cellular component thought to initiate gene transcription for the formation of lymphokines such as interleukin-2 (IL-2) and interferon-γ. Tacrolimus also inhibits the transcription for genes that encode IL-3, IL-4, IL-5, granulocyte-macrophage colony-stimulating factor (GM-CSF), and tumor necrosis factor–α (TNF-α), all of which are involved in the early stages of T-cell activation. In addition, it inhibits the release of preformed mediators from skin mast cells and basophils, as well as potentiating the effects of corticosteroids.

Pharmacokinetics

The pharmacokinetic profile of tacrolimus has been studied extensively in adults and children. Bioavailability after oral administration averages 17% to 22%. The presence of food, particularly a high-fat meal, decreases the rate and extent of tacrolimus absorption. Peak whole-blood levels are achieved within 1.5 to 3 hours after oral dosing.[7,8] Tacrolimus is highly protein bound and also binds to erythrocytes and lymphocytes. The volume of distribution in adults is 1.4 to 1.9 L/kg; in children, it is 2.6 L/kg. Tacrolimus is primarily metabolized in the liver via cytochrome P-450 isoenzymes CYP3A4 and CYP3A5. The metabolites are eliminated in the bile at a rate of 0.04 to 0.08 L/kg/hr in adults and 0.14 L/kg/hr in children. The elimination of tacrolimus is not affected by renal or mild hepatic dysfunction; however, in patients with severe hepatic dysfunction or hepatitis C, the clearance rate is prolonged.[7-11]

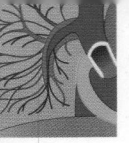

Tacrolimus is available in the United States and Canada in three formulations: oral, parenteral, and a topical ointment. Dosage varies and is based on body weight. Typically for adults, teenagers, or children, the oral dose will be 0.1 to 0.3 mg/kg/day. The parenteral dose is 0.01 to 0.05 mg/kg/day.

DRUG INTERACTIONS

The metabolism of tacrolimus by CYP3A increases the risk of drug interactions when it is used with drugs that are also metabolized via the cytochrome P-450 enzyme system. A variety of drug classes cause increased tacrolimus concentrations, including antifungal agents, corticosteroids, calcium channel blockers, macrolide antibiotics, and gastrointestinal (GI) prokinetic agents. Other substances such as cyclosporine, metronidazole, cimetidine, and grapefruit juice may lead to decreased tacrolimus concentrations. Nephrotoxicity has been reported in patients taking tacrolimus; the concomitant use of other nephrotoxins such as amphotericin, aminoglycosides, cisplatin, or nonsteroidal anti-inflammatory agents (NSAIDs) may place the patient at increased risk for this adverse effect.[7,8]

Toxicology

CLINICAL MANIFESTATIONS

Data are limited on cases of overdoses with tacrolimus. However, chronic overdose is known to cause nephrotoxicity. This usually is manifested early in therapy as an increase in serum creatinine and a decrease in urine output. Dosage adjustment or discontinuation of therapy will usually reverse the nephrotoxic effect. Neurotoxicity, which appears more commonly in patients with elevated tacrolimus concentrations or hepatic dysfunction, has also been reported. In severe cases, it may manifest as seizures, delirium, or coma. Some individuals may have a genetic predisposition to developing tacrolimus-induced neurotoxicity.[6]

ADVERSE EFFECTS

The most common adverse effects associated with tacrolimus are listed in Box 57-1. Type 1 diabetes mellitus develops in approximately 20% of patients taking tacrolimus. It appears to be more common in African Americans, in patients receiving high-dose corticosteroids, and in patients with elevated tacrolimus levels.[7,8]

Management

Supportive care is the mainstay of therapy. A single dose of charcoal should be given after an acute overdose to help decrease absorption. Benzodiazepines can be used to treat agitation and seizures if they develop. Currently, no robust data support the use of multiple-dose activated charcoal or hemodialysis as treatment for tacrolimus overdose.

BOX 57-1	MOST COMMON ADVERSE EFFECTS ASSOCIATED WITH TACROLIMUS

CNS	**Pulmonary**
Tremor	Pleural effusion
Confusion	Edema
Headache	Atelectasis
Hallucinations	
Dizziness	**GI**
Asthenia	Nausea
Insomnia	Diarrhea
Agitation	Pain
Seizures	Constipation
Metabolic	**Dermatologic**
Hyperkalemia	Rash
Hypomagnesemia	Pruritus
Hyperglycemia	Alopecia
Hypertension	

AZATHIOPRINE

Pharmacology

Azathioprine was originally approved by the Food and Drug Administration (FDA) in 1968 for use as an adjunct immunosuppressant agent. It was often used in combination with corticosteroids for solid organ transplantation. In recent years, azathioprine use has markedly declined and has been replaced by mycophenolate. Azathioprine is a pro-drug that is converted in the body to 6-mercaptopurine (6-MP). 6-MP is a purine analog that acts as an antimetabolite immunosuppressive agent inhibiting T-cell proliferation by interfering with the synthesis of nucleotides. Azathioprine is also used to treat Crohn's disease, lupus nephritis, rheumatoid arthritis, psoriasis, myasthenia gravis, and other autoimmune diseases.

Pharmacokinetics

Orally, azathioprine is well absorbed. Azathioprine is rapidly eliminated from the blood and converted in the liver by xanthine oxidase to 6-MP, which is then metabolized to 6-thiourate and several other metabolites. These metabolites are excreted in the urine; no azathioprine or 6-MP can be detected in the urine after 8 hours. The plasma half-life of azathioprine is less than 15 minutes, and the half-life of 6-MP is 1 to 3 hours. Azathioprine is 30% protein bound and only partially dialyzable.

The drug is available in two forms: an oral 50 mg tablet and an injectable solution of 100 mg/20 mL vial. The intravenous and oral doses are equivalent. Intramuscular injection is not advised. The initial recommended dose is 3 to 5 mg/kg once a day, and the maintenance dose is reduced to 1 to 2 mg/kg once a day. Dose reduction is necessary in patients with impaired renal function.

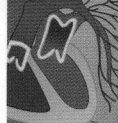

DRUG INTERACTIONS

The use of azathioprine with drugs including cotrimoxazole, carbamazepine, and ganciclovir affects leukocyte production and thus may induce hematologic toxicity in patients. The use of angiotensin-converting enzyme (ACE) inhibitors in patients taking azathioprine has been reported to cause anemia and severe leukopenia.[12] Severe leukopenia can develop particularly in renal transplant patients. Allopurinol inhibits xanthine oxidase, the enzyme responsible for the inactivation of 6-MP to 6-thiouric acid and other metabolites. The use of azathioprine and allopurinol in combination causes 6-MP to accumulate and places the patient at risk for marked immunosuppressive effects from azathioprine. Therefore, the dose of azathioprine should be reduced by 50% when used with allopurinol.[13] Prolonged use of azathioprine with corticosteroids may cause muscle wasting. Azathioprine also is known to impair fertility by reducing sperm counts in males. When azathioprine is used with tubocurarine, it decreases the effect of tubocurarine and other nondepolarizing neuromuscular blocking agents.[12]

Toxicology

CLINICAL MANIFESTATIONS

The principal and potentially serious toxic effects of azathioprine are hematologic and gastrointestinal. There also is an increased risk of secondary infection and cancer. Large overdoses of azathioprine may acutely cause abdominal pain, nausea, vomiting, and diarrhea. In general, patients undergoing azathioprine therapy experience nausea and vomiting for the first few months. Vomiting and abdominal pain may also be associated with hypersensitivity pancreatitis that rarely develops in these patients. Hepatotoxicity, manifested by elevated serum transaminases, alkaline phosphatase, and bilirubin, also is known to occur. Discontinuation of azathioprine therapy usually reverses the hepatotoxic effects. A rare but life-threatening hepatic veno-occlusive disease associated with chronic use of azathioprine has been reported.[12] Periodic measurements of serum transaminases, alkaline phosphatase, and bilirubin are indicated to detect hepatotoxicity early. Leukopenia and thrombocytopenia are dose dependent but may occur with chronic therapy. Dose reduction or temporary withdrawal will reverse these toxicities. In addition, macrocytic anemia and bleeding are known to occur with azathioprine therapy. A single case has been reported of a renal transplant patient who ingested a large dose (7500 mg) of azathioprine. The immediate toxic reactions were nausea, vomiting, and diarrhea, followed by mild leukopenia and mild abnormalities in liver function. The white blood cell count, serum glutamic oxaloacetic transaminase (SGOT), and bilirubin returned to normal 6 days after the overdose.[14]

ADVERSE EFFECTS

The most common adverse effects associated with azathioprine are listed in Box 57-2.

> **BOX 57-2   MOST COMMON ADVERSE EFFECTS ASSOCIATED WITH AZATHIOPRINE**
>
> **Hematologic**
> Leukopenia
> Pancytopenia
> Macrocytic anemia
>
> **GI**
> ↓ Appetite
> Nausea
> Vomiting
> Diarrhea
> Pancreatitis
>
> **Renal**
> Interstitial nephritis
>
> **Dermatologic**
> Rash
> Alopecia
> Skin cancer
> Jaundice
> Bruising
>
> **Systemic**
> Fatigue
> Fever
> Serum Sickness

Management

Overdose with azathioprine is rare; therefore, data regarding management in overdose are lacking. Supportive care seems to be the mainstay of treatment for GI manifestations. Protection from falls or injury seems prudent to avoid bruising or bleeding. Alanine transaminase (ALT), aspartate transaminase (AST), bilirubin, and alkaline phosphatase should be monitored. Hemodialysis may serve as an adjunct to supportive care with large ingestions, since it has been shown to remove up to 45% of azathioprine.[12] No data support the use of multiple-dose activated charcoal for azathioprine overdose. Single-dose activated charcoal may prove useful but may be complicated by the GI manifestations that preclude its successful administration.

CYCLOSPORINE

Cyclosporine is an 11–amino acid cyclic polypeptide produced by *Beauveria nivea* and *Tolypocladium inflatum Gams*. The amino acids at the 1, 2, 3, and 11 positions form an active site; experimental modifications of the drug have resulted in decreased immunosuppressive activity. Cyclosporine was introduced in the early 1980s and brought with it significant improvements to the field of organ transplantation. It has improved both initial and long-term allograft survival. The use of cyclosporine has also decreased the initial length of stay and the rate of readmission after transplantation. Cyclosporine is used in solid organ transplantation of heart, liver, and kidney as well as for treatment of rheumatoid arthritis and psoriasis. Minimal change, focal segmental, and immunoglobulin A (IgA) nephropathy may also be treated with cyclosporine.[15] It has shown benefit in the initial treatment of type 1 diabetes mellitus. There have been reports of significant decreases in the patient's insulin requirement if cyclosporine therapy is initiated within the first 2 months.[15]

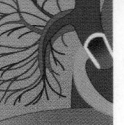

Pharmacology

Cyclosporine reversibly inhibits the proliferation of immunocompetent lymphocytes in G_0 and G_1 phases of the cell cycle, specifically, the T-cell lines. This inhibition of immune activity is accomplished by cyclosporine forming a complex with cyclophilin that binds to and inhibits the activity of the phosphatase, calcineurin. This in turn inhibits the production of the lymphokine, IL-2. IL-2 is a growth factor for the immune system and stimulates the replication of activated immunocompetent lymphocytes. This inhibition is greater in T-helper cells than in T-suppresser cells. The immunosuppressant activity of cyclosporine is largely due to the parent compound, because its metabolites have little pharmacologic activity.

Pharmacokinetics

Two forms of cyclosporine are currently available: Neoral, a microemulsion formulation, and Sandimmune, the conventional formulation. Neoral has significantly better bioavailability and less variability in absorption, both intra- and interindividual. It allows for more consistent dosing. The interindividual oral biovariability can still be quite significant, between 20% and 50% of the area under the curve. This great variability in absorption necessitates frequent drug monitoring to establish and maintain a stable dosing regime. Both forms of cyclosporine are highly lipid soluble, with absorption significantly affected by diet; high-fat meals increase absorption. Cyclosporine has a large volume of distribution, between 3 and 5 L/kg, and is up to 90% protein bound. Cyclosporine is metabolized by the cytochrome P-450 system, specifically CYP3A4, with 94% of metabolites excreted in the bile. A small portion, 6%, is excreted by the kidney, and 0.1% is excreted unchanged. Because excretion mainly is via the bile, there is a potential for enterohepatic recirculation. Cyclosporine has approximately 25 metabolites, none with significant immunosuppressive activity.

SPECIAL POPULATIONS

The pediatric population is notably different from the adult population in the metabolism and excretion of cyclosporine. Clearance has been reported to be enhanced significantly in the pediatric population—up to 40% greater.[15] This difference in clearance may be related to differences in body composition and an apparent decrease in the volume of distribution (Vd) in children. Cyclosporine is classified by the FDA as pregnancy class C but has been used during pregnancy. Placental transfer is estimated to be between 37% and 64%. There is little evidence that cyclosporine adversely affects fetal outcome. Although there does seem to be an increased rate of prematurity and a trend toward fetal malformation and low birth weight, only prematurity reached statistical significance in one meta-analysis.[16]

Cyclosporine clearance is decreased in the geriatric population. It is unclear whether this decrease relates to a decrease in hepatic function or a change in Vd or lipid transport.[15] Cyclosporine clearance has also been found to be decreased in patients with decreased levels of low-density lipoproteins. This most likely represents a decrease in the ability to transport the drug to the liver for metabolism and excretion. Since there is minimal renal excretion of cyclosporine, patients with poor but stable renal function do not require dose adjustment. Greater than 90% of cyclosporine is metabolized in the liver, particularly the cytochrome P-450 system, and then excreted in the bile. A patient with significantly decreased hepatic function requires changes in the dosing regime.

DRUG INTERACTIONS

Owing to the extensive number of drugs that are metabolized via the cytochrome P-450 system, the potential interactions are numerous. Many commonly prescribed therapeutics are metabolized at CYP3A, increasing the risk of potential drug–drug interactions. The macrolides, azole antifungals (e.g., fluconazole), antiretroviral protease inhibitors, and many calcium channel blockers are also known inhibitors of CYP3A. These drugs have the potential to elevate a patient's cyclosporine level either through competition for the active site as a competitive inhibitor or through inhibition of the cytochrome via a secondary allosteric site as a noncompetitive inhibitor.[17] Carbamazepine, a substrate of CYP3A, potentially acts as a competitive inhibitor. Many anticonvulsants such as carbamazepine, phenobarbital, phenytoin, and the glucocorticoids also interact with this cytochrome as inducers, increasing the amount of the enzyme and potentially leading to decreased cyclosporine levels and ineffective immunosuppression. Aminoglycosides, antineoplastics, antifungals such as amphotericin B, NSAIDs, and colchicines are known to cause renal dysfunction; concomitant use with cyclosporine may increase this risk.

Toxicology

Generally, acute toxicity from an oral ingestion is minimal. However, neonates and patients who receive unintentional parenteral overdoses are of concern, for they can develop significant toxicity. Parenteral overdose produces significant morbidity although the number of reported cases is limited. Reported effects, mainly in premature neonates, include worsening renal failure, metabolic acidosis, cyanosis, coma, hyponatremia, and hyperbilirubinemia.[18] There is also a case report of cerebral edema with uncal herniation due to an intravenous cyclosporine overdose.[19] When cyclosporine is used with other drugs that cause nephrotoxicity, synergistic effects could lead to rejection of an allograft. The pattern of nephrotoxicity has been broken down into three classes, all defined by a decrease in glomerular filtration rate (GFR) of 25%. The three classes are defined by the time course as acute (onset within the first 7 days of initiation of treatment), subacute (onset within 7 to 60 days of initiation of treatment), and chronic (onset >30 days after initiation of treatment). Increased serum creatinine, reduced glomerular filtration, and

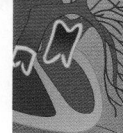

decreased renal plasma flow rates are believed to be secondary to alterations in intrarenal hemodynamic function. Cyclosporine is thought to cause increases in Ca^{2+} influx in response to vasoconstrictors, particularly in the afferent arteriole. Cyclosporine also increases levels of thromboxane A_2. Thromboxane A_2 increases vascular tone in the renal arterioles and myocyte proliferation in the intima of the vessel wall. Alternatively, an alteration in the ratio of thromboxane A_2 to prostacyclin could cause this effect, since thromboxane A_2 is a vasoconstrictor and prostacyclin is a vasodilator.

Many patients taking cyclosporine report neurologic side effects. The complaints consist mainly of paresthesias and numbness, although visual disturbances and coma have been reported. Many symptoms improve upon discontinuation of cyclosporine; however, they often recur upon rechallenge. GI disturbances including nausea and vomiting have been reported. Dysfunction of the biliary tree has been observed, with patients developing cholestasis, cholelithiasis, and hyperbilirubinemia.

Multiple endocrine effects have been noted with cyclosporine use, particularly hyperglycemia. The hyperglycemia is not associated with ketosis, and there is no change in the amount of secreted insulin or in the number of insulin receptors. Hyperglycemia is thought to be related to impaired glycogen synthesis with resulting accumulation of substrate.

Management

Decontamination of the GI tract with activated charcoal is suggested following acute toxic ingestion, particularly since cyclosporine has limited oral bioavailability. Some case reports suggest that multiple-dose activated charcoal decreases the half-life of cyclosporine although it is unclear whether these reported declines in serum levels represent redistribution to the tissues or elimination of the drug.[20,21] In the setting of parenteral overdose, various therapies have been attempted, some being more effective and having a better rationale than others. Plasmapheresis was used in an adult who developed hyperbilirubinemia after a 30 mg/kg unintentional intravenous overdose.[22] Although this therapy would help eliminate drug that was either free or bound to serum proteins, most of the circulating cyclosporine is bound to red blood cells (up to 50%) and 10% is bound to lymphocytes. Consequently, there appears to be little theoretic benefit to this intervention. Exchange transfusion has been used to treat neonatal cyclosporine overdose. In one case report, it produced a 30% reduction in cyclosporine level. In another case report, exchange transfusion was unsuccessful in changing the clinical outcome, and the patient died.[18] The timing of the transfusion in relation to the overdose was unclear. At autopsy, there was significant tissue accumulation of cyclosporine, suggesting sufficient time had elapsed for redistribution to the tissues to occur.

LABORATORY MONITORING

Several methods are used to measure serum cyclosporine concentration. High-performance liquid chromatography

(HPLC) and radioimmunoassay techniques are the most common; these tests have variable sensitivity for the detection of cyclosporine metabolites. Little evidence suggests that measuring acute serum cyclosporine concentrations is helpful in management, particularly since peak levels can be delayed by up to 4 hours. The value in serial cyclosporine levels is more to determine when to resume immunosuppression than to aid in acute management. Serum blood urea nitrogen (BUN), creatinine, transaminases, and bilirubin should be monitored in patients with underlying renal or hepatic dysfunction.

ELIMINATION

Cyclosporine is not effectively removed by hemodialysis or hemoperfusion. It is not known whether charcoal, either in single or multiple doses, is effective in enhancing elimination although multiple-dose activated charcoal has been suggested as an effective means of elimination enhancement. It has also been suggested that CYP3A inducers might be useful therapeutic adjuncts, but little evidence supports its efficacy.

MYCOPHENOLATE MOFETIL

Mycophenolate mofetil is a prodrug that is rapidly metabolized to the active metabolite mycophenolic acid (MPA). MPA is a reversible, noncompetitive inhibitor of inosine monophosphate dehydrogenase, an essential enzyme in the production of purines. B and T lymphocytes have a greater reliance on the de novo pathway of purine synthesis, while other cell lines can use scavenger pathways to meet their metabolic needs. MPA is thus cytostatic in respect to lymphocytes.

Pharmacokinetics

Mycophenolate mofetil is rapidly absorbed and converted to MPA. MPA has a large Vd—3.6 to 4 L/kg—and is up to 97% protein bound. MPA is then metabolized to the phenolic glucuronide (MPAG) form. MPAG is largely excreted by the kidney; 93% is eliminated either by glomerular filtration or secretion from the renal tubule. The remaining MPAG is eliminated in the GI tract via biliary excretion, or it is excreted unchanged. MPAG that has been secreted in the bile and eliminated into the GI tract undergoes enterohepatic recirculation.

The absorption, metabolism, and area under the curve for children are similar to those of adults. Pharmacokinetics have not been studied in the geriatric population.

Because mycophenolate mofetil requires metabolic activation, patients with significantly impaired hepatic function have lower levels of the active form of the drug and less immunosuppressive activity.

Renal elimination is required for the excretion of the inactivated metabolite, and patients with impaired renal function have a prolonged exposure to the active form of the drug. Patients with significantly decreased renal excretion have similar peak drug levels but a decreased

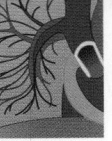
rate of excretion, leading to an enlarged area under the curve compared with that of patients with normal renal function.

Although mycophenolate mofetil has been shown to be teratogenic in animal experiments, it is classified as pregnancy class C.[23]

DRUG INTERACTIONS

Only a few drug–drug interactions have been studied with this agent. Antacids with magnesium and aluminum hydroxides decrease the amount of MPA absorbed. Cholestyramine lowers the area under the curve by interrupting the enterohepatic recirculation, leading to increased drug excretion. MPA decreases the amount of hormone absorbed from oral contraceptives, but what effect that has on suppression of ovulation is unknown. MPAG is excreted through glomerular filtration and tubular secretion; drugs that block this secretion such as probenecid will increase the area under the curve. Alterations in gut flora have the potential to alter the enterohepatic circulation and change the absorption and excretion characteristics of the drug, with less hydrolysis of MPAG, leaving less MPA for reabsorption. There are no reported significant drug interactions with cyclosporine, acyclovir, or ganciclovir. In patients with renal dysfunction, trimethoprim-sulfamethoxazole may compete with MPAG in the renal tubule for secretion into the tubular lumen.

Toxicology

Toxic manifestations of MPA are exaggerated therapeutic effects, consisting primarily of neutropenia.

Adverse effects that have been noted include an increased incidence of GI disturbance, GI bleeding, herpesvirus infection, and neutropenia.

Determination of drug levels is made either by enzyme-mediated immunofluorescence or HPLC.

Management

There are currently no case reports of acute MPA overdose in humans. Rats have been able to tolerate up to 4 g/kg and monkeys up to 1 g/kg; typical adult dosing is 2 to 4 g/day. Since many of therapeutic effects are dose dependent, the toxic manifestations would most likely be exaggerated clinical responses.

As for any overdose, supportive care is essential, with protection of the airway and evaluation of other toxic co-ingestants. Activated charcoal as a single dose may be useful in decreasing absorption of the drug. Evaluating serum drug concentration probably has more utility in determining when to restart MPA than in acute management. Secondary to the large Vd and protein binding of the drug, it is unlikely that either hemodialysis or hemoperfusion would be of significant benefit in enhancing elimination. There is significant enterohepatic recirculation, and animal studies suggest that cholestyramine can interrupt this circulation and possibly enhance elimination. There is also a theoretic rationale for the use of multiple-dose activated charcoal to interrupt enterohepatic recirculation.

REFERENCES

1. Braza TJ, DiCarlo JB, Soon SL, McCall CO: Tacrolimus 0.1% ointment for seborrhoeic dermatitis: an open-label pilot study. Br J Dermatol 2003;148:1242–1244.
2. Walker SL, Kirby B, Chalmers RJ: The effects of topical tacrolimus on severe recalcitrant chronic discoid lupus erythematous. Br J Dermatol 2002;147:405–406.
3. Assmann T, Becker-Wegerich P, Grewe M, et al: Tacrolimus ointment for the treatment of vulvar lichen sclerosus. J Am Acad Dermatol 2003;48:935–937.
4. Travis LB, Weinberg JM, Silverberg NB: Successful treatment of vitiligo with 0.1% tacrolimus ointment. Arch Dermatol 2003;139:571–574.
5. Boumpas DT, Kritikos HD, Daskalakis NG: Perspective on future therapy of vasculitis. Curr Rheumatol Rep 2000;2:423–429.
6. Yamauchi A, Ieiri I, Kataoka Y, et al: Neurotoxicity induced by tacrolimus after liver transplantation: relation to genetic polymorphisms of the ABCB1 (MDR1) gene. Transplantation 2002;74:817–821.
7. Prograf product information. Fujisawa, May 2002. Available at www.fujisawa.com/medinfo/pi/pi_page_pg.htm. Accessed January 6, 2005.
8. Tacrolimus. In Burnham TH (ed): Drug Facts and Comparisons. St. Louis, Facts and Comparisons, 2003, pp 1568c–1570a.
9. Spencer CM, Goa KL, Gillis JC: Tacrolimus: an update of its pharmacology and clinical efficacy in the management of organ transplantation. Drugs 1997;54:925–975.
10. Macphee IAM, Fredericks S, Tai T, et al: Tacrolimus pharmacogenetics: polymorphisms associated with expression of cytochrome P4503A5 and P-glycoprotein correlate with dose requirement. Transplantation 2002;74:1486–1489.
11. Wallemacq PE, Verbeeck RK: Comparative clinical pharmacokinetics of tacrolimus in pediatric and adult patients. Clin Pharmacokinet 2001;49:283–295.
12. Imuran product insert. September 2003 Available at webarchive.org/web/20030901170715/pharmacynetworkgroup.com/imuran-side-effects.htm. Accessed January 6, 2005.
13. Chan GL, Canafax DM, Johnson CA: The therapeutic use of azathioprine in renal transplantation. Pharmacotherapy 1987;7(5):165–177.
14. Schusziarra V, Ziekursch V, Schlamp R, et al: Pharmacokinetics of azathioprine under hemodialysis. Int J Clin Pharmacol Biopharm 1976;14:298–302.
15. Kahan BD, Oates JA, Wood AJ: Cyclosporine. N Engl J Med 1989;321:1725–1738.
16. Bar Oz B, Hackman R, Einarson T, Koren G: Pregnancy outcome after cyclosporine therapy during pregnancy: a meta-analysis. Transplantation 2001;71:1051–1055.
17. Ngheim DD: Role of pharmacologic enhancement of P-450 in cyclosporine overdose. Transplantation 2002;74:1355–1356.
18. Arellano F: Acute cyclosporine overdose: a review of present clinical experience. Drug Saf 1991;6:266–276.
19. De Perrot M, Spiliopoulos A, Cottini S, et al: Massive cerebral edema after IV cyclosporine overdose. Transplantation 2000;70:1259–1260.
20. Honcharik N, Anthone S: Activated charcoal in acute cyclosporine overdose. Lancet 1985;1:1051.
21. Qureshi ST, Smolinske S: Cyclosporin pharmokinetics with multidose charcoal after a ten-fold dosing error. J Toxicol Clin Toxicol 2003;41:747.
22. Kokado Y, Takahara S, Ishibashi M, Sonoda T: An acute overdose of cyclosporine. Transplantation 1989;47:1096–1097.
23. Tendron A, Gouyon JB, Decramer S: In utero exposure to immunosuppressive drugs: experimental and clinical studies. Pediatr Nephrol 2002;17:121–130.

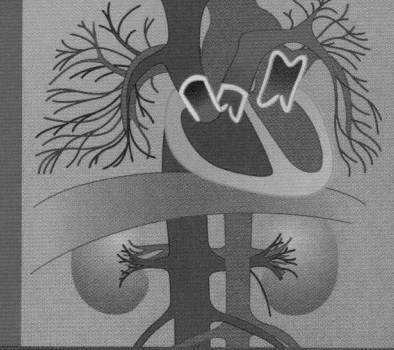

58 *Digitalis*

FRÉDÉRIC LAPOSTOLLE, MD, DMC ■ STEPHEN W. BORRON, MD, MS

At a Glance...

■ Digitalis glycosides (digoxin and digitoxin) are drugs with small therapeutic indices.

■ Digoxin is eliminated primarily via the kidneys, digitoxin by hepatic metabolism.

■ Symptoms of toxicity may be vague, particularly in the elderly, and may involve multiple organ systems.

■ Patients presenting with hyperkalemia, underlying cardiac disease, and advanced age have a poor prognosis.

■ Digitalis Fab fragments may be lifesaving and should be administered early in case of serious poisoning or in the presence of poor prognostic factors.

■ Cardiac conduction abnormalities, gastrointestinal disturbances, and both hypokalemia and hyperkalemia associated with digitalis toxicity are rapidly corrected by the administration of Fab fragments, obviating the need for other therapy.

Digitalis was introduced into clinical medicine by William Withering in 1785, after his investigation of a home remedy used by herbalists in the English countryside.[1,2] He reported therapeutic efficacy and toxicity of leaves of *Digitalis purpurea*, commonly named foxglove. He recommended that digitalis "be continued until it acts either on the kidneys, the stomach, the pulse, or the bowel . . . let it be stopped upon the first appearance of any of these effects and I will maintain that the patient will not suffer from its exhibition, nor the practitioner be disappointed in any reasonable effects."

Thereafter, cardiac glycosides, including digoxin, digitoxin, and ouabain, were extracted from plants and largely prescribed. Nowadays, indications for cardiac glycosides are restricted to the treatment of heart failure with or without associated supraventricular arrhythmia.

Due to a narrow therapeutic index (40% to 60% of the lethal dose is required to achieve the maximal therapeutic effect), digitalis toxicity remains frequent in patients with chronic heart diseases.[3] Less frequently,

digitalis toxicity results from acute overdose in suicide attempts. Digitalis poisoning treatment strategy has been dramatically modified since 1976, with the introduction of digoxin-specific Fab fragments by Smith and colleagues.[4]

SCOPE OF PROBLEM

Digitalis intoxication was once considered the most common adverse drug reaction in U.S. medical practice. Studies from the 1960s and 1970s showed that as many as 15% of all patients in medical admissions were taking digitalis, and 20% to 30% of these patients would have signs of toxicity.[5] Prescribing habits and the incidence of toxicity have begun to change because of (1) better appreciation of digitalis pharmacodynamics and drug interactions, (2) more appropriate maintenance dosage, (3) easy and rapid availability of serum digoxin determinations, and (4) expanded drug therapy for congestive heart failure, eliminating the need to push digitalis to higher, more potentially toxic concentrations. Nevertheless, the number of patients receiving maintenance digitalis therapy remains high, and the numerous common untoward effects still demand attention and understanding. Recently, toxicity associated with chronic digoxin treatment has been reported in 6% to 23% of patients, especially in the elderly.[3,6]

The mortality rate of poisoned patients is poorly documented in cases of chronic intoxications but reaches 25% in cases of acute overdose.[7] Neither pacing nor antidotal treatment has significantly reduced this mortality rate.[7,8]

PHARMACOLOGY

The preparations of cardiac glycosides now used in clinical practice were initially derived from the leaves of plants from the species *D. purpurea*. Other plants that contain cardiac glycosides (e.g., strophanthus, red squill,

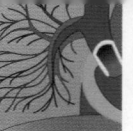

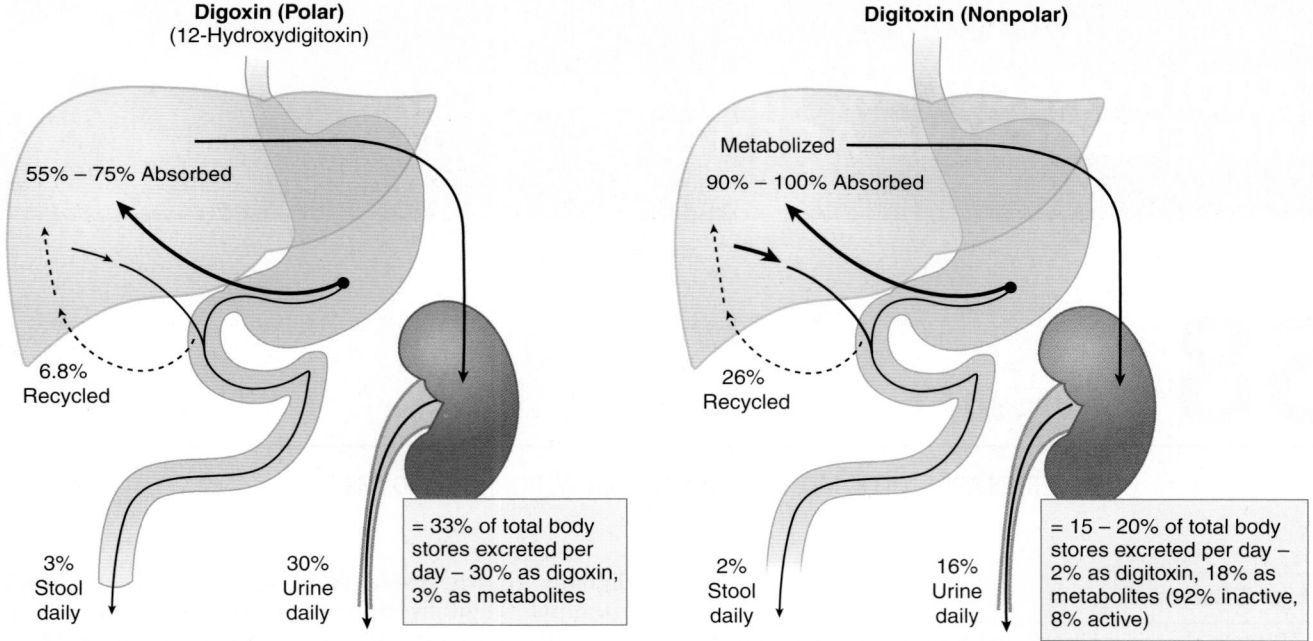

FIGURE 58-1 Digoxin and digitoxin pharmacokinetics, showing average values for absorption, excretion, enterohepatic circulation, and half-life. (From Doherty JE: Digitalis glycosides: pharmacokinetics and their clinical implications. Ann Intern Med 1973;79:229.)

TABLE 58-1 Digoxin and Digitoxin Main Phamacologic Characteristics

	DIGOXIN	DIGITOXIN
Absorption	55%–75% for tablets 90%–100% for liquid or encapsulated liquid	90%–100%
Volume of distribution	5.6 L/kg	0.56 L/kg
Protein binding	25%	95%
Half-life	33–34 hr	6–7 days
Clearance	Renal	Hepatic

and derivatives) have occasionally led to unsuspected cardiac complications. Recently, accidental contamination of dietary supplements by *Digitalis lanata* has been reported.[9]

Several preparations of digitalis are available. However, because of their ease of oral administration and duration of action, only two preparations are used in clinical practice today: digoxin and digitoxin. Their main pharmacologic characteristics are reported in Figure 58-1 and Table 58-1. Digoxin and digitoxin are both passively absorbed from the small intestine. Detailed pharmacodynamic studies have shown that drug action depends on tissue concentration, which is relatively constant in relation to serum concentrations, and that the major depot in humans is skeletal muscle.[10,11] These findings lead to two conclusions: (1) the constant relationship of myocardial digoxin concentration to serum concentration supports measuring serum concentrations to monitor patients' compliance

and toxicity, and (2) dosage requirements and the likelihood of toxicity can be anticipated on the basis of muscle mass and not overall body weight. Digoxin and digitoxin are eliminated differently (see Fig. 58-1). Digoxin is excreted primarily via the renal route, whereas digitoxin is eliminated primarily via metabolic inactivation. Because enterohepatic circulation has a role in the metabolism of both drugs, biliary production affects digitalis elimination. Bioavailability of the drug may vary with different manufacturing processes and malabsorption syndromes and because of inactivation of gut flora, which can be altered by antibiotics.[12] Furthermore, digoxin is one of the breakdown products of digitoxin metabolism (about 8%) (Figs. 58-1 and 58-2).

Basic Mechanism

Digitalis acts at the subcellular level by altering the sodium/potassium-adenosine triphosphatase (Na^+/K^+-ATPase) transport system (Fig. 58-3). The effect is an intracellular gain of Na^+ and loss of K^+ and a corresponding extracellular gain in K^+. Through interaction with Na^+ and Ca^{2+} membrane transporters, an associated intracellular gain of Ca^{2+} is observed. In short, the net effect is a decreased intracellular K^+ concentration and an increased Na^+ and Ca^{2+} concentration. The increased Ca^{2+} augments myofibril interaction in cardiac muscle and leads to positive inotropic action responsible for digitalis's usefulness in clinical practice.[13]

In an intact heart, the effects of digitalis can be separated into mechanical and electrophysiologic actions, with toxicity related to its excessive therapeutic effects and the status of the patient at the time of drug administration.

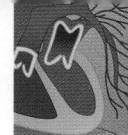

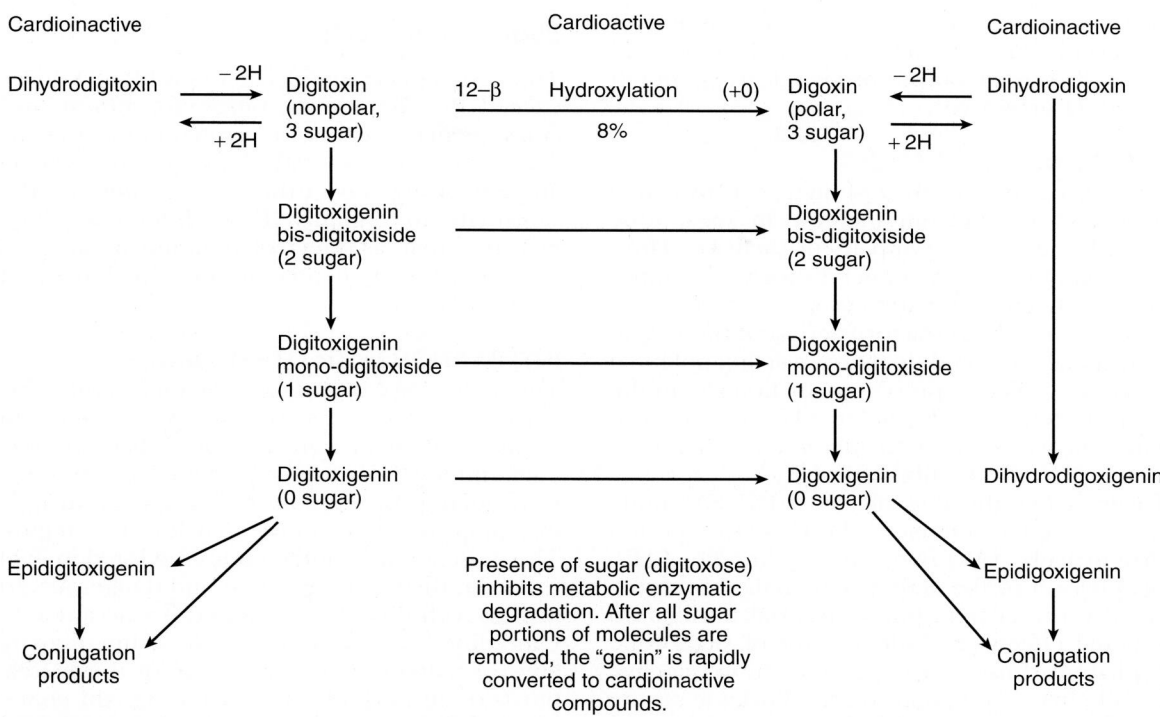

FIGURE 58-2 Metabolic pathways of digoxin and digitoxin. Note that digoxin is part of the metabolic pathway of digitoxin. (From Doherty JE: Digitalis glycosides: pharmacokinetics and their clinical implications. Ann Intern Med 1973;79:229.)

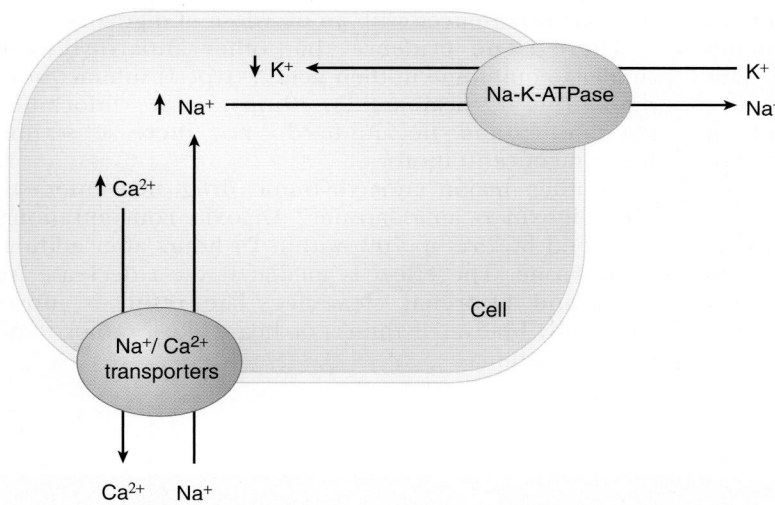

FIGURE 58-3 Cellular interactions between Na⁺/K⁺-ATPase pump and digoxin. Digitalis alters the Na⁺/K⁺-ATPase transport system. The net effect is an intracellular loss of K⁺ and gain of Na⁺ and Ca²⁺. The increased Ca²⁺ augments myofibril interaction in cardiac muscle and leads to positive inotropic action.

Normal Therapeutic Effects on Intact Heart (Summary of Actions)

DIGITALIS INOTROPIC EFFECT

A major therapeutic use for digitalis is for its inotropic effect. Digitalis augments the force of myocardial contraction by increasing the velocity of shortening and the velocity of developed tension of cardiac muscle.[13] Therefore, there is less encroachment on compensatory mechanisms, allowing greater cardiac reserve. In patients with heart failure, digitalis causes a decrease in end-diastolic pressure and volume, increasing cardiac output and stroke work. The usefulness of digoxin for congestive heart failure in patients in sinus rhythm has been the subject of some controversy. However, most conclude that digoxin is a weak inotropic agent.[14,15] The Digitalis Investigators' Group trial and the study by Krum and colleagues demonstrated the usefulness of digoxin in congestive heart failure.[16,17] More precisely, in 1997, The Digitalis Investigators' Group trial[17] showed that although, in comparison with placebo, digitalis treatment did not reduce the mortality rate, it did reduce the rate of hospitalization, including hospitalization for worsening heart disease. In a nonfailing heart, the effects

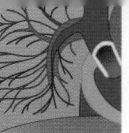

of digitalis are more controversial. Positive inotropic action may occur, but it is not manifested by a measurable change in cardiac output or by a decrease in left ventricular filling pressure.[18]

DIGITALIS CHRONOTROPIC EFFECT

The negative chronotropic effect of digitalis is primarily central, mediated through an increase in vagal tone associated with decreased sympathetic activity. Thus, effects of digitalis may vary, depending on the interaction of drug concentration and autonomic tone.

Digitalis decreases the refractory period of both atrial and ventricular cells and tends to increase action potential amplitude and V_{max}. This improves conduction within the muscle, as reflected in a shortened QT interval. The same mechanism accounts for the increased atrial rate in atrial flutter or atrial flutter-fibrillation.[13]

Digitalis decreases the rate of sinoatrial (SA) node depolarization. Digitalis increases the refractory period of the atrioventricular (AV) node and the bundle of His. It prolongs phase 3 of the action potential, accounting for decreased ventricular response in atrial fibrillation. Some AV nodal effects are independent of vagal tone and affect phase 0, thus decreasing conduction velocity.[1] Most if not all effects of digitalis on the Purkinje system and ventricular muscle are direct effects and do not depend on autonomic interaction.[13]

Digitalis causes significant effects on myocardial automaticity (ability of tissue to undergo spontaneous depolarization) and excitability (ability of tissue to respond to a given stimulus). Inhibition of the Na^+ pump leads to an influx of Na^+ into the cell (see Fig. 58-3). This Na^+ influx increases phase 4 depolarization in all cardiac tissue except the SA node and leads to the appearance of new or latent pacemakers, thus increasing automaticity. This influx also lowers the resting membrane potential threshold, thus increasing excitability.[19]

Na^+ influx also causes delayed afterpotentials (oscillations in transmembrane potentials that follow full repolarizations of the membrane), and this effect provides a logical basis for understanding digitalis-induced arrhythmias.[1,13]

Digitalis Toxicity

The toxic effects that occur when blood concentrations exceed the therapeutic range are almost uniformly a consequence of excessive normal physiologic responses. They can occur in any condition that increases the amount of digitalis in the body or modifies the cardiac sensitivity to digitalis. Drug interactions and other factors, such as electrolyte abnormalities, renal or hepatic failure, ischemia, or inflammation, predispose to digitalis toxicity.

INTERACTION WITH OTHER DRUGS

The importance of drug interactions in the development of digitalis toxicity was not truly appreciated until reliable assays of digoxin concentrations became widespread. Such interactions are important to consider, because introducing or discontinuing these drugs without changing the digoxin dose may lead to a digitoxic state. The most common interactions are listed in Table 58-2.

By far, the most important and dangerous drug interactions with digoxin are caused by the antiarrhythmics. Quinidine[20] causes an increase in serum digoxin in up to 90% of patients. The magnitude of the increase varies but is often twofold. The serum digoxin concentration begins to increase with the onset of quinidine therapy, and the concentration remains elevated as long as both drugs are continued. The adverse effects of elevated digoxin concentrations caused by quinidine are similar to those experienced with an overdose of digoxin.

There is no evidence that other antiarrhythmics similar to quinidine in their action (type I) interact with digoxin.[21-23] Procainamide, disopyramide, lidocaine, mexiletine, and flecainide do not increase serum digoxin concentrations.

Another major antiarrhythmic drug that interacts with digoxin is amiodarone.[24] Digoxin concentrations increased by 25% to 70% within 24 hours after adding amiodarone. The effect is mediated via a decrease in renal and nonrenal clearance. The result is more frequently bradyarrhythmias or heart block rather than tachyarrhythmias.

TABLE 58-2 Agents Affecting Digitalis Pharmacology

ALTERATION	AGENTS
Decreased absorption	Antacids, antibiotics (neomycin, sulfasalazine, p-aminosalicylic acid), bran, cholestyramine, cytotoxic, kaolin-pectin
Increased absorption (less of a problem when the capsule form is used)[12]	Antibiotics inhibiting gut flora (erythromycin and tetracycline), anticholinergics
Inhibited protein binding	Clofibrate, phenobarbital, phenylbutazone, prazosin, warfarin
Increased renal excretion	Hydralazine, levodopa, nitroprusside
Decreased extra renal clearance	Diatiazem, quinidine, verapamil
Decreased volume of distribution	Quinidine
Increased serum digitalis concentration	Amiodarone, aspirin, bepridil, diltiazem, flecainide, ibuprofen, indomethacin, nefidipine, nicardipine, nosoldipine, nitrendipine, propafenone

From Mooradian AD: Digitalis: an update of clinical pharmacokinetics, therapeutic monitoring techniques and treatment recommendations. Clin Pharmacokinet 1988;15(3):165–179.

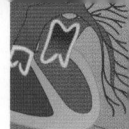

The interaction between Ca^{2+} channel–blocking drugs and digoxin varies greatly.[20-22] The dihydropyridines (nifedipine, amlodipine, isradipine, nicardipine) have minimal or no effect, and diltiazem has such a small effect that toxicity is unlikely. On the other hand, verapamil increases serum digoxin concentrations as much as 70% by altering renal and extrarenal clearance, which can lead to lethal cardiac toxicity.[21,25]

Other antiarrhythmics, such as sotalol, aprindine, ajmaline, and moricizine, do not affect digoxin concentrations.[21,22]

Potentially toxic interaction may also occur with potassium-sparing diuretics (such as spironolactone), which inhibit tubular secretion of digoxin; with antihypertensive agents, which can significantly alter renal reperfusion and glomerular filtration rate; and with anti-inflammatory drugs, especially indomethacin, in neonates or patients with renal dysfunction.

Some antiadrenergic agents, such as clonidine, methyldopa, reserpine, and β blockers, in combination with digitalis, may lead to severe bradyarrhythmias, especially in patients with SA node disease.[21,22]

Reports have shown toxicity in patients with myocarditis when cyclosporine is added to digoxin in patients who have heart failure.[26] Aside from the drug interactions discussed earlier, renal dysfunction leading to decreased renal excretion of digitalis is the major factor leading to the increased total of digitalis throughout the body. Neither dialysis nor cardiopulmonary bypass causes much body loss of digitalis.

ALTERING SENSITIVITY TO DIGITALIS

Toxicity from digitalis is not limited to situations that increase total body concentration of the drug but can develop with any condition that modifies the cardiac sensitivity to digitalis. These include myocardial infarction or ischemia, myocarditis, cardiomyopathy, amyloidosis, and other trauma, including surgery. A healthy heart tolerates large amounts of digitalis, whereas diseased myocardium appears to develop arrhythmias at lower serum concentrations.[27] The myocardial disease leads to local areas of altered electrophysiology, which in turn can cause variation in digitalis uptake by cardiac tissue. The concentration differences and local ischemia lead to variation of cellular recovery times and set the stage, once again, for reentry phenomena. Intrinsic cardiac disease alone may produce similar rhythm disturbances, several of which are common in acute myocardial infarction. These rhythm disturbances have no specific distinguishing feature. However, digitalis toxicity can be implicated in most instances when withdrawal of the drug is followed by resolution of the arrhythmia. This increased sensitivity does not preclude careful use of digitalis when clinically indicated.[28]

ALTERING METABOLISM

Metabolic factors are important in myocardial sensitivity to digitalis.[22,29] Electrolyte abnormalities, especially hypokalemia and hypocalcemia, are well known, but aberrations of magnesium are important to consider. Other metabolic abnormalities, including acidosis,

---

BOX 58-1 FACTORS PREDISPOSING TO DIGITALIS INTOXICATION

Patient-related Factors
Old age
Severe heart disease
Myocardial infarction
Myocarditis
Recent cardiac surgery
Cor pulmonale
Renal failure
Hemodialysis
Hypothyroidism
Anoxia
Amyloidosis

Electrolyte Abnormalities
Hypokalemia
Hypernatremia
Hypercalcemia
Hypomagnesemia
Alkalosis

Drugs
Diuretics
Steroids
Reserpine
Catecholamines
Quinidine
Verapamil
Amiodarone
Cyclosporine

---

alkalosis, hypoxemia, and hyperthermia, may alter digitalis's effect but are probably not independent risk factors. Diseases of other organ systems, especially chronic lung disease and hypothyroidism, predispose patients to digitalis toxicity. Acute cerebrovascular events may lead to toxicity by large sympathetic discharge, which may lower the arrhythmia threshold. Boxes 58-1 and 58-2 contain a more complete list.

CLINICAL PRESENTATION

Pathophysiology

Digitalis toxicity represents the result of the interactions of the drug on the transmembrane potentials and ionic current flows of the cardiac cells (direct effects) and those effects related to the autonomic nervous system (indirect). These interactions have various results depending on which cells are affected; they are expressed as abnormalities of atrial, AV nodal, or ventricular pathology. The mechanism of digitalis cardiotoxic rhythms may result from depression of conduction or alteration of impulse formation, with increased heterogeneity of refractory periods.

Manifestations

CARDIAC

Cardiac manifestations are frequent and dangerous presentations of digitalis toxicity.[7,29] A healthy heart rarely has any signs of toxicity unless the ingested quantity is high. Therefore, accidental overdoses, especially in children, rarely present any cardiac findings but may show AV conduction disturbances. On the other hand, a diseased heart is prone to lethal arrhythmias. No arrhythmias are pathognomonic of digitalis toxicity because similar rhythms may represent underlying disease. A change in the rhythm, especially decreased pulse rate, may be the most important clue. Never-

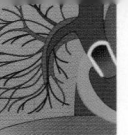

BOX 58-2	DIGOXIN PHARMACOKINETIC INTERACTIONS

Bioavailability

Decreased
Cathartics
Antacids
Cholesterol-binding agents
Malabsorption syndromes
Bowel edema
Eubacterium lentum
Gastric hyperacidity

Increased
Lanoxicaps or elixir
Antibiotics (*E. lentum*)
Omeprazole

Distribution

Decreased
Renal failure
Hyperkalemia
Aging
Hypothyroidism
Amiodarone

Increased
Hypokalemia
Hyperthyroidism
Pregnancy
Physical activity

Elimination

Decreased
Renal failure
Excessive diuretics
Aging
Indomethacin
Cyclosporine
Spironolactone
Verapamil
Quinidine
Propafenone

Increased
Diarrhea
Vasodilators

From Lewis RP: Clinical use of serum digoxin concentrations. Am J Cardiol 1992;69:97G.

BOX 58-3	RHYTHM AND CONDUCTION DISTURBANCES IN DIGITALIS INTOXICATION

Excitant

Atrial premature beats
Atrial tachycardia
Atrial flutter (rare)
Atrial fibrillation (rare)
Junctional premature beats
Accelerated junctional rhythms
Ventricular premature beats, bigeminy and multiformed
Ventricular tachycardia
Bidirectional tachycardia
Ventricular fibrillation

Suppressant

Sinus bradycardia
Sinoatrial block
Type I second-degree AV block (Wenckebach)
Bundle branch block
Complete AV block
Type II second-degree AV block (?)

Combination Excitant and Suppressant

Atrial tachycardia with AV block
Sinus bradycardia with junctional tachycardia
Wenckebach with junctional premature beats
Regularization of ventricular rhythm with atrial fibrillation

AV, atrioventricular.

theless, toxicity should be suspected in any patient receiving the medication and exhibiting evidence of depressed conduction, alteration of impulse formation (automaticity), or both.

Depressed conduction is related to slowing of SA and AV nodal conduction and prolonged nodal refractoriness from high vagal tone, but at high concentrations, digitalis may directly prolong AV nodal refractoriness. Thus, blocks of all types may be observed[30] (Box 58-3).

SA nodal block is relatively common since impulse-forming alterations from digitalis toxicity are often manifested as suppression of atrial pacemakers, primarily the SA node. SA nodal block may range from sinus pauses to the SA nodal Wenckebach phenomenon or to total SA nodal exit block. The resultant arrhythmia is frequently sinus bradycardia, which may be quite severe, especially in elderly patients and in those with SA node disease (Fig. 58-4).

First-degree AV block (i.e., with prolonged PR interval), from digitalis is indistinguishable from other causes (Fig. 58-5).

Second-degree AV block, with intermittent dropped beats, may be Mobitz type I (Wenckebach) or Mobitz type II (see Fig. 58-5). The resultant heart rhythm may be complicated by accelerated junctional escape beats.

Third-degree block, or complete AV dissociation, is usually associated with a narrow QRS escape focus at adequate rates, and hemodynamic alterations are rare in the absence of other cardiac abnormalities (Fig. 58-6).

Alterations of impulse formation may be divided into those that suppress higher pacemakers or those that excite lower pacemakers. Suppression of higher pacemakers is limited primarily to direct effect on the sinus node. Excitation is due to increased frequency of discharge of junctional or ventricular pacemakers, taking the form of accelerated junctional or accelerated ventricular tachycardias. The combination of suppressant and excitant effects should be considered digitalis toxicity until proven otherwise (Fig. 58-7). However, as

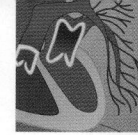

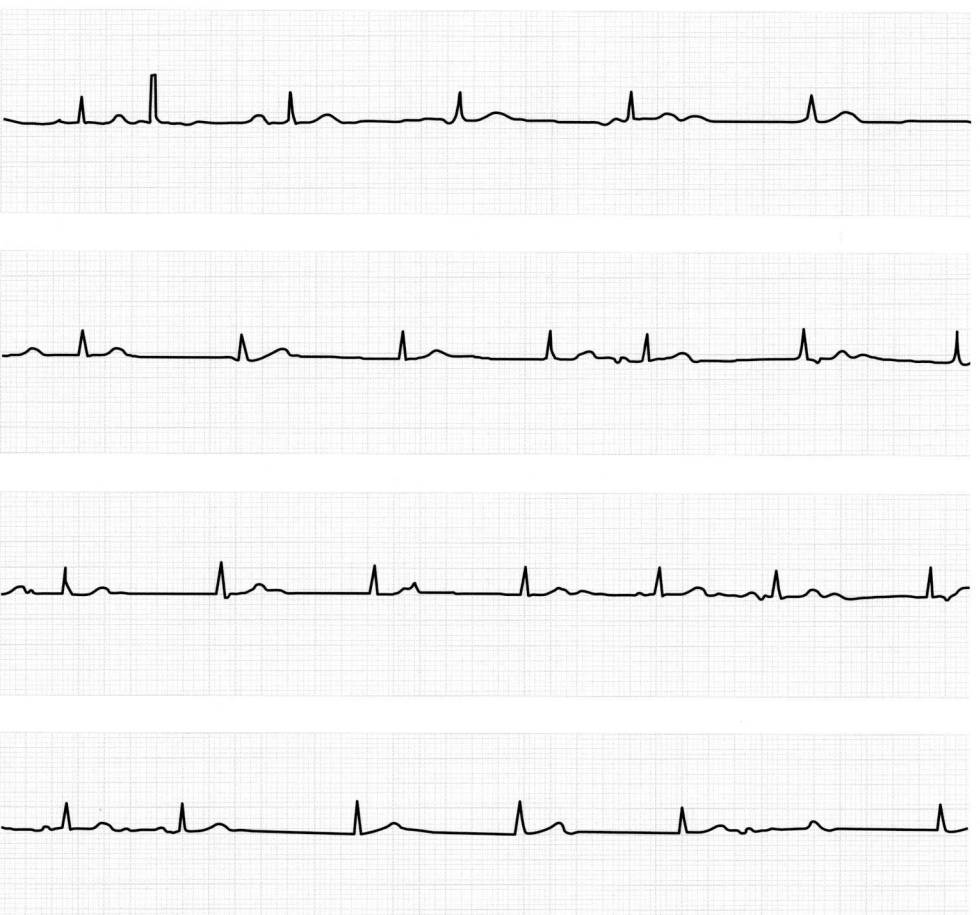

FIGURE 58-4 The electrocardiogram of an 82-year-old woman recently begun on digitalis shows sinus rhythm with sinus arrest and atrioventricular dissociation with slow atrial escape and faster junctional escape rhythm.

the number of older patients with intrinsic cardiac disease increases, these arrhythmias are not specific for digitalis toxicity. Digitalis toxicity results in an exacerbation of the drug's normal effects on refractory periods of the conduction system and myocardial cells. Increased heterogeneity of the refractory periods allows for the development of reentry phenomena, which are the probable mechanisms for the development of tachyarrhythmias. Myriad extrasystoles may be seen, such as premature ventricular contractions (PVCs) (see Fig. 58-7), ventricular parasystole, or ventricular or bidirectional tachycardia. The PVCs may be multiformed, bigeminal, paired, or in couplets. Before more current therapy, ventricular tachycardia related to digitalis toxicity carried a 50% mortality rate. Bidirectional tachycardia was almost always fatal.

Conduction and rhythm disturbances can be seen in combination, resulting in various electrocardiographic presentations. The rhythms are usually manifested by an increased sinus rate with block or second-degree AV block with accelerated lower pacer. Examples are atrial fibrillation with slow ventricular response rate resulting in irregular bradycardia, or Wenckebach block with accelerated junctional escape beats (Fig. 58-8). Even

though nonspecific, digitalis toxicity should always be considered when this type of arrhythmia is encountered.

NONCARDIAC

Digitalis intoxication induces noncardiac as well as cardiac clinical effects.[3,31,32] Gastrointestinal manifestations are present in both acute and chronic intoxication. Anorexia, nausea, and vomiting are common. These symptoms often occur early and may be the presenting complaint. In patients on chronic digitalis treatment, onset of these symptoms has to be considered a possible overdose symptom. Other gastrointestinal complaints are less common. Neurologic and visual manifestations are also frequent and range from headache and fatigue and weakness, to depression, confusion, disorientation, aphasia, delirium, and hallucinations. The visual disturbances of blurring and alteration in color are less common. A more complete list and incidence can be found in Table 58-3. In this study, vigorous attempts were made to establish digitalis as the cause of these symptoms.[31] Digitalis intoxication should always be considered in patients, particularly in the elderly, who are receiving digitalis therapy and present with vague gastrointestinal complaints, malaise, or altered mental status.[6,32]

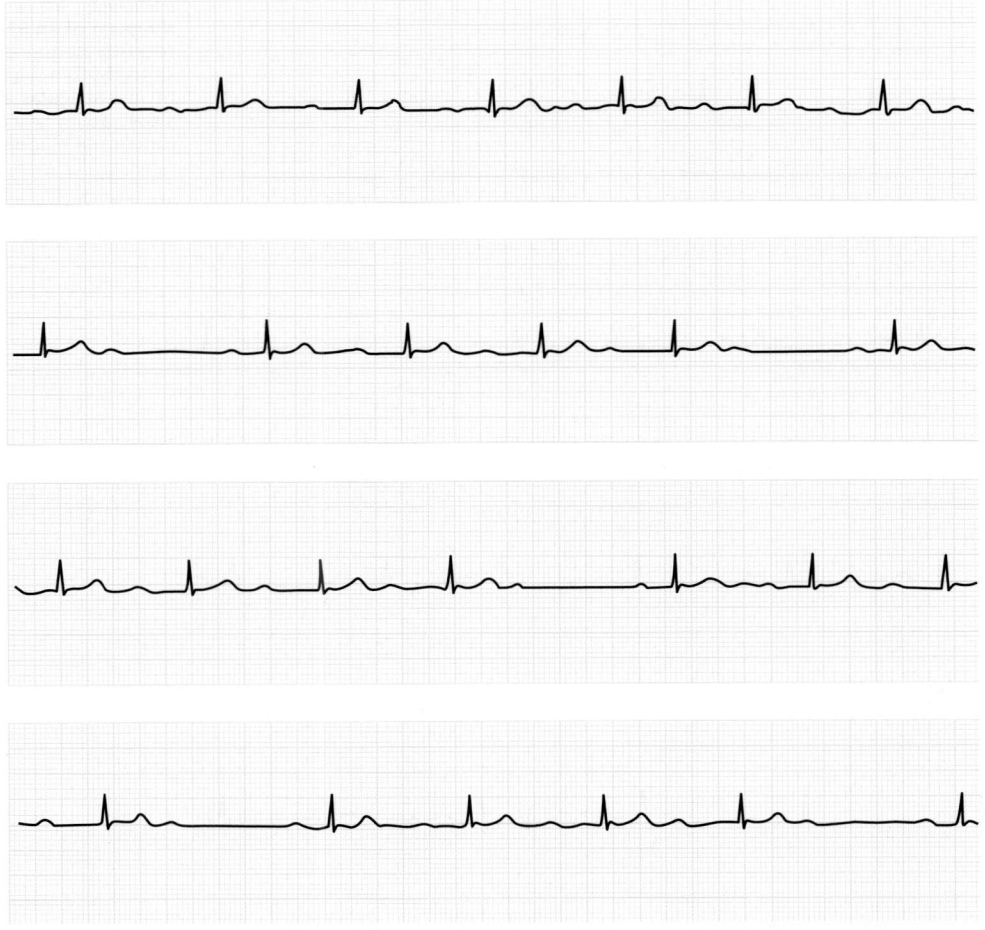

FIGURE 58-5 An 82-year-old man was referred for slow pulse. An electrocardiogram (ECG) 1 day before the present ECG showed 2:1 heart block. The patient was taking digoxin, 0.25 mg/day. Strips show first-degree atrioventricular (AV) block and 5:4 AV nodal block with a narrow QRS complex.

LABORATORY DERANGEMENTS

As previously mentioned, the mechanism of cellular digitalis toxicity directly induces hyperkalemia, which is significantly correlated with digitalis poisoning severity and mortality. Mortality rates are greater in patients with serum potassium greater than 4.5 mEq/L, approaching 35% in patients with serum potassium greater than 5 mEq/L, and 100% in patients with concentrations greater than 6.4 mEq/L.[33] A recent retrospective review has confirmed the importance of hyperkalemia as a poor prognostic indicator in digitalis poisoning.[34]

DIAGNOSIS

Acute overdose may result from accidental or suicidal overdose in patients, whether or not previously treated by digitalis.[7,35,36] In such cases, the main challenge is early detection of digitalis toxicity. Recognition of chronic digitalis toxicity requires a high index of suspicion among patients manifesting any of the cardiac or noncardiac symptoms mentioned earlier. In both cases, definitive diagnosis is via serum digitalis determinations.

Digitalis Concentrations

The concentration of digitalis in the serum is the net result of whole body absorption, distribution, and excretion. Measurement of serum concentrations is currently the cornerstone of digitalis poisoning diagnosis.

The range of therapeutic concentration is 0.5 to 2.0 ng/mL for digoxin and 10 to 30 ng/mL for digitoxin. Due to the lack of specificity of digitalis poisoning symptoms, serum concentrations must be liberally obtained

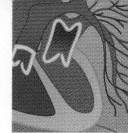

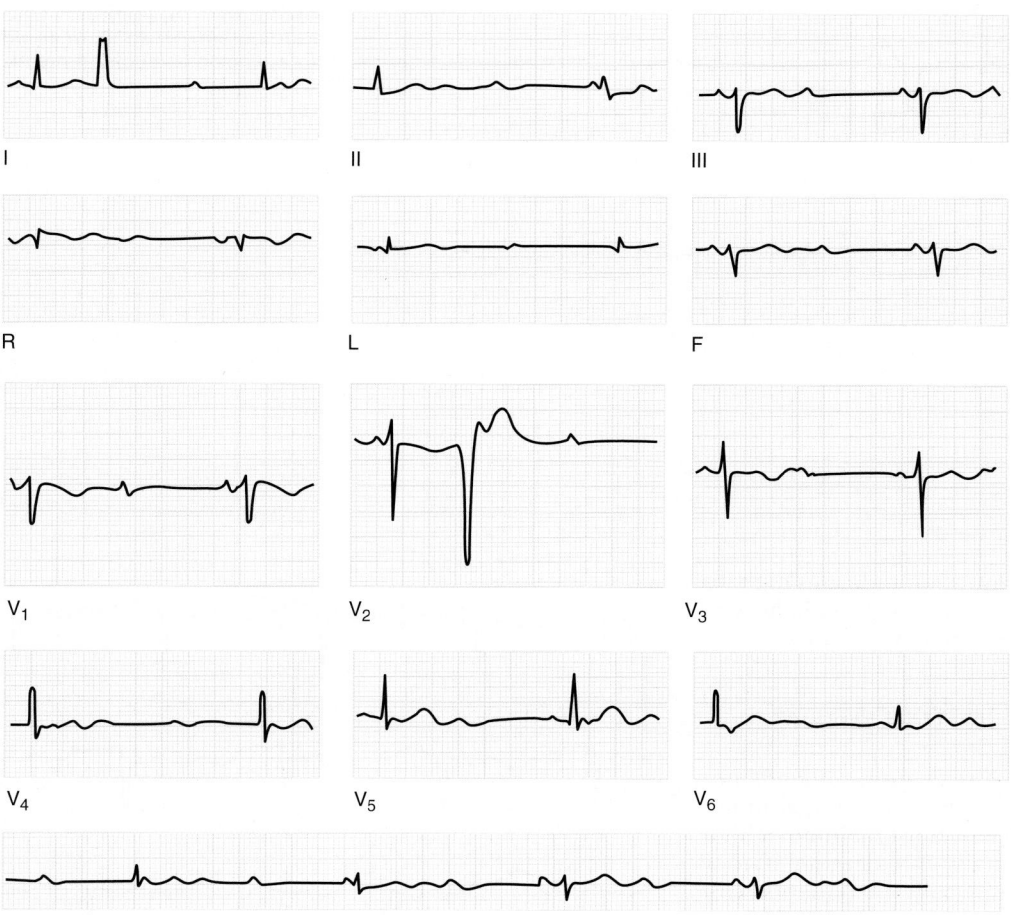

FIGURE   58-6 Electrocardio-gram (ECG) of a 79-year-old woman admitted with shortness of breath and weight loss. She was receiving maintenance digoxin therapy. The ECG shows atrioven-tricular (AV) dissociation secondary to a high-grade AV block with a narrow QRS complex.

in chronically treated patients who experience gastro-intestinal symptoms, malaise, or any change from baseline rhythm disturbances. However, serum concentrations are not always diagnostic; major problems remain in diag-nosing toxicity.

Assays of different digitalis preparations often overlap, and accurate interpretation of results is possible only if the exact preparation is known.

False-positive elevations may occur for several reasons. For example, spironolactone and hyperbilirubinemia interfere with the test. Far more frequent is a false-positive assay result in patients with chronic renal failure. This elevation is thought to be caused by an endogenous circulating digoxin-like substance, which has been reported in more than 60% of patients with chronic renal insufficiency.[37]

Clinical correlations of therapeutic and toxic concentrations all have been made at steady-state concentrations. These concentrations are reached 6 to 8 hours after administration, and any measurements made before this time may give values two to three times greater than at steady-state concentrations. Digoxin undergoes bimodal elimination; thus, measurements made in the first few hours of administration (α elimi-nation phase) do not correspond with toxicity. As the

α elimination phase begins, concentrations more closely approach steady-state concentrations and correspond better with toxicity.

Defining a toxic digitalis concentration is difficult because serum concentrations of patients with and without clinical toxicity overlap considerably. Figure 58-9 demonstrates this problem in an older study, but a more complete list is found in the review by Smith.[38]

Multiple factors, previously detailed, predispose patients to toxicity at concentrations well below 2 ng/mL, usually considered the upper limit of normal. Hypokalemia is the most important of these. Hypoxia caused by chronic pulmonary disease or advanced forms of heart disease is also important. Factors enhancing digitalis sensitivity are listed in Boxes 58-1 and 58-2.[22]

In summary, serum concentrations should be used as a guide to appropriate therapeutic doses and as an indication of toxicity. Serum concentrations also may verify drug compliance and aid dose regulation in patients with changing renal function, those who have undergone cardiac surgery, or those with severe congestive heart failure. It must be emphasized that toxicity cannot be diagnosed from serum concentrations alone. Special consideration must be given to those patients with underlying problems. In general, an

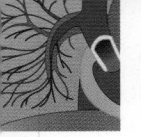

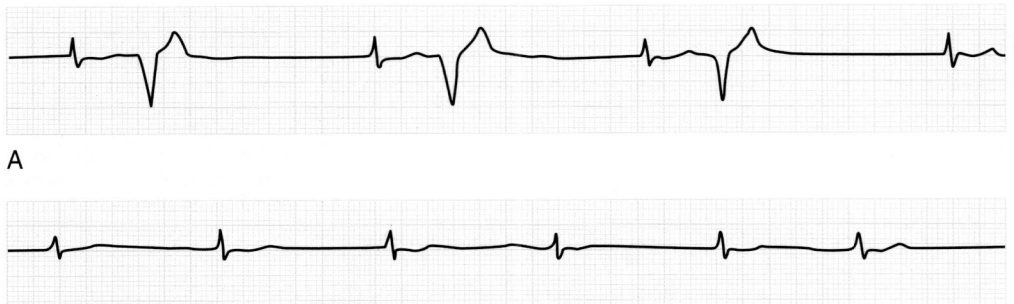

FIGURE 58-7 **A,** Admission electrocardiogram of an 89-year-old with a digoxin level of 2.4 ng/mL. **B,** One day later.

increased serum digitalis concentration indicates digitalis toxicity in patients chronically treated with digitalis who are manifesting cardiac or noncardiac symptoms.

THERAPY OF DIGITALIS INTOXICATION

Successful therapy of digitalis intoxication depends not only on early recognition but also on early and, at times, aggressive management. Physicians must maintain a high index of suspicion about digitalis intoxication if they are to make this diagnosis, especially in patients with predisposing factors, such as old age, renal disease, chronic lung disease, or quinidine use. Most of these patients suffer from chronic overdose, rather than severe suicidal or accidental acute ingestion. In unusual circumstances, such as involuntary plant poisoning or poisoning through herbal supplements, the diagnosis may be particularly elusive.[9,32,39-42] It should be remembered that gastrointestinal manifestations, such as anorexia, nausea, or vomiting, are often the first clinical signs in these rare poisonings. In these circumstances, electrocardiographic manifestations and hyperkalemia should strongly increase the suspicion of digitalis poisoning, calling for measurement of serum digitalis concentrations.

When digitalis poisoning is diagnosed, precocious treatment, including antidotal therapy, should be considered.

Conventional Therapy

GASTROINTESTINAL DECONTAMINATION

A single dose of activated charcoal should be used in patients with acute poisoning if the patient has ingested a potentially toxic dose of digitalis and if charcoal can be administered during the first 2 hours following ingestion.[43] Neither repeated charcoal administration in acute poisoning nor single-dose charcoal administration in patients with chronic overdose has been demonstrated to be of value.[44]

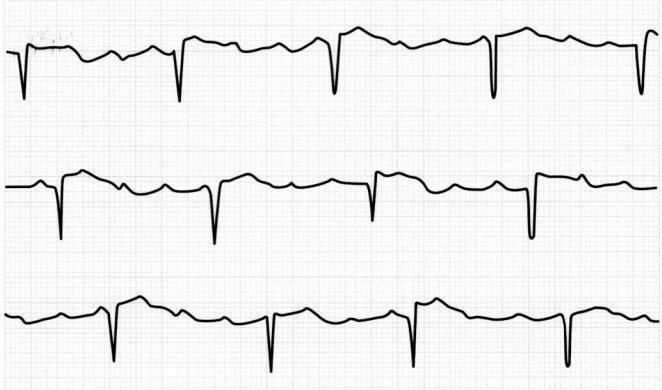

FIGURE 58-8 This rhythm strip shows atrial tachycardia with block. There is an atrial rate of approximately 150 beats/min with a 3:1 block.

TABLE 58-3 Noncardiac Symptoms of Digitalis Toxicity

	DEFINITE INTOXICATION (%)	POSSIBLE INTOXICATION (%)	NO INTOXICATION (%)
Vomiting	48	30	27
Anorexia	34	27	18
Dizziness	14	19	23
Fatigue	14	16	11
Visual disturbances	9	5	7
Syncope	6	3	2
Abdominal pain	6	4	0
Diarrhea	2	2	2
Headache	0	2	0
Delirium	0	1	0

Modified from Mahdyoon H, Battilana G, Rosman H, et al: The evolving pattern of digoxin intoxication: observations at a large urban hospital from 1980 to 1988. Am Heart J 1990;120:1189

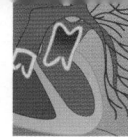

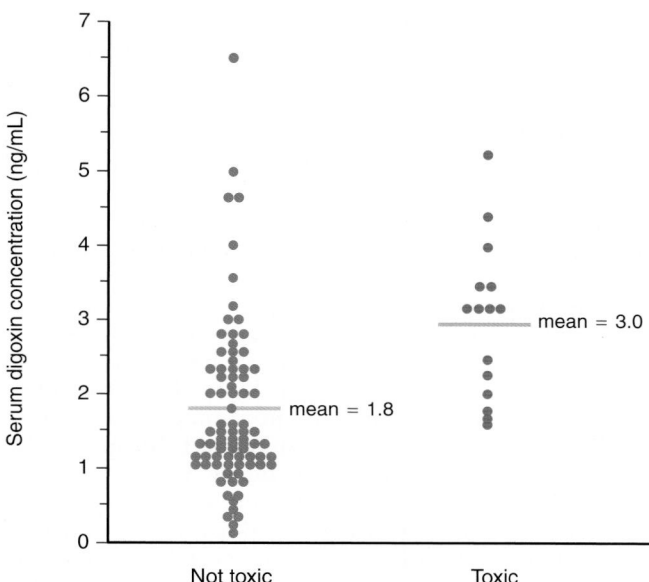

FIGURE 58-9 Results of 100 serum digoxin radioimmunoassay measurements. Sixteen patients were believed to be clinically toxic; their mean serum level was 3.0 ng/mL. Seven patients thought to be nontoxic also had serum levels of more than 3.0 ng/mL. Overlap of normal toxic values does occur; therefore, judgment must be used when evaluating results. (From Doherty JE: Digitalis glycosides: pharmacokinetics and their clinical implications. Ann Intern Med 1973;79:229.)

EXTRACORPOREAL REMOVAL TECHNIQUES

There are no data to support the use of any extracorporeal removal techniques in acute or chronic digitalis poisoning.

CORRECTION OF ELECTROLYTE DISORDERS

Correction of hypokalemia and dehydration are important in cases of chronic toxicity. However, the pathophysiologic mechanism of hypokalemia should be kept in mind, and care should be taken to avoid secondary hyperkalemia. It is generally recommended that calcium be avoided in the treatment of hyperkalemia in digitalis poisoning, due to concerns that intracellular calcium concentrations are already elevated and that administration of further calcium may lead to life-threatening dysrhythmias. This notion has been called into question by Kuhn, who cites a study by Nola and colleagues in dogs, which demonstrated that calcium could safely be administered in digitalis toxicity, so long as the serum calcium did not exceed 20 mg/dL.[44] A more recent paper by Hack and colleagues[45] demonstrated that calcium can be safely administered in a pig model of acute digitalis intoxication. Caution should be exercised, however, in overinterpretation of these studies, which involved acute contemporaneous digitalis and calcium administration, rather than administration of calcium in a model with extant digitalis intoxication (with sufficient time to observe poisoning of the Na/K-ATPase pump). More importantly, it should also be remembered that antidotal treatment with Fab

fragments corrects hyperkalemia,[35] so that administration of calcium for hyperkalemia should probably be reserved (if ever used) for those situations in which digitalis Fab fragments are not available.

TREATING BRADYCARDIA OR OTHER BRADYARRHYTHMIAS

Severe bradycardia and bradyarrhythmias are often related to increased vagal tone. Treatment is crucial, because bradyarrhythmias increase the risk for life-threatening ventricular arrhythmias.

Atropine is the treatment of first choice. A trial of 0.5 mg atropine may be given intravenously and repeated up to a total dose of 2.0 mg. Large cumulative doses of atropine may lead to anticholinergic encephalopathy.

Adrenergic agonists, such as isoproterenol, should be avoided, because the risk for precipitating more severe arrhythmias is high due to their dromotropic effects.

TREATING ECTOPY

One half to three fourths of patients developing high-grade ventricular tachyarrhythmias from digitalis toxicity will die. Early, aggressive therapy is essential in these situations. The following agents should be considered:

Cardiac pacing. Cardiac pacing can be used to treat bradycardia and bradyarrhythmias and to prevent ventricular arrhythmias.[7,8] But pacing is not immediately available everywhere and is associated with life-threatening ventricular arrhythmias and with other nonfatal complications, such as infection. As a rule, it should be performed only if treatment by Fab fragments is not rapidly available. A recent article by Chen and colleagues suggests that pacing can be safely performed in patients with chronic digitalis poisoning. The authors caution against its use in digitalis intentional overdose.[46]

Magnesium. The use of intravenous magnesium sulfate in digitalis toxicity has theoretical indications, especially if the magnesium concentration is low. Magnesium may be considered even when the magnesium concentration is normal or high if, as is often the case, the potassium concentration is elevated.[47] Magnesium potentiates Na/K-ATPase activity without affecting binding of proteins. Hypermagnesemia and related side effects may occur, particularly in patients with renal dysfunction. It is unlikely to appear, however, with an initial bolus of 10 to 20 mmol. Magnesium sulfate generally is packaged as 1.5 to 3 g of magnesium sulfate in 10 or 20 mL. Intravenous use for a cardiac emergency is 3 g diluted to 100 mL and given over 10 minutes. This is often repeated once, followed by maintenance intravenous drips, while monitoring the magnesium and potassium concentrations.

Other antiarrhythmic drugs, such as lidocaine and phenytoin, quinidine, procainamide, disopyramide, calcium channel blockers, and β blockers, have been previously used. Efficacy was poor and

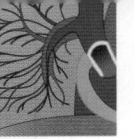

the risk for side effects high. Nowadays, antidotal treatment is the first-line treatment for digitalis poisoning.

Cardioversion. Direct current countershock should be the last resort in life-threatening arrhythmias, and if used, the lowest effective energy level for cardioversion is suggested. Even at low energy levels, the highest mortality rates for direct current cardioversion occur in digitalis toxicity. It should be performed only if treatment by Fab fragments is not rapidly available.

ANTIDOTAL THERAPY

The most immediate decision for the physician treating suspected digitalis overdose concerns the need for antidotal therapy. Digitalis in massive doses may be lethal after suicidal or accidental overdoses, which are not uncommon. Resultant ventricular arrhythmias are responsible for a high mortality rate, reaching 25% in recent studies.[4,35,36] The end result is asystole and finally a complete loss of any cardiac electric activity.

The best method for treating very high concentrations of digitalis poisoning is the use of digoxin-specific polyclonal antibody fragments (Fab). The first report of their use appeared in 1976 (Fig. 58-10).[4] Efficacy and safety have since been clearly demonstrated

in acute and chronic poisonings in adults and in children. The fragments (molecular weight 50,000 Daltons) neutralize digoxin and digitoxin toxicity by reversing tissue binding of digitalis. Bound digitalis reaches high concentrations in the plasma, but the relatively small molecular size allows glomerular filtration and rapid excretion.

Two methods of antidotal treatment with Fab fragments have been proposed,[48] equimolar neutralization in patients with life-threatening poisoning and semiequimolar neutralization in patients with less severe intoxication and/or poor prognostic risk factors, although the latter has not been subjected to clinical trial. In effect, survival of patients who experience cardiac arrest due to digitalis poisoning is very poor. Smolarz and colleagues first suggested "prophylactic" neutralization to prevent secondary ventricular life-threatening arrhythmias.[49] Woolf and colleagues recommended the same strategy in poisoned children.[50] Taboulet and colleagues recently suggested the following approach. Once again, it should be emphasized that "semimolar neutralization" has not been subjected to controlled clinical trials, although it has been routinely employed in France for several years.[48]

In patients with life-threatening intoxication, immediate equimolar neutralization:

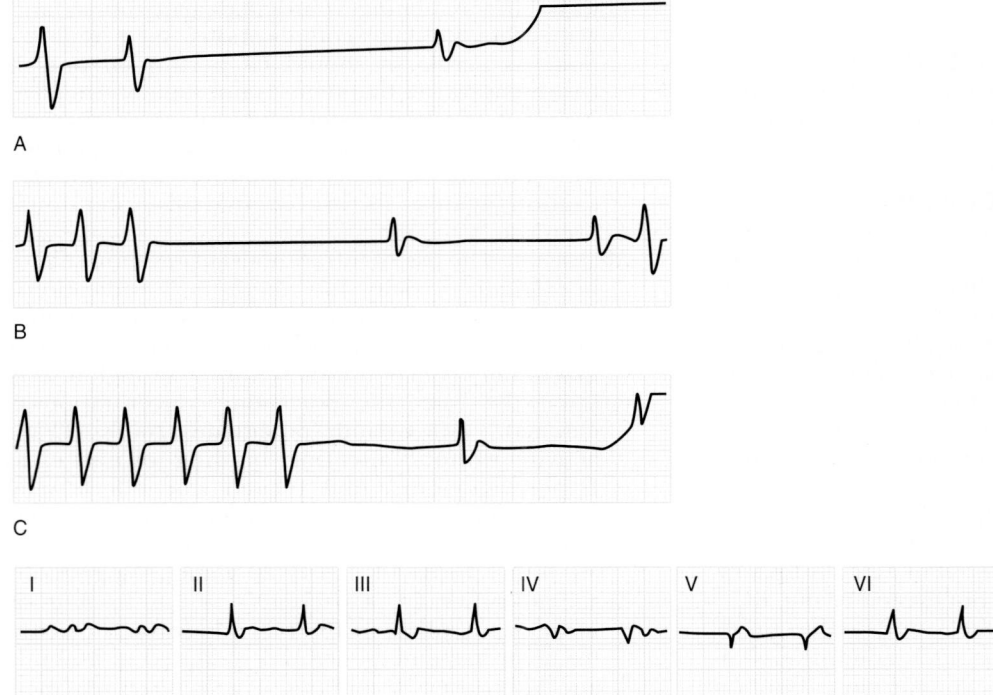

FIGURE 58-10 Sequential electrocardiograms recorded before, during, and after treatment with digoxin-specific Fab fragments. **A,** In the tracing recorded immediately before the start of Fab infusion, serum potassium level is 8.7 mEq/L; the escape interval when pacer stimulus is reduced below threshold is 4.60 seconds. **B,** In the tracing recorded 15 minutes after the start of Fab infusion, serum potassium level is 8.0 mEq/L; the escape interval is 3.96 seconds. **C,** In the tracing recorded 30 minutes after the start of Fab infusion, the escape interval is 2.76 seconds. **D,** In the tracing recorded 2 hours after the start of Fab infusion, the serum potassium level is 7.4 mEq/L; a sinus mechanism is present at a rate of 75 beats/min, with first-degree atrioventricular block (P-R interval of 0.24 second). (From Smith TW, Haber E, Yeatman L, Butler VP Jr: Reversal of advance digoxin intoxication with Fab fragments of digoxin-specific antibodies. N Engl J Med 1976;294:797.)

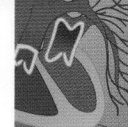

1. Asystole
2. Ventricular arrhythmia (fibrillation or tachycardia)
3. Bradycardia: heart rate less than 40 beats/min (after atropine venous infusion)
4. Serum potassium greater than 5.0 mmol/L

In patients with severe intoxication and/or bad prognostic risk factors, semimolar neutralization:

1. Patients older than 55 years
2. Patients with cardiac disease
3. Bradycardia: heart rate less than 60 beats/min (after intravenous atropine)
4. Second- or third-degree SA or AV blocks
5. Serum potassium greater than 4.5 mmol/L

Antidotal treatment is efficacious in the treatment of digitalis-induced cardiac as well as noncardiac disturbances. Hyperkalemia is best treated by Fab fragments. All others symptoms, including gastrointestinal symptoms, disappear after Fab fragment infusion.

The dose of Fab fragments to administer is determined by calculating digitalis body load.[7,8] Digitalis body load may be estimated, based on supposed ingested digitalis amount (in acute poisoning) or by measured digitalis blood concentrations. When these data are not available, in cases of acute toxicity, empirical dosing recommendations are that 20 vials (760 mg) of Digibind (GloxoSmithkline, Research Triangle Park, NC) is adequate to treat most life-threatening ingestions in both adults and children. However, in children it is important to monitor for volume overload. The physician may consider administering 10 vials, observing the patient's response, and following with an additional 10 vials if clinically indicated.

In cases of chronic intoxication, for adults, six vials (228 mg) usually is adequate to reverse most cases of toxicity. This dose can be used in patients who are in acute distress or for whom a serum digoxin or digitoxin concentration is not available. In infants and small children (weighing less than or equal to 20 kg), a single vial usually should suffice.

Total digitalis body load is calculated in Box 58-4. The rate of Fab fragment administration is determined on the basis of the presence of life-threatening toxicity: the fragments are given over a few minutes in cases of ventricular disturbances and over 1 hour in cases of prophylactic indications. Resolution of digitalis poisoning symptoms after Fab fragment infusion is rapid. Reversal, including correction of serum potassium concentration, has been obtained in 75% of the patients within 1 hour.[35] Vital signs, electrocardiogram, and serum potassium monitoring during Fab fragment infusion are means of assessing treatment efficacy and safety. It is important to understand that serum digitalis concentrations measured by routine methods rise dramatically after administration of digitalis Fab fragments. Free digitalis concentrations may be measured to distinguish bound from unbound fractions, but such measurements are technically more difficult to perform and generally less available.

Prior history of allergy after Fab fragment administration is the sole contraindication to Fab fragment

---

BOX 58-4   **CALCULATION OF DIGITALIS FAB FRAGMENT DOSAGE**

Calculation of digitalis body load based on ingested digitalis amount:

Digoxin body load (mg) = 0.8 × suspected ingested amount (mg)
Digitoxin body load (mg) = 1 × suspected ingested amount (mg)

NB: 0.8 and 1 are digoxin and digitoxin bioavailability. In case of elixirs and gel tablets, the value is 0.95.

Calculation of digitalis body load based on serum digitalis concentration:

Digoxin body load (mg) = [digoxin serm concentration (ng/mL)] × 5.6 (L/kg) × weight (kg)/1000
Digitoxin body load (mg) = [Digitoxin serum concentration (ng/mL)] × 0.56 (L/kg) × weight (kg)/1000

NB: 5.6 and 0.56 (L/kg) are digoxin and digitoxin's respective volumes of distribution

NB: Digoxin serum concentration (nmol/L) × 0.781 = digoxin serum concentration (ng/mL or μg/L)

Digitoxin serum concentration (nmol/L) × 0.765 = digoxin serum concentration (ng/mL or μg/L)

Thus, the dose of Fab fragments to administer is determined as follows:

One vial of 40 mg of Fab fragments (Digibind) neutralizes 0.6 mg of digitalis (digoxin or digitoxin).
One vial of 80 mg of Fab fragments (Digidot) neutralizes 1 mg of digitalis (digoxin or digitoxin).

To obtain equimolar neutralization, dose of Fab fragments to administer equals the total body load of digitalis: 1.7 vials of Digibind or 1 vial of Digidot for 1 mg of digitalis body load.

---

administration. Adverse effects associated with Fab fragment administration are rare and minor. The adverse effects potentially observed are (1) exacerbation of congestive heart failure, resistant to digoxin administration; (2) allergy; and (3) "overshoot" hypokalemia. Allergic reactions are reported in less than 1% of cases.[35]

SUMMARY

Digitalis intoxication is a common problem in medicine today. Toxicity is manifested by many systemic symptoms, the most important of which, clinically, are cardiac arrhythmias. Virtually every known arrhythmia has been reported to be caused by digitalis excess. Finally, the most important aid in the successful treatment of digitalis intoxication is prevention through patient education. Patients' awareness of potential problems enables them to recognize problems early. Patient education is especially important in view of the length of digitalis use.

When prevention fails, in patients with chronic treatment experimenting digitalis toxicity and in patients with acute poisoning, early diagnosis is crucial is in order to rapidly undertake appropriate treatment measures. Antidotal treatment using Fab fragments is the first-line treatment. Fab fragments can be used to obtain equimolar neutralization in patients with life-threatening symptoms in order to prevent life-threatening symptom complications.

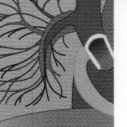

REFERENCES

1. Schwartz A: Is the cell membrane Na+, K+-ATPase enzyme system the pharmacological receptor for digitalis? Circ Res 1976;39(1):1–7.
2. Silverman ME: William Withering and an account of the foxglove. Clin Cardiol 1989;12(7):415–418.
3. Ordog GJ, Benaron S, Bhasin V, et al: Serum digoxin levels and mortality in 5,100 patients. Ann Emerg Med 1987;16(1):32–39.
4. Smith TW, Haber E, Yeatman L, Butler VP Jr: Reversal of advanced digoxin intoxication with Fab fragments of digoxin-specific antibodies. N Engl J Med 1976;294(15):797–800.
5. Beller GA, Smith TW, Abelmann WH, Haber E, Hood WB Jr: Digitalis intoxication. A prospective clinical study with serum level correlations. N Engl J Med 1971;284(18):989–997.
6. Borron SW, Bismuth C, Muszynski J: Advances in the management of digoxin toxicity in the older patient. Drugs Aging 1997;10(1):18–33.
7. Taboulet P, Baud FJ, Bismuth C, Vicaut E: Acute digitalis intoxication—is pacing still appropriate? J Toxicol Clin Toxicol 1993;31(2):261–273.
8. Bismuth C, Motte G, Conso F, Chauvin M, Gaultier M: Acute digoxin intoxication treated by intracardiac pacemaker: experience in sixty-eight patients. Clin Toxicol 1977;10:443–456.
9. Slifman NR, Obermeyer WR, Aloi BK, et al: Contamination of botanical dietary supplements by *Digitalis lanata*. N Engl J Med 1998;339(12):806–811.
10. Doherty JE: Digitalis glycosides. Pharmacokinetics and their clinical implications. Ann Intern Med 1973;79(2):229–238.
11. Doherty JE, de Soyza N, Kane JJ, et al: Clinical pharmacokinetics of digitalis glycosides. Prog Cardiovasc Dis 1978;21(2):141–158.
12. Lindenbaum J, Rund DG, Butler VP Jr, et al: Inactivation of digoxin by the gut flora: reversal by antibiotic therapy. N Engl J Med 1981;305(14):789–794.
13. Smith TW: Digitalis. Mechanisms of action and clinical use. N Engl J Med 1988;318(6):358–365.
14. Arnold SB, Byrd RC, Meister W, et al: Long-term digitalis therapy improves left ventricular function in heart failure. N Engl J Med 1980;303(25):1443–1448.
15. Mulrow CD, Feussner JR, Velez R: Reevaluation of digitalis efficacy. New light on an old leaf. Ann Intern Med 1984;101(1):113–117.
16. Krum H, Bigger JT Jr, Goldsmith RL, Packer M: Effect of long-term digoxin therapy on autonomic function in patients with chronic heart failure. J Am Coll Cardiol 1995;25(2):289–294.
17. Digitalis Investigation Group: The effect of digoxin on mortality and morbidity in patients with heart failure. N Engl J Med 1997;336(8):525–533.
18. Braunwald E: Effects of digitalis on the normal and the failing heart. J Am Coll Cardiol 1985;5(5 Suppl A):51A–59A.
19. Rosen MR: Cellular electrophysiology of digitalis toxicity. J Am Coll Cardiol 1985;5(5 Suppl A):22A–34A.
20. Bigger JT Jr: The quinidine-digoxin interaction: what do we know about it? N Engl J Med 1979;301(14):779–781.
21. Marcus FI: Pharmacokinetic interactions between digoxin and other drugs. J Am Coll Cardiol 1985;5(5 Suppl A):82A–90A.
22. Pentel PR, Salerno DM: Cardiac drug toxicity: digitalis glycosides and calcium-channel and beta-blocking agents. Med J Aust 1990;152(2):88–94.
23. Leahey EB Jr, Reiffel JA, Giardina EG, Bigger JT Jr: The effect of quinidine and other oral antiarrhythmic drugs on serum digoxin. A prospective study. Ann Intern Med 1980;92(5):605–608.
24. Nademanee K, Kannan R, Hendrickson J, et al: Amiodarone-digoxin interaction: clinical significance, time course of development, potential pharmacokinetic mechanisms and therapeutic implications. J Am Coll Cardiol 1984;4(1):111–116.
25. Klein HO, Lang R, Di Segni E, Kaplinsky E: Verapamil-digoxin interaction. N Engl J Med 1980;303(3):160.
26. Robieux I, Dorian P, Klein J, et al: The effects of cardiac transplantation and cyclosporine therapy on digoxin pharmacokinetics. J Clin Pharmacol 1992;32(4):338–343.
27. Iesaka Y, Aonuma K, Gosselin AJ, et al: Susceptibility of infarcted canine hearts to digitalis-toxic ventricular tachycardia. J Am Coll Cardiol 1983;2(1):45–51.
28. Muller JE, Turi ZG, Stone PH, et al. Digoxin therapy and mortality after myocardial infarction. Experience in the MILIS Study. N Engl J Med 1986;314(5):265–271.
29. Marchlinski FE, Hook BG, Callans DJ: Which cardiac disturbances should be treated with digoxin immune Fab (ovine) antibody? Am J Emerg Med 1991;9(2 Suppl 1):24–34.
30. Da Costa D, Brady WJ, Edhouse J: Bradycardias and atrioventricular conduction block. BMJ 2002;324(7336):535–538.
31. Mahdyoon H, Battilana G, Rosman H, et al: The evolving pattern of digoxin intoxication: observations at a large urban hospital from 1980 to 1988. Am Heart J 1990;120(5):1189–1194.
32. Brunner G, Zweiker R, Krejs GJ: A toxicological surprise. Lancet 2000;356(9239):1406.
33. Gaultier M, Welti JJ, Bismuth C, et al: [Severe digitalis intoxication. Prognostic factors. Value and limitations of electrosystolic pacemaking (apropos of 133 cases).] Ann Med Interne (Paris) 1976;127(10):761–766.
34. Pap C, Zacher G, Karteszi M [Prognosis in acute digitalis poisoning.] Orv Hetil 2005;146(11):507–513.
35. Antman EM, Wenger TL, Butler VP Jr, et al: Treatment of 150 cases of life-threatening digitalis intoxication with digoxin-specific Fab antibody fragments. Final report of a multicenter study. Circulation 1990;81(6):1744–1752.
36. Hickey AR, Wenger TL, Carpenter VP, et al: Digoxin Immune Fab therapy in the management of digitalis intoxication: safety and efficacy results of an observational surveillance study. J Am Coll Cardiol 1991;17(3):590–598.
37. Graves SW, Brown B, Valdes R Jr: An endogenous digoxin-like substance in patients with renal impairment. Ann Intern Med 1983;99(5):604–608.
38. Smith TW: Pharmacokinetics, bioavailability and serum levels of cardiac glycosides. J Am Coll Cardiol 1985;5(5 Suppl A):43A–50A.
39. Gowda RM, Cohen RA, Khan IA: Toad venom poisoning: resemblance to digoxin toxicity and therapeutic implications. Heart 2003;89(4):e14.
40. Kwan T, Paiusco AD, Kohl L: Digitalis toxicity caused by toad venom. Chest 1992;102(3):949–950.
41. Newman LS, Feinberg MW, LeWine HE: Clinical problem-solving. A bitter tale. N Engl J Med 2004;351(6):594–599.
42. Wamboldt FS, Jefferson JW, Wamboldt MZ: Digitalis intoxication misdiagnosed as depression by primary care physicians. Am J Psychiatry 1986;143(2):219–221.
43. Chyka PA, Seger D, Krenzelok EP, Vale JA: Position paper: Single-dose activated charcoal. Clin Toxicol (Phila) 2005;43(2):61–87.
44. American Academy of Clinical Toxicology; European Association of Poisons Centres and Clinical Toxicologists: Position statement and practice guidelines on the use of multi-dose activated charcoal in the treatment of acute poisoning. J Toxicol Clin Toxicol 1999;37(6):731–751.
45. Hack JB, Woody JH, Lewis DE, et al: The effect of calcium chloride in treating hyperkalemia due to acute digoxin toxicity in a porcine model. J Toxicol Clin Toxicol 2004;42(4):337–342.
46. Chen JY, Liu PY, Chen JH, et al: Safety of transvenous temporary cardiac pacing in patients with accidental digoxin overdose and symptomatic bradycardia. Cardiology 2004;102(3):152–155.
47. Reisdorff EJ, Clark MR, Walters BL: Acute digitalis poisoning: the role of intravenous magnesium sulfate. J Emerg Med 1986;4(6):463–469.
48. Taboulet P, Baud FJ, Bismuth C: Clinical features and management of digitalis poisoning—rationale for immunotherapy. J Toxicol Clin Toxicol 1993;31(2):247–260.
49. Smolarz A, Roesch E, Lenz E, et al: Digoxin specific antibody (Fab) fragments in 34 cases of severe digitalis intoxication. J Toxicol Clin Toxicol 1985;23(4–6):327–340.
50. Woolf AD, Wenger T, Smith TW, Lovejoy FH Jr: The use of digoxin-specific Fab fragments for severe digitalis intoxication in children. N Engl J Med 1992;326(26):1739–1744.

59 *Calcium Channel Antagonists*

STEVEN D. SALHANICK, MD

At a Glance...

- Calcium channel antagonist overdose can cause severe and prolonged toxicity resulting in a high degree of morbidity and mortality.
- Calcium channel antagonists are structurally diverse and vary greatly with regard to central versus peripheral cardiovascular effects.
- Toxicity is primarily an extension of therapeutic effects.
- Many xenobiotics interact with calcium channel antagonists, particularly those that are oxidized by the cytochrome P-450 system including grapefruit juice and digoxin. Care should be exercised when prescribing calcium channel antagonists in association with other xenobiotics.
- Early aggressive decontamination is warranted given the severity of toxicity.
- Virtually all forms of supportive care have been successful.
- Antidotes include calcium salts, but their effectiveness is debated.
- A promising recent development is high-dose insulin therapy, which is thought to be effective owing to correction of insulin deficiency and to its effects on myocardial energy metabolism.

Cytosolic calcium increase due to influx of calcium from the extracellular matrix has important physiologic consequences in both cardiac and vascular smooth muscle. As early as the 1960s, the negative chronotropic, inotropic, and vasodilatory effects of drugs that blocked calcium influx through cell membrane calcium channels was recognized, leading to the development of these pharmaceuticals as antiarrhythmic and antihypertensive agents.[1] Subsequently, a wide variety of indications for calcium channel antagonists has been realized, including tocolysis and cerebral vasospasm following aneurysmal subarachnoid hemorrhage. Given the prevalence of hypertensive disease, as well as the variety of indications that have been found for antagonists of calcium channels, these drugs are widely prescribed. Furthermore, given the lethal nature of these drugs in overdose, they are a frequent cause of morbidity and mortality.[2] Consequently, clinicians caring for patients exposed to overdose or potential overdose of calcium channel antagonists need to be familiar with the management of such patients.

STRUCTURE

Calcium channel antagonists are a structurally diverse group of drugs (Fig. 59-1). They are organized on the basis of structure and pharmacologic activity into five classes.

Phenylalkylamines

Verapamil is the prototypical phenylalkylamine. Verapamil depresses sinoatrial and atrioventricular conduction, decreases myocardial contractility, and decreases peripheral vascular resistance. Verapamil is widely prescribed for the treatment of hypertension and is frequently used to control supraventricular tachyarrhythmias. It is often prescribed in extended-release form. Verapamil undergoes *N*-demethylation by CYP3A3 to norverapamil, which has approximately 20% of the activity of the parent compound.

Benzothiazepines

Diltiazem is the prototypical benzothiazepine. Diltiazem is notable for its depressive effects on cardiac chronotropy and contractility. Diltiazem relaxes peripheral vascular smooth muscle to a lesser extent than do other calcium channel antagonists. It is metabolized to desacetyldiltiazem, which has 25% to 50% of the pharmacologic activity of the parent drug. Diltiazem is frequently sold as a sustained-release preparation.

Dihydropyridines

Nifedipine is the prototypical dihydropyridine. Dihydropyridines are the largest group of calcium channel antagonists in clinical use. Dihydropyridines are notable for their predominant effect on vascular smooth muscle. They generally have little effect on cardiac inotropy or chronotropy. They uniformly decrease peripheral vascular resistance and coronary artery blood flow. Because of its high lipid solubility, nimodipine is indicated for the prevention of cerebral artery vasospasm following aneurysmal subarachnoid hemorrhage. Nisoldipine is marketed as an antihypertensive agent.[3] It is notable for low bioavailability and marked peripheral vascular selectivity. Amlodipine, felodipine, and isradipine are remarkable for delayed time to peak plasma level and delayed onset of action. Dihydropyridines frequently cause reflex tachycardia owing to their peripheral vascular selectivity.

Diarylaminopropylethers

Bepridil is the prototypical diarylaminopropylether. It reduces blood pressure and heart rate in patients with stable angina. An adverse side effect profile including rate-related QT_c prolongation and torsades de pointes limits its use to refractory cases of angina.[4,5]

Tertraline Derivatives

Mibefradil is the prototypical tertraline derivative. Mibefradil is unique in that it has effects on the T-type as well as the L-type calcium channel, which is the site of action of other calcium channel antagonists.[6,7] T-type channels are thought to be involved in the control of

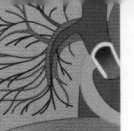

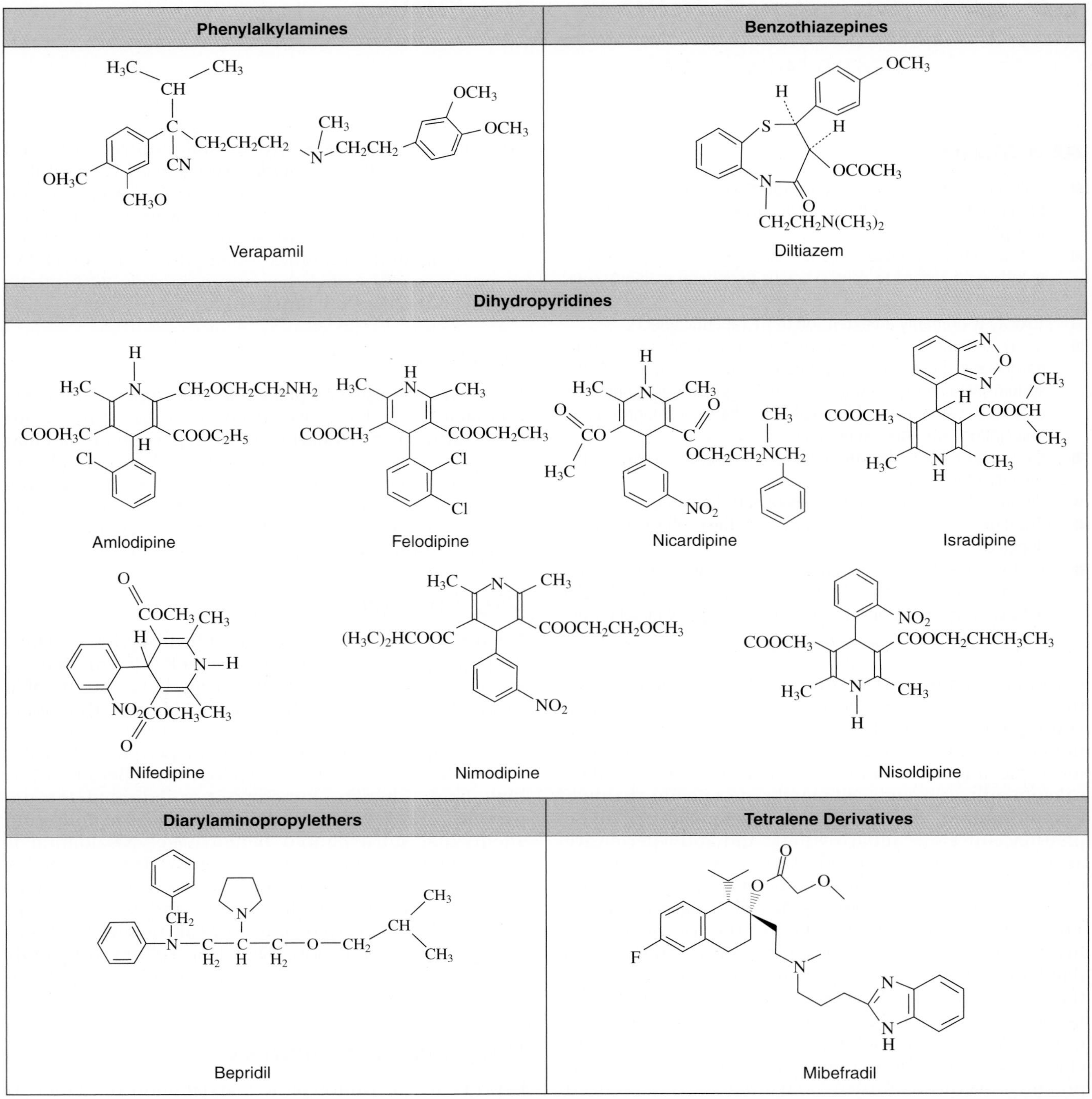

FIGURE 59-1 Chemical structures of the major calcium channel antagonists by class. (From Salhanick SD, Shannon MW: Management of calcium channel antagonist overdose. Drug Saf 2003;26[2]:65–79.)

supraventricular arrhythmias. They have been identified in cardiac pacemaker cells but are rare in myocytes.[6,8,9] They are involved in growth regulation of fibrosis and hypertrophy following myocardial infarction, and animal data suggest that mibefradil has beneficial effects on cardiac remodeling following myocardial infarction.[10-12] Mibefradil also binds at the verapamil binding site, but it has effects similar to those of dihydropyridines, affecting

vascular smooth muscle without exhibiting negative inotropic effect.[7,13] Mibefradil also acts at coronary vascular smooth muscle to increase coronary blood flow.[13]

Mibefradil has high oral bioavailability and a long serum half-life (17 to 25 hours); it does not produce precipitous hemodynamic changes.[7] It is metabolized by the cytochrome P-450 (CYP) 3A4 and 2D6 isoenzymes. Consequently, it interacts with many other drugs including several cardiovascular agents. Because of the large number of potential and actual drug interactions, mibefradil was voluntarily removed from the market in the United States in 1998, despite its desirable profile.[14]

PHARMACOLOGY

Calcium flux across cell membranes provides electrical signaling in cells and coupling of these signals to changes in cytosolic calcium.[15] Given the multitude of functions of cytosolic calcium, transmembrane calcium channels are of tremendous physiologic importance.

Several types of calcium channel have been described. They are primarily distinguished as low voltage activated or high voltage activated. Low-voltage-activated channels are poorly understood and found primarily in cells exhibiting repetitive electrical change. They are involved in pacemaker activity of cells, including the inflow of calcium into cardiac pacemaker cells during the first phase of depolarization.[16]

High-voltage-activated channels respond to relatively larger changes in the transmembrane potential. They function to couple electrical signals with increases in intracellular calcium. Five types of high-voltage channels have been described; classification is based on pharmacologic properties. The first described were the L-type channels classified on the basis of their sensitivity to dihydropyridines. Later, N-type channels were described in nervous tissue based on sensitivity to ω-conotoxin, a peptide isolated from the venom of the cone snail.[17] The

P-type channels of cerebellar Purkinje neurons, Q-type channels, and aforementioned T-type channels have all been subsequently identified.

Molecular structures of the different types of calcium channels have been identified and correlate well with the pharmacologic classification (Fig. 59-2). All calcium channels (low and high voltage) share the α_1 subunit that contains the calcium pore and voltage sensors. The α_1 subunit contains four homologous domains, each with six transmembrane subunits that come together to form a pore in the cell membrane. There are six known α_1 subunits among the various types of channels. Other protein subunits include at least four β subunits and α_2, γ, and δ subunits.[18,19] The β subunits are nonlinked cytoplasmic proteins that affect ionic gradients, rates of activation and inactivation, and dihydropyridine binding affinity of the L-type channels.[20] The α_2 and δ subunits are linked to one another and affect the rate of channel activation as well as increasing the ionic gradient across the channel. The function of the γ subunit may be to amplify the actions of the β subunit.[20] Because of the complex nature of the L-type calcium channel, multiple receptor sites exist for the structurally diverse calcium channel antagonists.[21]

The calcium channel antagonists currently available act on the L-type channels of cardiac and vascular smooth muscle cells. While L-type channels exist in skeletal muscle, the current classes of calcium channel antagonists have not shown an effect on skeletal muscle. The intracellular release of relatively large amounts of calcium from mitochondrial and sarcolemmal stores in

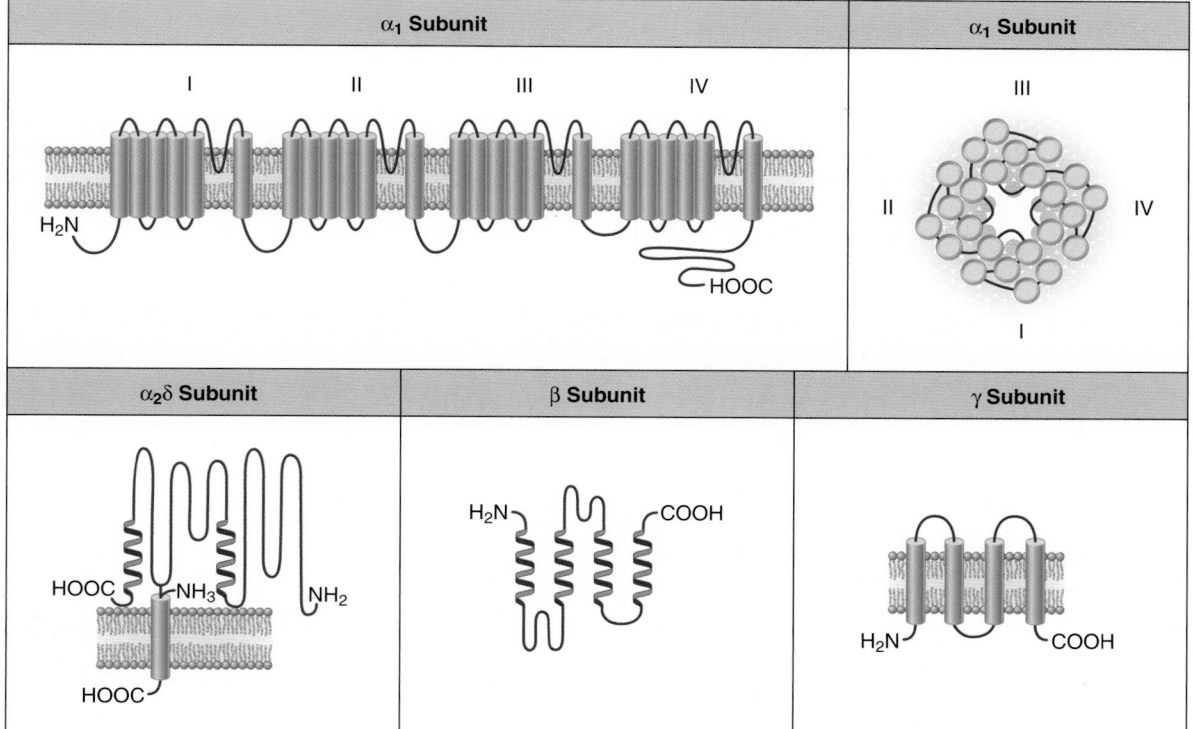

FIGURE 59-2 Molecular structure of the L-type calcium channel. (From Salhanick SD, Shannon MW: Management of calcium channel antagonist overdose. Drug Saf 2003;26[2]:65–79.)

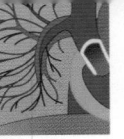

skeletal muscle is less dependent on a transmembrane calcium increase as a signaling mechanism.[22] L-type channels are also found in nervous tissue, but their function there is not well understood.[23]

Antagonism of susceptible L-type channels results primarily in effects on the heart and peripheral vascular smooth muscle. Cardiac effects include negative inotropy due to a decrease in available calcium to facilitate excitation-contraction coupling in the myocardial cells as well as negative chronotropy due to blockade of L-type channels in pacemaker cells in the sinoatrial and atrioventricular nodes. Relaxation of vascular smooth muscle results in decreased afterload, decreased systemic blood pressure, and increased coronary vascular dilatation. The effect is primarily on arterial smooth muscle and thus does not affect venous capacitance and preload.

The selectivity of the various calcium channel antagonists for cardiac versus peripheral vascular effects has long been recognized. The mechanism of this selectivity is not entirely clear. Charged drugs (e.g., verapamil) appear to block calcium channels preferentially in the open state, whereas nonpolar drugs block the channel in both open and closed states. This has been invoked to explain the selectivity of verapamil and other charged compounds for rhythmically depolarizing cardiac cells and why the effects may be more pronounced on pacemaker cells, which have a relatively depolarized diastolic membrane potential.[24] Additionally, as stated above, there is a degree of variability in the molecular structures of the α_1 subunit and the other subunits.[18,19] Consequently, calcium channel antagonists act at the particular L-type channel with the α_1 subunit that has the greatest affinity for the particular drug.[21]

PHARMACOKINETICS

The pharmacokinetics of calcium channel antagonists is summarized in Table 59-1. The calcium channel antagonists are rapidly and nearly completely absorbed from the gastrointestinal tract but have extensive first pass metabolism. Times to peak serum levels are typically rapid. Several have been formulated as extended-release preparations. Time to peak plasma concentration with extended-release preparations is 3 to 7 hours.

Several conditions as well as xenobiotics may affect the pharmacokinetics of the calcium channel antagonists. CYP3A3/4 isoenzymes and CYP1A2 isoenzyme are involved in phase one metabolism of all calcium channel antagonists.[25] Diltiazem and verapamil inhibit P glycoprotein–mediated drug transportation in the gut and peripheral tissues.[25] Consequently, interactions with other xenobiotics are extensive (Table 59-2).

Certain examples are notable. Verapamil and diltiazem both decrease digoxin clearance and reduce its distribution to peripheral tissues. Cyclosporin and carbamazepine bioavailability are also increased.[26] Lithium toxicity has been reported during verapamil therapy, but the mechanism is not known.[27] Cimetidine increases diltiazem, felodipine, nicardipine, nifedipine, and nisoldipine bioavailability as a result of interactions with CYP3A3/4.[26] Importantly, grapefruit juice contains spiro ortho esters that are powerful inhibitors of the intestinal CYP3A enzymes, leading to increased bioavailability of felodipine, nifedipine, and verapamil.[25,28]

Given the extensive hepatic metabolism of calcium channel antagonists, it is not surprising that disease states of the liver affect the pharmacokinetics of calcium channel antagonists. Verapamil has an increased half-life with both concomitant hepatic disease and reductions in hepatic blood flow.[29,30] Furthermore, nifedipine clearance is linearly related to hepatic blood flow in animals.[31]

TOXICOLOGY

Acute Toxicity

Acute effects following calcium channel antagonist overdose are both exaggerations of the therapeutic effects due to action at the therapeutically targeted L-type channels of the vascular system as well as other pathophysiologic effects due to cross-reactivity with lower affinity L-type channels in other tissues.

TABLE 59-1 Pharmacokinetics of Calcium Channel Blockers

	ABSORPTION (%)	BIOAVAILABILITY (%)	VOLUME OF DISTRIBUTION (L/kg)	PROTEIN BINDING (%)	TERMINAL HALF-LIFE (hr)
Verapamil	>90	10–22	4.7	90	3–7
Diltiazem	>90	30–60	5.3	80–90	4
Nifedipine	>90	65–70	0.8–1.4	90	5
Amlodipine	100	60-65	21.4	>95	35
Felodipine	–	10–25	9.7	>99	10.2
Isradipine	–	15–20	69–161 L	>95	8
Nicardipine	–	15–43	–	98	5
Mibefradil	>90	70–90	369	799	17–25
Nimodipine	–	6.6	0.94	–	1–2
Nisoldipine	–	8.4	2.3	–	4
Nitrendipine	>80	10–30	6.6	98	12
Bepridil	100	60	8.0	>99	33–48

Adapted from Pearigen PD, Benowitz NL: Poisoning due to calcium antagonists: experience with verapamil, diltiazem and nifedipine. Drug Saf 1991;6:418.

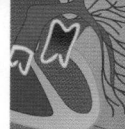

TABLE 59-2 Drug Interactions Involving Calcium Channel Blockers

DRUG	INTERACTING DRUG	EFFECT	PROBABLE MECHANISM	COMMENT
Verapamil Bepridil (other calcium channel blockers possible, but less likely)	β blockers	Heart block, cardiac failure, asystole (after IV verapamil)	Additive depression of AV conduction, myocardial contractility	Primarily seen with verapamil; use with caution in patients taking β blockers
	Digitalis	Aggravates heart block; asystole	Additive depression of cardiac conduction	Avoid use of calcium channel blockers in patients with digitalis toxicity
Verapamil Diltiazem	Propranolol	Reduced oral clearance with increased levels of propranolol	Inhibition of first pass metabolism	Propranolol dose may need to be reduced
Verapamil Diltiazem Bepridil (possibly)	Digoxin	Reduced digoxin clearance, increased digoxin levels	Inhibition of metabolism and renal excretion of digoxin	Reduce digoxin dose after starting verapamil or diltiazem; monitor serum digoxin concentration
Verapamil Diltiazem	Cyclosporine	Increased cyclosporine levels	Uncertain	Reduce cyclosporine dose after starting verapamil or diltiazem; monitor cyclosporine level
Verapamil	Quinidine	Hypotension (after IV verapamil)	Additive α-adrenergic blockade	Use IV verapamil cautiously in patients taking quinidine or other drugs with α-blocking activity
Verapamil	Prazosin	Increased prazosin levels; greater hypotensive effect	Reduced clearance; additive α-blocking effect	Use combination cautiously; may need to decrease prazosin dose
Verapamil	Halothane	Bradycardia Hypotension	Additive depression of sinus node function and myocardial contractility	Avoid coadministration
Verapamil Diltiazem	Disopyramide Flecainide	Cardiac failure	Additive depression of myocardial contractility	Avoid use if possible, particularly in patients with impaired myocardial function
Bepridil	Quinidine Disopyramide Procainamide Sotalol	Ventricular arrhythmias Torsades de pointes	Additive prolongation of QT interval	Avoid coadministration
Verapamil Diltiazem	Amiodarone Flecainide	Sinus arrest Heart block	Additive depression of sinus node function and AV nodal conduction	Use combination with extreme caution
All calcium channel blockers	Oral hypoglycemic agents	Hyperglycemia	Inhibition of insulin release usually stimulated by sulfonylurea drugs	May need to increase oral hypoglycemic doses or use insulin to maintain glucose control; beware of hypoglycemia when calcium channel blockers are discontinued
All calcium channel blockers	Cimetidine	Increased oral bioavailability of calcium channel blockers	Inhibition of metabolism; reduced presystemic metabolism	Reduce calcium channel blocker dose by 30% to 40%
Verapamil	Rifampin Sulfinpyrazone	Reduced oral bioavailability of verapamil	Accelerated metabolism; increased presystemic metabolism	Increase verapamil dose; use alternative calcium channel blocker with less presystemic metabolism

The pharmacokinetics is affected by the overdose state. All calcium channel antagonists undergo some degree of first pass metabolism. Several reports describe increased drug half-lives following overdose of verapamil, nifedipine, and diltiazem.[32-35] The mechanism is thought to be saturation of the microsomal CYP system enzymes. Sustained-release products may have delayed absorption that results in altered pharmacokinetics. Case reports describing overdose of sustained-release preparations describe a delay in symptoms by as long as 15 to 24 hours.[36-38]

In overdose, cardiac versus vascular selectivity is decreased but not abolished.[39,40] Vasodilatation, particularly associated with agents preferentially affecting vascular smooth muscle, results in decreased systemic vascular resistance, hypotension, and shock. The patient may appear warm and well perfused owing to a lack of vasomotor tone. Negative inotropic and chronotropic effects lead to decreased cardiac output contributing to the shock state. Cardiac ejection fractions as low as 10% have been reported in poisoned patients.[40,41] Depression

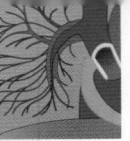

of myocardial conduction may cause depression of the sinus rate and any degree of atrioventricular block. Increased ventricular rate has been reported following overdose as a result of increased conduction across the accessory pathway in Wolff-Parkinson-White syndrome.[42] Mortality is high and is preceded by worsening shock and acidosis, culminating in cardiac arrest.

Effects not directly attributable to antagonism of L-type channels of the cardiovascular system are frequently noted. Some are due to effects on calcium channels in other tissues, while others may be attributable to the shock state.

Pulmonary edema not consistent with the degree of myocardial depression has been reported following overdose with verapamil and amlodipine.[43-49] Precapillary vasodilatation resulting in increase in transcapillary pressure is thought to be the mechanism.[50-52] Other proposed mechanisms include change in endothelial permeability due to a direct effect of calcium antagonism, prostaglandin effects, and effects secondary to the sympathetic discharge associated with toxicity.[53-56]

Delirium, agitation, seizures, and depressed level of consciousness have been described with calcium channel antagonist overdose.[57-59] Bowel infarction and ileus have been reported; however, they may be due entirely to the shock state.[41,60-64]

Hyperglycemia has been well documented with calcium channel antagonist toxicity.[43,65,66] Calcium influx into pancreatic islet cells via L-type channels stimulates insulin release. Nonselective blockade following calcium channel antagonist overdose with resulting hypoinsulinemia is the cause of hyperglycemia.[65,67,68] The decrease in insulin production produces ketoacidosis in addition to the lactic acidosis due to shock.[69]

Chronic Toxicity

Calcium channel antagonists are essentially free of chronic toxicity.

Adverse Effects

Prolongation of the QT interval, first-degree atrioventricular block, transient elevation of transaminases, and near syncope are reported. Most calcium channel antagonists are excreted in breast milk.[70] Levels in breast milk may approach plasma levels; however, there are no reports of neonatal toxicity.[70] Inhibition of sperm acrosomal activity resulting in reversible infertility in males taking calcium channel antagonists therapeutically has been reported.[71]

DIAGNOSIS

Diagnosis of calcium channel antagonist overdose includes the patient's history. If the patient is not cooperative, medication lists should be reviewed to determine if the patient has had access to calcium channel antagonists. Prehospital care providers may have seen medication containers or prescriptions. If the patient's pharmacy can be identified, the pharmacist may provide information. Family members should be questioned regarding medications available to the patient. Many reports of calcium channel antagonist toxicity describe co-ingestants with additive or synergistic effects. Consequently, a careful search for co-ingestants via history and laboratory analysis should be conducted as well. The physical examination may be notable for a warm, peripherally dilated patient who is hypotensive and bradycardic.

Serum levels of calcium channel antagonists are rarely available to the clinician treating the overdosed patient. An elevated serum glucose level may be present and support the diagnosis. The presence of ketoacidosis should be determined, since it also supports the diagnosis.

An electrocardiogram should be obtained to diagnose the presence of bradyarrhythmia that may be amenable to therapy. In cases of severe shock, invasive hemodynamic monitoring may confirm the decreased systemic resistance and provide evidence of response to therapy.

The differential diagnosis includes anything that may cause peripheral vasodilatation or bradyarrhythmia including myocardial infarction, insult to the cardiac conduction system, and ingestion of other vasoactive xenobiotic (e.g., β-adrenergic antagonists, clinidine, guanfacine, and digoxin).

MANAGEMENT

Supportive Measures

Initial supportive care should be aggressive owing to the high mortality associated with calcium channel antagonist overdose and the potential for rapid progression of symptoms. Large-bore intravenous access must be obtained. Continuous cardiac monitoring should be initiated. Airway and ventilatory support should be provided early because of the difficulties associated with intubation in the profoundly hypotensive patient.

No clear consensus exists regarding the optimal regimen for supportive care of the patient. Nearly every form of cardiovascular support has been tried, all with some reported success. Intravenous fluid therapy is typically initiated early following calcium channel antagonist overdose. Care should be exercised, however, given the aforementioned propensity of patients to develop pulmonary edema. Furthermore, these patients are not necessarily volume depleted; consequently, administration of large volumes of fluid should be avoided in favor of early administration of pharmacologic support or an antidote to avoid the complications of fluid overload.

The choice of pharmacologic supportive agents is best guided by the hemodynamic picture, since no single agent is clearly more beneficial than the others. Adrenergic agents such as dopamine, norepinephrine, or epinephrine should be initiated in the setting of significant toxicity. The choice of agent should be determined by the clinician's comfort with the agent administered and the clinical picture, with α-adrenergic agents administered to treat peripheral toxicity and

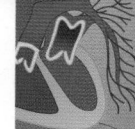

β-adrenergic agents administered to treat cardiac manifestations of toxicity. Atropine may be given to treat bradycardia likely to be responsive. Obtaining adequate hemodynamic data may require invasive hemodynamic monitoring, including the placement of arterial lines, central venous catheters, or pulmonary artery catheters.

Amrinone deserves special mention in the treatment of calcium channel antagonist toxicity. Amrinone inhibits phosphodiesterase III (found in cardiac and vascular tissues), resulting in decreased cyclic adenosine monophosphate (cAMP) breakdown. The increase in cAMP results in greater phosphorylation of L-type calcium channels, which increases their permeability to calcium ions. Amrinone does not increase myocardial oxygen demand as the catecholamines do. Data supporting the use of amrinone are limited, however. Amrinone has been shown to reverse myocardial depression in rats and dogs with verapamil toxicity.[72-74] Human case reports describing beneficial effect of amrinone also have been published.[75,76] Caution should be exercised, since amrinone can induce relaxation of vascular smooth muscle, potentially worsening the peripheral effects of calcium channel antagonists. Phosphodiesterase inhibitors thus have attractive properties for use in the management of calcium channel antagonist toxicity.

Mechanical inotropic supportive measures may be necessary if pharmacologic measures fail. Transvenous pacing has been reported in several cases with varying results.[59,77-84] Balloon pump and bypass have been successful therapies.[41,69,81,83,85] Given the limited data, these therapies should be reserved for cases in which pharmacologic measures have failed.

Decontamination

Following performance of initial supportive measures (airway control, intravenous access), appropriate decontamination measures should be instituted. Activated charcoal is generally the best option, since it likely will absorb the greatest amount of ingested drug, is less invasive, and has fewer complications than gastric emptying procedures. Emesis induction should not be attempted given the risk for rapid deterioration in hemodynamic status, the difficulty of airway control and other therapeutic measures, and risk of aspiration in the patient with uncontrollable emesis. Gastric lavage with a No. 36 to 40 French tube (24 to 28 for children) should be considered with caution. Lavage should be considered only after life-threatening ingestions within 1 hour of the ingestion. Importantly, gastric lavage may cause vagal stimulation, leading to death in patients with heart block or other bradyarrhythmias. Patients with a bradyarrhythmia should not undergo lavage. Whole-bowel irrigation with polyethylene glycol solution is recommended following overdose of sustained-release preparations.[86-88] Many calcium channel antagonists are formulated as sustained-release preparations, and these are frequently implicated in toxicity.[2] Whole-bowel irrigation should not be performed when the patient has ileus. Furthermore, nursing care is made more difficult when the unstable patient is producing a large amount of liquid stool. Vomiting is a risk, and airway control to protect from aspiration should be strongly considered. If whole-bowel irrigation is not feasible, multiple doses of activated charcoal may be considered although evidence of the clinical value of this intervention is lacking.

Laboratory Monitoring

As mentioned above, levels of calcium channel antagonists are generally not available in time to be useful. Several laboratory studies may be helpful, however. Serum electrolytes should be monitored to prevent arrhythmogenic abnormalities that may occur during therapy. Serum calcium concentrations are imperative when therapy with calcium salts is performed. Arterial blood gasses may be used to monitor acidosis. Serum digoxin concentrations should be obtained in anticipation of administration of calcium salts. Calcium channel blocker overdose has no effect on total or ionized serum calcium concentrations.

Antidotes

Several antidotes have been used for the treatment of calcium channel antagonist toxicity.

4-AMINOPYRIDINE

4-Aminopyridine is a potassium channel antagonist that causes an increase in intracellular calcium concentration by increasing calcium inflow across the L-type channel and an increase in calcium release from intracellular stores in the sarcoplasmic reticulum.[88] 4-Aminopyridine has improves hemodynamic parameters in cats and dogs.[89,90] Human use has been reported, but safety and efficacy remain in question.[91]

CALCIUM SALTS

Calcium salts are frequently employed in the management of calcium channel antagonist overdose.[38,92] Calcium salts are a reasonable first agent, since they are readily available and easily administered. Reports of this use of calcium salts date to the mid-1970s, and thus calcium is the first antidote reported in the English literature.[93]

The use of calcium salts is controversial, however. Animal data generally have been positive. Rats and rabbits given 5 to 15 mg/kg/min calcium chloride or gluconate with concurrent administration of nifedipine showed increased survival time, blood pressure, stroke volume, and cardiac output over controls; however, conduction disturbances were not affected.[94] Furthermore, serum calcium concentrations correlated with increases in blood pressure and cardiac output following calcium chloride administration to verapamil-poisoned dogs.[95]

Human case reports show conflicting results. Several authors report minimal or no response to the administration of calcium salts to treat severe calcium channel antagonist toxicity.[48,66,96-98] Proponents of the use of calcium argue that most of the reports of failed therapy are due to underdosing and that high doses of calcium are effective as antidote and without adverse effects.[45]

Several recommendations have been published for the administration of calcium salts. Calcium chloride has

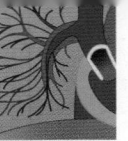

been administered in bolus doses of 1 g every 15 to 20 minutes for a total of four doses or more aggressively as 1 g every 2 to 3 minutes until clinical effect is achieved.[45] Continuous infusion of 0.2 to 0.4 mg/kg/hr calcium chloride (0.6 to 1.2 mg/kg/hr calcium gluconate) has been recommended.[40,99] Buckley and colleagues reported giving 30 g calcium chloride over 12 hours resulting in a plasma calcium level of 23.8 mg/dL with hemodynamic improvement and no adverse clinical effects.[45] Lam and colleagues advocate titrating calcium infusion to maintain a serum calcium level of 8 mg/dL.[100] Howarth and associates recommend continuous infusion titrated to improvement in hemodynamic parameters.[48]

Initial bolus administration of calcium salts followed by measurement of serum calcium at a minimum of every 12 hours is reasonable practice. Serum calcium levels should be maintained in the normal range because of the lack of evidence for efficacy of above-normal concentrations. Other modes of therapy should be added if calcium therapy does not rapidly improve hemodynamic parameters.

Several precautions should be taken during calcium therapy. Careful maintenance of intravenous sites is essential to prevent tissue damage due to extravasation of calcium chloride. Continuous cardiac monitoring and at least daily electrocardiograms should be performed to prevent arrythmias.[100] Calcium should not be administered if there is an elevated digoxin level or if the clinician has reason to believe that digoxin ingestion may have occurred, because of the concern for resulting life-threatening arrythmias.[101-103] The effect of administering exogenous calcium to patients with therapeutic digoxin serum concentrations and calcium channel antagonist toxicity is unknown. It is prudent to obtain the digoxin concentration before initiation of calcium therapy and to withhold calcium therapy if a measurable digoxin concentration is present, because of the potential for concurrent overdose of digoxin, the unclear interaction between calcium and therapeutic digoxin concentrations, and the availability of other therapies.

INSULIN

Insulin as an antidote for calcium channel antagonist poisoning is based on several observations.[104] Hyperglycemia in calcium channel antagonist toxicity is due to blockade of pancreatic L-type channels that results in decreased insulin production.[66] Furthermore, calcium channel antagonist toxicity results in decrease in uptake of insulin or free fatty acids by the myocardium as well as a shift from oxidation of fatty acids to carbohydrates for the production of energy.[69]

Insulin increases cellular uptake of glucose and lactate and improves hemodynamic parameters in verapamil-poisoned dogs.[104] Furthermore, measurement of the myocardial respiratory quotient and the ratio of myocardial oxygen delivery to myocardial work indicates that insulin therapy of verapamil-poisoned dogs causes an increase in energy efficiency of myocardial metabolism.[104] Insulin improves survival in critically ill patients owing to a variety of causes regardless of degree of hyperglycemia or insulin resistance.[105]

Human data support the use of insulin as an antidote for calcium channel antagonist toxicity. Yuan and associates reported on three patients with verapamil toxicity and one with amlodipine and atenolol toxicity refractory to calcium salts, fluids, and vasopressors. Patients received bolus doses of 10 to 20 IU of regular insulin followed by a continuous insulin infusion of 0.1 to 1.0 IU/kg/hr. All patients showed improvement in hemodynamic parameters temporally associated with insulin administration.[69] Serum verapamil concentrations obtained from two of these patients were markedly elevated, yet all patients survived without sequelae.[69] Boyer and Shannon reported on two patients who failed to respond to calcium or glucagon and aggressive supportive care, yet responded rapidly to insulin administration at 0.5 IU/kg/hr.[106] Supplemental glucose was required for only one of the patients. Insulin therapy with supplemental glucose as needed should therefore be initiated early in the treatment of calcium channel antagonist toxicity.

The preferred regimen at the author's institution for insulin therapy is as follows. Adult patients with serum glucose levels greater than 200 mg/dL receive one ampule (50 mL of 50% solution) of D-glucose (0.25 g/kg D-glucose for children). A serum potassium concentration of less than 2.5 mEq/dL is treated with 40 mEq orally or 20 mEq of potassium intravenously. A bolus dose of insulin, 1.0 U/kg, is given followed by an infusion at 0.5 to 1.0 IU/kg/hr titrated to clinical response. Therapeutic targets include a systolic blood pressure greater than 100 mm Hg and a sinus rhythm of greater than 50 beats per minute. Capillary glucose is checked every 20 minutes for 1 hour and then hourly thereafter. Serum potassium is checked hourly. Fluid therapy is half-normal saline with 10% dextrose at an infusion rate equal to 80% of maintenance. Insulin infusion is weaned as toxicity resolves. k Hyperinsulinemia, euglycemia (HIE) is the term applied to the use of insulin as an antidote given the large doses of insulin administered.

GLUCAGON

Glucagon has been recommended as an antidote for calcium channel antagonist therapy in prior editions of this and in other standard texts. Glucagon has a specific receptor on the surface of the myocyte.[107] Binding results in the stimulation of adenyl cyclase via G proteins followed by increased intracellular cyclic AMP, phosphorylation of L-type calcium channels, and influx of calcium.[108] In addition, the C-terminal portion of glucagon is cleaved to miniglucagon, which releases calcium from the sarcoplasmic reticulum.[109] Miniglucagon increases inotropy in embryonic chick ventricular myocytes. In vitro administration of both glucagon and miniglucagon produced a synergistic positive inotropic effect, thought to be due to effects on the L-type channel and the sarcoplasmic reticulum.[109]

Multiple studies show increased inotropy, chronotropy, and dromotropy following glucagon administration to animals poisoned by calcium channel antagonists.[110-114] Human case reports are less conclusive, since they are confounded by multiple treatment regimens and uncontrolled conditions. The majority, however, describe

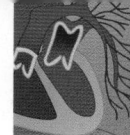

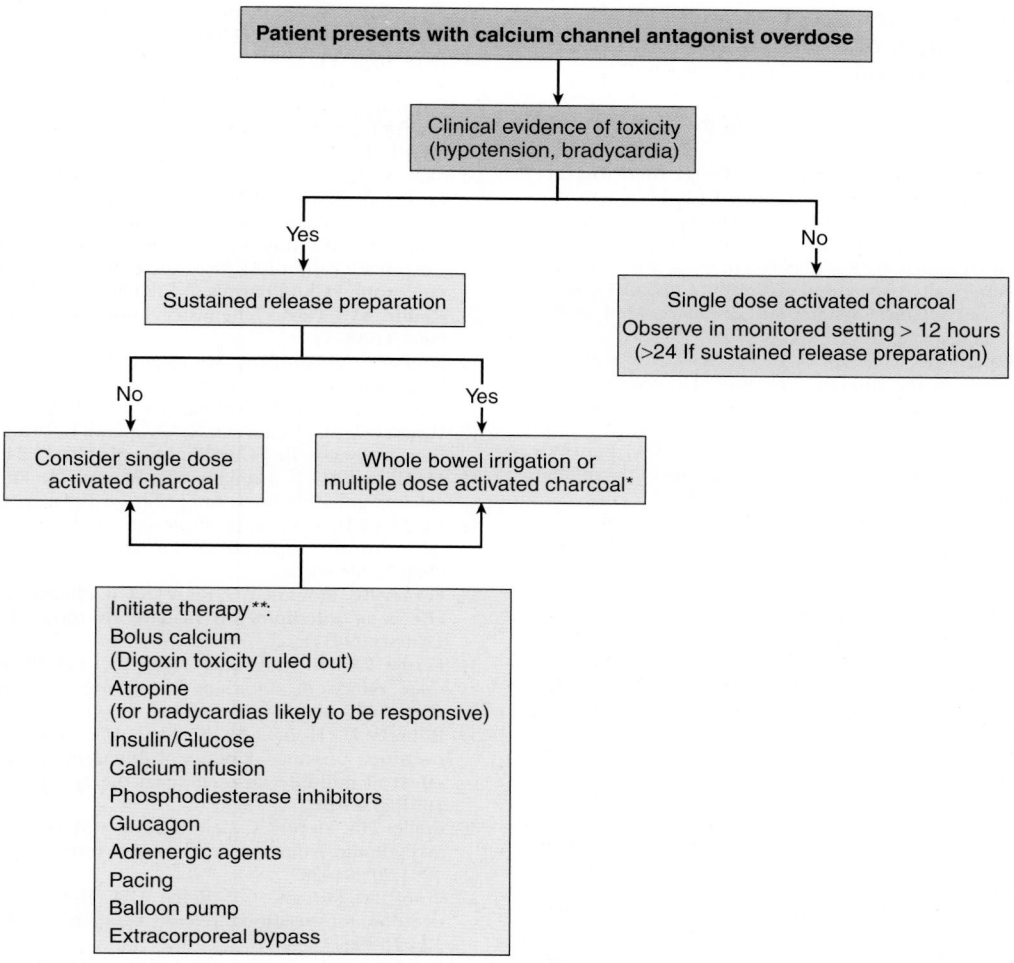

FIGURE 59-3 Algorithmic approach to the management of the patient with calcium channel antagonist toxicity.

beneficial effects on hemodynamic parameters following glucagon administration.[76,115,116]

The effects of glucagon begin within 1 to 3 minutes, peak at 5 to 7 minutes, and decline by 15 minutes.[117] Doses between 0.5 and 14 mg intravenously have been reported, but typical dosing is 1 to 10 mg as an intravenous bolus followed by infusions of 3 to 6 mg/hr.[115,116,118] The maintenance dose is determined by the initial effective dose, with the initial dose required to obtain response given as continuous infusion over 1 hour. The initial recommended pediatric dose is 50 to 150 μg/kg.[119] Adverse effects of glucagon include nausea, vomiting, flushing, hyperglycemia, smooth muscle relaxation, and intestinal ileus.

Elimination

No methods are known to enhance the elimination or metabolism of calcium channel antagonists. The high degree of protein binding and volumes of distribution generally larger than 1 L/kg make dialysis unlikely to be beneficial, and no benefit has ever been reported.

Significant enterohepatic circulation has not been demonstrated. Furthermore, gut dialysis with multiple-dose charcoal is not known to occur.

Disposition

Given the severity of calcium channel antagonist toxicity and the potential for delayed toxicity, patients with a history of ingestion should be observed in a monitored setting for a minimum of 12 hours. If there is a question whether a sustained-release preparation is involved, the period of observation should be extended to 24 hours. Patients exhibiting signs of toxicity should be treated in an intensive care unit. Following resolution of toxicity, a careful search should be conducted for sequelae of prolonged hypotension including bowel infarction, stroke, and subendocardial myocardial infarction and those issues treated accordingly. An algorithmic approach to the care of the patient suffering calcium channel antagonist toxicity is shown in Figure 59-3. As always, psychiatric evaluation is prudent following intentional ingestion. The causes of therapeutic mis-

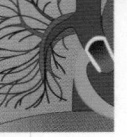

adventure should be investigated as well. Finally, a nonjudgmental evaluation of home safety should occur in cases of pediatric ingestion.

REFERENCES

1. Kerins DM, Robertson RM, Robertson D: Drugs used for the treatment of myocardial ischemia. In Limbard LE, Hardman JG, Gilman AG (eds): Goodman and Gilman's The Pharmacological Basis of Therapeutics. New York, McGraw-Hill, 2001, p 853.
2. Litovitz TL, Klein-Schwartz W, Rodgers GC Jr, et al: 2001 Annual report of the American Association of Poison Control Centers Toxic Exposure Surveillance System. Am J Emerg Med 2002; 20:391–452.
3. Godfraind T, Salomone S, Dessy C, et al: Selectivity scale of calcium antagonists in the human cardiovascular system based on in vitro studies. J Cardiovasc Pharmacol 1992;20(Suppl 5): S34–S41.
4. Zusman RM, Higgins J, Christensen D, Boucher CA: Bepridil improves left ventricular performance in patients with angina pectoris. J Cardiovasc Pharmacol 1993;22:474–480.
5. Hollingshead LM, Faulds D, Fitton A: Bepridil: a review of its pharmacological properties and therapeutic use in stable angina pectoris. Drugs 1992;44:835–857.
6. Mishra SK, Hermsmeyer K: Selective inhibition of T-type Ca2+ channels by Ro 40-5967. Circ Res 1994;75:144–148.
7. Fang LM, Osterrieder W: Potential-dependent inhibition of cardiac Ca2+ inward currents by Ro 40-5967 and verapamil: relation to negative inotropy. Eur J Pharmacol 1991;196:205–207.
8. Bean BP: Classes of calcium channels in vertebrate cells. Ann Rev Physiol 1989;51:367–384.
9. Tseng GN, Boyden PA: Multiple types of Ca2+ currents in single canine Purkinje cells. Circ Res 1989;65:1735–1750.
10. Sandmann S, Bohle RM, Dreyer T, Unger T: The T-type calcium channel blocker mibefradil reduced interstitial and perivascular fibrosis and improved hemodynamic parameters in myocardial infarction-induced cardiac failure in rats. Virchows Archiv 2000;436:147–157.
11. Sandmann S, Claas R, Cleutjens JP, et al: Calcium channel blockade limits cardiac remodeling and improves cardiac function in myocardial infarction-induced heart failure in rats. J Cardiovasc Pharmacol 2001;37:64–77.
12. Sandmann S, Spitznagel H, Chung O, et al: Effects of the calcium channel antagonist mibefradil on haemodynamic and morphological parameters in myocardial infarction-induced cardiac failure in rats (comment). Cardiovasc Res 1998;39:339–350.
13. Osterrieder W, Holck M: In vitro pharmacologic profile of Ro 40-5967 a novel Ca2+ channel blocker with potent vasodilator but weak inotropic action. J Cardiovasc Pharmacol 1989;13:754–759.
14. Glasser SP: The relevance of T-type calcium antagonists: a profile of mibefradil. J Clin Pharmacol 1998;38:659–669.
15. Hille B: Ionic channels in excitable membranes. Current problems and biophysical approaches. Biophys J 1978;22:283–294.
16. Perez-Reyes E, Lee JH, Cribbs LL: Molecular characterization of a neuronal low-voltage-activated T-type calcium channel (comment). Nature 1998;391(6670):896–900.
17. Plummer MR, Logothetis DE, Hess P: Elementary properties and pharmacological sensitivities of calcium channels in mammalian peripheral neurons. Neuron 1989;2:1453–1463.
18. Mitterdorfer J, Grabner M, Kraus RL, et al: Molecular basis of drug interaction with L-type Ca2+ channels. J Bioenerg Biomembr 1998;30:319–334.
19. Catterall WA: Molecular properties of sodium and calcium channels. J Bioenerg Biomembr 1996;28:219–230.
20. Clusin WT, Anderson ME: Calcium channel blockers: current controversies and basic mechanisms of action. Adv Pharmacol 1999;46:253–296.
21. Welling A, Ludwig A, Zimmer S, et al: Alternatively spliced IS6 segments of the alpha 1C gene determine the tissue-specific dihydropyridine sensitivity of cardiac and vascular smooth muscle L-type Ca2+ channels. Circ Res 1997;81:526–532.
22. Braunwald E: Mechanism of action of calcium-channel-blocking agents. N Engl J Med 1982;307:1618–1627.
23. Siesjo BK: Calcium-mediated processes in neuronal degeneration. Ann N Y Acad Sci 1994;747:140–161.
24. Bers DM, Perez-Reyes E: Ca channels in cardiac myocytes: structure and function in Ca influx and intracellular Ca release. Cardiovasc Res 1999;42:339–360.
25. Abernethy DR, Schwartz JB: Calcium-antagonist drugs. N Engl J Med 1999;341:1447–1457.
26. Shah S, Shah AN, Shaw LM: Calcium channel blockers: an overview. In Kwon T, Shaw LM, Rosano TG, et al (eds): The Clinical Toxicology Laboratory Contemporary Practice of Poisoning Evaluation. Washington, DC, AACC Press, 2001, pp 291–:328.
27. Price WA, Giannini AJ: Neurotoxicity caused by lithium-verapamil synergism. J Clin Pharmacol 1986;26:717–719.
28. Rouhi AM: Citrus chemistry boosts drugs. Chem Eng News 2003;81:38–39.
29. Somogyi A, Albrecht M, Kliems G, et al: Pharmacokinetics, bioavailability and ECG response of verapamil in patients with liver cirrhosis. Br J Clin Pharmacol 1981;12:51–60.
30. Woodcock BG, Rietbrock N: Verapamil bioavailability and dosage in liver disease. Br J Clin Pharmacol 1982;13:240–241.
31. McAllister RG Jr, Hamann SR, Blouin RA: Pharmacokinetics of calcium-entry blockers. Am J Cardiol 1985;55:30B–40B.
32. Buckley CD, Aronson JK: Prolonged half-life of verapamil in a case of overdose: implications for therapy. Br J Clin Pharmacol 1995;39:680–683.
33. Ferner RE, Monkman S, Riley J, et al: Pharmacokinetics and toxic effects of nifedipine in massive overdose. Hum Exp Toxicol 1990;9:309–311.
34. Ferner RE, Odemuyiwa O, Field AB, et al: Pharmacokinetics and toxic effects of diltiazem in massive overdose. Hum Toxicol 1989;8:497–499.
35. Roberts D, Honcharik N, Sitar DS, Tenenbein M: Diltiazem overdose: pharmacokinetics of diltiazem and its metabolites and effect of multiple dose charcoal therapy. J Toxicol Clin Toxicol 1991;29:45–52.
36. Spiller HA, Meyers A, Ziemba T, Riley M: Delayed onset of cardiac arrhythmias from sustained-release verapamil. Ann Emerg Med 1991;20:201–203.
37. Tom PA, Morrow CT, Kelen GD: Delayed hypotension after overdose of sustained release verapamil. J Emerg Med 1994; 12:621–625.
38. Ramoska EA, Spiller HA, Winter M, Borys D: A one-year evaluation of calcium channel blocker overdoses: toxicity and treatment. Ann Emerg Med 1993;22:196–200.
39. Proano L, Chiang WK, Wang RY: Calcium channel blocker overdose. Am J Emerg Med 1995;13:444–450.
40. Pearigen PD, Benowitz NL: Poisoning due to calcium antagonists: experience with verapamil, diltiazem and nifedipine. Drug Saf 1991;6:408–430.
41. Salhanick SD, Wax PM: Treatment of atenolol overdose in a patient with renal failure using serial hemodialysis and hemoperfusion and associated echocardiographic findings. Vet Hum Toxicol 2000;42:224–225.
42. McGovern B, Garan H, Ruskin JN: Precipitation of cardiac arrest by verapamil in patients with Wolff-Parkinson-White syndrome. Ann Intern Med 1986;104:791–794.
43. Brass BJ, Winchester-Penny S, Lipper BL: Massive verapamil overdose complicated by noncardiogenic pulmonary edema. Am J Emerg Med 1996;14:459–461.
44. Stanek EJ, Nelson CE, DeNofrio D: Amlodipine overdose (comment). Ann Pharmacother 1997;31:853–856.
45. Buckley NA, Whyte IM, Dawson AH: Overdose with calcium channel blockers (comment). BMJ 1994;308(6944):1639.
46. Gelbke HP, Schlicht HJ, Schmidt G: Fatal poisoning with verapamil. Arch Toxicol 1977;37:89–94.
47. Herrington DM, Insley BM, Weinmann GG: Nifedipine overdose. Am J Med 1986;81:344–346.
48. Howarth DM, Dawson AH, Smith AJ, et al: Calcium channel blocking drug overdose: an Australian series. Hum Exp Toxicol 1994;13:161–166.
49. Leesar MA, Martyn R, Talley JD, Frumin H: Noncardiogenic pulmonary edema complicating massive verapamil overdose. Chest 1994;105:606–607.

50. Humbert VH Jr, Munn NJ, Hawkins RF: Noncardiogenic pulmonary edema complicating massive diltiazem overdose. Chest 1991;99:258–259.

51. Gustafsson D: Microvascular mechanisms involved in calcium antagonist edema formation. J Cardiovasc Pharmacol 1987; 10(Suppl 1):S121–S131.

52. Low RI, Takeda P, Mason DT, DeMaria AN: The effects of calcium channel blocking agents on cardiovascular function. Am J Cardiol 1982;49:547–553.

53. Green K, Cheeks L, Hull DS: Effects of calcium channel blockers on rabbit corneal endothelial function. Curr Eye Res 1994;13:401–408.

54. Payne DK, Fuseler JW, Owens MW: Modulation of endothelial cell permeability by lung carcinoma cells: a potential mechanism of malignant pleural effusion formation. Inflammation 1994;18: 407–417.

55. Fedorak RN, Empey LR, Walker K: Verapamil alters eicosanoid synthesis and accelerates healing during experimental colitis in rats. Gastroenterology 1992;102(4 pt 1):1229–1235.

56. Simon RP: Neurogenic pulmonary edema. Neurol Clin 1993; 11:309–323.

57. Malcolm N, Callegari P, Goldberg J, et al: Massive diltiazem overdosage: clinical and pharmacokinetic observations. Drug Intell Clin Pharm 1986;20:888.

58. Wells TG, Graham CJ, Moss MM, Kearns GL: Nifedipine poisoning in a child. Pediatrics 1990;86:91–94.

59. Horowitz BZ, Rhee KJ: Massive verapamil ingestion: a report of two cases and a review of the literature. Am J Emerg Med 1989;7:624–631.

60. Fauville JP, Hantson P, Honore P, et al: Severe diltiazem poisoning with intestinal pseudo-obstruction: case report and toxicological data. J Toxicol Clin Toxicol 1995;33:273–277.

61. Goglin WK, Elliott BM, Deppe SA: Nifedipine-induced hypotension and mesenteric ischemia. South Med J 1989;82:274–275.

62. Gutierrez H, Jorgensen M: Colonic ischemia after verapamil overdose. Ann Intern Med 1996;124:535.

63. Sporer KA, Manning JJ: Massive ingestion of sustained-release verapamil with a concretion and bowel infarction. Ann Emerg Med 1993;22:603–605.

64. Wax PM: Intestinal infarction due to nifedipine overdose. J Toxicol Clin Toxicol 1995;33:725–728.

65. Devis G, Somers G, Van Obberghen E, Malaisse WJ: Calcium antagonists and islet function. 1. Inhibition of insulin release by verapamil. Diabetes 1975;24:247–251.

66. Enyeart JJ, Price WA, Hoffman DA, Woods L: Profound hyperglycemia and metabolic acidosis after verapamil overdose. J Am Coll Cardiol 1983;2:1228–1231.

67. Lebrun P, Malaisse WJ, Herchuelz A: Nutrient-induced intracellular calcium movement in rat pancreatic B cell. Am J Physiol 1982;243:E196–E205.

68. Malaisse WJ: Role of calcium in insulin secretion. Isr J Med Sci 1972;8:244–251.

69. Yuan TH, Kerns WP II, Tomaszewski CA, Ford MD, et al: Insulin-glucose as adjunctive therapy for severe calcium channel antagonist poisoning. J Toxicol Clin Toxicol 1999;37:463–474.

70. Briggs GG, Freeman RK, Yaffe SJ: Drugs in Pregnancy and Lactation, 5th ed. Baltimore, Williams & Wilkins, 1998.

71. Benoff S, Cooper GW, Hurley I, et al: The effect of calcium ion channel blockers on sperm fertilization potential. Fertil Steril 1994;62:606–617.

72. Tuncok Y, Apaydin S, Gidener S, et al: The effects of amrinone and glucagon on verapamil-induced myocardial depression in a rat isolated heart model. Gen Pharmacol 1997;28:773–776.

73. Alousi AA, Canter JM, Fort DJ: The beneficial effect of amrinone on acute drug-induced heart failure in the anaesthetised dog. Cardiovasc Res 1985;19:483–494.

74. Makela VH, Kapur PA: Amrinone and verapamil-propranolol induced cardiac depression during isoflurane anesthesia in dogs. Anesthesiology 1987;66:792–797.

75. Goenen M, Col J, Compere A, Bonte J: Treatment of severe verapamil poisoning with combined amrinone-isoproterenol therapy. Am J Cardiol 1986;58:1142–1143.

76. Wolf LR, Spadafora MP, Otten EJ: Use of amrinone and glucagon in a case of calcium channel blocker overdose. Ann Emerg Med 1993;22:1225–1228.

77. Ramoska EA, Spiller HA, Myers A: Calcium channel blocker toxicity. Ann Emerg Med 1990;19:649–653.

78. Snover SW, Bocchino V: Massive diltiazem overdose. Ann Emerg Med 1986;15:1221–1224.

79. Watling SM, Crain JL, Edwards TD, Stiller RA: Verapamil overdose: case report and review of the literature. Ann Pharmacother 1992;26:1373–1378.

80. Hofer CA, Smith JK, Tenholder MF: Verapamil intoxication: a literature review of overdoses and discussion of therapeutic options. Am J Med 1993;95:431–438.

81. Hendren WG, Schieber RS, Garrettson LK: Extracorporeal bypass for the treatment of verapamil poisoning. Ann Emerg Med 1989;18:984–987.

82. Ishikawa T, Imamura T, Koiwaya Y, Tanaka K: Atrioventricular dissociation and sinus arrest induced by oral diltiazem. N Engl J Med 1983;309:1124–1125.

83. Frierson J, Bailly D, Shultz T, Sund S, Dimas A, et al: Refractory cardiogenic shock and complete heart block after unsuspected verapamil-SR and atenolol overdose. Clin Cardiol 1991;14:933–935.

84. Orr GM, Bodansky HJ, Dymond DS, Taylor M: Fatal verapamil overdose. Lancet 1982;2(8309):1218–1219.

85. Holzer M, Sterz F, Schoerkhuber W, et al: Successful resuscitation of a verapamil-intoxicated patient with percutaneous cardiopulmonary bypass. Crit Care Med 1999;27:2818–2823.

86. Tenenbein M, Cohen S, Sitar DS: Whole bowel irrigation as a decontamination procedure after acute drug overdose. Arch Intern Med 1987;147:905–907.

87. Tenenbein M: Whole bowel irrigation and activated charcoal. Ann Emerg Med 1989;18:707–708.

88. Kirshenbaum LA, Mathews SC, Sitar DS, Tenenbein M: Whole-bowel irrigation versus activated charcoal in sorbitol for the ingestion of modified-release pharmaceuticals. Clin Pharmacol Ther 1989;46:264–271.

89. Agoston S, Maestrone E, van Hezik EJ, et al: Effective treatment of verapamil intoxication with 4-aminopyridine in the cat. J Clin Invest 1984;73:1291–1296.

90. Gay R, Algeo S, Lee R, et al: Treatment of verapamil toxicity in intact dogs. J Clin Invest 1986;77:1805–1811.

91. ter Wee PM, Kremer Hovinga TK, Uges DR, van der Geest S: 4-Aminopyridine and haemodialysis in the treatment of verapamil intoxication. Hum Toxicol 1985;4:327–329.

92. Belson MG, Gorman SE, Sullivan K, Geller RJ: Calcium channel blocker ingestions in children (comment). Am J Emerg Med 2000;18:581–586.

93. Perkins CM: Serious verapamil poisoning: treatment with intravenous calcium gluconate. BMJ 1978;2(6145):1127.

94. Strubelt O, Diederich KW: Experimental investigations on the antidotal treatment of nifedipine overdosage. J Toxicol Clin Toxicol 1986;24:135–149.

95. Hariman RJ, Mangiardi LM, McAllister RG Jr, et al: Reversal of the cardiovascular effects of verapamil by calcium and sodium: differences between electrophysiologic and hemodynamic responses. Circulation 1979;59:797–804.

96. Crump BJ, Holt DW, Vale JA: Lack of response to intravenous calcium in severe verapamil poisoning. Lancet 1982;2(8304): 939–940.

97. MacDonald D, Alguire PC: Case report: fatal overdose with sustained-release verapamil. Am J Med Sci 1992;303:115–117.

98. Haddad LM: Resuscitation after nifedipine overdose exclusively with intravenous calcium chloride. Am J Emerg Med 1996;14: 602–603.

99. Kenny J: Treating overdose with calcium channel blockers (comment). BMJ 1994;308(6935):992–993.

100. Lam YM, Tse HF, Lau CP: Continuous calcium chloride infusion for massive nifedipine overdose. Chest 2001;119:1280–1282.

101. Gold H, et al: The effects of ouabain on the heart in the presence of hypercalcemia. Am Heart J 1927;3:45–50.

102. Nola GT, Pope S, Harrison DC: Assessment of the synergistic relationship between serum calcium and digitalis. Am Heart J 1970;79:499–507.

103. Smith PK, et al: Calcium and digitalis synergism: the toxicity of calcium salts injected intravenously into digitalized animals. Arch Intern Med 1939;64:322–328.

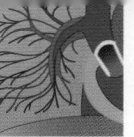

104. Kline JA, Leonova E, Raymond RM: Beneficial myocardial metabolic effects of insulin during verapamil toxicity in the anesthetized canine. Crit Care Med 1995;23:1251–1263.

105. van den Berghe G, Wouters P, Weekers F, et al: Intensive insulin therapy in the critically ill patients (comment). N Engl J Med 2001;345:1359–1367.

106. Boyer EW, Shannon M: Treatment of calcium-channel-blocker intoxication with insulin infusion. N Engl J Med 2001;344:1721–1722.

107. Levey GS, Fletcher MA, Klein I, et al: Characterization of 125I-glucagon binding in a solubilized preparation of cat myocardial adenylate cyclase: further evidence for a dissociable receptor site. J Biol Chem 1974;249:2665–2673.

108. Mery PF, Fischmeister R: Glucagon stimulates the cardiac Ca2+ current by activation of adenylyl cyclase and inhibition of phosphodiesterase. Nature 1990;345(6271):158–161.

109. Sauvadet A, Rohn T, Pecker F, Pavoine C: Synergistic actions of glucagon and miniglucagon on Ca2+ mobilization in cardiac cells. Circ Res 1996;78:102–109.

110. Stone CK, Thomas SH, Koury SI, Low RB: Glucagon and phenylephrine combination vs glucagon alone in experimental verapamil overdose (comment). Acad Emerg Med 1996;3:120–125.

111. Stone CK, May WA, Carroll R: Treatment of verapamil overdose with glucagon in dogs. Ann Emerg Med 1995;25:369–374.

112. Zaritsky AL, Horowitz M, Chernow B: Glucagon antagonism of calcium channel blocker-induced myocardial dysfunction. Crit Care Med 1988;16:246–251.

113. Sabatier J, Pouyet T, Shelvey G, Cavero I: Antagonistic effects of epinephrine, glucagon and methylatropine but not calcium chloride against atrio-ventricular conduction disturbances produced by high doses of diltiazem, in conscious dogs. Fundam Clin Pharmacol 1991;5:93–106.

114. Jolly SR, Kipnis JN, Lucchesi BR: Cardiovascular depression by verapamil: reversal by glucagon and interactions with propranolol. Pharmacology 1987;35:249–255.

115. Doyon S, Roberts JR: The use of glucagon in a case of calcium channel blocker overdose. Ann Emerg Med 1993;22:1229–1233.

116. Walter FG, Frye G, Mullen JT, et al: Amelioration of nifedipine poisoning associated with glucagon therapy. Ann Emerg Med 1993;22:1234–1237.

117. Parmley WW, Glick G, Sonnenblick EH: Cardiovascular effects of glucagon in man. N Engl J Med 1968;279:12–17.

118. Love JN, Sachdeva DK, Bessman ES, et al: A potential role for glucagon in the treatment of drug-induced symptomatic bradycardia. Chest 1998;114:323–326.

119. DeRoos F: Calcium channel blockers. In Goldfrank LR, Howland MA, Flomenbaum NE, et al (eds): Goldfrank's Toxicologic Emergencies. New York, McGraw-Hill, 2002, p 768.

60 β-Adrenergic Antagonists

STEVEN B. BIRD, MD

At a Glance...

- The classic presentation of overdose is bradycardia, hypotension, hypoglycemia, and decreased mental status.
- Some agents may produce tachycardia and hypertension.
- Glucagon is the treatment of choice for bradycardia and hypotension.
- Combined pharmacologic therapy is often needed in moderate-to-severe poisoning.
- Invasive measures such as transvenous pacing, intra-aortic balloon counterpulsion, and cardiopulmonary bypass should be considered if pharmacotherapy is ineffective.

INTRODUCTION AND RELEVANT HISTORY

Since the first use of β-adrenergic antagonists ("β blockers") for angina and hypertension in the early 1960s, the clinical indications for their use and number of prescriptions filled per year have increased dramatically. Currently, β-adrenergic antagonists are indicated for cardiac dysrhythmias, angina pectoris, hypertension, idiopathic hypertrophic subaortic stenosis, after myocardial infarction, for management of stable congestive heart failure, aortic dissection, thyroid storm, essential tremors, glaucoma, migraine prophylaxis, anxiety states, withdrawal states, and pheochromocytoma.[1,2]

EPIDEMIOLOGY

Not unexpectedly, increased use of these agents has led to increased incidence of toxicity. Frishman and colleagues[3] published the first review of β-adrenergic toxicity in 1979. The American Association of Poison Control Centers (AAPCC) reported a nearly sixfold increase in β-adrenergic exposures from 1984 to 2002, and an increase in mortality from 6 to 39 during the same time period.[4,5]

It has been estimated that by the year 2030, more than 20% of the U.S. population will be aged 65 years or older[6] and that the number of people with congestive heart failure will increase to nearly 6 million.[7] One may expect with an aging population, combined with ever-increasing indications for β-adrenergic antagonists, that the number of poisonings (as well as the severity of the poisonings) will continue to increase. Therefore, an understanding of the pharmacology, toxicology, and clinical presentation of patients after β-adrenergic antagonist poisoning is essential.

PHARMACOLOGY

β Blockers are generally classified on the basis of their cardioselectivity or the type of β-adrenergic receptor that is antagonized. These agents may also be classified according to the degree to which they possess partial agonist properties and also their membrane stabilization and antidysrhythmic effects (Table 60-1). As with many pharmaceutical agents, receptor selectivity is largely lost upon overdose.

A thorough understanding of β-adrenergic receptor antagonist toxicity requires a brief review of these receptors. The distinction between α and β receptors was elucidated and published in 1948 by Ahlquist.[8] Binding of epinephrine and norepinephrine to β receptors results in the phosphorylation of a G-protein complex on the cytoplasmic side of the cell membrane. Conformational changes in the G protein allow adenylate cyclase to catalyze the formation of cyclic adenosine monophosphate (cAMP) in the cytoplasm. In the myocyte, cAMP stimulates various protein kinases that phosphorylate calcium channels, thereby resulting in calcium entry into the cell and calcium-dependent calcium release from the sarcoplasmic reticulum. This calcium is responsible for the excitation-contraction coupling of myocytes.[9] Nonspecific phosphodiesterases then hydrolyze cAMP and prevent further downstream effects.[10]

Further characterization of the β_1 and β_2 receptors was published in 1967 by Lands and associates.[11] It was not until 1989 that a third β-adrenergic receptor was characterized,[12] although this β_3 receptor is primarily located on adipose cells and has no significant cardiovascular effects. A fourth type of β receptor that is responsible for partial agonist activity, termed the *cardiac putative β_4 adrenoreceptor*, has been proposed.[13]

β_1-Adrenergic specific receptors are found primarily in the myocardium, kidneys, and eyes, and they demonstrate roughly equal binding affinities for epinephrine and norepinephrine.[11] β_1-Receptor stimulation leads to increases in myocardial contractile force (inotropy) and rate (chronotropy) as a result of increased sinoatrial node firing as well as action potential conduction velocity.[14] β_1-Receptor activation also increases renin secretion by the kidney and aqueous humor production in the anterior chamber of the eye. β_2 Receptors are found predominantly in vascular smooth and skeletal muscle, the pancreas, the liver, and adipose tissue. Agonism of β_2 receptors leads to relaxation of smooth muscle in the lungs, blood vessels, uterus, and intestines. Metabolic effects of β_2-receptor stimulation include lipolysis, glycogenolysis, and increased insulin secretion (Table 60-2).

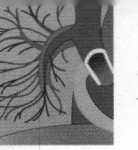

XTABLE 60-1 Classification of β Blockers

NAME	ADRENERGIC RECEPTOR ANTAGONISM	PARTIAL AGONIST	MEMBRANE STABILIZATION	LIPID SOLUBILITY	ORAL BIOAVAILABILITY (%)	PROTEIN BINDING (%)	VD (L/kg)	ELIMINATION	HALF-LIFE (hr)
Acebutolol	β_1	Yes	Yes	Moderate	40	25	2.3	Renal	3–6
Atenolol	β_1	No	No	Low	50	15	0.7	Renal	6–9
Betaxolol	β_1	No	Yes	Low	90	50	6.0	Hepatic	14–22
Bisoprolol	β_1	No	No	Low	80	30–50	2.7–3.1	Hepatic	9–12
Carteolol	β_1, β_2	No	No	Low	85	23–30	4.0	Renal	6
Carvedilol	$\beta_1, \beta_2, \alpha_1$	Yes	No	High	25–35	95	1.6	Hepatic	6–10
Esmolol	β_1	No	No	Low	N/A	55	3.4	Esterase	0.15
Labetalol	β_1, β_2	Yes	No	Low	30–40	50	10	Hepatic	3–6
Metoprolol	β_1	No	No	Moderate-high	40–50	12	5.5	Hepatic	3–4
Nadolol	β_1, β_2	No	No	Low	30–50	30	2.1	Renal	14–24
Penbutolol	β_1, β_2	Yes	No	High	100	90–98	>30	Hepatic	20
Pindolol	β_1, β_2	Yes	Yes	Moderate	99	40–60	2.0	Renal	3–12
Propranolol	β_1, β_2	No	Yes	High	30	90	3.6	Hepatic	3–5
Sotalol	β_1, β_2	No	No	Low	90–100	0	0.2	Renal	5–12
Timolol	β_1, β_2	No	No	Low	75	10	1.5	Renal	4

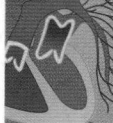

TABLE 60-2 β-Receptor Effects

β₁-RECEPTOR EFFECTS		β₂-RECEPTOR EFFECTS	
ORGAN	**EFFECT**	**ORGAN/SYSTEM**	**EFFECT**
Eye	Increased aqueous humor production	Lung	Bronchial dilation
Kidney	Increase renin production	Vascular system	Arteriole dilation
Heart	Increased inotropy and chronotropy		Increased insulin secretion
			Increased lipolysis
			Increased glycogenolysis
		Metabolic system	Increased lactic acid production
		Other	Intracellular potassium shift

PATHOPHYSIOLOGY

The antagonism of β receptors and subsequent derangements in catecholamine physiologic effects cannot account for all the observed toxicity following β-receptor antagonist overdose. That is, if β-receptor antagonism alone were responsible for the observed clinical effects, then β-receptor agonism should provide adequate means to overcome the receptor blockade. However, experimental evidence and clinical experience suggest other mechanisms are at work. For instance, in isolated rat hearts depleted of catecholamines, the addition of β blockers produces toxicity. Additionally, in a canine model of acute β-blocker toxicity, Kerns and associates demonstrated no improvement in survival with the addition of high-dose epinephrine.[15]

PHARMACOKINETICS

β Blockers are generally rapidly absorbed after ingestion, with peak effects occurring after 1 to 4 hours.[16] Sustained-release formulations, however, produce prolonged absorption. It is prudent to keep in mind that pharmacokinetics may be altered greatly in the setting of overdose.[17] The volume of distribution for β blockers varies widely: only atenolol and sotalol have volumes of distribution of less than one (see Table 60-1). Half-lives of these agents are generally brief (approximately 6 hours) but vary from a low of 10 minutes for esmolol, to 24 hours for nadolol. Low cardiac output states, hepatic dysfunction, and inducers of hepatic enzymes may alter the duration of action for those β blockers, which are metabolized by the liver. Similarly, renal dysfunction and low cardiac output may increase the duration of action for agents that are excreted unchanged in the urine (see Table 60-1).

After acute oral overdose of immediate-release preparations, signs of toxicity usually begin within 30 minutes and peak by 2 hours. Toxicity after ingestion of sustained-release preparations or sotalol may be delayed until 20 hours after ingestion.[18-21] Toxicity after β-blocker overdose may persist as long as several days.[22]

The lipid solubility of β blockers can significantly influence the degree of clinical toxicity observed after overdose owing to penetration of the blood-brain barrier. The agents with the highest degree of lipophilicity include metoprolol, penbutolol, propranolol, and carvedilol. The concentration of propranolol in the central nervous system (CNS) may exceed that seen in plasma by as much as 20-fold.[23]

Acebutolol, carteolol, penbutolol, pindolol, and timolol uniquely possess partial β-adrenergic agonist properties (also known as intrinsic sympathomimetic activity, or ISA), leading to a normal heart rate or even tachycardia. Therefore, bradycardia should not be viewed as invariably present after β-blocker poisoning.

The decreased cAMP formation following β-blocker administration also leads to inhibition of sodium and calcium influx currents during phase 0 of the cardiac action potential, thereby classifying β blockers as Vaughn Williams class II antidysrhythmics.[24] This effect is termed *membrane stabilization.*

Special Populations

Clinical effects observed with β-blocker toxicity may differ according to the age of the patient. Symptomatic hypoglycemia may be more common in children than in adults. The baseline cardiovascular disease present in many elderly patients may make overdoses or unintentional poisonings more severe in this age group.

Drug Interactions

Drugs that induce hepatic mixed-function oxygenases may increase metabolism of betaxolol, bisoprolol, carvedilol, labetalol, metoprolol, penbutolol, and propranolol. Notable examples include phenytoin, phenobarbital, isoniazid, and rifampin. Other drugs (e.g., erythromycin, clarithromycin, cimetidine) may inhibit hepatic metabolism of these agents and therefore produce toxicity at unexpected doses. The other β blockers listed in Table 60-1 (except esmolol) undergo primarily renal elimination and can therefore be affected by agents that decrease renal clearance (e.g., nonsteroidal anti-inflammatory drugs). It is unknown whether the new cyclooxygenase II inhibitors sufficiently perturb β-blocker elimination.

Owing to their significant effects on myocardial physiology, the principal drugs that interact with β blockers are other antihypertensive and antidysrhythmic agents. In both therapeutic doses and overdoses, the combination of a β blocker and a calcium channel blocker may lead to hypotension, bradycardia, and death.[25-27] Combination treatment with peripheral

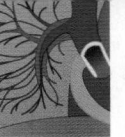

vasodilators such as hydralazine may lead to significant hypotension as a result of β-blocker inhibition of the usual reflex tachycardia. Administration of exogenous catecholamines, or the presence of any drug that leads to release or accumulation of catecholamines (e.g., cocaine, amphetamines, monoamine oxidase inhibitors), may lead to "unopposed α-adrenergic" stimulation and resultant hypertension, cardiac ischemia, or stroke.[28-30]

TOXICOLOGY

Clinical Manifestations

Cardiac conduction abnormalities are common. First-degree atrioventricular (AV) block, intraventricular conduction abnormalities, high-grade AV block, non-specific ST segment and T wave changes, QT prolongation, and asystole have all been recorded. Varying degrees of ventricular depolarization and repolarization abnormalities may occur, particularly with membrane stabilization agents and sotalol.[31-33] Most patients with overdose present with hypotension and bradycardia.[21] Ingestion of agents with ISA, however, may lead to tachycardia and hypertension.[34,35] Sotalol is particularly toxic, with frequent reporting of ventricular tachycardia, torsades de pointes, and ventricular fibrillation[19,36] owing to its effect on action potential duration and subsequent QT prolongation.[37,38]

CNS depression, ranging from drowsiness to coma, is a relatively common effect of β-blocker toxicity[32] and generally reflects the severity of the poisoning.[17,20] CNS toxicity may occur in the absence of bradycardia, hypotension, or hypoglycemia,[21] particularly with the lipid-soluble agents.[3,39,40] CNS depression also is exacerbated by β blocker–associated cerebral hypoperfusion, acidemia, and hypoxia.[32]

While bronchospasm has been traditionally been a concern following therapeutic use or overdose of β blockers, it remains an unusual complication of β-blocker toxicity. When it does occur, bronchospasm is more likely to occur in patients with preexisting pulmonary disease. More common is respiratory depression, usually due to CNS toxicity.[41] Central cyanosis may be present. Peripheral cyanosis due to antagonism of vascular β_2 receptors with the accompanying "unopposed α_1" effects may be evident[21,32,42] and has led to mesenteric ischemia.[43]

Frank hypoglycemia is infrequently seen with β-blocker toxicity, but normal serum glucose in the setting of significant β-blocker poisoning may in fact be relative hypoglycemia. Hypoglycemia is more common in children, persons with diabetes, and patients with uremia. The typical tachycardia seen during hypoglycemia may be diminished after β-blocker ingestion although other symptoms of hypoglycemia are relatively unchanged. Hyperkalemia is variably present and may be a clue to β-blocker poisoning.

Renal effects after β-blocker poisoning are unusual, although oliguric renal failure has been reported rarely.[44]

TABLE 60-3 Adverse Effects of β-Adrenergic Antagonists	
SYSTEM	**EFFECTS**
Cardiovascular	Hypotension
	Hypertension (partial agonists)
	Bradycardia, atrioventricular block, asystole
	Tachycardia (partial agonists)
	Prolonged PR interval
	Prolonged QT interval (sotalol)
	Prolonged QRS complex (membrane-stabilizing agents)
	Ventricular dysrhythmias (membrane-stabilizing agents, sotalol)
CNS	Decreased level of consciousness
(lipid-soluble and membrane-stabilizing agents)	Seizures
	Depression
	Insomnia
Respiratory	Bronchospasm
	Respiratory depression
Gastrointestinal	Esophageal spasm
	Mesenteric ischemia
Metabolic	Hypoglycemia
Other	Renal failure

The adverse effects observed after therapeutic doses of β blockers are listed in Table 60-3. Chronic therapeutic use of β blockers leads to an increase in adrenergic receptor expression and a resultant increase in catecholamine sensitivity upon withdrawal of β blockers. This may in part explain the degree to which high doses of β blockers are tolerated, so long as the dose is increased slowly, and why acute ingestion of a similar dose may produce toxicity in patients not accustomed to β-blocker use.[45]

DIAGNOSIS

Laboratory Testing

β Blockers are not detected by current enzyme immunoassays. Routine serum or urine β-blocker concentrations are not available. Additionally, owing to interindividual variations in metabolism and protein binding and variations in dosing, determination of serum concentrations in the acute setting generally are not helpful[22] but can be used as a confirmatory test when overdose is suspected.

Other Diagnostic Testing

All patients with confirmed or suspected β-blocker overdose or symptoms consistent with β-blocker toxicity should be placed on continuous cardiac monitoring and have a 12-lead electrocardiogram (ECG) interpreted. Frequent recording of vital signs should be routine. Symptomatic patients should have determination of electrolytes, blood urea nitrogen (BUN), creatinine, glucose, and complete blood count. Determination of serum drug concentrations as indicated (e.g., digoxin)

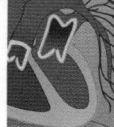

should be performed. For patients with abnormal vital signs, a chest radiograph and arterial blood gas measurement should be assessed.

Differential Diagnosis

Other causes of cardiovascular collapse with hypotension and bradycardia (except with the possibility of tachycardia after poisoning with β blockers that possess partial agonist activity) include shock of anaphylactic, cardiogenic (including pulmonary embolism), septic, and hypovolemic etiologies. Additionally, other toxicologic sources must be considered, particularly poisoning with calcium channel blockers, organophosphorus or carbamate agents, antidysrhythmics, centrally acting antihypertensives, cardiac glycosides, cyanide, hydrogen sulfide, narcotics, chloroquine, sedative-hypnotics, and tricyclic antidepressants. β-Blocker poisoning should be suspected in any patient with hypotension, bradycardia, and seizures. Differentiation between β-blocker and calcium channel blocker toxicity may be aided by measurement of the serum glucose: hypoglycemia may be present with β-blocker poisoning, whereas hyperglycemia is often seen after poisoning by calcium channel blockers. The presence of hyperkalemia may also be a clue to β-blocker toxicity.

MANAGEMENT

Supportive Measures

When possible, historical data regarding the time of ingestion, agents involved, quantity ingested, other medications, and a medical history should be obtained. One should also pay particular attention to the vital signs and examination of the cardiopulmonary and neurologic systems

As for any patient, priority should be given to establishment of adequate airway, breathing, and circulation. In at least two animal studies, the primary determinant of β-blocker toxicity and death was respiratory arrest.[46,47] Therefore, early establishment of adequate ventilation is essential.

All patients should have continuous cardiac monitoring, continuous pulse oximetry, an ECG, and frequent assessment of vital signs. Determination of the complete blood count, bedside finger-stick glucose, serum electrolytes, BUN, and serum creatinine should be performed. A chest radiograph and arterial blood gas measurement should be obtained in all symptomatic patients. If the diagnosis is uncertain, a comprehensive toxicology screen may be of benefit.

Decontamination

Gastrointestinal decontamination with activated charcoal 1 g/kg (maximum, 50 to 60 g) should be done as soon as possible after initiation of supportive care. The use of syrup of ipecac to induce emesis cannot be advocated because of the risk of vomiting and aspiration,

particularly if respiratory or CNS depression follow. At least one author has suggested that prophylactic atropine may be beneficial to inhibit vagally mediated bradycardia during endotracheal or gastric intubation.[24]

In an effort to decrease any enterohepatic circulation, repeated doses of activated charcoal are recommended for symptomatic patients. Additionally, in patients poisoned with sustained-release formulations, placement of a nasogastric or orogastric tube and whole-bowel irrigation with a polyethylene glycol solution (20 to 30 mL/kg/hr in adults and 10 to 20 mL/kg/hr in children) should be considered.

Laboratory Monitoring

Continuous cardiac monitoring and frequent ECGs are indicated for all patients. Serial determinations of serum potassium and glucose also are prudent, as is the determination of serum magnesium, particularly for agents known to cause torsades de pointes.

Antidotes

GLUCAGON

Glucagon is the most consistently effective agent for β-blocker poisoning in both laboratory studies and in humans[21,32] and is the therapeutic drug of choice. Glucagon is a pancreatic polypeptide whose inotropic and chronotropic effects were first discovered in 1960.[30] Glucagon is thought to activate adenylate cyclase independently of the β-adrenergic receptor, thereby increasing cAMP synthesis with the resultant increase in myocardial heart rate and contractility.[48-54] It increases mean arterial pressure, cardiac index, and contractility without altering the left ventricular end-diastolic pressure.[55-57] Glucagon is more effective in reversing hypotension than either epinephrine or isoproterenol.[32] However, therapy with several agents simultaneously may be required.

Glucagon has a half-life of roughly 20 minutes. After an initial IV bolus dose of 5 to 10 mg for adults (50 to 150 μg/kg in children), a continuous infusion of 1 to 5 mg/hr (10 to 50 μg/kg/hr in children) should be used, if effective. Continuous IV infusion of glucagon is preferred to intermittent bolus dosing owing to the more sustained increase in blood pressure observed after the former.[58] Clinical effects begin in as few as 1 to 3 minutes, with peak effects seen at 5 to 7 minutes.[48] It is recommended that glucagon be reconstituted in normal saline or 5% dextrose, because the diluent provided by the manufacturer contains 2 mg of phenol per 1 mg of glucagon, which may be toxic in doses of 25 mg or more.[59,60]

Nausea and vomiting (occurring in nearly one third of patients) are the most common side effects after glucagon therapy.[61,62] Hyperglycemia may occur and is the basis for administration of glucagon for hypoglycemia; however, the stimulation of pancreatic insulin secretion by glucagon may also lead to hypoglycemia. As a result of insulin-mediated intracellular ion shifts, hypokalemia may occur. Rare but more significant

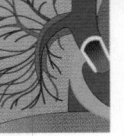

adverse effects after glucagon therapy include Stevens-Johnson syndrome, erythema multiforme minor, and acute allergic reaction.[63] The few contraindications to glucagon therapy that exist are the presence of insulinoma, pheochromocytoma, or glucagon hypersensitivity.[30] Because of limited hospital pharmacy stocking of glucagon, additional sources should be sought soon after initiation of continuous IV therapy.[64,65]

CALCIUM

Presumably owing to the derangements in calcium-mediated myocardial contraction and vascular tone, IV calcium is variably effective in reducing hypotension.[66-69] Calcium chloride 1 to 2 g intravenously every 5 to 10 minutes as necessary is commonly used, but it must be administered cautiously because of its highly irritating effects. One must give serious consideration to delivery via central venous access. Calcium gluconate may also be used but contains only one third the calcium of calcium chloride on a gram-for-gram basis. Hypercalcemia may be a theoretical concern. However, severely poisoned patients who receive several doses of calcium chloride should be intubated, thereby mitigating concerns about hypercalcemia-induced CNS and respiratory depression.[70]

CATECHOLAMINE AGENTS

Because β blockers bind to the adrenergic receptors in a competitive fashion, one might expect that β agonists and vasopressors alone would reverse toxicity. Unfortunately, therapeutic response to these agents alone is limited and variable. Doses of catecholamines needed to achieve a significant response may be four or more times greater than doses generally used.[20,21,71] The pro-dysrhythmic potential of these agents when used in high doses, particularly isoproterenol, mitigates some of the enthusiasm for their use. Nevertheless, catecholamines remain a vital part of the multitherapy strategy for severely poisoned patients.

PHOSPHODIESTERASE INHIBITORS

Inamrinone (formerly named amrinone) may produce an increase in contractility independently of the β receptor by inhibiting phosphodiesterase and thus slowing the breakdown of cAMP. Inamrinone increased inotropy in a canine model of β-blocker poisoning,[72] but was of no additional benefit (and may have been detrimental) when added to glucagon therapy.[73] The recommended dose of inamrinone for congestive heart failure is a 0.75 mg/kg IV bolus over 2 to 3 minutes, followed by a continuous infusion of 5 to 10 µg/kg/min. If needed, a repeat bolus dose may be given 30 minutes after the initiation of therapy.

ATROPINE

Although frequently ineffective, patients with bradycardia and hypotension warrant a trial of atropine therapy and may receive modest benefit.

TREATMENT OF SEIZURES

Seizures that are not responsive to glucose should be managed with benzodiazepines, barbiturates, and possibly phenytoin.

Treatment of Bronchospasm

Bronchospasm may be induced by β-blocker toxicity, particularly in patients with a history of reactive airway disease. Treatment should proceed much as for other nontoxicologic causes of asthma, including inhaled β_2 agonists and anticholinergic agents and subcutaneous epinephrine as needed.

Nonpharmacologic Therapies

External or transvenous cardiac pacing should be considered after failure of pharmacotherapy alone.[74,75] However, electrical capture is not always possible after severe poisoning, and while the heart rate may respond to pacing, a consistent increase in blood pressure is not always achieved.[21,76] Transvenous cardiac pacing may be most useful in treating refractory torsades de pointes due to sotalol poisoning.[19,36]

Other invasive measures that have been used with varying degrees of success in severe poisoning include intra-aortic balloon counterpulsion, cardiopulmonary bypass, and extracorporeal membrane oxygenation.[18,76,77]

Sotalol Intoxication

The unique pharmacology and pharmacokinetics of sotalol warrant special attention. Patients may have significant tachycardia and hypertension due to sotalol toxicity. If no end-organ dysfunction is present, however, close monitoring in the hospital setting may be all that is required. If end-organ toxicity exists, then short-acting agents such as nitroprusside and esmolol should be used. As mentioned above, ventricular dysrhythmias, QT prolongation, and subsequent torsades de pointes may be more frequent with sotalol poisoning. Treatment of sotalol-induced ventricular tachydysrhythmias includes magnesium, lidocaine, phenytoin, and "overdrive" pacing with either transvenous electrical pacing or isoproterenol.[78-81]

Elimination

Although the use of charcoal hemoperfusion after β-blocker poisoning has been reported,[74] the pharmacokinetic properties of most β blockers would appear to limit the usefulness of extracorporeal elimination. Owing to their low degree of protein binding and low volumes of distribution, atenolol and sotalol would be expected to be most responsive to extracorporeal elimination.[20,82]

Disposition

All symptomatic patients after β-adrenergic antagonist ingestion or overdose, and patients with a history of sotalol ingestion should be admitted to the hospital. Patients with significant signs or symptoms of toxicity (including but not limited to altered mental status, bradycardia, hypotension, and dysrhythmias) should be managed in an intensive care unit. While no prospective studies exist, patients who do not ingest a sustained-release formulation and who remain asymptomatic with a normal ECG and normal vital signs should be observed for at least 6 hours. Ingestion of a sustained-release formulation necessitates admission or observation for at least 24 hours.

From 30% to 40% of β-adrenergic receptor antagonist overdose patients remain asymptomatic.[83] However, other authors have reported a mortality rate as high as 26%.[84] In one review of the literature, 75% of deaths due to propranolol occurred at home.[83] Therefore, it would appear that if a patient arrives in the emergency department alive and appropriate treatment is initiated early, the prognosis is good. Attempts at prolonged resuscitation after β-blocker overdose are warranted, since survival without neurologic sequelae has been reported.[85]

REFERENCES

1. Hoffman BB: Catecholamines, sympathomimetic drugs, and adrenergic receptor antagonists. In Hardman JG, Limbird LE (eds): Goodman & Gilman's The Pharmacological Basis of Therapeutics, 10th ed. New York, McGraw-Hill, 2001, pp 215–268.
2. Packer M, Coats AJ, Fowler MB, et al: Effect of carvedilol on survival in severe chronic heart failure. N Engl J Med 2001;344:1651.
3. Frishman W, Silverman R, Strom J, et al: Clinical pharmacology of the new beta-adrenergic blocking drugs. 4. Adverse effects: choosing a beta-adrenoreceptor blocker. Am Heart J 1979;98:256.
4. Litovitz T, Veltri JC: 1984 annual report of the American Association of Poison Control Centers National Data Collection System. Am J Emerg Med 1985;3:423–450.
5. Watson WA, Litovitz TL, Rodgers GC Jr, et al: 2002 annual report of the American Association of Poison Control Centers toxic exposure surveillance system. Am J Emerg Med 2003;21:353.
6. U.S. Census Bureau: Statistical Abstract of the United States: 2001, 121st ed. Washington, DC, U.S. Department of Commerce, 2001.
7. Field JL: Beyond four walls: research summary for clinicians and administrators on CHF management. In Cardiology Preeminence Round Table, Advisory Board. Washington, DC, 1994.
8. Alquist R: Study of adrenotropic receptors. Am J Physiol 1948;153:586.
9. Colucci WS, Wright RF, Braunwald E: New positive inotropic agents in the treatment of congestive heart failure: mechanisms of action and recent clinical developments. N Engl J Med 1986;314:290.
10. Insel PA: Seminars in medicine of the Beth Israel Hospital, Boston: adrenergic receptors—evolving concepts and clinical implications. N Engl J Med 1996;334:580.
11. Lands AM, Arnold A, McAuliff JP, et al: Differentiation of receptor systems activated by sympathomimetic amines. Nature 1967;214(88):597.
12. Emorine LJ, Marullo S, Briend-Sutren MM, et al: Molecular characterization of the human beta 3-adrenergic receptor. Science 1989;245(4922):1118.
13. Kaumann AJ, Molenaar P: Modulation of human cardiac function through 4 beta-adrenoceptor populations. Naunyn Schmiedebergs Arch Pharmacol 1997;355:667.
14. Cirillo LA: Commonly used emergency cardiac medications. In Aghababian RV (ed): Emergency Management of Cardiovascular Disease. Boston, Butterworth-Heinemann, 1994, p 371.
15. Kerns W II, Schroeder D, Williams C, et al: Insulin improves survival in a canine model of acute beta-blocker toxicity. Ann Emerg Med 1997;29:748.
16. Hoffman B: Adrenoreceptor-blocking drugs. In Katzung B (ed): Basic and Clinical Pharmacology, 6th ed. Norwalk, CT, Appleton & Lange, 1995, p 137.
17. Jackson CD, Fishbein L: A toxicological review of beta-adrenergic blockers. Fundam Appl Toxicol 1986;6:395.
18. Love JN, Litovitz TL, Howell JM, Clancy C: Characterization of fatal beta blocker ingestion: a review of the American Association of Poison Control Centers data from 1985 to 1995. J Toxicol Clin Toxicol 1997;35:353.
19. Neuvonen PJ, Elonen E, Vuorenmaa T, Laakso M: Prolonged Q-T interval and severe tachyarrhythmias, common features of sotalol intoxication. Eur J Clin Pharmacol 1981;20:85.
20. Heath A: Beta-adrenoceptor blocker toxicity: clinical features and therapy. Am J Emerg Med 1984;2:518.
21. Weinstein RS: Recognition and management of poisoning with beta-adrenergic blocking agents. Ann Emerg Med 1984;13:1123.
22. Frishman W, Jacob H, Eisenberg E, Ribner H: Clinical pharmacology of the new beta-adrenergic blocking drugs. 8. Self-poisoning with beta-adrenoceptor blocking agents: recognition and management. Am Heart J 1979;98:798.
23. Cruickshank J: The clinical importance of cardioselectivity and lipophilicity in β-blockers. Am Heart J 1980;100:160.
24. Linden CH: Beta-blocker poisoning. In Harwood-Nuss A (ed): The Clinical Practice of Emergency Medicine, 3rd ed. Philadelphia, Lippincott Williams & Wilkins, 2001, p 1439.
25. Benaim ME: Asystole after verapamil. BMJ 1972;2(806):169.
26. Wayne VS, Harper RW, Laufer E, et al: Adverse interaction between beta-adrenergic blocking drugs and verapamil—report of three cases. Aust N Z J Med 1982;12:285.
27. Opie LH, White DA: Adverse interaction between nifedipine and beta-blockade. BMJ 1980;281(6253):1462.
28. Billman GE: The effect of adrenergic receptor antagonists on cocaine-induced ventricular fibrillation: alpha but not beta adrenergic receptor antagonists prevent malignant arrhythmias independent of heart rate. J Pharmacol Exp Ther 1994;269:409.
29. Tseng CC, Derlet RW, Albertson TE: Acute cocaine toxicity: the effect of agents in non-seizure-induced death. Pharmacol Biochem Behav 1993;46:61.
30. Wolf LR: Beta-adrenergic blocker toxicity. In Haddad LM, Shannon MW, Wionshester JF (eds): Clinical Management of Poisoning and Drug Overdose, 3rd ed. Philadelphia, WB Saunders, 1998, p 1031.
31. Frishman WH: Beta-adrenergic receptor blockers: adverse effects and drug interactions. Hypertension 1988;11(3 pt 2):II21.
32. Critchley JA, Ungar A: The management of acute poisoning due to beta-adrenoceptor antagonists. Med Toxicol Adverse Drug Exp 1989;4:32.
33. Gwinup GR: Propranolol toxicity presenting with early repolarization, ST segment elevation, and peaked T waves on the ECG. Ann Emerg Med 1988;17:171.
34. Love JN: Acebutolol overdose resulting in fatalities. J Emerg Med 2000;18:341.
35. Thorpe P: Prindolol in hypertension. Med J Aust 1971;1:1242.
36. Totterman KJ, Turto H, Pellinen T: Overdrive pacing as treatment of sotalol-induced ventricular tachyarrhythmias (torsade de pointes). Acta Med Scand Suppl 1982;668:28.
37. Baliga BG: Beta-blocker poisoning: prolongation of Q-T interval and inversion of T wave. J Indian Med Assoc 1985;83:165.
38. Beattie JM: Sotalol induced torsade de pointes. Scott Med J 1984;29:240.
39. Koella WP: CNS-related (side-)effects of beta-blockers with special reference to mechanisms of action. Eur J Clin Pharmacol 1985;28(Suppl):55.
40. Buiumsohn A, Eisenberg ES, Jacob H, et al: Seizures and intraventricular conduction defect in propranolol poisoning: a report of two cases. Ann Intern Med 1979;91:860.
41. Weinstein RS, Cole S, Knaster HB, Dahlbert T: Beta blocker overdose with propranolol and with atenolol. Ann Emerg Med 1985;14:161.
42. Lund-Johansen P: The hemodynamic effects of adrenergic blocking agents. Cleve Clin J Med 1992;59:193.
43. Pettei MJ, Levy J, Abramson S: Nonocclusive mesenteric ischemia associated with propranolol overdose: implications regarding splanchnic circulation. J Pediatr Gastroenterol Nutr 1990;10:544.

44. Snook CP, Sigvaldason K, Kristinsson J: Severe atenolol and diltiazem overdose. J Toxicol Clin Toxicol 2000;38:661.

45. Lifshitz M, Zucker N, Zalzstein E: Acute dilated cardiomyopathy and central nervous system toxicity following propranolol intoxication. Pediatr Emerg Care 1999;15:262.

46. Langemeijer J, de Wildt D, de Groot G, Sangster B: Respiratory arrest as main determinant of toxicity due to overdose with different beta-blockers in rats. Acta Pharmacol Toxicol (Copenh) 1985;57:352.

47. Toet AE, te Biesebeek JD, Vleeming W, et al: Reduced survival after isoprenaline/dopamine in d,l-propranolol intoxicated rats. Hum Exp Toxicol 1996;15:120.

48. Parmley WW, Glick G, Sonnenblick EH: Cardiovascular effects of glucagon in man. N Engl J Med 1968;279:12.

49. Murad F: Effect of glucagon on heart. N Engl J Med 1968;279:434.

50. Jolly SR, Kipnis JN, Lucchesi BR: Cardiovascular depression by verapamil: reversal by glucagon and interactions with propranolol. Pharmacology 1987;35:249.

51. Levey GS, Epstein SE: Activation of adenyl cyclase by glucagon in cat and human heart. Circ Res 1969;24:151.

52. Kosinski EJ, Malindzak GS Jr: Glucagon and isoproterenol in reversing propranolol toxicity. Arch Intern Med 1973;132:840.

53. Robson RH: Glucagon for beta-blocker poisoning. Lancet 1980;1(8182):1357.

54. Peterson CD, Leeder JS, Sterner S: Glucagon therapy for beta-blocker overdose. Drug Intell Clin Pharm 1984;18:394.

55. Abel FL: Action of glucagon on canine left ventricular performance and coronary hemodynamics. Circ Shock 1983;11:45.

56. Manchester JH, Parmley WW, Matloff JM, et al: Effects of glucagon on myocardial oxygen consumption and coronary blood flow in man and dog. Circulation 1970;41:579.

57. Diamond G, Forrester J, Danzig R, et al: Acute myocardial infarction in man. Comparative hemodynamic effects of norepinephrine and glucagon. Am J Cardiol 1971;27:612.

58. Illingworth RN: Glucagon for beta-blocker poisoning. Practitioner 1979;223(1337):683.

59. Brancato DJ: Recognizing potential toxicity of phenol. Vet Hum Toxicol 1982;24:29.

60. Cronholm LS, Fishel CW: Bordetella pertussis-induced alteration of the normal hyperglycemic response of mice to 3',5'-adenosine phosphate. J Bacteriol 1968;95:1993.

61. Vander Ark CR, Reynolds EW Jr: Clinical evaluation of glucagon by continuous infusion in the treatment of low cardiac output states. Am Heart J 1970;79:481.

62. Williams JF, Childress RH, Chip JN: Hemodynamic effects of glucagon in patients with heart disease. Circulation 1969;39:38.

63. Zavras GM, Papadaki PJ, Kounis NG, Dimopoulos JA: Glucagon-induced severe anaphylactic reaction. Rofo Fortschr Geb Rontgenstr Neuen Bildgeb Verfahr 1990;152:110.

64. Love JN, Tandy TK: Beta-adrenoceptor antagonist toxicity: a survey of glucagon availability. Ann Emerg Med 1993;22:267.

65. Smith RC, Wilkinson J, Hull RL: Glucagon for propranolol overdose. JAMA 1985;254:2412.

66. Henry M, Kay MM, Viccellio P: Cardiogenic shock associated with calcium-channel and beta blockers: reversal with intravenous calcium chloride. Am J Emerg Med 1985;3:334.

67. Pertoldi F, D'Orlando L, Mercante WP: Electromechanical dissociation 48 hours after atenolol overdose: usefulness of calcium chloride. Ann Emerg Med 1998;31:777.

68. Brimacombe JR, Scully M, Swainston R: Propranolol overdose—a dramatic response to calcium chloride. Med J Aust 1991;155:267.

69. Brimacombe J: Use of calcium chloride for propranolol overdose. Anaesthesia 1992;47:907.

70. Pearigen PD: Calcium channel blocker poisoning. In Haddad JJ, Shannon MW, Winchester JF (eds): Clinical Management of Poisoning and Drug Overdose. Philadelphia, WB Saunders, 1998, p 1020.

71. Avery GJ II, Spotnitz HM, Rose EA, et al: Pharmacologic antagonism of beta-adrenergic blockade in dogs. 1. Hemodynamic effects of isoproterenol, dopamine, and epinephrine in acute propranolol administration. J Thorac Cardiovasc Surg 1979;77:267.

72. Alousi AA, Canter JM, Fort DJ: The beneficial effect of amrinone on acute drug-induced heart failure in the anaesthetised dog. Cardiovasc Res 1985;19:483.

73. Love JN, Leasure JA, Mundt DJ: A comparison of combined amrinone and glucagon therapy to glucagon alone for cardiovascular depression associated with propranolol toxicity in a canine model. Am J Emerg Med 1993;11:360.

74. Anthony T, Jastremski M, Elliott W, et al: Charcoal hemoperfusion for the treatment of a combined diltiazem and metoprolol overdose. Ann Emerg Med 1986;15:1344.

75. Saitz R, Williams BW, Farber HW: Atenolol-induced cardiovascular collapse treated with hemodialysis. Crit Care Med 1991;19:116.

76. McVey FK, Corke CF: Extracorporeal circulation in the management of massive propranolol overdose. Anaesthesia 1991;46:744.

77. Lane AS, Woodward AC, Goldman MR: Massive propranolol overdose poorly responsive to pharmacologic therapy: use of the intra-aortic balloon pump. Ann Emerg Med 1987;16:1381.

78. Adlerfliegel F, Leeman M, Demaeyer P, et al: Sotalol posoning associated with asystole. Intensive Care Med 1993;19:57.

79. Arstall M, Mii J, Lehman R, Horowitz JD: Sotalol-induced torsades de pointes: management with magnesium infusion. Postgrad Med 1992;68:289.

80. Perrot D, Bui-Xuan B, Lang J, et al: A case of sotalol poisoning with fatal outcome. J Toxicol Clin Toxicol 1988;26:389.

81. Kenyon CJ, Aldinger GE, Joshipura P: Successful resuscitation using external cardiac pacing in beta-adrenergic antagonist-induced bradyasystolic arrest. Ann Emerg Med 1988;17:711.

82. Singh S, Lazin A, Cohen A, et al: Sotalol-induced torsades de pointes successfully treated with hemodialysis after therapy of conventional therapy. Am Heart J 1991;2:601.

83. Taboulet P, Cariou A, Berdeaux A, Bismuth C: Pathophysiology and management of self-poisoning with beta-blockers. J Toxicol Clin Toxicol 1993;31:531.

84. Langemeijer JJ, de Wildt DJ, de Groot G, Sangster B: Intoxication with beta-sympathicolytics. Neth J Med 1992;40:308.

85. Alderfliegel F, Leeman M, Demaeyer P, Kahn RJ: Sotalol poisoning associated with asystole. Intensive Care Med 1993;19:57.

61 Nitroprusside, ACE Inhibitors, and Other Cardiovascular Agents

WILLIAM H. RICHARDSON, MD ■ DAVID P. BETTEN, MD ■ SARALYN R. WILLIAMS, MD ■ RICHARD F. CLARK, MD

At a Glance...

■ Early cyanide poisoning from nitroprusside may manifest with central nervous system effects and tachyphylaxis.

■ Thiocyanate poisoning, in contrast to cyanide poisoning, occurs most frequently in the setting of renal insufficiency and does not cause a metabolic acidosis.

■ Supportive care including intravenous fluids and inotropic agents are the mainstay of treatment in hydralazine and minoxidil poisoning.

■ Nonspecific T-wave and ST-segment ECG abnormalities are commonly described in overdose and with therapeutic use of hydralazine and minoxidil.

■ Nitrates/nitrites are contraindicated in the setting of sildenafil use even in the setting of acute coronary syndrome.

■ The presence of angioedema is classically described with ACE inhibitors but can also occur with angiotensin receptor blockers.

■ The use of alpha-1 antagonists may result in symptomatic hypotension in the absence of tachycardia due to isolated effects on the alpha-1 adrenergic receptor.

■ In diuretic abuse and overdose, care should be directed toward identification and correction of fluid and electrolyte abnormalities.

NITROPRUSSIDE

Sodium nitroprusside (SNP) is a potent vasodilator widely used due to its rapid onset of action, short half-life, and ease of titration. It is approved for reduction of blood pressure in hypertensive emergencies and for controlled hypotension during surgical procedures to reduce the risk for hemorrhage.[1] The first human use of nitroprusside was reported in 1928,[2] but its regular use in humans was not established until 1955 when a short-term infusion was used to treat severe hypertension.[3] Approval for clinical use in the United States occurred in 1974 after a lyophilized preparation became available. In 1991 the Food and Drug Administration (FDA) approved new labeling for SNP to highlight the risk for cyanide toxicity associated with prolonged infusion at rates that exceed $2 \mu g/kg/min$.[1]

Structure

Each SNP molecule is composed of an iron center that is complexed with five cyanide molecules and one nitrosyl group. Cyanide comprises about 44% of the molecular weight of the compound. After infusion, the compound undergoes degradation and the cyanide molecules and the nitric oxide are released. Nitric oxide acts as an endothelium-relaxing factor that results in the desired vasodilatory effects of SNP (Fig. 61-1).[4]

SNP is soluble in water but is unstable when exposed to sunlight. Photodegradation may result in release of up to 40% of the cyanide into solution and reduced efficacy of the vasodilatory effect. Exposure to laboratory flourescent light does not result in the same degree of photodegradation.[5] Even after mild to moderate photodegradation, SNP remains biologically active and is able to reduce blood pressure.[6] Nitroprusside solutions that are protected from the sunlight are quite stable. Prevention of this photochemical reaction involves covering the infusion bag with aluminum foil or other opaque material to minimize the exposure to ultraviolet light.

Pharmacokinetics and Pathophysiology

Nitroprusside is a nonselective vasodilator of both arteriolar and capacitance vasculature. Regional distribution of blood flow is not affected, and there is preservation of flow to all organs as long as hypotension is avoided. Renal blood flow is maintained, and pulmonary vasoconstriction due to hypoxia is reduced.[4]

After infusion of SNP solution, spontaneous dissociation of the compound occurs. The breakdown of the molecule is triggered by contact between nitroprusside and sulfhydryl groups that are found along vessel walls.[7] Nitric oxide is released and is the active mediator of vasodilatory effects. Nitric oxide activates soluble guanylate cyclase resulting in increased intracellular concentrations of cyclic guanosine monophosphate (cGMP). Increased cGMP induces protein phosphorylation that reduces calcium influx into the cell. With less calcium movement, the smooth muscles are less likely to contract, resulting in relaxation. Vasodilation occurs with the reduced tone of the smooth muscles of blood vessels.[8]

Along with the release of nitric oxide, cyanide molecules are liberated into tissues or serum and can later be absorbed into erythrocytes.[6] Cyanogenesis most likely occurs in the extracellular space[9] rather than in the erythrocytes as previously thought.[10,11] Cyanide is cleared via transulfuration within the liver. The primary sulfur donor is thiosulfate, which is the rate-limiting step. Healthy adults usually have adequate thiosulfate to clear the cyanide released from about 50 mg of SNP.[12] Poor nutrition, recent surgery, and diuretic medications are considered risk factors for reduced thiosulfate stores.

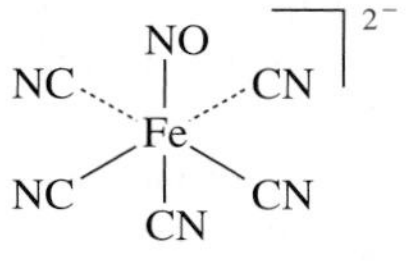

Nitroprusside

FIGURE 61-1 Nitroprusside.

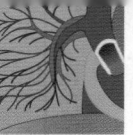

Children, and especially neonates, can have lower thiosulfate stores and may be more susceptible to elevated levels of cyanide.[12]

Cyanide acts as a nucleophilic acceptor for the transfer of sulfur from thiosulfate. Once thiocyanate is formed, the reaction is irreversible. The mechanism by which thiocyanate is formed is not entirely clear. Kinetic studies would suggest that cyanide detoxification occurs in a volume of distribution that is similar to the blood volume. A commonly accepted enzyme in the detoxification of cyanide is rhodanese; however, rhodanese may be restricted to the mitochondria in various tissues, including liver, kidney, and skeletal muscle. Thiosulfate may not be able to penetrate into the inner mitochondrial membrane. One theory suggests that sulfurtransferases including rhodanese may actually form sulfane sulfur that complexes with albumin. The sulfane–sulfur albumin complex reacts with cyanide to form thiosulfate.[13] In contrast to this theory, an experiment in bloodless rats demonstrated that available thiosulfate reduces cyanide in the absence of blood proteins.[14]

Because thiocyanate is produced from thiosulfate, there is no further degradation of the thiocyanate. It is eliminated from the body primarily through renal excretion. The half-life of thiocyanate in an adult with normal renal function is about 2.7 days. The half-life in patients with renal insufficiency may be prolonged to 9 days.[7] The elimination constants for thiocyanate were inversely proportional to the renal creatinine clearances when measured in patients with renal failure.[15]

In the first few minutes after infusion, SNP is found primarily in the serum compartment with minimal amounts in blood cells. The volume of distribution is the same as the extracellular space. The nonenzymatic breakdown of SNP occurs in minutes with the release of cyanide molecules and nitric oxide.[7] The rapid breakdown of SNP correlates with the short half-life and clinical effect. Onset of action is within 30 seconds of the infusion, with peak hypotensive effects within 2 minutes. The effect on blood pressure dissipates within 3 minutes after discontinuation of the infusion.

Toxicology

The amount of SNP that results in cyanide toxicity is variable, depending on the rate infused, amount infused, and thiocyanate stores of the individual. Cyanide clearance is a first order process when adequate thiosulfate is available; however, since thiocyanate stores are limited, the kinetics of detoxification are saturable. There is also interindividual variation in the ability to transulfurate the cyanide molecule into thiocyanate.[16] In the average adult patient, erythrocyte cyanide levels rise rapidly when the infusion of SNP exceeds 1 to 2 µg/kg/min.

Red blood cell cyanide levels from SNP tend to be higher than symptom equivalent levels from direct cyanide poisoning. There is a higher erythrocyte–plasma cyanide ratio during SNP-induced cyanogenesis.[17,18] Those individuals with less reserves or low thiosulfate stores will accumulate the cyanide more quickly and may manifest signs and symptoms at lower doses.

As cyanide accumulates during an SNP infusion, it distributes into tissues and plasma and will concentrate in erythrocytes. Cyanide binds and inhibits a number of enzymes in the body. The metalloenzyme most sensitive to the binding of cyanide is probably cytochrome aa_3, the last enzyme in the cytochrome system of oxidative phosphorylation. Cyanide has an affinity for the ferric iron that composes cytochrome aa_3. As a result of cyanide binding, electron transport via the cytochromes is halted, causing cessation of oxidative phosphorylation. Adenosine triphosphate (ATP) can no longer be produced by this route. Electrons are not able to associate with oxygen as the final electron acceptor, so oxygen consumption diminishes as well. As cells shift to anaerobic metabolism, accumulation of lactate occurs, and a lactate-dependent acidosis develops.[19]

Cyanide inhibits other enzymes, including xanthine oxidase, succinate dehydrogenase, and Schiff base intermediates. The central nervous system (CNS) appears to be the most sensitive organ to the cytotoxicity of cyanide.[19] Cyanide also inhibits glutamate decarboxylase, resulting in reduced production of γ-aminobutyric acid. This may cause an increased risk for convulsions.[20]

Thiocyanate toxicity rarely occurs during SNP infusion in the setting of normal renal function since it is cleared primarily through renal elimination. When thiocyanate was used as an antihypertensive in the early 1900s, cases of toxicity were described. Older literature reports mild toxicity characterized by abdominal pain, vomiting, tinnitus, weakness, and agitation. These early symptoms may progress to more profound CNS effects, including encephalopathy, delusions, lethargy, coma, and, rarely, death.[21-23] The pathophysiology of CNS effects is not delineated.

Thiocyanate does not affect the function of metalloenzymes such as cytochrome oxidases. Oxygen utilization is also not affected. As a result, thiocyanate toxicity does not result in a metabolic acidosis. When thiocyanate was used as an oral antihypertensive, cases of hypothyroidism were reported. The mechanism proposed for this observation was that thiocyanate interfered with thyroidal uptake of iodine.

Diagnosis

In the setting of SNP infusions, close monitoring of patients for clinical evidence of cyanide toxicity must occur. The organ systems usually first affected are the ones most sensitive to histotoxic anoxia: the central nervous and cardiovascular systems.

Early cyanide-induced CNS effects include agitation and restlessness. As cyanide poisoning progresses, encephalopathy may develop and may be misinterpreted as worsening hypertensive encephalopathy. This can progress to coma, and convulsions may occur. Cerebral death may occur simultaneously with terminal cardiovascular effects.

The initial cardiovascular effects are tachycardia and worsening hypertension. Tachyphylaxis to SNP develops and may not be recognized initially as a manifestation of cyanide toxicity. Late findings include hypotension,

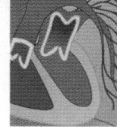

shock, and bradydysrhythmias. Tachypnea may be seen early in the poisoning and can be followed by apnea.

Since cyanide reduces oxygen utilization by the tissues, the mixed venous oxygen content will rise with a decline in the arteriovenous oxygen difference provided cardiac output has not dimished. Elevated venous oxygen concentrations may result in reddish skin coloration; however, cyanosis has also been reported in the setting of cyanide poisonings due to low cardiac output and intrapulmonary shunting.[24]

Due to disruption of oxidative phosphorylation and inability to produce ATP, an anion-gap metabolic acidosis ensues. A worsening metabolic acidosis is a sensitive marker for the presence of cyanide poisoning, although it is not specific for cyanide. Absence of a metabolic acidosis would infer that despite the body burden of cyanide from SNP, the cyanide is being effectively detoxified and is exerting minimal effects on the capacity of oxidative phosphorylation to manufacture ATP.

Blood cyanide levels are usually not available in an expedient manner to assist in the diagnosis of cyanide poisoning. Plasma cyanide concentrations are a better reflection of tissue cyanide levels because cyanide in the plasma is in equilibrium with tissue levels[25]; however, erythrocyte cyanide levels are more commonly measured. In the setting of SNP infusion, cyanide accumulates in erythrocytes, so the red blood cell to plasma cyanide concentrations will be higher than after acute poisoning from inorganic cyanide.[18,26]

Thiocyanate levels do not correlate with the degree of cyanide poisoning.[27] Likewise, an elevated thiocyanate level does not infer that the patient has high levels of cyanide. Thiocyanate levels correlate only with thiocyanate toxicity. Toxicity does not occur until thiocyanate levels have exceeded 100 mg/L. Thiocyanate levels will increase when thiosulfate is concurrently infused with the SNP.[28]

Management

If cyanide toxicity is suspected in a patient receiving an SNP infusion, the infusion must be discontinued while the patient is administered maximal oxygen therapy. Patients with evidence of severe poisoning may require induction of methemoglobinemia with intravenous infusion of sodium nitrite. The dose may need to be adjusted to accommodate a patient with anemia. Sodium thiosulfate should be administered to provide substrate for the production of thiocyanate. In those patients who may not tolerate a reduction in oxygen carrying capacity from methemoglobinemia, sodium thiosulfate should be administered alone. In an animal model, simultaneous infusion of thiosulfate during SNP infusion provided protection against cyanide toxicity.[29] Recommendations have included the mixing of thiosulfate into the SNP solution at a 10 to 1 ratio. This would require 1 g of thiosulfate for each 100 mg of SNP.[25] The coadministration of thiosulfate with SNP reduces the rise in cyanide concentrations in circulation.[7,17]

Hydroxycobalamin is another treatment for cyanide poisoning since it binds to cyanide to form cyanocobal-

amin, a nontoxic compound. Hydroxycobalamin has been used to prevent accumulation of cyanide after SNP administration. Concurrent infusion of hydroxycobalamin resulted in lower erythrocyte and plasma cyanide levels in patients receiving SNP compared with controls who received a similar rate of nitroprusside infusion.[30] One animal model compared infusion of thiosulfate to infusion of hydroxycobalamin during administration of SNP and measured the red blood cell and plasma cyanide levels. Thiosulfate appeared to be more effective in lowering cyanide levels; however, the amount of hydroxycobalamin that could be infused was a limiting factor, so smaller doses were used.[31] Side effects from the use of hydroxycobalamin may include a transient reddish discoloration of the skin and mucous membranes. Anaphylaxis has rarely been reported. The use of hydroxycobalamin may be limited by availability and cost of the product.[32]

Thiocyanate toxicity due to accumulation of thiocyanate from renal failure may be easily removed with hemodialysis. Rapid decline in levels correlates with improvement in the CNS effects.[33]

NITRATES

As a class, organic nitrates are commonly used for treatment of ischemic heart disease. Their effect of dilating coronary arteries and improving coronary blood flow in addition to reducing myocardial oxygen demand led to their use as a cornerstone of therapy in patients with ischemic heart disease.

Nitroglycerin was first synthesized in 1846 by Sobrero and was developed 1 year later into a formulation for sublingual administration. In the 1850s, amyl nitrite was found to relieve angina when given inhalationally; however, its clinical effects had a short duration.[34] In the 1870s, Murrell described the successful use of 1% nitroglycerin solutions in three patients who had symptoms consistent with angina pectoris. The patients would administer the solution orally via drops on a scheduled basis and if the symptoms occurred. Murrell also described the side effect of a severe headache that was associated with the administration of nitroglycerin, both from his patient's experiences and his own self-administration.[35] Subsequent use of nitrates became widespread as a treatment modality for angina pectoris.

Pharmacokinetics and Pharmacology

Nitroglycerin is a polyol ester of nitric acid and is known as glyceryl trinitrate. Organic nitrates of low molecular weight such as nitroglycerin tend to be volatile oily liquids. Organic nitrates such as isosorbide dinitrate are high-molecular-weight esters and are found in solid form.

Organic nitrates are biotransformed in the liver via reductive hydrolysis. The reduction of nitrates results in the formation of water-soluble metabolites that have less vasodilatory activity than the parent compound. Nitro-

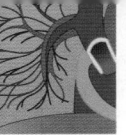

glycerin given sublingually reaches peak concentrations within 4 minutes after administration. The half-life of the parent compound is about 1 to 3 minutes. The dinitrate metabolites have a half-life of 40 minutes and have 10 times less potency as vasodilators.[34] Isosorbide dinitrate also undergoes denitration after reacting with glutathione. The parent compound has a half-life of about 45 minutes but the metabolites have half-lives of 3 to 6 hours. Isosorbide-5-mononitrate has a longer half-life than the dinitrate formulation and has increased bioavailability since it does not undergo first pass metabolism.[34]

Organic nitrates release nitric oxide via denitration when exposed to vascular smooth muscle. The release of nitric oxide stimulates soluble guanylate cyclase, causing increased cGMP. Increased cGMP activates cGMP-dependent protein kinase, culminating in dephosphorylation of the myosin light chain and subsequent vascular smooth muscle relaxation vasodilation.[36]

The mechanism for release of nitric oxide is not well elucidated. Nitroglycerin requires a three-electron reduction to release nitric oxide from its third carbon. This release occurs when nitroglycerin is exposed to mammalian vascular smooth muscle. Initial theories suggested that cellular thiols were needed to accomplish this biotransformation. Nonenzymatic release of nitric oxide may occur in the presence of large concentrations of thiol-containing compounds such as cysteine; however, the most abundant source of thiols, glutathione, does not release nitric oxide from nitroglycerin via this nonenzymatic process. Additional evidence in an experiment with bovine coronary smooth muscle cells suggests that nitroglycerin releases nitric oxide via an enzymatic process that is attached to cellular surface membrane. Glutathione may be required for this reaction as a cofactor, rather than a substrate.[37,38]

Nitroglycerin is also processed via enzymatic pathways that utilize glutathione S-transferases. Instead of releasing nitric oxide, this reaction releases inorganic nitrite (NO_2^-).[38] The inorganic nitrite is not vasoactive unless at very high concentrations; however, it may oxidize ferrous iron in hemoglobin to ferric iron, resulting in methemoglobinemia.

Tolerance to the antianginal effects may occur with continued use of organic nitrates. It is not a uniform phenomenon, since some individuals may develop only partial tolerance. The mechanisms of tolerance are not well understood and may be multifactorial. Tolerance may involve the reduced efficiency of the vascular wall to biotransform nitrates to nitric oxide. In addition, there has been a link between nitroglycerin tolerance and superoxide production from the endothelium. The superoxide may react with the nitric oxide to produce peroxynitrite. Peroxynitrite has a shorter half-life than nitric oxide and is less effective in activating guanylate cyclase.[39] Removal of endothelium of the aorta in animal models markedly reduces the development of tolerance to nitroglycerin. The role of endothelium in promoting tolerance has been confirmed in another animal model and was associated with the activation of nitric oxide synthase and protein kinase C as well as the production of superoxide and peroxynitrite free radicals.[40]

Toxicology

Since organic nitrates affect all smooth muscle beds, their effects extend beyond the coronary arteries. Low concentrations of nitroglycerin may result in venodilation that precedes the arteriodilation. Higher doses result in venous pooling and may reduce arteriolar resistance. A resulting decrease in systolic and diastolic blood pressure may result in dizziness, weakness, and postural hypotension. Syncope has even been described from the transgingival absorption of nitroglycerin paste that was inadvertently used as toothpaste.[41] Dilation of meningeal vessels is thought to result in the commonly reported side effect of headache.

Although rare, induction of methemoglobin has been reported in the setting of organic nitrate use. Nitrite is formed from the breakdown of the nitroglycerin and acts as the oxidizer of ferrous iron to the ferric state. One case of methemoglobinemia was reported after an oral overdose of nitroglycerin tablets, although the methemoglobin level was only 7% with a hemoglobin of 14 g/dL.[42] Intravenous nitroglycerin has been reported to result in methemoglobinemia, but the dose required is not clear. Higher infusions of nitroglycerin may be more likely to produce higher levels of methemoglobin than lower infusion rates.[43]

Cerebral vessel vasodilation from nitroglycerin infusion has been associated with a rise in intracranial pressure. Intracranial hypertension from therapeutic doses of nitroglycerin has been associated with oculomotor palsies, headache, vomiting, and coma. Reversal of these abnormalities occurred upon discontinuation of the nitroglycerin.[44,45]

Most preparations of nitroglycerin include propylene glycol as a diluent. Toxicity may occur in patients who accumulate propylene glycol. Since a large portion of propylene glycol is excreted by the kidneys, patients with renal insufficiency may be at greater risk for diminished clearance. Manifestations of toxicity may include hyperosmolality from the propylene glycol and a metabolic acidosis from its metabolism to lactate. Coma, stupor, and dysconjugate eye movements may occur. Hemolysis with subsequent hemoglobinuria has also been reported.[46]

Another potential interaction with nitroglycerin infusion is an interference with the efficacy of heparin infusion. Col and colleagues noticed a resistance to anticoagulation with heparin when nitroglycerin was concomitantly infused, and they performed in vitro and in vivo studies that supported their observation. These investigators found that the propylene glycol diluent alone could reduce the activated partial thromboplastin time (aPTT) prolongation induced by heparin. Infusion of nitroglycerin prepared with propylene glycol reduced the aPTT even more dramatically than just the propylene glycol.[47] Another study suggested that patients on nitroglycerin infusions require more heparin to maintain their anticoagulation. In addition, two patients in this study were administered nitroglycerin infusion prepared without propylene glycol. Heparin resistance still occurred comparably with those patients who received the standard nitroglycerin preparation with propylene

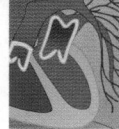

glycol.[48] In another study in patients with acute coronary syndromes, only nitroglycerin infusions that exceeded 350 µg/min had an effect on the aPTT and heparin requirements.[49] The mechanism of this potential drug interaction is not clear.

Drug interactions with medications that inhibit the cGMP phosphodiesterase-5 enzyme such as sildenafil may occur. In the presence of these inhibitors, nitrates cause a profound increase in cGMP. As a result, increased vasodilatory effects and hypotension results. Nitrates should be used with great caution in patients who have used sildenafil or one of its analogs in the previous 24 hours.[50]

Diagnosis

The diagnosis of nitroglycerin-induced hypotension requires the association of abnormal vital signs with a recent exposure. Medications that are orally administered may have longer half-lives as opposed to the intravenous formulations of organic nitrates.

The diagnosis of methemoglobinemia is suggested by the presence of cyanosis and reduced pulse oximetry in the setting of a relatively normal partial pressure of oxygen on arterial blood gas. Methemoglobin levels are measured using co-oximeter readings on heparinized blood samples. Levels that exceed 1.5 g/dL may induce cyanosis; however, levels below this threshold may still impact the oxygen-carrying capacity of critically ill patients, particularly if they are anemic.

During a rapid nitroglycerin infusion, the presence of a persistant metabolic acidosis that may also be associated with hyperosmolality would suggest propylene glycol toxicity. A patient with significant renal insufficiency may be at high risk for propylene glycol toxicity due to diminished renal elimination. Many other medications that utilize propylene glycol, such as lorazepam, phenytoin, diazepam, and intravenous formulations of sulfamethoxazole and trimethoprim, may be associated with formation of a lactate-dependent acidosis.[51]

Management

Cardiovascular effects and side effects from organic nitrates will resolve with discontinuation of the infusion. Hypotension may require fluid boluses of crystalloid or additional inotropic support given the clinical scenario.

Methemoglobinemia that is symptomatic may be treated with the infusion of a 1% methylene blue solution. The infusion rate is usually a 1- to 2-mg/kg bolus with a repeat dose if no response occurs in 30 minutes. If the patient has underlying glucose 6-phosphate dehydrogenase deficiency, then the administration of methylene blue will not be efficacious and could potentially be deleterious. These patients may benefit from a transfusion of packed red blood cells to provide additional oxygen-carrying capacity.

If a patient develops a severe metabolic acidosis from the accumulation of propylene glycol, hemodialysis will effectively remove the diluent. Reduction in the half-life of propylene glycol has been reported with hemodialysis.[46]

HYDRALAZINE

Hydralazine was introduced to the United States in the 1950s as an oral antihypertensive medication and has subsequently been approved for intramuscular and intravenous administration. Although labeled a class C medication during pregnancy, it is commonly used to treat hypertensive crisis in late gestation. Hydralazine is seldom the primary treatment for chronic hypertension because of tachyphylaxis and sympathetic discharge effects.

Despite its use as an oral treatment agent for hypertension, reports of acute severe poisoning with hydralazine are rare. The American Association of Poison Control Centers (AAPCC) reported 212 exposures to the Toxic Exposure Surveillance System (TESS) in 2002. No deaths were reported of the 103 hydralazine exposures subsequently treated in a health care facility.[52]

Structure

1-Hydrazinophthalazine, or hydralazine (Apresoline, [Ciba Pharmaceuticals Summit, NJ]), has a hydrazine moiety in the 1-position of the hydrazine ring that is believed to produce the vasodilatory effects of the drug.[53] The structure of hydralazine is shown in Figure 61-2.

Pharmacology and Pharmacokinetics

Hydralazine directly relaxes arteriolar smooth muscle through its effects on cGMP. Venous smooth muscle is not affected. Hydralazine-induced vasodilation frequently stimulates an increase in heart rate and myocardial contractility. This sympathetic surge is primarily a baroreceptor-mediated reflex, but hydralazine may directly stimulate the release of norepinephrine from sympathetic neurons.[54]

Absorption of hydralazine from the gastrointestinal tract is rapid, with peak plasma levels occurring between 30 and 120 minutes. The volume of distribution (Vd) is 1.6 L/kg with approximately 90% protein binding. Hydralazine is primarily metabolized by N-acetylation in the liver. With therapeutic dosing, the half-life is approximately 1 hour, although the duration of clinical effects usually lasts longer. The rate of elimination is dependent on genetically established N-acetyl-transferase activity. Approximately 50% of patients in the United States are fast acetylators. Fast acetylators produce an inactive metabolite more rapidly; therefore, slow

FIGURE 61-2 Hydralazine.

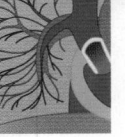

acetylators may have a greater or longer antihypertensive effect. Slow acetylators are also more likely to develop a hydralazine-induced lupus erythematosus–like syndrome and antinuclear antibodies.

Toxicology

Common side effects related to therapeutic use of hydralazine include tachycardia, hypotension, palpitations, headache, flushing, nausea, and dizziness. Many of these side effects may be minimized by administering a β-adrenergic receptor blocker and diuretic in conjunction with hydralazine. Chest pain and myocardial injury may occur with hydralazine administration, especially in patients with significant coronary artery disease or angina. Electrocardiogram (ECG) abnormalities, including reversible ST-segment depression, have been reported in a young female intentionally overdosing on hydralazine.[55] Caution should be used when considering hydralazine use in elderly patients and those with coronary artery disease. A coronary artery blood flow steal phenomenon, increased myocardial oxygen demand from greater sympathetic output, and lack of epicardial coronary artery vasodilation may precipitate myocardial ischemia.

The second type of hydralazine-related side effects appears to be immunologically mediated through production of autoantibodies. The exact mechanism of this reaction is uncertain. Most commonly described is a drug-induced lupus-like syndrome manifesting as fever, myalgias, arthralgias, and rash. This reaction usually resolves after discontinuation of the medication but may require corticosteroids for refractory symptoms. Less commonly reported are pleuritis, pericarditis, vasculitis, hemolytic anemia, and nephritis. Patients can also rarely develop a pyridoxine-responsive polyneuropathy from hydrazone formation when hydralazine binds to pyridoxine.[56]

Diagnosis and Management

Treatment of hydralazine poisoning is primarily supportive. Because no antidote exists, care should be directed toward improving hemodynamic status. Intravenous fluids are the initial management for hypotension. Additional vasopressor support with direct-acting α-adrenergic receptor agonists such as norepinephrine and phenylephrine should be considered for refractory hypotension. Administration of inotropic agents should be cautiously titrated because hydralazine-induced sympathetic discharge may already contribute to tachycardia. For recent oral ingestions where the airway is stable, consideration may be given to the administration of a single dose of activated charcoal. No additional gastrointestinal decontamination is indicated. Due to the rarity of overdose and lack of significant morbidity, few data exist regarding the benefit of enhanced elimination. Presently, there is no indication for hemodialysis or other methods of enhanced elimination in the management of hydralazine toxicity.

Cardiac telemetry for symptomatic patients is warranted until supportive care measures are no longer required, and clinical recovery has occurred. ECG and complete cardiac evaluation for myocardial injury may be necessary in the setting of chest pain from hypotension-induced cardiac ischemia in certain patient populations.

MINOXIDIL

The hypotensive effects of minoxidil were discovered in 1965, and the oral tablet formulation became available as Loniten (Pharmacia and Upjohn, Peapack, NJ) in October 1979.[57] It is primarily used to treat hypertension refractory to multiple other regimens. In 1988, a 2% Rogaine (Pharmacia and Upjohn, Peapack, NJ) formulation (topical minoxidil preparation) became available by prescription to enhance hair growth in male-pattern baldness. Hypertrichosis with minoxidil therapy was first described in 1980.[58] In November 1997, the FDA approved the over-the-counter (OTC) sale of 5% Rogaine Extra Strength for Men. This topical formulation contains minoxidil 50 mg/mL in excipients of 30% ethanol vol/vol, 50% propylene glycol vol/vol, and purified water.[57] Minoxidil overdose is uncommon today, and this is likely a reflection of its diminished use in the treatment of hypertension. However, the topical minoxidil preparations are frequently purchased OTC and provide an easy source of exposure for pediatric and intentional ingestions.[57,59,60]

Structure

6-Amino-1,2-dihydro-1-hydroxy-2imino-4-piperidinopyrimidine, or minoxidil, must be metabolized to minoxidil N-O sulfate by hepatic sulfotransferase to manifest vasodilatory properties.[61] The parent compound is not active, and the active metabolite produced from sulfate conjugation may explain the prolonged effects of the drug. The structure of minoxidil is shown in Figure 61-3.

Pharmacology and Pharmacokinetics

Minoxidil is rapidly and completely absorbed from the gastrointestinal tract, with peak plasma concentrations within 1 hour postingestion. The Vd is 2.8 to 3.3 L/kg, minimal plasma protein binding occurs, and the drug does not cross the blood-brain barrier. The large Vd is hypothesized to reflect an accumulation of the active drug in the vascular smooth muscle.[62] While the half-life of minoxidil is 3 to 4 hours, the duration of action is

Minoxidil

FIGURE 61-3 Minoxidil.

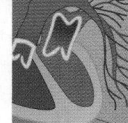

typically 24 hours and may extend to 3 days. The pharmacokinetics of minoxidil N-O sulfate are less clear but may explain the longer duration of action.

The primary route of elimination is hepatic glucuronide conjugation at the N-oxide position in the pyrimidine ring. The production of the active metabolite, minoxidil N-O sulfate, is a minor pathway. Twenty percent of the drug is excreted unchanged in the urine. Although minoxidil and its glucuronidation products are hemodialzyable, this does not reverse clinical effects from tissue sequestration of the active metabolite in the vascular smooth muscle.

Minoxidil sulfate activates ATP-sensitive potassium channels, enhancing channel opening and subsequent potassium efflux. This causes hyperpolarization and subsequent vascular smooth muscle relaxation.[63] While arteriolar vasodilation causes decreased peripheral vascular resistance and blood pressure, there is little effect on capacitance vessels. Hypertrichosis is also probably a consequence of potassium channel augmentation.

A baroreceptor-mediated sympathetic response can sometimes occur even with therapeutic dosing of minoxidil.[64] Sympathomimetic medications should be avoided due to excess cardiac stimulation with reflex tachycardia and baroreceptor activation from minoxidil therapy. Although renin and aldosterone secretion are increased during minoxidil therapy, it is thought that fluid retention occurs primarily from increased proximal renal tubular reabsorption secondary to reduced renal perfusion. Some side effects of minoxidil therapy, specifically fluid retention and reflex tachycardia, can be minimized by administering a diuretic and β-receptor antagonist in conjunction.

Toxicology

Typical adult therapeutic dosing is 10 to 40 mg orally once a day up to a maximum of 100 mg per day. Pediatric dosing is 0.25 to 1.0 mg/kg to a maximum of 50 mg per day. The manufacturer package insert states it is difficult to establish an exact minoxidil serum toxic level due to patient variation, but levels above 2000 ng/mL are likely representative of an overdosage.[65] An average adult consumption of 30 mg orally would produce a serum minoxidil level of 40 ng/mL 3 hours postingestion[59]; however, a 2-year-old was reported to consume 100 mg of minoxidil and developed significant tachycardia with a 3-hour postingestion serum minoxidil level of 150 ng/mL.[66]

The highest reported serum minoxidil concentration was 3140 ng/mL in a 20-year-old woman who developed tachycardia, labile hypotension, ST-segment depression, and T-wave inversion after an unknown quantity of minoxidil was ingested in a suicide attempt. She was stabilized with intravenous fluids and supportive care and eventually discharged from the hospital.[67]

Common pharmacologic side effects related to therapeutic administration of minoxidil include tachycardia, hypotension, and hypertrichosis. Because heart rate, myocardial contractility, and myocardial oxygen consumption are increased, chest pain and myocardial injury may develop in patients with significant coronary artery disease or angina. Worsening left ventricular systolic and diastolic dysfunction can develop in patients with congestive heart failure and pulmonary hypertension. While ECG abnormalities such as flattened and inverted T waves are commonly reported in therapeutic dosing or overdose of minoxidil from potassium channel activation,[67] myocardial infarction has also been reported.[60]

In addition to sodium and fluid retention, pericardial effusions and pericarditis have been reported with minoxidil use, primarily in hemodialysis patients.[68] Other rarely described complications include rashes, thrombocytopenia, nausea, headache, gynecomastia, polymenorrhea, and breast tenderness. Increased hair growth occurs on the scalp, face, back, arms, and legs. There are no reports of hypertrichosis occurring from a single ingestion or overdose.

Diagnosis and Management

Cardiac and hemodynamic monitoring is warranted in the symptomatic patient. Additional cardiac evaluation and serial ECGs may be indicated if chest pain or other symptoms of cardiac ischemia develop. A serum radioimmunoassay is available through the manufacturer, but serum concentrations generally do not correlate with therapeutic response and are often delayed and unlikely to assist in management.

Treatment of minoxidil poisoning is primarily supportive. No antidote exists, and a single dose of activated charcoal is only indicated in recent ingestions when airway reflexes are intact. Intravenous fluids are the initial management for hypotension. Additional vasopressor support with norepinephrine and phenylephrine should be considered for refractory hypotension. Cautious administration of inotropic support is necessary to avoid excessive tachycardia and cardiac stimulation. Although intravenous fluids should be used judiciously in the setting of hypotension, congestive heart failure in patients with reduced left ventricular function can develop. Enhanced elimination is not indicated.

Cardiac telemetry and hemodynamic monitoring is necessary in these cases until clinical recovery has occurred. Serial ECGs and evaluation of cardiac markers for myocardial injury may be necessary in the setting of hypotension-induced cardiac ischemia, especially in the elderly or patients with coronary artery disease ingesting minoxidil. T wave changes from minoxidil-induced potassium channel activation usually resolve once the metabolites are eliminated.

SILDENAFIL

Sildenafil (Viagra [Pfizer, New York, NY]) is the first oral drug approved by the FDA, in March 1998, for the treatment of male erectile dysfunction.[69] This condition affects more than 30 million men in the United States alone. While the development of this agent has significantly improved the lifestyle of many patients, concerns for medication interaction and drug abuse have arisen. Over 6 million outpatient prescriptions were

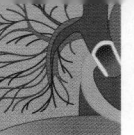

written during its initial marketing phase from March to November 1998, and it is estimated that sildenafil has been prescribed to over 10 million men worldwide.[70] Excessive consumer demand has created a black market, and sildenafil or similar agents are now commonly available over the Internet, in adult sex shops, and on the street due to its increasing use as a recreational drug.

Structure and Mechanism of Action

Sildenafil is a selective inhibitor of phosphodiesterase type 5 (PDE5), which is responsible for degradation of the second messenger cGMP. Normally, sexual stimulation enhances release of nitric oxide, activating guanylate cyclase with conversion of GTP to cGMP. cGMP acts as a smooth muscle relaxant and increases arterial blood flow in the penis to enhance tumescence. Although sildenafil is not a direct smooth muscle relaxer, it inhibits the breakdown of cGMP, culminating in prolonged blood flow to the corpora cavernosa and ultimately sustained penile erection. Because nitric oxide is essential to initiate this cascade, sexual stimulation is necessary and sildenafil acts more as a facilitator of tumescence rather than as a direct vasodilatory agent.[71] The structure of sildenafil is shown in Figure 61-4.

Pharmacology and Pharmacokinetics

Sildenafil is rapidly absorbed after oral administration, with peak effects in 60 minutes. There is only 40% bioavailability of this agent due to extensive first pass metabolism. The volume of distribution is approximately 1.5 L/kg in the average adult, with 96% protein binding. Metabolism is primarily via the hepatic P-450 CYP3A4 pathway to N-desmethyl sildenafil, an active metabolite responsible for up to 20% of the pharmacologic effect.[50] The majority of side effects from sildenafil are a result of CYP3A4 inhibition by cimetidine, macrolide antibiotics, antifungals, and protease inhibitors. The elimination half-life of sildenafil and its active metabolite is about 4 hours. While 13% of the drug is renally excreted and 80% fecally eliminated, significantly prolonged increased sildenafil concentrations can occur in the setting of severe renal dysfunction, hepatic insufficiency, and cytochrome P-450 inhibitors.

Toxicology

The average therapeutic dose of sildenafil is 25 to 100 mg, with a maximum of one dose per day. Lower

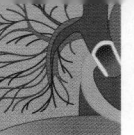

Sildenafil

FIGURE 61-4 Sildenafil.

dosing is advocated for patients older than 65 years and in those with renal or hepatic impairment. Although many side effects of sildenafil may be attributed to its inhibitory effect on other PDEs, the high selectivity it has for PDE5 may explain the low morbidity reported in overdose. There are few reports of serious side effects from isolated ingestion of sildenafil. One case reported a 42-year-old woman who developed weakness, flushing, headache, dizziness, tremor, and palpitations after ingestion of almost 2 g of sildenafil. While nasogastric tube irrigation and activated charcoal lavage occurred early after this ingestion, all symptoms rapidly resolved, and the patient was discharged in 12 hours.[72] However, another case of presumed sildenafil ingestion leading to death reported a postmortem blood sildenafil concentration of 6.27 µg/mL by high-pressure liquid chromatography/mass spectroscopy. Although this concentration was four times higher than previously reported therapeutic levels, the patient had extensive baseline medical problems, including severe cardiomyopathy.[70] While there is significant controversy regarding the interpretation of FDA postmarketing data, 1473 major adverse events, including 522 deaths, were reported within 13 months of sildenafil availability.[73,74] In summarizing TESS data, despite inherent underreporting and reporting bias, it seems that most pediatric exposures to sildenafil are well tolerated, whereas older men with preexisting cardiovascular disease and potential drug-drug interactions are more likely to experience adverse side effects.[71]

The most recognized drug interaction involving sildenafil use is with the administration of nitrates or nitrites. Sildenafil synergistically potentiates the hypotensive effects of medications that promote vasodilatory mechanisms via nitric oxide pathways. This may also be seen when amyl or butyl nitrite are recreationally inhaled while using sildenafil. Due to excessive morbidity and mortality associated with combined use of sildenafil with nitrates or nitrites in men with cardiovascular disease, sildenafil is contraindicated in patients requiring those medications. In addition, nitrates are contraindicated up to 24 hours after the last sildenafil use should angina or myocardial infarction occur in this time frame.[50] Other antihypertensives should also be used cautiously in this setting because sildenafil is known to produce small decreases in systolic and diastolic blood pressure. Common drug interactions include inhibitors of P-450 CYP3A4, such as cimetidine, ketoconazole, itraconazole, erythromycin, and clarithromycin. Starting doses of sildenafil should be no greater than 25 mg when patients are prescribed these other medications. The antiretroviral protease inhibitors also inhibit first pass metabolism of sildenafil, thus increasing its serum half-life and delaying peak concentrations.

The most common side effects reported in clinical trials of therapeutic sildenafil use were headache, flushing, dyspepsia, and nasal congestion.[69,75] Many of these effects, like dyspepsia due to lower esophageal sphincter relaxation, can be explained as a consequence of PDE5 inhibition. Because sildenafil is also a weak inhibitor of PDE6 in the retina, visual disturbances

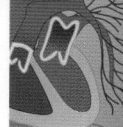

including blurred vision, light perception abnormalities, and color perception distortions can also develop with therapeutic dosing. Higher doses of sildenafil can increase the frequency of visual disturbances, but these symptoms are usually transient, lasting less than a few hours. Although rarely reported, myocardial infarction has occurred in close temporal proximity to sildenafil usage,[76] although this is likely a result of a transient decrease in blood pressure culminating in decreased coronary blood flow. These effects can be more significant in the setting of concomitant nitrate use. While a decrease in systemic vascular resistance may develop, sildenafil use is not thought to directly cause tachycardia.[69] Effective treatment of erectile dysfunction might intuitively increase the risk for priapism, but no cases of priapism were reported in the initial clinical trials.[69] More recently, a patient with sickle cell trait was reported to develop priapism while using sildenafil.[77] Another case of priapism, successfully treated with aspiration and intracorporal injection of α-receptor agonists, was described in a 28-year-old man taking a 100-mg dose of sildenafil-citrate for prior penile trauma-induced mild erectile dysfunction.[78]

Diagnosis and Management

In the setting of isolated sildenafil overdose, supportive care including intravenous fluids, cardiac monitoring, and direct-acting α agonists for refractory hypotension are indicated. Obtaining serum concentration results via the manufacturer are not likely to assist in clinical management of overdose. Although few gastrointestinal decontamination data exist, a single dose of activated charcoal is appropriate in the setting of recent ingestion and adequate airway protection.

The American College of Cardiology and the American Heart Association have several management recommendations for sildenafil-induced hypotension due to nitrate interaction. Discontinuing nitrate use, Tredelenberg positioning, intravenous fluid resuscitation, direct-acting α-agonist vasopressors, and intra-aortic balloon pump have all been advocated depending on the severity of hypotension.[50] In the setting of acute coronary syndrome in a patient using sildenafil, recommendations include avoiding nitrates if sildenafil has been used in the past 24 hours. Administering other non-nitrate antianginal agents like β-receptor antagonists is more appropriate under those circumstances. Otherwise, standard therapy for acute coronary syndrome is indicated.

ACE INHIBITORS

With the introduction of captopril in 1981, angiotensin-converting enzyme (ACE) inhibitors have gained widespread popularity due to their proven effectiveness in the treatment of hypertension and congestive heart failure.[79] Those populations that appear to derive benefit are diabetics and patients with recent myocardial infarctions.[80,81] With increasing use and various clinical indications, the potential for increased frequency of both intentional and unintentional poisonings exists. Despite their widespread use, however, the number of reported cases of toxicity related to overdose with ACE inhibitors remains relatively small. As a class, the ACE inhibitors have proven to be relatively safe with a high therapeutic index and infrequently reported poor outcomes secondary to overdose.

Pharmacology and Pharmacokinetics

There are currently 11 available ACE inhibitors approved for use by the FDA, including captopril, benazepril, enalapril, enaliprilat, fosinopril, lisinopril, moexipril, perinodpril, quinapril, ramipril, and trandolapril. While all contain a similar 2-methyl propanolol-L-proline moiety, the pharmacokinetic profiles differ considerably based on variations in this common core structure (Fig. 61-5).[82]

ACE inhibitors are generally well absorbed, reaching peak serum concentrations in the first 1 to 4 hours. The level of protein binding is low (25% to 60%), with the exception of benazepril (98%).[83] Drug half-lives of these agents range from 2 to 12 hours. With the exception of lisinopril and captopril, ACE inhibitors are administered as prodrugs with good bioavailability. In the liver, each of the prodrugs are converted to active metabolites following the cleavage of an ester moiety. These active metabolites may demonstrate effects for several days due to slow dissociation from the ACE. With the exception of fosinopril, which is eliminated both renally and hepatically, ACE inhibitors are cleared predominantly via the kidneys. Dosage adjustments should be considered in those with impaired renal function.[83]

The effectiveness of ACE inhibitors lies in their ability to directly bind to the active site of the ACE and inhibit the production of angiotensin II (see Fig. 61-6). In the lung and vascular endothelium, ACE is responsible for converting inactive angiotensin I to the highly active compound angiotensin II. Angiotensin II is a potent vasoconstrictor having direct effects on vascular smooth muscle. In addition, angiotensin II stimulates aldosterone release that acts at the distal and collecting tubules of the kidney by increasing sodium retention while excreting potassium and hydrogen ions. By inhibiting the production of angiotensin II, ACE inhibitors are able to decrease peripheral vascular resistance, lower sodium and water retention, and decrease blood pressure.

Other effects of ACE inhibitors include inhibiting bradykinin inactivation. Kininase II is responsible for the inactivation of bradykinin and is identical in structure to ACE. By inhibiting kininase II, ACE inhibitors allow bradykinin to accumulate, leading to a further decrease

$$HS-CH_2-CH-C-N \quad COO^-$$

Captopril

FIGURE 61-5 Captopril.

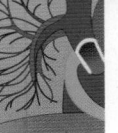

in blood pressure through direct vasodilation and stimulation of prostaglandin biosynthesis.[84] This accumulation of bradykinin also contributes to side effects of cough and angioedema commonly described with therapeutic ACE inhibitor usage.[85] The renin-angiotensin system plays a vital role in regulating perfusion to the kidney in states of reduced renal flow. In the setting of bilateral renal artery stenosis, the ability of angiotensin II to maintain adequate post–glomerular efferent arteriolar tone by way of its vasoconstrictive properties ensures adequate glomerular perfusion. By inhibiting the production of angiotensin II, ACE inhibitors are capable of decreasing glomerular perfusion leading to prerenal azotemia. While bilateral renal artery stenosis may primarily cause a small percentage of hypertension, acute renal decompensation following the administration of an ACE inhibitor should raise suspicion for this particular etiology.[86]

Toxicity

Hypotension is the most pronounced toxic effect of ACE inhibitor action. A "first dose phenomenon" similar to that described with α_1-antagonists following initiation of treatment can result in lightheadedness, dizziness, and syncope. One study described a systolic blood pressure decrease of greater than 50 mm Hg in 10% of healthy volunteers after initiation of captopril therapy.[87] Hypotension can be most pronounced in therapeutic and excessive dosing in patients with fluid depletion, renovascular disease, and congestive heart failure. Tachycardia is rarely reported in ACE inhibitor toxicity, and more frequently a relative bradycardia develops.

Noncardiovascular effects in overdose include drowsiness, lethargy, and confusion. Renal and electrolyte abnormalities may occur as a result of renal insufficiency related to profound hypotension.[88] In addition, decreased production of aldosterone may cause worsening hyperkalemia and hyponatremia. Hyperkalemia is more commonly seen in individuals with prior renal impairment or those taking potassium supplements or potassium-sparing diuretics such as spironolactone.[89] The presence of oliguria and electrolyte abnormalities are generally short lived and improve with discontinuation of the inciting agent. Cases of ACE inhibitor overdose are frequently complicated by the presence of co-ingestants that may contribute to the clinical presentation.[90] Death as a result of isolated ingestion of ACE inhibitors is exceedingly rare.[91,92] Interestingly, children seem to be particularly resistant to the effects of ACE inhibitors, remaining asymptomatic in most cases despite large accidental ingestions.[93]

Angioedema is a frequently reported side effect of ACE inhibitor therapy with the potential for significant morbidity and mortality. The overall incidence is estimated to be approximately 0.1% to 0.2%. African Americans have a 4.5 times greater risk of ACE inhibitor–induced angioedema compared with those of European descent.[94,95] Angioedema occurs as a result of increased perfusion in the capillary beds located in subcutaneous tissue and dermis with leakage of fluid into the interstitium. With fluid accumulation comes swelling, most prominently in the periorbital, perioral, and oropharyngeal tissue, that can rapidly progress to airway obstruction. The mechanism behind angioedema in the setting of ACE inhibitor administration is thought to involve increased levels of bradykinin, substance P, and other inflammatory intermediates such as histamines, prostaglandin D, and leukotrienes.[85]

The onset of angioedema resulting from ACE inhibitor therapy is classically described to occur in two thirds of patients within the first week of therapy, with the remaining one third developing this potentially life-threatening side effect weeks to years after initiation of the drug.[96] ACE inhibitors should not be prescribed to patients who have a history of hereditary or acquired angioedema.[97] Accumulation of bradykinin is felt to also be responsible for the persistent and often debilitating cough described in 5% to 10% of patients taking ACE inhibitors.

Management

Initial management of ACE inhibitor poisoning should focus on aggressive supportive care with cardiac monitoring and ensuring adequate urine output. Hypotension is often responsive to intravenous fluid administration alone. Vasopressors have been used with success in cases of refractory hypotension.[98] The presence of hyperkalemia should prompt urgent potassium-lowering intervention. Activated charcoal should be administered after recent ingestions in compliant and awake patients. Orogastric lavage, with its inherent risks, should not be routinely recommended due to the relatively low rates of morbidity and mortality associated with ACE inhibitors and the effectiveness of supportive care alone.

Reports of asymptomatic patients following large ingestions of ACE inhibitors are relatively common.[89,99] A study by Spiller and colleagues evaluated 48 children with ingestions not greater than adult therapeutic dosages of captopril and enalapril and found no adverse outcomes with close home monitoring and telephone follow-up.[100] Maximum hemodynamic effects following ingestion should occur within the first 1 to 6 hours, depending on the particular ACE inhibitor ingested.[101] Individuals manifesting hypotension at the time of evaluation should be monitored closely for at least 24 hours given the prolonged effects of many of these agents and their active metabolites.

Other treatment options that have found limited yet sometimes dramatic effects in reversing hypotension seen with ACE inhibitor overdose include naloxone and angiotensin II administration. Naloxone is felt to work through inhibition of the naturally occurring endorphins that can inhibit angiotensin II activity. Success has been demonstrated in both animal models and in limited case reports.[102,103] Angiotensin II administration has been effective in treating refractory hypotension from ACE inhibitor poisoning, but its lack of availability makes this intervention an unlikely treatment option.[104] Particular ACE inhibitors such as captopril, enalapril, and lisinopril may be amenable to dialysis; however, it would be rarely

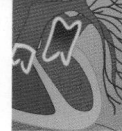

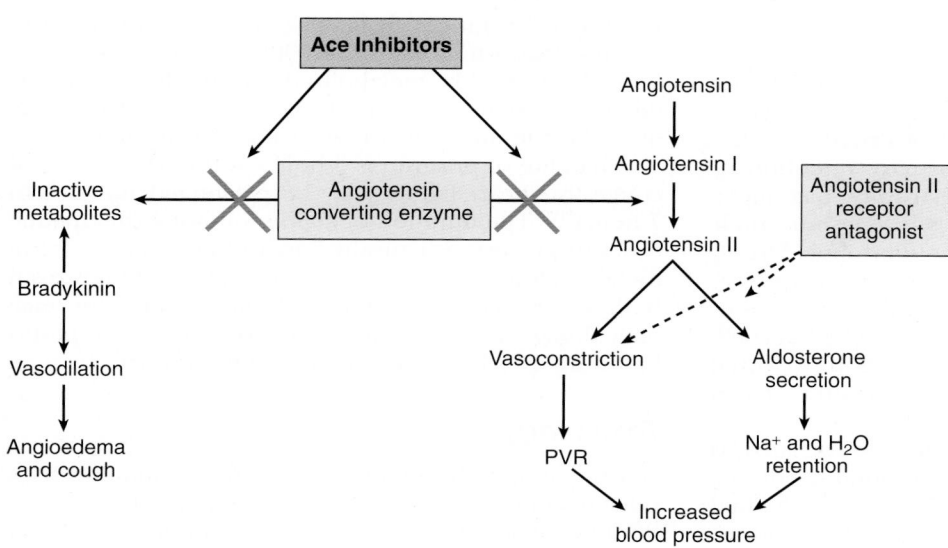

FIGURE 61-6 Sites of action of ACE inhibitors in the metabolism of angiotensin II and bradykinin and the site of action of the angiotensin II receptor antagonists.

necessary given the effectiveness of other treatment options and the lack of clinical symptoms in most cases.

Figure 61-6 shows the sites of action of ACE inhibitors in the metabolism of angiotensin II and bradykinin.

ANGIOTENSIN II RECEPTOR ANTAGONISTS

Currently, seven angiotensin II receptor antagonists are available in the United States: losartan, valsartan, irbesartan, telmisartan, olmesartan, candesartan, and eprosartan. This new class of antihypertensive agent was introduced in 1995 and has gained popularity due to its outstanding side effect profile and effectiveness in treating hypertension and heart failure.[105,106] These drugs are rapidly absorbed in the gastrointestinal tract and reach peak serum levels in 1 to 4 hours. Protein binding is greater than 90%, while bioavailability is generally low (less than 50%). Many of these drugs have active metabolites with effects lasting longer than their parent drug half-life, ranging from 6 to 24 hours. As a class, the angiotensin receptor antagonists and their metabolites are eliminated predominantly through biliary and fecal excretion and to a lesser degree by the kidneys.

The angiotensin II receptor antagonists are similar to ACE inhibitors in their ability to reduce the effects of angiotensin II. Rather than decreasing the production of angiotensin II through inhibition of the ACE, angiotensin receptor blockers competitively antagonize angiotensin II at the type I angiotensin receptors. These receptors are located in the adrenal gland and peripheral vasculature. Inhibition results in a loss of the vasoconstrictive properties and aldosterone-promoting effects of angiotensin II. Type II angiotensin receptors are not affected by angiotensin II receptor antagonists. In contrast to stimulation of type I angiotensin receptors, stimulation of uninhibited type II antiotension receptors by angiotensin II results in a vasodilatory response, further contributing to blood pressure reduction.[107]

This high specificity that angiotensin II antagonists have for the renin-angiotensin system is felt to be responsible for their favorable side effect profile. Angiotensin receptor antagonists block the effects of angiotensin II; however, they do not interfere with the metabolism of bradykinins. Due to a lack of bradykinin accumulation, cough, a side effect frequently reported with ACE inhibitors, is less likely to occur.[108] Decreased accumulation of bradykinin would also be expected to decrease the incidence of angioedema; however, numerous cases of angioedema in the setting of angiotensin receptor antagonists have been reported.[109,110] This challenges the previously held belief that bradykinin excess is responsible for angioedema. While the incidence of angioedema in patients taking angiotensin receptor antagonists is lower than that seen with ACE inhibitors, the use of these agents in patients with previous angioedema should be undertaken with caution. Patients with previous episodes of angioedema related to ACE inhibitors have had similar reactions when later given an angiotensin receptor antagonist.[109,110]

In individuals with severe renal artery stenosis or diffuse intrarenal vascular sclerosis, angiotensin receptor antagonists should be avoided because they can cause deleterious effects to renal function similar to that seen with ACE inhibitors.[111] In addition, given their effect on aldosterone production, hyperkalemia can occur in individuals with normal renal function. Recent case reports have also noted a relationship between angiotensin receptor blockers and pancreatitis.[112,113] Similar to ACE inhibitors, angiotensin receptor antagonists should be avoided in pregnancy because of teratogenic potential.[114]

There are no published reports of overdose involving this relatively new class of antihypertensive medication. Given the mechanism of action, hypotension and reflexive tachycardia would be anticipated to occur. Treatment with activated charcoal in individuals with recent ingestions is appropriate. Hypotension should be addressed with aggressive administration of intravenous fluid as well as vasopressors in cases of persistent hypotension.

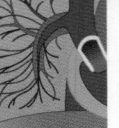

α₁-ADRENERGIC ANTAGONISTS

With the introduction of prazosin in the early 1970s, the selective α₁-adrenergic antagonists have gained acceptance as effective agents in the treatment of essential hypertension. Their ability to improve urinary retention in men with benign prostatic hypertrophy has more recently increased their popularity.[115] Despite their increased use, overdose with these quinazoline-derived α₁-receptor antagonists, including prazosin, doxazosin, and terazosin, is infrequently reported. Only 1555 cases of exposure were reported to the AAPCC's TESS in 2002, with major effects requiring hospitalization reported in only 26 patients.[52] The structure of prazosin is shown in Figure 61-7.

The α₁-antagonist nonspecific predecessors, such as phentolamine and phenoxybenzamine, inhibit both α₁ and α₂ receptors and continue to be used in limited circumstances. These nonspecific antagonists are attractive agents for the treatment of high catecholamine states such as pheochromocytomas, extravasation of vasopressors, and MAO inhibitor toxicity. Given their limited in-hospital administration, toxicity with these drugs is exceedingly rare.

Pharmacology and Pharmacokinetics

Located on the smooth muscle of arterioles and veins in the peripheral circulation, α₁ receptors respond to circulating catecholamines with vascular constriction leading to increased vascular tone and a resultant increase in blood pressure. Alpha-1 antagonists competitively inhibit these postsynaptically located adrenergic receptors. Unlike α₂ receptors, which are located both in the periphery and centrally, α₁ receptors appear to be present solely in the peripheral vascular system. α₂ Receptors lie presynaptically and inhibit the release of norepinephrine when stimulated. In a similar fashion, stimulation of central α₂ receptors will cause a decrease in sympathetic outflow. Phentolamine, capable of causing peripheral vasodilation via α₁-antagonistic effects, acts antagonistically at α₂ receptors as well producing an increase in sympathetic tone and a resultant tachycardia.

The selectivity that agents such as prazosin, doxazosin, and terazosin have for the α₁ receptor site is evident in the fact that tachycardia rarely occurs. In addition, α₁-antagonists have demonstrated the ability to depress sinus node sensitivity, further inhibiting a reflexive tachycardic response from the heart.[116] However, like many agents in the setting of overdose, the selectivity that α₁-antagonists have for particular receptors may be lost.[117]

The α₁-adrenergic antagonists are rapidly absorbed with peak plasma levels reached in the first 1 to 3 hours.

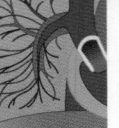

Prazosin

FIGURE 61-7 Prazosin.

Bioavailability ranges from 43% to 69% with prazosin and doxazosin to greater than 90% with terazosin.[118,119] Prazosin is highly metabolized in the liver, with its demethylated metabolite possessing a slower rate of excretion and the ability to cause prolonged hypotension.[119] The half-life of prazosin is 3 hours, but in the setting of congestive heart failure may be prolonged up to 6 to 7 hours.[120] The duration of action following therapeutic doses of prazosin is typically 7 to 10 hours due to active metabolites and tissue binding. Doxasozin and terazosin both possess half-lives of 9 to 12 hours allowing for once daily dosage and the potential for prolonged symptoms following overdose when compared to prazosin.

Toxicology

Not surprisingly, hypotension is the most commonly seen side effect in therapeutic dosing as well as with overdose. Postural hypotension can be seen following treatment initiation, an increase in dose, or with the addition of other antihypertensive medications. Frequently referred to as the "first dose phenomenon," lightheadedness, dizziness, palpitations, diaphoresis, and syncope may occur within 30 to 90 minutes of the initial dose. This symptomatic hypotension is felt to be secondary to selective antagonism of α₁ receptors, causing peripheral vasodilation without a compensatory sympathetic response. To avoid this effect and potential complications, current recommendations include administration of medication prior to sleeping, low starting doses, and slow upward titration of the dose.[121]

Transient hypotension responsive to intravenous fluid is the most common presentation of symptomatic α₁-antagonist overdose.[122-125] One elderly man who ingested 120 mg of prazosin had a prolonged course of hypotension, CNS depression, and respiratory failure secondary to pulmonary edema requiring vasopressor support and mechanical ventilation for 48 hours prior to recovery.[123] Hypotension was accompanied by tachycardia in a 19-year-old male who ingested approximately 10 times the maximum therapeutic dose of prazosin, with symptoms resolving after several hours of observation and hydration.[122] While tachycardia in overdose has been described, hypotension will more frequently be present with normocardia or mild bradycardia, consistent with isolated α₁ receptor antagonism.[123-125]

Priapism has been reported with both therapeutic administration and overdose and is likely related to the sympatholytic effects from α₁-adrenergic blockade. By inhibiting α₁ receptors, a parasympathetically mediated erection can occur while inhibiting ejaculation and detumescence.[126] Other symptoms described in overdose include headache, vertigo, paresthesias, and weakness.[123] In one small series of patients with chronic renal insufficiency taking prazosin, neuropsychiatric effects were reported and felt to be secondary to poor drug clearance. These symptoms included delusions of grandeur, visual hallucinations, confusion, as well as electroencephalography findings consistent with metabolic encephalopathy. These symptoms resolved within 2 months of medication cessation.[127]

Management

Supportive care and observation following overdose with α-adrenergic agents should include blood pressure and urine output monitoring to ensure adequate perfusion of vital organs. Aggressive intravenous hydration should be administered to hypotensive patients. Placement of a symptomatic patient in a supine or Trendelenburg position may be effective in correcting mild hypotension. The administration of a single dose of activated charcoal in a timely fashion is appropriate in patients with preserved mental status. Given the benign nature of most overdoses of α₁-antagonists, the risks associated with orogastric lavage in nearly all cases outweigh the potential benefit.

If vasopressor support is required, direct-acting α agents such as norepinephrine and vasopressin would be preferred over nonspecific α- and β-agonists such as epinephrine. Stimulation of vascular β₂ receptors by epinephrine could theoretically lead to worsened hypotension and tachycardia given the isolated α₁ receptor blockade. Drug levels can be obtained; however, it is unlikely that these levels would be useful in the acute management of overdose.[123,125] The occurrence of priapism warrants emergent urology consultation and the need for possible surgical intervention. Hemodialysis has not been reported after α₁-antagonist overdose and would likely be of little benefit given the high rate of protein binding and large volume of distribution.

DIURETICS

Diuretics make up the most commonly prescribed class of medications in the United States. One study found that 28% of individuals older than 70 years were taking diuretics at the time of hospital admission.[128] Despite their widespread use, the frequency of intentional or accidental overdose remains relatively small. With overdose and therapeutic use, potential complications related to volume depletion and electrolyte abnormalities may occur. Those most susceptible appear to be the elderly and the malnourished, and patients with renal failure. Intentional overuse of diuretics has also been described in individuals with anorexia and bulimia, with up to one third of bulimic patients reporting diuretic abuse in an attempt to decrease body weight.[129]

Diuretics used for the treatment of hypertension can be divided into three major classes: thiazide diuretics, loop diuretics, and potassium-sparing diuretics.

THIAZIDE DIURETICS

The thiazides were the first class of diuretics to be introduced in the 1950s when chlorothiazide was noted to be effective in decreasing blood pressure by reducing extracellular fluid volume and sodium in hypertensive patients. Other commonly used thiazide diuretics today include metolazone, chlorothalidone, indapamide, and hydrochlorothiazide. Thiazides act on the proximal

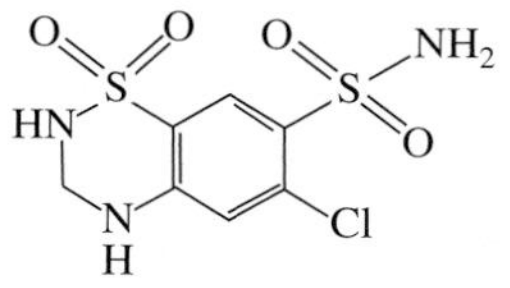

Hydrochlorothiazide

FIGURE 61-8 Hydrochlorothiazide.

portion of the distal tubule and the distal portion of the ascending loops of Henle by inhibiting the sodium/chloride symporter. The result is a decrease in renal sodium absorption and increase of sodium excretion into the urine. With less sodium uptake, the distal tubule is exposed to high sodium concentrations resulting in potassium excretion via the Na^+/K^+ pump. The structure of hydrochlorothiazide is shown in Figure 61-8.

The most serious effects of thiazide diuretics at therapeutic dosing, chronic overuse, and intentional overdose are related to fluid and electrolyte imbalance. With the loss of large amounts of sodium comes a decreased uptake of free water from distal tubules, leading to the potential for volume depletion and hypotension. Symptomatic dehydration appears most commonly in the elderly, who possess limited physiologic reserve.[128] Other evidence of decreased end-organ perfusion secondary to volume depletion includes cerebrovascular incidents and renal failure, often when used in conjunction with an ACE inhibitor or nonsteroidal anti-inflammatory drugs.[130-132] The presence of hyponatremia (less than 135 mmol/L) has been seen in one fifth of elderly patients taking thiazide diuretics.[133] The level of hypokalemia that may be induced appears to be dose dependent and more significant with thiazide diuretics when compared with loop diuretics.[134] In addition to hyponatremia and hypokalemia, other electrolyte abnormalities such as hypochloremia, hypomagnesemia, hypercalcemia, hyperuricemia, and metabolic alkalosis can be seen.

Thiazide-induced hypokalemia, while often mild at therapeutic dosing, becomes more concerning with diuretic abuse and in the setting of concomitant use of other potassium-wasting agents. The presence of significant hypokalemia and the potential for cardiac dysrhythmias warrants aggressive electrolyte replacement. The presence of hypokalemia in the setting of digoxin use is especially problematic because hypokalemia appears to enhance the effects of digoxin on the myocardium and predisposes the heart to additional dysrhythmias.

Other symptoms, including nausea, vomiting, diarrhea, anorexia, and abdominal pain, have been described with thiazide diuretic overdose. CNS depression ranging from mild transient lethargy to coma has been reported in the setting of overdose and after therapeutic administration. CNS depressant effects have also occurred in the absence of significant hypotension, suggesting a direct-acting CNS depressant effect. Grand mal seizures have been reported with the use of high-dose thiazide-type diuretics in the pediatric and adult population.[135,136] Other effects associated with thiazide use include pancreatitis,

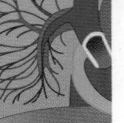

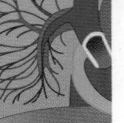

FIGURE 61-9 Furosemide.

cholecystitis, erectile dysfunction, thrombocytopenia, and hemolytic anemia.[130,137-140]

LOOP DIURETICS

Four loop diuretics are currently approved for use in the United States: furosemide, bumetanide, ethacrynic acid, and torsemide. Their effectiveness lies in their ability to inhibit the Na^+-K^+-Cl^- symporter found on the thick ascending limb of the loop of Henle, resulting in loss of sodium, chloride, and potassium ions in the urine. Loop diuretics also act as direct vasodilators that can reduce left ventricular filling pressures via increased systemic venous capacitance.[141] The structure of furosemide is shown in Figure 61-9.

Toxicity related to loop diuretic abuse in many ways is similar to that observed with thiazide diuretics, with the potential for developing hyponatremia, hypokalemia, hypocalcemia, hypomagnesemia, and fluid depletion. In addition to the potential risk for cardiac dysrhythmias, hypokalemia in the setting of furosemide overuse has led to significant muscular weakness and rhabdomyolysis. Hyponatremia can also be severe, resulting in seizures, lethargy, and coma. Rapid correction of hyponatremia following furosemide abuse resulted in central pontine myelinolysis in one report.[142] Symptoms such as tetany and peripheral sensory and motor dysfunction resulting from loop diuretic abuse improve rapidly following electrolyte correction.[136,143]

The use of loop diuretics has also been associated with auditory nerve damage. This dose-dependent phenomenon is reported with furosemide and bumetadine use but is more frequently described with the use of ethacrynic acid. The intravenous administration of high doses of loop diuretics concomitantly with other potentially ototoxic drugs such as aminoglycosides is associated with the highest risks of ototoxicity.[144,145] With discontinuation of treatment, hearing loss and tinnitus frequently improve.

POTASSIUM-SPARING DIURETICS

While relatively weak in diuretic activity, potassium-sparing diuretics such as triamterene and amiloride are frequently administered in combination with loop and thiazide diuretics to decrease the amount of potassium excreted into the urine. These agents, in addition to spironolactone and eplerenone, act on the distal renal tubule to decrease sodium reabsorption and limit excretion of potassium. While reports of toxicity related to overdose are exceedingly rare with potassium-sparing diuretics, the development of life-threatening hyperkalemia can occur with therapeutic dosing, frequently in patients with renal insufficiency or with coadministration of other potassium-elevating medications. One report found that 8.6% of patients treated with spironolactone developed hyperkalemia.[146]

The coadministration of a potassium-sparing diuretic with a loop or thiazide diuretic often obviates the need for supplemental potassium administration.[147] Two cases of life-threatening hyperkalemia were reported in individuals who were taking potassium-containing salt substitutes while concurrently taking spironolactone.[148] In overdose of these agents, gastrointestinal irritation and central nervous depression have also been reported. Spironolactone has other unique side effects related to its steroid structure, including development of gynecomastia, impotence, hirsutism, and menstrual irregularities. Use of triamterene is unique in its association with interstitial nephritis and nephrolithiasis.[149]

Management

Treatment of diuretic toxicity is supportive with close monitoring and correction of electrolyte abnormalities and hypovolemia. The administration of activated charcoal should take place shortly after drug ingestion in order to limit absorption. Aggressive fluid administration is indicated in cases of diuretic-induced hypotension and shock. The possibility of co-ingestion with potassium supplements must be considered. Large potassium tablets may be visible on radiography, and although poorly adsorbed by activated charcoal, whole bowel irrigation may be an appropriate intervention to decrease absorption. An initial ECG should be performed in patients with diuretic overdose followed by continuous cardiac monitoring when electrolyte abnormalities are suspected. Significant hyperkalemia in the presence of ECG abnormalities should be corrected with insulin and dextrose, calcium, sodium bicarbonate, and cation-exchange resins.

REFERENCES

1. Food and Drug Administration: New labeling for sodium nitroprusside emphasizes the risk of cyanide toxicity. JAMA 1991;265:847.
2. Johnson CC: Mechanisms of actions and toxicity of nitroprusside. Proc Soc Exp Biol Med 1928;26:102–103.
3. Page IH, Corcoran AC, Dustan HP, Koppanyi T: Cardiovascular actions of sodium nitroprusside in animals and hypertensive patients. Circulation 1955;11:188–198.
4. Friederich JA, Butterworth JF: Sodium nitroprusside: twenty years and counting. Anesth Analg 1995;81:152–162.
5. Frank MJ, Johnson JB, Rubin SH: Spectrophotometric determination of sodium nitroprusside and its photodegradation products. J Pharm Sci 1976;65:44–48.
6. Arnold WP, Longnecker DE, Epstein RM: Photodegradation of sodium nitroprusside: biologic activity and cyanide release. Anesthesiology 1984;61:254–260.
7. Schulz V: Clinical pharmacokinetics of nitroprusside, cyanide, thiosulphate, and thiocyanate. Clin Pharmacokinet 1984;9:239–241.
8. Moncada S, Palmer RMJ, Higgs EA: Nitric oxide: physiology, pathophysiology, and pharmacology. Pharmacol Rev 1991;43:109–142.

9. Kreye VAW, Reske SN: Possible site of the in vivo disposition of sodium nitroprusside in the rat. Naunyn Schmiedebergs Arch Pharmacol 1982;320:260–265.

10. Smith PR, Kruszyma H: Nitrprusside produced cyanide poisoning via a reaction with hemoglobin. J Pharmacol Exp Ther 1974;191:557–563.

11. Vesey CJ, Krapez JR, Cole PV: The effects of sodium nitroprusside and cyanide on haemoglobin function. J Pharm Pharmacol 1980;32:256–261.

12. Ivankovich AD, Braverman M, Stephens TS, et al: Sodium thiosulfate disposition in humans. Relation to sodium nitroprusside toxicity. Anesthesiology 1983;58:11–17.

13. Way JL: Cyanide intoxication and its mechanism of antagonism. Ann Rev Pharmacol Toxicol 1984;24:451–481.

14. Piantadose CA, Sylvia AL: Cerebral cytochrome a,a$_3$ inhibition by cyanide in bloodless rats. Toxicology 1984;33:67–79.

15. Schulz V, Bonn R, Kindler J: Kinetics of elimination of thiocyanate in seven healthy subjects and in eight subjects with renal failure. Klin Wochenscher 1979;57:243–247.

16. Vesey CJ, Wilson J: Red cell cyanide. J Pharm Pharmacol 1978;30:20–26.

17. Schulz V, Gross R, Patsch T, et al: Cyanide toxicity of sodium nitroprusside in therapeutic use with and without sodium thiosulfate. Klin Wochenschr 1982;60:1393–1400.

18. Vesey CJ, Cole PV: Blood cyanide and thiocyanate concentrations produced by long-term therapy with sodium nitroprusside. Br J Anaesth 1985;57:148–155.

19. Way JL, Sylvester D, Morgan RL, et al: Recent perspectives on the toxicodynamic basis of cyanide antagonism. Fundam Appl Toxicol 1984;4(Suppl):231–239.

20. Turský T, Šajter V: The influence of potassium cyanide poisoning on the γ-aminobutyric acid level in the rat brain. J Neurochem 1962;9:519–523.

21. Domalski CA, Kolk LC, Hines EA: Delirious reactions secondary to thiocyanate therapy of hypertension. Proc Mayo Clin 1953;28:272–280.

22. Garvin CF: The fatal toxic manifestations of the thiocyanates. JAMA 1939;112:1125.

23. Wald MH, Lindberg HA, Barker MH: The toxic manifestations of the thiocyanates. JAMA 1939;112:1120–1124.

24. Peters CG, Mundy JVB, Rayner PR: Acute cyanide poisoning. Anaesthesia 1982;37:582–586.

25. Curry SC, Arnold-Capell P: Nitroprusside, nitroglycerin, and angiotensin-coverting enzyme inhibitors. Crit Care Clin 1991;7:555–581.

26. Vesey CJ, Simpson PJ, Adams L, Cole PV: Metabolism of sodium nitroprusside and cyanide in the dog. Br J Anaesth 1979;51:89–97.

27. Vesey CJ, Cole PV, Simpson PJ: Cyanide and thiocyanate concentrations following sodium nitroprusside infusion in man. Br J Anaesth 1976;48:651–660.

28. Cole PV, Vesey CJ: Sodium thiosulfate decreases blood cyanide concentrations after the infusion of sodium nitroprusside. Br J Anaesth 1987;59:531–535.

29. Michenfelder JD, Tinker JH: Cyanide toxicity and thiosulfate protection during chronic administration of sodium nitroprusside in the dog. Anesthesiology 1977;47:441–448.

30. Cottrell JE, Casthely P, Brodie JD, et al: Prevention of nitroprusside-induced cyanide toxicity with hydroxocobalamin. N Engl J Med 1978;298:809–811.

31. Krapez JR, Vesey CJ, Adams L, Cole PV: Effects of cyanide antidotes used with sodium nitroprusside infusions: sodium thiosulphate and hydroxocobalamin given prophylactically to dogs. Br J Anaesth 1981;53:793–804.

32. Zerbe NF, Wagner BKJ: Use of vitamin B$_{12}$ in the treatment and prevention of nitroprusside-induced cyanide toxicity. Crit Care Med 1993;21:465–467.

33. Pahl MV, Vaziri ND: In-vivo and in-vitro hemodialysis studies of thiocyanate. J Toxicol Clin Toxicol 1982–1983;19:965–974.

34. Kerins DM, Robertson RM, Robertson D: Drugs used for the treatment of myocardial ischemia. In Hardman JG, Limbird LE, Gilman AG (eds): Goodman and Gilman's The Pharmacological Basis of Therapeutics, 10th ed. New York, McGraw-Hill, 2001.

35. Murrell W: Nitro-glycerine as a remedy for angina pectoris. Lancet 1879;1:234–236, 284–288.

36. Murad F: Cyclic guanosine monophosphate as a mediator of vasodilation. J Clin Invest 1986;78:1–5.

37. Chung SH, Fung HL: Identification of subcellular site for nitroglycerin metabolism to nitric oxide in bovine coronary smooth muscle cells. J Pharmacol Exp Ther 1990;253(2):614–619.

38. Harrison DG, Bates JN: The nitrovasodilators. New ideas about old drugs. Circulation 1993;87:1461–1467.

39. Münzel T, Sayegh H, Freeman BA, et al: Evidence for enhanced vascular superoxide anion production in nitrate tolerance. A novel mechanism underlying tolerance and cross-tolerance. J Clin Invest 1995;95:187–194.

40. Abou-Mohamed G, Johnson JA, Jin L: Roles of superoxide, peroxynitrite, and protein kinase C in the development of tolerance to nitroglycerin. J Pharmacol Exp Ther 2004;308(1):289–299.

41. O'Keefe JH, Kwong EM, Tangredi RG: Transgingival nitrate syncope. N Engl J Med 1986;315:1030.

42. Marshall JB, Ecklund RE: Methemoglobinemia from overdose of nitroglycerin. JAMA 1980;244:330.

43. Kaplan KJ, Taber M, Teagarden JR, et al: Association of methemoglobinemia and intravenous nitroglycerin administration. Am J Cardiol 1985;55:181–183.

44. Alexander J, Kaplan K, Davidson R, et al: Intravenous nitroglycerin-induced abducens nerve palsy. Am Heart J 1983;106:1159–1160.

45. Ohar JM, Fowler AA, Selhorst JB, et al: Intravenous nitroglycerin-induced intracranial hypertension. Crit Care Med 1985;13:867–868.

46. Demey HE, Daelemans RA, Verpooten GA, et al: Propylene glycol-induced side effects during the intravenous nitroglycerin therapy. Intensive Care Med 1988;14:221–226.

47. Col J, Col-Debeys C, Lavenne-Pardonge E, et al: Propylene glycol-induced heparin resistance during nitroglycerin infusion. Am Heart J 1985;110:171–173.

48. Habbab MA, Haft J: Heparin resistance induced by intravenous nitroglycerin: a word of caution when both drugs are used concomitantly. Arch Intern Med 1987;147:857–860.

49. Becker RC, Corrao JM, Bovill EG, et al: Intravenous nitroglycerin-induced heparin resistance: a qualitative antithrombin III abnormality. Am Heart J 1991;121(6 Pt 1):1849–1850.

50. Cheitlin MD, Hutter AM, Brindis RG, et al: Use of silfenafil (Viagra) in patients with cardiovascular disease. ACC/AHA Expert Consensus Document. Circulation 1999;99:168–177.

51. Kelner MJ, Bailey DN: Propylene glycol as a cause of lactic acidosis. J Anal Toxicol 1985;9:40–42.

52. Watson WA, Litovitz TL, Rodgers GC, et al: 2002 annual report of the American association of poison control centers toxic exposure surveillance system. Am J Emerg Med 2003;21(5):353–421.

53. Reece PA: Hydralazine and related compounds: chemistry, metabolism, and mode of action. Med Res Rev 1981;1:73–96.

54. Azuma J, Sawamura A, Harada H, et al: Mechanism of direct cardiostimulating actions of hydralazine. Eur J Pharmacol 1987;135:137–144.

55. Smith BA, Ferguson DB: Acute hydralazine overdose: marked ECG abnormalities in a young adult. Ann Emerg Med 1992;21(3):326–330.

56. Raskin NH, Fishman RA: Pyridoxine-deficiency neuropathy due to hydralazine. N Engl J Med 1965;273(22):1182–1185.

57. Farrell SE, Epstein SK: Overdose of Rogaine® Extra Strength for Men topical minoxidil preparation. J Toxicol Clin Toxicol 1999;37(6):781–783.

58. Zappacosta AR: Reversal of baldness in patient receiving minoxidil for hypertension. N Engl J Med 1980;303:1480–1481.

59. McCormick MA, Forman MH, Manoguerra AS: Severe toxicity from ingestion of a topical minoxidil preparation. Am J Emerg Med 1989;7:419–421.

60. MacMillan AR, Warshawski FJ, Steinberg RA: Minoxidil overdose. Chest 1993;103:1290–1291.

61. McCall JM, Aiken JW, Chidester CG, et al: Pyrimidine and triazine 3-oxide sulfates: a new family of vasodilators. J Med Chem 1983;26:1791–1793.

62. Gottlieg TB, Thomas RC, Chidsey CA: Pharmacokinetic studies of minoxidil. Clin Pharmacol Ther 1972;13:436–441.

63. Leblanc N, Wilde DW, Keef KD, Hume JR: Electrophysiologic mechanisms of minoxidil sulfate-induced vasodilation of rabbit portal vein. Circ Res 1989;65:1102–1111.

64. Allon MA, Hall WD, Macon EJ: Prolonged hypotension after initial minoxidil dose. Arch Intern Med 1986;146:2075–2076.

65. Manufacturer's information, Upjohn Company, Kalamazoo, MI.

66. Isles C, MacKay A, Barton PJM, Mitchell I: Accidental overdosage of minoxidil in a child. Lancet 1981;1:97.

67. Poff SW, Rose SR: Minoxidil overdose with ECG changes: case report and review. J Emerg Med 1992;10:53–57.

68. Krehlik JM, Hindson DA, Crowley JJ, Knight LL: Minoxidil-associated pericarditis and fatal cardiac tamponade. West J Med 1985;143:527–529.

69. Goldstein H, Lue TF, Padma-Nathan H, et al: Oral sildenafil in the treatment of erectile dysfunction. N Engl J Med 1998;338:1397–1404.

70. Tracqui A, Miras A, Tabib A, et al: Fatal overdosage with sildenafil citrate (Viagra®): first report and review of the literature. Hum Exp Toxicol 2002;21(11):623–629.

71. Krenzelok EP: Sildenafil: clinical toxicology profile. J Toxicol Clin Toxicol 2000;38(6):645–651.

72. Hung DZ, Yang DY: Sildenafil overdose in a female patient. J Toxicol Clin Toxicol 2001;39(4):423–424.

73. Kloner RA, Zusman RM: Cardiovascular effects of sildenafil citrate and recommendations for its use. Am J Cardiol 1999;84:11N–17N.

74. Azarbal B, Mirocha J, Shah PK, et al: Adverse cardiovascular events associated with the use of Viagra. J Am Coll Cardiol 2000;35(Suppl 1):553A–554A.

75. Morales A, Gingell C, Collins M, et al: Clinical safety of oral sildenafil citrate (Viagra) in the treatment of erectile dysfunction. Int J Impot Res 1998;10:69–74.

76. Muniz AE, Holstege CP: Acute myocardial infarction associated with sildenafil (Viagra) ingestion. Am J Emerg Med 2000;18(3):353–355.

77. Kassim AA, Fabry ME, Nagel RL: Acute priapism associated with the use of sildenafil in a patient with sickle cell trait. Blood 2000;95:1878–1879.

78. Sur RL, Cane CJ: Sildenafil-citrate associated priapism. Urology 2000;55(6):950.

79. Swedberg K, Held P, Kjekshus L, et al: Effects of enalapril on mortality in severe congestive heart failure: results of the Cooperative North Scandinavian Enalapril Survival Study (CONSENSUS). N Engl J Med 1992;327:685–691.

80. Lewis EJ, Hunsicker LG, Bain RP, Rohde RD: The effect of angiotensin-converting enzyme inhibition on diabetic nephropathy. The Collaborative Study Group. N Engl J Med 1993;329(20):1456–1462.

81. Michaels AD, Maynard C, Every NR, Barron HV: Early use of ACE inhibitors in the treatment of acute myocardial infarction in the United States: experience from the National Registry of Myocardial Infarction. Am J Cardiol 1999;84(10):1176–1181.

82. Gavras H, Gavras I: Angiotensin-converting enzyme inhibitors. Properties and side effects. Hypertension 1988;11(3 Pt 2):37–41.

83. Song JC, White CM: Clinical pharmacokinetics and selective pharmacodynamics of new angiotensin converting enzyme inhibitors: an update. Clin Pharmacokinet 2002;41(3):207–224.

84. Gainer JV, Morrow JD, Loveland A, et al: Effect of bradykinin-receptor blockade on the response to angiotensin-converting-enzyme inhibitor in normotensive and hypertensive subjects. N Engl J Med 1998;339(18):1285–1292.

85. Israili ZH, Hall WD: Cough and angioneurotic edema associated with angiotensin-converting enzyme inhibitor therapy. A review of the literature and pathophysiology. Ann Intern Med 1992;117(3):234–242.

86. Parker SC, Hannah A, Brooks M, et al: Renal artery stenosis: a disease worth pursuing. Med J Aust 2001;175(3):149–153.

87. Hodsman GP, Isles CG, Murray GD, et al: Factor related to first dose hypotensive effect of captopril: prediction and treatment. BMJ 1983;286(6368):832–834.

88. Verughese AA, Taylor AA, Nelson EB: Consequnces of angiotensin-converting enzyme inhibitor overdose. Am J Hypertens 1989;2(5 Pt 1):355–357.

89. Lau CP: Attempted suicide with enalapril. N Engl J Med 1986;315(8):197.

90. Lip GY, Ferner RE: Poisoning with anti-hypertensive drugs: angiotensin converting enzyme inhibitors. J Hum Hypertens 1995;9(9):711–715.

91. Park H, Purnell GV, Mirchandani HG: Suicide by captopril overdose. Clin Toxicol 1990;28(3):379–382.

92. Everson GW: Angiotensin converting enzyme inhibitor overdoses: a multicenter study. Vet Hum Toxicol 1990;32(4):352.

93. Spiller HA, Udicious TM, Muir S: Angiotensin converting enzyme inhibitor ingestion in children. Clin Toxicol 1989;27(6):435–353.

94. Brown NJ, Ray WA Snowden M, Griffin MR: Black Americans have an increased rate of angiotensin converting enzyme inhibit-associated angioedema. Clin Pharmacol Ther 1996;60(1):8–13.

95. Gibbs CR, Lip GYH, Beevers DG: Angioedema due to ACE inhibitors: increased risk in patients of African origin. Br J Clin Pharmacol 1991;48(6):861–865.

96. Chin HL, Buchan DA: Severe angioedema after long-term use of an angiotensin-converting enzyme inhibitor. Ann Intern Med 1990;112(4):312–313.

97. Orfan N, Patterson R, Dykewicz MS: Severe angioedema related to ACE inhibitors in patients with a history of idiopathic angioedema. JAMA 1990;264(10):1287–1289.

98. Augenstein WL, Kulig KW, Rumack BH: Captopril overdose resulting in hypotension. JAMA 1988;259:3302–3305.

99. Lechleitner P, Dzien A, Haring C, Glossmann H: Uneventful self-poisoning with a very high dose of captopril. Toxicology 1990;64(3):325–329.

100. Spiller HA, Udicious TM, Muir S: Angiotensin converting enzyme inhibitor ingestion in children. Clin Toxicol 1989;27:345–353.

101. Olin BR: Drug Facts and Comparisons. St. Louis, Facts and Comparisons, 2000.

102. Geh SL, Nott MW, Majewski H, et al: Effect of captopril on blood pressure responses to enkephalins in chloralose-anaesthetized rats. Arch Int Pharmacodyn Ther 1986;279(2):282–290.

103. Varon J, Duncan SR: Naloxone reversal of hypotension due to captopril overdose. Ann Emerg Med 1991;10:1125–1127.

104. Trilli LE, Johnson KA: Lisinopril overdose and management with intravenous angiotensin II. Ann Pharmacother 1994;28(10):1165–1168.

105. Mazzolai L, Burnier M: Comparative safety and tolerability of angiotensin II receptor antagonists. Drug Saf 1999;21(1):23–33.

106. Pitt B, Segal R, Martinez FA, et al: Randomized trail of losartan versus captopril in patients over 65 with heart failure (Evaluation of Losartan in the Elderly Study, ELITE). Lancet 1997;349(9054):747–752.

107. Sosa-Canache B, Cierco M, Gutierrez CI, et al: Role of bradykinins and nitric oxide in the AT2 receptor-medicated hypotension. J Hum Hypertens 2000;14(Suppl 1):40–46.

108. Lacourciere U, Brunner HR, Irwing R, et al: Effects of modulators of the rennin-angiotensin-aldosterone system on cough. J Hypertens 1994;12(12):1387–1393.

109. van Rijnsoever EW, Kwee-Zuiderwiju WJM, Feenstra J: Angioneurotic edema attributed to use of losartan. Arch Intern Med 1998;158(18):2063–2065.

110. Warner KK, Visconti JA, Tschampel MM: Angiotensin II receptor blockers in patients with ACE inhibitor-induced angioedema. Ann Pharmacother 2000;34(4):526–528.

111. Mimran A, Ribstein J, DuCailar G: Comparison of the acute renal effect of losartan and captopril in atheromatous renovascular disease. Am J Hypertens 1998;11:47A.

112. Birck R, Keim V, Fiedler F, et al: Pancreatitis after losartan. Lancet 1998;351(9110):1178.

113. Bosch X: Losartan-induced acute pancreatitis. Ann Intern Med 1997;127(11):1043–1044.

114. Barr M Jr: Teratogen update: angiotensin-converting enzyme inhibitors. Teratology 1994;50(6):399–409.

115. Cooper KL, McKeirnan JM, Kaplan SA: Alpha-adrenoceptor antagonists in the treatment of benign prostatic hyperplasia. Drugs 1999;57(1):9–17.

116. Sasso EH, O'Connor DT: Prazosin depression of baroreflex function in hypertensive man. Eur J Clin Pharmacol 1982;22(1):7–14.

117. Bateman DN, Hobbs DC, Twomey TM, et al: Prazosin, pharmacokinetics and concentration effect. Eur J Clin Pharmacol 1979;16(3):177–181.

118. Sonders RC: Pharmacokinetics of terazosin. Am J Med 1986;80(5B):20–24.

119. Piotrovskii VK, Veiko NN, Ryabokon OS, et al: Identification of a prazosin metabolite and some preliminary data on its kinetics in hypertensive patients. Eur J Clin Pharmacol 1984;27(3):275–280.

120. Baugham RA Jr, Arnold S, Benet LZ, et al: Altered prazosin pharmacokinetics in congestive heart failure. Eur J Clin Pharmacol 1980;17:425.

121. Hasford J, Bussmann WD, Delius W, et al: First dose hypotension with enalapril and prazosin in congestive heart failure. Int J Cardiol 1991;31(3):287–293.

122. McClean WJ: Prazosin overdose. Med J Aust 1976;1(16):592.

123. Lenz K, Druml W. Kleinberger G, et al: Acute intoxication with prazosin: case report. Hum Toxicol 1985;4(1):53–56.

124. Gokel Y, Dokur M, Paydas S: Doxazosin overdosage. Am J Emerg Med 2000;18(5):638–639.

125. Rygnestad TK, Dale O: Self-poisoning with prazosin. Acta Med Scand 1983;213(2):157–158.

126. Robbins DN, Crawford ED, Lackner LH: Priapism secondary to prazosin overdose. J Urol 1983;130(5):975.

127. Chin DK, Ho AK, Tse CY: Neuropsychiatric complications related to use of prazosin in patients with renal failure. BMJ 1986;293(6558):1347.

128. Baglin A, Boulard JC, Hanslick T, Prinseau J: Metabolic adverse reactions to diuretics. Clinical relevance to elderly. Drug Saf 1995;12(3):161–171.

129. Mitchell JE, Hatsukami D, Eckert ED, Pyle RL: Characteristics of 275 patients with bulimia. Am J Psychiatry 1985;142(4):482–485.

130. Garratty G, Houston M, Petz LD, Webb M: Acute immune intravascular hemolysis due to hydrochlorthiazide. Am J Clin Pathol 1981;76(1):73–78.

131. Rubinstein I: Fatal thrombosis of left internal carotid artery following diuretic abuse. Ann Emerg Med 1985;14(3):275.

132. O'Doherty NJ: Thiazide and cerebral ischemia. Lancet 1965;2(7425):1297.

133. Sunderam SG, Mankikar GD: Hyponatremia in the elderly. Age Ageing 1983;12(1):77–80.

134. Morgan DB, Davidson C: Hypokalemia and diuretics: an analysis of publications. BMJ 1980;280(6218):905–908.

135. Srivastava RN, Travis LB, Dodge WF, Kaye M: Prolonged coma and visual loss; unusual reaction to chlorthiazide. J Pediatr 1969;74(1):126–128.

136. Brucato A, Bonati M, Gaspari F, et al: Tetany and rhabdomyolysis due to surreptitious furosemide—importance of magnesium supplementation. Clin Toxicol 1993;31(2):341–344.

137. Vila JM, Blum L, Dosik H: Thiazide-induced immune hemolytic anemia. JAMA 1976;236(15):1723–1724.

138. Eckhauser ML, Dokler MA, Imbenbo AL: Diuretic-associated pancreatitis: a collective review and illustrative cases. Am J Gastroenterol 1987;82(9):865–870.

139. Grimm RH Jr, Grandtis GA, Prineas RJ, et al: Long-term effects on sexual function of five antihypertensive drugs and nutritional hygienic treatment in hypertensive men and women. Treatment of Mild Hypertension Study (TOMHS). Hypertension 1997;29 (1 Pt 1):8–14.

140. Eisner EV, Crowell EB: Hydrochlorothiazide-dependent thrombocytopenia due to IgM antibody. JAMA 1971;215(3):480–482.

141. Dormans TP, van Meyel JJM, Gerlag PGG, et al: Diuretic efficacy of high dose furosemide in severe heart failure: bolus injection versus continuous infusion. J Am Coll Cardiol 1996;28(2): 376–382.

142. Copeland PM: Diuretic abuse and central pontine myelinolysis. Psychother Psychosom 1989;52(1–3):101–105.

143. Kaufmann H, Elijovich F, Yahr MD: An unusual cause of tetany: surreptitious use of furosemide. Mt Sinai J Med 1984;51(5): 625–628.

144. Whitworth C, Morris C, Scott V, Rybak LP: Dose-response relationships for furosemide ototoxicity in rat. Hear Res 1993;71(1–2):202–207.

145. Bates DE, Beaumont SJ, Baylis BW: Ototoxicity induced by gentamicin and furosemide. Ann Pharacother 36(3):446–451.

146. Greenblatt DJ, Koch-Weser J: Adverse reactions to spironolactone. A report from the Boston Collaborative Drug Surveillance Program. JAMA 1973;225(1):40–43.

147. Hollenberg NK, Mickiewicz CW: Postmarketing surveillance in 70,898 patients treated with a triamterene/hydrochlorothiazide combination (Maxzide). Am J Cardiol 1989;63:37B–41B.

148. Yap V, Patel A, Thomsen J: Hyperkalemia with cardiac arrhythmia. Induction by salt substitutes, spironolactone and azotemia. JAMA 1976;236:2275–2276.

149. Carr MC, Prien EL, Babayan RK: Triamterene nephrolithiasis: renewed attention is warranted. J Urol 1990;144(6):1339–1340.

62 *Clonidine and Related Imidazoline Derivatives*

JAMES F. WILEY II, MD, MPH

At a Glance...

- Clonidine and related imidazolines act at central and peripheral α_2-adrenergic receptors and at imidazoline receptors.
- In overdose, imidazolines produce central nervous system depression, bradycardia, hypotension, and respiratory depression.
- As little as 0.1 mg or 1 clonidine tablet may cause major poisoning effects in young children.
- Pediatric clonidine exposure is increasing and reflects greater use of this drug for behavioral problems in children.
- Management of clonidine poisoning should focus on respiratory support and maintenance of hemodynamic stability.
- No antidote exists for clonidine toxicity, although reports of clinical improvement after naloxone or yohimbine administration have been described.

INTRODUCTION AND RELEVANT HISTORY

Clonidine and related drugs, including apraclonidine, brimonidine, dexmedetomidine, guanabenz, guanfacine, methyldopa, naphazoline, oxymetazoline, tetrahydrozoline, tizanidine, and xylometazoline, share similar toxicity. Clonidine, guanabenz, guanfacine, and methyldopa have been used primarily as antihypertensive medications, although new indications have been developed for clonidine and guanfacine. Tetrahydrozoline, oxymetazoline, naphazoline, and xylometazoline are over-the-counter topical vasoconstrictors. Apraclonidine and brimonidine are prescribed for ocular hypertension and open-angle glaucoma. Tizanidine is a new muscle relaxant used for the spasticity associated with cerebral and spinal disorders. Dexmedetomidine is a new imidazole used for intravenous sedation and analgesia.[1] Most examples of severe toxicity attributable to this class of drugs have occurred with clonidine.

Clonidine was initially developed as a topical nasal decongestant in 1962. Subsequently, it was found to be a potent antihypertensive agent with sympatholytic effects not attributable to ganglionic blocking.[2] Clonidine is synergistic in antihypertensive effect with diuretics and has been employed as a second or third agent in the treatment of essential hypertension. The advent of converting enzyme inhibitors has decreased the use of clonidine as an antihypertensive agent. Alternative off-label indications in adults include anesthetic premedication, induction of spinal anesthesia, ultrashort opiate detoxification, alcohol withdrawal, smoking cessation, and alleviation of postmenopausal hot flashes.[3-8] In children, treatment of attention-deficit hyperactivity disorder (ADHD) accounts for the greatest off-label use.[9] Refractory conduct disorder, Tourette's syndrome, and diagnosis of growth hormone deficiency make up other potential uses in children.[10,11] Guanfacine has been evaluated for the treatment of children with both ADHD and Tourette's syndrome[12] and has been shown to induce growth hormone secretion without the concomitant hypotension or sedation common with clonidine.[13]

EPIDEMIOLOGY

Clonidine exposure occurs in about 1 in 1000 poisonings and is notable for serious signs and symptoms after many ingestions.[14-16] In 2004, there were 5802 clonidine and 1579 tetrahydrozoline exposures reported to U.S. poison centers. Major toxicity and death occurred in only 3.6% and 0.2% of clonidine exposures and in 0.1% and 0% of tetrahydrozoline exposures, respectively.[17] Moderate toxicity, however, was observed in 22.8% of all clonidine exposures. Total clonidine exposures in children younger than 19 years have almost doubled in recent years.[14] Many pediatric exposures involve the child's own medication or that of another child in the household. This pattern contrasts with the previously reported situation of young toddlers ingesting a grandparent's clonidine.[16,18] Exposure to over-the-counter nose drops and eye drops is an another important cause of imidazoline poisoning but tends to be uneventful.[19] Guanabenz, guanfacine, and methyldopa are rarely prescribed or ingested and appear to cause similar but lesser effects than clonidine.[20-22]

STRUCTURE AND STRUCTURE–ACTIVITY RELATIONSHIPS

Clonidine and some related imidazolines are depicted in Figure 62-1.

PHARMACOLOGY

Clonidine, guanabenz, guanfacine, oxymetazoline, tetrahydrozoline, naphazoline, xylometazoline, tizanidine, and dexmedetomidine are related imidazolines with central and peripheral α_2-adrenergic agonist effects. In addition, some of the central antihypertensive effects may be attributable to binding of specific imidazoline receptors. As sympathomimetic agents, imidazolines have little to no β-adrenergic effect and have peripheral vasoconstrictive properties similar to specific α_1-adrenergic agonists. However, imidazolines differ markedly from most sympathomimetics in their central inhibition of sympathetic outflow.[23] Developed as an analog of 3,4-dihydroxyphenlyalanine (DOPA), methyldopa is chemically

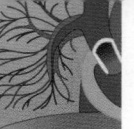

FIGURE 62-1 Structure of clonidine and some other imidazolines.

unrelated to the imidazolines but stimulates α_2-adrenergic receptors centrally through its metabolite, α-methyl norepinephrine.[24]

The imidazolines produce effects by a complex interaction with central α_2-adrenergic receptors, peripheral α_2-adrenergic receptors, and central imidazoline receptors. The α_2-adrenergic receptors have subtypes A, B, and C, which are structurally distinct and have varying affinity for α_2-adrenergic receptor agonists and antagonists. α_{2A}-Adrenergic receptors are found predominantly in the brainstem, whereas α_{2B}-adrenergic receptors are found on vascular smooth muscle cells.[25] Central α_{2A}-adrenergic receptors have a higher affinity for agonists (e.g., clonidine) than do peripheral α_{2B}-adrenergic receptors.[25] Binding at each of these receptors reduces the intracellular activity of adenyl cyclase through a pertussin toxin-sensitive G protein.[26] Elucidation of the receptor-binding properties for the drugs under discussion have involved radioligand studies using [³H]clonidine. Clonidine strongly binds to central α_{2A}-adrenergic receptors located in the brainstem (nucleus tractus solitarii). This binding has an inhibitory effect on norepinephrine release centrally, resulting in decreased sympathetic outflow.[27-29] Therapeutically, this action causes reduced blood pressure, bradycardia, and sedation. The hypotensive changes are not seen in quadriplegic patients who receive clonidine.[26] Clonidine also inhibits acetylcholine release. Clinically, this effect is manifest as dry mouth in therapeutic doses. In the hypothalamus, clonidine stimulates the release of growth hormone and has varying effects on sympathetic tone and blood pressure. In the spinal cord, clonidine decreases sympathetic tone and blood pressure and has analgesic properties that are similar to those of narcotic medications.[26,30]

The similarity in effects found upon stimulation of central α_2-adrenergic receptors and opiate receptors has prompted much investigation into a possible molecular link between these sites. Clinical evidence supporting such a link includes the use of clonidine for ultrashort opiate detoxification,[4,5] the successful use of clonidine for spinal analgesia,[30] the likeness of toxicity found after overdose with narcotics and clonidine, the reversal of clonidine toxicity with naloxone in some patients,[16] and the decreased density of central α_2-adrenergic receptors in heroin addicts.[31] Both opiate and central α_2-adrenergic receptors act through G proteins. The possibility of "cross-talk" between these receptors through the G-protein complex has been raised, although initial studies in a neuroblastoma-glioma cell line were not supportive.[32]

Other proposed mechanisms for α_2-agonist inhibitory effects, such as hyperpolarization of neuronal cells by activation of potassium channels, inhibition of N-type voltage-gated calcium channels, and increased Na^+/H^+ exchange, may hold the answer regarding the relationship between imidazolines and opiates.[24] Improved understanding concerning the relationship of central α_2-adrenergic and opiate receptors must await further study.

Specific imidazoline (I) receptors of multiple types exist and have been identified in a variety of tissues and animal species. Current nomenclature delineates I_1 and I_2 receptors, with a further breakdown of I_2 receptors into I_{2a} (amiloride-sensitive) and I_{2b} (amiloride-insensitive) receptors.[33] These receptors do not act through G proteins.[34] Clonidine has strong affinity at I_1 receptors, which are located in the ventrolateral medulla in humans. Binding at these sites leads to decrease in blood pressure independent of central α_2-adrenergic effects.[35] An endogenous substance with imidazoline receptor affinity called *clonidine-displacing substance* has also been discovered, but its physiologic role has yet to be elucidated. Guanabenz is an agonist at I_2 imidazoline receptors, which are strongly linked to monoamine oxidase A and B expression, but the mechanism of action and function of I_2 receptors is uncertain and requires further study.[36]

Peripheral imidazoline effects are varied, relate to agonist effects at α_{2B}-adrenergic receptors, and are usually overshadowed by central α_{2A}-adrenergic receptor effects. Agonist activity at peripheral α_{2B}-adrenergic receptors located on vascular smooth muscle cells causes vasoconstriction. Effects at these receptors typically require a higher serum concentration of agonist, as occurs after overdose and intravenous administration of agonist.[25] Thus, intravenous administration of clonidine and supratherapeutic levels of clonidine are associated with hypertension and pallor in some patients. Stimulation of presynaptic peripheral α_2-adrenergic receptors, however, reduces vasomotor tone in other blood vessel sites and inhibits renin release, which would lead to synergism with central effects.[35] The net effect is a reduction of blood pressure and sympathetic outflow in both hypertensive and normotensive patients who receive clonidine. By reducing sympathetic outflow, imidazolines lower arterial pressure through reduction in both cardiac output and peripheral vascular resistance. Reduced cardiac output is from a decrease in heart rate and myocardial contractility.

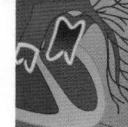

PATHOPHYSIOLOGY

In overdose, the sympatholytic effects of imidazolines predominate. The organs most commonly affected are the brain and the heart. Decreased norepinephrine release in the central nervous system (CNS) causes lethargy, coma, miosis, hypotonia, respiratory depression, apnea, and hypothermia.[14-18] Cardiac consequences of imidazoline toxicity include bradycardia (sinus or first-degree atrioventricular [AV] block) and hypotension related to central α_2-adrenergic and imidazoline receptor stimulation.[14-18] Peripheral α_2-adrenergic effects may cause vasoconstriction with hypertension. Rarely, malignant hypertension and seizures occur, particularly in patients with renal insufficiency who ingest large doses of clonidine.[37] Children are particularly sensitive to the toxic effects of the imidazolines. As little as 0.1 mg of clonidine and 2.5 mL ($\frac{1}{2}$ teaspoon) of 0.05% tetrahydrozoline eye drops have caused significant toxicity.[14,38,39]

PHARMACOKINETICS

Rapid absorption follows oral clonidine administration, with drug bioavailability of 75% to 96% after a single dose.[40] Bioavailability falls with chronic administration to 65%.[41] Maximal hypotensive effect coincides with peak plasma concentration 1 to 3 hours after ingestion. Therapeutic clonidine levels range from 0.5 to 2 ng/mL, with a close relationship between plasma concentration and clinical effects.[23] Clonidine is 20% to 40% protein bound and has a volume of distribution of 2.9 to 5.3 L/kg.[40] Clonidine undergoes hepatic metabolism to inactive compounds, but about half of a single oral dose is excreted unchanged in the urine. The elimination half-life is 12 to 16 hours and is prolonged in patients with renal insufficiency, often necessitating decreased dosing.[41] In preoperative patients, clonidine may be given sublingually or rectally, with pharmacokinetics similar to oral administration.[43,44]

Clonidine patch formulations range from 2.5 to 7.5 mg of drug within a timed matrix delivery system. These systems provide a constant rate of transdermal clonidine administration over 7 days. Maximum plasma concentration occurs 2 to 3 days after application and peaks at 0.1 to 0.5 ng/mL. Elimination half-life ranges from 26 to 55 hours while the patch is applied. Drug delivery varies by application site, with highest absorption from the left arm and lowest from the thigh.[45] Twenty to 75% of residual clonidine may remain in the patch after 7 days of use.[46]

Pharmacokinetic comparisons of certain imidazolines are shown in Table 62-1. α-Clonidine, brimonidine, naphazoline, tetrahydrozoline, oxymetazoline, and xylometazoline are approved and intended only for topical use; pharmacokinetic data based on ingestion are not available for these agents.

Special Populations

PEDIATRIC

Despite the frequent use of imidazolines (clonidine and guanfacine) in children, no controlled pharmacokinetic data exist.

HEPATIC AND RENAL IMPAIRMENT

Hepatic disease necessitates careful monitoring and possible dose reduction in patients receiving dexmedetomidine and guanabenz. Patients with renal disease should have a proportionate reduction in clonidine dose. Methyldopa is contraindicated in patients with active hepatic disease and in those who have experienced liver disorders attributable to prior methyldopa administration.[47]

PREGNANCY AND LACTATION

Methyldopa and guanfacine have category B designation for use in pregnancy. However, a great deal of human experience with methyldopa suggests that the chance of fetal harm is very low and that the benefit of controlling hypertension in pregnancy using methyldopa far outweighs potential teratogenic risks. No human reproductive data exist for guanfacine. Clonidine, guanabenz, and dexmedetomidine all have category C designation in pregnancy, with some evidence of adverse fetal effects in animals. Clonidine is also excreted in breast milk; its safety for use while breast-feeding is unknown.[47]

Pharmacologic Agents

Table 62-2 lists the most common imidazoline formulations available.

TABLE 62-1 Pharmacokinetics of Clonidine, Guanfacine, and Guanabenz						
DRUG	**BIOAVAILABILITY (%)**	**T_{max} (hr)**	**$t_{1/2}$ (hr)**	**Vd (L/kg)**	**PROTEIN BINDING (%)**	**ELIMINATION**
Clonidine	75–96	1–3	12–16	3–5	20–40	Renal
Clonidine patch	25–80*	40–80	26–55	3–5	20–40	Renal
Guanfacine[67,68]	95–100	1–3	17–24	4–6	20–30	Renal
Guanabenz[69]	75	2–5	7–14	7–17	90	Hepatic
Dexmedetomidine	100	0.1	2–3	1.3	94	Hepatic
Tizanidine	20–40	1–2	2–4	8–16	30	Hepatic

*Twenty percent to 75% of drug remains in the patch after 7 days.[26]
T_{max}, maximum plasma concentration; $t_{1/2}$, half-life of drug; Vd, volume of distribution.

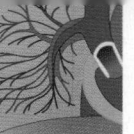

TABLE 62-2 Imidazoline Formulations

DRUG	FORM	DOSE/CONCENTRATION	BRAND NAME
Clonidine	Tablet	0.25 mg	Dixarit
		0.1, 0.2, or 0.3 mg	Catapres
		0.1, 0.2, or 0.3 mg with 15 mg chlorthalidone	Combipres
	Patch	2.5 (3 cm²)	Catapres-TTS 1
		5.0 (7 cm²)	Catapres-TTS 2
		7.5 mg (10 cm²)	Catapres-TTS 3
	Intravenous	100 µg/mL, 500 µg/mL	Duraclon
Guanfacine	Tablet	1, 2 mg	Tenex
Guanabenz	Tablet	4, 8 mg	Generic
Methyldopa	Tablet	125, 250, 500 mg	Generic
	Oral solution	250 mg/5 mL	
	IV solution	50 mg/mL	
Dexmedetomidine	IV solution	100 µg/mL	Precedex
Briminodine	Topical ophthalmic	0.15%, 0.2%, 0.5%	Alphagan-P
Naphazoline	Topical ophthalmic	0.1%	Naphcon Forte, Vasocon, and others
Tetrahydrozoline	Topical nasal and ophthalmic	0.05%, 0.1%	Tyzine, Visine, and others
Tizanidine	Tablet	2, 4 mg	Sirdalud, Ternelin, Zanaflex
Oxymetazoline	Topical nasal and ophthalmic	0.01%, 0.025%, 0.05%	Dristan, Afrin, Neosynephrine, Visine LR, and others
Xylometazoline	Topical nasal	0.05%, 0.1%	Otrivin

Drug Interactions

Significant drug interactions are rare with imidazolines. They may combine with other antihypertensive medications (e.g., α_1-adrenergic, β-adrenergic, and calcium channel antagonists) to produce hypotension or bradycardia. All forms of imidazolines may cause malignant hypertension in patients taking monoamine oxidase inhibitors. Methyldopa may alter lithium levels and has decreased bioavailability when ingested with iron formulations.[47] Three sudden deaths were reported in children taking the combination of clonidine and methylphenidate for ADHD. Circumstances in each case led the U.S. Food and Drug Administration to conclude that both clonidine and methylphenidate have potential cardiotoxicity, but there was no convincing evidence for a lethal drug interaction involving these two medications.[48,49] Cyclic antidepressants potentially interfere with the antihypertensive effect of clonidine. Clonidine may potentiate CNS depression when combined with ethanol, barbiturates, or other sedative-hypnotic medications. Klonopin (clonazepam) and clonidine sound alike and may be inadvertently substituted for each other and result in accidental toxicity.

TOXICOLOGY

Clinical Manifestations

Clinical findings of clonidine and other imidazoline poisonings appear soon after ingestion. In one series of clonidine poisoning in children, 75% of patients had signs of toxicity within 1 hour of ingestion, and no patient had any new findings occur more than 4 hours after poisoning.[16] Topical imidazoline exposure by unintentional oral ingestion or nasal administration in infants and young children can cause lethargy and coma within 1 hour.[50] One case report describes the intentional poisoning with clonidine eye drops for criminal purposes resulting in prolonged coma, respiratory depression, and hemodynamic instability.[51] The potential for rapid decompensation in patients who ingest imidazolines makes close observation of these patients imperative.

About 60% of clonidine exposures reported to poison control centers are symptomatic.[14] The relative frequency of clinical findings in symptomatic children and adults who ingest clonidine are shown in Table 62-3. Lethargy and coma typically accompany serious clonidine toxicity and occur soon after ingestion. Miosis, hyporeflexia, and hypotonia are common associated findings, particularly in children. This constellation of neurologic findings closely mimics opiate toxicity. Frequently, children with clonidine intoxication and coma have transient responsiveness to a painful stimulus, such as intravenous line placement or phlebotomy, but quickly revert back to profound CNS depression. Irritability, dilated pupils, and the presence of extensor plantar responses (i.e., positive Babinski's sign) occur less frequently in children and are rarely seen in adults.

Bradycardia and hypotension follow clonidine ingestion in a significant number of children and adults. Sinus bradycardia is the most common rhythm in these patients, with first-degree AV block seen occasionally. Although complete AV block and supraventricular tachycardia complicated clonidine ingestion in a 22-year-old woman with systemic lupus erythematosus and renal insufficiency,[52] second-degree block or complete AV dissociation should prompt the consideration of toxicity

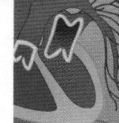

TABLE 62-3 Clinical Findings in Children and Adults after Clonidine Poisoning

FINDING	CHILDREN, HOSPITAL BASED* (<10 yr)	CHILDREN, POISON CONTROL CENTER (<19 yr)	ADULT, HOSPITAL BASED (>18 yr)
N (number)	180	6042	37
Central Nervous System			
Lethargy/coma	87%	82%	78%
Miosis	16%	3%	3%
Hypotonia	12%	—	2%
Irritability	11%	2%	1%
Hyporeflexia	10%	—	1%
Unreactive pupils	6%	—	—
Babinski's sign present	4%	—	—
Mydriasis	4% (2/47)	—	—
Ataxia/dizziness	—	4%	—
Cardiovascular System			
Bradycardia	32%	17%	49%
Hypotension	25%	15%	32%
Arrhythmia	11%	—	—
Hypertension	7%	2%	11%
Cardiac arrest	0%	0.01%	3%
Respiratory System			
Respiratory depression	16%	5%	5%
Apnea	7%	—	—
Other Findings			
Pallor	22%	—	16%
Hypothermia	17% (8/47)	—	—
Dry mouth	2%	—	11%

*Age-specific definitions of bradycardia, hypotension, and hypertension were used for pediatric findings in the hospital-based pediatric reports.
Adapted from Klein-Schwartz W: Trends and toxic effects from pediatric clonidine exposures. Arch Pediatr Adolesc 2002;156:392–396; Stein B, Volans GN: Dixarit overdose: the problem of attractive tablets. BMJ 1978;2:667–668; and Wiley JF II, Wiley CC, Torrey SB, Henretig FM: Clonidine poisoning in young children. J Pediatr 1980;116:654–658.

from other drugs, such as digoxin, calcium channel blockers, and β-adrenergic blockers. Hypotension may be quite profound but usually responds readily to rapid intravenous fluid administration.[16] Hypertension is associated with a large ingested dose of clonidine and is usually an early transient finding.[53] Severe hypertension with encephalopathy or seizures attributed to clonidine exposure has been described in a patient with renal insufficiency.[37] Hypertension may also be precipitated by naloxone administration.[16,53] Cardiac arrests have been described in adults with clonidine poisoning, and one pediatric death has been reported.[14,15]

Apnea and respiratory depression occur more commonly after clonidine exposure in children but also complicate clonidine poisoning in adults. In many patients, the degree of respiratory compromise necessitates endotracheal intubation. Stimulation of the child often increases respiratory rate and effort transiently. This finding may be useful in differentiating apnea caused by clonidine poisoning from the apnea associated with opiate intoxication. Occasional findings with clonidine intoxication include dry mouth, hypothermia, and pallor. The duration of toxic manifestations after ingestion of clonidine tablets is less than 24 hours, with an averaged reported duration of 9 to 16 hours.[15,16]

Other imidazolines could potentially cause any of the clinical findings seen with clonidine poisoning. Most topical imidazoline exposures result in no symptoms. Guanabenz, guanfacine, and methyldopa are rarely used or ingested. The most commonly reported adverse findings in symptomatic patients who have been exposed to imidazolines other than clonidine are variable CNS depression (i.e., lethargy to coma), miosis, bradycardia, and respiratory depression.[19-22,38,50,54] Similar to clonidine, tizanidine overdose has been associated with first-degree and Wenckebach's type II AV block.[55] Dexmedetomidine may cause profound bradycardia or hypotension but does not cause significant respiratory depression.[26]

Adverse Effects

Common adverse effects after oral clonidine, guanfacine, or guanabenz administration include dry mouth, lethargy, and dizziness. Methyldopa is notable for its ability to cause Coombs' test–positive hemolytic anemia and liver disorders. Reversible granulocytopenia and thrombocytopenia may also follow methyldopa therapy. Fever, eosinophilia, elevated serum liver transaminase levels, and jaundice may occur in the first month of treatment. Rarely, fatal hepatic necrosis may transpire. Dexmedetomidine infusion has been associated with transient hypertension, bradycardia, and hypotension. Overuse of topical nasal vasoconstrictors may result in

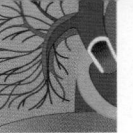

rebound congestion with chronic nasal redness and swelling.[47]

A withdrawal syndrome can occur after sudden cessation of clonidine. This state is characterized by hypertension, tachycardia, sweating, anxiety, insomnia, abdominal pain, nausea, and palpitations. Rarely, clonidine withdrawal can cause malignant hypertension and cardiac dysrhythmias in patients with heart disease. Clonidine withdrawal occurs 1 to 3 days after the abrupt termination of chronic clonidine therapy and coincides with elevated urine and plasma catecholamine levels.[56,57] Patients receiving concomitant β-blocker therapy at the time clonidine is stopped are at higher risk for serious effects. Reinstitution of clonidine therapy usually suffices to treat clonidine withdrawal, but occasionally patients may require nitroprusside infusion for control of hypertension.[58] β Blockers should be avoided because they could produce unopposed α-adrenergic effects that may worsen hypertension in the setting of withdrawal. Abrupt cessation of guanabenz and guanfacine may also cause mild withdrawal symptoms but to a lesser degree than clonidine.[59]

DIAGNOSIS

The diagnosis of imidazoline poisoning is based on a positive history of ingestion coupled with suggestive physical findings. When the history is unknown, imidazoline exposure should be suspected in any patient who has the appearance of opiate intoxication but does not respond to high doses of naloxone. A positive clinical response to naloxone and negative workup for opioid intoxication may occasionally be consistent with imidazoline poisoning. In addition, hypertension that occurs after naloxone administration may be suggestive of imidazoline poisoning, especially clonidine. No routine laboratory or other ancillary tests (e.g., electrocardiogram) can be used to identify imidazoline toxicity, but they are helpful to exclude other disease processes or poisonings. Imidazolines are not detected on routine comprehensive toxicology screening evaluations. Quantitative and qualitative tests are available for clonidine, guanabenz, and methyldopa to confirm the diagnosis, but they usually take several days to perform and are not helpful for patient management.

Differential Diagnosis

The clinical manifestations of imidazoline poisoning are similar to many toxicologic and nontoxicologic entities. Toxicity from imidazolines may be clinically indistinguishable from that produced by opioids. The CNS and cardiovascular manifestations of imidazolines may also be similar to effects produced by alcohols, antiarrhythmics, antiepileptics, barbiturates, α- and β-adrenergic antagonists, calcium channel antagonists, cardiac glycosides, carbon monoxide, cyanide, ergot alkaloids, lithium, sedative-hypnotics, γ-hydroxybutyrate, and skeletal muscle relaxants. CNS infection, traumatic head injury, cerebrovascular accidents, and metabolic disturbances should be considered and excluded with appropriate testing.

TREATMENT

Immediate Supportive Measures

The treatment for imidazoline overdose is primarily supportive. Patients with significant CNS or respiratory depression should have their airway protected, breathing assisted, and cardiovascular support provided as necessary. In one series, 12% of children who ingested clonidine required endotracheal intubation because of apnea, deep coma, or respiratory depression.[16] Although naloxone administration may reverse symptoms of respiratory depression, it has not prevented the need for endotracheal intubation in most reported patients.[16,60] When performing endotracheal intubation in these patients, atropine and muscle relaxant administration should precede laryngoscopy to avoid bradycardia and difficulty due to patient agitation, respectively.

All symptomatic patients suspected of imidazoline overdose should have continuous cardiac monitoring, an intravenous line established, and an electrocardiogram performed. Supplemental oxygen, continuous pulse oximetry, and parenteral thiamine, dextrose (or rapid fingerstick glucose determination), and naloxone should be considered for patients with altered mental status. Bradycardia typically responds well to administration of a routine dose of atropine (0.02 mg/kg, up to 1 mg). Hypotension should be treated with rapid infusion of 20 to 40 mL/kg of isotonic crystalloid, either normal saline or Ringer's lactate. Dopamine infusion has been used successfully in the minority of patients who do not improve after fluid administration.[16] Hypertension after clonidine ingestion is usually transient and frequently requires no treatment. If treatment is instituted, a short-acting agent such as sodium nitroprusside is recommended. β-Adrenergic blockers should be avoided for imidazoline-induced hypertension to prevent unopposed effects and worsening of hypertension. A search for an adherent clonidine patch should occur during skin exposure and examination of patients in whom imidazoline poisoning is suspected.[61]

Suggested laboratory analysis for symptomatic patients includes a complete blood count; blood gas analysis; measurement of electrolytes, blood urea nitrogen, creatinine, and glucose concentrations; and pregnancy testing for women of child-bearing age. Serum acetaminophen and salicylate concentrations should be measured in all intentional overdose patients.

Decontamination and Prevention of Systemic Absorption

The most useful method of decontamination after imidazoline overdose varies based on the type of exposure and the drug formulation. A single dose of activated charcoal is indicated after the oral ingestion of clonidine pills or imidazoline topical preparations. Gastric

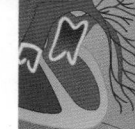

emptying with syrup of ipecac is contraindicated because of the potential for rapid onset of CNS depression. Gastric lavage before administration of activated charcoal may be useful in patients who have ingested a large amount of pills within 1 hour of hospital presentation. Toxicity after nasal or ocular administration of imidazoline drops in young children is unlikely to be significantly altered by any means of gastric decontamination.

Ingestion of a clonidine patch preparation presents a special challenge. Two reports highlight the beneficial use of cathartics in this situation. In one case, a 29-month-old girl had persistent findings of clonidine intoxication 26 hours after presumed ingestion of a patch. Administration of magnesium citrate led to passage of the patch 30 hours later.[62] Another patient had spontaneous passage of a clonidine patch after 4 hours of whole bowel irrigation with polyethylene glycol at 500 mL/hr.[63] Based on this experience, administration of a single dose of activated charcoal followed by whole bowel irrigation may be an effective method for the prevention of clonidine absorption after transdermal patch ingestion.

Antidotes

There is no true antidote for imidazoline poisoning. Naloxone, however, has reversed signs of imidazoline toxicity in some patients. The mechanism by which naloxone works in imidazoline poisoning is unknown. The response rate is about 15% to 40% in patients receiving up to 0.1 mg/kg of naloxone.[16] A total dose of 10 mg of naloxone may need to be administered before determining that naloxone is ineffective.[62] Naloxone infusion after an initial response is rarely needed in patients who ingest clonidine. Given the low risk of naloxone administration in the emergency setting, it should be given to patients with significant CNS, cardiovascular, or respiratory compromise. Patients with severe imidazoline poisoning often need immediate supportive care, such as endotracheal intubation, atropine administration, and rapid crystalloid infusion despite having received naloxone.[16]

Yohimbine, a central α_2-adrenergic antagonist, has reversed lethargy, miosis, and bradycardia due to clonidine ingestion. The oral dose used was 0.1 mg/kg. It has not been used to reverse respiratory depression. Furthermore, it is only available in oral form, thus limiting its efficacy as an antidote for clonidine toxicity.[64]

Tolazoline, a central and peripheral α_2-adrenergic antagonist, was initially used in the treatment of clonidine poisoning, but was frequently ineffective.[65] In addition, it has adverse effects of tachycardia, hypertension, and dysrhythmias. Given the excellent outcome in patients poisoned with imidazolines who receive supportive care alone, the risk of tolazoline outweighs the potential benefit.

Elimination Enhancement

The imidazolines are not amenable to any form of elimination enhancement.

Disposition

Small accidental dosing errors in patients already maintained on the medication may be managed outside of health care facilities with close phone follow-up.[14] Children younger than 6 years with any imidazoline exposure should be referred to a health care facility, as should any patient with intentional ingestion. Those patients who ingest imidazolines but remain asymptomatic can be watched for 4 to 6 hours from the time of ingestion and medically cleared if no physical findings of imidazoline poisoning are seen. Those patients who ingest a clonidine patch, however, should be admitted and monitored for 12 to 24 hours due to the potential for delayed clinical effects. Symptomatic patients who respond to naloxone should be admitted and monitored to ensure no recrudescence of toxicity. These patients often can receive adequate treatment on a regular inpatient ward. Symptomatic patients who do not respond to naloxone require immediate supportive care and admission to an intensive care unit. In most instances, patients fully recover from imidazoline poisoning within 1 to 2 days. There is one case report of permanent neurologic sequelae in a child who was repeatedly poisoned with clonidine by his mother.[66]

REFERENCES

1. Hall JE, Uhrich TD, Barney JA, et al: Sedative, amnestic, and analgesic properties of small-dose dexmedetomidine infusions. Anesth Analg 2000;90:699–705.
2. Lowenstein J: Clonidine. Ann Intern Med 1980;92:74–77.
3. Kahoru N, Katsuya M, Takanobu U, et al: Efficacy of clonidine for prevention of perioperative myocardial ischemia: a critical appraisal and meta-analysis of the literature. Anesthesiology 2002;96:323–329.
4. Gold MS, Redmond DE Jr, Kleber HD: Clonidine blocks acute opiate-withdrawal symptoms. Lancet 1978;2:599–602.
5. Riordan CED, Kleber HD: Rapid opiate detoxification with clonidine and naloxone. Lancet 1980;1:1079–1080.
6. Stanley KM, Worrall CL, Lunsford SL, et al: Experience with an adult alcohol withdrawal syndrome practice guideline. Pharmacotherapy 2005;25:1073–1083.
7. Glassman AH, Stetner F, Walsh T, et al: Heavy smokers, smoking cessation, and clonidine: results of a double-blind, randomized trial. JAMA 1988;259:2863–2866.
8. Clayden JR, Bell JW, Pollard P: Menopausal flushing: double-blind trial of a non-hormonal medication. BMJ 1974;9:490.
9. Connor DF, Fletcher KE, Swanson JM: A meta-analysis of clonidine for symptoms of attention-deficit hyperactivity disorder. J Am Acad Child Adolesc Psychiatry 1999;38:1551–1559.
10. Cohen DJ, Young JG, Nathanson JA, Shaywitz BA: Clonidine in Tourette's syndrome. Lancet 1979;2:551–553.
11. Gil-Ad I, Topper E, Laron Z: Oral clonidine as a growth hormone stimulation test. Lancet 1979;2:278–280.
12. Chappell PB, Riddle MA, Scahill L, et al: Guanfacine treatment of comorbid attention-deficit hyperactivity disorder and Tourette's syndrome: preliminary clinical experience. J Am Acad Child Adolesc Psychol 1995;34:1140–1146.
13. Balldin J, Berggren U, Eriksson E, et al: Guanfacine as an alpha-2-agonist inducer of growth hormone secretion—a comparison with clonidine. Psychoneuroendocrinology 1993;18:45–55.
14. Klein-Schwartz W: Trends and toxic effects from pediatric clonidine exposures. Arch Pediatr Adolesc 2002;156:392–396.
15. Stein B, Volans GN: Dixarit overdose: the problem of attractive tablets. BMJ 1978;2:667–668.
16. Wiley JF II, Wiley CC, Torrey SB, Henretig FM: Clonidine poisoning in young children. J Pediatr 1980;116:654–658.

17. Watson WA, Litovitz TL, Klein-Schwartz W, et al: 2003 annual report of the American Association of Poison Control Centers Toxic Exposure Surveillance System. Am J Emerg Med 2004;22:335–404.

18. Nichols MH, King WD, James LP: Clonidine poisoning in Jefferson County, Alabama. Ann Emerg Med 1997;29:511–517.

19. Lewis S, Giffen SL: Pediatric imidazoline exposures: incidence of serious effects. Vet Hum Toxicol 1992;34:333.

20. Hall AH, Smolinske SC, Kulig KW, Rumack BH: Guanabenz overdose. Ann Intern Med 1985;102:787–788.

21. Rogers SJ: Guanabenz overdose. Ann Intern Med 1986;104:445.

22. Shnaps Y, Almog S, Halkin H, et al: Methyldopa poisoning. J Toxicol Clin Toxicol 1982;19:501–503.

23. Langer SZ, Cavero I, Massingham R: Recent developments in nor-adrenergic neurotransmission and its relevance to the mechanism of action of certain antihypertensive agents. Hypertension 1980;2:372–382.

24. Bobik A, Jennings G, Jackman G, Oddie C, Korner P: Evidence for a predominantly central hypotensive effect of alpha-methyldopa in humans. Hypertension 1986;8:16–23.

25. Oates JA, Brown NJ: Antihypertensive agents and the drug therapy of hypertension. In Hardman JG, Limbird LE, Gilman AG (eds): Goodman & Gilman's the Pharmacological Basis of Therapeutics, 10th ed. New York, McGraw-Hill, 2001, pp 879–882.

26. Maze M, Scarfini C, Cavaliere F: New agents for sedation in the intensive care unit. Crit Care Clin 2001;17:881–897.

27. Reid JL: Alpha-adrenergic receptors and blood pressure control. Am J Cardiol 1986;57:6E–12E.

28. Van Zwieten PA: Overview of alpha2-adrenoceptor agonists with a central action. Am J Cardiol 1986;57:3E–5E.

29. Hoffman BB, Lefkowitz RJ: Alpha-adrenergic receptor subtypes. N Engl J Med 1980;302:1390–1396.

30. Niemi L: Effects of intrathecal clonidine on duration of bupivacaine spinal anaesthesia, haemodynamics, and postop-erative analgesia in patients undergoing knee arthroscopy. Acta Anaesth Scand 1994;38:724–728.

31. Gabilondo AM, Meana JJ, Barturen F, et al: Mu-opioid receptor and alpha 2-adrenoceptor agonist binding sites in the postmortem brain of heroin addicts. Psychopharmacology 1994;115:135–140.

32. Graeser D, Neubig RR: Compartmentation of receptors and guanine nucleotide-binding proteins in NG108-15 cells: lack of cross-talk in agonist binding among the alpha 2-adrenergic, mus-carinic, and opiate receptors. Mol Pharmacol 1993;43:434–443.

33. Ernsberger PR, Westbrooks KL, Christen MO, Schafer SG, et al: A second generation of centrally acting antihypertensive agents act on putative I1-imidazoline receptors. J Cardiovasc Pharmacol 1992;20(4):S1–S10.

34. Bricca G, Greney H, Zhang J, et al: Human brain imidazoline receptors: further characterization with [3H]clonidine. Eur J Pharmacol 1994;266:25–33.

35. Bousquet P, Feldman J, Tibirica E, et al: Imidazoline receptors: a new concept in central regulation of the arterial blood pressure. Am J Hypertens 1992;5(4):47S–50S.

36. Hudson A: Imidazoline receptors. Tocris Cookson Monograph January 1996.

37. Hunyor SN, Bradstock K, Somerville PJ, Lucas N: Clonidine overdose [letter]. BMJ 1975;4:23.

38. Higgins GL, Campbell B, Wallace K, Talbot S: Pediatric poisoning from over-the-counter imidazoline-containing products. Ann Emerg Med 1991;20:655–658.

39. Bamshad MJ, Wasserman GS: Pediatric clonidine intoxications. Vet Hum Toxicol 1990;32:220–223.

40. Dollery CT, Davies DS, Draffan GH, et al: Clinical pharmacology and pharmacokinetics of clonidine. Clin Pharmacol Ther 1976;19:11–17.

41. Frisk-Holmberg M, Paalzow L, Edlund PO: Clonidine kinetics in man-evidence for dose dependency and changed pharmacokinetics during chronic therapy. Br J Clin Pharmacol 1981;12:653–658.

42. Pettinger WA: Pharmacology of clonidine. J Cardiovasc Pharmacol 1980;1(Suppl):S21–S28.

43. Cunningham FE, Baughman VL, Peters J, Laurito CE: Comparative pharmacokinetics of oral versus sublingual clonidine. J Clin Anesth 1994;6:430–433.

44. Lonnqvist PA, Bergendahl HT, Eksborg S: Pharmacokinetics of clonidine after rectal administration in children. Anesthesiology 1994;81:1097–1101.

45. Ebihara A, Fujimura A, Ohashi K, et al: Influence of application site of a new transdermal clonidine, M-5041T, on its pharmaco-kinetics and pharmacodynamics in healthy subjects. J Clin Pharmacol 1993;33:1188–1191.

46. MacGregor TR, Matzed KM, Keirns JJ, et al: Pharmacokinetics of transdermally delivered clonidine. Clin Pharmacol Ther 1985;38:278–284.

47. Nissen D (ed): 2004 Mosby's Drug Consult. St. Louis: Mosby, 2004. Available at: http://www.mdconsult.com.

48. Fenichel RR: Post-marketing surveillance identifies three cases of sudden death in children during treatment with clonidine and methylphenidate. J Child Adolesc Psychopharmacol 1995;5:157–166.

49. Popper CW: Combining methylphenidate and clonidine: news reports about sudden death. J Child Adolesc Psychopharmacol 1995;5:155–156.

50. Mack RB: "Pack up the moon and dismantle the sun"—imidazoline overdose. Contemp Pediatr 1996;13:67–79.

51. Lusthof KJ, Lameijer W, Zweipfenning PG: Use of clonidine for chemical submission. J Toxicol Clin Toxicol 2000;38:329–332.

52. Williams PL, Krafcik JM, Potter BB, et al: Cardiac toxicity of clonidine. Chest 1977;72:784–785.

53. Yagupsky P, Gorodischer R: Massive clonidine ingestion with hypertension in a 9-month-old infant. Pediatrics 1983;72:500–502.

54. Adamson LA, Spiller HA, Bosse GM: Tizanidine (Zanaflex®) exposure [abstract]. J Toxicol Clin Toxicol 2003;41:664.

55. Luciani A, Brugioni L, Serra L, et al: Sino-atrial and atrio-ventricular node dysfunction in a case of tizanidine overdose. Vet Hum Toxicol 1995;37:556–557.

56. Ram CVS, Engelman K: Abrupt discontinuation of clonidine therapy. JAMA 1979;242:2104–2105.

57. Planz G, Beckenbauer U, Bundschu HD: Response of plasma catecholamines and blood pressure to clonidine and to sudden withdrawal of the drug in subjects with essential hypertension. Int J Clin Pharmacol Ther Toxicol 1982;29:474–478.

58. Campbell BC, Reid JL: Regimen for the control of blood pressure and symptoms during clonidine withdrawal. Int J Clin Pharmacol Res 1985;5:215–222.

59. Zamboulis C, Reid JL: Withdrawal of guanfacine after long-term treatment in essential hypertension: observations on blood pressure and plasma and urinary noradrenaline. Eur J Clin Pharmacol 1981;19:19–24.

60. Banner W, Lund ME, Clawson L: Failure of naloxone to reverse clonidine toxic effect. Am J Dis Child 1983;137:1170–1171.

61. Reed MT, Hamburg EL: Person-to-person transfer of transdermal drug delivery systems: a case report [letter]. N Engl J Med 1986;314:1120.

62. Knapp JF, Fowler MA, Wheeler CA, Wasserman GS: Case 01-1995: a two-year-old female with alteration of consciousness. Pediatr Emerg Care 1995;11:62–65.

63. Henretig FM, Wiley JF II, Brown L: Clonidine patch toxicity: the proof's in the poop! [abstract]. J Toxicol Clin Toxicol 1995;33:520.

64. Shannon M, Neuman MI: Yohimbine. Pediatr Emerg Care 2000;16:49–50.

65. Olsson JM, Pruitt AW: Management of clonidine ingestion in children. J Pediatr 1983;103:646–650.

66. Tessa C, Mascalchi M, Matteucci L, Gavazzi C, Domenici R: Permanent brain damage following acute clonidine poisoning in Munchausen by proxy. Neuropediatrics 2001;32:90–92.

63

Class IA Antiarrhythmics: Quinidine, Procainamide, and Disopyramide

KRISTINE A. NAÑAGAS, MD ■ R. BRENT FURBEE, MD

At a Glance...

- Life-threatening effects of IA antiarrhythmic overdose are cardiac.
- Sodium channel blockade leads to QRS widening and ventricular tachycardia, which is often responsive to sodium bicarbonate.
- Potassium efflux blockade causes widened QT_c and torsades de pointes and may respond to magnesium sulfate and correction of hypokalemia.
- Torsades de pointes usually develops in patients with bradycardia.
- Anticholinergic and hypoglycemic effects are seen with disopyramide > procainamide > quinidine.
- Extracorporeal drug removal may be of some use for procainamide and N-acetylprocainamide but is of minimal benefit for other IA antiarrhythmics.
- Peak plasma levels for therapeutic doses occur at 1 to 3 hours but may be delayed in overdose.
- Symptomatic patients should be admitted for cardiac monitoring.

The class IA antiarrhythmics include quinidine, procainamide, and disopyramide. Although dissimilar in structure (Fig. 63-1), all three drugs suppress cardiac dysrhythmias via the same mechanisms and produce adverse effects typical of the group. In the past, these drugs were widely used for the control of both atrial and ventricular arrhythmias, but because of the high incidence of adverse effects with therapeutic use and overdose, newer, safer agents have largely replaced them.

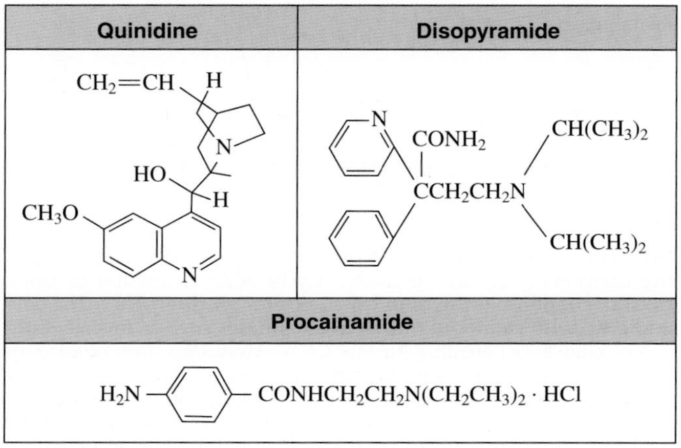

FIGURE 63-1 Although dissimilar in structure, all class IA antiarrhythmic agents share therapeutic and toxic effects.

HISTORY

Quinidine and its optical isomer quinine are extracted from the South American cinchona tree. Centuries ago, it was noted that patients with both malaria and atrial fibrillation, when treated with cinchona for malaria, were sometimes also cured of their arrhythmia. Jean-Baptiste de Senac, of Paris, recorded using cinchona in the treatment of atrial fibrillation in 1749. In 1936, Mautz demonstrated procaine to be effective in decreasing ventricular irritability, but this compound was rapidly metabolized and was too neurotoxic to be of clinical value. Procainamide, a congener of procaine, was introduced in 1955. Disopyramide was introduced in 1978.[1]

PHARMACOKINETICS

Quinidine is well absorbed after ingestion, with a bioavailability of between 70% and 80%. Quinidine sulfate levels peak at 1.5 hours. The gluconate, sulfate, and polygalacturonate salts are sustained-release preparations, and blood levels of these may not peak until 4 hours after ingestion. Peak levels may be significantly prolonged in overdose.[2,3] Quinidine is 75% to 95% protein bound and is metabolized by the liver via hydroxylation, with a half-life of approximately 6 hours.[4] Quinidine has two metabolites with antiarrhythmic properties: 2'-quinidinone and 3-hydroxyquinidine. Its apparent volume of distribution is 3 L/kg. Approximately 20% of quinidine is excreted unchanged in the urine.[2]

Oral procainamide is absorbed well from the small intestine; levels peak 1 to 2 hours after ingestion. After intravenous administration, the drug distributes to the tissue within 30 minutes. Procainamide diffuses well into tissue and has a volume of distribution of 2 L/kg. Protein binding is approximately 15% to 20%.[5] Procainamide is hydrolyzed by the liver into several active metabolites, the most significant being 1,4,2,-N-acetylprocainamide (NAPA).[6] Procainamide has a half-life of 3 hours, and NAPA of 6 hours. Fifty percent of procainamide is excreted in the urine unchanged.[7]

Disopyramide is well absorbed orally, with peak levels occurring 2 to 3 hours after ingestion.[8] Protein binding is 30%, and the volume of distribution is 0.8 L/kg. Disopyramide is partially metabolized by the liver, with 55% being excreted unchanged in the urine. The half-life of disopyramide is approximately 8 hours.[9]

PATHOPHYSIOLOGY

A summary of reported adverse effects of these agents is found in Table 63-1.

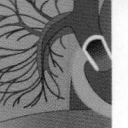

TABLE 63-1 Noncardiac Effects of Class IA Antiarrhythmics

SYSTEM	EFFECTS
Central nervous	Giddiness, depression, hallucinations* Blurred vision, sedation[†]
Pulmonary	Pleural fibrosis*, pneumonitis[‡]
Gastrointestinal	Nausea, vomiting, diarrhea Hepatitis*[,‡]
Genitourinary	Urinary retention
Muscloskeletal	Myopathy with muscle weakness*
Skin	Rashes Lichen planus[‡]
Hematologic	IgG-mediated agranulocytosis,*[,‡] thrombocytopenia*[,‡] IgM-mediated hemolysis (most often in patients with G6PD)[‡]
Rheumatologic	SLE*[,‡]
Other	Hypoglycemia[†]

*Primarily procainamide
[†]Primarily disopyramide
[‡]Primarily quinidine

Anticholinergic Effects

Many symptoms associated with class IA antiarrhythmics are related to the anticholinergic activity of these compounds. Disopyramide is the most anticholinergic, followed by procainamide and then quinidine. Confusion, hallucinations, tachycardia, decreased gastrointestinal motility, urinary retention, and dry mucous membranes all may occur with their use.[3] Because some patients may suffer from cinchonism, the clinical presentation may be a confusing combination of the two syndromes.

Immune System Effects

Hypersensitivity reactions most commonly occur with quinidine but may also occur with procainamide and disopyramide. Hypersensitivity may be manifested as fever, rash, thrombocytopenia, neutropenia, agranulocytosis, hepatitis, hemolytic anemia, or lymphadenopathy.[3,10-12] These reactions frequently are unrelated to dose.

Procainamide is the most common cause of drug-induced lupus. Antinuclear antibodies occur in 50% to 75% of patients treated with procainamide, and 20% to 30% of those patients develop components of drug-induced lupus.[7] Patients suffer from arthralgias, myalgias, malar rash, fever, pleuritis, pleural effusion, and pericarditis. Renal involvement is rare.[13] The mechanism responsible for the development of drug-induced lupus remains under investigation. Metabolic products of procainamide have been found to inhibit the covalent binding of C4 to C2 in the complement cascade, which is thought to decrease the clearance of immune complexes.[14,15]

Thrombocytopenia has been reported to occur with therapeutic use of quinidine and procainamide.[16,17] Drug-induced thrombocytopenia is an immune-mediated reaction. The sensitizing drug induces antiplatelet antibodies, which cause the rapid destruction of platelets.

Recovery is usually complete within 5 days of removal of the drug.[17]

Metabolic Effects

Symptomatic hypoglycemia has been reported to occur after therapeutic doses of disopyramide. Goldberg and colleagues demonstrated hypoglycemia with administration of disopyramide. Hypoglycemia could be reproduced on readministration of the drug.[18] Quinidine and disopyramide, like the sulfonylureas, have the ability to block potassium efflux from pancreatic β-cells, thus leading to increased insulin secretion resulting in hyperinsulinemia (Fig. 63-2).[19] Hyperinsulinemia is well documented with use of quinine, a stereoisomer of quinidine, and with disopyramide, but its occurrence in the presence of other class IA antiarrhythmics has not been clearly documented.[18,20,21]

Cardiac Effects

The class IA antiarrhythmics, although structurally dissimilar, produce similar effects on the heart. These agents cause numerous cardiac arrhythmias, including heart block, atrial tachycardia, premature ventricular contractions, torsades de pointes, ventricular tachycardia, and ventricular fibrillation.[3,10,22] The drug actions responsible for these arrhythmias are sodium channel blockade, potassium efflux blockade, and inhibition of the sodium/potassium–adenosine triphosphatase (Na^+/K^+-ATPase) pump. Other drug effects may play a role in the development of arrhythmia, but these are not as well described. Dysrhythmias can occur at therapeutic as well as toxic serum concentrations of these drugs. The cardiac effects of quinidine are the most studied, but all

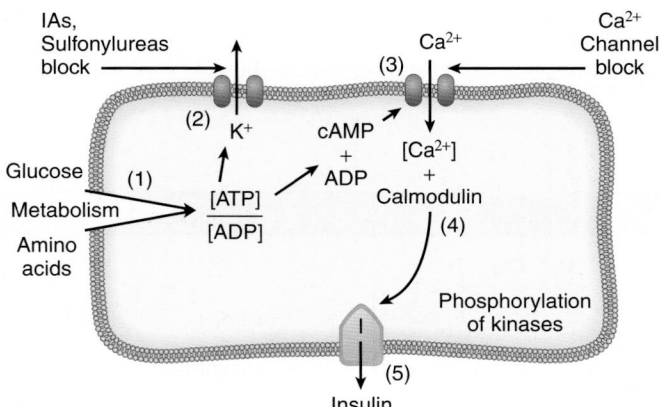

FIGURE 63-2 The presence of glucose or amino acids triggers the conversion of ATP to cAMP.[1] Cyclic AMP is needed to open calcium channels in the beta cell. Calcium ions then enter the cell[3] and bind with calmodulin to activate kinases such as myosin–light chain kinase or protein kinase C[4] to stimulate the release of insulin.[5] The initial depolarization of the beta cell triggers potassium efflux.[2] The IA antiarrhythmics are thought to block the potassium efflux out of beta cells in the pancreas. This would prolong "depolarization" of the cell and increase secretion of insulin. (Adapted from Gerich JE: Oral hypoglycemic agents. New Engl J Med 1989;321:1231–1245.)

agents in this class act in a similar manner. Procainamide has less cardiotoxicity than quinidine and disopyramide at therapeutic doses.[3]

Effects on Ion Channels

In a normal Purkinje cell, the rapid influx of sodium ions in phase 0 causes the interior of the cell to become more positive (Fig. 63-3 and 63-4). Phase 1 is associated with slow leakage of potassium out of the cell, causing a decrease in positive charge within the cell, which brings the cell slightly closer to its resting potential. During phase 2, voltage-dependent calcium channels open, allowing calcium ions to enter. This calcium influx, which sustains the positive charge within the cell, is reflected as the plateau of phase 2. The slow leak of potassium from the cell during phase 2 balances the inward flow of calcium, and the net result is little change in the membrane potential. In phase 3, however, further leakage of potassium out of the cell (potassium efflux) repolarizes the cell. In phase 4, the charge within the cell has returned to its resting potential and sodium begins to enter into the cell. This moves the cell membrane potential toward threshold again, and the next action potential can occur. Late phase 4 and phase 0 represent *depolarization* of the cardiac cell, whereas phases 1, 2, and 3 represent *repolarization*. Phases 0 to 3 correspond to systole, and phase 4 corresponds to diastole. Similar processes occur in other cardiac cells; however, each type of cardiac tissue has different concentrations of each kind of ion channel and thus has slightly varied patterns of depolarization and repolarization.

Sodium Channel Blockade

The IA antiarrhythmic agents can produce widening of the QRS, ventricular tachycardia, and decreased inotropy by blocking fast sodium channels in cardiac cells. Electrical conductance is dependent on the rapid influx of sodium through fast sodium channels. In terms of the action potential, this slows the rate of rise of phase 0 (V_{max}). Because phase 0 of the action potential corresponds to the QRS complex on the electrocardiogram (ECG), any toxin that slows the influx of sodium ions through the fast channels produces a widened QRS complex (Figs. 63-4 and 63-5). The class IA antiarrhythmics' ability to block Na^+ channels is dose dependent and is clinically significant only with high drug levels.[22,23] At toxic serum concentrations, QRS widening, bundle branch block, and sinoatrial or atrioventricular block may be present.

The sodium channel blockade caused by class IA antiarrhythmics increases as the heart rate increases. Normally, as the heart rate increases, both action potential duration and effective refractory period shorten.[24] Studies using these agents have shown that the

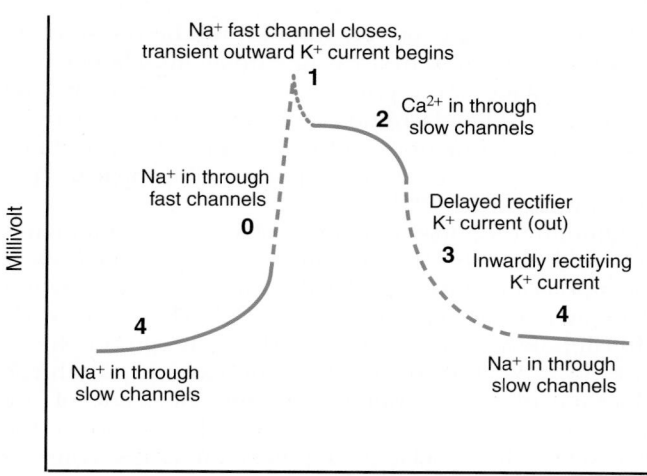

FIGURE 63-3 Ion flow during Purkinje cell action potential.

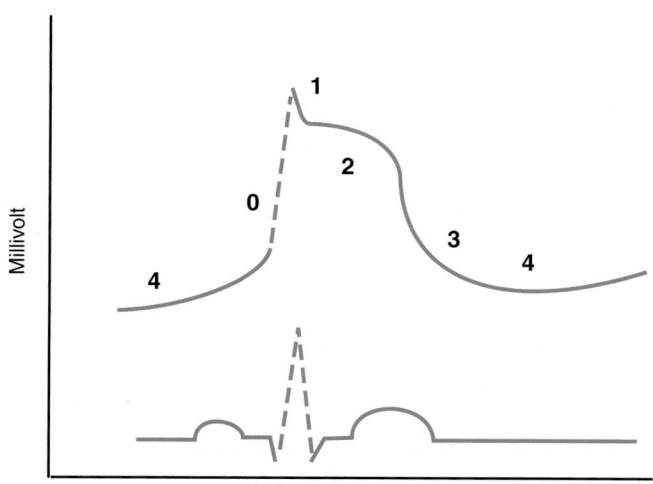

FIGURE 63-4 Normal Purkinje cell action potential and corresponding electrocardiographic pattern.

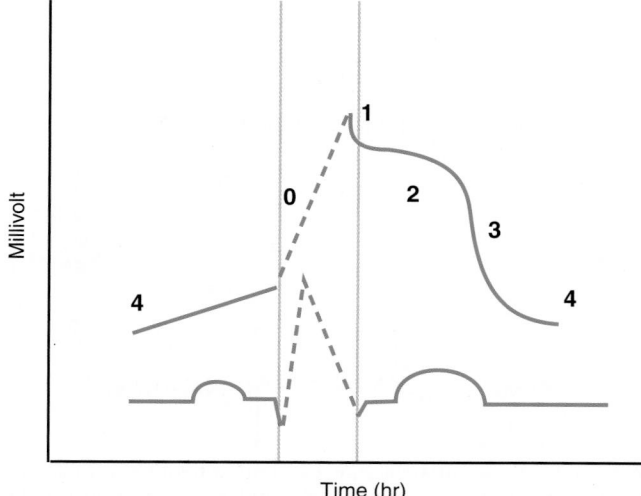

FIGURE 63-5 When sodium channels are blocked, the rate of rise of phase 0 (V_{max}) is decreased. This corresponds to a widening of the QRS complex.

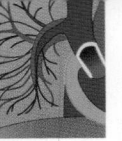

action potential duration and effective refractory period have a greater relative increase at higher heart rates.[24-27] Thus, they exhibit time-dependent suppression of excitability, and this effect is more pronounced at higher heart rates. This effect may be explained by the tendency of these drugs to bind to sodium channels in their open state. When heart rates are higher, there are more open sodium channels, and therefore more channels susceptible to blockade.[28] It may then be theorized that patients experiencing ventricular tachycardia secondary to procainamide and quinidine (and possibly disopyramide) toxicity may not respond favorably to overdrive pacing.[24]

Potassium Channel Blockade

Repolarization in the heart is largely due to efflux of potassium out of the cells. When potassium channels are blocked, as with the class IA antiarrhythmics, repolarization is prolonged. Prolongation of repolarization is reflected by prolonged QT on the ECG. Blockade of the delayed rectifier current, I_{Kr}, is most often associated with drug-induced prolonged QT[29-31] (Fig. 63-6). With potassium efflux blockade, prolonged QT, premature ventricular contractions, and torsades de pointes can be seen. Development of torsades de pointes is most likely dependent on both repolarization abnormalities and triggered activity. When repolarization is disorganized, the possibility of reentrant circuits is increased, and reentrant circuits are responsible for torsades de pointes.[28-30,32-37]

Afterdepolarization means electric oscillations of the conductive cell membrane that occur late in phase 2, throughout phase 3, or early in phase 4 of the action potential. This activity appears to occur primarily in Purkinje cells or deep subendocardial regions of the ventricular wall.[38] Afterdepolarization that occurs in phase 2 or 3 is known as *early afterdepolarization*. Early afterdepolarizations might be caused by calcium (L-type) current or sodium currents[29,33,39] or might be due to

adrenergic effects.[40-42] Afterdepolarization occurring in early phase 4 is termed *delayed afterdepolarization*.[39] Early afterdepolarization–triggered activity tends to result in torsades de pointes. Delayed afterdepolarization activity tends to be more closely associated with premature ventricular contractions.[26,43] The IA antiarrhythmics are capable of producing both.

Not all afterdepolarizations lead to dysrhythmias. Because they occur during the relative refractory period of cellular repolarization, some of these membrane oscillations do not cause the cell to fire again. If the cell has sufficiently repolarized, some afterdepolarizations are capable of reaching threshold and causing abnormal firing and dysrhythmias. Action potentials produced by afterdepolarizations that reach threshold are called *triggered activity* (Fig. 63-7). Triggered activity is partly responsible for the tachyarrhythmias that occur at therapeutic levels of the IA antiarrhythmics.[28,29,36,43]

The development of torsades de pointes also revolves around heterogeneity of repolarization in the ventricles. If the triggered activity reaches area of muscle that is sufficiently repolarized, the impulse will be transmitted. As a result of different areas of cardiac muscle being in differing stages of repolarization, some areas will be refractory to depolarization from the triggered activity. The area of functional block creates the possibility for reentry, and reentrant circuits will propagate the arrhythmia.[28,29,32,37,39,44,45]

Quinidine's potassium efflux blockade predominates at lower heart rates.[46,47] This phenomenon is called *reverse use dependence*, meaning the duration of repolarization is greater at slower heart rates.[28,48,49] Therefore, early afterdepolarization is more likely at slower heart rates.[33,49] As the heart rate increases, quinidine's blockade of Na⁺ channels is greater. Blockade of the movement of these positive ions into the interior of the cell keeps the blockade of potassium efflux counterbalanced.[27] The inside of the cell remains relatively more negative, making early afterdepolarization activity less likely and decreasing the risk of development of torsades de pointes.[46]

Some patients may be at greater risk of developing torsades de pointes than others owing to a genetic

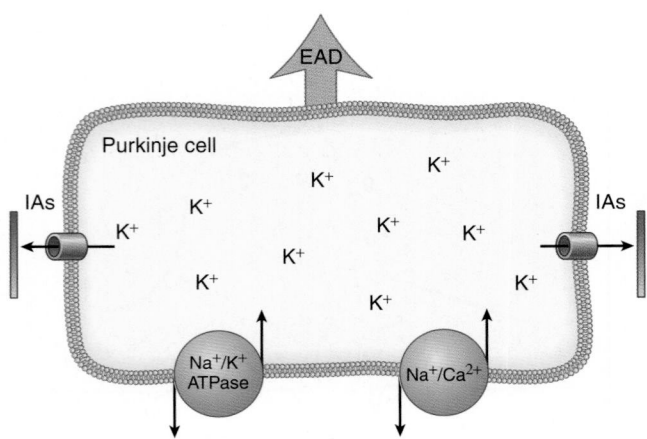

FIGURE 63-6 IA antiarrhythmics and other toxins may block the efflux of K+ from the cardiac cell, driving the charge on the interior of the cell membrane in a less negative direction, toward threshold. This change in charge leads to early afterdepolarization (EAD) formation.

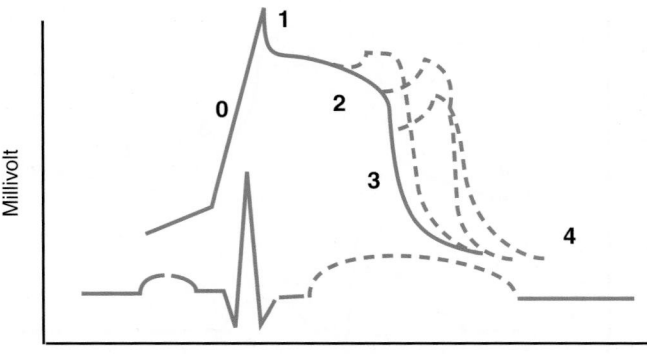

FIGURE 63-7 Blockade of potassium efflux out of the cells leads to membrane oscillations or afterdepolarizations. If they attain threshold voltage, "triggered activity" will occur.

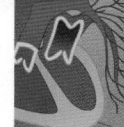

predisposition of arrhythmia. Inherited defects of ion channels resulting in prolonged QT have variable penetrance, and not every carrier will manifest changes on a baseline ECG; however, this patient population may be at increased risk when exposed to agents that block potassium channels. This concept is termed *repolarization reserve*.[30,50,51,52]

Na⁺/K⁺-ATPase Blockade

The premature ventricular contractions observed in overdose may be caused by inhibition of the Na^+/K^+-ATPase pump in cardiac cells. The Na^+/K^+-ATPase pump functions to repolarize the cell after contraction by transporting intracellular Na^+ ions out of the cell in exchange for K^+ ions transported into the cell. Class IA agents, in a fashion similar to digoxin, inhibit the Na^+/K^+-ATPase pump, resulting in intracellular Na^+ accumulation.[53] The intracellular Na^+ is exchanged for extracellular Ca^{2+} by the Na^+/Ca^{2+} pump, causing an increase in intracellular Ca^{2+} (Fig. 63-8). Normally, the sarcoplasmic reticulum takes up cytoplasmic Ca^{2+} and stores it; however, excessive intracellular Ca^{2+} is thought to overload the sequestration mechanism of the sarcoplasmic reticulum. The increased intracellular Ca^{2+} then activates the Na^+/Ca^{2+} pump, which stimulates the exchange of intracellular Ca^{2+} for extracellular Na^+. This creates an inward current of Na^+ ions and results in delayed afterdepolarizations[33,39,43] (Fig. 63-9). These delayed afterdepolarizations can result in triggered activity, usually manifested by premature ventricular contractions. Afterdepolarizations reach threshold more frequently as the heart rate accelerates.

Dzimiri and Almotrefi demonstrated increasing inhibition of the Na^+/K^+-ATPase pump with decreasing serum potassium levels,[53] which may explain the exacerbation of arrhythmias caused by class IA antiarrhythmics by hypokalemia. Low serum potassium levels further inhibit the Na^+/K^+-ATPase pump, worsening intracellular Ca^{2+} overload and resulting in an increased frequency of delayed afterdepolarization with resultant arrhythmia

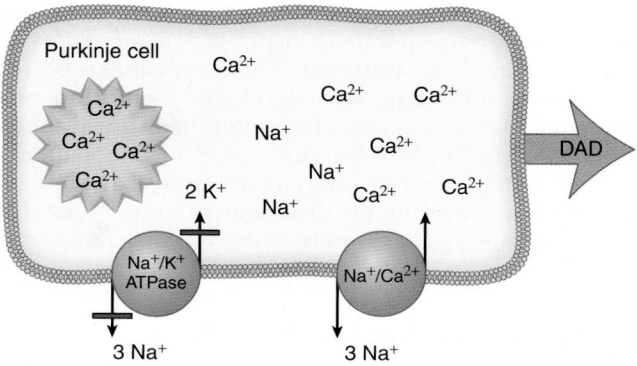

FIGURE   63-9 Delayed afterdepolarizations resulting in premature ventricular contraction (PVC).

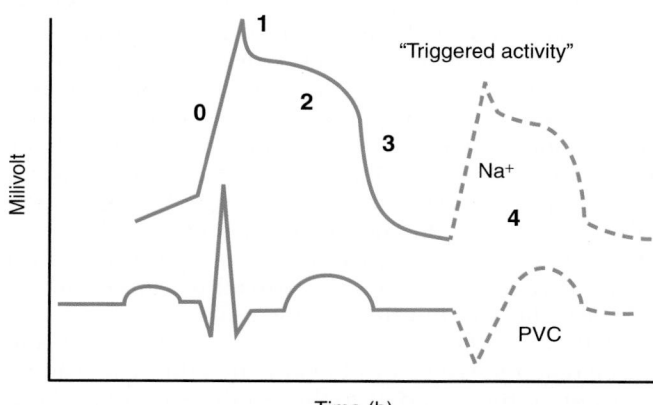

FIGURE 63-10   If the inhibition of the Na^+/K^+-ATPase pump leads to Ca^{2+} overload of the cell, the sarcoplasmic reticulum is unable to compensate by sequestration and the internal charge begins to increase, leading to delayed afterdepolarization (DAD) formation.

(Fig. 63-10). Conditions associated with exacerbation of this process include digitalis toxicity, hypernatremia, hypokalemia, and catecholamine excess.[53]

TOXICOLOGY

Significant ingestion of these drugs produces primarily neurologic and cardiovascular consequences.[10,54] Ingestion of more than 1 g of quinidine by an adult has been reported to produce symptoms. As little as 7 g of procainamide or 1.5 g of disopyramide is potentially toxic. In assessing the severity of a toxic ingestion, it is important to remember that the reported history of the amount of a drug ingested is very unreliable and individual responses to these drugs vary greatly. Underlying cardiac disease may make some patients symptomatic at lower than expected doses.

Central Nervous System Toxicity

Toxicity from class IA antiarrhythmics may cause mydriasis and blurred vision. A patient's mental status

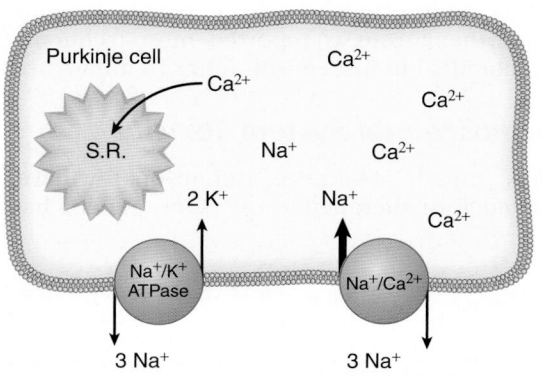

FIGURE 63-8   Inhibition of the Na^+/K^+-ATPase pump leads to an increase in intracellular Na^+. This, in turn, leads to an exchange of Na^+ for Ca^{2+} via the Na^+/Ca^{2+} pump. The excess intracellular Ca^{2+} is sequestered in the sarcoplasmic reticulum (SR).

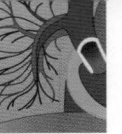

may range from lethargy and confusion to coma. Convulsions independent of hypotension secondary to quinidine have been reported.[54] Summers et al reported on a 69-year-old man who developed confusion and hallucinations while receiving quinidine during hospitalization for myocardial infarction.[55] The patient's mental status cleared after the administration of physostigmine, leading the investigators to conclude that mental status changes were due to anticholinergic toxicity.

Cardiovascular System Toxicity

The cardiotoxic effects of this class of drugs are the most threatening. Although tachycardia may be present early in serious poisoning, bradycardia secondary to conduction delays and blocks is most common. Other arrhythmias reported in overdose include atrial tachyarrhythmias, ventricular tachycardia, and fibrillation.[54] Risk factors for developing torsades de pointes include female sex, hypokalemia, bradycardia, long QT syndrome, and hypomagnesemia.[30,33,37] Hypotension and shock associated with class IA antiarrhythmics are primarily related to depressive actions on the heart rather than to direct effects on the peripheral vasculature.[56,57] Disopyramide exhibits the greatest negative inotropic effect of the three and has been reported to cause congestive heart failure with therapeutic use.[3,58]

Quinidine syncope, which occurs at therapeutic and subtherapeutic levels, was initially thought to be caused by hypotension secondary to the vasodilatory effect of this drug. Ventricular tachyarrhythmias were ultimately determined to be responsible. Fifty percent of patients who develop torsades de pointes do so within the first 5 days of therapy; the remainder of the cases occurs weeks to years later, often after a dosage change.[59] Disopyramide and procainamide, although less frequently than quinidine, have also been reported to cause fatal arrhythmias in the therapeutic range.[60-63] The arrhythmias usually are nonsustained but occasionally have been fatal. Sudden death while on quinidine therapy has been estimated at 0.5%.[10] Both polymorphic ventricular tachycardia and torsades de pointes have been reported. Both rhythms can produce a rotating axis on an electrocardiogram but respond differently to various therapeutic interventions.[64] Torsades de pointes may be distinguished from polymorphic ventricular tachycardia by the following criteria: The initial complex follows a pause or sudden rate deceleration, which produces a long preceding RR interval. The initiating complex also has an accentuated U wave and occurs in the setting of a prolonged QT (Fig. 63-11).[27,29,32,33,37,39,42-44,65,66]

There have been efforts to determine who is at risk for arrhythmia based on ECG interpretation. A QT interval greater than 500 ms[37,39] or prolongation of the QT interval by greater than 50%[54] indicates greater risk for developing torsades de pointes. Not only does a long QT appear to have some prognostic value, but also QT dispersion may have some utility in stratifying high-risk patients who have quinidine-induced repolarization abnormalities. Several methods exist to measure QT dispersion, but in general it is calculated by measuring all QT segments, finding the shortest QT interval, and subtracting it from the longest QT segment. A value greater than 100 appears to predict arrhythmia.[37,39,63,65]

Gastrointestinal System Toxicity

Dry mouth is a frequent complaint of patients exposed to class IA antiarrhythmics. Nausea, vomiting, and diarrhea also are common, although decreased bowel sounds, constipation, and ileus may occur secondary to the anticholinergic effects of these drugs.

Cinchonism

First described in association with quinine, the complex of symptoms called cinchonism may occur in chronic overuse or acute overdose of quinidine, although it is more common with quinine. This syndrome is characterized by abdominal pain, diarrhea, nausea, vomiting, hearing loss, tinnitus, visual disturbances, encephalopathy, coma, and seizures.[10] Symptoms typically resolve after removal of the causative agent.

Genitourinary System Toxicity

Urinary retention and anuria have been reported. They are thought to be associated with the anticholinergic effects of these drugs.

Immune System Toxicity

Thrombocytopenic purpura, angioedema, exfoliative dermatitis, livedo reticularis, and photodermatitis have all been reported. Urticaria, flushing, pruritus, bullous reactions, lichen planus, psoriasis, erythroderma, and erythema multiforme have been seen.[67] Drug-induced lupus erythematosus is reported most frequently with procainamide, but is seen with other IA antiarrhythmics.

Musculoskeletal System Toxicity

Myositis, muscle weakness, and myopathy have been associated with therapeutic use. One patient has been

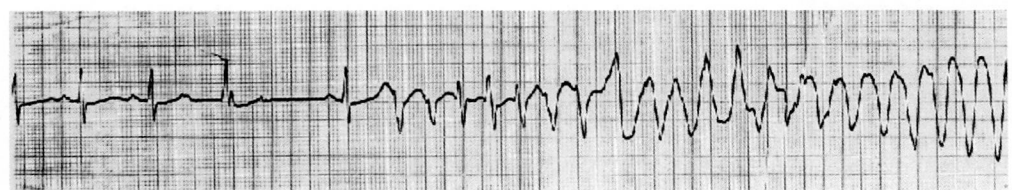

FIGURE 63-11 Rhythm strip of a patient with torsades de pointes suffering from chronic procainamide toxicity. Procainamide level was 27.5 µg/mL, and NAPA level was 62.4 µg/mL.

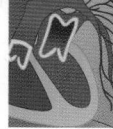

described with diaphragmatic paralysis while taking 750 mg of procainamide twice daily.[68]

Pregnancy

The class IA antiarrhythmic agents clearly cross the placenta. No evidence shows that they are teratogenic. Disopyramide has been associated with premature uterine contractions, which resolved on discontinuance of the drug.[69]

DRUG INTERACTIONS

A particular form of cytochrome P-450 inhibition has been described with quinidine use. Debrisoquin, an antihypertensive agent used in Europe, is metabolized by the cytochrome P-450 isozyme CYP2D6 (debrisoquin hydroxylase). A number of other drugs are metabolized by the same isozyme. Ten percent of the Western population is genetically deficient in this enzyme and metabolizes debrisoquin slowly. Quinidine, although not metabolized by this isozyme, binds to CYP2D6, interfering with its function. Commonly prescribed medications metabolized by this pathway, when taken with quinidine, are metabolized more slowly, causing higher than expected serum concentrations.[70] Drugs metabolized by CYP2D6 and potentially affected by quinidine are listed in Box 63-1.

Quinidine and Digitalis

Quinidine is thought to decrease the volume of distribution of some cardiac glycosides. This seems particularly true in the presence of digoxin. When these drugs are given concomitantly, the usual digoxin dose should be reduced by 50%.[71]

LABORATORY STUDIES

Serum quinidine levels of 1 to 4 µg/mL are considered therapeutic. Toxic symptoms are expected at levels greater than 5 µg/mL. Combined serum levels of both procainamide and its active metabolite, NAPA, must be measured for evaluation of procainamide toxicity. A combined level greater than 30 µg/mL is potentially cardiotoxic. Combined levels greater than 60 µg/mL are likely to cause lethargy and hypotension. Disopyramide levels greater than 5 µg/mL are considered toxic.

TREATMENT

General Management

Treatment of an overdose of a class IA antiarrhythmic should include early and aggressive management of the airway. The possibility of rapid decline in mental status and the onset of cardiac arrhythmias place these patients at very high risk of aspiration and pulmonary compromise. Once the airway is controlled, gastrointestinal

---

BOX 63-1	**DRUG METABOLIZED BY CYP2D6**

β-Blockers
Timolol
Propranolol
Metoprolol
Propafenone

Tricyclic Antidepressants
Nortriptyline
Amitriptyline
Desipramine
Imipramine
Clomipramine

Neuroleptics
Thioridazine
Fluphenazine
Perphenazine
Trifluperidol

MAO Inhibitors
Amiflamine
Methoxyphenamine

Antiarrhythmics
Flecainide
Encainide

Other
Codeine
Dextromethorphan
Phenformin
Methamphetamine

---

decontamination with oral activated charcoal may be considered. Repeat doses of charcoal are of minimal clinical benefit and may be harmful to patients with decreased gastrointestinal motility. Admission to an intensive care setting for cardiac monitoring is appropriate for all symptomatic patients.

Seizures secondary to use of class IA antiarrhythmics respond readily to administration of benzodiazepines. Loading with other anticonvulsants is not indicated unless the seizures are recurrent or prolonged. Phenobarbital, 15 mg/kg intravenously, should be used for persistent seizure activity. Higher doses may occasionally be required and can be associated with respiratory depression. Monitoring of creatine phosphokinase levels for evidence of rhabdomyolysis should be carried out for any patient "found down" (obtunded) for an unknown period.

Cardiac Toxicity

Class IA antiarrhythmics' strong cardiac sodium channel blocker activity is responsible for the intraventricular conduction delays in overdose.[55] *Wide complex rhythms may respond to intravenous administration of a sodium bicarbonate bolus.*[72,73] The exact mechanism of action of

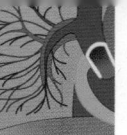

sodium bicarbonate in the treatment of ventricular tachycardia secondary to Na- blockade may be related to either the physical displacement of the drug from the Na- channel by increased serum Na- concentration[72] or decreased binding to the channel by increasing the serum pH.[73,74] Bradycardia unresponsive to atropine may require transcutaneous or transvenous pacing.[54] Hypotension should initially be treated with IV fluids. Patients with a history of cardiac dysfunction should be closely monitored for signs of fluid overload and may need placement of a Swan-Ganz catheter for continued evaluation of fluid status. Both epinephrine and dopamine are effective in treating associated hypotension.[75,76]

Torsades de pointes is usually preceded by a relatively slow heart rate and a prolonged QT interval.[1,3] Antiarrhythmics routinely used for ventricular tachycardia are often ineffective in its treatment. *Patients presenting with torsades de pointes of any origin should be given 2 g of intravenous magnesium sulfate followed by a 1- to 2-g/hr infusion.*[64,77] Although the exact mechanism by which magnesium sulfate terminates torsades de pointes is not understood, research suggests it suppresses early afterdepolarization activity by shortening the plateau phase of cardiac depolarization.[3] Hypokalemia also should be corrected. If these measures are ineffective, transvenous overdrive pacing may convert torsades de pointes.[59,78-81] Isoproterenol may be considered but must be used with caution in patients with underlying cardiac disease.

Extracorporeal Drug Removal

Hemodialysis and hemoperfusion have been reported[82-84] but are generally considered ineffective in the treatment of acute quinidine poisoning because of this drug's large volume of distribution and extensive protein binding.[2] The half-life of disopyramide is significantly reduced in patients undergoing hemodialysis, and this should be considered in patients not responding to supportive therapy.[85] Hemodialysis doubles the clearance of procainamide and provides a fourfold increase in elimination of NAPA, the active metabolite of procainamide.[86] Braden and associates demonstrated that hemoperfusion is superior to hemodialysis in the clearance of procainamide and NAPA.[87] Domoto et al showed that continuous arteriovenous hemofiltration provides even higher clearance than episodic hemoperfusion.[88] Dialysis equipment now capable of high flow rates may provide drug clearance that is equal if not superior to that of both hemofiltration and continuous arteriovenous hemofiltration.

Extracorporeal membrane oxygenation (ECMO) has been reported in a 16-month-old child. The ECMO course lasted 11 days with the toddler surviving neurologically intact.[89] Although ECMO is a consideration, the logistics make its use difficult and rare.

REFERENCES

1. Bigger JT Jr, Hoffman B: Antiarrhythmic drugs, in Gilman AG, Roll TW, Nies AS, et al (eds): Goodman and Gilman's The Pharma-cological Basis of Therapeutics. New York, Pergamon Press, 1990, pp 848–850.
2. Ochs HR, Greenblatt DJ, Woo E: Clinical pharmacokinetics of quinidine. Clin Pharmacokinet 1980;5:50–168.
3. Kim SY, Benowitz NL: Poisoning due to class IA antiarrhythmic drugs: quinidine, procainamide and disopyramide. Drug Saf 1990;5:393–420.
4. Palmer KH, Martin B, Baggett B, Wall ME: The metabolic fate of orally administered quinidine gluconate in humans. Biochem Pharmacol 1969;18:8145–8160.
5. Karlsson E: Clinical pharmacokinetics of procainamide. Clin Pharmacokinet 1978;3:97–107.
6. Giardina EG, Dreyfuss J, Bigger JT Jr, et al: Metabolism of procainamide in normal and cardiac subjects. Clin Pharmacol Ther 1976;19:339–351.
7. Galeazzi RL, Sheiner LB, Lockwood T, Benet LZ: The renal elimination of procainamide. Clin Pharmacol Ther 1976;19:55–62.
8. Bryson SM, Whiting B, Lawrence JR: Disopyramide serum and pharmacologic effect kinetics applied to the assessment of bioavailability. Br J Clin Pharmacol 1978;6:409–419.
9. Hinderling PH, Garrett ER: Pharmacodynamics of the anti-arrhythmic disopyramide in healthy humans: correlation of the kinetics of the drug and its effects. J Pharmacokinet Bio-pharmaceutics 1976;4:231–242.
10. Tiliakos N, Waites TF: Multiform quinidine toxicity. South Med J 74:1981;1267–1268.
11. Cohen IS, Jick H, Cohen SI: Adverse reactions to quinidine in hospitalized patients: findings based on data from the Boston Collaborative Drug Surveillance Program. Prog Cardiovasc Dis 1977;20:151–163.
12. Danielly J, DeJong R, Radke-Mitchell LC, Uprichard AC: Procainamide-associated blood dyscrasias [see comment]. Am J Cardiol 1994;74:1179–1180.
13. Heyman MR, Flores RH, Edelman BB, Carliner NH: Pro-cainamide-induced lupus anticoagulant. South Med J 1988;81:934–936.
14. Yung RL, Quddus J, Chrisp CE, et al: Mechanism of drug-induced lupus. 1. Cloned Th2 cells modified with DNA methylation inhibitors in vitro cause autoimmunity in vivo. J Immunol 1995;154:3025–3035.
15. Yung RL, Richardson BC: Drug-induced lupus. Rheum Dis Clini North Am 1994;20:61–86.
16. Chong BH, Berndt MC, Koutts J, Castaldi PA: Quinidine-induced thrombocytopenia and leukopenia: demonstration and charac-terization of distinct antiplatelet and antileukocyte antibodies. Blood 1983;62:1218–1223.
17. Landrum EM, Siegert EA, Hanlon JT, Currie MS: Prolonged thrombocytopenia associated with procainamide in an elderly patient. Ann Pharmacother 1994;28:1172–1176.
18. Goldberg IJ, Brown LK, Rayfield EJ: Disopyramide (Norpace)-induced hypoglycemia. Am J Med 1980;69:463–466.
19. Horie M, Mizuno N, Tsuji K, et al: Disopyramide and its metabolite enhance insulin release from clonal pancreatic beta-cells by blocking K(ATP) channels. Cardiovasc Drug Ther 2001;15:31–39.
20. Croxson MS, Shaw DW, Henley PG, Gabriel HD: Disopyramide-induced hypoglycaemia and increased serum insulin. N Z Med J 1987;100:407–408.
21. Strathman I, Schubert EN, Cohen A, Nitzberg DM: Hypoglycemia in patients receiving disopyramide phosphate. Drug Intell Clin Pharm 1983;17:635–638.
22. Hoffman BF, Rosen MR, Wit AL: Electrophysiology and pharma-cology of cardiac arrhythmias. 7. Cardiac effects of quinidine and procaine amide. B. Am Heart J 1975;90:117–122.
23. Ribeiro C, Longo A: Procainamide and disopyramide. Eur Heart J 1987;8:11–19.
24. Lee RJ, Liem LB, Cohen TJ, Franz MR: Relation between repolarization and refractoriness in the human ventricle: cycle length dependence and effect of procainamide. J Am Coll Cardiol 1992;19:614–618.
25. Kirchhof PF, Fabritz CL, Franz MR: Postrepolarization refractoriness versus conduction slowing caused by class I antiarrhythmic drugs: antiarrhythmic and proarrhythmic effects. Circulation 1998;97:2567–2574.
26. The Sicilian gambit: a new approach to the classification of antiarrhythmic drugs based on their actions on arrhythmogenic

mechanisms. Task Force of the Working Group on Arrhythmias of the European Society of Cardiology [see comment]. Circulation 1991;84:1831–1851.

27. Wyse KR, Bursill JA, Campbell TJ: Differential effects of antiarrhythmic agents on post-pause repolarization in cardiac Purkinje fibres. Clin Exp Pharmacol Physiol 1996;23:825–829.

28. Grace AA, Camm AJ: Quinidine. N Engl J Med 1998;338:35–45.

29. Roden DM: Acquired long QT syndromes and the risk of proarrhythmia [see comment]. J Cardiovasc Electrophysiol 2000;11:938–940.

30. Roden DM: Drug-induced prolongation of the QT interval. N Engl J Med 2004;350:1013–1022.

31. Shieh CC, Coghlan M, Sullivan JP, Gopalakrishnan M: Potassium channels: molecular defects, diseases, and therapeutic opportunities. Pharmacol Rev 2000;52:557–594.

32. el-Sherif N, Turitto G: Torsade de pointes. In Zipes DP, Jalife J (eds): Cardiac Electrophysiology. Philadelphia, WB Saunders, 2000, pp 662–673.

33. Lazzara R: Antiarrhythmic drugs and torsade de pointes. Eur Heart J 1993;14:88–92.

34. Woosley RL, Roden DM: Pharmacologic causes of arrhythmogenic actions of antiarrhythmic drugs. Am J Cardiol 1987;59:19E–25E.

35. De Ponti F, Poluzzi E, Montanaro N: Organising evidence on QT prolongation and occurrence of torsades de pointes with non-antiarrhythmic drugs: a call for consensus. Eur J Clin Pharmacol 2001;57:185–209.

36. Mathis AS, Gandhi AJ: Serum quinidine concentrations and effect on QT dispersion and interval. Ann Pharmacother 2002;36:1156–1161.

37. Al-Khatib SM, LaPointe NM, Kramer JM, Califf RM: What clinicians should know about the QT interval [see comment]. [Erratum in JAMA 2003;290(10):1318]. JAMA 2003;289:2120–2127.

38. Sicouri S, Antzelevitch C: Drug-induced afterdepolarizations and triggered activity occur in a discrete subpopulation of ventricular muscle cells (M cells) in the canine heart: quinidine and digitalis. J Cardiovasc Electrophysiol 1993;4:48–58.

39. Anderson ME, Al-Khatib SM, Roden DM, Califf RM: Duke Clinical Research Institute/American Heart Journal Expert Meeting on Repolarization C—Cardiac repolarization: current knowledge, critical gaps, and new approaches to drug development and patient management. Am Heart J 2002;144:769–781.

40. Martins JB: How do I prolong QT? Let me count the ways [comment]. J Cardiovasc Electrophysiol 2001;12:15–16.

41. Darbar D, Fromm MF, Dellorto S, Roden DM: Sympathetic activation enhances QT prolongation by quinidine [see comment]. J Cardiovasc Electrophysiol 2001;12:9–14.

42. Miyamoto S, Zhu B, Teramatsu T, et al: QT-prolonging class I drug, disopyramide, does not aggravate but suppresses adrenaline-induced arrhythmias: comparison with cibenzoline and pilsicainide. Eur J Pharmacol 2000;400:263–269.

43. Binah O, Rosen MR: Mechanisms of ventricular arrhythmias. Circulation 1992;85:I25–31.

44. Habbab MA, el-Sherif N: Drug-induced torsades de pointes: role of early afterdepolarizations and dispersion of repolarization. Am J Med 1990;89:241–246.

45. Roden DM, Anderson ME: The pause that refreshes, or does it? Mechanisms in torsades de pointes. Heart (British Cardiac Society) 2000;84:235–237.

46. Salata JJ, Wasserstrom JA: Effects of quinidine on action potentials and ionic currents in isolated canine ventricular myocytes. Circ Res 1988;62:324–337.

47. Sosunov EA, Anyukhovsky EP, Rosen MR: Effects of quinidine on repolarization in canine epicardium, midmyocardium, and endocardium: 1. In vitro study. Circulation 1997;96:4011–4018.

48. Anyukhovsky EP, Sosunov EA, Feinmark SJ, Rosen MR: Effects of quinidine on repolarization in canine epicardium, midmyocardium, and endocardium: 2. In vivo study. Circulation 1997;96:4019–4026.

49. Yao JA, Trybulski EJ, Tseng GN: Quinidine preferentially blocks the slow delayed rectifier potassium channel in the rested state. J Pharmacol Exp Ther 1996;279:856–864.

50. Roden DM: Taking the "idio" out of "idiosyncratic": predicting torsades de pointes. Pacing Clin Electrophysiol 1998;21:1029–1034.

51. Donger C, Denjoy I, Berthet M, et al: KVLQT1 C-terminal missense mutation causes a forme fruste long-QT syndrome. Circulation 96:2778–2781, 1997.

52. Priori SG, Barhanin J, Hauer RN, et al: Genetic and molecular basis of cardiac arrhythmias: impact on clinical management.1 and 2. Circulation 1999;99:518–528.

53. Dzimiri N, Almotrefi AA: Interaction between potassium concentration and inhibition of myocardial Na^+/K^+-ATPase by two class 1A antiarrhythmic drugs: quinidine and procainamide. Arch Int Pharmacodyn Ther 1991;314:34–43.

54. Kerr F, Kenoyer G, Bilitch M: Quinidine overdose: neurological and cardiovascular toxicity in a normal person. Br Heart J 1971;33:629-631.

55. Summers WK, Allen RE, Pitts FN Jr: Does physostigmine reverse quinidine delirium? West J Med 1981;135:411–414.

56. Grant AO, Starmer CF, Strauss HC: Antiarrhythmic drug action: blockade of the inward sodium current. Circ Res 1984;55:427–439.

57. Li GR, Ferrier GR: Effects of quinidine on arrhythmias and conduction in an isolated tissue model of ischemia and reperfusion. J Cardiovasc Pharmacol 1991;17:239–248.

58. Podrid PJ, Schoeneberger A, Lown B: Congestive heart failure caused by oral disopyramide. N Engl J Med 1980;302:614–617.

59. Jackman WM, Friday KJ, Anderson JL, et al: The long QT syndromes: a critical review, new clinical observations and a unifying hypothesis. Prog Cardiovasc Dis 1988;31:115–172.

60. Riccioni N, Castiglioni M, Bartolomei C: Disopyramide-induced QT prolongation and ventricular tachyarrhythmias. Am Heart J 1983;105:870–871.

61. Olshansky B, Martins J, Hunt S: N-acetyl procainamide causing torsades de pointes. Am J Cardiol 1982;50:1439–1441.

62. Strasberg B, Sclarovsky S, Erdberg A, et al: Procainamide-induced polymorphous ventricular tachycardia. Am J Cardiol 1981;47:1309–1314.

63. Hohnloser SH, Klingenheben T, Singh BN: Amiodarone-associated proarrhythmic effects: a review with special reference to torsade de pointes tachycardia [see comment]. Ann Intern Med 1994;121:529–535.

64. Tzivoni D, Banai S, Schuger C, et al: Treatment of torsade de pointes with magnesium sulfate. Circulation 1988;77:392–397.

65. Malik M, Batchvarov VN: Measurement, interpretation and clinical potential of QT dispersion. J Am Coll Cardiol 2000;36:1749–1766.

66. Waldo AL, Wit AL: Mechanisms of cardiac arrhythmias. Lancet 1993;341:1189–1193.

67. Sun D, Reiner D, Frishman W, et al: Adverse dermatologic reactions from antiarrhythmic drug therapy. J Clin Pharmacol 1994;34:953–966.

68. Javaheri S, Logemann TN, Corser BC, et al: Diaphragmatic paralysis. Am J Med 1989;86:623–624.

69. Leonard RF, Braun TE, Levy AM: Initiation of uterine contractions by disopyramide during pregnancy. N Engl J Med 1978;299:84–85.

70. Caporaso NE, Shaw GL: Clinical implications of the competitive inhibition of the debrisoquin-metabolizing isozyme by quinidine. Arch Intern Med 1991;151:1985–1992.

71. Thatcher SK, Lemberg L: Digitalis-quinidine interaction. Heart Lung 1980;9:352–357.

72. Ranger S, Sheldon R, Fermini B, Nattel S: Modulation of flecainide's cardiac sodium channel blocking actions by extracellular sodium: a possible cellular mechanism for the action of sodium salts in flecainide cardiotoxicity. J Pharmacol Exp Ther 1993;264:1160–1167.

73. Wasserman R, Brodsky L, Kathe J, et al: The effect of molar sodium lactate in quinidine intoxication. Am J Cardiol 1959;4:294.

74. Bellet S, Hamdan G, Somlyo A, et al: The reversal of cardiotoxic effects of quinidine by molar sodium lactate: an experimental study. Am J Med Sci 1959;237:177–189.

75. Nolan MT, Prichard JS: Non-fatal overdose with disopyramide. Irish Med J 1984;77:209.

76. Villalba-Pimentel L, Epstein LM, Sellers EM, et al: Survival after massive procainamide ingestion. Am J Cardiol 1973;32:727–730.

77. Vukmir RB: Torsades de pointes: a review. Am J Emerg Med 1991;9:250–255.

78. el-Sherif N, Bekheit SS, Henkin R: Quinidine-induced long QTU interval and torsade de pointes: role of bradycardia-dependent early afterdepolarizations. J Am Coll Cardiol 1989;14:252–257.

79. Bauman JL, Bauernfeind RA, Hoff JV, et al: Torsade de pointes due to quinidine: observations in 31 patients. Am Heart J 1984; 107:425–430.

80. Kaseda S, Gilmour RF Jr, Zipes DP: Depressant effect of magnesium on early afterdepolarizations and triggered activity induced by cesium, quinidine, and 4-aminopyridine in canine cardiac Purkinje fibers. Am Heart J 1989;118:458–466.

81. Swiryn S, Kim SS: Quinidine-induced syncope. Arch Intern Med 1983;143:314–316.

82. Shub C, Gau G, Sidell P, Brennan L: The management of acute quinidine intoxication. Chest 1978;73:173–178.

83. Woie L, Oyri A: Quinidine intoxication treated with hemodialysis. Acta Med Scand 1974;195:237–239.

84. Reinmold E, Reynolds W, et al: Use of hemodialysis in the treaaatment of quinidine poisoning. Pediatrics 1973;52:95–99.

85. Horn J, M H: Disopyramide dialysability (letter). Lancet 1978;2:214.

86. Aitchison JD, Campbell RW, Higham PD: Time dependent variability of QT dispersion after acute myocardial infarction and its relation to ventricular fibrillation: a prospective study. Heart (British Cardiac Society) 2000;84:504–508.

87. Braden GL, Fitzgibbons JP, Germain MJ, Ledewitz HM: Hemoperfusion for treatment of N-acetylprocainamide intoxication. Ann Intern Med 1986;105:64–65.

88. Domoto DT, Brown WW, Bruggensmith P: Removal of toxic levels of N-acetylprocainamide with continuous arteriovenous hemofiltration or continuous arteriovenous hemodiafiltration. Ann Intern Med 1987;106:550–552.

89. Tecklenburg F, Thomas N, Webb S, et al: Pediatric ECMO for severe quinidine cardotoxicity. Pediatr Emerg Care 1997;13:111–113.

64 *Diabetic Control Agents*

MICHAEL J. BURNS, MD ■ MICHAEL LEVINE, MD

At a Glance...

- Overdose of hypoglycemic agents (e.g., insulin, sulfonylureas, and meglitinides) is likely to produce hypoglycemia, whereas overdose of antihyperglycemic agents (e.g., α-glucosidase inhibitors, biguanides, and thiazolidinediones) is unlikely to result in hypoglycemia.

- Biguanide-associated lactic acidosis is associated with a high mortality rate and should be suspected in any critically ill patient taking metformin.

- Biguanide-associated lactic acidosis occurs most commonly in patients with renal, hepatic, or cardiac dysfunction or alcohol abuse.

- After treating hypoglycemia due to sulfonylurea ingestion with dextrose, octreotide should be given to prevent rebound hypoglycemia.

- All patients with intentional sulfonylurea overdoses, sulfonylurea exposures in children, and sulfonylurea ingestions associated with symptomatic hypoglycemia should be admitted for a 12- to 24-hour period of observation.

- Patients with inadvertent insulin reactions can usually be safely discharged after several hours of emergency department observation, whereas patients with intentional insulin overdose should be admitted for inpatient observation.

INTRODUCTION AND RELEVANT HISTORY

In recent years, the incidence of diabetes mellitus, especially type 2 diabetes, has dramatically increased in the United States and other Western countries. Currently, about 125 million people worldwide and 20 million Americans live with diabetes.[1-4] In patients with type 2 or non–insulin-dependent diabetes mellitus (NIDDM) (also known as *adult-onset diabetes*), insulin resistance is the primary abnormality, which often necessitates treatment with an oral hypoglycemic agent to achieve euglycemia. In patients with type 1 or insulin-dependent diabetes (IDDM), impaired insulin secretion is the primary abnormality, which necessitates treatment with exogenous insulin to maintain euglycemia.

Agents used to treat diabetes can be divided into two general categories: hypoglycemic agents (e.g., insulin, sulfonylureas, and meglitinides) and antihyperglycemic agents (e.g., biguanides, α-glucosidase inhibitors, and thiazolidinediones or glitazones).[2] Although these agents may be used alone, they are often used in combination to treat patients with both types of diabetes mellitus (see Chapter 16).

Insulin was first used to treat a patient with diabetes mellitus in 1921.[3] Since that time, it has been the mainstay of treatment for type 1 diabetes patients and is some-

times part of the treatment regimen for those with type 2 diabetes.

In 1942, it was observed that certain sulfonamides were associated with hypoglycemia in animals.[2] Subsequently, a number of first-generation sulfonylurea compounds (i.e., tolbutamide, acetohexamide, tolazamide, and chlorpropamide) were created and marketed specifically for their hypoglycemic effect. In the 1950s, tolbutamide was the first sulfonylurea to be widely used for patients with type 2 diabetes.[2] In the 1980s, the second-generation agents (i.e., glyburide, gliclazide, glipizide, and glimepiride) became commercially available. These agents are significantly more potent than the first-generation agents. Currently, chlorpropamide, glyburide, and glipizide account for most prescriptions of oral hypoglycemic agents.

The biguanides, phenformin and buformin, became available for use as antihyperglycemic agents in the late 1950s.[2] Phenformin was subsequently withdrawn from the market in the United States and Europe in 1977 because of an association with lactic acidosis; it is still available in other areas of the world.[5] Metformin, another biguanide less frequently associated with lactic acidosis, became available for use in Europe in 1970 and the United States in 1995.

Several other, novel classes of diabetes control agents were introduced in the late 1990s. In 1996, a new type of antihyperglycemic agent, referred to as an *α-glucosidase inhibitor*, became available for clinical use in the United States. Acarbose and miglitol are two agents in this class. In 1997, troglitazone was the first of the thiazolidinediones introduced to the U.S. market.[6] Although troglitazone was removed from the U.S. market in 2000 because of its ability to cause a rare, idiosyncratic hepatocellular injury,[7] other drugs in the glitazone class (i.e., rosiglitazone and pioglitazone) have become available and are frequently used.

The meglitinides, repaglinide and nateglinide, are in the latest class of antihyperglycemic agents to obtain approval for clinical use in the United States. Repaglinide became available for use in 1997, and nateglinide became available in 2000. Common diabetes control agents that are currently available for clinical use are listed in Table 64-1.

EPIDEMIOLOGY

Toxicity from diabetes control agents may be dose related, occurring after unintentional or intentional overdose, or idiosyncratic, occurring as unanticipated adverse effects during therapeutic administration. For the hypoglycemic agents, toxicity manifests largely as hypoglycemia or an overextension of the pharmacologic effects. Although

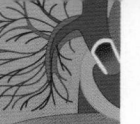

TABLE 64-1 Oral Hypoglycemic and Antihyperglycemic Agents

CLASS	GENERIC NAME	TRADE NAME	DURATION OF ACTION (hr)*
α-Glucosidase inhibitors	Acarbose	Precose	2
	Miglitol	Glyset	2
Biguanides	Metformin	Glucophage	1.5–4.9
Meglitinides	Nateglinide	Starlix	2–4
	Repaglinide	Prandin	1–3
Sulfonylureas (first generation)	Acetohexamide	Dymelor	12–18
	Chlorpropamide	Diabinese	24–72
	Tolazamide	Tolinase	16–24
	Tolbutamide	Orinase	6–12
Sulfonylureas (second generation)	Glyburide	Micronase, Glynase, Diaβeta	18–24
	Glipizide	Glucotrol, Glucotrol XL	16–24
Sulfonylureas (third generation)	Glimepiride	Amaryl	24
Thiazoldinediones	Pioglitazone	Actos	16–24
	Rosiglitazone	Avandia	12–24

*The pharmacokinetic data are based on therapeutic dosing and may change after agent overdose.
Adapted from Davis SN, Granner DK: Insulin, oral hypoglycemic agents, and the pharmacology of the endocrine pancreas. In Hardman JG, Limbrid LE, Gilman AG (eds): Goodman and Gilman's The Pharmacological Basis of Therapeutics, 10th ed. New York, McGraw-Hill, 2001, pp 1679–1714; Banting FG, Best CH, Collip JB, et al: Pancreatic extracts in the treatment of diabetes mellitus. Can Med Assoc J 1922;12:141–146; and Gerich JE: Oral hypoglycemic agents. N Engl J Med 1989;321:1123–1145.

agents from the antihyperglycemic class do not produce hypoglycemia when used alone, they can potentiate the hypoglycemic effect of the hypoglycemic agents when dosed with them.

The toxic effects occur commonly but are infrequently reported to U.S. poison control centers. Infrequent reporting of toxicity is likely due to the familiarity of most clinicians with the toxicity from these agents and its treatment. Most exposures are unintentional (78%) and occur in adults (68%), whereas most deaths follow acute exposure with suicidal intent.[8] In 2003, 12,736 diabetes control agent exposures were reported to U.S. poison centers, of which 4019 (32%) were due to sulfonylureas, 3811 (30%) to biguanides, 2914 (23%) to insulin, and 1586 (12%) to thiazolidinediones. The remainder of the exposures were uncharacterized.[8] Major toxicity and death occurred in 2.5% and 0.2% of all diabetes control agent exposures, respectively.[8]

STRUCTURE AND CLASSIFICATION

Sulfonylureas

The sulfonylureas are classified into two main groups: the first-generation agents include chlorpropamide, tolbutamide, acetohexamide, and tolazamide; the second-generation agents include glyburide (or glibenclamide), glipizide, and glimepiride. Glimepiride has sometimes been referred to as a third-generation agent. Additional agents available outside the United States include gliclazide and gliquidone. The sulfonylureas are *para*-substituted arylsulfonamides derived from sulfonic acid and urea. Sulfonylureas are closely related in structure to the sulfonamide antibiotics and thiazide diuretics. Differing side-chain substitutions on the *para* position of the benzene ring (R) and nitrogen on the urea moiety

(R_1) result in varying potency and duration of action[2] (Fig. 64-1). Second-generation agents are 100 to 150 times more potent than the first-generation agents owing to dif-fering binding affinity at the sulfonylurea receptor.[2] Comparative characteristics of selected sulfonylureas are found in Table 64-2.

Biguanides

The biguanides contain two guanidine molecules linked together with the elimination of an amino group. Metformin is N-1,1-dimethylbiguanide hydrochloride and is the only biguanide currently available in the United States (see Fig. 64-1). Phenformin and buformin are still available in other countries.

α-Glucosidase Inhibitors

The α-glucosidase inhibitors are a relatively new class of drug used to treat diabetes. Acarbose, the first drug in this class approved for use in the United States, is a large, complex oligosaccharide derived from the microorganism *Actinoplanes utahensis* (see Fig. 64-1). Miglitol, which is considered a second-generation glucosidase inhibitor, has subsequently been approved. Meglitol is a small monosaccharide derivative that resembles glucose. Voglibose is currently pending U.S. Food and Drug Administration approval but is available in other countries.

Thiazolidinediones

Two thiazolidinedione derivatives are available for clinical use in the United States: rosiglitazone and pioglitazone[9] (see Fig. 64-1). The thiazolidinediones are structurally unrelated to other diabetes control agents. These drugs are also available in a combination with other agents, such as metformin.

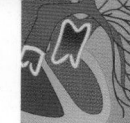

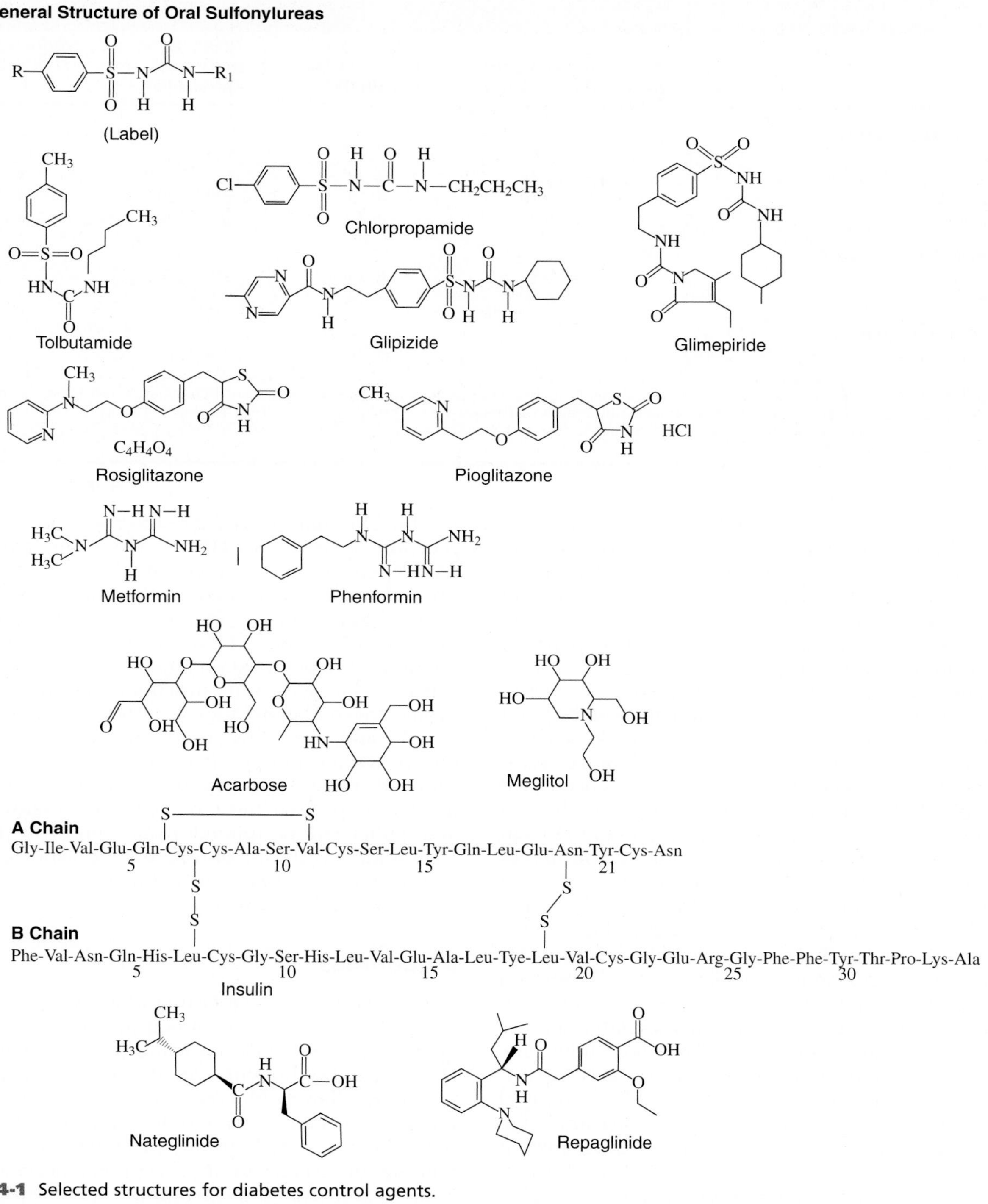

General Structure of Oral Sulfonylureas

(Label)

Tolbutamide

Chlorpropamide

Glipizide

Glimepiride

Rosiglitazone $C_4H_4O_4$

Pioglitazone   HCl

Metformin

Phenformin

Acarbose

Meglitol

A Chain
Gly-Ile-Val-Glu-Gln-Cys-Cys-Ala-Ser-Val-Cys-Ser-Leu-Tyr-Gln-Leu-Glu-Asn-Tyr-Cys-Asn
　　　　　5　　　　　　　　　　10　　　　　　　　　15　　　　　　　　　21

B Chain
Phe-Val-Asn-Gln-His-Leu-Cys-Gly-Ser-His-Leu-Val-Glu-Ala-Leu-Tye-Leu-Val-Cys-Gly-Glu-Arg-Gly-Phe-Phe-Tyr-Thr-Pro-Lys-Ala
　　　　　　5　　　　　　　　　10　　　　　　　　　15　　　　　　　　20　　　　　　　　25　　　　　　　　30
Insulin

Nateglinide

Repaglinide

FIGURE 64-1 Selected structures for diabetes control agents.

Meglitinides

The meglitinides are a novel class of insulin secretagogues that are structurally distinct from the sulfonylureas (see Fig. 64-1). They include repaglinide, which is a benzoic acid derivative, and nateglinide, which is a D-phenylalanine derivative.[2]

Insulin

Insulin is an endogenous protein hormone consisting of two polypeptide chains (A and B chains) connected by two intersubunit disulfide bonds (see Fig. 64-1 and Chapter 16). The β cells of the pancreatic islets synthesize insulin initially as the polypeptide precursor,

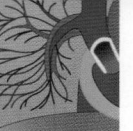

TABLE 64-2 Properties of Selected Sulfonylureas

DRUG	RELATIVE POTENCY	ELIMINATION HALF-LIFE (hr)	DURATION OF HYPOGLYCEMIC ACTION (hr)	THERAPEUTIC DAILY DOSE RANGE (mg)	FREQUENCY OF HYPOGLYCEMIA (%)
First-Generation Agents					
Acetohexamide	2.5	1–2	12–18	250–1500	4
Chlorpropamide	6	24–48	24–72	100–500	9
Tolbutamide	1	3–28	6–10	500–3000	3
Tolazamide	5	4–7	16–24	0.1–1000	4
Second-Generation Agents					
Glipizide	100	1–5	16–24	2.5–40	6
Glyburide	150	1.5–3	18–24	1.25–20	7
Third-Generation Agents					
Glimepiride	150	2–8	12–24	1–4	1

Adapted from Davis SN, Granner DK: Insulin, oral hypoglycemic agents, and the pharmacology of the endocrine pancreas. In Hardman JG, Limbrid LE, Gilman AG (eds): Goodman and Gilman's The Pharmacological Basis of Therapeutics, 10th ed. New York, McGraw-Hill, 2001, pp 1679–1714; Gerich JE: Oral hypoglycemic agents. N Engl J Med 1989;321:1123–1145; and Baselt RC: Disposition of Toxic Drugs and Chemicals in Man, 7th ed. Foster City, CA, Biomedical Publications, 2004.

preproinsulin.[2] In the rough endoplasmic reticulum, a portion of preproinsulin is cleaved to form proinsulin. Subsequent proteolytic cleavage of proinsulin in the Golgi apparatus forms insulin and a connecting segment or C peptide. Insulin is stored in secretory granules (along with equimolar amounts of the inert C peptide) in β cells until release into the circulation.

Insulins may be classified according to their species of origin as porcine, bovine, or human and by their duration of action as short-, intermediate-, and long-acting (or regular, Lente, and Ultralente).[2,10-12] Since 1921, insulin derived from beef or pork pancreas has been used therapeutically. During the past decade, however, human insulin has become the standard form of therapy. Human insulin is either derived enzymatically from pork insulin or produced from *Escherichia coli* using recombinant deoxyribonucleic acid techniques.[2] More recently, insulin analogs have also become commercially available.[13]

Insulin is prepared as an injectable solution for subcutaneous or intravenous administration. Doses and concentrations of insulin are expressed in units (U). Short-acting and rapid-acting insulins available for use include the readily soluble, regular (crystalline zinc insulin) formulation or the analogs lispro and aspart.[2] Intermediate-acting insulins include NPH (neutral protamine Hagedorn, an isophane suspension) and Lente (zinc suspension) formulations. Long-acting insulin preparations include Ultralente (extended insulin zinc suspension), protamine zinc suspension, and the analog glargine. The types of insulin and their pharmacokinetic properties are listed in Table 64-3.

PHARMACOLOGY AND PATHOPHYSIOLOGY

Sulfonylureas

The major mechanism of action of the sulfonylureas is to stimulate endogenous insulin secretion by pancreatic β cells. The sulfonylureas bind to a specific sulfonylurea receptor type 1 (SUR1) of adenosine triphosphate (ATP)–sensitive potassium channels (K_{ATP}). These potassium channels are located on the plasma membrane of β cells. Sulfonylurea binding to the receptor results in closure of the ATP-sensitive potassium channel, membrane depolarization, opening of voltage-sensitive calcium channels, and subsequent exocytic release of insulin. Second-generation agents have higher binding affinity and are, thus, more potent in their clinical effects. Other minor effects of sulfonylureas include reduced hepatic gluconeogenesis and clearance of insulin, suppressed glucagon and somatostatin secretion, and enhanced peripheral tissue sensitivity to insulin (stimulate synthesis of glucose transporters).[2] The extrapancreatic effects of sulfonylureas are not likely clinically significant in vivo.[2,14,15]

Biguanides

The biguanides reduce fasting blood glucose levels and insulin concentrations by suppressing basal hepatic gluconeogenesis and improving peripheral tissue (i.e., fat, muscle) insulin sensitivity, thus enhancing peripheral insulin-mediated glucose uptake.[2] The biguanides potentiate insulin and are only effective in the presence of this hormone. Specifically, the biguanides increase the binding of insulin to its receptors, increase tyrosine kinase activity, and promote the synthesis and translocation of glucose transporters to the cell surface. The biguanides may also decrease blood glucose levels by impairing glucose absorption from the small intestine.[16] The biguanides are not insulin secretagogues and do not cause hypoglycemia, even at large doses.[2] The biguanides also do not alter secretion of glucagon, cortisol, or somatostatin. Biguanides reduce blood triglycerides and free fatty acids.

The pathophysiology of lactic acidosis from biguanides is largely due to inhibition of gluconeogenesis.[17-22] At supratherapeutic levels, biguanides inhibit pyruvate

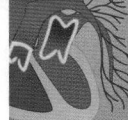

TABLE 64-3 Properties of Insulin Preparations Currently Available*

TYPE OF INSULIN	BRAND NAME	TIME TO ONSET (hr)	TIME TO PEAK EFFECT (hr)	DURATION OF ACTION (hr)
Rapid				
Regular (soluble crystalline zinc)	Novolin R	0.5–1	1.5–4	5–8
Lispro	Humalog	0.25	0.5–1.5	2–5
Aspart	NovoLog	0.17–0.33	1–3	3–5
Intermediate				
NPH (isophane insulin suspension)	Novolin N	1–1.5	4–12	24
Insulin zinc suspension	Lente	1–2	6–12	18–24
Slow				
Extended insulin zinc suspension	Ultralente	4–8	16–18	20–36
Glarginine	Lantus	2–5	5–24	18–24

*The pharmacokinetic data listed are for therapeutic doses with subcutaneous administration; times will vary with route of administration (intravenous versus subcutaneous administration and dose (therapeutic versus excessive doses).
NPH, neutral protamine Hagedorn.
Adapted from Davis SN, Granner DK: Insulin, oral hypoglycemic agents, and the pharmacology of the endocrine pancreas. In Hardman JG, Limbrid LE, Gilman AG (eds): Goodman and Gilman's The Pharmacological Basis of Therapeutics, 10th ed. New York, McGraw-Hill, 2001, pp 1679–1714; Hirsch IB: Drug therapy: insulin analogues. N Engl J Med 2005;352:174–183; Baselt RC: Disposition of Toxic Drugs and Chemicals in Man, 7th ed. Foster City, CA, Biomedical Publications, 2004; and Insulin preparations: drug information. UpToDate. Version 13.2. Accessed July 2, 2005.

carboxylase, the enzyme responsible for converting pyruvate to oxaloacetate (first step of gluconeogenesis). Elevations of pyruvate subsequently lead to lactate accumulation. Any condition that leads to elevated blood concentrations of biguanides (i.e., biguanide overdose, impaired excretion from hepatic and renal dysfunction) may precipitate lactate accumulation. Any medical condition that impairs lactate clearance (i.e., hepatic, renal, and cardiac dysfunction) will also lead to lactate accumulation and increase the risk for lactic acidosis. In addition, ethanol facilitates the accumulation of lactate; ethanol inhibits gluconeogenesis itself, and its metabolism results in an accumulation of reduced nicotinamide adenine dinucleotide (NADH), which inhibits conversion of lactate to pyruvate.

Biguanide-induced lactic acidosis is primarily type B, or that which occurs in the absence of tissue hypoxia or hypoperfusion, and results from impaired clearance of lactate. Type A lactic acidosis, or that which occurs in the presence of hypoxia or hypoperfusion, is from the increased production of lactate. Type A lactic acidosis may also be operative in the lactic acidosis induced by biguanides. Respiratory, cardiac, and renal dysfunction or polydrug overdoses that produce seizures, hypoxia, or tissue hypoperfusion lead to lactic acid accumulation. In addition, phenformin, unlike metformin, has the added ability to inhibit cellular oxidative phosphorylation directly and increase the tissue generation of lactate.[20,22,23]

α-Glucosidase Inhibitors

α-Glucosidase inhibitors have a unique mechanism of action, in that they are the only class of drug that is not directly designed to combat a specific pathophysiologic defect of type 2 diabetes.[6] Rather, these agents competitively inhibit the activity of α-glucosidase, a brush-border enzyme responsible for breaking down disac-

charides (e.g., sucrose, maltose) and polysaccharides (e.g., starch) into monosaccharide. Therefore, the α-glucosidase inhibitors delay intestinal glucose absorption and diminish postprandial glucose elevations.[24] Acarbose also competitively inhibits the action of pancreatic α-amylase. These drugs are not insulin secretagogues and do not result in hypoglycemia.

Thiazolidinediones

The thiazolidinediones improve insulin sensitivity (largely in adipose tissue) and result in a reduction of fasting plasma glucose, insulin, and free fatty acids. These agents regulate gene expression and are associated with a delay of 4 to 12 weeks from initiation of dosing to therapeutic effects. The thiazolidinediones are selective agonists for the nuclear hormone receptor known as *peroxisome-proliferation–activated receptor-γ* (PPAR-γ).[2] After binding, there is activation of transcription of a variety of genes that regulate lipid and carbohydrate metabolism.[6,25] Thus, similar to biguanides and α-glucosidase inhibitors, the thiazolidinediones do not stimulate the pancreatic β cells to secrete more insulin.

Meglitinides

Similar to sulfonylureas, meglitinides are insulin secretagogues that directly stimulate first-phase insulin release in pancreatic β cells. Although the meglitinides bind to a different receptor than the sulfonylureas, their mechanism of action is identical; their binding results in closure of K_{ATP} channels, membrane depolarization, opening of voltage-sensitive calcium channels, and subsequent exocytic release of insulin.[2,26]

Unlike the sulfonylureas, however, the meglitinides do not stimulate insulin secretion in the absence of glucose. In addition, these agents (particularly nateglinide) induce a more rapid but less sustained secretion of

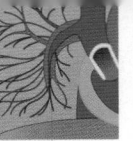

insulin than sulfonylureas.[6] Although the magnitude of the glucose-lowering effects of repaglinide is similar to that of the sulfonylureas, it is associated with a significantly reduced risk for delayed hypoglycemia owing to a shorter duration of action.[10] As compared with repaglinide, nateglinide has a higher binding affinity and quicker offset kinetics at the K_{ATP} channel. Thus, nateglinide has the more rapid onset and offset of insulinotropic effects of the two meglitinides.

Insulin

Insulin stimulates the uptake, utilization, and storage of glucose, amino acids, and fatty acids by peripheral tissues[2] (see Chapter 16). As an anabolic hormone, insulin impairs the catabolism of glycogen, proteins, and fats in all tissues. Insulin release by the pancreas is primarily regulated by and inversely correlated to blood glucose concentrations. Once released into the systemic circulation, insulin binds to specific membrane-bound receptors in peripheral tissues, which are ligand-activated protein kinases. Insulin binding stimulates tyrosine kinase activity, receptor autophosphorylation, and a cascade of phosphorylation and dephosphorylation reactions intracellularly, which serve to activate other intracellular signaling molecules.[2] The downstream effects of insulin binding are multiple. One such effect is the translocation of glucose transport proteins to the cell surface and subsequent enhanced glucose uptake by peripheral tissues (e.g., skeletal muscle and adipose tissue). In addition to stimulating the uptake of glucose by peripheral tissues, insulin also impairs hepatic gluconeogenesis and glycogenolysis. Insulin further promotes hypoglycemia by inhibiting protein degradation and lipolysis. The usual substrates for hepatic gluconeogenesis (e.g., alanine, glutamine, pyruvate, glycerol, nonesterified fatty acids) are reduced in the presence of insulin. In addition to its effects on carbohydrate, protein, and lipid metabolism, insulin promotes cellular uptake of potassium and magnesium.

PHARMACOKINETICS

Sulfonylureas

The sulfonylureas are available for oral administration only. These drugs are well absorbed from the gastrointestinal (GI) tract, with bioavailabilities greater than 80%.[27] Food and hyperglycemia reduce absorption. Once absorbed, all sulfonylureas are extensively (90% to 99%) bound to plasma proteins (predominantly albumin) and have small volumes of distribution (about 0.2 L/kg).[2,27] With the exception of acetohexamide, all sulfonylureas are metabolized in the liver to inactive or less active metabolites; metabolites and small amounts of unchanged drug are eliminated in the urine. Acetohexamide is metabolized to hydroxyhexamide, which is more active and more slowly eliminated than the parent drug. Up to 20% of chlorpropamide is excreted unchanged in the urine.[2]

With therapeutic dosing, the hypoglycemic effects of these agents begin within 1 to 2 hours of oral dosing and peak by 4 to 6 hours; the first-generation agents may have a more delayed time to peak effect. Relative potencies, elimination half-lives, duration of hypoglycemic action, and therapeutic dose range are found in Table 64-2. With therapeutic dosing, the first-generation agents have variable elimination half-lives and a long duration of hypoglycemic action (12 to 24 hours), whereas the second-generation agents have short elimination half-lives and a long duration of hypoglycemic action (12 to 24 hours).[2,27] After overdose, the duration of hypoglycemic action may last days.[11]

Biguanides

After oral administration, metformin has a bioavailability of 30% to 60%; significant concentrations (27%) of unabsorbed drug are recovered from feces.[27] Peak plasma concentrations of metformin occur within 1 to 3 hours of a therapeutic dose. The antihyperglycemic effects of metformin begin in 1 hour and last about 12 hours after standard oral dosing. Metformin is not bound to plasma proteins, has a volume of distribution of 3.7 L/kg, and is largely excreted unchanged in the urine (50%) by both glomerular filtration and tubular secretion. At therapeutic doses, the plasma elimination half-life is estimated at 1.5 to 4.9 hours in subjects with normal renal function.[28] Geriatric patients or those with renal impairment have prolonged elimination half-lives. The recommended daily oral doses for normal adult patients range from 500 to 2500 mg, either as a single dose of the extended-release preparation or twice daily with the normal-release preparation. Metformin can be used either as a single agent or in combination with a sulfonylurea or insulin in the management of diabetes.

α-Glucosidase Inhibitors

Less than 2% of acarbose is absorbed from the GI tract, and more than 50% is excreted unchanged in the feces. Acarbose is metabolized in the GI tract by intestinal bacteria and digestive enzymes. Acarbose is mostly absorbed (34% of a dose) as metabolites of the parent drug. Elimination half-life of acarbose activity is normally about 2 hours in adults. Thus, bioaccumulation of the drug does not occur with dosing three times a day. Unlike acarbose, which has minimal absorption from the small intestine, miglitol is well absorbed from the small intestine. Both of these drugs have a small volume of distribution, and little to no protein binding at therapeutic doses. Miglitol is excreted unchanged by the kidney. The recommended oral dose for adult patients ranges from 25 to 100 mg three times daily, just before each meal.[2]

Thiazolidinediones

Rosiglitazone and pioglitazone are rapidly absorbed (peak blood concentrations within 1 to 2 hours), with a bioavailability of 99% and 50%, respectively. These drugs

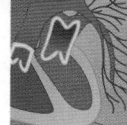

are highly protein bound (99%) and have similar small volumes of distribution (0.2 to 1.0 L/kg) and elimination half-lives (2.7 to 7 hours). Both drugs are extensively metabolized by the liver cytochrome P-450 system. Pioglitazone is metabolized by CYP2C8 to metabolites with pharmacologic activity similar to and elimination half-lives longer than the parent drug. Rosiglitazone is metabolized by CYP3A4 to very weakly active compounds. No clinically significant drug interactions have been described with the thiazolidinediones.[9,29] Although both thiazolidinediones are absorbed within 2 hours of oral administration, maximal clinical effect is not observed for 6 to 12 weeks. Pioglitazone is dosed from 15 to 45 mg once daily in adults, whereas rosiglitazone is administered as 4 to 8 mg daily in one or two divided doses.

Meglitinides

The meglitinides are rapidly absorbed from the GI tract, with peak blood concentrations observed within 0.5 to 1 hour of an oral therapeutic dose. The onset and duration of clinical effects are rapid, occurring within 1 and 4 hours, respectively. Bioavailability is about 60% for both agents. These drugs are highly protein bound (more than 98%) and have small volumes of distribution (0.4 L/kg). In addition, both drugs are metabolized by CYP3A4 to inactive metabolites.[2] Elimination half-lives are only 1 to 2 hours.[26] Drugs that enhance or inhibit CYP3A4 enzyme may decrease or increase the clinical effects of these drugs, respectively.[2,30] Small amounts of each drug are excreted by the kidney unchanged (10% to 16%).[2] The recommended adult dose is 60 to 120 mg for nateglinide or 0.5 to 4 mg for repaglinide, three times daily, each dose administered within 10 minutes of a meal.

TOXICOLOGY: CLINICAL MANIFESTATIONS AFTER OVERDOSE

Sulfonylureas

The principal effect of overdose of any of the sulfonylurea agents, whether in a diabetic or nondiabetic individual, is hypoglycemia. Although hypoglycemia has been defined in absolute terms as a plasma glucose concentration of less than 2.78 mmol/L (50 mg/dL),[31] it is perhaps more usefully defined in functional terms as a depressed concentration of blood or plasma glucose producing evidence of a physiologic counter-regulatory hormone response or evidence of neurologic dysfunction (neuroglycopenia). As the plasma glucose concentration decreases to about 4 mmol/L (72 mg/dL), there is an increase in the secretion of counter-regulatory hormones (e.g., glucagon, epinephrine, growth hormone, and cortisol) and activation of the autonomic nervous system. If the plasma glucose concentration reaches 3.2 mmol/L (58 mg/dL), this increase in autonomic activity is normally of a sufficient magnitude to result in symptoms. This response may be modified in patients with diabetic autonomic neuropathy or in those who are receiving β-blocker therapy. Glucose is the principal energy substrate for the brain. The brain does not produce glucose and can only store a few minutes' supply. Therefore, the brain is extremely sensitive to hypoglycemia. Concentrations of circulating glucose below 3 mmol/L (54 mg/dL) impair cerebral function, whereas more severe and prolonged hypoglycemia can cause convulsions, permanent neurologic damage, or death.[32]

The onset of hypoglycemia after acute sulfonylurea overdose occurs after a variable time interval; the latency is dependent on the size of the ingestion, the particular agent involved, and individual host factors (i.e., age, comorbid illness [hepatic or renal disease], presence of insulin resistance). It usually occurs within 6 to 8 hours of ingestion but may be delayed for 16 to 18 hours.[33,34] In one study of sulfonylurea ingestion in children, 50% and 96% of patients developed hypoglycemia within 2 and 8 hours, respectively.[34] A single tablet is sufficient to produce symptomatic hypoglycemia in children.[33,34] The duration of hypoglycemia is dose related and ranges from several hours to several days. In one case, hypoglycemia lasted for 27 days after intentional chlorpropamide overdose.[11]

The signs and symptoms of sulfonylurea-induced hypoglycemia are identical to those associated with hypoglycemia from other causes. Signs and symptoms are manifestations of neuroglycopenia or are the consequence of the autonomic response to hypoglycemia (Box 64-1). Long-lasting or permanent neurologic dysfunction may occur if hypoglycemia is severe or prolonged before treatment.

BOX 64-1	SIGNS AND SYMPTOMS OF HYPOGLYCEMIA

Central Nervous System Effects (Neuroglycopenia)

Lethargy to coma
Dizziness
Slurred speech, blurred vision, ataxia
Irritability, anxiety, agitated delirium
Headache
Confusion, cognitive dysfunction, memory loss
Seizures (single or multiple; focal or generalized)
Focal neurologic deficits
Hallucinations, altered personality
Generalized weakness
Paresthesias

Autonomic and Other Effects

Diaphoresis
Tachycardia, palpitations, tachyarrhythmias
Syncope
Hypertension
Hunger
Nausea, vomiting
Tremor
Piloerection
Tachypnea
Peripheral vasoconstriction, pallor
Hypothermia

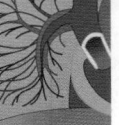

Biguanides

Acute biguanide overdose is usually well tolerated. GI effects occur most commonly and include nausea, vomiting, anorexia, hematemesis, metallic taste, abdominal pain, and diarrhea.[35-37] Although hypoglycemia virtually never occurs in association with therapeutic doses of biguanides, it has rarely been described after overdose with these agents.[38] Biguanide-induced lactic acidosis is the most serious complication of biguanide treatment. It is most commonly associated with therapeutic dosing of biguanides (see "Adverse Effects") but has also been described after acute, large, intentional overdose in adults.[39-46] Lactic acidosis has not been described after accidental ingestion of 1 or 2 tablets of metformin in children.[47] Patients with biguanide-associated lactic acidosis typically present with relatively nonspecific symptoms, such as vomiting, somnolence, agitation, nausea, epigastric pain, anorexia, hyperpnea, lethargy, diarrhea, and thirst.[22] Coma, hypothermia, seizures, and cardiovascular collapse may rapidly ensue.

α-Glucosidase Inhibitors

Overdose of the α-glucosidase inhibitors has not been reported in the literature. Signs and symptoms of overdose would be expected to include nausea, abdominal bloating and pain, flatulence, and diarrhea. Because these agents do not stimulate endogenous insulin release, they should not produce hypoglycemia with overdose.

Thiazolidinediones

There are no published data describing the effects of overdose with the thiazolidinediones. Supratherapeutic doses of these agents ingested over a week have not been associated with acute toxicity.[3] Because this class of drugs does not stimulate insulin secretion, hypoglycemia is not expected to occur with overdose.

Meglitinides

As insulin secretagogues, meglitinides are expected to produce hypoglycemia after overdose. Unlike the sulfonylureas, however, these agents have a very short duration of action. Thus, the hypoglycemic effect should not be delayed in onset or prolonged in effect. Limited clinical overdose experience with meglitinides, however, precludes confident clinical predictions at this time. Nakayama and colleagues reported a case of a 30-year-old nondiabetic woman who presented to the emergency department 1 hour after ingesting 3420 mg of nateglinide in a suicide attempt.[48] Her initial blood glucose was 2 mmol/L (36 mg/dL) 1 hour after ingestion, which was treated with 50 mL of 50% dextrose. Four hours after ingestion, rebound hypoglycemia occurred, which necessitated further dextrose administration. The patient remained hypoglycemic for 6 hours after nateglinide ingestion. Surreptitious doses of repaglinide have been associated with severe hypoglycemia in an 18-year-old man.[49]

Insulin

Insulin overdose manifests primarily as hypoglycemia (see Box 64-1). Other effects include various metabolic abnormalities, such as hypokalemia, hypomagnesemia, hypophosphatemia, and hypocalcemia. Cardiac effects are uncommon but include tachyarrhythmias (i.e., atrial fibrillation, premature atrial and ventricular contractions, and ventricular tachycardia), bradyarrhythmias (i.e., sinus bradycardia, heart block), repolarization abnormalities on the electrocardiogram (i.e., T-wave flattening, ST-T changes, and QTc prolongation), angina and myocardial infarction, congestive heart failure, and hypertension. Hypothermia may occur with prolonged hypoglycemia. As for sulfonylureas, prolonged hypoglycemia may be associated with prolonged or permanent neurologic deficits.[50]

Insulin-induced hypoglycemia occurs very commonly as an unintentional adverse effect (see "Adverse Effects") but may also occur as an intentional overdose (self-poisoning with suicidal intent, poisoning of others with homicidal intent, or as part of Munchausen syndrome or Munchausen syndrome by proxy). Although intentional insulin overdose is uncommon, it likely occurs more frequently than is recognized or reported. In 2003, 2914 insulin exposures were reported to U.S. poison control centers, of which 493 (17%) were categorized as intentional.[8] The time of onset and duration of hypoglycemia that occur with insulin overdose depend on the type and dose of insulin preparation used, the blood glucose of the patient, the caloric intake of the patient just before and after the overdose, and the presence of insulin antibodies (insulin resistance) in the patient. The onset of hypoglycemia may be delayed after overdose with extended-release preparations (e.g., NPH and Lente).[51] The duration of hypoglycemia may be prolonged and last for days after massive subcutaneous overdose of insulin.[52]

ADVERSE EFFECTS

Sulfonylureas

Sulfonylureas are generally well tolerated; adverse effects occur in 2% to 4% of patients, with less than 2% of patients discontinuing therapy because of side effects.[15,53]

As for sulfonylurea overdose, the most common and severe complication of sulfonylurea therapeutic dosing is hypoglycemia. Hypoglycemia is simply an extension of the therapeutic objective and effects of these agents. Hypoglycemia occurs in 2% to 4% of patients; severe hypoglycemia requiring patient hospitalization occurs in 0.4 cases per 10,000 patient-years of treatment.[53,54] Clinically significant hypoglycemic reactions occur more commonly with agents that have a longer duration of action[2] (see Table 64-2). Risk factors for sulfonylurea-induced hypoglycemia include an age older than 60 years, impaired renal and hepatic function, poor nutrition, and multidrug therapy.[55,56] The use of other diabetes control agents may result in inadvertent hypoglycemia from syn-

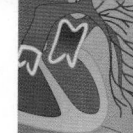

ergistic effects (pharmacodynamic interaction). Alternatively, hypoglycemia may occur with the coadministration of drugs that interfere with sulfonylurea protein binding, metabolism, or excretion (pharmacokinetic interaction). The concurrent use of sulfonylureas with the histamine-2 (H_2) receptor antagonists cimetidine and ranitidine, or with the antifungal azole derivatives ketoconazole and fluconazole, is associated with increased incidence of hypoglycemia.[29] In addition, the antibiotics doxycycline, ciprofloxacin, and gatifloxacin have been associated with increased incidence of hypoglycemia in patients taking sulfonylureas.[57-59] Furthermore, clofibrate, dicumarol, sulfonamides, sulfamethoxazole, angiotensin-converting enzyme inhibitors, nonsteroidal anti-inflammatory drugs (e.g., phenylbutazone, salicylates), β blockers, and ethanol may potentiate the hypoglycemic activity of these agents.[2,29,60]

Other adverse effects of sulfonylureas include hematologic (e.g., hemolytic anemia, bone marrow aplasia) and dermatologic (e.g., rashes, pruritus, erythema nodosum, erythema multiforme, and exfoliative dermatitis) complications. These effects are rare hypersensitivity reactions and usually occur during the first 6 weeks of therapy. Their incidence is less than 0.1% with all agents. GI side effects include nausea, vomiting, cholestatic jaundice, and liver function test abnormalities; they occur with a frequency of 1% to 3%. Weight gain is common in patients who achieve improved glycemic control and is probably the result of reduced caloric loss associated with the diminution in glycosuria.[9,61] Chlorpropamide, unique among the sulfonylureas, has been associated with a disulfiram-type reaction. Some sulfonylureas (e.g., chlorpropamide, glyburide, and glipizide) may produce hyponatremia by inducing increased renal sensitivity to antidiuretic hormone (syndrome of inappropriate antidiuretic hormone, or SIADH).[2,9,53] The sulfonylureas may be associated with an increased risk for cardiovascular mortality, but the data supporting this theory are conflicting.[2,62] In addition, some sulfonylureas can precipitate acute porphyria in susceptible individuals.[9]

Biguanides

When used at therapeutic doses, the most common side effects associated with metformin are GI and include anorexia, nausea, abdominal discomfort, and diarrhea. These symptoms occur in up to 20% of patients shortly after initiating therapy with metformin, but only rarely persist.[2] Nonetheless, about 10% of patients cannot tolerate the drug at any dose.[9] A metallic taste can also be observed in about 3% of patients taking metformin.[63]

The most serious adverse effect of metformin is lactic acidosis, which occurs in 0.06 cases per 1000 patient-years.[17] The incidence is significantly less with metformin therapy than with phenformin. Lactic acidosis is defined as a metabolic acidosis due to an accumulation of lactic acid in the blood in excess of 5 mmol/L with an accompanying blood pH of less than 7.35.[18,19] Biguanide-associated lactic acidosis is initially a type B lactic acidosis (not associated with tissue hypoxia or hypoperfusion).

BOX 64-2	CONTRAINDICATIONS TO BIGUANIDE THERAPY

- Renal impairment (plasma creatinine > 1.5 mg/dL [132 µmol/L] for men, > 1.4 mg/dL [124 µmol/L] for women)
- Cardiac or respiratory failure of sufficient magnitude to cause central hypoxia or reduced peripheral perfusion
- History of lactic acidosis
- Acute or chronic metabolic acidosis
- Severe infection that could lead to decreased tissue perfusion
- Liver dysfunction (demonstrated by abnormal liver function tests)
- Alcohol abuse with binge drinking sufficient to cause acute hepatotoxicity
- Use of iodinated radiographic contrast material (within 48 hours)
- Pregnancy

Adapted from Bailey CJ, Turner RC: Metformin. N Engl J Med 1996;334:574–579.

Type A lactic acidosis, however, is often superimposed on type B lactic acidosis in patients who are critically ill.

Biguanide-associated lactic acidosis has a mortality rate of 12% to 50%.[22] When this complication occurs at therapeutic doses, it usually is in the context of having been prescribed in patients for whom the drug was initially contraindicated (Box 64-2). It appears that a critical blood level of biguanide, as yet undefined, is required to produce the metabolic abnormalities that lead to lactic acidosis.[64] The listed contraindications, especially impaired renal function, are likely to result in impaired elimination and excessive blood levels of metformin, thus increasing the likelihood of the critical blood level and accumulation of lactic acid (see "Pharmacology and Pathophysiology"). As already stated, significant lactic acidosis may also occur after metformin overdose in the absence of established risk factors.[39,40]

In patients with metformin-associated lactic acidosis, there are frequently additional factors that increase blood lactate concentrations, such as major illness causing tissue hypoperfusion or liver disease.[28,65] Thus, an elevated plasma lactate concentration in someone who regularly takes metformin may primarily represent an underlying systemic process (e.g., septic shock) and not a direct complication of metformin therapy.[28] Iodinated contrast materials may create a predisposition to metformin-induced lactic acidosis. Current consensus recommendations are to withhold metformin for 24 to 48 hours before a planned procedure that necessitates administration of iodinated contrast. The metformin should not be reinstituted until at least 48 hours after the iodinated contrast administration.[66] Finally, treatment with metformin should be withheld if plasma lactate levels exceed 3 mmol/L (more than 3 mEq/L).[2]

α-Glucosidase Inhibitors

Adverse effects associated with the α-glucosidase inhibitors are primarily GI and include dose-related increases in flatulence, abdominal discomfort and bloating, and diarrhea.[2] Adverse effects tend to diminish with continued use.[67] Thus, side effects can be minimized by

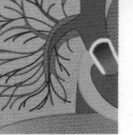

starting with low doses and titrating the dose upward at 4- to 8-week intervals.[2] Although approved for monotherapy, this class of drug rarely is used alone owing to its mild efficacy. More frequently, the α-glucosidase inhibitors are used in combination with sulfonylureas or insulin. This class of drugs is associated with dose-dependent hepatotoxicity (elevations of hepatic transaminases).[68] Hepatic transaminase elevations are usually asymptomatic and reversible with drug cessation.

Thiazolidinediones

The thiazolidinediones are relatively well tolerated. Side effects, when they occur, include anemia, edema, headache, myalgia, and weight gain. On average, the thiazolidinediones cause an increase of 2 to 3 pounds for every 1% decrease in glycosylated hemoglobin value.[25] Thus, these agents should be given cautiously, if at all, to patients with advanced heart failure or anemia. In Europe, the presence of congestive heart failure is considered a contraindication to the use of thiazolidinediones.[9] Idiosyncratic hepatotoxicity has rarely been associated with pioglitazone or rosiglitazone therapy.[69,70] The presence of hepatic dysfunction is considered a contraindication to treatment with thiazolidinediones. Hypoglycemia does not occur with thiazolidinedione monotherapy but has been described during combination therapy with sulfonylureas or insulin.

Meglitinides

The most common adverse effects from meglitinides include GI symptoms, weight gain, and hypoglycemia. Repaglinide has an incidence of adverse reactions similar to that observed with sulfonylureas, whereas nateglinide appears to be better tolerated.[2,6,26,30] Nateglinide appears to have a hypoglycemic effect that is more mild.[30]

Insulin

The primary adverse reaction from insulin is hypoglycemia.[2] Hypoglycemia may occur from an increase in insulin dose, change in insulin preparation, decreased food intake, increased exercise, or impaired insulin clearance (in those with renal dysfunction). The time of onset of hypoglycemia and time to peak hypoglycemic effect after therapeutic doses of insulin have been established and are listed in Table 64-3. The duration of hypoglycemia is less than that observed with insulin overdoses. Hypokalemia, hypomagnesemia, and hypophosphatemia may also occur as adverse effects of insulin, particularly if insulin is administered at high therapeutic doses.

DIAGNOSIS

The diagnosis of acute toxicity from diabetes control agents often occurs in the setting of symptomatic hypoglycemia and a positive history of exposure. Hypoglycemia should be considered in every patient who

TABLE 64-4 Dosing of Dextrose	
AGE	**DEXTROSE**
Adults	0.5–1.0 g/kg or 1–2 mL/kg D-50 (50% dextrose)
Children	2–4 mL/kg D-25
Infants/newborns	5–10 mL/kg D-10

presents after a seizure or with an alteration in mental status. The diagnosis should be rapidly excluded or confirmed on the basis of a bedside test for blood glucose concentration. When this cannot be done rapidly, or when the result is equivocal, an intravenous bolus of 50% dextrose (0.5 to 1 g/kg or 1 to 2 mL/kg D-50-W; Table 64-4) should be administered empirically. The diagnosis of hypoglycemia typically requires symptoms and a positive response to supplemental dextrose. A lack of response, however, does not exclude the diagnosis because prolonged, severe hypoglycemia can result in permanent neurology deficits that will not respond to correction of hypoglycemia. If a diagnosis of hypoglycemia is made, a patient history may help to establish whether toxicity from a diabetes control agent (e.g., sulfonylurea, meglitinides, insulin) is the likely cause. If the history does not suggest the diagnosis, other drug-associated and medical causes of hypoglycemia should be considered and addressed (Box 64-3).

Specific drug levels are rarely necessary to make the diagnosis. When no explanation for hypoglycemia is initially apparent, however, measurements of serum insulin, C peptide, proinsulin, and sulfonylurea concentrations and a urine screen for sulfonylureas may be helpful to establish a diagnosis, particularly in the setting of accidental, surreptitious, or felonious poisoning. Standard blood and urine toxic screens should be performed to rule out the presence of other drugs associated with hypoglycemia (e.g., ethanol, salicylate). Because therapeutic doses of sulfonylureas can produce hypoglycemia, the qualitative presence of this class of agents in blood or urine of patients not regularly prescribed these drugs is sufficient to confirm the diagnosis. In the presence of exogenous insulin injection, C peptide and proinsulin levels are low. In the presence of sulfonylurea or meglitinide toxicity (insulin secretagogues) or an insulinoma, the proinsulin, insulin, and C-peptide levels should be elevated. Insulinomas can be differentiated from ingestion of insulin secretagogues by the presence of very high proinsulin levels in patients with insulinomas, with an increased ratio of proinsulin to insulin.[71]

The diagnosis of biguanide-induced lactic acidosis should be suspected in any patient receiving therapeutic or taking excessive doses of biguanides who becomes ill. Laboratory analysis in these patients should include measurements of blood glucose, blood urea nitrogen, creatinine, electrolytes, and lactate and urinalysis. The diagnosis is confirmed by documentation of an anion-gap metabolic acidosis and an elevated serum lactate level (more than 5 mmol/L). For patients with an elevated

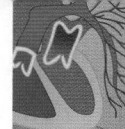

BOX 64-3	CAUSES OF HYPOGLYCEMIA

Gastrointestinal

Diarrhea (especially in children)
Pancreatitis
Postgastrectomy
Short gut syndrome

Hepatic

Alcoholism
Cirrhosis
Fulminant hepatic failure
Reye's syndrome

Metabolic/Endocrine

Adrenal insufficiency
Beckwith-Wiedemann syndrome
Carnitine deficiency
Fructose intolerance
Galactose intolerance
Glucagon deficiency
Glycogen storage diseases
Growth hormone deficiency
Hyperinsulinemia (neonates of diabetic mothers)
Hypothyroidism
Panhypopituitarism (Sheehan's syndrome)

Miscellaneous

Acquired immunodeficiency syndrome (AIDS)
Autoimmune disorders
Pregnancy

Oncologic

Insulinoma
Extrapancreatic/mesenchymal neoplasm

Systemic Illness

Burns
Hyperthermia
Severe renal or cardiac dysfunction
Sepsis
Starvation (or anorexia nervosa)

Toxin

Ackee fruit (hypoglycin A)
β-Adrenergic blockers (especially propranolol)
Disopyramide
Ethanol (especially in children)
Insulin
Meglitinides
Mushrooms
Opioids
Pentamidine
Quinine/quinidine
Salicylates
Sulfonylurea
Sulfonamides
Valproic acid

anion gap or blood lactate level, an arterial blood gas should be performed. The hallmark of biguanide-associated lactic acidosis is severe acidosis without evidence of hypotension or hypoxia.

TREATMENT

Overview

Treatment of diabetes control agent poisoning is largely directed at evaluating for and treating hypoglycemia. Although patients with significant central nervous system or respiratory depression may sometimes need airway protection, breathing assistance, and cardiovascular support, correction of hypoglycemia may be sufficient to normalize neurologic or cardiopulmonary function. In addition to fingerstick glucose determination and dextrose administration as necessary, supplemental oxygen, continuous pulse oximetry, and parenteral thiamine and naloxone should be considered in patients with altered mental status or seizures. All symptomatic patients should have an intravenous line established and continuous cardiac monitoring performed. Frequent neurologic evaluation and vital sign and fingerstick determinations should be performed in the initial several hours of evaluation. Fluid and electrolyte abnormalities should be corrected as necessary. Therapy (e.g., antidotal treatment, enhanced elimination) that is unique to each class of agents is discussed below.

After initial patient stabilization, GI decontamination is recommended for patients who present after acute oral overdose of most diabetes control agents. Single-dose administration of activated charcoal (1 g/kg orally or by nasogastric tube) is the preferred method of GI decontamination. Orogastric lavage is not routinely recommended because the risk for death after acute diabetes control agent overdose is very low. If performed, gastric lavage should be followed by the administration of activated charcoal.

Sulfonylurea Poisoning

Treatment with dextrose should be reserved for patients with symptomatic hypoglycemia and withheld from patients with low blood glucose values in the absence of symptoms. The administration of dextrose to an asymptomatic patient with numeric hypoglycemia may necessitate further treatment with dextrose and force a prolonged period of observation. Even in the absence of sulfonylurea exposure, exogenous dextrose administration can stimulate further insulin secretion, particularly when associated with transient hyperglycemia (overshoot). Rebound euglycemia or hypoglycemia often occurs and requires further treatment with dextrose. This pattern of cyclical hypoglycemia often results in a longer period of observation that would not have been necessary if dextrose had not been administered initially.

Treatment with oral dextrose may be sufficient for patients with mild hypoglycemia, whereas those with significant symptoms should receive an intravenous bolus of concentrated dextrose (see Table 64-4). It is advisable to give no more dextrose than is necessary to achieve euglycemia; overshoot may precipitate rebound hypoglycemia. Frequent fingerstick blood glucose determinations help to guide initial and continued dextrose supplementation. Once euglycemia is achieved, patients

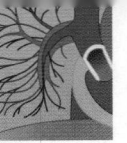

should be given a meal if oral intake is feasible and not contraindicated. A continuous infusion of 10% to 20% dextrose in water (D-10 to D-20) may be necessary to maintain euglycemia in patients with an intentional sulfonylurea overdose. If concentrations of 20% dextrose or greater are used, the infusion should be given through a central venous catheter to avoid damage to peripheral veins.

If oral dextrose is not an option (owing to patient altered mental status) and intravenous dextrose cannot be administered because of difficulty with intravenous access, glucagon can be administered to produce a temporary elevation in blood glucose. Glucagon is particularly helpful in the preadmission setting. Glucagon is administered by intramuscular or subcutaneous injection (1 mg for adults and children greater than 20 kg; 0.5 mg for children less than 20 kg). Glucagon increases blood glucose by promoting glycogenolysis and gluconeogenesis. It is usually effective only when adequate glycogen stores exist. Glucagon stimulates insulin release and, thus, needs to be followed by the parenteral administration of glucose.[72] Glucagon is only a bridging therapy before successful intravenous access and dextrose administration. Glucagon administration may be associated with nausea and vomiting.

In the setting of sulfonylurea toxicity, a profound rebound or recurrent hypoglycemia often occurs within 30 minutes of initial dextrose administration.[73] Although dextrose is the recommended initial treatment for all episodes of symptomatic hypoglycemia, a number of additional drugs can be used as adjuncts in the management of sulfonylurea-induced hypoglycemia.

The antihypertensive diazoxide effectively inhibits insulin secretion from the pancreatic β cells and has been used successfully in the management of refractory sulfonylurea-induced hypoglycemia.[74] Specifically, diazoxide may bind at the sulfonylurea binding site to prevent membrane depolarization and insulin release. Diazoxide is given by slow intravenous infusion over 30 minutes (3 mg/kg in adults; 1 to 3 mg/kg in children); the dose may be repeated every 4 hours. Diazoxide is complicated by orthostatic hypotension, tachycardia, and sodium and water retention.

Octreotide, a long-acting synthetic analog of somatostatin, is a potent inhibitor of insulin, glucagon, and growth hormone secretion. It has been reported to effectively inhibit excessive insulin secretion and significantly reduce dextrose requirements after sulfonylurea overdose. With octreotide treatment, insulin levels are reduced to baseline values, and there are fewer episodes of rebound hypoglycemia.[73-79] It appears that octreotide is superior to diazoxide for reducing the subsequent amount of glucose needed after the initial dextrose treatment.[73,74] The use of dextrose followed by octreotide should be considered first-line therapy in patients with sulfonylurea-induced hypoglycemia. Octreotide should be dosed in all individuals with a single episode of symptomatic hypoglycemia; it is not necessary to wait for recurrent hypoglycemia. Octreotide can be given by subcutaneous or intravenous injection (1 to 2 μg/kg in children and 50 to 100 μg in adults).[76] The dose can be

repeated in 6 to 12 hours, if clinically necessary. No significant side effects occur with octreotide therapy.

Activated charcoal has been demonstrated to bind effectively to chlorpropamide, tolbutamide, tolazamide, glibenclamide, and glipizide in vitro,[80] and to tolbutamide, chlorpropamide, and glipizide in vivo.[81-83] Although there has not previously been a study demonstrating clinical benefit from the administration of activated charcoal to patients who overdose on sulfonylureas, its administration is recommended in the overdose setting. The role of whole bowel irrigation is unknown after ingestion of sustained-release agents (e.g., Glucotrol XL) from this class.

Most cases of sulfonylurea overdoses are adequately managed with dextrose supplementation, and attempts at enhanced elimination are not indicated. Alkalinization of the urine has been demonstrated to enhance the excretion of chlorpropamide (a weak acid, pKa 4.8), reducing its elimination half-life from 50 to 13 hours.[81] However, in their position statement on urinary alkalinization, the American Academy of Clinical Toxicology and the European Association of Poison Centers and Clinical Toxicologists state "as the administration of dextrose alone is effective treatment in the majority of patients with chlorpropamide poisoning, which is now rare, urine alkalinization is only likely to be employed very occasionally.[84] Urinary alkalinization is not expected to enhance urinary excretion of other sulfonylureas.

Charcoal hemoperfusion was demonstrated to enhance elimination of chlorpropamide after overdose by a man with chronic renal failure.[85] In general, the use of extracorporeal methods to enhance removal of sulfonylureas is not recommended; most agents are metabolized in the liver. Repeat-dose activated charcoal is ineffective in enhancing elimination of chlorpropamide, and therefore is not recommended.[86] The use of multidose activated charcoal has not been investigated for other sulfonylureas.

Metformin Poisoning

The treatment of biguanide toxicity is supportive. Initial management should focus on stabilization of the airway, breathing, and circulation. Adequate and early volume expansion is essential and may improve lactic acidosis. Hypoglycemia, although rarely present or profound, should be corrected with intravenous dextrose administration.

The administration of intravenous bicarbonate to those with biguanide-induced lactic acidosis is controversial. Sodium bicarbonate may be detrimental by resulting in paradoxical acidification of cerebrospinal and intracellular fluid; increased hemoglobin affinity for oxygen, leading to impaired oxygen delivery to the tissues; hypernatremia and volume overload; severe hypokalemia and hypocalcemia; and increased cellular membrane permeability to biguanides, resulting in further increases in cellular lactate production.[87,88] Sodium bicarbonate therapy is not recommended because it has not been associated with clinical benefit in patients with biguanide-induced or other forms of lactic acidosis.[88-91]

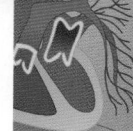

Hemodialysis with a bicarbonate dialysate has been reported to dramatically increase the survival rate of patients with metformin-induced lactic acidosis. Lalau and associates reported on five patients with severe metformin-induced lactic acidosis, whose clinical status and metabolic abnormalities rapidly responded to bicarbonate hemodialysis despite incomplete removal of metformin as determined by serum sampling. All patients had acute renal failure, and three were in cardiovascular collapse at the time of presentation.[92] In addition, Teale and colleagues reported on two patients with intentional metformin overdose with cardiovascular collapse, who were successfully managed with continuous venovenous hemodiafiltration.[39] Hemodialysis is recommended as first-line treatment in patients with severe biguanide-induced lactic acidosis.

α-Glucosidase Inhibitor and Thiazolidinedione Poisoning

The initial management of toxicity associated with α-glucosidase inhibitors and thiazolidinediones is supportive. Adequate volume expansion should be commenced early, if indicated. Hypoglycemia, which should only occur when these agents are ingested in combination with insulin secretagogues, should be treated with intravenous dextrose administration. In addition to standard laboratory analysis in poisoned patients, liver function tests should be obtained in patients who overdose on α-glucosidase inhibitors.

Meglitinide Poisoning

Treatment is aimed at correcting symptomatic hypoglycemia with administration of intravenous dextrose as necessary. The risk for and duration of hypoglycemia should last only a few hours after ingestion of meglitinides. Thus, a 4-hour period of observation is sufficient for patients who ingest meglitinides, even for those who required initial treatment with dextrose for symptomatic hypoglycemia.

Insulin Toxicity

The mainstay of treatment for insulin toxicity is the administration of supplemental dextrose for symptomatic hypoglycemia and correction of coexisting metabolic abnormalities (e.g., hypokalemia) as necessary. As for sulfonylurea toxicity, patients with mild hypoglycemia may be given an oral, rapidly acting dextrose formulation followed by a small meal. Patients who develop significant symptomatic hypoglycemia should receive an intravenous bolus of concentrated dextrose (see Table 64-4) followed by a continuous infusion of 10% or 20% dextrose. As for sulfonylurea overdose, overzealous administration of dextrose may precipitate rebound hyperinsulinemia (for patients without type 1 diabetes). Thus, the dextrose infusion should be titrated to just maintain euglycemia.

Oral overdose of insulin will not produce clinical effects because of rapid breakdown in the stomach.

Prolonged hypoglycemia (lasting days) has occurred in patients who have intentionally injected large subcutaneous overdoses of insulin.[93] Although surgical excision of skin and subcutaneous tissue insulin depots has been described for such patients, the clinical utility of this approach is unknown and cannot be recommended.[94,95,96]

DISPOSITION

Because of the potential for prolonged hypoglycemic effects, all patients who develop symptomatic hypoglycemia from sulfonylureas require admission for ongoing blood glucose monitoring and therapy with intravenous dextrose and octreotide, as necessary. The onset of hypoglycemia after sulfonylurea overdose may be delayed for up to 18 hours; therefore, all patients with deliberate overdose and all children with suspected ingestion must be admitted for up to 24 hours. A hospitalized patient is ready for medical discharge when euglycemia has been maintained for a period of 8 to 12 hours after the last dose of octreotide and supplemental parenteral dextrose. Appropriate psychiatric evaluation in cases of deliberate self-overdose should take place before final discharge. When the overdose was inadvertent, appropriate educational intervention should occur before discharge.

Evidence of lactic acidosis associated with biguanide therapy or after biguanide overdose mandates hospital admission. Lactic acidosis is unlikely to develop in individuals with normal renal function after relatively small ingestions of metformin, but because a dose–response relationship has not been well characterized, all patients with metformin overdose should be observed for at least 6 hours. If there is no evidence of acidosis or hypoglycemia, and the patient remains asymptomatic at that time, then the patient may be discharged after appropriate psychiatric evaluation and educational intervention.

For patients who ingest excessive doses of the thiazolidinediones, α-glucosidase inhibitors, or meglitinides, a 4- to 6-hour observation period is appropriate. The observation period may need to be extended if hypoglycemia occurs.

The duration of hospital observation necessary after insulin toxicity depends on the quantity and type of insulin injected, patient intent, and duration of symptomatic hypoglycemia. Patients who experience an unintentional hypoglycemic episode associated with therapeutic dosing (an insulin reaction) typically require only several hours emergency department observation. These patients can be safely discharged provided they have eaten a small meal, do not develop recurrent hypoglycemia during their period of observation, are at their baseline mental and health status at the time of discharge, are reliable or are discharged with reliable caretakers, and have been observed in the emergency department beyond the time of expected peak effects from the injected insulin preparation (see Table 64-3). Patients who have intentionally overdosed on insulin

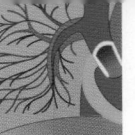

should be admitted for inpatient observation (24 hours) because of the possibility for delayed and prolonged hypoglycemia. Most of these patients are symptomatic within 12 hours of overdose.[93] Patients who require dextrose infusion after intentional insulin overdose should be observed for recurrent hypoglycemia for 8 to 12 hours after the dextrose infusion has been stopped. Intensive care unit admission is required for patients with significant and persistent central nervous system or cardiovascular abnormalities or those requiring large supplemental dextrose infusions to maintain euglycemia.

ACKEE FRUIT

Ackee (*Blighia sapida*), the national fruit of Jamaica, was originally imported to the Caribbean from West Africa in the 18th century (see Chapter 24). The ackee tree is a tall, evergreen, fruit-producing tree and is found in various parts of the world, including the Caribbean, the Antilles, Central America, and parts of Florida.[97] The fruit is yellow and opens while still attached to the tree to reveal three glassy black seeds surrounded by a thick, oily, yellow aril.

The ackee fruit was first associated with Jamaican vomiting sickness (also called *toxic hypoglycemic syndrome*) in 1875. Risk factors associated with the development of Jamaican vomiting sickness are threefold: (1) consumption of raw or unripe ackee fruit; (2) consumption of ackee that is forcibly opened; and (3) consumption of water in which unripe ackee was cooked.[98] The unripe ackee fruit contains hypoglycin A, which is a water-soluble liver toxin that causes profound hypoglycemia by interfering with certain cofactors and enzymes necessary for hepatic gluconeogenesis.[99] Hypoglycin A, or cyclo-propylaminoproprionic acid, interferes with carnitine-acyl CoA transferase and β oxidation of long-chain fatty acids.[100] Accumulations of serum carboxylic acids results in metabolic acidosis and leads to Jamaican vomiting sickness. Jamaican vomiting sickness is characterized by the onset of epigastric pain, which begins a few hours after eating the fruit. Shortly thereafter, there is a sudden onset of profuse vomiting and hypoglycemia. Seizures, coma, and metabolic acidosis are common, as is death.[97] Death typically occurs by 12 hours after ingestion. The hypoglycemia is profound, often with blood sugars as low as 3 mg/dL.[97]

The fruit is illegal in the United States, but nonetheless, there have been at least two reported cases in the United States in the 1990s. The first known case of Jamaican vomiting sickness occurred in Ohio, in a Jamaican female, after the consumption of canned Ackee.[101] The only other known case in the United States was a 27-year-old Jamaican man, residing in Connecticut, who presented with 2 months of jaundice, intermittent diarrhea, pruritus, right upper quadrant pain, and markedly elevated bilirubins.[102] This patient with cholestatic jaundice had resolution of his symptoms after he ceased consumption of the ackee fruit.

Treatment for poisoning from the ackee fruit is supportive, with correction of hypoglycemia, dehydration, acidosis, and metabolic abnormalities provided as necessary.

REFERENCES

1. Winer N, Sowers JR: Epidemiology of diabetes. J Clin Pharmacol 2004;44:397–405.
2. Davis SN, Granner DK: Insulin, oral hypoglycemic agents, and the pharmacology of the endocrine pancreas. In Hardman JG, Limbrid LE, Gilman AG (eds): Goodman & Gilman's the Pharmacological Basis of Therapeutics, 10th ed. New York, McGraw-Hill, 2001, pp 1679–1714.
3. Banting FG, Best CH, Collip JB, et al: Pancreatic extracts in the treatment of diabetes mellitus. Can Med Assoc J 1922;12:141–146.
4. Amos AF, McCarty DJ, Zimmet P: The rising global burden of diabetes and its complications: estimates and projections to the year 2010. Diabet Med 1997;14(Suppl 5):S1–S85.
5. Williams RH, Palmer JP: Farewell to phenformin for treating diabetes mellitus. Ann Intern Med 1975;83:567–568.
6. Inzucchi SE: Oral antihyperglycemic therapy for type 2 diabetes: scientific review. JAMA 2002;287:360–372.
7. Murphy EJ, Davern TJ, Shakil AO, et al: Troglitazone-induced fulminant hepatic failure: Acute Liver Failure Study Group. Dig Dis Sci 2000;45:549–553.
8. Watson WA, Litovitz TL, Klein-Schwartz W, et al: 2003 Annual report of the American Association of Poison Control Centers Toxic Exposure Surveillance System. Am J Emerg Med 2004;22:335–404.
9. Krentz AJ, Bailey CJ: Oral antidiabetic agents: current role in type 2 diabetes mellitus. Drugs 2005;65:385–411.
10. Hirsch IB: Insulin analogues. N Engl J Med 2005;352:174–183.
11. Ciechanowski K, Borowiak KS, Potocka BA, et al: Chlorpropamide toxicity with survival despite 27-day hypoglycemia. J Toxicol Clin Toxicol 1999;37:869–871.
12. Rosenfeld L: Insulin: discovery and controversy. Clin Chem 2002;48:2270–2288.
13. Hirsch IB: Drug therapy: insulin analogues. N Engl J Med 2005;352:174–183.
14. Beck-Nielsen H, Hother-Nielsen O, Pedersen O: Mechanism of action of sulfonylureas with special reference to the extra-pancreatic effect: an overview. Diabet Med 1988;5:613–620.
15. Gerich JE: Oral hypoglycemic agents. N Engl J Med 1989;321:1123–1145.
16. Czyzyk A, Tawecki J, Sadowski J, et al: Effect of biguanides on intestinal absorption of glucose. Diabetes 1968;17:492–498.
17. Wilholm BE, Myrhed M: Metformin-associated lactic acidosis in Sweden 1977–1991. Eur J Clin Pharmacol 1993;44:589–591.
18. Arieff AI: Pathogenesis of lactic acidosis. Diabetes Metab Rev 1989;5:637–649.
19. Luft FC: Lactic acidosis update for critical care clinicians. J Am Soc Nephrol 2001;12:S15–S19.
20. Misbin RI: Phenformin-associated lactic acidosis: pathogenesis and treatment. Ann Intern Med 1984;87:591–595.
21. Lalau JD, Race JM: Lactic acidosis in metformin therapy. Drugs 1999;58(Suppl 1):55–60.
22. Luft D, Schmulling RM, Eggstein M: Lactic acidosis in biguanide-treated diabetics: a review of 330 cases. Diabetologia 1978;14:75–87.
23. Bernier GM, Miller M, Sporingate CS: Lactic acid and phenformin hydrochloride. JAMA 1963;184:43–46.
24. Lebovitz HE: *Alpha* glucosidase inhibitors. Endocrinol Metab Clin North Am 1997;539–551.
25. Yki-Jarvinen HY: Thiazolidinediones. N Engl J Med 2004;351:1106–1118.
26. Landgraf R: Meglitinide analogues in the treatment of type 2 diabetes mellitus. Drugs Aging 2000;17:411–425.
27. Baselt RC: Disposition of Toxic Drugs and Chemicals in Man, 7th ed. Foster City, CA, Biomedical Publications, 2004.
28. Bailey CJ, Turner RC: Metformin. N Engl J Med 1996;334:57–579.
29. Scheen A: Drug interactions of clinical importance with anti-hyperglycaemic agents: an update. Drug Safety 2005;28:601–631.
30. Mikko N, Backman JT, Neuvonen M, et al: Rifampin decreases the plasma concentration and effects of repaglinide. Clin Pharmacol Ther 2000;68:495–500.

31. Field LB: Hypoglycemia: Definition, clinical presentations, classification, and laboratory tests. Endocrin Metabol Clin North Am 1989;18:27–43.
32. Gerich JE: Control of glycaemia. Ballieres Clin Endocrinol Metabol 1993;7:551–586.
33. Quadrani DA, Spiller HA, Widder P: Five year retrospective evaluation of sulfonylurea ingestion in children. J Toxicol Clin Toxicol 1996;34:267–270.
34. Spiller HA, Villalobos D, Krenzelok EP, et al: Prospective multicenter study of sulfonylurea ingestion in children. J Pediatr 1997; 131:141–146.
35. Dobson HL: Attempted suicide with phenformin. Diabetes 1965;14:811–812.
36. Pashley NRT, Felix RH: Phenformin overdose. BMJ 1972;1: 112–113.
37. Spiller HA: Management of antidiabetic medications in overdose. Drug Safety 1998;19:411–424.
38. Bingle JP, Storey GW, Winter JM: Fatal self-poisoning with phenformin. BMJ 1970;3:752.
39. Teale KFH, Devine A, Stewart H, Harper NJH: The management of metformin overdose. Anaesthesia 1998;53:691–701.
40. Lacher M, Hermanns-Clausen M, Haeffner K, et al: Severe metformin intoxication with lactic acidosis in an adolescent. Eur J Pediatr 2005;164:362–365.
41. Bismuth C, Gaultier M, Conso F, et al: Acidose lactique induite par l'ingestion excessive de metformine. Nouv Presse Med 1976;5: 261–263.
42. McLelland J: Recovery from metformin overdose. Diabet Med 1985;2:410–411.
43. Assan A, Heuelin C, Ganeval D, et al: Metformin-induced lactic acidosis in the presence of acute renal failure. Diabetologia 1977;13:211–217.
44. Barrueto F, Meggs WH, Barchman JM: Clearance of metformin by hemofiltration in overdose. J Toxicol Clin Toxicol 2002;40:177–180.
45. Larcan A, Lambert H, Ginsbourger F: Acute intoxication by phenformine hyperlactatemia reversible with extra-renal purification. Vet Hum Toxicol 1979;21(Suppl):19–22.
46. Brady WJ, Carter CT: Metformin overdose. Am J Emerg Med 1997;15:107–108.
47. Spiller HA, Weber JA, Winter ML, et al: Multicenter case series of pediatric metformin ingestion. Ann Pharmacother 2000;34: 1385–1388.
48. Nakayama S, Hirose T, Watada H, et al: Hypoglycemia following a nateglinide overdose in a suicide attempt. Diabetes Care 2005;28:227–228.
49. Hirshberg B, Skarulis MC, Pucino F, et al: Repaglinide-induced factitious hypoglycemia. J Clin Endocrinol Metab 2001;86: 475–477.
50. Cooper AJ: Attempted suicide using insulin by a non diabetic: a case study demonstrating the acute and chronic consequences of profound hypoglycemia. Can J Psychiatry 1994;39:103–107.
51. Stapczynski JS, Haskell RJ: Duration of hypoglycemia and need for intravenous glucose following intentional overdoses of insulin. Ann Emerg Med 1984;13:505–511.
52. Roberge R, Martin TG, Delbridge TR: Intentional massive insulin overdose: recognition and management. Ann Emerg Med 1993;22:228–234.
53. Paice BJ, Paterson KR, Lawson DH: Undesired effects of sulphonylurea drugs. Adverse Drug React Acute Poisoning Rev 1985;4:23–26.
54. DeFronzo RA: Pharmacologic therapy for type 2 diabetes mellitus. Ann Intern Med 2000;133:73–74.
55. Veitch PC, Clifton-Bligh RJ: Long-acting sulfonylureas-long acting hypoglycaemia. Med J Aust 2004;180:84–85.
56. Harrower ADB: Comparative tolerability of sulfonylureas in diabetes mellitus. Drug Safety 2000;22:313–320.
57. Odeh M, Oliven A: Doxycycline-induced hypoglycaemia. J Clin Pharmacol 2000;40:1173–1174.
58. Roberge RJ, Kaplan R, Frank R, et al: Glyburide-ciprofloxacin interaction with resistant hypoglycemia. Ann Emerg Med 2000;36:160–163.
59. Menzies DJ, Dorsainvil PA, Cunha BA, et al: Severe and persistent hypoglycemia due to gatifloxacin interaction with oral hypoglycemic agents. Am J Med 2002;113:232–234.
60. Kubacka RT, Antal EJ, Juhl RP, et al: Effects of aspirin and ibuprofen on the pharmacokinetics and pharmacodynamics of glyburide in healthy subjects. Ann Pharmacother 1996;30:20–26.
61. Welle S, Nair KS, Lockwood D: Effect of sulfonylurea and insulin on energy expenditure in type II diabetes mellitus. J Clin Endocrinol Metab 1988;6:593–597.
62. Aronow WS: Oral sulfonylureas and CV mortality. Geriatrics 2004;59:45–49.
63. Slagle M: Medication update. South Med J 2002;95:50–55.
64. Gan SC, Barr J, Arieff AI, Pear RG: Biguanide-associated lactic acidosis: case report and review of the literature. Arch Intern Med 1992;152:2333–2336.
65. Stades AME, Heikens JT, Erkelens DW, et al: Metformin and lactic acidosis: cause or coincidence? A review of the case reports. J Intern Med 2004;255:179–187.
66. Nisbet J, Sturtevant JM, Prins JB: Metformin and serious adverse effects. Med J Aust 2004;180:53–54.
67. Martin AE, Montgomery PA: Acarbose: an alpha-glucosidase inhibitor. Am J Health Syst Pharm 1996;53:2277–2290.
68. Carrasosa M, Pascual F, Aresti S. Acarbose-induced acute severe hepatotoxicity. Lancet 1997;349:698–699.
69. Al-Salaman J, Arjomand H, Kemp D, et al: Hepatocellular injury in a patient receiving rosiglitazone: a case report. Ann Intern Med 2000;132:121–124.
70. Maeda K: Hepatocellular injury in a patient receiving pioglitazone. Ann Intern Med 2001;135:306.
71. Hampton SM, Beyzavi K, Teale D, et al: A direct assay for proinsulin and its application in hypoglycemia. Clin Endocrinol 1988;29:9–16.
72. Thoma ME, Glauser J, Genuth S: Persistent hypoglycemia and hyperinsulinemia: caution in using glucagon. Am J Emerg Med 1996;14:99–101.
73. Boyle PJ, Justice K, Krentz AJ: Octreotide reverses hyperinsulinemia and prevents hypoglycemia induced by sulfonylurea overdoses. J Clin Endocrinol Metab 1993;76:752–756.
74. Palatnick W, Meatherall RC, Tenenbein M: Clinical spectrum of sulfonylurea overdose and experience with diazoxide. Arch Intern Med 1991;151:1859–1862.
75. Crawford BA, Perera C: Octreotide treatment for sulfonylurea-induced hypoglycemia. Med J Aust 2004;180:540–541.
76. McLaughlin SA, Crandall CS, McKinney PE: Octreotide: an antidote for sulfonylurea-induced hypoglycemia. Ann Emerg Med 2000;36:133–138.
77. Carr R, Zed PJ: Octreotide for sulfonylurea-induced hypoglycemia following overdose. Ann Pharmacother 2002;36:1727–1732.
78. Green RS, Palatnick W: Effectiveness of octreotide in a case of refractory sulfonylurea-induced hypoglycemia. J Emerg Med 2003;25:283–287.
79. Krentz AJ, Boyle PJ, Justice KM, et al: Successful treatment of severe refractory sulfonylurea-induced hypoglycemia with octreotide. Diabetes Care 1993;16:184–186.
80. Kannisto H, Neuvonen PJ: Adsorption of sulfonylureas onto activated charcoal. J Pharmacol Sci 1984;73:253–256.
81. Neuvonen PJ, Karhainen S: Effects of charcoal, sodium bicarbonate, and ammonia chloride on chlorpropamide kinetics. Clin Pharmacol Ther 1983;33:386–393.
82. Neuvonen PJ, Kannisto H, Hirvisalo EL: Effect of activated charcoal on absorption of tolbutamide and valproate in man. Eur J Clin Pharmacol 1983;24:243–246.
83. Kivisto KT, Neuvonen PJ: The effect of cholestyramine and activated charcoal on glipizide absorption. Br J Clin Pharmacol 1990;30:733–736.
84. Proudfoot AT, Krenzelok EP, Vale JA: Position paper on urine alkalinization. J Toxicol Clin Toxicol 2004;42:1–26.
85. Ludwig SM, McKenzie J, Faiman C: Chlorpropamide overdose in renal failure: Management with charcoal hemoperfusion. Am J Kidney Dis 1987;10:457–460.
86. American Academy of Clinical Toxicology; European Association of Poison Centres and Clinical Toxicologists: Position statement and practice guidelines on the use of multi-dose activated charcoal in the treatment of acute poisoning. J Toxicol Clin Toxicol 1999;37:731–751.
87. Arieff AJ: Indications for use of bicarbonate in patients with metabolic acidosis. Br J Anaesth 1991;67:165–177.

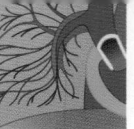

88. Forsythe SM, Schmidt GA: Sodium bicarbonate for the treatment of lactic acidosis. Chest 2000;117:260–267.

89. Fulop M, Hoberman HD: Phenformin-associated metabolic acidosis. Diabetes 1976;25:292–296.

90. Cooper JD, Walley KR, Wiggs BR, Russell JA: Bicarbonate does not improve hemodynamics in critically ill patients who have lactic acidosis. Ann Intern Med 1990;112:492–498.

91. Ryder RE: The danger of high dose sodium bicarbonate in biguanide-induced lactic acidosis: the theory, the practice and alternative therapies. Br J Clin Pract 1987;41:730–737.

92. Lalau JD, Westeel PF, Debussche X, et al: Bicarbonate hemodialysis: an adequate treatment for lactic acidosis in diabetics treated by metformin. Intensive Care Med 1987;13:383–387.

93. Arem R, Zoghbi W: Insulin overdose in eight patients: insulin pharmacokinetics and review of the literature. Medicine 1985;64:323–332.

94. Tofade TS, Liles EA: Intentional overdose with insulin glargine and insulin aspart. Pharmacotherapy 2004;24:1412–1418.

95 McIntyre AS, Woolf VJ, Burnham WR: Local excision of subcutaneous fat in the management of insulin overdose. Br J Surg 1986;73:538.

96 Campbell IW, Ratcliffe JG: Suicidal insulin overdose managed by excision of insulin injection site. BMJ 1982;285:408–409.

97. Toxic hypoglycemic syndrome—Jamaica, 1989–1991. MMWR Morb Mortal Wkly Rep 1992;41:53–55.

98. Ashcroft MT: Some noninfective diseases endemic in the West Indies. Trop Geogr Med 1978;30:5–21.

99. Feng PC, Patrick SJ: Studies of the action of hypoglycin-A, an hypoglycemic substance. Br J Pharmacol 1958;13:125–130.

100. Addae JR, Melvill GN: A re-examination of the mechanism of ackee induced vomiting sickness. West Ind Med J 1988;37:6–8.

101. McTague JA, Forney R: Jamaican vomiting sickness in Toledo, Ohio. Ann Emerg Med 1994;23:1116–1118.

102. Larson J, Vender R, Camuto P: Cholestatic jaundice due to ackee fruit poisoning. Am J Gastroenterol 1994;89:1577–1578.

65

Theophylline and Caffeine

MICHAEL W. SHANNON, MD, MPH

At a Glance...

- Methylxanthines are purine derivatives structurally related to adenosine.
- Methylxanthines have a narrow therapeutic index. Adverse effects can appear even at therapeutic doses and serum concentrations.
- Manifestations of theophylline intoxication vary according to mechanism of overdose (acute, chronic, or acute on therapeutic).
- The major life-threatening events of theophylline intoxication are seizures and cardiac arrhythmias.
- Metabolic consequences include hypokalemia, hyperglycemia, and metabolic acidosis.
- Management strategies for theophylline intoxication include supportive care, administration of multiple-dose activated charcoal, and, in severe cases, hemodialysis.
- Hemodialysis is preferred over hemoperfusion in the treatment of severe theophylline intoxication, because it is safer, more available, and equally effective.

Theophylline, caffeine, and theobromine are the major members of a group of pharmacologic agents known as *methylxanthines*. These drugs continue to have a ubiquitous position in society: Caffeine is used around the world for the pleasure that its mild stimulation provides. For almost a century, theophylline has been used for the treatment of respiratory ailments. Although theophylline use has fallen dramatically in recent years, it enjoys continued use as a therapeutic agent.

THEOPHYLLINE

Theophylline is used to treat various illnesses. At one time, it was the primary therapy for asthma, considered valuable both for treatment of acute exacerbations and for long-term prophylactic therapy.[1] Over the past two decades, β-adrenergic agonists have largely replaced theophylline for this indication, having a more favorable profile of safety and efficacy. However, theophylline is still used as a primary agent in areas where β-adrenergic agonists are less available and for individuals who have asthma that is resistant to β-adrenergic agonist and corticosteroid therapy.[2] Moreover, data that suggest that theophylline has anti-inflammatory properties have led to a slight increase in its use.[3,4] Besides asthma, theophylline is used for other syndromes of airway obstruction including chronic obstructive pulmonary disease in adults and bronchiolitis in infants, although there remains controversy about its efficacy in these diseases.[5-8] Theophylline is prescribed for neonates, particularly premature neonates, who have apnea and bradycardia.[9,10] Recent data suggest benefit in cardiac resuscitation, in renal protection after exposure to nephrotoxic agents, and in the treatment of acute mountain sickness.[11-14]

Individuals develop theophylline intoxication by two general mechanisms. First, its general availability makes theophylline an agent that can be ingested by curious toddlers or suicidal adolescents or adults, producing *acute intoxication*. Second, because of its highly variable pharmacokinetics and narrow therapeutic index, theophylline is often responsible for unintentional *chronic intoxication*. By either mechanism, theophylline poisoning leads to a host of clinical and metabolic complications that often result in disastrous consequences, including death. A thorough understanding of theophylline intoxication, including rational and effective treatment algorithms (Box 65-1), is therefore necessary for management of this overdose.

BOX 65-1   TREATMENT ALGORITHM FOR ACUTE THEOPHYLLINE INTOXICATION

Supportive Care

Airway control, respiratory support, and vascular access as needed; cardiorespiratory monitoring

Treatment of Life-Threatening Events

Seizures
  Give benzodiazepines. Add barbiturates if necessary. Avoid phenytoin.
  Paralyze if necessary. Provide electroencephalogram monitoring.
Cardiac arrhythmias
  Supraventricular—administer adenosine. Consider β blocker or calcium channel blocker.
  Ventricular—treat specific rhythm disturbance according to advanced cardiac life support protocols.

Laboratory Assessment

Electrolytes, arterial blood gas
Serum theophylline concentration (obtain serial measures until plateau is documented)
Electrocardiogram

Gastrointestinal Decontamination

Administer activated charcoal.
No established role for gastric emptying, e.g., ipecac or lavage. No role for cathartic administration.

Correction of Metabolic Disturbances

Hyperglycemia does not require treatment.
Hypokalemia should not be treated unless severe.
Metabolic acidosis is typically modest and requires no treatment.

Elimination Enhancement

Administer activated charcoal every 2–4 hours.
Consider hemodialysis for severe cases.
Hemoperfusion is also efficacious.

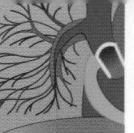

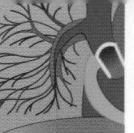

FIGURE 65-1 Theophylline and related compounds.

Structure and Structural Relationships

As illustrated in Figure 65-1, the methylxanthines are purines that are structurally related to the nucleotides adenine and guanine. Theophylline is 1,3-dimethylxanthine. It is closely related to caffeine (1,3,7-trimethylxanthine) and theobromine (3,7-dimethylxanthine). Caffeine is found in high concentration in coffee and certain teas. Theobromine is primarily found in cocoa. A related drug, pentoxifylline, is prescribed for treatment of peripheral vascular disease. Adenosine, which is an adenine-ribose nucleoside, is closely related to theophylline in structure and appears to have an important role in theophylline's pharmacologic actions and toxic effects.

Theophylline products are available as solutions, tablets, and sustained-release capsules. Because of its poor solubility in water, theophylline has an intravenous form, aminophylline, which is about 80% theophylline by weight.[15]

Pharmacology

PHARMACOKINETICS

In its oral form, theophylline is most commonly prescribed as a sustained-release capsule. Sustained-release theophylline is designed to provide stable serum concentrations by having a gastrointestinal (GI) absorption rate that approximates that of drug elimination. These agents are not completely absorbed until 6 to 8 hours after ingestion. Overdoses of sustained-release theophylline can be associated with 15- to 24-hour delays to peak absorption. There is no significant presystemic clearance (first-pass effect) of the drug.

Once absorbed, theophylline is distributed throughout the body with a relatively small volume of distribution (average, 0.45 L/kg, with a range of 0.3 to 0.7 L/kg).[15] Young infants and elderly people tend to have larger volumes of distribution. Plasma protein binding is 40% to 65%. The therapeutic serum concentration of theophylline is generally considered to be 10 to 20 µg/mL, although lower serum concentrations can produce the desired therapeutic effect. As a general rule, 1 mg/kg of administered theophylline raises serum theophylline concentration by 2 µg/mL. Theophylline freely crosses the placenta and enters breast milk.[15]

The metabolism of theophylline occurs through its biotransformation by the cytochrome P-450 system. The specific isoenzymes of this superfamily responsible for theophylline metabolism are CYP1A2, CYP2E1, and CYP3A3. The primary metabolic step is *N*-demethylation by the enzyme CYP1A2, producing the pharmacologically active agent 3-methylxanthine. The secondary metabolic pathway is hydroxylation, forming inactive 1,3-dimethyluric acid. Neonates also have the ability to metabolize theophylline by its methylation, producing caffeine. Moreover, neonates excrete about 50% of theophylline in urine unchanged (versus only 10% in children and adults).[15]

The rate of theophylline metabolism is variable; age is a very important influence (Table 65-1), with neonates

TABLE 65-1 Theophylline Elimination Patterns by Age			
POPULATION	**AGE**	**HALF-LIFE (hr)**	**CLEARANCE (mL/kg/min)**
Neonates and Infants			
Premature neonates	1 wk	30	0.29
Premature neonates	41 d	20	0.64
Term infants	18 wk	6.9	0.80
Term infants	34 wk	3.7	2.0
Children and Adolescents	4–15 yr	3.0	1.55
Adults			
Asthmatic nonsmokers	31 yr	9.4	0.65
Healthy nonsmokers	22–35 yr	8.1	0.86
Healthy elderly nonsmokers	67 yr	7.4	0.59
Healthy elderly nonsmokers	>70 yr	9.8	NA

NA, not available.

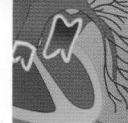

and elderly people eliminating the drug relatively slowly.[16] Theophylline clearance is maximal between the ages of 1 and 9 years; it decreases by about 50% in adults.[15] The reason for such age-dependent elimination rates is unclear but may be related to the relative activity of cytochrome P-450 enzymes.

Theophylline also exhibits Michaelis-Menten (saturable) kinetics. As a result, across a narrow range, increments in dose are associated with corresponding increments in serum theophylline concentration. At high doses, however, increments lead to disproportionate elevations in serum concentration.[17] Conversely, with severe theophylline intoxication, initial drug elimination rates are extremely slow, following zero order (dose-dependent) kinetics. With decreasing serum theophylline concentration, first order (dose-independent) kinetics eventually appear, leading to abrupt increases in elimination rate. These kinetics are often responsible for inadvertent theophylline intoxication, for example, if a clinician mistakenly assumes that a 50% increase in dose will always result in a 50% increase in serum theophylline concentration.

DRUG–DRUG INTERACTIONS

Theophylline is a drug whose metabolism is highly subject to alteration by concomitant drug use. A growing list of drugs, when prescribed with theophylline, can result in either increased or decreased clearance. Chronic theophylline intoxication is often a result of unrecognized drug interactions.

The drugs that have been associated with increased theophylline clearance are relatively few; all are known to be inducers of cytochrome P-450 enzymes. Such agents include phenobarbital, phenytoin, carbamazepine, and tobacco smoke. Patients who are taking these drugs often have difficulty maintaining therapeutic serum theophylline concentrations, requiring inordinately high doses because of their high drug clearance rate. If these patients discontinue their medications or quit smoking because they feel unwell, theophylline elimination rates can quickly revert to normal. For example, theophylline clearance falls by about 40% within 1 week of abstinence from cigarette smoking.[15] Passive smoking also appears to increase theophylline clearance.[18]

The list of agents that decrease theophylline clearance is extensive (Box 65-2). It is also notable that among drug classes, one member may inhibit clearance while others do not; for example, cimetidine, a histamine-2 (H_2) antagonist, is a potent inhibitor of theophylline metabolism. However, the H_2 antagonists ranitidine and famotidine do not appear to have this action. Other common drugs that diminish theophylline clearance include the macrolide antibiotics (e.g., erythromycin or clarithromycin) and the quinolone antibiotics (e.g., ciprofloxacin or norfloxacin). The erythromycin–theophylline interaction has been characterized as appearing between days 3 and 7 of their concomitant use, with serum theophylline concentrations rising by an average of 30% to 35% if dosing adjustments are not made.

BOX 65-2 **DRUGS COMMONLY REPORTED TO REDUCE THEOPHYLLINE METABOLISM**

Allopurinol
Cimetidine
Ciprofloxacin
Clarithromycin
Diltiazem
Disulfiram
Enoxacin
Erythromycin
Fluvoxamine
Interferon (recombinant α)
Methotrexate
Mexiletine
Nifedipine
Norfloxacin
Ofloxacin
Roxithromycin
Tacrine
Thiabendazole
Troleandomycin
Verapamil

Adapted from American Academy of Pediatrics Committee on Drugs: Precautions concerning the use of theophylline. Pediatrics 1992;89:781; and Hendeles L, Jenkins J, Temple R: Revised FDA labeling guidelines for theophylline oral dosage forms. Pharmacotherapy 1995;15:409.

DRUG–DISEASE INTERACTIONS

Several medical conditions have significant impact on theophylline pharmacokinetics. In young children, febrile illness can markedly reduce theophylline elimination; it is recommended that the dose of theophylline be reduced by half in children who are febrile for more than 24 hours.[10] Influenza and respiratory syncytial virus have also been reported as infectious agents that can reduce theophylline elimination.[10] Cardiac disease, particularly congestive heart failure, can reduce theophylline clearance by as much as 50%, presumably through hepatic congestion and secondary alterations in pharmacokinetic profile.[15] Primary hepatic disease can also reduce theophylline clearance by as much as 50%. Both cystic fibrosis and hyperthyroidism have been associated with increased theophylline clearance, resulting in larger dosing requirements. Renal disease has no important effect on theophylline pharmacokinetics.

PHARMACOLOGIC ACTIONS

Methylxanthines have a number of pharmacologic actions that give them therapeutic value. They relax smooth muscles, including those of the bronchi, esophagus, and gastroesophageal sphincter. They are central nervous system (CNS) stimulants that can reduce fatigue and improve concentration. Physiologic dependence may occur with this action: Acute abstinence from caffeine is associated with malaise, headaches, emotional lability, and depression. Other CNS actions include stimulation of the CNS respiratory center, producing

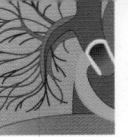
tachycardia. Cardiovascular effects include reduced peripheral vascular resistance with increased cardiac chronotropy and inotropy. Improved muscle function can enhance racing performance and improve pulmonary dynamics. Evidence indicates that theophylline is a potent inhibitor of renal erythropoietin production.[19] Methylxanthines are also diuretics.

MECHANISM OF ACTION

Four major hypotheses have been advanced to explain theophylline's pharmacologic effects. First is the theory that theophylline acts as an inhibitor of phosphodiesterase, the enzyme that breaks down intracellular cyclic adenosine monophosphate (cAMP). According to current theories, cAMP is created by the membrane-bound enzyme adenylate cyclase in response to a number of receptor-linked stimuli. cAMP effects a number of actions, including regulation of gated potassium channels. These actions are terminated when cAMP is metabolized by phosphodiesterase. Theophylline was once thought to be a potent inhibitor of phosphodiesterase. However, data now suggest that phosphodiesterase inhibition is negligible at therapeutic serum concentrations of theophylline, indicating that this mechanism alone cannot account for its actions.[20,21] The extent of phosphodiesterase inhibition has not been studied in victims of theophylline intoxication.

A second theory proposed for theophylline's actions is that of secondary sympathetic nervous system stimulation. In therapeutic doses, theophylline produces marked increases in the level of circulating catecholamines, particularly epinephrine and norepinephrine.[22-25] Theophylline's actions of bronchodilation, cardiac and respiratory stimulation, and even metabolic changes such as depression in serum potassium may result from augmented plasma catecholamine activity. In a canine model of theophylline poisoning, hypokalemia, increased oxygen consumption, metabolic acidosis, and cardiac disturbances have been directly related to plasma catecholamine activity.[22,23]

The third potential mechanism of theophylline's action is competitive antagonism of adenosine receptors. Adenosine, which is a bronchoconstrictor, anticonvulsant, and regulator of cardiac rhythm, interacts closely with theophylline through its competition for adenosine receptors.[19,26] The structural similarity between these chemicals and their opposite physiologic functions supports this theory of adenosine receptor antagonism.

Finally, theophylline's actions may result directly from changes in intracellular calcium transport. For example, caffeine has been shown to inhibit the uptake and storage of calcium by the sarcoplasmic reticulum of striated muscle, thereby producing increased strength in skeletal muscle. In animal models, administration of a calcium channel blocker appears to protect against theophylline-induced toxicity and death.[6]

Clinical Toxicity

Having a narrow therapeutic index, theophylline is associated with a high rate of adverse effects. For example, as many as 15% of patients complain of adverse effects when their serum theophylline concentration is in the therapeutic range. Once serum theophylline concentrations exceed the therapeutic range (>20 μg/mL), the prevalence of adverse effects exceeds 65% to 70%.[27] More than 90% of patients with serum theophylline concentrations greater than 30 μg/mL demonstrate signs of toxicity.[15] It is also notable that theophylline intoxication has a high rate of iatrogenic origin; Schiff and colleagues found that in 68% of patients hospitalized with theophylline intoxication, inpatient or emergency department drug administration was responsible or contributed to toxicity.[28]

CLINICAL MANIFESTATIONS

The signs and symptoms of theophylline intoxication can be placed into five categories: GI, musculoskeletal, cardiovascular, neurologic, and metabolic.[15,29-31]

Gastrointestinal

The GI tract seems most sensitive to theophylline's toxicity. The most common complaints associated with theophylline use are abdominal pain, heartburn, and vomiting.[32] In some cases, hemorrhagic gastritis can occur. These effects result from GI actions that include increased production of gastric acid and pepsin as well as relaxation of the lower esophageal sphincter. With moderate to severe theophylline intoxication, vomiting can be difficult to control despite antiemetic therapy.[33]

Musculoskeletal

Victims of theophylline intoxication often complain of generalized muscle aches. With moderate toxicity, muscular hypertonicity with frank myoclonus may develop. Coarse tremor has also been reported as a manifestation of toxicity.[32] These effects have been attributed to the potassium disturbances that accompany theophylline intoxication or disturbances in intracellular calcium transport. Elevations in serum creatine phosphokinase levels have been reported with severe intoxication.

Cardiovascular

Theophylline has several cardiovascular effects, some of which can be life threatening. Even when serum theophylline concentrations are in the therapeutic range, sinus tachycardia is often present. Greater toxicity has effects on vascular tone and cardiac rhythm.

Peripheral vasodilation is invariable with significant theophylline intoxication. This results in a widened pulse pressure and a fall in systemic vascular resistance.[34] Hypotension is generally present rather than hypertension.[22,23] The mechanism of vascular disturbances is thought to be vascular β-adrenergic receptor stimulation, produced by circulating plasma catecholamines.

Theophylline is arrhythmogenic.[35] Myocardial irritability appears with mild to moderate theophylline intoxication; electrocardiograms most often reveal ventricular premature beats. These are usually of no consequence. However, more severe myocardial irritability occurs with serious intoxication, producing bigeminy

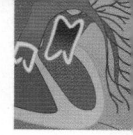

and other potentially unstable rhythms. These dysrhythmias may be a prelude to life-threatening cardiac arrhythmias such as ventricular tachycardia.

Although sinus tachycardia is one of the most common of manifestations of toxicity, appearing in as many as 82% of cases,[32] rhythm disturbances are a sign of severe theophylline intoxication and the most common cause of theophylline-induced fatalities. Sinus tachycardia can quickly progress to life-threatening rhythms, which can be either ventricular or supraventricular in origin.[36] Supraventricular disturbances reported after theophylline intoxication include supraventricular tachycardia, atrial fibrillation, atrial flutter, and multifocal atrial tachycardia.[37] Many of these rhythms, such as multifocal atrial tachycardia, are characteristic of theophylline intoxication.[38] Supraventricular tachyarrhythmias result in increased myocardial oxygen demand, compromised cardiac output, shock, metabolic acidosis, and myocardial ischemia or infarction. Life-threatening arrhythmias of ventricular origin consist of ventricular tachycardia and ventricular fibrillation.

The mechanism of cardiac rhythm disturbances is unclear. They may be secondary to elevated plasma catecholamine activity. Other data now suggest that the mechanism of rhythm disturbances is theophylline inhibition of cardiac adenosine receptors.

Neurologic

Neurologic manifestations of theophylline intoxication appear at relatively low serum concentration; users of theophylline may complain of anxiety and insomnia. In children, theophylline may produce behavioral disturbances (e.g., agitation and motor restlessness) that interfere with school function.[39,40] Although results of clinical investigations have been mixed, most data have failed to demonstrate a consistent effect on learning, although some children are likely to have a detrimental neurobehavioral response to the medication.[41,42]

With moderate theophylline intoxication, more striking signs of neurologic disturbance appear. An early sign of intoxication is tachypnea, representing stimulation of CNS respiratory centers and often resulting in respiratory alkalosis. Worsening clinical toxicity is attended by anxiety, agitation, and delirium or hallucinosis.[32]

The single most serious neurologic consequence of theophylline intoxication is the appearance of seizures. Theophylline-induced seizures can present in many patterns. These seizures are usually generalized, although focal seizures have been described.[43] In young infants, seizures may be subtle, consisting of generalized hypertonicity, posturing, eye deviation, and lip smacking without a clonic component. Theophylline-induced seizures can be single or repeated. They can appear without warning, although irritability, vomiting, and headache may be premonitory signs.[10] Seizures may occur at serum theophylline concentrations less than 20 μg/mL.[10] Once they appear, seizures can be extremely difficult to treat, being resistant to standard anticonvulsant therapy. Seizures due to theophylline use often predict a poor outcome; earlier case series reported a mortality rate of 50% to 100% among those who developed

seizures.[44,45] Numerous case reports and case series have reported disabling, permanent neurologic sequelae in those who develop theophylline-induced seizures.[10,46-51] Neurologic and neurobehavioral complications can include amnesia, personality changes, quadriplegia, and intractable seizure disorder. In young infants, associated intracerebral hemorrhage has been reported.[47] Neurologic sequelae are more common after long-term theophylline overmedication rather than acute single overdose.

The mechanism of theophylline-induced seizures is not completely understood and is likely multifactorial. However, in one series, as many as 34% of children and 12% of adults developed abnormalities on electroencephalogram while taking the medication.[46] Theophylline-induced seizures have been linked to dysfunction of GABAergic inhibitory neurons and depressed serum pyridoxal levels[52]; in an animal model, pyridoxine, which promotes γ-aminobutyric acid (GABA) synthesis, was found to ameliorate theophylline-induced seizures.[6,53]

Theophylline's relationship to CNS adenosine receptors has received considerable attention in recent years. The CNS has a dense population of adenosine receptors. These modulate the activity of various populations of neurons (e.g., cholinergic and glutaminergic). In vitro and in vivo studies have proved the importance of endogenous adenosine in regulating neuronal depolarization. For example, adenosine antagonists lead to marked alterations in seizure pattern after experimental administration of proconvulsant agents, producing uninterrupted electric discharge. Studies with radiolabeled theophylline have also shown it can displace adenosine from its receptor sites. In an animal model of theophylline-induced seizures, Shannon and Maher demonstrated that direct CNS administration of adenosine could forestall theophylline-induced seizures.[54]

In addition to its direct neuroexcitatory effects, theophylline has marked effects on cerebral vascular tone, an action that is also related to adenosine activity.[55] Adenosine is a potent stimulator of cerebral vasodilation; marked increases in CNS adenosine activity occur in response to cerebral ischemia, representing another cerebroprotective effect. Theophylline antagonizes this action, producing sustained cerebrovasoconstriction, which compromises CNS delivery of oxygen and nutrients as well as removal of toxic metabolic wastes.

Metabolic

Metabolic complications of theophylline intoxication are many.[56,57] Even in therapeutic doses, theophylline can produce depressions in serum potassium and elevations in blood glucose levels. With more severe intoxication, profound hypokalemia can result. Serum potassium concentrations as low as 1.7 mEq/L have been reported after theophylline poisoning.[34,58]

The mechanism of theophylline-induced hypokalemia is well defined. Although early theories attributed it to potassium losses as a result of vomiting or diuresis, these are unlikely to be the cause.[59] For example, Amitai and Lovejoy demonstrated that the hypokalemia often precedes vomiting.[60] The current belief is that hypokalemia results from increased intracellular transport of potassium ion,

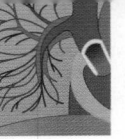

produced by amplification of sodium-potassium adenosine triphosphatase (Na^+/K^+-ATPase) or opening of calcium-linked potassium channels. This effect occurs secondary to catecholamine-induced β_2-adrenergic stimulation.[59,61-63] As a result, total-body potassium is preserved. Theophylline-induced hypokalemia promptly reverses as serum theophylline concentration declines, without potassium supplementation. The clinical consequences of theophylline-induced hypokalemia are unclear. Although hypokalemia has been implicated in the genesis of theophylline-induced cardiac arrhythmias, this is only speculative and is not supported by available data. Blood glucose elevations also appear to be a result of circulating plasma catecholamines. Serum blood glucose can rise to levels greater than 400 mg/dL; theophylline intoxication can mimic diabetic ketoacidosis.[34,64]

Metabolic acidosis with depression of serum bicarbonate levels is usually modest but can be severe, resulting in a high anion gap. Serum bicarbonate concentrations as low as 5 mEq/L have been reported after serum theophylline poisoning. Acidosis appears to result from the combination of increased lactate production and lipolysis with increased free fatty acid circulation.[65]

Other metabolic disturbances associated with theophylline intoxication include hypercalcemia, which has been reported in as many as 15% of patients.[66] Hypomagnesemia, hypophosphatemia, and respiratory alkalosis have also been reported.[56,58]

Theophylline has not been proved to have significant human genotoxicity or fetotoxicity, although such effects have been observed in experimental models.[6,15,67] However, it is listed as a pregnancy category C drug by the U.S. Food and Drug Administration.

Acute vs. Chronic Intoxication

The clinical course of patients with theophylline poisoning is highly variable and often unpredictable. The reasons for such wide variations in reaction to a drug whose toxic manifestations are so clearly recognized have been an enigma that continues to challenge clinicians who must provide immediate and appropriate care to theophylline-poisoned patients in order to prevent disastrous outcomes. During the past 20 years, a series of important modulators of theophylline poisoning have been identified.

Early descriptions of the clinical course of theophylline intoxication suggested that serum theophylline concentrations were highly predictive of outcome. For example, in a study of 28 children with acute theophylline intoxication, Gaudreault and colleagues demonstrated that life-threatening toxicity did not appear with serum theophylline concentrations less than 70 µg/mL and that the lower the serum theophylline concentration, the less likely the risk for major toxicity.[68] Bertino, Aitken, and others subsequently published case series indicating that serum theophylline concentration was not always predictive of clinical course and that patients with relatively low serum theophylline concentrations often had fatal outcomes.[46,69-71]

In 1985, Olson and colleagues were the first to clearly demonstrate that the clinical course of patients with theophylline intoxication was largely influenced by the mechanism of their poisoning.[72] This study found that victims of acute theophylline intoxication, although they were more likely to have metabolic consequences such as hypokalemia and hyperglycemia, seemed to tolerate elevated serum theophylline concentrations better than those with chronic overmedication. Those in the latter category had a lower incidence of metabolic disturbances but were more likely to have life-threatening seizures or cardiac disturbances. Moreover, these life-threatening events occurred at lower serum theophylline concentrations than in those with acute intoxication who developed life-threatening events.[72]

Subsequent studies have attempted to clarify differences in outcome as influenced by method of intoxication.[6] Consequently, three types of patients with theophylline intoxication have been identified: those with acute overdose, those with chronic overmedication, and those with acute-on-therapeutic intoxication. According to current definitions, the victim of acute theophylline overdose is one who has not been taking or receiving theophylline but is then exposed to a single dose exceeding 10 mg/kg. A patient who suffers an acute toxic overdose and who has been taking theophylline for only 1 or 2 days, not having reached steady-state concentrations (which require 4 to 5 half-lives), is also considered a victim of acute overdose. Common causes of acute overdose include ingestion by children, attempted suicide by young adults, and inadvertent administration of an excess dose by clinicians (physician, nurse, or pharmacist). Tenfold errors in drug administration are a common cause of acute intoxication in children.

The findings of Gaudreault and colleagues have been borne out by larger, subsequent clinical investigations: Patients with acute theophylline overdose generally exhibit signs of minor toxicity at serum theophylline concentrations of 20 to 40 µg/mL, moderate toxicity with concentrations of 40 to 80 µg/mL, and severe toxicity with concentrations of greater than 70 to 80 µg/mL. In the absence of prompt, aggressive care, serum theophylline concentrations of greater than 100 µg/mL are often fatal (although survival with only supportive care has been reported with serum theophylline concentrations of 203 and 300 µg/mL.[73,74]

Victims of chronic theophylline overmedication differ from those with acute poisoning in several respects. First, epidemiologically, these patients are more likely to be very young (i.e., neonates) or elderly. They invariably have preexisting cardiorespiratory disease, which is the reason they are taking the medication. Unintentional overmedication can result from a number of causes, most commonly inappropriate dosing by the patient or health care provider (Table 65-2). Those with chronic overmedication have a substantially higher risk for major toxicity than those with acute intoxication (49% versus 10% in one study[37]). This higher incidence occurs despite lower serum theophylline concentrations in those with chronic overmedication.[75]

The most distinctive feature of chronic theophylline overmedication is the complete loss of predictive value provided by serum theophylline concentration. Victims

TABLE 65-2 Common Causes of Chronic Theophylline Overmedication

CAUSE	PERCENTAGE OF CASES
Increased dosing by patient or parent	31
Physician dosing error	14
Drug interaction	7
Cardiac disease	10
Viral illness	3
Hepatic disease	1
Unknown	35

Adapted from Shannon M, Lovejoy F: The influence of age vs. peak serum concentration of life-threatening events after chronic theophylline intoxication. Arch Intern Med 1990;150:2045.

of chronic overmedication may have seizures, arrhythmias, and fatalities at serum theophylline concentrations as low as 20 to 30 µg/mL.[49] Conversely, patients may survive serum concentrations as high as 100 µg/mL. Olson and coworkers suggested that among those with chronic overmedication, serum theophylline concentrations have some predictive value; however, others have not found this. Studies now indicate that age rather than peak serum theophylline concentration is most predictive of major toxicity after chronic theophylline overmedication; proportional increases in the risk of a life-threatening event occur with advancing age.[37,76] In the pediatric age group, the opposite is true; the younger the patient, the greater the risk for major toxicity.[75,76] Age is not a risk factor in the development of major toxicity for those with acute theophylline overdose.

Acute-on-therapeutic theophylline intoxication acts in an intermediate fashion, with metabolic disturbances and clinical consequences occurring in a pattern that lies between the other two populations.[37,75,77]

Differences between those with acute versus chronic theophylline intoxication are also evident in patients' metabolic profile. For example, in those with acute intoxication, 85% to 95% develop hypokalemia, in contrast to 25% to 32% of those with chronic overmedication.[72,77] Serum glucose level is typically higher and serum bicarbonate level lower in those with acute theophylline overdose.

Diagnosis of Theophylline Poisoning

The diagnosis of theophylline poisoning is made in various ways. With acute overdose, patients, friends, or caretakers offer a history of recent use. In those with chronic overmedication, the diagnosis may be more elusive, with vague and nonspecific presenting complaints. Complaints of nausea, vomiting, and diarrhea may be erroneously diagnosed as gastroenteritis. In elderly patients, the presenting complaint is often respiratory decompensation; in such cases, the development of chronic theophylline overmedication has likely resulted from improper self-medication (i.e., taking extra doses). In many cases of theophylline

intoxication, seizures may be the presenting feature. Various presenting signs require a high index of suspicion as well as a detailed review of medications that the patient is taking. Because increasing numbers of drugs are being found to inhibit cytochrome P-450 activity, close attention should be paid to those patients taking theophylline in combination with another drug.

In those who receive inadvertent intravenous theophylline overdoses, representing either acute or acute-on-therapeutic poisoning, the error is often discovered when the clinical status deteriorates and tachycardia, agitation, or frank seizures appear.

Serum theophylline concentrations are readily measured. However, theophylline may not be a part of a general toxic screen, and thus the test must be specifically requested. Because serum theophylline concentrations may be of limited value in patients with chronic theophylline overmedication, it is essential that a thorough clinical assessment be performed. After an acute toxic ingestion, theophylline concentrations should be measured every 2 to 4 hours until a plateau is documented because of the risk for delayed peak absorption after ingestion of sustained-release theophylline preparations.[15,77,78]

Ancillary laboratory tests that are important in the treatment of patients with theophylline intoxication include an electrocardiogram; chest radiograph; measurement of arterial blood gas, serum electrolytes, calcium, and blood sugar; and occasionally liver function tests. Because seizures may be associated with a cerebrovascular accident, cranial tomography should be considered for those who develop convulsions.

Management of Theophylline Poisoning

SUPPORTIVE MEASURES

General management principles are key in the care of patients with theophylline poisoning. For those with respiratory compromise, cardiac disturbances, or seizures, initial interventions must include airway control, assisted ventilation, and vascular access. Patients who present with respiratory failure as a result of exacerbation of their pulmonary disease or seizure require immediate endotracheal intubation. Hypotension may reflect theophylline-induced vasodilation, dehydration, or myocardial infarction. In such cases, based on clinical assessment and, ideally, central venous pressure monitoring, modest fluid boluses should be administered. If vasopressor therapy is needed, there are theoretic advantages to using phenylephrine, a potent peripheral vasoconstrictor. However, more conventional vasopressors, including dopamine, dobutamine, and norepinephrine, are also effective for blood pressure support.

Cardiac arrhythmias also require immediate intervention and can be treated according to advanced cardiac life support algorithms. Isolated ventricular premature beats without hemodynamic compromise require no treatment. More significant signs of myocardial irritability should be treated with appropriate doses of lidocaine. Although the proconvulsant actions of lidocaine pose

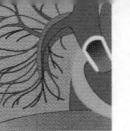

theoretic risks, no evidence shows that lidocaine is detrimental when used in appropriate doses. Supraventricular arrhythmias can be treated with agents including β blockers, verapamil, or adenosine. Propranolol has been shown to reverse peripheral vasodilation, hypotension, tachycardia, hypokalemia, and hypercalcemia after theophylline poisoning.[34,63,66,79] It may, however, produce bronchoconstriction in susceptible individuals. Esmolol, a very short-acting β_1-specific antagonist, has been used successfully for reversal of tachycardia.[80,81] The calcium channel blocker verapamil, although effective in the treatment of supraventricular tachycardia, carries the risk for exacerbating hypotension.[82]

The intimate relationship between theophylline and adenosine justifies the use of adenosine (Adenocard) as first-line treatment for theophylline-induced tachyarrhythmias. Supraventricular tachycardia is very responsive to adenosine therapy. If the basis of theophylline-induced tachyarrhythmias is cardiac adenosine receptor antagonism, exogenous adenosine can be considered an "antidote" in reversing this effect. The dose of adenosine is 6 to 20 mg for adults and 0.1 mg/kg for children. Adenosine is effective only if delivered into the central circulation by rapid bolus. Having an elimination half-life of about 10 seconds, adenosine may not produce sustained control of arrhythmias. Like propranolol, adenosine has been associated with the occurrence of bronchoconstriction.

Seizures are an ominous occurrence with theophylline intoxication because they are often multiple, are highly resistant to anticonvulsant therapy, and are associated with permanent neurologic disability. This recognition has led some physicians to recommend prophylactic anticonvulsant therapy to those patients who present with severe theophylline intoxication.[15] In many victims, however, particularly those with chronic theophylline overmedication (who have the greatest likelihood of seizures), high-risk patients are difficult to identify, making it unclear who should receive preventive anticonvulsant therapy. Certainly, once they appear, seizures should be treated aggressively. The initial anticonvulsant should be a benzodiazepine (e.g., diazepam or lorazepam). Benzodiazepines are considered agents of choice because the benzodiazepine receptor is linked to GABAergic neurons. Large doses of benzodiazepines may be necessary to control seizures. The second anticonvulsant choice is a barbiturate such as phenobarbital.[83] Like the benzodiazepines, barbiturates have actions at the GABA receptor; they are effective at terminating theophylline-induced seizures. Barbiturates do, however, have two disadvantages. First, they have a delayed onset of action. Also, being CNS depressants, they may produce severe respiratory depression if administered in conjunction with benzodiazepines. Phenytoin is relatively contraindicated in the treatment of theophylline-induced seizures, based on both empirical observation that it is ineffective in terminating theophylline-induced seizures and animal data that suggest that phenytoin increases the risk for theophylline-induced seizures.[83] If anticonvulsants are ineffective in terminating seizures, skeletal muscle paralysis may be

necessary to prevent the complications of prolonged tonic–clonic activity. However, with theophylline intoxication, paralysis carries the risk for masking continued seizure activity. Because experimental data suggest that continued electric discharge and resulting metabolic disturbances are pivotal in theophylline-induced neurologic injury, every effort should be made to provide electroencephalographic monitoring.

GI disturbances, although generally not considered life threatening, have a critical role in the management of theophylline intoxication because they prevent both successful GI decontamination and elimination enhancement with multiple-dose activated charcoal. Therefore, a treatment priority is control of vomiting. Vast clinical experience indicates that conventional interventions, including antiemetic suppositories and low-dose metoclopramide, are ineffective therapies. Phenothiazines are also disappointing as antiemetics; they also may precipitate seizures because of their ability to lower seizure threshold.

Several agents are effective in control of theophylline-induced emesis. Parenteral H_2 antagonists, particularly ranitidine, control gastric acid secretion and reduce the mucosal irritation that contributes to vomiting[84] (Fig. 65-2). Metoclopramide is an effective antiemetic if given in adequate doses. For control of theophylline-induced vomiting, the recommended dose is 0.1 to 1 mg/kg; lower doses are unlikely to be effective. Because metoclopramide doses of this magnitude have been associated with the development of acute dystonic

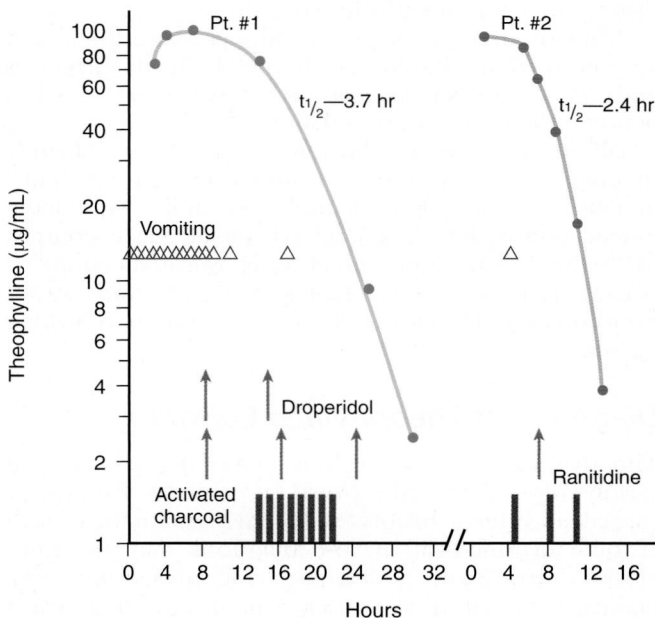

FIGURE 65-2 Serum theophylline concentrations and frequency of vomiting in two patients before and during treatment with ranitidine, droperidol, and repetitive activated charcoal. $t_{1/2}$, elimination half-life of theophylline. (From Amitai Y, Yeung AC, Moye J, Lovejoy FH: Repetitive oral activated charcoal and control of emesis in severe theophylline toxicity. Ann Intern Med 1986;105:386.)

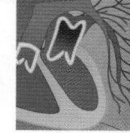

reaction, diphenhydramine should be made readily available or administered prophylactically. Ondansetron, a nonsedating antiemetic that acts as an inhibitor of CNS serotonergic neurons, has also been successfully used to control theophylline-induced vomiting.[85] Another agent that may be effective is droperidol.[84]

Aggressive GI decontamination is important because sustained-release theophylline tablets can coalesce, forming bezoars.[86] Activated charcoal should be administered as soon as possible. Whole bowel irrigation has been advocated for the treatment of sustained-release theophylline ingestion; however, whole bowel irrigation fluids may promote theophylline desorption from activated charcoal. One study has suggested that whole bowel irrigation offers no additional benefit over activated charcoal.[87] If confirmed by additional studies, these data would support omission of whole bowel irrigation as an adjunct to use of activated charcoal after theophylline ingestion.

Metabolic disturbances generally do not require aggressive management. Insulin therapy is not recommended for hyperglycemia because blood glucose elevations are transient and inconsequential.[34] Significant metabolic acidosis should be treated with administration of sodium bicarbonate.

The most significant metabolic abnormality is hypokalemia, which can be profound. Because total-body potassium is unchanged, exogenous potassium theoretically is not needed. However, because hypokalemia may be a risk factor for cardiac disturbances, it is appropriate to treat severe depressions of serum potassium concentration. Potassium supplementation should be provided cautiously and with close monitoring of serum potassium values to prevent iatrogenic hyperkalemia. D'Angio and Sabatelli described a patient with theophylline intoxication who was treated with aggressive potassium replacement. As the patient's serum theophylline concentration fell, however, serum potassium level rose, resulting in a hyperkalemic cardiac disturbance.[88]

ELIMINATION ENHANCEMENT

Having a favorable pharmacokinetic profile, theophylline can be removed by a number of methods; because of its life-threatening toxicity, the drug should be removed as quickly as possible once the need has been determined.[89]

Multiple-dose activated charcoal is very effective at enhancing the elimination of theophylline from the body, even if toxic doses have been administered intravenously.[84,90] Theophylline has the unusual property of diffusibility across the gut mucosa, such that if activated charcoal is present in the GI lumen, theophylline adsorbs to charcoal and is eliminated in the stool. This action is referred to as *GI dialysis* or *enterocapillary exsorption* (see Chapter 2). Animal models and case reports have demonstrated the efficiency with which repeat oral charcoal doses can eliminate theophylline that has been administered intravenously. Theophylline clearance rates as high as 100 mL/min, corresponding to serum elimination half-lives as low as 1 to 2 hours, have been reported with use of multiple-dose activated charcoal.[15,78,91] Because it is so effective yet noninvasive, multiple-dose activated charcoal is the cornerstone of elimination enhancement procedures in patients with theophylline intoxication.[92]

For treatment of theophylline intoxication, activated charcoal should be administered in a dose of 1 g/kg (maximum 50 g) every 4 hours. If vomited, the dose should be repeated. Alternative administration strategies include 20 g every 2 hours or continuous nasogastric infusion of activated charcoal.[93,94] Aggressive antiemetic therapy is usually necessary to permit retention of charcoal. Continuous assessment of bowel motility is important because of the risk for intestinal pseudo-obstruction, which has been associated with use of multiple-dose activated charcoal in theophylline intoxication.[95] Repeat doses of charcoal can be safely administered to young infants.[96]

In 1979, Russo demonstrated that theophylline could be rapidly removed from the body by hemoperfusion.[91] Theophylline clearance rates that were four to six times greater than endogenous clearance could be produced by hemoperfusion, making this procedure extremely valuable in treating theophylline intoxication.[48] With hemoperfusion, theophylline extraction ratios as high as 0.75, corresponding to elimination half-lives of 1 to 2 hours, were initially reported. Three hours of hemoperfusion removed more than 65% of a theophylline dose in early experiences.[97] In contrast, hemodialysis, an alternative to hemoperfusion, could only double theophylline clearance rates.[78]

Hemoperfusion has become widely considered to be the definitive treatment for theophylline intoxication. However, because newer high-flux hemodialysis machines are capable of increasing theophylline clearance rates greater than 300 mL/min, comparable to the rates achieved with hemoperfusion,[78] hemodialysis is now considered an option equal to charcoal hemoperfusion for serious theophylline intoxication.

The criteria for hemodialysis (or hemoperfusion; HD/HP) after theophylline intoxication are controversial. Park and colleagues proposed the criterion of peak serum theophylline concentration greater than 60 µg/mL or a concentration of greater than 30 µg/mL in patients older than 60 years.[50] Olson and coworkers have recommended hemoperfusion in those with acute intoxication and serum theophylline concentrations of greater than 100 µg/mL and in those with chronic overmedication and peak concentrations greater than 40 to 60 µg/mL.[72] Greenberg and associates recommended that hemoperfusion be performed only in those with intractable hypotension, ventricular ectopy, or resistant seizures.[82] Notably, all investigators have emphasized that a criterion for HD/HP is the appearance of seizures or arrhythmias, suggesting that HD/HP is also effective in reducing morbidity and mortality once major toxicity is manifested. However, data now suggest that most patients who received HD/HP *after* they had a seizure or cardiac arrhythmia continued to have these life-threatening events. In contrast, as few as 5% of patients who receive HD/HP before major toxicity eventually develop a life-threatening event.[37] Therefore, HD/HP is

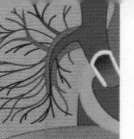

<table>
<tr><td>**BOX 65-3**</td><td>**RECOMMENDATIONS FOR ELIMINATION ENHANCEMENT AFTER THEOPHYLLINE INTOXICATION**</td></tr>
</table>

Acute Intoxication

1. Multiple-dose activated charcoal for all patients
2. HD/HP for patients with peak serum [theo] > 80–100 µg/mL*
3. HD/HP for patients with peak serum [theo] > 60–80 µg/mL and intractable vomiting
4. HD/HP for those with seizures or cardiac arrhythmias and serum [theo] > 100 µg/mL

Chronic Overmedication

1. Multiple-dose activated charcoal for all patients
2. HD/HP for all patients younger than 6 mo or older than 65 yr with serum [theo] > 30–40 µg/mL

*Exchange transfusion may be used as an alternative therapy for neonates.
HD/HP, hemodialysis or hemoperfusion.

---

best considered a preventive intervention rather than a procedure that offers great benefit after major toxicity has developed.

Based on the growing data that have analyzed major toxicity and its predictors as a function of method of intoxication, the following recommendations are rational (Box 65-3): For all patients with theophylline intoxication (serum theophylline concentration > 20 to 30 µg/mL), treatment should be initiated with multiple-dose oral charcoal. For those with acute theophylline intoxication, HD/HP should be performed in patients with a serum theophylline concentration of greater than 80 to 100 µg/mL. If uncontrolled vomiting prevents successful charcoal administration, HD/HP should be performed in all those with serum theophylline concentrations that exceed 60 to 80 µg/mL.

The decision to perform HD/HP after chronic theophylline intoxication is more difficult for several reasons. First, the patients at greatest risk for seizures and cardiac arrhythmias cannot be identified on the basis of peak serum theophylline concentration. Second, these victims are usually very young or very old, ages at which HD/HP is technically more difficult. Finally, patients with chronic theophylline intoxication often have seizures and cardiac arrhythmias as their presenting manifestations, making the value of HD/HP less clear. Nonetheless, because of the evidence that high-risk patients are those at extremes of age, hemodialysis should be considered in all patients with a serum theophylline concentration of greater than 30 µg/mL, particularly those younger than 6 months or older than 65 years.

HD/HP is technically difficult to perform in neonates, although it has been proved successful.[98] Consequently, alternative methods of extracorporeal drug removal have been evaluated. Among these, exchange transfusion is the procedure with the greatest promise. Although an early case report found no benefit of exchange transfusion in infants with severe acute theophylline intoxication,[74] two recent case reports have demonstrated that significant amounts of theophylline can be removed with exchange transfusion, making this therapy a viable option in acutely poisoned neonates.[99,100]

Plasmapheresis has also been successfully used in the treatment of theophylline intoxication, reducing elimination half-life to 1.7 hours.[101,102]

CAFFEINE

Caffeine is a plant alkaloid found in a wide variety of foods and beverages. Coffee, tea, and chocolate have the largest natural concentrations of caffeine. Caffeine is also added to carbonated beverages and a large number of over-the-counter medications including weight control aids, "alertness" tablets, pain relievers, diuretics, and cold remedies (Table 65-3). Finally, caffeine is prescribed for the treatment of apnea-bradycardia in newborns and as adjunctive therapy for cerebrovascular (migraine) headache.

Clinical Pharmacology

Found in the most popular beverages in the world (coffee and soft drinks), caffeine is a widely consumed drug. Significant increases in caffeine use among children and adolescents has been observed in recent years and has been attributed to increased rates of hypertension, insomnia, chronic headache, motor tics, irritability, learning difficulties, and other adverse health effects.[103-107]

Caffeine can be administered by a number of routes, including oral, intravenous, subcutaneous, and rectal.

TABLE 65-3 Average Caffeine Content of Beverages, Foods, and Pharmaceuticals

	DOSE RANGE (mg)
Beverages	
Coffee (5 oz)	
Brewed	40–200
Instant	30–150
Decaffeinated	1–5
Tea (5 oz)	
Brewed	20–100
Instant	25–50
Iced (12-oz glass)	65–80
Carbonated beverages, 12 oz	25–200
Chocolate milk	2–10
Food	
Dark chocolate, 1 oz	5–30
Nonprescription Pharmaceuticals	
Weight control aids	100–200
Alertness agents	100–200
Analgesics	30–65
Diuretics	100–200
Cold remedies	15–30

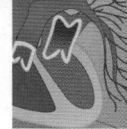

After ingestion, it is well absorbed, with an absorption pattern relatively unaffected by the presence of food. Peak plasma concentrations are achieved 30 to 60 hours after ingestion.[108] Absorption after rectal and subcutaneous administration is equally rapid. It has an apparent volume of distribution of 1 L/kg. As with theophylline, caffeine metabolism occurs through biotransformation in the cytochrome P-450 system. The primary metabolic pathway for caffeine is its demethylation. 1-Demethylation produces theobromine (3,7-dimethylxanthine), a pharmacologically active methylxanthine found widely in chocolate. 7-Demethylation of caffeine produces theophylline; as a result, caffeine ingestion produces measurable serum theophylline concentrations. The elimination half-life of caffeine is variable and highly age dependent; the average half-life in a nonsmoking adult is 3 to 6 hours. In contrast, premature neonates can have elimination half-lives that range from 1.5 to 6 days.[108] Agents associated with induction of cytochrome P-450 enzymes (e.g., smoking) produce shorter half-lives. About 5% of caffeine is excreted unchanged in the urine. Significant amounts of caffeine are excreted into breast milk.

Caffeine has a number of pharmacologic actions. Its most important property, mild CNS stimulation, is the basis for the worldwide enjoyment of caffeinated beverages, particularly coffee. This CNS stimulation is associated with increased alertness and concentration as well as mood elevation. In excessive doses, undesirable effects, including hyperactivity (particularly in children), anxiety, and insomnia, appear.[41]

Caffeine has become extremely valuable therapy in the treatment of the neonatal apnea-bradycardia syndrome. Newborns with this syndrome have recurrent hypoventilation, often accompanied by bradycardia. Both theophylline and caffeine are effective in treating this syndrome; stimulation of central respiratory centers by methylxanthines results in decreased apnea, increased minute ventilation, normalization of breathing pattern, increased ventilatory response to carbon dioxide, and reduction in both the need for and duration of mechanical ventilation. Another beneficial effect in newborns is increased cardiac output.[109] Caffeine offers the advantages of excellent absorption after ingestion and a longer elimination half-life; these provide more sustained serum concentrations and more predictable pharmacokinetics. The therapeutic serum concentration of caffeine is 8 to 20 µg/mL.

Caffeine is also a cardiotonic agent, producing positive inotropy and chronotropy. However, it does not consistently produce significant increases in pulse or blood pressure.[110,111] In susceptible individuals, caffeine occasionally leads to the development of premature ventricular contractions, which are usually of no clinical consequence. Important vascular effects of caffeine include cerebral vasoconstriction and renal vasculature relaxation. Because cerebral vasodilation often contributes to the pathophysiology of headache, constriction of cerebral blood vessels by caffeine can be therapeutic. Enhanced renal blood flow is associated with a modest diuretic effect.

Caffeine has two important GI effects: smooth muscle relaxation and stimulation of gastric secretion. Smooth muscle relaxation is most pronounced at the lower esophageal sphincter, where gastroesophageal reflux can result from caffeine use. In concert with increased secretion of both gastric acid and digestive enzymes, reflux can result in esophagitis (heartburn). These GI effects are also noted after ingestion of decaffeinated coffee, suggesting they are mediated by alkaloids other than caffeine. Metabolic effects of caffeine include increased fatty acid oxidation and glycogenolysis. According to one study, typical doses of caffeine, unlike theophylline, do not usually produce marked increases in circulating plasma catecholamines.[112] However, catecholamine elevations have been reported in victims of caffeine intoxication.[113]

Caffeine exhibits all the properties of an addictive drug (tolerance, dependence, and an abstinence syndrome on immediate withdrawal). Tolerance to all its pharmacologic effects develops after repeated use.

Clinical Toxicology

Undesirable effects of caffeine can appear after ingestion of as little as 50 mg; at these doses, anxiety, GI upset, and insomnia may occur. More significant toxicity appears after ingestion of 15 to 30 mg/kg. At this range, moderate toxicity is marked by vomiting, myoclonus, and myocardial irritability. Vomiting may be severe; frank hematemesis may occur.[114] Fatal oral doses of caffeine have ranged from 5 to 50 g, with a mean of 10 g; the lethal dose is estimated to be 100 to 200 mg/kg.[115] Clinical toxicity correlates with serum caffeine concentrations. Several cups of coffee yield a serum caffeine level of 5 to 10 µg/mL. Agitation and myoclonus occur at levels of 15 to 30 µg/mL; cardiac arrhythmias and seizures develop at 50 to 100 µg/mL. Fatalities have been associated with serum caffeine concentrations as low as 80 µg/mL to as high as 1560 µg/mL,[116] although concentrations as high as 200 µg/mL have been associated with survival. Deaths have also been reported from the use of coffee enemas as a naturopathic therapy.[117]

Many of the consequences of caffeine poisoning are identical to those of theophylline, although they are associated with comparably higher serum caffeine concentrations. Seizures can appear without warning and are often repeated. Opisthotonos, decerebrate posturing, and generalized muscular hypertonicity are also common.[118] Cardiac arrhythmias can be supraventricular or ventricular (ventricular tachycardia or fibrillation). Other manifestations of severe intoxication are rhabdomyolysis with resultant acute renal failure and pulmonary edema.[119] Rhabdomyolysis has been attributed to increased muscular activity. Pulmonary edema is a frequent occurrence with severe poisoning and is thought to result, in part, from pulmonary vasculature dilation.[108,118] Victims of caffeine intoxication develop the metabolic disturbances of hyperglycemia, hypokalemia, leukocytosis, ketosis, and metabolic acidosis.

Chronic caffeine intoxication (caffeinism) is manifested by irritability, insomnia, anxiety, emotional lability, and

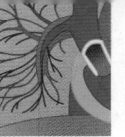

chronic abdominal pain. Cardiovascular disease, myocardial irritability, and fibrocystic disease of the breast all have been associated with long-term caffeine consumption.[112,120,121] However, for all these diseases, the association with caffeine has been controversial and inconsistent in clinical investigations.

Caffeine is both mutagenic and teratogenic in laboratory animal species.[108] A study of women suggested that more than 600 mg of caffeine daily could result in an increased incidence of spontaneous abortion and premature birth.[108] A causal link between caffeine use and birth defects remains tenuous[122]; however, the Food and Drug Administration has advised pregnant women to avoid or limit caffeine intake.

Caffeine has now been proved to produce a physiologic abstinence syndrome (withdrawal). Although it has been well recognized that abrupt termination of caffeine consumption could produce insomnia, malaise, and headache, little scientific investigation has addressed these phenomena. Silverman[123] and Strain[124] and their colleagues have shown that withdrawal from caffeine can produce an increase in depressive symptoms, anxiety, fatigue, headache, and decreased performance. Abstinence was also associated with a marked increase in the use of medications (e.g., headache relievers).

Management

In patients with an acute caffeine overdose, initial attention should be directed to airway, breathing, and circulation. The sudden appearance of airway compromise and hypoxia as a result of seizures, cardiac disturbances, or pulmonary edema should be anticipated, particularly in patients who ingest more than 30 to 50 mg/kg of caffeine.

Management of seizures and cardiac disturbances parallels their treatment in patients with theophylline intoxication. Therefore, seizures are preferably treated with a benzodiazepine (e.g., diazepam) or phenobarbital. There is no evidence that phenytoin is ineffective or harmful in the treatment of caffeine-induced seizures; however, because all methylxanthines are presumed to have similar mechanism of toxicity, phenytoin's lack of efficacy in theophylline-induced seizures argues against its use. Cardiac disturbances should be treated according to standard management strategies. Adenosine, verapamil, and β-blocking agents all are effective treatments for supraventricular arrhythmias.[114,125] Ventricular arrhythmias should be treated initially with intravenous lidocaine.

GI decontamination measures should include administration of activated charcoal with a cathartic. Vomiting is likely in those with significant ingestion. Although this provides gastric evacuation, it thwarts efforts at activated charcoal administration. Aggressive antiemetic therapy should therefore be provided. Antiemetic therapy should include the administration of H_2 antagonists, which reduce gastric hypersecretion. Other beneficial agents include metoclopramide, 0.1 to 1.0 mg/kg intravenously, and ondansetron, 0.6 mg/kg intravenously.

Laboratory evaluation should include electrolytes, blood glucose, creatine phosphokinase, arterial blood gas, and an electrocardiogram. Hypokalemia should be treated with modest potassium supplementation (because total-body potassium is preserved). Insulin is not recommended for treatment of hyperglycemia, although it has been suggested by others.[126]

Enhanced elimination is the final component of managing caffeine poisoning. A number of measures have been shown to be effective, including multiple-dose activated charcoal, peritoneal dialysis,[114,119] and HD/HP.[118,127] Although a proportion of caffeine is excreted from the urine unchanged, forced diuresis has no role in management. Diuresis should be provided only if patients have clinical evidence of severe rhabdomyolysis.

Multiple-dose activated charcoal has not been clearly shown to enhance caffeine elimination but does eliminate any theophylline that is generated; it is therefore considered an integral component of treatment. Use of several antiemetic agents may be necessary to end vomiting. Peritoneal dialysis has been used but is unlikely to be more helpful than multiple-dose activated charcoal. Hemodialysis is the procedure that provides greatest efficacy with the lowest complication rate. Indications for hemodialysis are not clearly established but should include a serum caffeine concentration of greater than 100 μg/mL and life-threatening seizures or cardiac arrhythmias, regardless of serum caffeine concentration. Because it is both invasive and unlikely to be more effective than hemodialysis, hemoperfusion has little to no role in the management of caffeine intoxication.

REFERENCES

1. Szefler SJ, Bender BG, Jusko WJ, et al: Evolving role of theophylline for treatment of chronic childhood asthma. J Pediatr 1995;127:176–185.
2. Yurdakul A, Taci N, Eren A, Sipit T: Comparative efficacy of once-daily therapy with inhaled corticosteroid, leukotriene antagonist or sustained-release theophylline in patients with mild persistent asthma. Respir Med 2003;97:1313–1319.
3. Epstein PE: Hemlock or healer? The mercurial reputation of theophylline. Ann Intern Med 1993;119:1216–1217.
4. McFadden ER: Methylxanthines in the treatment of asthma: the rise, the fall, and the possible rise again. Ann Intern Med 1991;115:323–324.
5. Barr R, Rowe B, Camargo C: Methylxanthines for exacerbations of chronic obstructive pulmonary disease: meta-analysis of randomized trials. BMJ 2003;327:643.
6. Shibata M, Wachi M, Kagawa M, et al: Acute and subacute toxicities of theophylline are directly reflected by its plasma concentration in dogs. Methods Find Exp Clin Pharmacol 2000;22:173–178.
7. Murciano D, Auclair M-H, Pariente R, Aubier M: A randomized, controlled trial of theophylline in patients with severe chronic obstructive pulmonary disease. N Engl J Med 1989;320:1521–1525.
8. Drazen JM, Gerard C: Reversing the irreversible. N Engl J Med 1989;320:1555–1556.
9. Henderson-Smart D, Steer P: Methylxanthine treatment for apnea in preterm infants. Cochrane Database Syst Rev 2001;3:CD000140.
10. American Academy of Pediatrics Committee on Drugs: Precautions concerning the use of theophylline. Pediatrics 1992;89:781–782.

11. Thomas N, Carcillo J: Theophylline for acute renal vaso-constriction associated with tacrolimus: a new indication for an old therapeutic agent? Pediatr Crit Care Med 2003;4:392–393.
12. Kapoor A, Kumar S, Gulati S, et al: The role of theophylline in contrast-induced nephropathy: a case-control study. Nephrol Dial Transplant 2002;17:1936–1941.
13. Huber W, Ilgmann K, Page M, et al: Effect of theophylline on contrast material-nephropathy in patients with chronic renal insufficiency: controlled, randomized, double-blinded study. Radiology 2002;223:772–779.
14. Fischer R, Lang SM, Steiner U, et al: Theophylline improves acute mountain sickness. Eur Respir J 2000;15:123–127.
15. Hendeles L, Jenkins J, Temple R: Revised FDA labeling guidelines for theophylline oral dosage forms. Pharmacotherapy 1995;15:409–427.
16. Lowry JA, Jarrett RV, Wassermann G, et al: Theophylline toxicokinetics in premature newborns. Arch Pediatr Adolesc Med 2001;155:934–939.
17. Weinberger M, Ginchansky E: Dose-dependent kinets of theophylline disposition in asthmatic children. J Pediatr 1977;91:820–824.
18. Mayo P: Effect of passive smoking on theophylline clearance in children. Ther Drug Monit 2001;23:503–505.
19. Bakris GL, Sauter ER, Hussey JL, et al: Effects of theophylline on erythropoietin production in normal subjects and in patients with erythrocytosis after renal transplantation. N Engl J Med 1990;323:86–90.
20. Fredholm BB: On the mechanism of action of theophylline and caffeine. Acta Med Scand 1985;217:149–153.
21. Polson JB, Krzanowski JJ, Goldman AL, Szentivanyi A: Inhibition of human pulmonary phosphodiesterase activity by therapeutic levels of theophylline. Clin Exp Pharm Physiol 1978;5:535–539.
22. Curry SC, Vance MV, Requa R, Armstead R: The effects of toxic concentrations of theophylline on oxygen consumption, ventricular work, acid base balance and plasma catecholamine levels in the dog. Ann Emerg Med 1985;14:554–561.
23. Curry SC, Vance MV, Requa R, Armstead R: Cardiovascular effects of toxic concentrations of theophylline in the dog. Ann Emerg Med 1985;14:547–553.
24. Higbee MD, Kumar M, Galant SP: Stimulation of endogenous catecholamine release by theophylline: a proposed additional mechanism of action for theophylline effects. J Allergy Clin Immunol 1982;70:377–382.
25. Vestal RE, Eiriksson CE, Musser B, et al: Effect of intravenous aminophylline on plasm plasma levels of catecholamines and related cardiovascular and metabolic responses in man. Circulation 1983;67:162–171.
26. Feoktistov I, Biaggioni I: Role of adenosine in asthma. Drug Dev Res 1996;39:333–336.
27. Visitsunthorn N, Udomittipong K, Punnakan L: Theophylline toxicity in Thai children. Asian Pac J Allergy Immunol 2001;19:177–182.
28. Schiff GD, Hegde HK, LaCloche L, Hryhorczuk DO: Inpatient theophylline toxicity: preventable factors. Ann Intern Med 1991;114:748–753.
29. Paloucek FP, Rodvold KA: Evaluation of theophylline overdoses and toxicities. Ann Emerg Med 1988;17:135–144.
30. Shannon MW, Lovejoy FH, Woolf A: Prediction of serum theophylline concentration after acute theophylline intoxication [abstract]. Ann Emerg Med 1990;19:627.
31. Stavric B: Methylxanthines: toxicity to humans. Food Chem Toxicol 1988;26:541–565.
32. Baker MD: Theophylline toxicity in children. J Pediatr 1986;109:538–542.
33. Amitai Y, Lovejoy FH: Characteristics of vomiting associated with acute sustained release theophylline poisoning: implications for management with oral activated charcoal. Clin Toxicol 1987;25:539–554.
34. Biberstein MP, Ziegler MG, Ward DM: Use of beta-blockade and hemoperfusion for acute theophylline poisoning. West J Med 1984;141:485–490.
35. Lin CK, Chuand IN, Cheng KK, Chiang BN: Arrhythmogenic effects of theophylline in human atrial tissue. Int J Cardiol 1987;17:289–297.
36. Sessler CN, Cohen MD: Cardiac arrhythmias during theophylline toxicity: a prospective continuous electrocardiographic study. Chest 1990;98:672–678.
37. Shannon M: Predictors of major toxicity after theophylline overdose. Ann Intern Med 1993;119:1161–1167.
38. Bittar G, Friedman HS: The arrhythmogenicity of theophylline: a multivariate analysis of clinical determinants. Chest 1991;99:1415–1420.
39. Rachelefsky GS, Wo J, Adelson J, et al: Behavior abnormalities and poor school performance due to oral theophylline use. Pediatrics 1986;78:1133–1138.
40. Rappaport L, Coffman H, Guare R, et al: Effects of theophylline on behavior and learning in children with asthma. Am J Dis Child 1989;143:368–372.
41. Stein M, Krasowski M, Leventhal BL, et al: Behavioral and cognitive effects of methylxanthines: a meta-analysis of theophylline and caffeine. Arch Pediatr Adolesc Med 1996;150:284–288.
42. Schlieper A, Alcock D, Beaudry P, et al: Effect of therapeutic plasma concentrations of theophylline on behavior, cognitive processing and affect in children with asthma. J Pediatr 1991;118:449–455.
43. Nakada T, Keww IL, Lerner AM, Remler MP: Theophylline-induced seizures: clinical and pathophysiologic aspects. West J Med 1983;138:371–374.
44. Zwillich CW, Sutton FD, Neff TA, et al: Theophylline-induced seizures in adults. Ann Intern Med 1975;82:784–787.
45. Phung ND: Theophylline toxicity in ambulatory elderly patients. Immunol Allergy Practice 1986;8:17–20.
46. Richards W, Church JA, Brent DK: Theophylline-associated seizures in children. Ann Allergy 1985;54:276–279.
47. Woody RC, Laney M: A second case of infantile intracranial hemorrhage and severe neurological sequelae following theophylline overdose. Dev Med Child Neurol 1986;28:120–121.
48. Sahney S, Abarzua J, Sessums L: Hemoperfusion in theophylline neurotoxicity. Pediatrics 1983;71:615–619.
49. Bahls F, Ma KK, Bird TD: Theophylline-associated seizures with "therapeutic" or low toxic serum concentrations: risk factors for serious outcome in adults. Neurology 1991;41:1309–1312.
50. Park GD, Spector R, Roberts RJ, et al: Use of hemoperfusion for treatment of theophylline intoxication. Am J Med 1983;74:961–966.
51. Parish RA, Haulman NJ, Burns RM: Interaction of theophylline with erythromycin base in a patient with seizure activity. Pediatrics 1983;72:828–830.
52. Seto T, Inada H, Kobayashi N, et al: Depression of serum pyridoxal levels in theophylline-related seizures. Brain Dev 2000;32:295–300.
53. Glenn GM, Krober MS, Kelly P, et al: Pyridoxine as therapy in theophylline-induced seizures. Vet Human Toxicol 1995;37:342–344.
54. Shannon M, Maher T: Anticonvulsant effects of intracerebroventricular Adenocard in theophylline-induced seizures. Ann Emerg Med 1995;26:65–68.
55. Pinard E, Riche D, Puiroud S, Seylaz J: Theophylline reduces cerebral hyperaemia and enhances brain damage induced by seizures. Brain Res 1990;511:303–309.
56. Hall KW, Dobson KE, Dalton JG, et al: Metabolic abnormalities associated with intentional theophylline overdose. Am J Emerg Med Ann Intern Med 1984;101:457–462.
57. Sawyer WT, Caravati EM, Ellison MJ, Krueger KA: Hypokalemia, hyperglycemia, and acidosis after intentional theophylline overdose. Am J Emerg Med 1985;3:408–411.
58. Robertson NJ: Fatal overdose from a sustained-release theophylline preparation. Ann Emerg Med 1985;14:154–158.
59. Buckley BM, Braithwaite RA, Vale JA: Theophylline poisoning. Lancet 1983;2:618.
60. Amitai Y, Lovejoy FH: Hypokalemia in acute theophylline poisoning. Am J Emerg Med 1988;6:214–218.
61. Clausen T, Flatman JA: Beta-2 adrenoceptors mediate the stimulating effect of adrenaline on active electrogenic Na-K-transport in rat soleus muscle. Br J Pharmacol 1980;68:749–755.
62. Clausen T: Adrenergic control of Na-K-homeostasis. Acta Med Scand 1983;672(Suppl):111–115.
63. Kearney TE, Manoguerra AS, Curtis GP, Ziegler MG: Theophylline toxicity and the beta-adrenergic system. Ann Intern Med 1985;102:766–769.

64. Polak M, Rolon MA, Chouchana A, Czernichow P: Theophylline intoxication mimicking diabetic ketoacidosis in a child. Diabetes Metab 1999;25:513–515.

65. Ryan T, Coughlan G, Mc Ging P, Phelan D: Ketosis, a complication of theophylline toxicity. J Int Med 1989;226:277–278.

66. McPherson ML, Prince SR, Atamer ER, et al: Theophylline-induced hypercalcemia. Ann Intern Med 1986;105:52–54.

67. Neff RD, Leviton A: Maternal theophylline consumption and the risk of stillbirth. Chest 1990;97:1266–1267.

68. Gaudreault P, Wason S, Lovejoy F: Acute pediatric theophylline overdose: a summary of 28 cases. J Pediatr 1983;102:474–476.

69. Aitken ML, Martin TR: Life-threatening theophylline toxicity is not predictable by serum levels. Chest 1987;91:10–14.

70. Bertino JS, Walker JW: Reassessment of theophylline toxicity-serum concentrations, clinical course, and treatment. Arch Intern Med 1987;147:757–760.

71. Covelli HD, Knodel AR, Heppner BT: Predisposing factors to apparent theophylline-induced seizures. Ann Allergy 1985;54:411–415.

72. Olson KR, Benowitz NL, Woo OF, Pond SM: Theophylline overdose: acute single ingestion versus chronic repeated overmedication. Am J Emerg Med 1985;3:386–394.

73. Dean LS, Brown JW: Massive theophylline overdose: survival without hemoperfusion. JAMA 1982;248:1742.

74. Wells DH, Ferlauto JJ: Survival after massive aminophylline overdose in a premature infant. Pediatrics 1979;64:252–253.

75. Shannon M, Lovejoy F: Effect of acute versus chronic intoxication on clinical features of theophylline poisoning in children. J Pediatr 1992;121:125–130.

76. Shannon M, Lovejoy F: The influence of age vs. peak serum concentration of life-threatening events after chronic theophylline intoxication. Arch Intern Med 1990;150:2045–2048.

77. Shannon M, Lovejoy F: Hypokalemia after theophylline intoxication: the effects of acute vs. chronic poisoning. Arch Intern Med 1989;149:2725–2729.

78. Heath A, Knudsen K: Role of extracorporeal drug removal in acute theophylline poisoning: a review. Med Toxicol 1987;2:294–308.

79. Amin DN, Henry JA: Propranolol administration in theophylline overdose. Lancet 1985;1:520–521.

80. Gaar GG, Banner W, Laddu AR: The effects of esmolol on the hemodynamics of acute theophylline toxicity. Ann Emerg Med 1987;16:1334–1339.

81. Seneff M, Scott J, Friedman B, Smith M: Acute theophylline toxicity and the use of esmolol to reverse cardiovascular instability. Ann Emerg Med 1990;19:671–673.

82. Greenberg A, Piraino BH, Kroboth PD, Weiss J: Severe theophylline toxicity—role of conservative measures, antiarrhythmic agents and charcoal hemoperfusion. Am J Med 1984;76:854–860.

83. Blake KV, Massey KL, Hendeles L, et al: Relative efficacy of phenytoin and phenobarbital for the prevention of theophylline-induced seizures in mice. Ann Emerg Med 1988;17:1024–1028.

84. Amitai Y, Yeung AC, Moye J, Lovejoy FH: Repetitive oral activated charcoal and control of emesis in severe theophylline toxicity. Ann Intern Med 1986;105:386–387.

85. Roberts JR, Carney S, Boyle SM, Lee D: Ondansetron quells drug-resistant emesis in theophylline poisoning. Am J Emerg Med 1993;11:609–611.

86. Bernstein G, Jehle D, Bernaski E, Braen GR: Failure of gastric emptying and charcoal administration in fatal sustained-release theophylline overdose: pharmacobezoar formation. Ann Emerg Med 1992;21:1388–1390.

87. Burkhart KK, Metcalf S, Shurnas E, et al: Exchange transfusion and multidose activated charcoal following vancomycin overdose. Clin Toxicol 1992;30:285–294.

88. D'Angio R, Sabatelli F: Management considerations in treating metabolic abnormalities associated with theophylline overdose. Arch Intern Med 1987;147:1837–1838.

89. Borkan S: Extracorporeal therapies for acute intoxications. Crit Care Clin 2002;18:393–420.

90. Kulig KW, Bar-Or D, Rumack BH: Intravenous theophylline poisoning and multiple-dose charcoal in an animal model. Ann Emerg Med 1987;16:842–846.

91. Russo ME: Management of theophylline intoxication with charcoal-column hemoperfusion. N Engl J Med 1979;300:24–26.

92. Anonymous: Position statement and practice guidelines on the use of multi-dose activated charcoal in the treatment of acute poisoning. J Toxicol Clin Toxicol 1999;37:731–751.

93. Ohning BL, Reed MD, Blumer JL: Continuous nasogastric administration of activated charcoal for the treatment of theophylline intoxication. Pediatr Pharmacol 1986;5:241–245.

94. Park GD, Radomski L, Goldberg MJ, et al: Effect of size and frequency of oral doses of charcoal on theophylline clearance. Clin Pharmacol Ther 1983;34:664–666.

95. Longdon P, Henderson A: Intestinal pseudo-obstruction following the use of enteral charcoal and sorbitol and mechanical ventilation with papaveretum sedation for theophylline poisoning. Drug Safety 1992;7:74–77.

96. Shannon M, Amitai Y, Lovejoy FH: Multiple-dose activated charcoal for theophylline poisoning in young infants. Pediatrics 1987;80:368–370.

97. Goldberg MJ, Park GD, Berlinger WG: Treatment of theophylline intoxication. J Allergy Clin Immunol 1986;78:811–817.

98. Gitomer J, Khan A, Ferris M: Treatment of severe theophylline toxicity with hemodialysis in a preterm neonate. Pediatr Nephrol 2001;16:784–786.

99. Osborn HH, Henry G, Wax P, et al: Theophylline toxicity in a premature neonate-elimination kinetics of exchange transfusion. Clin Toxicol 1993;31:639–644.

100. Shannon M, Wernovsky B, Morris C: Exchange transfusion in the treatment of severe theophylline poisoning. Pediatrics 1992;89:145–147.

101. Laussen P, Shann F, Butt W, Tibballs J: Use of plasmapheresis in acute theophylline toxicity. Crit Care Med 1991;19:288–290.

102. Gaudreault P, Guay J: Theophylline poisoning—pharmacological considerations and clinical management. Med Toxicol 1986;1:169–191.

103. Nawrot P, Jordan S, Eastwood J, et al: Effects of caffeine on human health. Food Addit Contam 2003;20:1–30.

104. Pollak C, Bright D: Caffeine consumption and weekly sleep patterns in US seventh-, eighth-, and ninth-graders. Pediatrics 2003;111:42–46.

105. Hering-Hanit R, Gadoth N: Caffeine-induced headache in children and adolescents. Cephalalgia 2003;23:332–335.

106. Savoca M, Evans CD, Wilson ME, et al: The association of caffeinated beverages with blood pressure in adolescents. Arch Pediatr Adolesc Med 2004:158:473–477.

107. Davis R, Osorio I: Childhood caffeine tic syndrome. Pediatrics 1998;101:E4.

108. Dalvi R: Acute and chronic toxicity of caffeine: a review. Vet Hum Toxicol 1986;28:144–150.

109. Walther FJ, Erickson R, Sims M: Cardiovascular effects of caffeine therapy in preterm infants. Am J Dis Child 1990;144:1164–1166.

110. Lovallo W, Wilson MF, Vincent AS, et al: Blood pressure response to caffeine shows incomplete tolerance after short-term regular consumption. Hypertension 2004;43:760–765.

111. Myers M: Effects of caffeine on blood pressure. Arch Intern Med 1988;148:1189.

112. Chelsky L, Cutter JE, Griffith K, et al: Caffeine and ventricular arrhythmias—an electrophysiological approach. JAMA 1990;264:2236–2240.

113. Benowitz N, Osterloh J, Goldschlager N: Massive catecholamine release from caffeine poisoning. JAMA 1982;248:1097–1098.

114. Walsh I, Wassermann GS, Mestad P, Lanman RC: Near fatal caffeine intoxication treated with perineal dialysis. Pediatr Emerg Care 1987;3:244–246.

115. Holmgren P, Norden-Pettersson L, Ahlner J: Caffeine fatalities—four case reports. Forensic Sci Int 2004;139:71–73.

116. Mrvos R, Reilly PE, Dean BS, Krenzelok EP: Massive caffeine ingestion resulting in death. Vet Hum Toxicol 1989;31:571–573.

117. Eisele J: Deaths related to coffee enemas. JAMA 1980;244:1608–1609.

118. Dietrich AM, Mortensen M: Presentation and management of an acute caffeine overdose. Pediatr Emerg Care 1990;6:296–298.

119. Wrenn K, Oschner I: Rhabdomyolysis induced by a caffeine overdose. Ann Emerg Med 1989;18:94–97.

120. Lubin F, Ron E, Wax P, et al: A case-control study of caffeine and methylxanthines in benign breast disease. JAMA 1985;253:2388–2392.

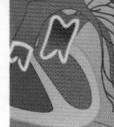

121. Minton J: Caffeine and benign breast disease. JAMA 1985;254: 2408–2409.
122. Signorello L, McLaughlin J: Maternal caffeine consumption and spontaneous abortion: a review of the epidemiologic evidence. Epidemiology 2004;15:229–239.
123. Silverman K, Evans SM, Strain EC, Griffiths RR: Withdrawal syndrome after the double-blind cessation of caffeine consumption. N Engl J Med 1992;327:1109–1114.
124. Strain E, Mumford GK, Silverman K, Griffiths RR: Caffeine dependence syndrome: evidence from case histories and experimental evaluations. JAMA 1994;272:1043–1048.
125. Price K, Fligner D: Treatment of caffeine toxicity with esmolol. Ann Emerg Med 1990;19:44–46.
126. Sullivan J: Caffeine poisoning in an infant. J Pediatr 1977;90: 1022–1023.
127. Holstege C, Hunter Y, Baer AB, et al: Massive caffeine overdose requiring vasopressin infusion and hemodialysis. J Toxicol Clin Toxicol 2003;41:1003–1007.

66 *Anticoagulants*

MELISA W. LAI, MD ■ MICHELE BURNS EWALD, MD

At a Glance...

- There are two main anticoagulant medication mechanisms of action: (1) platelet aggregation inhibition, involving the glycoprotein IIb/IIIa receptor inhibitors eptifibatide and abciximab and the cyclooxygenase inhibitor aspirin; and (2) disruption of the coagulation cascade, involving the vitamin K inhibitors warfarin and superwarfarins, antithrombin III acceleration through factors II and X, the heparins, and fondaparinux, and direct thrombin (factor II) inhibition through leech-derived anticoagulants (hirudins) and ximelagatran.
- Even in overdose situations, anticoagulants rarely precipitate life-threatening hemorrhage.
- Treatment should be based on clinical assessment supported by the results of bleeding time studies (partial thromboplastin time, prothrombin time, International Normalized Ratio, hematocrit concentration, and platelet concentration).

Anticoagulation has become a fundamental basis of medical therapy for patients with cardiovascular and thromboembolic disease. Medications that disrupt or block platelet aggregation and fibrin cross-linkage are now the standard of care in management and prevention of vaso-occlusive events.

The results of multiple studies on the treatment of acute coronary syndrome, deep vein thrombosis (DVT), and pulmonary embolism have led to the development, introduction, and implementation of new anticoagulant and antiplatelet medications as well as their dosing protocols. This increase in the number of available agents, in conjunction with the widespread use of anticoagulants, may explain the changing profile of anticoagulant overdose and exposure. Although anticoagulants have also had long-standing use as rodenticides, Toxic

Exposure Surveillance System (TESS) data from 2000 to 2004 show that the number of rodenticide anticoagulant exposures in the United States stayed constant at about 17,000 per year; the number of anticoagulant overdoses from medical therapeutic use increased each year during the same time period, from 2871 overdoses in 2000 to 4786 in 2004 (Table 66-1).

Anticoagulation medications targeted toward various components of the coagulation cascade and platelet aggregation systems continue to be developed, and new trials to prove efficacy in vaso-occlusive events continue to be held. As such, the scope of the material in this chapter is constantly evolving, and specific product information data sheets should be referred to when encountering new anticoagulant therapies.

REVIEW OF COAGULATION

Understanding the mechanism of coagulation is key to understanding the mechanism of action of various anticoagulants and therapies for overdose. The two components of the coagulation pathway are the platelet system and the coagulation cascade.

The Platelet System

Platelet coagulation is mediated by both vascular wall adhesion through von Willebrand factor (vWF) and platelet aggregation through glycoprotein IIb/IIIa (gpIIb/IIIa) receptors. Vascular injury exposes collagen and releases tissue factor. Circulating inactive platelets adhere to the site of injury by binding either directly to collagen or indirectly through vWF, and then are "activated" by locally generated thrombin. Soluble

---

TABLE 66-1 Anticoagulant Exposures and Overdoses in the United States

Therapeutic Anticoagulant Overdoses		2000	2001	2002	2003	2004
Glycoprotein IIb/IIIa inhibitor overdoses		Not reported	3	9	11	14
Other antiplatelet/anticoagulant overdoses		Not reported	993	1298	1490	1842
Herparin overdosesNot reported		138	149	164	176	198
Warfarin overdoses		2139	2304	2684	2718	2732
	TOTAL	2277	3449	4155	4395	4786
Anticoagulant-type Rodenticide Exposures						
Rodenticide exposures (warfarin-type)		1181	492	462	341	337
Rodenticide exposures (long-acting, superwarfarin)		16,006	16,423	17,100	16,481	16,054
	TOTAL	17,187	16,915	17,562	16,822	16,391
Total Anticoagulant Overdoses/Exposures		19,464	20,364	21,717	21,217	21,177

Compiled from Annual Reports of the American Association of Poison Control Centers Toxic Exposure Surveillance System, 2000–2002.

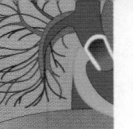

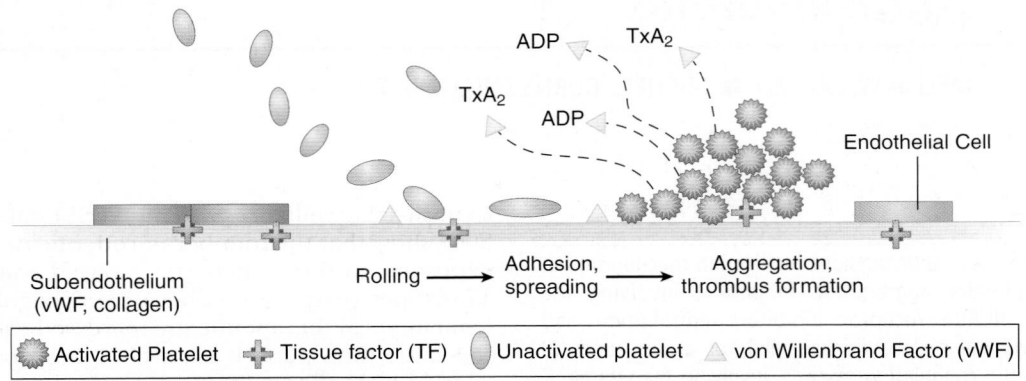

FIGURE 66-1 Platelet adhesion and aggregation to injured vascular wall. Platelets bind directly to collagen or to von Willebrand factor (vWF) and are "activated" by locally generated thrombin. Adenosine diphosphate (ADP) and thromboxane A_2 (TxA_2) are released by active platelets to recruit further platelets. Activated platelets bind to each other through fibrinogen linkages to gpIIb/IIIa receptors up-regulated to platelet membrane surface.

factors such as adenosine diphosphate (ADP) and thromboxane A_2 (TxA_2) are released by activated platelets to recruit nonadherent platelets.

Platelets then aggregate by adhering to each other through fibrinogen linkages. Fibrinogen molecules bind to the gpIIb/IIIa receptor, the most abundant platelet surface protein. The gpIIb/IIIa receptors can undergo up-regulation to effectively double in number on the surface of activated platelets (Fig. 66-1).

The Coagulation Cascade

The coagulation cascade is a chain of events that starts with dormant enzymes (proteases) called *coagulation factors* and ends with the activation of the protein thrombin. Thrombin is needed for platelet activation and to cleave fibrinogen into fibrin for cross-linkage (Fig. 66-2). By having this chain of activations rather than one single activation, modifications made early in the cascade can quickly be amplified, leading to timely changes in thrombin production.

Coagulation factor nomenclature uses Roman numerals; many also have eponyms or "given" labels (Table 66-2). An inactive factor will be written as simply the Roman numeral, whereas an activated factor has a small Roman alphabet letter "a" appended to it (e.g., inactive factor VII, when activated is written as factor VIIa).

Although most coagulation factors are made by the liver, factor XIII is derived from platelets and factor VIII from endothelial cells. Factors II (prothrombin), VII (Stable), IX (Christmas), and X (Stuart) and anticoagulant proteins C and protein S are dependent on γ-carboxylase, a vitamin K–dependent liver enzyme.

Intrinsic and Extrinsic Pathways

The coagulation cascade is triggered by either factors intrinsic to circulating blood (leading down the intrinsic pathway) or tissue-based factors extrinsic to blood (leading down the extrinsic pathway). The intrinsic system is activated when high-molecular-weight kininogens (precursors of bradykinin) and the enzyme kallikrein activate factor XII in the presence of collagen exposed from an injury. Its major factors are XII, XI, IX, and VIII. Factor VIII, normally complexed to vWF, is activated upon dissociation. Factor X is not activated until both activated factors VIIIa and IXa are in the presence of calcium and platelet phospholipids (PLs). This pathway is measured by the partial thromboplastin time (PTT). The extrinsic pathway is initiated when thromboplastin (i.e., tissue factor [TF]), a lipid-rich protein released on tissue injury, directly activates factor VII, which in turn triggers IX with subsequent activation of factor X. This pathway is measured by the prothrombin time (PT).

After convergence of the cascade at factor X, active factor Xa complexes with factor Va and Ca^{2+} in the presence of PLs to create the factor Va + Xa + calcium + PL complex that cleaves prothrombin (II) to thrombin (IIa).

Control of the Coagulation Cascade

There are two "brakes" that control the coagulation cascade: the thrombolytic system and coagulation factor inhibition. In the thrombolytic system, the inactive precursor protein plasminogen is cleaved into the serum protease plasmin after coming into contact with thrombin. Plasmin then cleaves fibrin to break up the clot and, in doing so, creates fibrin degradation products that inhibit further thrombin formation.

Coagulation factor inhibitors include antithrombin III (ATIII), protein C, and protein S. Protease inhibitor ATIII physically blocks the action of coagulation factors in the coagulation cascade (thrombin, IX, X, XI, and XII). This blockade is accelerated up to 2000 times by heparin. Protein C is activated by thrombin to cleave factor Va into its inactive form, preventing the factor Va + Xa + calcium + PL complex from cleaving prothrombin to thrombin. Protein S is a necessary cofactor of protein C.

Vitamin K and Coagulation

Vitamin K is discussed in detail elsewhere in this text. Because of its important role in coagulation and the

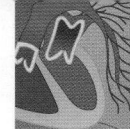

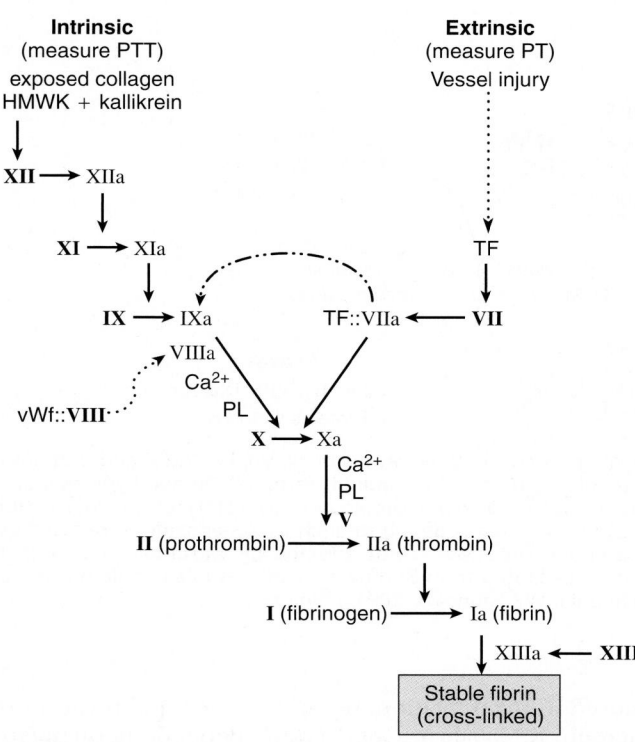

FIGURE 66-2 The coagulation cascade. HMWK, high-molecular-weight kininogens (bradykinin precursors); PL, platelet phospholipids; PT, prothrombin time; PTT, partial thromboplastin time; TF, tissue factor (thromboplastin); vWF, von Willebrand factor.

mechanism of action for some anticoagulants, it is reviewed here.

Vitamin K is a lipid-soluble vitamin found and manufactured in a synthetic and two natural forms. Natural vitamin K_1 (phytonadione, phylloquinone) is synthesized

TABLE 66-2 Coagulation Factors and Their Eponymous Names

FACTOR*	EPONYM/"TRIVIAL" NAME
I	Fibrinogen
II	Prothrombin
III	Tissue factor
IV	Calcium
V	Proaccelerin, labile†
VI	Accelerin
VII	Stable, proconvertin, serum prothrombin conversion accelerator (SPCA)
VIII	Antihemophiliac factor A
IX	Christmas, antihemophiliac factor B
X	Stuart-Power factor
XI	Plasma thromboplastin antecedent (PTA)
XII	Hageman factor
XIII	Fibrin stabilizing factor (FSF)

*Activated factors append a letter "a" to the Roman numeral (e.g., inactive factor *VII* becomes activated factor *VIIa*).
†Note that *Labile* is the eponym for factor V, while "factor V Leiden" refers to the gene defect in factor V resulting in diminished anticoagulation and consequent hypercoagulable state.
Adapted from King MW: Blood coagulation. Retrieved July 12, 2004, from http://web.indstate.edu/theme/mwking/blood-coagulation.html.

Vitamin K₃ (menadione)   **Vitamin K₂ (menaquinone)**

Vitamin K₁ (phytonadione)

FIGURE 66-3 Structure of vitamin K subtypes. All subtypes have a recognizable two-ring basic structure.

by plants and algae. Natural vitamin K_2 (menaquinone) is produced by bacteria. Vitamin K_3 (menadione) is synthetic and converted to active K_2 in vivo. All vitamin K subtypes are two-ring structures with variable carbon side chains (Fig. 66-3).

Vitamin K is required for γ-carboxylation of glutamate residues to activate factors II, VII, IX, and X. Vitamin K produces γ-carboxylase (γ-carboxyglutamate), which chelates Ca^{2+}, allowing binding of vitamin K–dependent clotting factors to phospholipid membranes during activation of the coagulation cascade. Reduction or absence of vitamin K leaves factors II, VII, IX, and X in their inactive states, halting the coagulation cascade. With an estimated plasma half-life of 1.7 hours,[1] vitamin K_1 depletion resulting in clinically significant change within the coagulation cascade is not expected for at least 24 hours; that is, five half-lives of vitamin K *plus* five half-lives of the vitamin K–dependent clotting factor with the shortest half-life ($t_{1/2}$[factor VII] = 6 hours[2]):

$$= 5(t_{1/2}[\text{vitamin K}]) + 5(t_{1/2}[\text{factor VII}])$$

ANTICOAGULANTS BY MECHANISMS OF ACTION

Vitamin K Inhibition

Warfarins and superwarfarins (4-hydroxycoumarins and inandiones) disrupt the vitamin K cycle by primarily inhibiting vitamin K 2,3-epoxide reductase and, to a lesser degree, vitamin K quinone reductase (Fig. 66-4). These drugs prevent the regeneration of active vitamin K_1 (quinol) with subsequent depletion of vitamin K–dependent coagulation factors (II, VII, IX and X) and disruption of the coagulation cascade.

WARFARIN
Background
Warfarin was developed after the discovery of the agent responsible for a hemorrhagic bovine disorder in which cows that ingested spoiled sweet clover silage would develop internal bleeding associated with plasma

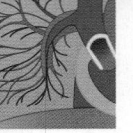

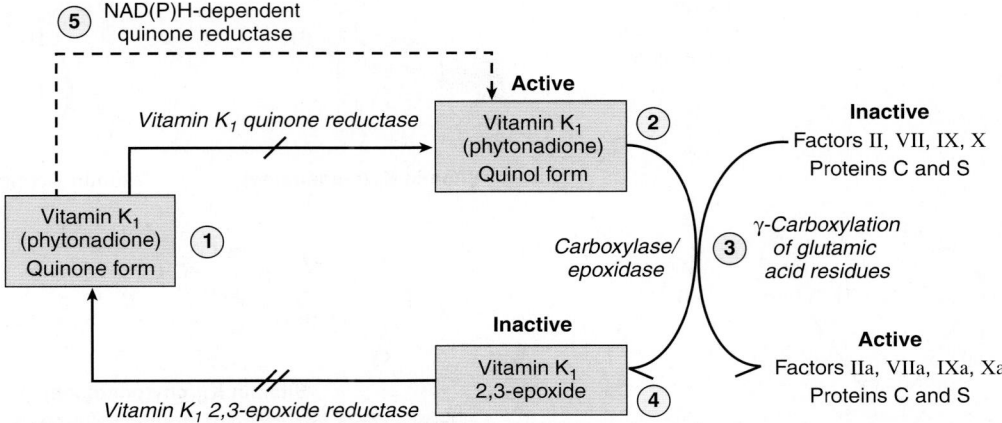

FIGURE 66-4 The vitamin K cycle. Inactive vitamin K–dependent prozymogens are coagulation factors II, VII, IX, and X and proteins C and S. (1) Vitamin K_1 (quinone form) is reduced by vitamin K_1 quinone reductase to its active (quinol) form. (2) Quinol (hydroquinone, vitamin KH_2) exists in hepatic microsomes. (3) Carboxylase-epoxidase (coupled) enzyme simultaneously catalyzes γ-carboxylation coagulation factors to active form *and* converts quinol to the inactive vitamin K_1 2,3-epoxide. (4) Vitamin K_1 2-3-epoxide → recycled via epoxide reductase to quinone. (5) *Alternatively,* NAD(P)H-dependent quinone reductase is not affected by warfarins → vitamin K administered exogenously may still be reduced and counter anticoagulation. (Adapted from Burkhart K: Anticoagulant rodenticides. In Ford MD, Delaney KA, Ling LJ, Erickson T [eds]: Clinical Toxicology. Philadelphia, WB Saunders, 2001, p 849.)

prothrombin reduction.[3] From this clover, the natural bishydroxywarfarin (dicoumarol) was eventually derived in 1939; later, the Wisconsin Alumni Research Foundation synthesized and named the pharmaceutical agent warfarin, which became commercially available in 1955.[3] In 2002, warfarin was the 64th-most frequently prescribed drug based on the number of prescriptions written.[4]

Usage and Indications

Warfarin is a racemic mixture of R- and S-enantiomers. The S-enantiomer is five times more potent than the R orientation at producing hypoprothrombinemia (decreased prothrombin slows the coagulation cascade) in rats[5] and 1.8 times more potent in humans.[6] The S-enantiomer is also eliminated more slowly than the R-enantiomer in rats, but is more rapidly eliminated in humans.[7] This difference in enantiomer potency and rate of elimination makes warfarin an appealing rodenticide. As a therapeutic anticoagulant in humans, warfarin is used for treatment of pulmonary embolism and DVT, to prevent atrial thrombus formation in atrial fibrillation, and for patients with severe peripheral vascular disease and arterial stenoses.

Pharmacokinetics

Warfarin's only route of administration is oral, and it is almost completely absorbed from the gastrointestinal tract.[4] Maximum plasma concentrations are reached within 20 minutes to 4 hours after ingestion.[4,8] Wafarin is highly protein bound (99%), but only the free fraction of the drug is active.[4] Warfarin's half-life is 36 to 42 hours,[9] and its duration of action after a single dose is 2 to 5 days[8]; it takes about 6 days to reach a steady state. Inhibition of vitamin K regeneration is almost immediate, but effects are delayed until existing stores of vitamin K are depleted and active coagulation factors re-

moved from circulation. Because of the rapid turnover of vitamin K, warfarin's effects are dependent on factor half-life, and PT prolongation is not seen until factors are reduced to 25% of their normal values. For example, factor VII, which is depleted most rapidly, has a half-life of 5 hours; hence, it takes at least 15 hours until PT prolongation is evident.

Metabolism

Warfarin is metabolized in the liver through the cytochrome P-450 system. The R-enantiomer is primarily metabolized by isoenzymes CYP1A2 and CYP3A4[10] and excreted in the kidney. The S-enantiomer is metabolized more rapidly by CYP2C9[10] and secreted into bile. Elimination half-life is 24 to 36 hours. Drugs that inhibit the P-450 system, and subsequently prolong warfarin's action, include erythromycin, metronidazole, thyroxine, isoniazid, and trimethoprim-sulfamethoxazole. Substances that enhance the P-450 system to induce warfarin's metabolism, thus decreasing its effectiveness, include barbiturates, penicillin, carbamazepine, charbroiled foods, and tobacco smoke.

Dosage and Therapeutic Monitoring

Warfarin is dosed once daily orally and titrated to an appropriate international normalized ratio (INR) for different conditions. Warfarin use is monitored by measuring PT and calculating the INR. The INR "normalizes" variations in PT measurement due to different sensitivities of reagents used by different laboratories.

Most clinicians opt for a goal INR of 2.0 to 2.5 in patients with atrial fibrillation; an INR of 2.5 to 3.0 for patients being treated for venous thromboses; and an INR as elevated as 2.5 to 3.5 in patients with mechanical prosthetic heart valves.[9] The optimal children's dose has been calculated to be 0.07 × [weight in kg] + 0.54 mg,[11]

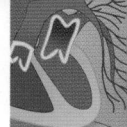

whereas nomograms have been developed to guide initial dosage in adults based on clinical situation and target INR.[12]

Warfarin in Pregnancy

Warfarin is a pregnancy category X drug (adverse effects reported, contraindicated in pregnancy) and is a teratogen that leads to a particular constellation of congenital defects after ingestion during the first trimester, particularly between weeks 6 and 9 of gestation. About one third of infants exposed to warfarin during this time period develop fetal warfarin syndrome (FWS; also known as *warfarin embryopathy* or *fetal Coumarin syndrome*).[13] Infants with FWS display a range of physical and central nervous system anomalies, including nasal hypoplasia, stippling of uncalcified epiphyses (particularly of the axial skeleton), mild hypoplasia of nails and shortened fingers, low birth weight, and varying degrees of mental retardation.

Patients who are breast-feeding may use warfarin for anticoagulation therapy. An inactive form of warfarin is excreted into breast milk,[8] but several researchers have confirmed that active warfarin is not detectable in human milk, and there is no evidence of detectable warfarin levels, altered coagulation, or other adverse events in infants exposed to breast milk from mothers taking warfarin.[14,15]

Overdose

In therapeutic overmedication, warfarin should be held and indications for vitamin K administration should be reviewed in consultation with those monitoring therapeutic dosing. Patients with an abnormally elevated INR or intentional warfarin overdose should be admitted to a hospital and placed on bed rest to minimize the risk for trauma with subsequent internal or intracranial bleeding. Often, depending on a patient's INR, withholding warfarin administration for several days is sufficient to bring an INR down to therapeutic levels. Vitamin K is indicated for those with a significantly elevated INR that does not decrease when warfarin is withheld or when there is evidence of hepatic synthetic dysfunction (e.g., a significant increase in liver transaminase concentrations or in the INR). Fresh frozen plasma is indicated for those with active bleeding. In the absence of recent changes in dosing regimen, clinicians should investigate reasons for an increased INR, such as the use of other medications that may inhibit the cytochrome P-450 system, infection, or misuse or mislabeling.

In acute overdose of warfarin, treating practitioners should determine the nature of the ingestion: unintentional (accidental) or intentional. In most accidental single ingestions, the amount of warfarin ingested is highly unlikely to result in a clinically apparent coagulopathy, and most patients may be monitored safely at home with appropriate caveats to avoid contact sports and situations increasing the likelihood of traumatic injury for several days. Intentional ingestions present the dilemma that a patient may ingest further warfarin when not being monitored. Repetitive

ingestions can lead to a clinically significant coagulopathy. These patients should be dispositioned after consultation with a poison control center (the American Association of Poison Control Centers national poison control center hotline is 1-800-222-1222; www.aapcc.org) and appropriate psychiatric services.

Nonbleeding Complications

Warfarin use has been implicated in the rare development of nonhemorrhagic skin lesions ranging from simple ecchymosis and purpura to urticaria, purple toes, and skin necrosis.[16] Warfarin skin necrosis usually appears over fatty tissues (breasts, buttocks, thighs) 3 to 6 days after warfarin therapy initiation; patients with protein C, protein S, and antithrombin III deficiency appear to be at greater risk for development of this condition.[17] Warfarin should be discontinued in patients who acquire skin necrosis, and alternative anticoagulation should be started to prevent postcapillary thrombosis. Purple toe syndrome is thought to be caused by anticoagulant-induced bleeding into atherosclerotic plaques releasing cholesterol crystal emboli.[18] Changing anticoagulation agents is thus unlikely to prevent or reverse progression.

SUPERWARFARINS
Background

The superwarfarins, 4-hydroxycoumarins and inandiones, were developed in response to genetic resistance to warfarin in rats.[19-21] They are primarily used as rodenticides and have no role in human medical therapeutic anticoagulation. In fact, warfarin ingestions were deemed "clinically insignificant" until 1976 when the superwarfarins were developed for use as rodenticides. The 4-hydroxycoumarins in use today are difenacoum, brodifacoum (D-Con), bromadiolone, and coumatetralyl. Inandiones include chlorophacinone, diphacinone, and pindone.

Both the hydroxycoumarins and inandiones have a two-ring base structure similar to warfarin (Figs. 66-5 and 66-6). Both groups function just as warfarin does, by inhibiting vitamin K 2,3-epoxidase.

Toxicokinetics

Superwarfarins are highly lipid soluble and are mostly concentrated in the liver. On a mole-for-mole basis, they are 100 times more potent than warfarin.[22] In overdose, their elimination half-life is weeks to months,[22] up to 60 times longer than warfarin's half-life of 35 hours. They also have a considerably longer duration of action: a rat that dies after a single superwarfarin ingestion would require 21 days of warfarin before meeting the same fate.

FIGURE 66-5 Warfarin.

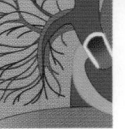

4-Hydroxycoumarin   Inandione

FIGURE 66-6 Structures of 4-hydroxycoumarin (*left*) and indanedione (*right*). Note the two-ring base structure, similar to that of warfarin in Figure 66-3.

Ingestion

Superwarfarin ingestions illustrate the toxicologist's adage that "it is only the dose which makes a thing a poison" (Aureolus Paracelsus, 1493–1541). Given that repetitive dosing is necessary to achieve therapeutic anticoagulation with warfarin alone, it stands to reason that small single acute ingestions (e.g., a mouthful) are unlikely to produce a clinically significant coagulopathy: a 10-kg child would need to ingest 3000 mg/kg of a 0.005% warfarin-based rodenticide for coagulopathy to develop.[23]

Management of superwarfarin ingestion should be based on amount ingested as related to circumstance of ingestion. Most cases of superwarfarin exposure are either intentional ingestions by adults or unintentional ingestions by children (including ingestion of rat feces from poisoned rodents[24]). Case reports have also described warfarin and superwarfarins as agents of ingestion for Munchausen syndrome and Munchausen syndrome by proxy.[25-31]

Regardless of amount of superwarfarin ingested, clinically significant anticoagulation in a patient not already taking an anticoagulant agent is not anticipated for about 24 hours, that is, until there is both the depletion of existing vitamin K stores and subsequent loss of vitamin K–dependent clotting factor regeneration (factors II, VII, IX, and X). Table 66-3 lists half-lives of vitamin K and vitamin K–dependent clotting factors.[32]

Patients who have ingested superwarfarins intentionally should undergo routine decontamination and have their PT and INR monitored 24 and 48 hours after ingestion. In the acute phase, PT and INR should be reassessed every 6 hours if prolongation is observed.

There are no means of enhanced elimination of superwarfarins, and multidose activated charcoal has not shown any clear benefit.[33] In asymptomatic patients, vitamin K_1 (phytonadione) may be administered orally at an initial dose of 5 to 15 mg/day, although an ideal dose has not been established. Bruno and colleagues reported that weight-based dosing of 7 mg/kg over 24 hours divided every 6 hours was needed to treat brodifacoum-induced coagulopathy from 344 g of rodenticide containing 0.005% brodifacoum (17.2 mg brodifacoum).[34] Administration of vitamin K_1, 100 to 125 mg/day for several months, has been reported in cases of severe overdose without ill effect; hence, oral dosing of up to 40 to 50 mg three times daily should be considered in those with clinically significant coagulopathy.

Historical recommendations for management of symptomatic patients using parenteral administration of vitamin K_1 are changing[35] (Table 66-4). Although intravenous (IV) administration of vitamin K_1 may reverse anticoagulation more quickly than oral administration,[36] IV administration remains controversial because it has been associated with anaphylactoid reactions.[37-39] Lubetsky and associates reported that oral administration of vitamin K_1 is as safe and efficacious in reversal of excessive anticoagulation as when administered intravenously,[40] making the argument for IV administration of vitamin K_1 a less appealing alternative.

With unintentional single ingestions, PT prolongation is unlikely, owing to the relatively small doses ingested. In Thacker's 14-year case series of children ingesting superwarfarins (1986 to 2000), PT and INR prolongation was seen in less than 0.5% of 11,751 exposures, and only 11 patients developed hemorrhage, all of minimal clinical significance (epistaxis [3], hemarthrosis [2], heme-positive stool [2], vomiting [2], minor bleeding not specified [1]).[41] A prospective study of pediatric superwarfarin poisoning by Smolinske and colleagues showed that PT value prolongation was not seen until 48 hours after suspected ingestion and that clinically significant ingestion was apparent in only 2 of 110 patients.[42]

Children who ingest a small dose of a warfarin-based rodenticide (0.01%–0.005% strength) do not need to

---

TABLE 66-3 Half-Lives of Vitamin K and Its Dependent Clotting Factors*

VITAMIN/FACTOR	HALF-LIFE ($t_{1/2}$)
Vitamin K_1	1.7 hr
Factor II	50–80 hr
Factor VII	6 hr
Factor IX	24 hr
Factor X	25–60 hr

*Disruption of the clotting cascade following warfarin or superwarfarin ingestion is expected when vitamin K is depleted and its dependent clotting factors cease regeneration[32]
From Makris M, Watson HG: The management of coumarin-induced over anticoagulation. Br J Haematol 2001;114(2):271–280.

TABLE 66-4 American College of Chest Physicians' Recommended Dosing of Subcutaneous Vitamin K_1 for Reversal of Warfarin/Superwarfarin-induced Coagulopathy in 1995

INR	BLEEDING	DOSE OF VITAMIN K_1 ADMINISTERED INTRAVENOUSLY OR SUBCUTANEOUSLY*
Any	Serious	10 mg
<6	None	None
6–10	None	0.5–1 mg
10–20	None	3–5 mg
>20	None	10 mg

*Intravenous or subcutaneous administration is in addition to oral vitamin K_1 administration. Single oral route of administration of vitamin K_1 has since proven equally effective.

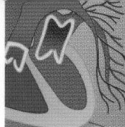

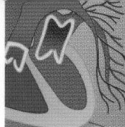

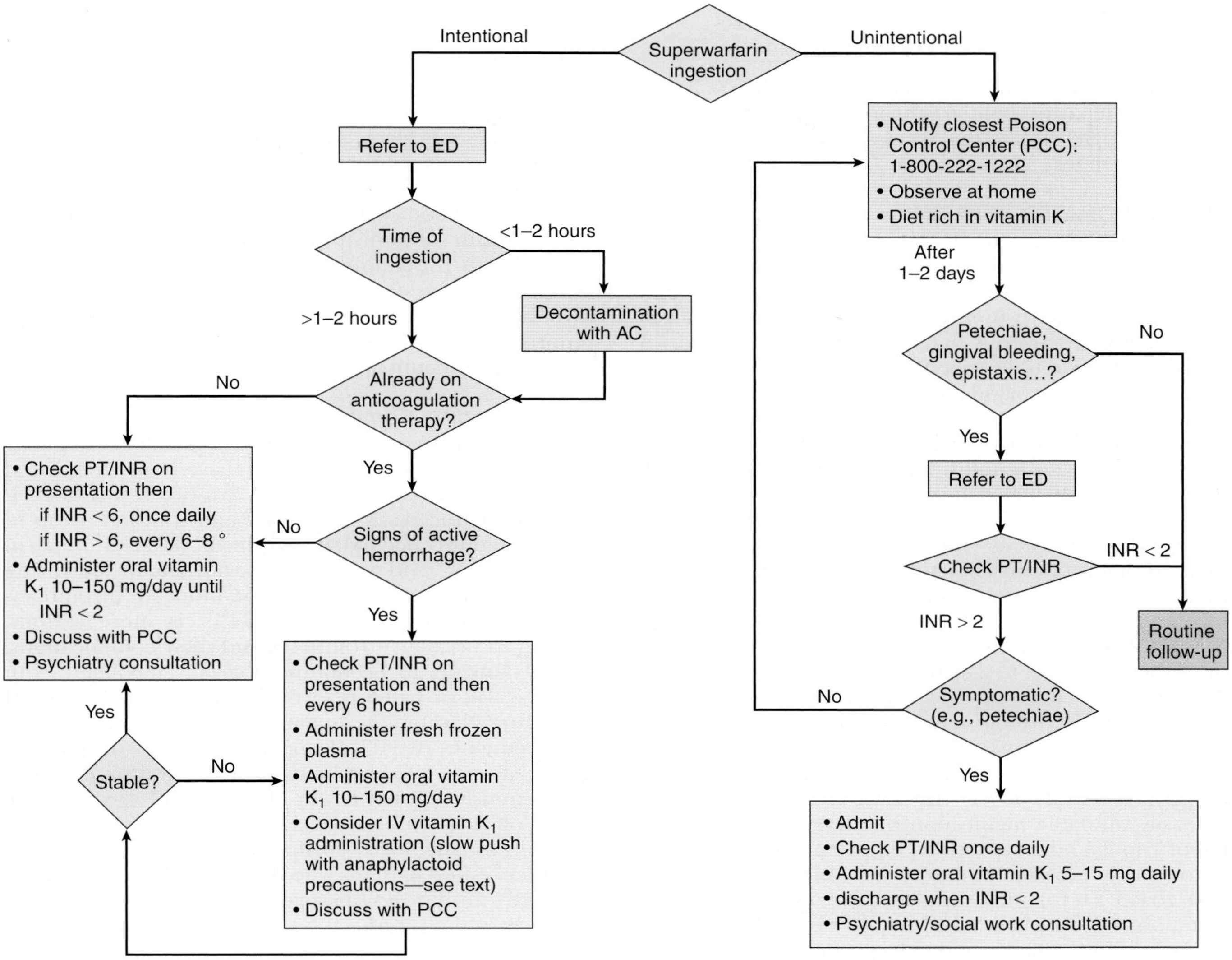

FIGURE 66-7 Proposed general guideline for management of superwarfarin ingestion. Clinicians should take care to assess whether the ingestion is intentional or unintentional. Intentional ingestions are generally by adults; unintentional ingestions are generally by children.

Unintentional ingestions are usually small (fewer than two are three mouthfuls) and are unlikely to cause clinically significant anticoagulation. The local poison control center should always be contacted, and the superwarfarin product should be reviewed for concentration of active ingredient and other possible toxins.

Patients who have ingested intentionally may present hours to days after their ingestion, usually to a local emergency department (ED) secondary to symptoms such as ecchymosis development or petechiae. Active bleeding (e.g., melena, expanding hematoma, bright red blood from rectum, oozing wounds) requires immediate reversal with fresh frozen plasma (FFP). Lubetsky and colleagues concluded in 2003 that oral administration of vitamin K is as effective as IV administration for warfarin anticoagulation reversal,[40] but patients unable to take vitamin K orally may require it intravenously. Note that IV administration of vitamin K remains controversial, with several reports of anaphylactoid reactions upon administration. In the event of anaphylaxis, IV vitamin K should be discontinued immediately and epinephrine administered in conjunction with antihistamines and steroids. Oral vitamin K may be continued unless a similar reaction is observed. AC, activated charcoal; INR, International Normalized Ratio; PT, prothrombin time. (Courtesy of M. W. Lai, MD, and M. W. Shannon, MD, MPH, Massachusetts/Rhode Island Poison Control Center [M. Burns Ewald, MD, Director], Boston.)

present to an emergency department.[43] However, patients and parents should be advised to watch for signs of bleeding diatheses; asymptomatic patients can be observed at home if the history is certain that the ingestion was unintentional. If any symptoms develop, the child should have a routine medical screening examination and PT and INR drawn. Increases in PT and INR should be followed weekly until a downward trend is seen. Oral

vitamin K_1, 5 to 10 mg, or a diet rich in vitamin K–containing vegetables can be encouraged in the interim.

A proposed guideline for superwarfarin ingestion management is shown in Figure 66-7.

Clinicians should take care to assess whether the ingestion is intentional or unintentional. Intentional ingestions are generally by adults; unintentional ingestions are generally by children.

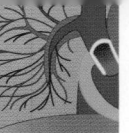

Antithrombin III Acceleration through Factor II and Factor X Inhibition

Antithrombin III blocks coagulation factors II, IX, X, XI, and XII. Heparins bind to thrombin (factor IIa) and factor Xa to accelerate the anticoagulant effect of ATIII up to 2000 times.

UNFRACTIONATED HEPARIN

Unfractionated heparin (UFH) is a naturally occurring, negatively charged mucopolysaccharide (glycosaminoglycan) primarily synthesized and secreted by mast cells. Deriving its name from its particular abundance in liver, heparin was discovered by a medical student who, in studying ether-soluble procoagulants, stumbled on this water-soluble anticoagulant instead. Heparin is manufactured through extraction from bovine lung tissue and porcine intestines. Because UFH has varying polysaccharide side-chain lengths, its molecular weight ranges from 3000 to 30,000 daltons.[44] UFH accelerates ATIII protease inhibition of thrombin by binding to thrombin (factor IIa) and factor Xa. When ATIII complexes to heparin that is bound to factors IIa and Xa, the complex causes conformational changes in these factors and inactivates them.

UFH is only administered parenterally (intravenously or subcutaneously). Dosing is weight based, and depending on the reason for administration, patients may receive 50 to 80 U/kg IV boluses followed by continuous infusions of 12 to 18 U/kg/hour or subcutaneous injections ranging from 7500 U (for DVT prophylaxis) to 20,000 U (for DVT treatment). UFH is an easily titratable medication because of its short half-life of 1 to 2.5 hours and short duration of action of 1 to 3 hours. Therapeutic monitoring is through the PTT.[45] The goal PTT for most vaso-occlusive events as well as thrombosis prophylaxis when heparin is used as a single agent is 60 to 80 seconds. Heparin is a pregnancy category C drug and the anticoagulant of choice during pregnancy; its negative charge and large size prevent its passage across the placenta.

Overdose

Because UFH is predominantly administered in the acute care setting, overdose is most often iatrogenic and may reflect transcription errors of the physician's or other health care provider's orders. Initial treatment is discontinuation of the heparin infusion. For patients with active bleeding requiring quick reversal, protamine sulfate (derived from salmon sperm and testes) should be administered. Protamine forms ionic bonds with heparin, preventing its attachment to factors II and Xa, with neutralization of heparin's effects within 5 minutes of administration.[46] Protamine should be dosed as follows:

- 1 mg protamine per 100 U heparin
  - Administer up to 50 mg intravenously over 10 minutes (more rapid administration may result in hypotension or anaphylactoid reaction).[47,48]
  - Half the dose of protamine for each half-life of heparin (about 90 minutes) that has passed since initial administration.

- Watch for "rebound" hemorrhage: the half-life of protamine is shorter than that of heparin.

Patients previously given protamine for heparin reversal, such as after cardiac bypass surgery, are at risk for becoming sensitized to protamine. Insulin-dependent diabetic patients face a similar risk because protamine is also used to extend the absorption rate of some insulin preparations. (e.g., neutral protamine Hagedorn [NPH] insulin). Antibodies to protamine that develop from NPH insulin administration or from prior heparin reversal with protamine predispose patients to anaphylactoid reactions from future heparin anticoagulation reversal with protamine.[49-53] There are no published reports of concurrent NPH insulin use interfering with heparin therapeutic goals.

Nonbleeding Complications

Patients who experience a drop in platelet count after initiation of heparin therapy may have heparin-induced thrombocytopenia (HIT). There are two forms of HIT. HIT I is characterized by a mild and transient drop in platelet count occurring within 2 days of heparin administration and is usually asymptomatic, resolving spontaneously.[54] HIT II (heparin-induced thrombocytopenia and thrombosis, or HITT) is more serious, leading to vascular thromboses and their complications. HIT II appears to be immunologically mediated, with 0.5% to 3% of patients given UFH developing HIT II after first developing heparin-induced antibodies.[55,56] The frequency of HIT II appears to be less in patients administered UFH subcutaneously compared with intravenously.[57] Patients who develop HIT II should be taken off heparin immediately and should not have heparin in any form readministered. Clinicians may consider testing patients who develop HIT I for heparin-induced antibodies before administering heparin products in the future.

LOW-MOLECULAR-WEIGHT HEPARINS

Low-molecular-weight heparins (LMWHs) are the fractionated active pentasaccharide segment of heparin. Commonly used LMWHs in the United States include enoxaparin (Lovenox), dalteparin (Fragmin), and ardeparin (Normiflo). Average molecular weights run from 4000 to 6000 Daltons. Because binding to factor IIa requires the heparin molecule to have at least 18 saccharide units, LMWHs display targeted factor Xa activity rather than the factor IIa and Xa binding seen with unfractionated heparin. LMWHs have fixed weight-based dosing and are generally administered either once or twice daily, depending on their reason for administration.

Pharmacokinetics

LMWHs have a higher bioavailability than unfractionated heparin owing to a lower affinity for and decreased binding to endothelium, macrophages, and heparin-binding proteins. Their plasma half-life is 4 to 6 hours, with hepatic metabolism and renal elimination. Patients receiving LMWH therapy do not routinely undergo therapeutic monitoring. Relative effectiveness

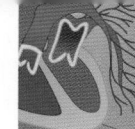

and concentration of LMWHs can be determined from serum anti–factor Xa concentrations, as measured in IU/mL, if needed. Because of its fixed-dosing regimen, overdoses of LMWHs are infrequent. Because of its renal elimination, patients with renal insufficiency may experience more potentiated effects if weight-based dosing does not take renal function into account. If a patient does suffer an overdose and has active bleeding, protamine should be administered using the same guidelines as for overdose of unfractionated heparin. Since 1 mg of available LMWHs equals approximately 100 anti-Xa units, 1 mg of protamine should be given for every 1 mg of LMWH for Xa neutralization. Protamine does not completely neutralize the anti-Xa activity of LMWH. This is likely due to decreased binding of protamine to LMWHs.[58]

DIRECT FACTOR XA INHIBITORS (FONDAPARINUX)

Similar to LMWHs, selective factor Xa inhibitors catalyze Xa inactivation by ATIII without inhibiting thrombin. These medications are essentially heparin derivatives, displaying similar structural features as UFH and LMWHs (Fig. 66-8). Fondaparinux (Arixtra) selectively binds ATIII and potentiates ATIII's neutralization of factor Xa by a factor of 300.[59] Currently, only fondaparinux has been approved for therapeutic anticoagulation in humans by targeting this stage in the coagulation cascade.

Representative of this emerging anticoagulant class, fondaparinux demonstrates 100% bioavailability and is 94% bound to ATIII. Peak plasma levels are seen in 2 hours. The volume of distribution (Vd) is 100 mL/kg. At least half of the drug is excreted unchanged in urine, and its elimination half-life is 17 to 21 hours. Fondaparinux is administered once daily by either IV or subcutaneous routes at a fixed non–weight-based dose. Presently, fondaparinux is approved for DVT prophylaxis, particularly after lower extremity surgery. Once-daily subcutaneous injection without monitoring has been shown to be as safe as adjusted-dose IV heparin for treatment of pulmonary embolus.[60] Administration in patients who weigh less than 50 kg is contraindicated because of doubling of the incidence of major bleeding.[59] Patients receiving fondaparinux therapy do not routinely undergo therapeutic monitoring. Plasma concentration of the drug can be quantified by serum anti–factor Xa activity when the anti–factor Xa assay is calibrated with fondaparinux. Hence, fondaparinux activity is expressed as milligrams of fondaparinux calibrator. The anti-Xa activity of the drug is enhanced by increasing drug concentration, reaching maximum values in about 3 hours.[59] No specific reversal agent has been developed yet for fondaparinux. Because of its small volume of distribution, however, this anti–factor Xa drug is amenable to hemodialysis. Further direct factor Xa inhibitors are being developed, including idraparinux, a "depo" fondaparinux requiring only once-weekly administration.[61]

Direct Thrombin Inhibition

LEECH-DERIVED ANTICOAGULANTS (HIRUDINS)

Background

Leech-derived anticoagulants are small molecules that directly inhibit thrombin (factor IIa). Halting the coagulation cascade at this stage prevents fibrinogen cleavage into fibrin, which is necessary for cross-linkage and subsequent clot formation. Hirudin is the actual 65–amino acid anticoagulant protein found in leech salivary glands. Recombinant DNA hirudins such as desirudin (Revasc) and lepirudin (Refludan) have been developed, as well as hirudin analogs such as bivalirudin (Angiomax). Hirudins are primarily used as heparin substitutes for patients unable to tolerate heparins because of HIT. To date, no published studies have indicated that hirudin use for acute coronary syndrome offers long-term advantage over heparin, but hirudins have been shown to be more effective in preventing postoperative DVT when compared with UFH.[62]

Hirudins can be administered by either intravenous or subcutaneous routes. Recombinant hirudins are pregnancy category B drugs. Animal studies have not shown teratogenic effects, but hirudins can cross the placental barrier in rats; it is unknown whether hirudins cross the human placenta.[63] Effectiveness of hirudin anticoagulation may be assessed through measuring the PTT. Although overdose is rare, hemodiafiltration has been successfully used to manage a 30-fold overdose of lepirudin without bleeding complications.[64]

XIMELAGATRAN AND MELAGATRAN

Melagatran is a direct thrombin inhibitor with a low molecular weight (429 Daltons). It has poor oral absorption (3% to 7% alone, 1% with food), but its prodrug, ximelagatran (Exanta), possesses better absorptive properties. Rapid hydrolysis and reduction of ximelagatran to melagatran increases melagatran's oral bioavailability to 25%. At present, melagatran and ximelagatran are primarily being used for DVT prevention and anticoagulation for patients with atrial fibrillation. Early studies suggest that it is "superior" to warfarin for prevention of DVTs while maintaining a similar hemorrhagic complication profile,[65] as well as the advantage of fixed dosing.

FIGURE 66-8 *Top,* Representative repeat unit of unfractionated heparin and low-molecular-weight heparin (LMWH). LMWH contains five repeating units. *Bottom,* fondaparinux.

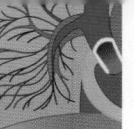

Melagatran and ximelagatran reach peak plasma levels in 2 hours and are 0% to 15% protein bound. Their Vd is 200 mL/kg, and they are renally excreted with an elimination half-life of 3.5 hours. Fixed dosing of melagatran, 2 to 3 mg subcutaneously, is followed by oral doses of ximelagatran at either 24 mg twice daily or 36 mg twice daily, depending on the reason for administration. Dose adjustments are made empirically for patients with renal insufficiency. Although there is no monitoring for therapeutic levels of these direct thrombin inhibitors, the PTT may be tested in patients with renal impairment in order to titrate to an appropriate fixed dose.

Overdose

There is no specific melagatran or ximelagatran antagonist in the event of an overdose. Patients with active hemorrhage should be administered fresh frozen plasma for replacement of coagulation proteins or prothrombin concentrate. Although there have been no reports of hemodialysis to remove the drug, its small molecular weight and volume of distribution suggest that it could be effectively hemodialyzed.

Inhibition of Platelet Aggregation (Antiplatelet Anticoagulation Therapies)

GLYCOPROTEIN IIB/IIIA INHIBITION

The gpIIb/IIIa receptor is the most prevalent cell surface protein on platelets. Activation of platelets from their exposure to thrombin at the site of endothelial injury up-regulates gpIIb/IIIa receptors, doubling or even tripling their number. Fibrin cleaved from fibrinogen in the coagulation cascade cross-links to itself as well as between platelets by adhering to the gpIIb/IIIa receptor. Inhibition of the gpIIb/IIIa receptor arrests platelet aggregation through these fibrin connections.

Since their development in the mid-1990s, there are now multiple gpIIb/IIIa inhibitors in use, primarily for the treatment of acute coronary syndromes. Multiple studies have shown the effectiveness of gpIIb/IIIa antagonists in reducing the incidence of death or myocardial infarction in patients who undergo percutaneous coronary intervention (PCI, or cardiac catheterization) for unstable angina (UA) or non–ST elevation myocardial infarction (NSTEMI).[66] Table 66-5 compares the three gpIIb/IIIa inhibitors used in the United States today.[67-71] Others are xemilofiban, sibrafiban, orbofiban, and lamifiban.

When used concomitantly with heparin, gpIIb/IIIa inhibitors should lower the PTT goal (to a range of either 50–70 or 40–60 seconds). In overdose, the gpIIb/IIIa infusion should be discontinued, and platelets should be administered for active bleeding or a platelet count of less than $20 \times 10^9/L$.

ADENOSINE DIPHOSPHATE–INDUCED PLATELET AGGREGATION INHIBITION

Platelet activation leads to release of ADP, a soluble factor that induces further platelet aggregation through their recruitment and activation.

Drugs in the thienopyridine class (ticlopidine [Ticlid] and clopidogrel [Plavix]) are platelet aggregation inhibitors that work by irreversibly inhibiting ADP-induced platelet aggregation. They selectively and noncompetitively inhibit the binding of ADP to its platelet receptor (P_2 receptors) by irreversibly modifying the receptor. Doing so halts the ADP-mediated activation of the gpIIb/IIIa complex necessary for platelet linkage.[72-74] The thienopyridine derivatives have similar chemical structures (clopidogrel adds a carboxymethyl side group). Both are metabolized by CYP1A to active metabolites that have not yet been isolated.[74] They affect

TABLE 66-5 Comparison of Properties of Three Major gpIIb/IIIa Inhibitors*

	EPTIFIBATIDE[67]	TIROFIBAN[68]	ABCIXIMAB[69]
Trade name	Integrelin	Aggrastat	ReoPro
Manufactured by/from	Solution-based peptide synthesis	Nonpeptide	Chimeric (human-murine) monoclonal antibody Fab fragment
Complete platelet inhibition	1–2 hr	Unclear; inhibition as early as 5 min	Within 2 hr
Return to platelet function after d/c of infusion	30 min	3–8 hr	48 hr
Elimination half-life	1–2.5 hr	1.5–3 hr	Phase 1 < 10 min Phase 2 ~ 30 min
Molecular weight	832	495.1	47455.4
Vd	185 mL/kg	22–42 L	Unknown
Excretion	Renal 50%	Renal 65%	Renal and protein catabolism[70]
Dose adjustment in renal failure?	Yes	Yes	No
Provides benefit in PCI?	Clear benefit	Benefit	No change
Hemodialyzable?	Yes	Yes	N/A

*Drugs used in the United States in 2003. gpIIb/IIIa, glycoprotein IIb/IIIa[71]; PCI, percutaneous coronary intervention (coronary artery catheterization).

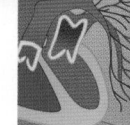

only P$_2$ receptors and do not inhibit ADP-induced changes in platelet shape.

Thienopyridines are being used as alternative antiplatelet agents in acute coronary syndromes. A single dose of 375 mg of clopidogrel achieves maximal platelet aggregation inhibition of 40% to 50% 2 to 6 hours after ingestion.[74] The same level of platelet inhibition is achieved in 3 to 7 days when clopidogrel is dosed at 75 mg once daily. Peak response is expected 5 days after the initial dose, and a return to baseline platelet function comes 5 days after discontinuation. Ninety-four percent to 98% protein bound, thienopyridines undergo about 50% to 60% renal excretion and 30% to 50% excretion in bile.[75,76] Table 66-6 summarizes the pharmacokinetic parameters of clopidogrel and ticlopidine.

Thienopyridine use in patients undergoing PCI has become increasingly popular. This drug class has become an effective alternative antiplatelet medication for aspirin-intolerant patients with atherosclerotic cardiac disease. However, the one exception for thienopyridine use in patients suffering an acute coronary event is when a patient is likely to undergo a coronary artery bypass graft. The delay in recovery of platelet function may complicate intraoperative and postoperative care.

There is no therapeutic monitoring for thienopyridine use. However, routine quantitative platelet analysis (e.g., through a complete blood count) is indicated for patients taking thienopyridines because they can cause neutropenia and thrombocytopenia. The platelet function analyzer (PFA 100, Dade Behring, Illinois) may be used to assess platelet aggregation, although the gold standard for this measurement is optical aggregometry.

Overdose of thienopyridines remains a rare occurrence compared with other anticoagulant overdoses. Ingestion of up to 6000 mg clopidogrel has been reported.[77] Animal studies have reported dyspnea, seizures, gastrointestinal bleeding, and ultimately death after single acute ingestions of 500 mg/kg ticlopidine in mice and 2000 mg/kg clopidogrel in rats.[78] Although no thienopyridine antiplatelet reversal agent has yet been developed, DDAVP (desmopressin) administration may temporarily improve primary hemostasis by stimulating release of vWF factor from storage in endothelial cells and platelets.[74] Patients who overdose with clopidogrel or ticlopidine should undergo routine decontamination with activated charcoal and receive supportive measures.

Because thienopyridines irreversibly change the ADP platelet receptor, return of platelet function is dependent on new platelet formation; platelet transfusion may be indicated for patients with active hemorrhage.

ASPIRIN

Acetylsalicylic acid (aspirin) has become a routine and ubiquitous agent in the treatment and prevention of unstable angina and myocardial infarction. Aspirin acetylates and irreversibly inhibits platelet cyclooxygenase to inhibit thromboxane production and hence interfere with platelet aggregation. A single 81-mg dose of aspirin or as little as 10 mg taken daily for 1 week will impair platelet function for the lifetime of a cohort of affected platelets.

Overdose

Hematologic complications of aspirin overdose are rarely seen, probably because the more active issues of metabolic derangement and subsequent central nervous system depression from salicylate toxicity must first be addressed. PT prolongation is fairly common, whereas disseminated intravascular coagulation, thrombocytopenia, and acute hemorrhage from aspirin overdose are uncommon.[79] Management of aspirin toxicity is addressed in greater depth elsewhere in this text (see Chapter 48).

BOTANICALS WITH ANTICOAGULANT PROPERTIES

Several botanicals have been demonstrated to show anticoagulant synergy with existing synthetic agents as well as when used as single agents. Garlic has been shown to inhibit platelet aggregation, and patients with previously stable INRs on warfarin have had elevated INRs after adding garlic to their diets.[80,81] Ginger may inhibit platelet aggregation, but ingestion of up to 40 g of cooked ginger does not seem to affect platelet function. Gingko may also affect platelet aggregation and has been implicated in increased bleeding complications in patients taking anticoagulants.[82] It has been suggested that ginseng can possibly inhibiting platelet aggregation; however, a decreasing INR was noted in one case report, and animal studies show no effect of ginseng on INR.[83]

SNAKE VENOM

Almost all snakes of the Crotalidae, Viperidae, and Crotalinae families have heparin-like substances that can lead to coagulopathy.[84] Elapidae bites rarely lead to hematologic disturbances; exceptions include *Naja nigricollis*, *Ophiophagus hannah* (king cobra), and the *Naja atra* (Chinese cobra).[85,86] All patients with snake envenomations should have PT, PTT, INR, and fibrin split products monitored for development of coagulopathies. Detailed management of snake envenomations is discussed in elsewhere in this text (See Chapters 21A and 21B).

SUMMARY

Anticoagulant medications play an important role in the treatment and prevention of thromboembolic and

TABLE 66-6   Pharmacokinetics of the Thienopyridines*

	CLOPIDOGREL	TICLOPIDINE
Trade name	Plavix	Ticlid
Oral bioavailability	50%	80%
Metabolism	CYP1A	CYP1A
Clearance	Linear	Nonlinear
Elimination half-life	8 hr	12.6 hr after single dose 4–5 days with repeated dosing
Protein bound	94%–98%	98%

*Available in 2004.

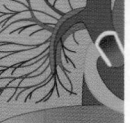

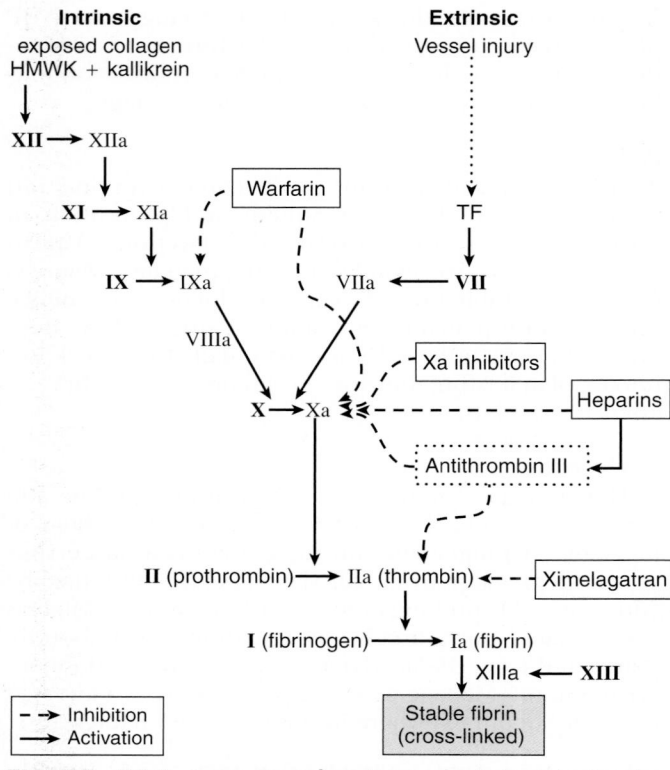

FIGURE 66-9 Summary of anticoagulant targets in the coagulation cascade. HMWK, high-molecular-weight kininogens.

cardiovascular disease (Fig. 66-9). Even in overdose, they rarely precipitate life-threatening hemorrhage.

In overdose, treatment should be based on clinical assessment of the patient, consideration of the nature of the overdose (unintentional versus intentional), and evaluation of bleeding time studies, hematocrit, and platelet concentration. Reversal agents, if available, should be administered for active exsanguination. In supratherapeutic administration of anticoagulants, most patients still need to maintain a certain degree of anticoagulation. In these cases, expectant management should be coordinated in conjunction with clinicians familiar with a patient's therapeutic monitoring trends. All overdoses of anticoagulants merit consultation with a poison control center.

REFERENCES

1. Park BK, Scott AK, Wilson AC, Haynes BP, Breckenridge AM: Plasma disposition of vitamin K1 in relation to anticoagulant poisoning. Br J Pharmacol 1984;18:655–662.
2. Makris M, Watson HG: The management of coumarin-induced over-anticoagulation. Br J Haematol 2001;114(2):271–280.
3. Top 200 most prescribed drugs 2002. In Nissen D (ed): Mosby's Drug Consult. Retrieved July 12, 2004, from http://www.mosbys drugconsult.com/DrugConsult/Top_200/.
4. Wittkowsky AK: Warfarin and other coumarin derivatives: pharmacokinetics, pharmacodynamics, and drug interactions. Semin Vasc Med 2003;3(3):221–230.
5. Breckenridge A: Oral anticoagulant drugs: pharmacokinetic aspects. Semin Hematol 1978;15(1):19–26.
6. Choonara IA, Haynes BP, Cholerton S, Breckenridge AM, Park BK: Enantiomers of warfarin and vitamin K1 metabolism. Br J Clin Pharmacol 1986;22(6):729–732.
7. Breckenridge A: Oral anticoagulant drugs: pharmacokinetic aspects. Semin Hematol 1978;15(1):19–26.
8. Luer J, Patterson LE: Warfarin (drug evaluation). In Klasco RK (ed): DRUGDEX System. Greenwood Village, CO, Thomson MICROMEDEX, 2004.
9. Hirsh J, Dalen JE, Anderson DR, et al: Oral anticoagulants: mechanism of action, clinical effectiveness, and optimal therapeutic range. Sixth ACCP Consensus Conference on Antithrombotic Therapy. Chest 2001;119(1):8S–21S.
10. Kaminsky LS, Zhang Z: Human P450 metabolism of warfarin. Pharmacol Ther 1997;73(1):67–74.
11. Tait RC, Ladusans EJ, El-Metaal M, Patel RG, Will AM: Oral anticoagulation in paediatric patients: dose requirements and complications. Arch Dis Child 1996;74(3):228–231.
12. Schulman S: Care of patients receiving long-term anticoagulant therapy. N Engl J Med 2003;349(7):675–683.
13. Jones KL: Smith's Recognisable Patterns of Human Malformation, 5th ed. Philadelphia, WB Saunders, 1997, pp 568–569.
14. Clark SL, Poerter TF, West FG: Coumarin derivatives and breast-feeding. Obstet Gynecol 2000;96(6 Pt 1):938–940.
15. Orme ML, Lewis PJ, de Swiet M, et al: May mothers given warfarin breast-feed their infants? BMJ 1977;1(6076):1564–1565.
16. Chan YC, Valenti D, Mansfield AO, Stansby G: Warfarin induced skin necrosis. Br J Surg 2000;87(3):266–272.
17. Yang Y, Algazy KM: Warfarin-induced skin necrosis in a patient with a mutation of the prothrombin gene. N Engl J Med 1999;340(9):735.
18. Raj K, Collins B, Rangarajan S: Purple toe syndrome following anticoagulant therapy. Br J Haematol 2001;114(4):740.
19. Kruse JA, Carlson RW: Fatal rodenticide poisoning with brodifacoum. Ann Emerg Med 1992;21(3):331–336.
20. Chua JD, Friedenberg WR: Superwarfarin poisoning. Arch Intern Med 1998;158(17):1929–1932.
21. Breckenridge A: Oral anticoagulant drugs: pharmacokinetic aspects. Semin Hematol 1978;15(1):19–26.
22. Kruse JA, Carlson RW: Fatal rodenticide poisoning with brodifacoum. Ann Emerg Med 1992;21(3):331–336.
23. Parsons BJ, Day LM, Ozanne-Smith J, Dobbin M: Rodenticide poisoning among children. Aust N Z J Public Health 1996;20(5):488–492.
24. Watts RG, Castleberry RP, Sadowski JA: Accidental poisoning with a superwarfarin compound (brodifacoum) in a child. Pediatrics 1990;86(6):883–887.
25. White ST, Voter K, Perry J: Surreptitious warfarin ingestion. Child Abuse Neglect 1985;93(3):349–352.
26. Lazarus A, Kozinn WP: Munchausen's syndrome with hematuria and sepsis: an unusual case. Int J Psychiatry Med 1991;21(1):113–116.
27. Souid AK, Korins K, Keith D, Dubansky S, Sadowitz PD: Unexplained menorrhagia and hematuria: a case report of Munchausen's syndrome by proxy. Pediatr Hematol Oncol 1993;10(3):245–248.
28. Babcock J, Harman K, Pedersen A, Murphy M, Alving B: Rodenticide-induced coagulopathy in a young child: a case of Munchausen syndrome by proxy. Am J Pediatr Hematol Oncol 1993;15(1):126–130.
29. Stanziale SF, Christopher JC, Fisher RB: Brodifacoum rodenticide ingestion in a patient with shigellosis. South Med J 1997;90(8):833–835.
30. Zahner J, Schneider W: Munchausen syndrome in hematology: case reports of three variants and review of the literature. Ann Hematol 1994;68(6):303–306.
31. Ayass M, Bussing R, Mehta P: Munchausen syndrome presenting as hemophilia: a convenient and economical "steal" of disease and treatment. Pediatr Hematol Oncol 1993;10(3):241–244.
32. Makris M, Watson HG: The management of coumarin-induced over-anticoagulation. Br J Haematol 2001;114(2):271–280.
33. Donovan JW: Brodifacoum therapy with activated charcoal: effect on elimination kinetics. Vet Hum Toxicol 1990;32:50.
34. Bruno GR, Howland MA, McMeeking A, Hoffman RS: Long-acting anticoagulant overdose: brodifacoum kinetics and optimal vitamin K dosing. Ann Emerg Med 2000;36(3):262–267.

35. Becker RC, Ansell J: Antithrombotic therapy: an abbreviated reference for clinicians. Arch Intern Med 1995;155(2):149–161.

36. Watson HG, Baglin T, Laidlaw SL, Makris M, Preston FE: A comparison of the efficacy and rate of response to oral and intravenous vitamin K in reversal of over-anticoagulation with warfarin. Br J Haematol 2001;115(1):145–149.

37. de la Rubia J, Grau E, Montserrat I, Zuazu I, Paya A: Anaphylactic shock and vitamin K1. Ann Intern Med 1989;110(11):943.

38. O'Reilly RA, Kearns P: Intravenous vitamin K1 injections: dangerous prophylaxis. Arch Intern Med 1995;155(19):2127–2128.

39. Wjasow C, McNamara R: Anaphylaxis after low dose vitamin K. J Emerg Med 2003;24(2):169–172.

40. Lubetsky A, Yonath H, Olchovsky D, et al: Comparison of oral vs intravenous phytonadione (vitamin K1) in patients with excessive anticoagulation: a prospective randomized controlled study. Arch Intern Med 2003;163(20):2469–2473.

41. Thacker JL: Long-acting anticoagulant rodenticides. Minnesota Poison Control System, Hennepin County Medical Center. Retrieved December 13, 2003, from http://www.mnpoison.org/index.asp.

42. Smolinske SC, Scherger DL, Kearns PS, et al: Superwarfarin poisoning in children: a prospective study. Pediatrics 1989;84(3):490–494.

43. Shaw S, Anderson J: Warfarin rodenticide poisoning treatment in children. Centre for Clinical Effectiveness, Institute for Public Health and Health Services Research Southern Health Care Network, Monash University, Evidence Centre Report, 1999.

44. Weitz JI: Low-molecular-weight heparin. N Engl J Med 1997;337(10):688–698.

45. Bates SM, Ginsberg JS: Treatment of deep-vein thrombosis. N Engl J Med 2004;351(3):268–277.

46. Protamine sulfate (drug evaluation). In Klasko RK (ed): DRUGDEX System. Greenwood Village, CO, Thomson MICROMEDEX, 1996.

47. Wakefield TW, Hantler CB, Wrobleski SK, Crider BA, Stanley JC: Effects of differing rates of protamine reversal of heparin anticoagulation. Surgery 1996;119(2):123–128.

48. Horrow JC: Protamine: a review of its toxicity. Anesth Analg 1985;64(3):348–361.

49. Ellerhorst JA, Comstock JP, Nell LJ: Protamine antibody production in diabetic subjects treated with NPH insulin. Am J Med Sci 1990;299(5):298–301.

50. Weiss ME, Chatham F, Kagey-Sobotka A, Adkinson NF Jr: Serial immunological investigations in a patient what had a life-threatening reaction to intravenous protamine. Clin Exp Allergy 1990;20(6):713–720.

51. Hakala T, Suojaranta-Ylinen R: Fatal anaphylactic reaction to protamine after femoropopliteal by-pass surgery. Ann Chir Gynaecol 2000;89(2):150–152.

52. Porsche R, Brenner ZR: Allergy to protamine sulfate. Heart Lung 1990;28(6):418–428.

53. Kim R: Anaphylaxis to protamine masquerading as an insulin allergy. Del Med J 1993;65(1):17–23.

54. Fabris F, Luzzatto G, Stefani PM, et al: Heparin-induced thrombocytopenia. Haematologica 2000;85(1):72–81.

55. Chong BH, Chong JH: Heparin-induced thrombocytopenia. Exp Rev Cardiovasc Ther 2004;2(4):547–559.

56. Mattioli AV, Bonetti L, Sternieri S, Mattioli G: Heparin-induced thrombocytopenia in patients treated with unfractionated heparin: prevalence of thrombosis in a 1 year follow-up. Ital Heart J 2000;1(1):39–42.

57. Girolami B, Prandoni P, Stefani PM, et al: The incidence of heparin-induced thrombocytopenia in hospitalized medical patients treated with subcutaneous unfractionated heparin: a prospective cohort study. Blood 2003;101(8):2955–2959.

58. Sugiyama T, Itoh M, Ohtawa M, Natsuga T: Study on neutralization of low molecular weight heperin by protaminesulfate and its neutralization characteristics. Thromb Res 1992;68:119–129.

59. Arixtra prescribing information 2003. Retrieved December 14, 2003, from http://www.sanofi synthelabous.com/products/pi_arixtra/pi_arixtra.html.

60. The Matisse Investigators: Subcutaneous fondaparinux versus IV unfractionated heparin in the initial treatment of pulmonary embolism. N Engl J Med 2003;349(18):1695–1702.

61. Drouet L: New and future antithrombotic agents in thromboembolic venous disease [French]. Rev Prat 2003;53(1):58–61.

62. Eriksson BI, Ekman S, Kabelo P, et al: Prevention of deep-vein thrombosis after total hip replacement: direct thrombin inhibition with recombinant hirudin, CGP 39393. Lancet 1996;347(9002):635–639.

63. Refludan product information 2003.

64. Bauersachs RM, Lindhoff-Last E, Ehrly AM, et al: Treatment of hirudin overdosage in a patient with chronic renal failure. Thromb Haemost 1999;81(2):323–324.

65. Francis CW, Berkowitz SD, Comp PC, et al: Comparison of ximelagatran with warfarin for the prevention of venous thromboembolism after total knee replacement. N Engl J Med 2003;349(18):1703–1712.

66. Braunwald E: Application of current guidelines to the management of unstable angina and non-ST-elevation myocardial infarction. Circulation 2003;108(Suppl III):28–37.

67. Kaufman M: Eptifibatide (drug evaluation). In Klasco RK (ed): DRUGDEX System. Greenwood Village, CO, Thomson MICROMEDEX, 2004.

68. Heath J, Bunch C: Tirofiban (drug evaluation). In Klasco RK (ed): DRUGDEX System. Greenwood Village, CO, Thomson MICROMEDEX, 2004.

69. Brueggman J: Abciximab (drug evaluation). In Klasco RK (ed): DRUGDEX System. Greenwood Village, CO, Thomson MICROMEDEX, 2004.

70. Abciximab. Retrieved July 21, 2004, from http://www.drugs.com/MMX/Abciximab.html.

71. Hurlbut KM: Glycoprotein IIb-IIIa receptor antagonists. POISINDEX Managements, Healthcare Series, Vol. 118. Greenwood Village, CO, Thomson MICROMEDEX, 2003.

72. Clopidogrel (Plavix) product information, 5 July 2002.

73. Ticlopidine (Ticlid) product information, March 2001.

74. Kam PCA, Nethery CM: The thienopyridine derivatives (platelet adenosine diphosphate receptor antagonists), pharmacology and clinical developments. Anaesthesia 2003;58(1):28–35.

75. Brunch C: Clopidogrel (drug evaluation). In Klasco RK (ed): DRUGDEX System. Greenwood Village, CO, Thomson MICROMEDEX, 2004.

76. Falcao A, Hunter M, Raasch R: Ticlopidine (drug evaluation). In Klasco RK (ed): DRUGDEX System. Greenwood Village, CO, Thomson MICROMEDEX, 2004.

77. Clopidogrel (drug evaluation). In Klasko RK (ed): DRUGDEX System. Greenwood Village, CO, Thomson MICROMEDEX, 2004.

78. Hurlbut KM, Waksman J, Kulig K: Ticlopidine and related agents. POISINDEX Managements, Healthcare Series, Vol. 118. Greenwood Village, CO, Thomson MICROMEDEX, 2003.

79. Hurlbut KM, Fish S, Kulg K, et al: Salicylates. POISINDEX Managements, Healthcare Series, Vol. 118. Greenwood Village, CO, Thomson MICROMEDEX, 2003.

80. Spoerke DG, Hulko KM, Rumack BH, and the POISINDEX Editorial Staff: Plants: allium species. In Klasco RK (ed): POISINDEX System. POISINDEX Managements, Healthcare Series, Vol. 118. Greenwood Village, CO, Thomson MICROMEDEX, 2003.

81. Luer J, Patterson LE, for the DRUGDEX Editorial Staff. DRUGDEX Drug evaluations. Warfarin. Drug-Drug interactions. Ginger.

82. Luer J, Patterson LE, and the DRUGDEX Editorial Staff: DRUGDEX drug evaluations. Warfarin. Drug–drug interactions. Gingko.

83. Luer J, Patterson LE, and the DRUGDEX Editorial Staff: DRUGDEX drug evaluations. Warfarin. Drug–drug interactions. Ginseng.

84. Editorial staff: African snakes: Viperidae. In Klasko RK (ed): POISINDEX System. POISINDEX Managements, Healthcare Series, Vol. 118. Greenwood Village, CO, Thomson MICROMEDEX, 2004.

85. Editorial staff: African snakes: Elapidae. In Klasko RK (ed): POISINDEX System. POISINDEX Managements, Healthcare Series, Vol. 118. Greenwood Village, CO, Thomson MICROMEDEX, 2004.

86. Editorial staff: Asian snakes: Elapidae. In Klasko RK (ed): POISINDEX System. POISINDEX Managements, Healthcare Series, Vol. 118. Greenwood Village, CO, Thomson MICROMEDEX, 2004.

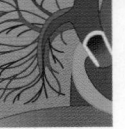

SUGGESTED READING

Brass LF: 2000. The molecular basis for platelet activation. In Hoffman R, Benz EJ Jr, Shattil SJ, et al (eds): Hematology: Basic Principles and Practice, 3rd ed. New York, Elsevier Science, 2000, pp 1753–1770.

Davis WE, Monet DM: Thrombolytic agents and anticoagulants. In Haddad LM, Shannon MW, Winchester JF (eds): Clinical Management of Poisoning and Drug Overdose, 3rd ed. Philadelphia, WB Saunders, 1988.

Quader MA, Stump LS, Sumpio BE: Low molecular weight heparins: current use and indications. J Am Coll Surg 1998;187(6):641–658. Retrieved December 11, 2003, from http://www.facs.org/jacs/articles/sumpio.html.

Su M, Hoffman RS: Anticoagulants. In Goldfrank LR, Flomenbaum NE, Lewin NA, et al (eds): Goldfrank's Toxicologic Emergencies, 7th ed. New York, McGraw-Hill Professional, 2002, pp 631–654.

67 Thyroid Agent Toxicity

LUKE YIP, MD

At a Glance...

- Toxicity from thyroid preparations may result in a hyper-adrenergic state with primary effects on the cardiovascular and central nervous systems.

- Although acute thyroid hormone overdose has been associated with moderate thyrotoxicosis and thyroid storm, most patients develop only mild signs and symptoms and do not require hospitalization.

- There does not appear to be a reported pediatric death due to acute thyroid hormone toxicity in the literature.

- Accidental acute ingestions of less than 5 mg of thyroxine may be managed at home and do not require emergent medical assessment and gastrointestinal decontamination.

- Patients with signs of thyroid hormone toxicity should be admitted to the hospital for close observation and expectant treatment.

- Treatments for exogenous thyroid storm include supportive care, hydration, antipyretics, β-adrenergic antagonists, iodine-containing contrast agents, corticosteroids, and gastrointestinal decontamination, as necessary.

- Iodide, propylthiouracil, and methimazole have minimal efficacy in the management of exogenous thyroid hormone toxicity.

Thyroid hormones are essential in normal growth and development, in many metabolic processes, and in the treatment of thyroid disorders. The clinical uses of thyroid hormones include replacement therapy for hypothyroidism, suppressive therapy to abolish thyroid-stimulating hormone (TSH) secretion in patients with differentiated thyroid carcinoma after total thyroidectomy or with diffuse and nodular nontoxic goiter. However, thyroid hormones are also abused by patients with thyrotoxicosis factitia, a syndrome due to surreptitious excess thyroid hormone ingestion because of psychopathologic disorders.[1-6] Acute thyroid hormone overdose has been associated with either few signs and symptoms that do not require hospitalization,[7-11] a mild to moderate thyrotoxicosis (e.g., flushing, tachycardia, fever, diarrhea, irritability, and insomnia),[12-15] or a thyroid storm.[16-18] Most cases follow a generally benign clinical course.[7-11] The incidence of life-threatening reactions that require treatment has been low,[2,12,14-16,19-22] and morbidity[5,18,23-28] and mortality[26,29,30] have rarely been reported after an acute single or repeated thyroid hormone overdose. Adverse reactions or toxicity during therapeutic use may occur.[23,31-34]

EPIDEMIOLOGY

Thyroid hormone–containing tablets are commonly prescribed drugs. Despite the fact that large numbers of thyroid hormone-containing drugs are prescribed each year in the United States to an estimated 4% of the adult population, only a small proportion of patients suffer accidental or intentional poisoning.[14,35] In 2004, there were 10,647 thyroid preparation exposures reported to U.S. poison centers, of which 89% were unintentional.[35] Moderate to major toxicity occurred in 445 (4.2%) and death occurred in 3 (0.3%) exposures. Deaths could generally be attributed to the effects of co-ingestants and not to the thyroid preparations themselves.

THYROID HORMONE PHYSIOLOGY AND PHARMACOLOGY

The mature thyroid gland contains follicles composed of thyroid follicular cells that surround secreted colloid, a proteinaceous fluid that contains large amounts of thyroglobulin, the glycoprotein precursor of thyroid hormones. The basolateral surface of the thyroid follicular cells is apposed to the bloodstream, and an apical surface faces the follicular lumen.

Dietary iodine is reduced to iodide and is absorbed in the small intestine. Thyroid follicular cells actively transport plasma iodide into their cytoplasm, and it is oxidized to iodine before binding to tyrosyl residues present in the thyroglobulin molecules. Iodination of the tyrosyl residues within thyroglobulin, a process called *organification of the iodine*, is catalyzed by thyroid peroxidase. If one iodine atom replaces a hydrogen atom, then monoiodotyrosine is formed; if two iodine atoms are joined in the tyrosyl ring, diiodotyrosine is the resultant product. Monoiodotyrosine and diiodotyrosine then undergo oxidative condensation to yield various iodothyronines. These include 3,5,3′,5′-tetraiodothyronine (thyroxine, T_4) and 3,5,3′-triiodothyronine (triiodothyronine, T_3) (Fig. 67-1). Iodine makes up 66% of T_4 and 58% of T_3 by weight.

Thyroid hormone secretion from the thyroid gland is regulated by the hypothalamic-pituitary-thyroid axis, which begins in the supraoptic nucleus cells of the hypothalamus. These cells secrete thyrotropin-releasing hormone (TRH), a tripeptide, and it is carried through the pituitary portal circulation to the anterior pituitary gland. TRH stimulates the pituitary gland to secrete TSH into the general circulation, which binds to its receptor on the basolateral surface of the follicular cells, resulting in thyroglobulin reabsorption from the follicular lumen and proteolysis within the cell to yield T_4 and T_3 for secretion into the bloodstream.

T_4 and T_3 are reversibly bound to plasma proteins synthesized by the liver. Transthyretin (TTR) has a low affinity and rapid dissociation constant and has a greater role in delivering iodothyronines to various tissues. In

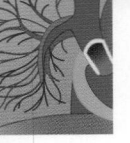

3', 5, 3-Triiodothyronine (T₃)

3, 5, 3', 5'-Thyroxine (Tetraiodothyronine, T₄)

FIGURE 67-1 Chemical structure of thyroxine (T_4) and triiodothyronine (T_3).

contrast, thyroxine-binding globulin (TBG), with its relatively high binding affinity and slower dissociation constant, serves as a stable hormone reservoir in the circulation. Albumin has low binding affinity and may act similarly to TTR to provide tissue delivery of the hormone.

Circulating T_4 is almost entirely bound (99.97%) to these plasma proteins and is predominantly bound to T_4-binding globulin (75% to 80%). TTR binds 15% to 20% and albumin binds 5% to 10%. In contrast, plasma T_3 is bound to a lesser extent. Target tissue responses are related principally if not exclusively to these free fractions of circulating T_4 and T_3. After thyroid hormones overdoses, there is little change in TBG concentration, and free hormone levels increase directly or even disproportionately with the total serum thyroid hormone concentrations.

T_3 is metabolically more active than T_4 and is generated by removal of either iodine atom from the outer ring (at 3' or 5' position) of the T_4 molecule. Peripheral deiodination contributes 80% to 85% of the daily T_3 production and most total daily T_3 production

results from extrathyroidal deiodination in such tissues as the liver and kidneys.

The principal actions of thyroid hormones in target tissues are initiated by the binding to specific nuclear receptors, T_3 receptors, which were first identified as cellular homologs of the avian erythroblastosis virus oncogene (c-*erb*A). These receptors have properties of (1) binding T_3 with high affinity; (2) binding specific oligonucleotide sequences, called T_3 regulatory elements, which are present in the regulatory regions of thyroid hormone-responsive genes; and (3) binding one another to form dimers; an important aspect of T_3 action. Within hours of thyroid hormone administration, T_3 binding to these receptors stimulates transcription of certain messenger RNAs that are then translated into proteins (e.g., β-myosin heavy chain in myocardium), which are ultimately responsible for effecting thyroid hormone actions in various tissues. Those actions include increases in metabolic rate, body temperature, heart rate, and myocardial contractility.

PHARMACOKINETICS

Dosing

The commercially available thyroid preparations and their approximate equivalent dosages are provided in Table 67-1. Recommended therapeutic T_4 and T_3 dosing is listed in Table 67-2.

Absorption

The average T_4 bioavailability is 80% after an oral therapeutic dose, and the time to maximal absorption is 2 hours. The serum T_4 level reaches its peak 4 hours after ingestion of 3 mg T_4.[36] Gastrointestinal diseases such as sprue, diabetic diarrhea, short bowel syndrome, and ileal-jejunal bypass surgery may reduce absorption.

TABLE 67-1 Thyroid Preparations*				
GENERIC NAME	**BRAND NAME**	**SUBSTRATE**	**APPROXIMATE EQUIVALENT DOSE**	**AVAILABLE ORAL DOSES†**
Liothyronine sodium	Cytomel	3,3,5'-triiodo-L-thyronine sodium T_3 (synthetic)	25 µg	5, 25, and 100 µg
Levothyroxine sodium	Synthroid Levoxyl Levothyroid Eltroxin	3,5,3',5'-tetraiodothyronine, T_4 (thyroxine sodium)	100 µg	25 to 300 µg
Liotrix	Thyrolar	T_4:T_3 sodium salts in ratio of 4:1	50/12.5 µg	12.5/3.1 to 150/37.5 µg
Thyroid extract	Armour Thyroid	Desiccated pork thyroid with T_4 and T_3 in approximate ratio of 4:1 38 µg T_4 and 9 µg T_3 per grain	60–65 mg (1 grain)	¼ to 5 grains (15 to 300 mg)
Thyroglobulin			65 mg	

*Only the preparations available in the United States are listed. Preparations other than the ones mentioned in this table may be available in other countries.
†Levothyroxine and liothyronine (Triostat, 10 µg/mL, 1 mL vial) are also available commercially as parenteral preparations.

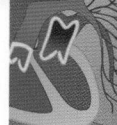

TABLE 67-2 Therapeutic T_4 and T_3 Dose			
	ORAL T_4 DAILY DOSE	**ORAL T_3 DAILY DOSE**	**INTRAVENOUS T_3 DOSE**
ADULT	100–200 µg	10 µg every 8 hr; may increase to 20 µg every 8 hr	5–20 µg every 8–12 hr
PEDIATRIC	25 µg; increase gradually to 3–5 µg/kg/day	0.2 µg/kg/dose (up to 10 µg) every 8 hr; may be increased to 0.4 µg/kg/dose (up to 20µg) every 8 hr	0.1–0.4 µg/kg/dose (up to 20 µg) every 8–12 hr

Cholestyramine, calcium carbonate, sucralfate, aluminum hydroxide, ferrous sulfate, soybean formula, lovastatin, and dietary fiber supplements may also impair T_4 absorption from the gastrointestinal (GI) tract. The maximum effects of T_4 are apparent 1 to 3 weeks after initiating oral therapy, and the effects persist for the same amount of time after discontinuing the drug.

T_3 is 95% absorbed from the GI tract after an oral therapeutic dose, and the serum T_3 level begins to rise at 1.5 to 2.5 hours.[37] The serum T_3 level peaks 2 hours after ingestion of 6 grains (360 mg) of desiccated thyroid and 4 hours after ingestion of 75 µg T_3.[36]

Distribution

T_4 has a 10-L volume of distribution (Vd) and is distributed into most body tissues and fluids, with highest concentrations in the liver and kidneys. T_3 has a volume distribution of 38 L. T_4 and T_3 are primarily bound to thyroxine-binding globulin and to a lesser extent to thyroxine-binding prealbumin and albumin. T_4 is more extensively and tightly bound than T_3. It is estimated that 0.04% of T_4 and 0.5% of T_3 are unbound (free) hormone, which is available to elicit a physiologic effect.

Elimination

Endogenously secreted T_4 (35%) is enzymatically monodeiodinated by type I 5′-monodeiodinase to T_3 in the peripheral tissues (e.g., liver and kidney) and accounts for 80% of total daily T_3 production. T_4 is also enzymatically monodeiodinated to reverse T_3 (rT_3). In the liver, T_4 may undergo glucuronidation and sulfation, which is eliminated in bile; some is hydrolyzed in the intestine and reabsorbed, and the remainder is hydrolyzed in the colon and eliminated unchanged in the feces. After an oral 3-mg T_4 dose, a significant increase in serum T_3 level is evident at 4 hours, and peak level is achieved between 2 and 4 days.[36] The elimination half-life of T_4 is 6 to 7 days. Drugs that increase nondeiodinative T_4 clearance include rifampin, carbamazepine, and phenytoin. Selenium deficiency and amiodarone may block T_4 conversion to T_3.

One metabolic pathway for T_3 and rT_3 is peripheral monodeiodination. The half-life of T_3 is 1 to 2 days. The maximum effects of T_3 are apparent within 24 to 72 hours after initiating oral therapy, and the effects persist

for up to 72 hours after discontinuing the drug. Urinary T_3 elimination increases linearly with the rise in urine flow rate and is doubled or tripled when urine flow rate is increased by fivefold to eightfold during acute hydration.[38]

TOXICOKINETICS

Adult

In a thyroidectomized patient who had ingested an estimated 2000 µg T_4, the serum concentrations of most thyroid hormones reached a peak on the second day.[39] The serum T_3 level peaked 1 day later and did not exceed the upper limit of the reference range. The serum T_4 and rT_3 levels returned to the reference range 13 to 17 days after ingestion. The serum TSH level was rapidly suppressed and reached nadir on the 6th day after ingestion. The serum T_4 half-life and metabolic clearance rate were 10.4 days and 0.64 L/day, respectively. An acute single oral ingestion of a large amount of T_4 does not induce a proportional increase in the serum T_3 level in an athyreotic person. The serum T_4 metabolic clearance rate is decreased, and the serum T_4 half-life is prolonged. This is consistent with D1 deiodinase activity in the thyroid being one of the major determinants in the metabolic clearance of serum T_4.

Two hours after an acute oral T_4 overdose, the serum T_4, free T_4, and free T_3 levels were 2.27, 7.17, and 2.85 times the upper limit of the reference range, respectively.[40] Two hours after an acute oral triiodothyronine overdose, the serum total T_4 and T_3 levels were 1.83 and 25 times the upper limit of the reference range, whereas the T_3 resin uptake (T_3RU) remained in the reference range.[19]

Pediatric

Two previously healthy female pediatric patients were hospitalized, treated with ipecac, gastric lavage, propranolol, prednisone, cholestyramine, and propylthiouracil (PTU) after inadvertent ingestion of 2500 µg T_4. The patients remained asymptomatic throughout their hospital course.[41] Serial serum T_4, T_3, rT_3, and thyroglobulin levels were obtained during the 20 days after ingestion. Serum T_4 concentrations were elevated 2 hours after ingestion and returned to the reference range after 13 days. The serum

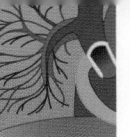
TSH levels reached their nadir 14 hours after ingestion and remained low until the fourth day, after which they rose gradually. However, the TSH levels remained below their initial values at 20 days after ingestion. The serum T_3 concentrations peaked 11 hours after ingestion and decreased to reference values after 3 days. Both T_3 production and degradation constants were significantly increased. The serum rT_3 concentration peaked on the second day after ingestion and decreased to reference values on the fourth day. Both rT_3 production and degradation constants were below reference values. The T_3/rT_3 ratio decreased from a reference value of 3 to 1 and then increased after 13 days to as high as 8. The serum thyroglobulin concentration continuously decreased, with a half-life of 1 to 5 days, and began rising after 2 to 13 days.

The toxicokinetics data from 15 previously healthy patients aged 12 to 49 months who were treated with GI decontamination within 6 hours of the overdose showed elevation in serum T_4 concentration as early as 1 to 2 hours after ingestion.[8] In 71% of patients, peak serum T_4 level was reached within 12 hours, whereas the serum T_3 concentration did not peak until after 24 hours after ingestion. The mean elimination half-life of T_4 was 2.8 ± 0.4 days (range, 1.5–4.5 days), and the mean elimination half-life of T_3 was 6 ± 1.7 days (range, 2.2–12.3 days), which is five times longer than that observed in physiologic conditions. Also, in physiologic conditions, the elimination half-life of T_3 is shorter than that of T_4.

The toxicokinetics data from a 13-year-old boy who was treated with activated charcoal, propranolol, and dexamethasone showed his serum T_4 level began to decline 48 to 72 hours after ingestion, whereas the serum T_3 level began to decline 24 to 36 hours after ingestion.[22] The calculated total T_4 and T_3 half-lives were 5.7 and 5.3 days, respectively. The serum TSH concentration was undetectable 19 hours after ingestion and remained suppressed for 10 days after the overdose. Administration of two additional doses of charcoal, 4 hours apart on the second day after ingestion, did not significantly change the T_4 or T_3 half-life. The patient's free T_4 and TSH returned to the normal range 2 weeks later.

Serum T_4 levels may be elevated as early as 30 minutes after an acute overdose[21]; T_3 and rT_3 levels may be elevated after 1.5 hours,[42] and serum TSH level may be undetectable after 19 hours.[22]

DRUG INTERACTIONS

In patients with endogenous thyrotoxicosis, there is a significant increase in serum free T_4 and T_3 levels after intravenous heparin (5000–30,000 U) administration.[43] This effect may be due to a hormonal shift from the cellular to the intravascular compartment when both cellular and intravascular hormonal binding sites are blocked by heparin. However, the metabolic significance of this is unknown. Certain drugs may interfere with the GI absorption of T_4, including sucralfate, cholestyramine resin, iron and calcium supplements, and aluminum hydroxide.[44] In addition, certain drugs that induce cytochrome P-450 enzymes may enhance biliary excretion of T_4 (e.g., phenytoin, carbamazepine, and rifampin) and necessitate increased oral T_4 dosing.

THYROID HORMONE TOXICOLOGY

Thyroid hormones regulate normal growth and development and act to maintain normal metabolic homeostasis. Some of the principal effects of thyroid hormones are to stimulate metabolic activity and oxygen consumption of numerous peripheral tissues (e.g., heart, skeletal muscle, liver, kidney) and to enhance the effects of other hormones (e.g., catecholamines). Thyrotoxicosis is the state produced by an excess of thyroid hormone. Although thyrotoxicosis occurs largely as a result of hyperthyroidism, or an overactive thyroid gland, the condition may also occur from ingestion of excess thyroid hormone.

Toxicity from excessive exposure to thyroid preparations manifests as an exaggeration of the physiologic effects of thyroid hormone and results in a hyperadrenergic state with primary effects on the GI, cardiovascular, and central nervous systems.

Thyroid hormone intoxication may occur after accidental or intentional and acute or chronic exposure. Acute thyroid hormone overdose occurs most commonly in children and is generally benign; major morbidity or mortality occurs very rarely in this setting.[9,11,26,29,30] Chronic exposure to excessive doses of thyroid hormone is more commonly associated with more severe illness and may present with thyroid storm. Mortality, however, is still rare with chronic overdose. Accidental chronic overexposure occurs from medication error (by physician, pharmacists, nurses, or patients) or from continued administration with therapeutic intent in patients with decreased thyroid hormone dose requirements. Intentional chronic overingestion of thyroid hormone is often referred to as *factitious thyrotoxicosis.*[45] Individuals with factitious thyrotoxicosis are often health care workers who ingest the hormone for weight reduction. "Hamburger thyrotoxicosis" is an unusual cause of exogenous thyrotoxicosis that follows the ingestion of ground beef contaminated with thyroid tissue.[46] Cooking the contaminated beef does not inactivate iodothyronines. Although inclusion of the thyroid gland in meat product preparations is now banned in the United States, this entity should still be considered in the differential diagnosis of thyrotoxicosis presenting with elevated serum T_3 and T_4, especially in a cluster pattern. Acute toxicity from thyroid hormone may also occur during the initial stages of thyroid hormone replacement therapy in those with hypothyroidism (see "Adverse Effects").

CLINICAL MANIFESTATIONS

Acute Overdose

The temporal relation between acute overdose and the onset of signs and symptoms is delayed by hours to days.

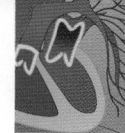

The latency is longer (3 to 7 days) after ingestion of T_4 because of the time it takes for peripheral conversion to T_3, the bioactive hormone. Clinical signs and symptoms after acute T_3 ingestion or desiccated thyroid (both T_3 and T_4 present) may occur within a few hours but usually appear after 2 to 3 days. Adult patients primarily present with cardiovascular and central nervous system manifestations.[14,15,18,40] Vomiting may be evident as soon as 2 hours after ingestion, tachycardia may be noted after 2 to 6 hours, and fever has been reported after 6 hours.[15,19,40] However, cardiovascular signs and symptoms usually do not become apparent until 16 hours to 4 days after ingestion, and neurologic manifestations may not occur until 2 to 6 days after ingestion.

Cardiovascular effects include tachycardia, shortness of breath, palpitations, vasodilation, systolic hypertension, and increased cardiac contractility. Hypotension, congestive heart failure, tachyarrhythmias, and cardiovascular collapse may occur.[17] Common tachyarrhythmias include sinus tachycardia, atrial fibrillation, paroxysmal atrial tachycardia, and atrial flutter.[17] Electrocardiographic changes are nonspecific.

Common neurologic effects are the result of sympathetic nervous system overactivity and include anxiety, agitation, restlessness, diaphoresis, hyperthermia, tachypnea, mydriasis, hyperactive bowel sounds, vomiting, diarrhea, and tremor.[17,18] Other neurologic manifestations may include a lack of energy, confusion, acute psychosis, mutism, combativeness, slurred or unintelligible speech, hyperreflexia, seizures, and coma.[17,18]

Other effects have included acute abdominal pain, peptic ulcer disease, muscle weakness and pain, malaise, weight loss, and delayed onset laminar desquamation of palms and soles and alopecia areata.[17]

Laboratory abnormalities include leukocytosis, hyperglycemia, hepatic aminotransferase abnormalities, and elevations of blood urea nitrogen, creatinine, and creatine phosphokinase (rhabdomyolysis). Fluid and electrolyte disturbances may include hypokalemic alkalosis and sodium and water retention.[17]

Acute thyroid hormone overdoses are well tolerated by children; there are no reported deaths due to acute toxicity in the literature. In one retrospective review of 92 children (ages 6 years or younger) with acute T_4 ingestion, no significant symptoms developed in those who ingested doses up to 3.75 mg T_4 with GI decontamination and 2.0 mg T_4 without GI decontamination.[11] In this study, clinical effects occurred in 8.7% and included irritability, hyperactivity, increased appetite, vomiting, diarrhea, fever, flushing, and rash. In this study, researchers concluded that ingestion of less than 5.0 mg T_4 equivalent of thyroid hormone is not associated with significant toxicity. Other toxic effects reported in children include supraventricular tachycardia, extrasystoles, hypertension, diaphoresis, abdominal pain, lethargy, extremity jerking, and seizures.[7-9,12,20-22,24,42,47-54] Although children usually tolerate relatively large doses of thyroid hormone without major toxicity, significant toxicity may rarely occur. For instance, Kulig and colleagues reported on a 30-month-old boy who had two grand mal seizures 7 days after acute ingestion of an estimated 18 mg of T_4.[24] GI decontamination was performed with 3.5 hours of ingestion. There is not consistently a close correlation between the severity and type of symptoms and the ingested amount or serum T_4 levels shortly after ingestion. Tenenbein and colleagues reported an overdose of 30 mg of T_4 in a child with no significant toxicity.[10] The time course of signs and symptoms of toxicity is similar for both children and adults.

Chronic Overdose

As for acute overdose, signs and symptoms of chronic overdose primarily affect the cardiovascular and sympathetic and central nervous systems. Clinical effects may begin within a few days of the first dose.[6,26,30] Unlike those following acute overdose, cardiovascular and neurologic effects tend to be more severe. For instance, there is a greater incidence of unstable arrhythmias (e.g., atrial and ventricular fibrillation), left ventricular heart failure, and serious neurologic effects (e.g., stupor, coma, aphasia, hemiparesis, and seizures).[5,26,28] When death occurs, it usually results from a lethal ventricular arrhythmia (e.g., ventricular fibrillation).[26,30] Other clinical effects noted with chronic excessive exposure include insomnia, heat intolerance, asthenia, sialorrhea, arthromyalgia, diarrhea, weight loss, fatigability, dyspnea on exertion, anxiousness, apprehension, hostility, restlessness, anorexia, jitteriness, depression, heat intolerance, warm moist palms, and generalized muscle weakness.[2,5,28]

The natural history of signs and symptoms of chronic toxicity is illustrated in one series of six adult patients (ages 46–74 years) who were erroneously administered between 70 and 1200 mg of T_4 for 2 to 12 days.[26] All patients developed tachycardia, fever, nervousness, insomnia, heat intolerance, asthenia, arthromyalgia, and diarrhea within 3 days of ingesting the first T_4 dose. Severe neurologic signs and symptoms occurred in all patients between day 7 and 10 after ingestion; coma developed in five patients, stupor in one patient, and aphasia with hemiparesis occurred in one patient. Left ventricular failure, atrial fibrillation, and ventricular fibrillation developed between days 8 and 11 in five patients. One patient developed diffuse ST-T wave changes on electrocardiogram on day 29. Intense laminar desquamation of the palms and soles developed between days 17 and 37 in five patients. One patient died; the other patients recovered completely.

ADVERSE EVENTS

The adverse drug effects associated with chronic thyroid hormone therapy include sinus tachycardia, nonsinus supraventricular tachycardias (e.g., atrial flutter and fibrillation), premature atrial contractions, coronary artery spasm, acute myocardial infarction, left ventricular hypertrophy, cardiac failure, reduced bone density and mass, thyroid storm, coma, and death.[23,31-34] Tachycardia is often out of proportion to fever. Adverse effects may also occur during acute exposure to thyroid hormones

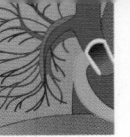

with therapeutic intent. Initiation of thyroid hormone replacement therapy in hypothyroid patients has been rarely associated with arrhythmias and death.[44] Thus, in patients older than 60 years and in those with known cardiac disease, thyroid hormone replacement is initiated at a lower daily dose of levothyroxine (e.g., 12.5 to 25 µg/day) and increased slowly to avoid cardiac adverse effects. Idiosyncratic or allergic reactions may occur with animal-derived products such as desiccated thyroid and thyroglobulin.

DIAGNOSIS

There are no essential tests recommended after thyroid hormone exposure. However, serum T_4, T_3, and thyroglobulin levels may have some diagnostic and prognostic value. Elevated serum T_4 and T_3 levels help to confirm excessive ingestion of thyroid preparations. In children, a serum T_4 concentration greater than 75 µg/dL within 7 hours after ingestion may be predictive of who will develop toxicity (e.g., fever, tachycardia, and agitation) 12 to 48 hours after ingestion.[8] Despite this study, measurements of serum T_4 and T_3 do not always correlate with the severity of illness and need for therapy, particularly in those with chronic thyroid preparation overdose. With acute thyroid hormone overdose, the initial serum TSH may not be suppressed until pituitary thyrotrophs respond to thyroid hormone excess and circulating TSH is metabolically cleared.

The serum T_4/T_3 ratio and thyroglobulin concentration may be helpful in distinguishing those patients with thyrotoxicosis factitia from those with endogenous causes of thyrotoxicosis.[55] The serum T_4/T_3 ratio in patients taking exogenous, excessive doses of T_4 is higher than in patients with endogenous thyrotoxicosis, in whom there is a marked T_3 secretion. In patients with thyrotoxicosis from Graves' disease, the mean T_4/T_3 ratio is 28 (range, 11–57), whereas patients with thyrotoxicosis factitia have a mean ratio of 70 (range, 48–114). Ordinarily, small amounts of thyroglobulin are released into the serum during normal T_4 release from the thyroid gland. Thus, patients with thyrotoxicosis factitia have either low or undetectable serum thyroglobulin levels,[3] as compared with those with endogenous thyrotoxicosis, in which thyroglobulin levels are normal or increased. Endogenous hyperthyroidism due to Graves' disease or nodular thyroid disease can also be differentiated from thyroid hormone overdose by measuring thyroidal uptake of iodine-123 or technetium-99m. The uptake is increased in hyperthyroidism due to Graves' disease or nodular thyroid disease, whereas it is suppressed with overdose. However, it should be understood that the uptake is also suppressed in hyperthyroidism associated with thyroiditis, metastatic thyroid cancer, and struma ovarii.

The dynamic pattern of a patient's serial thyroid function tests may provide evidence for diagnosis of exogenous T_3 ingestion.[6] The serum T_3 concentration will most likely far exceed that observed in endogenous causes of hyperthyroidism. The rapid fall in serum T_3 concentration indicates that T_3 toxicosis is a transient event rather than a sustained physiologic process. The serum T_4/T_3 ratio will be expected to consistently be less than 20, which is less than that observed in conditions of endogenous hyperthyroidism associated with T_3 toxicosis. This ratio reflects the extreme elevation of serum T_3 concentration and the decreased T_4 concentration with T_3 suppression of TSH.

An increased serum T_4/T_3 ratio may be observed in thyrotoxic states other than ingestion of excess amounts of T_4. Patients receiving amiodarone therapy have elevated T_4/T_3 ratios (mean, 57; range, 27–120), and it has been associated with increased serum thyroglobulin concentration (mean, 118 ng/dL; range, 17–460 ng/dL).[56]

In addition to thyroid function testing, routine laboratory analysis in patients who have taken excessive doses of thyroid hormones should include a complete blood count and measurement of serum electrolyte, blood urea nitrogen, creatinine, glucose, creatine phosphokinase (CPK), calcium concentrations, and pregnancy testing in women of childbearing age. Serum acetaminophen and salicylate concentrations should be performed in all intentional overdose patients. In patients with chest pain or cardiovascular toxicity, an electrocardiogram should be performed, and laboratory evaluation should include serial measurements of serum CPK and troponin concentrations. Other studies that may be helpful include head computed tomography, lumbar puncture, and toxicology studies of blood and urine.

Differential Diagnosis

The sympathomimetic effects of thyroid hormone overdose may present similarly to many other toxicologic and nontoxicologic entities (Box 67-1). Other toxic etiologies to consider include anticholinergic, neuroleptic-malignant, serotonin, and sedative-hypnotic withdrawal syndromes; and poisoning by hallucinogens, lithium, monoamine oxidase inhibitors, strychnine, sympathomimetics (e.g., cocaine, amphetamines, methylxanthines, cough and cold preparations, decongestants), salicylates, dinitrophenol and pentachlorophenol, and nicotine. Occasionally, thyrotoxicosis may be associated with ingestion of amiodarone, lithium, and excessive doses of iodine. Nontoxicologic conditions that should be considered in the differential diagnosis include endogenous thyrotoxicosis, traumatic head injury, intracranial hemorrhage, heatstroke, systemic infection, pheochromocytoma, hypoglycemia, malignant hyperthermia, and lethal catatonia.

As mentioned, specific thyroid function laboratory testing helps differentiate endogenous thyrotoxicosis from exogenous thyrotoxicosis (overdose). In addition, the relatively short duration of symptoms and the absence of exophthalmos, pretibial myxedema, onycholysis of fingernails, thyroid bruit, and goiter are helpful in ruling out endogenous hyperthyroidism.

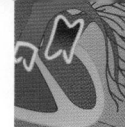

BOX 67-1 DIFFERENTIAL DIAGNOSIS OF THYROID HORMONE OVERDOSE

Hyperthyroidism
- Endogenous hyperthyroidism due to Graves' disease, multinodular goiter, solitary functioning adenoma, thyroiditis
- Hyperthyroidism associated with drug use such as thyroid hormone preparations, amiodarone, iodide-containing compounds, interferon, lithium

Acute disorders associated with sympathetic nervous system activation: infection, heatstroke, hemorrhage, trauma, pheochromocytoma, conditions associated with severe pain, and drug withdrawal states

Toxic drug ingestion
- Amphetamine, cocaine, methylxanthines, and other sympathomimetic agents
- Cyclic antidepressants and monoamine oxidase inhibitors
- Salicylates
- Dinitrophenol and pentachlorophenol
- Nicotine overdose
- Central hallucinogens
- Lithium and other psychotropic agents
- Toxic syndromes (e.g., neuroleptic malignant syndrome and serotonin syndrome)

MANAGEMENT

Overview

The treatment plan of patients who have ingested thyroid hormone is dependent on the intent of the exposure (suicidal or accidental), estimated dose ingested, time since ingestion, associated ingestion of other compounds, toxic effects present on presentation, and the patient's age, comorbid conditions, and reliability (when considering outpatient treatment). As noted already, healthy adults and children may tolerate even relatively large doses of thyroid hormone without serious consequences.[7,8,11,12,52,57,58] On the other hand, life-threatening toxicity can occur in elderly patients or those with underlying cardiac disease.[44,58-60] Indications for inpatient observation and treatment include (1) signs and symptoms of toxicity; (2) elderly age or the presence of underlying cardiopulmonary disease; (3) ingestion of more than 100 µg/kg of T_4 or 30 µg/kg of T_3; (4) serum T_4 concentrations greater than 75 µg/dL and/or T_3 levels greater than 350 ng/dL; and (5) unreliable patients or caretakers. Patients with mild to moderate signs of toxicity can be admitted to a monitored floor bed, whereas those patients manifesting significant cardiovascular or neurologic signs and symptoms should be managed in an intensive care unit.

Emergent medical assessment and GI decontamination are not recommended for every patient exposed to thyroid hormones. Most cases of accidental ingestion can be managed with home observation and telephone follow-up by health care professionals for a period of 7 days. Gastrointestinal decontamination is unnecessary for children younger than 12 years who accidentally ingest an estimated 2 mg or less of T_4 and may not be necessary for ingestions up to 5 mg.[9,11] These patients may be observed at home pending the onset of symptoms. Although the absence of initial symptoms does not preclude the possibility for delayed significant toxicity (e.g., seizures),[24] prophylactic treatment with antithyroid agents (e.g., propranolol, PTU, and corticosteroids) is not recommended in the absence of toxic effects.[7-11]

Patients who have ingested thyroid hormone with suicidal intent should be emergently assessed in a hospital, receive GI decontamination, and be observed for signs and symptoms of thyroid hormone toxicity or coingestants. After GI decontamination and an emergency department observation period of several hours, it may be acceptable to transfer an otherwise healthy, asymptomatic patient who ingested thyroid hormone with suicidal intent to an inpatient psychiatric facility. This is provided that the receiving facility is knowledgeable of the delayed toxic effects that can occur from thyroid hormone, can monitor for these effects, and will transfer the patient back to an acute care facility should these effects occur. Otherwise, it is more prudent to admit these patients to the hospital for close observation for a period of 3 to 5 days.

Decontamination

GI decontamination is recommended after intentional or accidental thyroid hormone overdose (greater than 5 mg T_4 equivalent), provided it can be initiated within a few hours of ingestion. Although it has not been well studied, single-dose administration of activated charcoal (1 g/kg orally or by nasogastric tube) is the preferred method of gastrointestinal decontamination. The bile acid sequestrant, cholestyramine, is an acceptable alternative agent for GI decontamination. Clinical studies have shown that cholestyramine significantly interferes with T_4 absorption from the GI tract and interrupts T_4 and T_3 enterohepatic circulation.[61,62] One in vitro study showed that 50 mg of cholestyramine resin is capable of irreversibly binding 3 mg of T_4.[61] The typical cholestyramine dose is 50 to 150 mg/kg/dose (adult, 3–9 g), and this dose can be repeated every 6 to 8 hours. Neither cathartic nor whole bowel irrigation has been formally studied as a decontamination method after thyroid hormone overdose.

Supportive Care

Supportive measures should include treatment of hyperthermia; correction and maintenance of fluid, electrolyte, and acid–base balance; and monitoring of cardiac rhythm and respiratory status. Intravenous fluid should be administered such that urine output is at least 1 to 2 mL/kg/hr. Hyperthermia should be managed using standard measures. Case reports suggest that dantrolene may be effective adjunct therapy for endogenous thyrotoxicosis,[63-65] but its efficacy remains to

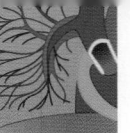
be established in exogenous thyroid hormone toxicity. Dantrolene inhibits the effects of high circulating T_4 levels on calcium flux across the sarcoplasmic reticulum.[63] Hypertension requiring medical treatment is rare and, if clinically indicated, should be managed as a hypertensive emergency.

Specific Treatment Measures

Specific treatment measures for exogenous thyroid storm include the administration of β-adrenergic antagonists to suppress the signs and symptoms and administration of agents that block conversion of T_4 to T_3 (active hormone) and block the release of thyroid hormone from the thyroid gland.

β-ADRENERGIC ANTAGONISTS
Agents in this class (e.g., propranolol and esmolol) rapidly reduce catecholamine-dependent signs and symptoms, such as tachycardia, supraventricular tachyarrhythmias, hypertension, tremor, palpitation, tension, and psychomotor agitation.[14,15,20,21,28,34,47,49,54] Propranolol, and possibly other β blockers, also partially inhibit the conversion of T_4 to T_3.[66] The typical oral propranolol dose is 0.2 to 0.5 mg/kg/dose (adult, 10–40 mg) every 4–6 hours; the dose should be adjusted according to the response, and large doses (240–280 mg/day) may be required in severely toxic patients. The intravenous propranolol dose is 0.1 mg/kg (adult, 2–10 mg) over 10 minutes and may be repeated up to three times as clinically indicated. An esmolol infusion can be initiated by administering 0.5 mg/kg over 1 minute, then 50 μg/kg/min for 4 minutes; if the response is inadequate, rebolus with 0.5 mg/kg and then 50 to 200 μg/kg/min for up to 48 hours.

CALCIUM CHANNEL ANTAGONISTS
Diltiazem appears to be an effective alternative therapy in controlling thyrotoxic symptoms in patients in whom β-blocker therapy may be contraindicated.[67,68] The oral diltiazem dose is 1 to 3 mg/kg/dose (adult, 60–180 mg) every 6 to 8 hours. Diltiazem may be administered intravenously as a bolus injection (0.25 mg/kg), typically 20 mg intravenously given initially followed by 5 to 10 mg/hr.

IODINATED RADIOCONTRAST AGENTS
Oral iodinated radiocontrast agents (e.g., sodium ipodate and iopanoic acid) are potent inhibitors of peripheral T_4 bioconversion to T_3 and appear to be effective adjunct treatment for patients with either exogenous[8,42,47,69] or endogenous thyrotoxicosis.[70-73] After administration of these contrast agents, there is marked prolongation in serum T_4 half-life, with a concurrent sharp increase in serum rT_3 level and a marked decrease in serum T_3 level.[42,47,69] Although not important for exogenous thyroid hormone overdose, these agents also release large amounts of iodide with their metabolism, which subsequently blocks the release of T_4 and T_3 from the thyroid. The typical sodium ipodate and iopanoic acid dose for adults is 3 g and that for children is 150 mg/kg/dose, and may be repeated for recurrence of symptoms. Sodium ipodate, 250 mg/kg/dose every 3 days for 18 days followed by 500 mg/kg/dose every 3 days for 21 days, has been successfully used to treat a patient with moderately severe neonatal Graves' disease.[71]

CORTICOSTEROIDS
The major effect of corticosteroids, particularly dexamethasone (2 mg every 6 hours for four doses), is to alter peripheral T_4 metabolism such that conversion from T_4 to T_3 is diminished and to rT_3 is enhanced.[74-76] In those with endogenous thyroid storm, relative adrenal insufficiency is often present, and corticosteroid administration (hydrocortisone at 200 to 400 mg daily) is important as part of treatment to reduce mortality. The presence of relative adrenal insufficiency in exogenous thyroid storm is unclear.

PROPYLTHIOURACIL AND METHIMAZOLE
The antithyroid thionamide drugs PTU and methimazole (MMI) inhibit the synthesis of both T_4 and T_3. These agents interrupt thyroid peroxidase–catalyzed inorganic iodide oxidation and thyroidal T_4 secretion.[66,77] PTU and MMI have limited to no efficacy in the management of exogenous thyroid hormone toxicity (see below for toxicity from these agents).

IODIDE
Iodide acutely inhibits thyroid hormone biosynthesis and release, and, like the thionamides, has no proven clinical utility in the treatment of exogenous thyroid hormone exposure.

Enhancement of Elimination

Multiple doses of activated charcoal have been used and case reports suggest it does not appreciably alter serum thyroid hormone levels or improve clinical outcome.[8,22] However, multiple doses of cholestyramine may be an effective means of decreasing the body's exogenous hormone load by binding GI tract T_4 and disrupting enterohepatic recirculation. Cholestyramine has been used successfully to treat iatrogenic thyrotoxicosis (Fig. 67-2).[61,62]

Hemodialysis is ineffective because of the high protein binding and limited renal excretion of thyroid hormones. Exchange transfusion,[40,48] plasmapheresis,[26,40,78] and hemoperfusion[26] have been used in the management of acute and nonacute thyroid hormone poisoning, but conclusive studies are lacking. Observations suggest that these extracorporeal techniques do not remove significant amount of thyroid hormones relative to the total ingestion and that their efficacy decreases with time.

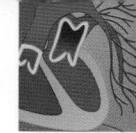

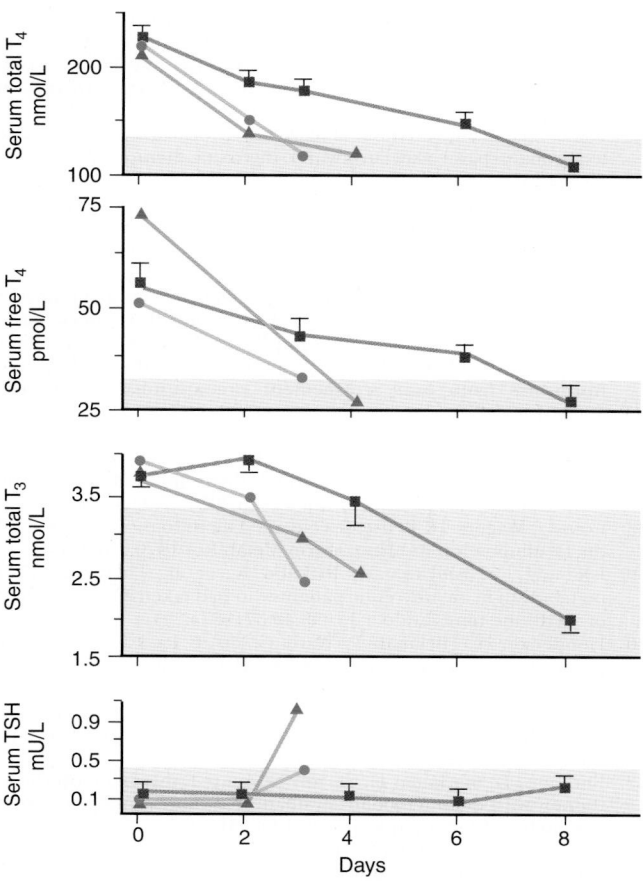

FIGURE 67-2 The use of the bile acid sequestrant cholestyramine to lower serum thyroid hormones in iatrogenic hyperthyroidism. Two patients with iatrogenic hyperthyroidism were administered 4 g of cholestyramine four times a day. The alterations in serum total T_4, free T_4, total T_3, and thyroid-stimulating hormone (TSH) levels in the two subjects (●—●; ▲—▲) and one control (■—■) (n = 3, values = mean ± SE) are shown. The normal serum values are as follows: total T_4, 51 to 142 nmol/L; free T_4, 10 to 36 pmol; total T_3, 1.2 to 3.4 nmol/L; and TSH, 0.4 values for T_4 and T_3 and the lower normal range values for TSH. (From Shakir KMM, Michaels RD, Hays JH, et al: The use of bile acid sequestrants to lower serum thyroid hormones in iatrogenic hyperthyroidism. Ann Intern Med 1993;118:113.)

TOXICOLOGY OF THYROID ANTAGONISTS

Thyroid antagonists are drugs that interfere with one or more steps in iodine metabolism, thyroid hormone synthesis, or hormone release by the thyroid gland. Drugs that prevent the secretion of thyroid hormones include iodides and lithium. The toxicity of iodine (see Chapter 96) and lithium (see Chapter 30) are discussed elsewhere. Amiodarone may produce both hyperthyroidism and hypothyroidism; its toxicity is discussed in Chapter 63. The toxicity of the thionamides, PTU and MMI (Tapazol), is discussed here. Another thionamide available in Great Britain, carbimazole (Neo-Mercazole), is converted to MMI after absorption.

PTU and MMI inhibit organification of iodide and the coupling of iodotyrosines for hormonally active iodo-thyronines. PTU also partially inhibits the peripheral deiodination of T_4 to T_3. Both agents are readily absorbed from the GI tract within an hour, and inhibition of thyroid iodine organification begins within 20 to 30 minutes.[44] The Vd for PTU is about 0.3 L/kg, and 75% is protein bound. The Vd for MMI is 0.6 L/kg, and protein binding is minimal. The plasma elimination half-lives of PTU and MMI are 1 to 2 hours and 4 to 6 hours, respectively. Intrathyroidal accumulation of drug occurs. Both PTU and MMI cross the placental barrier and appear in human breast milk.

There is a paucity of information regarding acute PTU or MMI overdose. Acute ingestion of an estimated 5 to 13 g of PTU in a 12-year-old patient did not result in any clinically significant effects.[82] A low incidence of adverse effects (3% to 7%) has been associated with therapeutic use of both PTU and MMI.[16,44,79-85] Most toxic reactions to thionamides occur with a few weeks or months of beginning therapy. Adverse drug events associated with PTU use include skin rash (purpuric or urticarial), granulocytopenia, eosinophilia, lupus-like syndrome, acute hepatitis, cholestatic hepatotoxicity, hepatic necrosis, liver failure, and death. Diagnostic laboratory studies may reveal complete blood count and liver function test abnormalities, hepatocellular necrosis around the central veins with moderate to severe lymphocytes and neutrophils infiltration in the portal areas and lobules on liver biopsy, positive migration inhibition factor test to PTU, and PTU-induced peripheral lymphocyte transformation.[81,85,86] PTU may traverse the placenta and cause neonatal hepatitis and lymphocyte sensitization.[86] Management of PTU toxicity includes immediate discontinuation of the drug, supportive care, steroid therapy, and, in cases of fulminant liver failure, orthotopic liver transplantation.[16,80,81,87,88]

Adverse drug events associated with MMI use include agranulocytosis, pancytopenia, plasmocytosis, serum sickness, acute include hepatitis, cholestatic jaundice, granulomatous hepatitis, hepatocellular necrosis, and death.[79,89-94] Diagnostic laboratory studies may reveal abnormalities in the complete blood count, liver function tests, liver biopsy, and bone marrow biopsy.[89,90,92] Management of MMI toxicity includes immediate discontinuation of the drug, supportive care, and, in cases of severe bone marrow toxicity, reverse isolation, antibiotics, dexamethasone, and granulocyte colony-stimulating factor therapy.[89,92]

Agranulocytosis from both agents has an overall incidence of about 1 in 500 patients. Like other adverse effects, agranulocytosis occurs with greatest incidence in the first few weeks of treatment. Agranulocytosis is usually heralded by fever and a sore throat. This adverse drug effect is reversible upon discontinuation of the offending thionamide.

The treatment of thionamide overdose is entirely supportive. Previously euthyroid patients who ingest these agents are not expected to become hypothyroid, as because these agents have a relatively short duration of action (<24 hours).

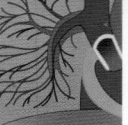

REFERENCES

1. Bogazzi F, Bartalena L, Scarcello G, et al: The age of patients with thyrotoxicosis factitia in Italy from 1973 to 1996. J Endocrinol Invest 1999;22:128–133.
2. Braunstein GD, Koblin R, Sugawara M, et al: Unintentional thyrotoxicosis factitia due to a diet pill. West J Med 1986;145:388–391.
3. Mariotti S, Martino E, Cupini C, et al: Low serum thyroglobulin as a clue to the diagnosis of thyrotoxicosis factitia. N Engl J Med 1982;307:410–412.
4. Matsubara S, Inoh M, Tarumi Y, et al: An outbreak (159 cases) of transient thyrotoxicosis without hyperthyroidism in Japan. Intern Med 1995;34:514–519.
5. Rose E, Sanders TP, Webbs WL Jr, et al: Occult factitial thyrotoxicosis. Thyroxine kinetics and psychological evaluation in three cases. Ann Intern Med 1969;71:309–315.
6. Sylvia Vela B, Dorin RI: Factitious triiodothyronine toxicosis. Am J Med 1991;90:132–134.
7. Golightly LK, Smolinske SC, Kulig KW, et al: Clinical effects of accidental levothyroxine ingestion in children. Am J Dis Child 1987;141:1025–1027.
8. Lewander WJ, Lacouture PG, Silva JE, et al: Acute thyroxine ingestion in pediatric patients. Pediatrics 1989;84:262–265.
9. Litovitz TL, White JD: Levothyroxine ingestions in children: an analysis of 78 cases. Am J Emerg Med 1985;3:297–300.
10. Tenenbein M, Dean HJ: Benign course after massive levothyroxine ingestion. Pediatr Emerg Care 1986;2:15–17.
11. Tunget CL, Clark RF, Turchen SG, et al: Raising the decontamination level for thyroid hormone ingestions. Am J Emerg Med 1995;13:9–13.
12. Funderburk SJ, Spaulding JS: Sodium levothyroxine (Synthroid) intoxication in a child. Pediatrics 1970;45:298–301.
13. Kirkland RT, Kirkland JL, Greger NG, et al: Thyroid hormone poisoning: therapy questioned. Pediatrics 1984;74:901.
14. Nystrom E, Lindstedt G, Lundberg PA: Minor signs and symptoms of toxicity in a young woman in spite of massive thyroxine ingestion. Acta Med Scand 1980;207:135–136.
15. Von Hofe SE, Young RL: Thyrotoxicosis after a single ingestion of levothyroxine. JAMA 1977;237:1361.
16. Levy R, Gilger WC: Acute thyroid poisoning. Report of a case. N Engl J Med 1957;255:456–460.
17. Schottstaedt ES, Smoller M: "Thyroid storm" produced by acute thyroid hormone poisoning. Ann Intern Med 1966;64:847–849.
18. Hack JB, Leviss JA, Nelson LS, et al: Severe symptoms following a massive intentional L-thyroxine ingestion. Vet Hum Toxicol 1999;41:323–326.
19. Dahlberg PA, Karlsson FA, Wide L: Triiodothyronine intoxication. Lancet 1979;2:700.
20. Mandel SH, Magnusson AR, Burton BT, et al: Massive levothyroxine ingestion. Conservative management. Clin Pediatr 1989;28:374–376.
21. Roesch C, Becker PG, Sklar S: Management of a child with acute thyroxine ingestion. Ann Emerg Med 1985;14:1114–1115.
22. Shilo L, Kovatz S, Hadari R, et al: Massive thyroid hormone overdose: kinetics, clinical manifestations and management. Isr Med Assoc J 2002;4:298–299.
23. Bergeron GA, Goldsmith R, Schiller NB: Myocardial infarction, severe reversible ischemia, and shock following excess thyroid administration in a woman with normal coronary arteries. Arch Intern Med 1988;148:1450–1453.
24. Kulig K, Golightly LK, Rumack BH: Levothyroxine overdose associated with seizures in a young child. JAMA 1985;254:2109–2110.
25. Vlase H, Lungu G, Vlase L: Cardiac disturbances in thyrotoxicosis: diagnosis, incidence, clinical features and management. Endocrinologie 1991;29:155–160.
26. Binimelis J, Bassas L, Marruecos L, et al: Massive thyroxine intoxication: evaluation of plasma extraction. Intensive Care Med 1987;13:33–38.
27. Petit WA Jr, Barrett EJ: Chronic thyroxine ingestion leading to thyroid storm and accelerated thyroxine turnover. Conn Med 1987;51:291–292.
28. van Huekelom S, Kinderen LH, der Vingerhoeds PJ: Plasmapheresis in L-thyroxine intoxication. Vet Hum Toxicol 1979;21(Suppl):7.
29. Bacci V, Schussler GC, Bhogal RS, et al: Cardiac arrest after intravenous administration of levothyroxine. JAMA 1981;245:920.
30. Bhasin S, Wallace W, Lawrence JB, et al: Sudden death associated with thyroid hormone abuse. Am J Med 1981;71:887–890.
31. Bartalena L, Bogazzi F, Martino E: Adverse effects of thyroid hormone preparations and antithyroid drugs. Drug Saf 1996;15:53–63.
32. Hiasa Y, Ishida T, Aihara T, et al: Acute myocardial infarction due to coronary spasm associated with L-thyroxine therapy. Clin Cardiol 1989;12:161–163.
33. Locker GJ, Kotzmann H, Frey B, et al: Factitious hyperthyroidism causing acute myocardial infarction. Thyroid 1995;5:465–467.
34. Redahan C, Karski JM: Thyrotoxicosis factitia in a post-aortocoronary bypass patient. Can J Anaesth 1994;41:969–972.
35. Watson WA, Litovitz TL, Rogers GC Jr, et al: 2004 annual report of the American Association of Poison Control Centers Toxic Exposure Surveillance System. Am J Emerg Med 2005;22:589–666.
36. LeBoff MS, Kaplan MM, Silva JE, et al: Bioavailability of thyroid hormones from oral replacement preparations. Metabolism 1982;31:900–905.
37. Wenzel KW, Meinhold H: Evidence of lower toxicity during thyroxine suppression after a single 3 mg L-thyroxine dose: comparison to the classical L-triiodothyronine test for thyroid suppressibility. J Clin Endocrinol Metab 1974;38:902–905.
38. Loos U, Wagner H, Bellstedt G, et al: The influence of hydration on T3 elimination in urine. Horm Metab Res 1976;8:154–155.
39. Ishihara T, Nishikawa M, Ikekubo K, et al: Thyroxine (T4) metabolism in an athyreotic patient who had taken a large amount of T4 at one time. Endocr J 1998;45:371–375.
40. Henderson A, Hickman P, Ward G, et al: Lack of efficacy of plasmapheresis in a patient overdosed with thyroxine. Anaesth Intensive Care 1994;22:463–464.
41. Kaiserman I, Avni M, Sack J: Kinetics of the pituitary-thyroid axis and the peripheral thyroid hormones in 2 children with thyroxine intoxication. Horm Res 1995;44:229–237.
42. Berkner PD, Starkman H, Person N: Acute L-thyroxine overdose; therapy with sodium ipodate: evaluation of clinical and physiologic parameters. J Emerg Med 1991;9:129–131.
43. Herrmann J, Rudorff KH, Gockenjan G, et al: Charcoal haemoperfusion in thyroid storm. Lancet 1977;1:248.
44. Farwell AP, Braverman LE: Thyroid and antithyroid drugs. In Hardman JG, Limbrid LE, Gilman AG (eds): Goodman & Gilman's the Pharmacological Basis of Therapeutics, 10th ed. New York, McGraw-Hill, 2001, p 1577.
45. Hamolsky MW: Truth is stranger than factitious. N Engl J Med 1982;307:436–437.
46. Hedberg CW, Fishbein DB, Janssen RS, et al: An outbreak of thyrotoxicosis caused by the consumption of bovine thyroid gland in ground beef. N Engl J Med 1987;316:993–998.
47. Brown RS, Cohen JH, Braverman LE: Successful treatment of massive acute thyroid hormone poisoning with iopanoic acid. J Pediatr 1998;132:903–905.
48. Gerard P, Malvaux P, De Visscher M: Accidental poisoning with thyroid extract treated by exchange transfusion. Arch Dis Child 1972;47:981–982.
49. Gorman RL, Chamberlain JM, Rose SR, et al: Massive levothyroxine overdose: high anxiety—low toxicity. Pediatrics 1988;82:666–669.
50. Jacobziner H, Raybin HW: Thyroid intoxication. N Y State J Med 1958;58:408–409.
51. Jahr HM: Thyroid "poisoning" in children. Nebr State Med J 1936;21:388.
52. Lehrner LM, Weir MR: Acute ingestions of thyroid hormones. Pediatrics 1984;73:313–317.
53. Levy M: Propylthiouracil hepatotoxicity. A review and case presentation. Clin Pediatr (Phila) 1993;32:25–29.
54. Singh GK, Winterborn MH: Massive overdose with thyroxine: toxicity and treatment. Eur J Pediatr 1991;150:217.
55. Pearce CJ, Himsworth RL: Thyrotoxicosis factitia. N Engl J Med 1982;307:1708–1709.
56. Mariotti S, Martino E, Aghini F, et al: Thyrotoxicosis factitia. N Engl J Med 1982;307:1709.
57. Dahl IL: Thyroid crisis in a three year old. Acta Paediatr Scand 1968;57:55.
58. Matthews SJ: Acute thyroxine overdose: two cases of parasuicide. Ulster Med J 1993;63:170.

59. Likoff WB, Levine SA: Thyrotoxicosis as the sole cause of heart failure. Am J Med Sci 1943;206:425.

60. Ridgway ED, McCammon JA, Benotti J, et al: Acute metabolic responses in myxedema to large doses of intravenous L-thyroxine. Ann Intern Med 1972;77:549.

61. Northcutt RC, Stiel JN, Hollifield JW, et al: The influence of cholestyramine on thyroxine absorption. JAMA 1969;208:1857–1861.

62. Shakir KMM, Michaels RD, Hays JH, et al: The use of bile acid sequestrants to lower serum thyroid hormones in iatrogenic hyperthyroidism. Ann Intern Med 1993;118:112–113.

63. Bennett MH, Wainwright AP: Acute thyroid crisis on induction of anaesthesia. Anaesthesia 1989;44:28–30.

64. Christensen PA, Nissen LR: Treatment of thyroid storm in a child with dantrolene. Br J Anaesth 1987;59:523.

65. Ebert RJ: Dantrolene and thyroid crisis. Anaesthesia 1994;49:924.

66. Perrild H, Hansen JM, Skovsted L, et al: Different effects of propranolol, alprenolol, sotalol, atenolol and metoprolol on serum T_3 and serum rT_3 in hyperthyroidism. Clin Endocrinol 1983;18:139–142.

67. Milner MR, Gelman KM, Phillips RA, et al: Double-blind crossover trial of diltiazem versus propranolol in the management of thyrotoxic symptoms. Pharmacotherapy 1990;10:100–106.

68. Roti E, Montermini M, Roti S, et al: The effect of diltiazem, a calcium channel-blocking drug, on cardiac rate and rhythm in hyperthyroid patients. Arch Intern Med 1988;148:1919–1921.

69. Lacouture PG, Lewander WJ, Silva E, et al: Pharmacokinetics of T3 and T4 after iopanoic acid. Pediatr Res 1987;21:249A.

70. Bal C, Nair N: The therapeutic efficacy of oral cholecystographic agent (iopanoic acid) in the management of hyperthyroidism. J Nucl Med 1990;31:1180–1183.

71. Karpman BA, Rapoport B, Filetti S, et al: Treatment of neonatal hyperthyroidism due to Grave's disease with sodium ipodate. J Clin Endocrinol Metab 1987;64:119–123.

72. Sharp B, Reed AW, Tamagna EI, et al: Treatment of hyperthyroidism with sodium ipodate (Oragrafin) in addition to propylthiouracil and propranolol. J Clin Endocrinol Metab 1981;53:622–625.

73. Wu SY, Shyh TP, Chopra IJ, et al: Comparison of sodium ipodate (Oragrafin) and propylthiouracil in early treatment of hyperthyroidism. J Clin Endocrinol Metab 1982;54:632–634.

74. Duick DS, Warren DW, Nicoloff JT, et al: Effect of single dose dexamethasone on the concentration of serum triiodothyronine in man. J Clin Endocrinol Metab 1974;39:1151–1154.

75. Croxson MS, Hall TD, Nicoloff JT, et al: Combination drug therapy for treatment of hyperthyroid Grave's disease. J Clin Endocriol Metab 1977;45;623–630.

76. Chopra IJ, Williams DE, Orgiazzi J, et al: Opposite effects of dexamethasone on serum concentrations of 3,3′,5′-triiodothyronine (reverse T3) and 3,3′5-triiodothyronine (T3). J Clin Endocrinol Metab 1975;41:911–920.

77. Furth ED, Rives K, Becker DV: Nonthyroidal action of propylthiouracil in euthyroid, hypothyroid and hyperthyroid man. J Clin Endocrinol Met 1966;26:239–246.

78. May ME, Mintz PD, Lowry P, et al: Plasmapheresis in thyroxine overdose: a case report. J Toxicol Clin Toxicol 1983;20:517–520.

79. Baker B, Shapiro B, Fig LM, et al: Unusual complications of antithyroid drug therapy: four case reports and review of literature. Thyroidology 1989;1:17–26.

80. Deidiker R, deMello DE: Propylthiouracil-induced fulminant hepatitis: case report and review of the literature. Pediatr Pathol Lab Med 1996;16:845–852.

81. Ichiki Y, Akahoshi M, Yamashita N, et al: Propylthiouracil-induced severe hepatitis: a case report and review of the literature. J Gastroenterol 1998;33:747–750.

82. Jackson GL, Flickinger FW, Wells LW: Massive overdose of propylthiouracil. Ann Intern Med 1979;91:418–419.

83. Lock DR, Sthoeger ZM: Severe hepatotoxicity on beginning propylthiouracil therapy. J Clin Gastroenterol 1997;24:267–269.

84. Pacini F, Sridama V, Refetoff S: Multiple complications of propylthiouracil treatment: granulocytopenia, eosinophilia, skin reaction and hepatitis with lymphocyte sensitization. J Endocrinol Invest 1982;5:403–407.

85. Seidman DS, Livni E, Ilie B, et al: Propylthiouracil-induced cholestatic jaundice. J Toxicol Clin Toxicol 1986;24:353–360.

86. Hayashida CY, Duarte AJ, Sato AE, et al: Neonatal hepatitis and lymphocyte sensitization by placental transfer of propylthiouracil. J Endocrinol Invest 1990;13:937–941.

87. Garty BZ, Kauli R, Ben-Ari J, et al: Hepatitis associated with propylthiouracil treatment. Drug Intell Clin Pharm 1985;19:740–742.

88. Kirkland JL: Propylthiouracil-induced hepatic failure and encephalopathy in a child. Drug Intell Clin Pharm 1990;24:470–471.

89. Breier DV, Rendo P, Gonzalez J, et al: Massive plasmocytosis due to methimazole-induced bone marrow toxicity. Am J Hematol 2001;67:259–261.

90. Di Gregorio C, Ghini F, Rivasi F: Granulomatous hepatitis in a patient receiving methimazole. Ital J Gastroenterol 1990;22:75–77.

91. Fischer MG, Nayer HR, Miller A: Methimazole-induced jaundice. JAMA 1973;223:1028–1029.

92. Luther AL, Wade JS, Slaughter JM: Agranulocytosis secondary to methimazole therapy: report of two cases. South Med J 1976;69:1356–1357.

93. Schwab GP, Wetscher GJ, Vogl W, et al: Methimazole-induced cholestatic liver injury, mimicking sclerosing cholangitis. Langenbecks Arch Chir 1996;381:225–227.

94. Van Kuyk M, Van Laethem Y, Duchateau J, et al: Methimazole-induced serum sickness. Acta Clin Belg 1983;38:68–69.

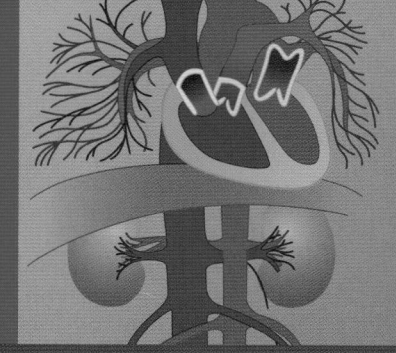

68 *Herbal, Traditional, and Alternative Medicines*

RICHARD L. KINGSTON, PHARMD ■ CHRIS FOLEY, MD

At a Glance...

- Alternative medicines, which include herbal, traditional, and many other dietary supplements, are used or relied on by more than half of the world's population.

- Despite an inherently wide margin of safety, selected alternative medicines have been associated with significant adverse effects.

- DSHEA, the law that regulates most commercially available alternative medicines, does not require manufacturers to undergo a premarket approval process for safety or efficacy. Despite this fact, relatively few serious adverse events involving most alternative medicines have been reported.

- The most serious concerns with alternative medicines have been related to adulterated products, selected herbs often used in traditional applications, and misidentification and inadvertent use of various botanicals.

- The greatest challenge for the future will likely relate to identifying which herbs or other alternative medicines possess the potential to pharmacokinetically alter or otherwise adversely affect the use of mainstream pharmacologic interventions.

- Absent a more stringent premarket approval process for safety, a national system of postmarket surveillance must be developed and embraced by regulators, manufacturers, health professionals, and the general public.

HERBAL MEDICINE AND MISCELLANEOUS AGENTS

Despite the continued development of medical and pharmacologic therapies for the treatment of illness, as many as 50% of people worldwide use alternative treatments, including herbal and traditional medicines.[1] Even in industrial nations, where there is no dearth of pharmaceutical agents, many seek "natural" products for their ailments. In one of the few studies of its kind, Eisenberg and colleagues, investigating the prevalence of use of unconventional medicine in the United States, found that one third of a sample population had used at least one unconventional therapy in the prior year.[2] Highest use was found among those with relatively more education and higher incomes. Annual prevalence was 3% for herbal medicines, 1% for homeopathy, and almost 1% for folk remedies. Reasons for using these therapies were extensive, including treatment of back pain, anxiety, headaches, cancer, and insomnia. In a similar pediatric study, 11% of children were found to have received one or more forms of alternative therapy since birth.[3] Parents stated that they chose alternative medicines after hearing about them from a friend, because of a fear of drug side effects, because they were dissatisfied with conventional medicine, or because they received more personal attention from alternative medicine practitioners. In a study conducted in a New York emergency department near the Chinatown district, Pearl and associates found that 43% of patients had used a traditional Chinese therapy within 1 week of their emergency department visit.[4] Fifty-eight percent of these had used at least one oral herbal preparation. Eleven patients reported using therapies that included unidentified tablets, nose drops, or topical preparations and animal preparations such as deer antler. Finally, although it may be of some epidemiologic importance that psychoactive plant materials such as jimsonweed, nutmeg, and morning glory seeds are often ingested as substances of abuse, most botanical and supplement use is generally benign. The major areas of concern will continue to be the potential for drug interactions when combined with conventional therapies and sorting out those substances, the dosing, and the routes of administration that are of true therapeutic value. Despite the relative wide margin of safety with most herbal products, in those rare circumstances in which a product is adulterated with unlabeled and unauthorized ingredients, there will be an opportunity for adverse consequences.

The increasing interest in alternative medicines as well as their proven therapeutic value[5-8] led in 1992 to the establishment of the Office of Alternative Medicine at the National Institutes of Health and subsequently the

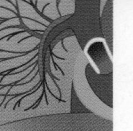

Office of Dietary Supplements. Through these organizations, investigators can obtain support for research designed to determine the range of benefit that alternative medicines or dietary supplements offer, with the goal of "integrating validated alternative medical practice with current conventional medical procedures."[9] Additional evidence of the public's interest in alternative medicine was shown in a survey that found that 10% of American pharmacies carry herbal remedies.[10] The potential routes of administration of alternative medicines include topical, rectal, and vaginal application as well as ingestion, injection, and inhalation.[11]

Nonetheless, alternative medicines, including herbs and other "dietary supplements," have been associated with examples of toxicity. The U.S. Food and Drug Administration (FDA) is given responsibility for protecting the public from dietary, nutritional, and pharmaceutical hazards. Oftentimes, however, the FDA has fallen short in terms of its capacity to offer the appropriate amount of regulation enforcement. Some have argued that this happens because substances in the dietary supplement classification fall into an ambiguous category.[12] When Congress passed the Dietary Supplement Health and Education Act (DSHEA), some felt that the FDA's ability to regulate alternative medicines was further weakened.[9,10] Seven major features of this law are as follows:

1. Dietary supplements can be marketed without any premarket efficacy studies.
2. Companies bear the burden of insuring product safety before marketing and sale. FDA must prove that the product is unsafe in order to remove a product from market.
3. Until recently, there were no guidelines for Good Manufacturing Procedures (GMPs) related to dietary supplements. New guidelines have since been promulgated by the FDA and will likely improve manufacturing accountability substantially.
4. Although specific health claims have been strictly regulated, certain product claims are permitted. For example, products cannot be claimed to cure a disease, but the label can discuss how a supplement affects the body's function. These are referred to as *structure function claims* and typically are more loosely defined than health claims.
5. Structure function labeling statements do not require extensive supportive evidence.
6. The FDA must be notified of proposed labeling, but no approval process is required. Accordingly, each label must contain a disclaimer related to any claims that states, "This statement has not been evaluated by the Food and Drug Administration. This product is not intended to diagnose, treat, cure, or prevent any disease."
7. Although there was a recommendation related to the establishment of a viable system of postmarket surveillance, none has been implemented. In the wake of reports of adverse consequences associated with ephedra, which resulted in its removal from the market, Congress has begun to consider options for mandatory adverse event reporting by manufacturers

of dietary supplements. Currently, dietary supplement manufacturers are not required to collect, document, and report to the FDA any reports of adverse consequences potentially associated with their products.

Although there is a clear need for the full implementation and enforcement of DSHEA as regards the manufacture, standardization, and postmarketing surveillance of dietary supplements, some of the risks and hazards claimed to be associated with this class of product are probably exaggerated. Despite their inherently wide margin of safety, monitoring for herb safety should remain a high priority, especially as pertains to interactions with mainstream pharmaceuticals, unexpected adverse effects during routine use, or potential contamination or adulteration issues. Although practitioners have been encouraged to report adverse effects directly to the FDA MedWatch system for both drugs and dietary supplements, it is believed that most events are underreported. Still, serious adverse reactions from alternative medications can and should be reported immediately to the FDA (telephone: 1-800-332-1088).[12] The dietary supplement industry has been examining options for the establishment of a voluntary system of adverse event management and reporting. This may provide an alternative system of surveillance that practitioners can participate in and utilize when assessing herbal product safety. Whether or not the overall system of postmarket surveillance for herbs and dietary supplements is improved remains to be seen.

Herbal Medicines

An herbal medicine can be defined as a plant extract that is used in various forms of refinement to achieve a preventive or therapeutic effect. For example, crude extracts of mushrooms and other fungi are considered to be herbal medicines alongside much more definitive formulations of ginseng and hawthorn extract. There is no controversy that many of these medicines have potent pharmacologic action, nor that they may provide some very useful benefits.[13-16] It is this same potency that often makes them responsible for inadvertent adverse effects as well as very useful alternatives to more toxic drugs.

The use of herbs and medicinal plants spans history and has been universal, occurring in every culture on earth. For example, Egyptian writings chronicled the use of medicinal herbs more than 4000 years ago; at that time, for example, poppy extracts were used to quiet crying children. Ayurvedic medicine (literally, "knowledge of how to live") emphasized the value of herbal medicines in texts dating back to 2500 BC. The Chinese *Materia Medica* lists about 5800 medicinal plants; about 2500 medicinal herbs are listed in Indian medical texts, and at least 800 are used in tropical Africa. As a general rule, herbalists regularly use a repertoire of 150 to 200 plants. Herbalists uncommonly prescribe animal parts, metals, and minerals.

One of the most widely practiced and enduring herbal traditions has been that of Chinese herbal medicine.

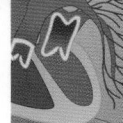

This form of herbal medicine has been traced back to about 2500 BC. In Chinese culture, herbs are considered basic to the treatment of all illness, in conjunction with aids such as acupuncture or acupressure. Generally speaking, among all alternative medical practices, Chinese herbal medicine has become a form familiar to many practitioners as a result of its incorporation into traditional Chinese medicine and acupuncture as practiced in many Western countries.

Herbs are prescribed in a number of different contexts. Standard formulas created by a trained herbalist or an individual with limited knowledge of herbal medicine are often used as an exclusive method of treatment by unlicensed practitioners. These typical prescriptions often may consist of 10 to 15 herbs.[17] When herbs are used to make herbal remedies, any or all parts of the plant can be used. These include flowers, leaves, seeds, roots, sap and resins, fruit, bark, or bulbs. These herbs can be administered in a number of tea forms (decoctions or infusions); they can be eaten in isolation or with food. Common terminology for how herbal remedies may be applied includes the following[14]:

Infusion—herbs that are steeped in hot water, similar to tea

Decoction—a technique that extracts more of the plant's ingredients by soaking and then boiling the plant in water

Tincture—an herb extract prepared by steeping the herb in a 25% solution of alcohol in water

Syrup—an herb extract prepared in honey or sugar in order to make its taste less unpleasant

Compress—a cloth pad soaked in a hot herbal extract and applied to a painful area

Poultice—similar to a compress, except that the entire herb is applied rather than an extract

Herbal Preparations and Adverse Effects

Despite the fact that the Western press often sensationalizes adverse reactions to certain specific herbals, systematic studies of poisoning due to herbal remedies are few. In a study conducted in China, 0.2% of all hospital admissions were the result of adverse reactions to Chinese herbal medicines.[17] Another Chinese study reviewed 33 hospitalizations resulting from toxicity related to herbal medicine.[17,18] The most common herb leading to toxic reactions was aconitine (accounting for 61%). In nine patients, adverse effects were life threatening; one fatality was reported. These numbers are hardly daunting when compared with typical adverse events histories from many over-the-counter drugs. Even in the United States, the reporting of the adverse reactions to ephedra—notwithstanding its dangers—greatly exaggerated its risks when properly used. For example, the investigational review of ephedra with respect to clinical efficacy and side effects done by the RAND organization and prepared by the Southern California Evidence-based Practice Center concluded that scientific studies are necessary to assess the possible

association between consumption of ephedra-containing dietary supplements and serious adverse events. Given the rarity of such events, they suggested that a properly designed case-control study would be necessary before drawing any additional conclusions.[19] Recently, Federal courts in Utah have agreed that the risk analysis relied on by the FDA to remove ephedra from the market needs to be reevaluated. Whether or not this will result in ephedra being returned to the supplement market remains to be seen, but it does suggest that data documenting its risk may not be as conclusive as previously believed.

Another issue that complicates the monitoring for adverse effects relates to the ability to standardize herbal products for both potency and quality. Although substantial strides have been made with the promulgation of GMPs for herbal products by the FDA, there are still challenges associated with ensuring potency and quality from product to product and brand to brand.

DOSE

Unlike the pharmaceutical industry, in which the quantity of active agent is consistent from pill to pill, quantities of active drug in a plant can be highly variable. Also, the content of active constituent is influenced by the particular species of plant, the growing conditions, the part of the plant, and its form when used (wet versus dry). Knowledgeable experts in the field of pharmacognosy have argued that this specific variability in diversity is actually desirable. Nonetheless, it can be problematic, particularly with respect to certain classes of substances such as those that might otherwise affect blood pressure, cardiac rhythm, level of consciousness, and so forth. Standards should be applied when possible, but these will likely never be uniformly achieved.

ROUTE OF EXPOSURE

Many herbs are applied topically, particularly those used to treat skin and musculoskeletal conditions. Although topical herbs occasionally produce systemic toxicity, their adverse effects are usually confined to development of contact dermatitis or phytodermatitis.[20] There are several herbals that have been traditionally smoked as substitutes for tobacco, but these play very minor roles in the overall medicinal application. Most botanicals are taken orally in the forms of extracts, tinctures, teas, and so forth. Inhalation is generally restricted to very traditional or illicit uses that usually do not find their way into medical practice. However, when dealing with a culturally diverse population, one must always be knowledgeable of the potential for toxic or hallucinatory effects of these. Examples include yohimbine, lobelia, cannabis, and others.[20]

DURATION OF USE

Many herbs with little to no toxicity after short-term use can produce adverse effects if they are ingested for a considerable time. For example, chronic use of pyrrolizidine alkaloids produces hepatic veno-occlusive disease, whereas short-term ingestion has no apparent hazards. Chronicity is also an important factor in the development of malignancies after use of carcinogenic

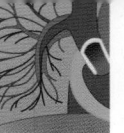

teas such as sassafras and comfrey.[21,22] As with any drug, botanicals must be used properly to maximize safety and efficacy. In an unsupervised environment with no professional oversight, botanicals with otherwise fairly safe therapeutic margins could become toxic over a period of time. The traditional benefits of comfrey, which contains pyrrolizidine alkaloids, include the management of inflammation, diarrhea, and gout. Generally, it should not be used for more than a few days. This is a good example of the potential for toxicity when individuals with poor professional advice seek to apply a botanical over a longer period of time.

PREEXISTING DISEASE

As the study by Eisenberg and colleagues illustrates,[2] herbal remedies are often sought as alternative treatments for illness or disease. Therefore, those using them may have preexisting disease that modulates the effect of that agent. For example, there are any number of botanicals that reportedly have or theoretically can affect the kinetics of warfarin. This is a good example of the necessity for professional supervision when a botanical is consumed with an anticoagulant therapeutic agent. However, that is not to say that botanicals might not be otherwise applied in a setting that involves anticoagulation. Pharmacists and physicians skilled in the chemistry of botanicals are necessary to help with the sorting-out process. Increasingly, it is becoming evident that there may be value in the application of functional foods, nutraceuticals, and botanicals in the context of prescription drug use. As a matter of fact, there are cases in which the simple application of a *nutraceutical* (defined as a naturally occurring dietary, microbiologic, mineral, or botanical substance exhibiting an inherently wide margin of safety when administered in doses or quantities that possess either functional or therapeutic value) may actually allow the more liberal use of a drug. Combining coenzyme Q with statin drugs appears to be advantageous. The knowledgeable application of probiotics will likely greatly reduce some of the side effects on the lower gastrointestinal (GI) tract from any number of antibiotics. There are numerous other examples for which the application of botanicals or nutraceuticals is not only desirable but perhaps will eventually become a standard of care as companions to certain drugs.

IMPROPER IDENTIFICATION

In circumstances in which crude herbs or other botanicals are harvested or used by individuals, there is a possibility of misidentification. Although trained herbalists can confidently prescribe herbs, an untrained or poorly trained herbalist sometimes misidentifies an herb and prescribes it, with disastrous consequences. For example, comfrey is similar to foxglove in appearance. Ingestion of foxglove, from which digitalis is derived, could lead to severe cardiac disturbances. The same risk for misidentification can occur when names are confused. Cohosh, a common herb used as a sedative and anti-inflammatory agent, generally refers to *Cimicifuga racemosa* (black cohosh) or *Caulophyllum thalictroides* (blue

cohosh). However, in other regions, cohosh refers to the toxic baneberry.[21]

HERB PREPARATION

How an herb is prepared has the most important influence on both the pharmacologic and toxicologic actions of the herb. Again, it is highly unlikely that an untrained herbalist might prescribe the wrong part of a plant when a standardized preparation that uses the appropriate part is available. The bark of the elder has considerable therapeutic value, but its stem is extremely toxic, containing cyanogenic alkaloids.[21] Equally important, an herb may be administered according to its dry weight rather than wet weight. Because the dried product almost always has a higher concentration of active agent than the fresh form, inadvertent overdose can occur. As the application of botanicals comes under the supervision of trained professionals, it becomes less likely that these types of errors will be made. In addition, with standardization and commercialization of products, individual preparation of remedies from crude botanicals will occur less and less. However, it will certainly still be possible for crude herbs or other botanicals to be provided directly to consumers or through an unlicensed practitioner.

CONTAMINATION

Herbs can become contaminated by toxins or toxicants through a number of means. The herbs sold by herbalists, as well as those that are picked in the wild, can be contaminated by agents including metals if they are grown in regions with contaminated soil, particularly if the plant is capable of incorporating the toxin. Teas prepared from herbs have been reported to contain lead, cadmium, mercury, copper, zinc, fluoride, and arsenic.[22]

Another means by which contamination can occur is by using plant products from improper sources. For example, commercial plant seeds may be used to prepare an herbal remedy. However, these seeds often contain pesticides or fungicides designed to lengthen their shelf life. If these seeds are ingested, serious toxicity can result. Finally, because herbs are often processed into tablets, capsules, and other pharmaceutical forms (commonly referred to as *Chinese proprietary medicine*), accidental or intentional adulteration by pharmaceutical agents can occur. Table 68-1 summarizes the clinical toxicity of popular herbs.

Herbal Teas

The preparation of teas is the most common use of herbal medicines. The illnesses associated with the use of herb teas can be placed into system categories of GI (including hepatic), hematologic, autonomic, neurologic, cardiac, allergic, and carcinogenic.

GASTROINTESTINAL

GI upset is the most common adverse effect associated with the use of herb teas. Although this is generally mild, severe vomiting and diarrhea can be produced by ingestion of poke root (*Phytolacca americana*), buckthorn (*Hippophae rhamnoides*), and senna (*Cassia augustifolia*).

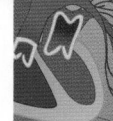

TABLE 68-1 Clinical Toxicity of Selected Herbs

COMMON NAME	BOTANIC NAME	THERAPEUTIC USES	POTENTIAL TOXICITY
Aconite (monkshood, wolfsbane)	*Aconitum* spp	Sedative, analgesic, antihypertensive	Cardiac arrhythmias
Aloe	*Aloe* spp	Burns, skin diseases	Nephritis, GI upset
Betel nut	*Areca catechu*	Mood elevation	Bronchoconstriction, oral cancers
Bloodroot	*Sanguinaria canadensis*	Emetic, cathartic, eczema	GI upset, vertigo, visual disturbances
Chaparral (greasewood)	*Larrea tridentata*	Aging, free radical scavenging	Hepatitis
Compound Q	*Trichosanthes kirilowi*	Antihelminthic, cathartic	Diarrhea, hypoglycemia, CNS toxicity
Dandelion	*Taraxacum officinale*	Diuretic, heartburn remedy	Anaphylaxis
Figwort (xuan shen)	*Scrophularia* spp	Anti-inflammatory, antibacterial	Cardiac stimulation
Ginseng	*Panax quinquefolium*	Antihypertensive, aphrodisiac, stimulant, mood elevation, digestive aid	Ginseng abuse syndrome
Goldenseal	*Hydrastis canadensis*	Digestive aid, mucolytic, anti-infective	Uterine, cardiac stimulation; GI upset, leukopenia
Hellebore	*Veratrum* spp	Antihypertensive	Vomiting, bradycardia, hypotension
Hyssop	*Hyssopus officinalis*	Asthma, mucolytic	Seizures
Juniper	*Juniperus communis*	Hallucinogen	GI upset, seizures, renal injury, hypotension, bradycardia
Kava kava	*Piper methysticum*	Sedative	Inebriation
Kombucha		Stimulant	Metabolic acidosis, hepatotoxicity, death
Licorice	*Glycyrrhiza* spp	Indigestion	Mineralocorticoid effects
Lily-of-the-valley	*Convallaria* spp	Cardiotonic	GI (nausea, vomiting), cardiac arrhythmias
Linn	*Salix caprea*	Purgative	Hemolysis with glucose-6-phosphate dehydrogenase deficiency
Lobelia (Indian tobacco)	*Lobelia* spp	Stimulant	Nicotine intoxication
Ma Huang	*Ephedra sinica*	Stimulant	Sympathetic crisis, especially with monoamine oxidase inhibitors
Mandrake	*Mandragora officinarum*	Hallucinogen	Anticholinergic syndrome
Mormon tea	*Ephedra nevadensis*	Stimulant, asthma, antipyretic	Hypertension, sympathomimetic
Nutmeg	*Myristica fragrans*	Hallucinogen, abortifacient	Hallucinations, GI upset
Oleander	*Nerium oleander*	Cardiac stimulant	Cardiac arrhythmias
Passion flower	*Passiflora caerulea*	Hallucinogen	Hallucinations, seizures, hypotension
Periwinkle	*Vinca* spp	Anti-inflammatory, diabetes	Alopecia, seizures, hepatotoxicity
Pokeweed	*Phytolacca* spp	Arthritis, chronic pain	GI upset, seizures, death
Sabah	*Sauropus androgynus*	Weight loss, vision	Pulmonary injury
Sage	*Salvia* spp	CNS stimulant	Seizures
Snakeroot	*Rauwolfia serpentina*	Sedative, antihypertensive	Bradycardia, coma
Squill	*Urginea maritima*	Arthritis, cardiac stimulant	Seizures, arrhythmias, death
Thorn apple	*Datura stramonium*	Hallucinations	Anticholinergic
Tonka bean	*Dipteryx odoratum*	Anticoagulant	Bleeding diathesis
Valerian root	*Valeriana* spp	Sedative	Sedation, obtundation
Wild (squirting) cucumber	*Ecbalium elaterium*	Constipation, anti-inflammatory, rheumatic disease	Airway obstruction
Wormwood (mugwort)	*Artemisia* spp	Stimulant, hallucinogen	Hallucinations, seizures, uterine stimulation
Yohimbine	*Coryanthe yohimbe*	Aphrodisiac, stimulant	Hypertension, sympathetic crisis

CNS, central nervous system; GI, gastrointestinal.

The term *herbal hepatitis* has been coined to describe the relatively frequent occurrence of herb-associated liver injury.[23] For example, fatal hepatitis has been associated with ingestion of wild germander (*Teucrium chamaedrys*).[24] Use of "chaparral" teas was associated with development of hepatitis (leading to the need for liver transplantation in one patient). This tea, which is derived from the ground leaves of the creosote bush (*Larrea tridentata*), has been promoted as an antioxidant, a blood purifier, and an inhibitor of aging.[25,26] Another reported outbreak of hepatitis was associated with the use of Chinese herbs[27]; in this case, the responsible toxin was not identified. As training and public awareness have increased, fewer of these problems have occurred. The herbs mentioned above are not used nearly as much as they were 20 years ago. Many pharmaceutical companies have taken the lead in producing highly standardized forms of botanicals. This has helped a great deal with respect to purity, labeling, and minimizing side effects.

HEMATOLOGIC

Herbs may contain alkaloids that are toxic to red blood cells. Among these are salicylate-containing agents such as willow bark; these can lead to hemolysis if ingested by

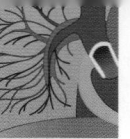
an individual with glucose-6-phosphate dehydrogenase deficiency. Other herbs contain Coumadin-like agents, including Tonka beans (*Coumarouna oppositifolia*), melilot (*Melilotus officinalis*), and woodruff (*Galium odoratum*); excess consumption can produce a coagulopathy.[22] This is no different from what can occur when certain drugs are taken injudiciously. However, oftentimes there is no package insert to the botanical regardless of its quality. This emphasizes the role of trained professionals in the application of these substances.

AUTONOMIC

Herbs that affect the autonomic nervous system include those containing the anticholinergic drugs atropine, scopolamine, and hyoscyamine.[22] These include mandrake (*Mandragora officinarum*), thorn apple (*Datura* spp), lobelia (*Lobelia inflata*), burdock root (*Arctium lappa*), and jimson root (*Datura stramonium*).[28] Other agents acting on the autonomic nervous system include sympathomimetics, such as Mormon tea (*Ephedra nevadensis*), which contains ephedrine; snakeroot tea (*Rauwolfia serpentina*), which contains reserpine; and yohimbe bark (*Corynanthe yohimbe*), which contains yohimbine, a central nervous system α_2-adrenergic antagonist.

NEUROLOGIC

A large number of herbal teas contain psychoactive substances that are the basis of their use (e.g., those containing caffeine). Although many, such as kava kava or chamomile, possess valuable and desirable therapeutic effects, excess dosing can produce toxicity. Teas associated with central nervous system toxicity include kava kava (*Piper methysticum*), jimson root (*Datura* spp), and nutmeg (*Myristica fragrans*).[22,29]

CARDIAC

Herbal teas associated with cardiotoxicity include those prepared from squill (*Urginea maritima*), lily-of-the-valley (*Convallaria majalis*), and oleander (*Thevetia* and *Nerium* spp). Some cardiac glycosides (e.g., those in oleander) produce toxic manifestations that resemble digitalis poisoning and that, like digitalis, respond to the administration of digoxin antibody fragments (Digibind).[30]

ALLERGIC

Chamomile (from *Chamomilla* spp) is a popular sedative. However, it is closely related to the ragweed and chrysanthemum families. Exposure to this tea can therefore produce a variety of reactions, although they are uncommon.

CARCINOGENIC

Sassafras is a popular tea that was once prescribed for a number of therapeutic effects. However, its active principal, safrole, is a recognized hepatic carcinogen. As a result, safrole has been banned from use by the FDA.[31] At this point, it is exceptional to find sassafras sold as an herb.

PYRROLIZIDINE TOXICITY

Many herbal teas contain pyrrolizidine alkaloids. These are a group of about 200 distinct substances found widely among plants.[32] The teas, such as comfrey, are prescribed as sedatives and as treatment for amenorrhea. However, since the first description of *Senecio* species disease (hepatic veno-occlusive syndrome) in 1920, small outbreaks of pyrrolizidine-associated hepatic disease have occasionally occurred. These alkaloids are highly hepatotoxic and, in some cases, carcinogenic.[33]

The hallmark of pyrrolizidine intoxication is the development of veno-occlusive disease, a hepatic disorder that is similar but not identical to the Budd-Chiari syndrome. The mechanism of pyrrolizidine toxicity appears to be formation of toxic pyrroles by cytochrome P-450 enzymes; these pyrroles alkylate nucleophilic groups on cell macromolecules.[34] Pyrrolizidine alkaloids can be transmitted across the placenta; in one case in which a woman ingested an herbal tea during her pregnancy, her newborn developed fatal hepatic veno-occlusive disease.[35] Because of their well-characterized toxicity, which can occur after ingestion of as little as 85 mg of pyrrolizidine alkaloid, pyrrolizidine-containing teas are not nearly as widely available in herbal and health food stores as they were 20 years ago.[33] The herbs most commonly associated with hepatic veno-occlusive disease are *Heliotropium*, *Crotalaria*, *Senecio*, and *Symphytum* species. Other herbs containing pyrrolizidine are listed in Table 68-2. Plant roots can contain 10 times more alkaloid than the leaf. Other toxicities associated with pyrrolizidine alkaloids include disturbances of GI, pancreatic, and renal function. Interestingly, inadvertent exposure to pyrrolizidine agents can also occur through their contamination of dietary staples. For example, as a result of contaminated grain, epidemics of hepatic veno-occlusive disease occurred in both Afghanistan and India in 1976, affecting more than 2000 persons and causing more than 30 deaths.[32,34] Epidemiologically, consumption of pyrrolizidine-containing plants is widespread in Africa, South and Central America, and Jamaica.[34] Jamaican bush tea, a popular drink, is largely prepared with *Crotalaria* species, making veno-occlusive disease endemic on this island.[34] Pyrrolizidine poisoning has also been blamed for major cases of livestock loss in the Pacific Northwest.[32,34]

The clinical presentation of hepatic veno-occlusive disease begins with severe abdominal pain and vomiting. Physical examination reveals hepatomegaly, abdominal distention, and ascites. In children, the clinical picture can mimic Reye's syndrome.[34] On biopsy, characteristic histopathology consists of perivenular congestion,

TABLE 68-2 Pyrrolizidine-Containing Teas	
COMMON NAME	**BOTANIC NAME**
Coltsfoot	*Tussilago farfara*
Comfrey	*Symphytum officinale*
Gordolobo	*Senecio longilobus*
Groundsel	*Senecio vulgaris*
Mate	*Ilex paraguayensis*
Tansy ragwort	*Senecio jacobea*
T'u-san-chi	*Gynura segetum*

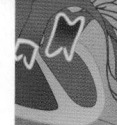

sinusoidal dilation, and occlusion of terminal venules by connective tissue. This is also the pattern seen in the Budd-Chiari syndrome, but course and outcome in Budd-Chiari syndrome are much more severe and life threatening without treatment.

The diagnosis of pyrrolizidine hepatotoxicity is made on the basis of history, clinical evidence of veno-occlusive disease, and pathognomonic histopathology. This disorder is restricted to those areas in which the traditional use of pyrrolizidine teas is commonplace. Treatment is supportive.

Clinical Toxicity of Specific Herbs

ARISTOLOCHIA SPECIES BOTANICALS

Chinese-herb nephropathy (CHN) was observed among women after the intake of weight-reducing pills containing a Chinese herb labeled as *Stephania tetrandra*.[36] Phytochemical analyses of the herb revealed the presence of aristolochic acids instead of tetrandrine.[37] *Aristolochia fangchi* (guang fangji) had been substituted for the *Stephania tetrandra*, leading to aristolochic acid exposure and nephropathy. Aristolochic acids are known for their nephrotoxic effects in rodents as well as for their carcinogenic and mutagenic properties.[38] Exposure in humans that resulted in nephropathy has been reported when contamination of herbal products with the *Aristolochia* species botanicals has occurred. The FDA took action in 2001 to ban all products containing any *Aristolochia* species so as to avoid exposure to aristolochic acids. Subsequent to the identification of nephrotoxic effects leading to kidney failure in humans, a study conducted in Belgium reported 18 cases of urothelial carcinoma among 39 patients with end-stage renal failure associated with *Aristolochia* toxins.[39]

GINSENG

Ginseng is a Chinese word meaning "the essence of man."[40] This herb has been used for centuries to treat a broad range of illnesses.[21] From the botanic genus *Panax*, ginseng is promoted as a respiratory, digestive, and central nervous system stimulant; a cure for fatigue; a treatment for ulcers; and a cholesterol-lowering agent. Ginseng's most active principals are alkaloids known as *saponins* (also referred to as *panaxosides* or *ginsenosides*). Scientific investigations have shown that these agents can release histamine; block calcium mobilization in smooth muscle, producing hypotension; stimulate α_2-adrenergic receptors; stimulate erythropoiesis; increase adrenocorticotropic hormone, antidiuretic hormone, and cortisol secretion; raise sperm count; increase glucose utilization; increase levels of circulating immunoglobulins; and inhibit the cells of tumor cells cultivated in vitro.[40] Therapeutically, ginseng has been prescribed for the treatment of shock, hypertension, hyperlipidemia, diabetes mellitus, depression, cough, headaches, and fever.

Excessive use of ginseng (more than 3 g daily) is associated with a ginseng abuse syndrome consisting of diarrhea, anxiety, insomnia, nonspecific dermatitis, depression, amenorrhea, and hypertension.[21] However,

as we have learned more and more about this beneficial botanical, it is rarely used in these doses. The wide therapeutic margin makes toxicity unlikely. Treatment of this transient, self-limited condition is supportive.

ACONITE

Aconites are among the most popular yet toxic herbs. At one time, execution of criminals was performed by the administration of aconite decoctions. The *Aconitum* genus includes many species, the most common being *Aconitum napellus*, popularly referred to as monkshood, wolfsbane, or friar's cap. Aconite is found in Chinese decoctions or soups, including Fu Zi, Wu Tao, Cao Wu, Chuan Wu, Ts'ao Wu, Futxu, Xue Shang Yi Zhi Gao, Shi-I, Fu Zi, and Sen Fu. Herbalists generally prescribe aconite for treatment of musculoskeletal complaints, angina, and congestive heart failure and as a sedative. The active principals of aconite have been shown to have pharmacologic properties that include stimulation of adrenocorticotropic hormone secretion.[41]

With the GI tract, nervous system, and heart as target organs, aconites, when taken in overdose, produce a distinctive clinical picture. GI effects occur initially, consisting of nausea, vomiting, and hypersalivation. These are followed by neurologic effects, including paresthesias, blurred vision, skeletal muscle weakness or frank paralysis,[42] coma, and seizures. Cardiac disturbances, which can be fatal,[43,44] include bradycardia, hypotension, ectopy, cardiac conduction disturbances (prolonged QRS or QT interval), and intractable ventricular tachyarrhythmias.

Treatment of aconite poisoning consists of stabilization of the airway, aggressive treatment of cardiac disturbances, and early GI decontamination. Subsequent treatment is supportive because there are no known antidotes and no identified mechanism for enhanced elimination of the toxin.

NUTMEG

The mood-elevating, aphrodisiac, narcotic, and hallucinogenic effects of nutmeg have been exploited for centuries. This spice remains popular, particularly as a hallucinogen. Prepared from the fruit of the evergreen tree *Myristica fragrans*, nutmeg is an easily obtained spice. The nutmeg seed contains a number of alkaloids, including myristicin, eugenol, isoeugenol, methyleugenol, methylisoeugenol, safrole, geraniol, borneal, and elemicin. Among these, myristicin is the most psychoactive compound. Myristicin is metabolized to the hallucinogen 3-methoxy-4,5-methylenedioxyamphetamine (MMDA), a substance closely related to methylenedioxymethamphetamine (MDMA, "Ecstasy"). Another alkaloid in nutmeg, elemicin, is metabolized to a hallucinogen.

Ingestion of 5 to 30 g of nutmeg produces symptoms promptly, with GI upset predominating. Within 3 hours, hallucinogenic effects appear, consisting of vivid visual hallucinations. The duration of this action can be as long as 2 to 3 days. Chronic abuse of this potent hallucinogen is limited by the GI disturbances it produces. Treatment of acute nutmeg intoxication consists of reducing environmental stimuli and attempting to calm the patient. Benzodiazepines may be valuable as adjunctive therapy.

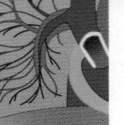

KOMBUCHA MUSHROOM

Kombucha is a plant that has recently gained popularity as a "fountain of youth." It has been promoted as a treatment for cancer, hypertension, fatigue, declining T-cell counts, arthritis, wrinkles, constipation, and gray hair. Prescribed and marketed by naturopathic healers in the United States, kombucha is often cultivated at home and passed on to friends.[45] Not a true mushroom, the plant is a yeast-bacterial aggregate surrounded by a membrane. Use of this mushroom has been blamed for sporadic cases of hepatotoxicity and severe metabolic acidosis, which was fatal in one case.[45,46] The toxic principals have not been identified; toxicity may result from kombucha contamination by other yeasts or bacteria.

SABAH

Marketed in the United States under the name "Defat," this vegetable has been associated with an epidemic of pulmonary disease in Taiwan. One report described 44 individuals, primarily women, who developed respiratory distress, insomnia, and obstructive pulmonary disease after consumption of the Sabah vegetable (*Sauropus androgynus*).[47] This vegetable, which is a regular part of the diet in many parts of the world, was being ingested in large daily quantities as a means of improving vision, reducing lipids, and treating constipation and hemorrhoids, or as a weight loss measure. An epidemiologic investigation was undertaken after repeated reports to the Taiwan Poison Center of illness related to ingestion of this vegetable. Victims were primarily females who had been taking the vegetable whole or in juice form. The average duration of consumption before the appearance of disease was 35 days. Initial symptoms consisted of insomnia and excitation, followed by difficulty in breathing, cough, and chest tightness. In many cases, illness developed after consumption of the vegetable had ceased. In a patient who underwent a lung biopsy, histopathology suggested bronchiolitis obliterans with organizing pneumonia. Four fatalities occurred. By December 1, 1995, 169 cases of Sabah-associated illness had been reported. An exact cause has yet to be determined.[48]

Chinese Patent (Proprietary) Medicines

In addition to herbs being prescribed and sold in their unadulterated form, herbs are often combined to form Chinese patent medicines. Chinese patent medicines, unlike Chinese herbal medicines, are mass-produced in a fashion similar to pharmaceutical manufacture.

The potential problems with these medicines are several. First, Chinese proprietary medicines are often sold in unlabeled or poorly labeled packages. Second, they typically contain a combination of products such that a distinctive clinical syndrome may not be present after intoxication. Jin Bu Huan tablets, prescribed for muscle spasm, pain, and insomnia, were associated with the poisoning of three children when they were discovered to contain an herb not usually a part of them.[49] In a later report, hepatitis was also associated with Jin Bu Huan.[12] Third, combining herbs from various sources poses a greater probability of product contamination. Fourth, because of sometimes relatively poor quality control in production, proprietary medicines can be entirely mislabeled, containing a product completely different from what is stated. Finally, these products can be adulterated with pharmaceutical agents. Several cases of intoxication have been attributed to these preparations.[50] For example, Gan Mao Tong Pian, a remedy prescribed for viral illness, produced aplastic anemia in a child as a result of its adulteration by phenylbutazone.[50] One Chinese proprietary product, *Chui-Fong-Tou-Gen-Wan*, has been found to contain agents including phenacetin, phenylbutazone, mercuric sulfide, lead, cadmium, and arsenic.[17,18,50,51] In one study, eight of nine Chinese patent medicines tested were found to be contaminated with arsenic and mercury.[51] In a 5-year study of hospital admissions resulting from use of Chinese proprietary medicines, Chan and colleagues identified 71 patients, of whom 42 were found to have elevated serum concentrations of aspirin or acetaminophen.[52] Products containing acetaminophen included Superior Yinchiao, Chieh, Tu Pien, Yinchiao Chieh Tu Pien, Ganyanquing Pian, and Suxiaao Shangfeng.

TRADITIONAL ("FOLK") MEDICINE

A *folk remedy* can be defined as an unrefined product that is taken for medicinal purposes. Unlike herbal medicines, folk remedies are regularly derived from animals, plants, or minerals. The use of folk medicines has a strong component of religious ritual (e.g., shamanism). Folk treatments may consist of physical modalities (e.g., "coining" or "cupping"), widely practiced in Asian cultures, as well as religious practices.[53] The use of so-called ethnomedical therapies is most prevalent among minority groups, especially among families who have either recently emigrated or who have a family member who has inherited knowledge about folk remedies. In many cases, the basis of therapies is an unorthodox belief about disease processes (e.g., the humoral [hot–cold] theory).[54] However, folk medicines are also used to treat well-defined Western diseases. These diseases may be referred to by archaic names such as rheumatism (musculoskeletal inflammation), dropsy (congestive heart failure), or consumption (tuberculosis). Folk medicines are also sought by those under the care of physicians because of frustration with the inability of Western medicine to cure a disease or because of the understandable desire to use natural remedies rather than pharmaceutical agents. With increasing frequency, these traditional medicines can be purchased in the United States. For example, in Hispanic populations, local *botanicas* usually provide religious objects as well as folk remedies.[54]

A list of folk medicines associated with clinical toxicity is found in Table 68-3. For example, the remedy alcanfor contains 20% camphor, sufficient to produce toxic manifestations.[54] Several folk remedies used in the treatment of GI disturbances contain lead. In some cases,

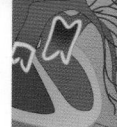

TABLE 68-3   Common Folk Medicines by Cultural Origin

NAME	CONTENTS	POTENTIAL TOXICITY
Hispanic		
Siete jarabes	Almond, castor oil, tolu, wild cherry licorice, cocillana, honey	GI upset, catharsis, electrolyte disturbances
Agua maravilla	Witch hazel, ethanol	Ethanol toxicity
Jarabe maguey	Maguey (*Agave* spp)	GI upset
Alcanfor	Camphor	Camphor toxicity
Azarcon	Lead	Lead intoxication
Greta	Lead	Lead intoxication
Azogue	Elemental mercury	Mercury intoxication
Ipecacuanha	Ipecac	Vomiting, myopathy
Southeast Asian		
Paylooah	Lead	Lead intoxication
Indian and Ayurvedic		
Surma	Lead	Lead intoxication
Deshi Dawa	Lead	Lead intoxication

GI, gastrointestinal.

use of these agents can produce lead-induced abdominal pain (lead colic), resulting in further use and more severe lead poisoning.

Identifying the ingredients in folk remedies is often assisted by knowledge of the cultural origins of the disease being treated. For example, empacho, one of the most common illnesses among Hispanic cultures, is treated by various means, including massages with olive oil (or other type of oil or grease), laxatives, conventional stomach remedies (e.g., bismuth subsalicylate [Pepto-Bismol]), chamomile tea, and antacids, as well as the folk remedies *greta* and *azarcon* (both of which contain up to 90% lead).[55] Other lead-containing folk medicines are listed in Table 68-3.

Pachter and associates described other potential toxicities from traditional medicines.[54] For example, azogue, which contains elemental mercury, is generally used as a talisman. However, if it is dispersed about the room to ward off evil spirits, inhalation of toxic mercury vapors could occur.

Ayurvedic Medicine

Ayurveda is a traditional system of medicine practiced primarily in Asian countries (Tibet, Burma, Pakistan, Sri Lanka, India, Bangladesh). Practitioners of Ayurvedic medicine not only rely on herbal remedies but also sometimes prescribe animal products, metals, and minerals as well. Increasingly, Ayurvedic remedies are being used in Western areas, including Europe and North America. Also, in becoming a commercial industry, Ayurvedic medicine has begun to include large-scale distribution of these herbals.

Because Ayurvedic medicine includes therapy with metals and minerals, inadvertent metal intoxication is the most significant potential occurrence. Ayurvedic medicines are typically sold in an "ash" powder form, packaged in capsules, and produced by the repeated pyrolysis of the metal. Zinc, iron, lead, tin, mercury, and silver are among the metals that may be contained in an Ayurvedic "tonic." As such, both consumers and manufacturers of these products are at risk for metal intoxication. Lead intoxication has been reported with the use of these medicines.[56,57]

ALTERNATIVE MEDICINES

Practices that can be placed in this category include homeopathy, naturopathy (the science of applying natural substances that enable the body to heal itself and maintain natural homeostasis), nutritional supplementation for medicinal purposes, and novel therapies, such as hyperoxygenation and oligotherapy (the administration of trace elements to improve health).[3]

Homeopathy

Homeopathy is a popular alternative therapy that advocates the use of toxic substances in small amounts. It is extremely popular in Europe, Latin America, and Asia and has been used by an estimated 1% of the American population.[8] The concept was introduced by Samuel Hahnemann in the late 18th century. Treatments in homeopathic medicine are based on three principles: "like cures like," "efficacy improves with increasing dilution," and "treatments need to be individualized."[58] Under these rules, a toxin, when administered in small doses, can have therapeutic value. Such a theory is not a great departure from Western medicine because it is the basis of desensitization therapy for allergies. However, the theory that the smaller the dose of medicine, the more effective, has not been well documented in scientific study. Homeopathy also requires that therapy be individualized; therefore, in principle, homeopathic medications should not be shared with another person.

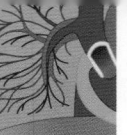

Homeopathic medicines are generally toxins derived from plants, animals, or minerals.[8] Common agents include strychnine, ipecac, arsenic, mercury, podophyllin, and sulfur.[8] Preparations of accepted therapeutic value are recorded in the *U.S. Homeopathic Pharmacopoeia*, published by the American Institute of Homeopathy.[58] Homeopathic products often are packages of capsules or tablets with the ingredients listed by their Latin names. Scientifically rigorous studies have suggested efficacy of some of these medicines.[5,7,8]

Homeopathic tinctures are generally made by adding 1 part of a toxin to 20 parts of alcohol. This tincture is diluted as needed to 1:1000, 1:10,000, and even further dilutions. A homeopathic product may therefore contain on its label a symbol of 1× (1:10 dilution), 2× (1:100 dilution), 3×, and so forth. Another dilution technique is the centidecimal ("c" or "cH"), in which 1 part of active substance is diluted in 99 parts of an alcohol mixture.[58] Therefore, a substance labeled 30C has had the active substance diluted 1:100 in a water/alcohol solution 30 times, yielding a final concentration of 1×10^{-60}.[8]

Because of the minute quantities of toxin, ingestion of homeopathic medications should rarely produce toxicity, even if as many as 100 tablets are ingested. Important exceptions to this rule would be if the product were homemade, thereby potentially having dilutions less than planned, or in the potential case of an allergic reaction, which could occur after exposure to small quantities of the active agent. Reports have described homeopathic products adulterated with active agents.[5]

Nutrition Supplements

In addition to using herbal and alternative medications, the public commonly takes substances that are promoted as nutrition supplements, designed to improve health or treat disease. Additionally, the concept of adding or supplementing with so-called "native molecules," now known as *natural medicines*, seems to be gaining validity. Ames postulates that individuals can be "tuned up" metabolically with the strategic use of nutraceuticals based on an understanding of their individual metabolic genetics.[59] By adding orthomolecular amounts of specific vitamins, amino acids, minerals, and other cofactors, the K_m of specific metabolic reactions can be normalized in individuals who might otherwise have metabolic defects as a result of genes or aging. The validation of this concept may have a significant impact regarding the value of using higher doses of specific nutraceuticals in restoring or maintaining optimal human health.[59]

In the past, the use of nutritional supplements for these purposes has been widespread and in some instances less responsible. For example, an examination of advertisements in 12 health and bodybuilding magazines disclosed 311 supplements, containing 235 unique ingredients. Most common among these were amino acids, followed by herbs, vitamins, minerals, and steroids.[60] The toxicity of vitamins is discussed in Chapter 69. The few specific nutritional supplements that have been reported to have clinical toxicity are discussed next. Based on the volume of use, there is remarkably little toxicity reported other than the specific cases outlined below.

γ-HYDROXYBUTYRATE

γ-Hydroxybutyrate (GHB) is a health food supplement that became popular in 1990 after its promotion as a bodybuilding and diet aid. Shortly after widespread use began, cases of a toxic syndrome related to its ingestion were reported. Dyer described a series of 16 cases of GHB toxicity reported to the San Francisco Regional Poison Center; manifestations included coma and seizures.[61] Other signs of toxicity were confusion, agitation, hallucinations, and bradycardia. These effects occurred after ingestions of as little as 1 to 4 tsp of GHB (sold as a white powder). Shortly after similar reports throughout the country, individual states banned the product.[61] GHB is now sold as a controlled substance as the drug Xyrem. It now has an FDA-approved indication for the management of narcolepsy. Other indications may follow. This is a good example of a natural molecule that does possess a much more narrow therapeutic margin and therefore should not be considered a nutraceutical.

L-TRYPTOPHAN

L-Tryptophan is an essential amino acid. As a precursor to the neurotransmitter serotonin, it has been touted as an effective treatment for ailments including insomnia, depression, and premenstrual syndrome. Its use, however, has been associated with at least two syndromes of intoxication.

An epidemic of multisystem disease occurred in the fall of 1989, when patients who had been ingesting L-tryptophan developed eosinophilia and severe myalgia. During the course of 6 to 9 months, an estimated 5000 to 10,000 developed this syndrome, and more than 36 fatalities occurred. Eighty-four percent of victims were female. Prominent symptoms were peripheral eosinophilia (with eosinophil counts $> 1000/mm^3$), severe diffuse myalgias, and dermatologic changes resembling scleroderma. Termed the *eosinophilia-myalgia syndrome* (EMS), this disease had other features that included pulmonary disturbances (dyspnea, cough, pulmonary infiltrates, and pulmonary hypertension, which occurred in about 60%), peripheral neuropathy, alopecia, edema, coronary artery spasm, and cardiac arrhythmias.[48,62] The illness bore a striking resemblance to the unexplained "toxic oil" epidemic that occurred in Spain in 1981.[48,63] When it was found that all cases of EMS could be traced to L-tryptophan synthesized by a single manufacturer, analysis revealed that owing to changes in the manufacturing method, the tryptophan was contaminated with an impurity, 1,1′-ethylidenebis [L-tryptophan].[48] There is still controversy about whether the true cause of EMS was discovered. Nonetheless, after the FDA's ban of tryptophan-containing products, the disease quickly and almost completely disappeared. This important mass poisoning has been extensively reviewed by others.[62,64-69]

Adverse effects have also occurred with the simultaneous use of tryptophan and antidepressants of the

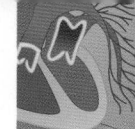

monoamine oxidase (MAO) inhibitor or serotonin reuptake inhibitor classes. In the case of MAO inhibitors, tryptophan was once recommended as adjunctive therapy for those who had a poor response to MAO therapy.[70] However, after this combination began being used more consistently, reports began to describe hypertensive crises, myoclonus, and delirium after their combined use.[71] This syndrome, now referred to as a *serotoninergic syndrome* (see Chapter 10A), appears to result from excess stimulation of central nervous system serotonin receptors and can include other features such as myoclonus, hyperreflexia, diaphoresis, priapism, and tremor. At its extreme, the serotoninergic syndrome can produce seizures, coma, and death. In addition to MAO inhibitors, the newer serotonin reuptake inhibitors (e.g., fluoxetine, paroxetine, and sertraline) have the potential to produce this syndrome after ingestion of tryptophan, although there has not been a sudden increase in reports of these cases. Tryptophan has been reintroduced to the market as an amino acid supplement following a great deal of diligence in improving its manufacturing. Thus far, there have been no new cases of EMS, nor a rise in the incidence of so-called serotoninergic syndrome since it has become more readily available.

CALCIUM SUPPLEMENTS

Use of calcium supplements has increased considerably during the past decade as the diminishing calcium intake of Americans is documented and the relationship between deficient calcium intake and osteoporosis, particularly in women, is recognized. Some calcium supplements that are derived from bone meal are reported to contain lead.

Hyperoxygenation Therapy

Hyperoxygen therapy is being increasingly promoted as a health aid. It has become particularly popular as an alternative treatment for AIDS. Acting in a fashion similar to white blood cells in their destruction of microbial agents, ingestion of oxygen-liberating agents is thought to augment host defense mechanisms. Hydrogen peroxide is the most common agent used for hyperoxygenation therapy. Hydrogen peroxide used for this purpose is generally sold in a 25% to 50% concentration, in contrast to the 3% to 5% concentration of household hydrogen peroxide. The user is directed to ingest several drops daily. Because the agent is refrigerated, the potential for inadvertent ingestion is increased.[72]

Toxicity from hyperoxygen therapy has been reported after ingestion of excess amounts. The two major consequences of this ingestion are corrosive injury of the GI tract and excess liberation of oxygen, resulting in the formation of gas emboli. One milliliter of a concentrated hydrogen peroxide solution can liberate about 115 mL of oxygen; ingestion of 2 ounces of 35% hydrogen peroxide could release 6.9 L of oxygen in the stomach.[72,73] Several researchers have described life-threatening or fatal gas emboli after ingestion of concentrated hydrogen peroxide.[72-74]

Treatment of concentrated hydrogen peroxide therapy includes supportive care, assessment of the esophagus and stomach for corrosive injury, and anticipation of air emboli. Diluting agents should not be administered because of their potential to enhance oxygen liberation.

Other Therapies

The promotion of tonics, extracts, and elixirs has a consistent ability to entice consumers. Their list is constantly changing. In rare circumstances, these alternative medicines prove to have therapeutic value. In most cases, they have no beneficial action but also no toxicity. These agents can occasionally be highly toxic, however. For example, laetrile was promoted in the early 1980s as an alternative treatment for cancer. Prepared from crushed apricot pits, this agent contained high concentrations of amygdalin, a cyanogenic alkaloid. Although it was not proved to have therapeutic value, laetrile did result in cases of cyanide intoxication after overdose.[75]

Other therapies, including ingestion of shark cartilage, boiled urchin, and algae, continue to be promoted without clear, scientifically proven benefit.

REFERENCES

1. Verhoef M, Sutherland L, Brkich L: Use of alternative medicine by patients attending a gastroenterology clinic. Can Med Assoc J 1990;142:121.
2. Eisenberg D, Kessler R, Foster C, et al: Unconventional medicine in the United States: prevalence, cost, and patterns of use. N Engl J Med 1993;328:246.
3. Spigelblatt L, Laine-Ammara G, Pless I, et al: The use of alternative medicine by children. Pediatrics 1994;94:811.
4. Pearl W, Leo P, Tsang WO: Use of Chinese therapies among Chinese patients seeking emergency care. Ann Emerg Med 1995;26:735.
5. Sampson W, London W: Analysis of homeopathic treatment of childhood diarrhea. Pediatrics 1995;96:961.
6. Weizman Z, Alkrinawi S, Goldfarb D, et al: Efficacy of herbal tea preparation in infantile colic. J Pediatr 1993;122:650.
7. Kleijnen J, Knipschild P, ter Riet G: Clinical trials of homeopathy. BMJ 1991;302:316.
8. Jacobs J, Jimenez L, Gloyd S, et al: Treatment of acute childhood diarrhea with homeopathic medicine. A randomized clinical trial in Nicaragua. Pediatrics 1994;93:719.
9. Delbanco T: Bitter herbs: mainstream, magic and menace. Ann Intern Med 1994;121:803.
10. Reports C: Herbal roulette. Consumer Reports 1995;(Nov):698–705.
11. Pereira C, Nishioka S: Poisoning by the use of Datura leaves in a homemade toothpaste. Clin Toxicol 1994;32:329.
12. Woolf G, Petrovic L, Rojter S, et al: Acute hepatitis associated with the Chinese herbal product Jin Bu Huan. Ann Intern Med 1994;121:729.
13. Bakhiet A, Adam S: Therapeutic utility, constituents and toxicity of some medicinal plants: A review. Vet Hum Toxicol 1995;37:255.
14. Ody P: The Complete Medicinal Herbal. London, Dorling Kindersley, 1993.
15. Vuksan V, Sievenpiper J, Koo V, et al: American ginseng (Panax quinquefolium L) reduces postprandial glycemia in nondiabetic subjects and subjects with type 2 diabetes mellitus. Arch Intern Med 2000;160:1009.
16. Tauchert M: Efficacy and safety of crataegus extract WS 1442 in comparison with placebo in patients with chronic stable New York Heart Association class-III heart failure. Am Heart J 2002;143:910.
17. Chan T, Chan J, Tomlinson B, et al: Poisoning by Chinese herbal medicines in Hong Kong: a hospital-based study. Vet Hum Toxicol 1994;36:546.
18. Chan T, Critchley J: The spectrum of poisonings in Hong Kong: An overview. Vet Hum Toxicol 1994;36:135.

19. Southern California Evidence-Based Practice Center R: Evidence Report/Technology Assessment Number 76 Task Order Number Nine. Rockville, Md: Agency for Healthcare Research and Quality, 2003.

20. Lee T, Lam T: Allergic contact dermatitis to Yunnan Paiyao. Contact Dermatitis 1987;17:59.

21. Saxe T: Toxicity of medicinal herbal preparations. Am Fam Physician 1987;35:135.

22. Ridker P: Toxic effects of herbal teas. Arch Environmental Health 1987;42:133.

23. Katz M, Saibil F: Herbal hepatitis: Subacute hepatic necrosis secondary to chaparral leaf. J Clin Gastroenterol 1990;12:203.

24. Mostefa-Kara N, Pauwels A, Pines E, et al: Fatal hepatitis after herbal tea. Lancet 1992;340:674.

25. Gordon D, Rosenthal G, Hart J, et al: Chaparral ingestion—the broadening spectrum of liver injury caused by herbal medications. JAMA 1995;273:489.

26. Centers for Disease Control and Prevention (CDC): Chaparral-induced toxic hepatitis—California and Texas. MMWR Morb Mortal Wkly Rep 1992;41:812.

27. Perharic L, Shaw D, Leon C, et al: Possible liver damage with the use of Chinese herbal medicine for skin disease. Vet Hum Toxicol 1995;563:563.

28. Chan TY: Anticholinergic poisoning due to Chinese herbal medicines. Vet Hum Toxicol 1995;37:156.

29. Coremans P, Lambrecht G, Schepens P, et al: Anticholinergic intoxication with commercially available thorn apple tea. Clin Toxicol 1994;32:589.

30. Eddleston M, Rajapakse S, Rajakanthan: Anti-digoxin Fab fragments in cardiotoxicity induced by ingestion of yellow oleander: a randomised controlled trial. Lancet 2000;355:967.

31. Segelman A, Segelman F, Karliner J, et al: Sassafras and herb tea—potential health hazards. JAMA 1976;236:477.

32. Ridker P, Ohkuma S, McDermott W, et al: Hepatic venocclusive disease associated with the consumption of pyrrolizidine-containing dietary supplements. Gastroenterology 1985;88:1050.

33. Huxtable R, Luthhyy J, Zweifel U: Toxicity of comfrey-pepsin preparations. N Engl J Med 1986;315:1095.

34. Huxtable R: Herbal teas and toxins: novel aspects of pyrrolizidine poisoning in the United States. Perspect Biol Med 1980;24:1.

35. Roulet M, Laurini R, Rivier L, et al: Hepatic veno-occlusive disease in newborn infant of a woman drinking herbal tea. J Pediatr 1988;112:433.

36. Vanherweghem J, Depierreux M, Tielemans C, et al: Rapidly progressive interstitial renal fibrosis in young women. Association with slimming regimen including Chinese herbs. Lancet 1993;174:174.

37. Vanhaelen M, Vanhaelen-Fastre R, But P, et al: Identification of aristolochic acid in Chinese herbs. Lancet 1994;343:174.

38. Schmeiser H, Pool B, Wiessler M: Identification and mutagenicity of metabolites of aristolochic acid formed by rat liver. Carcinogenesis (Lond) 1986;7:59.

39. Nortier JL, Martinez MC, Schmeiser HH, et al: Urothelial carcinoma associated with the use of a Chinese herb (Aristolochia fangchi). N Engl J Med 2000;342:1686.

40. Huang K: The Pharmacology of Chinese Herbs. Boca Raton, FL, CRC Press, 1993, p 388.

41. Bisset N: Arrow poisons in China. Part II. Aconiturn—botany, chemistry, and pharmacology. J Ethnopharmacol 1981;4:247.

42. Chan T, Tomlinson B, Critchley J, et al: Herb-induced aconitine poisoning presenting as tetraplegia. Vet Hum Toxicol 1994;36:133.

43. Fatovich D: Aconite: a lethal Chinese herb. Ann Intern Med 1992;21:309.

44. Tai Y-T, But P-H, Young K, et al: Cardiotoxicity after accidental herb-induced aconite poisoning. Lancet 1992;340:1254.

45. Perron A, Patterson J, Yanofsky N: Kombucha "mushroom" hepatotoxicity. Ann Emerg Med 1995;26:660.

46. Centers for Disease Control and Prevention (CDC): Unexplained severe illness possibly associated with consumption of kombucha tea—Iowa. MMWR Morb Mortal Wkly Rep 1995;44:892.

47. Lin T-J, Lu C-C, Chen K-W, et al: Outbreak of obstructive ventilatory impairment associated with consumption of sauopus androgynus vegetable. Clin Toxicol 1996;34:1.

48. Spyker D, Love L, Brooks S: An outbreak of pulmonary poisoning. Clin Toxicol 1996;34:15.

49. Centers for Disease Control and Prevention (CDC): Jin Bu Huan toxicity in children—Colorado. MMWR Morb Mortal Wkly Rep 1993;42:633.

50. Nelson L, Shih R, Hoffman R: Aplastic anemia induced by an adulterated herbal medication. Clin Toxicol 1995;33:467.

51. Espinoza E, Mann M-J, Bleasdell B: Arsenic and mercury in traditional Chinese herbal balls. N Engl J Med 1995;333:803.

52. Chan T, Lee K, Chan A, et al: Poisoning due to Chinese proprietary medicines. Hum Exp Toxicol 1995;14:434.

53. Pachter L: Culture and clinical care—folk illness beliefs and behaviors and their implications for health care delivery. JAMA 1994;271:690.

54. Pachter L, Cloutier M, Bernstein B: Ethnomedical (folk) remedies for childhood asthma in a maintained Puerto Rican community. Arch Pediatr Adolesc Med 1995;149:982.

55. Risser A, Mazur L: Use of folk remedies in a Hispanic population. Arch Pediatr Adolesc Med 1995;149:978.

56. McElvaine M, Harder E, Johnson L, et al: Lead poisoning from the use of Indian folk medicines. JAMA 1990;264:2212.

57. Kulshrestha M: Lead poisoning diagnosed by abdominal x-rays. Clin Toxicol 1996;34:107.

58. Spoerke D: Toxicity of homeopathic products. Vet Hum Toxicol 1989;31:259.

59. Ames B: A role for supplements in optimizing health: the metabolic tune-up. Arch Biochem Biophys 2004;423:227.

60. Philen R, Ortiz D, Auerbach S, et al: Survey of advertising for nutritional supplements in health and body building magazines. JAMA 1992;268:1008.

61. Dyer J: Gamma-hydroxybutyrate—a health-food product producing coma and seizurelike activity. Am J Emerg Med 1991;9:321.

62. Swygert L, Maes E, Sewell L, et al: Eosinophilia-myalgia syndrome—results of national surveillance. JAMA 1990;264:1698.

63. Hertzman P, Falk H, Kilbourne E, et al: The eosinophilia-myalgia syndrome: the Los Alamos Conference. J Rheumatol 1991;18:867.

64. Hertzman P, Blevins W, Mayer J, et al: Association of the eosinophilia-myalgia syndrome with the ingestion of tryptophan. N Engl J Med 1990;322:868.

65. Belongia E, Hedberg C, Gleich G, et al: An investigation of the cause of the eosinophilia-myalgia syndrome associated with tryptophan use. N Engl J Med 1990;323:357.

66. Kamb M, Murphy J, Jones J, et al: Eosinophilia-myalgia syndrome in L-tryptophan-exposed patients. JAMA 1992;267:77.

67. Centers for Disease Control and Prevention (CDC): Analysis of L-tryptophan for etiology of eosinophilia-myalgia syndrome. MMWR Morb Mortal Wkly Rep 1990;39:789.

68. Centers for Disease Control and Prevention (CDC): Eosinophilia-myalgia syndrome: follow-up survey of patients—New York. MMWR Morb Mortal Wkly Rep 1991;40:401.

69. Slutsker L, Hoesly F, Miller L, et al: Eosinophillia-myalgia syndrome associated with exposure to tryptophan from a single manufacturer. JAMA 1990;264:1213.

70. Pope H, Jonas J, Hudson J, et al: Toxic reactions to the combination of monoamine oxidase inhibitors and tryptophan. Am J Psychiatr 1985;142:491.

71. Blackwell B: Monoamine oxidase inhibitor interactions with other drugs. J Clin Psychopharmacol 1991;11:55.

72. Luu T, Kelley M, Strauch J, et al: Portal vein gas embolism from hydrogen peroxide ingestion. Am J Emerg Med 1992;21:1391.

73. Giberson T, Kern J, Pettigrew D, et al: Near-fatal hydrogen peroxide ingestion. Ann Emerg Med 1989;18:778.

74. Rackoff W, Merton D: Gas embolism after ingestion of hydrogen peroxide. Pediatrics 1990;85:593.

75. Hall A, Linden C, Kulig K, et al: Cyanide poisoning from Laetrile ingestion: Role of nitrite therapy. Pediatrics 1986;78:269.

69

The Vitamins

ALLISON A. MULLER, BS, PHARMD ■ FRED M. HENRETIG, MD

At a Glance...

■ The most crucial specific intervention for vitamin A poisoning is immediate discontinuation of vitamin A; this measure alone suffices in most cases.

■ Prompt withdrawal of vitamin D supplements and implementation of a diet low in calcium and vitamin D are sufficient therapy for mild to moderate cases of vitamin D poisoning.

■ It probably is prudent to caution against the use of high-dose vitamin C therapy for patients with known nephrolithiasis, G6PD deficiency, iron overload conditions, pregnancy, and perhaps for women taking oral contraceptives.

INTRODUCTION AND RELEVANT HISTORY

The vitamins are a defined group of essential organic micronutrients that are required in the human diet for optimal nutrition and to prevent specific deficiency syndromes.[1,2] This requirement is due to either a complete inability to synthesize these nutrients de novo or an inadequate rate of synthesis to maintain optimal health. Medical uses for the vitamins include the prevention or treatment of deficiency states and the treatment of rare vitamin-responsive inborn errors of metabolism.

A less accepted current usage of vitamins has been routine high-dose consumption by healthy adults. This practice has gained popularity with the lay public and some health care workers in an effort to enhance appearance, longevity, or athletic performance or to prevent or ameliorate nondeficiency-specific disease states. The clinically significant vitamin exposures occur most often under these circumstances of intentional chronic overdose. The water-soluble vitamins typically are excreted renally when ingested in excess, although very large doses taken chronically have resulted in adverse effects. The fat-soluble vitamins are stored in tissues, and excessive consumption is thus more likely to result in toxicity. Accidental overdose of pediatric multivitamin preparations by children also occurs frequently, although this is rarely a cause for significant concern aside from co-ingested iron in combination products. Serious iron toxicity is rare even in this context. Occasionally, vitamins are chosen as an intentional acute overdose agent. An unfortunately not uncommon scenario is the acute overdose by a young pregnant woman of her prescribed prenatal vitamin and mineral supplement. In this context, with a typical elemental iron content of 62.5 mg per tablet, serious iron poisoning may occur, although toxicity related to co-ingested vitamins is again rarely of significance (see also Chapter 72).

The medical use of vitamins can be traced to the 1753 discovery by British naval surgeon James Lind of the protection from scurvy afforded to sailors by the addition of fresh citrus fruits to their diets during long voyages.[1] Ascorbic acid (vitamin C) was, of course, subsequently identified as the antiscorbutic factor and became the first of the 13 named vitamins. Vitamins are currently classified as water soluble (nine vitamins: ascorbate, thiamine, riboflavin, niacin, pyridoxine, biotin, pantothenic acid, folate, and cyanocobalamin) or fat soluble (four vitamins: A, D, E, and K). Several of the vitamins exist in nature or in vivo as different but closely related chemical compounds or precursors and are referred to as *vitamers*. Many vitamins require processing in vivo to become biologically active. The water-soluble vitamins or their derivatives function primarily as coenzymes for apoenzymes. An example is pyridoxine (when converted to pyridoxal phosphate) as coenzyme to the glutamic acid decarboxylase apoenzyme, forming a holoenzyme that synthesizes γ-aminobutyric acid from glutamic acid. The fat-soluble vitamins A and D interact with specific intracellular receptors and have hormonal or prohormonal effects.[2]

Amounts of vitamins necessary daily to protect normal, healthy persons from vitamin deficiency states range from micrograms to milligrams and are designated the *minimum daily requirements* (MDRs). Currently in the United States, recommendations on daily intake are expressed as reference daily intakes (RDIs) for vitamins and minerals (Table 69-1). These replace the U.S. recommended daily allowance (RDA) and are based on average RDI values for the U.S. population over the age of 4 years.[2,3] Megadose usage typically involves self-administration of doses 20 to 660 times these recom-

TABLE 69-1 Reference Daily Intakes (RDIs)[3]	
VITAMIN	**RDI**
A	5000 IU
C	60 mg
D	400 IU
E	30 IU
B$_6$	2 mg
B$_{12}$	6 μg
Thiamine	1.5 mg
Riboflavin	1.7 mg
Niacin	20 mg
Folic acid	0.4 mg

IU, international units.

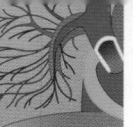

mended amounts. In the United States, efforts to regulate vitamin usage have had a complex and politically charged history. Currently, the U.S. Food and Drug Administration (FDA) has the authority to regulate the labeling of vitamin and mineral supplements. Currently, the FDA does not regulate the nutrient content of vitamin supplements, except those intended for use by children less than 12 years of age and by pregnant or lactating women, despite the well-recognized hazards of megadose vitamin usage.[2]

A number of vitamin-responsive metabolic disorders have been described, involving at least eight of the nine water-soluble vitamins and vitamin D.[1,4,5] Classic examples include pyridoxine-dependent infantile convulsions, pernicious anemia, and vitamin D–sensitive rickets. Pyridoxine dependency was first described in the early 1950s,[1] and the same era witnessed the observation that the dementia associated with pellagra (niacin deficiency) was similar in some ways to that of schizophrenia.[4,5] Early studies in the psychiatric literature suggested beneficial results in treating schizophrenia with massive doses of niacin, prompting further extension of this concept to other vitamins and to other illnesses.[4,6]

Pauling's 1970 monograph *Vitamin C and the Common Cold*[7] helped popularize the use of megadoses of vitamins for prevention and treatment of a number of illnesses ranging from viral infections to cancer. The increased interest in personal fitness and preventive health of the 1970s provided fertile ground for the expansion of this concept of vitamin megadosing. By the 1980s, more than 70% of Americans believed that vitamins could prevent fatigue, and 21% believed that diseases such as cancer and arthritis were caused by vitamin deficiency.[4,8] A 1987 survey found that half of adult Americans took occasional vitamin supplements, and more than 20% took vitamins daily.[9] The popularity of vitamin supplements is a reflection of broad media coverage of studies detailing the roles of vitamins in preventing and treating cancer, cardiovascular disease, ocular disorders, respiratory disorders, and osteoporosis.[10-12] Nutritional authorities caution that insufficient scientific evidence exists to support the megadosing of dietary antioxidants to prevent chronic illnesses such as cardiovascular disease or cancer.[13] It has been recommended that all adults take one multivitamin daily, since most people do not obtain a sufficient amount of all vitamins from dietary consumption alone.[14]

FAT-SOLUBLE VITAMINS

In general, toxic effects of vitamins are most often related to overdosing of the fat-soluble vitamins and have been observed particularly with excessive ingestion of vitamins A and D (Table 69-2). Adverse effects ascribed to vitamins E and K have been uncommon and noted primarily with parenteral use. In view of the prominent place afforded to vitamin A toxicity in reported medical literature, this vitamin is reviewed in some detail relative to the other vitamins covered in this chapter.

Vitamin A

INTRODUCTION AND RELEVANT HISTORY

Vitamin A has a long and fascinating history. As early as 1500 BC, night blindness that could be remedied by the topical application of roasted liver was described in Egypt, and Hippocrates later recommended the ingestion of cow liver as a cure.[15] In 1865, ophthalmia brasiliana, an eye disorder of poorly nourished slaves, was described. Further linkage of keratomalacia to nutritional deficiency was provided in the 1880s with descriptions of night blindness among Russian Orthodox Catholics who fasted during Lent and particularly with the description of corneal sloughing in breast-fed infants of fasting mothers.[15] Perhaps the oldest and largest recorded experience with vitamin toxicity is associated with both acute and chronic exposure to excess vitamin A. The 19th-century Arctic explorer Elisha Kane described a syndrome of severe headache, vomiting, drowsiness, and irritability occurring a few hours after the ingestion of polar bear liver.[16] This syndrome is recognized today as being quite likely due to acute hypervitaminosis A–induced pseudotumor cerebri. Modern authors continue to describe similar phenomena, for example, the 1984 report of a 25-year-old Sri Lankan woman who developed pseudotumor and markedly elevated serum vitamin A levels 1 week after consuming a meal of shark liver (see Toxicology).[17]

STRUCTURE

The vitamin A family consists of several related compounds, with their respective stereoisomers, which exhibit the vitamin's biologic effects. Retinol, also referred to as vitamin A_1, is the alcohol form, which is found primarily as an ester in the liver of many animals and saltwater fish (Fig. 69-1). Retinal, which is the vitamin A aldehyde, functions as the chromophore of the retina when it combines with the protein opsin to form rhodopsin. β-Carotene, or provitamin A, is a dimer of retinal that occurs in many pigmented plants. Retinoic acid, the carboxylic acid of retinol, is believed to be the relevant vitamer at the cellular level for most functions of vitamin A other than in the visual cycle.

Vitamin A is classically quantified by bioassay in rats, although purified preparations may also be determined spectrophotometrically.[15] The "retinol equivalent" is equal to 1 μg of all-*trans*-retinol (3.3 IU) or 6 μg of dietary β-carotene (10 IU).

PHARMACOLOGY AND PATHOPHYSIOLOGY

Vitamin A is believed to act through hormone-like activity on intracellular receptors, in addition to the well-understood specific effect of one of its vitamers, retinal, as the chromophore in the visual light-sensing cells. Vitamin A is essential in the visual cycle, in the maintenance of the functional and structural integrity of epithelium in mucus-secreting or keratinizing tissues, in bone growth, and in reproduction and embryologic development. It has an important role in enhancing immune function and reducing sequelae of some

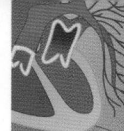

TABLE 69-2 Vitamin Toxicity Overview

VITAMIN	TOXIC DOSE	PRINCIPAL TOXIC EFFECTS
A	Acute: 　75,000–100,000 IU (P) 　>1 million IU (A) Chronic: 　18,000 IU/day (P) 　20,000–50,000 IU/day (A) Teratogenic: 　>10,000 IU/day	Initial: CNS; increased ICP with headache, irritability, lethargy, ophthalmoplegia, papilledema Later: hair loss, peeling skin, hepatomegaly CNS: increased ICP, pseudotumor cerebri Mucocutaneous: dry, scaly, peeling skin; hair loss, brittle nails; cheilitis, stomatitis, gingivitis Hepatic: early–hepatomegaly, anorexia, vomiting, +/– abnormal LFTs; late–hepatic fibrosis, ascites, cirrhosis, esophageal varices Skeletal: bone pain, cortical hyperostoses; premature epiphyseal closure (P) Reproductive: teratogenic effects on face, ears; occasional CNS, cardiac (less so than with isotretinoin)
D	1600–2000 IU/day (P) 60,000 IU/day (A) Teratogenic: 　(?) 2000–4000 IU/day Probably variable, with idiosyncratic hypersensitivity	Metabolic: hypercalcemia Renal: hypercalciuria, nephrocalcinosis CV: metastatic calcifications in heart, vessels CV: infantile hypercalcemia, supravalvular aortic stenosis syndrome
E	(?) 400–3000 IU/day	CNS: headache, weakness GI: nausea, cramps, diarrhea Heme: increased effect of anticogulants
K	(?) (Occurs with therapeutic IV dose)	Anaphylactoid reaction Heme: hemolysis, jaundice in newborns (especially with G6PD deficiency)
Pyridoxine	117–500 mg/day	Peripheral sensory neuropathy
Niacin	3.0–4.5 mg/day	Cutaneous: flushing, pruritus GI: cholestatic jaundice, hepatitis Heme: thrombocytopenia CV: atrial fibrillation Misc: gout, myopathy
Thiamine	Acute: (?) (rare, occurs with therapeutic IV dose) Chronic: 5 mg/day	Anaphylactic reaction Misc: headache, irritability, tachycardia
C	(?), probably > 4 g/day	GI: nausea, cramping, diarrhea Renal: nephrolithiasis (especially in predisposed patients) Heme: hemolysis with G6PD deficiency Misc: rebound scurvy after withdrawal

A, adult; CNS, central nervous system; CV, cardiovascular; GI, gastrointestinal; G6PD, glucose-6-phosphate dehydrogenase; Heme, hematologic; ICP, intracranial pressure; LFTs, liver function tests; Misc, miscellaneous; P, pediatric.

infections (e.g., measles in young children[18]) and may play a significant role in anticarcinogenesis. Several synthetic analogs of vitamin A have been developed as pharmaceutical agents for dermatologic applications.

In the visual system, both rods and cones utilize 11-*cis*-retinal as the chromophore. In the photoreceptor cells of the rods, especially sensitive to low-intensity light, this vitamer combines with the membrane protein opsin to form rhodopsin, which is the light-absorbing holoreceptor. The cones, which are the color-sensitive photoreceptor cells, are of three types, each having a separate protein that when combined with 11-*cis*-retinal responds optimally to red, green, or blue wavelengths of light. The visual cycle involves an interaction of the photon-activated rhodopsin with a G protein and interconversions of 11-*cis*-retinal to several stereoisomers.[19]

The basal mucus-secreting cells of many epithelia depend on vitamin A for normal structure and mucus secretion. These influences appear to be mediated primarily by retinoic acid, via changes in nuclear transcription. Retinoic acid receptors have been described that belong to a receptor "superfamily" that includes receptors for calcitriol as well as thyroid and steroid hormones.[15]

Possible anticarcinogenic effects of vitamin A have been attributed to its ability to induce differentiation of malignant cells and to function in the synthesis of cell-surface glycoproteins and glycolipids that may play an important role in cell adherence and communication. Splenic lymphocyte proliferation and killer cell cytotoxic activity is impaired in vitamin A deficiency. Therefore, differentiation of these immune cells may play a role in the vitamin's beneficial effect on immunity and resistance to infection.[20]

The primary food sources for vitamin A are liver, dairy products, egg yolk, and fish (providing retinol or retinol esters) and yellow and green vegetables (providing β-carotene).[15] In the average American diet, about 50% of the vitamin intake comes from animal-based products and 50% from vegetable sources. Absorption and

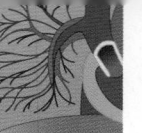
Vitamin A	Vitamin D$_3$
β-Carotene Retinol (CH$_2$OH)	Cholecalciferol

Vitamin K	Vitamin E
(structure with R)	CH$_3$ structure with CH$_2$[CH$_2$—CH$_2$—CH—CH$_2$]$_3$H

A

Pyridoxine	Niacin	Thiamine	Ascorbic acid
CH$_2$OH, CH$_2$OH, OH	COOH	NH$_2$, CH$_2$CH$_2$OH	O=C—C=C—C—C—CH$_2$OH with OH OH OH

B

FIGURE 69-1 Fat-soluble (**A**) and water-soluble (**B**) vitamins reported to have toxic effects in humans.

utilization of the vitamin is complex and varies with the source. Most animal-derived vitamin A is consumed in the form of retinol esters, typically retinyl palmitate, and when vitamin A is ingested in usual dietary amounts, absorption is virtually complete. These esters are hydrolyzed in the intestinal lumen and brush border and then taken up by the intestinal cells bound to a cellular retinol-binding protein (CRBP). There they are re-esterified and incorporated into chylomicrons for transport to the liver, where they are stored. Hepatic vitamin A storage capacity is considerable (average content of retinyl esters is 100 to 300 μg/g), with reserves sufficient to withstand several months of a vitamin A–free diet before the plasma concentration decreases markedly or deficiency symptoms appear. The liver normally releases vitamin A after hydrolysis to retinol, 95% of which is bound to an α_1-globulin, the retinol-binding protein (RBP). When the liver becomes saturated with vitamin A as a result of excessive ingestion or hepatic disease or both, retinyl esters may appear in the blood, eventually accounting for as much as 65% of the total circulating retinoids. Circulating retinol is carried to cells of various target organs, where it is taken up by a membrane-bound protein very similar to CRBP, re-esterified, then hydrolyzed and delivered to the appropriate intracellular sites by a cytosolic CRBP. The

fate of ingested carotenoids is slightly different.[15,21] Only about one third of the carotene content of a meal is absorbed. Some β-carotene is cleaved in the intestinal mucosa and esterified and transported to the liver via the lymphatics, while some is absorbed intact. When carotenoids are present in large amounts in the diet, they may cause an elevated blood carotene level (normal range, 50 to 200 μg/dL), associated with a benign and reversible yellowish (or "golden suntan") discoloration of the skin (but not the sclera, as occurs in jaundice). In most cases, excessive consumption of carotene does not lead to hypervitaminosis A, presumably because only limited conversion to retinol occurs. However, this occasionally occurs, as it did in a 20-year-old Japanese woman whose diet consisted mainly of pumpkin for 2 years. She subsequently developed vitamin A poisoning with hepatotoxicity, confirmed via liver needle biopsy.[22] In addition to hepatic storage and tissue uptake, some retinol is glucuronidated. Other water-soluble metabolites are also excreted, with no retinol normally found unchanged in the urine.[15]

SPECIAL POPULATIONS
In adults, vitamin A deficiency is usually related to chronic illnesses associated with fat malabsorption such as inflammatory bowel disease, biliary or pancreatic

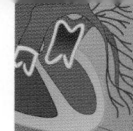

insufficiency, and cirrhosis. Children suffering from general malnutrition are especially susceptible, and it is believed that vitamin A deficiency is responsible for more than 250,000 cases per year worldwide of irreversible pediatric blindness, in addition to greatly enhanced mortality from infectious diseases, especially measles.[15,18] Features characteristic of vitamin A deficiency include night blindness and keratomalacia progressing to permanent blindness, keratinization and drying of the skin with follicular hyperkeratosis, increased incidence of respiratory infections, urinary calculi due to associated changes in the urinary tract epithelium, diarrhea, and occasional impairment of hearing, taste, and smell.[15]

TOXICOLOGY

With excessive vitamin A intake, hepatic storage capacity is exceeded, and the previously noted normal pattern of almost all circulating vitamin A existing as retinol bound to RBP is altered, with an increasing proportion of plasma retinoids being present as retinyl esters loosely associated with lipoproteins. Clinical case reports of vitamin A toxicity typically involve normal or only slight elevation of retinol (normal range, 30 to 70 µg/dL), with markedly elevated retinyl esters (normal, <7 µg/dL, or 5% to 8% of plasma retinol).[23,24] In more advanced cases of hypervitaminosis A, one may find an elevation of retinol to more than 100 µg/dL, and some authors suggest that excess circulating free retinol (e.g., a molar ratio of retinol to RBP of greater than 1) is important to clinical toxicity.[25] However, most reviews suggest that retinyl esters, which exhibit surfactant properties, are more likely responsible for toxic effects.[24] Retinyl esters—and perhaps free retinol—probably cause cellular toxicity via altered membrane lipoprotein phenomena. The precise mechanism of the increased intracranial pressure that is so characteristic of vitamin A toxicity is unclear, but it may relate to such altered membrane function in the choroid plexus.[26] As hepatic stores of vitamin A become saturated, another characteristic feature, hepatotoxicity, is observed when marked accumulation of retinyl esters and lipid develops in the perisinusoidal fat storage cells (Ito cells in the space of Disse). This process may stimulate transformation of these cells to fibroblasts[24]; clinically, progression is observed to sinusoidal fibrosis, portal fibrosis, central vein sclerosis, and eventually cirrhosis.

Toxicity may occur as the result of either acute or chronic overdose.[24] In children, single doses of 75,000 to 100,000 IU are necessary to produce toxicity, whereas in adults the range is usually in excess of 1 million IU. Chronic exposures of 18,000 to 60,000 IU/day in infants and children, and 50,000 to 100,000 IU/day in adults will result in toxicity. One adult patient has been reported with hepatotoxicity resulting from habitual daily ingestion of 20,000 IU.[27] Clinical manifestations of chronic toxicity may vary in terms of total dosage and duration of exposure; most case reports observe periods of excessive intake of months to years, although infants treated with 18,000 IU/day became symptomatic within 6 weeks.[28] Persons with underlying liver disease, or who develop acute hepatitis, are at increased risk. For acute intoxication, most reported cases are due to the ingestion of liver with high vitamin A content (e.g., bear, seal, or fish livers), with iatrogenic cases representing another sizable group. With chronic exposures, the most common cause is excessive intake via self-medication or food faddism in adults, or overzealous vitamin treatment of children by their parents.[15,24,28,29]

CLINICAL MANIFESTATIONS

Classically, vitamin A intoxication is stratified by age of patient and chronicity of exposure, although there is considerable overlap of symptomatology. The target body areas most typically affected are the central nervous system (CNS), liver, bone, and skin and mucous membranes.

Accounts of acute vitamin A toxicity are relatively uncommon, but typical early features are primarily neurologic. These include irritability, tiredness with intense sleep desire progressing to somnolence, increased intracranial pressure that may manifest as a bulging fontanelle in infants or signs of acute pseudotumor cerebri in older children and adults, anorexia, and vomiting.[24] Within a few days, cheilitis, hair loss and skin peeling, hepatomegaly, and epistaxis or miscellaneous hemorrhages may ensue. Laboratory abnormalities may include increased serum retinyl esters (and retinol in severe cases), hypercalcemia, and slight changes in liver function tests. An illustrative case report was provided by Misbah and colleagues.[17] A 25-year-old Sri Lankan woman ingested a meal of cooked shark liver and presented after several days of headache, vomiting, and diplopia. The examination was notable for bilateral florid papilledema, enlarged blind spots, and bilateral partial abducens palsies. Routine serum chemistry, liver function, and hematology values were normal, but total serum vitamin A level (retinol versus retinyl esters not specified) was elevated at 177 µg/dL. She recovered over an 8-week period, becoming asymptomatic with only residual but receding papilledema.

Far more common is the occurrence of chronic vitamin A toxicity, which tends to involve all four of the major target organ systems. The CNS and ophthalmologic effects include headache, fatigue but difficulty sleeping, visual disturbances, anorexia and weight loss, and signs of increased intracranial pressure with bulging fontanelles in infancy and pseudotumor cerebri in older children and adults. Changes of the integument and mucous membranes, including dry, pruritic, scaly, and peeling skin; hair loss; and brittle nails; and cheilitis, stomatitis, and gingivitis are regular and often early signs. Involvement of the liver is manifested as hepatosplenomegaly, nausea, abdominal pain, ascites, esophageal varices, and cirrhosis. Liver function tests may be abnormal, but patients with severe hepatic involvement and ascites and without jaundice have been reported, as have patients with minimally altered or normal liver function tests, although prothrombin time may be increased owing to hypoprothrombinemia.[23,25,28,29] A vicious cycle may be conceptualized wherein early vitamin A hepatotoxicity results in decreased liver

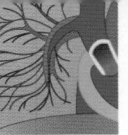

storage capacity or RBP synthesis or both; continued chronic excessive ingestion results in escalating release of retinyl esters, and in some cases unbound retinol, with resultant systemic toxicity. The skeletal system is also frequently affected, particularly in children with growing long bones. Bone pain and tenderness is often noted, and children may manifest painful swelling of overlying soft tissues.[29] Radiographic findings may include areas of osteoporosis or hypermineralization, periosteal calcifications and cortical hyperostosis of the cranium, clavicles, long bones, and metatarsals, as well as cup-shaped deformity of the metaphyses.[30,31] Permanent deformity and growth retardation may occur in children owing to partial or complete premature epiphyseal closure. Associated laboratory abnormalities of hypercalcemia and increased alkaline phosphatase are noted on occasion; these may represent effects of stimulation of osteoclastic resorption or inhibition of osteoblastic activity or both.[31]

Another area of concern related to vitamin A and its derivatives involves potential *teratogenic* effects. Isotretinoin, 13-*cis*-retinoic acid, has been used widely in the United States and Europe as a systemic agent for the treatment of nodulocystic acne vulgaris. A specific embryopathy has been well characterized for this agent, with a calculated relative risk of 26.5%.[32] Typical malformations include those related to four main structural areas: the brain, head and face, heart and great vessels, and thymus. These include hydrocephalus with or without areas of cerebral agenesis or hypoplasia; micrognathia, cleft palate, microtia with or without anotia; transposition of the great vessels, Fallot's tetralogy, or truncus arteriosus; and thymic hypoplasia or aplasia. Further studies have found that the crucial exposure period occurs during the first trimester (especially the second to fifth postconceptional weeks), and that the prevalence of malformations averages 85% for involvement of the brain, 70% for the ears, and 50% for the cardiovascular system.[33] Although used with caution in pregnant women, topical tretinoin has not been shown to achieve sufficient serum levels to cause teratogenic effects in humans to date.[33] Acitretin is an oral retinoid used for the treatment of severe or refractory psoriasis. This drug is contraindicated not only in pregnant women but also in women who are planning to become pregnant sooner than 2 years following discontinuation of the drug. Those women who used an older oral retinoid for psoriasis, etretinate, are advised by some physicians to avoid pregnancy indefinitely, as it may take 2 years, or longer, for the drug to be eliminated. Congenital malformations noted after high-dose maternal vitamin A therapy have also been reported; these tend to primarily involve facial and otic defects, with less frequent neurologic and cardiac involvement.[24,34] An attempt to calculate relative risks for vitamin A prenatal exposure has been reported from data collected on more than 20,000 pregnant women in the United States as part of a large prospective cohort study of congenital malformations.[35] These researchers compared outcomes in women taking supplements of more than 10,000 IU/day with those taking less than 5,000 IU/day and found a relative risk for cranial–neural crest defects of 4.8 (95% CI 2.2 to 10.5). They concluded that doses of supplemental vitamin A in excess of 10,000 IU/day pose a significant risk of teratogenicity.

DIAGNOSIS

Recognizing the characteristic clinical syndromes of acute or chronic hypervitaminosis A, along with finding a history of exposure, are the most important steps in diagnosis. As noted above, routine serum chemistries and liver function tests may be normal or only minimally elevated. Some patients manifest hypercalcemia or hypoprothrombinemia. Characteristic radiographic findings have been described and may be present in patients with chronic toxicity. Patients may be symptomatic at a time when serum vitamin A levels are normal. However, a retinol serum level exceeding 100 μg/dL is highly suggestive of toxicity, as is an elevated proportion of retinyl esters (more than 5% to 8% of total, or over 7 μg/dL), if specific tests are available. Characteristic liver pathology and an elevated liver vitamin A content may be found on biopsy in occult cases.

MANAGEMENT

The most crucial specific intervention is immediate discontinuation of vitamin A; this measure alone suffices in most cases. Most symptoms resolve over several weeks to months. Routine principles of gastrointestinal decontamination are probably appropriate in the uncommon situation of a patient seen soon after an acute overdose exceeding 75,000 to 100,000 IU in children or 1 million IU in adults. Patients with severe hepatotoxicity obviously require significant supportive care. Vitamin K may be of value for patients with hypoprothrombinemia. Associated increased intracranial pressure may occasionally require intervention depending on duration and severity. Neurologic consultation is probably advised prior to instituting a regimen that might include repeated lumbar punctures; diuretics (e.g., furosemide, initial IV dose 0.5 to 1 mg/kg up to 40 mg); mannitol (initial IV dose 0.25 g/kg); acetazolamide (5 mg/kg, up to 250 mg PO or IV every 6 hr); and/or steroids (e.g., prednisone 0.5 to 1.0 mg/kg up to 40 mg PO per day) as necessary. Hypercalcemia may also require specific treatment, although initial management with intravenous normal saline to enhance hydration usually suffices.[31] If hypercalcemia is severe or persistent, additional treatment may be warranted. Adjuvant therapy has included diuretics such as furosemide to enhance renal calcium excretion. Corticosteroids (e.g., prednisone in doses of 0.5 mg/kg/day, up to 20 mg/day) may also lower serum calcium by increasing renal excretion as well as decreasing intestinal calcium absorption and bone resorption.[36]

Vitamin D

INTRODUCTION

Vitamin D is another fat-soluble vitamin that produces a classic toxic syndrome following excessive ingestion. Vitamin D shares with vitamin A the properties of a

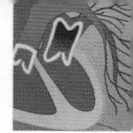

hormone. However, in some respects it is not truly a vitamin because, for most persons living in tropical or temperate geographic zones, cutaneous photobiosynthesis of the nutrient is sufficient to supply optimal nutritional needs.[37,38]

PHARMACOLOGY

Vitamin D congeners are secosterol (split sterol) derivatives of the cholesterol precursor 7-dehydrocholesterol.[37] Vitamin D_3 (cholecalciferol) is formed when this precursor absorbs ultraviolet light in the skin and splits the C9–C10 bond in the B ring of the sterol skeleton. Preformed vitamin D congeners with biologic equivalency to endogenous skin-derived vitamin D_3 may be absorbed from the diet, especially fish liver oils. Vitamin D_3 from all sources enters the circulation bound to a specific α_1-globulin, the vitamin D–binding protein, and is transported to the liver where it undergoes hydroxylation to 25-hydroxyvitamin D_3 [$25(OH)D_3$]. The production of $25(OH)D_3$ is influenced by feedback inhibition but is not tightly controlled, and levels of this congener rise dramatically in states of excess vitamin D exposure (normal range, 5 to 80 ng/mL). At physiologic levels, $25(OH)D_3$ is not thought to exhibit significant biologic activity, but it appears to be active at very elevated concentrations and may be responsible for much of the toxicity associated with hypervitaminosis D. The $25(OH)D_3$ is transported to the kidneys bound to the vitamin D–binding protein, where under the influence of parathyroid hormone, it is further hydroxylated to $1,25(OH)_2 D_3$, also known as *calcitriol.*

The synthesis of calcitriol is closely regulated by fluctuations in serum calcium. Hypocalcemia stimulates parathyroid hormone secretion and thus the synthesis of calcitriol, which is believed to be the significant biologically active congener at physiologic levels. Calcitriol is carried to target organs—particularly the intestine and bone—by the vitamin D–binding protein. (Normal serum concentration of total calcitriol ranges from 16 to 65 pg/mL.) Free calcitriol is taken up by cells and exhibits its hormone-like effect by complexing with a specific nuclear receptor, a member of the same receptor superfamily that includes receptors for retinol, steroids, and thyroid hormone. The calcitriol-receptor complex activates transcription of genes for the synthesis of an intestinal calcium-binding protein and bone osteocalcin, which increase intestinal calcium absorption and bone resorption, respectively, and result in increased serum calcium. Thus, vitamin D plays a central role in calcium homeostasis. Receptors for calcitriol have been identified in several other tissues, but their function is less well understood.

Daily requirements for vitamin D range from 200 to 400 IU (5 to 10 μg) per day.[2] In latitudes where and during seasons when sunlight intensity is limited, this MDR must be met by dietary intake, which was difficult to achieve in the era before widespread fortification of milk and bread products. The classic nutritional vitamin D deficiency state manifests as rickets in infants and growing children and as osteomalacia in adults. Several disorders in synthesis or response to calcitriol may require treatment with supraphysiologic doses of vitamin D analogs (e.g., vitamin D–resistant and vitamin D–dependent rickets and renal osteodystrophy). Today, most persons in the United States receive adequate vitamin D through their diet, unless they suffer from a primary intestinal malabsorption syndrome or from hepatic or biliary dysfunction. Rickets and osteomalacia have also been observed in patients on chronic anticonvulsant therapy with phenobarbital or phenytoin, although the mechanism is not well understood.

TOXICOLOGY

Hypervitaminosis D has been recognized for decades,[26] principally in persons treated with pharmacologic doses for diseases unrelated to vitamin D deficiency but thought likely to benefit from such treatment, such as rheumatoid arthritis. Occasional acute vitamin D exposures may occur from ingestion of vitamin D–containing rodenticides or massive ingestions of multivitamins. Chronic vitamin D consumption in excess of even four times the RDI may be hazardous to young infants; adults may experience toxicity at doses of 60,000 IU/day for weeks to months. Large numbers of infants were oversupplemented in England during World War II, typically with daily intakes of 2000 to 4000 IU/day. A number of such children developed hypercalcemia, a nonfamilial congenital syndrome related to maternal hypervitaminosis D, and abnormal fetal or infantile vitamin D sensitivity was also described with cerebral, cardiovascular, and renal anomalies, particularly supravalvular aortic stenosis.[39] Vieth and colleagues reported cases of vitamin D poisoning within a family following the mixing of crystalline vitamin D_3 into their table sugar.[40] The toxicity of excess vitamin D is thought to be due primarily to its exaggerated physiologic effects, resulting in hypercalcemia, hypercalciuria, and metastatic soft tissue calcification.

CLINICAL MANIFESTATIONS

Classically described clinical effects include initial symptoms of systemic hypercalcemia, including weakness, headache, fatigue, nausea, and vomiting. Subsequently, manifestations of soft tissue calcification may occur, including hypertension, polyuria, and polydipsia related to nephrocalcinosis, which may progress to uremia, as well as signs referable to calcifications in myocardium, vessels, muscle, lung, and skin; death may result. An outbreak of hypervitaminosis D due to overfortification of milk (up to 200,000 IU per quart) by a dairy in Massachusetts in 1988 to 1991 has allowed for case-control studies that have reinforced the association of these effects with excess vitamin D exposure.[41,42]

DIAGNOSIS AND TREATMENT

The clinical findings and exposure history may be characteristic. Observed laboratory abnormalities include hypercalcemia with variable phosphate levels, decreased renal function with albuminuria and anemia,

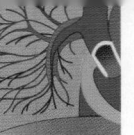
and elevated levels of 25(OH)D$_3$ and free calcitriol. (Total calcitriol is usually normal or only slightly elevated.[43]) Radiographic findings may include ectopic calcifications in kidneys, heart, and vessels as well as skeletal changes of periosteal thickening.

Prompt withdrawal of vitamin D supplements and implementation of a diet low in calcium and vitamin D are sufficient therapy for mild to moderate cases. In the acute overdose situation, as of a vitamin D–based rodenticide, appropriate gastrointestinal decontamination is warranted. Patients with persistent hypercalcemia may benefit from further measures as detailed above for vitamin A toxicity. Renal failure may require dialysis for a period of time. The induction of hepatic enzymes with glutethimide to facilitate degradative metabolism of vitamin D has been reported successful in one case.[44] Other case series have suggested a benefit in treating hypercalcemia and hypercalciuria with the biphosphonates, clodronate,[45] and pamidronate.[46,47]

Vitamin E

INTRODUCTION

Although vitamin E was isolated in 1936, its role in human nutrition is still controversial, and there is currently little unequivocal evidence that a specific deficiency state exists for it in otherwise normal full-term infants, in children, or in adults.[15] In premature babies, persons with severe fat malabsorption, and those with the rare genetic disease abetalipoproteinemia, vitamin E seems to protect against hemolytic anemia, although other nutrients may play a role. In animals, particularly rodents, vitamin E appears vital for normal reproduction and neuromuscular function. α-Tocopherol (see Fig. 69-1) is believed to be the most important vitamer and displays the most biologic activity in most bioassays. The vitamin has come under intense scrutiny in recent years because of its known antioxidant properties and the publicity surrounding studies evaluating its possibly protective effect from atherosclerosis and carcinogenesis.[10,11]

TOXICOLOGY

Case series of persons taking large doses of vitamin E (400 IU to more than 3000 IU) have reported a variety of symptoms, including fatigue, headache, muscle weakness, nausea, intestinal cramps, and diarrhea.[48] In addition, vitamin E may antagonize vitamin K, with resulting increased clotting time and effect of oral anticoagulants.[48,49] However, most large controlled studies (typical dose, 400 to 800 IU) have failed to find significant differences in the incidence of adverse effects between treated cases and controls.[11,50] Of historical interest was the tragic epidemic of morbidity (pulmonary deterioration, hepatic and renal failure, and thrombocytopenia) and 38 deaths in premature infants treated in the winter of 1983–1984 with an intravenous preparation of vitamin E (E-Ferol). This syndrome was subsequently determined to be due to the carrier, a mixture of polysorbate 80 and polysorbate 20 (oleate and laurate esters of sorbitol condensed with ethylene oxide).[51]

Vitamin K

PHARMACOLOGY

Vitamin K activity is found in two natural sources: a plant-derived form (phytonadione, vitamin K$_1$) and the form synthesized by intestinal bacteria (menaquinone, vitamin K$_2$).[15] Both are utilized as essential cofactors in the hepatic biosynthesis of blood coagulation factors II, VII, IX, and X. Other vitamin K–dependent proteins include the anticoagulant proteins C and S, as well as bone osteocalcin. Deficiency of vitamin K results in a hemorrhagic diathesis. A coumarin embryopathy has been described for skeletal abnormalities that may represent the effects of fetal vitamin K deficiency on osteocalcin synthesis.

TOXICOLOGY

Chronic ingestion of excess vitamin K is unusual because it is not available in the typical multivitamin supplements subject to abuse.[26] Large amounts may inhibit the desired effects of anticoagulant medications.[48] Water-soluble congeners (menadiones) given to newborns for hemorrhagic disease prophylaxis, particularly if there is glucose-6-phosphate dehydrogenase (G6PD) deficiency, may cause hemolysis and jaundice; phytonadione is rarely associated with this effect.[26,48,46] Intravenous administration of phytonadione may result in an anaphylactoid reaction of flushing, chest pain, hypotension, and death; it is unclear whether this is due to the vitamin itself or the vehicle. Concern has been raised about a potential association between the routine use of prophylactic vitamin K in healthy newborns and increased risk of subsequent childhood cancer; however, careful controlled studies have failed to substantiate this association, and authorities continue to recommend this use of vitamin K.[52]

WATER-SOLUBLE VITAMINS

Significant toxicity is well established for chronic excessive consumption of pyridoxine and niacin (see Table 69-2). Adverse effects have also been ascribed to thiamine and ascorbate and are briefly reviewed.

Pyridoxine

INTRODUCTION

The pyridoxamine congeners are utilized by mammals after hepatic conversion to the active form, pyridoxal phosphate, which in turn is an important coenzyme in numerous metabolic reactions of amino acids.[53] Pyridoxine is supplied by meats, whole grains, soybeans, and various vegetables. A deficiency state has been observed with mucocutaneous manifestations (seborrhea-like lesions and stomatitis) and seizures due to diminished γ-aminobutyrate (GABA) production. This role of pyridoxine as a cofactor in GABA synthesis underlies its use as an antidote in the treatment of isoniazid overdose and hydrazine-mushroom poisoning (see Chapter 23), as well as its previously noted use in pyridoxine dependency, an inherited disorder of pyridoxine metabolism resulting in

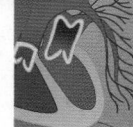

neonatal seizures. Pyridoxine has found similar use in the treatment of xanthurenic aciduria and homocystinuria.

TOXICOLOGY

Pyridoxine toxicity is most likely to occur with chronic ingestion in excess of 500 mg/day, often taken for self-treatment of premenstrual syndrome or as a body-building adjunct. Toxic effects have been reported with consumption of average total doses as low as 117 mg/day for 3 years.[54] The toxic syndrome manifests as a striking sensory axonal neuropathy, typically without weakness or CNS involvement.[55] Patients have an unsteady gait and difficulty in handling small objects. Neurologic findings include ataxia, severely impaired position and vibration sense, and less dramatic effects on light touch, pain sensation, and temperature. Diminished deep tendon reflexes and Lhermitte's sign (neck pain and tingling that shoots down the spine to the legs and feet after neck flexion) are also present. Dose response characteristics were studied in five healthy volunteers administered 1 or 3 g/day and closely followed for clinical symptoms and sural nerve electrophysiology.[56] Subjects receiving higher doses became symptomatic earlier, and symptoms persisted for 2 to 3 weeks after discontinuation of pyridoxine, a phenomenon termed *coasting* by the authors. An infant exposed to pyridoxine in utero (maternal dose 50 mg/day) was born with amelia of one leg.[57] At least one patient has been reported who developed motor weakness after 5 years of 10 g/day consumption.[58] An unusual episode of acute toxicity occurred in two patients who received an iatrogenic parenteral, massive (exceeding 100 g) pyridoxine overdose during treatment of *Gyromitra* mushroom poisoning.[59] These patients manifested weakness, lethargy, nystagmus, and respiratory depression in addition to severe sensory neuropathy. At follow-up 4 years after exposure, one of these patients had persistent profound sensory loss, although the motor abnormalities had disappeared.[60] Chronic pyridoxine intake at doses as low as 25 mg/day have been reported to antagonize the antiparkinsonian effect of L-dopa, and similar antagonisms have been observed for barbiturates and phenytoin.[48] The treatment of pyridoxine toxicity consists of its withdrawal, which usually results in gradual recovery,[54] although some patients may have long-term or permanent sequelae.

Niacin

INTRODUCTION AND RELEVANT HISTORY

Niacin has been long recognized as the antipellagra factor missing in diets based largely on corn.[53] The vitamin exists as nicotinic acid (niacin) and nicotinamide (niacinamide) (see Fig. 69-1), with equivalent biologic vitamin activity but different pharmacologic effects. In both forms, niacin is converted to either nicotinamide adenine dinucleotide (NAD) or its phosphate (NADP), which are vital coenzymes for a variety of enzymes involved in oxidation-reduction reactions necessary for tissue aerobic metabolism. Tryptophan may also be utilized in the biosynthesis of NAD, and diets rich in tryptophan

will offset low niacin intake in preventing deficiency. Pellagra is rare in the United States today, where dietary intake of animal protein tends to be high, but is classically manifested by cutaneous, gastrointestinal, and neurologic abnormalities. This clinical syndrome is often recalled with a mnemonic, the "three Ds": dermatitis, diarrhea, and dementia.[53] Typical clinical findings include desquamating skin rash; sialorrhea, stomatitis, and diarrhea; and headache, depression, memory loss, hallucinations and dementia, and motor and sensory changes.

Niacin toxicity has been primarily associated with the chronic therapeutic use of large doses of nicotinic acid as a lipid-lowering agent, although an epidemic has been reported in 17 persons after an acute "overdose" of pumpernickel bagels.[48,61-65] A 56-year-old man, attempting to treat his schizophrenia with high doses of niacin (19,500 mg), developed severe, persistent hypotension requiring intensive care management and dopamine.[66] Clinical effects predominate in the skin and gastrointestinal tract. Cutaneous manifestations of flushing and pruritus are common and classically have been attributed to histamine release[48] although more recent work suggests that prostaglandin E_2 is responsible and that pretreatment with prostaglandin inhibitors such as aspirin ameliorate this effect.[63] Hyperkeratosis and acanthosis nigricans have also been described in chronic users. Gastrointestinal effects include those that are likely mediated by prostaglandin, such as exacerbation of peptic ulcer disease, and hepatotoxicity, which may range from mild cholestatic jaundice to severe hepatitis with fulminant hepatic failure.[63-65] Hepatitis is typically associated with dosages ranging from 3 to 4.5 g/day for 1 to 18 months, although a patient has been reported to have developed hepatic dysfunction after 10 years of treatment without apparent prior side effects.[64] Recent studies suggest that time-release forms of niacin are more hepatotoxic.[63,64] Occasional additional findings include thrombocytopenia,[64] increased serum uric acid and gouty arthritis, glucose intolerance,[61] skeletal muscle myopathy,[62] and increased incidence of atrial fibrillation and other arrhythmias.[26,61] In most cases, all these effects have regressed with discontinuation of the niacin.

Thiamine

INTRODUCTION AND RELEVANT HISTORY

Thiamine was the first identified of the B-complex vitamins. Its history is traced back to the 19th-century Japanese navy; it was shown that adding fish, meat, and vegetables to the sailors' poor diet of polished rice reduced the incidence of beriberi.[53] Today thiamine deficiency is still common in Western societies among chronic alcoholics and is observed in patients with other malnourished states including AIDS, cancer, hyperemesis gravidarum, and eating disorders. It is also endemic among breast-fed infants in developing countries where rice consumption is high. Thiamine deficiency is classically associated with neurologic and cardiovascular abnormalities and includes the neurologic syndromes of alcoholic neuritis, Wernicke's encephalopa-

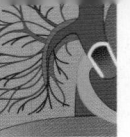
thy, and Korsakoff's psychosis[53,67,68] and the cardiovascular effects of peripheral vasodilation, biventricular heart failure, and peripheral edema. Thiamine pyrophosphate, the biologically active form of the vitamin, is a vital coenzyme in numerous metabolic pathways involving carbohydrate metabolism. It has been observed that rapid infusion of hypertonic glucose solutions to treat endogenous hypoglycemia may precipitate both neurologic and cardiac deterioration in thiamine-deficient patients, and concomitant thiamine administration is recommended.[68]

TOXICOLOGY

Oral absorption of thiamine is relatively limited, and large doses (e.g., 100 mg, or almost 100 times the RDI) are usually administered intravenously for the emergency treatment of suspected thiamine deficiency. In this context, a few severe anaphylactic reactions have been described,[69] while in a series of more than 1000 IV thiamine treatments given to 989 consecutive patients over a 6-month period only one patient with generalized pruritus was considered to have a possible precursor of anaphylaxis (less than 0.1%) and 11 patients with localized burning at the infusion site.[70] Of note, any patient with a history of thiamine reaction (number not stated) was excluded. The incidence of local reactions may be decreased if thiamine is administered slowly via relatively larger veins.[67,70] While thiamine is no longer used commonly in chronic therapeutic regimens, there are reports from the 1940s of headache, irritability, insomnia, tachycardia, and weakness said to resemble hyperthyroidism with doses as low as 5 mg/day for 4 to 5 weeks.[61,70]

Vitamin C (Ascorbic Acid)

INTRODUCTION AND RELEVANT HISTORY

Scurvy, the vitamin C deficiency state, has been recognized as a disease since the Middle Ages, and its relation to diets lacking fresh fruit and vegetables has been understood since the 16th to 18th centuries.[53] The human (along with other primates, guinea pigs, and Indian fruit bats) is one of the few mammals unable to synthesize vitamin C from glucose. This vitamin functions as an important cofactor for numerous hydroxylation and amidation reactions and has antioxidant properties. It is vital to normal synthesis of collagen, proteoglycans, and other components of the intercellular matrix, and therefore the structural integrity of tooth, bone, and capillary endothelium.[53] Scurvy is rarely encountered today, but occasional cases are still reported in malnourished persons, especially shut-ins and those espousing exaggerated food faddism.[71] One of the authors recalls from his medical school days a patient who developed scurvy by eating only at a fast-food restaurant. He felt this food would be free from contaminants, since it had been sold to millions of customers. Cutaneous findings include perifollicular hemorrhages, hyperkeratotic papules, petechiae, ecchymoses, and poor wound healing.[53,71] Additional effects include bone pain with subperiosteal hemorrhage, gingivitis and loosening of the teeth, and anemia.

TOXICOLOGY

The antioxidant (or free radical scavenger) effects of vitamin C effects have prompted widespread and largely unsupervised experimentation with megadose treatment (e.g., in excess of 1 g/day).[48,50,61] Numerous adverse effects have been ascribed to such usage, although with little controlled study.[72] These effects may include diarrhea and urinary calculi from oxalates or cysteine.[73] Rebound scurvy has been seen in persons abruptly discontinuing long-term high-dose therapy and also occurs in infants of mothers taking such doses.[48,53] Concern has been raised about increased blood estradiol levels noted in women taking oral contraceptive pills and high-dose vitamin C, as well as about this vitamin's potential to increase iron absorption in patients with iron overload states such as hemolytic anemia and hemochromatosis.[48,72] In contrast, most recent reviews have found that dosages of up to 4 g/day are actually unlikely to result in significant toxicity in otherwise healthy persons.[49,50,74] In particular, a prospective cohort study on over 45,000 men aged 40 to 75 years compared those taking 1500 mg/day or more with those taking less than 250 mg/day, and found no increased incidence of kidney stones in the high-dose patients.[75] Withdrawal of vitamin C (with surveillance for rebound scorbutic effects) and supportive care should suffice for treatment of presumed toxicity. It is probably prudent to caution against the use of high-dose vitamin C therapy for patients with known nephrolithiasis, G6PD deficiency, iron overload conditions, pregnancy, and perhaps for women taking oral contraceptives.

REFERENCES

1. Rudman D, Williams PJ: Megadose vitamins—use and misuse. N Engl J Med 1983;309:488.
2. Marcus R, Coulston AM: The vitamins: introduction. In Hardman JG, Limbard LE, Gilman AG (eds): Goodman and Gilman's The Pharmacologic Basis of Therapeutics, 10th ed. New York, McGraw-Hill, 2001, pp 1745–1752.
3. U.S. Food and Drug Administration: Reference daily intakes. Available at http://www.fda.gov/fdac/special/foodlabel/rdichrt.html. Accessed 12/22/03.
4. Davidson RA: Complications of megavitamin therapy. South Med J 1984;77:200.
5. Evans CDH, Lacey JH: Toxicity of vitamins: complications of a health movement. BMJ 1986;292:509.
6. Hoffer A, Osmond H: Treatment of schizophrenia with nicotinic acid: a ten-year follow-up. Acta Psychiatr Scand 1964;40:171.
7. Pauling L: Vitamin C and the Common Cold. San Francisco, WH Freeman, 1970.
8. Jukes TH: Revolution and counterrevolution in nutrition. Ann Nutr Health 1973;28:8.
9. Subar AF, Block G: Use of vitamin and mineral supplements: demographics and amounts of nutrients consumed. The 1987 Health Interview Survey. Am J Epidemiol 1990;132:1091.
10. Rapola JM, Virtamo J, Haukka JK, et al: Effect of vitamin E and beta-carotene on the incidence of angina pectoris: a randomized, double-blind, controlled trial. JAMA 1996;275:693.
11. Stephens NG, Parsons A, Schofield PM, et al: Randomised controlled trial of vitamin E in patients with coronary disease: Cambridge heart antioxidant study (CHAOS). Lancet 1996;347:781.

12. McDermott JH: Antioxidant nutrients: current dietary recommendations and research update. J Am Pharm Assoc (Wash) 2000; 40:785–799.

13. Johnson LJ, Meacham SL, Kurskall LJ:The antioxidants—vitamin C, vitamin E, selenium, and carotenoids. J Agromed 2003;9:65–82.

14. Fletcher RH, Fairfield KM: Vitamins for chronic disease prevention in adults—clinical applications. JAMA 2002;287:3127–3129.

15. Marcus R, Coulston AM: Fat-soluble vitamins. In Hardman JG, Limbard LE, Gilman AG (eds): Goodman & Gilman's The Pharmacologic Basis of Therapeutics, 9th ed. New York, McGraw-Hill, 2001, pp 1773–1791.

16. Kane EK: Arctic Explorations in the Years 1853, 1854, 1855. Vol. 1. Philadelphia, Childs & Peterson, 1856, p 392.

17. Misbah SA, Peiris JB, Atukorala TMS: Ingestion of shark liver associated with pseudotumor cerebri due to acute hypervitaminosis A. J Neurol Neurosurg Psychiatry 1984;47:216.

18. Hussey GD, Klein M: A randomized, controlled trial of vitamin A in children with severe measles. N Engl J Med 1990;323:160.

19. Stryer L: Visual excitation and recovery. J Biol Chem 1991; 266:10711–10714.

20. Ross AC: Vitamin A status: relationship to immunity and the antibody response—minireview. Proc Soc Exp Biol Med 1992;200:303.

21. Olson JA: The irresistible fascination of carotenoids and vitamin A: the 1992 Atwater lecture. Am J Clin Nutr 1993;57:833.

22. Nagai K, Hosaka H, Jubo S, et al: Vitamin A toxicity secondary to excessive intake of yellow-green vegetables, liver and laver. J Hepatol 1999;31:142–148.

23. Carpenter TO, Pettifor JM, Russell RM, et al: Severe hypervitaminosis A in siblings: evidence of variable tolerance to retinol intake. J Pediatr 1987;111:507.

24. Biesalski HK: Comparative assessment of the toxicology of vitamin A and retinoids in man. Toxicology 1989;57:117.

25. Mendoza FS, Johnson F, Kerner JA, et al: Vitamin A intoxication presenting with ascites and a normal vitamin A level. West J Med 1988;148:88.

26. Dipalma JR, Ritchie DM: Vitamin toxicity. Annu Rev Pharmacol Toxicol 1977;17:133.

27. Kowalski TE, Falestiny M, Furth E, Malet PF: Vitamin A hepatotoxicity: a cautionary note regarding 25,000 IU supplements. Am J Med 1994;97:523.

28. Persson B, Tunell R, Ekengran K: Chronic vitamin A intoxication during the first half year of life: description of 5 cases. Acta Pediatr Scand 1965;54:49.

29. James MB, Leonard JC, Fraser JJ, Stuemky JH: Hypervitaminosis A: a case report. Pediatrics 1982;69:112.

30. Rosenberg HK, Berezin S, Heyman S, et al: Pleural effusion and ascites: unusual presenting features in a pediatric patient with vitamin A intoxication. Clin Pediatr 1982;21:435.

31. Baxi SC, Dailey GE: Hypervitaminosis A: a cause of hypercalcemia. West J Med 1982;137:429.

32. Lammer EJ, Chen DT, Hoar RM, et al: Retinoic acid embryopathy. N Engl J Med 1985;313:837.

33. Kochlar DM, Christian MS: Tretinoin: a review of the nonclinical developmental toxicology experience. J Am Acad Dermatol 1997;36:S47–S59.

34. Rosa FW, Wilk AL, Kelsey FO: Teratogen update: vitamin A congeners. Teratology 1986;33:355.

35. Rothman KJ, Moore LL, Singer MR, et al: Teratogenicity of high vitamin A intake. N Engl J Med 1995;333:1369.

36. Bergman SM, O'Malia J, Krane NK, Wallin JD: Vitamin A induced hypercalcemia: response to corticosteroids. Nephron 1988;50:362.

37. Marcus R: Agents affecting calcification and bone turnover: calcium, phosphate, parathyroid hormone, vitamin D, calcitonin, and other compounds. In Hardman JG, Limbard LE, Gilman AG (eds): Goodman & Gilman's The Pharmacologic Basis of Therapeutics, 10th ed. New York, McGraw-Hill, 2001, pp 1715–1723.

38. Haddad JG: Vitamin D: solar rays, Milky Way or both? N Engl J Med 1992;326:1213.

39. British Paediatric Association: Hypercalcemia in infants and vitamin D. BMJ 1956;2:149.

40. Vieth R, Pinto T, Reen B, Wong M: Vitamin D poisoning by table sugar. Lancet 2002;359:672.

41. Jacobus CH, Holick MF, Shao Q, et al: Hypervitaminosis D associated with drinking milk. N Engl J Med 1992;326:1173.

42. Blank S, Scanlon KS, Sinks TH, et al: An outbreak of hypervitaminosis D associated with the overfortification of milk from a home-delivery dairy. Am J Public Health 1995;85:656.

43. Pettifor JM, Bikle DD, Caveleros M, et al: Serum levels of free 1,25-dihydroxyvitamin D in vitamin D toxicity. Ann Intern Med 1995; 122:511.

44. Iqbal SJ, Taylor WH: Treatment of vitamin D_2 poisoning by induction of hepatic enzymes. BMJ 1982;285:541.

45. Rizzoli R, Stoermann C, Ammann P, Bonjour JP: Hypercalcemia and hyperosteolysis in vitamin D intoxication: effects of clodronate therapy. Bone 1994;15:193.

46. Selby PL, Davies M, Marks JS, Mawer EB: Vitamin D intoxication causes hypercalcaemia by increased bone resorption which responds to pamidronate. Clin Endocrinol 1995;43:531.

47. Lee DC, Lee GY: The use of pamidronate for hypercalcemia secondary to acute vitamin D intoxication. J Toxicol Clin Toxicol 1998;36:719–721.

48. Toxic effects of vitamin overdosage. Med Lett Drugs Ther 198426:73.

49. Garewal HS, Diplock AT: How safe are antioxidant vitamins? Drug Saf 1995;13:8.

50. Diplock AT: Safety of antioxidant vitamins and β-carotene. Am J Clin Nutr 1995;62:1510S.

51. Alade SL, Brown RE, Paquet A: Polysorbate 80 and E-Ferol toxicity. Pediatrics 1986;77:593.

52. Brousson MA, Klein MC: Controversies surrounding the administration of vitamin K to newborns: a review. Can Med Assoc J 1996;154:307.

53. Marcus R, Coulston AM: Water-soluble vitamins: the vitamin B complex and ascorbic acid. In Hardman JG, Limbard LE, Gilman AG (eds): Goodman & Gilman's The Pharmacologic Basis of Therapeutics, 10th ed. New York, McGraw-Hill, 2001, pp 1753–1771.

54. Dalton K, Dalton MJ: Characteristics of pyridoxine overdose neuropathy syndrome. Acta Neurol Scand 1987;76:8.

55. Schaumberg H, Kaplan J, Windebank A, et al: Sensory neuropathy from pyridoxine abuse: a new megavitamin syndrome. N Engl J Med 1983;309:445.

56. Berger AR, Schaumberg HH, Schroeder C, et al: Dose response, coasting and differential fiber vulnerability in human toxic neuropathy: a prospective study of pyridoxine neurotoxicity. Neurology 1992;42:1367.

57. Gardner LI, Welsh-Sloan J, Cady RB: Phocomelia in infant whose mother took large doses of pyridoxine during pregnancy. Lancet 1985;1:636.

58. Morra M, Philipszoon HD, D'Andrea G, et al: Sensory and motor neuropathy caused by excessive ingestion of vitamin B6: a case report. Funct Neurol 1993;8:429.

59. Albin RL, Albers JW, Greenberg HS, et al: Acute sensory-neuropathy-neuronopathy from pyridoxine overdose. Neurology 1987;37:1729.

60. Albin RL, Albers JW: Long-term follow-up of pyridoxine-induced acute sensory neuropathy-neuronopathy. Neurology 1990;40:1319.

61. Alhadeff L, Gualtieri T, Lipton M: Toxic effects of water-soluble vitamins. Nutr Rev 1984;42:33.

62. Litin SC, Anderson CF: Nicotinic acid-associated myopathy: a report of three cases. Am J Med 1989;86:481.

63. Rader JI, Calvert RJ, Hathcock JN: Hepatic toxicity of unmodified and time-release preparations of niacin. Am J Med 1992;92:77.

64. Reimund E, Ramos A: Niacin-induced hepatitis and thrombocytopenia after 10 years of niacin use. J Clin Gastroenterol 1994; 18:270.

65. Gibbons LW, Gonzalez V, Gordon N, Grundy S: The prevalence of side effects with regular and sustained-release nicotinic acid. Am J Med 1995;99:378.

66. Santoni L, Strother JS, Grazer RE, et al: Critically ill niacin overdose. J Toxicol Clin Toxicol 2003;41:678.

67. Doyon S, Roberts JR: Reappraisal of the "coma cocktail": dextrose, flumazenil, naloxone, and thiamine. Emerg Med Clin North Am 1994;12:301.

68. Wrenn KD, Slovis CM: Neurologic complications of alcoholism. Emerg Med Clin North Am 1990;8:835.

69. Stephen JM, Grant R, Yeh CS: Anaphylaxis from administration of intravenous thiamine. Am J Emerg Med 1992;10:61.

70. Wrenn KD, Murphy F, Slovis CM: A toxicity study of parenteral thiamine hydrochloride. Ann Emerg Med 1989;18:867.

71. Kronauer CM, Buhler H: Skin findings in a patient with scurvy. N Engl J Med 1995;332:1611.

72. Sestili MA: Possible adverse health effects of vitamin C and ascorbic acid. Semin Oncol 1983;10:299.

73. Hamilton RJ: Vitamins. In Goldfrank LR, Flomenbaum NE, Lewin NE, et al (eds): Toxicologic Emergencies, 7th ed. Norwalk, CT, Appleton & Lange, 2002, pp 563–570.

74. Meyers DG, Maloney PA, Weeks D: Safety of antioxidant vitamins. Arch Intern Med 1996;156:925.

75. Curhan GC, Willett WC, Rimm EB, Stampfer MJ: A prospective study of the intake of vitamins C and B_6, and the risk of kidney stones in men. J Urol 1996;155:1847.

70 Performance Enhancers (Steroids, Creatine, DHEA)

DUNG THAI, MD, PHD ■ CHRISTINE A. HALLER, MD

At a Glance...

■ Use of anabolic steroids, steroid precursors, and other performance enhancers violates antidoping policies of the IOC and most collegiate and professional athletic associations; creatine supplementation is permitted.

■ Anabolic steroids are structural relatives of testosterone and have virilizing effects in females, cause gynecomastia and testicular atrophy in males, and produce short stature in children.

■ Organ system effects of anabolic steroids include hepato-toxicity, left ventricular (LV) hypertrophy, unfavorable blood lipid profiles, polycythemia, infertility, and aggression.

■ Steroid precursors such as androstenedione and DHEA are sold as dietary supplements because they are produced "naturally" in the body.

■ Steroid precursors do not increase strength or lean muscle mass in healthy users.

■ Short-term creatine supplementation is generally well tolerated but may produce muscle cramping and diarrhea; cases of compartment syndrome, rhabdomyolysis, and renal failure have been described.

Use of performance-enhancing drugs and supplements among amateur and professional athletes is widespread. Because the majority of drugs with performance-enhancing effects are banned by the International Olympic Committee (IOC) and other sports organizations, athletes may use oral sports supplements containing steroid precursors, amino acids, creatine, and herbal stimulants to gain a competitive edge and circumvent antidoping policies. Many of these commonly used substances have little or no proven benefits for improving athletic performance, and safety data are lacking. In addition, because these supplements are inadequately regulated, athletes may unknowingly ingest and test positive for a banned substance because of adulteration or improper labeling of the supplement. Some commonly used and potentially harmful performance enhancers including anabolic steroids, steroid precursors, and creatine are the focus of this chapter (Table 70-1). Sympathomimetics, erythropoietin, human growth hormone, and amino acid or protein supplements also are used by athletes but are not discussed here.

ANABOLIC STEROIDS

Anabolic steroids (ASs) are a class of synthetic molecules that are structurally related to testosterone and exert anabolic (i.e., muscle building) properties. ASs are most commonly prescribed by clinicians to treat disease-related wasting and disorders of testosterone deficiency.

They are abused by athletes seeking greater physical strength, ability, or appearance. Unfortunately, these steroids are not purely anabolic and, in fact, possess androgenic properties as well. Their androgenic qualities influence a number of different organ systems including the reproductive, cardiovascular, hematologic, central nervous, and hepatobiliary systems. The effects are most pronounced in athletes who tend to take suprapharmacologic doses.

Testosterone was first isolated, synthesized, and characterized in Europe in 1935.[1] Modern use as athletic performance enhancers began with Russian power-lifters in the early 1950s and peaked in the 1970s with the athletic programs in Germany. ASs have been banned by the IOC since 1964, yet their use is still widespread. In 1990, the Anabolic Steroids Control Act was enacted, putting ASs on Schedule III of the Controlled Substance Act and making them illegal without a prescription.[2] Despite these restrictions, use among athletes and teenagers continues. The Monitoring the Future (MTF) study, which has tracked anabolic steroid use among 8th, 10th, and 12th graders in the United States since 1989, reported that use of these substances was between 2.2% and 2.8% in 2000.[3] The majority of users were males. A 2001 National Collegiate Athletic Association (NCAA) study of substance use among college student-athletes revealed that anabolic steroid abuse had increased since 1997 and that the main reason for use was to improve athletic performance or appearance.[4]

Structure

All ASs currently available are structural analogs of testosterone. The core structure contains four fused rings with potential for modification in the A, B, or C rings as well as at carbon 17 (Fig. 70-1). Each structural modification imparts unique properties to the steroid derivative such as enhanced oral bioavailability, improved pharmacokinetics, or altered anabolic-to-androgenic activity. When testosterone is administered orally or by parenteral injection, the native molecule is rapidly degraded by the liver and does not achieve significant levels in the systemic circulation. For this reason, a number of formulations and structural derivatives have been prepared.

Testosterone is delivered as an injectable, transdermal patch, dermal gel, or micronized oral preparation. Wilson has presented an excellent review of the various formulations and structural properties,[5,6] which are described below.

1. Esterification of the 17-β hydroxyl group increases the lipophilicity of the steroid molecule and slows its release into the circulation. The ester must

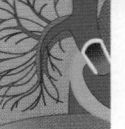

TABLE 70-1 Summary of Potential Adverse Effects of Common Performance Enhancers

ORGAN SYSTEM AND SPECIFIC HEALTH CONCERNS	ANABOLIC STEROIDS	STEROID HORMONE PRECURSORS	CREATINE
Cardiovascular	Hypertension, LVH, CHF, decreased HDL cholesterol	Decreased HDL	None known
Gastrointestinal/liver	Increased LFT, cholestatic jaundice, peliosis hepatis	None known	Diarrhea, gastromitestinal, pain, concern for suppression of hepatic creatine synthesis
Musculoskeletal	Increased muscle strength and mass	No different from placebo	Osmotic cell swelling, muscle cramping, rhabdomyolysis
Neurologic/psychiatric	Mood lability, euphoria, increased libido, withdrawal symptoms	None known	None known; rare reports of seizures
Reproductive/pregnancy/lactation	Amenorrhea, testicular atrophy, decreased or morphologically abnormal sperm, feminization in men, masculinization in women	Transient rise in testosterone or estradiol	Effects on testicular creatine production unknown
Hematologic	Polycythemia	None known	None known
Renal	None known	None known	Elevated serum and urinary creatinine; long-term effects on GFR unknown
Mutagenic/carcinogenic	Heptoma, hepatocellular carcinoma	None known	None known
Pediatric/adolescent	Precocious puberty, early closure of epiphyseal plates	None known	Theoretical concerns about effects on developing kidneys and immature musculature

CHF, congestive heart failure; GFR, glomerular filtration tate; HDL, high-density lipoprotein; LFT, liver function test; LVH, left ventricular hypertrophy.

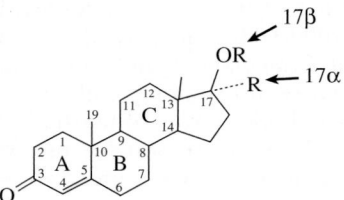

FIGURE 70-1 Core structure of anabolic steroids.

undergo hydrolysis before the steroid can act at its target receptor. Except for the undecenoate, these steroid esters are injectable.

2. Alkylation of the 17-α position renders the steroid resistant to hepatic degradation. These derivatives are orally active.

3. Alteration of the A, B, or C rings slows metabolism, increases or decreases affinity for the androgen receptor, or imparts resistance to aromatization.

The pharmacologic and toxicologic effects of the various steroid analogs can be predicted based on its chemical alteration. The 17-α alkylated androgens are more resistant to portal hepatic metabolism but are also more hepatotoxic. Fluoxymesterone, 19-nortestosterone, and 1-methyl-substituted steroids are not aromatized at the A ring to form estrogen-like compounds. Consequently, they lack the feminizing properties of testosterone. A final example is 7α-methyl-19-nortestosterone, which is a poor substrate for 5α-reductase and possesses minimal activity in prostate tissue.

Pharmacology[7]

The biosynthesis of testosterone from cholesterol is a multistep process involving enzymes in both the adrenal glands and the testis or ovaries. Cholesterol undergoes side chain cleavage and A-ring oxidation to form pregnenolone, which has two potential pathways to testosterone (Fig. 70-2). The pathway shown in bold arrows represents the predominant pathway and includes dehydroepiandrosterone (DHEA) as an intermediate. Alternatively, progesterone can be converted to androstenedione via 17-hydroxyprogesterone. Androstenedione and testosterone are reversibly interconverted.

Testosterone can be metabolized to active and inactive metabolites by extraglandular tissue. It can be reduced at the 5-α position to dihydrotestosterone, which influences male sexual development and virilization. Testosterone is also a substrate for adipose tissue aromatase, which synthesizes estrogens. These estrogens are responsible for testosterone's feminizing properties. The major inactive urinary metabolites include etiocholanolone and androsterone, which exist as free steroids or water-soluble conjugates.

PHARMACOLOGIC AGENTS

A list of the most commonly abused ASs is shown in Box 70-1. They are all classified as class III agents by the DEA and are banned by the IOC.

Several different dosing regimens are utilized to enhance the anabolic effects, to minimize side effects,

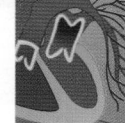

FIGURE 70-2 Biosynthesis of androgens and estrogens.

and to avoid detection of steroids in urine and blood.[8] "Stacking steroids" involves using two agents at once. This may include injectable forms taken with oral agents, or short-acting forms taken with long-acting agents. "Stacking the pyramid" is a regimen similar to "stacking steroids" except that doses of ASs are progressively escalated until halfway through the cycle at which point doses are then decreased to zero. Cycles last from 6 to 12 weeks. Another regimen termed *cycling* involves alternating between periods of use and nonuse. Periods vary between 6 and 14 weeks. It is not known whether continuous or intermittent regimens exert greater adverse effects on the body.

Toxicology

ANABOLIC EFFECTS

The anabolic properties of androgens in women and hypogonadal men are undisputed. East German sports programs reported impressive performances by their female athletes during the clandestine doping experiments of the 1970s and 1980s.[1] Testosterone replacement has also been shown to increase lean body mass in hypogonadal HIV patients.[9]

Despite these positive results in women and hypogonadal males, there was long-standing controversy regarding the anabolic potential of androgens in eugonadal males. Much of the debate arose because only slight and transient positive nitrogen balance was observed after modest doses of androgens were given. In addition, athletic performance did not improve when testosterone or other ASs were added to a training regimen. Critics argued that many of the studies were not standardized in terms of steroid dosing or training regimens, lacked proper controls, were unblinded, and relied on case studies or small study populations.[10] When suprapharmacologic doses of steroids were used to assess upper-body weight-lifting tasks in highly trained athletes, a statistically significant increase in muscle mass and strength was seen relative to placebo.[11] Bhasin and

BOX 70-1	COMMONLY ABUSED ANABOLIC STEROIDS
Oral	**Injectable**
Oxymetholone	Nandrolone decanoate
Oxandrolone	Nandrolone phenpropionate
Methndrostenolone	Testosterone cypionate
Stanozolol	Boldenone undecylenate
	Tetrahydrogestrinone

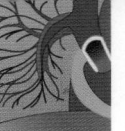

associates were able to demonstrate increases in fat-free mass and muscle size and strength in normal men on supraphysiologic doses of testosterone.[12]

VIRILIZING EFFECTS

All currently available ASs possess some androgenic properties. These virilizing properties are most apparent in women and children, whose testosterone levels increase several-fold from baseline. Elevations of up to 30-fold from normal have been reported in women self-administering testosterone and ASs.[13] Masculinization is one of the first effects seen in female athletes given ASs.[14,15] Deepening of the voice, clitoral hypertrophy, amenorrhea, hirsutism, and decreased body fat are reported in a majority of female athletes. In addition, approximately half these women experience acne, male pattern balding, and change in breast size. Deepening of the voice and clitoral hypertrophy are often irreversible after prolonged therapy. The other signs and symptoms may regress when the androgens are withdrawn.

Children taking ASs experience precocious puberty in the form of acne, early growth of pubic hair, penile enlargement, and frequent erections. ASs can also stunt the growth of children and adolescents. A 1956 study by Sobel and colleagues on the use of methyltestosterone as a growth stimulant in children noted profound discrepancy between height age and bone age.[16] Keele and Worley conducted a double-blind, placebo-controlled study on the effects of oxymetholone on growth in children and found that 12 months of treatment caused a mean increase in height relative to placebo without significant differences in bone age.[17] Thus, while short-term accelerated growth of bone is seen during early administration of ASs, long-term use leads to early closure of the epiphyseal plates and decreased stature compared with predicted height. Stunted growth is irreversible and is seen mainly with oxandrolone.

FEMINIZATION

Under physiologic conditions, a small percentage of naturally produced testosterone is metabolized to estradiol. The enzyme responsible for this reaction is aromatase and is found predominantly in adipose tissue. Male athletes administered parenteral testosterone esters in supraphysiologic doses have elevated plasma estradiol levels.[18] Consequently, they can develop gynecomastia and increased fatty deposition. The occurrence of gynecomastia is unpredictable but is more commonly observed in children or in adult males taking high doses of androgen. Feminization in male athletes is a phenomenon observed with steroids susceptible to aromatization (i.e., C_{19} steroids with a Δ^4, 3-keto configuration). Poor substrates for aromatase such as 19-nortestosterone and fluoxymesterone do not cause these side effects. Treatment of gynecomastia includes antiestrogens such as tamoxifen and clomiphene.[19]

REPRODUCTIVE SYSTEM EFFECTS

High doses of ASs are known to interrupt the hypothalamic-pituitary-gonadal axis in healthy men and women. ASs suppress gonadotropin (leutinizing hormone [LH] and follicle-stimulating hormone [FSH]) production, which normally acts on gonadal tissue to produce estrogen, progesterone, and testosterone. As mentioned above, women taking high-dose steroids frequently report irregular menses or amenorrhea. The hormonal perturbations resulting from ASs in healthy male athletes have been extensively studied.[20] Testicular atrophy, decreased sperm count, and increase in morphologically abnormal sperm paralleled reduction in serum FSH and LH.[21,22] The resulting infertility often remains long after the androgens are stopped but is reversible. Treatment with recombinant human chorionic gonadotropin can expedite return of normal sperm count and morphology.[23]

ERYTHROPOIESIS

Discrepancies in hemoglobin concentration between adult males and females appear to be related to differences in testosterone levels. Stimulation of erythropoiesis is a common effect of testosterone and other ASs. For this reason, ASs have had some therapeutic use in treating anemia. ASs in healthy athletes without anemia can cause profound polycythemia. Urhausen and coworkers[24] compared hemoglobin and hematocrit values in former and current male AS users and found significantly higher values in current users. Leukocyte and platelet counts were also increased. The average increase in hemoglobin concentration with pharmacologic doses of testosterone esters is 1 g/dL in men and 4.3 g/dL in women. Like many other effects of anabolic steroid use, erythropoiesis is reversible if the drug is discontinued.

HEPATOTOXICITY

ASs alkylated at the 17-α position are orally bioavailable and resist portal hepatic metabolism. These 17-α derivatives are also more hepatotoxic and are associated with elevated liver enzymes, peliosis hepatis, cholestatic jaundice, and hepatic neoplasms. Dickerman and colleagues observed that the incidence of hepatotoxicity may be overestimated if measured in terms of elevation in aspartate aminotransferase (AST) and alanine aminotransferase (ALT) in male resistance trainers.[25] Resistance training alone can cause elevations of AST and ALT, which are released from skeletal muscle. For this reason, the authors advocate measuring γ-glutamyl transferase (GGT) levels to assess specific hepatic damage along with creatine phosphokinase (CPK) levels to assess skeletal muscular damage. Despite these claims, Urhausen and coworkers have shown that plasma AST and ALT levels are higher in bodybuilders taking ASs than in body builders not taking these drugs.[24] GGT and bilirubin in the two groups were not above the normal reference range. In fact, GGT was lower in current abusers. The authors also point out that AST/ALT ratios are less than 1, which is more consistent with a hepatic rather than a skeletal muscular source of AST and ALT. Transaminase concentrations normalized after cessation of steroid use.

Cholestatic Jaundice

Numerous reports of cholestatic jaundice suggest that its development is dependent on the dose and duration

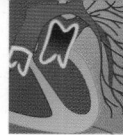

of exposure to 17-α substituted steroids. This condition is more common when high doses are used or in the presence of preexisting liver disease.[26,27] The doses and regimens of ASs used in the setting of sports enhancement likely pose potential risk of cholestatic liver disease. Jaundice, anorexia, malaise, and nausea develop in a minority of individuals. The liver is often cholestatic without frank inflammation. While some individuals have isolated elevations in AST, ALT, and bilirubin, rarely do they experience liver failure or necrosis as a result of 17-α steroid use. The cholestasis resolves when the drugs are discontinued.

Peliosis Hepatis

Peliosis hepatitis is a rare condition characterized by multiple small hemorrhagic cysts randomly distributed throughout the liver. Several cases associated with anabolic steroid use have been reported including one young athlete who was a long-term intermittent steroid user.[28] Fibrosis and portal hypertension as well as life-threatening hemorrhagic rupture of the cysts may occur. The cysts may recede when ASs are stopped.

Hepatic Adenomas and Carcinomas

Benign adenomas and malignant hepatocellular carcinoma have been reported in users of 17-α alkyl steroids.[29] Evidence for a strong cause–effect relationship comes from reports of hepatic adenoma regression upon discontinuation of the 17-α substituted steroid.[30] A more serious consequence of abuse of these androgens is hepatocellular carcinoma.[31] Athletes who use higher doses of oral androgens for long periods of time are particularly susceptible. The average time interval between initiation of oral ASs and detection of hepatocellular carcinoma is approximately 6 years. These highly vascularized tumors also can rupture, causing serious bleeding. Interestingly, the hepatocellular carcinoma associated with 17-α alkylated steroid abuse tends not to metastasize and regresses after withdrawal of medication.[32]

CARDIOVASCULAR EFFECTS

The cardiovascular effects of ASs are numerous and include alterations of serum lipid profiles, change in LV dimension, and increase in diastolic blood pressure. Studies examining serum cholesterol profiles in AS abusers have revealed a marked decline in high-density lipoprotein (HDL), which is not dose-dependent.[33] Serum low-density lipoprotein (LDL) and cholesterol effects were less consistent. While some studies have demonstrated statistically significant elevations of LDL levels, others have shown no LDL increases in AS users as compared with nonusers. Several case reports have described myocardial infarction and sudden cardiac death in young bodybuilders taking ASs.[34,35]

Ass have been reported to increase blood pressure in athletes. Comparison of blood pressure in weight-lifting AS users and nonusers revealed that resting and exertional systolic and diastolic values were higher in AS users.[36] However, after adjusting for biceps size, the authors concluded that differences in blood pressure may be an artifact of larger arm circumference in AS subjects. In a double-blind, crossover study of ASs in five body builders given nandrolone or placebo, diastolic blood pressures were higher during nandrolone treatment.[37] Values returned to baseline 6 weeks after cessation of AS use. Systolic blood pressures were not altered. Effects of ASs on blood pressure are thus not clear-cut.

Echocardiographic evaluations of LV size and function in elite body builders using ASs have yielded mixed results. Two studies showed increased LV wall and ventricular septal thickening associated with decreased ventricular compliance in weight lifters using versus not using ASs.[38,39] Greater LV mass and septal thickness were demonstrated in the same users on-versus-off AS dosing cycles. De Piccoli and associates[40] assessed LV morphology and function in AS-abusing bodybuilders, non-AS-abusing body builders, and sedentary individuals and found that AS could induce LV enlargement and thickening, leading to decreased diastolic compliance. Echocardiographic findings in sedentary controls and nonusers were similar. In contrast, a study by Salke and colleagues[41] concluded that weight lifting alone could cause myocardial hypertrophy and that AS does not potentiate this effect. In all of the above studies, there was no demonstrable impairment of LV function.

The risk of congestive heart failure may be increased in AS abusers because of the well-documented fluid-retaining properties of these androgens.[42] Niemenen and associates[43] reported two cases of male steroid-abusing weight trainers who exhibited signs and symptoms of congestive heart failure. These patients had echocardiographic evidence of LV hypertrophy and diastolic dysfunction both of which reversed with cessation of AS use. In individuals with myocardial changes from weight training and AS use, the added effect of fluid retention may be the determinant in exacerbating congestive heart failure. Despite these reports, the occurrence of heart failure in a population of healthy young AS-abusing athletes is rare.

PSYCHOLOGICAL EFFECTS

Behavioral effects of ASs include direct psychoactive effects such as psychosis and aggression as well as withdrawal-related symptoms such as depression. Because androgens play an important role in the development of secondary sexual characteristics, it is no surprise that many abusers who take supraphysiologic doses report increased libido. Other effects include euphoria, increased energy, and greater confidence as well as aggression, irritability, and mood lability. A phenomenon known as "steroid rage" has been described and may be responsible for criminal acts carried out by AS abusers, who prior to taking these drugs, did not have criminal records.[44] Several examples of manic behavior are also reported. Pope and Katz[45] conducted a controlled study of 88 athletes using ASs and 68 control athletes and found that 23% of steroid users reported mania, hypomania, or depression versus 6% of controls. Another study comparing aggression and mood changes in AS-abusing and nonabusing male weight lifters found

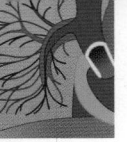

that supraphysiologic testosterone concentrations were associated with aggressive tendencies.[46]

Symptoms associated with withdrawal from steroids include depression, insomnia, anorexia, decreased libido, and fatigue. Kashkin and Kleber[47] compared the delayed depressive syndrome resulting from a fall in serum steroids to that observed in withdrawing cocaine-dependent individuals. Along with the above symptoms, the loss of physical prowess and muscular physique may have profound psychological effects on the steroid user. Dramatic changes in body image and performance often drive these athletes to resume use of ASs.

STEROID PRECURSORS

Androstenedione and DHEA are two important steroid precursors that are widely used and readily available in health food stores and pharmacies and via the Internet. Under the 1994 Dietary Supplement and Health Education Act, these agents can be sold over-the-counter because they occur "naturally" in the body. However, use of these supplements is currently banned by the IOC and several other athletic associations. Despite these bans, androstenedione and DHEA sales are on the rise. Androstenedione became popular after major league baseball player Mark McGwire admitted to taking it during the 1998 baseball season when he broke the major league home run record. DHEA has been touted as a "fountain-of-youth" remedy and has also been embraced by athletes as a "natural" precursor to testosterone.

Structure and Pharmacology

Androstenedione and DHEA are androgen precursors, that is, intermediates in the synthesis pathway of testosterone from cholesterol (see Figure 70-2). Strictly speaking, they are *androgenic* steroids and have not been proven to be *anabolic* steroids, and therefore they remain available as over-the-counter supplements instead of Schedule III Controlled Substances.

Androstenedione is produced by the adrenal glands and gonads and can be converted to either estrone or testosterone. It is currently marketed as a "natural" alternative to ASs, with claims that it increases serum testosterone levels and enhances muscle growth when combined with resistance training. In healthy women, a 100-mg dose of androstenedione resulted in a six- to sevenfold increase in serum testosterone levels.[48] Variable results were reported in healthy males taking androstenedione 100 to 300 mg/day. Statistically significant increases in serum testosterone levels were achieved within the first week of treatment at 200 to 300 mg/day relative to placebo,[49] but levels returned to baseline at 12 weeks of treatment.[50] Estradiol levels were significantly elevated at all doses. In addition, statistically significant decreases in HDL cholesterol were observed at 2, 5, and 8 weeks after initiation of androstenedione along with resistance training. Investigators have failed to demonstrate skeletal muscle adaptation to resistance

training or favorable changes in lean body mass when androstenedione is taken at recommended doses.[49,50]

DHEA is produced by the adrenal glands and is the most abundant steroid hormone in the blood. DHEA has been similarly studied to evaluate its role in altering serum testosterone levels and resistance training in healthy young males.[51] While DHEA supplementation does produce a rise in serum androstenedione, it does not affect serum testosterone or estrogen levels. In addition, DHEA does not increase strength or lean body mass in men compared with placebo treatment. Interestingly, a dose of 1600 mg/day (recommended dose, 30 to 90 mg/day) has been shown to reduce serum LDL and body fat in five healthy men with no reported side effects.[52] However, a similar evaluation of 1600 mg/day DHEA in eight healthy men did not demonstrate LDL or body fat alterations.[53]

CREATINE

Oral creatine supplementation has become a popular practice among athletes of all ages, and creatine is probably the best-studied sports supplement. Surveys on creatine use report that 28% of collegiate athletes use this supplement regularly, and creatine use has been reported by athletes as young as 10 years of age.[54] Typical use of creatine involves a loading period of 20 g/day for 5 days, followed by a maintenance dose of 2 to 5 g/day,[55] although continued high-dose use is not uncommon.

Structure and Pharmacology

Creatine is a nitrogenous amino-acid derivative that is ingested at the rate of 1 to 2 g/day in diets that include fish and meat (Fig. 70-3). An equal amount of creatine is synthesized endogenously in the liver, kidney, and pancreas. Creatine is found in numerous body tissues including skeletal muscle, heart, brain, and testes. It is entirely excreted by the kidneys after conversion to creatinine, and creatine supplementation can cause a small dose-dependent rise in serum creatinine.[56] Creatine has a single physiologic role (i.e., reversible equilibrium with phosphocreatine in generation of ATP during skeletal muscle contraction under anaerobic conditions). This reaction generates adenosine triphosphate (ATP) for 10 to 20 seconds. Creatine supplementation is claimed to enhance athletic performance by raising phosphocreatine muscle stores and increasing the duration of burst-exercise capacity.

Limited human pharmacologic data suggest that creatine exhibits saturable kinetics.[57] Both the volume of distribution and clearance decrease with increasing oral dose, possibly owing to limitations in skeletal muscle

$$H_2N-\overset{\displaystyle |}{\underset{\displaystyle NH}{C}}-\overset{\displaystyle CH_3}{\underset{}{N}}-CH_2-\overset{\displaystyle O}{\underset{}{C}}-OH$$

FIGURE 70-3 Chemical structure of creatinine.

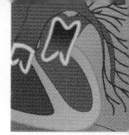

uptake and storage of creatine. With loading doses of 20 g/day, maximal intramuscular creatine levels appear to be achieved in about 2 days.[58] Continued high-dose creatine intake may be of no benefit beyond this time. Creatine levels remain elevated for as long as 1 month after supplementation owing to slow turnover of creatine to creatinine.[59]

A recent meta-analysis[60] of 96 published investigations concluded that creatine supplementation improves lean body mass and upper-body and repetitive-bout tasks lasting less than 30 seconds, such as stationary cycling sprints and weight lifting repetitions, but does not improve longer duration exercises such as running and swimming. Effect sizes were greater for loading than for maintenance creatine supplementation regimens, and there were no gender differences in effects of creatine. Creatine supplementation has also been demonstrated, in limited human studies, to improve the symptoms and slow the progression of certain neuromuscular diseases including muscular dystrophy, amyotrophic lateral sclerosis, and gyrate atrophy.[57]

Toxicology

Concerns about the safety of creatine supplementation have arisen from anecdotal case reports of dehydration, muscle cramping, rhabdomyolysis, and acute renal failure, as well as theoretical concerns about long-term use and effects on children and adolescents. One case of interstitial nephritis has been described in a 20-year-old male creatine user.[61] Creatine supplementation was also implicated in a case of relapsing nephrotic syndrome in a 25-year-old man.[62] Acute quadriceps compartment syndrome and rhabdomyolysis, necessitating bilateral thigh fasciotomy, was reported in a 24-year-old previously healthy male taking creatine 25 g/day for 1 year.[63]

Published studies indicate that short-term creatine use (<28 days) at recommended doses is not associated with significant adverse effects such as gastrointestinal, renal, or muscle dysfunction, although these were all performance studies involving fewer than 12 subjects.[64] Studies on side effects are limited, but one survey of NCAA Division I male baseball and football players who voluntarily took creatine revealed that of 52 athletes 16 (31%) reported having diarrhea, 13 (25%) experienced muscle cramps, and 7 (13%) complained of dehydration.[65] Rapid weight gain (within 24 hours of dosing) has been observed in several studies and is believed to be related to osmotic fluid retention in the muscle cell, which may account for reports of dehydration. Creatine has been shown to increase muscle compartment pressure both at rest and under exercise conditions.[66] No large-scale safety studies have been conducted on the long-term effects of chronic creatine supplementation.

Diagnosis

Adverse effects related to performance enhancers may go unrecognized because patients are reluctant to admit use of banned substances. Nonetheless, there are clinical signs and symptoms that suggest performance-enhancing drug and supplement use that could potentially be confirmed by serum and urine testing.

Evidence of masculinization in females, feminization in males, or short stature in young athletes suggests anabolic steroid use. Infertility, polycythemia, and abnormal liver function tests in athletes and body builders are other clinical clues of steroid use.

A thorough review of steroid drug testing is beyond the scope of this chapter, but basic principles of AS detection may be relevant for toxicologic diagnosis.[67] Testing for AS abuse has been controversial since its institution by the IOC in the early 1980s. Currently, the most widely used method for detecting ASs involves quantitative measurement of the parent compound or its metabolite in urine by gas chromatography (GC-MS). For compounds that are not naturally present in the body, such as nandrolone, diagnosis is straightforward. The detection of nandrolone or its metabolite in the urine of athletes strongly suggests that they have taken these ASs.

Testing for testosterone is more complicated because it is produced physiologically. For this reason, a urinary ratio of testosterone (T) to its 17-α epimer epitestosterone (E) is determined. T and E are produced in the body in relatively equivalent amounts and do not interconvert. Among healthy subjects not using ASs, the urinary ratio of T to E is approximately 1:1. Individuals who take T show a rise in their urinary T-to-E ratio. The IOC considers a result greater than 6:1 to be indicative of exogenous T use.[68] False-negative results can be obtained by coadministering E or using a short-acting T preparation that leaves the body quickly enough that the ratio falls below 6:1.[69] Other methods for detecting T have also been developed that evaluate T-to-E ratio over time, T-to-LH ratio, and T metabolite to other T metabolite ratios. Because these tests are time consuming and expensive, they are rarely utilized.

Androstenedione and DHEA supplementation cannot be confirmed by drug testing because these substances are produced endogenously. Occasionally, these products contain trace steroid contaminants, such as 19-noradrostenedione, that cause positive urine test results for metabolites of banned steroids such as nandrolone.[70]

Creatine can be measured in serum and urine, but such testing has little clinical utility. Creatine supplementation can increase serum creatinine in the absence of renal dysfunction owing to increased metabolic production and potential cross-reactivity of creatine with some creatinine assays.

Management

Treatment of adverse effects of performance-enhancing products is primarily supportive. Significant toxicity resulting from acute overdoses of oral steroids, androstenedione, DHEA, and creatine has not been described. No specific antidotes exist, and there is no role for enhanced elimination techniques in such cases. Because of reports of compartment syndrome and rhabdomyolysis with creatine, complaints of muscle pain or cramping by athletes warrant medical examination.

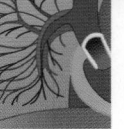
Rhabdomyolysis should be managed with aggressive hydration and alkalinization of the urine. Severe, persistent pain of the lower extremities may necessitate measurements of muscle compartment pressures.

Persons reporting long-term use of ASs may require evaluation of cardiac and hepatic function, including echocardiography and serum liver function tests. Athletes and body builders who report use of performance enhancers should be informed of the potential health risks associated with the use of such products, as well as the possibility of testing positive for banned substances.

REFERENCES

1. Yesalis C, Courson S, et al: History of anabolic steroid use in sport and exercise. In Yesalis C (ed): Anabolic Steroids in Sport and Exercise. Champaign, IL, Human Kinetics, 2000, pp 51–71.
2. Pub. L. 101-647, title XIX, Sec. 1902(a), Stat. 4851, Nov. 29, 1990, amending 21 U.S. Code 812(c) (1981) to include anabolic steroids.
3. Johnston L, O'Malley P, et al: Vol I: Secondary school students. NIH Publication No. 03-5375. Bethesda, MD, National Institute on Drug Abuse, 2003.
4. Green GA, Uryasz FD, Petr TA, Bray CD: NCAA study of substance use and abuse habits of college student-athletes. Clin J Sport Med 2001;11:51–56.
5. Wilson J: Androgens. In Hardman L, Limbird P, Molinoff R, et al (eds): Goodman and Gilman's Experimental Basis of Therapeutics. New York, McGraw-Hill, 1996, pp 1441–1457.
6. Wilson JD: Androgen abuse by athletes. Endocr Rev 1988;9:181–199.
7. Griffin J, Wilson J: Disorders of the testes. In Fauci A, Braunwald E, Isselbacher K, et al (eds): Harrison's Principles of Internal Medicine. New York, McGraw-Hill, 1998, pp 2087–2097.
8. Taylor W: Anabolic steroid regimens used by athletes. In Taylor W (ed): Anabolic Steroids and the Athlete. Jefferson, NC, McFarland and Company, 2002, pp 59–64.
9. Bhasin S, Storer TW, Javanbakht M, et al: Testosterone replacement and resistance exercise in HIV-infected men with weight loss and low testosterone levels. JAMA 2000;283:763–770.
10. Kuhn CM: Anabolic steroids. Recent Prog Horm Res 2002;57:411–434.
11. Giorgi A, Weatherby RP, Murphy PW: Muscular strength, body composition and health responses to the use of testosterone enanthate: a double blind study. J Sci Med Sport 1999;2:341–355.
12. Bhasin S, Storer TW, Berman N, et al: The effects of supraphysiologic doses of testosterone on muscle size and strength in normal men. N Engl J Med 1996;335:1–7.
13. Malarkey WB, Strauss RH, Leizman DJ, et al: Endocrine effects in female weight lifters who self-administer testosterone and anabolic steroids. Am J Obstet Gynecol 1991;165(5 pt 1):1385–1390.
14. Kennedy BJ, Nathanson IT: Effects of intensive sex steroid hormone therapy in advanced breast cancer. JAMA 1953;152:1135–1141.
15. Fruehan AE, Frawley TF: Current status of anabolic steroids. JAMA 1963;184:527–532.
16. Sobel EH, Raymond CS, Quinn KV, Talbot NB: The use of methyltestosterone to stimulate growth: relative influence on skeletal maturation and linear growth. J Clin Endocrinol Metab 1956;16:241–248.
17. Keele DK, Worley JW: Study of an anabolic steroid: certain effects of oxymetholone on small children. Am J Dis Child 1967;113:422–430.
18. Cunningham GR, Silverman VE, Thornby J, Kohler PO: The potential for an androgen male contraceptive. J Clin Endocrinol Metab 1979;49:520–526.
19. Khan HN, Blamey RW: Endocrine treatment of physiological gynaecomastia. BMJ 2003;327(7410):301–302.
20. Knuth UA, Maniera H, Nieschlag E: Anabolic steroids and semen parameters in bodybuilders. Fertil Steril 1989;52:1041–1047.
21. Inigo MA, Arrimadas E, Arroyo D: [43 cycles of anabolic steroid treatment studied in athletes: the uses and secondary effects.] Rev Clin Esp 2000;200:133–138.
22. Torres-Calleja J, Gonzalez-Unzaga M, DeCelis-Carrillo R, et al: Effect of androgenic anabolic steroids on sperm quality and serum hormone levels in adult male bodybuilders. Life Sci 2001;68:1769–1774.
23. Menon DK: Successful treatment of anabolic steroid-induced azoospermia with human chorionic gonadotropin and human menopausal gonadotropin. Fertil Steril 2003;79(Suppl 3):1659–1661.
24. Urhausen A, Torsten A, Wilfried K: Reversibility of the effects on blood cells, lipids, liver function and hormones in former anabolic-androgenic steroid abusers. J Steroid Biochem Mol Biol 2003;84:369–75.
25. Dickerman RD, Pertusi RM, Zachariah NY, et al: Anabolic steroid-induced hepatotoxicity: is it overstated? Clin J Sport Med 1999;9:34–39.
26. Evely RS, Triger DR, Milnes JP, et al: Severe cholestasis associated with stanozolol. BMJ (Clin Res Ed) 1987;294(6572):612–613.
27. Gurakar A, Caraceni P, Fagiuoli S, Van Thiel DH: Androgenic/anabolic steroid-induced intrahepatic cholestasis: a review with four additional case reports. J Okla State Med Assoc 1994;87:399–404.
28. Cabasso A: Peliosis hepatis in a young adult bodybuilder. Med Sci Sports Exerc 1994;26:2–4.
29. Balazs M: Primary hepatocellular tumours during long-term androgenic steroid therapy: a light and electron microscopic study of 11 cases with emphasis on microvasculature of the tumours. Acta Morphol Hung 1991;39:201–216.
30. Lowdell CP, Murray-Lyon IM: Reversal of liver damage due to long term methyltestosterone and safety of non-17 alpha-alkylated androgens. BMJ (Clin Res Ed) 1985;291(6496):637.
31. Ishak KG, Zimmerman HJ: Hepatotoxic effects of the anabolic/androgenic steroids. Semin Liver Dis 1987;7:230–236.
32. Shahidi NT: A review of the chemistry, biological action, and clinical applications of anabolic-androgenic steroids. Clin Ther 2001;23:1355–1390.
33. Glazer G: Atherogenic effects of anabolic steroids on serum lipid levels: a literature review. Arch Intern Med 1991;151:1925–1933.
34. Sullivan ML, Martinez CM, Gennis P, Gallagher EJ: The cardiac toxicity of anabolic steroids. Prog Cardiovasc Dis 1998;41:1–15.
35. Fineschi V, Baroldi G, Monciotti F, et al: Anabolic steroid abuse and cardiac sudden death: a pathologic study. Arch Pathol Lab Med 2001;125:253–255.
36. Riebe D, Fernhall B, Thompson PD: The blood pressure response to exercise in anabolic steroid users. Med Sci Sports Exerc 1992;24:633–637.
37. Kuipers H, Wijnen JA, Hartgens F, Willems SM: Influence of anabolic steroids on body composition, blood pressure, lipid profile and liver functions in body builders. Int J Sports Med 1991;12:413–418.
38. Sachtleben TR, Berg KE, Elias BA, et al: The effects of anabolic steroids on myocardial structure and cardiovascular fitness. Med Sci Sports Exerc 1993;25:1240–1245.
39. Dickerman RD, Schaller F, Zachariah NY, McConathy WJ: Left ventricular size and function in elite bodybuilders using anabolic steroids. Clin J Sport Med 1997;7:90–93.
40. De Piccoli B, Giada F, Benettin A, et al: Anabolic steroid use in body builders: an echocardiographic study of left ventricle morphology and function. Int J Sports Med 1991;12:408–412.
41. Salke RC, Rowland TW, Burke EJ: Left ventricular size and function in body builders using anabolic steroids. Med Sci Sports Exerc 1985;17:701–704.
42. Friedl K: Effect of anabolic steroid use on body ocmposition and physical performance. In Yesalis C: Anabolic Steroids in Sport and Exercise. Champaign, IL, Human Kinetics, 2000, pp 139–174.
43. Nieminen MS, Ramo MP, Viitasalo M, et al: Serious cardiovascular side effects of large doses of anabolic steroids in weight lifters. Eur Heart J 1996;17:1576–1583.
44. Corrigan B: Anabolic steroids and the mind. Med J Aust 1996;165:222–226.
45. Pope HG Jr, Katz DL: Psychiatric and medical effects of anabolic-androgenic steroid use: a controlled study of 160 athletes. Arch Gen Psychiatry 1994;51:375–382.
46. Perry PJ, Kutscher EC, Lund BC, et al: Measures of aggression and mood changes in male weightlifters with and without androgenic anabolic steroid use. J Forensic Sci 2003;48:646–651.
47. Kashkin KB, Kleber HD: Hooked on hormones? An anabolic steroid addiction hypothesis. JAMA 1989;262:3166–3170.

48. Mahesh V, Greenblatt R: The in vivo conversion of dehydroepiandrosterone and androstenedione to testosterone in the human. Acta Endrocrinol 1962;41:400–406.

49. King DS, Sharp RL, Vukovich MD, et al: Effect of oral androstenedione on serum testosterone and adaptations to resistance training in young men: a randomized controlled trial. JAMA 1999;281:2020–2028.

50. Broeder CE, Quindry J, Brittingham K, et al: The Andro Project: physiological and hormonal influences of androstenedione supplementation in men 35 to 65 years old participating in a high-intensity resistance training program. Arch Intern Med 2000;160:3093–3104.

51. Brown GA, Vukovich MD, Sharp RL, et al: Effect of oral DHEA on serum testosterone and adaptations to resistance training in young men. J Appl Physiol 1999;87:2274–2283.

52. Nestler JE, Barlascini CO, Clore JN, Blackard WG: Dehydroepiandrosterone reduces serum low density lipoprotein levels and body fat but does not alter insulin sensitivity in normal men. J Clin Endocrinol Metab 1988;66:57–61.

53. Welle S, Jozefowicz R, Statt M: Failure of dehydroepiandrosterone to influence energy and protein metabolism in humans. J Clin Endocrinol Metab 1990;71:1259–1264.

54. Metzl JD, Small E, Levine SR, Gershel JC: Creatine use among young athletes. Pediatrics 2001;108:421–422.

55. Juhn MS, Tarnopolsky M: Oral creatine supplementation and athletic performance: a critical review. Clin J Sports Med 1998;8:286–297.

56. Graham AS, Hatton RC: Creatine: a review of efficacy and safety. J Am Pharm Assoc 1999;39:803–810.

57. Persky AM, Brazeau GA, Hochhaus G: Pharmacokinetics of the dietary supplement creatine. Clin Pharmacokinet 2003;42:557–574.

58. Terjung RL, Clarkson P, Eichner ER, et al: American College of Sports Medicine roundtable: the physiological and health effects of oral creatine supplementation. Med Sci Sports Exer 2000; 32:706–717.

59. Hultman E, Soderlund K, Timmons JA, et al: Muscle creatine loading in men. J Appl Physiol 1996;81:232–237.

60. Branch JD: Effect of creatine supplementation on body composition and performance: a meta-analysis. Int J Sport Nutr Exerc Metab 2003;13:198–226.

61. Koshy KM, Griswold E, Schneeberger EE: Interstitial nephritis in a patient taking creatine. N Engl J Med 1999;340:814–815.

62. Pritchard NR, Kalra PA: Renal dysfunction accompanying oral creatine supplements. Lancet 1998;351:1252–1253.

63. Robinson SJ: Acute quadriceps compartement syndrome and rhabdomyolysis in a weight lifter using high-dose creatine supplementation. J Am Board Fam Pract 2000;13:134–137.

64. John MS, Tarnopolsky M: Potential side effects of oral creatine supplementation: a critical review. Clin J Sport Med 1998;8:298–304.

65. Juhn MS, O'Kane JW, Vinci DM: Oral creatine supplementation in male collegiate athletes: a survey of dosing habits and side effects. J Am Diet Assoc 1999;99:593–595.

66. Schroeder C, Potteiger J, Randall J, et al: The effects of creatine dietary supplementation on anterior compartment pressure in the lower leg during rest and following exercise. Clin J Sport Med 2001;11:87–95.

67. Taylor W: Limits of urine drug testing. In Taylor W (ed): Anabolic Steroids and the Athlete. Jefferson, NC, McFarland and Company, 2002, pp 147–167.

68. Dehennin L: Detection of simultaneous self-administration of testosterone and epitestosterone in healthy men. Clin Chem 1994;40:106–109.

69. Dehennin L: On the origin of physiologically high ratios of urinary testosterone to epitestosterone: consequences for reliable detection of testosterone administration by male athletes. J Endocrinol 1994;142:353–360.

70. Catlin DH, Leder BZ, Ahrens B, et al: Trace contamination of over-the-counter andostenedione and positive urine test results for a nandrolone metabolite. JAMA 2000;284:2618–2621.

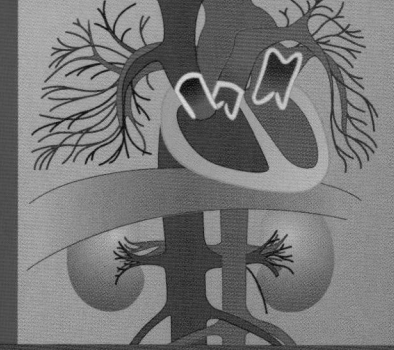

71 *Mercury: Heavy Metals and Inorganic Agents*

CARL R. BAUM, MD

At a Glance...

- Mercury exists in three forms: elemental, inorganic, and organic. Each of these forms produces a unique profile of toxicity. However, interconversion among the three forms of mercury can occur in situ, producing overlap in the spectrum of clinical manifestations associated with each.
- Mercury is ubiquitous; blood concentrations in the general US population are typically 1-5 µg/L.
- Exposure to toxic amounts of mercury can occur from a number of sources including occupation, diet, polluted air, and complementary/alternative remedies.
- The primary target organs of mercury toxicity are the brain, lungs and kidney.
- Mercury exposure is assessed through its measurement in blood and/or urine.
- The primary treatment of mercury intoxication is to end exposure; having a relatively short elimination half-life, mercury is readily excreted in urine or bile. In rare cases, chelation therapy may be warranted to treat severe intoxication. Dimercaprol and succimer are the most effective chelating agents for mercury intoxication.

Mercury, a heavy metal, exists in the environment in three major forms: elemental, inorganic, and organic.[1] As with most toxic heavy metals, human poisonings have been associated with mercury for centuries. In the 1800s, there were many reports in which chronic occupational exposure to elemental mercury fumes caused a dementia-like syndrome among hat felters. This central nervous system toxicity led to the coining of the phrase "mad as a hatter."[1-4] Individuals who attempt to vacuum spilled liquid mercury, or to extract gold or silver from alloys, risk acute inhalation exposure to the vaporized elemental mercury.[5-8] The approved use of mercury-containing medicinals in the form of antisyphilitic agents, diuretics, cathartics, topical salves, teething compounds, and diaper powders has, fortunately, been eliminated in the United States. Historically, however, these compounds were responsible for numerous outbreaks of mercurialism. The most widely known outbreaks were in children exposed to products containing calomel (mercurous chloride, an inorganic form). In the 1940s and 1950s, it became known that these products caused acrodynia, or so-called "pink disease." The manifestations of acrodynia include pain and erythema of the palms and soles, irritability, insomnia, anorexia, diaphoresis, photophobia, and skin rash.[9] Human exposure to methylmercury, the most common environmental form of organic mercury, has resulted in massive environmental disasters. One such massive exposure occurred in the 1950s in Japan, where effluent from an industrial plant contaminated Minamata Bay and led to more than 1000 deaths among area residents who consumed methylmercury-contaminated seafood.[10] Other mass exposures have been associated with grain contaminated with methyl- and ethylmercury.[11,12]

Sources of mercury are numerous. Mercury-containing minerals such as cinnabar (HgS) exist in the earth's crust, and erosion, volcanic eruptions, and natural degassing release mercury into the environment. Mining (cinnabar is the major ore), smelting, and fossil fuel combustion represent non-natural sources. Independent of the initial source (natural or industrial), mercury undergoes extensive transformation once it is released into the environment.[13] For example, aquatic microorganisms transform inorganic mercury via methylation into methylmercury, which accumulates in sea animals. Consumption of methylmercury-contaminated seafood is the major source of nonoccupational mercury exposure in humans. In addition, certain environmental conditions oxidize elemental mercury to divalent inorganic mercury; conversely, in vivo reduction reactions may convert inorganic mercury to the elemental form.[1,13]

Mercury is used in the production of chloralkali (caustic soda), batteries, and measuring devices (thermometers, barometers, and sphygmomanometers) (Fig. 71-1), and it is used as a fungicide in the agricultural industry. Indoor latex paint once contained a mercury-containing antimildew agent, but federal law prohibited further production (but not sales) in the United States after

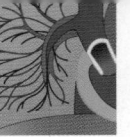

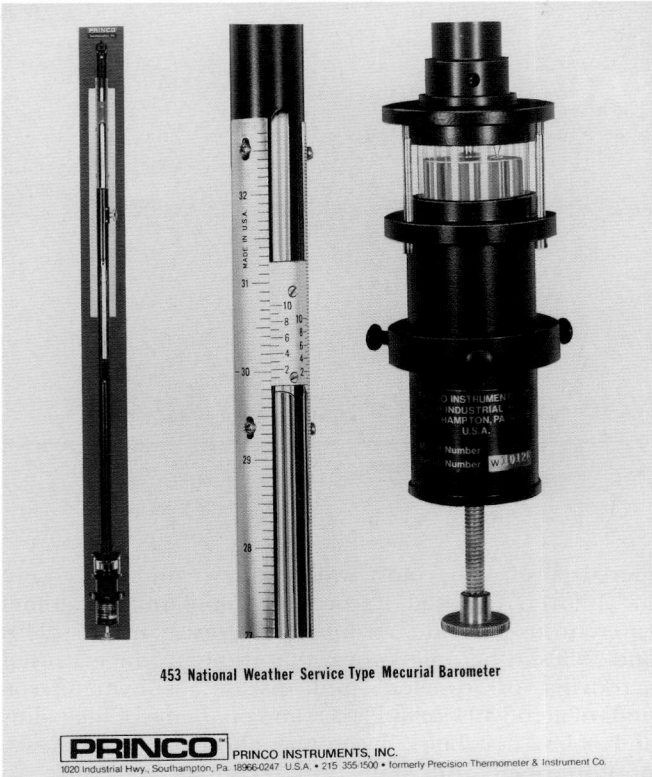

453 National Weather Service Type Mecurial Barometer

PRINCO PRINCO INSTRUMENTS, INC.
1020 Industrial Hwy., Southampton, Pa. 18966-0247 U.S.A. • 215 355-1500 • formerly Precision Thermometer & Instrument Co.

FIGURE 71-1 A Princo mercurial barometer. (Courtesy of Robert E. White Instruments, Inc., Boston, MA.)

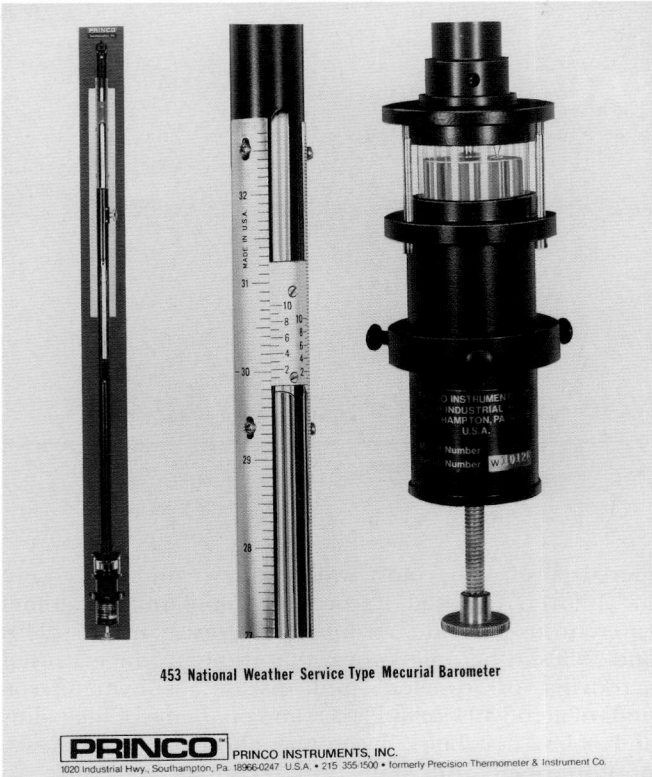

BOX 71-1   MERCURY-CONTAINING PRODUCTS AND OTHER SOURCES OF MERCURY

Elemental	**Inorganic**	**Organic**
Barometers	Acetaldehyde production	Antiseptics
Batteries	Antisyphilitic agents	Bactericidal agents
Bronzing	Chemical laboratory workers	Embalming agents
Calibration instruments	Cosmetics	Farming industry
Chloralkali production	Disinfectants	Fungicides
Dental amalgams	Embalming preparations	Germicidal agents
Electroplating	Explosives	Insecticidal products
Fingerprinting products	Fur hat processing	Laundry/diaper products
Fluorescent, mercury lamps	Ink manufacturing	Paper manufacturing
Infrared detectors	Mercury vapor lamps	Pathology/histology products
Jewelry industry	Mirror silvering	Seed preservatives
Manometers	Perfume industry	Wood preservatives
Neon lamps	Photography	
Paints	Spermicidal jellies	
Paper pulp production	Tattooing inks	
Photography	Taxidermy products	
Thermometers	Vinyl chloride production	
Semiconductor cells	Wood preservatives	
Silver and gold production		

August 1990.[14] Various medicinal and antiseptic agents, as well as dental amalgams, contain mercury.[13] Box 71-1 lists many sources and uses of mercury.

The occupational and environmental use of mercurial agents is regulated, and guidelines exist to limit exposure to these products. The Environmental Protection Agency includes mercury on its list of hazardous air pollutants and regulates its emission from industrial plants. Also, threshold limit values, permissible exposure limits, and short-term exposure limits have been established for various forms of mercury.[13]

PHARMACOLOGY

The chemical symbol for mercury, Hg, is derived from the Greek word *hydrargyros,* or "water silver."[13] This description is appropriate because mercury is the only metal that is liquid at room temperature. The three forms of mercury (elemental, inorganic, and organic) have different biologic and toxicologic properties. In general, however, mercury forms covalent bonds to sulfide groups; thus, it interferes with the function of sulfhydryl enzymes, disrupting many important metabolic cellular functions.[15]

Elemental Mercury

Elemental mercury (Hg^0) is liquid at room temperature. Commonly known as quicksilver, elemental mercury

transforms at room temperature from the liquid to an easily inhaled vapor; consequently, the lung is the major target organ of acute exposure. Elemental mercury is lipid soluble and, once inhaled, passes rapidly through the alveoli into the bloodstream and red blood cells. Once absorbed, most of the elemental mercury is oxidized to the inorganic divalent, or mercuric, form (Hg^{2+}) through the action of catalase enzymes; after intense inhalation exposures, therefore, symptoms and signs of subacute or chronic inorganic mercurialism predominate.[16] Although nonexcreted elemental mercury may accumulate to some degree in the kidney, it does not usually produce renal damage. The mercuric ion is not lipid soluble and does not readily cross the blood-brain barrier; however, a small but potentially significant amount of nonoxidized elemental mercury persists and penetrates readily into the central nervous system, where significant toxicity does occur. Most of the circulating mercuric ion is excreted in feces, urine, and, to a small degree, saliva. The intact gastrointestinal tract absorbs elemental mercury poorly, and ingestions of the metal from, for example, a thermometer are generally nontoxic.[1,13]

Inorganic Mercury

Historically, inorganic forms of mercury in topical medicines, cathartic agents, and diuretics were important sources of human poisonings; however, most of these

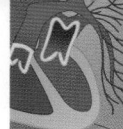

agents have been banned in the United States. Of interest, mercury-containing creams and soaps (used for skin lightening), although banned in the United States, continue to be manufactured and distributed in some European countries and have been discovered in areas in which their use is banned.[17] Currently, the occupational inhalation of elemental mercury with in vivo conversion to inorganic mercury is probably the most common source of inorganic mercury poisoning.[18] Inorganic mercury exists primarily as a salt of divalent (mercuric) and monovalent (mercurous) forms. The bichloride ($HgCl_2$) form of inorganic mercury, corrosive sublimate, is one of the most common of these salts, and as its name suggests, is directly toxic to the mucosa.[15] This corrosive property constitutes the major initial toxicity associated with acute exposure to inorganic mercury. The gastrointestinal tract absorbs approximately 2% to 15% of an ingested dose, which accumulates in the kidney and causes renal cell damage.[1] Cutaneous absorption of inorganic mercurials also occurs, and chronic exposure to topical inorganic mercurials may lead to significant toxicity.

Plasma proteins transport absorbed inorganic mercury (red blood cell:plasma ratio, 1:2.5) to the kidneys, where it undergoes glomerular filtration, tubular secretion and reabsorption, and eventual elimination.[1,15] However, because renal excretion is inefficient, mercury accumulates unless it binds to a chelating agent. Although inorganic mercury's lipid solubility is poor, chronic exposure leads to gradual accumulation of the mercuric ions in the cerebellar and cerebral cortices of the brain, and to eventual central nervous system disease.[19] Mercuric ions do not readily cross the placenta, and fetotoxicity, if it occurs, is rare.[15]

Organic Mercury

Organic mercurials are used extensively in agriculture as fungicides and seed dressings. Organic mercury exists in three major forms: aryl (phenylmercuric acetate), long-chain, and short-chain alkyl (methyl- and ethyl-) compounds. These forms are grouped according to absorption, distribution, and elimination into two classes: the aryl and long-chain organic mercurials, once absorbed, are converted rapidly to inorganic forms, and their toxicity is similar to that of inorganic mercury; the alkyl mercurials, methyl- and ethylmercury, are quite stable after absorption, with only a small amount of the parent compound converted to the mercuric form. Organic methylmercury is the most widely distributed and toxic form of organic mercury in the environment and is responsible for most of the mass toxic exposures. The gastrointestinal tract absorbs 90% to 95% of ingested alkyl forms, which rapidly penetrate red blood cells; this results in a large red blood cell:plasma ratio. Organic mercury binds avidly to and inactivates sulfhydryl-group enzymes.[1,15] Because of its lipid solubility, alkyl mercury is distributed throughout the entire body, accumulating in the brain, kidney, liver, hair, and skin; toxic effects are evident primarily in the brain. Methylmercury also passes readily through the placenta and is of major concern in pregnant women because of its profound fetotoxicity.[10] Methylmercury is acetylated or conjugated to cysteine or glutathione in the liver, and is then excreted in the bile. The N-acetyl-homocysteine-methylmercury metabolite undergoes enterohepatic recirculation and is excreted ultimately in the feces (approximately 90%) and in the urine.[20]

CLINICAL PRESENTATION

The manner in which patients present with mercury poisoning depends on the form of mercury, the duration and intensity of the exposure, and certain conditions of the patient. Inhalation of elemental mercury vapor and ingestion of inorganic mercurial compounds may lead to acute toxicity, while exposure to organic mercury generally causes chronic toxicity.

Elemental Mercury

Exposure to high concentrations of vaporized elemental mercury may cause acute pulmonary symptoms. Initial symptoms consist of fever, chills, shortness of breath, and a metallic taste in the mouth—all consistent with metal fume fever. Other symptoms and signs include stomatitis, lethargy, confusion, vomiting, and colitis. These clinical findings usually abate within 1 week; however, in some instances, they worsen and progress to pulmonary edema, respiratory failure, and death.[5-7] Young children are particularly susceptible to the acute pulmonary effects of elemental mercury vapor. Following exposure, usually from the melting of metals or vacuuming of elemental mercury in the home, the child may develop severe pulmonary disease, including alveolar dilation, interstitial emphysema, and pneumatocele, pneumothorax, and pneumomediastinum formation. Small airway obstruction from cellular desquamation may occur, and pulmonary fibrosis, granuloma formation, and respiratory failure often ensue.[6,7]

Elemental mercury-containing dental amalgams are another potential source of exposure. If appropriate guidelines for use and handling are not followed, dental workers may be exposed to toxic amounts of aerosolized elemental mercury.[21] The effects of vaporized dental amalgam fillings within patients' mouths is a subject of controversy. Although chewing does release elemental mercury vapor, and urinary mercury levels of patients with mercury fillings are slightly higher than those in people without mercury fillings, to date no scientifically rigorous studies have identified clinical evidence of associated disease.[22]

Ingestion of elemental mercury is usually of no concern because of poor gastrointestinal absorption. However, abnormal gastrointestinal function or anatomy (e.g., decreased gut motility or fistulous tracts) may allow elemental mercury into the bloodstream and the peritoneal space.[23] The common scenario of a child who has a small amount of elemental mercury from a broken thermometer in the mouth or rectum is of no concern unless direct trauma from the broken glass is evident.

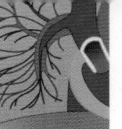

After intentional intravenous injection (usually as a suicide attempt), elemental mercury may embolize to the lungs and cause symptoms and signs of acute pulmonary embolus, including shortness of breath, dyspnea, chest pain, hypoxemia, and death.[24] In addition, elemental mercury may be transformed to its inorganic form and subsequently lead to renal disease. Accidentally or intentionally injected inorganic mercury may be absorbed gradually, leading to systemic symptoms unless the mercury is surgically removed.[25]

Intense acute or chronic exposure to elemental mercury fumes causes cutaneous and central nervous system dysfunction. The classic description is a triad of tremor, gingivitis, and erethism. Erethism is a constellation of findings that includes insomnia, shyness, memory loss, emotional lability, anorexia, and depression. Signs of oral toxicity include gingivitis, stomatitis, and loose dentition. Additional findings may include headaches, visual disturbances (constricted or tunnel vision), peripheral neuropathy with sensory or motor abnormalities (or both), anosmia, and ataxia.[2,4,18] If the medical and occupational history is not thorough, chronic mercurialism may be misdiagnosed as parkinsonism, depression, or Alzheimer's disease. Inhalation exposures have also been misdiagnosed as pheochromocytoma and toxic shock syndrome.[26,27]

Inorganic Mercury

Inorganic mercury poisoning occurs primarily via the oral route. Acute symptoms and signs of inorganic mercury poisoning are related to direct caustic effects, and depend to some degree on the concentration and type of salt (mercuric forms are more toxic than mercurous forms).[28] At high concentrations, symptoms are usually immediate and include pain, vomiting, and hematemesis. Necrosis of any portion of the gastrointestinal tract may occur with subsequent luminal pooling of body fluids, hypovolemia, electrolyte imbalance, acute tubular necrosis, and death. In those who survive the acute phase of toxicity, renal failure may develop. Home accidents involving the preservative in stool collection kits (mercuric chloride 4.5%) are not uncommon and should be considered in patients presenting with signs of corrosive gastrointestinal injury.[29,30] Ingestion of disk batteries, many of which contain mercury, is relatively common among pediatric patients; although these batteries are very unlikely to break apart and spill inorganic mercury into the gastrointestinal tract, complications are usually related to local corrosive injury. Ingestion of button batteries with subsequent clinical signs of systemic toxicity is very rare.[31]

Prolonged inhalation exposure to elemental mercury in an occupational setting is the most likely cause of chronic inorganic mercury poisoning.[18] Historically, the topical application of inorganic mercurial salves and the chronic ingestion of diuretics or cathartics were common sources of inorganic mercury poisoning, causing renal failure, dementia, and acrodynia. Acrodynia, which means "painful extremities" and is also known as "pink disease," presents as erythema and edema of the hands and feet, skin rash, diaphoresis, tachycardia, hypertension, photophobia, irritability, and decreased proximal muscle tone.[32] In addition, subtle neuropsychiatric disturbances have been reported in patients chronically exposed to inorganic mercury.[33] In the 1940s and 1950s, exposure to mercurous chloride was responsible for numerous cases of pediatric acrodynia.[9] Fortunately, federal regulations that have limited or banned many inorganic mercurial compounds have rendered chronic poisoning rare outside the occupational setting. However, new cases have been associated with exposures to broken mercury-containing light bulbs and spilled elemental mercury.[8,34,35] Of importance, acrodynia does not develop in everyone exposed to mercurial compounds; consequently, its presence is often a marker for a more widespread problem. In 1980, three cases of acrodynia led to the discovery that a commercial diaper service using a a phenylmercuric fungicide had exposed up to 12,000 infants.[36]

Organic Mercury

Ingestion of contaminated food products is the usual route of organic mercury exposure, although inhalation and dermal exposure may cause toxicity. The aryl and long-chain organic compounds may cause findings similar to those of chronic inorganic mercury. Depending on the amount ingested, symptoms of short-chain alkyl organic mercurial poisoning begin days to weeks after ingestion. This delay occurs primarily because organic mercury targets enzymes that must be depleted before clinical signs develop. The major symptoms and signs of alkyl mercury poisoning are neurologic, consisting of visual field constriction, ataxia, paresthesia, neurasthenia, hearing loss, dysarthria, mental deterioration, muscle tremor, movement disorders, and even death.[15] Dermal exposure to these products may cause dermatitis or burns. Ingestion of methylmercury rarely, if ever, causes gastrointestinal symptoms; however, the ingestion of ethylmercury may induce vomiting, cramping, and diarrhea. Organic mercurials have been reported to cause thrombocytopenia and agranulocytosis.[1,10] Symptoms of acute and chronic exposures to organic mercury are similar, with the central nervous system abnormalities predominating. Pathologic and magnetic resonance imaging findings include damage to the cerebral cortex—specifically the visual cortex (calcarine region), the motor and sensory centers (pre- and postcentral cortex), and the auditory center (temporal cortex)—and to the cerebellar cortex. Destruction and demyelination of the sensory nerve fibers and dorsal roots of the peripheral nervous system also occur.[37]

Organic mercurials are extremely toxic to the fetus. Although all forms of mercury cross the placenta, organic mercury passes most readily. Maternal exposure may lead to spontaneous abortion or severe mental retardation of the child, with global developmental delay, cerebellar ataxia, tremor, nystagmus, dysmetria, limb deformities, and seizure disorders, as in Minamata disease.[10]

More recent studies have described cognitive deficits in a cohort of children born in the Faroe Islands (located

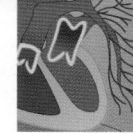

halfway between Iceland and Norway), where pilot whale meat is a staple of the diet. Mercury concentrations of cord blood and maternal hair served as indicators of prenatal exposure to methylmercury from whale meat. At 7 years of age, nearly 90% of members of the cohort underwent extensive neurodevelopmental examination, which revealed dysfunction most notably in language, attention, and memory.[38] In contrast, neurodevelopmental studies of children in the Republic of Seychelles (an island group in the Indian Ocean), where consumption of a variety of ocean fish is the only source of methylmercury, found no risk from prenatal exposure.[39]

A chemistry professor at Dartmouth who spilled liquid dimethylmercury inadvertently onto her gloved hand presented to medical attention 5 months later with acute deterioration in balance, gait, and speech. Despite aggressive therapy, she became unresponsive within 3 weeks. Life support was eventually withdrawn, and she died 10 months after the exposure. Autopsy revealed diffuse disease of the cortices, and remarkable atrophy of the cerebellum.[40]

Considerable debate has arisen over the vaccine preservative thimerosal, its active component ethylmercury, and their causal roles in neurodevelopmental disorders, such as autism, attention-deficit hyperactivity disorder, and speech and language delay. In an extensive review, the Institute of Medicine concluded that although the hypothesis, based primarily on analogies to methylmercury, is biologically plausible, there is inadequate evidence "to accept or reject a causal relationship between thimerosal exposure and neurodevelopmental disorders. . . ."[41]

DIAGNOSIS

A thorough occupational and environmental history may reveal exposure to a mercurial compound, particularly after an acute inhalation exposure to elemental mercury or an ingestion of inorganic mercury. The latter should be considered in the patient who presents after a suicide attempt with symptoms and signs of caustic ingestion. The diagnosis of chronic or subacute mercury poisoning may be more difficult. Because the major target organs of toxicity include the central nervous system, the kidneys, and skin and mucous membranes, any patient with an altered mental status and renal failure, with or without cutaneous findings, should be evaluated for mercury intoxication. The constellation of findings of acrodynia should also alert the physician to the possibility of exposure to mercurial compounds. Probably the most important tool in the diagnosis of chronic mercury poisoning is a very thorough occupational and environmental history.

If mercury poisoning is suspected, confirmatory laboratory evaluation is usually necessary, particularly in cases of chronic exposure. Measurement of urine mercury levels is generally considered the best method for determining whether exposure to inorganic or elemental mercury has occurred, and whether chelation therapy is effective. Concentrations of mercury in urine greater than 20 to 25 µg/L should be considered elevated.

Although no absolute correlation exists between urinary mercury concentrations and symptoms, levels greater than 150 µg/L have been associated with nonspecific symptoms after chronic exposure to mercury vapors; levels greater than 300 µg/L are usually associated with overt symptoms. Urine levels are helpful in confirming exposure to elemental and inorganic mercury. However, because organic mercury is poorly excreted in urine, organic mercurial exposure should not be ruled out on the basis of urinary mercury determination.

Blood (not serum) mercury levels in the normal population are usually less than 5 µg/L. Mercury levels in the blood may accurately reflect inorganic mercury exposure if they are obtained soon after exposure. However, because of redistribution to other body tissues, these levels may become less accurate as the exposure becomes more remote. Following methylmercury exposure, however, blood levels may remain elevated and are relatively accurate in determining the body's burden of organic mercury.[15]

Mercury accumulates in hair, and levels in hair may be used to document exposure. However, environmental mercury contaminates hair easily; therefore, measurements may be inaccurate following aerosol or other extraneous exposures. Thus, hair analysis alone should never be used to confirm exposure to mercury.[1]

For ingested, intravenous, or subcutaneous exposures to elemental mercury, radiographs may be necessary to document both the presence and the efficacy of removal of these compounds. X-ray fluorescence techniques have been used to estimate body burdens of mercury. However, these techniques remain experimental and are not used routinely.[42]

TREATMENT

Initial treatment of the mercury-poisoned patient is the same as that for any intoxicated patient. Assessment and management of the patient's *a*irway, *b*reathing, and *c*irculation (ABCs) are of primary importance. Prehospital or hospital providers should remove contaminated clothing and flush contaminated skin and eyes. All patients with signs of acute mercurialism should undergo continuous cardiac monitoring and pulse oximetry.

Acute inhalation exposure to elemental mercury may cause, as discussed earlier, symptoms of metal fume fever, pneumonitis, and respiratory failure. Humidified supplemental oxygen should be provided; endotracheal intubation may be necessary for those with signs of respiratory failure. There are no known aerosolized antidotes for acute inhalation exposures; therefore, respiratory support is the mainstay of treatment. Infants with severe respiratory compromise after inhalation of elemental mercury have survived with vigorous respiratory support, including the use of high-frequency ventilation when conventional mechanical ventilation has failed.[7] Patients with acute inhalation exposure to mercury may develop systemic poisoning once transformation of elemental mercury to inorganic mercury has occurred;

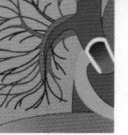

thus, they may require chelation therapy (see below in this section).

Ingestion of caustic inorganic mercury requires rapid assessment and treatment to prevent circulatory collapse. Rapid vascular access should be established, and vigorous replacement of fluid losses should be instituted. Caustic injury to the oropharyngeal mucosa may cause severe local edema, and endotracheal intubation or tracheostomy may be required to prevent obstruction of the airway. Decontamination procedures should be instituted early to prevent further corrosive injury and systemic absorption. The induction of emesis is, as with any caustic ingestion, contraindicated. The role of antiemetics has not been studied specifically, but they may be of benefit. Gastric lavage is no longer recommended routinely and is contraindicated if gastric or esophageal perforation is a possibility. Anecdotal evidence indicates that lavage with milk or egg whites may help bind mercurial compounds; thus, their use may be considered, especially since there is no evidence that these materials cause harm. If perforation is suspected or radiopaque objects remain present, direct endoscopic removal should be considered. Activated charcoal does not bind appreciably to metallic compounds. (However, some evidence indicates that some binding may occur; therefore, it may be considered unless perforation is suspected.[23]) Finally, whole bowel irrigation with polyethylene glycol may be administered until the rectal effluent is clear and the radiopaque material is absent. Extracorporeal methods of mercury removal are not recommended; however, hemodialysis may be necessary if renal failure ensues.

Initial laboratory tests should include serum chemistry assessments and a complete blood count. Type and cross-matching of blood should be performed if exposure to caustic inorganic mercury is suspected. Because elemental mercury is radiopaque, appropriate radiographs should be obtained. Blood and urine should be obtained for appropriate evaluation for the presence of mercury (see section on Diagnosis) and other toxins, as indicated.

Following initial management, chelation therapy should be instituted if systemic absorption is expected, if the patient is symptomatic, or if elevated mercury levels in the blood or urine are discovered. Effective chelating agents include oral D-penicillamine (D-PCN), parenteral dimercaprol (British antilewisite [BAL]) and its oral congeners meso-2,3-dimercaptosuccinic acid (DMSA) and sodium 2,3-dimercapto-1-propanesulfonate (DMPS). Each of these agents contains thiol groups that compete with endogenous sulfhydryl groups for mercury.[15,43]

After the acute ingestion of caustic inorganic mercury, chelation is best limited to the use of BAL. BAL is administered intramuscularly at a dose of 2.5 to 5 mg/kg every 6 to 12 hours. Common side effects of BAL include transient hypertension, tachycardia, pain at the injection site, nausea and vomiting, headache, and diaphoresis. Hemolysis may be induced if the patient has glucose-6-phosphate dehydrogenase deficiency. BAL should not be used for the treatment of alkyl organic mercury poisoning because it may actually worsen neurotoxicity.[44]

TABLE 71-1 Clinical Characteristics of Mercury Exposure

	ELEMENTAL	INORGANIC	ORGANIC
Major Route of Exposure	Inhalation	Inhalation (chronic), oral dermal	Oral
Clinical Effects			
CNS	Tremor	Erethism, tremor	Minamata disease
Pulmonary	+++	−	−
GI	+	+++	+
Renal	+	+++	+
Acrodynia	+	+	−
Treatment	BAL, DMSA	BAL, DMSA	DMSA

BAL, British antilewisite; DMSA, 2,3,-dimercaptosuccinic acid; +, pressent; −, absent.

If the patient is able to tolerate oral medications, PCN or DMSA may be used instead of or in addition to BAL. D-PCN forms a complex with mercury that is excreted in the urine. Therefore, it should not be used if the patient has renal failure. It is administered four times a day at 250 mg per dose (20 to 30 mg/kg/day for children). One- to 2-week courses of D-PCN therapy are given until the 24-hour urine mercury level is within an acceptable range. Side effects of D-PCN therapy include gastrointestinal upset, rash, leukopenia, thrombocytopenia, proteinuria, and hematuria. If mercury remains in the gastrointestinal tract, D-PCN should not be administered because it may increase absorption.[15,23]

DMSA is an oral, water-soluble congener of BAL. Its use in mercury-poisoned patients is increasing, and it seems to be more effective than D-PCN at increasing urinary mercury levels in chronically exposed patients. DMSA has a better side effect profile than those of D-PCN and BAL; its adverse effects are usually limited to mild transient elevations in hepatic transaminase levels and mild gastrointestinal upset. DMSA is administered at a dose of 10 mg/kg three times per day for the first 5 days of treatment, and two times per day for the next 14 days. Repeated administrations may be necessary, with a 2-week interval between treatments.[45] Table 71-1 summarizes the clinical effects and treatment for the three forms of mercury poisoning.

REFERENCES

1. Goyer RA: Toxic effects of metals. In Klaassen CD, Amdur MO, Doull J (eds): Casarett and Doull's Toxicology: The Basic Science of Poisons, 5th ed. New York, McGraw-Hill, 1996, pp 691–736.
2. Buckell M, Hunter D, Milton R, Perry KM: Chronic mercury poisoning: 1946 classic article. Br J Ind Med 1993;50:97–106.
3. Hamilton A: Exploring the dangerous trades. J Ind Hyg 1992;4:219.
4. Neal PA, Jones RR: Chronic mercurialism in the hatter's fur cutting industry. JAMA 1938;110:337.

5. Zelman M, Camfield P, Moss M, et al: Toxicity from vacuumed mercury: a household hazard. Clin Pediatr 1991;30:121–123.

6. Rowens B, Guerrero-Betancourt D, Gottlieb CA, et al: Respiratory failure and death following acute inhalation of mercury vapor: a clinical and histologic perspective. Chest 1991;99:185–90.

7. Moromisato DY, Anas NG, Goodman G: Mercury inhalation poisoning and acute lung in a child: use of high-frequency oscillatory ventilation. Chest 1994;105:613–615.

8. Schwartz J, Snider T, Montiel MM: Toxicity of a family from vacuumed mercury. Am J Emerg Med 1992;10:258–261.

9. Warkany J, Hubbard DM: Acrodynia and mercury. J Pediatr 1953;42:365–386.

10. Harada M: Minamata disease: methylmercury poisoning in Japan caused by environmental pollution. Crit Rev Toxicol 1995;25:1–24.

11. Clarkson TW, Amin-Zaki L, Al-Tikriti SK: An outbreak of methylmercury poisoning due to consumption of contaminated grain. Fed Proc 1976;35:2395–2399.

12. Bakir F, Damluji SF, Amin-Zaki L, et al: Methyl mercury poisoning in Iraq. Science 1973;181:230–241.

13. Campbell D, Gonzales M, Sullivan JB: In Sullivan JB Jr, Krieger GR (eds): Hazardous Materials Toxicology: Clinical Principles of Environmental Health. Baltimore, Williams & Wilkins, 1992, pp 824–833.

14. Agocs MM, Etzel RA, Parrish RG, et al: Mercury exposure from interior latex paint. N Engl J Med 1990;323:1096–1101.

15. Klaassen CD: Heavy metals and heavy-metal antagonists. In Hardman JG, Limbird LE, Molinoff PB, Ruddon RW (eds): Goodman & Gilman's The Pharmacological Basis of Therapeutics, 9th ed. New York, McGraw-Hill, 1996, pp 1649–1671.

16. Magos L, Halbach S, Clarkson TW: Role of catalase in the oxidation of mercury vapor. Biochem Pharmacol 1978;27:1373–1377.

17. The International Programme on Chemical Safety: Environmental Health Criteria, No. 118: Mercury, inorganic (1991). Available at http://www.who.int/ipcs/publications/ehc. Accessed October 18, 2006.

18. Bluhm RE, Bobbitt RG, Welch LW, et al: Elemental mercury vapour toxicity, treatment, and prognosis after acute, intensive exposure in chloralkali plant workers: Part I. History, neuropsychological findings and chelator effects. Hum Exp Toxicol 1992;11:201–210.

19. Williamson AM, Teo RK, Sanderson J: Occupational mercury exposure and its consequences for behaviour. Int Arch Occup Environ Health 1982;50:273–286.

20. Graef JW: Mercury. I. Clin Toxicol Rev 1980;2(7).

21. Pohl L, Bergman M: The dentist's exposure to elemental mercury vapor during clinical work with amalgam. Acta Odontol Scand 1995;53:44–48.

22. Eti S, Weisman R, Hoffman R, Reidenberg MM: Slight renal effect of mercury from amalgam fillings. Pharmacol Toxicol 1995;76:47–49.

23. Sue YJ: Mercury. In Goldfrank LR, Flomenbaum NE, Lewin NA, et al (eds): Goldfrank's Toxicologic Emergencies, 7th ed. New York, McGraw-Hill, 2002, pp 1239–1248.

24. Anderson WJ: Intravenous mercury: a three-year follow-up. Ulster Med J 1993;62:180–183.

25. Cole JK, Holbrook JL: Focal mercury toxicity: a case report. J Hand Surg 1994;19:602–603.

26. Henningsson C, Hoffmann S, McGonigle L, Winter JSD: Acute mercury poisoning (acrodynia) mimicking pheochromocytoma in an adolescent. J Pediatr 1993;122:252–253.

27. Mohan SB, Tamilarasan A, Buhl M: Inhalational mercury poisoning masquerading as toxic shock syndrome. Anaesth Intensive Care 1994;22:305–306.

28. Gosselin RE, Smith RP, Hodge HC: Mercury. In Gosselin RE, Smith RP, Hodge HC (eds): Clinical Toxicology of Commercial Products, 5th ed. Baltimore, Williams & Wilkins, 1984, pp 262–275.

29. Seidel J: Acute mercury poisoning after polyvinyl alcohol preservative ingestion. Pediatrics 1980;66:132–134.

30. Wang RY, Henry GC, Fine J, et al: Mercuric chloride poisonings from stool fixative ingestion. Vet Hum Toxicol 1992;34:341.

31. Litovitz T, Schmitz BF: Ingestion of cylindrical and button batteries: an analysis of 2382 cases. Pediatrics 1992;89:747–757.

32. Matheson DS, Clarkson TW, Gelfand EW: Mercury toxicity (acrodynia) induced by long term injection of gammaglobulin. J Pediatr 1980;97:153–155.

33. Andersen A, Ellingsen DG, Morland T, Kjuus H: A neurological and neurophysiological study of chloralkali workers previously exposed to mercury vapour. Acta Neurol Scand 1993;88:427–433.

34. Tunnessen WW, McMahon KJ, Baser M: Acrodynia: exposure to mercury from fluorescent light bulbs. Pediatrics 1987;79:786–789.

35. Foulds DM, Copeland KC, Franks RC: Mercury poisoning and acrodynia. Am J Dis Child 1987;141:124–125.

36. Clarkson TW: Mercury: an element of mystery. N Engl J Med 1990;323:1137–1139.

37. Korogi Y, Takahashi M, Shinzato J, Okajima T: MR findings in seven patients with organic mercury poisoning (Minamata disease). Am J Neuroradiol 1994;15:1575–1578.

38. Grandjean P, Weihe P, White RF, et al: Cognitive deficit in 7-year-old children with prenatal exposure to methylmercury. Neurotoxicol Teratol 1997;19:417–428.

39. Myers GJ, Davidson PW, Cox C, et al: Prenatal methylmercury exposure from ocean fish consumption in the Seychelles child development study. Lancet 2003;361:1686–1692.

40. Nierenberg DW, Nordgren RE, Chang MB, et al: Delayed cerebellar disease and death after accidental exposure to dimethylmercury. N Engl J Med 1998;338:1672–1676.

41. Stratton K, Gable A, McCormick MC (eds): Immunization Safety Review: Thimerosal-Containing Vaccines and Neurodevelopmental Disorders. Institute of Medicine. Washington, National Academy Press, 2001.

42. Borjesson J, Barregard L, Sallsten G, et al: In vivo XRF analysis of mercury: the relation between concentrations in the kidney and the urine. Phys Med Biol 1995;40:413–426.

43. Baum CR: Treatment of mercury intoxication. Curr Opin Pediatr 1999;11:265–268.

44. Howland MA: Antidotes in depth: dimercaprol (BAL). In Goldfrank LR, Flomenbaum NE, Lewin NA, et al (eds): Goldfrank's Toxicologic Emergencies, 7th ed. New York, McGraw-Hill, 2002, pp 1196–1199.

45. Howland MA: Antidotes in depth: Succimer. In Goldfrank LR, Flomenbaum NE, Lewin NA, et al (eds): Goldfrank's Toxicologic Emergencies, 7th ed. New York, McGraw-Hill, 2002, 1228–1234.

72 *Iron*

ERICA L. LIEBELT, MD

At a Glance...

- Acute iron poisoning is primarily a clinical diagnosis, supported by laboratory data.
- Gastrointestinal symptoms—vomiting, hematemesis, diarrhea, and abdominal pain—characterize the early signs of toxicity.
- Shock, metabolic acidosis, and decreased level of consciousness characterize serious systemic toxicity.
- Aggressive gastrointestinal decontamination measures, particularly whole bowel irrigation, may be necessary to decrease toxicity.
- Deferoxamine is the antidote for iron toxicity.

Acute iron poisoning continues to be a common and potentially lethal toxicologic problem, especially in the pediatric population. In 2002, there were more than 24,000 reported exposures to iron-containing products in children younger than 6 years of age; fortunately, most resulted in either minor or no adverse outcomes. However, in the 1990s, iron was the leading cause of unintentional poisoning deaths among children in the United States who ingested pharmaceutical preparations. Although there have been no reported deaths in the United States in the past 2 years, many factors account for this high incidence of exposures and past history of deaths. First, iron-containing compounds, such as multivitamins with iron or iron tablets, are readily available and widely used in households as nutritional supplements during childhood and adulthood, particularly during pregnancy. Second, many iron preparations are brightly colored, are sugar coated, and look like candy, making them attractive to curious young children. Finally, parents and the general public do not recognize the potential toxicity of a product that is regarded as promoting health.

Preventing iron exposures is necessary to decrease the morbidity and mortality associated with its toxicity. In 1997, the U.S. Food and Drug Administration (FDA) required warning labels on all iron-containing preparations and mandated unit-dose packaging for iron-containing dietary supplements and drug products that contained 30 mg or more of elemental iron per dosage unit. In October 2003, the mandate for unit-dose packaging was removed because of a court ruling, which stated that the FDA did not have the authority to require manufacturers of iron-containing dietary supplements and drug products to use unit-dose packaging for poison prevention purposes.[1] The ramifications of this ruling are yet to be seen.

PHARMACOLOGIC AGENTS

Three major categories of iron preparations are available, each with varying potential for toxicity based on their content of elemental iron (Table 72-1). Children's chewable multivitamins have a low concentration of elemental iron (10–18 mg per tablet packaged in bottles of 60–100 tablets) and are rarely associated with serious toxicity. Nonprescription iron products (adult multivitamins with iron and iron supplements) and prescription iron supplements (i.e., prenatal vitamins) contain substantially higher concentrations of iron in the form of ferrous salts. The toxicity of iron results from the amount of elemental iron ingested, which, in turn, depends on the type of iron preparation. Ferrous fumarate contains 33% elemental iron; ferrous sulfate, 20%; and ferrous gluconate, 12%. These iron products are responsible for the moderate and serious toxicity and fatal outcomes that are reported with exposures. Carbonyl iron is another formulation that has not been reported to cause the same corrosive injury to the gastrointestinal tract seen with iron salt formulations (50–66 mg/tablet or capsule).

PHARMACOLOGY AND PHARMACOKINETICS

The average healthy adult body contains 3 to 5 g of iron, of which 70% is present in the ferrous state (Fe^{2+}) in

TABLE 72-1 Elemental Iron Content in Different Preparations			
IRON PREPARATION	ELEMENTAL IRON CONTENT (%)	TABLET SIZE (mg)	ELEMENTAL IRON CONTENT/ UNIT DOSE
Iron Supplements			
Ferrous fumurate	33	200	65 mg
Ferrous sulfate	20	300	60 mg
		325	65 mg
Ferrous gluconate	12	300	36 mg
Feosol Elixir			44 mg/5 mL
Multivitamins			
Adult multivitamins with iron			10–110 mg/tablet
Children's multi- vitamins with iron			10–18 mg/tablet

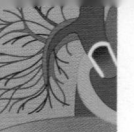

hemoglobin and myoglobin and 25% occurs in the ferric state (Fe^{3+}) in the form of ferritin and stored as hemosiderin. The remainder is found attached to transferrin or in heme and flavin enzymes. Dietary iron is absorbed in the ferrous form in the duodenum and upper jejunum. A transferrin-like protein facilitates the energy-dependent carrier-mediated transport across intestinal mucosal cells. This mucosal receptor-dependent process acts as a limiting barrier for normal iron absorption, thus regulating iron balance. Free iron is toxic to many cellular processes; however, the body has many protective mechanisms to prevent this toxicity. Once absorbed, iron is either stored within ferritin or prepared for release to transferrin, an iron-binding protein carrier. The constant sloughing of intestinal cells provides the main mechanism of physiologic iron excretion.

Plasma iron is bound to transferrin in the ferric state, with 30% to 40% of the iron-binding sites usually saturated. Transferrin is a protein carrier that transports either dietary or storage iron that is entering the plasma for redistribution and utilization. Total iron-binding capacity (TIBC) is a measurement of the total amount of iron that transferrin can bind and normally exceeds serum iron concentration by twofold to threefold.

Most iron is transported to the reticuloendothelial system and hepatocytes, where it is stored within the protein ferritin after ferrous ions are oxidized to the ferric state and complexed with apoferritin. With increasing iron storage, some of the ferritin is transformed into hemosiderin. The small percentage of iron not stored as ferritin is incorporated into iron-containing enzymes or proteins such as hemoglobin and cytochrome enzymes. Humans can eliminate only a small fixed amount of iron per day (1 mg in adult males and 1 to 2 mg in adult females) primarily through exfoliation of gastrointestinal (GI) mucosal cells or menstrual blood loss, which can increase up to only 2 mg/day when excess iron accumulation occurs.

PATHOPHYSIOLOGY

It is evident from the description of normal iron metabolism that the body is poorly equipped to handle excessive amounts of iron. Regulation of iron absorption does not occur in the presence of excessive iron ingestions. Iron may continue to be absorbed passively down a concentration gradient in overdose because of its oxidative and corrosive effects on the GI mucosa, leading to dysfunction of the regulatory balance seen in therapeutic settings. In acute iron poisoning, iron absorption may occur along the entire length of the small and large intestine rather than just the duodenum and upper jejunum. Furthermore, the normal protective mechanisms (transport and storage proteins) become saturated, resulting in more free circulating iron, the agent responsible for cellular toxicity.

Iron toxicity is manifested as both local and systemic effects. Excess free iron catalyzes redox reactions, producing secondary toxicity from lipid peroxidation and free radical formation.[2,3] Iron has effects on the GI and cardiovascular systems as well as on the central nervous system.

Gastrointestinal Tract

Iron has direct corrosive effects on the GI mucosa, resulting in ulceration, edema, bleeding, venous thrombosis, infarction, and perforation.[4] Deposition of iron can be demonstrated histologically in mucosal collagen and basement membranes as well as vascular tissues supplying the small intestine. These effects can lead to severe fluid losses both by direct hemorrhage and the "third spacing" of fluids, both contributing to systemic hypovolemia. The severity of these local corrosive effects depends on the quantity of elemental iron ingested, the concentration of iron in the preparation, the duration of its contact with the mucosa, and the amount of mucosal protection provided by food in the stomach at the time of ingestion; greatest mucosal damage occurs on an empty stomach. Gastric scarring may follow severe iron ingestion, resulting in stenosis of the gastric outlet and small bowel.[5]

Cardiovascular System

Multiple cardiovascular manifestations of iron excess are evident on the heart and blood vessels.[3,6–8] Both free iron and ferritin (whose release is stimulated by free iron) are potent vasodilators that can cause hypotension as a result of venodilation. Iron also directly injures blood vessels, resulting in postarteriolar dilation and decreased venous tone. Capillary membrane permeability increases from direct toxic effects of iron, resulting in diffusion of fluids from the vascular compartment into the interstitium, exacerbating hypovolemia and hypotension. Cardiac output is ultimately decreased as a result of decreased filling pressures from fluid losses, decreased systemic vascular resistance, and probably metabolic acidosis and its depression of myocardial contractility. Iron infiltrates myocardial cells and produces fatty degeneration, which can produce a cardiomyopathy.

Liver

Circulating free iron accumulates initially in the Kupffer cells of the reticuloendothelial system and then in the hepatocytes, localizing in the mitochondria, where its toxicity is exerted. The liver is probably the organ most susceptible to injury because it is the first organ to receive portal blood containing toxic amounts of iron; the liver also has the greatest capacity to sequester iron that is not bound to transferrin.[9] Histopathologically, the demonstrated effects of excess iron in the liver include cloudy swelling of the hepatocytes, portal iron deposition, fatty metamorphosis, and massive periportal necrosis.[10] Formation of reactive oxygen species in the hepatocytes is most likely responsible for the hepatocellular damage. Hepatocellular toxicity is manifested by elevated bilirubin concentrations 3 to 4 days after ingestion, hypoglycemia, hyperammonemia, coagulation

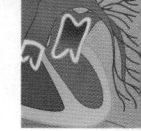

defects, and, ultimately, encephalopathy. Acute hepatic failure is rare except in massive iron overdoses.

Hematopoietic System

Several mechanisms are responsible for the coagulation disturbances often noted with iron intoxication. Free iron inhibits the thrombin-induced conversion of fibrinogen to fibrin, resulting in a direct and early effect on coagulation that precedes liver dysfunction.[11] The bleeding from this iron-induced coagulopathy may contribute to the early GI blood loss. In addition, experimental iron poisoning has been associated with decreased thrombin production, thrombocytopenia, hypoprothrombinemia, and synthetic disturbances at several stages in the coagulation cascade.[12] In the later stages of iron poisoning, impaired synthesis of clotting factors occurs as a result of hepatotoxicity.

Metabolic Acidosis

The metabolic acidosis of acute iron poisoning can be explained by a number of different mechanisms. Lactic acidosis may result from hypovolemia, hypotension, and anemia, producing tissue hypoperfusion that causes increased anaerobic metabolism. Iron also disrupts oxidative phosphorylation through interference of the electron transport system, promoting anaerobic metabolism. Lipid peroxidation, catalyzed by ferrous ions, alters the membrane permeability of the mitochondria, allowing greater intramitochondrial accumulation of iron.[13] The in situ conversion of iron from the ferrous (Fe^{2+}) to ferric (Fe^{3+}) state releases hydrogen ions that contribute to the metabolic acidosis. A buildup of unused hydrogen ions generated from nonbound ferric ions contributes to marked acidosis. Finally, iron directly inhibits enzymatic processes of the Krebs cycle, with the resultant accumulation of organic acids. Thus, metabolic acidosis is multifactorial in etiology and must be aggressively managed from all aspects.

Central Nervous System

Neurologic manifestations from iron toxicity are probably a result of the systemic manifestations of hypoperfusion, metabolic acidosis, hepatic toxicity, and coagulopathy. Iron can produce cerebral edema by an unknown mechanism that manifests itself as lethargy, coma, and seizures.

TOXICOLOGY

Clinical Manifestations

The clinical presentation of acute iron toxicity has traditionally been divided into four stages, which were first described in 1964, and based on the pathophysiology of iron poisoning.[14] Progression of signs and symptoms may occur rapidly depending on the severity of the ingestion; thus, this clinical staging should be determined primarily by the patient's clinical manifestations and not solely by the time since the ingestion. Some authors have suggested that there are five clinical stages, distinguishing hepatic necrosis as a separate stage.[15] Nevertheless, clinical stages usually overlap in severe poisonings.

STAGE I (30 MINUTES TO 6 HOURS AFTER INGESTION) OR GASTROINTESTINAL PHASE

This stage is characterized by the acute GI effects of iron toxicity: nausea, abdominal pain, vomiting, and diarrhea. Local corrosive effects of iron to the stomach and intestinal tract may result in hematemesis, hematochezia, and melena. The vomitus and stools may also be dark gray, green, or black owing to the presence of disintegrating iron tablets. Vomiting is the most sensitive indicator of serious ingestions. Most patients with mild to moderate iron toxicity do not progress beyond this stage, with symptoms resolving within 6 to 8 hours. In severe ingestions, cardiovascular toxicity may also appear at this stage as pallor, tachycardia, and hypotension. Central nervous system toxicity may include lethargy and coma. The presence of shock and lethargy on initial presentation are poor prognostic signs. If no GI symptoms develop within 6 hours of a presumed iron ingestion, it is unlikely that iron toxicity will develop. Ingestion of enteric-coated iron tablets is an exception to the 6-hour rule.

STAGE II (6 TO 24 HOURS AFTER INGESTION)

This second phase of iron poisoning is sometimes referred to as the latent or quiescent period and is characterized by a transient resolution of GI symptoms. However, there may be subclinical hypoperfusion and metabolic acidosis if adequate fluid resuscitation has not been performed in the initial stage. The abatement of GI symptoms is presumed to occur as circulating free iron is redistributed into the reticuloendothelial system. Some patients may be prematurely discharged from a health care facility despite potentially life-threatening ingestions because of the false reassurance of clinical improvement. Thus, clinical reassessment and observation should occur if GI symptoms have improved to determine whether the patient has truly recovered or may progress to further clinical deterioration. This phase may be transient or not appear at all in those with severe iron ingestions.

STAGE III (12 TO 48 HOURS AFTER INGESTION) OR SYSTEMIC TOXICITY

Life-threatening systemic symptoms predominate during this stage. Fortunately, only a small percentage of patients with iron ingestions progress to this phase. Some patients with severe ingestions will progress to this phase of multisystem failure without experiencing a "quiescent phase." Recurrence of GI hemorrhage, hematemesis, melena, and bowel perforation may be seen. Acute circulatory shock characterized by tachycardia, tachypnea, pallor, hypotension, and cyanosis may recur. Cardiogenic shock may occur several days later owing to direct effects of iron on the myocardium. Metabolic

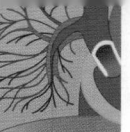
acidosis and coagulopathy are present. However, the hallmark of this phase is progressive pulmonary dysfunction with a radiologic appearance of adult-type respiratory distress syndrome or shock lung. The etiology is multifactorial: iron generation of free radicals that disrupt alveolar membranes in addition to the hypotension and metabolic acidosis. Hepatotoxicity usually occurs within 48 hours but does not develop in all iron-poisoned patients. It is the second most common cause of death after shock. Renal and neurologic dysfunction all may occur during this time. Death from iron toxicity is common in this phase, typically from respiratory failure and shock; thus, aggressive supportive treatment in addition to antidotal treatment is mandatory for survival.

STAGE IV (4 TO 6 WEEKS AFTER INGESTION) OR BOWEL OBSTRUCTION

Patients with severe poisoning who survive, as well as those who do not develop systemic toxicity, may go on to have gastric outlet obstruction or pyloric stenosis as a result of GI scarring. Vomiting is the presenting symptom of these late sequelae.

Range of Toxicity

The minimum toxic dose and the lethal dose of iron are not well established. Ingestions of less than 20 mg/kg of elemental iron have little risk for toxicity and require no specific treatment, although ingestion of 20 mg/kg in an adult human volunteer study resulted in nausea, malaise, and diarrhea in all six subjects.[16] Ingestions of greater than 60 mg/kg can be associated with serious toxicity and require immediate referral to a health care facility for evaluation. Death from iron toxicity has been reported with a wide range of doses, from 60 to 300 mg/kg. Ingestions of 20 to 60 mg/kg may or may not produce symptoms of serious toxicity and require other historical factors in making a decision regarding triage and referral. In a retrospective study of iron ingestions in children, 28% of 380 children who ingested 40 to 60 mg/kg of iron had symptoms of vomiting, diarrhea, and abdominal pain that resolved.[17] A retrospective review of 199 acute iron exposures revealed that only a small percentage of patients who ingested between 40 and 60 mg/kg of iron developed clinical symptoms (vomiting, diarrhea, abdominal pain), and no one developed serious toxicity.[18] No patient in this study who ingested between 20 and 60 mg/kg of elemental iron had a serum iron level of more than 385 µg/dL, and no one developed serious manifestations. Adult and adolescent overdoses should be considered as intentional and require immediate referral regardless of the dose assessment.

DIAGNOSIS

The relative infrequency of deaths associated with the large number of iron exposures suggests that a wide range of clinical toxicity exists in iron poisoning.

Evaluation, diagnosis, and subsequent management of the patient requires a knowledge of the pathophysiology and clinical presentation as well as the factors that can guide in predicting the severity of toxicity. Acute iron poisoning is a clinical diagnosis, supported by laboratory data. It is unlikely that a patient who does not have clinical signs and symptoms within 6 hours of reported ingestion will develop iron toxicity. There are many ancillary diagnostic tests that can help to confirm the diagnosis, although none of these should be used independently to determine disposition and treatment. It is important to accurately interpret and understand the limitations of these diagnostic tests in assessing a patient with suspected or known iron poisoning.

History

An important component of the history is the type of iron formulation and amount of elemental iron ingested because the likelihood of iron toxicity can be predicted based on this information. Ingestions of children's multivitamins with iron are rarely associated with significant clinical toxicity and have never been reported to cause death. The content of elemental iron is relatively small (10–18 mg/tablet), and thus an enormous number of pills must be ingested for toxicity to occur. On the other hand, pure iron preparations that contain ferrous salts (found in prenatal vitamins and nonprescription iron supplements) contain significantly more elemental iron per tablet. Very few tablets can produce toxicity when accidentally ingested by a small child.

Determining the estimated amount of elemental iron ingested on a milligram per kilogram basis can help predict iron toxicity, thereby directing the triage and management of patients with unintentional ingestions. The reliability of estimating the number of tablets ingested depends on an accurate history, which may not always be possible in every scenario, assuming the worst-case scenario in estimating total number of pills available. When determining the potential dose of iron ingested, it is important to calculate the amount of *elemental iron* present in the iron preparation by multiplying the milligram amount of the preparation times the percentage of elemental iron in that preparation. For example, each 325-mg tablet of ferrous sulfate contains 20% (65 mg) elemental iron. Thus, if a 12-kg child ingests 15 325-mg ferrous sulfate tablets, the dose ingested is 15 tablets × 65 mg per 12 kg body weight = 81 mg/kg of elemental iron.

Laboratory Testing

SERUM IRON CONCENTRATION

Serum iron concentrations cannot always be correlated with the severity or the clinical stage of iron intoxication because it is the intracellular iron, not the free circulating iron in the blood, that is responsible for systemic toxicity. The serum iron concentration is useful in confirming an ingestion and may be useful in predicting serious toxicity only if blood samples are

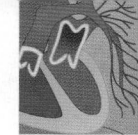

drawn at the appropriate time. The most valuable time to assess potential toxicity with an iron concentration is 4 to 6 hours after ingestion because this time reflects the peak absorption for most preparations, with the exception of slow-release iron. A serum iron measured after this time may be "normal" and inappropriately interpreted as "nontoxic" in the presence of a potentially toxic ingestion because of the intracellular distribution of iron. If the time of the ingestion is unknown, serial iron concentrations should be obtained to determine the peak iron concentration.

Serum iron concentrations less than 300 μg/dL (4–6 hours after ingestion) are associated with little to no toxicity, concentrations greater than 500 μg/dL are associated with definite serious toxicity, and concentrations greater than 1000 μg/dL have resulted in death. Iron concentrations between 300 and 500 μg/dL may be associated with mild, moderate, or no toxicity. Such concentrations must be used in conjunction with the patient's history and symptom complex to assess toxicity and the need for further intervention.

Iron concentrations are occasionally difficult to obtain on an emergency basis at many health care facilities. Thus, many studies have attempted to identify clinical symptoms and other laboratory data that would predict toxic iron concentrations. Invariably, these studies have been limited by their retrospective design and have not resulted in consistent identifiers. In one study, a white blood cell count greater than 15,000/mm[3] or a serum glucose concentration greater than 150 mg/dL had a high positive predictive value identifying the child with an iron concentration of more than 300 μg/dL.[19] Both parameters had very low specificity; thus, their absence did not exclude a high iron concentration. Vomiting was the most sensitive indicator for an iron concentration greater than 300 μg/dL. A subsequent study concluded that neither white blood cell count nor glucose concentration was accurate in identifying significant iron toxicity.[20] In a retrospective study of 92 children with iron poisoning, a serum iron concentration exceeding 500 μg/dL was associated with one single variable: coma.[21] Concurrent coma, radiopacities on abdominal radiographs, leukocytosis, and an elevated anion gap had a positive predictive value of 100%, and the absence of all the variables had a negative predictive value of 95% for a serum iron concentration higher than 500 μg/dL. These studies highlight the importance of inability to use a single laboratory test to predict iron toxicity.

A serum iron concentration should be obtained from every patient who has a history of ingesting more than 60 mg/kg elemental iron as well as anyone with significant clinical symptoms or an intentional overdose. Serial iron concentrations may be necessary if the time of ingestion is unknown. Serum iron concentrations may be falsely low in the presence of deferoxamine (DFO) because this chelator interferes with the standard colorimetric and radioimmunoassay methods for iron measurement.[22] When a patient is receiving DFO therapy, iron concentrations should be measured by atomic absorption spectrophotometry.

TOTAL IRON-BINDING CAPACITY

In the past, a serum iron concentration that exceeded the TIBC was considered an indication for chelation therapy and was believed to be a necessary laboratory test in the evaluation of the patient with iron poisoning. This was based on the assumption that the binding of iron to plasma proteins prevents any toxicity—when a serum iron concentration is less than the TIBC, there is little risk for toxicity. However, clinical experience has shown this maxim is untrue. No data have shown that iron toxicity only occurs when the serum iron concentration exceeds the TIBC. Also, TIBC measurements may be unreliable in the presence of excess serum iron or deferoxamine.[23,24] An in vitro study demonstrated that adding iron to pooled serum resulted in an artifactual rise in the TIBC.[25] This same study showed that TIBC determinations varied substantially among different laboratories. Another study demonstrated that even though the TIBC increased and remained above the serum iron concentration in patients with iron ingestions, symptoms of iron toxicity still occurred.[16] Because of the unreliability of the measured TIBC, this measurement is neither a useful nor a clinically indicated laboratory test in the evaluation of iron poisoning.

OTHER LABORATORY TESTS

Other laboratory studies that should be obtained in a patient with a significant iron ingestion include an arterial blood gas analysis; complete blood cell count; electrolytes, blood urea nitrogen, creatinine, glucose, and coagulation studies; serum transaminase determinations; and blood sampling for type and crossmatch.

Other Diagnostic Testing

ABDOMINAL RADIOGRAPHS

Because certain iron-containing preparations are radiopaque, an abdominal radiograph can be useful in confirming an iron ingestion and in determining the quantity and location of undissolved iron tablets in the intestinal tract (Fig. 72-1). However, the radiopacity of these tablets depends on the type of formulation and content of elemental iron. Thus, many liquid iron preparations and chewable vitamins with iron (which have low concentrations of iron) are not visible.[26] Also, the usefulness of the radiograph in determining the presence of iron pills may be limited if it is obtained more than 2 hours after the ingestion because the iron preparations may have dissolved and may not appear radiopaque despite their remaining in the GI tract. Thus, negative radiographs, especially 2 or more hours after ingestion, do not exclude iron overdose. Serial abdominal radiographs may be useful in determining the efficacy of GI decontamination.

Differential Diagnosis

The differential diagnosis should include infectious and metabolic etiologies for the GI symptoms and acid–base abnormalities. Similar clinical presentations from other

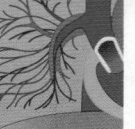

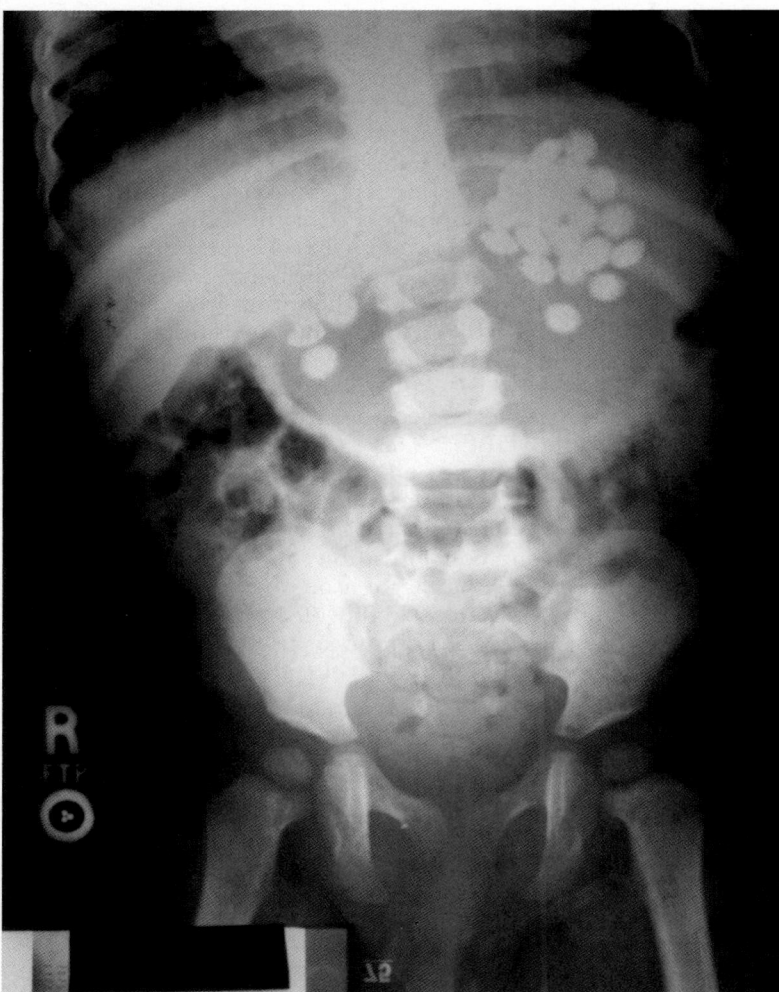

FIGURE 72-1. Abdominal radiograph of a 20-month-old child with a history of ingesting prenatal iron tablets.

poisonings include salicylates, theophylline, colchicine, organophosphates, arsenic, mercury, paraquat, and mushrooms. Fortunately, with pediatric ingestions, the history or abdominal radiograph confirms the diagnosis most of the time.

MANAGEMENT

Gastric decontamination, laboratory studies, and an abdominal radiograph are indicated for significant iron ingestions and clinical toxicity. For those unintentional ingestions between 40 and 60 mg/kg of elemental iron, the reliability of the history, reliability of the caretaker, and presence of clinical symptoms should dictate whether further diagnostic studies are necessary. Unintentional ingestions of less than 40 mg/kg of elemental iron require observation only (Fig. 72-2). Initial management should focus on ensuring an adequate airway, ventilation, and circulation. Hypovolemia and metabolic acidosis should be aggressively managed with isotonic fluid and bicarbonate.

Gastrointestinal Decontamination

Of major importance in limiting the severity of iron poisoning is preventing its absorption by removing as much as possible from the GI tract. Decisions regarding the optimal method for GI decontamination in iron ingestions are complicated by many issues. Many patients have already vomited, reducing the need for further gastric evacuation. This issue is addressed by obtaining an abdominal radiograph. Also, many adult iron preparations are too large to be removed from the holes in a gastric lavage tube, limiting the value of lavage in this setting. Finally, iron is not adsorbed by charcoal, increasing the overall importance of gastric evacuation efforts.

Gastric lavage with a large-bore orogastric tube may be indicated for intentional overdoses of iron and unintentional ingestions of more than 60 mg/kg of iron in those who have not vomited or who have visible pills in the stomach on abdominal radiograph. Normal saline is recommended as the lavage fluid. After lavage, a repeat abdominal radiograph should be obtained to assess the efficacy of gastric evacuation and determine whether further decontamination measures are necessary.

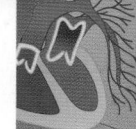

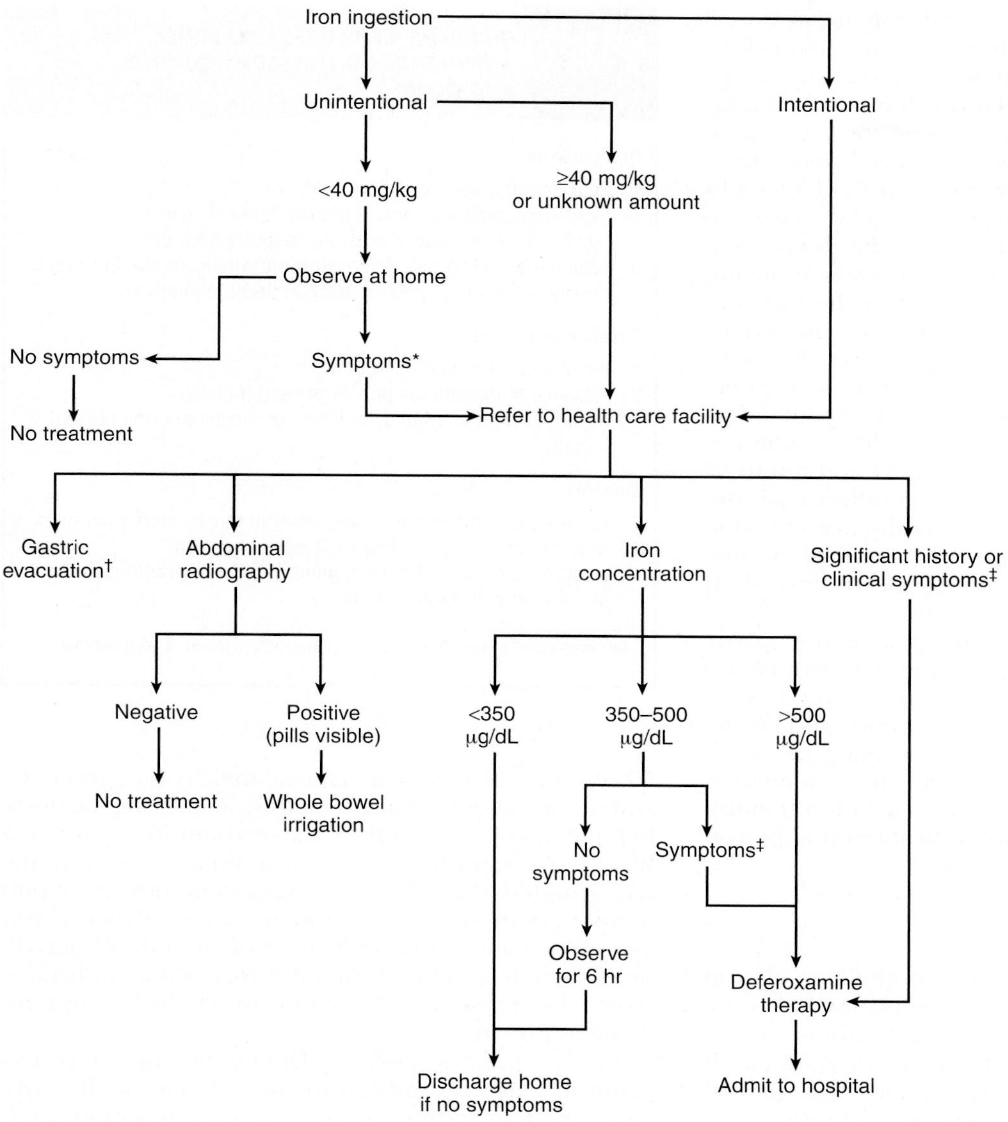

Iron ingestion

Unintentional — Intentional

<40 mg/kg — ≥40 mg/kg or unknown amount

Observe at home

No symptoms ← Symptoms*

No treatment → Refer to health care facility ←

Gastric evacuation†   Abdominal radiography   Iron concentration   Significant history or clinical symptoms‡

Negative → No treatment

Positive (pills visible) → Whole bowel irrigation

<350 µg/dL   350–500 µg/dL   >500 µg/dL

No symptoms   Symptoms‡

Observe for 6 hr

Deferoxamine therapy

Discharge home if no symptoms

Admit to hospital

FIGURE 72-2 Algorithm for evaluation and management of iron poisoning.
*Persistent vomiting, diarrhea, hematemesis, abdominal pain, and lethargy.
†See text regarding indications for gastric lavage and whole bowel irrigation.
‡Persistent vomiting, lethargy, coma, hypotension, and metabolic acidosis.

The use of complexing agents in lavage fluid is an interesting historical issue in iron poisoning. Sodium bicarbonate and phosphate solutions have been used on the theoretical assumption that insoluble ferrous salts will be formed in the stomach, limiting iron's systemic absorption.[27] However, multiple human and in vitro studies have failed to demonstrate benefits from these solutions. Moreover, toxicity from administration of phosphate solutions (hyperphosphatemia, hypocalcemia, and hypernatremia) contraindicates their use.[28] Complexing iron in the GI tract using oral DFO as a lavage fluid has also been advocated. Although some human and animal studies have suggested benefit from enterally administered DFO, others have shown it does not substantially reduce the amount of iron available for absorption.[29,30] Furthermore, some investigators have suggested that the iron–DFO complex ferrioxamine can be absorbed and contribute to increases in serum iron

concentrations; there is potential toxicity from the ferrioxamine compound as well.[31] From a clinical standpoint, oral DFO is impractical because of the large volumes required in overdose to have any appreciable effect (100 mg of DFO will bind only 8 or 9 mg of iron). Thus, no agent has proven advantage over normal saline; these alternatives are therefore not recommended.

Other measures to decrease the GI absorption of iron have been studied. Animal studies have demonstrated a marked reduction of iron absorption after administration of oral magnesium hydroxide preparations such as milk of magnesia, in a dose five times the amount of elemental iron ingested.[32] In addition, this solution may also provide a protective effect against the local corrosive effects of iron in the stomach and intestine. No human studies using magnesium hydroxide have been published. The use of an oral charcoal–DFO mixture has been shown in preliminary experimental studies to

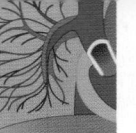

effectively decrease the amount of GI iron absorption.[33] Further studies are needed with this combination before it can be routinely recommended for GI decontamination.

If iron tablets persist in the GI tract despite vomiting, or gastric lavage and serum iron concentrations continue to rise, whole bowel irrigation with a polyethylene glycol electrolyte solution such as Colyte or GoLYTELY should be initiated. Whole bowel irrigation is an effective method of GI decontamination, decreasing the passage time of iron through the GI tract and thereby reducing the time available for absorption.[34] Given the fact that iron preparations may not be completely removed by emesis or lavage, as well as the fact that iron is poorly adsorbed to charcoal, whole bowel irrigation is theoretically the most effective means of GI decontamination. Polyethylene glycol solutions should be administered at a rate of 2 L/hr in adolescents and adults, 1 L/hr in children, and 500 mL/hr in toddlers until the rectal effluent is clear and there is an absence of visible iron on abdominal radiograph. If vomiting occurs, administration rate should be reduced and then gradually increased to the desired rate.

Iron tablets may become embedded in the gastric wall, forming bezoars or pseudo-concentrations that are resistant to normal methods of decontamination. In such cases, endoscopy or surgical gastrotomy should be considered, especially when clinical toxicity persists.[35] Aggressive decontamination measures, in combination with supportive care and appropriate chelation therapy, should obviate the need for the surgical removal of iron tablets except in rare circumstances.

Antidote

Deferoxamine is a relatively selective chelator of iron produced by the organism *Streptomyces pilosus* and is the antidote of choice for serious iron poisonings. Guidelines for DFO's use, route of administration, duration of therapy, and dosing are not clearcut, although general recommendations can be gleaned from clinical experience and several studies[30,31,36] (Box 72-1).

DFO combines with iron to form the iron–DFO complex known as ferrioxamine, which is then excreted through the kidneys. Ferrioxamine gives urine the classically described "vin rose" color, which actually is orange to reddish brown. DFO has a volume of distribution of 0.6 L/kg and a half-life of 10 to 30 minutes and is rapidly metabolized in the liver to inactive products. It binds iron in a 1:1 molar ratio, with 100 mg of DFO binding 9 mg of iron. Ferrioxamine has a volume of distribution of 0.2 L/kg. DFO binds circulating free iron in the ferric state. DFO also chelates ferric iron from ferritin and hemosiderin. DFO does not bind iron present in hemoglobin, myoglobin, transferrin, or cytochromes. However, there are other mechanisms that are probably responsible for DFO's protective effect; because it has a volume of distribution of 0.6 L/kg (indicating intracellular diffusion), it likely binds both cytosolic and intramitochondrial iron, preventing mitochondrial injury.

Indications for DFO chelation therapy are (1) peak serum iron concentration greater than or equal to

---

BOX 72-1   **GUIDELINES FOR DEFEROXAMINE ADMINISTRATION, DISCONTINUATION, AND DOSING**

Indications

1. Peak serum iron level ≥ 500 µg/dL, *or*
2. Significant clinical symptomatology: lethargy, coma, hypovolemia, metabolic acidosis, coagulopathy, *or*
3. Abdominal radiograph demonstrating significant number of pills despite attempts at gastrointestinal decontamination

Discontinuation*

1. Resolution of clinical symptoms
2. Absence of radiopaque pills (if present initially)
3. Return of normal urine color if vin rose–colored urine present initially

Dosing

1. Continuous intravenous infusion starting at 15 mg/kg per hour
2. May titrate dose according to severity of clinical symptomatology and development of hypotension (maximum infusion rate 30 mg/kg per hour)

*All three criteria should be present before deferoxamine is discontinued.

---

500 µg/dL; (2) significant clinical toxicity (i.e., severe GI symptoms, altered mental status, metabolic acidosis, hypoperfusion, cardiovascular instability); and (3) history of significant ingestion and an abdominal radiograph that demonstrates significant number of pills despite attempts at GI decontamination. Patients with peak iron concentrations between 350 and 500 µg/dL must be evaluated for chelation therapy on an individual basis; the presence of significant clinical symptoms mandates treatment.

In the past, a positive DFO challenge test was proposed as an indication for chelation therapy, particularly in settings where iron concentration levels are not readily obtainable. This test was performed by administering an intramuscular dose of DFO and then observing urine for the vin rose color. The ability to detect this urine color change is subjective, is qualitative, and requires prechelation urine samples for comparison. Several studies had found this urine color change to be an insensitive marker for the presence of significantly elevated serum iron concentrations or serious iron poisoning.[18,37] Thus, the absence of vin rose urine does not rule out severe iron toxicity. The DFO challenge test is therefore no longer recommended as a guide to determine the need for further chelation therapy.

Although DFO can be administered intravenously, intramuscularly, or subcutaneously, the preferred method for treatment of acute iron intoxication is a continuous intravenous infusion. Because of DFO's short half-life, the benefits of constant exposure to both the free circulating iron and the labile iron pool, this route is more advantageous. Intravenous administration of DFO has also been shown to be more efficient in removing iron than intramuscular administration.

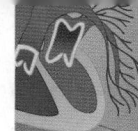

DFO should be administered at a starting rate of 15 mg/kg/hr. There has been considerable debate about the maximum dose of DFO that should be administered. This results from concerns about DFO-induced hypotension and about its possible relationship to the development of adult respiratory distress syndrome.[38] Although the package insert states that the maximum dose should be 6 g/day, there have been numerous cases in which doses up to 35 to 45 mg/kg/hr or 16 to 20 g/day were administered to seriously ill patients without complications.[39] The limiting factor in DFO use is development of hypotension; dosing should be titrated according to patient response and the development of side effects. With severe intoxication, blood pressure support with fluid and vasopressors may be necessary to give high-dose DFO. Dosing of DFO is based on the amount of "free iron"; theoretically, then, higher doses should be administered in the first 24 hours. Some investigators have recommended intermittent boluses of DFO or an initial "loading dose" followed by a reduced infusion rate.[40] Adequate hydration before and during DFO therapy is necessary because acute administration of DFO may lower glomerular filtration rate.[41]

Duration of DFO therapy is variable, and published guidelines for discontinuing DFO therapy are vague, occasionally being misleading or unsupported by scientific data. Rational criteria for termination of DFO are (1) resolution of clinical signs and symptoms of systemic iron poisoning, specifically anion-gap acidosis and shock; (2) disappearance of radiopaque iron pills on repeat abdominal radiographs; and (3) return of normal urine color if vin rose urine was initially present. Some investigators had advocated use of a urine iron-to-creatinine ratio to determine the end point of chelation; however, this measurement needs further clinical validation and is unavailable in most clinical settings.[42]

Potential adverse effects from DFO administration in acute iron poisoning are hypotension, rash, and *Yersinia enterocolitica* sepsis. Although the mechanism of hypotension is unknown, it may be caused by histamine release and is related to the rate of DFO infusion. The maximum rate of administration before hypotension develops is reported to be 45 mg/kg/hr; human reports have demonstrated infusion rates up to 35 mg/kg/hr without hypotension.[43] *Yersinia enterocolitica* sepsis has been reported in patients receiving DFO therapy.[44,45] DFO acts as a siderophore, supplying iron to the bacteria and thereby increasing its virulence. Any patient presenting with fever, nausea, diarrhea, or pulmonary symptoms during or after DFO therapy needs an assessment of infection, including blood and stool cultures for this pathogen.

Continuous DFO infusion for greater than 24 hours has been associated with the development of adult respiratory distress syndrome.[38] However, the validity of this association remains controversial because iron poisoning itself has been reported to cause similar pulmonary sequelae. The mechanism of action for this adverse effect is postulated to be production of free radicals in the lungs after prolonged exposure to DFO. However, iron can also generate free radicals that are capable of producing alveolar damage. The possibility of producing the adult respiratory distress syndrome in a patient with serious iron intoxication should not limit the use of DFO. Aggressive supportive therapy, careful monitoring, and appropriate discontinuation of DFO therapy should prevent this complication. One author has suggested administering the initial 24 hours of continuous deferoxamine infusion, followed by alternating 12 hours of DFO infusion with a 12-hour hiatus to allow for excretion of ferrioxamine.

The same guidelines for DFO administration should be applied to the pregnant patient without concern for adverse fetal effects from the DFO. Animal and human studies have demonstrated that neither toxic amounts of iron nor DFO cross the placenta.[46,47] Fetal death results from maternal death, not from the effects of iron or DFO on the fetus.

A new oral iron chelator, 1,2-dimethyl-3-hydroxypyrid-4-one (L1, deferiprone) is being investigated for treatment in chronically iron-overloaded patients.[48] Oral deferiprone recently was shown to be effective in reducing mortality in a rodent model of acute iron poisoning.[49] Its safety and efficacy in human iron overdose has not been studied.

Elimination Enhancement

Extracorporeal methods for enhancing the elimination of iron have been studied, although their potential effectiveness is quite limited because they only remove free circulating iron and must be initiated before significant intracellular transport of iron has occurred. Exchange transfusion is theoretically useful in removing a larger burden of free and bound iron from the blood, although there are no data to support its routine use.[50] Because the volume of distribution of ferrioxamine is low (0.2 L/kg), hemodialysis is effective in removing it should the patient develop renal failure.[51] Continuous arteriovenous hemofiltration has been investigated in experimental iron poisoning for removing ferrioxamine.[52] None of these therapies has been shown to decrease morbidity or mortality of iron intoxication.

Disposition

Unintentional ingestions of less than 20 mg/kg elemental iron may be observed at home. Unintentional exposures in patients who develop no signs and symptoms after 6 hours and have no iron seen on abdominal radiograph may be discharged from the emergency department. Patients who intentionally ingest iron may be cleared medically if the above criteria are met and other medical evaluation for co-ingestants does not necessitate intervention. Patients who develop significant clinical toxicity, including severe GI symptoms, metabolic acidosis, decreased level of consciousness, hemodynamic instability, or serum iron concentrations higher than 500 µg/dL, should be monitored and treated in an intensive care unit.

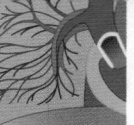

REFERENCES

1. U.S. Food and Drug Administration, HHS: Iron-containing supplements and drugs; label warning statements and unit-dose packaging requirements; removal of regulations for unit-dose packaging requirements for dietary supplements and drugs. Final rule: removal of regulatory provisions in response to court order. Fed Regist 2003;68:59714–59715.
2. Ryan TP, Aust SD: The role of iron in oxygen-mediated toxicities. CRC Crit Rev Toxicol 1992;22:119–141.
3. Whitten CF, Brough AJ: The pathophysiology of acute iron poisoning. Clin Toxicol 1971;4:585–595.
4. Tenenbein M, Littman C, Stimpson RE: Gastrointestinal pathology in adult iron overdose. J Toxicol Clin Toxicol 1990;28:311–320.
5. Ghandi R, Robarts F: Hourglass stricture of the stomach and pyloric stenosis due to ferrous sulfate poisoning. Br J Surg 1962;49:613–617.
6. Vernon DD, Banner W, Dean JM: Hemodynamic effects of experimental iron poisoning. Ann Emerg Med 1989;18:863–866.
7. Whitten CF, Chen YC, Gibson GW: Studies in acute iron poisoning. III. The hemodynamic alterations in acute experimental iron poisoning. Pediatr Res 1968;2:479–485.
8. Tenenbein M, Kopelow ML, deSa DJ: Mycardial failure and shock in iron poisoning. Hum Toxicol 1988;7:281–284.
9. Gleason WA, de Mello DE, deCastro FJ, et al: Acute hepatic failure in severe iron poisoning. J Pediatr 1979;95:138–140.
10. Bonkovsky HL: Iron and the liver. Am J Med Sci 1991;301:32–43.
11. Tenenbein M, Israels SJ: Early coagulopathy in severe iron poisoning. J Pediatr 1988;113:695–697.
12. Rosenmund A, Haeberli A, Straub PW: Blood coagulation and acute iron toxicity. J Lab Clin Med 1984;103:524–533.
13. Halliwell B, Gutteridge JMC: Oxygen free radicals and iron in relation to biology and medicine: some problems and concepts. Arch Biochem Biophys 1986;246:501–514.
14. Covey TJ: Ferrous sulfate poisoning: a review, case summaries, and therapeutic regimen. J Pediatr 1964;64:218–226.
15. Banner W, Tong TG: Iron poisoning. Pediatr Clin North Am 1986;33:393–409.
16. Burkhart KK, Kulig KW, Hammond KB, et al: The rise in the total iron-binding capacity after iron overdose. Ann Emerg Med 1991;20:532–535.
17. Oderda GM, Gorman RL, Rose SR, et al: When is referral to the hospital necessary in acute iron ingestion? [abstract]. Vet Hum Toxicol 1987;29:465.
18. Klein-Schwartz W, Oderda GM, Gorman RL, et al: Assessment of management guidelines: acute iron ingestion. Clin Pediatr 1990;29:316–321.
19. Lacouture PG, Wason S, Temple AR, et al: Emergency assessment of severity in iron overdose by clinical and laboratory methods. J Pediatr 1981;99:89–91.
20. Knasel AL, Collins-Barrow AL: Applicability of early indicators of iron toxicity. J Natl Med Assoc 1986;78:1037–1040.
21. Chyka PA, Butler AY: Assessment of acute iron poisoning by laboratory and clinical observations. Am J Emerg Med 1993;11:99–103.
22. Helfer RE, Rodgerson DO: The effect of deferoxamine on the determination of serum iron and iron binding capacity. J Pediatr 1986;68:804–806.
23. Bentur Y, St. Louis P, Klein J, Koren G: Misinterpretation of iron-binding capacity in the presence of deferoxamine. J Pediatr 1991;118:139–142.
24. Siff JE, Meldon SW, Tomassoni AJ: Usefulness of the total iron binding capacity in the evaluation and treatment of acute iron overdose. Ann Emerg Med 1999;33:73–76.
25. Tenenbein M, Yatscoff RW: The total iron-binding capacity in iron poisoning: Is it useful? Am J Dis Child 1991;145:437–439.
26. Everson GW, Oukjhane K, Young LW, et al: Effectiveness of abdominal radiographs in visualizing chewable iron supplements following overdose. Am J Emerg Med 1989;7:459–463.
27. Czajka PA, Konrad JD, Duffy JP: Iron poisoning: an in vitro comparison of bicarbonate and phosphate lavage solutions. J Pediatr 1981;98:491–494.
28. Geffner ME, Opas LM: Phosphate poisoning complicating treatment for iron ingestion. Am J Dis Child 1980;134:509–510.
29. Henretig FM, Karl SR, Weintraub WH: Severe iron poisoning treated with enteral and intravenous deferoxamine. Ann Emerg Med 1983;12:306–309.
30. McEnery JT, Greengard J: Treatment of acute iron ingestion with deferoxamine in 20 children. J Pediatr 1966;68:773–779.
31. Whitten CF, Chen YC, Gibson GW: Studies in acute iron poisoning. II. Further observations on desferrioxamine in the treatment of acute experimental iron poisoning. Pediatrics 1966;38:102–110.
32. Corby DG, McCullen AH, Chadwick EW, Decker WJ: Effect of orally administered magnesium hydroxide in experimental iron intoxication. J Toxicol Clin Toxicol 1985–1986;23:489–499.
33. Gomez HF, McClafferty H, Flory D, et al: Prevention of gastrointestinal iron absorption by chelation from an orally administered premixed deferoxamine/charcoal mixture. Ann Emerg Med 1997;30:587–592.
34. Tenenbein M: Whole bowel irrigation in iron poisoning. J Pediatr 1987;111:142–145.
35. Foxford R, Goldfrank L: Gastrotomy: a surgical approach to iron overdose. Ann Emerg Med 1985;14:1223–1226.
36. Whitten CF, Gibson GW, Good MH, et al: Studies in acute iron poisoning. I. Desferrioxamine in the treatment of acute iron poisoning: clinical observations, experimental studies and theoretical considerations. Pediatrics 1965;36:322–335.
37. Villalobos D: Reliability of urine color changes after deferoxamine challenge [abstract]. Vet Hum Toxicol 1992;34:330.
38. Tenenbein M, Kowalski S, Sienko A, et al: Pulmonary toxic effects of continuous desferrioxamine administration in acute iron poisoning. Lancet 1992;339:699–701.
39. Shannon M: Desferrioxamine in acute iron poisoning. Lancet 1992;339:1601.
40. Cheney K, Gumbiner C, Benson B, Tenenbein M: Survival after a severe iron poisoning treated with intermittent infusions of deferoxamine. Clin Toxicol 1995;33:61–66.
41. Koren G, Bentur Y, Strong D, et al: Acute changes in renal function associated with deferoxamine therapy. Am J Dis Child 1989;143:1077–1080.
42. Yatscoff RW, Wayne EA, Tenenbein M: An objective criterion for the cessation of deferoxamine therapy in the acutely iron poisoned patient. Clin Toxicol 1991;29:1–10.
43. Bentur Y, McGuigan M, Koren G: Deferoxamine: new toxicities for an old drug. Drug Saf 1991;6:37–46.
44. Melby K, Slorhahl S, Gutteberg TJ, Mordbo SA: Septicemia due to Yersinia enterocolitica oral doses of iron. BMJ 1982;285:487–488.
45. Mofenson HC, Caraccio TR, Sharieff N: Iron sepsis: Yersinia enterocolitica septicemia possibly caused by an overdose of iron. N Engl J Med 1987;316:1092–1093.
46. Curry SC, Bond GR, Raschke R, et al: An ovine model of maternal iron poisoning in pregnancy. Ann Emerg Med 1990;19:632–638.
47. McElhatton PR, Roberts JC, Sullivan FM: The consequences of iron overdose and its treatment with desferrioxamine in pregnancy. Hum Exp Toxicol 1991;10:251–259.
48. Kontoghiorghes GJ: New concepts of iron and aluminum chelation therapy with oral L1 (deferiprone) and other chelators: a review. Analyst 1995;120:845–851.
49. Berkovitch M, Livne A, Lushkov G, et al: The efficacy of oral deferiprone in acute iron poisoning. Am J Emerg Med 2000;18:36–40.
50. Movassaghi N, Purugganan GG, Leikin S: Comparison of exchange transfusion and deferoxamine in the treatment of acute iron poisoning. J Pediatr 1969;75:604–608.
51. Richardson JR, Sugerman DL, Hulet WH: Extraction of iron by chelation with desferrioxamine and hemodialysis. Clin Res 1967;15:368.
52. Banner W, Vernon DD, Ward RM, et al: Continuous arteriovenous hemofiltration in experimental iron intoxication. Crit Care Med 1989;17:1187–1190.

73 *Lead*

MICHAEL W. SHANNON, MD, MPH

At a Glance...

- Lead is a potent biologic toxin that possesses no physiologic benefit.
- Anthropogenic activity has placed enormous amounts of lead in the environment, resulting in almost universal exposure in humans.
- The major organ systems affected by lead are the brain, kidneys, bone marrow, skeleton, and reproductive tract.
- Lead is particularly harmful to young children, producing permanent effects to the brain and kidneys.
- Adults with lead poisoning can develop effects including emotional lability, memory difficulties, loss of libido, difficulty concentrating, and peripheral neuropathy.
- Treatment of lead poisoning in children consists of termination of exposure and nutritional supplementation; chelation therapy may also be necessary.
- Treatment of lead poisoning in adults consists of termination of exposure; chelation therapy is typically reserved for those with blood lead levels greater than 60 to 100 µg/dL.

Lead was once prized as one of the most valuable elements on earth. Because it has a number of highly desirable properties (low melting point, malleability, durability, low cost, octane-boosting), lead is ubiquitous in the environment. Both industrial and developing nations have found beneficial uses for lead. However, lead is also a potent toxin. In the past century, an explosion of scientific data has demonstrated the toxic effects of lead on the human body. This has been highlighted by the growing body of evidence that even small amounts of lead can produce permanent harm, particularly in young children. Lead poisoning (plumbism) is now considered one of the most common diseases of environmental origin.[1]

This chapter reviews the toxicology of lead poisoning. Because of unique differences in the epidemiology, clinical toxicity, and treatment strategies of lead poisoning in adults compared with children, the chapter is later subdivided into lead poisoning in adults and then children.

HISTORY

Lead has been mined for thousands of years; the earliest recorded lead mine reportedly existed in Turkey in 6500 BC.[2,3] Evidence of high lead use can be found in the skeletons of ancient Egyptians. By the Greek Bronze Age, lead was widely used in the manufacture of brass and cosmetics. Also, because lead geologically coexisted with silver, the mining of silver resulted in a marked increase in lead exposure. It is estimated that as long as 2200 years ago, 25,000 tons of lead were produced annually.[2] Reflecting the increased use of lead over time, contemporary skeletons have bone lead concentrations 500 times higher than skeletons from ancient societies.[2,4]

The fall of the Roman Empire is thought to have resulted from lead intoxication.[3-5] During this era, lead-induced gout was endemic. Romans used lead in their plumbing (the word *plumbing* is derived from the traditional use of lead in water conduits), in their cooking utensils, and in the vessels that concentrated grape juice for wine. Lead was popular in wine because it enhanced color, wetness, and bouquet. The lead content of wine in the Roman era may have been as high as 15 to 30 mg/L. In fact, well into the 20th century, wines contained added lead. Lead poisoning was described at the same time that the metal became popular. Hippocrates wrote descriptions of lead colic. Similar descriptions have been recorded throughout history by Benjamin Franklin and others.

Initial interest in the illnesses caused by lead poisoning has been attributed to an 1839 publication by Tanquerel des Plances in which he described the clinical course of workers, primarily painters, who developed lead colic.[4] In 1860, corresponding with the industrialization of Europe, epidemiologists described widespread reproductive toxicity in those with lead-related occupations as well as their spouses. In the 20th century, these occurrences, which were also being identified in the United States, led to regulations that protected workers from occupational exposure to lead. At an extreme, laws were passed to exclude women from lead-related occupations; the U.S. Supreme Court later reversed such laws.[4]

The increasing desire to reduce exposure to lead also resulted in legislation to protect not only workers but also the public at large from the hazards of lead exposure. Establishment of the Environmental Protection Agency (EPA) and passage of important laws including the Clean Air Act, the Clean Water Act, the Lead Poisoning Prevention Act, and the Housing and Community Development Act (Title X) all have served to dramatically reduce nonoccupational exposure to lead.

EPIDEMIOLOGY

Population Rates

The blood lead level of Americans has been monitored through the periodic conductance of the National Health and Nutrition Examination Survey (NHANES). The results of the most recent surveillance indicate that mean blood lead level has declined more than 80% since the performance of NHANES II (1976–1980), from 12.8 µg/dL to a current level of about 2 µg/dL.[6-8] In

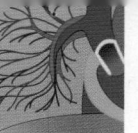

males, blood lead levels begin to rise in adolescence, continuing through most of adulthood, reflecting occupational exposure.[9] In both elderly men and women, blood lead levels rise again, representing remobilization of lead as bone resorption occurs.

No particular blood lead level clearly defines lead poisoning in adults. In the past, the reference range for blood lead in adults was up to 60 μg/dL. The normal range is now considered to be less than 40 μg/dL. However, many clinicians continue to believe that lead poisoning in adults is defined only by the presence of clinical symptoms, not by any particular blood lead level. The increasing evidence of subclinical effects at low blood levels in adults argues for defining lead intoxication as a blood lead level of greater than 25 μg/dL.

Sources

Lead can be found throughout the environment. Exposure to lead therefore usually occurs from a number of sources (Fig. 73-1). Many of these sources are highly age dependent. For example, most (but not all) lead-based occupations expose adults but not children to excess lead. Although lead exposure can occur after a single event—for example, after inhalation of lead fumes during welding—it is usually chronic.

OCCUPATIONAL

In adults, the most significant exposures to lead usually occur in the workplace. The list of occupations associated with lead exposure is large (Box 73-1). Occupation-specific tasks including demolition, radiator repair, home remodeling, burning, blasting, firearm instruction (indoor and outdoor), grinding, and sanding all can result in frank lead poisoning.[10-12]

Occupational lead standards were introduced by the Occupational Safety and Health Administration (OSHA) in 1978 and have not been significantly revised.[13] Under these guidelines, the permissible exposure limit for lead is 50 μg/m³ for an 8-hour time-weighted average. Employers are responsible for maintaining proper working conditions, as well as for environmental and medical monitoring.[13] Workers with blood lead levels of 60 μg/dL or greater must be removed from the workplace; those with blood lead levels of 50 μg/dL or greater on three occasions at 1-month intervals in the prior 3 months must also be removed from work. Those with blood lead levels of 40 μg/dL or greater must undergo medical evaluation.[11] Employers are responsible for paying the salaries of employees who are removed from work for lead-related reasons.[13] Because of the reproductive effects of lead at lower lead levels, recommendations have been made that the permissible blood lead level in workers be reduced to 10 μg/dL.[1]

LEAD PAINT

Lead has been added to paint for centuries in order to make pigments more vivid, colors more stable, and the paint more durable. For the years that these beneficial properties were exploited, the addition of lead to paint was an industry standard. It is because of its durability under adverse weather conditions that lead-based paint became most popular in the northeastern United States. Interestingly, in Canada, which has even harsher climatic conditions, lead was banned from residential paint early in the 20th century. In the United States, however, lead was added to paint until 1978, when, in an effort to reduce lead exposure, particularly among young children, lead was effectively banned (restricted to a concentration of no more than 0.06%) from use in

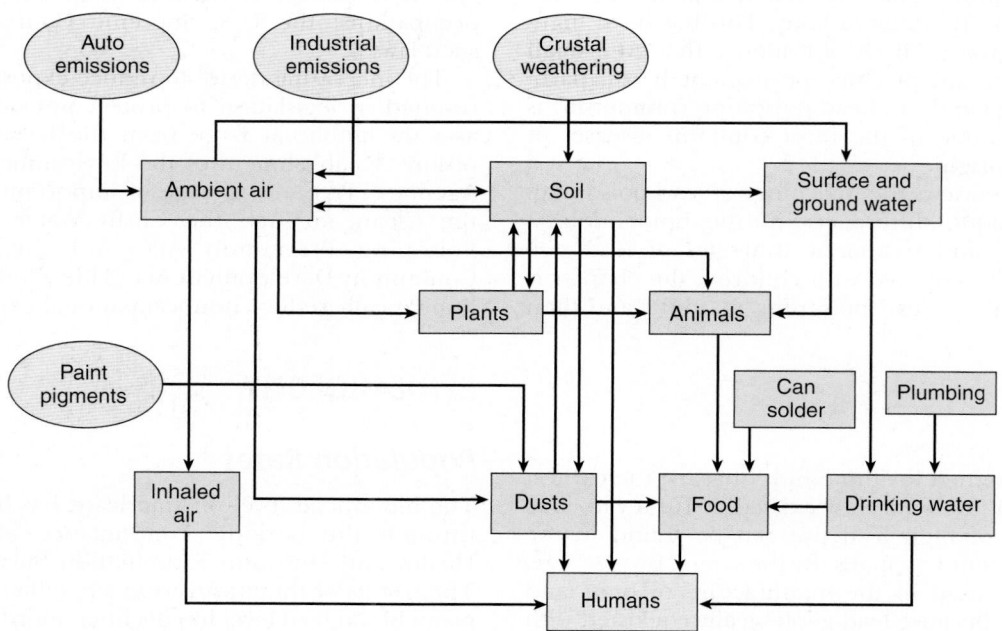

FIGURE 73-1 Sources and pathways of lead from environment to humans. (From U.S. Environmental Protection Agency: Air Quality Criteria for Lead. EPA-600/08_83/028aF-dF. Research Triangle Park, NC, Author, 1986.)

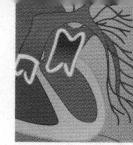

BOX 73-1   **SITES, INDUSTRIES, AND ACTIVITIES ASSOCIATED WITH LEAD EXPOSURE**

Sites

Firing ranges
Lead smelters
Homes and communities near lead smelters

Industries

Battery manufacture
Cooper smelting
Gasoline additive production
Ore crushing and grinding
Paint and pigment manufacture
Plastics industry
Printing industry
Rubber industry
Solid waste combustion
Zinc smelting

Activities

Auto repair
Construction and demolition
Firearm instruction
Home renovation
Professional painting
Plumbing
Radiator repair
Soldering of lead products
Welding and cutting operations

From Keogh JP, Boyer LV: Lead. In Sullivan JB, Krieger GR (eds): Hazardous Materials Toxicology, 2nd ed. Baltimore, Williams & Wilkins, 2001.

residential paint. Lead-containing paint is still used in nonresidential settings.[11] As a result of its extensive application, lead paint can be found in more than 38 million housing units in the United States.[14]

The presence of lead-based paint in homes has led to several problems. First, the natural decay of paint results in both chipping and the creation of lead dust. Also, when lead-containing homes undergo renovation of any type (e.g., scraping, demolition, window or wall removal), lead is released into the environment.[15] Certain types of renovation, particularly paint removal with a heat gun, are extremely hazardous, resulting in the creation of highly toxic lead fumes.[16] Even when homes are undergoing deleading in an effort to reduce lead hazards, improper techniques can result in lead poisoning in all family members.[17] The EPA has established guidelines for safe levels of lead in household dust as follows: maximum lead concentration in uncarpeted floors, 40 μg/ft^2; interior window wells, 250 μg/ft^2; and window wells, 400 μg/ft^2 (www.epa.gov).

AIR

Industrial and automobile emissions are historically a major source of lead exposure. In the United States, leaded gasoline released more than 30 million tons of lead into the air before it was banned.[4] The extent of airborne lead's contribution to lead levels is seen in the

effect of its removal from gasoline; when lead was phased out of gasoline in the 1970s, the mean blood lead of all Americans promptly declined by 35%. In the United States, the phase-out of leaded gasoline was completed in December 1995.

WATER

Water has become an increasingly important source of lead exposure, particularly as the contributions of paint, dust, food, and air diminish. Lead has contaminated many bodies of water as it has settled from the atmosphere. The increasing acidity of fresh water, due to acid rain, increases the solubility of waterborne lead. Soft water presents more of a lead hazard than hard water.[18]

Regulation of lead in public water supplies is the responsibility of the EPA. In a 1991 revision of the Clean Water Act, the maximum contaminant level of lead in water, which had been 50 parts per billion (ppb, μg/L), was replaced by an action level of 15 ppb. Under these new regulations, water suppliers must implement measures to reduce the level of lead in water if a significant number of homes are found to have elevated levels of lead.

Plumbing is an important cause of lead contamination in residential water. When public plumbing systems became widespread in the early 20th century, lead pipes served as the primary conduits directing water from public water sources into the home. In the 1950s, the use of lead pipes declined considerably. However, old public water systems continue to have extensive networks of lead pipe plumbing. Lead pipes have been largely replaced by copper or polyvinylchloride (PVC) pipes. The use of lead-based solder to join copper pipe joints was permitted until 1986. Therefore, homes with copper plumbing can be assumed to have lead in their water circuit. Because of the continued presence of lead pipes and copper pipes with lead solder joints, many cities in the United States have a high prevalence of lead-contaminated water.

Bottled water, which is under the regulation and oversight of the U.S. Food and Drug Administration, must have a lead content of no more than 5 ppb.

SOIL

Lead in soil can result either from its natural occurrence or contamination. The latter is responsible for most surface water lead in the United States. For example, studies of soil surrounding lead-emitting industries (e.g., smelters) have revealed soil lead concentrations higher than 60,000 parts per million (ppm, mg/L). In homes, lead contamination of soil occurs as painted exterior surfaces deteriorate.

Lead in soil is an important vector for human exposure. The EPA, in conjunction with the U.S. Department of Housing and Urban Development, has sought to reduce lead exposure through the development of guidelines on safe levels in soil. Under these standards, a safe concentration of lead in soil is considered to be less than 400 ppm.

HOBBIES

Certain household hobbies can result in lead exposure. These include any work that involves the use of solder

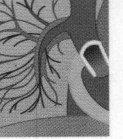

(which, when volatilized, produces highly absorbable lead fumes), the manufacture of fishing weights, and various aspects of artisanship. In the latter category, ceramic glazes occasionally contain lead. Although the use of lead glaze has been markedly reduced, it still occurs.

FOLK AND ALTERNATIVE MEDICINES

As discussed in Chapter 68, lead is sometimes found in alternative medicines, including Ayurvedic and folk remedies.[19-23] Dolomite, clamshell powder, and other calcium supplements may contain lead, particularly if their source is pulverized bone.[20-28]

FOOD

Food can be another source of chronic lead exposure. Lead enters the food chain through various routes. Vegetables, particularly homegrown vegetables that are grown in lead-contaminated soil, can introduce lead into the diet. Storage cans ("tin cans") were previously manufactured with a lead-solder seam. This seam, coming into direct contact with food, could readily release lead, particularly into acidic foods. In some studies, the solder seam raised the lead content of food as much as 4000-fold. The use of lead solder for the seam was banned in November 1991.[8] However, its widespread use has left many lead-containing cans still available.[8] Also, cans brought from other areas of the world are likely to contain lead.

Kitchenware can also be a source of lead. Previous reports have identified frank lead poisoning from the use of lead-containing vessels. These include samovars (heating urns), plates, bowls, cups, pots, and containers made of pewter.[29]

OTHER

Lead exposure can result from various types of substance abuse. First, the age-old practice of "moonshining"—that is, making illicit ethanol—has long been associated with lead poisoning from the use of lead-containing vessels such as discarded automobile radiators.[30,31] Lead poisoning can be caused by sniffing leaded gasoline; this is one of the few causes of organic lead exposure. Finally, the synthesis of methamphetamine may involve lead acetate. Sporadic reports have described lead intoxication from the injection of lead-contaminated methamphetamine.

Lead absorption from retained bullets can occur in those with gunshot wounds.[32,33] However, the kinetics of lead absorption from soft tissue have not been well characterized. For example, in animal models, lead appears to be poorly absorbed from muscle and fat; lead absorption from pleura and synovial fluid is most efficient.[34] Data from armed conflicts since the Civil War have documented lead poisoning in troops.[34]

TOXICOKINETICS

Lead is variably absorbed after ingestion. Its absorption is active, mediated by the same mucosal transport proteins that mediate calcium transport.[35] However, absorption is dependent on several factors, including the form of lead, particle size, gastrointestinal (GI) transit time, nutritional status, and chronologic age. Lead absorption is inversely proportional to size; the smaller the particle, the more complete the absorption. This is why exposure to lead dust results in higher lead concentrations than ingestion of an equal amount of lead from a paint chip.

Nutritional status is being increasingly shown to influence the extent of lead absorption. For example, iron deficiency results in increased lead absorption, probably because these atoms are linked to the same transport system.[35,36] Iron deficiency also alters lead distribution within the body.[37] The prevalence of lead intoxication in childhood results, in part, from the relatively high incidence of iron deficiency in this population. Similarly, calcium deficiency is associated with increased lead absorption. High fat intake and inadequate calories have also been associated with enhanced lead absorption. Lead absorption is increased when the stomach is empty; small frequent meals reduce absorption, probably through lead binding by dietary phytates and other complexing agents.[35] Finally, lead absorption is inversely proportional to chronologic age. As a general rule, 30% to 50% of ingested lead is absorbed from the gut of a child, compared with less than 10% in an adult.[11,35] This may be related to a higher density of intestinal transport proteins during periods of rapid growth.[35] Lead is also readily absorbed after inhalation of dust or fumes. Generally speaking, lead particles must be less than 0.5 μm to be absorbed from the respiratory tract.[38] Although inorganic lead is not absorbed through intact skin, organic lead compounds are.[11]

After absorption, lead circulates in blood, having a half-life of about 30 days in adults.[39] However, half-life is related to the duration of exposure. Those with short-term exposure experience more rapid disappearance of lead from blood than those with long-term exposure.[40] In the blood, 95% of lead is attached to (or within) the erythrocyte; thus, it is *blood lead* and not serum lead levels that are measured. The volume of distribution of lead is unclear but is presumed to be large; only 1% to 5% of the body's lead burden is in the circulation.[1] Lead readily crosses the placenta; fetal blood lead levels are typically 30% to 35% higher than maternal blood levels.[11,41-43]

The distribution kinetics of lead follows a three-compartment model. From blood, lead diffuses into soft tissues, including the liver, kidneys, bone marrow, and brain. This compartment is the primary site of lead's cellular toxicity. After a period that corresponds to a half-life of 1 to 2 months, lead diffuses from these tissues into bone. In bone, lead is incorporated into the hydroxyapatite lattice.[11] Lead is similarly incorporated into teeth. Once it is a part of bone, lead is presumed to be inert and nontoxic; however, this issue has been revisited as it becomes clear that conditions associated with bone mobilization (e.g., zero gravity, complete bed rest, medications, advancing years, and thyrotoxicosis) can also result in mobilization of lead.[44] Several researchers have described recurrent lead intoxication in children

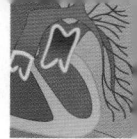

with a prior history of lead intoxication when they suffer conditions producing bone mobilization.[45,46] Concerns have been expressed that pregnancy, another state of bone resorption, can result in increased lead mobilization with the potential for fetal exposure to excess lead.[47-49]

Because of lead's incorporation into bone, most lead is retained in the body with very little elimination (in the absence of chelation); only about 30 μg/day is excreted by the kidneys.[11] Therefore, declining blood lead levels in those with lead poisoning not undergoing chelation represent only lead's distribution into soft tissues, not its excretion. In occupational monitoring, urinary lead excretion of less than 50 μg/g of creatinine is within normal limits. Lead's overall half-life is about 10,000 days (20–30 years).[1,3,50]

MECHANISMS OF TOXICITY

The cellular mechanisms of lead's toxicity are multiple and involve many different physiologic actions. Lead is particularly toxic to enzymes, particularly zinc-dependent enzymes. The blood lead levels at which adverse health effects occur are variable (Table 73-1).

Organs most sensitive to lead's toxicity are the kidneys, hematopoietic system, and nervous system. In the kidneys, lead interferes with the heme-containing hydroxylase enzyme, which converts 25-vitamin D to 1,25-vitamin D, an effect that is reversible.[11,51] In addition, a toxic action affects the renal tubules, producing a tubulopathy characterized by selective proteinuria. At blood levels as low as 40 μg/dL, lead produces dense intranuclear inclusion bodies in renal

tubules.[1] More advanced stages of lead nephropathy are associated with interstitial fibrosis, as well as tubular atrophy, with relative sparing of the glomeruli.[1]

Lead has a high affinity for sulfydryl groups, particularly those of metalloenzymes. Such enzymes include those in the heme synthetic pathway, particularly δ-aminolevulinic acid dehydratase, coproporphyrinogen oxidase, and ferrochelatase.[40] δ-Aminolevulinic acid dehydratase activity is inhibited at blood lead levels as low as 5 μg/dL.[40,52] This results in accumulation of δ-aminolevulinic acid, a putative neurotoxin.[43,53] Inhibition of ferrochelatase, which is responsible for incorporating iron into the porphyrin core, leads to elevated levels of erythrocyte protoporphyrin (EP).

Lead also affects neurotransmitter production.[48] This may be related to its ability to inhibit calmodulin, pyruvate kinase, and other enzymes essential to neuronal function. Many of lead's neurotoxic effects appear to result from its inhibition of cellular functions requiring zinc and calcium (which are also divalent cations).[53,54] Lead interferes with normal calcium metabolism, causing intracellular calcium buildup; it binds to most calcium-activated proteins with 100,000 times greater affinity.[4]

LEAD POISONING IN ADULTS

Clinical Manifestations

Acute lead intoxication in adults is rare but can occur after high-dose respiratory exposure, such as use of a heating gun, acetylene torching of lead-coated metal, or organic lead exposure.[11] Acute intoxication can produce

LOWEST OBSERVED EFFECT PbB (µg/dL)	HEME SYNTHESIS AND HEMATOLOGIC EFFECTS	NEUROLOGIC EFFECTS	EFFECTS ON THE KIDNEYS	REPRODUCTIVE FUNCTION EFFECTS	CARDIOVASCULAR EFFECTS
100–120		Encephalopathic signs and symptoms	Chronic nephropathy		
80	Frank anemia				
60				Female reproductive effects	
50	Reduced hemoglobin production	↑ Subencephalopathic neurologic symptoms		Altered testicular function	
40	Increased urinary ALA and elevated coproporphyrins	↓ Peripheral nerve dysfunction (slowed nerve conduction)			
30					Elevated blood pressure (white males, ages 40–49)
25–30	Erythrocyte protoporphyrin elevation in males				
15–20	Erythrocyte protoporphyrin elevation in females				
<10	ALA-D inhibition				

TABLE 73-1 Significant Health Effects of Lead at Lowest Observed Blood Lead (PbB) Levels in Adults

ALA-D, δ-aminolevulinic acid dehydratase.

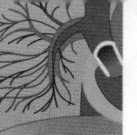

encephalopathy, severe GI upset, and renal failure. More commonly, lead intoxication results from long-term exposure.

Central nervous system (CNS) manifestations predominate in lead-poisoned adults. Signs and symptoms include fatigue, irritability, lethargy, insomnia, headache, difficulty concentrating, memory loss, and tremor.[11,55] Other symptoms include myalgias, vomiting, constipation, and loss of libido.[11] Severe lead intoxication can result in an encephalopathy characterized by depressed consciousness, seizures, and coma, in association with cerebral edema. Life-threatening neurotoxicity usually develops with blood lead levels exceeding 150 μg/dL. Another CNS effect of lead poisoning is an abnormal auditory brainstem evoked potential.[11,56]

Lead is also toxic to the peripheral nervous system, producing an axonopathy that results in motor disturbances.[13,56] The distinctive pattern of lead-induced peripheral neuropathy affects the upper extremities more than the lower extremities, the extensors more than the flexors, and the dominant more than the non-dominant arm. Painter's wristdrop is a once-endemic syndrome of upper extremity paresis found in painters who regularly used or removed lead-based paint. The initial segmental demyelination eventually leads to injury of both the axon and cell body.[3] Nerve conduction studies have shown that ulnar nerve conduction is disturbed at lead levels as low as 30 μg/dL.[1,11,50,56]

The kidneys are a third major site of lead's clinical toxicity. After lead exposure, lead concentrations are highest in the kidneys, particularly in the proximal tubules. As a result, lead, like cadmium, produces a renal injury characterized by excretion of β_2-microglobulin and N-acetylglucosidase.[57,58] These proteins have been suggested as early markers of subacute lead-induced renal injury. Finally, chronic exposure to lead can result in hypertension; animal models suggest that hypertension results from disturbances in vasomotor tone.[3,58-60]

Lead's effect on the hematopoietic system is one of its most described toxicities and has been used as a measure of its lead-induced physiologic dysfunction. *Basophilic stippling of erythrocytes, the precipitation of nuclear material, is a hallmark of severe lead exposure.* In fact, before laboratory techniques were available for measuring blood lead levels, the degree of basophilic stippling served as a diagnostic tool. Lead is also a potent suppressor of heme synthesis, producing anemia once lead levels exceed 50 μg/dL; the anemia can be either normochromic or hypochromic.[1]

Lead's effects on reproduction are profound and multiple. For example, because of lead's diffusibility across the placenta, pregnant women with lead intoxication invariably have lead-poisoned offspring.[49] Also, because pregnancy is a condition associated with bone mobilization, women with a past history of lead poisoning may have elevated lead levels during pregnancy. Other reproductive effects of lead poisoning in women include a higher rate of spontaneous abortion and stillbirth.[3,4,49] Lead is one of the few toxins in which paternal exposure is also associated with adverse reproductive outcomes.[1,61]

Lead-poisoned men have decreased sperm counts and a higher number of abnormal sperm; these effects can appear at blood lead levels as low as 40 μg/dL.[11,13,62]

Other complications of lead intoxication include hypertension, GI disturbances, mild liver function abnormalities, gingival lead lines (blue discolorations of the gingiva), muscle and joint aches, and gouty arthritis.[3,11,63]

Assessment

The diagnostic evaluation of lead intoxication focuses on identification and quantification of those disturbances that can be readily diagnosed. The most important test is measurement of blood lead level. Because of lead's 30-day half-life and large volume of distribution, blood lead level is a relatively poor measure of total body burden; however, because blood is easy to obtain and provides useful information after recent exposure, blood lead determination remains valuable. Blood lead levels can currently be measured by a number of techniques, including atomic absorption spectrometry, anodic strip voltammetry, thermal-ionization mass spectrometry, and inductively coupled plasma–mass spectrometry (ICP-MS).[4] All of these, when performed with appropriate quality control measures, are extremely accurate.

Because blood lead levels can be a poor representation of body lead burden, better methods of assessing lead exposure are being sought. With lead ultimately deposited in bone, and the skeleton serving as the primary in situ reservoir, diagnostic tools that measure lead in the skeleton are being developed. One of the most promising of these is x-ray fluorescence (XRF).[64-66] XRF works by emitting x-rays at bone in order to activate electrons in valence shells, a process that produces energy that can be measured. L-line XRF stimulates electrons in the L electron shell, whereas K-line XRF acts only at electrons in the K shell. The latter technique appears to have greater accuracy in assessing total bone lead concentration. Studies are demonstrating that XRF analysis of bone assesses body lead burden far more accurately than does blood lead determination. For example, Hu and colleagues showed that among carpenters with long-term lead exposure, lead burden as assessed by XRF correlated more closely with lead suppression of heme synthesis than did blood lead level.[66] Although promising, XRF has been difficult to develop in children because they have relatively little bone calcification and because lead incorporation into bone appears to occur at less predictable rates; however, the procedure has been used in several pediatric studies. XRF has the potential to replace blood lead measurement as a method of assessing lead exposure.

EP measurement remains important in the evaluation of lead exposure. Because it is not only the quantity of lead in blood that is important but also the effect of that lead burden on body function, EP measurement serves to provide information on lead's organ toxicity. EP is easily measured through hematofluorometry.[27] As a general rule, adults with lead poisoning have less EP disturbance than children. It is also notable that rises in

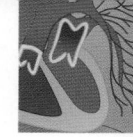

EP lag behind lead exposure by several days; therefore, if measured shortly after exposure, EP levels may not yet be abnormal.

Other laboratory tests useful in the evaluation of lead exposure include abdominal radiographs, renal function tests, complete blood count, and δ-aminolevulinic acid dehydratase activity. Abdominal radiographs are useful only if acute lead ingestion is suspected. Blood urea nitrogen and serum creatinine levels should be measured, and a urinalysis should be performed. Although investigators have suggested that N-acetylglucosidase can be used as a marker of lead-induced renal injury, the clinical utility of this test has not yet been proved. A complete blood count (CBC) serves to identify either preexisting iron deficiency anemia or lead suppression of hematopoiesis; also, basophilic stippling can be identified on blood smear.

Methods of assessing nervous system function after lead intoxication include measurement of auditory brainstem evoked potentials and nerve conduction velocity.[67] Lumbar puncture should not be performed in patients with altered mental status from suspected lead poisoning because the underlying cerebral edema can lead to herniation.

Treatment

Treatment of adult lead poisoning begins with cessation of further exposure. For those exposed in the workplace, OSHA standards must be implemented, if the business falls under OSHA regulations. Even for non-occupationally exposed adults (e.g., artisans or family members with lead poisoning due to home renovation), the primary intervention is prevention of further exposure.

CHELATION THERAPY

Parenteral Agents

Chelators are agents that form stable ligands with metal, effecting enhanced renal or biliary excretion of the drug–chelate complex. Many chelators have been discovered during the past century. However, it was only after the mid-20th century that chelation therapy flourished. More than five lead chelators have been identified.

The most important lead chelator developed is *dimercaprol*. This agent was created in England during World War II after the search for an antidote to the deadly arsenic-containing gas lewisite. The resulting antidote was an arsenic chelator termed *British antilewisite* (BAL). Since its creation, BAL has proved to be one of the most potent heavy-metal chelators.[68] In addition to lead, BAL chelates mercury, arsenic, and gold. BAL forms a stable dithiol bond with lead; the resulting complex is eliminated in both bile and urine.

BAL has a significant adverse effect profile; as many as half of those who receive this drug develop an adverse reaction. Part of this results from BAL's required preparation in a peanut oil vehicle; having such an excipient, the drug can only be administered intra-muscularly. BAL has oxidant properties that can produce hemolysis in those with glucose-6-phosphate dehydrogenase (G6PD) deficiency. Other adverse effects include hypotension, rash, vomiting, and a metallic taste in the mouth.[69] Toxic reactions occur when BAL is administered to those taking oral iron supplements.

BAL should be administered to any patient with encephalopathy or a whole blood lead level greater than 100 μg/dL.[9] The dose is 4 to 6 mg/kg per dose (maximum 300 mg per dose). Because of its vehicle, BAL should not be administered to patients with a history of peanut allergy.[69]

Another effective lead chelator is calcium disodium ethylene diamine tetraacetic acid (CaNa2EDTA, *calcium edetate*). Developed in the 1950s, this chelator became an important intervention in the treatment of childhood lead intoxication. Like BAL, EDTA forms a stable bond with the lead atom. The resulting complex is excreted in urine. EDTA can be administered intravenously or intramuscularly; it is not administered orally, both because this route is less effective and because evidence suggests that oral EDTA can enhance GI absorption of ingested lead. EDTA has a very short half-life (about 65 minutes). As a result, it is ideally administered by continuous intravenous infusion. Alternative administration strategies include intramuscular or intravenous administration two to three times daily. The dose of EDTA given to adults is 1 to 2 g daily.

As with BAL, adverse effects of EDTA limit its use. EDTA chelates nutrients, particularly zinc, in addition to lead. Therefore, in order to avoid zinc deficiency, courses of EDTA are limited to 5 days, followed by at least a 48-hour hiatus for nutritional recovery. EDTA courses are also limited to minimize its nephrotoxicity (manifested by proteinuria, hematuria, or glycosuria).[69] A limitation of EDTA is its relative ineffectiveness with blood lead levels less than 30 to 35 μg/dL, which narrows its range of utility.

Oral Chelators

Oral chelators have been developed to permit out-patient therapy for those with significant lead intoxication. These include succimer and D-penicillamine. They are discussed in the section on childhood lead poisoning.

INDICATIONS

Because adults, compared with children, are considered relatively resistant to the toxic effects of lead, indications for chelation therapy are controversial. In occupational medicine practice, treatment of lead poisoning is typically reserved for symptomatic adults, independent of blood lead level. Therefore, chelation therapy is often withheld until blood lead levels exceed 70 μg/dL, the range at which adults typically develop overt signs of lead intoxication. In such patients, hospitalization for EDTA chelation is recommended. Experience with childhood lead poisoning has demonstrated that EDTA chelation can exacerbate CNS toxicity when it is used as sole therapy in those with blood lead levels greater than 70 to 100 μg/dL; this CNS toxicity probably represents EDTA

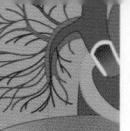

promotion of lead penetration into the brain. To prevent this, dual therapy with EDTA and BAL should be considered for adults with blood lead levels greater than 100 μg/dL. BAL can be discontinued once the blood lead level has fallen below the range of 70 to 80 μg/dL.

As the subclinical toxicity of lead becomes more appreciated, a growing opinion is that in adults, chelation therapy should be provided before overt clinical symptoms appear in order to prevent long-term sequelae, such as renal injury, as well as to reduce overall lead burden. Therefore, clinically asymptomatic adults can be considered candidates for chelation therapy even at lead levels of 25 to 40 μg/dL. Pregnant lead-poisoned women, unless their plumbism is severe, should not undergo chelation because of the possibility that the chelating agent will enhance lead movement across the placenta and be teratogenic.[13]

CHILDHOOD LEAD POISONING

History

The history of childhood lead intoxication is comparatively brief. Childhood lead poisoning was first reported in Brisbane, Australia, in 1899, when, after extensive epidemiologic investigation, A. J. Turner and J. L. Gibson associated the poisoning of young children with the ingestion of paint in their homes. Through the 20th century, increasing reports described catastrophic illness in children related to their ingestion of lead paint. Clinical features included basophilic stippling, abdominal pain, irritability, and often coma, seizures, and death. In 1943, Byers and Lord published a seminal article indicating that although childhood lead poisoning had been thought of as an illness that, among survivors, produced no obvious sequelae, many children suffered cognitive disturbances or frank mental retardation. Since that paper, many additional studies have reported that lead poisoning in children can lead to subnormal intelligence, hyperactivity, aggression, and school failure.[4,70]

In the 1950s and 1960s, many areas of the United States were found to have endemic rates of lead poisoning. These so-called lead belts were synonymous with large inner-city slums.[40] This observation led to public outcries until, in 1959, the U.S. Public Health Service recommended that blood lead levels of 60 to 80 μg/dL be considered evidence of increased lead absorption in children; levels below this were not thought to have any clinical effect.[40] In 1970, the Surgeon General reduced the level of concern to 40 μg/dL and for the first time shifted the focus from case finding to prevention through mass screening for childhood lead poisoning. Mass screening was facilitated through passage of the 1971 Lead-Based Paint Poisoning Prevention Act.[40] In 1975, the Centers for Disease Control (CDC) began to establish classifications and risk categories for childhood lead poisoning. The blood lead level of concern was reduced to 30 μg/dL in 1975, to 25 μg/dL in 1985, and to 10 μg/dL in 1991.

According to the 1991 CDC guidelines, the redefinition of childhood lead intoxication as a blood lead of 10 μg/dL or greater was based on increasing scientific data indicating that toxic effects of lead were demonstrable at this level.[40,71] Subsequent studies have suggested that neurodevelopmental harm can be demonstrated in children with blood lead levels below 10 μg/dL.[72,73] The 1991 CDC guidelines also moved from a single definition of lead poisoning to a tiered approach that recommended interventions based on a range of lead levels.[71]

The most important preventive legislative action to occur was the banning of lead from residential paint in 1978. However, with decades of use, the problem of lead poisoning from exposure to paint and dust continues.

Epidemiology

Childhood lead poisoning is currently defined as a blood lead level of 10 μg/dL or greater. The new classification of lead poisoning establishes degrees of lead exposure as a means of prioritizing interventions (Table 73-2).

Data from NHANES on the epidemiology of childhood lead poisoning indicate that the average lead level of American children is 2 μg/dL, which is 80% less than mean blood lead levels in 1976. This blood lead level represents "background" exposure, the sum of different environmental sources. An estimated 450,000 U.S. children have lead poisoning.[74] Childhood lead intoxication is more prevalent in minority groups and among those living in the Northeast. The peak onset of lead poisoning in children is the second year of life, although de novo lead poisoning can appear in later childhood years.[75] Refugee children and those adopted from foreign countries can have prevalence rates of lead poisoning as high as 10% to 15%.[76,77]

As with exposure to lead in adults, childhood lead exposure can result from many sources, including lead paint or dust, air, soil, water, and food.[4,40,71] However, there are significant differences in the etiology of frank lead poisoning according to age. For example, in children, lead paint and dust are the primary source of lead poisoning (in contrast to vocational or avocational exposure in adults). Also, children can develop congenital lead intoxication.[41,78]

Lead paint remains the most common cause of lead poisoning in children.[71] The singular importance of paint results from several factors: (1) lead-containing paint chips are relatively sweet; (2) the small size and color of paint chips make them attractive to curious young children; (3) containing up to 50% lead by weight, paint chips are a high-dose source of lead, capable of producing fatal degrees of exposure[79,80]; (4) pica, or repeated ingestion of nonfood objects, is most prevalent in early childhood, and in infants, hand-to-mouth activity is a completely normal developmental process; (5) children are more likely to have their hands dirtied by dust from the window well, the floor, or outdoor soil[81]; (6) household renovation of homes with lead generally results in greater contamination of the environment, a particular risk factor for lead poisoning in infancy[82]; and (7) even household deleading can

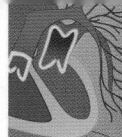

TABLE 73-2 Interpretation of Blood Lead Test Results and Recommended Follow-up for Children

CLASS	BLOOD LEAD CONCENTRATION (μg/dL)	COMMENT
I	≤9	A child in class I is not considered to be lead poisoned.
IIA	10–14	Many children (or a large proportion of children) with blood lead levels in this range should trigger community-wide childhood lead poisoning prevention activities. Children in this range may need to be rescreened more frequently.
IIB	15–19	A child in class IIB should receive nutritional and educational interventions and more frequent screening. If the blood lead level persists in this range, environmental investigation and intervention should be done.
III	20–44	A child in class III should receive environmental evaluation and remediation and a medical evaluation. Such a child may need pharmacologic treatment of lead poisoning.
IV	45–69	A child in class IV needs both medical and environmental interventions, including chelation therapy.
V	≥70	A child with class V lead poisoning poses a medical emergency. Medical and environmental management must begin immediately.

From the Centers for Disease Control and Prevention: Preventing Lead Poisoning in Children. Atlanta, Author, 1991.

result in greater exposure to lead if not performed properly. Children who live with an adult who has a lead-related occupation are at greater risk for lead intoxication as a result of dust importation by the adult.[83]

Exposure to lead in water has greater impact on young children because of their relatively small size, their greater daily water consumption, and the greater proportion of dietary lead absorbed by a child's gut. Lead poisoning from lead-contaminated water has been reported by several researchers.[82,84] In all these cases, water was being used to prepare infant formula. Water can become highly contaminated if warmed or boiled in a vessel that contains lead.[85,86]

Although soil has not been clearly associated with the development of lead poisoning, it clearly contributes to background lead levels in children. Also, in areas with highly contaminated soil (e.g., homes near smelter), children tend to have higher blood lead levels.[87] In a study of the impact of soil lead abatement on blood lead levels in children, Weitzman and colleagues[88] showed that elimination of lead in soil could effect a reduction in blood lead of about 1 μg/dL, an amount insufficient to justify large-scale soil abatement measures.

Other potential causes of lead poisoning in children include administration of folk remedies (e.g., greta, azarcon, or Paylooah), congenital exposure, and ingestion of foreign bodies.[4,42,71,89] A reported case of fatal childhood lead intoxication (blood lead level, 283 μg/dL) occurred after a child ingested a lead curtain weight, which was retained in the GI tract for several weeks.[90] Finally, lead intoxication has been reported in newborns who receive a blood transfusion from lead-poisoned donors.[91,92]

All children are not at equal risk for lead intoxication; rather, it is the unique relationship between the individual child and his or her environment that results in lead exposure. This explains the common phenom-enon of one child's developing lead poisoning while living in a house that contains lead, although other children in the same environment do not have increased lead exposure. The most important risk factor is generally the oral habits of the child, particularly the presence of pica. Another risk factor for childhood lead poisoning is developmental delay. Children with significant delays—for example, those with autism—are more likely to develop lead poisoning.[71,93-95] Moreover, the pattern of lead poisoning in these children has atypical features, including its appearance at an older age and the tendency for recurrent exposure, despite environmental hazard reduction.[96] Finally, for reasons that are not clearly explained, childhood lead poisoning is more prevalent in summer than winter.

Toxicokinetics

The kinetics of lead in children have not been extensively analyzed but are thought, with some exception, to parallel the kinetics in adults.[4] However, certain differences have been well characterized. For example, the extent of lead absorption is greater in children than in adults (30% to 50% versus 10%). Also, nutritional factors have a greater role in the development of childhood plumbism. Inadequate intake of iron, calcium, and total calories, all of which are more prevalent in children, are associated with higher blood lead levels.[35,96]After its absorption, lead is distributed through soft tissues before its deposition into bone. The half-life of lead in the soft tissues of children may be longer, probably because children have less bone available for lead incorporation. As with adults, the estimated body elimination half-life of lead is 20 years.

Lead toxicokinetics in the pregnant and lactating woman have significant effects on children.[97] During both pregnancy and lactation, women mobilize skeletal

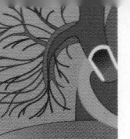

calcium.[47,98-100] In the process, lead is mobilized as well. Because lead freely crosses the placenta, the fetus invariably receives some amount of maternal lead, presumably in association with the degree of skeletal lead in the mother, reflecting her lifelong exposure. Maternal bone lead has been correlated with fetal neurotoxicity.[101] Lead is also mobilized with calcium during lactation.[102-105] However, several studies indicate that the amount of lead excreted into breast milk is negligible unless maternal blood lead level is greater than 40 to 50 μg/dL.[106,107]

Clinical Toxicity

Although the mechanisms of toxicity for lead poisoning in childhood are similar to those in adults, clinical manifestations are different. Also, the lead level at which these toxic manifestations appear is lower in children (Table 73-3). Children, for example, are more susceptible to all of lead's neurotoxic effects.

Lead encephalopathy in children has presenting features that are comparable to the disease in adults. However, encephalopathy appears in children at blood lead levels as low as 50 to 60 μg/dL.[40,108] Prominent features are irritability, anorexia, apathy, listlessness, abdominal pain, obtundation, and, if untreated, cerebral edema, seizures, and death.[108,109]

The CNS effects of lead have caused the greatest concern about childhood plumbism.[40,71,110] Exposure to lead during critical periods of neurodevelopment can produce permanent changes in cerebral architecture. The mechanisms of these changes have been described by Goldstein, Silbergeld, and others[53,111]: During the first 2 years of life, synaptic density and complexity are markedly increased such that by the third year of life, neuronal arborization exceeds the normal adult pattern almost twofold.[111,112] The enzymes that have an important role in mediating this process, including protein kinase C and calmodulin, are inhibited at very low concentrations of lead. Another critical factor in normal dendritic arborization is the activity of neural cell adhesions molecules; these proteins are also impaired by lead. The consequences of childhood lead exposure are thus reduced synaptogenesis and imprecise synaptic "pruning." Functional changes, including decreased neurotransmitter synthesis, also occur.[53,111,112] The hippocampus is thought to be the primary anatomic site for these effects, this being an area with a high zinc content.[48] Severe lead exposure can disturb the integrity of the already immature, permeable blood-brain barrier of a child.[40,113]

The clinical consequences of lead neurotoxicity are vast. At an extreme, children with severe lead intoxication can be left with profound cognitive disturbances (mental retardation). Estimates from several population-based studies are that children can lose about 5 points (95% confidence intervals ranging from 2 to 14) in intelligence quotient (IQ) for every 10 μg/dL elevation in their blood lead level.[13,69,114-116] Although a loss of 5 IQ points is arguably insignificant in any child, the potential left shift of the normal distribution of IQ among children would result in greater numbers of children with low IQ and a reduction in the number of children with superior IQ.[38] It is this principle that has, in part, maintained public health momentum to reduce blood lead levels in children to the lowest range possible. Other adverse developmental outcomes in lead-poisoned children include aggression, hyperactivity, school failure, and antisocial behaviors.[117-123] Childhood lead poisoning has been associated with juvenile delinquency and even homicidal tendencies.[124,125] Another

---

TABLE 73-3 Health Effects of Lead at Lowest Observed Blood Lead (PbB) Levels in Children

LOWEST OBSERVED EFFECT PbB (μg/dL)	NEUROLOGIC EFFECTS	HEME SYNTHESIS EFFECTS	OTHER EFFECTS
<10 (postnatal)	Deficits in neurobehavioral development		
10–15 (prenatal and postnatal)	Deficits in neurobehavioral development; electrophysiologic changes	ALA-D inhibition	Reduced gestational age and weight at birth; reduced size up to age 7–8 yr
15–20		Erythrocyte protoporphyrin elevation	Impaired vitamin D metabolism; pyrimidine-5'-nucleotidase inhibition
<25	Lower IQ, slower reaction time (studied cross-sectionally)		
30	Slowed nerve conduction velocity		
40		Reduced hemoglobin; elevated EP and ALA-U	
70	Peripheral neuropathies	Frank anemia	
80–100	Encephalopathy		Colic, other gastrointestinal effects; kidney effects

ALA, aminolevulinic acid; EP, erythrocyte protoporphyrin.
Adapted from Agency for Toxic Substances and Disease Registry: The Nature and Extent of Lead Poisoning in Children in the United States: A Report to Congress. Atlanta, U.S. Public Health Service, 1988.

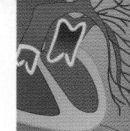

relatively common consequence of lead poisoning is the development of a learning disability in which overall IQ is normal by standardized testing but the child demonstrates discrete learning weaknesses such as impairment in memory, auditory processing, and visual-motor integration.[70,115,126-128] Attentional weaknesses can give the appearance of attention-deficit hyperactivity disorder (ADHD).[129] These effects, which have been demonstrated in children with blood lead levels as low as 6 µg/dL, can persist through the preadolescent and adolescent years.[72,73,119,121,122,130,131] Recent data suggest that there is the potential for some reversibility in lead neurotoxicity, challenging assumptions that all neurodevelopmental effects of lead poisoning are reversible.[132,133] Some researchers believe that there is no clear evidence that lead poisoning causes learning problems in children[134,135]

Peripheral neuropathy can occur in children with lead intoxication[136]; children with sickle cell disease may be at higher risk for this complication.[136,137] Children can develop subclinical peripheral neuropathy at lead levels as low as 30 µg/dL.[137] Hearing is also significantly depressed by low levels of lead exposure[138,139] (Fig. 73-2). Motor disturbances, including reduced scores on bilateral coordination, upper limb speed, and dexterity tests, may also occur.[140,141]

Renal toxicity due to childhood lead poisoning includes impairment of vitamin D activation[51,140,141]; this appears to be a reversible effect. A 50-year follow-up of lead-poisoned children suggests that they have a sevenfold greater risk for adult hypertension.

Hematopoietic effects of lead poisoning in children include suppression of erythropoiesis with resulting anemia. Children are more sensitive to lead suppression of heme synthesis, as evidenced by their higher EP concentrations. However, the anemia that accompanies lead poisoning is sometimes cause rather than effect because iron deficiency results in greater lead absorption.[71]

Lead can disturb bone development, leading to the formation of growth arrest, or "lead lines." Lead lines are best identified at the metaphyses of long bones, particularly the distal radius and proximal fibula. These lines generally appear 3 to 6 weeks after a period of significant lead exposure and generally correlate with a peak blood lead level of greater than 45 to 50 µg/dL.[142] Childhood lead poisoning has also been associated with the development of dental caries.[143,144]

Diagnosis

Assessment of children with known or suspected lead intoxication requires a careful physical evaluation that includes investigation of clinically overt signs and symptoms such as irritability and abdominal pain. The laboratory evaluation is an important adjunct. All children with lead intoxication should receive a venous blood lead and EP level, a CBC, measurement of blood urea nitrogen and creatinine, urinalysis, and measures of iron status (serum iron with total iron-binding capacity, serum ferritin, or reticulocyte hemoglobin). The need for radiographs should be individualized. If recent ingestion of lead-containing material is suspected, an abdominal radiograph should be obtained. Radiographs of the long bones can be useful as an assessment of timing and magnitude of exposure.[71] In children with blood lead level less than 45 to 50 µg/dL, long bone radiographs are usually valueless. As a general rule, long bone films never alter clinical management.

Newer means of assessing lead burden are being explored. For example, the research use of deciduous teeth has the potential to be clinically valuable. Also, XRF in children may ultimately prove to have the same value that is being found in the assessment of adult lead intoxication.[122,145]

Treatment

Treatment of lead intoxication in children focuses on three components, in descending order of importance: environmental inspection/hazard reduction, nutritional supplementation, and, if necessary, chelation therapy.[71,146]

Whenever a child is found to have lead poisoning, its etiology must be identified. Unless the source is clearly known, a complete environmental inspection is necessary. This inspection is guided by data obtained from an environmental history, including previous lead tests of the child, the age and condition of the child's housing, recent renovations, water intake, use of kitchenware that may contain lead, time spent elsewhere (including daycare, school, and relatives' homes), occupations of adult family members, oral habits of the child, and

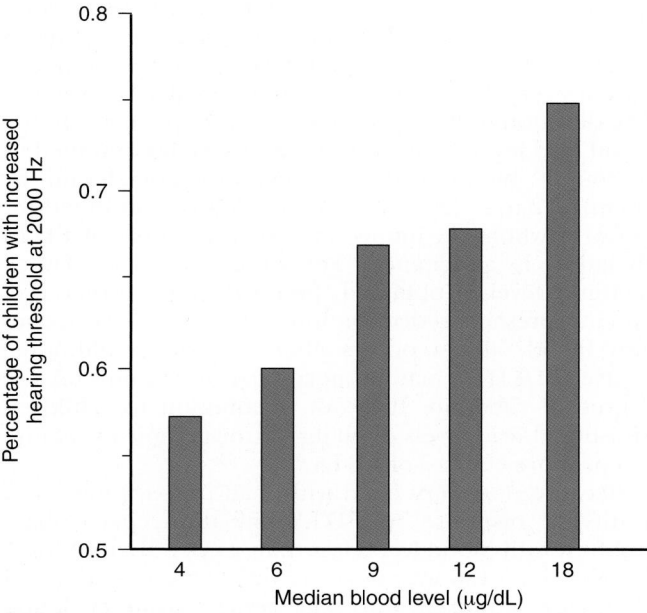

FIGURE 73-2 Fraction of children with hearing worse than a reference group stratified by quintiles of blood lead concentration, after adjustment for covariates. (From Schwartz J, Otto D: Lead and minor hearing impairment. Arch Environ Health 1991;46:300–305.)

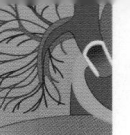

siblings or playmates with lead intoxication. The results of the history should guide inspection of areas that may include the home interior and exterior, water, and alternate housing.[71,146] Inspections for lead are generally performed using either a sodium sulfide test (the reaction between this solution and lead produces gray-black lead sulfide) or XRF. The latter test is best able to detect lead paint that is covered by a nonlead surface. Interior home inspection should include dust wipings, especially when there are children younger than 1 year, who are more likely to have dust-laden hands because of their crawling. Household lead hazards, if found, should be reduced or fully abated (i.e., deleaded). In one study, deleading alone was shown to reduce blood lead levels by as much as 30%.[147] On the other hand, deleading has the potential to result in greater lead exposure if not conducted properly.[148] Therefore, it is important that work be done with minimal environmental contamination, with the family living elsewhere and with final inspection before reoccupancy. Methods of reducing without removing household lead hazards include use of trisodium phosphate detergent and the application of encapsulants, which are chemical polymers that effectively (albeit temporarily) cover lead surfaces.

Nutritional supplementation focuses on eliminating iron and calcium deficiency, both of which result in greater absorption of ingested lead.[35,71,149,150] Because there are no consistently accurate measures of iron status in children,[35,71] iron supplementation should be empirically initiated; iron sulfate elixir or drops can be prescribed in a dose of 3 to 6 mg/kg per day for a period of 4 to 6 weeks. Although evidence in animal models suggests that iron supplementation promotes the elimination of lead from the body, in human subjects, its only proven effect is reduction of further lead absorption.[35,71] Calcium deficiency is uncommon in children who have a varied diet with regular milk intake. If there is any question about calcium intake, however, the diet should be enhanced with calcium-rich foods (e.g., yogurt, cheese, milk) or calcium supplementation should be prescribed.[35,71] The combination of environmental abatement and nutritional supplementation is often sufficient to produce prompt reductions in blood lead level. However, the diminution in blood lead level may not be sufficient or may not occur rapidly enough to reduce the risk for multisystem injury. In these cases, chelation therapy is warranted.

Chelation Therapy

Chelation therapy for lead intoxication was initially developed to reduce the mortality associated with childhood lead poisoning. Increasing emphasis is being placed on its use to prevent morbidity as well. Therefore, although the same agents are available for both adults and children with lead intoxication, the greater focus, particularly the development of oral chelators, has been directed to pediatric treatment.

Increasing options in both parenteral and oral chelation therapy have brought into question the indications for hospitalization of lead-poisoned children. Decisions for hospitalization should be individualized. However, the goals of hospitalization are at least threefold: (1) to provide environmental protection so that the child has no further lead exposure, (2) to provide close monitoring for evidence of clinical toxicity, and (3) to provide aggressive chelation therapy.[60] With these principles, hospitalization should be considered for all children who are younger than 6 years and who have a blood lead level exceeding 45 to 55 μg/dL. Children who are hospitalized for lead intoxication should never be returned to the environment in which their lead poisoning occurred unless hazard reduction measures have been completed.

PARENTERAL CHELATING AGENTS

Parenteral agents for lead intoxication in childhood are BAL and EDTA. However, both of these agents are used in different fashions in the pediatric population. For example, because of the risk for CNS deterioration or death when EDTA alone is given to children with severe lead intoxication,[151] dual therapy with both BAL and EDTA should be instituted for children with blood lead levels of 70 μg/dL or greater.[69] EDTA is begun about 4 hours after the first dose of BAL. BAL is given every 6 to 8 hours until the blood lead level is less than 70 μg/dL. Adverse reactions and cautions are the same in children as in adults, although children appear to have a higher prevalence of febrile reactions.[69] BAL should be used cautiously in those with G6PD deficiency, and oral iron therapy must be discontinued. Peanut allergy is a contraindication to the use of BAL.[69]

EDTA is given in a daily dose of 35 to 50 mg/kg per day (1000 to 1500 mg/m^2). Although the agent can be given intramuscularly, intravenous administration is preferred because intramuscular EDTA is extremely painful and because brisk urine output, necessary to prevent EDTA nephrotoxicity, is better achieved with intravenous hydration. Because of EDTA's short half-life, continuous intravenous infusion is preferred; however, administration every 8 to 12 hours is an acceptable alternative. The duration of therapy is 3 to 5 days, depending on the blood lead level.[69] Thereafter, therapy is discontinued. A "rebound" blood lead level measurement should be obtained 2 to 3 days after the EDTA is discontinued for those in whom an immediate second course of EDTA chelation is anticipated. For others, a 2- to 3-week rebound level is obtained. Some degree of rebound, which represents redistribution of lead from soft tissues into blood, always occurs after chelation. Additional courses of EDTA may be necessary, depending on the degree of rebound. It is not uncommon for children with blood lead levels of 60 μg/dL or greater to require two or more courses of EDTA.[69]

Because not every child with lead intoxication has a gratifying response to EDTA chelation, particularly children with blood levels less than 45 μg/dL, the EDTA mobilization test was once a widely used method of identifying children who will benefit from chelation therapy.[152,153] To perform the test, a child is given a single dose of EDTA followed by an 8-hour collection of urine, which is analyzed for total lead excretion. A positive mobilization test is considered a ratio of greater than 0.6

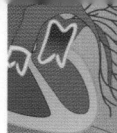

between the dose of EDTA administered (in milligrams) and the quantity of urine excreted (in micrograms). The lead mobilization test, although valuable, has shortcomings.[69,154] First, it is difficult to collect 8 hours of urine in small children in the absence of catheterization, which is traumatic. Spilled or lost urine makes test interpretation difficult if not impossible.[155] The performance of the test is labor intensive and requires an 8- to 10-hour health care visit (or brief hospitalization).[156] Finally, there is little likelihood of a positive mobilization test result in children with blood lead levels less than 25 to 35 μg/dL.[153] Collectively, these factors have made the mobilization test relatively useless.[69]

ORAL CHELATING AGENTS

Numerous oral chelating agents have been used or are in current use for the treatment of lead poisoning. The two most commonly used agents are D-penicillamine and succimer.

D-Penicillamine was fortuitously discovered in 1953 by Walshe[157] and, because of its copper-chelating ability, was quickly used in the treatment of Wilson's disease. Its efficacy at chelating lead initially resulted in suggestions that penicillamine be used to treat lead-exposed workers without their removal from work.

D-Penicillamine has unique, incompletely understood chelating properties.[151] For example, it does not appear to be capable of forming stable bonds with the lead atom. Nonetheless, it does enhance urinary lead excretion, possibly by forming a heterocyclic ring (sulfur and nitrogen atoms binding the lead).[158] Like BAL, penicillamine is capable of chelating other metals, including arsenic and mercury.

The efficacy of D-penicillamine in childhood lead intoxication has been demonstrated in studies by Sachs, Vitale, Marcus, Shannon, and others.[151,159-164] Data from these studies have shown that penicillamine can reduce blood levels, even in children with blood lead levels of 20 to 35 μg/dL. Blood lead levels as low as 3 μg/dL can be achieved using this drug.[163] D-Penicillamine can be considered for children with blood lead levels in the range of 2 to 35 μg/dL.[69]

D-Penicillamine is given in a dose of about 15 mg/kg daily.[159] Its use is initiated after baseline CBC. Available only in capsules or tablets of 125 and 250 mg, the tablets must usually be crushed or the capsules opened and placed in food or drink. Having an unpleasant odor and taste, penicillamine must often be concealed in juice or food. Because iron may decrease D-penicillamine absorption by as much as 65%, iron supplementation should be discontinued during penicillamine therapy.[158] The agent is given twice a day at home by the parents. During treatment, children must be monitored every 2 to 4 weeks for evidence of adverse effects. Monitoring laboratory tests include CBC, urinalysis, blood lead, and EP determinations. Typical courses of D-penicillamine therapy are 2 to 3 months in length.

Penicillamine has an overall adverse effect rate of 5% to 10%, a rate that has led to considerable reluctance to use it. The most common adverse effect is GI upset.

More serious effects occur in about 7% of children and include rash white blood cell count depression. The occurrence of adverse effects should prompt discontinuation of therapy.[159] In all reported experience with D-penicillamine use for childhood lead poisoning in otherwise healthy children, these effects have been mild and reversible.

Succimer is an oral chelating agent that was discovered in the 1950s; in 1991, it became the first oral chelating agent ever approved for the treatment of lead intoxication.[158,165-167] An oral congener of BAL, succimer has, interestingly, not been approved for adult lead intoxication, in part because of the ever-present risk for its abuse by workers, employers, or physicians.[168]

Succimer is has been approved for use in children with blood lead levels exceeding 45 μg/dL. However, studies have demonstrated that its safety and efficacy extend to children with blood lead levels between 25 and 45 μg/dL[167,169,170]; it is therefore a therapeutic option for these patients. Although there is no clearly defined upper limit of lead level for which succimer can be used, it is prudent to use conventional, dual parenteral therapy (EDTA and BAL) in children with blood lead levels of 70 μg/dL or greater.

Succimer is available in 100-mg capsules. The current treatment protocol is administration of 10 mg/kg per dose. For the first 5 days of succimer therapy, it is given three times daily. For the next 14 days, treatment is twice a day. A complete course of DMSA chelation is therefore 19 days. An alternative regimen is 10 mg/kg/dose, given twice a day for 28 days. Adverse effects associated with succimer, which occur in about 5% of patients, include rash and minor elevations in hepatic transaminases; monitoring should include periodic liver function testing.[158,162] Succimer, unlike BAL, does not produce hemolysis in those with G6PD deficiency. Also, succimer can be administered concomitantly with iron therapy. Mean reductions in blood lead with succimer are as great as 70% to 80%.[158,165,166] However, in contrast to penicillamine, succimer discontinuation is followed by a robust rebound in blood lead level, appearing 2 to 4 weeks after completion of therapy. It is not unusual to experience rebound lead values that approximate the pretreatment value. As a result, multiple courses of succimer are usually necessary to produce enduring reductions in blood lead levels. Because lead rebounds can be confused with reexposure to lead, it is important to monitor EP levels. Lead reexposure is associated with increases in EP values; lead rebound is not.

Additional agents that have been used for the treatment of lead intoxication are dimercaptopropane-sulfonate (DMPS) and trientine.[171,172] Neither of these agents has moved beyond the investigational stage.

INDICATIONS AND GOALS FOR CHELATION THERAPY

The indications for initiating chelation therapy in children are controversial. For children with blood lead levels of 10 to 20 μg/dL (the majority of lead-poisoned children in the United States), chelation therapy is not

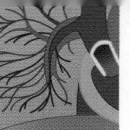

recommended, primarily because it is difficult to identify a single source of lead to abate and because for lead levels in this range, the risk for adverse effects from chelation therapy may outweigh the potential benefits.[71] Instead, education, hazard reduction (if a lead source is found), and nutritional supplementation are provided. For those children with blood lead levels of 20 µg/dL or greater, consultation with a lead specialist is recommended.[71] Among these children, chelation therapy should be considered. The decision to begin therapy should be based on (1) evidence that the blood lead level is not declining despite environmental abatement and nutritional supplementation, (2) the age of the child (evidence strongly suggests that the most neurodevelopmentally vulnerable age is the first 24 months of life[131], (3) evidence of biochemical disturbances (i.e., an elevated EP level), (4) the assumption that reducing lead burden does reverse some toxicity (e.g., renal and hematopoietic) and may reverse neurodevelopmental disturbances,[53,132,173] and (5) the desire to reduce lead burden to prevent its deposition in bone, where recrudescence later in life could occur. In initiating chelation therapy, the goals of treatment must also be established. Although this is also an area of some controversy, it is rational to have a goal of reducing blood lead level to the range of 10 to 15 mg/dL, if not lower. This requires long-term treatment strategies and frequent monitoring.

In children with more serious lead poisoning (blood lead > 30 to 35 µg/dL), formal cognitive or neuropsychological testing should be performed to identify neurodevelopmental weaknesses and initiate remedial programs as soon as possible. Because these weaknesses are generally not identifiable with gross developmental assessment (e.g., the Denver Developmental Screening Test) and may not be evident in the first few years of life, formal testing is recommended after the ages of 4 to 6 years of age, with close neurodevelopmental monitoring through adolescence.[174]

Prevention

Prevention of childhood lead poisoning has led to both primary and secondary prevention strategies.[71,110,175] Primary prevention consists of environmental inspection and abatement before a child develops lead intoxication. Because the cost of identifying and abating all homes (or other sources) with lead is prohibitive, primary prevention efforts have been difficult to implement. However, federal and state legislation that includes lead notification before home renting or purchase is being passed to ensure safe housing. Other primary preventive measures, including lead removal from soil, were attempted in a pilot study by Weitzman and colleagues, with little success.[88]

Prevention has focused primarily on secondary efforts. Under this philosophy, because lead poisoning is asymptomatic in its early phases, the goal is to identify children who have developed lead poisoning, in order to prevent their lead levels from rising further and to protect their siblings and playmates from lead exposure.

Secondary prevention forms the basis of routine lead screening in children.

Secondary prevention through screening initially consisted of capillary (fingerstick) measurement of EP levels. This test was used both because EP level rises with lead intoxication and because capillary lead tests are easily contaminated by lead on the fingertip, leading to a high rate of false-positive results. When the definition of lead poisoning was reduced to 10 µg/dL in 1991, EP screening had to be abandoned because EP does not consistently rise until blood lead level exceeds 30 to 35 µg/dL.[176] Therefore, with a desire to identify all children who have blood lead levels of 10 µg/dL or greater, the current recommendation is to measure blood lead only. Although capillary lead testing can produce false-positive results, making it less useful, it is an acceptable means of screening children if performed properly.[177,178]

Another strategy for secondary prevention is universal lead screening. Because lead intoxication is present throughout the United States and there are no completely reliable means of case finding, recommendations have been that all children receive periodic lead screening, regardless of where they live or their socioeconomic status. This recommendation has been strongly criticized because it is costly and because, in many areas, its yield is extremely low.[177] Opponents believe that lead screening in areas that have a low incidence of lead poisoning are a financial waste.[179] Targeted screening—that is, screening of children thought to be at risk for lead exposure—may be a more cost-effective strategy.[180,181] Selective screening, if used, should target siblings and close playmates of lead-poisoned children. Lead poisoning in domestic pets may signal lead intoxication in the child.[182] Other children at risk for exposure include those with developmental delays, those with a history of foreign body ingestion or insertion, and those with a history of physical abuse.[71,183-185] Risk assessment questions have been created by the CDC and other researchers to use in identifying children at risk for lead exposure.[186,187]

REFERENCES

1. Landrigan PJ, Todd AC: Lead poisoning. West J Med 1994;161:153–159.
2. Ericson JE, Shirahata H, Patterson C: Skeletal concentrations of lead in ancient Peruvians. N Engl J Med 1979;300:946–951.
3. Ibels LS, Pollock CA: Lead intoxication. Med Toxicol 1986;1:387–410.
4. National Research Council: Measuring Lead Exposure in Infants, Children, and Other Sensitive Populations. Washington, DC, National Academy Press, 1993, p 337.
5. Gilfillan SC: Lead poisoning and the fall of Rome. J Occup Med 1965;7:53–60.
6. Brody DJ, Pirkle JL, Kramer RA, et al: Blood lead levels in the US population: phase 1 of the Third National Health and Nutrition Examination Survey (NHANES III, 1988 to 1991). JAMA 1994; 272:277–283.
7. Pirkle JL, Brody DJ, Gunter EW, et al: The decline in blood lead levels in the United States: the National Health and Nutrition Examination Surveys (NHANES). JAMA 1994;272:284–291.
8. Pirkle JL, Kaufman RB, Brody DJ, et al: Exposure of the US population to lead, 1991–1994. Environ Health Perspect 1998; 106:745–750.

9. Centers for Disease Control and Prevention (CDC): Adult blood lead epidemiology and surveillance. MMWR Morb Mortal Wkly Rep 2002;53:578–582.

10. Goldman RH, Baker EL, Hannan M, et al: Lead poisoning in automobile radiator mechanics. N Engl J Med 1987;317:214–218.

11. Keogh JP: Lead. In Sullivan J, Kreiger G (eds): Hazardous Materials Toxicology: Clinical Principles of Environmental Health. Baltimore, Williams & Wilkins, 1992, pp 834–844.

12. Tripathi RK, Shereretz PC, Lewellyn GC, Armstrong CW: Lead exposure in outdoor firearm instructors. Am J Public Health 1991;81:753–755.

13. Rempel D: The lead-exposed worker. JAMA 1989;262:532–534.

14. Jacobs DE, Clickner RP, Zhou JY, et al: The prevalence of lead-based paint hazards in U.S. housing. Environ Health Perspect 2002;110(10):A599–A606.

15. Schneitzer L, Osborn HH, Bierman A, et al: Lead poisoning in adults from renovation of an older home. Ann Emerg Med 1990;19:415–420.

16. Fischbein A, Anderson KE, Sassa S, et al: Lead poisoning from "do-it-yourself" heat guns for removing lead-based paint: report of two cases. 1981;24:425–443.

17. Amitai Y, Graef JW, Brown MJ, et al: Hazards of deleading homes of children with lead poisoning. Am J Dis Child 1987;1411:758–760.

18. Beattie D, Moore MR, Devenay WT, et al: Environmental lead pollution in an urban soft-water area. BMJ 1972;2:491–493.

19. Centers for Disease Control and Prevention (CDC): Lead poisoning associated with Ayurvedic medications: five states, 2000–2003. MMWR Morb Mortal Wkly Rep 2004;53:582–584.

20. Bayly GR, Braithwaite RA, Sheehan TM, et al: Lead poisoning from Asian traditional remedies in the West Midlands: report of a series of five cases. Hum Exp Toxicol 1995;14:24–28.

21. Bose A, Vashistha K, O'Loughlin BJ: Azarcon por Empacho—another cause of lead toxicity. Pediatrics 1983;72:106–108.

22. Markowitz SB, Nuñez CM, Klitzman S, et al: Lead poisoning due to Hai Ge Fen—the porphyrin content of individual erythrocytes. JAMA 1994;271:932–934.

23. Smitherman J, Harber P: A case of mistaken identify: herbal medicine as a cause of lead toxicity. Am J Ind Med 1991;20:795–798.

24. Scelfo GM, Flegal AR: Lead in calcium supplements. Environ Health Perspect 2000;108:309–313.

25. Gulson BL, Mizon KJ, Palmer JM, et al: Contribution of lead from calcium supplements to blood lead. Environ Health Perspect 2001;109(3):283–288.

26. Bourgoin BP, Evans DR, Cornett JR, et al: Lead content in 70 brands of dietary calcium supplements. Am J Public Health 1993;83:1155–1160.

27. Lamola AA, Joselow M, Yamane T: Zinc protoporphyrin (ZPP): a simple, sensitive, fluorometric screening test for lead poisoning. Clin Chem 1975;21:93–97.

28. Miller SA: Lead in calcium supplements. JAMA 1987;257:1810.

29. Matte TD, Proops D, Palazuelos E, et al: Acute high-dose lead exposure from beverage contaminated by traditional Mexican pottery. Lancet 1994;344:1064–1065.

30. Morgan BW, Todd KH, Moore B: Elevated blood lead levels in urban moonshine drinkers. Ann Emerg Med 2001;37(1):51–54.

31. Mangas S, Visvanathan R, van Alphen M: Lead poisoning from homemade wine: a case study. Environ Health Perspect 2001;109(4):433–435.

32. Farrell SE, Vandevander P, Schoffstall JM, et al: Blood lead levels in emergency department patients with retained lead bullets and shrapnel. Acad Emerg Med 1999;6(3):208–212.

33. Lees RE, Scott GD, Miles CG: Subacute lead poisoning from retained lead shot. Can Med Assoc J 1988;138:130–131.

34. Magos L: Lead poisoning from retained lead projectiles. A critical review of case reports. Hum Exp Toxicol 1994;13:735–742.

35. Sargent JD: The role of nutrition in the prevention of lead poisoning in children. Pediatr Ann 1994;23:636–642.

36. Bradman A, Eskenazi B, Sutton P, et al: Iron deficiency associated with higher blood lead in children living in contaminated environments. Environ Health Perspect 2001;109(10):1079–1084.

37. Wright RO, Hu H, Maher TJ, et al: Effect of iron deficiency anemia on lead distribution after intravenous dosing in rats. Toxicol Ind Health 1998;14(4):547–551.

38. Goyer RA: Toxic effects of metals. In Amdur MO, Doull J, Klaassen CD (eds): Casarett and Doull's Toxicology: The Basic Science of Poisons. New York, Pergamon, 1991.

39. Rabinowitz MB, Wetherill GW, Kopple JD: Kinetic analysis of lead metabolism in healthy humans. J Clin Invest 1976;58:260–270.

40. Chisolm JJ, O'Hara DM: Lead absorption in children: management, clinical and environmental aspects. Baltimore, Munich, Urban & Schwarzenberg, 1982, p 229.

41. Ryu JE, Ziegler EE, Fomon SJ: Maternal lead exposure and blood lead concentration in infancy. J Pediatr 1978;93:476–478.

42. Timpo AE, Ain JS, Casalino MB, et al: Congenital lead intoxication. J Pediatr 1979;94:765–766.

43. Wong GP, Ng TL, Martin TR, et al: Effects of low-level lead exposure in utero. Obstet Gynecol 1992;47:285–289.

44. Goldman RH, White R, Kales SN, et al: Lead poisoning from mobilization of bone stores during thyrotoxicosis. Am J Ind Med 1994;25:417–424.

45. Shannon M, Landy H, Anast C, et al: Recurrent lead poisoning in a child with immobilization osteoporosis. Vet Hum Toxicol 1988;30:586–588.

46. Markowitz ME, Weinberger HL: Immobilization-related lead toxicity in previously lead-poisoned children. Pediatrics 1990;86:455–457.

47. Mahaffey KR: Biokinetics of lead during pregnancy. Fund Appl Toxicol 1991;16:15–16.

48. Silbergeld EK: Lead in bone: implications for toxicology during pregnancy and lactation. Environ Health Perspect 1991;91:63–70.

49. Shannon M: Severe lead poisoning in pregnancy. Ambul Pediatr 2003;3(1):37–39.

50. Landrigan PJ: Lead in the modern workplace. Am J Public Health 1990;80:907–908.

51. Rosen JF, Chesney RW, Hamstra A, et al: Reduction in 1,25-dihydroxyvitamin D in children with increased lead absorption. N Engl J Med 1980;302:1128–1130.

52. Hernberg S, Nikkanen J: Enzyme inhibition by lead under normal urban conditions. Lancet 1970;1:63–64.

53. Silbergeld EK: Mechanisms of lead neurotoxicity, or looking beyond the lamppost. FASEB J 1992;6:3201–3206.

54. Sandhir R, Gill KD: Lead perturbs calmodulin dependent cyclic AMP metabolism in rat central nervous system. Biochem Mol Biol Int 1994;33:729–742.

55. Stollery BT, Broadbent DE, Banks HL, et al: Short term prospective study of cognitive functioning in lead workers. Br J Ind Med 1991;48:739–749.

56. Murata K, Araki S, Yokoyama K, et al: Assessment of central, peripheral, and autonomic nervous system functions in lead workers: neuroelectrophysiological studies. Environ Res 1993;61:323–336.

57. Kumar BD, Krishnaswamy K: Detection of occupational lead nephropathy using early renal markers. Clin Toxicol 1995;33:331–335.

58. Staessen JA, Lauwerys R, Buchet J-P, et al: Impairment of renal function with increasing blood lead concentrations in the general population. N Engl J Med 1992;327:151–156.

59. Hu H: A 50-year follow-up of childhood plumbism: hypertension, renal function and hemoglobin levels among survivors. Am J Dis Child 1991;145:681–687.

60. Schwartz J: Lead, blood pressure, and cardiovascular disease in men. Arch Environ Health 1995;50:31–37.

61. Levine F, Muenke M: VACTERL association with high prenatal lead exposure: similarities to animal models of lead teratogenicity. Pediatrics 1991;87:390–392.

62. Alexander BH, Checkoway H, Faustman EM, et al: Contrasting associations of blood and semen lead concentrations with semen quality among lead smelter workers. Am J Ind Med 1998;4(5):464–469.

63. Nash D, Magder L, Lustberg M, et al: Blood lead, blood pressure, and hypertension in perimenopausal and postmenopausal women. JAMA 2003;289(12):1523–1532.

64. Hu H, Rabinowitz M, Smith D: Bone lead as a biological marker in epidemiologic studies of chronic toxicity: conceptual paradigms. Environ Health Perspect 1998;106(1):1–8.

65. Kosnett MJ, Becker CE, Osterloh J, et al: Factors influencing bone lead concentration in a suburban community assessed by noninvasive K X-ray fluorescence. JAMA 1994;271:197–203.

66. Hu H, Watanabe H, Payton M, et al: The relationship between blood lead and hemoglobin. JAMA 1994;272:1512–1517.

67. Holdstein Y, Pratt H, Goldsher M, et al: Auditory brainstem evoked potentials in asymptomatic lead-exposed subjects. J Laryngol Otol 1986;100:1031–1036.

68. Vilensky JA, Redman K: British anti-Lewisite (dimercaprol): an amazing history. Ann Emerg Med 2003;41(3):378–383.

69. American Academy of Pediatrics and Committee on Drugs: Treatment guidelines for lead exposure in children. Pediatrics 1995;96:155.

70. delaBurde B, Choate MS: Does asymptomatic lead exposure in children have latent sequelae? J Pediatr 1972;81:1088–1091.

71. Centers for Disease Control and U.S. Department of Health and Human Services: Preventing Lead Poisoning in Young Children. Washington, DC, U.S. Department of Health and Human Services, 1991, p 105.

72. Canfield RL, Henderson CR, Cory-Slechta DA, et al: Intellectual impairment in children with blood lead concentrations below 10 microg per deciliter. N Engl J Med 2003;348(16):1517–1526.

73. Lanphear B, Dietrich KN, Auinger P, et al: Cognitive deficits associated with blood lead concentrations < 10 μg/dl in US children and adolescents. Public Health Rep 2000;115:521–529.

74. Centers for Disease Control and Prevention (CDC): Children's Blood Lead Levels in the US. Atlanta, CDC, 2004.

75. Brown MJ, DeGiacomo JM, Gallagher G, et al: Lead poisoning in children of different ages. N Engl J Med 1990;323:135–136.

76. Geltman PL, Brown MJ, Cochran J: Lead poisoning among refugee children resettled in Massachusetts, 1995 to 1999. Pediatrics 2001;108(1):158–162.

77. Centers for Disease Control and Prevention (CDC): Elevated blood lead levels among internationally adopted children: United States, 1998. MMWR Morb Mortal Wkly Rep 2000;49:97–100.

78. Shannon MW, Graef JW: Lead intoxication in infancy. Pediatrics 1992;89(1):87–90.

79. McElvaine MD, DeUngria EG, Matte TD, et al: Prevalence of radiographic evidence of paint chip ingestion among children with moderate to severe lead poisoning, St. Louis, Missouri, 1989 through 1990. Pediatrics 1992;89:740–742.

80. Centers for Disease Control and Prevention (CDC): Fatal pediatric poisoning from leaded paint–Wisconsin 1990. MMWR Morb Mortal Wkly Rep 1991;40:193–195.

81. Lanphear BP, Hornung R, Ho M, et al: Environmental lead exposure during early childhood. J Pediatr 2002;140(1):40–47.

82. Shannon M, Graef JW: Lead intoxication in infancy. Pediatrics 1992;89:87–90.

83. Baker EL, Folland DS, Taylor TA, et al: Lead poisoning in children of lead workers—house contamination with industrial dust. N Engl J Med 1977;296:260–261.

84. Shannon M, Graef JW: Lead intoxication from lead-contaminated water used to reconstitute infant formula. Clin Pediatr 1989;28:380–382.

85. Lockitch G, Berry B, Roland E, et al: Seizures in a 10-week-old infant: lead poisoning from an unexpected source. Can Med Assoc J 1991;145:1465–1468.

86. Shannon MW: Lead poisoning from an unexpected source in a 4-month-old infant: case records of the Children's Hospital Pediatric Environmental Health Clinic. Environ Health Perspect 1998;106:313–316.

87. Levallois P, Lavoie M, Goulet L, et al: Blood lead levels in children and pregnant women living near a lead-reclamation plant. Can Med Assoc J 1991;144:877–885.

88. Weitzman M, Aaschengrau A, Bellinger D, et al: Lead-contaminated soil abatement and urban children's blood lead levels. JAMA 1993;269:1647–1654.

89. American Academy of Pediatrics and Committee on Environmental Health: Lead poisoning: from screening to primary prevention. Pediatrics 1993;92:176–183.

90. Hugelmeyer CD, Moorhead JC, Horenblas L, et al: Fatal lead encephalopathy following foreign body ingestion: case report. J Emerg Med 1988;6:397–400.

91. Bearer CF, O'Riordan MA, Powers R: Lead exposure from blood transfusion to premature infants. J Pediatr 2000;137(4):549–554.

92. Bearer CF, Linsalata N, Yomtovian R, et al: Blood transfusions: a hidden source of lead exposure. Lancet 2003;362(9380):332.

93. Accardo P, Whitman B, Calu J, et al: Autism and plumbism—a possible association. Clin Pediatr 1988;27:41–44.

94. Cohen DJ, Johnson WT, Caparulo BK: Pica and elevated blood lead level in autistic and atypical children. Am J Dis Child 1976;130:47–48.

95. Shannon MW, Graef JW: Lead intoxication in children with pervasive developmental delays. Clin Toxicol 1996;34:177–182.

96. Mahaffey KR: Environmental lead toxicity: nutrition as a component of intervention. Environ Health Perspect 1990;89:75–78.

97. Chuang HY, Schwartz J, Gonzales-Cossio T, et al: Interrelations of lead levels in bone, venous blood, and umbilical cord blood with exogenous lead exposure through maternal plasma lead in peripartum women. Environ Health Perspect 2001;109(5):527–532.

98. Han S, Pfizenmaier DH, Garcia E, et al: Effects of lead exposure before pregnancy and dietary calcium during pregnancy on fetal development and lead accumulation. Environ Health Perspect 2000;108(6):527–531.

99. Gulson BL, Mahaffey KR, Jameson CW, et al: Impact of diet on lead in blood and urine in female adults and relevance to mobilization of lead from bone stores. Environ Health Perspect 1999;107(4):257–263.

100. Mushak P: New findings on sources and biokinetics of lead in human breast milk: bone lead can target both nursing infant and fetus. Environ Health Perspect 1998;106(10):629–631.

101. Gomaa A, Hu H, Bellinger D, et al: Maternal bone lead as an independent risk factor for fetal neurotoxicity: a prospective study. Pediatrics 2002;110(1 Pt 1):110–118.

102. Ettinger AS, Tellez-Rojo MM, Amarasiriwardena C, et al: Effect of breast milk lead on infant blood lead levels at 1 month of age. Environ Health Perspect 2004;112(14):1381–1385.

103. Ettinger AS, Tellez-Rojo MM, Amarasiriwardena C, et al: Levels of lead in breast milk and their relation to maternal blood and bone lead levels at one month postpartum. Environ Health Perspect 2004;112(8):926–931.

104. Osterloh JD, Kelly TJ: Study of the effect of lactational bone loss on blood lead concentrations in humans. Environ Health Perspect 1999;107(3):187–194.

105. Gulson BL, Jameson CW, Mahaffey KR, et al: Relationships of lead in breast milk to lead in blood, urine, and diet of the infant and mother. Environ Health Perspect 1998;106(10):667–774.

106. Baum CR, Shannon MW: Lead in breast milk. Pediatrics 1996;97:932.

107. Gundacker C, Pietschnig B, Wittmann KJ, et al: Lead and mercury in breast milk. Pediatrics 2002;110(5):873–878.

108. Yaish HM, Niazi GA, Soby AA: Lead poisoning among Saudi children. Ann Saudi Med 1993;13:395–401.

109. Dietrich KN, Berger OG, Bhattacharya A: Symptomatic lead poisoning in infancy: a prospective case analysis. J Pediatr 2000;137(4):568–571.

110. American Academy of Pediatrics and Committee on Environmental Health: Screening for elevated blood lead levels. Pediatrics 1998;101:1072–1078.

111. Goldstein GW: Lead poisoning and brain cell function. Environ Health Perspect 1990;89:91–94.

112. Goldstein GW: Neurologic concepts of lead poisoning in children. Pediatr Ann 1992;21:384–388.

113. Dyatlov VA, Platoshin AV, Lawrence DA, Carpenter DO: Lead potentiates cytokine- and glutamate-mediated increases in permeability of the blood-brain barrier. Neurotoxicology 1998;19:283–292.

114. Baghurst PA, McMichael AJ, Wigg NR, et al: Environmental exposure to lead and children's intelligence at the age of seven years: the Port Pirie cohort study. N Engl J Med 1992;327:1279–1284.

115. Faust D, Brown J: Moderately elevated blood lead levels: effects on neuropsychologic functioning in children. Pediatrics 1987;80:623–629.

116. McMichael AJ, Baghurst PA, Wigg NR, et al: Port Pirie cohort study: environmental exposure to lead and children's abilities at the age of four years. N Engl J Med 1988;319:468–475.

117. Wasserman GA, Staghezza-Jaramillo B, Shrout P: The effect of lead exposure on behavior problems in preschool children. Am J Public Health 1998;88:481–486.

118. Burns J, Baghurst P, Sawyer M, et al: Lifetime low-level exposure to environmental lead and children's emotional and behavioral development at ages 11-13 years. Am J Epidemiol 1999;149:740–749.

119. Bellinger D: Teratogen update: lead. Teratology 1994;50:367–373.

120. Naeser MA: Outline guide to Chinese herbal patent medicines in pill form. Boston, Boston Chinese Medicine, 1990, p 372.

121. Needleman HL, Gatsonis CA: Low-level lead exposure and the IQ of children—a meta-analysis of modern studies. JAMA 1990;263:673–678.

122. Needleman HL, Reiss JA, Tobin MJ, et al: Bone lead levels and delinquent behavior. JAMA 1996;275:363–369.

123. Sciarillo WG, Alexander G, Farrell KP: Lead exposure and child behavior. Am J Public Health 1992;82:1356–1360.

124. Dietrich KN, Ris MD, Succop PA, et al: Early exposure to lead and juvenile delinquency. Neurotoxicol Teratol 2001;23(6):511–518.

125. Stretesky PB, Lynch MJ: The relationship between lead exposure and homicide. Arch Pediatr Adolesc Med 2001;155(5):579–582.

126. Counter SA, Buchanan LH, Rosas HD, et al: Neurocognitive effects of chronic lead intoxication in Andean children. J Neurol Sci 1998;160(1):47–53.

127. Baghurst PA, McMichael AJ, Tong S, et al: Exposure to environmental lead and visual-motor integration at age 7 years: the Port Pirie cohort study. Epidemiology 1995;6:104–109.

128. Fergusson DM, Horwood LJ: The effects of lead levels on the growth of word recognition in middle childhood. Int J Epidemiol 1993;22:891–897.

129. Morgan RE, Garavan H, Smith EG, et al: Early lead exposure produces lasting changes in sustained attention, response initiation, and reactivity to errors. Neurotoxicol Teratol 2001;23(6):519–531.

130. Bellinger D, Leviton A, Waternaux C, et al: Longitudinal analyses of prenatal and postnatal lead exposure and early cognitive development. N Engl J Med 1987;316:1037–1043.

131. Bellinger DC, Stiles KM, Needleman HL: Low-level lead exposure, intelligence and academic achievement: a long-term follow-up study. Pediatrics 1992;90:855–861.

132. Liu X, Dietrich KN, Radcliffe J, et al: Do children with falling blood lead levels have improved cognition? Pediatrics 2002;110(4):787–791.

133. Tong S, Baghurst PA, Sawyer MG, et al: Declining blood lead levels and changes in cognitive function during childhood: the Port Pirie Cohort Study. JAMA 1998;280(22):1915–1919.

134. Greene T, Ernhart CB: Dentine lead and intelligence prior to school entry: a statistical sensitivity analysis. J Clin Epidemiol 1993;46:323–339.

135. Pocock SJ, Smith M, Baghurst P: Environmental lead and children's intelligence: a systematic review of the epidemiological evidence. BMJ 1994;309:1189–1197.

136. Schwartz J, Landrigan PJ, Feldman RG, et al: Threshold effect in lead-induced peripheral neuropathy. J Pediatr 1988;112:12–17.

137. Erenberg G, Rinsler SS, Fish BG: Lead neuropathy and sickle cell disease. Pediatrics 1974;54:438–441.

138. Schwartz J, Otto D: Blood lead, hearing thresholds, and neurobehavioral development in children and youth. Arch Environ Health 1987;42:153–160.

139. Schwartz J, Otto D: Lead and minor hearing impairment. Arch Environ Health 1987;46:300–305.

140. Dietrich KN, Berger OG, Succop PA: Lead exposure and the motor developmental status of urban six-year-old children in the Cincinnati prospective study. Pediatrics 1993;91:301–307.

141. Needleman HL, Gunnoe C, Leviton A, et al: Deficits in psychologic and classroom performance of children with elevated dentine lead levels. N Engl J Med 1979;300:689–695.

142. Blickman JG, Wilkinson RH, Graef JW: The radiologic "lead band" revisited. Am J Radiol 1986;146:245–247.

143. Gemmel A, Tavares M, Alperin S, et al: Blood lead level and dental caries in school-age children. Environ Health Perspect 2002;110(10):A625–A630.

144. Dye BA, Hirsch R, Brody DJ: The relationship between blood lead levels and periodontal bone loss in the United States, 1988–1994. Environ Health Perspect 2002;110(10):997–1002.

145. Hoppin JA, Aro AC, Williams PL, et al: Validation of K-XRF bone lead measurement in young adults. Environ Health Perspect 1995;103(1):78–83.

146. Centers for Disease Control and Prevention and U.S. Department of Health and Human Services: Management of elevated blood lead levels in children. Washington, DC, U.S. Public Health Service, 2002.

147. Amitai Y, Brown MJ, Graef JW, et al: Residential deleading: effects on the blood lead levels of lead-poisoned children. Pediatrics 1991;88:893–897.

148. Amitai Y, Lovejoy FH: Characteristics of vomiting associated with acute sustained release theophylline poisoning: implications for management with oral activated charcoal. Clin Toxicol 1987;25:539–554.

149. Wright RO, Shannon MW, Wright RJ, et al: Association between iron deficiency and low-level lead poisoning in an urban primary care clinic. Am J Public Health 1999;89(7):1049–1053.

150. Gallicchio L, Scherer RW, Sexton M: Influence of nutrient intake on blood lead levels of young children at risk for lead poisoning. Environ Health Perspect 2002;110(12):A767–A772.

151. Chisolm JJ: The use of chelating agents in the treatment of acute and chronic lead intoxication in childhood. J Pediatr 1968;73:1–38.

152. Markowitz ME, Rose JF: Assessment of lead stores in children: validation of an 8-hour CaNa2EDTA provocative test. J Pediatr 1984;104:337–341.

153. Markowitz ME, Rosen JF: Need for the lead mobilization test in children with lead poisoning. J Pediatr 1991;119:305–310.

154. Weitzman M, Glotzer D: Lead poisoning. Pediatr Rev 1992;13:461–468.

155. Shannon M, Grace A, Graef J: Use of urinary lead concentration in interpretation of the EDTA mobilization test. Vet Hum Toxicol 1989;31:140–142.

156. Kassner J, Shannon M, Graef J: Role of forced diuresis of urinary lead excretion after the ethylenediaminetetraacetic acid mobilization test. J Pediatr 1990;117:914–916.

157. Walshe JM: Penicillamine, a new oral therapy for Wilson's disease. Am J Med 1956;21:487–495.

158. Liebelt EL, Shannon MW: Oral chelators for childhood lead poisoning. Pediatr Ann 1994;23:616–626.

159. Shannon MW, Townsend MK: Efficacy of reduced-dose D-penicillamine in children with mild to moderate lead poisoning. Ann Pharmacother 2000;34:15–18.

160. Marcus SM: Experience with D-penicillamine in treating lead poisoning. Vet Hum Toxicol 1982;24:18–20.

161. Sachs HK, Blanksma LA, Murray EF, et al: Ambulatory treatment of lead poisoning: report of 1155 cases. Pediatrics 1970;46:389–396.

162. Vitale LF, Rosalinas-Bailon A, Folland D, et al: Oral penicillamine therapy for chronic lead poisoning in children. J Pediatr 1973;83:1041–1045.

163. Shannon M, Grace A, Graef JW: Use of penicillamine in children with small lead burdens. N Engl J Med 1989;321:979–980.

164. Shannon M, Graef J, Lovejoy FH: Efficacy and toxicity of D-penicillamine in low-level lead poisoning. J Pediatr 1988;112:799–804.

165. Graziano JH, Lolacano NJ, Moulton T, et al: Controlled study of meso-2,3-dimercaptosuccininc acid for the management of childhood lead intoxication. J Pediatr 1992;120:133–139.

166. Graziano JH, Lolacono NJ, Meyer P: Dose-response study of oral 2,3-dimercaptosuccinic acid in children with elevated blood lead concentrations. J Pediatr 1988;113:751–757.

167. Liebelt EL, Shannon M, Graef JW: Efficacy of oral meso-2, 3 dimercaptosuccinic acid therapy for low-level childhood plumbism. J Pediatr 1994;124:313–317.

168. Royce S, Rosenberg J: Chelation therapy in workers with lead exposure. West J Med 1993;158:372–375.

169. Besunder JB, Anderson RL, Super DM: Short-term efficacy of oral dimercaptosuccinic acid in children with low to moderate lead intoxication. Pediatrics 1995;96:683–687.

170. Rogan W and Treatment of Lead-Exposed Children (TLC) Group: Safety and efficacy of succimer in toddlers with blood lead levels of 20–44 μg/dl. Pediatr Res 2000;48:593–599.

171. Chisolm JJ, Thomas DJ: Use of 2,3-dimercaptopropane-1-sulfonate in treatment of lead poisoning in children. J Pharm Exp Ther 1985;235:665–669.

172. Chisolm JJ: BAL, EDTA, DMSA and DMPS in the treatment of lead poisoning in children. Clin Toxicol 1992;30:493–504.

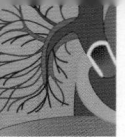

173. Ruff HA, Bijur PE, Markowitz M, et al: Declining blood lead levels and cognitive changes in moderately lead-poisoned children. JAMA 1993;269:1641–1646.

174. Centers for Disease Control and Prevention (CDC): Managing elevated blood lead levels among young children. Atlanta, U.S. Dept of Health and Human Services, Public Health Service, 2002.

175. American Academy of Pediatrics Committee on Environmental Health: Lead exposure in children: prevention, detection, and management. Pediatrics 2005;116:1036–1046.

176. Rolfe PB, Marcinak JF, Nice AJ, et al: Use of zinc protoporphyrin measured by the Protofluor-Z hematofluormeter in screening children for elevated blood lead levels. Am J Dis Child 1993;147:66–68.

177. Gellert GA, Wagner GA, Maxwell RM, et al: Lead poisoning among low-income children in Orange County, California—a need for regionally differentiated policy. JAMA 1993;270:69–71.

178. Schlenker TL, Fritz CJ, Mark D, et al: Screening for pediatric lead poisoning—comparability of simultaneously drawn capillary and venous blood samples. JAMA 1994;271:1346–1348.

179. Schoen EJ: Lead toxicity in the 21st century: will we still be treating it? Pediatrics 1992;90:481.

180. Rolnick SJ, Nordin J, Cherney LM: A comparison of costs of universal versus targeted lead screening for young children. Environ Res 1999;80(1):84–91.

181. Kemper AR, Bordley WC, Downs SM: Cost-effectiveness analysis of lead poisoning screening strategies following the 1997 guidelines of the Centers for Disease Control and Prevention. Arch Pediatr Adolesc Med 1998;152(12):1202–1208.

182. Dowsett R, Shannon M: Childhood plumbism identified after lead poisoning in household pets. N Engl J Med 1994;331:1661–1662.

183. Bithoney WG, Vandeven AM, Ryan A: Elevated lead levels in reportedly abused children. J Pediatr 1993;122:719–720.

184. Flaherty EG: Risk of lead poisoning in abused and neglected children. Clin Pediatr 1995;34:128–132.

185. Wiley JF, Henretig FM, Selbst SM: Blood lead levels in children with foreign bodies. Pediatrics 1992;89:593–596.

186. Binns HJ, Le Bailly SA, Fingar AR, et al: Evaluation of risk assessment questions used to target blood lead screening in Illinois. Pediatrics 1999;103(1):100–106.

187. Centers for Disease Control and Prevention (CDC): Screening young children for lead poisoning. Atlanta, U.S. Public Health Service, 1997.

74 *Arsenic and Arsine*

DAVID C. PIGOTT, MD ■ ERICA L. LIEBELT, MD

At a Glance...

- Acute inorganic arsenic toxicity is characterized by severe gastroenteritis, cardiovascular instability, seizures, acute respiratory distress syndrome, and renal failure.
- Survivors of acute inorganic arsenic toxicity develop peripheral neuropathy and Mees' lines.
- Chronic inorganic arsenic toxicity is characterized by sensorimotor peripheral neuropathy, pancytopenia, palmar and plantar hyperkeratoses, liver disease, and cancers.
- Seafood can contain large amounts of organic arsenic, a relatively nontoxic form.
- Laboratory diagnosis utilizing measurement of urinary arsenic concentrations supports the diagnosis; speciation to distinguish inorganic from organic arsenics is useful in identifying the type and source of arsenic.
- Treatment of arsenic toxicity may include the use of chelating agents—BAL, DMSA, or DMPS.
- Clinical signs and symptoms of arsine poisoning are abdominal pain, hematuria, and bronze-pigmented skin.
- Acute massive hemolytic anemia and renal failure characterize severe arsine toxicity.
- Treatment of severe arsine intoxication includes exchange transfusion.

ARSENIC

Introduction

Arsenic is a metalloid that exists in multiple forms—gaseous (arsine), organic, and inorganic (arsenite and arsenate). The name *arsenic*, which is derived from the Greek word *arsenikon*, meaning potent, has become synonymous with poison. The gaseous form, arsine, is the most toxic of arsenic species. Of the remaining forms, inorganic arsenate (pentavalent arsenic) and arsenite (trivalent arsenic) are the most toxic, while organoarsenical compounds ("fish arsenic") are generally considered to have little toxicity.

Arsenic has had various medicinal and industrial uses throughout history, which have led to the recognition of both its acute and chronic toxicities (Box 74-1). It also has been a popular homicidal or suicidal agent, the result of its availability, low cost, and tasteless and odorless characteristics. For similar reasons, arsenic has been included on lists of possible chemical substances that could be used as chemical warfare agents by terrorists.

History

Arsenic and arsenic poisoning have been recurring themes in history and literature for centuries. Aristotle referred to sandarach (arsenic trisulfide) in the 4th century BC. The first isolation of a free form of arsenic is generally credited to Albertus Magnus (c. 1206–1280), the famed theologian, philosopher, and scientist. The longtime use of arsenic and arsenical compounds in common household items has likewise been well documented. An arsenic-based pigment known as Paris green or Scheele's green was developed around 1775 by Carl Scheele, a Swedish chemist. It was used in paints, wallpaper, and fabrics (and also as an insecticide) until the end of the 19th century, when its toxic effects became known. Its bright green color was derived from a combination of copper arsenate and copper acetate.

The use of arsenical compounds for poisoning has also had a long and storied career. From the Borgias of the Middle Ages, who were rumored to have treated their unfortunate guests to arsenic-laced wine, to Napoleon, whose death has been argued by some to be the result of repeated arsenic poisoning, arsenic has long been the poison of choice for those bent on toxicologic malfeasance.

Famous epidemics of arsenic poisoning include the "Staffordshire Beer Epidemic" at the turn of the last century, the poisoning of a cohort of Japanese infants with arsenic-laced formula in 1955, and chronic arsenic poisoning in Singapore from a contaminated herbal preparation in 1972 and 1973. Millions of victims in India and Bangldesh have been chronically exposed to toxic levels of arsenic from their water supply and are suffering from arsenicalism.[1-3] This epidemic has been called the largest mass poisoning in recorded history. Recently, several incidents of mass arsenic poisoning have been reported, with the perpetrators adding arsenic to communal food or drink at public gatherings.[4]

Uses/Sources

Arsenic is an element that occurs naturally in the earth's crust. Environmental sources of arsenic include underground aquifers and volcanoes. Water coursing along geologic belts of arsenic (as in the Bangladesh epidemic) can become highly contaminated. The major source of environmental arsenic for the general population in the United States is food. In marine environments, inorganic arsenic can be made organic by microorganisms. The shellfish that ingest these microorganisms contain the highest concentrations of this nontoxic arsenic species in the form of organic arsenic or arsenobetaine. Other dietary sources of arsenic (usually inorganic) include grains, meats, and drinking water. The World Health Organization (WHO) guideline value for arsenic in drinking water is 0.01 mg/L.[5] In 2002, the U.S. Environmental Protection Agency (EPA)'s rule for new standards for arsenic in drinking water became effective,

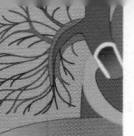

BOX 74-1   **SOURCES OF ARSENIC**

Inorganic Arsenic

Pesticides
Insecticides
Herbicides
Fungicides/algicides
Wood preservatives (chromium-copper-arsenate)

Occupation/Sites/Industries
Smelting/mining of nonferrous ores (copper and gold)
Microelectronic manufacture
Fossil fuel combustion
Forestry
Agriculture (cotton harvesting)
Decorative glass making
Metallurgy

Medicinals/Contaminated Drugs
Ayurvedic medications
Trisenox (arsenic trioxide)
Homeopathic remedies
Herbals
"Moonshine" ethanol
Opium and cocaine

Other
Contaminated well water

Organic Arsenic

Seafood (particularly shellfish)
Melarsoprol (trypanocide)

Arsine

Occupation/Sites/Industries
Semiconductors (gallium arsenide)
Galvanizers
Solderers
Etching
Lead plating
Microchip processing

---

decreasing the maximum contaminant level (MCL) from 50 ppb to 10 ppb in public water systems.[6] Water systems must meet this standard by January 2006. This change is estimated to prevent between 19 and 31 cases of bladder cancer and 19 to 25 cases of lung cancer each year as well as numerous cases of skin cancers and heart disease. However, it is still projected to lead to a cancer mortality rate as high as 1 per 100,000 people.

For centuries arsenic has been used for medicinal purposes. In the 1800s, Fowler's solution (1% potassium arsenite) was used to treat a variety of infectious and malignant diseases. In the past it was also used as a treatment for syphilis. It is still prescribed for African sleeping sickness (melarsoprol). In 2000, arsenic trioxide (Trisenox) was U.S. Food and Drug Administration (FDA)–approved as a chemotherapeutic agent for acute promyelocytic leukemia.

Industrial sources and uses of arsenic are numerous. It has been used in agriculture as an insecticide,

herbicide, defoliant, fungicide, and growth regulator. It has also been used as rat and ant poison. Arsenic is used in metallurgy for hardening alloys of copper and lead, as a dopant in semiconductor production, and in the manufacturing of pigments for paints, ceramics, and some types of glass.

Until recently, the most common use of arsenic in industry was as a wood preservative in combination with copper and chromium (copper chromium arsenate, or CCA). CCA protects wood from rotting due to insects and fungi, greatly extending the wood's life span. It has been used to pressure-treat the lumber used for decks, picnic tables, and playground and other outdoor equipment since the 1930s. Burning and sanding of arsenic-treated wood has resulted in clinical toxicity.[7,8] In 2003, the EPA finalized an agreement to phase out use of CCA-treated lumber in residential settings; as of January 2004, pressure-treated wood containing CCA could no longer be sold in the United States for home use. However, industrial uses of treated lumber such as for guardrails and utility poles are still allowed.

In 2002, arsenic exposures (including arsenic-based pesticides) represented 1621 of the over 2 million total poison exposures reported to the American Association of Poison Control Centers Toxic Exposure Surveillance System.[9] Of these exposures, 519 were reported in children younger than 6 years of age. Of these 1621 exposures, 1290 were unintentional. Nine patients developed life-threatening symptoms; one death was reported. These data almost certainly underrepresent the total number exposures in this country, particularly those resulting from occupational and environmental sources.

Pharmacology

Arsenic compounds exist primarily in two chemical states: trivalent (As^{3+}, arsenite, the most toxic and carcinogenic) and pentavalent (As^{5+}, arsenate). The basis of toxicity for trivalent arsenic stems largely from its affinity for sulfur, particularly sulfhydryl group–containing cellular enzymes.[10] Pentavalent arsenic compounds are less toxic but can uncouple oxidative phosphorylation via a process known as "arsenolysis." Organoarsenical compounds have no well-defined toxicity. However, organoarsenate toxicity has been reported in animals exposed to monosodium methyl arsenate, a common herbicide.[11]

Trivalent arsenic inhibits the conversion of dihydrolipoate to lipoate in the pyruvate dehydrogenase reaction, resulting in decreased production of acetyl coenzyme A, an essential cofactor in the ATP-generating Krebs cycle (Fig. 74-1). Through its affinity for sulfhydryl groups, trivalent arsenic interferes with multiple other cellular enzymes. It blocks the production of glutathione, an important endogenous antioxidant, thereby subjecting cells to greater risk of oxidative damage.[12,13]

The toxicity of pentavalent arsenic largely results from its in vivo conversion to trivalent arsenic. In addition, pentavalent arsenic has a molecular structure similar to that of inorganic phosphate; it therefore can substitute for phosphate in glycolysis and cellular respiration

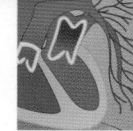

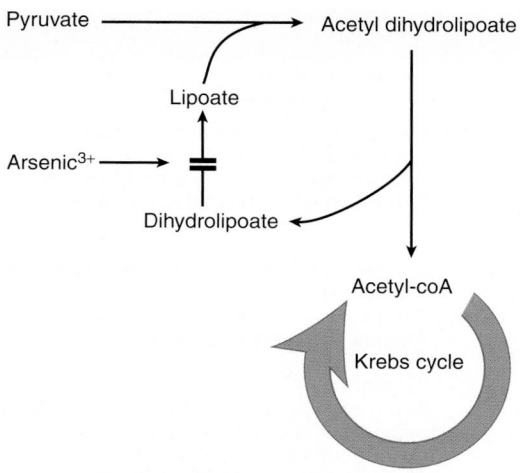

FIGURE 74-1 Pathophysiologic effects of trivalent arsenic, As(III). Trivalent arsenic interferes with the transformation of dihydrolipoate to lipoate, thereby inhibiting the formation of acetyl coenzyme A, an essential cofactor in the ATP-generating Krebs cycle.

processes. High-energy phosphate bonds are not made, leading to uncoupling of oxidative phosphorylation. Finally, adenosine diphosphate (ADP) binds to pentavalent arsenic, leading to the production of ADP-arsenate rather than the usual high-energy ATP molecule (Fig. 74-2).[12]

Pharmacokinetics and Toxicokinetics

The gastrointestinal (GI) absorption of most trivalent and pentavalent arsenic compounds dissolved in water exceeds 90%. Poorly soluble compounds, such as arsenic trioxide, are less well absorbed. The volume of distribution is 0.21 L/kg, with 90% being eliminated from the blood within 2 hours. For the remaining arsenic, a more gradual decline occurs, with a half-life of about 30 hours. Metabolism of arsenic is achieved primarily through its methylation. Pentavalent arsenic compounds are converted to the more toxic trivalent arsenic prior to their methylation. Trivalent arsenic undergoes methylation to monomethylarsenate and dimethylarsenate.[12,13]

Normal oxidative phosphorylation

$$ADP + P_i \longrightarrow ATP$$

In presence of Arsenic^{5+},
oxidative phosphorylation is uncoupled

$$ADP + As^{5+} \longrightarrow ADP\text{--}Arsenate \text{ (unstable)}$$

FIGURE 74-2 Pathophysiologic effects of pentavalent arsenic, As(V), termed *arsenolysis*. Pentavalent arsenic can substitute for inorganic phosphate in the formation of ATP, instead creating the unstable byproduct ADP-arsenate and thereby decoupling oxidative phosphorylation, an essential process in cellular respiration.

Urinary arsenic excretion is rapid, with 46% to 69% of arsenic eliminated with 4 to 5 days. However, continued excretion can occur for weeks to months.[14,15]

Dermal absorption is minimal unless arsenic is present in a lipid-soluble form or skin integrity is damaged; however, absorption can occur through the mucous membranes. The potentially fatal human dose of arsenic trioxide (arsenite) following an acute exposure is estimated to be between 1 and 4 mg/kg.

Special Population: Children

In the past several years, arsenic been increasingly scrutinized as a poisonous substance because of concerns about the potential health risks to children who play on arsenic-treated playground equipment. When exposed to outdoor elements, especially acidic rainwater, the arsenic in CCA can leach out of the wood. Several studies have documented significantly higher concentrations of arsenic in the soil immediately under pressure-treated wood compared with control samples.[16,17] In many samples, the concentrations were several-fold higher than state limits and EPA regulatory guidelines. Because of their normal hand-to-mouth activity, children can be exposed to high concentrations of arsenic from contaminated surfaces or soil over their lifetime, increasing their risk for cancer and chronic toxicity. Children's susceptibility to the toxic effects of arsenic may also be increased owing to differences in GI absorption; metabolism; higher body surface area, resulting in greater absorption per pound of body weight; higher respiratory rate; and different breathing zones. As mentioned above, commencing January 2004, the EPA no longer allows pressure-treated wood containing CCA to be used for residential applications. However, several thousand tons of existing lumber will remain on porch decks and playground equipment, and children will continue to be exposed.

Clinical Toxicology

Arsenic can affect nearly every major organ system and is also a well-known carcinogen.[18] Trivalent arsenic compounds are known to cause tracheal and bronchogenic carcinomas, hepatic angiosarcomas, and various skin cancers, such as intraepidermal carcinomas, squamous cell carcinomas, and basal cell carcinomas.[19] An increased risk of myelogenous leukemia has also been demonstrated after arsenic exposure.[20] Bladder, renal, lung, and liver cancers have all been associated with chronic internal exposure to arsenic-containing solutions or arsenic-contaminated drinking water.[19,21]

The toxic effects of arsenic depend largely on the degree and duration of exposure. A single large exposure can produce rapid and even fatal effects; a smaller chronic dose of arsenic leads to delayed or gradual effects that occur over months to years (Table 74-1).

Acute arsenic toxicity usually follows ingestion, but significant toxicity can also be seen following inhalation or dermal exposure. Initial symptoms affect the GI tract, causing oral irritation and burning in the oropharynx

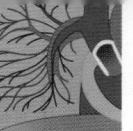

TABLE 74-1 Acute vs. Chronic Arsenic Toxicity

SYSTEM	ACUTE TOXICITY	CHRONIC TOXICITY
Central nervous	Confusion, delirium, encephalopathy, seizures	Encephalopathy, headache, seizures, psychosis, personality changes
Peripheral nervous	Peripheral neuropathy appears early	Sensorimotor neuropathy develops/persists
Cardiovascular	Hypotension, conduction delays (prolonged QT_c), dysrhythmias (bradycardia, ventricular fibrillation, torsades de pointes)	Prolonged QT_c and conduction delays
Gastrointestinal	Nausea, vomiting, intense thirst, watery or bloody diarrhea, abdominal pain, acute hepatitis	May be absent, stomatitis, cirrhosis, portal hypertension
Pulmonary	Cough, dyspnea, chest pain, pulmonary edema	Cough
Hemtologic	Hemolytic anemia	Anemia, leukopenia, pancytopenia
Renal	Acute tubular necrosis, acute renal failure	
Otolaryngologic	Mucous membrane irritation, metallic taste	Laryngitis
Dermatologic	Mees' lines, transverse lines in hair	Hypo- or hyperpigmentation, hyperkeratosis (palms and soles), skin cancers, facial/peripheral edema, alopecia
Other		Multiple cancers, blackfoot disease

and esophagus, followed by nausea, vomiting, and severe diarrhea. This diarrhea has been described as analogous to the "rice water" stools associated with cholera. Hemorrhagic gastroenteritis may occur, or necrosis of the GI mucosa leading to perforation. Increased vascular permeability and endothelial damage with "third spacing" of interstitial fluid are characteristic; adequate volume resuscitation of patients suffering from acute arsenic exposure is essential but may not prevent a fatal outcome.

Central nervous system (CNS) symptoms may also occur, including seizures or acute encephalopathy. Encephalopathic symptoms may include headache, confusion, decreased memory, personality change, irritability, hallucinations, and delirium. Development of peripheral neuropathy due to axonal degeneration, as in other heavy metal exposures, can occur relatively rapidly after acute arsenic ingestion.[22] Sensory symptoms predominate early in the course, with patients complaining of "pins and needles" primarily in the lower extremities. Progression of the neuropathy is characterized by numbness and tingling to absent sensation of pain, touch, temperature, and deep tendon reflexes in a stocking-glove distribution. Motor weakness may develop and sometimes progress to an ascending flaccid paralysis similar to Guillain-Barré syndrome. The peripheral neuropathy usually occurs within 1 to 3 weeks following exposure, but in one series, nine patients developed maximal neuropathy within 24 hours.[23]

Cardiac dysrhythmias such as torsades de pointes and ventricular fibrillation have been described, as well as sudden bradycardia leading to cardiac arrest.[24] Prolongation of the QT interval has also been well reported. Multisystem organ dysfunction is described, with hepatic involvement leading to acute hepatitis and renal failure.[25] Fetal demise is a documented complication of acute maternal arsenic poisoning.[26]

Less severe presentations of acute arsenic poisoning may result in persistent GI symptoms requiring hospitalization and intravenous fluid replacement. A garlicky breath odor may be present. Dermatologic findings are not characteristic early in the clinical course of acute arsenic toxicity. However, transverse lines across the finger and toenails (Mees' lines) appear after 1 to 2 weeks and are one of the most characteristic signs of acute arsenic poisoning. Mees' lines do not appear after chronic arsenic exposure.

In chronic arsenic toxicity, the fulminant presentations associated with a single acute arsenic ingestion are not seen. Rather, the gradual development of skin pigmentation changes, palmar and plantar hyperkeratoses, GI symptoms, anemia, and liver disease are common.[27]

Skin findings, such as hyperpigmentation and hyperkeratoses, are often among the first symptoms of chronic arsenic toxicity. Later, the development of skin cancers such as Bowen's disease (intraepithelial squamous cell carcinoma) is seen.[27] Hepatomegaly is a common finding in patients with chronic arsenic exposure.[28] Other hepatic abnormalities including cirrhosis and noncirrhotic portal hypertension have been linked to chronic arsenic exposure. Increased incidence of diabetes mellitus in arsenic-exposed populations has also been described, the result of arsenic's endocrine-disrupting effects.[29] GI volume losses as seen in acute arsenicalism are less common.

Arsenic has a deleterious effect on both red and white blood cell populations, leading to anemia, aplastic anemia, and agranulocytosis. Arsenic's adverse effect on white blood cell levels was first documented with the use of Fowler's solution on leukemia patients in the late 1800s; recently, arsenic trioxide (Trisenox, Cephalon, Inc., Frazer, PA) has surfaced as a potential therapy for patients with acute promyelocytic leukemia.[30,31]

Chronic encephalopathy, headache, and peripheral sensorimotor neuropathy can be seen with long-standing arsenic exposure because arsenic is primarily a peripheral neurotoxin.[32] Overt CNS toxicity, however, is rare. Chronic cough may develop. A syndrome of lower extremity vascular insufficiency (blackfoot disease) has been documented in Taiwanese populations exposed to elevated arsenic levels in well water.[33]

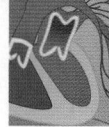

Diagnosis

The diagnosis of acute or chronic arsenic poisoning is made primarily on the basis of history and clinical presentation. In cases of homicide or environmental exposure, the patient or health care provider may not even know that arsenic poisoning has occurred. Medical history taking should address the patient's home heating methods (burning of arsenic-treated wood in stoves or fireplaces); drinking water source; gardening, farming or forestry activities; use of folk, herbal, or homeopathic remedies; location of residence in relation to agricultural or industrial activities; diet; and occupational history. Physical examination may provide the characteristics as described above. The utility of laboratory diagnostic studies depends on whether the exposure is acute, chronic, or remote, with residual clinical effects such as cancers.

LABORATORY TESTING
Arsenic Levels

To interpret blood and urine tests accurately, it is important to understand the pharmacology of arsenic, particularly its metabolism and clearance, as well as sources of organic arsenic. The most useful test for confirming excessive arsenic exposure is a 24-hour urine collection and analysis. An elevated arsenic level confirms the diagnosis of arsenic exposure but not the type of arsenic; a low level does not exclude the diagnosis of arsenic toxicity. Normal urine levels of arsenic in an unexposed person should be less than 25 µg per 24 hours or 10 to 30 µg/L of urine.[34] In infants and children, a 6- to 8-hour timed urine specimen can be substituted for a full 24-hour collection. Urinary levels of inorganic arsenic, both trivalent and pentavalent, peak within 10 hours and normalize as soon as 20 to 30 hours after ingestion. Levels of urinary methylarsonic acid and dimethyarsinic acid peak within 40 to 50 hours after ingestion and normalize approximately 6 to 20 days after ingestion.[35]

In an emergency, a single urine void or "spot" urine may be collected as a substitute for a 24-hour collection. In these specimens, arsenic should be measured per gram of creatinine. Because creatinine excretion is so variable in children, a "spot" urine is completely unreliable. In one study, initial spot urine arsenic levels ranged from 192,000 to 198,450 µg/L in patients with symptoms of acute toxicity.[36] Because urinary excretion of arsenic is intermittent, definitive diagnosis relies on finding a concentration of greater than 50 µg/L arsenic, 100 µg/g of creatinine, or a total of greater than 100 µg arsenic in a 24-hour urine collection, again taken in the context of the patient's history and clinical presentation. Urinary arsenic excretion varies inversely with the postexposure time period, but low-level excretion may continue for months after exposure. In one study of patients with arsenic-induced peripheral neuropathy, for 4 to 8 weeks' duration, patients had total 24-hour urinary arsenic measurements of 100 to 400 µg.[37]

When seafood is ingested, urinary arsenic levels may transiently increase to 200 to 1700 µg/L.[38] Therefore, laboratory arsenic speciation into organic arsenobetaine (predominant arsenic in seafood) versus inorganic levels is needed to determine the actual type and source of the exposure. Alternatively, patients can abstain from fish consumption for 1 week prior to testing; in this instance, all arsenic excreted can be presumed to be inorganic. All urine should be collected in metal-free containers. Most hospital laboratories do not routinely measure heavy metals; thus, it is important that specimens from acutely ill patients be sent to a reference laboratory.

A serum arsenic level is highly variable. It will usually be elevated in a recent acute exposure but is rapidly cleared after several hours. Serum levels of arsenic in unexposed persons are less than 3 µg/dL.[39] If there is a significant delay between ingestion and presentation, diagnosis of arsenic poisoning based on serum concentrations may be erroneous. Concentrations are often normal in cases of chronic toxicity.

Analysis of arsenic in hair or nails generally is not useful. Although arsenic may begin to accumulate in these areas within hours of exposure, these samples may also be contaminated by environmental deposition of arsenic. Analyzing pubic hair may be useful. Laboratories offering hair and nail analysis have demonstrated inconsistent results and fail to establish appropriate normal reference ranges.[40] However, such testing may be helpful to confirm exposure in populations.

Other Laboratory Studies

Because inorganic arsenic is radiopaque, an abdominal radiograph may demonstrate the material in the GI tract after an acute ingestion.[41] The rapid absorption of arsenic may limit the usefulness of this test after several hours.

Other laboratory tests to include in the evaluation are a complete blood count with peripheral smear, seeking the presence of anemia, leukopenia, thrombocytopenia, and/or basophilic stippling[42]; a chemistry panel that identifies renal insufficiency; liver function tests for elevated aminotransferases and bilirubin; and an electrocardiogram for prolongation of the QT_c interval and torsades de pointes. Urinalysis may show proteinuria, hematuria, and pyuria. Cerebrospinal fluid analysis in patients with CNS findings due to arsenic may be normal or exhibit mild protein elevation.[37] This is in contrast to patients with Guillain-Barré syndrome, who typically have an elevated protein concentration after the first week of the illness.

DIFFERENTIAL DIAGNOSIS

The differential diagnosis for inorganic arsenic toxicity depends on the particular symptom or combination of symptoms being manifested. Infectious gastroenteritis may mimic acute inorganic arsenic poisoning initially; however, the more prolonged course of clinical symptoms and persistent need for intravenous fluids with arsenic toxicity is atypical for most viral and bacterial enteric illnesses and should alert the health care provider to consider arsenic toxicity. Other toxic agents may present with acute GI symptoms (Box 74-2). Guillain-Barré syndrome and arsenic toxicity may present with very similar peripheral neuropathies,

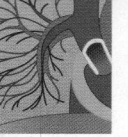

BOX 74-2	DIFFERENTIAL DIAGNOSIS OF INORGANIC ARSENIC TOXICITY

Gastrointestinal Disorders	Peripheral Neuropathies
Infectious gastroenteritis	Guillain-Barré syndrome
Hepatitis	Alcohol
Toxin-induced gastroenteritis	Diabetes
Mercury, iron	Thallium
Aspirin, colchicine	Lead
Marine toxins	
Organophosphorus	
compounds	
Ricin	

although the former is not associated with persistent GI symptoms. Peripheral neuropathies associated with diabetes, alcohol, thallium, and chronic lead poisoning should also be considered.

Management

SUPPORTIVE MEASURES

Acute arsenic toxicity can be life threatening and necessitates aggressive supportive therapy (Table 74-2). Hypotension should be treated with crystalloid fluids initially and may require blood products if GI hemorrhage is ongoing. Vasopressor and inotropic therapy may be necessary if fluids alone do not provide hemodynamic stability. All patients should be placed on a cardiac monitor and evaluated for cardiac dysrhythmias or conduction abnormalities. Ventricular tachycardia and fibrillation can be treated with lidocaine and/or amiodarone, and defibrillation.[24,43] Torsades de pointes can be treated with isoproterenol, magnesium, and/or overdrive pacing.

Patients with evidence of chronic arsenic toxicity should be removed from the arsenic source. If homicidal intent is suspected for hospitalized patients, visitors should be monitored closely and outside food forbidden.

GASTROINTESTINAL DECONTAMINATION

If radiopaque material is seen on abdominal radiograph, gastric lavage may be useful. However, its efficacy is likely to be limited because of rapid GI absorption of arsenic. Although arsenic poorly adsorbs to activated charcoal, it should be administered when there is suspicion for co-ingestants. Whole-bowel irrigation may be necessary to decontaminate the GI tract of any radiopaque material remaining after gastric lavage.[44] Continuous nasogastric suction may be important in removing arsenic resecreted in gastric or biliary secretions.[45] One study reported detectable arsenic in gastric aspirates of three patients 5 to 7 days following ingestion.[46]

ANTIDOTES

Chelating agents are the antidotes for severe arsenic poisoning. Chelation therapy should be initiated as soon as possible if acute inorganic arsenic toxicity is suspected; organic arsenic exposure does not require chelation. For cases of suspected chronic toxicity, therapy can wait until laboratory verification of the diagnosis is made unless the patient's clinical status is deteriorating. Four chelating agents are available in the United States, each with their own efficacy and safety profile.

British antilewisite (BAL), or 2,3-dimercaptopropanol, has been the standard therapy for acute inorganic toxicity. BAL was developed during World War II because of concern that lewisite, a toxic dichlorovinyl arsenic-

TABLE 74-2 Treatment

TOXIN	SUPPORTIVE CARE	GI DECONTAMINATION	CHELATION THERAPY	TRANSFUSION	HEMODIALYSIS
Inorganic arsenic	Intravenous crystalloids	Orogastric lavage (if radiopaque material is seen on abdominal radiograph)	BAL: 3 to 5 mg/kg IM every 4 hours		Hemodialysis for renal failure
	Monitor for hypotension, dysrhythmias, seizures	Whole-bowel irrigation until radiopaque material is gone	*or* DMPS: 3 to 5 mg/kg IV (maximum, 250 mg) every 4 hours; 4 to 8 mg/kg PO every 6 to 8 hours		
		Continuous nasogastric suction to interrupt enterogastric recirculation	DMSA: 10 mg/kg/dose PO tid for 5 days, then bid		
Arsine	Oxygen Intravenous crystalloids Red blood cell transfusion Monitor for hyperkalemia, oliguria/anuria, and dysrhythmias			Exchange transfusion for severe hemolysis/anemia	Hemodialysis for acute renal failure

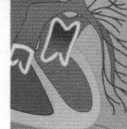

containing vesicant, would be used as a chemical weapon. BAL was used clinically for the treatment of arsenical dermatitis caused by diphenylamine chlorasine and organoarsenical antisyphilitic agents.

BAL is a lipid-soluble dithiol chelator formulated in peanut oil; it can be administered only as a deep intramuscular injection. It binds to arsenic to form a BAL-thioarsenite compound that is readily eliminated by the kidneys. Case series have demonstrated that BAL is efficacious and can reduce mortality of acute toxicity if given early (i.e., within 6 hours of exposure). In one study of 15 patients with encephalopathy, all but one patient improved clinically within 24 hours of BAL initiation.[47] Some reports suggest that neuropathy can be prevented if BAL therapy is instituted within hours of ingestion, whereas others have found that BAL is not effective in treating the neuropathy.[23,37,48] In these studies, however, treatment was not instituted in many patients until 4 to 6 weeks after ingestion.

Dosing for BAL is 3 to 5 mg/kg every 4 hours until the 24-hour urinary arsenic excretion is less than 50 µg/L or until another chelating agent is substituted. In some animal models, BAL appears to worsen arsenic toxicity by enhancing its redistribution in the brain.[49] Because BAL is lipid soluble, it may be more efficacious than DMSA and DMPS (see below), both of which are water soluble, in removing tissue arsenic.[50] Potential adverse effects of BAL include tachycardia, elevated temperature and blood pressure, nausea, vomiting, headache, burning sensation of the lips, and seizures. BAL can be administered parenterally to critically ill patients.

DMPS, or 2,3-dimercaptopropanol-sulfonic acid (Unithiol, Dimaval), is a water-soluble analog of BAL used in the treatment of mercury, arsenic, and lead poisoning. DMPS was first developed in the former Soviet Union in the 1950s but was not available outside that country until 1978, when it was approved in Germany for use in mercury and lead poisoning. Although not approved by the FDA, DMPS can be obtained for compassionate use through an Investigational New Drug (IND) Application Process from Heyl, a German pharmaceutical company. As of 2005, it is no longer distributed in the United States in bulk quantities for compounding.

Animal studies demonstrate that DMPS is equal to or better than DMSA and BAL in reducing toxic effects of arsenic.[51-53] It has also been associated with a reduction in tissue levels of arsenic in experimental animals and increased excretion of arsenic in human studies.[54,55] One randomized clinical trial found that DMPS significantly improved clinical scores and urinary excretion of arsenic compared with placebo in 21 patients with chronic arsenicalism.[56] An additional case report found that DMPS administration was associated with recovery from severe arsenic-induced peripheral neuropathy.[57]

DMPS can be administered by oral, intramuscular, or intravenous routes. The intravenous route should be reserved for those patients with a compromised cardiovascular or GI status (GI erosions) that would impair oral absorption. For severe acute toxicity, 3 to 5 mg/kg (maximum dose 250 mg) are given every 4 hours by slow intravenous infusion over 20 minutes. Once the patient

has been stabilized, oral DMPS, 4 to 8 mg/kg every 6 to 8 hours, is administered. Most of the reported adverse reactions to DMPS are allergic and include skin reactions (rash, urticaria), mucous membrane reactions, and elevated body temperature. Rapid intravenous administration may be associated with vasodilatation and transient hypotension. Although DMPS increases the urinary excretion of copper and zinc, this effect should not be clinically significant in patients without preexisting deficiency of these trace elements.

DMSA, 2,3-dimercaptosuccinic acid, is an oral analog of BAL and approved by the FDA for treatment of lead poisoning in children. Animal studies demonstrate that DMSA is equal or superior to BAL in urinary and fecal elimination of arsenic as well as decreasing concentration of arsenic in liver, kidneys, spleen, and brain.[58,59] DMSA has been used successfully to chelate arsenic in humans.[60] The dimercaptan-arsenic complex is water soluble, resulting in significant excretion of arsenic. The optimal dosing is unknown, and some clinicians follow the treatment guidelines established for lead (see Chapter 73). If urinary concentrations of arsenic remain elevated, prolonged therapy may be necessary. DMSA may be substituted for BAL once GI injury has resolved and gut motility has returned in acutely ill patients. For patients with chronic toxicity, DMSA may be the treatment of choice if DMPS is not available.

D-Penicillamine is an oral monothiol chelator originally developed as a chelator for copper but useful for other heavy metal poisonings. It has been used as a chelating agent for arsenic poisoning, although little experimental evidence validates its efficacy.[61,62] Animal models comparing D-penicillamine, BAL, DMSA, and DMPS found D-penicillamine ineffective in treating arsenic toxicity.[63] It should be used only when BAL, DMPS, and DMSA are unavailable. The recommended dose is 25 mg/kg dose (maximum, 1 g/24 hr) every 6 hours until the urinary arsenic is less than 50 µg/L/ 24 hours. Adverse effects include rashes, leukopenia, thrombocytopenia, and nephrotoxicity.

EXTRACORPOREAL ELIMINATION

Hemodialysis has been reported to eliminate arsenic at clearance rates ranging from 76 to 87 mL/min with or without concomitant BAL therapy.[64-66] It may be an effective adjunctive therapy in patients with renal insufficiency and should be instituted for patients with renal failure.

DISPOSITION

Patients exhibiting symptoms of acute arsenic toxicity should be admitted to the hospital for supportive care and chelation therapy. Patients with cardiovascular instability and significant symptoms should be managed in an intensive care unit. Appropriate law enforcement should be notified if homicidal intent is suspected. It is imperative that the source of arsenic exposure be identified by public health officials so that reexposure does not recur after discharge. If the exposure was suspected to be occupational, a workplace evaluation should be undertaken along with notification of the

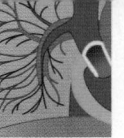

proper authorities. Long-term follow-up including physical therapy and rehabilitation may be necessary for patients with neurologic sequelae. Neurologic injury may be permanent.

ARSINE

Introduction

Arsine (arsenous hydride, or AsH_3) was identified in 1775 and its toxic properties discovered in the early 1800s when a German chemist died after inhaling the gas in his laboratory. It is the most toxic form of arsenic. Arsine is a colorless, odorless, nonirritating gas that is denser than air and has an odor of garlic. Arsine is produced when acids come into contact with arsenic residues or when water acts on metallic arsenide compounds. It is used as a dopant gas in the semiconductor industry. Occupational exposure may occur for workers involved in galvanizing, soldering, etching, lead plating, and computer microchip processing (see Box 74-1).

Pathophysiology

Arsine poisoning is characterized by rapid and fulminant hemolysis of red blood cells. Several mechanisms of red blood cell toxicity have been proposed.[67] Hemoglobin fixes arsine in a nonvolatile form within the red blood cell.[68] It has been suggested that the arsenic dihydride and elemental arsenic resulting from oxidation of arsine are the hemolytic agents. The inhibition of catalase by arsenic or arsenic compounds with the formation of hydrogen peroxide has also been proposed as a mechanism of hemolysis. Others have postulated that arsine depletes erythrocyte gluatathione stores, resulting in cell membrane instability, thereby causing hemolysis.[69] Explanations of the mechanisms by which very low levels of arsine gas induce severe hemolysis remain speculative.

Many theories have been advanced to explain arsine nephrotoxicity.[67] Deposition of erythrocyte breakdown products in the renal tubules may result in renal failure. Necrotic renal tubules containing hemoglobin casts are characteristically observed in tissue specimens obtained at autopsy in cases of fatal arsine poisoning. Further impairment results from a decrease in renal perfusion that is inversely proportionate to the degree of hemolysis. However, severe tubular damage has been described in arsine poisoning in the absence of extensive hemoglobinuria. Thus, it is unlikely that the nephrotoxic effects of arsine are entirely due to the lysis of red blood cells and blockage of renal tubules by products of red blood cell breakdown. Limited experimental evidence suggests a direct toxic effect of arsine on the kidneys, perhaps by inhibition of renal tubular-cell respiration.[70]

Cardiac effects, presenting as conduction disturbances, are most likely related to hyperkalemia as a result of massive hemolysis. Arsine may also exert direct toxicity on myocardial tissue.

Toxicokinetics

Arsine concentrations of 3 to 10 ppm for several hours have produced minimal symptoms, whereas exposure to 16 to 300 ppm for 30 to 60 minutes is dangerous.[71] Inhalation of an airborne concentration of 150 ppm or greater may cause death within 30 minutes after exposure, while lengthy exposure to 10 to 50 ppm may still cause death owing to hemolytic anemia and renal failure. The U.S. Occupational Safety and Health Administration (OSHA) permissible exposure limit (PEL) of arsine in an 8-hour time-weighted average is 0.05 ppm. The odor threshold of arsine is 10-fold greater than this limit. Following arsine absorption, the compound is oxidized to elemental trivalent arsenic and arsenous oxide, compounds known to be human carcinogens.

Toxicology

CLINICAL MANIFESTATIONS

The interval between arsine exposure and the onset of symptoms is variable, depending on concentration of the gas and duration of exposure. There usually is a delay of 2 to 24 hours. Clinical symptoms may include headache, malaise, weakness, dizziness, dyspnea, nausea, vomiting, abdominal and flank pain, and thirst. Excretion of dark-red urine frequently develops 4 to 6 hours after exposure. Bronzing of the skin that looks like jaundice may be observed 24 to 48 hours later. A unique triad of symptoms—abdominal pain, hematuria, and jaundice—has long characterized the clinical features of arsine poisoning.

Physical examination may reveal fever, tachycardia, tachypnea, and the peculiar bronze tinting of the skin and mucous membranes that is more often described as jaundice. Abdominal tenderness and rigidity, enlargement and tenderness of the liver, and costovertebral tenderness have been observed. A garlic odor may be present on the patient's breath or in the patient's sweat.

Acute renal failure may develop secondary to kidney damage by mechanisms described above. Oliguria or anuria may manifest before 72 hours. Renal failure is the usual cause of death in cases of lethal arsine poisoning. Pulmonary edema and congestive heart failure may occasionally occur. Electrocardiographic abnormalities have been noted. Delayed neurologic sequelae such as peripheral polyneuropathy and encephalopathy have been described.

Diagnosis

LABORATORY TESTS

The most characteristic laboratory finding of arsine poisoning is a Coombs' test–negative hemolytic anemia. Hemoglobin concentrations of less than 10 g/dL are not unusual. Reticulocytosis and leukocytosis are also observed. The peripheral blood smear may show red-cell fragments, ghost cells, anisocytosis, poikilocytosis, and basophilic stippling. It has been reported that unstained preparations of white cells demonstrate a blue-green cast to the nuclei.[72] The red-cell fragility test is normal.

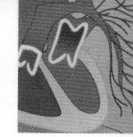

Serum bilirubin and lactate dehydrogenase are usually elevated.

Urinalysis may reveal hemoglobinuria and sometimes tubular casts containing erythrocytes and hemoglobin. Serum potassium usually is elevated because of hemolysis and decreasing renal function. Electrocardiographic findings may include high-peaked T waves, nonspecific ST-T wave changes, and various degrees of heart block. Chronic exposure to arsine gas may result in anemia, mild elevation in total bilirubin, and high concentration of urinary arsenic.

DIFFERENTIAL DIAGNOSIS

The differential diagnosis of arsine poisoning includes poisoning by other agents that cause hemolytic anemia, that is, potassium chlorate and stibine (antimony dihydride); infectious diseases such as leptospirosis and malaria; and the rare hematologic disorder paroxysmal nocturnal hemoglobinuria. Lead poisoning may mimic chronic low-level arsine exposure, since both may produce anemia and basophilic stippling.

Treatment

Decontamination must include removal from the environment where arsine exposure occurred, removal of clothing, and skin irrigation. Oxygen, intravenous crystalloids, and cardiac monitoring are included in the initial stabilization. The goal of further treatment for arsine toxicity is stopping the ongoing hemolysis and monitoring for renal failure.

ELIMINATION

Exchange transfusion is the only therapy that will remove the arsine-hemoglobin complexes and restore the red cell population without fluid overload.[73] It may be indicated when plasma free hemoglobin levels are greater than 1.5 g/dL or when exposure to high levels of arsine is suspected. Simple transfusion of packed red blood cells, however, may be adequate treatment for mild hemolysis. Hemodialysis is required for acute renal failure. Supportive care includes monitoring for hyperkalemia, urine output, and cardiac dysrhythmias. The role of urine alkalinization and forced diuresis with sodium bicarbonate to minimize precipitation of hemoglobin and prevent kidney damage is controversial.

ANTIDOTES

The role of chelation therapy in acute arsine poisoning is unestablished. BAL therapy does not prevent or reduce hemolysis even when administered soon after exposure.[74] One published case of chronic arsine exposure reports that D-penicillamine was associated with resolution of clinical symptoms.[75] Unlike in acute inorganic arsenic poisoning, chelation therapy should not be used routinely for acute arsine poisoning.

DISPOSITION

Asymptomatic patients should receive basic decontamination and be observed for 4 to 6 hours. Because of the rapid and significant toxicity after exposure to arsine gas, any patient with mild symptoms or a history of significant exposure should be admitted for observation and supportive care for a minimum of 24 to 48 hours. Patient with evidence of hemolysis should be admitted to an intensive care unit because of the potential for rapid and fulminant progression of hemolysis and the probable need for exchange transfusion.

Patients should have outpatient follow-up to monitor renal function and anemia. In addition, counseling and monitoring for the possible development of late-onset peripheral neuropathy and encephalopathy should be initiated.

REFERENCES

1. Rahman MM, Chowdhury UK, Mukherjee SC, et al: Chronic arsenic toxicity in Bangladesh and West Bengal, India. J Toxicol Clin Toxicol 2001;39:683–700.
2. Frisbie SH, Ortega R, Maynard DM, Sarkar B: The concentrations of arsenic and other toxic elements in Bangladesh's drinking water. Environ Health Perspect 2002;110:1147–1153.
3. Khan MM, Sakauchi F, Sonoda T, et al: Magnitude of arsenic toxicity in tube-well drinking water in Bangladesh and its adverse effects on human health including cancer: evidence from a review of the literature. Asian Pac J Cancer Prev 2003;4:7–14.
4. Uede K, Furukawa F: Skin manifestations in acute arsenic poisoning from the Wakayama curry-poisoning incident. Br J Dermatol 2003;149:757–762.
5. World Health Organization: Guidelines for drinking-water quality: health criteria and other supporting information, 2nd ed. Vol 2. Geneva, World Health Organization, 1996, pp 940–949.
6. Available at http://www.eap.gov/safewater/arenic.html. Accessed 12/20/2003.
7. Peters HA, Croft WA, Woolson EA, et al: Seasonal arsenic exposure from burning chromium-copper-arsenate-treated wood. JAMA 1984;251:2393–2396.
8. Geschke AM, Lynch V, Rouch GJ, et al: Arsenic poisoning after a barbecue. Med J Austr 1996;165:296.
9. Watson WA, Litovitz TL, Rodgers GC, et al: 2002 annual report of the American Association of Poison Control Centers Toxic Exposure Surveillance System. Am J Emerg Med 2003;21:353–421.
10. Hall AH: Chronic arsenic poisoning. Toxicol Lett 2002;128(1–3):69–72.
11. Shum S, Whitehead J, Vaughn L, et al: Chelation of organoarsenate with dimercaptosuccinic acid. Vet Hum Toxicol 1995;37:239–242.
12. Hughes MF: Arsenic toxicity and potential mechanisms of action. Toxicol Lett 2002;133(1):1–16.
13. Aposhian HV, Zakharyan RA, Avram MD, et al: Oxidation and detoxification of trivalent arsenic species. Toxicol Appl Pharmacol 2003;193:1–8.
14. Johnson LR, Farmer JG: Use of human metabolic studies and urinary arsenic speciation in assessing arsenic exposure. Bull Environ Contam Toxicol 1991;46:53–61.
15. Buchet JP, Lauwerys R, Roels H: Comparison of the urinary excretion of arsenic metabolites after a single oral dose of sodium arsenite, monomethylarsonate, or dimethylarsinate in man. Int Arch Occup Environ Health 1981;48:71–79.
16. Stilwell DE, Gorny KD: Contamination of soil with copper, chromium and arsenic under decks built from pressure treated wood. Bull Environ Contam Toxicol 1997;58:22–29.
17. Chirenje T, Ma LQ, Clark C, et al: Cu, Cr, and As distribution in soils adjacent to pressure-treated decks, fences, and poles. Environ Pollut 2003;124:407–417.
18. Rossman TG: Mechanism of arsenic carcinogenesis: an integrated approach. Mutat Res 2003;533:37–65.
19. Bates MN, Smith AH, Hopenhayn-Rich C: Arsenic ingestion and internal cancers: a review. Am J Epidemiol 1992;135:462–476.
20. Kjeldsberg CR, Ward HP: Leukemia in arsenic poisoning. Ann Intern Med 1972;77:935–937.
21. Chiou HY, Hsueh YM, Liaw KF, et al: Incidence of internal cancers and ingested inorganic arsenic: a seven-year follow-up study in Taiwan. Cancer Res 1995;55:1296–1300.

22. Hessl SM, Berman E: Severe peripheral neuropathy after exposure to monosodium methyl arsonate. J Toxicol Clin Toxicol 1982; 19:281–287.

23. Chuttani PN, Chawla LS, Sharma TD: Arsenical neuropathy. Neurology 1967;17:269–274.

24. Beckman KJ, Bauman JL, Pimental PA, et al: Arsenic-induced torsade de pointes. Crit Care Med 1991;19:290–292.

25. Bolliger CT, van Zijl P, Louw JA: Multiple organ failure with the adult respiratory distress syndrome in homicidal arsenic poisoning. Respiration 1992;59:57–61.

26. Lugo G, Cassady G, Palmisano P: Acute maternal arsenic intoxication with neonatal death. Am J Dis Child 1969;117: 328–330.

27. Wong SS, Tan KC, Goh CL: Cutaneous manifestations of chronic arsenicism: review of seventeen cases. J Am Acad Dermatol 1998;38(2 pt 1):179–185.

28. Santra A, Das Gupta J, De BK, et al: Hepatic manifestations in chronic arsenic toxicity. Indian J Gastroenterol 1999;18:152–155.

29. Lai MS, Hsueh YM, Chen CJ, et al: Ingested inorganic arsenic and prevalence of diabetes mellitus. Am J Epidemiol 1994;139: 484–492.

30. Kwong YL, Todd D: Delicious poison: arsenic trioxide for the treatment of leukemia. Blood 1997;89:3487–3488.

31. Soignet SL, Maslak P, Wang Z-G, et al: Complete remission after treatment of acute promyelocytic leukemia with arsenic trioxide. N Engl J Med 1998;339:1341–1348.

32. Beckett WS, Moore JL, Keogh JP, Bleecker ML: Acute encephalopathy due to occupational exposure to arsenic. Br J Ind Med 1986 Jan;43(1):66–67.

33. Liu CW, Lin KH, Kuo YM: Application of factor analysis in the assessment of groundwater quality in a blackfoot disease area in Taiwan. Sci Total Environ. 2003 Sep 1;313(1-3):77–89.

34. Basalt RC: Disposition of Toxic Drugs and Chemicals in Man, 5th ed. Chicago, Year Book, 2000, pp 61–66.

35. McKinney JD: Metabolism and disposition of inorganic arsenic in laboratory animals and humans. Environ Geochem Health 1992;14:43–48.

36. Kersjes MP, Maurer JR, Trestrail JH: An analysis of arsenic exposures referred to the Blodgett regional poison center. Vet Hum Toxicol 1987;29:75–78.

37. Heyman A, Pfeiffer JB, Willett RW: Peripheral neuropathy caused by arsenic intoxication: a study of 41 cases with observations of the effects of BAL (2,3-dimercaptopropanol). N Engl J Med 1956; 254:401–409.

38. Arbouine MW, Wilson HK: The effect of seafood consumption on the assessment of occupational exposure to arsenic by urinary arsenic speciation measurements. J Trace Elem 1992;6: 153–160.

39. Franzblau A, Lilis R: Acute arsenic intoxication from environmental arsenic exposure. Arch Environ Health 1989;11:385–390.

40. Seidel S, Kreutzer R, Smith D, et al: Assessment of commercial laboratories performing hair mineral analysis. JAMA 2001;285: 67–72.

41. Hilfer RM, Mandel A: Acute arsenic intoxication diagnosed by roentgenograms. N Engl J Med 1962;266:663–664.

42. Kyle RA, Pease G: Hematologic aspects of arsenic intoxication. N Engl J Med 1965;273:18–23.

43. Goldsmith S, From AH: Arsenic-induced atypical ventricular tachycardia. N Engl J Med 1980;303:1096–1098.

44. Lee DC, Roberts JR, Kelly JJ, et al: Whole-bowel irrigation as an adjunct in the treatment of radiopaque arsenic. Am J Emerg Med 1995;13:244–245.

45. Reichl F, Hunder G, Liebl B, et al: Effect of DMPS and various adsorbents on the arsenic excretion in guinea-pigs after injection with As$_2$O$_3$. Arch Toxicol 1995;69:712–717.

46. Manieu P, Buchet JP, Roels HA, Lauwerys R: The metabolism of arsenic in humans acutely intoxicated by As$_2$O$_3$: its significance for the duration of BAL therapy. Clin Toxicol 1981;18:1067–1075.

47. Eagle H, Magnuson HJ: The systemic treatment of 227 cases of arsenic poisoning (encephalitis, dermatitis,blood dyscrasias, jaundice, fever) with 2,3-dimercaptopropanol (BAL). Am J Syph Gonor Ven Dis 1946;30:420–441.

48. Jenkins RB: Inorganic arsenic and the nervous system. Brain 1966;89:479–98.

49. Snider TH, Wientjes MJ, Joiner RL, et al: Arsenic distribution in rabbits after Lewisite administration and treatment with British anti-Lewisite (BAL). Fundam Appl Toxicol 1990;14:262–272.

50. Muckter H, Liebl B, Reichl FX, et al: Are we ready to replace dimercaprol (BAL) as an arsenic antidote? Hum Exp Toxicol 1997;16:460–465.

51. Schafer B, Kreppel H, Reichl FX, et al: Effect of oral treatment with BAL, DMPS or DMSA arsenic in organs of mice injected with arsenic trioxide. Arch Toxicol Suppl 1991;14:228–230.

52. Flora SJ, Dube SN, Arora U, et al: Therapeutic potential of meso 2,3-dimercaptosuccinic acid or 2,3-dimercaptopropane 1-sulfonate in chronic arsenic intoxication in rats. Biometals 1995;8:111–116.

53. Inns RH, Rice P, Bright JE, Marrs TC: Evaluation of the efficacy of dimercapto chelating agents for the treatment of systemic organic arsenic poisoning in rabbits. Hum Exp Toxicol 1990;9:215–220.

54. Aposhian HV, Arroyo A, Cebrian ME, et al: DMPS-arsenic challenge test. 1. Increased urinary excretion of monomethylarsonic acid in humans given dimercaptopropane sulfonate. J Pharmacol Exp Ther 1997;282:192–200.

55. Aphosian HV: Mobilization of mercury and arsenic in humans by sodium 2,3-dimercapto-1-propane sulfonate (DMPS). Environ Health Perspect 1998;106(Suppl 4):1017–1025.

56. Guha Mazumder DN, De BK, Santra A, et al: Randomized placebo-controlled trial of 2,3-dimercapto-1-propanesulfonate (DMPS) in therapy of chronic arsenicosis due to drinking arsenic-contaminated water. J Toxicol Clin Toxicol 2001;39:665–674.

57. Wax PM, Thornton CA: Recovery from severe arsenic-induced peripheral neuropathy with 2,3-dimercapto-1-propaneslphonic acid. J Toxicol Clin Toxicol 2000;28:777–780.

58. Graziano JH: Rose of 2,3-dimercaptosuccinic acid in the treatment of heavy metal poisoning. Med Toxicol 1986;1:155–162.

59. Schafer B, Kreppel H, Reichl FX, et al: Effect of oral treatment with BAL, DMPS or DMSA. Arch Toxicol 1991;14(Suppl):228–230.

60. Lenz K, Hruby K, Druml W, et al: 2,3-diimercaptosuccinic acid in human arsenic poisoning. Arch Toxicol 1981;47:241–243.

61. Peterson RG, Rumack BH: D-Penicillamine therapy of acute arsenic poisoning. J Pediatr 1977;91:661–666.

62. Watson WA, Veltri JC, Metcalf TJ: Acute arsenic exposure treated with oral D-penicillamine. Vet Hum Toxicol 1981;23:164–166.

63. Kreppel H, Reichl FX, Forth W, et al: Lack of effectiveness of D-penicillamine in experimental arsenic poisoning. Vet Hum Toxicol 1989;31:1–5.

64. Giberson A, Dabir Vaziri N, Mirahamadi K, et al: Hemodialysis of acute arsenic intoxication with transient renal failure. Arch Intern Med 1976;136:1303–1304,

65. Vaziri ND, Upham T, Barton CH: Hemodialysis clearance of arsenic. Clin Toxicol 1980;17:451–456.

66. Kruszewska S, Wiese M, Kolacinski Z, et al: The use of haemodialysis and 2,3 propanesulphonate (DMPS) to manage acute oral poisoning by lethal dose of arsenic trioxide. Int J Occup Med Environ Health 1996;9:111–115.

67. Fowler BA, Weissberg JB: Arsine poisoning. N Engl J Med 1974; 291:1171–1174.

68. Graham AF, Crawford TBB, Marrian GF: The action of arsine on blood: observations on the nature of the fixed arsenic. Biochem J 1946;40:256–260.

69. Levinsky WJ, Smalley RV, Hillyer PN, et al: Arsine hemolysis. Arch Environ Health 1970;20:436–440.

70. Muehrcke RC, Pirani CL: Arsine-induced anuria: a correlative clinicopathological study with electron microscopic observations. Ann Intern Med 1968;68:853–866.

71. Peterson DP, Bhattacharyya MH: Hematological response to arsine exposure: quantitation of exposure response in mice. Fundam Appl Toxicol 1985;5:499–505.

72. Teitelbaum DT, Kier LC: Arsine poisoning: report of five cases in the petroleum industry and a discussion of the indications for exchange transfusion and hemodialysis. Arch Environ Health 1969;19:133–143.

73. McKinstry WJ, Hickes JM: Arsine poisoning. Arch Indust Health 1957;16:32–41.

74. Pinto SS, Petronella SJ, Johns DR, et al: Arsine poisoning: a study of thirteen cases. Arch Indust Hyg 1950;1:437–451.

75. Risk M, Fuortes L: Chronic arsenicalism suspected from arsine exposure: a case report and literature review. Vet Hum Toxicol 1991;33:590–595.

75 *Other Heavy Metals*

ALAN H. HALL, MD ■ MICHAEL W. SHANNON, MD, MPH

At a Glance...

- Aluminum was responsible for dialysis-associated encephalopathy, which has largely disappeared due to elimination of aluminum from dialysate solutions.
- Ingested antimony may result in a cholera-like illness. Inhalation of stibine (SbH_3) gas may result in massive intravascular hemolysis.
- Soluble barium compounds may cause significant gastrointestinal symptoms and potentially fatal hypokalemia.
- Beryllium, an irritant in acute respiratory exposures, causes a systemic granulomatous disease that has a radiological appearance similar to that of sarcoidosis.
- Long-term exposure to bismuth salts may cause encephalopathy with characteristic EEG changes.
- Cadmium is responsible for a potentially fatal pneumopathy when inhaled as the oxide. In the 1940s in Japan, it was responsible for *itai-itai* disease, characterized by leg and low back pain, chest pain, and difficulty walking with severe, diffuse osteopenia and physical deformities.
- In its hexavalent form, chromium is a bronchial and nasal carcinogen. Chromium is also extremely irritant, causing nasal perforation, "chrome holes" in the skin, and pulmonary irritation with sometimes delayed pulmonary edema. It is toxic to numerous organs.
- Cobalt is cardiotoxic and has been responsible for beer-drinker's cardiomyopathy due to its former use as a foaming agent in beer.
- Copper, an essential nutrient, has been associated with eye disease and cirrhosis of the liver in overdose.
- Gold, used in rheumatic disease, causes significant toxicity in skin and kidneys due to the formation of immune complexes.
- Magnesium is an essential nutrient. In overdose, central nervous system depression with lethargy, coma, neuromuscular paralysis, hypotonia, hyporeflexia, and ECG changes may be observed.
- Manganese is one of several metals (including zinc and copper) that are responsible acutely for metal fume fever. When chronically inhaled, it may cause a Parkinson-like syndrome.
- Nickel comes in numerous forms. It is a frequent cause of skin allergy. Like hexavalent chromium, nickel carbonyl is a nasal and lung carcinogen. Nickel carbonyl is a gas encountered in the petroleum industry and may be rapidly fatal.
- Acute selenium poisoning may result from ingestion of gun bluing solution. Death may ensue rapidly, associated with metabolic acidosis, ARDS, and myocardial depression.
- Colloidal silver has been widely promoted as an alternative medicine. It has no proven benefits and may cause argyria, a permanent pigmentation of skin, nails, and mucous membranes.
- Thallium is an extremely toxic metal employed as a pesticide. Toxic ingestion produces a practically pathognomic clinical triad of gastroenteritis, polyneuropathy, and alopecia.
- Trialkyltins are responsible for sometimes severe gastrointestinal, CNS, and renal toxicity.
- When ingested, zinc may cause significant local GI effects.
- Metal fume fever (most often occurring during welding) may result from inhalation of zinc, copper, magnesium, cadmium, manganese, and antimony. It is a self-limited illness with no demonstrated long-term sequelae.
- Chelators are available for treatment of some of the toxic metals.

SPECIFIC AGENTS

Aluminum

Aluminum is the most abundant metal in the earth's crust. It has no known human function. Exposure occurs from contaminated drinking water and aluminum cans, containers, and cooking utensils. Dermal exposure occurs from aluminum-containing deodorants. Aluminum silicate and magnesium aluminum silicate are generally safe as ingredients in topical cosmetic products; they are not significantly toxic, but may cause mild eye irritation.[1] Magnesium aluminum silicate application to human skin for 1 week did not cause adverse effects.[1] Some aluminum-containing cosmetic products cause dermal hypersensitivity reactions. Two patients developed multiple pruritic nodules that contained aluminum and persisted for several years after immunization with vaccines adsorbed on aluminum hydroxide.[2] Workers who mine and process aluminum silicate have developed pulmonary fibrosis and pneumoconiosis.[1]

The body absorbs less than 1% of an ingested aluminum dose. The body burden of 30 to 40 mg is kept low by renal homeostatic mechanisms. Normal plasma aluminum level is 5 to 10 μg/L. Aluminum is concentrated in the bones and liver. Because excretion of aluminum is primarily renal, poisoning is a risk for persons with renal insufficiency who take aluminum-containing antacids, and infants who do not have renal failure may have elevated plasma concentrations after such antacid administration.[3] Aluminum inhibits metabolic turnover of calcium, phosphorus, and iron. Its salts can bind to DNA and RNA, and inhibit a number of enzymes. Neurotoxicity may be due to substitution of magnesium ions in adenosine triphosphate (ATP).[4]

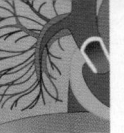

In gerbils, administration of aluminum trichloride caused biphasic stimulation of superoxide dismutase activity in various brain regions, indicating that oxidative stress is involved in aluminum central nervous system (CNS) toxicity.[5] Aluminum toxicity was formerly suggested to be implicated in development of Alzheimer's disease. However, patients treated with long-term hemodialysis and aluminum-containing medications had dialysis-associated encephalopathy but *not* Alzheimer's disease morphology in the brain at autopsy.[6]

Aluminum toxicity is characterized by encephalopathy, microcytic anemia, and osteomalacia. *Dialysis encephalopathy* is attributed to accumulation of aluminum from the dialysate, as is dialysis osteodystrophy. These illnesses have largely disappeared since aluminum was removed from water used to prepare dialysate.

Two fatalities due to aluminum poisoning were reported when a cement containing aluminum-calcium fluorosilicate was used for bone reconstruction after middle ear surgery. In both cases, refractory status epilepticus occurred and death resulted despite deferoxamine chelation.[7]

Urinary excretion of aluminum was unchanged after administration of 2,3-meso-dimercaptopropane-1-sulfonate (DMPS).[8]

Aluminum phosphide is a fumigant pesticide[9] that causes phosphine poisoning rather than aluminum toxicity (see Chapter 80).

Supportive care is all that is usually required for patients with aluminum toxicity. Hemodialysis and deferoxamine chelation may be considered in some cases.

Antimony

Antimony is a silver-gray metal and resembles arsenic in its toxic effects.[10] Antimony exists primarily in two valence states, Sb^{+3} and Sb^{+5}. Stibine (antimony hydride, SbH_3) is an extremely toxic gas. Antimony is used in the textile industry, to harden lead, as an alloy with tin or copper, and in glass manufacture. Occupational antimony exposure may occur in metallurgy, welding, and zinc etching.

Antimony tartrate and sodium stibogluconate are antibiotics for the treatment of leishmaniasis and schistosomiasis. Cumulative sodium stibogluconate toxicity has resulted in fatality.[11] Urticaria has been described during pentavalent antimony leishmaniasis treatment.[12]

Antimony compounds are rapidly and completely absorbed from the lungs after inhalation. Gastrointestinal (GI) absorption is less efficient; only 10% to 20% of an oral dose is absorbed. Distribution and organ concentration depend on valence. Pentavalent antimony has no significant binding to blood elements and is concentrated in the heart, liver, and thyroid. Trivalent antimony is more than 90% bound to erythrocytes.[13] After a single dose, more than 95% of pentavalent antimony can be recovered in the urine within 24 hours, and the elimination half-life is 2 to 4 hours. Trivalent antimony is primarily excreted in the feces, and only about 25% of a dose can be recovered in the urine. The distribution half-life of trivalent antimony is 30 hours, and the terminal half-life is 40 days.[14]

The mechanism of toxicity is unclear, but may be related to inhibition of thiol-containing enzymes.[10] After ingestion, the most prominent manifestations are vomiting, diarrhea, and abdominal pain (*cholera stibie*). Severe fluid and electrolyte disturbances can quickly ensue. After acute inhalation, both forms of antimony can produce severe respiratory tract irritation; high-concentration exposures can result in noncardiogenic pulmonary edema. Cardiovascular disturbances (QT prolongation and T-wave abnormalities) and liver function abnormalities may occur with acute poisoning.

Epistaxis is a common presenting complaint in chronic antimony poisoning. Occupational exposure produces a pneumoconiosis resembling silicosis. Cardiomyopathy can develop. *Antimony spots* are white spots on a pustular base on parts of the skin with a high concentration of sweat glands. Death due to either acute or chronic antimony poisoning results from multiorgan system failure.

Stibine is an odorless, colorless gas. Similar to arsine gas, it is capable of producing massive intravascular hemolysis with resultant hemoglobinuria and acute renal failure.

Diagnosis is based on urinary measurement for pentavalent antimony exposure and blood measurement for trivalent compounds (although urinary trivalent antimony levels have some value). Twenty-four-hour urine collections should be obtained. Laboratory assessment includes pulmonary function tests and chest x-ray (after inhalation exposure), electrocardiogram (ECG), and liver function tests.

Supportive care is the mainstay of treatment. Activated charcoal administration has been recommended after ingestion, although it is doubtful that significant adsorption occurs.[10] Fluid and electrolyte status should be monitored because of the risk for excessive GI losses. Chelation therapy with dimercaprol (BAL), dimercaptosuccinic acid (DMSA), or DMPS, if initiated early, appears to improve the clinical course.[10] Treatment of stibine exposure consists of immediate removal from the toxic site, supportive care, and exchange transfusion.

Barium

Barium is a radiopaque heavy metal used as a radiographic contrast agent. Barium sulfate is insoluble and is not toxic when ingested. It has also been used as a pesticide. Safer pesticides have replaced barium carbonate, but it is still used in countries outside the United States, where it continues to pose a hazard of inadvertent food contamination.[15] Barium compounds used industrially include barium hydroxide, barium chlorate, barium chloride, barium fluoride, barium acetate, and barium sulfide. Barium hexafluorosilicate is used in the manufacture of matches, explosives, and glass. Barium styphnate is used as a propellant. After an explosion involving this material, a patient had both traumatic injury and severe acute barium toxicity with prolonged GI dysfunction, severe and relapsing hypokalemia, cardiac arrhythmias, flaccid paralysis, myoclonus, respiratory failure, profound lactic acidosis, and hypertension.[16]

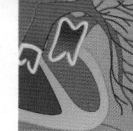

Soluble barium compounds are well absorbed after ingestion or inhalation, with peak serum levels occurring within 2 hours. The elimination half-life in serum is about 4 days. As much as 93% of an absorbed barium dose is ultimately sequestered in bone.

Symptom onset is rapid. The first signs are GI: epigastric pain, nausea, vomiting, and watery diarrhea.[15,17]

Barium intoxication is characterized by severe, potentially fatal hypokalemia. Serum potassium concentrations of less than 0.8 mEq/L may occur.[15,17] In one fatal case, barium levels at autopsy were as follows: blood, 9.9 mg/L; bile, 8.8 mg/L; urine, 6.3 mg/L; and gastric contents, 10.0 g/L.[18] Patients usually have hypokalemic paralysis.[17] Hypokalemia results from a shift of potassium into cells due to a specific potassium efflux channel blocking effect. Without affecting potassium uptake, hypokalemia results. Barium has no identified action on the sodium-potassium pump.[19]

The clinical presentation is initial GI toxicity followed by the sudden onset of areflexia and motor weakness.[20] Consciousness is not altered, and anal sphincter tone is typically preserved.[17] Trismus has also been described.[21] The degree of hypokalemia does not correspond to the extent of weakness,[17] which is better correlated with plasma barium levels.[20] ECG changes may occur, including atrioventricular dissociation, QRS widening, or U waves. Fatal ventricular fibrillation[19] or torsades de pointes polymorphic ventricular tachycardia[20] may occur. Other clinical features include bradycardia, premature ventricular beats, rhabdomyolysis, hypophosphatemia, and acute renal failure. Paralysis may persist from 8 hours to 5 days.[17] One case of prolonged (3 months) superior esophageal sphincter contracture and sequelae of extrapyramidal syndrome with bilateral hyperdense lesions in the basal ganglia and thalamus on magnetic resonance imaging has been reported.[22]

The estimated lethal dose of barium is 900 mg, although doses of 0.2 to 0.5 mg/kg have resulted in life-threatening toxicity.[17] Children seem to have greater tolerance than adults and typically only have GI symptoms.[19]

Long-term barium inhalation can produce a benign pneumoconiosis (*baritosis*).[17]

The triad of GI upset, weakness, and profound hypokalemia evokes the diagnosis of barium intoxication. Other causes of hypokalemia—including β$_2$-adrenergic agonists, theophylline, and chloroquine—do not have the other clinical signs as prominent features. Abrupt paralysis due to toxins including tetrodotoxin and tick paralysis is not associated with profound hypokalemia. A complete blood count and measurement of serum electrolytes, blood urea nitrogen, blood glucose, serum creatinine, calcium, and phosphorus should be done. Determinations of urinary potassium, arterial blood gases, muscle enzymes (creatinine phosphokinase and aldolase), and liver function tests are recommended.[17] ECG may reveal hypokalemic cardiac disturbances. Exposure can be confirmed with serum barium levels (normal: 3 to 29 μg/dL).[19] Because barium salts are radiopaque, they can be visualized on plain abdominal x-rays after ingestion.[20]

Assess respiration and support circulation. After barium inhalation, move the victim to fresh air and administer supplemental oxygen if hypoxia is present. Severe skeletal muscle weakness may lead to respiratory depression, and the need for assisted ventilation should be anticipated. Cardiac disturbances should be treated according to advanced cardiac life support algorithms. GI decontamination should be done after ingestion of soluble barium compounds. Gastric lavage with the cathartics sodium sulfate or magnesium sulfate may precipitate soluble compounds as insoluble barium sulfate and might prevent further absorption. Activated charcoal does not adsorb significant amounts of barium and should not be administered.[19] Whole bowel irrigation may be considered. Decontamination efficacy can be guided by plain abdominal x-rays.

Patients with significant hypokalemia, particularly those with ECG abnormalities, require potassium supplementation; doses up to 400 mEq may be required within the first 24 hours.[19] Because total-body potassium is preserved, serum levels should be monitored frequently to prevent hyperkalemia.[19] Parenteral administration of magnesium sulfate to render circulating barium insoluble risks precipitation in the renal tubules. Barium can be removed by hemodialysis.[17] In one patient, continuous venovenous hemofiltration improved motor function and allowed better control of serum potassium levels and acid–base status.[20]

Beryllium

Coal combustion is the principal source of environmental beryllium exposure.[23] Occupational exposure is the most common cause of beryllium sensitivity and chronic beryllium disease. From 1958 to 1989, the Rocky Flats, Colorado, nuclear weapons facility released beryllium into the air from normal operations and three accidental fires.[24] Beryllium-coated products such as computer components, telecommunications equipment, and consumer and automotive electronic products pose little risk.[25]

Beryllium was used in the manufacture of fluorescent lights in the 1930s, and beryllium-related pneumonitis with lesions resembling those of sarcoidosis became epidemic. Beryllium is currently used primarily in the aerospace and nuclear industries. Toxic forms include elemental beryllium, beryllium oxide, beryllium fluoride, and beryllium-copper alloys. Observed acute experimental pulmonary lesions after intratracheal administration of beryllium-copper alloys are most likely due to the copper rather than the beryllium.[26]

ACUTE EXPOSURE

Beryllium is an irritant that can cause conjunctivitis, periorbital edema, pharyngitis, tracheobronchitis, and pneumonitis. Skin exposure can produce a marked dermatitis. Pulmonary signs are most prominent with dyspnea, productive cough, chest pain, rales, and cyanosis. Infiltrates may be seen on chest x-ray, and hypoxia may occur at rest.[23]

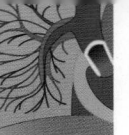

LONG-TERM EXPOSURE

Berylliosis is a systemic granulomatous disease resulting from long-term exposure.[23] It can appear anytime from a few months to 25 years after regular exposure. Noncaseating granulomas may appear in the liver, spleen, lymph nodes, heart, kidneys, bone, salivary glands, and skin. However, the primary target organ is the lung. Pulmonary manifestations include dyspnea, rales, and chest pain. Clubbing may be noted. Patients may present with right ventricular heart failure (*cor pulmonale*). Pulmonary function tests reveal either restrictive or obstructive lung disease. Chest x-rays characteristically demonstrate diffuse infiltrates and hilar adenopathy. The pulmonary toxicity of beryllium almost certainly represents a type IV immune-mediated hypersensitivity phenomenon.[23] A unique aspect of beryllium toxicity is its extremely slow elimination from the lungs.[23] CD4+ T cells likely play a critical role in the development of chronic beryllium disease, whereas CD8+ T cells do not.[27]

The diagnosis of berylliosis is based on a history of beryllium exposure. However, berylliosis can be identical to sarcoidosis in appearance, and an extensive evaluation is required to distinguish the two. The peripheral blood lymphocyte proliferation test is the most sensitive and specific test available to identify patients with chronic beryllium disease and those with beryllium sensitivity who may go on to develop the disease and require corticosteroid treatment to arrest progression.[28-31]

Although chelating agents such as DMPS, D-penicillamine, tiron, and calcium disodium EDTA and antioxidants such as selenium and glutathione have been effective in experimental animal models,[32,33] the treatment of berylliosis in humans is largely supportive. Corticosteroids may improve pulmonary symptoms and may prevent patients with beryllium sensitivity from progressing to chronic beryllium disease. Lung transplantation could be considered in patients with progressive respiratory failure.

Bismuth

Bismuth is in the Vb group of elements with antimony and arsenic. Its current therapeutic use is limited to antidiarrheal effects (bismuth subsalicylate; Pepto-Bismol). Because it is water insoluble, poorly absorbed from the gut, and rapidly excreted in the urine, bismuth accumulation rarely occurs despite excessive use.[34]

Although poorly absorbed, bismuth is measurable in blood after ingestion. The highest concentrations are found in the kidneys and liver. Bismuth also concentrates in the placenta.[35] Excretion of bismuth is primarily renal. It is rapid, being complete within 24 hours. Only about 10% of an absorbed dose is found in the feces.[35]

The symptoms of bismuth poisoning have been compared with those of lead and mercury poisoning.[35] Early signs are hypersalivation and a characteristic blue discoloration of the gums resulting from deposition of bismuth sulfide in fibrous tissue.[35] Stomatitis may also occur. Renal injury has been reported[36] and presents as acute renal failure, reversible nephropathy, or Fanconi's syndrome. Hepatic injury and peripheral neuritis have also been reported.[35] Skeletal disturbances, including osteoarthropathy, osteomalacia, and osteoporosis, have been associated with chronic bismuth intoxication and may result in pathologic fractures.[35] Nicolau's syndrome, characterized by a livedoid pattern on the skin followed by necrosis and scar formation, has followed intramuscular injection of bismuth salts.[37] Skin reactions, including erythema, exanthema, angioedema, and small-patch or maculopapular rashes, have been reported in patients treated with bismuth oxide.[38]

Encephalopathy has been reported after long-term high-level exposure to bismuth salts. Manifestations include altered mental status, ataxia, myoclonus, and distinctively abnormal electroencephalogram (EEG) findings.[34,35] Outbreaks of bismuth encephalopathy have been reported. Between 1973 and 1980, about 1,000 cases of bismuth poisoning with 72 fatalities were identified.[39] However, in a placebo-controlled clinical trial that included EEG evaluation, neurotoxicity was not demonstrated when bismuth was administered.[39]

The diagnosis of bismuth poisoning is made on the basis of history, characteristic clinical findings, and laboratory evaluation. The normal serum bismuth level is less than 50 μg/L.[39]

Supportive care is usually all that is required. Bismuth elimination can be enhanced by administration of BAL, DMPS, and DMSA; D-penicillamine and deferoxamine are inefficacious.[35,40]

Cadmium

Cadmium is one of the most common causes of environmentally associated renal injury. The major environmental sources of cadmium are industrial use and food contamination. Cadmium is a component of cigarette smoke.[41] Cadmium is used in alloy fabrication, metal plating, pigments, and the manufacture of rechargeable (nickel-cadmium) batteries. Cadmium's high volatility makes it particularly hazardous to welders.[42]

Cadmium is well absorbed after inhalation (up to 50% of an inhaled dose). In contrast, only about 5% of an ingested dose is absorbed.[41,42] GI absorption is enhanced by low intake of calcium, protein, or iron. Cadmium is circulated and stored bound to metallothionein. The main storage organs are the liver and kidneys. The biologic half-life in the liver is 5 to 10 years; it is twice that in the kidney. The overall biologic human half-life of cadmium is 30 years.[42]

Progressive accumulation occurs, and there is no effective endogenous cadmium elimination mechanism. Cadmium stimulates metallothionein production and reduces its overall toxicity. However, metallothionein binding is associated with selective cadmium accumulation, leading to renal injury.

Acute cadmium ingestion causes nausea, excessive salivation, abdominal pain, and diarrhea. Fatality results from cardiovascular collapse. The acute lethal oral dose is estimated at 350 to 8900 mg. Acute inhalation of cadmium oxide fumes as a result of welding, smelting, or soldering can produce a severe, sometimes fatal,

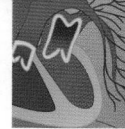

pneumonitis associated with elevated urinary cadmium concentrations.[43]

With long-term cadmium exposure, the major target organs are the kidneys, expressed as proximal tubulopathy with excretion of proteins weighing less than 40,000 daltons (β_2-microglobulin, lysozyme, retinol binding protein). Cadmium prevents tubular reabsorption of these proteins. Elevated urinary concentrations of N-acetyl-β-D-glucosaminidase (NAG) are an indicator of cadmium-induced proximal tubule disease. β_2-Microglobulin is a sensitive indicator of early cadmium-induced renal disease. Marked excretion of calcium and phosphorus also occurs, leading to osteopenia or nephrolithiasis. Effects on calcium and phosphorus homeostasis result in part from cadmium inhibition of vitamin D hydroxylation. Chronic cadmium exposure has been linked to essential hypertension. Renal disturbances may first manifest more than 10 years after chronic cadmium exposure. Nonrenal clinical effects include ulceration of the nasal mucosa, anemia, and hepatitis.[42]

An epidemic illness occurred in Japan during the 1940s called *itai-itai* (ouch-ouch) disease. Clinical characteristics were leg and low back pain, chest pain, and difficulty walking. Severe, diffuse osteopenia occurred, resulting in fractures after minor trauma and often producing physical deformities. Proteinuria, glycosuria, and aminoaciduria were common. Autopsy revealed marked renal tubular atrophy and degeneration. This epidemic was confined to the Jinzu River system, which suggested water contamination of rice, beans, fish, and other foodstuffs. The low-protein and low-calcium diet of the victims seemed to contribute to the development of the disease. Itai-itai occurred primarily in multiparous women, perhaps because they were already deficient in calcium and phosphorus. Vitamin D supplementation resulted in clinical improvement. Cadmium contamination of drinking water was ultimately identified as the cause, due to discharge from a zinc mine.[42]

The diagnosis of chronic cadmium poisoning can be made not only by urinary β_2-microglobulin excretion but also by measurement of blood cadmium. The normal blood cadmium level is less than 5 µg/L. The normal urinary excretion of cadmium is less than 1 µg/g creatinine. Twenty-four-hour urine collections for measurement of cadmium, creatinine, low-molecular-weight proteins, and amino acids should be done.

Cadmium chelation is difficult because of its high affinity for metallothionein. BAL treatment has been associated with increased renal accumulation and accelerated renal injury. All treatment is therefore supportive.

Chromium

Chromium is abundant in the earth's crust. It is an essential micronutrient and acts as a cofactor in insulin function. Chromium is used for the manufacture of stainless steel and in tanning, photography, and electroplating. Chromium has three main valence states: bivalent,[+2] trivalent,[+3] and hexavalent.[+6] Hexavalent compounds include chromic acid, potassium and ammonium dichromates, and chromium trioxide that is extremely corrosive when ingested.

Trivalent chromium is poorly absorbed (<1%) from the GI tract; however, more than 50% of ingested hexavalent chromium can be absorbed from the gut. Organ accumulation of chromium is extensive and includes the brain, liver, spleen, testes, bone marrow, and reticuloendothelial system. Serum half-life is 15 to 41 hours. About 80% of a chromium dose is excreted in the urine. Chromium toxicity results from its ability to penetrate cell membranes, inciting events resulting in cell death. Chromium VI (hexavalent) is carcinogenic and mutagenic, but it is reduced intracellularly to stable chromium III (trivalent). Chromium IV and V are produced in intracellular reduction pathways, and cellular damage may be at least partly due to these species.[44] Chromium is a redox-active metal that depletes cellular antioxidants.[45]

Ingestion of trivalent chromium picolinate dietary supplement has caused systemic contact dermatitis and acute generalized exanthematous pustulosis.[46,47]

Exposure to hexavalent chromium is associated with widespread organ toxicity. Respiratory tract effects include acute noncardiogenic pulmonary edema that can be delayed in onset up to 72 hours, nasal septal perforation, and diffuse pulmonary inflammation. Dermal exposure to chromium in felt produces eczematous changes referred to as *blackjack disease*, and painless ulcers can develop on the hands, periumbilical region, axillae, and forearms (*chrome holes*).[48] GI toxicity includes hemorrhagic gastroenteritis with characteristic yellow-green emesis. Hepatitis progressing to fulminant hepatic failure may result. Acute tubular necrosis and glomerulonephritis may occur, as well as methemoglobinemia, thrombocytopenia, anemia, and intravascular hemolysis. Circulatory collapse and shock may be seen, usually secondary to extensive GI corrosion or perforation. Corneal opacification, keratitis, and conjunctivitis may occur after ocular exposure. As little as 500 mg of ingested chromium can produce life-threatening toxicity; 1 to 2 g is potentially lethal.

A 2-year-old child ingested about 1 g of ammonium dichromate crystals.[49] Profuse diarrhea developed in association with coagulopathy, liver function disturbances, obtundation, and respiratory failure. Ascorbic acid was administered, and exchange transfusion was performed. Anuria, hypotension, and noncardiogenic pulmonary edema developed within 24 hours. Despite hemodialysis, progressive coagulopathy and hepatic failure occurred, resulting in death. The peak plasma concentration was 4163 µg/L.

Nasal insertion of a potassium dichromate crystal foreign body caused systemic chromium poisoning with diarrhea, vomiting, nasal obstruction, acute renal failure, pancreatitis, hepatitis, and drowsiness in a 3-year-old child.[50]

Occupational hexavalent chromium exposure has been associated with an increased incidence of nasal cancers and bronchial carcinoma.

Normal serum chromium concentrations are 0.3 to 1.0 µg/L. Normal urinary chromium concentration should be less than 40 µg/L. The 95% upper fractile level for urine chromium in normal individuals is 13 nmol/L.[51]

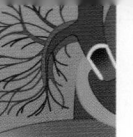

Treatment of hexavalent chromium ingestion includes management of hypotension or shock, forced diuresis (furosemide administration may be required), and treatment of corrosive GI injury. Ascorbic acid (vitamin C) reacts with hexavalent chromium to form the poorly absorbed trivalent form. Oral doses of 2 to 4 g per 1 g of ingested chromium have been recommended if there are no symptoms of severe gastroesophageal injury. However, even doses as high as 10 g given intravenously, although not toxic, are unlikely to reduce the mortality in patients with systemic hexavalent chromium poisoning.[52] Larger doses could be harmful because ascorbic acid is a metabolic precursor of oxalate that can cause nephropathy, especially if renal failure is already present.[52] N-Acetylcysteine (NAC) has been advocated to maintain chromium in its less toxic trivalent state.[49] DMPS chelation does *not* increase the urinary excretion of chromium.[8]

Treatment of chromium inhalation includes movement to fresh air. The possibility of late-onset noncardiogenic pulmonary edema should be considered. Dermal exposures should be treated by cleansing the skin with copious amounts of soap and water. Early excision of burned skin remains the best method to decrease the body hexavalent chromium load and risk for systemic toxicity after dermal contact with hot hexavalent chromic acid because systemic poisoning may occur when as little as 1% to 10% of the total-body surface area is involved.[53] Topical ascorbic acid may be useful to decrease dermal absorption of hexavalent chromium.[52] Ocular exposures require copious irrigation and ophthalmology consultation.

Chromium dietary supplement ingestions are generally nontoxic. Chronic overdosing with chromium picolinate has resulted in systemic chromium toxicity.[54] Additional ingredients in chromium dietary supplements (e.g., niacin and pyridoxine) also have the potential to produce toxicity. Death occurred in one patient who developed systemic chromium poisoning after ingesting a leather tanning solution containing 48 g of basic chromium sulfate.[55]

Cobalt

Cobalt is an essential trace element as a component of vitamin B$_{12a}$ (hydroxocobalamin). It has been used to treat selected anemias because it stimulates erythropoiesis. Normal serum cobalt levels are 2 to 17 nmol/L.[56]

Long-term excessive cobalt exposure has been associated with development of flushing, chest pain, tinnitus, nausea, vomiting, nerve deafness, thyroid hyperplasia, congestive heart failure, and renal disease. Frank hypothyroidism can result. Alopecia is a manifestation of cobalt poisoning found with only a few other toxicants such as thallium.

In the past, cobalt was responsible for recurring epidemics of cardiomyopathy (*beer-drinkers' cardiomyopathy*), which occurred when cobalt salts were added to beer as a foam stabilizer.[57]

Hard metal disease has occurred in workers who chronically inhale particulate matter during cutting or grinding operations on cobalt-containing metal alloys.

The interstitial pulmonary lesions seem to be due to inhalation of cobalt metal dust mixed with tungsten carbide particles, and not cobalt dust alone.[58]

In normal individuals, urinary cobalt levels are 23 nmol/L in men and 31 nmol/L in women.[51] Calcium disodium EDTA chelation has been used for the treatment of cobalt poisoning.[57] Administration of DMPS does not increase the urinary excretion of cobalt.[8]

Copper

Copper is an essential micronutrient. Catalase, peroxidase, and cytochrome oxidase require copper for their activity. Dietary copper deficiency is associated with microcytic anemia, leukopenia, and pathologic effects on the skeletal, cardiovascular, and nervous systems.

Copper is rapidly absorbed from the proximal GI tract. Copper is transported both by albumin and the specific α_2-globulin carrier protein, ceruloplasmin. Copper is concentrated in the liver, kidneys, heart, and brain. Stored copper is bound to metallothionein. The primary route of copper excretion is in the feces.[59] Copper undergoes redox cycling that can produce reactive oxygen species and oxidant stress in cells.[45]

Wilson's disease (hepatolenticular degeneration) is an inherited disease associated with systemic copper excess characterized by accumulation in the viscera and cornea.[60] *Indian childhood cirrhosis* also seems to be caused by copper excess. It is associated with elevated liver copper levels, early feeding with milk boiled or stored in copper-containing brass containers, a dramatic decrease in prevalence when milk preparation and storage vessels are changed to those not containing copper, and successful treatment with D-penicillamine.[60]

Copper sulfate was previously used as an emetic, but resulted in serious copper toxicity and death. Ingestion of such copper salts has caused severe GI toxicity with blue-green emesis, hematemesis, hypotension, centrilobular hepatic necrosis, coma, seizures, and death. Hemolytic anemia and methemoglobinemia are also prominent features. Chronic exposure to copper either occupationally or as a result of excessive dietary copper intake (e.g., from storing or cooking foodstuffs in copper-containing pans or from acidic water in copper pipes) has been associated with development of hepatic injury and cirrhosis.[59,61,62]

Alveolitis, interstitial inflammation, type II epithelial cell hyperplasia, and centriacinar fibrosis seen with intratracheal instillation of beryllium-copper alloy in experimental animals are due to the copper rather than the beryllium component.[26]

Copper poisoning diagnosis is based on an elevated serum level (normal: 50 to 120 mg/dL).[62] Copper elimination can be enhanced by chelation with either D-penicillamine or BAL. DMPS administration can produce a 2- to 119-fold increase in urinary copper excretion, whereas DMSA does not increase urinary copper excretion.[8,63]

Gold

Gold is a precious metal with no known biologic function. Exposure can occur from environmental sources

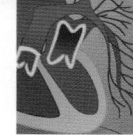

including seafood, but most human gold exposure results from medicinal use (chrysotherapy) for rheumatoid arthritis treatment. Gold-containing pharmaceuticals include aurothioglucose, gold sodium thiomalate, and auranofin.[64]

Medicinal gold salts are administered orally or parenterally. Circulating gold is mostly albumin bound.[64] Gold concentrations in synovial fluid are about one half those found in plasma. Gold has about a 7-day half-life, which lengthens during prolonged therapy because of avid tissue binding; blood gold levels remain measurable for up to 10 months after treatment termination.[65] Gold elimination is 60% to 90% fecal and 10% to 40% renal.[64]

Despite its beneficial effects in rheumatoid arthritis patients, gold has significant dermatologic and renal toxicity resulting from formation of immune complexes. Dermatitis is the most common adverse effect and may be associated with elevated immunoglobulin E levels.[61,65] Mucositis (stomatitis, tracheitis, gastritis, colitis, vaginitis) is a common adverse effect. Renal adverse effects may occur in 5% to 10% of patients treated with gold salts and consists of proteinuria, frank nephrosis, and immune complex glomerulonephritis. Thrombocytopenia, leukopenia, and (rarely) aplastic anemia may occur. Other adverse effects can include encephalitis, peripheral neuropathy, hepatitis, and pneumonitis.[64]

One case of gold poisoning without cyanide toxicity resulted from suicidal ingestion of 5 mL of a gold potassium cyanide solution.[66] This patient developed vomiting, hyperamylasemia, hepatic dysfunction, and centrilobular cholestasis with eosinic degeneration. Whole-blood gold level was 4361 µg/L, serum gold level was 6011 µg/L, and 24-hour urinary gold excretion was 429 µg/day on day 4 after ingestion.[66]

Allergic manifestations are at least partly responsible for the mucocutaneous adverse effects of therapeutic gold compounds. The peripheral venous blood lymphocyte proliferation test, when cultured with gold compounds, may be useful in diagnosis.[67] A patient with known allergy to gold jewelry developed gold allergy symptoms after drinking Goldschlager, a schnapps liquor product that contains gold particles.[68]

Treatment of gold toxicity is primarily symptomatic. Dermatitis and mucositis can be treated with antihistamines and corticosteroids. Corticosteroids can also be used to treat gold-induced nephrosis. Gold elimination can be enhanced with *N*-acetylcysteine, BAL, and D-penicillamine.[64,69]

Magnesium

Magnesium is found in ores such as dolomite, in seawater, and as a component of asbestos. It is an essential nutrient involved in glycolysis and formation of cyclic adenosine monophosphate. More than 300 enzymes are known to be activated by magnesium. Renal homeostatic mechanisms maintain serum magnesium concentrations within a narrow physiologic range.

Hypermagnesemia has several causes, with excessive ingestion of magnesium-containing antacids or excessive administration of magnesium-containing cathartics being most common (see Chapter 2A). Magnesium is administered intravenously for such conditions as pre-eclampsia, ischemic heart disease, asthma, and cardiac arrhythmias. Significantly elevated serum magnesium levels after therapeutic administration are usually seen only in patients with renal dysfunction.[70] Inhalation of magnesium oxide fumes can cause metal fume fever (MFF; see later). Dermal exposure to magnesium dust or fumes can cause contact dermatitis. Hypermagnesemia can result when the renal glomerular filtration rate decreases to less than 30 mL/min and magnesium intake is not reduced.[71]

Acute magnesium toxicity results in central nervous system depression with lethargy, coma, neuromuscular paralysis, hypotonia, and hyporeflexia. ECG changes may include prolonged QRS and PR and QT intervals. Inhalation exposure can cause respiratory tract irritation and noncardiogenic pulmonary edema.

Serum magnesium levels can confirm the diagnosis, although they may not correlate with clinical symptoms. In general, manifestations of magnesium toxicity according to serum concentrations are as follows: 3 to 9 mEq/L, vomiting, bradycardia, hypotension, hyporeflexia, lethargy; greater than 10 mEq/L, muscle paralysis, hypoventilation, stupor, cardiac conduction disturbances, ventricular arrhythmias; greater than 14 mEq/L, cardiac arrest, and death.[71]

Calcium administration ameliorates many toxic manifestations. Forced diuresis enhances magnesium elimination. Hemodialysis is effective for magnesium removal from the circulation but is rarely necessary in the absence of renal failure. Magnesium urinary excretion increased by 1.75- to 42.7-fold with DMPS chelation.[8]

Manganese

Manganese is an essential nutrient that crosses both the blood-brain and blood–cerebrospinal fluid barriers. Transferrin may be involved in this process.[72] Several enzymes, including decarboxylases, kinases, and transferases, are activated by manganese. Pyruvate carboxylase and superoxide dismutase contain manganese.

Manganese is used in the manufacture of batteries and as an ingredient in paints and varnishes, bleaching agents, laboratory reagents, motor oils, and disinfectants. It is used for decolorizing glass and ceramics and as a fertilizer for grapes and tobacco.

Occupational and environmental manganese exposures occur in steel manufacturing, welding, and ingestion of contaminated water. The unleaded gasoline antiknock additive, methylcyclopentadienyl manganese tricarbonyl (MMT), can release manganese to the atmosphere.[71] Manganese may occur in the Mn^{+2}, Mn^{+3}, and Mn^{+4} oxidation states after combustion of motor fuels containing the MMT additive.[73] Mn^{+2} is more toxic than Mn^{+3}.

Manganese can be absorbed from the GI tract as well as the lungs. Its absorption is enhanced by iron deficiency and calcium or phosphorus intake. Once absorbed, manganese is transported by transmagnin, a specific β_1-globulin.[71] The primary excretion route is fecal. Less than 6% of a dose is excreted in the urine.

Chronic poisoning causes neurologic toxicity,[72] although manganese penetrates into the CNS poorly.

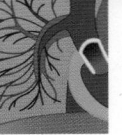

Manganese is concentrated in the globus pallidus and corpus striatum, resulting in decreased synthesis and depletion of catecholamines, including dopamine. Initial complaints are anorexia, insomnia, and fatigue. Delirium (*manganese madness*) may occur with inappropriate laughter, hallucinations, and confusion. Patients report vivid hallucinations and may commit violent acts. Marked diminution of spontaneous motor acts, ataxia, slurred speech, limb stiffness, tremor, paresthesias, amnesia, dysphagia, and a metallic taste in the mouth may develop. Impaired tandem gait and loss of associated movements may ensue, as well as masked facies, micrographia, and torticollis. Manganese poisoning mimics parkinsonism, and levodopa therapy may be effective.[74] Polymorphism of various metabolic genes may play a role in susceptibility to chronic manganese neurotoxicity.[75]

Other manifestations include marked hypocalcemia and reduced spermatogenesis. Birth defects, including talipes equinovarus and cleft lip, have been associated with chronic manganese exposure.[71]

Acute inhalation of manganese oxide can produce either MFF (see later) or a distinct manganese pneumonitis.[71] Unlike MMF, manganese pneumonitis is more severe and may have sequelae including persistent bronchospastic disease.

Manganese poisoning should be suspected on the clinical presentation (particularly a parkinsonian-like syndrome) and can be confirmed by measuring blood manganese levels. Normal mean whole blood manganese concentrations are 3 to 15 $\mu g/L$; normal mean serum concentrations are 1 to 3 $\mu g/L$.

Treatment of MMF is discussed later. Manganese pneumonitis may be treated with antibiotics and bronchodilators. For manganese-induced parkinsonian-like syndrome, therapy with either levodopa or a diet high in tryptophan may improve motor activity. No chelating agents are efficacious.

Nickel

Nickel exists in three major forms: elemental, inorganic (water soluble and water insoluble), and organic (including nickel carbonyl). Nickel is used in production of stainless steel, in electroplating, in the manufacture of nickel-cadmium (rechargeable) batteries and magnetic tape, and as a catalyst for the hydrogenation of soaps, fats, and oils.

Nickel carbonyl is an extremely toxic gas used as a catalyst in the petroleum, plastic, and rubber industries. This gaseous organometal is heavier than air and has a musty odor. With the exception of nickel allergic contact dermatitis, nearly all cases of acute nickel poisoning have resulted from nickel carbonyl exposure.[76] Nickel carbonyl readily oxidizes in air and is highly explosive.[77]

Most exposures occur through water contamination or by dermal contact with nickel-plated jewelry. Nickel is poorly absorbed (<1% of a dose) from the gut. In the blood, it is bound to albumin and α_2-microglobulin. Nickel induces metallothionein synthesis.[77]

Rashes from wearing nonrusting jewelry usually are due to nickel allergic contact dermatitis.[77] Chronic nickel exposure may also induce asthma and conjunctivitis. Other respiratory effects include chronic restrictive lung disease (nickel pneumoconiosis), sinusitis, nasal polyps, and nasal septum perforation.[78,79] Parenteral injection of nickel-containing medications can cause anaphylaxis.[79] Nickel's reactivity and ability to participate in free radical reactions are thought to be the basis of its apparent carcinogenicity.[79]

Inhalation of nickel carbonyl at 30 ppm for more than 30 minutes is lethal.[79] Death can be immediate but is typically delayed for several days.

Because it is highly lipophilic, nickel carbonyl readily penetrates into the CNS, producing delirium and coma. Hepatic injury, hyperglycemia, glycosuria, mucositis, and dermatitis may occur. Fatalities from acute nickel carbonyl poisoning result from respiratory and neurologic toxicity. Chronic nickel carbonyl exposure has been associated with lung cancer. Metallic nickel exposure does not increase the cancer risk, and exposure to carcinogenic forms of nickel does not pose a cancer risk other than to the lungs and nasal cavities.[76]

The diagnosis of nickel intoxication is made on clinical suspicion and urine or serum nickel levels. Severity can be determined by 8-hour urinary elimination results: mild toxicity corresponds to a urinary nickel concentration less than 100 $\mu g/L$; moderate toxicity is seen with 100 to 500 $\mu g/L$; and severe toxicity is associated with urinary concentrations exceeding 500 $\mu g/L$. The 95% fractile upper reference limit for urinary nickel concentration in normal individuals is 52 nmol/L.[51] Nickel carbonyl is metabolized by the liver, liberating carbon monoxide. Carboxyhemoglobin levels may be useful.

After ingestion, GI decontamination should include activated charcoal administration for organic nickel compounds; ingestion of inorganic or elemental nickel should require only gastric emptying. Nickel compounds can be chelated with sodium diethyldithiocarbonate (dithiocarb). This agent has substantially reduced morbidity and mortality after nickel carbonyl exposure, but its efficacy after elemental nickel exposure is not established.[80] However, dithiocarb enhances cerebral uptake of elemental nickel.[77] A potential dithiocarb alternative is disulfiram (Antabuse), which is metabolized to two molecules of dithiocarb, but 500 mg/kg of disulfiram offered no protection in acute rodent nickel carbonyl poisoning, and 1500 mg/kg was associated with increased mortality.[80] Currently available data are not sufficient to recommend disaffirm use.[80]

Selenium

Selenium is an essential micronutrient. It is an active part of the enzyme glutathione peroxidase that catalyzes oxygen radical scavenging.[81,82] Selenium deficiency is associated with *Keshan's cardiomyopathy*.[81] Dietary selenium supplements have become popular because of evidence suggesting they are helpful in preventing cancer, cardiovascular disease, cataracts, and arthritis.[83]

Normal serum selenium concentrations are about 100 ng/mL. Organic selenium compounds are more

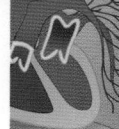

bioavailable and less toxic that the inorganic selenites and selenates.[81]

Selenium is used in paints, dyes, semiconductors, photoelectric cells, fertilizers, ceramics manufacture, rectifiers, steel production, and rubber manufacturing.[82] Gun bluing preparations contain highly toxic selenious acid as well as nitric acid, copper nitrate, and, occasionally, methanol and other solvents.

Selenium can penetrate through the skin, can be inhaled as dust, or can be absorbed after ingestion. Most of an absorbed selenium dose is excreted within 2 weeks.[83]

Excessive dietary selenium produces fingernail abnormalities, peripheral neuropathy, fatigue, muscle spasms, nausea, vomiting, alopecia, and a garlic breath odor.[82,84] Liver function abnormalities, prolonged QT interval, and hypotension (from decreased cardiac contractility and systemic vascular resistance) may occur.[85] Low-grade occupational exposure has been associated with abdominal pain, chronic diarrhea, alopecia, garlicky breath, a metallic taste in the mouth, and transverse nail creases similar to Mees' lines.[83] Occupational exposure can result in chemical pneumonitis.

Acute selenium poisoning from ingestion of gun bluing can result in death.[86,87] Gun bluing compounds produce severe burns of the stomach and esophagus with hypersalivation and vomiting, followed by metabolic acidosis, leukocytosis, myocardial depression, hepatitis, renal injury, pulmonary dysfunction (including adult respiratory distress syndrome), and seizures.[86] Ingestion of 15 mL of gun bluing solution has been fatal.[83]

The diagnosis of chronic selenium poisoning is based on clinical suspicion. Alopecia with a garlic odor of the breath is suggestive. Urinary selenium concentrations of 150 µg/L or less are normal.

Treatment of consists of general supportive measures and appropriate management of corrosive ingestion or toxic inhalation.

Case reports have suggested a beneficial role for forced diuresis and BAL administration. DMPS can increase urinary selenium excretion 30- to 42.7-fold.[8]

Silver

Silver was used medicinally in the past. Silver nitrate is an astringent and is used for treatment of burns and granulation tissue and as prophylaxis for *ophthalmia neonatorum*. Topical silver nitrate treatment may result in hyperpigmentation.[88]

Skin exposure may occur during the extraction of precious metals. Silver is used in jewelry manufacture and as a component of films, inks, and ceramics. Occupational exposure produces irritation of the mucous membranes and conjunctiva and respiratory complaints including coughing, wheezing, chest tightness, respiratory insufficiency, and epistaxis.[89]

Argyria is a condition with discoloration of the skin, nails, mucous membranes, and organs as a result of silver deposition.[90] Hyperpigmentation is pathognomonic for this otherwise asymptomatic condition.[89] The most vivid

areas of discoloration are on sun-exposed skin (e.g., face, hands).[91] Corneal deposition of silver can result in nyctalopia (disturbed night vision).[89]

Colloidal silver proteins have been promoted as mineral supplements and for the prevention of a variety of diseases. There is no evidence for the efficacy of colloidal silver proteins, and they can result in toxic effects, including argyria.[90]

The diagnosis of argyria can be made by skin biopsy showing silver deposits. Normal silver concentrations in unexposed individuals are 1 to 2 µg/L in urine and less than 0.27 µg/dL in blood.[89] There is no effective treatment for argyria and the pigmentation is permanent.[91]

Thallium

Thallium compounds are odorless, colorless, and tasteless and were formerly widely used as rodenticides. Thallium is used in the optical, electronic, and chemical research industries.[92]

Thallium is rapidly absorbed from the GI tract after ingestion and from the lungs after inhalation. Once absorbed, its distribution is extensive; no significant protein binding occurs. The estimated volume of distribution is 20 L/kg. There is significant enterohepatic recycling. Elimination half-life ranges from 3 to 8 days, although half-lives as long as 15 days have been reported. About two thirds of a thallium dose is excreted in the feces, and the remainder is excreted in the urine. Seventy percent of a single dose is excreted within 1 month.[93]

Thallium's toxicity results from its similarity to potassium.[94] It depolarizes excitable membranes and disturbs the function of sodium-potassium ATP. Mitochondria are particularly susceptible. Severe toxicity occurs with ingestions exceeding 200 mg, and the average lethal adult dose is 1 g.[95]

Thallium poisoning produces the triad of gastroenteritis, polyneuropathy, and alopecia. The immediate phase of intoxication consists of GI effects that appear within 3 to 4 hours, with nausea, vomiting, diarrhea, abdominal pain, and hematochezia. An intermediate phase appears within 1 week, consisting of hypertension, tachycardia, and chest pain. At this stage, signs of central and peripheral nervous system toxicity appear. CNS signs include optic neuritis, ptosis, confusion, coma, and psychosis. Peripheral neuropathy is more striking, with intense hyperesthesia of the soles making walking difficult. Weakness and ataxia may also occur.[92] Respiratory failure may ensue.[96] Gingival hyperpigmentation and pigmentation of the hair may appear. Severe, intractable constipation may develop. The late stage of thallium poisoning, appearing 2 to 4 weeks after exposure, consists of marked alopecia, a diffuse nonspecific rash, palmar erythema, perioral lesions, and Aldrich-Mees lines on the fingernails.[93,95-97] A "residual" stage, occurring more than 4 weeks after exposure, consists of memory loss, ataxia, tremor, and foot drop. Death generally occurs 10 to 15 days after severe exposure. Neurologic sequelae may occur in survivors.[98] Laboratory abnormalities consist of

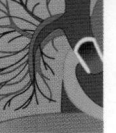

anemia, thrombocytopenia, increased levels of hepatic transaminases, and decreased complement levels.[95] Flat or inverted T waves may be seen on ECG.[95] Axonal destruction and demyelination may be present on sural nerve biopsy.[95]

Twelve cases of combined thallium and arsenic poisoning in a group of workers were reported by Rusyniak and colleagues.[99] Of these, 89% had myalgias and arthralgias, 78% had paresthesias and synesthesias, 67% had joint stiffness and insomnia, and 52% had alopecia and joint pain. Diarrhea and constipation were uncommon. Seven of 11 patients tested had blackened or darkened hair roots. Eight of 11 tested patients had sensorimotor peripheral neuropathies ranging from mild to moderate-severe. Two patients with both elevated thallium and arsenic blood levels had the most severe peripheral neuropathies. Eleven of the 12 patients were reevaluated 6 months later, and all had improvement of peripheral neuropathies. However, 6 of 11 still complained of dysesthesias, mainly involving the feet. Five developed early complete alopecia that began about 14 days after exposure and resolved over 4 months. Sequelae of anxiety and depression were common. None had Mees' lines.

Thallium poisoning during pregnancy has resulted in a wide range of fetal effects from severe toxicity and residual sequelae to apparently normal development.[100] There is a trend toward low birth weight and prematurity. Thallium crosses the placental barrier and is excreted in the breast milk.

Diagnosis is made on the basis of clinical manifestations and confirmed by measurement of thallium in serum or urine. Serum levels greater than 50 μg/dL suggest poisoning, but because 70% of thallium is bound to erythrocytes, whole-blood measurements are likely to be more accurate.[97] Urinary excretion of greater than 10 to 20 mg per 24 hours is considered excessive. Other potential methods for identifying thallium poisoning are electroretinography and electromyography (which demonstrates decreased distal motor units and membrane instability). Thallium poisoning may be misdiagnosed as Guillain-Barré syndrome, selenosis, arsenic poisoning, or acute porphyria.[96,97]

Treatment goals are enhancing fecal excretion, enhancing urinary excretion, and, when necessary, extracorporeal elimination. Early GI decontamination may decrease absorption. Fecal elimination may be enhanced by administration of Prussian blue (ferric ferrocyanide). Activated charcoal should be administered initially because there is no pharmaceutical preparation of Prussian blue available in the United States, and obtaining it from a chemical supply company may take an inordinately long time; 250 mg/kg of Prussian blue daily should be given orally in 4 divided doses with a cathartic.[99]

Administration of sodium iodide can form an insoluble thallium-iodine complex that is poorly absorbed.[96] Forced diuresis also has potential benefit; human studies have suggested that it increases thallium urinary elimination two- to sixfold.[101] Forced diuresis with potassium chloride supplementation has also been advocated; however, exogenous potassium may displace thallium

into the serum and thus provide greater opportunity for nervous system penetration.[97]

Dithiocarb is a chelating agent that enhances urinary elimination of thallium; however, the resulting thallium chelate is highly lipophilic, crosses the blood-brain barrier, and exacerbates neurologic toxicity. Therefore, dithiocarb administration is *not* recommended.

Extracorporeal removal techniques including peritoneal dialysis are unlikely to be efficacious.

Tin

Tin is a ubiquitous trace element. It exists in three forms (metallic, inorganic, organic), with the metallic and inorganic forms being the least toxic.[102] Organotins are used as stabilizers in polymers and as catalysts.

Most tin salts are insoluble, with less than 5% absorbed from the GI tract. Once absorbed, tin is distributed and deposited in the kidneys, lungs, and bone. Most circulating tin is bound to erythrocytes.

Trialkyltins are the most toxic organotins. Being highly lipophilic, they readily penetrate into the CNS.[103,104] Organotin exposure has been associated with altered mental status, confusion, and amnesia.[103] Ingestion results in abdominal pain, diarrhea, and vomiting.[105] Other complaints include headache, tinnitus, deafness, disorientation, syncope, and loss of consciousness; EEG changes may be present.[105] Triethyltin, unlike trimethyltin, may also produce acute cerebral edema. Ingestion of triphenyltin acetate has caused nephropathy with proteinuria, azotemia, polyuria, hematuria, and pyuria.[106] Hepatitis and pancreatitis may develop.[106] Delayed onset of sensorimotor peripheral neuropathy may occur.[105] Long-term tin inhalation can produce a benign pneumoconiosis (*stannosis*).[102] Delayed bullous irritant contact dermatitis has occurred after skin contact with a marine antifouling paint containing bis-tributyltin oxide.[107]

De-butylated metabolites of tributyltin chloride, particularly dibutyltin chloride, are responsible for observed hepatotoxicity. Cytochrome P-450 plays some role in metabolism.[108,109]

Diagnosis is based on the clinical presentation, history, and elevated serum tin levels. In a case of trimethyltin exposure, urinary excretion was 52 μg/dL, compared with a normal urine tin concentration of about 0.1 μg/dL.[103]

Treatment is supportive. No chelating agents alter the course of tin poisoning.

Zinc

Zinc is an essential micronutrient. More than 70 metalloenzymes require zinc for proper function. There is also a strong relationship between zinc and copper metabolism. Zinc has been used to treat copper accumulation associated with Wilson's disease.[110] Zinc dietary supplements are widely promoted, but their use can result in toxic manifestations.[111] Overexposure can occur in the workplace and in patients being hemodialyzed with water stored in galvanized steel tanks.[112]

Acute ingestion of 2 g or more results in GI irritation and vomiting. Continual excessive zinc intake results in

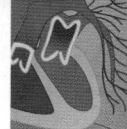

reductions in serum copper levels, (hypocupremia), sideroblastic anemia, and neutropenia.[110,111] A child with long-term zinc ingestion developed listlessness, anemia, neutropenia, poor weight gain, and sideroblastic anemia, indicative of copper deficiency.[111] A child who ingested an acid soldering flux solution with a zinc chloride concentration of 30% to 60% and a pH of 3.0 developed severe corrosive injury of the stomach and an antral stricture, but not systemic zinc poisoning.[113]

The diagnosis of zinc poisoning is confirmed by an elevated serum zinc level (normal: 9.2 to 23 μmol/L).

Treatment of zinc poisoning is supportive. After ingestion, GI decontamination measures include administration of activated charcoal. Chelation is very effective for reducing elevated zinc levels. Options include calcium disodium EDTA, BAL, D-penicillamine, and *N*-acetylcysteine.[112,114]

METAL FUME FEVER

MFF is an occupational disease caused by inhalation of freshly oxidized metal fumes with a particle size smaller than 0.5 to 1.0 μm.[115-117] MFF is also referred to as *Monday morning fever, the smothers, brass founder's ague, brazier's disease, foundry fever, galvanizer's poisoning, smelter's chills, zinc chills, zinc fume fever, brass chills,* and *copper fever.*[118] Although welding is the occupation most often associated with the disease,[119] MFF is encountered after soldering, forging, melting, and metal casting.

MFF is associated with a number of metals, including zinc, copper, magnesium, cadmium, manganese, and antimony (Box 75-1). Zinc, iron, and copper are the most common causes of MFF. Inhalation exposure to a powder catalyst containing vanadium used in production of maleic anhydride has caused an MMF-like syndrome with associated neutrophilic alveolitis.[120] Cadmium and tin, although associated with MFF, produce a more severe respiratory illness that shares some features with MFF; urinary cadmium levels may be elevated, and there can be associated transient renal impairment.[43]

The clinical presentation consists of chills, fever, leukocytosis, myalgias, chest pain, nonproductive cough, dry throat, intense thirst, and a metallic taste in the mouth.[118] These symptoms usually appear 4 to 12 hours after acute exposure. Temperature may be as high as 104° F (40° C), accompanied by sinus tachycardia and

rales. Chest x-rays may appear normal or may reveal a diffuse patchy infiltrate.[121] These findings characteristically appear to be more severe than the patient's clinical presentation would suggest. Bronchoalveolar lavage, if performed, may reveal inflammatory cells. Other clinical features include elevated lactate dehydrogenase levels and hypoxia.[122] Tolerance to MFF often develops. As a result, workers often complain of illness developing at the beginning of the week, improving by the end of the week, and completely resolving during the weekend. The benign clinical course of MFF distinguishes it from acute cadmium or tin pneumonitis.[122]

The cause of MFF is unclear, although it has been attributed to release of endogenous pyrogens or production of antigenic metal proteinates.[122] Delayed hypersensitivity pneumonitis and allergic reaction have been suggested as mechanisms.[118] MFF might result from a direct toxic effect on alveolar cells. Inhalation of purified zinc oxide fumes results in a dose-dependent increase in polymorphonuclear cells and proinflammatory cytokines in the lungs, indicating a role for cytokine networking in MFF development.[123]

MFF is self-limited and usually resolves within 48 hours. Bed rest and antipyretics are recommended. Corticosteroids have been recommended for patients with interstitial infiltrates on chest x-ray after a history of zinc fume exposure. A history of exposure to cadmium or tin fumes warrants hospitalization for observation and supportive care. No permanent sequelae of MFF have been identified. Elevated serum zinc levels and increased urinary copper levels have been reported, but their significance is unclear.[115]

CHELATORS

Exogenous

A number of chelating agents have been explored as potentially effective treatments for exposure to toxic metals. Table 75-1 summarizes their potential roles. A complete review of the pharmacology of these agents is beyond the scope of this chapter.

Endogenous

A number of endogenous metal-carrying proteins have been identified in humans and animals, such as transferrin, ferritin, ceruloplasmin, and transmagnin, that carry iron, copper, and manganese. Because they form stable bonds with metals, these agents have been referred to as *endogenous chelators.*

Metallothionein is a low-molecular-weight protein transport molecule, but its exact role has not been fully defined.[124] Its high sulfur content permits the formation of several types of stable bonds with metals.[124,125] Although found primarily in intracellular sites, it is also secreted into the bile, urine, and plasma. Zinc has a profound influence on metallothionein production, and synthesis decreases with zinc deficiency. Zinc excess produces a marked increase in metallothionein production.

BOX 75-1	METALS COMMONLY ASSOCIATED WITH METAL FUME FEVER

Zinc
Magnesium
Manganese
Iron
Copper
Cadmium
Tin

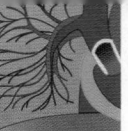

TABLE 75-1 Metal Chelators				
CHELATOR	**USEFUL**	**POSSIBLY EFFICACIOUS**	**UNLIKELY TO BE EFFICACIOUS**	**POTENTIALLY HARMFUL**
Calcium disodium EDTA	Zinc Cobalt		Chromium Nickel Thallium	Selenium
Dimercaprol (BAL)	Lead Nickel Copper Antimony Bismuth Gold Zinc Arsenic Mercury	Chromium	Thallium	Selenium Cadmium
Dithiocarb (sodium diethyldithio-carbamate)	Nickel carbonyl	Cadmium		Thallium Elemental Nickel
D-Penicillamine (currently not often used except for treatment of chronic copper accumulation)	Copper Lead Arsenic Mercury Zinc Gold		Nickel	Selenium
Dimercaptosuccinic acid (DMSA)	Antimony Lead Arsenic			
Dimercaptopropane sulfonic acid (DMPS)	Antimony Lead Mercury			
Deferoxamine	Iron Aluminum			
N-acetylcysteine (NAC)	Gold Zinc			

Metallothionein synthesis can also be induced by exposure to toxic metals, including cadmium, mercury, silver, platinum, gold, and bismuth. Cadmium is a particularly potent inducer of metallothionein synthesis. Very little is known about the degradation of this protein, although its loss is directly related to the bound metal. In experimental animal models, the half-lives, of cadmium-, zinc-, and copper-induced metallothioneins are 80, 20, and 17 hours, respectively.[125] Cadmium toxicity is reduced by the presence of metallothionein.[61]

REFERENCES

1. Elmore AR, for the Cosmetic Ingredient Review Expert Panel: Final report of the safety assessment of aluminum silicate, calcium silicate, magnesium aluminum silicate, magnesium silicate, sodium magnesium silicate, zirconium silicate, attapulgite, bentonite, Fuller's earth, hectorlite, kaolin, montmorillonite, pyrophyllite, and zeolite. Int J Toxicol 2003;22(Suppl 1):37–102.
2. Nagore E, Martinez-Escribano JA, Tato A, et al: Subcutaneous nodules following treatment with aluminum-containing allergen extracts. Eur J Dermatol 2001;11:138–140.
3. Tsou VM, Young RM, Hart MH, et al: Elevated plasma aluminum levels in normal infants receiving antacids containing aluminum. Pediatrics 1991;87:148–151.
4. Ochmanski W, Barabasz W: Aluminum—occurrence and toxicity for organisms [in Polish]. Przegl Lek 2000;57:665–668.
5. Micic DV, Petronijevic ND, Vucetic SS: Superoxide dismutase activity in the Mongolian gerbil brain after acute poisoning with aluminum. J Alzheimers Dis 2003;5:49–56.
6. Reusche E, Koch V, Lindner B, et al: Alzheimer morphology is not increased in dialysis-associated encephalopathy and long-term hemodialysis. Acta Neuropathol (Berl) 2001;101:211–216.
7. Hantson P, Nahieu P, Gersdorff M, et al: Fatal encephalopathy after otoneurosurgery procedure with an aluminum-containing biomaterial. Clin Toxicol 1995;33:645–648.
8. Torris-Alanis O, Garza-Ocanas L, Bernal MA, et al: Urinary excretion of trace elements in humans after sodium 2,3-dimercaptopropane-1-sulfonate challenge test. J Toxicol Clin Toxicol 2000;38:697–700.
9. Flinn PA, Hagstrum DW, Reed C, et al: United States Department of Agriculture—Agricultural Research Service stored-grain area wide integrated pest management program. Pest Manag Sci 2003;59:614–618.
10. Lauwers LF, Roelants A, Rosseel PM, et al: Oral antimony intoxications in man. Crit Care Med 1990;18:324–326.
11. Cesur S, Bahar K, Erekul S: Death from cumulative sodium stibogluconate toxicity on Kala-Azar. Clin Microbiol Infect 2002;8:606.
12. Oliveira MR, Marsden PD: A case of urticaria during pentavalent antimony use in a patient with mucous leishmaniasis [Portuguese]. Rev Soc Bras Med Trop 1995;28:287.
13. Agency for Toxic Substances and Disease Registry: Toxicological Profile for Antimony. Atlanta, U.S. Public Health Service, 1992.
14. Rees PH, Kager PA, Keating MI, et al: Renal clearance of pentavalent antimony (sodium stibogluconate). Lancet 1980;2:226–229.
15. Deng JF, Jan IS, Cheng HS: The essential role of a poison center in handling an outbreak of barium carbonate poisoning. Vet Human Toxicol 1991;33:173–175.
16. Jacobs IA, Taddeo J, Kelly K, et al: Poisoning as a result of barium styphnate explosion. Am J Ind Med 2002;41:285–288.
17. Agarwal AK, Ahlawat SK, Gupta S, et al: Hypokalaemic paralysis secondary to acute barium carbonate toxicity. Trop Doct 1995;25:101–103.

18. Jourdan S, Bertoni M, Sergio P, et al: Suicidal poisoning with barium chloride. Forensic Sci Int 2001;119:263–265.

19. Johnson CH, Van Tassell VJ: Acute barium poisoning with respiratory failure and rhabdomyolysis. Ann Emerg Med 1991;20:1138–1142.

20. Koch M, Appoloni O, Haufroid V, et al: Acute barium intoxication and hemofiltration. J Toxicol Clin Toxicol 2003;41:363–367.

21. Gupta S: Barium carbonate, hypokalemic paralysis and trismus. Postgrad Med J 1994;70:938–939.

22. Fogliani J, Giraud E, Henriquet D, et al: Voluntary barium poisoning [in French]. Ann Fr Anesth Reanim 1993;12:508–511.

23. Kriebel D, Brain JD, Sprince NL, et al: The pulmonary toxicity of beryllium. Am Rev Respir Dis 1988;137:464–473.

24. McGavran PD, Rood AS, Till JE: Chronic beryllium disease and cancer risk estimates with uncertainty for beryllium released to the air from the Rocky Flats Plant. Environ Health Perspect 1999;107:731–744.

25. Willis HH, Florig HK: Potential exposures and risks from beryllium-containing products. Risk Anal 2002;22:1019–1033.

26. Benson JM, Holmes AM, Barr EB, et al: Particle clearance and histopathology in lungs of C3H/HeJ mice administered beryllium/copper alloy by intratracheal instillation. Inhal Toxicol 2000;12:733–749.

27. Fontenot AP, Canavera SJ, Gharavi L, et al: Target organ localization of memory CD4$^+$ T cells in patients with chronic beryllium disease. J Clin Invest 2002;110:1473–1482.

28. Strange AW, Furman FJ, Hilmas DE: Rocky Flats beryllium health surveillance. Environ Health Perspect 1996;104(Suppl 5):981–986.

29. Newman LS: Significance of the blood beryllium lymphocyte proliferation test. Environ Health Perspect 1996;104(Suppl 5):953–956.

30. Newman LS, Lloyd J, Daniloff E: The natural history of beryllium sensitization and chronic beryllium disease. Environ Health Perspect 1996;104(Suppl 5):937–943.

31. Clarke SM, Thurlow SM, Hilmas DE: Application of beryllium antibodies in risk assessment and health surveillance: two case studies. Toxicol Ind Health 1995;11:399–411.

32. Johri S, Shukla S, Sharma P: Role of chelating agents and antioxidants in beryllium induced toxicity. Indian J Exp Biol 2002;40:575–582.

33. Sharma P, Johri S, Shukla S: Beryllium-induced toxicity and its prevention by treatment with chelating agents. J Appl Toxicol 2000;20:313–318.

34. Mendelowitz PC, Hoffman RS, Weber S: Bismuth absorption and myoclonic encephalopathy during bismuth subsalicylate therapy. Ann Intern Med 1990;112:140–141.

35. Winship KA: Toxicity of bismuth salts. Adv Drug React Acute Poisoning Rev 1983;2:103–121.

36. Islek I, Uysal S, Dundaroz R, et al: Reversible nephropathy after overdose of colloidal bismuth subcitrate. Pediatr Nephrol 2001;16:510–514.

37. Corazza M, Capossi O, Virgilit A: Five cases of livedo-like dermatitis (Nicolau's syndrome) due to bismuth salts and various other non-steroidal anti-inflammatory drugs. J Eur Acad Dermatol Venerol 2001;15:585–588.

38. Ottervanger JP, Stricker BH: Skin disorders caused by bismuth oxide (De-Nol) [in Dutch]. Ned Tijdschr Geneeskd 1994;138:152–153.

39. Noach LA, Eekhof JL, Bour LJ, et al: Bismuth salts and neurotoxicity: a randomized single-blind and controlled study. Hum Exp Toxicol 1995;14:349–355.

40. Slikkerveer A, Jong HB, Helmich RB, et al: Development of a therapeutic procedure for bismuth intoxication with chelating agents. J Lab Clin Med 1992;119:529–537.

41. Kowal NE, Johnson DE, Draemer DF, et al: Normal levels of cadmium in diet, urine, blood, and tissues of inhabitants of the United States. J Toxicol Environ Health 1979;5:995–1014.

42. Bernard A, Lauwerys R: Cadmium in human population. Experientia 1984;40:136–152.

43. Ando Y, Shibata E, Tsuchiyama F, et al: Elevated urinary cadmium concentrations in patients with acute cadmium pneumonitis. Scand J Work Environ Health 1996;22:150–153.

44. das Neves RP, Santos TM, Pereira Mde L, de Jesus JP: Comparative histological studies on liver of mice exposed to Cr(VI) and Cr(V) compounds. Hum Exp Toxicol 2002;21:365–369.

45. Ercal N, Gurer-Orhan H, Aykin-Burns N: Toxic metals and oxidative stress part I: Mechanisms involved in metal-induced oxidative damage. Curr Top Med Chem 2001;1:529–539.

46. Fowler JF: Systemic contact dermatitis caused by oral chromium picolinate. Cutis 2000;65:116.

47. Young PC, Turiansky GW, Bonner MW, et al: Acute generalized exanthematous pustulosis induced by chromium picolinate. J Am Acad Dermatol 1999;41(5 Pt 2):820–823.

48. Deng J-F, Fleeger AK: An outbreak of chromium ulcer in a manufacturing plant. Vet Human Toxicol 1990;32:142.

49. Meert KL, Ellis J, Aronow R, et al: Acute ammonium dichromate poisoning. Ann Emerg Med 1994;24:748–750.

50. Andre N, Paut O, Arditti J, et al: Severe potassium dichromate poisoning after accidental nasal introduction [in French]. Arch Pediatr 1998;5:145–148.

51. Kristiansen J, Christensen JM, Iversen BS, et al: Toxic trace element reference levels in blood and urine: influence of gender and lifestyle factors. Sci Total Environ 1997;204:147–160.

52. Bradberry SM, Vale JA: Therapeutic review: is ascorbic acid of value in chromium poisoning and chromium dermatitis? J Toxicol Clin Toxicol 1999;37:195–200.

53. Matey P, Allison KP, Sheehan TM, et al: Chromic acid burns: early aggressive excision is the best method to prevent systemic toxicity. J Burn Care Rehabil 2000;21:241–245.

54. Cerulli J, Grabe DW, Gauthier I, et al: Chromium picolinate toxicity. Ann Pharmacother 1998;32:428–431.

55. van Heerden PN, Jenkins IR, Woods WP, et al: Death by tanning—a case of fatal chromium sulphate poisoning. Intensive Care Med 1994;20:145–147.

56. Mucklow ES, Griffin SJ, Delves HT, et al: Cobalt poisoning in a 6-year-old. Lancet 1990;335:981.

57. Morin Y, Daniel P: Quebec beer-drinker's cardiomyopathy: Etiological considerations. Can Med Assoc J 1967;97:926–928.

58. Lasfargues G, Lardot C, Delos M, et al: The delayed lung response to single and repeated intratracheal administration of pure cobalt and hard metal powder in the rat. Environ Res 1995;69:108–121.

59. Walsh FM, Crosson FJ, Bayley M, et al: Acute copper intoxication. Am J Dis Child 1977;131:149–151.

60. Pankit AN, Bhave SA: Copper metabolic defects and liver disease: Environmental aspects. J Gastroenterol Hepatol 2002;17(Suppl 3):S403–S407.

61. Ringenberg QS, Doll DC, Patterson WP, et al: Hematologic effects of heavy metal poisoning. South Med J 1988;81:1132–1139.

62. Schwartz E, Schmidt E: Refractory shock secondary to copper sulfate ingestion. Ann Emerg Med 1986;15:952–954.

63. Chisolm JJ: Safety and efficacy of meso-2,3-dimercaptosuccinic acid (DMSA) in children with elevated blood lead concentrations. J Toxicol Clin Toxicol 2000;38:365–375.

64. Insel PA: Analgesic-antipyretic and anti-inflammatory agents and drugs employed in the treatment of gout. In Hardman JG, Limbird LE, Molinoff PB, et al (eds): Goodman & Gilman's the Pharmacological Basis of Therapeutics. New York, McGraw-Hill, 1996, pp 617–657.

65. Goyer RA: Toxic effects of metals. In Klaassen CD (ed): Casarett and Doull's Toxicology: The Basic Science of Poisons, 5th ed. New York, McGraw-Hill, 1996, pp 691–736.

66. Wu ML, Tsai WJ, Ger J, et al: Cholestatic hepatitis caused by acute gold potassium cyanide poisoning. J Toxicol Clin Toxicol 2001;39:739–743.

67. Rasanen L, Kaipiainen-Seppanen O, Myllykangas-Luosujarri R, et al: Hypersensitivity of gold in gold thiomalate-induced dermatosis. Br J Dermatol 1999;141:683–688.

68. Guenthner T, Stork CM, Cantor RM: Goldschlager allergy in a gold allergic patient. Vet Human Toxicol 1999;41:246.

69. Vilensky JA, Redman K: British anti-Lewisite (dimercaprol): an amazing history. Ann Emerg Med 2003;41:378–383.

70. Garcia MC, Byrd RP, Roy TM: Lethal iatrogenic hypermagnesemia. Tenn Med 2002;95:334–336.

71. Gilmore DA, Bronstein AC: Manganese and magnesium. In Sullivan J, Krieger G (eds): Hazardous Materials Toxicology—Clinical Principals of Environmental Health. Baltimore, Williams & Wilkins, 1992.

72. Takeda A: Manganese action in brain function. Brain Res Brain Res Rev 2003;41:79–87.

73. Reaney SH, Kwik-Uribe CL, Smith DR: Manganese oxidation state and its implications for toxicity. Chem Res Toxicol 2002;15:1119–1126.

74. Cook DG, Fahn S, Brait KA: Chronic manganese intoxication. Arch Neurol 1974;30:59–64.

75. Zheng YX, Chan P, Pan ZF, et al: Polymorphism of metabolic genes and susceptibility to occupational chronic manganism. Biomarkers 2002;7:337–346.

76. Barceloux DG: Nickel. J Toxicol Clin Toxicol 1999;37:239–258.

77. Leach CN, Sunderman FW: Nickel contamination of human serum albumin solutions. N Engl J Med 1985;313:1232.

78. Maibach HI, Menne T: Nickel and the Skin: Immunology and Toxicology. Boca Raton, FL, CRC Press, 1989.

79. Siegers C-P, Sullivan JB: Organometals and reactive metals. In Sullivan JB, Krieger GR (eds): Hazardous Materials Toxicology—Clinical Principals of Environmental Health. Baltimore, Williams & Wilkins, 1992, pp 928–936.

80. Bradberry SM, Vale JA: Therapeutic review: do diethyldithio-carbamate and disulfiram have a role in acute nickel carbonyl poisoning? J Toxicol Clin Toxicol 1999;37:259–264.

81. Tinggi U: Essentiality and toxicity of selenium and its status in Australia: a review. Toxicol Lett 2003;137:103–110.

82. Barceloux DG: Selenium. J Toxicol Clin Toxicol 1999;37:145–172.

83. Alderman LC, Ergin JJ: Hydrogen selenide poisoning: an illustrative case with review of the literature. Arch Environ Health 1986;41:354–358.

84. Ruta DA, Haider S: Attempted murder by selenium poisoning. BMJ 1989;299:316–317.

85. Civil IDS, McDonald MJA: Acute selenium poisoning: a case report. N Z Med J 1978;87:354.

86. Nantel AJ: Acute poisoning by selenious acid. Vet Human Toxicol 27:531, 1985.

87. Quadrani DA, Spiller HA, Steinhorn D: A fatal case of gun blue ingestion in a toddler. Vet Human Toxicol 2000;42:96–98.

88. Rauber A, Bruner B: Ingestion of concentrated silver nitrate: a report of two cases. Vet Human Toxicol 1987;29:321–322.

89. Rosenman KD, Seixas N, Jacobs J: Potential nephrotoxic effects of exposure to silver. Br J Ind Med 1987;44:267–272.

90. Fung MC, Bowen DL: Silver products for medical indications: risk-benefit assessment. J Toxicol Clin Toxicol 1996;34:119–126.

91. Gulbranson SH, Hud JA, Hansen RC: Agyria following the use of dietary supplements containing colloidal silver protein. Cutis 2000;66:373–374.

92. Desenclos J-CA, Wilder MH, Coppenger GW, et al: Thallium poisoning: an outbreak in Florida, 1988. South Med J 1992;85:1203–1206.

93. Pai V: Acute thallium poisoning. West Indian Med J 1987;36:256–258.

94. Mulkey JP, Oehme FW: A review of thallium toxicity. Vet Human Toxicol 1993;35:445–453.

95. Schwartz JG, Stuckey JH, Kunkel SP, et al: Poisoning from thallium. Tex Med 1988;84:46–48.

96. Vergauwe PL, Knockaert DC, Van Tittleboom TJ: Near fatal subacute thallium poisoning necessitating prolonged mechanical ventilation. Am J Emerg Med 1990;8:548–550.

97. Insley BM, Grufferman S, Ayliffe HE: Thallium poisoning in cocaine abusers. Am J Emerg Med 1986;24:545–548.

98. Atsmon J, Taliansky E, Landau M, et al: Thallium poisoning in Israel. Am J Med Sci 2000;320:327–330.

99. Rusyniak DE, Furbee RB, Kirk MA: Thallium and arsenic poisoning in a small Midwestern town. Ann Emerg Med 2002;39:307–311.

100. Hoffman RS: Thallium poisoning during pregnancy: a case report and comprehensive literature review. J Toxicol Clin Toxicol 2000;38:767–775.

101. Pedersen RS, Olesen AS, Freund LG, et al: Thallium intoxication treated with long-term hemodialysis, forced diuresis, and Prussian blue. Acta Med Scand 1978;204:429–432.

102. Wax PM, Dockstader L: Tributyltin use in interior paints: a continuing health hazard. Clin Toxicol 1995;33:239–241.

103. Yanofsky NN, Nieerenberg D, Turco JH: Acute short-term memory loss from trimethyltin exposure. J Emerg Med 1991;9:137–139.

104. Chang LW: The neurotoxicity and pathology of organomercury, organolead, and organotin. J Toxicol Sci 1990;15(Suppl 4):125–151.

105. Wu RM, Chang YC, Chiu HC: Acute triphenyltin intoxication: a case report. J Neurol Neurosurg Psychiatry 1990;53:356–357.

106. Lin JL, Hsueh S: Acute nephropathy of organotin compounds. Am J Nephrol 1993;13:124–128.

107. Lewis PG, Emmett EA: Irritant dermatitis from tri-butyl tin oxide and contact allergy from chlorocresol. Contact Dermatitis 1987;17:129–132.

108. Ueno S, Suzuki T, Susa N, et al: Effect of SKF-525A on liver metabolism and hepatotoxicity of tri- and dibutyltin compounds in mice. Arch Toxicol 1997;71:513–518.

109. Ueno S, Susa N, Furukawa Y, et al: Rome of cytochrome P450 in hepatotoxicity induced by di- and tributyltin compounds in mice. Arch Toxicol 1995;69:655–658.

110. Botash AS, Nasca J, Dubowy R, et al: Zinc-induced copper deficiency in an infant. Am J Dis Child 1992;146:709–711.

111. Broun ER, Greist A, Tricot G, et al: Excessive zinc ingestion—a reversible cause of sideroblastic anemia and bone marrow depression. JAMA 1990;264:1441–1443.

112. Domingo JL, Llobet JM, Paternain JL, et al: Acute zinc intoxication: comparison of the antidotal efficacy of several chelating agents. Vet Human Toxicol 1988;30:224–227.

113. Yamataka A, Pringle KC, Wyeth J: A case of zinc chloride ingestion. J Pediatr Surg 1998;33:660–662.

114. Fisher D: Zinc. In Sullivan JB, Krieger GR (eds): Hazardous Materials Toxicology—Clinical Principals of Environmental Health. Baltimore, Williams & Wilkins, 1992, pp 865–868.

115. Vogelmeier C, Konig G, Bencze K, et al: Pulmonary involvement in zinc fume fever. Chest 1987;92:946–948.

116. Kaye P, Young H, O'Sullivan I: Metal; fume fever: a case report and review of the literature. Emerg Med J 2003;19:268–269.

117. Merchant J, Webby R: Metal fume fever: a case report and literature review. Emerg Med (Fremantle) 2001;13:373–375.

118. Noel NE, Ruthman JC: Elevated serum zinc levels in metal fume fever. Am J Emerg Med 1988;6:609–610.

119. Van Pee D, Vandenplas O, Gillet JB: Metal fume fever. Eur J Emerg Med 1998;5:465–466.

120. Vandenplas O, Binard-van Cangh F, Gregoire J, et al: Fever and neutrophilic alveolitis caused by a vanadium based catalyst. Occup Environ Med 2002;59:785–787.

121. Ebran B, Quieffin J, Bedaneau G, et al: Radiological evidence of lung involvement in metal fume fever [in French]. Rev Pneumol Clin 2000;56:361–364.

122. Offerman PV, Finley C: Metal fume fever. Ann Emerg Med 1992;21:872–875.

123. Kuschner WG, D'Alessandro A, Wintermeyer SF, et al: Pulmonary response to purified zinc oxide fume. J Invest Med 1995;43:371–378.

124. Bremner I, Beattie JH: Metallothionein and the trace mineral. Annu Rev Nutr 1990;10:63–83.

125. Vallee BL: The function of metallothionein. Neurochem Int 1995;27:23–33.

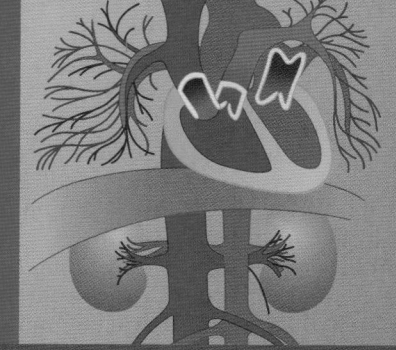

76 *Organophosphates and Carbamates*

CYNTHIA K. AARON, MD

At a Glance...

- Organophosphate and carbamate compounds produce toxic effects largely from inhibition of acetylcholinesterase.

- Manifestations of poisoning are variable but commonly include muscarinic signs (e.g., salivation, diaphoresis, abdominal cramps, vomiting, diarrhea, bronchorrhea, bradycardia, miosis, coma, seizures, apnea) and nicotinic signs (e.g., fasciculations, flaccid paralysis, tachycardia).

- The most common cause of death is respiratory failure associated with refractory hypotension.

- Treatment for poisoning from these agents includes health care provider self-protection and patient airway protection; administration of atropine, oximes, and benzodiazepines; and decontamination.

- Atropine is frequently underdosed in serious poisonings and should be titrated to clearing of pulmonary secretions and adequate oxygenation.

- Atropine should be administered rapidly and in escalating doses.

- Benzodiazepines may be cerebroprotective and should be used liberally in all severely ill patients.

- Oxime therapy should be used in all patients requiring atropine.

- Oxime therapy is recommended for all carbamate poisonings with the exception of carbaryl.

- Clinical findings suggestive of severe organophosphate poisoning warrant immediate treatment presumptively, before the results of lab testing are available.

RELEVANT HISTORY

Pesticides are the leading cause of fatality from acute poisoning worldwide.[1,2] In 1990, the World Health Organization (WHO) estimated that 3 million severe pesticide poisonings occur annually and are associated with up to 200,000 deaths.[3] To better characterize and track the epidemiology of these exposures, the WHO established the International Programme on Chemical Safety Poison Information Database Management (IPCS INTOX) Pesticide Project in 2002.[4] In the United States alone, the Environmental Protection Agency (EPA) estimates 10,000 to 20,000 physician-documented pesticide exposures annually among 3,380,000 agricultural workers. The EPA has instituted the Sentinel Event Notification System for Occupational Risk (SENSOR) Pesticides Program to monitor the incidence of these exposures.[5]

Pesticides are a diverse group of chemicals designed to kill and control various insects, animals, fungi, or plants. Insecticides, or chemicals designed to kill insects, are within the class of pesticides. Organophosphorus compounds, organophosphates (OPs), and carbamates, or other cholinesterase inhibitors, are the most commonly used insecticides worldwide and account for more human poisonings and death annually than any other pesticide class.[6] In 2004, there were 10,994 OP and carbamate exposures reported to U.S. poison centers; 70 (0.6%) resulted in major toxicity and 3 (0.3%) in death.[7] As potent eukaryotic toxins, OPs have been used broadly, serving as both military-based nerve agents and agricultural pesticides. Nerve agents have been in military arsenals since World War II. One of these agents, sarin, achieved international notoriety after its release by terrorists in Matsumoto and Tokyo in 1995[8] (see Chapter 105A).

OP and carbamate insecticides are a mixed group of chemicals. OPs are derived from phosphoric acid–containing compounds.[9] The OPs achieved great popularity after World War II because of their effectiveness and lack of environmental persistence. For the most part, they have an unstable chemical structure and disintegrate into harmless by-products within days under the influence of sunlight, oxygen, and reactive soil chemicals.[10] Except for the highly fat-soluble agents, OPs are less persistent in body tissues and the environment than dichlorodiphenyltrichloroethane (DDT) and other organochlorines. Because of their lack of persistence, OPs have replaced DDT as the insecticide agent of

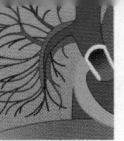

choice. Carbamates are commonly used both as insecticides and medicinals for the treatment of human disease. Pyridostigmine and neostigmine are both used to treat myasthenia gravis, neostigmine has been effective for adynamic ileus, and physostigmine is most often used to treat the anticholinergic syndrome. Donepezil and memantine, central nervous system (CNS) reversible inhibitors of acetylcholinesterase, are used to treat the relative acetylcholine deficiency existing in Alzheimer's disease.

The first OP, tetraethyl pyrophosphate (TEPP), was synthesized in 1854, but the class was not actively used commercially until World War II when the Germans used TEPP as a substitute for the scarce botanic insecticide nicotine. The human toxicity of OPs was exploited by the Germans at the end of World War II with the development of the nerve agents tabun, sarin, and soman (GA, GB, and GD). The allies developed VX after the war (see Chapter 105A).

OP poisoning can occur in various settings. Occupational exposures occur during application in farm workers and pest control workers and during their manufacture, storage, and transport. Children are accidentally exposed to these agents through domestic use or inappropriate home storage. Intentional or unintentional misuse and suicide gestures and attempts account for the remainder of civilian cases. The toxicity of OPs varies greatly. The most highly toxic group is used primarily for agricultural and military purposes. Those with lower toxicity are available for use by households and commercially around populated areas. Table 76-1 lists some of the better-known commercial OPs, their uses, and their relative human toxicity. Table 76-2 lists some common commercial carbamates (in decreasing order of toxicity).

STRUCTURE

OPs are a heterogeneous group of compounds but share some common chemical properties. OPs contain a central phosphorus atom with a double bond to either oxygen (P=O) or sulfur (P=S), two organic side chains (R_1 and R_2), and an additional side chain that becomes the leaving group (X). The leaving group is specific to the individual OP and may be a cyanide, thiocyanate, halide, phosphate, phenoxy, thiophenoxy, or carboxylate group (Fig. 76-1). The R_1 and R_2 groups are aryl or alkyl groups and, in most of the common pesticides, are either two methyl or two ethyl ester groups that form the dimethyl (dimethoxy) or diethyl (diethoxy) OPs. Carbamates are similar but have nitrogen bound to oxygen or sulfur instead of a phosphoric acid residue (Fig. 76-2).

TABLE 76-1 Examples of Organophosphate Insecticides

COMMON NAME	PRODUCT EXAMPLE	CHEMICAL NAME	ESTIMATED FATAL ORAL DOSE (g/70 kg)
Agricultural Insecticides (high toxicity)			
Tetraethyl pyrophosphate	Miller Kilmite 40	Tetraethyl pyrophosphate	0.05
Phorate	Thimet (American Cyanamid)	0,0,-Diethyl (S-ethylmercaptomethyl) dithiophosphate	
Parathion	Niagara Phoskil Dust	0,0,-Diethyl-0-p-nitrophenyl phosphorothioate	0.1
Phosdrin	Mevinphos (Shell)	Dimethyl-0-(1-methyl-2-carbomethoxy-vinyl) phosphate	0.15
Disulfoton	Disyston	Diethyl-S-2-ethyl-2-mercaptoethyl phosphorodithioate	0.2
Animal Insecticides (intermediate toxicity)			
Coumaphos	Co-Ral Animal Insecticide	Diethyl-0-(3-chloro-4-methyl-7-coumarinyl) phosphorothioate	
Chlorpyrifos (Dursban)	Rid-A-Bug (Kenco)	0,0-Diethyl-0-(3,5,6-trichloro-2-pyridyl) phosphorothioate	
Trichlorfon	Trichlorfon Pour On (Hess & Clark)	Dimethyl trichlorohydroxyethyl phosphonate	
Ronnel	Korlan Livestock Spray (Dow)	0,0-dimethyl-0-(2,4,5-trichlorophenyl) phosphorothioate	
Household Use or Golf Course/Community Spray (low toxicity)			
Diazinon	Security Fire Ant Killer (Woolfolk)	Diethyl-0-(2-isopropyl-4-methyl-6-pyrimidyl) phosphorothioate	25.0
Malathion	Ortho Malathion 50 Insect Spray	Dimethyl-S-(1,2-bis-carboethoxy) ethyl phosphorodithioate	60.0
Vapona (dichlorvos, DDVP)	Shell No-Pest Strip	0,0-Dimethyl-0-2,2-dichlorovinyl phosphate	
Acephate	Chevron Orthene	0,S-Dimethylacetylphosphoramidothioate	

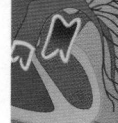

TABLE 76-2 Carbamate Insecticides

COMMERCIAL NAME	CHEMICAL
Temik	Aldicarb
Matacil	Aminocarb
Vydate	Oxamyl
Isolan	Isolan
Furadan	Carbofuran
Lannate	Methomyl
Zectran	Mexacarbate
Mesurol	Methiocarb
Dimetilan	Dimetilan
Baygon	Propoxur
Sevin	Carbaryl

From Coye MJ, Barnett PJ, Midtling JE, et al: Clinical confirmation of organophosphate poisoning by serial cholinesterase analyses. Arch Intern Med 1987;147:438.

FIGURE 76-1 Organophosphorus compound.

R$_1$ and R$_2$ = alkyl or aryl groups
X = leaving group and may be linked via O or S
Y = O or S or absent

FIGURE 76-2 Carbamate.

PHARMACOKINETICS

Organophosphorus agents are a diverse group of agents with widely variable human toxicity. The toxicity is largely determined by the individual agent, formulation, dose, route of exposure, duration of contact, and health status of exposed individuals. Estimates of relative human toxicity are typically based on the acute oral LD_{50} measured in rats. The WHO updated its toxicity ratings in 2002 and classified agents as extremely hazardous (Ia) (liquid state: $LD_{50} < 20$ mg/kg); highly hazardous (Ib) (20–200 mg/kg); moderately hazardous (II) (200–2000 mg/kg); and slightly hazardous (III) (>2000 mg/kg).[11] Extremely and highly hazardous agents are designated as "Poison or Toxic" on commercial labels. The WHO classification is different from that promulgated by the EPA, which classifies OP compounds as high toxicity (rat $LD_{50} < 50$ mg/kg), intermediate or moderate toxicity (LD_{50}, 50–1000 mg/kg) and low toxicity ($LD_{50} > 1000$ mg/kg)[12] (see Table 76-1). Thus, lethal doses for human

adults may vary from a few milligrams for the highly toxic agents (e.g., TEPP) to 50 g for the low-toxicity agents (e.g., malathion). Nerve agents are even more potent, with as little as 1 mg of sarin or soman being lethal to adult humans after inhalation of its vapors.[13] For nerve agents and other highly volatile or aerosolized OPs, toxicity is designated by a concentration time (Ct) variable that is a better measure of exposure by inhalation. For nerve agents, the lethal Ct_{50} ranges from 10 to 400 mg/min/m^3 (see Chapter 105A).[14]

Most OPs are effectively absorbed by all routes—dermal, respiratory, gastrointestinal, and conjunctival. The rapidity of onset and severity of effects may vary after exposure by different routes. The most common route of exposure is dermal, as occurs from most occupational and accidental poisonings. Most suicide attempts result from ingestion. Inhalation exposure may occur when agricultural pesticides (malathion and parathion) are dispersed as aerosols of solids in a liquid carrier or as a dust. Liquids may be mixed in a hydrocarbon vehicle for easy dispersal. The latter may facilitate absorption and add to the toxic effects (e.g., pulmonary toxicity). Aerosols can be absorbed through the skin, mucous membranes, and lungs, whereas liquids can be absorbed through the skin or ingested. Breaks in the skin may enhance absorption, and hot, humid environments or persistent skin contact can enhance toxicity. Gaseous, aerosolized, or dust forms of OPs have a rapid onset of action because they are taken immediately into the pulmonary circulation, leading to shortness of breath, bronchorrhea, bronchoconstriction, and rapid development of systemic signs and symptoms. Liquid and aerosolized forms can be absorbed through the skin; absorption depends on agent volatility, ambient temperature, and lipophilicity. These agents may show immediate local effects (local fasciculations and diaphoresis) or have delayed systemic effects. Ingested agents tend to have a rapid onset of action. Many OPs are highly lipophilic, which enhances their dermal absorption. High lipophilicity may also lead to agent sequestration in body fat stores and result in delayed and erratic toxicity that could occur for several days to weeks after initial exposure.

After absorption, OPs are commonly metabolized by hepatic oxidation, hydrolysis, and conjugation with glutathione. Some agents may undergo glucuronidation and demethylation. Oxidation occurs through the cytochrome P-450 system and often leads to bioactivation, or production of a more reactive oxon metabolite. Serum enzymes such as paraoxonase 1 (PON1) contribute to endogenous hydrolysis of several OPs, lipids, and other prodrugs.[15] Most OPs are rapidly degraded and eliminated in the urine; some may be detectable more than 48 hours after exposure.[16] OPs that are metabolized to para-nitrophenol, however, can be detected by measuring this metabolite in the urine. There is a rough correlation between the excretion of para-nitrophenol and the occurrence of illness.[17] Because the effect of cholinesterase inhibition is cumulative, toxicity may be evident after complete elimination of the OP, particularly with the fat-soluble agents.

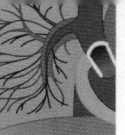
Although OP and carbamate insecticides are rapidly absorbed through dermal, respiratory, gastrointestinal (GI), and conjunctival routes, all OPs must be in the oxon formation (P=O) to inhibit acetylcholinesterase. Those agents that do not initially have the phosphorus bound to oxygen, such as the phosphorothioate (P=S), are metabolized by the hepatic cytochrome P-450 system into the activated oxon.[9] Parathion and malathion are examples of oxon activation; they must first be converted to paraoxon and malaoxon, respectively (by substitution of an oxygen for sulfur), to be physiologically active. Because of this activation step, the rapidity of symptom onset after OP exposure is partially dependent on the OP's initial state. Rate of activation and rate of enzyme inhibition may be equally important for toxicity. For example, in Sri Lanka, patients with dimethoate ingestions presented extremely ill but had acetylcholinesterase levels about one third to one fourth of normal, whereas patients similarly ill from chlorpyrifos and fenthion had almost no detectable cholinesterase levels. Most deaths from dimethoate occurred 24 to 36 hours after ingestion, at a time when their enzyme activity was continuing to decrease. All agents shared similar solvents, and the difference may reflect the low fat solubility of dimethoate, leading to a higher blood concentration.[18]

OPs that are already in the oxon form may cause symptoms earlier than those that need metabolic activation. However, some agents, such as parathion, are rapidly activated and can produce symptoms in less than 30 minutes.[19] Most OPs are readily lipid soluble, but certain agents (i.e., azinophos-ethyl, bromophos-ethyl, chlorpyrifos, coumaphos, diazinon, parathion, phosalone, sulfotep, and fenthion and chlorfenthion) are highly lipid soluble and tend to accumulate in adipose tissue.[15] Initial exposure may not lead to acute signs and symptoms of toxicity. After agent bioaccumulation and a time delay, the signs and symptoms of toxicity become evident.[9]

Carbamates have rapid onset but are less fat soluble. They may significantly inhibit acetylcholinesterase but undergo spontaneous hydrolysis with resumption of enzyme activity, usually within 24 hours. This is not an absolute, as some carbamates, such as carbosulfan, may have prolonged systemic effects.[20]

PHARMACOLOGY AND PATHOPHYSIOLOGY

OPs and carbamates produce toxicity by binding to and inhibiting the action of acetylcholinesterase at its serine active site. Acetylcholine accumulates at nerve terminals, initially stimulating, then paralyzing, cholinergic neurotransmission at both central and peripheral nicotinic and muscarinic receptors. Under normal physiologic conditions, acetylcholinesterase hydrolyzes acetylcholine into two primary inert fragments, acetic acid and choline, decreasing postsynaptic effect and neurotransmission and generating choline for reuptake and resynthesis. When acetylcholinesterase is inhibited, acetylcholine cannot be broken down and accumulates at the nerve or myoneural terminal, leading initially to

postsynaptic excitation followed by inactivation of the synapse or myoneural junction.[21] Inactivation occurs from depolarizing blockade at postsynaptic receptors.

True acetylcholinesterase (E.C. 3.1.1.7) is important for physiologic neurotransmission and is found primarily in nervous tissue but is also expressed on the surface of red blood cells (erythrocyte or red blood cell cholinesterase). Pseudocholinesterase or butyrylcholinesterase is found in serum and the liver and is important in the metabolism of xenobiotics. Erythrocyte acetylcholinesterase activity closely mimics neuronal acetylcholinesterase and is a more accurate measure of its physiologic activity.[22-24] Because butyrylcholinesterase (EC 3.1.1.8) measurements are technically simpler to perform, this is the more readily available assay in hospitals and in the field.[25]

Acetylcholinesterase is a convoluted protein structure with a pit containing a serine binding site and a catalytic site. Initially, the electrophilic OP oxon forms a reversible Michaelis-Menten complex, binding to the serine enzymatic active site followed by rapid phosphorylation of the serine residue. Once this happens, the leaving group (X) on the OP is released. As this reaction occurs, the OP becomes covalently bound to the enzyme, sitting in the pit and changing the conformation of the enzyme, preventing the active site from binding acetylcholine, and subsequently inhibiting catalytic activity.[26] The organophosphorylated enzyme can then undergo two different reactions. The enzyme can become "aged" or irreversibly bound and inactivated by cleavage of one of the R groups. This dealkylation process leads to a monosubstituted phosphoric acid residue that remains firmly attached to the enzyme. The rate of aging depends on the specific OP agent. Alternatively, reactivation of the enzyme can occur when the bond between the serine and organophosphorus moiety hydrolyzes. Enzyme reactivation occurs spontaneously at an extremely slow rate for diethyl-containing organophosphates or may be markedly accelerated with the addition of a nucleophilic oxime. The rate of reactivation and irreversible inactivation by aging is highly dependent on the attached R groups. Smaller side groups allow for more rapid reactivation and aging, whereas the presence of branched side chains provides steric hindrance and greater bond stability, thereby delaying reactivation and aging.[27] For instance, dimethyl OPs have significantly faster rates of spontaneous reactivation and aging (half-lives of about 0.7 hours and about 3.7 hours, respectively) than diethyl OPs (half-lives of 31 hours and 33 hours, respectively). Although dimethyl phosphorylated OPs age more rapidly than diethyl OPs, they are relatively resistant to oxime therapy, particularly pralidoxime. Although there is more time to reactivate diethyl OPs, they require significantly more oxime to achieve this reactivation.[9,28] Regardless of these differences, however, once the enzyme has "aged," it is no longer susceptible to reactivation by endogenous hydrolysis or oxime therapy.[9,29]

Carbamates bind to the same binding site of acetylcholinesterase by carbamylation (C-O bond). The carbamate–acetylcholinesterase covalent bond is not as

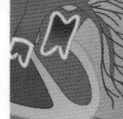

strong as that produced by OPs (P-O or P-S bond). Because of this, spontaneous hydrolysis or decarbamylation occurs more readily, usually reactivating acetylcholinesterase within 24 hours. Some carbamates may take longer to spontaneously hydrolyze. For example, in Sri Lanka, carbofuran-poisoned patients required ventilatory support for up to 48 to 72 hours.[17] Carbamylated acetylcholinesterase does not undergo irreversible binding or "aging" and can be reactivated using oximes.[24,30,31]

Acetylcholinesterase inhibition is not an equilibrium-dependent reaction and is most sensitive to the concentration of OP present at the enzyme interface. After a person is exposed to an OP, the formation of oxon peaks and then declines in the serum. However, even with a declining OP and oxon serum concentration, acetylcholinesterase inhibition continues to increase because this reaction proceeds by covalent binding. Physiologically, the exposed individual can continue to function normally until a minimum amount of functioning acetylcholinesterase is left unbound. Once this threshold has been reached, even removal of circulating OP will not enhance enzyme function. Enzyme catalysis then becomes entirely dependent on the restoration of a critical mass of uninhibited acetylcholinesterase. However, if the phosphorylated acetylcholinesterase can undergo a rapid endogenous reactivation such as with some dimethoxy OPs, then removal of the offending agent may contribute to recovery, but this is not true for dimethoate. The ability of a nucleophilic oxime to reactivate the enzyme depends then on the structure of the OP bound to acetylcholinesterase, the time that the reactivator is present at the site, and the concentration of the reactivator.[9,28]

The actual process of reactivating the phosphorylated acetylcholinesterase with a nucleophilic oxime involves formation of an intermediate step. At some point, a transient complex forms consisting of the phosphorylated enzyme and oxime. Because formation of this complex undergoes saturation kinetics, further increases in oxime concentration does not enhance reactivation. After the oxime has pulled off the OP from the enzyme, the phosphorylated oxime complex becomes a strong inhibitor of acetylcholinesterase. In addition, oximes themselves can inhibit acetylcholinesterase. The net effect is that even during treatment of an OP-inhibited enzyme with an oxime, there may be a transient, but undocumented, increase in inhibited acetylcholinesterase and worsening of symptoms.[9] This has not been shown to occur with pralidoxime because the phosphorylated oxime formed is very unstable, transiently present, and likely without clinical effect. More likely, there is no net difference. If the oxime removes the organophosphate from acetylcholinesterase and forms an active phosphorylated oxime, it can still only react with one acetylcholinesterase molecule so the stoichiometry remains unchanged (personal communication, Peter Eyer, 2006). Obidoxime produces a much more stable phosphorylated oxime and could have clinical consequences. This, however, has not yet been documented in vivo in humans.[32]

Despite oxime treatment, poisoning with highly fat-soluble agents (e.g., fenthion) or large exposures to agents that require bioactivation or prolonged elimination (e.g., fenthion) may lead to recurrent or delayed clinical toxicity. This is because the newly regenerated enzyme becomes reinhibited as the OP leaches out of the fat tissue or is bioactivated over a longer period of time.

The signs and symptoms of OP intoxication result from the overabundance of acetylcholine. This leads to initial excitation followed by paralyzed neurotransmission at cholinergic synapses.[26] Cholinergic neurotransmission occurs throughout the CNS, at the parasympathetic nerve endings, at a few sympathetic nerve endings such as the sweat glands (muscarinic effects), and in the somatic nerves (e.g., neuromuscular junction) and ganglionic synapses of autonomic ganglia (nicotinic effects). The signs and symptoms of OP poisoning are an expression of acetylcholine excess at numerous different nerve terminals (Table 76-3) and can manifest predominantly as muscarinic or nicotinic effects, or as a combination of both. The effects of OPs on acetylcholinesterase affect m-receptors differently than n-receptors and may account for some of the clinical variation. The OP effect on cholinesterase affecting m-receptors appears to be long-lasting, whereas n-receptors rapidly desensitize. Acetylcholine overstimulation at the neuromuscular junction leads to depolarization inactivation of myocytes; repolarization and, thus, recontraction are inhibited. This leads to muscle paralysis. In addition, the cholinergic nervous system has significant interplay with other neurotransmitters (i.e., γ-aminobutyric acid [GABA]) and results in additional toxic effects. CNS effects result largely from m-receptor stimulation but also occur from activation of n-receptors and *N*-methyl-*d*-

TABLE 76-3 Clinical Effects of Organophosphate Poisoning (Acetylcholine Excess)

ANATOMIC SITE OF ACTION	SIGNS AND SYMPTOMS
Muscarinic Effects	
Sweat glands	Sweating
Pupils	Constricted pupils
Lacrimal glands	Lacrimation
Salivary glands	Excessive salivation
Bronchial tree	Wheezing
Gastrointestinal	Cramps, vomiting, diarrhea, tenesmus
Cardiovascular	Bradycardia, decrease in blood pressure
Ciliary body	Blurred vision
Bladder	Urinary incontinence
Nicotinic Effects	
Striated muscle	Fasciculations, cramps, weakness, twitching, paralysis, respiratory embarrassment, cyanosis, arrest
Sympathetic ganglia	Tachycardia, elevated blood pressure
Central Nervous System Effects	Anxiety, restlessness, ataxia, convulsions, insomnia, coma, absent reflexes, Cheyne-Stokes respirations, respiratory and circulatory depression

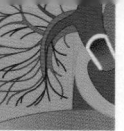

aspartate (NMDA) glutamate receptors and inhibition of central GABA neurotransmission.[19,33,34]

After the OP–acetylcholinesterase complex has undergone complete aging, enzyme resynthesis is the only means to restore acetylcholinesterase function. This may take weeks to months and necessitate prolonged pulmonary support for patients until sufficient enzyme resynthesis has occurred.[9]

TOXICOLOGY

Clinical Presentation

The onset and severity of clinical effects is variable and depends on the identity of the agent, its formulation, and the dose, duration, and route of exposure. Initial symptoms may range from mild to immediately life threatening. The most rapid onset of symptoms occurs with inhalation, and the slowest with dermal exposure. The onset of clinical effects may take up to 24 hours after skin exposure to highly lipophilic agents that require bioactivation. In contrast, systemic effects and respiratory arrest can occur within minutes of inhalation of an aerosol or vapor of nerve agents. After OP ingestion, clinical effects usually occur within 30 to 90 minutes. Although OP toxicity generally occurs within 4 to 12 hours, full-blown toxicity may not manifest for 24 hours.[35]

Stimulation of the muscarinic parasympathetic system will cause miosis, bradycardia, hypotension, bronchoconstriction, hyperactivity of GI smooth muscle, and oversecretion of the exocrine glands (salivary, lacrimal, bronchial, and pancreatic). Stimulation of the autonomic ganglia (nicotinic effects) produces sympathomimetic effects that include tachycardia, hypertension, and mydriasis. Nicotinic effects at the neuromuscular junction lead to muscle weakness, fasciculations, and muscle paralysis. This is also known as type I paralysis.[18] (see Table 76-3). GI symptoms are the most common manifestations early after ingestion of OPs. Aerosol exposure typically presents with respiratory and ocular complaints, whereas dermal exposure may cause localized fasciculations and sweating. The wide and mixed spectrum of clinical effects that occur with significant exposures may lead to misdiagnosis. In one study, 16 of 20 transfer patients were incorrectly diagnosed as having other conditions.[36] The presence of excessive salivation, lacrimation, fasciculations, noncardiogenic rales or rhonchi, and muscle weakness during the initial phase of poisoning is suggestive of OP poisoning. Miosis, a typical muscarinic sign, is not always present because mydriasis may result from concomitant and overriding nicotinic stimulation. Senanayake and colleagues developed a nonvalidated scoring system for organophosphorus intoxications called the Peradeniya Organophosphorus Poisoning Scale (POP Scale).[37] This system ranks the severity of poisonings using five clinical signs (miosis, bradycardia, heart rate, level of consciousness, and respiratory rate). Each sign is graded on a scale from 0 to 2, with an additional point given for those that seize. Based on results from the initial study, severe intoxications (score of 8 to 11) have a higher mortality rate, greater need for ventilatory support, and higher dose of atropine in the first 24 hours.

CNS effects generally include anxiety, restlessness, agitation, slurred speech, ataxia, confusion, lethargy, stupor, coma, seizures, and centrally mediated respiratory depression.[38] In addition, chorea, psychosis, depression, and choreoathetosis have been described.[39] Muscle weakness and paralysis develop in severe exposures. The most common cause of death is primary respiratory failure with subsequent cardiac arrest.[40] Early respiratory failure is largely mediated by CNS respiratory center depression from increased, uncoordinated CNS muscarinic neuronal activity.[19,26] In animal studies, such early respiratory depression can be prevented by anticholinergic agents that cross the blood-brain barrier.[26] Peripheral nicotinic and muscarinic effects contribute to respiratory failure and include excessive oral and tracheobronchial secretions, laryngospasm, bronchoconstriction, and paralysis of the diaphragm and intercostal muscles. There may be additional noncholinergic-mediated effects.[34]

Other findings associated with acute OP intoxication include hyperamylasemia with or without clinical pancreatitis.[41] Electrocardiogram abnormalities have been reported and include conduction disturbances (e.g., atrioventricular block, ST-segment elevation, QTc prolongation) and arrhythmias (e.g., supraventricular and ventricular dysrhythmias, including torsades de pointes).[42,43]

Diagnosis

The diagnosis of acute OP poisoning is made clinically and based on history and suggestive physical findings. The diagnosis should be considered whenever a patient presents with the cholinergic toxidrome or muscarinic signs and symptoms such as miosis, increased airway secretions, lacrimation, bradycardia, and GI complaints. The added presence of nicotinic findings such as muscle fasciculations and weakness further suggests the diagnosis of OP poisoning. A history of exposure is helpful but not often available. The simultaneous presence of muscarinic and nicotinic findings on physical exam are characteristic of organophosphorus poisoning and often warrant empiric treatment with atropine and oxime therapy. Clinical findings suggestive of severe OP poisoning (i.e., mental status changes, coma, seizures, bronchorrhea, bronchoconstriction, fasciculations, autonomic instability, and paralysis) warrant immediate treatment presumptively. When multiple victims become comatose or seize within minutes of an inhalational exposure, a terrorist incident with nerve agents should be suspected and empiric antidotal treatment given provided that supportive physical findings are present[14] (see Chapter 105A). When the diagnosis of OP poisoning is not evident or when toxicity is mild or chronic, a depressed serum or red blood cell cholinesterase level may be obtained to assist diagnosis. Cholinesterase levels, however, are rarely available in a timely manner.

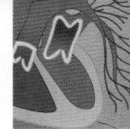

Thus, if OP poisoning is suspected, therapy should be initiated before confirmation by laboratory values.

Laboratory confirmation of poisoning is demonstrated by depressed erythrocyte or butyrylcholinesterase activity. Because non–hemoglobin normalized acetylcholinesterase levels are extremely variable between individuals, a mild intoxication may not be confirmed until serial levels document a steady increase in enzyme activity over time.[22,23] Erythrocyte acetylcholinesterase that is standardized to hemoglobin does not exhibit the same interindividual variability. As erythrocyte acetylcholinesterase is expressed on the erythrocyte membrane, in the absence of reactivation, restitution of normal, preintoxication enzyme activity levels are dependent on formation of new erythrocytes, a process that takes about 90 to 120 days and mimics neurologic function.[23,24] However, erythrocyte acetylcholinesterase regenerates more slowly than neuromuscular junction acetylcholinesterase. Butyrylcholinesterase is an acute-phase reactant and may normalize in 14 to 30 days. There is a genetic variant in about 3% of the population, causing baseline depression of butyrylcholinesterase activity level. Other conditions that may depress butyrylcholinesterase include parenchymal liver disease, secondary hepatic insufficiency from congestive heart failure, metastatic carcinoma, reduced levels of serum albumin, pregnancy, and several medications.[44,45]

The remainder of diagnostic studies are nonspecific and include elevated leukocyte count and hyperglycemia.[46] Occasionally, elevated levels of urinary p-nitrophenol may be found in cases of OP intoxication in which para-nitrophenol is the leaving group (e.g., parathion).[19,47]

Management

Treatment of OP poisoning consists of aggressive supportive care and antidotal therapy.

Initial management of the OP- or carbamate-poisoned patient requires immediate attention to the airway. Cyanosis or other evidence of hypoxia, rales, excessive oral secretions, or bronchorrhea should be treated with oxygen and rapid atropinization. Although most texts state that the patient should be oxygenated before atropine administration, it may be impossible to oxygenate until secretions are controlled. In a large cohort of OP-poisoned patients, Eddleston successfully administered early atropine without evidence of enhanced cardiovascular toxicity.[48] Atropine should be dosed until the secretions have dried and evidence of pulmonary fluid has diminished. During rapid atropinization, respiratory paralysis or excessive secretions should be managed by controlling the airway with intubation, ventilation, and continuous suctioning. When rapid sequence intubation (RSI) is necessary to control the airway of an OP- or carbamate-poisoned patient, the use of a depolarizing paralytic (e.g., succinylcholine), although not contraindicated, is discouraged. In such cases, succinylcholine may result in prolonged paralysis because it is metabolized through butyrylcholinesterase.[49] In one patient poisoned with chlorpyrifos, the use of succinylcholine resulted in neuro-muscular paralysis that lasted 192 minutes.[49] There are no data on the effect of prolonged chemical paralysis with a nondepolarizing agent in the OP-poisoned patient.[50] Thus, the use of rocuronium or other rapidly acting nondepolarizing agents is preferable for RSI in these patients. Concomitant with atropinization, patients should be resuscitated with intravenous (IV) fluids. OP pesticides result in significant GI fluid losses and probably cause nitric oxide–induced vasodilation.[51] Rapid IV administration of 2 L or more of an isotonic solution may be necessary to return the patient to euvolemia. Vasopressors are indicated when hypotension is unresponsive to atropine and fluids. A direct-acting α-adrenergic agent (e.g., phenylephrine) is preferred because poisoned patients have a reduced systemic vascular resistance and relatively normal inotropic state.[38,43,52-54] Dopamine and norepinephrine may increase the heart rate, which could prove beneficial or detrimental, depending on the initial pulse. These pressor recommendations, however, are based on pharmacologic principles and not animal or clinical data.

Seizure activity should be rapidly controlled with an IV GABAergic agent such as diazepam, midazolam, or lorazepam. Aggressive use of benzodiazepines may improve survival and prevent cardiac and CNS injury in OP-poisoned patients with seizures.[34,55-62] Many dosing regimens have been suggested. Initial dosing recommendations include the use at least 10 mg IV diazepam or 5 to 10 mg intramuscular (IM) midazolam in adults (pediatric dosing, diazepam 0.1–0.2 mg/kg IV or midazolam, 0.1–0.3 mg/kg IM) and then titrate upward as needed. There is some evidence to suggest that OP-induced seizures involve NMDA-glutamate receptors in addition to GABA, suggesting that propofol may be a useful adjunct for continued seizure activity. Both central GABA and NMDA-glutamate receptor pathways are likely involved with seizure production and delayed CNS neuropathology associated with significant poisoning with these agents (personal communication, M. Eddleston and A. Dawson, 2004).[58-61,63,64]

After initial stabilization, patient decontamination becomes a priority. Patients with liquid contamination of skin and clothing may have ongoing percutaneous absorption of a pesticide. In addition, they may pose a skin contact risk to health care personnel. Interestingly, there have been almost no reports of clinically significant healthcare worker secondary contamination coming from the South Asian and Indian continents, where OP intoxicaation is extremetly common.[65,66] Thus, as soon as possible, the patient should be disrobed completely and the skin thoroughly washed with alkaline soap and water. This should not delay initial life-saving treatment and administration of antidotes. The removal of clothing eliminates 85% to 90% of a contamination hazard.[67] Although hypochlorite solutions deactivate OPs in vitro, their use on human tissues is discouraged and may lead to corneal burns and other toxicity.[68] A standard hypochlorite solution (5%) can be used to decontaminate equipment.[69-72] Alternatively, the U.S. Military has adopted dry agents for field decontamination.[68] In civilian use, agents such as soil, flour, or

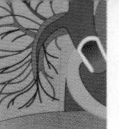

talcum powder may be applied to the skin and then mechanically removed.[71]

One of the first priorities in OP and nerve agent treatment is health care provider self-protection and decontamination. Medical personnel participating in the decontamination process should have adequate personal protective equipment (PPE) and training. Ideally, the patient should have undergone initial decontamination at the scene by appropriate personnel trained in Hazardous Materials in Level A or Level B protection. At the Health Care Facility, medical staff should be dressed at the minimum in Level C PPE, including impermeable gowns and shoe covers; butyl, neoprene, or nitrile gloves; and facial splash protection[70,73] (see Chapter 103). Standard latex gloves are readily permeable to and do not protect from transdermal absorption of OP agents. Solutions or dry agents used for decontamination are considered hazardous materials, and arrangements for their disposal should be prearranged. Further discussion on appropriate PPE and training should be directed to the local Poison Control Center, Metropolitan Medical Response System, HazMat team, Hospital Disaster Plan, or State Department of Health.[72]

The utility of GI decontamination after ingestion of an organophosphorus ester pesticide is controversial. Because these agents are highly emetogenic, most patients have vomited before presentation. If a patient presents early (less than 30–60 minutes) after ingestion, empiric nasogastric aspiration of an ingested solution seems appropriate. There are, however, no published randomized controlled trials (RCTs) that have evaluated the efficacy of this modality. Some OP agents are known to bind activated charcoal. Thus, the administration of oral activated charcoal is usually recommended after oral OP pesticide exposure. As for gastric lavage and aspiration, the efficacy of activated charcoal for OP poisoning by ingestion has been not been adequately studied. Because many of the OP agents are dissolved in hydrocarbon solvents that can result in significant pneumonitis when aspirated, the potential benefits of gastric decontamination must be balanced against the risk for enhanced morbidity from aspiration for each patient treated.[50] Currently, there is an ongoing large RCT in Sri Lanka investigating these issues.[73,74] Gastrointestinal decontamination is rarely necessary after nerve agent exposure because these patients have been poisoned by inhalation or dermal contact (see Chapter 105A).

ANTIDOTAL THERAPY

The accepted mainstays of antidotal therapy in OP poisoning are adequate use of atropine to treat muscarinic symptoms and an oxime to regenerate the acetylcholinesterase.[9,28] Atropine, a competitive antagonist at muscarinic cholinergic receptors, inhibits the postsynaptic binding of acetylcholine. As a tertiary amine structure, atropine crosses the blood-brain barrier and works at both peripheral and central muscarinic sites. It has no effect at nicotinic cholinergic receptors. Although there have been no RCTs to demonstrate the efficacy of

atropine for OP and carbamates poisoning, there are innumerable case reports that substantiate its efficacy and usefulness for this poisoning.[50] Atropine is indicated for muscarinic symptoms, primarily bronchorrhea and, sometimes, bradydysrhythmias and hypotension. The dosing of atropine is variable, and the dosing regimen used by Eddleston and colleagues is recommended. From their experience with OP poisonings in Sri Lanka, Eddleston and colleagues have shown that the administration of rapid, escalating doses of atropine ("rapid atropinization") followed by an atropine infusion is successful in controlling the airway and other muscarinic symptoms.[48,50] With this approach, patients with evidence of muscarinic excess are initially given 1 to 2 mg IV atropine, and doses are then doubled every 5 minutes as needed. This dosing regimen will rapidly yield a cumulative dose of 25 mg by 20 minutes and 75 mg by 25 minutes.[48] Patients with severe toxicity may require 75 to 100 mg atropine. The adequacy of atropine dosing is determined clinically by clearing secretions from the pulmonary tract as assessed by resolution of crepitus and rales, a heart rate greater than 80 beats/minute, dry skin, and a reasonable blood pressure (mean arterial pressure > 60 mm Hg or evidence of end-organ perfusion). Pupil dilation can be delayed up to 30 minutes and is not a useful sign initially, but the eventual aim is to have nonpinpoint pupils. However, in the Sri Lankan experience, patients with severe OP poisoning had mid to large but mildly reactive pupils after an adequate atropine dose had been administered (personal communication, M. Eddleston and A. Dawson, 2004).[48,50] After the patient has been stabilized, an atropine drip is established to maintain the patient at the appropriate level of atropinization, usually around 20% of the total loading dose per hour, and is titrated as needed. More than 5 mg/hr of atropine is rarely needed.[75] Glycopyrrolate has been suggested as an alternative to atropine. However, because it does not cross the blood-brain barrier, it should be reserved for patients with a purely peripheral muscarinic syndrome.[33,76-79] The use of inhaled atropine or ipratropium bromide has been recommended when pulmonary symptoms predominate to minimize systemic side effects produced by intravenous atropine administration.[33,34]

Although "rapid atropinization" is life saving, this method of atropine administration may occasionally overshoot and produce an anticholinergic delirium. In this situation, the atropine infusion should be halted and the patient closely observed until signs of cholinergic excess begin to reappear. At this point, the atropine can be restarted.[48] When this occurs, the patient may need sedation until the delirium recedes. Benzodiazepines appear to be the safest option in this situation.

Nerve agent intoxication does not appear to require similar atropine dosing (see Chapter 105A). Experience from the Matsumoto and Tokyo sarin incidents and declassified case reports suggest that 2 to 20 mg atropine appears to be adequate.[13,14,71,80,81] In the Tokyo sarin attacks, only 19% of poisoned patients required more than 2 mg of atropine.[7] Topical ocular homatropine or

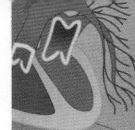

atropine preparations may be effective for focal ocular cholinergic toxicity (e.g., eye pain, dim vision) produced by aerosol nerve agent exposures.[71]

Oximes are used early after OP poisoning to regenerate active acetylcholinesterase. The use of oximes has become somewhat controversial after several Asian studies failed to demonstrate their efficacy for OP poisoning.[82-84,85] The conclusions of these studies, however, have been questioned because of flawed trial design and other reasons.[28,29] In Western countries, use of oxime therapy is fairly well accepted, and there are multiple animal studies and human case reports supporting its efficacy.[24,28,30,86-92] Pralidoxime (2-PAM chloride, Protopam) and obidoxime (Toxogonin) are the most commonly used agents, although P2S (pralidoxime mesylate), pralidoxime methiodide, TMB-4, HI-6 and HLö-7 (experimental use only) are used in other parts of the world. The H-series oximes (e.g., HI-6 and HLö-7) have greater efficacy against certain nerve agents (e.g., soman) and may be preferable for such poisoning. Multiple textbooks and the package insert for Protopam suggest that oxime therapy should be reserved for nicotinic signs and symptoms. There is no scientific basis for this because oximes will regenerate acetylcholinesterase at both muscarinic and nicotinic receptors. Many patients who were treated with only atropine may have had adequate endogenous hydrolysis of the phosphorylated acetylcholinesterase. Use of oxime therapy in carbamate poisoning is another area of uncertainty. On average, carbamylated acetylcholinesterase will spontaneously hydrolyze within 24 hours. Patients poisoned with carbamates, however, may become severely ill and require ventilatory support for greater than 24 hours, similar to an OP poisoning. There is good evidence to suggest that oximes are effective for treating these carbamate-poisoned patients and shortening intensive care unit time.[24,31,87,93-97] The exception to this may be carbaryl (Sevin), for which there is animal evidence to suggest that oxime use may worsen the cholinesterase block. There are no human data that demonstrate enhanced toxicity from oxime use in carbaryl-poisoned patients.[93,94,97] Currently, oxime therapy is recommended for all carbamate poisonings with the exception of carbaryl.

The apparent ineffectiveness of oximes for OP poisoning has several possible explanations. First, reactivation of acetylcholinesterase may be slowed and ineffective because of steric effects of certain OP compounds at the active site. Second, the rate of acetylcholinesterase inhibition may be greater than its rate of reactivation because of insufficient oxime dosing relative to the degree of OP exposure. Third, formation of phosphoryloximes during the reactivation process may paradoxically inhibit acetylcholinesterase to a greater extent and longer duration than would be present without oxime therapy. This is more significant with obidoxime than pralidoxime. Finally, oxime therapy may not be provided for a long enough time in instances in which OP metabolic activation or tissue redistribution occurs. Similarly, oxime therapy may not be initiated for patients who present late because of the belief that all the cholinesterases will have aged. Aging is a process,

and it is believed that as the acetylcholine accumulates at the receptor, acetylcholinesterase competes with the OP for the binding site.[27]

Most oxime controversy relates to appropriate dosing. Most U.S. textbooks suggest a pralidoxime dose of 1 to 2 g IV or IM followed by 1 g every 6 to 12 hours. This dose has not been subjected to rigorous scrutiny and may lead to low serum oxime concentrations. A serum concentration of 4 mg/L has been suggested as the minimum oxime "therapeutic level" for OP poisoning; this value was derived from animal data.[98,99] A subsequent pharmacokinetic study by Medicis used a pralidoxime infusion in human volunteers to maintain this serum concentration.[100] Further study has suggested that 1 g pralidoxime every 6 to 8 hours or the infusion rate from the Medicis study are inadequate to treat significantly poisoned patients and that larger oxime doses are necessary.[32,98,101-103] There are a number of reasons for this, which include poor affinity of oximes for the phosphorylated enzyme complex, overwhelming inhibition by a large OP exposure, reinhibition of the enzyme by sustained or high levels of OP, OP persistence in a deep compartment such as seen with extremely fat-soluble agents (duration of treatment), and aging of the enzyme.[9,28] The WHO has recommended an initial dose of 30 mg/kg pralidoxime IV followed by an IV infusion of 8 mg/kg/hr. Alternatively, if a continuous infusion is not possible, 30 mg/kg pralidoxime should be administered IM or IV every 4 hours. Obidoxime is dosed at 4 mg/kg initially then 0.5 mg/kg/hr or 4 mg/kg initially then 2 mg/kg every 4 hours. Both agents may be administered IV or IM.[104] Based on computer kinetic modeling, Eyer and associates have determined that an ideal plasma concentration of 50 to 100 μmol/L for pralidoxime and 10 μmol/L for obidoxime should produce an acceptable half-life of reactivation of about 10 minutes.[19] These can be achieved with a pralidoxime dosing of 1 g IV followed by 0.5 g/hr or an obidoxime dosing of 250 mg initially followed by 750 mg over 24 hours.[27] Regardless, the ideal oxime dose has not yet been established and will probably depend on the OP agent, time since exposure, body load, pharmacogenetics, and other variables. The South Asian Clinical Toxicology Research Collaboration initiated a study in 2004 that compares the WHO pralidoxime regimen versus placebo in the treatment of OP poisoning in Sri Lanka (personal communication, M. Eddleston and A. Dawson, 2004). These data should help to clarify the optimal pralidoxime dosing strategy.

It is important to be aware of the treatment distinction between diethyl and dimethyl phosphoryl OPs. Dimethyl-poisoned patients have a shorter window of opportunity for oxime treatment and necessitate higher doses. This discrepancy may be partially responsible for the variable results reported in the literature. Treatment of nerve agent poisoning follows similar precepts but uses a different dosing strategy. Because the G nerve agents age extremely rapidly, treatment must be started immediately (see Chapter 105A).

Adverse reactions from oxime therapy include hypertension, transient increases in neuromuscular block, and projectile vomiting after bolus administration of pral-

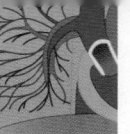

idoxime (personal communication, M. Eddleston and A. Dawson, 2004).[29,100,104] There are no good data on the effects of pralidoxime in the first trimester of pregnancy.[106,107] Pralidoxime is categorized by the U.S. Food and Drug Administration as a pregnancy category C medication. Thus, it should only be used with initial careful consideration of the relative risks and benefits to the mother and child.[108,109]

INTERMEDIATE SYNDROME

In 1987, Senanayake described a syndrome of proximal muscle weakness, weak neck flexors, and respiratory failure, which he designated as the intermediate syndrome (IMS) or type II paralysis.[110,111] The IMS has onset within 24 to 72 hours after the acute cholinergic crisis and can last several days to weeks.[112-116] Many authors have debated the existence of IMS versus continued neuromuscular junction (NMJ) acetylcholinesterase depression in the face of inadequate oxime therapy.[117-119] The syndrome has been characterized by absent muscarinic symptoms but continued severe acetylcholinesterase inhibition as measured by cholinesterase activity, and there is no therapy other than supportive care.[112,120-122] Electromyograms—Nerve Conduction Velocity Studies done during IMS have shown decrement pattern in neuromuscular transmission with repetitive stimulation at low rates consistent with presynaptic and postsynaptic impairment at the NMJ and desensitization.[123,124] At this time, there is no consensus on etiology; the pralidoxime study in Sri Lanka may provide some insight on this problem. Treatment of IMS is primarily supportive. Some recommend the administration of additional oxime, but few data support this recommendation.

DELAYED POLYNEUROPATHY (ORGANOPHOSPHATE-INDUCED DELAYED NEUROPATHY OR POLYNEUROPATHY)

Several classes of OPs (phosphates, phosphoramidates, and phosphonates) inhibit both acetylcholinesterase and neuropathy target esterase (NTE).[125,126] NTE is found on the Schwann cells lining the axons and, when aged, causes loss of the myelin sheath with a "dying back" axonopathy that is unresponsive to atropine and pralidoxime.[125,127-129] This leads to a symmetric demyelinating process with the patient complaining about cramping pain, paresthesias, and distal limb weakness. Patients notice the onset of weakness and paresthesias about 3 to 6 weeks after initial illness, with subsequent progression over weeks to months.[130,131] A lymphocyte NTE assay has been developed to assist diagnosis; depression of lymphocyte NTE correlates with development of organophosphate-induced delayed neuropathy (OPIDN).[132-138] There is no known treatment for OPIDN. Resolution may occur over 6 months to a year for those with mild symptoms, whereas those with severe OPIDN usually have persistent deficits.[125,130-136]

CHRONIC NEUROPSYCHIATRIC SEQUELAE

A number of other neurologic sequelae that have been associated with OP intoxication. Acutely, patients may develop severe encephalopathy.[139] Long-term effects have included short-term memory loss, fatigue, confusion, depression, psychosis, parkinsonism, and other extrapyramidal findings.[139-144] Some of these findings may resolve over time.

NEW TREATMENT DEVELOPMENTS

One of the difficulties in treating OP-poisoned patients is determining when to stop oxime therapy. Eyer and associates have started to assay whole blood for the ability of oximes to reactivate red blood cell cholinesterase before and during treatment. Ongoing acetylcholinesterase inhibition, recrudescent poisoning, and response to therapy could be recognized and diagnosed from a decrease in the ability to reactivate red blood cell cholinesterase in patient whole blood.[19] The increasing importance of pharmacogenomics is also being investigated. Depending on the paraxon concentration, studies in liver microsomal studies have shown that paraoxon has variable effects on the cytochrome P-450 enzymes (e.g., CYP1A2, 2B6, and 3A4). During parathion desulfuration, an electrophilic sulfur is released, which inactivates the cytochromes, leading to significant effects on other metabolic processes and detoxification of xenobiotics.[19]

Research on the use of hydrolases to treat OP toxicity has led to the potential for use of bacterial phosphotriesterases to cleave OPs.[145-147] The discovery of polymorphism in the *PON1* genetic coding suggests that there is a variable sensitivity to toxicity of OPs.[14,148] This may help to explain why some people exhibit a higher degree of toxicity when exposed to the same agents.

Other promising novel therapies for OP pesticide poisoning are being researched. There has been at least 10 years of work on the Hagedorn agents HI-6 and HLö-7. These two agents and others continue to show promise as the preferred oximes for nerve agent toxicity (see Chapter 105A).[28,86,89,90,149-152] Alkalinization with sodium bicarbonate has increased survival in animal models and may be useful in humans.[153,154] A recent Cochrane review of alkalinization for the treatment of OP intoxication suggested that it may be useful clinically, but there is insufficient evidence for routine use.[152] A promising new line of investigation is the use of OP hydrolases to break down OPs before they can covalently bind to acetylcholinesterase. Data from in vitro and animal models have demonstrated that the combined use of bacterial OP hydrolases and oxime therapy has been successful in preventing reinhibition of acetylcholinesterase.[155-157] Finally, human butyrylcholinesterase has been used to increase survival in soman-poisoned rats.[158,159]

ACKNOWLEDGMENTS

Special thanks to Drs. Darren Roberts, Peter Eyer, and Michael Eddleston for their editing contributions to this chapter.

REFERENCES

1. Eddleston M, Phillips MR: Self-poisoning with pesticides. BMJ 2004;328:42–44.

2. Gunnell D, Eddleston M: Suicide by intentional ingestion of pesticides: a continuing tragedy in developing countries. Int J Epidemiol 2003;32:902–909.
3. Jeyaratnam J: Acute pesticide poisoning: a major global health problem. World Health Stat Q 1990;43:139–144.
4. International Programme of Chemical Safety (IPCS INTOX): Pesticide Project: Collection of Human Case Data Exposures to Pesticides, 2002, http://www.intox.org/firstpage.htm.
5. CDC National Institute for Occupational Safety and Health: NIOSH Safety and Health Topic: Pesticide Illness and Injury Surveillance, http://www.cdc.gov/niosh/topics/pesticides/2004.
6. Watson WA, Litovitz TL, Rodgers CG Jr, et al: 2002 annual report of the American Association of Poison Control Centers Toxic Exposure Surveillance System. Am J Emerg Med 2003;21(5):353–421.
7. Watson WA, Litovitz TL, Rodgers GC, et al: 2004 annual report of the American Association of Poison Control Centers Toxic Exposure Surveillance System. Am J Emerg Med 2005;23:589–666.
8. Okumura T, Takasu N, Ishimatsu S et al: Report on 640 victims of the Tokyo subway sarin attack. Ann Emerg Med 1996;28(2):129–135.
9. Johnson MK, Jacobsen D, Meredith TJ, et al: Evaluation of antidotes for poisoning by organophosphorus pesticides. Emerg Med 2000;12:22–37.
10. Buttler T, Martinkovic W, Nesheim N: Factors influencing the movement of pesticides to ground water. In Pesticide Information Office (ed): University of Florida Cooperative Extension Service (EDIS), 1998, http://edas.ifas.ufl.edu/pdffiles/PI/P100200.pdf.
11. World Health Organization: The WHO recommended classification of pesticides by hazard. In International Programme on Chemical Safety (eds): Inter-organization Programme for the Sound Management of Chemicals, 2004, http:www.who.int/ipcs/publications/pesticides_hazards_rev_3.pdf.
12. Morgan DP: Recognition and management of pesticide poisonings, 4th ed, Vol. EPA-540/9-88-001. Washington, DC, U.S. Environmental Protection Agency, 1989.
13. Zajtchuk R, Bellamy RF (eds): Textbook of Military Medicine: Medical Aspects of Chemical and Biological Warfare. Part I. Washington, DC, Office of the Surgeon General, U.S. Dept of the Army, 1997, pp 129–179.
14. Sidell FR: Nerve agents. In Zajtchuk R, Bellamy RF (eds): Textbook of Military Medicine. Part 1. Warfare, Weaponry and the Casualty: Medical Aspects of Chemical and Biological Warfare. Washington, DC, Office of the Surgeon General, U.S. Army, 1997.
15. Costa LG, Cole TB, Furlong CE: Polymorphisms of paraoxonase (PON1) and their significance in clinical toxicology of organophosphates. J Toxicol Clin Toxicol 2003;41(1):37–45.
16. Temple WA, Smith NA: Organophosphorus pesticides (PIM G001). In IPCS INTOX Databank, http://www.intox.org/databank/documents/chemical/organpho/PIMG001.htm.
17. Hayes WJ Jr: Pesticides Studied in Man. Baltimore, Williams & Wilkins, 1982.
18. Eddleston M, Dawson A, Karalliedde L, et al: Early management after self-poisoning with an organophosphate or carbamate pesticide. A treatment protocol for junior doctors. Crit Care 2004;8:R391–R397.
19. Eyer F, Meichsner V, Kiderlen D, et al: Human parathion poisoning: a toxicokinetic analysis. Toxicol Rev 2003;22:143–163.
20. Paul N, Mannathukkoran TJ: Intermediate syndrome following carbamate poisoning. Clin Toxicol 2005;43:867–868.
21. Namba T, Nolte CT, Jackrel J, Grob D: Poisoning due to organophosphate insecticides. Acute and chronic manifestations. Am J Med 1971;50(4):475–492.
22. Coye MJ, Barnett PG, Midtling JE, et al: Clinical confirmation of organophosphate poisoning of agricultural workers. Am J Ind Med 1986;10(4):399–409.
23. Coye MJ, Barnett PG, Midtling JE, et al: Clinical confirmation of organophosphate poisoning by serial cholinesterase analyses. Arch Intern Med 1987;147(3):438–442.
24. Lifshitz M, Rotenberg M, Sofer S, et al: Carbamate poisoning and oxime treatment in children: a clinical and laboratory study. Pediatrics 1994;93(4):652–655.
25. Reigart JR, Roberts JR: Organophosphate insecticides. In Recognition and Management of Pesticide Poisoning, 5th ed.

Washington, DC, U.S. Environmental Protection Agency 735-R98-003, 1999, p 7, http://www.epa.gov/pesticides/safety/healthcare, http://npic.orst.edu/rmpp.htm.
26. Aldridge WN, Reiner E: Enzyme Inhibitors as Substrates. London, North Holland, 1972, pp 8–52.
27. Eyer P: The role of oximes in the management of organophosphorus pesticide poisoning. Toxicol Rev 2004;22:143–163.
28. Jacobsen D, Meredith TJ, Haines J: Poisoning with organophosphorus compounds. Emerg Med (Fremantle) 2001;13:260.
29. Eddleston M, Szinicz L, Eyer P, Buckley N: Oximes in acute organophosphorus pesticide poisoning: a systematic review of clinical trials. Q J Med 2002;95:275–283.
30. Lifshitz M, Shahak E, Sofer S: Carbamate and organophosphate poisoning in young children. Pediatr Emerg Care 1999;15(2):102–103.
31. Dawson RM, Poretski M: Carbamylated acetylcholinesterase: acceleration of decarbamylation by bispyridinium oximes. Biochem Pharmacol 1985;34(24):4337–4340.
32. Worek F, Backer M, Thiermann H, et al: Reappraisal of indications and limitations of oxime therapy in organophosphate poisoning. Hum Exp Toxicol 1997;16(8):466–472.
33. Bird SB, Gaspari RJ, Dickson EW: Early death due to severe organophosphate poisoning is a centrally mediated process. Acad Emerg Med 2003;10(4):295–298.
34. Dickson EW, Bird SB, Gaspari RJ, et al: Diazepam inhibits organophosphate-induced central respiratory depression. Acad Emerg Med 2003;10(12):1303–1306.
35. Haddad LM: Organophosphate poisoning [editorial]. J Toxicol Clin Toxicol 1992;30:331–332.
36. Zwiener RJ, Ginsburg CM: Organophosphate and carbamate poisoning in infants and children. Pediatrics 1988;81:121.
37. Senanayake N, de Silva HJ, Karalliedde L: A scale to assess severity in organophosphorus intoxication: POP scale. Hum Exp Toxicol 1993;12:297–299.
38. Asari Y, Kamijyo Y, Soma K: Changes in the hemodynamic state of patients with acute lethal organophosphate poisoning. Vet Hum Toxicol 2004;46(1):5–9.
39. Joubert J, Joubert PH, van der Spuy M, van Graan E: Acute organophosphate poisoning presenting with choreoathetosis. Clin Toxicol 1984;22:187–191.
40. Karalliedde L, Henry JB: Effects of organophosphates on skeletal muscle. Hum Exp Toxicol 1993;12:289–296.
41. Moore PG, James OF: Acute pancreatitis induced by acute organophosphate poisoning. Postgrad Med J 1981;57:660–662.
42. Kiss Z, Fazekas T: Organophosphates and torsades de pointes ventricular tachycardia. J R Soc Med 1983;76(11):984–985.
43. Saadeh AM: Metabolic complications of organophosphate and carbamate poisoning. Trop Doct 2001;31(3):149–152.
44. Henry JB: Clinical Diagnosis and Management by Laboratory Methods. Philadelphia, WB Saunders, 1996.
45. Yager J, McLean H, Hudes M, Spear RC: Components of variability in blood cholinesterase assay results. J Occup Med 1976;18(4):242–244.
46. Meller D, Fraser I, Kryger M: Hyperglycemia in anticholinesterase poisoning. Can Med Assoc J 1981;124(6):745–748.
47. Barr DB, Turner WE, DiPietro E, et al: Measurement of p-nitrophenol in the urine of residents whose homes were contaminated with methyl parathion. Environ Health Perspect 2002;110(Suppl 6):1085–1091.
48. Eddleston M, Buckley N, Checketts H, et al: Speed of initial atropinisation in significant organophosphorus pesticide poisoning—a comparison of recommended regimens. J Toxicol Clin Toxicol 2004;42:865–875.
49. Selden BS, Curry SC: Prolonged succinylcholine-induced paralysis in organophosphate insecticide poisoning. Ann Emerg Med 1987;16(2):215–217.
50. Eddleston M, Singh S, Buckley N: Acute organophosphorus poisoning. Clin Evid (BMJ) 2003;9:1542–1553.
51. Chang AY, Chan JY, Kao FJ, et al: Engagement of inducible nitric oxide synthase at the rostral ventrolateral medulla during mevinphos intoxication in the rat. J Biomed Sci 2001;8(6):475–483.
52. Buckley NA, Dawson AH, Whyte IM: Organophosphate poisoning: peripheral vascular resistance—a measure of adequate atropinization. J Toxicol Clin Toxicol 1994;32(1):61–68.

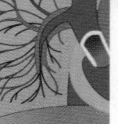

53. Yen DH, Yen JC, Len WB, et al: Spectral changes in systemic arterial pressure signals during acute mevinphos intoxication in the rat. Shock 2001;15(1):35–41.

54. Yeo V, Young K, Tsuen CH: Anticholinesterase-induced hypotension treated with pulmonary artery catheterization-guided vasopressors. Vet Hum Toxicol 2002;44(2):99–100.

55. Martin LJ, Doebler JA, Shih TM, Anthony A: Protective effect of diazepam pretreatment on soman-induced brain lesion formation. Brain Res 1985;325(1–2):287–289.

56. McDonough JH Jr, Dochterman LW, Smith CD, Shih TM: Protection against nerve agent-induced neuropathology, but not cardiac pathology, is associated with the anticonvulsant action of drug treatment. Neurotoxicology 1995;16(1):123–132.

57. McDonough JH Jr, Jaax NK, Crowley RA, et al: Atropine and/or diazepam therapy protects against soman-induced neural and cardiac pathology. Fundam Appl Toxicol 1989;13(2):256–276.

58. McDonough JH Jr, McMonagle J, Copeland T, et al: Comparative evaluation of benzodiazepines for control of soman-induced seizures. Arch Toxicol 1999;73(8–9):473–478.

59. McDonough JH Jr, Zoeffel LD, McMonagle J, et al: Anticonvulsant treatment of nerve agent seizures: anticholinergics versus diazepam in soman-intoxicated guinea pigs. Epilepsy Res 2000;38(1):1–14.

60. Shih T, McDonough JH Jr, Koplovitz I: Anticonvulsants for soman-induced seizure activity. J Biomed Sci 1999;6(2):86–96.

61. Shih TM, Duniho SM, McDonough JH: Control of nerve agent-induced seizures is critical for neuroprotection and survival small star, filled. Toxicol Appl Pharmacol 2003;188(2):69–80.

62. Shih TM, Koviak TA, Capacio BR: Anticonvulsants for poisoning by the organophosphorus compound soman: pharmacological mechanisms. Neurosci Biobehav Rev 1991;15(3):349–362.

63. Johnson PS, Michaelis EK: Characterization of organophosphate interactions at N-methyl-D-aspartate receptors in brain synaptic membranes. Mol Pharmacol 1992;41(4):750–756.

64. Rump S, Kowalczyk M: Management of convulsions in nerve agent acute poisoning: a Polish perspective. J Med Chem Def 2003–2004;1.

65. Little M, Murray L: Consensus statement: Risk of nosocomial organoposphate poisoning in the emergency departments. Emergency Medicine Australasia 2004;16:456–458.

66. Roberts D, Senarathna L: Secondary contamination in organophoshate poisoning. Q J Med 2004;97:1–2.

67. Kales SN, Christiani DC: Acute chemical emergencies. N Engl J Med 2004;350(8):800–808.

68. U.S. Army Medical Research Institute for Chemical Defense (ed): Medical Management of Chemical Casualties Handbook, 3rd ed. USAMRICD MCMR-UV-ZM, Aberdeen Proving Ground, MD, 2000, http://www.gmha.org/bioterrorism/usamricd/yellow_book_2000.pdf.

69. Stewart C, Sullivan JB Jr: Military munitions and antipersonnel agents. In JB Sullivan Jr, GR Krieger (eds): Hazardous Materials Toxicology: Clinical Principles of Environmental Health. Baltimore, Williams & Wilkins, 1992, p 986.

70. Macintyre AG, Christopher GW, Eitzen E Jr, et al: Weapons of mass destruction events with contaminated casualties: effective planning for health care facilities. JAMA 2000;283(2):242–249.

71. Sidell FR, Borak J: Chemical warfare agents. II. Nerve agents. Ann Emerg Med 1992;21(7):865–871.

72. Wetter DC, Daniell WE, Treser CD: Hospital preparedness for victims of chemical or biological terrorism. Am J Public Health 2001;91(5):710–716.

73. Agency for Toxic Substances Disease Registry: Appendix C: levels of protection. In Managing Hazardous Materials Incidents, Vol. II: Hospital Emergency Departments, 2001, www.atsdr.cdc.gov/mhmi-v2-c.pdf.

74. University of Oxford: Acute organophosphate pesticide poisoning in Sri Lanka: management, complications, and pharmacogenetics, 2004.

75. Eddleston M, et al: Emergency management of acute severe self-poisoning with an unknown pesticide. 1. A protocol. South Asian Clinical Toxicology Research Collaborative, 2004, p 1. Personal communication.

76. Choi PT, Quinonez LG, Cook DJ, et al: The use of glycopyrrolate in a case of intermediate syndrome following acute organophosphate poisoning. Can J Anaesth 1998;45(4):337–340.

77. Bardin PG, Van Eeden SF: Organophosphate poisoning: grading the severity and comparing treatment between atropine and glycopyrrolate. Crit Care Med 1990;18(9):956–960.

78. Kanto J, Klotz U: Pharmacokinetic implications for the clinical use of atropine, scopolamine and glycopyrrolate. Acta Anaesthesiol Scand 1988;32(2):69–78.

79. Lau WM: Protection by tacrine and some adjuncts against the depressant effects of soman in guinea-pig atrium. Gen Pharmacol 1993;24(6):1513–1519.

80. U.S. Army Medical Research Institute of Chemical Defense: Nerve agents. In Medical Management of Chemical Casualties Handbook. Aberdeen, MD, Aberdeen Proving Grounds—Edgewood Area, 1999.

81. Dunn MA: Progress in medical defense against nerve agents. JAMA, 1989;262:649.

82. Cherian AM, et al: Effectiveness of pralidoxime in the treatment of organophosphorus poisoning: a randomised, double-blind, placebo-controlled clinical trial. In International Clinical Epidemiology Network (ed): Monograph series on Critical International Health Issues, 1997, http//www.inclentrust.org/images/stories/mono 7_organophosphorus_poisoning[1].pdf.

83. Cherian AM, et al: Effectiveness of P2AM (PAM-pralidoxime) in the treatment of organophosphorus poisoning. A randomised, double-blind, placebo controlled trial. J Assoc Physicians India 1997;45:22–24.

84. Sungur M: Intensive care management of organophosphate insecticide poisoning. Crit Care 2001;5(4):211–215.

85. de Silva HJ, Wijewickrema R, Senanayake N: Does pralidoxime affect outcome of management in acute organophosphorus poisoning? Lancet 1992;339(8802):1136–1138.

86. Jovic R, Boskovic B: Antidotal action of pyridinium oximes in poisoning by O,O-diethyl-S-(2-(N-methyl-N-phenylamino)ethyl) thiophosphonate methylsulfomethylate (GT-45) and its two new analogs. Toxicol Appl Pharmacol 1970;16(1):194–200.

87. Kurtz PH: Pralidoxime in the treatment of carbamate intoxication. Am J Emerg Med 1990;8(1):68–70.

88. Petroianu G, Ruefer R: Poisoning with organophosphorus compounds. Emerg Med (Fremantle) 2001;13(2):258–260.

89. Shih TM: Comparison of several oximes on reactivation of soman-inhibited blood, brain and tissue cholinesterase activity in rats. Arch Toxicol 1993;67(9):637–646.

90. Simeon V, Wilhelm K, Granov A, et al: 1,3-Bispyridinium-dimethylether mono- and dioximes: synthesis, reactivating potency and therapeutic effect in experimental poisoning by organophosphorus compounds. Arch Toxicol 1979;41(4):301–306.

91. Vale JA: Toxicokinetic and toxicodynamic aspects of organophosphorus (OP) insecticide poisoning. Toxicol Lett 1998;102–103:649–652.

92. Shih TM, McDonough JH Jr: Organophosphorus nerve agents-induced seizures and efficacy of atropine sulfate as anticonvulsant treatment. Pharmacol Biochem Behav 1999;64(1):147–153.

93. Harris LW, Talbot BG, Lennox WJ, Anderson DR: The relationship between oxime-induced reactivation of carbamylated acetylcholinesterase and antidotal efficacy against carbamate intoxication. Toxicol Appl Pharmacol 1989;98(1):128–133.

94. Dawson RM: Rate constants of carbamylation and decarbamylation of acetylcholinesterase for physostigmine and carbaryl in the presence of an oxime. Neurochem Int 1994;24(2):173–182.

95. Lotti M: Treatment of acute organophosphate poisoning. Med J Aust 1991;154(1):51–55.

96. Sterri SH, Rognerud B, Fiskum SE, Lyngaas S: Effect of toxogonin and P2S on the toxicity of carbamates and organophosphorus compounds. Acta Pharmacol Toxicol (Copenh) 1979;45(1):9–15.

97. Lieske CN, Clark JH, Maxwell DM, et al: Studies of the amplification of carbaryl toxicity by various oximes. Toxicol Lett 1992;62(2–3):127–137.

98. Schexnayder S, James LP, Kearns GL, Farrar HC, et al: The pharmacokinetics of continuous infusion pralidoxime in children with organophosphate poisoning. J Toxicol Clin Toxicol 1998;36(6):549–555.

99. Sundwall A: Minimum concentrations of N-methylpyridinium-2-aldoxime methane sulphonate (P2S) which reverse neuromuscular block. Biochem Pharmacol 1961;8:413–417.

100. Medicis JJ, Stork CM, Howland MA, et al: Pharmacokinetics following a loading plus a continuous infusion of pralidoxime

compared with the traditional short infusion regimen in human volunteers. J Toxicol Clin Toxicol 1996;34(3):289–295.

101. Thiermann H, Szinicz L, Eyer F, et al: Modern strategies in therapy of organophosphate poisoning. Toxicol Lett 1999; 107(1–3):233–239.

102. Thiermann H, Mast U, Klimmek R, et al: Cholinesterase status, pharmacokinetics and laboratory findings during obidoxime therapy in organophosphate poisoned patients. Hum Exp Toxicol 1997;16(8):473–480.

103. Willems JL, De Bisschop HC, Verstraete AG, et al: Cholinesterase reactivation in organophosphorus poisoned patients depends on the plasma concentrations of the oxime pralidoxime methylsulphate and of the organophosphate. Arch Toxicol 1993;67(2):79–84.

104. Feldmann RJ, Szajewski J: Cholinergic syndrome. In International Programme on Chemical Safety Poison Information Database Management Databank, 1998.

105. Thompson DF, Thompson GD, Greenwood RB, Trammell HL: Therapeutic dosing of pralidoxime chloride. Drug Intell Clin Pharm 1987;21(7–8):590–593.

106. Bailey B: Are there teratogenic risks associated with antidotes used in the acute management of poisoned pregnant women? Birth Defects Res Part A Clin Mol Teratol 2003;67(2):133–140.

107. Bailey B: Organophosphate poisoning in pregnancy. Ann Emerg Med 1997;29(2):299.

108. Rotenberg JS, Newmark J: Nerve agent attacks on children: diagnosis and management. Pediatrics 2003;112(3 Pt 1):648–658.

109. U.S. Food and Drug Administration: FDA approves pediatric doses of AtroPen. Available at http://www.fda.gov.

110. Massachusetts Department of Public Health Office of Emergency Medical Services: Nerve agent exposure protocol. In Emergency Medical Services Pre-Hospital Treatment Protocols, 5th ed, version 5.1, January 1, 2004, http://www.cmemsc.org/protocols-state/wmd-protocols-intro.pdf.

111. Senanayake N, Karalliedde L: Neurotoxic effects of organophosphorus insecticides. An intermediate syndrome. N Engl J Med 1987;316(13):761–763.

112. De Bleecker J, Van Den Neucker K, Willems J: The intermediate syndrome in organophosphate poisoning: presentation of a case and review of the literature. J Toxicol Clin Toxicol 1992; 30(3):321–329; discussion, 331–332.

113. Karademir M, Erturk F, Kocak R: Two cases of organophosphate poisoning with development of intermediate syndrome. Hum Exp Toxicol 1990;9(3):187–189.

114. Khan S, Hemalatha R, Jeyasselan L, et al: Neuroparalysis and oxime efficacy in organophosphate poisoning: a study of butyrylcholinesterase. Hum Exp Toxicol 2001;20(4):169–174.

115. Routier RJ, Lipman J, Brown K: Difficulty in weaning from respiratory support in a patient with the intermediate syndrome of organophosphate poisoning. Crit Care Med 1989;17(10): 1075–1076.

116. Samal KK, Sahu CS: Organophosphorus poisoning and intermediate neurotoxic syndrome. J Assoc Physicians India 1990;38(2):181–182.

117. Curry SC: Organophosphate-associated "intermediate syndrome": for real? AACT Clin Toxicol Update 1994;7:1–2.

118. De Bleecker JL: The intermediate syndrome in organophosphate poisoning: an overview of experimental and clinical observations. J Toxicol Clin Toxicol 1995;33(6):683–686.

119. Sudakin DL, Mullins ME, Horowitz BZ, et al: Intermediate syndrome after malathion ingestion despite continuous infusion of pralidoxime. J Toxicol Clin Toxicol 2000;38(1):47–50.

120. Aygun D, Doganay Z, Altintop L, et al: Serum acetylcholinesterase and prognosis of acute organophosphate poisoning. J Toxicol Clin Toxicol 2002;40(7):903–910.

121. De Bleecker J, Willems J, Van Den Neucker K, et al: Prolonged toxicity with intermediate syndrome after combined parathion and methyl parathion poisoning. J Toxicol Clin Toxicol 1992;30(3):333–345; discussion, 347–349.

122. De Bleecker JL: Intermediate syndrome: prolonged cholinesterase inhibition. J Toxicol Clin Toxicol 1993;31(1):197–199.

123. De Wilde V, Vogelaers D, Colardyn F, et al: Postsynaptic neuromuscular dysfunction in organophosphate induced intermediate syndrome. Klin Wochenschr 1991;69(4):177–183.

124. De Bleecker J, Van den Abeele K, De Reuck J: Electromyography in relation to end-plate acetylcholinesterase in rats poisoned by different organophosphates. Neurotoxicology 1994; 15(2):331–340.

125. Jokanovic M, Stukalov PV, Kosanovic M: Organophosphate induced delayed polyneuropathy. Curr Drug Target CNS Neurol Disord 2002;1(6):593–602.

126. Lotti M, Moretto A, Bertolazzi M, et al: Organophosphate polyneuropathy and neuropathy target esterase: studies with methamidophos and its resolved optical isomers. Arch Toxicol 1995;69(5):330–336.

127. Johnson MK: Organophosphorus esters causing delayed neurotoxic effects: mechanism of action and structure activity studies. Arch Toxicol 1975;34(4):259–288.

128. Johnson MK, Glynn P: Neuropathy target esterase (NTE) and organophosphorus-induced delayed polyneuropathy (OPIDP): recent advances. Toxicol Lett 1995;82–83:459–863.

129. Weiner ML, Jortner BS: Organophosphate-induced delayed neurotoxicity of triarylphosphates. Neurotoxicology 1999;20(4): 653–673.

130. Gutmann L, Bodensteiner JB: Organophosphate-induced delayed polyneuropathy. J Pediatr 1993;123(5):837.

131. Lotti M: The pathogenesis of organophosphate polyneuropathy. Crit Rev Toxicol 1991;21(6):465–487.

132. Lotti M, Becker CE, Aminoff MJ: Organophosphate polyneuropathy: pathogenesis and prevention. Neurology 1984;34(5):658–662.

133. Singh S, Sharma N: Neurological syndromes following organophosphate poisoning. Neurol India 2000;48(4):308–313.

134. Abou-Donia MB: Toxicokinetics and metabolism of delayed neurotoxic organophosphorus esters. Neurotoxicology 1983;4(1): 113–129.

135. Metcalf RL: Historical perspective of organophosphorus ester-induced delayed neurotoxicity. Neurotoxicology 1982;3(4):269–284.

136. Wadia RS, Chitra S, Amin RB, et al: Electrophysiological studies in acute organophosphate poisoning. J Neurol Neurosurg Psychiatry 1987;50(11):1442–1448.

137. Bertoncin D, Russolo A, Caroldi S, Loth M: Neuropathy target esterase in human lymphocytes. Arch Environ Health 1985;40(3):139–144.

138. Lotti M, Moretto A, Zoppellari R, et al: Inhibition of lymphocytic neuropathy target esterase predicts the development of organophosphate-induced delayed polyneuropathy. Arch Toxicol 1986;59(3):176–179.

139. Shahar E, Andraws J: Extra-pyramidal parkinsonism complicating organophosphate insecticide poisoning. Eur J Paediatr Neurol 2001;5(6):261–264.

140. Senanayake N, Sanmuganathan PS: Extrapyramidal manifestations complicating organophosphorus insecticide poisoning. Hum Exp Toxicol 1995;14:600–604.

141. Rosenstock L, Daniell W, Burnhart S, et al: Chronic neuropsychological sequelae of occupational exposure to organophosphate insecticides. Am J Ind Med 1990;18(3):321–325.

142. Rosenstock L, Keifer M, Daniell WE, et al: Chronic central nervous system effects of acute organophosphate pesticide intoxication. The Pesticide Health Effects Study Group. Lancet 1991;338(8761):223–227.

143. Steenland K, Jenkins B, Ames RG, et al: Chronic neurological sequelae to organophosphate pesticide poisoning. Am J Public Health 1994;84(5):731–736.

144. Wadia RS: The neurology of organophosphorus insecticide poisoning newer findings a view point. J Assoc Physicians India 1990;38(2):129–131.

145. Raushel FM: Bacterial detoxification of organophosphate nerve agents. Curr Opin Microbiol 2002;5:288–295.

146. Raushel FM, Holden HM: Phosphotriesterase: an enzyme in search of its natural substrate. Adv Enzymol Relat Areas Mol Biol 2000;74:51–93.

147. Tuovinen K, Kaliste-Korhonen E, Raushel FM, Hanninen O: Phosphotriesterase—a promising candidate for use in detoxification of organophosphates. Fundam Appl Toxicol 1994;23:578–584.

148. Berwick P: 2,4-Dichlorophenoxyacetic acid poisoning in man. Some interesting clinical and laboratory findings. JAMA 1970;214(6):1114–1117.

149. de Jong LP, Verhagen MA, Langenberg JP, et al: The bispyridinium-dioxime HLo-7. A potent reactivator for acetylcholinesterase inhibited by the stereoisomers of tabun and soman. Biochem Pharmacol 1989;38(4):633–640.

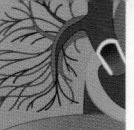

150. de Jong LP, Wolring GZ: Stereospecific reactivation by some Hagedorn-oximes of acetylcholinesterases from various species including man, inhibited by soman. Biochem Pharmacol 1984;33(7):1119–1125.

151. Hagedorn I, Gundel WH, Schoene K: Reactivation of phosphorylated acetylcholine esterase with oximes: contribution to the study of the reaction course. Arzneimittelforschung 1969;19(4):603–606.

152. Kuhnen-Clausen D, Hagedorn I, Gross G, et al: Interactions of bisquaternary pyridine salts (H-oximes) with cholinergic receptors. Arch Toxicol 1983;54(3):171–179.

153. Balai-Mood M, Ayati MH, Ali-Akbarian H: Effect of high doses of sodium bicarbonate in acute organophosphorus pesticide poisoning. Clin Toxicol 2005;43(6):571–574.

154. Roberts M, Buckley NA: Alkalinisation for organophosphorus pesticide poisoning: A review. Cochrane Database Syst Rev 2005:CD004897.

155. Ashani Y, Leader H, Rothschild N, Dosoretz C: Combined effect of organophosphorus hydrolase and oxime on the reactivation rate of diethylphosphoryl-acetylcholinesterase conjugates. Biochem Pharmacol 1998;55(2):159–168.

156. Ashani Y, Rothschild N, Segall Y, et al: Prophylaxis against organophosphate poisoning by an enzyme hydrolysing organophosphorus compounds in mice. Life Sci 1991;49(5):367–374.

157. Raveh L, Segall Y, Leader H, et al: Protection against tabun toxicity in mice by prophylaxis with an enzyme hydrolyzing organophosphate esters. Biochem Pharmacol 1992;44(2):397–400.

158. Raveh L, Grunwald J, Marcus D, et al: Human butyrylcholinesterase as a general prophylactic antidote for nerve agent toxicity. In vitro and in vivo quantitative characterization. Biochem Pharmacol 1993;45(12):2465–2474.

159. Guven M, Sungur M, Eser B, et al: The effects of fresh frozen plasma on cholinesterase levels and outcomes in patients with organophosphate poisoning. J Toxicol Clin Toxicol 2004;42(5):617–623.

77 *Pyrethrins, Repellants, and Other Pesticides*

STEPHEN W. BORRON, MD, MS

At a Glance...

■ Pyrethrins, pyrethroids, and newer compounds are rapidly replacing the organochlorines, organophosphates, and carbamates in many geographic areas, particularly in the consumer pesticide market.

■ Pyrethrins and pyrethroids have low mammalian toxicity, even in overdose, compared with the aforementioned pesticide families.

■ Amitraz exposure is generally benign; however, large overdoses may result in central nervous system depression, bradycardia, and hypotension. It is an α_2-adrenoceptor agonist.

■ The avermectins may induce coma, metabolic acidosis, and rhabdomyolysis after large ingestions.

■ Two newer pesticides, imidacloprid and fipronil, are discussed. Serious toxicity has been rarely reported in humans.

■ DEET is the most widely used insect repellant. Neurotoxicity has been reported with topical application and with ingestion, but the incidence of serious adverse reactions is small in comparison with the widespread use of these products.

■ The chemical and physical characteristics (e.g., volatility) of the active ingredients of pesticides and of the adjuvants and solvents associated with them should be considered in any evaluation of their toxicity and approach to treatment.

The relatively high mammalian (including human) toxicity of the organophosphates and carbamates (see Chapter 76) and environmentally persistent organochlorines (see Chapter 81) has led regulators and manufacturers of pesticides to search for safer alternatives. This chapter covers the family of pyrethrins and pyrethroids, as well as a number of other established and more recent compounds used as pesticides or repellants of biting insects. These include DEET, amitraz, imidacloprid, fipronil, and the avermectins. The pesticides covered here represent the present and near future of pesticides, owing to improved safety of these products relative to organophosphates, carbamates, and organochlorines. These compounds, in general, have limited toxicity in humans, animals, and the food supply but nonetheless require respect in their application and an understanding of the risks they pose in acute overexposure.

Although most life-threatening human poisonings have been reduced by the move away from the more traditional pesticides, there is concern among some that the pyrethroids and newer pesticides also pose unnecessary human risk. This chapter briefly examines the concerns for potential long-term and subtle forms of toxicity but focuses on the acute toxicity of these compounds in unintentional and intentional overexposure.

No discussion of the risks associated with chemical agents is appropriate without a balancing view of their benefits. We are continually placed at significant risk for disease and death by infectious disease vectors. Malaria continues to kill millions of people throughout the world, particularly in developing nations. The World Health Organization (WHO) estimated the worldwide incidence at 213 million cases in 1998.[1] Snow and colleagues believe that the number is much higher, about 515 million cases of *Plasmodium falciparum* malaria alone.[2] The developed world is not spared from vector-borne diseases. The United States has seen significant numbers of cases of West Nile Fever, dengue fever, Lyme disease, encephalitides, and other arthropod-borne illnesses in recent years (see www.cdc.gov/ncidod/dvbid/). The judicious use of pesticides and repellants has a significant effect on the incidence of these diseases. For example, Alten and colleagues showed a reduction of malaria from 8.29% to 1.57% in a test city when mosquito nets impregnated with deltamethrin (a pyrethroid) were employed, whereas malaria incidence slightly increased in a control area (no intervention) and in two areas where nonimpregnated nets were employed.[3] Flea- and tick-borne diseases have also been diminished by the appropriate use of insecticides and repellants by humans and their pets. Pesticides also decrease the amount of food that is wasted.

In any evaluation of pesticide safety, it is critical to remember the roles of solvents in which the pesticides are dissolved and any adjuvants used to increase their efficacy or ease of use. It is not uncommon, particularly among the newer "insect-selective" pesticides, that the solvent has greater acute toxicity to the patient than the active ingredient. This is important to recall not only in caring for patients but also when reporting cases in the medical literature. Furthermore, some cases of reported "pesticide poisoning" occurring through inhalation are probably solvent exposures because many pesticides have low vapor pressures and are unlikely to be inhaled unless dispersed as droplets or mists.

In addition to their accepted mechanisms of action, which often involve alteration of neural transmission, most of the pesticides show evidence of inducing oxidative stress, which naturally raises concern about long-term effects, such as the induction of cancer and other chronic adverse events. This issue is generally of greater concern to scientists and risk assessors on a population basis, rather than at the individual level. The reader is referred to the article by Abdollahi and associates[4] for a current review of the issue of oxidative stress induced by various pesticides.

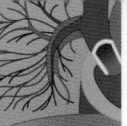

PYRETHRUM, PYRETHRINS, AND PYRETHROIDS

Substances and Mechanisms of Action

Pyrethrum is an oleoresin mixture derived from the common chrysanthemums, *Chrysanthemum cinerariifolium* and *Tanacetum cinerariifolium*. The natural pesticide pyrethrins are derived from pyrethrum. To enhance certain characteristics, particularly resistance against degradation by ultraviolet light, synthetic analogous compounds have been developed, which are referred to as *pyrethroids*. Pyrethroids constitute more than 30% of worldwide pesticide use, based on their efficacy in knockdown and killing of insects, low mammalian toxicity, and limited environmental persistence.[5] For reasons of simplicity and because the use of synthetic compounds now outweighs that of natural compounds, the term *pyrethroids* is used hereafter as a collective term for this family of pesticides when further precision is not required.

Pyrethroids act by altering the voltage dependence and rate of activation of the gated sodium channel and by inhibiting inactivation of the channel, increasing the likelihood that the channel opens or remains open. Although insect and mammalian voltage-gated channels share morphologic features and physiologic characteristics, natural toxins have developed that are highly specific for insect channels. The pyrethrins and pyrethroids are believed to be relatively specific based in part on their greater affinity for insect channels. Furthermore, body temperature differences between mammals and insects predispose the insect to greater effects from a pyrethroid of given toxicity because degradative metabolism is faster in mammals. Additionally, the insect's smaller size means that the toxicant is more likely to reach its target before deactivation by the organism.[5]

Uses

Pyrethroids are applied by a variety of methods. They are applied directly to fabrics, such as mosquito netting and curtains, to serve as insect repellants. Their efficacy in reducing disease-carrying insects for malaria and Chagas' disease has been demonstrated.[3,6] They are used in smoke coils and intermittent and total release sprays. Permethrin is applied in humans as a 5% cream for treatment of scabies and as a 1% cream rinse or lotion for the treatment of pediculosis capitis.

Toxicology

Gamnon (cited in Zlotkin) has divided the pyrethroids into two classes, which differ based on the absence (type I) or presence (type II) of an α-cyano group and which provide them with distinct toxicologic activities[5] (Fig. 77-1). Type I pyrethroids induce a tremor syndrome, composed of hyperexcitation, ataxia, and convulsions, followed by flaccid paralysis. Type II pyrethroids have greater effects in mammals and may cause a writhing syndrome (hypersensitivity, tremors, hypersalivation, and paralysis).

EXPOSURE ROUTES

Pyrethroids may enter the body by ingestion, inhalation, or dermal absorption, although the first two routes are certainly of greatest potential consequence. The "no observed adverse effect level" (NOAEL) for ingestion in animals is 1 mg/kg/day, above which neurotoxic effects may be seen.[7] The "acceptable daily intake" of permethrin and cypermethrin, as established by the WHO, is 0.05 mg/kg/day.[8] Schettgen and colleagues[9] have provided evidence that most pyrethroid body burden is due to ingestion of food-borne residues, based on an earlier experimental study by Woollen and colleagues.[10] Inhalation of pyrethroids is likely of significant concern only during the actual spray application of the products, owing to the low volatility of these compounds. For example, permethrin has a vapor pressure of only 45 µPa at 25° C (3.4×10^{-7} mm Hg).[9] Barlow and colleagues recently assessed the risk involved with the use of deltamethrin-impregnated bed nets for prevention of malaria.[7] They identified a NOAEL of 1000 mg/kg/day in animals. Applying safety factors, an "acceptable exposure level" (AEL) of 10 mg/kg/day was established for humans. Tests using the nets revealed that actual exposures incurred in use are less than one tenth of the AEL. The authors concluded that the risk-to-benefit ratios for mosquito net use are quite favorable.[7] The WHO has determined that the use of pyrethroid-treated bed nets reduces malaria mortality and morbidity, particularly in children and newborns, and may reduce transmission of malaria when used on a large scale.[11]

Pyrethroids

Permethrin (Type I)	Cyfluthrin (Type II)

A   B

FIGURE 77-1 Pyrethroids. **A**, Permethrin (type I). **B**, Cyfluthrin (type II). Note the α-cyano group.

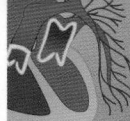

METABOLISM

Pyrethroids are rapidly hydrolyzed by esterases in the liver.[12] The metabolites are then eliminated in the urine. There is no correlation between urinary metabolite concentrations and symptoms. According to Leng and associates, the unchanged pyrethroids must be determined in plasma to explain clinical effects, but pyrethroids are detectable in plasma for only a few hours after exposure.[13]

ACUTE TOXICITY

Ray and Forshaw have published a useful review of the acute toxicity of pyrethroids, particularly as applies to animal studies.[14] The toxicity can be reduced to two clinical syndromes, type I (tremor syndrome) and type II (choreoathetosis/salivation syndrome), although some pyrethroids may produce a superimposed combination of both types. Type I syndrome is compared to the toxicity of DDT (see Chapter 81). The tremor may be severe, increasing the metabolic rate, and can lead to prostration and death in animals. Type II pyrethroids induce much longer delays in sodium channel conduction (>10 msec, the normal time constant of the unmodified sodium channel being about 0.5 msec). The effects of this prolongation include incoordination, choreoathetosis, seizures, and direct effects on skeletal and cardiac muscles and salivary glands, as well as reflex hyperexcitability.[14] Most human case reports of acute poisoning refer to type II (α-cyano) pyrethroids. Descriptions of acute poisoning in humans are relatively rare. An International Programme on Chemical Safety document cited three cases of deltamethrin poisoning, including a report by Rousselin[15] of a 13-year-old who ingested 5 g of deltamethrin (LD_{50} in rats, 30–140 mg/kg[16]) in a suicide attempt. The patient developed loss of consciousness, muscle cramps, miosis, and tachycardia. She received gastric lavage, 2-pyridine aldoxime methiodide (2-PAM), sodium nitrite, sodium thiosulfate, and high doses of diazepam and had complete recovery at 48 hours. The same document further cited an unpublished case of a 23-year-old man who ingested 1.75 g of deltamethrin with no neurologic signs or symptoms. Digestive and hepatic signs were attributed to the xylene used as a solvent.[17] He and colleagues reported on 573 cases of acute pyrethroids poisoning in China. Deltamethrin was involved in 325 cases.[18] About one third of cases were of occupational origin and due to poor utilization conditions and lack of personal protection. Two of 158 occupational cases died of convulsions, whereas the remainder of the 573 total cases survived with 1 to 6 days of treatment. Burning skin and paresthesias were the most common symptoms reported in a group of unprotected cotton workers in China in the 1980s.[19] Diarrhea, severe headaches, dizziness, fatigue, nausea, and anorexia were also reported. Transient electroencephalogram changes and fasciculations were noted, as well as convulsions in one case, with all patients making a complete recovery.

Yang and colleagues reported on 48 cases of acute ingestion of mixtures of permethrin, xylene, and surfactant.[20] Ten of these were accidental and 38 intentional attempts at suicide. Gastrointestinal symptoms predominated, with sore throat, mouth ulcerations, dysphagia, epigastric pain, and vomiting being common findings. Pulmonary abnormalities occurred in 29% and aspiration pneumonitis in 8 cases, with 1 fatality. Confusion (13%), coma (21%), and seizures (8%) were observed as well. A small percentage (3 of 48) had arrhythmias or shock. Mild renal and liver function abnormalities were seen in, respectively, 10% and 6% of patients. The authors concluded that this combination was responsible for significant poisonings, but that the relative contributions to toxicity were uncharacterized. Clearly, a number of these symptoms may have been attributable to the xylene carrier. LoVecchio and Knight recently reported on the case of a 36 year-old man who injected 6 mL of Real Kill Ant and Roach Killer 2 into the antecubital fossa and another 2 mL subcutaneously in a suicide attempt.[21] This product contains tralomethrin 0.01% and D-*trans*-allethrin 0.05%, as well as mineral spirits, a glycol ether, and simple hydrocarbons. The patient suffered pain and erythema at the injection site during a 4-hour observation period with resolution. No further symptoms were noted during a 3-day psychiatric evaluation.

Allergic Phenomena

Both acute exacerbations of hypersensitivity pneumonitis[22] and asthma, including fatalities,[23,24] have been described after pyrethroid exposures. A report from the New York City Department of Health and the Centers for Disease Control and Prevention (CDC), however, revealed that widespread spraying of urban pesticides for control of West Nile Virus in 2000 did not increase the incidence of emergency department asthma visits.[25] Allergic contact dermatitis[26,27] and irritant contact dermatitis[28] have also been reported. Amer and colleagues found that 70% of pesticide workers exposed to pyrethroids had positive patch tests.[29]

Skin Hyperesthesia

Paresthesia may be produced by dermal exposure to these compounds. This is apparently a dose-related phenomenon and is reversible. It represents local effects on skin nerve terminals rather than systemic toxicity. Vitamin E cream has been shown to ameliorate the unpleasant sensation.[30]

CHRONIC TOXICITY

Chronic toxicity from pyrethroids is not a generally accepted clinically recognized entity, although it is a hotly contested concern in Germany. Altenkirch reported in 1996 on 64 cases of "chronic pyrethroid toxicity" referred to the Federal Health Office.[31] Twenty-three of these patients underwent examination in a neurologic department on an inpatient basis, using clinical neurologic, neuroradiologic, and laboratory investigations, including the examination of pyrethroid concentrations in blood and urine. The presumed sources of chronic exposure included carpets, moth repellants, pesticide sprays, and wood preservatives. Nine patients were found to have severe somatic or psychiatric

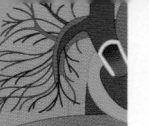

disorders determined to be unrelated to pesticide exposure, including Guillain-Barré syndrome, pituitary tumor, and spinal muscle atrophy. An additional eight were determined to meet criteria for "multiple chemical sensitivities" (see Chapter 85). In six of those cases, "a causal link between acute complaints and pyrethroid exposure could be established or not ruled out." However, the authors found no evidence for irreversible central or peripheral nervous system lesions. Muller-Mohnssen and Hahn published a series of cases of cerebro-organic dysfunction, locomotory disorders reminiscent of multiple sclerosis or Parkinson's disease, polyneuropathy, and immunosuppression, which they ascribed to chronic pyrethroid toxicity.[32] They have recently updated their findings.[33] The methodology of their findings has been sharply criticized.[34] Hildebrand and colleagues speculated that effects of pyrethroids on voltage-gated calcium channels may be responsible for "chronic effects of low-level pyrethroids poisoning."[35] This issue will likely not be settled in the near future but warrants careful analysis. Kolaczinski and Curtis have reviewed the literature and provide a useful summary of this contentious debate.[36]

Laboratory Studies and Biologic Monitoring

Biologic monitoring of manufacturing workers and pesticide applicators of pyrethroids is possible, employing either measurement of the intact compounds in the blood (possibly useful for very recent high exposures) or measurement of the intact compounds or their metabolites in the urine. Hydrolysis of the ester bond of permethrin, cypermethrin, deltamethrin, cyfluthrin, and fenvalerate produces acid metabolites and 3-phenoxybenzyl alcohol (4-fluoro-3 phenoxybenzyl alcohol in the case of cyfluthrin). These metabolites may be measured in urine shortly after oral or dermal exposure, up to a maximum of 5 days. A variety of methods of detection are described.[37] For plasma analysis, gas chromatography with electrochemical detection (GC-ECD) has been employed.[38] Measurement of deltamethrin and fenvalerate has been carried out using both high-performance liquid chromatography (HPLC) and GC-ECD.[39,40] Although useful for monitoring workers, these tests have little applicability to acute poisoning because they are not widely available and are unlikely to alter therapy.

Treatment

Treatment of pyrethroid overdose is generally supportive because there are no specific antidotes. Because of the risk for aspiration related to the associated hydrocarbon solvents and surfactants, careful attention to the airway must be ensured, particularly in the case of intentional oral overdose. Seizures are rare and may be expected to respond to benzodiazepines. The proconvulsant effects of pyrethroids are believed to be due to binding to peripheral-type benzodiazepine receptor ligands, to which diazepam has significant affinity.[41]

FORMAMIDINE COMPOUNDS

Substances and Mechanisms of Action

Chlordimeform and amitraz (Fig. 77-2) are the two representative compounds of this group of pesticides. Chlordimeform was voluntarily withdrawn from the U.S. market because of concerns of increased incidence of bladder cancer in manufacturing workers.[42] Amitraz is an insecticide and acaricide. Both of these agents act on the α_2 adrenoreceptors as agonists. Amitraz is available as an emulsifiable concentrate in an aromatic hydrocarbon solvent.

Uses

Amitraz is used in the United States to control red spider mites, leaf miners, scale insects, and aphids. On cotton, it is used to control bollworms, white fly, and leaf worms. On animals, it is used to control ticks, mites, lice, and other animal pests. It is approved for use on pears, cotton, hogs, and cattle.[43] It is used in some countries as treatment of generalized demodicosis of dogs and for control of ticks and mites on sheep.[44]

Toxicology

Both amitraz and chlordimeform are thought to exert their principle acute toxicity by agonism of α_2 adrenoceptors, in a manner similar to clonidine. These effects are discussed later. In addition, chlordimeform has been implicated in the production of symptomatic methemoglobinemia (probably through one of its metabolites, an aromatic amine) and also hematuria (hemorrhagic cystitis). Although amitraz has not been associated with either of these in case reports, Garnier and coworkers pointed out that amitraz also has as one of its main metabolites 2,4-dimethylaniline and that methemoglobinemia is a possibility.[45] The oral LD_{50} of amitraz in rats is 800 mg/kg.[46]

ACUTE TOXICITY

Amitraz poisoning is typically benign[45] and requires only supportive care, but there are reported cases of significant toxicity, described later. A NOAEL of 0.125 mg/kg

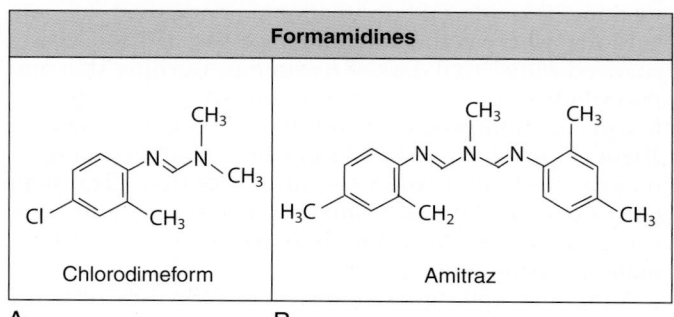

FIGURE 77-2 Formamidines. **A**, Chlordimeform. **B**, Amitraz.

has been established in healthy male volunteers.[47] The acute toxicity of amitraz is characterized by central nervous system (CNS) depression, bradycardia, and hypotension. In some cases, miosis is observed. Hyperglycemia may also be present. Most of these symptoms are attributable to α_2-adrenoceptor stimulation. Mydriasis may be seen with great stimulation of these receptors. The vomiting commonly seen has been attributed to the solvent, most often a petroleum distillate, as has aspiration pneumonitis and CNS depression. Agin and colleagues[42] published a series of seven cases of poisoning admitted to a children's hospital in Turkey between 1999 and 2001. Six cases were of oral route and one dermal. Amounts ingested were small (25–30 mL) in two cases and unknown in the rest. Dermal poisoning resulted from its misuse as a treatment for lice. Four children presented in coma, two with somnolence. CNS depression resolved within 6 to 20 hours. One was hypotensive, responding to intravenous fluids. Respiratory failure was noted in four cases, two requiring brief mechanical ventilation support (<10 hours). Mild increases in blood glucose were seen. Laboratory studies were otherwise normal. Some patients received up to four doses of atropine for bradycardia and miosis. All cases recovered within 3 days.

Doganay and colleagues previously reported two cases, one of which resulted in severe hypotension and bradycardia.[48] One case involved a 35-year-old man who drank between 50 and 100 mL (6.25–12.5 g) of amitraz in a suicide attempt. On arrival at the hospital, about 3 hours after ingestion, his heart rate was 35 beats/minute, and his blood pressure was unobtainable. The patient was in respiratory arrest. His Glasgow Coma Scale score was 3, and his body temperature was 34.5° C. He was intubated and ventilated, and atropine and dopamine were administered, along with intravenous fluids. He became conscious 22 hours after ingestion and was extubated after 24 hours. Hyperglycemia, with blood glucose as high as 500 mg/dL, persisted over a 5-day period. He was discharged without sequelae.[48]

Laboratory Studies

The presence of cyanosis should prompt obtaining of arterial blood gases and methemoglobin levels. Garnier and colleagues reported plasma amitraz concentrations of 100 ng/mL 2 hours after ingestion in an asymptomatic patient and of 500 ng/mL after 2 hours in a patient with drowsiness.[45] Plasma levels are generally unlikely to be of clinical use because of their limited availability. The reader is reminded that manufacturers can often be of assistance in quantifying or at least confirming the presence of particular compounds when there is doubt about the diagnosis or when forensic issues exist.

Treatment

As in all poisonings, supportive care is vital. Given the generally limited toxicity of amitraz and the presence of petroleum distillates, gastric emptying is generally not recommended, except in cases of massive exposure or if other, more toxic compounds are ingested. The airway should be protected if a decision is made to undertake gastric emptying by any means. A number of α_2-adrenoceptor antagonists have been proposed as potential "antidotes" against amitraz. Yohimbine and atipamezole have been successfully employed in dogs,[49] but human experience is lacking. Phentolamine has likewise been suggested in case of ingestion of a large amount of amitraz.[50] Chen and Lu[51] have recommended dimethylpropane sulfonate (DMPS) for treatment of chlordimeform poisoning and cite Chinese animal literature demonstrating its efficacy in mice, rats, and pigeons. They also report efficacy in clinical treatment of two patients poisoned with chlordimeform. The mechanism of supposed antidotal efficacy is not clearly explained.

AVERMECTINS

The avermectins are natural compounds produced by fermentation of the actinomyces, *Streptomyces avermitilis*.[52] This species produces eight macrocyclic lactones identified as members of "A" and "B" series. The B series has been shown effective against helminths and arthropods.[53] Chemical modification of the natural lactones resulted in the production of ivermectin (Fig. 77-3), which is approved for use in humans and animals as an antihelminthic. It is effective against *Onchocerca volvulus*, the nematode responsible for river blindness. The U.S. Food and Drug Administration (FDA) has approved its use for strongyloidiasis and onchocerciasis. It is subject to widespread off-label use and is effective against ectoparasites (scabies and lice) and cutanea larva migrans. Its use is restricted to adults and children older than 5 years.[54,55] Ivermectin has also been shown to improve the therapeutic response to chemotherapy drugs (paclitaxel [Taxol] and vincristine) by inhibiting multidrug resistance.[56]

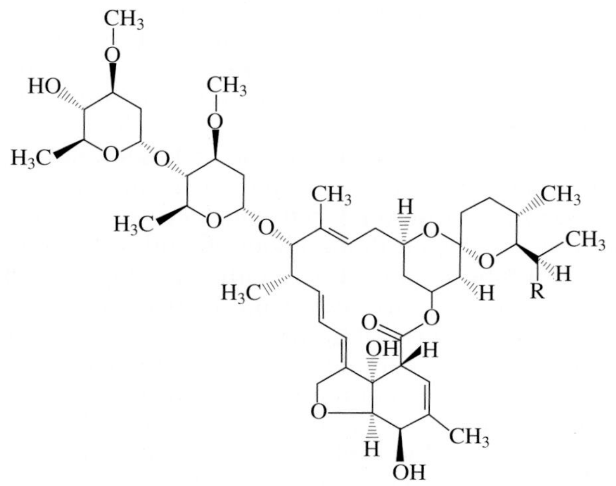

Ivermectin

FIGURE 77-3 Ivermectin.

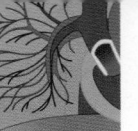

An additional compound, abamectin, is used in agriculture as an insecticide on vegetables and in fruit trees. It is widely used in the control of parasites and insects, and its use is increasing, particularly as ectoparasites develop resistance to pyrethroids. The avermectins have complex effects on both vertebrate and invertebrate γ-aminobutyric acid (GABA) channels and invertebrate glutamate gated chloride channels. The net increase in intracellular chloride ions leads to paralysis and death in the target organism.[57] A more recently developed product, emamectin, is also employed as an insecticide. This product is approved in the United States on fruiting vegetables (tomatoes and peppers), leafy vegetables, and leafy brassica (cole) vegetables, as well as head and stem cole crops, head lettuce, and celery, along with aerial application.

The incidence of avermectin poisonings appears to be low. None are identified specifically in the 2003 Annual Report of the American Association of Poison Control Centers (AAPCC) Toxic Exposure Surveillance System (TESS). Because these agents are used both as insecticides and as antiparasitics, they are likely classified under "other" categories in the database and are difficult to discern. Clinical use of ivermectin has resulted in itching, edema, malaise, cephalgia, and hypotension, as well as dyspnea, in a few patients. According to Elgart and Meinking, ivermectin has been therapeutically used in millions of patients without major adverse effects.[54] Overdose experience has been extremely limited. Chung and colleagues reported on the experience in Taiwan with two forms of avermectin, a 2% wt/wt or 2.5% wt/vol preparation of abamectin, used as an insecticide, and a 1% wt/vol preparation of ivermectin, used as an antiparasitic in hogs.[57] The authors report on the management of 19 patients seen between 1993 and 1997. Eighteen of the patients were exposed to abamectin and 1 to ivermectin. There were 15 ingestions, only 1 of which was accidental. Four of these patients remained asymptomatic, 8 had minor symptoms after a mean ingestion of 23 mg/kg or after dermal or inhalation occupational exposures. Seven patients had severe symptoms: coma (7), aspiration and respiratory failure (4), and hypotension (3), after a mean ingestion of 100 mg/kg. Metabolic acidosis was observed in four patients and rhabdomyolysis in three. One of 19 patients went on to die; his death attributed to multi-organ failure 18 days after exposure.

More recently, Yen and Lin, also of Taiwan, published a case report of an acute suicidal ingestion exposure to emamectin, a substituted benzoate salt of abamectin.[58] The 67-year-old man drank about 500 mL of a fourfold diluted solution. He subsequently developed gastrointestinal upset, with esophagoscopy-proven gastric erosions and superficial gastritis, mild CNS depression, and aspiration pneumonitis. It is worthy of mention that the 2.15% concentrate is dissolved in a substituted phenol (butylated hydroxyl toluene) and 1-hexanol, which may be responsible for the erosive lesions and mild CNS depression noted. He left the hospital on day 7 with no sequelae.

Drug Interactions

Avermectins have been shown to be potent inhibitors of the multidrug-resistant proteins [P-glycoprotein (Pgp) and others].[56] This is probably of little concern in an isolated avermectin overdose; however, other antiparasitic drugs, like colchicine, are largely dependent on elimination by Pgp.[59] This results in a theoretical increased risk if the drugs are taken in combination.

Laboratory Studies

Given the reports of metabolic acidosis and rhabdomyolysis in suicidal overdose, it seems prudent to obtain arterial blood gases and serum creatine phosphokinase concentrations in patients with significant ingestions.

Treatment

Treatment of avermectin poisonings is supportive. Given the propensity of the agents to cause CNS depression (whether due to the active ingredient or the carrier solvents), careful attention to the airway is in order. Rhabdomyolysis may necessitate urinary alkalinization, which may also correct the metabolic acidosis sometimes observed. Hypotension may respond to catecholamines and judicious use of crystalloids. Hsu and coworkers demonstrated in a rat model that the hypotension sometimes associated with abamectin is due to an increase in baroreflex sensitivity and to increased serum nitric oxide levels. The latter responds to treatment with epinephrine, whereas the baroreflex sensitivity does not.[60]

FIPRONIL

Fipronil (Fig. 77-4) is an *N*-phenylpyrazole, which competitively antagonizes the β subunit of the GABA α receptor. The binding to insect GABA is 1000-fold greater than that in human brain,[61] likely accounting for the low toxicity in humans.

Absorption and Metabolism

Fipronil appears to be poorly absorbed from the gastrointestinal tract, based on a rat model, with 45% to 75% being excreted in the feces.[62] Jennings and associates warned of possible human adverse effects due to skin absorption after repeated exposures to dogs treated with fipronil.[63] This conclusion was based on a

FIGURE 77-4 Fipronil.

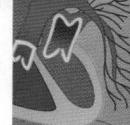

study of fipronil concentrations in gloves after petting treated dogs. Metabolism is by the liver, with CYP3A4 the major isoform responsible for fipronil oxidation in humans. CYP2C19 is considerably less active. Other human CYP isoforms have minimal or no activity toward fipronil.[64]

Toxicology

The oral LD_{50} in rats is 97 mg/kg, and the dermal LD_{50} is more than 2000 mg/kg. The no observed effect level (NOEL) in rats for neurologic effects is 0.5 mg/kg, and the lowest observed adverse effect level (LOAEL) is 5 mg/kg.[65] Fung and colleagues reported the accidental ingestion of a single ant bait (0.14 mg) of fipronil by a 77-year-old woman, who mistook it for a biscuit.[65] She had transient subjective impairment of sensorium 30 minutes after ingestion, which resolved about 30 minutes later. She had no other symptoms and no sequelae. Chodorowski and Anand reported on a 50-year-old man with occupational exposure while spraying with a solution of fipronil (Regent 200 SC) over a 5-hour period.[66] He complained of headache, nausea, vertigo, and weakness. All symptoms resolved over a 5-hour period.[66] The largest series of cases published so far comes from Mohamed and colleagues in Sri Lanka,[67] where seven patients taking intentional overdoses were described. Two patients suffered nonsustained generalized tonic–clonic seizures, which were responsive to treatment with diazepam. One patient with very high plasma concentration (1040 mg/L) remained entirely asymptomatic. There are no other reports of serious toxicity in humans.

IMIDACLOPRID

Imidacloprid (Fig. 77-5) is an insecticide of the chloronicotinyl neonicotinoid family. It has been suggested that mammalian toxicity should be low, as compared with insects, because of differences in nicotinic receptor subtypes. There have been very few reports of overdose from these compounds. Wu and colleagues have published a single clinical case involving a 64-year-old man who ingested an insecticide formulation (Tie-Boo-Tzang) containing 9.6% imidacloprid, less than 2% surfactant, and the balance a solvent, N-methyl pyrrolidone.[68] The patient experienced drowsiness, disorientation, dizziness, oral and esophageal erosions, hemorrhagic gastritis, productive cough, fever, leukocytosis, and hyperglycemia. Despite this, the patient recovered without sequelae and was discharged on

hospital day 4. Follow-up revealed no persistent gastrointestinal lesions on barium studies. The authors concluded that the solvent was likely responsible for the CNS depression, gastrointestinal irritation, and hyperglycemia. More recently, Proença and colleagues reported two fatalities involving presumed suicidal ingestions of imidacloprid.[69] Both patients were found dead at home, thus clinical details are lacking. The authors provide technical information on the liquid chromatography/mass spectrometry (LC/MS) analysis of the compound.

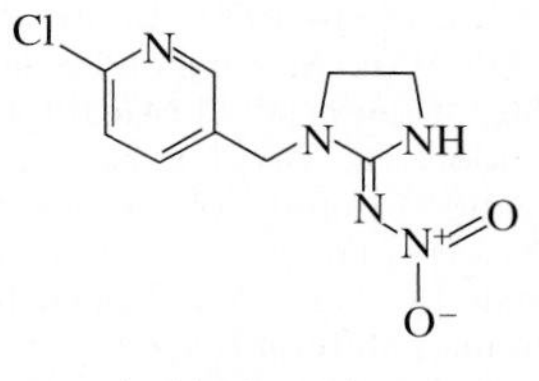

DEET

DEET is N,N-diethyl-m-toluamide (Fig. 77-6) and is one of the most widely employed insect repellants worldwide. It was developed in 1946 by the U.S. Department of Agriculture for use by the military and approved for civilian use in 1957. DEET has a colorful history in terms of its reported human toxicity, having been implicated, along with pyrethrins and organophosphates, in the development of Gulf War syndrome.[70] This issue has been studied intensively and reviewed by the Institute of Medicine, which reached no definitive conclusions about the involvement of DEET or other pesticides in the syndrome.[71] However, research continues in this area.[72] The complexity of this matter (multifactorial etiologies, problems with case definitions) does not permit its further discussion here.

The U.S. Environmental Protection Agency (EPA) issued a Reregistration Eligibility Decision (RED) in 1998 for DEET. After completing a comprehensive reassessment of DEET, the EPA concluded that, as long as consumers follow label directions and take proper precautions, insect repellents containing DEET do not present a health concern. Human exposure is expected to be brief, and long-term exposure is not expected. Based on extensive toxicity testing, the EPA believes that the normal use of DEET does not present a health concern to the general population.

Uses

DEET is widely employed as a mosquito and tick repellant in concentrations varying from 5% to 100%. The American Academy of Pediatrics previously recommended application of only dilute (<10%) products in children but now states that the safety of DEET does not appear to relate to differences in concentrations between 10% and 30%, recommending selection of the lowest concentration effective for the amount of time spent outdoors and no more than one application per day. The Academy does not recommend DEET for use in children younger than 2 months of age.[73]

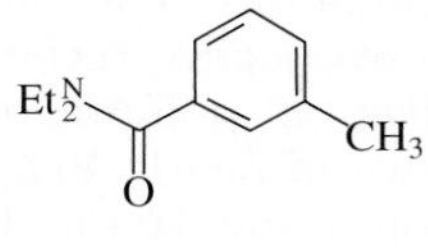

FIGURE 77-5 Imidacloprid.

FIGURE 77-6 DEET.

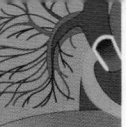

Routes of Entry

DEET may be toxic by ingestion, inhalation, or skin or eye absorption, although most cases of significant toxicity and death have followed multiple applications to the skin. Studies in normal male adult volunteers found dermal absorption in the range of 5.63% to 16.7% after single-dose applications.[74]

Metabolism

DEET is metabolized through cytochromes P-450 by an oxidation process (CYP2B6 and CYP1A2) to N,N-diethyl-m-hydroxymethylbenzamide (BALC) or by dealkylation by CYP2C19 and CYP3A4 to N-ethyl-m-toluamide (ET).[74]

Toxicity

Osimitz and Murphy reviewed the literature, clinical reports, and poison center records with regard to neurotoxicity.[75] They identified 14 reports concerning 20 individuals with reported adverse effects. These included 1 report of manic psychosis, 1 of anaphylaxis, a cardiovascular event, and 3 cases of alleged teratogenicity. The remaining 14 reports were of neurologic symptoms, including headaches, ataxia, seizures (n = 7), opisthotonos, disorientation and encephalopathy, myoclonus, and a movement disorder. Most were in children younger than 8 years of age, and three children died. Alternative diagnoses were proposed by the authors, including idiopathic seizures and various forms of infectious diseases and encephalopathy. The authors concluded that, given the widespread use of DEET, the paucity of such reports of neurologic toxicity and the case records of poison control centers, that the risk for adverse events was low. They recommended a prospective evaluation, in the form of a DEET registry, which was established by manufacturers and marketers. Bell and associates subsequently summarized the reports of DEET human exposures to the TESS database of the AAPCC from 1993 to 1997.[76] Of 20,764 reported exposures (oral, inhalation, dermal, ocular, and multiple routes), most had no effect, an unknown effect judged nontoxic, or minimal toxicity. There were two deaths associated with dermal exposures and none with other routes. Major effects were reported in just 26 cases (0.1%). Interestingly, the percentage of moderate effects involving adults (50%) exceeded that in children (38%) despite 64% of exposures being reported in children. Sudakin and Trevathan also recently reviewed the human toxicity of DEET.[74] They concluded that reports of adverse effects from topical application are rare, compared with their widespread use. They pointed out that the mechanisms for neurotoxic effects remain elusive, and advised prudent compliance with label directions and reporting of adverse events and careful identification of the implicated formulations. They also underlined the limitations of the retrospective review of poison center data by Bell and colleagues, pointing out that the medical outcome was unknown in nearly 40% of exposure cases, making interpretation of the dataset difficult.

Ingestion of DEET may result in rapid and severe toxicity. Petrucci and Sardini reported on a case of ingestion of 80 mg/kg (4 mL of a 20% solution) in a 10-kg, 3-year-old girl.[77] The child developed coma, with a Glasgow Coma Scale score of 6 and left horizontal nystagmus. She subsequently became hypertonic with opisthotonic episodes and three brief (<1 minute) generalized seizures. She received 15 mg of rectal diazepam and assisted ventilation with 100% oxygen. The level of consciousness improved over 4 hours, and the child was alert and responsive 10 hours later. She was discharged after 24 hours, without sequelae.[74] Tenenbein had previously reported on five ingestions of DEET. Each patient ingested large amounts of concentrated (47.5%–95%) products. Their common symptoms and signs were coma, seizures, and hypotension occurring within 1 hour of ingestion. Two patients died; three survivors had no sequelae.[78]

In summary, toxic neurologic complications have been reported after skin exposures (generally repeated) and ingestions of DEET. Toxicity with recommended use appears to be rare.

Laboratory Studies

DEET may be quantified in plasma and urine by an HPLC technique.[79] This test is not generally available in hospital laboratories and therefore is unlikely to guide therapy, but it may be useful for forensic purposes.

Treatment

Treatment of suspected DEET-related toxicity is supportive. Careful attention to the airway is necessary in the case of CNS depression or seizures. Seizures may be treated with benzodiazepines, when necessary. Refractory seizures may be treated with phenobarbital.

REFERENCES

 1. The World Health Report 1999: Making a Difference. Geneva, World Health Organization, 1999.
 2. Snow RW, Guerra CA, Noor AM, et al: The global distribution of clinical episodes of *Plasmodium falciparum* malaria. Nature 2005;434(7030):214–217.
 3. Alten B, Caglar SS, Simsek FM, Kaynas S: Effect of insecticide-treated bednets for malaria control in Southeast Anatolia-Turkey. J Vector Ecol 2003;28(1):97–107.
 4. Abdollahi M, Ranjbar A, Shadnia S, et al: Pesticides and oxidative stress: a review. Med Sci Monit 2004;10(6):RA141–RA147.
 5. Zlotkin E: The insect voltage-gated sodium channel as target of insecticides. Annu Rev Entomol 1999;44:429–455.
 6. Herber O, Kroeger A: Pyrethroid-impregnated curtains for Chagas' disease control in Venezuela. Acta Trop 2003;88(1):33–38.
 7. Barlow SM, Sullivan FM, Lines J: Risk assessment of the use of deltamethrin on bednets for the prevention of malaria. Food Chem Toxicol 2001;39(5):407–422.
 8. Pesticide residues in food—1999. Evaluations—1999. Part II. Toxicology. Joint FAO/WHO Meeting on Pesticide Residues. Report No. WHO/PCS/00.4. Geneva, World Health Organization, 2000.
 9. Schettgen T, Heudorf U, Drexler H, Angerer J: Pyrethroid exposure of the general population: is this due to diet? Toxicol Lett 2002;134(1–3):141–145.
10. Woollen BH, Marsh JR, Laird WJ, Lesser JE: The metabolism of cypermethrin in man: differences in urinary metabolite profiles following oral and dermal administration. Xenobiotica 1992;22(8):983–991.

11. World Health Organization: 1995 Vector control for malaria and other mosquito-borne diseases. Report of a WHO Study Group. Geneva, Author, 1995.

12. Leng G, Lewalter J: Role of individual susceptibility in risk assessment of pesticides. Occup Environ Med 1999;56(7):449–453.

13. Leng G, Lewalter J, Rohrig B, Idel H: The influence of individual susceptibility in pyrethroid exposure. Toxicol Lett 1999;107(1–3):123–130.

14. Ray DE, Forshaw PJ: Pyrethroid insecticides: poisoning syndromes, synergies, and therapy. J Toxicol Clin Toxicol 2000;38(2):95–101.

15. Rousselin X: Toxicité des dérivés du pyrèthre. Paris, Faculté de Médecine Lariboisière-Saint-Louis, Université Paris VII, 1983.

16. Kavlock R, Chernoff N, Baron R, et al: Toxicity studies with decamethrin, a synthetic pyrethroid insecticide. J Environ Pathol Toxicol 1979;2(3):751–765.

17. Environmental Health Criteria 97: Deltamethrin. Geneva, International Programme on Chemical Safety, 1990.

18. He F, Wang S, Liu L, et al: Clinical manifestations and diagnosis of acute pyrethroid poisoning. Arch Toxicol 1989;63(1):54–58.

19. Chen SY, Zhang ZW, He FS, et al: An epidemiological study on occupational acute pyrethroid poisoning in cotton farmers. Br J Ind Med 1991;48(2):77–81.

20. Yang PY, Lin JL, Hall AH, et al: Acute ingestion poisoning with insecticide formulations containing the pyrethroid permethrin, xylene, and surfactant: a review of 48 cases. J Toxicol Clin Toxicol 2002;40(2):107–113.

21. LoVecchio F, Knight J: Injection of pyrethroids without significant sequelae. Am J Emerg Med 2005;23(3):406.

22. Carlson JE, Villaveces JW: Hypersensitivity pneumonitis due to pyrethrum: report of a case. JAMA 1977;237(16):1718–1719.

23. Wagner SL: Fatal asthma in a child after use of an animal shampoo containing pyrethrin. West J Med 2000;173(2):86–87.

24. Wax PM, Hoffman RS: Fatality associated with inhalation of a pyrethrin shampoo. J Toxicol Clin Toxicol 1994;32(4):457–460.

25. Karpati AM, Perrin MC, Matte T, et al: Pesticide spraying for West Nile virus control and emergency department asthma visits in New York City, 2000. Environ Health Perspect 2004;112(11):1183–1187.

26. Spettoli E, Silvani S, Lucente P, et al: Contact dermatitis caused by sesquiterpene lactones. Am J Contact Dermat 1998;9(1):49–50.

27. Lisi P: Sensitization risk of pyrethroid insecticides. Contact Dermatitis 1992;26(5):349–350.

28. Flannigan SA, Tucker SB, Key MM, et al: Primary irritant contact dermatitis from synthetic pyrethroid insecticide exposure. Arch Toxicol 1985;56(4):288–294.

29. Amer M, Metwalli M, Abu el-Magd Y: Skin diseases and enzymatic antioxidant activity among workers exposed to pesticides. East Mediterr Health J 2002;8(2–3):363–373.

30. Malley LA, Cagen SZ, Parker CM, et al: Effect of vitamin E and other amelioratory agents on the fenvalerate-mediated skin sensation. Toxicol Lett 1985;29(1):51–58.

31. Altenkirch H, Hopmann D, Brockmeier B, Walter G: Neurological investigations in 23 cases of pyrethroid intoxication reported to the German Federal Health Office. Neurotoxicology 1996;17(3–4):645–651.

32. Muller-Mohnssen H, Hahn K: [A new method for early detection of neurotoxic diseases (exemplified by pyrethroid poisoning)]. Gesundheitswesen 1995;57(4):214–222.

33. Muller-Mohnssen H: Chronic sequelae and irreversible injuries following acute pyrethroid intoxication. Toxicol Lett 1999;107(1–3):161–176.

34. Nasterlack M, Chr Dietz M: [Comment on Muller-Mohnssen H, Hahn K: A method for early detection of neurotoxic diseases]. Gesundheitswesen 1996;58(1):49–50.

35. Hildebrand ME, McRory JE, Snutch TP, et al: Mammalian voltage-gated calcium channels are potently blocked by the pyrethyroid insecticide Allethrin. J Pharmacol Exp Ther 2004;308(3):805–813.

36. Kolaczinski JH, Curtis CF: Chronic illness as a result of low-level exposure to synthetic pyrethroid insecticides: a review of the debate. Food Chem Toxicol 2004;42(5):697–706.

37. Aprea C, Colosio C, Mammone T, et al: Biological monitoring of pesticide exposure: a review of analytical methods. J Chromatogr B Analyt Technol Biomed Life Sci 2002;769(2):191–219.

38. Leng G, Kuhn KH, Idel H: Biological monitoring of pyrethroids in blood and pyrethroid metabolites in urine: applications and limitations. Sci Total Environ 1997;199(1–2):173–181.

39. He F, Sun J, Han K, et al: Effects of pyrethroid insecticides on subjects engaged in packaging pyrethroids. Br J Ind Med 1988;45(8):548–551.

40. Zhang ZW, Sun JX, Chen SY, et al: Levels of exposure and biological monitoring of pyrethroids in spraymen. Br J Ind Med 1991;48(2):82–86.

41. Soderlund DM, Clark JM, Sheets LP, et al: Mechanisms of pyrethroid neurotoxicity: implications for cumulative risk assessment. Toxicology 2002;171(1):3–59.

42. Reigart JR, Roberts JR: Recognition and Management of Pesticide Poisoning. Washington, DC, U.S. Environmental Protection Agency, 1999.

43. Amitraz. In Extoxnet: Pesticide Information Profiles. Corvallis, OR, Oregon State University, 1995.

44. Agin H, Calkavur S, Uzun H, Bak M: Amitraz poisoning: clinical and laboratory findings. Indian Pediatr 2004;41(5):482–486.

45. Garnier R, Chataigner D, Djebbar D: Letter to the Editor. Hum Exp Toxicol 1998;17:294.

46. Jones RD: Xylene/amitraz: a pharmacologic review and profile. Vet Hum Toxicol 1990;32(5):446–448.

47. Cockburn A, Harvey PW, Needham D, et al: Double blind human dose tolerance study of amitraz with evaluation of autonomic, sensory and psychomotor function. Hum Exp Toxicol 1993;12:571.

48. Doganay Z, Aygun D, Altintop L, et al: Basic toxicological approach has been effective in two poisoned patients with amitraz ingestion: case reports. Hum Exp Toxicol 2002;21(1):55–57.

49. Hugnet C, Buronrosse F, Pineau X, et al: Toxicity and kinetics of amitraz in dogs. Am J Vet Res 1996;57(10):1506–1510.

50. Harvey PW, Cockburn A, Davies WW: Commentary on 'an unusual poisoning with the unusual pesticide amitraz' with respect to the pharmacology of amitraz. Hum Exp Toxicol 1998;17(3):191–192.

51. Chen ZK, Lu ZQ: Sodium dimercaptopropane sulfonate as antidote against non-metallic pesticides. Acta Pharmacol Sin 2004;25(4):534–544.

52. Prieto JG, Merino G, Pulido MM, et al: Improved LC method to determine ivermectin in plasma. J Pharm Biomed Anal 2003;31(4):639–645.

53. Campbell WC, Fisher MH, Stapley EO, et al: Ivermectin: a potent new antiparasitic agent. Science 1983;221(4613):823–828.

54. Elgart GW, Meinking TL: Ivermectin. Dermatol Clin 2003;21(2):277–282.

55. Heukelbach J, Feldmeier H: Ectoparasites: the underestimated realm. Lancet 2004;363(9412):889–891.

56. Korystov YN, Ermakova NV, Kublik LN, et al: Avermectins inhibit multidrug resistance of tumor cells. Eur J Pharmacol 2004;493(1–3):57–64.

57. Chung K, Yang CC, Wu ML, et al: Agricultural avermectins: an uncommon but potentially fatal cause of pesticide poisoning. Ann Emerg Med 1999;34(1):51–57.

58. Yen TH, Lin JL: Acute poisoning with emamectin benzoate. J Toxicol Clin Toxicol 2004;42(5):657–661.

59. Borron SW, Scherrmann JM, Baud FJ: Markedly altered colchicine kinetics in a fatal intoxication: examination of contributing factors. Hum Exp Toxicol 1996;15(11):885–890.

60. Hsu DZ, Chiang PJ, Hsu CH, et al: The elucidation of epinephrine as an antihypotensive agent in abamectin intoxication. Hum Exp Toxicol 2003;22(8):433–437.

61. Ratra GS, Kamita SG, Casida JE: Role of human GABA(A) receptor beta3 subunit in insecticide toxicity. Toxicol Appl Pharmacol 2001;172(3):233–240.

62. Hamernik KL: Pesticide residues in food. Geneva, International Programme on Chemical Safety, 1997.

63. Jennings KA, Canerdy TD, Keller RJ, et al: Human exposure to fipronil from dogs treated with Frontline. Vet Hum Toxicol 2002;44(5):301–303.

64. Tang J, Amin Usmani K, Hodgson E, Rose RL: In vitro metabolism of fipronil by human and rat cytochrome P450 and its interactions with testosterone and diazepam. Chem Biol Interact 2004;147(3):319–329.

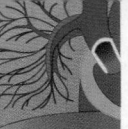
65. Fung HT, Chan KK, Ching WM, Kam CW: A case of accidental ingestion of ant bait containing fipronil. J Toxicol Clin Toxicol 2003;41(3):245–248.

66. Chodorowski Z, Anand JS: Accidental dermal and inhalation exposure with fipronil: a case report. J Toxicol Clin Toxicol 2004;42(2):189–190.

67. Mohamed F, Senarathna L, Percy A, et al: Acute human self-poisoning with the N-phenylpyrazole insecticide fipronil: a GABAA-gated chloride channel blocker. J Toxicol Clin Toxicol 2004;42(7):955–963.

68. Wu IW, Lin JL, Cheng ET: Acute poisoning with the neonicotinoid insecticide imidacloprid in N-methyl pyrrolidone. J Toxicol Clin Toxicol 2001;39(6):617–621.

69. Proença P, Teixeira H, Castanheira F, et al: Two fatal intoxication cases with imidacloprid: LC/MS analysis. Forensic Sci Int 2005;153:75–80.

70. Haley RW, Kurt TL: Self-reported exposure to neurotoxic chemical combinations in the Gulf War: a cross-sectional epidemiologic study. JAMA 1997;277(3):231–237.

71. Committee on Gulf War and Health: Gulf War and Health. 2. Insecticides and Solvents. Washington, DC, National Academy Press, 2003.

72. Abdel-Rahman A, Abou-Donia S, El-Masry E, et al: Stress and combined exposure to low doses of pyridostigmine bromide, DEET, and permethrin produce neurochemical and neuropathological alterations in cerebral cortex, hippocampus, and cerebellum. J Toxicol Environ Health A 2004;67(2):163–192.

73. AAP Committee on Environmental Health A: Follow safety precautions when using DEET on children. AAP News 2003;22(5):99.

74. Sudakin DL, Trevathan WR. DEET: a review and update of safety and risk in the general population. J Toxicol Clin Toxicol 2003;41(6):831–839.

75. Osimitz TG, Murphy JV: Neurological effects associated with use of the insect repellant N,N-diethyl-toluamide (DEET). J Toxicol Clin Toxicol 1997;35(5):435–441.

76. Bell JW, Veltri JC, Page BC: Human Exposures to N,N-diethyl-m-toluamide insect repellents reported to the American Association of Poison Control Centers 1993–1997. Int J Toxicol 2002;21(5):341–352.

77. Petrucci N, Sardini S: Severe neurotoxic reaction associated with oral ingestion of low-dose diethyltoluamide-containing insect repellent in a child. Pediatr Emerg Care 2000;16(5):341–342.

78. Tenenbein M: Severe toxic reactions and death following the ingestion of diethyltoluamide-containing insect repellents. JAMA 1987;258(11):1509–1511.

79. Abu-Qare AW, Abou-Donia MB: Development of a high-performance liquid chromatographic method for the quantification of chlorpyrifos, pyridostigmine bromide, N,N-diethyl-m-toluamide and their metabolites in rat plasma and urine. J Chromatogr B Biomed Sci Appl 2001;754(2):533–538.

78 *Herbicides*

SALLY M. BRADBERRY, BSc, MB, ChB ■ ALEX T. PROUDFOOT, BSc, MB ■ J. ALLISTER VALE, MD

At a Glance...

■ Herbicides form a diverse group of compounds designed to selectively or indiscriminately kill plants.

■ While use of herbicides far outweighs that of insecticides, significant poisoning by herbicides is relatively rare.

■ Herbicide toxicity varies significantly, and may be attributable to both active ingredients and adjuvants, such as solvents and surfactants.

■ The bipyridyls, diquat and paraquat, are highly toxic when ingested, through their production of highly reactive oxygen species. Diquat is primarily toxic to the kidneys, while paraquat causes often irreversible pulmonary injury. Plasma paraquat concentrations are helpful in predicting outcomes. Various antioxidant therapies have been proposed, but are unproven.

■ Chlorphenoxy herbicide ingestions likewise may result in severe toxicity. This is characterized by early persistent vomiting, metabolic acidosis, cardiac conduction and rhythm disturbances, and in severe cases, development of coma. Hemodialysis enhances removal of these compounds from the blood.

■ Glyphosate is widely used and is available as four different salts in association with various surfactants. Discerning the toxicity of the active ingredient from the surfactant is thus difficult. Severe poisonings may result in corrosive effects on the gastrointestinal tract with hemorrhage, hypovolemia, and cardiogenic shock, as well as aspiration pneumonitis. Pulmonary edema, metabolic acidosis, and hyperkalemia are poor prognostic indicators. Treatment is generally supportive.

■ Triazine herbicides rarely result in serious toxicity.

■ Urea herbicides may induce methemoglobinemia.

■ Bentazon poisoning is rare but may be fatal.

Herbicides comprise a diverse group of chemicals that kill plants either selectively or indiscriminately. They may be applied to clear ground of weeds before planting the crop to be grown, on ground so that weeds are killed as they emerge, and to weeds after they have emerged (called *preplanting, pre-emergence,* and *postemergence application,* respectively). Herbicides can also be classed according to chemical groups, as shown in Table 78-1. Although the tonnage of herbicides manufactured worldwide annually outweighs that of insecticides several-fold, herbicide poisoning in humans, both acute and chronic, is of considerably less importance than that caused by insecticides, especially in the developing world. Indeed, acute poisoning of humans with herbicides is uncommon. Therefore, despite the long list of herbicides available, this chapter considers only those that are likely to be of clinical importance today.

BIPYRIDYL HERBICIDES

Diquat

Diquat contains a bipyridyl ring (Fig. 78-1) and exists as a divalent cation associated with anions such as bromide and chloride. Diquat is classed as a nonselective, contact herbicide and is used as a preharvest desiccant on seed and fodder crops such as rice and sunflower.[1] Potential toxic effects on the environment are minimized by swift photochemical degradation and rapid adsorption to aquatic weeds and clay particles in soil.[2] Although there are many formulations containing diquat alone, it is also found in formulations with paraquat.

Most cases of diquat poisoning reported to date have resulted from the intentional, usually suicidal, ingestion of concentrated solutions, and rarely, accidental ingestion has occurred as a consequence of decanting diquat concentrates into soft drink bottles.[3] During the period from 1968 to 2004, only 34 cases of diquat poisoning were reported in detail in the literature,[4-8] of which 13 (43%) were fatal.

MECHANISMS OF TOXICITY

Diquat is a potent redox cycler, and its toxic effects depend on its ability to undergo a single electron addition to form a free radical. This occurs in the presence of

---

TABLE 78-1 Chemical Classification of Herbicides

CLASS	PRINCIPAL HERBICIDES
Aryphenoxypropionic acids	Diclofop and related compounds
Benzoic acids	Dicamba
Bipyridyl*	Paraquat, diquat*
Chloroacetanilides	Alachlor, propachlor
Chlorophenoxy*	2, 4-D*
Dinitrophenols	Dinoseb, di-nitro-orthocresol
Hydroxybenzonitriles	Bromoxynil, ioxynil
Organophosphonate*	Glyphosate*
Sulfonylureas	Triasulfuron
Triazines*	Atrazine, simazine, terbutryn*
Triazoles	Amitrole
Ureas*	Diuron, monolinuron*
Others	Bentazon(e)*

*Most likely to be of clinical importance today.

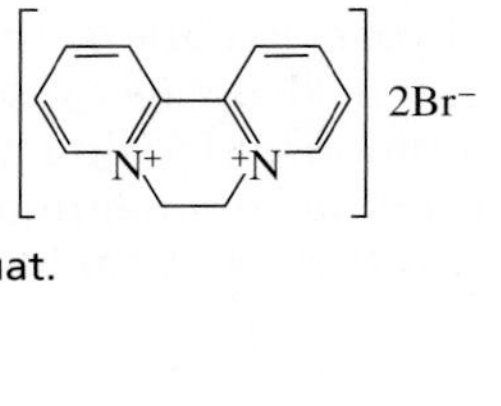

FIGURE 78-1 Diquat.

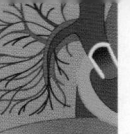

nicotinamide adenine dinucleotide phosphate (NADPH) and cytochrome P-450 reductase.[9] The diquat radical formed in this step is highly unstable and transfers an electron to molecular oxygen to form a superoxide anion radical, a highly reactive species. In this way, diquat is cycled in a continuous process of oxidation and reduction, hence the term *redox cycling*. The superoxide anion radicals produced react with each other, forming hydrogen peroxide and molecular oxygen, a reaction that may occur spontaneously or through the enzyme superoxide dismutase. Under normal circumstances, hydrogen peroxide is detoxified by catalase and glutathione peroxidase, but when such protective mechanisms are overwhelmed, it is free to cause devastating effects on cells.[10] In the presence of iron, the superoxide anion radical reacts with hydrogen peroxide, generating the even more potent hydroxyl radical, which can attack the lipid chains of biologic membranes, initiating lipid peroxidation that results in membrane damage and ultimately cell death.[10]

The oxidative stress induced by diquat is associated with the release of iron from hepatic ferritin[11,12] and the depletion of reducing equivalents, including glutathione and NADPH.[9,11] In experimental studies, protection against the toxic effects of diquat is provided by catalase, especially in the presence of the iron chelator, deferoxamine.[13] This suggests that hydrogen peroxide and transition metal ions may have important roles in the cytotoxicity of diquat. Unlike paraquat, diquat is not accumulated by the lung,[14] where it has a half-life 5 times shorter than paraquat.[15]

TOXICOKINETICS

In rats, less than 10% of an orally administered dose was absorbed, the unabsorbed portion being excreted in the feces.[16] Intact human skin is a very effective barrier against diquat absorption, and only 0.3% of an applied dose was absorbed in one study.[17]

CLINICAL FEATURES

Local Toxicity

Local toxicity has been reported after oral, dermal, inhalational, eye, and vaginal exposure to diquat-containing formulations. Corrosive damage to the oral mucosa, leading to burning in the mouth and painful hemorrhagic ulceration, is a common early feature of diquat ingestion. Mucosal edema of the tongue and oropharynx[18,19] may also develop and be severe enough to necessitate endotracheal intubation.[18] A male worker developed full-thickness burns of the feet after diquat dibromide leaked into his boots from a backpack sprayer[20]; skin grafting was required. Nail growth disturbances have been observed after contact of the nail base with diquat solutions for a few minutes, and shedding of the nail was reported after prolonged contact with concentrated diquat.[21]

Epistaxis and throat irritation have followed the inhalation of splashes or droplets caused by the careless mixing of diquat solutions.[21] Conjunctivitis and corneal scarring may occur if diquat-containing formulations are splashed directly into the eye.[22] Rudez and colleagues[23]

described extensive mucosal necrosis of the vagina and vulva after the intravaginal application of a 6% diquat solution.

Systemic Toxicity

Because skin absorption is poor, exposure by this route is unlikely to lead to systemic toxicity. The latter is usually associated with the ingestion of diquat, although it has followed the installation of 6% diquat solution intravaginally.[23]

Diquat may cause severe and extensive mucosal damage not only to the mouth but also to the esophagus, stomach, and small intestine.[19,24-26] As a consequence, generalized abdominal pain, vomiting, and diarrhea can occur within a few minutes of ingestion.[18,23,24,26-33] At endoscopy, severe panesophagitis and hemorrhagic gastritis at the fundus have been observed,[24] together with first- and second-degree burns of the esophagus and stomach.[19] Paralytic ileus may develop 1 to 4 days after ingestion[3,30,34] and is thought to be responsible for the accumulation or "sequestration" of large amounts of fluid in the gut, leading to hypovolemic shock.[30] Deranged liver function, as shown by a rise in hepatic aminotransferase/transaminase (SGOT, SGPT) activities, is reported commonly but is usually mild and transient and resolves spontaneously.[18,25,26,30-35]

Nephrotoxicity has been reported frequently and ranges from transient proteinuria[24,34] to acute renal failure.[3,18,19,23,26-30,32,33,35,35-39] Renal failure has developed between 1 hour[26] and 5 days[38] after ingestion and was invariably present in patients who died.

Bronchopneumonia has been reported at autopsy in four patients,[3,29,30,32] although it was diagnosed clinically in only two.[3,30] However, the radiologic appearances of pulmonary infiltration and exudates observed are similar to those in the adult respiratory distress syndrome, which may be the etiology of these features.

Coma has also been reported[3,30,32] and developed between 18 hours[30] and 4 days after ingestion.[3] It has been observed in association with pontine hemorrhages, and sometimes infarction, in life[3] and at autopsy.[3,29,30,32] Grand mal seizures, which progressed to status epilepticus, were observed in two patients.[18,26]

Of all the clinical features described, the rapid onset of acute renal failure, intestinal ileus, and subsequent fluid sequestration, pulmonary complications requiring ventilation and coma herald a poor prognosis.

MANAGEMENT

The use of methods to reduce diquat absorption may be considered. Gastric lavage and the administration of activated charcoal may be considered within 1 hour of a potentially life-threatening ingestion, although no controlled studies have been performed to support the value of this approach. If it is considered appropriate to undertake lavage, this must be done with extreme caution because there is a risk for perforation in the presence of corrosive mucosal damage. Oropharyngeal ulceration may be severe, and topical preparations, including local anesthetics, should be used to alleviate discomfort. Skin burns should be treated conventionally.

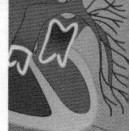

Because vomiting, diarrhea, and massive fluid sequestration in the gut can cause clinically significant hypovolemia, vigorous attention should be paid to fluid and electrolyte replacement, if necessary with the aid of central venous pressure or pulmonary capillary wedge pressure measurements. Hemofiltration or hemodialysis will need to be employed if acute renal failure supervenes.

Hemodialysis does not remove clinically and toxicologically relevant quantities of diquat[37,38] at the serum concentrations encountered in acute poisoning.

Paraquat

Paraquat contains a bipyridyl ring (Fig. 78-2) and exists as a divalent cation associated with anions such as chloride. From an agricultural point of view, it is the most important of the bipyridyl herbicides and is marketed in many countries either in granular form or as a water-soluble concentrate.

Although paraquat can be absorbed through the skin if improperly handled, poisoning much more commonly follows ingestion or, rarely, injection. Occasionally, food and drink may be adulterated with paraquat with intent to harm[40] or murder.[41] Less commonly, poisoning may follow careless handling of paraquat during occupational use. Normally, the surface epithelium of the skin is an excellent barrier to paraquat,[42] but prolonged skin contact with the herbicide may cause not only a chemical burn with blistering and ulceration but also serious and even fatal poisoning. Systemic toxicity is more likely to result if the paraquat solution is concentrated, exposure is prolonged, and the skin traumatized.[43] These conditions have been encountered as the result of poor occupational practice, including the use of leaking spray apparatus,[44-48] the nonuse of protective clothing,[43] prolonged wearing of contaminated clothing and failure to wash contaminated skin,[48] carelessness as with a farmer from Belize who fell off his bicycle with a bottle of paraquat in his pocket,[49] cleaning the perineum with paraquat by mistake,[50] and a mistaken belief that paraquat can be used as a treatment for lice and scabies.[47,51,52]

Systemic toxicity has followed the subcutaneous,[53] intraperitoneal, and intravenous[54,55] injection of paraquat. There is no conclusive evidence that systemic toxicity has ever followed inhalational exposure to paraquat.

MECHANISMS OF TOXICITY

Paraquat is thought to exert its cellular toxicity by, first, undergoing oxidation and reduction in a cyclical manner (redox cycling) to produce free radicals such as superoxide anion ($O_2^{\bullet-}$) and, second, depleting NADPH. Under anaerobic conditions, NADPH-dependent microsomal flavoprotein reductase reduces paraquat from its cation (PQ^{2+}) to form a stable free radical ($PQ^{\bullet\bullet}$).[56] In the presence of oxygen, the radical will immediately reform the cation,[57] with the concomitant production of superoxide anion ($O_2^{\bullet-}$). Provided there is a continuous supply of electrons to paraquat and that oxygen is present, paraquat will rapidly cycle from oxidized to reduced forms with the continuous production of superoxide anions.

The mechanism by which the redox cycling of paraquat leads to lung damage has not been established with certainty. There is indirect in vitro evidence that superoxide anions directly or indirectly, through the formation of more reactive species of oxygen such as hydroxyl radicals ($OH^{\bullet}$), cause peroxidation of vital lipid membranes.[58,59] However, some experiments have failed to demonstrate lipid peroxidation in vivo,[60] although there is a report that suggests that such a process can occur in humans after paraquat poisoning.[61]

An alternative or additional explanation for cellular toxicity of paraquat is that significant depletion of NADPH occurs by two mechanisms. First, redox cycling occurs to such an extent that NADPH levels within cells are decreased. Second, NADPH is used in the detoxification of hydrogen peroxide and lipid hydroperoxides through the glutathione peroxidase and reductase enzyme systems. It is postulated that depletion of NADPH not only disrupts essential physiologic and biochemical functions but also renders cells more susceptible to lipid peroxidation.[62] Baker and colleagues[62] have postulated that if the glutathione peroxide or reductase systems, together with endogenous levels of antioxidant, are inadequate to defend against peroxidation, it is possible that cell damage may occur. The depletion of NADPH by the redox cycling of paraquat leads to additional use of the remaining NADPH in an attempt to provide reduced glutathione for the glutathione enzyme activity. Thus, NADPH will be depleted both in the production of superoxide anion and in a defense to it. Consequently, the pentose phosphate pathway is stimulated in an attempt to regenerate NADPH.

The pathways dependent on NADPH appear to be inhibited either as a compensatory mechanism or because NADPH is depleted within the cell. With further generation of NADPH, this cofactor is available either to regenerate reduced glutathione or to further reduce paraquat cycling with oxygen. On balance, the evidence suggests that the concentration of paraquat in lung cells causes a severe redox stress that leads eventually to sustained depletion in NADPH levels. This by itself, or in combination with lipid peroxidation, initiates the cascade of biochemical events that lead to cell death.[62]

The biochemical effects described previously probably also occur in other organs in addition to the lung. It is likely that death occurring within a few hours of paraquat ingestion is due to massive depletion of NADPH with consequent destruction of energy metabolism, particularly in the liver. On the other hand, the clinical course observed in those suffering from less severe intoxication is in keeping with cell membrane destruction initiated by lipid peroxidation.

$$\left[H_3C-{}^+N \bigcirc\!\!-\!\!\bigcirc N^+ -CH_3 \right] 2Cl^-$$

FIGURE 78-2 Paraquat.

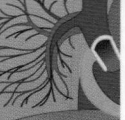

TOXICOKINETICS

Paraquat is absorbed incompletely from the gut, and in humans, it has been estimated that less than 10% of an ingested dose is absorbed over a 1- to 6-hour period.[63,64] Although absorption from the gut may be incomplete, it is rapid; paraquat may be detected in the urine as early as 1 hour after ingestion, and peak concentrations in humans are attained within 4 hours.[65]

CLINICAL FEATURES

Local Toxicity

Paraquat, especially in concentrated solutions, strongly irritates various types of epithelia. Thus, it causes erythema, blistering, and ulceration of the skin, and eczematous dermatitis has been reported.[66] Concentrated solutions may also cause localized discoloration or a white transverse band affecting the nail plate, although the latter may not become apparent for several weeks. Transverse ridging and furrowing progressing to gross deformity and nail loss may also occur.[66-68] Severe inflammation of the cornea and conjunctiva may follow the accidental splashing of paraquat concentrate into the eye. The inflammation develops gradually, reaches a maximum after 12 to 24 hours, and may lead to ulceration[69] with the risk for secondary infection. Lachrymal duct stenosis has also been described.[70] Inhalation of fine spray droplets through careless use can cause epistaxis and sore throat.

The corrosive action of paraquat when ingested causes patients who are moderately or severely poisoned to develop a burning sensation, soreness, and pain in the mouth, throat, chest (retrosternally), and abdomen (usually epigastric and sometimes associated with guarding). Ulceration in the mouth, sloughing of the oropharyngeal mucosa, inability to swallow saliva ("pseudo-hypersalivation"), dysphagia, and dysphonia are common. Prominent pharyngeal membranes ("pseudo-diphtheria") have been reported,[71] and perforation of the esophagus may result in mediastinitis, surgical emphysema, and pneumothorax. Most patients develop a cough, which may be productive and blood stained.

Systemic Toxicity

Three degrees of intoxication may usefully be distinguished.[72]

GROUP 1. Mild poisoning follows the ingestion or injection of less than 20 mg of paraquat ion per kilogram body weight. Patients are asymptomatic or develop vomiting and diarrhea. Full recovery occurs, but there may be a transient fall in the gas transfer factor and vital capacity.

GROUP 2. Moderate to severe poisoning follows the ingestion or injection of 20 to 40 mg/kg of paraquat ion. Patients suffer vomiting and diarrhea and develop generalized symptoms indicative of systemic toxicity. Pulmonary fibrosis develops in all cases, but recovery may occur. In addition, renal failure and, sometimes, hepatic dysfunction may supervene. Death occurs in most cases but can be delayed for 2 or 3 weeks.

GROUP 3. Acute fulminant poisoning follows the ingestion of more than (usually considerably in excess of) 40 mg/kg of paraquat ion. In addition to nausea and vomiting, there is marked ulceration of the oropharynx with multiple organ (cardiac, respiratory, hepatic, renal, adrenal, pancreatic, neurologic) failure. In this group, at least in our experience, the mortality rate is 100%. Death commonly occurs within 24 hours of ingestion of paraquat and is never delayed for more than 1 week.

Within 24 hours of ingestion, patients in groups 2 and 3 develop lethargy, a widespread burning sensation, generalized weakness, myalgia, giddiness, headache, anorexia, and fever. Fear and apprehension are prominent features, and restlessness is sometimes observed.

Oliguria or nonoliguric renal failure may supervene and is due usually to acute tubular necrosis, although, exceptionally, glomerular and tubular hemorrhage may be found.[73] Proximal tubular dysfunction, which results in proteinuria, microscopic hematuria, glycosuria, aminoaciduria, phosphaturia, and excessive leaking of sodium and urate, is common.[74] Jaundice, hepatomegaly, and central abdominal pain due to pancreatitis, together with associated biochemical abnormalities, are frequent complications in patients severely poisoned with paraquat. Centrilobular hepatic necrosis and cholestasis are seen at postmortem examination in these patients.

Dyspnea is a prominent feature and occurs early in those patients who have ingested a substantial amount and, in these circumstances, is due to the development of the adult respiratory distress syndrome. In less severely poisoned patients, the onset of dyspnea may be delayed and is then caused by pulmonary fibrosis. Rarely, pneumothorax (in association with mediastinitis), pleural effusion, and iatrogenic pulmonary edema, may precipitate dyspnea.

In addition to a falling gas transfer factor and vital capacity (which may return to normal in patients in group 1 and, less commonly, in those in group 2), severely poisoned patients will have a low and falling Po_2 with resultant central cyanosis. Radiologic changes do not always parallel the severity of clinical symptoms. Thus, the chest x-ray may be normal, particularly in those dying early from multiorgan failure. More usually, patchy infiltration occurs, which may progress to an opacification of one or both lung fields.

Except for sinus tachycardia, cardiovascular complications are not usually observed until the terminal phase of intoxication. Then, ventricular tachycardia, intraventricular conduction disturbances, and nonspecific T-wave changes on electrocardiogram (ECG) occur. Sinus bradycardia, hypotension, and cardiac arrest may supervene. The chest x-ray may show massive cardiomegaly, and at autopsy, toxic myocarditis is found histologically.

Coma is a common and terminal event, although other neurologic features, such as ataxia and facial paresis,[53] are observed occasionally. Convulsions have been reported[75-77] and may be due to cerebral edema[78] precipitated by fluid overload.[79]

A polymorphonuclear leucocytosis is a frequent finding, but rarely, erythrocyte aplasia leading to a normochromic anemia[80] has been reported. Metabolic acidosis, probably secondary to cardiovascular collapse and hypoxia, is a common complication. Hypocalcemia,

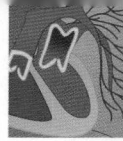

which sometimes results in tetany, is usually iatrogenic after either inappropriate attempts at forced diuresis in the presence of renal impairment[79] or charcoal hemoperfusion.[81] In addition, elevation of serum creatine kinase activity is seen, secondary to paraquat-induced muscle damage.

MANAGEMENT

Management has several aspects:

1. If the patient presents early (<1 hour after paraquat ingestion), attempts should be made to reduce paraquat absorption by the administration of activated charcoal.
2. Fluid loss induced by vomiting and diarrhea should be replaced.
3. The diagnosis should be confirmed and the prognosis determined by measurement of paraquat in blood.
4. Symptoms due to ulceration of the oropharynx must be relieved.
5. The use of specific therapy should be considered.
6. Appropriate supportive care for the patient and relatives must be provided.

Methods to Reduce Absorption

Gastric lavage and the administration of activated charcoal may be considered within 1 hour of a potentially life-threatening ingestion, although no controlled studies have been performed to support the value of these approaches. If it is considered appropriate to undertake lavage, this must be done with extreme caution because there is a risk for perforation in the presence of corrosive mucosal damage.

Supportive Measures

There is good evidence that, as a result of vomiting and diarrhea and the administration of purgatives, many patients poisoned with paraquat are fluid depleted.[82] An intravenous infusion should therefore be commenced on admission to reduce the risk for renal dysfunction and diminished renal excretion of paraquat.

Confirmation of the Diagnosis and Assessment of Prognosis

A qualitative urine test should be performed with alkaline sodium dithionite on presentation. If this test is negative within 4 hours of the overdose, there is no clinical need for a quantitative assay on the blood and the patient may be reassured accordingly. If, however, the urine test is positive, measurement of the plasma paraquat concentration is extremely helpful in determining prognosis[83] and may be interpreted by reference to published data,[65,84,85] which are summarized in Table 78-2.

Specific Therapy

Based on an understanding of the mechanism of paraquat toxicity, further management should theoretically be directed toward preventing the accumulation of paraquat in the lungs and reducing the acute alveolitis

TABLE 78-2 Predictive Plasma Paraquat Concentration Separating Surviving Patients and Fatalities	
TIME AFTER INGESTION (hr)	PLASMA PARAQUAT CONCENTRATION (µg/L)
4	2000
5	800
6	600
7	480
8	330
10	290
12	230
15	170
20	120
24	100
48	47
72	31
96	23
120	18
144	15
168	13
192	11
216	10
240	9
264	8
288	7
360	6

Based on Proudfoot AT, Stewart MS, Levitt T, et al: Paraquat poisoning: Significance of plasma-paraquat concentrations. Lancet 1979; 2:330; and Scherrmann JM, Houze P, Bismuth C, et al: Prognostic value of plasma and urine paraquat concentration. Hum Toxicol 1987; 6:91.

and pulmonary fibrosis that develop in severe cases of intoxication. However, there is no current clinical evidence that superoxide dismutase, propranolol, vitamin E, ascorbic acid, riboflavin, niacin, deferoxamine, clofibrate, acetylcysteine, cyclophosphamide, or corticosteroids are effective clinically.[86,87]

Use of Techniques to Increase Paraquat Elimination

Excretion of paraquat is almost exclusively renal; biliary excretion is very small.[16,64,88] The renal clearance of nontoxic doses of paraquat exceeds the glomerular filtration rate because of an active transport process[89] and may be in excess of 200 mL/min when renal function is normal.[89-92] As a result, more than 1000 mg/L paraquat ion may be excreted within the first few hours after ingestion.[93] Because renal failure supervenes early in severely poisoned patients, dialysis and hemoperfusion have been employed to increase paraquat elimination.

The clearance values achieved by hemodialysis are impressive (as much as 150 mL/min[94]), yet the amount removed is disappointingly small (often only a few milligrams of paraquat ion), in comparison to both the dose ingested and the contemporaneous renal clearance of paraquat.[64,95,96] The very small fraction of the dose eliminated by dialysis could not be expected to influence outcome in the more severely poisoned.

Similarly, despite impressive clearance data, the amount of paraquat removed by hemoperfusion is very small[94,97-100] and falls in parallel with the decrease in plasma paraquat concentrations.[101] Okonek and asso-

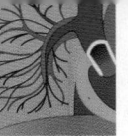

ciates[102] have proposed that hemoperfusion be performed for several days (8 hours per day for 2–3 weeks), and the authors claim that this approach has reduced the mortality from paraquat; their observations have not been confirmed.

Pond and colleagues[103] assessed the value of continuous arteriovenous hemofiltration (CAVH) in a patient whose presenting plasma paraquat concentration 4 hours after ingestion was 3 mg/L. CAVH was commenced 180 hours after paraquat ingestion (plasma concentration, about 0.34 mg/L). Over 46 hours of CAVH, 1.1 mg paraquat ion was removed, and a paraquat clearance of 6.1 mL/min was achieved.

In summary, there is no irrefutable evidence[95,101] that extracorporeal techniques used alone or together remove sufficient paraquat to alter the outcome in those patients who present with plasma paraquat concentrations above the predictive lines of Proudfoot and colleagues[65] and Bismuth and coworkers.[101]

Terminal Care: Relief of Local Pain and General Distress

No discussion of paraquat poisoning would be complete without considering how best to manage patients who are dying from this condition. It is of vital importance that the patient is not neglected or isolated. Frequent visits from medical and nursing staff are mandatory because bad or infrequent communication increases the suffering of the patient. Those who are dying reach out for support and companionship not only from their friends and relatives but also from their medical advisers. If asked, one should be honest about the prognosis while at the same time offering some hope.

Attention should be directed away from incurable organ damage to the alleviation of symptoms because there is always something that can be done to provide symptomatic relief. Pain and distress should be reduced to a minimum. It is difficult to abolish the severe pain produced by local ulceration. Mouth washes, ice-cold fluids (e.g., ice cream, lemon mucilage), local anesthetic sprays, and lozenges have all been employed with varying degrees of success. Opiates will be required in most patients to relieve general, as well as local, pain and distress. Above all, inappropriate treatment should be avoided. Thus, for example, the repeated use of cathartics when the outlook is hopeless is therapeutically irrelevant and clinically harmful. Although oxygen administration is theoretically harmful in paraquat poisoning, it should not be withheld in the terminal patient with air hunger.

CHLOROPHENOXY HERBICIDES

Chlorophenoxy herbicides are chemical analogs of auxins, a type of plant growth hormone, and produce uncontrolled and lethal growth in target plants. Because they are very effective selective weed killers, chlorophenoxy herbicides are used widely for the control of broad-leaved weeds in pastures, lawns, cereal crops, and public rights of way. In addition, closely related compounds are used as the active ingredients in rooting powders.

Structurally, chlorophenoxy herbicides comprise an aliphatic carboxylic acid moiety attached to a chlorine- or methyl-substituted aromatic ring. The most common is 2,4-D (2,4-dichlorophenoxyacetic acid); its formula and that of related compounds are shown in Figure 78-3. Dicamba is not a phenoxyacetate but is often considered with the chlorophenoxy compounds because it is an organic acid. 2,4,5-T has been largely withdrawn from worldwide use because of concerns that arose from contamination of some formulations with dioxin, the most notorious of which was Agent Orange, used as a defoliant in Vietnam.

Chlorophenoxy herbicides often are coformulated with ioxynil, bromoxynil, or both, which generally are more toxic and similarly uncouple oxidative phosphorylation. Formulations may also contain hydrocarbon solvents.

Chlorophenoxy herbicide poisoning is uncommon but may produce severe sequelae. Most cases of serious poisoning involve deliberate ingestion of 2,4-D either alone or in combination with other chlorophenoxy herbicides or ioxynil/bromoxynil.

Among more than 11.2 million human toxic exposures reported by U.S. Regional Poisons Centers to the American Association of Poison Control Centers (AAPCC) Toxic Exposure Surveillance System (TESS) between

2,4-Dichlorophenoxy acetic acid (2,4-D)

2,4,5-Trichlorophenoxy acetic acid (2,4,5-T)

4-Chloro-2-methylphenoxy propionic acid (Mecoprop)

4-Chloro-2-methylphenoxyacetic acid (MCPA)

2-(2,4-Dichlorophenoxy) propionic acid 2(2,4-DP, DCPP, dichlorprop)

3,6-Dichloro-2-methoxybenzoic acid (Dicamba)

4-(2,4-Dichlorophenoxy) butyric acid (2,4-DB)

4-Chloro-2-methylphenoxy butyric acid (MCPB)

FIGURE 78-3 Chemical structure of some chlorophenoxy herbicides.

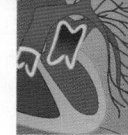

1998 and 2002,[104-108] 11,385 involved chlorophenoxy herbicides; at least 30% involved children younger than 6 years old and may not have been toxic exposures. Thirty-three exposures resulted in life-threatening or significant residual effects, and there were two deaths.

Mechanisms of Toxicity

Dose-dependent cell membrane damage is likely to be important in the mediation of chlorophenoxy-induced central nervous system (CNS) toxicity, for example by damage to the blood-brain barrier and disruption of neuronal and mitochondrial membranes. Mitochondrial membrane damage may trigger apoptosis.[109] In addition, chlorophenoxy herbicides are related structurally to acetic acid and can form analogs of acetyl coenzyme A (CoA; such as 2,4-D-CoA) or enter the acetylcholine (ACh) synthetic pathway to form choline esters (e.g., 2,4-D-ACh). Thus, they can disrupt metabolic pathways and act as "false" neurotransmitters. Uncoupling of oxidative phosphorylation is a further likely mechanism of toxicity.

Toxicokinetics

Chlorophenoxy compounds are absorbed rapidly after oral administration in humans,[110,111] but absorption dermally[17,111,112] and by inhalation[113] is limited. They bind extensively to serum albumin[114,115] and have relatively high volumes of distribution (between 0.1 L/kg[116] and 0.2 L/kg[110] for 2,4-D in humans). Some 82% of an administered dose is eliminated unchanged in urine.[110] Clearance occurs by first-order processes,[110] although at high doses, the organic anion secretory system may be overwhelmed, and elimination then follows Michaelis-Menten kinetics, at least in animals.[111]

Substantial interindividual and interspecies variation in elimination of chlorophenoxy herbicides is apparent.[117] The elimination half-life in humans of 2,4-D 5 mg/kg orally varies between 11.6[110] and 33 hours.[116]

Clinical Features

INGESTION

Nearly all reported cases of chlorophenoxy herbicide ingestion have involved 2,4-D, either alone or with other chlorophenoxy herbicides, such that it is difficult to distinguish between members of this pesticide class in terms of toxicity.[118] Vomiting is a prominent early feature and may be accompanied by burning in the mouth, abdominal pain, diarrhea, and occasionally gastrointestinal hemorrhage. Severe corrosive damage is rare and probably due to surfactants or solvents in the formulation. Gastrointestinal fluid loss, vasodilation, and direct myocardial toxicity contribute to the development of hypotension, which is common. Electrocardiogram abnormalities such as T-wave flattening or inversion,[119] QT-interval prolongation,[120,121] supraventricular or ventricular tachycardia, and rarely, sinus bradycardia[122] have been reported.

In severe cases, gastrointestinal features are followed frequently by the onset of coma, which is an almost invariable feature in fatal cases and often lasts several days in those who survive.[118] Hypertonia, hyperreflexia, clonus, and occasionally extensor plantar responses suggest upper motor neuron involvement.[119,123-128] Cerebral edema,[120] miosis, nystagmus, ataxia, alterations in color vision, memory loss, hallucinations, and convulsions have also been reported.[118]

Coma is associated frequently with respiratory distress, tachypnea, inadequate ventilation, and occasionally pulmonary edema. Hypoventilation secondary to CNS depression is the primary cause of hypoxia, although respiratory muscle weakness may contribute also as part of a generalized myopathy.[119,129] The latter is characterized by limb weakness, reduced or absent tendon reflexes,[119,123,127,130,131] and increased creatine kinase activity.[119,130,132] Aspiration of gastric contents may contribute to pulmonary complications.[123,131] Hemoptysis is a rare complication.[133]

Some degree of peripheral neuromuscular involvement is common, as evidenced by loss of tendon reflexes, muscle twitching, fasciculation, weakness, or myotonia.[118] Nerve damage with electromyographic evidence of a peripheral neuropathy has been reported rarely.[119,134] These effects may persist for several weeks in patients who survive.

Other reported features of chlorophenoxy herbicide ingestion include metabolic acidosis,[119,120,122] hyperthermia in the absence of infection (possibly reflecting uncoupling of oxidative phosphorylation),[119,122,129] renal failure,[126,135] rhabdomyolysis,[132] increased transaminase and aminotransferase activities (SGOT, SGPT), and lactate dehydrogenase,[130,136] thrombocytopenia,[132,137] hemolytic anemia, and hypocalcemia.[125]

Although the prognosis is poor in patients who rapidly become shocked and comatose, full recovery can ensue over weeks to months despite initial severe toxicity and prolonged neuromuscular effects.

It is not possible to derive a dose–response relationship from published cases because the dose was rarely, if ever, known with accuracy. Flanagan and coworkers[122] suggested that a total plasma chlorophenoxy concentration in excess of 500 mg/L was associated with severe toxicity. This view is supported by the postmortem findings in a 61-year-old woman who ingested a formulation containing 2,4-D, mecoprop, and dicamba: the blood concentrations for 2,4-D, mecoprop, and dicamba were, respectively, 520 mg/L, 530 mg/L, and 170 mg/L,[138] but more data are required.

DERMAL EXPOSURE

Because dermal absorption of chlorophenoxy herbicides is poor, acute poisoning through this route is uncommon. Local skin irritation may occur, but there are few reports of systemic toxicity following such exposures. Interpretation of cases in which systemic effects are described is complicated, and the etiologic role of chlorophenoxy herbicides in many has been challenged.[139] Five cases were published between 1959 and 1963.[140-142] All patients recovered, although mild weakness was present at 2- to 3-year follow-up in three cases.[141,142] It is noteworthy that there have been no published reports of

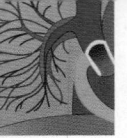

systemic chlorophenoxy herbicide poisoning following dermal exposure for more than 20 years, and no reported fatalities from such exposures in the history of chlorophenoxy herbicide use.

INHALATION

Gastrointestinal and peripheral neuromuscular symptoms have been reported also following occupational exposure in which inhalation was an important route, either alone or in combination with skin exposure.[143-146] Features described included nausea and vomiting, constipation, abdominal pain, limb paresthesias and pain, myalgia, weakness, hypertonia, dizziness, vertigo, loss of consciousness, nodal tachycardia, chest pain, and palpitation. In some cases, features persisted for several weeks after a single exposure. Again, a causative association in these cases cannot be confirmed.

OCULAR EXPOSURE

McMillin and Samples[147] reported the accidental exposure of a previously healthy 30-year-old man to a 2,4-D-containing herbicide. Within 3 hours, he developed decreased visual acuity, ocular discomfort, photophobia, and loss of accommodation in the exposed eye. The symptoms persisted despite topical treatment with prednisolone and scopolamine, but resolved over the ensuing 3 weeks. Whether this toxic iritis was due to 2,4-D or to some other component in the commercial formulation is unknown.

Management

The administration of oral activated charcoal, 50 to 100 g, to an adult may be considered in patients who have ingested a potentially toxic amount of a chlorophenoxy herbicide within 1 hour because in vitro studies demonstrate that chlorophenoxy herbicides are adsorbed to activated charcoal.[148]

Urine alkalinization and hemodialysis to enhance herbicide elimination should be considered in severely poisoned patients. However, despite several reports claiming enhanced elimination with urine alkalinization,[122,149,150] only for one patient[119,151] are there sufficient data to justify the claim. This 39-year-old man developed features of severe poisoning after ingestion of 2,4-D, 6.8 g, and mecoprop, 13.6 g (calculated).[119,151] The admission urine pH was 6.4, the plasma 2,4-D concentration 400 mg/L, and the plasma mecoprop concentration 751 mg/L. An "alkaline diuresis" comprising 14 L of fluid containing 69.3 g sodium bicarbonate (825 mmol) over 48 hours[119] was instituted some 42 hours after ingestion, although a urine pH greater than 7.5 was not achieved until after 70 to 75 hours. Increased renal clearance of both herbicides was achieved with alkalinization, but to an extent that was highly dependent on urine flow rate. Clinical improvement paralleled the fall in 2,4-D and mecoprop concentrations, and consciousness was regained on the fourth day after ingestion when the plasma 2,4-D and mecoprop concentrations were about 100 mg/L. When clearance data were corrected for urine flow rate, urine alkalinization without high

urine flow was markedly less efficient than hemodialysis as a means of removing 2,4-D.

Durakovic and associates[121] treated four patients with 2,4-D poisoning by hemodialysis, of whom two also had resin hemoperfusion. The dialysis clearance in one patient was 68.7 mL/min, and in the two patients receiving combined therapy, the clearances were 56.3 mL/min and 72.9 mL/min, suggesting that hemodialysis with or without hemoperfusion is more efficient than urine alkalinization, although urine alkalinization, combined with a high urine flow (600 mL/hour), produces similar clearance values.[119,151] Nonetheless, in all severe cases, hemodialysis is the preferred elimination treatment because it greatly enhances clearance without the need for urine pH manipulation and the administration of substantial amounts of intravenous fluid to compromised patients. The final choice may be dictated by the availability of hemodialysis.

GLYPHOSATE

Glyphosate (*N*-phosphonomethyl glycine) is a phosphorus-containing organic compound (Fig. 78-4) used extensively as an herbicide by both professionals and amateurs. It is one of the first herbicides against which crops have been genetically modified to increase their tolerance.

Commercial formulations range from concentrates containing 41% or more glyphosate as the isopropylamine (IPA) salt to 1% glyphosate formulations marketed for domestic use. They generally include a surfactant, antifoaming and color agents, biocides, and inorganic ions to produce pH adjustment.[152]

The attractiveness of glyphosate is due to several factors, including its plant-specific action, inactivation on contact with soil, and suitability for no-till conservation of crops. In addition, it has a favorable environmental safety profile.

In the 3-year period from 2001 to 2003, there were 13,318 reports to the AAPCC TESS relating to glyphosate exposure.[107,108,153] Of these, 3622 involved children younger than 6 years. There was a "moderate" outcome in 291 patients, a life-threatening outcome in 18, and death in 5. Case series of glyphosate ingestions[154-158] have reported mortality rates of 8% to 16%; of the 377 cases reported, 38 died.

Most glyphosate-related reports to the California Environmental Protection Agency Pesticide Illness Surveillance Program for 1982 to 1997 involved topical irritation of the eye or skin without systemic symptoms. Systemic features were present in 187 cases, but only in 22 were they probably or definitely related to glyphosate alone.[152]

$$HO-\overset{\displaystyle O}{\overset{\|}{C}}-CH_2-\underset{\displaystyle H}{N}-CH_2-\overset{\displaystyle O}{\overset{\|}{\underset{\displaystyle OH}{P}}}-OH$$

FIGURE 78-4 Chemical structure of glyphosate.

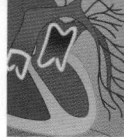

Mechanisms of Toxicity

The mechanisms of toxicity of glyphosate formulations are complex, not least because glyphosate is used as four different salts in combination with surfactants, which vary in nature and concentration. It is therefore difficult to separate the toxicity of glyphosate from that of the formulation as a whole or to determine the contribution of surfactants to overall toxicity.

GLYPHOSATE

Glyphosate alone is of very low toxicity orally (LD_{50} > 5000 mg/kg) and dermally (LD_{50} > 2000 mg/kg). It may enhance adenosine triphosphatase activity and uncouple mitochondrial oxidative phosphorylation,[159-162] although this has been disputed.[156] In rats, it decreases hepatic cytochrome P-450 and monooxygenase activities and the intestinal activity of aryl hydrocarbon hydroxylase.[163] Although at high concentrations in vitro, glyphosate inhibits acetylcholinesterase, there is no evidence that it inhibits acetylcholinesterase in vivo.

There is very limited evidence that products containing glyphosate trimesium are more toxic than those with other glyphosate salts.[164]

SURFACTANTS

Surfactants in concentrations of up to 50% are added to nearly all glyphosate preparations. In general, they interfere with the walls of mitochondria, destroying the proton gradient required for energy production, effects consistent with the poorly responsive multiple-organ failure generally seen after surfactant ingestions. Because some are strongly alkaline, adjustment to a neutral pH is required when they are coformulated with glyphosate.

The most widely used surfactant is polyoxyethyleneamine (POEA), although this name refers to a group of compounds rather than a single chemical entity. The concentration of polyoxyethyleneamine ranges from less than 1% in ready-to-use glyphosate formulations to 21% in some concentrated professional products.

Other surfactants used in glyphosate-containing herbicides include those derived from plant fats, alkyl polyoxyphosphate amine, polyethoxylated-alkyletheramine, trimethylethoxypolyoxypropyl–ammonium chloride, and ethoxylated phosphate ester.

The main controversy regarding the toxicity of glyphosate formulations is whether toxicity is due to the herbicide itself or to coformulants, notably surfactants. The evidence suggests that the toxicity of the surfactant, POEA, is greater than the toxicity of glyphosate alone. There is insufficient evidence to conclude that glyphosate preparations containing polyoxyethyleneamine are more toxic than those containing alternative surfactants. However, the weight of evidence is against surfactants potentiating the toxicity of glyphosate; indeed, the reverse may be more likely.

Toxicokinetics

The existing knowledge of the toxicokinetics of glyphosate is mainly derived from animal studies and has been reviewed recently.[165] Only some 30% is absorbed after oral administration to rats[165,166]; peak plasma concentrations are attained within 1 to 2 hours[165,167,168] and decline quickly.[169] Most absorbed glyphosate is then rapidly excreted unchanged in the urine.

A similar pattern of absorption, metabolism, and elimination after ingestion is seen in humans, although the data are limited. Absorption of glyphosate through human skin is poor (<1%).[165,170] Two poisoned patients reached peak plasma glyphosate concentrations within 4 hours of ingestion, the concentrations being almost undetectable by 12 hours.[171] Severe poisoning is associated with plasma glyphosate concentrations exceeding 1000 mg/L,[171] and occasionally, concentrations as high as 1600 mg/L have been encountered.[172]

Only a small proportion of glyphosate is metabolized to aminomethylphosphonic acid (AMPA): the ratios of glyphosate to AMPA in serum at 8 and 16 hours after ingestion were 126:1 and 147:1, respectively.[173]

Absorption after inhalation does not appear to have been studied but would not be expected to be significant.

Clinical Features

Regardless of the route of exposure, most reports of human poisoning with severe features generally involve concentrated formulations containing 41% glyphosate as the isopropylamine salt and 15% polyoxyethyleneamine. Accidental exposure usually causes only mild, transient features.

INGESTION

Nausea, vomiting, and diarrhea are the only likely features following ingestion of glyphosate ready-to-use amateur formulations. Up to 30 mL of the 41% glyphosate plus 5% to15% polyoxyethyleneamine formulations may also cause these symptoms, together with burning in the mouth and throat and hypersalivation, but has not caused severe systemic effects in adults.[155,156] Ingestion of more than 85 mL of the 41% glyphosate plus 5% to 15% polyoxyethyleneamine formulations is likely to cause significant toxicity in adults,[155] including gastrointestinal corrosive effects with mouth, throat, and epigastric pain and dysphagia.[156,174] The corrosive damage is predominantly gastric and esophageal rather than duodenal.[174] Patients with grade 2 or 3 (multiple ulcerations with necrosis) esophageal lesions were more likely to have ingested more than 200 mL of glyphosate concentrate and to manifest severe systemic sequelae, including gastrointestinal hemorrhage, hypotensive shock (not always in association with hypovolemia), or aspiration pneumonia. The latter complication is particularly likely if laryngeal corrosive injury occurs during ingestion.[175]

Lower gastrointestinal corrosive injury is rare,[155] but small bowel infarction has been reported, probably secondary to hypotension.[176] A 44-year-old man developed acute colitis 1 week after consuming glyphosate-contaminated wine.[177]

Aspiration of glyphosate-containing products contributes to ventilatory insufficiency in severely poisoned

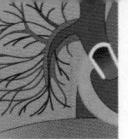

patients,[156] but noncardiogenic pulmonary edema is the underlying pathologic process in some cases.[155,176] Acute bronchospasm, followed by pneumomediastinum, tension pneumothorax, and subcutaneous emphysema, has been described in a man who ingested 500 mL of a glyphosate-containing product.[178]

Renal and hepatic impairment (increased amino-transferase and transaminase activities) and impaired consciousness are not uncommon in more severe cases[154,176] and usually reflect reduced organ perfusion, although a direct toxic effect of glyphosate or surfactant may contribute. Similarly, hypovolemia is an important factor in cases complicated by cardiogenic shock or acidosis, although direct toxicity, may contribute.[179] Glyphosate- or surfactant-induced myocardial depression may also occur.[180]

Other reported features include dilated pupils,[156,179,181] convulsions,[156] confusion, coma, fever,[154] neutrophil leucocytosis,[154,155] increased serum amylase activity,[155] metabolic acidosis,[154] and ECG abnormalities.[154,158] In a recent case,[176] broad complex tachycardia (140 beats/minute) was a presenting feature after ingestion of 1 L of glyphosate concentrate; it may be relevant that the patient also had a marked metabolic acidosis (pH, 7.25; HCO_3, 13 mmol/L) and a serum potassium concentration of 8.2 mmol/L. Bradycardia and ventricular arrhythmias may occur as preterminal events.[155,156,179,181]

Table 78-3 lists proposed criteria for classification of severity of poisoning resulting from glyphosate formulation ingestion.

There is a reasonable correlation between the amount of glyphosate ingested, the severity of damage,[155] and the likelihood of serious systemic sequelae[155,156] or death.[154,156] When a large quantity is ingested, death typically ensues within 72 hours.[154] Not surprisingly, not all cases conform to these prognostic criteria.[155,181] Other features significantly more likely in patients who die include the presence of respiratory distress, impaired consciousness, pulmonary edema, infiltration on chest x-ray, shock, arrhythmias, and renal failure requiring hemodialysis.[154] The triad of pulmonary edema, metabolic acidosis, and hyperkalemia is also a poor prognostic indicator,[176] as is advancing age.[154,156]

SKIN EXPOSURE

Skin contact with glyphosate formulations can cause irritation,[182] and contact dermatitis has been reported occasionally.[183] Severe skin burns are rare.[184] Transfer by contaminated hands to the face may lead to swelling, paresthesias, and periorbital edema.[181] Generalized pompholyx was reported in a man who was accidentally drenched with horticultural-strength glyphosate-containing product.[181] Although photosensitivity to glyphosate was claimed to have developed in a 64-year-old man,[185] the authors later concluded that the responsible agent was not glyphosate but the coformulant.[186]

INHALATION

Inhalation is a minor route of exposure to glyphosate,[187] but spray mist may cause oral or nasal discomfort, an unpleasant taste in the mouth, tingling, and throat

TABLE 78-3 Proposed Criteria for Classification of the Severity of Poisoning Resulting from Ingestion of Glyphosate Formulations

GRADE OF SEVERITY	CRITERIA
Asymptomatic	Absence of symptoms and abnormal clinical or laboratory findings
Mild	Short-lived (<24 hr) buccal or alimentary tract features
Moderate	*At least one of the following:* Buccal ulceration Endoscopically confirmed esophagitis Alimentary tract features lasting > 24 hr Gastrointestinal hemorrhage Transient hypotension Transient oliguria Transient renal impairment Transient acid–base abnormalities Transient hepatic damage
Severe	*At least one of the following:* Hypotension requiring intervention Loss of consciousness Recurrent convulsions Renal failure requiring replacement therapy Respiratory abnormalities requiring endotracheal intubation Cardiac arrest Death

Based on Talbot AR, Shiaw M, Huang J, et al: Acute poisoning with a glyphosate-surfactant herbicide ("Round-up"): a review of 93 cases. Hum Exp Toxicol 1991;10:1; and Tominack RL, Yang G, Tsai W, et al: Taiwan national poison center survey of glyphosate-surfactant herbicide ingestions. J Toxicol Clin Toxicol 1991; 29:91.

irritation. A single case of acute pneumonitis alleged to be due to inhalation of Roundup in a warm, confined space over a 4-hour period has been reported.[188] Whether the features were due to glyphosate including polyoxyethyleneamine or to some other cause was subsequently debated but not resolved.[189,190]

EYE EXPOSURE

Eye contact may lead to mild conjunctivitis, and superficial corneal injury is possible if irrigation is delayed or inadequate. One man who accidentally rubbed glyphosate into one eye developed chemosis, palpitations, raised blood pressure, headache, and nausea.[181] Permanent eye damage is most unlikely.[191]

Management

INGESTION

Management is symptomatic and supportive. Because ingestion of ready-to-use amateur products is unlikely to cause systemic toxicity, gut decontamination is unnecessary. Gastric lavage may be considered if a life-threatening amount of a concentrated glyphosate formulation has been ingested within 1 hour (unless there is evidence of buccal irritation or burns), but there

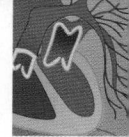

is no evidence that this procedure reduces absorption of either glyphosate or polyoxyethyleneamine. Alternatively, if there is no buccal irritation or burns, oral activated charcoal, 50 to 100 g for an adult, may be considered.

Hypotension secondary to fluid loss should be treated conventionally. Dopamine or dobutamine may be required in severe cases. Early upper alimentary endoscopy should be considered in patients with features suggesting significant gastrointestinal corrosive effects.

Intubation and mechanical ventilation are likely to be required in the most severely poisoned patients. Significant acidosis that persists despite adequate oxygenation and perfusion should be corrected by intravenous sodium bicarbonate. An ECG should be performed in all symptomatic cases.

SKIN EXPOSURE

Thorough skin decontamination is the priority with removal of contaminated clothing, and washing with soap and water. Management is otherwise symptomatic and supportive. Severe lesions should be managed as burns.

INHALATION

Removal from exposure is the priority. Management is otherwise symptomatic and supportive.

EYE EXPOSURE

Eye contamination should be managed as a chemical exposure, with attention particularly to adequate irrigation.

TRIAZINE HERBICIDES

The triazine herbicides are a class of compounds based on a symmetric six-member ring containing three carbon and three nitrogen atoms. Some 15 different triazines have been marketed and are still used widely as amateur and professional herbicides, often formulated with other pesticides. The Spanish Poison Control Centre found that 9% of all enquiries relating to occupational exposure to pesticides involved triazines.[192]

Clinical Features

Serious toxicity has not been reported,[193] except in one case in which it is probable that the observed features were due to other constituents of the formulation.[194] Any features directly attributable to triazines are likely to be nonspecific. Exposure to dusts or sprays may cause mucous membrane and eye irritation. Contact dermatitis may develop in sensitized individuals.[195-197]

Management

Gastric lavage and activated charcoal administration are unnecessary. Management is symptomatic and supportive. The possibility of features developing due to coformulated pesticides or from other constituents, most notably solvents, should be considered. In one case, the

clearance of atrazine by hemodialysis was 250 mL/min over 4 hours, and the dialysance was 76%.[194]

UREA HERBICIDES

Substituted urea compounds are used as pre-emergence and postemergence herbicides and as soil sterilants and generally are referred to as urea herbicides. Those that have caused clinical illness include diuron (1-[3,4-dichlorophenyl]-3,3 dimethylurea), monolinuron, and metobromuron (Fig. 78-5). They are often marketed in formulations containing other active ingredients. The toxicity of these compounds is probably due to their metabolism to aniline derivatives, which can cause methemoglobinemia. They also induce microsomal enzymes in animals.[198]

During the 10-year period from 1994 to 2003, 716 exposures to urea herbicides were reported to the AAPCC. There were no fatalities, but 46 cases were classified as being of moderate severity, and 3 were life threatening.[104-108,153,199-202] Release into the atmosphere of an estimated ton of isoproturon did not cause adverse effects in the inhabitants of a nearby residential area, probably because biomonitoring revealed that exposure was below the acceptable daily intake.[203]

Toxicokinetics

Diuron is absorbed from both the gastrointestinal and respiratory tracts. It undergoes hydroxylation, dealkylation, or both of the terminal nitrogen atom, the urea moiety generally remaining unchanged. Several metabolites have been identified in humans after suicidal ingestion of diuron[204-206] and are excreted in the urine with low concentrations of diuron.[204] Similarly, several metabolites were detected in the plasma and urine of a patient who had ingested metobromuron.[207]

Clinical Features

Urea herbicides are generally of low acute toxicity, and serious poisoning is only likely after ingestion of large quantities; four deaths have been recorded (Table 78-4). However, it is unlikely that three of these can be attributed to the urea herbicide. One was almost certainly

FIGURE 78-5 Chemical structure of two urea herbicides.

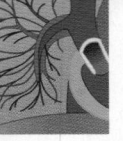

TABLE 78-4 Deaths from Formulations Containing Urea Herbicides

ACTIVE INGREDIENTS*	ESTIMATED DOSE OF UREA HERBICIDE	AGE AND SEX	MAIN FEATURES	METHEMOGLOBIN (%)	REFERENCE
Monolinuron (14%) + paraquat (10%)	40 mg/kg bw	59 M	Central cyanosis, renal, respiratory, and hepatic failure	52	Casey et al (1994)[208]
Diuron	Several grams	77 ?	Severe sedation	Unknown	Verheij et al (1989)[204]
Diuron + parathion	Unknown	38 F	Coma	Unknown	van Boven et al (1990)[205]
Diuron + atrazine + aminotriazole + propylene glycol	200 g	35 M	Metabolic acidosis	3	Brinquin et al (1993)[209]

*Urea herbicide in bold.

due to the paraquat coingested,[208] one to the solvent (propylene glycol) in the formulation,[209] and one to parathion.[205]

Nausea, vomiting, diarrhea, and abdominal pain are the initial features. Later, as the aniline-related metabolites appear, hemoglobin is oxidized to methemoglobin, accumulation of which is the principal cause of urea herbicide toxicity. The onset of clinically detectable methemoglobinemia may be delayed for 6 to 10 hours.[210] It was present in 5 of the 10 published cases.[207,208,210-212] Significant intravascular hemolysis followed in four.[207,210-212] For that reason, Heinz body formation, reticulocytosis, a positive Schumm's test, and brownish discoloration of the plasma and urine due to the presence of free hemoglobin may be observed. Plasma lactate dehydrogenase activity may be increased. Acute renal failure and metabolic acidosis may ensue.

A slate-gray color of the skin not reversed by supplemental oxygen may be seen when methemoglobin concentrations exceed 10% to 15%. The patient often appears unduly well for the degree of "cyanosis." As methemoglobin concentrations increase, features of hypoxia develop, with headache, fatigue, weakness, dizziness, syncope, tachycardia, dyspnea, and increasing respiratory distress. Methemoglobin concentrations in excess of 60% are life threatening, with coma, convulsions, cardiac arrhythmias, and cardiorespiratory arrest.

Chest discomfort and cough have been reported after heavy occupational inhalation of a mixture of diuron and 2,4-D,[214] but there are no reports relating to a urea herbicide alone. Similarly, there are no reports of toxicity after topical exposure, although skin may be irritated.

Management

Although gastric lavage may be considered if a life-threatening amount of a urea herbicide has been ingested within 1 hour, there is no evidence that it reduces absorption. The same is true of oral activated charcoal, although administration of 50 to 100 g to an adult may be considered in the same situation. Patients should be observed for several hours if substantial exposure is suspected because the onset of toxicity may be delayed. Arterial blood gas tensions and methemoglobin concentrations should be measured.

Methylthioninium chloride (methylene blue), 1 to 2 mg/kg given intravenously, is indicated if the methemoglobin concentration exceeds 30%. The plasma potassium concentration should be monitored frequently if hemolysis develops, and hyperkalemia is treated conventionally. Red blood cell transfusion should, if possible, be avoided until the toxic metabolites have been eliminated. Plasmapheresis may have a role in removing circulating free hemoglobin and red blood cell fragments. Renal function will also need to be monitored and failure treated conventionally.

BENTAZON (BENTAZONE)

Bentazon (bentazone) is a selective contact herbicide with the chemical structure shown in Figure 78-6.

Mechanisms of Toxicity

Its mechanism of action in humans is unknown, although the clinical features of poisoning suggest that bentazon may uncouple oxidative phosphorylation. It is likely that coformulants will be responsible for some of the toxic effects of some products.

Toxicokinetics

What little is known of the toxicokinetics of bentazon in humans indicates that it is rapidly and extensively absorbed after oral administration and excreted largely unchanged in urine. A possible hydroxylated metabolite was present in the blood of a farmer who died after ingestion of bentazon, the concentration of the parent compound in plasma being of the order of 1500 mg/L.[215] In another case, the postmortem blood concentration of bentazon was 625 mg/kg.[216]

FIGURE 78-6 Bentazon.

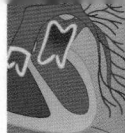

Clinical Features

The three reported cases of acute poisoning in humans involve ingestion. Analytic confirmation of the presence of bentazon was present in two,[215,216] but not in the third case.[217] The emerging pattern of bentazon poisoning is that the time required for onset of features may be less than 1 hour and that death may result within as little as 2 hours. Upper and lower gastrointestinal irritation is common, and although bentazon is said not to cross the blood-brain barrier in rats, drowsiness, agitation, talking nonsense, and loss of consciousness in these patients suggest that it may do so after consumption of very large amounts. Other features include sweating, hyperpyrexia, increased heart rate, tachypnea, and difficulty in breathing. Limb rigidity was a prominent feature in two patients, and one had clear evidence of rhabdomyolysis and several other features; those who cared for him proposed that acute bentazon poisoning mimicked neuroleptic malignant syndrome.[217] Leucocytosis and minor disturbances of liver and renal function have been reported.[217]

Management

The management of acute bentazon poisoning is symptomatic and supportive. Gastric lavage or oral activated charcoal (100 g for an adult) may be employed, although there are no data to indicate that they might be effective. Indeed, it is unlikely that they would be effective because absorption is so rapid. Liver and renal function and the ECG should be monitored. Dantrolene may be indicated if muscle rigidity is a problem.[217] Respiratory and renal failure should be managed conventionally. Antiemetics may be given if vomiting persists.

REFERENCES

1. Tomlin CDS (ed): The Pesticide Manual, 11th ed. Farnham, Surrey, UK, British Crop Protection Council, 1997.
2. IPCS: Health and Safety Guide No. 52. Diquat. Geneva, World Health Organization, 1991.
3. Powell D, Pond SM, Allen TB, et al: Hemoperfusion in a child who ingested diquat and died from pontine infarction and hemorrhage. J Toxicol Clin Toxicol 1983;20:405.
4. Jones GM, Vale JA: Mechanisms of toxicity, clinical features, and management of diquat poisoning: a review. J Toxicol Clin Toxicol 2000;38:123.
5. Van Berlo-van de Laar IRF, Tromp YH, Sluiter HE, et al: Klinisch verloop na een fatale inname van diquat. Suicide met onkruidbestrijdingsmiddel. Pharmaceutisch Weekblad 2003;138:720.
6. Hantson P, Wallemacq P, Mahieu P: A case of fatal diquat poisoning: toxicokinetic data and autopsy findings. J Toxicol Clin Toxicol 2000;38:149.
7. Ruha A-M, Wallace K, Tanen DA, et al: Dilute diquat death. Am J Emerg Med 2001;19:527.
8. Saeed SAM, Wilks MF, Coupe M: Acute diquat poisoning with intracerebral bleeding, Postgrad Med J 2001;77:329.
9. Rawlings JM, Wyatt I, Heylings JR: Evidence for redox recycling of diquat in rat small intestine. Biochem Pharmacol 1994;47:1271.
10. Niesink JM, de Vries J, Hollinger MA (eds): Toxicology: Principles and Applications. Boca Raton, FL, CRC Press, 1996.
11. Reif DW, Beales ILP, Thomas CE, et al: Effect of diquat on the distribution of iron in rat liver. Toxicol Appl Pharmacol 1988;93:506.
12. Samokyszyn VM, Thomas CE, Reif DW, et al: Release of iron from ferritin and its role in oxygen radical toxicities. Drug Metab Rev 1988;19:283.
13. Sandy MS, Moldeus P, Ross D, et al: Cytotoxicity of the redox cycling compound diquat in isolated hepatocytes: involvement of hydrogen peroxide and transition metals. Arch Biochem Biophys 1987;259:29.
14. Litchfield MH, Daniel JW, Longshaw S: The tissue distribution of the bipyridylium herbicides diquat and paraquat in rats and mice. Toxicology 1973;1:155.
15. Charles JM, Abou-Donia MB, Menzel DB: Absorption of paraquat and diquat from the airways of the perfused rat lung. Toxicology 1978;9:59.
16. Daniel JW, Gage JC: Absorption and excretion of diquat and paraquat in rats. Br J Indust Med 1966;23:133.
17. Feldmann RJ, Maibach HI: Percutaneous penetration of some pesticides and herbicides in man. Toxicol Appl Pharmacol 1974;28:126.
18. Schmidt DM, Neale J, Olson KR: Clinical course of a fatal ingestion of diquat. J Toxicol Clin Toxicol 1999;37:881.
19. Tanen DA, Curry SC, Laney RF: Renal failure and corrosive airway and gastrointestinal injury after ingestion of diluted diquat solution. Ann Emerg Med 1999;34:542.
20. Manoguerra AS: Full thickness skin burns secondary to an unusual exposure to diquat dibromide. J Toxicol Clin Toxicol 1990;28:107.
21. Clark DG, Hurst EW: The toxicity of diquat. Br J Indust Med 1970;27:51.
22. Cant JS, Lewis DRH: Ocular damage due to paraquat and diquat. BMJ 1968;2:59.
23. Rudez J, Sepcic K, Sepcic J: Vaginally applied diquat intoxication. J Toxicol Clin Toxicol 1999;37:877.
24. Valiante F, Farinati F, Dal Santo P, et al: Upper gastrointestinal injury caused by diquat. Gastrointest Endosc 1992;38:204.
25. Zilker T, Clarmann MV, Felgenhauer N, et al: Comparison of paraquat and diquat intoxications. Hum Toxicol 1987;6:103.
26. McCarthy LG, Speth CP: Diquat intoxication. Ann Emerg Med 1983;12:394.
27. Fél P, Zala I, Szüle E, et al: Haemodialysisse gyógyított diquat-dibromid (Reglone) mérgezés. Orvosi Hetilap 1976;117:1773.
28. Williams PF, Jarvie DR, Whitehead AP: Diquat intoxication: treatment by charcoal haemoperfusion and description of a new method of diquat measurement in plasma. J Toxicol Clin Toxicol 1986;24:11.
29. Van Den Heede M, Heyndrickx A, Timperman J: Thin layer chromatography as a routine appropriate technique for the determination of bipyridylium herbicides in post mortem human tissues. Med Sci Law 1982;22:57.
30. Vanholder R, Colardyn F, de Reuck J, et al: Diquat intoxication: report of two cases and review of the literature. Am J Med 1981;70:1267.
31. Buckley DA, McKiernan J: Survival after accidental ingestion of a fatal dose of diquat. Irish Med J 1991;84:134.
32. Schönborn H, Schuster HP: Klinik und Morphologie der akuten peroralen Diquatintoxikation (Reglone). Arch Toxikol 1971;27:204.
33. Weirich J: Intoxikation mit Diquat ("Reglone"). Deutsche Gesundheitswesen 1969;24:1986.
34. Mahieu P, Bonduelle Y, Bernard A, et al: Acute diquat intoxication interest of its repeated determination in urine and the evaluation of renal proximal tubule integrity. J Toxicol Clin Toxicol 1984;22:363.
35. Ferguson AH, Jacobsen JB, Nielsen H: Severe diquat poisoning. Ugeskrift for Laeger 1982;144:2293.
36. Narita S, Motojuku M, Sato J, et al: Autopsy in acute suicidal poisoning with diquat dibromide. Nippon Igakkai Zasshi 1978;27:454.
37. Okonek S, Hofmann A, Henningsen B: Efficacy of gut lavage, hemodialysis and hemoperfusion in the therapy of paraquat or diquat intoxication. Arch Toxicol 1976;36:43.
38. Okonek S, Hofmann A: On the question of extracorporeal hemodialysis in diquat intoxication. Arch Toxicol 1975;33:251.
39. Okonek S: Vergiftungen durch Paraquat oder Deiquat. Medizinische Welt 1976;27:1401.
40. Watts D: Poisoning highlights crime rise. The Times, 1985.

41. Teare D, Brown JS: Poisoning by paraquat. Medico-Legal J 1976;44:33.

42. Walker M, Dugard PH, Scott RC: Absorption through human and laboratory animal skins: in vitro comparisons. Acta Pharmaceutica Suecica 1983;20:52.

43. Newhouse M, McEvoy D, Rosenthal D: Percutaneous paraquat absorption. Arch Dermatol 1978;114:1516.

44. Jaros F: Acute percutaneous paraquat poisoning. Lancet 1978;1:275.

45. Levin PJ, Klaff LJ, Rose AG, et al: Pulmonary effects of contact exposure to paraquat: a clinical and experimental study. Thorax 1979;34:150.

46. Withers EH, Madden JJ, Lynch JB: Paraquat burn of the scrotum and perineum. J Tenn Med Assoc 1979;72:109.

47. Wohlfahrt DJ: Fatal paraquat poisonings after skin absorption. Med J Aust 1982;1:512.

48. Athanaselis S, Qammaz S, Alevisopoulos G, et al: Percutaneous paraquat intoxication. J Toxicol Cutan Ocular Toxicol 1983;2:3.

49. Waight JJJ: Fatal percutaneous paraquat poisoning. JAMA 1979;242:472.

50. Tungsanga K, Israsena S, Chusilp S, et al: Paraquat poisoning: evidence of systemic toxicity after dermal exposure. Postgrad Med J 1983;59:338.

51. Ongom VL: Paraquat ("Gramoxone") Used as a Pediculocide: Uses and Abuses of Drugs in Tropical Africa. Nairobi, East Africa Literature Bureau, 1974.

52. Binns CW: A deadly cure for lice: a case of paraquat poisoning. Papua New Guinea Med J 1976;19:105.

53. Almog CH, Tal E: Death from paraquat after subcutaneous injection. BMJ 1967;3:721.

54. Harley JB, Grinspan S, Root RK: Paraquat suicide in a young woman: results of therapy directed against the superoxide radical. Yale J Biol Med 1977;50:481.

55. Hendy MS, Williams PS, Ackrill P: Recovery from severe pulmonary damage due to paraquat administered intravenously and orally. Thorax 1984;39:874.

56. Gage JC: The action of paraquat and diquat on the respiration of liver cell fractions. Biochem J 1968;109:757.

57. Farrington JA, Ebert M, Land EJ, et al: Bipyridylium quaternary salts and related compounds. V pulse radiolysis studies of the reaction of paraquat radical with oxygen. Implications for the mode of action of bipyridyl herbicides. Biochim Biophys Acta 1973;314:372.

58. Bus JS, Aust SD, Gibson JE: Superoxide and singlet oxygen catalyzed lipid peroxidation as a possible mechanism for paraquat (methyl viologen) toxicity. Biochem Biophys Res Commun 1974;58:749.

59. Oh SJ, Kim JM: Giant axonal swelling in "huffer's" neuropathy. Arch Neurol 1976;33:583.

60. Trush MA, Mimnaugh EG, Ginsburg E, et al: In vitro stimulation by paraquat of reactive oxygen-mediated lipid peroxidation in rat lung microsomes. Toxicol Appl Pharmacol 1981;60:279.

61. Situnyake RD, Crump BJ, Thurnham DI, et al: Evidence for lipid peroxidation in man following paraquat ingestion. Hum Toxicol 1987;6:94.

62. Baker EL, Smith TJ, Landrigan PJ: The neurotoxicity of industrial solvents: a review of the literature. Am J Indust Med 1985;8:207.

63. Connign DM, Fletcher K, Swan AAB: Paraquat and related bipyridyls. Br Med Bull 1969;245.

64. van Dijk A, Maes RAA, Drost RH, et al: Paraquat poisoning in man. Arch Toxicol 1975;34:129.

65. Proudfoot AT, Stewart MS, Levitt T, et al: Paraquat poisoning: significance of plasma-paraquat concentrations. Lancet 1979;2:330.

66. Botella R, Sastre A, Castells A: Contact dermatitis to paraquat. Contact Dermatitis 1985;13:123.

67. Samman PD, Johnston ENM: Nail damage associated with handling of paraquat and diquat. BMJ 1969;818.

68. Hearn CED, Keir W: Nail damage in spray operators exposed to paraquat. Br J Indust Med 1971;28:399.

69. Joyce M: Ocular damage caused by paraquat. Br J Ophthalmol 1969;53:688.

70. Karai I, Nakano H, Horiguchi S: A case of lacrimal duct stenosis due to a herbicide paraquat. Jap J Indust Health 1981;23:552.

71. Stephens DS, Walker DH, Schaffner W, et al: Pseudodiphtheria: prominent pharyngeal membrane associated with fatal paraquat ingestion. Ann Intern Med 1981;94:202.

72. Vale JA, Meredith TJ, Buckley BM: Paraquat poisoning clinical features and immediate general management. Hum Toxicol 1987;6:41.

73. Kodagoda N, Jayewardene RP, Attygalle D: Poisoning with paraquat. Forensic Sci 1973;2:107.

74. Vazari ND, Ness RI, Fairshter RD, et al: Nephrotoxicity of paraquat in man. Arch Intern Med 1979;139:172.

75. Mickleson KNP, Fulton DB: Paraquat poisoning treated by a replacement blood transfusion: case report. N Z Med J 1971;74:26.

76. Conradi SE, Olanoff LS, Dawson WT: Fatality due to paraquat intoxication: confirmation by postmortem tissue analysis. Am J Clin Pathol 1983;80:771.

77. Addo E, Ramdial S, Poon-King T: High dosage cyclophosphamide and dexamethasone treatment of paraquat poisoning with 75% survival. West Indian Med J 1984;33:220.

78. Grant HC, Lantos PL, Parkinson C: Cerebral damage in paraquat poisoning. Histopathology 1980;4:185.

79. Fennelly JJ, Fitzgerald GR, Fitzgerald O: Recovery from severe paraquat poisoning following forced diuresis and immuno-suppressive therapy. J Irish Med Assoc 1971;64:69.

80. Fairshter RD, Rosen SM, Smith WR, et al: Paraquat poisoning: new aspects of therapy. Q J Med 1976;180:551.

81. Siefkin AD: Combined paraquat and acetaminophen toxicity. J Toxicol Clin Toxicol 1982;19:483.

82. Williams PS, Hendy MS, Ackrill P: Early management of paraquat poisoning. Lancet 1984;1:627.

83. Braithwaite RA: Emergency analysis of paraquat in biological fluids. Hum Toxicol 1987;6:83.

84. Hart TB, Nevitt A, Whitehead A: A new statistical approach to the prognostic significance of plasma paraquat concentration. Lancet 1984;1:1222.

85. Scherrmann JM, Houze P, Bismuth C, et al: Prognostic value of plasma and urine paraquat concentration. Hum Toxicol 1987;6:91.

86. Bateman DN: Pharmacological treatments of paraquat poisoning. Hum Toxicol 1987;6:57.

87. Suntres ZE: Role of antioxidants in paraquat toxicity. Toxicology 2002;180:65.

88. Hughes RD, Millburn P, Williams T: Biliary excretion of some diquaternary ammonium cations in the rat, guinea pig and rabbit. Biochem J 1973;136:979.

89. Davis DS, Hawksworth GM, Bennett PN: Paraquat poisoning. Proc Eur Soc Toxicol 1977;18:21.

90. Hawksworth GM, Bennett PN, Davies DS: Kinetics of paraquat elimination in the dog. Toxicol Appl Pharmacol 1981;57:139.

91. Bismuth C, Garnier R, Dally S, et al: Prognosis and treatment of paraquat poisoning: a review of 28 cases. J Toxicol Clin Toxicol 1982;19:461.

92. Webb DB: Nephrotoxicity of paraquat in the sheep and the associated reduction in paraquat secretion. Toxicol Appl Pharmacol 1983;68:282.

93. Scherrmann JM, Galliot M, Garnier R, et al: Acute paraquat poisoning: prognostic and therapeutic utility of determining the content in the blood. Toxicol Eur Res 1983;3:1.

94. Van de Vyver FL, Giuliano RA, Paulus GJ, et al: Hemoperfusion-hemodialysis ineffective for paraquat removal in life-threatening poisoning. J Toxicol Clin Toxicol 1985;23:117.

95. Proudfoot AT, Prescott LF, Jarvie DR: Haemodialysis for paraquat poisoning. Hum Toxicol 1987;6:69.

96. Spector D, Whorton D, Zachary J, et al: Fatal paraquat poisoning: tissue concentrations and implications for treatment. Johns Hopkins Med J 1978;142:110.

97. Bismuth C, Fournier PE: Biological evaluation of hemoperfusion in acute poisoning. In Holmstedt B, Lauwerys R, Mercier M, et al (eds): Mechanisms of Toxicity and Hazard Evaluation, Amsterdam, Elsevier/North Holland Biomedical Press, 1980.

98. De Groot G: Haemoperfusion in paraquat intoxication. In: Haemoperfusion in Clinical Toxicology. A Pharmacokinetic Evaluation (Thesis). Utrecht, University of Utrecht, 1982.

99. Mascie-Taylor BH: Haemoperfusion ineffective for paraquat removal in life-threatening poisoning. Lancet 1983;1:1376.

100. Vale JA: MD thesis. London, University of London, 1980.

101. Bismuth C, Scherrmann JM, Garnier R, et al: Elimination of paraquat. Hum Toxicol 1987;6:63.

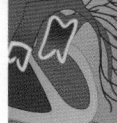

102. Okonek S, Weilemann LS, Majdandzic J, et al: Successful treatment of paraquat poisoning: activated charcoal per os and "continuous hemoperfusion." J Toxicol Clin Toxicol 1982;19:807.

103. Pond SM, Johnston SC, Schoof DD, et al: Repeated hemoperfusion and continuous arteriovenous hemofiltration in a paraquat poisoned patient. J Toxicol Clin Toxicol 1987;25:305.

104. Litovitz TL, Klein-Schwartz W, Caravati EM, et al: 1998 Annual report of the American Association of Poison Control Centers Toxic Exposure Surveillance System. Am J Emerg Med 1999;17:435.

105. Litovitz TL, Klein-Schwartz W, White S, et al: 1999 Annual report of the American Association of Poison Control Centers Toxic Exposure Surveillance System. Am J Emerg Med 2000;18:517.

106. Litovitz TL, Klein-Schwartz W, White S, et al: 2000 Annual report of the American Association of Poison Control Centers Toxic Exposure Surveillance System. Am J Emerg Med 2001;19:337.

107. Litovitz TL, Klein-Schwartz W, Rodgers GC Jr., et al: 2001 Annual report of the American Association of Poison Control Centers Toxic Exposure Surveillance System. Am J Emerg Med 2002;20:391.

108. Watson WA, Litovitz TL, Rodgers GC Jr., et al: 2002 Annual report of the American Association of Poison Control Centers Toxic Exposure Surveillance System. Am J Emerg Med 2003;21:353.

109. Tuschl H, Schwab C: Cytotoxic effects of the herbicide 2,4-dichlorophenoxyacetic acid in HepG2 cells. Food Chem Toxicol 2003;41:385.

110. Sauerhoff MW, Braun WH, Blau GE, et al: The fate of 2,4-dichlorophenoxyacetic acid (2,4-D) following oral administration to man. Toxicology 1977;8:3.

111. Arnold EK, Beasley VR: The pharmacokinetics of chlorinated phenoxy acid herbicides: a literature review. Vet Hum Toxicol 1989;31:121.

112. Harris SA, Solomon KR: Percutaneous penetration of 2,4-dichlorophenoxyacetic acid and 2,4-D dimethylamine salt in human volunteers. J Toxicol Environ Health 1992;36:233.

113. Grover R, Cessna AJ, Muir NI, et al: Factors affecting the exposure of ground-rig applicators to 2,4-D dimethylamine salt. Arch Environ Contam Toxicol 1986;15:677.

114. Rosso SB, Gonzalez M, Bagatolli LA, et al: Evidence of a strong interaction of 2,4-dichlorophenoxyacetic acid herbicide with human serum albumin. Life Sci 1998;63:2343.

115. Koschier FJ, Hong SK, Berndt WO: Serum protein and renal tissue binding of 2,4,5-trichlorophenoxyacetic acid. Toxicol Appl Pharmacol 1979;49:237.

116. Kohli JD, Khanna RN, Gupta BN, et al: Absorption and excretion of 2,4-dichlorophenoxyacetic acid in man. Xenobiotica 1974;4:97.

117. Piper WN, Rose JQ, Leng ML, et al: The fate of 2,4,5-trichlorophenoxyacetic acid (2,4,5-T) following oral administration in rats and dogs. Toxicol Appl Pharmacol 1973;26:339.

118. Bradberry SM, Watt BE, Proudfoot AT, et al: Mechanisms of toxicity, clinical features, and management of acute chlorophenoxy herbicide poisoning: a review. J Toxicol Clin Toxicol 2000;38:111.

119. Prescott LF, Park J, Darrien I: Treatment of severe 2,4-D and mecoprop intoxication with alkaline diuresis. Br J Clin Pharmacol 1979;7:111.

120. Brahmi N, Ben Mokhtar H, Thabet H, et al: 2,4-D (chlorophenoxy) herbicide poisoning. Vet Hum Toxicol 2003;45:321.

121. Durakovic Z, Durakovic A, Durakovic S, et al: Poisoning with 2,4-dichlorophenoxyacetic acid treated by hemodialysis. Arch Toxicol 1992;66:518.

122. Flanagan RJ, Meredith TJ, Ruprah M, et al: Alkaline diuresis for acute poisoning with chlorophenoxy herbicides and ioxynil. Lancet 1990;335:454.

123. Jones DIR, Knight AG, Smith AJ: Attempted suicide with herbicide containing MCPA. Arch Environ Health 1967;14:363.

124. Dudley AW Jr, Thapar NT: Fatal human ingestion of 2,4-D, a common herbicide. Arch Pathol 1972;94:270.

125. Kancir CB, Andersen C, Olesen AS: Marked hypocalcemia in a fatal poisoning with chlorinated phenoxy acid derivatives. J Toxicol Clin Toxicol 1988;26:257.

126. Popham RD, Davies DM: A case of MCPA poisoning. BMJ 1964;1:677.

127. Johnson HRM, Koumides O: A further case of MCPA poisoning. BMJ 1965;2:629.

128. O'Reilly JF: Prolonged coma and delayed peripheral neuropathy after ingestion of phenoxyacetic acid weedkillers. Postgrad Med J 1984;60:76.

129. Berthelot-Moritz F, Daudenthun I, Goullé J-P, et al: Severe intoxication following ingestion of 2,4-D and MCPP. Intensive Care Med 1997;23:356.

130. Friesen EG, Jones GR, Vaughan D: Clinical presentation and management of acute 2,4-D oral ingestion. Drug Saf 1990;5:155.

131. de Larrard J, Barbaste M: Intoxication suicidaire mortelle agro-chimique à l'hormone desherbante 2,4-D. Arch Mal Prof Med Trav Secur Soc 1969;30:434.

132. Meulenbelt J, Zwaveling JH, van Zoonen P, et al: Acute MCPP intoxication: report of two cases. Hum Toxicol 1988;7:289.

133. Davies MK, Jung RT: Lung involvement with "Verdone." Lancet 1976;2:370.

134. Lankosz-Lauterbach J, Kaczor Z, Kacinski M, et al: Severe polyneuropathy in a 3-year-old child after dichlorophenoxyacetic herbicide—Chwastox—intoxication, treated successfully with plasmapheresis (PF). Przeglad Lekarski 1997;54:750.

135. Keller T, Skopp G, Wu M, et al: Fatal overdose of 2,4-dichlorophenoxyacetic acid (2,4-D). Forensic Sci Int 1994;65:13.

136. Wells WDE, Wright N, Yeoman WB: Clinical features and management of poisoning with 2,4-D and mecoprop. J Toxicol Clin Toxicol 1981;18:273.

137. Jorens PG, Heytens L, De Paep RJ, et al: A 2,4-dichlorophenoxyacetic acid induced fatality. Eur J Emerg Med 1995;2:52.

138. Fraser AD, Isner AF, Perry RA: Toxicologic studies in a fatal overdose of 2,4-D, mecoprop, and dicamba. J Forensic Sci 1984;29:1237.

139. Mattsson JL, Eisenbrandt DL: The improbable association between the herbicide 2,4-D and polyneuropathy. Biomed Environ Sci 1990;3:43.

140. Berkley MC, Magee KR: Neuropathy following exposure to a dimethylamine salt of 2,4-D. Arch Intern Med 1963;111:351.

141. Goldstein NP, Jones PH, Brown JR: Peripheral neuropathy after exposure to an ester of dichlorophenoxyacetic acid. JAMA 1959;171:1306.

142. Todd RL: A case of 2,4-D intoxication. J Iowa Med Soc 1962;52:663.

143. Tsapko VG: On the probable harmful action of the herbicide 2,4-D on agricultural workers. Gigiena i Sanitariia 1966;31:79.

144. Kolny H, Kita K: Zatrucie Aminopielikiem D. Medycyna Pracy 1978;29:61.

145. Paggiaro PL, Martino E, Mariotti S: Su un caso di intossicazione da acido 2,4-diclorofenossiacetico. Medicina del Lavoro 1974;65:128.

146. Bezuglyi VP, Fokina KV, Komarova LI, et al: Clinical manifestations of long-term sequels of acute poisoning with 2,4-dichlorophenoxyacetic acid. Gigiena Truda i Professionalnye Zabolevaniia 1979;3:47.

147. McMillin RB, Samples JR: Iritis after herbicide exposure. Am J Ophthalmol 1985;99:726.

148. Grover R, Smith AE: Adsorption studies with the acid and dimethylamine forms of 2,4-D and dicamba. Can J Soil Sci 1974;54:179.

149. Schmoldt A, Iwersen S, Schlüter W: Massive ingestion of the herbicide 2-methyl-4-chlorophenoxyacetic acid (MCPA). J Toxicol Clin Toxicol 1997;35:405.

150. Proudfoot AT, Krenzelok EP, Vale JA: Position paper on urine alkalinization. J Toxicol Clin Toxicol 2004;42:1.

151. Park J, Darrien I, Prescott LF: Pharmacokinetic studies in severe intoxication with 2,4-D and mecoprop. Proceedings of an EAPCCT Meeting 1977;18:154.

152. Goldstein DA, Acquavella JF, Mannion RM, et al: An analysis of glyphosate data from the California Environmental Protection Agency Pesticide Illness Surveillance Program. J Toxicol Clin Toxicol 2002;40:885.

153. Watson WA, Litovitz TL, Klein-Schwartz W, et al: 2003 Annual report of the American Association of Poison Control Centers Toxic Exposure Surveillance System. Am J Emerg Med 2004;22:335.

154. Lee H-L, Chen K-W, Chi C-H, et al: Clinical presentations and prognostic factors of a glyphosate-surfactant herbicide intoxication: a review of 131 cases. Acad Emerg Med 2000;7:906.

155. Talbot AR, Shiaw M, Huang J, et al: Acute poisoning with a glyphosate-surfactant herbicide ("Round-up"): a review of 93 cases. Hum Exp Toxicol 1991;10:1.

156. Tominack RL, Yang G, Tsai W, et al: Taiwan national poison center survey of glyphosate-surfactant herbicide ingestions. J Toxicol Clin Toxicol 1991;29:91.

157. Sawada Y, Nagai Y: Roundup poisoning: its clinical observation. Possible involvement of surfactant. J Clin Exp Med 1987;143:25.

158. Sawada Y, Nagai Y, Ueyama M, et al: Probable toxicity of surface-active agent in commercial herbicide containing glyphosate. Lancet 1988;1:299.

159. Olorunsogo OO, Bababunmi EA, Bassir O: Effect of glyphosate on rat liver mitochondria. Bull Environ Contam Toxicol 1979;22:357.

160. Olorunsogo OO, Bababunmi EA: Inhibition of succinate-linking reduction of pyridine nucleotide in rat liver mitochondria "in vivo" by N-(phosphonomethyl)glycine. Toxicol Lett 1980;7:149.

161. Olorunsogo OO: Inhibition of energy-dependent transhydrogenase reaction by N-(phosphonomethyl)glycine in isolated rat liver mitochondria. Toxicol Lett 1982;10:91.

162. Bababunmi EA, Olorunsogo OO, Bassir O: The uncoupling effect of N-(phosphonomethyl)glycine on isolated rat liver mito-chondria. Biochem Pharmacol 1979;28:925.

163. Hietanen E, Linnainmaa K, Vainio H: Effects of phenoxy-herbicides and glyphosate on the hepatic and intestinal bio-transformation activities in the rat. Acta Pharmacol Toxicol 1983;53:103.

164. Sørensen FW, Gregersen M: Rapid lethal intoxication caused by the herbicide glyphosate-trimesium (Touchdown). Hum Exp Toxicol 1999;18:735.

165. Williams GM, Kroes R, Munro IC: Safety evaluation and risk assessment of the herbicide Roundup and its active ingredient, glyphosate, for humans. Regul Toxicol Pharmacol 2000;31:117.

166. Chan PC, Mahler JF: NTP technical report on toxicity studies of glyphosate (CAS No. 1071-83-6) administered in dosed feed to F344/N rats and B6C3F$_1$ mice. Research Triangle Park, NC, NIH, 1992.

167. Chan PC, Mahler JF: NTP technical report on toxicity studies of glyphosate (CAS No. 1071-83-6) administered in dosed feed to F344/N rats and B6C3F$_1$ mice. Research Triangle Park, NC, NIH, 1992.

168. Brewster DW, Warren J, Hopkins WE II: Metabolism of glyphosate in Sprague-Dawley rats: tissue distribution, identification, and quantitation of glyphosate-derived materials following a single oral dose. Fund Appl Toxicol 1991;17:43.

169. Chan PC, Mahler JF: NTP technical report on toxicity studies of glyphosate (CAS No. 1071-83-6) administered in dosed feed to F344/N rats and B6C3F$_1$ mice. Research Triangle Park, NC, NIH, 1992.

170. Franz JE, Mao MK, Sikorski JA: Glyphosate: A Unique Global Herbicide. Washington, DC, American Chemical Society, 1997.

171. Talbot A, Ku TS, Chen CL, et al: Glyphosate levels in acute Roundup herbicide poisoning. Ann Emerg Med 1995;26:717.

172. Tominack RL: Glyphosate: contemporary clinical features. J Toxicol Clin Toxicol 1999;37:374.

173. Hori Y, Fujisawa M, Shimada K, et al: Determination of the herbicide glyphosate and its metabolite in biological specimens by gas chromatography-mass spectrometry. A case of poisoning by Roundup(r) herbicide. J Anal Toxicol 2003;27:162.

174. Chang C-Y, Peng Y-C, Hung D-Z, et al: Clinical impact of upper gastrointestinal tract injuries in glyphosate-surfactant oral intoxication. Hum Exp Toxicol 1999;18:475.

175. Hung D-Z, Deng J-F, Wu T-C: Laryngeal survey in glyphosate intoxication: a pathophysiological investigation. Hum Exp Toxicol 1997;16:596.

176. Stella J, Ryan M: Glyphosate herbicide formulation: a potentially lethal ingestion. Emerg Med Australas 2004;16:235.

177. Delcenserie R, Yzet T, Duchmann JC, et al: Syndrome pseudo-appendiculaire tardif après intoxication au Roundup. Gastroenterol Clin Biol 1997;21:435.

178. Yang C-C, Lin T-J, Ger J, et al: Possible bronchial asthma necessitating prolonged mechanical ventilation in a patient with Roundup poisoning. 1994 Toxicology World Congress Abstracts. Ann Emerg Med 1995;26:722.

179. Menkes D, Temple WA, Edwards IR: Intentional self-poisoning with glyphosate-containing herbicides. Hum Exp Toxicol 1991;10:103.

180. Lin C-M, Lai C-P, Fang T-C, et al: Cardiogenic shock in a patient with glyphosate-surfactant poisoning. J Formosan Med Assoc 1999;98:698.

181. Temple WA, Smith NA: Glyphosate herbicide poisoning experience in New Zealand. N Z Med J 1992;105:173.

182. Maibach HI: Irritation, sensitization, photoirritation and photosensitization assays with a glyphosate herbicide. Contact Dermatitis 1986;15:152.

183. Rodríguez A, Echechipia S, Olaguibel JM, et al: Occupational contact allergy to herbicide glyphosate. J Allergy Clin Immunol 1997;99:S336.

184. Amerio P, Motta A, Toto P, et al: Skin toxicity from glyphosate-surfactant formulation. J Toxicol Clin Toxicol 2004;42:317.

185. Hindson C, Diffey B: Phototoxicity of glyphosate in a weedkiller. Contact Dermatitis 1984;10:51.

186. Hindson TC, Diffey BL: Phototoxicity of glyphosate in a weedkiller: a correction. Contact Dermatitis 1984;10:260.

187. IPCS: Environmental health criteria 159. Glyphosate. Geneva, World Health Organization, 1994.

188. Pushnoy LA, Avnon LS, Carel RS: Herbicide (Roundup) pneumonitis. Chest 1998;114:1769.

189. Goldstein DA, Johnson G, Farmer DR, et al: Pneumonitis and herbicide exposure. Chest 1999;116:1139.

190. Carel RS, Pushnoy LA: Pneumonitis and herbicide exposure. Chest 1999;116:1139.

191. Acquavella JF, Weber JA, Cullen MR, et al: Human ocular effects from self-reported exposures to Roundup herbicides. Hum Exp Toxicol 1999;18:479.

192. Martinez-Arrieta R, Ballesteros S, Ramón MF, et al: Spanish poison control centre survey of herbicide occupational exposures. J Toxicol Clin Toxicol 2003;41:522.

193. Loosli R: Epidemiology of atrazine. Rev Environ Contam Toxicol 1995;143:47.

194. Pommery J, Mathieu M, Mathieu D, et al: Atrazine in plasma and tissue following atrazine-aminotriazole-ethylene glycol-formaldehyde poisoning. J Toxicol Clin Toxicol 1993;31:323.

195. Elizarov GP: [Occupational skin diseases caused by simazine and propazine]. Vestn Dermatol Venerol 1972;46:27.

196. Schlicher JE, Beat VB: Dermatitis resulting from herbicide use: a case study. J Iowa Med Soc 1972;62:419.

197. Schuman SH, Dobson RL, Fingar JR: Dyrene dermatitis. Lancet 1980;2:1252.

198. Kinoshita FK, DuBois KP: Induction of hepatic microsomal enzymes by herban, diuron, and other substituted urea herbicides. Toxicol Appl Pharmacol 1970;17:406.

199. Litovitz TL, Felberg L, Soloway RA, et al: 1994 Annual report of the American Association of Poison Control Centers Toxic Exposure Surveillance System. Am J Emerg Med 1995;13:551.

200. Litovitz TL, Felberg L, White S, et al: 1995 Annual report of the American Association of Poison Control Centers Toxic Exposure Surveillance System. Am J Emerg Med 1996;14:487.

201. Litovitz TL, Klein-Schwartz W, Dyer KS, et al: 1997 Annual report of the American Association of Poison Control Centers Toxic Exposure Surveillance System. Am J Emerg Med 1998;16:443.

202. Litovitz TL, Smilkstein M, Felberg L, et al: 1996 Annual report of the American Association of Poison Control Centers Toxic Exposure Surveillance System. Am J Emerg Med 1997;15:447.

203. Heudorf U, Peters M: Isoproturon-Störfall am 27.1.1996 in einer Produktionsanlage der AgrEvo in Frankfurt am Main. Gesundheitswesen 1997;59:661.

204. Verheij ER, van der Greef J, La Vos GF, et al: Identification of diuron and four of its metabolites in human postmortem plasma and urine by LC/MS with a moving-belt interface. J Anal Toxicol 1989;13:8.

205. Van Boven M, Laruelle L, Daenens P: HPLC analysis of diuron and metabolites in blood and water. J Anal Toxicol 1990;14:231.

206. Geldmacher-von Mallinckrodt M, Schüssler F: Zu Stoffwechsel und Toxizität von 1-(3,4-Dichlorphenyl)-3,3-dimethylharnstoff (Diuron) beim Menschen. Arch Toxikol 1971;27:187.

207. Turcant A, Cailleux A, Le Bouil A, et al: Acute metobromuron poisoning with severe associated methemoglobinemia. Identification of four metabolites in plasma and urine by LC-DAD, LC-ESI-MS, and LC-ESI-MS-MS. J Anal Toxicol 2000;24:157.

208. Casey PB, Buckley BM, Vale JA: Methemoglobinemia following ingestion of a monolinuron/paraquat herbicide (Gramonol). J Toxicol Clin Toxicol 1994;32:185.

209. Brinquin L, Rousseau JM, Corbe H, et al: Intoxication aiguë volontaire par herbicide à base de diuron, d'atrazine et

d'aminotriazole. Toxicité du solvant, le propylène-glycol? JEUR 1993;6:20.

210. Ng LL, Naik RB, Polak A: Paraquat ingestion with methaemoglobinaemia treated with methylene blue. BMJ 1982;284:1445.

211. Proudfoot AT: Methaemoglobinaemia due to monolinuron—not paraquat. BMJ 1982;285:812.

212. Anic B, Plestina S, Radonic R, et al: Methemoglobinemija uzrokovana akcidentalnom intoksikacijom metolaklorom i metobromuronom. Arhiv za Higijenu Rada i Toksikologiju 1999;50:193.

213. Casey P, Vale JA: Deaths from pesticide poisoning in England and Wales: 1945–1989. Hum Exp Toxicol 1994;13:95.

214. Torrington KG: Herbicide exposure and pulmonary disease. J Occup Med 1983;25:354.

215. Turcant A, Harry P, Cailleux A, et al: Fatal acute poisoning by bentazon. J Anal Toxicol 2003;27:113.

216. Müller IB, Petersen HW, Johansen SS, et al: Fatal overdose of the herbicide bentazone. Forensic Sci Int 2003;135:235.

217. Lin TJ, Hung D-Z, Hu W-H, et al: Acute basagran poisoning mimicking neuroleptic malignant syndrome. Hum Exp Toxicol 1999;18:493.

79 *Rodenticides*

HOLLY E. PERRY, MD

At a Glance...

■ All rodenticides possess some human toxicity when taken in overdose.

■ High-toxicity rodenticides include thallium, sodium monofluoroacetate, strychnine, aluminum and zinc phosphide, vacor, naphthylthiourea (ATNU), and cholecalciferol. Low-toxicity agents include superwarfarins and red squill.

■ Originating from multiple classes of compounds, the rodenticides produce a broad range of toxicities.

■ The treatment of rodenticide overdose is generally supportive. For select agents, such as vacor and superwarfarins, specific therapies are available.

Competition between humans and lower animals for food and shelter, whether real or imagined, is a constant struggle. In an attempt to gain the ecologic upper hand, humans have endeavored to develop ways to curb rodent populations. The rodenticides encompass a diverse group of chemicals with a wide variety of actions. Whether organic or inorganic, mildly or highly toxic, all these agents are designed to kill in a cost-effective manner. A problem arises when humans or nontarget animals come into contact with these chemicals.

Rodenticides are designed to kill rodents considered a nuisance, such as rats, mice, gophers, moles, voles, ground squirrels, and prairie dogs. These animals damage crops in the field and foods in storage, host human diseases, bite people, and are capable of causing material damage by gnawing. It makes sense from both an economic and health perspective to attempt to control populations of these animals.[1,2]

Historically, a wide variety of inorganic and organic compounds have been used as rodenticides. Early rodenticides were agents derived from plant material such as strychnine and red squill or were inorganic chemicals such as arsenic trioxide and thallium. Newer agents tend to be synthetic organic compounds. Regardless of type, virtually all rodenticides are referred to as "rat poisons" by the lay public.

Some substances used as rodenticides proved to be nearly as dangerous to humans and other animals as they are to rodents. Thallium and vacor are no longer marketed in the United States because of severe toxicity. Efforts have been made to lessen the risk of using rodenticides by restricting the use of some substances and by requiring premarketing studies of potential new products. Still, all rodenticides are toxic if misused.[1]

The many chemical agents used as rat poisons are listed in Table 79-1. When possible, the container label should be used to identify a particular product. Even labeling can be a problem if not read carefully. For example, bromethalin, a neurotoxin, can be confused with bromadiolone or brodifacoum, which are long-acting anticoagulants. It is generally worth the effort to find the container and positively identify the ingredients in order to know what effects might be expected and how to approach treatment.

Rodenticides are regulated by the U.S. Environmental Protection Agency (EPA) in accordance with two acts. The Federal Insecticide, Fungicide and Rodenticide Act (FIFRA) of 1947 regulates distribution, use, and sale of these products within the United States. In 1972, the Federal Pesticide Control Act was passed as an amendment to the FIFRA. This is the act that most pesticide legislation is based on. According to this act, licensed exterminators must undergo a rigorous application procedure as well as ongoing training. This act also regulates labeling of pesticides. All pesticides must have a signal word clearly displayed on the front panel that reflects the highest possible toxicity of the product. The signal word "Danger" is indicative of a product that has an LD_{50} of 0 to 50 mg/kg; "Warning" indicates LD_{50} of 50 to 500 mg/kg; "Caution" indicates an LD_{50} of 500 to 5000 mg/kg. Under this categorization, a taste (one seventh of a teaspoon) of a rodenticide with signal word "Danger" would be enough to kill 50% of children weighing 10 kg. The corresponding lethal dose for a rodenticide with the signal word "Warning" would be 1 teaspoon.[3] There are a variety of ways that rodenticides may be classified, but for the purposes of this chapter, they are classified according to the severity of their toxicity.

HIGHLY TOXIC RODENTICIDES (SIGNAL WORD: "DANGER")

Thallium

AVAILABLE PRODUCTS
No thallium rodenticides are sold in the United States, but they are available in Mexico. Exposures rarely still occur in the United States as a result of homicide attempts,[4,5] from contaminated herbal preparations,[6] and from illicit drugs.[7]

DESCRIPTION
Thallium sulfate is a tasteless and odorless powder. Exposure can occur by absorption through intact skin, inhalation, or ingestion. It was introduced in the United States as a rodenticide in the 1920s.[8,9] The use of thallium as a pesticide was restricted in the United States to commercial exterminators in 1965[8,9] and was completely banned in 1975 because of continued accidental exposures. The LD_{50} in humans is 8 to 12 mg/kg.[10] Thallium is rapidly absorbed. Cell membranes do not differentiate between thallium and potassium because

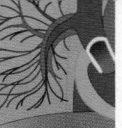
TABLE 79-1 Alphabetical List of Rodenticides by Trade Name and Type of Agent*

TRADE NAME	ACTIVE INGREDIENTS	TYPE OF RODENTICIDE
Acme Mole and Gopher Killer	Zinc phosphide	Phosphides
Anchor Rat and Mouse Bait Packet	Warfarin	Warfarin
Assault Rat Pellets	Bromethalin	Bromethalin
Assault Rat Place Pack	Bromethalin	Bromethalin
Assault Rat WR	Bromethalin	Bromethalin
Bantu	ANTU	ANTU
Bengal Mouse Bait	Chlorophacinone	Long-acting anticoagulant
Black Magic Rat Killer	Pivalyl	Long-acting anticoagulant
Blue Ball Rat Killer	Arsenous oxide	Arsenic
Bromone Mouse Killer	Bromodiolone	Long-acting anticoagulant
Caid	Chlorphacinone	Long-acting anticoagulant
Chopped Poison Peanuts	Strychnine	Strychnine
College Brand Rodenticide	ANTU	ANTU
Compound 1080	Sodium monofluoroacetate	Sodium monofluoroacetate
Compound 1081	Sodium monofluoroacetate	Sodium monofluoroacetate
Contrac	Brodifocoum	Long-acting anticoagulant
D-Con Mouse Prufe (no longer sold)	Warfarin	Warfarin
D-Con Mouse Prufe II	Brodifacoum	Long-acting anticoagulant
Death to Gophers	Strychnine	Strychnine
Deathdiet	Red squill	Red squill
Dipaxin	Diphacinone	Long-acting anticoagulant
Diphacin	Diphacinone	Long-acting anticoagulant
DLP 787 Tracking Powder	Pyriminil	Pyriminil
Dr. Hess Anturat	ANTU	ANTU
Drat	Chlorphacinone	Long-acting anticoagulant
Eagles 7 Final Bite	Diphacinone	Long-acting anticoagulant
El Ray Mouse Bait	Strychnine	Strychnine
Endox	Coumatetral	Long-acting anticoagulant
Endrocide	Coumatetral	Long-acting anticoagulant
Enforcer Rat and Mouse Killer	Chlorophacinone	Long-acting anticoagulant
Enforcer Mouse Kill III	Bromodiolone	Long-acting anticoagulant
Enforcer Rat and Mouse Bars II	Diphacinone	Long-acting anticoagulant
Final Bite	Diphacinone	Long-acting anticoagulant
Finis Rat and Mouse Killer	Diphacinone	Long-acting anticoagulant
Fluorakil 3	Sodium monofluoroacetate	Sodium monofluoroacetate
Fluorakil 100	Sodium monofluoroacetate	Sodium monofluoroacetate
Fluoroacetamide	Sodium monofluoroacetate	Sodium monofluoroacetate
Formula 163 Rat Kill	Diphacinone	Long-acting anticoagulant
Fratol	Sodium monofluoroacetate	Sodium monofluoroacetate
Fussol	Sodium monofluoroacetate	Sodium monofluoroacetate
Gopha Rid	Zinc phosphide	Phosphides
Gopher and Mole Killer Pellets	Zinc phosphide	Phosphides
Gopher Corn	Strychnine	Strychnine
Gopher Getter Bait	Strychnine	Strychnine
Gopher Getter Pills	Strychnine	Strychnine
Gopher Go	Strychnine	Strychnine
Gopher Gone	Diphacinone	Long-acting anticoagulant
Gopher Killer Pellets	Zinc phosphide	Phosphides
Gopher Mix	Strychnine	Strychnine
Gopher Poison Grain Bait	Strychnine	Strychnine
Gopher Probe Mix	Strychnine	Strychnine
Gopher Tabs	Strychnine	Strychnine
Gopher-Rodent Killer	Strychnine	Strychnine
Guardian Rat Bait	Diphacinone	Long-acting anticoagulant
Havoc Rodenticide Bait Pack	Brodifacoum	Long-acting anticoagulant
Hot Shot Sudden Death Mouse Killer	Bromethalin	Bromethalin
Isotrac Tracking Powder	Isovaleryl	Long-acting anticoagulant
Just One Bite Rat and Mouse Bait	Bromodiolone	Long-acting anticoagulant
Kil-Ko Rat Killer	Diphacinone	Long-acting anticoagulant
Kill Kantz	ANTU	ANTU
Klerat	Brodifacoum	Long-acting anticoagulant
Krysid	ANTU	ANTU
Maki Rat and Mouse Meal Bait	Bromodiolone	Long-acting anticoagulant
Maki Rat and Mouse Bait Packs Pellets	Bromodiolone	Long-acting anticoagulant
Megarox	Sodium monofluoroacetate	Sodium monofluoroacetate
Milo Gopher Bait	Strychnine	Strychnine
Miracle Mouse Bait	Strychnine	Strychnine
Mouse-B-Gon, Ortho	Cholecalciferol	Cholecalciferol
Mouse-Con No. 2	Zinc phosphide	Phosphides

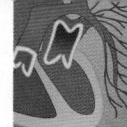

TABLE 79-1 Alphabetical List of Rodenticides by Trade Name and Type of Agent*–(Cont'd)

TRADE NAME	ACTIVE INREDIENTS	TPYE OF RODENTICIDE
Mouse Feast	Strychnine	Strychnine
Mouse Maize	Strychnine	Strychnine
Mouse Nots	Strychnine	Strychnine
Mouse Prufe II	Brodifacoum	Long-acting anticoagulant
Mouse Sault	Strychnine	Strychnine
Mouse Rid	Strychnine	Strychnine
Mr. Rat Guard	Zinc phosphide	Phosphides
Nott's	ANTU	ANTU
Packet Mouse Seed Bait	Strychnine	Strychnine
Patterson Mole Killer	Strychnine	Strychnine
PCQ Rat and Mouse Bait	Diphacinone	Long-acting anticoagulant
Phostoxin Fumigant	Aluminum phosphide	Phosphides
Phosvin	Zinc phosphide	Phosphides
Phosyin	Zinc phosphide	Phosphides
Piper Mouse Bait Packet	Strychnine	Strychnine
Pivalyl	Pindone	Long-acting anticoagulant
Pival	Pindone	Long-acting anticoagulant
Poison Peanut	Strychnine	Strychnine
Prolin	Warfarin	Warfarin
Promar Bait Pellets	Diphacinone	Long-acting anticoagulant
Purina Rat Kill	Pindone	Long-acting anticoagulant
Quick Ravac	Chlorphacinone	Long-acting anticoagulant
Quintox	Cholecalciferol	Cholecalciferol
Ramik Bait Pack	Diphacinone	Long-acting anticoagulant
Ramik Brown	Diphacinone	Long-acting anticoagulant
Ramik Green	Diphacinone	Long-acting anticoagulant
Rampage	Cholecalciferol	Cholecalciferol
Ratangle II	Warfarin	Warfarin
Rat-A-Rest	Bromodiolone	Long-acting anticoagulant
Ratak Bait Pack	Diphenicoum	Long-acting anticoagulant
Rat Bait Meat Bits	Warfarin	Warfarin
Rat Busters	Warfarin	Warfarin
Rat Death Liquid	Sodium arsonite	Arsenic
Rat Doom	Warfarin	Warfarin
Rat Dragon	Warfarin	Warfarin
Rat End	Warfarin	Warfarin
Rat-Fix	Warfarin	Warfarin
Rat Free Rat and Mouse Bait Pack	Bromodiolone	Long-acting anticoagulant
Rat-I-Cide	Warfarin	Warfarin
Raticate	Norbromide	Norbromide
Ratindan	Ratindan	Long-acting anticoagulant
Ratimus	Bromodiolone	Long-acting anticoagulant
Rat Kakes	Warfarin	Warfarin
Rat Kill Formula 163	Diphacinone	Long-acting anticoagulant
Rat Lunches	Strychnine	Strychnine
Ratmort	Warfarin	Warfarin
Rat Nip (Nip-Co)	Red squill	Red squill
Rat Nots	Red squill	Red squill
Rat-O-Cide	Warfarin	Warfarin
Rat-Ola	Diphacinone	Long-acting anticoagulant
Ratorex	Warfarin	Warfarin
Rat Poison (Pearson)	Zinc phosphide	Phosphides
Rat Snak	Arsenic trioxide	Arsenic
Rat Snax	Red squill	Red squill
Rat Squill	Red squill	Red squill
Rattrach	ANTU	ANTU
Rat-tu	ANTU	ANTU
Rat War	Warfarin	Warfarin
Real-Kill Ratex	Bromethalin	Bromethalin
Reardon Mouse Seed	Strychnine	Strychnine
Ro-Dex	Strychnine	Strychnine
Rodentin	Coumatetral	Long-acting anticoagulant
Rodent Kill	Diphacinone	Long-acting anticoagulant
Rodent Pellets	Zinc phosphide	Phosphides
Rodere Paraffinized Rat Bait	Diphacinone	Long-acting anticoagulant
Rodine	Red squill	Red squill
Ropax	Brodifacoum	Long-acting anticoagulant
Rozol	Chlorphacinone	Long-acting anticoagulant
Rumetan	Zinc phosphide	Phosphides

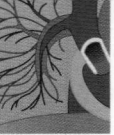

TABLE 79-1 Alphabetical List of Rodenticides by Trade Name and Type of Agent*–(Cont'd)

TRADE NAME	ACTIVE INREDIENTS	TPYE OF RODENTICIDE
S.L. Cowley & Sons Rat and Mouse Poison	Arsenic trioxide	Arsenic
Shoxin	Norbromide	Norbromide
Sla-Rat	Warfarin	Warfarin
Sodium fluoroacetate	Sodium monofluoroacetate	Sodium monofluoroacetate
Sodium monofluoroacetate	Sodium monofluoroacetate	Sodium monofluoroacetate
Stearn's Electric Brand Paste	Phosphorus	Phosphorus
Strike	Warfarin	Warfarin
Super Caid	Bromodiolone	Long-acting anticoagulant
Sweeney's Ready Mixed	Warfarin	Warfarin
Sweeney's Mouse Bait	Warfarin	Warfarin
T&C Gopher Pellets from Sears	Strychnine	Strychnine
Talon	Brodifacoum	Long-acting anticoagulant
Talon G	Brodifacoum	Long-acting anticoagulant
Thro Pac Rat and Mouse Killer Pellets	Diphacinone	Long-acting anticoagulant
Trax-one	Bromodiolone	Long-acting anticoagulant
Tri-Ban	Pindone	Long-acting anticoagulant
Trounce	Bromethalin	Bromethalin
True Grit Tracking Powder	Zinc phosphide	Phosphides
True Grit Gopher Rid	Zinc phosphide	Phosphides
Vacor Rat Bait	Pyriminil	Pyriminil
Vam-o	Warfarin	Warfarin
Vengeance	Bromethalin	Bromethalin
Yancock	Sodium monofluoroacetate	Sodium monofluoroacetate
Zinc-Tox	Zinc phosphide	Phosphides
ZP	Zinc phosphide	Phosphides
ZP AG	Zinc phosphide	Phosphides
ZP Tracking Powder	Zinc phosphide	Phosphides

ANTU, α-naphthyl-thiourea.
*Many trade names sound similar. Package labels should always be checked to verify the type of rodenticide when possible.

their ionic radii are similar: 1.47 Angstroms versus 1.33 Angstroms. Thus, thallium is distributed to tissues with a high potassium concentration such as the nervous system, muscle, and liver. Elimination is primarily by feces,[11] with significant enterohepatic circulation.[12] Its volume of distribution is estimated to be 3.6 L/kg.[13]

Thallium poisoning causes a distinct constellation of symptoms. Immediately after exposure, patients experience gastrointestinal (GI) symptoms, including vomiting, abdominal pain, or constipation. Within 24 to 48 hours, exquisitely painful paresthesias of the hands and feet occur. Alopecia begins by 10 days after the exposure and is complete within 1 month, although facial hair, axillary hair, and the inner one third of the eyelashes may be spared.[14] The amount ingested determines the severity of symptoms and the rapidity of onset. The GI symptoms tend to be relatively mild in comparison to other heavy-metal intoxication, unless the ingestion was large. Other symptoms that occur within days of an exposure include autonomic instability, cranial nerve palsies, and altered mental status—specifically confusion, delirium, and psychosis. Optic neuritis and Mees' lines may be late findings. Patients are at risk for sudden cardiac death for many weeks after an exposure.[15] Persistent neurologic sequelae such as impaired memory and weakness are common.[14]

MANAGEMENT
Agreement on a treatment protocol is lacking. Gastric lavage should be considered if exposure is recent unless the patient has vomited. A dose of activated charcoal should be given immediately. Thallium undergoes enterohepatic circulation; therefore, multiple doses of an absorbent should be continued. Prussian blue is the preferred decontamination strategy based on animal data[16-20] and in vitro models.[21,22] The safety and efficacy of Prussian blue in humans have not been systematically tested, although no adverse effects have been recorded. The release of cyanide ions is negligible.[23] The recommended dose for adults is 3 g orally three times a day and for children 2 to 12 years old is 1 g orally three times a day. The recommended duration of treatment is 6 weeks.[24] Prussian blue (Radiogardase) was not available in the United States until 2003, when it was approved by the U.S. Food and Drug Administration (FDA), because of concerns of terrorists deploying "dirty bombs." Radiogardase is approved for use in decontamination of patients exposed to radioactive cesium, radioactive thallium, and nonradioactive thallium. (For information: 1-888-CALL-FDA.) If it is not available, laboratory reagent grade Prussian blue may be used. Activated charcoal has also been shown to bind a significant amount of thallium[21]; therefore, multi-dose activated charcoal may be an acceptable alternative.

Other treatment modalities are of questionable benefit. In the past, forced potassium diuresis had been used and was shown to decrease the half-life of thallium from 30 days to 8 to 10 days.[25-27] However, potassium diuresis was noted to worsen symptoms in humans[4,28-31]

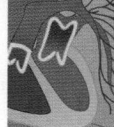

and increase central nervous system (CNS) toxicity and lethality in animals.[15,32] The use of hemoperfusion or hemoperfusion alternating with hemodialysis may enhance the elimination of thallium to some degree[25,33,34] and may be useful in certain patients such as those with renal insufficiency or if combined with other therapies.

Sodium Monofluoroacetate and Fluoroacetamide

DESCRIPTION

Sodium monofluoroacetate is a white powder that is usually mixed with a black dye when used as a rodenticide. Its use is restricted to commercial exterminators. It is odorless, tasteless, and highly water soluble and remains stable for a long period of time. It is readily absorbed through the GI tract, respiratory tract, mucous membranes, and abraded skin. In humans, doses of 0.5 to 2 mg/kg should be considered highly dangerous, and 5 mg/kg is estimated to be the lethal dose.[35] The fluoroacetate metabolite, fluorocitric acid, inhibits aconitase, a necessary cofactor in the Krebs cycle, resulting in lactic acidosis, accumulation of citrate in the cells, and chelation of serum calcium.[36] It has recently received more attention because of its potential use in biochemical warfare. Its lethality was highlighted in 2004 when it was implicated in the mass poisoning of zoo animals in São Paulo, Brazil.

There is a latent period before symptoms develop because sodium monofluoroacetate must first be metabolized to fluorocitrate for toxicity to occur, Typically, the lag time is between 30 and 180 minutes, but symptoms can be delayed for up to 20 hours.[37] Fluoroacetamide has essentially the same actions as fluoroacetate but is less toxic.[1] It has a slightly higher fatal dose (13–14 mg/kg) and a more delayed onset.[38]

The clinical effects are variable, although nausea, vomiting, and abdominal pain occur in most patients.[39] CNS effects and cardiac effects predominant. CNS effects include agitation, muscle spasm, stupor, and seizures. Apprehension, auditory hallucinations, and facial paresthesias often precede seizures. Cardiac effects include ectopic beats, ventricular tachycardia, ventricular fibrillation, and sudden cardiac arrest. Hypocalcemia, hypokalemia, and acidosis are frequent metabolic aberrations. Most deaths occur within hours of ingestion and are due to ventricular tachycardia or fibrillation; all fatalities occur by 72 hours.[39] In survivors, delayed effects include renal dysfunction, liver dysfunction, cerebellar degeneration, and cerebral atrophy. Paresthesia, neuropathies, and weakness may be permanent sequelae.[36]

MANAGEMENT

Treatment of sodium monofluoroacetate and fluoroacetamide toxicity is supportive. A dose of activated charcoal should be given if the exposure is recent. The patient should be placed on a continuous cardiorespiratory monitor and monitored for hypocalcemia, hypokalemia, and acidosis. Seizures should be treated with benzodiazepines. Arrhythmias may respond to

procainamide or calcium. Asymptomatic patients should be observed for at least 24 hours.

There is no known antidote, but a number of potential therapies have been studied. Ethanol, which is metabolized to acetate, has been shown to be an effective antidote in animals but has not been studied in humans.[36] Glycerol monoacetate (monacetin), which acts as an acetate substrate in the Krebs cycle, has been used experimentally in monkeys.[40]

Strychnine

DESCRIPTION

Strychnine is a plant alkaloid found in the seeds of *Strychnos nux-vomica*, a tree native to India. It was first used as a rat poison during the 16th century in Germany and is still used worldwide today.[41] Strychnine-impregnated bait is also used to control pests such as pigeons, rabbits, porcupines, and wild carnivores. Strychnine is available to the public in concentrations ranging from 0.3% to 0.5%. Licensed exterminators may obtain preparations that are 5% strychnine by weight. For the past 5 years, there have consistently been more than 100 exposures reported to the American Association of Poison Control Centers Toxic Exposures Surveillance System (AAPCC-TESS).[42-46] Strychnine has also been reported to be an adulterant in both cocaine and heroin.[47-49]

The mechanism of strychnine poisoning is well understood. Strychnine blocks uptake of glycine, an inhibitory neurotransmitter. Inhibition occurs primarily at the level of the postsynaptic spinal cord motor neurons and to a lesser extent in the brainstem and higher centers.[50] Thus, strychnine poisoning causes an increase in motor impulses reaching the spinal cord.

Toxic amounts are rapidly absorbed,[51] with convulsions occurring within 15 to 20 minutes. Because strychnine's effects occur primarily at the level of the spinal cord, the patient typically is awake both during and after the convulsions. In massive ingestions, the patient may be unconscious.[52] Characteristic convulsions are trismus or facial grimacing (*risus sardonicus*) and extensor spasm or frank opisthotonus. Convulsive episodes are brief but very painful. They can be precipitated by any sensory stimuli. Convulsions generally decrease within 12 to 24 hours. Respiratory arrest secondary to spasm of respiratory muscles is the usual fatal event.[50] Animal studies have shown that artificial ventilation protects from otherwise fatal doses of strychnine. Other complications of strychnine poisoning are due to the violent muscle activity. Profound lactic acidosis, rhabdomyolysis, hyperthermia, and compartment syndrome have been reported.[50]

MANAGEMENT

The primary goals are prevention or control of convulsions[41,53-55] and ensuring adequate ventilation. Because any stimulation may precipitate convulsions, the patient should be placed in a nonstimulating environment and given benzodiazepines prophylactically. Large amounts of benzodiazepines (>1 mg/kg) may be needed to control seizures. If seizures are not controlled by these measures, pentobarbital or a neuromuscular blocking

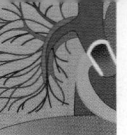

agent should be considered. Gastric lavage is not recommended because strychnine is rapidly absorbed and stimulation can precipitate convulsions. If symptoms are minimal or absent, activated charcoal should be considered. The patient should be monitored for lactic acidosis and rhabdomyolysis. The prognosis is generally favorable if the patient can be supported for the first 24 hours.[47]

Aluminum Phosphide, Zinc Phosphide

DESCRIPTION

Phosphides are used throughout the world to protect stored grains from rodents and other pests.[56] They are also available as mole and gopher killers. Phosphine gas is rapidly formed when zinc or aluminum phosphide comes in contact with dilute acids or with water[57] and is thought to be primarily responsible for their toxicity.[56-60] The exact mechanism of action is unclear, but phosphine is thought to produce toxicity by blocking cytochrome-c oxidase, which inhibits oxidative phosphorylation and eventually results in cell death.[56] Phosphine is heavier than air and has an odor of rotten fish, which can be detected at levels of 2 ppm.[56,61] Unfortunately, odor cannot be relied on as either a warning sign or diagnostic aid because toxicity can occur below the olfactory threshold.[61] Oral exposures to phosphides have become more numerous, with more than 100 exposures being reported to the AAPCC-TESS in 2001 and 2002.[45,46] Phosphides are reported to be a common suicidal agent in northern India.[56,62-64] The lethal dose in humans is not known, but patients ingesting zinc phosphide have died after ingesting as little as 4 to 5 g and have survived ingestion of 25 to 50 g. Toxic exposures to phosphine gas by inhalation have been reported.[58,59,65] The threshold limit value for phosphine gas is 0.3 ppm.[61]

Phosphides cause severe GI irritation. Nausea and vomiting with epigastric pain is universal and occurs within 10 to 15 minutes[56] in the case of aluminum phosphide and within 20 to 40 minutes for zinc phosphide.[63] Other frequent symptoms include hypotension, tachypnea, metabolic acidosis, palpitations, and hypocalcemic tetany. Pulmonary edema, jaundice, and widened QRS on the electrocardiogram occasionally occur.[64] Except for the universal occurrence of anxiety and restlessness, CNS symptoms are not prominent, although convulsions and coma have occurred in fatal cases.[59,60] Most deaths occur about 30 hours after ingestion but may be delayed up to 14 days. Death is most likely due to myocardial damage.[61]

MANAGEMENT

Treatment is symptomatic and supportive. A dose of activated charcoal is given if the exposure is recent. The patient should be placed on a cardiorespiratory monitor. Electrolytes and calcium should be followed closely and treated as necessary. Renal and liver function tests should be monitored daily. Phosphine can be off-gassed from emesis, feces, or lavage solution, and these fluids should be cleaned up immediately and disposed of properly.

The prognosis for patients with severe cardiovascular and pulmonary problems is grave.

Phosphorus

DESCRIPTION

Elemental phosphorus exists in two forms. The red form, used in manufacturing matches, is not absorbed and is nontoxic. In contrast, the yellow (also called white) form is a highly toxic protoplasmic poison and is available as a rat or roach paste.[66] The acute lethal dose has been reported to be about 1 mg/kg.[67]

Symptoms have classically been divided into three stages. In stage 1 occurring minutes to hours after the ingestion, severe oral burns, vomiting, stomach pain, garlic-like odor on the breath, and diarrhea may be noted. The feces or vomitus may appear phosphorescent in a darkened room, and hence phosphorus poisoning has been called the *smoking stool syndrome.*[68] Death in stage I has been attributed to ventricular dysrhythmia and cardiovascular collapse.[68] If the patient survives, a quiescent period of several weeks ensues (stage II). The third stage represents systemic toxicity caused by phosphorus. Organ systems primarily affected are the GI tract, liver, heart, kidneys, and CNS.[69]

MANAGEMENT

Treatment is primarily directed toward removing and preventing absorption of the phosphorus, as well as symptomatic and supportive care of patient. Emesis should be avoided. Dilution with milk is not recommended because digestible fat increases the absorption of phosphorous. Gastric lavage with 1:5000 potassium permanganate or a 2% solution of hydrogen peroxide may be useful if begun before onset of symptoms; these solutions oxidize phosphorus to the less harmful phosphate. Care must be taken to protect both the patient and caregivers from contact with phosphorous, which may be present in emesis or feces.

The patient should be observed for damage to the GI tract, liver, kidneys, heart, and cardiovascular system. Hypoglycemia, hypoprothrombinemia, and clotting abnormalities may be noted with liver damage, and clotting studies should be performed in seriously affected patients. Hypocalcemia has been reported. Asymptomatic patients should be monitored for 24 to 36 hours.

Arsenic

DESCRIPTION

Although more commonly used as a pesticide or herbicide, arsenic finds some limited use as a rodenticide. Arsenites are salts of arsenous acid (from arsenic trioxide). Arsenites are more soluble and have a faster onset of toxicity than other forms of arsenic, thus making them likely choices for rodenticides, herbicides, and pesticides.[1]

For effects and treatment of exposure to arsenic, see Chapter 74.

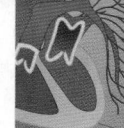

Barium Carbonate

DESCRIPTION

Barium carbonate is one of several soluble barium salts, including sulfide, chloride, chlorate, and nitrate. All are highly toxic. On the other hand, barium sulfate, an insoluble salt, is harmless and is used in medicine as a radiopaque contrast medium. In the past, rodenticides were used that contained 20% to 25% barium carbonate. No barium rodenticides are currently in use, although other forms used for poisoning are available.[70,71] The lethal dose is estimated to be 2 g. Acute toxicity may occur with 200 mg.[1]

Barium apparently produces a depolarizing neuromuscular blockade resulting in weakness of striated, cardiac, and smooth muscle. Hypokalemia, often profound, may occur. Symptoms include paresthesias around the mouth; this may spread to the hands and feet. Vomiting and diarrhea with colicky abdominal pain may ensue 1 to 8 hours after ingestion. Tightness in the throat, dysarthria, headache, muscle twitching, general weakness, and paralysis may be noted. Paralysis can range from weakness of one limb to complete paralysis with respiratory failure.[71] Many of the reported cases have resulted from contamination of food. In such cases, the rapidity of onset and absence of eye signs can help rule out botulism.[71]

MANAGEMENT

Treatment should start with emptying the stomach by emesis or lavage unless substantial vomiting has already occurred. A lavage solution of magnesium or sodium sulfate (30 g in 250 mL of water) should be used to precipitate the barium as insoluble barium sulfate. The patient's fluids and electrolytes should be monitored. Hypokalemia is common and should be treated aggressively.[72,73] Muscle tone and respiratory effort should be followed closely and mechanical ventilation instituted as needed.

The prognosis is favorable if patients are stabilized and are maintained for 24 hours. Recovery is usually complete.

Pyriminil (Vacor, PNU)

DESCRIPTION

This agent was released in 1975 as a one-feeding, acutely toxic rodenticide. Because of its severe toxicity, it was withdrawn as a general-use pesticide in 1979. The manufacturer asked for return of unsold packages but did not request a general recall of packages sold to the public. As a result, rare exposures continued to occur as recently as 2002.[46]

Pyriminil destroys the β cells of the islets of Langerhans in the pancreas, resulting in inadequate production of insulin. Patients may present within hours of exposure with diabetic ketoacidosis. Death may result from dysrhythmias or diabetic ketoacidosis. Sequelae are significant and includes brittle diabetes mellitus; postural hypotension, which can be difficult to control; and sensory and motor neuropathies.[74-76] Death has been reported with a dose of 780 mg, and symptoms have been noted after ingestion of as little as 390 mg (5.6 mg/kg).[76]

The exact mechanism of action of pyriminil is not known, but in animals, it seems to act as a niacinamide antagonist, interfering with the pentose phosphate shunt, particularly in liver, brain, and islet cells, and resulting in defects in RNA production.

MANAGEMENT

A dose of activated charcoal is given if the exposure is recent. Although niacinamide (nicotinamide) may be an antidote, it is no longer available, and therefore niacin (nicotinic acid) has been substituted. Of note is that the vasodilation caused by niacin may exacerbate the existing postural hypotension. The recommended dose is 500 mg administered intravenously (slow push), followed by 100 to 200 mg every 4 hours for 48 hours. If symptoms of poisoning are present, the dosing interval should be decreased to every 2 hours.

Monitoring should include glucose, ketones, electrolytes, and liver function tests. Diabetic ketoacidosis should be treated with insulin and fluid as necessary.

MODERATELY TOXIC RODENTICIDES (SIGNAL WORD: "WARNING")

α-Naphthyl-Thiourea (ANTU)

DESCRIPTION

ANTU produces pulmonary edema and pulmonary effusion in adult Norway rats. Young Norway rats, roof rats, and most other animals except dogs are resistant to its effects.[1]

Animal studies suggest the lethal dose for humans may be between 0.5 and 5 mg/kg.[77] Expected effects after ingestion include vomiting, dyspnea, cyanosis, and pulmonary rales or edema. Exposures are rare but continue to be reported. There have been no recorded human fatalities.

MANAGEMENT

Treatment is supportive. Routine decontamination should be performed. The patient should be monitored for pulmonary edema and treated symptomatically if it occurs.

Cholecalciferol

DESCRIPTION

A rodenticide first marketed in 1984, cholecalciferol (vitamin D_3) takes advantage of the fact that rodents are extremely sensitive to small percentage changes in the calcium balance in their blood. Cholecalciferol causes hypercalcemia both by mobilizing calcium from bone and by increasing absorption of calcium by the gut. The hypercalcemic state results in calcification of the organs, blood vessels, and soft tissue. It may also lead to nerve and muscle dysfunction as well as cardiac rhythm disturbances.[78]

Cholecalciferol is commonly used by the general public as well as licensed exterminators. Pellets are available in 30-g packs and in bulk containers. Each pellet contains 0.0577 mg, or 2308 IU, of vitamin D.[79] There is wide individual variation in the amount of

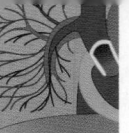

cholecalciferol required to produce hypervitaminosis D in humans, with most reported poisonings a result of chronic excess of vitamin D. Continued ingestion of 50,000 IU or more per day can cause toxicity.[80] No serious toxicity or death has been reported from the rodenticide form of D_3. However, there are several reports of toxicity due to hypervitaminosis D_3 when added in error to milk[81] and nutritional supplements[82] or when industrial concentrates of vitamin D_3 were used as a cooking oil.[83,84] No information is available on acute exposures. Because of the long elimination half-life (>30 days), however, a very large single dose might produce the same effects as long-term exposures.

Symptoms of hypercalcemia are common with levels above 11.5 to 12 mg/dL. These include anorexia, weight loss, weakness, fatigue, disorientation, vomiting, polyuria, and constipation.[81] Levels exceeding 13 mg/dL may produce seizures and renal insufficiency. Calcification in the kidneys, skin, vessels, lungs, heart, and stomach also may occur at this level. In children, one episode of moderately severe hypercalcemia may result in growth retardation. Six months or more may pass before growth resumes.[85]

MANAGEMENT

Several bait pellets or a small amount of the mouse seed should not be toxic, and no treatment is necessary. Patients who have ingested a single large dose of cholecalciferol should be given a dose of activated charcoal. Serum calcium levels must be monitored for 24 to 48 hours after ingestion. Normal serum calcium by 48 hours excludes significant toxicity. Serum potassium and magnesium levels should also be monitored frequently.

Hypercalcemia should be treated aggressively. Forced diuresis using normal saline and furosemide increases the elimination of calcium. Prednisone (5–15 mg every 6 hours by mouth) is effective in vitamin D intoxication to lower calcium levels. Calcitonin (4–8 IU/kg subcutaneously or intramuscularly every 12 hours) may significantly lower calcium levels over the course of hours. In severe hypercalcemia (>15 mg/dL), or for those patients not responding to other measures, the use of mithramycin should be considered. All patients should be placed on a low calcium diet.

LOW-TOXICITY RODENTICIDES (SIGNAL WORD: "CAUTION")

Warfarin and Long-Acting Anticoagulants (Second-Generation Anticoagulants, Superwarfarins)

DESCRIPTION

Warfarin and the long-acting anticoagulants (brodifacoum, bromadiolone, difenacoum, and chlorophacinone) act by inhibiting vitamin K epoxide reductase and vitamin K reductase. However, the long-acting anticoagulants differ from warfarin in two important ways: they are more potent, and they have longer half-lives. They thus have advantages as rodenticides in that they are

effective in single or limited feedings (warfarin requires repeated feeding for 4 to 5 days), and they are effective against animals that are resistant or more tolerant to warfarin.[5] Since their introduction during the mid to late 1970s as a second generation of anticoagulants, these agents have essentially replaced the older warfarin-containing products.

The long-acting anticoagulants are responsible for more than 80% of the human rodenticide exposures reported in the United States. Most of these exposures are reported in children younger than 6 years as a consequence of exploratory behavior.[46] Significant clinical toxicity has never been shown in this subset of patients.[86-91] In contrast, both single ingestions of a large amount and multiple ingestions of small amounts either through occupational exposure[92,93] or surreptitious exposure[94-96] can result in toxicity with symptoms lasting for months.

For effects and treatment of warfarin and the long-acting anticoagulants, see Chapter 66.

Bromethalin

DESCRIPTION

Bromethalin is one of the newer rodenticides, having entered the market in 1985 but not widely available until the late 1990s with significant numbers of exposures only reported in 2001.[45] Bromethalin acts as a neurotoxin. It is metabolized to desmethylbromethalin, which has much more potent neurotoxic activity.[97] The CNS effects appear to be secondary to the uncoupling of mitochondrial oxidative phosphorylation. A resultant decrease in the production of adenosine triphosphate causes the development of fluid-filled vacuoles between the myelin sheaths covering the central nerves. Increased CNS pressure and pressure on nerve axons result in decreased nerve impulse conduction. Resulting paralysis is followed by eventual death.[98] Bromethalin is a nonselective mammalian poison. All animals, including humans, are vulnerable to its toxic effects. Its effectiveness as a rodenticide is based on smaller rodents consuming larger quantities per kilogram of body weight than larger animals.[99] One possible exposure has been reported in which the patient presented unconscious with severe myoclonic jerks when touched. This patient had almost complete neurologic recovery within 48 hours.[100]

Treatment of a bromethalin ingestion should be symptomatic and supportive.[99,101-103] Effects in animals are typically noted within 2 to 4 hours but may be delayed up to 12 to 24 hours. Therefore, massive ingestions should be observed for at least 12 hours.

Red Squill

DESCRIPTION

Red squill is a botanic rodenticide derived from the red variety of *Urginea maritima*, or sea onion. Red squill contains two cardiac glycosides, scillaren A and scillaren B.[104]

Red squill is very bitter and has a powerful emetic action; hence, much of the material may be spontaneously removed from the stomach before it is

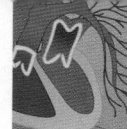

absorbed. The scillaren A and B produce effects similar to digitalis, and treatment is the same as for digitalis toxicity, including the use of Digibind (see Chapter 68). A polyclonal assay for digoxin may confirm a significant ingestion. However, signs and symptoms may exceed what would be predicted from the level because the assay does not have equivalent cross-reactivity for all cardiac glycosides.[105]

Norbromide

DESCRIPTION

Norbromide is selectively toxic to Norway rats, in which it acts to produce smooth muscle constriction. Death is a result of intense peripheral vasoconstriction.[106] Other rats, rodents, and animals, including humans, are resistant because they do not have the receptor for this compound in their blood vessels. Human volunteers given 20 to 300 mg had no symptomatic complaints but at the higher doses demonstrated slight decreases in temperature and blood pressure. Lowest values were seen 1 hour after ingestion, and values returned to normal by 2 hours.

MANAGEMENT

After large exposures, activated charcoal should be given. Treatment is rarely needed but would be symptomatic and supportive.

CONCLUSION

A number of groups of persons are poisoned by rodenticides. Children are especially at risk. Of 20,507 calls about rodenticides recorded by members of the AAPCC-TESS in 2002, 85% involved children younger than 6 years.[46] Other exposures occur in suicide attempts, victims of attempted homicide, exterminators and others putting out rodenticides, intoxicated individuals, psychiatric or mentally impaired patients, and people who accidentally eat rodenticides that are stored in containers normally used for edible products.

REFERENCES

1. Hayes WJ: Pesticides Studied in Man. Baltimore, Williams & Wilkins, 1982.
2. Public Health Study Team: Pest Control and Public Health, Vol. 5. Washington, DC, National Academy of Sciences, 1976, p 81.
3. Spann MF, Blondell JM, Hunting KL: Acute hazards to young children from residential pesticide exposures. Am J Public Health 2000;90:971.
4. Meggs WJ, Hoffman RS, Shih RD, et al: Thallium poisoning from maliciously contaminated food. Clin Toxicol 1994;32:723.
5. Desenclos JA, Wilder MH, Coppenger GW, et al: Thallium poisoning: an outbreak in Florida, 1988. S Med J 1992;85:1203.
6. Schaumberg HH, Berger A: Alopecia and sensory polyneuropathy from thallium in a Chinese herbal medicine. JAMA 1992;268:3430.
7. Insley BM, Grufferman S, Ayliffe HE: Thallium poisoning in cocaine abusers. Am J Emerg Med 1986;4:545.
8. Mack RB: Schemes Gang Aft Agley, thallium poisoning. N C Med J 1990;51:156.
9. Saddique A, Peterson CD: Thallium poisoning: a review. Vet Hum Toxicol 1983;25:16.
10. Fergusson JE: The Heavy Elements: Chemistry, Environmental Impact and Health Effects. New York, Pergamon, 1990.
11. Lund A: The effect of various substances on the excretion and the toxicity of thallium in the rat. Acta Pharmacol Toxicol 1956;33:260.
12. Thompson DF: Management of thallium poisoning. Clin Toxicol 1981;18:979.
13. De Groot G, van Heijst ANP, van Kesteren RG, et al: An evaluation of the efficacy of charcoal hemoperfusion in the treatment of three cases of acute thallium poisoning. Arch Toxicol 1985;57:61.
14. Reed D, Crawley J, Faro SN, et al: Thallotoxicosis: acute manifestations and sequelae. JAMA 1963;183:96.
15. Grand Rounds—Guy's Hospital: Thallium poisoning. BMJ 1993;306:1527.
16. Meggs WJ, Goldfrank LR, Hoffman RS: Effects of potassium in a murine model of thallium poisoning [abstract]. Clin Toxicol 1995;33:559.
17. Krazov J, Rios C, Altagracia M, et al: Relationship between physiochemical properties of Prussian blue and its efficacy as antidote against thallium poisoning. J Appl Toxicol 1993;13:213.
18. Heydlauf H: Ferric-cyanoferrate (II): an effective antidote in thallium poisoning. Eur J Pharmacol 1969;6:340.
19. Meggs WJ, Morasco RC, Shih RD, et al: Effects of Prussian blue and N-acetylcysteine on thallium toxicity in mice. Clin Toxicol 1997;35:163.
20. Rios C, Monroy-Noyola A: D-penicillamine and Prussian blue as antidotes against thallium intoxication in rats. Toxicology 1992;74:69.
21. Hoffman RS, Stringer JA, Feinberg RS, et al: Comparative efficacy of thallium adsorption by activated charcoal, Prussian blue, and sodium polystyrene sulfonate. Clin Toxicol 1999;37:833.
22. Lehmann PA, Favare L: Parameters for the adsorption of thallium ions by activated charcoal and Prussian blue. Clin Toxicol 1984;22:331.
23. Moore D, House I: Thallium poisoning: diagnosis may be elusive but alopecia is the key. BMJ 1993;306:1527.
24. Pai V: Acute thallium poisoning. Prussian blue therapy in 9 cases. W I Med J 1987;36:256.
25. Nogue S, Mas A, Pares A, et al: Acute thallium poisoning: an evaluation of different forms of treatment. Clin Toxicol 1982–83;19:1015.
26. Chamberlain PH, Stavinoha WB, Davis H, et al: Thallium poisoning. Pediatrics 1958;22:1170.
27. Reed D, Crawley J, Faro SN, et al: Thallotoxicosis. JAMA 1963;183:516.
28. Gastel B: Clinical conferences at Johns Hopkins Hospital. Thallium poisoning. Johns Hopkins Med J 1978;142:27.
29. Papp JP, Gay PC, Dodson VN, et al: Potassium chloride treatment in thallotoxicosis. Ann Intern Med 1969;71:119.
30. Bank WJ, Pleasure DE, Suzuki K, et al: Thallium poisoning Arch Neurol 1972;26:456.
31. Roby DS, Fein AM, Bennet RH, et al: Cardiopulmonary effects of acute thallium poisoning. Chest 1984;84:236.
32. Hasan M, Chandra S, Dua PR, et al: Biochemical and electrophysiological effects of thallium poisoning on the rat corpus striatum. Toxicol Appl Pharmacol 1977;41:353.
33. Moeschlin MD: Thallium poisoning. Clin Toxicol 1980;17:133.
34. DeBaker W, Zachee P, Verpooten GA, et al: Thallium intoxication treated with combined hemoperfusion-hemodialysis. Clin Toxicol 1982;19:259.
35. Proctor NH, Hughes JP: Chemical Hazards of the Workplace. Philadelphia, JB Lippincott, 1978.
36. Robinson RF: Intoxication with sodium monofluoroacetate (compound 1081). Vet Human Toxicol 2002;44:93.
37. Reigart JR, Brueggerman JL, Keil JE: Sodium fluoroacetate poisoning. Am J Dis Child 1975;129:1224.
38. Hayes WJ: Pesticides studied in man. Baltimore, Williams & Wilkins, 1982.
39. Chi C, Chen K, Chan S, et al: Clinical presentation and prognostic factors in sodium monofluoroacetate intoxication. J Toxicol Clin Toxicol 1996;34:707.
40. Chenworth MB: Fluoroacetate: still a portal to comparative toxicology. Fed Proc 1967;26:1074.
41. Teitlebaum DT, Ott JE: Acute strychnine intoxication. Clin Toxicol 1970;267:3.

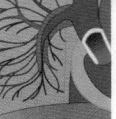

42. Litovitz TL, Klein-Schwartz W, Caravati EM, et al: 1998 Annual report of the American Association of Poison Control Centers toxic exposure surveillance system. Am J Emerg Med 1999;17:435.

43. Litovitz TL, Klein-Schwartz W, White S, et al: 1999 Annual report of the American Association of Poison Control Centers toxic exposure surveillance system. Am J Emerg Med 2000; 18:517.

44. Litovitz TL, Klein-Schwartz W, White S, et al: 2000 Annual report of the American Association of Poison Control Centers toxic exposure surveillance system. Am J Emerg Med 2001;19:337.

45. Litovitz TL, Klein-Schwartz W, Rodgers GC, et al: 2001 Annual report of the American Association of Poison Control Centers toxic exposure surveillance system. Am J Emerg Med 2002;20:391.

46. Watson WA, Litovitz TL, Rodgers GC, et al: 2002 Annual report of the American Association of Poison Control Centers toxic exposure surveillance system. Am J Emerg Med 2003;21:353.

47. Boyd RE, Brennan PT, Deng J, et al: Strychnine poisoning: recovery from profound lactic acidosis, hyperthermia and rhabdomyolysis. Am J Med 1983;74:507.

48. Decker WJ, Baker HE, Tamulinus SH: Two deaths resulting from apparent parenteral injection of strychnine Vet Hum Toxicol 1982;24:161.

49. O'Callaghan WG, Joyce N, Counihan HE, et al: Unusual strychnine poisoning and its treatment: report of eight cases. Clin Res Ed 1982;285:478.

50. Smith BA: Strychnine poisoning. J Emerg Med 1990;8:321.

51. Blain PG, Nightingale S, Stoddart JC: Strychnine poisoning: abnormal eye movements. Clin Toxicol 1982;19:215.

52. Heiser JM, Daya MR, Magnussen AR, et al: Massive strychnine intoxication: serial blood levels in a fatal case. Clin Toxicol 1992;30:269.

53. Edmunds M, Sheehan TMT, Van't-Hoff W: Strychnine poisoning: clinical and toxicological observations on a non-fatal case. Clin Toxicol 1986;24:245.

54. Maron BJ, Krupp JR, Tune B: Strychnine poisoning successfully treated with diazepam. J Pediatr 1971;78:697.

55. Sgaragli GP, Mannaioni PF: Pharmacokinetic observations on a case of massive strychnine poisoning. Clin Toxicol 1973;6:533.

56. Gupta S, Ahlawat SK: Aluminum phosphide poisoning—a review. Clin Toxicol 1995;33:19.

57. Stephenson JBP: Zinc phosphide poisoning. Arch Environ Health 1967;15:83.

58. Wilson R, Lovejoy FH, Jaeger RJ, Landrigan PL: Acute phosphene poisoning aboard a grain freighter. JAMA 1980;244:148.

59. Garry VF, Good PF, Manivel C, et al: Investigation of a fatality from nonoccupational aluminum phosphide exposure: measurement of aluminum in tissue and body fluids as a marker of exposure. J Lab Clin Med 1993;122:139.

60. Johnson HD, Voss E: Toxicological studies of zinc phosphide. J Am Pharm Assoc 1952;41:468.

61. Rodenberg HD, Chang CC, Watson WA: Zinc phosphide ingestion: a case report and review. Vet Hum Toxicol 1989;31:559.

62. Banjaj R, Wasir HS: Epidemic aluminum phosphide poisoning in northern India. Lancet 1988;1:820.

63. Jayaraman KS: Death pills from pesticide. Nature 1991;353:377.

64. Chugh SN, Aggarwal HK, Mahajan SK: Zinc phosphide intoxication symptoms: analysis of 20 cases. Int J Clin Pharmacol Ther 1998;36:406.

65. Feldstein A, Heumann M, Barnett M: Fumigant intoxication during transport of grain by railroad. J Occup Med 1991;33:377.

66. Simon FA, Pickering LK: Acute yellow phosphorus poisoning. JAMA 1976;235:1343.

67. Diaz-Rivera RS, Callazo PJ, Pons ER, et al: Acute phosphorous poisoning in man: a study of 56 cases. Medicine 1950;29:269.

68. Simon FA, Pickering LK: Acute yellow phosphorus poisoning: "smoking stool syndrome." JAMA 1976;235:1343.

69. McCarron MM, Trotter AT: Acute yellow phosphorus poisoning from pesticide pastes. Clin Toxicol 1981;18:693.

70. Jourdan S, Bertoni M, Pelligrino S: Case report: suicidal poisoning with barium chloride. Forensic Sci Int 2001;119:263.

71. Lewi Z, Bar-Khayim Y: Food poisoning from barium carbonate. Lancet 1964;2:342.

72. Phelan DM, Hagley SR: Is hypokalemia the cause of paralysis in barium poisoning? BMJ 1984;289:882.

73. Bering J: Hypokalemia of barium poisoning [letter]. Lancet 1975;1:110.

74. Prosser PR, Karam JH: Diabetes mellitus following rodenticide ingestion in man. JAMA 1978;239:1148.

75. Pont A, Rubino JM, Bishop D, Peal R: Diabetes mellitus and neuropathy following vacor ingestion in man. Arch Intern Med 1979;139:185.

76. LeWitt PA: The neurotoxicity of the rat poison vacor. N Engl J Med 1980;301:73.

77. Gosselin RE, Smith RP, Hodge H: Clinical Toxicology of Common Products. Baltimore, Williams & Wilkins, 1984.

78. Product Information: True Grit Rampage Rat and Mouse Bait. Overland Park, KS, Ceva Laboratories, 1986.

79. Production Information: Quintox Rat and Mouse Bait, Quintox Mouse Seed. Rodent control product and label catalog. Madison, WI, Bell Laboratories, 1985.

80. Paterson CR: Vitamin D poisoning: survey of causes in 21 patients with hypercalcemia. Lancet 1980;1:1165.

81. Blank S, Scanlon KS, Sinks TH, et al: An outbreak of hypervitaminosis D associated with the over fortification of milk from a home-delivery dairy. Am J Public Health 1995;85:656.

82. Koutjia P, Chen TC, Holik MF: Vitamin D intoxication associated with an over-the-counter supplement. N Eng J Med 2002; 345:66.

83. Down, PF, Polak A, Regan RJ: A family with massive acute vitamin D intoxication. Postgrad Med J 1979;55:897.

84. Pettifor JM, Bikle DD, Cavaleros M, et al. Serum levels of free 1,25-dihydroxyvitamin D in vitamin D toxicity. Ann Intern Med 1995;122:511.

85. Haynes RC, Murad F: Agents affecting calcification. In Gilman AG, Goodman LS, Rall TW, Murad F (eds): The Pharmacological Basis of Therapeutics, 7th ed. New York, Macmillan, 1985.

86. Smolinske SC, Scherger DL, Kearns PS, et al: Superwarfarin poisoning in children: a prospective study. Pediatrics 1989;84:490.

87. Ingels M, Lai C, Tai W, et al: A prospective study of acute, unintentional pediatric superwarfarin ingestions managed without decontamination. Ann Emerg Med 2002;40:73.

88. Morrissey B, Burgess JL, Robertson WO: Washington's experience and recommendations re: anticoagulant rodenticides. Vet Human Toxicol 1995;37:362.

89. Mullins ME, Brands CL, Daya MR: Unintentional pediatric superwarfarin exposures: do we really need a prothrombin time? Pediatrics 2000;105:402.

90. Shepherd G, Klein-Schwartz W, Anderson BD: Acute, unintentional pediatric brodifacoum ingestions. Pediatr Emerg Care 2002;18:174.

91. Kanabar D, Volans G: Accidental superwarfarin poisoning in children—less treatment is better. Lancet 2002;360:963.

92. Svendson SW, Kolstad HA, Steesby E: Bleeding problems associated with occupational exposure to anti-coagulant rodenticides. Int Arch Occup Environ Health 2002;75:515.

93. Spiller HA, Gallenstein GL, Murphy MJ: Dermal absorption of a liquid diphacinone rodenticide causing coagulopathy. Vet Human Toxicol 2003;45:313.

94. Poovalingam V, Kenoyer DG, Mahomed, et al: Superwarfarin poisoning—a report of 4 cases. S Afr Med J 2002;92:874.

95. Berry RG, Morrison JA, Watts JW, et al: Surreptitious superwarfarin ingestion with brodifacoum. South Med J 2000;93:74.

96. Greef MC, Mashile O, MacDougall LG: "Superwarfarin" (bromadiolone) poisoning in two children resulting in prolonged anti-coagulation. Lancet 1987;2:1269.

97. Cherry JT, Gunnoe MD, VanLier RBL: The metabolism of bromethalin and its effects on oxidative phosphorylation and cerebral fluid pressure. Toxicologist 1982;2:108.

98. Technical Bulletin: Assault (bromethalin). St. Louis, Purina Mills, 1988.

99. VanLier RBL, Cherry LD: The toxicity and mechanism of toxicity of bromethalin: a new single-feeding rodenticide. Fund Appl Toxicol 1988;11:664.

100. Buller G, Heard J, Gorman S: Possible bromethalin-induced toxicity in a human, a case report [abstract]. Clin Toxicol 1996;34:572.

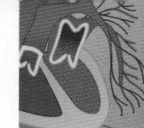

101. Dreikorn BA, O'Doherty OP: The discovery of bromethalin, an acute rodenticide with a unique mode of action. American Chemical Society Symposium Series 1984;255:45.

102. Jackson WB, Spaulding SR, VanLier RBL, et al: Bromethalin—a promising new rodenticide. In Proceedings of the Material Safety Data Sheet: Bromethalin Concentrate 2%. Indianapolis, Elanco Products, 1987.

103. Grant R, Dickerson C: Verbal communication. St. Louis, Purina Mills, May 1995.

104. Klaassen CD: Nonmetallic environmental toxicants: air pollutants, solvents and vapors and pesticides. In Gillman AG, Goodman LS, Rall TD, Murad F (eds): The Pharmacological Basis of Therapeutics, 7th ed. New York, Macmillan, 1985.

105. Gittelman MA, Stephan M, Perry H: Acute pediatric digoxin ingestion. Pediatr Emerg Care 1999;15:359.

106. Morgan DP: Recognition and Management of Pesticide Poisonings, 3rd ed. Washington, DC, U.S. Environmental Protection Agency, 1982.

80

Fumigants

JUDITH M. EISENBERG, MD, MS ■ MICHAEL I. GREENBERG, MD, MPH

At a Glance...

- Fumigants exist in the gaseous state as nonselective pesticides. They pose significant risks to humans when conditions of safe use are not observed.
- Some fumigants may be explosive as well as toxic. Depending on their molecular weight, they may be heavier or lighter than air, and thus tend to accumulate in corresponding (low or high) areas of confined spaces
- Phosphine has been responsible for numerous human poisonings. Patients may complain of headache, dizziness, tremors, cough, chest pain, shortness of breath, nausea, vomiting, and abdominal pain. Clinical signs include depressed mental status, pulmonary edema, hypotension, cardiac dysrhythmias. Seizures have been reported.
- Methyl bromide is a neurotoxicant and may cause status epilepticus. It is also a potent vesicant.
- Sulfuryl fluoride may cause bronchospasm, mucosal irritation, nausea, vomiting, and abdominal pain, as well as paresthesias, refractory seizures, and coma. Fluoride toxicity may result in profound shock, life-threatening cardiac dysrhythmias, and pulmonary edema.

Fumigants are chemical pesticides that exist as gases at specific ambient temperatures and atmospheric pressures. In their gaseous state, these chemicals are able to easily penetrate into treated agricultural product stores as well into the crevices of structural materials that would be difficult to reach with conventional liquid spray techniques. Fumigants are generally not selective with regard to target pests, and human exposure to these agents may under specific circumstances result in significant human morbidity. Individuals who use these chemicals must have special training in how to work with these chemicals safely before becoming certified fumigators.

This chapter summarizes the chemical and biomedical characteristics of the fumigants currently available for use in the United States. In addition, several fumigants no longer approved for use are discussed because important lessons have been learned from their prior use.

1,3-DICHLOROPROPENE (CAS: 542-75-6) (TELONE II)

1,3-Dichloropropene (DCP) is a chlorinated aliphatic hydrocarbon with a strong chloroform odor. Its chemical formula is $C_3H_4Cl_2$. Used as a soil fumigant, it is useful as a fungicidal and nematocidal agent in vegetable and tobacco crops. At room temperature, this chemical is a yellow liquid, which is applied by injection into soil. After injection, it quickly vaporizes.

Data regarding human exposure to 1,3-dichloropropene are limited. A study of commercial fumigant applicators in the potato fields of the Netherlands revealed no nephrotoxicity or hepatotoxicity after 117 days of exposure to an 8-hour time-weighted average (TWA) of 2 ppm.[1] The current TWA standard of the Occupational Safety and Health Administration (OSHA) is 1 ppm for dermal exposure.[2]

Animal studies have demonstrated that DCP is metabolized in the liver by the glutathione transferase enzyme. A study of DCP in rats showed that the main excreted product in the urine is *N*-acetyl-S-(cis-3-chloro-2-propenyl)-L-cysteine, a mercapturic acid metabolite.[3] Human studies involving biologic monitoring of commercial applicators have used this same mercapturic acid metabolite as a marker of exposure to DCP.[4]

Symptoms of acute exposure are primarily the result of mucosal irritation and include eye burning, tearing, coughing, difficulty breathing, and skin rashes.[5] There are also reports of contact dermatitis arising from chronic use of this product.[6] Treatment is primarily supportive after decontamination measures appropriate for the route of exposure have been completed. Pulmonary edema, acute renal and hepatic failure, and adult respiratory distress syndrome have been described after ingestion of this product. Activated charcoal may be beneficial after oral ingestion. Copious irrigation using normal saline solution or water is recommended for ocular and dermal exposures.[7,8]

DCP has been listed as a possible human carcinogen by the U.S. Environmental Protection Agency (EPA). Multiple animal studies showed an increase in tumors of the stomach, liver, lung and bladder.[9]

PHOSPHINE (CAS 7803-51-2) (PH₃)

Phosphine gas is produced when pellets of aluminum, calcium, magnesium, or zinc phosphide are exposed to water vapor. Aluminum phosphide is used primarily to treat grain and tobacco stores. Its formulation as pellets lends itself for use in treating transport containers. Phosphine gas is described as having a garlic or rotten fish odor. The OSHA threshold limit value (TLV) for phosphine gas is 0.3 ppm. The odor is detectable at a concentration of 2 ppm. However, this odor threshold does not give adequate warnings regarding possible dangerous gas concentrations. For this reason, manu-facturers of aluminum phosphide include ammonia-producing agents in the pellets as the more noxious ammonia odor may allow for better detection of possible phosphine gas release. This gas is highly explosive, and additives are placed within the pellets to slow the rate of gas formation to reduce the risk for explosion.

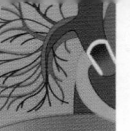

Multiple mechanisms of action have been proposed for phosphine gas. Animal studies demonstrated inhibition of the mitochondrial cytochrome oxidase system as well as interference with amino acid incorporation into proteins. Small vessels appear to be affected to a greater degree than the major vessels, which may explain the extensive third spacing and profound cardiovascular collapse that may occur with phosphine poisoning.[10] Numerous cases have been reported of human exposures both as accidental exposures in a commercial fumigation setting and as reports of these agents being used in suicidal gestures. One in vitro study showed that phosphine induces the formation of excess superoxide radicals in red blood cells. This resulted in the production of denatured hemoglobin aggregates (Heinz bodies) in the erythrocyte in the course of a hemolytic anemia.[11] Another case report of a 25-year-old man who ingested 6 g of aluminum phosphide pellets describes the development of methemoglobinemia (32%) occurring 32 hours after ingestion.[12]

Numerous deaths have been reported when stowaways attempt to use grain cars on trains and ships as transportation, not realizing that these containers have been treated with one of the phosphide chemicals to prevent pest and fungi destruction of the grain during transport. One report described three adults who became ill and a 12-year-old boy who died after spending 18 hours in a railroad boxcar containing lima beans that had been fumigated with aluminum phosphide. At time of discovery, the child was dead, and the adults were complaining of nausea, vomiting, abdominal pain, headache, and dizziness. Another report describes the discovery of a 23-year-old man who was found dead after he had broken the plastic seal in a rice-filled boxcar in order to gain entry. Postmortem toxicologic analysis of this individual showed phosphine levels in all tissue samples taken.[13]

Clinical findings in acute phosphine poisoning may include depressed mental status, pulmonary edema, hypotension, cardiac dysrhythmias, liver and kidney failure, and severe gastritis.[14] Inhalation of low levels of phosphine gas may produce symptoms of headache, dizziness, tremors, cough, chest pain, shortness of breath, nausea, vomiting, and abdominal pain. Seizures have been reported.

OSHA exposure limits for phosphine gas are 3 ppm for an 8-hour TWA; exposure to 500 ppm for 30 minutes is expected to be fatal, whereas only "a few breaths" of phosphine at a concentration of 1000 ppm can be lethal.[15] Treatment for phosphine toxicity includes removing the victim from the source of exposure and supportive care. Patients must be closely observed for the development of hypoxia due to pulmonary edema or methemoglobinemia. Patients who develop hemolytic anemia may require the administration of blood products. The electrocardiogram may show nonspecific ST-T changes, but no one pattern is pathognomonic for phosphine toxicity. One study done on rats showed some improvement in cardiovascular status and overall survival after administration of N-acetylcysteine.[16]

Tachycardia, both supraventricular and atrial fibrillation, has been reported, as well as ST changes and various conduction delays and blocks. Reports of patients who manifested electrocardiographic changes due to their phosphine exposure show that these changes resolve within 25 days if the patient survives the first 24 hours after exposure.[17] There are also reports of hypokalemia after acute exposure; serum magnesium levels may also be elevated or decreased. Although blood phosphine levels have been studied, they are not routinely used to manage patients. One author examined blood phosphine levels in 40 cases of oral ingestion and found that blood phosphine levels correlated with severity of clinical symptoms. This study demonstrated that patients with a blood phosphine concentration of 1.067 mg/dL or less survived the ingestion.[18] Anger and colleagues were able to detect elevated levels of both aluminum and phosphorous in blood and tissue samples of a 39-year-old man who committed suicide by ingestion of aluminum phosphide.[19] The authors were unable to detect any phosphine in the blood or urine samples; however, the phosphine was present in tissue samples from the brain, liver, and kidney.

Decontamination for oral ingestion may include the use of activated charcoal. Patients who vomit may risk exposing hospital staff to phosphine by means of off-gassing from the vomitus. Emesis should be suctioned and placed in sealed containers as soon as possible. Overdose victims also run a significant risk for chemical pneumonitis if they aspirate.[7,8]

Phosphine gas is not listed as a possible carcinogen with the International Agency for Research on Cancer. However, there are studies suggesting that fumigators who have chronic exposure to phosphine may have an increased risk for non-Hodgkin's lymphoma. One investigation found consistent chromosomal abnormalities in the pesticides applicator group as compared with the nonexposed control group.[20]

METHYL BROMIDE (CAS 74-83-9)

Methyl bromide is a colorless and odorless liquid that quickly volatilizes. The gaseous form is heavier than air. It is used for pest control in agriculture and home fumigation. A lacrimating agent, chlorpicrin, is usually added to provide some warning of exposure. Methyl bromide has a TLV of 5 ppm, and the concentration which is immediately dangerous to life and health (IDLH) is 2000 ppm. Aside from use as a fumigant, this chemical has also been used in the past in fire extinguishers. The primary route of exposure is by inhalation, although dermal absorption may also result in significant morbidity.

Methyl bromide is a severe vesicant. Dermal exposure to the gas can result in severe blistering of the skin. It can irritate the mucosa of the oropharynx; coughing may be sufficiently intense to produce post-tussive emesis. The central nervous system is the most profoundly affected in cases of methyl bromide poisoning. Early neurologic symptoms of an acute exposure may vary from tremors, headache, ataxia, blurred or double vision, and vertigo

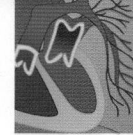

to grand mal seizure, status epilepticus, and coma. The onset of symptoms after an acute exposure may be delayed up to 24 hours. Both acute and chronic exposures may result in psychosis, hallucinations, or delirium.[21] Chronic exposures of methyl bromide are associated with extremity paresthesia, hearing or vision loss, balance disturbances, and syncopal episodes. One study found symmetric midbrain and cerebellar lesions on magnetic resonance imaging of a 30-year-old man who worked in a warehouse that was regularly fumigated with methyl bromide. His presenting complaints were foot paresthesia and a gait disturbance.[22]

Exposures to methyl bromide occur under a variety of circumstances. Some cases are the result of fumigators who did not follow proper procedures or had faulty protective equipment. Other reports involve use of the chemical in an area that had previously unknown venting sources. Underground sewer pipes and other similar conduits have been implicated in several deaths. In Norway, a newborn infant was killed when the methyl bromide that was used to fumigate a house in another part of the housing subdivision leaked into the victim's home through the sewer pipes.[23] In the United States, there is a case report of a 36-year-old woman who died from methyl bromide exposure. This woman lived in a guesthouse that was connected to the main house by eight hidden conduit pipes of which the property owner was unaware. Aside from these abandoned pipes, the guesthouse was not structurally connected to the main house. The property owner had the main house fumigated with methyl bromide, and that evening, the woman told friends she felt ill. The next morning, she was found in status epilepticus, which persisted despite multiple anticonvulsants and being placed on a pentobarbital infusion. She remained in a persistent vegetative state until she died 19 days after fumigation. At autopsy, the heart showed areas of edema and hemorrhage, the lungs had severe edema with infiltrates of neutrophils and macrophages, the liver had areas of centrilobular necrosis, and the brain had bilateral hippocampal necrosis which was thought to be consistent with status epilepticus and anoxia. All tested tissue samples, blood, bile, liver, and adipose tissue had detectable levels of methyl bromide.[24]

Several mechanisms have been postulated for the severity of the neurotoxic effects of methyl bromide. Its overall toxicity is believed to be the result of alkylation of sulfhydryl groups of numerous enzymes involved in routine physiologic functioning. Methyl bromide is metabolized into methyl glutathione by the enzyme glutathione transferase. The methyl glutathione is then converted into the neurotoxic metabolites of methanethiol and formaldehyde. Animal studies have shown that those species with decreased glutathione stores manifest lesser neurotoxic effects when exposed to methyl bromide.[25] This may be one of the few instances when treatment with N-acetylcysteine may be detrimental.

Treatment of methyl bromide exposure consists of thorough decontamination and supportive care. Seizures should be treated aggressively with anticonvulsants, benzodiazepines, and barbiturates if needed. Although it is possible to obtain blood and urine methyl bromide levels, these assays are not routinely used and have little bearing on the management of the patient. Serum bromide levels may be used as a marker for exposure. Methyl bromide is not listed as a possible carcinogen.

Under the Clean Air Act passed in 1993, methyl bromide was declared to be an ozone-depleting agent. Therefore, manufacture and importation of this substance was set to be phased out by 2001. However, in 2003, the EPA announced the phase-out would not be completed until 2005. Methyl bromide may still be used under a critical use exemption as alternative fumigants are still being investigated. Unfortunately, methyl bromide has been an effective agricultural fumigant for more than 30 years, and some of its uses have no good alternative treatments at this time. It is expected that total cessation of methyl bromide use will be met with some resistance, and the phase-out is expected to take longer than expected.[26]

SULFURYL FLUORIDE (CAS 2699-79-8)

Sulfuryl fluoride gas is colorless, odorless, and heavier than air. It has a threshold limit value of 5 ppm for an 8-hour TWA, a 15-minute short-term exposure limit (STEL) of 10 ppm, and an IDLH value of 1000 ppm.[27] Aside from agricultural uses, it is also used to eradicate termites. The mechanism of action of sulfuryl fluoride was shown in a termite study that revealed excretion of inorganic sulfate when these insects were exposed to a nonlethal dose.[28] This is consistent with signs and symptoms of fluoride toxicity seen in sulfuryl fluoride exposure across many different species. Fluoride is rapidly absorbed in the body and quickly binds any available calcium ion, resulting in profound hypocalcemia, which can precipitate cardiac dysrhythmias.

Exposure to this substance can cause severe bronchospasm, which is why it is shipped as a compressed gas. Symptoms of exposure begin with mucosal irritation, nausea, vomiting, and abdominal pain. Clinical symptoms then shift to its central nervous system effects, which may then predominate with paresthesias, refractory seizures, and coma. Finally, effects of the fluoride toxicity itself may result in profound shock, life-threatening cardiac dysrhythmias, and pulmonary edema. Sulfuryl fluoride exposure in some animal studies has resulted in symptoms consistent with parasympathetic toxidromes, including salivation, lacrimation, vomiting, and diarrhea.[29]

This gas leaves behind a large amount of residue of sulfuryl fluoride on the foods it was used to fumigate. When heated, this residue may give off dangerous gases, such as hydrofluoric acid.[30]

Treatment of ingestion of this substance includes gastric lavage with a 0.15% calcium hydroxide solution or with any available calcium salt to bind the fluoride ion before it is absorbed. In cases of inhalational toxicity or after absorption for ingestion, the mainstay of treatment is to be aggressive with calcium replacement to prevent the life-threatening cardiac dysrhythmias that may result

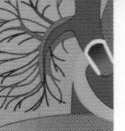
if a hypocalcemic state is untreated. Calcium may be replaced with a calcium gluconate solution through a peripheral intravenous line, whereas calcium chloride may only be administered through a central venous catheter because of the irritation it may cause when delivered into a small blood vessel. Because the fluoride ion is excreted primarily in the urine, fluid resuscitation should be delivered to maintain a steady urine output.[7,8]

METHYL ISOTHIOCYANATE (CAS 556-61-6)

Methyl isothiocyanate (MITC) has a solid crystalline structure at room temperature, which sublimes directly to a gaseous state. It has a sharp horseradish odor and is a severe skin irritant.

Although it has been restricted from use as a pesticide or a fumigant since 1992, this agent is still encountered in a variety of sources. It is only available as MITC as a wood preservative at this time. This compound should not be confused with methyl isocyanate (MIC), which was involved in the Union Carbide disaster in Bhopal, India. MITC is a breakdown product of two pesticides that are still in use: metam sodium, and dazomet.[31] This substance has been described as a breakdown product of many of the carbamate pesticides.[32] MITC was noted in 30 name-brand cigarettes after the company discovered strange odors appearing to originate from the filters. This finding launched a recall of more than 8 billion cigarettes in the U.S. market starting in 1995. The Centers for Disease Control and Prevention could not definitively link this finding as a causative agent in complaints regarding respiratory symptoms made by 72 consumers.[33,34] Also, Italian wine producers were discovered placing MITC in their products to prevent secondary fermentation during shipping.[35]

MITC is metabolized through glutathione pathways, and animal studies in rats and mice show the major excretion product is a mercapturic acid derivative found in the urine.[36] Clinical signs of exposure are skin and mucosal irritation from the vesicant effects. MITC can also produce severe bronchospasm. Exposure to metam sodium results in similar symptoms of mucosal and dermal irritation. There are reports of blistering, papular eruptions, and skin discoloration, which responded to topical corticosteroids.[37] There are no minimal exposure limits for MITC, and it is unknown whether this compound is carcinogenic. The treatment of exposure to MITC is primarily supportive.[7,8]

MITC was first registered in 1987 as a preventative treatment for wood-destroying fungi. It is currently under restricted use for this purpose. This substance may only be handled by those who have been certified in its use. MITC had been used as a soil fumigant until 1992, when the producer voluntarily withdrew this application from its registration. This withdrawal allowed 1 year for the remaining stocks to be destroyed and for retailers to use up the stock they already had on hand.[31]

REFERENCES

1. Verplanke AJW, Bloeman LJ, VanSittert NJ, et al: Occupational exposure to cis-1,3-dichloropropene: biological effect monitoring of kidney and liver function. Occup Environ Med 2000;57:745–751.
2. Lewis RJ Sr: Hazardous Chemicals Desk Reference, 5th ed. New York, John Wiley & Sons, 2002, p 401.
3. Climie IJG, Hutson DH, Morrison BJ, et al: Glutathione conjugation in the detoxification of (Z)-1,3-dichloropropene (a component of the nematocide D-D) in the rat. Xenobiotica 1979;9:149–156.
4. Brouwer EJ, Verplanke AJW, Boogaard PJ, et al. Personal air sampling and biological monitoring of occupational exposure to the soil fumigant cis-1,3-dichloropropene. Occup Environ Med 2000;57:738–744.
5. Cox C: 1,3,-Dichloropropene. J Pesticide Reform 1992;12(1):33–37.
6. Corazza M, Zinna G, Virgili A: Allergic contact dermatitis due to 1,3-dichloropropene soil fumigant. Contact Dermatitis 2003;48:341–342.
7. Rumack BH: POISINDEX® Information System. CCIS Vol. 118, edition expires November 2003. Englewood, Colo, Micromedex, 2003.
8. Hall AH, Rumack BH (eds): TOMES® Information System. CCIS Volume 118, edition expires November 2003. Englewood, Colo, Micromedex, 2003.
9. U.S. Environmental Protection Agency's Integrated Risk Information System (IRIS) on 1,3-dichloropropene(542-75-6). Available at: http://www.epa.gov/ngispgm3/iris on the Substance File List as of May 25, 2000.
10. Schelble DT: Phosgene and phosphine. In Haddad LM, Shannon MW, Winchester J (eds): Clinical Management of Poisoning and Drug Overdose, 3rd ed. Philadelphia, WB Saunders, 1998, pp 960–963.
11. Potter WT: Phosphine-mediated Heinz body formation and hemoglobin oxidation in human erythrocytes. Toxicol Lett 1991;57(1):37–45.
12. Lakshmi B: Methemoglobinemia with aluminum phosphide poisoning. Am J Emerg Med 2002;20(2):130–132.
13. Perrotta D, Willis T, Salzman D, et al: Deaths associated with exposure to fumigants in railroad cars—United States. MMWR Morb Mortal Wkly Rep 1994;43(27):489–491.
14. Misra UK, Tripathi AK, Pandy R, Bhargwa B: Acute phosphine poisoning following ingestion of aluminum phosphide. Hum Toxicol 1988;7(4):343–345.
15. Spencer EY: Guide to the Chemicals Used in Crop Protection, 7th ed. Publication No. 1093. Research Institute, Agriculture Canada. Ottawa, Information Canada, 1982, p 458.
16. Azad A: Effect of N-acetylcysteine and L-NAME on aluminum phosphide induced cardiovascular toxicity in rats. Acta Pharmacol Sin 2001;22(4):298–304.
17. Chugh SN, Chugh K, Ram S, et al. Electrocardiographic abnormalities in aluminum phosphide poisoning with special reference to its incidence, pathogenesis, mortality and histopathology. J Indian Med Assoc 1991;89:32–35.
18. Chugh SN: Serial blood phosphine levels in acute aluminum phosphide poisoning. J Assoc Physicians India 1996;44(3):184–185.
19. Anger F, Brousse F, Le Normand I, et al. Fatal aluminum phosphide poisoning. J Anal Toxicol 2000;24(2):90–92.
20. Garry VF: Chromosome rearrangements in fumigant appliers: possible relationship to non-Hodgkin's lymphoma risk. Cancer Epidemiol Biomarkers Prev 1992;1(4):287–291.
21. Sullivan JB, Kreiger GR: Clinical Environmental Health and Toxic Exposures, 2nd ed. Philadelphia, Lippincott, Williams & Wilkins, 2001, pp 1088–1090.
22. Ichikawa H: A case of chronic methyl bromide intoxication showing symmetrical lesions in the basal ganglia and brain stem on magnetic resonance imaging. Rinsho Shinkeigaku 2001;47(7):423–427.
23. Langard S, Rognum T, Flotterod O, et al. Fatal accident resulting from methyl bromide poisoning after fumigation of a neighboring

house; leakage through sewer pipes. J Appl Toxicol 1996;16: 445–448.

24. Horowitz BA, Albertson TE, O'Malley M, et al. An usual exposure to methyl bromide leading to fatality. J Tox Clin Toxicol 1998;36(4):353–355.

25. Lifshitz M, Gavrilov V: Central nervous system toxicity and early peripheral neuropathy following dermal exposure to methyl bromide. Clin Toxicol 2000;38(7):799–801.

26. U.S. Environmental Protection Agency. 2003 U.S. nomination for the methyl bromide critical use exemption executive summary. Available at: http://www.epa.gov/ozone/.

27. National Institute of Occupational Safety and Health: Pocket Guide to Chemical Hazards. DHHS (NIOSH) Publication No. 2002-140. Washington, DC, U.S. Government Printing Office, 2002.

28. Hayes WJ Jr, Laws ER Jr (eds): Handbook of Pesticide Toxicology, Vol. 2. Classes of Pesticides. New York, Academic Press, 1991, p 564.

29. Scheuerman E: Suicide by exposure to sulfuryl fluoride. J Forensic Sci 1986;31(3):1154–1158.

30. Sullivan JB, Kreiger GR: Clinical Environmental Health and Toxic Exposures, 2nd ed. Philadelphia, Lippincott, Williams & Wilkins, 2001, p 1089.

31. U.S. Environmental Protection Agency: Pesticides: topical and chemical fact sheets. Available at: http:www.epa.gov.

32. Kassie F, Laky B, Nobis E, et al. Genotoxic effects of methyl isothiocyanate. Mutat Res 2001;490:1–9.

33. Anonymous: Philip Morris cigarettes recall, May 1995–March 1996. JAMA 1996;275(16):1225.

34. Anonymous: Recall of Phillip Morris cigarettes, March 1996. MMWR Morb Mortal Wkly Rep 1996;45:251–254.

35. Roston C: Methyl isocyanate in wine. Fd Chem Toxicol 1992;30:821–828.

36. Lam W, Kim J, Sparks S, et al: Metabolism in rats and mice of the soil fumigants metham, methyl isothiocyanate and dazomet. J Agric Food Chem 1993;41(9):1497–1502.

37. Burgess JL, Morrissey B, Keifer MC, et al. Fumigant related illnesses: Washington State's five year experience. Clin Toxicol 2000;38(1):7–14.

81 *Organochlorine Insecticides*

JAMES W. RHEE, MD ■ STEVEN E. AKS, DO

At a Glance...

- Most organochlorine insecticides are widely restricted or banned.
- The major effect of acute toxicity is central nervous system excitation.
- Chronic exposure may result in persistent neurologic disability.
- Treatment of acute toxicity centers on supportive care and control of seizure activity.

INTRODUCTION AND RELEVANT HISTORY

Organochlorine insecticides (sometimes referred to as *chlorinated hydrocarbon insecticides*) were introduced in the 1940s with Paul Müller's effective demonstration of dichlorodiphenyltrichloroethane (DDT).[1] Before this time, available insecticides were limited to arsenicals, petroleum oils, nicotine, pyrethrum, rotenone, sulfur, hydrogen cyanide gas, and cryolite.[2] The organochlorine insecticides proved to be nonvolatile, inexpensive to manufacture, environmentally stable, and relatively less toxic than previous insecticides. These properties led to the widespread use of this class of insecticides.

Utilization of DDT has had a tremendous impact on human health. DDT was used in worldwide mosquito abatement programs and is credited for saving millions of lives from malaria and typhus. This success led to the development of other organochlorine insecticides.

However, although these organochlorine compounds were very effective as insecticides, there were subsequent ecological repercussions that developed from their use. In 1962, Rachel Carson, in her book *Silent Spring*, described the reduction of the eagle and osprey population as result of DDT's persistence in the environment and its ability to bioconcentrate within certain animals.[3] These properties eventually led to a ban on DDT in the United States, and subsequent bans on other organochlorine insecticides that demonstrated these properties of environmental persistence and bioconcentration. The 2001 Stockholm Convention on Persistent Organic Pollutants (POPs) targeted a number of pollutants, including many organochlorine pesticides, and recommended a worldwide ban on these compounds. This agreement became legally binding on May 17, 2004.[4]

EPIDEMIOLOGY

Because organochlorine insecticides are strictly restricted or banned in North America and Europe, exposures to them are rare in these regions. In 2003, of about 2.4 million exposures reported to U.S. poison centers, only 1435 exposures involved chlorinated hydrocarbon insecticides. There were only 13 major outcomes, and no reported deaths.[5] However, because organochlorine insecticides are very effective and cheap, they are still widely used in developing countries, despite the Stockholm Convention agreement. In 2002, evidence of continued poisoning episodes with organochlorine insecticides in developing countries occurred in India where, due to food contamination, 36 people were poisoned by endosulfan, resulting in the deaths of three children.[6]

Although chlorinated hydrocarbons are no longer in agricultural use in the United States, the organochlorine γ-hexachlorocyclohexane, better known as *lindane*, is still used for medicinal purposes, as a scabicide. As a result, in the United States, lindane is probably the most common source of toxicity from a chlorinated hydrocarbon insecticide. As safer agents for scabies treatment have been developed, lindane has become a second-line agent. The U.S. Food and Drug Administration (FDA), in 2003, issued a public health advisory regarding the risk for potential toxicity from treatment with lindane by misuse or therapeutic use. The FDA also required a boxed warning, product size limitation, and distribution of a medication guide with each prescription. In 2001, California banned the use and sale of lindane in the state. Texas poison control centers found that accounts of lindane exposure declined from 132 to 75 between 1998 and 2002 as newer, safer therapies became available and regulations on lindane increased.[7]

STRUCTURE AND STRUCTURE–ACTIVITY RELATIONSHIPS

Organochlorine insecticides represent a diverse group of compounds that contain carbon, hydrogen, and chlorine. However, unlike the volatile chlorinated hydrocarbons found in solvents, organochlorine insecticides have higher molecular weights and are consequently less volatile.

Organochlorine insecticides belong to four distinct structural classes: diphenyl aliphatics (e.g., DDT and related compounds), cyclodienes (e.g., aldrin, dieldrin, endrin, endosulfan, heptachlor), cyclohexanes (e.g., γ-hexachlorocyclohexane, known more commonly as lindane), and polychloroterpenes (e.g., toxaphene). The organochlorine pesticides chlordecone and mirex are also called *cage compounds*; they do not fall into a distinct category, although they are sometimes classified with the cyclodienes.

The activity and toxicity of these insecticides do not necessarily correlate with structure. In fact, some structurally similar compounds can have vastly different

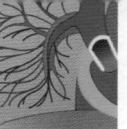
activities and toxicities. For instance, the γ-isomer of hexachlorocyclohexane has insecticidal properties and will cause central nervous system excitation, whereas other isomers have no insecticidal properties and will cause central nervous system depression.[8]

PHARMACOLOGY

Pathophysiology

In general, the primary means by which organochlorine insecticides kill insects is through their neurotoxicity. As such, when toxic to humans, the predominant system affected is the nervous system. The mechanism of toxicity, however, varies among the different organochlorine insecticides.

Simplistically, DDT acts on the central nervous system by interfering with the movement of ions through neuronal membranes. There appear to be multiple mechanisms by which DDT affects this ion movement. DDT delays the closing of the sodium ion channel and prevents the full opening of potassium channels.[9] It also appears to affect a specific neuronal adenosine triphosphatase (ATPase) involved in sodium, potassium, and calcium movement through the nerve membrane.[10] DDT may inhibit the neuron's ability to transport calcium ions by binding to calmodulin and affecting a Ca/Mg ATPase; however, this theory has not been confirmed.[11]

The combined effect of these actions would lead to sustained depolarization of the neuronal membrane, resulting in continued release of neurotransmitters and central nervous system excitation.

There is also some evidence to suggest that DDT may also have the effect of increasing serotonin and norepinephrine breakdown as well as increasing levels of aspartate and glutamate in the central nervous system.[12-14] Because serotonin and norepinephrine modulate (and sometimes inhibit) central nervous system activity, and aspartate and glutamate act as excitatory transmitters, the subsequent imbalance that results may lead to central nervous system excitation.

Lindane and the cyclodienes, although structurally different, seem to have a similar mechanism of neurotoxicity, further demonstrated by the development of cross-tolerance between these two classes of organochlorines in insects.[15] Both lindane and cyclodienes inhibit γ-aminobutyric acid (GABA) activity by interacting with the picrotoxin binding site of the GABA$_A$ receptor–ionophore complex and subsequently blocking the influx of chloride through the complex.[16-28] As a result of this action, a major inhibitory neurotransmitter is antagonized. Toxaphene seems to antagonize GABA at the GABA$_A$ receptor–ionophore complex as well.[29]

Although chlordecone antagonizes the GABA receptor at the picrotoxin binding site in cockroaches,[30] it does not appear to do the same in humans. The mechanism of chlordecone neurotoxicity in humans is poorly understood.

Organochlorines cause sensitization of the myocardium to endogenous catecholamines and predispose test animals to dysrhythmias, presumably in a fashion similar to the chlorinated hydrocarbon solvents.

Pharmacokinetics

In varying degrees, the absorption of organochlorine insecticides occurs after ingestion, inhalation, or dermal absorption. The efficiency of dermal absorption is variable. Lindane and most of the cyclodienes are well absorbed across the skin, whereas DDT and its analogs, along with toxaphene and mirex, have low dermal absorption.

Most of the solid organochlorines are not highly volatile; however, inhalational exposure can still occur with pesticide-laden aerosol or dust particles. They can then become trapped in respiratory mucus and subsequently swallowed, leading to significant gastrointestinal absorption.

Once absorbed, some organochlorines are stored in adipose tissue as the unchanged parent compound; however, the degree to which this occurs is variable. Those compounds that undergo slow metabolism tend to be stored in body fat to a greater extent than those compounds that undergo rapid metabolism. As a result, the organochlorines that are metabolized slowly are likely detected in breast milk because of their lipophilic nature.

Most organochlorines are metabolized to some degree, being dechlorinated, oxidized, and then conjugated. The primary mode of elimination is through biliary excretion, although nearly all organochlorines yield measurable urinary metabolites. Because many of the unmetabolized pesticides are excreted into the bile, these organochlorines often undergo enterohepatic and enteroenteric circulation, substantially retarding fecal excretion.[31] The kinetics of elimination after lindane ingestion appear to have two phases: a rapid distributive phase and a slower elimination phase. The second phase parallels the elimination seen with dermal exposure. These pharmacokinetics may be due to ingestion that results in more rapid absorption and is followed by a distributive phase that is not seen with dermal administration.[32]

Special Populations

Children are particularly susceptible to toxicity from organochlorines, as highlighted by an episode of mass endosulfan poisoning that recently occurred in India. Although 36 victims of all ages became ill from the exposure, the illness first became manifest in children. Children were also more severely ill and accounted for the only fatalities; only children had electroencephalogram abnormalities, although their serum endosulfan concentrations were comparable to adults.[6] Children may also be more susceptible to developing toxicity from topical application of lindane, presumably because of their less keratinized, more permeable skin.

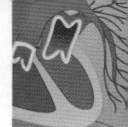

Elderly people may also be predisposed to toxicity from topical application of lindane, as highlighted by seizures that developed in 3 of 19 geriatric patients who were being treated with topical 1% lindane. These victims may have been given greater than the normal dose and received their applications following hot baths. Atrophic skin and age-related sensitivity may have had a role as well.[33]

Pharmacologic Agents

The only pharmacologic agent among the organochlorine insecticides that has been approved by the FDA for medicinal use is lindane.

Drug Interactions

Organochlorines have been shown to induce hepatic microsomal drug-metabolizing enzymes.[34] Although this liver enzyme induction will accelerate the metabolism of the insecticide itself, other theoretical consequences include the enhanced metabolism of certain drugs. However, there are a few anecdotal case reports describing this and no definitive reports of enhanced metabolism of therapeutic drugs or adverse reactions because of microsomal enzyme induction in humans.

TOXICOLOGY

Clinical Manifestations

Most victims of acute ingestion of organochlorines develop nausea, vomiting, and abdominal pain. There may be evidence of dermal irritation if the exposure is cutaneous.

The major acute effects of organochlorine pesticides are primarily related to central nervous system stimulation. These effects manifest primarily as convulsions; motor overactivity may be limited to myoclonic jerking but is often expressed as seizures, which is sometimes the only clinical manifestation of organochlorine toxicity. Other less severe signs of neurologic toxicity include paresthesias, tremor, ataxia, and hyperreflexia. Seizures are more characteristic of acute toxicity to lindane and the cyclodienes. DDT and its analogs, as well as chlordecone, tend to cause neurosensory and mild motor abnormalities.

The clinical effects of chronic exposure to chlordecone have been well described after the "Hopewell epidemic" that came to light during the summer of 1975.[35-38] Because of poor industrial hygiene, more than 100 employees at a chlordecone manufacturing plant were chronically exposed to chlordecone during its synthesis. Patients with prolonged exposure developed toxic effects that included tremors, weight loss, arthralgias, skin rashes, chest pains, mental changes, opsoclonus, muscle weakness, ataxic gait, incoordination, and slurred speech. Patients characteristically had an intention tremor and, in severe cases, a resting tremor.[38] Although

the hands were chiefly involved, fine tremors of the head and trembling of the entire body were also noted. This condition was termed "Kepone shakes" by the workers. An exaggerated startle response was also observed in some severely affected patients. Other prominent features included visual difficulties with an inability to fixate and focus, and bursts of erratic movements of the eye. Personality changes were also observed, with irritability, poor short-term memory, and mild depression being the most common. In a few cases, frank disorientation was also observed.[35] Nerve biopsies have demonstrated that chlordecone causes degenerative nerve changes predominantly affecting the unmyelinated and smaller myelinated fibers.[37]

There has been an increased interest in the potential hazards posed by certain substances that may affect the endocrine system because of the ability of these chemicals to mimic or block endogenous hormones; such agents are known as *environmental endocrine disrupters*. In vitro assays have demonstrated that a number of organochlorine insecticides have estrogen-like activity.[39,40] As a result of this characteristic of organochlorines, they have been examined very closely for potential associations with certain developmental and reproductive disorders as well as cancers of reproductive organs—breast, testicular, and prostate.

Although some case-control studies have implicated organochlorines as having a possible etiologic role in the development of breast cancer,[41-43] more recent studies have found no increased risk due to organochlorine exposure.[44,45] The International Agency for Research on Cancer (IARC) reviewed DDT and its metabolite DDE as a potential carcinogen, and although evidence for carcinogenesis was found in a murine model, there is no convincing evidence that these compounds are carcinogenic in humans.

Adverse Effects

Organochlorine insecticides have been associated with a number of other adverse effects. A small number of case reports have associated lindane and chlordane with certain hematologic disorders, including aplastic anemia and megaloblastic anemia.[46-49] Disseminated intravascular coagulation has also been reported in association with chlordane ingestion.[50] Rhabdomyolysis and profound lactic acidosis have been described with lindane ingestion.[51] Although not definitive, there may also be an association between organochlorine insecticides and the development of chronic motor neuron diseases, such as amyotrophic lateral sclerosis.[52]

DIAGNOSIS

Laboratory Testing

Gas chromatography analysis of biologic specimens can be used to identify organochlorine levels.[53] However, such testing is usually not necessary for the management

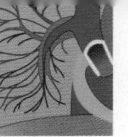

of acute toxicity. Because many of the organochlorines are stored in lipids, adipose tissue biopsies and human breast milk have been used to measure organochlorine residues. The value of measuring organochlorine concentrations in these tissues is primarily to confirm past exposure.

Other Diagnostic Testing

There are no other specific biomarkers that confirm organochlorine exposure. Certain laboratory testing may be helpful to help rule out other causes of a patient's clinical manifestations, or to evaluate for possible sequelae of toxicity from organochlorines. This evaluation may include determination of complete blood count, renal function, serum electrolytes, creatine phosphokinase, urine myoglobin, lactic acid, computed tomography of the brain, electroencephalograms, and coagulation studies.

Differential Diagnosis

The diagnosis of organochlorine toxicity should be made primarily by history because there are no pathognomonic features. The common presenting symptoms after acute exposures include nausea, vomiting, abdominal pain, agitation, irritability, dizziness, drowsiness, lethargy, and seizures. However, these are fairly nonspecific. Other potential toxic agents that can produce similar neurologic symptoms include any toxin that produces central nervous system excitation, such as strychnine.

Other medical causes are numerous and include underlying seizure disorder, meningitis, encephalitis, trauma, electrolyte derangements, cancer, and hypoglycemia.

MANAGEMENT

Supportive Measures

Initial supportive measures include airway protection, ventilatory support, and maintenance of adequate circulation. Meticulous attention to these supportive measures is likely the only intervention needed for treatment of the acute manifestations of organochlorine toxicity because these symptoms are usually self-limited.

If needed, seizure control can be achieved by the administration of GABA agonists such as benzodiazepines and barbiturates. The use of benzodiazepines or barbiturates is rational, given that the underlying mechanism of neurotoxicity of many of the organochlorines revolves around the antagonism of GABA.

Phenytoin, in general, is not a first-line agent for toxicant-induced seizures. In fact, for lindane-induced seizures, phenytoin may worsen seizures. However, phenytoin has been shown in experimental models to decrease DDT-induced tremor.[13,54] This makes mechanistic sense because DDT will keep a sodium channel open, leading to sustained or repetitive nerve firing, and phenytoin acts as a sodium channel blocker. In the same model, phenytoin administered to rats

exacerbated the neurologic symptoms in those who were dosed with chlordecone or lindane.[54]

Decontamination

For dermal exposures, contaminated clothing should be removed and the skin decontaminated with copious amounts of soap and water.

Gastric lavage may be considered after ingestion if the patient presents in a timely manner. As organochlorine insecticides are often found in a liquid form, nasogastric aspiration of stomach contents may be less traumatic to the patient. However, all precautions should be taken to avoid aspiration because a chemical pneumonitis may develop, particularly because the insecticides are often formulated in a hydrocarbon vehicle.

Activated charcoal can be administered after an acute ingestion in an effort to decrease absorption. However, there is some evidence that suggests activated charcoal does not adsorb to organochlorine insecticides well.[55,56]

Cholestyramine has been found in a murine model to adsorb lindane, decreasing absorption better than activated charcoal.[56]

Laboratory Monitoring

There are no standard laboratory tests to monitor. However, measurement of creatine phosphokinase, blood cell counts, renal function, liver function, and coagulation studies should identify evidence of the serious sequelae that have been associated with organochlorine toxicity.

Antidotes

No specific therapies have been reported effective in blocking the toxicities of organochlorine insecticides. Treatment centers primarily on supportive care and prevention of future exposures.

Elimination

Because organochlorine insecticides are highly lipophilic and undergo extensive tissue distribution, methods to enhance elimination through extracorporeal techniques, such as hemodialysis, hemoperfusion, exchange transfusion, and peritoneal dialysis, are unlikely to be efficacious.

However, for certain organochlorines that undergo enterohepatic and enteroenteric recirculation, prolonged administration of cholestyramine may be helpful in enhancing the fecal elimination and subsequent decrease in body burden. This was demonstrated during the Hopewell epidemic, when cholestyramine (16 g/day) was administered to adult patients who were heavily exposed to chlordecone. In this setting, cholestyramine was associated with a sevenfold increase in the fecal excretion of chlordecone, a significant decrease in the half-life of the compound in the body, subsequent improvement of neurologic symptoms, and increased motile sperm.[36] Cholestyramine has also been found to be effective in adsorbing to lindane in the murine model and may potentially have a role in the enhanced elimination of this compound, but this has not been well investigated.[56]

Disposition

Patients who are exposed to an organochlorine insecticide, either through ingestion or inhalation, should develop symptoms immediately because these compounds are absorbed very quickly. After an observation period of several hours, asymptomatic patients can be discharged home safely.

REFERENCES

1. Nobelstiftelsen: Physiology or medicine. In Nobel Lectures, Including Presentation Speeches and Laureates' Biographies. Amsterdam, New York, Elsevier, 1964, pp 227–237.
2. Ware GW, Whitcare DM: An introduction to pesticides. Retrieved October 31, 2004, from http://ipmworld.umn.edu/chapters/ware.htm.
3. Carson R: Silent Spring. Boston, Houghton Mifflin, 1962.
4. Stockholm Convention on Persistent Organic Pollutants (POPs). Retrieved October 31, 2004, from http://www.pops.int.
5. Watson WA, Litovitz TA, Klein-Schwartz W, et al: 2003 Annual report of the American Association of Poison Control Centers Toxic Exposure Surveillance System. Am J Emerg Med 2004; 22(5):335–404.
6. Dewan A, Bhatnagar VK, Mathur ML, et al: Repeated episodes of endosulfan poisoning. J Toxicol Clin Toxicol 2004;42(4):363–369.
7. Forrester MB, Sievert JS, Stanley SK: Epidemiology of lindane exposures for pediculosis reported to Poison Centers in Texas, 1998–2002. J Toxicol Clin Toxicol 2004;42(1):55–60.
8. Hayes WJ: Chlorinated hydrocarbon insecticides. In Pesticides Studied in Man. Baltimore, Williams & Wilkins, 1982.
9. Narahashi T, Haas HG: DDT: interaction with nerve membrane conductance changes. Science 1967;157(795):1438–1440.
10. Matsumura F, Patil KC: Adenosine triphosphatase: sensitive to DDT in synapses of rat brain. Science 1969;166(901):121–122.
11. Rashatwar SS, Matsumura F: Interaction of DDT and pyrethroids with calmodulin and its significance in the expression of enzyme activities of phosphodiesterase. Biochem Pharmacol 1985.;34(10): 1689–1694.
12. Hwang EC, Van Woert MH: p,p′-DDT-induced neurotoxic syndrome: experimental myoclonus. Neurology 1978;28(10):1020–1025.
13. Hong JS, Herr DW, Hudson PM, Tilson HA: Neurochemical effects of DDT in rat brain in vivo. Arch Toxicol Suppl 1986;9:14–26.
14. Pratt JA, Rothwell J, Jenner P, Marsden CD l: Myoclonus in the rat induced by p,p′-DDT and the role of altered monoamine function. Neuropharmacology 1985;24(5):361–373.
15. Busvine JR: Houseflies resistant to a group of chlorinated hydrocarbon insecticides. Nature 1954;174(4434):783–785.
16. Lawrence LJ, Casida JE: Interactions of lindane, toxaphene and cyclodienes with brain-specific t-butylbicyclophosphorothionate receptor. Life Sci 1984;35(2):171–178.
17. Abalis IM, Eldefrawi ME, Eldefrawi AT: Effects of insecticides on GABA-induced chloride influx into rat brain microsacs. J Toxicol Environ Health 1986;18(1):13–23.
18. Bloomquist JR: Intrinsic lethality of chloride-channel-directed insecticides and convulsants in mammals. Toxicol Lett 1992;60(3): 289–298.
19. Cole LM, Casida JE: Polychlorocycloalkane insecticide-induced convulsions in mice in relation to disruption of the GABA-regulated chloride ionophore. Life Sci 1986;39(20):1855–1862.
20. Gant DB, Eldefrawi ME, Eldefrawi AT: Cyclodiene insecticides inhibit GABAA receptor-regulated chloride transport. Toxicol Appl Pharmacol 1987;88(3):313–321.
21. Narahashi T, Frey JM, Ginsburg KS, Roy ML: Sodium and GABA-activated channels as the targets of pyrethroids and cyclodienes. Toxicol Lett 1992;64–65:429–436.
22. Pomes A, Rodriguez-Farre E, Sunol C: Disruption of GABA-dependent chloride flux by cyclodienes and hexachlorocyclohexanes in primary cultures of cortical neurons. J Pharmacol Exp Ther 1994;271(3):1616–1623.
23. Ikeda T, Nagata K, Shono T, Narahashi T: Dieldrin and picrotoxinin modulation of GABA (A) receptor single channels. Neuroreport 1998;9(14):3189–3195.
24. Liu J, Morrow AL, Devaud LL, et al: Regulation of GABA (A) receptor subunit mRNA expression by the pesticide dieldrin in embryonic brainstem cultures: a quantitative, competitive reverse transcription-polymerase chain reaction study. J Neurosci Res 1997;49(5):645–653.
25. Nagata K, Narahashi T: Differential effects of hexachlorocyclohexane isomers on the GABA receptor-chloride channel complex in rat dorsal root ganglion neurons. Brain Res 1995; 704(1):85–91.
26. Narahashi T, Ginsburg KS, Nagata K, et al: Ion channels as targets for insecticides. Neurotoxicology 1998;19(4–5):581–590.
27. Nagata K, Narahashi T: Dual action of the cyclodiene insecticide dieldrin on the gamma-aminobutyric acid receptor-chloride channel complex of rat dorsal root ganglion neurons. J Pharmacol Exp Ther 1994;269(1):164–171.
28. Anand M, Agrawal AK, Rehmani BN, et al: Role of GABA receptor complex in low dose lindane (HCH) induced neurotoxicity: neurobehavioural, neurochemical and electrophysiological studies. Drug Chem Toxicol 1998;21(1):35–46.
29. Saleh MA: Toxaphene: chemistry, biochemistry, toxicity and environmental fate. Rev Environ Contam Toxicol 1991;118:1–85.
30. Matsumura F: Involvement of picrotoxinin receptor in the action of cyclodiene insecticides. Neurotoxicology 1985;6(2):139–163.
31. Reigert JR, Roberts JR: Solid organochlorine insecticides. In Recognition and Management of Pesticide Poisonings. Washington, DC, U.S. Environmental Protection Agency, 1999, pp 55–62.
32. Aks SE, Krantz A, Hryhrczuk DO, et al: Acute accidental lindane ingestion in toddlers. Ann Emerg Med 1995;26(5):647–651.
33. Tenenbein M: Seizures after lindane therapy. J Am Geriatr Soc 1991;39(4):394–395.
34. Hunter J, Maxwell JD, Stewart DA, et al: Increased hepatic microsomal enzyme activity from occupational exposure to certain organochlorine pesticides. Nature 1972;237(5355):399–401.
35. Cannon SB, Veazey JM Jr, Jackson RS, et al: Epidemic kepone poisoning in chemical workers. Am J Epidemiol 1978;107(6): 529–537.
36. Cohn WJ, Boylan JJ, Blanke RV, et al: Treatment of chlordecone (Kepone) toxicity with cholestyramine. Results of a controlled clinical trial. N Engl J Med 1978;298(5):243–248.
37. Martinez AJ, Taylor JR, Dyck PJ, et al: Chlordecone intoxication in man. II. Ultrastructure of peripheral nerves and skeletal muscle. Neurology 1978;28(7):631–635.
38. Taylor JR, Selhorst JB, Houff SA, Martinez AJ: Chlordecone intoxication in man. I. Clinical observations. Neurology 1978; 28(7):626–630.
39. Soto AM, Sonnenschein C, Chung KL, et al: The E-SCREEN assay as a tool to identify estrogens: an update on estrogenic environmental pollutants. Environ Health Perspect 1995;103(Suppl. 7): 113–122.
40. Soto AM, Chung KL, Sonnenschein C: The pesticides endosulfan, toxaphene, and dieldrin have estrogenic effects on human estrogen-sensitive cells. Environ Health Perspect 1994;102(4):380–383.
41. Falck F Jr, Ricci A Jr, Wolff MS, et al: Pesticides and polychlorinated biphenyl residues in human breast lipids and their relation to breast cancer. Arch Environ Health 1992;47(2):143–146.
42. Wassermann M, Nogueira DP, Tomatis L, et al: Organochlorine compounds in neoplastic and adjacent apparently normal breast tissue. Bull Environ Contam Toxicol 1976;15(4):478–484.
43. Wolff MS, Toniolo PG, Lee EW, et al: Blood levels of organochlorine residues and risk of breast cancer. J Natl Cancer Inst 1993;85(8):648–652.
44. Hunter DJ, Hankinson SE, Laden F, et al: Plasma organochlorine levels and the risk of breast cancer. N Engl J Med 1997;337(18): 1253–1258.
45. Krieger N, Wolff MS, Hiatt RA, et al: Breast cancer and serum organochlorines: a prospective study among white, black, and Asian women. J Natl Cancer Inst 1994;86(8):589–599.

46. Rauch AE, Kowalsky SF, Lesar TS, et al: Lindane (Kwell)-induced aplastic anemia. Arch Intern Med 1990;150(11):2393–2395.

47. Furie B, Trubowitz S: Insecticides and blood dyscrasias. Chlordane exposure and self-limited refractory megaloblastic anemia. JAMA 1976;235(16):1720–1722.

48. Epstein SS, Ozonoff D: Leukemias and blood dyscrasias following exposure to chlordane and heptachlor. Teratog Carcinog Mutagen 1987;7(6):527–540.

49. Infante PF, Epstein SS, Newton WA Jr: Blood dyscrasias and childhood tumors and exposure to chlordane and heptachlor. Scand J Work Environ Health 1978;4(2):137–150.

50. Sunder Ram Rao CV, et al: Disseminated intravascular coagulation in a case of fatal lindane poisoning. Vet Hum Toxicol 1988;30(2):132–134.

51. Munk ZM, Nantel A: Acute lindane poisoning with development of muscle necrosis. Can Med Assoc J 1977;117(9):1050–1054.

52. McGuire V, Longstreth WT Jr, Nelson LM, et al: Occupational exposures and amyotrophic lateral sclerosis. A population-based case-control study. Am J Epidemiol 1997;145(12):1076–1088.

53. Saady JJ, Poklis A: Determination of chlorinated hydrocarbon pesticides by solid-phase extraction and capillary GC with electron capture detection. J Anal Toxicol 1990;14(5):301–304.

54. Tilson HA, Hong JS, Mactutus CF: Effects of 5,5-diphenyl-hydantoin (phenytoin) on neurobehavioral toxicity of organo-chlorine insecticides and permethrin. J Pharmacol Exp Ther 1985;233(2):285–299.

55. Morgan DP, Dotson TB, Lin LI: Effectiveness of activated charcoal, mineral oil, and castor oil in limiting gastrointestinal absorption of a chlorinated hydrocarbon pesticide. Clin Toxicol 1977;11(1):61–70.

56. Kassner JT, Maher TJ, Hull KM, Woolf AD: Cholestyramine as an adsorbent in acute lindane poisoning: a murine model. Ann Emerg Med 1993;22(9):1392–1397.

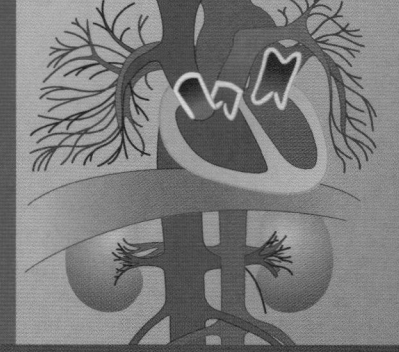

82 *Occupational Toxicology*

MICHAEL G. HOLLAND, MD

At a Glance...

- Occupational diseases from toxicant exposures often mimic or present as common nonoccupational conditions.
- Occupational diseases and illnesses are underreported because of poor recognition.
- The occupational history is the crucial part of a workup for any patient presenting with new onset of symptoms.
- Occupational toxicants primarily affect the skin and respiratory tract.
- Soluble irritant gases cause primarily upper airway irritation, whereas poorly soluble gases can lead to alveolar injury.
- Systemic absorption following dermal or respiratory exposures can lead to other end-organ toxicities.
- Electronic databases and Poison Control Centers are valuable resources for information on the toxicity of the more than 70,000 chemicals in commercial use.
- Passage of the Occupational Safety and Health Act of 1970 has greatly reduced the incidence of occupational poisonings in the United States.

The U.S. Bureau of Labor Statistics (BLS) reported 5559 occupational fatalities in private industry for the year 2003, most due to physical hazards, accidents, homicides, and falls. However, 9.0% were due to exposure to harmful substances or environments, and 4% were due to fires and explosions.[1] The BLS report for the year 2003 (most current year available) reveals there were about 269,500 newly reported cases of nonfatal occupational illnesses in private industry, of which 4.9%, or 43,400, were skin disorders; 2.2%, or 19,000, were listed as respiratory conditions; and 0.4%, or 3900, were due to poisoning.[2] These numbers may be misleading because illnesses or exposures requiring only first-aid treatment are not generally reported. Also, the connection between work and the illness is often missed because of latent onset of symptoms or disease; thus, the actual incidence is probably much higher.

On a global scale, the World Health Organization (WHO) estimates more than 200 million workers are affected by occupational diseases worldwide.[3] The overwhelming majority of these diseases are seen in developing nations, where workers often do not wear personal protective equipment (PPE) and where regulatory bodies to ensure worker safety often do not exist or are grossly underfunded and understaffed. In addition to the human suffering involved, economic costs of these occupational diseases constitute a significant percentage of each country's gross national product.[4]

There are millions of chemical substances in existence and more than 70,000 in common commercial use. About 3300 of these are designated high-production-volume (HPV) chemicals by the U.S. Environmental Protection Agency (EPA), signifying that they are produced in excess of 1 million tons per year. These HPV chemicals are listed by the EPA as part of the Inventory Update Rule of the Toxic Substances Control Act of 1986, and the list is revised every 4 years.[5] Given these large numbers of potential toxicants, it is not surprising that relevant toxicology data regarding human health effects are not available for most of these chemicals. As an example, the Hazardous Substances Data Bank (HSDB) operated by the National Library of Medicine's (NLM) Toxicology Data Network (TOXNET) has comprehensive data on less than 4800 chemicals. Therefore, treating physicians need to know what available resources can help when confronted with exposures to chemical hazards with which they are not familiar. Often, toxicity must be extrapolated from the knowledge of familiar chemicals with known toxicities that may share similar properties or structure–activity relationships with the new chemical.

HISTORICAL PERSPECTIVES

Physicians have long recognized the connection between workplace and environmental exposures and disease

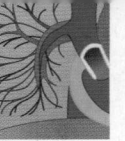

states. Georgius Agricola described the diseases associated with mining as early as the 16th century.[6] Bernardo Ramazzini, generally regarded as the father of occupational medicine, in 1713 recognized the connection of disease to work in many occupations, noting that the route of exposure was usually inhalational. He also described numerous occupational diseases, including lead and mercury poisoning. He emphasized the critical need to delve into the work history when evaluating a patient's symptoms.[7] Alice Hamilton was the first American physician who dedicated her career to industrial medicine. She described the effects of lead poisoning in workers, as well as "phossy" jaw of matchmakers, and hematologic effects of benzene exposure.[8]

Occupational medicine became a recognized specialty of the American Board of Medical Specialties in 1955. With the passage of the Occupational Safety and Health Act in 1970, the specialty experienced remarkable growth. With the creation of the Occupational Safety and Health Administration (OSHA) and the National Institute of Occupational Safety and Health (NIOSH), the United States has since witnessed a marked decrease in classic occupational diseases and deaths. However, developing nations are experiencing dramatic increases in some of these classic occupational diseases. In any event, workers everywhere will continue to be exposed to chemicals and toxicants, and knowledge of the health effects of these exposures is important not only in occupational medicine but also in primary care and other medical specialties.

RECOGNITION OF OCCUPATIONAL DISEASES

The diagnosis of industrial poisoning is important not only for the care of the patient but also because accurate diagnosis makes it possible to identify potential workplace hazards that may affect the patient's coworkers or the community at large. Emergency physicians and primary care specialists should maintain a high index of suspicion for the possibility of industrial poisoning, familiarize themselves with industrial processes and toxic substances used locally, maintain an adequate reference library or have on-line access to toxicology databases, and obtain occupational histories from their patients. In addition, potential hazardous releases can be prevented if inadequate engineering controls are identified.[9] However, there are problems with recognition and diagnosis of occupational diseases for numerous reasons, discussed next.

Similarity to Common Diseases

Many occupational illnesses caused by toxic exposures will mimic or duplicate nonoccupational diseases. Unless a proper history is taken, along with the knowledge that similarly exposed workers were experiencing similar effects, the connection of the disease to the work exposure might be missed. An example is occupational asthma, by far the most common occupational disease in the United

States. Asthma is also a very common condition in the general population. Exposures to certain industrial chemicals (toluene diisocyanate [TDI], maleic anhydride) can cause occupational asthma. Knowing the job a patient performs and the chemicals used there (e.g., polyurethane foam manufacturing and TDI use) may help identify the cause as occupational in origin.

Latency

Recognition of industrial poisoning may be obvious when the acutely ill person is transported directly from the workplace where an unprotected exposure to a known toxic substance has occurred. However, many toxicants have a latent period between the time of exposure and the onset of clinical illness. This can involve several hours for acute effects, such as acute lung injury from phosgene or oxides of nitrogen exposure, to weeks for the peripheral neuropathy seen after exposure to hexacarbons like n-hexane and methyl-n-butyl ketone, to years for dust exposure and pneumoconioses like silicosis and asbestosis.

Toxicants That Exist as Mixtures or Are Contaminated with Other Chemicals

If there are multiple or unknown potential toxicants, recognition of the link to work may be missed or underestimated. For instance, methyl ethyl ketone (MEK), a widely used industrial solvent, does not produce peripheral neuropathy. However, when MEK is mixed with small amounts of n-hexane, a peripheral neurotoxicant, it potentiates the effects of the n-hexane. Also, some toxicants may be present only as contaminants of the chemical in use, and therefore are not listed on ingredient labels. The herbicide mixture 2,4-dinitrochlorophenoxyacetic acid (2,4-D) and 2,4,5-trinitrochlorphenoxyacetic acid (2,4,5-T) was known as Agent Orange because of the color of the containers in which it was shipped to Vietnam. This mixture contained a significant amount of 2,3,7,8-tetrachlorodibenzo-p-dioxin (TCDD, or simply "dioxin"). Dioxin was previously an unknown contaminant produced when manufacturing the 2,4,5-T component of the mixture (but not 2,4-D). Because of the chloracne caused by dioxin in 2,4,5-T manufacturing workers, and other alleged health effects in exposed soldiers in Vietnam, the use of 2,4,5-T in the United States has been discontinued.

Unavailable Information Regarding the Chemical in Use

As mentioned previously, comprehensive toxicologic information is available for only a small fraction of chemicals in use. Also, many chemical mixtures are patented, proprietary mixtures. As such, the ingredients may not be listed on the material safety data sheet (MSDS), and manufacturers may be hesitant to release this information. Also, the fear of litigation may prevent an employer from admitting to using a hazardous

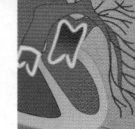

chemical, that proper engineering controls were not in place, or that personal protective equipment was not provided to their exposed employees.

Other Nonoccupational Conditions That May Affect the Response to Industrial Toxicants

Certain nonoccupational conditions or ingestions can exacerbate or ameliorate the effects due to occupational exposures. For example, degreaser's flush only occurs after exposure to trichloroethylene and subsequent ethanol ingestion. Conversely, it has been demonstrated that smokers have a decreased incidence of hypersensitivity pneumonitis after exposures to appropriate antigens when compared with nonsmokers, possibly owing to effects on cytokine populations and antigen handling.[10]

Inadequate Physician Training Regarding Occupational Illnesses

Medical schools have very few courses or electives in occupational health and other preventive medicine disciplines. This is true in American,[11] British,[12] Australian, and New Zealand medical schools.[13] In addition, most primary care residency programs lack formal rotations in occupational medicine, and sadly, the number of residents and programs in occupational medicine in the United States is declining.[14]

CLASSIFICATION OF HAZARDOUS MATERIALS

The U.S. Department of Transportation requires all shipping papers to have classifications as well as identification numbers.[8] This classification and numbering system is used by many other regulatory agencies and authorities for identifying potentially hazardous substances[9] (Box 82-1).

The National Fire Protection Association (NFPA) Committee on Fire Hazards of Materials developed a hazard signal system: NFPA-704[10] (Fig. 82-1). This includes a numeric rating scale to identify the degree of hazard in the categories of health, fire, and reactivity (Box 82-2). This system is frequently used for labeling by chemical manufacturers; however, this system is rarely employed for chemicals in transport. Under this system, the term *health hazard* refers specifically to the capacity of a material to cause personal injury from contact with or absorption into the body of a chemical. In fire fighting or other emergency conditions, the term *health hazard* refers to a single exposure, which may vary in duration from a few seconds to 1 hour. It is not applicable to the situation of an industrial worker who is exposed on as routine basis. The NFPA-704 system's use of the five ratings of the degree of hazard of a specific chemical is defined as follows:

BOX 82-1   LABELING AND CLASSIFICATION SYSTEMS

US Department of Transportation
1. Class A explosives
2. Class B explosives
3. Blasting agent
4. Poison A
5. Flammable gas
6. Nonflammable gas
7. Nonflammable gas (chlorine)
8. Nonflammable gas (oxygen, pressurized liquid)
9. Flammable liquid
10. Combustible liquid
11. Flammable solid
12. Flammable solid (dangerous when wet)
13. Oxidixer
14. Organic peroxide
15. Poison B (nonflammable gas—fluorine)
16. Radioactive material
17. Corrosive material
18. Irritating material

United Nations Classification Numbers
1. Explosives
2. Gases
3. Flammable and combustible liquids
4. Flammable solids, spontaneous combustion substances
5. Oxidizers and organic peroxides
6. Poisonous materials
7. Radioactive materials
8. Corrosives
9. Miscellaneous hazardous materials

0—Materials that on exposure under fire conditions would present no hazard beyond that of ordinary combustible materials
1—Materials that on exposure would cause irritation but only minor residual injury even if no treatment were given
2—Materials that on intense or continued exposure could cause temporary incapacitation or possible residual injury unless prompt medical treatment is given
3—Materials that on short exposure could cause serious temporary or residual injury even if prompt medical treatment is given
4—Materials that on very short exposure could cause death or major residual injury even if prompt medical treatment is given

The MSDS contains detailed information about specific chemicals and their toxicity. Because of their standard format and availability, these sheets have become required by many fire department HAZMAT (hazardous materials) units and in right-to-know ordinances. Since 1986, OSHA has required that an MSDS be readily available for any chemical used in the workplace. It is the responsibility of the importer or manufacturer of each chemical to prepare these forms in a standardized format. In 29CFR1910.120, OSHA defines what min-

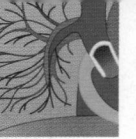

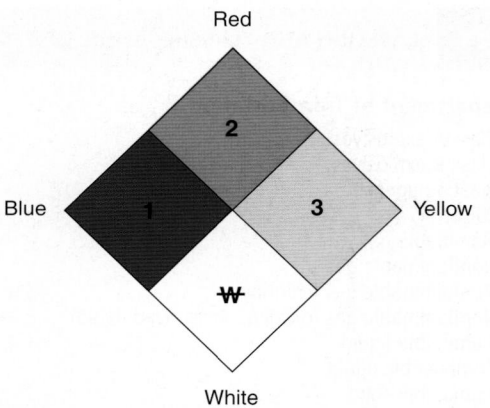

FIGURE 82-1 Symbol of the National Fire Protection 704 Hazard Signal System. See Box 82-2 for explanation.

imum information must be included in these sheets. The employer is required to provide an MSDS to the treating physician when an employee is involved in an acute exposure. The quality of the medical treatment guidelines of an MSDS varies widely, but in general is poor, because these documents are generally produced without input by physicians or toxicologists. However, they contain useful information regarding the chemical content of the material and its reactivity and explosive nature, and advice on the proper method to be used for decontamination, environmental cleanup, and fire control.

BOX 82-2   NFPA HAZARD SIGNAL SYSTEM "704"

Flammable (Red)

4—Extremely flammable
3—Ignites at normal temperatures below 37.8° C (100° F)
2—Ignites at temperatures below 93.3° C (200° F)
1—Must be preheated to burn
0—Will not burn

Health Hazard (Blue)

4—Too dangerous to enter vapor or liquid
3—Extreme danger
2—Hazardous
1—Slightly hazardous
0—Normal material

Reactivity (Yellow)

4—May detonate
3—Shock and heat may detonate
2—Violent chemical change
1—Unstable if heated
0—Stable

Specific Hazard (White)

OXY—Oxidizer
ACID—Acid
ALK—Alkali
COR—Corrosive
 —Use no water
☢ —Radiation hazard

OCCUPATIONAL HISTORY

Obtaining a detailed occupational history on every patient presenting to an emergency department or primary care office may not be practical and often is too time consuming for use as a screening instrument. Goldman and Peters developed a systematic approach (Fig. 82-2) for evaluating hazardous exposures.[15] The algorithm begins with a quick survey that can be performed routinely on all patients. The clinician may then proceed to a more detailed line of questioning to follow any indications of toxic exposure.

Routine Survey

The first step includes asking questions about three essential topics that are easily incorporated into routine history taking: (1) current and past job titles; (2) known exposure to fumes, chemicals, dusts, or radiation; and (3) any temporal relationship of the chief complaint to work activities or other contributory factors. The work and exposure history acts as a broad screen to elicit potentially hazardous exposures at home or work. When conditions with short latency periods are under evaluation, such as occupational asthma, the emphasis should be on the current job and exposures. For conditions of longer latency, such as asbestosis, the history must focus on jobs and exposures in the past. Allergic responses to agents may develop even after years of asymptomatic exposure.

A temporal relationship between the onset of symptoms and work or home activities can provide an important clue to recent sources of exposure. In general, symptoms that recede on the weekend or at vacation time and return at the start of the workweek indicate some current job-related exposure. For example, acute systemic solvent toxicity, which includes the symptoms of headache, gastrointestinal disturbances, and lightheadedness, usually occurs within a short time of exposure and lessens within hours after removal from exposure. The expression of toxic symptoms also is influenced by the use of medications, preexisting medical diseases, and exposure to other hazardous substances. In addition, some personal habits (e.g., the use of tobacco or alcohol) represent significant environmental exposures that may interact with or add to occupational exposures.

If, after the initial screening survey, there appears to be a possible link between the illness and work exposures, further investigation is necessary. This will consist of a comprehensive occupational and environmental history as well as an in-depth past medical history.

Current Occupation

In assessing the likelihood of the workplace as a source of toxic exposure, the physician should obtain a complete description of all jobs that the patient has had, beginning with the current job and working backward in time to prior jobs. Necessary information includes the chemicals used, the products manufactured, and the processes involved. Many workers are well informed

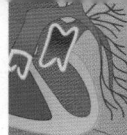

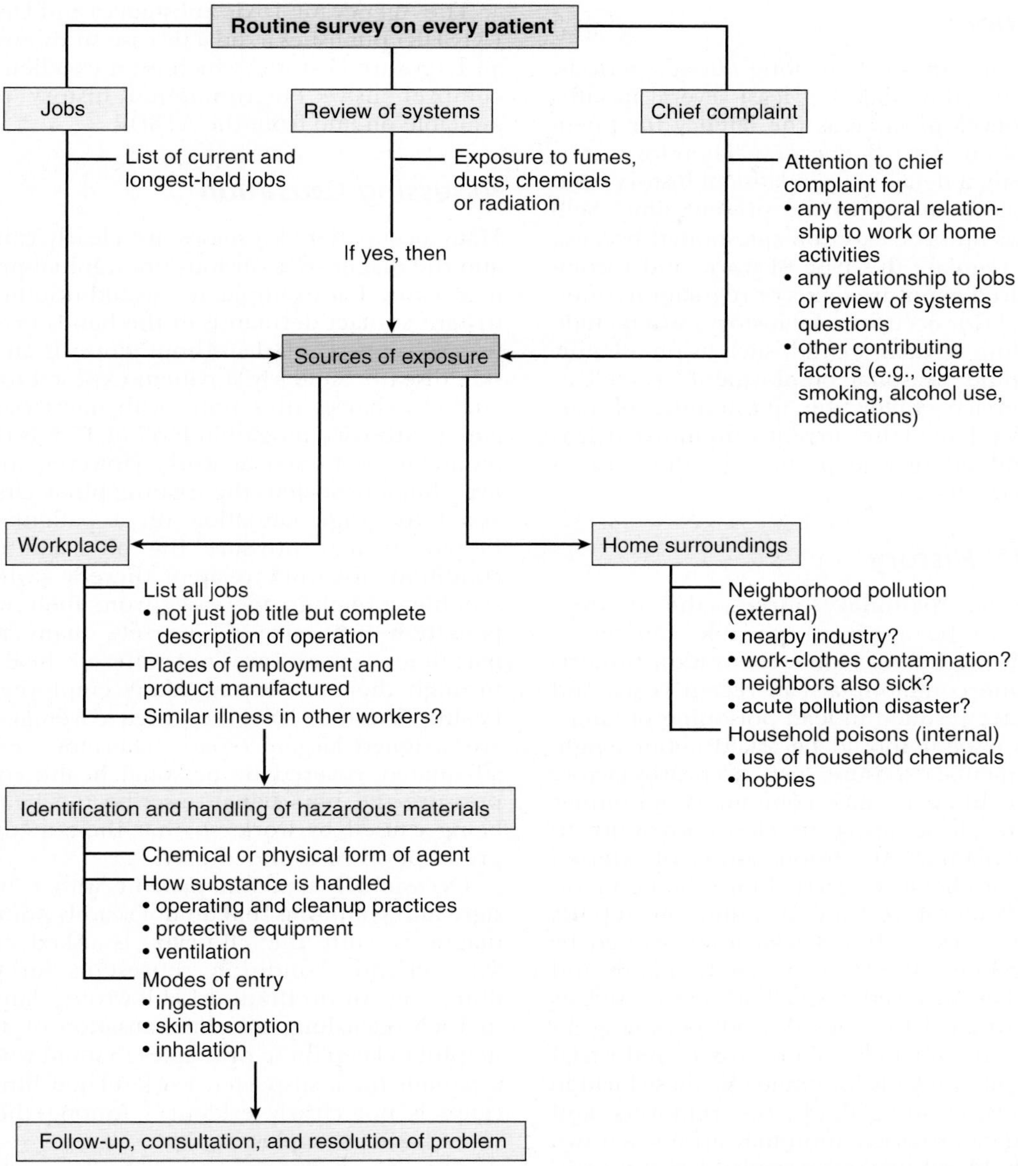

Routine survey on every patient

Jobs
— List of current and
longest-held jobs

Review of systems
— Exposure to fumes,
dusts, chemicals
or radiation

If yes, then

Chief complaint
— Attention to chief
complaint for
• any temporal relation-
ship to work or home
activities
• any relationship to jobs
or review of systems
questions
• other contributing
factors (e.g., cigarette
smoking, alcohol use,
medications)

Sources of exposure

Workplace
— List all jobs
• not just job title but complete
description of operation
— Places of employment and
product manufactured
— Similar illness in other workers?

Home surroundings
— Neighborhood pollution
(external)
• nearby industry?
• work-clothes contamination?
• neighbors also sick?
• acute pollution disaster?
— Household poisons (internal)
• use of household chemicals
• hobbies

Identification and handling of hazardous materials
— Chemical or physical form of agent
— How substance is handled
• operating and cleanup practices
• protective equipment
• ventilation
— Modes of entry
• ingestion
• skin absorption
• inhalation

Follow-up, consultation, and resolution of problem

FIGURE 82-2 Systematic approach to history taking and diagnosis of occupational illness. (From Goldman RH, Peters JM: The occupational and environmental health history. JAMA 1981;246:2831–2836. Copyright 1981, American Medical Association.)

about specific exposures at the workplace, and the information that they provide is sufficient for documentation. Often, however, obtaining an exposure history requires further detective work for identification of specific components of products and for documentation of exposure levels. Most jobs have their own jargon for processes performed and materials used. Patients may know the chemical only by its trade name or process name (e.g., "blanket wash" for ink press solvent cleaner) and do not know the generic or chemical name. Whenever possible, workers should be urged to bring the MSDS for all chemicals with which they work to the emergency department or clinic visit. Many times a simple phone request from the treating physician to the worksite will prompt the MSDS to be faxed to the clinical site. In the case of multiple casualty incidents, prehos-

pital medical care personnel or HAZMAT team members may be helpful in locating chemical labels, manifest sheets, MSDS, shipping papers, or knowledgeable personnel who can identify the agent involved.

Patients should be asked whether fellow workers have similar complaints; the cluster of symptoms among employees may be the first clue to identifying the presence of an occupational hazard, and Hill's criteria require that similarly exposed workers should have similar medical conditions.[27] The workplace industrial hygienist, occupational medicine physician or nurse, or plant manager can often provide the most useful information on working conditions and chemicals in use, as well as PPE employed and the extent of engineering controls employed. In addition, OSHA requires that the employer provide a copy of the MSDS.

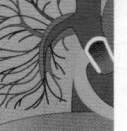

Prior Occupations

Many occupational illnesses have long latency periods. Sensitizer-induced asthma takes at least several months of exposure to develop, whereas the latency for pneumoconioses is often 2 to 3 decades. Therefore, it is important to obtain a detailed occupational history from the start of employment up to the present time. Self-employed persons must be carefully questioned because OSHA does not regulate this type of work, and recommended or required exposure limits or regulations often are not followed. Prior occupational history must include questions regarding work as a child, such as on a family farm, and part-time, seasonal employment, as well as prior military service. Tailor the questioning of past exposures as they relate to the current symptoms, such as prior irritant and allergen exposures in the case of possible pulmonary disease.

Environmental History

In addition to occupational sources, the treating physician needs to be aware of possible sources of contamination in the home. Home renovation projects have become quite commonplace in recent years, and these activities have resulted in lead poisoning of family members.[17] The patient should be asked about neighborhood environmental exposure, such as a nearby factory or chemical waste dump, because community poisonings have occurred in those living in close proximity to certain industrial plants.[18] An obvious source of external pollution is dust or chemicals carried into the home on work clothes. The literature contains numerous reports of children with excessive blood lead levels caused by parents bringing home the toxicant on the hands and clothing[19-21]; workers involved in small businesses such as radiator repair shops have caused lead poisoning in multiple family members.[22] Many toxic industrial chemicals are readily available for home use; these include pesticides, solvents, cleaning fluids, rust removers, and disinfectants. A dangerous situation may arise when two common household substances are mixed together in the hope of producing a more potent compound (e.g., chloramine, a soluble irritant gas, is produced when ammonia and household bleach [sodium hypochlorite] are mixed; chlorine gas is produced when acid toilet bowl cleaners and bleach are mixed).

The growth and diversification of hobbies have introduced a multitude of hazardous substances into the household. Artists are generally self-employed, and their studios exist in their homes, placing them and their families at risk for exposure to toxic chemicals, metals, and dusts. Artists and craftspeople, depending on their medium of choice, can face daily exposure to diverse toxic substances such as solvents, paints, inks, and thinners[23,24]; lead, cadmium, and other metals in pigments, pottery glazes, copper enamels, solders, and other metalworking materials[25]; and dusts such as silica and asbestos in clays, talcs, and glazes.[26] Further compounding this problem is the inadequate labeling of many art materials and the relative naiveté of the artists to the potential risks they face.

The Agency for Toxic Substances and Disease Registry (ATSDR) publishes a didactic case study entitled "Taking an Exposure History," which is an excellent source for a comprehensive environmental history form, and is available on-line from the ATSDR.[27]

Assessing Causation

Many occupational diseases are clearly caused by work, and the diagnosis is obvious upon initial presentation in most cases. For example, few would dispute the fact that irritant contact dermatitis of the hands in a patient who uses solvents regularly without gloves is an occupational skin disease. Similarly, a patient exposed to unventilated engine exhausts presenting with nausea and headache and a carboxyhemoglobin level of 15% is clearly carbon monoxide poisoned at work. However, in our increasingly litigious society, the treating physician is frequently asked to assign causation on a patient's initial visit. Employers may pressure the physician to deem the condition not work related, thereby saving money by avoiding premium increases from their worker's compensation insurance. Conversely, many temporary or part-time workers are not offered health insurance through their employers. Many employees covered by health insurance have seen their coverage reduced and are assigned larger co-pays. Therefore, employees not adequately covered by personal health insurance may pressure the physician to ascribe the health effects as being caused by work, so that their medical bills and prescription costs are covered.

Occasionally, a patient presents with a constellation of signs and symptoms that do not readily point to a specific diagnosis, and the clinician is asked to determine whether this condition represents an occupational illness. Sir Austin Bradford Hill wrote a landmark article in 1965 regarding assessing causation of a disease. It is helpful to keep these principles in mind when evaluating a patient for a suspected work-related illness when the cause is not clearly evident.[16] Among the criteria are seven basic principles:

1. *Strength of association:* The rate of increase in a disease in the exposed population over that seen in the unexposed, and disease seen in specific organ systems of the exposed population.

As an example, nylon flock worker's lung is seen only in random-cut flock workers at two plants using this process, not in other flock workers exposed to precision-cut flocking process, and not in other nylon workers.[28,29]

2. *Consistency:* The relationship is seen in multiple studies of workers with similar exposures at other locations studied by different investigators.

Workers with similar exposures should have similar effects. This is why it is especially helpful to survey an individual patient's coworkers to determine whether similar symptoms or physical findings are present. In the example cited earlier, nylon flock workers in the other random-cut plant had similar findings, and rat studies

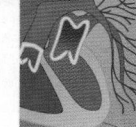

had revealed pulmonary toxic effects due to the nylon particles.[30]

3. *Specificity:* The exposure causes a specific disease or related group of diseases, not a constellation of unrelated, vague, multisystem symptoms.

Symptoms such as cough and dyspnea and chest tightness after exposure to animal dander at work, along with measurable decrements in FEV_1 on pulmonary function testing, is excellent presumptive evidence for diagnosing occupational asthma. However, vague, multisystem symptoms such as headache, fatigue, mental fogging, and body aches in an office worker are more difficult to definitively diagnose as an occupational illness.

4. *Temporality:* Exposure must precede the disease.

This seems obvious, but often a review of a patient's past medical history and old charts reveals that similar symptoms preceded the exposure. This emphasizes the need for a comprehensive past medical history in all patients suspected of having an occupational illness.

5. *Dose–response, or the biologic gradient:* The risk for the disease increases as the dose of the exposure increases.

As an example, low-level toluene vapor exposures can cause eye and upper respiratory tract irritation. As exposures become more intense, central nervous system (CNS) effects such as lightheadedness and dizziness can be seen. Higher exposures can cause frank ataxia and CNS impairment (feeling drunk or "high"), and overwhelming exposure such as that which occurs in an unventilated confined space can cause loss of consciousness. The biologic effect exhibits a definable, recognizable dose–response relationship.

The dose–response criterion is also subject to the experimentation test: reducing the exposure causes a concomitant reduction in the disease. As a historical example, carbon disulfide, a volatile organic solvent, is used in the viscose rayon industry. In the early 1900s, levels in the workplace were so high that workers experienced acute CNS effects, ranging from mood changes to frank delirium and psychosis. Workplaces even had to have bars across windows to prevent affected employees from jumping out. Through the efforts of pioneers like Dr. Alice Hamilton, much of the process was contained with engineering controls to greatly reduce workplace exposure levels (i.e., dose reduction), so that this effect of carbon disulfide is no longer seen. As a more recent example, reduction of TDI levels by the use of engineering controls has reduced the incidence of occupational asthma in polyurethane foam production workers.

6. *Biologic plausibility:* The associated disease and the exposure make sense (i.e., it is plausible); the subjective and objective findings are explained by the exposure. The association should be analogous to other well-characterized diseases.

For example, suppose that a new organic solvent comes into use, and a worker develops a peripheral neuropathy after using it for several months. If you find that this solvent has a metabolite with a gamma diketone structure, it is plausible that this new solvent could be the causative agent. Known peripheral neurotoxicants *n*-hexane and methyl *n*-butyl ketone both have the common gamma diketone metabolite 2,5-butanedione. Knowledge of this structure–activity relationship makes it biologically plausible that this exposure could cause this disease.

Conversely, attributing neuropsychiatric symptoms in workers to toxigenic fungi and molds found growing on wallboard in an office building with indoor air quality issues is not biologically plausible, given the known scientific facts of mold growth, mycotoxin production, and bioavailability through the inhalational route.[31-34]

7. *Coherence:* The association is consistent with other established scientific evidence regarding the disease and the toxicant and requires that other known common causes of the disease not be ignored.

For instance, a known clinical syndrome caused by mycotoxin ingestion is alimentary toxic aleukia (ATA), which was seen in Russia in the 1930s when people ate overwintered wheat that had been contaminated by mold growth of *Fusarium* species that produced the trichothecene mycotoxin T-2. This syndrome consisted of bone marrow suppression and gastrointestinal hemorrhage and resulted in thousands of deaths. Similarly, aflatoxins are contaminants found in food products and are produced by *Aspergillus* species. Aflatoxins are known acute hepatotoxins at high doses, and at lower doses are carcinogens contained in the human diet, with daily exposure limits set by regulatory bodies. All these effects are seen with ingestion of the mycotoxins, none by inhalation.

However, ascribing the vague symptoms seen in some sick building syndrome evaluations to mycotoxin exposure due to indoor fungi is not coherent with the known scientific evidence regarding mycotoxins. Mycotoxins are not produced to any significant quantity when growing on environmental surfaces, and because the contaminated wallboard and carpeting are not ingested, employees cannot receive any measurable dose of mycotoxin from inhalational exposure in the workplace.[32,33] In other words, this association is not consistent with known established scientific evidence regarding the toxins and the diseases they produce. Other factors that can cause these symptoms, such as elevated volatile organic compounds, poor air exchange levels (as evidenced by high ambient CO_2 levels), high job dissatisfaction, and high work stress levels would have to be ignored.

Exposure Characterization

In characterizing the health effects of a chemical exposure, it is important to determine not only the generic ingredients of the compound involved but also

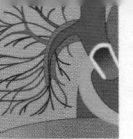

its physical state and the process employed at the time of exposure. For example, chlorinated hydrocarbon solvents or chlorofluorocarbon refrigerants are simple asphyxiants, which can cause CNS depression and may precipitate cardiac arrhythmias when inhaled in sufficient concentrations. However, when these compounds are heated or burned, such as in torch cutting or welding activities, phosgene is produced.[35] This low-solubility irritant gas can then cause acute lung injury and adult respiratory distress syndrome.[36] Knowledge of processes occurring near the patient's workspace is important because gases can diffuse and travel to other areas of the worksite. In the previous example, phosgene has a vapor density that is 3.4 times the density of air, and as such will settle in low areas. Therefore, employees working below the welder and unaware of the inadvertent production of phosgene can nonetheless be poisoned.

In addition to the character of an exposure, the quantity and concentration as it exists is often a crucial determinant of toxicity. As Paracelsus taught centuries ago, the "dose makes the poison." Simply being at a workplace where a certain chemical is used does not imply poisoning. If the process is completely contained or if the material is not in an absorbable form, then toxicity is not likely. Whenever possible, engineering controls and personal protective equipment should be used to reduce exposures. Workplace monitoring of chemical levels will determine exposure risks and dictate the need for personal protective equipment.

Workplace Exposure Levels and Monitoring

Many employers using potentially hazardous chemicals will have exposure monitoring programs in place. These include general workplace air monitoring and personal breathing space monitoring. Air monitoring is also performed because certain toxicants have OSHA-regulated permissible exposure limits (PELs). These air-monitoring samples are taken during normal work processes and are irrespective of PPE being worn. Those that do not have OSHA-mandated PELs often have NIOSH-recommended exposure limits (RELs), which employers can use as a guide to reduce exposures. In addition, the American Conference of Governmental Industrial Hygienists (ACGIH) develops threshold limit values (TLVs) and biologic exposure indices (BEIs) that can also be helpful (see later). Workplace air monitoring is performed using various methods for a specified time period, and then expressed as an 8-hour time-weighted average (TWA). The goal of setting exposure limits is to find a level to which it is safe to be exposed for 8 hours per day, 40 hours per week.

With the passage of the Occupational Safety and Health Act of 1970, the U.S. Congress created two new federal agencies, OSHA, the regulatory arm, and NIOSH, the research and training arm. OSHA has published mandatory PELs for a number of chemical agents. These are available at the OSHA website.[37] Several hazardous substances also have their own standards regarding PELs,

action levels, and medical monitoring requirements. These are listed in the Code of Federal regulations, CFR 1910 subpart Z, and are available at the OSHA website.[38] For most of these chemicals, workplace air monitoring must be performed to determine the exposure level. If the airborne concentration is above the mandated "action level," then compliance with airborne monitoring, employee biologic monitoring, and necessary PPE is required. Many of these regulations also mandate pre-exposure and periodic medical examinations, as well as when biologic monitoring indicates excess employee exposure or absorption (e.g., elevated blood lead level).

OSHA levels are a balance between recommended safe levels and practicality of achieving these levels, and the cost and industry lobbying efforts. However, NIOSH recommended levels, like the ACGIH TLVs, are levels that are believed to be safe based on best available science and toxicologic data, and are not particularly influenced by economic or political concerns. This explains the frequent discrepancy whereby the NOISH RELs or ACGIH TLVs are lower than the OSHA PELs.

The ACGIH, formed in 1938, publishes the TLVs on 642 chemical substances and physical agents, and BEIs on 38 different chemicals. The ACGIH developed their TLVs and BEIs as guidelines to assist in the control of health hazards, not to be used as legal standards, and ACGIH does not advocate their use as such. The TLVs and BEIs represent conditions under which ACGIH believes that nearly all workers may be repeatedly exposed without adverse health effects.[39]

NIOSH publishes the *NIOSH Pocket Guide to Chemical Hazards (NPG)*, which is intended as a source of general industrial hygiene information for workers, employers, and occupational health professionals. The *NPG* presents key information and data in abbreviated tabular form for 677 chemicals or substance groupings (e.g., manganese compounds, tellurium compounds, inorganic tin compounds) that are found in the work environment. The current version contains information on all substances for which NIOSH has recommended exposure limits (RELs) and those for which OSHA has established PELs.[40]

NIOSH has also defined exposure levels that are considered immediately dangerous to life or health. The current NIOSH definition for an immediately dangerous to life or health (IDLH) condition is a situation "that poses a threat of exposure to airborne contaminants when that exposure is likely to cause death or immediate or delayed permanent adverse health effects or prevent escape from such an environment." It is also stated that the purpose of establishing an IDLH is to "ensure that the worker can escape from a given contaminated environment in the event of failure of the respiratory protection equipment." These levels are published in the *NPG* as well at the NIOSH IDLH home page.[41]

Exposure Route

The normal routes of exposure in the occupational setting are inhalation and dermal. The most common effects are the dermatoses, consisting mainly of irritant

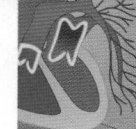

contact dermatitis and allergic contact dermatitis. Most of these effects are confined to the skin and are not usually an acute problem. Systemic absorption may occur and cause systemic effects when large skin areas are exposed, or when prolonged contact occurs, such as when clothing becomes soaked and is not removed, or when the skin is not decontaminated. Certain toxicants, such as phenol, are very well absorbed dermally, and significant systemic toxicity from skin spills can occur in these cases.[42]

Inhalation exposures to toxic fumes, vapors, and gases pose the greatest danger to life and health. Irritant gases cause airway and pulmonary injury depending on the length of exposure and the water solubility of the gas. Simple asphyxiants displace oxygen from ambient air and cause hypoxia due to decreased FIO_2. Systemic asphyxiants cause toxicity either by interfering with hemoglobin's ability to carry oxygen (CO, methemoglobin-forming agents), or interfering with mitochondrial ability to utilize molecular oxygen (CN, H_2S, azides). Also, in the case of gaseous releases, the potential to affect many people simultaneously is very real, both in the industrial setting and after a hazardous chemicals (HAZMAT) incident. See Chapter 9 for more detailed description of inhalational toxicity of specific agents and recommended management.

Accidental or intentional toxic ingestions occur much less commonly in the occupational setting. However, eating or smoking in the workplace may put the worker at increased risk for absorption of toxicants, such as metallic dusts (lead, cadmium). Smoking at work when fingers are contaminated with certain chemicals can cause systemic effects, like polymer fume fever in the case of polytetrafluoroethylene (PTFE, Teflon).

PATHOPHYSIOLOGY OF WORKPLACE EXPOSURES

The pathologic effects that may occur with exposure to a specific hazardous substance include direct injury, sensitization, asphyxiation, or systemic toxicity. Effects such as carcinogenesis, mutagenesis, and teratogenesis have long latency periods and thus are not considered in the category of toxicologic emergencies.

Dermal Exposures

Irritant contact dermatitis is the most common occupational skin disorder and is associated with a wide variety of chemical and physical agents. The chemical agents involved may be acids, alkalis (caustics), certain metal compounds, detergents, or solvents. Strong corrosives may incite an acute injury that manifests as a vesicular (blistering) or ulcerative injury. Milder irritants, such as soaps, detergents, and solvents, remove surface lipids and cause dryness and cracking of the skin. Chronic exposure to these agents can result in the skin becoming thickened (lichenified) along with erythema, dryness, and fissuring due to the chronic irritation. Workers commonly affected are metalworkers who use

degreasing solvent and metalworking fluids, as well as printers using ink solvents. Mechanical irritation, heat, cold, and low humidity are important contributing factors in many cases. An example is the hand dermatitis seen in health care workers in northern states that occurs during the winter months as a result of the frequent hand washing and the associated low-humidity winter air. Exposures predominantly to oils and greases can incite acneiform lesions as well. After avoidance and corticosteroid treatment, most workers can resume work with the substance as long as barrier creams or gloves are used to minimize future contact. Specific toxicants are addressed in their respective chapters of this textbook.

Allergic contact dermatitis is a delayed type IV, cell-mediated hypersensitivity reaction. The prototypical, common example of this type of reaction is ivy poison dermatitis due to urushiol resins found in poison ivy, poison oak, and poison sumac. Chemicals commonly associated with allergic contact dermatitis include permanent hair dyes (p-phenylenediamine), epoxy resins, and rubber accelerants, which can occur with both natural and synthetic rubber gloves and products. Allergic contact dermatitis requires prior sensitization, which takes a minimum of a few days of contact to occur, but can occur even after years of asymptomatic exposures. The reaction in sensitized individuals takes place within 1 to 2 days after contact with the allergen and manifests as intensely pruritic erythema followed by papular lesions and vesicles. Treatment consists of drying the weeping areas, and topical corticosteroids can be helpful. Rarely, systemic glucocorticoids are necessary when large areas are involved. Contact urticaria can occur in sensitized individuals using natural rubber latex gloves and may progress to systemic anaphylaxis (see later).

The amounts of toxic chemicals absorbed systemically from dermal exposure of intact skin are usually minimal. Exceptions include chlorinated hydrocarbons, warfarin, organophosphates, organic mercury, tetraethyl lead, and dimethylsulfoxide.[20] However, systemic effects can occur under certain circumstances, and because of recent improvements in airborne toxicant reductions and respiratory protection, the relative importance of dermal exposure has increased. Certain toxicants are listed by the regulatory bodies of several countries as having skin designation in addition to their allowable airborne exposure levels. The most common systemic poisoning from dermal exposure is cholinergic excess, occurring in the agricultural setting as a result of carbamate and organophosphorus pesticide exposures. Significant effects can also be seen after dermal contamination by aromatic amines, chlorinated hydrocarbons, and polycyclic aromatic hydrocarbons.[43] Concentrated hydrofluoric acid can cause systemic fluoride poisoning from even relatively small body surface area burns. Topical phenol can cause systemic poisoning as mentioned above.

Inhalation Exposures and Pulmonary Toxicity

Highly water-soluble irritant gases cause upper airway burning immediately, and if exposure continues, they

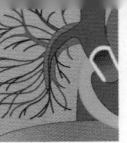

can cause lower airway and alveolar injury as well. Low-solubility gases such as phosgene and oxides of nitrogen cause little upper airway burning, so that workers tolerate prolonged exposures, only to suffer delayed acute lung injury hours later. Late effects can include reactive airway dysfunction syndrome/irritant-induced asthma, bronchiectasis, bronchiolitis obliterans fibrosa, and pulmonary fibrosis (for a more in-depth discussion, see Chapter 9).

Hypersensitivity reactions are caused by repeated exposure to specific organic and inorganic agents. Occupational asthma can occur after exposure to various high-molecular-weight antigens encountered in the workplace, most commonly animal and plant antigens such as bird feathers, animal excreta, and serum proteins. Plant antigens include wheat flour proteins, natural rubber latex, and wood dusts.

Most recently, latex allergy has become a significant problem among health care workers. Exposures to natural rubber latex have increased since 1980 because of increased glove use for protection from blood-borne pathogens. This has caused many workers to become sensitized, with an estimated prevalence of 2% to 17%. Natural rubber latex gloves can induce an immediate type I hypersensitivity reaction to the protein allergens, or a type IV delayed hypersensitivity reaction to the chemicals used to process the rubber gloves. Cornstarch powders used as donning agents act as vectors to increase inhalation and mucosal exposures to the allergens, and gloves with higher protein contents correlate with higher allergenicity. The use of powder-free, low-protein gloves has been shown to be effective in reducing symptoms and decreasing markers of systemic sensitization. As a minimum, all latex gloves in use should be low protein and powder free. Whenever possible, nonlatex gloves, such as those made of nit rile or vinyl, should be used. Use of these safer products will likely decrease the incidence of latex sensitization in health care workers.[44]

Certain low-molecular-weight antigens can induce occupational asthma as well, most notably isocyanates and trimellitic anhydride. The basic mechanism involved is type I, immunoglobulin E–mediated hypersensitivity reactions. Low-molecular-weight antigens and chemicals (TDI, TMA) can also cause occupational asthma. They sensitize by acting as a hapten and combining with serum proteins to become a complete antigen.

Hypersensitivity pneumonitis, also known as *extrinsic allergic alveolitis*, is an immunologic reaction probably involving type I and type IV mechanisms, and occurs after exposures to various antigens in the occupational setting. The most common is the prototypical disease Farmer's lung, caused by exposure to the antigens from thermophilic actinomyces from moldy hay (see Chapter 9).

Numerous gases encountered in the workplace act as asphyxiants. Simple asphyxiants exert their toxic effects by decreasing available oxygen concentration of inspired air. These include carbon dioxide, methane, propane, chlorinated hydrocarbons, and the noble gases. This usually occurs in confined spaces. The hydrocarbons also carry significant explosive risks as well. Chemical asphyxiants cause systemic poisoning by either disrupting natural hemoglobin's ability to carry oxygen (methemoglobin-forming agents such as nitrites; carbon monoxide causing carboxyhemoglobin) or by interfering with cellular utilization of oxygen (cytochrome oxidase poisoning by cyanide, hydrogen sulfide, or azide).

Inhalation absorption of toxicants is very rapid owing to the huge alveolar absorptive surface and the rich pulmonary capillary blood supply. In fact, inhalational absorption approaches the rapidity of intravenous administration. Once an agent has been absorbed, the clinical manifestations depend on many factors, including the inherent toxicity of the chemical, the total dose, and the duration of exposure. Exposure to other agents such as alcohol or drugs may modify the response (Table 82-1). The clinical spectrum is accordingly very broad.

OTHER ORGAN-SPECIFIC TOXICITY

Hepatotoxicity

The liver is the primary organ involved in the detoxification of xenobiotics, both from orally ingested drugs and toxicants and from inhaled or dermally absorbed toxicants. Hepatic enzyme systems metabolize lipid-soluble xenobiotics through phase I biotransformation reactions, usually through oxidation and reduction or hydration. Phase II reactions involve conjugation with glucuronides or glutathione, causing them to become more polar and excretable in the urine. In some instances, the oxidation system converts inactive chemicals to highly reactive electrophiles that can then cause hepatocellular necrosis (carbon tetrachloride). The most potent hepatotoxicants are chlorinated hydrocarbons (e.g., CCl_4, $CHCl_3$), white phosphorus, and dimethylformamide. Table 82-2 lists the common occupational hepatotoxicants.

Renal Toxicity

The kidneys will be exposed to most excreted toxicants because they receive 20% of the cardiac output. There are numerous P-450 metabolic enzymes present in renal tissue, and therefore certain toxicants can cause nephrotoxicity through reactive intermediates. Because renal excretion is the major elimination pathway, the kidneys will have significant exposure to these reactive species. The most common nephrotoxicants are metals and chlorinated solvents, but any agent that produces rhabdomyolysis or hemolysis can induce acute renal failure by pigment precipitation in the renal tubules. In such cases, adequate intravenous fluids and diuretics as needed to maintain high urine flow rates, as well as urinary alkalinization with intravenous sodium bicarbonate to prevent precipitation, can prevent renal injury. Table 82-3 lists industrial toxicants that can cause renal toxicity.

Cardiac Toxicity

Numerous industrial chemicals can cause cardiovascular toxicity. The most common acute toxicity is from in-

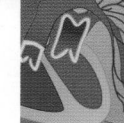

TABLE 82-1 Factors that Modify Risk for Occupationally Related Illness

MODIFYING FACTOR	KNOWN OR PROBABLE EFFECT
General	
Age	Youth—latency for cancer; elderly—more susceptible to toxicity
Sex	Sex differences exist for some toxicity states; reproductive effects
Smoking status	
Current smoker	Confers additive risk in some situations
Smoker at time of exposure	Confers synergistic risk in some situations
Smoking during exposure	Modifies toxic exposure in some situations, such as polymer fume fever
Family history	Hereditary conditions or predispositions may be exacerbated or triggered, such as in cancer-prone families
Exercise	
Conditioning	Fitness may reduce susceptibility in some situations
At time of exposure	Generally increased susceptibility
Metabolic states	Activity of certain enzyme systems involved in activation, detoxification, and adaptation to toxic exposures may modify response bout within range of normal
Medical	Generally, any debilitating condition may enhance clinical susceptibility
Atopy	
Asthma	Tendency toward easy sensitization
Eczema	Increased bronchial reactivity
Chronic respiratory disease	
Respiratory insufficiency	Diminished pulmonary reserve
Bronchitis	Increased bronchial reactivity; exacerbated bronchial irritation
Chronic cardiovascular disease	
Cardiac insufficency	Increased susceptibility
Coronary artery disease	Angina in some situations, such as carbon monoxide, methylene chloride exposure
Infection	
Acute viral illness	Increased susceptibility to bronchial irritation; possibly synergistic effect
Exposure to infectious agents	Certain exposures may depress host defenses
Immune deficiency states	Increased susceptibility to infections
Hereditary	
Immunosuppressive therapy	
Renal disease	Additive or synergistic effects may occur with exposure to nephorotoxic agents
Renal insufficiency	Increased susceptibility to toxic agents excreted via renal route
Chronic renal disease	Immunodeficiency; increased susceptibility to toxic effects
Neurologic conditions	
Diminished mental capacity	May affect judgement and response to exposure situation
Neurologic disease	Toxic effects may be additive; increased clinical susceptibility
Seizure disorder	Certain toxic exposures may alter threshold
Impaired perceptive ability (visual or hearing impairment, anosmia)	Impaired ability to avoid hazard
Dermatologic conditions	Skin rashes may increase dermal absorption; may condition response
Subtance abuse	Concomitant alcohol and drug abuse may have additive or synergistic effects in some situations
Hepatic insufficiency	Increased susceptibility to toxic agents detoxified by liver; increased susceptibility to hepatotoxic agent; reduced hepatic reserve
Systemic conditions	
Malnutrition (general)	Increased susceptibility to toxic effects
Vitamin deficiency (selective)	Diminished host defenses againts toxic effects
Inborn errors of metabolism	Selective susceptibility (depending on abnormality)
Genetic diseases	Certain genetic diseases associated with increased susceptibility to mutagenic effects
Mental status	Stress may increase susceptibility to some toxic exposure. Stress, affective disorders, neuroses, or psychoses may mask, mimic, or subtly modify the clinical presentation

(From Occupational and Environmental Health Committee of the American Lung Association of San Diego and Imperial Counties: Taking the occupational history. Ann Intern Med 1983;99:641–651.)

halation of hydrocarbons, especially halogenated hydrocarbons. They can sensitize the myocardium to endogenous as well as exogenous catecholamines, and ventricular arrhythmias can result. Historically, occupational toxicology studies showed carbon disulfide to be atherogenic, but newer data have called this effect into question.[45] Chronic exposure to nitrates can precipitate angina in workers when they withdraw from the chronic vasodilatory effects. Any systemic asphyxiants (H_2S, CO, CN, methemoglobin formers) can precipitate acute coronary syndromes in workers with preexisting atherosclerotic disease.

Neurotoxicity

Any of the simple asphyxiants can cause CNS depression and even death by displacing oxygen from the inspired air. Very high concentrations can cause rapid uncon-

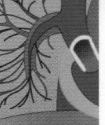

TABLE 82-2 Occupational Illnesses, Selected Associated Agents, and Associated Uses and Occupations and Industries[i–v],*

ILLNESS	AGENT	USE/OCCUPATION/INDUSTRY
Pulmonary injury ALI, ARDS, RADS/IIA, BOF Degree of injury, injury type, and sequelae, depend on exposure duration and agent. See text for discussion.	Irritant gases *Soluble* HCl, HF, H_2SO_4, HNO_3, NH_3, and other alkali and acid mists	Acid, alkali production workers; manure pits (NH_3 + H_2S)
	SO_2	Sulfuric acid production; air pollutant
	Tear gas	Law enforcement
	Isocyanates	
	Insoluble	Polyurethane industry, firefighters
	Phosgene	Polymer industry, welders—burning chlorinated metal degreasers
	Ozone	Any worker exposed to air pollution: city workers, bus drivers, cab drivers, etc.
	NO_2	Silo fillers, high temp arc welders, nitric acid workers
	Medium solubility	
	Chlorine	Water purification, paper pulp, swimming pool workers
	Acrolein	Polymer industry, firefighters (component of smoke)
	Smoke inhalation	Firefighters
	Pesticides Organophosphates (OP), carbamates, type II pyrethroids, dinitrophenol, pentachlorophenol (wood preservative), paraquat	Farmers, exterminators, crop dusters, pest control workers, lumber industry
	Metals and metal compounds	
	Cd, Hg, Mn	Smelters, welders
	Nickel carbonyl—$Ni(CO)_4$	Mond process of nickel refining
Occupational asthma (see Chapter 9 for expanded detail)	High-molecular-weight antigens Animal proteins (danders, feathers, excreta, serum)	Animal handlers, lab workers, farmers, many others
	Plant proteins	
	Natural rubber latex	Health care workers
	Wheat flour	Bakers (Baker's asthma)
	Low-molecular-weight antigens	
	Certain antibiotics, drugs	Pharmaceutical industry
	Metals: Cr, Co Ni, Pt, various others	Metal plating, metal workers, others
	Chemicals: Inorganic	
	Ammonium persulfate	Beauticians
	Fluoride	Aluminum pot-room workers
	Chemicals: Organic	
	Plicatic acid (Western red cedar)	Lumberjacks, sawmill workers
	Abeitic acid (colophony: pine rosin)	
	Isocyanates: TDI, MDI	Polyurethane foam workers
	Many others	See Chapter 9
Popcorn worker's lung	Diacetyl from artificial butter flavor	Microwave popcorn workers
Nylon flock worker's lung	Random-cut nylon flock	Nylon flock workers in random-cut factories
Pneumoconioses	Asbestos fibers: asbestosis	Asbestos miners, shipbuilders, insulators, brake linings
	Coal dust: coal workers' pneumoconiosis	Coal miners
	Silica: silicosis	Miners, sandblasters, foundries, quarries, stone carvers, ceramics
	Mica: combination of asbestosis and silicosis	Miners
Lung cancer[vi] (IARC Class I carcinogens)	Asbestos	Asbestos miners, shipbuilders, insulators, brake linings, vermiculite miners
	Arsenic (mainly arsenic trioxide)	Smelting lead, copper, gold, others; Arsenical pesticides; coal burning
	Beryllium	Beryllium extraction and processing; aircraft and aerospace industries; electronics and nuclear industries; jewelers
	Cadmium	Cadmium-smelter workers; battery production workers; cadmium-copper alloy workers; dyes and pigments
	Chloromethyl ethers *bis*(chloromethy) ether (BCME) and chloromethyl methyl ether (technical grade)	Production; chemical intermediate; alkylating agent laboratory reagent; plastic manufacturing; ion-exchange resins and polymers
	Chromium (Cr VI)	Chromium mining, chromate production
	Crystalline silica	Granite and stone industries; ceramics, glass, and related industries; foundries; and metallurgical industries; abrasives; construction; farming
	Enviromental tobacco smoke (ETS)	Bartenders, waitresses, etc.; other workers exposed to ETS

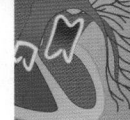

TABLE 82-2 Occupatinal Illnesses, Selected Associated Agents, and Associated Uses and Occupations and Industries[i–v],*—(Cont'd)

ILLNESS	AGENT	USE OCCUPATION INDUSTRY
Lung cancer (IARC Class 1 carcinogens) cont'd.	Ionizing radiation	Radiologists; technologists; nuclear workers; radium-dial, painters; plutonium workers; cleanup workers following nuclear accidents; aircraft crew
	Mustard gas	Mustard gas production; used in research laboratories; military personnel
	Nickel	Nickel refining
	Polycyclic aromatic hydrocarbons (PAHs)	Fossil fuel burning, exhaust smoke
	Radon	Uranium miners, other underground mining
	Talc (containing asbestos fibers)	Manufacture of pottery, paper, paint, and cosmetics
	Wood dusts	Loggers, carpenters, sawmills, etc.
Acute toxic encephalopathy	Acrylamide monomer	Wastewater treatment, grouting
	Azides	Lab reagent, preservative, weed control; inflates automobile air bags
	Carbon disulfide	Viscose rayon workers, rubber manufacture*
	Carbon monoxide	Any exposure to incomplete burning, improper ventilation, or exhaust: garage workers, firefighters; paint strippers (methylene chloride)
	Cyanide (CN)	Metal plating, jewelers, firefighters (smoke inhalation)
	Hydrogen sulfide	Farmers (manure pits), sewer workers, petroleum refineries
	Mercury	Chlor-alkali workers (electrolytic production of chlorine and caustic soda), manufacturing mercury-containing instruments, fungicide users, topical antiseptics*
Seizures	Simple asphyxiant gases (CO_2, CH_4, propane)	Gas production, various industries with confined space issues
	Toluene, xylene, other hyrocarbon solvent vapors	Painters, chemical production, solvent use (confined space)
	Metals	
	Arsenic	Smelting lead, copper, gold, others; arsenical pesticides
	Copper	Coal burning, leather tanning, pesticides
	Lead	Copper smelters, miners
		Lead-acid battery, HAZMAT site cleanup, automobile radiator repair, lead reclamation, solder
	Manganese	Mn miners, chemical industry, metal refining
	Nickel carbonyl	Model nickel refining process
	Pesticides	
	Organochlorines* (lindane, cyclodienes, DDT)	Farmers, agriculture, forestry, landscapers, pest control
	Organophosphates	
	Paraquat, Diquat (herbicides)	
	Pentachlorophenol (PCP)	
	Dinitrophenol	
	Chlorophenoxyacetic acid herbicides	
	Rodenticides* (thallium, SMFA, strychnine, Zn phosphide, As, methyl bromide)	Rodenticide users: graineries, longshoremen, exterminators (many of these rodenticides are no longer in use in the United States)
	Phosphine, methyl bromide (fumigants)	Grain workers
	Any general CNS depressant producing hypoxia	
	Toxic inhalants (CN, H_2S, CO)	See Acute Toxic Encephalopathy, above
	Simple asphyxiants (hydrocarbons, CO_2, He, N_2, etc.)	
	See also Toxic Encephalopathy, above	
	Chlorinated HC solvent vapors	
Peripheral neuropathy	Acrylamide monomer	Wastewater treatment, grouting
	Arsenic	Smelting lead, copper, gold, others; arsenical pesticides; coal burning, leather tanning, pesticides
	Carbon disulfide	Viscose rayon, rubber manufacturing
	Lead	Lead-acid battery, HAZMAT site cleanup, automobile radiator repair, lead reclamation, solder
	Mercury	Chlor-alkali workers (electrolytic production of chlorine and caustic soda), manufacturing mercury-containing instruments, fungicide users, topical antiseptics*
	Methyl bromide	Fumigation
	n-Hexane, methyl n-butyl ketone	Solvent users, glues
	Organophosphates	Pesticide users
	Thallium	Rodenticide users
	Trichloroethylene	Solvent, degreasers

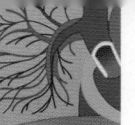

TABLE 82-2 Occupatinal Illnesses, Selected Associated Agents, and Associated Uses and Occupations and Industries[i–v,*]—(Cont'd)

ILLNESS	AGENT	USE OCCUPATION INDUSTRY
Cyanosis	Methemoglobin-forming agents: organic amino and nitro compounds*	Synthetic dyes, leather and shoe industry, fabric dyeing*
	CNS depressants causing hypoventilation and hypoxia	Various industries; see Toxic Encephalophathy, above
Hyperthermia/fever	Pentachlorophenol (wood preservative)	Lumber production, landscaping
	Nitrophenol pesticides	Exterminators, pest control, agriculture, farmers, forestry workers
	Chlorophenoxyacetic acid herbicides	Landscapers
	Inhalational fever syndromes	See Fume Fever Syndromes, below
Hematologic toxicants	Methemoglobin (MetHgb) producers	
	Aniline, nitroaniline, *p-chloroaniline* dyes	Rubber industry, dye manufacturing, dye users, pharmaceuticals
	Toluidine	Dyes
	Napthalene	Clothing fumigant (mothballs)
	Paradichlorobenzene	Clothing fumigant (mothballs)
	Nitrates	Fertilizers
	Trinitrotoluene (TNT)	Explosives
	Hemolytic agents	
	Any methemoglobin- producing agent (above) in G6PD-deficient workers, or with large exposures in normal workers	As above
	Arsine (AsH$_3$), stibine (SbH$_3$)	Dopant gases for n-type semi-conductors in the microelectronics industry; zinc smelting
	Chlorate salts (MetHgb unresponsive to methylene blue antidote, denatures hemoglobin)	Match and explosive production, dye manufacture, paper pulp bleach manufacturing (ClO$_2$), pesticides, herbicides
	Organic nitro and amino compounds	Synthetic dyes, leather and shoe industry, fabric dyeing
	Toxic porphyrias (acquired)	
	Hexachlorobenzene	Herbicide (accidental ingetion)
	2,4-D, 2-4-5-T herbicides (? due to TCCD contaminant	Herbicide
	Lead (when whole blood level > 60 µg/dL)	Lead-acid battery, HAZMAT site cleanup, automobile radiator repair, lead reclamation, soldering
	Vinyl chloride monomer	PVC production
	Bone marrow toxicants	
	Leukemogen	
	Benzene (acute myelogenous leukemia AML)	Chemical intermediate, glues, solvents, inks, paints; components of gasoline-petrochemical workers
	Ionizing radiation	Military exposures, uranium miners, nuclear power personnel
	Ethylene oxide (possible leukemogen)	Health care industry gas sterilizers; chemical intermediate
	Multiple myeloma (increased risk suggested, causation not proven)	
	Benzene	Chemical intermediate, glues, solvents, inks, paints; component of gasoline-petrochemical workers
	Ionizing radiation	Military exposures, uranium miners, nuclear power personnel
	Myelodysplastic syndromes (implicated toxicants);	
	Benzene	Chemical intermediate, glues, solvents, inks, paints; component of gasoline-petrochemical workers
	Ionizing radiation	Military exposures, uranium miners, nuclear power personnel
	Chemotherapeutic agents (association seen, risk not proved)	Nurses, oncologists, pharmacists
Rhabdomyolysis	Any agent causing seizures (see above)	See above
	Any agent causing hyperthermia associated with hypermetabolic state such as pentachlorophenol, dinitrophenol, chlorophenoxy herbicides	Farmers, lumber industry, pest control, exterminators
	CO (direct cellular toxicity)	Any exposure to incomplete burning, improper ventilation, or exhaust: garage workers, firefighters; paint strippers (methylene chloride)
	Any CNS depressants causing coma and thereby inducing rhabdomyolysis from pressure	See Toxic Encephalopathy, above

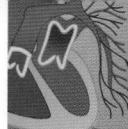

TABLE 82-2 Occupatinal Illnesses, Selected Associated Agents, and Associated Uses and Occupations and Industries[i–v],*—(Cont'd)

ILLNESS	AGENT	USE OCCUPATION INDUSTRY
Fume fever syndromes	Metal fume fever: Zn, Cu	Welders (galvanized metal), foundries, smelting, metal refining
	Polymer fume fever (PTFE)	Welders (cutting through Teflon coatings or polymer pipes), polymer workers
Organic dust toxic syndrome (ODTS) and other inhalation fevers	ODTS: Bio-aerosols of fungi, bacteria, exotoxins	
	Moldy hay, moldy silage, compost	Farmers (silo-unloader's disease)
	Sewage sludge	Sewer workers, plumbers
	Grain dust	Grain mills ("grain fever")
	Cotton dust	Cotton mills ("mill fever")
	Animal confinement buildings	Veterinary, laboratory workers
	Other inhalation fevers	
	Contaminated humidifiers	Any building with contaminated humidifiers (humidifier fever)
	Contaminated water cooling systems, spas, fountains	Any building with contaminated cooling system or fountain (Pontiac fever)
	Contaminated wood dusts/chips/bark (moldy wood chip exposure)	Sawmills, pulp and paper mills, landscapers (wood trimmer's disease)
Hypersensitivity pneumonitis (HP)	Organic antigen exposures	Farmers (farmer's lung)
	Moldy hay	Mushroom workers (mushroom worker's lung)
	Moldy compost	Office workers (any contaminated building)–humidifier lung
	Contaminated humidifiers, dehumidifiers, HVACs	Sugarcane workers (bagassosis)
	Bagasse (moldy pressed sugarcane)	Animal handlers, etc. (pigeon breeder's disease, duck fever)
	Animal products (excreta, serum, feathers, dander)	
	Chemicals	
	Trimellitic anhydride (TMA), phthalic anhydride	Painters, epoxy resin users
	Diisocyanates	Polyurethane foam industry
	Plicatic acid (red cedar)	Red cedar workers, lumber industry, carpenters
	Pyrethrum insecticides	Exterminators, pest control, insecticide manufacturing
	Sodium diazobenzene-sulfonate (Pauli's reagent)	Chromatography
	Many others (see Chapter 9)	Varied industries
Cardiovascular disease (atherosclerosis, myocardial infarction, and ischemia)	CO: acute MI and/or angina due to carboxyhemoglobin formation	Jobs with exposure to exhaust or poorly ventilated combustion: miners, forklift operators, mechanics, firefighters, etc.
	Methylene chloride (metabolized to CO)	Paint strippers, solvent use
	Carbon disulfide (CS_2) (recent evidence weak)	Viscose rayon workers,* rubber industry workers, chemical intermidiate
	Organic nitrates:	
	Ethylene glycol dinitrate	Explosive industry (TNT)
Cardiac arrhythmias		
Tachydysrhythmias	Chlorinated HC	Mechanics, degreasers, dry cleaners
	Hydrocarbon (HC) solvents	Printers, painters, mechanics, degreasers, dry cleaners
	CO	Paint strippers (CH_3Cl), jobs with exposure to exhaust or poorly ventilated combustion: miners, forklift operators, mechanics, firefighters, etc.
Bradydysrythmias	Organophosphates, carbamates	Farmers, pest control applicators
Nephrotoxicants	Arsine, stibine (due to massive hemolysis)	Semiconductor industry
	Halogenated hydrocarbon solvents (CCl_4, $CHCl_3$, ethylene dichloride, trichlorethylene, tetrachloroethane, others)	Dry cleaning, degreasers, plastics industry, other solvent use
	Vinylidene chloride	Monomer used in polymer industry
	Ethylene glycol ethers	Solvents, paints, coatings
	Ethylene chlorohydrin	Solvent, chemical intermediate; penetrates skin readily
	Toluene (ATN)	Painters
	White phosphorus	Match production (historical); military exposures
	Any agent associated with rhabdomyolysis	See above
	Beryllium (granulomatous renal disease, only seen with concomitant lung disease)	Beryllium extraction and processing; aircraft and aerospace industries; electronics and nuclear industries; jewelers
	Cadmium	Cadmium-smelter workers; battery production workers; cadmium-copper alloy workers; dyes and pigments, welders
	Lead	Lead-acid battery, HAZMAT site cleanup, automobile radiator repair, lead reclamation, soldering

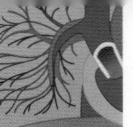

TABLE 82-2 Occupatinal Illnesses, Selected Associated Agents, and Associated Uses and Occupations and Industries[i-v,]*—(Cont'd)

ILLNESS	AGENT	USE OCCUPATION INDUSTRY
	Mercury	Chlor-alkali workers (electrolytic production of chlorine and caustic soda), manufacturing mercury-containing instruments, fungicide users, topical antiseptics*
Acute hepatoxicants[vii]	Anesthetic gases (halothane)	Anesthesiologists, nurses
	Hydrazine (steatosis)	Rocket fuels
	Halogenated hydrocarbons: CCl_4, CBr_4, $CHCl_3$, bromobenzene, others	Mechanics, degreasers, dry cleaners, plastics industry, solvents
	White phosphorus	Match production (historical); military exposures
	Methylene dianiline (MDA): cholestatic "Epping jaundice"	Epoxy resins
	Trinitrotoluene (TNT)	Explosives
	Dimethylacetamide	Textile workers
	Dimethylformamide (DMF)	Solvents, chemical manufacturing
	2-Nitropropane	Painters
Chronic hepatotoxicants	Cirrhosis	
	Arsenic	Smelting lead, copper, gold, others; arsenical pesticides; coal burning, leather tanning, pesticides
	CCl_4	Chemical intermediate
	Tetrachloroethane	Solvent
	Trinitrotoluene	Explosives
	Granulomatous hepatic disease	
	Beryllium (only seen with concomitant lung disease)	Beryllium extraction and processing; aircraft and aerospace industries; electronics and nuclear industries; jewelers
	Copper	Copper smelting, production workers
Hepatic carcinogens	Arsenic: hepatic angiosarcoma, hepatocellular carcinoma	Smelting lead, copper, gold, others; arsenical pesticides; coal burning, leather tanning, pesticides
	Vinyl chloride monomer: hepatic angiosarcoma	Polyvinyl chloride industry
	Dimethylnitrosamine: hepatocellular carcinoma	Rocket manufacturing
Skin disorders		
Chloracne	Chlorinated herbicides (2,4-D, 2,4,5-T)	Herbicide use (probably due to TCDD contaminant)
	PCBs	Electrical transformer insulators
	TCDD ("dioxin")	As above
Occupational acne	Lubricating oils	Metalworkers, mechanics
	Petroleum oils	Refinery workers, highway workers
	Vegetable oils	Fry cooks
Contact dermatitis	Irritant contact dermatitis	
	Solvents, oils	Solvent users, metalworkers, mechanics
	Soaps, frequent hard washing	Health care workers, food workers
	Allegic contact dermatitis	
	Biocides	Water treatment, pool workers
	Chromate	Inks, dyes, paints, corrosion inhibitors
	Epoxy resins	Epoxy resin manufacturers
	Formaldehyde	Formaldehyde workers, pathologists, deniers, morticians
	p-Phenylenediamine (hair dye)	Beauticians, rubber workers, rubber workers
	Para-aminobenzoic acid (PABA) sunscreens	Outdoor workers
Skin cancer	Arsenic	Smelting lead, copper, gold, others; arsenical pesticides; coal burning, leather tanning, pesticides
	Ionizing radiation	Radiologists; technologists; nuclear workers; radium-dial, painters; plutonium workers; claenup workers following nuclear accidents; aircraft crew
	Polycyclic aromatic hydrocarbons	Coal tar workers, petroleum products, chimney sweeps
	Ultraviolet radiation (sunlight)	Outdoor workers
Reproductive toxicants		
Female reproductive system	Chemotherapeutic agents anesthetic gases	Health care workers, nurses, anesthesiology
	Chlorinated hydrocarbon solvents	Solvent users
	Ionizing radiation	Radiologists; technologists; nuclear workers; radium-dial, painters; plutonium workers; cleanup workers following nuclear accidents
	Environmental tobacco smoke (ETS)	Bartenders, waitresses, etc.; other workers exposed to ETS
	Mercury	Chlor-alkali workers (electrolytic production of chlorine and caustic soda), manufacturing mercury-containing instruments, fungicide users, topical antiseptics*
	Lead	Lead-acid battery, HAZMAT site cleanup, automobile radiator repair, lead reclamation, soldering

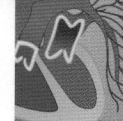

TABLE 82-2 Occupatinal Illnesses, Selected Associated Agents, and Associated Uses and Occupations and Industries[i-v],*—(Cont'd)

ILLNESS	AGENT	USE OCCUPATION INDUSTRY
Male reproductive toxicants	Carbon disulfide	Viscose rayon workers,* rubber industry workers, chemical intermediate
	Dibromochloropropane (DBCP)	Nematocide users, applicators; DBCP production workers
	Ionizing radiation	Radiologists; technologists; nuclear workers; radium-dial, painters; plutonium workers; cleanup workers following nuclear accidents; aircraft crew
	Lead	Lead-acid battery, HAZMAT site cleanup, automobile radiator repair, lead reclamation, soldering
	Pesticides (chlordecone, carbaryl, 2,4-D, ethylene dibromide)	Farmers, pest control applicators

*Many of the chemicals/toxicants may no longer be used or manufactured in the United States but still are in common use in other parts of the world. U.S. industries with modern IH practices have limited or eliminated many exposures to industrial toxicants, but workers in developing nations may remain at substantial risk.

[i]Hazardous Substances Database (HSDB). Available at: http://toxnet.nlm.nih.gov/.
[ii]McCunney RJ (ed): A Practical Approach to Occupational and Environmental Medicine, 3rd ed. Philadelphia, Lippincott Williams & Wilkins, 2003.
[iii]Rom WN (ed): Environmental and Occupational Medicine, 3rd ed. Philadelphia, Lippincott-Raven, 1998.
[iv]Zenz C (ed): Occupational Medicine, 3rd ed. St. Louis, Mosby, 1994.
[v]LaDou J (ed): Occupational and Environmental Medicine, 3rd ed. New York, Mc Graw-Hill, 2004.
[vi]Siemiatycki J, Richardson L, Straif K, et al: Listing occupational carcinogens. Environ health Perspect 2004;9112(15):1447–1459.
[vii]Leikin JB, Davis A, Klodd DA, Thunder T, et al: Selected topics related to occupational exposures. Part IV. Occupational liver disease. Dis Mon 2000;46(4): 295–310.
ALI, acute lung injury; AML, acute myelogenous leukemia; ARDS, adult respiratory distress syndrome; BOF, bronchiolitis obliterans fibrosa; G6PD, glucose 6-phosphate dehydrogenase; IARC, International Agency for Research on Cancer; IIA, irritant-induced asthma; MDI, methyl diphenyl diisocyanate; MI, myocardial infarction; PCB, polychlorinated biphenyl; PTFE, polytetrafluoroethylene; PVC, polyvinyl chloride; RADS, reactive dysfunction airway dysfunction syndrome; SMFA, sodium monofluoroacetate; TCDD, 2,3,7,8-tetrachlorodibenzo-p-dioxin; TDI, toluene diisocyanate. Chart adapted from Holland MG: The critically poisoned worker. In Brent J, Wallace KL, Burkhart KK, et al (eds): Critical Care Toxicology. St. Louis, Mosby, 2005, used with permission.

sciousness. Numerous volatile hydrocarbons, both aliphatic and aromatic, as well as halogenated hydrocarbons, can have general anesthetic effects when inhaled, leading to CNS depression and even to coma in high doses. Lower doses cause dizziness, lightheadedness, or a drunk or "high" feeling. Chemical asphyxiants cause CNS depression by interfering with oxygen transport or utilization (discussed previously).

Peripheral neuropathies can be induced by *n*-hexane and methyl *n*-butyl ketone, which share the common toxic metabolite 2,5-hexanedione. This effect is potentiated when these hexacarbons exist in mixtures containing MEK. Acrylamide monomer can induce both CNS effects in high concentrations and a peripheral neuropathy following an acute high-dose exposure or chronic exposure. These hexacarbons, as well as carbon disulfide, ethylene oxide, and heavy metals (arsenic, thallium, lead, mercury), are commonly cited as causes of peripheral neuropathy. Certain organic phosphorus compounds (e.g., tri-ortho cresyl phosphate) can induce peripheral neuropathy through inhibition of the enzyme neuropathic target esterase, which is independent of its acetylcholinesterase inhibition.

Reproductive Toxicology

Few toxicants have been definitively shown to adversely affect female reproduction, mainly because few have been adequately investigated. Those that have shown strong associations with an increased incidence of spon-

taneous abortions are environmental tobacco smoke, ionizing radiation, chemotherapeutic agents, mercury, and lead. In addition, chlorinated hydrocarbon solvents, anesthetic gases, and chemotherapeutic agents have been associated with birth defects.

There exists slightly more evidence for male reproductive toxicants. The most notable historically is dibromochloropropane (DBCP), a nematocide. DBCP production workers developed dose-dependent decreased sperm counts, with azoospermia in the highest exposure groups. Lead can cause oligospermia and decreased libido. Other reproductive toxicants include carbon disulfide, ionizing radiation, and other pesticides (chlordecone, carbaryl, 2,4-D, ethylene dibromide).

LABORATORY EVALUATION

The current role of the clinical laboratory in the medical management of industrial poisoning is to help provide effective supportive care (e.g., arterial blood gases, acid–base status, complete blood count). Blood and urine levels of most occupational toxicants are not available acutely and are used primarily to document exposures. Some are obtained as mandatory medical monitoring and, if elevated to a certain level, may require medical removal from further exposure. Twenty-four-hour urine collections and blood levels for some metals can guide the need for chelation therapy. Elevated BEIs can indicate overexposure in the workplace, or improper use of PPE.

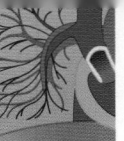

TABLE 82-3 Internet Sources of Information on Toxicologic Properties of Various Chemical Agents

INTERNET SERVICE	WEBSITE COMMON NAME	WEB ADDRESS	DESCRIPTION
Toxicology Data Network The following databases are all included in TOXNET and can be searched individually or simultaneously via TOXNET.	TOXNET	http://toxnet.nlm.nih.gov	Allows searching of nine different databases below all at once
Hazardous Substances Data Bank	HSDB	http://toxnet.nlm.nih.gov/cgi-bin/sis/htmlgen?HSDB	Included in TOXNET search; broad scope in human and animal toxicity, safety and handling, environmental fate, and more. Scientifically peer-reviewed.
Integrated Risk Information System	IRIS	http://toxnet.nlm.nih.gov/cgi-bin/sis/htmlgen?IRIS	Data from the EPA in support of human health risk assessment, focusing on hazard identification and dose–response assessment.
International Toxicity Estimates for Risk	ITER	http://toxnet.nlm.nih.gov/cgi-bin/sis/htmlgen?iter	Provides chemical risk information from authoritative groups worldwide (EPA, ATSDR, Health Canada, IARC, etc.) peer-reviewed.
Genetic Toxicology (Mutagenicity)	Gene-Tox	http://toxnet.nlm.nih.gov/cgi-bin/sis/htmlgen?GENETOX	Peer-reviewed mutagenicity test data from the EPA
Chemical Carcinogenesis Research Information System	CCRIS	http://toxnet.nlm.nih.gov/cgi-bin/sis/htmlgen?CCRIS	Carcinogenicity, mutagenicity, tumor promotion, and tumor inhibition data from the National Cancer Institute
Toxicology Bibliographic Information	Toxline	http://toxnet.nlm.nih.gov/cgi-bin/sis/htmlgen?TOXLINE	Biochemical, pharmacologic, physiologic, and toxicologic effects of drugs, chemicals
Developmental and Reproductive Toxicology and Environmental Teratology Information Center	DART/ETIC	http://toxnet. nlm.nih.gov/cgi-bin/sis/htmlgen?DARTETIC	Current and older literature on developmental and reproductive toxicology
Toxica Release Inventory	TRI	http://toxnet.nlm.nih.gov/cgi-bin/sis/htmlgen?TRI	Annual estimated releases of toxic chemicals to the environment—EPA's TRI (Toxics Release Inventory)—reporting years, 1995–2000.
Chemical Identification Plus	ChemID plus	http://chem.sis.nlm.nih.gov/chemidplus/chemidlite.jsp	Numerous chemical synonyms, structures, regulatory list information, and links to other databases containing information about the chemicals.
Haz-Map	Haz-Map	http://hazmap.nlm.nih.gov/	Chemicals and biologic agents in Haz-Map are linked to industrial processes and other activities such as hobbies. Occupational diseases and their symptoms are associated with hazardous job tasks and possible exposure to hazardous agents.
MSDS online	MSDSonline	http://www.msdsonline.com/	On-line access to millions of MSDS
Agency for Toxic Substances and Disease Registry	ATSDR ToxFAQ	http://www.atsdr.cdc.gov/toxfaq.html	Series of summaries about hazardous subtances developed by the ATSDR Division of Toxicology
Agency for Toxic Subtances and Disease Registry	ATSDR toxicologic Profiles	http://www.atsdr.cdc.gov/toxpro2.html	ATSDR produces "toxicologic profiles" for hazardous substances found at National Priorities List (NPL) sites.Ranked based on frequency of occurrence at NPL sites, toxicity, and potential for human exposure. Developed from a priority list of 275 substances.
National Pesticide Information Center	NPIC	http://npic.orst.edu/	Cooperative effort between Oregon State University and the EPA, offers objective, science-based pesticide information
New Jersey Department of Health	Hazardous Substances Fact Sheets	http://www.state.nj.us/health/eoh/rtkweb/rtkhsfs.htm	Brief fact sheets containing physical, chemical, toxicologic, and medical data on hundreds of substances

EPA, U.S. Environmental Protection Agency.

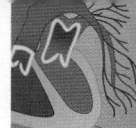

Acutely, some tests are helpful after inhalation exposures to toxic gases, such as carboxyhemoglobin and methemoglobin levels. Whole blood lead levels can often be obtained acutely, and guide therapy. Central to the evaluation of pulmonary problems are chest radiography and pulmonary function testing. Radiography may reveal aspiration pneumonitis, noncardiogenic pulmonary edema, pleural effusions, or interstitial fibrosis. High-resolution computed tomography of the chest is more sensitive in detecting subtle opacities in many occupational lung diseases, such as hypersensitivity pneumonitis (HP), coal worker's pneumoconiosis (CWP), and other pneumoconioses. A xenon ventilation-perfusion lung scan may be useful in patients with suspected inhalation injury.

Electrocardiography is neither very sensitive nor specific for diagnosing occupational exposures or illnesses. Chemical asphyxiants or arsenic may produce an ECG picture of myocardial ischemia by interfering with cellular respiration, and the ECG may reveal ischemic changes. Both arsine and antimony have been associated with abnormalities of the T waves. Overexposure to phosphorous, hydrofluoric acid (due to subsequent hypocalcemia), or arsenic can cause QT-segment prolongation.

INFORMATION SOURCES

The clinician is often faced with incomplete toxicologic data on which to base treatment. If adequate information on the toxic agent is not available on site or from the manufacturer, the nearest poison control center should be contacted once the chemical has been identified. Poison control centers rely on a wide variety of information sources and specialty consultants to assess toxicity and can offer treatment advice. The Regional Poison Control Center can be accessed by the national toll-free number at 1-800-222-1222.

There is no comprehensive database available anywhere that will have information on every chemical that is in commercial use. Information on the toxicologic properties of chemical agents is available in various forms and from various agencies and organizations. Therefore, the clinician should be familiar with the readily available sources of information for chemicals and how to readily access them. Table 82-3 lists useful websites that have information regarding toxicologic properties of various agents.

SUMMARY

Legislative measures, such as the Toxic Substances Control Act of 1976, alone may not be sufficient to reduce occupational disease significantly. Millions of chemicals exist, about 70,000 chemical substances are in common use, and several hundred new compounds are added by industrial processes each year. Unpredicted health hazards from new processes continue to emerge, and "well-known" occupational exposures still escape

surveillance and control.[15] As a result, any patient presenting with an unusual symptom or group of symptoms should always prompt suspicion of an occupationally related disease. A systematic approach to recording the occupational history serves as a guide to discovering a specific toxic exposure that may be the cause of the presenting symptoms. Even when such a history is unavailable, a thorough physical examination and initial laboratory analysis may suggest a toxidrome that can lead the clinician to an early toxicologic diagnosis.

The predominant route of exposure to toxicants in the occupational setting is through inhalation. Irritant gases, metal dusts or fumes, and chemicals of extreme pH or reactivity may produce mucosal damage to the respiratory tract. The location of injury depends on the water solubility and particle size of the substance. The highly water-soluble gases—ammonia, hydrogen chloride, and hydrogen fluoride—dissolve readily in the moisture associated with the mucous membranes of the eyes, nose, and upper respiratory tract. Inflammation, ulceration, edema, and necrosis may acutely obstruct the upper airway. Recovery may be incomplete, and reactive airways dysfunction syndrome, also known as *irritant-induced asthma*, may result. Gases with a low solubility in water, such as ozone, nitrogen dioxide, and phosgene, reach the lower airway and can produce acute lung injury pneumonitis and pulmonary edema. Potential late effects from the inhalation of these substances include bronchiolitis obliterans fibrosa, bronchiectasis, chronic bronchitis, and varying degrees of pulmonary fibrosis.

Most respiratory irritants are gases or vapors, but they may also exist as particulates (e.g., mist) or may be absorbed onto particulates (e.g., sulfur dioxide).[46] The particle size largely determines the extent of accessibility to small airways. Particles measuring between 1 and 5 μm can reach the alveoli. Pneumoconiosis is the result of chronic exposure to dusts (e.g., asbestos) and leads to the development of fibrorestrictive disease. Systemic absorption of inhaled occupational toxicants can lead to effects on many other organ systems.

Occupational dermatoses are the most common occupational diseases, with irritant contact dermatitis and allergic contact dermatitis predominating. Dermal absorption can also lead to systemic poisoning, especially with certain toxicants such as phenol, hydrofluoric acids, and pesticides. Table 82-2 lists some common occupational illnesses and their causative agents seen in various industrial and occupational settings.

REFERENCES

1. U.S. Department of Labor, Bureau of Labor Statistics, Census of Fatal Occupational Injuries: 2003 Data. Available at: http://www.bls.gov.
2. U.S. Department of Labor, Bureau of Labor Statistics, Census of Non-Fatal Occupational Injuries: 2003 Data. Available at: http://www.bls.gov.
3. World Health Organization (WHO). Available at: http://www.who.int.
4. World Health Organization Global strategy on Occupational Health. Available at: http://www.who.int.
5. U.S. EPA Inventory Update Rule. Available at: http://www.epa.gov.

6. Weber LW: Georgius Agricola (1495–1555): scholar, physician, scientist, entrepreneur, diplomat. Toxicol Sci 2002;69(2):292–294.

7. Ramazzini B: Diseases of Workers. New York, Hafner, 1964.

8. Hamilton A: Exploring the Dangerous Trades. Beverly Farms, Mass, OEM Press, 1995.

9. Linz DH, Barker AF, Morton WE, et al: Occupational toxic inhalations. Top Emerg Med 1985;7:21–33.

10. Israel-Assayag E, Dakhama A, Lavigne S, et al: Expression of costimulatory molecules on alveolar macrophages in hyper-sensitivity pneumonitis. Am J Respir Crit Care Med 1999; 159(6):1830–1834.

11. Levy B: The teaching of occupational health in American medical schools: five year follow-up of initial study. Am J Public Health 1985;75:79–80.

12. Wynn PA, Aw TC, Williams NR, Harrington M: Teaching of occupational medicine to undergraduates in UK schools of medicine. Occup Med (Lond) 2003;53(6):349–353.

13. Shanahan EM, Murray AM, Lillington T, Farmer EA: The teaching of occupational and environmental medicine to medical students in Australia and New Zealand. Occup Med (Lond) 2000; 50(4):246–250.

14. LaDou J: The rise and fall of occupational medicine in the United States. Am J Prev Med 2002;22:285–295.

15. Goldman RH, Peters JM: The occupational and environmental health history. JAMA 1981;246:2831–2836.

16. Hill AB: The environment and disease: association or causation. Proc R Soc Med 1965;58:295–300.

17. Centers for Disease Control and Prevention (CDC): Children with elevated blood lead levels attributed to home renovation and remodeling activities—New York, 1993–1994. MMWR Morb Mortal Wkly Rep 1997;45(51–52):1120–1123.

18. Morales Bonilla C, Mauss EA: A community-initiated study of blood lead levels of Nicaraguan children living near a battery factory. Am J Public Health 1998;88(12):1843–1845 [erratum in Am J Public Health 1999;89(2):256].

19. Whelan EA, Piacitelli GM, Gerwel B, et al: Elevated blood lead levels in children of construction workers. Am J Public Health 1997;87(8):1352–1355.

20. O'Tuama LA, Rogers JF, Rogan W: Lead absorption by children of battery workers. JAMA 1979;241(18):1893.

21. Gerson M, Van den Eeden SK, Gahagan P: Take-home lead poisoning in a child from his father's occupational exposure. Am J Ind Med 1996;29(5):507–508.

22. Aguilar-Garduno C, Lacasana M, Tellez-Rojo MM, et al: Indirect lead exposure among children of radiator repair workers. Am J Ind Med 2003;43(6):662–667.

23. Lesser SH, Weiss SJ: Art hazards. Am J Emerg Med 1995; 13(4):451–458.

24. Spandorfer M, Curtiss D, Snyder JW: Health hazards in drawing and painting. Occup Med 2001;16(4):535–555.

25. Weiss SJ, Lesser SH: Hazards associated with metalworking by artists. South Med J 1997;90(7):665–771.

26. Dorevitch S, Babin A: Health hazards of ceramic artists. Occup Med 2001;16(4):563–575.

27. ATSDR Case studies in Environmental Medicine: Taking an exposure history. Available at: http://www.atsdr.cdc.gov.

28. Kern DG. Kuhn C 3rd, Ely EW, et al: Flock worker's lung: broadening the spectrum of clinicopathology, narrowing the spectrum of suspected etiologies. Chest 2000;117(1):251–259.

29. Centers for Disease Control and Prevention (CDC): Chronic interstitial lung disease in nylon flocking industry workers—Rhode Island, 1992–1996. MMWR Morb Mortal Wkly Rep 1997;46:897–901.

30. Porter DW, Castranova V, Robinson VA, et al: Acute inflammatory reaction in rats after intratracheal instillation of material collected from a nylon flocking plant. J Toxicol Environ Health 1999; 57:25–45

31. Kuhn DM, Ghannoum MA: Indoor mold, toxigenic fungi, and Stachybotrys chartarum: infectious disease perspective. Clin Microbiol Rev 2003;16(1):144–172.

32. Evidence Based Statements: Adverse human health effects associated with molds in the indoor environment. 2002 American College of Occupational and Environmental Medicine. Available at: http://www.acoem.org.

33. Assoulin-Daya Y, Leong A, Shoenfeld Y, Gershwin ME: Studies of sick building syndrome. IV. Mycotoxicosis. J Asthma 2002; 39(3):191–201.

34. Bardana EJ Jr: Indoor air quality and health: does fungal contamination play a significant role? Immunol Allergy Clin North Am 2003;23(2):291–309.

35. Nieuwenhuizen MS, Groeneveld FR: Formation of phosgene during welding activities in an atmosphere containing chlorinated hydrocarbons. AIHAJ 2000;61(4):539–543.

36. Sjogren B, Plato N, Alexandersson R, et al: Pulmonary reactions caused by welding-induced decomposed trichloroethylene. Chest 1991;99(1):237–238.

37. OSHA Toxic and Hazardous Substances: Air borne contaminants, CFR 1910.10000. Available at: http://www.osha.gov.

38. Occupational Safety and Health Administration (OSHA): CFR 1910 Occupational Safety and Health Standards. Available at: http://www.osha.gov.

39. American Conference of Industrial Hygienists (ACGIH). Available at: http://www.acgih.org.

40. National Institute for Occupational Safety and Health (NIOSH): Pocket Guide to Chemical Hazards. Available at: http://www.cdc.gov.

41. National Institute for Occupational Safety and Health (NIOSH): IDLH listing. Available at: http://www.cdc.gov.

42. Bentur Y, Shoshani O, Tabak A, et al: Prolonged elimination half-life of phenol after dermal exposure. J Toxicol Clin Toxicol 1998;36(7):707–711.

43. Sartorelli P: Dermal exposure assessment in occupational medicine. Occup Med (Lond) 2002;52(3):151–156.

44. Ahmed SM, Aw TC, Adisesh A: Toxicological and immunological aspects of occupational latex allergy. Toxicol Rev 2004;23(2): 123–134.

45. Sulsky SI, Hooven FH, Burch MT, Mundt KA: Critical review of the epidemiological literature on the potential cardiovascular effects of occupational carbon disulfide exposure. Int Arch Occup Environ Health 2002;75(6):365–380.

46. Smith DC: Acute inhalation injury. Clin Pulm Med 1999;6(4): 224–235.

83 *Environmental Toxicology*

EDWIN M. KILBOURNE, MD ■ JEFFREY B. NEMHAUSER, MD

At a Glance...

- Environmental exposure pathways include the ambient air, water, dust, soil and other solids, and other living organisms.

- In situations of chemical environmental contamination, an obvious and clearcut relationship of an exposure and a health impact is relatively uncommon.

- When the health impact of an environmental exposure is unclear, public health and environmental authorities are the clinician's best source of guidance.

- Risk assessment is the process used to determine the relationship between toxicant exposure and the development of adverse health effects.

- Risk assessment requires: (1) identification of the hazard; (2) assessment of the toxicity of the hazard (e.g., dose–response relationship); (3) characterization of the exposure of the population; and (4) characterization of the risk (e.g., risk quantification).

- Risk management includes plans to separate people from the substances that may harm them.

- Certain federal agencies have developed standards for nonoccupational exposure limits, which represent an estimated daily human exposure below which there is a minimal risk for developing adverse health effects.

- Knowledge of the various environmental and public health agencies and their responsibilities can facilitate the care of patients exposed to environmental contaminants.

Environmental toxicology is the study of adverse effects that occur in living organisms from exposure to hazardous substances or pollutants in the surrounding ecosystem. The impact of these chemicals on human health is one focus of this discipline. Environmental toxicology is defined by context and not by a specific set of toxicants or agents. Toxicology is "environmental" by virtue of the routes, doses, and contexts underlying the exposures. Generally, the term *environmental* is applied to exposures that occur outside the workplace and in the area where a patient lives. Exposures are usually either unavoidable or difficult to avoid.

The concept of environmental toxicology as it relates to humans may be more easily understood from examples: Exposure to silica dust in a facility specializing in finishing quarried stone would be considered "occupational" rather than environmental, since the silica in inspired air can be reduced by adequate personal protective equipment, by a change in work practices, by relocating workers, or by other means. Indeed, one can avoid the exposure entirely by choosing other employment. On the other hand, the airborne mercury exposure of populations located downwind of coal-fired power plants is not easily controlled by the individual. Likewise, where arsenic is present in higher than recommended

levels in finished drinking water or polychlorinated biphenyls (PCBs) are present in fish sold for human consumption, these are exposures in a person's physical surroundings or environment.

Environmental media or exposure pathways include all of the principal classes of substances with which people regularly come in contact and which may convey environmental toxicants. These media include the ambient air (both indoor and outdoor), recreational water and drinking water, dust, soil and other solids, and other living organisms. Food and drink should be considered environmental media unless the toxins or toxicants they may contain are sufficiently familiar for them to be easily identified and avoided. For example, it is possible to avoid exposure to nicotine and to the carcinogens in cigarettes or to abstain from ingestion of ethanol in beer and other alcoholic beverages. Rarely, the clinical, social, and political contexts concerning certain parenteral exposures allow them, too, to be considered "environmental." Recent concerns about thimerosal in pediatric vaccines fall into this category.[1]

HISTORY

Environmental health in the United States arose as an active field of endeavor in the 19th century. Indeed, it was the principal component of public health during that era. However, early environmental health was concerned primarily with the control of infectious diseases. The field was based on the work of such scientists as Joseph Lister, who used disinfectants (carbolic acid or phenol) in medical procedures to decrease the incidence of (and mortality from) wound infection and sepsis.[2] In 1854, another leader in the environmental control of infections, John Snow, interrupted transmission of cholera in London by identifying and restricting access to a source of contaminated drinking water.[3]

Based on the work of these and many other public health leaders, the "sanitary revolution" of the late 19th and early 20th centuries transformed the spectrum of health and disease in Europe and North America, resulting in substantial decreases in the deaths of newborns and infants from diarrhea and consequent dehydration.[4] The availability of pure drinking water was a major contributor to the dramatic increases in overall life expectancy that occurred during this period.[5]

The possible admixture of toxic substances into food, water, and other ingested products has caused public concern since at least the early 20th century. After World War II, however, the continuing increase in the industrialization of North America and the burgeoning use of a wide variety of chemical products brought noninfectious environmental problems to the forefront. Chemical

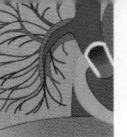

pollution generated increased concern about water quality. Air pollution, previously a safety concern in the workplace, became a major health concern in the general environment, although concerns about outdoor and indoor air differed. By the late 1970s, the documentation of many instances of extensive land and soil-surface pollution from highly toxic substances located in close proximity to residential areas (as occurred at Love Canal in Niagara Falls, New York) generated worry about human proximity to highly toxic environmental solids.

CLINICAL CONSIDERATIONS

Situational Factors

The special considerations pertaining to toxicants found in the environment are most relevant to physicians attending or consulting on individual cases in two broad sets of circumstances:

1. *Active Community Discussion.* There may be ongoing discussions and concern in the larger community or region about a particular environmental exposure or set of exposures. Such concerns may or may not represent a realistic view of the risks involved.
2. *Individual Concern.* Fears about the consequences of a particular exposure or perceived exposure may be patient specific and independent of any particular community concern about the environment. Patients develop such concerns (a) on their own, (b) based on interactions with other health practitioners, (c) based on findings of laboratories specializing in biomonitoring of various substances, or (d) based on their interactions with advocacy groups.

Under any of these sets of circumstances, the physician should be mindful of the broader set of societal issues that likely constitute the patient's frame of reference. Where an active community discussion exists about a specific environmental exposure or set of exposures, there are typically broader social, economic, and political forces at work. For example, concerns about decreased residential property values may energize assertions of a negative health impact. On the other hand, the threat to bottom line corporate profits may lead a company to disclaim responsibility for any illness. The practitioner should be aware that assertions made on either side of an environmental debate often lack clear-cut scientific support.

To the extent possible, the physician should determine the patient's individual relationship to these larger processes. He or she should attempt to understand how community concerns of all types may serve as stressors or otherwise influence the clinical presentation at hand. It is particularly important for the physician not to prejudge the medical importance of the presenting complaints. A relationship of the symptoms to an environmental exposure should not be assumed, nor should it be summarily discounted. The diagnostic workup should involve a careful history and physical examination, with due weight given to all reasonably possible causes of the presenting symptoms, whether or not they relate to the community concerns about the environment.

Nor should the clinician assume that the lay press has described a possible environmental exposure or the type(s) of environmental contamination either accurately or completely. Press stories may be unduly influenced by the unverified assertions of interested parties. Where specific data about the environment are needed to properly evaluate the patient, the physician should contact the relevant public health officials or environmental authorities who will likely have detailed and reliable information.

Clear-cut Exposures

There are few doubts about the clinical status of patients who present with a typical history of an exposure and matching clinical findings. However, in situations of chemical environmental contamination, an obvious and clear-cut relationship of an exposure and a health impact is relatively uncommon. It occurs, for example, in the context of abrupt releases of toxic environmental contaminants causing familiar syndromes with short latencies (e.g., the abrupt onset of respiratory findings following chlorine gas exposure due to derailment and rupture of a chlorine-containing tanker car). At such times, the authorities responsible for handling acute contamination events should convey information regarding the nature of the contamination to local health care providers. The means for this notification should be written into local emergency management plans. Ideally, local environmental officials will communicate this information to departments of public health and to relevant health care organizations, including those responsible for emergency medical services and also to the directors of poison control centers in the affected areas. If they do not receive information about the exposure through their hospitals or health care organizations, clinicians may wish to contact environmental or public health officials directly in an emergency.

Less commonly, typical illness from an environmental exposure will emerge over a period of days to weeks (or even months) as an ongoing intoxication epidemic comes to medical attention. Such retrospective identification of an environmentally mediated epidemic occurred in the eosinophilia-myalgia syndrome episode that occurred in the United States in 1989.[6] More recently, hundreds of residents of Libby, Montana, who did not necessarily have any direct occupational exposure to asbestos were found to have clinical findings consistent with asbestosis, apparently from exposure to asbestos-containing mineral tailings distributed widely throughout the community.[7]

Poorly Defined Exposures

Because of the evident danger to people potentially affected by the environmental exposures with a clear-cut etiologic and demonstrable health impact, such occurrences are typically treated as emergencies. The immediacy of an unambiguous threat prompts an unequivocal call for environmental remediation and for appropriate treatment or management of affected persons.

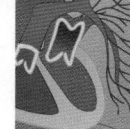

Commonly, however, the health impact of environmental exposures is less clear. Whether a putative environmental toxicant is capable of causing the reported health complaints may be at issue. Alternatively, there may be questions as to whether a dose sufficient to cause the health effects has actually reached the population that is potentially at risk. There may be inconsistent or contradictory data or assertions regarding the nature of the health impact at a population level. In these and similar circumstances, the appropriate clinical approach to individual patients may be unclear, especially if expert opinion is divided as to whether there are sufficient data of the kinds required to infer a causal link (see Chapter 82). Again, public health and environmental authorities are the clinician's best source of guidance.

Roles of Clinical Toxicologists

With increasing frequency, clinical toxicologists also function as public health officials and may have to balance the competing demands of clinical work and public health. The American College of Medical Toxicology has designated particular individuals as points of contact and referral into the medical toxicologic community for situations in which environmental and health authorities in government need specific clinically based advice. Currently, at least two states (Iowa and Pennsylvania) have given specific physicians the title of State Medical Toxicologist. In some states, entire poison control centers operate in an official or quasi-official manner, representing state, local, or regional health authorities.

Clinical toxicologists filling these roles must be aware that public health officials' responsibilities differ somewhat from those of their clinical colleagues. Public health organizations serve the community as a whole, whereas clinical toxicologists typically act on behalf of their specific patients. Nevertheless, supporting clinical health care professionals is one of the most important duties of public health officers. Clinicians require—and should expect public health officials to provide—up-to-date and accurate information about environmental exposures that may affect their patients.

Clinicians' primary concerns are individual patients, on whose behalf they must advocate. Where available information is inadequate for clinical decision making or for optimal clinical care, they can and should advocate for better information to be obtained or developed. Although clinicians will be best served if they understand the constraints and context within which public health officials operate, they should not necessarily accept those limitations as their own. Where necessary for the benefit of their patients, clinicians should advocate for further studies and for the means to care properly for patients who may have been affected by environmental contamination.

Clinicians also have a duty to oppose the practices of providers and laboratories that exploit current fears regarding environmental contamination. For example, some practitioners use chelating agents extensively with neither a recognized indication nor a proper basis in scientific theory that would stand up to careful scrutiny. When such agents are used for extended periods, they may be harmful. The overuse of chelating agents and other similar excesses in medical practice tend to undercut the trust of both the public and the medical community in clinical toxicologists who undertake a more judicious and scientifically based approach to the assessment and treatment of the health impacts of environmental agents.

BACKGROUND FOR THE CLINICAL ENCOUNTER

Formal Approach to Risk

In the years following World War II, the U.S. public became sensitized to the potential dangers of long-term low-dose exposure to the many new chemicals being developed, manufactured, and introduced into commerce. Repeated announcements warning of pesticides in food, pollutants in the air, chemical contaminants in drinking water, and toxicants emanating from hazardous waste sites generated increasing levels of concern. In particular, the likelihood emerged—now well established—that environmental chemicals could cause cancer. The practical expression of this concern was legislation to limit the exposure of people to potential chemical carcinogens. The landmark "Delaney clause," enacted within the Food Additive Amendments of 1958, forbade the use in food of any additives that were "known to cause cancer."

Implementation of the Amendment was complicated by the fact that established and accepted procedures for distinguishing carcinogens from noncarcinogens did not exist. Nevertheless, following Delaney, science and law developed in parallel. In vitro and in vivo tests were devised to identify and characterize carcinogens. Based on these tests, regulations were devised, applied, and tested in the courts. Over time, a process for characterizing the danger posed by specific chemicals, now called risk assessment, was developed. The steps involved in both assessing and managing environmental risk are diagrammed in Figure 83-1.

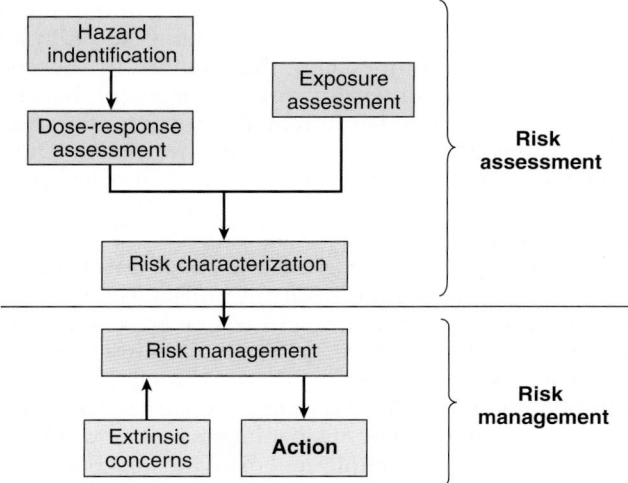

FIGURE 83-1 Outline of current procedures for risk assessment and risk management in regulatory toxicology.

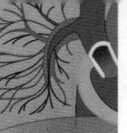

As currently conceived, risk assessment involves the identification of a hazard and then an assessment of the likely human dose response for the impact of concern (e.g., cancer). Hazard toxicity assessment also includes an attempt to identify the threshold dose, or dose below which no adverse effect is observed. Unfortunately, human data are often insufficient, particularly for assessing dose response. Thus, animal studies are required. Procedures have been developed for extrapolation of animal findings to human beings and are widely used. In addition, the risk estimate derived from animal data is modified by uncertainty factors. The final risk assessment must also include a detailed assessment of the exposure. The magnitude, frequency, duration, and routes of exposure have a significant impact on the risk assessment. The final risk characterization, which is based on toxicity and exposure assessments, is a quantitative estimate of the health risk of the hazard. Risk management decisions are made from the results of the risk characterization and other factors.

Of the current sources of systematic reviews and expert judgments on the carcinogenic potential of particular chemical exposures, three stand out:

1. The International Agency for Research on Cancer (IARC), an arm or the World Health Organization (WHO)[8]
2. The Report on Carcinogens (ROC), the development and revisions of which are staffed by the National Toxicology Program (NTP) of the National Institute for Environmental Health Sciences (NIEHS)[9]
3. The Integrated Risk Information System (IRIS) of the U.S. Environmental Protection Agency (EPA).

There are certain features common to each of the three programs.[10] Although the procedures differ for each, all three sources periodically update their conclusions to take into account new information.

The current model for regulating both cancer and other risks maintains a strict distinction between actual management of the risk (actions taken) and assessment of the risk itself (see Fig. 83-1). Risk management decisions involve more than the mere fact or level of risk. In addition, there are logistical, economic, and political considerations. Certain ways of tackling a pollution problem may be more likely than others to succeed. Community values enter into risk management, because some solutions to environmental contamination may be unacceptable to the communities involved. Other aspects of public policy, such as overall land use plans and competing needs for resources, may also modify the actions taken.

Risk management decisions, in their essence, are plans to separate people from the substances that may harm them. This may be done in several ways. Removing or relocating the hazard is generally the most desirable plan from the point of view of those affected. However, it is frequently expensive. Polluting industries, hazardous wastes, and other foci of environmental concern are not very mobile. Thus, techniques to isolate the hazard or diminish the intensity of exposure are used. This may involve the improvement of industrial pollution controls,

barriers to prevent the spread of noxious substances in air and water, or other means. An extreme measure available to the risk manager is the relocation of an entire community. At Love Canal, an exposure situation described in more detail below, many houses were bought so that the owners could move out. At Times Beach, Missouri, the entire town was bought from its owners by the federal government as a risk management measure. The relocation of large numbers of people (or of entire communities) is disruptive to community life and extremely expensive and is a last resort.

Occupational Exposure Limits

In 1946, the American Conference of Governmental Industrial Hygienists (ACGIH) published its first list of 148 exposure limits. In 1956, the ACGIH adopted the term *threshold limit values for chemical substances* (TLV-CS).[11] Currently, seven U.S. organizations publish and maintain systematic guidance on toxicant exposures on the basis of which the risk for adverse health effects from specific hazardous substances can be assessed. Measurements of occupational exposures are commonly compared with one or more of three sets of criteria:

1. Permissible exposure limits (PELs), established by the Occupational Safety and Health Administration (OSHA)[12]
2. Recommended exposure limits (RELs), established by the National Institute for Occupational Safety and Health (NIOSH)[13]
3. TLVs, established by the ACGIH[14]

In general, workers' risks for experiencing adverse health effects are increased to the extent that their levels of exposure exceed published criteria or standards (see also Chapter 82). The activities of these organizations are described in detail below.

The goal of the criteria for workplace exposures established by these organizations is to prevent adverse health effects in most workers exposed up to 10 hours per day, 40 hours per week for a working lifetime. The emphasis is on a "most workers" basis; the limits are not formulated to protect highly sensitive individuals. Thus, some small proportion of workers may be adversely affected despite adherence to the guidelines. Individual susceptibility, preexisting medical conditions, prescription or illicit drug use, and/or hypersensitivity (allergy) are often cited as examples of factors increasing the susceptibility of workers and leading to toxicity.

To facilitate access to information on occupational exposure limits and supporting material, NIOSH publishes numerous documents and databases that may be useful to clinical toxicologists. Current Intelligence Bulletins, Criteria Documents, and NIOSH Alerts all highlight the current state of knowledge of various chemical and physical toxins. *The NIOSH Pocket Guide to Chemical Hazards* is a comprehensive listing of general industrial hygiene information on several hundred chemicals and chemical classes for workers, employers, and occupational health professionals. Detailed information about chemical exposures may be found in the U.S. version of *NIOSH's*

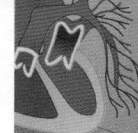

International Chemical Safety Cards and the *Occupational Safety and Health Guidelines for Chemical Hazards.*

Occupational exposure limits are sometimes used in the evaluation of community environmental hazards, in part because there are many potential toxicants for which occupational exposure guidance is available but on which guidance on exposures of the general population is lacking. Although sometimes unavoidable, there are pitfalls to this practice because the general population has many more sensitive individuals than the typical workplace. Moreover, a higher level of safety is typically required. Limits for occupational exposure are suggested maximum levels of exposures based on an 8- to 10-hour time-weighted average workday exposure, designed only to protect an ideal "normal, healthy adult."[15]

Nonoccupational Exposure Limits

Certain federal agencies have developed standards for exposures in nonoccupational environments. Like occupational exposure standards, the nonoccupational exposure limits represent an estimated daily human exposure below which there is a minimal risk for developing adverse health effects. Where sufficient human exposure data do not exist to establish exposure limits for a given toxicant, they are typically based on animal studies using a no observed adverse effect level/uncertainty factor (NOAEL/UF) approach. Test animals are exposed to varying concentrations of a toxicant by different routes and over varying periods in order to identify the organ and lowest threshold for toxicity in the most sensitive organ. This level is called the lowest observable adverse effect level (LOAEL). At some exposure level below this, there will be a level at which there is no evidence of an adverse effect, the no observable adverse effect level (NOAEL). Once a NOAEL has been determined among test animals, a standard set of calculations and decision making are used to derive an initial exposure limit based on the NOAEL. To assure protection of vulnerable subpopulations of people (e.g., infants and the elderly) and to account for other points of uncertainty (e.g., establishing a value for the protection of humans on the basis of animal data), the initial NOAEL-based value may be decreased by (divided by) one or more uncertainty factors with values of from 2 to 10, inclusive. Thus, the final value of the minimal risk level (MRL) is often as much as two orders of magnitude lower than the NOAEL.[16]

Because of slight differences in their procedures, the different agencies use different terms for their exposure limits. The Agency for Toxic Substances and Disease Registry (ATSDR) derives MRLs. The EPA develops exposure limits termed the *reference dose* (RfD) for oral exposures and the reference concentration (RfC) for air. The FDA's guidance values are termed *action levels.*

FEDERAL AGENCIES

Because of the number of persons involved, significant environmental exposures frequently involve environ-

mental and public health authorities, and clinicians should expect to deal with them. At the very least, clinicians will need to understand their deliberations and pronouncements. Interactions with environmental and health authorities can be greatly facilitated by a working knowledge of the various agencies (particularly the federal agencies) with responsibilities in the field. Moreover, an understanding of the procedures followed by these agencies, together with knowledge of their historical underpinnings, assists in comprehension, allowing the clinician to serve both (1) as interpreter of government agencies' actions for his or her patients and (2) as effective advocate on behalf of patients to the government agencies involved.

U.S. environmental public health at the federal level is divided into various functional components and falls under the jurisdictions of a number of departments and agencies. These include the Departments of Health and Human Services (DHHS), Labor (DOL), and Agriculture (USDA), as well as several independent agencies, including the EPA and the Consumer Product Safety Commission (CPSC).*

Environmental Protection Agency

On July 9, 1970, President Richard Nixon submitted to Congress plans to establish the EPA.[17] As the principal "watchdog" of the nation's environment, the EPA is responsible for both shaping and enforcing the environmental laws enacted by Congress. The EPA oversees compliance with a lengthy list of laws and regulations written to fulfill them. Among the most important environmental laws protecting human health and overseen by the EPA are:

National Environmental Policy Act of 1969
Clean Air Act (CAA, 1970)
Federal Insecticide, Fungicide, and Rodenticide Act (FIFRA, 1972)
Safe Drinking Water Act (1974)
Toxic Substances Control Act (1976)
Resource Conservation and Recovery Act (RCRA, 1976)
Clean Water Act (1977)
Comprehensive Environmental Response, Compensation and Liability Act (CERCLA, 1980)
Superfund Amendments and Reauthorization Act (SARA, 1986; amendment to CERCLA)
Emergency Planning and Community Right-to-Know Act (EPCRA, 1986)

A substantial proportion of the EPA's resources have been divided among 10 regional offices for the purposes of administering these laws. The regions correspond to the 10 regions under which the DHHS administers some of its programs, providing a context by which federal agencies can integrate activities in the field. Under the

---

*Independent agencies report to the president but are not directly affiliated with an executive department headed by a cabinet secretary. Agency heads may or may not sit with the cabinet.

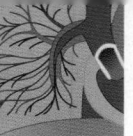

EPA's stewardship, the air, water, and soil are notably cleaner, particularly with respect to toxicants with an impact on human health.

The EPA protects people from water-borne toxicants by formulating and enforcing the National Primary Drinking Water Regulations. These standards regulate the content of microbiologic, radiologic, and toxicologic contamination of water destined for human consumption. In addition, the required frequency of monitoring and the definitions of compliance are set by the EPA.

Two laws constitute the EPA's principal authorization for activities related to the safe management of environmental hazardous wastes. CERCLA (also known as Superfund), enacted in 1980, was designed to manage the clean-up of closed or abandoned hazardous waste sites.[18] Although the RCRA of 1976 had authorized the EPA to hold industrial polluters responsible for the clean-up of hazardous waste sites,[19] CERCLA strengthened the procedures for holding polluters accountable and outlined provisions for clean-ups at sites where directly responsible parties cannot be identified.[18]

Under the CAA, the EPA formulated a series of regulations. Among them are regulations identifying and setting National Ambient Air Quality Standards (NAAQS). The six pollutants for which the NAAQS currently exist are:

1. Ozone
2. Particulate matter
3. Carbon monoxide
4. Sulfur dioxide
5. Nitrogen oxides
6. Lead

These six air contaminants are termed priority pollutants and are monitored widely throughout the United States. The measurements made in local areas are judged against the NAAQS, and the areas are determined to be attainment or nonattainment areas accordingly. Based on these determinations, corrective action is taken. The 1990 amendments also identified 188 chemicals as hazardous air pollutants (also known as air toxics) because these chemicals are reasonably common pollutants and are particularly toxic.

The tragic deaths of thousands of people from a massive unintentional release of toxic methyl isocyanate (MIC) gas in Bhopal, India, aroused concern about the possibility of a similar event occurring in the United States.[20] This concern was reinforced less than a year later by a release of toxic chemicals into the air by a plant in West Virginia that also handled MIC.[21] Thus, in 1986, Congress passed the SARA.[22] The EPCRA, part of the SARA, required all businesses storing hazardous chemicals to provide their area's local emergency planning committee (LEPC) with information concerning the location and quantity of these chemicals. LEPCs may develop response plans for potential environmental and public health emergencies in anticipation of inadvertent releases. Moreover, the EPCRA mandates annual data collection concerning actual releases of hazardous chemicals. This information, designed to make companies accountable for their handling of toxic chemicals, is known as the toxic release inventory (TRI).[23,24] The TRI covers toxic releases from various industrial sectors, including manufacturing, metal and coal mining, electrical utilities, and commercial hazardous waste treatment.

Consumer Product Safety Commission

The CPSC was created in 1972 as an independent, freestanding federal regulatory agency responsible for protecting the public "against unreasonable risks of injuries associated with consumer products."[25] Currently, the CPSC ensures the public's safety from over 15,000 consumer products. Among the laws enforced by the CPSC are the Federal Hazardous Substances Act (FHSA) and the Poison Prevention Packaging Act (PPPA). Passed in 1970, the PPPA requires the use of child-resistant packaging as a means of preventing accidental childhood poisoning.

The term *special packaging* means packaging that is designed or constructed to be significantly difficult for children younger than 5 years of age to open or for them to obtain a toxic or harmful amount of the substance contained therein within a reasonable time [12 U.S.C. § 1471 (4)].

Over-the-counter medications, prescription drugs, household cleaners, beauty aids and cosmetics, prepackaged fuels, and FHSA-designated hazardous substances are subject to the packaging legislation. Even solder with a lead content in excess of 0.2% is considered hazardous. Currently, 28 classes of products are included on the list of agents requiring child-resistant packaging.[26-28] The CPSC also regulates the use of certain radioactive substances, as well as products involving electrical, mechanical, or thermal hazards. Although considered hazardous under the CPSC's legislation, pesticides are subject to regulation by the EPA under the FIFRA and are not regulated by the CPSC.

Knowledge of specific words on product labels, required under the FHSA, may be of use to clinicians: extremely flammable, corrosive, or highly toxic substances must be labeled with the signal word *DANGER*; all other hazardous substances must carry one of two signal words, *WARNING* or *CAUTION*. In addition, descriptions of the principal hazard and any precautionary measures to be employed when handling the substance must be included on the label. Substances may also be banned under the FHSA; these include toys or other articles intended for children that are determined to be hazardous substances and any products found to be too hazardous for household use, regardless of labeling.

In addition to its regulatory function, the CPSC runs the National Electronic Injury Surveillance System.[29,30] This surveillance system relies on data collected from a sample of 100 hospital emergency departments to provide a national estimate of injuries (including poisonings) caused by consumer products. Available for query, this database includes information about the drug or drugs implicated in poisoning incidents.

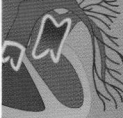

Food and Drug Administration and U.S. Department of Agriculture

By the latter half of the 19th century, concerns about the purity of medications resulted in attempts by the government to enforce standards of safety. In 1848, for example, to combat the influx of "counterfeit, contaminated, diluted, and decomposed" drugs entering the country, Congress passed the Import Drugs Act.[31] Congress became acutely aware of the impact of tainted drugs when, during the course of the U.S.-Mexican war (1847 to 1848), an estimated 11,000 U.S. soldiers died of disease and illness (out of 13,000 who lost their lives).[32] Many of the men who died of malaria had been dispensed ineffective or sham medicines. Under the 1848 law, laboratories set up by the U.S. Customs Service were given the responsibility for ensuring the purity and potency of drugs imported into the country.[31] By the early 1900s, however, popular and financial support for this initiative had waned and the program ended.

During the same period, so-called "patent medicines" also drew Congress's attention. Despite containing such now-illicit substances as opium, heroin, and cocaine, these products were sold without restriction, and labels failed to fully disclose the active ingredients.[31] The labels typically made fabulous (and usually fictitious) claims about the medicine's efficacy, advertising cures for ailments as diverse as fatigue, toothache, gout, and diabetes.

Congress responded to the commonplace use of "patent" medicines and food adulterants by passing the Pure Food and Drug Act in 1906. This law was the first of its kind and required all food and drug labels to reflect package contents accurately.[33] Any food, drink, or drug being shipped across state lines and found to be improperly labeled (i.e., lacking a complete accounting of its contents) was subject to seizure; persons found responsible for the products could be prosecuted. Drugs had to be manufactured according to the standard set forth in the U.S. Pharmacopoeia.[33] Ingredients like alcohol, heroin, and cocaine had to be identified clearly on the label.

By 1862, the wholesomeness of foods came into question. Chemists within the USDA began to analyze food products for the presence of adulterants. Within a decade, USDA chemists were debating possible adverse effects of the arsenic- and copper-based pesticide residues then found in foods.[31] Other food additives of the time included boric acid, potassium nitrate, saccharin, salicylic acid, sulfuric acid, benzoic acid, and formaldehyde.[31,34]

The USDA Bureau of Chemistry had the responsibility of enforcing the Pure Food and Drug Act. To reflect its role more accurately, the Bureau was renamed the Food, Drug, and Insecticide Administration. In 1930, it became the Food and Drug Administration.[31] During the rest of the 20th century, Congress continued to broaden the powers of the FDA by enacting other laws, many in response to public health disasters.

Today, according to its mission statement, the FDA is "responsible for protecting the public health by assuring the safety, efficacy, and security of human and veterinary drugs, biological products, medical devices, our nation's food supply, cosmetics, and products that emit radiation."[35,36]

Within the FDA, there are five regulatory centers. The Center for Veterinary Medicine evaluates the safety and efficacy of drugs used to treat livestock and companion animals such as dogs, cats, and horses.[37] Livestock drugs are also tested to make sure that residues, where they exist, do not pose a risk to the people who consume them. The Center for Food Safety and Applied Nutrition is responsible for ensuring the safety of the nation's entire food supply, with the exception of fresh meat, poultry, and some egg products.[38] (Responsibility for the latter rests with the USDA. Protecting food in the United States from adulteration by terrorists is a role shared by the USDA and FDA.)

The Center for Drug Evaluation and Research conducts premarketing evaluation of all prescription and over-the-counter drugs and provides the lay public and health care providers with drug use information.[39] Oversight of the manufacture, marketing, and use of biologic products for health care (e.g., blood and blood products, vaccines, and protein-based drugs such as monoclonal antibodies) is provided by the Center for Biologics Evaluation and Research (CBER).[40] The FDA's Center for Devices and Radiological Health (CDRH) regulates the safety of all medical devices marketed and used in the United States, including everything from tongue depressors and thermometers to contact lenses, pacemakers, orthopedic implants, heart valves, dialysis machines, and the computerized robotic arms used in surgery.[41] The CDRH is also responsible for ensuring public safety from excessive and unnecessary radiation exposure from both medical and nonmedical devices. Thus, not only must radiology equipment and lasers meet safety standards, but household items such as microwave ovens, television sets, and cell phones are also subject to FDA regulation.

National Institute for Occupational Safety and Health

In 1970, Congress passed the Occupational Safety and Health Act (OSH Act, Williams-Steiger Act), creating both OSHA and NIOSH.[42] The stated goal of the OSH Act was to ensure that workers are provided a "place of employment free from recognized hazards to safety and health." In order to achieve this goal, Congress created the two agencies to serve dual functions: regulatory and research. OSHA, situated within the DOL, has the regulatory function. This agency is responsible for the creation and enforcement of workplace safety and health regulations. NIOSH, by contrast, conducts research to propose science-based standards designed to minimize work-related injuries and illnesses. NIOSH, part of the Centers for Disease Control and Prevention (CDC), is under the DHHS.

In addition to research aimed at preventing workplace injuries, NIOSH conducts injury surveillance and develops worker training and communication programs.[43]

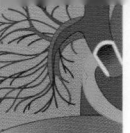

At the request of employers, employees (or their representatives), or government agencies, NIOSH investigators in the Health Hazard Evaluation Program conduct on-site workplace evaluations to identify potential or actual hazards, whether physical, chemical, or biological. The National Personal Protective Technology Laboratory conducts research that establishes standards of safety and protection for personal protective equipment such as respirators, gloves, and hard hats. The Sentinel Event Notification System for Occupational Risks (SENSOR) program, a collaborative effort with state health departments, has established ongoing surveillance programs to rapidly identify cases of exposures and injuries, including occupational asthma, pesticide poisoning, silicosis, amputations, burns, occupational dermatitis, and noise-induced hearing loss. Surveillance for occupational lead poisoning is conducted under a separate program, the Adult Blood Lead Epidemiology and Surveillance Program.

Agency for Toxic Substances and Disease Registry

In August 1978, the New York State Department of Health, the governor of New York, and President Jimmy Carter declared a state of emergency at the community of Love Canal, New York,[44] located near Niagara Falls. The houses and local public school of Love Canal were built on a former chemical waste dump site. Ultimately, families were evacuated, the school was closed, and state and federal funding was applied to the clean-up. Two years later (December 1980), Congress passed the Superfund law and in doing so, both expanded the powers of the EPA (as described above) and created a new agency, the ATSDR. The ATSDR was directed to assist the EPA in determining the exposure levels at which hazardous chemicals may result in adverse health effects.[45]

The ATSDR conducts public health assessments at all sites proposed for or listed on the EPA's National Priorities List of sites for investigation and possible remediation.[46] The results of these public health assessments are made available to city, state, and federal agencies, and to the affected communities. In those situations where the ATSDR identifies exposure to hazardous substances at levels at or above those known to cause adverse health effects, they provide the EPA with recommendations to guide potential appropriate actions or interventions. In the event that a survey identifies an urgent public health threat, the ATSDR may warn the community by issuing a public health advisory.[46]

The ATSDR is also legally required to develop and compile health information on hazardous substances. The ATSDR's Toxicological Profiles are a mandated health consultation activity and serve a broad purpose as key reference documents on specific substances. Each Toxicological Profile is based on comprehensive reviews of the toxicologic and epidemiologic literature available for a given chemical.[47]

The ATSDR also conducts surveillance and registers exposed individuals for possible later follow-up. The Hazardous Substances Emergency Events Surveillance System was created to gather information about both acute and threatened releases of hazardous substances that require some form of environmental or public health intervention.[48] Information concerning approximately 9000 events is captured annually. Of interest, only 25% to 30% of acute or threatened releases of hazardous substances are transportation related; the vast majority are "fixed facility" events that involve the release or threatened release of only a single hazardous substance. The National Exposure Registry is a database kept by the ATSDR of people who have been exposed to trichloroethylene, trichloroethane, benzene, or dioxin. The health of these individuals is then tracked.[49] The database thus serves as a tool to help facilitate epidemiologic studies of chemical exposures, generally at low levels and over long periods.

As part of its "Managing Hazardous Material Incidents" series, the ATSDR has developed medical management guidelines (MMGs), reference materials designed to assist emergency physicians and other emergency health care personnel to manage acute chemical and hazardous material exposures.[50] In addition to including basic chemical and exposure information and a summary of potential health effects that may result from exposure, MMGs provide prehospital management information, emergency department management information, and information concerning proper decontamination and use of personal protective equipment.[51] Information for patients is also included in these documents. As part of its educational mission, the ATSDR publishes *Case Studies in Environmental Medicine*, a series of monographs written to provide health care providers with guidance concerning the management of exposed (and potentially exposed) individuals who present in an office setting.[52]

National Center for Environmental Health

The National Center for Environmental Health (NCEH) of the CDC hosts a wide variety of scientific and programmatic activities in preventive toxicology. The NCEH has one of the foremost analytical toxicology laboratories in the world. The chemists and toxicologists of the NCEH laboratory have pioneered analyses for chemicals found at extremely low levels but which are nevertheless so potent that harm may result. Some analytical techniques are so sensitive that they yield measurements expressed in units of parts per quadrillion, that is, femtograms of analyte per gram of the matrix. To provide reliable analyses at this level of sensitivity, a program of intensive quality control with statistical checking on essentially every run has been put in place. The laboratory has become a center of reference for quality control techniques for measurement of specific chemicals in biologic matrices. The laboratory runs national programs of standardization for measurement of such analytes as cholesterol and lead. In the current era of concerns about terrorism, the laboratory has developed the capacity to measure rapidly and definitively some 200 analytes of concern for both

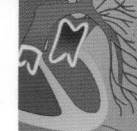

chemical warfare agents and toxic industrial chemicals that might be used by terrorists.

Another laboratory project, the periodically updated and expanded *National Report on Human Exposure to Environmental Chemicals*,[53] is of particular importance for clinical toxicologists. The project involves blood and urine samples collected as part of the National Health and Nutrition Examination Survey. The CDC's National Center for Health Statistics designed the survey such that appropriate statistical analysis yields estimates of the mean or median values (with confidence limits) of U.S. residents' levels of the chemicals measured in the specimens. The exposure of the U.S. population to an increasing number of substances is described in successive iterations of the report. The concept of "normal levels" is problematic when applied to xenobiotics. Nevertheless, the report provides a basis for comparison for the same analytes measured in individual cases. Although no xenobiotic level is "normal," a particularly high level may reflect "unusual" exposure.

Other programs of the NCEH include a program of targeted surveillance for high blood lead levels in children. This program also supports interventions designed to protect children from undue lead exposure. The asthma and respiratory diseases group investigates the factors involved in the gradually increasing levels seen in the United States in recent years of disease involving hyper-reactive airways.

A particularly strong asset of the NCEH is the capability to investigate new or unusual syndromes of chemical (or other environmental) origin. Although such investigations are typically supported by the very capable NCEH laboratory, a key part of the success of such investigations involves "old fashioned shoe leather epidemiology," requiring investigators to go to the field, ascertain key facts, organize data, and come to conclusions, supported (where possible) by laboratory analyses. The CDC's Epidemic Intelligence Service plays a key role in this activity.

National Institute of Environmental Health Sciences

The NIEHS, a component institute of the National Institutes of Health (NIH), supports and conducts research into the underlying mechanisms of disease caused by chemical and biologic agents found in the air, ground, food, and water, and develops appropriate interventions based on an understanding of those mechanisms.[54] The NIEHS is the lead agency in the National Toxicology Program (NTP), which conducts toxicologic testing programs within the DHHS. NTP also involves NIOSH and the FDA's National Center for Toxicologic Research.[55] In addition, the NTP provides administrative oversight to two centers: the Center for the Evaluation of Risks to Human Reproduction (CERHR) and the Center for Phototoxicology, a function it shares with the FDA (described above). Established in 1998, the CERHR assesses chemicals for their potential to affect human reproduction and development adversely.[56] The CERHR convenes independent panels to review all available scientific literature concerning chem-

icals that are nominated for review by industry, federal, state, and local governments, academia, environmental groups, and private citizens. The NIEHS/Environmental Genome Project conducts research designed to improve current knowledge of human genetic susceptibility to environmental exposures.[57] The research goals of the NIEHS/National Center for Toxicogenomics include improved understanding of the relationship between environmental exposures and human susceptibility to disease, identification of bio-markers of exposure to and disease caused by toxic substances, and creation of a public database of the effects of toxic substances in biologic systems.[58]

NONGOVERNMENTAL ORGANIZATIONS

American Conference of Governmental Industrial Hygienists

The ACGIH was born out of the need to provide standards and guidance for managing occupational exposures to protect workers from health effects of harmful substances encountered in the workplace. Although the original members were largely government employees and its guidance is highly influential, the ACGIH is a private, not-for-profit, nongovernmental organization.[59] Members work as volunteers on committees to review the existing published, peer-reviewed literature. Experts in various scientific disciplines arrive at their judgments and guidance regarding the likely health impacts of exposures to chemicals and physical agents at specific levels. The members work to develop the guidance ultimately issued by the parent organization.

The bulk of this guidance ultimately developed by the ACGIH is issued as TLVs and biological exposure indices (BEIs). The TLV is meant to be the maximum permissible concentration of a material, generally expressed in parts per million in air, for some defined period of time (often 8 hours, but sometimes for 40 hours per week over an assumed working lifetime). TLVs and BEIs are guidelines, not standards. The ACGIH states that they are only two of multiple factors to be considered in evaluating specific workplace situations and conditions.

BEIs are intended for use in the practice of industrial hygiene as guidelines or recommendations to assist in the control of potential workplace health hazards and for no other use. Biologic monitoring entails measurement of the concentration of a chemical determinant in the biologic media of the exposed person and is an indicator of the uptake of the substance. The determinant (analyte) used to establish the BEI may be the chemical itself, one or more metabolites, or a characteristic reversible biochemical change induced by the chemical. The BEI is meant to correspond to the level of the determinant in a worker exposed at the level of the TLV.

Agencies of the United Nations

Established on April 7, 1948, the World Health Organization (WHO) is the United Nations' specialized

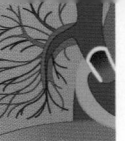

agency for health. The goal of WHO is to attain the highest possible level of health in all of the peoples of the world. Of interest, "health" is defined by WHO as state of complete physical, mental, and social well-being, and not merely the absence of disease or infirmity. A number of special units and subcomponents of WHO's program are dedicated to environmental health. Two deserve specific mention.

The International Programme on Chemical Safety (IPCS) is sponsored jointly by the United Nations Environment Programme, the International Labour Organisation, and WHO. The main objective of the IPCS is to carry out and disseminate evaluations of the effects of chemicals on human health and on the quality of the environment. Its activities include the development of epidemiologic, experimental laboratory, and risk assessment methods. The IPCS develops its methods with the specific aim of producing internationally comparable results. A further goal of the IPCS is the development of more person power in the field of toxicology. Other activities include developing the know-how to cope with chemical accidents, coordinating laboratory testing, conducting or supporting epidemiologic studies, and promoting research on the mechanisms of the biologic action of chemicals.

The IARC is also part of WHO. The IARC's mission is to coordinate and conduct research on the causes of human cancer and the mechanisms of carcinogenesis, and to develop scientific strategies for cancer control. The IARC is involved in both epidemiologic and laboratory research and disseminates scientific information through publications, meetings, courses, and fellowships.

REFERENCES

1. Institute of Medicine, Immunization Safety Review Committee: In Stratton K, Gable A, McCormick M, eds. Immunization Safety Review: Thimerosal-Containing Vaccines and Neurodevelopmental Disorders. Washington, DC, National Academies Press, 2001.
2. Newsom SW: Pioneers in infection control—Joseph Lister. J Hosp Infect 2003;55(4):246–253.
3. Centers for Disease Control and Prevention: 150th Anniversary of John Snow and the pump handle. MMWR 2004;53(34):783.
4. Guerrant RL, Carneiro-Filho BA, Dillingham RA: Cholera, diarrhea, and oral rehydration therapy: triumph and indictment. Clin Infect Dis 2003;37(3):398–405.
5. Cutler D, Miller G: The role of public health improvements in health advances: the twentieth-century United States. Demography 2005;42(1):1–22.
6. Swygert LA, Maes EF, Sewell LE, et al: Eosinophilia-myalgia syndrome. Results of national surveillance. JAMA 1990;264(13):1698–1703.
7. Whitehouse AC: Asbestos-related pleural disease due to tremolite associated with progressive loss of lung function: serial observations in 123 miners, family members, and residents of Libby, Montana. Am J Ind Med 2004;46(3):219–225.
8. International Agency for Research on Cancer: Lists of IARC evaluations. Accessed March 1, 2005, at http://monographs.iarc.fr/monoeval/grlist.html.
9. U.S. Department of Health and Human Services, Public Health Service, National Toxicology Program: Report on Carcinogens, 11th ed. Accessed March 1, 2005, at http://ntp.niehs.nih.gov/ntp/roc/toc11.html.
10. U.S. Environmental Protection Agency–Integrated Risk Information System: IRIS Database for Risk Assessment. Accessed March 1, 2005, at http://www.epa.gov/iriswebp/iris/index.html.
11. American Conference of Governmental Industrial Hygienists: History of the ACGIH. Accessed July 26, 2005, at http://www.acgih.org/About/history.htm.
12. Code of Federal Regulations: 29 CFR 1910.1000. Washington, DC, U.S. Government Printing Office, Office of the Federal Register, 2002.
13. Centers for Disease Control and Prevention: Recommendations for occupational safety and health: compendium of policy documents and statements. DHHS (NIOSH) Publication No. 92-100. Cincinnati, OH, U.S. Department of Health and Human Services, Public Health Service, Centers for Disease Control and Prevention, National Institute for Occupational Safety and Health, 1992.
14. American Conference of Governmental Industrial Hygienists: 2004 TLVs® and BEIs®: Threshold Limit Values for Chemical Substances and Physical Agents. Cincinnati, OH, American Conference of Governmental Industrial Hygienists, 2004.
15. American Conference of Governmental Industrial Hygienists: Statement of Position Regarding the TLVs® and BEIs®. Accessed March 1, 2005, at http://www.acgih.org/TLV/PosStmt.htm.
16. Agency for Toxic Substances and Disease Registry: Minimal Risk Levels (MRLs) for Hazardous Substances. Accessed February 11, 2005, at http://www.atsdr.cdc.gov/mrls.html.
17. Environmental Protection Agency: Reorganization Plan No. 3 of 1970. U.S. Environmental Protection Agency—History. Accessed March 1, 2005, at http://www.epa.gov/history/org/origins/reorg.htm.
18. Environmental Protection Agency: CERCLA Overview. Accessed March 1, 2005, at http://www.epa.gov/superfund/action/law/cercla.htm.
19. Environmental Protection Agency: New Law to Control Hazardous Wastes, End Open Dumping, Promote Conservation of Resources. U.S. Environmental Protection Agency—History. Accessed March 1, 2005, at http://www.epa.gov/history/topics/rcra/05.htm.
20. Mehta PS, Mehta AS, Mehta SJ, Makhijani AB: Bhopal tragedy's health effects. A review of methyl isocyanate toxicity. JAMA 1990;264(21):2781–2787.
21. Coppock R: Improving Risk Communication: Working Papers. Communicating Corporate Disaster: The Aldicarb Oxime Release at the Union Carbide Plant at Institute, West Virginia, on August 11, 1985. Washington, DC, National Academies Press, 1989, pp 29–52. (Also available at http://www.nap.edu/openbook/POD289/html/29.html.)
22. Environmental Protection Agency: SARA Overview. Accessed March 1, 2005, at http://www.epa.gov/superfund/action/law/sara.htm.
23. U.S. Environmental Protection Agency–Toxics Release Inventory (TRI) Program: What is the Toxics Release Inventory (TRI) Program? Accessed March 1, 2005, at http://www.epa.gov/tri/whatis.htm.
24. U.S. Environmental Protection Agency–Toxics Release Inventory (TRI) Program: Toxics Release Inventory (TRI) Program Fact Sheet. Accessed March 1, 2005, at http://www.epa.gov/tri/tri_program_fact_sheet.htm.
25. U.S. Consumer Product Safety Commission: Who We Are—What We Do for You. Accessed March 1, 2005, at http://www.cpsc.gov/cpscpub/pubs/103.html.
26. U.S. Consumer Product Safety Commission: Poison Prevention Packaging Act. Accessed March 1, 2005, at http://www.cpsc.gov/businfo/pppa.html.
27. U.S. Consumer Product Safety Commission: Poison Prevention Packaging Act [15 U.S.C. 1471-1476: Public Law 91-601; 84 Stat. 1670, December 30, 1970, as amended]. Accessed March 1, 2005, at http://www.cpsc.gov/businfo/pppa.pdf.
28. U.S. Consumer Product Safety Commission: Poison Prevention Packaging: A Text for Pharmacists & Physicians. Accessed March 1, 2005, at http://www.cpsc.gov/cpscpub/pubs/384.pdf.
29. U.S. Consumer Product Safety Commission: National Electronic Injury Surveillance System [CPSC Document #3002]. Accessed March 1, 2005, at http://www.cpsc.gov/cpscpub/pubs/3002.html.
30. Committee on Poison Prevention and Control, Board on Health Promotion and Disease Prevention: Forging a Poison Prevention and Control System. Washington, DC, Institute of Medicine of the National Academies, National Academies Press, 2004.

31. Janssen WF: The story of the laws behind the labels, part I: 1906 Food and Drugs Act. FDA Consumer Magazine, June 1981. Accessed March 1, 2005, at http://vm.cfsan.fda.gov/~lrd/history1.html.

32. Descendants of Mexican War Veterans: Mexican War Veteran Research, An Introduction. Accessed March 1, 2005, at http://www.dmwv.org/mwvets/howto.htm.

33. U.S. Department of Health and Human Services, Food and Drug Administration: History of the FDA: The 1906 Food and Drugs Act and Its Enforcement. Accessed March 1, 2005, at http://www.fda.gov/oc/history/historyoffda/section1.html.

34. Lewis C: The "Poison Squad" and the advent of food and drug regulation. FDA Consumer Magazine, November–December 2002. Accessed March 1, 2005, at http://www.fda.gov/fdac/features/2002/602_squad.html.

35. U.S. Department of Health and Human Services, Food and Drug Administration: FDA's Mission Statement. Accessed March 1, 2005, at http://www.fda.gov/opacom/morechoices/mission.html.

36. U.S. Department of Health and Human Services, Food and Drug Administration: FDA Overview. Accessed March 1, 2005, at http://www.fda.gov/oc/opacom/fda101/sld001.html.

37. U.S. Department of Health and Human Services, Food and Drug Administration: Safeguarding Animal Health to Protect Consumers. Accessed March 1, 2005, at http://www.fda.gov/opacom/factsheets/justthefacts/6cvm.pdf.

38. U.S. Department of Health and Human Services, Food and Drug Administration: Keeping the Nation's Food Supply Safe: FDA's Big Job Done Well. Accessed March 1, 2005, at http://www.fda.gov/opacom/factsheets/justthefacts/2cfsan.pdf.

39. U.S. Department of Health and Human Services, Food and Drug Administration: Improving Public Health: Promoting Safe and Effective Drug Use. Accessed March 1, 2005, at http://www.fda.gov/opacom/factsheets/justthefacts/3cder.pdf.

40. U.S. Department of Health and Human Services, Food and Drug Administration: FDA's Center on the Front Line of the Biomedical Frontier. Accessed March 1, 2005, at http://www.fda.gov/opacom/factsheets/justthefacts/4cber.pdf.

41. U.S. Department of Health and Human Services, Food and Drug Administration: Better Health Care with Quality Medical Devices: FDA on the Cutting Edge of Device Technology. Accessed March 1, 2005, at http://www.fda.gov/opacom/factsheets/justthefacts/5cdrh.pdf.

42. Occupational Safety and Health Administration: Public Law 91-596, 84 STAT. 1590, 91st Congress, S.2193, December 29, 1970, as amended through January 1, 2004. Accessed February 11, 2005, at http://www.osha-slc.gov/pls/oshaweb/owadisp.show_document?p_table=OSHACT&p_id=2743.

43. U.S. Department of Health and Human Services, Centers for Disease Control and Prevention, National Institute for Occupational Safety and Health: About NIOSH. Accessed March 1, 2005, at http://www.cdc.gov/niosh/about.html.

44. Beck EC: The Love Canal Tragedy. EPA Journal, January 1979. U.S. Environmental Protection Agency—History. Accessed March 1, 2005, at http://www.epa.gov/history/topics/lovecanal/01.htm.

45. U.S. Department of Health and Human Services, Agency for Toxic Substances and Disease Registry: ATSDR Background and Congressional Mandates. Accessed March 1, 2005, at http://www.atsdr.cdc.gov/congress.html.

46. U.S. Department of Health and Human Services, Agency for Toxic Substances and Disease Registry: ATSDR Public Health Assessments. Accessed March 1, 2005, at http://www.atsdr.cdc.gov/HAC/PHA/foreword.html.

47. U.S. Department of Health and Human Services, Agency for Toxic Substances and Disease Registry: Toxicological Profile Information Sheet. Accessed March 1, 2005, at http://www.atsdr.cdc.gov/toxpro2.html.

48. U.S. Department of Health and Human Services, Agency for Toxic Substances and Disease Registry: Hazardous Substances Emergency Events Surveillance. Accessed March 1, 2005, at http://www.atsdr.cdc.gov/HS/HSEES/.

49. U.S. Department of Health and Human Services, Agency for Toxic Substances and Disease Registry: What Is the National Exposure Registry (NER)? Accessed March 1, 2005, at http://www.atsdr.cdc.gov/NER.

50. U.S. Department of Health and Human Services, Agency for Toxic Substances and Disease Registry: HazMat Emergency Preparedness Training and Tools for Responders. Accessed March 1, 2005, at http://www.atsdr.cdc.gov/hazmat-emergency-preparedness.html.

51. U.S. Department of Health and Human Services, Agency for Toxic Substances and Disease Registry: Medical Management Guidelines (MMGs) for Acute Chemical Exposures. Accessed March 1, 2005, at http://www.atsdr.cdc.gov/mmg.html.

52. U.S. Department of Health and Human Services, Agency for Toxic Substances and Disease Registry: Case Studies in Environmental Medicine. Accessed March 1, 2005, at http://www.atsdr.cdc.gov/HEC/CSEM/.

53. Department of Health and Human Services, Centers for Disease Control and Prevention: National Report on Human Exposure to Environmental Chemicals Nation. July 2005, Atlanta, Georgia. Accessed July 26, 2005, at http://www.cdc.gov/exposurereport/3rd/pdf/thirdreport.pdf.

54. U.S. Department of Health and Human Services, National Institutes of Health, National Institute of Environmental Health Sciences: Introduction to NIEHS. Accessed March 1, 2005, at http://www.niehs.nih.gov/external/intro.htm.

55. U.S. Department of Health and Human Services, National Institutes of Health, National Institute of Environmental Health Sciences: National Toxicology Program. Accessed March 1, 2005, at http://ntp-server.niehs.nih.gov/.

56. U.S. Department of Health and Human Services, National Institutes of Health, National Institute of Environmental Health Sciences, National Toxicology Program: About CERHR. Accessed March 1, 2005, at http://cerhr.niehs.nih.gov/aboutCERHR/index.html.

57. U.S. Department of Health and Human Services, National Institutes of Health, National Institute of Environmental Health Sciences: Environmental Genome Project. Accessed March 1, 2005, at http://www.niehs.nih.gov/envgenom/home.htm.

58. U.S. Department of Health and Human Services, National Institutes of Health, National Institute of Environmental Health Sciences, National Center for Toxicogenomics: Concept Statement. Accessed March 1, 2005, at http://www.niehs.nih.gov/nct/concept.htm.

59. American Conference of Governmental Industrial Hygienists: History of the American Conference of Governmental Industrial Hygienists. Accessed March 1, 2005, at http://www.acgih.org/about/history.htm.

84 *Pediatric Environmental Health for Toxicologists*

ROBERT J. GELLER, MD

At a Glance...

■ Pediatric environmental health is a relatively new discipline that examines the effects of environmental agents on the health of children.

■ Children have greater risk of exposure to environmental agents, as well as greater susceptibility to toxic effects, than adults.

■ A number of environmental pollutants are more likely to produce clinical toxicity in children than in adults. These include lead, mercury, and polychlorinated biphenyls.

■ There is a growing list of environmental agents that act as endocrine disrupters with the potential to affect critical aspects of organogenesis in young children.

■ Environmental regulations have recently begun to consider the unique susceptibilities of children in risk assessments and the establishment of exposure tolerances.

The field of pediatric environmental health may be unfamiliar to many. It is a relatively new discipline, one that attempts to combine the principles of environmental medicine with observations about metabolic pathways and toxicant-induced insults during the fetal, infant, and childhood periods of growth and development.

Many substances have the potential to affect children adversely. They range from organophosphate and carbamate pesticides to industrial chemicals such as polychlorinated biphenyls (PCBs) and by-products such as dioxins, from heavy metals such as mercury and lead to arsenic (Box 84-1). Even seemingly benign materials such as iodinated antiseptics and vaccine preservatives have become agents of concern.

This chapter provides an introduction to the principles of pediatric environmental health and discusses them in the context of several compounds. The chapter does not cover any of these issues exhaustively; the reader is referred to the chapter covering the specific compound and to published monographs on pediatric environmental health for more information.[1-3] The reader also should recognize that our knowledge about many issues in pediatric environmental health remains fragmentary; consequently, different clinicians, scientists, and policy makers may reach differing conclusions even while using the same data.

ASSESSING RISK

For some compounds, injury occurs after a certain threshold concentration of the compound is exceeded in the target organ. For others, toxicity results from accumulation of one or more metabolites of the parent compound. When the concentration of the compound and its metabolites remain below the threshold level, toxic injury does not occur. This is often referred to as a *threshold,* or *deterministic* effect.

Other substances appear to pose a risk for toxic effect at any concentration. The risk at low concentrations is usually below the risk posed by other causes, but is not zero. As the intensity of exposure increases, the risk for adverse effect also increases. In some circumstances, intensity of exposure may reflect both dose and length of exposure. Effects displaying this pattern often are mediated by injury to DNA of a single cell or a few cells. This pattern can be called a *no-threshold,* or *stochastic,* effect.

Toxicologic effects usually follow deterministic patterns, whereas mutagenic and carcinogenic effects usually fit a stochastic model. Both deterministic and stochastic effects may display linear or curvilinear relationships between the risk for toxicity and the concentration of the substance. The slope of the line and the shape of the curve display the relative susceptibility of the individual to the compound. These concepts are illustrated in Figure 84-1.

In the science of risk assessment, the level below which toxicity cannot be demonstrated is often referred to as the *no observable adverse effect level* (NOAEL). This level is determined using available data, which are ideally human; in the absence of robust human data, data from various animal species at varying ages are used. It is always uncertain to what extent animal-derived NOAEL concentrations can be applied to humans across the age spectrum—humans may ultimately prove to be more susceptible (such as to thalidomide embryopathy), equally susceptible, or less susceptible than experimental animals. To account for these uncertainties, different expert and regulatory bodies take different approaches in establishing risk thresholds. One of the most widely used approaches is that of the U.S. Environmental

BOX 84-1	ENVIRONMENTAL TOXINS RELEVANT TO CHILDREN'S HEALTH
Air particulates	Mercury
Arsenic	Ozone
Asbestos	Perchlorates
Carbon monoxide	Pesticides
Environmental tobacco smoke (ETS)	Polybrominated diphenyl ethers (PDBE)
Indoor air pollutants	Polychlorinated biphenyls (PCBs)
Lead	Radon
M-tert-butyl ether (MTBE)	Trichloroethylene

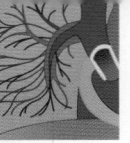

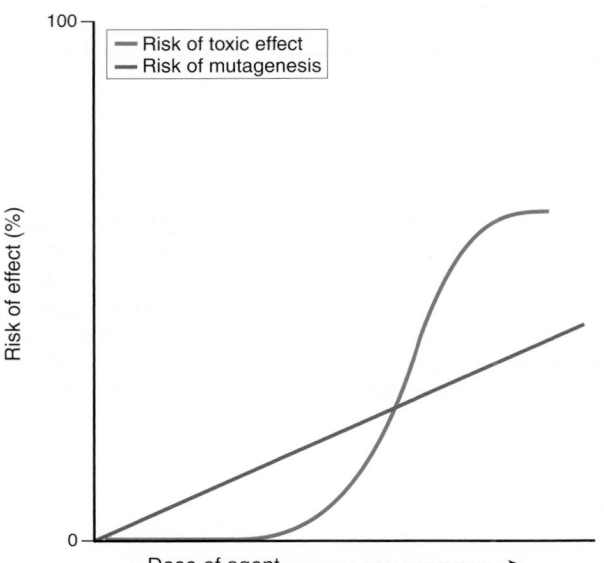

FIGURE 84-1. The dose–response curve of potential toxins, including drugs, chemicals, and physical agents, can have threshold deterministic and stochastic effects. Whether the curve is linear or curvilinear for stochastic phenomena can be debated, but it traverses 0. Toxicologic phenomena often follow an S-shaped curve, with a threshold below which no increased risks are expected. (From Brent RL, Tanski S, Weitzman M: A pediatric perspective on the unique vulnerability and resilience of the embryo and the child to environmental toxicants: the importance of rigorous research concerning age and agent. Pediatrics 2004;113[Suppl 4]:935–944.)

Protection Agency (EPA), which establishes a *reference dose* (RfD) or *reference concentration* (RfC) by starting with the NOAEL, adding a safety factor of 10 to account for interspecies difference, and adding another safety factor of 10 to account for interindividual differences. Since 1996, an additional safety factor of 10 is added to account for differences between humans of various ages, having the primary goal of establishing safe tolerances for children.[4] Existing data do not provide enough information to be certain that a factor of 10 is the best number to account for each of these differences.[1,5] It is therefore important to remember that this strategy produces reasonable approximations for safe use in the absence of actual substance-specific data. It is desirable to obtain actual data, which can then be used to provide more accurate guidance. However, there is considerable controversy about the research ethics of intentionally exposing humans to toxic agents (e.g., pesticides) in an effort to firmly establish a NOAEL.

Some of the differences among infants, children, and adults in their response to substances can be attributed to the differences in pharmacodynamics and pharmacokinetics at different ages, which are addressed by the field of study called *developmental pharmacology*. Other differences in response between children and adults are related to physiologic differences between them. Table 84-1 summarizes these concepts.

DEVELOPMENTAL PHARMACOLOGY

Different enzyme systems mature at different rates during fetal development and childhood. Although drug dose estimations derived from adult doses per kilogram of body weight have been used for many years, we have learned that such dosing strategies sometimes do not produce the expected results. Toxic outcomes, such as the "gray-baby syndrome" following chloramphenicol use in neonates and increased neonatal sensitivity to opioids and benzodiazepines,[6,7] have been observed when neonatal pharmacologic differences are not taken in account. Alternatively, dosing interpolated from adult doses to children may lead to decreased drug efficacy.

TABLE 84-1 Overview of Children's Developmental Features that Can Affect Toxicokinetics		
DEVELOPMENTAL FEATURE	**RELEVANT AGE PERIOD**	**TOXICOKINETICS IMPLICATIONS**
Body composition: lower lipid content, greater water content	Birth through 3 mo	Less partitioning and retention of lipid-soluble chemicals; larger Vd for water-soluble chemicals
Larger liver weight/body weight	Birth through 6 yr but largest ratios in first 2 yr	Greater opportunity for hepatic extraction and metabolic clearance; however, also greater potential for activation to toxic metabolites
Immature enzyme function: phase I reactions, phase II reactions	Birth through 1 yr but largest differences in first 2 mo	Slower metabolic clearance of many drugs and environmental chemicals; less metabolic activation but also less removal of activated metabolites
Larger brain weight/body weight; greater blood flow to CNS; higher BBB permeability	Birth through 6 yr but largest differences in first 2 yr	Greater CNS exposure, particularly for water-soluble chemicals that are normally impeded by BBB
Immature renal function	Birth through 2 mo	Slower elimination of renally cleared chemicals and their metabolites
Limited serum protein-binding capacity	Birth through 3 mo	Potential for greater amount of free toxicant and more extensive distribution for chemicals that are normally highly bound

BBB, blood-brain barrier; CNS, central nervous system; Vd, volume of distribution.
Adapted from Ginsberg G, Hattis D, Miller R, Sonawane B: Pediatric pharmacokinetic data: implications for environmental risk assessment for children. Pediatrics 2004;113 (Suppl 4):973–983.

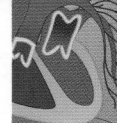

Compounds dependent for their metabolism on cytochrome isoforms such as CYP1A2 and CYP2A4 may undergo minimal biotransformation in utero because of the immaturity of cytochrome isoenzyme function in the fetus. CYP3A7 is present in large quantities during late fetal development and growth, fading rapidly after birth. To the extent that CYP3A7 metabolizes substrates similar to CYP3A4, the behavior of compounds principally metabolized in adulthood by CYP3A4 can be predicted. However, even this remains an approximation because the metabolic patterns of CYP3A4 and CYP3A7 are not identical.[8-12] Developmental differences in cytochrome function also have implications in how children are affected by environmental toxicants. For example, poly-aromatic hydrocarbons are metabolized to carcinogenic metabolites by CYP2A1. The relative immaturity of this enzyme in infants potentially confers protection from the carcinogenicity of these compounds. These concepts of developmental pharmacology are illustrated in Figure 84-2.

Other pharmacokinetic parameters also change as the child develops and matures. Total-body water decreases from about 0.8 L/kg (80% of body weight) to about 0.6 L/kg (60% of body weight) by 5 months of age.[8] Albumin binding sites may be present in lesser quantities, owing either to lower albumin levels or to these sites being occupied by bilirubin, which is normally present in higher concentrations in neonates and young infants than in adults. Lipid content may be lower in the young infant, resulting in increased deposition of lipophilic compounds in lipophilic organs such as the central nervous system (CNS).

PHYSIOLOGIC SUSCEPTIBILITIES

Infants and young children differ from adults in other ways that make them more susceptible to exposure and are more likely to develop exaggerated responses when exposed to environmental toxicants.

Infants display rapid growth. Their weight typically doubles by 3 months of age and triples by the end of their first year of life. Their length increases by 50% in the first year. To fuel this rapid growth, infants consume large amounts of food relative to their body weight. Initially, this comes from breast milk or infant formula. Environmental toxicants may have an impact on both. For example, breast milk can contain contaminants such as dichlorodiphenyltrichloroethane (DDT), PCBs, and polybrominated diphenyl ethers (PDBE). Infant formula is typically used in a powder or concentrated form, both of which require the addition of water. A formula-fed infant may ingest more than 100 mL/kg/day of water. Consequently, even the smallest degree of water contamination can lead to significant exposures in infants. As newborns become infants, a small number of foods make up a disproportionate amount of their solid intake. For example, compared with adults, young children eat significantly more fruits, particularly apples and grapes; they also consume disproportionately greater amounts of potatoes and beef (Figure 84-3).

Infant skin is less keratinized and more permeable than adult skin, which may lead to higher absorption of substances across the skin. As an example, premature infants exposed to topical povidone-iodine antiseptic agents have had elevations of plasma iodine levels, with resultant impact on thyroid function.[13] Melanocytes, the pigmented cells of the skin, are postulated to be more sensitive to the carcinogenic effects of exposure to ultraviolet light.[13]

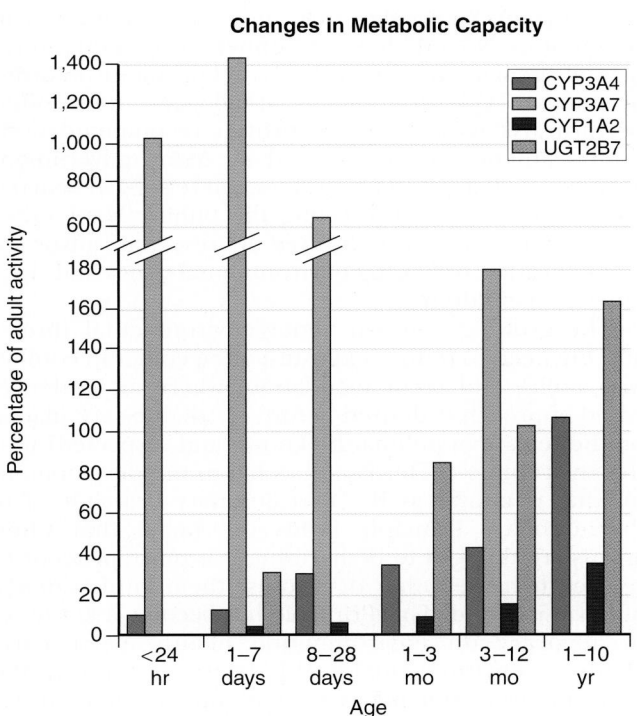

FIGURE 84-2. Changes in the activity of cytochrome systems at various ages. (Adapted from Kearns GL, Abdel-Rahman SM, Alander SW, et al: Developmental pharmacology: drug disposition, action, and therapy in infants and children. N Engl J Med 2003;349:1157–1167, and Lacroix D, Sonnier M, Moncion A, et al: Expression of CYP3A in the human liver: evidence that the shift between CYP3A7 and CYP3A4 occurs immediately after birth. Eur J Biochem 1997;247:625–634.)

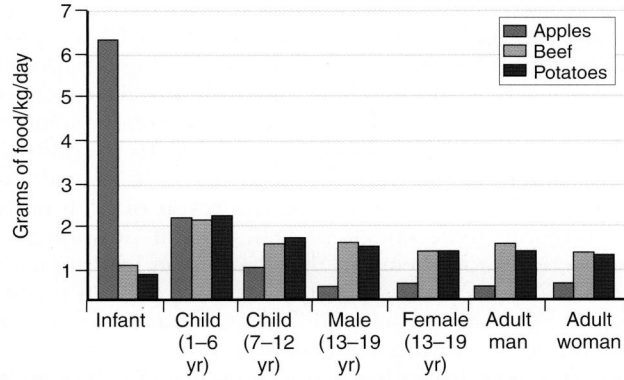

FIGURE 84-3. Differences in intake of selected food choices at various ages. (From Etzel RA, Balk SJ (eds): Pediatric Environmental Health, 2nd ed. Elk Grove Village, IL, American Academy of Pediatrics Committee on Environmental Health, 2003, p 14.)

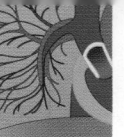

The infant immune system is still maturing and is not fully functional for at least the first few months of life. Various compounds may affect the immature immune system's development differently than they affect a mature immune system. In terms of infant lymphocyte maturation, infant exposure to environmental agents in the current era is postulated to be biased toward developing immune systems with a predominance of Th2-type CD4 T cells; these favor the development of an atopic state, away from Th1-type cellular immune responses (the so-called hygiene hypothesis).[14]

During their first year of life, infants and young children have a relatively higher minute ventilation (500 mL/kg/min versus 140 mL/kg/min in adults). Moreover, they breathe air that is closer to the ground because they crawl rather than walk upright (the "personal breathing zone"). This combination of factors predisposes them to toxicity from inhaled substances, particularly those present in higher concentration in air close to the ground. Settling of heavier-than-air compounds can particularly occur when air is stagnant or has uneven circulation.

The immaturity of the child's gastrointestinal and renal systems also has potential impact on the effects of exposure to environmental agents. The gastrointestinal tract of the child has greater permeability than that of the adult. For example, the gastrointestinal tract of the child absorbs up to 50% of ingested lead, whereas the gut of an adult absorbs about 10%. The glomerular filtration rate of children does not achieve adult capacity before 6 months of postnatal age, thereby reducing the ability of children to excrete toxicants.

Several aspects of brain development place the child at significantly increased risk for adverse neurodevelopmental effects after exposure to CNS neurotoxins. First, dendritic arborization, the process by which neuronal dendrites proliferate extensively, occurs primarily in the first 3 years of life. Second, the critical process of neuronal pruning, which eliminates useless and redundant neuronal connections, occurs during the same period. Third, myelination of neurons in the CNS occurs progressively during the first few years of life. Finally, the blood-brain barrier, which is designed to protect the CNS by preventing the intrusion of xenobiotics, is not completely formed until the second or third year of life. As a consequence of these critical aspects of development, children have a much greater risk for CNS injury, which could be permanent, when they are exposed during early childhood to environmental toxicants known to have any of these effects. The greater toxicity of lead, mercury, and other CNS neurotoxins to children is presumed to be the result of these CNS vulnerabilities.[15] Lead toxicity may be the result of both early and ongoing toxic effects of lead.[16] Lead poisoning is discussed in more detail in the chapter on lead toxicity, and has also been the subject of several excellent recent reviews.[15-17] The fetus and young infant are more susceptible to adverse neurodevelopmental outcomes after exposure to both organic mercury and inorganic mercury vapor. Severe methylmercury poisoning afflicted more than 3000 humans, many of them infants, in Minamata and Niigata, Japan, in the 1950s, as a result of industrial discharges into coastal waters that were the source of fish eaten by local residents. Although their mothers remained asymptomatic, 22 infants exposed in utero to the methylmercury displayed severe developmental disabilities.[18] A similar poisoning event occurred after the consumption of bread made from grain treated with a methylmercury fungicide.[18] The brain of the fetus has been estimated to be 10 to 15 times more sensitive to mercury effects than the brain of infants and children.

The endocrine system of children may also be more susceptible to harm from environmental agents. So-called *environmental endocrine disrupters* (EED) are chemical that in vitro possess an ability to act on the endocrinologic system. The list of putative EEDs is long and includes herbicides, fungicides, and plasticizers. Agents of great concern are bisphenol-A (a weak estrogen found in many plastics), phthalates (an agent commonly used in plastics with suspected spermatotoxic effects), PCB (which can affect the duration of lactation in women and the age of menarche in young girls), arsenic (which appears to have toxicity on the adrenal cortex), and perchlorates, dioxin, and PDBE (all of which have suspected effects on the thyroid). The clinical significance of these compounds remains controversial.[19,20]

GOVERNMENTAL AND NONGOVERNMENTAL APPROACHES

Our current knowledge does not always permit firm conclusions. Nonetheless, governmental and nongovernmental agencies, having a need to act prudently in order to mitigate risks to humans at all ages, must often perform risk assessments and provide recommendations in the absence of complete data. Many government agencies, at federal, state, and local levels, have enacted legislation aimed at protecting the public. Many other organizations also are involved in research, advocacy, and education regarding environmental issues and their impact on children.

The growing concern about environmental threats and the need to reduce exposure often comes in conflict with policy and recommendation, where an evidence-based approach is desired before restrictions are placed on the release of pollutants (known and suspected) into the environment. This issue has led to the development of what is known as the Precautionary Principle. The Precautionary Principle holds the belief that when agents are thought to be harmful, it is more prudent to restrict their use rather than to use them until evidence of harm is found. This Principle has become a key tenet in advocacy on environmental health, particularly children's environmental health. However, although the Precautionary Principle as been adopted by may nations and organizations (e.g., the European Union), it has met considerable resistance elsewhere. The basis of this resistance is that the Principle would produce undue restraint on the development of new products that help to advance society. Consequently, the Precautionary Principle remains controversial among both scientists and policy makers.

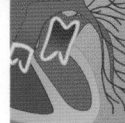

Many organizations, governmental and nongovernmental, have taken a lead role in protecting children from environmental threats. The American Academy of Pediatrics, for example, created its Committee on Environmental Health (COEH) in 1947 as a response to concerns about the impact of radioactive fallout from nuclear testing. The COEH has produced educational material and policy statements on issues in pediatric environmental health since its inception. Recently, the Committee produced a manual, *The Handbook on Pediatric Environmental Health,* designed to be a current, thorough resource on environmental health issues; a second edition of the handbook was released in 2003.[1] The EPA and the U.S. Agency for Toxic Substances and Disease Registry (ATSDR) jointly created the Pediatric Environmental Health Specialty Units (PEHSUs) in 1998, having the goal of creating a national network of environmental health clinical programs where parents and pediatricians could refer children for evaluation. A PEHSU is now located in each of the 10 U.S. EPA regions as well as in Mexico and Canada. The PEHSUs respond to inquiries from parents and professionals. They also educate the local population through education and outreach efforts. Additionally, EPA and the National Institute for Environmental Health Sciences (NIEHS) have created pediatric environmental health research units that are actively involved in performing and sponsoring research that improves understanding of pediatric environmental issues. Finally, in 1997, EPA created an Office of Child Health Protection whose goal is to ensure that EPA, as the nation's primary regulatory agency around environmental pollutants, consistently includes pediatric issues in all of its rulemaking.

CONCLUSIONS

The vulnerability and sensitivity of children to environmental agents is significantly different from that in adults. Because of the unique susceptibility of children to environmental toxicants, risk assessments and the subsequent policies they create now commonly include these pediatric issues.

A large of group of environmental pollutants affects children much more than adults. Pollutants in this category include lead, mercury, endocrine disrupters, and pesticides. Because of marked differences in the effects of these toxicants between children and adults, clinical management is significantly different.

These principles of children's environmental health are rapidly evolving into a new and unique clinical discipline.

REFERENCES

1. Etzel RA, Balk SJ (eds): Pediatric Environmental Health, 2nd ed. Elk Grove Village, IL: American Academy of Pediatrics Committee on Environmental Health, 2003.
2. Brent R, Weitzman M (eds): The vulnerability, sensitivity, and resiliency of the developing embryo, infant, child, and adolescent to the effects of environmental chemicals, drugs, and physical agents as compared to the adult. Pediatrics 2004;113(Suppl 4): 933–1172.
3. Schettler T, Stein J, Reich F, et al: In harm's way: toxic threats to child development. Boston, Greater Boston Physicians for Social Responsibility, 2000. Retrieved January 30, 2005, from http://www.igc.org.
4. Brent RL, Tanski S, Weitzman M: A pediatric perspective on the unique vulnerability and resilience of the embryo and the child to environmental toxicants: the importance of rigorous research concerning age and agent. Pediatrics 2004;113(Suppl 4):935–944.
5. Samet JM: Risk assessment and child health. Pediatrics 2004; 113(Suppl 4):954–955.
6. Mandelli M, Tognoni G, Garattini S: Clinical pharmacokinetics of diazepam. Clin Pharmacokinet 1978;3:72–91.
7. Coffey B, Shader RI, Greenblatt DJ: Pharmacokinetics of benzodiazepines and psychostimulants in children. J Clin Psychopharmacol 1983;3:217–225.
8. McCarver DG: Applicability of the principles of developmental pharmacology to the study of environmental toxicants. Pediatrics 2004;113(Suppl 4):969–972.
9. Ginsberg G, Hattis D, Miller R, Sonawane B: Pediatric pharmacokinetic data: implications for environmental risk assessment for children. Pediatrics 2004;113(Suppl 4):973–983.
10. DeWildt SN, Kearns GL, Leeder JS, et al: Cytochrome P450 3A: ontogeny and drug disposition. Clin Pharmacokinet 1999;37(6): 485–505.
11. Kearns GL, Abdel-Rahman SM, Alander SW, et al: Developmental pharmacology: drug disposition, action, and therapy in infants and children. N Engl J Med 2003;349:1157–1167.
12. Lacroix D, Sonnier M, Moncion A, et al: Expression of CYP3A in the human liver: evidence that the shift between CYP3A7 and CYP3A4 occurs immediately after birth. Eur J Biochem 1997;247:635–634.
13. Mancini AJ: Skin. Pediatrics 2004;113(Suppl 4):1114–1119.
14. McGeady SJ: Immunocompetence and allergy. Pediatrics 2004; 113(Suppl 4):1107–1113.
15. Canfield RL, Henderson CR Jr, Cory-Slechta DA, et al: Intellectual impairment in children with blood lead concentrations below 10 micrograms per deciliter. N Engl J Med 2003;248:1517–1526.
16. Chen A, Dietricj KN, Ware JH, et al: IQ and blood lead from 2 to 7 years of age: are the effects in older children the residual of high blood leads in 2 year olds? Environ Health Perspect 2005;113:597–601.
17. Koller K, Brown T, Spurgeon, Levy L: Recent developments in low-level lead exposure and intellectual impairment in children. Environ Health Perspect 2004;112(9):987–994.
18. Davidson PW, Myers GJ, Weiss B: Mercury exposure and child development outcomes. Pediatrics 2004;113(Suppl 4):1023–1029.
19. Greim HA: The endocrine and reproductive system: adverse effects of hormonally active substances. Pediatrics 2004;113(Suppl 4): 1070–1075.
20. Colborn T: Neurodevelopment and endocrine disruption. Environ Health Perspect 2004;112(9):944–949.
21. Weiss B, Amler S, Amler RW: Pesticides. Pediatrics 2004; 113(Suppl 4):1030–1036.

85 Common Perceived but Unproven Toxic Syndromes

JEFFREY BRENT, MD, PHD ■ LAURA J. KLEIN, MD

At a Glance...

■ Patients with a number of psychiatric diagnoses may present with signs and symptoms they attribute to being poisoned.

■ The determination of whether a chemical substance can cause a particular condition requires the application of appropriate methodology.

■ The conduction of an epidemiologic study that applies the criteria promulgated by Hill can be used to clarify whether there is a statistically significant relationship between an exposure and outcome in question.

■ Common perceived toxicologic syndromes for which application of appropriate methodology has failed to confirm a causal relationship are allegations of mercury toxicity from dental amalgam, systemic and cognitive symptoms from mold, childhood developmental disorders caused by the organomercurial preservative thimerosal in vaccines, and idiopathic environmental intolerance from low level exposures.

INTRODUCTION AND RELEVANT HISTORY

Matter, the tangible stuff of which biologic organisms and the world in which they live are made, is by definition composed of chemical substances. In the absence of a true vacuum, the entire world around us, both perceived and nonperceived (e.g., air), is a complex mixture of chemical substances. However this scientific depiction of our chemical world differs from the public perception that chemical substances, by their intrinsic nature, are harmful. Thus, for example, patients with the condition referred to as *idiopathic environmental intolerance* (IEI), formerly *multiple chemical sensitivity* (MCS), frequently complain that they develop symptoms when exposed to "chemicals."

The fundamental misconception regarding our exposure to chemical substances in the minds of the lay public, and too often in that of some health care practitioners, is easily fueled by nonscientific, non–peer-reviewed information disseminated by the popular press and Internet. These misconceptions and popularizations of nonsupportable scientific myths can create the perception of being poisoned by chemical substances, particularly in those individuals whose psychological constitution renders them vulnerable to these beliefs. This chapter critically examines a number of these so-called toxic syndromes and assesses whether or not there is scientific support for concluding that they have a true toxicologic etiology.

PSYCHOPATHOLOGY AND THE PERCEPTION OF TOXIC INJURY

The understanding of the etiologic nature of these syndromes is of fundamental importance in patient care because the misattribution of a toxicologic etiology to a patient's complaints may divert clinical attention from their psychiatric issues or medical diagnoses by reinforcing the belief that they are suffering a toxin-induced condition. Appreciation of the emotional features that may render an individual vulnerable to the development of these disorders is important for their appropriate treatment. Patients who attribute symptoms to a physical illness, when the true etiology is predominantly psychological in nature, are most commonly diagnosed with somatoform disorders, personality disorders, and mood disorders (i.e., depression and bipolar disorder). Alternatively, in cases in which secondary gain issues are present, such as in litigation, patients may engage in feigning of symptoms due to toxic exposure. This is diagnosed as malingering. When the sole purpose of the conscious, false presentation is to assume the so-called "sick role," the diagnosis is factitious disorder. Somatoform disorders are a cluster of psychiatric conditions in which bodily perceptions or functions are influenced by a mental disorder. According to the American Psychiatric Association's *Diagnostic and Statistical Manual of Mental Disorders* (DSM-IV-TR), somatoform disorders exist when "physical symptoms that suggest a general medical condition are not fully explained by a general medical condition, the direct effects of a substance or by another mental disorder."[1] The symptoms must cause significant distress or impairment in important areas of functioning and are not intentionally feigned. The key feature of the somatoform disorders is that psychological factors and conflicts are deemed important in initiating, exacerbating, or maintaining the disturbance. These patients characteristically are highly suggestible and are vulnerable to becoming convinced that they are experiencing serious physical problems. As such, they are frequently characterized as "reliable historians." This may result in the institution of medical treatment that may further reinforce their belief system or lead to iatrogenic conditions. Frequently, this leads to a vicious cycle of overinterpreting symptoms, development of increased anxiety, and creation of additional physical symptoms.[2] Addition of medication to treat anxiety may lead to adverse effects, including those affecting cognition, a frequent complaint in toxic exposures.

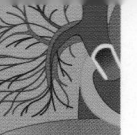

If patient symptoms are limited to the neurologic realm (i.e., motor and sensory function deficits) the diagnosis of conversion disorder is made. This is the most common type of somatoform disorder. Historically, the term *conversion* was first used by Sigmund Freud to describe the substitution of a somatic symptom for a repressed thought. Today, the *DSM-IV-TR* definition is more limited, yet the historical basis still continues to have importance in arriving at treatment recommendations. Treatment is aimed at focusing on the patient's psychological issues and, when possible, gaining insight into the meaning of the patient's symptoms. Direct confrontation of the patient's physical symptoms is discouraged, and this approach most commonly results in increased somatic complaints.

ASSESSMENT OF TOXICOLOGIC CAUSATION

To assess whether a specific medical condition is potentially caused by a toxic exposure, it is necessary to formally assess the likelihood of the existence of a true causal nexus between the chemical exposure and the condition in question. Doing so requires a formal scientific analysis of the relevant data using appropriate methodology.

The determination of whether a causal nexus exists between a toxic exposure and a subsequent medical illness is necessary to assess the likelihood of causation. Often, the possibility of such an association is raised by animal studies or anecdotal observations, such as those originating from case reports or uncontrolled case series. In many circumstances, these kinds of observations cannot truly assess the risk, if any, of developing a specific medical condition after an exposure. Thus, these observations are primarily useful for generating hypotheses about a potential causal relationship. In most instances, a controlled study, such as an epidemiologic investigation or a prospective trial, constitutes the primary source of evidence supporting causal hypotheses. If an association between a chemical exposure is demonstrated to exist in an epidemiologic study, the likelihood that this association represents a true causal nexus can be assessed by using the criteria promulgated by Hill.[3] This methodology is graphically illustrated in Figure 85-1.

A poignant example of anecdote versus epidemiology unfolded throughout the 1990s in the scientific investigation concerning the possible association between silicone breast implants and systemic rheumatologic conditions. Based on anecdotal observations of women with silicone breast implants who developed various rheumatologic conditions, it was hypothesized that there was a relationship between these devices and autoimmune or connective tissue diseases in these women. This was sensationalized in 1990 by a television broadcast by a major U.S. network suggesting that women were being harmed from these implants. The ensuing years were characterized by a flurry of litigation based on this hypothesized relationship, resulting in the bankruptcy of a major U.S. corporation. However, starting in 1993, and continuing throughout the next decade, at least 30 epidemiologic studies were published that evaluated the relationship between breast implants and systemic medical diseases or symptoms potentially referable thereto. This subsequent large number of studies has conclusively demonstrated that these implants do not confer any risk for having either these diseases or associated symptoms. Finally, in 1999, the U.S. National Academy of Sciences, Institute of Medicine (IOM) published a report concluding that there was no demonstrable association between silicone breast implants and the conditions that they were alleged to have caused.[4] Since the publication of the IOM report, further epidemiologic studies have been published, adding yet additional data supporting the lack of relationship between silicone breast implants and systemic disease.[5,6]

The scientific landscape is replete with other examples of overreaction to preliminary observations, which were subsequently proven wrong. It is interesting to note that there is a predictable evolutionary course for unfounded toxicologic notions. First, observations that lack scientific surety, such as anecdotes or rodent studies, generate a hypothesis that, before subject to the proper scrutiny described previously, becomes a widely held notion, often associated with considerable litigation. This attention leads to epidemiologic studies, which, if negative, generates an in-depth examination by the IOM, which finally puts the matter to rest. The tragedy of this repeating theme is that it consumes large amounts of societal resources, simply because of the sensationalism of preliminary observations.

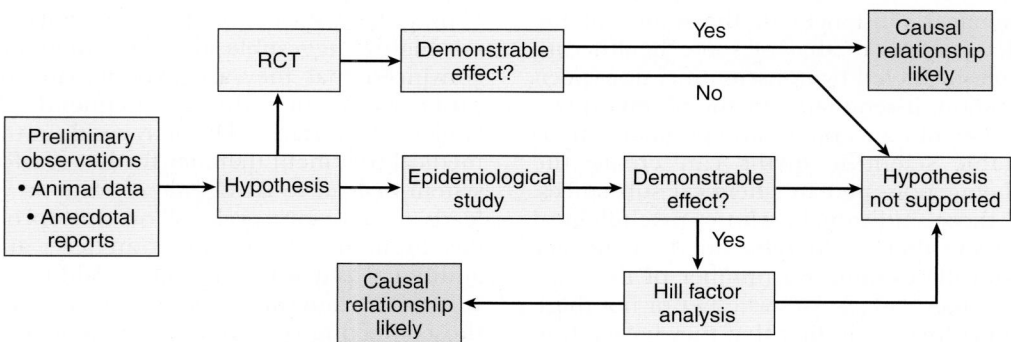

FIGURE 85-1 Steps in the formal methodology for assessing whether a causal nexus exists between a chemical exposure and a medical condition. This methodology employs Hill factor analysis.[3] RCT, randomized clinical trial.

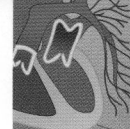

This chapter critically evaluates allegations of disease related to chemical exposures by focusing on four prototypical examples of alleged harm supported more by nonconventional sources than rigorous scientific studies. Yet these are perceived by a significant proportion of the population as representing true chemical hazards. Specifically, this chapter focuses on claims of systemic mercury poisoning from dental amalgam, autism from mercurial preservatives in vaccines, mold as a cause of systemic disease, and IEI.

DENTAL AMALGAMS AND MERCURY TOXICITY

Dental caries are a major form of oral morbidity, and their repair is essential to the maintenance of the masticatory function, which is important for ensuring normal human nutrition. The treatment of simple caries involves restoration with nonbiologic materials. Reports of the use of mercury for dental restoration can be found in 7th century Chinese literature. However, starting about 150 years ago, Western literature began to promote mercury-containing amalgams for this purpose. These are still used widely, although they are being replaced by other composites. The reason for the phasing out of mercury amalgams is primarily to reduce exposure to dental personnel and concern for environmental mercury contamination. However, there is an additional concern raised by advocacy groups who believe that systemic toxicity from mercury may occur as a result of having amalgams. Remarkably similar to the situation with breast implants, the discourse on this topic was further stimulated by a 1990 segment on the popular yet sensationalistic television program *60 Minutes* called "Is there Poison in Your Mouth?"

The controversy about potential adverse effects of amalgam stems from findings of concentrations of mercury in the oral cavity of amalgam-containing patients that might exceed occupational air level guidelines. These data generally derive from experiments using either vapor collectors, such as those that absorb mercury on gold or silver, or spectrophotometers. However, these instruments are designed to detect mercury leaks in large spaces. For example, accurate spectrophotometric analysis requires a constant flow rate, a condition that cannot be satisfied during intraoral measurements. In 1985, there were two reports of measurements of mercury intraoral mercury vapor, which incorrectly treated the concentration in their collection vessel as if it were representative of intraoral levels.[7,8] Such an assumption introduced a large overestimation of oral mercury concentration.[9-11] In order to avoid this kind of error, it is important to avoid equating concentration measurements with dose. Dose is best determined by the release rate of mercury from the amalgams. As discussed subsequently, this has been done and found not to be toxicologically consequential.

Standard dental amalgams contain about 50% mercury in its elemental form (Hg^0), combined with other metals such as copper or silver. Mercury has a small but measurable ability to volatilize (vapor pressure, 0.0013 mm at 20° C) (see Chapter 71). During normal wear and tear, small amounts of elemental mercury are vaporized into the oral cavity, where it can be inhaled or solubilized in saliva and swallowed. Microparticles may also be generated during the chewing process. It is this small amount of mercury that constitutes a systemic dose and has led to the concerns about alleged mercury poisonings from amalgams.

About 80% of mercury vapor that is inhaled is subsequently absorbed.[12] The amount of mercury released in patients with amalgam is less than 10 μg/day.[13] For patients with few restorations, the ultimate pulmonary absorption may be as low as 1 μg/day; the absorption is greater in those with a larger number of amalgam surfaces.[11] In contrast, only 0.01% to 0.04% of evaporated mercury vapor that is swallowed will be absorbed.[12] This also amounts to about 1 μg/day, but it is in the form of mercuric ion, which does not appreciably cross the blood-brain barrier. The amount of mercury absorbed is, thus, significantly less than the World Health Organization (WHO) acceptable daily limit of mercury ingestion of 40 μg. Once absorbed into the circulation, mercury has a blood half-life of about 2 days[14] but a total-body half-life of about 60 days.[15] There is some pulmonary clearance of circulating mercury; up to 15% of the absorbed dose is exhaled by 1-week after exposure[16,17] (Fig. 85-2). To put these doses in context, the total mercury exposure from all sources in nonoccupationally exposed individuals is estimated to be between 2.3 to 5.8 μg/day.[18] Thus, in non–fish-eating populations, dental amalgam is potentially the largest source of mercury exposure. Heavy fish or seafood eaters may ingest larger amounts of mercury, but in the form of the organomercurial methyl mercury.

Being lipid soluble, Hg^0 may bidirectionally diffuse across the blood-brain barrier (see Fig. 85-2) and has the potential to be neurotoxic in sufficient doses. Once in the brain, elemental mercury that does not diffuse out may be oxidized to Hg^{2+} (mercuric ion). The mercuric ion has a very high affinity for sulfhydryl groups, such as those found on glutathione (GSH), cysteine, metallothioneins, polypeptides, and proteins.[19] Mercury can also bind to selenium. It is likely that binding to GSH, metallothioneins, and selenium represents protective pathways, whereas binding to sulfhydryl groups of structural proteins and enzymes may be either protective or result in functional alterations. Although the kidney is the major storage organ for Hg^0, about 7% of an absorbed dose is stored in the brain.[16,20] Studies on human cadavers indicate that occipital lobe mercury concentrations in the absence of amalgams are about 7 ng/g.[21] Each amalgam surface adds only about 0.24 ng/g to this value.[10,22] Occipital lobe is chosen for these studies because it is a primary target of mercury toxicity, explaining the characteristic constriction of visual fields seen in mercurialism. Most of the elemental mercury absorbed is systemically oxidized by catalase to Hg^{2+}, which can be excreted. Although there is some biliary mercury clearance, most (60%) is renally

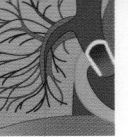

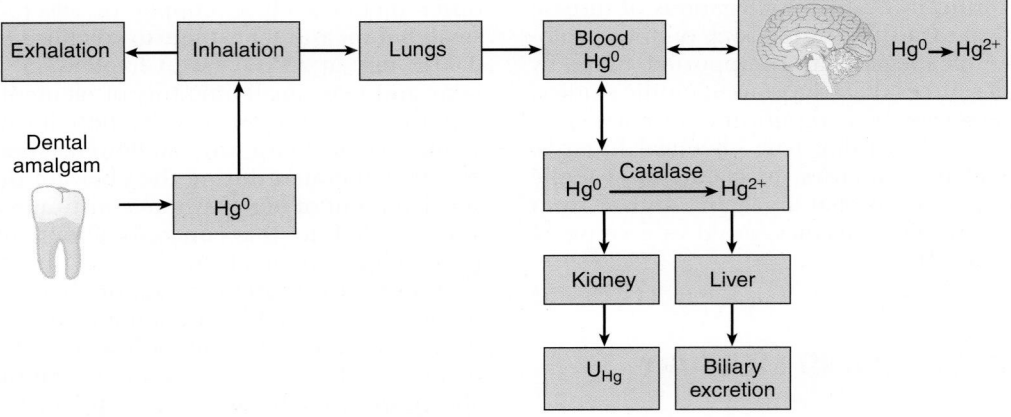

FIGURE 85-2 Body handling of mercury released from dental amalgam.

eliminated.[23] Thus, urine mercury concentrations are an excellent quantitative biomarker for Hg^0 exposure.[24]

Because mercury vapor is released from amalgams, there is a relationship between the number of amalgam surfaces and the blood and urine mercury concentration (U_{Hg}).[24] However, the U_{Hg} of amalgam-bearing patients is in the 2- to 4-μg/L range, which is 12- to 25-fold lower than the acceptable U_{Hg} for occupationally exposed workers.[15] The combined urinary and biliary excretion of mercury is sufficient to clear an absorbed daily amalgam-derived dose.[13]

Elemental mercury has been implicated as causing immune dysfunction, antibiotic resistance, autoimmune diseases such as systemic lupus erythematosus and multiple sclerosis, and vague symptoms of neurotoxicity. Like most chemical substances, elemental mercury can cause hypersensitivity reactions in predisposed individuals. These are very rare; about 50 cases have been reported. The literature contains descriptions of a few cases of type I (anaphylactic) reactions.[25] More commonly, when hypersensitivity reactions occur from dental amalgam, they represent a type IV reaction and are manifested by oral lichenoid manifestations.[26-29] However, there is little to support allegations of alterations in normal flora, systemic immunologic abnormalities, or autoimmune disease resulting from amalgams. Among the most studied of the effects of amalgam have been those relating to mood and to neurocognitive and neuropsychological function. The most comprehensive study to date broadly assessed health effects related to any body system, evaluated neurologic effects in great detail, and assessed for renal disease because the kidney is a major end organ for mercury poisoning.[30] No amalgam-related adverse effects were found. However, a high frequency of psychiatric diagnoses has been reported in patients who attribute their symptoms to amalgams.[31,32] In a dedicated multidisciplinary clinic for patients with concern about amalgam, it was found that among 379 patients evaluated, the presence of symptoms, as measured by the Standard Symptom Checklist-90 (SCL-90) questionnaire, was very high, with 20 or

more symptoms commonly reported.[33] The most common symptoms were myalgias, arthralgias, weakness, fatigue, dizziness, difficulty in concentrating, headache, anxiety, and depression. More than 70% of the patients had serious psychological trauma in the past year, and nearly 10% of patients were found to have previously undiagnosed significant medical problems. The results of the SCL-90 showed a tendency to somatization in almost 70% of the patients. Elevated parameters for anxiety, depression, and obsessive tendencies were common. No patient had mercury toxicity.[33] A number of other recent studies have similarly suggested psychological etiologies for amalgam-related symptoms.[34-36] A recent in-depth review commissioned by the U.S. government found that the existing data of this body of literature fail to support amalgam-related health effects.[37]

Poisoning from elemental mercury is well described and is characterized by tremor, constriction of visual fields, alterations in renal function, ataxia, psychological syndrome known as erethism, and gingivitis-stomatitis (see Chapter 71). This characteristic spectrum of mercurialism is markedly different than the aforementioned complaints of individuals with symptoms they attribute to dental amalgam.[38,39]

Further support for the notional, rather than physiologic, basis for complaints related to mercury from dental amalgams comes from the study of the effects of chelation therapy on symptoms in patients who have attributed their illnesses to their amalgams. In a double-blinded randomized trial on patients ascribing their symptoms to dental amalgam, there was improvement reported after chelation therapy. Improvement was similar, however, in the group that received placebo.[40] The significant placebo effect demonstrable in these patients might indicate that they have heightened suggestibility.

Subsequent to concern raised by advocacy groups, governmental agencies in Europe,[41] Canada,[42,43] Australia,[44] and the United States,[37,45,46] as well as nongovernmental organizations such as WHO,[47] the

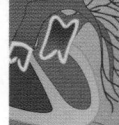

American[18] and Canadian Dental Associations,[18] and the National Multiple Sclerosis Society[48] studied the strength of the association between dental amalgams and human mercury poisoning. These groups have all concluded that, in the absence of demonstrable hypersensitivity reactions, there are insufficient scientific data to conclude that there is a relationship between mercury exposure from dental amalgams and their various alleged effects.

AUTISM FROM THIMEROSAL IN VACCINES

The organomercurial preservative thimerosal has been used in a number of biologic preparations since the 1930s. At that time, various mercurials were used for a number of purposes, including the treatment of infectious diseases and as diuretics. Nonorganomercurials are no longer used for these purposes because of their relatively low margin of safety and the introduction of more efficacious agents. However, organomercurials were found to have minimal toxicity and a favorable safety profile. Based on this, ethyl mercury salicylate (thimerosal) was developed and ultimately became widely used as a pharmaceutical under the brand name of Merthiolate. A number of early papers indicated that relatively large doses of Merthiolate did not cause toxicity to humans or animals.[49] The first major clinical use of Merthiolate use was reported in 1930, which involved intravenous administration of large doses of thimerosal as an "antiseptic solution" for the treatment of meningococcal meningitis.[50] Thimerosal was also administered intranasally to people with positive nasopharyngeal cultures for meningococcus. No significant toxicity from thimerosal administration to either the patient or the carriers was reported.

Widespread use of Merthiolate blossomed during World War II when large amounts of serum and plasma were used for resuscitation and volume support. Despite its widespread use, no significant toxicity was associated with Merthiolate except for possible allergic reactions. Throughout this time period, and for the balance of the 20th century, thimerosal was widely used.

Because of the tremendous public health benefit of vaccines, the number and types of vaccinations steadily rose throughout the 1990s. Coincident with the increased intensity of childhood vaccination, there has been a rise in the incidence of autism spectrum disorder (ASD), largely due to changes in diagnostic practices. This temporal relationship has led to speculation that there may be a relationship between the administration of vaccines and childhood ASD. A number of advocacy groups that have embraced the concept that vaccines are causally related to the increase in ASD have focused on the thimerosal in these vaccines and have suggested that this compound may cause autism. These claims have been widely distributed on a number of Internet sites. As a result, many families have opted to attempt to forgo vaccination or even subject their children to chelation therapy. Speculation about the role of thimerosal in the etiology of ASD was fueled by a widely quoted analysis that inappropriately applied the U.S. Environmental Protection Agency (EPA) reference dose (RfD) for *methyl mercury* to thimerosal.[51] Restriction of the analysis to the first 6 months of life and a full vaccination schedule leads to the potential for exceeding this dose based on vaccine administration. However, this is an illogical comparison for a number of important reasons. The EPA RfD, as noted previously, is for methyl mercury. Thimerosal is known to quickly dissociate to ethyl mercury. Ethyl mercury and methyl mercury are markedly different in their toxicologic and pharmacokinetic properties. Thus, the methyl mercury RfD should not be considered applicable to thimerosal or ethyl mercury.[52] Further, the RfD for methyl mercury is based on a study of a fish-eating population in the Faroe Islands, where subtle decrements on neurocognitive testing in children have reported an inverse correlation between blood and hair mercury concentrations and testing results.[53] A very similar study, done on another predominantly fish-eating population in the Seychelles Islands, however, has failed to find a similar effect based on hair mercury concentrations.[54] Thus, the Faroe data, on which the EPA RfD is based, are questionable. It should also be noted that the effects reported in the Faroese cohort are very subtle and based strictly on sensitive neurocognitive testing. There were no clinically discernible mercury-related effects based on physical examinations or maternal reports. Thus, the EPA RfD is based on very subtle and questionable effects that have nothing at all to do with ASD. The concentration of mercury from vaccines, which before the removal of thimerosal in 1999 was generally 12.5 or 25 µg per vaccination, is extremely small and therefore would not be expected to cause toxicity of any kind.

Because of the allegations of ASD being caused by thimerosal from childhood vaccination, a number of epidemiologic studies have evaluated whether an association exists between mercury administration from thimerosal and ASD. These studies have failed to find a relationship between the administration of mercury-containing vaccines and ASD.[55] Based on these epidemiologic studies, the considerations described previously, and other factors, the IOM published a report in 2003 formally rejecting the hypothesis of an association between thimerosal administration and the subsequent development of ASD.[55]

MOLD AS A SOURCE OF SYSTEMIC DISEASE

The term *mold*, as used in this chapter, refers to a ubiquitous subgroup of fungi that grow as multicellular visible colonies containing large numbers of intertwined hyphae. Fungi are a group of spore-forming eukaryotic organisms that some put in their own unique kingdom. Other nonmold fungi of toxicologic interest are mushrooms, which are discussed in detail in Chapter 23. An additional group of nonmold fungi is responsible for human morbidity, including opportunistic organisms

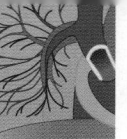

(e.g., coccidioides, histoplasma) and superficial integumental infections such as tinea pedis and onychomycosis.

Mold tends to grow in damp environments, a condition satisfied by virtually all buildings some, or most, of the time. Concern for environmental mold as a source of major human disease to the nonimmunocompromised host was fueled in the early 1990s when investigators initially implicated the mold *Stachybotrys chartarum* in several cases of infantile pulmonary hemorrhage in Cleveland.[56] Although these cases focused attention on potential systemic disease caused by environmental mold exposure, particularly *Stachybotrys* species, subsequent reanalysis of these cases by both the IOM and the U.S. Centers for Disease Control and Prevention have failed to verify the link between mold exposure and these cases.[57,58] In the interim, however, there has been an explosion of allegations on the Internet, fueled by advocacy groups and other interested parties, linking environmental mold exposure and multiple systemic symptoms or diseases, a phenomenon that one editorialist deemed "mold madness."[59]

There are a number of health problems that are potentially attributable to molds; therefore, any complaint of mold-related illness must consider these diagnoses. Most prominent are allergic reactions, which may be either immunoglobulin E (IgE)- or IgG-mediated. The former causes atopic effects, such as rhinosinusitis, atopic asthma, or dermatitis. IgE is generally reactive with fungal proteins of either hyphal or spore origin. The most prominent indoor molds that cause immediate hypersensitivity are *Aspergillus* and *Penicillium* species.[60] Typical outdoor molds of interest are *Alternaria* and *Cladosporium* species.[60] Individuals who have IgE-mediated immediate hypersensitivity to molds tend to be more generally atopic and thus respond to other common environmental allergens. Much less common is IgG-mediated hypersensitivity in the form of extrinsic allergic alveolitis (EAA), formally referred to as hypersensitivity pneumonitis. Individuals with mold-related EAA have generally been exposed to large amounts of mold-derived protein and develop an exaggerated IgG response. Because this is due to inhalation, the antibody–antigen interaction occurs in the lung. A more detailed discussion of mold-related EAA can be found in other references.[57] Ingestion of the plant fungus *Claviceps purpurea* caused the vasospastic syndrome known as *St. Anthony's fire* from ergot alkaloids produced by the fungus.[61]

Molds may also produce mycotoxins, which are large molecules elaborated from fungi. Because of their size, they have a low vapor pressure and are thus not a significant airborne threat. However, when ingested, mycotoxins may cause aflatoxicosis and manifest as liver or renal disease. Mold is also found as a commensal organism colonizing the human vagina and gastrointestinal tract.

A number of adverse health outcomes have been associated with exposure to indoor mold. These have primarily been related to the respiratory system but have also involved allegations of dermatologic, gastrointestinal, connective tissue, immune, and neuropsychiatric syndromes, including fatigue. Patients who complain of mold-related systemic symptoms do not generally test positive for allergic responses to these fungi, nor can a relationship between symptoms and dose be demonstrated.[62] Because of the profound public concern for adverse effects from moldy environments, the IOM undertook a detailed evaluation of the potential adverse effects of damp indoor spaces.[63] Their methodology involved four levels of scientific certainty, the highest being sufficient evidence of a causal relationship and the lowest being inadequate or insufficient evidence to determine whether an association exists between damp indoor environment or mold and adverse health outcomes. There was no health effect that was considered to be documented well enough to meet the sufficient evidence of a causal relationship standard. Some upper respiratory effects were through to be characterized by sufficient evidence of an association, and others were characterized by limited or suggestive evidence of an association. All the other effects were found to characterize the lowest level of surety, indicating that there was not evidence to determine an association. Although the IOM report is the most comprehensive to date, other professional societies, including the American College of Occupational and Environmental Medicine and the Texas Medical Association, have taken similar positions.[57,64]

Thus, based on currently available information, other than the allergic and opportunistic effects described previously, there are few data to support the widespread notion of more diffuse toxic effects of exposure to mold.

IDIOPATHIC ENVIRONMENTAL INTOLERANCE

Originally referred to as multiple chemical sensitivity (MCS), this syndrome is now more properly referred to as idiopathic environmental intolerance (IEI). The former designation, invoking the concept of sensitization, has an etiologic implication. Sensitization is properly viewed as an immunologic phenomenon. In fact, early proponents of a physiologic basis for this syndrome evoked such an immunologic ideology. However, with the subsequent evolution of a significant body of data refuting an immunologic basis for MCS, this designation became obsolete. As the designation for this syndrome has morphed, so has the nomenclature of its proponents. Formally called "clinical ecologists," the group of physicians advocating a physiologic basis for IEI now designate themselves "environmental medicine" physicians. However, environmental medicine is not an accepted medical specialty in the United States. It is important to distinguish this group from the recognized specialty of Occupational and Environmental Medicine. The ethos of the latter group is directly contrary to that of "environmental physicians." The American College of Occupational and Environmental Medicine has formally rejected a physiologic basis for IEI.[65]

In 1996, a WHO/German Government Conference suggested that idiopathic environmental intolerance was a more appropriate designation.[66] The 1996 Conference

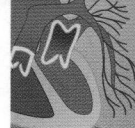

determined that IEI was a symptom complex experienced by people after exposure to nonspecific environmental chemicals at concentrations and doses that do not affect most people with a repetitive pattern of symptom occurrence, not explainable by any well-accepted medical condition.

There have been two major categories of theories proposed to explain the occurrence of these symptoms in the absence of a medical explanation. Toxicogenic theories posit that low-level "chemical" exposures in a hypothesized physiologic vulnerable population trigger these repetitive symptoms in an as yet scientifically unexplainable fashion. In contrast, psychogenic theories are based on the concept of an overvalued belief of toxic harm based on psychological factors. A recent in-depth critical analysis of these two disparate theories strongly concluded that the psychogenic explanation is most consistent with the current state of scientific knowledge.[67,68]

The optimum methodologic approach to the study of IEI uses exposure chambers, where the subject is exposed to either filtered room air or substances they have previously identified as "provocants." The odor properties are masked by innocuous substances such as peppermint, which is also added to the air in placebo trials. Pioneering work in this field by Staudenmayer and colleagues has shown with this methodology that patients complaining of IEI cannot identify their provocants in anything more than chance fashion.[69] The WHO has assessed IEI and recommended that the existence of this condition could best be verified by exposure chamber experiments.[66] The results of exposure chamber studies, therefore, provide strong support for the psychogenic theory of IEI symptoms. The diagnoses that apply would most commonly be in the realm of somatoform disorders, although individual psychiatric evaluation is mandatory before such a diagnosis can be established. Many patients with IEI symptoms have overlap syndromes with other conditions that are often explainable by a somatoform disorder, such as the mold or dental amalgam syndromes discussed earlier in this chapter. Examples of other conditions commonly explainable by the presence of a somatoform disorder are some cases of fibromyalgia, sick-building syndrome, and chronic fatigue syndrome.

Disclaimer: Dr. Brent has served as a consultant to SmithKline Glaxo, a vaccine manufacturer.

REFERENCES

1. American Psychiatric Association: Diagnostic and Statistical Manual of Mental Disorders, 4th ed. Washington, DC, American Psychiatric Association, 2000.
2. Lees-Haley PR, Brown RS: Biases in perception and reporting following a perceived toxic exposure. Percept Mot Skills 1992;-75:531–544.
3. Hill AB: The environment and disease: association or causation? Proc R Soc Med 1965;58:295–300.
4. Bondurant S, Ernster V, Herdman R (eds): Safety of Silicone Breast Implants. Washington DC, National Academy Press, 1999.
5. Janowsky EC, Kupper LK, Hulka BS: Meta-analysis of the relation between silicone breast implants and the risk of connective-tissue diseases. N Engl J Med 2000;342:781–790.
6. Lipworth L, Tarone RE, McLaughlin JK: Silicone breast implants and connective tissue disease: an updated review of the epidemiologic evidence. Ann Plastic Surg 2004;52:598–601.
7. Vimy MJ, Lorscheider FL: Intra-oral mercury released from dental amalgam. J Dent Res 1985;64:1069–1071.
8. Vimy MJ, Lorscheider FL: Serial measurements of intra-oral mercury: estimation of daily dose from dental amalgam. J Dent Res 1985;64:1072–1075.
9. Berglund A, Pohl L, Olsson S, et al: Determination of the rate of release of intra-oral mercury vapor from amalgam. J Dent Res 1988;57:1235–1242.
10. Mackert IR Jr: Factors affecting estimation of dental amalgam mercury exposure from measurements of mercury vapor levels in intra-oral and expired air. J Dent Res 1987;66:1775–1780.
11. Eley BM: The future of dental amalgam: a review of the literature. Part 4: Mercury exposure hazards and risk assessment. Br Dental J 1997;182:373–381.
12. Clarkson TW: The three modern faces of mercury. Environ Health Perspect 2002;110(Suppl 1):11–23.
13. Halbach S: Amalgam tooth fillings and man's mercury burden. Hum Exp Toxicol 1994;13:496–501.
14. Magos L, Halbach S, Clarkson TW: Role of catalase in the oxidation of mercury vapor. Biochem Pharmacol 1978;27:1373–1377.
15. Clarkson TW: The toxicology of mercury: current exposures and clinical manifestations. N Eng J Med 2003;349:1731–1737.
16. Hursh JB, Cherian MG, Clarkson TW, et al: Clearance of mercury (Hg-197, Hg-203) vapor inhaled by human subjects. Arch Environ Health 1976;31:302–309.
17. Sandborgh-Englund G, Elinder CG, Johanson G, et al: The absorption, blood levels, and excretion of mercury after a single dose of mercury vapor in humans. Toxicol Appl Pharmacol 1998;150:146–153.
18. Levy M: Dental amalgam: toxicological evaluation and health risk assessment. J Can Dent Assoc 1995;61:667–674.
19. Rahola T, Hattula T, Korolainen A, et al: Elimination of free and protein-bound ionic mercury ($^{203}Hg^{2+}$) in man. Ann Clin Res 1973;5:214–219.
20. Kaga M, Seale NS, Hanawa T, et al: Cytotoxicity of amalgams. J Dent Res 1988;67:1221–1224.
21. Eggleston DW, Nylander M: Correlation of dental amalgam with mercury in brain tissue. J Prosthet Dent 1987;58:704–707.
22. Nylander M, Friberg L, Lind B: Mercury concentrations in the human brain and kidneys in relation to exposure from dental amalgam fillings. Swed Dent J 1987;11:179–187.
23. Clarkson TW, Hursh JB, Sager PR, et al: Mercury. In Clarkson TW, Friberg L, Nordberg Gf, Sager PR (eds): Biological Monitoring of Toxic Metals. New York, Plenum Press, 1988:199–246.
24. Agency for Toxic Substances and Disease Registry: Toxicological profile for mercury. Available at: http://www.atsdr.cdc.gov.
25. Enestrom S: Does amalgam affect the immune system? A controversial issue. Int Arch Allergy Immunol 1995; 1–6:180–203.
26. Ellingsen DG, Efskind J, Haug E, et al: Effects of low mercury vapour exposure on the thyroid function in chloralkali workers. J Appl Toxicol 2000;20:483–489.
27. Soleo L, Vacca A, Vimercati L, et al: Minimal immunological effects on workers with prolonged low exposure to inorganic mercury. Occup Environ Med 1997;54:437–442.
28. Ibbotson SH, Speight El, Macleod RI, et al: The relevance and effect of amalgam replacement in subjects with oral lichenoid reactions. Br J Dermatol 1996;134:420–423.
29. Koch P, Bahmer FA: Oral lesions and symptoms related to metals used in dental restorations: a clinical, allergological, and histologic study. J Am Acad Dermatol 1999;41:422–430.
30. Bates MN, Fawcett J, Garrett N, et al: Health effects of dental amalgam exposure: a retrospective cohort study. Intl J Epidemiol 2004;33:894–902.
31. Bratel J, Haraldson T, Ottosson JO: Potential side effects of dental amalgam restorations. II. No relation between mercury levels in the body and mental disorders. Eur J Oral Sci 1997; 105:244–250.
32. Bratel J, Haraldson T, Meding B, et al: Potential side effects of dental amalgam restorations. I. An oral and medical investigation. Eur J Oral Sci 1997;105:234–243.

33. Langworth S: Experiences from the amalgam unit at Huddinge hospital: somatic and psychosomatic aspects. Scand J Work Environ Health 1997;23(Suppl 3):65–67.
34. Bailer J, Rist F, Rudolf A, et al: Adverse health effects related to mercury exposure from dental amalgam fillings: toxicological and psychological causes? Psychol Med 2001;31:255–263.
35. Gottwald B, Traenckner I, Kupfer J, et al: "Amalgam disease": poisoning, allergy, or psychic disorder? Int J Hyg Environ Health 2001;204:223–229.
36. Zimmer H, Ludwig H, Bader M, et al. Determination of mercury in blood, urine and saliva for the biological monitoring of an exposure from amalgam fillings in a group with self-reported adverse health effects. Int J Hyg Environ Health 2002;205:205–211.
37. Review and Analysis of the Literature on the Potential Adverse Effects of Dental Amalgam. Bethesda, MD, Life Sciences Research Office, 2004.
38. Ask K, Akesson A, Berglund M, et al: Inorganic mercury and methylmercury in placentas of Swedish women. Environ Health Perspect 2002;110:523–526.
39. Vahter M, Akesson M, Lind B, et al: Longitudinal study of methylmercury and inorganic mercury in blood and urine of pregnant and lactating women, as well as in umbilical cord blood. Environ Res 2000;84:186–194.
40. Grandjean P, Guldager B, Larsen IB, et al: Placebo response in environmental disease: chelation therapy of patients with symptoms attributed to amalgam fillings. J Occup Environ Med 1997;39:707–714.
41. Commission of the European Union Ad Hoc Working Group in Amalgam. Ad Hoc Working Group Report on Amalgam. Available at: http://www.nordiskadental.se.
42. Health Canada: Mercury and human health. Available at: http://www.hc-sc-gc.ca.
43. Counseil d'Evaluation des Technologies de la Sante du Quebec (CETS): Reports from the Counseil d'Evaluation des Technologies de la Sante du Quebec (CETS). The safety of dental amalgam: a state-of-the-art review. Int J Technol Assess Health Care 1997; 13:639–642.
44. National Health and Medical Research Council: Dental amalgam and mercury in dentistry. http://www.health.gov.au.
45. U.S. Department of Health and Human Services: Dental amalgam: a scientific review and recommended public health service strategy for research, education and regulation. Available at: http://www.health.gov.
46. U.S. Department of Health and Human Services. Dental amalgam and alternative restorative materials. Available at: http://www.health.gov.
47. FDI World Dental Federation: WHO consensus statement on dental amalgam. FDI World 1997;6:9.
48. Slater R, Calvano M: Silver amalgam fillings and multiple sclerosis. Memorandum No. 115-83, National Multiple Sclerosis Society, 1983.
49. Powell HM: Merthiolate as a germicide. Am J Hyg 1931;13:296–310.
50. Smithburn, et al: Meningococcic meningitis. JAMA 1930;95: 776–779.
51. Ball L, Ball R, Pratt RD: An assessment of thimerosal use in childhood vaccines. Pediatrics 2001;107:1147–1154.
52. Brent J: Toxicologists and the assessment of risk: the problem with mercury. J Toxicol Clin Toxicol 2001;39:707–710.
53. Grandjean P, Budtz-Jorgensen E, White RF, et al: Methylmercury exposure biomarkers as indicators of neurotoxicity in children aged 7 years. Am J Epidemiol 1999;150:301–305.
54. Myers GJ, Davidson PW, Cox C, et al: Prenatal methylmercury exposure from ocean fish consumption in the Seychelles child development study. Lancet 2003;361:1686–1692.
55. Institute of Medicine: Immunization Safety Review. Vaccines and Autism. Washington, DC, National Academies Press, 2004.
56. Centers for Disease Control and Prevention (CDC): Acute pulmonary hemorrhage/hemosiderosis among infants—Cleveland, January 1993–November 1994. MMWR Morb Mortal Wkly Rep 1994;43:881–883.
57. American College of Occupational and Environmental Medicine (ACOEM): Adverse Human Health Effects Associated with Molds in the Indoor Environment. Elk Grove Village, IL, ACOEM, 2002.
58. Centers for Disease Control and Prevention (CDC). Availability of case definition for acute idiopathic pulmonary hemorrhage in infants. MMWR 2001;50:494–495.
59. Zacharisen MC, Fink JN: Is indoor "mold madness" upon us? Ann Allergy Asthma Immun 2005;94:12–13.
60. Solomon WR, Platts-Mills TAE: Aerobiology and inhalant allergens. In Middleton E Jr, Ellis EF, Yunginger JW, et al (eds): Allergy: Principles and Practice. St. Louis, Mosby, 1998, pp 367–403.
61. Kulig K: Ergot alkaloids. In: Brent J, Burkhart K, Donovan W, et al (eds): Critical Care Toxicology: Diagnosis and Management of the Critically Poisoned Patient. Philadelphia, Elsevier Mosby, 2005, pp 723–728.
62. Bobbitt, Jr RC, Crandall MS, Venkataraman MS, et al: Characterization of a population presenting with suspected mold-related health effects. Ann Allergy Asthma Immunol 2005; 94:39–44.
63. Institute of Medicine: Damp Indoor Spaces and Health. Washington, DC, National Academies Press, 2004.
64. McClusky OE: Report of Council on Scientific Affairs of the Texas Medical Association on "Black mold and human illness." (CSA Report 1-I-02, September, 2002), Austin, TX, Texas Medical Association, 2002.
65. American College of Occupational and Environmental Medicine: Multiple chemical sensitivities: idiopathic environmental intolerance. Position statement. ACOEM Report 1999; June 1–3.
66. International Programme on Chemical Safety/World Health Organization (PPCS/WHO): Conclusions and recommendations of a workshop on multiple chemical sensitivities (MCS). Regul Toxicol Pharmacol 1996;24:S188–189.
67. Staudenmayer H, Binkley KE, Leznoff A, et al: Idiopathic environmental intolerance. 1. A causation analysis applying Bradford Hill's criteria to the toxicogenic theory. Toxicol Rev 2003;22:235–246.
68. Staudenmayer H, Binkley KE, Leznoff A, et al: Idiopathic environmental intolerance. 2. A causation analysis applying Bradford Hill's criteria to the psychogenic theory. Toxicol Rev 2003;22:247–261.
69. Staudenmayer H: Clinical consequences of the EI/MCS "diagnosis": two paths. Regul Toxicol Pharmacol 1996;24:S96–110.

86 *Smoke Inhalation*

CHRISTOPHER H. LINDEN, MD

At a Glance...

■ Smoke inhalation accounts for more than 80% of fire-related fatalities, most of which result from residential fires.

■ The pathophysiology of smoke inhalation is multifactorial and involves additive or synergistic toxicity from hypoxia, thermal injury, and numerous chemical toxins (e.g., carbon monoxide, hydrogen cyanide, irritant gases).

■ The ultimate cause of death in patients with smoke inhalation is asphyxia (i.e., tissue hypoxia and consequent acidosis).

■ The carboxyhemoglobin fraction is elevated in virtually all patients exhibiting signs and symptoms of asphyxia.

■ Unexplained coma, severe metabolic (lactic) acidosis, and refractory hypotension victims suggests cyanide poisoning.

■ Urgent endotracheal intubation is indicated in patients with cyanosis or hypoxemia despite oxygen therapy, respiratory depression or acute hypercarbia, pulmonary edema, altered mental states, full-thickness burns of the face or neck, and respiratory distress due to upper airway obstruction.

■ Intubation should also be considered for patients with upper airway pathology on laryngoscopy or a respiratory rate of more than 30 breaths/min who do not improve with oxygen or other pharmacologic therapy.

■ Hyperbaric oxygen can be effective in treating carbon monoxide or cyanide poisoning, cerebral edema, and thermal burns; it should also be considered for patients with refractory hypoxemia.

■ When cyanide poisoning is suspected in smoke inhalation victims, sodium thiosulfate may be administered without nitrates.

Smoke is a complex mixture of liquid and solid aerosols, fumes, gases, and vapors resulting from thermal decomposition or pyrolysis.[1,2] Although commonly defined as the visible cloud emitted from a material that has been ignited, smoke is not always visible. In fires, pyrolysis usually begins as flaming combustion (oxidative pyrolysis or thermo-oxidation) resulting from the application of an igniting source (e.g., spark or flame) to a flammable material. As heat is generated and oxygen is consumed, smoldering combustion (oxidative pyrolysis without flame) and nonoxidative or anaerobic pyrolysis become the dominant processes. Pyrolysis can also result from the application of intense heat without fire or flame. Metal fume fever and polymer fume fever, which result from the inhalation of products generated when metals and synthetic polymers (e.g., fluorocarbons and other plastics) are heated above their melting points, are classic examples.[3,4] Hence, the adage, "where there's smoke, there's fire," is not always true.

Although not often appreciated, the scene of smoldering combustion is more far more hazardous than that of flaming combustion.[2] Not only is less oxygen available, more toxic gases are present, and the potential for flare-up is greater. Because combustion is less complete, more carbon monoxide (CO), a product of incomplete combustion, is evolved during smoldering combustion than during flaming combustion, where carbon dioxide (CO_2) is the predominant product of combustion. In addition, combustible gases generated under conditions of oxygen depletion can suddenly ignite, particularly when enclosed spaces are subsequently opened (i.e., supplied with oxygen). Examples include "flashover" (the simultaneous ignition of all surfaces of a room or structure without the progressive spread of flame) and explosive "flare-up," as exemplified in the 1991 movie *Backdraft*. Preventing such events explains the "C" in the fire response acronym RACE (rescue, alarm, close all doors and windows, extinguish) and the recommendation that a person attempting to escape a fire scene not open a door if it is hot.

Thousands of potentially toxic organic and inorganic chemicals are generated when materials undergo pyrolysis.[1,2,5-11] Their identity, amount, and rate of production depend on the source material and the temperature, rate, and mode of pyrolysis. However, technical limitations and lack of knowledge of the materials and conditions involved, which vary with time and space, make it impossible to determine precisely what chemicals (and physical factors) are present at the scene of naturally occurring events such as fires. Those most widely studied and thought to be most responsible for morbidity and mortality in human smoke inhalation are listed in Table 86-1.

Although smoke invariably contains CO, the pathophysiology and management of smoke inhalation are far more complex than of pure CO poisoning (see Chapter 87). In contrast to CO poisoning, morbidity and mortality from smoke inhalation are due to multiple chemical and physical factors (see Table 86-1). CO poisoning is often involved, but other causes of asphyxia, particularly inhalation (respiratory tract) injury, must also be evaluated and treated.

EPIDEMIOLOGY AND HISTORY

In the United States, more than 4000 people die from fire-related injuries each year (about 2.3 deaths per 100,000 population).[12] Smoke inhalation is the primary cause of death in more than 80% of cases, with surface burns and other trauma accounting for the remainder.[1,2,13] Of note, in some commercial aircraft crashes, more people die from smoke inhalation secondary to postcrash fire than from injuries sustained on impact.[14]

Eighty percent of smoke inhalation deaths occur within 6 hours of exposure and 93% within 24 hours.[12,15]

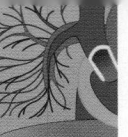

TABLE 86-1 Factors Involved in the Pathophysiology of Smoke Inhalation

MECHANISM OF ASPHYXIA	CAUSE	SOURCE
Oxygen deficiency (simple asphyxia)	Ambient hypoxia Carbon dioxide Multiple other gases	All combustible materials
Functional anemia (abnormal hemoglobin)	Carbon monoxide Methemoglobin inducers	All combustible materials Unknown
Cytochrome oxidase inhibition (cellular asphyxia)	Carbon monoxide Hydrogen cyanide	All combustible materials Animal products, acrylics, acrylonitrile-butadiene-styrene plastics, melamine resins, nylons, urea-formaldehyde foam insulation, wool
Airway or lung injury (corrosive effects)	Acrolein, other aldehydes and hydrocarbons, organic acids, nitrogen oxides	Most combustible materials
	Ammonia, isocyanates	Same as for hydrogen cyanide
	Carbonyl fluoride	Fluorocarbons (e.g., Teflon)
	Halogen acids, phosgene	Fire extinguishers, flame retardants, acrylics, films, polyvinylchloride plastic, resins
	Heat, flame, steam Sulfur oxides	Most combustible materials Animal and petroleum products, rubber, wool
Mechanical airway obstruction Central nervous system depression	Soot Alchohol Drugs Cellular asphyxiants Hypoxemia Trauma	All combustible materials

In victims who are dead when discovered, death has historically been attributed to asphyxia due to CO poisoning or severe upper- and lower-airway obstruction and pneumonitis. Environmental oxygen depletion, heat, and cyanide poisoning are now considered contributing factors.[16] In those who are found alive but moribund, early death results from respiratory failure due to progressive airway and lung injury. Delayed deaths primarily result from anoxic brain damage, pulmonary edema, bacterial pneumonia, sepsis, and pulmonary embolism.

About 75% of fire-related fatalities in the United States result from residential fires.[12] Carelessness with cigarettes, matches, flammable liquids (e.g., fuels and cooking oils), wood stoves, and other heating devices and malfunctioning appliances and heating systems are the underlying causes in most instances. In multiperson-dwelling fires, children younger than 5 years of age, the elderly, those with physical or cognitive disabilities, and those impaired by alcohol or other drugs are at higher risk for death than able-bodied, unimpaired adults.[12] More than half of home fire deaths result from fires in the 5% of homes with no smoke alarms. Despite stricter building codes, increased use of smoke detectors, and improvements in medical care, the annual number of fire-related fatalities has changed little in the past 60 years.

Before World War II, most fire-related fatalities were due to surface burns rather than smoke inhalation.[1,2] During the next two decades, the incidence of death due to smoke inhalation tripled.[17] In 1951, Zapp, considered the father of combustion toxicology, first reported that more fatalities were caused by smoke inhalation than by surface burns.[18] It was not initially recognized that pyrolysis products of plastics or synthetic polymers, which were introduced during the previous two decades and increasingly used in the construction and furnishing of buildings, were responsible for these observations. When first introduced, plastics were promoted by manufacturers as nonburning and self-extinguishing.[1]

In 1962, Zapp was again the first to report that pyrolysis products of synthetic polymers (e.g., polyamine, polyethylene, polypropylene, polystyrene, polyurethane, polyvinyl chloride) were different from and more toxic than those from natural materials (e.g., cotton, wood, and wool).[19] Subsequent research confirmed these findings. Plastics manufacturers, however, continued to deny responsibility. In 1972, the Federal Trade Commission initiated a complaint charging the plastics industry with failing to disclose, misrepresenting, and falsifying evidence.[1]

It is now known that, compared with natural materials, plastics (and other synthetics) spread flame faster, make flare-ups and flashover more likely, and generate more heat more quickly, more and denser visible smoke, and greater amounts of more toxic invisible products of pyrolysis.[1] Paradoxically, although newer structures are less likely to catch fire, building construction materials and contents have become more dangerous when subjected to thermal decomposition. This, along with population increases, most likely explains why the annual number of fire-related fatalities has remained relatively constant.

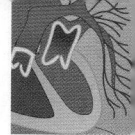

In most countries, every fire death is subject to investigation by a coroner or medical examiner and nonmedicolegal authorities. Forensic investigations have attempted to define the role or contribution of individual chemical and physical factors in causing death by analyzing autopsy data and by fire dynamics modeling. Infamous single events that have been studied include fires at the Cleveland Clinic in 1929,[20] the Coconut Grove (Boston) night club in 1942,[21,22] the Maura County (Tennessee) jail in 1977,[23] the Las Vegas MGM Grand hotel in 1980,[24] the Westchase (Houston) Hilton hotel in 1982,[25] the aircraft crash in Manchester (England) in 1985,[14] the Dupont Plaza Hotel (San Juan, Puerto Rico) in 1986,[26] and the Happy Land Social Club (New York City) in 1990.[16] Data from multiple fire locations have been reported from Wayne County (Detroit area),[27] Cuayhoga County (Case Western Reserve University, Cleveland),[28,29] the Foundation for Fire Safety (16 jurisdictions in the United States and Canada),[30] Maryland,[31] Mississippi (University of Southern Mississippi),[32] Glasgow (Scotland),[33-35] Munich (Germany),[36] New York City,[5,37,38] Oslo (Norway),[39] and Paris (France).[40] In many instances, victims were found dead in areas remote from the fire, sometimes without evidence of heat, smoke, or soot, emphasizing the fact that in enclosed spaces, fatal smoke inhalation can occur without palpable or visible warning.

Despite such investigations, the specific toxicants responsible for morbidity and mortality in human smoke inhalation remain uncertain and unpredictable.[16] For example, in many fires, victims have lethal carboxyhemoglobin (COHb) fractions,[5,27,37,38] lethal blood cyanide (CN) levels,[30] or both,[16,40] but a correlation between the two is not necessarily present.[14,29,30] In other fires, nonlethal COHb fractions and CN levels are found, and death is attributed to respiratory tract injury from irritant gases[24,28] or to heat shock and oxygen depletion.[25] Even in a single fire, factors responsible for death vary from individual to individual.[16]

One objective of forensic investigations is to determine whether death resulted from smoke inhalation or whether fire was used to conceal a prior death (e.g., a homicide or suicide). Historically, COHb has been used as a biomarker of smoke inhalation. Multiple studies have shown that COHb fractions in victims of fatal smoke inhalation are lower than in nonfire CO fatalities (e.g., from exposure to pyrolysis products of fossil fuels).[27,31,38] In fire exposures, a COHb fraction of 50% or greater is considered evidence that CO was the principal cause of death and that the victim died from smoke inhalation.[16] In contrast, in nonfire exposures, a COHb fraction of 60% or greater is generally used when assessing whether, "more likely than not," death was due to CO poisoning. Again, the reason for this difference is that multiple other factors are involved in the pathogenesis of smoke inhalation. It is now clear that fire victims can have COHb fractions well below 50%, yet their death can clearly be attributed to smoke inhalation. Analysis of fire fatality data shows that COHb fractions have declined over time. It follows that other chemical or physical factors have become relatively more important.

One such factor is hydrogen cyanide gas (HCN). In contrast to CO, the definition of a lethal blood CN level is controversial, with 1 to 3 μg/mL considered potentially lethal after the inhalation of HCN.[16] Interestingly, in the first study to measure CN levels in fire victims, none had potentially lethal levels.[26] Also in contrast to CO, analysis of fire fatality data shows that blood CN levels in fire fatalities and the fraction of victims with potentially lethal CN levels have been increasing with time.[16] Irritant gases are also considered to have an increasing role in morbidity and mortality from smoke inhalation. Increased use of synthetic materials in the construction and furnishing of buildings is again the likely explanation for these trends.

Nitrogen oxides produced by burning nitrocellulose x-ray film were implicated as the cause of inhalation injury in victims of the 1929 Cleveland Clinic fire.[19] It is now known that ammonia, HCN, isocyanates, methemoglobin inducers, and other respiratory tract irritants are also generated when nitrogen-containing compounds undergo pyrolysis. Inhalation injuries in victims of the 1942 Coconut Grove night club fire were described as similar to those caused by "certain war gases," presumably referring to chlorine and phosgene, the gases used in World War I.[20] It is now appreciated that these gases, along with many other irritants (see Table 86-1), are indeed found in smoke.

The toxicity of the individual chemical and physical factors that contribute to morbidity and mortality is well known. Recent research has focused on the effect of combinations of factors. Most significantly, these studies show additive or synergistic toxicity when oxygen depletion and irritant gas exposure is combined with CO and HCN (see later), again emphasizing the fact that the pathophysiology of smoke inhalation is multifactorial.

Attempts to find practical, nontoxic fire retardants have met with limited success.[1,2] When applied or added to materials, a variety of chemicals (e.g., antimony oxide; aluminum, boron, bromine, chlorine, molybdenum, and organophosphorus compounds; halogenated polymers) make them more difficult to ignite and less likely to propagate flame. None is completely effective or safe. Fire retardants themselves can produce toxic products when thermally degraded.

Smoke alarms decrease the risk for death from fire by up to 60%.[12,41] Both ionization smoke alarms, which contain material that ionizes the air and creates an electrical path when products of combustion enter the device, and photoelectric alarms, which contain a light source that activates a photocell when light is reflected off smoke particles, provide a warning well before life-threatening conditions develop. Sprinkler systems are also advocated for the prevention of fire-related morbidity and mortality, but data regarding their efficacy are limited, particularly in residential settings.[12,41] Sprinkler systems typically require an air temperature of 150° C at the ceiling level for activation. Although such temperatures are reached before immediately lethal conditions develop, they do not occur until many minutes after conditions become sufficient to activate smoke alarms or cause inhalation injury.[16] Hence, it is unlikely that sprinkler systems will be shown to be as effective as smoke alarms in preventing morbidity and mortality from smoke inhalation.

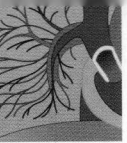

PATHOPHYSIOLOGY

Chemical and physical agents most commonly implicated in the pathophysiology of smoke inhalation are listed in Table 86-1. The severity of injury varies with both time and space. Those victims with longer exposure time and shorter distance to the source (i.e., greater toxicant concentrations) will have more severe effects. There is a hyperbolic relationship between the time of onset and severity of effects and exposure conditions: the greater the exposure, the more rapid and pronounced the effects, and vice versa.

In a closed space, potential lethal conditions can develop within minutes of fire ignition.[42] Smoke initially accumulates in a hot layer at the ceiling level and subsequently descends toward the floor.[16] This explains why those attempting escape a fire scene are advised to crawl or stay close to the floor (i.e., "fall and crawl"). Indeed, there are anecdotal reports of survivors collapsing or fainting, falling to the floor (where they breathe cooler and less contaminated air), regaining consciousness, and subsequently crawling to safety.

Victims succumb because of incapacitation (cognitive and physical dysfunction) and escape impairment that results from smoke inhalation, other fire scene factors, and preexisting or concurrent illness or infirmity.[8,16] Factors that contribute to incapacitation and escape impairment include asphyxia; coughing, choking, and dyspnea; impaired vision due to smoke, darkness, and ocular irritation; surface burns and traumatic injuries; physical obstacles such as debris, fire, heat, and slippery surfaces; and alcohol or drug intoxication, extremes of age, cardiovascular or pulmonary disease, and physical handicaps. Incapacitation and escape impairment increase smoke exposure and result in further cognitive and physical dysfunction. A progressive downward spiral ensues, ending with physical collapse, loss of consciousness, apnea, and cardiac arrest. Natural reactions to a fire, such as attempting to extinguish it and attempting to warn and rescue others, also prolong exposure. Indeed, many victims appear to have been attempting to escape before their death, and significant numbers die upon reentering the fire scene.[12]

Regardless of contributing factors, the ultimate cause of death in patients with smoke inhalation is asphyxia (i.e., tissue hypoxia, hypercarbia, and acidosis). Asphyxia may be due to oxygen deficiency (i.e., breathing air rarified by combustion or containing gases that lower the partial pressure of oxygen), impaired oxygen transport and delivery (e.g., by COHb and methemoglobin), inhibition of cellular respiration (e.g., by CO and CN), central respiratory depression (e.g., by CO, CN, and carbon dioxide), and direct or indirect obstruction of air passages and alveoli (e.g., by heat, humidity, irritant gases, and soot).

CO, heat, and oxygen deficiency are produced by all fires and are the primary causes of death due to enclosed-space fuel fires under experimental conditions.[18] Historically, CO poisoning (see Chapter 87) has been considered the primary cause of death in human smoke inhalation.[34] However, when a COHb fraction of 50% or greater is used as the criterion for death from CO due to smoke inhalation, this conclusion is no longer true. Since about 1970, fewer than half of the fatalities in multiple fire databases (primarily residential fires) have COHb fractions of 50% or greater. For example, in the Maryland study, 40% of victims dead at the scene had COHb fractions less than 50%, 24% had COHb fractions less than 30% (the fraction associated with incapacitation and escape impairment but not death), and 9% had COHb fractions less than 10%.[31] Similar findings have been reported by others.[27-30,34,39] The data from single mass casualty incidents is even more impressive. Most victims in the MGM Grand Hotel, the Dupont Plaza Hotel, and the Manchester aircraft fires had COHb fractions less than 50% (88%, 95%, and 92%, respectively), and a greater percentage had COHb fractions less than 30% (41%, 40%, and 28%, respectively).[14,24,26]

For a variety of reasons, assessing the contribution of CO to morbidity and mortality from smoke inhalation is difficult. Although COHb fractions generally correlate with the severity of inhalation injury, victims of smoke inhalation can have high COHb fractions without significant pulmonary toxicity, and vice versa.[15,31,38,43-48] Because manifestations of CO poisoning are virtually identical to other causes of asphyxia, the relative contribution of CO cannot be determined by clinical assessment. In addition, COHb fractions correlate with clinical toxicity only after relatively brief exposures. The longer the duration of exposure, the greater the effect at a given COHb fraction.[30] This suggests that it takes time for blood and tissues levels of CO to equilibrate and that the area under the time–concentration curve (AUC) must be considered when interpreting COHb fractions. The effect of CO also depends on the extent of its binding to and inhibition of cytochrome oxidase, the mechanism of CO-induced cellular asphyxia. Binding of CO to cytochrome oxidase depends on the oxidation state of this enzyme, with binding to the reduced (deoxygenated) form being greater than it is to the oxidized form. The same is true for CN. This is the rationale for oxygen therapy in CO and CN poisoning. It also explains why the lethality of CO is enhanced when combined with oxygen depletion or HCN exposure. In experimental animals, these three agents act synergistically, with time to death and lethal levels of CO and CN decreasing as much as 10-fold in combined exposures.[16,49] In contrast, the effect of combining irritant gases with oxygen depletion, CO, or HCN appears to be simply additive.[50-54] These findings probably explain why sublethal levels of both COHb and CN and insignificant inhalation injury are observed in some fire fatalities.

The higher the ambient air temperature and humidity, the greater the morbidity and mortality from smoke inhalation in experimental animals.[55] Exposure of animals to dry air heated to 200° C for 5 minutes or to 125° C for 15 minutes is potentially lethal.[5] Shorter exposures to dry air at temperatures of 350° C to 500° C result in tracheitis.[56] Exposure to steam, which has much greater heat capacity, results in bronchitis and pul-

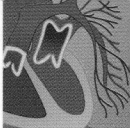

monary parenchymal damage in addition to tracheitis at such temperatures. High skin surface temperature and hyperthermia undoubtedly contribute to incapacitation and escape impairment. Surprisingly, however, respiratory tract injury secondary to heat and humidity is relatively uncommon in human exposures and occurs primarily in those with concomitant surface burns.[25,57]

Decreased ambient oxygen fractions, which occur as oxygen is progressively consumed during combustion, result in hypoxic asphyxia. At sea level, the normal oxygen fraction is about 21%. An acute reduction in the inspired oxygen reduction to 15% to 18% results in dyspnea on exertion, and a reduction to 10% to 14% results in confusion and dyspnea at rest.[1] At fractions of 6% to 8%, loss of consciousness followed by death occurs within 5 to 8 minutes. Experimentally, lethal oxygen fractions do not occur until the temperature is quite high (about 315° C).[16] This combination, however, is rapidly lethal. In addition, as noted earlier, oxygen depletion enhances the toxicity of both CO and CN. Although the effects of ambient hypoxia are indistinguishable from those of other causes of asphyxia and cannot be assessed clinically, circumstantial and experimental evidence suggest that it plays a significant role in causing fire scene deaths. Because this condition is readily reversible and ceases to exist after removal from the fire scene, its only subsequent effects are those related to anoxic organ damage.

HCN is produced when materials containing nitrogen (e.g., acrylonitrile plastics, melamine resins, nylon, wool, urea-formaldehyde foam insulation) are burned. The pathophysiology of cyanide poisoning is discussed in Chapter 88. HCN is more potent and produces more rapid incapacitation and death than CO in experimental animals.[16] Potentially toxic CN blood levels have been noted in as many as 30% of survivors and 100% of fatalities, and potentially lethal levels have been reported in up to 10% of survivors and 70% of fatalities.[11,29,30,35,40,46,58,59] Data are difficult to interpret, however, because the technique and time of blood sampling, storage, and analysis and definitions of potentially toxic and potentially fatal blood CN concentrations vary from study to study. Using cutoffs of 1 µg/mL or greater and 3 µg/mL or greater, potentially toxic and potentially lethal blood CN levels were found in 7% to 74% and 0% to 46% of multiple fire fatalities, respectively.[16] In single-casualty incidents, potentially toxic and potentially lethal levels were noted in 48% to 87% and 5% to 33%, respectively. As noted earlier, the highest blood CN levels are noted in victims of recent fires.

For a number of other reasons, the contribution of CN to death from smoke inhalation is difficult to quantify.[16] The kinetics of CN are much more complex than for CO, and few data exist regarding its kinetics after HCN inhalation. Such exposure results in a rapid rise in the blood CN level, which may not be in equilibrium with those in mitochondria, and thus not reflect tissue toxicity. As with CO, CN binding to cytochrome oxidase and its toxicity are enhanced by oxygen depletion, and CN, CO, and oxygen depletion have synergistic effects in experimental animals. Although blood CN levels usually correlate with the both the COHb fraction[16,35,40] and the severity of inhalation injury,[46,58,59] this is not always true. In some fires, high CN levels with low COHb fraction are seen,[14] and vice versa.[16] Such apparently "antagonistic" findings could result if high concentrations of either HCN or CO (but not both) were present, with respiratory depression caused by one agent preventing the uptake of the other agent. In those found dead at the fire scene, levels of CN and CO tend to be lower when both are present, consistent with an additive or synergistic effect in humans. The interpretation of such data depends on the level of CN assumed to be lethal.[16] As with other factors, manifestations of CN poisoning are indistinguishable from other causes of asphyxia, preventing clinical assessment of its role in human morbidity. Furthermore, blood CN levels are not routinely available and cannot be rapidly measured. Finally, the short half-life of CN, about 1 hour,[40] suggests that its role in nonfatal smoke inhalation is minor.

Smoke contains a variety of chemicals that are directly toxic to the mucosal surfaces of the eyes and respiratory tract (see Table 86-1). Differences in pyrolysis products explain why smoke from natural materials is more irritating or corrosive than that from synthetic ones. Smoke from materials of animal (e.g., fur, hide, silk, wool) or plant (e.g., cotton, paper, wood) origin contains mostly aldehydes (e.g., acetaldehyde, formaldehyde, acrolein) and lesser amounts of organic acids (e.g., formic and acetic acid), alcohols, and aliphatic and aromatic hydrocarbons.[2,5-10] Smoke from animal products also contains appreciable amounts of ammonia (NH_3), nitrogen oxides (primarily NO_2), and sulfur oxides (primarily SO_2). With the exception of NH_3, these chemicals are considered mildly to moderately corrosive to tissues. Because they also have low water solubility, they tend to travel to the distal respiratory tract and cause bronchial, bronchiolar, and alveolar injury.

Smoke from synthetic materials contains a greater amount and variety of mildly to moderately corrosive organic compounds (e.g., acids, alcohols, aldehydes, aliphatic and aromatic hydrocarbons, amines and nitriles, halogenated hydrocarbons, ketones, and polymer monomers such as acrylates, esters, carbonates, phenols, and styrene) along with ammonia, and nitrogen and sulfur oxides.[2,5-11,60] Most important, smoke from halogenated materials (e.g., acrylics, fire extinguishers and retardants, solvents, and polyvinylchloride) contains hydrogen bromide (HBr), hydrogen chloride (HCl), hydrogen fluoride (HF), phosgene (CCl_2O), and carbonyl fluoride (CF_2O or fluophosgene). CCl_2O and CF_2O are instantly hydrolyzed to their respective acids and CO_2 on contact with water.[3] All these compounds are inorganic acids, which, in contrast to organic ones, are considered highly corrosive to mucosal tissues. Remarkably, the inhalation of HCl causes incapacitation faster than CO (but slower than HCN) in experimental animals.[16] Acids and bases (e.g., NH_3) have high water solubility and tend to dissolve in the moist tissues of the

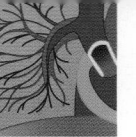

upper airway, causing nasopharyngeal, laryngeal, and tracheal injury. They can also cause immediate or delayed pulmonary toxicity. Persistent or permanent respiratory dysfunction can occur after acute inhalation injury (see later) or with chronic exposure to smoke (e.g., in tobacco smokers or firefighters).[61]

Delayed pulmonary effects are characteristic of polymer fume fever.[4] This syndrome is a flulike illness that occurs several hours after the inhalation of products generated when fluorocarbon polymers such as polytetrafluoroethylene (PTFE, Teflon) are heated to about 400° C. This can occur during manufacturing processes (when ventilation fails or is insufficient), when workers smoke contaminated cigarettes (e.g., without first washing their hands), when lubricants are heated by friction, and when coated cookware is overheated in the home. Fine particulates are thought to cause the pyrogenic reaction, and vapors (e.g., carbonyl fluoride) are thought to be responsible for respiratory effects. The inhalation of smoke from the combustion of PTFE or its pyrolysis at higher temperatures results in more fulminant and typical inhalation injury. Metal fume fever is discussed in Chapter 75.

The tissue toxicity of smoke, like other inflammatory reactions, appears to be mediated by arachidonic acid metabolites (e.g., leukotrienes, prostacyclins, and thromboxanes), cytokines (e.g., platelet-activating factor), free radicals (e.g., superoxide, peroxide, hydroxyl), and activated polymorphonuclear leukocytes.[62] In experimental animals, smoke inhalation causes mucosal edema, necrosis and pseudomembrane formation, and obstruction in the trachea and bronchi, followed by pulmonary vascular congestion, alveolar edema, atelectasis, and bronchopneumonia.[63] Respiratory tract inflammation also results in bronchospasm, loss of ciliary function, destruction of surfactant, and increased microvascular permeability.[47,64,65] Increased shunting (secondary to pulmonary vasoconstriction), loss of lung compliance, and ventilation-perfusion mismatching may ensue. Although concentrations of irritants (in air and tissues) are difficult to measure, their contribution to morbidity and mortality in human smoke inhalation can be assessed both clinically and pathologically.

CO_2, along with CO, constitutes most of the gaseous fraction of smoke.[2] An increased CO_2 fraction in inspired air causes simple asphyxia by physically displacing oxygen. Increasing blood levels of CO_2 initially stimulate and subsequently depress brainstem respiratory centers. High levels also cause generalized central nervous depression. These actions could increase exposure to smoke by increasing ventilation and causing incapacitation, and potentially contribute to fire scene deaths. As with oxygen depletion, except for postanoxic organ dysfunction, the effects of CO_2 are readily reversible when exposure ends, and thus probably contribute little to subsequent morbidity and mortality.

Methemoglobinemia is an infrequently reported complication of smoke inhalation.[66] It is not clear whether this is due to infrequent occurrence or infrequent recognition. The identity of the offending toxicants is also unknown. Aromatic amino (-NH₂), nitro (-NO₂) and nitroso (-NO) compounds and oxides of nitrogen have been suggested as etiologies. The pathophysiology of methemoglobinemia is discussed in Chapter 14. Effects are similar to those of anemia and difficult to distinguish from other causes of asphyxia. Although COHb fractions are usually elevated when methemoglobinemia is present, there does not appear to be a direct correlation between the two. Given that the oxygen binding and delivery by hemoglobin are decreased by both COHb and methemoglobin (MetHb), their combined effects are likely to be additive.

Soot, the particulate fraction of smoke, is similar to activated charcoal and relatively inert.[2,5-11] Large amounts can cause mechanical airway obstruction. Although this usually occurs at the bronchiolar level (resulting in atelectasis and subsequent pneumonia), in extreme situations (e.g., volcanic eruptions), it can result in upper airway obstruction. More significantly, however, soot can adsorb toxic gases and liquids and act as vehicle for delivering them to various locations along the respiratory tract. Where a particle settles depends on its size.[2] Those smaller than 1 μm reach the alveoli (primarily by diffusion), those 1 to 5 μm in size settle on tracheal, bronchial, and bronchiolar surfaces (as a result of sedimentation), and those measuring 5 to 30 μm are trapped in the nasopharynx (by inertial impaction). The same is true for aerosolized liquid particles of similar size.

Smoke also contains carcinogens, which are primarily of concern in those with chronic exposure.[2,7,61] All fires generate benzopyrene, the classic chemical initiator of carcinogenesis, as well as hundreds of other polyaromatic hydrocarbons (PAHs), some of which are known to be promoting agents. Such chemicals appear to be responsible for the increased incidence of lung cancer in tobacco smokers and have been linked with an increased risk for lung cancer in foundry workers.[67] Interestingly, PAHs present in soot were probably also responsible for the high incidence of scrotal cancer in chimney sweeps, described more than 200 years ago by the English surgeon Percivall Pott and considered to be the first recognized occupational cancer. Whether or not others with occupational exposure to smoke (e.g., blackmiths, firefighters) are at increased risk for cancer is unknown.

Fires involving plastics, especially polyvinyl chloride, can emit acrylonitrile, arsenic, benzene, chromium, and vinyl chloride. Those involving transformers may result in exposure to polychlorinated biphenyls, polychlorinated dibenzofuran contaminants, and pyrolysis products such as polychlorinated dibenzofurans, chlorinated biphenylenes, and dioxin. Finally, smoke from both natural and synthetic materials may contain formaldehyde. All these chemicals are known or suspected human carcinogens.

TOXICOLOGY

Clinical Manifestations

The clinical course of smoke inhalation can be divided into early, intermediate, and late stages.[47,68] During the first 36 hours, the systemic effects of asphyxia and the local (i.e., respiratory tract) effects of irritant gases, heat,

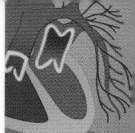

humidity, and soot predominate. Six hours to 5 days after exposure, pulmonary edema, cerebral edema, and the multiple-organ dysfunction syndrome develop in patients with prolonged or severe hypoxia. Complications that occur or become apparent days to weeks after exposure include permanent central nervous system (CNS) damage (e.g., coma, encephalopathy) due to anoxia, bronchiectasis and subglottic stenosis due to airway injury or its treatment (e.g., endotracheal intubation), pneumonia and sepsis due to impaired defense mechanisms, and malnutrition, pressure sores, and thromboembolism in those with prolonged critical illness. Chronic sequelae such as asthma (reactive airways dysfunction syndrome), bronchiolitis obliterans, chronic bronchitis and obstructive pulmonary disease, and pulmonary fibrosis can develop days to years after the original insult.

Victims of smoke inhalation may present with signs and symptoms of asphyxia or inhalation injury.[15,44,47,48,62,64,65,68-75] Both are typically present in those with significant exposures, but isolated inhalation injury is common in those with mild exposures. Surface burns, other trauma, and alcohol or drug intoxication may also be present. The larger the surface burn, the more likely there will be concomitant inhalation injury.[62,68-70,74] Respiratory failure and mortality from smoke inhalation is higher in those with concomitant surface burns than in those without them. Traumatic injuries may results from falling objects, jumping to escape, and structural collapse. Intoxicating levels of ethanol have been reported in 30% to 53% of fatalities due to residential fires.[12,46]

Asphyxia is manifested primarily by CNS and cardiovascular dysfunction.[44,48,64,69,72,74,75] Nausea, vomiting, and diarrhea may also be noted. Manifestations of asphyxia are present at the time of exposure and again later, if inhalation injury worsens with time. CNS effects range from agitation, anxiety, confusion, dizziness, and transient loss of consciousness to coma with seizures or abnormal posturing. Headache is a prominent, sensitive, and relatively specific manifestation of CO poisoning. It can also be seen in CN poisoning and with methemoglobinemia. Cardiovascular manifestations may include dysrhythmias, heart failure, hypotension, and myocardial ischemia or infarction. Underlying cardiovascular disease increases the risk for cardiac complications and may be a contributing factor in as many as 20% of smoke inhalation fatalities.[46]

The COHb fraction is elevated in virtually all patients exhibiting signs and symptoms of asphyxia. It may also be elevated in patients with isolated or predominantly respiratory complaints and findings. Blood CN levels may also be elevated, particularly in those with CNS and cardiovascular dysfunction, but methemoglobinemia appears to be rare. Findings that are relatively uncommon yet specific to CO poisoning include retinal hemorrhages and cherry-red skin color. Lack of a color difference between retinal arterioles and venules (i.e., an equally red appearance) has been described in CN poisoning. An elevated plasma lactate concentration (>10 mEq/L) correlates with the presence of high blood CN levels.[40] However, lactic acidosis invariably accompanies severe or prolonged tissue hypoxia or shock regardless of the underlying cause. Hypoxemia and respiratory acidosis (hypercapnia, $P_{CO_2} > 40$ mm Hg) may be seen in patients with CNS depression or severe inhalation injury. Cyanosis from methemoglobinemia usually appears more gray or brown than that due to hypoxemia, which is purplish. Blood containing a high MetHb fraction has a milk-chocolate color.

Inhalation injury may involve the upper (laryngotracheal) or lower (bronchopulmonary) respiratory tract.[15,44,47,62,64,65,68-72,74,75] The lower respiratory tract is affected more often than the upper. Cutaneous burns of more than 15% body surface area, a history of exposure in an enclosed space, an altered level of consciousness, and carbonaceous sputum production are associated with a high incidence of bronchopulmonary injury. Facial and neck burns are associated with a high incidence of both upper and lower respiratory tract injury. Those with preexisting pulmonary disease are more susceptible to the respiratory effects of smoke.

Nonspecific manifestations of inhalation injury include cough, dyspnea, tachycardia, tachypnea, retractions, and hypoxemia. Hypoxemia is usually defined as an oxygen saturation less than 95% by pulse oximetry or arterial blood gas (ABG) analysis (SpO_2 and SaO_2, respectively), a partial pressure of oxygen (PO_2) less than 85% in an arterial sample, or an arterial oxygen tension–to–inspired oxygen fraction ratio (PaO_2/FiO_2) of less than 400 in an otherwise healthy person breathing room air. Cyanosis, which corresponds to 5 g/dL of reduced or deoxyhemoglobin or an oxygen saturation of about 60% in a healthy adult with a normal hemoglobin level, and respiratory acidosis may be seen in severe cases.

In most patients with smoke exposure, some degree of conjunctivitis, lacrimation, pharyngitis, and rhinitis is also present. Corneal abrasions caused by soot are also relatively common. Exposure to fire or extreme heat may result in corneal burns or desiccation with superficial sloughing. Examination of the nose, mouth, and throat may reveal erythema, edema, or soot. In severe cases, singed nasal hair and mucosal ulcerations and hemorrhage may be seen.

Signs and symptoms of laryngotracheal involvement include drooling, dysphasia, hoarseness, neck pain, and stridor.[15,44,47,64,68-78] Complete obstruction of the upper airway can occur in severe cases. Mucosal edema, erythema, blistering, ulceration, and sloughing; laryngospasm; increased secretions; and soot may be seen on laryngoscopy.[68-70] Laryngeal, epiglottic, and periglottic edema may be visible on soft tissue neck radiographs. A chest radiograph may reveal tracheal narrowing. A sawtoothed or plateau pattern of the inspiratory curve and an expiratory-to-inspiratory ratio greater than 1 may be seen on flow-volume loop spirometry.[77]

Complaints and physical findings indicative of bronchopulmonary injury include chest burning or tightness, carbonaceous sputum production, rhonchi, rales, and wheezing.[15,44,47,64,68-75] In some symptomatic patients, no auscultatory abnormalities are noted. Rales or crackles may be localized (e.g., from atelectasis

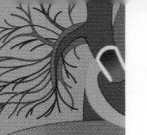

or pneumonia) or diffuse (e.g., from pneumonitis or pulmonary edema). Fever and leukocytosis may accompany atelectasis, pneumonitis, or pneumonia. When they occur within 2 days of exposure, atelectasis or inflammation rather than infection is the likely cause. Fever is also a characteristic feature of polymer fume fever.[4] A chest radiograph may reveal peribronchial cuffing (due to airway edema) and patchy or diffuse infiltrates (due to atelectasis, pneumonitis, pneumonia, or pulmonary edema).[44,79-83] It may appear normal, however, when obtained soon after exposure.[44,79] High-resolution thin-section chest computed tomography can detect late complications such as bronchiectasis, bronchiolitis obliterans, and interstitial lung disease.[47]

Bronchial and bronchiolar obstructions cause decreased peak expiratory flow rate (PEFR), forced expiratory volume in the first second (FEV_1), and forced vital capacity (FVC) on bedside spirometry.[70,78,79] An increased expiratory-to-inspiratory ratio on flow-volume loop spirometry is more sensitive in detecting increases in small airway resistance. Radionuclide (xenon or technetium) ventilation-perfusion imaging may show segmental delayed washout (retention of gas for more than 90 seconds) in areas of small airway obstruction before abnormalities appear on plain films.[70,78,84,85] Formal spirometry may reveal a restrictive pattern in patients with decreased lung compliance due to pulmonary parenchymal damage. Unventilated areas on lung scanning and decreased CO_2 diffusing capacity usually indicate parenchymal injury but can also be seen with severe airway obstruction. Bronchoscopy may reveal crusts, casts, and plugs (mucus or soot) along with mucosal injury.[37,69,86]

Pulmonary edema and bacterial pneumonia are common complications in patients with significant inhalation injury.[15,44,47,68-73,75] Pulmonary edema occurs in 5% to 30% of hospitalized patients and is associated with a mortality rate as high as 70%. It can be acute or insidious in onset and progress to fulminant adult respiratory distress syndrome (ARDS). It can also occur in patients with extensive cutaneous burns in the absence of significant smoke inhalation. Bacterial pneumonia is even more common, occurring in 15% to 60% of hospitalized patients and associated with mortality rates of 50% or greater. Pneumonia that develops within 3 to 4 days of exposure is usually due to *Staphylococcus aureus*. When it occurs later, gram-negative organisms such as *Escherichia coli* and *Enterobacter, Klebsiella,* and *Pseudomonas* species are the likely etiology.

DIAGNOSIS AND EVALUATION

The history should include details of exposure; symptoms, condition, and treatment before arrival; and past medical history. If the patient is unable to provide details, rescuers or other witnesses should be questioned. The nature of the material that generated the smoke (e.g., natural or synthetic); the presence or absence of flame, heat, steam, or explosion; a description of the smoke (e.g., density, color, odor); and the duration of exposure and the time elapsed since exposure should be noted. Of particular importance is whether the exposure occurred indoors or out in the open. The possibility of concomitant drug or alcohol use, trauma, and attempted arson, murder, or suicide should also be explored. How and where a comatose victim was found may provide valuable clues. Firefighters should be asked about mask use, its fit and functioning, and its method of oxygen delivery (e.g., by demand valve or by continuous positive pressure). Exposure to invisible gases may occur when they remove their masks after a fire has been extinguished (e.g., during the clean-up or cool-down period). Firefighters should also be asked about the duration and intensity of exertion, the type and amount of protective gear, and environmental conditions. Answers to these questions may suggest additional or alternative diagnoses such as dehydration and hypothermia or hyperthermia.

The nature of symptoms at the time of exposure or discovery, as well as at the time of arrival, is important in assessing the severity of an exposure. Altered mental status, collapse, or syncope at the scene suggests significant CO or CN poisoning or inhalation injury. These events may be overlooked if clinical improvement has occurred by the time of arrival (e.g., if oxygen was administered or presentation was delayed). Cyanosis unresponsive to oxygen suggests severe inhalation injury or methemoglobinemia. The presence of preexisting disease must be considered when interpreting clinical events and determining disposition and treatment.

Vital signs should be carefully evaluated. Particular attention should be given to the respiratory rate. Body temperature should be measured as soon as possible for all patients. This vital sign is often not measured until very late in the evaluation of critically ill patients (i.e., those at greatest risk for hyperthermia or hypothermia). Oxygen saturation measured by ear or finger pulse oximetry (SpO_2) should be considered a fifth vital sign and obtained in all patients.

The physical examination should first focus on assessing the patency of the airway and adequacy of respirations. Cardiovascular stability, CNS function (mental status as well as level of consciousness), and skin color and integrity should then be evaluated. A trauma survey should be included in the evaluation of those with a history of trauma or altered mental status. Patients with respiratory symptoms must be frequently reevaluated for signs of upper airway obstruction, hypoxia, and hypercapnia. Those with abnormal vital signs, altered mental status, hypoxemia, hypercapnia, chest pain, or respiratory distress should have continuous cardiac monitoring. Those who have eye signs or symptoms or are unresponsive should have an ophthalmologic evaluation that includes fluorescein examination to check for corneal injury. Those who are unresponsive should also have a funduscopic examination to assess for papilledema and to compare the color of retinal arterioles and venules.

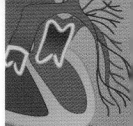

The SpO_2 may be falsely elevated and near normal when COHb and MetHb are present (see Chapters 14 and 87). Hence, unless the history suggests trivial exposure and the patient is asymptomatic and has normal results on physical examination, COHb and MetHb fractions should be measured. In those who are awake and who have mild respiratory symptoms and normal cardiopulmonary findings, venous blood, placed in a heparinized ABG collection syringe, can be used instead of an arterial sample for measuring COHb and MetHb fractions.[41] If COHb and MetHb fractions cannot readily be measured, a decreased oxygen saturation measured directly by co-oximetry in conjunction with a normal PO_2 (and hence normal calculated oxygen saturation) suggests the diagnosis of either CO poisoning or methemoglobinemia. The oxygen saturation gap, the difference between the calculated and measured oxygen saturation, can be used to estimate the fraction of COHb or MetHb, but it cannot differentiate the two.

The SpO_2 is also less sensitive than the PO_2 in detecting mild hypoxemia because the oxygen–hemoglobin dissociation curve, which relates oxygen saturation to the PO_2, is S shaped and nearly flat above a PO_2 of 60 mm Hg (corresponding to an SpO_2 of 90%), and a relatively large decrease in the PO_2 occurs before the SpO_2 changes appreciably. Measuring the PO_2 in an arterial sample may therefore be helpful in confirming or excluding inhalation injury when the diagnosis is not clear (e.g., the patient with dyspnea, normal SpO_2, and normal exam who may simply be anxious). Both the SpO_2 and PO_2 can be normal in patients with inhalation injury, however, and pulmonary function testing may also be necessary.

In patients treated with oxygen, assessing the degree of hypoxemia and severity of inhalation injury can be accomplished by calculating the PO_2/FIO_2 ratio, with FIO_2 expressed as a decimal fraction rather than as a percentage (e.g., room air has an FIO_2 of 0.21, not 21%). Although the FIO_2 is known with certainty only when the patient is intubated and on a ventilator, Venturi masks deliver oxygen at fairly reliable and known concentrations. In patients receiving oxygen by nasal cannula, the FIO_2 can be estimated by adding 0.04 to the room air FIO_2 for each liter per minute of oxygen administered (up to a maximum of 6 L/min, after which the FIO_2 will not increase, unless a mask is also used). For example, 4 L/min of nasal O_2 will provide an FIO_2 of about 0.37 (= 0.21 + 4 × 0.04). A mask with a reservoir bag will deliver an FIO_2 of about 0.6 at an oxygen flow rate of 10 L/min or greater. As noted earlier, the normal PO_2/FIO_2 ratio is about 400 in a healthy adult. In patients with smoke inhalation, a PO_2/FIO_2 ratio of less than 200 indicates severe bronchopulmonary injury and a potentially fatal outcome.

Patients with altered mental status, cardiovascular abnormalities, respiratory distress, or significant hypoxemia should be assessed for acid–base disturbances and hypercapnia by ABG analysis. If metabolic (lactic) acidosis is present, COHb and MetHb fractions are not elevated, and the PO_2 is normal, CN poisoning should be suspected. Unexplained coma and refractory hypotension also suggest CN poisoning. Although CN levels are not widely available and results will not be known in time to alter therapy, obtaining a blood CN level may retrospectively confirm the diagnosis of cyanide poisoning.

Calculating the alveolar-arterial PO_2 (A-A) gradient may sometimes be helpful in patients with hypoxemia and hypercapnia. The A-A gradient ($150 - 1.25 \times PCO_2 - PO_2$, where 150 is the alveolar PO_2) is normally $2.5 + 0.21 \times$ age (in years). It is increased in patients with inhalation injury but not in those with extrapulmonary causes of hypoxemia and hypercapnia (e.g., hypoventilation secondary to muscular weakness or CNS depression). Patients with signs and symptoms of inhalation who are not in acute distress should have bedside pulmonary function testing. Those who have persistent symptoms and are otherwise normal should be referred for comprehensive pulmonary function testing.

Patients with altered mental status, cardiovascular abnormalities, respiratory distress, or significant hypoxemia should also have a chest radiograph and electrocardiogram. A chest x-ray is also suggested for patients with respiratory complaints or abnormal lung sounds. Those with chest pain, palpitations, or an abnormal cardiac rhythm, and those with other signs or symptoms and a history of cardiopulmonary disease should also have an electrocardiogram.

The evaluation of patients with upper respiratory tract signs and symptoms who do not have respiratory distress or other indications for immediate endotracheal intubation (see later) is best accomplished by fiberoptic laryngoscopy. Alternatively, soft tissue radiographs of the neck and flow-volume loop spirometry can be used to detect upper airway narrowing. Bronchoscopy can be performed to assess the lower airway. Although it is said to be the best test for confirming the diagnosis of inhalation injury,[47,73,85] it will not detect small airway or pulmonary parenchymal injury, and the prognostic value of abnormal findings remains controversial.[87]

The possibility of occult alcohol or drug intoxication and trauma should also be considered in patients with abnormal mental status or vital signs. Depending on the history and clinical presentation, toxicology testing and additional imaging studies (e.g., cervical spine films, computed tomography of the head) may be indicated. Women of childbearing age who have findings suggestive of significant smoke exposure, particularly those with elevated COHb fractions, should have a pregnancy test.

MANAGEMENT

Prehospital care should begin with the prompt but safe removal of the patient from the smoky environment. Rescue attempts should left to fire department personnel. Rescuers should never enter a fire scene without respiratory, eye, and skin protection. All patients exposed to smoke should receive supplemental oxygen. Decontamination measures such as irrigation of the eyes

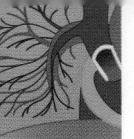

and skin may also be indicated. Blankets should be provided if the patient is wet or cold, or if clothing removal is necessary.

Basic and advanced cardiac and trauma life support measures should be instituted as necessary. Urgent endotracheal intubation is indicated for patients with respiratory distress due to upper airway obstruction, cyanosis or hypoxemia ($SpO_2 < 90\%$, $Po_2 < 60$ mm Hg, or Po_2/FIO_2 ratio < 100) despite oxygen therapy by reservoir mask, respiratory depression (respiratory rate < 12 breaths/min), acute hypercarbia (Pco_2 45–50 mm Hg or greater), pulmonary edema, altered or depressed mental status, and full-thickness burns of the face or neck.[68-70,72,76,78] Intubation should also be considered for patients with upper airway pathology on laryngoscopy or a respiratory rate of more than 30 breaths/min who do not improve with oxygen or other pharmacologic therapy. Assisted ventilation using continuous positive airway pressure by mask (CPAP or BiPAP) is a reasonable alternative to endotracheal intubation for the treatment of hypoxemia and hypercapnia due to bronchopulmonary injury.[88,89]

When performing endotracheal intubation, the largest possible endotracheal tube should be used so that bronchoscopy can subsequently be accomplished. Nasotracheal intubation, alternative airways (e.g., laryngeal mask or Combitube, surgical procedures), or use of a fiberoptic laryngoscope or bronchoscope may be necessary in those with constricting perioral or neck burns or if airway edema prevents visualization of the larynx. If the history or physical examination suggests the possibility of head or neck trauma, cervical spine injury precautions should be taken until radiographs preclude this possibility.

After intubation, the airway should be suctioned aggressively to remove secretions and inhaled debris. Oxygen should be humidified to prevent drying of secretions. Positive end-expiratory pressure at 5 to 10 cm H_2O should be routinely administered to prevent or treat atelectasis.[68,85] Higher pressures may be necessary for patients who remain hypoxic despite administration of 100% oxygen. Chest physiotherapy and postural drainage may also be helpful.

Bronchoscopy is indicated for therapeutic purposes in intubated patients with inhalation injury because it allows for more effective and directed removal of inhaled debris and bronchial secretions. It may be especially useful in patients with lobar atelectasis or focal infiltrates on chest radiographs. For those with inspissated mucous plugs or bronchial casts, repeated bronchoscopy may be necessary. Tracheostomy should be reserved for those who require prolonged intubation (3 weeks or more) because it is associated with significant complications and increased mortality.[90]

Inhaled (aerosolized) racemic epinephrine or albuterol may be tried patients who have upper airway signs and symptoms but who do not require immediate endotracheal intubation. Such patients must be carefully monitored for deterioration. Inhaled and parenteral bronchodilators (e.g., albuterol, isoproterenol, terbutaline) should be administered to patients with wheezing or other evidence of lower airway obstruction. Incentive spirometry and encouragement of coughing may also be helpful.

Corticosteroids are of potential benefit for laryngeal edema and small airways dysfunction. They may also be useful in the treatment of cerebral edema, irritant-induced bronchiolitis obliterans, and postextubation stridor. However, corticosteroids may increase mortality from infection, particularly in patients with pulmonary parenchymal injury and surface burns.[69,91] In patients with inhalation injury, a single large dose of corticosteroid administered at the time of presentation is reasonable. Reserving subsequent doses for those with severe upper airway obstruction and refractory wheezing is suggested.

Positive-pressure ventilation with positive end-expiratory pressure (PEEP) is the treatment of choice for pulmonary edema secondary to smoke inhalation.[92] Complications include decreased cardiac output and pulmonary barotrauma. High-frequency ventilation may reduce the incidence of pneumonia and decrease mortality.[93,94] Inhaled nitric oxide and arteriovenous or venovenous extracorporeal membrane oxygenation (ECMO) should be considered for patients with hypoxemia refractory to other measures.[95,96] Experimental evidence suggests that nonsteroidal anti-inflammatory drugs (e.g., ibuprofen), antioxidants and free radical scavengers (e.g., superoxide dismutase, catalase, deferoxamine, butylated hydroxytoluene/piperonyl butoxide, mannitol), endotracheal fluorocarbons and exogenous surfactant, heparin, and hyperbaric oxygen may be beneficial in the treatment of pneumonitis and pulmonary edema.[97-102] Hyperbaric oxygen (HBO) can also be effective in treating CO poisoning, CN poisoning, cerebral edema, and thermal burns.[103] It should also be considered for patients with refractory hypoxemia.

Patients with concomitant surface burns and inhalation injury may require more fluids for circulatory support than those with either alone.[94,104] The assertion that excessive fluid resuscitation may worsen airway and pulmonary edema and should be avoided[69,70,78] has recently been challenged.[105] Worsening edema may simply be the natural course of inhalation injury. The use of fluid restriction and diuretics for the treatment of edema due to inhalation injury is also controversial.[94,104,105] They are potentially dangerous, particularly in those with surface burns or shock. The goal of fluid therapy should be to maintain normal cardiac output. In critically ill patients, Swan-Ganz catheterization with hemodynamic monitoring may help optimize such therapy.

Antibiotic therapy should be reserved for patients with documented pulmonary infection. Prophylactic use of antibiotics is of no benefit and may foster the development of infection by drug-resistant organisms. The choice of agent should be guided by the results of sputum Gram stain, culture, and sensitivity. In patients with fever and leukocytosis persisting or developing more than 2 days after exposure, empirical therapy with an agent effective against *S. aureus* (e.g., cefazolin or nafcillin), as well as gram-negative bacteria including *Pseudomonas* species (e.g., gentamicin, cefotaxime, or ticarcillin), can be initiated if laboratory results are not immediately available.

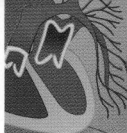

CO poisoning and methemoglobinemia should generally be treated according to usual guidelines (see Chapters 14 and 87). HBO will not be effective in CO (or CN) poisoning unless a high P_{O_2} level can be achieved. Hence, patients with severe inhalation injury (i.e., hypoxemia despite the administration of 100% oxygen by endotracheal tube) may not benefit from HBO. In addition, the indications for its use in these conditions remain controversial.

The treatment of CN poisoning (see Chapter 88) in victims of smoke inhalation is also controversial. Although sodium thiosulfate and hydroxycobalamin can be given safely, an effective formulation of hydroxycobalamin is not yet available in the United States, and nitrites, which induce methemoglobinemia, could cause additional asphyxia in patients with hypoxemia or elevated COHb fractions. Hence, it is suggested that nitrites be reserved for those in extremis or those who remain critically ill with persistent coma, seizures, cardiac dysrhythmias, shock, and lactic acidosis despite intubation and 100% oxygen.[105] Sodium thiosulfate alone may be administered when CN poisoning is suspected because it will enhance the metabolism of CN (enhances conversion of CN to thiocyanate) and is safe (see Chapter 88 for recommended dosing). Because HBO therapy provides enough dissolved oxygen to sustain life in the absence of hemoglobin and obviates concerns over the induction of methemoglobin, it has also been suggested that nitrites be withheld until after HBO therapy has been begun. However, the short half-life of CN and the length of time usually required to arrange for HBO therapy makes it unlikely that nitrites will be necessary or effective in those who survive long enough to receive HBO therapy.

Disposition

The disposition of patients with smoke inhalation depends on its severity. Patients who are asymptomatic on arrival or who become asymptomatic with oxygen therapy alone can be discharged if they have normal findings on physical examination and ancillary testing. Those with mild symptoms and minor abnormalities on clinical evaluation or ancillary testing can also be discharged if they are otherwise healthy and their condition remains stable after a period of observation. Depending on clinical findings, observation for 1 to 6 hours is recommended before discharge. All discharged patients should be instructed to call or return immediately if symptoms develop, recur, or worsen. Patients who do not meet discharge criteria should be admitted. Depending on the nature and severity of injury and the presence or absence of preexisting disease, an observation area, regular floor, or telemetry, intermediate, or critical care unit may be appropriate. Critically ill patients are best managed at a tertiary care facility or burn center and should be transferred if necessary. Although patients with severe CO or CN poisoning may benefit from HBO therapy, HBO treatment centers do not necessarily provide adult or pediatric intensive care or burn services. Hence, the level of care available at such facilities, as well as patient stability and the nature of other injuries, should be considered when deciding if transfer for HBO therapy is appropriate.

REFERENCES

1. Landrock AH: Handbook of Plastics Flammability and Combustion Toxicology. Park Ridge, NJ, Noyes Publications, 1983.
2. Gad SC, Anderson RC: Combustion Toxicology. Boca Raton, FL, CRC Press, 1990.
3. Gordon T, Fine JM: Metal fume fever. Occup Med 1993;8(3):505–517.
4. Shusterman DJ: Polymer fume fever and other fluorocarbon pyrolysis-related syndromes. Occup Med 1993;8(3):519–531.
5. Terrill JB, Montgomery RR, Reinhardt CF: Toxic gases from fires. Science 1978;200:1343.
6. Packham SC, Hartzell GE: Fundamentals of combustion toxicology in fire hazard assessment. J Test Eval 1981;9:341.
7. Kaplan HL, Grand AF, Hartzell GE: Combustion Toxicology: Principles and Test Methods. Lancaster, PA, Technomic Publishing, 1983.
8. Hartzell GE, Packam SC, Switzer WG: Toxic products from fires. Am Ind Hyg Assoc J 1983;44:248–255.
9. Lowry WT, Jaurez L, Petty CS, Roberts B: Studies of toxic gas production during actual structural fires in the Dallas area. J Forensic Sci 1985;30:59–72.
10. Hartzell GE: Overview of combustion toxicology. Toxicology 1996;115:7–23.
11. Orzel RA: Toxicological aspects of firesmoke: polymer pyrolysis and combustion. Occup Med 1993;8(3):415–429.
12. Marshall SW, Runyun CW, Bangdiwala SI, et al: Fatal residential fires: who dies and who survives. JAMA 1998;279:1633–1637.
13. Harwood B, Hall JR: What kills in fires: smoke inhalation or burns? Fire J 1989;84:29–34.
14. Mayes RW: The toxicological examination of the victims of British Air Tours Boeing 737 accident at Manchester in 1985. J Forensic Sci 1985;36:179–184.
15. Haponik EF, Munster AM: Respiratory injury: smoke inhalation and burns. New York, McGraw-Hill, 1990.
16. Alarie Y: Toxicity of fire smoke. Crit Rev Toxicol 2002;32:259–289.
17. Bowes PC: Smoke and toxicity hazards of plastics in fire. Ann Occup Hyg 1974;17:143–157.
18. Zapp JA: The Toxicology of Fire. Medical Division Special Report No. 4. Aberdeen, MD, U.S. Army Chemical Center, 1951.
19. Zapp JA: Toxic and health effects of plastics and resins. Arch Environ Health 1962;4:335.
20. Disaster at the Cleveland Hospital Clinic, Cleveland, OH on May 15, 1929. In Proceedings of the Board of Chemical Warfare Service. Washington, DC, U.S. Government Printing Office, 1929.
21. Cope O: Management of the Cocunut Grove burns at the Massachusetts General Hospital. Ann Surg 1943;117:801–802.
22. Findland M, Davison CS, Levinson SM: Clinical and therapeutic aspects of conflagration injuries to respiratory tract sustained by victims of Coconut Grove disaster. Medicine 1946;25:215.
23. Birky MM, Paabo M, Brown JE: Correlation of autopsy data and materials involved in the Tennessee jail fire. Fire Saf J 1980;2:17–22.
24. Birky MM, Brown JE: Study of biological samples obtained from victims of MGM Grand Hotel fire. J Anal Toxicol 1983;7:265–271.
25. National Fire Protection Agency: Twelve die in fire at Westchester Hilton Hotel, Houston, Texas. Fire J 1983;Jan:10–56.
26. Levin BC, Rechani PR, Gurman JL, et al: Analysis of carboxyhemoglobin and cyanide in blood from victims of the Dupont Plaza Hotel fire in Puerto Rico. J Forensic Sci 1990;35:151–168.
27. Wetherell JR: The occurrence of cyanide in the blood of fire victims. J Forensic Sci 1966;11:167–173.
28. Hirsch CS, Bost RO, Gerber SR, et al: Carboxyhemoglobin concentrations in flash fire victims without elevated carboxyhemoglobin. Am J Clin Pathol 1977;68:317–320.
29. Debane SM, Rowland DY: Carbon monoxide and fatalities: secular trends. In Hirschler MM (ed): Carbon Monoxide and Human Lethality: Fire and Non-fire Studies. New York, Elsevier, 1993, pp 179–196.

30. Alarie Y, Memon R, Esposito F: Role of hydrogen cyanide in human deaths in fires. In Nelson GL (ed): Fire and Polymers. Washington, DC, American Chemical Society, 1990, pp 21–34.

31. Birky MM, Halpin BM, Caplan YH, et al: Fire fatality study. Fire Mater 1979;3:211.

32. Nelson G: Effects of carbon monoxide in man: exposure fatalities studies. In Hirschler MM (ed): Carbon Monoxide and Human Lethality: Fire and Non-fire Studies. New York, Elsevier, 1993, pp 3–60.

33. Anderson RA, Watson AA, Harland WA: Fire deaths in the Glasgow area I: general considerations and pathology. Med Sci Law 1981;21:51–59.

34. Anderson RA, Watson AA: Fire deaths in the Glasgow area II: the role of carbon monoxide. Med Sci Law 1981;21:288.

35. Anderson RA, Harland WA: Fire deaths in the Glasgow area III: the role of hydrogen cyanide. Med Sci Law 1982;22:35.

36. Von Meyer L, Drasch G, Kauert G: Significance of hydrocyanic acid formation during fires. Z Rechtsmed 1979;84:69–73.

37. Barillo DJ, Goode R, Esch V: Cyanide poisoning in victims of fire: analysis of 364 cases and review of the literature. J Burn Care Rehabil 1994;15:46–57.

38. Zikria BA, Weston GC, Chodoff M, et al: Smoke and carbon monoxide poisoning in fire victims. J Trauma 1972;12:641.

39. Teige B, Lundeval J, Fleischer E: Carboxyhemoglobin concentrations in fire victims and in cases of fatal carbon monoxide poisoning. Z Rechtsmed 1977;80:17–21.

40. Baud FJ, Barriot P, Toffis V, et al: Elevated blood cyanide concentrations in victims of smoke inhalation. N Engl J Med 1991;325:1761.

41. AMA Council on Scientific Affairs. Preventing death and injury from fires with automatic sprinklers and smoke detectors. JAMA 1987;257:1618–1620.

42. Purser DA: Behavioral impairment in smoke environments. Toxicology 1996;115:25–40.

43. Zarem HA, Rattenborg CC, Harmel MH: Carbon monoxide toxicity in human fire victims. Arch Surg 1973;107:851.

44. Clark WR, Bonaventura M, Myers W: Smoke inhalation and airway management at a regional burn unit: 1975–1983. Part I: Diagnosis and consequences of smoke inhalation. J Burn Care Rehabil 1989;10:52.

45. Shusterman D, Alexeff G, Hargis C, et al: Predictors of carbon monoxide and hydrogen cyanide exposure in smoke inhalation patients. Clin Toxicol 1996;34:61.

46. Halpin BM, Berl WG: Human fatalities from unwanted fires. Fire J 1979;73:105.

47. Haponik EF: Clinical smoke inhalation injury: pulmonary effects. Occup Med 1993;8(3):431–468.

48. Shusterman DJ: Clinical smoke inhalation injury: systemic effects. Occup Med 1993;8(3):469–504.

49. Esposito FM, Alarie Y: Inhalation toxicity of carbon monoxide and hydrogen cyanide gases released during thermal decomposition of polymers. J Fire Sci 1988;6:195–242.

50. Levin BC, Paabo M, Gurman JL, et al: Effects of exposure to single or multiple combinations of the predominant toxic gases and low oxygen atmospheres produced in fires. Fund Appl Toxicol 1987;9:236–250.

51. Hartzell GE: Toxic products from fires. In Cote AE, Linville JL (eds): Fire Protection Handbook. Quincy, MA, National Fire Protection Association, 1991, pp 3–14.

52. Hartzell GE: Overview of combustion toxicology. Toxicology 1996;115:7–23.

53. Levin BC: New research in toxicology: 7-gas N-gas model, toxicant suppressants, and genetic toxicology. Toxicology 1996;115:89–106.

54. Speitel LC: Fractional effective dose model for post-crash aircraft survivability. Toxicology 1996;115:167–177.

55. Stone HH: Respiratory burns: a correlation of clinical and laboratory results. Ann Surg 1967;165:157.

56. Moritz AR, Henriques FC, McLean R: The effects of inhaled heat on the air passages and lungs. Am J Pathol 1945;21:311.

57. Fein A, Leff A, Hopewell PC: Pathophysiology and management of complications resulting from fire and the inhaled products of combustion. Crit Care Med 1980;8:94.

58. Birky MM, Clark FB: Inhalation of toxic products from fires. Bull N Y Acad Med 1981;57:997.

59. Clark CJ, Campbell D, Reid WH: Blood carboxyhemoglobin and cyanide levels in fire survivors. Lancet 1981;1:1332.

59. Zikria BA, Ferrer JM, Floch HF: The chemical factors contributing to pulmonary damage. Surgery 1972;71:704.

60. Peterson JE: Toxic pyrolysis products of solvents, paints, and polymer films. Occup Med 1993;8(3):533–547.

61. Morse LH, Owen DH, Fujimoto G, et al: Toxic hazards of firefighters and combustion toxicology. In Sullivan JB, Drieger GR (eds): Clinical Environmental Health and Toxic Exposures. Baltimore, Lippincott Williams & Wilkins, 2001, pp 630–636.

62. Traber DI, Linares HA, Herndon DN: The pathophysiology of inhalation injury: a review. Burns 1988;14:357.

63. Hubbard GB, Langlinais PC, Shimazu T, et al: The morphology of smoke inhalation in sheep. J Trauma 1991;31:1477–1486.

64. Clark WR, Nieman GF: Smoke inhalation. Burns 1988;14:473.

65. Kinsella J: Smoke inhalation: the James Ellsworth Laing prize-winning essay for 1988. Burns 1988;14:2698.

66. Hoffman RS, Santer D: Methemoglobinemia resulting from smoke inhalation. Vet Hum Toxicol 1989;31:168.

67. International Agency for Research on Cancer: Polynuclear aromatic compounds. IARC Monogr Eval Carcinog Risks Chem Hum 1984;34:27.

68. Herndon DN, Thompson PB, Traber DL: Pulmonary injury in burned patients. Crit Care Clin 1985;1:79.

69. Robinson L, Miller RH: Smoke inhalation injuries. Am J Otolaryngol 1986;7:375.

70. Haponik EF, Summer WR: Respiratory complications in burned patients: diagnosis and management of inhalation injury. J Crit Care 1987;2:121.

71. Mosley S: Inhalation injury: a review of the literature. Heart Lung 1988;17:3.

72. Clark WR: Smoke inhalation: diagnosis and treatment. World J Surg 1992;16:24.

73. Ruddy RM: Smoke inhalation injury. Pediatr Clin North Am 1994;41:317–336.

74. Monafo WW: Current concepts: initial management of burns. N Engl J Med 1996;335:1581–1586.

75. Ramzi PI, Barret JP, Herndon DN: Thermal injuries. Crit Care Clin 1999;15:333–352.

76. Wroblewski DA, Bower FC: The significance of facial burns in acute smoke inhalation. Crit Care Med 1979;7:335–338.

77. Haponik EF, Munster AM, Wise RA, et al: Upper airway function in burn patients: correlation of flow volume curves and nasopharyngoscopy. Am Rev Respir Dis 1984;129:251.

78. Haponik EF, Meyers DA, Munster AM, et al: Acute upper airway injury in burn patients. Am Rev Respir Dis 1987;153:360–366.

79. Whitener DR, Whitener LM, Robertson J, et al: Pulmonary function measurements in patients with thermal injury and smoke inhalation. Am Rev Respir Dis 1980;122:731.

80. Teixidor HS, Rubin E, Novick GS, et al: Smoke inhalation: radiologic manifestations. Radiology 1983;149:383–387.

81. Lee MJ, O'Connell DJ: The plain chest radiograph after acute smoke inhalation. Clin Radiol 1988;39:33.

82. Peitzman AB, Shires GT, Teixidor S, et al: Smoke inhalation injury: evaluation of radiographic manifestations and pulmonary dysfunction. J Trauma 1989;29:1232.

83. Whittram C, Kenney JB: The admission chest radiograph after acute inhalation injury and burns. Br J Radiol 1994;67:751–754.

84. Moylan JA, Wilmore DW, Mouton DE, et al: Early diagnosis of inhalation injury using [133]xenon lung scan. Ann Surg 1972;176:477.

85. Sheridan RL: Airway management and respiratory care of the burn patient. Int Anesthesiol Clin 2000;38:129–145.

86. Hunt JL, Agee RN, Pruitt BA: Fiberoptic bronchoscopy in acute inhalation injury. J Trauma 1975;15:641.

87. Bingham HG, Gallagher TJ, Powell MD: Early bronchoscopy as a predictor of ventilatory support for burned patients. J Trauma 1987;27:1286.

88. Davies LK, Poulton TJ, Modell JH: Continuous positive airway pressure is beneficial in treatment of smoke inhalation. Crit Care Med 1983;11:726.

89. Delelaux C, L'Her E, Alberti C, et al: Treatment of acute hypoxemic respiratory insufficiency with continuous positive

airway pressure delivered by face mask. JAMA 2000;284:
2352–2360.

90. Lund T, Goodwin CW, McManus WF, et al: Upper airway sequelae
in burn patients requiring endotracheal intubation or tracheostomy. Ann Surg 1985;201:304.

91. Robinson NB, Hudson LD, Riem M, et al: Steroid therapy
following isolated smoke inhalation injury. J Trauma 1982;22:876.

92. Cox CS, Zwischenberger JB, Traber DL, et al: Immediate positive
pressure ventilation with positive end expiratory pressure
(PEEP) improves survival in ovine smoke inhalation. J Trauma
1992;33:821.

93. Cioffi WG, Graves TA, McManus WF, et al: High-frequency
percussive ventilation in patients with inhalation injury. J Trauma
1989;29:350–354.

94. Pruitt BA, Cioffi WG, Shimazu T, et al: Evaluation and management of patients with inhalation injury. J Trauma 1990;30:563.

95. Sheridan RL Hurford WE, Kacmarek RM, et al: Inhaled nitric
oxide in burn patients with respiratory failure. J Trauma
1997;42:629–634.

96. O'Toole G, Peek G, Jaffe W, et al: Extracorporeal membrane
oxygenation in the treatment of inhalational injuries. Burns
1998;24:562–565.

97. Shinozawa Y, Hales C, Jung W, et al: Ibuprofen prevents synthetic
smoke-induced pulmonary edema. Am Rev Respir Dis 1986;
134:1145.

98. Stewart RJ, Yamaguchi KT, Knost PM, et al: Effects of ibuprofen on
pulmonary oedema in an animal smoke inhalation model. Burns
1990;16(6):409–413.

99. Stewart RJ, Mason SW, Taira MT, et al: Effect of radical scavengers
and hyperbaric oxygen on smoke-induced pulmonary edema.
Undersea Hyperb Med 1994;21(1):21–30.

100. Demling R, LaLonde C, Ikegami K: Fluid resuscitation with
deferoxamine hetastarch complex attenuates the lung and systemic
response to smoke inhalation. Surgery 1996;119:340–348.

101. Jeng MJ, Kou YR, Sheu CC, et al: Effects of exogenous surfactant
supplementation and partial liquid ventilation on acute lung
injury induced by wood smoke inhalation in newborn piglets. Crit
Care Med 2003;31(4):166–174.

102. Cox CS, Zwischhenberger JB, Traber, et al: Heparin improves
oxygenation and minimizes barotrauma after severe smoke
inhalation in an ovine model. Surg Gynecol Obstet 1993;176:
339–349.

103. Hart GB, Strauss MB, Lennon PA, et al: Treatment of smoke
inhalation by hyperbaric oxygen. J Emerg Med 1985;3:211.

104. Navar PD, Saffle JR, Warden GD: Effect of inhalation injury
on fluid requirements after thermal injury. Am J Surg 1985;150:
716–720.

105. Holm C, Tegeleer J, Mayr M, et al: Effect of crystalloid
resuscitation and inhalation injury on extravascular lung water:
clinical implication. Chest 2002;121:1956–1962.

87 *Carbon Monoxide Poisoning*

ERIC J. LAVONAS, MD

At a Glance...

■ Carboxyhemoglobin levels confirm the diagnosis of carbon monoxide poisoning, but severity of illness, rather than levels, determines the type and intensity of treatment.

■ Treatment consists of patient removal from exposure environment and administration of high-flow, high-concentration oxygen at normobaric or hyperbaric pressure.

■ Hyperbaric oxygen therapy is most likely to benefit patients with severe carbon monoxide poisoning, such as those with loss of consciousness, persistent altered mental status, seizures, ataxia, hypotension, myocardial injury, and significant symptoms that do not resolve with surface pressure oxygen.

■ Pregnant patients with acute carbon monoxide poisoning should be treated with hyperbaric oxygen therapy if they meet criteria defined for nonpregnant patients or if there are signs of fetal distress; treatment with normobaric oxygen should be prolonged because of the slower elimination of carbon monoxide from the fetus.

INTRODUCTION AND RELEVANT HISTORY

Carbon monoxide (CO), a colorless, odorless, nonirritating gas created by incomplete burning of carbonaceous fossil fuels, is a ubiquitous toxin. Mild CO poisoning often masquerades as nonspecific headache or is misdiagnosed as viral illness, whereas moderate to severe CO poisoning produces significant morbidity (e.g., delayed neurologic dysfunction) and mortality and provokes treatment controversy. With more than 2000 annual deaths and at least 15,000 to 40,000 diagnosed cases of nonfatal acute CO poisoning occurring annually in the United States, this poison affects the practice of all physicians.

EPIDEMIOLOGY

Carbon monoxide poisoning is the third leading cause of accidental poisoning death in the United States.[1] Although CO death rates have declined by 80% since the introduction of the catalytic converter in 1975, CO was still responsible for 2379 deaths in the United States in 1998.[2] Most of these deaths were due to suicide, but a large number of accidental poisonings also occurred (Tables 87-1 and 87-2). In addition to those listed, common sources of accidental CO poisoning include small engines (i.e., electrical generators and power washers), propane-powered fork lifts, boats, ice skating rink resurfacers (Zambonis), paint strippers (methylene chloride), and fires (i.e., victims of smoke inhalation).[3,4] About 40,000 people are diagnosed with CO poisoning in emergency departments in the United States annually.[3] Among emergency department patients with headache or "flulike symptoms," the incidence of occult CO poisoning (defined as venous carboxyhemoglobin [COHb] level of 10%) may range from 0.2% to 23.6%.[5-11] Outbreaks of CO poisoning occur after storm-related power outages, in both warm and cold weather.[12] During these outages, charcoal and electrical generators predominate as sources of CO. Poor and immigrant populations are at highest risk.

STRUCTURE AND STRUCTURE–ACTIVITY RELATIONSHIPS

Carbon monoxide is colorless, odorless, and tasteless. Because it has almost the same density as air, CO dis-

TABLE 87-1 Sources of Carbon Monoxide in Fatal Poisoning, 1998

CARBON MONOXIDE	NO. OF FATALITIES
All carbon monoxide–related deaths	2379
Unintentional deaths	*491*
Motor vehicle related	238
Non–motor vehicle related	93
Mechanism undetermined	160
Suicide deaths	*1747*
Motor vehicle related	1330
Non–motor vehicle related	4
Mechanism undetermined	413
Homicides and deaths of undetermined or other intent	*141*

Modified from Mott JA, Wolfe MI, Alverson CJ, et al: National vehicle emissions policies and practice and declining US Carbon monoxide-related mortality. JAMA 2002;288:988–995.

TABLE 87-2 Sources of Carbon Monoxide in Unintentional, Nonfire Carbon Monoxide Poisoning Deaths Due to Consumer Products, 1994–2000

CARBON MONOXIDE	PERCENT AGE OF FATALITIES
Heating systems	52
Engine-powered tools	16
Charcoal grills and charcoal	12
Other or multiple appliances	9
Gas ranges and ovens	8
Camp stoves and lanterns	6
Gas water heaters	2

Modified from Vagts SA: Non-fire Carbon Monoxide Deaths Associated with the Use of Consumer Products: 1999 and 2000 Annual Estimates. Bethesda, MD, U.S. Consumer Products Safety Commission, 2003.

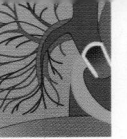

tributes equally throughout an enclosed area. Because CO is a small, nonpolar molecule, it penetrates through standard drywall and can disperse throughout separate units of a multifamily dwelling.

PHARMACOLOGY

Pathophysiology

Carbon monoxide enters the body through the lungs, where it binds to hemoglobin with an affinity 200 to 240 times that of oxygen.[13] The binding of CO to one of the four binding sites on the hemoglobin tetramer shifts hemoglobin to its high-affinity conformation. This shifts the oxyhemoglobin dissociation curve to the left, greatly impairing the ability of hemoglobin to deliver oxygen to tissues. This enhanced affinity and impaired unloading of oxygen is referred to as the *Haldane effect.*

COHb plays only a partial role in the pathogenesis of CO poisoning. This is suggested by the clinical observation that COHb levels do not correlate with the severity of clinical effects and can be low in the face of coma from CO poisoning.[14] Further evidence is provided by a canine study that revealed markedly differing mortality rates for dogs with similar blood COHb levels but differing tissue CO levels.[15] In this study, death occurred uniformly in dogs that breathed air containing 13% CO for 15 minutes resulting in COHb blood levels of about 65%. In contrast, death did not occur in other groups of dogs that were transfused with enough COHb red blood cells to produce blood COHb levels of 60%. In addition, death did not occur in a third group of dogs that had their blood hemoglobin content reduced by 68% through phlebotomy. Thus, animals spontaneously breathing CO had a higher total-body content of CO from its tissue redistribution. Redistributed or "tissue" CO accounts for 10% to 15% of total-body CO stores but is critical to the pathophysiology of CO.[16]

CO produces tissue toxicity from its avid binding to other heme proteins (cytochromes), such as myoglobin, the cytochrome a-a_3 complex (cytochrome oxidase) of the mitochondrial respiratory chain, and guanylate cyclase. Myoglobin's affinity for CO is about 30 to 60 times greater than that for oxygen.[17] CO binding to myoglobin impairs myocardial oxygen uptake from blood into the mitochondria of tissues. Binding of CO to cytochrome oxidase disrupts cellular respiration and oxygen utilization in all tissues, including the brain. Although cytochrome oxidase binds oxygen with greater affinity than CO, CO competes with oxygen for binding sites under conditions of cellular hypoxia and dissociates slowly from cytochrome oxidase once binding has occurred.[18]

In addition to direct cytochrome oxidase blockade, CO promotes the production of reactive nitrogen species that further inhibit cellular cytochrome oxidase and electron transport.[19,20] Cellular hypoxia causes free radical release from vascular endothelial cells and platelets. Concurrently, CO displaces nitric oxide (NO) from heme-containing proteins in endothelial cells and platelets.[21] Once released from cells, NO reacts with free radicals to produce peroxynitrate (ONOO⁻), which further inhibits cytochrome oxidase, injures DNA and cell membranes, and triggers apoptosis in neuronal tissue.[19,21]

In addition to cellular hypoxia, CO produces smooth muscle relaxation and vasodilation. CO binds to and stimulates the activity of the heme protein, guanylate cyclase.[22] This results in an increased production of the smooth muscle relaxant, cyclic guanosine monophosphate (cGMP). The displacement of NO from platelets and endothelial cells by CO also results in vasodilation.[21,23] NO, also known as *endothelial derived relaxation factor*, is a potent smooth muscle relaxant. Headache from CO poisoning is likely mediated by extracerebral and intracerebral vasodilation. Hypotension and syncope from CO poisoning may be mediated by some combination of peripheral vasodilation, with COHb-induced myocardial ischemia, direct myocardial depressant effects, and loss of central control of vasomotor tone. Clinically, hypotension and syncope (even if transient) signify serious CO exposure and are ominous predictors of serious neurologic sequelae.[24,25] Brain areas that have high oxygen requirements or are watershed regions of perfusion (e.g., basal ganglia, hippocampus, and subcortical white matter) are particularly susceptible to CO-mediated injury. In monkeys, cerebral white matter lesions correlated better with decreases in blood pressure than with COHb levels, and it has been suggested that an episode of hypotension may be required for severe neurologic deficits to occur.[26] In essence, cellular hypoxia is often accompanied by tissue ischemia. These primary CO-induced pathophysiologic processes (hypoxia and ischemia) induce a cascade of secondary events (ischemia reperfusion effects) that are integral to short- and long-term central nervous system (CNS) toxicity associated with CO.

The histopathology of CO poisoning is similar to that of postanoxic encephalopathy, or so-called reperfusion injury. Brain reperfusion injury patterns are largely mediated by oxidative damage initiated by oxygen free radicals and sustained by second-generation lipid radicals. Current evidence suggests that xanthine oxidase activity is largely responsible for the generation of free radicals associated with CO-mediated lipid peroxidation and brain injury.[27] When CO exposure is associated with tissue hypoxia, adenosine dinucleotide triphosphate (ATP) stores are depleted in tissues. Simultaneously, the cells have a greatly increased demand for ATP to repair oxidative damage. In a series of steps, ATP is converted to uric acid and an oxygen free radical.

Investigations by Thom and colleagues indicate that significant CO exposure produces a cascade of biochemical events responsible for delayed neurologic sequelae.[19,21,23,24,27] Significant CO exposure promotes release of NO from endothelial cells and platelets. Concurrently, impaired mitochondrial function and oxidative stress promotes production and release of oxygen free radicals from these cells. NO reacts with oxygen radicals to form peroxynitrite. Peroxynitrite binds to perivascular tissue proteins causing endothelial

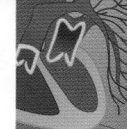

injury. Endothelial injury provokes expression of adherence molecules (e.g., β-integrin) on cell surfaces, which promotes leukocyte binding to injured endothelial cells. Leukocytes release proteases that further augment the activity of xanthine oxidase and production of oxygen free radicals. Subsequently, brain lipid peroxidation and delayed CNS toxicity ensue. Brain injury is also mediated by additional mechanisms, such as activation of excitatory amino acids (e.g., glutamate) and apoptosis-related enzymes (e.g., caspase-1).[23,28]

Pharmacokinetics

Carbon monoxide uptake and elimination occur through the lungs and are dependent on minute volume. Only a small amount of CO is metabolized by oxidation to carbon dioxide. Because CO diffusion through the alveoli is rapid and complete, the amount of CO dissolved in arterial blood is directly related to the concentration of CO in the air of the patient's environment. Depending on conditions, whole-body equilibrium may only be reached after 4 to 6 hours of exposure. Conversely, measurements of CO concentration in expired air correlate well with venous CO levels. Overall, the amount of CO absorbed by the body depends on ambient air CO and oxygen concentrations, minute ventilation, and duration of exposure. In human volunteer studies, the elimination of CO in room air (21% oxygen) ranges from 249 to 320 minutes.[29,30] Administration of 100% oxygen shortens the elimination half-life to 47 to 80 minutes at normal atmospheric pressure and to about 20 minutes at 2.5 to 3 atmospheric pressure.[31,32]

Methylene chloride (see Chapter 93), found in paint strippers, degreasers, and other solvents, is another potential source of CO poisoning. It is readily absorbed from the lungs and gastrointestinal tract; lesser amounts may also be absorbed from the skin. Once absorbed, methylene chloride is slowly metabolized in the liver to CO and carbon dioxide. Peak CO levels from methylene chloride depend on the route of exposure but may not occur for over 8 hours. Because of ongoing CO production through metabolism of methylene chloride, the half-life of CO may appear to be prolonged, up to 13 hours, in these cases.[33,34]

Special Populations

Because of their rapid respiratory rate, children may be more susceptible to CO poisoning than adults. Advanced age may be a risk factor for adverse neurologic outcomes after CO poisoning.[35] Although fetal hemoglobin has a higher affinity for CO than hemoglobin A in similar pH and P_{O_2} conditions, this effect is largely counteracted by the acidemic, hypoxic milieu of the normal fetus. As a result, fetal COHb levels are expected to be within 10% of maternal levels.[36] Based on animal data and mathematical models, the elimination half-life of fetal COHb is significantly longer (up to 3.5 times greater) than that of adult COHb.[37,38]

TOXICOLOGY

Clinical Manifestations

ACUTE EFFECTS

Signs and symptoms of mild CO poisoning include headache, nausea, vomiting, diarrhea, dizziness, weakness, dyspnea, and fatigue (Table 87-3). Misdiagnoses, such as viral illness and benign headache, are common. In one study, the diagnosis of CO poisoning was initially missed in up to 30% of cases; the most common incorrect diagnosis, "food poisoning" was made in 43% of these cases. The diagnosis of CO poisoning should be considered for patients presenting with one or more of the listed symptoms in the absence of fever.[39] A history of exposure to possible CO sources (e.g., fossil fuel heat, engines, propane and natural gas appliances, grills) or groups of patients with similar complaints should suggest occult CO poisoning and prompt blood or breath testing for CO.[8] With more severe exposure, patients can present with signs of neurologic, cardiovascular, and pulmonary dysfunction. These effects include confusion, irritability, ataxia, coma, focal neurologic deficits, seizures, syncope, hypotension, arrhythmias, myocardial ischemia or infarction, tachycardia, tachypnea, noncardiogenic and cardiogenic pulmonary edema, and respiratory and cardiac arrest.

In general, any organ can be affected by CO. Table 87-4 lists the spectrum of complications that can be associated with CO poisoning. Unusual complications include retinal hemorrhages, compartment syndromes, rhabdomyolysis and renal failure, skin blisters, bowel ischemia, and peripheral neuropathy. Although patients with more severe signs of acute CO poisoning (e.g., syncope, hypotension, coma) are more likely to develop delayed and long-lasting morbidity, this is not uniformly true. Patients with mild toxicity may develop delayed neurologic sequelae, and those with severe toxicity may have complete recovery.

CHRONIC EFFECTS

Some CO-poisoned patients develop lasting signs of brain injury, most commonly cognitive and personality

---

TABLE 87-3 Acute Symptoms in 1144 Patients with Carbon Monoxide Poisoning

SYMPTOM	PERCENTAGE OF PATIENTS
Headache	85
Dizziness	69
Fatigue or generalized weakness	67
Nausea or vomiting	52
Trouble thinking or confusion	37
Loss of consciousness	35*
Dyspnea	7
Chest pain	2

*Patients with loss of consciousness (LOC) were excluded from Thom's series (N = 65 without LOC; number with LOC excluded not stated).
Data from references 35, 41–43, 64, 68, and 90.

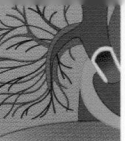

TABLE 87-4 Spectrum of Complications Due to Carbon Monoxide Poisoning

SYSTEM	COMPLICATIONS
Central nervous	Impaired cognition, memory dysfunction, vertigo, ataxia, parkinsonism, muscle rigidity, gait disturbance, disorientation, mutism, urinary incontinence, fecal incontinence, cortical blindness, hearing loss, tinnitus, nystagmus, seizures, coma, electroencephalographic abnormalities, cerebral edema, leukoencephalopathy, diabetes insipidus, globus pallidus necrosis
Psychiatric	Personality changes, depression, flattened affect, Tourette's syndrome, anxiety, agitation, poor impulse control
Cardiovascular	Tachycardia, easy fatigue, hypotension, ischemic electrocardiographic changes, arrhythmias, new-onset angina or exacerbation of existing angina, myocardial infarction
Pulmonary	Shortness of breath, pulmonary edema, hemoptysis
Gastrointestinal	Nausea, vomiting, abdominal cramps, diarrhea, gastrointestinal bleeding
Ophthalmologic	Decreased acuity, retrobulbar neuritis, paracentral scotomata, papilledema, flame-shaped retinal hemorrhages
Dermatologic	Erythematous patches, cherry-red skin, bullae, alopecia, sweat gland necrosis
Muscular	Rhabdomyolysis, compartment syndrome
Hematologic	Disseminated intravascular coagulation, thrombotic thrombocytopenic purpura, leukocytosis
Metabolic	Lactic acidosis, hyperglycemia, hypocalcemia, hyperamylasemia (salivary origin)

changes and parkinsonism. These may develop at the time of CO poisoning and continue (persistent neurologic sequelae) or develop after an asymptomatic interval of 3 to 21 days (delayed neurologic sequelae, or DNS). Longer latent periods have been reported. DNS manifest with a variety of neurologic and psychiatric signs and symptoms. Commonly described findings include memory loss, confusion, ataxia, incontinence, emotional lability, hallucinations, personality changes, blindness, and parkinsonism. There are no established diagnostic criteria for this disorder, and the observed incidence varies widely, from 12% to 74% for CO poisoning victims in recently published clinical trials.[35,40-45] One recent study, which paired 32 CO poisoning victims (8 of whom had loss of consciousness and 24 of whom received hyperbaric oxygen [HBO]) with gender, age, and educationally matched controls, found no evidence of the syndrome at all.[44] Many patients recover to normal over several weeks to months.[45,46]

DIAGNOSIS

Laboratory Testing

The diagnosis of CO poisoning is based on suggestive history and physical findings coupled with confirmatory COHb testing (Table 87-5). CO levels can be tested in either whole blood or exhaled air. In hospitals, the most commonly used technique is to measure COHb as a percentage of total hemoglobin using a multiple wavelength spectrophotometer. Blood is collected in a closed, heparinized container (a blood gas syringe or "green-top" tube) and analyzed on a co-oximeter. Because there is no significant difference between venous and arterial COHb levels, either type of sample is appropriate.[47] Because of endogenous CO production, some COHb is present in the blood of healthy subjects. Normal COHb levels are 0.5% to 2% in nonsmokers and up to 10% to 12% in smokers. Levels are somewhat

higher in pregnant women, infants, and patients with hemolytic anemia. COHb is often misinterpreted as oxyhemoglobin by simple bedside pulse oximetry. Pulse oximetry overestimates oxyhemoglobin measurements by the approximate amount of COHb that is present.[48] Thus, co-oximetry is required to measure COHb levels accurately.

TABLE 87-5 Relationship of Carbon Monoxide Levels in Air and Carboxyhemoglobin Levels at Steady State

CARBON MONOXIDE CONCENTRATION IN AIR (PPM)	CARBOXYHEMOGLOBIN (%) ACHIEVED AT STEADY STATE	NOTES
10	1.5	Approximate upper limit of normal in nonsmokers
35	5	NIOSH-recommended exposure level for 8-hr workday
50	7	Current OSHA 8-hr permissible exposure level for 8-hr workday
70	10	Approximate upper limit of normal in smokers
350	35	NIOSH recommends supplied-air respirator use
1200	65	Immediately dangerous to life and health level (NIOSH)

NIOSH, National Institute of Occupational Safety and Health; OSHA, Occupational Safety and Health Administration. Calculated from formulas in reference 36, assuming adult patients with normal hemoglobin. Interindividual variability exists.

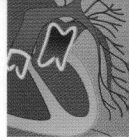

An alternative method, more commonly used in Europe, is to measure CO directly. A blood sample is diluted and mixed with a reagent to liberate CO from hemoglobin. The CO content of head-space gas is then measured with gas chromatography or infrared spectrophotometry.[49,50] Although this method is more accurate for measuring low CO levels, there is no clear advantage in the assessment of acute poisoning.

COHb "spot tests," performed by adding sodium hydroxide or ammonia to a tube of blood and observing for a persistent pink color, are neither sensitive nor specific.[51]

Breath analysis is a valid alternative to blood testing.[52,53] However, because patient cooperation is necessary, breath analysis may be impractical in young children and patients with significantly altered mental status. Models vary greatly in their ease of use, and some give false-positive results in the presence of ethanol. Normal levels of CO in exhaled air are 0 to 6 ppm in nonsmokers and up to 70 ppm in smokers. Most analyzers automatically convert these levels to predicted COHb levels for medical use.

A promising new technology is noninvasive pulse co-oximetry. These devices, which are essentially a technological improvement on pulse oximetry, use multiple wavelengths of light to directly measure oxyhemoglobin, deoxyhemoglobin, and COHb (and, in some models, methemoglobin) through a probe applied to the finger or ear. Because this procedure is rapid and noninvasive and does not require patient cooperation, it has the potential to replace exhaled breath and blood co-oximetry analysis for the diagnosis of CO poisoning.

COHb levels do not correlate well with clinical severity, outcome, or response to therapy.[41-43,46,54] The role of a COHb measurement is to confirm or exclude that a CO exposure has occurred. The diagnosis of CO poisoning is made when an elevated COHb level is documented concurrently with history, signs, and symptoms suggestive of poisoning. In order to interpret COHb measurements, it is important to know the time since cessation of exposure and whether the patient was on oxygen during this time. Although COHb elimination varies considerably between individuals, a reasonable estimate is to assume that COHb levels fall by half every 4 to 5 hours in patients breathing air and every 1 hour in patients breathing oxygen by mask. If calculations reveal a "predicted peak" COHb level of less than 10%, symptomatic CO poisoning is unlikely, and an alternative diagnosis should be sought. If the diagnosis of CO poisoning is confirmed, the history and physical examination guide the choice of therapy. Depending on the route of exposure, patients with methylene chloride poisoning may need serial measurements of blood COHb to rule out significant CO poisoning.

Arterial blood gas measurements are not useful to make the diagnosis of CO poisoning. They provide useful information with regard to the adequacy of ventilation and presence and degree of metabolic acidosis.[55]

Although elevated blood lactate levels may occur in severe CO poisoning, most patients in published case series have normal lactate levels. It is not clear whether elevated lactate is an independent risk factor in CO victims who otherwise appear well. CO poisoning rarely causes a lactate level greater than 4 mmol/L; an alternate explanation for lactic acidosis, such as cyanide poisoning or shock, should be sought. In particular, the measurement of blood lactate may be a useful surrogate for cyanide poisoning for smoke inhalation victims (see Chapters 86 and 88).

Carbon monoxide poisoning can cause myocardial infarction. In one case series, patients who demonstrated clinical evidence of myocardial injury (elevated CK-MB, elevated troponin I, and/or diagnostic ECG changes) were followed prospectively.[56] Survivors had a significant increase in cardiac and all-cause mortality over several years after the poisoning, compared with CO-poisoned patients who did not have myocardial injury.

Unfortunately, it is difficult to extrapolate from this study to a management strategy for patients with CO-induced myocardial infarction. All patients in this study were treated with HBO; HBO did not prevent the increased mortality, and it is speculative to say whether the rate would have been different had HBO not been employed. Patients with myocardial infarction were older and more severely poisoned than those without such injury, potentially confounding these results. Because CO can cause diffuse myocardial injury in the absence of coronary artery disease, it unclear whether evidence of myocardial infarction indicates a need for coronary angiography in the CO-poisoned patient or whether cardiac stress testing is safe or accurate in the immediate aftermath of CO poisoning.

Any patient who suffers a prolonged period of unconsciousness or shock may develop complications such as rhabdomyolysis, compartment syndrome, renal failure, or disseminated intravascular coagulopathy. Testing for these conditions should be performed when clinical suspicion is high.

Other Diagnostic Testing

All women with childbearing potential who are suspected of having CO poisoning should have a pregnancy test. Although this topic is controversial, many experts recommend a prolonged period of oxygen therapy and a lower threshold for hyperbaric oxygen treatment if the CO poisoning victim is pregnant. An assessment of fetal status, such as a fetal heart rate, nonstress test, or ultrasound, should be performed when practical.

An ECG should be performed on individuals with a history of chest pain, dyspnea, or hypotension. Other testing, such as head computed tomography (CT) or lumbar puncture, may be needed to exclude other causes of altered mental status when the diagnosis of CO poisoning is inconclusive.

A special neuropsychological battery has been developed to detect subtle impairment in CO poisoning victims that might be missed by routine neurologic testing.[57] Performance on this battery is altered with CO poisoning and improves with therapy. However, the test is designed only to detect neuropsychological impairment and does not distinguish CO poisoning from other

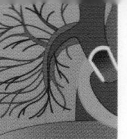

causes of encephalopathy, including alcohol. The battery is somewhat cumbersome, requires 30 to 45 minutes to administer, must be administered in a quiet area, requires fluency and literacy in English, assumes normal intelligence, is not valid for children younger than 15 years, and does not predict patients at risk for developing delayed neurologic sequelae.[43,57] A standard focused neurologic examination, including mini-mental status examination and testing for ataxia, is adequate for routine clinical use.

Chest radiography is recommended for all seriously poisoned patients and those with cardiopulmonary signs and symptoms. Noncardiogenic pulmonary edema may be evident on chest radiograph. Brain CT is recommended for seriously poisoned patients. Brain CT may show signs of cerebral infarction secondary to hypoxia or ischemia. Symmetric low-density lesions of the globus pallidus, putamen, and caudate may be detected as early as 12 hours after CO poisoning and are associated with a poorer prognosis.[58,59] Brain magnetic resonance imaging (MRI) is able to detect basal ganglia lesions with greater sensitivity than head CT. In addition, other abnormal findings demonstrated on head MRI in CO-poisoned patients include diffuse, symmetric white matter lesions of the periventricular areas.[60]

Differential Diagnosis

Just as CO poisoning can mimic other illnesses, many other conditions cause encephalopathy, headache, nausea, weakness, or hypotension. When the diagnosis of CO poisoning is excluded or uncertain, testing for occult trauma, stroke, infection, drug intoxication, or metabolic derangement may be necessary. Rapid bedside tests should be used to exclude hypoglycemia and hypoxemia in almost all patients. Victims of smoke inhalation who have significant lactic acidosis should be suspected of having associated cyanide poisoning.

MANAGEMENT

Supportive Measures

All patients should receive aggressive supportive care while the diagnosis of CO poisoning is established. Patients with significant CNS or respiratory depression should have their airway protected, breathing assisted, and cardiovascular support provided as necessary. The administration of high-concentration, high-flow oxygen by tight-fitting face mask or endotracheal tube is fundamental. Severely poisoned patients should have continuous cardiac monitoring, an intravenous (IV) line established, and an ECG performed. Continuous pulse oximetry and parenteral thiamine, dextrose (or rapid fingerstick glucose determination), and naloxone should be considered for patients with altered mental status or seizures because of the potential for concurrent illness. Hypotension may be treated with IV fluids and, if necessary, vasoactive infusions.

Decontamination

Immediate removal from the contaminated environment is critical. Except for methylene chloride exposures, CO absorption ceases as soon as the patient is removed from the poisoned environment. Although CO victims have elevated amounts of CO in exhaled air, the amount involved poses no danger to health care workers. Although placing the patient on oxygen speeds the elimination of CO from the body, no form of decontamination is required.

Laboratory Monitoring

Serial measurements of COHb or breath CO are not helpful in management unless the exposure was to methylene chloride. Once the diagnosis of CO poisoning is established, further lab monitoring is only indicated as required by other medical conditions (e.g., cyanide poisoning, shock, trauma, and metabolic acidosis).

Antidotes

The antidote for CO poisoning is oxygen, which should be administered at a concentration as close to fiO_2 1.0 as reasonably achievable and for a period of at least 4 hours. High-concentration oxygen is delivered by a tight-fitting, reservoir-containing (non-rebreather) face-mask or by endotracheal tube. Oxygen is delivered at ambient (atmospheric) pressure or elevated ambient pressure. Although the practice of administering oxygen has never been tested to see if it improves outcome, oxygen therapy is safe, inexpensive, and convenient and greatly improves the rate of CO elimination. The 4-hour duration of therapy is chosen for practicality and because it allows even the most severely poisoned patients (i.e., COHb > 40%) to eliminate CO to negligible levels.

Many experts recommend HBO or administration of oxygen at 2 to 3 atmospheres pressure absolute (ATA) in a hyperbaric chamber. Although HBO is reasonably safe, it is considerably more expensive and less convenient than administration of oxygen at ambient pressure ("normobaric" oxygen, or NBO), particularly if transfer to another facility is required.

In experimental animal models of severe CO poisoning, HBO therapy decreases brain injury by a variety of mechanisms, including improved mitochondrial oxidative metabolism, inhibition of leukocyte adherence to injured vasculature, and reduced lipid peroxidation. In this setting, HBO has a paradoxical, and beneficial, antioxidant effect.[23,28,61-63] However, although treatment with HBO eliminated hippocampal cell death in a mouse model of CO poisoning, there was no difference in learning and memory testing.[64]

At least seven case series and nonrandomized clinical trials of HBO for CO poisoning have been published.[65-71] Few of these studies assessed outcomes by objective measures, and none were blinded. All reported a benefit from HBO over standard NBO therapy. five randomized clinical trials studying the effect of HBO on neuropsychological outcomes have been published and are listed in Table 87-6. Three of these trials reported a

TABLE 87-6 Randomized Trials of Neuropsychological Outcomes in Carbon Monoxide Poisoning Treated with HBO versus Normobaric Oxygen

STUDY	PATIENTS INCLUDED	BLINDED?	NEUROPSYCHO-LOGICAL TESTS?	NO. OF TREATMENTS	LOST TO FOLLOW-UP (%)	NO. NBO PATIENTS	NO. (%) NBO PATIENTS WITH POOR OUTCOME*	NO. HBO PATIENTS	NO. (%) HBO PATIENTS WITH POOR OUTCOME*	HBO BENEFIT REPORTED	NO. NEEDED TO TREAT TO BENEFIT ONE PATIENT
Raphael, 1989[41]	No LOC	No	No	1	10	170	58 (34)	173	55 (32)	No	50.0
Thom, 1995[43]	No LOC	No	Yes	1	14	30	7 (22)	30	0 (0)	Yes	4.5
Mathieu, 1996[45]	Non-comatose	No	No	1	Unk.	276	42 (15)	299	26 (9)	Yes	15.4
Scheinkestel, 1999[42]	All	Yes	Yes	3–6	54	87	59 (68)	104	82 (79)	No (trend toward harm)	N/A (harm: 1 in 9.1)
Weaver, 2002[35]	All	Yes	Yes	3	3	76	35 (46)	76	19 (25)	Yes	2.9
Total*						639	201 (31)	682	182 (27)		21.0

*Some authors did not report the number of patients lost to follow-up by treatment group, making totals approximate.
LOC, loss of consciousness; NBO, normobaric oxygen; Unk., unknown.

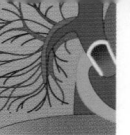

benefit to HBO, and two showed NBO to be equally efficacious. These trials have differed greatly in entry criteria, blinding, time from poisoning to experimental therapy, and outcome measures studied. Only two were double-blinded, employed sham "hyperbaric" therapy in the NBO arm, and measured outcomes by objective neuropsychological testing.[42,43] These studies produced conflicting results; one study found a strong advantage to HBO, whereas the other showed no benefit and a nonsignificant trend toward harm. A fifth randomized trial used a nonclinical end point, which makes interpretation of results and extrapolation to clinical practice virtually impossible.[54] Methodologic differences between studies and missing data make formal meta-analysis of these trials impossible. A crude summary of the results suggests that HBO provides an advantage over NBO that is nearly statistically significant ($P = 0.056$; Chi-squared, 1 degree of freedom), but clinically very modest; only 1 of every 21 patients receiving HBO appeared to benefit from the therapy.

If HBO does prevent neurologic injury, it must do so by a mechanism other than enhancing CO elimination from the blood. In all trials for which the data are reported, COHb had declined to negligible levels in almost all patients by the time HBO therapy could be initiated, and COHb levels did not correlate with neurologic outcome or response to therapy. From animal studies, HBO appears to displace CO from mitochondrial cytochromes, has antioxidant effects that minimize ischemic-reperfusion injury, and prevents cellular apoptosis.

Although expensive and inconvenient, HBO therapy is reasonably safe; chamber-related complications occur in 0 to 8% of patients.[35,43,72] Complications include middle ear or sinus barotrauma (most common), seizures (1%), pneumothorax, gas embolism, and intolerable claustrophobia. HBO therapy is not available in most American hospitals. Transport to a center that can deliver HBO may contribute greatly to expense, inconvenience, and treatment delay.

Unfortunately, no single or combination of factors has been shown to reliably predict which CO poisoning patients will develop DNS. Most CO-poisoned patients recover completely with NBO alone, and therefore would not benefit from or need HBO therapy. In addition, no trial of HBO therapy has included children. Although outcomes are generally worse in elderly people, regardless of treatment, it is unclear whether the benefits of HBO are any greater in this group. Despite the lack of reliably identifying patients with CO poisoning at high risk for developing DNS, criteria have been proposed to use as indications for HBO in patients with CO poisoning[73,74] (Box 87-1). These indications have not been prospectively evaluated and validated, but their presence should provoke strong consideration for HBO treatment.

Almost all experts recommend HBO therapy for pregnant women with significant CO poisoning, regardless of stage of pregnancy or severity of clinical signs and symptoms. A landmark study in pregnant ewes showed that COHb levels in the fetus rise more slowly than in the mother, ultimately reaching a level 98% higher than the

---

BOX 87-1 **INDICATIONS AND CONSIDERATIONS FOR HYPERBARIC OXYGEN TREATMENT IN CARBON MONOXIDE POISONING**

Accepted Indications

Altered mental status
History of loss of consciousness or syncope
Coma
Seizures
Focal neurologic deficits
Pregnancy with evidence of fetal distress

Considerations

Metabolic acidosis
Cardiac end-organ effects (severe arrhythmia, ischemia, or infarction)
Extremes of age
COHb level > 25%–40%
Abnormal neuropsychometric testing
Persistent neurologic symptoms after 4–6 hr of high-flow normobaric oxygen
Pregnancy with COHb level > 15%–20%

COHb, carboxyhemoglobin.
Adapted from references 73, 74, and 85.

---

maternal level.[75] When CO exposure was discontinued, CO was eliminated from the fetus at about half the maternal rate. However, these results cannot be extrapolated directly to humans. Sheep hemoglobin A has a lower affinity for CO than human hemoglobin A, whereas sheep fetal hemoglobin has a much higher affinity for CO than human fetal hemoglobin.[76] During human poisoning, the peak fetal COHb percentage should be within 1% to 4% of maternal peak levels.[36,76] CO poisoning interferes with oxygen delivery to the fetus, but because the normal fetus is profoundly hypoxic and acidotic by postnatal standards, it unclear at what threshold this would lead to injury. Although unclear, pregnant patients likely need longer treatment with oxygen because of the slower elimination of CO across the placenta, particularly when the CO exposure occurred over several hours or more.[75]

It is known that severe maternal CO poisoning can cause intrauterine fetal demise, limb and vertebral anomalies, cranial deformities, brain injury, transient hepatomegaly, and congestive heart failure in the newborn.[77-79] It is unclear, however, whether mild to moderate maternal CO poisoning can produce adverse fetal outcomes. Three case series have examined pregnancy outcomes in CO-poisoned women.[77-79] In all cases, women with minor CO poisoning (no loss of consciousness and normal mental status) delivered healthy babies, despite not receiving HBO. Animal studies suggest that a single CO exposure can lead to intrauterine hypoxia, fetal brain injury, and increased rates of fetal death.[80-82] It is unclear from these studies, however, whether exposures that lead to adverse fetal

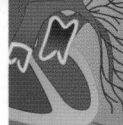

outcome can occur in the absence of significant maternal poisoning. The efficacy of NBO or HBO for preventing adverse fetal outcomes for pregnant patients with CO poisoning has not been determined. To date, pregnant women have been excluded from all published trials of HBO in CO poisoning.

HBO is generally considered safe for the fetus and has been used safely in pregnant women with CO poisoning.[83] The results in these patients were similar to those of the pregnant women treated without HBO. When the mothers had normal mentation, the fetuses universally did well, whereas maternal coma or loss of consciousness carried a poor prognosis despite HBO.

Patients who develop cardiac arrest as a result of CO poisoning have very poor outcomes. In one series of such patients, none (0 of 18) survived to hospital discharge despite aggressive therapy, including HBO.[84]

A reasonable algorithm for managing CO-poisoned patients is presented in Figure 87-1. This management strategy is in keeping with a recent position statement of the Undersea and Hyperbaric Medical Society and the consensus report of a panel of CO-poisoning experts.[73,85] Unresolved issues include which subgroups of CO poisoned patients are most likely to benefit from HBO, the optimum HBO treatment pressure and number of sessions, the necessary intensity of NBO therapy in patients not receiving HBO, and the "window of opportunity" after which brain injury is irreversible even with therapy.[73]

In addition to oxygen therapy, several novel neuroprotective strategies have been evaluated in a mouse model of CO poisoning. Glutamate antagonists (riluzole), caspase-inhibitors (disulfiram), nitric oxide synthase inhibitors (N-nitro-L-arginine methyl ester, or L-NAME), adenosine agonists (2-chloro-N^6-cylopentyl-adenosine, or CCPA), and adenosine deaminase inhibitors (erythro-9-2-hydroxy-3-nonyl-adenine, or EHNA), have all been shown to prevent hippocampal damage and learning and memory defects in mice.[86-88] HBO did not prevent neurologic injury in the same model.[64] Although riluzole and disulfiram have been found to be safe and effective treatment for other human diseases, neither has been tested in human victims of CO poisoning.

Elimination

DISPOSITION
Victims of CO poisoning can be released from the hospital after 4 to 6 hours of oxygen therapy (whether NBO or a combination of HBO) if they are neuro-logically normal, have no more than mild symptoms, and have no unmet medical or psychiatric needs. NBO may be discontinued before 4 hours for patients with mild CO poisoning whose symptoms have resolved and who have COHb levels below 5%.[89] Patients who do not recover fully after initial therapy should receive further high-flow oxygen treatment and consideration for HBO referral and treatment. Patients with moderate to severe CO poisoning should be considered for HBO treatment upon arrival and subsequently admitted to the hospital, preferably to an intensive care unit.

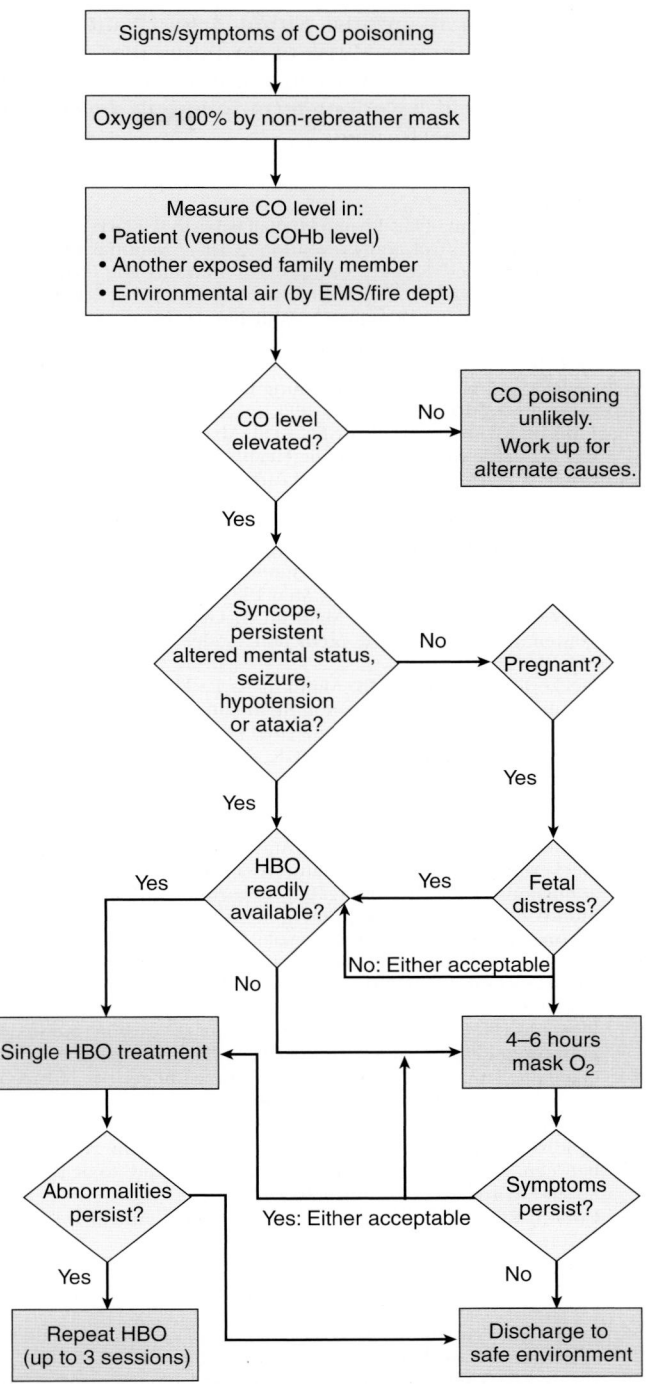

FIGURE 87-1 Suggested management algorithm for carbon monoxide poisoning.

Upon hospital discharge, patients should be warned of the possibility of delayed neuropsychological complications and provided with instructions about what to do if these occur. All patients diagnosed with CO poisoning who are discharged from the emergency department after NBO treatment should also have mandatory medical follow-up within 1 to 2 weeks so that repeat neurologic evaluation can be conducted. Most

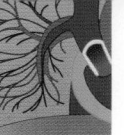

patients return to normal within 3 to 12 months.[13,21] Because of the increased risk of cardiovascular mortality, patients who suffer myocardial infarction due to CO poisoning should have long-term follow-up and cardiac risk assessment performed.[56]

REFERENCES

1. U.S. Department of Health and Human Services (USDHHS), Centers for Disease Control and Prevention (CDC), National Center for Health Statistics (NCHS), Compressed Mortality File (CMF) compiled from CMF 1999–2002, Series 20, No. 2H 2004 on CDC WONDER On-line Database. Available at http://wonder.gov/mort SQL.htm, accessed January 13, 2005.
2. Mott JA, Wolfe MI, Alverson CJ, et al: National vehicle emissions policies and practices and declining US carbon monoxide-related mortality. JAMA 2002;288:988–995.
3. Johnson EJ, Moran JC, Paine SC, et al: Abatement of toxic levels of CO in Seattle rinks. Am J Public Health 1975;65:1087–1090.
4. Cobb N, Etzel RA: Unintentional carbon monoxide-related deaths in the United States, 1979 through 1988. JAMA 1991;266:659–663.
5. Chisholm CD, Reilly J, Berejan B: Carboxyhemoglobin levels in patients with headache. Ann Emerg Med 1987;16(4):170.
6. Heckerling PS; Occult carbon monoxide poisoning: a cause of winter headache. Am J Emerg Med 1987;5:201–204.
7. Heckerling PS, Leikin JB, Maturen A: Occult carbon monoxide poisoning: validation of a prediction model. Am J Med 1988;84: 251–256.
8. Heckerling PS, Leikin JB, Maturen A, Perkins JT: Predictors of occult carbon monoxide poisoning in patients with headache and dizziness. Ann Intern Med 1987;107:174–176.
9. Turnbull TL, Hart RG, Strange GR, et al: Emergency department screening for unsuspected carbon monoxide exposure. Ann Emerg Med 1988;17:478–484.
10. Dolan MC, Haltom TL, Barrows GH, et al: Carboxyhemoglobin levels in patients with flu-like symptoms. Ann Emerg Med 1987;16:782–786.
11. Heckerling PS, Leikin JB, Maturen A, et al: Screening hospital admissions from the emergency department of occult carbon monoxide poisoning. Am J Emerg Med 1990;8:301–304.
12. Lavonas EJ, Kerns WP, Tomaszewski CA, et al: Epidemic carbon monoxide poisoning despite a CO alarm law: Mecklenburg County, NC, December, 2002. MMWR Morb Mortal Wkly Rep 2004;53: 189–192.
13. Piantadosi CA: Diagnosis and treatment of carbon monoxide poisoning. Respir Care Clin North Am 1999;5:183–202.
14. Okeda R, Funata N, Takano T, et al: The pathogenesis of carbon monoxide encephalopathy in the acute phase: physiological and morphological correlation. Acta Neuropathol 1981;54:1–10.
15. Goldbaum LR, Orellano T, Dergal E: Studies on the relationship between carboxyhemoglobin concentration and toxicity. Aviat Space Environ Med 1977;48:969–970.
16. Coburn RF: The carbon monoxide body stores. Ann N Y Acad Sci 1970;174:11–22.
17. Coburn RF, Mayers LB: Myoglobin oxygen tension determines from measurements of carboxyhemoglobin in skeletal muscle. Am J Physiol 1971;220:66–74.
18. Brown SD, Piantadosi CA: In vivo binding of carbon monoxide to cytochrome C oxidase in rat brain. J Appl Physiol 1990;69:604.
19. Hardy KR, Thom SR: Pathophysiology and treatment of carbon monoxide poisoning. J Toxicol Clin Toxicol 1994;32:613–629.
20. Zhang J, Piantadosi CA: Mitochondrial oxidative stress after carbon monoxide hypoxia in the rat brain. J Clin Invest 1992;90:1193–1199.
21. Thom SR, Ohnishi TS, Ischiropoulos H: Nitric oxide release by platelets inhibits neutrophil B₂ integrin function following acute carbon monoxide poisoning. Toxicol Appl Pharmacol 1994;128: 105–110.
22. Verma A, Hirsch DJ, Glatt CE, et al: Carbon monoxide: a putative neural messenger. Science 1993;259:381–384.
23. Thom SR, Fisher D, Xu YA, et al: Role of nitric oxide-derived oxidants in vascular injury from carbon monoxide in the rat. Am J Physiol 1999;276(3 Pt 2):H984–H992.
24. Thom SR: Carbon monoxide-mediated brain lipid peroxidation in the rat. J Appl Physiol 1990;68:997–1003.
25. Choi HS: Delayed neurological sequelae in carbon monoxide intoxication. Arch Neurol 1982;40:433–435.
26. Ginsberg MD, Myers RE, McDonaugh BF: Experimental carbon monoxide encephalopathy in the primate. II. Clinical aspects, neuropathology and physiologic correlation. Arch Neurol 1974;30:209–216.
27. Thom SR: Dehydrogenase conversion to oxidase and lipid peroxidation in brain after carbon monoxide poisoning. J Appl Physiol 1992;73:1584–1589.
28. Thom SR, fisher D, Xu YA, et al: Adaptive responses and apoptosis in endothelial cells exposed to carbon monoxide. Proc Natl Acad Sci U S A 2000;97:1305–1310.
29. Pace N, Stajman E, Walker EL: Acceleration of carbon monoxide elimination in man by high pressure oxygen. Science 1950;111: 652–654.
30. Peterson JE, Stewart RD: Absorption and elimination of carbon monoxide by inactive young men. Arch Environ Health 1970;21:165–171.
31. Jay GD, McKindley DS: Alterations in pharmacokinetics of carboxyhemoglobin produced by oxygen under pressure. Undersea Hyperb Med 1997;24:165–173.
32. Langehennig PK, Seeler RA, Berman E: Paint removers and carboxyhemoglobin. N Engl J Med 1976;295:1137.
33. Leiken JB, Kaufman D, Lipscomb JW, et al: Methylene chloride report of 5 exposures and 2 deaths. Am J Emerg Med 1990; 8:534–537.
34. Ratney RS, Wegman DH, Elkins HB: In vivo conversion of methylene chloride to carbon monoxide. Arch Environ Health 1974;28:223–236.
35. Weaver LK, Hopkins RO, Chan KJ, et al: Hyperbaric oxygen for acute carbon monoxide poisoning. N Engl J Med 2002;347: 1057–1067.
36. Tikuisis P: Modeling the uptake and elimination of carbon monoxide. In Penney DG (ed): Carbon Monoxide. Boca Raton, FL, CRC Press, 1996, pp 45–67.
37. Longo LD: Carbon monoxide effects on oxygenation of the fetus in utero. Science 1976;194:523–525.
38. Hill EP, Hill JR, Power GG, et al: Carbon monoxide exchanges between the human fetus and mother: a mathematical model. Am J Physiol 1977;232:H311–H323.
39. Barret L, Danel V, Faure J: Carbon monoxide poisoning: a diagnosis frequently overlooked. Clin Toxicol 1985;23:309–313.
40. Parkinson RB, Hopkins RO, Cleavinger HB, et al: White matter hyperintensities and neuropsychological outcome following carbon monoxide poisoning. Neurology 2002;58:1525–1532.
41. Raphael J-C, Elkharrat D, Jars-Guincestre M-C, et al: Trial of normobaric and hyperbaric oxygen for acute carbon monoxide intoxication. Lancet 1989;414–419.
42. Scheinkestel CD, Bailey M, Myles PS, et al: Hyperbaric or normobaric oxygen for acute carbon monoxide poisoning: a randomised controlled clinical trial. Med J Aust 1999;170:203–210.
43. Thom SR, Taber RL, Mendiguren II, et al: Delayed neuropsychologic sequelae after carbon monoxide poisoning: prevention by treatment with hyperbaric oxygen. Ann Emerg Med 1995; 25:474–480.
44. Deschamps D, Geraud C, Julien H, et al: Memory one month after acute carbon monoxide intoxication: a prospective study. Occup Environ Med 2003;60:212–216.
45. Mathieu D, Wattel F, Mathieu-Nolf M, et al: Randomized prospective study comparing the effect of HBO versus 12 hours of NBO in non comatose CO poisoned patients. Undersea Hyperbar Med 1996;23(Suppl.):7–8.
46. Weaver LK, Howe S, Hopkins R, Chan KJ: Carboxyhemoglobin half-life in carbon monoxide-poisoned patients treated with 100% oxygen at atmospheric pressure. Chest 2000;117:801–808.
47. Touger M, Gallagher EJ, Tyrell J: Relationship between venous and arterial carboxyhemoglobin levels in patients with suspected carbon monoxide poisoning. Ann Emerg Med 1995;25:481–483.
48. Buckley RG, Aks SE, Eshom JL, et al: The pulse oximetry gap in carbon monoxide intoxication. Ann Emerg Med 1994;24:252–255.
49. Moureu H, Chovin P, Truffer L, Lebbe J: Nouvelle micromethode pour la determination rapide et precise de l'oxycarbonemie par absorption selective dans l'infrarouge [New micromethod for the rapid and precise determination of blood carbon monoxide by

selective absorption in the infrared spectrum (French)]. Arch Mal Prof 1957;18:116–124.

50. Widdop B: Analysis of carbon monoxide. Ann Clin Biochem 2002; 39:378–391.

51. Otten EJ, Rosenberg JM, Tasset JT: An evaluation of carboxyhemoglobin spot tests. Ann Emerg Med 1985;14:850–852.

52. Cunnington AJ, Hormbrey P: Breath analysis to detect recent exposure to carbon monoxide. Postgrad Med J 2002;78:233–237.

53. Kurt TL, Anderson RJ, Reed WG: Rapid estimation of carboxyhemoglobin by breath sampling in an emergency setting. Vet Hum Toxicol 1990;32:227–229.

54. Ducasse JL, Celsis P, Marc-Vergnes JP: Non-comatose patients with acute carbon monoxide poisoning: hyperbaric or normobaric oxygenation? Undersea Hyperbar Med 1995;22:9–15.

55. Myers RAM, Britten JS: Are arterial blood gases of value in treatment decisions fro carbon monoxide poisoning? Crit Care Med 1989;17:139–142.

56. Henry CR, Satran D, Lindgren B, et al: Myocardial injury and long-term mortality following moderate to severe carbon monoxide poisoning. JAMA 2006;295:398–402.

57. Messier LD, Myers RAM: A neuropsychological screening battery for emergency assessment of carbon-monoxide-poisoned patients. J Clin Psychol 1991;47:675–684.

58. Silver DA, Cross M, Fox B, Paxton RM: Computed tomography of the brain in acute carbon monoxide poisoning. Clin Radiol 1996;51:480–483.

59. Sawada Y, Takahashi M, Ohashi N, et al: Computerised tomography as an indication of long-term outcome after acute carbon monoxide poisoning. Lancet 1980;1:783–784.

60. Parkinson RB, Hopkins RO, Cleavinger HB, et al: White matter hyperintensities and neuropsychological outcome following carbon monoxide poisoning. Neurology 2002;58:1525–1532.

61. Brown SD, Piantodosi CA: Recovery of energy metabolism in rat brain after carbon monoxide hypoxia. J Clin Invest 1991;89: 666–672.

62. Thom SR: Antagonism of carbon monoxide-mediated brain lipid peroxidation by hyperbaric oxygen. Toxicol Appl Pharmacol 1990; 105:340–344.

63. Thom SR: Functional inhibition of leukocyte B2 integrins by hyperbaric oxygen in carbon monoxide-mediated brain injury in rats. Toxicol Appl Pharmacol 1993;123:248–256.

64. Gilmer B, Kilkenny J, Tomaszewski C, Watts JA: Hyperbaric oxygen does not prevent neurologic sequelae after carbon monoxide poisoning. Acad Emerg Med 2002;9:1–8.

65. Ely EW, Moorehead B, Haponik EF: Warehouse workers' headache: emergency evaluation and management of 30 patients with carbon monoxide poisoning. Am J Med 1995;98:145–155.

66. Gorman DF, Clayton D, Gilligan JE, Webb RK: A longitudinal study of 100 consecutive admissions for carbon monoxide poisoning to the Royal Adelaide Hospital. Undersea Hyperb Med 1992;20:311–316.

67. Goulon M, Barios A, Rapin M: Carbon monoxide poisoning and acute anoxia due to breathing coal gas and hydrocarbons. J Hyperbar Med 1986;1:23–41.

68. Mathieu D, Nolf M, Durocher A: Acute carbon monoxide poisoning: risk of late sequelae and treatment by hyperbaric oxygen. J Toxicol Clin Toxicol 1985;23:315–324.

69. Myers RAM, Snyder SK, Emhoff TA: Subacute sequelae of carbon monoxide poisoning. Ann Emerg Med 1985;14:1167.

70. Roche L, Bertoye A, Vincent P: Comparison de deux groupes de vingt intoxications oxycarbonees traitees par oxygenennormobare et hyperbare [French]. Lyon Med 1968;220:1483–1499.

71. Wilms SJ, Turner F, Kerr J: Carbon monoxide or smoke inhalations treated with oxygen (hyperbaric vs normobaric): 118 reviewed. Undersea Biomed Res 1985;S56.

72. Scheinkestel CD, Bailey M, Myles PS, et al: Hyperbaric or normobaric oxygen for acute carbon monoxide poisoning: a randomized controlled clinical trial. Undersea Hyperb Med 2000;27:163–164.

73. Hampson NB, Mathieu D, Piantadosi CA, et al: Carbon monoxide poisoning: interpretation of randomized clinical trials and unresolved treatment issues. Undersea Hyperb Med 2001; 28:157–164.

74. Kao LW, Nanagas KA: Carbon monoxide poisoning. Emerg Med Clin North Am 2004;22:985–1018.

75. Longo LD, Hill EP: Carbon monoxide uptake in fetal and maternal sheep. Am J Physiol 1977;232:H324–H330.

76. Longo LD: Carbon monoxide poisoning in the pregnant mother and fetus and its exchange across the placenta. Ann N Y Acad Sci 1970;174:313–341.

77. Caravati EM, Adams CJ, Joyce SM, Schafer NC: Fetal toxicity associated with maternal carbon monoxide poisoning. Ann Emerg Med 1988;17:714–717.

78. Koren G, Sharav T, Pastuszak A, Garrettson LK, et al: A multicenter, prospective study of fetal outcome following accidental carbon monoxide poisoning in pregnancy. Reprod Toxicol 1991;5:397–403.

79. Norman CA, Halton DM: Is carbon monoxide a workplace teratogen? A review and evaluation of the literature. Ann Occup Hyg 1990;34:335–347.

80. Ginsberg MD, Myers RE: Fetal brain damage following maternal carbon monoxide intoxication: an experimental study. Acta Obstet Gynecol Scand 1974;53:309–317.

81. Ginsberg MD, Myers RE: Fetal brain injury after maternal carbon monoxide intoxication: clinical and neuropathologic aspects. Neurology 1976;26:15–23.

82. Singh J: Early behavioral alterations in mice following prenatal carbon monoxide exposure. Neurotoxicology 1986;7:475–482.

83. Elkharrat D, Raphael JC, Korach JM, et al: Acute carbon monoxide intoxication and hyperbaric oxygen in pregnancy. Intens Care Med 1991;17:289–292.

84. Hampson NB, Zmaeff JL: Outcome of patients experiencing cardiac arrest with carbon monoxide poisoning treated with hyperbaric oxygen. Ann Emerg Med 2001;28:36–41.

85. Thom SR, Weaver LK: Carbon monoxide poisoning. In Feldmeier JJ (ed): Hyperbaric Oxygen 2003 Indications and Results: The Hyperbaric Oxygen Therapy Committee Report. Kensington, MD: Undersea and Hyperbaric Medical Society, 2003, pp 11–17.

86. Tomaszewski C, Gilmer B, Watts JA: The neuroprotective effects of dimethyl sulfoxide on memory following acute carbon monoxide poisoning in mice. Ann Emerg Med 2000;36:S69.

87. Gilmer B, Thompson C, Tomaszewski C, Watts JA: The protective effects of experimental neurodepressors on learning and memory following carbon monoxide poisoning. J Toxicol Clin Toxicol 1999; 37:606.

88. Thompson C, Gilmer B, Tomaszewski C, Watts JA: The neuroprotective effects of glutamate antagonism on memory following acute carbon monoxide poisoning. J Toxicol Clin Toxicol 1999;37:608.

89. Ilano AL, Raffin TA: Management of carbon monoxide poisoning. Chest 1990;7:165–169.

90. Vagts SA: Non-fire Carbon Monoxide Deaths Associated with the Use of Consumer Products: 1999 and 2000 Annual Estimates. Bethesda, MD, U.S. Consumer Products Safety Commission, 2003.

91. Burney RE, Wu SC, Nemiroff MJ: Mass carbon monoxide poisoning: clinical effects and results of treatment in 184 victims. Ann Emerg Med 1982;11:399.

88 Cyanide and Related Compounds—Sodium Azide

ALAN H. HALL, MD

At a Glance...

- Severe acute cyanide poisoning can be seen in a wide variety of settings, including enclosed-space fire smoke inhalation.
- Cyanide is a credible toxic terrorism threat agent.
- Whole-blood cyanide levels require several hours or longer to obtain.
- Emergent suspicion of the diagnosis and the decision to administer specific antidotes must be made on clinical and screening laboratory grounds.
- Elevated plasma lactate levels are a specific and sensitive indicator of the presence of significant cyanide poisoning in both smoke inhalation and pure cyanide poisoning cases.
- Several specific cyanide antidotes are available throughout the world.
- In the United States, only the cyanide antidote kit containing amyl nitrite for inhalation administration and sodium nitrite/sodium thiosulfate for intravenous administration is available as of June 2006.
- Amyl nitrite inhalation is an effective first-aid measure, especially in cases of hydrogen cyanide gas exposure.
- Growing evidence indicates that hydroxocobalamin may be the cyanide antidote of choice because of its efficacy and superior safety and adverse effects profile.
- The nitrite and thiosulfate antidote kit is not efficacious for sodium azide poisoning; hydroxocobalamin may be of theoretical benefit based on limited in vitro data.

INTRODUCTION AND RELEVANT HISTORY

Cyanide poisoning may be encountered in a wide variety of settings. Cyanide salts and hydrocyanic acid are used in common industrial processes such as electroplating, jewelry and metal cleaning, precious metal extraction, laboratory assays, and photographic processes.[1-4] Hydrogen cyanide is a chemical intermediate for the manufacture of synthetic fibers, plastics, and nitriles.[5] Criminal tampering by replacement of the ingredients in over-the-counter capsules with cyanide salts has resulted in a number of deaths.[6,7] Victims of enclosed-space fire-smoke inhalation may have both cyanide and carbon monoxide poisoning.[8,9]

Cyanide and carbon monoxide are synergistic toxicants[10] (see Chapters 86 and 87). Nontraumatic deaths in aircraft accidents may be due to inhalation of carbon monoxide and cyanide combustion products.[11] A number of compounds can liberate cyanide on spontaneous or thermal decomposition or by chemical reaction with acids (e.g., cyanogen, cyanogen bromide, cyanogen iodide, cyanogen chloride, calcium cyanide).[1] Cyanogen halides and hydrogen cyanide are potential chemical warfare agents.[12] At low concentrations, however, cyanogen halides are primarily lacrimating and pulmonary irritant agents.[3]

Cyanogenic compounds (laetrile, amygdalin from plant sources, nitrile compounds such as acetonitrile or propionitrile) can release cyanide during metabolism, chemical reaction in the gut, or bacterial degradation after ingestion.[3,13-17] Acute cyanide poisoning from apricot or peach kernels is unusual because the pits are usually swallowed whole and simply pass through the gastrointestinal tract; rare cases have been reported.[18] Severe or fatal cyanide poisoning with symptom onset delay of several hours has followed accidental acetonitrile ingestion from glue-on artificial nail–removing compounds.[19,20]

Acrylonitrile is a special case. After inhalation or dermal exposure, it both undergoes hepatic metabolism releasing cyanide and is itself hepatotoxic. Whole blood cyanide levels as high as 4.3 µg/mL have been found in patients with acrylonitrile poisoning.[17] In addition to supportive care and cyanide antidotes, treatment with N-acetylcysteine in a manner similar to that for acetaminophen poisoning has been recommended to prevent hepatotoxicity[17] (see Chapter 47).

Sodium nitroprusside releases cyanide during metabolism, which can result in elevated whole blood cyanide levels, and, occasionally, clinical cyanide poisoning.[21-24]

Coadministration of sodium thiosulfate or hydroxocobalamin can prevent cyanide toxicity, especially in patients receiving sodium nitroprusside infusions at rates greater than 2 µg/kg/minute[24,25] (see Chapter 61). The frequent lack of correlation between blood cyanide levels and cyanide poisoning symptoms during nitroprusside administration suggests that the decision of whether to administer antidote therapy must be made on clinical grounds (e.g., presence of lactic acidosis or signs and symptoms consistent with cyanide poisoning). Clinical symptoms in this setting may, however, be due to thiocyanate accumulation.[26]

Chronic exposure to low levels of cyanide has been postulated to cause retrobulbar optic atrophy (in heavy smokers) and ataxic peripheral neuropathy (tropical ataxic neuropathy), as well as konzo (spastic upper motor neuron paraparesis) in people who consume large amounts of improperly prepared cassava, which contains the cyanogenic glycosides linamarin and lotaustralin in both roots and leaves.[27,28] Development of these neuropathies seems to require both chronic low-level cyanide exposure and either a deficiency of the endogenous cyanide-detoxifying enzyme rhodanese or protein-calorie malnutrition with dietary sulfur deficiency. A condition resembling acute cyanide poisoning treatable with hydroxocobalamin has resulted from acute ingestion of improperly prepared cassava.[29]

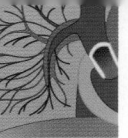

Mild disorders of vitamin B_{12} and folate levels and some subclinical thyroid function abnormalities were noted in one group of workers with chronic cyanide salt exposure.[2]

Thyroid enlargement (goiter) and altered iodine-131 uptake have also been described in workers chronically exposed to cyanide[3] and in populations eating an iodine-deficient monotonous cassava diet.[30]

EPIDEMIOLOGY

Despite widespread cyanide and cyanogenic compound use, serious acute cyanide poisoning is rare. Of a total of 2,267,979 human poison exposures reported to the American Association of Poison Control Centers Toxic Exposure Surveillance System (TESS) during 2001, only 303 involved cyanide poisoning; of these, 17 were in children younger than 6 years of age, 17 were in patients 6 to 19 years of age, and 263 were in patients older than 19 years of age (the remainder were in patients of unknown age).[31]

Of the 295 cases in which the reason for exposure was known, 237 were unintentional exposures, 37 were intentional exposures, and 21 were classified as other.

A total of 199 (65%) of these patients were treated in a health care facility.[31] Of cyanide antidotes available in the United States, amyl nitrite was not listed in the 2001 TESS database, sodium nitrite administration was recorded in 27 instances, and sodium thiosulfate administration was recorded in 57 instances.

Of the 303 cyanide exposures, clinical outcome was known in only 194 (64%).[31] In 64 cases (21%), no signs or symptoms of cyanide poisoning developed; 116 patients (38%) became symptomatic, and 7 (2.3%) developed major symptoms (life-threatening signs or symptoms; significant residual disability or disfigurement).[31] Fourteen TESS-reported patients (4.6%) died of cyanide poisoning during 2001.[31]

Some details of these 14 fatal cyanide poisonings were available.[31] One involved combined carbon monoxide and cyanide poisoning from smoke inhalation (carboxyhemoglobin level, 35%; whole blood cyanide level, 40 µg/mL).

Of the 13 "pure" fatal cyanide poisoning cases, all were adults.[31] Ingestion of the involved cyanide compound was intentional in 12, and 1 case was classified as unintentional misuse. In three of these cases, whole blood cyanide levels were more than 20 µg/mL, 66 µg/mL, and 26.7 µg/mL; times after ingestion were not specified.

An adult man who worked in a jewelry shop drank from an already-open bottle of soda and rapidly developed fatal cardiac arrest. The soda was subsequently found to have a pH of 7 and a cyanide concentration of 100 mg/L.[31]

An elderly retired chemist accidentally ingested a swallow of sodium cyanide–copper cyanide etching solution. He was apparently successfully resuscitated from the initial severe cyanide poisoning, but subsequently developed fatal liver, renal, and pancreatic damage, suggesting that copper poisoning contributed to the fatal outcome.[31]

PHARMACOLOGY

Pathophysiology

Cyanide produces histotoxic hypoxia by binding with the ferric iron (Fe^{3+}) of mitochondrial cytochrome oxidase, thus disrupting the normal functioning of the electron transport chain and the ability of cells to utilize O_2 in oxidative phosphorylation.[1] The result is a shift to anaerobic metabolism, a substantial decrease in adenosine triphosphate synthesis, depletion of cellular energy stores, and greatly increased lactic acid production, which causes an elevated anion-gap metabolic acidosis. Numerous iron- or copper-containing enzymes are inhibited by cyanide, but cytochrome oxidase inhibition is the major intracellular toxic mechanism in cyanide poisoning.[3]

The tissue hypoxia of cyanide poisoning has several causes. Those tissues most dependent on oxidative phosphorylation—heart and brain—are the most severely and rapidly affected. Central inhibition of the respiratory centers leads to hypoventilation, which in turn produces hypoxic hypoxia.

Myocardial depression with decreased cardiac output produces stagnation hypoxia. Until the stage of respiratory depression or arrest, the blood is relatively normally oxygenated. However, the tissues are unable to extract and utilize this O_2, which leads to a greater than normal amount of O_2 in venous blood and an increased venous O_2 percent saturation.

Cyanide binding to cytochrome oxidase is a reversible process. The endogenous enzyme, rhodanese, is a natural defense against cyanide exposure. This enzyme complexes cyanide with sulfane sulfur, forming much less toxic thiocyanate. The body's sulfur pool is small, however, and the availability of sulfane sulfur constitutes the rate-limiting factor in natural cyanide detoxification. In the absence of an exogenous source of sulfur, rhodanese activity is too slow to prevent serious toxicity or death in significant cyanide poisoning.

The central nervous system is a primary target organ in cyanide poisoning.[32,33] The mechanism by which cyanide exposure causes neurotoxicity is not completely understood. An increase in intraneuronal calcium levels and lipid peroxidation, perhaps initiated by cyanide-induced decreased adenosine triphosphate levels, which impairs sodium and calcium extrusion processes, might be a mechanism of nerve injury.[34] Cyanide-induced apoptosis is mediated by cytochome-*c* release from mitochondria.[35] Generation of reactive oxygen species (ROS) also plays an important role in cyanide-induced apoptosis in cortical neurons.[33]

Pharmacokinetics

TOXICOKINETICS

The toxicokinetics of cyanide are not well understood. Available data are either from animal experiments or

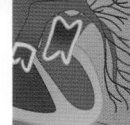

anecdotal human case reports. In dog plasma in vitro, cyanide is about 60% protein bound.[36] In vivo, whole blood cyanide levels may be four or more times greater than serum levels because of the concentration of cyanide in erythrocytes.[1]

The volume of distribution (Vd) of cyanide in dogs is 0.498 L/kg.[37] A similar Vd of 0.41 L/kg was estimated in a single case of human potassium cyanide poisoning.[38] In this same case, estimates of other toxicokinetic parameters were area under the curve (AUC) 48 µg/mL/hr, clearance 163 mL/min, initial phase half-life ($t_{1/2\alpha}$) 20 to 30 minutes, and terminal-phase elimination half-life ($t_{1/2\beta}$) 19 hours.[38] The last value is consistent with findings in dogs showing only minimal excretion within the first 3 hours after oral administration, despite absorption of about 95%.[36] In victims of human cyanide poisoning from smoke inhalation, blood cyanide half-life was about 60 minutes.[9]

TOXICODYNAMICS

In a single patient not treated with specific antidotes, the average urinary cyanide excretion over nearly 40 hours was 0.64 mg/hr after a probable ingestion of between 117 and 511 mg of potassium cyanide.[6] In this same patient, the mean whole blood cyanide level 1 hour after ingestion was 8.2 µg/mL. This level increased to a mean of 19.7 µg/mL at 3 hours and to 23.4 µg/mL at 9 hours after ingestion. Despite intensive supportive treatment, this patient died about 40 hours after ingestion.

In contrast, in a patient who survived ingestion of 1 g of potassium cyanide after treatment with sodium nitrite and sodium thiosulfate, the highest whole blood cyanide level was 15.68 µg/mL at 1.75 hours after ingestion; this level decreased to 0.82 µg/mL at 5 hours after ingestion.[38] In another patient who survived cyanide poisoning secondary to dermal and inhalation exposure to propionitrile, treatment with hydroxocobalamin–sodium thiosulfate was associated with a decrease in the whole blood cyanide level from 5.71 µg/mL at 2 hours after exposure to 0.93 µg/mL 30 minutes later.[13] Specific cyanide antidote administration is associated with more rapid decreases in whole blood cyanide levels than is seen in patients not administered antidotes.[1]

TOXICOLOGY

Clinical Manifestations

The natural history of severe acute cyanide poisoning is a rapid progression (faster with inhalation than ingestion) to coma, shock, respiratory failure, and death.[1] Less severely poisoned patients administered only intensive supportive care have survived,[6,39] whereas patients also administered specific antidotes have survived with whole blood cyanide levels as high as 40 µg/mL.[40] Most patients who recover from acute cyanide poisoning do not have permanent sequelae, although rare cases of parkinsonian-like states with bilaterally symmetric lesions in the basal ganglia (putamen or globus pallidus) or memory deficits and personality changes have been reported.[16,41-43]

The clinical presentation depends on the route, dose, and time elapsed since exposure. Patients with inhalation exposure to high concentrations may experience sudden loss of consciousness after only a few breaths.[3,44] Combined inhalation and dermal or pure dermal exposure to a gas containing 19% hydrogen cyanide caused severe acute cyanide poisoning in two workers with whole blood cyanide levels of 5.3 and 6.75 µg/mL, respectively.[45] Patients who ingest potentially fatal amounts of cyanide salts may not develop life-threatening symptoms for up to 0.5 to 1 hour after exposure.[38] Delayed onset of symptoms (after 1 to 12 or more hours) may follow exposure to cyanogens such as laetrile, amygdalin, and nitrile compounds.[6,15,19,20]

In patients who do not experience sudden collapse, the initial signs and symptoms can resemble those of anxiety or hyperventilation.[1] Early signs include central nervous system stimulation (giddiness, headache, anxiety), tachycardia, hyperpnea, mild hypertension, and palpitations.[6]

Late signs are nausea, vomiting, tachycardia or bradycardia, hypotension, seizures (rare), coma, apnea, dilated pupils, and a variety of cardiac effects, including erratic supraventricular or ventricular arrhythmias, atrioventricular blocks, ischemic changes on electrocardiography, and asystole.[1] Noncardiogenic pulmonary edema may rarely occur, even after ingestion of cyanide salts.[39]

Of 21 acute cyanide poisoning victims, the following effects were noted: loss of consciousness ($N = 15$), metabolic acidosis ($N = 14$), cardiopulmonary failure ($N = 9$), anoxic encephalopathy ($N = 6$), and diabetes insipidus or conditions mimicking this condition ($N = 1–3$), which may be an ominous sign.[16]

The smell of "bitter almonds" (often described as "musty") may be appreciated in some cases, but the ability to detect this odor is genetically determined, and many people cannot do so.[1] Cyanosis is a late sign usually only noted at the stage of apnea and circulatory collapse.[1]

Dermal exposure to cyanide can result in systemic cyanide poisoning due to serious burns from molten cyanide salts, immersion in vats of cyanide salt solutions (with the potential for ingestion and vapor inhalation as well as dermal exposure), or total-body contamination with cyanide salts in confined spaces. Severe acute cyanide poisoning can rarely result from dermal exposure to hydrogen cyanide gas.[45]

Diagnosis

The initial physical examination focuses on the vital signs and the respiratory, cardiovascular, and central nervous systems. Continuous vital signs and electrocardiographic monitoring should be done. Whole blood cyanide levels are available, but generally take hours to obtain and cannot be used to guide emergent diagnosis or therapy.[1] They can, however, document the diagnosis and response to treatment.

LABORATORY TESTING

Plasma lactate, serum electrolytes, and arterial blood gases should be monitored as frequently as necessary to

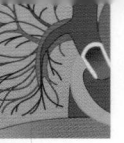

guide fluid, electrolyte, sodium bicarbonate, and respiratory therapy. Pulse oximetry may be unreliable in cases of smoke inhalation with combined carbon monoxide and cyanide poisoning and after administration of methemoglobin-inducing cyanide antidotes.

Based on anecdotal case reports and animal experiments, certain screening laboratory values may help suggest the diagnosis when no history is available.[1] Cyanide produces lactic acidosis, which can be confirmed by plasma lactate measurements.[15,46] Normal plasma lactate levels are 1.0 mEq/L (mmol/L) or less. Lactic acidosis is present when serum lactate levels are more than 2.0 mEq/L (mmol/L). In combined poisoning with carbon monoxide and cyanide from smoke inhalation, plasma lactate levels may be the best marker of the presence and severity of a cyanide poisoning component.[9] Plasma lactate levels of 10 mEq/L (mmol/L) or greater in smoke inhalation victims without severe burns or levels of 8 mEq/L (mmol/L) or greater in patients with "pure" cyanide exposure are sensitive and specific indicators of cyanide poisoning.[47,48]

If the patient is still breathing or is receiving assisted ventilation, the arterial partial pressure of O_2 may be relatively normal. Cyanide inhibits the extraction of O_2 from the blood at the tissue level. Thus, more O_2 than normal is present in the venous blood; this may be reflected by an increased (>40 mm Hg) peripheral venous partial pressure of O_2, an increased measured peripheral venous O_2 percent saturation (>70%), or a narrowing of the normal difference between the measured arterial O_2 percent saturation and the measured central venous or pulmonary artery O_2 percent saturation (the normal central venous O_2 percent saturation is about 70%).[1,16] However, a mixed venous O_2 percent saturation less than 90% does not, in itself, exclude acute cyanide poisoning.[15]

OTHER DIAGNOSTIC TESTING

If pulmonary edema develops, a chest radiograph should be obtained periodically.

A smoke inhalation clinical scoring system (scale from 1 to 10) based on the following clinical findings has been proposed: hoarseness (1 point); stridor (1 point); carbonaceous sputum (1 point); soot in the airways (1 point); singed nasal hairs (1 point); facial burns (1 point); abnormal chest auscultation findings (1 point); mental status change (1 point); and abnormal findings on chest radiography (2 points). In one case series, this clinical scoring system was predictive of a fatal outcome after smoke inhalation exposure from enclosed-space fires; it was also the strongest predictor of measured carboxyhemoglobin and whole blood cyanide levels.[49]

DIFFERENTIAL DIAGNOSIS

Other cytochrome oxidase inhibitors such as hydrogen sulfide and sodium azide may produce clinical and laboratory findings similar to those seen in cyanide poisoning (see Chapter 91 and later discussion in this chapter on Sodium Azide). Although sodium nitrite might have some efficacy in the treatment of hydrogen sulfide poisoning, it is ineffective for treating sodium azide poisoning.[50]

MANAGEMENT

Supportive Measures

Cyanide-exposed patients with only restlessness, anxiety, or hyperventilation do not require antidote therapy. Such patients should be administered supplemental O_2 and undergo a few hours of clinical monitoring. Antidotes should be administered only if more serious symptoms develop.

Rescuers must not enter areas with high airborne concentrations of cyanide without a self-contained breathing apparatus or air-supplied respirators. Mouth-to-mouth breathing should be avoided if at all possible, and care must be taken by rescuers not to inhale the victim's exhaled breath. Appropriate prehospital care consists of airway management, including endotracheal intubation if required, administration of 100% supplemental O_2 by tight-fitting mask or endotracheal tube, placement of at least one large-bore intravenous line, administration of sodium bicarbonate if shock (with presumed metabolic acidosis) is present, decontamination of exposed skin or eyes, administration of standard antiarrhythmic or anticonvulsant medications if necessary, and administration of amyl nitrite by inhalation.

Amyl nitrite pearls may be broken in gauze and held close to the nose and mouth of patients who are spontaneously breathing. Alternatively, they may be placed into the lip of the facemask or inside the resuscitation bag in patients with apnea or hypoventilation. Amyl nitrite should be inhaled for 30 seconds of each minute, and a used pearl should be replaced with a fresh one every 3 to 4 minutes. Amyl nitrite and supplemental O_2 administration alone have been efficacious in treating hydrogen cyanide–poisoned patients in one occupational exposure setting.[51] Supportive measures alone may sometimes prove to be satisfactory,[39,44] although patients administered specific antidotes together with supportive therapy have survived with higher whole blood cyanide levels, awakened sooner from coma, and had more rapid resolution of acidosis.[6,38,39]

Standard antiarrhythmic and anticonvulsant medications are appropriate for the treatment of cyanide-induced arrhythmias and seizures. Atropine or vasopressors may be required if symptomatic bradycardia or hypotension unresponsive to less aggressive measures are present.

Normobaric O_2 is synergistic with cyanide antidotes. Although not proved, hyperbaric oxygen (HBO) may be efficacious in patients not responsive to supportive and antidotal therapy, and some severely cyanide-poisoned patients treated with HBO have survived.[14,46] Smoke inhalation victims with serious known carbon monoxide poisoning and suspected cyanide toxicity may be treated with HBO when available.[8]

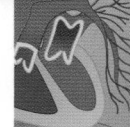

Decontamination

Exposed skin and eyes should be copiously flushed with water or normal saline. Contaminated clothing should be removed and isolated in impervious containers. Inducing emesis is contraindicated because of the potential for rapid progression to coma or seizures. Gastric aspiration might be beneficial within about 30 minutes after ingestion of cyanide salts. Although older references question the efficacy of activated charcoal administration, a single dose of about 1 g of activated charcoal per kilogram of body weight may be administered to patients who have ingested cyanide salts and related compounds.

Antidotes

In the United States and some other countries, specific therapy consists of the administration of the antidotes found in the cyanide antidote kit. Once intravenous access has been established, amyl nitrite inhalation should be discontinued and sodium nitrite administered intravenously. The usual adult dose is 300 mg (one 10-mL ampoule of 3% solution). The pediatric dose for the average child is 0.12 to 0.33 mL/kg administered over absolutely no less than 5 minutes intravenously.

Sodium nitrite is a potent vasodilator, and rapid administration may cause significant hypotension, which can be avoided by initial slow administration, either (1) by slow intravenous push over absolutely no less than 5 minutes, or (2) by diluting the dose in 50 to 100 mL of 5% dextrose in water, initially beginning with a slow infusion rate, and then increasing to the most rapid rate possible without causing hypotension. Frequent blood pressure monitoring should be done during sodium nitrite administration.

Another potentially serious, although rare, adverse effect of sodium nitrite administration is induction of excessive methemoglobin levels. Induction of some level of methemoglobinemia has long been thought to be the mechanism of action of sodium nitrite because methemoglobin has a greater affinity for cyanide than cytochrome oxidase. This hypothesis has been questioned.

Excessive methemoglobin induction occurs most often in patients given excessive amounts of sodium nitrite, but it is rarely seen with therapeutic doses. Methemoglobin levels should be monitored, especially when multiple doses of sodium nitrite are required. Inducing levels greater than 30% to 40% must be avoided. The determinant of when "enough" sodium nitrite has been infused is the patient's clinical response.

Sodium nitrite is followed by intravenous administration of sodium thiosulfate, in an adult dose of 12.5 g (one 50-mL ampoule of a 25% solution). The average pediatric dose is 1.65 mL/kg. No cases of significant adverse effects from sodium thiosulfate administration have been reported in humans, despite more than 50 years of clinical use of the drug. A continuous infusion of 1 g of sodium thiosulfate per hour for 24 hours was considered efficacious in one case of potassium cyanide ingestion poisoning.[52]

In cases of smoke inhalation with known carbon monoxide and suspected cyanide poisoning, sodium thiosulfate and 100% supplemental O_2 can be administered initially if hydroxocobalamin is not available. Sodium nitrite administration should be withheld until the patient is at pressure in an HBO chamber, where dissolved plasma O_2 can adequately compensate for induced methemoglobinemia.[8] When HBO was not immediately available for treatment of smoke inhalation patients, sodium nitrite was administered successfully without significant complications.[53]

Second doses of sodium nitrite and sodium thiosulfate at one half the initial amounts may be administered 30 minutes after the first doses if clinical response is inadequate. With exposure to certain nitrile compounds, continued metabolic release of cyanide may cause prolonged poisoning requiring multiple antidote doses. If producing a satisfactory clinical response, sodium thiosulfate alone could be used in such cases because its inherent toxicity is low.

Alternate antidotes in clinical use in other parts of the world such as hydroxocobalamin (Cyanokit), dicobalt–ethylenediaminetetra-acetic acid (Kelocyanor), and 4-dimethylaminophenol (4-DMAP) are not available in the United States as of June 2006. A growing body of evidence, primarily from patients with combined carbon monoxide and cyanide poisoning from enclosed-space fire smoke inhalation, but also from patients with aliphatic nitrile or cyanide salt poisoning, indicates that hydroxocobalamin may be the cyanide antidote of choice.[47,54,55]

Hydroxocobalamin is more rapidly acting than sodium thiosulfate, does not produce methemoglobinemia, which can impair oxygen transport as do 4-DMAP and the nitrites, does not cause hypotension as does sodium nitrite, and has a much better adverse effect and safety profile than do the nitrites, 4-DMAP and Kelocyanor.[47,54] It has been shown to be safe and effective for decreasing low whole blood cyanide levels in volunteer heavy smokers and is an effective and safe cyanide antidote in a variety of experimental animal species.[56,57] The only noted side effect in patients treated with hydroxocobalamin has been transient reddish-brown discoloration of the urine, sclera, mucous membranes, and skin from the color of the medication itself.[47,54] Hydrocobalamin can be combined with sodium thiosulfate in more severe poisoning cases because there is an antidotal synergy.[47,54,57]

Because of its intense reddish-brown color and peak light absorption at 352 and 525 nm, hydroxocobalamin can interfere with automated colorimetric clinical chemistry measurements of aspartate aminotransferase, total bilirubin, creatinine, magnesium, and serum iron.[58]

Elimination

Hemodialysis cannot be considered standard treatment for cyanide poisoning, but it has been efficaciously used as supportive therapy in a patient who developed renal failure secondary to rhabdomyolysis in the course of severe cyanide poisoning.[16] One patient with severe acute

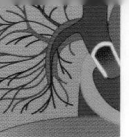

cyanide poisoning treated with supportive measures, antidotes, and charcoal hemoperfusion has also been reported.[4] This patient was improving after antidotal and supportive therapy at the time that hemoperfusion was begun. Hemoperfusion has no place in the treatment of acute cyanide poisoning.

Disposition

Asymptomatic patients with apparent minimal exposure should be observed in a controlled setting for 4 to 6 hours. If exposure was to a nitrile compound, the onset of symptoms may be delayed for 12 hours or longer; in this situation, a longer period of observation and monitoring is necessary.

Patients who have serious symptoms (coma, seizures, shock, metabolic acidosis, cardiac arrhythmias, ischemic electrocardiographic changes, or hypoventilation) and all those administered antidotes should be admitted to an intensive care unit for clinical monitoring until all symptoms have resolved, or for a minimum period of 24 hours. Outpatient follow-up at intervals for a period of weeks should be arranged to screen for the possible development of rare delayed central nervous system effects.

Given the acute shortage of suitable organ donors, brain-dead poisoning victims should not be excluded as donors, if: (1) clinical and laboratory evidence shows true brain death (*not* central nervous system depression or lack of central nervous system activity due to the continued presence of the poison); (2) the poison itself has not irretrievably damaged or destroyed the organ under consideration for transplantation; and (3) the organ being considered for transplantation is not a reservoir, such that the transplanted organ itself might secondarily poison the transplant recipient. Organs have been successfully transplanted from brain-dead acute cyanide poisoning victims without causing secondary cyanide poisoning.[59,60]

SODIUM AZIDE

Sodium azide is a white to colorless crystalline solid that is highly soluble in water and is used as a preservative in aqueous laboratory reagents and biologic fluids and in automobile airbags as a gas generator.[61] It has also been investigated for use as an herbicide, insecticide, nematocide, fungicide, and bacteriocide and is used in the manufacturing of rubber, latex, wine, and Japanese beer, and as a chemical intermediate in lead azide production.[61] Its use in automotive airbags has not resulted in sodium azide poisoning, but it has rarely caused relatively minor chemical burns by producing nitrogen gas and sodium oxide; the latter reacts with water to form corrosive sodium hydroxide.[61]

Sodium azide poisoning has most often occurred as a result of accidental or suicidal ingestion of colorless, odorless, tasteless laboratory solutions, which can be mistaken for water or normal saline, and has occurred in health care settings or laboratories.[61–63] Suicidal cases have generally been seen in individuals with access to the chemical in laboratories because otherwise it has limited availability.[63,64] One patient died after mistakenly ingesting 1 g of sodium azide obtained from a hospital but intended to be added as a preservative to a container for his 24-hour urine specimen.[65]

The 2001 American Association of Poison Control Centers TESS[31] does not have a specific listing for sodium azide. A recent systematic review covering the period of 1927 to 1999 found that a total of 38 publications constituted the knowledge base of sodium azide human health effects.[61] Of these, 32 publications were case reports, 5 were occupational studies, and 1 paper was an experimental study of the use of sodium azide as a potential antihypertensive agent (since abandoned because of significant side effects).[61,64] There were a total of 185 exposed people, with 116 from the experimental study.[61] Adults were involved in 183 cases and children in 2 cases.

Of the 69 acute poisoning cases, 43 followed ingestion (26 survivors; 17 fatalities), 12 followed inhalation from occupational exposure (all 12 patients survived), 9 were exposed by the intravenous route from sodium azide contamination of hemodialysis apparatus (all 9 survived), and 5 patients had dermal exposure (4 survivors; 1 fatality).[61] The dermal exposure fatality involved exposure to a metal azide during an explosion causing 45% total-body surface area burns.[61] The hemodialysis patients exposed by the intravenous route developed hypotension, blurred vision, headache, nausea, vomiting, syncope, and cramping when ultrafilters used for preparation of dialysis fluid were pretreated with a preservative consisting of 0.25% sodium azide and 25% glycerin and not flushed.[66]

Ingestion is the most common route of exposure in serious poisoning cases.[61] Fatality is usually associated with doses greater than 700 mg (or 10–13 mg/kg), whereas nonfatal poisoning has been seen with doses ranging from 0.3 to 150 mg (or 0.004–2 mg/kg).[61] In a series of four fatal and six nonfatal sodium azide poisoning cases, the lowest dose in survivors was 5 to 10 mg, and the highest dose was 80 mg.[67] The lowest fatal doses were 0.7 g in women and 1.2 to 2 g in men.[67]

Sodium azide is rapidly absorbed from the gastrointestinal and respiratory tracts (as hydrazoic acid vapor).[61] Its extent of dermal absorption is unclear, but a single fatal case from a warehouse accident has been reported.[61] Sodium azide is metabolized by the liver and excreted by the kidneys, but human absorption, distribution, metabolism, and excretion kinetics data are not available,[61] except for a half-life of about 2.5 hours calculated in a single fatal case.[68]

Hypotension is the most common clinical effect, and the time between exposure and the onset of hypotension is somewhat predictive of survival.[61] When hypotension occurs within minutes to 1 hour after exposure, it is a physiologic response, and the clinical course is most often benign. When the hypotension is delayed in onset more than 1 hour, it ". . . constitutes an ominous sign for death."[61]

Other common clinical effects are nausea, vomiting, diarrhea, headache, dizziness, temporary vision loss, pal-

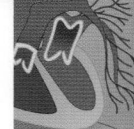

pitations, dyspnea, temporary loss of consciousness, and depressed sensorium.[61] Markedly depressed sensorium, seizures, coma, hypothermia, cardiac dysrhythmias, chest pain, tachypnea, cyanosis, noncardiogenic pulmonary edema, acute respiratory distress syndrome (ARDS), metabolic acidosis, oliguria, and cardiorespiratory arrest are seen in severe poisoning cases.[61,62,65,68]

The hypotensive effects are due to dilation of peripheral blood vessels, but it is unclear whether this effect is caused by the parent compound or its metabolism to nitric oxide.[61] Sodium azide does inhibit heme-containing enzymes such as catalase, peroxidase, and cytochrome oxidase,[61,69,70] but its lethality may be due instead to enhanced excitatory nervous transmission in the central nervous system, caused by the parent compound itself or by metabolically released nitric oxide.[61,71]

One case of cardiomyopathy presenting as an acute myocardial infarction was reported in a previously healthy 29-year-old female student who mistakenly ingested 700 mL of a buffering solution containing 0.1% sodium azide.[72] Nausea, weakness, and confusion occurred initially and prompted overnight observation in a hospital. These effects had resolved by the following morning, and she was discharged, only to develop exertional dyspnea over the following 24 hours and severe precordial chest pain radiating to the left arm 3 days after ingestion. Electrocardiogram and creatine kinase elevations indicated possible myocardial infarction. Cardiac catheterization and chest x-ray were consistent with cardiomyopathy. Over several hours, the patient developed episodes of ventricular tachycardia and refractory hypotension and died in asystolic arrest. At autopsy, histology of the left ventricle revealed cardiomyopathy but no monocellular infiltrates to suggest an inflammatory etiology.[72] Chest pain for 6 months after survival of acute sodium azide poisoning has been reported in one patient who ingested 80 mg.[67]

Sodium azide levels in blood are not readily available, and diagnosis and treatment decisions must be based on clinical grounds. Postmortem blood concentrations have ranged from 7.4 to 8.3 mg/L in one acutely fatal suicidal case to between 40 and 262 mg/L in other reported cases.[64] Interestingly, cyanide has been detected in the postmortem blood in three sodium azide fatalities (0.38 mg/L, 1.6 mg/L, and 9 mg/L), but it is not clear whether the cyanide production took place in vivo or in the postmortem remains.[64]

Severe hypotension may be unresponsive to volume expansion and vasopressors.[61] Phenobarbital had a protective effect against sodium azide poisoning in mice and rats, whereas diazepam and phenytoin did not.[71] Phenobarbital should thus be considered for patients with seizures after sodium azide exposure not responsive to other anticonvulsants.

There is no specific antidote for sodium azide poisoning in current clinical use[61,72] and only symptomatic and supportive treatment can be given.[63] The U.S. cyanide antidote kit containing amyl nitrite, sodium nitrite, and sodium thiosulfate has not been efficacious in human poisoning cases or in animal experiments.[61,67,71,73]

Kelocyanor (dicobalt EDTA) and sodium thiosulfate alone have been ineffective for prevention of sodium azide poisoning in experimental animals.[71]

Hydroxocobalamin has not been administered to sodium azide–poisoned humans. An in vitro study in isolated rat mitochondria found that when hydroxocobalamin was added to sodium azide–inhibited mitochondria, cytochrome-c oxidase was less inhibited than when sodium azide was added alone.[74] This gives a potential theoretical mechanism of action for hydrocobalamin in the treatment of sodium azide poisoning, and further studies should be pursued. When it is available, hydroxocobalamin could be administered to patients with life-threatening sodium azide poisoning because of its highly favorable safety profile. It is notably efficacious for reversing the severe hypotension seen in acute cyanide poisoning, and severe hypotension unresponsive to usual treatments is a hallmark of sodium azide poisoning.

REFERENCES

1. Hall AH, Rumack BH: Clinical toxicology of cyanide. Ann Emerg Med 1986;15:1067.
2. Blanc P, Hogan M, Mallin K, et al: Cyanide intoxication among silver-reclaiming workers. JAMA 1985;253:367.
3. Hartung R: Cyanides and nitriles. In Clayton GD, Clayton FE (eds): Patty's Industrial Hygiene and Toxicology, Vol. 11, 4th ed. New York, John Wiley, 1994, p 3119.
4. Krieg A, Saxena K: Cyanide poisoning from metal cleaning solutions. Ann Emerg Med 1987;16:582.
5. Hathaway GJ, Proctor NH, Hughes JP: Hydrogen cyanide. In Proctor and Hughes' Chemical Hazards of the Workplace, 4th ed. New York, Van Nostrand Reinhold, 1996, p 346.
6. Hall AH, Rumack BH, Schaffer MI, Linden CH: Clinical toxicology of cyanide: North American clinical experiences. In Ballantyne B, Marrs TC (eds): Clinical and Experimental Toxicology of Cyanides. Bristol, UK, John Wright, 1987, p 312.
7. Anonymous: Cyanide poisoning associated with over-the-counter medication—Washington State. MMWR Morb Mortal Wkly Rep 1991;40:161.
8. Hart GB, Strauss MB, Lennon PA, Whitcraft DD: Treatment of smoke inhalation by hyperbaric oxygen. J Emerg Med 1985;3:211.
9. Baud FJ, Barriot P, Toffis V, et al: Elevated blood cyanide concentrations in victims of smoke inhalation. N Engl J Med 1991;325:1761.
10. Norris JC, Moore SJ, Hume AS: Synergistic lethality induced by the combination of carbon monoxide and cyanide. Toxicology 1986;40:121.
11. Mayes RW: The toxicological examination of the British Air Tours Boeing 737 accident at Manchester in 1985. J Forensic Sci 1991;36:179.
12. Barr SJ: Chemical warfare agents. Top Emerg Med 1985;7:62.
13. Bismuth C, Baud FJ, Djeghout H, et al: Cyanide poisoning from propionitrile exposure. J Emerg Med 1987;5:191.
14. Scolnik B, Hamel D, Woolf AD: Successful treatment of life-threatening propionitrile exposure with sodium nitrite/sodium thiosulfate followed by hyperbaric oxygen. J Occup Med 1993;35:577.
15. Yeh MM, Becker CE, Arieff AI: Is measurement of venous oxygen saturation useful in the diagnosis of cyanide poisoning? Am J Med 1992;93:582.
16. Yen D, Tsai J, Wang L-M, et al: The clinical experience of acute cyanide poisoning. Am J Emerg Med 1995;13:524.
17. Peden NR, Taha A, McSorley PD, et al: Industrial exposure to hydrogen cyanide: implications for treatment. BMJ 1986;293:538.
18. Suchard JR, Wallace WL, Gerkin RD: Acute cyanide poisoning caused by apricot kernel ingestion. Ann Emerg Med 1998;32:724.
19. Kurt TH, Day LC, Reed WG: Cyanide poisoning from glue-on nail remover. Am J Emerg Med 1991;9:201.

20. Michaelis HC, Clemens C, Kijewski H, et al: Acetonitrile concentrations and cyanide levels in a case of suicidal oral acetonitrile ingestion. J Toxicol Clin Toxicol 1991;29:447.

21. Schulz V, Gross R, Pasch T, et al: Cyanide toxicity of sodium nitroprusside in therapeutic use with and without sodium thiosulfate. Klin Wochenschr 1982;60:1393.

22. Linakis JG, Lacouture PG, Woolf A: Monitoring cyanide and thiocyanate concentrations during infusion of sodium nitroprusside in children. Pediatr Cardiol 1991;12:214.

23. Vesey CJ, Cole PV, Linnell JC, Wilson J: Some metabolic effects of sodium nitroprusside in man. BMJ 1974;2:140.

24. Cottrell JE, Casthely P, Brodie JD, et al: Prevention of nitroprusside-induced cyanide toxicity with hydroxocobalamin. N Engl J Med 1978;298:809.

25. Vesey CJ, Cole PV: Blood cyanide and thiocyanate concentrations produced by long-term therapy with sodium nitroprusside. Br J Anaesthiol 1985;57:148.

26. Osuntokun BO: Chronic cyanide intoxication of dietary origin and a degenerative neuropathy in Nigerians. Acta Hortic 1994;375:311.

27. Tylleskar T, Howlett WP, Rwiza HT, et al: Konzo: a distinct disease entity with selective upper motor neuron damage. J Neurol Neurosurg Psychiatr 1993;56:638.

28. Ngudi DD, Kuo YH, Lambein F: Cassava cyanogens and free amino acids in raw and cooked cassava leaves. Food Chem Toxicol 2003;41:1193.

29. Espinoza OB, Perez M, Ramirez MS: Bitter cassava poisoning in eight children: a case report. Vet Hum Toxicol 1992;34:65.

30. Delange F, Ekpechi LO, Rosling H: Cassava cyanogenesis and iodine deficiency disorders. Acta Hortic 1994;375:289.

31. Litovitz TL, Klein-Schwartz W, Rodgers GC, et al: 2001 annual Report of the American Association of Poison Control Centers Toxic Exposure Surveillance System. Am J Emerg Med 2002;20:391.

32. Shou Y, Gunasekar PG, Borowitz JL, et al: Cyanide-induced apoptosis involves oxidative-stress-activated NF-kappaB in cortical neurons. Toxicol Appl Pharmacol 2000;164:196.

33. Bi QN, Sun PW, Gunasekar PG, Isom GE: Involvement of CA^{2+}/calmodulin-dependent protein kinase II in cyanide-induced cytotoxicity in cultured cerebellar granular cells [abstract]. Toxicologist 1996;30:186.

34. Shou Y, Li L, Prabhakaran K, et al: p38 Mitogen activated protein kinase regulates BAX translocation in cyanide-induced apoptosis. Toxicol Sci 2003;75:99.

35. Christel D, Eyer P, Hegemann M, et al: Pharmacokinetics of cyanide poisoning in dogs, and the effects of 4-dimethylaminophenol or thiosulfate. Arch Toxicol 1977;38:177.

36. Sylvester DM, Hayton WL, Morgan RL, Way JL: Effects of thiosulfate on cyanide pharmacokinetics in dogs. Toxicol Appl Pharmacol 1983;69:265.

37. Hall AH, Doutre WH, Ludden T, et al: Nitrite/thiosulfate treated acute cyanide poisoning: estimated kinetics after antidote. Clin Toxicol 1987;25:121.

38. Graham DL, Laman D, Theodore J, Robin ED: Acute cyanide poisoning complicated by lactic acidosis and pulmonary edema. Arch Intern Med 1977;137:1051.

39. Feihl F, Domenighetti G, Perret C: Intoxication massive au cyanure avec evolution favorable. Schweiz Med Wschr 1982;112:1280.

40. Jouglard J, Fagot G, Deguigne B, Arlaud J-A: L'intoxication cyanhydrique aigue et son traitement d'urgence. Mars Med 1971;9:571.

41. Rosenberg NL, Myes JA, Martin MRW: Cyanide-induced parkinsonism: clinical, MRI, and 6-fluorodopa PET studies. Neurology 1989;39:142.

42. Feldman JM, Feldman MD: Sequelae of attempted suicide by cyanide ingestion: a case report. Int J Psychiatr Med 1990;20:173.

43. Steffens W, Leng G, Bayer KB: Nitrile poisonings: cyanide formation, clinical course and treatment [abstract]. J Toxicol Clin Toxicol 2003;41:410.

44. Steffens W, Leng G, Pelster M: Percutaneous hydrocyanic acid poisoning [abstract]. J Toxicol Clin Toxicol 2003;41:483.

45. Goodhart GL: Patient treated with antidote kit and hyperbaric oxygen survives cyanide poisoning. South Med J 1994;87:814.

46. Megarbane B, Delahaye A, Goldgran-Toledano D, et al: Antidotal treatment of cyanide poisoning. J Chin Med Assoc 2003;66:193.

47. Baud FJ, Borron SW, Megarbane B, et al: Value of lactic acidosis in the assessment of the severity of acute cyanide poisoning. Crit Care Med 2002;30:2044.

48. Shusterman D, Alexeef G, Hargis C, et al: Predictors of carbon monoxide and hydrogen cyanide exposure in smoke inhalation patients. Clin Toxicol 1996;34:61.

49. Hall AH, Rumack BH: Hydrogen sulfide poisoning: an antidotal role for sodium nitrite? Vet Human Toxicol 1997;39:152.

50. Wurzburg H: Treatment of cyanide poisoning in an industrial setting. Vet Hum Toxicol 1996;38:44.

51. Heintz B, Bock TA, Kierdorf H, Sieberth HG: Cyanid Intoxikation: Behandlung mit Hyperoxigenation und Natriumthiosulfat. Dtsch Med Wochenschr 1990;115:1100.

52. Kirk MA, Gerace R, Kulig KW: Cyanide and methemoglobin kinetics in smoke inhalation victims treated with the cyanide antidote kit. Ann Emerg Med 1993;22:9.

53. Megarbane B, Baud F: Cyanide poisoning: diagnosis and antidote choice in an emergency situation [abstract]. J Toxicol Clin Toxicol 2003;41:438.

54. Santiago I: [Gas poisoning]. An Sist Sanit Navar 2003;26(Suppl 1):173.

55. Suchard JR, Wallace KL, Gerkin RD: Acute cyanide toxicity caused by apricot kernal ingestion. Ann Emerg Med 1998;32:724.

56. Forsyth JC, Mueller PD, Becker CE, et al: Hydroxocobalamin as a cyanide antidote: safety, efficacy and pharmacokinetics in heavily smoking normal volunteers. J Toxicol Clin Toxicol 1993;31:277.

57. Hall AH, Rumack BH: Hydroxycobalamin as a cyanide antidote. J Emerg Med 1987;5:115.

58. Curry SC, Connor DA, Rashke RA: Effect of the cyanide antidote hydroxocobalamin on commonly ordered serum chemistry studies. Ann Emerg Med 1994;24:65.

59. Swanson-Bierman B, Krenzelok EP, Snyder JW, et al: Successful donation and transplantation of multiple organs from a victim of cyanide poisoning. Clin Toxicol 1993;31:95.

60. Hantson P, Mahieu P, Hassoun A, Otte J-B: Outcome following organ removal from poisoned donors in brain death status: a report of 12 cases and review of the literature. Clin Toxicol 1995;33:709.

61. Chang S, Lamm SH: Human health effects of sodium azide exposure: a literature review and analysis. Int J Toxicol 2003;22:175.

62. Singh N, Singh CP, Brar CK: Sodium azide: a rare poisoning. J Assoc Physicians India 1994;42:755.

63. Wollenek G: Akute vergiftungen durch natriumazid. Wein Klin Wochenschr 1989;101:314.

64. Marquet P, Clément S, Lotfi H, et al: Analytical findings in a suicide involving sodium azide. J Anal Toxicol 1996;20:134.

65. Herbold M, Schmitt G, Aderjan R, Pedal I: Tödliche natriumazidvergiftung im krankenhaus: eine vermeidbarer zwischenfall. Arch Kriminol 1995;196:143.

66. Arduino MJ: CDC investigations of noninfectious outbreaks of adverse events in hemodialysis facilities, 1979–1999. Semin Dial 2000;13:86.

67. Chiba M, Ohmichi M, Inaba Y: [Sodium azide: a review of biological effects ad case reports] [Japanese]. Nippon Eiseigaku Zasshi 1999;53:572.

68. Senda T, Nishio K, Hori Y, et al: [A fatal case of fatal acute sodium azide poisoning] [Japanese]. Chudoku Kenkyu 2001;14:339.

69. Bennett MC, Mlady GW, Kwon Y-H, Rose GM: Chronic in vivo sodium azide infusion induces selective and stable inhibition of cytochrome c oxidase. J Neurochem 1996;66:2606.

70. Bennett CM, Mlady GW, Fleshner M, Rose GM: Synergy between chronic corticosterone and sodium azide treatments in producing a spatial learning deficit and inhibiting cytochrome oxidase activity. Proc Natl Acad Sci U S A 1996;93:1330.

71. Smith RP, Louis CA, Kruszyna R, Kruszyna H: Acute neurotoxicity of sodium azide and nitric oxide. Fundam Appl Toxicol 1991;17:120.

72. Judge KW, Ward NE: Fatal azide-induced cardiomyopathy presenting as acute myocardial infarction. Am J Cardiol 1989;64:830.

73. Klein-Schwartz W, Gorman RL, Oderda G, et al: Three fatal sodium azide poisonings. Med Toxicol Adverse Drug Exp 1989;4:219.

74. Vieira Lopes LC, Campello AP: Effect of hydroxocobalamin on the inhibition of cytochrome c oxidase by cyanide. I. In intact mitochondria. Res Comm Chem Pathol Pharmacol 1975;12:521.

89

Isocyanates and Related Compounds

JASON VENA, MD ■ CHARLES MCKAY, MD

At a Glance...

■ The isocyanates are widely used precursors to polyurethane products, as well as carbamate insecticides.

■ Methyl isocyanate was released at the worst industrial disaster in history on December 2 and 3, 1984, at Bhopal, India.

■ Isocyanates are chemical compounds consisting of R–N=C=O groups, which react with compounds containing reactive hydrogen atoms to form polymers.

■ Toxicity of the isocyanates varies inversely with molecular weight, related to volatility and vapor pressure.

■ The most common occupational illness associated with the isocyanates is diisocyanate asthma, which has a distinct mechanism of toxicity as compared with atopic asthma.

■ Management of isocyanate exposure is supportive; asthmatic symptoms should be managed as for atopic asthma.

The isocyanates are a diverse group of molecules that contain one or more R–N=C=O moieties, used most commonly in the synthesis of polyurethane plastics, foams, paints, and coatings, as well as in the production and degradation of carbamate insecticides. Regarding the latter, the isocyanates are known for the worst industrial disaster in history, in which thousands died in Bhopal, India in 1984 (discussed later).

Demand for polyurethanes, and thus their isocyanate precursors, is strong. Worldwide production of polyurethanes had been estimated at 2.2 to 3.4 million tons (2 to 3 million tonnes) in 2001; an automobile may contain 110 pounds (50 kg) of polyurethane and a residence 440 to 660 pounds (200–300 kg).[1]

Because of their commercial ubiquity, clinically relevant toxicity, and historical infamy, the isocyanates merit awareness by the medical toxicologist. This chapter discusses four isocyanates of commercial importance: methyl isocyanate (MIC), methylene diphenyl diisocyanate (MDI), toluene-2,4 and 2,6 diisocyanate (TDI, or 2,4-TDI or 2,6-TDI), and hexamethylene diisocyanate (HDI).

PHYSICOCHEMICAL PROPERTIES

MIC (CAS 624-83-9) is most commonly associated with production and degradation of carbamate insecticides. At ambient conditions, it is a colorless liquid with a pungent odor and a high vapor pressure (348 mm Hg). Its odor threshold of 2.1 parts per million (ppm) is two orders of magnitude greater than its recommended exposure limits (see "Regulations"). Water solubility is 10% at 59° F (15° C). MIC reacts violently with water in an exothermic reaction producing polymeric MIC gas (perhaps creating trimers of MIC under the conditions

seen at Bhopal[2]). Flammability is high, with a flash point of 19° F (−7° C). Pyrolysis results in decomposition to hydrogen cyanide and carbon dioxide. Environmental degradation of MIC is prolonged in air, with an atmospheric half-life estimated at 3 months; water degradation is shorter, at a half-life of about 2 days.[3]

MDI (CAS101-68-8), TDI (CAS 584-84-9 and 91-08-7), and HDI (CAS 822-06-0) are known as diisocyanates, that is, molecules containing two isocyanate moieties. Their use is predominantly in the formation of polymers, namely polyurethane plastics and foams, by means of reaction with alcohols (polyols). At ambient conditions, MDI and 2,4-TDI are white-yellow solids, whereas 2,6-TDI and HDI are clear to pale yellow liquids. The vapor pressures of the diisocyanates (0.000005–0.5 mm Hg) are low. Water solubilities are low to insoluble. Flammabilities are low, with flash points above 200° F (93° C). The diisocyanates are less reactive with water than MIC, and under conditions of controlled water addition, they have the desirable effect of producing foams.[4] In addition, the less toxic MDI has replaced TDI in many settings. Environmental degradation is more rapid than with MIC, with the diisocyanates having atmospheric half-lives of hours to 2 days, as well as "rapid" water degradation.[3] Table 89-1 provides a comparison of these agents.

SOURCES OF EXPOSURE

MIC is both a crop pesticide reagent and an ingredient, as well as a degradation product of the pesticide metam-sodium. Air concentrations of MIC were found to be up to 2.5 ppb in the 72 hours following ground injection of metam-sodium for field fumigation in California.[3] Cigarettes may contain four micrograms of MIC each, and workers who are in an environment at the threshold value for an 8-hour workday may be exposed to 460 μg daily.[3] On the night of December 2 and 3, 1984, the introduction of water into two MIC storage tanks at the Union Carbide plant in Bhopal (capital of Madhya Pradesh, India, population 900,000) overwhelmed multiple safety systems and released about 27 tons of MIC into the environment within 1 to 2 hours, resulting in a mean estimated air concentration 1350 times the U.S. Occupational Safety and Health Administration (OSHA) limit (see "Regulations").

The diisocyanates (MDI, TDI, HDI) are used in countless global industries, including adhesives, painting and varnishing, wire coating, vehicle building, mining, upholstery, plastics, rubber, insulation, and textiles.[4] The major group of workers potentially exposed are those in the foam and rubber industry, who use the isocyanate monomers during manufacturing.

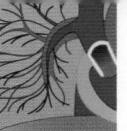

TABLE 89-1 Comparison of Common Isocyantes

COMPOUND	STRUCTURE	MOL. WT. (g/mol)	VAPOR PRESSURE (mm Hg) AT 77° F/25° C	ODOR THRESHOLD (ppm)	CONVERSION (ppm TO mg/m³)*
Methyl isocyanate	CH₃N=C=O	57.05	348	2.1	1 ppm = 2.3 mg/m³
Hexamethylene diisocyanate	OCN(C₆H₁₂)NCO	168.22	0.03	0.001	1 ppm = 6.9 mg/m³
Toluene diisocyanate (shown as 2,4-TDI)	NCO / H₃C—⬡—NCO	174.15	0.05	0.17	1 ppm = 7.12 mg/m³
Methylene diphenyl diisocyanate	[OCN(C₆H₆)]₂-CH₂	250.25	5×10^{-6}	0.4	1 ppm = 10.2 mg/m³

*mg/m³ = ppm × mol. wt./24.45, under conditions of 1 atmosphere and 25° C.

TOXICITY

Mechanisms of isocyanate toxicity are incompletely understood. Much of the literature regarding the cellular and molecular toxicity of MIC followed from the acute, high-dose exposure in Bhopal. Most of the literature available concerning the diisocyanates focuses on the occupational asthma phenomenon (see "Clinical Manifestations"), a predominantly chronic, low-dose exposure.

MIC toxicity, despite the horrible disaster of 1984, remains enigmatic for several reasons. Although the Bhopal incident released mostly MIC (probably in trimerized form), it is likely that decomposition products such as hydrogen cyanide, nitrogen oxides, carbon monoxide, and other molecules (including reagents, etc.) played a role in the toxicity experienced by the Bhopal victims.[5] Descriptions of "relief of symptoms" when sodium thiosulfate was administered to 30 Bhopal victims 2 months after the event prompted Indian authorities to recommend widespread thiosulfate treatment, although ultimately this was not carried out. Details of the reported response to delayed thiosulfate administration in these 30 victims are not known, and conclusions about efficacy cannot be drawn.

A two-part study conducted on rats by Jeevaratnam and Sriramachari[6,7] examined the histopathologic manifestations of pulmonary MIC toxicity both by inhalational (232, 465, and 930 ppm) and subcutaneous (164.3, 328.6, and 657.2 mg/kg) routes. In the acute phase, concentration- and dose-dependent necrotizing bronchitis and pulmonary edema were seen by inhalation, whereas subcutaneous administration resulted in vascular endothelial damage and pulmonary edema, apparently leaving normal bronchial epithelium.[6] The subacute and chronic phase (10 weeks) demonstrates a convergence of the inhalational and subcutaneous group tissue findings, both manifesting a diffuse interstitial pulmonary fibrosis.[6]

A burst of research activity in the immediate post-Bhopal era regarding the systemic toxicity of MIC appears to have been short-lived, but quite interesting. Jeevaratnam and Sriramachari[8] examined the non-pulmonary viscera of rats exposed to both inhalational and subcutaneous MIC and found vascular congestion, focal hepatocellular necrosis, and tubular rupture and degeneration in the kidney. Other authors have investigated in animal and in vitro models the inhibition of cardiac Na⁺/K⁺-ATPase in rabbits,[9] binding to erythrocyte membrane sulfhydryl groups in rats,[10] and changes in free amino acids in the brain and plasma of mice.[11] These data are not directly applicable to occupational exposures of much lower concentrations, particularly given the propensity of isocyanates to react with surface water and proteins, decreasing their absorption.

Issues of carcinogenicity and reproductive effects of MIC are unclear. The Agency for Toxic Substances and Disease Registry (ATSDR) of the Centers for Disease Control and Prevention (CDC) reports that MIC is not classified in terms of carcinogenicity, nor for reproductive effects, but makes mention of some of the observations at Bhopal, which included an apparent increase in stillbirths and spontaneous abortions.[12] Dhara and Dhara[2] cited a few epidemiologic, animal, and cytogenetic studies from the Bhopal experience that yielded no definitive conclusions for humans but do suggest the need for further observation.

The mechanisms of diisocyanate toxicity (see "Clinical Manifestations") are likewise incompletely understood. Asthma induced by the diisocyanates differs mechanistically, yet less so clinically, from atopic asthma. This form of occupational asthma is of great concern because sensitization to subsequent lower exposure levels has been demonstrated. Diisocyanate asthma, in contrast to atopic asthma, appears to lack a consistent immunoglobulin E (IgE)–associated mechanism. The prevalence of diisocyanate-specific IgE in symptomatic patients has been reported to be less than 20%; furthermore, these antibodies have been found in asymptomatic patients, indicating a weak association with the disease state.[4,13] Regarding the airway inflammatory

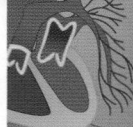

response, it appears that diisocyanate-induced asthma results in an increased neutrophil influx with increased interleukin-8 (IL-8) production, as compared with atopic asthma, which demonstrates relatively more eosinophils.[13] The cellular immune response differs as well. Diisocyanate-induced asthma seems to invoke more of a helper T-cell subset 1 (T$_H$1) response (with a subsequent neutrophil, IL-8, and interferon-γ [IFN-γ] response), as compared with atopic asthma, which has a predominantly T$_H$2-mediated response.[14] Transmigration of these inflammatory and immune cells across endothelial and epithelial basement membranes is, in part, mediated by enzymes known as matrix metalloproteinases (MMPs). In a recent murine model by Lee and colleagues,[15] in which bronchioalveolar lavage (BAL) fluid is examined after nebulized TDI exposure, MMP inhibitors are shown to blunt the migration of leukocytes and decrease the expression of adhesion molecules, interleukins, and tumor necrosis factor-α that are initiated after TDI exposure. Extrapulmonary sensitization (e.g., skin sensitization resulting in pulmonary effects) may also play a role in diisocyanate-induced asthma. As for immune recognition, the diisocyanates appear to haptenize with native protein in order to initiate a cellular response; in most models, albumin has been the carrier protein used. Wisnewski and coworkers[16] examined HDI-exposed volunteers, through inhalational (20–30 parts per billion [ppb]) and skin (0.1% v/v) routes, and found that keratin 18 and keratin 10, both type I (acidic) keratins of the respiratory epithelium and skin, respectively, were conjugated to HDI and might play a role in antigen presentation. Genetics also appear to play a role; allelic variations of glutathione S-transferase appear to alter susceptibility to isocyanate hypersensitivity.[17]

Carcinogenesis and reproductive issues regarding the diisocyanates are also being investigated, but current knowledge regarding these in humans is limited. Bolognesi and colleagues[18] provide a review of the evidence regarding TDI and MDI carcinogenesis and conclude that, although some short-term animal studies have shown gene mutations and chromosomal damage, the few epidemiologic studies produced have not been able to demonstrate that TDI and MDI are occupational carcinogens. As with MIC, the potential role of metabolic intermediates and adducts is undergoing continued study.

CLINICAL MANIFESTATIONS

The toxicity of the isocyanates will vary by the specific substance (e.g., MIC versus TDI), dose, route, and chronicity of the exposure. In humans, the predominant effects of the isocyanates are mucosal and respiratory, both upper and lower, consistent with an intermediate water solubility (see Chapter 9), and in some cases, dermal. A distinction should be made between the chronic effects of an acute exposure and the chronic effects of a chronic exposure, as provided by the examples of Bhopal and diisocyanate asthma, respectively (discussed subsequently).

Acute Exposure

Despite the confounders and limitations described, the largest acute human MIC exposure was the Bhopal incident. More than 200,000 people were exposed to MIC at this tragic event.[19] The immediate (1 week) death toll has been estimated at 2500, thought to be due predominantly to acute pulmonary edema.[20] Early autopsy results revealed severe necrotizing lesions of the upper and lower respiratory tract as well as pulmonary edema. In survivors, respiratory symptoms were described as rhinorrhea, throat irritation, cough with frothy expectoration, and dyspnea. Chest films obtained 2.5 to 3 months after exposure in 903 subjects revealed only 65 that were thought to be associated with acute gas exposure,[2] although the immediate radiographic appearance in these patients is unknown. Ocular toxicity in the acute phase included symptoms of severe burning and photophobia associated with chemosis and corneal ulceration; only a few cases of iritis were seen, and blindness was not known to have occurred.[2]

Chronic effects of acute exposure to MIC resulted (and continue to result by some accounts) in much morbidity and mortality. The death toll is recently said to be greater than 6000, and the number of victims with chronic health effects greater than 50,000.[5] Later pulmonary deaths may have been related to secondary infections,[20] as well as interstitial fibrosis and other structural changes,[2] consistent with findings from an animal model[7] (see "Toxicity"). Beckett[21] stratified 454 adults by distance from the incident site and found forced midexpiratory flow rate (FEF$_{25-75}$) reductions that correlate with distance from the incident, concluding that small airways obstruction may be attributed to gas exposure. Chronic ocular issues may include chronic conjunctivitis and corneal opacities.[22] Chronic neurologic effects are reported, but these are not well defined, and associations may be stronger with a mass casualty event than with the chemical itself.[2] Reproductive and pediatric effects of MIC are discussed later.

Acute diisocyanate toxicity is predominantly pulmonary and may be subdivided into four entities: chemical bronchitis, hypersensitivity pneumonitis, asthma, and acute nonspecific airways disease.[4] Chemical bronchitis is typically associated with an acute, higher-level exposure, resulting in marked upper respiratory and ocular irritation symptoms as well as cough, chest pain, and tightness; transitory or permanent changes in pulmonary function tests may be seen.[4] High-level exposures would be expected to produce symptoms as seen with MIC, including pulmonary edema and death. Hypersensitivity pneumonitis is a rare presentation; in one series by Baur,[23] 16 patients were diagnosed clinically from 1780 isocyanate workers based on their symptoms of repeated episodes of fever, dyspnea, and malaise after a latency period of several hours after isocyanate exposure. Of those selected, 14 agreed to participate in the study, yielding the confirmatory findings of decreased diffusion capacity (10 patients), reticulonodular pattern on chest film (9 patients), and the presence of serum IgG to TDI-albumin (10 patients). Five patients underwent lung biopsy, revealing lymphohistiocytic infiltrates in all.

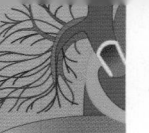

Diisocyanate asthma is the most common manifestation of diisocyanate-associated pulmonary disease,
with the initial description in 1951 by Fuchs and Valade.[4]
Asthma associated with the diisocyanates may be subdivided into immediate, late-onset, and dual-onset forms.
An interesting case series by Zammit-Tabona and
colleagues[24] provides insight into these presentations. In
their series, 11 foundry workers with exposure to MDI
and symptoms consistent with asthma were subjected to
a single inhalational MDI challenge at a concentration
less than 0.02 ppm for 60 minutes. Seven patients, two of
whom were atopic, developed asthmatic reactions as
measured by spirometry (>20% fall in forced expiratory
volume in 1 second [FEV$_1$]). One patient was discounted
owing to response to formaldehyde challenge. The
remaining six had late-onset reactions, with onset an
average of 5 hours after the exposure; two of these
patients also had immediate-onset reactions (before the
end of the challenge). Four of the six patients also
developed recurrent nocturnal asthmatic symptoms,
away from any known exposure, for a period of 3 to 7
days after the single-dose challenge.

Chronic Exposure

Chronic MIC exposure and resulting effects are not well
defined in the literature. In regard to chronic
pulmonary diisocyanate exposure, the clinical effects
may be divided into isocyanate-associated asthma and
chronic nonspecific airways disease.[4] Diisocyanate
asthma may be diagnosed after several years of potential
exposure; whether this phenomenon is due to the
chronicity of the exposure and disease latency or to a
delay in diagnosis[25] is unknown. Diisocyanate asthma
may develop within months after exposure[4]; however,
newer employees may have had exposures during
previous jobs, confounding the time course.[26] Loss of
sensitization after removal from exposure is a possibility
in diisocyanate asthma. Mapp and colleagues[27] found
that in a group of TDI-sensitized patients, provocation
after increasing intervals of time following TDI exposure
indicates a reversible increase in airway responsiveness.
In a recent 30-year follow-up of workers at a single TDI
factory unit, Ott and colleagues[26] reported an initial
decline in FEV$_1$ within the first 2 years of reporting
symptoms, but no acceleration of decline in lung
function thereafter. These two studies seem to be in
contrast to the findings of Padoan and associates,[28] in
which 87 subjects with TDI-induced asthma were
followed for 11 years. In this group, airway reactivity to
methacholine challenge persisted even after 10 years of
nonexposure, and the presenting FEV$_1$ and provocative
dose were among the factors predictive of subsequent
reactivity and decline in pulmonary function. All these
considerations highlight the importance of early
recognition of respiratory symptoms and removal of
employees from further isocyanate exposure.

Case reports exist for diisocyanate-associated skin
lesions in chronically exposed workers. Larsen and
colleagues[29] reported on 10 nurses in an outpatient
orthopedic clinic who worked with diisocyanate-

containing casting material. Patch testing to five types of
diisocyanates yielded one patient with a "doubtful"
reaction toward two types. Their conclusion that the
diisocyanates are predominantly irritants rather than
sensitizers stands in contrast to other animal studies and
case reports identifying positive patch testing or IgE
antibodies to isocyanates after dermal exposure.

Any potential carcinogenic risk after chronic diisocyanate exposure in humans is only theoretical at this
time and is based on very heavy (e.g., 6 mg/m^3) chronic
inhalation exposures in animal models.[18,30]

PRENATAL AND PEDIATRIC ISSUES

The reproductive effects of the isocyanates in humans
are largely undefined, but some evidence for adverse
effects exists at massive exposure doses. In the case of the
Bhopal disaster, Dhara and Dhara[2] reported on a study
indicating that a higher rate of miscarriages occurred in
the affected area, as well as higher perinatal and
neonatal mortality rates. In a recent letter,[19] Ranjan and
associates discussed their findings of a selective growth
retardation in boys exposed in utero or as young
children to the Bhopal disaster versus matched controls.
Reproductive toxicity data regarding the diisocyanates
are also limited, but reassuring. One study found a no
observed adverse effect level (NOAEL) of about 0.3 ppm
MDI in pregnant Wistar rats with regard to maternal and
developmental toxicity.[31] Other studies showed NOAELs
in the range of 0.1 to 0.3 ppm TDI in CD rats in regard
to reproductive toxicity.[32,33]

ASSESSMENT

Diagnosis of isocyanate-associated disease is best defined
in the occupational setting, particularly for diisocyanate-
induced asthma. Important historical components
include a suspected exposure and symptoms of airway
hyperreactivity, including cough, wheezing, and shortness
of breath; these may be delayed by several hours after
each exposure and therefore may present as nocturnal
asthma in day-shift workers. Fever and respiratory symptoms in exposed workers would suggest hypersensitivity
pneumonitis. A full medical, occupational, and social
history should be elicited, including personal and family
history of pulmonary disease, potential sources of previous
isocyanate exposure (and perhaps sensitization), and
smoking status.

Pulmonary function testing begins with sequential
peak expiratory flow measurements both during and
away from a potential exposure. Inhalational challenge
testing may be indicated and is divided into nonspecific
bronchial hyperresponsiveness (NSBH) and specific
bronchoprovocation testing (SBPT).[34] NSBH is performed
by challenging the patient with a known airway reactant
such as methacholine or histamine, whereas SBPT involves
the use of the suspect diisocyanate itself. Generally, a 20%
decrease in FEV$_1$ during either test supports a diagnosis
of reactive airways[4,28]; however, the SBPT is considered

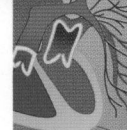

the gold standard.[34] Nonspecific testing is often performed in lieu of SBPT because of the lack of availability of such tests at many centers. Many organizations have published guidelines on the diagnosis of occupational asthma, including that of the diisocyanates, and are included in a review by Bernstein and Jolly.[34]

Laboratory evaluation for diisocyanate-associated asthma is not well-defined, although currently an area of research interest (see "Toxicity"). Other ancillary tests that may be useful include chest radiography, bronchoalveolar lavage, and biopsy, particularly in cases of suspected hypersensitivity pneumonitis.[23]

MANAGEMENT

Treatment of isocyanate-associated disease, regardless of the specific moiety or the acuity, requires removal of the patient from the source of exposure, followed by surface decontamination as needed (see Chapter 2). Management of the patient's airway and breathing takes precedence over further care. Co-inhalations should always be suspected, especially in the setting of fire (e.g., carbon monoxide, cyanide gas). Management in the disaster setting is addressed in Chapter 103. In cases of diisocyanate-associated asthma, acute treatment should follow that of standard principles for the atopic asthmatic. Removal of the worker from any further isocyanate exposure is required because the safe concentration for reexposure of sensitized individuals has not been defined.

PREVENTION

It is uncertain at what levels and duration of exposure diisocyanate-associated pulmonary disease develops.[4] Although there are mandated exposure guidelines (see "Regulations"), some authors believe these to be too lenient. Baur[35] advises that although occupational exposure limits for the various diisocyanates in most Western countries are placed at about 10 ppb, a more appropriate "health-based" level based on current research would be 2.5 to 5 ppb.

Environmental monitoring is an important component of exposure prevention. There are several methods for detecting the presence of isocyanates, including colorimetry (wet and dry) and chromatography (thin layer, gas, and high-performance liquid).[4] Each regulatory or advisory body, as discussed next, adopts an explicit method for standardizing detection of the environmental burden.

REGULATIONS AND EXPOSURE ADVISORIES

In the United States, multiple agencies, both governmental and private, dispense recommended worker exposure limits in multiple formats. In general, it is helpful to categorize these into "regulatory" (enforceable) and

TABLE 89-2 Regulatory and Advisory Limits for Representative Isocyanates

	OSHA PEL (ppb)	NIOSH REL (ppb)	NIOSH IDLH (ppb)	ACGIH TLV (ppb)	AIHA ERPG (ppb)
MIC	20 (TWA)	20 (TWA)	3000	20	25–5000
MDI	20 (C)	5 (C)	7500	5	N/A
TDI	20 (C)	None	2500	5	N/A
HDI	None	5 (TWA)	N/A	N/A	N/A

ACGIH, American Conference of Government and Industrial Hygienists; AIHA, American Industrial Hygiene Association; C, ceiling limit; ERPG, emergency response planning guidelines; HDI, hexamethylene diisocyanate; IDLH, immediate danger to life or health; MDI, methylene diphenyl diisocyanate; MIC, methyl isocyanate; N/A, not available; NIOSH, National Institute of Occupational Safety and Health; OSHA, Occupational Safety and Health Association; PEL, permissible exposure limit; ppb, parts per billion; REL, recommended exposure limit; TDI, toluene-2,4 and 2,6 diisocyanate; TLV, threshold limit value; TWA, threshold weighted average.

"advisory" types. OSHA provides regulatory values. The National Institute of Occupational Safety and Health (NIOSH), also a federal program, provides advisory limits. Private programs such as the American Conference of Government and Industrial Hygienists (ACGIH) and the American Industrial Hygiene Association (AIHA) also provide advisory limits. The AIHA guidelines are for emergency exposures only. These are summarized in Table 89-2 for MIC, MDI, TDI, and HDI.[36,37]

There are also regulations at the state level, superseded at all times by federal regulation. Other nations have their own regulations. Refer to Chapter 82 for definitions and further details on regulatory agencies and promulgations.

REFERENCES

1. Bakke JV (ed): Isocyanates: Risk assessment and preventive measures. Meeting of the Nordic Supervisory Authorities in Copenhagen, April 27, 2000. Norwegian Labor Inspection Authority. Available at: http://www.arbeidstilsynet.no.
2. Dhara VR, Dhara R: The Union Carbide disaster in Bhopal: A review of health effects. Arch Environ Health 2002;57(5):391–404.
3. Ontario Ministry of the Environment, Standards Development Branch. Information Draft on the Development of Air Standards, December 2002. Available at: http://www.ene.gov.on.ca.
4. Sullivan JB, Krieger GR: Clinical Environmental Health and Exposures, 2nd ed. Philadelphia, Lippincott Williams & Wilkins, 2001, pp 994–998.
5. Dhara VR, Gassert TH: The Bhopal syndrome: persistent questions about acute toxicity and management of gas victims. Int J Occup Environ Health 2002;8:380–386.
6. Jeevaratnam K, Sriramachari S: Comparative toxicity of methyl isocyanate and its hydrolytic derivatives in rats. I. Pulmonary histopathology in the acute phase. Arch Toxicol 1994;69(1):39–44.
7. Sriramachari S, Jeevaratnam K: Comparative toxicity of methyl isocyanate and its hydrolytic derivatives in rats. II. Pulmonary histopathology in the subacute and chronic phases. Arch Toxicol 1994;69(1):45–51.
8. Jeevaratnam K, Sriramachari S: Acute histopathological changes induced by methyl isocyanate in lungs, liver, kidneys and spleen of rats [abstract]. Indian J Med Res 1994;99:231–235.
9. Jeevaratnam K: Effect of methyl isocyanate on rabbit cardiac Na+, K+ ATPase. Arch Toxicol 1995;69(10):694–697.
10. Bhattacharya BK, Sharma SK, Jaiswal DK: Binding of [1-14C] methyl isocyanate to erythrocyte membrane proteins. J Appl Toxicol 1996;16(2):137–138.

11. Gupta M, Prabha V: Changes in brain and plasma amino acids of mice intoxicated with methyl isocyanate. J Appl Toxicol 1996; 16(6):469–473.

12. Retrieved February 13, 2004, from http://www.atsdr.cdc.gov/MHMI/mmg182.html.

13. Liu Q, Wisnewski AV: Recent developments in diisocyanate asthma. Ann Allergy Asthma Immunol 2003;90(Suppl):35–41.

14. Wisnewski A, Herrick CA, Liu Q, et al: Human γ/δ T-cell proliferation and IFN-γ production induced by hexamethylene diisocyanate. J Allergy Clin Immunol 2003;112:538–546.

15. Lee KS, Jin SM, Kim HJ, Lee YC: Matrix metalloproteinase inhibitor regulates inflammatory cell migration by reducing ICAM-1 and VCAM-1 expression in a murine model of toluene diisocyanate-induced asthma. J Allergy Clin Immunol 2003;111(6):1278–1284.

16. Wisnewski AV, Srivastava R, Herrick C, et al: Identification of human lung and skin proteins conjugated with hexamethylene diisocyanate in vitro and in vivo. Am J Respir Crit Care Med 2000;162:2330–2336.

17. Frew AJ: Advances in environmental and occupational disorders. J Allergy Clin Immunol 2003;111:S824–S828.

18. Bolognesi C, Baur X, Marczynski B, et al: Carcinogenic risk of toluene diisocyanate and 4,4′-methylenediphenyl diisocyanate: epidemiological and experimental evidence. Crit Rev Toxicol 2001;31(6):737–772.

19. Ranjan N, Saranji S, Padmanabhan V, et al: Methyl isocyanate exposure and growth patterns of adolescents in Bhopal [letter]. JAMA 2003;290(14):1856–1857.

20. Environmental Protection Agency: Air toxics. Available at http://www.epa.gov. Updated May 30, 2003.

21. Beckett WS: Persistent respiratory effects in survivors of the Bhopal disaster. Thorax 1998;53(Suppl 2):S43–S46.

22. Raizada JK, Dwivedi PC: Chronic ocular lesions in Bhopal gas tragedy [abstract]. Indian J Ophthalmol 1987;35(5–6):453–454.

23. Baur X: Hypersensitivity pneumonitis (extrinsic allergic alveolitis) induced by isocyanates. J Allergy Clin Immunol 1995;95(5 Part 1): 1004–1010.

24. Zammit-Tabona M, Sherkin M, Kijek K, et al: Asthma caused by diphenylmethane diisocyanate in foundry workers. Clinical, bronchial provocation, and immunologic studies. Am Rev Respir Dis 1983;128:226–230.

25. Mapp CE, Boschetto P, Dal Vecchio L, et al: Occupational asthma due to isocyanates. Eur Respir J 1988;1(3):273–279.

26. Ott MG, Klees JE, Poche SL, et al: Respiratory health surveillance in a toluene di-isocyanate production unit, 1967–1997: clinical observations and lung function analyses. Occup Environ Med 2000;57(1):43–52.

27. Mapp CE, Polato R, Maestrelli P, et al: Time course of the increase in airway responsiveness associated with late asthmatic reactions to toluene diisocyanate in sensitized subjects. J Allergy Clin Immunol 1985;75(5):568–572.

28. Padoan M, Pozzato V, Simoni M, et al: Long-term follow-up of toluene diisocyanate-induced asthma. Eur Respir J 2003; 21:637–640.

29. Larsen TH, Gregersen P, Jemec GB: Skin irritation and exposure to diisocyanates in orthopedic nurses working with soft casts. Am J Contact Dermat 2001;12(4):211–214.

30. U.S. National Library of Medicine: Integrated risk information system (IRIS). Available at: http://toxnet.nlm.nih.gov. Updated on December 16, 2002.

31. Gamer AO, Hellwig J, Doe JE, Tyl RW: Prenatal toxicity of inhaled polymeric methylenediphenyl diisocyanate (MDI) aerosols in pregnant Wistar rats [abstract]. Toxicol Sci 2000;54(2):431–440.

32. Tyl RW, Neeper-Bradley TL, Fisher LC, et al: Two-generation reproductive toxicity study of inhaled toluene diisocyanate vapor in CD rats. Toxicol Sci 1999;52(2):258–268.

33. Tyl RW, Fisher LC, Dodd DE, et al: Developmental toxicity evaluation of inhaled toluene diisocyanate vapor in CD rats. Toxicol Sci 1999;52(2):248–257.

34. Bernstein DI, Jolly A: Current diagnostic methods for diisocyanate induced occupational asthma. Am J Ind Med 1999;36:459–468.

35. Baur X: Are we closer to developing threshold limit values for allergens in the workplace? Ann Allergy Asthma Immunol 2003;90(Suppl):11–18.

36. National Institute for Occupational Safety and Health: Pocket Guide to Chemical Hazards. Available at: http://www.cdc.gov.

37. Olson KR, ed: Poisoning and Drug Overdose, 3rd ed. Stamford, CT, Appleton & Lange, 1999.

ANTHONY J. SCALZO, MD ■ CAROLYN M. BLUME-ODOM, RN, BSN

At a Glance...

- Hydrofluoric acid is highly toxic by the dermal, inhalation, ocular, and oral routes.
- Symptoms and tissue effects may be delayed.
- HF exposure can induce systemic toxicity related to electrolyte abnormalities.
    - Hypocalcemia
    - Hypomagnesemia
    - Hyperkalemia
- Treatment is directed at rapid and complete deactivation of absorbed fluoride ion.
- Treatment options vary by site of exposure.
    - Dermal: initial water irrigation and use of calcium gluconate via various routes
        - Topical calcium gluconate gel
        - Subcutaneous intralesional calcium infiltration
        - Regional intravenous calcium infusion—Bier block technique
        - Intra-arterial calcium infusion
    - Ocular: water/normal saline irrigation, 1% calcium gluconate drops
    - Inhalation: fresh air and nebulized 2.5% calcium gluconate
    - Ingestion: cautious lavage with calcium gluconate, support for systemic complications

INTRODUCTION AND EPIDEMIOLOGY

Hydrofluoric acid (HF) is an aqueous solution of the inorganic acid of elemental fluorine. HF will dissolve anything that has glass or silica content as well as various metals, rubber, leather, and most organic materials including human tissue. In the industrial setting, HF is used to etch and frost glass, clean metal parts before electroplating, and etch silicon wafers in electronic semiconductor materials. HF is used in the petroleum industry to manufacture high-octane gasoline and in various metal processes, including pickling stainless steel, producing aluminum and uranium, and cleaning and removing rust from iron, copper, and brass.

The majority of inhalation exposures and those involving high concentrations are nearly exclusive to industry. Industrial exposures, though less frequent than home exposures, normally account for the majority of severe exposures accompanied by long-term morbidity and mortality. An 11-year investigation by the U.S. Occupational Safety and Health Administration (OSHA) of nine deaths attributed to HF indicated that unsafe work practices were contributing factors in all nine.[1]

In the home setting, HF exposures can occur when rust removers are used with inadequate dermal protection. Consumer HF-containing products are most commonly rust removers and aluminum and chrome cleaning products. The majority of exposures in the home setting involve the distal extremities, primarily the hands and fingers. A case of hydrofluoric acid burns to the hand has been reported after ignition of a compressed air duster containing 1,1-difluoroethane, which decomposes to HF at high temperatures.[2] Other products of concern to the lay public are wire wheel cleaners, which contain ammonium bifluoride in a concentration of 15.9%. As little as 2 mL of this type of product has proved fatal in toddlers when ingested.[3]

STRUCTURE-ACTIVITY RELATIONSHIPS

Hydrofluoric acid is a colorless, corrosive liquid or gas, which fumes at concentrations greater than 40% to 48%,[4] boils at 19.5°C, and has an odor threshold in air of 0.5 to 3 ppm.[5] The vapor pressure of HF gas over a concentrated solution (70% HF at 80°F) is relatively high at 150 mm Hg and thus resembles acetone and other volatile liquids.[6] HF is miscible in water and in solution has virtually no odor as opposed to in gaseous form, where it has a strong, irritating odor. HF is manufactured from calcium fluoride (fluorospar), which is reacted with sulfuric acid to form HF gas[7]:

$$CaF_2 + H_2SO_4 \leftrightarrow 2\ HF + CaSO_4$$

where CaF_2 = fluorospar and H_2SO_4 = sulfuric acid.

The gas is then cooled to be stored as anhydrous HF liquid, which by definition refers to concentrations greater than 99%. Most injuries from HF do not involve anhydrous HF but varying concentrations of >20% used in diverse industry applications or household products with lower concentrations. HF and additional free fluoride ions are also generated when ammonium bifluoride dissociates in aqueous solution:

$$NH_4HF_2 \rightarrow HF + F^- + NH_4^+$$

where NH_4HF_2 = ammonium bifluoride.

PHARMACOLOGY AND TOXICOLOGY

Pathophysiology

Concentrated solutions of HF are strong proton (H^+) donors that can cause coagulative necrosis similarly to other strong inorganic acids (e.g., HCl), while dilute solutions of HF are weak acids. HF is referred to as a binary hydride, and it has the highest bond dissociation energy, so it requires more energy to dissociate compared with other halogen group series acids (i.e., HF > hydrochloric acid [HCl] > hydrobromic acid [HBr] or > hydriodic acid [HI]). The reverse is true with regard to

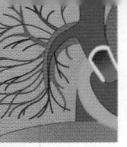

strength of acidity (ability to donate a proton, or H[+]). HF has a dissociation constant (K_d) of 3.53×10^{-4}, which is 1000 times less dissociated than HCl. It has a pKa of 3.8.[8] Cellular damage from the proton donated by HF causes initial tissue injury by dehydration and corrosion. It is the fluoride ion, however, that is responsible for the majority of tissue damage from HF. Fluoride ion has a permeability coefficient similar to that of water (P = 1.4×10^{-4} cm/sec).[4,9] HF in the systemic circulation may dissociate to H[+] and free fluoride ions, which may cause severe acidosis as well as systemic fluorosis.[8,10]

The presence of free fluoride ions results in a number of pathophysiologic effects. Fluoride ions are intensely electronegative and attract several cellular and systemic cations such as calcium and magnesium. In this process, biologically active calcium and magnesium are depleted at a rapid rate. Specifically, the binding of calcium may exceed the rate at which calcium can be mobilized from bone, and this process may lead to severe systemic hypocalcemia.[11] Fluoride ion exposure also results in low ionized calcium.[12,13] In general, low ionized or low total calcium may be associated with significant neurologic effects including tetany and seizures as well as cardiovascular instability and other effects.[14-16] Although the systemic depletion of calcium may be severe, in most cases of HF poisoning, clinical evidence of hypocalcemia such as tetany, Chvostek's sign, and Trousseau's sign may be absent.[17] Some authors have described patients with leg cramping.[18] Because of the rapid onset of hypocalcemia, early replacement of calcium is crucial in significant exposures and should not await laboratory confirmation. The electrocardiogram at the bedside may also offer clues, since hypocalcemia is a well-known cause of prolonged QT_c interval. One author described recurrent ventricular tachycardia in association with QT prolongation after an adult was exposed to 30% HF over 44% body surface area (BSA) and survived.[19] The hypomagnesemia seen with HF poisoning may also cause prolonged QT and atypical ventricular tachycardia.[20] According to the World Health Organization (WHO) guidelines, increased likelihood of significant hypocalcemia may be suspected if the patient has a dermal burn of 1% BSA from HF concentrations of 50% or greater, any dermal burn of 5% BSA regardless of the concentration of HF, inhalation of HF vapors from solutions of greater than or equal to 60%, or even small ingestions of HF solutions including more dilute household products.[21,22] In clinical practice, however, there are often exceptions to these guidelines.

Additionally, free fluoride ions inhibit many membrane and intracellular enzymes including those of the Krebs cycle and importantly the Na[+]/K[+]-ATPase pump[8,23] as well as enzymes that are magnesium or manganese dependent.[24] Inhibition of Krebs cycle enzymes may result in cellular energy failure, which contributes to cell death. Fluorides react with trace amounts of aluminum (Al[3−]) to form AlF[4−] complexes that have been shown to activate G proteins in cell membranes, which may alter cell-signaling processes and lead to inflammation.[25] Fluoride ions also stimulate phospholipase A_2, which may liberate arachidonic acid, the precursor for various inflammatory eicosanoids.[25] On a more emergent level, fluoride reportedly stimulates adenylate cyclase,[26] which in the myocardium results in increased cyclic adenosine monophosphate (AMP) and may increase the possibility of arrhythmias.[20] Direct myocardial tissue injury is also possible from high myocardial fluoride levels in cases of fatal systemic fluorosis from serious dermal burns.[10]

Changes in potassium flux across membrane channels have been implicated in fluoride poisoning and are the subject of recent research on the use of amiodarone for its potassium channel blocking effects.[27] The Na[+]/K[+]-ATPase system is responsible for pumping sodium ions out of the cell and potassium ions into the cell to maintain normal extracellular levels of each cation. When poisoned by fluoride ions, this pump will result in excess extracellular potassium, which exacerbates the hyperkalemic state. The resultant hyperkalemia is likely a contributory factor in enhancing myocardial irritability. The effects of hypocalcemia and dysfunction of the Na[+]/K[+]-ATPase system on potassium flux may not be immediate. Delayed ventricular fibrillation, frequently described in severe dermal exposure, ingestions, and inhalation exposures to concentrated HF may be due to late-onset hyperkalemia.[23] Others report this arrhythmia in the absence of hyperkalemia.[13,19] The mechanism of acute fluoride-induced sudden cardiac death from ventricular arrhythmias has been attributed to profound hypocalcemia, but in canine studies this lethal effect appears to be more temporally due to the elevation in serum potassium.[23] A large fraction of the increase in extracellular potassium may derive from transfer across the erythrocyte membrane of red blood cells in circulation that are exposed to the fluoride ion.[28] In vitro studies show that while fluoride ion decreases extracellular calcium, it increases intracellular calcium, which is believed to trigger calcium-dependent K[+] channels that allow for enhanced K[+] efflux and resultant hyperkalemia.[29] Moreover, in dogs this fluoride-induced hyperkalemia cannot be prevented by glucose, insulin, or bicarbonate.[23]

From a pathophysiologic standpoint, the treatment of fluoride-induced hyperkalemia may depend on removal of fluoride as well as potassium. This is problematic at best. To some extent, the treatment of HF-induced hypocalcemia with intravenous (IV) calcium should help correct some effects of hyperkalemia. Although sodium bicarbonate administration may lower extracellular potassium and correct the acidosis of systemic HF poisoning, it also may lower ionized calcium.[30] Maintaining normal to supranormal extracellular calcium levels may diminish the likelihood of ventricular arrhythmias (ventricular fibrillation, or VF) in severe HF exposure.[8] In one report, a 33-year-old man developed severe hypocalcemia (0.78 mmol/L ionized calcium), metabolic acidosis (pH 7.04), and several episodes of VF after ingesting HF. As much as 4 g of IV calcium chloride including 1 g/hr infusion were administered, yet the patient still had five episodes of VF. An ultrahigh dose of calcium at 200 mL/hr (20 g/hr calcium chloride) was subsequently infused and achieved an ionized calcium level of 4.34 mmol/L; no further VF was observed.[8]

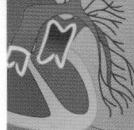

The delayed pain characteristic of HF dermal exposures can be attributed to some of these pathophysiologic effects on potassium flux across the membrane but likely is more complex. Some authors have attributed pain as secondary to the precipitation of calcium fluoride and magnesium fluoride in deep tissues as well as hyperkalemia, which leads to neural stimulation.[31,32] We question, however, the notion of attributing pain (nociceptive stimulus) to tissue deposition of insoluble calcium and magnesium salts of fluoride. The effective correction of pain due to fluoride toxicity employs calcium and possibly magnesium to complex with free fluoride ions. This process generates insoluble calcium fluoride or magnesium fluoride, yet is the very therapy that alleviates pain.

The authors believe that the neural stimulation theory from enhanced K^+ flux and in some cases extracellular hyperkalemia is more plausible. The stimulation of unmyelinated free nerve endings (C fibers) and later, slower conducting myelinated A-δ fibers in damaged tissue likely occurs after HF exposure. Fluoride-induced calcium deficiency at the cellular membrane allows enhanced outward K^+ flux through Ca^{2+}-dependent K^+ channels.[29,33] Extracellular hyperkalemia at the cell membrane surface may not always translate to abnormal serum potassium even in severe or fatal human HF poisoning,[22,34,35] but it may occur and be life threatening.[18,23] Hyperkalemia is associated with peripheral neural depolarization as well as depolarization in muscle and excitable cardiac tissue.[36-38] Mild to moderate hyperkalemia shifts the resting potential toward depolarization and there is an increase in conduction velocity in human atrial cells, whereas severe hyperkalemia may lead to a reduction in conduction velocity.[36] This discussion of potassium in no way diminishes the consequences of severe systemic hypocalcemia or hypomagnesemia seen in serious HF exposures. Hypocalcemia, especially in combination with hypomagnesemia, is a major contributing factor in myocardial irritability in many cases.

Enhanced potassium flux at the cellular level is probably insufficient explanation for the mechanism of pain. The molecular mechanism of pain, especially in damaged or inflamed tissue, is complex, and sodium channels, voltage-gated potassium channels (Kv), and a host of neuropeptides and excitatory amino acids are involved.[39] Protons (H^+) and lower tissue pH may stimulate a subpopulation of C fibers and contribute to pain.[40] Substance P (an 11–amino acid peptide), released from vesicles in sensory nerve fibers, also may contribute to pain.[41] Hyperkalemia may signal increases in calcitonin gene–related peptide (CGRP), a known nociceptive neuropeptide, as evidenced by in vitro release of CGRP by potassium chloride.[42] High extracellular potassium appears to enhance the release of glutamate in the central nervous system.[43,44] Glutamate receptors are localized in the peripheral nervous system on nociceptive, afferent, unmyelinated C-fiber type nerves.[45] Studies in animal models of pain have shown that peripheral glutamate is involved in nociceptive transmission under normal conditions and with

inflammation.[46] Thus, inflamed and injured tissue having suffered the initial burn effects of the H^+ ions and subsequently the effects of fluoride ions will likely have exposed free unmyelinated nerve endings that will signal the pain sensation.[47]

In summary, fluoride ion results in alterations of potassium flux with extracellular hyperkalemia, as well as hypocalcemia and hypomagnesemia, all of which contribute to altered membrane excitability of peripheral sensory nerves as well as cardiac tissue. These ion derangements, especially hyperkalemia, may herald the release of nociceptive peptides such as CGRP and glutamate, all of which play a role in the generation of pain. More research is needed at the molecular biologic level to further clarify these constructs.

Toxic Pathology and Clinical Effects

HF and related products may cause dermal, ocular, pulmonary, gastrointestinal (GI), and systemic injury. Unique exposure routes, however, include a case of intradermal injection of 5 mL of 7% HF in a suicide attempt with severe local and systemic effects including hypocalcemia,[48] and fulminant colitis following self-administration of an HF enema.[49] Nevertheless, most HF-related injuries that the emergency or occupational physician encounters are from dermal exposures with resultant injury largely dependent on the concentration of HF and extent of exposure. Oral and inhalation exposures, however, should be considered potentially fatal irrespective of HF concentration. Industrial exposures may involve exposure to anhydrous HF and varying concentrations below that to approximately 20% HF.

Household products usually contain HF in lower concentrations but may also cause injury from misuse or failure to use protective equipment. Household products used as rust removers and aluminum wheel cleaners for automobiles usually contain 6% to 12% and less than 20% HF.[50] Consumers may use these products without wearing gloves or protective garments, and the lack of immediate pain or irritation often is deceiving. Vinyl or rubber gloves are superior to latex, since HF attacks latex. Additionally, since moist skin appears to be more permeable to HF, a glove with a pinhole leak may allow HF to contact skin and the occlusive, moisture-retaining effect of the glove may enhance absorption.[6,51] Other forms of fluoride that dissociate to HF upon contact with water include ammonium bifluoride found in automobile alloy wheel cleaners. Exposures, both dermal and inhalational, to ammonium bifluoride–containing products has resulted in deaths and serious morbidity including marked hypocalcemia, hypomagnesemia, and ventricular fibrillation in several pediatric patients.[3,13,52]

Additional forms of fluoride that are significant for human health include sodium fluoride as found in fluoridated water supplies or dental products. Sodium fluoride tablets, which generally contain 0.25 to 1 mg of fluoride ion, have caused fluoride poisoning in children.[53,54] As opposed to HF in household and automobile cleaners, the fluoride contained in toothpaste usually is not consumed in quantities sufficient to cause

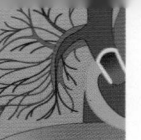

toxicity with common daily use. Dental preparations containing fluoride include toothpaste and gels as well as mouthwashes, topical fluoride gels, and dental rinses that may induce minimal toxicity in accidental overdoses. The forms of fluoride found in these products usually release only small amounts of free fluoride anion, thus reducing the risk of acute toxicity.

Nevertheless, cases of fluoride poisoning have occurred with ingestion of fluoride rinses as well as large ingestions of toothpaste (4.5 to 9 ounces with 0.15% fluoride ion w/v) in small children.[55] Some consider approximately 5 mg/kg of F[-] ion from dental products as "toxic," with nausea, vomiting, diarrhea, and abdominal cramping likely to occur at this dose,[53] whereas others believe the toxic range is 5 to 10 mg/kg.[56] The estimated lethal dose of fluoride is in excess of 30 mg/kg.[57]

In a series of 87 children, those who ingested up to 8.4 mg/kg from dental products had mild, self-limited primarily GI symptoms.[58] A 15-kg toddler who ingests a full 4.6-ounce tube of children's fruit-flavored toothpaste, however, could be at risk for significant toxicity. This exposure can be calculated as follows:

> A 4.6-ounce tube of a popular children's flavored toothpaste contains 2.4% sodium fluoride and has 0.15% w/v of fluoride ion.
> 4.6 ounces × 29.57 mL/oz = 136.02 mL in the tube.
> 136.02 mL × 0.15 g/100 mL (0.15% w/v fluoride) = 204.03 mg of fluoride.
> 204.03 mg fluoride in a 15-kg child = 13.6 mg/kg.

Serious poisoning due to fluoride-containing dental products has been reported. GI hemorrhage, hypocalcemia, hypomagnesemia, ventricular tachycardia, and ventricular fibrillation have been reported in a 43-year-old following an ingestion of up to 25 ounces of a topical fluoride gel containing 1.23% fluoride.[59] Death occurred following ingestion of 200 mg (16 mg/kg) of fluoride in a 3-year-old boy.[60] Subgingival irrigation of deep periodontal pockets with a 2% stannous fluoride (SnF_2) solution resulted in extensively erythematous mucosa of half of the hard palate and necrosis of the soft tissue close to the palatal aspect of two molars.[61]

Excessive fluoridation has also been associated with skeletal fluorosis.[5] The American Academy of Pediatrics Committee on Nutrition and Fluoridation recommends that the optimal daily dose of fluoride effective in preventing dental caries is 0.05 to 0.07 mg/kg/day.[62] Dental fluorosis, characterized by mottled teeth, has occurred with excessive fluoridation. There is evidence that levels of fluorosis have increased in part owing to widespread use of fluoridated water in food processing and dentifrices containing sodium fluoride used in combination with ingestion of fluoridated water.[5]

DERMAL TOXICITY

When in contact with skin, HF dissociates into hydrogen ions and free fluoride ions. There may be a latent period before a clinically evident burn is apparent, dependent on the concentration of the acid and the length of time it is in contact with the skin.[63-65] Other mineral acids are rapidly neutralized, whereas the process of tissue destruction may continue for days with HF.[66] Fluoride ions penetrate tissues deeply, causing tissue damage and the potential for systemic toxicity depending on the HF acid concentration.

In general, exposure to HF solutions of greater than 50% concentration results in immediate pain and tissue destruction.[4,21,67] The skin appears blanched, and within 1 to 2 hours the dermal lines are obliterated by edema.[65] Even a small cutaneous exposure to greater than 50% HF can be rapidly fatal.[17,68] Two cases of delayed death at 7 days and at 15 days resulting from multiple organ system failure have been reported following significant dermal burns from 70% HF.[69,70] Dermal contact with concentrations of 20% to 50% HF usually result in a burn that develops within a few hours.[31] In fact, concentrations greater than 20% HF have a potential for serious toxicity regardless of the degree of surface area involved.[71] Contact with solutions of less than 20% HF concentration results in dermal injury that usually develops with a latent period of about 24 hours.[72]

Hand and finger involvement is common in household product exposures[73-76] as well as industrial-strength solutions of HF.[4,77] The clinical presentation of exposure to strong HF solutions of greater than 20% begins with pain at the site that is characteristically intense[77] and often described by patients as "burning," "deep," "throbbing," or "exquisite."[64] Local erythema and edema may or may not be present initially, but later a pale, blanched appearance of the skin is apparent in more severe burns from concentrated HF (e.g., >50%).[24,65,77] Extensive bullae and maceration of tissue may be seen.[74] Gray areas may develop and progress to frank necrosis and deep ulceration within 6 to 24 hours.[24]

Since subungual tissue is lacking in stratum corneum, it is particularly susceptible to the penetration of fluoride ions, and exposure may result in a gray, black, or bluish discoloration of the nails.[21,78] This is of clinical importance, since the nail bed is generally inaccessible to administration of topical calcium therapy.

Tissue fluoride may be extremely high at the site of the burn, but such burns also result in elevated serum fluoride levels. In a fatal industrial exposure to 70% HF over 9% BSA, the burn site had 303 μg of fluoride per gram of dry tissue (normal, 0.2 to 0.8 μg/g) and serum fluoride was measured at 4.17 μg/mL (normal, 0.01 to 0.04 μg/mL).[10] In another case, a serum fluoride level of 21.3 μg/mL (normal, 0 to 0.5 μg/mL) was reported in a child who survived an 11% BSA burn from a combination product consisting of 8% hydrofluoric acid and 23% hydrochloric acid.[20] Urinary fluoride (toxic, >10 mg/L) is also used to document exposures.[13,79]

Secondary contamination attendants to the victims of HF exposure has been reported in two emergency department (ED) personnel who developed respiratory and skin irritation from patients who had not been decontaminated prior to arrival.[80] In another case, all three members of an operating room team developed marked conjunctival and nasal irritation from presumably unbound fluoride present in tissue that they were débriding on the fifth day postinjury.[69]

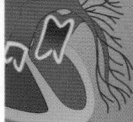

OCULAR TOXICITY

Ocular toxicity with concentrated HF solutions may be immediate or delayed.[67] Denuded corneal and conjunctival epithelium, corneal stromal edema, and conjunctival ischemia may be seen.[81] Severe eyelid edema and conjunctival chemosis with decreased visual acuity has also been described in a worker sprayed with aerosolized and solid particles of HF.[82] Even vapors of HF can cause ocular damage.[83,84] Anhydrous HF may result in immediate damage and globe perforation necessitating enucleation.[85] Lid deformities, uveitis, and glaucoma have also been described.[4]

Delayed effects may be seen, as evidenced by a 25-year-old sprayed in the eye with HF who was treated in an ER and released, only to return 5 days later with a foreign body sensation in his affected eye. Examination revealed a corneal erosion measuring 4×5 mm accompanied by marked conjunctival injection, chemosis, and subconjunctival hemorrhages.[82] In a 3-year-old child, initial symptoms of pain and redness resolved with irrigation alone after she had sprayed her eyes with a wire wheel cleaner containing an unknown percentage of phosphoric acid and hydrofluoric acid. Pain, however, returned in 4 days. She sustained bilateral corneal opacities, which were treated with topical antibiotics and corticosteroids under the care of an ophthalmologist. Her ocular examination was normal at 30 days postexposure.[86]

INHALATION TOXICITY

Upon inhalation, HF has resulted in local pulmonary as well as systemic effects. Acute lethal inhalation exposures in humans have resulted in congestion, edema, or necrosis in the liver, kidneys, and spleen, as noted on autopsy.[87] The American Conference of Governmental Industrial Hygienists' (ACGIH) threshold limit value (TLV) and the OSHA permissible exposure limit (PEL) have both been set at 3 ppm or 2.6 mg/m³.[88] Since TLV is a ceiling threshold level and PEL is a time-weighted average over 8 hours, these standards are not very useful to the emergency physician confronted with a worker who has been exposed in a factory accident to HF at 100 or 150 ppm for a short time. Thus, some researchers have sought to define a short-term exposure limit (STEL) at which brief (≤10 minutes) exposures at higher levels might produce irritation but not serious or irreversible effects on the respiratory tract. In one such study, rats were used to derive an STEL for humans of 130 ppm for a 10 minute or less exposure.[88]

Potroom workers in the aluminum smelting industry are at increased risk for inhalation of HF[89] and particulate fluoride salts,[90] which have caused inflammatory responses in the upper and lower respiratory tracts of healthy individuals at HF levels of less than 5 mg/m³.[25] In a volunteer study, 20 individuals exposed to HF at levels varying from 0.2 mg/m³ to 5.2 mg/m³ had elevated levels of plasma fluoride that correlated with increasing concentrations of HF. The authors also found that exposures above 2.5 mg/m³ were associated with pronounced upper respiratory tract symptoms and with increased neutrophils and tumor necrosis factor–α

(TNF-α) in nasal fluid.[25] In some cases, HF inhalation may result in pulmonary edema and severe lung injury[1] or death,[91] whereas others report an adult respiratory distress syndrome (ARDS)–like syndrome necessitating prolonged intubation but with normal pulmonary function at outcome.[92] Postmortem examination of tissue in fatal inhalation cases has revealed bronchi obstructed with mucus and blood and severely ulcerated, necrotizing tracheobronchitis with pseudomembrane formation.[91]

The sudden onset of asthma in an adult with no previous history has been reported immediately following an inhalation exposure to an 8% to 9% HF rust remover.[93] Chemical pneumonitis has been reported in a previously healthy 26-year-old woman who used three 10-ounce applications of an 8% HF-containing rust remover in an attempt to remove a stain in a bathtub. On presentation, she had shortness of breath, orthopnea, fever, nonproductive cough, severe right shoulder pain, and auscultated wheezes and crackles over her right thorax. A chest radiograph revealed a right lower lobe infiltrate. Over the ensuing 3 to 4 days, her respiratory status deteriorated and she was intubated, requiring a fraction of inspired oxygen (FIO_2) of 1.0 and positive end-expiratory pressure (PEEP) of 10 cm H_2O to maintain oxygen saturation above 70%. All cultures for bacteria, viruses, fungi, and mycobacteria were negative.[94]

Respiratory symptoms may be persistent for months to years following inhalation of HF.[91] While changes in respiratory function have been described with large exposures as mentioned above, there also appears to be an association between low-level HF exposure and a decline in chronic lung function as measured by forced vital capacity (FVC) and forced expiratory volume in 1 second (FEV_1).[25,89]

INGESTION TOXICITY

The toxicity of HF in oral ingestions is generally severe and rapid, with death occurring in less than 1 hour in some cases.[4,22] This route of exposure is not uncommon, as reported by one regional poison center over a 2-year period. The authors found 1172 HF exposures 99 of which were human cases of ingestion.[34] All these ingestions involved products which contained 6% to 8% HF. Hypocalcemia was found in 4 of 29 cases in which calcium was measured, and all four of these patients were adults who intentionally drank 3 oz or more in a suicide attempt. Two of these patients died.

GI symptoms after HF ingestion include throat pain, nausea, vomiting, gastric pain, and hematemesis.[8,34,35] Endoscopic studies show esophageal erythema and edema[35] as well as superficial ulcerations in the stomach in treated cases.[8] Systemic symptoms are also likely with HF ingestion and may be life threatening. A survivor of two swallows of an 8% HF-containing rust remover developed severe hypocalcemia and received 1100 mg of calcium gluconate in the first few hours. Despite calcium replacement, the patient became hypotensive (BP 62/40, HR 140) and developed ventricular fibrillation for which she was defibrillated as many as 30 times[35]; she ultimately survived neurologically intact.

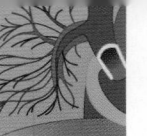

Ingestion of ammonium bifluoride (NH_4HF_2) resulting in death in two children has been reported[3,52] and survival in two others.[13] In one case, a 3-year-old girl ingested an unknown quantity of a wheel cleaner containing NH_4HF_2, which had been placed in a drinking cup. Within 20 minutes of ingestion she was obtunded, flaccid, and with circumoral cyanosis. She was intubated and treated with multiple doses of IV and nebulized calcium gluconate, but within 30 minutes of arrival she suffered bradyasystolic arrest. Curiously, the QT_c interval remained normal until the time of the arrest. She could not be resuscitated, and postmortem examination revealed severe pulmonary hemorrhage as well as hemorrhagic necrosis of the pharynx, esophagus, and stomach.[52] Both of two survivors of significant NH_4HF_2 ingestion displayed significant hypocalcemia (one, 4.2 mg/dL, and the other, 2.6 mg/dL; normal, 9 to 11 mg/dL) and one displayed severe hypomagnesemia (0.3 mg/dL; normal, 1.5 to 2.1 mg/dL). An electrocardiogram (ECG) available in the first case revealed a slightly prolonged QT_c (0.48 seconds) that prompted treatment with IV calcium. One patient developed delayed ventricular fibrillation at approximately 3.5 hours and the second at an estimated 6 to 7 hours postingestion.[13] Urinary fluoride levels confirmed the exposure in both cases (77 and 110 mg/L; toxic, >10 mg/L).

DIAGNOSIS

Laboratory and Other Diagnostic Testing

Diagnosis of acute fluoride toxicity is based on clinical presentation and history of exposure. The onset of systemic toxicity may be rapid and abrupt; hence, treatment is best initiated prior to definitive knowledge of the electrolyte status of the patient. Frequent monitoring of calcium, magnesium, potassium, and phosphorus as well as arterial blood gas (ABG) levels is essential during evaluation and treatment of HF exposure. Hypocalcemia, hypomagnesemia, hyperkalemia, and acidosis are suggestive of HF toxicity. Renal and hepatic functions are important parameters to monitor, since toxicity to these organs may accompany systemic fluorosis.[85]

Continuous cardiac monitoring and hourly serum calcium concentrations are essential during parenteral (i.e., subcutaneous, intravenous, or intra-arterial) calcium supplementation to guard against the risk of hypercalcemia associated with the inexact nature of dosing with calcium salts.[20]

Serum and urinary fluoride levels may be used as indicators of severity of exposure, since neutralized fluoride is eliminated primarily by the renal system. Fluoride levels are not very useful in the management of acute overdose, and normal or reference values vary in the literature. For serum, the generally accepted "normal" range is 0.01 to 0.04 µg/mL; some use an upper reference limit of no more than 2 µmol/L. The normal range for urine fluoride varies from 0.2 to 3.2 mg/L (toxic, >10 mg/L).

Differential Diagnosis

Phosphoric acid may be present in products used for etching metals and creating semiconductor products. It may also burn the skin but does not have the delayed effects characteristic of HF. If the patient has severe pain in the extremities or other areas of the skin without noticeable redness early following exposure to unknown chemicals, HF toxicity should be considered.

MANAGEMENT

Regardless of the route of HF exposure, initial management is aimed at thorough decontamination to reduce the absorption of fluoride. This is followed by attempts at rapid and complete deactivation and neutralization of absorbed fluoride ion to prevent or minimize tissue damage and systemic toxicity.

Dermal Exposure

First aid for dermal exposure to HF is immediate removal of contaminated clothing, taking extreme caution to protect attending personnel from cross-contamination, and irrigation of the exposed site with copious amounts of water for a minimum of 15 to 20 minutes. Decontamination is followed by careful débridement of vesicles and bullae to allow topical neutralization efforts to be optimally effective.[4]

A wide variety of treatment options have been devised to treat tissue hypocalcemia by deactivating free fluoride ions at the site of injury, thereby promoting formation of a nontoxic, insoluble calcium salt. Selection of a treatment modality is based on the history of the exposure and clinical status of the patient (Fig. 90-1).

Initial topical neutralization should include massage of a 2.5% to 5% calcium gluconate gel into the burn site.[64,75,85,95] An extemporaneous preparation of calcium gluconate gel 2.5% to 5% is formulated by adding 3.5 to 7 g of calcium gluconate powder to a 5-ounce tube of water-soluble surgical lubricant (e.g., K-Y Jelly).[4,21] Alternatively, the gel may be formulated by adding 10 1-g calcium carbonate tablets (e.g., Tums antacid tablets), which have been crushed into a fine powder, to 20 mL of water-soluble surgical lubricant to create a slurry.[95] The calcium carbonate will not be fully dissolved. Some authors advocate formulating the gel with dimethyl sulfoxide (DMSO), since it is thought to enhance the absorption of calcium into underlying tissues[20,96]; however, safety and efficacy of DMSO use have not been established.[66] Calcium chloride should not be used as a substitute for either the gluconate or the carbonate forms of calcium in topical applications owing to its potential for cellular toxicity and tissue irritation.[95] To facilitate application to the hands and digits, it is recommended to place 10 mL of the prepared gel inside a sterile surgical glove that is a half-size too large and insert the patient's hand into the glove.[4,75,95] Bending the fingers intermittently ensures optimal contact between the gel and the treatment area and facilitates main-

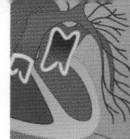

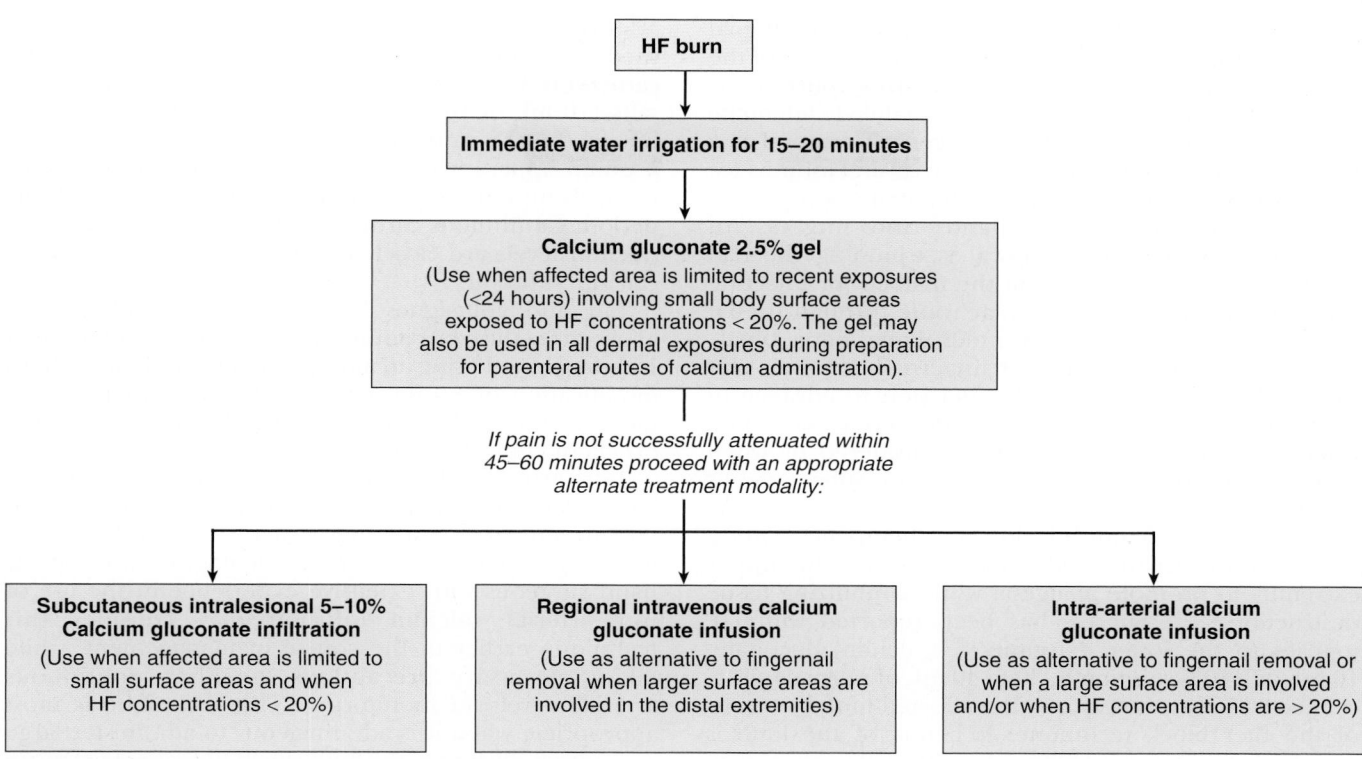

FIGURE 90-1 Dermal treatment of hydrofluoric acid burns.

tenance of joint mobility. If the patient obtains pain relief within 1 hour, liberal use of the gel can be continued for 3 to 4 days at 4- to 6-hour intervals[85] or whenever pain recurs.[21] It is hypothesized that topical treatment with calcium pulls fluoride ions back across the skin by a diffusion gradient.[95] This rationale suggests that topical administration of calcium is more efficacious in recent exposures (<24 hours), where the fluoride ion may not have penetrated deeper tissue layers, or in extensive exposures while preparing for more invasive means of calcium delivery to the tissues.[76,95]

Topical applications to neutralize the fluoride ion may have limited success in extremely late presentations (>24 hours) or when the skin shows evidence of altered integrity such as a toughened outer coagulum and blisters that may limit the access of subcutaneous tissues to administered calcium.[95]

When pain persists beyond 45 to 60 minutes of topical calcium neutralization[7,65,66] or if severe burns from solutions greater than 20% HF are present on initial consultation,[21,78,85,97] subcutaneous intralesional administration of calcium gluconate should be considered. Tissue destruction and associated pain may be minimized by subcutaneous intralesional administration of calcium gluconate, as introduced in 1932 by Freehagen and Wellmann,[98] with proven efficacy by Jones[99] in 1939.

A standard protocol in use, first described by Dibbell[78] in 1970, involves multiple subcutaneous intralesional injections of 10% calcium gluconate beneath the affected area by means of a 30-gauge needle to deliver a maximum volume of 0.5 mL/cm^2 of tissue, extending 5 mm beyond the injured site.[4,65,72,78,100] Each injection of

0.5 mL of 10% calcium gluconate solution delivers 4.2 mg of elemental calcium, which has been estimated to neutralize 0.025 mL of 20% HF.[101] A plastic surgeon or hand specialist should be consulted prior to attempting tissue infiltration. Subcutaneous injections into the tissues of the fingers must not be circumferential nor should they exceed 0.5 mL per affected digit owing to the possibility of the injection itself producing vascular impairment or of local compartment syndrome in already edematous tissue,[65] If local pain recurs, repeat injections[21,78] may be warranted, with extension of the treated site beyond the recommended 5 mm.[72,97] When tissues of the face are infiltrated, it is advised that a 5% calcium gluconate injection be used to reduce the risk of tissue irritation, potential scarring, and keloid formation.[4,85] Administering large volumes of subcutaneous calcium gluconate in single or repeated injections should be avoided because it may result in hypercalcemia, decreased tissue perfusion, local compartment syndrome, and ischemia-induced necrosis.[7,20,63] Calcium chloride should never be substituted for calcium gluconate in subcutaneous injections owing to the risk of tissue necrosis related to its hypertonicity.[4,11,21]

Velvart[102] recommends that subcutaneous calcium injections not be attempted when necrosis is apparent on presentation in favor of a more definitive treatment modality. The main disadvantage of subcutaneous infiltration is obvious discomfort to the patient. Since the end point of therapy is cessation of pain, the use of anesthesia has been discouraged during the infiltration procedure[21,65,78] although parenteral morphine is often required. Local calcium infiltration may require removal

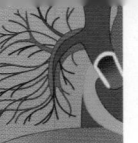

of fingernails to gain access to contaminated subungual structures that are easily penetrated by HF because of the lack of corneum stratum. In some instances, "burr holes" into the fingernails may be sufficient to deliver adequate calcium to underlying tissues.[7] Fingernail removal is a disfiguring process that requires up to several months for regrowth, causing extended disability in occupations requiring the use of the hands and fingers. An alternative to fingernail removal is trimming the nail plate back to its attachment at the nailbed[4] or injecting the nail bed via a lateral or volar route through the fat pad,[75] which is accomplished under digital nerve block. Instead of local injection and fingernail removal, one can infuse calcium locally. The decision to advance to more definitive modes of calcium delivery is warranted when fingernail removal is being considered or when there is lack of response to topical or subcutaneous injection.

Regional IV calcium infusion is a therapeutic option proposed for treatment of HF burns of the upper extremity to promote analgesia while minimizing tissue destruction.[103-107] Success has been reported with HF injuries to the lower extremity.[108] Calcium gluconate, 10 mL of a 10% solution in 30 to 40 mL of normal saline, is injected intravenously into the affected limb by means of the Bier block technique. Ischemia of the limb is maintained with a tourniquet for 20 to 25 minutes to allow calcium to accumulate in tissues at the site of injury.[106] Some clinicians utilize a second tourniquet proximal to the first to prevent inadvertent systemic calcium administration. In the event of failure of regional IV calcium infusion, a second infusion should be attempted.[103,107] Patients should have continuous cardiac monitoring and frequent serum calcium level measurements during Bier block–IV calcium infusion. Some authors advise regional IV calcium infusion as a viable alternative to subcutaneous intralesional infiltration owing to the discomfort imposed on the patient during infiltration without anesthesia and the need for fingernail removal in some instances.[106,107] Adverse effects reported with regional IV calcium infusion have been limited to minor complaints of warmth and burning during the calcium infusion and discomfort during maintenance of tourniquet inflation.[106] Transient forearm fasciculation for up to 1 hour has been reported in one case.[106]

An additional yet more invasive means of fluoride ion deactivation is delivery of calcium by an intra-arterial infusion method. This treatment modality is indicated for severe exposures to HF of greater than 20% concentration, late presentations (>24 hours) unresponsive to other therapies, extensive burn areas where available tissue space is limited for subcutaneous infiltration of calcium.[77] Aschinger and colleagues[109] introduced the procedure, specified for injuries to the distal extremities, in 1979, with modifications by Velvart[102] in 1983 and Vance[77] in 1986. The technique for intra-arterial infusion involves the percutaneous insertion of a long catheter into the radial, ulnar, or brachial artery, as determined by the site of injury. The origin of vascular supply to the injured area is identified by digital subtraction arteriography. A pressure transducer and monitor are used to confirm the position of the catheter; once the catheter is optimally in place, a dilute solution of calcium salts (10 mL of 10% calcium gluconate in 40 to 50 mL 5% dextrose) is infused over a 4-hour period by means of a pump apparatus. Treatments are repeated at 4-hour intervals until the patient remains pain free for a 4-hour period. Continuous cardiac monitoring, vital signs, and calcium levels are closely observed during intra-arterial calcium infusion.

Lin and colleagues[110] recommend modifying the above procedure by continuously infusing calcium over a 12-hour period using an ambulatory infusion pump. This modification offers the patient additional comfort and mobility during the treatment period while maintaining excellent clinical efficacy.

Intra-arterial calcium infusion enables the delivery of large volumes of calcium to the injured site without impairment of surrounding structures or induction of local tissue toxicity.[77,102] Some toxicologists and vascular hand surgeons with extensive experience in the use of intra-arterial calcium infusion may consider this technique earlier in the course of management, while taking necessary precautions including continuous arterial waveform monitoring. This technique is most appropriate when it is advantageous to administer large amounts of calcium to the burn site in the case of extensive burns from highly concentrated HF accompanied by a considerable risk of hypocalcemia and systemic toxicity.

A single 10-mL intra-arterial infusion of 10% calcium gluconate delivers 84 mg (4.7 mEq) of elemental calcium to tissues injured by HF.[77] The infusion is painless to the patient and avoids the need for fingernail removal. Case reports have demonstrated proven efficacy for pain relief up to 24 hours after the injury with intra-arterial infusion.[102] When intra-arterial infusion is employed early in the course of treatment, initial tissue débridement should be conservative, since rejuvenation of avital tissue has been noted.[102] Despite its advantages, intra-arterial infusion has significant drawbacks in that it requires hospitalization, specialized equipment, and coordination by a vascular surgeon experienced in the technique.[77] Complications include local arterial spasm, arteritis, and soft tissue loss.[77] Siegel and Heard[105] reported nerve palsies, carpal tunnel syndrome, and persistent increased sensitivity to cold and paresthesias from their experience in treating 38 extremities in 28 patients.

Ocular Exposure

The speed with which irrigation is instituted is the most important factor in preventing damage from ocular exposure to HF. An immediate *single* irrigation with tap water or isotonic NaCl for 15 to 20 minutes is the best initial first aid and should be instituted immediately at the scene. Multiple or prolonged irrigations are discouraged on the basis of studies in rabbit eyes which indicate that multiple irrigations can increase the rate of corneal ulceration from 6% to 40%.[81] Although the pH of the burn surface may rapidly return to normal after initial irrigation, deeper tissues may remain at con-

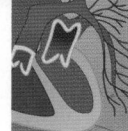

siderable risk for serious injury. Some clinicians recommend that once the patient is in the ED, an additional 5 to 10 minutes of irrigation with a 1% calcium gluconate solution should be instituted to ensure that adequate decontamination has been achieved and that remaining fluoride ion on the surface of the eye is neutralized.[21,85] Calcium gluconate 1% drops should be instilled every 2 to 3 hours for up to 2 to 3 days,[82,84,85] accompanied by conventional use of cycloplegics and antimicrobial agents when necessary. Efficacy of this treatment has been demonstrated in several cases involving HF concentrations of up to 49%.[84] The use of corticosteroid agents is proposed by some clinicians to lessen fibroblast formation in the cornea.[85,111] Systemic analgesic agents are helpful in controlling the pain associated with ocular exposure to HF. An ophthalmology consultation and examination are highly advisable for all patients with ocular exposure to HF.

It is not feasible to extrapolate treatment for dermal HF burns to the eye.[81,86] Many irrigants that have been suggested as immediate first aid in dermal exposures (e.g., Hyamine 0.2% and Zephiran 0.05%) can induce additional toxicity to the eye.[81]

Other irrigant solutions have been proposed for the treatment of ocular exposure to HF. Hatai[86] suggested the use of milk or lactated Ringer's solution as appropriate eye irrigants, since both have physiologic compatibility with the eye and both have a divalent calcium ion. Further research is needed to evaluate their efficacy.

Water, isotonic sodium chloride (NaCl), and isotonic magnesium chloride ($MgCl_2$) when available are the best irrigating solutions for HF exposures to the eye in an experimental rabbit model.[81]

Inhalation Exposure

Inhalation exposure to HF is most common in industrial settings. Multiple organ systems are at risk, since HF fumes at concentrations greater than 40% to 48%. Rapid removal from the contaminated environment is key to reducing morbidity and mortality. Rescue personnel should wear self-contained breathing apparatus (SCBA) and containment suits to prevent exposure. To patients in respiratory distress, 100% humidified oxygen should be administered immediately, followed by administration of a 2.5% to 3% calcium gluconate solution in normal saline with 100% oxygen via nebulization.[7,85] HF inhalation is accompanied by a significant risk for immediate or delayed-onset pulmonary edema, especially with prolonged exposure or exposure to high concentrations. If there is evidence of pulmonary edema, the patient should be placed on intermittent positive pressure breathing (IPPB) with PEEP and calcium should be delivered per nebulization.[85] In a reported case, 5% calcium gluconate per IPPB was employed utilizing a nebulizer after an inhalation exposure to 100% HF. Chest films and computed tomographic (CT) scan were normal at 21 days postexposure when the patient was discharged.[92] Patients exposed to HF by inhalation may require intubation and mechanical ventilation, especially when exposed to concentrations exceeding 60%.[6] Inhaled HF

is rapidly introduced into the liver and kidneys via the blood stream and is accompanied by a high risk for systemic toxicity.[85] It is essential to maintain an adequate airway and closely monitor serum calcium, magnesium, and potassium levels; arterial blood gases (ABGs); and O_2 saturation. Continuous observation for 24 to 48 hours after inhalation exposure to HF in a health care facility is suggested.

Some clinicians recommend the early use of corticosteroids to prevent noncardiogenic pulmonary edema and to control the inflammatory response.[85,98] Since there is not complete agreement about this recommendation, the use of steroids as a standard regimen remains controversial.

Oral Exposure

Oral exposure to HF results in rapid systemic absorption even with dilute solutions and is associated with a high risk for systemic toxicity. Simple dilution with a demulcent will not arrest the progression of tissue damage or the development of systemic toxicity when HF preparations are ingested. Induced emesis is contraindicated, as is neutralization with oral sodium bicarbonate.[21] Recommended first aid is oral administration of 1 to 2 cupfuls of milk or water. Milk is preferred owing to the presence of calcium ions,[35] though milk of magnesia may be given for its available magnesium ions and its demulcent effect on oral and gastric mucosa. To the authors' knowledge, there are no reports of benefit from activated charcoal in the management of oral exposures to HF.

Treatment in the ED may include cautious nasogastric lavage with a small-bore nasogastric tube to remove residual HF if this can be performed within 60 to 90 minutes of ingestion and perforation has not occurred.[4,21] It has been advocated to add 10% calcium gluconate to the lavage fluid to help bind fluoride present in the GI tract.[4,13] Lavage with 20 mL of calcium chloride in 1000 mL of normal saline has been initiated after ingestion of 10% HF.[8] Chan and Duggin[8] contend that it does not matter which form of calcium is used for lavage so long as enough calcium is provided to bind available fluoride. In a rare case of a self-administered concentrated HF enema, calcium carbonate enemas were given to bind intraluminal fluoride ion.[49] A gastroenterology/surgery consultation and examination are highly advisable for all patients with significant or symptomatic oral exposure to HF.

Systemic Toxicity: Flouride-induced Electrolyte and Cardiac Abnormalities

Systemic toxicity should be anticipated with any ingestion or inhalation of HF and with any dermal exposure involving a large surface area or a high concentration of HF. Continuous cardiac monitoring, hourly electrolyte values, and frequent ABG determinations are essential during the acute phase of systemic toxicity. IV access is essential for the supplementation of depleted electrolytes and sodium bicarbonate.

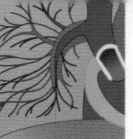
HYPOCALCEMIA

Hypocalcemia has been associated with a prolonged QT_c interval and ventricular fibrillation. In adults, a slow IV, prophylactic infusion of 20 mL of 10% calcium gluconate is recommended when systemic toxicity is anticipated.[85] Continuous cardiac monitoring is indicated, since too rapid calcium administration may induce cardiac arrhythmias, most notably bradycardia. Prior to calcium administration, a serum calcium level should be drawn but the initial prophylactic infusion should not be delayed pending results. Calcium should be infused until the level reaches the upper limit of normal in an effort to prevent ventricular fibrillation related to hypocalcemia in myocardial tissue.[20,21,24] Some clinicians propose the substitution of chloride salt for calcium gluconate, since it provides increased amounts of calcium ion. Calcium chloride however, has a potential for irritation and is best delivered by a central line. In addition, calcium chloride is acidifying and so should not be used when acidosis coincides with hypocalcemia. It is important to note that attempts to increase extracellular calcium through supplementation may exacerbate potassium efflux, so treatment of hypocalcemia may confound hyperkalemia in the setting of systemic fluorosis.[23]

HYPERKALEMIA

Hyperkalemia may precipitate the development of peaked T waves and cardiac arrhythmias. Aggressive measures such as hemodialysis may be required to achieve normalization of potassium levels.[23,35] Although there are recent reports of the use of cation exchange resins (e.g., Kayexalate) for hyperkalemia,[112] no one has reported such use to treat the hyperkalemia of HF exposure. Considering the time delay in rise of extracellular potassium, this may be an intervention to consider in advance of the anticipated hyperkalemia seen in significant HF exposures.

HYPOMAGNESEMIA

Hypomagnesemia is associated with QT prolongation and ventricular arrhythmias. Correction of hypomagnesemia is achieved with IV magnesium sulfate.

ACIDOSIS

Sodium bicarbonate may be used to correct acidosis. Inducing a slight metabolic alkalosis with sodium bicarbonate is indicated to enhance the excretion of fluoride ions in the urine.[31]

ALTERNATE FORMS OF FLUORIDE AND RELATED TOXICITY

With exposures to oral forms of fluoride including toothpastes, oral rinses, dentifrices, and oral supplements, it is important to establish the type and the amount of the fluoride salt present in the product as well as the amount ingested. Table 90-1 gives a partial listing of fluoride salts and the amount of elemental fluoride in each.

When ingested amounts of elemental fluoride exceed 5 to 8 mg/kg,[58] provision of calcium in the form of milk

TABLE 90-1 Elemental Fluoride Amounts in Common Fluoride Salts

SALTS OR PRODUCT	ELEMENTAL FLUORIDE
Sodium fluoride (NaF), 2.2 mg	1 mg
Stannous fluoride (SnF₂), 4.1 mg	1 mg
Sodium monofluorophosphate (MFP) 7.6 mg	1 mg
Fluoride toothpaste	Maximum of 1 mg per gram of toothpaste The maximum allowable amount of elemental fluoride in a tube of toothpaste is 260 mg
Oral nutritional supplements	0.25 to 1.0 mg per tablet or milliliter of product

and dairy products or calcium-containing antacid tablets will bind fluoride in the stomach. Fluoride salts dissociate in the acidic environment of the stomach to form HF acid, which causes GI irritation. When large amounts of fluoride salts are ingested, there is a risk of systemic fluoride toxicity, but this is rarely the case in accidental ingestion.

REFERENCES

1. Blodgett DW, Suruda AJ, Crouch BI: Fatal unintentional occupational poisonings by hydrofluoric acid in the U.S. Am J Ind Med 2001;40:215–220.
2. Foster KN, Jones L, Caruso DM: Hydrofluoric acid burn resulting from ignition of gas from a compressed air duster. J Burn Care Rehabil 2003;24:234–237.
3. Klasner AE, Scalzo AJ, Blume CM, Johnson P: Ammonium bifluoride causes another pediatric death (letter). Ann Emerg Med 1998;31:525.
4. Caravati EM: Acute hydrofluoric acid exposure. Am J Emerg Med 1988;6:143–150.
5. Agency for Toxic Substance and Disease Registry: Toxicologic Profiles for Fluorides. U.S. Department of Health and Human Services, 2002.
6. Mayer L, Guelich J: Hydrogen fluoride inhalation and burns. Arch Environ Health 1963;7:445–447.
7. MacKinnon MA: Hydrofluoric acid burns. Dermatol Clin 1988;6:67–74.
8. Chan BSH, Duggin GG: Survival after a massive hydrofluoric acid ingestion. J Toxicol Clin Toxicol 1997;35:307–309.
9. Gutknecht J, Walter A: Hydrofluoric and nitric acid transport through lipid bilayer membranes. Biochem Biophys Acta 1981;644:153–156.
10. Mayer TG, Gross PL: Fatal systemic fluorosis due to hydrofluoric acid burns. Ann Emerg Med 1985;14:149–153.
11. Greco RJ, Hartford CE, Haith LR Jr, Patton ML: Hydrofluoric acid–induced hypocalcemia. J Trauma 1988;28:1593–1596.
12. Mullet T, Zoeller T, Bingham H, et al: Fatal hydrofluoric acid cutaneous exposure with refractory ventricular fibrillation. J Burn Care Rehabil 1987;8:216–219.
13. Klasner AE, Scalzo AJ, Blume CM, et al: Marked hypocalcemia and ventricular fibrillation in two pediatric patients exposed to a fluoride-containing wheel cleaner. Ann Emerg Med 1996;28:713–718.
14. Lynch RE: Ionized calcium: pediatric perspective. Pediatr Clin North Am 1990;37:373–389.
15. Jankowski S, Vincent SL: Calcium administration for cardiovascular support in critically ill patients: when is it indicated? J Intensive Care Med 1995;10:91–100.

16. Riggs JE: Neurologic manifestations of fluid and electrolyte disturbances. Neurol Clin 1989;7:509–523.

17. Dowbak G, Rose K, Rohrich RJ: A biochemical and histologic rationale for the treatment of hydrofluoric acid burns with calcium gluconate. J Burn Care Rehabil 1994;15:323–327.

18. Yu-Jang S, Li-Hua L, Wai-Mau C, Kuo-Song C: Survival after a massive hydrofluoric acid ingestion with ECG changes (letter). Am J Emerg Med 2001;19:458–460.

19. Yamaura K, Kao B, Iimori E, et al: Recurrent ventricular tachyarrhythmias associated with QT prolongation following hydrofluoric acid burns. J Toxicol Clin Toxicol 1997;35:311–313.

20. Bordelon BM, Saffle JR, Morris SE: Systemic fluoride toxicity in a child with hydrofluoric acid burns: case report. J Trauma 1993;34:437–443,.

21. Upfal M, Doyle C: Medical management of hydrofluoric acid exposure. J Occup Med 1990;32:726–731.

22. Manoguerra AS, Neuman TS: Fatal poisoning from acute hydrofluoric acid ingestion. Am J Emerg Med 1986,4:362–363.

23. McIvor ME, Cummings CE, Mower MM, et al: Sudden cardiac death from acute fluoride intoxication: the role of potassium. Ann Emerg Med 1987;16:77–81.

24. Kirkpatrick JJR, Enion DS, Burd DAR: Hydrofluoric acid burns: a review. Burns 1995;21:483–493.

25. Lund K, Ekstrand J, Boe J, et al: Exposure to hydrogen fluoride: an experimental study in humans of concentrations of fluoride in plasma, symptoms, and lung function. Occup Environ Med 1997;54:32–37.

26. McIvor ME: Acute fluoride toxicity: pathophysiology and management. Drug Saf 1990;5:79–85.

27. Su M, Chu J, Howland MA, et al: Amiodarone attenuates fluoride-induced hyperkalemia in vitro. Acad Emerg Med 2003;10:105–109.

28. Danowski TS: The transfer of potassium across the human red blood cell membrane. J Biol Chem 1941;139:693–705.

29. Cummings CC, McIvor ME: Fluoride-induced hyperkalemia: the role of Ca^{2+}-dependent K^+ channels. Am J Emerg Med 1988;6:1–3.

30. Cooper DJ, Walley KR, Wiggs BR, Russell JA: Bicarbonate does not improve hemodynamics in critically ill patients who have lactic acidosis: a prospective, controlled clinical trial. Ann Intern Med 1990;112:492–498.

31. Bertolini JC: Hydrofluoric acid: a review of toxicity. J Emerg Med 1992;10:163–168.

32. Bracken WM, Cuppage F, McLaury RL, et al: Comparative effectiveness of topical treatments for hydrofluoric acid burns. J Occup Med 1985;27:733–739.

33. Gofa A, Davidson RM: NaF potentiates a K(+)-selective ion channel in G292 osteoblastic cells. J Membr Biol 1996;149:211–219.

34. Kao W, Dart RC, Kuffner E, Bogdan G: Ingestion of low-concentration hydrofluoric acid: an insidious and potentially fatal poisoning. Ann Emerg Med 1999;34:35–41.

35. Stremski ES, Grande GA, Ling LJ: Survival following hydrofluoric acid ingestion. Ann Emerg Med 1992;21:1396–1399.

36. Nygren A, Giles WR: Mathematical simulation of slowing of cardiac conduction velocity by elevated extracellular. Ann Biomed Eng 2000;28:951–957.

37. Bradberry SM, Vale JA: Disturbances of potassium homeostasis in poisoning. J Toxicol Clin Toxicol 1995;33:295–310.

38. Seneviratne KN, Peiris OA, Weerasuriya A: Effects of hyperkalaemia on the excitability of peripheral nerve. J Neurol Neurosurg Psychiatry 1972;35:149–155.

39. Rasband MN, Park EW, Vanderah TW, et al: Distinct potassium channels on pain-sensing neurons. Proc Natl Acad Sci U S A 2001;98:13373–13378.

40. Steen KH, Reeh PW, Anton F, Handwerker HO: Protons selectively induce lasting excitation and sensitization to mechanical stimulation of nociceptors in rat skin, in vitro. J Neurosci 1992;12:86–95.

41. Onuoha GN, Alpar EK: Levels of vasodilators (SP, CGRP) and vasoconstrictor (NPY) peptides in early human burns. Eur J Clin Invest 2001;31:253–257.

42. Hoogerwerf WA, Zou L, Shenoy M, et al: The proteinase-activated receptor 2 is involved in nociception. Neuroscience 2001;21:9036–9042.

43. Wu A, Fujikawa DG: Effects of AMPA-receptor and voltage-sensitive sodium channel blockade on high potassium-induced glutamate release and neuronal death in vivo. Brain Res 2002;946:119–129.

44. Katayama Y, Becker DP, Tamura T, Hovda DA: Massive increases in extracellular potassium and the indiscriminate release of glutamate following concussive brain injury. J Neurosurg 1990;73:889–900.

45. Carlton SM, Zhou S, Coggeshall RE: Evidence for the interaction of glutamate and NK1 receptors in the periphery. Brain Res 1998;790:160–169.

46. Carlton SM: Peripheral excitatory amino acids. Curr Opin Pharmacol 2001;1:52–56.

47. Messlinger K: What is a nociceptor? Anaesthesist 1997;46:142–153.

48. Gallerani M, Bettoli V, Peron L, Manfredini R: Systemic and topical effects of intradermal hydrofluoric acid. Am J Emerg Med 1998;16:521–522.

49. Cappell MS, Simon T: Fulminant acute colitis following a self-administered hydrofluoric acid enema. Am J Gastroenterol 1993;88:122–126.

50. Perry HE: Pediatric poisonings from household products: hydrofluoric acid and methacrylic acid. Curr Opin Pediatr 2001;13:157–161.

51. Kunkel DB: Hydrofluoric acid: a toxin on the rise. Emerg Med 1988(Feb 15):237–242.

52. Mullins ME, Warden CR, Barnum DW: Pediatric death and fluoride-containing wheel cleaner (letter). Ann Emerg Med 1998;31:524–525.

53. Mallatt ME, Smith CE: Acute fluoride ingestion: recognition and management. J Indiana Dent Assoc 1996;75:23–24, 26.

54. Monsour PA, Kruger BJ, Petrie AF, McNee JL: Acute fluoride poisoning after ingestion of sodium fluoride tablets. Med J Aust 1984;141:503–505.

55. Shulman JD, Wells LM: Acute fluoride toxicity from ingesting home-use dental products in children, birth to 6 years of age. J Public Health Dent 1997;57:150–158.

56. Spoerke DG, Bennett DL, Gullekson DJ: Toxicity related to acute low dose sodium fluoride ingestions. J Fam Pract 1980;10:139–140.

57. Whitford GM: Fluoride in dental products: safety considerations. J Dent Res 1987;66:1056–1060.

58. Augenstein WL, Spoerke DG, Kulig KW, et al: Fluoride ingestion in children: a review of 87 cases. Pediatrics 1991;88:907–912.

59. Fisher K, Picciotti M, Henretig F, et al: Fluoride (Fl) toxicity from a topical dental care product (TDCP) (abstract). Vet Human Toxicol 1991;33:365.

60. Eichler HG, Lenz K, Fuhrmann M, Hruby K: Accidental ingestion of NaF tablets by children: report of a poison control center and one case. Int J Clin Pharmacol Ther Toxicol 1982;20:334–338.

61. Sjostrom S, Kalfas S: Tissue necrosis after subgingival irrigation with fluoride solution. J Clin Periodontol 1999;26:257–260.

62. AAP Committee on Nutrition: Fluoride supplementation. Pediatrics 1986;77:758–761.

63. Dale RH: Treatment of hydrofluoric acid burns. BMJ 1952;1:728–732.

64. Browne TD: The treatment of hydrofluoric acid burns. J Soc Occup Med 1974;24:80–89.

65. Edelman P: Hydrofluoric acid burns. Occup Med 1986;1:89–103.

66. Anderson WJ, Anderson JR: Hydrofluoric acid burns of the hand: mechanism of injury and treatment. J Hand Surg [Am] 1988;13:52–57.

67. Bosse GM, Matyunas NJ: Delayed toxidromes. J Emerg Med 1999;17:679–690.

68. Tepperman PB: Fatality due to acute systemic fluoride poisoning following a hydrofluoric acid skin burn. J Occup Med 1980;22:691–692.

69. Gubbay AD, Fitzpatrick RI: Dermal hydrofluoric acid burns resulting in death. Aust N Z J Surg 1997;67:304–306.

70. Muriale L, Lee E, Genovese J, Trend S: Fatality due to acute fluoride poisoning following dermal contact with hydrofluoric acid in a palynology laboratory. Ann Occup Hyg 1996;40:705–710.

71. Rao RB, Hoffman, RS: Caustics and batteries. In Goldfrank's Toxicologic Emergencies, 7th ed. New York, McGraw-Hill, 2002, Chapter 87.

72. Matsuno K: The treatment of hydrofluoric acid burns. Occup Med 1996;46:313–317.

73. Mangion SM, Buelke SH, Braitberg G: Hydrofluoric acid burn from a household rust remover. Med J Aust 2001;175:270–271.

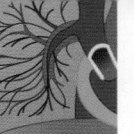

74. Asvesti C, Guadagni F, Anastasiadis G, et al: Hydrofluoric acid burns. Cutis 1997;59:306–308.

75. Roberts JR, Merigian KS: Acute hydrofluoric acid exposure (letter). Am J Emerg Med 1989;7:125–126.

76. El Saadi MS, Hall AH, Hall PK, et al: Hydrofluoric acid dermal exposure. Vet Hum Toxicol 1989;31:243–247.

77. Vance MV, Curry SC, Kunkel DB, et al: Digital hydrofluoric acid burns: treatment with intra-arterial calcium infusion. Ann Emerg Med 1986;15:890–896.

78. Dibbell DG, Iverson RE, Jones W, et al: Hydrofluoric acid burns of the hand. J Bone Joint Surg [Am] 1970;52:931–936.

79. Kono K, Yoshida Y, Watanabe M, et al: Urine, serum and hair monitoring of hydrofluoric acid workers. Int Arch Occup Environ Health 1993;65(1 Suppl):S95–S98.

80. Horton DK, Berkowitz Z, Kaye WE: Secondary contamination of ED personnel from hazardous materials events, 1995–2001. Am J Emerg Med 2003;21:199–204.

81. McCulley JP, Whiting DW, Petitt MG, Lauber SE: Hydrofluoric acid burns of the eye. J Occup Med 1983;25:447–450.

82. Rubinfeld RS, Silbert DI, Arentsen JJ, Laibson PR: Ocular hydrofluoric acid burns. Am J Ophthalmol 1992;114:420–423.

83. Rose L: Further evaluation of hydrofluoric acid burns of the eye. J Occup Med 1984;26:483–486.

84. Bentur Y, Tannenbaum S, Yaffe Y, Halpert M: The role of calcium gluconate in the treatment of hydrofluoric acid eye burn. Ann Emerg Med 1993;22:1488–1490.

85. Trevino MA, Herrmann GH, Sprout WL: Treatment of severe hydrofluoric acid exposure. J Occup Med 1983;25:861–863.

86. Hatai JK, Weber JN, Doizaki K: Hydrofluoric acid burns of the eye: report of possible delayed toxicity. J Toxicol Cutaneous Ocul Toxicol 1986;5:179–184.

87. Meldrum M: Toxicology of hydrogen fluoride in relation to major accident hazards. Regul Toxicol Pharmacol 1999;30:110–116.

88. Dalbey W, Dunn B, Bannister R, et al: Acute effects of 10-minute exposure to hydrogen fluoride in rats and derivation of a short-term limit for humans. Regul Toxicol Pharmacol 1998;27:207–216.

89. Radon K, Nowak D, Heinrich-Ramm R, Swzadkowski D: Respiratory health and fluoride exposure in different parts of the modern primary aluminum industry. Int Arch Occup Environ Health 1999;72:297–303.

90. Healy J, Bradley SD, Northage C, Scobbie E: Inhalation exposure in secondary aluminum smelting. Ann Occup Hyg 2001;45:217–225.

91. Braun J, Stob H, Zober A: Intoxication following the inhalation of hydrogen fluoride. Arch Toxicol 1984;56:50–54.

92. Kono K, Watanabe T, Dote T, et al: Successful treatments of lung injury and skin burn due to hydrofluoric acid exposure. Int Arch Occup Environ Health 2000;73(Suppl):S93–S97.

93. Franzblau A, Sahakian N: Asthma following household exposure to hydrofluoric acid. Am J Ind Med 2003;44:321–324.

94. Bennion JR, Franzblau A: Chemical pneumonitis following household exposure to hydrofluoric acid. Am J Ind Med 1997; 31:474–478.

95. Chick LR, Borah G: Calcium carbonate gel therapy for hydrofluoric acid burns of the hand. Plast Reconstr Surg 1990;86:935–940.

96. Zachary LS, Reus W, Gottlieb J, et al: Treatment of experimental hydrofluoric acid burns. J Burn Care Rehabil 1986;7:35–39.

97. Iverson RE, Laub DR, Madison MS: Hydrofluoric acid burns. Plast Reconstr Surg 1971;48:107–112.

98. Freehagen K, Wellman M: Atzwirkungen des Fluorwasserstoffs und Gegenmittel. Angew Chem 1932;45:537–538.

99. Jones AT: The treatment of hydrofluoric acid burns. J Ind Hyg Toxicol.1939;21:205–212.

100. Blunt CP: Treatment of hydrofluoric acid skin burns by injection with calcium gluconate. Ind Med Surg 1964;33:869–871.

101. Carney SA, Hall M, Lawrence JC, Ricketts CR: Rationale of the treatment of hydrofluoric acid burns. Br J Ind Med 1974;31: 317–321.

102. Velvart J: Arterial perfusion for hydrofluoric acid burns. Hum Toxicol 1983;2:233–238.

103. Henry JA, Hla KK: Intravenous regional calcium gluconate perfusion for hydrofluoric acid burns. J Toxicol Clin Toxicol 1992;30:203–207.

104. Wilkes GJ: Intravenous calcium gluconate for hydrofluoric acid burns of the digits. Emerg Med 1983;5:155–158.

105. Siegel DC, Heard JM: Intra-arterial calcium infusion for hydrofluoric acid burns. Aviat Space Environ Med 1992;63:206–211.

106. Graudins A, Burns MJ, Aaron CK: Regional intravenous infusion of calcium gluconate for hydrofluoric acid burns of the upper extremity. Ann Emerg Med 1997;30:604–607.

107. Ryan JM, McCarthy GM, Plunkett PK: Regional intravenous calcium—an effective method of treating hydrofluoric acid burns to limb peripheries. J Accid Emerg Med 1997;14:401–404.

108. Ryan JM, McCarthy GM, Plunkett PK: Regional intravenous infusion of calcium for hydrofluoric acid burns of the upper extremity (letter). Ann Emerg Med 1998;31:526.

109. Achinger R, Kohnlein HE, Jacobitz K: A new treatment method of hydrofluoric acid burns of the extremities. Chir Forum Exp Klin Forsch 1979;229–231.

110. Lin TM, Tsai CC, Lin SD, Lai CS: Continuous intra-arterial infusion therapy in hydrofluoric acid burns. J Occup Environ Med 2000;42:892–897.

111. Vaughn D, Asbury T: General Ophthalmology. Los Altos, CA, Lange, 1983, p 39.

112. Kim HJ, Han SW: Therapeutic approach to hyperkalemia. Nephron 2002;92(Suppl 1):33–40.

91 *Hydrogen Sulfide*

TEE L. GUIDOTTI, MD, MPH

At a Glance...

- Severe acute hydrogen sulfide poisoning can be seen in a variety of settings but is most commonly observed in the oil and gas industry.
- High concentrations of hydrogen sulfide may cause "knockdown," a sudden loss of consciousness, which may be accompanied by apnea.
- Unprotected rescuers are at high risk of death. Self-contained breathing apparatus should always be worn during rescue attempts.
- In addition to altered consciousness, hydrogen sulfide sometimes causes pulmonary edema and keratoconjunctivitis ("gas eye").
- Laboratory studies are rarely available for confirmation; therefore, the diagnosis is based on history and clinical grounds.
- Supportive care, with attention to the airway, is critical.
- Sodium nitrite, a component of the Taylor cyanide kit, is a useful antidote for hydrogen sulfide but only if given promptly. Hyperbaric oxygen may also be effective in severe cases.

Hydrogen sulfide (H_2S) has been recognized as an occupational hazard since the time of Ramazzini in the 18th century. H_2S is among the most common causes of fatal gas inhalation exposures in the workplace and is mostly a problem today in the oil and gas industry, in swine confinement facilities, and in manure collection systems. H_2S is generated in municipal sewers and sewage treatment plants, pulp and paper operations (in Kraft and especially sulfite mill technologies), construction zones in wetlands (such as marshes), asphalt roofing, and pelt processing (in which soaking in sulfide solution loosens hair for removal), and may be a hazard in confined spaces in which organic material, such as fish or offal, has decayed or in which inorganic sulfides may be reduced.[1-6] H_2S may be both an occupational and a potential community environmental health risk in areas with geothermal activity and hot springs, such as Rotorua, New Zealand.[7]

H_2S is the principal hazard in the "sour gas industry," that part of the natural gas industry extracting sulfur-containing natural gas. Organic sulfur is reduced to hydrogen sulfide during the prolonged degradation process of organic material underground that forms natural gas and petroleum. Sour gas is distributed in oil and gas fields worldwide but is concentrated in western Canada, Texas and the Gulf Coast, Michigan, the Middle East (including Saudi Arabia and Abu Dhabi), central Asia (including Kazakhstan, Iran, and Pakistan), and Russia. Most sour gas falls between 2% and 35% H_2S, but some wells in the Canadian province of Alberta exceed 98%.[8-12]

MECHANISM OF ACTION

The primary toxicity of H_2S is conventionally assumed to result from inhibition of cytochrome-*c* oxidase and possibly other heme-containing macromolecules by aqueous sulfide.[13,14] H_2S is classified as a cellular asphyxiant, together with carbon monoxide, cyanide, and azide. H_2S interacts with a number of enzymes and other macromolecules, including hemoglobin and myoglobin. The effect of H_2S in disrupting cytochrome-*c* oxidase activity is the same as oxygen deprivation or asphyxiation except that it may act more quickly. This is thought to be the primary mechanism of action of the characteristic reversible neurotoxicity associated with H_2S, the sudden loss of consciousness called "knockdown."[6]

The mechanism of action of H_2S is often attributed to inhibition of cytochrome-*c* oxidase and therefore to a mechanism identical to that of cyanide.[15] However, there are clearly other mechanisms.[16] One lethal end point of H_2S exposure is respiratory paralysis, a dose-dependent reduction in ventilatory drive resulting in apnea, which follows an initial hyperpnea.[17] Infusion of the sulfide ion alone into the circulation mimics the systemic effects of H_2S inhalation. The apneic response to H_2S is not enhanced by intra-arterial injection of sulfide into the carotid artery, which delivers blood directly to the brain, compared with intravenous injection into the femoral artery, in which mixing occurs in the general circulation. The apneic response can also be blocked by paralysis of the vagal nerve by lidocaine or by infusion of sodium bicarbonate solution, in the absence of acidosis. These findings strongly suggest that a peripheral receptor in the lung is responsible for the apneic response.[18] Hydrogen sulfide may also be a neuromodulator, and so toxic exposure may involve direct functional effects as well as cell toxicity.[16,19,20]

Pulmonary edema and mucosal irritation, particular of the eye, are nonspecific irritant effects of hydrogen sulfide, reflecting its chemical reactivity.[21]

TOXICOKINETICS

H_2S is poorly soluble in water. Exposure occurs exclusively by the inhalation route, and to date all described toxicity incidents have involved exposure in the gaseous phase. H_2S is inhaled and enters the circulation directly across the alveolar-capillary barrier. Once absorbed, H_2S dissociates in part into hydrosulfide ion, HS^-, then is spontaneously transformed into sulfide $[S^{2-}]$ and then sulfate $[SO_4^{2-}]$. Some H_2S remains as free H_2S in blood, and this fraction appears to interact with metalloproteins, disulfide-containing proteins, and thio-S-methyl-

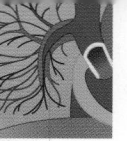

transferase, forming methyl sulfides. The sulfide ion binds to heme compounds and is itself metabolized by oxidation to sulfate. Sulfate is then excreted by the kidney or lost in intermediary metabolism. Little is known of the toxicokinetics of H_2S and sulfide.[22]

CLINICAL PRESENTATION

Pathophysiology

It has been known for many years that H_2S has potent neurotoxic properties. Respiratory paralysis may occur if exposure is prolonged, presumably as a direct consequence of sulfide toxicity inhibiting brainstem respiratory nuclei. However, the studies cited on apnea,[16,18] supported by studies suggesting a chemoreceptor response,[20] suggest that there are other pathways that affect central activity.

Animal studies of the toxicity of H_2S are often difficult to interpret. Exposure to H_2S is known to increase levels of taurine in cerebrospinal fluid, for example, but it is not clear whether this is a toxic effect or a protective effect because taurine may act on neurons to reduce the neurotoxicity of some agents.[23] Likewise, H_2S is known to increase serum glucose levels in postpartum rats, but an aggravating effect on diabetes has not been suggested in the literature on human toxicity.[24] Chronic low-level exposure to H_2S is associated with abnormal proliferation and ramification of Purkinje cells in the cerebellum of rats, but there is no comparable human exposure outcome with which to compare these observations.[24]

In healthy, fit human volunteers, exposure to H_2S as low as 5 ppm during exercise (30 minutes) is associated with an early shift from aerobic to anaerobic metabolism, as indicated by increasing blood lactate levels, but without symptoms.[25] This observation precipitated a review of occupational exposure levels in the United Kingdom.[26]

In the past, there was a controversy over whether sulfhemoglobin occurs after high-level H_2S exposure, but the weight of evidence is that it does not.[14]

Manifestations

ACUTE TOXICITY

Acute central neurotoxicity, pulmonary edema, and the mucosal effects are the characteristic features of acute toxicity of H_2S. Odor perception, olfactory paralysis, and keratoconjunctivitis are the characteristic effects of H_2S at lower concentrations.[3,5,6,9,11,21] In addition to the effect of olfactory paralysis, which is an effect at higher exposure levels (>100 ppm), olfactory fatigue occurs at lower, ambient levels, so that the person exposed may not be as aware of the odor because of habituation, even though there is no toxic effect on olfaction. See Table 91-1 for health effects of hydrogen sulfide at various exposure levels.

H_2S-induced acute central toxicity leading to reversible unconsciousness is sudden and is colloquially called a "knockdown."[6] Knockdowns can be acutely fatal as a consequence of respiratory paralysis and cellular anoxia. Very high concentrations (500–1000 ppm) are associated with a knockdown. This is an abrupt loss of

TABLE 91-1 Health Effects of Hydrogen Sulfide at Various Exposure Levels

CONCENTRATION (ppm)	EFFECTS
0.01–0.3	Odor threshold (highly variable)
1–5	Moderate offensive odor, may be associated with nausea, tearing of the eyes, headaches, or loss of sleep with prolonged exposure; healthy young male subjects experience no decline in maximal physical work capacity.
10	8-hour occupational exposure limit in Alberta, OSHA PEL
15	15-minute occupational exposure limit in Alberta
20	Ceiling occupational exposure limit evacuation level in Alberta; odor very strong
20–50	Keratoconjunctivitis (eye irritation) and lung irritation. Possible eye damage after several days of exposure; may cause digestive upset and loss of appetite
100	Eye and lung irritation; olfactory paralysis, odor disappears
150–200	Sense of smell paralyzed; severe eye and lung irritation
250–500	Pulmonary edema may occur, especially if prolonged
500	Serious damage to eyes within 30 minutes; severe lung irritation; unconsciousness and death within 4 to 8 hours; amnesia for period of exposure; knockdown
1000	Breathing may stop within one or two breaths; immediate collapse

OSHA, Occupational Safety and Health Administration; PEL, permissible exposure limit.
From Guidotti TL: Hydrogen sulfide. Occup Med 1996;46(5):367–371.

consciousness and collapse, described by those who witness it as appearing much like turning off the switch on a mechanical doll. A knockdown may be fatal if exposure is prolonged. If exposure is transient, as usually happens in the oil patch, recovery may be equally rapid and apparently complete.[9,27] Some veteran oilfield workers have returned to what they were doing without reporting the event and without treatment, considering the experience all in a day's work.

Central effects observed after a knockdown might represent primary toxicity of H_2S, secondary effects from low-level cellular anoxia, or the sequelae of acute brain injury. The long-term central effects of a knockdown in any given case may represent an episode of toxic anoxia, or even a secondary traumatic injury. In at least one case, focal cortical necrosis was documented following a knockdown in which the patient never recovered consciousness.

H_2S is irritating to mucous membranes, although this feature of H_2S exposure may have been overly emphasized in the literature.[26] H_2S penetrates deeply into the respiratory tract because its solubility is relatively low, rendering it capable of causing alveolar injury leading to acute pulmonary edema.

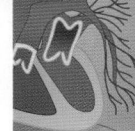

The irritant effect is also seen in the upper airway; experimental studies suggest that the olfactory mucosa do not recover as fast as the bronchial epithelium. Recently, this pattern of toxicity was demonstrated to be attributable to selective toxicity of olfactory mucosa in the nasal passages.[28] Human subjects exposed to transient high levels of H_2S have been reported to show deficits on standardized tests of smell and taste years later, suggesting that the effect may be a permanent sequela under some circumstances.[29]

Pulmonary edema is also a well-recognized acute effect of H_2S toxicity, especially when exposure is prolonged. Older studies suggest that 20% of cases of H_2S toxicity reaching the emergency department showed evidence of pulmonary edema.[9] Experimental studies have shown that although H_2S at high concentrations produces a marked alveolitis and profuse edema, it is only moderately cytotoxic for pulmonary cells and does not seem to disrupt the basement membrane of the alveolar endothelium. Thus, the ultimate prognosis for recovery and remodeling may be good if the patient can be supported through the acute episode.[9,30,31] Acute inhalation of H_2S may be fatal, depending on the concentration and duration of exposure and the duration of anoxia. In one series of 152 cases from China, an overall mortality rate of 5% was reported.[30,32]

It is not clear whether hydrogen sulfide exposure is associated with chronic respiratory sequelae. Exposure in the short term does not appear to be associated with reduced lung function or increased airways reactivity.[33,34] However, other studies have suggested that a reduction in residual volume is a subclinical effect.[35] Cross-sectional studies of sewer workers, who are exposed to hydrogen sulfide, suggest that after accounting for smoking, lung function is significantly reduced and may show an accelerated rate of decline among age groups.[31] A single case report has suggested interstitial fibrosis, but this has not been observed in other studies or case series.[36]

Prolonged anoxia, which might be due in these incidents to respiratory paralysis, pulmonary edema, or asphyxia in a confined space, results in a severe metabolic acidosis that further complicates resuscitation. Overwhelming exposure may be associated at autopsy with skin and organ discoloration, pulmonary edema, and renal tubular necrosis.[5,6]

Most standards for the protection of occupational and community populations are based on prevention of keratoconjunctivitis (eye irritation) and respiratory tract irritation. The slope of the exposure–response relationships for these conditions is not as steep as it is for central nervous system effects.[37]

"Gas eye," or keratoconjunctivitis, is a superficial inflammation of the cornea and conjunctiva that is often recurrent in workers in sour gas plant who are exposed for prolonged periods to relatively low concentrations. A peculiar feature of this effect is that it can be associated with reversible chromatic distortion and visual changes. It has been suggested that the corneal epithelium develops a fine punctate stain and becomes edematous, and that small vesicles form that act as a diffraction grating. This results in a colored halo surrounding the object. This effect is sometimes accompanied by blepharo-spasm, tearing, and photophobia. In the viscous rayon industry, this problem is encountered with carbon disulfide exposure.[5,21,37]

There are few data on teratogenicity, mutagenicity, or carcinogenicity for H_2S, largely because it is so toxic. In animal studies, H_2S appeared unlikely to cause reproductive toxicity after exposures that are plausible in occupational and workplace situations.[38,39] Exposure to 75 ppm is reported to prolong delivery time of gravid rat dams at the time of parturition, and rat pups exposed at the same level in utero or neonatally showed only minor delays in ear and hair development.[38] Exposure to lower levels, although still toxic in human context, has been shown to elevate circulating glucose in maternal rats, with secondary metabolic effects in the offspring.[24] H_2S appears to enhance the mutagenicity of peroxide but is not genotoxic alone.[40] Evidence for cancer in human populations is weak. Studies of residents of Rotorua, which is a largely Maori community and cultural center, have observed an excess of cancers of the sinus overall (which may be confounded by wood dust exposure in Rotorua's extensive native craft industry) and of lung cancer in Maori women, which was not completely explained by higher smoking rates but which was accompanied by a statistically significant deficit among Maori men.[41]

Laboratory Features

The management of H_2S toxicity does not depend on laboratory confirmation or monitoring sulfide levels.[42-50]

Sulfide measurements can be made on postmortem brain tissue, but this is currently a research tool that has not been validated for forensic use in humans.[51] Blood sulfide levels are not diagnostic of H_2S toxicity, must be performed within 2 hours of exposure, but are seldom available, are subject to many limitations, and are not available on an emergency basis.[5]

Urinary thiosulfate levels show promise as a biologic exposure indicator in the monitoring of occupational exposure but are profoundly influenced by diet and have not been validated for human toxicity.[5]

The partial pressure of oxygen in arterial blood may be normal in H_2S toxicity, unless there is pulmonary edema or another reason for respiratory compromise. Metabolic acidosis and a low arteriovenous oxygen difference may indicate anoxia at the cellular level and may correlate with severity of toxicity, but this has not been documented.

The chest film may show evidence of noncardiogenic pulmonary edema.[5]

TREATMENT

Treatment of transient exposures, and of knockdowns in which the worker has regained consciousness, is not specific.[52] Removal from exposure is critical, of course. Unlike cyanide intoxication, there is no evidence that H_2S intoxication would confer a risk on the rescuer during mouth-to-mouth resuscitation.[5]

Patients should be observed for pulmonary edema overnight, and metabolic acidosis should be treated.[13] Because workers may encounter H_2S while performing

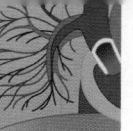

hazardous tasks, incidental injuries may require treatment.[53] Overwhelming exposures and prolonged knockdowns may require aggressive treatment, but the circumstances in which these exposures occur often lead to delays in transport and treatment.

Combined treatment with hyperbaric oxygen and nitrite has emerged as the treatment of choice, but the literature remains anecdotal, reflecting experience acquired one case at a time.[2,14,44,54-60] Increased oxygen tension may overcome some of the physiologic disadvantages of nitrite treatment.

Empirically, nitrite treatment alone has been used successfully in managing acute cases, but its mechanism of action remains uncertain. Nitrite treatment is based on the observation that H_2S resembles cyanide in that both bind reversibly to cytochromes, although there appear to be differences at a biochemical level.[13] The theory is that methemoglobin generated by nitrite would displace the sulfide, as it does cyanide, and regenerate the active cytochrome oxidase.[58] Although methemoglobin is more effective in binding sulfide than oxyhemoglobin, the complex between sulfide and methemoglobin does not last long enough to make much difference. The sulfide disappears quickly from the circulation under conditions of good oxygenation anyway. The evidence suggests that nitrite can only be effective within the first few minutes after exposure and may actually slow sulfide removal thereafter. There are also reasons to believe that the methemoglobin hypothesis is insufficient to explain the action of nitrite even in the first few minutes. A further practical problem with this approach is that it may add to the anoxic burden that already may exist from the cytochrome poisoning, respiratory paralysis due to central toxicity, and ventilation-perfusion mismatch associated with pulmonary edema. It may also induce hypotension and further complicate the anoxia with hypoperfusion. Administration of nitrites is usually begun with inhalation of amyl nitrite perles (for 30 seconds out of every minute) followed by sodium nitrite intravenously, in the same dosages as for cyanide poisoning. The literature suggests infusion of 300 mg of fluid containing 10 mL of 3% $NaNO_2$ over 4 minutes, titrating the drop in blood pressure to maintain systolic pressure above 80 mm Hg (10.6 kPa).[13,55-58] In children, the recommended intravenous treatment dose would be as for cyanide intoxication (see Chapter 88). Because of the potential for inducing hypotension in a child, however, such treatment should only be considered in cases in which the cause is indisputably hydrogen sulfide exposure and the patient is not already recovering. Because hydrogen sulfide is primarily an occupational exposure, occasional episodes of toxicity may occur in adolescents[30] but would be extremely rare in children.

Treatment with oxygen and supportive care alone has been recommended in order to avoid further complicating the toxic effects with iatrogenic anoxia and nitrite toxicity. However, confirmation that oxygen therapy alone works is limited to anecdotal reports and experimental studies with H_2S-exposed mice did not show increased survival with oxygen alone.

Hyperbaric oxygen therapy is an attractive and logical option for treating H_2S intoxication, and anecdotal evidence suggests that it may be effective.[59] The utility of oxygen is probably related to the oxygenation of marginally anoxic tissues and the displacement of sulfide from binding sites on cytochrome-c oxidase, but this has not been worked out. By the nature of such poisoning incidents, it is difficult to perform clinical trials and to compare therapies. A series of three treatments at 2.5 atmospheres for 90 minutes each has been recommended.[60] Given the low morbidity of hyperbaric oxygen treatment in skilled hands,[61] it is a prudent intervention if facilities are available.[62,63] Outcomes are not guaranteed, and neurologic sequelae may still occur following treatment.[46]

Decontamination is not required for the protection of health providers and bystanders. However, the foul odor of hydrogen sulfide may complicate management and cause anxiety among other patients. Removal of clothing and simple skin washing with soap and water should remove the odor from the patient. Airing outdoors should greatly reduce the odor from clothing.

Many antidotes to H_2S intoxication have been proposed, but few have shown efficacy. Ascorbate has been proposed to reverse methemoglobinemia, but because this is not the problem in sulfide toxicity, this intervention, although benign, is unlikely to be useful.[63]

Sodium thiosulfate has been proposed as a treatment for H_2S intoxication on analogy to its role in cyanide toxicity, but its efficacy has not been demonstrated, and the rationale is in question. Sulfide is oxidized and excreted sufficiently rapidly by the body that clearance is not the problem. Thiosulfate is a metabolite of sulfide and not a substrate for enzymatic oxidation, which destroys the toxic moiety, in the case of cyanide intoxication.[5,13]

There is evidence that the respiratory paralysis observed in some fatal knockdowns is associated with monoamine oxidase inhibition.[64] This inhibition is reversed by dithiothreitol (DTT), which also displaces sulfide from brain tissue in vitro after exposure in animals.[65] DTT has also been found to be protective if given to animals as pretreatment before exposure. These observations have led to efforts to use this agent and other thiol compounds as specific antidotes. In practice, however, these approaches have been disappointing.

Pretreatment with several agents is associated with increased survival in animals: pyruvate,[66] α-ketocarboxylic acids,[67] bicarbonate,[18] and glucose (unpublished observation). To date, these pretreatments have not led to successful therapeutic or prophylactic interventions.

DISPOSITION

Patients presenting to the emergency department after significant acute hydrogen sulfide exposure should be admitted or observed for several hours in most cases, owing to the substantial risk of development for pulmonary edema.

The prognosis for recovery after exposure to hydrogen sulfide is an area of controversy. The evidence is strong for neurologic sequelae following knockdown, in the context of acute high exposure, but weak for effects associated with chronic, low-level exposure.

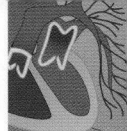

Chronic Sequelae of Acute Exposure

Chronic central nervous system effects after repeated or prolonged knockdowns have not been adequately studied. The available evidence strongly suggests that knockdowns are sometimes, if not usually, associated with chronic neurologic sequelae.[4,32,37,42-46] However, case series describing these effects may be confounded by effects of head trauma during falls, anoxia from apnea, or seizure activity. Extrapyramidal symptoms resembling Parkinson's diseases may appear during recovery from an H_2S-induced coma.[46-48]

Experimental studies on mice do suggest a cumulative effect in reducing brain cytochrome-c oxidase activity. Experimental studies also help to localize the effects of H_2S in the brain and appear to suggest anoxia as the mechanism. The available animal evidence points to injury to the cerebral cortex, cerebellum, and possibly brainstem and spinal cord at concentrations approaching those humans might encounter. The lesions are similar to those seen in oxygen deficiency and in poisoning by other cytochrome oxidase inhibitors.[17,42,47]

Chronic Effects of Lower-Level Exposure

Although there is sufficient evidence to conclude that a chronic toxicity syndrome exists as a sequela of knockdown, the evidence to date is weak for the conclusion that a chronic toxicity syndrome exists as a result of long-term, low-level exposure. Ecological studies of residents of Rotorua suggest some excess morbidity in both the central and peripheral nervous systems, but the pattern is not consistent, being strongest for mononeuritis. There was an elevated risk for cardiovascular disease but a reduced frequency of stroke and evidence for an elevated prevalence of high blood pressure. Other potential confounders include mercury (which was not measured) and other sulfides (not reported).[41]

Kilburn and colleagues have published data[48] suggesting neurobehavioral effects observed in populations exposed to low levels of H_2S, including single exposures below 1.0 or 0.5 ppm. The subjects consisted primarily of litigants, involved in a lawsuit for compensation for damages arising out of their exposure. The studies describe a pattern of poor recall, delayed reaction time, unilateral (not bilateral) changes in visual performance, and abnormal balance (requiring special technology to detect). The group has described similarly nonspecific patterns for other potential hazards. In these studies to date, the effects of litigation, posttraumatic stress, anticipation of compensation, and test bias cannot easily be ruled out. Neurobehavioral testing is also easily confounded by effects of learning, practice, motivation, sleep, education, distraction, depressed mood, and stress. The wide range of "normal" performance on these tests renders them rather insensitive and nonspecific in identifying neurotoxic outcomes, limitations freely acknowledged in the neurobehavioral literature. This literature is therefore difficult to interpret.

The Medical Diagnostic Review, a population-based prevalence survey and clinical screening conducted in southern Alberta in the mid-1980s, found no evidence of an excess in prevalence of neurologic signs and findings, both soft and hard, in populations living downwind of sour gas facilities.[49] Animal studies show no evidence of behavioral change after exposures of less than 80 ppm, a concentration that is effectively much higher in rats than humans because upper airway clearance is less in the rat.[50]

Other properties of H_2S have been difficult to assess because mucosal irritation and cellular anoxia dominate the clinical picture. Secondary effects may be overlooked in the more obvious acute toxicity profile of H_2S. Respiratory, cardiac, eye, and host defense disorders emerge as the most likely secondary effects to be associated with H_2S, but the evidence remains inconclusive.[11,37]

PREVENTION

H_2S is heavier than air. Workers entering a depression or confined space in which the gas has collected are likely to be at highest risk, although potentially lethal exposures can and do take place in the open air. Personal protection required is the self-contained breathing apparatus (SCBA).[68] In the past, tympanic membrane defects (perforated eardrums) excluded workers from certification for SCBA gear, on the grounds that H_2S could bypass the SCBA; this is not supported by the evidence and no longer recommended.[69]

H_2S is very odorous, with a low olfactory threshold, from less than 0.01 to 0.3 ppm. By 1 to 5 ppm, the odor is very offensive, like rotten eggs. However, the gas has poor warning properties at high exposure levels. As with most strong odors, workers may become accustomed to them in the short term, a phenomenon known as *olfactory fatigue*. There is also a specific mechanism known as olfactory paralysis that results in loss of the ability to perceive the odor, owing to neurotoxicity affecting the olfactory bulb and fibers. In relatively high concentrations (about 100 ppm), H_2S paralyzes the olfactory mechanism, preventing perception of any smell. This removes the primary warning sign of H_2S exposure and the principal warning to, say, oilfield workers caught in a plume.[5,6,14,27,69,70]

As in most such incidents, casualties usually occur in twos or more, as would-be rescuers rush to save their coworkers and in their haste neglect to protect themselves with an SCBA. Intensive training and ready availability of personal protective equipment are required to prevent such situations.[68]

Although there have been no documented cases of serious, irreversible injury or death in the public attributed to Alberta's sour gas industry, there have been a number of occupational fatalities arising from H_2S exposure in Alberta.[12] As a consequence, the oil and gas industry, the Alberta Government, and representatives of local residents and public agencies have developed an elaborate network of stakeholder organizations and public consultation mechanisms, which have been a model for other jurisdictions. Other locations where H_2S is a prominent hazard include Texas, Louisiana, and Iran. When a well blowout releases substantial quantities of sour gas, the usual management strategy is to ignite the gas, so that combustion converts the H_2S to less toxic

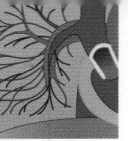

sulfur dioxide, notwithstanding the recognized irritant effects of this agent. This protects the community and nearby workers and allows crews to get closer to cap or shut down the well.

The OSHA Permissible Exposure Limit and the NIOSH Recommended Exposure Limit for H_2S are both 10 ppm, 8-hour time-weighted average. OSHA also has a short-term standard of 15 ppm. Alberta has adopted the same set of standards as occupational exposure levels and in addition has a ceiling of 20 ppm and an evacuation standard for the general population of 5 ppm.[6,71] Studies on normal volunteers during exercise suggest that 5 ppm of H_2S is easily tolerated and results in minimal detectable physiologic change.[25] In the absence of definitive studies of community residents or low-level exposure of workers, this is the best evidence available that current occupational exposure standards are probably adequate, bearing in mind that time-weighted averages are generally of less significance than peak exposures for this agent for neurotoxicity but may be more suitable for irritant effects.

The encroachment of communities on industrial sites and oil and gas fields that were once relatively isolated, together with economic incentives to site wells and facilities where deposits exist in urban locations, has resulted in many conflicts in land use and regulatory requirements for emergency planning to protect residents and create setbacks, or buffer zones, between gas facilities and populated areas. The Alberta Energy and Utilities Board and its predecessor agencies have been particularly proactive in emergency planning based on projected concentrations generated by computer models in the event of an uncontrolled release. Because of the nature of incidents involving H_2S, emergency response usually involves high levels in uncontrolled situations requiring rescue. Table 91-2 summarizes acute exposure levels proposed for both emergency planning and response purposes.

The exposure–response curve for lethality is extremely steep for hydrogen sulfide.[6,72] Among inhaled toxic substances, H_2S gives little margin of safety. One can visualize an encounter with concentrations of H_2S

TABLE 91-2 Guidelines for Emergency Planning and Response

GUIDELINE	CONCENTRATION (ppm)		INTERPRETATION
Emergency response planning guidelines (ERPGs)	Note: Concentrations are modeled for planning purposes.		Source: American Industrial Hygiene Association, 2004. ERPGs are intended to guide land use and resource planners and to determine appropriate emergency response contingencies for communities near facilities. They assume exposure of the general population, including more susceptible individuals.
ERPG-1	0.1		Exposure for up 1 hour without experiencing "other than mild transient adverse health effects or perceiving a clearly defined objectionable odor."
ERPG-2	30		Exposure for up to 1 hour without developing "irreversible or other serious health effects or symptoms that could impair an individual's ability to take protective action."
ERPG-3	100		Maximum airborne concentration "below which it is believed nearly all individuals could be exposed for up to one hour without experiencing or developing life-threatening health effects."
Acute exposure guideline levels (AEGLs)	Note: In actual uncontrolled incidents, it may not be possible to measure exposure.		Source: U.S. Environmental Protection Agency, Office of Pollution Prevention and Toxics, 2002. Intended to be guidelines in context of emergency response only: once-in-a-lifetime, short-term exposure to airborne chemicals that are acutely toxic. (Note: the significant figures in which AEGLs are given far exceed the accuracy of exposure assessment in most real uncontrolled incidents.)
AEGL 1	10 min	0.75	"Concentrations above which predicted that general population, including susceptible individuals, could experience notable discomfort, irritation or certain asymptomatic non-sensory effects that are not disabling and that are transient and reversible."
	30 min	0.60	
	60 min	0.51	
	4 hr	0.36	
	8 hr	0.33	
AEGL 2	10 min	41	"Concentrations above which predicted that general population, including susceptible individuals, could experience irreversible or other serious, long-lasting adverse health effects or an impaired ability to escape."
	30 min	32	
	60 min	27	
	4 hr	20	
	8 hr	17	
AEGL 3	10 min	76	"Concentrations above which predicted that general population, including susceptible individuals, could experience life-threatening health effects or death."
	30 min	59	
	60 min	50	
	4 hr	37	
	8 hr	31	

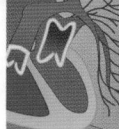

above 500 ppm as being much like hitting a wall, with the degree of damage having much more to do with concentration, analogous to the speed with which one hits the wall, than with the duration of contact with the wall. Concentration is much more important than duration of exposure. Fatal exposures to hydrogen sulfide in humans, for example, may in theory take place at 150 ppm for 6 hours (concentration-time product = 0.252) or 650 ppm for 8.5 minutes (0.005). This means that, for H_2S, higher concentrations are much more toxic, even with proportionally shorter exposure levels. This also appears to be true for experimental pulmonary edema induced in the rat. Many current models for risk assessment use a concentration-time constant for lethality of the general form $C^n \times t$, where n ranges from 1.43 to more than 4.36; the empirical evidence favors the higher exponents. Occupational exposure levels based on time-weighted averages do not take this into account.[6,72]

Sour gas, the accepted term in the oil patch for natural gas containing H_2S, contains more than natural gas and hydrogen sulfide. The process stream contains variable amounts of methyl mercaptans (CH_3SH, $[CH_3]_2S$, and $[CH_3]_2S_2$), carbonyl sulfide (COS) and carbon disulfide (CS_2), and some trace metals. Mercaptans are also added to natural gas as a safety measure to ensure detection of leaks. Production also involves exposure to a variety of production chemicals incidental to gas exposure.[8,73] Flaring introduces numerous other products of incomplete combustion and has become a particularly controversial issue in Alberta in recent years. A major study of downwind exposure to emissions from gas facilities and effects on animals is under way, and findings are expected to be available in the near future.

REFERENCES

1. Kangas J, Jäppinen P, Savoilainen H: Exposure to hydrogen sulphide, mercaptans and sulphur dioxide in the pulp industry. Am Ind Hyg Assoc J 1984;45:787–790.
2. Hoidal CR, Hall AH, Robinson MD, et al: Hydrogen sulphide poisoning from toxic inhalations of roofing asphalt. Ann Emerg Med 1986;15:826–830.
3. Osbern LN, Crapo RO: Dung lung: a report of toxic exposure to liquid manure. Ann Intern Med 1981;95:312–314.
4. Parra O, Mon E, Gallego M, Morera J: Inhalation of hydrogen sulphide: a case of subacute manifestations and long term sequelae. Br J Indust Med 1991;48:286–287.
5. Milby HT, Baselt RC: Hydrogen sulfide poisoning: clarification of some controversial issues. Am J Indust Med 1999;35:192–195.
6. Guidotti TL: Hydrogen sulfide. Occup Med 1996;46(5):367–371.
7. Bates MN, Garrett N, Graham B, Read D: Air pollution and mortality in the Rotorua geothermal area. Aust N Z J Public Health 1997;21(6):581–586.
8. Hoffman H, Guidotti TL: Natural gas. In Greenberg MI, Hamiton RJ, Phillips SD (eds): Occupational, Industrial and Environmental Toxicology. Philadelphia, Mosby, 1997, pp 359–366.
9. Burnett WW, King EG, Grace M, Hall WF: Hydrogen sulfide poisoning: review of 5 years' experience. Can Med Assoc J 1977;117:1277–1280.
10. Alberta Environment Sour-Gas Processing-Plant Applications: A Guide to Content. Calgary: Energy Resources Conservation Board, Guide G-26, 1981.
11. Arnold IMF, Dufresne RM, Alleyne BC, Stuart PJW: Health implications of occupational exposures to hydrogen sulfide. J Occup Med 1985;27:373–376.
12. Evans H: Occupational hygiene at an Alberta (Canada) natural gas processing plant. Ann Occup Hyg 1989;47:221–224.
13. Smith L, Kruszyna H, Smith RP: The effect of methemoglobin on the inhibition of cytochrome c oxidase by cyanide, sulphide or azide. Biochem Pharmacol 1977;26:2247–2250.
14. Smith RP, Gosselin RE: Hydrogen sulphide poisoning. J Occup Med 1979;21:93–97.
15. Roth SH, Skrajny B, Bennington R, Brookes: Neurotoxicity of hydrogen sulphide may result from inhibition of respiratory enzymes. Proc West Pharmacol Soc 1997;40:41–43.
16. Geer JJ, Reiffenstein R, Almeida AF, Carter JE: Sulfide-induced perturbations of the neuronal mechanisms controlling breathing in rats. J Appl Physiol 1995;78(2):433–440.
17. Haggard HW, Henderson Y: The influence of hydrogen sulphide upon respiration. Am J Physiol 1922;61:289–296.
18. Almeida AF, Guidotti TL: Differential sensitivity of lung and brain to sulfide exposure: a peripheral mechanism for apnea. Toxicol Sci 1999;50:287–293.
19. Boehning D, Snyder SH: Novel neural modulators. Annu Rev Neurosci 2003;26:105–131.
20. Klentz RD, Fedde MR: Hydrogen sulfide: effects on avian respiratory control and intrapulmonary CO_2 receptors. Respir Physiol 1978;32(3):55–67.
21. Tansy MF, Kendall FM, Fantasia J, et al: Acute and subchronic toxicity studies of rats exposed to vapors of methyl mercaptan and other reduced-sulphur compounds. J Toxicol Environ Health 1981;8:71–88.
22. Haggard HW: The toxicology of hydrogen sulphide. J Indust Hyg 1925;7:113–121.
23. Hayden LJ, Goeden H, Roth SH: Exposure to low levels of hydrogen sulfide elevates circulating glucose in maternal rats. J Toxicol Environ Health 1990;31:45–52.
24. Roth SH, Skrajny B, Reiffenstein RJ: Alteration of the morphology and neurochemistry of the developing mammalian nervous system by hydrogen sulphide. Clin Exp Pharmacol Physiol 1995;22(5):79–80.
25. Bhambhani Y, Burnham R, Snydmiller G, MacLean I: Effects of 10-ppm hydrogen sulfide inhalation in exercising men and women. Cardiovascular, metabolic, and biochemical responses. J Occup Environ Med 1997;39(2):22–29.
26. Costigan MG: Hydrogen sulfide: UK occupational exposure limits. Occup Environ Med 2003;60(12):918–928.
27. WHO International Programme on Chemical Safety. Environmental Health Criteria 19: Hydrogen Sulphide. Geneva, World Health Organization, 1983.
28. Brenneman KA, James RA, Gross EA, Dorman DC: Olfactory neuron loss in adult male CD rates following subchronic inhalation exposure to hydrogen sulfide. Toxicol Pathol 2000;28(2):26–33.
29. Hirsh AR, Zavala G: Long term effects on the olfactory system of exposure to hydrogen sulfide. Occup Environ Med 1999;56:284–287.
30. Nikkanen HE, Burns MM: Severe hydrogen sulphide exposure in a working adolescent. Pediatrics 2004;113(4):927–929.
31. Richardson DB: Respiratory effects of chronic hydrogen sulphide exposure. Am J Ind Med 1995;28:99–108.
32. Wang DX. A review of 152 cases of acute poisoning of hydrogen sulfide [in Chinese]. Chin J Prev Med 1989;23:330–332.
33. Bhambhani Y, Burnham R, Snydmiller G, et al: Effects of 10-ppm hydrogen sulfide inhalation on pulmonary function in health men and women. J Occup Environ Med 1996;38(10):1012–1017.
34. Jäppinen P, Vikka V, Marttila O, Haatela T: Exposure to hydrogen sulphide and respiratory function. Br J Ind Med 1990;47:824–828.
35. Buick JB, Lowry RC, Magee TRA: Is a reduction in residual volume a sub-clinical manifestation of hydrogen sulfide intoxication? Am J Ind Med 2000;37:296–299.
36. Duong TX, Saruda AJ, Maier LA: Interstitial fibrosis following hydrogen sulfide exposure. Am J Ind Med 2001;40(2):221–224.
37. Guidotti TL: Occupational exposure to hydrogen sulfide in the sour gas industry: some unresolved issues. Int Arch Occup Environ Health 1994;66:153–160.
38. Hayden LJ, Goeden H, Roth SH: Growth and development in the rat during sub-chronic exposure to low levels of hydrogen sulfide. Toxicol Ind Health 1990;6(3–4):389–401.
39. Dorman DC, Brenneman KA, Struve MF, et al: Fertility and developmental neurotoxicity effects of inhaled hydrogen sulfide in Sprague-Dawley rats. Neurotoxicol Teratol 2000;22:71–84.

40. Berglin EH, Carlsson J: Effect of hydrogen sulfide on the mutagenicity of hydrogen peroxide in Salmonella typhimurium strain TA102. Mutat Res 1986;175(1):5–9.

41. Bates MN, Garrett N, Graham B, Read D: Cancer incidence, morbidity and geothermal air pollution in Rotorua, New Zealand. Int J Epidemiol 1998;20(3):339–408.

42. Kilburn K: Case report: profound neurobehavioural deficits in an oil field worker overcome by hydrogen sulfide. Am J Med Sci 1993;306:301–305.

43. Snyder JW, Safir EF, Summerville GP, Middleberg RA: Occupational fatality and persistent neurological sequelae after mass exposure to hydrogen sulfide. Am J Emerg Med 1995;13:199–203.

44. Tvedt B, Edland A, Skyberg K, Forberg O: Delayed neuropsychiatric sequelae after acute hydrogen sulfide poisoning: affection of motor function, memory, vision, and hearing. Acta Neurol Scand 1991;84:348–351.

45. Tanaka S, Fujimoto S, Tamagaki Y, et al: Bronchial injury and pulmonary edema caused by hydrogen sulphide poisoning. Am J Emerg Med 1999;17(4):427–429.

46. Schneider JS, Tobe EH, Mozley PD Jr, et al: Persistent cognitive and motor deficits following acute hydrogen sulphide poisoning. Occup Med (Lond) 1998;48(4):255–260.

47. Inoue N. Extrapyramidal syndrome induced by chemical substances [in Japanese]. Nippon Rinsho 1993;51(11):2924–2928.

48. Kilburn KH: Exposure to reduced sulphur gases impairs neurobehavioral function. South Med J 1997;90(10):997–1006.

49. Spitzer WO, for the McGill Inter-University Research Group: The Southwestern Alberta Medical Diagnostic Review: Summary. Montreal, June 1986.

50. Struve MF, Brisbois JN, James RA, et al: Neurotoxicological effects associated with short-term exposure of Sprague-Dawley rats to hydrogen sulphide. Neurotoxicol 2001;22(3):375–385.

51. Smith RP, Kruszyna R, Kruszyna H: Management of acute sulfide poisoning: effects of thiosulfate, oxygen, and nitrite. Arch Environ Health 1976;31:166–169.

52. Goodwin LR, Francom D, Dieken FP, et al: Determination of sulphide in brain tissue by gas dialysis/ion chromatography: postmortem studies and two case reports. J Anal Toxicol 1989;13(2):105–109.

53. Gabbay DS, De Roos F, Perrone J: Twenty-foot fall averts fatality from massive hydrogen sulphide exposure. J Emerg Med 2001;20(2):141–144.

54. Stine RJ, Slosberg B, Beacham BE: Hydrogen sulfide intoxication: a case report and discussion of treatment. Ann Intern Med 1976;85:756–758.

55. Vannatta JB: Hydrogen sulfide poisoning: report of four cases and brief review of the literature. J Okla State Med Assoc 1982;75:29–32.

56. Mack RB: World enough and time: hydrogen sulfide poisoning. N C Med J 1987;48:33–34.

57. Ravizza AG, Carugo D, Cerchiari EL, et al: The treatment of hydrogen sulfide intoxication: oxygen versus nitrites. Vet Human Toxicol 1982;24:241–242.

58. Beck JF, Bradbury CM, Conors AJ, Donini JC: Nitrite as antidote for acute hydrogen sulfide intoxication? Am Ind Hyg Assoc J 1981;42:805–809.

59. Smilkstein MJ, Bronstein AC, Pickett HM, Rumack BH: Hyperbaric oxygen therapy for severe hydrogen sulphide poisoning. J Emerg Med 1985;3:27–30.

60. Whitcraft DD III, Bailey TD, Hart GB: Hydrogen sulfide poisoning treated with hyperbaric oxygen. J Emerg Med 1985;3:23–25.

61. Gorman DF: Problems and pitfalls in the use of hyperbaric oxygen for the treatment of poisoned patients. Med Toxicol Adverse Drug Exp 1989;4:393–399.

62. Peters JW: Hydrogen sulfide poisoning in a hospital setting. J Am Med Assn 1981;246:1558–1589.

63. Demaret D, Fialaire J: Les intoxications par l'hydrogène sulfuré dans une raffinerie de gaz naturel. J Eur Toxicol 1974;1:32–36.

64. Warenycia MW, Smith KA, Blashko CS, et al: Monoamine oxidase inhibition as a sequel of hydrogen sulfide intoxication: increase in brain catecholamine and 5-hydroxytryptamine levels. Arch Toxicol 1989;63:131–136.

65. Warenycia MW, Goodwin LR, Francom DM, et al: Dithiothreitol liberates non-acid labile sulfide from brain tissue of H_2S-poisoned animals. Arch Toxicol 1990;64(8):650–655.

66. Dulaney M Jr, Hume AS: Pyruvic acid protects against the lethality of sulfide. Res Commun Chem Pathol Pharmacol 1988;59:133.

67. Hume AS, Dulaney MD: The effectiveness of various ketocarboxylic acids in preventing sulfide-induced lethality. Toxicologist 1988;8:28.

68. Mattarano DA, Merinar T: Respiratory protection on offshore drilling rigs. Appl Occup Environ Hyg 1999;14:141–148.

69. Ronk R, White MK: Hydrogen sulphide and the probabilities of "inhalation" through a tympanic membrane defect. J Occup Med 1985;27(5):337–340.

70. Turner RM, Fairhurst S: Toxicology of substances in relation to major hazards: hydrogen sulphide. London, HMSO, 1990, pp 1–14.

71. Provincial Advisory Committee on Public Safety and Sour Gas: Public Safety and Sour Gas: Findings and Recommendations—Final Report. Calgary, Alberta, Energy and Utilities Board, 2000.

72. Prior MG, Sharma AK, Yong S, Lopez A: Concentration-time interactions in hydrogen sulphide toxicity in rats. Can J Vet Res 1988;52:375–379.

73. Cottle MKW, Guidotti TL: Process chemicals in the oil and gas industry: potential occupational hazards. Toxicol Ind Health 1989;6:41–56.

92 *Petroleum Distillates and Plant Hydrocarbons*

WILLIAM J. LEWANDER, MD ■ ALFRED ALEGUAS, JR., RPH, BSPharm, PHARMD

At a Glance...

- Patients should be evaluated for pulmonary, gastrointestinal, and CNS toxicity.
- Management is primarily symptomatic and supportive.
- Radiographic findings do not always correlate with clinical presentation.
- All symptomatic or suicidal patients should be admitted.
- Patients who remain asymptomatic for 6 hours with normal radiographic findings may be considered for discharge.

Hydrocarbons are a group of organic compounds composed primarily of hydrogen and carbon. Common hydrocarbons are derived either directly from plants (e.g., pine oil) or from petroleum distillates. Although often mixtures, petroleum distillates are of three basic types: aliphatic, halogenated, and aromatic hydrocarbons. Aromatic and halogenated hydrocarbons are discussed in other chapters. Petroleum distillates are produced from the fractional distillation of crude petroleum and contain various amounts of aliphatic (straight chain) and aromatic (cyclic) hydrocarbons. Those classified predominantly as aliphatic hydrocarbons are discussed here. Some examples are kerosene, gasoline, mineral spirits, naphtha, mineral seal oil, diesel oil, and fuel oil (see Table 73-1). Turpentine is a hydrocarbon made from pine oil.

EPIDEMIOLOGY

Hydrocarbon exposures are frequent and account for an inordinate number of health care visits and hospital admissions. The American Association of Poison Control Centers reported 59,132 hydrocarbon exposures in 2002.[1] Twenty-two percent of exposed individuals required treatment in a health care facility, and nearly 22% of these patients were considered to have suffered exposures of moderate or major severity. Nearly half of all exposures occur in children younger than 6 years of age, and the vast majority of exposures are unintentional. Nevertheless, intentional exposures are not uncommon and frequently have greater potential for toxicity. Fifteen deaths were reported as a result of hydrocarbon exposure in 2002.[1]

Petroleum distillates continue to be the most commonly reported cause of hydrocarbon poisoning, accounting for more than 39,000 exposures. Unmarked, poorly stored containers and an attractive aroma or color may account for the high percentage of exposures among young children. In adults, poisoning is most often by intentional ingestion, occupational exposure, or inadvertant aspiration when siphoning fuels. Adult ingestions generally involve larger volumes along with a greater likelihood of co-ingested toxins. The most common route of exposure is by ingestion, but inhalation, cutaneous, and intravenous exposures have been reported. Nearly one quarter require treatment in a health care facility. The most commonly ingested products in this group in order of frequency are (1) gasoline, (2) lubricating oil, (3) mineral spirits, (4) lighter fluid or naphtha, (5) lamp oil, and (6) kerosene.[1]

PATHOPHYSIOLOGY

Petroleum distillates are potent solvents, capable of destroying lipid-containing cell membranes. The toxicity of petroleum distillates is mainly a result of their potential to cause a fulminant and sometimes fatal pneumonitis when aspirated. Central nervous system (CNS), gastrointestinal (GI), hepatic, renal, cardiovascular, and hematologic toxicity may also occur. Cutaneous toxicity may occur with prolonged dermal exposure. After oral ingestion, pulmonary toxicity occurs from aspiration rather than by GI absorption. Aspiration may occur when the hydrocarbon is initially ingested or during vomiting. Although vomiting often precedes and results in aspiration, lack of vomiting does not preclude the possibility that aspiration has occurred. The potential for aspiration is determined by the physical properties of viscosity, surface tension, and volatility. The risk of aspiration involving any particular petroleum distillate increases with low viscosity, low surface tension, and high volatility.[2] However, the single most important property determining aspiration potential is viscosity, the tendency to resist flow. Low viscosity allows penetration further into the distal airways. Viscosity is measured in Saybolt seconds universal (SSU). Substances with an SSU value greater than 100 have a low aspiration potential (e.g., mineral and fuel oil), whereas those with an SSU value of less than 45 have a high potential for aspiration (e.g., gasoline, kerosene, mineral seal oil). Low surface tension may allow the petroleum distillate to spread from the upper GI tract to the trachea, and high volatility (i.e., tendency of a liquid to become a gas) increases the likelihood of pulmonary absorption and risk of CNS depression that can blunt the gag reflex. When aspirated, petroleum distillates dissolve surfactant, resulting in alveolar collapse, ventilation-perfusion mismatch, and subsequent hypoxemia.[2-4] Bronchospasm and direct capillary damage lead to a chemical pneumonitis and hemorrhagic bronchitis and alveolitis that peak in intensity at about 3 days.[5] A late process of alveolar proliferation and thickening may occur, peaking at about 10 days.[5] Upper airway injury may occur and includes hyperemia, mucosal irritation, and inflammation

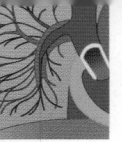

of the oropharynx. A case of epiglottitis has been reported after gasoline ingestion.[6]

Systemic toxicity is uncommon after ingestion or aspiration but may develop if a petroleum distillate contains toxic additives, if it is a vehicle for more toxic substances, or if a massive ingestion has occurred. The specific toxin involved determines whether cardiovascular, renal, hepatic, or hematologic toxicity ensues.[7] Petroleum distillate inhalation abuse (e.g., gasoline sniffing) does not produce a chemical pneumonitis but instead leads to complex CNS toxicity caused by the combined effects of its many constituents (e.g., aromatic hydrocarbons, naphthenes, and tetraethyl lead).[8,9]

Plant Hydrocarbons (Terpenes)

Terpenes are aliphatic or cyclic hydrocarbons and include turpentine, pine oil, and camphor. Pine oil, a component of many household cleaners, is a product of pine trees and is composed primarily of terpene alcohols. It is normally present in cleaners in concentrations of 20% to 35% and occasionally as high as 60% in products such as Pine Sol. Turpentine is a distillate from pine trees and is commonly used as a solvent for paints and varnishes. Camphor is discussed in Chapter 99.

Pine oil is well absorbed from the GI tract and is metabolized by the epoxide pathway and excreted in the urine.[10] The volume of distribution is thought to be quite large, with the highest concentrations found in the brain, lungs, and kidneys.

Turpentine is also readily absorbed through the GI tract and lungs[11] and distributed throughout the body. The highest concentrations are found in the liver, spleen, kidneys, and brain.[12] The details of turpentine metabolism remain unclear. Elimination of turpentine and its metabolites is primarily by the kidneys.

Because of the terpenes' lower volatility and higher viscosity, the risk of aspiration is somewhat less than with the more volatile or less viscous hydrocarbons. In addition to the aspiration risk, pine oil and turpentine produce more CNS and GI symptoms than do the aliphatic hydrocarbons. Ingestions of turpentine exceeding 2 mL/kg are potentially toxic.[11] Although adults have survived pine oil ingestions of up to 500 g,[13] the commonly cited lethal dose is 60 to 120 g. In children, the minimum lethal dose is probably 14 g.[10]

CLINICAL PRESENTATION

The initial signs and symptoms following petroleum distillate ingestion usually involve three main organ systems: pulmonary, GI, and CNS. The majority of children who present to health care facilities after a petroleum distillate exposure remain asymptomatic. Patients who aspirate generally demonstrate initial symptoms (e.g., coughing, gasping, and choking) within 30 minutes; these reach peak intensity between 24 and 48 hours after exposure.[14] During the first 24 hours, tachypnea with grunting respirations, nasal flaring, retractions, and

cyanosis may develop or may be delayed as long as 2 days.[4] The characteristic odor of the petroleum distillate may be apparent on the breath. Although auscultation may reveal rales, rhonchi, and wheezing, lower airway involvement cannot be predicted by initially normal findings on examination. Hemoptysis and pulmonary edema may be observed in severe cases. Laboratory evaluation (e.g., arterial blood gases, pulse oximetry) may reveal hypoxemia (from ventilation-perfusion mismatching) and early hypocarbia. This may progress to hypercarbia and acidosis. As many as 75% of hospitalized patients demonstrate chest film abnormalities. These abnormalities occur within 2 hours in up to 88% of patients and in 98% by 12 hours.[7,15,16] Common early changes include unilateral and bilateral basilar infiltrates, punctate perihilar densities, and localized areas of atelectasis.[15-18] Pneumatoceles are infrequent but when they occur are delayed in onset (e.g., 3 to 15 days) and resolution (e.g., 15 days to 21 months).[19] Pleural effusion, pneumothorax, pneumomediastinum, pneumopericardium, and subcutaneous emphysema may develop.[15,17,20,21] Symptoms correlate poorly with radiographic findings, and both may be delayed in onset.[7,22] It is best to treat patients rather than rely on the absence of or delayed resolution of radiographic findings. Although fever and leukocytosis may be noted in as many as 15% to 20% of victims during the first 48 hours, their persistence suggests bacterial superinfection.[14]

GI symptoms are common and include local irritation of the oropharynx, nausea, vomiting, and abdominal pain. Vomiting appears to increase the likelihood of aspiration.[17,23] CNS toxicity may occur in the presence of aspiration-induced hypoxemia, large ingestions, or toxic additives (e.g., aromatic hydrocarbons). Symptoms range from lethargy (91%) or somnolence (5%) to coma (3%) and seizures (1%).[7,24]

Cardiovascular toxicity is uncommon, but both fatal dysrhythmias and myocardial dysfunction have been reported.[25] Dysrhythmias and sudden death after siphoning gasoline may be attributed to hypoxia or absorption after aspiration resulting in myocardial sensitization to endogenous catecholamines.[7,22] A 19-month-old girl developed severe, reversible myocardial dysfunction after ingesting paint thinner.[24] Isolated case reports of acute renal tubular necrosis,[26,27] supraglottitis,[28] severe burns after prolonged immersion in gasoline,[29] and hemoglobinuria secondary to intravascular hemolysis have been reported.[28,30] One case report associated turpentine ingestion with hemorrhagic cystitis.[31] Both inhalation abuse and parenteral administration of petroleum distillates have been reported to cause toxicity. CNS manifestations of inhalation abuse include confusion, dizziness, agitation, incoordination, and coma.[7,8,32,33] Inhalation of leaded gasoline has also been associated with the development of organic lead poisoning.[8,9,32,33] Parenteral administration has resulted in thrombophlebitis, cellulitis, and necrotizing myositis with compartment syndrome. Systemic toxicity includes seizures, hemorrhagic pneumonitis, pulmonary edema, and febrile reactions.[34-36]

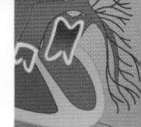

Systemic toxicity of pine oil and turpentine ingestion primarily consists of GI irritation and CNS depression. Signs and symptoms include nausea, vomiting, diarrhea, weakness, somnolence, or agitation. Severe cases may present as stupor or coma; seizures are uncommon.[37] When systemic toxicity occurs, it usually develops within 2 to 3 hours of the exposure. GI and CNS symptoms generally resolve within 12 hours in moderately severe exposures. Dysuria and hematuria thought to be secondary to hemorrhagic cystitis have been reported in a turpentine ingestion 12 to 72 hours after exposure.[31]

DIAGNOSTIC EVALUATION

All symptomatic patients should receive a medical evaluation. A thorough history should include product identification, approximate amount, concentration, time of ingestion, and symptoms before presentation. The physical examination should focus on the vital signs and mental status, and the pulmonary and GI systems. If significant aspiration has occurred, respiratory symptoms should develop within 6 hours and reach peak intensity 24 to 48 hours after exposure.[14] Pulse oximetry should be performed and a chest film obtained. Laboratory evaluation for symptomatic patients and for those who have ingested concomitant toxins may include arterial blood gas determination; complete blood count; determinations of electrolytes, glucose, blood urea nitrogen, and creatinine; urinalysis; and liver function tests. A directed toxic screen may help confirm the presence of toxic additives or other concomitant ingestions. Patients without symptoms for 6 hours after exposure remain asymptomatic.[14]

The distinctive odors of pine oil and turpentine and a thorough history and physical examination are the keys to diagnosis. The examination should focus on the pulmonary, GI, and central nervous systems. No specific laboratory tests help determine severity.[11] If aspiration is suspected, an arterial blood gas determination and appropriately timed chest radiograph should be obtained.

MANAGEMENT

Clinical and radiographic assessment of a patient's respiratory status determines initial management. Patients who remain asymptomatic with normal findings on chest films (obtained 4 or more hours after exposure) may be discharged after 6 hours of observation. Patients who are symptomatic, who have abnormal findings on chest films, or who have suicidal intent should be hospitalized. Gastric decontamination is not recommended for petroleum distillate ingestions because absorption and systemic toxicity are minimal, and spontaneous or induced vomiting increases the risk of aspiration and pneumonitis.[38-40]

Patients who have ingested toxic additives or other toxins with systemic toxicity should be considered for gastric decontamination. This decision is complex, often must be individualized, and should be made after con-

sultation with the regional poison center. The incidence of aspiration pneumonitis may be increased by either gastric lavage or ipecac-induced emesis. Either method is acceptable in an awake, alert patient.[16,38] When GI decontamination is indicated in patients with altered mental status, the airway should first be protected by endotracheal intubation. Activated charcoal is indicated only if an adsorbable toxic additive or concomitant ingestion has occurred. Clothing that has been contaminated should be carefully removed, and contaminated skin washed with soap and water.[7]

Patients with respiratory symptoms should be given oxygen, placed on cardiopulmonary and pulse oximetry monitors, and have intravenous access established. An arterial blood gas determination and chest film should be obtained. Findings on chest films do not always correlate with the clinical status of the patient. The need for intubation should be based on the clinical assessment of respiratory distress. Continuous positive airway pressure may be necessary to maintain oxygenation, and bronchospasm should be treated with noncardioselective bronchodilators because of potential myocardial sensitization to catecholamines.[41] Supportive care of serious petroleum distillate pneumonitis includes careful monitoring of fluid and electrolyte balance, continuous pulse oximetry, and serial chest films. Complete blood counts with differential and sputum Gram staining and cultures help identify bacterial superinfection. The regional poison center should be consulted. Fever and leukocytosis secondary to chemical pneumonitis are commonly noted during the first 24 to 48 hours, and prophylactic antibiotics should not be instituted.[39,42,43] Treatment with antibiotics should be provided only to patients with documented bacterial pneumonia (e.g., Gram staining or culture of sputum or tracheal aspirate) or worsening of chest film findings, chest pain, leukocytosis, and fever after the first 40 hours.[7,22] Several animal and clinical investigations have failed to demonstrate any benefit from corticosteroid treatment. Two animal studies indicate they may be harmful[42-45]; therefore, corticosteroids should not be administered.

Several reports document the efficacy of both extracorporeal membrane oxygenation and high-frequency jet ventilation as alternative therapies when conventional treatment for respiratory failure is unsuccessful.[46-49]

Most patients with petroleum distillate poisoning recover fully with supportive care. The majority have no significant sequelae despite the report of minor pulmonary function abnormalities in as many as 82% of asymptomatic survivors of aspiration pneumonitis.[20] Long-term follow-up with pulmonary testing should be considered. When indicated, psychiatric consultation should be obtained and poison prevention education given before discharge.

With plant hydrocarbons, the time and amount of ingestion, evidence of aspiration, and patient's level of consciousness largely determine treatment. A fully alert patient who is seen within 2 hours of ingesting greater than 2 mL/kg of turpentine should be considered for GI decontamination. Although not clearly defined

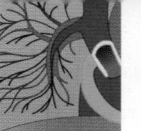

for pine oil, lavage is generally recommended for ingestions of greater than 5 mL in adults.[50] Airway protection is recommended for all but the alert patients because of the risk of aspiration. Activated charcoal is not useful, and the apparent large volume of distribution of terpenes precludes the use of hemodialysis or hemoperfusion.

Disposition

Medical disposition is based on clinical toxicity and time since ingestion. Patients who are either asymptomatic or who have only mild GI or CNS symptoms after 6 hours are unlikely to develop serious complications. All patients with evidence of significant toxicity (i.e., pulmonary or CNS) should be admitted for symptomatic and supportive care.

REFERENCES

1. Watson WA, Litovitz TL, Rodgers GC, et al: 2002 Annual Report of the American Association of Poison Control Centers Toxic Exposure Surveillance System. Am J Emerg Med 2003;21:353.
2. Gerarde HW: Toxicologic studies on hydrocarbons. 9. The aspiration hazard and toxicity of hydrocarbons and hydrocarbon mixtures. Arch Environ Health 1963;6:329.
3. Giammona ST: Effects of furniture polish on pulmonary surfactant. Am J Dis Child 1967;13:658.
4. Truemper E, DeLaRocha SR, Atkinson SD: Clinical characteristics, pathophysiology, and management of hydrocarbon ingestion: case report and review of the literature. Pediatr Emerg Care 1987;3:187.
5. Gross P, McNerney JM, Babyak MA: Kerosene pneumonitis: an experimental study with small doses. Am Rev Respir Dis 1963;88:656.
6. Grufferman S, Walker FW: Supraglottitis following gasoline ingestion. Ann Emerg Med 1982;11:368.
7. Ellenhorn MJ, Barceloux DG: Medical Toxicology, Diagnosis, and Treatment of Human Poisoning. New York, Elsevier, 1988, p 940.
8. Fortenberry JD: Gasoline sniffing. Am J Med 1985;79:740.
9. Edminster SC, Bayer MJ: Recreational gasoline sniffing: acute gasoline intoxication and latent organolead poisoning. J Emerg Med 1985;3:365.
10. Jill RM, Barer J, Leighton Hill L, et al: An investigation of recurrent pine oil poisoning in an infant by the use of gas-chromatographic mass spectrometric methods. J Pediatr 1975;87:115.
11. McGuigan MA: Turpentine. Clin Toxicol Rev 1985;8:1.
12. Sperling F: In vivo and in vitro toxicology of turpentines. Clin Toxicol 1969;2:21.
13. Koppel C, Tenczer J, Tennesmarm U, et al: Acute poisoning with pine oil: metabolism of monoterpenes. Arch Toxicol 1981;49:73.
14. Anas N, Narnasonthia V, Ginsburg CM: Criteria for hospitalizing children who have ingested products containing hydrocarbons. JAMA 1981;246:840.
15. Eade NR, Taussig LM, Marks MI: Hydrocarbon pneumonitis. Pediatrics 1974;54:351.
16. Beamon RF, Siegel CJ, Landers G, et al: Hydrocarbon ingestion in children: a six year retrospective study. JACEP 1976;5:771.
17. Foley JC, Dreyer NB, Soule AB Jr, et al: Kerosene poisoning in young children. Radiology 1954;62:817.
18. Ervin ME: Petroleum distillates and turpentine. In Haddad LM, Winchester JF (eds): Clinical Management of Poisoning and Drug Overdose. Philadelphia, WB Saunders, 1983, p 771.
19. Bergeson PS, Hates SW, Lustgarten MD, et al: Pneumatoceles following hydrocarbon ingestion. Am J Dis Child 1975;129:49.
20. Gurwitz D, Kattan M, Levison H, et al: Pulmonary function abnormalities in asymptomatic children after hydrocarbon pneumonitis. Pediatrics 1970;62:789.
21. Brunner S, Rovsing H, Wulf H: Roentgenographic changes in the lungs of children with kerosene poisoning. Am Rev Respir Dis 1964;89:250.
22. Klein BL, Simon JE: Hydrocarbon poisonings. Pediatr Clin North Am 1986;33:411.
23. Bratton L, Haddow JE: Ingestion of charcoal lighter fluid. J Pediatr 1974;87:633.
24. Myocardial dysfunction after hydrocarbon ingestion (abstract). Crit Care Med 1994;22:3.
25. Bass M: Death from sniffing gasoline (letter). N Engl J Med 1978;299:203.
26. Barrientos A, Ortuno MT, Morales JM, et al: Acute renal failure after use of diesel fuel as shampoo. Arch Intern Med 1977;137:1217.
27. Crisp AJ, Bhalla AK, Hoffbrand BI: Acute tubular necrosis after exposure to diesel oil. BMJ 1979;2:177.
28. Crisp AJ, Bhalla AK, Hoffbrand BI: Acute tubular necrosis after exposure to diesel oil. BMJ 1979;2:177.
29. Walsh WA, Scarpa FJ, Brown RS, et al: Gasoline immersion burn case report. N Engl J Med 1974;291:830.
30. Stockman JA: More on hydrocarbon-induced hemolysis. J Pediatr 1977;90:848.
31. Klein FA, Hackler RH: Hemorrhagic cystitis associated with turpentine ingestion. Urology 1980;16:187.
32. Poklis A, Burkett CD: Gasoline sniffing: a review. Clin Toxicol 1977;11:35.
33. Chessare JD, Wodarcyk K: Gasoline sniffing and lead poisoning in a child. Am Fam Physician 1988;38:181.
34. Wason S, Greiner PT: Intravenous hydrocarbon abuse. Am J Emerg Med 1986;4:543.
35. Neeld EM, Limacher MC: Chemical pneumonitis after the intravenous injection of hydrocarbons. Radiology 1978;129:36.
36. Tennenbein M: Hydrocarbon ingestion. Curr Probl Pediatr 1986;16:221.
37. Jacobziner H, Raybin HW: Turpentine poisoning. Arch Pediatr 1961;78:357.
38. Press E, Adams WC, Chittenden RF, et al: Report of the subcommittee on accidental poisoning: co-operative kerosene poisoning study. Pediatrics 1962;29:648.
39. Litovitz T, Green AE: Health implications of petroleum distillate ingestion. Occup Med 1988;3:555.
40. Cachia EA, Fenech FF: Kerosene poisoning in children. Arch Dis Child 1964;39:502.
41. James FW, Kaplan S, Benzing G: Cardiac complications following hydrocarbon ingestion. Am J Dis Child 1971;121:431.
42. Steele RW, Conklin RH, Mark HM: Corticosteroids and antibotics for the treatment of fulminant hydrocarbon aspiration. JAMA 1972;219:1424.
43. Brown J, Burke B, Dajani AS: Experimental kerosene pneumonia: evaluation of some therapeutic regimens. J Pediatr 1974;84:396.
44. Zieserl E: Hydrocarbon ingestion and poisoning. Compr Ther 1979;5:35.
45. Marks MI, Chicoine L, Legere G, et al: Adrenocorticosteroid treatment of hydrocarbon pneumonia in children: a cooperative study. J Pediatr 1972;81:366.
46. Scazo AJ, Weber TR, et al: Extracorporeal membrane oxyenation for hydrocarbon aspiration. Am J Dis Child 1990;144:867.
47. Weber TR, Tracey TF, et al: Prolonged extracorporeal support for nonneonatal respiratory failure. J Pediatr Surg 1992;27:1100.
48. Bysani GK, Rucoba RJ, et al: Treatment of hydrocarbon pneumonitis. Chest 1994;106:300.
49. Lee LK, Shannon M: The use of high frequency oscillatory ventilation in hydrocarbon pneumonitis. Int J Med Toxicol 2003;6(2):10.
50. Brook MP, McCarron MM, Mueller JA: Pine oil cleaner ingestion. Ann Emerg Med 1989;18:391.

93 *Chlorinated Hydrocarbons*

ROBERT B. PALMER, PHD ■ SCOTT D. PHILLIPS, MD

At a Glance...

- Chlorinated hydrocarbons generally share three acute health effects: dermatitis, narcosis, and the ability to induce cardiac arrhythmias.
- One of these compounds, carbon tetrachloride, was banned in the United States because of its propensity for hepatotoxicity and carcinogenesis.
- Trichloroethylene and tetrachloroethylene (perchloroethylene) continue to be employed as industrial solvents and the latter as a dry cleaning agent.
- Most of these compounds are highly volatile but generally not flammable—some have been used for fire extinguishing.
- CNS toxicity is prominent and may result from accidental exposure or intentional abuse. Seizures and coma are possible.
- Cardiac toxicity has been attributed to membrane stabilization and "sensitization" to catecholamines, although other mechanisms may play a role. Sudden sniffing deaths may occur.
- Carbon tetrachloride may cause hepatic necrosis. Other chlorinated hydrocarbons may cause fatty liver.
- Defatting of the skin may lead to chronic irritant dermatitis.
- Removal from exposure and supportive care is indicated in the treatment of disease caused by chlorinated hydrocarbons.

Compounds of only carbon, hydrogen, and chlorine are collectively known as *chlorinated hydrocarbons*. These compounds are used for a variety of industrial and medical purposes, including degreasing solvents in manufacture and topical anesthetics. Chlorinated hydrocarbons are not naturally occurring. Human exposures to these compounds are typically either the result of solvent abuse or occupational or environmental in nature. Although the specific toxicity profiles for the individual chlorinated hydrocarbons vary, essentially all these compounds share three fundamental acute effects: dermatitis, narcosis, and the potential to induce cardiac dysrhythmias. Literally hundreds of compounds are classifiable as chlorinated hydrocarbons, but the most commonly encountered are chlorinated derivatives of methane, ethane, and ethylene (Table 93-1). These compounds are the focus of this chapter.

Trichloromethane (chloroform) was first used as a veterinary anesthetic in 1847; its first reported use in human surgery came later that same year.[1,2] Chloroform was the anesthetic agent of choice for nearly a century until the post–World War II era when compounds less toxic to the heart and liver were developed. Chloroform has also gained notoriety as an anesthetic agent used for murder or to incapacitate people for nefarious purposes.[3] More recent medical applications of chloroform include topical use in herpes labialis, where it was shown to decrease time to scab formation when compared with control.[4] Warmed (40° C) chloroform has also been used to liquefy cholesterol gallstones.[4]

Other medical applications for chlorinated hydrocarbons include the use of small oral doses of carbon tetrachloride as an antihelminthic agent to treat hookworm infection in the 1920s. Despite its efficacy, use of carbon tetrachloride for this purpose was associated with hepatic necrosis, renal injury, and gastrointestinal hemorrhage, especially in alcoholics and malnourished children. Because of this, carbon tetrachloride was replaced with tetrachloroethylene for the management of both hookworm and pinworm. Tens of thousands of cases were treated with tetrachloroethylene, and only mild adverse effects, such as giddiness and lightheadedness, were reported. Chloroform, as part of "Hermann's mixture" (chloroform, eucalyptus oil, and castor oil), was also employed in the management of hookworm infestation.[5]

In addition to its former use as an antihelminthic agent, carbon tetrachloride saw widespread industrial use as a degreasing solvent, dry cleaning agent, grain fumigant, and as fire extinguisher component.[6] However, as a result of its potential toxicity, household use of carbon tetrachloride was banned in 1970, and its use as a grain fumigant was discontinued in the United States in 1985.[6] The principal contemporary use of carbon tetrachloride is as an intermediate in the synthesis of chlorofluorocarbon refrigerants.[7]

The two-carbon (ethane and ethene) chlorinated derivatives have been used extensively as degreasing solvents, in the preparation of many insecticidal fumigants, and in dry cleaning. Trichloroethylene is also used in the textile industry for removing basting threads and as a swelling agent for dying polyester as well as a diluent for paints and varnishes. Trichloroethylene has also seen use as an inhaled anesthetic and is known to have poor muscle relaxant but excellent analgesic properties.[4,6] In the past, trichloroethylene was used in the extraction of olive oil; however, the use of this solvent in the food industry was eliminated in 1975.[8] Tetrachloroethylene is still used in American veterinary medicine as an antihelminthic and is available in capsules ranging from 0.2 to 5.0 mL and marketed by Parke Davis as NemaWorm. The antihelminthic activity of tetrachloroethylene is reportedly due to the ability of the compound to interfere with the release of lysosomal enzymes in the gut of nematodes. This results in paralysis of the parasitic worms, breaking their adhesion to the intestinal wall.[9]

PHYSICOCHEMICAL PROPERTIES

The chlorinated hydrocarbons discussed in this chapter are small aliphatic (acyclic open chain) organic com-

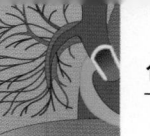

TABLE 93-1 Commonly Encountered Chlorinated Hydrocarbons

COMPOUND	PHYSICAL DESCRIPTION	EXPOSURE GUIDELINES	METABOLITES	POTENTIAL TOXICITIES	TARGET ORGANS	IARC CLASS
Dichloromethane (methylene chloride; DCM) Cl—C—Cl with H above and H below the central C MW: 84.9 g/mol Density: 1.320 g/mL Vapor pressure: 45 kPa CAS: 75–09-2	Colorless volatile nonflammable liquid with a sweet ether-like odor Odor threshold variable from 25–150 ppm	TLV (TWA): 50 ppm PEL (TWA): 25 ppm PEL (STEL): 125 ppm IDLH: 2300 ppm	Carbon monoxide Carbon dioxide Formaldehyde Formic acid	Irritant Burns with high concentrations CNS depression with high concentrations	CNS Skin Heart	2B
Trichloromethane (chloroform) Cl—C—Cl with H above and Cl below the central C MW: 119.4 g/mol Density: 1.492 g/mL Vapor pressure: 21 kPa CAS: 67-66-3	Heavy colorless volatile nonflammable liquid with a sweet taste and odor Odor threshold 85 ppm	TLV (TWA): 10 ppm PEL (STEL-C): 50 ppm IDLH: 500 ppm	Chloromethanol Hydrochloric acid Phosgene Carbon dioxide Diglutathionyl dithiocarbonate	Irritant Burns with high concentrations CNS depression with high concentrations Hepatorenal toxicity	CNS Skin Heart Liver Kidney	2B
Tetrachloromethane (carbon tetrachloride) Cl—C—Cl with Cl above and Cl below the central C MW: 153.8 g/mol Density: 1.594 g/mL Vapor pressure: 12 kPa CAS: 56–23–5	Heavy colorless volatile nonflammable liquid a sweet ether-like odor Odor threshold > 10 ppm	TLV (TWA): 5 ppm PEL (TWA): 10 ppm PEL (STEL-C): 25 ppm IDLH: 200 ppm	Trichloromethyl radical Phosgene Hydrochloric acid	Irritant Burns with high concentrations CNS depression with high concentrations Hepatorenal toxicity	CNS Skin Heart Liver Kidney	2B

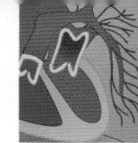

TABLE 93-1 Commonly Encountered Chlorinated Hydrocarbons (Cont'd)

COMPOUND	PHYSICAL DESCRIPTION	EXPOSURE GUIDELINES	METABOLITES	POTENTIAL TOXICITIES	TARGET ORGANS	IARC CLASS
1,1,1-Trichloroethane (methylchloroform; TCA) MW: 133.4 g/mol Density: 1.338 g/mL Vapor pressure: 13 kPa CA: 71-55-6	Colorless watery volatile nonflammable liquid a pleasant sweet ether-like odor	TLV (TWA): 350 ppm TLV (STEL): 450 ppm PEL (TWA): 350 ppm IDLH: 700 ppm	Trichloroethanol Trichloroacetic acid	Irritant Burns with high concentrations CNS depression with high concentrations	CNS Skin Heart	3
Trichloroethene (trichloroethylene; TCE) MW: 131.4 g/mol Density: 1.463 g/mL Vapor pressure: 8 kPa CAS: 79-01-6	Clear colorless volatile non-flammable liquid a pleasant sweet ether-like odor May be dyed blue Odor threshold 50–100 ppm	TLV (TWA): 50 ppm TLV (STEL): 100 ppm PEL (TWA): 100 ppm PEL (STEL-C): 200 ppm IDLH: 1000 ppm	Trichloroethanol Trichloroacetic acid Chloroform Chloroacetic acid Dichloroacetic acid	Irritant Burns with high concentrations CNS depression with high concentrations Hepatorenal toxicity	CNS Skin Heart Liver Kidney	2A
Tetrachloroethene (tetrachloroethylene; perchloroethylene; PCE) MW: 165.8 g/mol Density: 1.623 g/mL Vapor pressure: 1.9 kPa CAS: 127-18-4	Clear colorless volatile nonflammable liquid a sweet ether-like odor that will rapidly sink to the bottom when mixed with water	TLV (TWA): 25 ppm TLV (STEK): 100 ppm PEL (TWA): 100 ppm PEL (STEL-C): 200 ppm IDLH: 150 ppm	Trichloroethanol (TCE) Trichloroacetic acid (TCA) Dichloroacetic acid Trichloroacetic acid	Irritant Burns with high concentrations CNS depression with high concentrations Noncardiogenic pulmonary edema Hepatorenal toxicity	CNS Skin Heart Lung Liver Kidney	2A

CAS, chemical abstract service; IARC, International Agency for Research on Cancer; IDLH, immediate danger to life and health; MW, molecular weight; PEL, permissible exposure limit; STEL, short-term exposure limit; TLV, threshold limit value, TWA: time-weighted average.

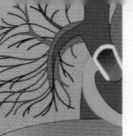

pounds. They are typically clear colorless liquids, although trichloroethylene may be dyed blue. As is typical of halogenated organic solvents, the chlorinated hydrocarbons are poorly miscible in water but highly miscible with other less polar organics such as diethyl ether. They are most often quite volatile, a property that led to their use as inhaled anesthetic agents, and have a characteristic sweet chloroform-like odor, which most patients did not find objectionable. Inhalation of high concentrations of chlorinated hydrocarbons is irritating to the mucosa. Although workers generally cannot detect concentrations of chlorinated hydrocarbons at the recommended workplace standard levels, they are typically able to smell these compounds at airborne concentrations at the immediate danger to life and health (IDLH) level.

In general, vapor pressure decreases and boiling point increases with increasing molecular weight. Therefore, in progressing from chloromethane (a gas), to dichloromethane, to chloroform, and ultimately to carbon tetrachloride, volatility steadily decreases. Despite their volatility (i.e., ease of going from liquid to vapor), the chlorinated hydrocarbons are generally not flammable. The exceptions to this rule are 1,2-dichloroethane and 1,2-dichloroethylene, which are flammable. Interestingly, although trichloroethane liquid is not flammable and no flashpoint has been defined using traditional methods, the vapor of this compound will burn. However, it takes an enormous amount of energy to ignite trichloroethane, and once ignited, the compound will not sustain combustion. In the presence of an open flame, chlorinated hydrocarbons such as methylene chloride decompose without burning and can be converted to phosgene and hydrogen chloride. Many of the chlorinated hydrocarbon solvents of industrial importance are photolabile. For example, chloroform is subject to photochemical decomposition to phosgene and hydrogen chloride. Chemical stabilizers such as small amounts of ethanol, triethylamine, or epichlorohydrin are often added to prevent degradation of the solvent in the presence of light.[10]

The number of chlorine atoms that can be added to a chlorinated hydrocarbon is determined by the number of hydrogen atoms on the unsubstituted hydrocarbon (i.e., the chlorine atoms replace only the hydrogen atoms of the hydrocarbon). The simplest chlorinated hydrocarbons are the chloromethanes. This series of compounds is created by progressively adding one to four chlorine atoms to methane (CH_4). The chloromethane series includes, in order of fewest to greatest number of chlorines, chloromethane, dichloromethane (methylene chloride), trichloromethane (chloroform), and tetrachloromethane (carbon tetrachloride) (see Table 93-1). The chloroethane series is based on substitution of ethane (CH_3CH_3) with chlorine. These compounds contain two carbon atoms connected by a single bond. The carbon skeleton of the chloroethylenes, although also composed of two carbons, is based on ethylene (ethene; CH_2CH_2), in which the two carbon atoms are joined with a double bond. Therefore, the chloroethane derivatives contain one to six chlorine atoms, whereas

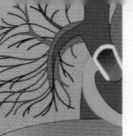

FIGURE 93-1 Chemical structures of *cis-* and *trans-* isomers of 1,2-dichloroethylene.

the chloroethylenes bear a maximum of four chlorine atoms. Chlorinated derivatives of three (propane), four (butane), and five (pentane) carbon chains also exist but are less commonly encountered and will therefore not be discussed further.

Various isomers (compounds with the same molecular formula but different arrangements of atoms) can be formed from the chloroethanes and chloroethylenes when two or more chlorine atoms are present on the molecule. Isomerism is not possible in the chloromethane series because there is only a single carbon atom. The chloroethane isomers may have the chlorine atoms distributed on one or both carbon atoms in any combination. This is also true in the chloroethylene series, in which up to four chlorine atoms may be added. Notably, within the chloroethylenes, an additional form of isomerism, "geometric" or "*cis-/trans-*" isomerism, is also possible because of the double bond prohibiting rotation about the carbon–carbon bond. This lack of available rotation results in the molecule having defined, noninterchangeable sides. In the 1,2-dichloroethylenes, both chlorines may be on the same side of the double bond (*cis-*) or on opposite sides of the double bond (*trans-*) (Fig. 93-1). Isomerism can result in differences in biologic activity. When examined in inhalation studies in rats, the *trans*-1,2-dichloroethylene isomer is twice as potent as an anesthetic than the *cis*-1,2-dichloroethylene isomer.[11] These two isomers cannot interconvert without breaking the carbon–carbon double bond. Further, subchronic dosing studies in animals indicate that 1,1-dichloroethane is about five times less injurious than 1,2-dichloroethane.[12] Geometric isomerism is not possible in the chloroethanes because there is free rotation around the carbon–carbon single bond.

EXPOSURE

Historically, significant exposures to chlorinated hydrocarbons occurred as a result of medicinal applications (e.g., as inhaled anesthetics and antihelminthic agents). However, this route of exposure has been largely mitigated by bans on the use of these agents as anesthetics, surgical disinfectants, and food extraction solvents. Currently, most exposures are the result of industrial contact from activities requiring large volumes of degreasing solvents (e.g., aircraft manufacture), in the manufacture and use of large volumes of paints and varnishes, or from work in the dry cleaning industry. Extensive industrial use of the chlorinated hydrocarbons has resulted in the release of these compounds into the environment where they may leach into ground water.

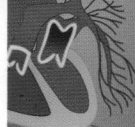

Most chlorinated hydrocarbon exposures generally fall into one of three broad categories: (1) very large acute exposure as a result of solvent abuse, (2) chronic higher concentration occupational exposure, and (3) chronic low-level exposure as a result of contamination of ground water supplies or other environmental sources.

TOXICOKINETICS

Absorption

Absorption of chlorinated hydrocarbons after ingestion is variable but can be significant. The one-carbon chloromethane compounds tend to be well-absorbed after ingestion. Absorption is increased further with physical exertion in the case of methylene chloride and with alcohol consumption after both inhalation and ingestion of carbon tetrachloride.[13,14] Serious toxicity from chlorinated hydrocarbon ingestion is typically the result of large volume deliberate (i.e., suicidal) ingestions. Ingestion of these compounds as a result of low-level drinking water contamination does not cause acute toxic effects.

Inhalation is the primary route of exposure to the chlorinated hydrocarbons both occupationally and as a result of abuse. Because of their volatility, the chlorinated hydrocarbons are easily inhaled, and because of their lipophilicity, they are typically well absorbed. In fact, about 70% of an inhaled dose of methylene chloride is absorbed.[15]

As a general rule, absorption through intact skin is inefficient, although transdermal penetration through damaged skin may be more efficient. Most chlorinated hydrocarbons are not transdermally absorbed to levels of clinical significance unless contact is prolonged and an impermeable barrier prevents evaporation. The most significant exception to this rule is carbon tetrachloride, for which amounts capable of causing adverse health effects may be absorbed through the skin.[16] Gastrointestinal effects, as well as liver damage and kidney failure, have been reported in individuals using a topically applied lotion containing carbon tetrachloride.[16] Chloroform and methylene chloride are also percutaneously absorbed to a somewhat greater extent than other chlorinated hydrocarbons, but to a lesser degree than is seen with carbon tetrachloride. Percutaneous absorption can also be increased by trapping the liquid against the skin with clothing or gloves. Tetrachloroethylene is absorbed through the skin only to a very limited degree.

Although a single dermal exposure to a chlorinated hydrocarbon may not represent a toxicologic hazard, repeated dermal exposures to certain substances may become significant.[17] This is illustrated by the observation that application of dichloroethane to the skin of guinea pigs causes blood levels of trichloroethylene to increase.[18]

Distribution

After absorption, chlorinated hydrocarbons are rapidly distributed to body tissues. As a result of their lipophilic character, large concentrations tend to be deposited in the fat, brain, and blood.[17] It is also notable that the lipophilic character of chlorinated hydrocarbon compounds such as chloroform and trichloroethylene allows some crossing of the placenta and potential exposure of the fetus.[17] Placental crossing is also known to occur with chloroform and dichloroethane exposure.[4,17] As expected from the partitioning of the chlorinated hydrocarbons into lipophilic tissues, their volumes of distribution are relatively large, ranging from about 2.6 L/kg for chloroform to about 10 L/kg for trichloroethylene.[19,20]

Metabolism and Elimination

The chlorinated hydrocarbons are eliminated from the body through two fundamental routes: exhaled air and hepatic metabolism. That portion eliminated from the lungs is largely as unchanged parent compound, although some is first metabolically converted to carbon dioxide. The extent of biotransformation is variable by compound and exposure dose. Species dependence also exists in the clearance of chlorinated hydrocarbons because some animals have more active metabolic pathways than others, which makes interspecies comparisons problematic.[21] For example, scaling of metabolic parameters for tetrachloroethylene determined in mice overestimates human metabolism.[22]

The main metabolic routes are oxidative transformation through the cytochrome P-450 systems and subsequent conjugation (Fig. 93-2). The P-450 enzymes involved exist primarily in the liver and kidneys, although they are also present to a lesser extent in the lungs and gastrointestinal tract. The initial oxidative transformation creates a reactive intermediate that is then conjugated with a polar moiety such as glutathione or glucuronic acid in order to create a more water-soluble compound that can be eliminated from the body. The kinetics of these enzymatic transformations is not always linear in humans.[22]

Other enzyme systems may also be involved with the biotransformation of chlorinated hydrocarbons. For example, ethanol changes the metabolism of trichloroethylene, suggesting that alcohol dehydrogenase may also be involved in its elimination.[20] The influences of aliphatic alcohols on the effects of chlorinated hydrocarbons containing a carbon–carbon double bond have been studied. It appears that the alcohols may influence the hepatotoxicity of some chlorinated hydrocarbons.[23] A secondary metabolic pathway also exists for methylene chloride and involves a glutathione transferase–dependent pathway, which produces carbon dioxide, formaldehyde, and formic acid.[24,25]

The initial metabolic activation is the proposed source of toxicity for many of the chlorinated hydrocarbons (see Fig. 93-2). Hepatic P-450 enzymes oxidatively convert the chlorinated hydrocarbon to free radicals. These reactive radicals may then combine with molecular oxygen to form peroxy radicals, or they may react with endogenous lipids to form lipid radicals. By their very nature, free radicals are highly unstable and react essentially as soon as they are created. Therefore, the toxic effects of these

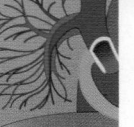

FIGURE 93-2 An abbreviated metabolic scheme for trichloroethylene.

reactive metabolites typically occur at or near their site of production. Additional significant clinical effects may result from the individual toxicities of the metabolites. For example, about 25% to 34% of an absorbed dose of methylene chloride is metabolically converted to carbon monoxide.[15] This biotransformation takes place primarily in the liver but also occurs to a lesser extent in the kidneys and lungs and is mediated by the 2E1 isozyme of the cytochrome P-450 system.[26,27] This pathway is also saturable in the presence of high substrate (methylene chloride) concentrations.[25] Carbon monoxide and carboxyhemoglobin may be formed for several hours after cessation of exposure.[25,28] The two-carbon compounds, 1,1,1-trichloroethane, trichloroethylene, and tetrachloroethylene, undergo biotransformation to form trichloroacetic acid and trichloroethanol, which are excreted in the urine in both free and conjugated forms.[29-31] In addition,

both trichloroacetic acid and dichloroacetic acid, which may be hepatotoxic, are produced.[32]

As a general rule, there is relatively little bioaccumulation of the chlorinated hydrocarbons in adipose tissues unless chronic high-concentration exposure has been maintained. Trichloroethylene's elimination follows a two-compartment model, with the first elimination half-life being about 0.5 to 3 hours and the second about 22 to 30 hours.[33,34] However, it is known that adipose tissues can act as a reservoir for trichloroethylene deposition.[35] The extent of significant adipose deposition seems to correlate well with long-term high-concentration occupational exposure; however, ongoing exposure could not be excluded. One report describes an individual with exhaled trichloroethylene breath concentrations of 135 ng/L (1.8 mg/day) 4 years after the last exposure to the compound following a 20-year

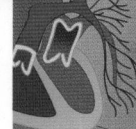

occupational exposure.[36] The elimination half-life of the chlorinated hydrocarbons may also vary by route of administration. A half-life of 72 hours is observed after inhalation of tetrachloroethylene, whereas the half-life is about doubled (144 hours) when the compound is ingested.[19,30]

The extended elimination profile seen with tetrachloroethylene actually affects the minority of the inhaled dose. With acute exposure to most chlorinated hydrocarbons, a large portion of the dose is excreted as unchanged parent compound in the air expired from the lungs.[37,38] In the case of methylene chloride, the saturability of the enzymatic conversion to carbon monoxide has a dramatic effect on the elimination of the compound. A dose-dependent elimination of methylene chloride is observed, with low-dose exposures being principally eliminated through the lungs as carbon monoxide while a greater proportion of unchanged parent methylene chloride is exhaled in the setting of larger exposures.[39]

EFFECTS ON BODY SYSTEMS

Central Nervous

Chlorinated hydrocarbons exert dose-dependent effects on the central nervous system (CNS), where the dose is a function of both the duration of exposure and the concentration of the substance. The effects of these compounds are not mediated by interaction with any specific CNS receptor. Rather, the mechanism of toxicity appears to be alteration of neurotransmission as a result of direct effect to nerve cell membranes by the chlorinated hydrocarbons,[40,41] which may be temporary or permanent.[42] In animal models, low-dose exposures to chlorinated hydrocarbons produce minimal histologic evidence of damage to nerve cells.[43] In high-dose exposure, the histologic results are equivocal.[43] No specific pathologic changes in the CNS are seen as a result of death from chlorinated hydrocarbon exposure. Rather, alterations in the CNS observed at autopsy are typically the result of underlying disease.[44]

Acute high-level exposures can be encountered in cases of solvent abusers or with large accidental releases of chlorinated hydrocarbon solvents in a workplace. Chronic high-level exposure is really only germane in the circumstance of long-term solvent inhalation abuse. Chronic low-level exposure is typically the result of routine occupational encounters with solvents in the course of normal work procedures. Chronic very-low-concentration exposures, as would be seen from drinking ground water contaminated with small amounts of chlorinated hydrocarbon solvents, are not expected to have any effects on the CNS.

Acute high-level exposure typically causes CNS depression, dizziness, narcosis, nausea, vomiting, seizures, coma, and possibly death from respiratory failure. Because there is no discrete receptor and no requirement for metabolic activation of the chlorinated hydrocarbon to exert effects on the CNS, onset of effects is rapid.

Likewise, because effects are not the result of a covalent drug-receptor interaction, recovery from intoxication is typically rapid and, except when very high doses are abused chronically or significant hypoxic insult is incurred, recovery is usually fairly prompt and complete. Most deaths associated with acute high doses are caused by either narcosis and apnea or cardiac arrest, which is discussed in greater detail under Cardiovascular.

Chronic high-dose exposure to chlorinated hydrocarbons, most frequently as a result of long-term solvent abuse, may have substantial effects on the CNS. The primary pathologic change to the CNS from solvent abuse is degeneration of the white matter (leukoencephalopathy).[45] Other CNS changes observed at autopsy in the brains of toluene abusers include substantial atrophy and mottling of the white matter, as well as myelin and oligodendrocyte loss with relative axonal preservation.[45] These conditions are characterized for toluene, not chlorinated hydrocarbon, abuse, and it is known from animal studies that some differences in specific neurologic effects may exist between the individual solvents.[46] However, a pathologic picture similar to that seen with toluene abuse may occur in cases of chronic chlorinated hydrocarbon abuse. Metabolites may also contribute to CNS effects, especially in the case of metabolically produced carbon monoxide from significant methylene chloride exposure.[47]

Chronic exposure to chlorinated hydrocarbons at lower levels is most frequently associated with occupational settings. The CNS depression and narcosis seen with acute high-dose exposure is generally not seen with chronic low-dose exposures. The occurrence of solvent-induced encephalopathy from low-dose exposure is a matter of some debate. Several epidemiologic studies have looked for cognitive dysfunction in workers exposed to individual and mixtures of solvents with batteries of psychometric tests.[48-50] However, these studies are often difficult to interpret because of confounders such as simultaneous exposure to multiple chemicals, including alcohol use, and have not consistently and definitively shown any predictable CNS dysfunction with this exposure paradigm.

Cardiovascular

The effects of chlorinated hydrocarbons on the cardiovascular system are visible on heart rate, contractility, and conduction. In general, the effects on all three of these parameters are dose-dependent depressive clinical effects. These depressant effects are likely at least twofold in etiology. First, the chlorinated hydrocarbons exert solvent-like effects that alter the fluidity of myocardial cell membranes, causing direct myocardial depression of contractility.[51,52] Second, because of their lipophilic character, the chlorinated hydrocarbons readily cross the blood-brain barrier and disrupt the neuronal control of both heart rate and contractility. In fact, trichloroethylene (TCE) was once used as an inhaled agent for human anesthesia but was abandoned because of its cardiac depressant effects, which caused excessive bradycardia and hypotension.[52]

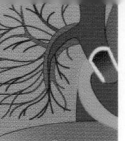

The effects of chlorinated hydrocarbons on cardiac conduction are slightly more complex but can be considered to fall into two basic categories: depression and sensitization. The depressant effects are the result of the solvents acting to stabilize the myocardial cell membranes to depolarization.[53] This increased membrane stability blocks conduction impulse transmission resulting in an increased risk for dysrhythmias. In vitro evidence also suggests that some depressant activity appears to be the result of the ability of the chlorinated hydrocarbons to attenuate calcium dynamics in cardiac myocytes during excitation-contraction coupling.[54] The potency of the tested compounds to inhibit calcium dynamics in the cardiac myocytes expressed as IC_{50} correlated strongly ($r = 0.9829$) with compound lipophilicity expressed as octanol:water partition coefficient.[54]

Sudden death in humans following large exposure to chlorinated hydrocarbons has been reported numerous times and is often referred to as "sensitization." Often, those afflicted by sudden death are solvent abusers, although death following occupational exposures to some solvents has occurred.[55,56] The strong link between solvent abuse and sudden death was the genesis of the descriptive term *sudden sniffing death*, which is sometimes used to refer to this condition. Postmortem examination of people who died under such circumstances is often without adequate anatomic abnormality to alternatively explain death. The demise is sudden and often without apparent neurologic involvement such as seizures, so it seems likely that the cause of death is a dysrhythmia-associated sudden cardiac arrest. As such, the concept of "myocardial sensitization" has been offered as an explanation. The actual pathophysiology of myocardial sensitization is poorly understood. The general theory is that the myocardium becomes more responsive to the effects of systemic catecholamines, including endogenously released epinephrine, and that any excess catecholamine exposure causes irritability of the myocardium, resulting in dysrhythmias. Hypoxia may be an alternative explanation.

Perhaps the most widely cited study of myocardial sensitization from halogenated hydrocarbon inhalation was reported in 1971 by Reinhardt and colleagues.[57] Due to the frequency with which it is cited in other works, this study deserves a brief discussion. In this investigation, the potential of 13 compounds to produce dysrhythmias in a dog model was examined. Nine of the test compounds were fluorocarbon derivatives (Freon), seven of which were also chlorinated; two compounds (isobutane and propane) were simple hydrocarbons; one was an aliphatic ether (dimethyl ether); and the last was vinyl chloride. Two exposure circumstances were used and designated "standard exposure" (test compound inhaled over 10 minutes) and "short-term exposure" (high concentration of test compound inhaled for 30 seconds accompanied by a stimulus to frighten the animal in order to stimulate endogenous epinephrine release).

In the standard exposure experiment, the animals were equipped with continuous electrocardiographic monitors and received an intravenous injection of epinephrine (0.008 mg/kg over 9 seconds) followed by the desired dose of test compound through mask inhalation. Midway through a 10-minute inhalation of test compound, a "challenge injection" of epinephrine was given, and the electrocardiogram was observed for the development of alterations in cardiac rhythm. The short-term exposure experiments were conducted in a similar fashion, except a high concentration of test compound was inhaled by the animal for only 30 seconds, and an external stimulus was applied to frighten the animal. The external stimulus used was a loud recording of noises such as sirens, gongs, and jet takeoffs. The authors examined the electrocardiographic data for the presence of marked responses, which they defined as development of a dysrhythmia considered to pose a serious threat or ending in cardiac arrest. In the standard exposure group, marked responses were seen only with higher concentrations of test compound, although not every animal who received the higher-dose test compound developed a marked response. The total number of dogs used in each phase of the experiment ranged from 6 to 13. Of the 367 dog exposures studied in the standard exposure experiments, 111 cases of marked response were reported, of which 14 were ventricular fibrillation and cardiac arrest. Alternatively stated, a cardiac arrest rate of only 3.8% was observed. In the short-term study, 66 dog exposures provided 9 marked responses, none of which were ventricular fibrillation or cardiac arrest. Notably, two animals manifested a bigeminal rhythm with areas of the electrocardiogram suggestive of multiple ventricular beats. The authors further indicated that the potential activity of a given compound depended at least partly on the specific halogen atoms present in the test compound. Those compounds that contained chlorine atoms produced the greatest degree of effect, whereas those halogenated only with fluorine were less effective. No brominated or iodinated compounds were studied. The nonhalogenated compounds produced a marked response rate similar to that seen with the halogenated compounds.

The authors suggested that smaller doses of epinephrine were required to induce life-threatening dysrhythmias or cardiac arrest following exposure to the test compounds. Other investigators have indicated that the concentrations of epinephrine required to cause cardiac dysrhythmias with exposure to inhaled chlorinated hydrocarbons are within the physiologic range.[58] However, even with the significantly higher doses of epinephrine used in Reinhardt's dog study, none of the animals in the short-term exposure group suffered cardiac arrest. The cardiotoxicity associated with inhaled chlorinated hydrocarbons appears to be exacerbated in the setting of hypoxia and hypercarbia.[57,59] A lack of protective effect against development of cardiac dysrhythmias because of tolerance with long-term use has been suggested as support for the theory of myocardial sensitization. Although the principle of myocardial sensitization has been proposed in human cases of sudden death from solvent abuse, definitive data are lacking.

Several other factors may be either responsible or at least contributory to sudden death in chlorinated hydro-

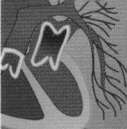

carbon exposures. For example, chronic solvent abuse is associated with the development of cardiomyopathy, which is a known substrate for dysrhythmias. This may explain the lack of tolerance to cardiac dysrhythmias in people with a long-standing history of solvent abuse. Hypoxia and hypercarbia also put patients at greater risk for potentially lethal cardiac dysrhythmias; and hypoxia, anoxia, and suffocation all result from excessive oxygen displacement or positioning following loss of consciousness when chlorinated solvents are inhaled in large quantities. Finally, depression of sinus node impulse generation can be induced, leading to profound bradycardia with subsequent ventricular escape rhythms. In short, sudden death associated with inhalation of high concentrations of chlorinated hydrocarbon solvents, especially solvent abuse, is probably multifactorial, and myocardial sensitization to endogenous catecholamines is likely not the sole etiology.

When victims of sudden sniffing death are examined at autopsy, both gross and microscopic examinations are frequently normal. This has been demonstrated not only in animals but also in human cases.[57,60] Two papers have also examined the postmortem tissue concentrations of trichloroethylene in cases of human death following acute occupational exposure.[55,56] In one of the listed cases, a brain trichloroethylene concentration of 2.5 mg/100 g was detected 33 days after death demonstrating the significant partitioning of the solvent into the CNS.[55]

Liver

Chlorinated hydrocarbons, especially carbon tetrachloride and chloroform, are known to cause centrilobular hepatic necrosis and hepatomegaly.[17] The destruction of liver cells, which may progress to involve the entire hepatic lobule, requires the metabolic activation of the chlorinated hydrocarbon (Fig. 93-3). The metabolically produced radicals are highly reactive, so the site of toxic effect is the liver because this is the site of radical production. The two most significant effects of free radical production are steatosis and carcinogenesis. Free radicals bind components of hepatocytes, resulting in inhibition of lipoprotein secretion.[17,43] This causes an accumulation of fatty tissues in the liver, resulting in steatosis. When radicals react with DNA, the resulting adducts may be carcinogenic.

Although other chlorinated hydrocarbons do not cause hepatic necrosis, many induce fatty changes in the liver. Even though the fatty changes are typically

FIGURE 93-3 Metabolic activation of carbon tetrachloride to form free radical species.

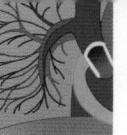

reversible, it is a matter of some discussion as to whether or not the fatty changes are a prelude to hepatocyte death. The significance of the damage and ultimate prognosis for recovery are based on several factors. Among these factors are the magnitudes of exposure, underlying liver health, and presence or absence of other hepatotoxins. It is also important to realize that the extent of CNS involvement is not necessarily predictive of liver or kidney injury.

Kidney

Renal damage may also be associated with exposure to some of the chlorinated hydrocarbons. Reported toxic effects of chlorinated hydrocarbon poisoning on the kidney include azotemia, oliguria, anuria, ketonuria, acute tubular necrosis, and renal failure.[61,62] Granular casts and red blood cells have also been seen in the urine after chloroform exposure.[37] Although inadequate to explain all cases of renal injury that have been reported after exposure to chlorinated hydrocarbons, at least part of the mechanism of injury in the kidney is likely the same as in the liver: production of reactive free radical and other reactive metabolites in the kidney by P-450–mediated oxidation.[63] It has been suggested that occupational exposure to chlorinated solvents is linked to glomerulonephritis, but this association has not been clearly defined.[61,62] Renal failure has been reported after dermal exposure to carbon tetrachloride.[16]

Dermal

Because chlorinated hydrocarbon solvents are very hydrophobic, they tend to dissolve the lipids in the epidermis. This defatting of the skin surface often leads to a chronic irritant dermatitis. Most chlorinated hydrocarbon solvents are mild irritants. However, repeated or prolonged dermal contact may produce inflammation or burns. Trapping of solvents such as chloroform and methylene chloride under jewelry like rings and watches results in an almost immediate burning sensation on the contacted skin. Skin exposed to chlorinated hydrocarbon solvents may become hyperkeratotic, scaly, or thickened, and painful cracks or fissures may also be present.[14] Tetrachloroethylene (perchloroethylene) is a much stronger irritant than the other chlorinated hydrocarbon solvents, and even brief contact with this compound can result in blistering and burns.[14]

Beyond simply the discomfort associated with solvent-caused dermatitis, the violation of the integrity of the skin as a barrier may also have significant clinical consequences. Dermal absorption of chlorinated hydrocarbon solvents alone is generally insufficient to cause systemic illness. However, when the skin is no longer intact, absorption of solvents may be greater, potentially leading to systemic effects. Dermal absorption of some important chlorinated hydrocarbon compounds may be clinically significant through the contribution of this route of exposure to the total-body burden of the compounds. In addition, although the chlorinated hydrocarbons are not themselves allergenic, it is possible that destruction of

the skin by these solvents may make the skin more permeable to sensitizing agents with which the exposed individual may be working.

Effects of chlorinated hydrocarbon exposure on the skin may also be systemic. Development of local scleroderma on the volar surfaces of the forearms and dorsal surfaces of the ankles in a 26-year-old woman with a history of working with tetrachloroethylene was reported, although this patient also worked with other solvents and this association remains elusive.[64]

Exposure to trichloroethylene is associated with a unique toxicity known as "degreaser's flush." This condition is manifested by flushing of the face after ingestion of ethanol in people with chronic exposure to trichloroethylene vapor. The flushing is a result of vasodilation of the superficial blood vessels on the face. The exact mechanism of this effect is unclear, but it may be due to the direct effects of the trichloroethylene metabolites chloral hydrate and trichloroacetic acid on the vasculature.

The time course of degreaser's flush is predictable. Typically, red blotches develop on the nose and malar eminences within about 30 minutes after the individual ingests alcohol. The blotches increase in size and then become confluent, resulting in a generalized flushing of the face and neck, which peaks within about an hour. The flushing then gradually diminishes to disappearance over the course of the subsequent hour. In daily drinkers of alcohol, degreaser's flush is generally not observed until after about 3 weeks of daily exposure to trichloroethylene vapor. Notably, once established, the flushing reaction may occur with ethanol ingestion as much as 3 weeks after the last trichloroethylene vapor exposure.

Ocular

Like the skin, damage to the eye as a result of ocular chlorinated hydrocarbon exposure is largely due to delipification. Most often, the result of ocular exposure is mild chemical conjunctivitis, although direct application of high-concentration liquid chlorinated solvents may cause pain or burning with corneal dulling.[14] Diplopia, visual blurring, and blindness have also been reported with contact with bulk chlorinated hydrocarbon solvents.[14] Punctate staining of the epithelium may be seen with fluorescent examination. Unless serious chemical burns result, the damage is generally reversible. Both carbon tetrachloride and tetrachloroethylene have been implicated in development of optic neuritis, although this is not universally supported in the literature.[42]

Blepharospasm has been reported after exposure to high concentrations of chloroform vapor.[6] However, most cases of exposure to airborne chlorinated hydrocarbons do not result in persistent ocular damage even when the solvent concentrations are quite high.

Systemically absorbed chlorinated hydrocarbons do not typically cause ocular toxicity. However, development of blue-gray corneal opacities was observed in a dog model after systemic, but not intraocular, administration

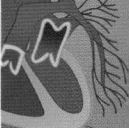

of dichloroethane.[17] No reports of similar systemically mediated ocular effects in humans exist.

Pulmonary

Exposure of the lungs to chlorinated hydrocarbons must be divided into two distinct situations: aspiration and inhalation. The effects on the lungs from these two different routes of exposure are quite different. With aspiration of liquid solvent, potentially severe chemical pneumonitis is the primary concern. This is largely due to the solubility of lung surfactant in the chlorinated hydrocarbon solvent leading to profound inflammation of the lung. In contrast, inhalation of solvent vapor does not typically cause this sort of injury, although massive inhalation has caused pulmonary hemorrhage.[14,65] Even though respiratory arrest may be seen with large inhalation exposures to chlorinated hydrocarbons, the mechanism is typically CNS depression (solvent narcosis) rather than direct damage to the lung.

Because of the volatility of the chlorinated hydrocarbon solvents, the lungs represent a major exposure pathway. Although metabolism by P-450 enzymes in the Clara cells may produce some reactive metabolites, the lungs are not a principal target organ for chlorinated hydrocarbon toxicity.[66] Pulmonary irritation is possible, and is expected with high-concentration exposures. Very large pulmonary exposures to some compounds, including methylene chloride, may produce chemical pneumonitis or noncardiogenic pulmonary edema.[14,67,68]

Teratogenicity and Carcinogenicity

The association of reproductive effects, including teratogenicity, and carcinogenicity with exposure to the chlorinated hydrocarbon compounds is a topic that is hotly debated. Vinyl chloride, which is not discussed in this chapter, is an International Association for Research on Cancer (IARC) class 1 compound, and knowledge of this association fuels concern about the cancer-causing potential of other chlorinated hydrocarbons. Conflicting data between studies, as well as significant species dependence in observed effects, make evaluation and comparison of much of the data difficult. Interpretation of the human epidemiologic data is further hindered by the presence of confounders such as simultaneous significant exposure to other potentially toxic compounds, poor quality of exposure measurements, and recall bias.

Perhaps the simplest case is that for 1,1,1-trichloroethane. Data suggest no teratogenic effects in laboratory animals or humans; further, carcinogenicity of this compound has not been demonstrated in humans. Animal data suggest that tetrachloroethylene is fetotoxic, and both tetrachloroethylene and trichloroethylene have been reported to cause developmental abnormalities in animals.[69,70] However, these observations do not seem to translate to human epidemiologic investigations. No adverse effects on reproduction have been shown in humans after exposure to tetrachloroethylene. Although trichloroethylene exposure is a suggested culprit in human cases of birth defects and

increased rates of spontaneous abortion, inadequate data regarding the amounts of other compounds to which the mothers were exposed is missing, making establishment of a link impossible.[69,70] Although associations between exposure to tetrachloroethylene and development of malignancy (leukemia as well as liver, esophageal, and urinary tract tumors) and also between trichloroethylene and other cancers (non-Hodgkin's lymphoma, hepatic and renal cancers) have been alleged, the epidemiologic data are not sufficient to establish a definitive connection.[71,72] Impurities in the chlorinated hydrocarbon solvents may significantly influence evaluation of cancer-causing potential. One study reported development of pulmonary tumors in mice exposed to trichloroethylene; however, the trichloroethylene used in the experiments may have been contaminated with trace amounts of the stabilizer epichlorohydrin, a known carcinogen.[73] Tetrachloroethylene and trichloroethylene are both classified as IARC 2A compounds, whereas 1,1,1-trichloroethane is IARC class 3 based on animal studies. Concerns about possible adverse health effects have resulted in published efforts describing methods to limit occupational exposure to chlorinated hydrocarbon solvents and influence both technologic innovation and legislation on industrial metal degreasing.[74]

The case of association is modestly stronger for adverse reproductive effects and carcinogenicity with exposure to the one-carbon chlorinated derivatives. Although methylene chloride and chloroform have not been shown to be teratogenic in some animal models, chloroform is highly embryotoxic and causes changes in sperm morphology in animals.[14,75] Chloroform readily crosses the placenta.[76] Two cases of eclamptic toxemia were reported in pregnant women who worked in a laboratory where chloroform was used, although the association was circumstantial.[77]

The situation for carbon tetrachloride is similar. This compound also crosses the placenta and has been detected in cord blood in exposed humans.[69,76] Carbon tetrachloride has been reported to be both fetotoxic and teratogenic in rats.[78] Other investigators have not observed teratogenic effects in rats or rabbits.[69] At carbon tetrachloride doses of 0.1 and 0.01 of the LD_{50} given to mice on days 1, 6, and 11 of gestation, no evidence of teratogenicity or fetotoxicity was observed.[79] Carcinogenicity of other compounds may be enhanced by exposure to carbon tetrachloride.[80] Methylene chloride, chloroform, and carbon tetrachloride are all classified as IARC class 2B. Except for vinyl chloride, the data in animals suggest an association with development of cancer; data in humans are inadequate to establish causality.

DIAGNOSIS

Although patients presenting with acute chlorinated hydrocarbon toxicity may be quite ill, the signs and symptoms are nonspecific. Further, specific laboratory assays for the detection of chlorinated hydrocarbons are not routinely available in most hospital laboratories but

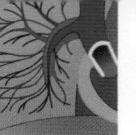

are from certain reference laboratories. Therefore, to diagnose chlorinated hydrocarbon toxicity, it is necessary to obtain a history of exposure. In cases of acute occupational exposure, container labels or material safety data sheets may be available. Additional helpful information, such as air monitoring results, may be available from local emergency medical services personnel or fire department hazardous materials teams who responded to the incident. Cases of chronic exposure in which no immediate life threats exist may be more challenging to reconcile. Such incidents require careful physical examination along with a detailed history and differential diagnosis. Although it is most often essentially impossible to determine exact dose, especially in chronic exposure circumstances, some topics that should be addressed include the conditions of use, temperature, ventilation systems and other workplace controls in place, use of personal protective equipment, and whether the agent is aerosolized or used as bulk solvent. In the evaluation of less critical patients presenting with possible chronic toxicity, the history must include not only workplace exposure but also potential household and hobby sources such as home improvement, automotive repair, art, and cleaning activities.

In general, chlorinated hydrocarbons are CNS depressants, although this diminished level of consciousness may be preceded by an initial brief period of CNS excitation. The exact effects on the CNS and the time course of onset are largely dose dependent. Dose is determined by duration of exposure, concentration of the solvent, and minute ventilation volume. Individual susceptibility may also play a role in the development of specific signs and symptoms.

Large inhalation exposures are typically manifested by headache, fatigue, lethargy, nausea, and abdominal discomfort. Continued exposure may result in a progression to ataxia, stupor, coma, and death. Higher concentration exposures are generally associated with more rapid onset of more significant signs and symptoms. In some rare cases, coma and death may occur within minutes. Fortunately, with removal from the source of exposure, recovery is typically rapid provided the victim has not suffered serious trauma or hypoxic insult. Because of its prolonged elimination time, recovery may be somewhat slower after exposure to high concentrations of tetrachloroethylene.

Clinical presentation after ingestion of chlorinated hydrocarbon solvents is analogous to that seen with inhalation. However, the CNS depression may be delayed in onset with ingestion as a result of the time lag required for systemic absorption. In cases of large ingestions of trichloroethylene or tetrachloroethylene, onset of neurologic signs and symptoms may be delayed for several hours. As previously stated, trichloroethylene is eliminated very slowly. Therefore, prolonged coma may result after significant ingestions. Furthermore, it is possible that cardiac dysrhythmias may develop hours after ingestion of trichloroethylene when CNS depression is present or after significant methylene chloride exposure as a result of carbon monoxide production. One other special case that must be kept in mind is the potential for metabolic production of carbon monoxide from significant exposures to dichloromethane. Although recovery may be slightly slower than with inhalation, recovery from chlorinated hydrocarbon poisoning as a result of ingestion is typically complete within about 24 hours in the absence of secondary effects such as aspiration, hypoxia, or carbon monoxide production.

MANAGEMENT

The initial approach to the medical management of acute chlorinated hydrocarbon toxicity is appropriate supportive care. As toxic exposure to this class of compounds is associated with substantial CNS and respiratory depression, as well as the possibility of oropharyngeal edema due to chemical burns, early and aggressive airway management is paramount. In these situations, as well as in cases of large ingestions, protection of the airway with endotracheal intubation is appropriate. Pulse oximetry and cardiac monitoring should be initiated and intravenous access obtained with crystalloid fluids. Baseline laboratory evaluation of acid–base status, electrolytes, and renal and hepatic function is appropriate. Chest radiography to assess endotracheal tube placement or the possibility of aspiration is indicated if clinically appropriate. Interestingly, some chlorinated hydrocarbons are radiopaque, which may assist in locating significant depots. In cases of significant methylene chloride exposure, absorption may be prolonged; therefore, serial carboxyhemoglobin determinations are appropriate until a definitive downward trend is demonstrated. Chlorinated hydrocarbon toxicity frequently causes profound diarrhea, which may exacerbate electrolyte imbalances. As such, fluid intake and output should be monitored closely as significant volumes of fluid and associated electrolytes may need to be replaced.

There is no specific antidotal therapy for chlorinated hydrocarbon intoxication. As such, treatment is symptomatic and supportive using standard basic and advanced life support interventions. Dysrhythmias resulting from chlorinated hydrocarbon toxicity should be managed according to standard advanced cardiac life support protocols. Many sources recommend that clinicians avoid the use of catecholamines such as epinephrine during the course of resuscitation of chlorinated hydrocarbon–induced cardiac arrest because of the possibility of myocardial sensitization to endogenous catecholamines. However, because myocardial sensitization has not been definitively shown to be the principal mechanism for sudden death associated with chlorinated hydrocarbon exposure and because administration of catecholamines such as epinephrine and dopamine is a standard resuscitative measure, complete avoidance of these therapies may be unwise.

Decontamination and Prevention of Absorption

External decontamination after exposure to chlorinated hydrocarbons is necessary to limit continued absorption by the victim as well as to protect the rescuers. Largely as

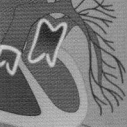

a result of the volatility of these compounds, simple decontamination techniques are quite effective. Removal of clothing followed by washing with copious amounts of water is the management of choice. Addition of soap to the decontamination rinse may assist in increasing the solubility of the chlorinated hydrocarbon compounds in the decontamination water. As with most liquid chemicals, the possibility of enhancement of absorption through vasodilation as a result of using scrubbing brushes or hot decontamination water exists with chlorinated hydrocarbon solvents. However, these compounds are sufficiently volatile and their percutaneous absorption generally low enough that this concern is largely theoretical. Special attention should be given to the decontamination of open wounds and mucous membranes.

Gastric decontamination after ingestion of chlorinated hydrocarbons should be undertaken on a carefully considered case-by-case basis. Induction of emesis is contraindicated because these compounds are commonly associated with CNS depression. Gastric aspiration may be considered in cases of large carbon tetrachloride or chloroform ingestion presenting shortly after ingestion in an attempt to limit the risk for hepatic damage. Administration of a single dose of activated charcoal may be considered, especially in cases of polysubstance ingestion. However, the clinician should remain mindful that the efficacy of activated charcoal has not been proved in cases of chlorinated hydrocarbon ingestion and that the potential for CNS depression, emesis, and aspiration exists.

There are no specific antidotes for toxic exposure to chlorinated hydrocarbons. *N*-acetylcysteine (NAC) is beneficial in preventing damage due to acetaminophen intoxication as well as in cases of fulminant hepatic failure.[81,82] There are several proposed mechanisms of action for the hepatoprotective effects of NAC, including acting as both a glutathione precursor and a glutathione surrogate. Based on this theory, case reports have suggested using NAC to assist in minimizing hepatic damage as a result of acute carbon tetrachloride exposure.[83] Additional case reports suggest benefit from hyperbaric oxygen therapy in cases of methylene chloride or carbon tetrachloride poisoning.[28,38]

Enhancement of elimination from the gastrointestinal tract using methods such as whole-bowel irrigation is not appropriate for toxic ingestions of chlorinated hydrocarbons. Because chlorinated hydrocarbons are eliminated largely through the lungs, hyperventilation may be beneficial. A case report of tetrachloroethylene poisoning suggested some benefit in accelerated clearance with hyperventilation.[30] Because of the large volumes of distribution, clearance of the chlorinated hydrocarbons using hemodialysis is generally ineffective. However, in cases of chlorinated hydrocarbon–induced renal failure, hemodialysis may be necessary and should be continued until renal function normalizes.

Disposition

In cases of toxicity after inhalation of chlorinated hydrocarbons, cessation of symptoms and complete recovery are expected shortly after termination of the exposure. Typically, if the patient is asymptomatic, discharge is appropriate as soon as any alterations in mental status clear. The oral pathway may require a longer observation period. Depending on the circumstances of the exposure, discussion of safety practices at the worksite or referral for psychiatric evaluation may be warranted.

Patients with persistent CNS depression, cardiac dysrhythmias, or pulmonary involvement should be admitted until the clinical picture resolves. Further, in the event of a significant exposure, admission, with serial clinical and laboratory evaluations, is recommended. Renal and hepatic injury typically resolves with generalized supportive care and returns to baseline within days to weeks.

REFERENCES

1. Beattie C: History and principles of anesthesiology. In Hardman JG, Limbird LE, Gilman AG (eds): Goodman and Gilman's The Pharmacological Basis of Therapeutics. New York, McGraw-Hill, 2001.
2. Dilger JP: Basic pharmacology of inhalational anesthetic agents. In Bowdle TA, Horita A, Kharasch EDe (eds): The Pharmacologic Basis of Anesthesiology: Basic Science and Practical Applications. New York, Churchill-Livingstone, 1994.
3. Nashelsky MB, Dix JD, Adelstein EH: Homicide facilitated by inhalation of chloroform. J Forensic Sci 1995;40:134–138.
4. Reynolds JEF: Martindale: The Extra Pharmacopoeia, 28th ed. London, The Pharmaceutical Press, 1982.
5. Dykes MH: Halogenated hydrocarbon ingestion. Int Anesthesiol Clin 1970;8:357–368.
6. Hathaway GJ, Proctor NH, Hughes JP, et al: Chemical Hazards of the Workplace, 4th ed. New York, Van Nostrand Reinhold, 1996.
7. Lewis RA: Lewis' Dictionary of Toxicology. Boca Raton, FL, Lewis, 1998.
8. American Conference of Industrial Hygienists: Documentation of the Threshold Limit Values and Biological Exposure Indices, 6th ed. Cincinnati, Author, 1996.
9. Hazardous Substances Data Bank, National Library of Medicine. Englewood, CO, Micromedex, 2000.
10. International Programme on Chemical Safety: Environmental Health Criteria 163—Chloroform. Geneva, World Health Organization, 1994.
11. Smyth HF: Hygiene standards for daily inhalation. The Donald E. Cummings Memorial Lecture. Am Ind Hyg Q 1956;17:129–185.
12. Hoffman HT, Birnstiel H, Jobst P: On the inhalation toxicity of 1,1- and 1,2-dichloroethane. Arch Toxicol 1971;27 :248–265.
13. New PS, Lubash GD, Scherr L: Acute renal failure associated with carbon tetrachloride intoxication. JAMA 1962;181:903–906.
14. Harbison RM: Hamilton and Hardy's Industrial Toxicology, 5th ed. St. Louis, Mosby, 1998.
15. DiVincenzo GD, Kaplan CJ: Uptake, metabolism, and elimination of methylene chloride vapor by humans. Toxicol Appl Pharmacol 1981;59:130–140.
16. Perez AJ, Courel M, Sobrado J, Gonzalez L: Acute renal failure after topical application of carbon tetrachloride. Lancet 1987; 1:515–516.
17. Barceloux DG: Halogenated solvents, trichloroethylene and methylene chloride. In Sullivan JB, Krieger GR (eds): Clinical Environmental Health and Toxic Exposures. Philadelphia, Lippincott Williams & Wilkins, 2001.
18. Jakobson I, Wahlberg JE, Holmberg B, Johansson G: Uptake via the blood and elimination of 10 organic solvents following epicutaneous exposure of anesthetized guinea pigs. Toxicol Appl Pharmacol 1982;63:181–187.
19. Baselt RC: Disposition of toxic drugs and chemicals in man, 6th ed. Foster City, CA, Chemical Toxicology Institute, Biomedical Publications, 2002.
20. Koppel C, Lanz HJ, Ibe K: Acute trichloroethylene poisoning with additional ingestion of ethanol: concentrations of trichloro-

ethylene and its metabolites during hyperventilation therapy. Intensive Care Med 1988;14:74–76.

21. Reitz RH, Gargas ML, Mendrala AL, Schumann AM: In vivo and in vitro studies of perchloroethylene metabolism for physiologically based pharmacokinetic modeling in rats, mice, and humans. Toxicol Appl Pharmacol 1996;136:289–306.

22. Ward RC, Travis CC, Hetrick DM, et al: Pharmacokinetics of tetrachloroethylene. Toxicol Appl Pharmacol 1988;93:108–117.

23. Cornish HH, Barth ML, Ling B: Influence of aliphatic alcohols on the hepatic response to halogenated olefins. Environ Health Perspect 1977;21:149–152.

24. Gargas ML, Clewell HJ 3rd, Andersen ME: Metabolism of inhaled dihalomethanes in vivo: differentiation of kinetic constants for two independent pathways. Toxicol Appl Pharmacol 1986;82:211–223.

25. Mahmud M, Kales SN: Methylene chloride poisoning in a cabinet worker. Environ Health Perspect 1999;107:769–772.

26. Kim NY, Park SW, Suh JK: Two fatal cases of dichloromethane or chloroform poisoning. J Forensic Sci 1996;41:527–529.

27. Guengerich FP, Kim DH, Iwasaki M: Role of human cytochrome P-450 IIE1 in the oxidation of many low molecular weight cancer suspects. Chem Res Toxicol 1991;4:168–179.

28. Rioux JP, Myers RA: Hyperbaric oxygen for methylene chloride poisoning: report on two cases. Ann Emerg Med 1989;18:691–695.

29. Barceloux DG, Rosenberg J: Trichloroethylene toxicity. J Toxicol Clin Toxicol 1990;28:479–504.

30. Koppel C, Arndt I, Arendt U, Koeppe P: Acute tetrachloroethylene poisoning: blood elimination kinetics during hyperventilation therapy. J Toxicol Clin Toxicol 1985;23:103–115.

31. Lash LH, Qian W, Putt DA, et al: Renal and hepatic toxicity of trichloroethylene and its glutathione-derived metabolites in rats and mice: sex-, species-, and tissue-dependent differences. J Pharmacol Exp Ther 2001;297:155–164.

32. Lash LH, Parker JC: Hepatic and renal toxicities associated with perchloroethylene. Pharmacol Rev 2001;53:177–208.

33. Mycroft FJ, Fan A: Trichloroethylene (TCE). Hazard Rev 1985;2:1–4.

34. Kostrzewski P, Jakubowski M, Kolacinski Z: Kinetics of trichloroethylene elimination from venous blood after acute inhalation poisoning. J Toxicol Clin Toxicol 1993;31:353–363.

35. Perbellini L, Olivato D, Zedde A, Miglioranzi R: Acute trichloroethylene poisoning by ingestion: clinical and pharmacokinetic aspects. Intensive Care Med 1991;17:234–235.

36. Kohlmuller D, Kochen W: Exhalation air analyzed in long-term postexposure investigations of acetonitrile and trichloroethylene exposures in two subjects. Clin Chem 1994;40:1462–1464.

37. Schroeder HG: Acute and delayed chloroform poisoning. Br J Anaeseth 1965;37:972–975.

38. Burkhart KK, Hall AH, Gerace R, Rumack BH: Hyperbaric oxygen treatment for carbon tetrachloride poisoning. Drug Saf 1991;6:332–338.

39. U.S. Department of Health and Human Services: ATSDR case studies in environmental medicine: methylene chloride toxicity. Atlanta, Agency for Toxic Substances and Disease Registry, 1990.

40. Bass M: Sudden sniffing death. JAMA 1970;212:2075–2079.

41. England A, Jones RM: Inhaled anaesthetic agents: from ether to halothane. Br J Hosp Med 1992;47:699–702.

42. Onofrj M, Thomas A, Paci C, et al: Optic neuritis with residual tunnel vision in perchloroethylene toxicity. Eur Neurol 1999;41:51–53.

43. Kalf GF, Post GB, Snyder R: Recent advances in the toxicology of benzene, the glycol ethers and carbon tetrachloride. Annu Rev Pharmacol Toxicol 1987;27:399–427.

44. Cohen MM: Central nervous system in carbon tetrachloride intoxication. Neurology 1957;7:238–244.

45. Kornfeld M, Moser AB, Moser HW, et al: Solvent vapor abuse leukoencephalopathy: comparison to adrenoleukodystrophy. J Neuropathol Exp Neurol 1994;53:389–398.

46. Rebert CS, Matteucci MJ, Pryor GT: Acute effects of inhaled dichloromethane on the EEG and sensory-evoked potentials of Fischer-344 rats. Pharmacol Biochem Behav 1989;34:619–629.

47. Barrowcliff DF, Knell AJ: Cerebral damage due to endogenous chronic carbon monoxide poisoning caused by exposure to methylene chloride. J Soc Occup Med 1979;29:12–14.

48. Edling C, Ekberg K, Ahlborg G Jr, et al: Long-term follow up of workers exposed to solvents. Br J Ind Med 1990;47:75–82.

49. Gregersen P: Neurotoxic effects of organic solvents in exposed workers: two controlled follow-up studies after 5.5 and 10.6 years. Am J Ind Med 1988;14:681–701.

50. Rasmussen K, Jeppesen HJ, Sabroe S: Solvent-induced chronic toxic encephalopathy. Am J Ind Med 1993;23:779–792.

51. Herd PA, Lipsky M, Martin HF: Cardiovascular effects of 1,1,1-trichloroethane. Arch Environ Health 1974;28:227–233.

52. Zakhari S: Cardiovascular toxicology of halogenated hydrocarbons and other solvents. In Acosta D (ed): Cardiovascular Toxicology. New York, Raven, 1992.

53. Henry J, Cassidy S: Membrane stabilizing activity: a major cause of fatal poisoning. 1986;1:1414–1417.

54. Hoffmann P, Heinroth K, Richards D, et al: Depression of calcium dynamics in cardiac myocytes—a common mechanism of halogenated hydrocarbon anesthetics and solvents. J Mol Cell Cardiol 1994;26:579–589.

55. Ford ES, Rhodes S, McDiarmid M, et al: Deaths from acute exposure to trichloroethylene. J Occup Environ Med 1995;37:749–754.

56. Coopman VA, Cordonnier JA, De Letter EA, Piette MH: Tissue distribution of trichloroethylene in a case of accidental acute intoxication by inhalation. Forensic Sci Int 2003;134:115–119.

57. Reinhardt CF, Azar A, Maxfield ME, et al: Cardiac arrhythmias and aerosol "sniffing." Arch Environ Health 1971;22:265–279.

58. Shepherd RT: Mechanism of sudden death associated with volatile substance abuse. Hum Toxicol 1989;8:287–291.

59. Ramsey JD, Flanagan RJ: The role of the laboratory in the investigation of solvent abuse. Hum Toxicol 1982;1:299–311.

60. Alha A, Korte T, Tenhu M: Solvent sniffing death. Z Rechtsmed 1973;72:299–305.

61. Bell GM, Gordon ACH, Lee P: Proliferating glomerulonephritis and exposure to organic solvents. Nephron 1985;40:161.

62. Harrington JM, Whitby H, Gray CN: Renal disease and occupational exposure to organic solvents: a case referent approach. Br J Ind Med 1989;46:643.

63. Boogaard PJ, Caubo ME: Increased albumin excretion in industrial workers due to shift work rather than to prolonged exposure to low concentrations of chlorinated hydrocarbons. Occup Environ Med 1994;51:638–641.

64. Czirjak L, Pocs E, Szegedi G: Localized scleroderma after exposure to organic solvents. Dermatology 1994;189:399–401.

65. Patel R, Janakiraman N, Johnson R, Elman JB: Pulmonary edema and coma from perchloroethylene. JAMA 1973;223:1510.

66. Nichols WK, Covington MO, Seiders CD, et al: Bioactivation of halogenated hydrocarbons by rabbit pulmonary cells. Pharmacol Toxicol 1992;71:335–339.

67. Garriott J, Petty CS: Death from inhalant abuse: toxicological and pathological evaluation of 34 cases. Clin Toxicol 1980;16:305–315.

68. Trense E, Zimmermann H: Fatal inhalation poisoning with chronically acting tetrachloroethylene vapors. Zentralbl Arbeitsmed 1969;19:131–137.

69. Barlow SM, Sullivan FM: Reproductive hazards of industrial chemicals: an evaluation of animal and human data. London, Academic Press, 1982.

70. Schardein JL: Chemically induced birth defects, 3rd ed. New York, Marcel-Dekker, 2000.

71. Chang YM, Tai CF, Yang SC, et al: A cohort mortality study of workers exposed to chlorinated organic solvents in Taiwan. Ann Epidemiol 2003;13:652–660.

72. Raaschou-Nielsen O, Hansen J, McLaughlin JK, et al: Cancer risk among workers at Danish companies using trichloroethylene: a cohort study. Am J Epidemiol 2003;158:1182–1192.

73. U.S. Department of Health and Human Services: ATSDR toxicological profile for trichloroethylene. Atlanta, Agency for Toxic Substances and Disease Registry, 1992.

74. von Grote J, Hurlimann C, Scheringer M, Hungerbuhler K: Reduction of occupational exposure to perchloroethylene and trichloroethylene in metal degreasing over the last 30 years: influences of technology innovation and legislation. J Expo Anal Environ Epidemiol 2003;13:325–340.

75. Clayton GD, Clayton FE: Patty's Industrial Hygiene and Toxicology, 4th ed. New York, John Wiley & Sons, 1994.

76. Dowty BJ, Laseter JL, Storer J: The transplacental migration and accumulation in blood of volatile organic constituents. Pediatr Res 1976;10:696–701.

77. Tylleskar-Jensen J: Chloroform—a cause of pregnancy toxemia? Nord Med 1967;77:841–842.

78. Registry of Toxic Effects of Chemical Substances: NIOSH. Englewood, CO, Micromedex, 1999.

79. Hamlin GP, Kholkute SD, Dukelow WR: Toxicology of maternally ingested carbon tetrachloride (CCl4) on embryonal and fetal development and in vitro fertilization in mice. Zool Sci 1993;10:111–116.

80. Takizawa S, Watanabe H, Naito Y, Inoue S: Preparative action of carbon tetrachloride in liver tumorigenesis by a single application of N-butylnitrosourea in male ICR/JCL strain mice. Gann 1975;66:603–614.

81. Smilkstein MJ, Knapp GL, Kulig KW, Rumack BH: Efficacy of oral N-acetylcysteine in the treatment of acetaminophen overdose: analysis of the national multicenter study (1976 to 1985). N Engl J Med 1988;319:1557–1562.

82. Harrison PM, Wendon JA, Gimson AE, et al: Improvement by acetylcysteine of hemodynamics and oxygen transport in fulminant hepatic failure. N Engl J Med 1991;324:1852–1857.

83. Valles EG, de Castro CR, Castro JA: N-acetyl cysteine is an early but also a late preventive agent against carbon tetrachloride-induced liver necrosis. Toxicol Lett 1994;71:87–95.

94 *Benzene and Related Aromatic Hydrocarbons*

DANA B. MIRKIN, MD

At a Glance...

- Being highly lipophilic, all can produce narcosis if inhaled in high concentration, with CNS depressant effects that compare with those of general anesthetics
- The major aromatic compounds of toxicologic importance are toluene, benzene, styrene, ethylbenzene, trimethylbenzene, and xylene.
- The toxicity of the aromatic hydrocarbons is variable. Some, such as benzene, are highly toxic, affecting the CNS, bone marrow, and other vital organs.
- Many of the aromatic compounds are metabolized by cytochrome P450 isozymes.
- Metabolites of aromatic compounds are excreted in urine, making biological monitoring for occupational exposures relatively simple. In contrast, analysis of aromatics and their metabolites in blood is difficult.
- Treatment of severe exposure is supportive and includes the provision of fresh air or oxygen. There is probably little role for gastrointestinal decontamination since aromatics are not well adsorbed by activated charcoal.

Aromatic hydrocarbons are benzene derivatives; they constitute more than 50% of the different chemicals in common use.[1,2] Aromatic solvents are found widely in many diverse occupations and products, in degreasing operations, lacquers manufacturing, printing, electronics and rubber (especially tire) manufacturing, paints, resins, pharmaceuticals, and glues and adhesives. They are liquids that typically exhibit high vapor pressures and low boiling points that rise with increasing molecular weight. This group of compounds has chemical structures of unsaturated cyclic compounds with the benzene ring as its basis. Benzene is the simplest homolog within the group.

Aromatic hydrocarbons are divided into the *benzene* group (one ring), the *naphthalene* group (two rings), and the *anthracene* group (three rings). *Polycyclic aromatic hydrocarbons* (polynuclear aromatic hydrocarbons) have multifused benzene rings.[3] This chapter reviews only the aromatic hydrocarbons in the benzene (single-ring) group, specifically benzene and its common derivatives, styrene, toluene, and xylene. These four compounds have historically been used as solvents, antiknock agents in motor fuel, and process intermediates and feedstock for chemical synthesis.

Although originally derived from coal tar, the main source of aromatic organic compounds today is petroleum.

The term *aromatic* originally stemmed from the pleasant odor characteristic of the earlier recognized compounds in the group; these substances were used in perfumes and flavorings. However, some aromatic hydrocarbons are odorless.

Aromatic solvents are characterized by nonpolarity and high lipid solubility. Structurally, their molecules are flat, with reactive electron clouds above and below the ring. The aromatic solvents have historically been found as mixtures in occupational settings, such as combinations of toluene, benzene, styrene, ethylbenzene, trimethylbenzene, and xylene.

Exposure to aromatic solvents occurs through contact with vapor or liquid with absorption through inhalation or the skin. Acute inhalational exposure to high airborne concentrations can produce dizziness, syncope, confusion, euphoria, respiratory irritation, and in some instances, coma through direct neurotoxicity (solvent narcosis). Inhalational exposure to high airborne concentrations may also sensitize the myocardium to catecholamines, both endogenous and exogenous, leading to potentially dangerous dysrhythmias, once dubbed "sudden sniffing death syndrome." Their individual toxicity correlates with physical chemical properties, inherent toxicity, and clinical pharmacokinetics, including metabolite production. Some aromatics, such as benzene and styrene, have metabolites that are their primary toxins.

BENZENE

Benzene, CAS registry 71-43-2, also referred to as annulene, benzeen (Dutch), benzen (Polish), benzol, benzole, benzolo (Italian), bicarburet of hydrogen, coal naphtha, cyclohexatriene, fenzen (Czech), phene, phenyl hydride, pyrobenzol, pyrobenzole, and Polystream, is a clear, colorless to yellow liquid. Its odor threshold is 1.54 to 4.68 ppm, with a taste threshold in water of 0.5 to 4.5 mg/L. The molecular weight is 78.11.[4,5] Benzene in mixtures deviates from Raoult's law. Its vapor concentration is frequently higher than would be expected based on the concentration of benzene found in a solvent or hydrocarbon mixture. This is especially true of mixtures of hydrocarbons or solvents containing more than 5% benzene, from which substantial exposures to benzene vapors might occur during routine use.[6]

Benzene, a highly flammable liquid, was first discovered in 1825 by Michael Faraday, who isolated it from a liquid condensed from compressed oil gas.[7] The heating of coal in a "by-product coke oven" resulted in the extraction of benzene, a significant by-product that, because of its low cost, excellent solvent properties, and rapid rate of evaporation, was used to make solutions of rubber or inks. Benzene was also involved in the chemical synthesis of dyes or halobenzene derivatives and other chemicals.[8] In the 19th century, benzene was a common household degreasing agent and used in the dry-cleaning industry until its flammability, rather than its toxicity, led to its replacement by chlorinated

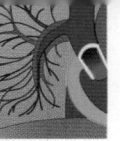

hydrocarbon solvents. Benzene was one of the first cancer chemotherapeutic agents recommended for the treatment of leukemia. The rationale for this astonishing treatment was that leukopenia occurred in some cases of benzene poisoning. However, "benzene therapy" was short-lived because of the complex action of the substance on the blood and the ensuing toxicity.[9]

Today, benzene is a widely used chemical with an annual production ranging from 10 to 30 billion pounds.[10,11]

Recently, the mandatory decrease of lead alkyls in gasoline has led to an increase in the aromatic hydrocarbon content of gasoline to maintain high octane levels and antiknock properties. In the United States, gasoline typically contains less than 2% benzene by volume, but in other countries, benzene concentrations can be as high as 5%.[11]

Human exposure to benzene takes place in factories, refineries, and other industrial settings. Although only a relatively small number of individuals are occupationally exposed to benzene, the general population is exposed to benzene contained in gasoline, automobile exhaust, and diesel fuel. Benzene is present in cigarette smoke, and smoking is the main source of benzene exposure for many people.[7] It is found naturally in the environment at low concentrations.[12] For example, a hen's egg contains 35 to 133 µg of benzene. Many other foods (haddock fillet, red beans, blue cheese, cheddar cheese, pineapple, roasted filberts, potato tubers, cooked chicken, tomatoes, strawberries, black currants, roasted peanuts, soybean milk, codfish) also contain benzene in minute quantities. However, the exposure to benzene through normal dietary intake is not considered to be significant for the general population. Intakes per day from other exposures include smoking (1800 µg), passive smoke (50 µg), filling a gas tank (10 µg), driving or riding in a car (40 µg), and breathing outdoor air (120 µg).[10,13]

In 1897, Santesson, a professor of pharmacology at the University of Stockholm, first reported the deaths from aplastic anemia of four female industrial workers who used a benzene-based rubber cement in the course of their work in a tire factory. Subsequently, Selling at Johns Hopkins (1910) substantiated his suspicion that benzene was the cause of aplastic anemia among workers in a canning factory, inducing leukopenia and marrow aplasia in rabbits by injecting them with benzene (subcutaneously, 1 mL/kg daily). Weiskotten (1920) at Syracuse University College of Medicine administered benzene by inhalation to rabbits (240 ppm) and produced similar results. Confirmed by subsequent studies, the direct relationship between benzene exposure and aplastic anemia was established.[14]

Acceptance of the cause-and-effect association between benzene exposure and leukemia was, however, slower in gaining acceptance after initial case reports by LeNoir and Claude in 1897 and Delore and Borgomano in 1928[7] because few cases of leukemia were observed compared with reports of aplastic anemia associated with benzene exposure during that period. Nevertheless, Vigliani (1938) described benzene toxicity and classified it into four groups: (1) typical aplastic anemia, (2) atypical aplastic anemia with the bone marrow appearing

to be quite active in the formation of undifferentiated cells, (3) atypical aplastic anemia in which the marrow appeared to be either "hyperplastic" or "metaplastic," and (4) aleukemic leukemia.[14]

A cottage industry in shoemaking existed in Turkey, with families making shoes in their poorly ventilated homes. A petroleum-based solvent was used as a base for the glue until 1955 to 1960, when a change was made to a benzene-based glue. Professor M. Aksoy of the Department of Hematology at the University of Istanbul recognized an unusual number of cases of aplastic anemia and leukemia among his clinic patients. Aware of Vigliani's work, he studied the shoemakers of Istanbul, a cohort that numbered 28,500, and initially described 217 cases of bone marrow depression and 26 cases of leukemia (1971). He detected several cases of "preleukemia" and subsequently reported that of 51 cases of pancytopenia, 13 developed leukemia (1972).[14]

U.S. agencies, such as the Occupational Safety and Health Administration (OSHA) and the National Institute of Occupational Safety and Health (NIOSH) conducted further studies that established benzene as a leukemogen; those agencies and others attempted to determine acceptable levels of workplace exposure.[15] A scientific consensus group (International Agency for Research on Cancer, IARC) concluded in 1982 that benzene was etiologically related to the development of acute nonlymphocytic leukemia based on epidemiologic studies.[16]

Later, a retrospective study was conducted on a well-defined cohort of workers in Ohio who were engaged in the manufacture of a rubberized material termed *Pliofilm*, in which benzene was used as a solvent for the rubber. The study showed elevated risks for leukemia associated with benzene exposure and argued that the risk was cumulative with prolonged exposure.[14]

Despite criticism of the Pliofilm study, subsequent analyses have supported the role of benzene as a leukemogen, and the argument has since revolved around estimates of risk.

An opportunity to use a larger cohort of benzene-exposed workers, which might be a better source of data for relating dose to leukemogenesis, arose in China where Dr. S-N. Yin of the Institute of Health of the Chinese Academy of Medical Sciences studied more than 500,000 workers demonstrating yet again the associations between benzene exposure and aplastic anemia and leukemia. Although the average benzene exposure concentration of the entire exposed cohort was determined to be 5.6 ppm, ranges of exposure among subcohorts of workers developing aplastic anemia and leukemia were found to be much higher, 29 to 361 ppm over varying periods of time.

A joint effort on the part of Dr. Yin's group and the U.S. National Cancer Institute (NCI) involving almost 75,000 exposed workers and 36,000 controls demonstrated significantly elevated levels of acute myelogenous leukemia (AML), myelodysplastic syndrome (MDS), and aplastic anemia associated with benzene exposure at levels below 10 ppm. However, the accuracy of exposure measurements and estimates in the Chinese cohorts

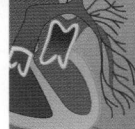

have since been questioned, and exposure levels may have been much higher than originally reported.[17] The controversy regarding a "safe" level for occupational exposure continues.

The benzene ring is not a structure that readily binds covalently to glutathione, proteins, DNA, and RNA. It requires metabolic activation to a more reactive structure beginning with conversion to an epoxide (i.e., benzene oxide). Benzene oxide, in equilibrium with its oxepin form, is further metabolized to hydroquinone and catechol, which can then be readily converted to a ben-zoquinone (*ortho*- or *para*-), the ultimate toxic metabolite of benzene. Another potentially toxic metabolite, muconaldehyde, may arise from opening of the benzene oxide ring.[9,15]

The mechanisms by which benzene produces bone marrow damage involve several targets of benzene metabolites. These include inhibition of spindle for-mation, which impairs mitosis; inhibition of the synthesis of interleukin-1, an essential factor in normal bone marrow function; covalent binding to proteins and DNA, forming adducts; inhibition of DNA polymerase con-tributing to irreversible changes in DNA; and chromo-some damage, observed in MDS. Although the impact of these and other possible effects may have differential significance in the development of benzene toxicity, all appear to occur in the course of the development of benzene-induced hemopathies.[8]

Upon inhalation of benzene vapors, respiratory uptake varies from 47% to 80%; dermal absorption from liquid ranges from 0.05% to 0.2%. Absorption data for oral exposure are not available for humans; however, in animals, absorption rates following oral ingestion of benzene have been found to be 90% to 100%.[11]

Benzene is distributed throughout the body after absorption into the blood. Because it is lipophilic, a high distribution to fatty tissue is expected. Benzene crosses the human placenta and is present in the cord blood in amounts equal to or greater than that in maternal blood.[4]

After inhalational exposure, most benzene is excreted unchanged in exhaled air. Absorbed benzene is rapidly detected in all organs. Its excretion involves a biphasic urinary excretion of conjugated derivatives (sulfates and glucuronides) with a half-life of 0.7 hours. The half-life of benzene in lipid tissues is about 24 hours.

Metabolism of benzene occurs primarily in the liver, although metabolism in bone marrow is also believed to play an important role in myelotoxicity. After rapid absorption from the lungs, benzene undergoes both phase I and II biotransformation in the liver. The primary phase I biotransformation of benzene involves cytochrome P-450 2E1-catalyzed (CYP2E1) conversion initially to phenol and subsequently to hydroquinone and catechol.[18]

The opening of the benzene ring, to eventually form muconic acid, appears to include a number of inter-mediates that arise from muconaldehyde.[19]

The many urinary metabolites of benzene include sulfate and glucuronic acid conjugates of the hydrox-ylated ring metabolites, several glutathione derivatives, and muconic acid. At least one residue of a DNA adduct (7-phenylguanine) has been reported.[19]

Factors that alter the metabolism of benzene have the potential to influence its hematopoietic toxicity and carcinogenicity. Current research centers on the identification of risk factors for susceptibility to benzene toxicity, and there is evidence that metabolic susceptibility and genetic predisposition may play a major role. Metabolism and disposition are among the most important determinants of benzene toxicity. This variability results from intrinsic differences in the activities of xenobiotic metabolizing enzymes (so-called genetic polymorphisms). Variable factors in sensitivity include (1) hepatic CYP2E1, a major enzyme of the cytochrome P-450 family involved in benzene oxidation; (2) conjugating enzymes such as glutathione transferases; and (3) comparative activity of myeloperoxidase and myeloreductase (NQO1) in bone marrow. Benzene toxicity is thought to be exerted through oxidation metabolites formed in the liver primarily through pathways mediated by the cytochrome P-450 family of enzymes; benzene oxide may be sufficiently stable to reach the bone marrow. Interindividual variations in benzene metabolism are related to CYP2E1 expression, possibly owing to polymorphism of the *CYP2E1* gene. CYP2E1 is found in both the liver and bone marrow. Another enzyme found to metabolize benzene is CYP1B1.[20]

An important protective mechanism against oxidative stress is the detoxification of lipid peroxidation products by glutathione S-transferase-theta (GSTT1) and -mu (GSTM1). Phase II metabolizing enzymes such as GSTT1 show genetic polymorphisms that correlate with GSTT1 activity. Studies have demonstrated an increased risk for myelodysplastic syndromes in individuals with a *GSTT1* gene defect or absence.[20]

Hydroxylated metabolites of benzene are activated to toxic and genotoxic species in the bone marrow through oxidation by myeloperoxidase (MPO). NAD(P)H:quinone oxidoreductase (NQO1) is an enzyme capable of reducing the oxidized quinone metabolites and thereby potentially reducing their toxicities. A polymorphism in NQO1, a C609T substitution, has been identified, and individuals homozygous for this change (T/T) have no detectable NQO1. A higher frequency of an inactivating polymorphism in NQO1 has been reported in a cohort of patients with myeloid leukemias, especially those with an abnormality of chromosome 5 or 7, a chromosomal aberration associated with benzene exposure. It has been postulated that homozygotes (who display a complete loss of enzyme activity), as well as heterozygotes (who are at risk for loss of the remaining wild-type allele in their hematopoietic stem cells), may be particularly vulner-able to leukemogenic changes induced by carcinogens such as benzene.[15,19,20] Limited gender comparisons suggest that males metabolize benzene at a higher rate then females, who retain benzene longer, owing to their higher body-fat content.

There is little evidence, however, that women and offspring are more susceptible to clastogenic or leu-kemogenic actions of benzene.

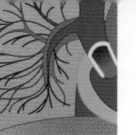

It remains unknown whether benzene affects reproductive function in humans.[21] A study of benzene-exposed female dental surgeons failed to show an adverse effect on fertility, whereas another study of aircraft maintenance workers exposed to solvents and fuel showed some adverse effects on sperm function, including a decline in sperm motility, but the finding could not be attributed solely to benzene exposure.[20]

It has been demonstrated that pretreatment of rats with ethanol, a CYP2E1 inducer, enhances metabolism of benzene and potentiates its acute myelotoxicity. Pretreatment of male B6C3F1 mice with acetone, another CYP2E1 inducer, increases benzene oxidation about five times. Pretreatment with diethyldithiocarbamate, a CYP2E1 inhibitor, completely abolishes benzene oxidation.

Pretreatment of mice with inducers of metabolism such as 3-methylcholanthrene and β-naphthoflavone increased both benzene metabolism and benzene toxicity.

Toluene inhibits benzene metabolism.[22] Workers exposed to a combination of benzene and toluene produced significantly lower urinary phenol (a biomarker for benzene exposure) than those exposed to either benzene or toluene alone; toluene has also been shown to lower the toxicity of benzene in animals. It should be noted that Aroclor 1254, a polychlorinated biphenyl (PCB) used as a coolant in electrical transformers, is also known to alter the toxicity and metabolism of benzene.[11] It is unclear what role phenobarbital plays; one author claims a negligible effect, whereas another states it alters the toxicity and metabolism of benzene.[11,15]

Benzene readily enters the central nervous system (CNS) and may cause immediate effects including headache, nausea, dizziness, confusion, convulsions, and coma leading to death.[21,23] It has even been used as a general anesthetic. CNS responses to airborne levels are generally as follows: 2.5 ppm, no effect regardless of duration; 50 to 150 ppm, headache and lassitude; 500 ppm, sleepiness after 3 to 4 hours; 3000 ppm, sleep within 30 minutes, then progressive stupor; 7000 ppm, stupor within 30 minutes. Oral ingestion of 9 to 12 g of benzene causes staggering gait, vomiting, delirium, tachycardia, hypotension, coma, and occasionally death.[23] Severe inhalation may lead to noncardiogenic pulmonary edema. Ventricular arrhythmias may result from increased sensitivity of the myocardium to catecholamines. Benzene can cause chemical burns to the skin with prolonged contact or massive topical exposure.[21]

Evidence of benzene poisoning may appear in a few weeks or only after many years of exposure, or it may not be discovered until the onset of infection from bone marrow suppression, long after exposure has ceased.

Benzene produces a continuum of effects on the bone marrow ranging from reversible abnormalities to AML. These effects appear to be dose dependent. Chronic exposure to benzene results in bone marrow depression and tissue damage, with effects ranging from decreases in selective blood elements (leukocytes, lymphocytes, or platelets) to aplastic anemia (decreases in all cell types). Pancytopenia, aplastic anemia, AML, and their variants may occur.[21] Findings are variable, especially in early examination of blood. The most common abnormality is a decrease in total white blood cell count, which may be accompanied by a relative lymphocytosis and a macrocytic, normochromic, or slightly hyperchromic anemia and thrombocytopenia. The bone marrow may reveal nonspecific changes initially. Depression of bone marrow function occurs after months or years of relatively low-level exposure. Myelotoxicity may initially manifest as stimulation of all three bone marrow elements, which is soon followed by progressive anemia and thrombocytopenia. As the disease progresses, the bone marrow may become aplastic or hyperplastic in a manner that does not always correlate with the peripheral blood picture.

In the early stages, bone marrow depression is reversible; continued exposure, however, has led to fatal aplastic anemia.[23] After benzene exposure, decreases in circulating blood cells may also be observed in the presence of a dysplastic marrow characterized by abnormal architecture, chromosomal damage in many cells, and inadequate hematopoiesis leading to MDS, a preleukemic state that usually proceeds to AML. MDS is now believed to be a result of benzene exposure. There is interest centering on the possibility that environmental benzene exposure in the general public (such as exposure to vehicle exhaust emissions) may be associated with a rise in the occurrence of non-Hodgkin's lymphoma (NHL).[20] Causality is also suspected for chronic myelogenous leukemia and chronic lymphocytic leukemia.[21] Benzene was formerly suspected of causing multiple myeloma, but subsequent studies have failed to confirm an association. In fact, the weight of the evidence, at present, leans against an association between benzene and multiple myeloma. There have been unproven associations between benzene exposure and acute lymphoblastic leukemia, myelofibrosis, and lymphomas.

The diagnosis of benzene poisoning is based on a history of exposure and typical clinical findings. With chronic hematologic toxicity, erythrocyte, leukocyte, and thrombocyte counts may first increase and then decrease before the onset of aplastic anemia. Such a pattern may signal a history of benzene exposure.

Biomarkers of exposure to benzene have been developed and carefully evaluated. Concentrations of the parent compound in exhaled breath parallel blood concentrations. This is confounded by smoking, which also causes elevations of benzene in exhaled breath. Urine benzene is quite specific and correlates well with concentrations between 32 and 800 µg/m³, but it is easily confounded by smoking. Moreover, measurements at these levels are at the limit of detection, rendering them unreliable.[24]

Urinary excretion of a variety of benzene metabolites (i.e., phenol, catechol, hydroquinone, 1,2,4-trihydroxybenzene, S-phenylmercapturic acid, and *t,t*-muconic acid) have shown correlation with benzene exposure in occupational settings. Phenol, catechol, and hydroquinone analyses are neither sensitive nor specific because relatively high levels are found in nonexposed

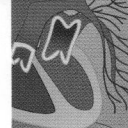

individuals. Similarly, *t,t*-muconic acid is not specific because it is a metabolite of sorbic acid, a common food additive. Nevertheless, urinary phenols have been useful for respiratory exposure greater than 5 ppm (16 mg/m^3). Testing for urinary phenol is required by OSHA in workers exposed to benzene in an emergency involving an unexpected significant release of benzene. Below this concentration, there is too much interference from food and medication and results are unreliable.

S-phenylmercapturic acid (SPMA), an end product of the conjugation of benzene oxide and glutathione (GSH), is a suitable urinary biomarker of low-level benzene exposure (0.01 ppm) because of its specificity and relatively long half-life (9 hours). It is very specific for benzene.

Adducts to hemoglobin and cysteine groups of proteins have been demonstrated in rodents, but not in humans. DNA damage manifested by chromosome abnormalities has been detected in benzene-exposed workers, although such measures have not yet found widespread acceptance as biomarkers of effect.

Blood benzene is useful for determining exposure to concentrations exceeding 0.25 ppm but is also confounded by smoking. The specimen must be collected at or immediately after exposure because the half-life of benzene in the blood has been reported to be as brief as 30 to 60 minutes.[24]

Potential etiologies for aplastic anemia include idiopathic, inborn (Fanconi's anemia), dose-related reactions (e.g., antineoplastic agents, benzene, chloramphenicol, inorganics, irradiation); idiosyncratic reactions (e.g., acetazolamide, arsenicals, barbiturates, chloramphenicol, gold, insecticides, phenothiazines, phenylbutazone, pyrimethamine, solvents, sulfa drugs, thiouracils); viral infections (e.g., hepatitis); pregnancy; and rheumatoid arthritis. Many medications can cause aplastic anemia.

For a summary of clinical management, refer to Box 94-1.

A spot urine phenol measurement of all exposed, including the victim, rescuers, and health care personnel, may serve as a useful indicator of high-level exposure to benzene. It is not immediately clinically useful because it may take days for the result to be reported, and it does not alter immediate therapy. Nevertheless, measurement should be made to ensure appropriate follow-up of those exposed. Acute high-level exposure to benzene may lead to hematotoxicity at a later date; thus, it is important to identify exposed individuals so that their blood indices can be followed to ensure appropriate diagnosis and treatment. This is mandated for occupational exposures by OSHA. OSHA (29CFR1910.1028) requires that after an emergency (unexpected) exposure to benzene, a urine phenol should be collected at the end of the work shift. The specimen's specific gravity must be corrected to 1.024 for proper adjustment of the phenol level. Levels of 75 mg/L or higher require complete blood counts with differentials every month for 3 months. A spot urine level higher than 20 mg/L suggests excessive occupational exposure, although the test is nonspecific and can be confounded by the presence of other aromatic com-

BOX 94-1	TREATMENT PROTOCOL FOR ACUTE EXPOSURE TO AROMATIC HYDROCARBONS

1. Avoid unprotected contact with liquid and vapor via appropriate skin and respiratory protection.
2. Decontaminate victim by removal from exposure, removal and disposal of contaminated clothing, and copious irrigation of contaminated eyes and skin.
3. Monitor O_2 and intravenous line.
4. Do not induce emesis; gastric lavage if recent (within 30 minutes) ingestion.
5. Protect airway from aspiration.
6. Provide supportive care to maintain airway, oxygenation, ventilation, and circulation.
7. Treat coma, seizures, arrythmias, and other complications if they occur.
8. Avoid sympathomimetics (e.g., epinephrine), if possible, to prevent potentially fatal tachyarrythmias. Tachyarrythmias may require treatment with β blockers (esmolol, metoprolol, or propranolol).
9. Perform chest roentgenogram, liver profile, urinalysis, serum electrolytes, blood urea nitrogen, creatinine, electrocardiogram, and complete blood counts with differential as necessary.
10. Do specific lab analyses as required, e.g., OSHA requires a urine phenol analysis for benzene exposure to determine the need to monitor for delayed hematotoxicity.
11. Monitor for 12–24 hours if exposure is substantial.

OSHA, Occupational Safety and Health Administration.

pounds both in the workplace and in the diet of those exposed. Over-the-counter cough and sore throat lozenges can cause an elevated urine phenol. Benzene can also be measured in expired air for up to 2 days after exposure.[21]

A baseline complete blood count with differential should be obtained along with the urine phenol. Other laboratory tests, including liver function studies, electrolytes, chest x-ray, and blood gases, may be ordered based on clinical findings.

There is no antidote.

Benzene overexposure requires prolonged (months to years) follow-up of hematologic parameters beyond the acute phase to monitor for changes in blood cell counts and differentials that may require hematology consultation and treatment (e.g., transfusion).

OSHA (29CFR1910.1028) requires that baseline and annual testing be made available to workers occupationally exposed to benzene. Workers are offered medical exams consisting of a medical and occupational history and complete blood count with differential. Abnormal findings trigger medical evaluations, which may lead to removal from exposure and evaluation by a hematologist or other appropriate specialist.

Urine S-phenylmercapturic acid measurement at the end of the work shift is a sensitive and specific marker of exposure to low levels of benzene and can be used to detect overexposure. The American Conference of Governmental Industrial Hygienists (ACGIH) has established a biologic exposure index (BEI) of 25 µg/g creatinine.

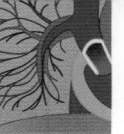

Recovery from acute benzene exposure depends on severity of symptoms. Symptoms may persist for 2 to 3 weeks. Chronic effects of benzene intoxication may arise and persist long after an acute exposure occurs. Benzene is a leukemogen; leukemia can occur before or after aplastic anemia. Individual response to either acute or chronic benzene exposure is variable.

STYRENE

Styrene, also known as cinnamene, phenylethylene, and vinyl benzene, is a high-production-volume chemical, with more than 10 billion pounds produced annually in the United States.[25] Styrene is a colorless to slightly yellow, oily liquid that spontaneously polymerizes unless inhibited. It is liquid at room temperature and highly flammable.[26,27] At low concentrations, it has a sweet odor; at concentrations above 100 ppm, it's odor is objectionable. Styrene has a low vapor pressure and is soluble in organic solvents, but only slightly soluble in water.[27]

Although styrene was discovered in 1831, it did not become commercially important until 1942, when it was used in the synthesis of unsaturated polyesters and reinforced plastics. Currently, styrene is widely used to make plastics and resins for surface coatings. It is also used as a chemical intermediate. Styrene-containing polymers are used to make tires, boat hulls, shower stalls, bath tubs, dental restorative plastics, and many other plastic products. Styrene can be synthesized but is also found naturally in storax, a gum derived from styracaceous trees. Primary exposures to styrene occur during its manufacture and polymerization, particularly in situations in which open polymerization processes are used, for example, in boat building or shower-stall manufacturing. Styrene is present in tobacco smoke and has been detected in ambient urban air samples.

Styrene is naturally present in foods such as strawberries, beef, and spices, and is naturally produced in the processing of foods such as wine and cheese. Styrene is permitted as a direct food additive in small quantities under the Food and Drug Act, and as an indirect food additive that migrates from packaging materials into food. It undergoes rapid biodegradation; styrene levels in surface water and groundwater are generally very low (<1 μg/L) or nondetectable.

Cancer bioassays and epidemiology studies have failed to identify the nervous system as a target, and they have failed to identify a cancer risk associated with styrene.[28]

Several epidemiologic studies on workers have shown that styrene affects color vision in a dose-dependent manner. These effects on color perception are in the blue-yellow axis, in contrast to congenital color-blindness, which is in the red-green axis. Alterations appear to be reversible when exposure conditions are improved. The Lanthony D15-d panel has proved the most efficient in detecting acquired deficiencies in color vision.[29]

The mechanism of styrene's effects on the nervous system is not known. It is likely that the effects of high-level, acute exposure are due to styrene itself because they appear shortly after exposure and before significant metabolism. However, it is unclear whether the parent compound or metabolites are neurotoxic at lower exposure levels. Because of its potential reactivity, styrene oxide is an obvious candidate metabolite for concern; its potential reactivity has implications for genotoxicity and carcinogenesis for styrene because it is mutagenic in vitro and carcinogenic in animal studies. However, neither animal studies nor human epidemiology studies have validated these concerns.

Styrene is absorbed after oral, inhalation, or dermal exposure. The primary route of human exposure is through the lungs. Average retention of styrene in the respiratory tract after inhalation of 4.6 to 46 ppm is 71% for humans. Once absorbed, styrene is widely distributed in the body.

Styrene requires metabolic activation to induce effects other than acute toxicity.[30] Metabolism of styrene includes, as an initial step, oxidation of styrene by cytochrome P-450 enzymes to form styrene oxide or styrene-7,8-epoxide, which may be responsible for some of the toxic effects observed after styrene exposure. The major metabolic and detoxication pathway involving styrene oxide results in the formation of styrene glycol, followed by mandelic acid and phenylglycolic acid, which are often used as biologic exposure indices.

Styrene oxide is further metabolized by epoxide hydrolase and GSH S-transferase activities. There are species differences, with humans showing little conversion to styrene oxide through CYP450, but enhanced conversion of styrene oxide by epoxide hydrolase, which suggests the human body burden of styrene oxide after either styrene or styrene oxide exposure is lower than in rats or mice.

Due to its relatively high lipid solubility, styrene may be retained in human fat for up to 5 weeks after exposure. The half-life of styrene in fat is 2.2 to 4 days for men exposed to 50 ppm styrene for 1 hour (30 minutes rest plus 30 minutes exercise).[27] The half-life of styrene in human blood is believed to be biphasic. There is a rapid elimination phase with a half-life of 0.57 to 0.68 hour and a second slow phase with a half-life of 13 hours.

The elimination of mandelic acid in urine is biphasic. The first-phase half-life is 2 to 4 hours, and the second-phase half-life is 25 to 30 hours. The elimination half-life of phenylglyoxylic acid in urine is 11 hours.

Styrene has been found in breast milk in U.S. cities. It has been suggested that styrene would be expected to be found in breast milk at higher concentrations than in blood or urine because of its lipophilicity.

Styrene has been subjected to extensive toxicologic investigation. Subchronic and chronic experimental studies with styrene have not clearly identified neurotoxic effects in animals beyond those effects that can be attributed to CNS depression.

Animal studies indicate that styrene may alter brain neurochemistry, although the pattern of effects is not well understood. The only long-lasting reproducible effect observed in animal studies is ototoxicity, which has not been clearly demonstrated in humans.

Ototoxicity has been found at styrene concentrations at and above 800 ppm for prolonged periods. These

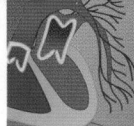

functional changes in laboratory animals have been correlated with morphologic changes, including deficits in outer hair cells in the basal and lower middle turns of the organ of Corti. Ototoxicity has not been observed at 50 or 200 ppm exposure levels. Studies in humans have generally been negative or failed to control for noise. However, a recent study funded by NIOSH found a dose-dependent effect of low-level styrene exposure on hearing thresholds, which acted independently of the effect of noise exposure. Levels of mandelic acid in urine correlated with hearing loss, lending credence to claims that low-level styrene exposure can contribute to elevated hearing thresholds independently.[31]

Several studies have reported impaired color vision among styrene workers.

Based on differences in metabolism between rodents and humans, no lung or nasal toxicity is expected in humans from styrene exposure.[32]

Although not thoroughly tested, styrene does not appear to be an important reproductive toxicant. Similarly, studies so far do not indicate that developmental toxicity is likely to be a major concern. Teratologic studies have shown fetotoxicity, fetal weight reduction, and reduced survival in rats, but only at doses that also produced maternal toxicity. No malformations have been reported.

There is no evidence that styrene is a teratogen. Styrene is not a developmental toxicant at nonmaternally toxic exposures in experimental animals. There are still no convincing indications of styrene-induced malformations. There is some evidence, from reliable studies, for slight embryo-fetal toxicity (primarily developmental delays; possible increases in skeletal variations) at maternally toxic exposures. There is a combined weight of evidence that suggests the developing CNS may be adversely affected by the neurotoxic effects of styrene at high doses.[33]

High-level styrene inhalation exposure of rabbits and oral administration to rats induce some changes in brain dopamine, which may affect the function of the hypothalamus and pituitary. Abnormalities of pituitary secretion in women exposed to styrene have also been suggested. These effects may be connected with putative effects on the menstrual cycle.

The current weight of evidence suggests that styrene is not likely to affect estrogenic or androgenic activity, and, thus, it would not appear to be a hormonally active agent.

Styrene irritates the mucosal membranes of the respiratory tract. It can cause sore throat, nasal irritation, and increased nasal secretion. Pulmonary edema may develop 24 to 72 hours after high-grade exposure.

It has been suggested that at 100 to 200 ppm, the irritant properties of styrene develop, and at concentrations between 150 and 200 ppm, impairment of reaction time and balance may occur. At 350 ppm, definite signs of impairment of reaction time and balance occur.

Styrene has irritating, drying, and defatting effects on the skin.

Occupational asthma due to exposure to styrene has been reported, and allergic contact dermatitis has also been reported.

At less than 10 ppm, styrene's odor is not detected. Between 50 and 100 ppm, styrene has a strong odor that is not objectionable. At 100 ppm, transient eye irritation may be observed, but tests of coordination and dexterity are unaffected. Reaction time is impaired at exposures of 350 ppm for 30 minutes, but perceptual speed and manual dexterity are unaffected. At 376 ppm for 25 minutes, performance on the Romberg test is impaired. At 800 ppm for a few hours, styrene is reported to cause listlessness, drowsiness, and impaired balance that lasts beyond the exposure period. Workplace exposures at more than 100 ppm styrene have resulted in the observation of similar acute effects. Subchronic and chronic experimental studies with styrene have not clearly identified neurotoxic effects in animals beyond those effects that can be attributed to CNS depression. Styrene vapor exposure at concentrations in excess of 50 ppm is irritating to the eyes and respiratory system.

Reports of clinically evident neurologic disease among styrene workers are uncommon. In general, the neurotoxicology literature for styrene consists of reports of subclinical effects among boat builders. The effects include changes in self-reported symptoms, psychomotor function, color vision, vestibular function, somatosensory evoked potentials, and nerve conduction velocity. Absence of clinical and neurobehavioral effects and nerve conduction changes following chronic workplace exposures have also been reported. Although fairly voluminous, the clinical literature does not allow conclusions about chronic neurotoxicity, particularly at levels recommended for workplace exposure, which are generally in the range of 20 to 50 ppm. Because the half-life of styrene in body fat is 2 to 4 days, many of the studies have failed to distinguish between acute toxicity due to peak exposures and chronic toxicity due to repeated low-level exposure. Also, workplace conditions are often not accounted for in sufficient detail. This is particularly important because boat building involves the use of many different materials, paints, solvents, and adhesives. Clean-up procedures to remove excess styrene from equipment and body surfaces may include neurotoxic solvents such as *n*-hexane and gasoline. Thus, the present database for styrene is inadequate to conclude that chronic low-level exposure to styrene provides a significant neurotoxic risk.

The metabolites of styrene, mandelic acid, phenylglyoxylic acid, hippuric acid, and styrene oxide can be analyzed in blood and urine as measures of exposure.

The differential diagnosis includes any acute condition that might affect the CNS, including cerebrovascular accident, trauma, alcohol, drug overdose, other chemicals, and so forth.

See Box 94-1 for appropriate management of acute exposure.

Patients with acute exposure to styrene should have baseline liver and renal function tests, urinalysis, complete blood count, and amylase and lipase levels performed. If significant respiratory tract irritation occurs, arterial blood gases should be monitored and a chest x-ray taken. Testing for metabolites of styrene, mandelic acid, phenylglyoxylic acid, and others may

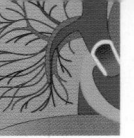

be useful for documentation of exposure but, otherwise, have no clinical utility and will not affect clinical outcome.

There is no antidote; care is supportive. For elimination, refer to Box 94-1. Dialysis and hemoperfusion are not useful. Disposition is described in Box 94-1.

TOLUENE

Toluene, also referred to as toluol, methylbenzene, methacide, and phenylmethane,[34] is an alkylbenzene derived from crude oil and coal tar during petroleum refining. It is a common component of gasoline, adhesives, paints, inks, and solvents.[1]

At room temperature, toluene is a volatile, flammable liquid with a sweet, pungent odor.[35] Its molecular weight is 92.15, and it has an odor threshold of 2.9 to 8 ppm.

Toluene has replaced benzene as the primary solvent in many commercial products such as oil paints and stains. It is readily available[3] and is a favorite of solvent abusers, who intentionally inhale high concentrations to induce a "sniffer's high."[15,36] The concentration of toluene inhaled by solvent abusers is 50 times the maximum permissible in industry.[37]

Toluene is also used in the production of other chemicals. Gasoline, which contains 5% to 7% toluene by weight, is the largest source of atmospheric emissions and exposure to the general population.

Volatile substance abuse involves children throughout the world.[35] In North America, inhalant solvent (toluene) abuse is especially prevalent in economically disadvantaged, neglected, or abused adolescents. Most are Hispanic immigrants, or children of immigrants, from Central America and Mexico. Males outnumber females ten to one. Native Americans also have an especially high prevalence of inhalant abuse. Much North American inhalant abuse ("sniffing," "huffing," or "bagging") involves paint or lacquer thinners that contain toluene as the principal constituent.

Owing to the CNS effects associated with toluene exposure, a number of researchers have attempted to measure subtle changes using neurobehavioral tests and measures of workers exposed to relatively low levels of toluene[34]; however, the studies have shown conflicting results with no clear indication of neurobehavioral effects resulting from workplace exposures.

The toluene molecule is devoid of actual or potential electrophilic centers. In this respect, it is similar to benzene and the xylene (dimethylbenzene) isomers.[38]

The desired effects of recreational toluene inhalation are euphoria and a sense of relaxation. Visual and auditory hallucinations may appear; they sometimes are frightening and provoke outbursts of antisocial behavior. Hallucinations usually abate after the initial months of abuse. Many chronic abusers inhale almost constantly from solvent-soaked rags or filled plastic bags and eventuate in a mildly stuporous, tranquilized state. Sudden death may occur from vomiting, aspiration, suffocation by plastic bags, or cardiac arrhythmias. Inhalant abusers experience tolerance to the acute effects. Sudden with-

drawal produces a syndrome similar to ethanol withdrawal. Addiction is common.

Little is known about mechanisms by which toluene and similar solvents produce acute or residual CNS effects. The acute effects of high-level toluene exposure (excitement followed by CNS depression) suggest a neurotransmitter-mediated mechanism similar to that of the hydrocarbon general anesthetics and ethanol. It has also been suggested that toluene and other volatile hydrocarbons may act by enhancing γ-aminobutyric acid A (GABA$_A$) receptor function, attenuating N-methyl-D-aspartate (NMDA) receptor-stimulated calcium flux, or activating dopaminergic systems.

Multifocal and diffuse leukoencephalopathy from prolonged high-level exposure (inhalant abuse) most likely reflects a direct effect on myelin or on the oligodendrocyte. The biochemical and morphologic similarities to adrenoleukodystrophy raise the possibility of an induced disorder of peroxisome or fatty acid metabolism.

Chronic toluene abuse can cause transient distal renal tubular acidosis (RTA) via an incompletely understood mechanism. Prolonged (years) of inhalant abuse may cause renal dysfunction and a secondary severe electrolyte imbalance; the usual profile includes metabolic acidosis, hypokalemia, and hypophosphatemia. This syndrome is secondary to toluene-induced renal tubular acidosis, *not* to increased urinary levels of hippuric acid; it is suggested that the site of primary dysfunction is the distal renal tubule. Renal potassium loss may be severe and can result in symptomatic hypokalemia, which may be so profound as to cause diffuse flaccid paralysis.

It is suggested that maternal toluene exposure, like maternal alcoholism, causes embryonic cell death resulting in deficiencies in early migrating neuroepithelial and mesodermal components.

Toluene toxicokinetics has been thoroughly characterized in humans and laboratory animals. Toluene is well absorbed from the lungs and gastrointestinal tract; dermal absorption may also occur but is less efficient.

Toluene rapidly accumulates in and affects the brain, owing to the brain's high rate of blood perfusion and high lipid content. The brainstem has the highest initial concentrations. Toluene is well metabolized, but a portion is exhaled unchanged. Circulating toluene is metabolized in hepatic microsomes, which contain CYP450s, particularly CYP2E1, that catalyze metabolism of toluene.

Toluene's metabolic products are cresol (less than 1%) and the intermediate metabolite benzaldehyde. Benzaldehyde is then metabolized to benzoic acid, which is conjugated with glycine to form hippuric acid. In humans, up to 75% of inhaled toluene is metabolized to hippuric acid and excreted in the urine within 12 hours of exposure. The remainder of the toluene is excreted unchanged, with a small percentage excreted as a sulfate or glucuronide of cresol. The metabolism and excretion of toluene are rapid, occurring within 12 hours of exposure. Elimination from the CNS is rapid; however, subcutaneous lipid may constitute a temporary storage site, and its concentration may continue to increase for

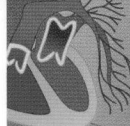

1 hour after exposure. Plasma concentrations generally parallel the lipid-stored fraction. The concentration of blood toluene drops rapidly during the first 10 minutes after termination of exposure; after 3 hours, very low concentrations are detectable in blood and in alveolar air.[35] The half-life of toluene in adipose tissue of humans has ranged from 0.5 to 3 days.

Toluene readily crosses the placenta.[39]

Recent genetic evidence suggests that some ethnic populations may be more at risk for the neurobehavioral effects of toluene than others because of metabolic differences.[40]

Toluene is initially metabolized to benzyl alcohol by the microsomal mixed-function oxidase system. Subsequently, oxidation to benzaldehyde and then to benzoic acid is carried out by the alcohol and aldehyde dehydrogenase, respectively. All populations appear to have two forms of aldehyde dehydrogenase, one having a high K_m and one with a much lower K_m. However, some Japanese and possibly other populations of Asian origin and Native Americans have a defective gene for the low K_m enzyme. When toluene-exposed Japanese workers (both male and female) were evaluated for the defective gene, it was found that those possessing the defective gene had lower levels of urinary hippuric acid and o-cresol than those with the normal or heterozygous gene. This observation suggests these individuals may be at a higher risk for toluene-induced CNS decrements owing to a decreased rate of toluene metabolism, leading to increased blood levels of benzaldehyde.

As toluene is metabolized by CYP450s (generally CYP2E1) and alcohol dehydrogenase, the chemical can interact with other xenobiotics metabolized by these enzymes. Concurrent exposure to solvents metabolized by the same CYP450 isozymes can result in competitive metabolic inhibition. Benzene and toluene suppress one another's metabolism in humans. Toluene greatly reduces manifestations of peripheral neuropathy caused by n-hexane in rats. Simultaneous exposure to high levels of toluene and xylene resulted in mutual metabolic suppression. Prior exposure to P450 inducers can result in increased rates of toluene metabolism and elimination and more rapid recovery from toluene-induced CNS depression.

In humans, occupational exposure to toluene is so low that it could not lead to the induction of P-450. However, the induction may be seen in toluene sniffers who are exposed to high concentrations.[41]

Contradictory effects of ethanol consumption on toluene metabolism are described; experimental animals given ethanol have elevated toluene blood levels, as do healthy human volunteers, whereas workers who regularly consume ethanol are reported to have lower plasma toluene measures than controls, presumably owing to enzyme induction. Phenobarbital stimulates hepatic side-chain hydroxylase, accelerating the metabolism of toluene to hippuric acid and yielding lower blood and tissue levels of toluene.

Human toxicity from toluene exposure occurs primarily by the inhalational and dermal routes, although ingestion is another absorption route. Toluene is mildly irritating to the mucous membranes, skin, and eyes. Short-term exposure to airborne toluene levels of less than 100 ppm has not been associated with discomfort. Humans exposed to concentrations of toluene of between 200 and 800 ppm may experience respiratory and ocular irritation. Prolonged contact between toluene and skin can produce irritation from solvent defatting of the skin, and direct splashing of the eyes may cause corneal injury. Dermal sensitization to toluene is extremely rare.

Ingestion of toluene may cause vomiting or diarrhea, and if pulmonary aspiration occurs, chemical pneumonitis may result. Systemic absorption may lead to CNS depression.

The CNS is the primary target organ of toluene and other alkylbenzenes. CNS neurotoxicity is the primary concern in toxic inhalational exposure.

Manifestations of exposure range from slight dizziness and headache to unconsciousness, respiratory depression, and death. Occupational inhalation exposure guidelines are established to prevent significant decrements in psychomotor functions.

Exposure to levels at 100 ppm for 4 hours causes eye irritation, headache, and lightheadedness but no consistent alterations in performance.[35] However, controlled studies with volunteers at 100 ppm showed decrements in vigilance, visual perception, motor performance, and ability to carry out functions. One extensive study claimed minor alterations in memory and dexterity following a 7-hour exposure at 150 ppm. Exposures at 200 ppm for 8 hours caused mild fatigue, confusion, lassitude, and lacrimation. At 600 ppm, euphoria and severe headache were prominent; at 800 ppm, all symptoms were more pronounced and were followed by 4 days of nervousness, fatigue, and insomnia.

Acute CNS effects are rapidly reversible upon cessation of exposure.

Prolonged high-level (1000–20,000 ppm) toluene exposure from inhalant abuse can cause symptomatic, disabling, multifocal leukoencephalopathy.

Toluene neurotoxicity has been clearly defined; it is most consistent in case descriptions of persons who daily spend their waking hours for years, nose-to-rag/bag, in a toluene-induced recumbent stupor. The daily dose from inhalation can exceed 350 mg of toluene; one individual "huffed" (orally inhaled) a gallon every 2 weeks of 99% pure toluene. Consumed at this rate, the shortest documented duration before onset of lasting symptoms is 1 year; most begin to show clinical manifestations after 2 to 4 years. Initial symptoms are behavioral changes (loss of initiative, depression, irritability), weight loss, impaired sense of smell, impaired concentration and memory, and mild unsteadiness of hand movements and gait. Subsequently, symptoms are slurred speech, head tremor, stiff-legged and staggering gait, poor vision, deafness, and dementia. Examination after 4 weeks of abstinence (avoiding the effects of acute intoxication) discloses sustained multidirectional nystagmus, titubation, ataxic tremor of all limbs, spasticity with hyperreflexia and Babinski's responses, broad-based and staggering stiff-legged gait, deafness, impaired vision and color dis-

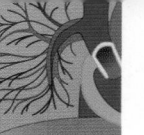

crimination, memory loss, inattention, apathy, and abulia. Even the most severely impaired display significant improvement after 6 months of abstinence; persons with mild or moderate dysfunction often recover completely. Infrequent abuse may cause no neurologically detectable CNS dysfunction; moderate frequency and intensity may cause a partial syndrome of mild cognitive dysfunction and slight tremor. Years of daily inhalation in the highest-level pattern described earlier almost inevitably leads to CNS dysfunction, and there is a predictable dose–effect relationship at these high levels.

Magnetic resonance imaging (MRI) has revealed permanent changes in brain structure, which correspond to the degree of brain dysfunction. Inhalational solvent abuse in particular has led to permanent neurologic sequelae and CNS lesions that have been described on both computed tomography (CT) and MRI.

Because of the accumulation of toluene in the anatomic areas of the CNS, symptoms can last hours beyond an exposure. Such impairments may be cognitive or involve coordination, motor control, intention tremor, and gait disturbances.

Decreased vision has been described in individuals chronically inhaling toluene-containing solvents. Optic neuropathy is manifest as decreased visual acuity but normal pupillary reactions along with associated cerebellar signs. Improvement in vision has occurred after discontinuation of toluene exposure.

Subtle neurologic effects have been reported in some groups of occupationally exposed individuals.[15]

Exposure to about 100 ppm of toluene for years may result in subclinical effects, as evidenced by altered brainstem auditory evoked potentials and changes in visual evoked potentials.

Chronic exposure to low toluene concentrations is associated with fatigue, headache, dizziness, shortness of breath, cough, throat irritation, nausea, and other constitutional symptoms. Disturbance of vestibulo-ocular responses has been demonstrated in subjects exposed to concentrations of toluene ranging from 103 to 140 ppm for more than 2 hours while doing light work. Color vision has also been shown to be impaired by occupational exposure to toluene.

It is claimed that chronic occupational exposure to low levels is associated with psychiatric change and mild cognitive dysfunction. There have been conflicting studies on the effect of chronic low-level (88–150 ppm) exposure of workers to toluene. Prolonged, low-level occupational inhalation of pure toluene is rare; most workers are exposed to solvent mixtures. There is one report of an anosmic lens cleaner who had chronic, intermittent exposure to toluene and developed, over a period of 3 months, poor concentration and memory, somnolence, slurred speech, and unsteady gait. Examination disclosed normal mental function, mild dysarthria, and gait-limb ataxia. He recovered completely within 1 month of abstinence. Although the data on this report (exposure and objective clinical findings) are limited, it suggests that intermittent, moderate- to high-level industrial exposure to toluene produces an illness that is a microcosm of the inhalant abuse syndrome.

Chronic exposure can lead to myopathy; hypokalemia and renal tubular acidosis are also common. Clinical findings are a hyperchloremic metabolic acidosis, hypokalemia, and aciduria. There is typically an associated transient renal azotemia, as well as proteinuria. Rarely, proximal RTA or the Fanconi's syndrome may occur. The metabolic acidosis is believed to be multifactorial, involving RTA, accumulation of toluene metabolites, and tissue hypoxia.

Toluene can cause nephrotoxicity in two forms: acute renal failure after massive ingestions and distal renal tubular acidosis. Clinical reports state that excess proteinuria, abnormal liver function test results, interstitial nephritis, and glomerulonephritis have also been related to toluene. Nephrotoxic effects that have been documented in chronic toluene abusers include hematuria, proteinuria, and type 1 renal tubular acidosis.

Patients with metabolic acidosis after toluene inhalational abuse have also exhibited associated hypokalemic muscular weakness and paralysis with neuropsychiatric manifestations.

Renal tubular function usually recovers during abstinence. Extreme cases of solvent inhalant abuse may also display evidence of hepatic failure. Studies with human volunteers and experimental animals have failed to demonstrate renal or hepatic dysfunction at levels encountered in the workplace.

Toluene is not a serious immunopathogen or carcinogen; previous reports of malignancy among exposed workers are now presumed to reflect the effects of benzene (formerly a component of commercial-grade toluene).

Toluene is a teratogen in humans and experimental animals. Children with microcephaly, minor craniofacial and limb anomalies, CNS defects, attention disorders, developmental delay, learning disorders, and language deficits were born to mothers who abused toluene by inhalation during pregnancy. These phenotypic and behavioral features strikingly resemble those associated with fetal alcohol syndrome.

There is report of a case of recurrent non–Q-wave myocardial infarction and cardiomyopathy associated with toluene abuse.[42]

Most hospital admissions for toluene abuse are for hepatic-renal failure or life-threatening cardiac arrhythmias.

Correct diagnosis is seldom difficult when presented with an intoxicated person. In the emergency room, solvent-smelling breath (persistent for hours) and a perioral rash ("huffer's rash") are often clues. Children who lack obvious neurologic deficits may develop hypokalemia and metabolic acidosis during early toluene abstinence. Occasionally, they are repeatedly admitted to renal medical units for treatment of distal renal tubular dysfunction of "obscure origin." Toxicologic screens in most commercial laboratories employing gas chromatography can detect toluene in the blood; hippuric acid analysis of urine is also widely available.

Hippuric acid is used as a biologic marker for occupational exposure to toluene. Minor toluene metabolites are o-cresol, p-cresol, and phenol. The minor

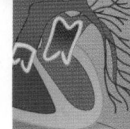

metabolites are conjugated with either sulfate or glucuronic acid and are excreted in the urine.

However, hippuric acid monitoring is especially unreliable in persons with low-level exposures. Individual variations with respect to metabolism of toluene and the correlation of occupational exposure to toluene and urinary excretion of hippuric acid and cresol can occur, especially if there is coexposure to other solvents or ethanol. Ethnic variations in toluene metabolism also are seen. Owing to this variability of metabolism among individuals, the biologic monitoring of hippuric acid and other metabolite excretions is merely a qualitative indication of exposure and not a quantitative indication of toluene toxicity. The average amount of hippuric acid excreted in the urine by persons not exposed to toluene is 0.7 to 1.0 g/L of urine.

Toluene in venous blood has been reported as the most reliable and sensitive marker of exposure. Although blood toluene, like other biomarkers, is influenced by smoking, exercise, alcohol ingestion, and sex differences, its usefulness as a surrogate of exposure is predicated on the multiphasic time course of elimination and a linear relationship at low levels of exposure. The initial elimination from blood upon termination of exposure is rapid, on the order of minutes; at an exposure level of 34 ppm, the blood level 16 hours after exposure was only 2% of the maximum blood level reached. Blood levels immediately after exposure reflect time-weighted average (TWA) exposure during the preceding 8 to 10 hours.[40]

Because of a slow release of toluene from adipose tissues (half-life is about 80 hours), blood toluene levels on Monday mornings before work or near the end of the workweek were observed to correlate with exposures during the preceding week. This slow decline in blood toluene has been demonstrated to result in detectable levels in workers who ceased exposure 2 weeks previously.

O-cresol has been used as a marker of toluene exposure in the workplace. It can be easily obtained by a noninvasive urine sampling procedure at the end of the work shift. One study reported that a value of 3 mg o-cresol per liter of urine correlates with an exposure level of 50 ppm, which also correlates with a value of 1000 µg/L toluene in blood.[43]

Laboratory studies of intoxicated persons may reveal evidence of renal tubular failure or mild hepatic dysfunction. Most hospitalizations of adolescents are for renal insufficiency and hypokalemia. Laboratory evidence of neuroendocrine effects is described in factory workers, whereas hypothalamic dysfunction (hyperprolactinemia, decreased testosterone and growth hormone) is reported in a boy whose toluene abuse was accompanied by central sleep apnea, diabetes insipidus, and poikilothermia.

CNS electrophysiologic studies reveal a characteristic abnormality of the brainstem auditory evoked response (BAER), namely, sparing of early components (wave I) and decrement or loss of late components (waves III–V). Abnormal BAERs appear to be among the most sensitive measures of toluene neurotoxicity; they may appear at a time when the neurologic exam is still unremarkable. Visual evoked responses appear less sensitive; they usually display diminished amplitudes throughout, with moderate delay in the late component. Electroencephalograms are frequently abnormal; even after 4 weeks of abstinence, they show mild diffuse slowing without paroxysmal, epileptiform activity. CT in severe cases almost always discloses mild to moderate cerebellar cortical and cerebral hemisphere atrophy. MRI in some advanced cases has provided solid evidence of white matter disease; this is evidenced by increased signal intensity on T2-weighted images in the periventricular, internal capsular, and brainstem pyramidal regions. MRI also reveals loss of differentiation between gray and white matter throughout the CNS and atrophy of cerebellum, cerebral hemispheres, and brainstem. These MRI findings are nonspecific; they may be seen in inflammatory demyelinating diseases, anoxic demyelination, and ischemic white matter disease. Neuroimaging studies show that CNS white matter changes due to toluene toxicity appear to be irreversible.

Neurologic lesions on MRI and CT scanning correlate with impairments on psychological tests in toluene abusers. MRI of the CNS in toluene vapor abusers has demonstrated multifocal CNS involvement and diffuse CNS demyelination. These findings correlated with a clinical presentation that included neurobehavioral, cerebellar, brainstem, and pyramidal tract abnormalities.

Neuropathologic changes that correlated with MRI and CT scanning in toluene abuse patients include diffuse cerebral demyelination, diffuse cerebellar demyelination, demyelination of subcortical white matter, degeneration and gliosis of ascending and descending long fiber tracts and nerves of the corpus callosum, and atrophy of the cerebrum, cerebellum, and corpus callosum. Necropsy showed myelin pallor in deep periventricular white matter, with axonal and neuronal loss combined with demyelination. Electroencephalogram abnormalities are reported in some cases.

Individuals exposed to long-term low concentrations of toluene, as compared with controls, showed abnormal visual evoked potentials.

Treatment of toluene exposure lies primarily in the correction of the resulting metabolic disorders. Most patients require parenteral hydration and attention to renal function. Recovery is usually rapid with the correction of the electrolyte disorders.[44]

Hypokalemia, cardiac arrhythmia, and metabolic acidosis require skilled medical management. Chronic toluene inhalational abuse can result in a normal anion-gap metabolic acidosis with hypokalemia, hypophosphatemia, and hyperchloremia. This type of acidosis was first described in association with glue sniffing and is termed *type 1 renal tubular acidosis*. Renal tubular acidosis is a derangement in the capacity of distal renal tubules to maintain a hydrogen ion gradient and usually is reversible within a few days once exposure to toluene ceases, although reversal of this disorder may require several weeks. Treatment ranges from observation to administration of sodium bicarbonate and potassium, depending on the severity of the acidemia and electrolyte loss.

Decontamination is described in Box 94-1.

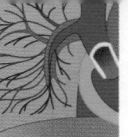

Other than abstinence, there is no specific treatment for the CNS effects.

In acute symptomatic exposures, toluene may be detectable in blood drawn with a gas-tight syringe, but usually only for a few hours. The metabolites hippuric acid and orthocresol are excreted in the urine and can be used to document exposure, but urine levels do not correlate with systemic effects.[36]

Other useful laboratory studies include electrolytes, glucose, blood urea nitrogen, creatinine, liver transaminases, creatine phosphokinase, and urinalysis.

There is no antidote. There is no role for enhanced elimination.

Consider hospitalizing the symptomatic patient who has significant inhalation or ingestion exposure with symptoms of CNS depression or respiratory distress.[45] Observe hospitalized patients for signs of acute tubular necrosis, encephalopathy, and arrhythmia. In addition, patients who have inhaled large amounts of toluene should be observed for signs of pulmonary edema, and those who have ingested toluene should be watched for signs of aspiration pneumonitis.

XYLENE

Xylene (dimethylbenzene) is a commonly used aromatic solvent with three isomeric forms: *ortho-*, *meta-*, and *para-*xylene. Xylenes are one of the highest-volume chemicals produced and used by industry. A mixture of all three isomers is termed *xylol*.[1] It is a colorless, flammable, liquid hydrocarbon with a characteristic aromatic odor. It is commonly found in products such as varnish, ink, paint thinners, degreasers, and insecticides.[46] Xylenes like benzene and toluene are major components of gasoline and fuel oil. The primary uses of xylenes industrially are as solvents and synthetic intermediates.[15] Commercial xylene is often contaminated with other organic compounds such as ethylbenzene, toluene, benzene, trimethylbenzene, phenol, thiophene, and pyridine. The volumes of these contaminants are very minor, making up less than a fraction of 1%.

The odor threshold of xylenes depends on the isomer. On average, the odor threshold appears to be about 1.0 ppm. *m*-Xylene has an airborne odor threshold of 3.7 ppm; *o*-xylene, 0.17 ppm; and *p*-xylene, 0.47 ppm.

Liquid xylene is irritating to the skin and eyes, causing local vasodilation by the liberation of histamine and 5-hydroxytryptamine. Direct xylene eye splash causes initial transient discomfort and hyperemia of the conjunctiva. The cornea may rapidly develop a visually significant central haze usually limited to the anterior portions of the stroma. A characteristic clinical feature reveals clear vacuoles resembling microcystic corneal epithelial edema but localized mostly in the anterior stroma. The stromal vacuoles are very characteristic and only mentioned in a few other entities such as *n*-butanol and nitronaphthalene exposure. In contrast, epithelial cystic changes differ from stromal vacuoles and are commonly seen in other keratopathies such as contact lens toxicity and increased intraocular pressure.

The CNS mechanism of toxicity is identical to that of toluene and other hydrocarbons.[36]

The toxicokinetics (TK) and acute toxicity of toluene, xylenes, and other aromatic solvents are quite similar. Xylenes and the others are well absorbed from the lungs and gastrointestinal tract, distributed to tissues according to tissue blood flow and lipid content, exhaled to some extent, well metabolized by hepatic P-450s, and largely excreted as urinary metabolites.

Dermal xylene absorption is low compared with respiratory tract absorption.

Xylene is metabolized through the P-450 mixed-function microsomal enzyme system in the endoplasmic reticulum of the liver. The biotransformation of xylene through side-chain oxidation and aromatic oxidation results in metabolites of methylbenzyl alcohols, methylbenzaldehyde, and methylbenzoic acids (toluic acids). Methylbenzoic acids are conjugated with glycine to form methyl hippuric acids, the main urinary metabolites of xylene. A minor (1%–4%) metabolic pathway of xylene metabolism is aromatic ring hydroxylation, which forms xylenol.

The major route of clearance is through the kidneys, with metabolites of xylene being excreted by a slow phase and a rapid phase. In humans, about 36% of xylene is excreted by the end of the daily working period, and about 70% to 80% of metabolites are excreted within 24 hours of cessation of exposure. Removal from fat occurs slowly over a period of days.[47]

The co-ingestion of ethanol will inhibit the metabolism of xylene through the pathway leading to methylhippuric acid, but not the path leading to 2,4-xylenol.

Coexposure to other solvents affects xylene metabolism. Exposure to both methyl ethyl ketone and xylene results in about a 50% increase in blood xylene concentrations. Also, urinary excretion of methyl hippuric acid decreases, indicating competition for enzyme metabolism. Coexposure to trichloroethylene, ethylbenzene, and toluene also inhibits xylene metabolism. Increased use of the minor aromatic ring hydroxylation pathway occurs when other solvents compete with CYP450 enzyme pathway metabolism.

Xylene is irritating to the eyes, skin, and mucous membranes. Exposure may cause dyspnea, anorexia, nausea, vomiting, and dermatitis. There are several ways in which xylene can be toxic, such as through inhalation, ingestion, or direct contact with the liquid. Ocular injuries such as irritation or conjunctivitis have been reported after exposure to vapors or accidental splashes. Additional ocular toxic changes may include vacuolar keratopathy, which has been reported in only a few cases with prolonged exposure to high vapor concentrations or to mixed solvents.

Owing to its high vapor pressure, most exposures to xylene and its isomers are by inhalation.

Acute CNS effects are identical to those of toluene and other volatile hydrocarbons. Workers rarely progress to the level of intoxication because the respiratory irritability and odor threshold limit of xylene are such that workers are unlikely to tolerate high exposures necessary to produce these effects.[49] Nevertheless, animal

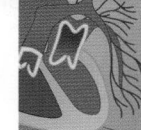

studies lend support to the theory that mixed xylene isomers are neurotoxic after inhalation.

Increased theta waves over occipital regions are seen in electroencephalogram results in subjects exposed to xylene peaks of 200 ppm for 4 hours.

Xylenes appear to have very limited capacity to adversely affect organs other than the CNS. Mild, transient liver or kidney toxicity has occasionally been reported in humans exposed to high vapor concentrations of xylenes.

Xylene does not appear to be genotoxic or carcinogenic.

For day-long working conditions, most experimentally exposed subjects have selected 100 ppm as the highest tolerable concentration, with considerable eye irritation in some individuals exposed to 200 ppm in air. Nose and throat irritation from xylene has been reported at 200 ppm for 3 to 5 minutes and 100 ppm for 1 to 7.5 hours per day for 5 days. Chronic occupational exposure to unspecified or unknown concentrations of xylene vapors has been associated with difficulty breathing and impaired pulmonary function. Nose and throat irritation has been reported with increased prevalence by workers who are exposed chronically to xylene vapors at a geometric mean TWA concentration of 14 ppm.

Death was reported in an individual exposed to paint solvents containing primarily xylene at an estimated atmospheric concentration of 10,000 ppm. Autopsy demonstrated severe pulmonary congestion with hemorrhage and pulmonary edema.

Liver necrosis and steatosis have been reported after xylene exposure.

Xylene vapors have a sweet odor that, in conjunction with irritation of the airways and respiratory tract, will cause most individuals to avoid exposure to the compound at high concentrations. Those who may be tolerant of the odor or who remain in the area of airborne xylene may develop headaches, nausea, vomiting, fatigue, dizziness, irritability, insomnia, a drunken feeling, impaired memory, loss of coordination, and unsteady gait, in addition to upper airway and ocular irritation.

Like toluene, xylene can also sensitize the myocardium to the arrhythmogenic effects of catecholamines.

Assays of blood and alveolar air can detect xylene, and its metabolites can be detected in urine. Blood levels of xylene can be affected by coexposure to other solvents. Coexposure to toluene, trichloroethylene, ethylbenzene, methyl ethyl ketone, or alcohol is known to increase xylene blood concentrations by competing for metabolic enzymes. Aspirin decreases methylhippuric acid urinary excretion.

Methylhippuric acid is not normally present in the urine, and methylhippuric acid concentration has, therefore, been proposed as a marker for the biologic monitoring of workers exposed to xylene. In general, methylhippuric acid levels appear to correlate linearly and significantly with the TWA exposure if urine is collected at the end of the daily working period and, preferably, in the latter half of the workweek when urinary metabolites are likely to reach maximum levels.[47]

The BEI for xylene is 1.5 g methylhippuric acid per gram of creatinine in urine collected at the end of the work shift.[48]

See Box 94-1 for acute clinical management.

After an acute splash in the eye, immediate and thorough irrigation with Ringer's lactate solution or saline is recommended. Delayed irrigation, especially in the presence of normal ocular pH, does not seem to be indicated. Removal of particulate chemical matter from ocular surfaces and conjunctival fornices is crucial. If significant corneal edema is present, topical steroids may shorten the course. Xylene keratopathy should be considered in the differential diagnosis of epithelial and stromal vacuolar keratopathy.

In acute symptomatic exposures, xylene may be detectable in blood drawn with a gas-tight syringe, but usually only for a few hours. The metabolite methylhippuric acid is excreted in the urine and can be used to document exposure, but urine levels do not correlate with systemic effects.

There is no antidote. There is no role for enhanced elimination. Disposition is the same as for toluene.

REFERENCES

1. Sullivan JB Jr, Van Ert MD: Aromatic solvents. In Clinical Environmental Health and Toxic Exposures, 2nd ed. New York, Lippincott Williams & Wilkins, 2001.
2. Aw T: Aromatic chemicals. In Hunter's Diseases of Occupations, 9th ed. New York, Oxford University Press, 2000.
3. Gummin DD, Hryhorczuk DO: Hydrocarbons. In Goldfrank's Toxicologic Emergencies, 7th ed. San Francisco, McGraw-Hill, 2002, pp 1303–1322.
4. Agency for Toxic Substances and Disease Registry: Toxicological Profile for Benzene. Public Health Service. Atlanta, U.S. Department of Health and Human Services, September 1997.
5. Hazardous Substances Data Bank. National Library of Medicine, National Toxicology Program (via TOXNET), Bethesda, MD, February 2003.
6. Cowell J, Johnston D: Other important and widely encountered chemicals. Selected petroleum-derived solvents. In Zenz C, Dickerson OB, Horvath EP Jr (eds): Occupational Medicine, 3rd ed. St. Louis, Mosby–Year Book, 1994.
7. Zhang L, Eastmond DA, Smith MT: The nature of chromosomal aberrations detected in humans exposed to benzene. Crit Rev Toxicol 2002;32(1):1–42.
8. Snyder R: Recent developments in the understanding of benzene toxicity and leukemogenesis. Drug Chem Toxicol 2000;23(1):13–25.
9. Golding WT, Watson WP: Chemistry: possible mechanisms of carcinogenesis after exposure to benzene. In Singer B, Bartsch B (eds): Exocyclic DNA Adducts in Mutagenesis and Carcinogenesis. IARC Scientific Publications No. 150, International Agency for Research on Cancer, Lyon, France, 1999.
10. Wester RC, Maibach HI: Benzene percutaneous absorption: dermal exposure relative to other benzene sources. Int J Occup Environ Health 2000;6(2).
11. Gist GL, Burg JR: Benzene: a review of the literature from a health effects perspective. Toxicol Indust Health 1997;13(6).
12. Duarte-Davidson R, Courage C, Rushton L, Levy L: Benzene in the environment: an assessment of the potential risks to the health of the population. Occup Environ Med 2001;58:2–13
13. Lovern MR, Cole CE, Schlosser PM: A review of quantitative studies of benzene metabolism. Crit Rev Toxicol 2001;31(3):285–311.
14. Snyder R: Benzene and leukemia. Crit Rev Toxicol 2002;32(3):155–210.
15. Bruckner JV, Warren DA: Toxic effects of solvents and vapors. In Klassen CD (ed): Casarett and Doull's Toxicology: The Basic Science of Poisons, 6th ed. San Francisco, McGraw-Hill, 2001, pp 869–916.
16. Hayes RB, Songnian Y, Dosemeci M, Linet M: Benzene and lymphohematopoietic malignancies in humans. Am J Indust Med 2001;40:117–126.

17. Wong O: Investigations of benzene exposure, benzene poisoning, and malignancies in China. Regul Toxicol Pharmacol 2002;35: 126–135.

18. Bolton JL, Trush MA, Penning TM, et al: Role of quinones in toxicology. Chem Res Toxicol 2000;13(3):135–160.

19. Ross D: The role of metabolism and specific metabolites in benzene-induced toxicity: evidence and issues. J Toxicol Environ Health [A] 2000;61:357–372.

20. Kacew S, Lemaire I: Recent developments in benzene risk assessment. J Toxicol Environ Health [A] 2000;61:485–498.

21. Buchwald A: Benzene. In Olson KR (ed): Poisoning and Drug Overdose, 3rd ed. Stamford, CT, Appleton & Lange, 1999, pp 104–105.

22. Krewski D, Snyder R, Beatty P, et al: Assessing the health risks of benzene: a report on the Benzene State-of-the-Science Workshop. J Toxicol Environ Health [A] 2000;61:307–338.

23. Schaumburg HH. Benzene. In Spencer PS, Schaumburg HH, Ludolph AC (eds): Experimental and Clinical Neurotoxicology, 2nd ed. New York, Oxford University Press, 2000, pp 228–229.

24. Dor F, Dab W, Empereur-Bissonnet P, Zmirou D: Validity of biomarkers in environmental health studies: the case of PAHs and benzene. Crit Rev Toxicol 1999;29(2):129–168.

25. Cohen JT, Carlson G, Charnley G, et al: A comprehensive evaluation of the potential health risks associated with occupational and environmental exposure to styrene. J Toxicol Environ Health [B] Crit Rev 2002;5(3):335.

26. Sherrington EJ, Routledge PA: The toxicity of styrene monomer. Adverse Drug React Toxicol Rev 2001;20(1):9–35.

27. O'Donoghue JL: Styrene. In Spencer PS, Schaumburg HH, Ludolph AC (eds): Experimental and Clinical Neurotoxicology, 2nd ed. New York, Oxford University Press, 2000, pp 1116–1120.

28. Greim H: Mechanistic and toxicokinetic data reducing uncertainty in risk assessment. Toxicol Lett 2003;138:1–8.

29. Iregren A, Andersson M, Nylen P: Color vision and occupational chemical exposures. I. An overview of tests and effects. Neurotoxicology 2002;23:719–733.

30. Feldman RG, Ratner MH: The pathogenesis of neurodegenerative disease: neurotoxic mechanisms of action and genetics. Curr Opin Neurol 1999;12(6):725–731.

31. Morata TC, Johnson AC, Nylen P, et al: Audiometric findings in workers exposed to low levels of styrene and noise. J Occup Environ Med 2002;44(9):806–814.

32. Cruzan G, Carlson GP, Johnson KA, et al: Styrene respiratory tract toxicity and mouse lung tumors are mediated by CYP2F-generated metabolites. Regul Toxicol Pharmacol 2002;35:308–319.

33. Brown NA, Lamb JC, Brown SM, Neal BH: A review of the developmental and reproductive toxicity of styrene. Regul Toxicol Pharmacol 2000;32:228–247.

34. Von Burg R: Toxicology update: toluene. J Appl Toxicol 1993; 13(6):441–446.

35. Schaumburg HH: Toluene. In Spencer PS, Schaumburg HH, Ludolph AC (eds): Experimental and Clinical Neurotoxicology, 2nd ed. New York, Oxford University Press, 2000, pp 1183–1189.

36. Weiss J: Toluene and xylene. In Olson KR (ed): Poisoning and Drug Overdose, 3rd ed. Stamford, CT, Appleton & Lange, 1999, pp 307–308.

37. Gupta RK, van der Meulen J, Johny KV: Oliguric acute renal failure due to glue-sniffing. Scand J Urol Nephrol 1991;25: 247–250.

38. McGregor D: The genetic toxicology of toluene. Mutat Res 1994;317:213–228.

39. Pearson MA, Hoyme HE, Seaver LH, Rimsza ME: Toluene embryopathy: delineation of the phenotype and comparison with fetal alcohol syndrome. Pediatrics 1994;93(2):211–215.

40. Greenberg MM: The central nervous system and exposure to toluene: a risk characterization. Environ Res 1997;72:1–7.

41. Nakajima T, Wang RS: Induction of cytochrome P450 by toluene. Int J Biochem 1994;26(12):1333–1340.

42. Hussain TF, Heidenreich PA, Benowitz N: Recurrent non-Q-wave myocardial infarction associated with toluene abuse. Am Heart J 1996;131:615–616.

43. Angerer J, Kramer A: Occupational chronic exposure to organic solvents XVI. Ambient and biological monitoring of workers exposed to toluene. Int Arch Occup Environ Health 1997; 69:91–96.

44. Baskerville JR, Tichenour GA, Rosen PB: Toluene induced hypokalaemia: case report and literature review. Emerg Med J 2001;18:514–516.

45. Agency for Toxic Substances and Disease Registry (ATSDR): Toluene. In Emergency Department Management, Managing Hazardous Materials Incidents, Vol. 3. Medical Management Guidelines for Acute Chemical Exposures, March 2001.

46. Trujillo F, Dang D, Starck T: Xylene keratopathy: a case report and review of the literature. Cornea 2003;22(1):88–90.

47. Langman J: Xylene: its toxicity, measurement of exposure levels, absorption, metabolism and clearance. Pathology 1994;26: 301–309.

48. American Conference of Governmental Industrial Hygienists (ACGIH): 2003 TLVs® and BEIs®. Cincinnati, ACGIH, 2003.

49. Low LK, Meeks JR, Mackerer CR: Health effects of the alkylbenzenes. II. Xylenes. Toxicol Indust Health 1989;5:1.

95

Freon and Other Inhalants

ANTONIO DUEÑAS-LAITA, MD, PHD

At a Glance...

- Fluorocarbons and chlorofluorocarbons (best known by the trade name Freon) are widely employed as refrigerants, aerosol propellants, and solvents. Because of their negative impact on the ozone layer, they are being gradually replaced by other compounds, including hydrogenated chlorofluorocarbons.

- Generally viewed as less toxic than other solvents, fluorocarbons are nonetheless responsible for numerous deaths due to occupational exposures and after intentional abuse.

- Narcosis and cardiac arrhythmias may occur after intense exposures. The pathophysiology of arrhythmia induction in humans is not clear.

- Decomposition of chlorofluorocarbons may lead to production of chlorine, hydrogen fluoride, phosphine, and chloride gases.

- Chlorofluorocarbons may cause eye, nose, and skin irritation as well as potentially severe cryogenic injuries (frostbite).

- Chronic chlorofluorocarbon exposures may lead to neuropsychiatric sequelae.

- Boron hydrides (boranes) are potent irritants that may induce pulmonary edema and central nervous system narcosis.

- Treatment of both fluorocarbons and boranes consists of removal from exposure and good supportive care.

- Hydrazines are potent alkaline compounds, are explosive, and interfere, through multiple mechanisms, with γ-aminobutyric acid production. As such, they may result in seizures that are poorly responsive to usual anticonvulsant therapy. Pyridoxine (vitamin B_6) administration may be life saving.

- Numerous hydrocarbons and substituted hydrocarbons, as well as nitrites, are abused by inhalation. Volatile inhalant abuse may lead to narcosis, seizures, arrhythmias, and sudden death. Chronic abuse of some compounds may result in encephalopathy. Treatment is supportive.

FREON AND OTHER FLUOROCARBONS

Introduction and Relevant History

Fluorocarbons are halogenated hydrocarbons. The best known is Freon, the commercial name given to the group most commonly used in industry some years ago. Fluorocarbons that contain chlorine are called chlorofluorocarbons (CFCs). CFCs have been used industrially since the 1930s and are generally known by commercial names such as Freon, Arcton, and Frigen. They were initially used by the armed forces in World War II and reached the civilian market in 1947. Because of their unique combination of nonflammability and general inertness, CFCs are used as refrigerants, aerosol propellants, foam-blowing agents, solvents, glass chillers, and polymer intermediates, as well as in fire extinguishers and anesthetics.

Their chemical stability, however, which makes them relatively safe and nontoxic, is also responsible for their potential damage to the environment. Since 1974, it has been believed that CFCs might indirectly affect the stratospheric ozone layer through their ability to transport halogens, particularly chlorine, to this level. By the mid-1980s, a consensus had emerged that atmospheric CFCs could contribute significantly to ozone depletion, and an annual thinning (a "hole") in the ozone layer over the Antarctic had been reported. Some of the atmospheric chemistry that is believed to occur and some of the measurements performed on the ozone layer are reviewed, together with the environmental regulatory actions that have been taken. These are leading to a controlled rapid phase-out of a number of industrial chemicals, including CFCs.

Production of CFCs ceased in the United States as of December 31, 1995, because of their destructive effect on the ultraviolet radiation shield (ozone) of the atmosphere.[1-3] However, these compounds are still available for sale, and some areas have stockpiled supplies. Hydrogenated chlorofluorocarbons (HCFCs), which can be used instead of CFCs, are currently being manufactured with a cease production date of the year 2020, again because their effect on the ozone layer. At that time, hydrogenated fluorocarbons (HFCs) will take the place of HCFCs and CFCs.[4]

CFCs were initially regarded as less toxic in terms of narcosis and other common solvent health effects, and thus higher levels of exposure were permitted. This led to a higher incumbent risk for problems. Many fatal cases associated with the inhalation of CFCs have been reported.[5-10] Most of these have occurred in work-related incidents or self-induced exposures. The autopsy reports of these cases reflect generic evidence of acute cardiorespiratory failure. It is believed that the toxic action of CFCs occurs through cardiac toxicity or by hypoxemic asphyxiation due to CFC saturation of the room atmosphere.[6,11]

CFCs are known irritants to the upper airway with ambient exposure. They may also cause cryogenic effects on tissue. Liquid CFCs with low boiling points or under pressure can cause freezing of the skin if they come into contact with the body for more than 3 to 5 seconds.[12]

It should be noted that Freon decomposes into chlorine, hydrogen fluoride, phosphine, and chloride gases, all of which are extremely toxic.[13]

Structure

Fluorocarbons are a group of synthetic halogen-substituted methane and ethane derivatives containing atoms of chlorine and fluorine. At least 36 commercially available fluorocarbons exist, of which 10 are produced

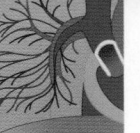

TABLE 95-1 Common Chlorofluorocarbons and Their Chemical Formulas

COMPOUND NUMBER	CHEMICAL FORMULA	CHEMICAL NAME
CFC 11	CCl_3F	Trichlorofluoromethane
CFC 12	CCl_2F_2	Dicholorodiflouromethane
HCFC 22	$CHClF_2$	Chlorodifluoromethane
CFC 13	$CClF_3$	Chlorotrifluoromethane
CFC 112	$Cl_2F—CCl_2F$	1,1,2,2-Tetrachloro-1,2 difluoroethane
CFC 113	$Cl_2F—CClF_2$	1,1,2-Trichloro-1,2,2 trifluoroethane
CFC 114	$ClF_2—CClF_2$	1,2-Dichloro-1,1,2,2 tetrafluoroethane
CFC 115	$ClF_2—CF_3$	1-Chloro-1,1,2,2,2 pentafluoroethane

Adapted from Aviado DM: Fluorine-containing organic compounds In Clayton GD, Clayton FE (eds): Patty's Industrial Hygiene and Toxicology, 4th ed. New York, John Wiley & Sons, 1994, pp 1177–1220, and American Conference of Governmental Industrial Hygienists, Inc.: Documentation of the Threshold Limit Values and Biological Exposure Indices, 5th ed. Cincinnati, OH, ACGIH, 1986

and used in significant amounts. The main CFCs and their chemical structures appear in Table 95-1.

Pathophysiology

Extensive animal studies have found a relationship between CFC inhalation and cardiac arrhythmias, even without evidence of asphyxiation.[10,14,15] Arrhythmias reported to occur in CFC exposure include ventricular arrhythmias, atrioventricular nodal block, and atrial fibrillation.[16,17] Reinhardt and associates also reported increased sensitization to arrhythmias when epinephrine was given to dogs with exposure to FC_{11}.[18] It has been postulated that CFCs decrease the ionic permeability of the cellular membranes, leading to transient and localized conduction blocks, altered refractory periods, and disturbance of the pacemaker ability of the heart.[19,20] Another theory suggests that CFCs do not sensitize the myocardium to endogenous catecholamines but have a depressant effect on the sinus atrioventricular and ventricular conduction systems, allowing other ectopic foci to produce arrhythmias.[21]

Despite the fatal exposures and reports of arrhythmia, the documentation of arrhythmias caused by CFCs in human subjects is ambiguous. Egeland and colleagues[22] found no significant difference in atrial or ventricular premature beats, heart rate, or PR intervals in a group of 16 aerospace workers with high and low exposures. Edling and coworkers[23] studied 89 refrigerator repairmen and concluded that CFCs do not induce arrhythmias in exposed workers. However, the frequency of arrhythmia was high in these men regardless of exposure. No clear connection was found by Antti-Poika and colleagues,[8] but one subject had ectopy that may have been related to exposure. Although ectopy or other arrhythmias occurring with CFC exposure have not been associated with underlying heart disease, increased circulating concentrations of catecholamines may make patients prone to arrhythmia.[5] Caffeine intake, physical

activity, and tobacco use have been suggested to have a proarrhythmic effect.[23]

Pharmacokinetics

CFCs are absorbed rapidly by inhalation, whereas oral absorption is slower and more complicated. The distribution half-life is rapid in comparison with elimination because of the slow release from fat stores. Clark and colleagues[24] reported three fatalities due to Freon exposure, and these patients had the highest concentrations in brain tissue, reflecting the high solubility of hydrocarbons. An individual who suffered a fatal exposure secondary to FC_{113} that had vaporized out of the sludge collection pit in glass lens manufacture also showed high levels in brain tissue.[9] High concentrations in heart tissue of people suffering fatal exposures have also been found.[6,7] Lung concentrations reported in all human cases are low, and this is probably a reflection of resuscitative efforts. Elimination half-life is 1.5 hours, probably as a result of its slow liberation from fat stores.

Clinical Manifestations

Transient low-concentration CFC exposures result in eye, nose, and throat irritation. Frostbite of the oral cavity has been described after deliberate inhalation of a propellant.[25] Pulmonary irritation, bronchial constriction, cough, dyspnea, and chest tightness may develop after inhalation. Pulmonary edema is an autopsy finding in fatal inhalation cases.[6,26] Edema may be secondary to aspiration or decomposition products of CFCs, which include chlorine, hydrogen fluoride, phosphine, and chloride gases.

Neurologic sequelae of CFCs involve a spectrum of symptoms that include headache, lightheadedness, dizziness, and disorientation. Workers with chronic exposure to CFC 113 were found to have impaired psychomotor speed, impaired learning and memory, and emotional lability.[27] Cerebral edema has been found at autopsy.[26]

Toxic exposures to CFCs have been associated with fatal ventricular arrhythmias, atrial fibrillation, and sudden death.[11,14-17,24] However, no clear connection with low-concentration exposure and cardiac arrhythmias has been documented.[8,22,23]

Freon exposure causing severe frostbite has been reported,[12] and a related case of compartment syndrome required amputation of the digits.[28] Direct accidental injections have also occurred, and these respond to conservative therapy with minimal tissue damage.[29,30]

Other rare toxic effects include gastric perforation secondary to ingestion, elevation of transaminase levels, jaundice, contact dermatitis, and rhabdomyolysis.[31-35]

Management

The first step in the management of CFC exposure is to remove the offending agent, avoiding exposure to other subjects. Attention to airway, breathing, and circulation with supplemental oxygen, symptomatic therapy, and a calming environment to avoid endogenous adrenergic stimulation are important. Use of adrenergic drugs should be avoided to prevent myocardial stimulation. Use of countershock or phenytoin may be indicated for ventricular arrhythmias. Digestive decontamination techniques (gastric lavage, activated charcoal) are not normally used because the ingestion of CFCs is exceptional. There is no antidote, and extrarenal purification techniques do not work.[36]

If frostbite occurs, the exposed area should be soaked in lukewarm water if possible within 20 to 30 minutes after exposure. Ice or heat should not be applied. A light coating of a bland ointment, such as petroleum jelly, should be applied and covered with a light bandage. Ocular injuries should be irrigated and assessed for injury.

BORON

Introduction and Relevant History

Boron hydrides are highly toxic chemical compounds composed of boron and hydrogen. Inhalation, ingestion, or percutaneous exposure to boranes can result primarily in pulmonary, gastrointestinal, or central nervous system (CNS) toxicity.

Boranes are used mainly in high-energy fuels such as rocket propellants but are also used in semiconductor manufacturing and welding and as fungicides and bactericides. They are also used as initiators of ethylene, styrene, vinyl, and acrylic polymerization and in the vulcanization of rubber. In recent years, they have also been employed in the automobile airbag industry.[37,38]

Structure

Boron hydrides are produced by the reaction of lithium aluminum hydride with boron fluoride to make diborane, and pyrolysis of diborane produces the remaining boranes. The three most commonly encountered in industry are diborane (B_2H_6), a colorless gas with a sickly sweet, nauseating smell, like rotten eggs; pentaborane (B_5H_9), a colorless volatile liquid with a sweetish, garlic-like, unpleasant odor; and decaborane ($B_{10}H_{14}$), a white crystal with an intense bitter chocolate odor. These compounds oxidize easily, are strong reducing agents that are highly flammable, and may ignite or explode in the presence of oxygen.

Pathophysiology

Boranes are highly toxic by inhalation, skin absorption, or ingestion. They may produce both acute and chronic poisoning.

Diborane gas is primarily a pulmonary irritant at 0.1 ppm. Inhalation exposure results in hydrolysis to boric acid and hydrogen.[39] Acute exposure causes pulmonary edema and hemorrhage as well as temporary damage to the liver and kidneys. Autopsies reveal rhinitis, pneumonia, and structural lung damage.[40,41]

Pentaborane and decaborane vapor affects the nervous system and causes signs of both hyperexcitability and narcosis.[42] Pentaborane is considered to be the most toxic of the boron hydrides when inhaled, although it is also readily absorbed through intact skin. CNS norepinephrine depletion, intracranial hypertension, and cortical atrophy have been demonstrated after exposure to pentaborane and decaborane. These agents also cause gastrointestinal toxicity, with fatty necrosis of the liver and elevation of transaminase levels.

Direct myotoxic effects of the boron hydrides as well as myoclonus and seizures can result in rhabdomyolysis and myoglobinuria.

Clinical Manifestations

Acute diborane poisoning in humans results in a syndrome like that of metal fume fever, with symptoms of tightness, heaviness, and burning in the chest; cough; shortness of breath; pericardial pain; nausea; shivering; and drowsiness. Signs of intoxication may occur soon after exposure or after a latent period of up to 24 hours and may persist for 1 to 3 days or more. Long-term exposure to low concentrations results in pulmonary irritation, dizziness, headaches, weakness, and tremors.

Drowsiness and nausea may occur with slight pentaborane toxicity. In moderate exposures, headaches, dizziness, nervous excitation, and hiccups may occur. Muscle pain and spasms of the muscles of the face and extremities may be noted. In more severe exposures, after 48 hours, patients may suffer loss of mental concentration, incoordination, disorientation, cramps, convulsions, and coma. On certain occasions, there have been reports of intense acidosis.[43,44]

Decaborane toxicity in humans produces symptoms of restlessness, aggressiveness, depressed breathing, incoordination, general weakness, spasmodic movements, and convulsions.

Sometimes, symptoms of acute toxic exposure may take several hours to develop and may persist for days. Chronic liver, kidney, and CNS impairments can result from significant exposures. Low-level exposures over time may cause CNS symptoms, including poor decision making and concentration, as well as apparent psychiatric symptoms of poor emotional control and personality change.

Management

People exposed to boron hydrides should be immediately removed from the exposure. After contaminated clothing has been removed, victims' skin should be thoroughly washed with water. There is no known antidote for borane poisoning. Treatment is symptomatic and supportive. If high-level inhalation has occurred, hospitalization for 48 to 72 hours is recommended to monitor cardiopulmonary function, acid–base balance, and neurologic status.

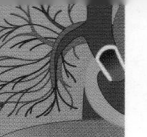

As regards preventive steps, it should be made clear that toxic levels of some boron hydrides are below the odor threshold for humans. Exposure to others with a scent, in higher concentration, may cause loss of ability to detect an odor. Therefore, great caution must be used when working around these substances. Personal protective equipment should be used to prevent inhalation, skin, or mucous membrane exposure.

HYDRAZINES

Introduction and Relevant History

Hydrazine (NH_2NH_2) is a colorless, oily, fuming liquid that is used in agricultural chemicals, the space industry, and medicine. It is also used in photographic developing and in the manufacturing of drugs, herbicides, dyes, textile treatments, explosives, and plastics.[45] Hydrazine is also a powerful explosive, used as a rocket fuel, and can self-ignite when adsorbed onto earth, cloth, wood, and asbestos. It emits toxic nitrogen compounds when heated to decomposition. Its vapors are heavier than air and have an ammonia or fishy odor.[46]

Pathophysiology

Hydrazines are poisonous by ingestion and by intravenous and dermal routes. Their toxicity occurs in multiple organ systems, and they are known carcinogens. Hydrazine and its metabolite monoacylhydrazine are hepatotoxic, causing nuclear and nucleolar enlargement, mitochondrial swelling, and increased formation of antibodies and free radicals.[47,48] Because acetylation is the pathway for metabolism, toxicity may be more common in people who are slow acetylators.

Hydrazine is also known to produce a functional pyridoxine deficiency through inhibition of synthesis or deactivation of coenzymes.[49] Pyridoxine may be useful for treatment.

Other toxicities caused by hydrazine include a direct CNS toxicity, a negative inotropic effect on the heart leading to cardiovascular depression and hypotension, and hemolysis leading to acute tubular necrosis or nephritis.

Clinical Manifestations

Hydrazines are local irritants causing ocular irritation, facial edema, salivation, and dermal irritation. Even low concentrations can cause bronchial mucous destruction and pulmonary edema. Other symptoms are nausea, vomiting, dizziness, and agitation.

Anemia due to hemolysis has been reported and can lead to renal dysfunction.[50] This blood loss can also worsen a patient's cardiovascular status and lead to progressive weakness and dyspnea.

Manifestations of the liver disease include hypoglycemia and hyperglycemia, depending on a patient's glycogen stores. In extreme situations, a fatal hepatorenal failure may result.[51]

Finally, among CNS manifestations, severe encephalopathy and seizures are the most significant disorders.[52,53]

Management

Prompt removal of the irritant and basic life support measures are key. Dermal exposure should be treated immediately with soap and water. Ocular exposure requires copious irrigation with tepid water.

Respiratory exposure should be treated with humidified supplemental oxygen and monitoring for respiratory distress. Chest radiographs, arterial blood gas determinations, and intubation may be clinically indicated.

Oral exposures may be treated with gastric lavage and activated charcoal. Emesis must be induced with caution because delayed neurologic effects, such as seizure and coma, may occur. This is dependent on the chemical ingested, the volume, and the duration of exposure.

Pyridoxine may be antidotal in hydrazine ingestions. The recommended dose for patients with neurologic symptoms is 70 mg/kg over 30 minutes intravenously, repeated as necessary, with a maximum of 15 g/day. These amounts should be respected because of the risk for peripheral neuropathy associated with the use of pyridoxine. Seizures are treated also with routine medications, including diazepam, lorazepam, or phenytoin, and phenobarbital. Other routine laboratory studies include monitoring blood glucose, liver function tests, and hemoglobin measurement. If methemoglobinemia exists at a level greater than 30%, methylene blue should be used, 1 to 2 mg/kg slowly every 4 hours as needed. The remaining treatment is supportive: fluid therapy, glucose in the case of hypoglycemia, conventional treatment of hepatic insufficiency if need be, and other maintenance measures.

ACROLEIN

Introduction and Relevant History

Acrolein, a colorless or yellowish liquid with a disagreeable odor, is ubiquitous in the environment. It is a highly toxic, reactive, and irritating aldehyde that occurs as a product of organic pyrolysis, as a metabolite of a number of compounds, and as a residue in water when used for the control of aquatic organisms. It is an intermediate in the production of acrylic acid, DL-methionine, and numerous other agents. Its major direct use is as a biocide for the control of aquatic flora and fauna. It is used also in the manufacturing of pharmaceuticals, food supplements, perfumes, plastics, and textiles. It is also present in cigarette smoke.[54]

It enters the environment through a variety of sources, including organic combustion such as automobile exhaust, cigarette smoke, and manufacturing and cooking emissions, as well as direct biocidal applications. Organic combustion from both fixed and mobile sources is the significant source of acrolein in the atmosphere;

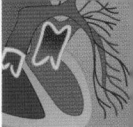

it represents up to 8% of all aldehydes generated by vehicles and residential fireplaces and 13% of all atmospheric aldehydes. This reactive aldehyde also occurs in organisms as a metabolite of allyl alcohol, allylamine, spermine, spermidine, and the anticancer drug cyclophosphamide, and as a product of ultraviolet radiation of the skin lipid triolein. Furthermore, small amounts are found in foods; when animal or vegetable fats are overheated. However, large amounts may also be produced. Most human contact occurs during exposure to smoke from cigarettes, automobiles, industrial processes, and structural and vegetation fires. Besides cigarette smoke, occupational exposures are a common mode of human contact, particularly in industries that involve combustion of organic compounds. Firefighters, in particular, are exposed to extremely high levels during the extinguishing and overhaul phases of their work.

Pathophysiology

Most exposures to acrolein occur through inhalation. Acrolein is a severe pulmonary irritant and lacrimating agent. The strong irritant effect usually prevents serious exposures, but fatalities have been reported.[55] Studies suggest that pulmonary insult from acrolein is due to alterations of the plasma membrane–dependent transport system in the pulmonary artery endothelial cells as well as to the intracellular generation of oxidants.[56,57]

Skin and corneal burns may result from direct contact with the liquid. Concentrations of 0.25 ppm may cause eye irritation.

Clinical Manifestations

Splash contact may cause irritation, erythema, edema, and actual burns. Difficulty breathing, chest congestion, delayed pulmonary edema, asthma, bronchiectasis, and permanent lung damage may result from acute exposures. Nausea and vomiting are common. Ingestion may produce severe irritation of the mouth and gastrointestinal tract. Hypertension and tachycardia may result from inhalation. Inhalation can also cause loss of consciousness and coma.[58,59]

Management

Because the primary toxic effects of acrolein involve irritation of the mucous membranes, lungs, and skin, removal of the agent is paramount. Washing with soap and water and irrigation of the eyes with tepid water are appropriate. If pain and burning persist, repeat examination is necessary.

Pulmonary support should be given as needed, including oxygen, intubation, and mechanical ventilation. Arterial blood gas measurement and chest radiograph are used to assess and monitor respiratory status. Patients with high-volume exposure may require hospitalization to be observed for delayed sequelae such as pulmonary edema.

Ingestion should be treated with gastric lavage followed by activated charcoal and cathartics. Gastric lavage should not be used in patients with neurologic deterioration without airway protection.

All other treatment is supportive and symptomatic. The use of steroids remains controversial. Antibiotic use should be aimed at treating specific infections and should not be used as a prophylactic measure.

VOLATILE INHALANT ABUSE

Introduction and Relevant History

Inhalants or volatile substances are a broad heterogeneous group of substances with differing structures and toxic effects. Their study as a toxicologic entity is determined by their abuse as inhalant drugs. All are volatile and liposoluble and have good pulmonary absorption, which avoids first pass metabolism in the liver; in addition, a small quantity produces a rapid effect on the CNS.

In general, these substances are cheap and legally obtainable. From an epidemiologic point of view, the rate of abuse of volatile substances varies greatly from country to country, although in the United States or Great Britain, for instance, this problem causes up to 100 deaths every year.[60] In those areas where the problem exists, 13- to 15-year-olds are mainly affected, yet there are cases involving 8- to 19-year-olds.[61,62]

Structure

The chief substances are (1) aerosols, including fluorocarbons (Freon) and isobutane; (2) aliphatic hydrocarbons, including n-hexane, ethane, acetylene, butane (lighter fuel), and isopentane; (3) general anesthetics, including nitrous oxide, ether, chloroform, enflurane, halothane, and isoflurane; (4) aromatic hydrocarbons, including benzene, toluene, xylene, styrene, and naphthalene; (5) esters, including ethylacetate, and isopropyl acetate; (6) fuels, including gasoline and naphthalene; (7) halogenated hydrocarbons, including carbon tetrachloride, trichloroethane, perchloroethylene, methylene chloride, methylchloroform, and fluorocarbons; (8) ketones, including acetone, methyl-n-butyl-ketone, and methylethyl ketone; and (9) nitrites, including amyl nitrite ("poppers" among the gay community), isobutyl nitrite, and butyl nitrite.[63]

Patients who abuse these substances normally obtain them as products containing them, such as acrylic paints, adhesives, propellants, aerosols, stain removers, degreasers, dry-cleaning agents, nail polish removers, gasoline, glues, paint thinners, room fresheners, lighter fluid, shoe polish, and correction fluids.

Pharmacokinetics

There are various ways of inhaling these products: (1) sniffing—breathing in directly from the container; (2) huffing—placing a rag soaked in solvent over the nose and mouth and inhaling; and (3) bagging—inhaling from a paper or plastic bag. The concentration of

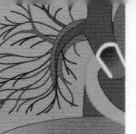

inhaled substances increases from sniffing to huffing to bagging. After one or two inhalations, the effects begin in a few seconds and last several minutes. Periodic inhalations, the most comman use pattern, maintain the effects over several hours.[64]

Volatile inhalants are rapidly absorbed by the alveolus and rapidly distributed to the central nervous system and lipid-rich tissues. Some of them can also be absorbed through the skin. Plasma concentrations are associated with the blood–air partition coefficient of each inhalant. Many inhalants are, in addition, eliminated mainly through the lungs. Several undergo hepatic transformation with the appearance of metabolites, which can be detected in the urine.

Clinical Manifestations

After inhaling for a few minutes, the user starts to notice a feeling similar to drunkenness, together with, among other effects, impaired perception, euphoria, a loss of inhibitions, and a pleasant dizziness. It has been pointed out that nitrites can increase the intensity of and prolong orgasm, as well as relax the muscles, thereby facilitating anal penetration. Such effects last between 15 and 45 minutes.

Acute toxicity requiring emergency room admission fundamentally involves arrhythmias or other serious cardiovascular manifestations, including ventricular fibrillation, ventricular and supraventricular tachycardia, bradycardia, myocardial depression, and hypotension. On occasions, these problems cause the patient to die, as a result of which *sudden death syndrome* by inhalants has come into modern-day parlance. Apparently, certain acute cardiac manifestations are caused by sensitivity to catecholamines produced by volatile substances.[65]

Acute disorders may also affect the CNS, producing incoordination, delirium, agitation, hallucinations, central depression (dizziness, blurred vision, headache, stupor, lethargy, ataxia, coma), respiratory depression, and seizures. On other occasions, patients present with digestive disorders, such as nausea, vomiting, abdominal pain, hematemesis, and necrosis of the liver (with trichloroethylene, among others). In exceptional cases, reports exist of laryngospasm, pulmonary aspiration with consequent chemical pneumonitis, methemoglobinemia (more commonly occurring with the ingestion rather than the inhaling of nitrites), and elevated carboxyhemoglobin (methylene chloride).

In addition to acute cases, there is evidence that chronic abuse of these substances may induce long-term neurologic toxicity in up to 65% of nonsporadic users. Neurologic alterations in heavy long-term abusers are probably due to the action of neurotoxins on neuronal membranes. Findings include spastic motor neuropathy, cognitive dysfunction, personality changes, problems with hearing and sense of smell, cerebellar dysfunction, Parkinson's disease, and optic neuropathy. Magnetic resonance imaging has revealed that toluene causes irreversible changes in brain white matter.[66] In certain instances of neurologic toxicity, there is peripheral neuropathy; this is the case of glues or adhesives containing n-hexane or methyl-n-butyl-ketone.

With regard to the digestive system, chronic abuse may bring about lack of appetite and weight loss. Hepatoxicity is associated with chronic exposure to carbon tetrachloride, toluene, and trichloroethylene. In the case of toluene, reports also exist of renal tubular acidosis, metabolic acidosis, hypokalemia, muscle weakness, and rhabdomyolysis; benzene can induce aplastic anemia.[66,67]

In recent years, there has been speculation that inhaling solvents during pregnancy produces fetal solvent syndrome, similar although not identical to fetal alcohol syndrome. Toluene is the agent most commonly related with this disorder.[68,69]

Diagnosis

A diagnosis of arrhythmia or any other acute complaint associated with the abuse of volatile substances is a simple one if the patient cites previous use; however, it is difficult if no such reference exists in the clinical history. The detection of substance remains around the mouth or the appearance of "glue sniffer's rash" can aid in the diagnosis.

Conventional toxicological analysis is seldom helpful, but one occasionally observes metabolic acidosis with hyperchloremia or anion gap, methemoglobinemia (nitrites), or elevated carboxyhemoglobin (methylene chloride). Certain special types of analysis may have an *a posteriori* clinical and legal interest but are rarely available in the hospital: hippuric acid (toluene), methyl hippuri acid (xylene), trichloroethanol, and trichloroacetic acid in urine.[70]

Management

Treatment should be strictly individual. General monitoring of the airway, respiratory support, electrocardiogram monitoring, pulse oximetry, and chest radiography (to watch for the appearance of aspiration pneumonitis) are applicable in many cases. There are no specific antidotes, with few exceptions (discussed later). In the case of contamination of the skin or mucosa, these should be washed with abundant water.

As regards arrhythmia management, adenosine has been proposed for supraventricular tachyarrhythmias and lidocaine for ventricular tachycardia, with countershock with or without defibrillation suggested if no response is achieved. In the case of bradycardia, initial treatment should be with atropine, and if this fails, an external or transvenous pacemaker should be used.

Care should be taken with sympathomimetic vasopressors because these could trigger arrhythmias as a result of sensitivity to catecholamines induced by solvents.

For cases of agitation or delirium and convulsions, intravenous benzodiazepines are recommended. If methemoglobinemia induced by nitrites is above 30%, methylene blue (1–2 mg/kg intravenously over 10 minutes) should be administered. Further management should be symptomatic.[71]

ACKNOWLEDGMENTS

Michelle Blanda, MD, and John V. Weigand, MD, contributed to this chapter in a previous edition.

REFERENCES

1. Wu L, Chen L, Li Y, et al: Study on the abundance of CFCs varying with the latitude at the bottom of the troposphere in the southern hemisphere. Environ Sci Technol 2001;35:2436.
2. Hayman GD: CFCs and the ozone layer. Br J Clin Pract 1997;(Suppl 89):2.
3. Noakes TJ: CFCs, their replacements, and the ozone layer. J Aerosol Med 1995;8(Suppl 1):S3.
4. Reizian-Fouley A, Dat Y, Rault S: Chlorofluorocarbon CFCs, potential alternative HCFCs and HFCs, and related chlorinated compounds: mass spectral study, part II. Ecotoxicol Environ Saf 1997;36:197.
5. Fitzgerald RL, Fishel CE, Bush LL: Fatality due to recreational use of chlorodifluoromethane and chloropentafluoroethane. J Forensic Sci 1993;38:477.
6. Groppi A, Polettini A, Lunetta P: A fatal case of trichloro-fluoromethane (Freon 11). J Forensic Sci 1994;39:871.
7. Kaufman JD, Silverstein MA, Moure-Eraso R: Atrial fibrillation and sudden death related to occupational solvent exposure. Am J Ind Med 1994;25:731.
8. Antti-Poika M, Heikkila J, Saarinen L: Cardiac arrhythmias during occupational exposure to fluorinated hydrocarbons. Br J Ind Med 1990;47:138.
9. McGee MB, Meyer RF, Jejurikar SG: A death resulting from trichlorotrifluorethane poisoning. J Forensic Sci 1990;35:1453.
10. Kintz P, Baccino E, Tracqui A, Mangin P: Headspace GC/MS testing for chlorodifluoromethane in two fatal cases. Forensic Sci Int 1996;82:171.
11. Morita M, Miki A, Kazama H, et al: Case report of deaths caused by Freon gas. Forensic Sci 1977;10:253.
12. Standefer JC: Death associated with fluorocarbon inhalation: report of a case. J Forensic Sci 1975;20:548.
13. Arena JM: Freon (dichlorodifluoromethane). In Kugelmass IN (ed): Poisoning, 4th ed. Springfield, IL, Charles C Thomas, 1979, pp 624–625.
14. Flowers NC, Horan LG: Nonanoxic aerosol arrhythmias. JAMA 1972;219:33.
15. Flowers NC, Horan LG: The electrical sequelae of aerosol inhalation. Am Heart J 1972;83:644.
16. Taylor GJ, Harris WS: Cardiac toxicity of aerosol propellants. JAMA 1970;214:81.
17. Aviado DM, Belez MA: Toxicity of aerosol propellants on the respiratory and circulatory systems. I. Cardiac arrhythmia in the mouse. Toxicology 1974;2:31.
18. Reinhardt CF, Mullin LS, Maxfield ME: Epinephrine-induced cardiac arrhythmia potential of some common industrial solvents. J Occup Med 1973;15:953.
19. Lessard Y, Begue J, Paulet G: Fluorocarbons and cardiac arrhythmia: does difluorodichloromethane (FC 12) inhibit cardiac metabolism? Acta Pharmacol Toxicol 1986;58:71.
20. Lessard Y, Paulet G: A proposed mechanism for cardiac sensitisation: electrophysiological study of effects of difluorodichloromethane and adrenaline on different types of cardiac preparations isolated from sheep hearts. Cardiovasc Res 1986;20:807.
21. Reinhardt CV, Azar A, Maxfield ME, et al: Cardiac arrhythmias and aerosol sniffing. Arch Environ Health 1971;22:265.
22. Egeland GM, Bloom TF, Schnorr TM, et al: Fluorocarbon 113 exposure and cardiac dysrhythmias among aerospace workers. Am J Ind Med 1992;22:851.
23. Edling C, Ohlson CG, Ljungkvist G, et al: Cardiac arrhythmia in refrigerator repairmen exposed to fluorocarbon. Br J Ind Med 1990;47:207.
24. Clark MA, Jones JW, Robinson JJ, et al: Multiple deaths resulting from shipboard exposure to trichlorotrifluoroethane. J Forensic Sci 1985;30:1256.
25. Elliott DC: Frostbite of the mouth: a case report. Milit Med 1991;156:18.
26. Lerman Y, Winkler E, Tirosh MS, et al: Fatal accidental inhalation of bromochlorodifluoromethane (Halon 1211). Hum Exp Toxicol 1991;10:125.
27. Rasmussen K, Jeppesen HJ, Arlien-Soborg P: Psychoorganic syndrome from exposure to fluorocarbon 13—an occupational disease? Eur Neurol 1988;28:205.
28. Wegener EE, Barraza KR, Das SK: Severe frostbite caused by Freon gas. South Med J 1991;84:1143.
29. Goetting AT, Carson J, Burton BT: Freon injection injury to the hand: a report of four cases. J Occup Med 1992;34:775.
30. Craig EV: A new high-pressure injection injury of the hand. J Hand Surg 1984;9A:240.
31. Haj M, Burstein Z, Horn E, et al: Perforation of the stomach due to trichlorofluoromethane (Freon 11) ingestion. Isr J Med Sci 1980;16:392.
32. Steadman C, Dorrington LC, Kay P, et al: Abuse of a fire-extinguishing agent and sudden death in adolescents. Med J Aust 1984;141:115.
33. Brady WJ, Stremski E, Eljaiek L, et al: Freon inhalational abuse presenting with ventricular fibrillation. Am J Emerg Med 1994;12:533.
34. Denborough MA, Hopkkinson KC: Firefighting and malignant hyperthermia. BMJ 1988;296:1442–1443.
35. Bircher AJ, Hampl K, Hirsbrunner P, et al: Allergic contact dermatitis from ethyl chloride and sensitization to dichlorodifluoromethane (CFC 12). Contact Dermatitis 1994;31:41.
36. Dueñas-Laita A: Freón (fluorocarbonos). In Dueñas Laita A (ed): Intoxicaciones agudas en medicina de urgencia y cuidados críticos. Barcelona, Masson SA, 1999, pp 139–140.
37. Hitt JM: Automobile airbag hazards. In Sullivan JB, Krieger GR (eds): Clinical Environmental Health and Toxic Exposures, 2nd ed. Philadelphia, Lippincott Williams & Wilkins, 2001, pp 489–495.
38. Harbison RD: Boron. In Harbison RD (ed): Hamilton & Hardy's Industrial Toxicology, 5th ed. St. Louis, Mosby–Year Book, 1998, pp 44–46.
39. Sullivan JB: Oxidizers, reducing agents and other highly reactive chemicals. In Sullivan JB, Krieger GR (eds): Clinical Environmental Health and Toxic Exposures, 2nd ed. Philadelphia, Lippincott Williams & Wilkins, 2001, pp 963–973.
40. Uemura T, Omae K, Nakashima H, et al: Acute and subacute inhalation toxicity of diborane in male ICR mice. Arch Toxicol 1995;69:397.
41. Nomiyama T, Omae K, Vemura T, et al: No-observed-effect level of diborane on the respiratory organs of male mice in acute and subacute inhalation experiments. Sangyo Eiseigaku Zasshi 1995;37:157.
42. Elinder C, Zenz C: Other metals and their compounds. In Zenz C, Dickerson O, Horvath E (eds): Occupational Medicine, 3rd ed. St. Louis, Mosby, 1994.
43. Silverman JJ, Hart RP, Garrettson LK, et al: Posttraumatic stress disorder from pentaborane intoxication: neuropsychiatric evaluation and short-term follow-up. JAMA 1985;254:2603.
44. Yarbrough BE, Garrettson LK, Zolet DI, et al: Severe central nervous system damage and profound acidosis in persons exposed to pentaborane. J Toxicol Clin Toxicol 1985–86;23:519.
45. Rumack BH (ed): Hydrazine. In Poisindex System. Englewood, CO, Micromedex, 2004.
46. Martin Ga, Cardinale MA, Taffer JR: Space operations. In Harbison RD (ed): Hamilton & Hardy's Industrial Toxicology, 5th ed. St. Louis, Mosby–Year Book, 1998, pp 589–596.
47. Albano E, Goria-Gatti L, Clot P, et al: Possible role of free radical intermediates in hepatotoxicity of hydrazine derivatives. Toxicol Ind Health 1993;9:529.
48. Ganote CE, Rosenthal AS: Characteristic lesions of methyla-zoxymethanol-induced liver damage. Lab Invest 1968;19:382.
49. Clark DA, Bairrington JD, Bitter HL, et al: Pharmacology and toxicology of propellant hydrazines. Aeromed Rev 1968;11:68.
50. Clayton GD, Clayton FE: Patty's Industrial Hygiene and Toxicology, 4th ed. New York, John Wiley & Sons, 1994.
51. Hainer MI, Tsai N, Komura ST, Chiu CL: Fatal hepatorenal failure associated with hydrazine sulfate. Ann Intern Med 2000;133:877.

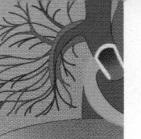

52. Nagappan R, Riddell T: Pyridoxine therapy in a patient with severe hydrazine sulfate toxicity. Crit Care Med 2000;28:2116.

53. Zelnick SD, Mattie DR, Stepaniak PC: Occupational exposure to hydrazines: treatment of acute central nervous system toxicity. Aviat Space Environ Med 2003;74:1285.

54. Ghilarducci DP, Tjeerdema RS: Fate and effects of acrolein. Rev Environ Contam Toxicol 1995;144:95.

55. Mahut B, Delacourt C, de Blic J, et al: Bronchiectasis in a child after acrolein inhalation. Chest 1993;104:1286.

56. Paten JM, Block ER: Acrolein-induced injury to cultured pulmonary artery endothelial cells. Toxicol Appl Pharmacol 1993;122:46.

57. Nardini M, Finkelstein EI, Reddy S, et al: Acrolein-induced cytotoxicity in cultured human bronchial epithelial cells. Modulation by alpha-tocopherol and ascorbic acid. Toxicology 2002;170:173.

58. Gosselin B, Wattel F, Chopin C, et al: Intoxication aiguë par l'acroleine. Une observation. Nouv Presse Med 1979;8:2469.

59. Azoyan P, Mahut B, Garnier R, et al: Intoxication aiguë par l'acroleine due a l'exposition aux produits de degradation thermique d'une graisse vegetale. J Toxicol Clin Exp 1992;12:285.

60. Lorenc JD: Inhalant abuse in the pediatric population: a persistent challenge. Curr Opin Pediatr 2003;15:204.

61. Kurtzman TL, Otsuka KN, Wahl RA: Inhalant abuse by adolescents. J Adolesc Health 2001;28:170.

62. Anderson CE, Loomis GA: Recognition and prevention of inhalant abuse. Am Fam Physician 2003;68:869.

63. Romanelli F, Smith KM, Thornton AC, Pomeroy C: Poppers: epidemiology and clinical management of inhaled nitrite abuse. Pharmacotherapy 2004;24:69.

64. Brouette T, Anton R: Clinical review of inhalants. Am J Addict 2001;10:79.

65. Williams DR, Cole SJ: Ventricular fibrillation following butane gas inhalation. Resuscitation 1998;37:43.

66. Filley CM, Halliday W, Kleinschmidt-DeMasters BK: The effects of toluene on the central nervous system. J Neuropathol Exp Neurol 2004;63:1.

67. Baskerville JR, Tichenor GA, Rosen PB: Toluene induced hypokalaemia: case report and literature review. Emerg Med J 2001;18:514.

68. Jones HE, Balster RL: Inhalant abuse in pregnancy. Obstet Gynecol Clin North Am 1998;25:153.

69. Wilkins-Haug L: Teratogen update: toluene. Teratology 1997;55:145.

70. Broussard LA: The role of the laboratory in detecting inhalant abuse. Clin Lab Sci 2000;13:205.

71. Flanagan RJ, Ives RJ: Volatile substance abuse. Bull Narc 1994;46:49.

96 Halogens (Bromine, Iodine, and Chlorine Compounds)

ALBERTO PEREZ, MD ■ CHARLES MCKAY, MD

At a Glance...

- The halogens are potent oxidizers and irritants, frequently used as antiseptics.
- Chronic bromide intoxication presents predominantly as a neuropsychiatric degenerative disorder.
- Acute ingestion of bromates found as neutralizers in cold-wave hair permanent kits can result in vascular collapse, renal failure, and sensorineural hearing loss.
- Acute iodine exposures result in severe skin, mucous membrane, and gastrointestinal injury.
- Chronic iodide toxicity can present as sialorrhea, coryza, bronchorrhea, and salivary gland enlargement, as well as hypothyroidism.
- Iodophors (organic iodine compounds) have little free iodine and are less toxic than iodine or iodide salts.
- Mixing chlorine-containing bleach (sodium hypochlorite) with acids or ammonia results in the release of chlorine gas or chloramine gas, respectively.
- Chlorine inhalation can produce delayed-onset pulmonary edema; early clinical presentation is predictive of short-term sequelae.
- Symptomatic severe chlorine inhalation can result in reactive airways dysfunction syndrome.
- Halogenated disinfection by-products are generated during disinfection of water containing large amounts of organic wastes.
- In large quantities, halogenated disinfection by-products cause reproductive abnormalities and bladder or rectal cancer in animals.
- Bromide and iodide can interfere with the analytic detection of chloride by certain instruments, resulting in pseudohyperchloremia.

Fluorine, chlorine, bromine, and iodine are collectively known as the *halogen elements,* and their ionic (salt) forms are known as fluoride, chloride, bromide, and iodide. They are strongly electronegative agents with potent oxidizing ability. Except for bromine, these are essential nutritional elements. This chapter reviews bromine, iodine, chlorine and their related compounds. Fluoride compounds are discussed in Chapter 90, whereas effects of and response to radioactive iodine compounds is covered in Chapter 104.

BROMINE COMPOUNDS: BROMIDE, BROMATE, AND BROMINE

Introduction and Relevant History

Bromides were historically prescribed as sedative-hypnotics and anticonvulsants in the mid 1800s.[1] They remained the mainstay anticonvulsant therapy until the advent of barbiturates in the 1920s. Their widespread use as anxiolytics led to the admonition to "take a bromide." Organic bromides, also known as *bromureides,* have been less commonly used.

In addition to acute sedative and anticonvulsant effects, chronic bromide ingestion produces a number of neuropsychiatric changes. In retrospective studies, it was found that many patients who were hospitalized in psychiatric institutions in the mid-20th century in fact had bromide intoxication.[2] Bromide psychosis has been described after prolonged use of bromide-containing medication (pyridostigmine, dextromethorphan).[3-5] Historically, Bromo-Seltzer and Miles Nervine were once associated with widespread cases of bromide intoxication.[1,6]

Dietary bromide exposure occurs in all humans because bromides can be found in trace amounts in natural soils and waters (e.g., igneous rock contains 0.02 mmol/kg bromide; fresh water contains 0.05 to 10 mmol/L, and seawater contains 0.4 to 0.8 mmol/L). Vegetables may contain bromide residues as a result of soil fumigation with methyl dibromide and ethylene dibromide.

Bromide salts are currently found in photographic chemicals (e.g., activators and developers), fire extinguishers, and refrigerants, as well as several medications (Table 96-1). Pharmaceutical bromides can be divided into inorganic bromide salts ($NaBr$, KBr, NH_4Br, and

TABLE 96-1 Bromide-Containing Medications

MEDICATION	% BROMIDE
Acecarbromal	29
Ammonium bromide	80
Bromisovalum	36
Bromodiphenhydramine	24
Carbromal	34
Dextromethorphan hydrobromide	23
Pyridostigmine bromide	31
Brompheniramine maleate	25
Halothane hydrobromide	81
Homatropine methylbromide	29
Neostigmine bromide	38
Bromocriptine	12
Pancuronium bromide	37
Potassium bromide	67
Propantheline bromide	18
Quinine hydrobromide	17
Vecuronium bromide	25
Scopolamine hydrobromide	29

Adapted from Bowers GN, Onoroski M: Hypochloremia and the incidence of bromism in 1990. Clin Chem 1990;36:1399–1403; and Rothenberg DM, Berns AS, Barkin R, Glantz RH: Bromide intoxication secondary to pyridostigmine bromide therapy. JAMA 1990;263: 1121–1122.

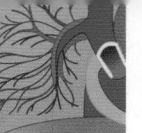

CaBr₂) and organic bromides (e.g., brompheniramine). Detectable serum bromide concentrations have been reported 3 weeks after prolonged anesthesia with halothane.[7] Ingestion of dextromethorphan, a common over-the-counter cough suppressant, has been associated with significant bromide absorption.[8] Unusual but significant exposures to bromide have resulted from consumption of large amounts of bromide-containing soft drinks and from exposure to cleansing compounds containing bromide and over-the-counter medications.[9-11]

Pharmacology

Bromine has a weight of 79.9 daltons. Daily bromide intake of more than 1 g may result in sedation, corresponding to serum concentrations of greater than 5 mEq/L (40 mg/dL). The primary pharmacologic action of bromide is a central nervous system (CNS) membrane-stabilizing effect that results in sedation and an elevated seizure threshold–anticonvulsant effect. This effect may result from the disturbance of active and passive transport of chloride across neuronal membranes.

Pharmacokinetics

Bromides are well absorbed from the gastrointestinal (GI) tract. Their oral bioavailability is about 96%, and peak serum concentrations are reached within 2 hours. Bromide has a low volume of distribution (0.35–0.48 L/kg) and tends to concentrate in erythrocytes and neurons.[12,13]

Serum bromide concentrations are expressed in several units, including mEq/L, mg/L, mg/dL, and mmol/L. The interpretation of recorded values is therefore subject to considerable confusion. Because of bromide's close relationship with chloride, its serum concentrations are best expressed in the equivalent mEq/L or mmol/L. Unit relationships are as follows:

$$0.1 \text{ mg/dL} = 1 \text{ mg/L} = 0.0125 \text{ mEq/L} = 0.0125 \text{ mmol/L}$$

Bromide is readily filtered by the glomeruli. Once in the tubular lumen, bromide competes with chloride for reabsorption with tubules having a higher affinity for bromide ion; therefore, chloride is preferentially excreted under typical circumstances. As a result, prolonged administration of bromide results in significant total-body loss of chloride. An intimate relationship exists between in situ chloride and bromide concentrations; the body maintains the molar sum of chloride and bromide ion at about 110 mmol/L.[12] The elimination half-life of bromide is 7 to 12 days; this half-life is increased with a salt-deficient diet.[1,11,12] Average renal bromide clearance is about 26 mL/kg per day. Bromide readily diffuses across the placenta and accumulates in fetal tissues. It is also secreted into breast milk.

Toxicology

Acute bromide intoxication is uncommon. Bromide salts are extremely irritating to the GI tract, generally resulting in spontaneous emesis. Although animal studies have reported LD₅₀ in the range of 2 to 5 g/kg, the reported human lethal dose is as low as 14 mg/kg. Nonetheless, experimental administration of up to 9 mg/kg/day of bromide for 12 weeks was reported to cause difficulty with concentration and sleepiness only. Bromide intoxication usually results from long-term overmedication, resulting in *bromism*.

Bromism is a clinical syndrome that consists of GI, dermatologic, and CNS manifestations (Box 96-1). GI manifestations include nausea, vomiting, a fetid odor on the breath, anorexia, and weight loss.[2] Dermatologic manifestations are found in as many as 30% of those with bromism[2]; *bromoderma* is the name given to the associated skin lesions. The most common lesion is an acneiform eruption on the face. Another frequent finding is an eruption resembling ecthyma, appearing on the lower extremities (nodose bromoderma). Other skin lesions include pemphigus-like, bromide-filled vesicles on the lower extremity, erythema multiforme, pyoderma gangrenosum, and bromoderma tuberosum (tumor-like lesions).

The neurobehavioral signs and symptoms of bromism are prominent. Behavioral disturbances include the appearance of a bromide dementia characterized by delirium, agitation, auditory and visual hallucinations, depression, and schizophrenic and manic-depressive psychosis. Hallucinosis may occur with an otherwise clear consciousness. Neurologic manifestations of bromism include dysarthria, hyporeflexia, and coma. An increased cerebrospinal fluid protein level occurs in 2% to 40% of patients.[14] Low-grade fever may be found in as many as 25% of cases.[2] Neurologic signs of bromism are slow to resolve and lag behind the decrease in serum bromide concentration because of the slow diffusion of bromide out of the CNS.[13] Among those who present with obtundation or coma, retrograde amnesia may develop. Ocular findings may also be striking in bromide intoxication and may consist of mydriasis, color disturbances, blurred vision, and micropsia or macropsia.

BOX 96-1	CLINICAL MANIFESTATIONS OF BROMISM	
Behavioral	**Neurologic**	**Laboratory**
Delirium	Dysarthria	Pseudohyperchloremia
Hallucinations	Hyporeflexia	Low or negative anion
Agitation	Encephalopathy	gap
Amnesia	Fever	
Depression	Papilledema	
Mania	Ataxia	
	Tremor	
Gastrointestinal	**Dermatologic**	**Ocular**
Nausea, vomiting	Facial acneiform	Mydriasis
Abdominal pain	eruption	Color disturbances
Halitosis	Nodose bromoderma	Blurred vision
Anorexia	Bromide-filled	Micropsia
Weight loss	vesicles	Ocular bobbing

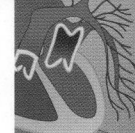

These latter two syndromes are perceptual distortions in which objects appear smaller or larger, respectively, than they actually are. Ocular bobbing (opsoclonus) has been described in a patient with bromide encephalopathy.[15] Papilledema is occasionally found on funduscopic evaluation.

Bromide ingestions of 9 mg/kg/day have been associated with modest increases in serum thyroxine and triiodothyronine concentrations.[16]

Because of its ready diffusion across the placenta, bromide accumulates in the fetus and can produce neonatal bromism. Clinical features of neonatal bromism are CNS depression, hypotonia, and weak suck and cry.[17,18] CNS manifestations of bromism are thought to be more prominent in neonates because their larger brains (15% of body weight versus 2% of body weight in an adult) are the storage site of a large bromide pool.[18] Bromide also appears to be teratogenic.[17]

Diagnosis

The diagnosis of bromide toxicity is clinical. Direct laboratory measurement of serum bromide concentrations supports the diagnosis but is not readily available. Serum bromide concentrations can be measured by a gold chloride colorimetric procedure, ion-exchange chromatography, and coupled plasma mass spectometry.[8,19,20] Normal "background" bromide serum concentrations in adults are 0.03 to 0.06 mEq/L. Although serum bromide concentrations do not consistently correlate with severity of intoxication, levels greater than 12.5 mEq/L are associated with important clinical toxicity. Serious toxicity occurs when serum concentrations exceed 25 mEq/L. Serum concentrations of greater than 37.5 mEq/L may be lethal. Elderly and debilitated patients, especially those on salt-restricted diets or with congestive heart failure, hypertension, or chronic renal failure, manifest toxicity at lower levels.

Although total-body chloride is decreased with chronic bromide use, measured serum chloride concentrations may be elevated after bromide intake (pseudohyperchloremia).[21] Serum chloride concentrations as high as 282 mEq/L have been reported with bromide intoxication.[22] Despite the artifactual chloride elevation, the degree of elevation cannot be used to estimate serum bromide concentration. The pseudohyperchloremia of bromide intoxication can result in a low, even negative, anion gap, which can be diagnostic.[23] With high bromide concentrations, negative anion gaps as low as −60 mEq/L can occur. The physician should be cognizant of potential significant analytic interference by other halogens.

Management

There is no role for GI decontamination in chronic intoxications. In the rare case of acute bromide ingestion, emesis will probably have occurred. Aggressive GI decontamination (ipecac, gastric lavage) is not warranted. We would not expect significant amounts of bromide ion to be adsorbed to activated charcoal.

Organic bromides may be well adsorbed to charcoal; thus, the administration of charcoal after organic bromide ingestion is reasonable.

Neutral diuresis with intravenous sodium chloride will accelerate renal excretion. Urine output should be maintained at 3 to 6 mL/kg/hr. Saline diuresis reduces bromide half-life to 2 to 3 days. The use of mannitol or furosemide can further reduce bromide half-life and is helpful in avoiding fluid overload. Hemodialysis is effective in removing bromide (elimination half-life of 2 hours), but the clinician must be aware of postdialysis redistribution rebound. The end point of treatment is symptomatic improvement and, if accessible, a bromide determination less than 6 mEq/L. Correction of pseudohyperchloremia, if present, could serve as a screen for bromide clearance, although true hyperchloremia as a result of overaggressive saline infusion may interfere with interpretation.

BROMATES

Introduction and Relevant History

Bromate salts ($KBrO_3$, $NaBrO_3$) are highly water-soluble oxidizing agents. These agents are used widely to bleach flour and produce explosives. Potassium bromate is almost completely converted to potassium bromide during the bread-baking process. Bromates are also found in the "neutralizers" that are part of cold-wave hair permanent kits, which contain either 2% potassium bromate or 10% sodium bromate.[24] A wave of bromate-containing hair permanent kit suicidal ingestions in the 1960s and 1970s that culminated in renal failure led to a clinical syndrome known as *hairdresser's anuria*.[25-27]

Pharmacology and Pharmacokinetics

Bromates are colorless, odorless, tasteless compounds that are readily absorbed from the GI tract. Once absorbed, a small amount of bromate ion may be reduced to bromide, and modestly elevated serum bromide concentrations result. Serum bromate concentrations are not readily measurable, and thus toxic serum bromate concentrations are unknown. Bromates are excreted unchanged in urine.

The lethal dose of potassium bromate has not been established in humans, but the LD_{50} in animal experiments range from 160 to 500 mg/kg. Life-threatening toxicity has occurred in children who ingested as little as 2 to 4 ounces of 2% potassium bromate solution.[25] Potassium bromate appears to be more toxic than sodium bromate.

Toxicology

Symptoms of bromate intoxication are diverse (Box 96-2). Manifestations appear within 2 hours of ingestion and begin with the GI effects of nausea, vomiting, diarrhea, and abdominal pain. These are thought to result from the formation of irritating hydrobromic acid

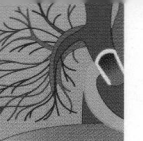

BOX 96-2	CLINICAL MANIFESTATIONS OF BROMATE INTOXICATION

Gastrointestinal	Renal	Auditory
Nausea	Acute renal	Sensorineural
Vomiting, diarrhea	failure	hearing loss
Abdominal pain	Uremia	

Central Nervous System	Cardiovascular
Encephalopathy	Hypotension
Seizures	

in the gut. Cardiovascular instability with hypotension may be an early manifestation with severe exposures.

Nephrotoxicity and ototoxicity are the hallmarks of bromate intoxication. Acute renal failure (ARF) varies from mild and transient to severe anuric form. ARF usually appears 1 to 3 days after ingestion. Renal failure occurs in 90% to 100% of patients with significant bromate intoxication and historically was the most common cause of death. In children, bromate-induced ARF typically resolves within 1 to 3 weeks of onset. In adult case series, however, many victims eventually develop chronic renal failure or persistent renal tubular acidosis.[14,24,27] Pathologic findings in the kidneys consist of acute tubular necrosis with relative glomerular sparing. Tubular histopathology consists of karyorrhexis, karyolysis, and lymphocytic interstitial infiltrates. Later changes consist of scarring, interstitial fibrosis, and glomerular sclerosis.[24]

Bromate ototoxicity can result in permanent sensorineural hearing loss with intact vestibular function. The mechanism of this effect is unclear; it may be related to damage of the stria vascularis with degenerative changes in the outer hair cells of the cochlea.[24] Deafness has been reported in as many as 85% of adults with significant bromate poisoning but is less frequent in children. Tinnitus and decreased hearing may appear as early as 4 to 6 hours after ingestion.[28]

Other toxicities of bromate poisoning include encephalopathy, myocarditis, and hepatitis.[24] Encephalopathy is typically manifested as agitation, delirium, seizures, and coma. A peripheral neuropathy with burning in the feet has also been described in adults. The neuropathy usually manifests 1 to 2 months after the ingestion and is self-limited, with typical duration of 1 month.[24] Anemia may also be seen, resulting from microangiopathy, a clinical picture resembling hemolytic-uremic syndrome.[26]

Management

General management principles apply to unstable patients who present after bromate intoxication. Fluid, acid–base, and electrolyte status should be carefully assessed, with particular attention to hyperkalemia. An electrocardiogram should be obtained in all cases of bromate ingestion. Acute renal failure, if present, should

be treated with judicious fluid restriction, fluid and electrolyte monitoring, and, if indicated, hemodialysis or peritoneal dialysis.

Because ototoxicity and nephrotoxicity are of rapid onset, prompt GI decontamination after recent ingestion is required. Gastric lavage with a 2% to 5% solution of sodium bicarbonate reduces bromate absorption and prevents the formation of irritant hydrobromic acid. The administration of activated charcoal is of unproven efficacy.

Bromate ion can be reduced to less toxic bromide by intravenous administration of sodium thiosulfate. Early therapy may be beneficial in reducing ototoxicity and nephrotoxicity. One to 5 g of sodium thiosulfate can be administered to adults (150 to 200 mg/kg to children) over 30 to 60 minutes. Administration of thiosulfate is associated with immediate elevations in serum bromide concentration, which confirm the conversion of bromate to the less toxic bromide.[28]

Early hemodialysis or peritoneal dialysis may remove bromate and prevent clinical toxicity. Therefore, these modalities should be strongly considered for patients who present within a few hours of a significant bromate ingestion.[28]

BROMINE

Bromine is a potent oxidizing agent. It is a highly hydrophilic reddish-brown gas that is heavier than air.[29] Elemental bromine is widely used in industry; its largest use is as an additive to gasoline.[30] Significant occupational exposure is controlled by an Occupational Safety and Health Administration (OSHA) permissible exposure limit for a time-weighted average 8-hour work day (PEL-TWA) of 0.1 ppm.

Bromine is very irritating to mucous membranes and produces pain and irritation of the upper airways and the eyes. Lacrimation, tearing, coughing, respiratory distress, and headaches all develop after inhalation exposures. High concentrations of bromine can cause inflammatory lesions of the upper airway as well as photophobia and blepharospasm.[29] Other clinical manifestations are dizziness, headache, and nosebleeds. Animal studies have shown that 3-hour exposures to bromine at 3 ppm can result in pulmonary edema.[30] Bromine gas at a concentration of 10 ppm is a severe irritant that cannot be tolerated. Death may occur secondary to bromine pneumonitis, which resembles adult respiratory distress syndrome. Necropsy revealed massive hemorrhagic alveolitis in one report. Direct skin exposure to liquid bromine can result in formation of vesicles and pustules, which develop into deep, painful ulcers with a brown discoloration of skin.[31] The manifestations of bromine exposure parallel those of chlorine exposure.

Exposure to elemental bromine is uncommon but has been reported after occupational or environmental disasters. In one of the most important such exposures, a chemical plant in Geneva, Switzerland released bromine gas in November 1984, and about 25,000 inhabitants

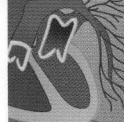

TABLE 96-2 Clinical Manifestations Reported After Bromine Gas Exposure in 59 Patients	
SYMPTOMS	**NUMBER OF PATIENTS (%)**
Eye irritation	53 (90)
Upper airway irritation	40 (68)
Cough	28 (47)
Expectoration	20 (34)
Headache	27 (46)
Photophobia	7 (12)
Weakness	7 (12)
Nausea	6 (10)
Dizziness	6 (10)
Abdominal pain	4 (7)
Itching	2 (3)
Sweating	2 (3)
Vomiting	2 (3)

From Morabia A, Selleger C, Landry JC, et al: Accidental bromine exposure in an urban population: An acute epidemiological assessment. Int J Epidemiol 1988;17:148–152.

were exposed to high concentrations of bromine. Clinical manifestations were extensive[29] (Table 96-2). Many of these symptoms persisted 1 month later, particularly eye and upper airway irritation, headache, and cough. Smaller mass exposures have occurred from swimming pools, where bromine compounds are used as sanitizers.[32]

Treatment of bromine exposure consists of ventilatory support and copious irrigation of eyes and skin with water or isotonic saline.[29] Corticosteroids have been administered in cases of severe respiratory distress without clear efficacy.[29] Prophylactic antibiotics are not recommended for bromine pneumonitis because they may promote the selection of resistant organisms.

IODINE

Introduction and Relevant History

Shortly after its identification in 1812, iodine's antiseptic and antimicrobial properties were recognized. Its essential role in thyroid hormone metabolism was also recognized early, with dietary supplementation begun in goitrous regions as early as 1920. An adult daily requirement of 150 µg is recommended. The threshold limit value for occupational iodine exposure is 0.1 ppm.

Uses of iodine include the manufacture of organic chemicals, pharmaceuticals such as contrast media for radiographic procedures, antiseptics and germicides, dyes and inks, and catalysts for photography, engraving, and lithography.

Medicinally, elemental iodine is used almost exclusively as a topical antiseptic or water-purifying agent. Iodine topical solution contains about 2 g of iodine and 2 g of sodium iodide per 100 mL. A tincture of iodine has the same composition, but in a 50% alcohol base. In aqueous solutions, iodine is present as seven different species: elemental iodine (I_2), hypoiodic acid (HOI), iodine cation ($[H_2OI]^+$), triiodide ion (I_3^-), iodide ion (I^-), hypoiodite ion (OI^-), and iodate ion (IO_3^-).[33]

Pharmacology

Elemental iodine, hypoiodic acid, and iodine cation are potent germicides, whereas triiodide and hypoiodite ions are relatively weak antiseptics. Topically applied iodide ion has no antimicrobial activity. Although the exact mechanism of its antimicrobial effect remains unclear, iodine compounds may work by (1) reacting with amine groups, (2) oxidizing the sulfhydryl group of cysteine, (3) disrupting protein synthesis, (4) reacting with the phenolic group of tyrosine, or (5) reacting with fatty acid double bonds, thereby disrupting the cell wall lipid bilayer.

Pharmacokinetics

Iodine is not absorbed through intact skin. Systemic absorption in the intestine of iodine requires reduction to iodide. Once absorbed, interconversion occurs between iodine and iodide. Both are renally excreted, with systemic accumulation seen in patients with renal impairment.

Toxicology

Topical use of 2% solution has minimal toxicity, although it may stain the skin and produce dermal injury (iodine burns). Iodine solutions of greater than 7% are corrosive to skin and mucous membranes. Sensitization may occur in susceptible individuals.[33] Tincture of iodine is more irritating than aqueous solution. Occlusive dressing increases the risk for dermal injury after iodine application. Ocular exposure results in intense pain and blepharospasm; staining of the corneal epithelium after prolonged occupational exposure has been reported. Severe inhalation exposure can lead to pneumonitis and pulmonary edema.

Iodine ingestion may result in perforation with peritonitis, metabolic acidosis, sepsis, and death. Two to 4 g of iodine is potentially fatal. Significant iodine ingestion also produces a clinical syndrome that includes tachycardia, parotitis, bronchitis, and insomnia.[30]

Diagnosis

The diagnosis is essentially based on the history of exposure and consistent clinical findings. Any starch-containing food complexes with iodine and blue emesis that is considered pathognomonic for iodine ingestion may be seen. Iodine compounds can produce false-positive test results for blood when orthotoluidine (Hematest) or guaiac reagents are used. When used as a topical antiseptic, iodine may also produce pseudohyperglycemia.[34] As with bromide, pseudohyperchloremia could be noted with exceptional iodide exposures.

Management

The unstable patient with potential GI perforation requires aggressive supportive care, endoscopic evalua-

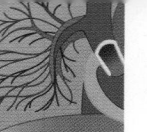

tion, and surgical consultation. As with any corrosive ingestion, ipecac, orogastric lavage, and activated charcoal (AC) are contraindicated. Immediate administration of dietary complex sugars (flour, starch) or milk may be effective by reducing iodine to the less toxic iodide; however, the specter of potential GI corrosion mitigates against their use in a symptomatic individual. The oral administration of sodium thiosulfate (100 mL of a 1% solution) can rapidly reduce iodine to iodide and may be of benefit if administered early. Thiosulfate can also be used to remove iodine stains from skin and clothing.[33]

IODIDES

Introduction and Relevant History

Iodides have also been used as antimicrobial agents. Tertiary syphilis was among the dozens of diseases that were treated with potassium iodide at the turn of the century.[35] The successful quasi-eradication of endemic goiter by the addition of iodide (100 μg/g) to table salt underlines the importance of iodide as an essential nutrient. Other important dietary sources include dairy products and seafood.

Clinical conditions treated with iodide salts are hyperthyroidism and sporotrichosis. Iodides are also encountered in iodoquinol, amiodarone, and in certain expectorants. Potassium iodide salts are also provided as protection after unintentional exposure to I^{131} (see Chapter 104).

Pharmacokinetics

Iodide is readily absorbed from the GI tract and transported into the thyroid. Blood concentrations of iodide are typically low (0.2–0.4 μg/dL), whereas the thyroid typically contains about 10 mg iodide. Iodide is renally excreted, with a usual clearance of 40 mL/min.

Toxicology

Iodism, a syndrome resulting from chronic iodide intoxication, consists of oral, respiratory, salivary, pulmonary, dermatologic, and GI effects (Box 96-3). Metallic taste, burning in the mouth, gum and teeth soreness, and sialorrhea make up the oral manifestations. Iodide toxicity can also simulate sinusitis or a head cold including fever.[36] Severe bronchorrhea can result in pulmonary edema. Other signs of iodism include iodide mumps[37] and iododerma—similar to bromism.

Iodide can significantly affect thyroid metabolism with both hypothyroidism and hyperthyroidism resulting from excess iodide. Iodide's potent inhibition of thyroid hormone synthesis[35] (the Wolff-Chaikoff effect) and hormone release is the basis of its use in the treatment of hyperthyroid states and why excess iodide intake during pregnancy can result in neonatal hypothyroidism (cretinism). Prolonged use of iodide salts produces thyroid gland hyperplasia, goiter, thyroid adenoma, or severe hypothyroidism or thyrotoxicosis.[38]

BOX 96-3	CLINICAL MANIFESTATIONS OF IODISM	
Oral Metallic taste Gingivitis Pharyngitis Laryngitis	**Salivary** Excess salivation Salivary gland enlargement	**Dermatologic** Acneiform eruption Vesicles Pustules
Nasal Nasal congestion Sneezing "Sinus" headache	**Pulmonary** Productive cough Pulmonary edema	**Gastrointestinal** Bloody diarrhea Anorexia
Thyroid Thyroid enlargement Hypothyroidism Cretinism Adenoma Myxedema	**Ocular** Eye irritation Periorbital edema	

Immune reactions include anaphylactoid reactions (particularly to iodinated contrast agents), serum sickness–like syndrome; attributed cases of thrombotic thrombocytopenic purpura and fatal periarteritis nodosa have been reported.[36]

Diagnosis

The diagnosis is essentially based on the history of exposure and clinical findings. As with bromide, elevated iodide concentrations may result in pseudohyperchloremia, rendering the anion gap calculation unreliable. The silver halide precipitation method of serum chloride measurement is not influenced by iodide elevation.[39] If clinically indicated, thyroid function tests should be ordered in cases of chronic exposure or follow-up to a large acute ingestion.

Management

The mainstay therapy is excretion enhancement through saline diuresis. Hemodialysis can increase excretion fourfold to fivefold but is rarely required in the presence of normal renal function.[40] Certain manifestations of iodism, particularly salivary gland inflammation and ioderma, may respond to corticosteroid therapy.[41,42]

IODOPHORS

Iodophors are substances that have elemental iodine attached to a high-molecular-weight moiety. As a general rule, iodophors enhance the bactericidal activity of iodine. Iodophors are found in solutions, ointments, and surgical scrubs. The most common iodophor, povidone-iodine (Betadine), is an iodine molecule linked to

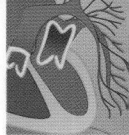

polyvinylpyrrolidone. Betadine is used most commonly as a 10% solution (which contains only 0.001% free iodine). Because iodine is tightly bound to the carrier, iodophors have very low rates of iodine release. These substances are therefore nonirritating after ingestion and generally have low toxicity. However, because they do contain substantial amounts of iodine, iodophors can result in significant iodine absorption in certain situations, particularly (1) when the integrity of the skin is compromised; (2) in infants, who have greater skin permeability; (3) after mucosal application (e.g., vaginal instillation); and (4) after excessive topical application.[39] Because of iodine diffusion into breast milk, vaginal or perirectal application of povidone-iodine and maternal treatment have been associated with elevated serum iodide levels in a breast-fed infant.[43,44] Neonates readily absorb iodine from topical povidone-iodine solutions, and their total plasma iodine levels remain elevated for 3 days after a single application. Goiter and hypothyroidism, dermatitis, liver function abnormalities, and neutropenia have also been described after prolonged exposure to povidone-iodine and other iodophors. Serum iodide concentrations can increase 100-fold in those who have iodophors applied to open wounds, burns, or decubitus ulcers, and iodide-related fatalities are reported.[45] In an unusual report, Kurt and colleagues described a 9-week-old infant who received 150 mL of povidone-iodine through a nasogastric tube and died of severe corrosive injury to the GI tract with a blood iodine level of 14,600 µg/dL.[46] Systemic absorption of iodophors has also been associated with the development of a metabolic acidosis. The cause of the acidosis has not been identified, although its etiology may be related to either the acidity of the povidone-iodine solution (pH < 3), bicarbonate complexation to iodine, or renal tubular acidosis. Both normal and elevated lactate levels have been described after iodine absorption from iodophors.[39] Other metabolic abnormalities associated with iodine absorption from iodophors include hypernatremia, hyperchloremia, renal insufficiency, and renal tubular acidosis.

Treatment of iodine intoxication resulting from iodophor exposure consists of basic interventions used to treat iodide toxicity. However, because iodophors have very low toxicity unless ingested in massive amounts, no specific intervention is recommended after ingestion. Activated charcoal has a potential role because iodophors are organic compounds; charcoal should be considered after ingestion of more than 6 to 8 ounces of Betadine (or other iodophor). Because of the potential disturbances in thyroid function, thyroid-stimulating hormone should be monitored weekly for up to 4 weeks after very large ingestions.

CHLORINE

Introduction and Relevant History

Chlorine (atomic weight of 35.45 daltons) is a gas at standard temperature and pressure. It has a vapor pressure of 4800 mm Hg at 20° C and a relative density to air of 2.5. It is commonly used in industrial processes as a reagent in plastics manufacturing and as a bleaching agent in the paper industry.[47] Chlorine-producing compounds are also used as disinfectants and water-purifying agents.

Although it was recognized in the 17th century that heating ammonium chloride and nitric acid together created an irritating gas, chlorine was first described and used as a bleaching agent in the 1770s. In 1774, chlorine was generated by oxygenation of hydrochloric acid, and it is currently produced by electrolysis of brine. Although chlorine was the first chemical warfare agent in World War I, only 1843 of the 70,552 reported Americans victims of gassing were reportedly exposed to chlorine.[48] Although initial clinical data linked these exposures with chronic pulmonary sequelae, lack of uniformity in evaluation and comorbidities prohibit any substantiated conclusions.

Chlorine is the most compressible element; it is shipped as a pressurized liquid. One pound of liquid chlorine generates about 5 cubic feet of gas when released. A typical rail tank car, containing more than 50 tons of liquid chlorine, would therefore be capable of releasing more than 500,000 cubic feet of gas.[49] It is this potential for massive release that results in such concern about transportation and storage accidents involving chlorine.

Chlorine is heavier than air (vapor density, 2.5) and is recognizable in concentrated releases as a yellow-green cloud. The noxious odor does not serve as a reliable warning. The odor threshold of chlorine is less than 3 ppm, whereas the OSHA threshold limit value–time-weighted average (TLV-TWA) for an 8-hour work day is 0.5 ppm. Extreme irritative symptoms can occur at levels as low as 1 ppm over 4 to 8 hours,[50] and levels of 30 ppm can lead to severe respiratory symptoms within minutes. Levels of 1000 ppm cause immediate death.[51]

From an epidemiologic perspective, the summary of poisonings in the United States reported to the American Association of Poison Control Centers (AAPCC) for 2003 documents 727 exposures to chlorine generated by the mixture of acid with bleach and 6090 other exposures to chlorine in the fume/gases/vapors section of the annual report. It is likely that other exposures are contained within the 57,790 exposures to hypochlorite-containing bleaches and disinfectants documented within the household cleaning substances category.[52] Clinical experience certainly suggests that the most common source of chlorine exposure resulting in emergent symptoms is the admixture of household cleaning agents. The combination of bleach (sodium hypochlorite) and acids or ammonia results in the formation of chlorine or chloramine gases, respectively.[53] Another common source of residential chlorine poisoning is from swimming pool disinfectant processes.[54-56] This is a particularly common exposure source for children. Hemodialysis patients may be exposed to chloramine toxicity if chloramines are inadequately removed after maintenance of hemodialysis machines.[57] Industrial and transportation incidents account for infrequent but large-scale releases of chlorine gas.[58,59]

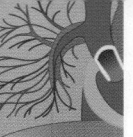

$$Cl_2 + H_2O \rightarrow HCl + HOCl$$

$$HOCl \rightarrow HCl + O^-$$

FIGURE 96-1 Irritant products from reaction of chlorine with water.

Structure and Structure–Activity Relationships

Chlorine itself is only moderately soluble in water, but when it comes in contact with water, hydrochloric acid and hypochlorous acid are generated (Fig. 96-1). Hypochlorous acid is thought to degenerate readily at physiologic pH to hydrochloric acid and oxygen free radicals with resultant coagulation necrosis and oxidative tissue damage. Hypochlorous acid is far more irritating than hydrochloric acid.[60] Chloramine gas, when exposed to moist surfaces, also releases hypochlorous acid.[61]

Pharmacology

Chlorine and chlorine-producing compounds primarily cause symptoms when inhaled in a closed space or in high concentrations. Contact of chlorine gas with moist surfaces such as the mucous membranes of the eyes, mouth, and respiratory tract produces both upper and lower airway symptoms. Upper airway irritation tends to be prominent and serves as a noxious warning preventing continued voluntary exposure; therefore, lower tract symptoms are less frequent. Nonetheless, severe lower airway damage can occur, particularly in settings of highly concentrated exposure or when victims are trapped. Persistent airways dysfunction and bronchiolitis obliterans have been described after acute exposure, although the true incidence of these chronic effects and their relation to smoking and preexisting atopy are uncertain.[59,62-64] Although repeated symptomatic chlorine exposures can also lead to persistent airways dysfunction, chronic exposure to controlled levels without acute symptomatic "gassing" episodes is unlikely to cause chronic pulmonary dysfunction.[65,66] Severe exposures may cause noncardiogenic pulmonary edema.

Diagnosis

Chlorine gas toxicity is primarily a clinical diagnosis suggested by the circumstances of exposure and clinical picture. Laboratory evaluation is nonspecific, often revealing leukocytosis, metabolic acidosis, and hypoxemia or respiratory alkalosis in those who are most symptomatic. Chest radiographs may demonstrate focal areas of consolidation, central pulmonary congestion, or diffuse increased interstitial markings.[67] Neumomediastinum has also been reported. All these abnormalities generally correlate with more severe clinically apparent disease. Laboratory studies other than pulse oximetry should have little if any role in the initial assessment and disposition of exposed individuals.

Triage can be performed on a clinical basis. The following triage guidelines were generated from available clinical data:

1. Mildly affected individuals improve with removal from exposure. Symptomatic treatment with humidified oxygen or bronchodilators may be beneficial. Asymptomatic individuals will not worsen.
2. Moderately affected individuals, if asymptomatic after a period of several hours after treatment, will not acutely worsen. Those with underlying pulmonary or atopic conditions may have persistence of reactive airways for weeks to months after the acute exposure. Rarely, chemical or infectious pneumonitis may develop over a few days after exposure.
3. Severely affected individuals demonstrate symptoms early and stabilize or suffer worsening of their condition; they require aggressive treatment and immediate hospitalization.

A triage algorithm is provided in Figure 96-2.

Toxicology

The clinical spectrum following acute chlorine exposure can include mucous membrane irritation with chemical conjunctivitis, corneal burns, orofacial burns, acute tracheobronchitis, chemical pneumonitis, pulmonary edema, and hypoxemia with metabolic acidosis. Initial symptoms after exposure to chlorine fumes include cough and eye, nose, and throat irritation. Chest heaviness/burning, dyspnea, wheezing, and hemoptysis or syncope can occur with more severe exposures. Nonspecific nausea and vomiting, headache, dizziness, and chills may also be reported.

The physical findings are often unremarkable, although initial tachypnea, conjunctival injection, tearing, and wheezing may be found. Tachycardia and both mildly elevated and depressed temperature may be noted.

Various pulmonary function abnormalities have been reported in the hours after an acute exposure, including both restrictive and obstructive deficits. These changes represent the variable effects of differing concentrations of chlorine and its by-products on the airways and parenchyma in patients with or without underlying lung diseases. In one study that evaluated 18 patients after exposure to a chlorine tank leak, all subjects had evidence of moderate pulmonary obstruction, which improved over 2 weeks.[62] None developed pulmonary edema, although all were described as showing a "worsening clinical picture during the first 2 days of hospitalization, with signs of recovery noted thereafter." Despite this assessment, only one patient in that case series was treated with bronchodilators or steroids. The authors described the presenting symptom of dyspnea as identifying individuals with a worse clinical course (slower recovery) than those with a primary complaint of paroxysmal dry cough. The former group was more likely to smoke (100% versus 25%) and to have a preexposure history of wheezing (50% versus 8%). This may serve as a useful triage tool in a multiple-patient encounter; however, prospective validation is lacking.

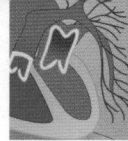

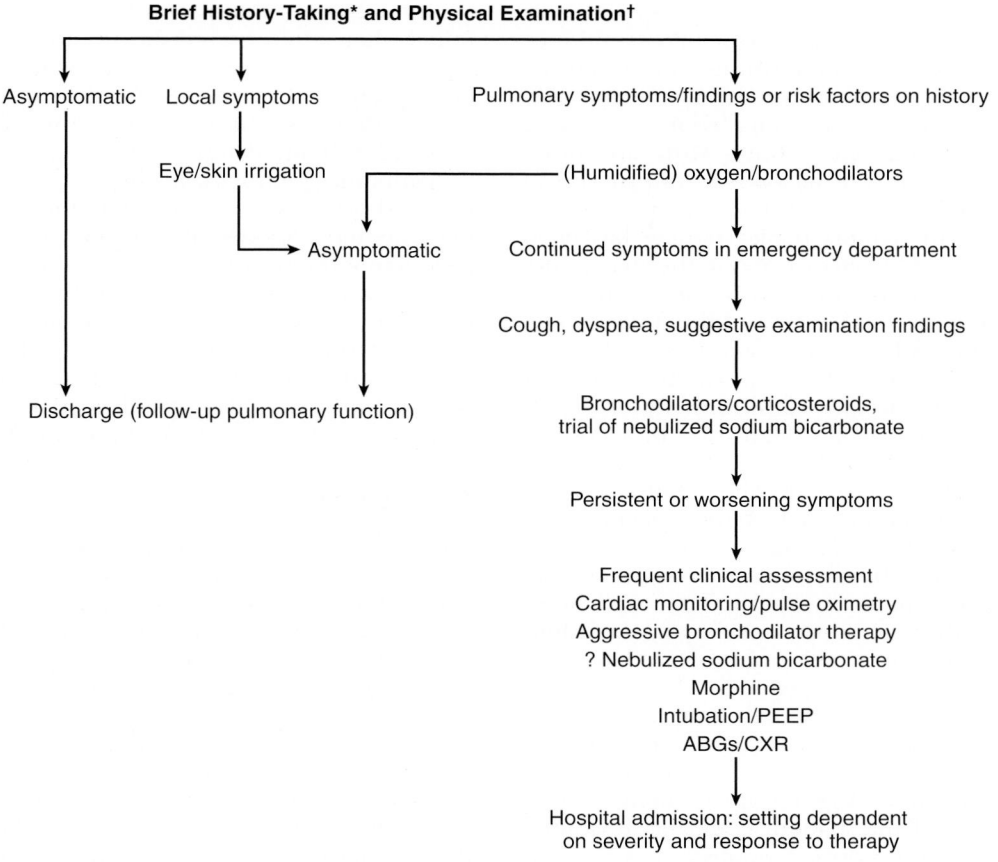

Brief History-Taking* and Physical Examination†

Asymptomatic   Local symptoms

Eye/skin irrigation

Asymptomatic

Discharge (follow-up pulmonary function)

Pulmonary symptoms/findings or risk factors on history

(Humidified) oxygen/bronchodilators

Continued symptoms in emergency department

Cough, dyspnea, suggestive examination findings

Bronchodilators/corticosteroids,
trial of nebulized sodium bicarbonate

Persistent or worsening symptoms

Frequent clinical assessment
Cardiac monitoring/pulse oximetry
Aggressive bronchodilator therapy
? Nebulized sodium bicarbonate
Morphine
Intubation/PEEP
ABGs/CXR

Hospital admission: setting dependent
on severity and response to therapy

*Brief history-taking: Focus on concurrent trauma, burns, symptoms referable to mucous membrane, pulmonary
signs (cough vs. dyspnea), nonspecific chest pain, nausea/vomiting, and mental status changes, as well as history of
atopy, asthma, cardiopulmonary disease, or smoking.

†Physical examination: Evaluate acute chlorine exposure. PEEP, positive end-expiratory pressure; ABGs, arterial
blood pressure.

FIGURE 96-2 Triage guidelines following acute chlorine exposure. ABGs, arterial blood gases (analysis); CXR, chest radiography; PEEP, positive end-expiratory pressure.

In one review of regional poison control center exposures, Mrvos and colleagues assessed symptoms in 216 individuals who were exposed to chlorine or chloramine gas from mixing household cleaners.[53] Symptoms were mild and did not require specific therapy. Most had early resolution of symptoms; only 16 had symptoms that persisted for more than 6 hours. One patient, who had underlying chronic pulmonary disease and a concurrent acute respiratory infection, was hospitalized. None developed pulmonary edema. This favorable experience can be contrasted with reports of acute pulmonary edema in two children immediately after brief exposures to vapors from containers of swimming pool chlorinator pellets.[55]

Management

After victims are removed from the source of exposure, involved skin or symptomatic eyes should be copiously irrigated with water. Attention should focus on a patient's airway and any respiratory complaints.

Aggressive treatment includes high-flow humidified oxygen, inhaled bronchodilators, and intravenous corticosteroids. Arrhythmias are not a prominent complication of chlorine fume inhalation; once supplemental oxygen has been provided, subcutaneous epinephrine, if it is the only β-adrenergic agent available, should not be withheld for fear of provoking arrhythmias. Patients with respiratory failure secondary to pulmonary edema or the rare individual with upper airway obstruction from chlorine-induced burns may require intubation with early administration of positive end-expiratory pressure.[68] Although opiates have not been used at times because of the risks for altered mental status, respiratory depression, and cough inhibition, judicious use of parenteral opiates with close observation may be beneficial.[69]

Some investigators have advocated nebulized sodium bicarbonate for patients with persistent cough or those with evidence of severe pulmonary injury. This therapy attempts to chemically neutralize the acid products of chlorine hydration. In one animal study, 10 sheep

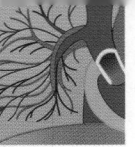

treated with this modality after 4 minutes of exposure to 500 ppm chlorine had statistically higher Po_2 and lower Pco_2 values than animals treated with nebulized normal saline, although there was no difference in the mortality rate of 30% at 24 hours.[70] It has been recommended and used in unselected patient cohorts with anecdotal reports of improvement, but its value is unproven; no reports have described clinical worsening with this therapy.[71,72] Although nebulized bicarbonate has been condemned because of concern about thermal injury from the heat of neutralization, this risk is theoretically minimized by the large surface area of the lungs as well as the small volumes of bicarbonate administered. Given the proposed mechanism, this therapy would seem most useful early in a patient with significant lower airway penetration of chlorine. It has been used in a dose of 3 mL of 8.4% sodium bicarbonate and 2 mL normal saline nebulized with oxygen or air. The nebulization can be repeated if beneficial; however, there is no rationale for its continued use long after the exposure.

Corticosteroids have been used to treat pulmonary edema and bronchospastic symptoms. As with many proposed uses of these anti-inflammatory agents, their efficacy in the treatment of chlorine toxicity has never been subjected to a randomized trial. Early inhaled budesonide (within 30 minutes of lung injury) was shown to be beneficial in a pig model.[73] One report of two sisters exposed to the same chlorine release suggested that the more rapid improvement in pulmonary parameters of one patient could be attributed to the combination of hospital admission, rest, and treatment with oxygen and corticosteroids compared with the sibling who received only brief oxygen therapy.[74] To date, this anecdotal report forms the basis for any recommended use of corticosteroids after chlorine exposure. Another potential treatment modality focuses on reducing the oxidative destruction that potentially follows chlorine-induced generation of oxygen radicals. Animal models of smoke inhalation, hydrochloric acid aspiration, and pulmonary macrophage allergic

response suggest that ibuprofen can reduce pulmonary injury when administered shortly after exposure to these agents.[75,76] Inhibition of thromboxane A_2 synthesis has been postulated to be the mechanism for these effects. No clinical reports have described the utility of this agent after chlorine inhalation.

Antibiotics, although historically used after chlorine-induced pulmonary injury, should be reserved for documented episodes of infection, which for the most part manifest days after exposure. The initial tachypnea, sputum production, pulmonary findings, and consolidation on chest radiographs are attributable to chemical tracheobronchopneumonitis or pulmonary edema. Prophylactic antibiotics are unlikely to alter the clinical course and may also predispose to infection with antibiotic-resistant or other opportunistic organisms.

Case Series

Important clinical findings from six relatively large case series of acute chlorine exposure are summarized in Table 96-3. In the poison center review mentioned earlier, Mrvos and coworkers[53] found a high prevalence of cough with little dyspnea, as well as rapid resolution of symptoms, after home exposures to mixed cleaning agents.

Fleta and associates[77] reported on 76 children (newborn to 14 years old) who were exposed to a leak of 300 L of chlorine gas from a pressurized canister used to purify municipal drinking water in Spain. Seventy of the 76 children were discharged from the hospital within 2 hours; the longest period of observation was 12 hours. No one developed pulmonary edema. Most symptoms resolved on removal from the source; those with "signs of irritation of the lower respiratory tract" were treated with oxygen and intramuscular corticosteroids.

Moulick and colleagues[64] described 82 adults (21–60 years old) who were within 20 yards of a chlorine storage tank leak in Bombay, India. An ambient chlorine concentration of 66 ppm was measured in the area

TABLE 96-3 Representative Distributions of Findings in Reported Exposures to Chlorine Gas

SYMPTOM/SIGN	% REPORTED OCCURRENCE					
	MRVOS et al[53]	FLETA et al[77]	MOULICK et al[64]	HEDGES AND MORRISSEY[58]	BOSSE[71]	WEILL et al[78]
Oropharyngeal irritation	6	66	100	23	14	—
Cough	84	91	100	30	52	81
Dyspnea	19	14	100	19	51	85
Chest pain	5	14	5	17	34	—
Headache	—	9	29	9	1	—
Vomiting	3	5	24	19	8	69
Abdominal pain	<1	—	27	—	1	—
Eye complaints	2	—	—	36	—	80
Hoarseness	—	14	—	—	—	—
Loss of consciousness	—	3	—	—	—	—
Tachypnea	—	20	100	—	2	—
Shock/stupor	—	—	—	—	—	62
Rhonchi/wheezing	4	—	100	—	21	—
Rales	—	—	30	—	—	—

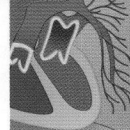

2 hours after the exposure. Sixty-two patients were hospitalized for 2 or more days. Two patients developed pulmonary edema within 6 to 8 hours; 5 had hypoxemia requiring ventilatory support. "Late" pneumonia developed in two patients. All 56 who underwent bronchoscopy had tracheobronchial mucosal congestion; 20 patients had hemorrhagic spots. Erosions or ulcerations were identified in 7 patients; the presence of these correlated with more severe symptoms. All patients were treated with oxygen, aminophylline, hydrocortisone, and ampicillin. Four of 16 patients who were observed for a year or more had persistent cough for 4 to 6 weeks; no residual symptoms or chest radiographic or pulmonary function abnormalities were found at the end of the follow-up.

Hedges and Morrissey[58] summarized findings in 64 patients evaluated after a leak of about 4 tons of liquid chlorine from storage tanks in Philadelphia. These patients represented about 60% of the people evaluated at one medical center; after triage, the others were found to be asymptomatic and were sent home from the waiting area. All six patients admitted to the hospital with "marked tracheobronchitis" complained of dyspnea, whereas this complaint was present in only 10% of those able to be discharged. There were no deaths or cases of pulmonary edema. Symptomatic patients were treated with humidified oxygen, a combination of bronchodilators, and antitussives. Triage and treatment recommendations for management of multiple-casualty chlorine exposures were made by these authors.

Bosse[71] reviewed 86 cases (24 adults) seen at 49 medical facilities in Kentucky with poison center recommendation of nebulized sodium bicarbonate treatment for symptomatic chlorine inhalation. Sixty-nine patients were discharged from the emergency department after one to two nebulized sodium bicarbonate treatments. Seven patients were treated with bronchodilators, and one received steroids. Seventeen patients were admitted to the hospital for 1 to 3 days. All improved; none developed pulmonary edema or required ventilatory support. Some received sodium bicarbonate; four were treated with inhaled bronchodilators, and one each received inhaled steroids and intravenous aminophylline.

Weill and colleagues[78] summarized initial symptoms and results of pulmonary function follow-up in those exposed to release of up to 30 tons of liquid chlorine after a freight train derailment in Louisiana. Ambient chlorine levels in some areas 7 hours after the derailment were in excess of 400 ppm, and levels at the fringe of contamination 3 hours after the event were 10 ppm.[79] Hundreds of animals in the area died; more than 100 people developed symptoms requiring treatment. The symptoms in the 17 admitted patients, of 75 who were treated at one hospital, are noted in the table. One infant died shortly after severe exposure. Therapy at that time (1961) relied mainly on oxygen, postural drainage, atropine, penicillin, chymotrypsin, Alevaire (a nonionic surfactant, sodium bicarbonate, and glycerin), and some narcotics and expectorants.

It is important to understand the circumstances of exposure when interpreting the relative prominence of findings such as those listed in Table 96-3. Symptoms demonstrated by any one individual depend heavily on the circumstances of exposure and individual predisposing characteristics such as smoking history and atopy.

Chronic Chlorine Exposure

Other areas of potential concern about chlorine toxicity include chronic effects from low-level ambient workplace exposure and the potential carcinogenic or teratogenic effects of oral exposure to chlorinated water supplies. As described earlier, reversible obstructive airways dysfunction in workers continually exposed to chlorine has been demonstrated,[65,66] although the effect of concurrent cigarette smoking, atopy, and the contribution of acute exposures above TLV-TWA levels ("gassing") made it difficult to sort out relative contributions. In one study, the effects of up to 2.3 ppm chlorine inhalation by rhesus monkeys for 6 hours daily for 1 year were evaluated. Conjunctival and focal tracheal irritative changes were seen only at the highest exposure levels, and not in all animals.[80] Most individuals do not suffer prolonged airway dysfunction after an acute exposure, although resolution of abnormal findings on pulmonary function tests can be prolonged, particularly in smokers and those with preexisting pulmonary function abnormalities.[81-83]

Some halogenated compounds are known to be mutagenic. The use of chlorine, chloramine, and chlorine dioxide as disinfecting and bleaching agents in municipal water supplies and the food industry has therefore generated concern about the tradeoff between convenience, markedly improved sanitation, and the risk for increased cancer incidence. Concern has focused on the generation of disinfection by-products known as trihalomethanes. These include chloroform, bromoform, dibromochloromethane, and bromodichloromethane. The water concentration of these by-products is increased by the higher concentration of nitrogen waste products in surface water and heat.[84,85] A small study demonstrated detectable chloroform in the blood of indoor competitive swimmers (mean, 0.89 ng/mL), which was not found in outdoor swimmers.[86] This was associated with a "significantly elevated" β_2-microglobulin urine concentration, possibly suggesting renal damage. Patients on long-term hemodialysis are another group exposed to increased concentrations of chlorine by-products.[87] Community-based population studies have also suggested a statistical increase in the relative risk (ranging from 1.2 to 2.2) of a number of cancers in those populations dependent on chlorinated surface water when compared with ground-water users.[88,89] The affected sites have included the bladder, kidneys, pancreas, stomach, and rectum; malignant melanoma has also been associated. These associations obviously do not equate with causality, particularly within the individual. Various confounding variables, including socioeconomic factors or the presence of other toxic compounds, could have a role.

Similar concerns have been raised about possible reproductive toxicity of disinfection by-products. Although severe acute chlorine exposures have resulted

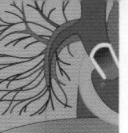

in fetal wastage in cows and decreased egg production in chickens,[79] low-level oral exposure to sodium hypochlorite in the drinking water of hens did not alter egg production until the chloride concentration exceeded 40 ppm.[90] Chlorine treatment of both male and female rats with up to 5 mg/kg per day resulted in no detectable reproductive or fetal changes.[91] It is only at exposures several thousand times those typically seen in humans that animal studies show reproductive abnormalities.[92] Despite these reassurances, there have been calls to ban the use of chlorine. Caution must be exercised before abandoning the use of a substance with at most uncertain low-level toxicity in favor of other agents that have not been studied as extensively.[93] Nonetheless, given the ubiquitous nature of chlorination processes, these issues will continue to be studied.[94]

ACKNOWLEDGMENTS

We gratefully acknowledge the contributions of the previous authors of chapters that covered these topics in the third edition of Haddad, Winchester, and Shannon's *Clinical Management of Poisoning and Drug Overdose*: Michael W. Shannon, MD, MPH, Jonathan Borak, MD, and Charles McKay, MD.

REFERENCES

1. Bowers GN, Onoroski M: Hypochloremia and the incidence of bromism in 1990. Clin Chem 1990;36:1399–1403.
2. Trump DL, Hochberg MC: Bromide intoxication. Johns Hopkins Med J 1976;138:119–123.
3. Rothenberg DM, Berns AS, Barkin R, Glantz RH: Bromide intoxication secondary to pyridostigmine bromide therapy. JAMA 1990;263:1121–1122.
4. Jinkins JR, Chaleby K: Acute toxic encephalopathy secondary to bromide sedative ingestion. Neuroradiology 1987;29:212.
5. Senecal P-E, Osterloh J: Confusion from pyridostigmine bromide: was there bromide intoxication? JAMA 1990;264:454–455.
6. McDanal CE, Owens D, Bolman WM: Bromide abuse: A continuing problem. Am J Psychiatry 1974;131:913–915.
7. Meldgaard OT, Cold GE: Serum bromide after general anaesthesia with halothane. Acta Anaesth Scand 1979;23:513–518.
8. Ng Y-Y, Lin W-L, Chen T-W, et al: Spurious hyperchloremia and decreased anion gap in a patient with dextromethorphan bromide. Am J Nephrol 1992;12:268–270.
9. Jih DM, Khanna V, Somach SC: Bromoderma after ingestion of Ruby Red Squirt. N Engl J Med 2003;348:1932.
10. Burn MJ, Linden CH: Another hot tub hazard to bromine and hydrobromic acid exposure Chest 1997;111:816.
11. Frances C, Hoizey G, Lamiable D, et al: Bromism from daily over intake of bromide salts J Toxicol Clin Toxicol 2003;41:181–183.
12. Rauws AG: Pharmacokinetics of bromide ion: an overview. Food Chem Toxicol 1983;21:379–382.
13. Iberti TJ, Patterson BK, Fisher CJ: Prolonged bromide intoxication resulting from a gastric bezoar. Arch Intern Med 1984;144:402–403.
14. Kuwahara T, Ikehara Y, Kanatsu K, et al: Two cases of potassium bromate poisoning requiring long-term hemodialysis therapy for irreversible tubular damage. Nephron 1984;37:278–280.
15. Paty DW, Sherr H: Ocular bobbing in bromism. Neurology 1971;22:526–527.
16. Sangster B, Blom JL, Sekhuis VM, et al: The influence of sodium bromide in man: a study in human volunteers with special emphasis on the endocrine and the central nervous system. Food Chem Toxicol 1983;21:409–419.
17. Mangurten HH, Kaye CI: Neonatal bromism secondary to maternal exposure in a photographic laboratory. J Pediatr 1982; 100:596–598.
18. Pleasure JR, Blackburn MG: Neonatal bromide intoxication: prenatal ingestion of a large quantity of bromides with transplacental accumulation in the fetus. Pediatrics 1975;55:503–506.
19. Miller ME, Cappon CJ: Anion-exchange chromatographic determination of bromide in serum. Clin Chem 1984;30:781–783.
20. Allain P, Mauras Y, Douge C, et al: Determination of iodine and bromide in the plasma and urine by inductively coupled plasma mass spectrometry. Analyst 1990;115:813–815.
21. Emancipator K, Kroll MH: Bromide interference: is less really better? Clin Chem 1990;36:1470–1473.
22. Kan K, Satowa S, Takeuchi I, et al: Unusual apparent hyperchloremia induced by long-term abuse of bromide-containing drugs. Int J Clin Pharmacol Ther Toxicol 1986;24:399–402.
23. Vasuvattakul S, Lertpattanasuwan N, Vareesangthip K, et al: A negative anion gap as a clue to diagnose bromide intoxication. Nephron 1995;69:311–313.
24. Matsumoto I, Morizono T, Paparella MM: Hearing loss following potassium bromate: two case reports. Otolaryngol Head Neck Surg 1980;88:625–629.
25. Kutom A, Bazilinshi NG, Magana L, Dunea G: Bromate intoxication: hairdressers' anuria. Am J Kidney Dis 1990;15:84–85.
26. Warshaw BL, Carter MC, Hymes LC, et al: Bromate poisoning from hair permanent preparations. Pediatrics 1985;7:975–978.
27. Lue JN, Johnson CE, Edwards DL: Bromate poisoning from ingestion of professional hair-care neutralizer. Clin Pharmacol 1988;7:66–70.
28. Lichtenberg R, Zeller WP, Gatson R, Hurley RM: Bromate poisoning. J Pediatr 1989;114:891–894.
29. Morabia A, Selleger C, Landry JC, et al: Accidental bromine exposure in an urban population: an acute epidemiological assessment. Int J Epidemiol 1988;17:148–152.
30. Broderick A, Schwartz DA: Halogen gases, ammonia, and phosgene. In Sullivan JB, Krieger GR (eds): Hazardous Materials Toxicology: Clinical Principles of Environmental Health. Baltimore, Williams & Wilkins, 1992, pp 792–793.
31. Sullivan JB Jr: Oxidizers, reducing agents, and other highly reactive chemicals. In Sullivan JB, Krieger GR (eds): Clinical Environmental Health and Toxic Exposures, 2nd ed. Baltimore, Williams & Wilkins, 2001, pp 967–968.
32. Woolf A, Shannon M: Reactive airway dysfunction and systemic complication after mass exposure to bromine. Environ Health Perspect 1999;107:507–509.
33. American Hospital Formulary Service: Iodine. In McEvoy GK (ed): Drug Information 95. Bethesda, MD, American Society of Health-System Pharmacists, 1995, pp 2427–2428.
34. Feingold KR, Sater B, Engle B: Iodine-induced artifacts in home blood glucose measurements. Diabetes Care 1983;6:317–318.
35. Haynes RC: Thyroid and antithyroid drugs. In Gilman AG, Rall TW, Nies AS, Taylor P (eds): Goodman and Gilman's the Pharmacological Basis of Therapeutics. New York, Pergamon Press, 1990, pp 1361–1383.
36. Beeson PB: Effects of iodides on inflammatory processes. Perspect Biol Med 1994;37:173–181.
37. Sussman RM, Miller J: Iodide "mumps" after intravenous urography. N Engl J Med 1956;255:433–434.
38. Robertson P, Fraser J, Sheild J, Weir P. Thyrotoxicosis related to iodine toxicity in a paediatric burn patient. Intensive Care Med 2002;28(9):1369.
39. Dela Cruz F, Brown DH, Leikin JB: Iodine absorption after topical administration. West J Med 1987;146:43–45.
40. Kanakiriya S, De Chazal I, Nath KA, et al: Iodine toxicity treated with hemodialysis and continuous venovenous hemodiafiltration. Am J Kidney Dis 2003;41(3):702–708.
41. Aquilina JT: Fungating ioderma treated with hydrocortisone. JAMA 1955;158:727–728.
42. Waugh WH: Use of cortisone by mouth in the prevention and therapy of severe iodism. Arch Intern Med 1954;93:299–303.
43. Postellon DC, Aronow R: Iodine in mother's milk. JAMA 1982;247:463.
44. L'Italien A, Starceski PJ, Dixit NM: Transient hypothyroidism in a breastfed infant after maternal use of iodoform gauze J Pediatr Endocrinol Metab. 2004;17(4):665–667.
45. D'Auria J, Lipson S, Garfield JM: Fatal iodine toxicity following surgical debridement of a hip wound: case report. J Trauma 1990;30:353–355.

46. Kurt TL, Morgan ML, Hnilica V: Fatal iatrogenic iodine toxicity in a 9-week old infant J Toxicol Clin Toxicol 1996;34(5):531–533.

47. Scone JS: Chlorine: Its Manufacture, Properties and Uses. New York, Reinhold, 1962.

48. Das R, Blanc PD: Chlorine gas exposure and the lung: a review. Toxicol Ind Health 1993;9:439–455.

49. Borak J: Chlorine. TEMIS 5.4. New Haven, CT, Jonathan Borak & Co, 1995.

50. Rotman HH, Fliegel MJ, Moore T, et al: Effects of low concentrations of chlorine on pulmonary function in humans. J Appl Physiol 1983;54:1120–1124.

51. Hathaway GJ, Proctor NH, Hughes JP, et al: Chemical Hazards of the Workplace, 3rd ed. New York, Van Nostrand Rinehold, 1991.

52. Watson WA, Litovitz TL, Klein-Schwartz W, et al: 2003 Annual report of the American Association of Poison Control Centers Toxic Exposure Surveillance System. Am J Emerg Med 2004;22:335–404.

53. Mrvos R, Dean BS, Krenzelok EP: Home exposure to chlorine/chloramines gas: review of 216 cases. South Med J 1993;86:654–657.

54. Sexton JD, Pronchik DJ: Chlorine inhalation: the big picture. J Toxicol Clin Toxicol 1998;36:87–93.

55. Wood BR, Colombo JL, Benson BE: Chlorine inhalation toxicity from vapors generated by swimming pool chlorinator tablets. Pediatrics 1987;79:427–429.

56. Martinez TT, Long C: Explosion risk from swimming pool chlorinators and review of chlorine toxicity. J Toxicol Clin Tox 1995;33:349–354.

57. Detorres JP, Strom JA, Jaber BL, Hendra KP: Hemodialysis associated methhemoglobinemia in acute renal failure. Am J Kidney Dis 2002;39:1307–1309.

58. Hedges JR, Morrissey WL: Acute chlorine gas exposure. JAMA 1979;8:59–64.

59. Horton DK, Berkowitz Z, Kaye WE: The public health consequences from acute chlorine releases, 1993–2000. J Occup Environ Med 2002;44:906–913.

60. Barrow CS, Alarie Y, Warrick JC, et al: Comparison of the sensory irritation response in mice to chlorine and hydrogen chloride. Arch Environ Health 1977;32:68–76.

61. Krenzelok E, Mrvos R: Chlorine and chloramines. J Toxicol Clin Toxicol 1995;33:255–357.

62. Jones R, Hughes JM, Glindmeyer H, Weill H: Lung function after acute chlorine exposure. Am Rev Respir Dis 1986;134:1190–1195.

63. Winder C: The toxicology of chlorine. Environ Res 2001;85:105–114.

64. Moulick ND, Banavali S, Abhyankar AD, et al: Acute accidental exposure to chlorine fumes. Indian J Chest Dis Allied Sci 1992;34:85–89.

65. Malo JL, Cartier A, Boulet LP, et al: Bronchial hyperresponsiveness can improve while spirometry plateaus two to three years after repeated exposure to chlorine causing respiratory symptoms. Am J Res Crit Care Med 1994;150:1142–1145.

66. Bherer L, Cusshman R, Courteau JP, et al: Survey of construction workers repeatedly exposed to chlorine over a three to six month period in a pulpmill. Follow up of affected workers by questionnaire, spirometry and assessment of bronchial responsiveness 18 to 24 months after exposure ended. Occup Environ Med 1994;51:225–228.

67. Beach FXM, Jones ES, Scarrow GD: Respiratory effects of chlorine gas. Br J Ind Med 1969;26:231–236.

68. Heidemann SM, Goetting MG: Treatment of acute hypoxemic respiratory failure caused by chlorine exposure. Pediatr Emerg Care 1991;7:87–88.

69. Pino F, Puerta H, D'Apollo R, et al: Effectiveness of morphine in noncardiogenic pulmonary edema due to chlorine gas inhalation. Vet Hum Toxicol 1993;35:36.

70. Chisholm CD, Sigletary EM, Okerberg CV, Langinais PC: Inhaled sodium bicarbonate for chlorine inhalation injuries [abstract]. Ann Emerg Med 1989;18:466.

71. Bosse GM: Nebulized sodium bicarbonate in the treatment of chlorine gas inhalation. J Toxicol Clin Toxicol 1994;32:233–241.

72. Vinsel PJ: Treatment of acute chlorine gas inhalation with nebulized sodium bicarbonate. J Emerg Med 1990;8:327–329.

73. Wang J, Zhang L, Walther S: Inhaled budesonide in experimental chlorine gas injury: influence of time interval between injury and treatment. Int Care Med 2003;28:352–357.

74. Chester EH, Kaimel PJ, Payne CB Jr, Kohn PM: Pulmonary injury following exposure to chlorine gas. Chest 72:247–250.

75. Tamaoki J: Possible contribution of lung macrophage to airway hypersensitivity. Jpn Thorac Dis 1990;28:1294–1298.

76. Shinozawa Y, Hales C, Jung W, et al: Ibuprofen prevents synthetic smoke-induced pulmonary edema. Am Rev Respir Dis 1986;134:1145–1148.

77. Fleta J, Calvo C, Zuniga J, et al: Intoxication of 76 children by chlorine gas. Hum Toxicol 1986;5:99–100.

78. Weill H, Geaorge R, Schwaz M, Ziskind M: Late evaluation of pulmonary function after acute exposure to chlorine gas. Am Rev Respir Dis 1969;90:374–379.

79. Joyner RE, Durel EG: Accidental liquid chlorine spill in a rural community. J Occup Med 1962;4:152–154.

80. Klonne DR, Ulrich CE, Riley MG, et al: One-year inhalation toxicity of chlorine in rhesus monkeys (Macaca mulatto). Fund Appl Toxicol 1987;9:557–572.

81. Abhyanker A, Bhambure N, Kamath NN, et al: Six month follow-up of fourteen victims with short term exposure to chlorine gas. J Soc Occup Med 1898;39:131–132.

82. Donnelly SC, FitzGerald MX: Reactive airway dysfunction syndrome (RADS) due to chlorine gas exposure. Ir J Med Sci 1990;159:275–276.

83. Gorguner M, Aslan S, Inandi T, Cakir Z. Reactive airways dysfunction syndrome in housewives due to a bleach-hydrochloric acid mixture. Inhal Toxicol 2004;16:87–91.

84. Weisel CP, Chen WJ: Exposure to chlorination by-products from hot water uses. Risk Anal 1994;14:101–106.

85. Espigares M, Lardelli P, Ortega P: Evaluating trihalomethane content in drinking water on the basis of common monitoring parameters: regression models. J Environ Health 2003;66(3):9–13, 20.

86. Aikink H, van Acker MB, Scholten RJ, et al: Swimming pool chlorination: a health hazard? Toxicol Lett 1994;72:375–380.

87. Smith RP, Willhite CC: Chlorine diozide and hemodialysis. Regul Toxicol Pharmacol 1990;11:42–62.

88. McGeehin MA, Reif JS, Becher JC, Mangione EJ: Case-control study of bladder cancer and water disinfection methods in Colorado. Am J Epidemiol 1993;138:492–501.

89. Morris RD, Audet AM, Angelillo IF, et al: Chlorination, chlorination by-products and cancer: a meta-analysis. Am J Public Health 1992;82:955–963.

90. Damron BL, Fluncker LK: Broiler chick and laying hen tolerance to sodium hypochlorite in drinking water. Poultry Sci 1993;72:1950–1655.

91. Carlton BD, Barlett P, Basaran A, et al: Reproductive effects of alternative disinfectants. Environ Perspect 1986;69:237–241.

92. Nieuwenhuijsen MJ, Toledano MB, Eaton NE, et al: Chlorination disinfection by-products in water and their association with adverse reproductive outcomes, a review. Occup Environ Med 2000;57:73–85.

93. Karol MH: Toxicologic principals do not support the banning of chlorine. A Society of Toxicology position paper. Fund Appl Toxicol 1995;24:1–2.

94. Cap AP: The chlorine controversy. Int Arch Occup Environ Health 1996;68:455–458.

97 *Ammonia and Nitrogen Oxides*

MARTIN BELSON, MD

At a Glance...

- Management of ammonia and nitrogen oxide poisonings involves supportive care, decontamination, and disposition.

- Supportive care includes removal from the source and rapid assessment of airway, breathing, and circulation; establishment of oxygen, the cardiac monitor, and intravenous access; administrations of nebulized β_2 agonists; and, as indicated, administration of endotracheal intubation and positive end-expiratory pressure.

- Decontamination includes removal of all contaminated clothing and irrigation of skin and eyes with water, if symptomatic. If ammonia or nitrogen oxide is ingested, do not induce vomiting or give activated charcoal.

- Disposition includes 2-hour observation in the emergency department for mild exposures without airway compromise; inpatient observation for anything more than mild symptoms; and intensive care unit admission for airway compromise or severe burns.

AMMONIA

Introduction and Relevant History

Ammonia (NH_3) is a highly irritating, water-soluble, colorless gas with a distinctive pungent odor. When ammonia gas (anhydrous) is dissolved in water, the resulting material is ammonium hydroxide (NH_4OH), or "aqueous" ammonia. Anhydrous ammonia is easily compressed and forms a clear, colorless liquid under pressure, which makes it ideal for storage and shipping in pressurized containers, such as tank cars and trucks.

Ammonia is widely used as a refrigerant, a fertilizer, and a household and commercial cleaning agent. Ammonia is also used as a solvent in the manufacture of textiles and leather, in pulp and paper processing, and in petroleum refining. Other applications include the synthesis of plastics, pesticides, cyanide, explosives, and rocket fuels.

Aqueous ammonia with concentrations of 5% to 10% is used as a household cleaner or bleaching agent. Industrial-strength aqueous ammonia at concentrations greater than 25% to 30% is considered an alkaline corrosive. Anhydrous ammonia may burn but does not ignite readily; however, a pressurized container of the gas may explode in heat or fire.

Epidemiology

The widespread use of ammonia greatly increases the possibility of accidental or intentional release and human exposure to toxic concentrations. In fact, ammonia is one of the most commonly spilled chemicals in the United States.[1] Human exposure to ammonia may occur after an industrial accident, such as the rupture of a tank, or after a transportation accident, which may result in large-scale environmental exposures to ammonia gas. Ammonia is one of the top five substances released in transit involving acute public health consequences.[2] However, most ammonia releases occur at fixed facilities (e.g., food manufacturing industry) rather than during transportation.[3]

In the household, exposure may occur if an *ammonia*-containing cleaner is mixed with a *chlorine*-containing bleach, leading to the release of *chloramine* fumes.[4,5] According to the American Association of Poison Control Centers Toxic Exposure Surveillance System, 2993 exposures to chloramine occurred in 2002, resulting in one death.[6]

In a 5% to 10% concentration, ammonia generally is considered an irritant and rarely is reported to cause burns when inhaled.[7] However, three patients who attempted suicide by ingesting household ammonia reportedly had esophageal burns. One of these patients had severe corrosive injury of the upper airway and esophagus with aspiration pneumonia and died. The death was attributed to adult respiratory distress syndrome and renal failure.[8]

Anhydrous ammonia accounts for a significant percentage of chemical burns in the occupational setting. In one review, 34% of the chemical burns admitted to University of Iowa hospitals were the result of ammonia exposure.[9]

Structure and Structure–Activity Relationships

Ammonia reacts with strong oxidizers, acids, and various heavy metals. It is corrosive to copper and galvanized surfaces. When ammonia is mixed inappropriately with sodium hypochlorite ($NaOCl$) bleach in an attempt to potentiate the chemicals' individual cleaning powers, chloramine gas, an irritant with properties similar to those of chlorine, is formed (see text box).[4]

(a) $3NaOCl + 2NH_3 \rightarrow NH_2Cl + NHCl_2 + 3NaOH$

(b) $NH_2Cl + H_2O \rightarrow HOCl + NH_3$

(c) $HOCl \rightarrow HCl + O^-$

(a) Sodium hypochlorite (bleach) plus ammonia form monochloramine and dichloramine. (b) Chloramine gas may decompose in water to form free ammonia and hypochlorous acid. (c) hypochlorous acid may combine with moisture to yield nascent oxygen, a potent oxidizing agent and mucous membrane irritant.

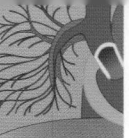

Pathophysiology

The extent of injury after exposure to ammonia depends on a number of factors. According to the National Institute of Occupational Safety and Health (NIOSH), the irritating effects of exposure to ammonia are more dependent on concentration than length of exposure[10,11] (Table 97-1). Although ammonia's odor threshold is low enough to provide adequate warning of its presence, the odor causes olfactory fatigue, making ammonia's presence difficult to detect when exposure is prolonged.

Anhydrous ammonia is highly water-soluble and rapidly produces an irritant and alkaline, corrosive effect on contact with mucosal membranes such as the eyes and upper respiratory tract. Ammonia and water combine to form ammonium hydroxide that dissociates to ammonium (NH_4^+) and hydroxyl (OH^-) ions. These ions cause a severe alkaline burn characterized by liquefaction necrosis.[12,13] The reaction is exothermic and produces thermal as well as chemical injury.[13,14] The deepest damage to the skin appears to occur in areas with the highest moisture content, such as the axilla and groin. Edema of all involved tissues is common, and laryngeal edema can be life threatening.[14,15]

In the airways, desquamation of the epithelial layer of the upper tracheobronchial tree (tracheobronchitis) with membrane formation is the usual pathology.[12] There tends to be relatively little effect on the lower airways because ammonia's high solubility prevents it from reaching the distal airways. With very high concentrations of the vapors, damage to the pulmonary endothelial and epithelial cells leads to increased permeability and exudation of fluid into the alveoli, producing the characteristic clinical findings of acute lung injury (ALI).[16,17] Experimental inhalation of nebulized high-dose ammonia causes ALI manifested by a fall in oxygen saturation and a rise in airway pressure within 2 minutes of initiation.[18]

Ammonium hydroxide penetrates the eye far more rapidly than other alkalis. Researchers have demonstrated that ammonium hydroxide can significantly increase anterior chamber pH within 15 seconds.[19]

Toxicology

CLINICAL MANIFESTATIONS

The clinical manifestations of ammonia poisoning depend on many factors, including the ammonia's physical state, the concentration and amount of ammonia, the depth of inhalation, the duration of exposure, and the route of exposure. Inhalation of ammonia gas results in rapid onset of irritation to the eyes, nose, throat, and upper respiratory tract. Prolonged exposures, or exposures to large amounts of ammonia, may result in irritation of the lower respiratory tract. Ingestion of aqueous ammonia results in immediate burning of the mouth and throat and could cause esophageal and gastric damage. Skin or eye contact with either ammonia gas or aqueous ammonia may cause serious alkaline, corrosive burns. Clinical manifestations of ammonia poisoning typically result from an acute exposure, but ammonia poisoning also can cause chronic, long-term adverse effects.

Acute Clinical Manifestations

After inhalation of ammonia fumes, immediate signs and symptoms include a burning sensation in the nose, throat, and eyes, followed by lacrimation, blurred vision, rhinorrhea, and possibly eyelid and lip edema. Headache and coughing also are typical early findings. Upper airway edema rapidly may cause airway obstruction, preceded by hoarseness and stridor. Lower airway involvement may cause chest tightness, dyspnea, bronchospasm with wheezing, and hypoxia. ALI, presenting with rales and rhonchi if the ammonia concentration was great enough to have penetrated the lower airways, eventually may develop. Copious amounts of tracheal secretions, hemoptysis, and fever are not uncommon. Pneumonia with consolidation may be evident on radiographs.[14,20,21]

Inhalation injury may follow a biphasic course. After the initial pneumonitis or ALI, a patient may experience relative improvement for 48 to 72 hours. Subsequently, there is the gradual onset of airway obstruction, and respiratory failure may develop.

Physical examination of the chest during the first 24 hours after exposure is the best predictor of subsequent hospital course.[20] In a report of 14 patients accidentally exposed to a high concentration of ammonia, all patients who exhibited respiratory symptoms and had a normal chest examination at the time of admission recovered quickly, without specific therapy. Patients who exhibited respiratory symptoms and significant findings on chest examination (i.e., rales, wheezing) had a more protracted and relatively more complicated hospital course. Also, among patients with a mild to moderate clinical illness, radiographic findings were rather

TABLE 97-1 Exposure Limits and Clinical Effects of Ammonia at Different Concentrations

CONCENTRATION (ppm)	EFFECTS
5	Odor threshold, tolerance may develop to the odor
25	NIOSH-REL
35	NIOSH-STEL
50	OSHA-PEL
<50	Eye and upper respiratory irritant
300	NIOSH-IDLH
1000	Direct caustic effects on the respiratory tract
2500	Death has been reported after 30 minutes of exposure
30,000	Lowest concentration leading to death after 5 minutes of exposure in human references[14,22]

IDLH, immediate danger to life or health; NIOSH, National Institute for Occupational Safety and Health; OSHA, Occupational Safety and Health Administration; PEL, permissible exposure limit; REL, recommended exposure limit; STEL, short-term exposure limit.

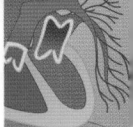

unremarkable. The report's authors concluded that the radiographic findings appear to offer little assistance in assessing the immediate status of respiratory tract involvement, or in predicting the future clinical course of patients suffering acute ammonia inhalation.[20]

After ingestion of liquid ammonia, common signs and symptoms include severe pain in the mouth, chest, and abdomen, accompanied by vomiting and possibly followed by shock. Severe local edema of the lips and mouth is present; burns of the soft palate also may occur. Twenty-four to 72 hours later, esophageal and gastric perforation with mediastinitis may occur. Victims with perforation have severe abdominal pain and rigidity and may have associated respiratory complications, including ALI.[22,23] Alkaline corrosive ingestions are discussed further in Chapter 98. Ingestion of ammonia does not normally result in systemic poisoning.

Dermal exposure to ammonia liquid or gas initially may result in a burning sensation, followed rapidly by blister or vesicle formation. Injuries may vary from mild erythema and edema after a low concentration exposure to severe edema and deep penetrating burns after a more concentrated exposure.[22] Skin exposure to ammonia liquid that has a temperature of −33° C produces frostbite-type injuries, with first- to third-degree burns.[14,22]

Chronic Clinical Manifestations

Repeated exposure to ammonia gas may cause chronic irritation of the conjunctiva and upper respiratory tract.[21] The potential effect of chronic exposure to ammonia on pulmonary function remains controversial because some authors have failed to find an effect[24] whereas others have shown an association.[25,26] The results of one large case-control study suggested that exposure to a high cumulative ammonia level (based on estimates only) produces a combined restrictive and obstructive ventilatory defect.[26]

Adverse Effects

Although complete pulmonary recovery is the usual outcome, acute ammonia inhalation injury has been associated with chronic pulmonary conditions such as bronchiectasis, reactive airways dysfunction syndrome (RADS), and chronic obstructive pulmonary disorder.[27-30] The association between exposure to high concentrations of ammonia and bronchiectasis is probably best documented, varying from 2 months to 2 years after the acute episode.[27,28] The patients usually had severe clinical disease immediately after the exposure, with bacterial superinfection documented or suspected in most cases.

One patient without a preexisting history of sinusitis or allergies exhibited chronic, relapsing sinusitis after being exposed acutely to gaseous ammonia.[31]

Permanent ocular damage may occur as a result of tissue destruction and elevations in intraocular pressure. Ammonium hydroxide is especially destructive to the eye because it penetrates far more rapidly than do other alkalis. Cataract formation and corneal opacification are common complications of severe ammonia exposure, particularly if the patient is not treated promptly.[12]

Late complications from ulcerative esophagitis include stricture formation.[22,23]

DIAGNOSIS

Laboratory Testing

Laboratory results generally are nonspecific and are not helpful after an ammonia exposure. It is important to obtain serial arterial blood gas values, both to monitor the progress of respiratory failure and because these patients may develop a metabolic acidosis. The serum ammonia level does not correlate with the degree of injury.[22]

Differential Diagnosis

Exposure to other acid- or base-forming irritant gases may result in a clinical picture similar to that of exposure to ammonia. Other highly water-soluble agents include the chloramines, hydrogen chloride (HCl), acrolein, formaldehyde, and sulfur dioxide/sulfuric acid (SO_2/H_2SO_4); intermediate water-soluble agents include chlorine (Cl_2). Exposure to oxidant gases, such as oxides of nitrogen, and riot-control agents or lacrimators (e.g., capsaicin, chloroacetone) also should be considered.

MANAGEMENT

Supportive Measures

Prehospital management must be started early and aggressively in patients suspected of having been exposed to ammonia. First and foremost, it is necessary to evacuate patients from the exposure site. An initial survey of the patient's airway, breathing, and circulation will identify immediately any life-threatening injuries.

For any patient with respiratory symptoms, respiratory support with 100% oxygen through a non-rebreathing face mask is indicated in the prehospital setting, although early intubation may be necessary. Early intubation should be considered whenever a patient develops stridor, second- or third-degree burns to the neck or throat, or central nervous system depression.

In the hospital, aggressive respiratory support should be continued or initiated as indicated. Positive end-expiratory pressure ventilation may be necessary to maintain an adequate Po_2.[14,20] Inhaled β_2 agonists are indicated for bronchospasm. In one study, nebulized 3.75% sodium bicarbonate was shown to improve oxygenation after chlorine exposure.[32] Nebulized 5% sodium bicarbonate was shown to be safe and potentially beneficial in a large retrospective study,[33] but has not been studied after ammonia exposure. In one case series, 22 patients exposed to chloramine gas were treated with a nebulized solution of 3.75% sodium bicarbonate with no significant statistical or clinical difference in outcome.[5] At this time, routine use of nebulized sodium bicarbonate as a neutralizing agent is not recommended after exposure to ammonia.

Fluids should be restricted early, unless the patient clearly is dehydrated or hypotensive, because excessive hydration may contribute to further airway edema. Central venous and pulmonary capillary wedge pressure monitoring may be required in seriously burned patients.

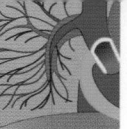

Decontamination

If the exposure involves aqueous ammonia, removal of contaminated clothing is imperative. Emergency medical service personnel should wash exposed skin with copious amounts of water and irrigate the eyes continuously, if the patient is symptomatic, until definitive medical care is reached. Contact lenses should be removed before flushing the eyes to prevent the concentration of ammonia beneath the lenses.

If aqueous ammonia is ingested, vomiting should not be induced, and charcoal should not be given because it does not adsorb ammonia and may obscure the view for endoscopy.

In the hospital, it is important to determine whether decontamination of any remaining ammonia from the patient's eyes or skin is warranted to prevent further absorption and to protect the health care staff. Irrigation of the eyes should continue until the patient is more comfortable and until a conjunctivae sac pH below 8.5 is achieved.[14] Irrigation of affected skin should continue for at least 15 to 20 minutes.

After the initial skin washing, irrigation with water should be continued at regular intervals for 24 hours. The use of greasy ointments is discouraged for at least 24 hours because they may promote increased penetration of anhydrous ammonia.[12] Nonviable skin should be débrided early, and wounds should be dressed with topical antibiotics. Alkaline corrosive injury to the skin is discussed further in Chapter 98.

Laboratory Monitoring

Serial arterial blood gas measurements and radiographs and continuous pulse oximetry may be indicated depending on the severity of illness.

Other Medical and Diagnostic Interventions

There is no specific antidote for poisoning from ammonia exposure. Use of systemic corticosteroids for inhalation injury is controversial, although many case reports include their use. In experimental studies, methylprednisolone was not shown to protect the lung from the acute physiologic consequences of inhalation injury,[34] and budesonide inhalation had no effect on ammonia-induced lung injury.[18] Prophylactic systemic antibiotics are not recommended. If mediastinitis develops, antibiotics are recommended.[14,20,22]

After the eyes have been adequately irrigated, slit-lamp evaluation with fluoroscein stain should be performed to evaluate for corneal burns. Immediate consultation with an ophthalmologist is essential for an abnormal slit-lamp examination. Use of ophthalmic antibiotics for corneal damage is recommended. A mydriatic agent (e.g., Atropine) and cycloplegic agent (e.g., Cyclogyl) can decrease the patient's discomfort and generally are recommended.[12] Ophthalmic corticosteroids frequently are recommended for use shortly after alkaline injury, but no controlled trials are available to support this recommendation. Alkaline corrosive injury to the eye is discussed further in Chapters 15 and 98.

If an aqueous ammonia solution of 10% or greater has been ingested, or there are symptoms of corrosive injury (e.g., drooling), flexible endoscopy is warranted to evaluate for serious esophageal or gastric injury. A chest film should be obtained to look for mediastinal air, which suggests esophageal perforation. The use of corticosteroids has been proven ineffective in alkaline corrosive ingestions and may be harmful to patients with serious infection.[35]

Bronchoscopy can be both a diagnostic and therapeutic aid by assisting with the removal of sloughed tissues.

Disposition

Patients with mild exposures, who have no evidence of airway compromise, may be discharged from the emergency department after 2 hours of observation, with instructions to seek medical attention if late symptoms present.[35] Any patient who has developed anything more than minor symptoms should be admitted for inpatient observation. Any patient with airway compromise or severe burns should be admitted to an intensive care unit. Because of the potential for chronic respiratory effects, hospitalized patients require outpatient follow-up.

NITROGEN OXIDES

Introduction and Relevant History

Nitrogen oxides are a series of oxidized nitrogenous compounds that are irritant gases with relatively low water solubility (Table 97-2). These compounds occur together in dynamic equilibrium. For example, below 21° C, NO_2 exists as a liquid in the form of N_2O_4; however, higher temperatures favor the formation of NO_2.[36]

Toxic gas inhalation involving nitrogen oxides has been reported in both single cases and mass exposures for the past 200 years. The earliest recorded case of toxic inhalation of these fumes involved a French merchant who died after breathing concentrated nitric acid fumes in 1804.[37] Nitrogen oxides were not recognized as the cause of silo filler's disease until 1956,[38] although the clinical entity was recognized as early as 1914.[39]

NO_2, in addition to hydrogen cyanide, is produced in the pyrolysis of nitrocellulose, a component of radiographic film. During the Cleveland Clinic disaster of 1929, NO_2 and cyanide poisoning caused 125 casualties.[37,40]

Missile silos, where nitrogen tetroxide is used as a fuel oxidizer, have been the site of accidental exposures, including three Apollo-mission astronauts.[41,42]

TABLE 97-2 Nitrogen Oxides	
NO	Nitric oxide (mononitrogen monoxide)
NO_2	Nitrogen dioxide
N_2O	Nitrous oxide
N_2O_2	Nitrogen peroxide
N_2O_3	Nitrogen trioxide (dinitrogen trioxide)
N_2O_4	Nitrogen tetroxide (dinitrogen tetroxide)
N_2O_5	Nitrogen pentoxide (dinitrogen pentoxide)

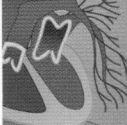

During one outbreak, there were reports of 116 cases of nitrogen dioxide–induced respiratory illness in high school students attending hockey games at a Minnesota arena. Of those surveyed, 69% of students who were on or near the ice developed acute symptoms. Authorities blamed a defective engine in the ice-resurfacing machine.[43]

Epidemiology

Nitrogen oxides are formed naturally, primarily as a result of bacterial metabolism of nitrogenous compounds. Combustion of fossil fuels (e.g., motor vehicle exhaust) is the chief human-made source of nitrogen oxides.

Common nonoccupational exposures to nitrogen oxides include kerosene heaters, gas appliances,[44] cigarette smoke, ice-skating rinks,[43,45] and ambient air pollution. Common occupational exposures include electric arc welding, manufacture of explosives, dyes and lacquers,[37] nitric acid production, firefighting,[46] and agriculture. NO_2 is produced during the decomposition of grain that has high nitrite content (i.e., corn) stored in silos. Inhalation of NO_2 generated from this source is responsible for silo filler's disease.[41,47-49] The decomposition process begins shortly after putting crops into a silo and continues for at least 10 days. Dangerous amounts of gas may remain in the silo for a month if the silo is not opened.[48] One case report involved a man who was exposed to NO_2 6 weeks after silage was stored.[49]

Because NO is useful as a vasodilator to treat such conditions as pulmonary hypertension and acute lung injury, health care workers in intensive care could be exposed to both NO and NO_2.[50,51]

Structure and Structure–Activity Relationships

Nitrogen oxides are a series of oxidized nitrogenous compounds that react violently with combustible and reducing materials (e.g., NH_3, carbon disulfide) (see Table 97-2). NO_2 is a reddish-brown gas or yellowish-brown liquid that reacts with water to produce nitric acid and nitric oxide. NO is a colorless gas that reacts with water to form nitric acid and rapidly is converted in air to NO_2.

Pathophysiology

Because nitrogen oxides are less soluble (hydrolyze more slowly) than most irritant gases, they penetrate the lower respiratory tract (the principal site of toxicity) more readily. Within the lungs, slow accumulation of nitrogen oxides and hydration to nitric acid (HNO_3) in the alveoli result in delayed onset of chemical pneumonitis. Pulmonary edema occurs when one inhales high concentrations of the gases.[41,52] Both increased airway resistance and decreased diffusion capacity occur. Inhalation of as little as 0.3 ppm of NO_2 has been shown to potentiate induced bronchospasm in asthmatic individuals.[53] The acute increase in airway resistance that occurs after nitrogen dioxide exposure, even at low

TABLE 97-3 Exposure Limits and Clinical Effects of Nitrogen Oxides at Different Concentrations

CONCENTRATION (ppm)	NITROGEN OXIDE	EFFECTS
1	NO_2	NIOSH-REL (15-minute STEL)
1–1.6	NO_2	Lowest level associated with measurable impairment of pulmonary function
0.04–5	NO_2	Odor detectable (acrid or bleach)
5	NO_2	OSHA-PEL (ceiling limit)
1–13	NO_2	Mucous membrane irritation
20	NO_2	NIOSH-IDLH
25	NO	NIOSH-REL (TWA) and OSHA-PEL (TWA)
50–150	NO_2	Mild irritant to eyes and upper airways
100	NO	NIOSH-IDLH
174	NO_2	LD_{50} at 1 hr

IDLH, immediate danger to life or health; NIOSH, National Institute for Occupational Safety and Health; OSHA, Occupational Safety and Health Administration; PEL, permissible exposure limit; REL, recommended exposure limit; STEL, short-term exposure limit; TWA, time-weighted average.

doses, appears to be mediated by histamine release.[37] According to NIOSH, the toxic effects associated with exposure to NO_2 are primarily determined by peak, and not average, concentrations of exposure[54,55] (Table 97-3).

The toxicity of the oxides of nitrogen may result from the initiation of lipid peroxidation and oxidation of cellular proteins, which leads to the generation of free radicals.[56] These free radicals damage the pulmonary epithelial cells, most notably type I alveolar and ciliated cells, principally at the juncture of the terminal airways and the gas exchange tissues.[56,57] Antioxidants, such as ascorbic acid, that act as a free radical scavenger help protect human endothelial cells exposed to NO_2. This implies an important role for free radicals in the toxicology of these agents.[56,58,59]

NO, whose affinity for hemoglobin is 1000 times greater than that of carbon monoxide, may be absorbed from the lung and bound to hemoglobin. As a result, hemoglobin is oxidized to nitrosylhemoglobin (NOHb) and subsequently to methhemoglobin.[36] Some absorbed NO_2 participates in other reactions, including nitrosation of amines to form nitrosamines, a reaction that may play a role in gastrointestinal cancers.

Toxicology

CLINICAL MANIFESTATIONS

The clinical presentation and progression of the disease depend on the concentration and duration of exposure, the patient's activity level, and perhaps the patient's predisposition to lung disease. Clinical presentation generally is divided into three clinical stages: acute, delayed, and subacute.[37] These stages may be observed in sequence or alone.

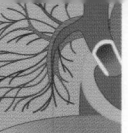

Acute Phase

Because of the poor water solubility of nitrogen oxides, upper respiratory irritation may not be evident after exposure to very low levels. With more concentrated exposures, upper respiratory symptoms such as burning eyes, sore throat, and cough may occur. Nonspecific signs and symptoms may include nausea, vomiting, headache, dizziness, a "choking sensation," and weakness. Bronchospasm may be present with wheezing and dyspnea. Radiographic findings soon after exposure may be normal and do not rule out the subsequent development of ALI. Many of the effects are self-limited if exposure has been only mild and brief. Symptoms may persist for 1 to 2 weeks, and complete recovery usually follows.

Delayed Phase

A symptom-free interval of 3 to 24 hours typically follows the acute phase. This asymptomatic phase, in turn, is followed by the development of chemical pneumonitis or ALI, characterized by dyspnea, tachypnea, hemoptysis, bronchospasm, rales, and hypoxia. Hypotension (direct effect of nitrate- or nitrite-induced vasodilation) is not common. Methemoglobinemia may occur in this stage, and levels have been reported from 2% to 44%.[36]

Radiographic findings generally begin with perihilar infiltrates and progress to ALI. In one study of 34 patients, 40% of the patients who developed ALI died.[37] Those who survived developed long-term complications, experienced a subacute phase, or recovered completely.

Subacute Phase

This phase, in which the patient develops bronchiolitis obliterans, usually appears 2 to 4 weeks after the delayed phase. It also may occur in the absence of a prior episode of ALI, about 10 to 30 days after the initial exposure. The patient becomes acutely ill with fever and chills, cough, dyspnea, rales, wheezing, and hypoxia. At this point, the chest radiographic findings again may resemble those characteristic of ALI or may show multiple discrete nodules (miliary pattern).[36] Pulmonary function testing reveals both obstructive and restrictive defects. This stage may prove fatal.[37,42,48]

Chronic Clinical Manifestations

In animals, long-term exposure to nitrogen oxides has caused emphysema, immunosuppression,[60] and increased incidence of pulmonary adenomas.[61] There have been reports of coal miners developing emphysema with long-term exposure to NO_2.[62] There is little evidence to implicate NO_2 directly as a pulmonary carcinogen in humans, but it could modify and influence the carcinogenic process in the lung.[63] One report of the mortality experience in a large cohort, from 1977 to 1992, found an association between mean ambient NO_2 concentrations and lung cancer in women.[64]

Because various indoor and outdoor sources release nitrogen oxides, the general public may experience persistent, low-level exposure to these compounds. Although epidemiologic studies have not identified an independent effect of long-term exposure to ambient NO_2, researchers hypothesize that several chronic health problems may occur as a result of this low-grade exposure, including increased incidence and severity of respiratory tract infections, reduced lung function, and increased symptoms in patients with asthma and chronic obstructive pulmonary disease.[65,66]

Adverse Effects

Persistent respiratory disease, including symptoms of chronic bronchitis and spirometric evidence of obstructive or restrictive disease, has been documented after acute exposure to nitrogen oxides.[41,67] In one study of 23 cases, of the 5 cases that progressed beyond the acute phase, all had some persistent pulmonary dysfunction several years later.[41] In another study, 6 cases of RADS were diagnosed among 234 patients exposed to dinitrogen tetroxide.[68]

It is difficult to predict who will have long-term complications from a single acute exposure, and meaningful numbers from studies are essentially nonexistent. Generally, a patient whose illness does not progress beyond the acute phase will not have subsequent problems, and patients who have pulmonary edema or whose illness evolves to bronchiolitis obliterans seem to have a high probability of developing long-term complications.

With regard to nonrespiratory symptoms, in one report 6 of 24 victims of a missile-silo accident developed chronic headaches and other subjective neuropsychiatric complaints after the accident.[69]

DIAGNOSIS

Laboratory Testing

Serial arterial blood gas measurements and radiographs, methemoglobin levels, and continuous pulse oximetry may be indicated, depending on the degree of the patients' illness. Patients with bronchiolitis obliterans may have a neutrophilic leukocytosis and an elevated sedimentation rate.

Differential Diagnosis

A latency period of several hours, followed by signs and symptoms consistent with ALI, is suggestive of this exposure. The differential diagnosis should include allergic lung disease due to molds (farmer's lung due to hypersensitivity reaction), asthma, pneumonia, miliary tuberculosis, viral influenza, carbon monoxide exposure, myocardial infarction, or ALI following exposure to other toxic products of combustion or respiratory irritants with low water solubility (e.g., phosgene).

MANAGEMENT

Supportive Measures

Treatment depends on a patient's phase of clinical illness and the symptomatic presentation. Oxygen and intubation with positive-pressure ventilation, as needed, are considered the mainstays of treatment.[37] Use of the minimum concentration of oxygen has been recommended to maintain arterial oxygenation because hyperoxia may exacerbate the oxidant injury induced by

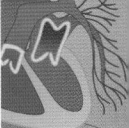

NO_2.[36] Inhaled bronchodilators are recommended for bronchospasm.

Because these patients are prone to infection, frequent sputum cultures should be obtained and antibiotics started when indicated.

Decontamination

Wet clothing should be removed, and any exposed skin flushed with water. Exposed eyes should be irrigated with copious amounts of water or saline.

Other Medical and Diagnostic Interventions

There is no specific antidote for nitrogen oxide poisoning. Methemoglobinemia should be treated with oxygen and methylene blue (1–2 mg/kg intravenously). Corticosteroids have been shown in many case reports to be beneficial, in both the treatment and prevention of ALI and bronchiolitis obliterans.[36,41,42,48,49,70] Many researchers report dramatic improvement in symptoms after use of corticosteroids and recurrence of the symptoms when the corticosteroids are abruptly stopped; the symptoms then respond to reinstitution of the corticosteroids.[36,41,42,48] High-dose corticosteroids have been recommended for a 6- to 8-week course, and tapered gradually to prevent relapses.[41,46]

Disposition

In all instances in which significant exposure may have occurred, affected patients should be observed for at least 24 to 48 hours after exposure, even if they are asymptomatic and exhibiting a normal chest radiograph. In-hospital observation for 6 hours is recommended for patients with potential or mild nitrogen oxide exposure. If a patient is asymptomatic after that time and has rapid access to medical care, he or she may be discharged for close follow-up.

REFERENCES

1. ATSDR: Hazardous Substances Emergency Events Surveillance (HSEES) Annual Reports. Atlanta: U.S. Department of Health and Human Services, Agency of Toxic Substances and Disease Registry; 1998–2001. Reports available at: http://www.atsdr.cdc.gov.
2. Horton KD, Berkowitz Z, Haugh GS, et al: Acute public health consequences associated with hazardous substances released during transit, 1993–2000. J Hazard Mater 2003;98:161–175.
3. Weisskopf MG, Drew JM, Hanrahan LP, et al: Hazardous ammonia releases: public health consequences and risk factors for evacuation and injury, United States, 1993–1998. J Occup Environ Med 2003;45:197–204.
4. Mrvos R, Dean BS, Krenzelok EP: Home exposures to chlorine/chloramines gas: review of 216 cases. South Med J 1993;86:654–657.
5. Pascuzzi TA: Mass casualties from acute inhalation of chloramine gas. Milit Med 1996;163:102–104.
6. Watson WA, Litovitz TL, Rodgers GC, et al: 2002 Annual report of the American Association of Poison Control Centers Toxic Exposure Surveillance System. Am J Emerg Med 2003;21:353–421.
7. Blanc PD, Galbo M, Hiatt P, Olson KR: Morbidity following acute irritant inhalation in a population-based study. JAMA 1991;266:664–669.
8. Klein J, Olsen KR, McKinney HE: Caustic injury from household ammonia. Am J Emerg Med 1985;3:320.
9. Wibbenmeyer LA, Morgan LJ, Robinson BK, et al: Our chemical burn experience: exposing the dangers of anhydrous ammonia. J Burn Care Rehabil 1999;20:226–231.
10. NIOSH: Toxicological review of selected chemicals—ammonia. Available at: http://www.cdc.gov.
11. NIOSH: Pocket guide to chemical hazards—ammonia. Available at: http://www.cdc.gov.
12. Amshel CE, Fealk MH, Phillips BJ, Caruso DM: Anhydrous ammonia burns case report and review of the literature. Burns 2000;26:493–497.
13. O'Kane GJ: Inhalation of ammonia vapor. Anaesthesia 1983;38:1208–1213.
14. Arwood R, Hammond J, Ward G: Ammonia inhalation. J Trauma 1985;25:444–447.
15. Close LG, Catlin FI, Cohn AM: Acute and chronic effects of ammonia burns of the respiratory tract. Arch Otolaryngol 1980;106:151–158.
16. Rabinowitz PM, Siegel MD: Acute inhalation injury. Clin Chest Med 2002;23:707–715.
17. McDonald DM, Thurston G, Baluk P: Endothelial gaps as sites for plasma leakage in inflammation. Microcirculation 1999;6:7–22.
18. Sjoblom E, Hojer J, Kulling PE, et al: A placebo-controlled experimental study of steroid inhalation therapy in ammonia-induced lung injury. J Toxicol Clin Toxicol 1999;37:59–67.
19. Grant WM, Schuman JS: Toxicology of the Eye, 4th ed. Springfield, IL, Charles C Thomas, 1993.
20. Montague TJ, MacNeil AR: Mass ammonia inhalation. Chest 1980;77:496–498.
21. Grook B, Robertson JF, Glass SA, et al: Airborne dust, ammonia, microorganisms and antigens in pig confinement houses and the respiratory health of exposed farm workers. Am Ind Hyg Assoc J 1991;52:271–279.
22. Proctor NH, Hughes JP: Chemical Hazards of the Workplace, 2nd ed. Philadelphia, JB Lippincott, 1988, pp 373–374.
23. Howell JM: Alkalinity of non-industrial cleaning products and the likelihood of producing significant esophageal burns. Am J Emerg Med 1991;9:560–562.
24. Holmes DL, Durdhan TT, Nethercott JR: Acute and chronic respiratory effect of occupational exposure to ammonia. Am Ind Hyg Assoc J 1989;50:646–650.
25. Dreller L, Heedrick D, Boleij JS, et al: Lung function and chronic respiratory symptoms of pig farmers: focus on exposure to endotoxin and ammonia and use of disinfectants. Occup Environ Med 1995;52:654–660.
26. Ali BA, Ahmed HO, Ballal SG, Albar AA: Pulmonary function of workers exposed to ammonia: a study in the eastern province of Saudi Arabia. Int J Occup Environ Med 2001;7:19–22.
27. Kass J, Zamel N, Dobry CA, et al: Bronchiectasis following ammonia burns of the respiratory tract: a review of two cases. Chest 1972;62:282–285.
28. Leduc D, Gris P, Lheureux P, et al: Acute and long term respiratory damage following inhalation of ammonia. Thorax 1992;47:755–757.
29. De la Hoz RE, Schlueter DP, Rom WN: Chronic lung disease secondary to ammonia inhalation injury: a report on three cases. Am J Indust Med 1996;29:209–214.
30. Bernstein IL, Bernstein DI: Reactive airway disease syndrome (RADS) after exposure to toxic ammonia fumes. J Allergy Clin Immunol 1989;83:173.
31. Brautbar N: Ammonia exposure: a common cause for sinusitis—a case report and review of the literature. Toxicol Indust Health 1998;14:891–895.
32. Vinsel PJ: Treatment of acute chlorine gas inhalation with nebulized sodium bicarbonate. J Emerg Med 1990;8:327–329.
33. Bosse GM: Nebulized sodium bicarbonate in the treatment of chlorine gas inhalation. Clin Toxicol 1994;32:233.
34. Nieman GF, Clark WR, Hakim T: Methylprednisolone does not protect the lungs from inhalation injury. Burns 1991;17:384–390.
35. Tharratt RS: Ammonia. In Olsen KR (ed): Poisoning and Drug Overdose. Stamford, CT, Appleton & Lange, 1999, pp 67–68.
36. Lipsett MJ: Oxides of nitrogen and sulfur. In Sullivan JB, Krieger GR (eds): Clinical Environmental Health and Toxic Exposures, 2nd ed. Philadelphia, Lippincott Williams & Wilkins, 2001, pp 818–832.
37. Guidotti TL: The higher oxides of nitrogen: inhalation toxicology. Environ Res 1978;15:443–472.
38. Grayson RR: Silage gas poisoning: nitrogen dioxide pneumonia, a new disease in agricultural workers. Ann Intern Med 1956;45:393–396.

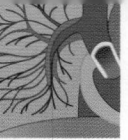

39. Hayhurst ER, Scott E: Four cases of sudden death in a silo. JAMA 1914;63:1570.

40. Gregory KL, Malinoski VF, Sharp CR: Cleveland Clinic fire survivorship study, 1929–1965. Arch Environ Health 1969;18:508–515.

41. Horvath EP, Dopico GA, Barbee RA, et al: Nitrogen dioxide-induced pulmonary disease: five new cases and review of the literature. J Occup Med 1978;20:103–110.

42. Jonas DO: Case for diagnosis. Milit Med 1984;149:481–485.

43. Hedburg K, Hedburg CW, Iber C, et al: An outbreak of nitrogen dioxide-induced respiratory illness among ice hockey players. JAMA 1989;262:3012–3017.

44. Jarvis D: Association of respiratory symptoms and lung function in young adults with use of domestic gas appliances. Lancet 1996;347:426–431.

45. Pelham TW, Holt LE, Moss MA: Exposure to carbon monoxide and nitrogen dioxide in enclosed ice arenas. Occup Environ Med 2002;59:224–233.

46. Tse RL, Bockman AA: Nitrogen dioxide toxicity-report of four cases in firemen. JAMA 1970;212:1341–1344.

47. Douglas WW, Hepper NGG, Colby TV: Silo-filler's disease. Mayo Clin Proc 1989;64:291–304.

48. Maurer WJ: Silo-filler's disease: a historical perspective and report of a case. Wisc Med J 1985;84:13–16.

49. Moskowitz RL, Lyons HA, Cottle HR: Silo filler's disease: clinical, physiological and pathologic study of a patient. Am J Med 1964;36:457–462.

50. Goldman AP, Cook PD, Macrae DJ: Exposure to intensive-care staff to nitric oxide and nitrogen dioxide. Lancet 1995;345:923–924.

51. Williams TJ, Salamonsen RF, Snell G, et al: Preliminary experience with inhaled nitric oxide for acute pulmonary hypertension after heart transplantation. J Heart Lung Transplant 1995;14:419–423.

52. Fleming GM, Chester EH, Montenegro HD: Dysfunction of small airways following pulmonary injury due to nitrogen dioxide. Chest 1979;75:720–721.

53. Bauer MA, Utell MJ, Morrow PE, et al: Inhalation of 0.30 ppm nitrogen dioxide potentiates exercise-induced bronchospasm in asthmatics. Am Rev Respir Dis 1986;134:1203–1208.

54. NIOSH: Toxicological review of selected chemicals—nitrogen dioxide. Available at: http://www.cdc.gov.

55. NIOSH: Pocket guide to chemical hazards—nitric oxide. Available at: http://www.cdc.gov.

56. Sagai M, Ichinose T: Lipid peroxidation and antioxidative protection mechanism in rat lungs upon acute and chronic exposure to nitrogen dioxide. Environ Health Perspect 1987;73:179–189.

57. Evans MJ: Oxidant gases. Environ Health Perspect 1984;55:85–95.

58. Velsor LW, Postlewait EM: NO$_2$-induced generation of extracellular reactive oxygen is mediated by epithelial lining layer antioxidants. Am J Physiol 1997;273:L1265–L1275.

59. Tu B, Wallin A, Moldeus P, Cotgreave I: The cytoprotective roles of ascorbate and glutathione against nitrogen dioxide toxicity in human endothelial cells. Toxicology 1995;98:125–136.

60. Azoulay-Dupuis E, Bouley G, Moreau J, et al. Evidence for humoral immunodepression in NO$_2$-exposed mice: influence of food restriction and stress. Environ Res 1987;42:446–454.

61. Victorin K: Genotoxicity in health risk evaluation of nitrogen oxides. Scand J Work Environ Health 1993;19(Suppl 2):50–56.

62. Robertson A, Dodgson J, Collings P, Seaton A: Exposure to oxides of nitrogen: respiratory symptoms and lung function in British coalminers. Br J Ind Med 1984;41:214–219.

63. Witschi H: Ozone, nitrogen oxide and lung cancer: a review of some recent issues and problems. Toxicology 1988;48:1–20.

64. Abbey DE, Nishino N, McDonnell WF, et al: Long-term inhalable particles and other air pollutants related to mortality in nonsmokers. Am J Respir Crit Care Med 1999;159:373–382.

65. Samet JM, Utell MJ: The risk of nitrogen dioxide: what have we learned from epidemiological and clinical studies? Toxicol Ind Health 1990;6:247–262.

66. Cushing AH, Samet JM: Indoor pollutants: How hazardous for children? Contemp Pediatr 1991;8:109–127.

67. Leib GMP, Davis WN, Brown T, McQuiggan M: Chronic pulmonary insufficiency secondary to silo-filler's disease. Am J Med 1958;24:471–474.

68. Conrad E, Lo W, DeBoisblanc BP, Shellito JE: Reactive airways dysfunction syndrome after exposure to dinitrogen tetroxide. South Med J 1998;91:338–341.

69. Yockey CC, Eden BM, Byrd RB: The McConnell missile accident. Clinical spectrum of nitrogen dioxide exposure. JAMA 1980;244:1221–1223.

70. Karlson-Stiber C, Hojer J, Sjoholm A, et al: Nitrogen dioxide pneumonitis in ice hockey players. J Intern Med 1996;239:451–456.

98 Corrosives

PAUL M. WAX, MD ■ MARK YAREMA, MD

At a Glance...

- Alkalis and acids can injure either the esophagus or the stomach.
- The potential for tissue injury is dependent on the duration of contact and on the concentration, volume, and pH of the product.
- No one symptom or group of symptoms can reliably predict the degree of esophageal injury after a corrosive ingestion.
- Upper gastrointestinal endoscopy is the only diagnostic test available that reliably detects the degree of esophageal injury.
- Patients who are asymptomatic after a corrosive ingestion can be safely discharged without the need for endoscopy.
- Corticosteroid therapy remains highly controversial. Corticosteroids may be beneficial for endoscopy-diagnosed second-degree burns.
- The risk for esophageal stricture is greatest after circumferential second- and third-degree burns.
- There is a long latency period between corrosive ingestion and esophageal or gastric carcinoma.

INTRODUCTION AND RELEVANT HISTORY

Corrosives are a group of chemicals that have the capacity to cause tissue injury on contact with multiple organ systems, most commonly the gastrointestinal, respiratory, ophthalmologic, and dermatologic systems. Examples of agents capable of causing chemical burn injuries include alkalis (e.g., NaOH, KOH), acids (e.g., HCl, H_2SO_4), and certain antiseptics, such as phenol, formaldehyde, iodine, and concentrated hydrogen peroxide. Hydrofluoric acid (HF), a relatively weak acid, is particularly known for its ability to cause necrotizing injury and life-threatening systemic toxicity as a result of the fluoride moiety chelating endogenous calcium (see Chapter 90). For the purpose of this chapter, the term *corrosive* (a term sometimes used interchangeably with *caustic*) refers to any of these agents capable of causing tissue injury on contact. The term *lye* refers to specific alkali, typically sodium hydroxide or potassium hydroxide.

Corrosives are widely available to the public, primarily as household cleaners (Table 98-1). More than 60,000 corrosive exposures were reported to poison centers in the United States in 2002.[1] The focus of this chapter is on alkalis and acids and their toxic effect on the previously mentioned systems, with special attention to the gastrointestinal tract.

Before 1950, strong lyes (concentration > 50%) made up most caustic ingestions in the United States. Not uncommonly, ingestions of strong lyes led to respiratory compromise, severe esophageal burns, perforation of the esophagus and stomach, mediastinitis, late stricture, and sometimes death.

Over the years, three legislative acts were passed by Congress to help reduce the occurrence of corrosive injuries in the United States, particularly in children. The first was the Federal Caustic Poison Act of 1927, which for the first time mandated that concentrated lye and acid-containing products clearly display a "poison" label.[2] The second was the Federal Hazardous Substances Act of 1960, which imposed mandatory standards for labeling of hazardous materials. Finally, in 1970, Congress enacted the Poison Prevention Pack-

TABLE 98-1 Sampling of Currently Manufactured Household Cleaning Products That Contain Caustic Chemicals

APPLICATION	PRODUCT	CHEMICAL
Drain cleaner, liquid	Heavy Duty Liquid Drain Opener (Share)	H_2SO_4 93%
	Drain Out Extra (Iron Out)	KOH 30%
	Liquid-Plumr (Clorox)	NaOH 0.5%–2%, NaOCl 10%
	Maximum Strength Drain Opener (Enforcer)	KOH 5%–15%
Drain cleaner, crystals	Crystal Drain Opener (Rohyme)	NaOH 74%
	Crystal, Drain Out (Iron Out)	NaOH 55%
	Drano Pipe Cleaner (Johnson)	NaOH 54%
Oven cleaner	Easy-Off Heavy Duty Oven Cleaner (Rickitt Benckiser)	NaOH < 5%
Rust remover	Rust Stain Remover (Whink)	HF 2.5%–3%
	Rust Stripper (Certified)	NaOH 50%–75%
	Naval Jelly Rust Remover (Loctite)	Phosphoric Acid 25%–30%
Toilet bowl cleaner	Instant Power Toilet Bowl Cleaner (Scotch)	HCl 26%
	Bowl and Porcelain Cleaner (Cleanline)	HCl < 10%
Swimming pool cleaner	Muriatic Acid, Aqua Chem (Recreational Water)	HCl 31%

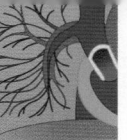

aging Act.[3] This legislation resulted in the mandatory packaging of corrosive agents in child-resistant containers if the concentration of the active agent was either greater than 10% or 2% by weight of free chemical.

Despite these legislative efforts, highly concentrated caustic products remain on the market, although they are typically less available as household products than in the past. Such products continue to be used in commercial industries, on farms, and as swimming pool cleansers. Household products that contain caustic chemicals include drain cleaners, toilet bowl cleaners, and general purpose anticorrosive cleaners. Although low lye (<10%) or no lye (enzymatic) drain cleaners have replaced some of the more highly concentrated caustic products, household liquid drain cleaners with high concentrations of alkali (30% KOH) or acid (93% H_2SO_4) may still be purchased in neighborhood hardware stores (e.g., Home Depot) in 2004 (see Table 98-1). Commercial industries and farms often use concentrated corrosives as chemical reagents and as cleansers.[3] Dairy farms use pipeline cleaners that contain liquid NaOH and KOH in concentrations of 8% to 25%.

Ingestion of crystal lye may be particularly problematic and result in severe burns because of the opportunity for prolonged tissue contact. Fortunately, most crystal lye ingestions are limited by immediate oral pain. The ingestion of granular automatic dishwashing detergents has been associated with devastating injuries.[4] Crystal drain cleaners have lye concentration as high as 74% NaOH and may cause proximal esophageal injury. Some liquid dishwashing detergents and laundry detergents have a pH greater than 12, but because the titratable base content is significantly lower, there is less risk for injury after ingestion.

Ingestion of liquid household bleach containing dilute (5.25%) sodium hypochlorite (NaOCl) rarely causes significant injury. Industrial-strength bleach may contain significantly higher concentrations of sodium hypochlorite, leading to esophageal necrosis. Toilet bowl cleaners contain hydrochloric acid as high as 26% HCl. General purpose anticorrosive cleaners, such as 31% muriatic acid (HCl), are sold in gallon containers for home use and as swimming pool cleaners.

Sodium hydroxide is also found as a constituent of hair perm relaxers. Excessive topical use of these relaxers may occasionally cause facial and oral burns, as well as esophageal burns and airway compromise, if ingested, although most exposures do not cause significant injuries.[5,6] The alkali powder in airbags has caused ocular burns. Perfumes accidentally sprayed into the eyes can cause burns.[7] Cement is alkaline and causes topical burns, typically on the knees.[8]

More than 70 different pills may cause damage when they come in contact with the esophageal mucosa for prolonged periods.[9] Patients who take medications in the supine position or take pills without water are at higher risk. Pills most likely to adhere are doxycycline, tetracycline, potassium chloride, and aspirin. Ingestion of potassium chloride pills has caused perforation into the aorta, left atrium, and bronchial artery.[9]

STRUCTURE AND STRUCTURE–ACTIVITY RELATIONSHIPS

Pathophysiology

The type of agent, formulation of the product, concentration of solution, volume, viscosity, pH, duration of contact, and presence or absence of food in the stomach are all factors that influence the extent of injury from a caustic exposure. The titratable alkaline reserve of an alkali or acid may be particularly correlative with the likelihood of burn injury.[10] Regarding alkalis, it has been suggested that the critical pH that causes esophageal ulceration is 12.5.[11] Corrosives may cause injury to any exposed tissue, including skin, mucous membranes, eyes, gastrointestinal tract, and lungs.

Alkalis

Alkalis, such as sodium hydroxide and potassium hydroxide, directly damage tissue by producing saponification of the fatty acids within cell membranes, resulting in the loss of membrane integrity. In addition, the reaction of hydroxide ions with collagen may cause protein disruption and considerable edema. The end result is liquefaction necrosis and a softening of the tissues. Unfortunately, the process of liquefaction necrosis allows for further penetrance of the alkali into the tissue and further injury.

The depth of the necrosis is dependent on the concentration of the lye.[12] Strong caustics cause their damage quickly. In one study, contact of the esophageal tissue with sodium hydroxide at 22.5% for only 10 seconds resulted in a full-thickness burn.[12] In another study, a solution of 30% sodium hydroxide in contact with tissue for 1 second resulted in a full-thickness burn.[13]

Acids

Acids, such as hydrochloric acid and sulfuric acid, dissociate on contact with water to release hydrogen ions. Contact of acids with tissue causes tissue destruction. Unlike alkalis, a coagulum or eschar may develop after acid contact, in some cases limiting the further spread of the acid and depth of necrosis. However, subsequent sloughing of the coagulum may still occur, extending the tissue injury sometimes in a delayed manner. Full-thickness burns resulting in perforation may result.[14]

Historically, acid-induced injury to the gastrointestinal tract was summarized in the phrase "lick the esophagus, bite the pyloric antrum."[15] However, reports indicate that acid ingestion may result in both esophageal and gastric injury.[16] Gastric injury is more likely to occur in the pylorus and antrum. This may be because of the preferential flow of liquids rapidly from the esophagus along the lesser curvature of the stomach to the pylorus rather than into the fundus and body, where solids tend to collect. Duodenal injury may also occur, but this is appears to be less common than gastric injury, possibly

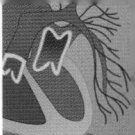

because of pylorospasm induced by the acid or the neutralization of the acid by duodenal contents.

In the past, it was thought that ingestion of strong acids was more likely to cause gastric necrosis and that ingestion of strong lyes was more likely to cause esophageal injury. In fact, it appears that acids cause a similar incidence of esophageal and gastric injury and may also cause laryngeal burns. Alkalis may cause gastric necrosis and perforation and small intestine injury, as well as esophageal injury.[17,18] Perforation from either acids or alkalis may result in extensive necrosis of abdominal viscera.

Time Course and Natural History

Typically, the damage from corrosives occurs in four stages. Initially, necrosis occurs with invasion by bacteria and polymorphonuclear leukocytes. Subsequently, vascular thrombosis occurs, increasing the damage. Over the next 2 to 5 days, superficial layers of injured tissues begin to slough. After the caustic exposure, the tensile strength of the healing tissue may be quite low for up to 3 weeks. In some cases, this loss of tissue integrity greatly increases the chance of delayed perforation and is the main reason patients remain at risk for deterioration for up to 14 days or longer after exposure. The formation of granulation tissue, collagen deposition, and re-epithelization signals the tissue recovery process and generally occurs between 1 week and several months after the exposure. Unfortunately, the wound healing itself may herald a constrictive phase, ultimately causing esophageal stricture formation because of scar contraction—a process that may occur over a period of weeks to years.

Morphology

Caustic injuries are categorized as first-, second-, and third-degree burns, similar to thermal burns, based on their appearance at endoscopy (Table 98-2). The initial depth of injury found on esophagoscopy correlates with the risk for stricture formation. First-degree (grade 1) burns consist of edema and hyperemia. In these cases,

the depth of involvement would be similar to a sunburn. Blisters do not occur, and strictures would not result from these superficial burns. Ulcers, whitish membranes, exudates, friability, and hemorrhage characterize second-degree (grade 2) burns. These partial-thickness burns are further subdivided into grade 2a—non-circumferential—and grade 2b—circumferential—burn injuries. Although overall about 15% to 20% of grade 2 esophageal burns develop strictures, 75% of grade 2b burns develop strictures.[19] Third-degree injuries involve the full thickness of the mucosa, often with necrosis. These injures are most likely to perforate. Of those who survive the acute injury, 90% develop strictures.

Special Populations

PEDIATRIC PATIENTS

Corrosive injury to the esophagus remains a serious health problem in children. Nearly 80% of reported caustic ingestions occur in children. At least 85% of reported ingestions are unintentional.[20] More than 125,000 ingestions of household cleaning products in 2002 occurred in children younger than 6 years, second only to cosmetics and personal care products in frequency.[1] Storage of corrosives in inappropriate containers, such as sports drink bottles, soda cans and bottles, and jars, contributes to unintentional ingestion. Although contact with the oral mucosa usually causes severe pain and vomiting that theoretically limits further damage, a small ingestion may be sufficient to result in serious morbidity and mortality. Given the long-term complications of stricture and esophageal and gastric carcinoma, prevention of exposure to these toxic agents is of paramount importance.

PSYCHIATRIC PATIENTS

Although unintentional ingestion of small amounts of a caustic agent may still cause devastating injuries, intentional ingestion among adolescents and adults accounts for a higher percentage of significant injuries. Among suicidal patients who ingest caustic agents, more than half have a history of psychiatric illness.[21] Many of these deliberate ingestions of caustic chemicals occur among individuals who are confined in psychiatric hospitals or prisons. This occurs because of the availability of a variety of cleansers in these facilities (and the lack of availability of pharmaceuticals and other toxic agents). Because some psychiatric patients have been known to attempt to mask their symptoms after caustic ingestion, a high suspicion of possibly corrosive injury should be considered in this population.

TOXICOLOGY

Clinical Manifestations

The acute and chronic (long-term) complications resulting from caustic ingestion may be devastating. Initially during the first few hours and days after the caustic exposure, the development of airway edema

GRADE OF INJURY	FINDINGS
	TABLE 98-2 Classification of Corrosive Burns to the GI Tract
0	Normal examination
1	Erythema, hyperemia
2a	Superficial ulceration, erosions, whitish membranes
2b	As for grade 2a, plus deep discrete or circumferential ulcerations
3	Multiple deep ulcerations, areas of necrosis

From Zargar SA, Kochlar R, Nagi B, et al: Ingestion of corrosive acids. Spectrum of injury to upper gastrointestinal tract and natural history. Gastroenterology 1989;97:702.

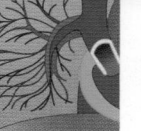

leading to a compromised airway and esophageal or gastric perforation is the most emergent issue. Over the long term, the ingestion of caustics may lead to esophageal or gastric strictures requiring repetitive dilatory procedures and in some cases esophageal bypass and colonic interposition. Patients with significant acute injuries are at significantly increased risk for esophageal carcinoma, a most unfortunate long-term sequela.

Acute Presentation

Small ingestions of a concentrated caustic can be as problematic as larger ingestions. More than 40% of patients reporting to have "only taken a lick" have esophageal burns.[22] Some of the most common complaints are oral pain (41%), abdominal pain (34%), vomiting (19%), and drooling (19%).[20] Other clinical features may include crying, dysphagia, odynophagia, hematemesis, wheezing, coughing, stridor, dysphonia, chest pain, and respiratory distress. Pain, crying, excessive salivation, and dysphagia tend to be associated with lesions of the buccal mucosa but do not accurately predict lesions elsewhere. Spontaneous vomiting is associated with a higher incidence of more severe esophageal injury. Visible burns to the face, lips, and oral cavity may be seen and appear as white or gray patches with an erythematous border.

Laryngeal edema often occurs over a matter of minutes to hours, requiring rapid intubation. Peritoneal signs suggest hollow viscus perforation or contiguous extension of the burn injury to adjoining visceral areas. Systemic toxicity, hypovolemic shock, and hemodynamic instability manifested as hypotension, tachycardia, fever, and acidosis may occur in these cases and are ominous findings. Emergency surgical intervention may be required in these cases.

Correlating clinical symptoms with the severity of esophageal burns can prove very difficult because different studies have presented conflicting data over the years.[19,20,23] Although there is a tendency to use the results of the oropharyngeal examination to predict more distal injury, such a strategy is not reliable. Oral burns on admission predicted burns of the esophagus with a sensitivity of 52.9% and specificity of 51%.[24] Prolonged drooling and dysphagia (12–24 hr) were much more predictive of significant lesions, with 100% sensitivity and 90% specificity.[24] Vomiting and stridor also appear more predictive than oropharyngeal burns in predicting burn injury.

Although acid ingestions are much less common than alkali ingestions in the United States, significant acid ingestions may also cause extensive tissue injury and result in a higher mortality rate than alkali ingestions. Massive upper gastrointestinal bleeding and aspiration pneumonia may also occur.[25,26] Systemic effects from acid ingestions include metabolic acidosis, disseminated intravascular coagulation, hyponatremia, and hypotension. The more fulminant course of some acid ingestions may be due to systemic absorption of the acid resulting in metabolic acidosis (which may also be the result of extensive tissue necrosis), hemolysis, and renal failure.

In Russia, concentrated acetic acid ingestions account for 64% of caustic ingestions.[27]

Patients with pill-associated caustic injury may present with less acute symptoms. They may not clearly relate their current symptoms to the pill ingestion, although they often recall a transient feeling of "something stuck." Most present with severe retrosternal pain. Dysphagia is not common. The pain lasts 3 days to a few weeks. Occasionally, more severe cases present with hematemesis, weight loss, or fever. Endoscopy generally reveals a sharply demarcated superficial ulcer. Deep ulcerations or even penetration may occur particularly with potassium tablets.

Long-Term Complications

Long-term consequences can be more damaging than the acute injury. The two major long-term concerns after alkali ingestion are the risk for stricture and esophageal carcinoma. Patients with significant esophageal burns, particularly those that are circumferential, develop esophageal stricture. Eighty percent of strictures first become apparent in 2 to 8 weeks. Symptoms include dysphagia and food impactions. Strictures that become symptomatic early are generally more severe.

The risk for stricture can be predicted based on the degree of burn visualized at endoscopy. First-degree burns do not progress to stricture. Second-degree burns may progress to stricture in at least 15% to 20% of cases. Third-degree burns carry the worst prognosis for stricture, with a risk for at least 90%.[19,22]

The latent period between corrosive ingestion and the development of squamous cell esophageal carcinoma may be as long as 40 to 50 years. Hence, adults with significant childhood exposures need lifelong surveillance. Patients have at least a 1000- to 3000-fold increased risk for esophageal cancer after corrosive ingestion.[28] A recent long-term study showed that 1.8% of patients who ingested caustic soda developed esophageal cancer.[29] Nearly 3% of esophageal cancer patients have a history of caustic ingestion.[28]

Sequelae of acid ingestion include esophageal stricture, pyloric and antral stenosis, duodenal atonicity, gastric metaplasia, and carcinoma. The risk for carcinoma after caustic acid ingestion is unknown.

DIAGNOSIS

Laboratory Testing

No specific laboratory tests are available that predict severity of poisoning after corrosive ingestion. General laboratory studies should include a complete blood count, serum electrolytes, blood type and screen, renal and liver function tests, and coagulation studies. An arterial blood gas measurement should be obtained if there is ongoing stridor or evidence of hemodynamic compromise. Arterial blood gas determination may be particularly useful after significant acid ingestions given the propensity for severe acid–base disturbances in these

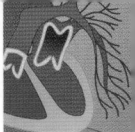

cases. A recent study suggested that pH less than 7.22 was correlative with severe injury requiring surgical intervention.[36] A white blood cell count greater than 20,000/mL may be predictive of death after caustic ingestion when combined with other parameters such as age, ingestion of strong acid, presence of deep gastric ulcers, or gastric necrosis.[31] In intentional overdoses, co-ingestants should be considered and a comprehensive urine drug screen obtained. However, the caustic chemical itself will not be detected on a urine drug screen.

Other Diagnostic Testing

In symptomatic patients, a chest x-ray and abdominal flat plate should be obtained to look for evidence of peritoneal and mediastinal air denoting perforation or pleural effusion, suggesting esophageal leak. It is important to note that the depth of esophageal burns cannot be predicted based on signs or symptoms. Noninvasive techniques, such as chest and abdominal x-rays, water-soluble contrast swallow, or computed tomography (CT) with contrast can suggest or detect perforation but do not provide sufficient information to gauge depth of burn injury.[32]

The test of choice for proper staging of burn severity is upper gastrointestinal endoscopy. Not only can endoscopy define the extent of disease after acute ingestion, but also it can document healing after ingestion. Endoscopy results will divide patients into four groups: no esophageal/gastric injury, gastric injury, linear burns of the esophagus, and circumferential burns. Those with gastric injury are at risk for pyloric ulceration and later gastric outlet obstruction. Linear burns of the esophagus often heal well; circumferential burns are likely to lead to stricture.

Much attention has been devoted to finding a single clinical feature or group of signs and symptoms that can reliably predict esophageal injury, and therefore which patients should go on to endoscopy. Studies to date have produced conflicting results. What is clear is that patients who are asymptomatic on presentation and are able to drink liquids without any discomfort can be assumed to have no significant esophagogastric injury and may be managed conservatively without the need for endoscopy.[33] As stated previously, the absence of external visible signs of exposure cannot be equated with absence of esophageal lesions.[23,34,35] In general, the greater the number of presenting signs and symptoms, the higher the like-lihood of significant esophageal burns.[34,36] Unfortunately, there is no pathognomonic group of presenting signs and symptoms that can identify all patients with potentially serious gastrointestinal burns.[33,34]

Based on the studies to date, the main indication for endoscopy is a symptomatic patient who exhibits vomiting, drooling, dysphagia, odynophagia, stridor, or dyspnea. Endoscopy may also be warranted in less symptomatic cases if the ingestion is intentional. Ideally, endoscopy should be performed within 12 to 24 hours after ingestion. Endoscopy performed before 12 hours may not delineate the extent of injury, and wound softening makes endoscopy initiated after 24 hours more hazardous.

In some cases, early endoscopy may help guide the need for corticosteroid therapy, which, if indicated, should be initiated within the first 24 hours. The gastroenterologist may also choose to place a soft feeding tube or silk string in the esophagus when burns are present at the time of endoscopy. The string provides a guide for future dilation. In the past, endoscopy was often terminated at the most proximal burn area because of worry about iatrogenic perforation. Although this concern was applicable to rigid esophagogastroscopy techniques, flexible endoscopes can be carefully passed beyond the area of burn (unless there is a perforation), allowing for a more complete examination including evaluation of the stomach, if possible.

Any suspicion of abdominal involvement should be studied by repeated abdominal CT or ultrasound.[37] Follow-up contrast studies are useful to evaluate for the presence of esophageal or gastric strictures.

MANAGEMENT

Supportive Measures

Protection of the airway supersedes all other interventions. Because oropharyngeal and laryngeal edema may rapidly ensue, making airway control considerably problematic, early endotracheal intubation is indicated when there is concern regarding compromise of the airway, especially in cases with stridor. Fiberoptic airway evaluation to determine the extent of injury may prove useful. Surgical cricothyrotomy may be required when the airway cannot be secured by less invasive means. Blind nasotracheal intubation is contraindicated. Intravenous access should be established and fluid resuscitation initiated. With significant exposures, vigorous fluid resuscitation may be required. It is essential to employ early and continuous hemodynamic monitoring to evaluate for evidence of shock and volume depletion secondary to hollow viscus perforation. Analgesics should be provided as clinically indicated, with care taken not to oversedate the patient.

On arrival in the emergency department, the patient should be fully unclothed and examined for evidence of dermal and ocular caustic exposures. Ongoing dermal exposure from a caustic spill may continue to be injurious until the clothing is removed and copious irrigation has taken place. Contaminated clothing should be treated as hazardous waste and disposed using proper precautions.

Decontamination

Treatment often begins at the scene of the ingestion. Sips of water or milk can dislodge solid particles and dilute material residing in the stomach, but may cause an exothermic reaction. In alert patients who are not vomiting and can tolerate liquids, small volumes (1–2

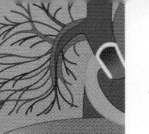

cups) of water or milk may be considered within the first few minutes after ingestion. Because injuries occur almost immediately, later dilution is not warranted. Forcing fluids is never indicated because the precipitation of emesis may lead to further caustic exposure. Experimentally, it has been shown that significant heat is generated by contact of the acid or alkali with the moist esophageal surface.[38] More recent studies have not generated significant amounts of heat.[39] Whether heat increases the injury has never been quantified, but has led to concerns regarding initial dilution or gastric lavage. Regardless of where treatment is initiated, those who come in contact with the patient should take proper precautions to protect themselves from secondary caustic exposure.

Over the years, neutralization approaches to caustic ingestions such as treating alkali ingestion with dilute acetic acid (vinegar) or treating acid ingestion with sodium bicarbonate have been frowned on. Such therapy may produce gas-forming exothermic reactions, potentially stressing already compromised tissues.

Gastrointestinal decontamination procedures, such as activated charcoal administration and gastric lavage, are usually not indicated. Activated charcoal would obscure endoscopic visualization of the mucosa and increase the risk for vomiting. Careful nasogastric aspiration may be useful in the setting of significant acid ingestions, however, given the ominous natural history of many of these ingestions and the somewhat lower risk for esophageal perforation. A nasogastric tube may be placed under fluoroscopy and used to drain the contents of the stomach and lavage with cold fluids. Polyvinyl chloride (PVC) nasogastric tubes harden with time and should not be used for long-term treatment.[40] Ipecac is always contraindicated.

Other Therapy

The initiation of corticosteroid therapy has remained controversial. Therapy with corticosteroids has been advocated to potentially limit the inflammatory response and prevent stricture formation. Studies to date have produced conflicting results on the effectiveness of these agents, and their use has not been validated in prospective clinical trials.[29,41-45] These trials have suffered from methodologic errors such as a lack of randomization, nonblinding of patients and investigators, small number of patients in study groups, different corticosteroids used, failure to perform endoscopy in all patients, or retrospective study design.

The natural history of corrosive injury can be of assistance in determining which patients, if any, may benefit. The nature of first-degree burns is such that they do not need to be treated with corticosteroids because stricture formation does not occur in these cases. Similarly, third-degree burns are unlikely to benefit from corticosteroid therapy because the extensive damage caused is not expected to respond to corticosteroid therapy.[46] Furthermore, third-degree burn injuries have a high incidence of perforation and fistula formation, and steroid therapy may potentially worsen these

injuries. Therefore, the controversy is in regard to their use in second-degree burns. A 20-year prospective clinical trial demonstrated no benefit with corticosteroids in the prevention of strictures after corrosive ingestion, including those patients with second-degree burns.[43] However, power limitations of the study limit these conclusions. Regardless, corticosteroids continue to be recommended by some individuals in the treatment of circumferential second-degree burn injuries of the esophagus.[41,47]

If the decision is made to treat with steroids based on endoscopic results, the choice of corticosteroid is largely left to the individual physician. The studies to date have included methylprednisolone, prednisolone, and prednisone. The recommended dose of prednisolone is 2 mg/kg/day in children or 40 mg three times daily in adults for 14 to 21 days, followed by a taper. Careful analysis of the benefits and risks of this therapy must be undertaken because corticosteroids may mask symptoms of a deteriorating clinical condition, and increase the risk for other infectious conditions because of their immunosuppressive effects.

Antibiotics are only indicated if there is clinical or endoscopic evidence of perforation or infection or if corticosteroid therapy is used. Prophylactic antibiotics can mask evidence of impending perforation. The antibiotics chosen should have coverage against a broad spectrum of oral and enteral pathogens because gram-positive and gram-negative pathogens and anaerobes can all be potentially encountered. Initial parenteral therapy with piperacillin-tazobactam or a third-generation cephalosporin plus clindamycin followed by oral therapy with a fluoroquinolone and clindamycin is one such regimen. Ampicillin and clindamycin have also been used in these cases.

Surgical Treatment

Immediate surgical intervention is indicated for the presence of free air, peritonitis, increasing and severe chest and abdominal pain, and hemorrhagic shock unresponsive to blood component therapy. Exploratory surgery may also be warranted in patients with suspected full-thickness burns. Early consultation with a gastroenterologist or general surgeon is recommended in any critically ill patient after corrosive ingestion.[48]

Esophageal stricture begins early and remains a lifelong problem. Treatment with repeated bougienage can be started as early as 3 weeks after ingestion. Although no randomized trials have studied the efficacy of repeated dilation, it is a widely used treatment and in some cases may eliminate the need for surgical intervention.[49,50] As with any esophageal dilating procedure, repeated trauma to the esophagus creates areas of weakness, increasing the chance of perforation. Recent animal studies and human case reports have suggested that esophageal stents have greater success long term.[51,52] Colonic interposition procedures may be performed in some patients requiring eventual esophageal replacement.[46,53,54] The development of cancer in the residual esophageal stump despite replace-

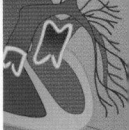

ment has been reported.[55] Gastric outlet obstruction may also require endoscopic balloon dilation or surgical correction.[56]

Disposition

Asymptomatic patients can be observed in the emergency department and subsequently discharged home if they are able to ingest fluids with no discomfort. Parents should be informed that development of signs and symptoms after discharge warrants further medical attention. All symptomatic patients require admission to the intensive care unit and should remain NPO pending gastrointestinal consultation. Psychiatric evaluation is warranted for patients with intentional ingestion.

REFERENCES

1. Watson WA, Litovitz TL, Rogers GC, et al: 2002 annual report of the American Association of Poison Control Centers Toxic Exposure Surveillance System. Am J Emerg Med 2003;21:351.
2. Boyd A: Chevalier Jackson: The father of American broncho-esophagoscopy. Ann Thorac Surg 1994;57:502.
3. Neidich G: Ingestion of caustic alkali farm products. J Pediatr Gastroenterol Nutr 1993;16:75.
4. Kynaston JA, Patrick MK, Shepherd RW, et al: The hazards of automatic-dishwasher detergent. Med J Aust 1989;151:5.
5. Aronow SP, Aronow HD, Blanchard T, et al: Hair relaxers: a benign caustic ingestion? J Pediatr Gastroenterol Nutr 2003;36:120.
6. Babl FE, Edelberg LH, Shannon M: Oral and airway sequelae after hair relaxer ingestion. Pediatr Emerg Care 2001;17:36.
7. White JE, McClafferty K, Orton RB, et al: Ocular alkali burn associated with automobile air-bag activation. CMAJ 1995;153:933.
8. Spoo J, Elsner P: Cement burns: a review 1960–2000. Contact Dermatitis 2001;45:68.
9. Kikendall JW: Pill-induced esophageal injury. Gastroenterol Clin North Am 1991;20:835.
10. Hoffman RH, Kamerow HN, Goldfrank LR: Comparison of titratable acid/alkaline reserve and pH in potentially caustic household products. J Toxicol Clin Toxicol 1989;27:241.
11. Vancura EM, Clinton JE, Ruiz E, et al: Toxicity of alkaline solutions. Ann Emerg Med 1980;9:118.
12. Krey H: On the treatment of corrosive lesions in the oesophagus. Acta Otolaryngol 1952;1:S102.
13. Kirsh MM, Ritter F: Caustic ingestion and subsequent damage to the oropharyngeal and digestive passages. Ann Thorac Surg 1976;21:74.
14. Fisher RA, Eckhauser ML, Radivoyevitch M: Acid ingestion in an experimental model. Surg Gynecol Obstet 1985;161:91.
15. Marks IN, Bank S, Werbeloff L, et al: The natural history of corrosive gastritis: Report of five cases. Am J Dig Dis 1963;8:509.
16. Zargar SA, Kochhar R, Nagi B, et al: Ingestion of corrosive acids. Spectrum of injury to upper gastrointestinal tract and natural history. Gastroenterology 1989;97:702.
17. Thompson J: Corrosive esophageal strictures. I. A study of nine cases of concurrent accidental caustic ingestion. Laryngoscope 1987;97:1060.
18. Zargar SA: Ingestion of corrosive acids. Gastroenterology 1989;97:702.
19. Christesen H: Prediction of complications following unintentional caustic ingestion in children. Is endoscopy always necessary? Acta Paediatr Scand 1995;84:1177.
20. Gorman RK, Khin-Maung-Gyi MT, Klein-Schwartz W, et al: Initial symptoms as predictors of esophageal injury in alkaline corrosive ingestions Am J Emerg Med 1992;10:189.
21. Christesen HB: Prediction of complications following caustic ingestion in adults. Clin Otolaryngol 1995;20:272.
22. Anderson KR, Randolph JG: A controlled trial of corticosteroids in children with corrosive injury of the esophagus. N Engl J Med 1990;323:637.
23. Gaudreault PP, Parent M, McGuigan M, et al: Predictability of esophageal injury from signs and symptoms: a study of caustic ingestion in 378 children. Pediatrics 1983;71:767.
24. Nuutinen MU, Karvali T, Kouvalainen K: Consequences of caustic ingestion in children. Acta Paediatr 1994;83:1200.
25. Tseng YL, Wu MH, Lin MY, et al: Massive upper gastrointestinal bleeding after acid-corrosive injury. World J Surg 2004;28:50.
26. Tseng YL, Wu MH, Lin MY, et al: Outcome of acid ingestion related aspiration pneumonia. Eur J Cardiothorac Surg 2002;21:638.
27. Kirichenko AS, Wax PM: Caustic ingestions in Russia: a perpetual problem demanding further study. J Toxicol Clin Toxicol 1997;35:514.
28. Isolauri JM: Ingestion and carcinoma of the esophagus. Acta Chir Scand 1989;155:269.
29. Mamede RC, de Mello Filho FV: Ingestion of caustic substances and its complications. Sao Paulo Med J 2001;119:10.
30. Cheng YJ, Kao EL: Arterial blood gas analysis in acute caustic ingestion injuries. Surg Today 2003;33:483.
31. Rigo GP, Camellini L, Azzolini F, et al: What is the utility of selected clinical and endoscopic parameters in predicting the risk of death after caustic ingestion? Endoscopy 2002;34:304.
32. Backer CL, Hartz RS, Donaldson JS, Shields T: Computed tomography in patients with esophageal perforation. Chest 1990;98:1078.
33. Lamireau T, Rebouissoux L, Denis D, et al: Accidental caustic ingestion in children: is endoscopy always mandatory? J Pediatr Gastroenterol Nutr 2001;33:81.
34. Crain EF, Gershel JC, Mezey AP: Caustic ingestions: symptoms as predictors of esophageal injury. Am J Dis Child 1984;138:863.
35. Middelkamp JN, Ferguson TB, Roper CL, et al: The management and problems of caustic burns in children. J Thorac Cardiovasc Surg 1969;57:341.
36. Gorman RL, Khin-Maung-Gyi MT, Klein-Schwartz W, et al: Initial symptoms as predictors of esophageal injury in alkaline corrosive ingestions. Am J Emerg Med 1992;10:189.
37. Guth AP, Albanese C, Kim U: Combined duodenal and colonic necrosis in an unusual sequela of caustic ingestion. J Clin Gastroenterol 1994;19:303.
38. Maull KO, Maull CD: Liquid caustic ingestions. An in vitro study of the effects of buffer, neutralization and dilution. Ann Emerg Med 1988;14:1160.
39. Homan CS, Singer AJ, Thomajan C, et al: Thermal characteristics of neutralizing therapy and water dilution for strong acid ingestion: an in-vivo canine model. Acad Emerg Med 1998;5:286.
40. Berkovits RB, Wijburg FA, Holzki J: Caustic injury of the oesophagus: sixteen years experience and introduction of a new model oesopheageal stent. Laryngol Otol 1996;11:1041.
41. Boukthir S, Fetni I, Mrad SM, et al: High doses of steroids in the management of caustic esophageal burns in children. Arch Pediatr 2004;11:13.
42. Ulman I, Mutaf O: A critique of systemic steroids in the management of caustic esophageal burns in children. Eur J Pediatr Surg 1998;8:71.
43. Anderson KD, Rouse TM, Randolph JG: A controlled trial of corticosteroids in children with corrosive injury of the esophagus. N Engl J Med 1990;323:637.
44. Keskin E, Okur H, Koltuksuz U, et al: The effect of steroid treatment on corrosive oesophageal burns in children. Eur J Pediatr Surg 1991;1:335.
45. Cakmak M, Nayci A, Renda N, et al: The effect of corticosteroids and pentoxifylline in caustic esophageal burns: a prospective trial in rats. Int Surg 1997;82:371.
46. Moazam F, Talbert JL, Miller D, et al: Caustic ingestion and its sequelae in children. South Med J 1987;80:187.
47. Howell JM, Dalsey WC, Hartsell FW, et al: Steroids for the treatment of corrosive esophageal injury: a statistical analysis of past studies. Am J Emerg Med 1992;10:421.
48. Andreoni B, Farina ML, Biffi R, et al: Esophageal perforation and caustic injury: emergency management of caustic ingestion. Dis Esophagus 1997;10:95.
49. Broto J, Asensio M, Jorro CS, et al: Conservative treatment of caustic esophageal injuries in children: 20 years of experience. Pediatr Surg Int 1999;15:323.

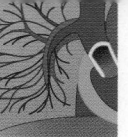

50. Saetti R, Silvestrini M, Cutrone C, et al: Endoscopic treatment of upper airway and digestive tract lesions caused by caustic agents. Ann Otol Rhinol Laryngol 2003;112:29.

51. Thompson J: Corrosive esophageal injuries. II. An investigation of treatment methods and histochemical analysis of esophageal strictures in a new animal model. Laryngoscope 1987;97:1191.

52. Wijburg FH, Urbanus NAM: Caustic esophageal lesions in childhood: prevention of stricture formation. J Pediatr Surg 1989;24:171.

53. Sugawa C, Lucas CE: Caustic injury of the upper gastrointestinal tract in adults: a clinical and endoscopic study. Surgery 1989;106:802.

54. Bassiouny IE, Bahnassy AF: Transhiatal esophagectomy and colonic interposition for caustic esophageal stricture. J Pediatr Surg 1992;27:1091.

55. Jung HY, Kim HJ, Kim SB, et al: Esophageal cancer in an esophagus remaining after colonic interposition for lye stricture. Endoscopy 1999;31:S1.

56. Tekant G, Eroglu E, Erdogan E, et al: Corrosive injury-induced gastric outlet obstruction: a changing spectrum of agents and treatment. J Pediatr Surg 2001;36:1004.

99

Baby Powder, Borates, and Camphor

YOUNG-JIN SUE, MD ■ HEIDI PINKERT, MD

At a Glance...

- Baby powder inhalation produces hypoxia by obstructing the airway and interfering with ciliary action. No systemic toxicity has been reported. Pulmonary manifestations range from cough to respiratory failure and apnea. Adult respiratory distress syndrome and long-term pulmonary impairment can occur.

- Management for baby powder inhalation includes establishing and maintaining the vital functions. Clear the airway, administer 100% oxygen, and give assisted ventilation and positive end-expiratory pressure if necessary. Obtain chest x-rays and monitor arterial blood gases if symptomatic. Corticosteroids may be useful. Admit to hospital in cases of hypoxemia or respiratory distress; the chest x-ray findings are sometimes delayed.

- After oral or dermal absorption of boric acid, the earliest symptoms are gastroenteritis with blue-green vomitus and diarrhea. Central nervous system stimulation may occur. An erythematous rash may develop within 6 hours after ingestion. Desquamation and exfoliation ("boiled lobster" appearance) can occur within 2 to 5 days after exposure. Blood levels of boric acid do not correlate well with toxicity.

- Management of boric acid toxicity consists of symptomatic and supportive care. Activated charcoal has limited utility. Hemodialysis may enhance elimination in severe cases.

- Onset of CNS stimulation (seizures) may begin within 5 minutes after camphor ingestion. It has a distinctive odor.

- Treat seizures with a benzodiazepine. Gastrointestinal decontamination is not advised, nor are extracorporeal measures. There is no specific antidote. Ingestions in children of more than 30 mg/kg or more than 3 g in an adult need medical evaluation and monitoring for at least 4 hours. Symptomatic patients should be placed in the intensive care unit.

BABY POWDER

Introduction and Relevant History

There are many formulations of baby powder, but the major ingredient is usually talc.[1] Historically, talcum powder had originally been reported as an ingredient in paints used by cave dwellers and in glazed pottery made by the Chinese more than 1300 years ago. Today, talcum powder is a commercially mined mineral that is primarily composed of hydrated magnesium silicate.[2,3] Talcum powder is used in the manufacture of a myriad of products, including animal feed, automobiles, cables, candles, ceramic tiles, chewing gum, cosmetics, wastewater treatment technology, fertilizers, paints, pharmaceuticals, plaster, putties, tires, and baby powder. Specific purity guidelines have been set forth to eliminate asbestos contamination of cosmetic and pharmaceutical grade talc.[3,4] Other common ingredients of baby powder may include calcium and zinc salts, petrolatum, and perfume. Cornstarch is a major ingredient in "talc free" baby powder.[3] All these substances can, when inhaled, produce a similar aspiration pneumonitis.[4-6] The routine use of nonmedicated powders in the skin care of infants can be hazardous and should be discouraged.[5,6] Most exposure to baby powder generally occurs either through accidental inhalation by infants and children or through its routine use by women as a dusting powder in the perineal area.[5,6] Workers are variably exposed to talc in the course of mining it.[7,8] Oral ingestion of talc is not likely to be toxic; it is contained in some pills, and there is no evidence to suggest adverse effects from moderate intake.[4]

Epidemiology

Data on the toxic effects of talc inhalation originally came from a few case reports of unintentional massive exposures in infants and children.[9-15] Many of the children in the older literature died as a result of the exposure. According to the Annual Report of the American Association of Poison Control Centers Toxic Exposure Surveillance System (TESS), there were 6291 powder exposures reported in 2002. Of these, 5719 (91%) cases were in children younger than 6 years, 259 (4.1%) were in patients between 6 and 19 years of age, and 301(4.8%) were in patients older than 19 years. There were 403 (6.4%) exposures managed in a health care facility. Only 81 (13%) exposures resulted in moderate effects, and no major morbidity or mortality was reported.[16] Most of the children who inhale baby powder recover well.[2,16]

A number of studies have attempted to ascertain whether perineal exposure to talc in women increases the risk for ovarian cancer.[8] Although the frequency and duration of use have also been examined, a clearcut relationship between perineal talc exposure and ovarian cancer has not been clearly established.[17]

Structure and Structure–Activity Relationships

The molecular formula of hydrous magnesium silicate is $Mg_3Si_4O_{10}(OH)_2$. It has a molecular weight of 96.49.[18]

Pharmacology

PATHOPHYSIOLOGY

The physical properties of talc account for its toxicity when inhaled. It is insoluble in water and not biodegrad-

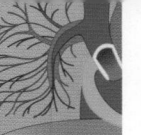

able; it thus may obstruct the airways to variable degrees.[14] The size of talc particles, which averages less than 5 μm,[19] would allow them to reach the alveoli; this has indeed been confirmed on pathologic specimens.[10] Other pathologic findings after talc inhalation consist of inflammatory changes in the airway and interstitium, bronchiolitis with bronchiolar obstruction, atelectasis, emphysema, and fibrosis.[10,11,14] These pathologic findings are in accord with the observation that the clinical picture may resemble severe bronchiolitis.[13]

PHARMACOKINETICS

Although widely used, baby powder has few, if any, indications. Its absorptive capacity is negligible compared with that of a diaper, its fragrance and friction-reducing effects are transient, and it is less effective than a cream or lotion, which cannot be inhaled. The kinetics of powders such as talcum has not been elucidated.

Toxicology

CLINICAL MANIFESTATIONS (ACUTE AND CHRONIC)

Acute aspiration of baby powder or talc can cause coughing, dyspnea, tachypnea, sneezing, vomiting, cyanosis, and pulmonary edema, which may be delayed up to several hours.[2] Respiratory acidosis, bronchitis, bronchiolitis, pulmonary edema, atelectasis, emphysema, and severe bronchiolar obstruction may develop.[11,14] Cardiorespiratory arrest may occur after severe aspiration.[13]

Chronic inhalation of industrial talc dusts or body talc produces talcosis due to talc, silica, and asbestos (talc pneumoconiosis) and is characterized by productive cough, dyspnea, rales, diminished breath sounds, limited chest expansion, interstitial fibrosis, and granulomas.[20] The extent and severity of fibrosis correlates with the length of exposure and dust concentration. Pneumoconiosis associated with obstructive and restrictive lung disease after chronic intentional inhalation of talcum powder has been reported. Chest x-ray has revealed a diffuse reticulonodular interstitial infiltrate with conglomerate masses in both mid-lung zones.[21] Chronic talc inhalation may increase the risk for bronchogenic carcinoma.[22] Chronic abuse of talc-contaminated cocaine by insufflation has resulted in pulmonary talc granulomatosis, with chest x-ray showing diffuse bilateral infiltrates.[23]

Intravenous injection of talc-containing tablets or capsules produces foreign-body vascular granulomas (microemboli) at the site of intramuscular or subcutaneous injection and widespread arterial wall granulomas.[20] Angiothrombotic pulmonary arterial hypertension and cor pulmonale may develop. Pulmonary effects include nonproductive cough, fever, dyspnea, and granulomatosis. Subtle x-ray changes may develop showing symmetric hilar and perihilar interstitial infiltrations, which are only minimally reversible.[24] Pulmonary infiltrates have been observed in intravenous drug abusers[25] and after therapeutic use for pleurodesis.[26]

Diagnosis

LABORATORY TESTING

If the patient is symptomatic, obtain baseline complete blood count, electrolytes, and chest x-ray. Monitor arterial blood gases regularly in patients with severe respiratory findings. Chest x-ray may show symmetric hilar and perihilar infiltrates.

OTHER DIAGNOSTIC TESTING

Diagnosis may be established by transbronchial biopsy using scanning electron microscopy and energy-dispersive x-ray analysis to establish the presence of and identify the particles.[14,15] Subtle pulmonary abnormalities such as decreased carbon monoxide diffusing capacity are an earlier indication of pulmonary damage rather than clinical or radiologic evidence.

DIFFERENTIAL DIAGNOSIS

The medical causes of aspiration pneumonia and pneumonitis are extensive and include all causes of respiratory distress, especially pulmonary embolism and cardiogenic pulmonary edema, as well as other aspiration syndromes (airway obstruction, lung abscess, exogenous liquid pneumonia, chronic interstitial fibrosis). Differentiation is largely dependent on clinical setting.

Toxin-mediated small airway disease has developed after exposure to nitrogen dioxide, sulfur dioxide, ammonia, chlorine, phosgene, chloropicrin, trichloroethylene, ozone, cadmium, methyl sulfate, hydrogen sulfide, hydrogen fluoride, zinc chloride, talcum powder, high-dose oxygen therapy, and free-base cocaine.[27]

Management

SUPPORTIVE MEASURES

Begin immediately to prevent complications from acute inhalation exposure of large amounts in an asymptomatic patient. Establish and maintain the vital functions. Clear the airway, and administer 100% oxygen.

DECONTAMINATION

Decontamination procedures are not useful in treating talcum inhalation.

LABORATORY MONITORING

Monitor blood gases in symptomatic patients for the development of respiratory acidosis. When the P_{CO_2} rises above 50 mm Hg, mechanical ventilation with positive end-expiratory pressure (PEEP) should be instituted.[12]

ANTIDOTES

N-Acetylcysteine

There is a case report in which the administration of N-acetylcysteine and oxygen in a mist tent appeared to be helpful in improving respiratory distress.[12] Aspiration of mucus secretions after tracheal instillation of 5 mL of normal saline may be preferred to N-acetylcysteine therapy at this time.

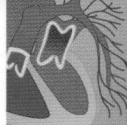

Corticosteroids

Prednisone, 1 to 2 mg/kg/day for 3 to 5 days, adult maximum 60 mg/day, may be administered to prevent inflammation and exudation of mucus secretions.[12] For symptomatic patients, dexamethasone, 0.1 to 0.2 mg/kg/day, adult maximum 10 mg.[9,28] Bronchodilators have been tried with only limited success and generally not used. Prophylactic antibiotics such as ampicillin may be indicated but are not generally recommended unless for cultured pathogens.[12,13]

Consider bronchoalveolar lavage with normal saline to remove aspirated powder. This will have limited value because of talc insolubility and is potentially dangerous, but it may remove excessive mucus secretions refractory to N-acetylcysteine therapy.[12,13] Bronchoalveolar lavage has been used for the differential diagnosis of talc-induced lung disease.[29,30]

Other

Chest physiotherapy and postural drainage may be helpful.

ELIMINATION

Elimination is not applicable.

DISPOSITION

Admit the patient to the hospital in cases of hypoxemia or respiratory distress. The chest x-ray findings are sometimes delayed.[31] Follow-up pulmonary function studies for long-term restrictive-obstructive sequelae are indicated in significant inhalations.

BORIC ACID

Introduction and Relevant History

The Babylonians allegedly used borax more than 4000 years ago as a flux for working gold, and there are data to suggest that the Egyptians used boron for mummifying, medicinal, and metallurgic purposes.[32] Today, borate-mineral concentrates are used in fertilizer, fire retardants, laundry bleaches, and glass and related vitreous applications.[32] The antiseptic effects of boric acid were first described by Lord Lister in 1875.[33] At one time, it was mixed with honey and glycerin and sold to treat topical mucosal sores in children.[34] Historically, significant toxicity and fatalities occurred after chronic exposure to boric acid preparations. In one series, 11 infants died when inadvertently fed a 2.5% boric acid solution over several days.[35] Because of its weak antiseptic properties and significant toxicity, it is no longer used in medicinal preparations.[34] A common cause of exposure today is related to unintentional ingestion of powdered boric acid used to kill cockroaches. Acute unintentional ingestions rarely result in significant toxicity, whereas chronic exposure results in more serious toxicity.[36-39] Suicidal ingestions of large amounts (280 g in one case) may be fatal.[38]

Epidemiology

There were a total of 2724 exposures to boric acid reported by TESS in 2002. Of those, 1317 (48.3%) patients were younger than 6 years, 315 (11.5%) were between the ages of 6 and 19 years, and 1071 (39.3%) were older than 19 years. There were 481 (18%) patients treated in a health care facility. Eighty-three (8.8%) of the patients were judged to have moderate outcomes; 5 patients suffered major morbidity, and 1 expired.[40]

Structure and Structure–Activity Relationships

Boric acid is an odorless, colorless compound that can occur in crystalline, granular, or white powder form. Borates and borate-mineral concentrates such as borax ($Na_2B_4O_7 \cdot 10\ H_2O$) are salts or esters of boric acid.

Pharmacology

PATHOPHYSIOLOGY

Autopsy findings in patients who have died as a result of boric acid poisoning have noted significant involvement of several organ systems, including the skin, gastrointestinal tract, kidneys, brain, and liver.[36,38,41,42] In those individuals with skin eruptions, pathologic specimens were consistent with an exfoliative dermatitis. The gastrointestinal tract demonstrates inflammatory changes, with congestion, edema, and mucosal exfoliation, although boric acid is not caustic. Renal changes have ranged from gross pallor to cloudy swelling and renal tubular degeneration. The CNS effects reported have included congestion and edema of the brain.[36] The liver rarely has demonstrated clinical manifestations of boric acid toxicity.[36,43,44] Pathologic findings consist of fatty change and congestion.

PHARMACOKINETICS

Absorption of boric acid occurs easily through abraded or excoriated skin,[38,41,45] but absorption through intact skin is negligible.[46,47] Oral ingestion results in rapid and complete absorption of boric acid from the gastrointestinal tract. Distribution occurs throughout body water and ranges from 0.17 to 0.50 L/kg. The highest concentrations occur in the brain, liver, and kidneys.[43,48,49] Most ingested boric acid is excreted unchanged by the kidneys; more than 50% of the oral dose is eliminated within 24 hours, and more than 90% is excreted within 96 hours of ingestion.[38,44] The half-life of boric acid has been reported to range from 5 to 21 hours.[38,48]

Special Populations (Pediatrics, Geriatrics, Liver Failure, Renal Failure, Pregnancy)

A case series of oral boric acid intoxications in a newborn nursery was reported by Wong and colleagues that

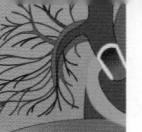

indicated the ingested dose by those infants who died ranged between 4.5 and 15.0 g of boric acid.[35] Deaths occurred as a result of drinking formula accidentally prepared with a 2.5% boric acid solution. Infants who survived the poisoning but were symptomatic ingested amounts ranging from 2.0 to 4.5 g. In general, a dose of 2 to 3 g in newborns and infants and 5 g in children is regarded as lethal. A significant amount of boric acid must be ingested for toxicity to occur because the solutions available with boric acid usually range in concentration from 2.5% to 5%. Of greater concern is the ingestion of boric acid powder, crystals, or granules; 1 teaspoonful of 100% boric acid in these forms contains 2.9 to 4.4 g.[50] The literature regarding adults describes four deaths due to acute boric acid or sodium borate ingestion since 1921.[51] Based on these data and other case series, it has been estimated that the adult human median lethal dose is likely to be greater than 30 g. Although case series reveal a wide range for toxicity,[36,38] ingestion of 15 to 20 g of boric acid is generally cited as the lethal dose for adults.[39]

Toxicology

CLINICAL MANIFESTATIONS (ACUTE AND CHRONIC)

Usually, symptoms develop within 4 to 6 hours. The initial manifestations may resemble gastroenteritis, with blue-green vomitus, diarrhea that may be bloody (hemorrhagic gastroenteritis), and colicky abdominal pain.[36,38] Solutions up to 5% do not cause gastrointestinal irritation. CNS stimulation, headache, agitation, delirium, hypertonia, hyperreflexia, meningeal irritation, and increased intracranial pressure may occur; in severe cases, seizures and coma may ensue.[36,38,51] Cardiovascular effects include hypotension and oliguria; anuria and renal failure may develop.[39,51,52]

An erythematous rash develops as early as 6 hours after ingestion in most patients, starting on the face, the inguinal creases, axillary creases, buttocks, and scrotum and then spreading to cover the entire surface, including the palms, soles, and oral and anal mucosa. Desquamation and exfoliation ("boiled lobster" appearance) can occur within 2 to 5 days after exposure. Anemia, abnormal liver function tests, and rarely alopecia totalis have been reported.[51]

Chronic boric acid poisoning occurs usually in infants from repeated topical application to diaper dermatitis. This may also be associated with renal impairment, hypothermia, or hyperthermia.[36,53]

Reversible upper respiratory tract irritation has been reported with exposure to boron oxide or boric acid dust concentrations of less than 10 mg/m³ and borax dust concentrations of 1.1 mg/m³ to 14.6 mg/m³ and 10 to 14 mg/m³.[54-56] Symptoms commonly included nasal irritation, mucous membrane dryness, dry or productive cough, and nose bleeds. Shortness of breath, chest pain, and chest tightness were reported less frequently.[54-56] A statistically significant increased risk for phlegm production and chronic bronchitis in nonsmokers was associated with exposure to 14.6 mg/m³ of borax dust.[55]

Diagnosis

The diagnosis of boric acid poisoning requires careful history taking with the appropriate clinical picture.

LABORATORY TESTING

Although levels of boric acid do not correlate well with toxicity, levels in seriously poisoned patients with acute exposure are generally above 34 mg/dL.[38] Seizures in one child with chronic exposure were associated with a serum boric acid level of 9.44 mg/dL.[34] A fatal case of acute boric acid poisoning in an adult had a 52-hour level of 42 mg/dL.[39] Boric acid levels in Wong's series of 11 fatal pediatric poisonings ranged from 40 to 160 mg/dL.[35] Because most hospital laboratories do not have the capability to quickly determine serum borate levels, this information cannot be relied on to make the diagnosis of borate toxicity. Two commercial laboratories that are able to quantitate serum borate levels are National Medical Services, Inc., 2300 Stratford Ave., P.O. Box 433A, Willow Grove, PA, 19090, telephone 215-657-4900, and West Coast Analytical Services, Inc., 9840 Alburtis Ave., Santa Fe Springs, CA 90670, telephone 310-948-2225. The U.S. Borax and Chemical Co. provides a 24-hour telephone number for medical emergencies related to borates: 800-228-5635.

OTHER DIAGNOSTIC TESTING

Urinary boron concentrations can indicate total-body burden of boron. The normal range of urinary boron has been reported as 0.004 to 0.66 mg/100 mL.[57]

DIFFERENTIAL DIAGNOSIS

The differential diagnosis of the "boiled lobster" appearance is Kawasaki disease, scarlet fever, and staphylococcal scalded skin syndrome.[58]

Management

SUPPORTIVE MEASURES

Treatment consists of symptomatic and supportive care and includes monitoring for the development of hypotension, fluid and electrolyte imbalance, seizures, renal failure, cardiac arrhythmias, and shock. Severe dehydration can occur and contribute to adverse renal and cardiovascular effects. Administer intravenous fluids to treat dehydration. Treatment of hypotension may include intravenous fluids, dopamine, or norepinephrine.

DECONTAMINATION

Syrup of ipecac is *not advised* for boric acid ingestion. Activated charcoal has limited ability to absorb boric acid. An in vitro study demonstrated that 30 g of charcoal was required to adsorb 38% of a 1-g boric acid dose.[59] The use of activated charcoal in potentially fatal ingestions of 5 g in a child and 20 g in an adult was considered impractical because 5 to 10 times the recommended doses of activated charcoal would be required to effectively adsorb the boric acid.

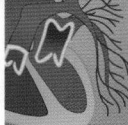

LABORATORY MONITORING

Monitor renal function tests, cardiovascular status, and fluid and electrolyte balance in symptomatic patients.

ANTIDOTES

No antidotes are available.

ELIMINATION

Hemodialysis, peritoneal dialysis, and exchange transfusion may enhance elimination. Exchange transfusion has been advocated and successful in cases of chronic exposure.[60,61] Hemodialysis and peritoneal dialysis have been advocated to increase excretion.[62] In comparison to renal elimination, the amount removed by peritoneal dialysis is small.[63]

DISPOSITION

Unintentional ingestions usually result in minimal toxicity. A lick or a taste of a topical powder of less than 5% may be observed at home. A teaspoonful of a 99% powder in a child should be evaluated in an emergency department. When an approximation of the amount ingested can be made, Table 99-1 can be used to determine the appropriate management. This table has been modified from a large series involving 784 boric acid ingestions.[38]

CAMPHOR

Introduction and Relevant History

Camphor was one of the therapeutic agents of the 19th-century pharmacopoeia used as an analgesic, expectorant, counterirritant, and abortifacient, as well as a stimulant.[64] Camphor is a naturally occurring essential oil (volatile oil). Historically, it has been claimed that camphor was mentioned by Marco Polo in the 13th century and Camoens in 1571, who called it the "balsam of disease."[65] Camphor is highly prized by the Chinese, who used it for embalming purposes and to scent soap.[65] In the 1930s, Ladislav Meduna induced seizures with intramuscular injections of camphor to treat catatonia, a therapeutic predecessor to electroconvulsive therapy.[66] This continued use persisted into the 1940s.

TABLE 99-1 Triage of Boric Acid Ingestions		
BODY WEIGHT	**AMOUNT INGESTED**	**MANAGEMENT**
<30 kg	<200 mg/kg	Observe at home.
	>200 mg/kg	Emergency department for gastrointestinal decontamination and evaluation
>30 kg	<6 g ingested	Observe at home.
	>6 g	Emergency department for gastrointestinal decontamination and evaluation

Most unintentional overdoses of camphor have occurred when it has been mistakenly administered for castor oil or cough syrup.[67] Often produced in similar packaging and stocked on adjacent shelves in pharmacies, the confusion of camphorated oil, a 20% mixture of camphor and cottonseed oil, for castor oil was predictable. In 1983, the U.S. Food and Drug Administration ruled that over-the-counter products cannot contain camphor in excess of 11%.[68] In 1994, the American Academy of Pediatrics recommended the removal of camphor from all medicinal products.[67] However, despite these efforts, camphor continues to be ubiquitous in over-the-counter preparations such as local anesthetics, antipruritics, rubefacients, antitussives, "chest cold" inhalants, and some herbal products despite a lack of therapeutic value and the availability of safer alternatives.

Epidemiology

According to the 2002 Annual Report of the American Association of Poison Control Centers TESS, there were a total of 8817 exposures to camphor reported. Of those, 6852 (77.7%) patients were younger than 6 years, 526 (5.9%) were between the ages of 6 and 19 years, and 1426 (16.2%) were older than 19 years. There were 922 (10.5%) cases treated in a health care facility. Seventy-seven patients were judged to have moderate outcomes, 9 suffered major morbidity, and 1 expired.[69]

Structure and Structure–Activity Relationships

Camphor is a crystalline ketone, related to the terpenes, that was originally steam-distilled from the bark of the camphor tree *Cinnamomum camphora*. Today, it is synthetically produced from α-pinene ($C_{10}H_{10}$), a hydrocarbon extracted from turpentine oil.[70] Chemically, it is described as a bicyclomonoterpenoid or 1,7,7-trimethybicyclo(2,1,1)-2-heptanone.[71,72]

Pharmacology

The mechanism of toxicity of camphor is unclear. Topically, camphor is a rubefacient, producing local hyperemia and warmth. It is thought to generate its perceived therapeutic benefits through the "counterirritant analgesic effect" in which moderate visceral pain is masked by a milder skin irritation.[73] Camphor's intense odor and sensation of warmth on application contributes to the feeling of relief from pain or congestion that may be greater than that actually physiologically present. Although the biochemical basis by which camphor leads to CNS excitation and seizures is not well understood, it is thought to act directly to stimulate nervous tissue. In 1954, Smith and Margolis reported a 19-month-old child who died 5 days after the ingestion of an estimated 1 teaspoon of camphorated oil.[64] They found "extensive degenerative changes" selectively involving the neurons of the cerebral cortex, basal ganglia, and hippocampus. The same investigators found

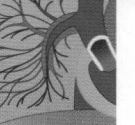

no neurologic pathologic lesions in mice when seizures were prevented by the concomitant administration of pentobarbital with camphor. These findings suggest that the neuronal damage found in camphor fatalities may result from seizures and anoxia rather than from a direct action of camphor on neurons.[64]

PATHOPHYSIOLOGY

See Box 99-1 for the pharmacokinetics of camphor ingestion.

Special Populations

After oral ingestion, camphor has been associated with spontaneous abortion. It has therefore been classified by the Food and Drug Administration as a Pregnancy Category C drug.[74]

Toxicology

CLINICAL MANIFESTATIONS (ACUTE AND CHRONIC)

Classically, seizures may occur suddenly and without warning within 5 minutes of an acute ingestion of camphor; these seizures may be followed by coma.[75] In Phelan's review of 748 patients, 42% had seizures after ingestion of 700 to 6000 mg of camphor.[76] Apnea and visual hallucinations, confusion, tremors, and myoclonic jerking may occur.[77] Other disturbances that may precede the seizures include anxiety, confusion, dizziness, and facial fasciculations. Death is due to respiratory arrest or secondary to status epilepticus.

BOX 99-1	**PHARMACOKINETICS**

Absorption

- Rapidly and readily absorbed through the skin and mucous membranes, including the gastrointestinal and respiratory tracts[71]

Distribution

- Camphor crosses the placenta.[86]
- Large volume of distribution: 1.2–4 L/kg[87]
- Camphor is highly lipid soluble, so significant toxic substances accumulate in fat tissue.
- Onset of action is 5–20 min with a peak effect within 90 min.[86]

Metabolism

- Camphor is rapidly oxidized to campherols (2-hydroxycamphor and 3-hydroxycamphor) and then conjugated in the liver to the glucoronide form.[86]

Excretion

- Campherol conjugated to glucuronic acid is eliminated mainly in the urine as an inactive compound.
- Pulmonary excretion of camphor and its metabolites causes an odor on the breath.[86]

Elimination Half-Life

- A plasma elimination half-life of 93–167 min was reported in a volunteer given 200 mg of camphor.[87]

Initial gastrointestinal symptoms usually include the feeling of warmth, thirst, nausea, spontaneous vomiting, epigastric burning, and abdominal pain. Aspiration of vomitus is a major complication. Urinary retention, anuria, and albuminuria (transient) have been described in some patients.

Chronic administration of camphor can cause an altered mental status with elevation of the liver enzymes, which may mimic Reye syndrome. The liver has showed fatty metamorphosis with no cell necrosis, inflammation, or biliary stasis.[77] Similar effects may occur in acute poisoning.

ADVERSE EFFECTS

Adverse effects associated with the topical use of any camphor-containing creams include dermal irritation when applied in excessive amounts or too vigorously.

Diagnosis

Because most instances of camphor intoxication occur after unintentional ingestion, patients usually promptly seek medical attention and willingly offer historical information relevant to the poisoning. Even in the absence of such historical information, however, the presence of camphor is readily apparent owing to its intense and characteristic odor, which may be detected on the breath, vomitus, clothes, and hair. This is further aided by the typical clinical picture of gastrointestinal distress, agitation, somnolence, and seizures. Hyperthermia and tachycardia usually accompany prolonged agitation and seizures. No laboratory derangements are specifically characteristic of camphor poisoning, although transient liver function abnormalities have been reported in some cases.[78,79]

LABORATORY TESTING

Camphor plasma concentrations are not readily available and do not correlate with symptoms. However, patients who had camphor plasma concentrations of 1.5 μg/mL were asymptomatic, and those who developed seizures have been reported to have levels of 19.5 μg/mL.[67]

OTHER DIAGNOSTIC TESTING

Complete blood count, electrolytes, liver function tests, and renal function tests should be monitored. Consider a chest radiograph to exclude aspiration. Obtain arterial blood gases if the patient is comatose or has respiratory symptoms. Abnormalities reported can include leukocytosis, albuminuria, and a transient rise in liver enzymes.

DIFFERENTIAL DIAGNOSIS

The differential diagnosis is any cause of afebrile seizures. The odor on the patient's body or clothes may be an important clue.

Management

SUPPORTIVE MEASURES

Monitor for hypotension, dysrhythmias, and respiratory depression. Treat respiratory depression with endotracheal intubation and ventilatory assistance as necessary.

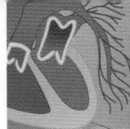

Intravenous access should be obtained; fluid and pressor support may become necessary. Seizure precautions should be established. Treat seizures with intravenous diazepam (adult: 5–10 mg, repeat every 10–15 minutes as needed; child: 0.2–0.5 mg/kg [maximum, 10 mg/dose], repeat every 15 minutes as needed) or intravenous lorazepam (adult: 2–4 mg [maximum, 8 mg/dose]; child: 0.05–0.1 mg/kg [maximum, 4 mg]). Consider phenobarbital if seizures recur after diazepam. The dose for intravenous phenobarbital in adults and children is 20 mg/kg at 50 to 100 mg/min.

DECONTAMINATION

Avoid the induction of emesis because of the potential for an early onset of seizures.[80] Activated charcoal has doubtful efficacy.[81] Some clinicians have advised early emesis, gastric lavage, and activated charcoal, but these forms of gastrointestinal decontamination are unreasonable in view of the potential for early onset of symptoms and danger of aspiration. *Avoid* giving fats, oils, alcohol, or milk, which increase absorption and increase the risk for aspiration.[80]

For dermal exposures, remove contaminated clothing and wash the exposed area extremely thoroughly with soap and water.

For inhalation exposures, move patient from the toxic environment to fresh air. Monitor for respiratory distress. If cough or difficulty in breathing develops, evaluate for hypoxia, respiratory tract irritation, bronchitis, or pneumonitis.

Provide symptomatic and supportive care as needed (100% humidified supplemental oxygen, endotracheal intubation, assisted ventilation, and inhaled β-adrenergic agonists).

LABORATORY MONITORING

See previous discussion. If prolonged seizures occur, monitor arterial blood gases, body temperature, renal function, creatinine kinase, and the urine for myoglobin.

ANTIDOTES

There are no specific antidotes for camphor toxicity, but *N*-acetylcysteine has been reported effective in preventing liver damage in chronic poisoning.[82]

ELIMINATION

Extracorporeal measures of elimination are not routinely used for camphor poisoning owing to the large distribution of camphor. There are, however, isolated case reports in which both lipid hemodialysis[79] and resin hemoperfusion[83] have been used to lower the blood camphor concentration in severely poisoned patients. Lipid dialysis, however, is no longer recommended because of complications of the therapy, and resin hemoperfusion is no longer available in the United States.[84]

DISPOSITION

Medical evaluation and monitoring for symptoms (CNS depression or seizures) with seizure precautions should be considered for *any* ingestion of camphor of more than 30 mg/kg in a child, more than 1 g in an adult, or

deliberate ingestion. If symptoms of intoxication are present, the patient should be admitted to an intensive care unit.[74,85] Patients who are asymptomatic or who have only mild gastrointestinal symptoms and are asymptomatic for 4 hours after ingestion are at low risk for serious complications.[74,86] Clinically significant camphor toxicity has not been reported below 30 mg/kg of camphor and is uncommon below 50 mg/kg of camphor in asymptomatic patients.[74] Patients who have developed either severe gastrointestinal or neurologic symptoms of poisoning should also be admitted regardless of the amount ingested. Patients should be observed in a monitored setting where immediate anticonvulsant therapy and respiratory support can be provided. Consider transportation by ambulance after any acute ingestion. Seizures may occur suddenly within minutes after ingestion while en route to the emergency department.[84]

REFERENCES

1. Cosmetic talc powder [editorial]. Lancet 1977;1:1348.
2. Mofenson HC, Greensher J, DiTomasso A, et al: Baby powder: a hazard. Pediatrics 1981;68:265.
3. Rohl AN, Langer AM, Selikoff IJ, et al: Consumer talcums and powders: mineral and chemical characterization. J Toxicol Environ Health 1976;2:255.
4. Wehner AP: Biological effects of cosmetic talc. Food Chem Toxicol 1994;32:1173.
5. Pairaudeau PW: Inhalation of baby powder: an unappreciated hazard. BMJ 1991;302:1200–1201.
6. Sparrow SA, Hallam LA: Talc granulomas. BMJ 1991;303:58.
7. Gamble JF: A nested case control study of lung cancer among New York talc workers. Int Arch Occup Environ Health 1993;64:449.
8. Hartge P, Stewart P: Occupation and ovarian cancer: a case-control study in the Washington, DC, metropolitan area, 1978–1981. J Occup Med 1994;36:924.
9. Hughes WT, Kalmer T: Massive talc aspiration: successful treatment with dexamethasone. Am J Dis Child 1966;111:653.
10. Molnar JT, Nathenson G, Edberg S: Fatal aspiration of talcum powder by a child: report of a case. N Engl J Med 1962;266:36.
11. Gould SR, Bernardo ED: Respiratory distress after talc inhalation. Br J Dis Chest 1972;66:230.
12. Pfenniger J, D'Apuzzo V: Powder aspiration in children: report of two cases. Arch Dis Child 1977;52:157.
13. Brouillette F, Weber ML: Massive aspiration of talcum powder by an infant. Can Med Assoc J 1978;119:354.
14. Motomatsu K, Adachi H, Uno T: Two infant deaths after inhaling baby powder. Chest 1979;75:448.
15. Cruthrids TP, Cole FH, Paul RN: Pulmonary talcosis as a result of massive aspiration of baby powder. South Med J 1977;70:626.
16. Watson WA, Litovitz TL, Rodgers GC, et al: 2002 Annual report of the American Association of Poison Control Centers Toxic Exposure Surveillance System. Am J Emerg Med 2003;21:353–421.
17. Harlow BL, Cramer DW, Bell DA, et al: Perineal exposure to talc and ovarian cancer risk. Obstet Gynecol 1992;80:19.
18. Hazardous Substances Data Bank. National Library of Medicine, Bethesda, MD (CD-ROM Version). Micromedex, Inc, Englewood, CO (expires October 31, 1999).
19. Abraham JL, Brambilla C: Particle size for differentiation between inhalation and injection pulmonary talcosis. Environ Res 1980;21:94.
20. Kleinfeld M, Giel CP, Majeranowski JF, et al: Talc pneumoconiosis: a report of six patients with postmortem findings. Arch Environ Health 1963;7:101–115.
21. Goldbach PD, Mohsenifar Z, Abraham JL, et al: Talcum powder pneumoconiosis: diagnosis by transbronchial biopsy using energy-dispersive x-ray analysis. West J Med 1982;136:439–442.
22. Vallyathan NV, Craighead JE: Pulmonary pathology in workers exposed to nonasbestiform talc. Human Pathol 1981;12:28–35.

23. Oubeid M, Bickel JT, Ingram EA, et al: Pulmonary talc granulomatosis in a cocaine sniffer. Chest 1990;98:237–239.

24. Davis LL: Pulmonary "mainline" granulomatosis: talcosis secondary to intravenous heroin abuse with characteristic x-ray findings of asbestosis. J Natl Med Assoc 1983;75:1225–1228.

25. Ben-Haim SA, Ben-Ami H, Edoute Y, et al: Talcosis presenting as pulmonary infiltrates in an HIV-positive heroin addict. Chest 1988;94:656–658.

26. Bouchama A, Chastre J, Gaudichet, A et al: Acute pneumonitis with bilateral pleural effusion after talc pleurodesis. Chest 1984;86:795–797.

27. Cruthirds TP, Cole FH, Paul RN: Pulmonary talcosis as a result of massive aspiration of baby powder. South Med J 1977;70:626–628.

28. Craig SA: Radiology. In Ford MD, Delaney KA, Ling LJ, Erickson T (eds): Clinical Toxicology. Philadelphia, WB Saunders, 2001, p 65.

29. Lund JS, Feldt-Rasmussen M: Accidental aspiration of talc: report of a case in a 2 year old child. Acta Pediatr Med Scand 1969;58:295–296.

30. Redondo AA, Ettensohn DB, Khan M, et al: Bronchoalveolar lavage in talc induced lung disease. Thorax 1988;43:1019–1021.

31. De Vuyst P, Dumortier P, Leophonte P: Bronchoalveolar lavage in talc induced lung disease [letter]. Thorax 1989;44:607.

32. Woods WG: An introduction to boron: history, sources, uses, and chemistry. Environ Health Perspect 1994;102S:5.

33. Lister J: The clinical use of boric acid. Surg Gynecol Obstet 1945;80:651–652.

34. Gordon AS, Prichard JD, Freedman MH: Seizure disorders and anemia associated with chronic borax intoxication. Can Med Assoc J 1973;108:719–724.

35. Wong LC, Heimbach, Truscott DR, Duncan BD: Boric acid poisoning: report of 11 cases. Can Med Assoc J 1964;90:1018–1023.

36. Goldbloom RB, Goldbloom A: Boric acid poisoning: report of four cases and a review of 109 cases from the world literature. J Pediatr 1953;43:631.

37. Linden CH, Hall AH, Kulig KW, et al: Acute ingestions of boric acid. Clin Toxicol 1986;24:269–279.

38. Litovitz TL, Klein-Schwartz W, Oderda GM, et al: Clinical manifestations of toxicity in a series of 784 boric acid ingestions. Am J Emerg Med 1988;6:209–213.

39. Restuccio A, Mortensen ME, Kelley MT: Fatal ingestion of boric acid in an adult. Am J Emerg Med 1992;10:545–547.

40. Watson WA, Litovitz TL, Rodgers GC, et al: 2002 Annual report of the American Association of Poison Control Centers Toxic Exposure Surveillance System. Am J Emerg Med 2003;21:353–421.

41. Skipworth GB, Goldstein N, McBride WP: Boric acid intoxication from "medicated talcum powder." Arch Dermatol 1967;95:83.

42. Ducey J, Williams DB: Transcutaneous absorption of boric acid. J Pediatr 1953;43:644.

43. Brooke C, Boggs T: Boric acid poisoning: report of a case and review of the literature. Am J Dis Child 1951;82:465.

44. Schillinger BM, Berstein M, Goldberg LA, et al: Boric acid poisoning. J Am Acad Dermatol 1982;7:667–673.

45. Jordon JW, Crissey JT: Boric acid poisoning: a report of a fatal adult case from cutaneous use. A critical evaluation of the use of this drug in dermatologic practice. Arch Dermatol 1957;75:720.

46. Fisher RS, Freimuth HC: Blood boron levels in human infants. J Invest Dermatol 1958;50:85.

47. Friis-Hansen B, Aggerbeck B, Aas Jansen J: Unaffected blood boron levels in newborn infants treated with a boric acid ointment. Food Chem Toxicol 1982;20:451.

48. Baker MD, Bogema SC: Ingestion of boric acid by infants. Am J Emerg Med 1986;4:358.

49. McNally WD, Rust CA: The distribution of boric acid in human organs in six deaths due to boric acid poisoning. JAMA 1928;90:382.

50. Toxicology update: boron, boric acid, borates, and boron oxide. J Appl Toxicol 1992;12:149–152.

51. Ishii Y, Fujizuka N, Takahashi T, et al: A fatal case of acute boric acid poisoning. Clin Toxicol 1993;31:345.

52. Teshima D, Taniyama T, Oishi R: Usefulness of forced diuresis for acute boric acid poisoning in an adult. J Clin Pharm Ther 2001;26:387–390.

53. Valdes-Depena MA, Arey JB: Boric acid poisoning: three fatal cases with pancreatic inclusions and a review of the literature. J Pediatr 1962;61:534–546.

54. Garabrant DH, Bernstein L, Peters JM, et al: Respiratory and eye irritation from boron oxide and boric acid dusts. J Occup Med 1984;26:584–586.

55. Garabrant DH, Bernstein L, Peters JM, et al: Respiratory effects of borax dust. Br J Ind Med 1985;42:831–837.

56. Hu X, Wegman DH, Eisen EA, et al: Dose related acute irritant symptom responses to occupational exposure to sodium borate dusts. Br J Indust Med 1992;49:706–713.

57. U.S. Department of Health and Human Services: Toxicological Profile for Boron and Compounds. Life Systems, Inc., for the Agency for Toxic Substances and Disease Registry, US PHS, 1992.

58. Rubinstein AD, Musher DM: Epidemic boric acid poisoning simulating staphylococcal toxic epidermolysis in a newborn Ritter's disease. J Pediatr 1970;77:884.

59. Oderda GM, Klein-Schwartz W, Insley BM: In vitro study of boric acid and activated charcoal. J Toxicol Clin Toxicol 1987;25:13–19.

60. Boggs TR, Anrode HG: Boric acid and exchange transfusion. Pediatrics 1955;16:109–114.

61. Segar WE: Peritoneal dialysis in the treatment of boric acid poisoning. N Engl J Med 1960;262:798–800.

62. Baliah T, MacLeish H, Drummond KN: Acute boric acid poisoning: report of an infant successfully treated by peritoneal dialysis. Can Med Assoc J 1969;101:166–168.

63. Martin GI: Asymptomatic boric acid intoxication. N Y State Med J 1971;71:1842–1844.

64. Smith AG, Margolis G: Camphor poisoning: anatomical and pharmacologic study. Report of a fatal case; experimental investigation of protective effect of barbiturate Am J Pathol 1954;30:857–868.

65. Grieve M: Camphor: A modern herbal. Available at http://botanical.com.

66. Fink M: Meduna and the origins of convulsive therapy. Am J Psychiatry 1984;141:1034.

67. Kauffman RE, Banner W, Berlin CM, et al: Camphor revisited: focus on toxicity. Pediatrics 1984;94:127–128.

68. Poison treatment drug products for over-the-counter human uses tentative final monograph. Fed Reg 1985;50:2244–2262.

69. Watson WA, Litovitz TL, Rodgers GC, et al: 2002 Annual report of the American Association of Poison Control Centers Toxic Exposure Surveillance System. Am J Emerg Med 2003;21:353–421.

70. Aronow R: Camphor poisoning [editorial]. JAMA 1976;235:1290.

71. Koppel C, Tenczer J, Scirop T, et al: Camphor poisoning. Arch Toxicol 1982;51:101.

72. Trestrail JH, Spartz ME: Camphorated and castor oil confusion and its toxic results. Clin Toxicol 1977;11:151.

73. Skoutakis VA, Koumbourlis TC: Camphor intoxication: diagnosis and management. Clin Toxicol Consultant 1981;3:131.

74. Briggs GG, Freeman RK, Yaffe SJ: Drugs in Pregnancy and Lactation, 5th ed. Baltimore, Williams & Wilkins, 1998, p 115.

75. Geller RJ, Spyker DA, Garretson LK, et al: Camphor toxicity: development of a triage strategy. Vet Hum Toxicol 1984;26 (Suppl 2):8–10.

76. Phelan WJ III: Camphor poisoning: the over-the-counter dangers. Pediatrics 1976;57:428–430.

77. Enez JF, Brown AL, Arnold WC, et al: Chronic camphor poisoning mimicking Reyes' syndrome. Gastroenterology 1983;84:394–398.

78. Weiss J, Catalano P: Camphorated oil. Pediatrics 1973;52:713.

79. Antman E, Jacob G, Volpe B, et al: Camphor overdosage. N Y State J Med 1978;78:896.

80. Camphor monograph. MICROMEDEX Healthcare Series Vol. 118 (expires December 2003).

81. Dean BS, Burdick JD, Goetz PD: In vivo evaluation of the adsorptive capacity of activated charcoal for Camphor. Vet Hum Toxicol 1992;34:297–299.

82. Riggs JR, Hamilton R, Homel S, et al: Camphorated oil intoxication in pregnancy. Obstet Gynecol 1965;25:255–258.

83. Kopelman R, Miller S, Kelly R, et al: Camphor intoxication treated by resin hemoperfusion. JAMA 1979;241:727–728.

84. Gibson DE, Moore GP, Pfaff JA: Camphor ingestion. Am J Emerg Med 1989;7:41–43.

85. Goium S, Patel H: Unusual cause of seizure. Pediatr Emerg Care 1996;12:298–300.

86. Kresel JJ: Camphor. Clin Toxic Rev 1982;7:1.

87. Koeppel C, Martens F, Schirop T, et al: Hemoperfusion in acute camphor poisoning. Intensive Care Med 1988;14:431–433.

100 Cosmetics and Toilet Articles

THOMAS R. CARACCIO, PHARMD, RPH ■ R. B. MCFEE, DO, MPH

At a Glance...

- Alcohols (hair spray, cologne) ingested by children can cause hypoglycemia and central nervous system (CNS) depression.
- Oxidizers and corrosives such as thioglycolic acid and sodium bromate (hair waving agents) can cause severe burns and erosions to the skin, gastrointestinal (GI) tract, or eyes depending on the route of exposure. Bromate ingestion produces GI symptoms within 30 minutes and can lead to profound, irreversible renal failure that can result in death.
- Acetonitrile (artificial nail remover), which is metabolized to cyanide, can cause respiratory failure, convulsions, and death.
- Nitroalkane or nitroethane (artificial nail removers) can cause methemoglobinemia and respiratory distress.
- Cosmetics, especially face and skin care products, cause approximately 10% of contact dermatitis cases. Reactions range from the irritant contact form of dermatitis to allergic contact dermatitis and contact urticaria.
- With the exception of acetonitrile (cyanide antidote kit), management of cosmetic toxicity primarily consists of symptomatic and supportive care.
- Decontamination of skin and ocular exposures should consist of copious irrigation guided by bidirectional pH paper until neutral pH is obtained and symptoms have resolved.

INTRODUCTION AND RELEVANT HISTORY

The term *cosmetics* refers to a broad range of products—synthetic and natural—used to enhance appearance or improve hygiene.[1-3] The ancient Egyptians and Romans used creams for beautification.[1] Queen Cleopatra was well known for her use of cosmetics and skin creams.[1] In the late 19th century, women used belladonna alkaloids to dilate their pupils to make their eyes appear more attractive.[3] Virtually all cultures have utilized a variety of powders, creams, and other preparations to enhance beauty and adorn and decorate the human body. Such preparations range from colorful makeup including henna, to hair dyes, tattoos, body paints, feathers, and skin piercing. Some of these applications are permanent, others temporary to suit a particular function. The cosmetic industry is a multi-billion-dollar per year enterprise. As society increasingly becomes preoccupied with youthful appearance, the demand for new products including topical applications has grown significantly. Although historically cosmetic products were developed from plants and herbs, most of these substances in contemporary society are synthetic.[1,3] Ingredients of synthetic cosmetics are contributing to the increasing incidence of skin reactions termed *cosmetic dermatitis*[1,4,5] (Table 100-1).

From a regulatory standpoint, according to the U.S. Food and Drug Administration (FDA) Federal Food, Drugs and Cosmetics Act (FDCA) of 1938, the term *cosmetic* is defined as "articles intended to be rubbed, sprinkled, sprayed, introduced into, or otherwise applied to the human body, or any part thereof, for cleansing, beautifying, promoting attractiveness, or altering the appearance without affecting the body's structure or functions."[1-3,6,7] Critical to an agent being classified as a cosmetic is the understanding that the product will not be toxic when used according to labeled instructions.[2,8] Cosmetics come not only under the auspices of the FDA; they must also follow requirements of the 1970 U.S. Poison Prevention Packaging Act, the Fair Packaging and Label Act of 1966, and the Color Additives Amendments to the FDCA of 1962.[7] The FDA in 21 CFR 720.4 describes 13 categories of products designated "cosmetics" that contain a total of 66 product types[7,9] (Table 100-2). These regulations notwithstanding, the manufacturer is responsible for assuring the safety of cosmetics. Of interest, premarket approval of cosmetics is not required. No product can be marketed if it contains "a poisonous or deleterious substance, which may render it injurious to health" (FDCA Section 601).[7] Some cosmetics, namely, hair-coloring preparations, are permitted to include dyes that are not on the FDA safety list.[2] The product packaging must clearly state, "Caution: this preparation contains ingredients that may cause skin irritation in certain individuals, and a preliminary test according to accompanying directions should first be made. This product must *not* be used for dyeing eyelashes or eyebrows; to do so may cause blindness." The

TABLE 100-1 Most Frequently Identified Ingredients Causing Cosmetic Dermatitis*

RANK	CATEGORY	NUMBER OF PREPARATIONS/ FORMULATIONS
1	Fragrance Ingredients	161
2	Preservatives	149
3	p-Phenylenediamine (PPD)	41
4	Lanolin and derivatives	29
5	Glyceryl thioglycolate	25
6	Propylene glycol	25
7	Toluene sulfonamide/formaldehyde resin	23
8	Sunscreen and other UV absorbers	20
9	Methacrylate	9
10	Others (≤3)	56
Total		536

*Data from Adams RM, Maibach IH: A five-year study of cosmetic reactions. J Am Acad Dermatol 1985;13:1062–1069.

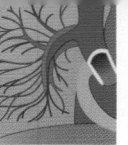

TABLE 100-2 Cosmetic Product Categories*

CATEGORY	PRODUCT TYPE	CATEGORY	PRODUCT TYPE
Baby products	Shampoos Lotions Oils Powders Creams Other baby products	Makeup preparations (not for eyes)	Blushers (all types) Face powders Foundations Leg and body paints Lipsticks Makeup bases
Bath preparations	Bath oils, tablets, salts Bubble bath preparations Bath capsules Other bath preparations		Rouges Makeup fixatives Other makeup preparations
Eye makeup preparations	Eyebrow pencil Eyeliner Eye shadow Eye lotion Eye makeup remover Mascara Other eye makeup preparations	Manicuring preparations	Basecoats and undercoats Cuticle softeners Nail creams and lotions Nail polishes and enamel Nail polish and enamel removers Other manicuring preparations
		Oral hygiene products	Dentrifices (aerosol, liquid, paste, and powder)
Fragrance preparations	Perfumes, colognes, and toilet waters Powders (dusting and talcum, excluding aftershave talc) Sachets Other fragrance preparations		Mouthwashes and breath fresheners (liquid and powder) Other oral hygiene products
		Personal cleanliness	Bath soaps and detergents Douches Feminine hygiene deodorants Other personal cleanliness products
Hair preparations (noncoloring)	Hair conditioners Hair sprays (aerosol fixatives) Hair straighteners Permanent wave solutions Rinses (noncoloring) Shampoos (noncoloring) Tonics, dressings, and other hair grooming aids Wave sets Other hair preparations	Shaving preparations	Aftershave lotions Beard softeners Men's talcum Preshave lotions (all types) Shaving cream (aerosol, brushless, lather) Shaving soap (cakes, sticks, etc) Other shaving preparations
Hair coloring preparations	Hair dyes and colors (*all* types require a caution statement and patch test) Hair tints Hair rinses (coloring) Hair shampoos (coloring) Hair color sprays (aerosol) Hair lighteners with color Hair bleaches Other hair coloring preparations	Skin care preparations (creams, lotions, powders, and sprays)	Cleansing (cold creams, cleansing lotions, liquids, and pads) Depilatories Face and neck (excluding shaving preparations) Body and hand (excluding shaving preparations) Foot powders and sprays Moisturizing Nighttime preparations Paste masks (mud packs) Skin fresheners Other skin preparations
		Suntan preparations	Suntan gels, creams, and liquids Indoor tanning preparations Other suntan preparations

*Data from Code of Federal Regulations, Title 21, Vol. 7 (21 CFR 710), Food and Drug Administration, Center for Food Safety and Applied Nutrition. Washington, DC, U.S. Government Printing Office, Rev. April 1, 2002.

instructions accompanying these products must include directions to perform a patch test 24 hours prior to applying the preparation.

In terms of product safety, producers rely heavily on historical safety data, structure-activity studies, and validated in vitro testing to demonstrate the safety of their products.[7]

Several resources are available to provide in-depth toxicity information on chemicals utilized in the production of cosmetics. These include the *International Journal of Toxicology*, which reports evaluations by the Cosmetic Ingredient Review (CIR) Expert Panel of the Cosmetic, Toiletry and Fragrance Association (CTFA).

The chemical ingredient can be identified in the CTFA Cosmetic Ingredient Dictionary, which is available through the Cosmetic Toiletry and Fragrance Association, located in Washington, DC.[2] Cosmetic manufacturers also file cosmetic ingredient composition with the FDA. The FDA Cosmetic Information Center can be accessed via a toll-free number: 1 (800) 270-8869. Labeling, ingredients, dyes, and sun care product information are available as well as instructions for reporting adverse reactions.

Historically, most categories of cosmetics are considered to pose a very low risk of toxicity beyond dermal reactions.[1,2,10,11] However, certain categories—notably, artificial nail removers and hair straightening products—

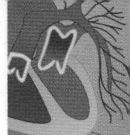

contain a variety of chemicals that pose a moderate to severe toxicity risk.[1-3,12-19] Alcohol-containing products also pose a serious poisoning risk.[18] Like most toxicants, primary routes of exposure are ingestion and topical exposures, which include the skin and the eyes.[2,11,19,20] Caution must always be exercised to prevent children from becoming exposed to cosmetics. Many of these products pose a greater health risk in overdose or unintentional ingestion to children than to adults. This is especially true of alcohol-containing products such as colognes and perfumes.

EPIDEMIOLOGY

Cosmetics and personal care products resulted in 224,792 calls to poison centers in 2004 according to the American Association of Poison Control Centers Toxic Exposure Surveillance System (TESS).[19] Of these calls, 38,081 involved adults; the majority—185,862—involved children and represented the leading category (13.4%) of toxicant affecting children 6 years of age and younger. Three deaths were associated with cosmetics, including that of a 72-year-old man who intentionally ingested a large amount of aftershave and a 39-year-old and a 54-year-old who both ingested mouthwash. Only ethanol-containing products were associated with fatalities. Overall, this category is associated with mostly mild to nontoxic exposures: 69,465 (96%) were considered mild to none in severity, and 14,334 were referred to a health-care facility (HCF). Contrast this with 279,955 analgesic category exposures, which were responsible for 658 deaths.

HAIR PRODUCTS

Hair care products include hair colors, hair lighteners, hair waving agents, hair straighteners, hair sprays, shampoos, and conditioners.[1-3] Most of these products, such as the shampoos, have low or virtually no risk of toxicity. The hair lighteners, straighteners, and waving agents that contain oxidizers and potential corrosives pose a greater risk to health especially when misused or ingested.[21]

Epidemiology

According to TESS[19] in 2004 there were 2347 hair coloring–related exposures, for which the following numbers of patients were sent to an HCF: 355 with no toxicity, 585 with mild toxicity, 135 with toxicity of moderate severity, 2 with major severity, and there were no deaths. Hair relaxing agents with sodium hydroxide (NaOH) accounted for 768 exposures. Of those referred to an HCF, 151 were relatively nontoxic, 268 were mildly toxic, 96 were of moderate severity, 1 was major, and there were no deaths. Hair relaxing agents with other alkaline ingredients accounted for 847 cases. Again, there were no deaths, and most cases were of mild to moderate severity. For the nonalkaline hair relaxers, there were 66 cases. Permanent wave solutions accoun-

ted for 397 cases. Of these, 68 were nontoxic, 117 mild, 52 moderate, and 0 severe. There were no deaths. Hair spray accounted for 2165 calls, but there were only nine major exposures and the rest were predominantly nontoxic or mildly toxic. Of the 6175 hair shampoo calls, 64 were moderately severe cases and 2 major.

HAIR COLORS

Hair color products are categorized as either permanent or semipermanent. Permanent hair colors contain oxidizing agents and dye intermediates in a 1:1 concentration. The oxidizer interacts with a dye intermediate to cause color molecules to adhere to the hair shaft. The oxidizer is usually hydrogen peroxide (H_2O_2)—most commonly a 6% solution by volume although 12% solutions are available. H_2O_2 oxidizes while lightening the hair. Usually greater than 10% H_2O_2 is associated with toxicity although large ingestions of 6% H_2O_2 can cause gastritis. Commonly used dyes include *p*-phenylenediamine, resorcinol, and aminophenols. *Para*-phenylenediamine (PPD) and *para*-aminophenol undergo oxidation to reactive imine compounds. Resorcinol reacts with imines to produce the final colors.

Toxicology

Para-phenylenediamine can cause local irritation, or urticaria. PPD toxicity can include angioneurotic edema presenting from 2 to 24 hours postexposure. A 20-year-old adult who ingested 40 mL of 4% solution experienced angioneurotic edema, hemolysis, and renal failure. The patient survived after 13 days of hemodialysis. Rhabdomyolysis, renal failure, acute tubular necrosis, and disseminated intravascular coagulation (DIC) can occur.[22] Aromatic nitro- and amino-compounds can become cyanogenic at toxic levels. These products also may contain soaps, water, isopropanol, ammonia, propylene glycol, and glycerin. These additional ingredients confer viscosity and enhance penetration. Hydrogen sulfide and ammonia are used to hasten the dying process. Ammonia can produce a pH of 9.5; scalp burns have resulted.

Other chemicals in hair dyes include toluene, diamine, ammonium hydroxide, sodium sulfite, and sodium hydroxide. Semipermanent hair colors contain propylene glycol, isopropanol, fatty acids, alkanolamines, and dyes. Permanent hair colors contain oxidizers; semipermanent hair colors do not. Some hair colors, such as "Grecian Formula" contain lead acetate.[2,3] These progressive hair dyes contain less than 0.6% elemental lead with elemental sulfur in an alcohol vehicle. Lead forms insoluble oxides and the sulfides impart a darker color to gray hair when exposed to air. Lead hair dyes produce lead-coated hands with 150 to 700 mg per hand. While the potential for lead exposure exists, to date lead toxicity has not been reported as a result of this residue.[17]

Diagnosis

The diagnosis of oxidizing agents is usually made by history.

Laboratory tests may assist management in terms of monitoring electrolytes, blood alcohol concentration, and cardiac and respiratory function.

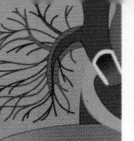

Management

If ingested, oxidizing agents are toxic. However, the ammonia or ethanolamine present in these products is highly emetogenic, making it unlikely that a quantity sufficient to cause toxicity would be ingested.[23] Nonetheless, if ingestion occurs, copious rinsing of the mouth is important. Symptomatic and supportive care are the mainstay of therapy.

Symptomatic patients and children with large ingestions should be referred to an HCF. Activated charcoal may mask erosions if endoscopic evaluation is necessary; its administration is discouraged. Some suggest drinking milk after rinsing the mouth with water as a method to alleviate GI irritation.[2] Syrup of ipecac (SOI) is not recommended. Beyond the fact many of these products are emetogenic, the potential for exacerbating gastric irritation and damage compared with the low potential for altering outcome militates against the use of SOI. Large-volume dilution may increase the likelihood of exothermic reactions. Since these products contain multiple ingredients, including alcohols, H_2O_2, and other chemicals, management should be directed at likely toxicants. For example, individuals with low hepatic glycogen reserve and impaired gluconeogenesis due to an alcohol-depleting nicotinamide adenine dinucleotide (NAD) may be at greater risk for hypoglycemia when exposed to hair-coloring products containing alcohols. Children, malnourished patients, and chronically ill patients are especially susceptible. Ingestions of greater than 1 mL of 50% ethanol/kg can produce a blood alcohol concentration of 50 mg/dL or greater. Since these patients may develop symptoms consistent with hypotension or hypoglycemia, they should be referred to an HCF.[24] H_2O_2 decomposes and liberates oxygen. Large ingestions of H_2O_2 can be expected to cause mild-to-moderate gastritis.[3] If a "Grecian Formula" product is ingested, it is prudent to obtain blood lead levels.[2,17]

Ocular exposures require immediate and copious eye irrigation. If the product contains 6% H_2O_2, injury usually is limited to burning and itching of the conjunctiva with no long-term sequelae if appropriate decontamination is initiated. Irrigation should continue for at least 15 to 20 minutes. If discomfort persists, continue irrigation and consider an ophthalmology consult. Higher H_2O_2 concentration exposures require immediate saline irrigation, ocular examination by a trained health care professional, and referral to an ophthalmologist. Skin exposure is unlikely to cause toxicity. However, some individuals may be hypersensitive to some of the ingredients or exhibit allergic reactions. A good outcome is expected with symptomatic and supportive care including washing the affected area completely with water and hypoallergenic soap. Antihistamines may be administered. No specific antidotes are available for hair-coloring products.

Disposition

With appropriate intervention, most patients survive the exposure to hair colors with good outcomes.

Prevention

Keeping these products out of the reach of young children is critical to reducing this pattern of pediatric exposure and injury. Using the product only as directed will also reduce the risk from hair colors.

HAIR LIGHTENERS

Hair lighteners—often referred to as "hair bleaches"—are used to give hair a lighter color or as preparation for dye applications. In addition to the oxidizer H_2O_2 found in hair colors, other oxidizers are used, including ammonia and potassium or sodium persulfate. These agents intensify and speed the lightening process. Additional ingredients including metasilicates and detergents may be present to thicken, disperse, or stabilize the color.

Toxicology

Lightener solutions usually have a pH in the range of 9.5 to 11.5. Alkaline agents are corrosive irritants and, depending on the dose and duration of exposure, can cause GI irritation and ocular injury. Concentrated solutions of persulfates are irritating to the skin and mucous membranes. Ammonium persulfate can cause urticaria and anaphylactoid reactions. Owing to the powerful and offensive odors (and presumably taste) of many of these products, unintentional ingestion is unlikely. Intentional ingestion can produce clinically significant toxicity manifested by vomiting, hematemesis, and diarrhea.

Diagnosis

Most exposures are readily identified by history.

Laboratory testing should be tailored to the clinical situation and ingredients present in the preparation.

Management

Ingestion of products containing corrosive alkali agents should be managed in the same way as for any highly irritating corrosive chemical. Referral to an HCF, availability of endoscopic evaluation, and access to an intensive care unit usually are advised if the patient is symptomatic. Allergic or anaphylactoid reactions to hair-coloring agents should be managed per standard protocol, which includes close attention to cardiovascular/respiratory function. Oxygen and antihistamines (H_1 and H_2), fluid support, and bronchodilators if the clinical situation warrants, are administered. Ocular exposures require immediate and copious saline irrigation. While Morgan lenses may not be necessary, testing with pH paper to determine the effectiveness of decontamination, ocular examination by a trained health care professional, and referral to an ophthalmologist are warranted.

Disposition

Hair-coloring products are generally considered low toxicity exposures. Appropriate intervention and minimal toxicity offer good long-term outcomes.

Prevention

Keeping these products away from children and using the preparations as directed are critical to reducing the pediatric injury pattern.

HAIR WAVING AGENTS

The process of hair waving involves altering the molecular structure of hair during the stepwise process

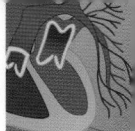

of softening, followed by reshaping or curling, then finally hardening. Most hair waving solutions contain thioglycolate, which softens and straightens hair by breaking the sulfhydryl bonds. Other softeners in addition to thioglycolate and thioglycolic acid salts include sodium sulfite and ammonium sulfite. Hydrogen peroxide or sodium bromate in dilute acidic solution are used to halt the process as desired results are approached. Some permanent wave products contain 2% to 8% (weight/volume) mercuric chloride.[3] Neutralizers in hair waving agents usually contain bromates. Sodium borate or perborate also is used (see Chapter 99).

Diagnosis

Most exposures are readily identified by history.

Laboratory testing should be tailored to the clinical situation and ingredients of the preparation. To obtain blood concentration of bromate in the serum, specify bromate exposure. However, serum bromate levels do not correlate with the severity of the intoxication. Intervention should not be delayed in lieu of laboratory results. Electrolytes, ethanol levels, complete blood count, methemoglobin, and renal function tests should be obtained.

Toxicology and Management

Thioglycolic acids are toxic corrosives. Ingestions can cause irritation of the mouth and throat accompanied by nausea, vomiting, and possibly diarrhea. Thioglycolate can cause immediate-type hypersensitivity reaction. In large amounts, it can cause hypoglycemia and cyanosis. Mercuric chloride as a toxicant can cause erosive oral and GI effects, which, if the exposure is significant, may cause hemorrhage and shock. A potentially lethal oral dose is 10 to 50 mg/kg.[20] The softening agents ammonium or sodium sulfite are alkaline with pH ranging from 7.0 to 8.5. They are GI irritants. Rinsing the mouth or exposed area is usually all that is necessary. Milk may provide symptomatic relief. Ocular exposure to any of these compounds requires immediate irrigation and possible referral to an ophthalmologist.

Bromates are very toxic. Contact between bromate-containing neutralizers and the skin or eyes can cause erythema, burning, and edema. Copious irrigation with soap and water usually is sufficient intervention. Very concentrated solutions (2%) at doses of 1 to 2 teaspoons (1.5 to 3 g) can produce serious toxicity in children between the ages of 1 to 3 years.[3] The toxic dose in children is estimated to be 250 to 500 mg/kg.[3] A 5-g ingestion can potentially lead to fatality with a 10-g ingestion representing a lethal dose in adults.[2,12] Fortunately, few fatalities have been reported. No fatalities were reported in 2002 TESS. GI symptoms can occur within 30 minutes postingestion. Upon ingestion, significant gastroenteritis may result from the production of hydrobromic acid. Hypotension can ensue. The route of elimination for bromates is renal, and renal failure is the primary cause of death.[12,13] Renal impairment may first present as anuria or oliguria within 24 hours. Bromate poisoning may present similarly to hemolytic uremic syndrome. Hemolysis and thrombocy-

topenias have been reported. Bromates may act as an oxidizing agent converting hemoglobin to methemoglobin, although this is infrequently reported. If methemoglobinemia occurs, do not use methylene blue because it may exacerbate bromate toxicity. Patients should respond to oxygen and symptomatic and supportive care. If toxicity is severe, exchange transfusion may be considered. Neurosensory hearing loss and tinnitus may occur within 24 hours. Irreversible otic and renal damage may occur. Central nervous system (CNS) depression and seizures may occur. Ocular exposure should be treated with copious water or saline irrigation. Ophthalmology referral is recommended owing to the significant alkalinity of bromates.

Sodium borate breaks down into borate and peroxide and is less toxic than bromates.[3,20] However, a 3- to 6-g ingestion is potentially lethal to children with 15 to 30 g being similarly lethal to adults. Skin manifestation to borates can lead to desquamation and erythematous rash commonly found over palms, soles, buttocks, and scrotum. This may progress to exfoliation. CNS symptoms include irritability, headache, and restlessness, seizures, and coma, depending on the exposure. GI symptoms include nausea, vomiting, and diarrhea. Acute tubular necrosis may lead to renal failure.[3,20]

Disposition

This category of cosmetic poses a greater threat to health owing to the toxicity of bromates and borates in addition to the oxidizer H_2O_2. Few deaths are reported. With rapid symptomatic and supportive care, benign outcomes can be expected.

HAIR STRAIGHTENERS

Of all the hair care products, hair straighteners pose the greatest threat to health and are extremely toxic.[1-3,19,20,25] They contain 1% to 3% sodium hydroxide, ammonium hydroxide, potassium carbonate, or bicarbonate. Precise adherence to application instruction is critical when using these products. They are highly alkaline and pose a risk for liquefaction necrosis. The typical pH is 13. Prolonged exposure with hair and scalp may cause injury.[2] Ingestion or ocular exposure must be considered a medical emergency.[2,20,25]

Diagnosis

Most exposures are readily identified by history.

Laboratory testing should be tailored to the clinical situation and ingredients of the preparation. No test is required if the ingestion is no more than a "sip."[20] Otherwise, complete blood count (CBC), serum electrolytes, and renal function tests should be obtained. In patients exhibiting respiratory symptoms, arterial blood gases and chest radiographs should be obtained. For patients with suspected perforation, abdominal radiographs should be obtained in addition to chest radiographs. Gastrointestinal endoscopy should be performed within 24 hours of a large ingestion or for patients who have diminished voice, stridor, drooling, or vomiting.

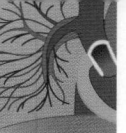

Toxicology and Management

Hair straighteners are highly toxic alkaline agents that can cause severe burns, irritation, and erosions. They should be treated as aggressively as any other caustic exposure. Ingestion requires immediate referral to an HCF. Treatment should focus on airway control, keeping in mind that severe GI damage including strictures and obstructions may occur. Hemodynamic function and assessment of burn function are critical.[2,3,20,25] Because the rate of GI and esophageal mucosal injury is rapid there is concern about using dilution as an intervention. Symptomatic and supportive care are critical, as is referral to gastroenterology and general surgery for evaluation. Steroids such as dexamethasone 0.1 mg/kg or prednisone 1 to 2.5 mg/kg for 3 weeks have been recommended for grade II burns to reduce stricture formation by some but are considered controversial. Steroids are not usually necessary for grade I burns and are to be avoided in grade III exposures because of the risk of perforation. Hypovolemia and shock, bleeding, tissue necrosis, metabolic acidosis, and renal failure are usual complications.

Disposition

Deliberate ingestions usually are large doses and result in complications or death.[19,20,25] Long-term sequelae include anatomic changes to the GI tract including pyloric stenosis, bleeding, stricture formation, fistula, or perforation. Patients who develop esophageal burns and stricture are at increased risk for esophageal cancer.[20] Children with small "sip" or "taste" exposures usually have benign outcomes.[19]

HAIR SPRAYS

Hair sprays are one of the least toxic categories of hair care product.[2,3,19,20] When ingested, quantities and concentrations usually are small. There are two delivery formulations: liquid pump and aerosols that rely on propellants such as butane, propane, or isobutane. Hair spray products contain a solvent—usually denatured ethanol—and resin polymers—vinyl acetate, methyl vinyl ether, and acrylamides.[2,3] The resins are delivered in the solvent. Ethyl alcohol can constitute up to 95% of the product preparation.

Diagnosis

Blood ethanol levels, CBC, electrolytes, and frequent glucose levels should be obtained in moderate- to large-dose ingestions of ethanol-containing products.

Toxicology and Management

Hair sprays are generally low toxicity products posing little risk when ingested in small quantities, sprayed on intact skin of nonsensitive individuals, or sprayed in the eye in a small amount. There are no specific antidotes. Symptomatic and supportive care is the mainstay of therapy. Ingestions of large volumes of ethanol-based hair sprays should be treated as any ethanol toxic exposure. Ethanol is metabolized by the enzyme alcohol dehydrogenase. Ethanol overdose can cause hypoglycemia and CNS depression in addition to electrolyte derangement. If hair spray is sprayed into the eyes, rinsing with clean warm water or saline is usually sufficient, and a benign outcome is expected. If symptoms persist, evaluation by an ophthalmologist is recommended.

Disposition

Most exposures are unintentional and thus low in dose with expected benign outcomes. Long-term sequelae are not expected.

SHAMPOOS, CONDITIONERS, SOAPS, AND BATH OILS

This category of cosmetics is of very low toxicity. Most shampoos are composed of anionic and nonanionic surfactants, perfumes, and high levels of water. They may contain small amounts of ethanol. Dry shampoos contain methanol or isopropyl alcohol. Bath salts are primarily inorganic salts—usually sodium chloride—which is nontoxic. Electrolyte derangements can occur in large ingestions. Soaps and bubble bath preparations are similar to shampoos and are generally considered nontoxic. Mild toxicity and GI irritation can occur in moderate ingestions. Bath oils are primarily composed of surfactants, emulsifiers, preservatives, and mineral or vegetable oils, which are nontoxic.[2,20] Aspiration of bath oils like other oils can cause a chemical lipoid pneumonia. Some bath oils have essential oils as ingredients, including eucalyptus or pennyroyal. Pennyroyal (pulegium) is an essential oil found in *Hedeoma pulegioides* and *Mentha pulegium* plants as well as some herbal teas. Skin exposure is rarely problematic unless the individual is sensitive to one or more of the ingredients in which case a hypersensitivity reaction or cosmetic dermatitis may occur.[1,2,20]

Epidemiology

There were 6175 exposures reported to TESS of which 4827 involved young children.[19] There were no deaths, and only 2 exposures were considered major toxicity exposures. The majority were considered nontoxic or minor toxicity exposures.[19]

Kinetics

Isopropyl alcohol is rapidly absorbed and distributed, with a volume of distribution of 0.6 L/kg. It is metabolized by alcohol dehydrogenase to acetone with a half-life of 2.5 to 3 hours. The toxic oral dose of 70% isopropyl alcohol is 0.5 to 1 mL/kg.

Diagnosis

Laboratory tests are unnecessary for most ingestions in this category. For essential oil or alcohol ingestions or symptomatic exposures, electrolytes, CBC, glucose monitoring, coagulation studies, liver and renal function tests, urinalysis, electrocardiogram (ECG), and aspirin and acetaminophen levels should be obtained. For patients who have ingested isopropyl alcohol, the following laboratory tests should be obtained: serum isopropyl alcohol, acetone level, serum osmolality and osmolar gaps, electrolytes, glucose, renal function tests, arterial blood gases, and oximetry. Cardiopulmonary function should be monitored.

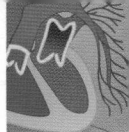

Toxicology and Management

Shampoos, conditioners, soaps, and bath salts are generally considered nontoxic products. If ingested, shampoo is nontoxic and will most likely cause mild GI discomfort and nausea. Large ingestions of isopropyl alcohol or other alcohol-containing products should be managed as any potential alcohol toxicity, with special attention to hypoglycemia, electrolytes, and airway management. Isopropyl alcohol is a significant CNS depressant that can lead to coma or respiratory arrest. Large ingestions can cause myocardial suppression and hypotension.[26] There are no antidotes. Owing to the rapidity of absorption and distribution, emesis is not likely to confer benefit and may be deleterious. Activated charcoal may be useful in spite of the fact that it has marginal adsorbing ability for alcohol; however, it is estimated that 1 g of activated charcoal can bind 1 mL of 70% alcohol[26] (see Chapter 31).

Ocular exposures usually require only copious irrigation with warm water or saline. Long-term damage to the eye is unlikely. Symptomatic and supportive care is the mainstay of therapy.

Bath oils containing essential oils such as safe, eucalyptus, turpentine, pine, pennyroyal, and cinnamon contain alcohols, esters, and ketones.[2,3] These can cause allergic contact dermatitis that begins within 12 hours.[3] Essential oils are mucosal irritants.[3] Concentrated preparations of essential oils can cause seizures and CNS depression at 10 mL doses. The alcohol content can cause hypoglycemia, especially in children.[1-3,20] Pennyroyal may pose a more significant toxicity.[20] Large ingestions can cause GI irritation accompanied by nausea, vomiting, and abdominal pain. CNS effects may occur. When pennyroyal is an ingredient, toxicity is possible. The active toxic volatile is pulegone, which is metabolized to a liver and lung toxin. Toxicity may develop at a dose of 5 mL and death is associated with a 15-mL ingestion. Hepatic injury and abdominal pain along with altered mental status occur early in a toxic exposure. Hypotension and metabolic acidosis along with protracted emesis, GI bleeding, and hematuria can occur. Renal failure is common in large pennyroyal ingestions. Although there is no specific antidote, since pennyroyal can deplete hepatic glutathione, use of N-acetylcysteine (NAC) has been suggested. The exact dosing regimen has not been determined.[20] Symptomatic and supportive care is critical (see Chapter 101).

Disposition

With the exception of pennyroyal and other essential oil products, the remaining products in this category are considered nontoxic; outcomes are expected to be benign.

COLOGNES AND PERFUMES

As for other categories of cosmetic products, toxicity depends on the ingredients and their concentration in the formulation.[1-3,20] Colognes and perfumes usually contain ethanol at concentrations ranging from 50% to 95% as well as oils, which can be either volatile or essential oils. The toxicity of these products is dependent on the ethanol concentration and amount ingested. Since skin is an intended area of application, these products are not expected to cause toxicity via the dermal route except in hypersensitive individuals. Cosmetics and perfumes can be irritating to the eyes but are not expected to cause long-term damage.

Epidemiology

There were 17,627 perfume and cologne exposures in 2004 reported to PCC, of which 14,917 involved young children.[19] There was only one death and 11 major toxicity cases, while the majority (7808) were considered nontoxic or of mild toxicity.

Diagnosis

Most acute exposures are readily identified by history. An elevated blood ethanol level and the development of hypoglycemia, especially in children, are important clues to significant toxic exposures.

Blood ethanol levels, CBC, electrolytes, anion gap, and renal function tests along with frequent monitoring of blood glucose are recommended. Attention should be paid to respiratory function, seizure precaution, and fluid status.

Toxicology and Management

Depending on the concentration and amount ingested, especially by young children owing to their increased risk of hypoglycemia from ethanol as well as CNS effects, perfumes and colognes should be managed like toxic ethanol exposures. Symptomatic and supportive care is the mainstay of intervention. There are no specific antidotes. For skin irritation, soap and water should be sufficient. Ocular exposures require copious irrigation with warm water or saline.

Disposition

Most cologne or perfume exposures are considered low toxicity events, and benign outcomes are expected

NAIL CARE PRODUCTS

This category comprises nail polishes and nail polish removers. Nail polish contains hydrocarbon solvents such as xylene, toluene and acetone, plasticizers, resins, and alcohol solvents. Methanol may also be used. The likelihood of toxicity from ingestion is generally small owing to the small volume contained in nail polish bottles. GI irritation is the most likely result of ingestion. Skin irritation is rare. In the event of an ocular exposure, copious irrigation with warm water or saline should be sufficient.

Nail polish removers are also solvents containing acetone or ethanol. These too are generally considered

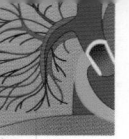

low toxicity products although bottles of nail polish remover are larger than nail polish bottles and thus pose a greater ingestion risk but still of low toxicity.

False or acrylic nails have been removed with acetonitrile, which is a highly toxic chemical (vinyl cyanide). Although these nail products have been reformulated by removal of acetonitrile, the potential of toxicity exists if older products are still available in a household. Artificial nail glue removers can also contain nitroalkane and nitroethane.

Epidemiology

There were 50 acrylic nail remover–related calls to American Association of Poison Control Centers in 2004.[19] There were no deaths; 27 cases involved young children. There were 10,876 nail polish–related calls, of which 9,775 involved young children. The majority of exposures were nontoxic or of mild toxicity, and there were no deaths. For nail polish removers, there were 2742 acetone preparation calls, 2114 with other ingredients and 8178 with unknown active ingredient. Most were nontoxic and involved children. There were no deaths.

Kinetics

Acetonitrile is metabolized by the cytochrome P-450 microsomal system to several metabolites, including cyanohydrin, which is subsequently metabolized to aldehyde and cyanide.[20,27,28]

Nitroethane is metabolized to aldehyde and nitrite. Nitrite is an oxidizer. Nitroethane has a half-life of 6 hours.

Diagnosis

The diagnosis of nail care products can usually be established by the history.

For exposures of old nail products containing acetonitrile, arterial and venous blood gas analysis and serum lactate levels are useful. An increased lactic acidosis suggests cyanide toxicity. Cyanide levels may not be readily available and may not correlate with severity; thus treatment should be based on the clinical situation.

For exposures of nail products containing nitroethane, electrolytes, renal function tests, and methemoglobin levels are useful to monitor. Cardiopulmonary monitoring maybe necessary in symptomatic patients.

For exposures to nail products containing ethanol, see above and Chapter 31. For exposures to nail products containing acetone, see Chapter 32.

Toxicology and Management

For acetone toxicity, see Chapter 32. For ethanol toxicity, see Chapter 31.

The clinical manifestations of acetonitrile are similar to those of cyanide although they may be delayed from 3 to 24 hours. Acetonitrile ingestion requires immediate medical attention. One swallow of acetonitrile-containing artificial nail glue remover can cause death in a toddler. The prudent clinician will be mindful that acetonitrile patients may be stable on presentation but can develop significant delayed toxicity. Clinical symptoms include respiratory distress and cyanosis. Cardiovascular symptoms including hypotension may occur. Headache, agitation, and CNS effects including altered mental status, seizures, and tremor may occur. Cherry red skin is usually a terminal event. Nausea and vomiting as well as abdominal pain occur with inhalation or ingestion. The cyanide antidote kit should be available, since it contains the three agents approved for cyanide intoxication by the FDA: amyl nitrate, sodium nitrate, and sodium thiosulfate. Activated charcoal has minimal binding affinity for cyanide. However, 1 g is considered adequate to bind 100 to 500 mg.[26]

Of note, acrylic fingernails that contain N,N-dimethyl-p-toluidine have been reported to produce methemoglobinemia.[15,16] Nitroalkane and nitroethane can also cause methemoglobinemia. Cyanosis, tachypnea, and chocolate-colored lips are manifestations. Methylene blue may be useful therapy.

Disposition

With most nail products, benign outcomes are expected. Acetonitrile ingestions can cause death. If the patient survives the exposure, unless anoxic brain injury has occurred, the long-term outcome is expected to be benign.[2,20,27,28]

ORAL HYGIENE PRODUCTS AND DENTIFRICES

Toothpastes, powders, liquids, and gels for cleaning teeth are generally considered nontoxic.[2,3,20] These products contain calcium phosphates, abradants such as silica or calcium carbonate, flavoring, and coloring. Some may contain stannous fluoride or sodium monofluorophosphate, which are low solubility/low toxicity chemicals. Most exposures can cause GI irritation. Although toothpaste may contain up to 1 mg fluoride per gram of toothpaste, generally the low concentration of fluoride in these products is unlikely to produce clinically significant toxicity.[29] Denture cleaners are similar products but may contain bleaching products such as potassium persulfate, sodium perborate, trisodium phosphate, and sodium carbonate.

At-home teeth whitening products contain peroxides, often in the form of 18% carbamide peroxide, which is the equivalent of 6.5% hydrogen peroxide.[30] Studies support the safety of this product for daily use as directed. Toxicity in a large ingestion would be referable to H_2O_2.

Mouthwashes contain alcohol, flavoring, and sweeteners. Toxicity is proportional to alcohol content but generally is considered low.

Epidemiology

According to 2004 TESS data,[19] there were 24,180 toothpaste with fluoride exposures of which 21,890

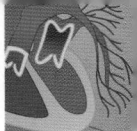

involved young children. There were few referrals to an HCF. There were no deaths and none developed major toxicity exposure, with the majority being mild to nontoxic. For toothpaste without fluoride, 1616 exposures were reported, with 1398 involving young children. No deaths were reported, and few were treated at an HCF. Denture cleaners resulted in 1440 exposures, with 288 involving children. There was one death.

Kinetics

Fluoride absorption peaks in approximately 1 hour. Volume of distribution is 0 .5 to 0.7 L/kg. Fluoride is not protein bound. Elimination half-life is 2 to 9 hours but is prolonged in patients with renal failure. Doses of 3 to 5 mg/kg elemental fluoride can cause GI symptoms including abdominal pain and vomiting. Death has been reported in a 3-year-old child who ingested 16 mg/kg and in adults with doses above 32 mg/kg.[29]

Diagnosis

The diagnosis of fluoride or borate intoxication is usually determined by obtaining a history of exposure to oral hygiene products.

Specific fluoride levels may be difficult to obtain and should not be relied on in the acute management of an ingestion. Albumin, magnesium, and calcium levels; renal function tests; cardiovascular status; fluid status; and electrolytes should be obtained. For nonfluoride ingestions, obtain tests based on ingredients. The basic assessments should include renal function tests and electrolytes with cardiorespiratory monitoring.

Toxicology and Management

Sodium perborate breaks down into sodium borate and peroxide. These are irritating agents. Borate poisoning can ensue, resulting in CNS irritability, acute tubular necrosis, and renal dysfunction and the classical finding of "boiled lobster appearance."[2,20] As discussed above, peroxide ingestion is strongly irritating to the GI tract and can cause vomiting, diarrhea, and hematochezia. Symptomatic and supportive care is the mainstay of therapy. Activated charcoal has limited ability to absorb boric acid. An in vitro study demonstrated that 30 g of charcoal was required to adsorb 38% of a 1-g boric acid dose. No specific antidotes are recommended.[31] Hemodialysis, peritoneal dialysis, and exchange transfusion may enhance elimination.

Mouthwash toxicity is directly proportional to the ethanol concentration. Large unintentional ingestions are unlikely. With large ingestions, management is consistent with treatment of ethanol overdose.[2,3]

Products involving fluoride pose a toxicity risk related to both cytoxicity and metabolic effects.[29] Fluoride is cytotoxic and binds to calcium and magnesium, which can lead to hypocalcemia and hypomagnesemia. Impaired oxidative phosphorylation and glycolysis, impaired blood coagulation, and myocardial irritability can result as well as impaired neurotransmission and possibly tetany.[29]

Disposition

Most exposures are of low toxicity. Benign outcomes are expected; however, there are exceptions: a 75-year-old woman unintentionally applied denture powder to her dentures while they were still in her mouth. On emergency department evaluation she was found to have severe burns to the lips, mouth, and oropharynx with swelling and drooling. She required endotracheal intubation for respiratory distress secondary to increased secretions and irritation. She developed profound hypotension and died.[19]

FACIAL/BODY PAINTS AND MAKEUP

Ingestions of facial makeup such as lipstick, rouge, mascara, blushers, and other products are considered nontoxic.[2,32] These preparations are composed of water, waxes, and vegetable oils. Some products contain talcs. The primary risk of talcs is to the respiratory system, but owing to their small volume, this risk is negligible. If ingestion of makeup occurs, the small packaging size precludes the likelihood of toxicity.[1-3,11,19,20] Of note, use of henna is increasing. Henna is a vegetable dye from dried leaves of *Lawsonia intermis*, which grows in Egypt, Tunisia, and India. Historically, henna has been used by Indian and Pakistani families to decorate the hands and feet as part of special celebrations such as weddings. Increasingly, henna is being adopted in Western cultures as a hair treatment and body makeup. The active ingredient is lawsone (2-hydroxy-1,4-napthoquinone). Contact dermatitis has not been documented unless henna is adulterated by other chemicals including purified protein derivative (PPD), which is believed to be causal.[1,33] One case report suggested that a woman experienced an allergic reaction including wheezing and coryza after handling henna.[33]

Body paints are similar to colognes and perfumes in that their predominant ingredients are ethanol, color additives, pigments, emulsifiers, and preservatives.[2,11,32] These are considered low toxicity products, with most of the risk associated with alcohol content.[2]

Lipstick is made with waxes, water, and occasionally camphor. The low dose of camphor in lipstick makes ingestion virtually nontoxic.

Epidemiology

According to TESS, there were 1192 lipstick with camphor exposures, of which more than 90% involved children; most ingestions were nontoxic or of minimal toxicity, and there were no deaths. Of the 4467 exposures involving lipstick without camphor, 4189 were in young children. Most exposures were nontoxic,[19] and again there were no deaths.

Kinetics

Ethanol is readily absorbed after ingestion, peaking in 30 to 120 minutes. Volume of distribution is 0.5 to 0.7 L/kg. Elimination is via hepatic oxidation following zero order kinetics.[34]

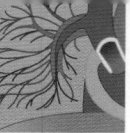

Diagnosis

Diagnosis is by history. A patient who exhibits signs and symptoms consistent with alcohol toxicity in whom pigmentation or a scent is present also suggests the diagnosis.

No specific laboratory studies are associated with makeup. However, serum ethanol levels, electrolytes, and renal function tests should be obtained. Additional studies should be guided by clinical presentation, including cardiopulmonary monitoring.

Toxicology and Management

Alcohol content is the primary toxicant in this category. Since 0.7 mg/dL ethanol will produce a blood ethanol level of 100 mg/dL (0.1 g/dL), which is considered legally intoxicated, and 300 mg/dL can cause coma in novice drinkers, ingestions of body paints would have to be considerable to achieve these ethanol levels. Toxic cases should be managed as any alcohol exposure (see Chapter 31). CNS depression and hypoglycemia are the primary manifestations of alcohol toxicity. Alcohol is hepatotoxic.

DISPOSITION

Most exposures are of low toxicity. Benign outcomes are expected.

HYGIENE PRODUCTS: DEODORANTS AND ANTIPERSPIRANTS

Deodorants, like most other cosmetic products, are considered nontoxic in spite of the fact the primary ingredients are alcohol, water, and a deodorizing agent. Antiperspirants are deodorants with a sweat-inhibiting agent, usually aluminum hydroxychloride.[2,3]

Deodorants and antiperspirants are found as sticks, roll-on products, and aerosols.

Epidemiology

As reported in 2004, there were 17,566 deodorant category exposures, of which 15,277 involved young children. There were no deaths; most exposures were nontoxic or minimally toxic.[19]

Diagnosis

The diagnosis of acute ethanol toxicity from hygiene products is usually determined by obtaining a history of exposure to these products.

No specific laboratory studies are associated with makeup. However, serum ethanol, serial glucose level, electrolytes, and renal function test should be obtained in exposures to alcohol-containing products, especially in children, Additional studies should be guided by clinical presentation, including cardiopulmonary monitoring.

Toxicology and Management

Skin and eye irritation as well as mild GI irritation are the primary effects. Contact dermatitis is possible.[3,35] Toxicity would be related to alcohol ingestion. However, owing to the small concentration and quantity contained within the package, toxicity is unlikely. Management depends on the ingredients of the product and should be guided by clinical presentation. Symptomatic and supportive care is the mainstay of treatment. Products with alcohol content should be managed as for other toxic alcohol exposures. Other than hypersensitivity, these products are safe as intended for dermal contact. Ocular exposures may cause mild and transient corneal epithelial irritation, but no persistent injury has been reported. These require copious irrigation, for at least 15 to 20 minutes, with benign outcome expected.[2,3,11,32]

Disposition

Most exposures are of low toxicity. Benign outcomes are expected.

DEPILATORIES

Unlike the majority of cosmetic products, which are considered nontoxic or mildly toxic, depilatories (otherwise known as hair removers) are considered moderately toxic because of their sodium hydroxide (1% to 10%) or calcium hydroxide content. These hydroxides are alkaline caustics. Thioglycolate may also be present and is alkaline, capable of toxicity similar to sodium hydroxide. Depilatories also contain water and other ingredients not dissimilar to those in soaps or skin lotions. These ingredients are relatively nontoxic.

These alkaline agents dissolve hair or damage the hair shaft, resulting in hair loss.

Epidemiology

There were 1959 depilatory related exposures reported to TESS, of which 541 involved young children. There were no deaths, and only 4 developed major toxicities.[19]

Toxicology

Depilatories are skin irritants because of the alkaline ingredients. Sodium hydroxide (NaOH) is a caustic alkali that can cause severe burns. Fumes or mists are irritating to mucosa, eyes, skin, and the respiratory tract.[2,36]

Ingestion of corrosives can cause burns of the esophagus as well as the oral cavity, resulting in dysphagia, drooling, and pain in the mouth, oropharynx, chest, or abdomen. The damage is dependent on the concentration and volume.[2,36] Ocular exposure can cause conjunctivitis and even blindness. Skin exposure results in pain, erythema, blistering, and penetrating necrosis.

Alkalies such as NaOH cause liquefaction necrosis with saponification such that continued penetration

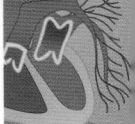

from the surface to deeper tissues occurs and results in significant damage.[36] While there is no generally accepted toxic dose of depilatory owing to the wide variety of concentrations and volumes of solutions, the concentration or pH of the product is indicatory of its potential for damage and toxicity. The concentration of the base, also referred to as the titratable alkalinity, is a good predictor of corrosive risk.[36]

Management

Unlike acids, which produce coagulation necrosis that can lead to an eschar, thereby limiting the damage somewhat, alkali burns can produce liquefaction necrosis. Exposure requires copious irrigation until a neutral pH is attained. Usually, this requires in excess of 20 minutes of irrigation with warm water or saline. Ocular involvement should be considered a medical emergency. Immediate irrigation for a minimum of 20 minutes and at least 1 L of warm water or saline should be initiated without delay. While the use of pH paper can help guide irrigation toward a neutral end point, extensive irrigation of the eye and consultation with immediate referral to ophthalmology are required. For skin exposures, the area should be washed with large volumes of warm water or saline (see Chapter 98).

Disposition

Minor, low concentration, and unintentional exposures generally result in minimal toxicity and benign outcomes. Larger exposures or ocular involvement can lead to scarring, blindness, or significant toxicity.

SUMMARY

Cosmetic products are generally considered nontoxic. There are ingredients, such as alcohol, peroxides, or other oxidizers, that when ingested in quantity can lead to toxicity and even death although this is generally rare. Some products such as hair straighteners and acrylic nail removal preparations contain highly toxic chemicals but in low dose. These nonetheless can cause significant symptoms. When used strictly as directed, they pose a low toxicity risk. With few exceptions, the management of toxic cosmetic exposures is symptomatic and supportive. Emesis is not recommended. Activated charcoal may confer benefit in specific situations. Antidotes are not readily available except for a few products.

Most unintentional cosmetic product exposures involve children. Caution must be exercised in storing these products, just as for other chemicals, toxicants, and household products.

REFERENCES

1. Mehta SS, Reddy BS: Cosmetic dermatitis—current perspectives. Int J Dermatol 2003;42:533–542.
2. Lucas JK: Cosmetics and toilet articles. In Haddad L, Shannon M, Winchester J (eds): Clinical Management of Poisoning and Drug Overdose, 3rd ed. Philadelphia, Saunders, 1998, pp 1169–1170.
3. Prathibha RS, Kulkarni SG, Mehendale HM: Cosmetics. In Wexler P (ed-in-chief): Encyclopedia of Toxicology. San Diego, Academic Press, pp 380–382.
4. Adams RM, Maibach IH: A five-year study of cosmetic reactions. J Am Acad Dermatol 1985;13:1062–1069.
5. Wilkinson JD: Cosmetic Dermatitis. In Champion RH, Burton JL, Burns DA, Breathnach SM (eds): Textbook of Dermatology, 6th ed. Vol. I. Oxford, Blackwell Scientific Publications, 1998, pp 785–787.
6. Larsen WG, Jackson EM, Barker MD, et al: A primer on cosmetics. J Am Acad Dermatol 1992;27:469–484.
7. Naas DJ: Regulatory Toxicology: Consumer Products. In Derelanko U, Hollinger MA (eds): Handbook of Toxicology, 2nd ed. Boca Raton, FL, CRC Press, 2002, pp 1195–1213.
8. Federal Food, Drug and Cosmetic Act, current as amended. Washington, DC, U.S. Government Printing Office, 1990.
9. Code of Federal Regulations, Title 21, Vol. 7 (21 CFR 710), Food and Drug Administration, Center for Food Safety and Applied Nutrition. Washington, D.C., U.S. Government Printing Office, Rev. April 1, 2002.
10. Berne B, Bostrom A, Grahnen AF, Tammela M: Adverse effects of cosmetics and toiletries reported to the Swedish Medical Products Agency 1989–1994. Contact Dermatitis 1996;34:359–362.
11. Weisman RS: Nontoxic ingestion. In Goldfrank L, Flomenbaum NE, Lewin NA, et al (eds): Goldfrank's Toxicological Emergencies, 7th ed. Norwalk, CT, Appleton & Lange, 2002, pp 40–43.
12. Hymes LC, Bruner BS, Rauber AP: Bromate poisoning from hair permanent preparations. Pediatrics 1985;76:975–977.
13. Quick CA, Chole RA, Mauer SM: Deafness and renal failure due to potassium bromate poisoning. Arch Otolaryngol 1975;101:494–495.
14. Geller RJ, Ekins BR, Iknoian RC: Cyanide toxicity from acetonitrile-containing false nail remover. Am J Emerg Med 1991;9:271–272.
15. Scherger DL, Wruk KM, Kulig KW, Rumack BH: Ethyl alcohol containing cologne, perfumes and after-shave ingestions in children. Am J Dis Child 1988;142:630.
16. Porter JL, Krill CF, Neal D, et al: Methemoglobinemia due to the ingestion of N,N-dimethyltoluidine: a component used in the fabrication of artificial nails. Ann Emerg Med 1988;17:1098–1100.
17. Mielke HW, Taylor MD, Gonzales CR, et al: Lead based hair-coloring products—too hazardous for household use. J Am Pharm Assoc 1997;57:85–89.
18. Cox AJ, Eisenbeis JF: Ingestion of caustic hair relaxer: is endoscopy necessary? Laryngoscope 1997;107:897–902.
19. Watson WA, Litovitz, TL, Rodgers GC Jr, et al: 2004 annual report of the American Association of Poison Control Centers Toxic Exposure Surveillance System. Am J Emerg Med 2005;23:588–666.
20. Agency for Toxic Substances and Disease Registry (ATSDR): Toxicological profiles for mercury. Atlanta, GA, U.S. Department of Health and Human Services, May 1999. Available at http://www.atsdr.cdc.gov/toxprofiles/tp46.html
21. Forsen JW, Muntz HR: Hair relaxer ingestion: a new trend. Ann Otol Rhinol Laryngol 1993;102:781–784.
22. Kent DA, Willis CA, Lepik KJ: Hair care products—dyes and lighteners. In Poison Management Manual, 4th ed. Vancouver, British Columbia, BC Drug and Poison Information Center, 1997, pp 261–263.
23. Gosselin RE, Hodge HD, Smith RP, et al: Clinical Toxicology of Commercial Products, 4th ed. Baltimore, Williams & Wilkins, 1976.
24. Vogel C, Caraccio TR, Mofenson HC, Hart S: Alcohol intoxication in young children. J Toxicol Clin Toxicol 1995;33:25–33.
25. Rao RB, Hoffman RS: Caustics and batteries. In Goldfrank L, Flomenbaum NE, Lewin NA, et al (eds): Goldfrank's Toxicological Emergencies, 7th ed. Norwalk, CT, Appleton & Lange, 2002, pp 1323–1345.
26. Roth B: Isopropyl alcohol. In Olson KR: Poisoning and Drug Overdose, 3rd ed. Stamford, CT, Appleton & Lange, 1999, pp 197–198.
27. Kurt TI, Day LC, Reed WGT, et al: Cyanide poisoning from sculptured nail remover. Vet Hum Toxicol 1989;31:339.
28. Caravati EM, Litovitz TL: Pediatric cyanide intoxication and death from acetonitrile containing cosmetic. JAMA 1988;260:3470–3473.

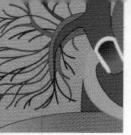

29. Meier KH: Fluoride. In Olson KR (ed): Poisoning and Drug Overdose, 4th ed. Stamford, CT, Appleton & Lange, 2004, pp 200–201.

30. Slezak B, Santarpia P, Xu T, et al: Safety profile of a new whitening gel. Compend Contin Educ Dent 2002;23(11 Suppl 1):4–11.

31. Oderda GM, Klein-Schwartz W, Insley BM: In vitro study of boric acid and activated charcoal. J Toxicol Clin Toxicol 1987;25:13–19.

32. Mofenson HC, Caraccio TR, Greensher J: Ingestions considered nontoxic. Pediatr Clin North Am 1984;2:159–174.

33. Cronin E: Immediate-type of hypersensitivity to henna. Contact Dermatitis 1979;5:198.

34. Horowitz BZ: Ethanol. In Olson KR (ed): Poisoning and Drug Overdose, 3rd ed. Stamford, CT, Appleton & Lange, 1999, pp 162–164.

35. DeGroot AC, Beverdam GA, Ayong CT, et al: The role of the contact allergy in the spectrum of adverse effects caused by cosmetics and toiletries. Contact Dermatitis 1988;19:195–201.

36. Mullen WH: Caustic and corrosive agents. In Olson KR (ed): Poisoning and Drug Overdose, 3rd ed. Stamford, CT, Appleton & Lange, 1999, pp 129–131.

101 *Essential Oils*

JACK MAYPOLE, MD ■ ALAN DAVID WOOLF, MD, MPH

At a Glance...

- Essential oils are a family of plant-derived hydrocarbons that possess (or are believed to possess) a broad range of therapeutic benefits.
- Essential oils of clinical and/or toxicologic importance include cinnamon, eucalyptus, pennyroyal, tea tree, peppermint, and clove.
- All essential oils contain concentrated amounts of volatile aromatic hydrocarbons, such that ingestion can result in aspiration which in turn results hydrocarbon pneumonitis.
- The same principles of treatment employed after hydrocarbon aspiration should be used in managing a patient with essential oil aspiration.

Since the early 1990s the use of herbal products by the general public has increased in North America, in parallel with the use of complementary and alternative medicines. Herbs that are used for medicinal purposes come in a variety of forms; active parts of a plant may include leaves, flowers, stems, roots, seeds, and/or berries. Herbal products may be taken internally as pills or powders, dissolved into tinctures or syrups, or brewed in teas and decoctions. Salves, ointments, shampoos, pessaries, suppositories, or poultices may be applied to wounds, the skin, scalp, or mucous membranes.

Many plants contain the so-called essential oils (EOs), aromatic hydrocarbon-based oils. The highly concentrated, volatile EOs, which have pungent odors and rapidly evaporate in room air, are distilled as extracts, packaged, and sold unregulated to the public for medicinal purposes. In terms of their therapeutic effects, herbalists believe EOs have pharmacologic, physiologic, and psychological actions on the body. Box 101-1 defines some terms useful in understanding herbal therapy involving EOs. The increasing accessibility and popularity of the therapeutic use of EOs have been mirrored by a rise in inadvertent poisonings, and toxicity associated with their use and misuse.

THERAPEUTIC USES

EOs from many spices and herbs have antimicrobial and antifungal properties, attributable in part to their monoterpene constituents. These properties underlie the ability of EOs to prevent food spoilage and treat health problems, although there is limited scientific data regarding the therapeutic benefits of EOs. The traditional individualized therapeutic approach conflicts with the scientific research demand for empiric, controlled studies. The distinctive aromatic nature of

EOs also contributes to methodologic problems in conducting blinded randomized controlled trials.

Antiseptic/Antimicrobial

A growing body of evidence supports the potential usefulness of EOs for their antimicrobial and antiseptic effects. Tea tree oil (TTO), lavender, mint, sandalwood, and thyme have been found to possess in vitro antibacterial and antifungal activity against such organisms as methicillin-resistant *Staphylococcus aureus*, vancomycin-resistant *Enterococcus faecium*, *Escherichia coli*, and *Candida albicans*.[1,2] Lavender, geranium, sandalwood, TTO, ylang ylang, patchouli, myrrh, and bergamot have demonstrated activity against both gram-positive and gram-negative microorganisms and *C. albicans* in laboratory studies. TTO contains terpinen-4-ol and other terpenes that may be responsible for its antimicrobial action. The mechanism is thought to be the disruption of the cell membrane, allowing potassium ion leakage, which leads to loss of chemiosmotic control and, therefore, causes rupture and destruction of the bacterial or fungal cell walls.[1] Terpinen-4-ol, has been demonstrated in vitro to suppress inflammatory mediator production by activated human monocytes.[3]

Such antimicrobial actions, as well as specific actions against *Staphylococcus mutans* (causing plaque and gingivitis) have led to the inclusion of EOs in dental

---

BOX 101-1　DEFINITIONS

Essential oils ("volatile oils," "ethereal oil"): Any of a class of highly concentrated, volatile oils composed of a mixture of complex hydrocarbons (usually terpenes) and other chemicals extracted from a plant, typically by a method of distillation. Essential oils give a plant its characteristic pungent or fragrant aroma and will evaporate quickly off skin or another surface.
Essence: A concentrated fragrance or perfume.
Fixed oil: A nonvolatile oil made of long-chain fatty acids (such as castor oil or safrole).
Carrier oils: Essential oils are too concentrated to be applied directly to the skin during therapeutic use. Frequently, only a few drops of the essential oil are diluted into the carrier oils, such as safflower oil.
Aromatherapy: The use of volatile oils via inhalation in the treatment of certain health problems.
Carminative: An agent that aids in expelling gas from the gastrointestinal tract.
Rubefacient: An agent that reddens the skin and causes a localized feeling of warmth via cutaneous vasodilation.
Emmenagogue: An agent that influences menstruation and addresses problems related to menstrual flow.
Abortifacient: An agent that induces abortion.

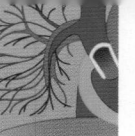

hygiene products, including mouthwash, toothpaste, rinses, implants, and temporary amalgams used in dental repairs.[4] TTO has purported antiseptic, antifungal, and antimicrobial properties when applied topically to mucous membranes and is used in the treatment of vaginal candidiasis, chronic cystitis, tinea pedis, genital herpes, and acne. TTO and other EOs have also been added to soaps, lotions, liniments, creams, and salves used to treat skin infections and improve wound healing.

Psychological Effects

EOs have been used in the management of behavior problems, stress reduction, relaxation therapy, and sleep disorders. Aromatherapy links EO odors to a healthy lifestyle by boosting awareness, stimulating the senses, and facilitating memory and learning.

Other Uses

EOs are used to enhance digestion, stimulate appetite, and lessen abdominal discomfort (e.g., inflammatory bowel disease or menstrual problems). EOs are used to manage muscle spasm or soreness after strain or injury and for nerve or dental pain. EOs have also been used for weight loss, although coriander and bergamot are reportedly appetite stimulants.

GENERAL TOXICITY

As food additives, essential oils are regulated by the Food and Drug Administration (FDA). A ceiling concentration limited to less than 300 ppm makes toxicity through ingestion of flavored foodstuffs unlikely, although allergic reactions are still possible.[5] All EOs contain concentrated amounts of volatile aromatic hydrocarbons, such that unintentional ingestion can result in aspiration and hydrocarbon pneumonia. As plant derivatives, EOs can cause allergic skin reactions as well, including allergic or irritant contact dermatitis, other skin eruptions, phototoxic reactions, and urticaria. Systemic anaphylactoid reactions are also possible. Occupational workers in settings where EOs are present, such as aromatherapists, dentists and dental hygienists, fruit pickers, beauticians, physiotherapists, and cosmeticians, are particularly vulnerable to such reactions.[6] Some EOs exhibit genotoxicity, with in vitro studies revealing chromosome aberrations (e.g., sister chromatid exchanges).[7]

SPECIFIC ESSENTIAL OILS

Cinnamon (Cinnamon cassia nees ex blume)

Cinnamon is harvested from the bark of the *Cinnamon cassia nees ex blume* plant, a member of the Lauraceae family. Besides its use as a spice, cinnamon's EO is promoted for a variety of medical conditions related to its properties as a stimulant, astringent, and carminative agent. Historically, it was used with other EOs and herbs

as a treatment for chronic bronchitis. Up to 80% of the fresh oil is cinnamic aldehyde, which can have sensitizing properties. Patients who develop cinnamon sensitivity usually develop an allergic, potentially "systemic" dermatitis or urticarial lesions upon reexposure. Cinnamic aldehyde is metabolized to cinnamic acid and excreted as benzoic and hippuric acids.

While ingestion of large amounts of cinnamon oil has been rarely reported, as little as 5 to 10 mL taken orally may cause central nervous system effects, possibly including seizures, and respiratory depression.[8,9] A 7-year-old child who ingested about 2.5 mL/kg developed gastrointestinal symptoms, dizziness, lethargy, and rectal burning, which resolved over a 5-hour period.[10]

In sensitive patients, the use of cinnamic aldehyde–containing products such as toothpaste may produce white mucosal lesions in the mouth similar to leukoplakia seen with squamous cell carcinoma—in fact, squamous cell carcinoma has been associated with chronic oral cinnamon use.[11,12]

Additionally, oral cheilitis, welts, erythema, ulcers, and vesicles may be observed. The patient may complain of burning pain from such lesions. The condition, known as *stomatitis venenata* and *mucositis*, can develop into orofacial granulomatosis and must be differentiated from lupus, lichen planus, oral candidiasis, lichenoid mucositis, cheek biting, and malignant conditions.[13,14] A history of chronic cinnamon exposure—noted in cases of occupational exposure of bakers, or in health care providers using cinnamon oils topically[15]—reveals the correct etiology of the lesions, and abstinence from cinnamon results in their resolution. Immunoglobulin E (IgE) and radioallergosorbent tests are unhelpful for the diagnosis. A skin biopsy reveals characteristic perivascular infiltrates.

The practice of sucking on cinnamon oil–dipped toothpicks or hard candy by adolescents as a recreational activity has been reported.[16] Self-limited signs of acute cinnamon toxicity, including facial flushing, oral burning, shortness of breath, tachycardia, dizziness, and abdominal pain, resulted. Typically, only supportive management is required.

Eucalyptus Oil (Eucalyptus globulus)

Eucalyptus oil has been recommended for the treatment of upper respiratory and other viral infections, and is also used in a liniment for muscle aches and strains. The yellowish oil has a distinctive camphor-like, pungent odor, which lingers on the breath of a poisoned patient. The active ingredient in the EO is eucalyptol, made of 1, 8-cineole plus tannins, in up to a 70% concentration. Hydrocyanic acid, present in lesser amounts, is also a contributor to the oil's toxicity.[17] Eucalyptus oil is capable of hepatic microsomal induction, and thus may affect the metabolism of other drugs and chemicals. It is rapidly absorbed and has primary neurotoxicity (seizures, coma). Elimination of eucalyptol may be largely via the pulmonary route.

Although 80% of 42 children with eucalyptus poisoning remained asymptomatic in one study,[18] two other case

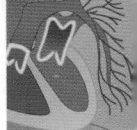

series have documented symptoms in 65%[19] and 59% of victims.[20] In one Australian telephone survey, eucalyptus oil was a leading agent associated with hospitalization for poisoning/ingestion among children younger than five years; 74% of preschoolers gained access to eucalyptus oil via a home vaporizer unit, most frequently placed at ground level.[21]

Diagnosis is evident after unintentional ingestion of eucalyptus oil because of its pungent odor on the breath. Small amounts may cause a rapid onset of nasal and epigastric burning, vomiting, gastrointestinal distress, miosis, weakness, headache, drowsiness, ataxia, or coma. In a review of fatalities caused by eucalyptus oil, oral burning, emesis, and abdominal pain were early symptoms of poisoning.[22] Bronchospasm, bronchorrhea, hyperpnea, dyspnea, and pneumonia are also associated with aspiration of the volatile oil.[22] Cyanosis, coma and seizures are sometimes seen, especially in infantile poisoning, and have been associated with respiratory depression and death.[19] As little as 0.6 to 5.0 mL of 100% eucalyptus oil causes severe illness in children. Seizures and death were reported in an 8-month-old child after ingestion of 30 mL of the oil.[19] In adults, symptoms may occur with an ingestion of as little as 1 to 2 teaspoons of eucalyptus oil, although an adult died after reportedly ingesting only 4 mL of eucalyptus oil.[23]

Topical application of eucalyptus oil may also cause toxicity. A 6-year-old girl presented with rapidly progressing slurred speech, ataxia, muscle weakness, and unconsciousness following the widespread application of a eucalyptus oil–containing home remedy for urticaria.[24]

Some victims of eucalyptus oil may only require close observation; however, in known large ingestions or when a poisoned patient presents early with clinical symptoms, the clinician may consider decontamination with activated charcoal, with elective intubation to protect the airway.[18–20] Respiratory support, antiemetics, and vasopressors are indicated in the management of some patients. Symptoms may be delayed for several hours, so the suspected victim deserves a longer period of monitoring than usual.

Nutmeg (Myristica fragrans)

Nutmeg is the seed kernel of the evergreen tree *Myristica fragrans*, the outer shell of which is also the source of the spice mace. Originally grown in the Malucca Island of the South Pacific, nutmeg was transplanted to Grenada, Trinidad, and other "spice islands" of the Caribbean, where it is grown commercially today. Besides its common culinary use as a spice, fresh nutmeg is recommended by herbalists as a gastrointestinal stimulant, as a carminative, for the treatment of rheumatism, for neurologic complaints, and as an emmenagogue. Nutmeg was introduced as a spice in the 12th century, and abuse of the spice was recorded as early as the 1500s. It is well known among sailors, jail inmates, and, more recently, adolescents as a cheap, readily available euphoriant. Unfortunately, the euphoria is short lived and is accompanied by such an array of unpleasant side effects, including severe headache and vomiting, that, after the first experiment, repetitive abuse is unlikely.

The oil of the nutmeg spice contains a mix of aromatic allylbenzenes, including the active principal, myristacin, as well as other complex hydrocarbons, including alamecin, borneol, safrole, isoeugenol, geraniol, and eugenol. Myristicin has been characterized as causing both hallucinogenic as well as amphetamine-like symptoms. It can be metabolized endogenously to 5-methoxy–3, 4-methylenedioxyamphetamine, which may be the proximal mediator of some of its toxic effects. Alamecin may also be metabolized to a hallucinogenic agent. These compounds have been described as having LSD-like and monoamine oxidase inhibitor properties as well.

Fresh nutmeg contains much higher concentrations of the EO than the dried, powdered spice. An estimated one to three whole nutmegs can cause moderate toxicity when ingested, which translates to 5 to 15 g of the freshly ground spice.[25] A dose of 18 g of fresh ground nutmeg has been associated with obtundation in a patient; such very large doses (14 to 21 g, or 280 to 420 mg/kg) may be associated with liver failure and death.[26,27]

Usually, ingestion of 10 to 50 g of fresh nutmeg produces clinical intoxication. Prominent nausea, vomiting, headache, and chest and abdominal pain are invariably an early part of the clinical picture and limit the abuse potential of the EO. Patients may experience a sense of impending doom, which precedes uncontrollable retching. Flushed skin, decreased salivation, tachycardia, and slightly elevated blood pressure may remind the clinician of the anticholinergic syndrome. But these patients differ from those with an anticholinergic syndrome in that they present early on with pinpoint rather than dilated pupils and a depressed body temperature rather than fever. Patients may develop other neurologic symptoms besides hallucinations, including agitation, tremors, lethargy, confusion, delirium, or psychosis. The hallucinations are said to be visual and auditory, with distortions in color, time, and space. Symptoms may persist for up to 2 to 3 days.

Many cases of nutmeg abuse have been described, but only one fatal case of poisoning has been reported. Myristicin (4 µg/mL) and flunitrazepam (0.072 µg/mL) were detected in the postmortem serum of a 55-year-old woman.[27] From 1996 to 1998, seven poisonings with nutmeg were recorded by the Erfurt Poison Information Centre. Even where higher doses (20 to 80 g of powder) had been ingested, a life-threatening situation was never observed. In one of these cases, a myristicin blood level of 2 µg/mL was measured 8 hours after ingestion of 2 to 3 tablespoons of nutmeg powder (approximately 14 to 21 g, or 280 to 420 mg/kg).[27] Management of nutmeg poisoning includes oral decontamination with activated charcoal, supportive care including antiemetics, and, where necessary, sedation with a benzodiazepine medication. Reduction of visual and auditory stimuli is also helpful in calming the agitated patient.

Pennyroyal (Squaw Mint) Oil (Hedeoma pulegiodes)

Pennyroyal oil is distilled from *Hedeoma pulegiodes* or *Mentha pulegium* and may be prescribed for a variety of

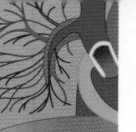

medical conditions, including for toothache, as a flea and tick repellent, for chronic bronchitis or asthma, as an anti-inflammatory agent, or for genitourinary complaints. Use of pennyroyal oil as an emmenagogue or as an abortifacient has been described in young women.[28] Yerba buena, an herbal tea made from mint leaves, is popular in Latino and other cultures as an indigenous cure for infantile abdominal pain and colic. However, when pennyroyal oil–containing mint is used, life-threatening poisoning among treated infants has been reported.[29]

Studies of pennyroyal oil in mice have established its ability to cause hepatic and pulmonary necrosis at doses of 400 mg/kg.[30] The active chemical in pennyroyal is pulegone, an aromatic ketone that undergoes bioactivation to menthofuran, a cyclohexanone. Both of these compounds, as well as other reactive intermediates derived from the metabolism of pulegone, can bind to subcellular proteins and cause cellular damage.[31,32] Pulegone and menthofuran also deplete cellular glutathione levels and make hepatocytes vulnerable to attack by oxidizing radicals.[32] Menthofuran can be detected by gas chromatography in the urine, blood, and other tissues of a poisoned patient.

Gastrointestinal symptoms, delirium, and seizures are noted at doses of pennyroyal oil as low as 3.5 mL, with cases of centilobular hepatitis following ingestion of 30 mL or more. Signs of poisoning are apparent soon after ingestion and may include a burning in the throat, nausea, vomiting, dizziness, abdominal pain, gastrointestinal bleeding, and hematuria.[33–36] Chemical hepatitis is usually detectable within 24 hours of ingestion. Later the patient will manifest liver dysfunction with secondary complications including coagulopathy, renal failure, seizure, and death.[36] One young woman who ingested 30 mL of pennyroyal oil to induce an abortion quickly developed a rash and repeated retching, followed by severe hepatorenal failure, disseminated intravascular coagulation, metabolic acidosis, pneumonia, and death 7 days later.[36] Autopsy confirmed the presence of pulmonary consolidation and widespread hepatic necrosis. A second case report of pennyroyal-induced death in a 24-year-old woman noted a variety of pathologic findings at autopsy, including hemolysis, renal tubular necrosis, pulmonary consolidation, and cerebral edema.[28]

Management of the affected patient includes oral decontamination by lavage if performed soon after ingestion and administration of activated charcoal, although charcoal's efficacy is unproven. The similarity of the pathogenesis of pennyroyal-induced centrilobular hepatic necrosis to that produced by acetaminophen suggests a prominent role for N-actylcysteine (NAC) as an antidote. Indeed, NAC was given to a child who had ingested life-threatening amounts of pennyroyal oil and the patient did not subsequently develop hepatitis.[28] Recent investigations of pulegone toxicity of a mouse model suggest some mitigation of liver damage when combination pretreatment with cytochrome CYP1A2 inhibitors (cimetidine and disulfuram) prevents formation of the toxic furan metabolite, although the clinical utility of such inhibitors has not been established.[30]

Tea Tree Oil (Melaleuca alternifolia)

TTO extract is derived from oil of the *Melaleuca alternifolia* tree, indigenous to Australia. Distillation of the leaves yields a pale, colorless oil that is approximately 50% terpenes and 6% to 8% cineol, with a variety of other compounds. Active ingredients include terpinen-4-ol, found also in eucalyptus oil. There are no clear data in humans to indicate a dose range associated with acute toxicity. TTO ingestion has also been reported in dogs and cats, with the primary symptoms appearing to be depression, weakness, incoordination, and muscle tremors. Acute oral toxicity in rats occurs at doses of 1.9 to 2.6 mL/kg.[37]

TTO shows promise as an effective treatment for a number of microorganisms commonly associated with otitis externa and otitis media, but its possible ototoxicity may discourage such uses. The ototoxicity of tea tree oil was examined in the guinea pig by measuring the thresholds of the compound auditory nerve action potential (CAP) to tone bursts before and after instillation of TTO into the middle ear. After 30 minutes of instillation, 100% TTO caused a partial CAP threshold elevation at 20 kHz, although a 2% concentration did not cause any significant lasting threshold change.[38]

Contact dermatitis and/or systemic hypersensitivity reactions have been seen after topical administration of TTO, although the incidence of such reactions is thought to be infrequent.[39] Topical administration has been associated with the formation of blisters and sores, as well as flare-ups in individuals with a history of eczema.[40] Australian TTO has been used as a veterinary antiseptic for many years and, more recently, this indication has been extended into human use. There have been many reports of allergic contact dermatitis and other dermal toxicity reactions, but TTO has never been implicated in immediate systemic hypersensitivity. A 38-year-old man experienced immediate flushing, pruritus, throat constriction, and lightheadedness after topical application of Australian TTO. The patient had a positive wheal and flare reaction on intradermal testing with TTO. No specific IgG or IgE was detected.[41]

Confusion, obtundation, coma, and a neutrophil leukocytosis have been associated with ingestion of TTO. Toxicity of the individual components of the oil has not been clearly established, but it is thought that terpenin-4-ol and other terpenes are responsible for its toxic effects. Symptoms may also include a strong mint-like aromatic odor to the breath.[42] A 23-month-old boy demonstrated mental status changes and ataxia after ingesting less than 10 mL of a TTO preparation. His symptoms lasted for approximately 5 hours.[42] Ingestion of half a cup of neat TTO by an adult caused coma that lasted about 48 hours.[43] Management of TTO poisoning consists of supportive care.

Peppermint/Mentha (Mentha piperit)

There are a wide variety of *Mentha* species of mint, all of which contain various amounts of the chemicals menthol and menthone. In two separate analyses, more than 30 other chemicals were identified from different mint

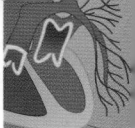

species, including pinene, limonene, menthofuran, pulegone, eugenol, menthyl acetate, diosphenol, and others.[44,45] Peppermint is not only an herbal remedy for abdominal pain and other discomforts, but also a ubiquitous flavoring in everything from gum to toothpaste. Peppermint is used as a breath freshener, decongestant, and antitussive. It is an intestinal antispasmodic, aiding in dyspepsia, flatulence, and colic and has been administered to patients to decrease symptoms in irritable bowel syndrome, inflammatory bowel disease, and biliary tract disorders. Menthol is used in shaving creams, mouthwash, lip balm, and many other personal hygiene products.

The actions of peppermint oil on the gut are complex. Some have found that it relaxes smooth muscle via effects on calcium channel receptors, whereas others have found that it stimulates intestinal smooth muscle and can cause cramps and the urge to defecate and urinate.[46] EOs from two different *Mentha* species produced central nervous system depression and hypothermia when fed to rats.[45] Seizures, ataxia, and respiratory depression were seen in rats after acute menthol dosing (median lethal dose [LD_{50}] 2.5 g/kg).[47] Chronic dosing at 40 to 100 mg/kg/day in rats over a 3-month period produced cystic lesions in the cerebellum and a progressive nephropathy.[48]

The clinical toxicity of peppermint includes a dermatitis associated with hypersensitivity to menthol. Chronic urticaria, "hot flashes," and gastrointestinal irritation are common in susceptible individuals. Diagnosis is possible by challenging the allergic individual with mint; besides eliciting the symptoms, a characteristic basopenia is observed in the blood count after provocative testing. Because a wide variety of everyday foods and household products contain mint flavoring, strict surveillance to avoid offending foodstuffs is difficult.

Acute *Mentha* reactions in humans can also include neurologic changes such as tremor, ataxia, drowsiness, or even coma. In one instance, menthol drops were mistakenly instilled into the nose of a 2-month-old infant, who subsequently developed dyspnea, unconsciousness, hyperextension of the extremities, and a metabolic acidosis.

A variety of other toxic effects are occasionally seen. Peppermint may precipitate hemolysis and jaundice in newborns with glucose-6-phosphate dehydrogenase deficiency,[49] and it was implicated in the development of pneumonia in an infant exposed to aerosolized peppermint.[50] Peppermint oil is also an irritant of the eyes and skin. It can cause burns of the skin or oral cavity and gingival and pharyngeal edema. It can cause gastrointestinal symptoms, perianal burning, cramps, and diarrhea. Myalgia and bradycardia have been reported. Management of peppermint poisoning consists of supportive care and may include activated charcoal for recent ingestions.

Clove Oil (*Clove Plant*)

Eugenol, a phenol, is the ingredient that makes up more than 90% of clove oil. Other ingredients of clove oil include caryophillin and vanillin. Clove oil is used widely as a fragrance or to flavor a variety of products, including foods, candles and incense, soaps, and toothpastes. Eugenol's disinfectant and analgesic properties have led to its use to treat dental pain and gingivitis, and it is commonly used during dental procedures and cleaning. According to Poisindex, the clinical effects of eugenol in clove oil resemble those of phenol, but are not as severe.[51] Clove oil may manifest its toxicity via direct injury to tissues, as seen when instilled directly into the trachea of rats, where eugenol caused interstitial hemorrhage, acute emphysema, and acute pulmonary edema.[52]

Toxicity of clove oil must be extrapolated from animal studies due to a lack of data defining specific toxic doses in humans. Dogs given oral doses of 0.25 g/kg of eugenol manifest with vomiting, weakness, lethargy, and ataxia.[53] In rat studies, eugenol was shown to cause coma and death within 24 hours with doses of 0.5 g/kg. The LD_{50} of eugenol has been determined to be 1.8 mL/kg (1.93 g/kg), with evidence of cardiovascular collapse.[53] The relatively low LD_{50} (11 mg/kg) of clove oil administered via the pulmonary route suggests the danger if clove oil is aspirated.[52]

In humans, a case of ingestion of oil of cloves by a young child was reported, which resulted in coma, seizures, a coagulopathy, and acute liver damage.[54] A reported case of accidental oral administration of clove oil resulted in central nervous system depression, urinary abnormalities, and large anion-gap acidosis.[55]

Topical exposure to clove oil can cause irritation to the skin, eyes, and oral mucosa. Clove oil splashed into the eye may cause acute pain, blepharospasm, lacrimation, and conjunctival edema, with loss of corneal epithelium.[56] It has been responsible for cases of contact dermatitis, stomatitis, and systemic allergic reactions. Orally, the initial stinging and irritation noted after topical exposure may progress to permanent local anesthesia and anhidrosis if contact is prolonged.[57]

Clove oil is also used in "bidi" cigarettes, an Indian product, which has been popularly used as a tobacco substitute. Clove cigarettes (approximately 40% dried clove and 60% tobacco) may also cause toxicity. Principally, bidi cigarettes are imported from Asia, and are available throughout the United States and Canada. Respiratory and systemic side effects of bidi cigarettes are numerous, and they include nausea, vomiting, dyspnea, bronchospasm, pulmonary edema, hemoptysis, and epistaxis. Side effects may be due to the direct effects of eugenol, including eugenol-induced anesthesia of the mucous membranes. In turn, this permits deeper inhalation of smoke and may result in greater tissue irritation and injury.[58]

Management of ingestion of clove oil may begin with dilution with water or milk prior to gastric evacuation. Concern for aspiration makes emesis undesirable, but activated charcoal may be indicated although direct evidence of its efficacy is lacking.[51] Topical exposures to the eye or mucous membranes should be addressed with vigorous and lengthy irrigation. Mild to moderate allergic reactions, including anaphylaxis, may be treated with antihistamines with or without inhaled β agonists, corticosteroids, or epinephrine.

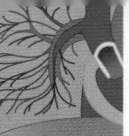

MANAGEMENT OF POISONING BY ESSENTIAL OILS

Exposure of the eyes or skin to undiluted EOs will likely cause pain and irritative reactions. Treatment of skin exposures should include immediate thorough washing with soap and water. Skin eruptions may necessitate steroid-containing creams or other local therapy. Generalized allergic rashes, urticaria, or anaphylaxis may require the use of oral or parenteral antihistamines, subcutaneous epinephrine, intravenous steroids, and other anti-inflammatory and resuscitative measures.

Eye exposures may cause pain, erythema, photophobia, lacrimation, blepharospasm, and even corneal clouding and more serious burns. Exposed eyes should be flushed with a cool stream of water or an eye wash solution for at least 15 to 20 minutes. Patients with lingering photophobia, conjunctival injection and irritation, or other symptoms despite initial dilution efforts will require ophthalmologic consultation and management.

Ingestion of EOs can lead to allergic symptoms or, depending on the specific EO, other toxic effects in target organ systems (Table 101-1). Patient assessment includes obtaining a careful history and performing a thorough physical examination, during which it should be determined whether a splash event for aspiration has also occurred. Gastric emptying using ipecac may increase the risk for aspiration during vomiting and is not recommended. Oral administration of activated charcoal, with care to avoid inducing emesis extending to elective endotracheal intubation to protect the airway, may be helpful if the patient presents to medical care in a timely fashion, although its value in improving patient outcome after EO ingestion is uncertain.

EOs contain aromatic or branched hydrocarbons with high volatility and low viscosity. Toxic effects of many EO also include central nervous system depression and a depressed gag reflex. These properties place the patient at high risk for aspiration. When aspirated, the effects of EOs are similar to those of hydrocarbon aspiration, with possible bronchospasm, pneumonia, and pulmonary edema. Patients who have aspirated an EO require and assessment for aspiration pneumonia, including serial chest radiographs and white blood cell counts, both of which may become progressively more abnormal as time goes on. Patients in respiratory distress may require transport to a facility with intensive care capabilities and expertise in advanced cardiovascular and respiratory medical care.

Patients in acute respiratory distress require close monitoring of arterial blood gases, with the administration of oxygen and supportive measures. In life-threatening aspirations, such measures may include endotracheal intubation and artificial ventilation. The value of steroids in such patients is controversial.[59] The use of bronchodilators may be necessary for patients who exhibit bronchospasm; antibiotics may be needed for patients who develop secondary pulmonary infections. High-frequency oscillatory ventilation and extracorporeal membrane oxygenation might be considered in patients with severe, life-threatening pulmonary failure due to aspiration unresponsive to conventional measures, but are still considered experimental measures.[60]

Other complications of oral EO poisoning include allergic reactions whose treatment is described above and EO-specific toxicities such as hepatitis or central nervous system depression. Treatment of hepatitis or coma requires frequent monitoring of the patient's status, with supportive measures as indicated. Hemodialysis may be indicated for patients in acute renal failure, but has not been shown to enhance elimination of a clinically significant amount of an EO. Ingestion of pennyroyal oil may require early consideration of administration of the antidote, NAC, to prevent hepatic injury.

RESOURCES

Box 101-2 provides information on Internet resources for herbs, dietary supplements, and essential oils.

TABLE 101-1 Selected Essential Oils and Their Toxicities

ESSENTIAL OIL	BOTANICAL NAME	PURPORTED INDICATIONS	TOXIC INGREDIENTS	SYMPTOMS/TOXIC EFFECTS
Chamomile	*Chamaemelum nobile*	Eczema, asthma	Tiglic oil	Somnolence, gastrointestinal upset, allergic reactions, bronchospasm, increased bleeding time, uterine stimulant
Absinthe	*Artemisia* species	Malaria, antihelminthic	Thujone	GI upset, seizures, coma, psychosis, memory loss
Chenopodium	American wormseed, Jerusalem oak	Anti-parasitic agent	Ascaridole, cymene, camphor, limonene	Nausea, vomiting, abdominal pain, dizziness, parethesias, seizures, coma, impaired vision, optic atrophy, hepatitis
Cinnamon	*Cinnamomum zeylanicum*	Flavoring, stimulant, carminative	Cinnamic aldehyde	Hypersensitivity reactions, dermatitis, stomatitis, nausea, vomiting, abdominal pain, facial flushing, dizziness, oral lesions, skin burning sensation

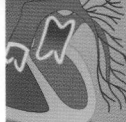

TABLE 101-1 Selected Essential Oils and Their Toxicities—*cont'd*

ESSENTIAL OIL	BOTANICAL NAME	PURPORTED INDICATIONS	TOXIC INGREDIENTS	SYMPTOMS/TOXIC EFFECTS
Clove	*Eugenia* species	Toothache, flavoring, disinfectant as used in dental procedures	Eugenol, caryophillin, vanillin	Oral and skin irritation, allergic reactions, nausea, vomiting, respiratory symptoms, hepatic necrosis, lethargy, ataxia, seizures
Eucalyptus	*Melaleuca alternifolia*	Antitussive	1,8 cineole (eucalyptol), hydrocyanic acid	Vomiting, abdominal pain, bronchospasm, bronchorrhea, pneumonitis, respiratory depression, dizziness, headaches, ataxia, obtundation, coma, seizures
Hyssop	*Hyssopus officinalis*	Nervous exhaustion, grief, emmenagogue	Pinocamphone	Seizures, hypertension
Juniper	*Juniperus communis*	Arthritis, antibacterial, carminative, diuretic	Terpinen-4-ol	Uterine spasm, tachycardia, dermatitis
Lavender	*Lavandula* species	Many dysfunctions, including sedative, anxiolytic, antimicrobial	Cintronellal, others	Allergies
Lemon grass	*Melissa oficinalis,* lemon balm, sweet balm	Flavoring, sedative, antidepressant	Citral	Dermatitis
Myrrh	*Comiphora molmol*	Anti-inflammatory, GI upset, asthma	Sesquiterpenes	Tachycardia, dermatitis, abortifacient
Nutmeg	*Myristica fragrans*	Toothache, GI upset, halitosis	Myristacin	Nausea, vomiting, abdominal pain, diarrhea, hallucinations, coma
Pennyroyal	*Hedeoma pulegiodies*	Abortifacient	Pulegone	Nausea, vomiting, abdominal pain, hepatitis, centrilobular hepatic necrosis, kidney failure, pneumonia
Peppermint	*Mentha* species	Antispasmodic, carminative, used in irritable bowel syndrome	Menthol, menthone	Hypersensitivity reactions, ataxia, myalgia
Pine	*Pinus* species	Disinfectant	Monoterpene, aromatic pine oil, other hydrocarbons	CNS effects, respiratory failure
Rose	*Rosa* species	Aphrodisiac, anxiety	Hydrocarbons	Aspiration pneumonia, nephrotoxic
Sandalwood	*Santalum album*	Flavor, anxiety	Santalol	CNS effects, mucous membrane irritant, GI upset, kidney pain
Sassafras	*Sassafras albidum*	Pediculosis capitis, abortifacient	Safrole, pinene, camphor	Vomiting, dizziness, stupor, shock, hepatocarcinoma
Tea tree	*Melaleuca alternifolia*	Antibacterial	Terpinen-4-ol	Stupor, ataxia, sores
Yarrow	*Achillea millefolium*	Anti-inflammatory, antispasmodic	Sesquiterpene lactones, polyacetylenes, simple coumarins, flavonoids	Allergy, antispermatogen

BOX 101-2   INTERNET RESOURCES ON HERBS, DIETARY SUPPLEMENTS, AND ESSENTIAL OILS

www.mcp.edu/herbal: Longwood Herbal Task Force Monographs and clinician and patient information sheets on over 80 selected herbs and dietary supplements.

www.holistickids.org: Website providing overview of complementary and alternative medicine use in children, including herbs and dietary supplements.

www.micromedex.com/products/poisindex/: Subscription-based database with documents providing data on clinical effects, range of toxicity, and treatment protocols for toxic exposure.

www.naturalstandard.com: Subscription-based website providing peer-reviewed monographs on herbs, dietary supplements, and complementary and alternative medicine.

www.herbalgram.org: Established in 1988, the American Botanical Council is an independent and not-for-profit member-based organization providing science-based and traditional information on herbal medicine.

ods.od.nih.gov/showpage.aspx?pageid=48: The International Bibliographic Information on Dietary Supplements database provides access to bibliographic citations and abstracts from published international scientific literature on dietary supplements. It is maintained by the Office of Dietary Supplements (ODS).

www.mskcc.org: Information on natriceuticals and complementary and alternative medicine (CAM) for oncologists and health care professionals, including a clinical summary for each agent and details about constituents, adverse effects, interactions, and potential benefits or problems.

www.mdanderson.org: University of Texas, Houston, M.D. Anderson Cancer Center overview of integrative therapies, including resources on herbs and dietary supplements.

www.fda.org: Source for updates from the Food and Drug Administration concerning possible interactions between commonly used herbs and drugs or new information concerning adverse effects of commonly used herbal preparations or dietary supplements.

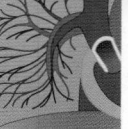
REFERENCES

1. Nelson RR: In-vitro activities of five plant essential oils against methicillin-resistant *Staphylococcus aureus* and vancomycin-resistant *Enterococcus faecium*. J Antimicrob Chemother 1997;40(2):305–306.
2. Maudsley F, Kerr KG: Microbiological safety of essential oils used in complementary therapies and the activity of these compounds against bacterial and fungal pathogens. Support Care Cancer 1999;7(2):100–102.
3. Hart PH, Brand C, Carson CF, et al: Terpinen-4-ol, the main component of the essential oil of *Melaleuca alternifolia* (tea tree oil), suppresses inflammatory mediator production by activated human monocytes. Inflamm Res 2000;49(11):619–626.
4. Seymour R: Additional properties and uses of essential oils. J Clin Periodontol 2003;30(suppl 5):19–21.
5. Rittenberry TJ, Feldman R: The volatile oils. In Hadadd LM (ed): Clinical Management for Poisoning and Drug Overdose. New York, WB Saunders, 1998, pp 1174–1179.
6. Bleasel N, Tate B, Rademaker M: Allergic contact dermatitis following exposure to essential oils. Aust J Dermatol 2002; 43(3):211–213.
7. Lazutka JR, Mierauskiene J, Slapsyte G, et al: Genotoxicity of dill (*Anethum graveolens L.*), peppermint (*Menthaxpiperita L.*) and pine (*Pinus sylvestris L.*) essential oils in human lymphocytes and *Drosophila melanogaster*. Food Chem Toxicol 2001;39(5):485–492.
8. Osal A: The Dispensatory of the United States of America. Philadelphia, Lippincott, 1955.
9. Rumack BH: POISINDEX. Greenwood Village, CO, Thomson Micromedex, 1989.
10. Pilapil VR: Toxic manifestation of cinnamon oil ingestion in a child. Clin Pediatr (Phil) 1989;28(6):276.
11. Westra WH, McMurray JS, Califano J, et al: Squamous cell carcinoma of the tongue associated with cinnamon gum use: a case report. Head Neck 1998;20(5):430–433.
12. Lamey PJ, Lewis MAO, Rees TD, et al: Sensitivity reaction to the cinnamonaldehyde component of toothpaste. Br Dent J 1990;168(3):115–118.
13. Mihail RC: Oral leukoplakia caused by cinnamon food allergy. J Otolaryngol 1992;21(5):366–367.
14. Miller RL, Gould AR, Bernstein ML: Cinnamon-induced stomatitis venenata. Clinical and characteristic histopathologic features. Oral Surg Oral Med Oral Pathol 1992;73(6):708–716.
15. Sachez-Perez J, Garcia-Diez NA: Occupational allergic contact dermatitis from eugenol, oil of cinnamon and oil of cloves in a physiotherapist. Contact Dermatitis 1999;41(6):346–347.
16. Perry PA, Dean BS, Krenzelok EP: Cinnamon oil abuse by adolescents. Vet Hum Toxicol 1990;32(2):162–164.
17. Whitman BW, Ghazizadeh H: Eucalyptus oil: therapeutic and toxic aspects of pharmacology in humans and animals. J Paediatr Child Health 1994;30(2):190–191.
18. Webb NJ, Pitt WR: Eucalyptus oil poisoning in childhood: 41 cases in south-east Queensland. J Paediatr Child Health 1993;29(5):368–371.
19. Spoerke DG, Vandenberg SA, Smolinske SC, et al: Eucalyptus oil: 14 cases of exposure. Vet Hum Toxicol 1989;31(2):166–168.
20. Tibballs J: Clinical effects and management of eucalyptus oil ingestion in infants and young children. Med J Aust 1995; 163(4):177–180.
21. Day LM, Ozanne-Smith J, Parsons BJ, et al: Eucalyptus oil poisoning among young children: mechanisms of access and the potential for prevention. Aust N Z J Public Health 1997;21(3): 297–302.
22. Gurr FW: Eucalyptus oil poisoning treated by dialysis and mannitol infusion. Aust Ann Med 1965;4:238–249.
23. MacPherson J: The toxicology of eucalyptus oil. Med J Aust 1925;1:313.
24. Darben T, Cominos B, Lee CT: Topical eucalyptus oil poisoning. Aust J Dermatol 1998;39(4):265–267.
25. Payne RB: Nutmeg intoxication. N Engl J Med 1963;269:36–39.
26. Anonymous: Toxic reactions to plant products sold in health food stores. Med Lett Drugs Ther 1979;21(7):29–32.
27. Stein U, Greyer H, Hentschel H: Nutmeg (myristicin) poisoning—report on a fatal case and a series of cases recorded by a poison information centre. Forensic Sci Int 2001;118(1):87–90.
28. Anderson IB, Mullen WH, Meeker JE, et al: Pennyroyal toxicity: measurement of toxic metabolite levels in two cases and review of the literature. Ann Intern Med 1996; 124(8):726–734.
29. Bakerink JA, Gospe SM, Dimand RJ, et al: Multiple organ failure after ingestion of pennyroyal oil from herbal tea in two infants. Pediatrics 1996;98(5):944–947.
30. Sztajnkrycer MD, Otten EJ, Bond GR, et al: Mitigation of pennyroyal oil hepatotoxicity in the mouse. Acad Emerg Med 2003; 10(10):1024–1028.
31. Gordon WP, Huitric AC, Seth CL, et al: The metabolism of the abortifacient terpene, (R)-(+)-pulegone, to a proximate toxin, menthoruran. Drug Metab Dispos 1987;15(5):589–594.
32. Thomassen D, Slattery JT, Nelson SD: Contribution of menthofuran to the hepatotoxicity of pulegone: assessment based on matched area under the curve and on matched time course. J Pharmacol Exp Ther 1988;244(3):825–829.
33. Early DF: Pennyroyal poisoning: rare case of epilepsy. Lancet 1961;2:580.
34. Holland GW: A case of poisoning from pennyroyal. Va Med Semimonthly 1902;7:319.
35. Kimball HW: Poisoning by pennyroyal. Atlanta Med Weekly 1898;9:397.
36. Sullivan JB Jr, Rumack BH, Thomas H, et al: Pennyroyal oil poisoning and hepatotoxicity. JAMA 1979;242(26):2873–2874.
37. Altman PM: Summary of safety studies concerning Australian tea tree oil. In Modern Phytotherapy—The Clinical Significance of Tree Oil and Other Essential Oils. Proceedings of a Conference. Surfer's Paradise, Australia, 1990.
38. Zhang SY, Robertson D: A study of tea tree oil ototoxicity. Audiol Neurootol 2000;5(2):64–68.
39. Carson CF, Riley TV: Safety, efficacy and provenance of tea tree (*Melaleuca alternifolia*)oil. Contact Dermatitis 2001;45(2):65–67.
40. Herbal/plant therapies: tea tree oil (*Melaleuca alternifolia* [Maiden & Betche] Cheel). In Review of Herbal Therapies. www.naturalstandard.com, 2002.
41. Mozelsio NB, Harris KE, McGrath KG, et al: Immediate systemic hypersensitivity reaction associated with topical application of Australian tea tree oil. Allergy Asthma Proc 2003;24(1):73–75.
42. Jacobs MR, Hornfeldt CS: Melaleuca oil poisoning. J Toxicol Clin Toxicol 1994;32(4):461–464.
43. Seawright A: Comment: tea tree oil poisoning. Med J Aust 1993;159:831.
44. Maffei M, Sacco T: Chemical and morphometrical comparison between two peppermint notomorphs. Planta Med 1987;53: 214–215.
45. Perez-Raya MD, Utrilla MP, Navarro MC, et al: CNS activity of *Mentha rotundifolia* and *mentha longifolia* essential oil in mice and rats. Phytother Res 1990;4:232–234.
46. Rogers J, Tay HH, Misiewicz JJ, Peppermint oil. Lancet 1988; 2(8602):98–99.
47. Eickholt TH, Box RH, Toxicities of peppermint and *Pycnanthemum albescens* oils, fam. Labiateae. J Pharm Sci 1965;54(7):1071–1072.
48. Spindler P, Madsen C: Subchronic toxicity study of peppermint oil in rats. Toxicol Lett 1992;62(2–3):215–220.
49. Olowe SA, Ransome-Kuti O: The risk of jaundice in glucose-6-phosphatase deficient babies exposed to menthol. Acta Paediatri Scand 1980;69:341–345.
50. Blake KD, Fertleman CR, Meates MA: Dangers of common cold treatments in children. Lancet 1993;341(8845):640.
51. Poisinex Managements: Eugenol. In Thomson Micromedex Healthcare Series, Vol 119. Greenwood Village, CO, Thomson, 2004.
52. LaVoie EJ, Adams J, Reinhardt J, et al: Toxicity studies on clove cigarette smoke and constituents of clove: determination of the LD50 of eugenol by intratracheal instillation in rats and hamsters. Arch Toxicol 1986;59(2):78–81.
53. Lauber FU, Hollander F: Toxicity of the mucigogue, eugenol, administered by stomach tube to dogs. Gastroenterology 1950; 15:481.
54. Hartnoll G, Moore D, Douek D: Near fatal ingestion of oil of cloves. Arch Dis Child 1993;69(3):392–393.
55. Lane BW, Ellenhorn MJ, Hulbert TV, et al: Clove oil ingestion in an infant. Hum Exp Toxicol 1991;10(4):291–294.
56. Libby GF: Ocular injury from oil of cloves. Opthalmic Rec 1912;21:189.
57. Isaacs G: Permanent local anaesthesia and anhidrosis after clove oil spillage. Lancet 1983;1(8329):882.
58. Centers For Disease Control and Prevention: Illnesses possibly associated with smoking clove cigarettes. MMWR 1985;34(21):297–299.
59. Klein BL, Simon JE: Hydrocarbon poisonings. Pediatr Clin North Am 1986;33(2):411–419.
60. Scalzo AJ, Weber TR, Jaeger RW, et al: Extracorporeal membrane oxygenation for hydrocarbon ingestion. Am J Dis Child 1990; 144(8):867–871.

102 Soaps, Detergents, and Bleaches

LEO J. SIORIS, PHARMD ■ HEATHER K. SCHULLER, PHARMD

At a Glance...

- Household cleaning products generally have a low level of toxicity.
- Toxicity is more often due to local effects than systemic effects.
- Personal care soaps, hand dishwashing detergents, household laundry detergents, and household bleaches may be irritants.
- Automatic dishwashing detergents and cationic disinfectants can be corrosive.
- Ocular tissues and respiratory mucosa tend to be more sensitive than gastrointestinal mucosa or skin to exposures by household products.
- Inhalation or aspiration of household products may warrant medical attention.
- Powdered products may cause mechanical irritation as well as chemical irritation, especially to the eye.

Exposures to household cleaning products account for a large proportion of calls to poison control centers in the United States. The 2003 Annual Report of the American Association of Poison Control Centers (AAPCC) reports that cleaning products, as a category, rank second (to analgesics) in number of exposures to humans of all ages (9.4% of exposures), second (to cosmetics and personal care products) in number of exposures to children younger than 6 years (9.7% of exposures), and third (to analgesics and sedative-hypnotics and antipsychotics) in number of exposures to adults older than 19 years (8.9% of exposures). Of these exposures to cleaning products, only 0.011% resulted in the death of the exposed individual.[1] As categorized by the AAPCC, household cleaning products include, but are not limited to, bleaches, soaps, detergents, ammonia, disinfectants, glass cleaners, acids, and alkalis. This chapter examines the toxicologic aspects of bleaches, soaps, and detergents. Tables 102-1 and 102-2 summarize the AAPCC 2003 Annual Report's age-related and outcome data for these types of cleaning products.

SOAPS AND DETERGENTS

A *soap* is defined as the salt of a fatty acid (most often the sodium or potassium salt) and is one of the simplest and earliest examples of a household cleaning agent. Soaps belong to the broader category of substances called *surface-active agents*, or *surfactants*. Surfactant molecules contain both polar and nonpolar regions, which effectively decreases the surface tension of water. This helps water to wet surfaces more effectively and results in more efficient cleaning and washing. Surfactants can also help remove dirt, disperse soil, and emulsify oil or grease in the wash water.[2] A major limitation of soap as a cleaning agent is its decreased effectiveness when used in hard water. Hard water contains minerals such as calcium, magnesium, iron, or manganese that can combine with the fatty acids in soap and form a precipitate known as soap scum or film. This film does not rinse away easily, leaving deposits on clothing and surfaces. In addition, because some of the soap is removed from the wash water in this precipitate, the amount of soap available for cleaning is reduced. The development of detergents that perform well under a variety of conditions has reduced this problem.[3]

Like soaps, detergents are surfactants, but are more variable in structure and function. Detergent surfactants fall into one of four categories corresponding to the electrical charge on the polar portion of the molecule: nonionic, anionic, cationic, and amphoteric. Box 102-1 lists common examples of each type of surfactant. Household detergents usually contain nonionic or anionic surfactants, or a combination of the two. Cationic and amphoteric surfactants are used to a lesser extent in household detergents.[2] Soaps are anionic surfactants and, therefore, could be considered a subtype of detergents. In its common usage, the term *detergent* encompasses cleaning products that contain detergent surfactants as well as additional ingredients that enhance the cleaning efficacy of the surfactants. This usage is employed for the remainder of this chapter, with detergent surfactants being referred to as *surfactants*.

In addition to surfactants, many detergent products contain alkaline builders that enhance or maintain the cleaning efficacy of the surfactants. The primary function of builders is to reduce water hardness by inactivating hardness minerals. Builders can also supply and maintain alkalinity, prevent redeposition of soil during washing, and emulsify oily and greasy soils. Common builders found in household detergents include complex phosphates, sodium carbonate, sodium silicate, and sodium metasilicate.[3] Due to concern that began building in the late 1960s over the contribution of phosphates to eutrophication of lakes, phosphates are now banned in most states in the United States. For manufacturing convenience and cost-effectiveness, the detergent industry phased out the use of phosphates in domestic laundry detergents by 1996.[4]

A few detergent products contain small amounts of enzymes such as proteases, amylases, lipases, and cellulases that catalyze the breakdown of organic stains. This improves detergent performance and reduces required wash temperature and cycle time.[5] Detergents may also contain whiteners, colorants, softeners, fragrances, and bleaches.[2] Concentrations of these additives are

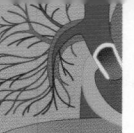

TABLE 102-1 Age-Related Statistics for Selected Household Products

			AGE (yr)			
		NO. OF EXPOSURES	**<6**	**6–19**	**>19**	**UNACCOUNTED**
Personal Care Soaps	Soap	17,265	13,475	1275	2465	50
	Percentage		78.05%	7.38%	14.28%	0.29%
Hand Dishwashing	Anionic/nonionic	5614	3609	423	1545	37
Detergents	Other/unknown	1885	1123	175	580	7
	Total	**7499**	**4732**	**598**	**2125**	**44**
	Percentage		63.10%	7.97%	28.34%	0.59%
Automatic Dishwasher	Granular	4310	3638	117	537	18
Detergents	Liquid or gel	4690	4001	120	561	8
	Tablet	787	714	17	54	2
	Rinse agent	1394	1306	13	74	1
	Other/unknown	1044	827	53	158	6
	Total	**12,225**	**10,486**	**320**	**1384**	**35**
	Percentage		85.78%	2.62%	11.32%	0.29%
Laundry Detergents	Granular	5448	4427	269	731	21
	Liquid	4683	3282	287	1097	17
	Soap	86	55	4	27	0
	Other/unknown	283	211	16	54	2
	Total	**10,500**	**7975**	**576**	**1909**	**40**
	Percentage		75.95%	5.49%	18.18%	0.38%
Bleaches	Borate	690	347	50	273	20
	Hypochlorite	54,284	20,839	5277	27,497	671
	Nonhypochlorite	703	307	62	322	12
	Other/unknown	468	170	46	239	13
	Total	**56,145**	**21,663**	**5435**	**28,331**	**716**
	Percentage		38.58%	9.68%	5046%	1.28%
Chlorine or Chloramine Gas	Chloramine	642	22	57	556	7
	Chlorine	727	32	68	620	7
	Total	**1369**	**54**	**125**	**1176**	**14**
	Percentage		3.94%	9.13%	85.90%	1.02%

Adapted from Watson WA, Litovitz TL, Klein-Schwartz W, et al: 2003 annual report of the American Association of Poison Control Centers Toxic Exposure Surveillance System. Am J Emerg Med 2004;22(5):335–404.

typically too low to result in clinically significant toxicity, but sensitization may occur. Medicinal soaps contain small amounts of antibacterial agents that do not contribute significant toxicity.[6]

Sources

The term *soap* generally refers to personal care soaps such as bar soaps and liquid hand and body soaps. The term *detergent* generally refers to, but is not limited to, hand dishwashing detergents, automatic dishwasher detergents, and laundry detergents. Some liquid hand and body soaps also contain mild detergents.

Personal care soaps and hand dishwashing detergents generally contain anionic, nonionic, or amphoteric surfactants. Laundry detergents generally contain anionic or nonionic surfactants. Automatic dishwasher detergents generally contain nonionic surfactants because they are lower sudsing than anionic surfactants.[3,7] Fabric softeners generally contain cationic surfactants, and some disinfectants contain cationic surfactants.[3,8,9] Builders are typically included in laundry and automatic dishwashing detergents and account for much of the toxicity related to these products.[2]

Toxicity

The surfactants and builders contained in these products are the major contributors to product toxicity. The relative toxicity of surfactants can be graded according to the type of surfactant involved. Nonionic and amphoteric surfactants have the lowest toxicity, anionic surfactants have intermediate toxicity, and cationic surfactants have the highest toxicity.[10] Nonionic, anionic, and amphoteric surfactants are irritating to the gastrointestinal (GI) mucosa and conjunctiva.[11,12] Cationics are classified as irritants at concentrations below 7.5%, but can be corrosive at concentrations above this. Cationic surfactants can also cause systemic toxicity if ingested at higher doses or concentrations (see later).[8,13] Surfactants of any type may cause or contribute to dermal irritation by increasing permeability of the skin.[14] Therefore, the surfactant itself may cause irritation, as well as contribute to increased sensitivity to other substances with which the skin may come in contact.

Builders are alkaline compounds that are irritants at low concentrations but can be corrosive at higher concentrations. For example, corrosive injury can result from a 0.5% solution of sodium metasilicate or a 15%

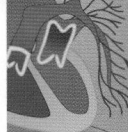

TABLE 102-2 Outcome-Related Statistics for Selected Household Products

			OUTCOME					
		NO. OF EXPOSURES	NONE	MINOR	MODERATE	MAJOR	DEATH	UNACCOUNTED
Personal Care Soaps	Soap	17,265	2732	2262	127	5	1	12,138
	Percentage		15.82%	13.10%	0.74%	0.029%	0.01%	70.30%
Hand Dishwashing	Anionic/nonionic	5614	772	1189	73	1	1	3578
Detergents	Other/unknown	1885	234	363	23	0	0	1265
	Total	**7499**	1006	1552	96	1	1	4843
	Percentage		13.42%	20.70%	1.28%	0.01%	0.013%	64.58%
Automatic Dishwasher	Granular	4310	1389	626	46	1	1	2247
Detergents	Liquid or gel	4690	1450	877	53	1	1	2308
	Tablet	787	271	101	4	0	0	411
	Rinse agent	1394	319	146	14	0	0	915
	Other/unknown	1044	250	134	18	1	0	641
	Total	**12,225**	3679	1884	135	3	2	6522
	Percentage		30.09%	15.41%	1.10%	0.025%	0.02%	53.35%
Laundry Detergents	Granular	5448	1262	1237	78	1	1	2869
	Liquid	4683	807	1162	97	5	0	2612
	Soap	86	21	16	4	0	0	45
	Other/unknown	283	77	51	8	0	0	147
	Total	**10,500**	2167	2466	187	6	1	5673
	Percentage		20.64%	23.49%	1.78%	0.057%	0.010%	54.03%
Bleaches	Borate	690	125	181	20	1	0	363
	Hypochlorite	54,284	7419	15,559	2530	60	1	28,715
	Nonhypochlorite	703	111	194	32	1	0	365
	Other/unknown	468	51	146	40	2	0	229
	Total	**56,145**	7706	16,080	2622	64	1	29,672
	Percentage		13.73%	28.64%	4.67%	0.11%	0.0018%	52.85%
Chlorine or Chloramine	Chloramine	642	42	243	106	0	0	251
Gas	Chlorine	727	54	340	137	2	1	193
	Total	**1369**	96	583	243	2	1	444
	Percentage		7.01%	42.59%	17.75%	0.15%	0.073%	32.43%

Adapted from Watson WA, Litovitz TL, Klein-Schwartz W, et al: 2003 annual report of the American Association of Poison Control Centers Toxic Exposure Surveillance System. Am J Emerg Med 2004;22(5):335–404.

solution of sodium carbonate.[13,15,16] Sodium silicate is less corrosive but can produce corrosive injury at concentrations of 20% to 40% or more. Complex phosphates are the least toxic builders; however, they can be corrosive at high concentrations with prolonged contact.[15,17] Systemic effects related to hyperphosphatemia can result from substantial ingestions of phosphate-containing detergents.[13]

If the concentration of a builder or other possibly corrosive substance in a product is unknown, the product's pH can be used to assess probable corrosiveness. A general rule is that corrosive injury becomes a risk at pH lower than 2 or higher than 12.[18] However, product pH should not be used as the sole determinant in the assessment of an exposed patient. In addition, it must be recognized that some substances with a neutral pH can cause tissue damage (such as quaternary ammonium cationic surfactants) and that the concentration and other physical properties of a substance also contribute to corrosiveness.

Enzymes exhibit a very low level of toxicity, with adverse effects being limited to the development of hypersensitivity and irritation of the skin, eye, and other mucosal sites. Enzymes have also been linked to occu-pational asthma in employees of detergent manufacturing plants; however, encapsulation of enzymes has decreased the inhaled dust and the associated incidence of asthma in the industry. If used as directed in laundry products, enzymes are not generally irritating.[19]

Manifestations

PERSONAL CARE SOAPS AND HAND DISHWASHING DETERGENTS

Personal care soaps and hand dishwashing detergents are of low toxicity. Ingestion may cause GI irritation with associated complaints of nausea, vomiting, and diarrhea.[2,7,12] There is a slight risk for aspiration of foam or vomitus after ingestion of these products, which can result in respiratory irritation, chemical pneumonitis, or pulmonary edema with associated coughing, gagging, dyspnea, or stridor.[11,12] Ocular exposure to these products is associated with irritation and mild conjunctivitis without damage to the corneal epithelium.[2] However, some heavy-duty personal care soaps contain abrasives that can cause mechanical injury to the corneal epithelium and conjunctiva. Although uncommon, some sensitive individuals may experience dermal irritation

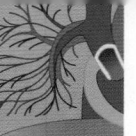

BOX 102-1	SURFACTANTS USED IN SYNTHETIC HOUSEHOLD DETERGENTS

Anionic

Alkyl sodium sulfates
Alkyl sodium sulfonates
Dioctyl sodium sulfosuccinate
Linear alkyl benzene sulfonate (Na⁺)
Sodium lauryl sulfate
Tetrapropylene benzene sulfonate (Na⁺)

Nonionic

Alkyl ethoxylate
Alkyl phenoxy polyethoxy ethanols
Polyethylene glycol stearate

Cationic

Quaternary ammonium compounds
  Benzalkonium chloride
  Benzethonium chloride
Pyridinium compounds
  Cetylpyridinium chloride
Quinolinium compounds
  Dequalinium chloride

Amphoteric

Imidazolines
Betaines

Adapted from Haddad LM, Shannon MW, Winchester JF: Clinical Management of Poisoning and Drug Overdose, 3rd ed. Philadelphia, WB Saunders, 1998.

with prolonged exposure, especially in cold, dry climates where the skin may already be compromised. This would manifest as dryness, pruritus, or erythema.[2]

LAUNDRY DETERGENTS

Laundry detergents contain builders as well as surfactants, adding another dimension of toxicity. However, most household laundry detergents, whether liquid or granular, do not generally contain high enough concentrations of builders to be considered corrosive. Like soaps and hand dishwashing detergents, laundry detergents are irritants, and ingestion is associated with nausea, vomiting, and diarrhea.[2,7,12] A small number of laundry detergents may contain high enough concentrations of builders to cause mucosal injury on ingestion, which, by law, should be indicated on the label. Aspiration of product or vomitus may lead to respiratory irritation or chemical pneumonitis with associated symptoms discussed previously. Ocular exposure typically results in irritation, stinging, and erythema of the conjunctiva, with granular laundry detergents contributing greater toxicity owing to the risk for abrasive injury.[2] Whether liquid or granular, formulations containing sodium carbonate have been shown to have greater potential for ocular irritation, possibly leading to corrosion and opacity of the cornea.[7] Dermal exposure may result in similar manifestations as those due to soaps and hand dishwashing detergents, with a small number of sensitive individuals experiencing irritation, pruritus, and erythema, especially in cold, dry climates where the skin may already be compromised.[2]

In countries other than the United States, phosphates may be a major ingredient of laundry detergents. Despite their low toxicity, there is a case report of a 30-year-old patient in the United Kingdom developing hyperphosphatemia as a result of the intentional ingestion of an unknown amount of a laundry detergent containing more than 30% phosphates. This was associated with hypocalcemia and hypomagnesemia due to chelation by the phosphate. The hypocalcemia resulted in ventilatory failure due to respiratory muscle spasm. Supportive measures were instituted, and the patient survived.[20]

A less common but potentially serious complication of ingestion or inhalation of *powdered* laundry detergents is respiratory distress. Case studies appearing in the literature describe the development of drooling, stridor, retractions, and respiratory distress in pediatric patients who ingested or inhaled non–phosphate powdered laundry detergents. Symptoms were often accompanied by erythema and edema of the vocal cords and epiglottis. There was no damage to the esophageal mucosa in most cases and only minimal damage in the remainder.[1] The irritant effect of powdered laundry detergents is of little clinical significance in the GI tract, but if the vocal cords or epiglottis are affected, erythema and edema may result in significant airway compromise.[21,22]

AUTOMATIC DISHWASHER DETERGENTS

Automatic dishwasher detergents are more alkaline than the other detergents described previously because of higher concentrations of alkaline builders, possibly up to 70% to 80%. The high alkalinity is required for product performance, but unfortunately, increases the risk for corrosive injury.[17] Ingestion of even small amounts of granular or liquid products is associated with nausea, immediate vomiting, and possibly diarrhea.[2] Corrosive injury to the upper GI tract is possible, symptoms of which may include burns to the mouth and oropharynx, coughing, drooling, vomiting, chest or throat pain, stridor, and dysphagia.[2,6] Endoscopy may reveal edema of the epiglottis and vocal cords as well as erosion of the esophageal mucosa. Development of strictures (although uncommon) may follow esophageal injury.[17] It is important to note that the presence of oral injury does not necessarily correlate with the presence of esophageal or gastric injury.[2,15,17] Additionally, it has been reported that a small number of asymptomatic individuals may have esophageal lesions revealed on endoscopy.[17] As with other soaps and detergents, aspiration of product or vomitus can result in chemical pneumonitis and respiratory distress. Because of the alkalinity of automatic dishwasher detergents, sequelae due to aspiration may be more severe, and death has been reported.[19]

Ocular exposure to automatic dishwasher detergents generally produces conjunctival irritation with the potential for corrosive injury. Because the tissues of the eye can be more sensitive to exposure than the tissue of the GI tract, the incidence of symptoms from ocular

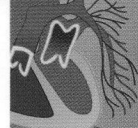

exposure is greater than that from ingestion. In a study of exposures to liquid automatic dishwasher detergents, most patients with eye exposures presented with minor corneal abrasions, whereas a minority of the patients had more severe abrasions. Because liquid automatic dishwasher detergents are aqueous slurries of solute, whether the exposure is to a liquid or granular product, it is difficult to determine if the ocular irritation is secondary to mechanical abrasion or to alkaline injury.[23]

Dermal exposure to automatic dishwasher detergents, like other detergents, may result in irritation, pruritus, erythema, and rash.[2] Blistering has been reported infrequently. Because of product alkalinity, symptoms are more frequent than with hand dishwashing and laundry detergents, yet only occur in a minority of exposures.[23] Contact with undiluted product has been rarely associated with contact dermatitis.[2]

CATIONIC DETERGENTS

Fabric softeners and some disinfectant cleaners contain cationic surfactants. Generally, the cationics used in household fabric softeners have a much lower order of toxicity than those in disinfectants. Fabric softeners and disinfectants with cationic surfactant concentrations below 7.5% are GI and dermal irritants, with manifestations similar to exposure to hand dishwashing or laundry detergents.[2,8] Ocular tissues are more sensitive to cationic surfactants, with even one drop of a 2% solution having the potential to cause corrosive injury and severe corneal damage.[8] Symptoms often include irritation, tearing, erythema, and burning. Disinfectants with cationic surfactant concentrations higher than 7.5% can cause corrosive injury to any tissue. Symptoms associated with ingestion include drooling; vomiting; hematemesis; burning pain in the mouth, throat, and abdomen; and possibly oral burns. Esophageal burns may be discovered on endoscopy.[8,13]

Because cationic surfactants are rapidly absorbed from the GI tract, ingestion can result in systemic symptoms that include hypotension, restlessness, confusion, central nervous system depression, renal insufficiency, circulatory collapse, convulsions, and coma. The mechanism of these toxic effects is unknown.[13,24] Because of a structural similarity to curare-type skeletal muscle relaxants, ingestion of quaternary ammonium-type cationics has been associated with muscle weakness and paralysis, possibly preceded by transient muscle fasciculation. This may progress to weakness of the respiratory muscles, dyspnea, and asphyxial death.[8,10,13,24] Death due to circulatory failure or asphyxia may occur within 1 to 2 hours of ingestion.[13] Human deaths due to benzalkonium chloride ingestion have been seen at doses of 100 to 400 mg/kg and at 1 to 3 g total.[24] Some observations of cholinesterase inhibition have been demonstrated in vitro by several cationic surfactants. A 50% inhibition of red cell, but not plasma, cholinesterase was observed after intraperitoneal injection of cationic surfactants in rats; however, no symptoms were observed. It was therefore concluded that toxicity due to cholinesterase inhibition is improbable,[13] especially after expected routes of household exposure.

Dermal exposure to concentrated cationic surfactants can cause dermal necrosis, exacerbated by occlusion of the skin.[8] Cationic surfactants have also been associated with occupational asthma, allergic contact dermatitis, and ocular hypersensitivity.[9,25]

Management

INGESTION

Most sources suggest that ingestion of soaps, hand dishwashing detergents, and laundry detergents can be managed at home by dilution with milk or water. If an animal is exposed, water is suggested because other fluids may cause further GI irritation. Oral fluid intake should be limited to 4 oz for children and 8 oz for adults, so as not to distend the stomach. Other sources advocate no oral dilution because of a possible risk for "sudsing" and aspiration. GI decontamination by any means is unnecessary, with spontaneous vomiting often occurring nonetheless. If vomiting or diarrhea is excessive, fluid and electrolytes should be replaced and monitored as necessary, possibly in a health care facility. Any patient who experiences spontaneous vomiting should be monitored for 6 to 8 hours for signs of aspiration of product or vomitus. Manifestations, including coughing, gagging, dyspnea, or stridor, warrant an emergency department visit for chest radiograph and supportive care. Management of ingestion or inhalation of *powdered* laundry detergent must also include careful monitoring of respiratory function. In cases of respiratory complications, the onset of symptoms may occur between 2 and 12 hours after exposure. Development of symptoms necessitates an immediate emergency department visit for supportive care and evaluation.[21] If a large concentration of a phosphate-containing laundry detergent is ingested, electrolyte levels should be monitored for 4 to 6 hours (including phosphorus, calcium, magnesium) and treated appropriately. Phosphate binders such as Sevelamer may be a better treatment than calcium supplementation because of the risk for precipitation of calcium phosphate crystals in soft tissues.[20]

Ingestions of automatic dishwasher detergents should be managed based on the properties of the particular detergent and on the individual's symptoms. GI decontamination is unwarranted in any exposure to automatic dishwasher detergents and could be harmful with corrosive ingestions. For detergents with pH lower than 12, which are less likely to cause corrosive injury, patient symptoms can guide treatment. If the exposed individual is asymptomatic, dilution at home with 4 to 8 oz of water or milk should suffice initially. The individual should then be observed for an additional 6 to 8 hours for symptoms of oral or esophageal injury. Symptom manifestation warrants emergency department care for corrosive injury (see Chapter 98). If the exposed individual is symptomatic at the outset, immediate evaluation for corrosive injury should be sought. Dilution with a small amount of water or milk (2–4 oz) may be beneficial in rinsing the product from the affected area. If detergent pH is higher than 12 and the

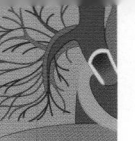

patient is symptomatic, emergency care for corrosive injury should be sought. Again, dilution with 2 to 4 oz of water or milk may be helpful in rinsing the product from the affected area. Animals exposed to automatic dishwasher detergent may not have the ability to display symptoms of corrosive injury nor vocalize their discomfort. Therefore, all ingestions of automatic dishwasher detergents in animals should be evaluated by a veterinarian for corrosive esophageal injury.

Ingestions of cationic detergents should be managed based on the concentration of the cationic compound in the product and the individual's symptoms. Small ingestions of products with concentrations below 7.5% can be managed similarly to hand dishwashing and laundry detergents. Ingestions of concentrated cationic detergents (>7.5%) should be managed as corrosive exposures. If a very large amount of a dilute product or more than a few swallows of a concentrated product has been ingested (fatal dose estimated to be 1 to 3 g), the individual should be observed in a health care facility for symptoms of systemic toxicity for an additional 2 to 4 hours with supportive care as necessary.

OCULAR EXPOSURE

Eye exposures to soaps and hand dishwashing detergents should be managed by gently irrigating the eye on-site with lukewarm water or saline continuously for 15 minutes. On the rare occasion that ocular irritation lasts longer than 2 to 3 hours after irrigation, or the exposure was to a product containing an abrasive, emergency department care is warranted, including a slit-lamp examination with fluorescein dye.

Ocular exposures to laundry detergents and very dilute cationic surfactants (<2%) should be irrigated as described previously. However, greater discretion is warranted in these cases, with immediate medical evaluation necessary if irritation persists for more than 1 to 2 hours after irrigation. It should be kept in mind that the presence of alkaline builders in laundry detergents or an exposure to granular detergent can be associated with an increased risk for corrosive or mechanical injury to the eye. Eye exposure to any laundry detergent with pH > 12 or to any cationic surfactant with a concentration of 2% or greater should be managed as a corrosive.

Because ocular exposure to automatic dishwasher detergents is associated with a high incidence of corneal abrasions as well as corrosive injury to the eye, all exposed patients should have an emergency department evaluation after thorough on-site irrigation for 20 minutes with lukewarm water or saline.[23]

DERMAL EXPOSURE

Management of dermal exposure to any of the above products should begin with irrigation of the exposed area for 5 to 10 minutes with lukewarm water. Exposed clothing should be removed to prevent further contamination. In the rare instances of irritation by noncorrosive products, application of cold packs, vitamin E lotions, or aloe vera gels or lotions may reduce discomfort. If irritation is due to a drying effect of the product,

moisturizing creams may be applied. Dermal exposure to potentially corrosive products can be managed similarly, although oil-based creams or ointments should be avoided. If skin becomes blistered or broken, or begins bleeding or oozing, the care of a physician should be sought. At the discretion of the physician, treatment may include topical corticosteroids in the early stages, topical antibiotics, and wet-to-dry dressings. The rare case of contact dermatitis is best referred to a dermatologist.

BLEACHES

The predominant types of bleach on the market are one of two types: chlorine-releasing aqueous solutions of sodium hypochlorite, or oxygen-releasing powders containing sodium percarbonate/sodium carbonate or sodium perborate/sodium carbonate.[2] Because the hypochlorite ion in chlorine bleach is unstable in acidic solutions, chlorine bleaches generally contain a small percentage of sodium hydroxide.[12] Some chlorine bleach may also contain a very small percentage of cationic surfactants that slightly increases product viscosity.

Sources

Chlorine bleaches are the most common and familiar bleaching agents for household use. Traditional household laundry bleach generally contains 4% to 6% sodium hypochlorite (most commonly, 5.25%) and up to 0.5% sodium hydroxide. The newer "ultra" or "advanced" household bleaches generally contain 5% to 10% sodium hypochlorite and 0.5% to 2% sodium hydroxide. Some hard surface cleaners contain 1% to 4% sodium hypochlorite in combination with surfactants.[26] Oxygen bleaches are all-fabric bleaches that generally contain 5% to 15% sodium percarbonate, sodium perborate, or both, plus up to 75% sodium carbonate. The newer "oxy"-type stain removers contain as much as 89% sodium percarbonate, with the remainder being sodium carbonate. Some of these stain removers may also contain up to 5% sodium metasilicate. Sodium percarbonate is more commonly used than sodium perborate in oxygen bleaches because sodium perborate does not dissolve as readily at cooler wash temperatures.

Toxicity

Although there has been much controversy in the literature during the past 40 years regarding the corrosiveness of chlorine bleaches, it is generally agreed that household chlorine bleach is a mild to moderate mucosal irritant.[11,27,28] The deleterious effects of bleach are related to both the sodium hypochlorite concentration and the pH (or hydroxyl ion concentration). When a sodium hypochlorite solution is ingested, the acidic environment of the stomach transforms the sodium hypochlorite to hypochlorous acid and chlorine gas. At the levels produced from household bleach, hypochlorous acid and chlorine gas are both irritants to

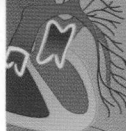

mucous membranes. Sodium hypochlorite solutions of less than 10% are mild to moderate mucosal irritants, whereas solutions of greater than 10% are considered corrosive.[26,27] Sodium hydroxide concentrations of less than 2% are considered irritants, whereas concentrations of greater than 2% may be corrosive.[29] Household bleach solutions generally do not exceed 10% sodium hypochlorite or 2% sodium hydroxide. Most household bleaches have a pH between 11 and 12, also supporting a lack of corrosiveness. Some sources state the critical pH for corrosive injury from bleaches is 12.5.[27,30] It must be noted that bleaches manufactured in countries outside the United States or bleaches manufactured with inadequate production controls may have higher sodium hypochlorite concentrations and higher sodium hydroxide concentrations.[6,27]

The extent of irritation from household chlorine bleach depends on the volume ingested, the concentration, viscosity, and duration of contact. Corrosive injury rarely results and is often due to ingestion of a very large quantity (>5 mL/kg) or a concentrated solution (>10%).[10,12] Dermal exposure may result in mild to moderate irritation, whereas ocular exposure can cause moderate irritation with superficial damage to the corneal epithelium at concentrations of 5.25% sodium hypochlorite or greater.[28,30]

If chlorine bleach is mixed with certain other household cleaning products, toxicity may result from inhalation of gaseous by-products. For example, if chlorine bleach is mixed with a strong acid, chlorine gas evolves. If chlorine bleach is mixed with ammonia, chloramine gas evolves. Both gases can be very irritating to the nasal and oral mucosa, respiratory tract, and ocular surfaces. When chlorine gas comes in contact with moist tissue, it is transformed to hydrochloric acid and nascent oxygen. When chloramine gas contacts moist tissue, it is transformed into hydrochloric acid, gaseous ammonia, and nascent oxygen. The oxygen radicals generated are strong oxidizing agents that, along with the acids and ammonia, can cause corrosive effects and cellular injury.[31,32]

Very little experimental data exist regarding the toxicity of the powdered all-fabric oxygen bleaches and oxygen stain fighters. The bleaching system in these products is commonly sodium percarbonate or sodium perborate, with stabilization and alkalinity contributed by sodium carbonate. A review of several manufacturers' material safety data sheets reveals that sodium percarbonate and sodium perborate powders are generally classified as mild to moderate mucosal, dermal, and respiratory irritants, and as moderate to severe eye irritants.

On contact with moisture, sodium percarbonate breaks down into hydrogen peroxide and sodium carbonate, whereas sodium perborate breaks down into hydrogen peroxide and sodium borate. The concentration of these by-products in the traditional all-fabric bleaches is generally of a level that may cause mucosal irritation on ingestion, although borates could cause systemic toxicity. (Borates are discussed in Chapter 99.) However, some of these all-fabric bleaches contain more than 70% sodium carbonate, which has been reported to be corrosive in solutions of 15% or more.[16] The concentration of by-products from the oxygen stain removers could theoretically be high enough to cause corrosive injury, but as of yet, this effect has not been reported. It would likely depend on the quantity of moisture available in the exposed area. In addition, some of these products contain up to 5% sodium metasilicate, which may be corrosive in solutions of 0.5% or more.[13,15] Further research and experience in this area are needed.

Manifestations

CHLORINE BLEACH

Ingestion of small amounts of household chlorine bleach is generally associated with nausea, vomiting, abdominal pain, diarrhea, and coughing.[26,27,33,34] Less common symptoms include dyspnea, drooling, temporary dysphagia, skin burns, and oral burns.[27] Most investigations in the literature show no evidence of esophageal injury, but a minority show self-limiting erythema and exudates, still without mucosal ulceration. If corrosive injury is present, symptoms may include vomiting, drooling, chest or throat pain, and dysphagia. Progression to stricture has been reported, but is very rare, as are fatalities. Such outcomes are generally due to large intentional ingestions or to co-ingestants.[12,26-28,35,36] Large ingestions of chlorine bleach have also been shown to lead to hyperchloremic acidosis and hypernatremia. The conversion in the stomach of sodium hypochlorite to hypochlorous acid and chlorine contributes to the hyperchloremic acidosis, whereas fluid loss and sodium overload (from the sodium salt of hypochlorite) contribute to the hypernatremia.[34,37]

Aspiration of bleach or bleach-containing vomitus can rarely lead to respiratory complications such as airway edema and pneumonitis manifested as wheezing, tachypnea, stridor, and retractions. These symptoms may be present without concomitant esophageal injury. It is speculated that respiratory epithelium may be more sensitive to household bleach than pharyngeal and esophageal mucosa.[12,28] This is similar to the inhalation of powdered laundry detergents discussed previously.

Ocular exposure to chlorine bleach can be associated with a burning sensation, tearing, erythema, injection, photophobia, and blepharospasm. If thorough irrigation is performed immediately, sequelae are limited to superficial loss of corneal epithelium, slight corneal epithelial haze, and conjunctival edema, all of which subside within 48 hours. If the bleach is left on the eye for a longer period time, tissue necrosis may spread through the entire thickness of the corneal epithelium, possibly leading to irreversible damage and infection.[30] Dermal exposure to chlorine bleach may infrequently cause irritation, erythema, and pruritus. Allergic contact dermatitis has been rarely reported.[26,38]

CHLORINE BLEACH MIXED WITH OTHER PRODUCTS

Exposure to chlorine or chloramine gas can cause irritation and cellular injury to the moist surfaces of the

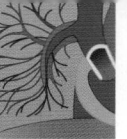

nasal passages, oral and respiratory mucosa, and eyes. The extent of injury depends on the concentration of gas, duration of exposure, and preexisting cardiopulmonary disease. With home exposure, it is very difficult to determine the amount or concentration of gas in the immediate area. Acute mild exposures to chlorine or chloramine gas are generally limited to the upper respiratory tract and may manifest as coughing, dyspnea, stridor, hoarseness, and sore throat. Other common symptoms include chest pain, dizziness, vomiting, ocular irritation, and nasal irritation. Severe exposure can progress to tracheobronchitis, pneumonitis, pulmonary edema, pneumomediastinum, and, ultimately, respiratory failure.[31,39] This is rare in the household setting, but may occur as a result of continued exposure long after initiation of respiratory and ocular irritation. Residual interstitial infiltrates, dyspnea on exertion, and reduced vital capacity have been reported after prolonged exposure.[40] Death occurs very rarely and may be more common in individuals with previous respiratory illness or dysfunction.[39]

OXYGEN BLEACHES

Ingestion of the powdered all-fabric oxygen bleaches and oxygen stain removers may result in nausea, vomiting, and diarrhea. Because these products are powders, mucosal contact time may be prolonged, which could result in epithelial damage to the mouth and esophagus.[2] Ocular exposure to these products can produce moderate irritation and erythema with the possibility of severe irreversible eye damage with prolonged contact.[41,42] The granular nature of the products may also contribute to abrasive injury. Dermal exposure to the dry product may be mildly irritating, with exposure to the wet product possibly producing mild to moderate irritation, erythema, and dryness. Allergic contact dermatitis has not been reported. Inhalation of dust from the products may cause mild respiratory irritation with associated coughing and dyspnea.[41,42]

Management

INGESTION

Management of chlorine bleach ingestion is dependent on the properties of the specific product and on the individual's symptoms. Ingestion of regular household bleach (4% to 6% sodium hypochlorite) can initially be managed at home by dilution with milk or water. If an animal is exposed, water should be used because other fluids may cause further GI irritation. Oral fluid intake should be limited to 4 oz for children and 8 oz for adults, so as not to distend the stomach. GI decontamination by any means is unnecessary, with spontaneous vomiting often occurring nonetheless. If vomiting or diarrhea is excessive, fluid and electrolytes should be replaced and monitored as necessary, possibly in a health care facility. Observation should continue at home for the next 8 hours for symptoms of esophageal damage or of aspiration. Symptoms such as drooling, dysphagia, chest or throat pain, and vomiting warrant emergency department investigation for corrosive injury. Symptoms

such as wheezing, tachypnea, stridor, and retractions warrant a chest x-ray and respiratory supportive care. Animals exposed to chlorine may not have the ability to display symptoms of corrosive injury nor vocalize their discomfort. Therefore, all ingestions of chlorine bleach in animals should be evaluated by a veterinarian for corrosive esophageal injury.

Ingestion of "ultra" or "advanced" bleach may require more diligent monitoring owing to the higher concentrations of sodium hypochlorite and sodium hydroxide, as well as the possibility of increased contact time with mucosal surfaces because of increased product viscosity. However, management still begins in the home and follows the same steps described previously. All ingestions of a large amount of chlorine bleach (>5 mL/kg), regardless of whether they are regular or ultra preparations, should be managed in a health care facility because of the possibility of systemic effects and a greater chance of local tissue injury. Management should include supportive care, investigation for corrosive injury, and 4 to 6 hours of monitoring of arterial blood gases, serum pH, and serum electrolytes, with appropriate treatment.

Despite the uncertainty over the true toxicity of powdered oxygen bleach products, it is suggested that ingestions be managed similarly to those of chlorine bleach, as described previously, with diligent monitoring for symptoms of esophageal injury.

OCULAR EXPOSURE

Eye exposures to regular household bleach should be managed by immediately irrigating the eye on-site with lukewarm water or saline continuously for 15 minutes. If irrigation cannot be performed immediately or if irritation persists immediately after irrigation, emergency department care is warranted, including a slit-lamp examination with fluorescein dye. Eye exposure is to an ultra or advanced chlorine bleach or powdered oxygen bleach–stain remover should be irrigated for 20 minutes on-site, followed by an emergency department evaluation for corneal injury. If exposure to chlorine or chloramine gas causes significant ocular irritation, eye irrigation should be performed for 20 minutes, followed by slit-lamp examination if irritation persists for 1 to 2 hours after exposure.

DERMAL EXPOSURE

Management of dermal exposure to any of the bleaches should begin with irrigation of the exposed area for 5 to 10 minutes with lukewarm water. Exposed clothing should be removed to prevent further contamination. Occlusive creams or ointments should be avoided in the early stages. If skin becomes blistered or broken, or begins bleeding or oozing, the care of a physician should be sought. The rare case of contact dermatitis to chlorine bleach is best referred to a dermatologist.

INHALATION

Inhalation of chlorine or chloramine gas can often be managed on-site or at home with fresh air, cool oral liquids, and inhaled steam. Most patients with exposure

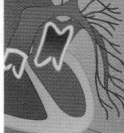

to chlorine or chloramine gas will have resolution of symptoms within 6 hours of exposure. If symptoms worsen at any time or persist for longer than 6 hours, emergency supportive care is warranted.[39] Patients with preexisting respiratory conditions may be more sensitive to exposure, but can still be monitored at home if symptoms are mild and air exchange is not compromised.[31] Anecdotal evidence has suggested that nebulized sodium bicarbonate may be an effective adjunct for chlorine gas exposure. Prospective, randomized, controlled trials have not been carried out. A nonrandomized, nonblinded investigation of its use in chloramine gas exposure did not find a significant difference compared with oxygen alone.[32] Inhalation of powdered oxygen bleach can be managed with fresh air and cool oral fluids. If symptoms persist for more than 6 hours after inhalation, emergency supportive care should be sought.

REFERENCES

1. Watson WA, Litovitz TL, Klein-Schwartz W, et al: 2003 annual report of the American Association of Poison Control Centers Toxic Exposure Surveillance System. Am J Emerg Med 2004;22(5):335–404.
2. Temple AR, Spoerke DG: Household Cleaning Products and Their Accidental Exposure. New York, Soap and Detergent Association, 1989.
3. The Soap and Detergent Association. Available at: http://sdahq.org (accessed June 2004).
4. Litke DW: Review of phosphorus control measures in the United States and their effects on water quality. U.S. Geological Survey National Water-Quality Assessment Program: Water Resources Investigations Report 99-4007. Denver, CO, U.S. Geological Survey, 1999.
5. Peters G, Johnson GQ, Golembiewski A: Safe use of detergent enzymes in the workplace. Applied Occup Environ Hygiene 2001;16(3):389–396.
6. Mofenson HC, Greensher J: The Nontoxic Ingestion. Pediatr Clin North Am 1970;17(3):583–590.
7. DiCarlo MA: Scientific reviews. Household products: a review. Vet Human Toxicol 2003;45(2):256–261.
8. Mack RB: Decant the wine, prune back your long-term hopes: cationic detergent poisoning. N C Med J 1987;48(11):593–595.
9. Kanerva L, Jolanki R, Estlander T: Occupational allergic contact dermatitis from benzalkonium chloride. Contact Derm 2000;42:357–358.
10. McGuigan MA: Bleach, soaps, detergents, and other corrosives. In Haddad LM, Shannon MW, Winchester JF (eds): Clinical Management of Poisoning and Drug Overdose, 3rd ed. Philadelphia, WB Saunders, 1998, pp 830–835.
11. Riordan M, Rylance G, Berry K: Poisoning in Children 4: Household products, plants, and mushrooms. Arch Dis Child 2002;87(5):403–406.
12. Bates N: Acute poisoning: bleaches, disinfectants and detergents. Emerg Nurse 2001;8(10):14–19.
13. Gosselin RE, Smith RP, Hodge HC, Braddock JE: Clinical Toxicology of Commercial Products, 5th ed. Baltimore, Williams & Wilkins, 1984.
14. Gloxhuber C: Toxicological properties of surfactants. Arch Toxicol 1974;32:245–270.
15. Krenzelok EP, Clinton JE: Caustic esophageal and gastric erosion without evidence of oral burns following detergent ingestion. J Am Coll Emerg Phys 1979;8(5):194–196.
16. Klasco RK (ed): POISINDEX System, Vol. 121. Thomson MICROMEDEX, Greenwood Village, CO (expires September 2004).
17. Kynaston JA, Patrick MK, Shepherd RW, et al: The hazards of automatic-dishwasher detergent. Med J Aust 1989;151:5–7.
18. Winter ML, Ellis MD: Automatic dishwashing detergents: their pH, ingredients, and a retrospective look. Vet Hum Toxicol 1986;28(6):536–538.
19. Schweigert MK, Mackenzie DP, Sarlo K: Occupational asthma and allergy associated with the use of enzymes in the detergent industry: a review of the epidemiology, toxicology, and methods of prevention. Clin Exp Allergy 2000;30:1511–1518.
20. Vincent JC, Sheikh A: Phosphate poisoning by ingestion of clothes washing liquid and fabric conditioner. Anaesthesia 1998;53:1004–1006.
21. Wheeler DS, Bonny AE, Ruddy RM, Jacobs BR: Late-onset respiratory distress after inhalation of laundry detergent. Pediatr Pulm 2003;35:323–325.
22. Einhorn A, Horton L, Altieri M, et al: Serious respiratory consequences of detergent ingestions in children. Pediatrics 1989;84(3):472–474.
23. Krenzelok EP: Liquid automatic dishwashing detergents: a profile of toxicity. Ann Emerg Med 1989;18(1):60–62.
24. van Berkel M, de Wolff FA: Survival after acute benzalkonium chloride poisoning. Hum Toxicol 1988;7:191–193.
25. Purohit A, Kopferschmitt-Kubler MC, Moreau C, et al: Quaternary ammonium compounds and occupational asthma. Int Arch Occup Environ Health 2000;73:423–427.
26. Racioppi R, Daskaleros PA, Besbelli N, et al: Household bleaches based on sodium hypochlorite: review of Acute Toxicology and Poison Center Experience. Food Chem Toxicol 1994;32(9):845–861.
27. Harley EH, Collins MD: Liquid household bleach ingestion in children: a retrospective review. Laryngoscope 1997;107:122–125.
28. Babl FE, Kharsch S, Woolf A: Airway edema following household bleach ingestion. Am J Emerg Med 1998;16:514–516.
29. Code of Federal Regulations. 16 CFR 1700.14(a)(5).
30. Ingram TA: Response of the human eye to accidental exposure to sodium hypochlorite. J Endodon 1990;16(5):235–238.
31. Mrvos R, Dean BS, Krenzelok EP: Home exposures to chlorine/chloramine gas: review of 216 cases. South Med J 1993;86(6):654–657.
32. Pascuzzi TA, Storrow AB: Mass casualties from acute inhalation of chloramine gas. Milit Med 1998;163(2):102–104.
33. Jakobsson SW, Rajs J, Jonsson JA, Persson H: Poisoning with sodium hypochlorite solution: report of a fatal case. Supplemented with an Experimental and Clinico-Epidemiological Study. Am J Forensic Med Pathol 1991;12(4):320–327.
34. Ward MJ, Routledge PA: Hypernaetremia and hyperchloraemic acidosis after bleach ingestion. Hum Toxicol 1988;7:37–38.
35. Kiristioglu I, Gurpinar A, Kilic N, et al: Is it necessary to perform an endoscopy after the ingestion of liquid household bleach in children? Acta Paediatr 1999;88:233–236.
36. French RJ, Tabb HG, Rutledge LJ: Esophageal stenosis produced by ingestion of bleach: report of two cases. South Med J 1970;63(10):1140–1144.
37. Ross M, Spiller H: Fatal ingestion of sodium hypochlorite bleach with associated hypernatremia and hyperchloremic metabolic acidosis. Vet Hum Toxicol 1999;41(2):82–86.
38. Eun HC, Lee AY, Lee YS: Sodium hypochlorite dermatitis. Contact Derm 1984;11(1):45.
39. Krenzelok E: Chlorine/chloramines. J Toxicol Clin Toxicol 1995;33(4):355–356.
40. Reisz GR, Gammon RS: Toxic pneumonitis from mixing household cleaners. Chest 1986;89(1):49–52.
41. U.S. Environmental Protection Agency: Sodium carbonate peroxyhydrate fact sheet (128860), 2002. Available at: http://www.epa.gov.
42. National Institutes of Health, National Library of Medicine Specialized Information Services: Household Products Database. Available at: http://householdproducts.nlm.nih.gov (accessed June 2004).

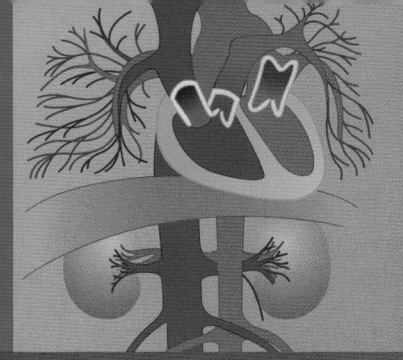

103

Principles of Emergency Management and Management of Hazardous Materials Incidents

JAMES CISEK, MD, MPH

At a Glance...

- Disaster preparedness and management should be based on an "all-hazards approach," leading to comprehensive, risk-based, and integrated responses.

- Immediate disaster response is local. Communities must plan an initial response to all disasters based on available resources. Regional and national response must not be relied on primarily, but disaster management plans should readily integrate components at all levels as they come into play, emphasizing partnership and flexibility.

- The disaster life cycle is composed of four elements: (1) mitigation (long-term efforts to prevent or reduce the probability of disasters or lessen the consequences of a disaster), (2) preparedness (establishment of authorities and responsibilities for emergency actions and collection of resources to support them), (3) response (prompt critical actions to save lives and property), and (4) recovery (restoration of vital infrastructure, assessment of damage, and timely restoration of economic activity and rebuilding of the community).

- Hazardous materials releases may be unintentional or intentional. Chemical terrorism has occurred and will likely reoccur.

- Although most hazardous materials releases result in few or no casualties, disastrous exceptions, such as the releases of methyl isocyanate in Bhopal, of radionuclides in Chernobyl, of hydrogen sulfide and natural gas in Gaoqiao, and of deadly explosive materials in Neyshabur, remind us of their terrifying potential for human tragedy.

- Although the all-hazards approach provides a base for response to chemical disasters, additional expertise and elements will be required, including hazard identification, exposure assessment, decontamination, and prehospital and hospital management, including the appropriate use of antidotes, which may be needed in large quantity.

- The approach to hazardous materials emergencies is multidisciplinary, requiring consultation and cooperation from all involved specialists.

PRINCIPLES OF EMERGENCY MANAGEMENT

This chapter begins with a generalized discussion of disaster management and then focuses on management aspects of a unique disaster involving hazardous materials. All disasters are unexpected events, require a rapid response to save life and property, generate more need than available resources can manage, and require unusual procedures for resolution. Disasters may be natural (e.g., infections, drought, hurricanes, floods, severe winter storms, earthquakes, wildfires), human made (e.g., industrial, transportation, power outage), or national security threats (attack, terrorism). It is important to remember that early disaster declaration by an appropriate local, state, or federal official is an essential step that allows authorities to suspend regulations, allows the expenditure of funds for purchasing and hiring of elements for disaster control, grants authority to order evacuations, puts extensive liability protections into place, and creates the expectation that the government is primarily responsible for controlling the impact of the event.

In 1979, The Federal Emergency Management Agency (FEMA) coined the term *comprehensive emergency management* (CEM) to reflect a change in orientation from preparedness for a single hazard toward an "all-hazards" approach to potential disasters that threaten life and property.[1] CEM strives to minimize the impact caused by an emergency in a locality. FEMA stresses the importance of disaster planning being integrated, comprehensive, risk based, and all-hazard in approach. The similarities among all types of disasters suggest strongly that many of the same management strategies will apply to all such emergencies. It is critical to remember that all disasters are initially a local event, so that all disaster management must begin at the local

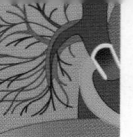

level. Effective disaster management requires a close partnership between all aspects of government (local, county, state, regional, federal) and the private sector. FEMA developed the Integrated Emergency Management System (IEMS) so as to integrate these critical partnerships into an all-hazards approach to emergency management. The IEMS as defined by FEMA focuses on four specific goals:

1. Promotion of a full federal, state, local, and tribal government partnership with emphasis on flexibility for achieving common goals
2. Emphasizing emergency management measures with known proven effectiveness
3. Achieving more complete integration of emergency management planning into policy-making and operational systems
4. Building on established emergency management plans, systems, and capabilities to enhance their applicability to the full spectrum of possible hazards

FEMA has defined a four-phase disaster life cycle for CEM that involves mitigation, preparedness, response, and recovery. These four phases appear in a circular association such that activities in one phase overlap those of the previous (Fig. 103-1).

Mitigation involves long-term efforts to prevent or reduce the probability of disasters or lessen the consequences of a disaster once it has occurred. Examples of mitigation activities include the issuance of flood insurance, flood hazard mapping with the prohibition of home building or the removal of homes within a flood plane, improved building safety for earthquakes or tornados, the opening of shelters in emergencies, and the relocation to temporary housing in the aftermath of a disaster.

Although mitigation can improve community safety, it does not eliminate susceptibility for all hazards. Disasters evolve rapidly and are too complex for effective extemporization. Localities must be prepared for disasters that cannot be mitigated away. Emergency management

mandates that preparedness actions be taken before an emergency has occurred. Preparedness establishes the authorities and responsibilities for emergency actions and collects the resources to support them. Preparedness mandates that jurisdictions have a plan for response, trained personnel to respond, and necessary structural and equipment resources with which to respond. FEMA states that preparedness planning covers three objectives:

1. Maintaining existing emergency management capability in readiness
2. Preventing emergency management capabilities from themselves falling victim to emergencies
3. Augmenting the jurisdiction's emergency management capability

The *preparedness* process begins with a comprehensive community hazard assessment done in collaboration with community, state, and federal personnel. This assessment begins with the accurate identification of community hazards and their potential consequences and then compares and prioritizes these risks. This is the approach required of all jurisdictions and agencies that intend to be compliant with the National Fire Protection Association's Standard on Disaster/Emergency Management and Business Continuity Programs.[2] It then proceeds through a capability analysis that evaluates personnel and equipment needs, and moves to the development of an operations plan. The most important aspect of preparedness is the creation of an all-hazards emergency operations plan (EOP). Training and exercises are clearly defined in the EOP. Training allows personnel to become familiar with their assigned responsibilities and to acquire the skills necessary to perform those tasks. Exercising allows for the testing of plans and the evaluation of skills acquired by response personnel. In addition, the EOP assists in the rapid response that is required for effective disaster relief. Response activities that are time sensitive are clearly defined so as to be performed most efficiently. The EOP includes a listing by position and organization of what kinds of tasks are to be performed. When more than one organization performs a task, one should be given primary responsibility, and the others should be given a supporting role. The EOP must be attentive to relevant local and state laws, federal regulations, and mutual aid agreements. Finally, the EOP provides an adaptable emergency management minimum set of procedures that can be relied on when responding to an unknown disaster. Hazard-specific appendices provide additional critical information relevant to a particular hazard (e.g., hazardous materials, hurricane).

Response is the third phase of emergency management and covers the period during and immediately after a disaster. The response phase of a disaster begins with a need for prompt critical actions to save lives and property. In addition, procedures must be initiated to stabilize the situation so that the locality can reorganize. Critical actions include emergency notification of emergency management personnel, warning and evacu-

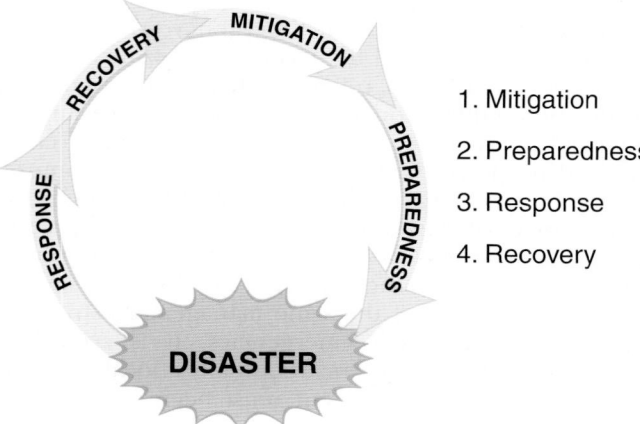

1. Mitigation
2. Preparedness
3. Response
4. Recovery

FIGURE 103-1 The disaster cycle.

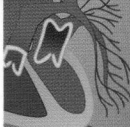

ating or sheltering the population, keeping the population informed, rescuing individuals, providing medical treatment, maintaining the rule of law, assessing damage, addressing mitigation issues that arise from response activities, and requesting help from outside the jurisdiction.

Recovery is the fourth and final phase of the emergency management cycle. It continues until all systems return to normal operation. Short-term recovery begins to restore vital utilities (e.g., power, water, sanitation, communications), transportation infrastructure, the removal of debris, and the assessment of damage. Once some stability is achieved, the jurisdiction can begin recovery efforts for the long term, restoring economic activity and rebuilding community facilities and family housing with attention to long-term mitigation needs. Recovery should incorporate mitigation as demonstrated by a town relocating portions of its flood-prone community and transforming the area into a park.

MANAGEMENT OF HAZARDOUS MATERIALS INCIDENTS

Epidemiology

Exposure to hazardous materials is unfortunately as much a fact of modern life as are such things as vehicular crashes and infectious diseases. The term *hazardous material* is used here to mean any substance that can be harmful to humans, animals, or the environment when released in any uncontrolled manner. This chapter focuses on the management principles applicable to acute exposure to hazardous materials, including large-scale incidents. It does not address the issues surrounding chronic lower-level exposure or terrorism-related events. It must be clearly understood that planning and responding to a hazardous materials incident has many similarities to those needed in a terrorism-related event. An attack on the United States might focus on the release of a toxic chemical from a fixed facility or during transportation. Prehospital providers must think about the potential for terrorism in their response to all hazardous materials events. The potential for a secondary device (e.g., explosive) with potential harm to first responders is a consideration at all hazardous materials events. Terrorism and weapons of mass destruction are discussed in other chapters of this book.

One need not live near a chemical manufacturing plant, heavy industry, or a chemical dump site to be at risk for exposure to hazardous materials. A source of potential exposure is the nearest road, railroad track, or waterway. In 2002, the U.S. Department of Transportation reported 15,399 hazardous materials incidents, with 515 that were considered serious.[3] During 2002, the Chemical Transportation Emergency Center (CHEMTREC) logged more than 121,809 telephone calls for hazardous materials emergency assistance.[4] Most of these voluntary calls were informational: Medical emergencies represented only 18% of the calls.

According to the Occupational Safety and Health Administration (OSHA), more than 575,000 chemicals are used in the workplace. More than 1.5 billion tons of hazardous cargo is shipped nationwide each year by air, rail, sea, and land. These include flammable liquids, pressurized gases, explosives, poisons, and radioactive material. The U.S. Department of Transportation indicates that about 800,000 shipments of hazardous materials are transported each day.[5] In regard to bulk rail shipments, the industry uses roughly 200,000 rail tank cars. A subset of these cars moves more than 275,000 shipments of chlorine, anhydrous ammonia, propane gas, and gasoline every year. The motor carrier industry dedicates more than 400,000 large trucks to the transportation of hazardous materials. A subset of this fleet participates in about 18 million shipments of gasoline and 125,000 shipments of explosives a year.

In 1990, the Agency for Toxic Substances and Disease Registry began an active, state-based Hazardous Substances Emergency Events Surveillance (HSEES) system to define the public health implications of the release of hazardous substances. The HSEES system collected data from 16 states in 2001.[6] This most recent information indicates that 75% of the events occurred at fixed facilities, with equipment failure (38%) and operator error (30%) being the most common factors associated with the release. Of the transportation events, 85% occurred during ground transport (e.g., truck, van), and 10% involved transport by rail. Fewer events involved water, air, pipeline, or other transportation modes. Most events involved the release of one substance (91%), whereas two substances were released in 4%. Air releases were involved in 42% of cases, followed by spill releases (40%), fires (4%), and threatened releases and explosions (0.8%). Ammonia, sulfur dioxide, and carbon monoxide were the substances most commonly released. Human victims were involved in 8% of the releases. Of the events with victims, 62% involved only one victim, and 79% involved one or two victims. Multiple-casualty events were uncommon. Of the total victims, 89% were injured in fixed-facility events. Employees (51%) were the population group most often injured, followed by the general public (21%), students (8%), and responders (13%). The substances released most often were not the most likely to result in victims. As an example, chlorine was released in only 1.2% of the events, but 19% of the chlorine releases resulted in injury. The most commonly reported injuries in fixed-facility events were respiratory irritation (31%), headache (12%), eye irritation (11%), and gastrointestinal problems (10%). Transportation-related events were associated with a greater incidence of trauma (32%) than fixed facilities (2%) were. In total, 1% of all victims died.

Hazardous Materials Events of Greatest Magnitude

Hazardous materials incidents occur with great frequency, and keeping up with the details of releases from across the United States can be very challenging. Previous hazardous materials events must be studied so that history does not repeat itself and for the development of better prevention strategies. The U.S.

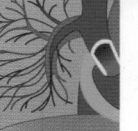

Chemical Safety Board is an excellent resource to facilitate the dissemination of objective information regarding larger-scale incidents. The U.S. Chemical Safety Board is an independent federal agency whose mission is to prevent industrial chemical accidents and save lives.[7] This is accomplished by investigating chemical incidents and hazards, determining fundamental causes of a release, and issuing safety recommendations to government agencies, industry, labor unions, trade associations, and other organizations. This organization determines the causes of accidents, but does not issue fines or penalties. The investigative staff includes chemical and mechanical engineers, industrial safety experts, and other specialists drawn from the private and public sectors. The board can be accessed at the website www.chemsafety.gov.

Four world events involving the release of hazardous materials deserve brief overview. The events involving Bhopal, Chernobyl, Gaoqiao, and Neyshabur are discussed here. The release of sarin in Tokyo is discussed in Chapter 105A.

BHOPAL

The events in Bhopal, India, represent the largest modern hazardous materials incident outside of warfare and terrorism. On the night of December 3, 1984, a cloud of methyl isocyanate gas leaked from a storage tank at the Union Carbide plant in Bhopal, India. Methyl isocyanate is used in the manufacture of carbamate insecticides. As a liquid, it has a low boiling point and is heavier than air in its gaseous form. It has a strong odor and is irritating to the eyes, skin, and respiratory tract. It may be toxic both by inhalation and cutaneous exposure. At the time of the incident, no plans existed to alert the local population in the event of a disaster. Population-based methods for protection and evacuation did not exist. The plant was located in a densely populated area, with poorly constructed housing adjacent to the plant. Knowledge of the hazardous materials being used and the products manufactured was lacking among the employees, and there were no standard operating practices and few engineering controls. About 50,000 lb of methyl isocyanate in liquid and vapor form was released into the atmosphere when a valve on a storage tank opened for about 2 hours. Light winds prevented rapid dispersal of the heavier-than-air cloud. The accident happened at night, when most of the residents were asleep. Because of the rapid onset of symptoms and the large numbers of people affected, local hospitals were rapidly overwhelmed. Many patients were treated in the hospital garden. Local citizens helped each other in the initial rescue attempt. No local medical authority on methyl isocyanate was immediately available.

More than 200,000 people were exposed, and about 500 people in the surrounding area were killed before reaching medical treatment. The total death count was about 2500. One hospital alone treated 25,000 patients in the first 24 hours. Immediate respiratory problems consisted of severe coughing, dyspnea, pharyngitis, and pulmonary edema. Severe conjunctival irritation and corneal ulceration developed. Gastrointestinal symptoms consisted of increased salivation, nausea, vomiting, abdominal pain, and defecation. Central nervous system symptoms were manifested by coma, seizures, dizziness, limb weakness, and tremors.[8]

Ninety-five percent of the dead and severely injured came from the neighborhood immediately adjacent to the plant. A crowded railway station situated 1 km from the plant had more than 100 dead: 200 people were unconscious, and 600 were lying about injured. Several studies of survivors were undertaken 3.5 months after the incident.[9] Patients in these studies were categorized according to their distance from the plant on the night of the accident. Group 1 consisted of those 0.5 to 2 km from the plant, and group 2 was composed of those at least 8 km from the plant. Both groups were matched socioeconomically and demographically. All of the group 1 sample and 42% of group 2 had symptoms at the time of the incident. At the time of the study, 80% of group 1 and 28% of group 2 had continued respiratory complaints consisting of cough, with or without sputum production; breathlessness; and chest pain. Fifty-seven percent of group 1 had abnormal chest radiographs, 49% had documented restrictive defects, and 21% had obstructive defects. Smokers constituted 12%. It is unclear whether previous pulmonary disease was present or whether some patients had both restrictive and obstructive pulmonary disease.

In a group of children categorized in the same manner, most symptoms occurred in the immediate area of the plant, although the more remote group was not without symptoms. Ninety-five percent of children from group 1 had immediate cough, and 74% experienced breathlessness.[10] Three months later, 84% noted persistent cough, and 48% suffered from continued breathlessness. Abnormal radiographs were found in 66% of group 1 children, compared with 8.1% of group 2 children. Pulmonary testing was performed on children older than 7 years. Obstructive defects were found in 28 of 33 children. Persistent abdominal pain and anorexia were found in the group 1 children only. Group 1 children experienced persistent conjunctivitis, and 10% demonstrated visual abnormalities. No persistent eye abnormalities were found in group 2. Persistent neurobehavioral symptoms consisted of poor memory and weakness. Comprehensive psychological testing was not performed. Some children who later developed obvious psychic disturbances had been classified as dead at the time of the accident and had been initially placed in morgues. Others had witnessed the deaths of parents or siblings.

A recent study found selective growth retardation in boys, but not girls, who were either exposed to the released gases as toddlers or born to exposed parents.[11] It is theorized that methyl isocyanate is quickly degraded into trimethylamine, which in mice has been reported to produce selective growth retardation of male progeny mice. This is associated with a decrease in the serum testosterone in the mice.

CHERNOBYL

Late in the evening of April 25, 1986, the fourth reactor at Chernobyl was shut down for routine maintenance

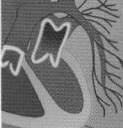

and testing. This electrical generating plant is located 130 km north of Kiev, near the current convergent borders of Ukraine, Belarus, and Russia. Inadequate safety precautions and operational errors during the testing resulted in a sudden increase in heat production, which ruptured part of the nuclear fuel. The water-cooled, graphite-moderated reactor did not have a concrete containment vessel. By 1:30 AM (April 26), hot fuel particles, reacting with water, had caused a steam explosion. Within seconds, this was followed by a second explosion. The explosions totally destroyed the Unit 4 reactor core and roof of the building. By 5:00 AM, although more than 100 local firefighters succeeded in extinguishing conventional fires, a graphite moderator fire began and was not extinguished until May 6. This fire was responsible for the dispersion of radionuclides into the atmosphere. Seven months later, the remains of the destroyed reactor and building were enclosed in a concrete sarcophagus designed to provide some containment of the damaged nuclear fuel and to reduce further releases of radioactivity until a more permanent containment facility could be designed and implemented. Thankfully, only 3% to 5% of the total amount of radiation was released. Fifty thousand people were evacuated from the nearby town of Pripyat after a delayed public announcement a day and a half after the release began. It is estimated that a total of 135,000 persons were evacuated and permanently rehoused outside of the 30-km exclusion zone; in addition, 500,000 mothers and children from the surrounding area were reportedly sent to resorts along the Black Sea, and another 300,000 were sent to other locations. It was estimated that 30 to 60 km^2 of topsoil and road surfaces would have to be removed to properly decontaminate the area.[12-15]

Firefighters and plant personnel suffered the highest radiation exposures and casualties. No members of the general public received sufficient radiation doses to induce acute radiation syndrome. Three deaths were immediately associated with the accident. Two hundred thirty-seven patients were admitted for acute radiation syndrome, of which 28 died. Bone marrow transplantation was performed in 13 patients, with death occurring in all but 2 of these patients.

Fifty tons of radioactive dust was dispersed over 140,000 square miles of mainly Belarus, Ukraine, and a part of Russia. Seventy percent of the radiation was deposited over Belarus. The doses to individuals outside of this area were small and varied depending on whether rainfall occurred during the passage of the radioactive cloud. The plume moved predominately northward and then over Western Europe. The initial international detection came from Sweden, when radiation alarms went off 2 days after the accident. The accident was announced that evening by the Soviet Union. The isotopes of greatest concern were iodine-131 (^{131}I) and cesium-137 (^{137}Cs). The affected area was large because of the dispersion of small particles into the upper atmosphere and the duration of the release. Almost 5 million people were exposed to either internal or external radiation. The major routes of human exposure were from the ingestion of cow's milk contaminated with ^{131}I (resulting in internal exposure), contact with γ/β radiation from the radioactive cloud, and contact with ^{137}Cs deposited on the ground (resulting in external exposure). Children who consumed fresh cow's milk in May and June 1986 received the highest doses to the thyroid.

Estimates of cancer increases were initially said to be "no more than 1000" and have risen in the past 10 years since the accident. Most of the pilots who helped to entomb the reactor are dead or have leukemia. More and more of the cleanup workers have required treatment for radiation-induced diseases. Thyroid cancer has increased a 100-fold in Belarus. The World Health Organization (WHO) predicts that one third of all the children from the area around Gomel who were between 0 and 4 years of age at the time of the accident will develop thyroid cancer during their lifetime—a total of 50,000 children in this group alone. The negative social and psychological consequences of this event have been profound. There was no identified increase in congenital anomalies, adverse pregnancy outcomes, or other radiation-induced disease in either the contaminated area or in Western Europe. The WHO established the International Program on the Health Effects of Chernobyl Accident to further define the long-term significance of this accident.

GAOQIAO

In December 2003, there occurred a release of natural gas and hydrogen sulfide at the Chuandongbei gas field in China. The gas field is run by the China National Petroleum Corporation. Although the exact cause of the release is unclear, it led to the evacuation of more than 41,000 people in a 25-km^2 area. The mountainous terrain and muddy roads made it difficult for villagers to flee and hindered rescue work. At least 233 people died, and more than 10,000 people were treated for hydrogen sulfide toxicity. Thousands of animals died as the gas devastated villages and poisoned farms.

NEYSHABUR

In February 2004, 48 rail cars derailed and caught fire outside of Neyshabur, Iran. This community is an ancient city of 170,000 people in a farming region 400 miles east of the capital, Tehran. Firefighters had nearly put out the blaze when an explosion occurred about 5 hours after the derailment. The cars contained sulfur, gasoline, fertilizer, and cotton. The explosion killed 320 people and injured 460 others. Nearly 200 of the dead were rescue workers who were fighting the fires when the blast occurred. The blast was so powerful that Iranian seismologists recorded a quake of magnitude 3.6 at the time of the explosion, and the blast shattered windows 6 miles away.

Hazardous Materials Preparedness

In planning for chemical, radiation, and biologic disasters, one must consider all the possibilities, from human error, to employee sabotage, to mentally ill workers, to

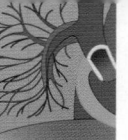

terrorism. A specific hazardous materials appendix to the EOP must be developed. This hazardous materials appendix must be updated regularly, simple to follow, and cost effective; must provide for resources that are immediately available; and should minimize manpower needs. This appendix should contain detailed instructions to follow, including emergency response operations; a roster of emergency assistance phone numbers; a description of each service's legal authority and responsibility during an emergency; a description of the structure and responsibility of the designated response organization; a section on resource laboratories for analysis of chemical and patient data; and a cleanup and disposal equipment resource section.

Hazardous materials planning begins with the Emergency Response Commission, established in each state under the Superfund Amendments and Reauthorization Act of 1986 (SARA). This commission, appointed by the governor of the state, must coordinate with the Local Emergency Planning Committees (LEPCs) in their development of plans for emergency response to hazardous materials emergencies. It is the responsibility of the LEPC to develop plans to define and coordinate contaminated areas, to decontamination and triage on scene, to optimize resource and information management, and for the transportation to definitive medical care. This preplanning begins with developing a clear understanding of the potential toxic chemicals stored, transported, and used within a community. A community's "right to know" is mandated by the Comprehensive Environmental Response, Compensation and Liability Act (CERCLA) amendments of 1986, otherwise known as SARA, Title III. Title III of SARA, the Emergency Planning and Community Right to Know Act, encourages state and local planning and provides planning groups with information concerning chemical releases and the potential chemical risks in their communities. A list of 402 extremely hazardous materials, published in the Federal Register (November 17, 1986), gave threshold planning quantities. If these materials are produced, used, or stored in quantities exceeding the thresholds, they become subject to the emergency planning requirements. Additionally, requirements were set for emergency notification whenever a release of hazardous material exceeded a reportable quantity.

In addition to community notification, workers are protected by the OSHA Hazard Communication Standard, which states that "hazards of all chemicals produced or imported by chemical manufacturers or importers [must be] evaluated, and information concerning their hazards [must be] transmitted to affected employers and employees within the manufacturing sector. This transmittal of information is to be accomplished by means of comprehensive hazard communication programs, which are to include container labeling and other forms of warning, material safety data sheets (MSDS), and employee training" (29 CFR 1910.1200). Workers must know the hazards of the chemicals with which they work and methods to protect themselves in the event of an accident or incident. There should also be some training in first aid and decontamination procedures at the plant.

Ideally, a plant's MSDS should be on file in the emergency department, and emergency physicians should be familiar with them. Additionally, patients should be transported from the plant to the department along with copies of the appropriate MSDS.

Surveying the major pipelines in one's area and knowing major road, rail, and water shipping routes in one's community are critical. Prevention strategies should include consideration of restricted transportation routes and times of access to these venues. Little regulation exists to limit the routes and times of day that may be used for hazardous materials transportation. The District of Columbia and New York City have enacted bills to require shippers of certain hazardous materials to obtain a permit and conform to routes, times, and other safety conditions when traveling into or out of these cities. This was in response to recent terrorism concerns.

Hazardous materials training of first responders is paramount.[16] Rescuers must be trained in the use of protective equipment and in decontamination procedures to minimize contamination of citizens, medical personnel, vehicles, medical facilities, and the environment. Persons using a self-contained breathing apparatus (SCBA) must be properly fit tested, be trained in their use, and understand the limitations of the equipment. Specifically, the time limitations of the supply tank and the reserve tank must be understood so that egress from the contaminated area can be accomplished before loss of supply air. Local hazardous materials response units with special training and equipment exist in many communities. These units are responsible for evaluation and management of scene hazards and decontamination before transport. With multiple casualties, the real possibility exists that many patients will present to local hospitals while still contaminated. All medical facilities should have plans to identify contaminated patients, protect personnel and the hospital environment, and provide for decontamination with protective equipment.[17,18] Sheltered off-site locations for treatment should be available if a hospital is overwhelmed or must be evacuated. Warning mechanisms and a plan for early evacuation will minimize injuries to hospital personnel.

Planning for the treatment of persons exposed to chemicals involves all levels of the health care team, from firefighters to hazardous materials teams to emergency medical services personnel to hospital providers. It is important to establish a unified command approach such that the prehospital plan seamlessly interfaces with that of the hospital. It is essential to ensure that exposure is limited to the smallest number of people possible. Guidelines must be established for triage, decontamination, and medical management.[19] Patients may require specialized care and early transportation to hospitals providing medical specialists in burn and trauma care, hyperbaric oxygen, and medical toxicology. Important resources may include an emergency physician, a medical toxicologist, a trauma surgeon, a pharmacologist, an industrial hygienist, an occupational medicine specialist, testing laboratories, and chemists. Plans must also include members from the mental health community,

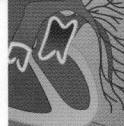

media relations, and security. Large amounts of antidotes specific to the potential exposures must be available at the scene and within the hospital.

Plans should include sources of specialized equipment that may be needed for a given hazard. Planning must include the provision of equipment for air sampling, decontamination, handling of spills (e.g., absorbent materials, diking equipment), and protective equipment for rescuers. This equipment must be strategically located in the community, and its location must be known to all responders. An adequate supply of air tanks and SCBAs and equipment to refill tanks with adequate-quality breathing air must be available.

Planning must include concerns for the environment. Environmental liability resulting from critical life-saving actions has been a concern for first responders. Section 107 of CERCLA addresses this issue. Section 107(d)(1), often known as the "Good Samaritan" provision, states: "No person shall be liable under this subchapter for costs or damages as a result of actions taken or omitted in the course of rendering care, assistance, or advice in accordance with the National Contingency Plan (NCP) or at the direction of an on-scene coordinator appointed under such plan, with respect to an incident creating a danger to public health or welfare or the environment as a result of any releases of a hazardous substance or the threat thereof." This does not preclude liability for costs or damages as a result of negligence. In addition, section 107(d)(2) provides that state and local governments are not liable under CERCLA "as a result of actions taken in response to an emergency created by the release or threatened release of a hazardous substance generated by or from a facility owned by another person." In response to a hazardous materials event, prehospital providers should undertake any necessary emergency actions to save lives and protect the public and themselves. Once any imminent threats to human health are addressed, first responders should immediately take all reasonable efforts to contain the contamination and avoid or mitigate environmental consequences. The Environmental Protection Agency (EPA) will not pursue enforcement actions against state and local responders for the environmental consequences of necessary and appropriate emergency response actions. The EPA cannot prevent a private person from filing suit under CERCLA. However, first responders can use CERCLA's Good Samaritan provision as a defense to such an action.

Hazardous Materials Response

In general terms, the sequence of events in a disaster is as follows: An accident occurs. Knowledge of it is transmitted to appropriate agencies; these agencies respond and gather more data. They may activate additional resources. Fire and the hazardous materials team assume charge and direct law enforcement to control and secure the scene. The scope of the problem is defined. The necessary plans for the solution of the problem are activated, and follow-up and evaluation are accomplished.

First and foremost is notification of appropriate agencies, that is, police, fire department, hazardous materials team, emergency medical system, local disaster coordinator, county and state officials, and federal agencies. It is beyond the scope of this chapter to indicate who must be notified in any given incident. This varies with the incident and with local and state regulations. Various local and state agencies may have jurisdiction over a particular kind of hazard. These interests may overlap, depending on the nature of the chemical, the location of a spill, and the various laws in a state. The fire chief and the hazardous materials team assume charge and usually have the police set up perimeters and evacuate the surrounding area, if necessary. If the hazardous materials release involves terrorism, the Federal Bureau of Investigation assumes charge of the scene. Crowd control and control of access to the site are also the responsibility of the police agency. A fire agency has responsibility to respond to the chemical or fire hazard and to initiate mitigation, extrication, decontamination, and first aid to casualties. An Emergency Medical Service (EMS) agency is responsible for medical decisions and treatment. Other agencies may have jurisdiction and authority or serve in an advisory capacity, such as the Agency for Toxic Substances and Disease Registry (ATSDR), the Centers for Disease Control and Prevention (CDC), the EPA, OSHA, FEMA, and the state health department. Local municipal authorities must know how to gain access to other sources of help, including state and federal agencies. At all times, it is critical for all responders to know who is in control. The agency that assumes control may change as more information concerning the exact nature of the hazard becomes available or during different phases of the entire operation, including cleanup.

Identification of the Release

Identification of the hazardous material should be attempted before approach to the spill. Community preplanning should identify the specific sites that contain hazardous materials. One can read the placarding on the truck or train car from afar (Fig. 103-2). Be aware that placarding may be wrong 40% of the time, and manifest papers may be wrong 35% of the time. Binoculars are an invaluable aid. The bill of lading (cargo manifest) is located in the cab of a truck, but it may not be accessible without full protective gear. The diamond-shaped placard on the side of a tank or rail car with the Department of Transportation (DOT) number on it will identify the specific material, and the DOT Emergency Response Guidebook will provide the hazard class and general emergency information as well as evacuation distances.[20] Some states also have numbered placards with emergency telephone numbers to call. These telephone numbers are a good first resource. Follow-up continues by contacting the shipper and confirming materials that are in the container or vehicle. The various symbols within the diamond-shaped placard should identify the general class of material being shipped. The absence of a placard should not lead one to believe that danger is absent. An empty tank car is considered to be one that

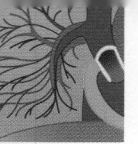

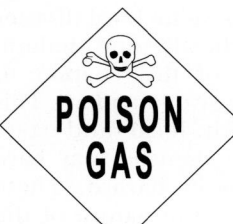

Guide 15

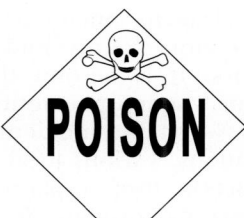

Guide 55

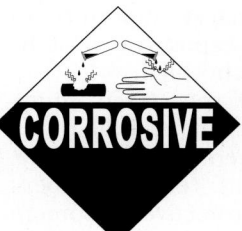

Guide 59

FIGURE 103-2 Table of placards and applicable response guide pages. (From Office of Hazardous Materials Regulation: Emergency Response Guidebook. Washington, DC, Materials Transportation Bureau, U.S. Department of Transportation, 1980.)

Guide 11

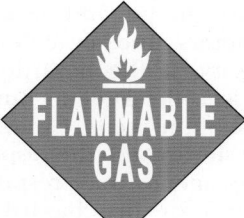

Guide 19

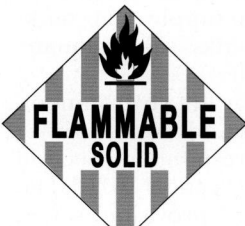

Guide 38

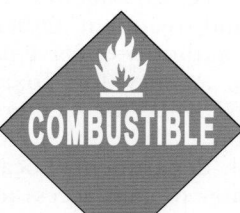

Guide 26

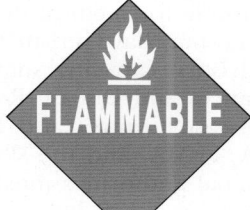

Guide 26

BLASTING AGENTS

Guide 46

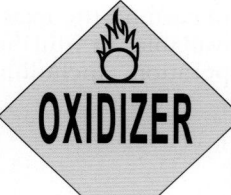

Guide 47

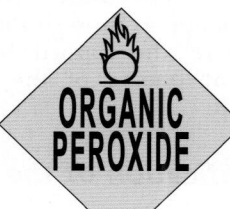

Guide 52

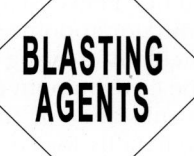

Guide 63

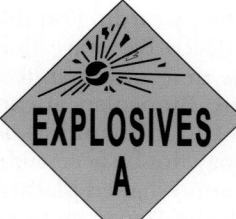

Guide 46

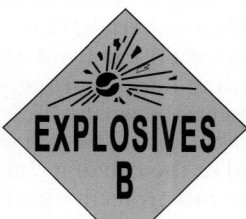

Guide 46

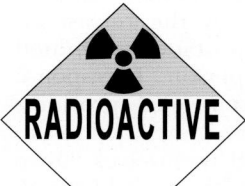

Guide 16

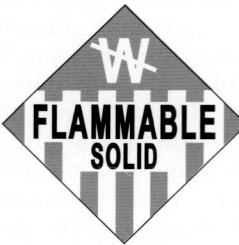

Guide 41

Guide 20

Class Number
A number 2 at the bottom of a placard without any name means that the material in the tank is a gas. Specific chemical group is at the center.

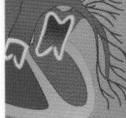

contains less than 300 gallons of material. One should treat a chemical spill and injuries from an unplacarded vehicle with the same caution. Identification of the shipper may be possible by reading the markings on the truck or train car from a distance. The shipper may be contacted to assist in chemical identification and provision of resources. On a train, the waybill can be found with the conductor. Call the nearest company trainmaster, relay the number of the car and the location, and get information and handling information from the tracking computer. The waybill contains a standard transportation code (STC) number that identifies the specific chemical. Chemicals whose numbers begin with 49 are classified as hazardous. The waybill contains specific chemical names and handling information. With train cars numbered from engine to caboose, one can thus learn what chemical the car contains.

Packaging configuration can provide valuable information for hazard identification. There are three categories of packaging: stationary bulk storage containers at fixed facilities that come in a variety of sizes and shapes; bulk transport vehicles for truck and rail transportation; and labeled fiberboard boxes, drums, or cylinders for smaller quantities of hazardous materials. The shape and configuration of the container can often be a useful clue to the presence of hazardous materials.

Rapid emergency information can be obtained by calling CHEMTREC at 800-424-9300 in an emergency situation and giving the name of the compound. In an emergency, CHEMTREC will connect emergency personnel with the manufacturer's and/or shipper's personnel, who can advise on emergency handling. CHEMTREC can then advise what sort of rescue gear may be needed and what decontamination, if any, is needed at the site. Injuries that involve human exposures and injuries will be referred to an appropriate poison control center. The Agency for Toxic Substances and Disease Registry can be accessed at any time by calling 404-498-0120. ATSDR can provide additional valuable information and also has physicians available to provide medical treatment recommendations.

EXPOSURE ASSESSMENT

The assessment of exposure risks in the hazardous materials scene environment requires equipment and methods from the field of industrial hygiene. The industrial hygienist can perform qualitative and quantitative studies both on site and in the laboratory. Members of the hazardous materials team perform exposure assessments in the setting of an acute release of a toxic substance. Before discussing actual monitoring methods, however, it would be useful to define some terms and review some fundamental industrial hygiene concepts.

First, any chemical can be handled safely if proper precautions are taken. In an uncontrolled chemical release, hazardous environments can be approached with proper personal protective equipment. In most major incidents and in some minor incidents, this includes full-body suits that are impermeable to the hazardous material, and a positive-pressure demand style of SCBA. Personnel wearing an SCBA must be fully trained in its use, limitations, and what to do if the equipment fails. These persons must be medically cleared for SCBA use before acceptance as part of an emergency response team. The SCBA must have been properly inspected, maintained, and cleaned at regular intervals. A full respirator program as required by OSHA (29 CFR 1910.134) must be in place. This includes periodic medical monitoring.

Second, any chemical, no matter now nontoxic, can be hazardous if handled inappropriately. For example, a release of methane or nitrogen in an enclosed space can cause asphyxiation. Numerous reports have been published of attempted rescues in such "nontoxic" environments, in which the initial victim and the rescuers all died of simple asphyxiation.

The identity of the specific agent is only one of a number of factors affecting the actual hazard. Other factors include the air concentration, potential for skin contact, duration of exposure, temperature of the material, and individual susceptibility of the exposed persons.

Inhalation of air contaminants is the most frequent route of exposure for hazardous materials. Air contaminants may be found in a variety of forms, such as gases, vapors (the gaseous form of a substance that is primarily liquid or solid at room temperature), dusts (solid particles entrained in air), fumes (tiny solid particles often formed when a metal is heated, as in welding), mists (liquid particles entrained in air), and smoke (carbon or soot particles from incomplete combustion). Fumes, dusts, and smokes are measured in mass units of contaminant per volume unit of air (e.g., milligrams per cubic meter or parts per million). These two units can be easily interconverted if molecular weight, temperature, and altitude are known. Because fumes are minute solid particles, respirators designed specifically for protection against fumes will have no efficacy against vapors or gases, and vice versa.

Once an air concentration is determined, several criteria exist for assessing the risk for exposure. The level that is immediately dangerous to life and health (IDLH) "represents a maximum concentration from which, in the event of respirator failure, one could escape within 30 minutes without experiencing any escape-impairing or irreversible health effects." The IDLH level is used to determine the unquestionable need for a reliable positive-pressure demand SCBA. Standby personnel with full protective gear and a lifeline should be available when the IDLH level is exceeded. Specific IDLH values can be found in the National Institute for Occupational Safety and Health (NIOSH) *Pocket Guide to Chemical Hazards.*[21]

The most widely used criteria for assessing exposure levels are the threshold limit values (TLVs) for hundreds of common industrial chemicals, which are updated and published annually by the American Conference of Governmental Industrial Hygienists.[22] They "represent conditions under which it is believed that nearly all

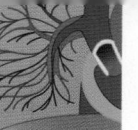

workers may be repeatedly exposed day after day without adverse effect." Most TLVs are established for 8-hour time-weighted average exposures (TWAs). In general, these values protect against the effects of a lifetime of chronic exposure. However, short-term exposure limits and ceiling limits for some substances are also included in the TLV list.

TLVs are designed to protect a population of healthy workers and are not meant to be applied to a general community population that may include infants, elderly people, and infirm people. Thus, care should be exercised when clinical interpretations based on TLVs are made at a hazardous materials scene. In addition to TLVs, a set of legally enforceable workplace standards, known as permissible exposure limits (PELs), has been established.

A common fallacy is the use of odor as a measure of exposure. Information about odor may sometimes be helpful in the qualitative identification of agents or as a crude guide to the exposure level. Odor thresholds for a wide variety of materials have been published. However, wide variations between reference sources and considerable individual variation in the ability to perceive specific odors may occur. For example, up to 40% of the population cannot detect the almond-like odor of cyanide. Some materials have excellent warning properties. For example, if the odor or irritation of ammonia is absent, one can be sure that there will be no toxic sequelae due to exposure to this agent. However, some materials, such as carbon monoxide, are odorless at lethal levels. Other agents, such as hydrogen sulfide, have a characteristic odor initially but induce olfactory fatigue. As a result, lethal exposures may result as exposed individuals perceive levels to be diminishing. Thus, quantitative assessments based on odor thresholds are quite unreliable and possibly dangerous.

Air concentrations can be measured at specific locations, and computer models can sometimes be used to predict worst-case ambient concentrations at downwind locations. Environmental monitoring can be performed with direct reading instruments providing real-time measurements of levels, or it can be performed by taking air samples that can be analyzed subsequently. Direct reading instruments include photoionization detectors, portable gas chromatographs, portable infrared spectrophotometers, portable carbon monoxide detectors, flammable gas detectors, and oxygen detectors. A simple direct reading method for instantaneous levels is the colorimetric detector tube.

In addition to monitoring the environment, it is important to provide medical surveillance for exposed victims and rescuers, both to assess potential health effects and to provide information about the exposure. Excellent documentation is essential because many of these incidents result in litigation. It is important to document subjective complaints and objective findings and assessments thoroughly and carefully. One should not document that symptoms are all due to a "toxic exposure" unless this is clearly the case. Describe actual clinical findings as they are manifest. The physician's initial charting may be a deciding factor in determining whether someone gets their deserved compensation. It may also determine whether abuses of the system occur, which cost public and private organizations large sums of money.

DIAGNOSTIC STUDIES

The diagnostic studies for each patient will depend on the clinical presentation and the specific agents to which they have been exposed. Please refer to specific chapters in this textbook for the discussion of specific toxins.

FIELD DECONTAMINATION AND TRIAGE

In the event that the chemical is unknown, the safest way to rescue any victim is for rescuers to enter the area in fully encapsulated suits (level A) with positive-pressure SCBA. The exact type of level A suit is determined by the nature of the chemical involved. Firefighters are trained in use of this gear, whereas many EMS rescue teams are not. Under medical guidance, the firefighters begin decontamination and rescue of casualties and begin first aid. The fire department is the most qualified to assess the potential for fires and explosions and to advise medical personnel of such.

The smallest number of rescuers possible should enter the contaminated area. At least two should go in together, employing a buddy system, to ensure each other's safety. A backup person with a similar level of protective gear should remain at the boundary to assist the rescuers in the event of an accident. Hyperthermia and dehydration can occur quickly in the fully encapsulated level A suites. Adequate hydration and close attention to rescuer vital signs are important.

Standard principles of triage apply in a chemical disaster. The sequence for field decontamination is illustrated by the following example: A truck transporting a concentrated liquid chemical turns over on a highway, and the tank begins to leak. A large pool of chemical is rapidly filling a low section of roadway, and a hazy cloud begins to form over the pool. The driver and companion, who are both injured, begin to move away under their own power. They begin to cough and choke, and then they pass out. Several bystanders enter to help and are overcome and lose consciousness. In the meantime, all the victims have chemical on their clothing. Without going into specific details of particular chemicals, how might rescue be accomplished? The first responders must attempt to identify the chemical from the placard on the truck. Especially note the logo W, which means USE NO WATER. The chemical may ignite, explode, or produce toxic fumes with water. The responders should notify central dispatching for fire department, police, and EMS backup and indicate that specialized resources or expertise may be required for a hazardous materials incident. If the placard can be read, the dispatcher can call CHEMTREC for specific handling information. Police, fire department, or EMS personnel should have access to the DOT *Emergency*

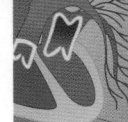

Response Guide: Emergency Handling of Hazardous Materials in Surface Transportation. Access to other guides, Poisindex, or a poison control center for further information should be available, if possible. A triage or medical station should be set up upwind from the site at a "safe" distance. Distances are listed in the DOT *Emergency Response Guidebook.* An area designated as contaminated or hot should be defined (Fig. 103-3). An intermediate or containment area should be established. Rescuers can continue decontamination and emergency treatment in this area.

Cutaneous decontamination is not required for all patients exposed to a hazardous material. Exposure to an inhaled toxicant (e.g., carbon monoxide or arsine gas) poses little risk for skin injury, mucous membrane injury, or secondary contamination such that decontamination

is not required. Many gases and vapors (e.g., isocyanates, chlorine) can cause skin and mucous membrane injury and necessitate formal decontamination. Any liquid or solid material must be removed promptly. If uncertainty exists, then prompt decontamination is mandatory.

The nature of the hazard and the necessary protective equipment must be determined before first responders enter an area of chemical spill (e.g., equipment for extrication and diking, decontamination showers, oxygen, protective gear, and transportation vehicles). Rescuers should enter the contaminated area with full protective gear unless the hazard assessment indicates otherwise. If the details of the release are uncertain, level A protective gear is essential. Level A suites are composed of various materials, and proper suit selection is important.

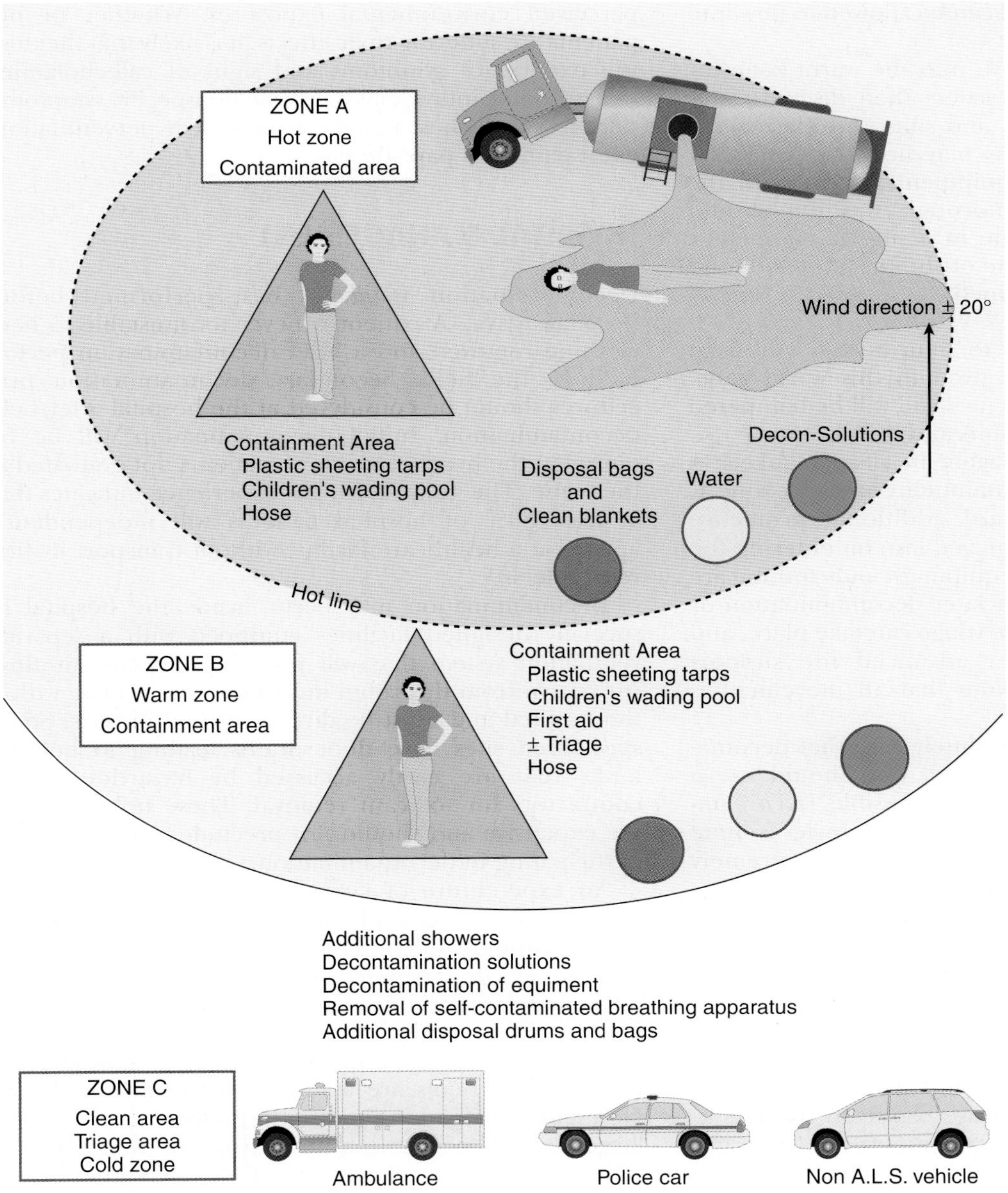

FIGURE 103-3 Sequence for field detonation.

ZONE A
Hot zone
Contaminated area

Wind direction ± 20°

Containment Area
Plastic sheeting tarps
Children's wading pool
Hose

Disposal bags
and
Clean blankets

Water

Decon-Solutions

Hot line

ZONE B
Warm zone
Containment area

Containment Area
Plastic sheeting tarps
Children's wading pool
First aid
± Triage
Hose

Additional showers
Decontamination solutions
Decontamination of equiment
Removal of self-contaminated breathing apparatus
Additional disposal drums and bags

ZONE C
Clean area
Triage area
Cold zone

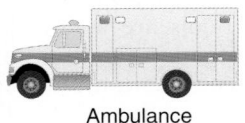
Ambulance

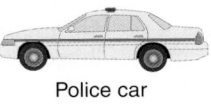
Police car

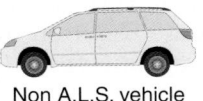
Non A.L.S. vehicle

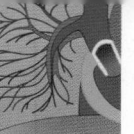

Only a minimum of first aid, such as attention to the cervical spine and exsanguinating hemorrhage, should be attempted in a highly toxic environment. Do not intubate or establish intravenous access in a highly toxic environment. Move victims from the immediate area of the spill. Remove all clothing. In general, wash the entire body, including the hair, quickly with water. Exceptions to this rule include contaminants that are elemental metals, such as sodium, which react violently with water. All the wash water should be contained (if possible). This can be done in a number of ways. Children's plastic wading pools or plastic sheeting may be used with an earthen dam or brick border to prevent used wash water from entering ground water. Three fire ladders may be laid sideways in a triangle and tarpaulins placed over them to form a pool. All waste water, hoses, tarpaulins, pools, and so on are left inside the "hot zone" for the environmental cleanup team (see Fig. 103-3). In the event of mass decontamination, the effluent water does not need to be contained and can be allowed to flow into the sewer or other location.

The victims may then move into the warm zone for further decontamination. Rescuers then discard outer layers of gloves, boot covers, and suits and place these in disposal containers. SCBAs may need to be left on and are the last piece of equipment removed. In the containment area, more thorough washing should take place. This may be done in a similar manner by setting up a hose or some type of shower. If possible, all waste water must be contained so as not to spread contamination.

More thorough attention to injuries and advanced airway management can be given in this warm zone. With very toxic materials, rescuers still will be hampered in their efforts by protective suits and SCBA.

The victims are wrapped again in clean blankets as they move from zone B (containment area) to zone C (cold zone). Rescuers discard additional protective clothing, and the SCBA is removed last, on entering the cold zone. All contaminated equipment and clothing are placed in bags and drums for later decontamination or disposal. Here, more extensive triage can take place, and intravenous lines and other advanced life support treatment can take place. Note that all movement is upwind from the spill.

Because one cannot be absolutely sure that decontamination is complete in the field, one should use a non–advanced life support vehicle if possible. Decontamination of an advanced life support vehicle is time consuming and costly, and availability is extremely limited. To have one out of service for decontamination imposes a hardship on the community.

The selection of receiving hospitals must be based on the number of victims and the hospital's ability to manage concomitant trauma, burns, contamination, and systemic toxicity. All equipment and gear in vehicles and in the emergency department should be protected from any contamination by layers of plastic and blankets, if possible.

Decisions about evacuation are based on the identification of the chemical, information from the transporter or manufacturer, chemical characteristics, explosive characteristics, danger of fire, means of safe evacuation, and weather conditions.

REGIONAL ASSESSMENT OF EXPOSURE

A major hazardous spill may raise fears in the general population of possible long-term toxic effects. Patients and workers immediately exposed to the chemical hazard, as well as firefighters, EMS personnel, and police, may require ongoing medical surveillance. The long-term environmental impact also must be assessed. If a survey of the immediate area and patient population shows no significant hazard, then the public may be reassured. In the event a persistent hazard is determined to exist, local and national authorities may need to expand testing in concentric circles from the exposure site.

The health care providers must be aware of the mass psychogenic component that is commonly present in perceived environmental exposures. Whether or not patients are suffering toxic effects, it is likely that they also will experience symptoms and signs of catecholamine release. Some individuals may have nonspecific symptoms, such as headaches, nausea, vomiting, hyperventilation, chest pain, and paresthesias.[23]

HOSPITAL MANAGEMENT

Decontamination is *always* best performed before hospital arrival. A patient is never too unstable to have clothing removed and a brief decontamination performed in the field. Secondary decontamination procedures should be considered at the hospital after field decontamination. Initial decontamination will be required at the hospital for those patients not evaluated at the scene. The Tokyo sarin gas experience indicates that at least 80% of hospital patients will independently appear at a healthcare facility, without transport by first responders.[24]

Decontamination may occur inside the hospital in specially designed facilities equipped with a separate ventilation system that will provide adequate air flow. Air return from this room must never recirculate within the hospital and must be directly vented outside. Some specialized sites have floor drains leading to holding tanks that are easily accessed by hazardous waste contractors for toxicant removal. These holding tanks are expensive and should not preclude a hospital from participating in decontamination.

An expenditure of large amounts of money is not necessary for the safe, efficient management of patients. Most hospitals decontaminate patients outside the emergency department. Portable curtains provide privacy, and warm water can be delivered outside in all weather. Portable decontamination stretchers allow for synchronous decontamination and resuscitation. Portable wading pools are an inexpensive means of containment of irrigation fluid for ambulatory patients. If a large-scale decontamination effort is needed, the effluent can be allowed to flow into the sewer.

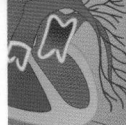

Contaminated patients must always be decontaminated before entry into the main emergency department. All hospital protocols must focus on efficient rapid patient processing. Hospitals must not rely on fire departments for decontamination because they will likely be deployed to the site of the release.

Cutaneous surface swipes before and after dermal cleansing can provide valuable information on the extent of contamination and efficacy of removal. Portable radiation detectors guide the duration and intensity of decontamination. Assessing the adequacy of chemical decontamination is more difficult in that the laboratory analysis takes more time. The physician will often not know "how clean is clean?" and will be forced to terminate decontamination based on less objective criteria.

Protection of hospital personnel is of primary importance.[25] Most health care facilities are poorly prepared to handle contaminated casualties. The medical team must always be equipped with a level of protection consistent with the contamination of the victim. Patient care must never be initiated before the donning of appropriated protection. There is a great deal of controversy regarding what level of personal protective equipment is appropriate for hospital personnel. Recent consensus opinions for health care facility–based personnel recommend level C personal protective equipment with OSHA operations-level training curricula modified to the health care environment.[26,27] Level C includes a nonencapsulating chemical-resistant suit and an air-purifying respirator. Hospitals may choose a powered air-purifying respirator (more expensive) because the work of breathing is much less with these devices, and fit testing is not required. An SCBA or air-supplied respirator is not required if the decontamination occurs outside of the hospital. Chemically resistant clothing and gloves are vital for the safe management of patients.

Water irrigation, mild soap, and gentle washing are the initial approach for all toxicants except elemental metals (e.g., sodium, lithium). These metals explode on contact with water and should be removed by other methods before the application of water. Occasionally, detergents are required to remove viscous materials. The irrigation of contaminated wounds should take priority to lessen system absorption of toxicants. Care must be taken not to allow irrigation runoff to contaminate clean skin.

A small number of dermal toxicants require special attention. Phenol is best removed with 200– to 400– molecular weight polyethylene glycol or isopropanol. Small amounts of water could increase dermal absorption of phenol. "Deluge" quantities of water are required when polyethylene glycol is not available. Limited data indicate that hexavalent chromium may be treated with topical ascorbic acid to allow reduction to the trivalent (less toxic) state. White phosphorus fumes or flames spontaneously on contact with air. Before débridement, the phosphorus should be covered with a moistened gauze. A Wood's lamp allows visualization of phosphorus in tissues. Copper sulfate irrigation of wounds for phosphorus visualization can cause copper

TABLE 103-1 Antidotes for Common Hazardous Materials Toxicants

ANTIDOTE	TOXIN
Lilly cyanide antidote kit	Cyanide
Methylene blue	Methemoglobin
Atropine or pralidoxime	Organophosphates, carbamates, nerve agents
Calcium	Hydrofluoric acid
Oxygen or hyperbaric oxygen	Carbon monoxide, cyanide, hydrogen sulfide
Prussian blue (Radiogardase)	Cesium, thallium
Chelators (DTPA, BAL, DMSA)	Heavy metals

toxicity and provides little benefit over a Wood's lamp. Calcium gluconate is the antidote in hydrofluoric acid (HF) exposures (Table 103-1). HF is a weak acid but causes systemic and local toxicity through its strong affinity for calcium and magnesium ions. Severe exposure to concentrated HF is associated with rapid hemodynamic compromise. Intravenous calcium must be administered early in these cases to control arrhythmias and shock. Dilute HF (<20%) typically causes delayed pain and tissue injury presenting as late as 24 hours after exposure. Topical application of a 2.5% calcium gluconate gel and parenteral narcotics constitute the initial management of dermal injury. If this fails to relieve pain, then calcium gluconate can be infiltrated into the wounds at a dose of 0.5 mL/cm^2. Hand wounds with persistent pain that do not respond to topical therapy are best managed with an intra-arterial infusion of calcium gluconate (10 mL of a 10% solution mixed with 40 mL of saline infused over 4 hours) until pain is resolved. Patients should not be discharged home with persistent pain. Table 103-1 provides specific commonly used antidotes in hazardous materials events that should be available to both prehospital and hospital health care providers.

REFERENCES

1. Federal Emergency Management Agency: Guide for All-Hazard Emergency Operations Planning, State and Local Guide 101, 1996.
2. National Fire Protection Association 1600: Standard for Disaster/ Emergency Management and Business Continuity Programs Current Edition, 2004.
3. U.S. Department of Transportation, Office of Hazardous Materials Safety, 2002.
4. CHEMTREC data, verbal communication, 2003.
5. Office of Hazardous Materials Safety Research and Special Programs Administration: Hazardous Materials Shipments. Washington, DC, U.S. Department of Transportation, 1998.
6. Hazardous Substances Emergency Events Surveillance: Annual Report 2001. Agency for Toxic Substances and Disease Registry, Division of Health Studies, Epidemiology and Surveillance Branch, 2001.
7. Available at: http://www.chemsafety.gov.
8. Dhara V, Dhara R: The Union Carbide disaster in Bhopal: a review of health effects. Arch Environ Health 2002;57:391–404.
9. Kamat SR, Mahashur AA, Twari AK, et al: Early observations on pulmonary changes and clinical morbidity due to the isocyanate gas leak at Bhopal. J Postgrad Med 1985;31:63–72.
10. Irani SF, Mahashur AA: A survey of Bhopal children affected by methyl isocyanate gas. J Postgrad Med 1986;32:195–198.

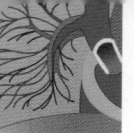
11. Ranjan N, Sarangi S, Padmanabhan V, et al: Methyl isocyanate exposure and growth patterns of adolescents in Bhopal. JAMA 2003;290:1856–1857.

12. Gale RP: Final Warning: The Legacy of Chernobyl. New York, Warner Books, 1988.

13. Mould RF: Chernobyl: The Real Story. Oxford, UK, Pergamon Press, 1988.

14. UNDP/UNICEF: The Human Consequences of the Chernobyl Nuclear Accident. A Strategy for Recovery, January 2002.

15. Nuclear Energy Agency: Chernobyl: Assessment of Radiological and Health Impacts 2002. Update of Chernobyl: Ten Years On, 2002.

16. Agency for Toxic Substances and Disease Registry: Volume I: Emergency Medical Services. A Planning Guide for the Management of Contaminated Patients. Washington, DC, U.S. Department of Health and Human Services, Public Health Service, 2001.

17. Agency for Toxic Substances and Disease Registry: Volume II: Hospital Emergency Departments. A Planning Guide for the Management of Contaminated Patients. Washington, DC, U.S. Department of Health and Human Services, Public Health Service, 2001.

18. Kirk MA, Cisek J, Rose SR: Emergency department response to hazardous materials incidents. Emerg Clin North Am 1994; 12:461–481.

19. Agency for Toxic Substances and Disease Registry: Volume III: Medical Management Guidelines (MMGs) for Acute Chemical Exposures. Washington, DC, U.S. Department of Health and Human Services, Public Health Service, 2001.

20. U.S. Department of Transportation: Hazardous Material—Emergency Response Guidebook. Washington, DC, U.S. Department of Transportation, 1994.

21. National Institute for Occupational Safety and Health (NIOSH): Pocket Guide to Chemical Hazards. NIOSH publication No. 97-140. Washington, DC, U.S. Department of Health and Human Services, 2003.

22. American Conference of Governmental Industrial Hygienists: 2004 Chemical Substances TLVs® and BEIs®, 2004.

23. Jones T, Crain A, Hoy D, et al: Mass Psychogenic Illness Attributed to Toxic Exposure at a High School. N Engl J Med 2000;342: 96–100.

24. Okumura T, Suzuki K, Fukuda A, et al. The Tokyo subway sarin attack: disaster management. 2. Hospital response. Acad Emerg Med 1998;5:618–624.

25. Horton DK, Berkowitz Z, Kaye W: Secondary contamination of emergency department personnel from hazardous materials events, 1995–2001 Am J Emerg Med 2003;21:199–204.

26. Hick J, Hanfling D, Burstein J, et al: Protective equipment for health care facility decontamination personnel: regulation, risks, and recommendations. Ann Emerg Med 2003;42:370–379.

27. Hicks J, Penn P, Hanfling D, et al: Establishing and training health care facility decontamination teams. Ann Emerg Med 2003;42: 381–390.

104 *Medical Management of Radiation Incidents*

RONALD E. GOANS, PHD, MD, MPH

At a Glance...

- Radiation incidents have historically been classified into five major categories:
  1. High-level external radiation exposure with late systemic symptoms, often neutropenia and sepsis 2 to 3 weeks postexposure.
  2. Low-level external exposure, with a normal physical examination.
  3. Local radiation injury to an extremity or other localized part of the body, generally with minimal systemic symptoms.
  4. Inhalation or ingestion of radioactive material accompanied by a normal physical examination.
  5. Hospital-related incidents, generally related to misadministration in brachytherapy, external dose, or in nuclear medicine studies.
- Victims of radiation-related terrorism require prompt treatment of medical and surgical conditions and initial evaluation for radiation exposure. Since radiation-related illness requires days to weeks to become clinically evident, patients should be triaged using traditional medical and trauma criteria, medically stabilized initially, and then assessed for radiation injury.
- An early estimation of the magnitude of the incident by the physician is crucial.
- Cobalt 60, cesium 137, iridium 192, and strontium 90 are major isotopes often involved in incidents of severe external exposure. High-level external exposure via a lost source in the public domain may cause patient death through neutropenic sepsis or multiorgan failure.
- Internal exposure rarely causes patient death, but significant regulatory issues and delayed radiation-related medical effects may ensue.
- External contamination is generally more of a nuisance issue and can be dealt with readily by removal of clothing and prompt decontamination, initially with soap and water.
- The lethal dose to 50% of an exposed population in 30 days (LD 50/30) in humans with only supportive treatment is approximately 3.5 to 4.0 Gy and may be extended to 6 to 8 Gy with modern critical care medicine. Rarely does a patient survive long-term with an acute whole body dose of 10 Gy or more, even with the most advanced medical care.

INTRODUCTION AND BACKGROUND

In the medical management of injury in a radiation terrorism event, it is important to remember that the "golden hour" is widely recognized by surgeons to be an hour of opportunity in which the lives of severely injured people may be saved if they are rapidly triaged by first response personnel and treated by trauma specialists. The presence of radiation issues must not interfere with rapid triage and removal of trauma victims from the field of injury.

Several excellent textbooks are available[1-9] in radiation medicine and in health physics that expand further on the topics in this chapter. Radiation accident medicine is often confusing to physicians and other medical personnel, mainly because the subject is not part of the traditional medical school curriculum. Common radiation terminology and radiation units are summarized in Appendix A. In addition, various examples are provided of the use of radioactive substances in medicine and in industry. Appendix B describes two additional resource organizations useful to assist in radiation accident analysis (Radiation Emergency Assistance Center/Training Site [REAC/TS] in Oak Ridge, Tennessee, and the Armed Forces Radiobiology Research Institute [AFRRI], located in Bethesda, Maryland). Several problems and medical case histories are also included in this chapter to illustrate various techniques useful in the practice of radiation medicine.

Many patients involved in radiation accidents may also be externally contaminated with radioactive particles. Removing contaminated clothing promptly will eliminate 80% to 90% of external contamination, and soap and water should be the first approach to removing remaining external contamination, particularly in exposed areas such as the face and hair. Irrigation of contaminated wounds is also readily performed using a saline jet under mild pressure. Ambient radiation levels from contaminated wounds are rarely medically significant, and hospital personnel attending the patient(s) should be reassured that their radiation dose will be minimal.

SOURCES OF RADIATION EXPOSURE

The most serious exposure scenario is high-level, high–dose rate, acute external whole body or partial body gamma irradiation. The patient may manifest significant systemic signs and symptoms associated with the acute radiation syndrome (ARS). Such an exposure could manifest from terrorist use of an improvised nuclear device or low-yield weapon (IND) or from close proximity to a radioactive dispersal device or high-level industrial source (Cs 137, Co 60, Ir 192, or Sr 90). Medical management of patients with moderate to severe radiation exposure (effective whole body dose > 3 Gy) should emphasize treatment of radiation-induced neutropenia and the prevention of infection. Initial care is directed toward reduction of pathogen acquisition through reverse isolation, low-microbial-content food and water, selective use of gastrointestinal (GI) decontamination, and consideration of antibiotic prophylaxis for opportunistic bacterial, viral, or fungal infections. Established or suspected infection in the neutropenic

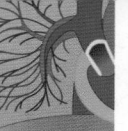

patient is managed in the same manner as for chemotherapy patients. Antibiotic prophylaxis should be considered in the severely neutropenic patient and in afebrile patients at the highest risk for infection.

Second, high-level local radiation injury occasionally arises from touching lost or covertly placed industrial radiation sources. These incidents often involve significant radiation burns to either the hands or other localized anatomic regions. However, the appearance of these lesions is usually delayed in time as noted below. Acute local irradiation events may occur separately or co-exist with the ARS. Deterministic thresholds exist as follows for certain ranges of localized skin radiation dose:

1. 3 Gy threshold for epilation, beginning 14 to 21 days postaccident.
2. 6 Gy for erythema, which may be observed transiently postaccident, and appears in permanent form 14 to 21 days thereafter. The pathophysiology for erythema involves arteriolar constriction with capillary dilation and local edema.
3. 10 to 15 Gy for dry desquamation of the skin secondary to irradiation of the germinal layer. Dry desquamation results from response of the germinal epidermal layer to radiation. There is diminished mitotic activity in cells of the basal and parabasal layers with thinning of the epidermis and desquamation of large macroscopic flakes of skin.
4. 20 to 50 Gy for wet desquamation (partial thickness injury) at least 2 to 3 weeks postexposure, depending on dose. In moist desquamation, microscopically, one finds intracellular edema, coalescence of vesicles forming macroscopic bulla, and a wet dermal surface, coated by fibrin.
5. For doses of more than 50 Gy to a localized area, overt radionecrosis and ulceration occurs secondary to endothelial cell damage and fibronoid necrosis of the arterioles and venules in the affected area. A cutaneous syndrome, arising from high-level whole body irradiation along with local injury, has also been described by various researchers.[10,11]

Third, accidents occur in either the industrial or government sector primarily involving inhalation or ingestion of radioactive material without overt systemic signs and symptoms. These accidents often involve medical misadministration of correctly prescribed radioisotopes or accidents involving nuclear medicine therapy or brachytherapy.

ACUTE RADIATION EXPOSURE

The correct diagnosis of acute radiation injury may be made approximately 85% of the time by a traditional, well-designed medical history. However, physicians often do not include radiation injury in the differential diagnosis of the usual radiation prodromal symptoms of nausea, vomiting, and diarrhea. Analysis of the recent history of radiation medicine shows many cases of delayed diagnosis.

In a review of four recent major radiation accidents[3] involving lost high-level gamma sources (Bangkok, Thailand [February, 2000]; Mit Halfa, Egypt [May, 2000]; Tammiku, Estonia [October, 1994]; Goiania, Brazil [September, 1987][12]), the average time from beginning of the accident until definitive diagnosis averaged approximately 22 days. However, in the recent nuclear criticality accident in Tokaimura, Japan[13] (September, 1999), awareness of the accident was essentially immediate because it occurred in an industrial environment with many witnesses.

Therefore, radiation accidents are recognized in a dichotomous fashion: either soon postaccident (industrial or medical setting), or 2 to 4 weeks or more postaccident when the patient becomes ill due to neutropenia and sepsis (misplaced sources found or stolen by a member of the public). The clinical presentation of the externally irradiated patient will be much different in these two scenarios. In addition, the patient presenting primarily with internal contamination will have few signs and symptoms and will generally have a normal physical examination.

In a terrorism event, radiation dose may be estimated early using rapid-sort, automated biodosimetry, employing such parameters such as the clinical history, the time to emesis (TE), and lymphocyte depletion kinetics.[14-20] For TE of less than 2 hours, the effective whole body dose is at least 3 Gy. If TE is less than 1 hour, the whole body dose most probably exceeds 4 Gy. Lymphocyte depletion follows dose-dependent, first-order kinetics after high-level gamma and criticality incidents. Patient radiation dose can be estimated very effectively from the medical history, serial lymphocyte counts, and TE, and subsequently confirmed with chromosome-aberration bioassay, the current U.S. and world gold standard. These data may be effectively analyzed using a computer tool developed at the Armed Forces Radiobiology Research Institute (Biodosimetry Assessment Tool [BAT]; http://www.afrri.usuhs.mil/). Input to BAT includes historical and clinical data, TE, and serial complete blood counts (CBCs), and the output provides a statistically weighted estimate of dose. It is possible therefore to determine the magnitude of the exposure within the first 12 to 18 hours postevent. The program is currently available free of charge for the personal computer (PC) laptop and will soon be available for the personal digital assistant (PDA).[17]

The medical management of patients with acute, moderate to severe radiation exposure (effective whole body dose greater than 3 Gy) should emphasize the rapid administration of colony-stimulating factors (CSF). All of these compounds decrease the duration of radiation-induced neutropenia and stimulate neutrophil recovery. For those patients developing febrile radiation-induced neutropenia, adherence to the current Infectious Diseases Society of America guidelines for high-risk neutropenia is recommended (IDSA; http://www.idsociety.org/).

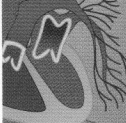

INDUSTRIAL TOXICOLOGY OF COMMON RADIOISOTOPES

Following an accidental intake of radioactive material, dose, toxicity, and treatment methods are dependent on various factors such as the identity of the radionuclide and its physical and chemical characteristics (physical and biological half-life, particle size, chemical composition, solubility, etc.). In the inhalation pathway, particle characteristics (size, chemical composition, chemical solubility in body fluids) are important determinants of dose. The fate of inhaled particles is critically dependent on particle physicochemical properties and the size of aerosol particles determines the region of the respiratory tract where most will be deposited. Highly insoluble particles may remain in the lung for long periods of time, and a small fraction will be transported to the tracheobronchial lymph nodes by pulmonary macrophages. Insoluble particles may be swallowed and therefore excreted primarily in the feces.

Treatment considerations for internal contamination of radioisotopes are very similar to traditional poison control measures and fall into several major categories[21]:

1. Reduce and/or inhibit absorption of the isotope in the GI tract.
2. Block uptake to the organ of interest.
3. Utilize isotopic dilution.
4. Alter the chemistry of the substance.
5. Displace the isotope from receptors.
6. Utilize traditional chelation techniques.

The most common isotopes seen in the management of internal contamination will now be presented along with selected case histories. It is hoped that these case histories will give the reader some idea of the decision-making process involved in management of internal contamination cases.

CASE HISTORY: ESTIMATING THE MAXIMUM CREDIBLE INHALATION ACCIDENT

Two scientists at a government facility accidentally break the integrity of a glovebox known to contain americium 241. Nasal swipes taken within 10 minutes postaccident read 10,000 dpm and 12,000 dpm alpha for the left and right nares, respectively. The presenting issue is to estimate the maximum credible accident.

Mansfield[22] has given a rough rule of thumb that the combined activity of both nasal swipes should approximate 5% of deep lung deposition, using the International Commission on Radiological Protection (ICRP) 30 lung model. Using this rule of thumb to estimate the magnitude of the incident, we have the total anterior nasal passage activity to be 22,000 dpm alpha = 9.9 nCi. The estimated lung deposition is therefore on the order of 200 nCi, or approximately 10 annual limits of intake (ALI; 1 ALI = 5 rem) for inhalation. Experience has shown that this is generally a very conservative overestimate, but useful for initial estimates, pending the results of bioassay.[23]

MEDICAL CONSIDERATIONS FOR SELECTED RADIONUCLIDES[23]

Tritium (^3H)

Dose to total body water is the critical issue in the management of tritium accidents. The ICRP 67 model for tritium[24] assumes two compartments for tritiated water, A and B, with age-dependent biologic half-lives ranging from 3 to 10 days for compartment A and 8 to 40 days for compartment B. In addition, organically bound tritium is treated in an age-dependent manner. For accident dosimetry purposes, tritium retention may be approximated by a single exponential with a half life of 10 days. For reference, the ALI for tritium is 80,000 μCi. Medical management of tritium intake is directed toward increasing body water turnover by increasing oral fluid intake, thereby diluting the tritium and increasing excretion by physiologic mechanisms.

An increase in oral fluids of 3 to 4 L/day reduces the biologic half-life of tritium by a factor of 2 to 3 and therefore reduces whole body dose in the same proportion.

CASE STUDIES: TRITIUM EXPOSURE

Six male teens at a government dormitory facility break an exit sign, releasing approximately 10 Ci of tritium gas. The highest levels of tritium are found on the public telephone (157,000 dpm). Urine samples are taken from all six teens and sent for tritium bioassay. From liquid scintillation counting at a national laboratory, the highest urine value is found to be 6.5 μCi/L in a 17-year-old boy.

Using the conservative rule of thumb from ICRP 65 that 1 μCi/L peak tritium concentration in urine corresponds to an integrated whole body dose of 10 mrem,[21] the maximum estimated dose is approximately 65 mrem (0.65 mSv) whole body. Prior to receiving the urine bioassay results, all teens were instructed to increase oral hydration to 3 to 4 L/day. There were no adverse medical events from this tritium intake.

Historically, tritium exposures have resulted in relatively low whole body dose, but Seelentag and Minder[25] have reported cases of two fatalities possibly related to high-level tritium intake in an industrial environment over a period of years. From these cases, they concluded that there is possible evidence that two people died secondary to radiation-induced bone marrow suppression, although there was also prior exposure to strontium and radium.

Strontium

Sr 90 is the predominant isotope of interest in this chemical series, and a comprehensive model for strontium

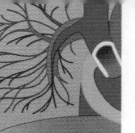

retention, developed by Snyder and colleagues[26] that indicates that 73% of material in the transfer compartment is eliminated with a 3-day half-life, 10% with a 44 day half-life, and 17% with a 4000-day half-life. All chemical forms except $SrTiO_3$ are considered relatively soluble (class D in the ICRP 30 formalism). $SrTiO_3$ is considered insoluble (class Y). In the ICRP 76 treatment[27] of alkaline earth distribution, an age-dependent biokinetic model is given, with transfer to soft tissue, cortical and trabecular bone volume and surface, two liver compartments, and the renal system. For most forms of strontium, except titanate, bone surface is the dose-limiting organ for both inhalation and ingestion. Because of the biologically significant rate of strontium transfer to the GI tract, it is also necessary to block intestinal absorption in those cases where intake is by inhalation. The following treatments are useful in the medical management of inhalation cases with strontium:

1. Intravenous (IV) calcium gluconate 2 g in 500 mL over 4 to 6 hours (competes for strontinum at bone binding sites).
2. Ammonium chloride (300 mg orally) to produce a moderate metabolic acidosis.
3. Barium sulfate 300 g orally as soon as possible postaccident to block intestinal absorption.

Iodine

The thyroid is the critical organ after intake of radioactive iodine. Retention in the thyroid is described by a three-component exponential with half-lives of 0.24 days, 11 days, and 120 days. In the ICRP 67 model, age-dependent elimination rate constants are given. In this model, uptake to the thyroid is 30%, with 70% of intake routed to prompt urinary excretion. The ICRP 67 model[24] for adults has a half-life of 80 days for iodine in the thyroid and 12 days for iodine in the rest of the body. For accident dosimetry, the effective half-life of iodine may be taken to be approximately 12 days.

Thyroid blocking in adults is accomplished by administering 130 mg potassium iodide (KI) orally as soon as possible postaccident and one tablet daily for 7 to 14 days. Another convenient way to administer stable iodide is five or six drops of saturated solution of KI (SSKI, 1 g/mL). In addition, potassium perchlorate (200 mg) may be used in patients with iodine sensitivity. The timing of iodine administration is as soon as possible postaccident, up to 6 hours. However, in a situation with continuing exposure, stable iodine may be 50% effective even 5 to 6 hours after exposure to radioiodine.

CASE STUDY: RADIOIODINE ADMINISTRATION IN PREGNANCY[23,28]

A 26-year-old female nurse presents with clinical hyperthyroidism.[23,28] During the laboratory analysis, a T_4 level is found to be 19.5 μg/dL (normal 5 to 12.5 μg/dL). She is given 9.2 mCi iodine 131 (NaI) for thyroid ablation, and the patient's hyperthyroid symptoms subside within 1 week. However, the patient is subsequently found to be 14 weeks pregnant at the time of iodine administration by ultrasound dating. The fetal self dose in this case is calculated to be 2.4 rad (0.024 Gy; dose conversion factor [DCF] = 0.068 mGy/MBq), but the fetal thyroid dose is calculated to be 88 Gy (DCF = 260 mGy/MBq). This is ablative to the fetal thyroid.

The mother and fetus were followed throughout the remainder of the pregnancy by a specialist in fetal-maternal medicine. The pregnancy was clinically uneventful, with a normal delivery. At birth, the infant was found to be profoundly hypothyroid and in the 6th percentile for growth on standard growth charts. At 1 year of age, the baby also exhibited minor developmental delay on standard neurocognitive tests.

Cesium

Following systemic uptake of cesium, the isotope is uniformly distributed in the body with distribution similar to potassium. Systemic retention for cesium is often represented by a two exponential retention function with retention half-lives of approximately 2 days and approximately 110 days. However, a range of retention half-lives has been noted.[12]

The most effective means for removing radioactive cesium is the oral administration of ferric ferrocyanate, commonly called Prussian blue (PB). Insoluble PB (ferric hexacyanoferrate, $Fe_4[Fe(CN)_6]_3$) is an orally administered drug that enhances excretion of isotopes of cesium and thallium from the body by means of ion exchange. One gram orally three times daily for 2 to 3 weeks reduces the biological half-life of radiocesium to about one third the normal value. PB has a high affinity for cesium, whose metabolism follows an entero-enteric cycle. Orally administered PB traps cesium in the gut, interrupts its reabsorption from the GI tract, and thereby increases fecal excretion. Thus, the biologic half-life of cesium is significantly reduced after decorporation therapy with PB.

CASE STUDY: CESIUM

The most famous case[12] involving cesium intake was the radiologic accident in Goiania, Brazil, in 1987. In September 1987, two men removed the rotating assembly of a cesium 137 teletherapy unit and breached the capsule containing 50.9 TBq (1375 Ci) of ^{137}Cs. The source was in the form of soluble ^{137}CsCl, which is highly dispersible in the environment. The teletherapy assembly was initially sold to a junkyard and the junkyard owner believed that it had mystical power since it glowed blue in the dark (Cherenkov radiation from the cesium beta decay). Samples of the material were given to many friends and relatives, resulting in widespread contamination to people and to the environment. Residual contamination levels near the initial breach of containment were on the order of 1.1 Gy/hr.

Approximately 112,000 persons were monitored for radioactive contamination, of whom 249 were contaminated externally or internally. Four individuals died of

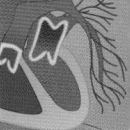

the acute radiation syndrome, with whole body dose in the range 4 to 7 Gy. These included the 38-year-old wife of the junkyard owner (5.7 Gy), 18- and 22-year-old employees (4.5 and 5.3 Gy, respectively), and a 6-year-old niece of the junkyard owner (6.0 Gy). The latter case represented a situation of extreme internal contamination (1×10^9 Bq) by ingestion, since the young girl was playing with a piece of the source while eating a sandwich.

Forty-six individuals, internally contaminated in this incident, were treated with PB in daily divided doses of 3 to 20 g. The use of PB reduced the average ^{137}Cs biologic half-life from 110 to 115 days to about 40 days, with a consequent reduction in dose.

Uranium

The two most common uranium isotopes seen in research and in industry are uranium 238 and 235. Acute toxicity is most closely related to chemical rather than radiologic properties, particularly with regard to the renal system. For uranium entering the transfer compartment, approximately 20% is transferred to mineral bone with a half-life of 20 days and 2.3% to bone with a half-life of 5000 days. In addition, 12% and 0.05% are transferred to the kidneys with half-lives of 6 and 1500 days, respectively. Systemic body retention of uranium is given by a five exponential retention function with half-lives of 0.25, 6, 20, 1500, and 5000 days.[19-31]

Uranium has an overall effective half-life of 15 days, and 85% of retained uranium resides in bone. Kidney toxicity is the basis of occupational exposure limits. In acidic urine, the uranyl ion binds with renal tubular surface proteins, and some of the bound UO_2^{2+} is therefore retained in the kidney. The kidney is the first organ to show chemical damage in the form of nephritis and proteinuria. Oral doses or infusions of sodium bicarbonate have historically been the treatment of choice and should be dosed to keep the urine alkaline by frequent pH measurements. The non-toxic uranium carbonate complex is increased by three to four orders of magnitude in alkaline urine and promptly excreted.[30,32]

Annual occupational limits for uranium are based on levels estimated to induce renal damage. The threshold for transient renal injury is estimated to be 0.058 mg U/kg body weight or intake of 4.06 mg in a 70-kg individual. Likewise, the threshold for permanent renal damage is estimated to be 0.3 mg U/kg body weight, or 21 mg U in a 70-kg person. Permanent renal damage is shown by a permanent increase in blood urea nitrogen and creatinine, along with proteinuria and a decrease in glomerular filtration rate. From animal research, the 50% lethality level is estimated to be 1.63 mg/kg body weight, or 114 mg in a 70-kg person. A very useful Internet calculator for determining organ levels of uranium from either ingestion or inhalation is found through Martindale's Online Center (http://www.martindalecenter.com/CalculatorsD_Rad.html). This very extensive calculator originated through the WISE Uranium Project in the Netherlands.

Current research on decorporation therapy of uranium and the actinides has evaluated analogs to siderophores.[30,31] Siderophores are agents produced by microorganisms to obtain Fe(III) from the environment. These compounds are good candidates for trial since actinide and uranium biokinetics are associated with Fe(III) transport and storage systems. The association rate constant for actinide-ligand and uranium-ligand binding is generally found to be much greater than that for diethylenetriamine-penta-acetic acid (DTPA) binding.

Durbin and colleagues[33,34] have considered a linear hydroxypyridinone derivative of deferoxamine: 3,4,3-LIHOPO, or simply LIHOPO. LIHOPO is readily given by IV injection in a rat model with low toxicity and has been found to be an effective chelator for both actinides and for uranium. Consider a rat model where plutonium and americium particulates are inhaled. The summary of experiments below shows relative improvement ratios for decorporation therapy using LIHOPO compared with traditional methods using DTPA.[23]

1. Plutonium: LIHOPO/DTPA = a factor of 6.7 improvement for plutonium deposition in lungs.
2. Americium: LIHOPO/DTPA = a factor of 2.0 improvement for americium deposition in lungs.
3. Plutonium: LIHOPO/DTPA = a factor of 4.8 improvement for plutonium deposition in skeleton.

In a plutonium wound model in rats, LIHOPO was found to be 2 to 40 times more effective than DTPA in chelation therapy, depending on the nature of the experiment and route of LIHOPO administration. In another series of experiments, small oral doses of LIHOPO mobilized more americium than plutonium from liver and bone. Furthermore, in rat experiments using injected uranium, LIHOPO was 3.6 times more effective in renal protection than $NaHCO_3$ and 1.7 times more effective in decreasing dose to bone volume.[32] These experiments appear to be quite promising for eventual human use.

Durbin and colleagues[33] have also recently presented experiments designed to identify the most effective multidentate 1,2-HOPO and Me-3,2-HOPO ligands for chelation of Pu(IV) in vivo. Nine HOPO ligands, when injected or given orally, were found to be superior to Ca-DTPA for reducing plutonium 238 retention in the mouse model. These tetradentate and hexadentate compounds are found to be highly effective, but moderately toxic, and deserve more intensive study prior to human studies. While these experiments to date appear quite promising, U.S. Food and Drug Administration (FDA) phase I human trials have not yet begun. Therefore, the compounds will not be available in the clinic for several years. A recent review article[34] provides additional details of this preclinical research.

Henge-Napoli and colleagues[35,36] have evaluated the efficacy of ethane-1-hydroxy-1,1 bisphosphonate (EHBP, etidronate, Didronel [Proctor and Gamble, Mason, OH]) in experiments to obtain com pounds that will reduce the fixation of uranium in its main target organs of bone and kidney. Etidronate, a synthetic analog of pyrophosphate, is used in the treatment of moderate to severe Paget's disease, heterotopic ossification, and hypercalcemia associated with malignant neoplasms. The

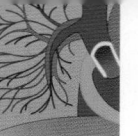

work of Henge-Napoli and colleagues showed that one injection of EHBP (50 to 100 mol/kg), given acutely after uranium inhalation in animals, reduced uranium deposition in the renal system by a factor of five, and still a factor of two when given 30 minutes postexposure.

This work is particularly important since Etidronate is currently approved by the FDA for reduction of bone resorption, is clinically accepted, and has a well-studied adverse reaction profile. Etidronate has pharmacologic actions that are similar to pyrophosphate, a salt of phosphoric acid, which occurs naturally in the body and acts to inhibit bone metabolism. In contrast to the endogenous compound, etidronate is resistant to enzymatic metabolism. The drug decreases both normal and abnormal bone resorption, thereby reducing bone turnover and slowing the remodeling of pagetic or heterotopic bone.

In another series of animal experiments, Destombes and colleagues[37] compared the carbonic anhydrase inhibitor acetazolamide (Diamox [Barr Pharmaceuticals, Pomona, NY]), with bicarbonate in the treatment of internal contamination with uranium. This work is quite important since acetazolamide is also currently approved by the FDA and could be adapted easily for use in cases of uranium contamination in a mass casualty terrorist incident.

Carbonic anhydrase is an enzyme responsible for forming hydrogen and bicarbonate ions from carbon dioxide and water. By inhibiting this reaction, acetazolamide reduces the availability of these ions for active transport. Hydrogen ion concentrations in the renal tubule lumen are therefore reduced by acetazolamide, leading to an alkaline urine and an increased excretion of bicarbonate, sodium, potassium, and water. A reduction in plasma bicarbonate results in a metabolic acidosis, which rapidly reverses the diuretic effect.

Acetazolamide is classically used for the prophylaxis and treatment of altitude sickness, and as an adjunct treatment for glaucoma and epilepsy. It has also long been approved by the FDA for use as a diuretic. Acetazolamide is rapidly absorbed from the GI tract, and peak serum concentrations for the tablets and extended-release capsules are achieved in 2 to 4 hours and 8 to 12 hours, respectively. For use in urinary alkalization, the adult dose is 5 mg/kg IV or as needed to maintain an alkaline diuresis. In their recent animal work, Destombes and colleagues[37] noted that acetazolamide is three times more effective than bicarbonate in reducing the renal content of uranium, but has no effect on skeletal content. These experiments appear quite promising clinically and deserve to be extended.

Actinides

Plutonium is the model element in this series. After plutonium enters the transfer compartment, approximately 45% translocates to the liver and 45% to bone. The retention time is assumed to be 20 years in the liver and 50 years in bone. The classical plutonium retention function is given by Durbin[38] based on her data and that of earlier work by Langham.[39] The Durbin model for plutonium uses a five-component exponential with half-lives of 1.2, 5.5, 42, 300, and 4000 days. The retention functions for other actinides are similar to that for plutonium.

Trisodium calcium diethylenetriaminepentaacetate (Ca-DTPA) and Zn-DTPA chelation therapy are the treatment of choice for inhalation accidents involving actinides. Ca-DTPA is a calcium salt of DTPA, and Zn-DTPA is similar, except for the substitution of Zn for Ca. Ca-DTPA appears to be approximately 10 times more effective than Zn-DTPA for initial chelation of transuranics; therefore, Ca-DTPA should be used whenever larger body burdens of transuranics are involved. Approximately 24 hours after exposure, Zn-DTPA is, for all practical purposes, as effective as Ca-DTPA. This comparable efficacy, coupled with its lesser toxicity, makes Zn-DTPA the preferred agent for protracted therapy. The route of administration may be either slow IV push of the drug over a period of 3 to 4 minutes, IV infusion (1 g in 100 to 250 mL D_5W, Ringer's lactate, or normal saline), or inhalation in a nebulizer (1:1 dilution with water or saline). The Centers for Disease Control and Prevention (CDC) has included both Zn- and Ca-DTPA in the Strategic National Stockpile.

THE RADON ISSUE

Radon (radon 222) is the sixth element in the radioactive decay chain of ^{238}U, one of the major natural isotopes on earth. Radon gas poses an environmental risk because of its potential carcinogenic properties (increases in small cell and squamous cell carcinomas of the lung). This risk is not primarily due to radon's chemical and radiologic characteristics (noble gas; physical half-life 3.825 days), but mostly to the short-lived, reactive alpha-emitting progeny that occur after radon in the decay chain.

Radon is formed in soil and rock from the radioactive decay of its parent, radium (radium 226, half-life 1622 years), and can easily diffuse from its source. Radon tends to accumulate in enclosed structures, including mines, buildings, and basements, as a combination of diffusion from the soil and flow from air pressure differentials. Most biologic damage in human lungs is caused by its alpha-emitting progeny, particularly polonium (polonium 218 and 210, half-lives 3.11 min and 138.4 days, respectively) and lead 214. The conventional radiologic units associated with radon dose are particularly confusing and derive from historical epidemiologic considerations of working populations in underground mines.

Radon activity may be expressed in pCi/L (equal to 37 Bq/m^3 in SI units) and one working level (WL) is equivalent to a radon concentration of 100 pCi/L at equilibrium and to approximately 200 pCi/L at 50% equilibrium, which is typical of many buildings. The working level is therefore a unit of radioactivity per liter of air or water. One working level month (WLM) is historically defined as a month of occupational exposure (170 hours) to one WL of airborne radon activity. One

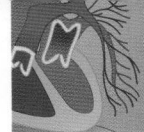

WLM equates to approximately 5 pCi/L-year under typical conditions of equilibrium and an assumption of 75% occupancy. In addition, one WLM (5 pCi/L-year) results in approximately 0.5 rad (0.5 cGy) of absorbed alpha dose to the lung.

The current Environmental Protection Agency (EPA) voluntary indoor air action level is 4 pCi/L air, and most recent documents[40-42] continue to use the correlation that 10,000 pCi/L of radon in water correlates to 1 pCi/L in air (transfer coefficient of 10^{-4}). In poorly ventilated residences, typical radon concentrations are in the range 0.5 to 1.5 pCi/L, somewhat dependent on weather, proximity to the basement substructures, and human use patterns. Typical residential exposures are about 0.2 WLM per year, equivalent to 1 pCi/L-year

PATIENT ASSESSMENT IN RADIATION TERRORISM EVENTS

Victims of radiation terrorism events require prompt diagnosis and treatment of medical and surgical conditions as well as conditions related to radiation exposure. Hospital emergency personnel should triage victims using traditional medical and trauma criteria. Radiation dose can be estimated early postevent using rapid-sort, automated biodosimetry and clinical parameters such as the clinical history, TE,[43,44] and lymphocyte depletion kinetics. Patient radiation dose can be estimated very effectively from the medical history, serial lymphocyte counts, and TE, and subsequently confirmed with chromosome-aberration bioassay, the current gold standard. These data are effectively analyzed using the Armed Forces Radiobiology Research Institute Biodosimetry Assessment Tool.

The medical management of patients with acute, moderate to severe radiation exposure (effective whole body dose greater than 3 Gy) should emphasize the rapid administration of granulocyte colony stimulating factor (G-CSF).[45] These compounds appear to decrease the duration of radiation-induced neutropenia and to stimulate neutrophil recovery in patients who have received myelotoxic insult. For those patients developing febrile radiation-induced neutropenia, adherence to the current Infectious Diseases Society of America guidelines for high-risk neutropenia is recommended (http://www.idsociety.org/).

CLINICAL MANIFESTATIONS OF HIGH-LEVEL EXTERNAL EXPOSURE

Radiation damage results from the inherent sensitivity of certain cell types to radiation, with mitotically active cells most sensitive to acute effects. The inherent sensitivity of these cells results in a constellation of clinical syndromes (ARS) that occur within a predictable range of dose (greater than 2 Gy) after whole body irradiation delivered at a relatively high dose rate. The clinical components of ARS include hematopoietic, GI, and cerebrovascular syndromes and are reviewed elsewhere.[14,43-45]

Symptoms of acute, high dose radiation are dependent on the absorbed dose and may appear within hours to days and follow a somewhat predictable course. Individuals suffering from a lethal dose of radiation may experience a compression of these phases over a period of hours, resulting in early death. Because of the rapid cell turnover of the lymphohematopoietic elements, these cells are among the most radiation-sensitive tissue in mammals. As such, irradiation of bone marrow stem and progenitor cells results in exponential death.

The onset of cytopenia is variable and dose dependent. In particular, the duration of neutropenia may be prolonged, requiring prolonged administration of hematopoietic growth factors, blood product support, and antibiotics. The primary goal of medical therapy is to shift the survival curve to the right by about 2 Gy. Many casualties in a terrorist-initiated weapon event (IND) whose dose exceeds 6 to 8 Gy will also have significant blast and thermal injuries that will preclude survival when combined with their radiation insult

The medical management of patients with acute, moderate to severe radiation exposure (effective whole body dose greater than 3 Gy) should emphasize early initiation of G-CSF, transfusion support as needed, antibiotic prophylaxis, and treatment of febrile neutropenia, which is discussed in more detail below. Additional supportive medications may include antiemetics, antidiarrheals, fluid and electrolytes replacement, and topical burn creams. In the case of coexisting trauma (combined injury), wound closure should be performed within 24 to 36 hours. In non-neutropenic patients, antibiotics should be directed toward the foci of infection and the most likely pathogens. For those who experience significant neutropenia (absolute neutrophil count [ANC] less than 500 cells/mm^3), broad-spectrum prophylactic antimicrobials should be given during the potentially long duration of neutropenia. Prophylaxis should include a fluoroquinolone, an antiviral agent (if indicated), and an antifungal agent.[43-45]

These antimicrobials should be continued until either the patient experiences a neutropenic fever and requires alternate coverage or experiences neutrophil recovery (ANC greater than 500 cells/mm^3). In patients who experience first fever, traditionally therapy is directed at gram-negative bacteria (in particular, *Pseudomonas aeruginosa*), because infections of this type may be rapidly lethal. Any focus of infection that develops during the neutropenic period will require a full course of therapy.

DELAYED EFFECTS OF RADIATION EXPOSURE

It is common to distinguish late organ effects from the acute effects of radiation exposure. Deterministic effects typically show a sigmoid dose–response curve above an appropriate threshold, and the severity of the harm from radiation exposure increases with dose. Effects are non-neoplastic and are expressed in the exposed individual. In contrast, stochastic effects represent a probabilistic tissue response to radiation exposure. Stochastic effects

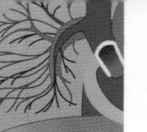

are nonthreshold and expressed in the exposed population. Damage in reproductive cells may give rise to inheritable genetic mutations, while damage in somatic cells may increase the chance of neoplasia. Leukemias and bone cancers have a minimum latency time of 2 to 5 years, while solid tumors have a minimum latency time of approximately 10 years. For carcinomas of normal adult onset, current evidence suggests that the latency period may be greater than 10 years.

From the adult atomic bomb data,[46] there is statistically significant evidence for all radiation-induced leukemia (except chronic lymphocytic leukemia [CLL]), as well as for breast, thyroid, colon, stomach, lung, and ovarian carcinoma, and borderline or inconsistent results for radiation-induced carcinoma of the esophagus, liver, skin, bladder, and central nervous system (CNS), as well as multiple myeloma and lymphoma. Regarding non-neoplastic disease,[46] there is strong evidence for radiation-induced cataracts, hyperparathyroidism, a decrease in the T cell–mediated and humoral immune response, and chromosomal aberrations in lymphocytes.

The International Agency for Research on Cancer Study Group[47] recently studied combined mortality data for 96,000 nuclear industry workers in the United States, Canada, and the United Kingdom. The exposure was primarily to low-level gamma radiation and the risk analysis was based on a constant linear relative risk model, excess relative risk (ERR) = 1 + b(dose). In this study, the ERR was found to be 2.2 per sievert for leukemia, with ERR for all other cancers, excluding leukemia, being essentially zero. Additional risk estimates for carcinoma from large epidemiologic studies have been published recently.[48,49]

The Biological Effects of Ionizing Radiation (BEIR) V[50] excess cancer mortality estimates are widely quoted in the radiation medicine literature. Consider, for example, the hypothetical risk for a single occupational or terrorist exposure to 10 rem (0.1 Sv). Risk is traditionally expressed as lifetime risk per 100,000 exposed persons. Approximately 20,000 cancer deaths would occur in the absence of radiation exposure. For the hypothetical acute dose of 0.1 Sv, 770 excess cancers (660 nonleukemia and 110 leukemia) would be expected in the male cohort and 810 excess cancers (730 nonleukemia and 80 leukemia) expected in the female cohort. The risk model as a function of dose D is of the form:

$$\text{risk}(D) = \text{risk}(0)[1 + f(D)g(\text{age,sex},...)]$$

BEIR V also estimated the genetic effects of 1 rem (0.01 Sv) per generation. The autosomal-dominant natural incidence is approximately 10,000 cases per million. For an additional dose of 1 rem above natural background, one would expect an additional 5 to 20 cases in the first generation and 25 cases at genetic equilibrium. Most cases would be clinically mild in a 3:1 mild:severe ratio. The natural incidence of X-linked disease is estimated in BEIR V at 400 cases per million. For a dose of 1 rem we expect less than one additional case in the first generation and fewer than five cases at equilibrium. Regarding translocations/trisomies, the natural incidence is approximately 600 translocations and 3800 trisomies per million. At 1 rem, we would expect fewer than an additional five translocations in the first generation and less than one additional trisomy.

If we consider congenital abnormalities as an entire entity, the current incidence is approximately 20,000 to 30,000 per million. Given 1 rem whole body dose-equivalent, it is expected that an additional 10 would occur in the first generation and 10 to 100 at equilibrium. In all of these calculations, BEIR V assumes a doubling dose of 100 rem (1 Sv). Risk analysis from radiation exposure is a complicated and controversial science.

PRENATAL AND PEDIATRIC ISSUES

Differential cell sensitivity to radiation damage is simply expressed by the law of Bergonie and Tribondeau (1906)[51] as follows: Cells are generally radiosensitive if they have a high mitotic rate, have a long mitotic future, and are of a primitive type. The developing embryo and fetus fit within these conditions. Pregnancy dating as taught in medical school is the gestational age calculated from beginning of the last menstrual period so that the average length of pregnancy is 280 days or 40 weeks (95% confidence interval [CI] 2 weeks), split into three trimesters. During the first 2 weeks following ovulation, successive developmental phases are fertilization of the ovum, formation of the free blastocyst, and implantation of the blastocyst into the uterus.[52]

Prior to comparing the effects of radiation on the fetus, it is interesting to compare risks that normally occur during pregnancy. For example, if the patient contracts maternal rubella in the first trimester, approximately 80% of cases will have a fetus with congenital infection. If infection occurs early in the second trimester, there is approximately a 54% incidence of congenital infection. By infection in the third trimester, approximately 25% of fetuses will be born with congenital syndrome. Additionally, if maternal alcohol consumption[52] is considered, two to three drinks per day will cause a risk of approximately 10% incidence of fetal alcohol syndrome (FAS). Heavy maternal drinking in pregnancy (more than five drinks per day) will also cause approximately a 30% incidence of FAS. The issue of maternal smoking is particularly important in the incidence of fetal growth retardation, and many experts consider intrauterine growth retardation directly proportional to number of cigarettes smoked.[52]

Deterministic effects[52-55] of radiation exposure to the embryo/fetus may be considered in stages. Preconception, generally no statistically significant effects are noted at low to moderate radiation doses. When the fetus receives a moderate dose in the preimplantation phase, generally an "all or none" effect is noted. If implantation succeeds, the pregnancy is often successful. At a threshold of 10 to 20 rad, transient growth retardation has been noted shortly after implantation. During the period of organogenesis (7 to 13 weeks' gestation), the embryo is sensitive to the lethal, teratogenic, and growth-retarding effects of radiation because of the

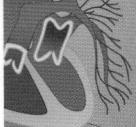

criticality of cellular activities and the high proportion of radiosensitive cells. Growth retardation, gross congenital malformations, microcephaly, and mental retardation are the predominant effects for a uterine dose of greater than 50 rad (0.5 Gy). For survivors of in utero exposure, important clinical sequelae are microcephaly, mental retardation, growth and development delay, and lower IQ and poorer school performance. The highest risk for mental retardation occurs during major neuronal migration in the 8- to 15-week period of time. There is no report of external irradiation inducing morphologic malformation in humans unless the individual also had growth retardation or a CNS anomaly.

Generally, there exist specific windows of opportunity for radiation damage in certain organs during fetal development:

Cataracts: 0 to 6 days (gestational)
Exencephaly: 0 to 37 days
Embryonic death: 4 to 11 days
Anencephaly or microcephaly: 9 to 90 days
Anophthalmia: 16 to 32 days
Cleft palate: 20 to 37 days
Skeletal dyscrasias: 25 to 85 days
Growth retardation: 50+ days

Occasionally the question arises regarding a clinical decision to terminate a pregnancy because of first trimester radiation exposure to the fetus. It is important in this regard to consider that the normal rate of first trimester preclinical loss is greater than 30%. For a fetal exposure of 0.1 Gy (10 rad), this risk is increased by less than 1%. A useful number to consider is that the lifetime risk for induction of childhood tumors is approximately 1 in 2000 per rad or 5% per sievert. Consider a case where a fetus received a 5-rad whole body dose in a nuclear medicine procedure where the mother was not known to be pregnant. At 5 rad, the maximal risk for childhood leukemia is 1 in 400. Conversely, the probability of not having a childhood cancer is greater than 99%. If the fetal absorbed dose is greater than 50 rad in the 7- to 13-week window, then there is a substantial risk for growth retardation and CNS damage. It is relatively unusual to have a fetal dose in the range of 25 to 50 rad during the organogenesis period of 7 to 13 weeks. However, if pregnancy termination is at issue for any fetal dose, it is important to have parental value input as well as scientific and clinical input from the physician of record. However, the ultimate decision belongs with the patient.

Childhood irradiation problems are of particular concern for the primary care physician. From the atomic bomb data, the doubling dose for childhood abnormalities is at least 1.7 to 2.2 Sv (170 to 220 rem), but these data reflect both a high dose and a high dose rate. According to the BEIR V report, the minimal doubling dose in humans for chronic exposure is at least 4 Sv (400 rem) and greater than 20 rad for children. In cases of childhood irradiation therapy for CNS tumors, depression and somnolence have been noted clinically as well as late development of cognitive dysfunction. For a tumor dose of 40 to 65 Gy, at long-term follow-up, mental retardation was found in 17% of patients, although 89% functioned at a satisfactory level. Behavioral disorders were found in 39% of this cohort. Mental retardation was greatest in those irradiated at less than 3 years of age or if the tumor was in the thalamus or hypothalamus.[54,55]

Childhood acute lymphoblastic leukemia (ALL) is the most common childhood neoplasm. Current therapy can be expected to produce remission in greater than 95% of children, and 70% do not have a recurrence. At least 2000 new cases occur each year in children under the age of 15 years. However, treatment including radiation therapy can be potentially carcinogenic. Second neoplasms are relatively common, especially for children younger than 5 years or who have received cranial irradiation.[56-58] The Children's Cancer Study Group[57] is an excellent retrospective cohort study of adverse effects from 9720 children exhibiting second neoplasms after ALL treatment. The median follow-up was 4.6 years (range 2 months to 16 years). The study results showed 43 second neoplasms, including 24 CNS neoplasms, 10 new leukemias and lymphomas, and 9 other neoplasms. These data represent a 7-fold excess of all cancers and a 22-fold increase of CNS neoplasms. All children with CNS tumors had undergone cranial irradiation with 18 to 24 Gy.

Late deaths and survival after childhood cancer were recorded in the U.K. National Register of Childhood Tumours.[57] In a retrospective cohort study, 9080 5-year survivors of childhood cancer were followed for variable periods of time. In this study, 781 deaths were recorded; 74% of these deaths were due to recurrent tumor with treatment-related effects in 15% of deaths, and a second primary tumor in 7% of cases. The important point for the primary care physician is that continued close medical monitoring of survivors of childhood cancer is very important.

Childhood thyroid cancer near Chernobyl[59] has been studied extensively after that accident. In the Gomel region of Belarus, north of Chernobyl, children are currently screened for thyroid cancer by physical examination, ultrasound imaging of the thyroid, and thyroid function tests. Prior to the accident, the thyroid cancer rate was 0.5 per million population. In the period 1991 to 1994, the corresponding rate was 96.4 per million. This represents almost a 200-fold increase.

Intracranial tumors after radium treatment for skin hemangioma during infancy have been studied through the Swedish Cancer Registry.[60] In this study, 11,805 infants treated with Ra 226 for hemangioma of the skin between 1930 and 1965 (402,958 person-years of risk) were followed through the Swedish Registry. In this relatively lose-dose study, 47 intracranial tumors developed in 46 people. The standard incidence ratio was 1.89 (95% CI 1.2 to 2.83), with a mean brain dose of 7 cGy.[49]

As can be seen, analysis of radiation risk is a rapidly changing and complicated issue, and current health physics references should be consulted for the latest information. In addition, Internet programs (e.g., National Institute for Occupational Safety and Health–Radio-Epidemiological Program, http://www.niosh-

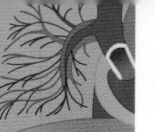

irep.com/irep_niosh/) are available to calculate the probability of causation of cancer development after either an acute or a chronic dose. Appendix C gives a hypothetical calculation for a nonradiation worker (secretary) who receives 0.5 Sv over the course of 6 months due to a lost source placed in her desk.

LABORATORY AND CLINICAL HISTORY

Upon admission to the emergency department after a radiation incident, it is always appropriate to obtain a CBC with differential, either as a baseline level or as a beginning step for lymphocyte kinetic analysis. Other laboratory tests should be considered as appropriate to the presenting medical situation.

The TE, measured from the irradiating event, decreases with increasing whole body dose. For TE of greater than 1 but less than 2 hours, the effective whole body dose is likely at least 3 Gy. If TE is less than 1 hour, the whole body dose likely exceeds 4 Gy. In a mass casualty incident, patients who experience emesis less than 4 hours postaccident should be triaged to professional medical care while those with emesis greater than 4 hours can be instructed to receive delayed medical attention, either with their private physician or with a peripheral center available to deal with minimally injured patients. Patients who experience radiation-induced emesis within 1 hour after a radiation incident will require extensive and prolonged medical intervention, and an ultimately fatal outcome will occur in many instances.

CASE STUDIES IN RADIATION MEDICINE

Clinical Example: Historical Radiation Burns (U.S. Surgery Cases, 1949)

The history of medicine is replete with examples of radiation burns,[61] either from incorrect implementation of a proper radiation procedure, or of improper use of radiation therapy to treat benign conditions. Viewed in a historical context, many early workers experimenting with the medical use of radiation therapy suffered burns to the hands that eventually required excision and grafting. Of interest are early radiologists performing various prolonged fluoroscopic examinations and dentists experiencing radiation burns to the fingers from holding films in the mouths of patients during exposure.

We will consider here only two cases, but many case reports are available describing the use of radiation therapy for treatment of acne, eczema, port-wine hemangiomas, plantar warts, epidermophytosis, and pruritus ani, among other benign conditions. Figure 104-1 illustrates atrophy and facial deformity following radium treatment of a hemangioma. Two operations eventually were required with excision and repair with a cross lip flap. Figure 104-2 presents a young female patient with multiple facial carcinomas throughout the nose and chin resulting from radium therapy for eczema. There was extreme involvement of the nose and chin with malignant loss of the nose. Repair (requiring four operations) was accomplished by complete excision and immediate free grafting with application of a prosthetic acrylic nose.

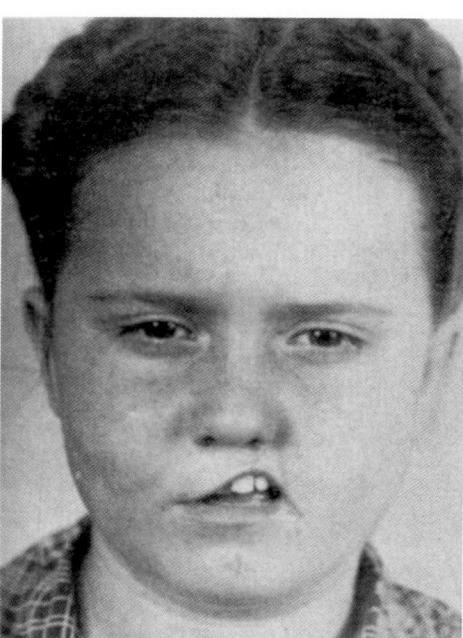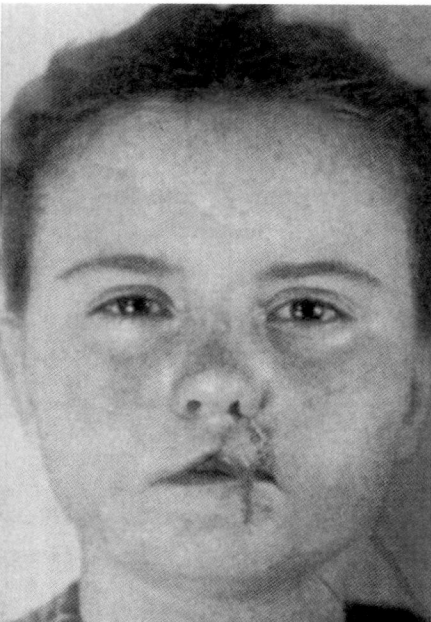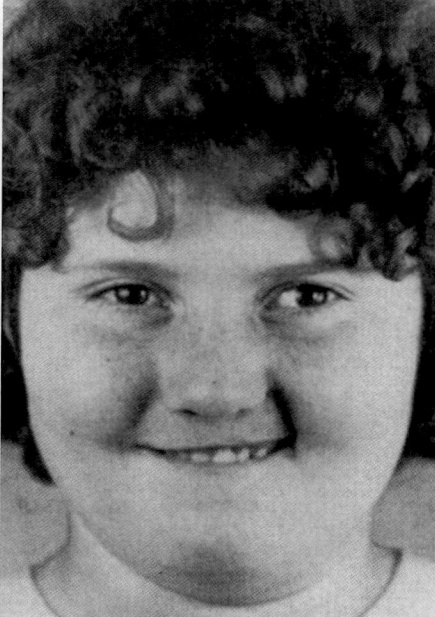

FIGURE 104-1 Atrophy and facial deformity following radium treatment of a hemangioma. Two operations eventually were required with excision and repair with a cross lip flap. (From Brown JB, McDowell F, Fryer MP: Surgical treatment of radiation burns. Surg Gynecol Obstet 1949;88:609–622. With permission of American College of Surgeons.)

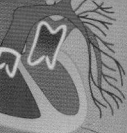

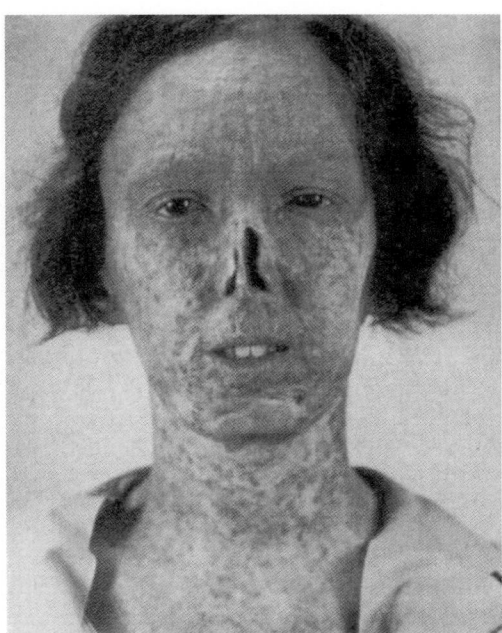 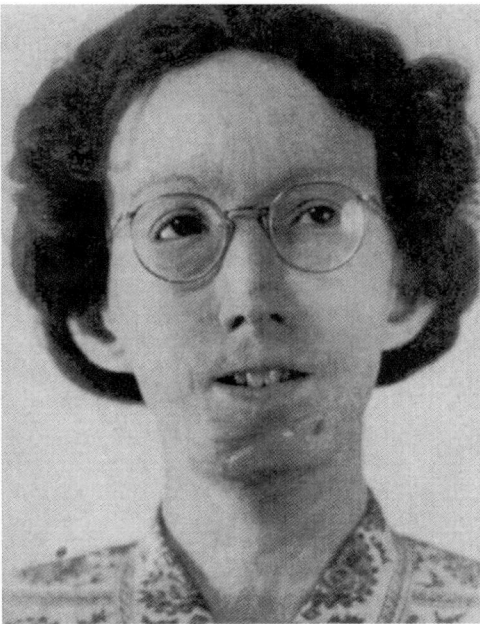

FIGURE 104-2 A patient with multiple facial carcinomas near the nose and chin resulting from radium therapy for eczema. There was extensive involvement of the nose and chin with malignant loss of the nose. Plastic repair (requiring four operations) was accomplished by complete excision and immediate free grafting with application of a prosthetic acrylic nose. (From Brown JB, McDowell F, Fryer MP: Surgical treatment of radiation burns. Surg Gynecol Obstet 1949;88:609–622. With permission of American College of Surgeons.)

Residential Radiation Accident Case Study (Estonia, 1994)

On October 21, 1994, an Estonian citizen, RIH, along with his two brothers, visit a radioactive waste facility to scavenge for scrap metal, overriding the electrical alarm system and cutting various padlocks.[62] RIH climbs into one of the vaults to obtain salvageable metal and passes a large Cs-137 source to his brothers. At this time, none of the brothers realize that this metallic object is highly radioactive. During the theft, RIH injures his leg slightly when an aluminum drum falls against it. Shortly after entry into the repository, RIH begins to feel ill and goes home. Other occupants of the house are the man's stepson (RT), the boy's mother, and the boy's great-grandmother. The cesium source is initially placed in the man's coat pocket that hangs in the hall. It eventually is placed in the kitchen drawer along with various tools.

RIH is hospitalized soon thereafter with severe injury to his leg. During the intake medical history, he claims that he received the injury while working in the nearby forest and he is therefore treated for crush injury. On November 2, 1994, RIH dies and medical authorities have no suspicion of radiation exposure as the etiology of the medical condition.

By November 9, 1994, it is clear that the stepson RT has come in contact with the source multiple times while living in the house and while working on his bicycle. Shortly thereafter, the 4-month-old pet dog dies. The dog had slept much of the time in the kitchen near the cesium source. RT is also eventually admitted to the hospital with severe hand burns, which physicians diagnose as radiation burns and the police are notified. A Russian medical delegation also arrives soon thereafter to provide medical and health physics consultation.

After an extensive radiation dose reconstruction, the deceased father, RIH, is thought to have received

approximately 1830 Gy local dose to his thigh and approximately 4 Gy whole body. Clinically, RIH experienced many of the effects of the hematopoietic subset of ARS along with severe, extensive local injury to his thigh (dose rate estimated to be 2000 to 3000 Gy/hr) (see Figure 104-3 for cell responses to irradiation). He died on day 12 postaccident from neutropenic sepsis and in acute renal failure. An autopsy showed acute radiation necrosis of the right thigh and hip, along with hemorrhage and intestinal thinning of the GI wall. The cause of death was ARS with both hematopoietic and GI components, along with severe local radiation necrosis.

The stepson, RT, is estimated to have received doses of 20 to 30 Gy to his left hand, 8 to 10 Gy to his right hand, and approximately 2.5 Gy whole body during various episodes of bicycle maintenance. Other family members received hand doses in the range 8 to 20 Gy and whole body doses in the range of 1 to 2.5 Gy. The cumulative dose was based on each individual's recollection of the degree of occupancy of various locations in the house. In addition, spatial computer analysis, chromosome aberration analysis, and other specialized assays were employed.

U.S. Fatal Criticality Accidents (Neutron-Gamma Exposures)

Two early criticality (weapons research) events occurred with a 6.2-kg plutonium sphere at Los Alamos National Laboratory.[63-66] The first incident occurred on August 21, 1945, when a worker was preparing a critical assembly by stacking tungsten carbide bricks around the plutonium core as a reflector. He moved the final block over the assembly but, noting that this block would make the assembly supercritical, he withdrew it. The brick fell onto the center of the assembly, resulting in a super-prompt critical state of approximately $6 \times E+15$ fissions. The worker sustained an average whole body dose of

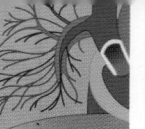

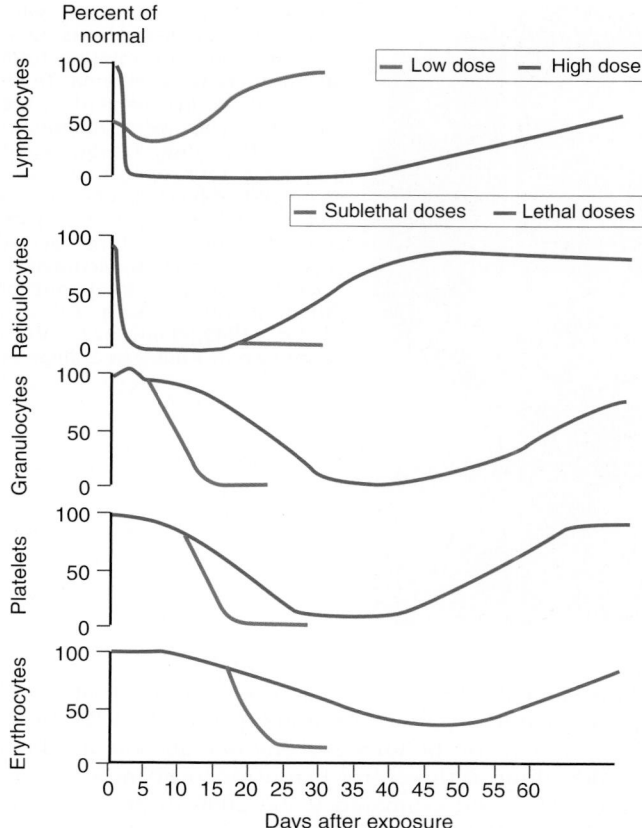

FIGURE 104-3 Hematopoietic response of various cell lines to an acute irradiation incident. The threshold is approximately 50 to 100 cGy.

approximately 5.1 Gy and a dose to the right hand of approximately 100 to 400 Gy.

Within 36 hours postaccident, blisters were noted on the volar aspect of the right third finger, and within 24 hours thereafter, extensive erythema and eventual blistering was noted on both palmar and volar surfaces of the hand. By the third week, the right hand had progressed to a dry gangrene. Desquamation of the epidermis involved almost all of the skin of the dorsum of the forearm and hand. In addition, epilation was almost complete at the time of death. The patient died of sepsis 28 days postaccident.

At autopsy, severe skin necrosis was observed as well overt dry gangrene. The cardiorespiratory system was significant for pericarditis, cardiac hypertrophy, pulmonary edema, and alveolar hemorrhage. The spleen was noted to have no germinal centers, and the mucosa of the large bowel was ulcerated, as was the buccal mucosa. The bone marrow was noted to be hypoplastic, and lymph nodes also showed significant lymphocyte depletion. A solitary ulcer was noted in the large colon, as was a right renal infarct. This case is an excellent example of the hematopoietic component of ARS with perhaps the beginning of the GI component.

The second criticality accident occurred in 1946 during an approach to criticality demonstration at which several observers were present. The operator used a screwdriver as a lever to lower a hemispherical beryllium shell reflector into place. While holding the top shell with his left thumb, the screwdriver slipped and caused a critical configuration. The fission yield in this accident was estimated at $3 \times E+15$ fissions. The operator received an estimated acute whole body dose of approximately 21 Gy, with a dose to the left hand of approximately 150 Gy and somewhat less to the right hand. Clinically, the patient complained of nausea in the hour prior to admission and vomited once in the first hour post-accident. On the fifth day post-accident there was a precipitous drop in his neutrophil count, and his condition began to decline rapidly. The patient rapidly lost weight, became mentally confused on day 7 post-event, became comatose, and died quietly on the ninth day in cardiovascular shock (GI and CNS syndrome). At the time of death, both hands showed extensive radiation damage.

At autopsy, the cardiorespiratory system was remarkable for cardiac hemorrhage and myocardial edema, and the terminal bronchi showed features of aspiration pneumonia. In addition, most of the GI tract showed sloughing, most pronounced in the jejunum and ileum. Widespread hyaline changes were also noted in the renal tubular epithelium.

The third major U.S. criticality accident occurred on December 30, 1958, during purification and concentration of plutonium. In the process, unexpected plutonium-rich solids were washed from two vessels into a single large vessel that contained layered, dilute aqueous and organic solutions. Accident analysis shows that the aqueous layer initially was slightly below delayed critical (approximately 203 mm thick, critical thickness 210 mm). When the stirrer was started, the central portion of the liquid system was thickened, changing system reactivity to super-prompt critical. The excursion yield was approximately $1.5 \times E+17$ fissions. Bubble generation was the negative feedback mechanism for terminating the neutron spike. The dose to the patient's upper extremity was estimated to be 120 Gy ± 50%.

The clinical course of this case has traditionally been divided into four separate phases of varying duration:

Phase 1 (20 to 30 minutes postevent): immediate physical collapse and mental incapacitation, progressing eventually into semiconsciousness

Phase 2 (90 minutes): signs and symptoms of cardiovascular shock accompanied by severe abdominal pain

Phase 3 (28 hours): subjective minimal clinical improvement

Phase 4 (2 hours): rapidly appearing irritability and mania, progressing to coma and death

The clinical course was remarkable for continuing, profound hypotension, tachycardia, and intense dermal and conjunctival hyperemia. The patient died 35 hours postexposure of the cardiovascular-CNS syndrome.

On autopsy, examination of the heart showed acute myocarditis, myocardial edema, cardiac hypertrophy, and a fibrinous pericarditis. Examination of the brain demonstrated cerebral edema, diffuse vasculitis, and

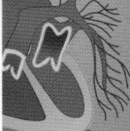

cerebral hemorrhage. The GI system showed necrosis of the anterior gastric wall parietal cells, acute upper jejunal distention, mitotic suppression throughout the entire GI tract, and acute jejunal and ileal enteritis.

The fourth fatal U.S. criticality accident occurred on July 24, 1964, at the United Nuclear Fuels Recovery Plant, Wood River Junction, Rhode Island. A chemical processing plant was designed to recover highly enriched uranium from scrap material left over from the production of fuel rods. The critical excursion occurred when nearly all of the uranium had been transferred, resulting in approximately 1.0 to $1.1 \times E+17$ fissions. The acute dose to the operator was estimated to be 100 Gy. Approximately 4 hours postaccident, the patient experienced transient difficulty in speaking, hypotension, and tachycardia. A portable chest x-ray 16 hours postadmission showed hilar congestion. On day 2, the patient became very disoriented, hypotensive, and anuric and died 49 hours postaccident in cardiovascular shock.

At autopsy, examination of the heart, lungs, and abdominal cavity revealed acute pulmonary edema, bilateral hydrothorax, hydropericardium, abdominal ascites, acute pericarditis, interstitial myocarditis, and inflammation of the ascending aorta. Examination of the GI tract showed severe subserosal edema of the stomach and of the transverse and descending colon.

Industrial Radiography Accident at the Yanango Hydroelectric Power Plant (1999)

Prior to hydrostatic testing of a pipe under repair at the Yanango hydroelectric power plant in the San Ramon District in Peru (300 km east of Lima, Peru), Ir 192 radiography was required to check welded repairs for defects. At 11:30 A.M. on February 20, 1999, an industrial radiographer and his assistant took their equipment to the area of a large, 2-m diameter pipe where repairs were underway. Their radiography equipment, a projection type camera designed to use a cable to drive a radiation source in and out through a guide tube, was reported to contain a 1.37 TBq (37 Ci) Ir 192 source. The welders had not yet completed their repairs, so the radiographer and his assistant left their locked camera (with the drive cable attached, but the guide tube not connected) in order to proceed with other tasks. They returned later that night to perform the radiography. On development of their x-ray films, the radiographer discovered that the film had not been exposed. He checked his radiography equipment around midnight and discovered that the iridium source was missing. A search was initiated, and at 1 A.M. on February 21 the radiographer recovered the source at the home of the welder.

The welder reported he had found the source in the pipe, had picked it up with his right hand, and put it into the right rear pocket of his loose fitting denim trousers. The welder then took a minibus and arrived home after a 30-minute ride. He experienced slight nausea earlier that evening and also noted some discomfort in his right thigh. On arrival home, he asked his wife to check a painful area on the back of his right thigh and she noted the area was reddened. A local physician was consulted and gave a diagnosis of "insect bite" and was told to use hot compresses on the inflamed area. Once aware of the accident, the company promptly notified the national authority for radiation safety and regulation, the Instituto Peruano de Energia Nuclear (IPEN).[67]

IPEN personnel then notified the head of the radiotherapy department of the Instituto de Enfermedades Neoplasicas (INEN) in Lima, where arrangements had previously been made for treatment of persons with radiation injury. Subsequently, IPEN personnel gathered information about the incident and arranged medical examinations for all potentially exposed persons, including the welder's three children (ages 10 and 7 years and 18 months), his wife, and his assistant. Arrangements were then made to facilitate transport of the welder and his family to INEN in Lima. The welder was admitted to the hospital on February 21, 1999, approximately 20 hours after the discovery of the accident. Extensive clinical and dosimetric details of this accident have been published elsewhere.[68,69]

Physical examination of the patient on admission revealed a 37-year-old, well-built Peruvian man weighing approximately 78 kg. A painful, erythematous area was noted on the right upper posterior thigh. Over the next few days, a very painful, bullous lesion surrounded by a large inflammatory halo developed, reaching 4 cm^2 in size by day 3. The right hip, buttock, and thigh became quite swollen over several days, and a computed tomography scan performed on February 26 showed generalized, marked edema involving all muscle groups in the right posterior thigh as well as in subcutaneous tissue. Swelling in the area diminished several days later, but extension, denudation, and necrosis of the lesion progressed rapidly.

By March 19, 1 month after the accident, the patient's deteriorating health was evident. He had lost 7 kg in weight and was in intense pain with clinical pain control increasingly difficult, and his lesion now involved an area of more than 10×12 cm. The lesion at this time had dark, firm necrotic edges, was partially covered with a fibrin crust, and appeared superficially infected. The wound later progressed to approximately 2 cm in depth, with necrosis of underlying fat and involvement down to the semitendinosus and biceps femoralis muscles. Nerve involvement was suspected and subsequently diagnosed using nerve conduction studies.

A team of experts, at the request of the IAEA, arrived on March 19 to consult with the Peruvian physicians regarding details of the accident, treatment protocols, lessons learned, and so forth. The team noted slightly depressed white blood cell counts indicating low-level whole body irradiation, estimated to be between 1 and 3 Gy. The team at this time discussed the potential need for a right hemipelvectomy. Also, in this time period, the source was calibrated and found to be somewhat less than the 1.37 TBq originally reported. Measurements indicated its activity was approximately 0.962 T.Bq (26 Ci). By the end of March, the thigh lesion had now extended to 20×15 cm, with a large area of central necrosis and a surrounding fibrotic rim. Electromy-

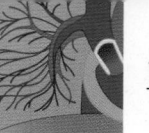

ography at this time confirmed signs of denervation of the sciatic nerve. Histologic studies of the necrotic lesions revealed microscopic hemorrhages, extensive areas of coagulation necrosis, edema, severe inflammation, and destruction of vascular structures. In addition, walls of small and moderate-sized arteries showed a distinct postradiation necrotizing vasculitis.

Subsequent surgical exploration and débridement of the area revealed that the lesion had extended to the femur and to the sciatic nerve. On August 16, the right hip was disarticulated and a left iliac colostomy was performed. The patient left the burn center on day 205 postaccident for transfer to a rehabilitation center. By late September, the radionecrosis and superficial infection was noted to extend to the perineum, including the anal sphincter and scrotum. In May 2000, the patient was transferred from Lima to an intensive care unit in a hospital near his home town. Because of severe psychological issues, close family contact proved to be of significant therapeutic value. At the last physical examination, the patient had some closure of the necrotic perineal area, with formation of granulation tissue and progressive fibrosis. The urethral fistula was still present and requires plastic reconstruction.

CONCLUSION

In evaluation of the magnitude of a radiation event (either an industrial accident or terrorist event), it is important for the health physicist, physician, and radiobiologist to work closely together and to evaluate many variables, particularly the initial patient medical history and physical examination and the timing of pro-dromal signs and symptoms (nausea, vomiting, diarrhea, transient incapacitation, hypotension), and other signs and symptoms suggestive of high-level exposure. The diagnosing physician charged with medical care of patients following a radiation accident is therefore likely to see at least two distinct patient presentations: (1) a normal-appearing patient with few signs or symptoms, or perhaps offering symptoms of unexplained nausea and vomiting, or of unexplained skin lesions, or (2) a very ill patient with stigmata of the acute radiation syndrome and/or local radiation injury. The astute diagnostician must be aware of these different presentations.

APPENDIX A. A BRIEF INTRODUCTION TO RADIATION PHYSICS AND TO RADIOLOGICAL UNITS

In order for the toxicologist or emergency medicine specialist to provide initial treatment and advice to the nuclear accident victim, it is necessary to consider only a few basic ideas from radiation physics. Radioactive materials are materials that emit ionizing radiation. They emit various types of energetic particles to reach a more stable quantum ground state. These radioisotopes are chemically and physically identical to their nonradioactive counterparts and behave metabolically in the human body only according to their chemical properties.

The fact that an isotope is radioactive does, however, determine the effective half-life in the body. As is well known in toxicology, the radioactive half-life is the time required for a radioactive substance to lose half of its radioactivity. Each radionuclide has a unique half-life. Half-lives range from extremely short fractions of a second to billions of years. A long half-life implies a low specific activity (activity per unit mass) and a short half-life implies a high specific activity. If TB is the biological half-life of the stable element as degraded via normal metabolic pathways and TR is the radioactive half-life, then the effective half-live T(eff) is the parallel combination:

$$1/T(eff) = 1/TB + 1/TR$$

From Equation 1, we can see, if the radioisotope is long-lived (TR >> TB), then the effective half-life is essentially the biologic or metabolic half-life TB. Conversely, if the isotope is short-lived (TB >> TR), the effective half-life is dominated by the radioactive half-life.

Ionizing radiation refers to radiation (alpha, beta, photons, and neutrons) whose energy is sufficient to strip electrons from atoms or molecules. Essentially all types of radiation from the atomic nucleus are ionizing. Nonionizing radiation includes visible light, microwaves, radio waves, ultrasound, and so forth and are not included for consideration here.

Alpha particles (energetic helium nuclei) generally do not pass through the keratinizing layer of skin and therefore are primarily of interest in situations involving inhalation or ingestion of radioactive material. Generally, alpha particles are emitted only from the very heavy nuclei. Beta particles (energetic electrons) have a greater range in air and in tissue. Beta particles therefore are of interest in estimation of skin dose and in situations involving internal deposition. Gamma rays are photons emitted from the nucleus that generally penetrate the skin, soft tissue, and bone. Gamma rays are involved in the vast majority of radiation accidents involving external irradiation. X-rays are relatively lower-energy photons arising from transitions between atomic energy levels and are occasionally involved in radiation accidents arising from improper use of industrial or medical equipment.

Generally, most of the lighter radioisotopes emit both beta and gamma rays while the very heavy elements typically emit alpha particles along with relatively low energy photons. However, given the large number of isotopes, it is difficult to generalize, and many isotopes have a large number of emissions.

Atomic nomenclature shows the abbreviation of the element and atomic number A (number of protons + neutrons) as shown:

$$^{A}(element) \text{ or } (element)\text{-}A$$

Examples are ^{60}Co or Co 60 and ^{137}Cs or Cs 137 (see Box 104-1). Radiation energies are typically measured in electron-volts (eV), kilo-electron volts (KeV) or million-electron volts (MeV). For example, the main gamma ray of interest in Cs 137 is 661 KeV or 0.661 MeV. Co 60 emits

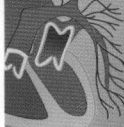

BOX104-1	RADIOISOTOPES OFTEN INVOLVED IN VARIOUS COMMERCIAL SECTORS

The University "Seven"	The Industrial "Four"
H 3	Ir 192
C 14	Co 60
P 32	Cs 137
Co 60	Sr 90
I 125/I 131	
Cf 252	**The Military "Three"**
	U 235
	Pu 239
	Am 241

two very penetrating gamma rays of energy, 1.17 MeV and 1.33 MeV.

Ir 192 (iridium) is widely used throughout the world in industrial radiography, and this radioisotope is probably the most significant isotope involved in localized radiation injury. In the United States, over a million high-level Ir 192 sources exist, and a few are unaccounted for at any point in time. It is an interesting phenomenon that specific isotopes tend to be involved in radiation accidents in certain industries. For example, only seven isotopes tend to appear in most university accidents as noted above, generally four isotopes in most accidents in the industrial sector, and essentially three in the military environment. The above list is somewhat of a generalization and there is certainly crossover between sectors, but this short list probably accounts for 90% of accidents in their respective sectors.

In radiation physics, "exposure" relates to the amount of ionization produced by x-rays or gamma rays in air under standard conditions. Exposure R is the quotient Q/m, where Q is the sum of the electrical charges on all the ions of one sign produced in air when electrons and positrons liberated by photons in a volume element of air whose mass is m, are completely stopped. The traditional unit of exposure is the roentgen (R) defined by 1 R $= 2.58 \times 10^4$ C/kg. The SI unit of exposure is the C/kg.

Dose refers to the absorption of radiation energy per unit mass of absorber (e.g., soft tissue, lung, bone, etc.). The conventional unit of radiation dose is the rad (1 rad = 100 ergs/g of absorbed energy). The SI unit of dose is the gray (Gy), equal to 100 rad, and also equal to 1 joule/kg. Dose may refer either to whole body dose, partial body dose, or to organ dose. Dose equivalent is dose multiplied by a factor to account for the varying effectiveness of various types of radiation. The traditional unit of dose equivalent is the rem, while the SI unit is the sievert (Sv), equal to 100 rem. Generally, it is not necessary to consider dose equivalent in the initial evaluation of the patient involved in a radiation accident. For soft tissue, it is quite acceptable medically to assume that 1 R is approximately numerically equal to 1 rad, which is approximately equal to 1 rem. This is not true for other organs such as bone or lung. However, such approximations are quite adequate in a mass casualty radiation event.

Activity is the number of disintegrations or nuclear transformations per unit of time occurring in radioactive material. The conventional unit of activity is the curie (Ci; 1 Ci $= 3.7 \times 10^{10}$ disintegrations per second. The SI unit of activity is the becquerel (Bq) equal to one disintegration per second. Therefore 1 Ci $= 3.7 \times 10^{10}$ Bq. The activity per unit mass (specific activity, SA) is another useful quantity defined as Ci/g or Bq/kg. SA is defined by Ci/g $= (1.3 \times 10^8)/$(half-life in days $\times$ atomic mass).

Example 1. Internal Dose from a Cardiac Scan

A patient is given 20 mCi technetium-99m as part of a cardiac stress test performed in a university teaching hospital. First, express this activity in SI units. We therefore have 20 × E-3 Ci × 3.7 E+10 Bq/Ci = 740 MBq. What is the patient dose from this medical procedure?

From the Radiation Internal Dose Information Center (RIDIC) and from CDC Dosimetry Services (http://www.internaldosimetry.com/linkedpages/doseestimates.html), we have a DCF (dose per unit input; 1.3 E-2 mSv/MBq for ^{99m}Tc). The effective dose equivalent is therefore 740 MBq × (1.3 E-2 mSv/MBq) = 9.6 mSv = 0.96 rad. Our patient has therefore received an effective dose of about 1 rad during the cardiac stress test. The key to effective and efficient internal dose calculations is proper determination of the DCF. Another very useful compilation of DCF data and health physics information in general is the Radiation Dose Assessment Resource, RADAR (http://www.ieo.it/radar/).

Assume that ^{99m}Tc has an effective half-life of 6 hours. After one half-life (6 hours), there is 10 mCi remaining, after two half-lives (12 hours), there is 5 mCi remaining, and so forth.

Example 2. Regulatory Limits

What are the current regulatory limits to the public and to occupational workers (Table 104-1)?

Example 3. Illustrations of Commonly Used Radioisotopes

Give some illustrations of commonly used radioisotopes and their uses (Table 104-2).

TABLE 104-1 Regulatory Limits

Members of the Public Occupational Limits	Limit 100 mrem
Total effective dose equivalent	5 rem
Lens of the eye	15 rem
Single organ dose equivalent	50 rem
Skin dose equivalent	50 rem
Extremity dose equivalent	50 rem

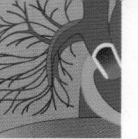

TABLE 104-2 Commonly Used Radioisotopes and Their Use

NUCLIDE	HALF-LIFE	SpA (Ci/g)	EMITS	USE
H-3	12.3 yr	9640	Beta	Luminous signs
Co-60	5.3 yr	1130	Beta, gamma	Medical therapy
I-131	8.05 days	1.23×10^5	Beta, gamma	Medical therapy
Cs-137	30 yr	87	Beta, gamma	Medical therapy
Ir-192	84 days	9170	Beta, gamma	Industrial radiography
Ra-226	1620 yr	0.99	Alpha, gamma	Medical therapy
U-235	7×10^8 yr	2.1×10^{-6}	Alpha, beta, gamma	Reactors/weapons
Pu-238	87 yr	17.2	Alpha	Thermoelectric generation
Pu-239	24,400 yr	0.061	Alpha	Reactors/Weapons
Pu-241	13.2 yr	112	Beta	Waste product
Am-241	458 yr	3.2	Alpha, gamma	Smoke detectors

SpA, specific activity.

Example 4. Typical Radiation Dose in Life Activities and in Common Medical Procedures

Provide some illustrative dose estimates for common life and medical activities (approximate doses) (Table 104-3).

Example 5. Common Industrial Applications of Radioactive Materials

Describe various common applications where radioactivity is used, and therefore where the possibility of an accident exists (not comprehensive).

IONIZING RADIATION: MEDICAL, INDUSTRIAL, AND CONSUMER PRODUCT APPLICATIONS

Radiography, analytical, and irradiation techniques (e.g., irradiation of food products)

Instrument calibration techniques using unsealed radioactive sources

Industrial gamma and x-ray industrial radiography (nondestructive testing)

Medical diagnostic radiography

Industrial beta and neutron radiography; x-ray fluorescence gauges such as instrumentation to detect residential lead levels

Photon switching gauges (level gauges)

Medical therapy: radiation beam therapy and brachytherapy for cancer treatment

High-level radiation sources for sterilization of food and medical products, food preservation, and crosslinking, curing, and grafting

Radioisotope tracer techniques in research and the therapeutic use of radiopharmaceuticals

Use of radioisotopes for self-luminous dials and devices

Radioisotopes for enhancement of electrical discharge, static elimination, and commercial and residential smoke (approximately 0.9 µCi of ^{241}Am in each residential smoke detector.

Use of radioisotopes for nuclear batteries, such as those used in spacecraft and in remote areas of the earth for instrumentation

APPENDIX B. ASSETS AVAILABLE TO ASSIST IN THE MEDICAL MANAGEMENT OF RADIATION ACCIDENTS

Two major U.S. organizations are available to assist the toxicologist in the initial medical management of the radiation victim. These are the Radiation Emergency Assistance Center/Training Site (REAC/TS; www.orau.gov/reacts/), a Department of Energy medical asset located in Oak Ridge, Tennessee, and the Armed Forces Radiobiology Research Institute (AFRRI) located in Bethesda, Maryland.

Since its formation in 1976, REAC/TS has provided medical support and advice in the medical management of many radiation accidents. A 24-hour emergency response team is available through the U.S. Department of Energy 24-hour number in Oak Ridge, Tennessee (865-576-1005). The Center's team of physicians, nurses, health physicists, radiobiologists, and emergency coordinators is prepared around the clock to provide medical and health physics assistance at the local, national, or international level.

TABLE 104-3 Dose Estimates for Common Life and Medical Activities

ACTIVITY	DOSE ESTIMATE
Natural background and manmade radiation (annual average dose equivalent, including radon)	360 mrem
Diagnostic chest x-ray	6–10 mrem
Flight from Los Angeles to Paris	5 mrem
Barium enema	800 mrem
Smoking 1.5 packs per day for 1 year	16,000 mrem = 16 rem
Heart catheterization	45,000 mrad = 45 rad = 0.45 Gy
Mild acute radiation syndrome	200 rad = 2 Gy
LD_{50} for acute whole body irradiation	450 rad = 4.5 Gy
Occupational limit for a radiation worker	5 rem = 0.05 Sv
Limit of a member of the public	0.1 rem = 0.001 Sv = 1 mSv

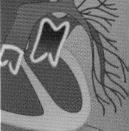

The AFRRI is a tri-service laboratory chartered in 1961 to conduct research in the field of radiobiology and related matters essential to the operational and medical support of the U.S. Department of Defense and the military services. The institute collaborates with other governmental facilities, academic institutions, and civilian laboratories in the United States and other countries. Its research findings have had broad military and civilian applications. The AFRRI Biodosimetry Team may be reached at 301-295-0484 and the Medical Radiobiology Advisory Team (MRAT) physician may be reached at 301-295-0530.

In particular, the Biodosimetry Assessment Tool (BAT) is a comprehensive software application developed by the AFRRI for recording diagnostic information in suspected radiologic exposures. The application, for use on the Microsoft Windows operating system, is available at www.afrri.usuhs.mil. A companion program, the First-responder Radiological Assessment Triage (FRAT) software application, is a complementary product under development for use on hand-held PDAs. It is being designed as templates into which first responders record clinical signs and symptoms, lymphocyte counts, physical dosimetry, radioactivity, and location-relevant dose estimates.

The FRAT and BAT applications compare collected data with known radiation dose response to provide triage and multiparameter dose assessment. The software allows the entry of exposure information based on multiple parameters (physical dosimetry, prodromal symptoms, hematology, radiation cytogenetics, etc.). Templates are available for recording exposure information based, for example, on physical dosimetry (e.g., personnel dosimeters) or contamination (e.g., radioactivity bioassay counting). An integrated, interactive human body map permits convenient documentation of the location of a personnel dosimeter, radiation-induced erythema, and radioactivity detected by an appropriate radiation detection device.

APPENDIX C. RADIATION RISK EXAMPLE

A 25-year-old secretary, while on vacation, is notified that an old radium source was found in the back of a desk drawer in her office. The source is traced to a hospital decommissioned some 20 years ago. A time and motion health physics analysis indicates that she may have received, at most, 50 rem (0.5 Sv) over the course of 6 months. The risk analysis was performed using the SURVRAD software,[70] which generally uses state of the art radiation epidemiology risk models. The SURVRAD computer output follows:

Run date	March 6, 2005
Title	25 year-old secretary with source in her desk
Sex	Female
Race	All races
Type vital statistic	Period-specific
Life table used	1990
Truncate last plateau	No
Risk coefficients	From Thompson et al (1994) and Preston et al (1994)
Type lifetime risks:	Incidence

Leukemia
  Minimal latency (yr) 2
  Plateau (yr) 40
Solid cancers
  Minimal latency (yr) 10
  Plateau (yr) 100
Leukemia plateau
  Beginning (age) 27
  End (age) 67
Solid cancer plateau
  Beginning (age) 35
  End (age) 100

DRREF	2.0
Age at first exposure	25
Age at last exposure	25
Total dose equivalent (SV)	0.5000000

		RADIATION-INDUCED CANCERS			BASELINE CANCERS	
MODEL	**SITE**	**PER 10⁵**	**90.0% CI**		**PER 10⁵**	**PC (90.0% CI)**
RR	Oral cavity	121	(52, 280)		826	0.13 (0.05, 0.30)
RR	Digestive	1653	(715, 3817)		11073	0.13 (0.06, 0.30)
RR	Esophagus	107	(46, 248)		245	0.30 (0.09, 1.00)
RR	Stomach	144	(62, 332)		937	0.13 (0.06, 0.31)
RR	Colon	683	(295, 1577)		5710	0.11 (0.05, 0.25)
RR	Rectum	151	(65, 349)		1095	0.12 (0.05, 0.28)
RR	Liver	0	(0, 0)		190	0.00 (0.00, 0.00)
RR	Pancreas	195	(84, 450)		1387	0.12 (0.05, 0.29)
RR	Respiratory	2369	(1025, 5470)		5779	0.29 (0.12, 0.69)
RR	Lung	2526	(1094, 5833)		5386	0.32 (0.13, 0.76)
RR	Nonmelanoma	42	(18, 98)		111	0.28 (0.07, 1.00)
RR	Breast	4122	(1785, 9518)		14569	0.22 (0.10, 0.51)
RR	Uterus	0	(0, 0)		53	0.00 (0.00, 0.00)
RR	Ovary	86	(37, 199)		1798	0.05 (0.02, 0.11)
RR	Bladder	865	(374, 1999)		1352	0.39 (0.15, 1.00)
RR	Kidney	514	(223, 1189)		828	0.38 (0.13, 1.00)
RR	CNS	23	(10, 54)		483	0.05 (0.02, 0.11)
RR	Thyroid	43	(18, 100)		492	0.08 (0.03, 0.19)
RR	Nonleukemia	7195	(3116, 16617)		47011	0.13 (0.06, 0.31)
AR	Leukemia	157	(67, 362)		203	0.44 (0.11, 1.00)
AR	ALL	40	(17, 93)		22	0.64 (0.00, 1.00)
AR	AML	48	(21, 112)		86	0.36 (0.07, 1.00)
AR	CML	52	(22, 120)		54	0.49 (0.04, 1.00)

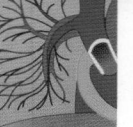

Probabilities of causation (PCs) represent the likelihood that either a cancer (for incidence) or cancer death (for mortality) is attributable to radiation exposure. PCs are based on the end of the plateau period for the last age at exposure. The probability of causation PC is defined as the (RR-1)/RR, where RR is the relative risk. As noted above, PC is only significant in this case for those cancers of hematopoietic origin (ALL, acute myeloid leukemia [AML], chronic myelogenous leukemia [CML]), although with large uncertainty. CLL is thought by most investigators not to be radiation-related.

REFERENCES

1. Gusev IA, Guskova AK, Mettler FA (eds): Medical Management of Radiation Accidents, 2nd ed. Boca Raton, FL, CRC Press, 2001.
2. Mettler FA, Upton AC: Medical Effects of Ionizing Radiation, 2nd ed. Philadelphia, WB Saunders, 1995.
3. Ricks RC, Berger ME, O'Hara FM Jr: The Medical Basis for Radiation-Accident Preparedness. The Clinical Care of Victims. Proceedings of the Fourth International REAC/TS Conference on the Medical Basis for Radiation-Accident Preparedness, Orlando, FL, March 2001. Pearl River, NY, Parthenon, 2002.
4. Fajardo LF, Berthrong M, Anderson RE: Radiation Pathology. New York, Oxford University Press, 2001.
5. Bevelacqua JJ: Basic Health Physics. Problems and Solutions. New York, Wiley Inter-Science, 1999.
6. Scleien B, Slaback LA, Birky BK (eds): Handbook of Health Physics and Radiological Health, 3rd ed. Baltimore, MD, Williams & Wilkins, 1998.
7. Shapiro J: Radiation Protection, 4th ed. Cambridge, MA, Harvard University Press, 2002.
8. Cember H: Introduction to Health Physics, 3rd ed. New York, McGraw-Hill, 1996.
9. Armed Forces Radiobiology Research Institute: Medical Management of Radiological Casualties. Military Medical Operations. Bethesda, MD, Armed Forces Radiobiology Research Institute, accessed November 21, 2006 at http://www.afrri.usuhs.mil.
10. Gottlober P, Krahn G, Peter RU: Cutaneous radiation syndrome: clinical features, diagnosis and therapy. Hautarzt 2000;51(8): 567–574.
11. Gottlober P, Steinert M, Weiss M, et al: The outcome of local radiation injuries: 14 years of follow-up after the Chernobyl accident. Radiat Res 2001;155(3):409–416.
12. International Atomic Energy Agency TECDOC-1009. Dosimetric and Medical Aspects of the Radiological Accident in Goiania in 1987. IAEA, Vienna, Austria, June 1998.
13. Tsujii H, Akashi M (eds): Proceedings of an International Symposium on the Criticality Accident in Tokaimura. Medical Effects of Radiation Emergency. Chiba, Japan, National Institute of Radiological Sciences, 2001.
14. Goans RE: Clinical care of the radiation accident patient: patient presentation, assessment, and initial diagnosis. In Ricks RC, Berger ME, O'Hara FM Jr (eds): The Medical Basis for Radiation-Accident Preparedness. The Clinical Care of Victims. Proceedings of the Fourth International REAC/TS Conference on the Medical Basis for Radiation-Accident Preparedness, Orlando, FL, March 2001. Pearl River, NY, Parthenon, 2002, pp 11–22.
15. Goans RE, Holloway EC, Berger ME, Ricks RC: Early dose assessment following severe radiation accidents. Health Phys 1996;72(4):513–518.
16. Goans RE, Holloway EC, Berger ME, et al: Early dose assessment in criticality accidents. Health Phys 2001;81(4):446–449.
17. Sine RC, Levine IH, Jackson WE, et al: Biodosimetry assessment tool: a post-exposure software application for management of radiation accidents. Milit Med 2001;166(12 Suppl):85–87.
18. Goans RE: Medical Lessons from US and International Radiation Accidents. Chapter 21. In Brodsky A, Johnson RH, Goans RE: Proceedings of the 2004 Health Physics Society Summer School. Madison, WI, Medical Physics Publishing, 2004, pp 373–393.
19. Brodsky A, Johnson RH, Goans RE, eds: Public Protection from Nuclear, Chemical, and Biological Terrorism. Health Physics Society 2004 Summer School. Medical Physics Publishing, 2004.
20. Koenig K, Goans RE, Hatchett RJ, et al: Medical treatment of radiological casualties: current concepts. Ann Emerg Med 2005; 45(6):643–652.
21. NCRP Report No. 65. Management of Persons Accidentally Contaminated with Radionuclides. Bethesda, MD, National Council on Radiation Protection and Measurements, 1980.
22. Mansfield WG: Nuclear Emergency and Radiological Decision Handbook. Livermore, CA, Lawrence Livermore National Laboratory, May 1997.
23. Goans RE: Update on the treatment of internal contamination. In Ricks RC, Berger ME, O'Hara FM Jr (eds): The Medical Basis for Radiation-Accident Preparedness. The Clinical Care of Victims. Proceedings of the Fourth International REAC/TS Conference on the Medical Basis for Radiation-Accident Preparedness, Orlando, FL, March 2001. Pearl River, NY, Parthenon, 2002.
24. ICRP Publication 67. Age-Dependent Doses to Members of the Public from Intake of Radionuclides: Parts 1,2. Atlanta, Elsevier, 1993.
25. Seelentag W: Two cases of tritium fatality. In Moghissi AA, Carter MW, eds. Tritium. Phoenix, AZ, Messenger Graphics, 1973.
26. Snyder WS, Cook MJ, Ford MR: Estimates of $(MPC)_w$ for occupational exposure to Sr^{90}, Sr^{89}, and Sr^{85}. Health Phys 1964; 10(3):171–182.
27. ICRP Publication 76. Strontium Biokinetic Model. New York, Pergamon, 1995.
28. Rubery E, Smales E: Iodine Prophylaxis Following Nuclear Accidents, Proceedings of a WHO/CEC Workshop. Geneva, World Health Organization, July 1988.
29. Durbin PW: Metabolic models for uranium. In: Biokinetics and Analysis of Uranium in Man F1-F62. US Uranium Registry Report USUR-05 HEHF 47. Springfield, VA, National Technical Information Service, 1984, pp 121–137.
30. Fong FH Jr: Acute effects of internal exposure to depleted uranium. In: Proceedings of the Depleted Uranium Health and Safety Information Exchange Meeting, November 30–December 1, 1993. U.S. Department of Energy. Oak Ridge, TN, Oak Ridge Associated Universities, 1993, pp 9–14.
31. Wrenn ME, Lipzstein J, Bertelli L: Pharmacokinetic models relevant to toxicity and metabolism for uranium in humans and animals. Radiat Protect Dosimetry 1989;26:243–248.
32. West CM: Depleted uranium processing and use. In Proceedings of the Depleted Uranium Health and Safety Information Exchange Meeting, November 30–December 1, 1993. U.S. Department of Energy. Oak Ridge, TN, Oak Ridge Associated Universities, 1993, pp 2–8.
33. Durbin PW, Kullgren B, Ebbe SN, et al: Chelating agents for uranium(VI): 2. Efficacy and toxicity of tetradentate catecholate and hydroxypyridinonate ligands in mice. Health Phys 2000;78(5): 511–521.
34. Durbin PW, Kullgren B, Xu J, Raymond KN: Multidentate hydroxypyridinonate ligands for Pu(IV) chelation in vivo: comparative efficacy and toxicity in mouse of ligands containing 1,2-HOPO or Me-3,2-HOPO. Int J Radiat Biol 2000;76(2):199–214.
35. Henge-Napoli MH, Stradling GN, Taylor DM, eds: Decorporation of radionuclides from the human body. Radiat Protect Dosimetry 2000;87(1 Special issue).
36. Henge-Napoli MH, Ansoborlo E, Chazel V, et al: Efficacy of ethane-1-hydroxl-1,2-bisphosphonate (EHBP) for the decorporation of uranium after intramuscular contamination in rats. Int J Radiat Biol 1999;75(11):1473–1477.
37. Destombes C, Laroche P, Cazoulat A, Gerasimo P: Reduction of renal uranium uptake by acetazolamide: the importance of urinary elimination of bicarbonate. Ann Pharm Fr 1999;57(5):397–400.
38. Durbin PW: Plutonium in man: a new look at old data. In Stover BJ, Lee WSS (eds): Radiobiology of Plutonium. Salt Lake City, UT, JW Press, 1972.
39. Langham WH, Bassett SH, Harris PS, Carter RE: Distribution and excretion of plutonium administered intravenously to man. Health Phys 1980;38(6):1031–1060.
40. Radon in Drinking Water: Risk Assessment by the National Academy of Sciences, 1998. Accessed November 21, 2006, at www.epa.gov.

41. National Research Council Staff: Health Risks of Radon and Other Internally Deposited Alpha-Emitters: BEIR IV. Washington, DC, National Research Council, January 1988.

42. National Research BEIR VI Committee: Health Effects of Exposure to Radon: BEIR VI. National Research Council, Washington, DC, June 1999.

43. Goans RE, Wald N: Radiation accidents with multi-organ failure—selected historical experience in the United States. Radiation-induced multi-organ involvement and failure: a challenge for pathogenetic, diagnostic and therapeutic approaches and research. Advanced Research Workshop. BJR 2005;27(Suppl):41–46.

44. Goans RE, Waselenko JK: Medical management of radiological casualties. Proceedings of the NCRP 2004. Health Phys 2005;89:505–512.

45. Waselenko JK, MacVittie TJ, Blakely WF, et al: Medical management of the acute radiation syndrome: recommendations of the Strategic National Stockpile Radiation Working Group. Ann Intern Med 2004;140:1037–1051.

46. Shigematsu I, Ito C, Kamade N, et al: In Hiroshima International Council for Medical Care of the Radiation-Exposed (ed): A-Bomb Radiation Effects Digest. Translated by Brian Harrison. Harwood Academic Publishers. Chuo University, Tokyo, Japan, 1995. Chur, Switzerland, Bunkodo Ltd/Harwood Academic Publishers.

47. IARC Study Group on Cancer Risk among Nuclear Industry Workers: Direct estimates of cancer mortality due to low doses of ionising radiation: an international study. Lancet 1994;344:1039–1043.

48. Ivanov VK, Gorski AI, Tsyb AF, et al: Solid cancer incidence among the Chernobyl emergency workers residing in Russia: estimation of radiation risks. Radiat Environ Biophys 2004 43:35–42. Epub 2004 Feb 5.

49. Sigurdson AJ, Doody MM, Rao RS, et al: Cancer incidence in the US radiologic technologists health study, 1983–1998. Cancer 2003;97(12):3080–3089.

50. Health Effects of Exposure to Low Levels of Ionizing Radiation: BEIR V. Washington, DC, National Research Council, December, 1990.

51. Casarett AP: Radiation Biology. Prentice-Hall. Prepared under the auspices of the Atomic Energy Commission, 1968.

52. Cunningham FG, MacDonald PC, Gant NF, et al: Williams Obstetrics, 19th ed. Norwalk, CT, Appleton & Lange, 1993.

53. Garcia-Algar O, Puig C, Vall O, et al: Effects of maternal smoking during pregnancy on newborn neurobehavior: neonatal nicotine withdrawal syndrome. Pediatrics 2004;113(3 Pt 1):623–624.

54. Kal HB, Struikmans H: Pregnancy and medical irradiation; summary and conclusions from the International Commission on Radiological Protection, Publication 84. Ned Tijdschr Geneeskd 2002;146(7):299–303.

55. Harding LK, Thomson WH: Radiation and pregnancy. Q J Nucl Med 2000;44(4):317–324.

56. Radiation and your patient: a guide for medical practitioners. Ann ICRP 2001;31(4):5–31.

57. Robertson CM, Hawkins MM, Kingston JE: Late deaths and survival after childhood cancer: implications for cure. BMJ 1994;309(6948):162–166.

58. Neglia JP, Meadows AT, Robison LL, et al: Second neoplasms after acute lymphoblastic leukemia in childhood. N Engl J Med 1991;325(19):1330–1336.

59. Niedziela M, Korman E, Breborowicz D, et al: A prospective study of thyroid nodular disease in children and adolescents in western Poland from 1996 to 2000 and the incidence of thyroid carcinoma relative to iodine deficiency and the Chernobyl disaster. Pediatr Blood Cancer 2004;42(1):84–92.

60. Karlsson P, Holmberg E, Lundberg LM, et al: Intracranial tumors after radium treatment for skin hemangioma during infancy—a cohort and case-control study. Radiat Res 1997;148(2):161–167.

61. Brown JB, McDowell F, Fryer MP: Surgical treatment of radiation burns. Surg Gynecol Obstet 1949;88:609–622.

62. International Atomic Energy Agency (IAEA): The Radiological Accident in Tammiku, Estonia. Vienna, Austria, IAEA, 1994.

63. McLaughlin TP, Monahas SP, Pruvost NL, et al: A Review of Criticality Accidents 2000 Revision. LA-13638. Los Alamos, NM, Los Alamos National Laboratory, May 2000.

64. Hempelmann LH, Lisko L, Hoffman JG: The acute radiation syndrome: a study nine cases and a review of the problem. Ann Intern Med 1952;36(2):279–510.

65. Shipman TL, Lushbaugh LL, Peterson DF, et al: Acute radiation death resulting from an accidental nuclear critical excursion. J Occup Med 1961;March(Special Suppl):145–192.

66. Karas JS, Stanbury JB: Fatal radiation syndrome from an accidental nuclear excursion. N Engl J Med 1965;272(15):755–776.

67. Goans RE: Project Sapphire. Health Phys 1995;68(3):296–298.

68. Zaharia M, Goans RE, Berger ME, et al: Industrial radiography accident at the Yanango hydroelectric power plant. In Ricks RC, Berger ME, O'Hara FM Jr, eds: The Medical Basis for Radiation-Accident Preparedness. The Clinical Care of Victims. Proceedings of the Fourth International REAC/TS Conference on the Medical Basis for Radiation-Accident Preparedness, Orlando, FL, March 2001. Pearl River, NY, Parthenon, 2002.

69. The Radiological Accident in Yanango. Vienna, Austria, International Atomic Energy Agency, 2000.

70. SURVRAD, V2.1. User's Guide. Tulsa, OK, Viking Software Corporation, 1995.

105 *Chemical Weapons*

A Nerve Agents

EDWARD W. CETARUK, MD

At a Glance...

- Nerve agents are highly toxic organophosphate compounds that inhibit the enzyme acetylcholinesterase as their mechanism of action.
- Their mechanism of action is identical to that of organophosphate pesticides, although they are more highly toxic.
- Historically, they have been manufactured and used by the military. However, more recently, they have been manufactured and used by nongovernmental terrorist groups as well.
- Nerve agents can be absorbed by multiple routes: inhalational, dermal, and ingestion.
- Patients present with a cholinergic syndrome that may include excessive salivation, lacrimation, incontinence of bowel and bladder, abdominal cramping, respiratory distress including wheezing and dyspnea, vomiting, miosis, muscular weakness, fasciculations, and paralysis, coma, and seizures.
- Antidotes for nerve agent poisoning include atropine (to block the effect of excess acetylcholine at muscarinic receptors), an oxime (to reactivate acetylcholinesterase), and a benzodiazepine (e.g., diazepam) for treatment of nerve agent–induced seizures.
- Early administration of antidotes and aggressive advanced life support measures can result in survival for even severely poisoned patients.
- Decontamination is extremely important in the treatment of nerve agent casualties.
- Nerve agents can be detected by a wide range of chemical detection equipment.
- Proper personal protection equipment is essential for those responding to a nerve agent release.

RELEVANT HISTORY

Nerve agents are extremely toxic organophosphate compounds that were initially developed by the German chemist Gerhard Schrader, who synthesized tabun in 1937 (GA) while researching new insecticides. Tabun was followed by the development of sarin (GB) in 1938, soman (GD) in 1944, and then VX (developed by Ghosh in England) in 1952. Although stockpiled in great quantities during both World War I and World War II, nerve agents were not employed in warfare until the Iran-Iraq War during the 1980s. Many additional nerve agents have been developed since the G agents, including derivatives of the G and V agents, newer binary agents, and others not described in the open scientific literature. However, resources are readily available that provide detailed information regarding the preparation of nerve agents, as well as other chemical weapons.[1]

The government of Iraq was responsible for the first large-scale use of nerve agents in warfare as well as against civilians. The Iraqi army use of tabun in a 1984 attack on Iranians near al-Basrah is the first documented use of a nerve agent in warfare. During the 1980s, Iraqi military forces also undertook an attempt to eradicate, relocate, and otherwise commit genocide against the Kurdish population of northern Iraq. The Kurds sought self rule for the ethnic region of Kurdistan, which encompasses geographic portions of northern Iraq, southeastern Turkey, and western Iran. During this war, they often allied themselves with the Iranians and were considered traitors and saboteurs by the Iraqi regime. *al-Anfal* was the name given to a series of eight military offensives, conducted in six geographic areas between February and September 1988. However, their first use of chemical weapons is reported to have occurred almost 1 year earlier, with the bombing of Sheikh Wasan and the Balisan Valley on April 16, 1987. Based on reports from survivors and medical care providers, both mustard and nerve agents were used. The operation was under the command of Saddam Hussein's cousin, Ali Hassan al-Majid, also known as "Chemical Ali," and officially began in February 1988 with conventional and chemical weapon attacks on 25 to 30 villages in the Jafati valley, including Sergalou, Bergalou, and Halabja, a town just a few miles from the Iranian border. The eighth and final Anfal operation was against the 300 to 400 Kurdish villages of Badinan, a 4000 square-mile area of the Zagros Mountains bounded to the east by the Greater Zab River and to the north by Turkey. The actual number of people killed during this genocide may never be known but has been estimated to be in the hundreds of thousands.

To date, the most significant uses of nerve agents against civilians by a terrorist group have been by the Aum Shinrikyo cult of Japan. This cult, led by Chizuo Matsumoto, who later took the name Shoko Asahara ("Bright Light") to attract followers, was well financed with assets estimated in the hundreds of millions of dollars. It subscribed to Asahara's "doomsday" philosophy that included causing catastrophic anarchy in Japan so that he could take power in the aftermath. The Aum chemical weapons program was able to produce significant quantities of VX and sarin, and lesser amounts of other nerve agents, mustard agent, phosgene, and cyanide. Nerve agents were used in a number of

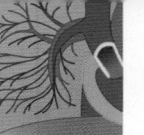

assassinations of cult "enemies,"[2,3] as well as two large-scale attacks.[4-7] The first was in Matsumoto, Japan on June 27, 1994, when the cult released about 20 kg of sarin vapor from a specially equipped van in an effort to assassinate three district court judges hearing a civil suit brought against the cult. This attack killed seven people and sent several hundred more to local hospitals, with 58 being admitted for treatment. The Aum subsequently perpetrated another, larger-scale nerve agent attack in Tokyo on March 20, 1995. In this attack, about 159 ounces of sarin was released from eight nylon-polyethylene bags (three additional bags were recovered intact) that were punctured by *Aum* cult members between 7:46 AM and 8:01 AM on five of Tokyo's main subway lines, causing 12 deaths. Ultimately, Tokyo hospitals and clinics saw 5510 patients: 17 critical, 37 severe, and 984 moderately ill. More than 70% of those presenting for treatment had no objective signs of nerve agent poisoning. Additional aspects of this event are addressed later under Management of Mass Casualties.

All nerve agents are organic ester derivatives of phosphoric acid, with varied chemical functional groups replacing the hydroxyl radical group of the basic phosphate structure. All are volatile liquids at room temperature, colorless, tasteless, and odorless. However, several of the G agents have been reported to have a fruity or sweet smell.[8] Their vapors are all heavier than air; hence, they tend to remain close to the ground, traveling downwind, downhill, and into geographic depressions. These physical characteristics make them ideal for controlled deployment and dissemination by either military forces or terrorists, although weather conditions can unpredictably disperse chemical agent releases, resulting in exposure to the terrorists who released the agent.[6]

The physiochemical properties affect their use as chemical weapons. Volatility and vapor pressure determine the likelihood that a chemical agent will be an inhalational threat. At room temperature, nerve agents exist as liquids and therefore must be aerosolized or evaporated to become inhalational threats. In traditional military munitions, nerve agents are disseminated by artillery shells or rockets using low-order bursting charges to disperse the agent on impact, or can be sprayed from aircraft. Binary and trinary nerve agents, whereby multiple separate chemical components combine during the flight of a projectile (e.g., partitioned 155-mm artillery shell, GB-2, M687) to deliver active agent on impact, have also been developed. In their attack on the Tokyo subway system, the Aum Shinrikyo simply allowed sarin that leaked from punctured nylon-polyethylene bags to evaporate. Because this dissemination method was relatively inefficient, affecting primarily nearby people, it caused only 12 fatalities out of potentially hundreds or thousands.

Another important characteristic of nerve agents is persistence: the ability to remain present and active in the environment after dissemination. Although nerve agents with high volatility pose significant inhalation hazard, they soon evaporate and dissipate, limiting their persistency. Agents with low volatility and vapor pressure,

such as the V agents, do not readily evaporate and therefore do not pose an inhalational threat, but they are persistent. Ambient temperature directly correlates with an agent's rate of evaporation and inversely correlates with its persistence. Generally speaking, sarin evaporates about as fast as water, cyclosarin about 20 times slower, and VX about 1500 times slower.[1] Heavily splashed tabun, soman, or cyclosarin (GF) will persist for 1 or 2 days and V agents for weeks to months.[1] As a result of their environmental persistence (creating a prolonged contact threat), the V agents have often been weaponized and deployed (e.g., land mines) to deny territory or the use of equipment to an enemy on the battlefield. Also, some of the G agents (e.g., soman) have been "thickened" to decrease their volatility and make them more persistent. Additional factors that affect an agent's persistence in the environment include hydrolysis (all agents undergo spontaneous hydrolysis) and density (higher-density liquids and aerosols remain in the environment longer).

PATHOPHYSIOLOGY OF INJURY

Nerve agents exert their primary toxicity at cholinergic synapses of the central and peripheral nervous systems and at neuromuscular junctions that use acetylcholine (ACh) as their neurotransmitter. It is released from presynaptic postganglionic parasympathetic nerve fibers (innervating exocrine glands and smooth muscle), somatic motor nerve endings (i.e., the neuromuscular junction), and both parasympathetic and sympathetic preganglionic nerve fibers, and at synapses within the central nervous system (CNS). Under normal physiologic conditions, ACh binds to specific receptors (AChRs) on the postsynaptic membrane of the cholinergic synapse. AChRs are divided into two major types: nicotinic (found at cholinergic synapses in the CNS, at parasympathetic and sympathetic autonomic ganglia, and at the neuromuscular junction) and muscarinic (found at cholinergic synapses in the CNS, at postganglionic parasympathetic nerve termini, and at the postganglionic sympathetic fibers that release acetylcholine rather than norepinephrine) of sweat glands. Binding of ACh to a nicotinic receptor results in opening of membrane sodium channels and depolarization of the postsynaptic neuron or skeletal muscle cell. Muscarinic AChRs modulate their effects through the G-protein secondary messenger system and are found on smooth muscle and exocrine glands and in the CNS.

The enzyme acetylcholinesterase (AChE, E.C. 3.1.1.7) is located on the postsynaptic membrane of all cholinergic synapses and the neuromuscular junction where it terminates or regulates cholinergic activity by hydrolyzing ACh within the synapse. AChE is a serine esterase that contains an active site composed of neighboring esteratic and anionic active sites that cooperate to catalyze the hydrolysis of acetylcholine. The choline quaternary nitrogen of ACh forms an electrostatic bond with a glutamate amino acid residue in the anionic site, essentially positioning the acetyl moiety of ACh in the esteratic active site. The carbonyl carbon of ACh binds to

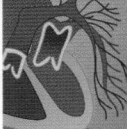

the hydroxyl group of serine-203 residue of the enzyme's esteratic site, forming an unstable tetrahedral enzyme-substrate intermediate (which is also stabilized by hydrogen bonding with other amino acid residue moieties within the esteratic site), which spontaneously collapses, releasing the choline moiety and leaving the acetyl group bound to the esteratic site. The acetyl–AChE bond is then quickly and spontaneously hydrolyzed by weakly nucleophilic H_2O, releasing acetic acid and regenerating AChE to its active form. Hydrolysis of ACh decreases its concentration in the synapse and at postsynaptic AChRs, terminating cholinergic stimulation of the postsynaptic cell.

Nerve agents are derivatives of phosphoric acid whose relative toxicity, as well as their toxicokinetics, is largely determined by the molecular substitutions on the organophosphate skeleton. Their primary mechanism of toxicity is the inhibition of AChE by acting as pseudosubstrates, occupying AChE's esteratic active site and inhibiting its hydrolysis of ACh in the synapse. The nucleophilic hydroxyl group of serine-203 (activated by the adjacent imidazole nitrogen of histidine) attacks this electrophilic phosphorous atom of the nerve agent (activated by the presence of an adjacent alkyl moiety, also called a "leaving group"), forming a stable covalent bond and phosphorylating the AChE serine residue. In contrast to the relatively unstable tetrahedral ACh–AChE intermediate, the nerve agent–AChE intermediate is extremely slow to spontaneously hydrolyze. This results in noncompetitive inhibition of AChE, leading to increased synaptic concentrations of ACh and continual stimulation of the postsynaptic acetylcholine receptors, producing a clinical cholinergic toxidrome.

Similar to the loss of acetylcholine's choline moiety, nerve agents bonded to AChE undergo dealkylation to release a functional group in a process referred to as "aging."[9,10] However, unlike acetylcholine, the loss of this leaving group results in an irreversible nerve agent–AChE bond that permanently inactivates AChE. Amino acid mutation studies have shown that the configuration and type of amino acids within the catalytic gorge of AChE containing the anionic and esteratic active sites is thought to have significant impact on AChE's interaction with each anticholinesterase compound, especially the alkyl functional (leaving) group.[10–13] This may explain why this aging can occur within minutes for some nerve agents (e.g., soman) or over many hours for others (e.g., VX).[9] In vitro studies have shown that soman irreversibly phosphonylates AChE within minutes (half-life of 2.2 ± 0.3 minutes).[10] Once aged, AChE cannot be reactivated by spontaneous hydrolysis or by an oxime antidote (see later).

Nerve agents inhibit a number of serine esterases, including acetylcholinesterase (red blood cell cholinesterase or true cholinesterase, E.C. 3.1.1.7), butyrocholinesterase (plasma cholinesterase or pseudocholinesterase, E.C. 3.1.1.8), carboxylesterase (EC 3.1.1.1), and neurotoxic esterase (NTE).[14] Nerve agents are also thought to exert toxic effects by inhibiting other noncholinesterase targets.[15,16] These include serine proteases, a large family of enzymes that also use a serine hydroxyl group in their

esteratic active site. These proteases are important in the formation, as well as breakdown, of many biologically active peptides (e.g., enkephalin, endorphin, substance P), that, in turn, modulate the activity of neurotransmitters. For example, substance P acts to modulate the nicotinic acetylcholine response. These noncholinesterase effects of anticholinesterase compounds may explain the clinical manifestations of nerve agent exposure not explained by acetylcholinesterase inhibition alone.[16] Van Meter and colleagues showed that sarin could induce seizures in rabbits, even though their AChE had already been profoundly inhibited by a prior dose of sarin (administered with atropine to prevent seizures).[17]

CLINICAL PRESENTATION

Nerve agents exert their toxic effects at peripheral muscarinic and nicotinic nerves by inhibiting acetylcholinesterase, resulting in excess acetylcholine at the postsynaptic acetylcholine receptors, and by multiple, and not completely understood, CNS effects (Table 105A-1). The clinical manifestations can be described in terms of organ systems, acetylcholine receptor distribution, routes of nerve agent exposure, and severity of exposure.

The characteristic clinical toxicity of nerve agents is a cholinergic toxidrome, which is a direct result of excess acetylcholine binding to nicotinic and muscarinic acetylcholine receptors in the CNS, the autonomic nervous system, and the neuromuscular junction. Muscarinic manifestations of nerve agent poisoning include excess exocrine secretions and smooth muscle contraction. These effects are often summarized in the mnemonics SLUDGE or DUMBELS, which include salivation, lacrimation, urination, gastrointestinal distress, defecation or diarrhea, emesis, bronchoconstriction and bronchorrhea, and miosis. The most clinically significant of these are the respiratory effects, bronchorrhea and bronchoconstriction, and should be the initial focus of clinical assessment, treatment, and antidote administration. Nicotinic manifestations of nerve agent poisoning are primarily the result of excess acetylcholine at the neuromuscular junction causing skeletal muscle fasciculations, weakness, and eventually, paralysis. Paralysis of the skeletal muscles involved in respiration, including the diaphragm, adds to muscarinic-mediated respiratory distress and can rapidly lead to respiratory failure or apnea. Excessive acetylcholine at autonomic ganglia may cause increased heart rate and hypertension. However, these manifestations are not typically clinically significant in the overall picture of nerve agent poisoning. Diaphoresis is also seen as a result of excessive cholinergic tone at the autonomic ganglia of sweat glands (Table 105A-2).

As mentioned previously, the respiratory system is the site of the most serious acute clinical manifestations of nerve agent poisoning. The direct effects of the nerve agent on the respiratory tract (bronchorrhea and bronchoconstriction), inhibition of the CNS medullary respiratory center, and paralysis of the diaphragm and

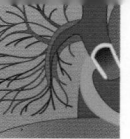

TABLE 105A-1 General Properties of Nerve Agents

COMMON NAME	CHEMICAL NAME	LCt50 (RESPIRATORY AT REST)	LD50 (DERMAL)	VAPOR PRESSURE (mmHg)	VOLATILITY (mg/m³)	VAPOR DENSITY*	PERSISTENCY†
Tabun (GA)	Ethyl N, N-dimethyl-phosphoroami-docyanidate (CAS 77-81-6)	400 mg/min/m³	1–1.5 mg/person	0.037 at 20° C	610 at 25° C	5.63	1–2 days
Sarin (GB)	Isopropyl methyl phosphono-fluoridate (CAS 107-44-8)	100 mg/min/m³	N/A	2.10 at 20° C	16,091 at 20° C	4.86	Hours
Cyclosarin (GF)	O-cyclohexyl phosphono-fluoridate (CAS 329-99-7)	N/A	N/A	0.044 at 20° C	438 at 20° C	6.2	1–2 days
Soman (GD)	Pinacolyl methyl phosphono-fluoridate (CAS 96-64-0)	0.16 mg/min/m³	N/A	0.40 at 25° C	3900 at 25° C	6.33	1–2 days
VX	O-ethyl-S-(2-isopropyl-aminoethyl) methyl phosphonothiolate (CAS 50782-69-9)	100 mg/min/m³	10 mg/person	0.0007 at 20° C	10.5 at 25° C	9.2	Days to weeks

*Air = 1.0.
†Persistency is highly dependent on weather conditions. As ambient temperature decreases, persistency increases. Persistency durations given are for "heavily splashed liquid" under "average weather conditions."
N/A, not available.
From U.S. Army Field Manual 3-9. Washington, DC, Department of the Army, 1990.

TABLE 105A-2 Signs and Symptoms Following Short-Term Nerve Agent Exposure

SITE OF ACTION	SIGNS AND SYMPTOMS
Ciliary body	Frontal headache, eye pain on focusing, blurred vision
Conjunctivae	Hyperemia
Nasal mucous membranes	Rhinorrhea, hyperemia, but this may also be present after systemic absorption
	Following systemic absorption of liquid and prolonged vapor expossure
Bronchial tree	Tightness in chest sometimes with prolonged wheezing, expiration suggestive of bronchoconstriction or increased secretion, dyspnea, slight pain in chest, increased bronchial secretion, cough, pulmonary edema, cyanosis
Gastrointestinal system	Anorexia, nausea, vomiting, abdominal cramps, epigastric and substernal tightness (cardiospasm) with "heartburn" and eructation, diarrhea, tenesmus, involuntary defecation
Sweat glands	Increased sweating
Salivary glands	Increased salivation
Lachrymal glands	Increased lachrymation
Heart	Bradycardia
Pupils	Slight miosis, sometimes unequal, later maximal miosis (pinpoint pupils); sometimes mydriasis is observed
Bladder	Frequent, involuntary microurination
Striated muscle	Easy fatigue, mild weakness, muscular twitching, fasciculation cramps, generalized weakness including muscles of respiration with dyspnea and cyanosis
Sympathetic ganglia	Pallor, occasional elevation of blood pressure
Central nervous system	Ataxia, generalized weakness, coma with absence of reflexes, Cheyne-Stokes respiration, convulsions, depression of respiratory and circulatory centers resulting in dyspnea and fall in blood pressure; emotional effects very often occur

From Grob D: Manifestations and treatment of nerve gas poisoning in man. US Armed Forces Med J 1956;7(6):781–789. Used with permission.

skeletal muscles associated with respiration[18,19] combine to cause respiratory failure. Neurologic symptoms include seizures, coma, muscular weakness and paralysis, and delayed neuropsychiatric effects, including depression and anxiety. Gastrointestinal symptoms include vomiting, abdominal cramping, and diarrhea. Respiratory failure is the ultimate cause of death after nerve agent poisoning.

The severity (i.e., acuity and dose) and route of exposure are also significant factors in determining the clinical presentation of nerve agent poisoning. Nerve agents are well absorbed by all routes (e.g., inhalation,

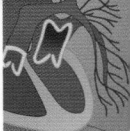

ingestion, and dermal route). Nerve agents absorbed through the inhalation route cause symptoms within seconds to minutes of exposure, whereas absorption by the dermal route may result in a delay in onset of symptoms because of the time required for the agent to be systemically absorbed. Victims of a vapor or aerosol nerve agent exposure may initially complain of eye pain exacerbated by accommodation, loss of dark adaptation, dim or blurred vision, conjunctival irritation, lacrimation, and miosis. These effects are thought to result both from direct exposure of the eye to the nerve agent vapor and CNS effects.[20-22] Upper respiratory tract symptoms (e.g., rhinorrhea and nasal congestion) are followed by progressive respiratory complaints, including chest tightness, dyspnea, wheezing, shortness of breath, cough, and increased bronchial secretions. If the exposure is significant or prolonged, other signs of respiratory toxicity rapidly develop, including severe bronchoconstriction, wheezing, bronchorrhea, respiratory distress, and apnea. Inhalational exposure to nerve agents results in the most rapid onset of symptoms because of rapid absorption of nerve agent through the large surface area of the pulmonary bed. Studies have shown that a high percentage of inhaled nerve agent is retained in the lungs, and the systemically absorbed dose is a factor of minute ventilation and the nerve agent vapor concentration.[23] Also, if the concentration of the inhaled nerve agent vapor is high, patients may not develop symptoms in a typical "respiratory route pattern," with dyspnea, wheezing, and bronchorrhea, but may rapidly

lose consciousness, become apneic, and have seizures due to the rapid absorption of the agent into the CNS (Table 105A-3).

Dermally absorbed nerve agent will initially cause localized symptoms at the site of exposure (e.g., fasciculations, diaphoresis). The rate of dermal absorption of nerve agent is dependent on the physical characteristics of the agent, environmental temperature, type, and condition of the skin exposed.[24,25] Absorption increases on damaged skin and varies with anatomic location.[26] As agent is systemically absorbed, victims develop other cholinergic symptoms, such as bronchorrhea and bronchoconstriction, gastrointestinal symptoms, muscle weakness, and seizures. Development of miosis is delayed[3] and is often absent following dermal absorption. It is important to note that dermal exposure to nerve agents may result in latent or progressive intoxication, even after appropriate skin decontamination, owing to deposition of the nerve agents in the skin and delayed systemic absorption.[24,25] Therefore, victims of dermal nerve agent exposure must be observed for a minimum of 18 hours after decontamination for the delayed development of toxicity.

Sidell reported a case in which a 33-year-old man was splashed in the face and mouth with about 1 mL of a 25% (v/v) soman solution.[27] He immediately rinsed his face and mouth with water and was asymptomatic until collapsing about 10 minutes after the exposure. He was immediately treated with atropine (4 mg intravenously, 8 mg intramuscularly) and 2-PAM (2 g intravenously over

TABLE 105A-3   Signs and Symptoms in Patients with Moderate to Severe Sarin Exposure

		PATIENTS	
	SIGN OR SYMPTOM	**NO. OF PATIENTS**	**PERCENTAGE (*N* = 111)**
Eye	Miosis	110	99.0
	Eye pain	50	45.0
	Blurred vision	44	39.6
	Dim vision	42	37.8
	Conjunctival injection	30	27.0
	Tearing	10	9.0
Chest	Dyspnea	70	63.1
	Cough	38	34.2
	Chest oppression	29	26.1
	Wheezing	7	6.3
	Tachypnea	28	31.8*
Gastrointestinal tract	Nausea	67	60.4
	Vomiting	41	36.9
	Diarrhea	6	5.4
Neurologic	Headache	83	74.8
	Weakness	41	36.9
	Fasciculations	26	23.4
	Numbness of extremities	21	18.9
	Decrease of consciousness level	19	17.1
	Vertigo and dizziness	9	8.1
	Convulsion	3	2.7
Ear, nose, and throat	Running nose	28	25.2
	sneezing	5	9.0
Psychological	Agitation	37	33.3

*N = 88.
From Okumura T, Takasu N, Ishimatsu S, et al: Report on 640 victims of the Tokyo subway sarin attack. Ann Emerg Med 1996;28(2):129–135. Used with permission.

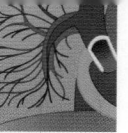

30 minutes). Endotracheal intubation was unsuccessful due to trismus. Signs and symptoms included miosis, coma, markedly injected conjunctiva, marked oral and nasal secretions, prominent muscular fasciculations, tachycardia, cyanosis, bronchoconstriction, and decreased respiratory rate and amplitude. He began to awaken after 30 minutes but continued to have fasciculations, tremor, nausea, vomiting, abdominal pain, and restlessness over the next 36 hours. Red blood cell cholinesterase activity was undetectable until 10 days after the exposure.

Sidell also reported a case of a 52-year-old man with an inhalational exposure to sarin.[27] Within minutes of noticing increased nasal and oral secretions and difficult breathing while wearing a protective gas mask (later determined to have been damaged), he developed seizures, respiratory distress, miosis, muscular fasciculations, cyanosis, wheezing, and copious secretions. His respirations were less labored, and cyanosis decreased within minutes of being treated with atropine (intravenously and intramuscularly), 2-PAM intravenously, and oxygen. He received a total of 14 mg of atropine, and 6 g of 2-PAM was administered over 1 hour. An electrocardiogram taken 1 hour after admission showed global ST-segment depression. Additional electrocardiograms obtained 18 and 42 hours after admission showed ST-segment elevation in leads I, aVL and V_{1-3} and ST-segment elevation in leads I, aVL, and V_{2-6} as well as T-wave inversion in leads I, II, aVL, and V_{2-6}. No cardiac enzymes were obtained, and the patient's electrocardiogram normalized within 4 months.[27]

PRENATAL AND PEDIATRIC ISSUES

Because of the relatively indiscriminant nature of terrorist attacks on civilians, children will likely be among the victims. A report of the sarin attacks in Matsumoto, Japan in 1994 lists the victims' ages as 3 to 86 years.[28] Although information regarding pediatric nerve agent poisoning is minimal, the release of a nerve agent could disproportionately affect children by several mechanisms. If the agent were aerosolized, the higher minute ventilation of children could result in a larger relative inhalational dose compared with adults. Further, the breathing zone for the typical adult is 4 to 6 feet above the floor, compared with a child's, which is much closer to the ground depending on the child's height. Because nerve agent vapor (e.g., sarin) is likely to be at its highest concentration closer to the ground, children potentially face a greater inhalational exposure compared with adults. Also, preambulatory infants, toddlers, or young children will not be able to remove themselves from the scene of a chemical agent release. Even if they were able to walk, they may not know in which direction to escape. These factors may leave proportionately more children poisoned at a scene than adults.

Pediatric victims of nerve agent poisoning may not present with the same pattern of clinical signs and symptoms typically seen in adults. Reports of pediatric organophosphate pesticide poisoning have noted that children are less likely to manifest muscarinic-mediated glandular hypersecretion and may present with more marked signs of central toxicity such as coma.[29] As is seen in other illnesses, pediatric patients often precipitously decompensate as their condition worsens, necessitating more careful assessment and closer monitoring of pediatric nerve agent victims compared with adults.

The more permeable skin of infants and children would also increase absorption of nerve agents because of dermal exposure. Also, because their larger surface-to–body mass ratio, children may absorb a larger relative dose of nerve agent than adults for a given exposure. Their relatively larger body surface area also increases the rate at which they will lose body heat when they undergo water decontamination. Skin decontamination with cold water, or in cold weather conditions, may result in hypothermia in children unless the decontamination water can be warmed or postdecontamination shower warming equipment is used (e.g., heating lamps, warm indoor environment). Because children have smaller bodies, they require smaller equipment (e.g., endotracheal tubes, needles and tubing, oxygen masks and ventilators). Additionally, the personal protective equipment (PPE) worn by first responders, which is essential for the safe response to a chemical terrorist event (e.g., level A), makes moving, working, and delivering care to victims much more difficult. These challenges are compounded when caring for small children, who present unique challenges of their own (e.g., obtaining intravenous access). Finally, the psychological impact that a terrorist attack will have on a child cannot be underestimated. The child will likely witness and experience events that are well beyond the child's scope of understanding and may be forced to do so without the comfort of a parent (who may indeed be a victim). Therefore, as much as is possible, provisions should be made to move children to places of safety where they can be appropriately medically observed, but spared ongoing exposure to the traumatic exposure of a terrorist incident and its aftermath. Ideally and if possible, they should also be reunited with their parents, or other family members, as soon as possible after all medical concerns have been properly attended to.

Adjustment of antidote dosing in children is also essential. In 2003, the U.S. Food and Drug Administration (FDA) approved a pediatric-dose atropine autoinjector. Although not yet widely available, it raises concerns regarding the use of adult-dose autoinjectors in children.[30] However, published experience with children receiving supratherapeutic doses of nerve agent antidote has not reported cases of significant poisoning.[30-32] Ideally antidotes should be administered in appropriate pediatric doses according to weight and severity of poisoning. The doses approved for use in children and adolescents with symptoms of nerve agent poisoning include 0.5 mg for children weighing between 15 and 40 lb, 1 mg for children weighing between 40 and 90 lb, and 2 mg doses for adults and children weighing more than 90 lb. These doses should be repeated and titrated according to clinical response (i.e., improvement and stabilization of respiratory function or control of seizures or other serious neurologic toxicity). A study of

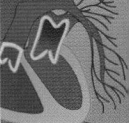

accidental atropine administration using atropine autoinjectors in 268 children found that many received higher than therapeutic doses, and in 20 children, the atropine was administered by an adult. However, only 8% experienced serious signs of atropinization, and no seizures of life-threatening cardiac arrhythmias were reported.[31] The administration of an oxime antidote is indicated for pediatric nerve agent poisoning and should be done using established pediatric doses: 25 to 50 mg/kg intravenously or intramuscularly. Benzodiazepines are also indicated for severe nerve agent poisoning and should be administered in the appropriate pediatric doses according to the benzodiazepine used. Pediatric dosing for nerve agent antidotes is summarized in Table 105A-4.

The initial assessment of any suspected nerve agent victim should include airway, breathing, and circulation. The initial assessment and triage of pediatric victims of nerve agent poisoning is also different from the approach used for adults. The clinical presentation of a child poisoned by nerve agent may differ from that of an adult. An effective response to a mass casualty incident (MCI) includes rapid assessment, triage, and treatment of victims. However, the typical parameters used for assessing adult victims of a nerve agent attack may not be appropriate for assessing the pediatric victims of the same attack.

Although there is no replacement for sharp clinical acumen is assessing and treating any patient, adult or pediatric, the Pediatric Assessment Triangle (PAT) is a tool developed for the assessment of pediatric patients that uses only visual and auditory clues to develop a first impression of the severity of the child's condition and to identify physiologic instability. It offers a quick (30–60 seconds) standardized approach to triage, resuscitation, treatment, and transport. The PAT includes assessment of appearance, work of breathing, and circulation to the skin. Appearance is assessed by generally observing the child (e.g., alertness, age-appropriate speech and behavior). Work of breathing is assessed by listening for abnormal breath sounds (e.g., wheezing) and looking for signs of increased work of breathing (e.g., grunting, retractions). Skin circulation is assessed by looking for signs of poor skin perfusion (e.g., pallor, mottling, cyanosis). The combination of all three components of the PAT should determine a child's degree of nerve agent poisoning and need for treatment.

In addition, the JumpSTART system is an adaptation of the START (Simple Triage and Rapid Treatment) algorithm developed as a more appropriate system for assessing children.[33] It should be considered another possible tool for the triage of children in a nerve agent mass casualty incident and is delineated in Figure 105A-1.

Similar to children, elderly victims with impaired mobility may find it difficult to escape from the scene of a nerve agent release. Therefore, it is theoretically possible that they may have prolonged exposure at the incident scene. Also, elderly individuals with preexisting medical conditions, especially cardiac and pulmonary disease, may have lower tolerance of the clinical manifestations of nerve agent poisoning (e.g., respiratory distress, hypoxia) or to the adverse effects of antidotes (e.g., atropine). However, the overall approach to triage and treatment of elderly victims is the same as for adults.

There are very few data regarding nerve agent poisoning in pregnancy. However, there were five pregnant women among the victims of the Tokyo sarin attack.[4,5] All had signs and symptoms of mild exposure and were admitted for observation, but none required antidotal treatment. Although one victim reportedly underwent an elective abortion as a result of the exposure (F. R. Sidell, personal communication), follow-up questionnaires sent to victims 1 month and 1 year after the incident reported no fetal malformations.[28]

TABLE 105A-4 Pediatric Nerve Antidote Indications and Doses

SYMPTOMS	TRIAGE LEVEL: DISPOSITION	ATROPINE*	PRALIDOXIME	BENZODIAZEPINES (E.G., DIAZEPAM, MIDAZOLAM)
Asymptomatic	Delayed: observe	None	None	None
Miosis, mind rhinorrhea	Delayed: admit or observe	None	None	None
Miosis and any other symptom	Immediate-moderate: admit	0.05 mg/kg IV or IM Repeat as needed q5–10 min until respiratory status improves	25–50 mg/kg IV or IM (may repeat q1h) Adverse effects: Muscle rigidity Hypertension Laryngospasm Tachycardia	For any neurologic effect 30 days to 5 years: 0.05 to 0.3 mg/kg IV (maximum of 5 mg/dose) May repeat q15–30 min 5 years and older: 0.05 to 0.3 mg/kg IV (maximum of 10 mg/dose) May repeat q15–30 min
Apnea, convulsions, cardiopulmonary arrest	Immediate-severe: admit critical care status	0.05–0.1 mg/kg IV, IM, per endotracheal tube No maximum Repeat q5–10 min as above	25–50 mg/kg IV or IM as above	See above

*Correct hypoxia before IV use due to increased risk for ventricular arrhythmias.
From Walter Reed Army Medical Center.

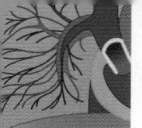

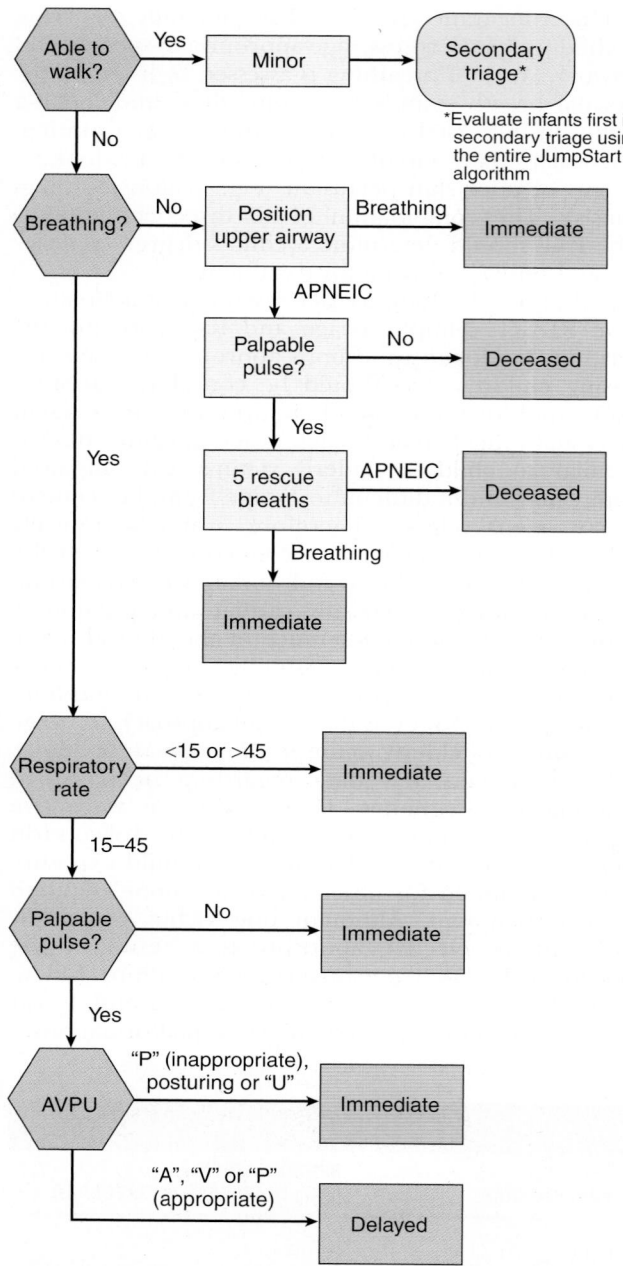

FIGURE 105A-1 JumpStart algorithm. AVPU: alert, verbal, painful, unresponsive (referring to neurologic function). (From Romig LE: Pediatric triage: a system to JumpSTART your triage of young patients at MCIs. JEMS 2002;27(7):52–58, 60–63. Used with permission.)

Therefore, in the absence of any additional data regarding nerve agent poisoning and its treatment during pregnancy, all therapeutic interventions recommended for adults should be used in pregnant patients as well.

ASSESSMENT

The diagnosis of nerve agent poisoning may be made on the basis of a single patient's presentation (i.e., a cholinergic toxidrome), and on a situational basis, in which multiple patients present with similar or identical symptoms that, collectively, suggest a diagnosis of nerve agent poisoning.[34] Regardless of how the diagnosis is determined, because of the extreme toxicity of nerve agents, victims must be evaluated as quickly as possible to determine their need for airway management (i.e., intubation) and the administration of antidotal therapy (e.g., atropine and oxime). Therefore, the clinical assessment of a nerve agent victim is based on the severity of their cholinergic toxidrome. Although useful retrospectively, the measurement of cholinesterase activity is not practical in the acute assessment of a nerve agent victim because of the delay in obtaining results. Further, in the case of an MCI, the initial assessment of victims must be accomplished in a rapid and efficient manner so as to triage victims for treatment.

Victims of a vapor nerve agent exposure will likely present with ocular and upper respiratory symptoms as described previously. Miosis is the earliest sign of a vapor nerve agent exposure but may be absent or delayed in a dermal exposure. Patients with only miosis and upper respiratory tract symptoms can be observed without treatment. Patients with lower respiratory tract manifestations (e.g., wheezing, dyspnea), neurologic symptoms (e.g., seizures, weakness) or multiple-organ system involvement should receive antidotal therapy with atropine and an oxime (see Treatment section). The assessment of victims of dermal nerve agent exposure should also be based on the severity of their clinical cholinergic toxidrome. However, it is important to note that initial symptoms can be localized to the site of nerve agent exposure and that severe or fatal toxicity can develop up to 18 hours after exposure. All patients should be reassessed frequently for worsening, or resolution, of symptoms, the effectiveness of antidote administration, or the need for additional antidote.

TREATMENT

The most immediate concern in the treatment of acute nerve agent poisoning is to establish an airway and provide adequate ventilation and oxygenation, using advance life support techniques including intubation and ventilation with supplemental oxygen. Mouth-to-mouth resuscitation is not recommended because of the high risk for rescuer contamination and poisoning. Note that oropharyngeal intubation may be difficult owing to trismus from muscular spasm and fasciculations or seizures.[24,27] Succinylcholine should be used with extreme caution and at lower doses because its pharmacologic half-life and duration of paralysis may be markedly prolonged as a result of nerve agent inhibition of plasma cholinesterase.[35] During the 1991 Persian Gulf War, military patients who had received pyridostigmine (a carbamate acetylcholinesterase inhibitor) as a nerve agent pretreatment and then underwent intubation using succinylcholine did not exhibit prolonged paralysis. However, they did have copious upper airway secretions requiring large amounts of atropine.[36] These

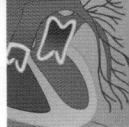

initial advanced life support measures should be accompanied by the earliest possible administration of nerve agent antidotes, including atropine, an oxime, and a benzodiazepine for the treatment of seizures. Initial ventilation may demonstrate marked airway resistance due to severe bronchoconstriction and bronchorrhea. Therefore, atropine should be administered as soon as possible by whatever route is available (e.g., intramuscular, intravenous, endotracheal) to reverse the respiratory effects of the nerve agent.

Decontamination is a critical step in the care of nerve agent victims. Continued absorption of agent will significantly undermine the effectiveness of advanced life support measures and antidotes administered to victims of nerve agent poisoning. Therefore, treatment plans and protocols should provide for decontamination taking place as early as possible. The key to successful mass casualty decontamination is to use the fastest approach that will cause the least harm and do the most good for the most people. The choice of decontamination methods depends on the route and intensity of exposure and available resources. Briefly, victims with dermal exposure require thorough decontamination, including undressing and full-body water decontamination. Large-volume, low-pressure water is the preferred method of decontamination. Soap is also recommended but has not been found to offer significant benefit over timely and adequate water decontamination. Victims with *only* vapor exposure (i.e., no possible contact with liquid agent) to nerve agent can be adequately decontaminated by removing them from the exposure and undressing them. If the exposure occurred indoors, moving the patient into outdoor fresh air and undressing them should be sufficient. If nerve agent is released outdoors in sufficient quantity to create toxic ambient concentrations, upwind evacuation from the plume of agent is necessary, as is respiratory protection for rescuers and victims if possible. See the Management of Mass Casualties section for a more complete discussion of decontamination.

Decontamination should begin with removal of the victim's clothing. It is estimated that removal of all clothing will provide about 80% of all possible decontamination after vapor exposure to a nerve agent. In addition, nerve agents from aerosols or vapors can adsorb into victims' clothing and then off-gas well after the victim has been removed from the site of exposure. Victims of the 1995 Tokyo subway sarin attack were transported from the scene of the attack without any form of decontamination. Prehospital first responders quickly became symptomatic until ambulances were ordered to keep all windows open to maximize ventilation during transport. Hospital-based care providers also became symptomatic after exposure to off-gassing victims who were brought into the hospital without decontamination.[4,5]

Atropine is a direct-acting competitive muscarinic receptor antagonist. It binds to muscarinic AChRs, preventing ACh from binding, thereby decreasing cholinergic tone at the postsynaptic cell or organ, including smooth muscle, exocrine glands, and muscarinic synapses within the CNS. Other potent antimuscarinic compounds have also been investigated as potentially effective organophosphate antidotes.[27,37,38] Atropine reverses muscarinic-mediated smooth muscle contraction and exocrine hypersecretion. This clinical effect is most important in the lungs, where excessive bronchorrhea and bronchoconstriction lead to hypoxemia, decreased ventilation, respiratory failure, and death. However, note that the respiratory failure is also the result of CNS nerve agent toxicity at the medullary respiratory center. Atropine does not bind to nicotinic receptors and therefore does not have any therapeutic effect at the neuromuscular junction or ganglia. Because the AChRs found at the neuromuscular junction are nicotinic, atropine does not reverse skeletal muscle paralysis. Atropine eye drops can be used to reverse nerve agent–induced miosis and paralysis of accommodation.[39]

Adverse effects of atropine are unlikely except if administered to a victim misdiagnosed with a cholinergic toxidrome (i.e., nerve agent or other organophosphate poisoning). These include increased heart rate, drying of secretions, mydriasis, loss of accommodation, and decreased sweating.[32] The last of these adverse effects is the most significant and can lead to severe hyperthermia, especially in the setting of a warm environment or physical exertion.[31,40] All patients who receive atropine should be monitored not only for therapeutic improvement but also for signs of anticholinergic effects.

The recommended adult dose of atropine is 2 mg, which can be administered intravenously, intramuscularly, endotracheally, or by autoinjector (e.g., Mark I kit). The autoinjector is an effective means of administering atropine expeditiously because it can quickly deliver antidote through clothing (including PPE). Animal studies have shown that atropine administered by autoinjector was absorbed at a rate intermediate between intravenous administration and intramuscular administration with a conventional syringe.[41,42] Atropine administration should be repeated in 2-mg doses every 5 to 10 minutes based on clinical response. The most critical indicator of antidotal response is pulmonary function (i.e., drying of bronchial secretions and decreased airway resistance). This can be assessed by the patient's self-reported ease of breathing or by improved compliance if the patient is being artificially ventilated. There is no dose limit for the total amount of atropine administered, and end of therapy should be determined by clinical stabilization. Patients who require continued antidotal treatment after initial improvement should suspected of having continued dermal nerve agent absorption and undergo repeat decontamination.

The early administration of antidotes is critical in the treatment of nerve agent poisoning. Antidotal therapy for nerve agent poisoning includes atropine, an oxime, and a benzodiazepine (each is discussed in detail later). The decision to administer an antidote is based on the severity of poisoning and route of exposure. Victims of an inhalational exposure that present with mild symptoms including miosis, eye pain, and rhinorrhea, but no other significant signs or symptoms, may be observed without the administration of antidote. Those with any complaints of respiratory distress, including

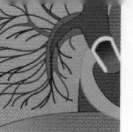

shortness of breath, complaints of chest tightness, wheezing, or dyspnea, should be treated with a initial administration of 2 mg of atropine plus pralidoxime, 600 mg through intramuscular autoinjector or 500 to 1000 mg/hour through intravenous infusion. If respiratory symptoms are significant (e.g., dyspnea, wheezing, shortness of breath), or the victim has additional symptoms such as weakness or vomiting, the initial doses of atropine and pralidoxime should be doubled to 4 mg of atropine through intramuscular or intravenous injection, and 1200 mg of pralidoxime (i.e., two 600-mg intramuscular autoinjectors). Victims with severe manifestations of nerve agent poisoning, including severe respiratory distress or apnea, seizures or coma, or significant skeletal muscle weakness, should receive initial doses of atropine and pralidoxime of 6 mg and 1800 mg, respectively, as well as a benzodiazepine to treat or prevent seizures.

OXIME ANTIDOTES

Oximes are the second important antidote in the treatment of nerve agent poisoning.[43] Their primary role is to reactivate AChE after it has been phosphorylated by a nerve agent by removing the nerve agent from its active site. Oximes reactivate AChE by acting as potent nucleophiles that attack the phosphorous moiety of the nerve agent, cleaving the nerve agent–serine-203 bond and displacing the nerve agent from the enzyme active site as an oxime–phosphate complex.[10] Because atropine effectively antagonizes the muscarinic effects of nerve agent poisoning, oximes are clinically most important because of their ability to reactivate AChE in nicotinic synapse, restoring neuromuscular function and reversing skeletal muscle paralysis.

In the United States, 2-pralidoxime chloride (2-PAM, pyridine-2-aldoxime methochloride, Protopam) is the only oxime currently approved by the FDA for the treatment of organophosphate or nerve agent poisoning. However, other oximes, including obidoxime, pralidoxime iodide (2-PAM iodide), pralidoxime mesylate (P2S), pralidoxime methylsulfate, and trimedoxime (TMB4), are available in other countries. The differences in the oxime effectiveness are mainly due to the variation in aging rates that the nerve agent, the oxime, and the animal model, including human, used.[44-47] The reactivation of AChE inhibited by VX, sarin, or GF is possible hours after the intoxication, whereas soman-inhibited AChE cannot be reactivated within minutes after intoxication because of its rapid aging of AChE.

Pralidoxime can be administered by repeat intramuscular injection (e.g., autoinjector), as described earlier, to reach the traditional therapeutic level of 4 µg/mL.[48,49] If pralidoxime is administered intravenously, a dosing regimen consists of an intravenous bolus of 500 to 1000 mg over 30 minutes, followed by an infusion of 500 mg/hour, appears to maintain a concentration of about 13 mg/L for a 70-kg person, which is above the previously reported minimum therapeutic level (4 µg/mL)[48,49] and below the level at which adverse effects are seen

(14 µg/mL).[50] The infusion should be continued until the patient's muscle weakness has resolved. As a general rule, any victim that receives atropine should also receive an oxime antidote.

Newer oximes under active development include the bisquaternary oxime Hagedorn agents (H oximes). HI-6 has been shown to as effective, or superior, to 2-PAM in the treatment of OP pesticide poisoning.[47,51] HI-6 plus atropine has been reported to produce a protective ratio of 42 against VR (O-isobutyl S-[2-(diethylamino) ethyl]methylphosphonothioate, a structural isomer of VX, also known as Russian VX), whereas pralidoxime plus atropine under identical conditions produced a protective ratio of 6 (P. M. Lundy, personal communication). Interestingly, although comparable to other oximes as a reactivator of AChE in in vitro studies,[46] HI-6 has been shown to be a more effective antidote in studies in which AChE was permanently and irreversibly inhibited (aged).[52,53] The newer bispyridinium oximes, including HI-6, have been found to have significant pharmacologic properties not associated with the reactivation of nerve agent–inhibited AChE.[52-55] However, HI-6 and HLö-7 chloride salts are unstable over time in aqueous solution and must be stored as lyophilized powder, complicating their use in autoinjectors.[56] Recent research has shown the HI-6 dimethanesulphonate salt (HI-6 DMS) to be stable in aqueous solution, as well as safe and effective against nerve agents, making it more attractive for use in autoinjectors.[57] Overall, HI-6 has shown potential advantages over other oximes and may eventually emerge as the oxime of choice.[55,58,59] Several countries, including Canada, Sweden, the former Yugoslav entities, and the Czech Republic, are investigating HI-6 as their oxime of choice for the treatment of nerve agent poisoning.

BENZODIAZEPINES

Victims with severe nerve agent poisoning are likely to also have seizures. The addition of a benzodiazepine has been shown to improve survival from nerve agent poisoning and to decrease the development of permanent brain damage.[60,61] Diazepam is available in an autoinjector and is issued (in addition to 3 Mark I autoinjectors) to U.S. military personnel as part of their nerve agent medical countermeasure kit. It is recommended that a benzodiazepine be administered for any seizure activity as well as for any moderate to severe manifestations of nerve agent poisoning (before the development of seizures). Although diazepam is most commonly recommended, other benzodiazepines should be considered if diazepam is not available, as might be the case in an MCI.

OTHER MEDICAL COUNTERMEASURES IN DEVELOPMENT

Atropine, oximes, and benzodiazepines have been the mainstay of therapy for nerve agent poisoning for almost

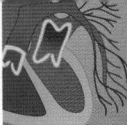

as long as nerve agents have been a threat. Additional therapeutic measures in development include other anticholinergic compounds such as biperiden, scopolamine, and trihexyphenidyl. The excitatory neurotransmitter glutamate and its stimulation of the *N*-methyl-D-aspartate (NMDA) receptors, has also been found to play a role in nerve agent–induced seizures. This work has lead to research in the development of NMDA receptor antagonists such as MK801 and gacyclidine (GK-11) that may find a place in nerve agent treatment in the future.[59,62]

MANAGEMENT OF MASS CASUALTIES

Decontamination and patient management priorities at the scene of a terrorist attack using nerve agents include collection of victims at a point upwind of the chemical hazard, the establishment of a clean–dirty line between the contaminated (i.e., "hot") and uncontaminated (i.e., "cold") zones, and the administration of initial medical treatment if necessary (i.e., antidotes, advanced life support). Plans should include means to decontaminate both ambulatory and nonambulatory victims and provide a way for emergent medical treatment to be administered as soon as possible once the patient exits the "warm" decontamination zone (Fig. 105A-2). If adequate PPE is available for medical personnel, treatment may be started earlier (i.e., before or during decontamination).

Basic principles of mass casualty decontamination include the following: (1) decontamination should take place as soon as possible—expect the ratio of unaffected to affected to be about 5:1; (2) disrobing *is* decontamination and should be the earliest step in the process; (3) high-volume, low-pressure water showers are the best mass decontamination method; and (4) after a known dermal exposure, first responders must be decontaminated as soon as possible.[63] Terrorist attacks using nerve agents in cold weather present additional decontamination challenges. If ambient temperatures are above 18.3° C (65° F), all methods of decontamination can be done outdoors. As ambient fall below 18.3° C (65° F), heated enclosures should be made available for postdecontamination shelter. As ambient temperatures fall further, water decontamination should take place in a heated enclosure, and under extreme weather conditions (e.g., below 1.7° C [35° F]), dry decontamination methods are recommended (e.g., removal of all outer garments and dry blotting of the skin with absorbents) until victims can be transported to a heated facility for water decontamination. However, regardless of the ambient temperature, people who have been exposed to a known life-threatening level of chemical contamination should disrobe, undergo decontamination with copious amounts of high-volume, low-pressure water or an alternative decontamination method, and be sheltered as soon as possible.[64] In 2003, the FDA approved a reactive skin decontamination lotion (RSDL) for use as a decontaminating liquid for dermal nerve agent exposure. It is an oximate-based skin decontaminant developed in Canada and currently in use worldwide.[65] In the absence of a water-flushing or showering system, it represents a viable method of portable decontamination.

Ideally, all victims would undergo adequate decontamination before leaving the incident scene. Historically, however, about 70% to 80% of victims of an MCI evacuate themselves and each other from the incident scene and then self-triage to nearby health care facilities. This creates the need for decontamination plans and equipment at the receiving health care facilities. This was the case during the 1995 Tokyo sarin attack, when there was no field decontamination of victims at the incident scene. Secondary contamination occurred at the receiving hospitals, with 23% of the Saint Luke's hospital staff developing signs and symptoms of

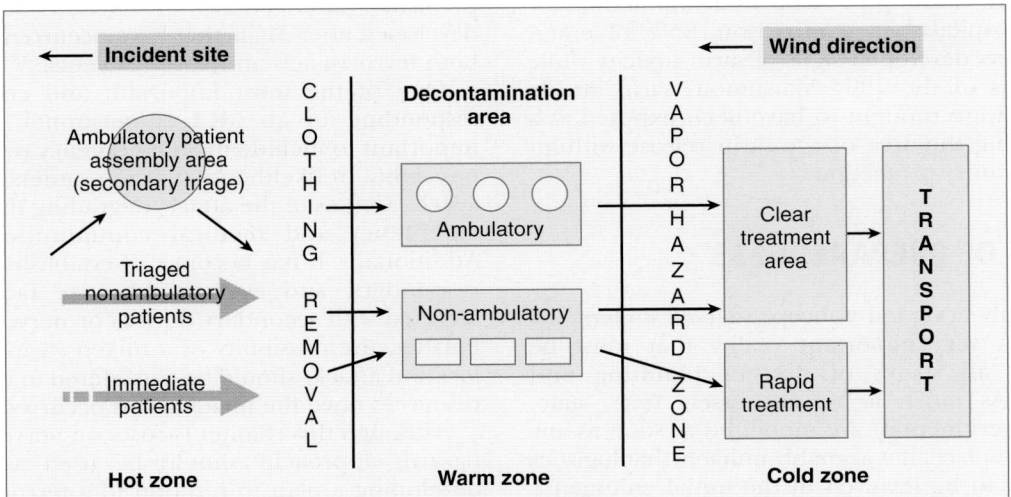

FIGURE 105A-2 The dual-corridor emergency decontamination system has two corridors for the triage, decontamination, and treatment of nerve agent victims. (From U.S. Army Soldier and Biological Chemical Command (SBCCOM): Guidelines for mass casualty decontamination during a terrorist chemical incident. Aberdeen, MD, Edgewood Chemical Biological Center, 2003.)

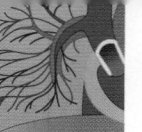

sarin poisoning while treating the hundreds of victims, many of whom were contaminated, who presented to the hospital. Forty-six percent of those working in a poorly ventilated hospital chapel became symptomatic. However, only one nurse was admitted, and no one required antidotal treatment.[4,5,34,66] An inhalational exposure is likely due to the use of a nerve agent aerosol or vapor, as in the Tokyo subway attacks of 1995. Victims exposed to nerve agent vapor adsorb the agent into their clothing and off-gas the agent after they have been removed from the exposure. The risks associated with off-gassing include continued inhalational exposure for the patient and medical care providers who will be in close proximity to the patient, especially indoors and in confined spaces (e.g., ambulances). This was seen after the Matsumoto and Tokyo sarin attacks, in which prehospital care providers became symptomatic from exposure to sarin off-gassing from victims transported to hospitals by ambulance. Hospital care providers also became symptomatic as a result of off-gassing from patients brought into the hospital without decontamination.

The hospital response to a terrorist nerve agent attack should anticipate mass casualties arriving unannounced, contaminated, and in a disorganized fashion. Saint Luke's Hospital's first victim arrived on foot 30 minutes after the attack and was followed by about 500 more within the next 30 minutes. Among 640 victims who presented to Saint Luke's Hospital on the day of the attack, 15% arrived by emergency vehicle (only 10% by ambulance), 48% by foot or private vehicle, and 25% by taxi. Radio-dispatched taxis played a significant role in transporting victims from the scene and were also important in communicating information.[4,5] Typically, because they are the most able to flee the incident scene and make their way to the hospital, most of the early presenters are less severely affected than those incapacitated at the scene.

Ten percent of first responders developed acute signs and symptoms of nerve agent poisoning (some requiring treatment) primarily as the result of sarin vapor off-gassing from the clothing of victims during ambulance transport to hospitals.[4] In comparison, 35% of emergency responders developed signs of sarin toxicity while rescuing victims of the 1994 Matsumoto sarin attack, although most were thought to have been exposed as a result of entering the area of the sarin release without adequate respiratory protection.[67]

PRINCIPLES OF PREPAREDNESS

It is a commonly accepted concept that *all disasters are local.* This is a very important reality that must be considered in all stages of disaster planning and preparedness. As much as outside assets (e.g., state, federal, nongovernmental) are mobilized as soon as any major MCI takes place, it is arguably unlikely that logistics will allow them to be involved in the initial emergency response at a significant level within 48 hours of the incident. Therefore, consumable supplies, medications, antidotes, personnel, and safe food and water should be stockpiled in quantities to suffice for at least 3 days or more, depending on the community's accessibility.

An important step in preparing to respond to a nerve agent terrorist attack is to perform community risk assessments to identify potential targets, their degree of vulnerability to attack, and when an attack would be likely to occur. By determining the maximum number of potential victims for a "worst case scenario" attack, preparations can be made to respond. Advance planning should include identifying potential staging areas, victim collection points, sites for decontamination stations, and sites for victim and responder sheltering in extreme weather conditions for all sites (e.g., sports arenas, mass transit systems) that are deemed at high risk for a terrorist MCI based on a community vulnerability analysis. Additionally, alternatives for all sites mentioned should also be determined.

Another essential step is to take inventory of any and all resources that are *available* in your community to respond to a terrorist attack. This assessment should include decontamination equipment, personnel, hospital beds, alternative health care facilities, ambulances, antidotes, ventilators, PPE, and additional items too numerous to list here. This should be followed be an estimation of what is *needed* to respond to an MCI in your community (based on a vulnerability assessment). In the event that a community's maximal response capability could not adequately respond to a worst case scenario, emergency preparations should include planning to rapidly access, or even predeploy in the case of a scheduled event (e.g., large sporting event), outside assets to close the gap between likely emergency response needs and those locally available. Access to outside assets can be facilitated by the advanced establishment of interagency and interjurisdictional memoranda of understanding that delineate how and when assets are brought in to assist with a local MCI or major disaster. The difference between the two is the *gap* that additional planning and preparation can lessen. Emergency planners should avail themselves of the many published after-action reports and "lessons learned" developed after MCIs that have occurred as the result of both terrorist acts and natural events.[4-7,66-71]

One of the most important and critical assets for responding to an MCI is personnel. However, it is important to include in an emergency response plan the possibility, or likelihood, that responders at all levels may also be victims of the attack, degrading the ability for the emergency and medical communities to respond. Additionally, it has become an established fact that first responders, and even health care facilities, may be targeted with secondary devices or nerve agent releases. Further, the possibility of a mixed weapon or multiple-location attacks should be considered in the allocation of resources once the incident has occurred.

Although this chapter focuses on nerve agents, an "all-hazards approach" should be used as the basis for developing a plan to respond to a terrorist nerve agent attack. By establishing robust plans and procedures for responding to any hazardous materials (Hazmat) event, additional measures (e.g., specific antidote availability,

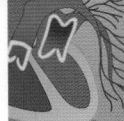

BOX 105A-1   NERVE AGENT–RELATED INTERNATIONAL CLASSIFICATION OF DISEASES CODES

ICD-9-CM

Toxic effect of organophosphate & carbamate	989.3
Accidental poisoning by other specified gases and vapors	E869.8
Suicide and self-inflicted poisoning using other specified gases and vapors	E952.8
Assault by poisoning using other gases and vapors	E962.2
Injury due to terrorism involving chemical weapons	E979.7
Injury due to war operations by gases, fumes, and chemicals	E997.2
Death due to terrorism involving chemical weapons	U01.7

ICD-10

Accidental poisoning by and exposure to other and unspecified chemicals and noxious substances	X49
Intentional self-poisoning (suicide) by and exposure to other gases and vapors	X67
Assault (homicide) by gases and vapors	X88
Assault (homicide) by other specified chemicals and noxious substances	X89
Assault (homicide) by unspecified chemical or noxious substance	X90
War operations involving chemical weapons and other forms of unconventional warfare	Y36.7

---

medical training for the recognition and treatment of nerve agent poisoning) can be developed and added. Moreover, it is of paramount importance that any and all emergency plans be exercised regularly using realistic scenarios.

See the International Classification of Diseases Codes in Box 105A-1.

REFERENCES

1. Ledgard J: The Preparatory Manual of Chemical Warfare Agents. Columbus, OH, The Paranoid Publications Group, 2003.
2. Morimoto F, Shimazu T, Yoshioka T: Intoxication of VX in humans. Am J Emerg Med 1999;17(5):493–494.
3. Nozaki H, Aikawa N, Fujishima S, et al: A case of VX poisoning and the difference from sarin. Lancet 1995;346(8976):698–699.
4. Okumura T, Takasu N, Ishimatsu S, et al: Report on 640 victims of the Tokyo subway sarin attack. Ann Emerg Med 1996;28(2):129–135.
5. Ohbu S, Yamashina A, Takasu N, et al: Sarin poisoning on Tokyo subway. South Med J 1997;90(6):587–593.
6. Tu A: Anatomy of Aum Shinrikyo's organization and terrorist attacks with chemical and biological weapons. Arch Toxicol Kinetics Xenobiotic Metabolism 1999;7(3):45–82.
7. Tu A: The first mass chemical terrorism using sarin in Matsumoto, Japan. Arch Toxicol Kinet Xenobiot Metab2001;9(3):65–93.
8. Neitlich H: Effect of percutaneous GD on human subjects. Report No.: CRDL Technical Memorandum 2-21,DTIC AD471794. Fort Belvoir, VA, Defense Technical Information Center, 1965.
9. Berends F, Posthumus CH, vd SI, Deierkauf FA: The chemical basis of the "ageing process" of DFP-inhibited pseudocholinesterase. Biochim Biophys Acta 1959;34:567–568.
10. Fleisher JH, Harris LW: Dealkylation as a mechanism for aging of cholinesterase after poisoning with pinacolyl methylphosphono-fluoridate. Biochem Pharmacol 1965;14(5):641–650.
11. Saxena A, Doctor BP, Maxwell DM, et al: The role of glutamate-199 in the aging of cholinesterase. Biochem Biophys Res Commun 1993;197(1):343–349.
12. Shafferman A, Ordentlich A, Barak D, et al: Aging of phosphylated human acetylcholinesterase: catalytic processes mediated by aromatic and polar residues of the active centre. Biochem J 1996;318(Pt. 3):833–840.
13. Sidell FR, Groff WA: The reactivatibility of cholinesterase inhibited by VX and sarin in man. Toxicol Appl Pharmacol 1974;27(2):241–252.
14. Vranken MA, De Bisschop HC, Willems JL: "In vitro" inhibition of neurotoxic esterase by organophosphorus nerve agents. Arch Int Pharmacodyn Ther 1982;260(2):316–318.
15. Duysen EG, Li B, Xie W, Schopfer LM, et al: Evidence for nonacetylcholinesterase targets of organophosphorus nerve agent: supersensitivity of acetylcholinesterase knockout mouse to VX lethality. J Pharmacol Exp Ther 2001;299(2):528–535.
16. O'Neill JJ: Non-cholinesterase effects of anticholinesterases. Fundam Appl Toxicol 1981;1(2):154–160.
17. Van Meter WG, Karczmar AG, Fiscus RR: CNS effects of anticholinesterases in the presence of inhibited cholinesterases. Arch Int Pharmacodyn Ther 1978;231(2):249–260.
18. Rickett DL, Glenn JF, Beers ET: Central respiratory effects versus neuromuscular actions of nerve agents. Neurotoxicology 1986;7(1):225–236.
19. Wright PG: An analysis of the central and peripheral components of respiratory failure produced by anticholinesterase poisoning in the rabbit. J Physiol 1954;126(1):52–70.
20. Rengstorff RH: Accidental exposure to sarin: vision effects. Arch Toxicol 1985;56(3):201–203.
21. Rubin LS, Krop S, Goldberg MN: Effect of sarin on dark adaptation in man: mechanism of action. J Appl Physiol 1957;11(3):445–449.
22. Rubin LS, Goldberg MN: Effect of sarin on dark adaptation in man: threshold changes. J Appl Physiol 1957;11(3):439–444.
23. Oberst FW, Koon WS, Christensen MK, et al: Retention of inhaled sarin vapor and its effect on red blood cell cholinesterase activity in man. Clin Pharmacol Ther 1968;9(4):421–427.
24. Blank IH, Griesemer RD, Gould E: The penetration of an anticholinesterase agent (sarin) into skin. I. Rate of penetration into excised human skin. J Invest Dermatol 1957;29(4):299–309.
25. Craig FN, Cummings EG, Sim VM: Environmental temperature and the percutaneous absorption of a cholinesterase inhibitor, VX. J Invest Dermatol 1977;68(6):357–361.
26. Duncan EJ, Brown A, Lundy P, et al: Site-specific percutaneous absorption of methyl salicylate and VX in domestic swine. J Appl Toxicol 2002;22(3):141–148.
27. Sidell F. Sarin and soman: observations on accidental exposures. Report No.: Edgewood Arsenal Technical Report 4747, DTIC AD769737. Fort Belvoir, VA, Defense Technical Information Center, 1973.
28. Morita H, Yanagisawa N, Nakajima T, et al: Sarin poisoning in Matsumoto, Japan. Lancet 1995;346(8970):290–293.
29. Rotenberg JS: Diagnosis and management of nerve agent exposure. Pediatr Ann 2003;32(4):242–250.
30. Aaron C: Safety of adult nerve agent autoinjectors in children. J Pediatr 2005;146(1):8–10.
31. Amitai Y, Almog S, Singer R, et al: Atropine poisoning in children during the Persian Gulf crisis. A national survey in Israel. JAMA 1992;268(5):630–632.
32. Kozer E, Mordel A, Haim SB, et al: Pediatric poisoning from trimedoxime (TMB4) and atropine automatic injectors. J Pediatr 2005;146(1):41–44.
33. Romig LE: Pediatric triage: a system to JumpSTART your triage of young patients at MCIs. JEMS 2002;27(7):52–58, 60–63.
34. Nozaki H, Hori S, Shinozawa Y, et al: Secondary exposure of medical staff to sarin vapor in the emergency room. Intensive Care Med 1995;21(1):1032–1035.
35. Selden BS, Curry SC: Prolonged succinylcholine-induced paralysis in organophosphate insecticide poisoning. Ann Emerg Med 1987;16(2):215–217.
36. Baker D, Rustick J: Anaesthesia for casualties of chemical warfare agents. In Anaesthesia and Perioperative Care of the Combat Casualty. Washington, DC, Office of the Surgeon General, U.S. Army Medical Center, 1995, p 850.
37. Sidell FR: Soman and sarin: clinical manifestations and treatment of accidental poisoning by organophosphates. Clin Toxicol 1974;7(1):1–17.

38. Bird SB, Gaspari RJ, Lee WJ, Dickson EW: Diphenhydramine as a protective agent in a rat model of acute, lethal organophosphate poisoning. Acad Emerg Med 2002;9(12):1369–1372.

39. Nozaki H, Aikawa N, Shinozawa Y, et al: Sarin poisoning in Tokyo subway. Lancet 1995;345(8955):980–981.

40. Robinson S, Buckingham R, Pearcy M, et al: 1952 Field test of atropine. In The Physiological Effects of Atropine and Potential Atropine Substitutes. Fort Belvoir, VA, Defense Technical Information Service, 1953.

41. Sidell FR, Markis JE, Groff W, Kaminskis A: Enhancement of drug absorption after administration by an automatic injector. J Pharmacokinet Biopharm 1974;2(3):197–210.

42. Friedl KE, Hannan CJ Jr, Schadler PW, Jacob WH: Atropine absorption after intramuscular administration with 2-pralidoxime chloride by two automatic injector devices. J Pharm Sci 1989;78(9):728–731.

43. Grob D, Johns RJ: Use of oximes in the treatment of intoxication by anticholinesterase compounds in patients with myasthenia gravis. Am J Med 1958;24(4):512–518.

44. Dawson RM: Review of oximes available for treatment of nerve agent poisoning. J Appl Toxicol 1994;14(5):317–331.

45. Lundy PM, Hansen AS, Hand BT, Boulet CA: Comparison of several oximes against poisoning by soman, tabun and GF. Toxicology 1992;72(1):99–105.

46. Worek F, Kirchner T, Backer M, Szinicz L: Reactivation by various oximes of human erythrocyte acetylcholinesterase inhibited by different organophosphorus compounds. Arch Toxicol 1996;70(8):497–503.

47. Worek F, Widmann R, Knopff O, Szinicz L: Reactivating potency of obidoxime, pralidoxime, HI 6 and HLo 7 in human erythrocyte acetylcholinesterase inhibited by highly toxic organophosphorus compounds. Arch Toxicol 1998;72(4):237–243.

48. Sidell FR, Groff WA: Intramuscular and intravenous administration of small doses of 2-pyridinium aldoxime methochloride to man. J Pharm Sci 1971;60(8):1224–1228.

49. Sundwall A: Minimum concentrations of N-methylpridinium-2-aldoxime methane sulphonate which reverse neuromuscular blockade. Biochim Pharmacol 1961;8:432–434.

50. Eyer P: The role of oximes in the management of organophosphorus pesticide poisoning. Toxicol Rev 2003;22(3):165–190.

51. Clement JG, Bailey DG, Madill HD, et al: The acetylcholinesterase oxime reactivator HI-6 in man: pharmacokinetics and tolerability in combination with atropine. Biopharm Drug Dispos 1995;16(5):415–425.

52. Kusic R, Jovanovic D, Randjelovic S, et al: HI-6 in man: efficacy of the oxime in poisoning by organophosphorus insecticides. Hum Exp Toxicol 1991;10(2):113–118.

53. Kassa J: Review of oximes in the antidotal treatment of poisoning by organophosphorus nerve agents. J Toxicol Clin Toxicol 2002;40(6):803–816.

54. van Helden HP, Busker RW, Melchers BP, Bruijnzeel PL: Pharmacological effects of oximes: how relevant are they? Arch Toxicol 1996;70(12):779–786.

55. Koplovitz I, Stewart JR: A comparison of the efficacy of HI6 and 2-PAM against soman, tabun, sarin, and VX in the rabbit. Toxicol Lett 1994;70(3):269–279.

56. Eyer P, Hell W, Kawan A, Klehr H: Studies on the decomposition of the oxime HI 6 in aqueous solution. Arch Toxicol 1986;59(4):266–271.

57. Lundy PM, Hill I, Lecavalier P, et al: The pharmacokinetics and pharmacodynamics of two HI-6 salts in swine and efficacy in the treatment of GF and soman poisoning. Toxicology 2005;208(3):399–409.

58. Kassa J, Cabal J, Bajgar J: The choice: HI-6, pralidoxime or obidoxime against nerve agents? ASA Newsletter 1997;97:4.

59. Aas P: Future considerations for the medical management of nerve-agent intoxication. Prehospital Disaster Med 2003;18(3):208–216.

60. Rump S, Kowaczyk M: Management of convulsions in nerve agent acute poisoning: a Polish perspective. J Med Chem Def 2003;1:1–14.

61. Martin LJ, Doebler JA, Shih TM, Anthony A: Protective effect of diazepam pretreatment on soman-induced brain lesion formation. Brain Res 1985;325(1–2):287–289.

62. Lallement G, Clarencon D, Galonnier M, et al: Acute soman poisoning in primates neither pretreated nor receiving immediate therapy: value of gacyclidine (GK-11) in delayed medical support. Arch Toxicol 1999;73(2):115–122.

63. U.S. Army Soldier and Biological Chemical Command (SBCCOM): Guidelines for mass casualty decontamination during a terrorist chemical incident. Aberdeen, MD, Edgewood Chemical Biological Center, 2003.

64. U.S. Army Soldier and Biological Chemical Command (SBCCOM): Guidelines for cold weather mass decontamination during a terrorist chemical agent incident, revision 1. Aberdeen, MD, Edgewood Chemical Biological Center, 2003.

65. Sawyer TW, Parker D, Thomas N, et al: Efficacy of an oximate-based skin decontaminant against organophosphate nerve agents determined in vivo and in vitro. Toxicology 1991;67(3):267–277.

66. Okumura T, Suzuki K, Fukuda A, et al: The Tokyo subway sarin attack: disaster management. 2. Hospital response. Acad Emerg Med 1998;5(6):618–624.

67. Nakajima T, Sato S, Morita H, Yanagisawa N: Sarin poisoning of a rescue team in the Matsumoto sarin incident in Japan. Occup Environ Med 1997;54(10):697–701.

68. Yokoyama K, Yamada A, Mimura N: Clinical profiles of patients with sarin poisoning after the Tokyo subway attack. Am J Med 1996;100(5):586.

69. Okumura T, Suzuki K, Fukuda A, et al: The Tokyo subway sarin attack: disaster management. 1. Community emergency response. Acad Emerg Med 1998;5(6):613–617.

70. Matsui Y, Ohbu S, Yamashina A: Hospital deployment in mass sarin poisoning incident of the Tokyo subway system: an experience at St. Luke's International Hospital, Tokyo. Jpn Hosp 1996;15:67–71.

71. Smithson AE: Stimson Center Report No. 35. Ataxia: The Chemical and Biological Terrorism Threat and the US Response. Washington, DC, The Henry L. Stimson Center, 2005.

B Vesicants

LAWRENCE STILWELL BETTS, MD, PHD ■ BRIAN CHRISTOPHER BETTS, MD

At a Glance...

- Sulfur mustard (or "mustard") is the most significant member of the vesicant agents. It is the only vesicant with known use in combat.
- Skin lesions produced by contact with vesicant agents are nonspecific and, alone, are of little diagnostic value in identifying the etiology in early cases. History of the use of, or presence of, a vesicant agent, or prior cases with similar presentations, is of great value in approaching the differential diagnosis.
- The most important preventive measure to control exposure is avoidance of contact; the most important treatment measure to limit injury is prompt decontamination.

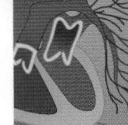

- Skin decontaminants available to the general public include a dilute hypochlorite solution (0.5%); military chemical agent decontaminants, such as the M291 kit, can be used as available.
- There is no specific antidote for mustard, and medical management of cases is based on treating signs and symptoms as they develop.
- Patient management ranges from very simple, for erythema or minor vesicles, to extremely complex, for immunosuppressed patients with multisystem derangements and extensive skin lesions.
- Disposition of casualties varies with intensity of exposure, delay and efficacy of decontamination, and severity of injuries.
- Repeated occupational exposures to mustard at levels that result in toxic effects are known to cause cancer of the upper airways.

RELEVANT HISTORY

A *vesicant* is a chemical that produces vesicles or blisters at the site of contact. This class of "military chemical agents," specifically sulfur mustard (also called *H; HD; CAS No. 505-60-2; mustard gas, mustard*), has been a major military threat agent since its introduction in combat in World War I. The vesicants constitute a hazard to exposed skin and mucous membranes in both the vapor and liquid states. Three groups of vesicants are considered useful for tactical military weapons as "chemical agents": the mustard agents, the arsenicals, and the halogenated oximes. The main vesicant agents and their short-hand military designations are listed in Table 105B-1.

Sulfur mustard (bis-[2-chloroethyl] sulfide) was first used as a weapon in World War I. Mustard was responsible for more battlefield casualties than caused by all of the other chemical agents. Mustard is the most important agent in the vesicant group and remains a current military threat today. Although chemical agents were not used on the battlefield in World War II, their

use by Iraq was reported during the 1980s during in the Iran–Iraq conflict. Some of the Iranian casualties were evacuated and treated in Belgium, the country where mustard was first used in warfare in 1915 and in France. An excellent discussion and color image presentation of the clinical findings and medical management of these casualties is provided by Jan L. Willems.[1] The images can also be found in the *Textbook of Military Medicine.*[2]

Lewisite, or dichloro-2-chlorovinylarsine, is an arsenical compound that produces toxic effects more rapidly than mustard. Lewisite has not been used in combat and has a low military threat potential. The widely known chelating agent, dimercaprol, or British Anti-Lewisite (BAL), was originally developed for use as an antidote for Lewisite. BAL currently finds therapeutic application in the treatment of some metal poisonings.

Phosgene oxime (dichloroformoxime) is the only representative of the halogenated oxime group with military application. It is not a true vesicant. Although it causes irritation and corrosion, reaction to contact results in a solid, urticaria-like lesion that is not filled with fluid. The military includes it as a vesicant agent, and a

TABLE 105B-1 Vesicant Groups*				
AGENT	**MILITARY SYMBOL**	**COMMON NAME**	**ONSET OF PAIN**	**TISSUE DAMAGE**
Mustard Agents				
bis-(2-chloroethyl) sulfide (Impure) (C₄H₈CL₂S and contaminants	*H*	*Mustard; sulfur mustard; Yperite; "lost"*	*Delayed—hours*	*Immediate*
bis-(2-chloroethyl) sulfide (distilled)† (C₄H₈CL₂S)	HD	Distilled mustard; sulfur mustard	Same	Same
60% bis-(2-chloroethyl) sulfide and 40% bis-(2-[2-chloroethylthio]-ethyl) ether mixture†	HT	—	Same	Same
mustard with Lewisite mixture	HL	—	Same	Same
nitrogen mustards: bis(2-chloroethyl)ethylamine (HN1) 2-Chloro-N-(2-chloroethyl)-N-ethylethanamine (HN2) 2,2',2" tri(chloroethyl)amine (HN3)	HN1, HN2, and HN3	Nitrogen mustard	Same	Same
Organic Arsenical Agents				
dichloro-2-chlorovinylarsine (C₂H₂AsCl₃)	*L*	*Lewisite*	*Immediate*	*Seconds to minutes*
methyldichloroarsine	MD	—	Same	Same
phenyldichloroarsine	PD	—	Same	Same
ethyldichloroarsine	ED	—	Same	Same
Halogenated Oxime Agents				
dichloroformoxime (Cl₂CNOH)	*CX*	*Phosgene oxime*	*Immediate*	*Seconds*

*Prototype agent in italics.
†Lewisite, or agent "T" (a vesicant chemically related to mustard), is added to decrease the freezing point and maintain the liquid form at lower ambient temperatures

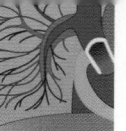

brief discussion is included in this chapter. Phosgene oxime has not been used in combat, and there is little information regarding its use and toxicity. Although it is considered to have a low military threat potential, its rapid penetration of protective garments and rapid onset of severe effects make it of military interest.[2]

Because of the amount of information available on the use and effects of mustard from World War I and the Iran–Iraq conflict, and the relative lack of information on Lewisite and phosgene oxime, this chapter discusses mustard as the prototype vesicant.

EXPOSURE SCENARIOS

Mustard can contaminate environmental surfaces, including food and water supplies. During World War I, exposure to mustard resulted in a large number of casualties, but relatively few deaths. These findings underlie the reasons vesicants have military application. The potential for their use, with the accompanying fear of injury and need to avoid exposure, requires personnel to carry or wear protective equipment and to be fearful when touching anything, including food and water supplies. The need for precautions and the use of protective equipment restricts and impairs the ability to maneuver and fight. The resulting casualties decrease the strength of the fighting force, require medical assets, and further affect morale. It is easy to understand why the mere threat to use a chemical agent can be a powerful military tactic. The potential to use a vesicant against an unprotected and unknowing civilian population could be an even greater weapon in the hands of a terrorist.

The volatility of a chemical agent and its persistence in the environment are inversely related: The more volatile agents have less persistence in the environment. They simply evaporate based on their vapor pressure. However, the vapor may still present a significant hazard! Temperature is the main environmental factor affecting persistence. Other environmental factors, such as terrain, wind, and rain, also affect dispersal and persistence. All these factors have been exploited in the past to obtain a military advantage. At temperatures below 57° F (14° C), mustard is a solid, but still biologically active, chemical. It forms a persistent, oily liquid at higher temperatures that may be detected by its garlic- or onion-like (mustard) odor. In areas such as the Middle East, where summer temperatures often exceed 100° F (38° C), evaporation into the vapor state becomes significant. Such temperatures increase the risk for exposure to mustard vapor, but they simultaneously decrease its persistence.[3] The finding of more casualties with eye and lung damage during the Iran–Iraq conflict than were observed in World War I has been attributed to the higher temperatures and increased volatilization in the hotter climate. Mustard vapor is also much denser than air and forms high vapor concentrations close to the ground or in low-lying areas. When an agent evaporates off the ground after dispersal, injuries may occur low on the body or in individuals in low-lying areas. To maintain mustard in the liquid state at lower temperatures, mustard has been mixed with other chemicals (including Lewisite) to decrease its freezing point.

Chemical warfare material (CWM), composed of stockpiled agents (Table 105B-2) and "nonstockpiled" materials (such as buried items and contaminated objects from former production and storage), are currently being destroyed under federal statute and the Chemical Weapons Convention demilitarization program.[4] Although extremely remote, there is a possibility of accidental release during storage, transportation, or destruction of the agent or its original container. Programs have been established to inform and educate adjacent communities regarding the potential risks and planned emergency response actions. In 2001, the Agency for Toxic Substances and Disease Registry released a draft toxicologic profile for "Mustard Gas" for review and comment. When officially released in 2003, the name of the profile was changed to "Sulfur Mustard." This profile provides a comprehensive review of the environmental release and public exposure concerns.[5]

Nonmilitary "environmental" exposures have been reported in the literature.[6,7] Often these reports involve adults or children finding undetonated shells. In some

TABLE 105B-2 Chemical Agents in the U.S. National Stockpile

AGENT	MILITARY SYMBOL/ NAME	CHEMICAL ABSTRACT SERVICE (CAS) NUMBER
bis-(2-chloroethyl) sulfide	H, HD; sulfur mustard	505-60-2
bis(2-chloroethylthioethyl)ether	HT	63918-89-8
dichloro-2-chlorovinylarsine	L; Lewisite	541-25-3
ethyl *N,N*-dimethyl phosphoroamidiocyanidate	GA; Tabun	77-81-6
isopropyl methylphosphonofluoridate	GB; Sarin	107-44-8
O-ethyl-S-(2-diisopropylaminoethyl)-methyl phosphonothiolate	VX	50782-69-9

The Convention on the Prohibition of the Development, Production, Stockpiling, and Use of Chemical Weapons and Their Destruction, also known as the Chemical Weapons Convention (CWC), was signed by the United States on January 13, 1993, and ratified by Congress on April 25, 1997. The CWC mandates that nonstockpile chemical warfare materials (CWM) be destroyed by 2007. Extensions to this deadline can be obtained.[4]
From National Center for Environmental Health: Final Recommendations for Protecting the Health and Safety against Potential Adverse Effects of Long-Term Exposure to Low Doses of Agents: GA, BV, VX, Mustard Agent (H, HD, V), and Lewisite (L). Public Health Service, Centers for Disease Control and Prevention. Washington DC, U.S. Department of Health and Human Services, 1988.

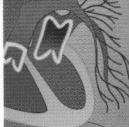

instances, the shells had remained under water or buried for many years before being found. The shells may leak or even detonate. Accidental exposures of this type still present possible patient scenarios that may be encountered by public service and medical personnel.

PATHOPHYSIOLOGY OF INJURY

The relationship between the toxic effects caused by mustard and the mechanism of cellular tissue injury that causes them is not well understood.[8] The liquid and vapor states of mustard pass rapidly through intact skin. As a potent alkylating agent, mustard reacts rapidly with structural and functional molecules of the cell, forming adducts. The altered molecules include nucleic acids, proteins, lipoproteins, and peptides, which affect various cell functions and lead to the observed injuries. Because of the rapid rate of these cellular reactions, mustard is quickly "fixed" after only a few minutes in a biologic milieu. Mustard is then no longer present as the "free," reactive agent. Blister fluid, blood, or other body fluids do not present a continuing exposure hazard to the individual or the caregiver. It must be remembered that mustard may contaminate inanimate objects (such as clothing or equipment) and remain "free" and biologically available for many days! These objects can result in a source of continued or accidental exposure to the vesicant.

As little as a 10-μg droplet of mustard on the skin can produce vesication. The LD_{50} from dermal contact to mustard is about 100 mg/kg. This is equivalent to about 7 g, or 5 to 8 mL, of the liquid agent for the average 70-kg person. When dispersed, this amount could cover about one fourth of the body surface with erythema or vesication.[2] The LD_{50} for human oral exposure is estimated to be 0.7 mg/kg.[9]

Exposure levels for aerosols or vapors are often expressed in the inhalation and military literature as the product of the substance's concentration ("C," in mg/m^3) and the duration of exposure ("t" in minutes)—the C $\cdot$ t (or Ct) value expressed as X mg $\cdot$ min/m^3. It has been stated that equal Ct values cause equal toxic effects; that is: C $\times$ t = k (constant effect) in a relationship known as *Haber's rule*.[10] Note that in the practical application of Haber's rule, caution must be used because departures from the rule are possible.[11] Table 105B-3 provides Ct values for injuries by different routes of exposure to mustard in the aerosol or vapor states. Although it is unlikely that quantitative exposure data will be available to the treating physician during the early phases of treatment, military chemical agent detectors are becoming more widely distributed. When available, these provide valuable exposure information in the assessment, treatment, and demonstration of contamination and decontamination of patients.

MANIFESTATIONS

Mustard is the only vesicant that does not cause immediate pain. The exposed individual is asymptomatic

TABLE 105B-3 Mustard Ct Values for Aerosol or Vapor Exposure and Injuries

CT VALUE (mg · min/m^3)	INJURY
>10	Eye damage (under laboratory conditions)
Estimated 12–70	Eye damage (under field conditions)
100–500	Airway damage
200–2000	Threshold for skin damage in eye- and respiratory-protected individuals
~1500	Estimated LCt_{50} through inhalation

From Sidell FR, Urbanetti JS, Smith WJ, Hurst CG: Vesicants. In Medical Aspects of Chemical and Biological Warfare. Textbook of Military Medicine. Washington, DC, Borden Institute, 1997; and U.S. Army Soldier and Biological Chemical Command (USASBCCOM): Distilled Mustard (HD) Material Safety Data Sheet. Aberdeen Proving Ground, MD, 1999.

until the effects become apparent after a period of delay—usually a few hours to 24 hours. Even in cases with severe (heavy) exposure, the onset of symptoms does not appear in the first hour. All body surfaces that come into contact with the liquid or vapor can be affected, but the eye is the most sensitive target organ, with effects ranging from mild conjunctivitis to severe eye damage. The warm, moist, and thin regions of the skin (such as the groin or axilla) are the most severely affected with erythema and vesicles, with the thicker sites (such as the palm or sole) being less affected. Respiratory tract injuries can range from mild irritation of the upper respiratory tract to severe bronchiolar damage with necrosis and hemorrhage of the mucosa and musculature. Acute, chronic, or delayed clinical effects can also be seen in the hematopoietic, gastrointestinal, and central nervous systems after severe exposures.[12] At very high doses, the systemic effects on the blood-forming tissues can result in leukopenia, thrombocytopenia, and anemia. After mild to moderate exposures, death from systemic effects is not anticipated.[13]

Erythema is an early, mild presentation of skin injury and may be the extent of response to a light (small or mild) exposure. The effects are delayed and do not become apparent until an hour or more after exposure; they may be delayed up to a day or more. The skin reaction resembles sunburn that may be present with itching, burning, or stinging. Frequently, small vesicles form in a linear array that may later join together into larger vesicles. The appearance of vesicles follows the erythema, and they may take several days to fully develop. Data from the early studies of mustard reveal variations in skin sensitivity between individuals with apparently the same, as well as differing, amounts of skin pigmentation. Highly pigmented individuals appear to be more resistant to the acute dermal effects.[14] The nonspecific skin lesions produced by mustard resemble those following contact with plants (Rhus family—poison ivy, oak, and sumac) or other contact irritants. Although difficult to differentiate from effects of typical exposures, suspicious circumstances and a corresponding history of exposure are invaluable in making the diagnosis of vesicant exposure. Often, the initial case or cases will not

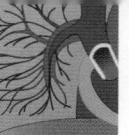

be attributed to a chemical vesicant agent. Melanoderma may develop after unroofing of the blisters, aiding in the physical diagnosis.

The latency period for ocular effects is shorter than that for the skin. Ocular effects may appear after exposure to mustard concentrations barely perceptible by odor. These levels are below those that cause effects on the skin or in the respiratory tract.[13] As the Ct increases (with direct contact of liquid mustard being the worst case), the effects progress to severe damage to the cornea and intraocular structures. Photophobia occurs with even minimal exposures, and it may persist for weeks.

Mustard produces varying degrees of inflammation to the respiratory tract, depending on the Ct. Coughing and shortness of breath are common. The onset and severity of symptoms correspond to the degree of injury, but the injury may develop over a period of several days. Because of the rapid reaction with moist tissues, injury is often confined to the airways and adjacent tissue. Necrosis and sloughing of these tissues may occur. Death from pulmonary insufficiency, due to airway injury and infection, is seen in a small percentage of personnel who reach a medical facility. These deaths commonly occur several days or more after exposure.[13]

Mustard is classified as a known human carcinogen based on human data from manufacturing experience and combat casualties.[15] The human evidence indicates a causal relationship with cancers of the respiratory tract and skin, and possibly leukemia.[12]

PRENATAL AND PEDIATRIC ISSUES

No specific information is available that directs exposure or treatment considerations different from those presented. From the clinical experience involving pediatric casualties during the Iran–Iraq conflict, the onset of symptoms in children was earlier and more severe than in adults.[16] Mustard is known to be a mutagen and a carcinogen.

ASSESSMENT

There is no specific laboratory test available for evaluating exposure to mustard. Analysis of a mustard metabolite, thiodiglycol, in the urine has been developed by the U.S. Army Medical Research Institute of Chemical Defense (USAMRICD) to verify that an exposure to mustard has occurred.[17] Additional methods for analyzing other mustard metabolites as exposure indicators have been developed and are undergoing evaluation.[18,19]

The current U.S. Army "Standards and Guidelines as of March 2006" give a general population limit (GPL: maximum concentration for long-term exposure to sulfur mustard by the civilian general population) of 0.00002 milligrams per cubic meter of air (0.00002 mg/m^3) and 0.0004 milligrams per cubic meter of air (0.0004 mg/m^3) for civilian and Department of Defense personnel who work with sulfur mustard (WPLs).[20] Incorporating the

National Advisory Committee's (NAC) acute exposure guideline levels (AEGLs)[21,22] into Army policy, the AEGLs are used as guidance to protect individuals from the harmful effects of a single, short-term (8 hours or less) exposure to sulfur mustard. The three AEGL exposure levels have time durations ranging from 10 minutes to 8 hours. The effects at the three levels range from minor discomfort at the lowest concentration and exposure duration (AEGL-1) to potentially life threatening at the highest and longest exposure level (AEGL-3) (Table 105B-4). The U.S. Army has also adopted an immediately dangerous to life or health (IDLH) level of 0.7 mg/m^3 and a short-term exposure limit (STEL) of 0.003 mg/m^3 for civilian and Department of Defense workers initially published as interim recommendations by the Centers for Disease Control and Prevention (CDC).[23] On the other end of the exposure spectrum, the Agency for Toxic Substances and Disease Registry (ATSDR) has adopted "minimum risk levels" (MRL: a level below which daily human exposure is likely to be without appreciable risk of untoward non-cancer health effects over a specified duration of time). The following MRLs for sulfur mustard have been established for acute inhalation (1–14 days): 0.0007 mg/m^3; intermediate duration inhalation (14–365 days): 0.00002 mg/m^3; and acute oral (1–14 days): 0.0005 mg/kg/day and intermediate duration oral: 0.00007 mg/kg/day. Chronic MRLs have not been established.[24]

TREATMENT

Decontamination involves the physical removal or chemical deactivation of the vesicant. Both fresh and sea water have been used for the mechanical removal and dissolution of solid or liquid vesicants. Although water (with or without soap) is not the ideal option, it may be the only available decontaminant, and it is a reasonable option.[25] However, at least one military guidance document cautions against the use of water for removing known mustard agent contamination from the skin.[26] Care should be taken to avoid spreading the agent during the decontamination process, and the use of absorbent powders (Fuller's earth, talcum powder, flour) has been recommended to prevent this from occurring.[27] A 0.5% hypochlorite solution (diluted household bleach in water [1:9]) has been used since World War I for decontaminating the skin. A freshly made (daily) solution of alkaline (pH = 10–11) hypochlorite is currently recommended by the U.S. military as the universal decontaminating solution for all liquid and solid agents on the skin.[28] Either solution should be rinsed off the intact skin and hair within 4 minutes, taking care to avoid contact with wounds or the eyes.[13] Poisindex recommends an alternate skin decontamination method of washing with water and a 2.5% sodium thiosulfate solution.[29] The use of a hypochlorite solution is not recommended for abdominal wounds, open chest wounds, wounds exposing nervous tissue, or the eye. These sites should be rinsed liberally with appropriate irrigation fluid (normal saline, lactated Ringer's solution). Vapor exposures are treated by simple removal from the

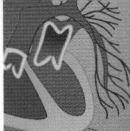

TABLE 105B-4 National Research Council Acute Exposure Guideline Levels (AEGLs) of Sulfur Mustard (adopted by the U.S. Army [in parts per million of air [ppm] and milligrams per cubic meter of air [mg/m³])

SINGLE, ACUTE EXPOSURE PERIOD IN MINUTES	AEGL-1 Conjunctival injection and minor discomfort; no functional decrement in humans		AEGL-2 General conjunctivitis with irritation, edema, photophobia, and eye irritation in humans		AEGL-3 Estimated lethal dose estimate in mice	
	ppm	mg/m³	ppm	mg/m³	ppm	mg/m³
10	0.6	0.40	0.09	0.60	0.59	3.9
30	0.02	0.13	0.03	0.20	0.41	2.7
60	0.01	0.067	0.02	0.10	0.32	2.1
240	0.003	0.017	0.004	0.025	0.08	0.53
480	0.001	0.008	0.002	0.013	0.04	0.27

All of the AEGL-1 and AEGL-2 levels, and the 240 minute and 480 minute AEGL-3 levels, are at or below the odor threshold for sulfur mustard.
From National Research Council of The National Academies: Acute Exposure Guideline Levels for Selected Airborne Chemicals, Vol. 3. Washington, DC, Subcommittee on Acute Exposure Guideline Levels, Committee on Toxicology, Board on Environmental Studies and Toxicology, 2003; National Advisory Council: Acute Exposure Guideline Levels (AEGLs) for Sulfur Mustard (Agent HD). Final Acute Exposure Guidance Levels (AEGLs). Washington, DC, National Advisory Committee on Exposure Guideline Levels for Hazardous Substances, 2001; and United States Army Center for Health Promotion and Preventive Medicine (USACHPPM): Chemical Agent Air Standards Status Table: Existing Standards and Guidelines as of March 2006. Environmental Medicine Program, 2006.

contaminated atmosphere.[30] There are additional skin decontaminants used by the military (M291 resin kit), which may become more generally available with increased homeland defense capabilities.

Sulfur mustard, in both the impure and pure forms (H and HD, respectively), has been a major military threat agent since its introduction in World War I. It is both a vapor and a liquid threat to all exposed skin and mucous membranes. The effects of mustard are delayed, appearing hours after exposure. This lack of early warning signs may result in a longer period of exposure before decontamination. There is no specific antidote for mustard, and management is based on symptomatic and supportive therapy for the lesions or systemic effects. (See also Chapters 2B, 9, and 15.) Immediate decontamination (within 2 minutes) prevents or maximizes the reduction of tissue damage.

BAL (2, 3-dimercapto-1-propanol; dimercaprol) was developed as an antidote for Lewisite. BAL is currently used in medicine as a chelating agent for heavy metals. There is evidence that BAL in oil, given intramuscularly, will reduce the systemic effects of Lewisite. However, caution should be taken because there are toxic effects associated with the use of BAL. BAL skin ointment and BAL ophthalmic ointment decrease the severity of skin and eye lesions when applied immediately after early decontamination. However, neither of these formulations is currently manufactured.

There is no antidote or specific treatment for phosgene oxime.

MANAGEMENT OF MASS CASUALTIES

Actual measurements of air concentrations of the liquid or vapor will not likely be available in most casualty situations. Based on history and clinical findings, prompt decontamination followed by symptomatic care is indicated. Topical decontamination is not effective once a chemical agent has been absorbed. For mustard, the greatest efficacy of this treatment is obtained if accomplished in less than 2 minutes after contact, but it may have some value even 15 minutes later.[31] As discussed previously, a dilute 0.5% hypochlorite solution is used by the military as the preferred decontaminating solution for removing mustard from the skin. If this solution is not available, water (with or without soap) can be used. Care should be taken during decontamination not to force a superficial chemical agent into the skin, or create a wound from a high-pressure water stream. High-volume, low-pressure water (with or without soap) should be used for decontaminating large numbers of exposed individuals. Further treatment for mustard exposure should be based on the clinical findings after decontamination.

PRINCIPLES OF PREPAREDNESS

Prevention of contact and prompt decontamination are the paramount public health measures. Individual exposures are difficult to recognize, and a high index of suspicion must be maintained by public service and medical personnel to recognize cases and avoid self-contamination. Butyl rubber provides a good barrier to mustard.[28] The National Institute for Occupational Safety and Health (NIOSH), the U.S. Army Soldier Biological and Chemical Command (SBCCOM), and the National Institute for Standards and Technology (NIST) are working to develop appropriate standards and test procedures for all classes of respirators that will provide respiratory protection from chemical, biological, radiological, and nuclear (CBRN) agent inhalation hazards. Further information can be obtained at http://www.cdc.gov. Contact with mustard does not cause immediate pain and, therefore, does not provide a

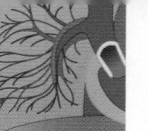

warning to decontaminate or use personal protective equipment (PPE). Contact with the other two groups of vesicants in either liquid or vapor state results in immediate irritation or pain and provides a warning to decontaminate immediately and don PPE. The immediate onset of irritation or pain may result in less severe lesions from these two groups.

Topically applied barrier and other decontamination creams, as well as decontamination powders, have been recently developed. Distribution will initially be limited to military applications.

REFERENCES

1. Willems JL: Clinical management of mustard gas casualties. Ann Med Milit Belg 1989;3S:1–61.
2. Sidell FR, Urbanetti JS, Smith WJ, Hurst CG: Vesicants. In Medical Aspects of Chemical and Biological Warfare. Textbook of Military Medicine. Washington, DC, Borden Institute, 1997.
3. Borak J, Sidell FR: Agents of chemical warfare: sulfur mustard. Ann Emerg Med 1992;21(3):303–308.
4. Committee on Review and Evaluation of the Army Non-Stockpile Chemical Materiel Disposal Program: Disposal of Neutralent Wastes Board on Army Science and Technology. Board on Army Science and Technology. National Research Council, 2001
5. Rosemond GA, Beblo DA, Amata R, authors and chemical managers: Toxicological Profile for Sulfur Mustard (formerly called Mustard Gas). Washington, DC, U.S. Department of Health and Human Services Public Health Service, Agency for Toxic Substances and Disease Registry (ATSDR), 2003.
6. Aasted A, Darre MD, Wulf HC: Mustard gas: clinical, toxicological, and mutagenic aspects based upon modern experience. Ann Plastic Surg 1987;19:330–333.
7. Ruhl CM, Park DJ, Danisa O, Morgan RP, et al: A serious skin sulfur mustard burn from artillery shell. J Emerg Med 1994;12(2):159–166.
8. Papirmeister B, Feister AJ, Robinson SI, Ford RD: Medical Defense Against Mustard Gas: Toxic Mechanisms and Pharmacological Implications. Baton Rouge, FL, CRC Press, 1991.
9. U.S. Army Soldier and Biological Chemical Command (USASBCCOM): Distilled Mustard (HD) Material Safety Data Sheet. Aberdeen Proving Ground, MD, 1999.
10. Rinehart WE, Hatch T: Concentration-time product (CT) as an expression of dose in sublethal exposures to phosgene. Ind Hyg J 1964;25:545–553.
11. Rozman KK, Doull J: The role of time as a quantifiable variable of toxicity and the experimental conditions when Haber's $c \times t$ product can be observed: implications for therapeutics. J Pharmacol Exp Ther 2001;296(3):663–668.
12. Pechura CM, Rall DP (eds): Veterans at Risk: The Health Effects of Mustard Gas and Lewisite. Institute of Medicine. Washington, DC, National Academy Press, 1993.
13. Departments of the Army, the Navy, and the Air Force, and Commandant, Marine Corps: Treatment of Chemical Agent Casualties and Conventional Military Chemical Injuries FM 8-285. Chapter 4: Vesicants. Washington, DC, Author, 1995.
14. Marshall EK, Lynch V, Smith HW: On dichlorethylsulfide (mustard gas) II: variations in susceptibility of the skin to dichlorethylsulfide: J Pharmacol Exp Ther1919;12:291–301.
15. U.S. Department of Health and Human Services (USDHHS): Report on Carcinogens, 10th ed. Washington, DC, Public Health Service, National Toxicology Program, 2002.
16. Momeni AZ, Aminjavaheri M: Skin manifestations of mustard gas in a group of 14 children and teenagers: a clinical study. Int J Dermatol 1994;33(3):184–187.
17. U.S. Army, Headquarters: Assay Techniques for Detection of Exposure to Sulfur Mustard, Cholinesterase Inhibitors, Sarin, Soman, GF, and Cyanide. Technical Bulletin Medical 296. Washington, DC, Author, 1996.
18. Black RM, Read RW: Improved methodology for the detection and quantization of urinary metabolites of sulphur mustard using gas chromatography-tandem mass spectrometry. J Chromatogr 1995;665:97–105.
19. Black RM, Read RW: Application of liquid chromatography-atmospheric pressure chemical ionization mass spectrometry, and tandem mass spectrometry, to the analysis and identification of degradation products of chemical warfare agents. J Chromatogr 1997;759:79–92.
20. United States Army Center for Health Promotion and Preventive Medicine (USACHPPM): Chemical Agent Air Standards Status Table: Existing Standards and Guidelines as of March 2006. Environmental Medicine Program, 2006, http://chppm-www.apgea.army.mil/chemicalagent/PDFFiles/CWA-AirTableMarch2006.pdf, accessed October 25, 2006.
21. National Advisory Council: Acute Exposure Guideline Levels (AEGLs) for Sulfur Mustard (Agent HD). Final Acute Exposure Guidance Levels (AEGLs). Washington, DC, National Advisory Committee on Exposure Guideline Levels for Hazardous Substances, 2001.
22. National Research Council of the National Academies: Acute Exposure Guideline Levels for Selected Airborne Chemicals, Vol 3. Subcommittee on Acute Exposure Guideline Levels, Committee on Toxicology, Board on Environmental Studies and Toxicology, Washington, DC, 2003, http://fermat.nap.edu/books/0309088836/html/R1.html, accessed October 25, 2006.
23. Department of Health and Human Services: Interim Recommendations for Airborne Exposure Limits for Chemical Warfare Agents H and HD (Sulfur Mustard). Centers for Disease Control and Prevention. Fed Reg 2004;69(86):24164–24168, http://a257.g.akamaitech.net/7/257/2422/14mar20010800/edocket.access.gpo.gov/2004/pdf/04-9946.pdf, accessed October 25, 2006.
24. Agency for Toxic Substances and Disease Registry (ATSDR): Minimal Risk Levels (MRLs) for Hazardous Substances. Atlanta, Author, 2005, http://www.atsdr.cdc.gov/mrllist 12 05.pdf, accessed October 25, 2006.
25. Hurst CG: Decontamination. In Medical Aspects of Chemical and Biological Warfare. Textbook of Military Medicine. Washington, DC, Borden Institute, 1997.
26. U.S. Army Center for Health Promotion and Preventive Medicine (USACHPPM). Chemical. In Medical NBC Battlebook; Technical Guide 244. Aberdeen Proving Ground, MD, Author, 2000.
27. Departments of the Army, the Navy, and the Air Force: Vesicants (blister agents). In Part 3: Chemicals; NATO Handbook on the Medical Aspects of NBC Defensive Operations AMedP-6(B). U.S. Army Field Manual 8-9. Washington, DC, Author, 1996.
28. U.S. Army Medical Research Institute of Chemical Defense (USAMRICD): Decontamination in Medical Management of Chemical Casualties Handbook, 3rd ed. Aberdeen Proving Ground, MD, Author, 1999.
29. Coppock R, Hurlbut KM: Mustard gas. In POISINDEX® Information System. Thomson Micromedex Healthcare Series Volume 118. Greenwood Village, CO, 2003.
30. Wartell MA, Kleinman MT, Huey BM, Duffy LM (eds): Decontamination. In Strategies to Protect the Health of Deployed U.S. Forces: Force Protection and Decontamination. Commission on Engineering and Technical Systems. National Research Council. Washington, DC, National Academy Press, 1999.
31. National Center for Environmental Health: Final Recommendations for Protecting the Health and Safety against Potential Adverse Effects of Long-Term Exposure to Low Doses of Agents: GA, BV, VX, Mustard Agent (H, HD, Y), and Lewisite (L). Public Health Service. Centers for Disease Control. Washington, DC, U.S. Department of Health and Human Services, 1988.

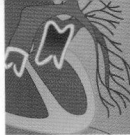

C Choking Agents

LAWRENCE STILWELL BETTS, MD, PHD ■ BRIAN CHRISTOPHER BETTS, MD

At a Glance...

■ Choking agents cause acute effects in the upper respiratory tract and lungs, including irritation, increased secretions, cough, dyspnea, chest tightness, and pulmonary edema.

■ Termination of inhalation exposure by removal of the victim to fresh air (and with copious skin irrigation for liquid exposure), while maintaining the safety of the rescuer, is the initial and most important postexposure action.

■ There is no specific, postexposure management for any of the choking agents.

■ Depending on the severity of exposure, a period of observation is necessary to fully assess and treat potential lung damage and the delayed development of pulmonary edema.

■ The development of several different chronic pulmonary sequelae is possible after acute exposure to agents in this class.

■ After even a mildly significant acute event, follow-up pulmonary function testing may reveal persistent changes.

RELEVANT HISTORY

In the classification of military chemical warfare agents, choking agents are often included in the larger category of "pulmonary" or "lung-damaging" agents. Smokes, as members of the choking agents, are among the oldest of the chemical agents. The use of smoke dates back to the time when humans first exploited this by-product of fire in warfare. Industrial process chemicals, namely, chlorine (military symbol: CL) and phosgene (CG), were used in World War I as simple, but large-scale, chemical weapons. Their use was intended to demoralize the enemy by causing widespread effects from an unseen, and unnatural, opposing force. These two chemicals are representative of the class of chemical warfare agents that cause choking and damage in the upper airways and lungs. The continuum of dose-related toxic effects is similar for all of the choking agents with differences in each agent's properties and potency. Chloropicrin (PS), diphosgene (DP), sulfur mustard (H, HD), and Lewisite (L) are also considered by the military as choking agents, but the latter two substances are primarily classified as vesicants. The choking agents also include chemicals that are used in conventional warfare, such as zinc-containing smoke (HC), as well as chemicals associated with industrial and agricultural processes. The United States does not consider nonlethal chemicals, such as riot control agents and herbicides, as "chemical warfare agents," which are controlled under the 1925 Geneva Convention.[1] Table 105C-1 provides data on selected choking agents and their sources. The riot control agents, such as tear gas and pepper spray, may cause choking and other temporary clinical features associated with the choking agents, but they are not discussed in this chapter.

Specific chemicals that cause choking and that are internationally classified as "chemical weapons (CW)," or feedstock, are listed under the Convention on the Prohibition of the Development, Production, Stockpiling and Use of Chemical Weapons and on their Destruction (Chemical Weapons Convention, CWC)," which entered into force in 1997.[2] This international treaty prohibits

TABLE 105C-1 Select Military Choking Agents				
CHEMICAL	**CHEMICAL SYNONYM**	**CHEMICAL ABSTRACT SERVICE (CAS) NUMBER**	**MILITARY CHEMICAL AGENT SYMBOL**	**INDUSTRIAL OR AGRICULTURAL PRODUCT USES OR BY-PRODUCT**
Phosgene	Carbonyl chloride	75-44-5	CG	Synthesis of drugs, plastics, adhesives, dyes, pesticides
Chlorine	Molecular chlorine	7782-50-5	CL	Chemical synthesis; bleaching agent; water/waste disinfection
Chloropicrin	Trichloronitromethane; nitrochloroform	76-06-2	PS	Fumigant; pesticide; organic synthesis; dyes
Diphosgene	Trichloromethylchloro formate	503-38-8	DP	Limited chemical synthesis
Military smoke*	HC/HC smokes, TiCl$_4$[†], others	Mixture of chemicals; 7550-45-0[†]	HC; FM[†]	Visualization of air movement in ventilation assessments; chemical synthesis; pigments[†]
Perfluoroisobutylene	PFIB	382-21-8	—	Pyrolysis product of organofluoride polymers
Oxides of nitrogen	Nitrogen oxides; NO$_x$	Numerous	—	Combustion of fuels; welding and other high-temperature operations; fermentation

*Military "HC" smoke contains a mixture of chemicals that cause choking. The military also generates smoke through the partial combustion of fuel.
[†]Titanium tetrachloride (TiCl$_4$).

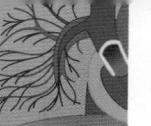

the development, production, stockpiling, and use of chemical weapons. However, it does not prohibit production, processing, consumption, or trade of related chemicals that are verified for use in peaceful purposes. Chlorine was the first lethal choking agent used as a chemical weapon in modern warfare. Chlorine was released in Ypres, Belgium in 1915, but it is not controlled as a potential chemical weapon under the CWC. The use of chlorine as a weapon is now obsolete, but its industrial use is enormous. In addition to the chemicals that have been used, or have the potential to be used, as military weapons, perfluoroisobutylene (PFIB), or 1,1,3,3,3-pentafluoro-2-(trifluoromethyl)-1-propene—a thermal decomposition product of tetrafluoroethylene (Teflon) and other organofluoride polymers—is also a controlled chemical under the CWC. Table 105C-2 provides a list of specifically identified ("named") chemicals that are controlled under the CWC.

The "oxides of nitrogen (NO_x)" comprise a group of compounds that are products of combustion and explosion generated from the discharge of munitions and propellants. These oxides are considered by the U.S. military as choking agents, but they are not used as chemical warfare agents. These compounds can also arise from sources unrelated to combat, including fires, internal combustion engine exhaust, food processing,

and biologic fermentation (see discussion of silo filler's disease in Chapter 9). Military smokes are also considered choking agents because of their use in military applications. They are not directly used in chemical warfare, and like PFIB and the oxides of nitrogen, excessive exposure can damage the airways or lungs.

The clinical features that follow exposure to any of these chemicals are similar—hence their collective grouping as "choking agents." Most important, this class contains chemicals that are associated with the development of potentially fatal pulmonary edema. The onset of this pulmonary edema may be delayed for many hours and is "permeability related," or noncardiogenic in origin.[3]

EXPOSURE SCENARIOS

The historical use of trench warfare, with the massing of large numbers of troops in interconnected, low-lying positions, made the use, or even the potential for use, of a chemical that could cause choking and lung damage a tactic that could be exploited to military advantage. Denser-than-air gases could be released and follow the pathway created by the defensive earthen channels. With a wind favorable to the user, the opposing forces would be forced to abandon their positions or be required to

---

TABLE 105C-2   Named Chemicals and Chemical Abstract Service (CAS) Numbers Scheduled under the Chemical Weapons Convention (CWC)

Schedule 1*	**Toxic chemicals:** sarin (107-44-8); soman (99-64-0); tabun (77-81-6); VX (50782-69-9); sulfur mustards (various); Lewisites (various); nitrogen mustards (various); saxitoxin (50782-69-9); ricin (9009-86-3) and related congeners
	Precursors: methylphosphonyldifluoride (676-99-3); O-ethyl O-2-diisopropylaminoethyl methylphosphonite (57856-11-8); chlorosarin: o-isopropyl methylphosphonochloridate (1445-76-7); chlorosoman: o-pinacolyl methylphosphonochloridate (7040-57-5); and related congeners
Schedule 2†	**Toxic chemicals:** amiton: O,O-diethyl S-[2(diethylamino)ethyl] phosphorothiolate (78-53-5); PFIB: 1,1,3,3,3-pentafluoro-2-(trifluoromethyl)-1-propene (382-21-8); BZ: 3-quinuclidinyl benzilate (6581-06-2); and related congeners
	Precursors: methylphosphonyl dichloride(676-97-1); Dimethyl methylphosphonate (756-79-6); N,N-dialkyl (Me, Et, n-Pr or i-Pr) phosphoramidic dihalides (various); dialkyl (Me, Et, n-Pr or i-Pr) N,N-dialkyl (Me, Et, n-Pr or i-Pr)-phosphoramidates (various); arsenic trichloride (7784-34-1); 2,2-diphenyl-2-hydroxyacetic acid (76-93-7); quinuclidin-3-ol (1619-34-7); N,N-dialkyl (Me, Et, n-Pr or i-Pr) aminoethyl-2-chlorides (various); N,N-dialkyl (Me, Et, n-Pr or i-Pr) aminoethane-2-ols (various); N,N-dialkyl (Me, Et, n-Pr or i-Pr) aminoethane-2-thiols (various); thiodiglycol: bis(2-hydroxyethyl)sulfide (111-48-8); pinacolyl alcohol: 3,3-dimethylbutan-2-ol (464-07-3); and related congeners
Schedule 3‡	**Toxic chemicals:** phosgene (75-44-5); cyanogen chloride (506-77-4); hydrogen cyanide (74-90-8); chloropicrin (76-06-2); and related congeners
	Precursors: phosphorus oxychloride (10025-87-3); phosphorus trichloride (7719-12-2); phosphorus pentachloride (10026-13-8); trimethyl phosphate (121-45-9); triethyl phosphate (122-52-1); dimethyl phosphate (868-85-9); diethyl phosphate (762-04-9); sulfur monochloride (10025-67-9); sulfur dichloride (10545-99-0); thionyl chloride (7719-09-7); ethyldiethanolamine (139-87-7); methyldiethanolamine (105-59-9); triethanolamine (102-71-6); and related congeners

*Criteria considered for listing chemical in schedule 1: chemical has been developed, produced, stockpiled, or used as a chemical weapon; chemical has a high potential for use in prohibited activities due to similarities in structure and toxicity as chemicals listed in Schedule 1; chemical has significant lethality or incapacitating properties that could have application as a chemical weapon; chemical could be used as a precursor in the final stage of production of a Schedule 1 chemical; and chemical has little or no use for nonprohibited purposes.
†Criteria considered for listing chemical in schedule 2: chemical poses a significant risk due to its lethality or incapacitating toxicity and other properties useful in chemical weapons; chemical may be used as a precursor in the final stages of making schedule 1 or 2 chemicals; chemical may be important in the production of schedule 1 or 2 chemicals; and chemicals is not produced in large quantities for purposes that are not prohibited.
‡Criteria considered for listing chemical in schedule 3: chemical has been produced, stockpiled, or used as a chemical weapon; chemical poses a risk due to its lethality or incapacitating toxicity and other properties useful in chemical weapons; chemical may be important in the production of one or more chemicals listed in schedule 1 or schedule 2; and chemical may be produced in large commercial quantities for non-prohibited purposes
Data from Organisation for the Prohibition of Chemical Weapons (OPCW): Convention on the Prohibition of the Development, Production, Stockpiling and Use of Chemical Weapons and on Their Destruction (Chemical Weapons Convention). The Hague, Netherlands, 1997. Available at http://www.opcw.org (updated 2003).

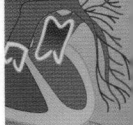

don cumbersome protective equipment. However, even before the end of World War I, the volatile choking agents were replaced with the more persistent (and more controllable) vesicants in order to deny terrain and maneuverability, harass the opposition, cause casualties, consume resources, and create fear. Although no longer a military threat on the battlefield, chemicals that can cause choking and pulmonary damage are found in large quantities in industrial and agricultural settings. The sizeable amounts and widespread availability of this group of chemical agents create the potential for an occupational or environmental catastrophe—or an attractive weapon to a terrorist for release into an enclosed structure. These choking agents do not need to be synthesized by a terrorist; they only need to be commandeered! Concern for the use of these agents by terrorists caused the Centers for Disease Control and Prevention to issue an alert through the Health Alert Network on New Year's Eve 2003.[4]

Phosgene replaced chlorine as a chemical weapon and accounted for 80% of all chemical fatalities during World War I.[5] Although phosgene was stockpiled in munitions for use in World War II, it was not used and is no longer stockpiled by the U.S. military.[6] Phosgene is extensively used as a feedstock in many chemical processes. It is also formed when chlorinated compounds are heated to decomposition. This can occur when a chlorinated compound—found in solvents, degreasers, and dry cleaning agents—contacts a high temperature source, such as a welding arc or flame. Plastic materials containing chlorinated compounds produce phosgene when they burn. Phosgene is considered a potential chemical weapon,[7] and the potential for individual or mass exposure from weaponized military use, industrial accidents, or acts of terror still presents a significant risk. The physiologic effects caused by exposure to phosgene and their medical management are representative of the general class of "choking agents."

Military smokes, or "obscurants," are used to conceal personnel and equipment. Exposure to obscurants may occur in training or combat situations, or the products or devices may be used by terrorists during an attack. HC smoke is produced from a reaction involving zinc oxide, hexachloroethane, and fine aluminum particles. HC smoke contains zinc chloride, as well as phosgene, carbon monoxide, and other chlorinated hydrocarbons. There are many other military obscurants, including chlorosulfonic acid (CSA); titanium tetrachloride (FM), and partially burned hydrocarbons. Although militarily useful in low concentrations, exposure to high or heavy concentrations of obscurants for extended periods can result in illness or death.[5,8]

Choking agents can be produced from nonmilitary processes or sources. PFIB results from the pyrolysis of materials containing organofluoride polymers, such as tetrafluoroethylene (Teflon). Modern military vehicles, aircraft, and vessels use significant amounts of these polymers. Fires in vehicles, aircrafts, ships, and structures present possible situations in which PFIB can be formed and inhaled. Oxides of nitrogen (NO_x) are formed as products of combustion and of fermentation (see Chapters 9 and 86). NO_x may be produced with carbon monoxide during combustion of a fuel in air (air is about 78% nitrogen and about 21% oxygen). In individuals with exposure to exhaust gases from internal combustion engines using various fuels, the physiologic effects of NO_x may be initially combined and masked with those caused by carbon monoxide.[9,10] Silo filler's disease is caused by the inhalation of nitrogen dioxide (one member of the family of NO_x compounds), which is formed during fermentation of corn and other green plants.[11]

PATHOPHYSIOLOGY OF INJURY

Choking agents can cause asphyxiation; irritation and damage to mucous membranes (affecting the airways, alveoli, or the tissues surrounding them); alteration of systemic processes; or an allergic response.[12] The toxic effects caused by exposure to a specific inhaled chemical are due to many factors, including the properties of the chemical, the chemical concentration, and the duration of exposure—the latter two factors comprise the "Ct" product discussed in Chapter 105B. Additional factors are related to the health status of the exposed individual, as well as the individual's level of activity during, and after, the exposure. Heavy activity during exposure results in deeper breathing and deeper penetration of the toxicant into the lungs. Heavy activity after exposure results in greater physiologic stress on the respiratory and circulatory systems—and perhaps a greater degree of tissue damage. The potential to cause delayed pulmonary edema through effects leading to membrane disruption at the alveolar–capillary bed is common to all the choking agents (see Chapters 8 and 9).

MANIFESTATIONS

Choking agents cause acute clinical effects in the upper respiratory tract and lungs, including irritation, increased secretions, cough, dyspnea, chest tightness, and pulmonary edema. One of the most important clinical features of agents in this class is the potential to cause pulmonary edema after a clinically unremarkable latent period. The period of time before the onset of pulmonary edema is related to the severity of the exposure (Ct) and to the prognosis. The onset of signs and symptoms of pulmonary edema within 4 hours of exposure is a sensitive indicator of a poor prognosis. Without intensive medical support, there is a high risk for death in patients with this early finding.[6] Acute exposure to choking agents may result in chronic bronchitis, emphysema, bronchiolitis obliterans, or reactive airway dysfunction syndrome (RADS) (see Chapters 8 and 9).

PRENATAL AND PEDIATRIC ISSUES

Clinically significant exposure to choking agents can result in acute hypoxia in the mother and an associated lowered PO_2 level available to the fetus. This may result in

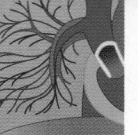

harm to the pregnancy or the fetus. Asthma, in any age group, may be nonspecifically initiated or exacerbated by exposure to the irritant effects of the choking agents.

ASSESSMENT

A history of exposure is essential to make and confirm an early diagnosis during the latent period. A period of observation is necessary as the dose-dependent clinical effects resulting from pulmonary damage become apparent over time. The prognosis for patients developing early pulmonary edema, cyanosis, and hypotension is poor. Survival is greater in patients developing these findings 4 to 6 hours or longer after exposure, and in those with immediate, intensive medical care.[6]

TREATMENT

The primary initial treatment consists of cessation of exposure. For inhalation exposure, moving the patient to fresh air and insuring an open airway and proper ventilation is essential, while taking precautions to prevent the rescuer or caregiver from also becoming a victim! For exposure to liquids, remove clothing and rinse liquid agents off the skin with copious soap or detergent and water irrigation. The eyes should be rinsed with running water or saline. Supplemental oxygen, intubation, suction, and mechanical ventilation are used as needed to treat respiratory distress. Based on the exposure history and clinical findings, a period of forced rest and observation is important in the medical management. The potential development of delayed, noncardiogenic pulmonary edema requires medical observation for a suitable period of time based on the severity of exposure and the clinical course. Treatment of pulmonary edema and other clinical findings, and the use of steroids and other therapeutic agents and modalities, are discussed elsewhere in this text. See Chapters 9, 86, 93, and 102.

A short latent period is a harbinger of a more severe clinical course. Patients developing pulmonary edema within 12 hours of exposure will usually require intensive pulmonary care. Based on U.S. Army triage recommendations, patients with dyspnea and no objective signs should be observed closely and reevaluated hourly. Asymptomatic patients with known exposures should be observed and reevaluated every 2 hours. If these patients remain asymptomatic for 24 hours, they may be considered for discharge. Patients with doubtful exposures, and no symptoms after 12 hours of observation, can also be considered for discharge at that time.[6] The chest radiograph is helpful in the assessment before discharge. If not available, Borak and Diller recommend an observation period of 24 hours for asymptomatic patients after suspected phosgene inhalation.[3]

MANAGEMENT OF MASS CASUALTIES

The activity of patients under evaluation after inhalation of any of the choking agents should be controlled. Physical activity[12] and emotional factors[3] can influence the development and severity of clinical findings.

PRINCIPLES OF PREPAREDNESS

The absence of early signs or symptoms involving mucous membrane irritation or respiratory distress, or a warning odor of a chemical, does not prove that an exposure was inconsequential. It is necessary to maintain vigilance for patients presenting with a reliable history of exposure to a choking agent, or with developing signs and symptoms consistent with such an exposure.

REFERENCES

1. Sidell FR: Riot control agents. In Textbook of Military Medicine: Medical Aspects of Chemical and Biological Warfare. Washington, DC, Office of the Surgeon General, Department of the Army, 1997.
2. Organisation for the Prohibition of Chemical Weapons (OPCW). Convention on the Prohibition of the Development, Production, Stockpiling and Use of Chemical Weapons and on their Destruction (Chemical Weapons Convention). The Hague, NL, 1997 Available at http://www.opcw.org (updated 2003).
3. Borak J, Diller WF: Phosgene exposure: mechanisms of injury and treatment strategies. J Occup Environ Med 2001;43:110–119.
4. Centers for Disease Control and Prevention (CDC): Update on Public Health Precautions related to Orange Threat Level. 2. Public Health Information and Resources for a Possible Chemical Emergency. Distributed via Health Alert Network. CDCHAN-00178-03-12-31-UPD-N. Atlanta, Author, December 31, 2003.
5. Departments of the Army, the Navy, and the Air Force: Lung damaging agents. In Part Three: Chemicals. NATO Handbook on the Medical Aspects of NBC Defensive Operations AMedP-6(B). U.S. Army Field Manual 8–9. Washington, DC, Author, 1996.
6. U.S. Army Medical Research Institute of Chemical Defense (USAMRICD): Pulmonary (Choking) Agents in Medical Management of Chemical Casualties Handbook, 3rd ed. Aberdeen Proving Ground, MD, Author, August 1999.
7. Sidell FR, Frantz D: Overview. Defense Against the Effects of Chemical and Biological Warfare Agents. In Textbook of Military Medicine: Medical Aspects of Chemical and Biological Warfare. Washington, DC, Office of the Surgeon General, Department of the Army, 1997.
8. Evans EH: Casualties following exposure to zinc chloride smoke. Lancet 1945;2:368–370.
9. Anderson DE: Problems created for ice arenas by engine exhaust. Am Ind Hyg Assoc J 1971;32:790–801.
10. Hedberg K, Hedberg CW, Iber C, et al: An outbreak of nitrogen dioxide-induced respiratory illness among ice hockey players: JAMA 1989;262:3014–3017.
11. Douglas WW, Hepper NGG, Colby TV: Silo-filler's disease. Mayo Clin Proc 1989;64:291–304.
12. Urbanetti JS: Toxic inhalational injury. In Textbook of Military Medicine: Medical Aspects of Chemical and Biological Warfare. Washington, DC, Office of the Surgeon General, Department of the Army, 1997.

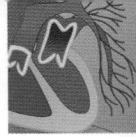

D Lacrimators

ANDIS GRAUDINS, MBBS (HONS), PHD

At a Glance...

- Lacrimators are also known as *irritant incapacitants, tear gas,* and *riot control* or *harassing agents.*
- Lacrimators are used primarily by law enforcement and military personnel for riot control.
- Lacrimators usually result in transient incapacitation with skin and mucosal membrane irritation.
- When used at high concentrations (i.e., enclosed, poorly ventilated spaces), lacrimators may produce significant respiratory and ocular effects.
- Following chronic, high concentration exposures, lacrimators may produce reactive airways dysfunction and dermatitis in sensitized individuals.
- Physical injury (i.e., cutaneous burns and trauma) may be sustained after exposure to exploding cartridges used to deploy lacrimators.
- Treatment is largely supportive; decontamination of the skin and mucosal surfaces is the mainstay of therapy.
- Medical staff should protect themselves with gloves, gowns, and eyewear and work in a well-ventilated environment to avoid secondary exposure to lacrimators from contaminated clothing.

INTRODUCTION AND RELEVANT HISTORY

Lacrimators, also known as *irritant incapacitants, tear gas,* and *riot control* or *harassing agents,* are aerosol-dispersed chemicals that produce near-immediate eye, skin, and upper respiratory tract irritation. Lacrimators have become widely accepted by law enforcement and military personnel as a method of controlling civilian crowds and criminal uprisings in correctional facilities. Virtually all police departments use tear gas as a nonlethal means of subduing suspected criminals. These agents are also advertised as nonlethal personal safety agents (in lieu of gun ownership). Ownership by civilians, however, is illegal in many countries. Large amounts of tear gas have been used worldwide. Tear gas has been used to suppress demonstrations and civil unrest in culturally diverse places, such as Chile, Panama, South Korea, and the Gaza strip and West Bank in Israel. The true incidence of complications associated with the use of these agents is unknown because of the difficulty in collecting epidemiologic information on victims of mass exposures to tear gas. Consequently, the overall safety of these agents has been questioned by the medical community.[1,2]

Although the modern use of irritant incapacitants is for riot control, historically these agents were used in warfare to incapacitate enemy forces. From antiquity to the Middle Ages, oxides of sulfur were combusted upwind of enemies with the aim of enveloping them in a cloud of smoke. Arsenical smoke was used sporadically from the 15th to 17th centuries. In the 20th century, the Paris police were the first to use chemical agents in 1912. Grenades filled with ethylbromoacetate (EBA) were deployed against "lawless gangs." EBA was also used in the early phases of World War I by French ex-police conscripts.[3,4] Modern tear gas agents were first used in the United States during the crime waves of the 1920s to combat gangsters and as personal protection agents.[5] Subsequently, many harassing agents have been developed. Dispersal systems have also been refined in the ensuing years to improve delivery of these agents.

As many as 15 different irritants have been developed during the course of this century. Of these, only four lacrimator agents remain in common use worldwide: 1-chloracetophenone (CN, Mace); 2-chlorobenzylidene malonitrile (CS); dibenz-1,4-oxazepine (CR); and capsaicin (pepper spray, "pepper Mace").[4]

CHLOROACETOPHENONE

CN is the oldest of the currently used lacrimators. The name "Mace" originally described this agent alone.[4] The eponym MACE was derived from a particular chemical formulation of CN: methylchloroform chloroacetophenone. CN is manufactured by chlorination of acetophenone with selenium oxychloride.[4,5] Its chemical formula is $C_6H_5COCH_2Cl$. Under normal atmospheric conditions, chloroacetophenone exists as a white solid or powder.[4] It can be delivered as a smoke from thermal grenades or artillery shells or as a solid or liquid aerosol. CN is heat stable, breaking down only when exposed to temperatures greater than 300° C for 15 minutes or more.[4] CN is poorly soluble in water, even when alkalinized; this characteristic predicts a moderate degree of environmental persistence and resistance to skin decontamination with soap and water.[4,6] When used in large amounts, CN can persist in the environment for hours to days, depending on prevailing meteorologic conditions.[4,7]

Although less potent than CS, CN is the most toxic of the currently used lacrimators.[3,4,6] The concentration-time product ($mg \cdot min/m^3$) of CN that will incapacitate 50% of exposed individuals (ICt_{50}) is about 10 times greater than that for CS, yet the concentration-time product that will be lethal to 50% of exposed individuals (LCt_{50}) is about 6 times less than that for CS[3,4,6] (Table 105D-1). At high concentrations, CN has produced permanent corneal epithelial damage, severe skin irritation with blistering, noncardiogenic pulmonary edema, and asphyxiation. At least five deaths have occurred from acute pulmonary injury or asphyxiation when CN grenades were used in enclosed spaces.[3,4,6,8,9]

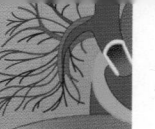

	CN	CS	CR
TC_{50} [eyes] (mg/m^3)	0.3	0.004	0.002
TC_{50} [airway] (mg/m^3)	0.4	0.023	0.002
ICt_{50} $(mg \cdot min/m^3)$	20–40	3–5	0.7
LCt_{50} $(mg \cdot min/m^3)$	7000–14,000	60,000	>100,000

TABLE 105D-1 Riot Control Agents: Comparison of Potency and Toxicity

TC_{50}, the concentration in air (mg/m^3) that will irritate the eyes of 50% of the population exposed; ICt_{50}, the concentration time product $(mg \cdot min/m^3)$ that incapacitates 50% of the population exposed; LCt_{50}, the concentration time product $(mg \cdot min/m^3)$ that is lethal to 50% of the population exposed.
Modified from Beswick FW: Chemical agents used in riot control and warfare. Hum Toxicol 1983;2:247–256; Sidell FR: Riot control agents. In Sidell FR, Takafuji ET, Frank DR (eds): Textbook of Military Medicine. I. Warfare, Weaponry, and the Casualty: Medical Aspects of Chemical and Biological Warfare. Washington DC, Office of the Surgeon General, 1997, pp 307–324; and Blain PG: Tear gases and irritant incapacitants: 1-chloroacetophenone, 2-chlorobenzylidene malonitrile and dibenz[B,F]-1,4-oxazepine. Toxicol Rev 2003;22(2):103–110.

CHLORBENZYLIDENE MALONITRILE

CS was first produced in 1928 by Corson and Stoughton (hence the designation CS).[4,6] Because it is more effective and less toxic than CN (see Table 105D-1), CS became the standard riot control agent used by military and law enforcement agencies in 1959.[4] CS is still the riot control agent most commonly used worldwide today.[4,6] Chemically, CS is a variant of an older, previously used irritant, bromobenzyl cyanide. It is a stable gas with a pepper-like odor.[10] CS exists as a crystalline powder and is dispersed by aerosol blowers, hand-held devices, or bursting thermal grenades.[4,7] The chemical formula of CS is $ClC_6H_4CHCCH(CN)_2$.[4,6] Vaporization of CS can be achieved by igniting a mixture of the powder with a fuel substance, producing clouds of white smoke containing CS vapor.[10] When detonated in the open, a CS grenade can produce a cloud 6 to 9 M in diameter. The concentration of CS at the center of the cloud can range from 2000 to 5000 mg/m^3, rapidly declining at the periphery.[2] Detonation in an enclosed space, or multiple-grenade-burst detonation, has the potential for producing much higher concentrations. High-temperature dispersal (>700° C) of CS has been shown to release small amounts of hydrogen cyanide and hydrochloric acid as air contaminants.[11] The clinical effects of this are unknown. CS is rapidly hydrolyzed in water and even more rapidly in aqueous alkaline solutions.[6] Unlike CN, CS is readily inactivated in soap and water.[4,6] The U.S. military has developed hydrophobic, microencapsulated formulations of CS (CS1 and CS2) that are resistant to water degradation.[4] These formulations have not been used by civilian authorities because of their environmental persistence.

DIBENZOXAZEPINE

CR was first synthesized in 1962.[4] It is the most potent and least toxic lacrimator currently used[4,6] (see Table 105D-1). CR is about 5 to 10 times more potent than CS and is effective at concentrations as low as 1 mg/m^3.[4,6] The lethal dose in humans is thought to be 2 times that of CS and more than 10 times that of CN.[3,4,6] CR is more stable than CN or CS because of a lower water solubility and vapor pressure.[6] CR is, thus, much more persistent in the environment than the other lacrimators.[3,4,6] CR is commonly deployed as a liquid but can also be aerosolized. Because CR is usually delivered in solution, its effects tend to be localized to the skin and eyes. Pulmonary effects are rare owing to its low vapor pressure. Compared with other lacrimators, skin and eye effects are not as persistent following CR exposure. Based on animal studies, CR appears to be less toxic than CN or CS, but few data exist to support or refute these observations in humans.[3]

CAPSAICIN

Capsaicin (8-methyl-N-vanillyl-6-nonenamide) is the active ingredient largely responsible for the irritating and pungent effects of the fruits of the various species of *Capsicum*. These include the Mexican chile pepper and the Hungarian red pepper.[12] The potent topical irritant effects of capsaicin have made its use as a personal protection and immobilizing device appealing for both law enforcement agencies and the civilian population. Repeated topical capsaicin application has been used for cutaneous counterirritant effects in chronic pain and inflammatory conditions.

In 1993, more than 6 million "pepper gas" spray units were sold in the United States alone.[13] When used as a harassing agent, capsaicin is used as a spray at close quarters. When used correctly, capsaicin can result in transient, severe skin and mucous membrane irritation, incapacitating an assailant rapidly. Improper use has resulted in significant morbidity in a small number of reported cases.

News reports in the lay press have raised the issue of deaths in custody temporally related to the use of capsaicin sprays. Extensive testing by the Federal Bureau of Investigation in the 1980s found no evidence of toxic problems with capsaicin use.[14] No firm scientific data currently substantiate any casual relationship between these deaths and capsaicin exposure. In these situations, victims are often in an agitated state requiring restraint, which may be implemented in a way that unintentionally produces postural asphyxia.[14] Victims are often under the influence of alcohol and drugs of abuse, which may increase aggression, mask occult trauma, and delay recognition of medical problems. In the absence of any definite link between capsaicin exposure and sudden death, law enforcement agencies currently continue to use capsaicin as a harassing agent.

EXPOSURE SCENARIOS

Riot control agents are generally dispersed as liquid or solid aerosols.[4,6] The circumstances of an exposure (i.e.,

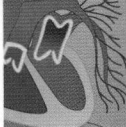

intended target and purpose) dictate the specific method of riot control agent delivery. Irritant smoke can be produced by combining the agent (CN or CS) with a pyrotechnic mixture containing chlorate and lactose. The igniter vaporizes the irritant, which then condenses into a cloud of solid or liquid particles 1 to 2 μm in diameter that can be easily inhaled.[7] This method is best used in the control of large-scale riots. CS also exists as a micropulverized powder that can be dispersed by mechanical force, using a vehicle- or aircraft-mounted "smoke" generator, or from a hand-held tank using carbon dioxide as a propellant.[7] This method does not require the use of a thermal agent to volatilize the irritant.

Most lacrimators have low water solubility, which necessitates their dissolution in a hydrocarbon organic solvent when used in pressurized, hand-held, delivery devices.[6] For instance, Mace is a 1% solution of CN in a solvent mixture containing kerosene, 1,1,1-trichloroethane, and Freon 113.[6] The United Kingdom police personnel carry hand-held CS spray devices that contain 5% CS in a methyl isobutyl ketone solvent.[6] Pepper spray devices contain tetrachloroethylene, Freon, or isopropyl alcohol as the hydrocarbon vehicle.[6] These organic solvent mixtures are irritants themselves and will potentiate lacrimator toxicity.[3,6]

CN and CS can also be delivered by a thermal grenade or a cartridge fired from a gun. Grenades are often launched into confined spaces by law enforcement agencies to incapacitate criminals in siege situations. Thermal grenades may produce fires.[7] There is a risk for mechanical trauma and burns to victims hit by projectiles or in close proximity to exploding grenades.[15,16]

In general, CS and CN used as a particulate smoke tend to affect the eyes and respiratory tract to a greater degree than the skin. Aerosols and liquid sprays are likely to produce more marked effects on the skin and eyes with less effect on the respiratory tract.

PATHOPHYSIOLOGY OF INJURY

The mechanism of tissue injury from CN and CS is not fully elucidated but likely results from alkylation of key tissue enzymes and direct reactivity of their respective chloride moiety with mucosal tissue.[6] Both CN and CS are SN_2 alkylating agents and likely produce tissue toxicity after binding and inhibiting key sulfhydryl-containing enzymes (e.g., lactic dehydrogenase and thioctic acid of the pyruvate decarboxylase complex).[6] Alkylation of cellular proteins also increases the potential for mutagenesis.[3] In addition, CS exposure has been shown to result in the production of bradykinin locally, which could produce tissue edema and inflammatory injury.[3,17] Animal studies and postmortem human data have demonstrated intra-alveolar hemorrhage, pulmonary exudation of protein and polymorphonuclear cells, and tissue necrosis after exposure to high concentrations of CN.[8,9] This is followed by suppressed phagocytic capability of immunocompetent cells. Increased susceptibility to infection is a potential consideration after large or repeated exposures to CN.[18,19] The actual risk for infection to humans after massive exposures to CN or other lacrimators is unknown. Additionally, little is known about the risk for chronic pulmonary toxicity, genotoxicity, or reproductive toxicologic effects associated with CN and CS exposure.

When animals are given lethal doses of CS by parenteral injection, CS is metabolized to cyanide, as evidenced by elevated levels of blood thiocyanate within hours.[6] Inhalation and cutaneous exposures, however, do not produce significant amounts of free cyanide in plasma because systemic absorption of CS by these routes is extremely small.[3,6] Thus, victims of CS poisoning do not need treatment for cyanide toxicity.[6]

The mechanism of action of capsaicin on cutaneous nerve endings has been extensively studied. Application of capsaicin to the skin or mucous membranes results in widespread excitation of cutaneous C-fiber polymodal nociceptor afferent nerve terminals. Capsaicin achieves this by nonspecifically opening nerve fiber sodium, calcium, and potassium channels and releasing substance P from nerve endings.[20] This produces an intense sensation of burning pain and marked hyperalgesia to skin heating and pressure. Symptoms may be exacerbated by the presence of sweat or the application of cold water. Hyperalgesia may persist for as long as 24 hours. Cutaneous vasodilation is also seen at the site of application and the surrounding skin through an axon flare reflex.[20]

MANIFESTATIONS

All lacrimators produce near-immediate stinging and burning of the skin and mucosal surfaces, lacrimation, blepharospasm, salivation, and rhinorrhea.[4,6,7,21] Inhalation produces a sensation of chest constriction with dyspnea, gagging, and burning of the respiratory tract.[4,6,22] The dermal irritant effects of all agents are enhanced in the presence of moisture or sweat on the skin. Hot, humid weather can produce a similar augmentation of irritant effects.[4,10] Sensitivity to tear gas is individual and age dependent.[6] Children appear to be more susceptible to the toxic effects.[6] In most instances, the effects of tear agents are transient and dissipate within 30 minutes of removal from the source of exposure.[23] More prolonged effects may be seen with higher-concentration, enclosed-space exposures. In addition, ocular effects may be prolonged. Conjunctivitis and blurred vision may persist for as long as 24 hours after exposure.[22]

The eye is the most sensitive organ to tear gas agents.[3,4,6] The threshold value for eye irritation is as low as 0.002 mg/m^3 for CR[3,4,6] (see Table 105D-1). An effective aerosol concentration of 5 mg/m^3 results in severe burning of the eyes, with lacrimation, blepharospasm, and conjunctival injection. Ocular injuries include mild conjunctival irritation, corneal and periorbital edema, focal corneal epithelial injury, iridocyclitis, and necrotizing, coagulative keratoconjunctivitis.[4,6,24] Permanent corneal damage has occurred from CN particles becoming embedded on the cornea, particularly after exposure to aerosolized particulates.[25] Epithelial recovery of the

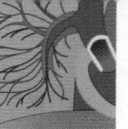

cornea may take months, leaving permanent corneal opacities and visual loss.[26] Direct spraying of CN, capsaicin, and similar agents onto the face from high-pressure aerosols has the potential to produce barotrauma to the eyes.

Cutaneous injury from tear agents is more likely to occur with aerosol or liquid spray exposures; prolonged, concentrated exposures; direct contact of an agent to skin or exposure through wet clothing; or exposure to skin that is thin, moist, abraded, or has preexisting disease.[4,6] Skin effects include simple stinging and burning, erythema, vesication, and allergic dermatitis. For instance, CN exposure has resulted in cutaneous allergic reactions and dermatitis, skin burns, and bullous eruptions from prolonged exposure or direct spraying of CN onto the skin.[27,28] Generalized papulovesicular rashes responding to treatment with systemic steroid therapy have also been reported.[28] Despite initial enthusiasm for the use of CS as a less toxic alternative to CN, reports of significant toxicity of CS have appeared in the medical literature. Severe reactions to CS have resulted from its direct spraying onto cutaneous surfaces. Vesicular dermatitis with blistering, crusting, and marked facial swelling has developed from 12 hours to 3 days after either single or repeated exposures to CS.[29] Allergic contact dermatitis has been documented in cases of recurrent exposure to CS, with allergy subsequently confirmed by patch testing.[29] Skin discomfort may recur up to 48 hours after CR exposure when exposed skin contacts water.[30,31] Cutaneous application of capsaicin over days to weeks can result in habituation to its irritant effects and hypalgesia of the skin.[20] In contrast, severe dermatitis, labeled *Hunan hand syndrome*, may result after skin exposure to capsaicin. This is particularly common in people who handle chile peppers with bare hands, resulting in severe pain and erythema of exposed surfaces.[32,33] Relief from symptoms may be difficult to achieve.

Respiratory effects from lacrimators include nasal irritation, rhinorrhea, sneezing, mouth burning, sore throat, cough, chest tightness, and bronchorrhea. Effects typically resolve within 30 minutes for most exposures.[4,6] Tidal volume and minute ventilation have been observed to decrease with experimental exposure to CS.[34] The reasons for this are uncertain. Inhalation of capsaicin by asthmatic and nonasthmatic volunteers resulted in coughing and transient increases in airway resistance. This is postulated to be due to stimulation of airway sensory nerves.

High-concentration, enclosed-space exposures to lacrimators have resulted in acute laryngotracheo-bronchitis, pulmonary edema, and death.[6] Pulmonary edema is delayed in onset, occurring 6 to 8 hours after exposure.[35] Death is extremely rare but has occurred from pulmonary edema 12 hours after exposure to CN.[8,36] Severe respiratory distress and bronchopneumonia were identified in a 4-month-old infant after exposure to CS for 2 to 3 hours in an enclosed space.[37,38] Respiratory symptoms may persist for days to weeks after exposure and include cough, dyspnea, hemoptysis, and wheezing.[2,39] Reactive airways dysfunction has been described after exposure to CS and CR.[6,40,41] Permanent lung damage is unlikely to occur from lacrimator exposure; long-term effects typically resolve by 12 weeks after exposure.[6]

Respiratory symptoms and signs are uncommon after exposure to capsaicin; effects are likely related to direct exposure of the respiratory tract to capsaicin. Laryngeal edema, stridor, and pulmonary edema requiring endo-tracheal intubation were observed in an 11-year-old boy 4 hours after the intentional inhalation of several sprays of a capsaicin in a hydrofluorocarbon vehicle. His clinical condition improved over 24 hours.[42] A 4-week-old infant accidentally sprayed in the face with a 5% capsaicin aerosol developed respiratory failure and pulmonary edema, requiring extracorporeal membrane oxygenation.[42] It is difficult to ascertain the degree of influence that inhaled capsaicin had in the evolution of pulmonary injury in both cases. Exposure to high concentrations of hydrocarbon propellant may have also had a role in the development of lung injury.[42]

Nausea and vomiting may result from swallowing saliva that contains CS. Oral ingestion of CS has resulted in oropharyngeal irritation and pain, nausea, vomiting, abdominal cramping, and diarrhea.[4,6,43] Increases in pulse and blood pressure often occur immediately after tear agent exposure. These cardiovascular responses are transient and are secondary to the anxiety and pain of exposure rather than the direct effects of tear agents.[6]

The risk for congenital anomalies, stillbirth, and spontaneous abortion was not increased in areas of heavy tear gas use in Londonderry during the late 1960s.[44] However, cytotoxic and mutagenic activity has been observed in mammalian cells in culture exposed to CS.[45] Animal studies have been unable to conclusively prove any carcinogenic or teratogenic effects after exposure to CR or CS tear gas.[46]

ASSESSMENT

The diagnosis of tear agent exposure is based on a suggestive history and physical findings. The acute onset of irritant effects to the eyes, nose, and respiratory tract in one or more patients following an airborne chemical exposure suggests tear agent toxicity. Similar effects may occur after exposure to other irritant or corrosive gases (i.e., choking agents, ammonia), allergic reactions, and exacerbations of asthma or chronic obstructive disease. The history should include details of the exposure (time, duration, nature), associated trauma, treatment before arrival, and symptoms and past medical history of the victim. Of particular importance is whether the exposure occurred in an enclosed space or out in the open. The physical examination should focus on the patency of the airway and adequacy of respirations, vital signs, mental status, and ocular and skin findings. Patients with eye symptoms should have fluorescein and slit-lamp examination to determine the presence of corneal injury. Patients with respiratory symptoms must be re-evaluated frequently. Although lacrimators may be identified by gas chromatography/mass spectrometry and other techniques,[6] laboratory identification of lacrimators is not possible or necessary at most hospitals.

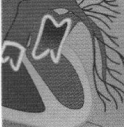

TREATMENT

Most victims exposed to lacrimators develop transient symptoms and signs of skin and mucosal irritation that usually subside within 15 to 30 minutes of removal from the source of the exposure.[4,6] Thus, medical treatment is often unnecessary. Treatment of victims after more significant exposure is supportive. The first priorities of treatment are health care provider self-protection and patient decontamination to reduce ongoing irritation. Health care personnel should protect themselves with gloves, gowns, and eyewear. Victims should be treated in a well-ventilated area to prevent atmospheric accumulation of the tearing agent. Contaminated clothing should be removed and discarded in plastic bags. Exposed skin areas should be washed with copious amounts of warm water and soap. Attempted orotracheal intubation of patients exposed to CS has resulted in severe blepharospasm and lacrimation in anesthesiologists performing the procedure owing to oropharyngeal contamination with tear gas.[47] This situation may result in difficulty or delay in airway control in a patient with otherwise normal airway anatomy.

The eyes should be irrigated for at least 30 minutes with normal saline in symptomatic patients. This should be followed by ophthalmologic assessment for ocular injury, including fluorescein and slit-lamp examination for corneal ulceration and abrasion. Particulate matter should be removed carefully with a cotton swab. Treatment with topical antibiotics, cycloplegics, and oral analgesics should be provided as necessary. Persisting symptoms and signs require formal ophthalmologic follow-up. Skin erythema alone does not usually require any treatment and usually diminishes within 24 hours. Severely affected skin areas that are denuded and oozing may be treated with wet compresses containing avena (colloidal oatmeal) or aluminum acetate (Burow solution).[4,6] Contact dermatitis due to CN or CS has responded to topical or systemic corticosteroid therapy and antipruritics.[4,27,48] Immersion of the hands in vinegar has been successful in providing relief if applied within 30 minutes of exposure to capsaicin.[49] Topical lidocaine gel has also been successful in relief of irritation.[32] Prolonged immersion of hands in vegetable oil after exposure to chile slurry has also been found to provide better long-term relief from the pain of Hunan hand than bathing in cool tap water.[50] Milk compresses and topical antacid suspensions have also been suggested as effective analgesics measures for the relief of capsaicin-induced dermal irritation.[51,52]

Respiratory symptoms due to CN or CS exposure are usually transient and should disappear within 15 to 30 minutes of removal from the exposure environment. Factors that may increase the risk for persisting pulmonary symptoms and development of pulmonary edema include prolonged exposure to CN or CS in an enclosed space, direct inhalation of capsaicin into the respiratory tract, or a history of asthma or other chronic lung disease. Humidified oxygen should be provided as necessary. Bronchospasm may respond to inhaled β-adrenergic agonists and oral or parenteral corticosteroids. Patients with persistent symptoms or signs of respiratory distress may be at risk for delayed pulmonary edema and require observation for 12 to 24 hours. Standard supportive measures and ventilatory support are indicated for pulmonary edema. Extracorporeal membrane oxygenation has been successfully used to support an infant with pulmonary edema after exposure to capsaicin aerosol.[42] Because reactive airways dysfunction may be a long-term consequence of patients presenting with significant acute respiratory symptoms, pulmonary specialist follow-up may be necessary for severely affected patients.

Finally, attention should also be paid to the potential for physical injury and burns to victims of harassing agents. Injury may be masked by the presence of alcohol or other drugs of abuse. Trauma may be due to the violent situations in which the individuals were involved or may be a direct consequence of ballistic trauma due to the projectiles used to propel harassing agents.

MANAGEMENT OF MASS CASUALTIES

Similar to other airborne toxicants, tear gas release can create a multiple-casualty incident. The priorities in management of mass casualties from tear gas include immediate removal of all victims from the source of exposure, decontamination of symptomatic patients, and the provision of supportive care as indicated. Fortunately, less than 1% of exposed patients require medical care because of the mild and transient nature of their symptoms.[6] In ideal situations, prehospital, hazardous material (Hazmat) personnel provide on-scene triage, initial patient assessment, decontamination, and symptomatic treatment. Hazmat personnel only transport patients with significant or persistent effects. In circumstances in which prehospital care does not occur and multiple victims present unannounced to the hospital, symptomatic care and patient decontamination (e.g., clothing removal, eye and skin irrigation) should be delivered in a predetermined, segregated area of the emergency department (see Chapter 103). Activation of a hospital's internal disaster plan is unlikely necessary for multiple casualties from a tear gas incident but will depend on the number and experience of hospital personnel, the number of victims, and the severity of their illness.

PRINCIPLES OF PREPAREDNESS

Preparation for casualties from tear gas exposure does not require any specialized equipment that would not already be present in most emergency departments (see Chapter 103). The presence of a decontamination area that is segregated from the rest of the emergency department and can treat multiple victims simultaneously is ideal. It is recommended that you be familiar with the treatment of chemical casualties and the principles of advanced Hazmat life support in order to optimize patient care.

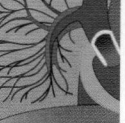

REFERENCES

1. Fraunfelder FT: Is CS gas dangerous? Current evidence suggests not but unanswered questions remain. BMJ 2000;320:458–459.
2. Hu H, Fine J, Epstein P, et al: Tear gas—harassing agent or toxic chemical weapon? JAMA 1989;262:660–663.
3. Beswick FW: Chemical agents used in riot control and warfare. Hum Toxicol 1983;2:247–256.
4. Sidell FR: Riot control agents. In Sidell FR, Takafuji ET, Frank DR (eds): Textbook of Military Medicine. I. Warfare, Weaponry, and the Casualty: Medical Aspects of Chemical and Biological Warfare. Washington DC, Office of the Surgeon General, 1997, pp 307–324.
5. Sanford JP: Medical aspects of riot control (harassing agents). Annu Rev Med 1976;27:421–429.
6. Blain PG: Tear gases and irritant incapacitants: 1-chloroacetophenone, 2-chlorobenzylidene malonitrile and dibenz[B,F]-1,4-oxazepine. Toxicol Rev 2003;22(2):103–110.
7. Compton AF: Chloracetophenone (CN). In Compton AF (ed): Military Chemical and Biological Agents—Chemical and Toxicological Properties. Caldwell, NJ, Telford Press, 1987.
8. Stein AA, Kirwan WE: Chloroacetophenone (tear gas) poisoning: a clinicopathologic report. J Forensic Sci 1964;9:374–382.
9. Chapman AJ, White C: Death resulting from lacrimatory agents. J Forensic Sci 1978;23:527–530.
10. Danto BL: Medical problems and criteria regarding the use of tear gas by police. Am J Forensic Med Pathol 1987;8:317–322.
11. Kluchinsky TA Jr, Savage PB, Fitz R, Smith PA et al: Liberation of hydrogen cyanide and hydrogen chloride during high-temperature dispersion of CS riot control agent. AIHA J 2002;63:493–496.
12. Virus RM, Gebhart GF: Pharmacologic actions of capsaicin: apparent involvement of substance P and serotonin. Life Sci 1979;25:1273–1283.
13. Wily J, Balmier D, Farina P: Severe pulmonary injury in an infant after pepper gas self defence spray exposure [abstract]. J Toxicol Clin Toxicol 1995;33:519.
14. Krolikowski FJ: Oleo capsicum (O.C.): the need for careful evaluation. Am J Forensic Med Pathol 1994;15:267.
15. Zekri AM, King WW, Yeung R, Taylor WR: Acute mass burns caused by O-chlorobenzylidene malononitrile (CS) tear gas. Burns 1995;21:586–589.
16. Clarot F, Vaz E, Papin F, et al: Lethal head injury due to tear-gas cartridge gunshots. Forensic Sci Int 2003;137:45–51.
17. Cucinell SA, Swentzel KC, Biskup R, et al: Biochemical interactions and metabolic fate of riot control agents. Fed Proc 1971;30:86–91.
18. Kumar P, Flora SJ, Pant SC, et al: Toxicological evaluation of 1-chloroacetophenone and dibenz[b,f]-1,4-oxazepine after repeated inhalation exposure in mice. J Appl Toxicol. 1994;14:411–416.
19. Kumar P, Vijayaraghavan R, Pant SC, et al: Effect of inhaled aerosol of 1-chloroacetophenone (CN) and Dibenz (b,f)-1,4 oxazepine (CR) on lung mechanics and pulmonary surfactants in rats. Hum Exp Toxicol 1995;14:404–409.
20. Lynn B: Capsaicin: actions on nociceptive C-fibres and therapeutic potential. Pain 1990;41:61–69.
21. Tominack RL, Spyker DA: Capsicum and capsaicin—a review: case report of the use of hot peppers in child abuse. J Toxicol Clin Toxicol 1987;25:591–601.
22. Punte CL, Gutentag PJ, Owens EJ: Inhalation studies with chloracetophenone, diphenylaminochlorasine and pelargonic morpholide. Eleven human exposures. Am Ind Hyg Assoc J 1962;23:199–202.
23. Holland P, White RG: The cutaneous reactions produced by O-chlorobenzyl-idenemalononitrile and -chloroacetophenone when applied directly to the skin of human subjects. Br J Dermatol 1972;86:150–154.
24. Vesaluoma M, Muller L, Gallar J, et al: Effects of oleoresin capsicum pepper spray on human corneal morphology and sensitivity. Invest Ophthalmol Vis Sci 2000;41:2138–2147.
25. Gaskins JR, Hehir RM, McCaulley DF, Ligon EW Jr : Lacrimating agents (CS and CN) in rats and rabbits. Acute effects on mouth, eyes, and skin. Arch Environ Health 1972;24:449–454.
26. Liss G: Reaction to Mace. J Am Intraocul Implant Soc 1982;8:371.
27. Treudler R, Tebbe B, Blume-Peytavi U, et al: Occupational contact dermatitis due to 2-chloracetophenone tear gas. Br J Dermatol 1999;140:531–534.
28. Thorburn KM: Injuries after use of the lacrimatory agent chloroacetophenone in a confined space. Arch Environ Health 1982;37:182–186.
29. Ro YS, Lee CW: Tear gas dermatitis. Allergic contact sensitization due to CS. Int J Dermatol 1991;30:576–577.
30. Holland P: The cutaneous reactions produced by dibenzooxazepine (CR). Br J Dermatol 1974;90:657–659.
31. Ballantyne B, Gazzard MF, Swanston DW, Williams P: The comparative ophthalmic toxicology of 1-chloroacetophenone (CN) and dibenz(b.f)-1,4-oxazepine(CR). Arch Toxicol 1975;34:183–201.
32. Williams SR, Clark RF, Dunford JV: Contact dermatitis associated with capsaicin: Hunan hand syndrome. Ann Emerg Med 1995;25:713–715.
33. Weinberg RB: Hunan hand. N Engl J Med 1981;305:1020.
34. Cole TJ, Cotes JE, Johnson GR: Ventilation, cardiac frequency and pattern of breathing during exercise in men exposed to O-chlorbenzylidene malonitrile (CS) and ammonia gas in low concentrations. Q J Exp Physiol 1977;62:341–351.
35. Vaca FE, Myers JH, Langdorf M: Delayed pulmonary edema and bronchospasm after accidental lacrimator exposure. Am J Emerg Med 1996;14:402–405.
36. Thomas RJ, Smith PA, Rascona DA, et al. Acute pulmonary effects from o-chlorobenzylidenemalonitrile "tear gas": a unique exposure outcome unmasked by strenuous exercise after a military training event. Mil Med 2002;167:136–139.
37. Park S, Giammona ST: Toxic effects of tear gas on an infant following prolonged exposure. Am J Dis Child 1972;123:245–246.
38. Fuller RW: Pharmacology of inhaled capsaicin in humans. Respir Med 1991;85(Suppl A):31–34.
39. Hill AR, Silverberg NB, Mayorga D, Baldwin HE: Medical hazards of the tear gas CS. A case of persistent, multisystem, hypersensitivity reaction and review of the literature. Medicine 2000;79:234–240.
40. Hu H, Christiani D: Reactive airways dysfunction after exposure to tear gas. Lancet 1992;339:1535.
41. Roth VS, Franzblau A: RADS after exposure to a riot-control agent: a case report. J Occup Environ Med 1996;38:863–865.
42. Winograd HL: Acute croup in an older child: an unusual toxic origin. Clin Pediatr 1977;16:884–887.
43. Solomon I, Kochba I, Eizenkraft E, MaharshakN: Report of accidental CS ingestion among seven patients in central Israel and review of the current literature. Arch Toxicol 2003;77:601–604.
44. Himsworth H: Report of the enquiry into the medical and toxicological aspects of CS (orthochlorbenzylidene malonitrile). II. Enquiry into toxicological aspects of CS and its use for civil purposes. London, Her Majesty's Stationary Office, 1971.
45. Ziegler-Skylakakis K, Summer KH, Andrae U: Mutagenicity and cytotoxicity of 2-chlorbenzylidene malonitrile (CS) and metabolites in V79 Chinese hamster cells. Arch Toxicol 1989;63:314–319.
46. Anonymous: NTP toxicology and carcinogenesis studies of 2-chloroacetophenone (CAS No. 532-27-4) in F344/N rats and B6C3F1 mice (inhalation studies). Natl Toxicol Program Tech Rep Ser 1990;379:1–191.
47. Bhattacharya ST, Hayward AW: CS gas—implications for the anaesthetist. Anaesthesia 1993;48:896–897.
48. Parneix-Spake A, Theisen A, Roujeau JC, Revuz J: Severe cutaneous reactions to self-defense sprays. Arch Dermatol 1993;129:913.
49. Vogl TP: Treatment of Hunan hand. N Engl J Med 1982;306:178.
50. Jones LA, Tandberg D, Troutman WG: Household treatment for "Chile burns" of the hands. J Toxicol Clin Toxicol 1987;25:483–491.
51. Herman LM, Kindschu MW, Shallash AJ: Treatment of Mace dermatitis with topical antacid suspension. Am J Emerg Med 1998;16:613–614.
52. Anderson W: Relief of capsaicin contact dermatitis. Ann Emerg Med 1995;26:659–660.

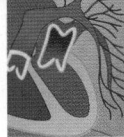

E Central Nervous System Disabling Agents

JEFFREY R. SUCHARD, MD

At a Glance...

- 3-Quinuclidinyl benzilate (BZ, QNB) or similar agents may disable by producing antimuscarinic effects, including visual impairment, ataxia, and delirium. Treatment consists of supportive care and the judicious use of restraints, sedation, and/or anticholinesterase agents (e.g., physostigmine) to reverse central antimuscarinic toxicity.
- Ultrapotent opioids (fentanyl derivatives) may be used as incapacitating agents, producing an opioid toxidrome with depressed mental status and respiratory drive. Treatment consists of airway management and opiate-receptor antagonists (e.g., naloxone).

RELEVANT HISTORY

Central nervous system (CNS) disabling or incapacitating agents are nonlethal compounds intended to temporarily disrupt an enemy's ability to fight. For over 2000 years, military planners have occasionally used chemical agents to alter the mental status of and temporarily incapacitate their enemy rather than cause death or permanent physical injury. In an era before aerosol dissemination of chemical agents was technically feasible, food or water contamination was the primary method used to disable the enemy; belladonna alkaloids were frequently used for this purpose. As early as 200 BCE, the Carthaginian officer Maharbal mixed wine with the antimuscarinic agent "mandragora" and then abandoned camp during a feigned retreat. Rebellious African forces discovered and drank the drugged wine and subsequently were easily taken prisoner or slaughtered when they fell into a stupor.[1]

According to the U.S. military, the ideal CNS disabling agent should be potent, effective, persistent, logistically feasible, predictable, treatable, unlikely to produce permanent injuries or death when used as intended (high therapeutic index), and affordable.[2] From 1953 to 1973, the U.S. Army investigated many methods of incapacitation to find one suitable for standardization.[1] Nonchemical agents, such as noise, high-intensity photostimulation, microwaves, and olfactory assault, generally proved impractical, potentially physically damaging, or too easy to thwart with routine respiratory protective measures. Although several types of chemical and biowarfare (CBW) agents (e.g., lacrimators, vomiting agents, staphylococcal enterotoxin B, mild exposures to nerve agents or vesicants) were considered for use as incapacitants by the U.S. military, the psychochemical agents—chemicals that disable by producing behavioral or direct CNS effects—were considered most suitable for study and investment.

The psychochemical agents were classified into four general categories: stimulants, depressants, psychedelics, and deliriants. The stimulants included amphetamines, cocaine, caffeine, nicotine, strychnine, and metrazole. None of the stimulants proved effective as airborne incapacitating agents. In addition, it was feared that stimulants could enhance performance rather than hinder it following low- to moderate-dose exposures.

CNS depressant agents were either insufficiently potent or had a relatively narrow therapeutic index (TI; median lethal dose ÷ lowest median effective dose), with lethal doses in the range of 10 to 20 times the effective incapacitating dose.

From 1959 to 1965, D-lysergic acid diethylamide (LSD) was the primary psychedelic agent studied by the U.S. military. LSD had an inhaled ID_{50} (the dose incapacitating 50% of those exposed) of only 5.6 μg/kg, but results were unpredictable, with exposed victims still occasionally capable of effective volitional activities.

The deliriants, anticholinergic drugs with prominent CNS effects, were considered most suitable for use as military incapacitating agents. Of the deliriants, 3-quinuclidinyl benzilate (U.S. military designation BZ) was considered the most ideal for use as a CNS disabling agent.[1] BZ is stable when delivered by a thermal munition, environmentally persistent, and more potent than a variety of widely recognized anticholinergic agents (e.g., atropine and scopolamine).[1] The U.S. military weaponized and stockpiled BZ as its only incapacitating agent in the 1960s. These stockpiles were subsequently destroyed. The drug, however, is still used in medical pharmacology research as a muscarinic receptor antagonist; it is designated QNB for such purposes.

Modern use of CNS disabling agents in warfare has been reported, but the veracity of such reports is not clear. In 1995, during the Balkan wars, Serbian military forces allegedly used BZ against civilians, who reported hallucinations associated with attacks by artillery shells that emitted smoke. Although BZ exposure has not been completely excluded, the hallucinations could be ascribed to exhaustion and other physical and psychological stressors.[3,4]

In contrast, the modern use of nonlethal agents as weapons against terrorists is well documented. In October 2002, the Russian Federal Security Service used CNS disabling agents to end a standoff with terrorists in a Moscow theater. Chechen rebels held more than 800 hostages and threatened to detonate explosives unless their political demands were met. After a 3-day siege, "gas" was introduced into the theater's ventilation system and quickly subdued both the terrorists and their hostages. More than 650 of the hostages were hospitalized, and 128 died; all but five apparently died of the effects of the "gas."[5] The identity of the agent used was not at first disclosed. Early reports suggested the use of BZ,[6] but the clinical findings and time course of

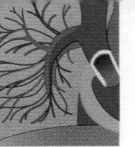

symptom onset were not consistent. Traces of halothane, however, were detected in two of the victims that were transported to Germany.[7,8] Several days after the incident, the Russian Health Minister stated that the agent used was a derivative of fentanyl,[7,9] which was not expected to cause fatalities Although expert opinion is not uniform, current consensus holds that the "knockout gas" was composed of an ultrapotent opioid aerosol (possibly carfentanil[9] or remifentanil[10]) probably along with halothane. The relatively high case fatality rate could be due to multiple factors, including variability in dose, displacement of oxygen by rapid introduction of gas into the building, failure to adequately notify health care teams and supply them with antidotes, and poor physical condition of the hostages due to limited food and water and to immobility during their captivity. This use of an incapacitant by the Russian military as an antiterrorist agent has rejuvenated U.S. military interest in developing an effective nonlethal chemical weapon.[9]

EXPOSURE SCENARIOS

Like most chemical and biological agents, CNS disabling agents would be most effective if disseminated as an aerosol, vapor, or gas. Incapacitating agents could be delivered outdoors as an aerosol from low-flying aircraft (e.g., crop dusters), vehicle-mounted or hand-held spray devices, or detonation of artillery, missiles, or bombs. If the agent is used outdoors, low-wind conditions would be preferable, to minimize rapid dissipation. The Moscow theater siege illustrates the prototypical exposure environment for effective delivery of CNS disabling agents: an enclosed space, which allows for near-simultaneous respiratory exposure to all building occupants (particularly if a ventilation system is available for agent delivery). An enclosed space allows for more accurate estimation of the appropriate dose of incapacitant to achieve rapid tranquilization of multiple persons while minimizing permanent harm. The Moscow siege also illustrates the grim reality that incapacitating agents can have unpredictable and lethal effects, even when conditions a priori are presumed to be ideal.

Because the general tactical goals of war are to kill combatants and destroy material goods, conventional weapons or physically injurious chemical or biological agents would have more utility. CNS disabling agents, however, could be used in operations in which casualties were to be minimized or avoided, such as capture scenarios or when civilians are present. Terrorist use of CNS disabling agents seems less probable because conventional weapons or other chemical agents would be easier to procure and because the diminished likelihood of casualties would lessen the imperative to respond to threats.

PATHOPHYSIOLOGY OF INJURY

The CNS disabling agents discussed do not possess unique pathophysiology. Like other anticholinergic agents, 3-quinuclidinyl benzilate is a potent competitive antagonist of both peripheral and central muscarinic receptors (see Chapter 39). A detailed review of opiate pathophysiology is found in Chapter 33 and of LSD in Chapter 45. The features distinguishing the CNS disabling agents from other members of their respective classes relate mostly to potency and time course of effects.

MANIFESTATIONS

BZ produces clinical effects similar to those of atropine, although it is more potent. The ID_{50} for BZ is 6.2 μg/kg (approximately 0.5 mg for adults), whereas the ID_{50} for atropine is 140 μg/kg (8 to 14 mg). Mild cognitive impairment is seen in 50% of individuals with BZ doses of approximately 2.5 μg/kg.[1]

BZ has a slower onset and longer duration of action than atropine does. The effects of BZ are barely measurable 1 hour after exposure to the ID_{50} dose. Central effects are seen after about 4 hours, peak at 8 to 10 hours, and then gradually subside over 24 to 72 hours. The duration of incapacitation from an ID_{50} dose is roughly 24 hours.[1,2] Doubling the dose increases the rate of onset of effects and produces incapacitation within 1 hour of exposure but also prolongs recovery an additional 48 hours.[1] In actual use, wide variation in dosing among exposed individuals is expected, with consequent variability in symptom onset and offset. It is estimated that the human ID_{50} is approximately 40-fold lower than the lethal dose (therapeutic index of 40).[1]

Although toxicity from BZ is most likely to occur after inhalation of vapor or liquid aerosol, symptoms may also result from intravenous or intramuscular injection or, to a small degree, from skin contact with liquid. Effects may be delayed up to 24 hours after dermal absorption.

The clinical signs and symptoms of BZ exposure are the typical antimuscarinic effects. Peripheral signs include tachycardia, mydriasis, and dry skin and mucous membranes. Mild exposures cause drowsiness, lapses of attention, and difficulty in following complex instructions. Moderate exposures ($\approx$ 4 μg/kg) cause somnolence or stupor, mumbling speech, ataxia, slowing of thought processes, and confusion. Higher exposures cause full delirium with staring, muttering, and hallucinations, with fluctuating lucid intervals.[1] Bizarre behaviors are often seen among individuals with antimuscarinic delirium, including undressing, crawling or climbing motions, and plucking or picking at the air or garments (carphology or "woolgathering").

As mentioned above, depressant psychochemical agents were found by the U.S. military either to be insufficiently potent or to have relatively narrow therapeutic indices, where lethal doses exceeded incapacitating doses by factors of only 10 to 20. In actual use, when precise dose control is not possible, unintentional lethal dosing would not be unexpected. A recent review by Wax et al, however, illustrates that some ultrapotent fentanyl derivatives have very high therapeutic indices and might therefore be considered as potential CNS disabling

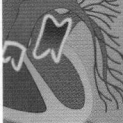

agents when aerosolized.[9] Morphine has a therapeutic index of 70. Fentanyl is roughly 300 times as potent as morphine and has a TI of 300, sufentanil is 4500 times as potent as morphine with a TI of 25,000, remifentanil is 220 times as potent as morphine with a TI of 33,000, and carfentanil is 10,000 times as potent as morphine with a TI of 10,600. Such figures, however, are usually based on animal data, often from a single animal species, and do not necessarily apply to humans.[9] Even if such agents were found to have remarkable safety margins in controlled settings, the doses required to induce rapid unconsciousness could also cause significant respiratory depression or apnea. With appropriate supportive care, such doses might be safe. Hypoxic brain injury might result, however, if exposed persons do not rapidly receive assisted ventilation or antidotal therapy; this is the likely reason for the "gas" fatalities in the Moscow theater incident. The aerosolized doses necessary to incapacitate humans and rate of onset and duration of clinical effects has not yet been elucidated. The clinical manifestations following opioid aerosolization, however, are similar to those experienced by other routes (see Chapter 33).

LSD is a difficult agent to disseminate and consequently is most likely to be used in a clandestine manner, such as food or water contamination.[2] An early stage of nausea is commonly seen, followed in 45 to 60 minutes by CNS effects (anxiety, euphoria, delusions, kaleidoscopic imagery, etc) and peripheral signs of sympathetic stimulation (see Chapter 45).

ASSESSMENT

The diagnosis of CNS disabling agent toxicity is based on a suggestive history coupled with toxidrome recognition on physical examination. Rapid identification of the chemical agents will not be possible by laboratory tests available at most hospitals. Diagnosis is further supported by the complete reversal of toxic effects following empiric antidotal therapy. Chemical warfare agent poisoning should be suspected when a group of patients have the acute onset of a similar constellation of signs or symptoms. Multiple casualties with altered mental status first require evaluation to rule out the more lethal chemical agents, such as nerve agents or cyanide. The presence of coma, miosis, and respiratory depression could occur with either nerve agents or opioids; the additional presence of seizures, fasciculations, and cholinergic findings suggests nerve agent toxicity. BZ will produce an anticholinergic toxidrome. Unintentional atropine overdose from nerve agent antidote autoinjectors may mimic BZ toxicity; multiple simultaneous atropine casualties may occur if a group believes it has been exposed to nerve agent, although clinical history should easily differentiate these exposures. Intoxication with LSD might be difficult to differentiate from intentional self-exposure to cannabinoids, but the treatment is similar and supportive for both. Anxiety reactions and malingering may mimic any potential CNS-disabling agent exposure, although peripheral signs of toxicity may be blunted or absent.

TREATMENT

For most CNS disabling agent casualties, only symptomatic and supportive treatment will be necessary. Victims should be rapidly removed from the exposure environment, and airway support should be provided as necessary. To avoid hyperthermia with BZ intoxication, restrictive clothing should be removed, especially in hot environments. Psychomotor agitation may respond to verbal assurance in mildly affected individuals, while restraints, nonspecific sedation (e.g., with benzodiazepines), or antidotal physostigmine may be indicated for more seriously poisoned patients. Physostigmine, a reversible carbamate acetylcholinesterase inhibitor, has been used safely to reverse antimuscarinic toxicity from BZ exposure.[1,2] Intravenous doses of 30 µg/kg (about 2 mg in 70- to 75-kg persons) are effective in reducing peripheral effects, but higher doses (at least 45 µg/kg) are often required to significantly reverse severe central cognitive effects. For unclear reasons, physostigmine appears to be ineffective if given during the first 4 to 6 hours after BZ exposure.[1,2] Physostigmine is primarily indicated for the treatment of agitated delirium or to confirm diagnosis (see Chapter 39). Physostigmine has a short duration of action (20 minutes to 2 hours) and may require repeated dosing every 1 to 2 hours for recurrent agitation. Careful patient monitoring is necessary during physostigmine administration to avoid inducing excess cholinergic effects.

Patients with suspected opioid agent toxicity may require emergent airway support and administration of an opiate-receptor antagonist (e.g., naloxone; see Chapter 33). Larger than usual doses of naloxone (up to 10 mg) may be needed to completely reverse the toxic effects from potent, synthetic, opioid agents. Data from animal studies suggest that repeated administration of naloxone may be necessary for a period of 2 to 24 hours following fentanyl derivative toxicity.[9,11,12] The high lipophilicity of fentanyl derivatives allows for their redistribution from tissues to the CNS, making recrudescent opiate toxicity (e.g., CNS and respiratory depression) a real possibility. The treatment of LSD intoxication is entirely supportive.

Because of the possibility of prolonged and recurrent clinical effects, patients exposed to BZ and high-potency opioid derivatives require a prolonged period of hospital observation (12 to 24 hours).

MANAGEMENT OF MASS CASUALTIES

With mass casualties from BZ exposure, control and containment of delirious victims is the primary concern. These victims may be capable of injuring themselves or others, so dangerous objects (e.g., weapons, small items that may be swallowed) should be removed.[2] Loose restraints or tethers are preferable to allowing victims to roam freely without supervision. Separation of affected individuals into small groups, rather than a single large group, may prevent a crowd control crisis induced by a few agitated victims.[1] Intravenous physostigmine dosing

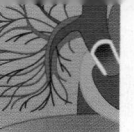

to multiple victims may not be feasible under field conditions. Intramuscular (1 to 2 mg) or oral (2 to 5 mg) dosing every 1 to 2 hours titrated as needed may help maintain victim comfort and manageability.[1,2] Physostigmine may be mixed into juice to mask its bitter taste for oral administration.[1]

Mass casualties from opioid toxicity can easily outstrip resources necessary to avoid complications from respiratory depression. Intramuscular or subcutaneous naloxone administration, as opposed to the intravenous route, should save time and minimize permanent injury or death when the number of victims greatly exceeds the number of rescuers.

PRINCIPLES OF PREPAREDNESS

CNS disabling agents appear less likely to be used than conventional weapons or other chemical warfare agents. Therefore, in preparing for chemical weapons casualties, it would be prudent to concentrate more on the agents intended to inflict fatalities or permanent injuries. If used as intended, the CNS disabling agents should temporarily incapacitate, and the victims may require only monitoring and supportive therapy. Nevertheless, agents with lower therapeutic indices can cause fatalities, since precise control of the administered dose is not possible and individuals may have varying susceptibilities to toxic effects. If time and resources permit, preparations for chemical casualties should include stockpiling and training in the use of physostigmine and naloxone, the antidotes for CNS disabling agents. Airway management equipment would likely already be part of the armamentarium for chemical casualty preparedness.

REFERENCES

1. Ketchum JS, Sidell FR: Incapacitating Agents. In Sidell FR, Takafuji ET, Frank DR (eds): Medical Aspects of Chemical and Biological Warfare. Washington DC, Office of the Surgeon General, 1997, pp 287–305.
2. Chemical casualties: centrally acting incapacitants. J R Army Med Corps 2002;148(4):388–391.
3. Hay A: Surviving the impossible: the long march from Srebrenica—an investigation of the possible use of chemical warfare agents. Med Confl Surviv 1998;14(2):120–155.
4. Sharp D: Alleged chemical warfare in Bosnia conflict. Lancet 1998;351:1500.
5. Russia: officials raise hostage death toll. NTI Global Security Newswire. November 8, 2002. Available at http://www.nti.org/d_newswire/issues/2002/11/8/7s.html, accessed October 27, 2006.
6. Lethal Moscow gas an opiate? CBSNEWS.com. October 29, 2002. Available at http://www.cbsnews.com/stories/2002/10/29/world/main527298.shtml, accessed October 27, 2006.
7. Enserink M, Stone R: Toxicology: questions swirl over knockout gas used in hostage crisis. Science 2002;298(5596):1150–1151.
8. Schiermeier Q: Hostage deaths put gas weapons in spotlight. Nature 2002;420(6911):7.
9. Wax PM, Becker CE, Curry SC: Unexpected "gas" casualties in Moscow: a medical toxicology perspective. Ann Emerg Med 2003;41:700–705.
10. Chemical and Biological Weapons Nonproliferation Program: The Moscow Theater hostage crisis: incapacitants and chemical warfare. Available at http://cns.miis.edu/pubs/week/02110b.htm, accessed October 27, 2006.
11. Shaw ML, Carpenter JW, Leith DE: Complications with the use of carfentanil citrate and xylazine hydrochloride to immobilize domestic horses. J Am Vet Med Assoc 206:833, 1995.
12. Miller MW, Wild MA, Lance WR: Efficacy and safety of naltrexone hydrochloride for antagonizing carfentanil citrate immobilization in captive Rocky Mountain elk (*Cervus elaphus nelsoni*). J Wildlife Dis 32:234, 1996.

INDEX

Note: Page number followed by the letter f refer to figures; those followed by letter t to tables, and the letter b to boxed material.

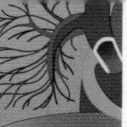

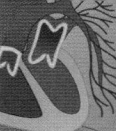

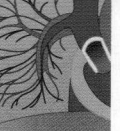

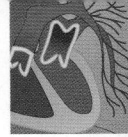

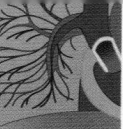

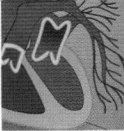

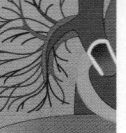

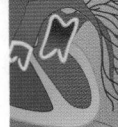

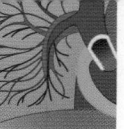

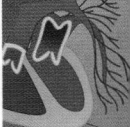

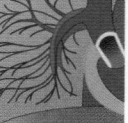

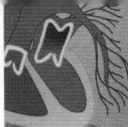

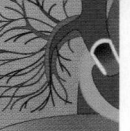

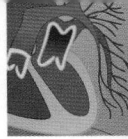

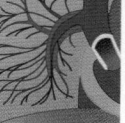

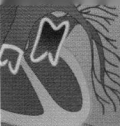

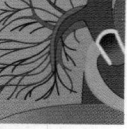

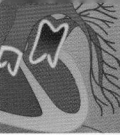

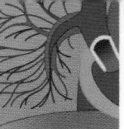

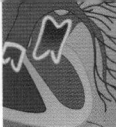

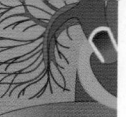

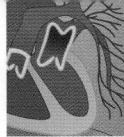

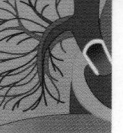

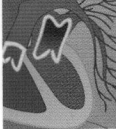

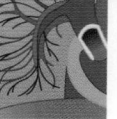

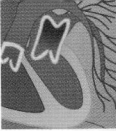

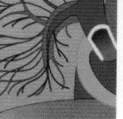

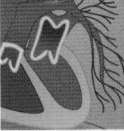

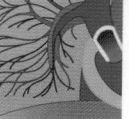

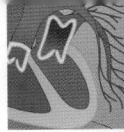

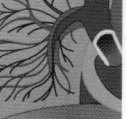

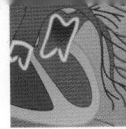

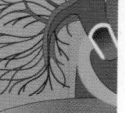

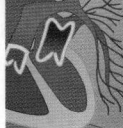

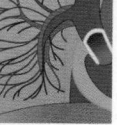

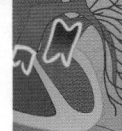

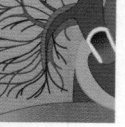

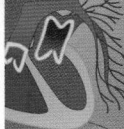